Preface

BNF for Children aims to provide prescribers, pharmacists, and other healthcare professionals with sound up-to-date information on the use of medicines for treating children.

A joint publication of the British Medical Association, the Royal Pharmaceutical Society, the Royal College of Paediatrics and Child Health, and the Neonatal and Paediatric Pharmacists Group, BNF for Children ('BNFC') is published under the authority of a Paediatric Formulary Committee which comprises representatives of these bodies, the Department of Health for England, and the Medicines and Healthcare products Regulatory Agency.

Many areas of paediatric practice have suffered from inadequate information on effective medicines. BNFC addresses this significant knowledge gap by providing practical information on the use of medicines in children of all ages from birth to adolescence. Information in BNFC has been validated against emerging evidence, best-practice guidelines, and crucially, advice from a network of clinical experts.

Drawing information from manufacturers' literature where appropriate, BNFC also includes a great deal of advice that goes beyond marketing authorisations (product licences). This is necessary because licensed indications frequently do not cover the clinical needs of children; in some cases, products for use in children need to be specially manufactured or imported. Careful consideration has been given to establishing the clinical need for unlicensed interventions with respect to the evidence and experience of their safety and efficacy; local paediatric formularies, clinical literature and national information resources have been invaluable in this process.

BNFC has been designed for rapid reference and the information presented has been carefully selected to aid decisions on prescribing, dispensing and administration of medicines. Less detail is given on areas such as malignant disease and the very specialist use of medicines generally undertaken in tertiary centres. BNFC should be interpreted in the light of professional knowledge and it should be supplemented as necessary by specialised publications. Information is also available from Medicines Information Services (see inside front cover).

It is **important** to use the most recent BNF or making clinical decisions. The print edition of *BNF for Children* is updated in September each year. Monthly updates are provided online via the BNF Publications website www.bnf.org, MedicinesComplete and the NHS Evidence portal. The more important changes listed under Changes p. xix are cumulative (from one print edition to the next), and can be printed off each month to show the main changes since the last print edition as an aide memoire for those using print copies.

The website (www.bnf.org) includes additional information of relevance to healthcare professionals. Other digital formats of BNFC—including versions for mobile devices and integration into local formularies—are also available.

BNF Publications welcomes comments from healthcare professionals. Comments and constructive criticism should be sent to:

British National Formulary,
Royal Pharmaceutical Society,
66–68 East Smithfield
London
E1W 1AW
editor@bnf.org

The contact email for manufacturers or pharmaceutical companies wishing to contact BNF Publications is manufacturerinfo@bnf.org

Contents

Preface	page iii
Acknowledgements	v
How BNF publications are constructed	ix
How to use BNF Publications in print	xii
Changes	xix
Guidance on Prescribing	1
Prescription writing	4
Supply of medicines	6
Emergency supply of medicines	7
Controlled drugs and drug dependence	8
Adverse reactions to drugs	11
Guidance on intravenous infusions	14
Prescribing in hepatic impairment	15
Prescribing in renal impairment	15
Prescribing in pregnancy	17
Prescribing in breast-feeding	17
Prescribing in palliative care	18
Drugs and sport	22
Prescribing in dental practice	23

NOTES ON DRUGS AND PREPARATIONS

1 Gastro-intestinal system	page 24
2 Cardiovascular system	69
3 Respiratory system	137
4 Nervous system	180
5 Infection	281
6 Endocrine system	403
7 Genito-urinary system	456
8 Malignant disease	483
9 Blood and nutrition	521
10 Musculoskeletal system	595
11 Eye	619
12 Ear, nose and oropharynx	643
13 Skin	665
14 Vaccines	724
15 Anaesthesia	757
16 Emergency treatment of poisoning	786

APPENDICES AND INDICES

Appendix 1 Interactions	799
Appendix 2 Borderline substances	926
Appendix 3 Cautionary and advisory labels for dispensed medicines	966
Dental Practitioners' Formulary	969
Nurse Prescribers' Formulary	970
Non-medical prescribing	973
Index of proprietary manufacturers	974
Special-order Manufacturers	979
Index	981
Medical emergencies in the community	inside back cover

BNF
for Children

2016
2017

September 2016–17

ROYAL
PHARMACEUTICAL
SOCIETY

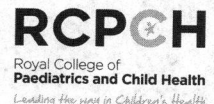

Royal College of
Paediatrics and Child Health
Leading the way in Children's Health

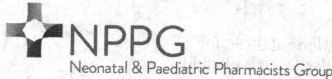

Neonatal & Paediatric Pharmacists Group

Published jointly by
BMJ Group
Tavistock Square, London, WC1H 9JP, UK

and

Pharmaceutical Press
Pharmaceutical Press is the publishing division of the Royal Pharmaceutical Society.
66-68 East Smithfield, London E1W 1AW, UK

RCPCH Publications Ltd
5–11 Theobalds Road, London, WC1X 8SH, UK

ISBN: 978 0 85711 247 7

ISBN: 978 0 85711 304 7 (NHS edition)

ISBN: 978 0 85711 306 1 (ePDF)

Printed by GGP Media GmbH, Pößneck, Germany

Typeset by Data Standards Ltd, UK

Text designed by Peter Burgess

A catalogue record for this book is available from the British Library.

Requesting copies of BNF publications
Paper copies may be obtained through any bookseller or direct from:

Pharmaceutical Press
c/o Macmillan Distribution (MDL)
Brunel Rd
Houndmills
Basingstoke
Hampshire
RG21 6XS
Tel: +44 (0) 1256 302 699
Fax: +44 (0) 1256 812 521
direct@macmillan.co.uk

For all bulk orders of more than 20 copies:
Tel: +44 (0) 207 572 2266
pharmpress@rpharms.com

BNFC is available online through MedicinesComplete and as mobile apps; a PDA version is also available. In addition, BNFC content can be integrated into a local formulary by using BNFC on FormularyComplete; see www.bnf.org for details.

BNFC is also available on www.evidence.nhs.uk and eligible users can download smartphone apps from the relevant app stores.

Distribution of printed BNFCs
In **England**, NICE purchases print editions of BNFC for distribution within the NHS. For details of who is eligible to receive a copy and further contact details, please refer to the NICE website:
www.nice.org.uk/mpc/BritishNationalFormulary.jsp. If you are entitled to an NHS copy of BNFC, please call (0) 1268 495 609 or email: bnf@binleys.com.

In **Scotland**, email:
nss.psd-bnf@nhs.net

In **Wales**, contact NHS Wales Shared Services Partnership—Contractor Services:
Tel: 01792 607420

In **Northern Ireland**, email:
ni.bnf@hscni.net

About BNFC content
The *BNF for Children* is for rapid reference by UK health professionals engaged in prescribing, dispensing, and administering medicines to children. *BNF for Children* has been constructed using robust procedures for gathering, assessing and assimilating information on paediatric drug treatment, but may not always include all the information necessary for prescribing and dispensing. It is expected that the reader will be relying on appropriate professional knowledge and expertise to interpret the contents in the context of the circumstances of the individual child. *BNF for Children* should be used in conjunction with other appropriate and up-to-date literature and, where necessary, supplemented by expert advice. Information is also available from Medicines Information Services.

Special care is required in managing childhood conditions with unlicensed medicines or with licensed medicines for unlicensed uses. Responsibility for the appropriate use of medicines lies solely with the individual health professional.

Please refer to digital versions of *BNF for Children* for the most up-to-date content. *BNF for Children* is published in print but interim updates are issued and published in the digital versions of *BNF for Children*. The publishers work to ensure that the information is as accurate and up-to-date as possible at the date of publication, but knowledge and best practice in this field change regularly. *BNF for Children's* accuracy and currency cannot be guaranteed and neither the publishers nor the authors accept any responsibility for errors or omissions. While considerable efforts have been made to check the material in this publication, it should be treated as a guide only. Prescribers, pharmacists and other healthcare professionals are advised to check www.bnf.org for information about key updates and corrections.

Pharmaid
Numerous requests have been received from developing countries for BNFCs. The Pharmaid scheme of the Commonwealth Pharmacists Association will dispatch old BNFCs to certain Commonwealth countries. For more information on this scheme see www.commonwealthpharmacy.org/about/projects/pharmaid/. If you would like to donate your copy email: admin@commonwealthpharmacy.org

Acknowledgements

The Paediatric Formulary Committee is grateful to individuals and organisations that have provided advice and information to the *BNF for Children* (BNFC).

The principal contributors for this update were:

M.N. Badminton, S. Bailey, G.D.L. Bates, H. Bedford, M.W. Beresford, R.M. Bingham, L. Brook, K.G. Brownlee, I.F. Burgess, A. Cant, R. Carr, T.D. Cheetham, A.G. Cleary, A.J. Cotgrove, J.B.S. Coulter, B.G. Craig, J.H. Cross, A. Dhawan, P.N. Durrington, A.B. Edgar, J.A. Edge, D.A.C. Elliman, N.D. Embleton, P.J. Goadsby, J. Gray, J.W. Gregory, P. Gringras, J.P. Harcourt, C. Hendriksz, R.F. Howard, R.G. Hull, H.R. Jenkins, S. Jones, B.A. Judd, E. Junaid, P.T. Khaw, J.M.W. Kirk, E.G.H. Lyall, P.S. Malone, S.D. Marks, D.F. Marsh, P. McHenry, P.J. McKiernan, L.M. Melvin, E. Miller, S. Moledina, R.E. Morton, P. Mulholland, C. Nelson-Piercy, J.M. Neuberger, K.K. Nischal, C.Y. Ng, L.P. Omerod, J.Y. Paton, G.A. Pearson, J. Puntis, M.M. Ramsay, J. Rogers, K.E. Rogstad, J.W. Sander, N.J. Scolding, M.R. Sharland, N.J. Shaw, O.F.W Stumper, A.G. Sutcliffe, E.A. Taylor, S. Thomas, M.A. Thomson, J.A. Vale, S. Vijay, J.O. Warner, N.J.A. Webb, A.D. Weeks, R. Welbury, W.P. Whitehouse, A. Wright, M.M. Yaqoob, Z. Zaiwalla, and S.M. Zuberi.

Members of the British Association of Dermatologists' Therapy & Guidelines Subcommittee, D.A. Buckley, N. Chiang, M. Cork, K. Gibbon, R.Y.P. Hunasehally, G.A. Johnston, T.A. Leslie, E.C. Mallon, P.M McHenry, J. Natkunarajah, C. Saunders, S. Ungureanu, S. Wakelin, F.S. Worsnop, A.G. Brain (Secretariat), and M.F. Mohd Mustapa (Secretariat) have provided valuable advice.

Members of the Advisory Committee on Malaria Prevention, R.H. Behrens, D. Bell, P.L. Chiodini, V. Field, F. Genasi, L. Goodyer, A. Green, J. Jones, G. Kassianos, D.G. Lalloo, D. Patel, H. Patel, M. Powell, D.V. Shingadia, N.O. Subair, C.J.M. Whitty, M. Blaze (Secretariat), and V. Smith (Secretariat) have provided valuable advice.

Members of the UK Ophthalmic Pharmacy Group have also provided valuable advice.

The MHRA have provided valuable assistance.

Correspondents in the pharmaceutical industry have provided information on new products and commented on products in BNFC.

Numerous doctors, pharmacists, nurses, and others have sent comments and suggestions.

BNFC interactions are provided by C.L. Preston, S.L. Jones, H.K. Sandhu, and S. Sutton.

The BNFC has valuable access to the *Martindale* data banks by courtesy of A. Brayfield and staff.

Valuable technical assistance provided by J. Macdonald, H. Benson, R. Calle, J. Cater, D. Granger, N. Judd, M. Mebrate, K. Parsons, B. Stephenson, J. Stott and I. White.

S. Frau, E. Laughton, P.D. Lee, J. Martin, L. Mistry, S. Sacranie, and A. Sparshatt provided considerable assistance during the production of this update of the BNFC.

BNF Staff

BNF DIRECTOR
Karen Baxter
BSc, MSc, MRPharmS

HEAD OF CONTENT
Kate Towers
BPharm (AU), GCClinPharm

CONTENT MANAGERS
Kristina Fowlie
MPharm, CertPharmPract, MRPharmS
Heenaben Patel
MPharm, DipClinPharm, MRPharmS

QUALITY AND PROCESS MANAGER
Angela M.G. McFarlane
BSc, DipClinPharm

CLINICAL WRITERS
Naimah Callachand
MPharm

Thomas F. Corbett
BScPharm (IRL), MPharm (IRL)

Joyce Donnelly
MPharm, MRPharmS

Belén Granell Villén
BSc, DipClinPharm

Basma Hossin
MPharm, PhD

Maeve A.M. Lynn
MPharm, CertClinPharm

Claire McSherry
BPharm (NZ), PGCertClinPharm (NZ)

Kere Odumah
MPharm

Paridhi K. Prashar
MPharm, MRPharmS

Dominique Shakir
MPharm, MRPharmS, IP, PGDip

Jacob M. Warner
BPharm (AU)

Sharyn Young
BPharm (NZ), PGDipClinPharm (NZ)

CLINICAL ASSISTANTS
Elizabeth King

EDITORIAL ASSISTANTS
Jaya Venkitachalam
BSc, MRes

SENIOR BNF ADMINISTRATOR
Heidi Homar
BA

MANAGING DIRECTOR, PHARMACEUTICAL PRESS
Alina Lourie
B.Ed, MSc

SENIOR MEDICAL ADVISER
Derek G. Waller
BSc, MB, BS, DM, FRCP

Paediatric Formulary Committee 2015-2016

CHAIR (ACTING)
David Tuthill
MB, BCh, FRCPCH

COMMITTEE MEMBERS
Indraneel Banerjee
MB BS, MD, FRCPCH

Neil A. Caldwell
BSc, MSc, MRPharmS, FFRPS

Martin G. Duerden
BMedSci, MB BS, DRCOG, MRCGP, DipTher, DPH

Sunit Godambe
MRCP, FRCPCH

Jessica Higson
BN, MSc, DipHE, RN (Adult), RN (Child), IP

James H. Larcombe
MB, ChB, PhD, FRCGP, DipAdvGP

John Marriott
BSc, PhD, MRPharmS, FHEA

E. David G. McIntosh
MB BS, MPH, LLM, PhD, FAFPHM, FRACP, FRCPCH, FFPM, DRCOG, DCH, DipPharmMed

Angeliki Siapkara
MSc, MD, CCST (Ortho)

Adam Sutherland
MPharm, MSc, FFRPS, MRPharmS

LAY MEMBER
Emily Lam

EXECUTIVE SECRETARY
Heidi Homar
BA

Dental Advisory Group 2015-2016

CHAIR
Sarah Manton
BDS, FDSRCS Ed, FHEA, PhD

COMMITTEE MEMBERS
Karen Baxter
BSc, MSc, MRPharmS

Andrew K. Brewer
BSc, BchD

Lesley P. Longman
BSc, BDS, FDSRCS Ed, PhD

Michelle Moffat
BDS, MFDS RCS Ed, M Paed Dent RPCS, FDS (Paed Dent) RSC Ed

SECRETARY
Arianne J. Matlin
MA, MSc, PhD

EXECUTIVE SECRETARY
Heidi Homar
BA

ADVICE ON DENTAL PRACTICE
The **British Dental Association** has contributed to the advice on medicines for dental practice through its representatives on the Dental Advisory Group.

Nurse Prescribers' Advisory Group 2015–2016

How BNF Publications are constructed

Overview

The BNF *for Children* (BNFC) is an independent professional publication that addresses the day-to-day prescribing information needs of healthcare professionals involved in the care of children. Use of this resource throughout the health service helps to ensure that medicines are used safely, effectively, and appropriately.

Hundreds of changes are made between print editions, and are published monthly in some digital formats. The most clinically significant updates are listed under Changes p. xix.

BNFC is unique in bringing together authoritative, independent guidance on best practice with clinically validated drug information.

Information in BNFC has been validated against emerging evidence, best-practice guidelines, and advice from a network of clinical experts. BNFC includes a great deal of advice that goes beyond marketing authorisations (product licences or summaries of product characteristics). This is necessary because licensed indications frequently do not cover the clinical needs of children; in some cases, products for use in children need to be specially manufactured or imported. Careful consideration has been given to establishing the clinical need for unlicensed interventions with respect to the evidence and experience of their safety and efficacy.

Validation of information follows a standardised process. Where the evidence base is weak, further validation is undertaken through a process of peer review. The process and its governance are outlined in greater detail in the sections that follow.

Paediatric Formulary Committee

The Paediatric Formulary Committee (PFC) is responsible for the content of BNFC. The PFC comprises pharmacy, medical and nursing representatives with a paediatric background, and lay representatives who have worked with children or acted as a carer of a paediatric patient; there are also representatives from the Medicines and Healthcare products Regulatory Agency (MHRA) and the Department of Health for England. The PFC decides on matters of policy and reviews amendments to BNFC in the light of new evidence and expert advice.

Dental Advisory Group

The Dental Advisory Group oversees the preparation of advice on the drug management of dental and oral conditions; the group includes representatives from the British Dental Association and a representative from the UK Health Departments.

Nurse Prescribers' Advisory Group

The Nurse Prescribers' Advisory Group oversees the list of drugs approved for inclusion in the Nurse Prescribers' Formulary; the group includes representatives from a range of nursing disciplines and stakeholder organisations.

Expert advisers

BNFC uses about 80 expert clinical advisers (including doctors, pharmacists, nurses, and dentists) throughout the UK to help with the clinical content. The role of these expert advisers is to review existing text and to comment on amendments drafted by the clinical writers. These clinical experts help to ensure that BNFC remains reliable by:

- commenting on the relevance of the text in the context of best clinical practice in the UK;
- checking draft amendments for appropriate interpretation of any new evidence;
- providing expert opinion in areas of controversy or when reliable evidence is lacking;
- advising on the use of unlicensed medicines or of licensed medicines for unlicensed uses ('off-label' use);
- providing independent advice on drug interactions, prescribing in hepatic impairment, renal impairment, pregnancy, breast-feeding, neonatal care, palliative care, and the emergency treatment of poisoning.

In addition to consulting with regular advisers, BNFC calls on other clinical specialists for specific developments when particular expertise is required.

BNFC also works closely with a number of expert bodies that produce clinical guidelines. Drafts or pre-publication copies of guidelines are often received for comment and for assimilation into BNFC.

Editorial team

BNFC clinical writers have all worked as pharmacists or possess a pharmacy degree and further, relevant post-graduate qualification, and have a sound understanding of how drugs are used in clinical practice. A number of the clinical writers have specific experience of paediatric practice. As a team, the clinical writers are responsible for editing, maintaining, and updating BNFC content. They follow a systematic prioritisation process in response to updates to the evidence base in order to ensure the most clinically important topics are reviewed as quickly as possible. In parallel the team of clinical writers undertakes a process of rolling revalidation, aiming to review all of the content in the BNF over a 3- to 4-year period.

Amendments to the text are drafted when the clinical writers are satisfied that any new information is reliable and relevant. A set of standard criteria define when content is referred to expert advisers, the Joint Formulary Committee or other advisory groups, or submitted for peer review.

Clinical writers prepare the text for publication and undertake a number of validation checks on the knowledge at various stages of the production.

Sources of BNFC information

BNFC uses a variety of sources for its information; the main ones are shown below.

Summaries of product characteristics

BNFC reviews the summaries of product characteristics (SPCs) of all new products as well as revised SPCs for existing products. The SPCs are a key source of product information and are carefully processed. Such processing involves:

- verifying the approved names of all relevant ingredients including 'non-active' ingredients (BNFC is committed to using approved names and descriptions as laid down by the Human Medicines Regulations 2012);
- comparing the indications, cautions, contra-indications, and side-effects with similar existing drugs. Where these are different from the expected pattern, justification is sought for their inclusion or exclusion;
- seeking independent data on the use of drugs in pregnancy and breast-feeding;
- incorporating the information into BNFC using established criteria for the presentation and inclusion of the data;
- checking interpretation of the information by a second clinical writer before submitting to a content manager; changes relating to doses receive a further check;
- identifying potential clinical problems or omissions and seeking further information from manufacturers or from expert advisers;
- constructing, with the help of expert advisers, a comment on the role of the drug in the context of similar drugs.

Much of this processing is applicable to the following sources as well.

Literature

Clinical writers monitor core medical, paediatric, and pharmaceutical journals. Research papers and reviews relating to drug therapy are carefully processed. When a difference between the advice in BNFC and the paper is noted, the new information is assessed for reliability (using tools based on SIGN methodology) and relevance to UK clinical practice. If necessary, new text is drafted and discussed with expert advisers and the Paediatric Formulary Committee. BNFC enjoys a close working relationship with a number of national information providers.

In addition to the routine process, which is used to identify 'triggers' for changing the content, systematic literature searches are used to identify the best quality evidence available to inform an update. Clinical writers receive training in critical appraisal, literature evaluation, and search strategies.

Consensus guidelines
The advice in BNFC is checked against consensus guidelines produced by expert bodies. The quality of the guidelines is assessed using adapted versions of the AGREE II tool. A number of bodies make drafts or pre-publication copies of the guidelines available to BNFC; it is therefore possible to ensure that a consistent message is disseminated. BNFC routinely processes guidelines from the National Institute for Health and Care Excellence (NICE), the Scottish Medicines Consortium (SMC), and the Scottish Intercollegiate Guidelines Network (SIGN).

Reference sources
Paediatric formularies and reference sources are used to provide background information for the review of existing text or for the construction of new text. The BNFC team works closely with the editorial team that produces *Martindale: The Complete Drug Reference*. BNFC has access to *Martindale* information resources and each team keeps the other informed of significant developments and shifts in the trends of drug usage.

Peer review
Although every effort is made to identify the most robust data available, inevitably there are areas where the evidence base is weak or contradictory. While the BNF has the valuable support of expert advisers and the Paediatric Formulary Committee, the recommendations made may be subject to a further level of scrutiny through peer review to ensure they reflect best practice.

Content for peer review is posted on bnf.org and interested parties are notified via a number of channels, including the BNF e-newsletter.

Statutory information
BNFC routinely processes relevant information from various Government bodies including Statutory Instruments and regulations affecting the Prescription only Medicines Order. Official compendia such as the British Pharmacopoeia and its addenda are processed routinely to ensure that BNFC complies with the relevant sections of the Human Medicines Regulations 2012.

BNFC maintains close links with the Home Office (in relation to controlled drug regulations) and the Medicines and Healthcare products Regulatory Agency (including the British Pharmacopoeia Commission). Safety warnings issued by the Commission on Human Medicines (CHM) and guidelines on drug use issued by the UK health departments are processed as a matter of routine.

Relevant professional statements issued by the Royal Pharmaceutical Society are included in BNFC as are guidelines from bodies such as the Royal College of Paediatrics and Child Health.

Medicines and devices
NHS Prescription Services (from the NHS Business Services Authority) provides non-clinical, categorical information (including prices) on the medicines and devices included in BNFC.

Comments from readers
Readers of BNFC are invited to send in comments. Numerous letters and emails are received by the BNF team. Such feedback helps to ensure that BNFC provides practical and clinically relevant information. Many changes in the presentation and scope of BNFC have resulted from comments sent in by users.

Comments from industry
Close scrutiny of BNFC by the manufacturers provides an additional check and allows them an opportunity to raise issues about BNFC's presentation of the role of various drugs; this is yet another check on the balance of BNFC advice. All comments are looked at with care and, where necessary, additional information and expert advice are sought.

Market research
Market research is conducted at regular intervals to gather feedback on specific areas of development.

Assessing the evidence
From January 2016, recommendations made in BNFC have been evidence graded to reflect the strength of the recommendation. The addition of evidence grading is to support clinical decision making based on the best available evidence.

The BNFC aims to revalidate all content over a rolling 3- to 4-year period and evidence grading will be applied to recommendations as content goes through the revalidation process. Therefore, initially, only a small number of recommendations will have been graded.

Grading system
The BNFC has adopted a five level grading system from A to E, based on the former SIGN grading system. This grade is displayed next to the recommendation within the text.

Evidence used to make a recommendation is assessed for validity using standardised methodology tools based on AGREE II and assigned a level of evidence. The recommendation is then given a grade that is extrapolated from the level of evidence, and an assessment of the body of evidence and its applicability.

Evidence assigned a level 1- or 2- score has an unacceptable level of bias or confounding and is not used to form recommendations.

Levels of evidence
- **Level 1++**
  High quality meta-analyses, systematic reviews of randomised controlled trials (RCTs), or RCTs with a very low risk of bias.
- **Level 1+**
  Well-conducted meta-analyses, systematic reviews, or RCTs with a low risk of bias.
- **Level 1–**
  Meta-analyses, systematic reviews, or RCTs with a high risk of bias.
- **Level 2++**
  High quality systematic reviews of case control or cohort studies; or high quality case control or cohort studies with a very low risk of confounding or bias and a high probability that the relationship is causal.
- **Level 2+**
  Well-conducted case control or cohort studies with a low risk of confounding or bias and a moderate probability that the relationship is causal.
- **Level 2–**
  Case control or cohort studies with a high risk of confounding or bias and a significant risk that the relationship is not causal.
- **Level 3**
  Non-analytic studies, e.g. case reports, case series.

- **Level 4**
  Expert advice or clinical experience from respected authorities.

Grades of recommendation

- **Grade A: High strength**
  NICE-accredited guidelines; or guidelines that pass AGREE II assessment; or at least one meta-analysis, systematic review, or RCT rated as 1++, and directly applicable to the target population; or a body of evidence consisting principally of studies rated as 1+, directly applicable to the target population, and demonstrating overall consistency of results.

- **Grade B: Moderate strength**
  A body of evidence including studies rated as 2++, directly applicable to the target population, and demonstrating overall consistency of results; or extrapolated evidence from studies rated as 1++ or 1+.

- **Grade C: Low strength**
  A body of evidence including studies rated as 2+, directly applicable to the target population and demonstrating overall consistency of results; or extrapolated evidence from studies rated as 2++.

- **Grade D: Very low strength**
  Evidence level 3; or extrapolated evidence from studies rated as 2+; or tertiary reference source created by a transparent, defined methodology, where the basis for recommendation is clear.

- **Grade E: Practice point**
  Evidence level 4.

How to use BNF Publications in print

How to use the BNF *for Children* in print
This edition of the BNF *for Children* (BNFC) continues to display the fundamental change to the structure of the content that was first shown in BNFC 2015-2016. The changes were made to bring consistency and clarity to BNFC content, and to the way that the content is arranged within print and digital products, increasing the ease with which information can be found.

For reference, the most notable changes to the structure of the content include:

- Drug monographs – where possible, all information that relates to a single drug is contained within its drug monograph, moving information previously contained in the prescribing notes. Drug monographs have also changed structurally: additional sections have been added, ensuring greater regularity around where information is located within the publication.
- Drug class monographs – where substantial amounts of information are common to all drugs within a drug class (e.g. macrolides p. 308), a drug class monograph has been created to contain the common information.
- Medicinal forms – categorical information about marketed medicines, such as price and pack size, continues to be sourced directly from the Dictionary of Medicines and Devices provided by the NHS Business Services Authority. However, clinical information curated by the BNF team has been clearly separated from the categorical pricing and pack size information and is included in the relevant section of the drug monograph.
- Section numbering – the BNF and BNFC section numbering has been removed. This section numbering tied the content to a rigid structure and enforced the retention of defunct classifications, such as mercurial diuretics, and hindered the relocation of drugs where therapeutic use had altered. It also caused constraints between the BNF and BNFC, where drugs had different therapeutic uses in children.
- Appendix 4 – the content has been moved to individual drug monographs. The introductory notes have been replaced with a new guidance section, Guidance on intravenous infusions p. 14.

Introduction
In order to achieve the safe, effective, and appropriate use of medicines, healthcare professionals must be able to use the BNFC effectively, and keep up to date with significant changes in the BNFC that are relevant to their clinical practice. This *How to Use the BNF for Children* is key in reinforcing the details of the new structure of the BNFC to all healthcare professionals involved with prescribing, monitoring, supplying, and administering medicines, as well as supporting the learning of students training to join these professions.

As with previous editions, the BNFC provides information on the use of medicines in children ranging from neonates (including preterm neonates) to adolescents. The terms infant, child, and adolescent are not used consistently in the literature; to avoid ambiguity actual ages are used in the dose statements in BNFC. The term neonate is used to describe a newborn infant aged 0–28 days. The terms child or children are used generically to describe the entire range from infant to adolescent in BNFC.

Structure of the BNFC
This BNFC edition continues to broadly follow the high level structure of earlier editions of the BNFC (i.e. those published before BNFC 2015-2016):

Front matter, comprising information on how to use the BNFC, the significant content changes in each edition, and guidance on various prescribing matters (e.g. prescription writing, the use of intravenous drugs, particular considerations for special patient populations).

Chapters, containing drug monographs describing the uses, doses, safety issues and other considerations involved in the use of drugs; drug class monographs; and treatment summaries, covering guidance on the selection of drugs. Monographs and treatment summaries are divided into chapters based on specific aspects of medical care, such as Chapter 5, Infections, or Chapter 16, Emergency treatment of poisoning; or drug use related to a particular system of the body, such as Chapter 2, Cardiovascular.

Within each chapter, content is organised alphabetically by therapeutic use (e.g. Airways disease, obstructive), with the treatment summaries first, (e.g. Asthma p. 138), followed by the monographs of the drugs used to manage the conditions discussed in the treatment summary. Within each therapeutic use, the drugs are organised alphabetically by classification (e.g. Antimuscarinics, Beta$_2$-agonist bronchodilators) and then alphabetically within each classification (e.g. Formoterol fumarate, Salbutamol, Salmeterol, Terbutaline sulfate).

Appendices, covering interactions, borderline substances, and cautionary and advisory labels.

Back matter, covering the lists of medicines approved by the NHS for Dental and Nurse Practitioner prescribing, proprietary and specials manufacturers' contact details, and the index. Yellow cards are also included, to facilitate the reporting of adverse events, as well as quick reference guides for life support and key drug doses in medical emergencies, for ease of access.

Navigating the *BNF for Children*
The contents page provides the high-level layout of information within the BNFC; and in addition, each chapter begins with a small contents section, describing the therapeutic uses covered within that chapter. Once in a chapter, location is guided by the side of the page showing the chapter number (the *thumbnail*), alongside the chapter title. The top of the page includes the therapeutic use (the *running head*) alongside the page number.

Once on a page, visual cues aid navigation: treatment summary information is in black type, with therapeutic use titles similarly styled in black, whereas the use of colour indicates drug-related information, including drug classification titles, drug class monographs, and drug monographs.

Although navigation is possible by browsing, primarily access to the information is via the index, which covers the titles of drug class monographs, drug monographs and treatment summaries. The index also includes the names of branded medicines and other topics of relevance, such as abbreviations, guidance sections, tables, and images.

Content types

Treatment summaries
Treatment summaries are of three main types;

- an overview of delivering a drug to a particular body system (e.g. Skin conditions, management p. 665),
- a comparison between a group or groups of drugs (e.g. beta-adrenoceptor blockers (systemic) p. 95),
- an overview of the drug management or prophylaxis of common conditions intended to facilitate rapid appraisal of options (e.g. Hypertension p. 90, or Malaria, prophylaxis p. 364).

In order to select safe and effective medicines for individual children, information in the treatment summaries must be used in conjunction with other prescribing details about the drugs and knowledge of the child's medical and drug history.

Monographs

Overview

In earlier editions (i.e. before BNFC 2015-2016), a systemically administered drug with indications for use in different body systems was split across the chapters relating to those body systems. So, for example, codeine phosphate p. 259 was found in chapter 1, for its antimotility effects and chapter 4 for its analgesic effects. However, the monograph in chapter 1 contained only the dose and some selected safety precautions.

Now, all of the information for the systemic use of a drug is contained within one monograph, so codeine phosphate p. 259 is now included in chapter 4. This carries the advantage of providing all of the information in one place, so the user does not need to flick back and forth across several pages to find all of the relevant information for that drug. Cross references are included in chapter 1, where the management of diarrhoea is discussed, to the drug monograph to assist navigation.

Where drugs have systemic and local uses, for example, chloramphenicol, and the considerations around drug use are markedly different according to the route of administration, the monograph is split, as with earlier editions, into the relevant chapters.

This means that the majority of drugs are still placed in the same chapters and sections as earlier editions, and although there may be some variation in order, all of the relevant information will be easier to locate.

One of the most significant changes to the monograph structure is the increased granularity, with a move from around 9 sections to over 20 sections; sections are only included when relevant information has been identified. The following information describes these sections and their uses in more detail.

Nomenclature

Monograph titles follow the convention of recommended international non-proprietary names (rINNs), or, in the absence of a rINN, British Approved Names. Relevant synonyms are included below the title and, in some instances a brief description of the drug action is included. Over future editions these drug action statements will be rolled out for all drugs.

In some monographs, immediately below the nomenclature or drug action, there are a number of cross references used to signpost the user to any additional information they need to consider about a drug. This is most common for drugs formulated in combinations, where users will be signposted to the monographs for the individual ingredients (e.g. senna with ispaghula husk p. 42) or for drugs that are related to a drug class monograph (see Drug class monographs, below).

Indication and dose

User feedback has highlighted that one of the main uses of the BNFC is identifying indications and doses of drugs. Therefore, indication and dose information has been promoted to the top of the monograph and highlighted by a coloured panel to aid quick reference.

The indication and dose section is more highly structured than in earlier editions, giving greater clarity around which doses should be used for which indications and by which route. In addition, if the dose varies with a specific preparation or formulation that dosing information has been moved out of the preparations section and in to the indication and dose panel, under a heading of the preparation name.

Doses are either expressed in terms of a definite frequency (e.g. 1 g 4 times daily) or in the total daily dose format (e.g.

6 g daily in 3 divided doses); the total daily dose should be divided into individual doses (in the second example, the child should receive 2 g 3 times daily).

Doses for specific patient groups (e.g. neonates) may be included if they are different to the standard dose. Doses for children can be identified by the relevant age range and may vary according to their age or body-weight.

Selecting the dose

The dose of a drug may vary according to different indications, routes of administration, age, body-weight, and body surface area. The right dose should be selected for the right age and body-weight (or body surface area) of the child, as well as for the right indication, route of administration, and preparation.

In earlier editions of the BNFC, age ranges and weight ranges overlapped. For clarity and to aid selection of the correct dose, wherever possible these age and weight ranges now do not overlap. When interpreting age ranges it is important to understand that a child is considered to be 11 up until the point of their 12th birthday, meaning that an age range of child 12 to 17 years is applicable to a child from the day of their 12th birthday until the day before their 18th birthday. All age ranges should be interpreted in this way. Similarly, when interpreting weight ranges, it should be understood that a weight of up to 30 kg is applicable to a child up to, but not including, the point that they tip the scales at 30 kg and a weight range of 35 to 59 kg is applicable to a child as soon as they tip the scales at 35 kg right up until, but not including, the point that they tip the scales at 60 kg. All weight ranges should be interpreted in this way.

A pragmatic approach should be applied to these cut-off points depending on the child's physiological development, condition, and if weight is appropriate for the child's age.

For some drugs (e.g. vancomycin p. 305) the neonatal dose varies according to the *corrected gestational* age of the neonate. Corrected gestational age is the neonate's total age expressed in weeks from the start of the mother's last menstrual period. For example, a 3 week old baby born at 27 weeks gestation is treated as having a corrected gestational age of 30 weeks. A term baby has a corrected gestational age of 37–42 weeks when born. For most other drugs, the dose can be based on the child's actual date of birth irrespective of corrected gestational age. However, the degree of prematurity, the maturity of renal and hepatic function, and the clinical properties of the drug need to be considered on an individual basis.

Many children's doses in BNFC are standardised by *body-weight*. To calculate the dose for a given child the weight-standardised dose is multiplied by the child's weight (or occasionally by the child's ideal weight for height). The calculated dose should not normally exceed the maximum recommended dose for an adult. For example, if the dose is 8 mg/kg (max. 300 mg), a child of 10 kg body-weight should receive 80 mg, but a child of 40 kg body-weight should receive 300 mg (rather than 320 mg). Calculation by body-weight in the overweight child may result in much higher doses being administered than necessary; in such cases, the dose should be calculated from an ideal weight for height.

Occasionally, some doses in BNFC are standardised by *body surface area* because many physiological phenomena correlate better with body surface area. In these cases, to calculate the dose for a given child, the body surface area-standardised dose is multiplied by the child's body surface area. The child's body surface area can be estimated from his or her weight using the tables for Body surface area in children, see inside back cover.

Wherever possible, doses are expressed in terms of a definite frequency (e.g. if the dose is 1 mg/kg twice daily, a child of body-weight 9 kg would receive 9 mg twice daily).

Occasionally, it is necessary to include doses in the total daily dose format (e.g. 10 mg/kg daily in 3 divided doses); in these cases the total daily dose should be divided into individual doses (in this example a child of body-weight 9 kg would receive 30 mg 3 times daily).

Most drugs can be administered at slightly irregular intervals during the day. Some drugs, e.g. antimicrobials, are best given at regular intervals. Some flexibility should be allowed in children to avoid waking them during the night. For example, the night-time dose may be given at the child's bedtime.

Special care should be taken when converting doses from one metric unit to another, and when calculating infusion rates or the volume of a preparation to administer. Where possible, doses should be rounded to facilitate administration of suitable volumes of liquid preparations, or an appropriate strength of tablet or capsule.

Other information relevant to Indication and dose
The dose panel also contains, where known, an indication of **pharmacokinetic considerations** that may affect the choice of dose, and **dose equivalence** information, which may aid the selection of dose when switching between drugs or preparations.

The BNFC includes **unlicensed use** of medicines when the clinical need cannot be met by licensed medicines; such use should be supported by appropriate evidence and experience. When the BNFC recommends an unlicensed medicine or the 'off-label' use of a licensed medicine, this is shown below the indication and dose panel in the unlicensed use section.

Minimising harm and drug safety
The drug chosen to treat a particular condition should minimise the patient's susceptibility to adverse effects and, where co-morbidities exist, have minimal detrimental effects on the patient's other diseases. To achieve this, the *Contra-indications*, *Cautions* and *Side-effects* of the relevant drug should be reviewed.

The information under Cautions can be used to assess the risks of using a drug in a patient who has co-morbidities that are also included in the Cautions for that drug—if a safer alternative cannot be found, the drug may be prescribed while monitoring the patient for adverse-effects or deterioration in the co-morbidity. Contra-indications are far more restrictive than Cautions and mean that the drug should be avoided in a patient with a condition that is contra-indicated.

The impact that potential side-effects may have on a patient's quality of life should also be assessed. For instance, in a child who has constipation, it may be preferable to avoid a drug that frequently causes constipation.

Clinically relevant *Side-effects* for drugs are included in the monographs or drug class monographs. Side-effects are listed in order of frequency, where known, and arranged alphabetically. The frequency of side-effects follows the regulatory standard:

- Very common — occurs more frequently than 1 in 10 administrations of a drug
- Common — occurs between 1 in 10 and 1 in 100 administrations of a drug
- Uncommon — between 1 in 100 and 1 in 1,000 administrations of a drug
- Rare — between 1 in 1,000 and 1 in 10,000 administrations of a drug
- Very rare — occurs less than 1 in 10,000 administrations of a drug
- Frequency not known

An exhaustive list of side-effects is not included, particularly for drugs that are used by specialists (e.g. cytotoxic drugs and drugs used in anaesthesia). The BNFC also omits effects that are likely to have little clinical consequence (e.g. transient increase in liver enzymes).

Recognising that hypersensitivity reactions can occur with virtually all medicines, this effect is generally not listed, unless the drug carries an increased risk of such reactions, when the information is included under *Allergy and cross sensitivity*.

The *Important safety advice* section in the BNFC, delineated by a coloured outline box, highlights important safety concerns, often those raised by regulatory authorities or guideline producers. Safety warnings issued by the Commission on Human Medicines (CHM) or Medicines and Healthcare products Regulatory Agency (MHRA) are found here.

Drug selection should aim to minimise drug interactions. If it is necessary to prescribe a potentially serious combination of drugs, patients should be monitored appropriately. The mechanisms underlying drug interactions are explained in Appendix 1, followed by details of drug interactions.

Use of drugs in specific patient populations
Drug selection should aim to minimise the potential for drug accumulation, adverse drug reactions, and exacerbation of pre-existing hepatic or renal disease. If it is necessary to prescribe drugs whose effect is altered by hepatic or renal disease, appropriate drug dose adjustments should be made, and patients should be monitored adequately. The general principles for prescribing are outlined under *Prescribing in hepatic impairment* p. 15, and *Prescribing in renal impairment* p. 15. Information about drugs that should be avoided or used with caution in hepatic disease or renal impairment can be found in drug monographs under *Hepatic impairment* and *Renal impairment* (e.g. fluconazole p. 352).

Similarly, drug selection should aim to minimise harm to the fetus, nursing infant, and mother. The infant should be monitored for potential side-effects of drugs used by the *mother during pregnancy or breast-feeding*. The general principles for prescribing are outlined under Prescribing in pregnancy p. 17 and Prescribing in breast-feeding p. 17. The Treatment Summaries provide guidance on the drug treatment of common conditions that can occur during pregnancy and breast-feeding (e.g. Asthma p. 138). Information about the use of specific drugs during pregnancy and breast-feeding can be found in their drug monographs under *Pregnancy*, and *Breast-feeding* (e.g. fluconazole p. 352).

A new section, *Conception and contraception*, containing information around considerations for females of childbearing potential or men who might father a child (e.g. isotretinoin p. 712) has been included.

Administration and monitoring
When selecting the most appropriate drug, it may be necessary to screen the patient for certain genetic markers or metabolic states. This information is included within a section called *Pre-treatment screening* (e.g. abacavir p. 390). This section covers one-off tests required to assess the suitability of a patient for a particular drug.

Once the drug has been selected, it needs to be given in the most appropriate manner. A *Directions for administration* section contains the information about intravenous administration previously located in Appendix 4. This provides practical information on the preparation of intravenous drug infusions, including compatibility of drugs with standard intravenous infusion fluids, method of dilution or reconstitution, and administration rates. In addition, general advice relevant to other routes of administration is provided within this section (e.g. fentanyl p. 262) and further details, such as masking the bitter taste of some medicines.

Whenever possible, intramuscular injections should be **avoided** in children because they are painful.

After selecting and administering the most appropriate drug by the most appropriate route, patients should be monitored to ensure they are achieving the expected benefits from drug treatment without any unwanted side-effects. The *Monitoring* section specifies any special monitoring requirements, including information on monitoring the plasma concentration of drugs with a narrow therapeutic index (e.g. theophylline p. 159). Monitoring may, in certain cases, be affected by the impact of a drug on laboratory tests (e.g. hydroxocobalamin p. 534), and this information is included in *Effects on laboratory tests*.

In some cases, when a drug is withdrawn, further monitoring or precautions may be advised (e.g. clonidine hydrochloride p. 93); these are covered under *Treatment cessation*.

Choice and supply
The prescriber, the child's carer, and the child (if appropriate) should agree on the health outcomes desired and on the strategy for achieving them (see *Taking Medicines to Best Effect*). Taking the time to explain to the child (and the child's carer if appropriate) the rationale and the potential adverse effects of treatment may improve adherence. For some medicines there is a special need for counselling (e.g. appropriate posture during administration of doxycycline p. 332, or recognising signs of blood, liver, or skin disorders with carbamazepine p. 184); this is shown in *Patient and carer advice*.

Other information contained in the latter half of the monograph also helps prescribers and those dispensing medicines choose medicinal forms (by indicating information such as flavour or when branded products are not interchangeable e.g. modified-release theophylline p. 159), assess the suitability of a drug for prescribing, understand the NHS funding status for a drug (e.g. sildenafil p. 111), or assess when a patient may be able to purchase a drug without prescription (e.g. loperamide hydrochloride p. 44).

Medicinal forms
In the BNFC, preparations follow immediately after the monograph for the drug that is their main ingredient.

In earlier editions, when a particular preparation had safety information, dose advice or other clinical information specific to the product, it was contained within the preparations section. This information has been moved to the relevant section in the main body of the monograph under a heading of the name of the specific medicinal form (e.g. peppermint oil p. 32).

The medicinal forms (formerly preparations) section provides information on the type of formulation (e.g. tablet), the amount of active drug in a solid dosage form, and the concentration of active drug in a liquid dosage form. The legal status is shown for prescription-only medicines and controlled drugs, as well as pharmacy medicines and medicines on the general sales list. Practitioners are reminded, by a statement under the heading of "Medicinal Form" that not all products containing a specific drug ingredient may be similarly licensed. To be clear on the precise licensing status of specific medicinal forms, practitioners should check the product literature for the particular product being prescribed or dispensed.

Details of all medicinal forms available on the dm+d for each drug in BNF Publications appears online on MedicinesComplete. In print editions, due to space constraints, only certain branded products are included in detail. Where medicinal forms are listed they should not be inferred as equivalent to the other brands listed under the same form heading. For example, all the products listed under a heading of "Modified release capsule" will be available as modified release capsules, however, the brands listed under that form heading may have different release profiles, the available strengths may vary and/or the

products may have different licensing information. As with earlier editions of the BNFC, practitioners must ensure that the particular product being prescribed or dispensed is appropriate.

As medicinal forms are derived from dm+d data, some drugs may appear under names derived from that data; this may vary slightly from those in earlier BNFC versions, e.g. sodium acid phosphate, is now sodium dihydrogen phosphate anhydrous.

Children should be prescribed a preparation that complements their daily routine, and that provides the right dose of drug for the right indication and route of administration. When dispensing liquid preparations, a sugar-free preparation should always be used in preference to one containing sugar. Patients receiving medicines containing cariogenic sugars should be advised of appropriate dental hygiene measures to prevent caries.

Earlier editions of the BNFC only included excipients and electrolyte information for proprietary medicines. This information is now covered at the level of the dose form (e.g. tablet). It is not possible to keep abreast of all of the generic products available on the UK market, and so this information serves as a reminder to the healthcare professional that, if the presence of a particular excipient is of concern, they should check the product literature for the particular product being prescribed or dispensed.

Cautionary and advisory labels that pharmacists are recommended to add when dispensing are included in the medicinal forms section. Details of these labels can be found in Appendix 3, Guidance for cautionary and advisory labels p. 966. These labels have now been applied at the level of the dose form.

In the case of compound preparations, the prescribing information for all constituents should be taken into account.

Prices in the BNFC
Basic NHS **net prices** are given in the BNFC to provide an indication of relative cost. Where there is a choice of suitable preparations for a particular disease or condition the relative cost may be used in making a selection. Cost-effective prescribing must, however, take into account other factors (such as dose frequency and duration of treatment) that affect the total cost. The use of more expensive drugs is justified if it will result in better treatment of the patient, or a reduction of the length of an illness, or the time spent in hospital.

Prices are regularly updated using the Drug Tariff and proprietary price information published by the NHS dictionary of medicines and devices (dm+d, www.dmd.nhs.uk). The weekly updated dm+d data (including prices) can be accessed using the dm+d browser of the NHS Business Services Authority (https://apps.nhsbsa.nhs.uk/DMDBrowser/DMDBrowser.do). Prices have been calculated from the net cost used in pricing NHS prescriptions and generally reflect whole dispensing packs. Prices for extemporaneously prepared preparations are not provided in the BNFC as prices vary between different manufacturers.

BNFC prices are not suitable for quoting to patients seeking private prescriptions or contemplating over-the-counter purchases because they do not take into account VAT, professional fees, and other overheads.

A fuller explanation of costs to the NHS may be obtained from the Drug Tariff. Separate drug tariffs are applicable to England and Wales (www.ppa.org.uk/ppa/edt_intro.htm), Scotland (www.isdscotland.org/Health-Topics/Prescribing-and-Medicines/Scottish-Drug-Tariff/), and Northern Ireland (www.hscbusiness.hscni.net/services/2034.htm); prices in the different tariffs may vary.

Typical layout of a monograph and associated medicinal forms

❶ Class Monographs and drug monographs
In most cases, all information that relates to an individual drug is contained in its drug monograph and there is no symbol. Class monographs have been created where substantial amounts of information are common to all drugs within a drug class, these are indicated by a flag symbol in a circle:

Drug monographs with a corresponding class monograph are indicated by a tab with a flag symbol: ⚑ 1234

The page number of the corresponding class monograph is indicated within the tab. For further information, see How to use BNF Publications

❷ Drug classifications
Used to inform users of the class of a drug and to assist in finding other drugs of the same class. May be based on pharmacological class (e.g. opioids) but can also be associated with the use of the drug (e.g. cough suppressants)

❸ Review date
The date of last review of the content

❹ Specific preparation name
If the dose varies with a specific preparation or formulation it appears under a heading of the preparation name

❺ Evidence grading
Evidence grading to reflect the strengths of recommendations will be applied as content goes through the revalidation process. A five level evidence grading system based on the former SIGN grading system has been adopted. The grades Ⓐ Ⓑ Ⓒ Ⓓ Ⓔ are displayed next to the recommendations within the text, and are preceded by the symbol: EvGr

For further information, see How BNF Publications are constructed

---

Class monograph ❶

CLASSIFICATION ❷   ⚑ 1234

❘ Drug monograph ❶   **❸** 1.6.2016

(Synonym) another name by which a drug may be known
● DRUG ACTION how a drug exerts its effect in the body

● **INDICATIONS AND DOSE**
Indications are the clinical reasons a drug is used. The dose of a drug will often depend on the indications
Indication
▸ ROUTE
▸ Age groups: [Neonate/Child]
   Dose and frequency of administration (max. dose)
SPECIFIC PREPARATION NAME ❹
Indication
▸ ROUTE
▸ Age groups: [Neonate/Child]
   Dose and frequency of administration (max. dose)
DOSE EQUIVALENCE AND CONVERSION information around the bioequivalence between formulations of the same drug, or equivalent doses of drugs that are members of the same class
PHARMACOKINETICS how the body affects a drug (absorption, distribution, metabolism, and excretion)
POTENCY a measure of drug activity expressed in terms of the concentration required to produce an effect of given intensity
DOSES AT EXTREMES OF BODY-WEIGHT dosing information for patients who are overweight or underweight

● **UNLICENSED USE** describes the use of medicines outside the terms of their UK licence (off-label use), or use of medicines that have no licence for use in the UK

> **IMPORTANT SAFETY INFORMATION**
> Information produced and disseminated by drug regulators often highlights serious risks associated with the use of a drug, and may include advice that is mandatory

● **CONTRA-INDICATIONS** circumstances when a drug should be avoided
● **CAUTIONS** details of precautions required
● **INTERACTIONS** when one drug changes the effects of another drug; the mechanisms underlying drug interactions are explained in Appendix 1
● **SIDE-EFFECTS** listed in order of frequency, where known, and arranged alphabetically
● **ALLERGY AND CROSS-SENSITIVITY** for drugs that carry an increased risk of hypersensitivity reactions
● **CONCEPTION AND CONTRACEPTION** potential for a drug to have harmful effects on an unborn child when prescribing for a woman of childbearing age or for a man trying to father a child; information on the effect of drugs on the efficacy of latex condoms or diaphragms
● **PREGNANCY** advice on the use of a drug during pregnancy
● **BREAST FEEDING** EvGr advice on the use of a drug during breast feeding Ⓐ ❺

- **HEPATIC IMPAIRMENT** advice on the use of a drug in hepatic impairment
- **RENAL IMPAIRMENT** advice on the use of a drug in renal impairment
- **PRE-TREATMENT SCREENING** covers one off tests required to assess the suitability of a patient for a particular drug
- **MONITORING REQUIREMENTS** specifies any special monitoring requirements, including information on monitoring the plasma concentration of drugs with a narrow therapeutic index
- **EFFECTS ON LABORATORY TESTS** for drugs that can interfere with the accuracy of seemingly unrelated laboratory tests
- **TREATMENT CESSATION** specifies whether further monitoring or precautions are advised when the drug is withdrawn
- **DIRECTIONS FOR ADMINISTRATION** practical information on the preparation of intravenous drug infusions; general advice relevant to other routes of administration
- **PRESCRIBING AND DISPENSING INFORMATION** practical information around how a drug can be prescribed and dispensed including details of when brand prescribing is necessary
- **HANDLING AND STORAGE** includes information on drugs that can cause adverse effects to those who handle them before they are taken by, or administered to, a patient; advice on storage conditions
- **PARENT AND CARER ADVICE** for drugs with a special need for counselling
- **PROFESSION SPECIFIC INFORMATION** provides details of the restrictions certain professions such as dental practitioners or nurse prescribers need to be aware of when prescribing on the NHS
- **NATIONAL FUNDING/ACCESS DECISIONS** details of NICE Technology Appraisals and SMC advice
- **LESS SUITABLE FOR PRESCRIBING** preparations that are considered by the Paediatric Formulary Committee to be less suitable for prescribing
- **EXCEPTION TO LEGAL CATEGORY** advice and information on drugs which may be sold without a prescription under specific conditions

---

- **MEDICINAL FORMS**
  Form
  CAUTIONARY AND ADVISORY LABELS if applicable
  EXCIPIENTS clinically important but not comprehensive [consult manufacturer information for full details]
  ELECTROLYTES if clinically significant quantities occur
  ▸ Preparation name (Manufacturer/Non-proprietary)
  Drug name and strength pack sizes PoM ❻ Prices

  Combinations available this indicates a combination preparation is available and a cross reference page number is provided to locate this preparation

❻ Legal categories

PoM This symbol has been placed against those preparations that are available only on a prescription issued by an appropriate practitioner. For more detailed information see *Medicines, Ethics and Practice*, London, Pharmaceutical Press (always consult latest edition)

CD1 CD2 CD3 CD4–1 CD4–2 These symbols indicate that the preparations are subject to the prescription requirements of the Misuse of Drugs Act

For regulations governing prescriptions for such preparations, see Controlled Drugs and Drug Dependence

Not all monographs include all possible sections; sections are only included when relevant information has been identified

Drug class monographs

In earlier editions of the BNFC, information relating to a class of drug sharing the same properties (e.g. tetracyclines p. 332), was contained within the prescribing notes. In the updated structure, drug class monographs have been created to contain the common information; this ensures such information is easier to find, and has a more regularised structure.

For consistency and ease of use, the class monograph follows the same structure as a drug monograph. Class monographs are indicated by the presence of a flag ○ (e.g. beta-adrenoceptor blockers (systemic) p. 95). If a drug monograph has a corresponding class monograph, that needs to be considered in tandem, in order to understand the full information about a drug, the monograph is also indicated by a flag ⌐1234 (e.g. metoprolol tartrate p. 98). Within this flag, the page number of the drug class monograph is provided (e.g. 1234), to help navigate the user to this information. This is particularly useful where occasionally, due to differences in therapeutic use, the drug monograph may not directly follow the drug class monograph (e.g. sotalol hydrochloride p. 74).

Evidence grading

The BNF has adopted a five level evidence grading system (see How BNF Publications are constructed p. ix). Recommendations that are evidence graded can be identified by a symbol appearing immediately before the recommendation. The evidence grade is displayed at the end of the recommendation.

Other content

Nutrition

Appendix 2 includes tables of ACBS-approved enteral feeds and nutritional supplements based on their energy and protein content. There are separate tables for specialised formulae for specific clinical conditions. Classified sections on foods for special diets and nutritional supplements for metabolic diseases are also included.

Other useful information

Finding significant changes in the BNFC

- *Changes*, provides a list of significant changes, dose changes, classification changes, new names, and new preparations that have been incorporated into the BNFC, as well as a list of preparations that have been discontinued and removed from the BNFC. Changes listed online are cumulative (from one print edition to the next), and can be printed off each month to show the main changes since the last print edition as an aide memoire for those using print copies. So many changes are made for each update of the BNFC, that not all of them can be accommodated in the *Changes* section. We encourage healthcare professionals to review regularly the prescribing information on drugs that they encounter frequently;

- *Changes to the Dental Practitioners' Formulary*, are located at the end of the Dental List;

- *E-newsletter*, the BNF & BNFC e-newsletter service is available free of charge. It alerts healthcare professionals to details of significant changes in the clinical content of these publications and to the way that this information is delivered. Newsletters also review clinical case studies, provide tips on using these publications effectively, and highlight forthcoming changes to the publications. To sign up for e-newsletters go to www.bnf.org.

- An e-learning programme developed in collaboration with the Centre for Pharmacy Postgraduate Education (CPPE), enables pharmacists to identify and assess how significant changes in the BNF affect their clinical practice. The module can be found at www.cppe.ac.uk.

Using other sources for medicines information

The BNFC is designed as a digest for rapid reference. Less detail is given on areas such as malignant disease and anaesthesia since it is expected that those undertaking treatment will have specialist knowledge and access to specialist literature. The BNFC should be interpreted in the light of professional knowledge and supplemented as necessary by specialised publications and by reference to the product literature. Information is also available from medicines information services.

Changes

Monthly updates are provided online via MedicinesComplete and the NHS Evidence portal. The changes listed below are cumulative (from one print edition to the next).

Significant changes

Significant changes that will appear in the print edition of *BNF for Children* 2016–2017:

- Abatacept p. 598, adalimumab p. 598, etanercept p. 600 and tocilizumab p. 597 for treating juvenile idiopathic arthritis [NICE guidance]
- Asthma: updated guidance on management of chronic asthma and acute asthma.
- Adalimumab p. 598: new indications [enthesitis-related arthritis and chronic plaque psoriasis].
- Bisphosphonates: risk of osteonecrosis of the external auditory canal [MHRA/CHM advice].
- Drug allergy (suspected or confirmed): new guidance.
- Intra-uterine contraception (intra-uterine contraceptive devices (copper) p. 471 and levonorgestrel p. 475): uterine perforation—updated information on risk factors [MHRA/CHM advice].
- Intravenous bisphosphonates: osteonecrosis of the jaw—further measures to minimise risk [MHRA advice].
- Isoflurane p. 761 is not recommended for induction of anaesthesia in infants and children of all ages [MHRA advice].
- Latanoprost (*Xalatan*®) p. 641 —increased reporting of eye irritation since reformulation [MHRA advice].
- Levonorgestrel releasing intra-uterine device p. 475: brand name prescribing [MHRA/CHM advice].
- Live attenuated vaccines [MHRA/CHM advice].
- Meningococcal group B vaccine, meningococcal groups A, C, W135 and Y vaccine, and influenza vaccine added to the childhood Immunisation Schedule (Summer 2015), see Vaccines p. 731.
- Mycophenolate mofetil p. 492: new pregnancy-prevention advice for women and men.
- Obesity: updated guidance on management.
- Proton pump inhibitors: very low risk of subacute cutaneous lupus erythematosus [MHRA advice].
- Sodium valproate p. 195 and risk of abnormal pregnancy outcomes [updated MHRA/CHM advice].
- Valproic acid p. 200 and risk of abnormal pregnancy outcomes [updated MHRA/CHM advice].

Dose changes

Changes in dose statements that will appear in the print edition of *BNF for Children* 2016–2017:

- Ceftriaxone p. 302
- Colistimethate sodium p. 326 [*Promixin*®]
- Diamorphine hydrochloride p. 261 [licensed intranasal dose]
- Hydroxyzine hydrochloride p. 169
- Insulin degludec p. 424 [licensed in children over 1 year]
- Nystatin p. 663
- Oseltamivir p. 399

Classification changes

Classification changes that will appear in the print edition of *BNF for Children* 2016–2017:

New names

Name changes that will appear in the print edition of *BNF for Children* 2016–2017:

Deleted preparations

Preparations discontinued in the print edition of *BNF for Children* 2016–2017:

- Phenoxybenzamine injection
- *TriNovum*® tablets [ethinylestradiol with norethisterone p. 471].

New preparations

New preparations that will appear in the print edition of *BNF for Children* 2016–2017:

- *Ayendi*® [diamorphine hydrochloride p. 261]
- *Intuniv*® [guanfacine p. 217]
- *Levosert*® [levonorgestrel p. 475]
- *Nuwiq*® [simoctocog alfa (factor VIII fraction, dried p. 78)]
- *Orphacol*® [cholic acid p. 60]
- *Tresiba*® [insulin degludec p. 424]

Guidance on prescribing

General guidance

Medicines should be given to children only when they are necessary, and in all cases the potential benefit of administering the medicine should be considered in relation to the risk involved. This is particularly important during pregnancy, when the risk to both mother and fetus must be considered.

It is important to discuss treatment options carefully with the child and the child's carer. In particular, the child and the child's carer should be helped to distinguish the adverse effects of prescribed drugs from the effects of the medical disorder. When the beneficial effects of the medicine are likely to be delayed, this should be highlighted.

Taking medicines to best effect

Difficulties in adherence to drug treatment occur regardless of age. Factors that contribute to poor compliance with prescribed medicines include:

- difficulty in taking the medicine (e.g. inability to swallow the medicine);
- unattractive formulation (e.g. unpleasant taste);
- prescription not collected or not dispensed;
- purpose of medicine not clear;
- perceived lack of efficacy;
- real or perceived adverse effects;
- carers' or child's perception of the risk and severity of side-effects may differ from that of the prescriber;
- instructions for administration not clear.

The prescriber, the child's carer, and the child (if appropriate) should agree on the health outcomes desired and on the strategy for achieving them ('concordance'). The prescriber should be sensitive to religious, cultural, and personal beliefs of the child's family that can affect acceptance of medicines.

Taking the time to explain to the child (and carers) the rationale and the potential adverse effects of treatment may improve adherence. Reinforcement and elaboration of the physician's instructions by the pharmacist and other members of the healthcare team can e improve adherence. Giving advice on the management of adverse effects and the possibility of alternative treatments may encourage carers and children to seek advice rather than merely abandon unacceptable treatment.

Simplifying the drug regimen may help; the need for frequent administration may reduce adherence, although there appears to be little difference in adherence between once-daily and twice-daily administration. Combination products reduce the number of drugs taken but at the expense of the ability to titrate individual doses.

Drug treatment in children

Children, and particularly neonates, differ from adults in their response to drugs. Special care is needed in the neonatal period (first 28 days of life) and doses should always be calculated with care; the risk of toxicity is increased by a reduced rate of drug clearance and differing target organ sensitivity. The terms infant, child and adolescent are used inconsistently in the literature. However, **for reference purposes only**, the terms generally used to describe the paediatric stages of development are:

Preterm neonate	Born at < 37 weeks gestation
Term neonate	Born at 37 to 42 weeks gestation
Post-term neonate	Born at $\geq$42 weeks gestation
Neonate	From 0 up to 28 days of age (or first 4 weeks of life)
Infant	From 28 days up to 24 months of age
Child	From 2 years up to 12 years of age
Adolescent	From 12 years up to 18 years of age

In BNF for *Children*, the term neonate is used to describe a newborn infant aged 0–28 days. The terms child or children are used generically to describe the entire range from infant to adolescent (1 month–17 years). An age range is specified when the dose information applies to a narrower age range than a child from 1 month–17 years.

Administration of medicines to children

Children should be involved in decisions about taking medicines and encouraged to take responsibility for using them correctly. The degree of such involvement will depend on the child's age, understanding, and personal circumstances.

Occasionally a medicine or its taste has to be disguised or masked with small quantities of food. However, unless specifically permitted (e.g. some formulations of pancreatin p. 66), a medicine should **not** be mixed with large quantities of food because the full dose might not be taken and the child might develop an aversion to food if the medicine imparts an unpleasant taste. Medicines should not be mixed or administered in a baby's feeding bottle.

Children under 5 years (and some older children) find a liquid formulation more acceptable than tablets or capsules. However, for long-term treatment it may be possible for a child to be taught to take tablets or capsules.

An oral syringe should be used for accurate measurement and controlled administration of an oral liquid medicine. The unpleasant taste of an oral liquid can be disguised by flavouring it or by giving a favourite food or drink immediately afterwards, but the potential for food-drug interactions should be considered.

Advice should be given on dental hygiene to those receiving medicines containing cariogenic sugars for long-term treatment; sugar-free medicines should be provided whenever possible.

Children with nasal feeding tubes in place for prolonged periods should be encouraged to take medicines by mouth if possible; enteric feeding should generally be interrupted before the medicine is given (particularly if enteral feeds reduce the absorption of a particular drug). Oral liquids can be given through the tube provided that precautions are taken to guard against blockage; the dose should be washed down with warm water. When a medicine is given through a nasogastric tube to a neonate, **sterile water** must be used to accompany the medicine or to wash it down.

The intravenous route is generally chosen when a medicine cannot be given by mouth; reliable access, often a central vein, should be used for children whose treatment involves irritant or inotropic drugs or who need to receive the medicine over a long period or for home therapy. The subcutaneous route is used most commonly for insulin administration. Intramuscular injections should preferably be **avoided** in children, particularly neonates, infants, and young children. However, the intramuscular route may be advantageous for administration of single doses of medicines when intravenous cannulation would be more problematic or painful to the child. Certain drugs, e.g. some vaccines, are only administered intramuscularly. The intrathecal, epidural and intraosseous routes should be used **only** by staff specially trained to administer medicines by these routes. Local protocols for the management of intrathecal injections must be in place.

Managing medicines in school

Administration of a medicine during schooltime should be avoided if possible; medicines should be prescribed for once or twice-daily administration whenever practicable. If the medicine needs to be taken in school, this should be discussed with parents or carers and the necessary arrangements made in advance; where appropriate, involvement of a school nurse should be sought. *Managing Medicines in Schools and Early Years Settings* produced by the Department of Health provides guidance on using medicines in schools (www.dh.gov.uk).

Patient information leaflets

Manufacturers' patient information leaflets that accompany a medicine, cover only the licensed use of the medicine. Therefore, when a medicine is used outside its licence, it may be appropriate to advise the child and the child's parent or carer that some of the information in the leaflet might not apply to the child's treatment. Where necessary, inappropriate advice in the patient information leaflet should be identified and reassurance provided about the correct use in the context of the child's condition.

Biosimilar medicines

A biosimilar medicine is a new biological product that is similar to a medicine that has already been authorised to be marketed (the biological reference medicine) in the European Union. The active substance of a biosimilar medicine is similar, but not identical, to the biological reference medicine. Biological products are different from standard chemical products in terms of their complexity and although theoretically there should be no important differences between the biosimilar and biological reference medicine in terms of safety or efficacy, when prescribing biological products, it is good practice to use the brand name. This will ensure that substitution of a biosimilar medicine does not occur when the medicine is dispensed. Biosimilar medicines have black triangle status at the time of initial marketing. It is important to report suspected adverse reactions to biosimilar medicines using the Yellow Card Scheme. For biosimilar medicines, adverse reaction reports should clearly state the brand name and the batch number of the suspected medicine.

The following biological medicines are available as biosimilar preparations and should therefore always be prescribed by brand name:

- Epoetin alfa p. 524
- Etanercept p. 600
- Filgrastim p. 538
- Infliximab p. 30
- Insulin glargine p. 424
- Somatropin p. 443

Complementary and alternative medicine

An increasing amount of information on complementary and alternative medicine is becoming available. Where appropriate, the child and the child's carers should be asked about the use of their medicines, including dietary supplements and topical products. The scope of *BNF for Children* is restricted to the discussion of conventional medicines but reference is made to complementary treatments if they affect conventional therapy (e.g. interactions with St John's wort). Further information on herbal medicines is available at www.mhra.gov.uk.

BNF for Children and marketing authorisation

Where appropriate the *doses, indications, cautions, contra-indications,* and *side-effects* in *BNF for Children* reflect those in the manufacturers' Summaries of Product Characteristics (SPCs) which, in turn, reflect those in the corresponding marketing authorisations (formerly known as Product Licences). *BNF for Children* does not generally include proprietary medicines that are not supported by a valid Summary of Product Characteristics or when the marketing authorisation holder has not been able to supply essential information. When a preparation is available from more than one manufacturer, *BNF for Children* reflects advice that is the most clinically relevant regardless of any variation in the marketing authorisation. Unlicensed products can be obtained from 'special-order' manufacturers or specialist importing companies.

As far as possible, medicines should be prescribed within the terms of the marketing authorisation. However, many children require medicines not specifically licensed for paediatric use. Although medicines cannot be promoted outside the limits of the licence, the Human Medicines Regulations 2012 do not prohibit the use of unlicensed medicines.

BNF for Children includes advice involving the use of unlicensed medicines or of licensed medicines for unlicensed uses ('off-label' use). Such advice reflects careful consideration of the options available to manage a given condition and the weight of evidence and experience of the unlicensed intervention. Where the advice falls outside a drug's marketing authorisation, *BNF for Children* shows the licensing status in the drug monograph. However, limitations of the marketing authorisation should not preclude unlicensed use where clinically appropriate.

Prescribing unlicensed medicines Prescribing unlicensed medicines or medicines outside the recommendations of their marketing authorisation alters (and probably increases) the prescriber's professional responsibility and potential liability. The prescriber should be able to justify and feel competent in using such medicines, and also inform the patient or the patient's carer that the prescribed medicine is unlicensed.

Drugs and skilled tasks

Prescribers and other healthcare professionals should advise children and their carers if treatment is likely to affect their ability to perform skilled tasks (e.g. driving). This applies especially to drugs with sedative effects; patients should be warned that these effects are increased by alcohol. General information about a patient's fitness to drive is available from the Driver and Vehicle Licensing Agency at www.dvla.gov.uk.

A new offence of driving, attempting to drive, or being in charge of a vehicle, with certain specified controlled drugs in excess of specified limits, came into force on 2nd March 2015. This offence is an addition to the existing rules on drug impaired driving and fitness to drive, and applies to two groups of drugs—commonly abused drugs, including amfetamines, cannabis, cocaine, and ketamine p. 773, and drugs used mainly for medical reasons, such as opioids and benzodiazepines. Anyone found to have any of the drugs (including related drugs, for example, apomorphine hydrochloride) above specified limits in their blood will be guilty of an offence, whether their driving was impaired or not. This also includes prescribed drugs which metabolise to those included in the offence, for example, selegiline hydrochloride. However, the legislation provides a statutory "medical defence" for patients taking drugs for medical reasons in accordance with instructions, *if their driving was not impaired*—it continues to be an offence to drive if actually impaired. Patients should therefore be advised to continue taking their medicines as prescribed, and when driving, to carry suitable evidence that the drug was prescribed, or sold, to treat a medical or dental problem, and that it was taken according to the instructions given by the prescriber, or information provided with the medicine (e.g. a repeat prescription form or the medicine's patient information leaflet). Further information is available from the Department for Transport at www.gov.uk/government/collections/drug-driving.

Oral syringes

An **oral syringe** is supplied when oral liquid medicines are prescribed in doses other than multiples of 5 mL. The oral syringe is marked in 0.5-mL divisions from 1 to 5 mL to measure doses of less than 5 mL (other sizes of oral syringe may also be available). It is provided with an adaptor and an instruction leaflet. The 5-*mL spoon* is used for doses of 5 mL (or multiples thereof).

Excipients

Branded oral liquid preparations that do not contain *fructose, glucose,* or *sucrose* are described as 'sugar-free' in *BNF for Children*. Preparations containing hydrogenated glucose syrup, mannitol, maltitol, sorbitol, or xylitol are also marked 'sugar-free' since they do not cause dental caries. Children receiving medicines containing cariogenic sugars, or their carers, should be advised of dental hygiene measures to prevent caries. Sugar-free preparations should be used whenever possible, particularly if treatment is required for a long period.

Where information on the presence of *alcohol, aspartame, gluten, sulfites, tartrazine, arachis (peanut) oil* or *sesame oil* is available, this is indicated in *BNF for Children* against the relevant preparation.

Information is provided on *selected excipients* in skin preparations, in vaccines, and on *selected preservatives* and *excipients* in eye drops and injections.

The presence of *benzyl alcohol* and *polyoxyl castor oil* (polyethoxylated castor oil) in injections is indicated in *BNF for Children*. Benzyl alcohol has been associated with a fatal toxic syndrome in preterm neonates, and therefore, parenteral preparations containing the preservative should not be used in neonates. Polyoxyl castor oils, used as vehicles in intravenous injections, have been associated with severe anaphylactoid reactions.

The presence of *propylene glycol* in oral or parenteral medicines is indicated in *BNF for Children*; it can cause adverse effects if its elimination is impaired, e.g. in renal failure, in neonates and young children, and in slow metabolisers of the substance. It may interact with metronidazole p. 313.

The *lactose* content in most medicines is too small to cause problems in most lactose-intolerant children. However in severe lactose intolerance, the lactose content should be determined before prescribing. The amount of lactose varies according to manufacturer, product, formulation, and strength.

Important In the absence of information on excipients in *BNF for Children* and in the product literature (available at www.medicines.org.uk/emc/), contact the manufacturer if it is essential to check details.

Health and safety

When handling chemical or biological materials particular attention should be given to the possibility of allergy, fire, explosion, radiation, or poisoning. Care is required to avoid sources of heat (including hair dryers) when flammable substances are used on the skin or hair. Substances, such as corticosteroids, some antimicrobials, phenothiazines, and many cytotoxics, are irritant or very potent and should be handled with caution; contact with the skin and inhalation of dust should be avoided. Healthcare professionals and carers should guard against exposure to sensitising, toxic or irritant substances if it is necessary to crush tablets or open capsules.

EEA and Swiss prescriptions

Pharmacists can dispense prescriptions issued by doctors and dentists from the European Economic Area (EEA) or Switzerland (except prescriptions for controlled drugs in Schedules 1, 2, or 3, or for drugs without a UK marketing authorisation). Prescriptions should be written in ink or otherwise so as to be indelible, should be dated, should state the name of the patient, should state the address of the prescriber, should contain particulars indicating whether the prescriber is a doctor or dentist, and should be signed by the prescriber.

Security and validity of prescriptions

The Councils of the British Medical Association and the Royal Pharmaceutical Society have issued a joint statement on the security and validity of prescriptions. In particular, prescription forms should:

- not be left unattended at reception desks;
- not be left in a car where they may be visible;
- when not in use, be kept in a locked drawer within the surgery and at home.

Where there is any doubt about the authenticity of a prescription, the pharmacist should contact the prescriber. If this is done by telephone, the number should be obtained from the directory rather than relying on the information on the prescription form, which may be false.

Patient group direction (PGD)

In most cases, the most appropriate clinical care will be provided on an individual basis by a prescriber to a specific child. However, a Patient Group Direction for supply and administration of medicines by other healthcare professionals can be used where it would benefit the child's care without compromising safety.

A Patient Group Direction is a written direction relating to the supply and administration (or administration only) of a licensed prescription-only medicine (including some Controlled Drugs in specific circumstances) by certain classes of healthcare professionals; the Direction is signed by a doctor (or dentist) and by a pharmacist. Further information on Patient Group Directions is available in Health Service Circular HSC 2000/026 (England), HDL (2001) 7 (Scotland), and WHC (2000) 116 (Wales); see also the Human Medicines Regulations 2012.

NICE and Scottish Medicines Consortium

Advice issued by the National Institute for Health and Care Excellence (NICE) is included in *BNF for Children* when relevant. *BNF for Children* also includes advice issued by the Scottish Medicines Consortium (SMC) when a medicine is restricted or not recommended for use within NHS Scotland. If advice within a NICE Single Technology Appraisal differs from SMC advice, the Scottish Executive expects NHS Boards within NHS Scotland to comply with the SMC advice. Details of the advice together with updates can be obtained from www.nice.org.uk and from www.scottishmedicines.org.uk.

Prescription writing

Shared care

In its guidelines on responsibility for prescribing (circular EL (91) 127) between hospitals and general practitioners, the Department of Health has advised that legal responsibility for prescribing lies with the doctor who signs the prescription.

Requirements

Prescriptions should be written legibly in ink or otherwise so as to be indelible (it is permissible to issue carbon copies of NHS prescriptions as long as they are signed in ink), should be dated, should state the name and address of the patient, the address of the prescriber, an indication of the type of prescriber, and should be signed in ink by the prescriber (computer-generated facsimile signatures do not meet the legal requirement). The age and the date of birth of the patient should preferably be stated, and it is a legal requirement in the case of prescription-only medicines to state the age for children under 12 years. These recommendations are acceptable for **prescription-only medicines**. Prescriptions for controlled drugs have additional legal requirements.

Wherever appropriate the prescriber should state the current weight of the child to enable the dose prescribed to be checked. Consideration should also be given to including the dose per unit mass e.g. mg/kg or the dose per m^2 body-surface area e.g. mg/m^2 where this would reduce error. The following should be noted:

- The strength or quantity to be contained in capsules, lozenges, tablets etc. should be stated by the prescriber. In particular, strength of liquid preparations should be clearly stated (e.g. 125 mg/5 mL).
- The unnecessary use of decimal points should be avoided, e.g. 3 mg, not 3.0 mg. Quantities of 1 gram or more should be written as 1 g etc. Quantities less than 1 gram should be written in milligrams, e.g. 500 mg, not 0.5 g. Quantities less than 1 mg should be written in micrograms, e.g. 100 micrograms, not 0.1 mg. When decimals are unavoidable a zero should be written in front of the decimal point where there is no other figure, e.g. 0.5 mL, not .5 mL. Use of the decimal point is acceptable to express a range, e.g. 0.5 to 1 g.
- 'Micrograms' and 'nanograms' should **not** be abbreviated. Similarly 'units' should **not** be abbreviated.
- The term 'millilitre' (ml or mL) is used in medicine and pharmacy, and cubic centimetre, c.c., or cm^3 should not be used. (The use of capital 'L' in mL is a printing convention throughout the BNF; both 'mL' and 'ml' are recognised SI abbreviations).
- Dose and dose frequency should be stated; in the case of preparations to be taken 'as required' a **minimum dose interval** should be specified. Care should be taken to ensure children receive the correct dose of the active drug. Therefore, the dose should normally be stated in terms of the mass of the active drug (e.g. '125 mg 3 times daily'); terms such as '5 mL' or '1 tablet' should be avoided except for compound preparations. When doses other than multiples of 5 mL are prescribed for *oral liquid preparations* the dose-volume will be provided by means of an **oral syringe**, (except for preparations intended to be measured with a pipette). Suitable quantities:
  - Elixirs, Linctuses, and Paediatric Mixtures (5-mL dose), 50, 100, or 150 mL
  - Adult Mixtures (10 mL dose), 200 or 300 mL
  - Ear Drops, Eye drops, and Nasal Drops, 10 mL (or the manufacturer's pack)
  - Eye Lotions, Gargles, and Mouthwashes, 200 mL
- The names of drugs and preparations should be written clearly and **not** abbreviated, using approved titles **only**;

avoid creating generic titles for modified-release preparations).
- The quantity to be supplied may be stated by indicating the number of days of treatment required in the box provided on NHS forms. In most cases the exact amount will be supplied. This does not apply to items directed to be used as required—if the dose and frequency are not given then the quantity to be supplied needs to be stated. When several items are ordered on one form the box can be marked with the number of days of treatment provided the quantity is added for any item for which the amount cannot be calculated.
- Although directions should preferably be in **English without abbreviation**, it is recognised that some Latin abbreviations are used.

Sample prescription

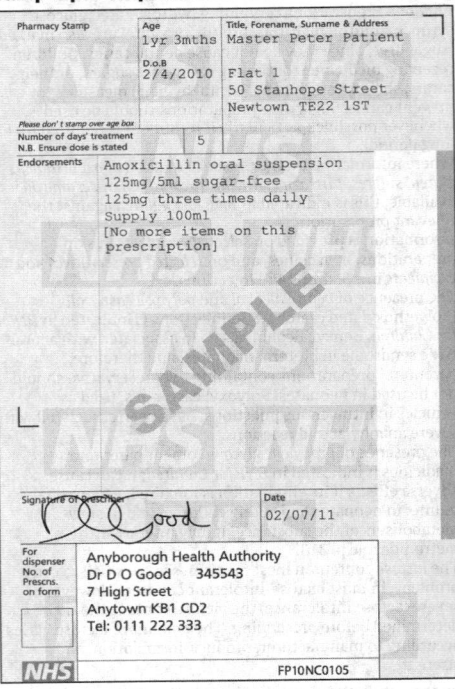

Pharmacy Stamp	Age 1yr 3mths	Title, Forename, Surname & Address Master Peter Patient
	D.o.B 2/4/2010	Flat 1 50 Stanhope Street Newtown TE22 1ST

Please don't stamp over age box

Number of days' treatment N.B. Ensure dose is stated   5

Endorsements

Amoxicillin oral suspension
125mg/5ml sugar-free
125mg three times daily
Supply 100ml
[No more items on this prescription]

Signature of Prescriber   Date 02/07/11

For dispenser No. of Prescns. on form

Anyborough Health Authority
Dr D O Good   345543
7 High Street
Anytown KB1 CD2
Tel: 0111 222 333

NHS   FP10NC0105

Abbreviation of titles In general, titles of drugs and preparations should be written *in full*. Unofficial abbreviations should **not** be used as they may be misinterpreted.

Non-proprietary titles Where non-proprietary ('generic') titles are given, they should be used for prescribing. This will enable any suitable product to be dispensed, thereby saving delay to the patient and sometimes expense to the health service. The only exception is where there is a demonstrable difference in clinical effect between each manufacturer's version of the formulation, making it important that the child should always receive the same brand; in such cases, the brand name or the manufacturer should be stated.

Non-proprietary names of compound preparations Non-proprietary names of **compound preparations** which appear in *BNF for Children* are those that have been compiled by the British Pharmacopoeia Commission or another recognised body; whenever possible they reflect the names of the active ingredients. Prescribers should avoid creating their own compound names for the purposes of generic prescribing; such names do not have an approved definition and can be misinterpreted.

Special care should be taken to avoid errors when prescribing compound preparations; in particular the hyphen in the prefix 'co-' should be retained. Special care should also be taken to avoid creating generic names for **modified-release** preparations where the use of these names could lead to confusion between formulations with different duration of action.

Supply of medicines

Overview
When supplying a medicine for a child, the pharmacist should ensure that the child and the child's carer understand the nature and identity of the medicine and how it should be used. The child and the carer should be provided with appropriate information (e.g. how long the medicine should be taken for and what to do if a dose is missed or the child vomits soon after the dose is given).

Safety in the home
Carers and relatives of children must be warned to keep all medicines out of the reach and sight of children. Tablets, capsules and oral and external liquid preparations must be dispensed in a reclosable *child-resistant container* unless:

- the medicine is in an original pack or patient pack such as to make this inadvisable;
- the child's carer will have difficulty in opening a child-resistant container;
- a specific request is made that the product shall not be dispensed in a child-resistant container;
- no suitable child-resistant container exists for a particular liquid preparation.

All patients should be advised to dispose of *unwanted medicines* by returning them to a pharmacy for destruction.

Labelling of prescribed medicines
There is a legal requirement for the following to appear on the label of any prescribed medicine:

- name of the patient;
- name and address of the supplying pharmacy;
- date of dispensing;
- name of the medicine;
- directions for use of the medicine;
- precautions relating to the use of the medicine.

The Royal Pharmaceutical Society recommends that the following also appears on the label:

- the words 'Keep out of the sight and reach of children';
- where applicable, the words 'Use this medicine only on your skin'.

A pharmacist can exercise professional skill and judgement to amend or include more appropriate wording for the name of the medicine, the directions for use, or the precautions relating to the use of the medicine.

Unlicensed medicines
A drug or formulation that is not covered by a marketing authorisation may be obtained from a pharmaceutical company, imported by a specialist importer, manufactured by a commercial or hospital licensed manufacturing unit, or prepared extemporaneously against a prescription.

The safeguards that apply to products with marketing authorisation should be extended, as far as possible, to the use of unlicensed medicines. The safety, efficacy, and quality (including labelling) of unlicensed medicines should be assured by means of clear policies on their prescribing, purchase, supply, and administration. Extra care is required with unlicensed medicines because less information may be available on the drug and any formulation of the drug.

The following should be agreed with the supplier when ordering an unlicensed or extemporaneously prepared medicine:

- the specification of the formulation;
- documentation confirming the specification and quality of the product supplied (e.g. a certificate of conformity or of analysis);
- for imported preparations product and licensing information should be supplied in English.

Extemporaneous preparations
A product should be dispensed extemporaneously only when no product with a marketing authorisation is available. Every effort should be made to ensure that an extemporaneously prepared product is stable and that it delivers the requisite dose reliably; the child should be provided with a consistent formulation regardless of where the medicine is supplied to minimise variations in quality. Where there is doubt about the formulation, advice should be sought from a medicines information centre, the pharmacy at a children's hospital, a hospital production unit, a hospital quality control department, or the manufacturer.

In many cases it is preferable to give a licensed product by an unlicensed route (e.g. an injection solution given by mouth) than to prepare a special formulation. When tablets or capsules are cut, dispersed, or used for preparing liquids immediately before administration, it is important to confirm uniform dispersal of the active ingredient, especially if only a portion of the solid content (e.g. a tablet segment) is used or if only an aliquot of the liquid is to be administered. In some cases the child's clinical condition may require a dose to be administered in the absence of full information on the method of administration. It is important to ensure that the appropriate supporting information is available at the earliest opportunity.

Preparation of products that produce harmful dust (e.g. cytotoxic drugs, hormones, or potentially sensitising drugs such as neomycin sulfate p. 675) should be **avoided** or undertaken with appropriate precautions to protect staff and carers.

The BP direction that a preparation must be *freshly prepared* indicates that it must be made not more than 24 hours before it is issued for use. The direction that a preparation should be *recently prepared* indicates that deterioration is likely if the preparation is stored for longer than about 4 weeks at 15–25°C.

The term **water** used without qualification means either potable water freshly drawn direct from the public supply and suitable for drinking or freshly boiled and cooled purified water. The latter should be used if the public supply is from a local storage tank or if the potable water is unsuitable for a particular preparation.

Emergency supply of medicines

Emergency supply requested by member of the public

Pharmacists are sometimes called upon by members of the public to make an emergency supply of medicines. The Human Medicines Regulations 2012 allows exemptions from the Prescription Only requirements for emergency supply to be made by a person lawfully conducting a retail pharmacy business provided:

a) that the pharmacist has interviewed the person requesting the prescription-only medicine and is satisfied:

   i) that there is immediate need for the prescription-only medicine and that it is impracticable in the circumstances to obtain a prescription without undue delay;

   ii) that treatment with the prescription-only medicine has on a previous occasion been prescribed for the person requesting it;

   iii) as to the dose that it would be appropriate for the person to take;

b) that no greater quantity shall be supplied than will provide 5 days' treatment of phenobarbital p. 203, *phenobarbital sodium*, or Controlled Drugs in Schedules 4 or 5 (doctors or dentists from the European Economic Area and Switzerland, or their patients, cannot request an emergency supply of Controlled Drugs in Schedules 1, 2, or 3, or drugs that do not have a UK marketing authorisation) or 30 days' treatment for other prescription-only medicines, except when the prescription-only medicine is:

   i) insulin, an ointment or cream, or a preparation for the relief of asthma in an aerosol dispenser when the smallest pack can be supplied;

   ii) an oral contraceptive when a full cycle may be supplied;

   iii) an antibiotic in liquid form for oral administration when the smallest quantity that will provide a full course of treatment can be supplied;

c) that an entry shall be made by the pharmacist in the prescription book stating:

   i) the date of supply;

   ii) the name, quantity and, where appropriate, the pharmaceutical form and strength;

   iii) the name and address of the patient;

   iv) the nature of the emergency;

d) that the container or package must be labelled to show:

   i) the date of supply;

   ii) the name, quantity and, where appropriate, the pharmaceutical form and strength;

   iii) the name of the patient;

   iv) the name and address of the pharmacy;

   v) the words 'Emergency supply';

   vi) the words 'Keep out of the reach of children' (or similar warning);

e) that the prescription-only medicine is not a substance specifically excluded from the emergency supply provision, and does not contain a Controlled Drug specified in Schedules 1, 2, or 3 to the Misuse of Drugs Regulations 2001 except for phenobarbital p. 203 or *phenobarbital sodium* for the treatment of epilepsy: for details see *Medicines, Ethics and Practice,* London, Pharmaceutical Press (always consult latest edition). Doctors or dentists from the European Economic Area and Switzerland, or their patients, cannot request an emergency supply of Controlled Drugs in Schedules 1, 2, or 3, or drugs that do not have a UK marketing authorisation.

Emergency supply requested by prescriber

Emergency supply of a prescription-only medicine may also be made at the request of a doctor, a dentist, a supplementary prescriber, a community practitioner nurse prescriber, a nurse, pharmacist, or optometrist independent prescriber, or a doctor or dentist from the European Economic Area or Switzerland, provided:

a) that the pharmacist is satisfied that the prescriber by reason of some emergency is unable to furnish a prescription immediately;

b) that the prescriber has undertaken to furnish a prescription within 72 hours;

c) that the medicine is supplied in accordance with the directions of the prescriber requesting it;

d) that the medicine is not a Controlled Drug specified in Schedules 1, 2, or 3 to the Misuse of Drugs Regulations 2001 except for phenobarbital p. 203 or *phenobarbital sodium* for the treatment of epilepsy: for details see *Medicines, Ethics and Practice,* London, Pharmaceutical Press (always consult latest edition); (Doctors or dentists from the European Economic Area and Switzerland, or their patients, cannot request an emergency supply of Controlled Drugs in Schedules 1, 2, or 3, or drugs that do not have a UK marketing authorisation).

e) that an entry shall be made in the prescription book stating:

   i) the date of supply;

   ii) the name, quantity and, where appropriate, the pharmaceutical form and strength;

   iii) the name and address of the practitioner requesting the emergency supply;

   iv) the name and address of the patient;

   v) the date on the prescription;

   vi) when the prescription is received the entry should be amended to include the date on which it is received.

Royal Pharmaceutical Society's guidelines

1. The pharmacist should consider the medical consequences of not supplying a medicine in an emergency.

2. If the pharmacist is unable to make an emergency supply of a medicine the pharmacist should advise the patient how to obtain essential medical care.

For conditions that apply to supplies made at the request of a patient see Medicines, Ethics and Practice, London Pharmaceutical Press, (always consult latest edition).

Controlled drugs and drug dependence

Regulations and classification

The Misuse of Drugs Act, 1971 prohibits certain activities in relation to 'Controlled Drugs', in particular their manufacture, supply, and possession. The penalties applicable to offences involving the different drugs are graded broadly according to the *harmfulness attributable to a drug when it is misused* and for this purpose the drugs are defined in the following three classes:

- **Class A** includes: alfentanil p. 772, cocaine, diamorphine hydrochloride (heroin) p. 261, dipipanone hydrochloride, lysergide (LSD), methadone hydrochloride p. 279, methylenedioxymethamfetamine (MDMA, 'ecstasy'), morphine, opium, pethidine hydrochloride p. 269, phencyclidine, remifentanil p. 772, and class B substances when prepared for injection.
- **Class B** includes: oral amfetamines, barbiturates, cannabis, cannabis resin, codeine phosphate p. 259, ethylmorphine, glutethimide, ketamine p. 773, nabilone p. 245, pentazocine, phenmetrazine, and pholcodine p. 176.
- **Class C** includes: certain drugs related to the amfetamines such as benzfetamine and chlorphentermine, buprenorphine p. 257, mazindol, meprobamate, pemoline, pipradrol, most benzodiazepines, tramadol hydrochloride p. 270, zaleplon, zolpidem tartrate, zopiclone, androgenic and anabolic steroids, clenbuterol, chorionic gonadotrophin (HCG), non-human chorionic gonadotrophin, somatotropin, somatrem, and somatropin p. 443.

The Misuse of Drugs Regulations 2001 (and subsequent amendments) define the classes of person who are authorised to supply and possess controlled drugs while acting in their professional capacities and lay down the conditions under which these activities may be carried out. In the regulations drugs are divided into five schedules each specifying the requirements governing such activities as import, export, production, supply, possession, prescribing, and record keeping which apply to them.

- **Schedule 1** includes drugs such as lysergide which is not used medicinally. Possession and supply are prohibited except in accordance with Home Office authority.
- **Schedule 2** includes drugs such as diamorphine hydrochloride (heroin) p. 261, morphine p. 265, nabilone p. 245, remifentanil p. 772, pethidine hydrochloride p. 269, secobarbital, glutethimide, the amfetamines, sodium oxybate and cocaine and are subject to the full controlled drug requirements relating to prescriptions, safe custody (except for secobarbital), the need to keep registers, etc. (unless exempted in Schedule 5).
- **Schedule 3** includes the barbiturates (except secobarbital, now Schedule 2), buprenorphine p. 257, mazindol, meprobamate, midazolam p. 210, pentazocine, phentermine, temazepam p. 774, and tramadol hydrochloride p. 270. They are subject to the special prescription requirements. Safe custody requirements do apply, except for any 5,5 disubstituted barbituric acid (e.g. phenobarbital), mazindol, meprobamate, midazolam p. 210, pentazocine, phentermine, tramadol hydrochloride p. 270, or any stereoisomeric form or salts of the above. Records in registers do not need to be kept (although there are requirements for the retention of invoices for 2 years).
- **Schedule 4** includes in Part I benzodiazepines (except temazepam p. 774 and midazolam p. 210, which are in Schedule 3), zaleplon, zolpidem tartrate, and zopiclone which are subject to minimal control. Part II includes androgenic and anabolic steroids, clenbuterol, chorionic gonadotrophin (HCG), non-human chorionic gonadotrophin, somatotropin, somatrem, and

somatropin p. 443. Controlled drug prescription requirements do not apply and Schedule 4 Controlled Drugs are not subject to safe custody requirements.
- **Schedule 5** includes those preparations which, because of their strength, are exempt from virtually all Controlled Drug requirements other than retention of invoices for two years.

Prescriptions

Preparations in Schedules 2, 3, and 4 of the Misuse of Drugs Regulations 2001 (and subsequent amendments) are identified throughout *BNF for children* using the following symbols:

CD2	for preparations in Schedule 2
CD3	for preparations in Schedule 3
CD4-1	for preparations in Schedule 4 (Part I)
CD4-2	for preparations in Schedule 4 (Part II)

The principal legal requirements relating to medical prescriptions are listed below (see also Department of Health Guidance).

Prescription requirements Prescriptions for Controlled Drugs that are subject to prescription requirements (all preparations in Schedules 2 and 3) must be indelible and must be *signed* by the prescriber, be *dated*, and specify the prescriber's *address*. A machine-written prescription is acceptable, but the prescriber's signature must be handwritten. Advanced electronic signatures can be accepted for Schedule 2 and 3 Controlled Drugs where the Electronic Prescribing Service (EPS) is used. All prescriptions for Controlled Drugs that are subject to prescription requirements must always state:

- the name and address of the patient;
- in the case of a preparation, the form (The dosage form e.g. tablets must be included on a Controlled Drugs prescription irrespective of whether it is implicit in the proprietary name e.g. *MST Continus* or whether only one form is available) and where appropriate the strength (when more than one strength of a preparation exists the strength required must be specified) of the preparation;
- for liquids, the total volume in millilitres (in both words and figures) of the preparation to be supplied; for dosage units, the number (in both words and figures) of dosage units to be supplied; in any other case, the total quantity (in both words and figures) of the Controlled Drug to be supplied;
- the dose (the instruction 'one as directed' constitutes a dose but 'as directed' does not);
- the words 'for dental treatment only' if issued by a dentist.

A pharmacist is **not** allowed to dispense a Controlled Drug unless all the information required by law is given on the prescription. In the case of a prescription for a Controlled Drug in Schedule 2 or 3, a pharmacist can amend the prescription if it specifies the total quantity only in words or in figures or if it contains minor typographical errors, provided that such amendments are indelible and clearly attributable to the pharmacist (implementation date for *N. Ireland* not confirmed). Failure to comply with the regulations concerning the writing of prescriptions will result in inconvenience to patients and delay in supplying the necessary medicine. A prescription for a Controlled Drug in Schedules 2, 3, or 4 is valid for 28 days from the date stated thereon (the prescriber may forward-date the prescription; the start date may also be specified in the body of the prescription).

Instalments and 'repeats'

A prescription may order a Controlled Drug to be dispensed by instalments; the amount of instalments and the intervals to be observed must be specified (A total of 14 days' treatment by instalment of any drug listed in Schedule 2 of the Misuse of Drugs Regulations, buprenorphine p. 257, and diazepam p. 207 may be prescribed in England. In *England*, forms FP10(MDA) (blue) and FP10H (MDA) (blue) should be used. In *Scotland*, forms GP10 (peach), HBP (blue), or HBPA (pink) should be used. In Wales a total of 14 days' treatment by instalment of any drug listed in Schedules 2–5 of the Misuse of Drugs Regulations may be prescribed. In *Wales*, form WP10(MDA) or form WP10HP(AD) should be used. Instalment prescriptions must be dispensed in accordance with the directions in the prescription. However, the Home Office has approved specific wording which may be included in an instalment prescription to cover certain situations; for example, if a pharmacy is closed on the day when an instalment is due. For details, see *Medicines, Ethics and Practice*, London, Pharmaceutical Press (always consult latest edition) or see *Drug Misuse and Dependence: UK Guidelines on Clinical Management* (2007), available at www.nta.nhs.uk/uploads/clinical_guidelines_2007.pdf. Prescriptions ordering 'repeats' on the same form are **not** permitted for Controlled Drugs in Schedules 2 or 3.

Private prescriptions

Private prescriptions for Controlled Drugs in Schedules 2 and 3 must be written on specially designated forms provided by Primary Care Trusts in England, Health Boards in Scotland, Local Health Boards in Wales, or the Northern Ireland Central Services Agency; in addition, prescriptions must specify the *prescriber's identification number*. Prescriptions to be supplied by a pharmacist in hospital are exempt from the requirements for private prescriptions.

Department of Health guidance

Guidance (June 2006) issued by the Department of Health in England on prescribing and dispensing of Controlled Drugs requires:

- in general, prescriptions for Controlled Drugs in Schedules 2, 3, and 4 to be limited to a supply of up to 30 days' treatment; exceptionally, to cover a justifiable clinical need and after consideration of any risk, a prescription can be issued for a longer period, but the reasons for the decision should be recorded on the patient's notes;
- the patient's identifier to be shown on NHS and private prescriptions for Controlled Drugs in Schedules 2 and 3.

Further information is available at www.gov.uk/dh.

See sample prescription:

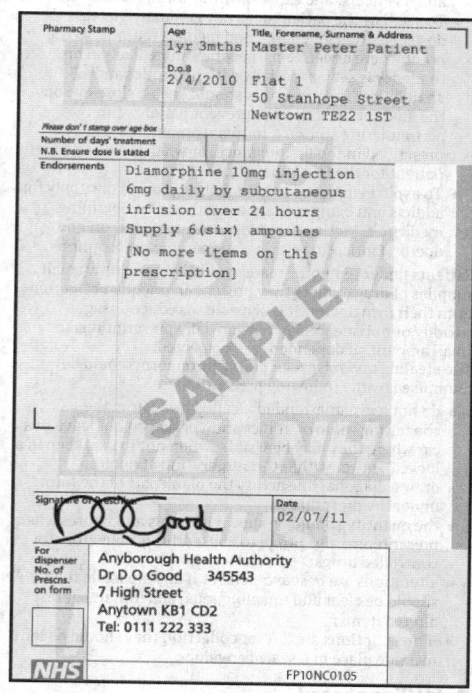

Dependence and misuse

The most serious drugs of addiction are **cocaine**, diamorphine hydrochloride (heroin) p. 261, morphine p. 265, and the **synthetic opioids**.

Despite marked reduction in the prescribing of **amfetamines**, there is concern that abuse of illicit amfetamine and related compounds is widespread. **Benzodiazepines** are commonly misused. However, the misuse of **barbiturates** is now uncommon, in line with declining medicinal use and consequent availability. **Cannabis** (Indian hemp) has no approved medicinal use and cannot be prescribed by doctors. Its use is illegal but widespread. Cannabis is a mild hallucinogen seldom accompanied by a desire to increase the dose; withdrawal symptoms are unusual. However, cannabis extract is licensed as a medicinal product. **Lysergide** (lysergic acid diethylamide, LSD) is a much more potent hallucinogen; its use can lead to severe psychotic states which can be life-threatening.

There are concerns over increases in the availability and misuse of other drugs with variously combined hallucinogenic, anaesthetic, or sedative properties. These include ketamine p. 773 and gamma-hydroxybutyrate (sodium oxybate, GHB).

Prescribing drugs likely to cause dependence or misuse

The prescriber has three main responsibilities:

- To avoid creating dependence by introducing drugs to patients without sufficient reason. In this context, the proper use of the morphine-like drugs is well understood. The dangers of other Controlled Drugs are less clear because recognition of dependence is not easy and its effects, and those of withdrawal, are less obvious.

- To see that the patient does not gradually increase the dose of a drug, given for good medical reasons, to the point where dependence becomes more likely. This tendency is seen especially with hypnotics and anxiolytics. The prescriber should keep a close eye on the amount prescribed to prevent patients from accumulating stocks. A minimal amount should be prescribed in the first instance, or when seeing a new patient for the first time.
- To avoid being used as an unwitting source of supply for addicts and being vigilant to methods for obtaining medicines. Methods include visiting more than one doctor, fabricating stories, and forging prescriptions.

Patients under temporary care should be given only small supplies of drugs unless they present an unequivocal letter from their own doctor. It is sensible to reduce dosages steadily or to issue weekly or even daily prescriptions for small amounts if dependence is suspected.

The stealing and misuse of prescription forms could be minimised by the following precautions:

- do not leave unattended if called away from the consulting room or at reception desks; do not leave in a car where they may be visible; when not in use, keep in a locked drawer within the surgery and at home;
- draw a diagonal line across the blank part of the form under the prescription;
- the quantity should be shown in words and figures when prescribing drugs prone to abuse; this is obligatory for controlled drugs;
- alterations are best avoided but if any are made they should be clear and unambiguous; add initials against altered items;
- if prescriptions are left for collection they should be left in a safe place in a sealed envelope.

Travelling abroad

Prescribed drugs listed in Schedule 4 Part II (CD Anab) and Schedule 5 of the Misuse of Drugs Regulations 2001 are not subject to export or import licensing. However, patients intending to travel abroad for more than 3 months carrying any amount of drugs listed in Schedules 2, 3, or 4 Part I (CD Benz) will require a personal export/import licence. Further details can be obtained at www.gov.uk/guidance/controlled-drugs-licences-fees-and-returns or from the Home Office by contacting licensing_enquiry.aadu@homeoffice.gsi.gov.uk (in cases of emergency, telephone (020) 7035 6330).

Applications must be supported by a covering letter from the prescriber and should give details of:

- the patient's name and address;
- the quantities of drugs to be carried;
- the strength and form in which the drugs will be dispensed;
- the country or countries of destination;
- the dates of travel to and from the United Kingdom.

Applications for licences should be sent to the Home Office, Drugs Licensing & Compliance Unit, Fry Building, 2 Marsham Street, London. SW1P 4DF.

Alternatively, completed application forms can be emailed to dlcucommsofficer@homeoffice.gsi.gov.uk with a copy of the covering letter from the prescriber as a pdf. A minimum of two weeks should be allowed for processing the application.

Patients travelling for less than 3 months do not require a personal export/import licence for carrying Controlled Drugs, but are advised to carry a letter from the prescribing doctor. Those travelling for more than 3 months are advised to make arrangements to have their medication prescribed by a practitioner in the country they are visiting.

Doctors who want to take Controlled Drugs abroad while accompanying patients may similarly be issued with licences. Licences are not normally issued to doctors who want to take Controlled Drugs abroad solely in case a family emergency should arise.

Personal export/import licences do not have any legal status outside the UK and are issued only to comply with the Misuse of Drugs Act and to facilitate passage through UK Customs and Excise control. For clearance in the country to be visited it is necessary to approach that country's consulate in the UK.

Notification of drug misusers

Doctors should report cases of drug misuse to their regional or national drug misuse database or centre.

In **England**, doctors should report cases where they are providing structured drug treatment for substance dependence to their local National Drug Treatment Monitoring System (NDTMS) Team. General information about NDTMS can be found at www.nta.nhs.uk/ndtms.aspx. Enquiries about NDTMS, and how to submit data, should initially be directed to:
EvidenceApplicationTeam@phe.gov.uk

In **Scotland**, doctors should report cases to the Substance Misuse Programme (SMP).

Tel: (0131) 275 6348

In **Northern Ireland**, the Misuse of Drugs (Notification of and Supply to Addicts) (Northern Ireland) Regulations 1973 require doctors to send particulars of persons whom they consider to be addicted to certain controlled drugs to the Chief Medical Officer of the Department of Health and Social Services. The Northern Ireland contacts are:

Medical contact:

Dr Ian McMaster, C3 Castle Buildings, Belfast, BT4 3FQ
Tel: (028) 9052 2421, Fax: (028) 9052 0718
ian.mcmaster@dhsspsni.gov.uk

Administrative contact:

Public Health Information & Research Branch, Annex 2, Castle Building, Belfast, BT4 3SQ
Tel: (028) 9052 2520

Public Health Information & Research Branch also maintains the Northern Ireland Drug Misuse Database (NIDMD) which collects detailed information on those presenting for treatment, on drugs misused and injecting behaviour; participation is not a statutory requirement.

In **Wales**, doctors should report cases where they are providing structured drug treatment for substance dependence on the Welsh National Database for Substance Misuse; enquiries should be directed to:
substance.misuse-queries@wales.nhs.uk.

Adverse reactions to drugs

Yellow card scheme

Any drug may produce unwanted or unexpected adverse reactions. Rapid detection and recording of adverse drug reactions is of vital importance so that unrecognised hazards are identified promptly and appropriate regulatory action is taken to ensure that medicines are used safely. Healthcare professionals and coroners are urged to report suspected adverse drug reactions directly to the Medicines and Healthcare products Regulatory Agency (MHRA) through the Yellow Card Scheme using the electronic form at www.mhra.gov.uk/yellowcard. Alternatively, prepaid Yellow Cards for reporting are available from the address below and are also bound in the inside back cover of *BNF for Children*. Send Yellow Cards to:

FREEPOST YELLOW CARD
(No other address details required).
Tel: 0800 731 6789

Suspected adverse drug reactions to any therapeutic agent should be reported, including drugs (*self-medication* as well as *prescribed*), blood products, vaccines, radiographic contrast media, complementary and herbal products. For biosimilar medicines and vaccines, adverse reaction reports should clearly state the brand name and the batch number of the suspected medicine or vaccine.

Suspected adverse drug reactions should be reported through the Yellow Card Scheme at www.mhra.gov.uk/yellowcard. Yellow Cards can be used for reporting suspected adverse drug reactions to medicines, vaccines, herbal or complementary products, whether self-medicated or prescribed. This includes suspected adverse drug reactions associated with misuse, overdose, medication errors or from use of unlicensed and off-label medicines. Yellow Cards can also be used to report medical device incidents, defective medicines, and suspected fake medicines.

Report all suspected adverse drug reactions that are:

- **serious, medically significant or result in harm**. Serious events are fatal, life-threatening, a congenital abnormality, disabling or incapacitating, or resulting in hospitalisation;
- associated with **newer drugs and vaccines**; the most up to date list of black triangle medicines is available at: www.mhra.gov.uk/blacktriangle

If in doubt whether to report a suspected adverse drug reaction, please complete a Yellow Card.

The identification and reporting of adverse reactions to drugs in children and neonates is particularly important because:

- the action of the drug and its pharmacokinetics in children (especially in the very young) may be different from that in adults;
- drugs may not have been extensively tested in children;
- many drugs are not specifically licensed for use in children and are used either 'off-label' or as unlicensed products;
- drugs may affect the way a child grows and develops or may cause delayed adverse reactions which do not occur in adults;
- suitable formulations may not be available to allow precise dosing in children or they may contain excipients that should be used with caution in children;
- the nature and course of illnesses and adverse drug reactions may differ between adults and children.

Even if reported through the British Paediatric Surveillance Unit's Orange Card Scheme, any identified suspected adverse drug reactions should also be submitted to the Yellow Card Scheme.

Spontaneous reporting is particularly valuable for recognising possible new hazards rapidly. An adverse reaction should be reported even if it is not certain that the drug has caused it, or if the reaction is well recognised, or if other drugs have been given at the same time. Reports of overdoses (deliberate or accidental) can complicate the assessment of adverse drug reactions, but provide important information on the potential toxicity of drugs.

A freephone service is available to all parts of the UK for advice and information on suspected adverse drug reactions; contact the National Yellow Card Information Service at the MHRA on 0800 731 6789. Outside office hours a telephone-answering machine will take messages.

The following Yellow Card Centres can be contacted for further information:

Yellow Card Centre Northwest
2nd Floor, 70 Pembroke Place, Liverpool, L69 3GF
Tel: (0151) 794 8122

Yellow Card Centre Wales
Cardiff University, Department of Pharmacology, Therapeutics and Toxicology, Heath Park, Cardiff, CF14 4XN
Tel: (029) 2074 4181

Yellow Card Centre Northern & Yorkshire
Regional Drug and Therapeutics Centre, 16/17 Framlington Place, Newcastle upon Tyne, NE2 4AB
Tel: (0191) 213 7855

Yellow Card Centre West Midlands
City Hospital, Dudley Road, Birmingham, B18 7QH
Tel: (0121) 507 5672

Yellow Card Centre Scotland
CARDS, Royal Infirmary of Edinburgh, 51 Little France Crescent, Old Dalkeith Road, Edinburgh, EH16 4SA
Tel: (0131) 242 2919
YCCScotland@luht.scot.nhs.uk

The MHRA's database facilitates the monitoring of adverse drug reactions. More detailed information on reporting and a list of products currently under additional monitoring can be found on the MHRA website: www.mhra.gov.uk.

MHRA Drug Safety Update

Drug Safety Update is a monthly newsletter from the MHRA and the Commission on Human Medicines (CHM); it is available at www.mhra.gov.uk/drugsafetyupdate.

Self-reporting

Patients and their carers can also report suspected adverse drug reactions to the MHRA. Reports can be submitted directly to the MHRA through the Yellow Card Scheme using the electronic form at www.mhra.gov.uk/yellowcard, by telephone on 0808 100 3352, or by downloading the Yellow Card form from www.mhra.gov.uk. Alternatively, patient Yellow Cards are available from pharmacies and GP surgeries. Information for patients about the Yellow Card Scheme is available in other languages at www.mhra.gov.uk/yellowcard.

Prescription-event monitoring

In addition to the MHRA's Yellow Card Scheme, an independent scheme monitors the safety of new medicines using a different approach. The Drug Safety Research Unit identifies patients who have been prescribed selected new medicines and collects data on clinical events in these patients. The data are submitted on a voluntary basis by general practitioners on green forms. More information about the scheme and the Unit's educational material is available from www.dsru.org.

Newer drugs and vaccines

Only limited information is available from clinical trials on the safety of new medicines. Further understanding about the safety of medicines depends on the availability of information from routine clinical practice.

The black triangle symbol identifies newly licensed medicines that require additional monitoring by the European Medicines Agency. Such medicines include new active substances, biosimilar medicines, and medicines that the European Medicines Agency consider require additional monitoring. The black triangle symbol also appears in the Patient Information Leaflets for relevant medicines, with a brief explanation of what it means. Products usually retain a black triangle for 5 years, but this can be extended if required.

Medication errors

Adverse drug reactions where harm occurs as a result of a medication error are reportable as a Yellow Card or through the local risk management systems into the National Reporting and Learning System (NRLS). If reported to the NRLS, these will be shared with the MHRA. If the NRLS is not available and harm occurs, report using a Yellow Card.

Adverse reactions to medical devices

Suspected adverse reactions to medical devices including dental or surgical materials, intra-uterine devices, and contact lens fluids should be reported. Information on reporting these can be found at: www.mhra.gov.uk.

Side-effects in the *BNF for Children*

The *BNF for Children* includes clinically relevant side-effects for most drugs; an exhaustive list is not included for drugs that are used by specialists (e.g. cytotoxic drugs and drugs used in anaesthesia). Where causality has not been established, side-effects in the manufacturers' literature may be omitted from the *BNF for Children*.

Description of the frequency of side-effects	
Very common	greater than 1 in 10
Common	1 in 100 to 1 in 10
Uncommon [formerly 'less commonly' in BNF publications]	1 in 1000 to 1 in 100
Rare	1 in 10 000 to 1 in 1000
Very rare	less than 1 in 10 000

Special problems

Symptoms Children may be poor at expressing the symptoms of an adverse drug reaction and parental opinion may be required.

Delayed drug effects Some reactions (e.g. cancers and effects on development) may become manifest months or years after exposure. Any suspicion of such an association should be reported directly to the MHRA through the Yellow Card Scheme.

Congenital abnormalities When an infant is born with a congenital abnormality or there is a malformed aborted fetus doctors are asked to consider whether this might be an adverse reaction to a drug and to report all drugs (including self-medication) taken during pregnancy.

Prevention of adverse reactions

Adverse reactions may be prevented as follows:
- never use any drug unless there is a good indication. If the patient is pregnant do not use a drug unless the need for it is imperative;
- allergy and idiosyncrasy are important causes of adverse drug reactions. Ask if the child has had previous reactions to the drug or formulation;
- prescribe as few drugs as possible and give very clear instructions to the child, parent, or carer;

- whenever possible use a familiar drug; with a new drug be particularly alert for adverse reactions or unexpected events;
- consider if excipients (e.g. colouring agents) may be contributing to the adverse reaction. If the reaction is minor, a trial of an alternative formulation of the same drug may be considered before abandoning the drug;
- obtain a full drug history including asking if the child is already taking other drugs *including over-the-counter medicines*; interactions may occur;
- age and hepatic or renal disease may alter the metabolism or excretion of drugs, particularly in neonates, which can affect the potential for adverse effects. Genetic factors may also be responsible for variations in metabolism, and therefore for the adverse effects of the drug;
- warn the child, parent, or carer if serious adverse reactions are liable to occur.

Drug allergy (suspected or confirmed)

Suspected drug allergy is any reaction caused by a drug with clinical features compatible with an immunological mechanism. All drugs have the potential to cause adverse drug reactions, but not all of these are allergic in nature. A reaction is more likely to be caused by drug allergy if:

- The reaction occurred while the child was being treated with the drug, or
- The drug is known to cause this pattern of reaction, or
- The child has had a similar reaction to the same drug or drug-class previously.

A suspected reaction is less likely to be caused by a drug allergy if there is a possible non-drug cause or if there are only gastro-intestinal symptoms present.

The following signs, allergic patterns and timing of onset can be used to help decide whether to suspect drug allergy:

Immediate, rapidly-evolving reactions (onset usually less than 1 hour after drug exposure)

- Anaphylaxis, with erythema, urticaria or angioedema, and hypotension and/or bronchospasm. See also Antihistamines, allergen immunotherapy and allergic emergencies p. 162
- Urticaria or angioedema without systemic features
- Exacerbation of asthma e.g. with non-steroidal anti-inflammatory drugs (NSAIDs)

*Non-immediate reactions, **without** systemic involvement* (onset usually 6–10 days after first drug exposure or 3 days after second exposure)

- Cutaneous reactions, e.g. widespread red macules and/or papules, or, fixed drug eruption (localised inflamed skin)

*Non-immediate reactions, **with** systemic involvement* (onset may be variable, usually 3 days to 6 weeks after first drug exposure, depending on features, or 3 days after second exposure)

- Cutaneous reactions with systemic features, e.g. drug reaction with eosinophilia and systemic signs (DRESS) or drug hypersensitivity syndrome (DHS), characterised by widespread red macules, papules or erythroderma, fever, lymphadenopathy, liver dysfunction or eosinophilia
- Toxic epidermal necrolysis or Stevens–Johnson syndrome
- Acute generalised exanthematous pustulosis (AGEP)

EvGr Suspected drug allergy information should be clearly and accurately documented in clinical notes and prescriptions, and shared among all healthcare professionals. Children and parents or carers should be given information about which drugs and drug-classes to avoid and encouraged to share the drug allergy status. Ⓐ

[EvGr] If a drug allergy is suspected, consider stopping the suspected drug and advising the child and parent or carer to avoid this drug in future. Symptoms of the acute reaction should be treated, in hospital if severe. Children presenting with a suspected anaphylactic reaction, or a severe or non-immediate cutaneous reaction, should be referred to a specialist drug allergy service. Children presenting with a suspected drug allergic reaction or anaphylaxis to NSAIDs, and local and general anaesthetics may also need to be referred to a specialist drug allergy service, e.g. in cases of anaphylactoid reactions or to determine future treatment options. Children presenting with a suspected drug allergic reaction or anaphylaxis associated with beta-lactam antibiotics should be referred to a specialist drug allergy service if their disease or condition can only be treated by a beta-lactam antibiotic or they are likely to need beta-lactam antibiotics frequently in the future (e.g. immunodeficient children). ⒶFor further information see Drug allergy: diagnosis and management. NICE Clinical Guideline 183 (September 2014) www.nice.org.uk/guidance/cg183.

Defective medicines

During the manufacture or distribution of a medicine an error or accident may occur whereby the finished product does not conform to its specification. While such a defect may impair the therapeutic effect of the product and could adversely affect the health of a patient, it should **not** be confused with an Adverse Drug Reaction where the product conforms to its specification.

The Defective Medicines Report Centre assists with the investigation of problems arising from licensed medicinal products thought to be defective and co-ordinates any necessary protective action. Reports on suspect defective medicinal products should include the brand or the non-proprietary name, the name of the manufacturer or supplier, the strength and dosage form of the product, the product licence number, the batch number or numbers of the product, the nature of the defect, and an account of any action already taken in consequence. The Centre can be contacted at:

The Defective Medicines Report Centre
Medicines and Healthcare products Regulatory Agency,
151 Buckingham Palace Road, London, SW1W 9SZ
Tel: (020) 3080 6574
dmrc@mhra.gsi.gov.uk

Guidance on intravenous infusions

Intravenous infusions for neonatal intensive care

Intravenous policy A local policy on the dilution of drugs with intravenous fluids should be drawn up by a multi-disciplinary team and issued as a document to the members of staff concerned.

Centralised additive services are provided in a number of hospital pharmacy departments and should be used in preference to making additions on wards.

The information that follows should be read in conjunction with local policy documents.

Guidelines

- Drugs should only be diluted with infusion fluid when constant plasma concentrations are needed or when the administration of a more concentrated solution would be harmful.
- In general, only one drug should be mixed with an infusion fluid in a syringe and the components should be compatible. Ready-prepared solutions should be used whenever possible. Drugs should not normally be added to blood products, mannitol, or sodium bicarbonate. Only specially formulated additives should be used with fat emulsions or amino-acid solutions.
- Solutions should be thoroughly mixed by shaking and checked for absence of particulate matter before use.
- Strict asepsis should be maintained throughout and in general the giving set should not be used for more than 24 hours (for drug admixtures).
- The infusion syringe should be labelled with the neonate's name and hospital number, the name and quantity of drug, the infusion fluid, and the expiry date and time. If a problem occurs during administration, containers should be retained for a period after use in case they are needed for investigation.
- Administration using a suitable motorised syringe driver is advocated for preparations where strict control over administration is required.
- It is good practice to examine intravenous infusions from time to time while they are running. If cloudiness, crystallisation, change of colour, or any other sign of interaction or contamination is observed the infusion should be discontinued.

Problems

Microbial contamination The accidental entry and subsequent growth of micro-organisms converts the infusion fluid pathway into a potential vehicle for infection with micro-organisms, particularly species of Candida, Enterobacter, and Klebsiella. Ready-prepared infusions containing the additional drugs, or infusions prepared by an additive service (when available) should therefore be used in preference to making extemporaneous additions to infusion containers on wards etc. However, when this is necessary strict aseptic procedure should be followed.

Incompatibility Physical and chemical incompatibilities may occur with loss of potency, increase in toxicity, or other adverse effect. The solutions may become opalescent or precipitation may occur, but in many instances there is no visual indication of incompatibility. Interaction may take place at any point in the infusion fluid pathway, and the potential for incompatibility is increased when more than one substance is added to the infusion fluid.

Common incompatibilities Precipitation reactions are numerous and varied and may occur as a result of pH, concentration changes, 'salting-out' effects, complexation or other chemical changes. Precipitation or other particle formation must be avoided since, apart from lack of control of dosage on administration, it may initiate or exacerbate adverse effects. This is particularly important in the case of drugs which have been implicated in either thrombophlebitis (e.g. diazepam) or in skin sloughing or necrosis caused by extravasation (e.g. sodium bicarbonate and parenteral nutrition). It is also especially important to effect solution of colloidal drugs and to prevent their subsequent precipitation in order to avoid a pyrogenic reaction (e.g. amphotericin).

It is considered undesirable to mix beta-lactam antibiotics, such as semi-synthetic penicillins and cephalosporins, with proteinaceous materials on the grounds that immunogenic and allergenic conjugates could be formed.

A number of preparations undergo significant loss of potency when added singly or in combination to large volume infusions. Examples include ampicillin in infusions that contain glucose or lactates.

Blood Because of the large number of incompatibilities, drugs should not be added to blood and blood products for infusion purposes. Examples of incompatibility with blood include hypertonic mannitol solutions (irreversible crenation of red cells), dextrans (rouleaux formation and interference with cross-matching), glucose (clumping of red cells), and oxytocin (inactivated).

If the giving set is not changed after the administration of blood, but used for other infusion fluids, a fibrin clot may form which, apart from blocking the set, increases the likelihood of microbial growth.

Intravenous fat emulsion These may break down with coalescence of fat globules and separation of phases when additions such as antibacterials or electrolytes are made, thus increasing the possibility of embolism. Only specially formulated products such as *Vitlipid N*® may be added to appropriate intravenous fat emulsions.

Other infusions Infusions that frequently give rise to incompatibility include amino acids, mannitol, and sodium bicarbonate.

Method

Ready-prepared infusions should be used whenever available. When dilution of drugs is required to be made extemporaneously, any product reconstitution instructions such as those relating to concentration, vehicle, mixing, and handling precautions should be strictly followed using an aseptic technique throughout. Once the product has been reconstituted, further dilution with the infusion fluid should be made immediately in order to minimise microbial contamination and, with certain products, to prevent degradation or other formulation change which may occur; e.g. reconstituted ampicillin injection degrades rapidly on standing, and also may form polymers which could cause sensitivity reactions.

It is also important in certain instances that an infusion fluid of specific pH be used (e.g. **furosemide** injection requires dilution in infusions of pH greater than 5.5).

When drug dilutions are made it is important to mix thoroughly; additions should not be made to an infusion container that has been connected to a giving set, as mixing is hampered. If the solutions are not thoroughly mixed, a concentrated layer of the drug may form owing to differences in density. **Potassium chloride** is particularly prone to this 'layering' effect when added without adequate mixing to infusions; if such a mixture is administered it may have a serious effect on the heart.

A time limit between dilution and completion of administration must be imposed for certain admixtures to guarantee satisfactory drug potency and compatibility. For admixtures in which degradation occurs without the formation of toxic substances, an acceptable limit is the time taken for 10% decomposition of the drug. When toxic substances are produced stricter limits may be imposed. Because of the risk of microbial contamination a maximum time limit of 24 hours may be appropriate for additions made elsewhere than in hospital pharmacies offering central additive service.

Certain injections must be protected from light during continuous infusion to minimise oxidation, e.g. sodium nitroprusside.

Drugs given by continuous intravenous infusion to neonates

The information provided in *BNF for Children* covers dilution with *Glucose intravenous infusion* 5% and 10% and *Sodium chloride intravenous infusion* 0.9%. Compatibility with glucose 5% and with sodium chloride 0.9% indicates compatibility with *Sodium chloride and glucose intravenous infusion*. Infusion of a large volume of hypotonic solution should be avoided, therefore care should be taken if water for injections is used.

Prescribing in hepatic impairment

Overview

Children have a large reserve of hepatic metabolic capacity and modification of the choice and dosage of drugs is usually unnecessary even in apparently severe liver disease. However, special consideration is required in the following situations:

- liver failure characterised by severe derangement of liver enzymes and profound jaundice; the use of sedative drugs, opioids, and drugs such as diuretics and amphotericin p. 351 which produce hypokalaemia may precipitate hepatic encephalopathy;
- impaired coagulation, which can affect response to oral anticoagulants;
- in cholestatic jaundice elimination may be impaired of drugs such as fusidic acid p. 336 and rifampicin p. 342 which are excreted in the bile;

- in hypoproteinaemia, the effect of highly protein-bound drugs such as phenytoin p. 193, prednisolone p. 413, warfarin sodium p. 89, and benzodiazepines may be increased;
- use of hepatotoxic drugs is more likely to cause toxicity in children with liver disease; such drugs should be avoided if possible;
- in neonates, particularly preterm neonates, and also in infants metabolic pathways may differ from older children and adults because liver enzyme pathways may be immature.

Where care is needed when prescribing in hepatic impairment, this is indicated under the relevant drug in *BNF for Children*.

Prescribing in renal impairment

Issues encountered in renal impairment

The use of drugs in children with reduced renal function can give rise to problems for several reasons:

- reduced renal excretion of a drug or its metabolites may produce toxicity;
- sensitivity to some drugs is increased even if elimination is unimpaired;
- many side-effects are tolerated poorly by children with renal impairment;
- some drugs are not effective when renal function is reduced;
- neonates, particularly preterm, may have immature renal function.

Many of these problems can be avoided by reducing the dose or by using alternative drugs.

Principles of dose adjustment in renal impairment

The level of renal function below which the dose of a drug must be reduced depends on the proportion of the drug eliminated by renal excretion and its toxicity.

For many drugs with only minor or no dose-related side-effects, very precise modification of the dose regimen is unnecessary and a simple scheme for dose reduction is sufficient.

For more toxic drugs with a small safety margin dose regimens based on glomerular filtration rate should be used.

When both efficacy and toxicity are closely related to plasma-drug concentration, recommended regimens should be regarded only as a guide to initial treatment; subsequent doses must be adjusted according to clinical response and plasma-drug concentration.

The total daily maintenance dose of a drug can be reduced either by reducing the size of the individual doses or by increasing the interval between doses. For some drugs, although the size of the maintenance dose is reduced it is important to give a loading dose if an immediate effect is required. This is because it takes about five times the half-life of the drug to achieve steady-state plasma concentration. Because the plasma half-life of drugs excreted by the kidney is prolonged in renal impairment, it can take many doses at the reduced dosage to achieve a therapeutic plasma concentration. The loading dose should usually be the same as the initial dose for a child with normal renal function.

Nephrotoxic drugs should, if possible, be avoided in children with renal disease because the consequences of nephrotoxicity are likely to be more serious when the renal reserve is already reduced.

Glomerular filtration rate is low at birth and increases rapidly during the first 6 months. Thereafter, glomerular filtration rate increases gradually to reach adult levels by 1–2 years of age, when standardised to a typical adult body surface area (1.73 m^2). In the first weeks after birth, serum creatinine falls; a single measure of serum creatinine provides only a crude estimate of renal function and observing the change over days is of more use. In the neonate, a sustained rise in serum creatinine or a lack of the expected postnatal decline, is indicative of a reduced glomerular filtration rate.

Dose recommendations are based on the severity of renal impairment. This is expressed in terms of **glomerular filtration rate** (mL/minute/1.73 m^2).

The following equations provide a guide to glomerular filtration rate.

Child over 1 year:
Estimated glomerular filtration rate (mL/minute/1.73 m^2)=
40 × height (cm)/serum creatinine (micromol/litre)

Neonate:
Estimated glomerular filtration rate (mL/minute/1.73 m^2)=
30 × height (cm)/serum creatinine (micromol/litre)

The values used in these formulas may differ according to locality or laboratory.

The serum-creatinine concentration is sometimes used as a measure of renal function but is only a **rough guide** even when corrected for age, weight, and sex.

Important The information on dose adjustment in *BNF for Children* is expressed in terms of estimated glomerular filtration rate. Renal function in adults is increasingly being reported as estimated glomerular filtration rate (eGFR) normalised to a body surface area of 1.73 m^2; however, eGFR is derived from the MDRD (Modification of Diet in Renal Disease) formula which is not validated for use in children. eGFR derived from the MDRD formula should **not** be used to adjust drug doses in children with renal impairment.

In *BNF for Children*, values for measures of renal function are included where possible. However, where such values are not available, the *BNF for Children* reflects the terms used in the published information.

Degrees of renal impairment defined using estimated glomerular filtration rate (eGFR)

Chronic kidney disease in adults: UK guidelines for identification, management and referral (March 2006) defines renal function as follows:	
Degree of impairment	eGFR[1] mL/minute/1.73 m^2
Normal: Stage 1	More than 90 (with other evidence of kidney damage)
Mild: Stage 2	60–89 (with other evidence of kidney damage)
Moderate[2]: Stage 3	30–59
Severe: Stage 4	15–29
Established renal failure: Stage 5	Less than 15

1. Estimated glomerular filtration rate (eGFR) derived from the Modification of Diet in Renal Disease (MDRD) formula for use in patients over 18 years
2. NICE clinical guideline 73 (September 2008)–Chronic kidney disease: Stage 3A eGFR = 45–59, Stage 3B eGFR = 30–44

Drug prescribing should be kept to the minimum in all children with severe renal disease.

If even mild renal impairment is considered likely on clinical grounds, renal function should be checked before prescribing **any** drug which requires dose modification. Where care is needed when prescribing in renal impairment, this is indicated under the relevant drug in *BNF for Children*.

Dialysis

For prescribing in children on renal replacement therapy consult specialist literature.

Prescribing in pregnancy

Overview

Drugs can have harmful effects on the embryo or fetus at any time during pregnancy. It is important to bear this in mind when prescribing for a woman of *childbearing age* or for men *trying* to *father* a child.

During the *first trimester* drugs can produce congenital malformations (teratogenesis), and the period of greatest risk is from the third to the eleventh week of pregnancy. During the *second* and *third trimesters* drugs can affect the growth or functional development of the fetus, or they can have toxic effects on fetal tissues.

Drugs given shortly before term or during labour can have adverse effects on labour or on the neonate after delivery.

Not all the damaging effects of intra-uterine exposure to drugs are obvious at birth, some may only manifest later in life. Such late-onset effects include malignancy, e.g. adenocarcinoma of the vagina after puberty in females exposed to diethylstilbestrol in the womb, and adverse effects on intellectual, social, and functional development. The BNF and *BNF for Children* identifies drugs which:

- may have harmful effects in pregnancy and indicates the trimester of risk
- are not known to be harmful in pregnancy

The information is based on human data, but information from *animal* studies has been included for some drugs when its omission might be misleading. Maternal drug doses may require adjustment during pregnancy due to changes in maternal physiology but this is beyond the scope of the *BNF* and *BNF for Children*.

Where care is needed when prescribing in pregnancy, this is indicated under the relevant drug in the BNF and *BNF for Children*.

Important

Drugs should be prescribed in pregnancy only if the expected benefit to the mother is thought to be greater than the risk to the fetus, and all drugs should be avoided if possible during the first trimester. Drugs which have been extensively used in pregnancy and appear to be usually safe should be prescribed in preference to new or untried drugs; and the smallest effective dose should be used. Few drugs have been shown conclusively to be teratogenic in humans, but no drug is safe beyond all doubt in early pregnancy. Screening procedures are available when there is a known risk of certain defects.

Absence of information does not imply safety. It should be noted that the BNF and *BNF for Children* provide independent advice and may not always agree with the product literature.

Information on drugs and pregnancy is also available from the UK Teratology Information Service. www.uktis.org. Tel: 0344 892 0909 (09.00–17:00 Monday to Friday; urgent enquiries only outside these hours).

Prescribing in breast-feeding

Overview

Breast-feeding is beneficial; the immunological and nutritional value of breast milk to the infant is greater than that of formula feeds.

Although there is concern that drugs taken by the mother might affect the infant, there is very little information on this. In the absence of evidence of an effect, the potential for harm to the infant can be inferred from:

- the amount of drug or active metabolite of the drug delivered to the infant (dependent on the pharmacokinetic characteristics of the drug in the mother);
- the efficiency of absorption, distribution, and elimination of the drug by the infant (infant pharmacokinetics);
- the nature of the effect of the drug on the infant (pharmacodynamic properties of the drug in the infant).

Most medicines given to a mother cause no harm to breast-fed infants and there are few contra-indications to breast-feeding when maternal medicines are necessary. However, administration of some drugs to nursing mothers can harm the infant. In the first week of life, some such as preterm or jaundiced infants are at a slightly higher risk of toxicity. Toxicity to the infant can occur if the drug enters the milk in pharmacologically significant quantities. The concentration in milk of some drugs (e.g. fluvastatin p. 124) may exceed the concentration in maternal plasma so that therapeutic doses in the mother can cause toxicity to the infant. Some drugs inhibit the infant's sucking reflex (e.g. phenobarbital p. 203) while others can affect lactation (e.g. bromocriptine). Drugs in breast milk may, at least theoretically, cause hypersensitivity in the infant even when concentration is too low for a pharmacological effect. *BNF for Children* identifies drugs:

- which should be used with caution or which are contra-indicated in breast-feeding for the reasons given above;
- which, on present evidence, may be given to the mother during breast-feeding, because they appear in milk in amounts which are too small to be harmful to the infant;
- which are not known to be harmful to the infant although they are present in milk in significant amounts.

Where care is needed when prescribing in breast-feeding, this is indicated under the relevant drug in the *BNF for Children*.

Important

For many drugs insufficient evidence is available to provide guidance and it is advisable to administer only essential drugs to a mother during breast-feeding. Because of the inadequacy of information on drugs in breast-feeding, absence of information does not imply safety.

Prescribing in palliative care

Overview

Palliative care is the active and total approach to the care of children and young adults with life-limiting and life-threatening conditions, embracing physical, emotional, social, and spiritual elements of their care. It focuses on enhancing the quality of life for the child and support for their family, and includes the management of distressing symptoms, provision of respite, and care following death and bereavement.

Effective palliative care requires a broad multidisciplinary approach that includes the whole family, and ideally should start as soon as possible after diagnosis or recognition of a life-threatening condition.

Drug treatment The number of drugs should be as few as possible. Oral medication is usually appropriate unless there is severe nausea and vomiting, dysphagia, weakness, or coma, when parenteral medication may be necessary.

Pain

Pain management in palliative care is focused on achieving control of pain by administering the right drug in the right dose at the right time. Analgesics can be divided into three broad classes: non-opioid (paracetamol p. 254, NSAID), opioid (e.g. codeine phosphate p. 259 'weak', morphine p. 265 'strong') and adjuvant (e.g. antidepressants, antiepileptics). Drugs from the different classes are used alone or in combination according to the type of pain and response to treatment. Analgesics are more effective in preventing pain than in the relief of established pain; it is important that they are given regularly.

Paracetamol or a NSAID given regularly will often be sufficient to manage mild pain. If non-opioid analgesics alone are not sufficient, then an opioid analgesic alone or in combination with a non-opioid analgesic at an adequate dosage, may be helpful in the control of moderate pain. Codeine phosphate or tramadol hydrochloride p. 270 can be considered for moderate pain. If these preparations do not control the pain then morphine is the most useful opioid analgesic. Alternatives to morphine, including transdermal buprenorphine p. 257, transdermal fentanyl p. 262, hydromorphone hydrochloride p. 265, methadone hydrochloride p. 279, or oxycodone hydrochloride p. 267, should be initiated by those with experience in palliative care. Initiation of an opioid analgesic should not be delayed by concern over a theoretical likelihood of psychological dependence (addiction).

Bone metastases In addition to the above approach, radiotherapy and bisphosphonates,, may be useful for pain due to bone metastases.

Neuropathic pain Patients with neuropathic pain may benefit from a trial of a tricyclic antidepressant, most commonly amitriptyline hydrochloride p. 224, for several weeks. An antiepileptic such as carbamazepine p. 184, may be added or substituted if pain persists. Ketamine p. 773 is sometimes used under specialist supervision for neuropathic pain that responds poorly to opioid analgesics. Pain due to nerve compression may be reduced by a corticosteroid such as dexamethasone p. 410, which reduces oedema around the tumour, thus reducing compression. Nerve blocks can be considered when pain is localised to a specific area. Transcutaneous electrical nerve stimulation (TENS) may also help.

Pain management with opioids

Oral route Treatment with morphine p. 265 is given by mouth as immediate-release or modified-release preparations. During the titration phase the initial dose is based on the previous medication used, the severity of the pain, and other factors such as presence of renal impairment or frailty. The dose is given either as an immediate-release preparation 4-hourly (for starting doses, see Morphine p. 265), or as a 12-hourly modified-release preparation, in addition to rescue doses. If replacing a weaker opioid analgesic (such as codeine phosphate p. 259), starting doses are usually higher.

If pain occurs between regular doses of morphine ('breakthrough pain'), an additional dose ('rescue dose') of immediate-release morphine should be given. An additional dose should also be given 30 minutes before an activity that causes pain, such as wound dressing. The standard dose of a strong opioid for breakthrough pain is usually one-tenth to one-sixth of the regular 24-hour dose, repeated every 2–4 hours as required (up to hourly may be needed if pain is severe or in the last days of life). Review pain management if rescue analgesic is required frequently (twice daily or more). Each child should be assessed on an individual basis. Formulations of fentanyl p. 262 that are administered nasally, buccally or sublingually are not licensed for use in children; their usefulness in children is also limited by dose availability.

Children often require a higher dose of morphine in proportion to their body-weight compared to adults. Children are more susceptible to certain adverse effects of opioids such as urinary retention (which can be eased by bethanechol chloride), and opioid-induced pruritus. When adjusting the dose of morphine, the number of rescue doses required and the response to them should be taken into account; increments of morphine should not exceed one-third to one-half of the total daily dose every 24 hours. Thereafter, the dose should be adjusted with careful assessment of the pain, and the use of adjuvant analgesics should also be considered. Upward titration of the dose of morphine stops when either the pain is relieved or unacceptable adverse effects occur, after which it is necessary to consider alternative measures.

Once their pain is controlled, children started on 4-hourly immediate-release morphine p. 265 can be transferred to the same total 24-hour dose of morphine given as the modified-release preparation for 12-hourly or 24-hourly administration. The first dose of the modified-release preparation is given with, or within 4 hours of the last dose of the immediate-release preparation. For preparations suitable for 12-hourly or 24-hourly administration see modified-release preparations under morphine. Increments should be made to the dose, not to the frequency of administration. The patient must be monitored closely for efficacy and side-effects, particularly constipation, and nausea and vomiting. A suitable laxative should be prescribed routinely.

Oxycodone hydrochloride p. 267 can be used in children who require an opioid but cannot tolerate morphine. If the child is already receiving an opioid, oxycodone hydrochloride should be started at a dose equivalent to the current analgesic. Oxycodone hydrochloride immediate-release preparations can be given for breakthrough pain.

Equivalent doses of opioid analgesics

This table is only an **approximate** guide (doses may not correspond with those given in clinical practice); children should be carefully monitored after any change in medication and dose titration may be required.

Analgesic/Route	Dose
Codeine: PO	100 mg
Diamorphine: IM, IV, SC	3 mg
Dihydrocodeine: PO	100 mg
Hydromorphone: PO	2 mg
Morphine: PO	10 mg
Morphine: IM, IV, SC	5 mg
Oxycodone: PO	6.6 mg
Tramadol: PO	100 mg

PO = by mouth; IM = intramuscular; IV = intravenous; SC = subcutaneous

Parenteral route Diamorphine hydrochloride p. 261 is preferred for injection because, being more soluble, it can be given in a smaller volume. The equivalent subcutaneous dose is approximately a third of the oral dose of morphine p. 265. Subcutaneous infusion of diamorphine hydrochloride via a continuous infusion device can be useful (for details, see Continuous Subcutaneous Infusions).

If the child can resume taking medicines by mouth, then oral morphine may be substituted for subcutaneous infusion of diamorphine hydrochloride. See the table *Approximate Equivalent doses of Morphine and Diamorphine*.

Rectal route Morphine p. 265 is also available for rectal administration as suppositories.

Transdermal route Transdermal preparations of fentanyl p. 262 and buprenorphine p. 257 [not licensed for use in children] are available; they are not suitable for acute pain or in those children whose analgesic requirements are changing rapidly because the long time to steady state prevents rapid titration of the dose. Prescribers should ensure that they are familiar with the correct use of transdermal preparations (see under fentanyl p. 262) because inappropriate use has caused fatalities.

The following 24-hour oral doses of morphine are considered to be *approximately* equivalent to the buprenorphine and fentanyl patches shown, however when switching due to possible opioid-induced hyperalgesia, reduce the calculated equivalent dose of the new opioid by one-quarter to one-half.

Buprenorphine patches are *approximately* equivalent to the following 24-hour doses of oral morphine

morphine salt 12 mg daily	≡ *BuTrans*® '5' patch: 7-day patches
morphine salt 24 mg daily	≡ *BuTrans*® '10' patch: 7-day patches
morphine salt 48 mg daily	≡ *BuTrans*® '20' patch: 7-day patches
morphine salt 84 mg daily	≡ *Transtec*® '35' patch: 4-day patches
morphine salt 126 mg daily	≡ *Transtec*® '52.5' patch: 4-day patches
morphine salt 168 mg daily	≡ *Transtec*® '70' patch: 4-day patches

Conversion ratios vary and these figures are a guide only. Morphine equivalences for transdermal opioid preparations have been approximated to allow comparison with available preparations of oral morphine.

72-hour Fentanyl patches are *approximately* equivalent to the following 24-hour doses of oral morphine

morphine salt 30 mg daily	≡ fentanyl '12' patch
morphine salt 60 mg daily	≡ fentanyl '25' patch
morphine salt 120 mg daily	≡ fentanyl '50' patch
morphine salt 180 mg daily	≡ fentanyl '75' patch
morphine salt 240 mg daily	≡ fentanyl '100' patch

Fentanyl equivalences in this table are for children on well-tolerated opioid therapy for long periods; fentanyl patches should not be used in opioid naive children. Conversion ratios vary and these figures are a guide only. Morphine equivalences for transdermal opioid preparations have been approximated to allow comparison with available preparations of oral morphine.

Symptom control

Unlicensed indications or routes Several recommendations in this section involve unlicensed indications or routes.

Anorexia Anorexia may be helped by prednisolone p. 413 or dexamethasone p. 410.

Anxiety Anxiety can be treated with a long-acting benzodiazepine such as diazepam p. 207, or by continuous infusion of the short-acting benzodiazepine midazolam p. 210. Interventions for more acute episodes of anxiety (such as panic attacks) include short-acting benzodiazepines such as lorazepam p. 209 given sublingually or midazolam given subcutaneously. Temazepam p. 774 provides useful night-time sedation in some children.

Capillary bleeding Capillary bleeding can be treated with tranexamic acid p. 76 by mouth; treatment is usually continued for one week after the bleeding has stopped but it can be continued at a reduced dose if bleeding persists. Alternatively, gauze soaked in tranexamic acid 100 mg/mL p. 76 or adrenaline/epinephrine solution 1 mg/mL (1 in 1000) p. 128 can be applied to the affected area.

Vitamin K may be useful for the treatment and prevention of bleeding associated with prolonged clotting in liver disease. In severe chronic cholestasis, absorption of vitamin K may be impaired; either parenteral or water-soluble oral vitamin K should be considered.

Constipation Constipation is a common cause of distress and is almost invariable after administration of an opioid analgesic. It should be prevented if possible by the regular administration of laxatives. Suitable laxatives include osmotic laxatives (such as lactulose p. 37 or macrogols), stimulant laxatives (such as co-danthramer p. 40 and senna p. 42) or the combination of lactulose and a senna preparation. Naloxone hydrochloride p. 796 given by mouth may help relieve opioid-induced constipation; it is poorly absorbed but opioid withdrawal reactions have been reported.

Convulsions Intractable seizures are relatively common in children dying from non-malignant conditions. Phenobarbital p. 203 by mouth or as a continuous subcutaneous infusion may be beneficial; continuous infusion of midazolam p. 210 is an alternative. Both cause drowsiness, but this is rarely a concern in the context of intractable seizures. For breakthrough convulsions diazepam p. 207 given rectally (as a solution), buccal midazolam p. 210, or paraldehyde p. 208 as an enema may be appropriate. See *Continuous subcutaneous infusions*, below, for the use of midazolam by subcutaneous infusion using a continuous infusion device

Dry mouth Dry mouth may be caused by certain medications including opioid analgesics, antimuscarinic drugs (e.g. hyoscine), antidepressants and some antiemetics; if possible, an alternative preparation should be considered. Dry mouth may be relieved by good mouth care and measures such as chewing sugar-free gum, sucking ice or pineapple chunks, or the use of artificial saliva, dry mouth associated with candidiasis can be treated by oral preparations of nystatin p. 663 or miconazole p. 663, alternatively, fluconazole p. 352 can be given by mouth.

Dysphagia A corticosteroid such as dexamethasone p. 410 may help, temporarily, if there is an obstruction due to tumour. See also *Dry mouth*, above.

Dyspnoea Breathlessness at rest may be relieved by regular oral morphine p. 265 in carefully titrated doses. Diazepam p. 207 may be helpful for dyspnoea associated with anxiety. Sublingual lorazepam p. 209 or subcutaneous or buccal midazolam p. 210 are alternatives. A nebulised short-acting beta₂ agonist or a corticosteroid, such as dexamethasone p. 410 or prednisolone p. 413, may also be helpful for bronchospasm or partial obstruction.

Excessive respiratory secretion Excessive respiratory secretion (death rattle) may be reduced by hyoscine hydrobromide patches or by subcutaneous or intravenous injection of hyoscine hydrobromide p. 250, however, care must be taken to avoid the discomfort of dry mouth. Alternatively, glycopyrronium bromide p. 765 may be given. Hyoscine hydrobromide can be administered by subcutaneous or intravenous infusion using a continuous infusion device.

Fungating tumours Fungating tumours can be treated by regular dressing and antibacterial drugs; systemic treatment with metronidazole p. 313 is often required to reduce malodour, but topical metronidazole is also used.

Gastro-intestinal pain The pain of bowel colic may be reduced by loperamide hydrochloride p. 44. Hyoscine hydrobromide p. 250 may also be helpful in reducing the frequency of spasms; it is given sublingually as *Kwells*® tablets and also by subcutanous infusion. Gastric distension pain due to pressure on the stomach may be helped by a preparation incorporating an antacid with an antiflatulent and a prokinetic such as domperidone before meals.

Hiccup Hiccup due to gastric distension may be helped by a preparation incorporating an antacid with an antiflatulent.

Insomnia Children with advanced cancer may not sleep because of discomfort, cramps, night sweats, joint stiffness, or fear. There should be appropriate treatment of these problems before hypnotics are used. Benzodiazepines, such as temazepam p. 774, may be useful.

Intractable cough Intractable cough may be relieved by moist inhalations or by regular administration of oral morphine p. 265 every 4 hours. Methadone hydrochloride linctus p. 279 should be avoided because it has a long duration of action and tends to accumulate.

Mucosal bleeding Mucosal bleeding from the mouth and nose occurs commonly in the terminal phase, particularly in a child suffering from haemopoeitic malignancy. Bleeding from the nose caused by a single bleeding point can be arrested by cauterisation or by dressing it. Tranexamic acid p. 76 may be effective applied topically or given systemically.

Muscle spasm The pain of muscle spasm can be helped by a muscle relaxant such as diazepam p. 207 or baclofen p. 603.

Nausea and vomiting Nausea and vomiting are common in children with advanced cancer. Ideally, the cause should be determined before treatment with an antiemetic is started. Nausea and vomiting with opioid therapy are less common in children than in adults but may occur particularly in the initial stages and can be prevented by giving an antiemetic. An antiemetic is usually necessary only for the first 4 or 5 days and therefore combined preparations containing an opioid with an antiemetic are not recommended because they lead to unnecessary antiemetic therapy (and associated side-effects when used long-term).

Metoclopramide hydrochloride p. 246 has a prokinetic action and is used by mouth for nausea and vomiting associated with gastritis, gastric stasis, and functional bowel obstruction. Drugs with antimuscarinic effects antagonise prokinetic drugs and, if possible, should not therefore be used concurrently.

Haloperidol p. 231 is used by mouth or by continuous intravenous or subcutaneous infusion for most metabolic causes of vomiting (e.g. hypercalcaemia, renal failure). Cyclizine p. 244 is used for nausea and vomiting due to mechanical bowel obstruction, raised intracranial pressure, and motion sickness.

Ondansetron p. 248 is most effective when the vomiting is due to damaged or irritated gut mucosa (e.g. after chemotherapy or radiotherapy).

Antiemetic therapy should be reviewed every 24 hours; it may be necessary to substitute the antiemetic or to add another one.

Levomepromazine p. 251 can be used if first-line antiemetics are inadequate. Dexamethasone p. 410 by mouth can be used as an adjunct.

See *Continuous subcutaneous infusions*, below, for the administration of antiemetics by subcutaneous infusion using a continuous infusion device.

Pruritus Pruritus, even when associated with obstructive jaundice, often responds to simple measures such as application of emollients. Ondansetron p. 248 may be effective in some children. Where opioid analgesics cause pruritus it may be appropriate to review the dose or to switch to an alternative opioid analgesic. In the case of obstructive jaundice, further measures include administration of colestyramine p. 120.

Raised intracranial pressure Headache due to raised intracranial pressure often responds to a high dose of a corticosteroid, such as dexamethasone p. 410, for 4 to 5 days, subsequently reduced if possible; dexamethasone should be given before 6 p.m. to reduce the risk of insomnia. Treatment of headache and of associated nausea and vomiting should also be considered.

Restlessness and confusion Restlessness and confusion may require treatment with haloperidol p. 231. Levomepromazine p. 251 is also used occasionally for restlessness.

Continuous subcutaneous infusions

Although drugs can usually be administered *by mouth* to control symptoms in palliative care, the parenteral route may sometimes be necessary. Repeated administration of *intramuscular injections* should be avoided in children, particularly if cachectic. This has led to the use of portable continuous infusion devices such as syringe drivers to give a *continuous subcutaneous infusion*, which can provide good control of symptoms with little discomfort or inconvenience to the patient.

Indications for the **parenteral route** are:

- inability to take medicines by mouth owing to *nausea and vomiting*, *dysphagia*, *severe weakness*, or *coma*;
- *malignant bowel obstruction* for which surgery is inappropriate (avoiding the need for an intravenous infusion or for insertion of a nasogastric tube);
- refusal by the child to take regular medication by mouth.

Syringe driver rate settings Staff using syringe drivers should be **adequately trained** and different rate settings should be **clearly identified** and **differentiated**; incorrect use of syringe drivers is a common cause of medication errors.

Bowel colic and excessive respiratory secretions Hyoscine hydrobromide p. 250 effectively reduces respiratory secretions and is sedative (but occasionally causes paradoxical agitation); it is given in a *subcutaneous* or *intravenous infusion*. Glycopyrronium bromide p.765 may also be used.

Hyoscine butylbromide p. 57 is effective in bowel colic, is less sedative than hyoscine hydrobromide, but is not always adequate for the control of respiratory secretions; it is given by *subcutaneous infusion* (**important**: *hyoscine butylbromide* must not be confused with *hyoscine hydrobromide*, above).

Confusion and restlessness Haloperidol p. 231 has little sedative effect. Levomepromazine p. 251 has a sedative effect. Midazolam p. 210 is a sedative and an antiepileptic that may be suitable for a very restless patient.

Convulsions If a child has previously been receiving an antiepileptic drug *or* has a primary or secondary cerebral tumour *or* is at risk of convulsion (e.g. owing to uraemia) antiepileptic medication should not be stopped. Midazolam p. 210 is the benzodiazepine antiepileptic of choice for *continuous subcutaneous infusion*.

Nausea and vomiting Levomepromazine p. 251 causes sedation in about 50% of patients. Haloperidol p. 231 has little sedative effect.

Cyclizine p. 244 is particularly likely to precipitate if mixed with diamorphine hydrochloride p. 261 or other drugs (see under *Mixing and compatibility*); it is given by *subcutaneous infusion*.

Pain control Diamorphine hydrochloride p. 261 is the preferred opioid since its high solubility permits a large dose to be given in a small volume (see under *Mixing and compatibility*). The table shows approximate equivalent doses of morphine and diamorphine hydrochloride.

Mixing and compatibility The general principle that injections should be given into separate sites (and should not be mixed) does not apply to the use of syringe drivers in palliative care. Provided that there is evidence of compatibility, selected injections can be mixed in syringe drivers. Not all types of medication can be used in a subcutaneous infusion. In particular, chlorpromazine hydrochloride p. 230, prochlorperazine p. 252, and diazepam p. 207 are **contra-indicated** as they cause skin reactions at the injection site; to a lesser extent cyclizine p. 244 and levomepromazine p. 251 also sometimes cause local irritation.

In theory injections dissolved in water for injections are more likely to be associated with pain (possibly owing to their hypotonicity). The use of physiological saline (sodium chloride 0.9% p. 547) however increases the likelihood of precipitation when more than one drug is used; moreover subcutaneous infusion rates are so slow (0.1– 0.3 mL/hour) that pain is not usually a problem when water is used as a diluent.

Compatibility with diamorphine Diamorphine can be given by *subcutaneous infusion* in a strength of up to 250 mg/mL; up to a strength of 40 mg/mL either *water for injections* or *physiological saline* (sodium chloride 0.9%) is a suitable diluent—above that strength only *water for injections* is used (to avoid precipitation).

The following can be mixed with *diamorphine*:

- **Cyclizine**, may precipitate at concentrations above 10 mg/mL *or* in the presence of sodium chloride 0.9% *or* as the concentration of diamorphine relative to cyclizine increases; mixtures of diamorphine and cyclizine are also likely to precipitate after 24 hours.
- **Dexamethasone**, special care is needed to avoid precipitation of dexamethasone when preparing it.
- **Haloperidol**, mixtures of haloperidol and diamorphine are likely to precipitate after 24 hours if haloperidol concentration is above 2 mg/mL.
- **Hyoscine butylbromide**
- **Hyoscine hydrobromide**
- **Levomepromazine**
- **Metoclopramide**, under some conditions infusions containing metoclopramide become discoloured; such solutions should be discarded.
- **Midazolam**

Subcutaneous infusion solution should be monitored regularly both to check for precipitation (and discolouration) and to ensure that the infusion is running at the correct rate.

Problems encountered with syringe drivers The following are problems that may be encountered with syringe drivers and the action that should be taken:

- if the subcutaneous infusion runs *too quickly* check the rate setting and the calculation;
- if the subcutaneous infusion runs *too slowly* check the start button, the battery, the syringe driver, the cannula, and make sure that the injection site is not inflamed;
- if there is an *injection site reaction* make sure that the site does not need to be changed—firmness or swelling at the site of injection is not in itself an indication for change, but pain or obvious inflammation is.

Equivalent doses of morphine sulfate and diamorphine hydrochloride given over 24 hours

These equivalences are *approximate only* and should be adjusted according to response

ORAL MORPHINE	PARENTERAL MORPHINE	PARENTERAL DIAMORPHINE
Oral morphine sulfate **over 24 hours**	Subcutaneous infusion of morphine sulfate **over 24 hours**	Subcutaneous infusion of diamorphine hydrochloride **over 24 hours**
30 mg	15 mg	10 mg
60 mg	30 mg	20 mg
90 mg	45 mg	30 mg
120 mg	60 mg	40 mg
180 mg	90 mg	60 mg
240 mg	120 mg	80 mg
360 mg	180 mg	120 mg
480 mg	240 mg	160 mg
600 mg	300 mg	200 mg
780 mg	390 mg	260 mg
960 mg	480 mg	320 mg
1200 mg	600 mg	400 mg

If breakthrough pain occurs give a subcutaneous injection equivalent to one-tenth to one-sixth of the total 24-hour subcutaneous infusion dose. With an intermittent subcutaneous injection absorption is smoother so that the risk of adverse effects at peak absorption is avoided (an even better method is to use a subcutaneous butterfly needle). To minimise the risk of infection no individual subcutaneous infusion solution should be used for longer than 24 hours.

Drugs and sport

Anti-doping

UK Anti-Doping, the national body responsible for the UK's anti-doping policy, advises that athletes are personally responsible should a prohibited substance be detected in their body. An advice card listing examples of permitted and prohibited substances is available from:

UK Anti-doping
Oceanic House
1a Cockspur Street
London
SW1Y 5BG
Tel: (020) 7766 7350
information@ukad.org.uk
www.ukad.org.uk

General Medical Council's advice

Doctors who prescribe or collude in the provision of drugs or treatment with the intention of improperly enhancing an individual's performance in sport contravene the GMC's guidance, and such actions would usually raise a question of a doctor's continued registration. This does not preclude the provision of any care or treatment where the doctor's intention is to protect or improve the patient's health.

Prescribing in dental practice

General guidance

Advice on the drug management of dental and oral conditions has been integrated into the main text. For ease of access, guidance on such conditions is usually identified by means of a relevant heading (e.g. Dental and Orofacial Pain) in the appropriate sections.

The following is a list of topics of particular relevance to dentists.

Prescribing by dentists, see Prescription writing p. 4

Oral side-effects of drugs, see Adverse reactions to drugs p. 11

Medical emergencies in dental practice, see BNF

Medical problems in dental practice, see BNF

Drug management of dental and oral conditions

Dental and orofacial pain, see Analgesics p. 252

Neuropathic pain p. 275

Non-opioid analgesics and compound analgesic preparations, see Analgesics p. 252

Opioid analgesics, see Analgesics p. 252

Non-steroidal anti-inflammatory drugs p. 604

Oral infections

Bacterial infections, see Antibacterials, principles of therapy p. 281

Phenoxymethylpenicillin p. 319

Broad-spectrum penicillins (amoxicillin p. 320 and ampicillin p. 321)

Cephalosporins (cefalexin p. 298 and cefradine p. 299)

Tetracyclines p. 332

Macrolides (clarithromycin p. 309, erythromycin p. 310 and azithromycin p. 308)

Clindamycin p. 307

Metronidazole p. 313

Fusidic acid p. 336

Fungal infections

Local treatment, see Oropharyngeal fungal infections p. 662

Systemic treatment, see Antifungals, systemic use p. 348

Viral infections

Herpetic gingivostomatitis, local treatment, see Oropharyngeal viral infections p. 663

Herpetic gingivostomatitis, systemic treatment, see Oropharyngeal viral infections p. 663 and Herpesvirus infections p. 380

Herpes labialis p. 674

Anaesthetics, anxiolytics and hypnotics

Sedation, anaesthesia, and resuscitation in dental practice p. 758

Hypnotics, see Hypnotics and anxiolytics p. 275

Sedation for dental procedures, see Hypnotics and anxiolytics p. 275

Local anaesthesia p. 776

Minerals

Fluorides p. 657

Oral ulceration and inflammation p. 659

Mouthwashes and gargles, see Mouthwashes and other preparations for oropharyngeal use p. 655

Dry mouth, see Treatment of dry mouth p. 654

Aromatic inhalations, see Aromatic inhalations, cough preparations and systemic nasal decongestants p. 176

Nasal decongestants, see Aromatic inhalations, cough preparations and systemic nasal decongestants p. 176

Dental Practitioners' Formulary p. 969

Chapter 1
Gastro-intestinal system

CONTENTS

1	**Chronic bowel disorders**	page 24
1.1	Inflammatory bowel disease	24
1.2	Irritable bowel syndrome	31
2	**Constipation and bowel cleansing**	32
2.1	Bowel cleansing	32
2.2	Constipation	34
3	**Diarrhoea**	43
4	**Disorders of gastric acid and ulceration**	46
4.1	Dyspepsia	46
4.2	Gastric and duodenal ulceration	49
4.3	Gastro-oesophageal reflux disease	55
4.4	*Helicobacter pylori* diagnosis	56

5	**Food allergy**	page 56
6	**Gastro-intestinal smooth muscle spasm**	56
7	**Liver disorders and related conditions**	59
7.1	Biliary disorders	59
7.2	Oesophageal varices	61
8	**Obesity**	62
9	**Rectal and anal disorders**	63
9.1	Haemorrhoids	64
10	**Reduced exocrine secretions**	66
11	**Stoma care**	67

1   Chronic bowel disorders

Chronic bowel disorders

Overview

Individual symptoms of chronic bowel disorders need specific treatment including dietary manipulation as well as drug treatment and the maintenance of a liberal fluid intake.

Irritable bowel syndrome

Irritable bowel syndrome can present with pain, constipation, or diarrhoea. Some children have important psychological aggravating factors which respond to reassurance. The **fibre** intake of children with irritable bowel syndrome should be reviewed. If an increase in dietary fibre is required, soluble fibre (e.g. oats, ispaghula husk p. 36, or sterculia p. 36) is recommended; insoluble fibre (e.g. bran) should be avoided. A **laxative** can be used to treat constipation. An osmotic laxative, such as a macrogol, is preferred; lactulose p. 37 may cause bloating. Loperamide hydrochloride p. 44 may relieve diarrhoea and antispasmodic drugs may relieve pain. Opioids with a central action, such as codeine phosphate p. 259, are better avoided because of the risk of dependence.

Clostridium difficile infection

Clostridium difficile infection is caused by colonisation of the colon with *Clostridium difficile* and production of toxin. It often follows antibiotic therapy and is usually of acute onset, but may become chronic. It is a particular hazard of ampicillin p. 321, amoxicillin p. 320, co-amoxiclav p. 323, second- and third-generation cephalosporins, clindamycin p. 307, and quinolones, but few antibacterials are free of this side-effect. Oral metronidazole p. 313 or oral vancomycin p. 305 are used as specific treatment; vancomycin may be preferred for very sick patients. Metronidazole can be given by intravenous infusion if oral treatment is inappropriate.

Malabsorption syndromes

Individual conditions need specific management and also general nutritional consideration. Coeliac disease (gluten enteropathy) usually needs a gluten-free diet and pancreatic insufficiency needs pancreatin supplements.

For further information on foods for special diets (ACBS), see Borderline substances.

1.1   Inflammatory bowel disease

Inflammatory bowel disease

Management of acute ulcerative colitis and Crohn's disease

Chronic inflammatory bowel diseases include *ulcerative colitis* and *Crohn's disease*. The treatment of inflammatory bowel disease in children should be initiated and supervised by a paediatric gastroenterologist. Effective management requires drug therapy, attention to nutrition, and in severe or chronic active disease, surgery.

Aminosalicylates (balsalazide sodium p. 26, mesalazine p. 26, olsalazine sodium p. 28, and sulfasalazine p. 29), **corticosteroids** (hydrocortisone p. 411, budesonide p. 30, and prednisolone p. 413), and **drugs that affect the immune response** are used in the treatment of inflammatory bowel disease.

Treatment of acute ulcerative colitis and Crohn's disease

Acute mild to moderate disease affecting the rectum (proctitis) or the recto-sigmoid (distal colitis) is treated initially with local application of an aminosalicylate; alternatively a local corticosteroid can be used but it is less effective. Foam preparations and suppositories are useful for children who have difficulty retaining liquid enemas.

Diffuse inflammatory bowel disease or disease that does not respond to local therapy requires oral treatment. Mild disease affecting the proximal colon can be treated with an oral aminosalicylate alone; a combination of a local and an oral aminosalicylate can be used in proctitis or distal colitis. Refractory or moderate inflammatory bowel disease usually requires adjunctive use of an oral corticosteroid such as prednisolone for 4–8 weeks. Modified-release budesonide is used for children with Crohn's disease affecting the ileum and the ascending colon; it causes fewer systemic side effects than oral prednisolone, but may be less effective. As an alternative to an oral corticosteroid, **enteral nutrition** may be used for 6–8 weeks in children with active Crohn's disease.

Severe inflammatory bowel disease or disease that is not responding to an oral corticosteroid requires hospital admission and treatment with an intravenous corticosteroid such as hydrocortisone or methylprednisolone p. 412; other therapy may include intravenous fluid and electrolyte replacement, and possibly parenteral nutrition. Children with ulcerative colitis that fails to respond adequately to these measures may benefit from a short course of ciclosporin p. 486. Children with unresponsive or chronically active Crohn's disease may benefit from azathioprine p. 485, mercaptopurine p. 505, or once-weekly methotrexate p. 506; these drugs have a slow onset of action.

Infliximab p. 30 is used in specialist centres for children with severe active Crohn's disease or severe active ulcerative colitis whose condition has not responded adequately to treatment with a corticosteroid and a conventional drug that affects the immune response, or who are intolerant of them. Adalimumab p. 598 is licensed for children with severe active Crohn's disease whose condition has not responded adequately to conventional therapy (including corticosteroids, other drugs that affect the immune response, and primary nutrition therapy) or who are intolerant of it. There are concerns about the long-term safety of infliximab and adalimumab in children; hepatosplenic T-cell lymphoma has been reported.

Crohn's disease of the mouth or of the perineum is more common in children than in adults and it is difficult to treat; elimination diets and the use of a topical corticosteroid may be beneficial, but a systemic corticosteroid and occasionally azathioprine may be required in severe cases.

Maintenance of remission of acute ulcerative colitis and Crohn's disease

Children should be advised not to smoke because smoking increases the risk of relapse in Crohn's disease. Smoking cessation should be encouraged when necessary.

Aminosalicylates are efficacious in the maintenance of remission of ulcerative colitis, but there is no evidence of efficacy in the maintenance of remission of Crohn's disease. Corticosteroids are **not** suitable for maintenance treatment because of their side-effects. In resistant or frequently relapsing cases either azathioprine or mercaptopurine may be helpful. Methotrexate is used in Crohn's disease when azathioprine or mercaptopurine are ineffective or not tolerated. Infliximab can be used for maintenance therapy in Crohn's disease or ulcerative colitis in children who respond to the initial induction course of this drug. Adalimumab is also licensed for maintenance therapy in Crohn's disease. There are concerns about the long-term safety of infliximab and adalimumab in children.

Fistulating Crohn's disease

Treatment may not be necessary for simple, asymptomatic perianal fistulas. Metronidazole p. 313 or ciprofloxacin p. 328 may be beneficial for the treatment of fistulating Crohn's disease [both unlicensed for this indication]. Metronidazole by mouth is usually given for 1 month but no longer than 3 months because of concerns about peripheral neuropathy. Ciprofloxacin by mouth is given twice daily. Other antibacterials should be given if specifically indicated (e.g. sepsis associated with fistulas and perianal disease) and for managing bacterial overgrowth in the small bowel. Fistulas may also require surgical exploration and local drainage.

Either azathioprine or mercaptopurine is used as a second-line treatment for fistulating Crohn's disease and continued for maintenance. Infliximab is used for fistulating Crohn's disease refractory to conventional treatments; maintenance therapy with infliximab should be considered for patients who respond to the initial induction course.

Adjunctive treatment of inflammatory bowel disease

Due attention should be paid to diet; high-fibre or low-residue diets should be used as appropriate.

Antimotility drugs such as codeine phosphate p. 259 and loperamide hydrochloride p. 44, and antispasmodic drugs may precipitate paralytic ileus and megacolon in active ulcerative colitis; treatment of the inflammation is more logical. Laxatives may be required in proctitis. Diarrhoea resulting from the loss of bile-salt absorption (e.g. in terminal ileal disease or bowel resection) may improve with colestyramine p. 120, which binds bile salts.

Drugs used in inflammatory bowel disease

Aminosalicylates

Sulfasalazine is a combination of 5-aminosalicylic acid ('5-ASA') and sulfapyridine; sulfapyridine acts only as a carrier to the colonic site of action but still causes side-effects. In the newer aminosalicylates, mesalazine (5-aminosalicylic acid), balsalazide sodium (a prodrug of 5-aminosalicylic acid) and olsalazine sodium (a dimer of 5-aminosalicylic acid which cleaves in the lower bowel), the sulfonamide-related side-effects of sulfasalazine are avoided, but 5-aminosalicylic acid alone can still cause side-effects including blood disorders and lupus-like syndrome also seen with sulfasalazine.

Drugs affecting the immune response

Azathioprine, mercaptopurine, or once weekly methotrexate are used to induce remission in unresponsive or chronically active Crohn's disease. Azathioprine or mercaptopurine may also be helpful for retaining remission in frequently relapsing inflammatory bowel disease; once weekly methotrexate is used in Crohn's disease when azathioprine or mercaptopurine are ineffective or not tolerated. Response to azathioprine or mercaptopurine may not become apparent for several months. Folic acid p. 533 should be given to reduce the possibility of methotrexate toxicity. Folic acid is usually given once weekly on a different day to the methotrexate; alternative regimens may be used in some settings.

Ciclosporin (ciclosporin) p. 486 is a potent immunosuppressant and is markedly nephrotoxic. In children with severe ulcerative colitis unresponsive to other treatment, ciclosporin may reduce the need for urgent colorectal surgery.

Cytokine modulators

Infliximab p. 30 and adalimumab p. 598 are monoclonal antibodies which inhibit the pro-inflammatory cytokine, tumour necrosis factor alpha. They are used in the treatment of severe refractory Crohn's disease. Infliximab is also used in the treatment of severe refractory ulcerative colitis. They should be used only when treatment with other immunomodulating drugs has failed or is not tolerated and for children in whom surgery is inappropriate. Cytokine modulators should be used under specialist supervision. Adequate resuscitation facilities must be available when infliximab is used.

AMINOSALICYLATES

Aminosalicylates

- ● **SIDE-EFFECTS**
  - ▸ **Rare** Acute pancreatitis · agranulocytosis · alopecia · aplastic anaemia · arthralgia · blood disorders · eosinophilia · fibrosing alveolitis · hepatitis · interstitial nephritis · leucopenia · lung disorders · lupus erythematosus-like syndrome · methaemoglobinaemia · myalgia · myocarditis · nephrotic syndrome · neutropenia · pericarditis · peripheral neuropathy · renal dysfunction · skin reactions · Stevens-Johnson syndrome · thrombocytopenia
  - ▸ **Frequency not known** Abdominal pain · diarrhoea · exacerbation of symptoms of colitis · headache · hypersensitivity reactions · nausea · rash · urticaria · vomiting

SIDE-EFFECTS, FURTHER INFORMATION
‣ Blood Disorders A blood count should be performed and the drug stopped immediately if there is suspicion of a blood dyscrasia.
● **ALLERGY AND CROSS-SENSITIVITY** Contra-indicated in salicylate hypersensitivity.
● **RENAL IMPAIRMENT**
Monitoring
Renal function should be monitored more frequently in renal impairment.
● **MONITORING REQUIREMENTS** Renal function should be monitored before starting an oral aminosalicylate, at 3 months of treatment, and then annually during treatment.
● **PATIENT AND CARER ADVICE**
Blood disorders Patients receiving aminosalicylates, and their carers, should be advised to report any unexplained bleeding, bruising, purpura, sore throat, fever or malaise that occurs during treatment.

F 25

Balsalazide sodium

● **INDICATIONS AND DOSE**
Treatment of mild to moderate ulcerative colitis, acute attack
‣ BY MOUTH
 ‣ Child 12-17 years: 2.25 g 3 times a day until remission occurs or for up to maximum of 12 weeks
Maintenance of remission of ulcerative colitis
‣ BY MOUTH
 ‣ Child 12-17 years: 1.5 g twice daily (max. per dose 3 g), adjusted according to response; maximum 6 g per day

● **UNLICENSED USE** Not licensed for use in children under 18 years.
● **CAUTIONS** History of asthma
● **SIDE-EFFECTS** Cholelithiasis
● **PREGNANCY** Manufacturer advises avoid.
● **BREAST FEEDING** Diarrhoea may develop in the infant. Monitor breast-fed infants for diarrhoea.
● **HEPATIC IMPAIRMENT** Avoid in severe impairment.
● **RENAL IMPAIRMENT** Manufacturer advises avoid in moderate to severe impairment.

● **MEDICINAL FORMS**
There can be variation in the licensing of different medicines containing the same drug.
Capsule
CAUTIONARY AND ADVISORY LABELS 21, 25
 ‣ Colazide (Almirall Ltd)
  Balsalazide disodium 750 mg Colazide 750mg capsules | 130 capsule PoM £30.42 DT price = £30.42

F 25

Mesalazine

● **INDICATIONS AND DOSE**
ASACOL® MR 400MG TABLETS
Treatment of mild to moderate ulcerative colitis, acute attack
‣ BY MOUTH
 ‣ Child 12-17 years: 800 mg 3 times a day
Maintenance of remission of ulcerative colitis and Crohn's ileo-colitis
‣ BY MOUTH
 ‣ Child 12-17 years: 400–800 mg 2–3 times a day

ASACOL® FOAM ENEMA
Treatment of acute attack of mild to moderate ulcerative colitis affecting the rectosigmoid region
‣ BY RECTUM
 ‣ Child 12-17 years: 1 g daily for 4–6 weeks, to be administered into the rectum
Treatment of acute attack of mild to moderate ulcerative colitis, affecting the descending colon
‣ BY RECTUM
 ‣ Child 12-17 years: 2 g once daily for 4–6 weeks, to be administered into the rectum

ASACOL® SUPPOSITORIES
Treatment and maintenance of remission of ulcerative colitis affecting the rectosigmoid region
‣ BY RECTUM
 ‣ Child 12-17 years: 250–500 mg 3 times a day, last dose to be administered at bedtime

IPOCOL®
Treatment of mild to moderate ulcerative colitis, acute attack
‣ BY MOUTH
 ‣ Child 6-17 years (body-weight 40 kg and above): 800 mg 3 times a day
Maintenance of remission of ulcerative colitis
‣ BY MOUTH
 ‣ Child 6-17 years (body-weight 40 kg and above): 1.2–2 g daily in divided doses

OCTASA®
Treatment of mild to moderate ulcerative colitis, acute attack
‣ BY MOUTH
 ‣ Child 6-17 years (body-weight 40 kg and above): 2.4–4 g daily in divided doses
Maintenance of remission of ulcerative colitis and Crohn's ileo-colitis
‣ BY MOUTH
 ‣ Child 6-17 years (body-weight 40 kg and above): 1.2–2 g once daily, alternatively daily in divided doses

PENTASA® GRANULES
Treatment of mild to moderate ulcerative colitis, acute attack
‣ BY MOUTH
 ‣ Child 5-17 years (body-weight up to 40 kg): 10–20 mg/kg 3 times a day
 ‣ Child 5-17 years (body-weight 40 kg and above): 1–2 g twice daily, total daily dose may alternatively be given in 3–4 divided doses
Maintenance of remission of ulcerative colitis
‣ BY MOUTH
 ‣ Child 5-17 years (body-weight up to 40 kg): 7.5–15 mg/kg twice daily, total daily dose may alternatively be given in 3 divided doses
 ‣ Child 5-17 years (body-weight 40 kg and above): 2 g once daily

PENTASA® RETENTION ENEMA
Treatment of acute attack of mild to moderate ulcerative colitis affecting the rectosigmoid region
‣ BY RECTUM
 ‣ Child 12-17 years: 1 g once daily, dose to be administered at bedtime

PENTASA® SUPPOSITORIES

Treatment of acute attack, ulcerative proctitis
▶ BY RECTUM
- Child 12–14 years: 1 g daily for 2–4 weeks
- Child 15–17 years: 1 g daily for 2–4 weeks

Maintenance, ulcerative proctitis
▶ BY RECTUM
- Child 12–14 years: 1 g daily
- Child 15–17 years: 1 g daily

PENTASA® TABLETS

Treatment of mild to moderate ulcerative colitis, acute attack
▶ BY MOUTH
- Child 5–17 years (body-weight up to 40 kg): 10–20 mg/kg 3 times a day
- Child 5–17 years (body-weight 40 kg and above): 1–2 g twice daily, total daily dose may alternatively be given in 3 divided doses

Maintenance of remission of ulcerative colitis
▶ BY MOUTH
- Child 5–17 years (body-weight up to 40 kg): 7.5–15 mg/kg twice daily, total daily dose may alternatively be given in 3 divided doses
- Child 5–17 years (body-weight 40 kg and above): 2 g once daily

SALOFALK® ENEMA

Treatment of acute attack of mild to moderate ulcerative colitis or maintenance of remission
▶ BY RECTUM
- Child 12–17 years: 2 g once daily, dose to be administered at bedtime

SALOFALK® GRANULES

Treatment of mild to moderate ulcerative colitis, acute attack
▶ BY MOUTH
- Child 5–17 years (body-weight up to 40 kg): 30–50 mg/kg once daily, dose preferably given in the morning, alternatively 10–20 mg/kg 3 times a day
- Child 5–17 years (body-weight 40 kg and above): 1.5–3 g once daily, dose preferably given in the morning, alternatively 0.5–1 g 3 times a day

Maintenance of remission of ulcerative colitis
▶ BY MOUTH
- Child 5–17 years (body-weight up to 40 kg): 7.5–15 mg/kg twice daily, total daily dose may alternatively be given in 3 divided doses
- Child 5–17 years (body-weight 40 kg and above): 500 mg 3 times a day

SALOFALK® RECTAL FOAM

Treatment of mild ulcerative colitis affecting sigmoid colon and rectum
▶ BY RECTUM
- Child 12–17 years: 2 g once daily, dose to be administered into the rectum at bedtime, alternatively 2 g daily in 2 divided doses

SALOFALK® SUPPOSITORIES

Treatment of acute attack of mild to moderate ulcerative colitis affecting the rectum, sigmoid colon and descending colon
▶ BY RECTUM
- Child 12–17 years: 0.5–1 g 2–3 times a day, adjusted according to response, dose to be given using 500 mg suppositories

SALOFALK® TABLETS

Treatment of mild to moderate ulcerative colitis, acute attack
▶ BY MOUTH
- Child 5–17 years (body-weight up to 40 kg): 10–20 mg/kg 3 times a day
- Child 5–17 years (body-weight 40 kg and above): 0.5–1 g 3 times a day

Maintenance of remission of ulcerative colitis
▶ BY MOUTH
- Child 5–17 years (body-weight up to 40 kg): 7.5–15 mg/kg twice daily, total daily dose may alternatively be given in 3 divided doses
- Child 5–17 years (body-weight 40 kg and above): 500 mg 3 times a day

DOSE EQUIVALENCE AND CONVERSION
There is no evidence to show that any one oral preparation of mesalazine is more effective than another; however, the delivery characteristics of oral mesalazine preparations may vary.

- **UNLICENSED USE**
  ▶ With oral use *Asacol*® (all preparations) not licensed for use in children under 18 years. *Pentasa*® tablets not licensed for use in children under 15 years. *Pentasa*® granules and *Salofalk*® tablets and granules not licensed for use in children under 6 years.
  ▶ With rectal use *Asacol*® (all preparations) and *Salofalk*® enema not licensed for use in children under 18 years. *Salofalk*® suppositories and *Pentasa*® suppositories not licensed for use in children under 15 years. *Salofalk*® rectal foam no dose recommendations for children (age range not specified by manufacturer). *Pentasa*® enema not licensed for use in children.

- **CONTRA-INDICATIONS** Blood clotting abnormalities
- **CAUTIONS** Pulmonary disease
- **INTERACTIONS** The manufacturers of some mesalazine gastro-resistant and modified-release medicines (*Asacol*® MR tablets, *Ipocol*®, *Salofalk*® granules) suggest that preparations that lower stool pH (e.g. lactulose) may prevent the release of mesalazine.
- **SIDE-EFFECTS**
  ▶ **Rare** Dizziness
  ▶ **Very rare** Oligospermia (reversible)
- **PREGNANCY** Negligible quantities cross placenta.
- **BREAST FEEDING** Diarrhoea reported in breast-fed infants, but negligible amounts of mesalazine detected in breast milk.
  Monitor breast-fed infant for diarrhoea.
- **HEPATIC IMPAIRMENT** Avoid in severe impairment.
- **RENAL IMPAIRMENT** Use with caution. Avoid if estimated glomerular filtration rate less than 20 mL/minute/1.73 m^2.
- **DIRECTIONS FOR ADMINISTRATION**
  PENTASA® TABLETS Tablets may be halved, quartered, or dispersed in water, but should not be chewed.
  SALOFALK® GRANULES Granules should be placed on tongue and washed down with water without chewing.
  PENTASA® GRANULES Granules should be placed on tongue and washed down with water or orange juice without chewing.
  Contents of one sachet should be weighed and divided immediately before use; discard any remaining granules.
- **PRESCRIBING AND DISPENSING INFORMATION** There is no evidence to show that any one oral preparation of mesalazine is more effective than another; however, the delivery characteristics of oral mesalazine preparations may vary.
  Flavours of granule formulations of *Salofalk*® may include vanilla.

Gastro-intestinal system

1

● PATIENT AND CARER ADVICE
If it is necessary to switch a patient to a different brand of mesalazine, the patient should be advised to report any changes in symptoms.

Some products may require special administration advice; patients and carers should be informed.

Medicines for Children leaflet: Mesalazine (oral) for inflammatory bowel disease www.medicinesforchildren.org.uk/mesalazine-oral-for-inflammatory-bowel-disease

Medicines for Children leaflet: Mesalazine foam enema for inflammatory bowel disease www.medicinesforchildren.org.uk/mesalazine-foam-enema-for-inflammatory-bowel-disease

Medicines for Children leaflet: Mesalazine liquid enema for inflammatory bowel disease www.medicinesforchildren.org.uk/mesalazine-liquid-enema-for-inflammatory-bowel-disease

Medicines for Children leaflet: Mesalazine suppositories for inflammatory bowel disease www.medicinesforchildren.org.uk/mesalazine-suppositories-for-inflammatory-bowel-disease

● MEDICINAL FORMS
There can be variation in the licensing of different medicines containing the same drug.

Modified-release tablet
CAUTIONARY AND ADVISORY LABELS 21 (does not apply to Pentasa® tablets), 25 (does not apply to Pentasa® tablets)
▸ Pentasa (Ferring Pharmaceuticals Ltd)
Mesalazine 500 mg Pentasa 500mg modified-release tablets | 100 tablet [PoM] £30.74 DT price = £30.74
Mesalazine 1 gram Pentasa 1g modified-release tablets | 60 tablet [PoM] £36.89 DT price = £36.89

Gastro-resistant tablet
CAUTIONARY AND ADVISORY LABELS 5 (does not apply to Octasa®), 25
▸ Asacol MR (Allergan Ltd)
Mesalazine 400 mg Asacol 400mg MR gastro-resistant tablets | 84 tablet [PoM] £27.45 DT price = £27.45 | 168 tablet [PoM] £54.90
Mesalazine 800 mg Asacol 800mg MR gastro-resistant tablets | 84 tablet [PoM] £54.90 DT price = £54.90
▸ Ipocol (Sandoz Ltd)
Mesalazine 400 mg Ipocol 400mg gastro-resistant tablets | 120 tablet [PoM] £17.68
▸ Octasa MR (Tillotts Pharma Ltd)
Mesalazine 400 mg Octasa 400mg MR gastro-resistant tablets | 90 tablet [PoM] £19.50 DT price = £19.50 | 120 tablet [PoM] £26.00
Mesalazine 800 mg Octasa 800mg MR gastro-resistant tablets | 90 tablet [PoM] £47.50 | 180 tablet [PoM] £95.00 DT price = £95.00
▸ Salofalk (Dr. Falk Pharma UK Ltd)
Mesalazine 250 mg Salofalk 250mg gastro-resistant tablets | 100 tablet [PoM] £16.19
Mesalazine 500 mg Salofalk 500mg gastro-resistant tablets | 100 tablet [PoM] £32.38

Modified-release granules
CAUTIONARY AND ADVISORY LABELS 25 (does not apply to Pentasa® granules)
EXCIPIENTS: May contain Aspartame
▸ Pentasa (Ferring Pharmaceuticals Ltd)
Mesalazine 1 gram Pentasa 1g modified-release granules sachets sugar-free | 50 sachet [PoM] £30.74 DT price = £30.74
Mesalazine 2 gram Pentasa 2g modified-release granules sachets sugar-free | 60 sachet [PoM] £73.78 DT price = £73.78
Mesalazine 4 gram Pentasa 4g modified-release granules sachets sugar-free | 30 sachet [PoM] £73.78
▸ Salofalk (Dr. Falk Pharma UK Ltd)
Mesalazine 500 mg Salofalk 500mg gastro-resistant modified-release granules sachets sugar-free | 100 sachet [PoM] £28.74
Mesalazine 1 gram Salofalk 1g gastro-resistant modified-release granules sachets sugar-free | 50 sachet [PoM] £28.74 DT price = £28.74
Mesalazine 1.5 gram Salofalk 1.5g gastro-resistant modified-release granules sachets sugar-free | 60 sachet [PoM] £48.85 DT price = £48.85
Mesalazine 3 gram Salofalk 3g gastro-resistant modified-release granules sachets sugar-free | 60 sachet [PoM] £97.70 DT price = £97.70

Foam
EXCIPIENTS: May contain Cetostearyl alcohol (including cetyl and stearyl alcohol), disodium edetate, hydroxybenzoates (parabens), polysorbates, propylene glycol, sodium metabisulfite

▸ Asacol (Allergan Ltd)
Mesalazine 1 gram per 1 application Asacol 1g/application foam enema | 14 dose [PoM] £26.72
▸ Salofalk (Dr. Falk Pharma UK Ltd)
Mesalazine 1 gram per 1 application Salofalk 1g/application foam enema | 14 dose [PoM] £30.17

Suppository
▸ Asacol (Allergan Ltd)
Mesalazine 250 mg Asacol 250mg suppositories | 20 suppository [PoM] £4.82 DT price = £4.82
Mesalazine 500 mg Asacol 500mg suppositories | 10 suppository [PoM] £4.82 DT price = £4.82
▸ Pentasa (Ferring Pharmaceuticals Ltd)
Mesalazine 1 gram Pentasa 1g suppositories | 28 suppository [PoM] £40.01 DT price = £40.01
▸ Salofalk (Dr. Falk Pharma UK Ltd)
Mesalazine 500 mg Salofalk 500mg suppositories | 30 suppository [PoM] £14.81
Mesalazine 1 gram Salofalk 1g suppositories | 30 suppository [PoM] £29.62

Enema
▸ Pentasa (Ferring Pharmaceuticals Ltd)
Mesalazine 10 mg per 1 ml Pentasa Mesalazine 1g/100ml enema | 7 enema [PoM] £17.73 DT price = £17.73
▸ Salofalk (Dr. Falk Pharma UK Ltd)
Mesalazine 33.9 mg per 1 ml Salofalk 2g/59ml enema | 7 enema [PoM] £29.92

▣ 25

Olsalazine sodium

● INDICATIONS AND DOSE
Treatment of acute attack of mild ulcerative colitis
▸ BY MOUTH
▸ Child 2–17 years: 500 mg twice daily, dose to be taken after food, then increased if necessary up to 1 g 3 times a day, dose to be increased over 1 week

Maintenance of remission of mild ulcerative colitis
▸ BY MOUTH
▸ Child 2–17 years: Maintenance 250–500 mg twice daily, dose to be taken after food

● UNLICENSED USE Not licensed for use in children under 12 years.

● SIDE-EFFECTS
▸ Common or very common Watery diarrhoea
▸ Frequency not known Blurred vision · palpitation · photosensitivity · pyrexia · tachycardia

● PREGNANCY Manufacturer advises avoid unless potential benefit outweighs risk.

● BREAST FEEDING
Monitoring
Monitor breast-fed infants for diarrhoea.

● RENAL IMPAIRMENT Use with caution; manufacturer advises avoid in significant impairment.

● DIRECTIONS FOR ADMINISTRATION Capsules can be opened and contents sprinkled on food.

● MEDICINAL FORMS
There can be variation in the licensing of different medicines containing the same drug. Forms available from special-order manufacturers include: oral suspension, oral solution

Tablet
CAUTIONARY AND ADVISORY LABELS 21
▸ Olsalazine sodium (Non-proprietary)
Olsalazine sodium 500 mg Olsalazine 500mg tablets | 60 tablet [PoM] £85.00–£161.00 DT price = £161.00

Capsule
CAUTIONARY AND ADVISORY LABELS 21
▸ Olsalazine sodium (Non-proprietary)
Olsalazine sodium 250 mg Olsalazine 250mg capsules | 112 capsule [PoM] £75.00–£144.00 DT price = £144.00

Sulfasalazine

F 25

(Sulphasalazine)

- **INDICATIONS AND DOSE**

Treatment of acute attack of mild to moderate and severe ulcerative colitis | Active Crohn's disease
- ▸ BY MOUTH
  - ▸ Child 2-11 years: 10–15 mg/kg 4–6 times a day (max. per dose 1 g) until remission occurs; increased if necessary up to 60 mg/kg daily in divided doses
  - ▸ Child 12-17 years: 1–2 g 4 times a day until remission occurs
- ▸ BY RECTUM
  - ▸ Child 5-7 years: 500 mg twice daily
  - ▸ Child 8-11 years: 500 mg, dose to be administered in the morning and 1 g, dose to be administered at night
  - ▸ Child 12-17 years: 0.5–1 g twice daily

Maintenance of remission of mild to moderate and severe ulcerative colitis
- ▸ BY MOUTH
  - ▸ Child 2-11 years: 5–7.5 mg/kg 4 times a day (max. per dose 500 mg)
  - ▸ Child 12-17 years: 500 mg 4 times a day
- ▸ BY RECTUM
  - ▸ Child 5-7 years: 500 mg twice daily
  - ▸ Child 8-11 years: 500 mg, dose to be administered in the morning and 1 g, dose to be administered at night
  - ▸ Child 12-17 years: 0.5–1 g twice daily

Juvenile idiopathic arthritis
- ▸ BY MOUTH
  - ▸ Child 2-11 years: Initially 5 mg/kg twice daily for 1 week, then 10 mg/kg twice daily for 1 week, then 20 mg/kg twice daily for 1 week; maintenance 20–25 mg/kg twice daily; maximum 2 g per day
  - ▸ Child 12-17 years: Initially 5 mg/kg twice daily for 1 week, then 10 mg/kg twice daily for 1 week, then 20 mg/kg twice daily for 1 week; maintenance 20–25 mg/kg twice daily; maximum 3 g per day

- **UNLICENSED USE** Not licensed for use in children for juvenile idiopathic arthritis.
- **CONTRA-INDICATIONS** Child under 2 years of age
- **CAUTIONS** Acute porphyrias p. 562 · G6PD deficiency · history of allergy · history of asthma · maintain adequate fluid intake · risk of haematological toxicity · risk of hepatic toxicity · slow acetylator status
- **INTERACTIONS** → Appendix 1 (aminosalicylates).
- **SIDE-EFFECTS**
- ▸ **Common or very common** Blood disorders · cough · dizziness · fever · Heinz body anaemia · insomnia · megaloblastic anaemia · proteinuria · pruritus · stomatitis · taste disturbances · tinnitus
- ▸ **Uncommon** Alopecia · convulsions · depression · dyspnoea · vasculitis
- ▸ **Frequency not known** Anaphylaxis · aseptic meningitis · ataxia · crystalluria · disturbances of smell · epidermal necrolysis · exfoliative dermatitis · gastro-intestinal intolerance · hallucinations · hypersensitivity reactions · leucopenia (especially in patients with rheumatoid arthritis) · loss of appetite · neutropenia (especially in patients with rheumatoid arthritis) · oligospermia · parotitis · photosensitivity · rashes · serum sickness · some soft contact lenses may be stained · thrombocytopenia (especially in patients with rheumatoid arthritis) · yellow-orange discoloration of other body fluids · yellow-orange discoloration of skin · yellow-orange discoloration of urine

SIDE-EFFECTS, FURTHER INFORMATION
- ▸ Gastro-intestinal side-effects Upper gastro-intestinal side-effects common over 4 g daily.

- ▸ Blood disorders Haematological abnormalities occur usually in the first 3 to 6 months of treatment and are reversible on cessation of treatment.
- **PREGNANCY** Theoretical risk of neonatal haemolysis in third trimester; adequate folate supplements should be given to mother.
- **BREAST FEEDING** Small amounts in milk (1 report of bloody diarrhoea); theoretical risk of neonatal haemolysis especially in G6PD-deficient infants.
- **HEPATIC IMPAIRMENT** Use with caution.
- **RENAL IMPAIRMENT** Risk of toxicity, including crystalluria, in moderate impairment—ensure high fluid intake. Avoid in severe impairment.
- **MONITORING REQUIREMENTS**
- ▸ Blood disorders Close monitoring of full blood counts (including differential white cell count and platelet count) is necessary initially, and at monthly intervals during the first 3 months.
- ▸ Renal function Although the manufacturer recommends renal function tests in rheumatic diseases, evidence of practical value is unsatisfactory.
- ▸ Liver function Liver function tests should be performed at monthly intervals for first 3 months.
- **PATIENT AND CARER ADVICE**
Contact lenses Some soft contact lenses may be stained.

- **MEDICINAL FORMS**
There can be variation in the licensing of different medicines containing the same drug. Forms available from special-order manufacturers include: oral suspension

Tablet
CAUTIONARY AND ADVISORY LABELS 14
- ▸ Sulfasalazine (Non-proprietary)
  Sulfasalazine 500 mg Sulfasalazine 500mg tablets | 112 tablet [PoM] £18.00 DT price = £6.13
- ▸ Salazopyrin (Pfizer Ltd)
  Sulfasalazine 500 mg Salazopyrin 500mg tablets | 112 tablet [PoM] £6.97 DT price = £6.13

Gastro-resistant tablet
CAUTIONARY AND ADVISORY LABELS 5, 14, 25
- ▸ Sulfasalazine (Non-proprietary)
  Sulfasalazine 500 mg Sulfasalazine 500mg gastro-resistant tablets | 100 tablet [PoM] no price available | 112 tablet [PoM] £27.00 DT price = £8.63
- ▸ Salazopyrin EN (Pfizer Ltd)
  Sulfasalazine 500 mg Salazopyrin EN-Tabs 500mg | 112 tablet [PoM] £8.43 DT price = £8.63
- ▸ Sulazine EC (Genesis Pharmaceuticals Ltd, Teva UK Ltd)
  Sulfasalazine 500 mg Sulazine EC 500mg tablets | 112 tablet [PoM] £8.00 DT price = £8.63

Oral suspension
CAUTIONARY AND ADVISORY LABELS 14
EXCIPIENTS: May contain Alcohol
- ▸ Sulfasalazine (Non-proprietary)
  Sulfasalazine 50 mg per 1 ml Sulfasalazine 250mg/5ml oral suspension sugar free sugar-free | 500 ml [PoM] £44.09 DT price = £43.42

Suppository
CAUTIONARY AND ADVISORY LABELS 14
- ▸ Salazopyrin (Pfizer Ltd)
  Sulfasalazine 500 mg Salazopyrin 500mg suppositories | 10 suppository [PoM] £3.30

1

Gastro-intestinal system

CORTICOSTEROIDS ⌦ 407

Budesonide

- **INDICATIONS AND DOSE**

BUDENOFALK® CAPSULES

Mild to moderate Crohn's disease affecting the ileum or ascending colon | Chronic diarrhoea due to collagenous colitis
- BY MOUTH
  - Child 12–17 years: 3 mg 3 times a day for up to 8 weeks, reduce dose for the last 2 weeks of treatment

ENTOCORT® CAPSULES

Mild to moderate Crohn's disease affecting the ileum or ascending colon
- BY MOUTH
  - Child 12–17 years: 9 mg once daily for up to 8 weeks; reduce dose for the last 2–4 weeks of treatment, to be taken in the morning

ENTOCORT® ENEMA

Ulcerative colitis involving rectal and recto-sigmoid disease
- BY RECTUM
  - Child 12–17 years: 1 enema daily for 4 weeks, to be administered at bedtime

- **UNLICENSED USE** Not licensed for use in children.
- **DIRECTIONS FOR ADMINISTRATION** Capsules can be opened and the contents mixed with apple or orange juice.
- **PRESCRIBING AND DISPENSING INFORMATION**
ENTOCORT® CAPSULES Dispense modified-release capsules in original container (contains desiccant).

- **MEDICINAL FORMS**
There can be variation in the licensing of different medicines containing the same drug.

Modified-release capsule
CAUTIONARY AND ADVISORY LABELS 5, 10, 25
- Entocort CR (Tillotts Pharma Ltd)
  Budesonide 3 mg Entocort CR 3mg capsules | 100 capsule PoM £99.00 DT price = £99.00

Gastro-resistant capsule
CAUTIONARY AND ADVISORY LABELS 5, 10, 22, 25
- Budenofalk (Dr. Falk Pharma UK Ltd)
  Budesonide 3 mg Budenofalk 3mg gastro-resistant capsules | 100 capsule PoM £75.05 DT price = £75.05

Enema
- Entocort (Tillotts Pharma Ltd)
  Budesonide 20 microgram per 1 ml Entocort 2mg/100ml enema | 7 enema PoM £39.60

IMMUNOSUPPRESSANTS > TUMOR NECROSIS FACTOR ALPHA (TNF-α) INHIBITORS

Infliximab   31.5.2016

- **INDICATIONS AND DOSE**

Severe active Crohn's disease
- BY INTRAVENOUS INFUSION
  - Child 6–17 years: Initially 5 mg/kg, then 5 mg/kg after 2 weeks, then 5 mg/kg after 4 weeks, then maintenance 5 mg/kg every 8 weeks, interval between maintenance doses adjusted according to response; discontinue if no response within 10 weeks of initial dose

Fistulating Crohn's disease
- BY INTRAVENOUS INFUSION
  - Child 6–17 years: Initially 5 mg/kg, then 5 mg/kg after 2 weeks, followed by 5 mg/kg after 4 weeks, if condition has responded consult product literature for guidance on further doses

Severe active ulcerative colitis
- BY INTRAVENOUS INFUSION
  - Child 6–17 years: Initially 5 mg/kg, then 5 mg/kg after 2 weeks, followed by 5 mg/kg after 4 weeks, then 5 mg/kg every 8 weeks, discontinue if no response within 8 weeks of initial dose

- **UNLICENSED USE** Not licensed for fistulating Crohn's disease in children.

> **IMPORTANT SAFETY INFORMATION**
> Adequate resuscitation facilities must be available when infliximab is used.

- **CONTRA-INDICATIONS** Moderate or severe heart failure · severe infections
- **CAUTIONS** Demyelinating disorders (risk of exacerbation) · dermatomyositis · development of malignancy · hepatitis B virus—monitor for active infection · history of malignancy · history of prolonged immunosuppressant or PUVA treatment in patients with psoriasis · mild heart failure (discontinue if symptoms develop or worsen) · predisposition to infection (discontinue if new serious infection develops) · risk of delayed hypersensitivity reactions if drug-free interval exceeds 16 weeks (re-administration after interval exceeding 16 weeks not recommended)

CAUTIONS, FURTHER INFORMATION
- Tuberculosis Manufacturer advises to evaluate patients for active and latent tuberculosis before treatment. Active tuberculosis should be treated with standard treatment for at least 2 months before starting infliximab. If latent tuberculosis is diagnosed, treatment should be started before commencing treatment with infliximab. Patients who have previously received adequate treatment for tuberculosis can start infliximab but should be monitored every 3 months for possible recurrence. In patients without active tuberculosis but who were previously not treated adequately, chemoprophylaxis should ideally be completed before starting infliximab. In patients at high risk of tuberculosis who cannot be assessed by tuberculin skin test, chemoprophylaxis can be given concurrently with infliximab. Patients should be advised to seek medical attention if symptoms suggestive of tuberculosis develop (e.g. persistent cough, weight loss and fever).
- Hypersensitivity reactions Hypersensitivity reactions (including fever, chest pain, hypotension, hypertension, dyspnoea, transient visual loss, pruritus, urticaria, serum sickness-like reactions, angioedema, anaphylaxis) reported during or within 1–2 hours after infusion (risk greatest during first or second infusion or in patients who discontinue other immunosuppressants). Manufacturer advises prophylactic antipyretics, antihistamines, or hydrocortisone may be administered.

- **INTERACTIONS** → Appendix 1 (infliximab).
- **SIDE-EFFECTS**
- **Common or very common** Alopecia · arthralgia · constipation · diarrhoea · dizziness · dry skin · dyspepsia · ecchymosis · epistaxis · flushing · gastro-intestinal haemorrhage · gastro-oesophageal reflux · hyperhydrosis · hypertension · hypoaesthesia · hypotension · myalgia · new onset or worsening psoriasis · palpitation · paraesthesia · rash · sleep disturbances · tachycardia
- **Uncommon** Abnormal skin pigmentation · agitation · amnesia · arrhythmia · bradycardia · bullous eruption · cheilitis · cholecystitis · confusion · eye disorders · heart failure · hepatitis · hyperkeratosis · impaired healing · intestinal perforation · nervousness · neuropathy · pancreatitis · peripheral ischaemia · pleurisy · pulmonary oedema · rosacea · seborrhoea · seizures · syncope · vaginitis

► **Rare** Demyelinating disorders · interstitial lung disease · leukaemia · lymphoma · melanoma · pericardial effusion · Stevens-Johnson syndrome · toxic epidermal necrolysis · vasospasm

► **Frequency not known** Abdominal pain · anaemia · antibody formation · aplastic anaemia · blood disorders · depression · fever · headache · hepatic failure · hepatosplenic T-cell lymphoma (more likely in inflammatory bowel disease) · hypersensitivity reactions · injection-site reactions · leucopenia · lupus erythematosus-like syndrome · Merkel cell carcinoma · nausea · pancytopenia · pruritus · thrombocytopenia · worsening heart failure · worsening symptoms of dermatomyositis

SIDE-EFFECTS, FURTHER INFORMATION
Associated with infections, sometimes severe, including tuberculosis, septicaemia, and hepatitis B reactivation.

● **CONCEPTION AND CONTRACEPTION** Manufacturer advises adequate contraception during and for at least 6 months after last dose.

● **PREGNANCY** Use only if essential.

● **BREAST FEEDING** Amount probably too small to be harmful.

● **PRE-TREATMENT SCREENING**
Tuberculosis Patients should be evaluated for tuberculosis before treatment.

● **MONITORING REQUIREMENTS**
► Monitor for infection before, during, and for 6 months after treatment.
► All patients should be observed carefully for 1–2 hours after infusion and resuscitation equipment should be available for immediate use (risk of hypersensitivity reactions).
► Monitor for symptoms of delayed hypersensitivity if re-administered after a prolonged period.
► Manufacturer advises periodic skin examination for non-melanoma skin cancer, particularly in patients with risk factors.

● **DIRECTIONS FOR ADMINISTRATION**
► With intravenous use For *intravenous infusion* reconstitute each 100-mg vial of powder with 10 mL Water for Injections; to dissolve, gently swirl vial without shaking; allow to stand for 5 minutes; dilute required dose with Sodium Chloride 0.9% to a final volume of 250 mL and give through a low protein-binding filter (1.2 micron or less) over at least 2 hours; start infusion within 3 hours of reconstitution.

● **PRESCRIBING AND DISPENSING INFORMATION** Products containing infliximab are not identical and although there should be no important differences in terms of safety and efficacy, when prescribing biological products it is good practice to use the brand name, see *Biosimilar medicines*, under Guidance on prescribing p. 1.

● **PATIENT AND CARER ADVICE** An alert card should be provided.
Tuberculosis Patients and carers should be advised to seek medical attention if symptoms suggestive of tuberculosis (e.g. persistent cough, weight loss, and fever) develop.
Blood disorders Patients and carers should be advised to seek medical attention if symptoms suggestive of blood disorders (such as fever, sore throat, bruising, or bleeding) develop.
Hypersensitivity reactions Patients and carers should be advised to keep Alert card with them at all times and seek medical advice if symptoms of delayed hypersensitivity develop.

● **NATIONAL FUNDING/ACCESS DECISIONS**

NICE technology appraisals (TAs)
► **Infliximab for Crohn's disease (May 2010)** NICE TA187
In children over 6 years of age, infliximab is recommended for the treatment of severe active Crohn's disease that has

not responded to conventional therapy (including corticosteroids and other drugs affecting the immune response, and primary nutrition therapy) or when conventional therapy cannot be used because of intolerance or contra-indications.
Infliximab should be given as a planned course of treatment for 12 months or until treatment failure, whichever is shorter. Treatment should be continued beyond 12 months only if there is evidence of active disease—in these cases the need for treatment should be reviewed at least annually. If the disease relapses after stopping treatment, infliximab can be restarted.
www.nice.org.uk/TA187

► **Infliximab, adalimumab and golimumab for treating moderately to severely active ulcerative colitis after the failure of conventional therapy (February 2015)** NICE TA329
Infliximab is an option for treating severely active ulcerative colitis in children whose disease has responded inadequately to conventional therapy including corticosteroids and mercaptopurine or azathioprine.
Infliximab should be given as a planned course of treatment until treatment fails (including the need for surgery) or until 12 months after starting treatment, whichever is shorter. Treatment should be continued only if there is clear evidence of a response. Patients who continue treatment should be reassessed every 12 months to determine whether ongoing treatment is still clinically appropriate.
www.nice.org.uk/TA329

● **MEDICINAL FORMS**
There can be variation in the licensing of different medicines containing the same drug.

Powder for solution for infusion
CAUTIONARY AND ADVISORY LABELS 10
► Inflectra (Hospira UK Ltd) ▼
Infliximab 100 mg Inflectra 100mg powder for concentrate for solution for infusion vials | 1 vial PoM £377.66 (Hospital only)
► Remicade (Merck Sharp & Dohme Ltd)
Infliximab 100 mg Remicade 100mg powder for concentrate for solution for infusion vials | 1 vial PoM £419.62 (Hospital only)
► Remsima (Napp Pharmaceuticals Ltd) ▼
Infliximab 100 mg Remsima 100mg powder for concentrate for solution for infusion vials | 1 vial PoM £377.66 (Hospital only)

1.2 Irritable bowel syndrome

> **Drugs used for Irritable bowel syndrome not listed below**
> Alverine citrate, p. 58 · Mebeverine hydrochloride, p. 58

ANTISPASMODICS

Mebeverine with ispaghula husk   4.2.2016

The properties listed below are those particular to the combination only. For the properties of the components please consider, mebeverine hydrochloride p. 58, ispaghula husk p. 36.

● **INDICATIONS AND DOSE**
Irritable bowel syndrome
► BY MOUTH
► Child 12-17 years: 1 sachet twice daily, in water, morning and evening, 30 minutes before food and 1 sachet daily if required, taken 30 minutes before midday meal

● **DIRECTIONS FOR ADMINISTRATION** Contents of one sachet should be stirred into a glass (approx. 150 mL) of cold water and drunk immediately.

- PATIENT AND CARER ADVICE Patients or carers should be given advice on how to administer ispaghula husk with mebeverine granules.

- MEDICINAL FORMS
There can be variation in the licensing of different medicines containing the same drug.
Effervescent granules
CAUTIONARY AND ADVISORY LABELS 13, 22
EXCIPIENTS: May contain Aspartame
ELECTROLYTES: May contain Potassium
  ▸ Fybogel Mebeverine (Reckitt Benckiser Healthcare (UK) Ltd)
  Mebeverine hydrochloride 135 mg, Ispaghula husk
  3.5 gram Fybogel Mebeverine effervescent granules sachets orange sugar-free | 10 sachet ℗ £4.22 DT price = £4.22

Peppermint oil

- INDICATIONS AND DOSE
COLPERMIN®
Relief of abdominal colic and distension, particularly in irritable bowel syndrome
  ▸ BY MOUTH
  ▸ Child 15-17 years: 1–2 capsules 3 times a day for up to 3 months if necessary, capsule to be swallowed whole with water

- CAUTIONS Sensitivity to menthol

- SIDE-EFFECTS
▸ **Rare** Allergic reactions · ataxia · bradycardia · headache · muscle tremor · rash
▸ **Frequency not known** Heartburn · perianal irritation

- PREGNANCY Not known to be harmful.

- BREAST FEEDING Significant levels of menthol in breast milk unlikely.

- DIRECTIONS FOR ADMINISTRATION Capsules should not be broken or chewed because peppermint oil may irritate mouth or oesophagus.

- MEDICINAL FORMS
There can be variation in the licensing of different medicines containing the same drug.
Modified-release capsule
CAUTIONARY AND ADVISORY LABELS 5, 22, 25
EXCIPIENTS: May contain Arachis (peanut) oil
  ▸ Colpermin (McNeil Products Ltd)
  Peppermint oil 200 microlitre Colpermin gastro-resistant modified-release capsules | 20 capsule GSL £3.33 | 100 capsule GSL £12.18 DT price = £12.18

2 Constipation and bowel cleansing

2.1 Bowel cleansing

Drugs used for Bowel cleansing not listed below
Bisacodyl, p. 40 · Docusate sodium, p. 43

DIAGNOSTIC AGENTS ❭ RADIOGRAPHIC CONTRAST MEDIA

Meglumine amidotrizoate with sodium amidotrizoate

(Diatrizoates)

- DRUG ACTION Meglumine amidotrizoate with sodium amidotrizoate is a radiological contrast medium with high osmolality.

- INDICATIONS AND DOSE
Uncomplicated meconium ileus
  ▸ BY RECTUM
  ▸ Neonate: 15–30 mL for 1 dose.

Distal intestinal obstruction syndrome in children with cystic fibrosis
  ▸ BY MOUTH, OR BY RECTUM
  ▸ Child 1-23 months: 15–30 mL for 1 dose
  ▸ Child (body-weight 15-25 kg): 50 mL for 1 dose
  ▸ Child (body-weight 26 kg and above): 100 mL for 1 dose
Radiological investigations
  ▸ Child: Dose to be recommended by radiologist

- UNLICENSED USE Not licensed for use in distal intestinal obstruction syndrome.

- CONTRA-INDICATIONS Hyperthyroidism

- CAUTIONS Asthma · benign nodular goitre · dehydration · electrolyte disturbance (correct first) · enteritis · history of allergy · in children with oesophageal fistulae (aspiration may lead to pulmonary oedema) · latent hyperthyroidism · risk of anaphylactoid reactions increased by concomitant administration of beta-blockers

- SIDE-EFFECTS
▸ **Common or very common** Diarrhoea · nausea · vomiting
▸ **Frequency not known** Abdominal pain · bowel necrosis · disturbances in consciousness · dizziness · electrolyte disturbances · headache · hypersensitivity reactions · hyperthyroidism · intestinal perforation · oral mucosal blistering · pyrexia · skin reactions · toxic epidermal necrolysis

- ALLERGY AND CROSS-SENSITIVITY Hypersensitivity to iodine.

- PREGNANCY Manufacturer advises caution.

- BREAST FEEDING Amount probably too small to be harmful.

- DIRECTIONS FOR ADMINISTRATION Intravenous prehydration is essential in neonates and infants. Fluid intake should be encouraged for 3 hours after administration. *By mouth*, for child bodyweight under 25 kg, dilute *Gastrografin*® with 3 times volume of water or fruit juice; for child bodyweight over 25 kg, dilute *Gastrografin*® with twice its volume of water or fruit juice. *By rectum*, administration must be carried out slowly under radiological supervision to ensure required site is reached. For child under 5 years, dilute *Gastrografin*® with 5 times its volume of water; for child over 5 years dilute *Gastrografin*® with 4 times its volume of water.

- MEDICINAL FORMS
There can be variation in the licensing of different medicines containing the same drug.
Oral solution
EXCIPIENTS: May contain Disodium edetate
  ▸ Gastrografin (Bayer Plc)
  Sodium amidotrizoate 100 mg per 1 ml, Meglumine amidotrizoate 660 mg per 1 ml Gastrografin oral solution sugar-free | 1000 ml ℗ £175.00 (Hospital only)

LAXATIVES > OSMOTIC LAXATIVES

Citric acid with magnesium carbonate

(Formulated as a bowel cleansing preparation)

- ● **INDICATIONS AND DOSE**

Bowel evacuation for surgery, colonoscopy or radiological examination
  - ▸ BY MOUTH
  - ▸ Child 5–9 years: One-third of a sachet to be given at 8 a.m. the day before the procedure and, one-third of a sachet to be given between 2 and 4 p.m. the day before the procedure
  - ▸ Child 10–17 years: 0.5–1 sachet, given at 8 a.m. the day before the procedure and 0.5–1 sachet, given between 2 and 4 p.m. the day before the procedure

- ● **CONTRA-INDICATIONS** Acute severe colitis · gastric retention · gastro-intestinal obstruction · gastro-intestinal perforation · toxic megacolon

- ● **CAUTIONS** Children · colitis (avoid if acute severe colitis) · debilitated · hypovolaemia (should be corrected before administration of bowel cleansing preparations) · impaired gag reflex or possibility of regurgitation or aspiration · patients with fluid and electrolyte disturbances

  CAUTIONS, FURTHER INFORMATION
  Adequate hydration should be maintained during treatment.

- ● **INTERACTIONS** Other oral drugs should not be taken one hour before or after administration of bowel cleansing preparations because absorption may be impaired.

- ● **SIDE-EFFECTS**
  - ▸ **Common or very common** Abdominal distention · abdominal pain · nausea · vomiting
  - ▸ **Uncommon** Dehydration · dizziness · electrolyte disturbances · headache

  SIDE-EFFECTS, FURTHER INFORMATION
  - ▸ Abdominal pain Abdominal pain is usually transient and can be reduced by taking preparation more slowly.

- ● **PREGNANCY** Use with caution.

- ● **BREAST FEEDING** Use with caution.

- ● **HEPATIC IMPAIRMENT** Avoid in hepatic coma if risk of renal failure.

- ● **RENAL IMPAIRMENT** Avoid if estimated glomerular filtration rate less than 30 mL/minute/1.73 m^2—risk of hypermagnesaemia.

- ● **MONITORING REQUIREMENTS** Renal function should be measured before starting treatment in patients at risk of fluid and electrolyte disturbances.

- ● **DIRECTIONS FOR ADMINISTRATION** One sachet should be reconstituted with 200 mL of hot water; the solution should be allowed to cool for approx. 30 minutes before drinking.

- ● **PRESCRIBING AND DISPENSING INFORMATION** Reconstitution of one sachet containing 11.57 g magnesium carbonate and 17.79 g anhydrous citric acid produces a solution containing magnesium citrate with 118 mmol Mg^{2+}.
    Flavours of oral powders may include lemon and lime.

- ● **PATIENT AND CARER ADVICE** Low residue or fluid only diet (e.g. water, fruit squash, clear soup, black tea or coffee) recommended before procedure (according to prescriber's advice) and copious intake of clear fluids recommended until procedure. Patient or carers should be given advice on how to administer oral powder.

- ● **MEDICINAL FORMS**
  There can be variation in the licensing of different medicines containing the same drug.

Effervescent powder
CAUTIONARY AND ADVISORY LABELS 13, 10
ELECTROLYTES: May contain Magnesium
  - ▸ Citramag (Sanochemia Diagnostics UK Ltd)
    Magnesium carbonate heavy 11.57 gram, Citric acid anhydrous 17.79 gram Citramag effervescent powder sachets sugar-free | 10 sachet ⓟ £18.92

Macrogol 3350 with anhydrous sodium sulfate, potassium chloride, sodium bicarbonate and sodium chloride

(Formulated as a bowel cleansing preparation)

- ● **INDICATIONS AND DOSE**

Bowel cleansing before radiological examination, colonoscopy, or surgery
  - ▸ INITIALLY BY MOUTH
  - ▸ Child 12–17 years: Initially 2 litres daily for 2 doses: first dose of reconstituted solution taken on the evening before procedure and the second dose on the morning of procedure, alternatively (by mouth) initially 250 mL every 10–15 minutes, reconstituted solution to be administered, alternatively (by nasogastric tube) initially 20–30 mL/minute, starting on the day before procedure until 4 litres have been consumed

Distal intestinal obstruction syndrome
  - ▸ BY MOUTH, OR BY NASOGASTRIC TUBE, OR BY GASTROSTOMY TUBE
  - ▸ Child 1–17 years: 10 mL/kilogram/hour for 30 minutes, then increased to 20 mL/kilogram/hour for 30 minutes, then increased if tolerated to 25 mL/kilogram/hour, max. 100 mL/kg (or 4 litres) over 4 hours, repeat 4 hour treatment if necessary

- ● **UNLICENSED USE** *Klean-Prep*® not licensed for use in children.

- ● **CONTRA-INDICATIONS** Acute severe colitis · gastric retention · gastro-intestinal obstruction · gastro-intestinal perforation · gastro-intestinal ulceration · toxic megacolon

- ● **CAUTIONS** Children · colitis (avoid if acute severe colitis) · debilitated patients · fluid and electrolyte disturbances · heart failure · hypovolaemia (should be corrected before administration of bowel cleansing preparations) · impaired gag reflex or possibility of regurgitation or aspiration

- ● **SIDE-EFFECTS**
  - ▸ **Common or very common** Abdominal distention · abdominal pain · nausea · vomiting
  - ▸ **Uncommon** Anal discomfort · dehydration · dizziness · electrolyte disturbances · headache

  SIDE-EFFECTS, FURTHER INFORMATION
  - ▸ Abdominal pain Abdominal pain is usually transient and can be reduced by taking preparation more slowly.

- ● **PREGNANCY** Manufacturers advise use only if essential—no information available.

- ● **BREAST FEEDING** Manufacturers advise use only if essential—no information available.

- ● **MONITORING REQUIREMENTS** Renal function should be measured before starting treatment in patients at risk of fluid and electrolyte disturbances.

- ● **DIRECTIONS FOR ADMINISTRATION** 1 sachet should be reconstituted with 1 litre of water. Flavouring such as clear fruit cordials may be added if required. After reconstitution the solution should be kept in a refrigerator and discarded if unused after 24 hours.

- **PRESCRIBING AND DISPENSING INFORMATION** Each *Klean-Prep*® sachet provides Na⁺ 125 mmol, K⁺ 10 mmol, Cl⁻ 35 mmol and HCO³⁻ 20mmol when reconstituted with 1 litre of water.

- **PATIENT AND CARER ADVICE** Solid food should not be taken for 2 hours before starting treatment. Adequate hydration should be maintained during treatment. Treatment can be stopped if bowel motions become watery and clear.

- **MEDICINAL FORMS**
  There can be variation in the licensing of different medicines containing the same drug.
  Powder
  CAUTIONARY AND ADVISORY LABELS 10, 13
  EXCIPIENTS: May contain Aspartame
  ELECTROLYTES: May contain Bicarbonate, chloride, potassium, sodium
  ▸ **Klean-Prep** (Norgine Pharmaceuticals Ltd)
  Potassium chloride 742.5 mg, Sodium chloride 1.465 gram, Sodium bicarbonate 1.685 gram, Sodium sulfate anhydrous 5.685 gram, Polyethylene glycol 3350 59 gram Klean-Prep oral powder 69g sachets sugar-free | 4 sachet Ⓟ £9.98

LAXATIVES ⟩ STIMULANT LAXATIVES

Magnesium citrate with sodium picosulfate

(Formulated as a bowel cleansing preparation)

- **INDICATIONS AND DOSE**
  PICOLAX® SACHETS
  Bowel evacuation on day before radiological procedure, endoscopy, or surgery
  ▸ BY MOUTH
  ▸ **Child 1 year:** 0.25 sachet taken before 8 a.m, then 0.25 sachet after 6–8 hours
  ▸ **Child 2-3 years:** 0.5 sachet taken before 8 a.m, then 0.5 sachet after 6–8 hours
  ▸ **Child 4-8 years:** 1 sachet taken before 8 a.m, then 0.5 sachet after 6–8 hours
  ▸ **Child 9-17 years:** 1 sachet taken before 8 a.m, then 1 sachet after 6–8 hours

  PHARMACOKINETICS
  Acts within 3 hours of first dose.

- **CONTRA-INDICATIONS** Acute severe colitis · ascites · congestive cardiac failure · gastric retention · gastro-intestinal obstruction · gastro-intestinal perforation · gastro-intestinal ulceration · toxic megacolon

- **CAUTIONS** Cardiac disease (avoid in congestive cardiac failure) · children · colitis (avoid if acute severe colitis) · debilitated patients · fluid and electrolyte disturbances · hypovolaemia (should be corrected before administration) · impaired gag reflex or possibility of regurgitation or aspiration · recent gastro-intestinal surgery

- **SIDE-EFFECTS**
  ▸ **Common or very common** Abdominal distention · abdominal pain (usually transient—reduced by taking more slowly) · nausea · vomiting
  ▸ **Uncommon** Dehydration · dizziness · electrolyte disturbances · headache
  ▸ **Frequency not known** Anal discomfort · fatigue · rash · sleep disturbances

- **PREGNANCY** Caution.

- **BREAST FEEDING** Caution.

- **HEPATIC IMPAIRMENT** Avoid in hepatic coma if risk of renal failure.

- **RENAL IMPAIRMENT** Avoid if estimated glomerular filtration rate less than 30 mL/minute/1.73 m²—risk of hypermagnesaemia.

- **DIRECTIONS FOR ADMINISTRATION** One sachet of sodium picosulfate with magnesium citrate powder should be reconstituted with 150 mL (approx. half a glass) of cold water; patients should be warned that heat is generated during reconstitution and that the solution should be allowed to cool before drinking.

  PICOLAX® SACHETS One sachet should be reconstituted with 150 mL (approx. half a glass) of cold water.

- **PRESCRIBING AND DISPENSING INFORMATION** Flavours of oral powder formulations may include lemon.

  PICOLAX® SACHETS One reconstituted sachet contains K⁺ 5 mmol and Mg²⁺ 87 mmol.

- **PATIENT AND CARER ADVICE** Low residue diet recommended on the day before procedure and copious intake of water or other clear fluids recommended during treatment. Patients or carers should be given advice on how to administer sodium picosulfate with magnesium citrate oral powder.

  PICOLAX® SACHETS Low residue diet recommended on the day before procedure and copious intake of water or other clear fluids recommended during treatment.

  Patients and carers should be given advice on how to administer oral powder; they should be warned that heat is generated during reconstitution and that the solution should be allowed to cool before drinking.

- **MEDICINAL FORMS**
  There can be variation in the licensing of different medicines containing the same drug.
  Powder
  CAUTIONARY AND ADVISORY LABELS 10, 13
  ELECTROLYTES: May contain Magnesium, potassium
  ▸ **Picolax** (Ferring Pharmaceuticals Ltd)
  Sodium picosulfate 10 mg, Magnesium oxide 3.5 gram, Citric acid anhydrous 12 gram Picolax oral powder 16.1g sachets sugar-free | 2 sachet Ⓟ £3.39

2.2 Constipation

Constipation

Overview

Before prescribing laxatives it is important to be sure that the child *is* constipated and that the constipation is *not* secondary to an underlying undiagnosed complaint. Laxatives should be prescribed by a healthcare professional experienced in the management of constipation in children. Delays of greater than 3 days between stools may increase the likelihood of pain on passing hard stools leading to anal fissure, anal spasm and eventually to a learned response to avoid defaecation.

In *infants*, increased intake of fluids, particularly fruit juice containing sorbitol (e.g. prune, pear, or apple), may be sufficient to soften the stool. In infants under 1 year of age with mild constipation, lactulose p. 37 can be used to soften the stool; either an oral preparation containing macrogols or, rarely, glycerol suppositories p. 41 can be used to clear faecal impaction. The infant should be referred to a hospital paediatric specialist if these measures fail.

The diet of *children over 1 year of age* should be reviewed to ensure that it includes an adequate intake of fibre and fluid. An osmotic laxative containing macrogols can also be used, particularly in children with chronic constipation; lactulose is an alternative in children who cannot tolerate a macrogol. If there is an inadequate response to the osmotic laxative, a **stimulant laxative** can be added.

Treatment of faecal impaction may initially increase symptoms of soiling and abdominal pain. In children over 1 year of age with faecal impaction, an oral preparation containing macrogol is used to clear faecal mass and to establish and maintain soft well-formed stools. If disimpaction does not occur after 2 weeks, a **stimulant laxative** can be added. If the impacted mass is not expelled following treatment with macrogols and a stimulant laxative, a sodium citrate enema can be administered. Although rectal administration of laxatives may be effective, this route is frequently distressing for the child and may lead to persistence of withholding. A **phosphate enema** may be administered under specialist supervision if disimpaction does not occur after a sodium citrate enema; a **bowel cleansing preparation** is an alternative. Manual evacuation under anaesthetic may be necessary if disimpaction does not occur after oral and rectal treatment, or if the child is afraid.

Long-term regular use of laxatives is essential to maintain well-formed stools and prevent recurrence of faecal impaction; intermittent use may provoke relapses. In children with chronic constipation, laxatives should be continued for several weeks after a regular pattern of bowel movements or toilet training is established. The dose of laxatives should then be tapered gradually, over a period of months, according to response. Some children may require laxative therapy for several years.

Laxatives are also of value in *drug-induced constipation*, in *distal intestinal obstruction syndrome* in children with cystic fibrosis, for the expulsion of *parasites* after anthelmintic treatment, and to clear the alimentary tract before *surgery and radiological procedures*.

Laxatives also have a role in the treatment of irritable bowel syndrome. Also see the prevention of opioid-induced constipation in palliative care.

Chronic constipation

For children with chronic constipation, it may be necessary to exceed the licensed doses of some laxatives. Parents and carers of children should be advised to adjust the dose of laxative in order to establish a regular pattern of bowel movements in which stools are soft, well-formed, and passed without discomfort.

Laxatives should be administered at a time that produces an effect that is likely to fit in with the child's toilet routine.

Pregnancy

If dietary and lifestyle changes fail to control constipation in pregnancy, moderate doses of poorly absorbed laxatives may be used. A bulk-forming laxative should be tried first. An osmotic laxative, such as lactulose, can also be used. Bisacodyl p. 40 or senna p. 42 may be suitable, if a stimulant effect is necessary.

Laxatives drugs

The laxatives that follow have been divided into 5 main groups. This simple classification disguises the fact that some laxatives have a complex action.

Bulk-forming laxatives

Bulk-forming laxatives are of value if the diet is deficient in fibre. During treatment with bulk-forming laxatives, adequate fluid intake must be maintained to avoid intestinal obstruction. Proprietary preparations containing a bulking agent such as ispaghula husk p. 36 are often difficult to administer to children.

Proprietary preparations containing a bulking agent such as ispaghula husk are often difficult to administer to children. Bulk-forming laxatives may be used in the management of children with *haemorrhoids*, *anal fissure*, and *irritable bowel syndrome*.

Stimulant laxatives

Stimulant laxatives include bisacodyl, sodium picosulfate p. 42, and members of the **anthraquinone** group, senna, co-

danthramer p. 40 and co-danthrusate p. 41. The indications for co-danthramer and co-danthrusate are limited by its potential carcinogenicity (based on rodent carcinogenicity studies) and evidence of genotoxicity. Powerful stimulants such as **cascara** (an anthraquinone) and **castor oil** are obsolete. Docusate sodium p. 43 probably acts both as a stimulant and as a softening agent.

Stimulant laxatives increase intestinal motility and often cause abdominal cramp; they should be avoided in intestinal obstruction. Stools should be softened by increasing dietary fibre and liquid or with an osmotic laxative before giving a stimulant laxative. In chronic constipation, especially where withholding of stool occurs, additional doses of a stimulant laxative may be required. Long-term use of stimulant laxatives is sometimes necessary, but excessive use can cause diarrhoea and related effects such as hypokalaemia.

Glycerol suppositories act as a lubricant and as a rectal stimulant by virtue of the mildly irritant action of glycerol.

Faecal softeners

Enemas containing arachis oil p. 43 (ground-nut oil, peanut oil) lubricate and soften impacted faeces and promote a bowel movement.

Bulk laxatives and non-ionic surfactant 'wetting' agents e.g. docusate sodium also have softening properties. Such drugs are useful for oral administration in the management of anal fissure; glycerol suppositories are useful for rectal use.

Osmotic laxatives

Osmotic laxatives increase the amount of water in the large bowel, either by drawing fluid from the body into the bowel or by retaining the fluid they were administered with.

Lactulose is a semi-synthetic disaccharide which is not absorbed from the gastro-intestinal tract. It produces an osmotic diarrhoea of low faecal pH, and discourages the proliferation of ammonia-producing organisms. It is therefore useful in the treatment of *hepatic encephalopathy*.

Macrogols are inert polymers of ethylene glycol which sequester fluid in the bowel; giving fluid with macrogols may reduce the dehydrating effect sometimes seen with osmotic laxatives. Macrogols are an effective non-traumatic means of evacuation in children with faecal impaction and can be used in the long-term management of chronic constipation.

Saline purgatives such as **magnesium hydroxide** are commonly abused but are satisfactory for occasional use; adequate fluid intake should be maintained. Magnesium salts are useful where rapid bowel evacuation is required. **Sodium salts** should be avoided as they may give rise to sodium and water retention in susceptible individuals. **Phosphate enemas** are useful in bowel clearance before radiology, endoscopy, and surgery. Enemas containing phosphate or **sodium citrate**, and oral **bowel cleansing preparations** should only be used on the advice of a specialist practitioner.

Bowel cleansing preparations

Bowel cleansing preparations are used before colonic surgery, colonoscopy, or radiological examination to ensure the bowel is free of solid contents. They are **not** treatments for constipation.

LAXATIVES 〉 BULK-FORMING LAXATIVES

Ispaghula husk

24.2.2016

- **DRUG ACTION** Bulk-forming laxatives relieve constipation by increasing faecal mass which stimulates peristalsis.

● INDICATIONS AND DOSE

Constipation
▶ BY MOUTH
- ▸ Child 1 month–5 years: 2.5–5 mL twice daily, dose to be taken only when prescribed by a doctor, as half or whole level spoonful in water, preferably after meals, morning and evening
- ▸ Child 6–11 years: 2.5–5 mL twice daily, dose to be given as a half or whole level spoonful in water, preferably after meals, morning and evening
- ▸ Child 12–17 years: 1 sachet twice daily, dose to be given in water preferably after meals, morning and evening

DOSE EQUIVALENCE AND CONVERSION
1 sachet equivalent to 2 level 5 ml spoonsful.

- **CONTRA-INDICATIONS** Colonic atony · faecal impaction · intestinal obstruction · reduced gut motility
- **CAUTIONS** Adequate fluid intake should be maintained to avoid intestinal obstruction
- **SIDE-EFFECTS** Abdominal distension · flatulence · gastro-intestinal impaction · gastro-intestinal obstruction · hypersensitivity
- **DIRECTIONS FOR ADMINISTRATION** Dose to be taken with at least 150 mL liquid.
- **PRESCRIBING AND DISPENSING INFORMATION** Flavours of soluble granules formulations may include plain, lemon, or orange.
- **HANDLING AND STORAGE** Ispaghula husk contains potent allergens. Individuals exposed to the product (including those handling the product) can develop hypersensitivity reactions such as rhinitis, conjunctivitis, bronchospasm and in some cases, anaphylaxis.
- **PATIENT AND CARER ADVICE** Manufacturer advises that preparations that swell in contact with liquid should always be carefully swallowed with water and should not be taken immediately before going to bed. Patients and their carers should be advised that the full effect may take some days to develop and should be given advice on how to administer ispaghula husk.

- **MEDICINAL FORMS**
There can be variation in the licensing of different medicines containing the same drug.

Granules
CAUTIONARY AND ADVISORY LABELS 13
EXCIPIENTS: May contain Aspartame
- ▸ Ispaghula husk (Non-proprietary)
Ispaghula husk 3.5 gram Ispaghula husk 3.5g granules sachets gluten free | 30 sachet GSL £2.48

Effervescent granules
CAUTIONARY AND ADVISORY LABELS 13
EXCIPIENTS: May contain Aspartame
- ▸ Ispaghula husk (Non-proprietary)
Ispaghula husk 3.5 gram Ispaghula husk 3.5g effervescent granules sachets gluten free sugar free sugar-free | 30 sachet P no price available DT price = £2.48
- ▸ Fybogel (Reckitt Benckiser Healthcare (UK) Ltd)
Ispaghula husk 3.5 gram Fybogel 3.5g effervescent granules sachets plain SF sugar-free | 30 sachet GSL £2.48 DT price = £2.48
Fybogel Orange 3.5g effervescent granules sachets SF sugar-free | 30 sachet GSL £2.48 DT price = £2.48
Fybogel Lemon 3.5g effervescent granules sachets SF sugar-free | 30 sachet GSL £2.48 DT price = £2.48
- ▸ Fybogel Hi-Fibre (Reckitt Benckiser Healthcare (UK) Ltd)
Ispaghula husk 3.5 gram Fybogel Hi-Fibre Orange 3.5g effervescent granules sachets sugar-free | 10 sachet GSL £2.26 sugar-free | 30 sachet GSL £4.85 DT price = £2.48

Fybogel Hi-Fibre Lemon 3.5g effervescent granules sachets sugar-free | 10 sachet GSL £2.26
- ▸ Ispagel (Bristol Laboratories Ltd)
Ispaghula husk 3.5 gram Ispagel Orange 3.5g effervescent granules sachets sugar-free | 10 sachet GSL £1.65 sugar-free | 30 sachet GSL £2.25 DT price = £2.48

Combinations available: *Senna with ispaghula husk,* p. 42

Methylcellulose

- **DRUG ACTION** Bulk-forming laxatives relieve constipation by increasing faecal mass which stimulates peristalsis.

● INDICATIONS AND DOSE

Constipation | Diarrhoea
▶ BY MOUTH USING TABLETS
- ▸ Child 7–11 years: 2 tablets twice daily
- ▸ Child 12–17 years: 3–6 tablets twice daily

- **UNLICENSED USE** No age limit specified by manufacturer.
- **CONTRA-INDICATIONS** Colonic atony · difficulty in swallowing · faecal impaction · infective bowel disease · intestinal obstruction
- **CAUTIONS** Adequate fluid intake should be maintained to avoid intestinal obstruction
- **SIDE-EFFECTS** Abdominal distension (especially during the first few days of treatment) · flatulence (especially during the first few days of treatment) · gastro-intestinal impaction · gastro-intestinal obstruction · hypersensitivity
- **DIRECTIONS FOR ADMINISTRATION** In constipation the dose should be taken with at least 300 mL liquid. In diarrhoea, ileostomy, and colostomy control, avoid liquid intake for 30 minutes before and after dose.
- **PATIENT AND CARER ADVICE** Patients and their carers should be advised that the full effect may take some days to develop. Preparations that swell in contact with liquid should always be carefully swallowed with water and should not be taken immediately before going to bed.

- **MEDICINAL FORMS**
There can be variation in the licensing of different medicines containing the same drug.
Tablet
- ▸ Celevac (AMCo)
Methylcellulose "450" 500 mg Celevac 500mg tablets | 112 tablet GSL £4.64 DT price = £4.64

Sterculia

19.2.2016

- **DRUG ACTION** Sterculia is a bulk-forming laxative. It relieves constipation by increasing faecal mass which stimulates peristalsis.

● INDICATIONS AND DOSE

Constipation
▶ BY MOUTH
- ▸ Child 6–11 years: 0.5–1 sachet 1–2 times a day, alternatively, half to one heaped 5-mL spoonful once or twice a day; washed down without chewing with plenty of liquid after meals
- ▸ Child 12–17 years: 1–2 sachets 1–2 times a day, alternatively, one to two heaped 5-mL spoonfuls once or twice a day; washed down without chewing with plenty of liquid after meals

- **CONTRA-INDICATIONS** Colonic atony · difficulty in swallowing · faecal impaction · intestinal obstruction
- **CAUTIONS** Adequate fluid intake should be maintained to avoid intestinal obstruction
- **SIDE-EFFECTS** Abdominal distension (especially during the first few days of treatment) · flatulence (especially

during the first few days of treatment) · gastro-intestinal impaction · gastro-intestinal obstruction · hypersensitivity

- **DIRECTIONS FOR ADMINISTRATION** May be mixed with soft food (e.g. yoghurt) before swallowing, followed by plenty of liquid.
- **PATIENT AND CARER ADVICE** Patients and their carers should be advised that the full effect may take some days to develop. Preparations that swell in contact with liquid should always be carefully swallowed with water and should not be taken immediately before going to bed.

- **MEDICINAL FORMS**
There can be variation in the licensing of different medicines containing the same drug.
Granules
CAUTIONARY AND ADVISORY LABELS 25, 27
  ▸ Normacol (Norgine Pharmaceuticals Ltd)
  Sterculia 620 mg per 1 gram Normacol granules 7g sachets | 60 sachet GSL £6.35 DT price = £5.77
  Normacol granules | 500 gram GSL £7.54 DT price = £6.85

Sterculia with frangula

The properties listed below are those particular to the combination only. For the properties of the components please consider, sterculia p. 36.

- **INDICATIONS AND DOSE**
Constipation
  ▸ BY MOUTH
  ▸ Child 6–11 years: 0.5–1 sachet 1–2 times a day, alternatively, 0.5–1 heaped 5-mL spoonful once or twice a day; washed down without chewing with plenty of liquid after meals
  ▸ Child 12–17 years: 1–2 sachets 1–2 times a day, alternatively, 1–2 heaped 5 mL spoonfuls once or twice a day; washed down without chewing with plenty of liquid after meals

- **PREGNANCY** Manufacturer advises avoid.
- **BREAST FEEDING** Manufacturer advises avoid.
- **PATIENT AND CARER ADVICE** Patients and their carers should be advised that the full effect may take some days to develop. Preparations that swell in contact with liquid should always be carefully swallowed with water and should not be taken immediately before going to bed.

- **MEDICINAL FORMS**
There can be variation in the licensing of different medicines containing the same drug.
Granules
  ▸ Normacol Plus (Norgine Pharmaceuticals Ltd)
  Frangula 80 mg per 1 gram, Sterculia 620 mg per 1 gram Normacol Plus granules 7g sachets | 60 sachet GSL £6.78 DT price = £6.16
  Normacol Plus granules | 500 gram GSL £8.05 DT price = £7.32

LAXATIVES ❭ OSMOTIC LAXATIVES

Lactulose

- **INDICATIONS AND DOSE**
Constipation
  ▸ BY MOUTH
  ▸ Child 1–11 months: 2.5 mL twice daily, adjusted according to response
  ▸ Child 1–4 years: 2.5–10 mL twice daily, adjusted according to response
  ▸ Child 5–17 years: 5–20 mL twice daily, adjusted according to response

Hepatic encephalopathy (portal systemic encephalopathy)
  ▸ BY MOUTH
  ▸ Child 12–17 years: Adjusted according to response to 30–50 mL 3 times a day, subsequently adjusted to produce 2–3 soft stools per day

PHARMACOKINETICS
Lactulose may take up to 48 hours to act.

- **UNLICENSED USE** Not licensed for use in children for hepatic encephalopathy.
- **CONTRA-INDICATIONS** Galactosaemia · intestinal obstruction
- **CAUTIONS** Lactose intolerance
- **INTERACTIONS** → Appendix 1 (lactulose).
- **SIDE-EFFECTS**
  ▸ **Common or very common** Abdominal discomfort · cramps · flatulence · nausea · vomiting
  SIDE-EFFECTS, FURTHER INFORMATION
  ▸ Nausea Nausea can be reduced by administration with water, fruit juice or meals.
- **PREGNANCY** Not known to be harmful.
- **PATIENT AND CARER ADVICE**
  Medicines for Children leaflet: Lactulose for constipation www.medicinesforchildren.org.uk/lactulose-for-constipation

- **MEDICINAL FORMS**
There can be variation in the licensing of different medicines containing the same drug.
Oral solution
  ▸ Lactulose (Non-proprietary)
  Lactulose 666.667 mg per 1 ml Lactulose 10g/15ml oral solution 15ml sachets sugar free sugar-free | 10 sachet P £2.50 DT price = £2.50
  Lactulose 680 mg per 1 ml Lactulose 3.1-3.7g/5ml oral solution | 300 ml P £2.73 | 500 ml P £4.55 DT price = £2.50
  ▸ Duphalac (BGP Products Ltd)
  Lactulose 680 mg per 1 ml Duphalac 3.35g/5ml syrup | 200 ml P £1.92
  ▸ Lactugal (Intrapharm Laboratories Ltd)
  Lactulose 680 mg per 1 ml Lactugal 3.1-3.7g/5ml oral solution | 500 ml P £4.56 DT price = £2.50 | 2000 ml P £16.42

Macrogol 3350 with potassium chloride, sodium bicarbonate and sodium chloride

- **INDICATIONS AND DOSE**
Chronic constipation (dose for non-proprietary 'full-strength' sachets)
  ▸ BY MOUTH
  ▸ Child 12–17 years: 1–3 sachets daily in divided doses usually for up to 2 weeks; maintenance 1–2 sachets daily

Faecal impaction (dose for non-proprietary 'full-strength' sachets)
  ▸ BY MOUTH
  ▸ Child 12–17 years: 4 sachets on first day, then increased in steps of 2 sachets daily, total daily dose to be drunk within a 6 hour period, after disimpaction, switch to maintenance laxative therapy if required; maximum 8 sachets per day

continued →

Gastro-intestinal system

1

MOVICOL-HALF®

Chronic constipation

▶ BY MOUTH

▸ Child 12–17 years: 2–6 sachets daily in divided doses usually for up to 2 weeks; maintenance 2–4 sachets daily

Faecal impaction

▶ BY MOUTH

▸ Child 12–17 years: Initially 8 sachets daily on first day, then increased in steps of 4 sachets daily, total daily dose to be drunk within 6 hours, after disimpaction, switch to maintenance laxative therapy; maximum 16 sachets per day

MOVICOL-PAEDIATRIC®

Chronic constipation | Prevention of faecal impaction

▶ BY MOUTH

▸ Child 1–11 months: 0.5–1 sachet daily
▸ Child 1 year: 1 sachet daily, adjust dose to produce regular soft stools; maximum 4 sachets per day
▸ Child 2–5 years: 1 sachet daily, adjust dose to produce regular soft stools; maximum 4 sachets per day
▸ Child 6–11 years: 2 sachets daily, adjust dose to produce regular soft stools; maximum 4 sachets per day

Faecal impaction

▶ BY MOUTH

▸ Child 1–11 months: 0.5–1 sachet daily
▸ Child 1–4 years: Initially 2 sachets daily on first day, then 4 sachets daily for 2 days, then 6 sachets daily for 2 days, then 8 sachets daily, total daily dose to be taken over a 12-hour period, after disimpaction, switch to maintenance laxative therapy
▸ Child 5–11 years: Initially 4 sachets daily on first day, then increased in steps of 2 sachets daily, total daily dose to be taken over a 12-hour period, after disimpaction, switch to maintenance laxative therapy; maximum 12 sachets per day

MOVICOL® LIQUID

Chronic constipation

▶ BY MOUTH

▸ Child 12–17 years: 25 mL 1–3 times a day usually for up to 2 weeks; maintenance 25 mL 1–2 times a day

MOVICOL® ORAL POWDER

Chronic constipation

▶ BY MOUTH

▸ Child 12–17 years: 1–3 sachets daily in divided doses usually for up to 2 weeks; maintenance 1–2 sachets daily

Faecal impaction

▶ BY MOUTH

▸ Child 12–17 years: Initially 4 sachets daily on first day, then increased in steps of 2 sachets daily, total daily dose to be drunk within 6 hour period, after disimpaction, switch to maintenance laxative therapy if required; maximum 8 sachets per day

● UNLICENSED USE
MOVICOL-PAEDIATRIC® *Movicol® Paediatric* not licensed for use in faecal impaction in children under 5 years, or for chronic constipation in children under 2 years.

● CONTRA-INDICATIONS Crohn's disease · intestinal obstruction · intestinal perforation · paralytic ileus · severe inflammatory conditions of the intestinal tract · toxic megacolon · ulcerative colitis
MOVICOL-PAEDIATRIC® Cardiovascular impairment · renal impairment

● CAUTIONS Cardiovascular impairment (should not take more than 2 'full-strength' sachets or 4 'half-strength' sachets in any one hour) · discontinue if symptoms of fluid and electrolyte disturbance

MOVICOL-PAEDIATRIC® Impaired consciousness (with high doses) · impaired gag reflex (with high doses) · reflux oesophagitis (with high doses)

● INTERACTIONS → Appendix 1 (macrogols).

● SIDE-EFFECTS Abdominal distention · abdominal pain · flatulence · nausea

● PREGNANCY Limited data, but manufacturer advises that it can be used.

● BREAST FEEDING Manufacturer advises that it can be used.

● RENAL IMPAIRMENT
MOVICOL-PAEDIATRIC® Contra-indicated in renal impairment.

● DIRECTIONS FOR ADMINISTRATION Contents of each 'full strength' sachet of oral powder to be dissolved in half a glass (approx. 125 mL) of water; after reconstitution the solution should be kept in a refrigerator and discarded if unused after 6 hours.
MOVICOL® LIQUID 25 mL of oral concentrate to be diluted with half a glass (approx. 100 mL) of water. After dilution the solution should be discarded if unused after 24 hours.
MOVICOL-PAEDIATRIC® Contents of each sachet to be dissolved in quarter of a glass (approx. 60–65 mL) of water; after reconstitution the solution should be kept in a refrigerator and discarded if unused after 24 hours.
MOVICOL® ORAL POWDER Contents of each sachet to be dissolved in half a glass (approx. 125 mL) of water; after reconstitution the solution should be kept in a refrigerator and discarded if unused after 6 hours.
MOVICOL-HALF® Contents of each sachet to be dissolved in quarter of a glass (approx. 60–65 mL) of water; after reconstitution the solution should be kept in a refrigerator and discarded if unused after 6 hours.

● PRESCRIBING AND DISPENSING INFORMATION Flavours of oral liquid formulations may include orange.
Flavours of oral powder formulations may include chocolate, lime and lemon, or plain.
MOVICOL® LIQUID 25 mL of oral concentrate when diluted with 100 mL water provides K^+ 5.4 mmol/litre.
MOVICOL® ORAL POWDER Amount of potassium chloride varies according to flavour of *Movicol®* as follows: plain-flavour (sugar-free) = 50.2 mg/sachet; lime and lemon flavour = 46.6 mg/sachet; chocolate flavour = 31.7 mg/sachet. 1 sachet when reconstituted with 125 mL water provides K^+ 5.4 mmol/litre.

● PATIENT AND CARER ADVICE
Medicines for Children leaflet: Movicol for constipation www.medicinesforchildren.org.uk/movicol-for-constipation
Patients or carers should be counselled on how to take the oral powder and oral solution.
MOVICOL® LIQUID Patients or carers should be counselled on how to take *Movicol®* oral solution.
MOVICOL® ORAL POWDER Patients or carers should be counselled on how to take *Movicol®* oral powder.
MOVICOL-HALF® Patients or carers should be given advice on how to administer *Movicol-Half®* oral powder.

● MEDICINAL FORMS
There can be variation in the licensing of different medicines containing the same drug.

Oral solution
CAUTIONARY AND ADVISORY LABELS 13
ELECTROLYTES: May contain Bicarbonate, chloride, potassium, sodium
▸ Macrogol 3350 with potassium chloride, sodium bicarbonate and sodium chloride (Non-proprietary)
Bicarbonate 17 mmol per 1 litre, Chloride 53 mmol per 1 litre, Macrogol '3350' 13.125 gram, Potassium 5.4 mmol per 1 litre, Sodium 65 mmol per 1 litre Macrogol compound oral liquid NPF sugar free sugar-free | 500 ml Ⓟ no price available

▸ **Movicol** (Norgine Pharmaceuticals Ltd)
Bicarbonate 17 mmol per 1 litre, Chloride 53 mmol per 1 litre, Macrogol '3350' 13.125 gram, Potassium 5.4 mmol per 1 litre, Sodium 65 mmol per 1 litre Movicol Liquid sugar-free | 500 ml [P] £5.15

Powder
CAUTIONARY AND ADVISORY LABELS 13
ELECTROLYTES: May contain Bicarbonate, chloride, potassium, sodium

▸ **Macrogol 3350 with potassium chloride, sodium bicarbonate and sodium chloride (Non-proprietary)**
Bicarbonate 17 mmol per 1 litre, Chloride 53 mmol per 1 litre, Macrogol '3350' 13.125 gram, Potassium 5.4 mmol per 1 litre, Sodium 65 mmol per 1 litre Macrogol compound oral powder sachets sugar free sugar-free | 20 sachet [P] £4.45 sugar-free | 30 sachet [P] £6.68 DT price = £4.27
Bicarbonate 17 mmol per 1 litre, Chloride 53 mmol per 1 litre, Macrogol '3350' 6.563 gram, Potassium 5.4 mmol per 1 litre, Sodium 65 mmol per 1 litre Macrogol compound half-strength oral powder sachets NPF sugar free sugar-free | 20 sachet [PoM] no price available sugar-free | 30 sachet [PoM] no price available

▸ **CosmoCol** (Stirling Anglian Pharmaceuticals Ltd)
Bicarbonate 17 mmol per 1 litre, Chloride 53 mmol per 1 litre, Macrogol '3350' 13.125 gram, Potassium 5.4 mmol per 1 litre, Sodium 65 mmol per 1 litre CosmoCol Orange Lemon and Lime oral powder sachets sugar-free | 20 sachet [P] £2.75 sugar-free | 30 sachet [P] £3.95 DT price = £4.27
CosmoCol Plain oral powder sachets sugar-free | 30 sachet [P] £3.95 DT price = £4.27
CosmoCol Orange Flavour oral powder sachets sugar-free | 20 sachet [P] £2.75 sugar-free | 30 sachet [P] £3.95 DT price = £4.27
CosmoCol Lemon and Lime Flavour oral powder sachets sugar-free | 20 sachet [P] £3.56 sugar-free | 30 sachet [P] £5.34 DT price = £4.27
Bicarbonate 17 mmol per 1 litre, Chloride 53 mmol per 1 litre, Macrogol '3350' 6.563 gram, Potassium 5.4 mmol per 1 litre, Sodium 65 mmol per 1 litre CosmoCol Half oral powder 6.9g sachets sugar-free | 30 sachet [P] £2.99
CosmoCol Paediatric oral powder 6.9g sachets sugar-free | 30 sachet [PoM] £2.99

▸ **Laxido** (Galen Ltd)
Bicarbonate 17 mmol per 1 litre, Chloride 53 mmol per 1 litre, Macrogol '3350' 13.125 gram, Potassium 5.4 mmol per 1 litre, Sodium 65 mmol per 1 litre Laxido Orange oral powder sachets sugar free sugar-free | 20 sachet [P] £2.85 sugar-free | 30 sachet [P] £4.27 DT price = £4.27
Bicarbonate 17 mmol per 1 litre, Chloride 53 mmol per 1 litre, Macrogol '3350' 6.563 gram, Potassium 5.4 mmol per 1 litre, Sodium 65 mmol per 1 litre Laxido Paediatric Plain oral powder 6.9g sachets sugar-free | 30 sachet [PoM] £2.99

▸ **Macilax** (Teva UK Ltd)
Bicarbonate 17 mmol per 1 litre, Chloride 53 mmol per 1 litre, Macrogol '3350' 13.125 gram, Potassium 5.4 mmol per 1 litre, Sodium 65 mmol per 1 litre Macilax oral powder 13.8g sachets sugar-free | 20 sachet [P] £3.20 sugar-free | 30 sachet [P] £4.81 DT price = £4.27 sugar-free | 50 sachet [P] £8.01
Bicarbonate 17 mmol per 1 litre, Chloride 53 mmol per 1 litre, Macrogol '3350' 6.563 gram, Potassium 5.4 mmol per 1 litre, Sodium 65 mmol per 1 litre Macilax Paediatric oral powder 6.9g sachets sugar-free | 30 sachet [P] £3.15

▸ **Molaxole** (Meda Pharmaceuticals Ltd)
Bicarbonate 17 mmol per 1 litre, Chloride 53 mmol per 1 litre, Macrogol '3350' 13.125 gram, Potassium 5.4 mmol per 1 litre, Sodium 65 mmol per 1 litre Molaxole oral powder sachets sugar-free | 20 sachet [P] £3.78 sugar-free | 30 sachet [P] £5.68 DT price = £4.27

▸ **Movicol** (Norgine Pharmaceuticals Ltd)
Bicarbonate 17 mmol per 1 litre, Chloride 53 mmol per 1 litre, Macrogol '3350' 13.125 gram, Potassium 5.4 mmol per 1 litre, Sodium 65 mmol per 1 litre Movicol Plain oral powder 13.7g sachets sugar-free | 30 sachet [P] £7.72 DT price = £4.27 sugar-free | 50 sachet [P] £12.85
Movicol Chocolate oral powder 13.9g sachets sugar-free | 30 sachet [P] £7.72 DT price = £4.27
Movicol oral powder 13.8g sachets lemon & lime sugar-free | 20 sachet [P] £5.15 sugar-free | 30 sachet [P] £7.72 DT price = £4.27 sugar-free | 50 sachet [P] £12.85
Bicarbonate 17 mmol per 1 litre, Chloride 53 mmol per 1 litre, Macrogol '3350' 6.563 gram, Potassium 5.4 mmol per 1 litre, Sodium 65 mmol per 1 litre Movicol-Half oral powder 6.9g sachets sugar-free | 20 sachet [P] £3.37 sugar-free | 30 sachet [P] £5.06

Movicol Paediatric Plain oral powder 6.9g sachets sugar-free | 30 sachet [PoM] £4.38
Movicol Paediatric Chocolate oral powder 6.9g sachets sugar-free | 30 sachet [PoM] £4.38

Magnesium hydroxide

● **INDICATIONS AND DOSE**
Constipation
▸ BY MOUTH
▸ Child 3–11 years: 5–10 mL as required, dose to be given mixed with water at bedtime
▸ Child 12–17 years: 30–45 mL as required, dose to be given mixed with water at bedtime

● **CONTRA-INDICATIONS** Acute gastro-intestinal conditions
● **INTERACTIONS** → Appendix 1 (antacids).
● **SIDE-EFFECTS** Colic
● **HEPATIC IMPAIRMENT** Avoid in hepatic coma if risk of renal failure.
● **RENAL IMPAIRMENT** Avoid or reduce dose. Increased risk of toxicity in renal impairment.
● **PRESCRIBING AND DISPENSING INFORMATION** When prepared extemporaneously, the BP states Magnesium Hydroxide Mixture, BP consists of an aqueous suspension containing about 8% hydrated magnesium oxide.
● **MEDICINAL FORMS**
There can be variation in the licensing of different medicines containing the same drug.
Oral suspension
▸ **Magnesium hydroxide (Non-proprietary)**
Magnesium hydroxide 83 mg per 1 ml Phillips' Milk of Magnesia 415mg/5ml oral suspension sugar-free | 200 ml [GSL] £3.22 DT price = £3.22

Sodium acid phosphate with sodium phosphate

● **INDICATIONS AND DOSE**
Constipation (using Phosphates Enema BP Formula B) | Bowel evacuation before abdominal radiological procedures, endoscopy, and surgery (using Phosphates Enema BP Formula B)
▸ BY RECTUM
▸ Child 3–6 years: 45–65 mL once daily
▸ Child 7–11 years: 65–100 mL once daily
▸ Child 12–17 years: 100–128 mL once daily

FLEET® READY-TO-USE ENEMA
Constipation | Bowel evacuation before abdominal radiological procedures | Bowel evacuation before endoscopy | Bowel evacuation before surgery
▸ BY RECTUM
▸ Child 3–6 years: 40–60 mL once daily
▸ Child 7–11 years: 60–90 mL once daily
▸ Child 12–17 years: 90–118 mL once daily

● **CONTRA-INDICATIONS** Conditions associated with increased colonic absorption · gastro-intestinal obstruction · inflammatory bowel disease
● **CAUTIONS** Ascites · congestive heart failure · electrolyte disturbances · uncontrolled hypertension
● **SIDE-EFFECTS** Electrolyte disturbances · local irritation
● **HEPATIC IMPAIRMENT** Use with caution in cirrhosis.
● **RENAL IMPAIRMENT** Use with caution.
● **PRESCRIBING AND DISPENSING INFORMATION** When prepared extemporaneously, the BP states Phosphates Enema BP Formula B consists of sodium dihydrogen phosphate dihydrate 12.8 g, disodium phosphate

dodecahydrate 10.24 g, purified water, freshly boiled and cooled, to 128 mL.

- **MEDICINAL FORMS**
There can be variation in the licensing of different medicines containing the same drug.
Enema
  - ▸ Sodium acid phosphate with sodium phosphate (Non-proprietary)
Disodium hydrogen phosphate dodecahydrate 80 mg per 1 ml, Sodium dihydrogen phosphate dihydrate 100 mg per 1 ml Phosphates enema (Formula B) 128ml long tube | 1 enema Ⓟ £27.93 DT price = £27.93
Phosphates enema (Formula B) 128ml standard tube | 1 enema Ⓟ £3.98 DT price = £3.98
  - ▸ Fleet Ready-to-use (Casen Recordati S.L.)
Disodium hydrogen phosphate dodecahydrate 80 mg per 1 ml, Sodium dihydrogen phosphate dihydrate 181 mg per 1 ml Fleet Ready-to-use 133ml enema | 1 enema Ⓟ £0.68

Sodium citrate

- **INDICATIONS AND DOSE**

MICOLETTE®

Constipation
- ▸ BY RECTUM
  - ▸ Child 3-17 years: 5-10 mL for 1 dose

MICRALAX®

Constipation
- ▸ BY RECTUM
  - ▸ Child 3-17 years: 5 mL for 1 dose

RELAXIT®

Constipation
- ▸ BY RECTUM
  - ▸ Child 1 month-2 years: 5 mL for 1 dose, insert only half the nozzle length
  - ▸ Child 3-17 years: 5 mL for 1 dose

- **CONTRA-INDICATIONS** Acute gastro-intestinal conditions
- **CAUTIONS** Sodium and water retention in susceptible individuals

- **MEDICINAL FORMS**
There can be variation in the licensing of different medicines containing the same drug.
Enema
  - ▸ Micolette Micro-enema (Pinewood Healthcare)
Sodium citrate 90 mg per 1 ml Micolette Micro-enema 5ml | 12 enema Ⓟ £3.40
  - ▸ Micralax Micro-enema (Focus Pharmaceuticals Ltd)
Sodium citrate 90 mg per 1 ml Micralax Micro-enema 5ml | 12 enema Ⓟ £4.87
  - ▸ Relaxit (Supra Enterprises Ltd)
Sodium citrate 90 mg per 1 ml Relaxit Micro-enema 5ml | 12 enema £5.21

LAXATIVES ⟩ STIMULANT LAXATIVES

Bisacodyl

- **INDICATIONS AND DOSE**

Constipation
- ▸ BY MOUTH
  - ▸ Child 4-17 years: 5-20 mg once daily, adjusted according to response, dose to be taken at night
- ▸ BY RECTUM
  - ▸ Child 2-17 years: 5-10 mg once daily, adjusted according to response

Bowel clearance before radiological procedures and surgery
- ▸ INITIALLY BY MOUTH
  - ▸ Child 4-9 years: 5 mg once daily for 2 days before procedure, dose to be taken at bedtime and (by rectum) 5 mg if required, dose to be administered 1 hour before procedure
  - ▸ Child 10-17 years: 10 mg once daily for 2 days before procedure, dose to be taken at bedtime and (by rectum) 10 mg if required, dose to be administered 1 hour before procedure
- **PHARMACOKINETICS**
Tablets act in 10-12 hours; suppositories act in 20-60 minutes.

- **CONTRA-INDICATIONS** Acute abdominal conditions · acute inflammatory bowel disease · intestinal obstruction · severe dehydration
- **CAUTIONS** Excessive use of stimulant laxatives can cause diarrhoea and related effects such as hypokalaemia · risk of electrolyte imbalance with prolonged use
- **SIDE-EFFECTS**
GENERAL SIDE-EFFECTS
Abdominal cramp · colitis · nausea · vomiting
SPECIFIC SIDE-EFFECTS
- ▸ With rectal use Local irritation
- **PREGNANCY** May be suitable for constipation in pregnancy, if a stimulant effect is necessary.

- **MEDICINAL FORMS**
There can be variation in the licensing of different medicines containing the same drug. Forms available from special-order manufacturers include: oral suspension, suppository, enema
Gastro-resistant tablet
CAUTIONARY AND ADVISORY LABELS 5, 25
  - ▸ Bisacodyl (Non-proprietary)
Bisacodyl 5 mg Bisacodyl 5mg gastro-resistant tablets | 60 tablet Ⓟ £3.25 DT price = £1.85 | 100 tablet Ⓟ £5.40 | 500 tablet Ⓟ £25.73 | 1000 tablet Ⓟ £51.45
Suppository
  - ▸ Bisacodyl (Non-proprietary)
Bisacodyl 10 mg Bisacodyl 10mg suppositories | 12 suppository Ⓟ £3.53 DT price = £3.53
Enema
  - ▸ Bisacodyl (Non-proprietary)
Bisacodyl 333.333 microgram per 1 ml Fleet Bisacodyl 10mg/30ml enema | 1 enema ⟨PoM⟩ no price available

Co-danthramer

- **INDICATIONS AND DOSE**

Constipation in terminally ill patients (standard strength capsules)
- ▸ BY MOUTH USING CAPSULES
  - ▸ Child 6-11 years: 1 capsule once daily, dose should be taken at night
  - ▸ Child 12-17 years: 1-2 capsules once daily, dose should be taken at night

Constipation in terminally ill patients (strong capsules)
- ▸ BY MOUTH USING CAPSULES
  - ▸ Child 12-17 years: 1-2 capsules once daily, dose should be given at night

Constipation in terminally ill patients (standard strength suspension)
- ▸ BY MOUTH USING ORAL SUSPENSION
  - ▸ Child 2-11 years: 2.5-5 mL once daily, dose should be taken at night
  - ▸ Child 12-17 years: 5-10 mL once daily, dose should be taken at night

Constipation in terminally ill patients (strong suspension)
▶ BY MOUTH USING ORAL SUSPENSION
▶ Child 12–17 years: 5 mL once daily, dose should be taken at night

DOSE EQUIVALENCE AND CONVERSION
Co-danthramer (standard strength) capsules contain dantron 25 mg with poloxamer '188' 200 mg per capsule.
Co-danthramer (standard strength) oral suspension contains dantron 25 mg with poloxamer '188' 200 mg per 5 mL.
Co-danthramer **strong** capsules contain dantron 37.5 mg with poloxamer '188' 500 mg.
Co-danthramer **strong** oral suspension contains dantron 75 mg with poloxamer '188' 1 g per 5 mL.
Co-danthramer suspension 5 mL = one co-danthramer capsule, **but** strong co-danthramer suspension 5 mL = two strong co-danthramer capsules.

● **CONTRA-INDICATIONS** Acute abdominal conditions · acute inflammatory bowel disease · intestinal obstruction · severe dehydration
● **CAUTIONS** Excessive use of stimulant laxatives can cause diarrhoea and related effects such as hypokalaemia · may cause local irritation · *rodent* studies indicate potential carcinogenic risk
  CAUTIONS, FURTHER INFORMATION
  ▶ Local irritation Avoid prolonged contact with skin (as in incontinent patients or infants wearing nappies—risk of irritation and excoriation).
● **SIDE-EFFECTS** Abdominal cramp · urine may be coloured red
● **PREGNANCY** Manufacturers advise avoid—limited information available.
● **BREAST FEEDING** Manufacturers advise avoid—no information available.

● **MEDICINAL FORMS**
There can be variation in the licensing of different medicines containing the same drug.
Oral suspension
CAUTIONARY AND ADVISORY LABELS 14 (urine red)
▶ Co-danthramer (Non-proprietary)
  Dantron 5 mg per 1 ml, Poloxamer 188 40 mg per 1 ml Co-danthramer 25mg/200mg/5ml oral suspension sugar free sugar-free | 300 ml PoM £146.39 DT price = £146.27
  Dantron 15 mg per 1 ml, Poloxamer 188 200 mg per 1 ml Co-danthramer 75mg/1000mg/5ml oral suspension sugar free sugar-free | 300 ml PoM £293.63 DT price = £293.39

Co-danthrusate

20.4.2016

● **INDICATIONS AND DOSE**
Constipation in terminally ill patients
▶ BY MOUTH USING CAPSULES
▶ Child 6–11 years: 1 capsule once daily, to be taken at night
▶ Child 12–17 years: 1–3 capsules once daily, to be taken at night
▶ BY MOUTH USING ORAL SUSPENSION
▶ Child 6–11 years: 5 mL once daily, to be taken at night
▶ Child 12–17 years: 5–15 mL once daily, to be taken at night

DOSE EQUIVALENCE AND CONVERSION
Co-danthrusate suspension contains dantron 50 mg and docusate 60 mg per 5 mL.
Co-danthrusate capsules contain dantron 50 mg and docusate 60 mg per capsule.

● **CONTRA-INDICATIONS** Acute abdominal conditions · acute inflammatory bowel disease · intestinal obstruction · severe dehydration

● **CAUTIONS** Excessive use of stimulant laxatives can cause diarrhoea and related effects such as hypokalaemia · may cause local irritation · *rodent* studies indicate potential carcinogenic risk
  CAUTIONS, FURTHER INFORMATION
  ▶ Local irritation Avoid prolonged contact with skin (as in incontinent patients or infants wearing nappies—risk of irritation and excoriation).
● **SIDE-EFFECTS** Abdominal cramp · urine may be coloured red
● **PREGNANCY** Manufacturers advise avoid—limited information available.
● **BREAST FEEDING** Manufacturers advise avoid—no information available.

● **MEDICINAL FORMS**
There can be variation in the licensing of different medicines containing the same drug.
Capsule
CAUTIONARY AND ADVISORY LABELS 14 (urine red)
▶ Co-danthrusate (Non-proprietary)
  Dantron 50 mg, Docusate sodium 60 mg Co-danthrusate 50mg/60mg capsules | 63 capsule PoM £52.50 DT price = £52.50
Oral suspension
CAUTIONARY AND ADVISORY LABELS 14 (urine red)
▶ Co-danthrusate (Non-proprietary)
  Dantron 10 mg per 1 ml, Docusate sodium 12 mg per 1 ml Co-danthrusate 50mg/60mg/5ml oral suspension sugar free sugar-free | 200 ml PoM £89.92

Glycerol

(Glycerin)

● **INDICATIONS AND DOSE**
Constipation
▶ BY RECTUM
▶ Child 1–11 months: 1 g as required
▶ Child 1–11 years: 2 g as required
▶ Child 12–17 years: 4 g as required

● **DIRECTIONS FOR ADMINISTRATION** Moisten suppositories with water before insertion.

● **PRESCRIBING AND DISPENSING INFORMATION** When prepared extemporaneously, the BP states Glycerol Suppositories, BP consists of gelatin 140 mg, glycerol 700 mg, purified water to 1 g.

● **PATIENT AND CARER ADVICE**
Medicines for Children leaflet: Glycerin (glycerol) suppositories for constipation www.medicinesforchildren.org.uk/glycerin-glycerol-suppositories-for-constipation

● **MEDICINAL FORMS**
There can be variation in the licensing of different medicines containing the same drug. Forms available from special-order manufacturers include: suppository
Suppository
▶ Glycerol (Non-proprietary)
  Gelatin 140 mg per 1 gram, Glycerol 700 mg per 1 gram Glycerol 2g suppositories | 12 suppository GSL £1.73 DT price = £1.67
  Glycerol 1g suppositories | 12 suppository GSL £1.69 DT price = £1.04
  Glycerol 4g suppositories | 12 suppository GSL £1.54 DT price = £1.39

Senna
13.6.2016

- **DRUG ACTION** Senna is a stimulant laxative. After metabolism of sennosides in the gut the anthrone component stimulates peristalsis thereby increasing the motility of the large intestine.

- **INDICATIONS AND DOSE**

Constipation
  - ▸ BY MOUTH USING TABLETS
  - ▸ Child 2-3 years: 3.75–15 mg once daily, adjusted according to response
  - ▸ Child 4-5 years: 3.75–30 mg once daily, adjusted according to response
  - ▸ Child 6-17 years: 7.5–30 mg once daily, adjusted according to response
  - ▸ BY MOUTH USING SYRUP
  - ▸ Child 1 month-3 years: 3.75–15 mg once daily, adjusted according to response
  - ▸ Child 4-17 years: 3.75–30 mg once daily, adjusted according to response

PHARMACOKINETICS
Onset of action 8–12 hours.

- **UNLICENSED USE** *Tablets* not licensed for use in children under 6 years. *Syrup* not licensed for use in children under 2 years.
  Doses in BNF adhere to national guidelines and may differ from those in product literature.

- **CONTRA-INDICATIONS** Intestinal obstruction · undiagnosed abdominal pain

- **SIDE-EFFECTS** Abdominal spasm · discoloration of urine · pruritus

  SIDE-EFFECTS, FURTHER INFORMATION
  Prolonged or excessive use of stimulant laxatives can cause diarrhoea and related effects such as hypokalaemia.

- **PREGNANCY** EvGr Specialist sources indicate suitable for use in pregnancy. ⟨D⟩

- **BREAST FEEDING** EvGr Specialist sources indicate suitable for use in breast-feeding in infants over 1 month. ⟨D⟩

- **PATIENT AND CARER ADVICE**
  Medicines for Children leaflet: Senna for constipation www.medicinesforchildren.org.uk/senna-for-constipation

- **NATIONAL FUNDING/ACCESS DECISIONS**
  NHS restrictions Senokot® tablets

- **EXCEPTIONS TO LEGAL CATEGORY** Senna is on sale to the public for use in children over 12 years; doses on packs may vary from those in BNF Publications.

- **MEDICINAL FORMS**
  There can be variation in the licensing of different medicines containing the same drug.
  Tablet
  - ▸ Senna (Non-proprietary)
    Sennoside B (as Sennosides) 7.5 mg Senna 7.5mg tablets | 20 tablet P £0.99 | 20 tablet GSL £0.99 | 60 tablet P £3.47 DT price = £3.01 | 60 tablet GSL £1.70 DT price = £3.01 | 100 tablet GSL £2.10 | 100 tablet P £2.10 | 1000 tablet GSL no price available

  Oral solution
  - ▸ Senokot (Forum Health Products Ltd, Reckitt Benckiser Healthcare (UK) Ltd)
    Sennoside B (as Sennosides) 1.5 mg per 1 ml Senna 7.5mg/5ml Syrup Pharmacy sugar free sugar-free | 500 ml P £3.99 DT price = £3.99
    Senokot 7.5mg/5ml syrup sugar free sugar-free | 150 ml GSL £3.49

Senna with ispaghula husk
24.2.2016

The properties listed below are those particular to the combination only. For the properties of the components please consider, senna above, ispaghula husk p. 36.

- **INDICATIONS AND DOSE**

Constipation
  - ▸ BY MOUTH
  - ▸ Child 12-17 years: 5–10 g once daily, to be taken at night, 5 g equivalent to one level spoonful of granules

- **SIDE-EFFECTS** Urine coloured yellow or red-brown

- **PREGNANCY** Manufacturer advises avoid during first trimester. To be used only intermittently and only if dietary and lifestyle changes fail.

- **DIRECTIONS FOR ADMINISTRATION** Take at night with at least 150 mL liquid..

- **MEDICINAL FORMS**
  There can be variation in the licensing of different medicines containing the same drug.
  Granules
  CAUTIONARY AND ADVISORY LABELS 25
  EXCIPIENTS: May contain Sucrose
  - ▸ Manevac (Meda Pharmaceuticals Ltd)
    Senna fruit 124 mg per 1 gram, Ispaghula 542 mg per 1 gram Manevac granules | 400 gram P £9.25 DT price = £9.25

Sodium picosulfate
6.5.2016

(Sodium picosulphate)

- **DRUG ACTION** Sodium picosulfate is a stimulant laxative. After metabolism in the colon it stimulates the mucosa thereby increasing the motility of the large intestine.

- **INDICATIONS AND DOSE**

Constipation
  - ▸ BY MOUTH
  - ▸ Child 1 month-3 years: 2.5–10 mg once daily, adjusted according to response
  - ▸ Child 4-17 years: 2.5–20 mg once daily, adjusted according to response

PHARMACOKINETICS
Onset of action 6–12 hours.

- **UNLICENSED USE** Sodium picosulfate doses in BNF Publications adhere to national guidelines and may differ from those in product literature.

- **CONTRA-INDICATIONS** Intestinal obstruction · undiagnosed abdominal pain

- **SIDE-EFFECTS**
  - ▸ **Common or very common** Abdominal cramp
  - ▸ **Uncommon** Dizziness · nausea · vomiting
  - ▸ **Frequency not known** Angioedema · pruritus · rash · syncope

  SIDE-EFFECTS, FURTHER INFORMATION
  Prolonged or excessive use can cause diarrhoea and related effects such as hypokalaemia.

- **PREGNANCY** Manufacturer states evidence limited but not known to be harmful.

- **BREAST FEEDING** EvGr Specialist sources indicate suitable for use in breast-feeding in infants over 1 month—not known to be present in milk. ⟨D⟩

- **PATIENT AND CARER ADVICE**
  Medicines for Children leaflet: Sodium picosulfate for constipation www.medicinesforchildren.org.uk/sodium-picosulfate-for-constipation

- MEDICINAL FORMS
There can be variation in the licensing of different medicines containing the same drug.

Oral solution

EXCIPIENTS: May contain Alcohol

▸ **Sodium picosulfate (Non-proprietary)**
Sodium picosulfate 1 mg per 1 ml Sodium picosulfate 5mg/5ml oral solution sugar free sugar-free | 100 ml Ⓟ £2.37 sugar-free | 300 ml Ⓟ £7.10 DT price = £7.10

▸ **Dulco-Lax (sodium picosulfate)** (Boehringer Ingelheim Self-Medication Division)
Sodium picosulfate 1 mg per 1 ml Dulcolax Pico 5mg/5ml liquid sugar-free | 100 ml Ⓟ £1.85 sugar-free | 300 ml Ⓟ £4.40 DT price = £7.10

SOFTENING DRUGS

Arachis oil

- **INDICATIONS AND DOSE**

To soften impacted faeces

▸ BY RECTUM

▸ Child 3–6 years (under close medical supervision): 45–65 mL as required

▸ Child 7–11 years (under close medical supervision): 65–100 mL as required

▸ Child 12–17 years (under close medical supervision): 100–130 mL as required

- UNLICENSED USE Licensed for use in children (age range not specified by manufacturer).

- CONTRA-INDICATIONS

▸ With rectal use Inflammatory bowel disease

- CAUTIONS Hypersensitivity to soya · intestinal obstruction

- ALLERGY AND CROSS-SENSITIVITY Contra-indicated if history of hypersensitivity to arachis oil or peanuts.

- DIRECTIONS FOR ADMINISTRATION Warm enema in warm water before use.

- MEDICINAL FORMS
There can be variation in the licensing of different medicines containing the same drug.

Enema

▸ **Arachis oil (Non-proprietary)**
Arachis oil 1 ml per 1 ml Arachis oil 130ml enema | 1 enema Ⓟ £37.50 DT price = £37.50

Docusate sodium

(Dioctyl sodium sulphosuccinate)

- **INDICATIONS AND DOSE**

Chronic constipation

▸ BY MOUTH

▸ Child 6 months–1 year: 12.5 mg 3 times a day, adjusted according to response, use paediatric oral solution

▸ Child 2–11 years: 12.5–25 mg 3 times a day, adjusted according to response, use paediatric oral solution

▸ Child 12–17 years: Up to 500 mg daily in divided doses, adjusted according to response

▸ BY RECTUM

▸ Child 12–17 years: 120 mg for 1 dose

Adjunct in abdominal radiological procedures

▸ BY MOUTH

▸ Child 12–17 years: 400 mg, to be administered with barium meal

▸ BY RECTUM

▸ Child 12–17 years: 120 mg for 1 dose

PHARMACOKINETICS

- With oral use or rectal use Oral preparations act within 1–2 days; response to rectal administration usually occurs within 20 minutes.

- UNLICENSED USE *Adult oral solution and capsules* not licensed for use in children under 12 years.

- CONTRA-INDICATIONS Avoid in intestinal obstruction

- CAUTIONS Do not give with liquid paraffin · excessive use of stimulant laxatives can cause diarrhoea and related effects such as hypokalaemia · rectal preparations not indicated if haemorrhoids or anal fissure

- SIDE-EFFECTS Abdominal cramp · diarrhoea (excessive use) · hypokalaemia · rash

- PREGNANCY Not known to be harmful—manufacturer advises caution.

- BREAST FEEDING

▸ With oral use Present in milk following oral administration— manufacturer advises caution.

▸ With rectal use Rectal administration not known to be harmful.

- DIRECTIONS FOR ADMINISTRATION For administration *by mouth*, solution may be mixed with milk or squash.

- MEDICINAL FORMS
There can be variation in the licensing of different medicines containing the same drug.

Capsule

▸ **Dioctyl (UCB Pharma Ltd)**
Docusate sodium 100 mg Dioctyl 100mg capsules | 30 capsule Ⓟ £2.09 DT price = £2.09 | 100 capsule Ⓟ £6.98

Oral solution

▸ **Docusol (Typharm Ltd)**
Docusate sodium 2.5 mg per 1 ml Docusol Paediatric 12.5mg/5ml oral solution sugar-free | 300 ml Ⓟ £5.29 DT price = £5.29
Docusate sodium 10 mg per 1 ml Docusol Adult 50mg/5ml oral solution sugar-free | 300 ml Ⓟ £5.49 DT price = £5.49

Enema

▸ **Norgalax (Essential Pharma Ltd)**
Docusate sodium 12 mg per 1 gram Norgalax 120mg/10g enema | 6 enema Ⓟ £28.00

3   Diarrhoea

Acute diarrhoea

Management of acute diarrhoea

The priority in acute diarrhoea, as in gastro-enteritis, is the prevention or reversal of fluid and electrolyte depletion— this is particularly important in infants. **Oral rehydration preparations** are used in the prevention or reversal of fluid and electrolyte depletion. Severe dehydration requires immediate admission to hospital and urgent replacement of fluid and electrolytes.

Adsorbents and bulk-forming drugs

Adsorbents such as kaolin are **not** recommended for *acute diarrhoeas*. Bulk-forming drugs, such as ispaghula husk p. 36, methylcellulose p. 36, and sterculia p. 36 are rarely effective in controlling faecal consistency in ileostomy and colostomy.

Colestyramine p. 120 binds unabsorbed bile salts and provides symptomatic relief of diarrhoea following ileal disease or resection.

Antibacterial drugs

Antibacterial drugs are generally unnecessary in simple gastro-enteritis because the complaint usually resolves quickly without such treatment, and infective diarrhoeas in the UK often have a viral cause. Systemic bacterial infection does, however, need appropriate systemic treatment.

Antimotility drugs

Antimotility drugs relieve symptoms of diarrhoea. They prolong the duration of intestinal transit by binding to opioid receptors in the gastro-intestinal tract. Loperamide hydrochloride below is used due to its action on opioid receptors in the gastrointestinal tract and because it does not cross the blood-brain barrier readily. Antimotility drugs have a role in the management of uncomplicated *acute diarrhoea* in adults but not in children under 12 years.

Antimotility drugs have a role in Inflammatory bowel disease p. 24 and are also used in Stoma care p. 67.

Antispasmodics
Antispasmodics are occasionally of value in treating abdominal cramp associated with diarrhoea but they should **not** be used for primary treatment. Antispasmodics and antiemetics should be **avoided** in young children with gastro-enteritis since they are rarely effective and have troublesome side-effects.

Enkephalinase inhibitors
Racecadotril p. 45 is a pro-drug of thiorphan. Thiorphan is an enkephalinase inhibitor that inhibits the breakdown of endogenous opioids, thereby reducing intestinal secretions. Racecadotril is licensed, as an adjunct to rehydration, for the symptomatic treatment of uncomplicated acute diarrhoea; it should only be used in children over 3 months of age when usual supportive measures, including oral rehydration, are insufficient to control the condition. Racecadotril does not affect the duration of intestinal transit.

> **Drugs used for Diarrhoea not listed below** Codeine phosphate, p. 259

ANTIDIARRHOEALS ›
ANTIPROPULSIVES

F 256

Co-phenotrope

● **INDICATIONS AND DOSE**
Adjunct to rehydration in acute diarrhoea
▸ BY MOUTH
▸ Child 2-3 years: 0.5 tablet 3 times a day
▸ Child 4-8 years: 1 tablet 3 times a day
▸ Child 9-11 years: 1 tablet 4 times a day
▸ Child 12-15 years: 2 tablets 3 times a day
▸ Child 16-17 years: Initially 4 tablets, followed by 2 tablets every 6 hours until diarrhoea controlled

Control of faecal consistency after colostomy or ileostomy
▸ BY MOUTH
▸ Child 2-3 years: 0.5 tablet 3 times a day
▸ Child 4-8 years: 1 tablet 3 times a day
▸ Child 9-11 years: 1 tablet 4 times a day
▸ Child 12-15 years: 2 tablets 3 times a day
▸ Child 16-17 years: Initially 4 tablets, then 2 tablets 4 times a day

● **UNLICENSED USE** Not licensed for use in children under 4 years.

● **CONTRA-INDICATIONS** Gastro-intestinal obstruction · intestinal atony · myasthenia gravis (but some antimuscarinics may be used to decrease muscarinic side-effects of anticholinesterases) · paralytic ileus · pyloric stenosis · severe ulcerative colitis · significant bladder outflow obstruction · toxic megacolon · urinary retention

● **CAUTIONS** Presence of subclinical doses of atropine may give rise to atropine side-effects in susceptible individuals or in overdosage · young children are particularly susceptible to **overdosage**; symptoms may be delayed and observation is needed for at least 48 hours after ingestion

● **INTERACTIONS** → Appendix 1 (antimuscarinics, opioid analgesics).

● **SIDE-EFFECTS**
▸ **Very rare** Angle-closure glaucoma

▸ **Frequency not known** Abdominal pain · anorexia · constipation · dilation of the pupils with loss of accomodation · dry mouth · dryness of the skin · fever · flushing · giddiness · nausea · photophobia · reduced bronchial secretions · transient bradycardia (followed by tachycardia, palpitation and arrhythmias) · urinary retention · urinary urgency · vomiting

● **PREGNANCY** Manufacturer advises caution.

● **BREAST FEEDING** May be present in milk.

● **HEPATIC IMPAIRMENT** Avoid in jaundice.

● **DIRECTIONS FOR ADMINISTRATION** For administration *by mouth* tablets may be crushed.

● **PRESCRIBING AND DISPENSING INFORMATION** A mixture of diphenoxylate hydrochloride and atropine sulfate in the mass proportions 100 parts to 1 part respectively.

● **EXCEPTIONS TO LEGAL CATEGORY** Co-phenotrope 2.5/0.025 can be sold to the public for children over 16 years (provided packs do not contain more than 20 tablets) as an adjunct to rehydration in acute diarrhoea (max. daily dose 10 tablets).

● **MEDICINAL FORMS**
There can be variation in the licensing of different medicines containing the same drug.
Tablet
▸ Co-phenotrope (Non-proprietary)
Atropine sulfate 25 microgram, Diphenoxylate hydrochloride 2.5 mg Lomotil 2.5mg/25microgram tablets | 100 tablet PoM no price available Schedule 5 (CD Inv)

Loperamide hydrochloride

● **INDICATIONS AND DOSE**
Symptomatic treatment of acute diarrhoea
▸ BY MOUTH
▸ Child 4-7 years: 1 mg 3–4 times a day for up to 3 days only
▸ Child 8-11 years: 2 mg 4 times a day for up to 5 days
▸ Child 12-17 years: Initially 4 mg, followed by 2 mg for up to 5 days, dose to be taken after each loose stool; usual dose 6–8 mg daily; maximum 16 mg per day

Chronic diarrhoea
▸ BY MOUTH
▸ Child 1-11 months: 100–200 micrograms/kg twice daily, to be given 30 minutes before feeds; increased if necessary up to 2 mg/kg daily in divided doses
▸ Child 1-11 years: 100–200 micrograms/kg 3–4 times a day (max. per dose 2 mg), increased if necessary up to 1.25 mg/kg daily in divided doses; maximum 16 mg per day
▸ Child 12-17 years: 2–4 mg 2–4 times a day; maximum 16 mg per day

● **UNLICENSED USE** Not licensed for use in children for chronic diarrhoea. *Capsules* not licensed for use in children under 8 years. *Syrup* not licensed for use in children under 4 years.

● **CONTRA-INDICATIONS** Active ulcerative colitis · antibiotic-associated colitis · conditions where abdominal distension develops · conditions where inhibition of peristalsis should be avoided

● **CAUTIONS** Not recommended for children under 12 years

● **INTERACTIONS** → Appendix 1 (loperamide).

● **SIDE-EFFECTS**
▸ **Common or very common** Dizziness · flatulence · headache · nausea
▸ **Uncommon** Abdominal pain · drowsiness · dry mouth · dyspepsia · rash · vomiting

▸ **Rare** Fatigue · hypertonia · paralytic ileus · Stevens-Johnson syndrome · toxic epidermal necrolysis · urinary retention

● **PREGNANCY** Manufacturers advise avoid—no information available.

● **BREAST FEEDING** Amount probably too small to be harmful.

● **HEPATIC IMPAIRMENT** Risk of accumulation—manufacturer advises caution.

● **PATIENT AND CARER ADVICE**
Medicines for Children leaflet: Loperamide for diarrhoea www.medicinesforchildren.org.uk/loperamide-for-diarrhoea

● **EXCEPTIONS TO LEGAL CATEGORY** Loperamide can be sold to the public, for use in children over 12 years, provided it is licensed and labelled for the treatment of acute diarrhoea.

● **MEDICINAL FORMS**
There can be variation in the licensing of different medicines containing the same drug. Forms available from special-order manufacturers include: oral suspension, oral solution

Tablet
▸ Loperamide hydrochloride (Non-proprietary)
Loperamide hydrochloride 2 mg Loperamide 2mg tablets |
30 tablet PoM £2.25 DT price = £2.15
▸ Norimode (Tillomed Laboratories Ltd)
Loperamide hydrochloride 2 mg Norimode 2mg tablets |
30 tablet PoM £2.15 DT price = £2.15
▸ Normaloe (Tillomed Laboratories Ltd)
Loperamide hydrochloride 2 mg Normaloe 2mg tablets |
12 tablet P £1.70

Orodispersible tablet
▸ Imodium (McNeil Products Ltd)
Loperamide hydrochloride 2 mg Imodium Instants 2mg orodispersible tablets sugar-free | 6 tablet GSL £2.45 sugar-free |
12 tablet GSL £3.76
Imodium Instant Melts 2mg orodispersible tablets sugar-free |
12 tablet P £3.75 sugar-free | 18 tablet P £5.02 DT price = £5.02

Capsule
▸ Loperamide hydrochloride (Non-proprietary)
Loperamide hydrochloride 2 mg Loperamide 2mg capsules |
6 capsule GSL no price available | 12 capsule P £1.94 |
30 capsule PoM £2.99 DT price = £1.39
▸ Imodium (McNeil Products Ltd)
Loperamide hydrochloride 2 mg Imodium LiquiCaps 2mg Soft capsules | 6 capsule GSL £2.45
Imodium 2mg Soft capsules | 12 capsule P £3.79
Imodium IBS Relief 2mg capsules | 12 capsule P £3.79
Imodium Classic 2mg capsules | 12 capsule P £3.31 |
18 capsule P £4.13
Imodium Original 2mg capsules | 6 capsule GSL £1.88

Oral solution
▸ Imodium (Janssen-Cilag Ltd)
Loperamide hydrochloride 200 microgram per 1 ml Imodium 1mg/5ml oral solution sugar-free | 100 ml PoM £1.17 DT price = £1.17

Loperamide with simeticone

The properties listed below are those particular to the combination only. For the properties of the components please consider, loperamide hydrochloride p. 44, simeticone p. 48.

● **INDICATIONS AND DOSE**

Acute diarrhoea with abdominal colic
▸ BY MOUTH
▸ Child 12–17 years: Initially 1 tablet, then 1 tablet, after each loose stool, for up to 2 days; maximum 4 tablets per day

● **MEDICINAL FORMS**
There can be variation in the licensing of different medicines containing the same drug.
Tablet
▸ Imodium Plus (McNeil Products Ltd)
Loperamide hydrochloride 2 mg, Dimeticone (as Simeticone)
125 mg Imodium Plus Comfort tablets | 6 tablet GSL £2.51
Imodium Plus caplets | 12 tablet P £3.66

ANTIDIARRHOEALS › ENKEPHALINASE INHIBITORS

Racecadotril

11.2.2016

● **INDICATIONS AND DOSE**

Adjunct to rehydration, for the symptomatic treatment of uncomplicated acute diarrhoea
▸ BY MOUTH USING GRANULES
▸ Child 3 months–17 years (body-weight up to 9 kg): 10 mg 3 times a day until diarrhoea stops; maximum duration of treatment 7 days
▸ Child 3 months–17 years (body-weight 9–12 kg): 20 mg 3 times a day until diarrhoea stops; maximum duration of treatment 7 days
▸ Child 3 months–17 years (body-weight 13–27 kg): 30 mg 3 times a day until diarrhoea stops; maximum duration of treatment 7 days
▸ Child 3 months–17 years (body-weight 28 kg and above): 60 mg 3 times a day until diarrhoea stops; maximum duration of treatment 7 days

● **CONTRA-INDICATIONS** Antibiotic-associated diarrhoea

● **SIDE-EFFECTS**
▸ **Uncommon** Erythema · rash
▸ **Frequency not known** Angioedema · pruritus · urticaria
SIDE-EFFECTS, FURTHER INFORMATION
▸ Skin reactions Severe skin reactions have been reported—discontinue treatment immediately.

● **PREGNANCY** Manufacturer advises avoid—no information available.

● **BREAST FEEDING** Manufacturer advises avoid—no information available.

● **HEPATIC IMPAIRMENT** Manufacturer advises avoid.

● **RENAL IMPAIRMENT** Manufacturer advises avoid.

● **DIRECTIONS FOR ADMINISTRATION** Granules may be added to food or mixed with water or bottle feeds and then taken immediately.

● **PATIENT AND CARER ADVICE** Patients and carers should be given advice on how to administer racecadotril granules.

● **NATIONAL FUNDING/ACCESS DECISIONS**

Scottish Medicines Consortium (SMC) Decisions
The *Scottish Medicines Consortium*, has advised (July 2014) that racecadotril (*Hidrasec*®) is **not** recommended for use within NHS Scotland for the treatment of acute diarrhoea in children because there is insufficient evidence that it improves the recovery rate.

● **MEDICINAL FORMS**
There can be variation in the licensing of different medicines containing the same drug.
Granules
EXCIPIENTS: May contain Sucrose
▸ Hidrasec (Lincoln Medical Ltd)
Racecadotril 10 mg Hidrasec Infants 10mg granules sachets |
20 sachet PoM £8.42
Racecadotril 30 mg Hidrasec Children 30mg granules sachets |
20 sachet PoM £8.42

4 Disorders of gastric acid and ulceration

4.1 Dyspepsia

Dyspepsia

Overview

Dyspepsia covers upper abdominal pain, fullness, early satiety, bloating, and nausea. It can occur with gastric and duodenal ulceration, gastro-oesophageal reflux disease, gastritis, and upper gastro-intestinal motility disorders, but most commonly it is of uncertain origin.

Patients with dyspepsia should be advised about lifestyle changes (avoidance of excess alcohol and of aggravating foods such as fats); other measures include weight reduction, smoking cessation, and raising the head of the bed. Some medications may cause dyspepsia—these should be stopped, if possible.

A compound alginate preparation may provide relief from dyspepsia; persistent dyspepsia requires investigation. Treatment with a H_2-receptor antagonist or a proton pump inhibitor should be initiated only on the advice of a hospital specialist.

Helicobacter pylori may be present in children with dyspepsia. *H. pylori* eradication therapy should be considered for persistent dyspepsia if it is ulcer-like. However, most children with functional (investigated, non-ulcer) dyspepsia do not benefit symptomatically from *H. pylori* eradication.

ANTACIDS

Antacids

Overview

Antacids (usually containing aluminium or magnesium compounds) can often relieve symptoms in *ulcer dyspepsia* and in *non-erosive gastro-oesophageal reflux* ; they are also sometimes used in functional (non-ulcer) dyspepsia but the evidence of benefit is uncertain.

Aluminium- and **magnesium**-containing antacids, being relatively insoluble in water, are long-acting if retained in the stomach. They are suitable for most antacid purposes. Magnesium-containing antacids tend to be laxative whereas aluminium-containing antacids may be constipating; antacids containing both magnesium and aluminium may reduce these colonic side-effects.

Complexes such as **hydrotalcite** confer no special advantage.

Calcium-containing antacids can induce rebound acid secretion; with modest doses the clinical significance of this is doubtful, but prolonged high doses also cause hypercalcaemia and alkalosis.

Simeticone

Simeticone (activated dimeticone p. 48) is used to treat infantile colic, but the evidence of benefit is uncertain.

Simeticone is added to an antacid as an antifoaming agent to relieve flatulence. These preparations may be useful for the relief of hiccup in palliative care.

Alginates

Alginates taken in combination with an antacid increases the viscosity of stomach contents and can protect the oesophageal mucosa from acid reflux. Some alginate-containing preparations form a viscous gel ('raft') that floats on the surface of the stomach contents, thereby reducing symptoms of reflux. Alginate-containing preparations are used in the management of mild symptoms of dyspepsia and gastro-oesophageal reflux disease.

The amount of additional ingredient or antacid in individual preparations varies widely, as does their sodium content, so that preparations may not be freely interchangeable.

ANTACIDS > ALGINATE

Alginic acid

● INDICATIONS AND DOSE

GAVISCON INFANT® POWDER SACHETS

Management of gastro-oesophageal reflux disease
▸ BY MOUTH

▸ Neonate (body-weight up to 4.5 kg): 1 dose as required, to be mixed with feeds (or water, for breast-fed infants); maximum 6 doses per day.

▸ Neonate (body-weight 4.5 kg and above): 2 doses as required, to be mixed with feeds (or water, for breast-fed infants); maximum 12 doses per day.

▸ Child 1–23 months (body-weight up to 4.5 kg): 1 dose as required, to be mixed with feeds (or water, for breast-fed infants); maximum 6 doses per day

▸ Child 1–23 months (body-weight 4.5 kg and above): 2 doses as required, to be mixed with feeds (or water, for breast-fed infants); maximum 12 doses per day

● **CONTRA-INDICATIONS** Intestinal obstruction · preterm neonates · where excessive water loss likely (e.g. fever, diarrhoea, vomiting, high room temperature)

● **INTERACTIONS** → Appendix 1 (antacids).
Not to be used with other preparations containing thickening agents.
Antacids should preferably not be taken at the same time as other drugs since they may impair absorption.
Antacids may damage enteric coatings designed to prevent dissolution in the stomach.

● **HEPATIC IMPAIRMENT** In patients with fluid retention, avoid antacids containing large amounts of sodium. Avoid antacids containing magnesium salts in hepatic coma if there is a risk of renal failure.

● **RENAL IMPAIRMENT** In patients with fluid retention, avoid antacids containing large amounts of sodium.

● **PRESCRIBING AND DISPENSING INFORMATION** Each half of the dual-sachet is identified as 'one dose'.
To avoid errors prescribe with directions in terms of 'dose'.

● **MEDICINAL FORMS**
There can be variation in the licensing of different medicines containing the same drug.

Powder
ELECTROLYTES: May contain Sodium
▸ Gaviscon Infant (Forum Health Products Ltd)
Magnesium alginate 87.5 mg, Sodium alginate 225 mg Gaviscon Infant oral powder sachets sugar-free | 15 dual dose sachet GSL
£4.39

Sodium alginate with potassium bicarbonate

The properties listed below are those particular to the combination only. For the properties of the components please consider, alginic acid p. 46.

- **INDICATIONS AND DOSE**

  Management of mild symptoms of dyspepsia and gastro-oesophageal reflux disease
  - ‣ BY MOUTH USING CHEWABLE TABLETS
  - ‣ Child 6–11 years (under medical advice only): 1 tablet, to be chewed after meals and at bedtime
  - ‣ Child 12–17 years: 1–2 tablets, to be chewed after meals and at bedtime
  - ‣ BY MOUTH USING ORAL SUSPENSION
  - ‣ Child 2–11 years (under medical advice only): 2.5–5 mL, to be taken after meals and at bedtime
  - ‣ Child 12–17 years: 5–10 mL, to be taken after meals and at bedtime

- **PRESCRIBING AND DISPENSING INFORMATION** Flavours of oral liquid formulations may include aniseed or peppermint.

- **MEDICINAL FORMS**
  There can be variation in the licensing of different medicines containing the same drug.
  Chewable tablet
  EXCIPIENTS: May contain Aspartame
  ELECTROLYTES: May contain Potassium, sodium
  - ‣ **Sodium alginate with potassium bicarbonate (Non-proprietary)**
    Potassium bicarbonate 100 mg, Sodium alginate 500 mg Sodium alginate 500mg / Potassium bicarbonate 100mg chewable tablets sugar free sugar-free | 60 tablet GSL no price available DT price = £3.07
  - ‣ Brands may include Gaviscon Advance

  Oral suspension
  ELECTROLYTES: May contain Potassium, sodium
  - ‣ **Gaviscon Advance** (Reckitt Benckiser Healthcare (UK) Ltd)
    Potassium bicarbonate 20 mg per 1 ml, Sodium alginate 100 mg per 1 ml Gaviscon Advance oral suspension aniseed sugar-free | 150 ml P £3.23 sugar-free | 300 ml P £5.82
    Gaviscon Advance oral suspension peppermint sugar-free | 300 ml P £5.82

ANTACIDS > ALUMINIUM AND MAGNESIUM

Co-magaldrox

The properties listed below are those particular to the combination only. For the properties of the components please consider, aluminium hydroxide p. 558, magnesium hydroxide p. 39.

- **INDICATIONS AND DOSE**
  MAALOX®
  Dyspepsia
  - ‣ BY MOUTH
  - ‣ Child 14–17 years: 10–20 mL, to be taken 20–60 minutes after meals, and at bedtime or when required

  MUCOGEL®
  Dyspepsia
  - ‣ BY MOUTH
  - ‣ Child 12–17 years: 10–20 mL 3 times a day, to be taken 20–60 minutes after meals, and at bedtime, or when required

- **PRESCRIBING AND DISPENSING INFORMATION** Co-magaldrox is a mixture of aluminium hydroxide and magnesium hydroxide; the proportions are expressed in the form x/y where x and y are the strengths in milligrams per unit dose of magnesium hydroxide and aluminium hydroxide respectively.

MUCOGEL® Mucogel® suspension is low in sodium.
MAALOX® Maalox® suspension is low in sodium.

- **MEDICINAL FORMS**
  There can be variation in the licensing of different medicines containing the same drug.
  Oral suspension
  - ‣ Maalox (Sanofi)
    Magnesium hydroxide 39 mg per 1 ml, Aluminium hydroxide gel dried 44 mg per 1 ml Maalox oral suspension sugar-free | 500 ml GSL £3.35
  - ‣ Mucogel (Chemidex Pharma Ltd)
    Magnesium hydroxide 39 mg per 1 ml, Aluminium hydroxide gel dried 44 mg per 1 ml Mucogel oral suspension sugar-free | 500 ml GSL £2.99

Co-simalcite

- **INDICATIONS AND DOSE**
  Dyspepsia
  - ‣ BY MOUTH
  - ‣ Child 8–11 years: 5 mL 4 times a day as required, to be taken between meals and at bedtime
  - ‣ Child 12–17 years: 10 mL 4 times a day as required, to be taken between meals and at bedtime

- **CONTRA-INDICATIONS** Hypophosphataemia · infants · neonates

  CONTRA-INDICATIONS, FURTHER INFORMATION
  - ‣ Aluminium-containing antacids Aluminium-containing antacids should not be used in neonates and infants because accumulation may lead to increased plasma-aluminium concentrations.

- **INTERACTIONS** → Appendix 1 (antacids).
  Antacids should preferably not be taken at the same time as other drugs since they may impair absorption. Antacids may damage enteric coatings designed to prevent dissolution in the stomach.

- **SIDE-EFFECTS**

  SIDE-EFFECTS, FURTHER INFORMATION
  - ‣ Constipation and diarrhoea Magnesium-containing antacids tend to be laxative whereas aluminium-containing antacids may be constipating; antacids containing both magnesium and aluminium may reduce these colonic side-effects.

- **HEPATIC IMPAIRMENT** Avoid; can cause constipation which can precipitate coma. Avoid in hepatic coma; risk of renal failure.

- **RENAL IMPAIRMENT** Antacids containing magnesium salts should be avoided or used at a reduced dose since there is an increased risk of toxicity. Aluminium-containing antacids should not be used in children with renal impairment, because accumulation may lead to increased plasma-aluminium concentrations.

- **PRESCRIBING AND DISPENSING INFORMATION** Altacite Plus® is low in Na⁺.

- **MEDICINAL FORMS**
  There can be variation in the licensing of different medicines containing the same drug.
  Oral suspension
  - ‣ Altacite Plus (Peckforton Pharmaceuticals Ltd)
    Simeticone 25 mg per 1 ml, Hydrotalcite 100 mg per 1 ml Altacite Plus oral suspension sugar-free | 100 ml P £4.00 sugar-free | 500 ml P £5.20 DT price = £5.20

1

Gastro-intestinal system

Simeticone with aluminium hydroxide and magnesium hydroxide

The properties listed below are those particular to the combination only. For the properties of the components please consider, simeticone below, aluminium hydroxide p. 558.

● **INDICATIONS AND DOSE**

Dyspepsia
▸ BY MOUTH
▸ Child 2–4 years: 5 mL 3 times a day
▸ Child 5–11 years: 5–10 mL 3–4 times a day
▸ Child 12–17 years: 5–10 mL 4 times a day, to be taken after meals and at bedtime, or when required

● **MEDICINAL FORMS**
There can be variation in the licensing of different medicines containing the same drug.

Oral suspension
▸ Maalox Plus (Sanofi)
  Simeticone 5 mg per 1 ml, Magnesium hydroxide 39 mg per 1 ml, Aluminium hydroxide gel dried 44 mg per 1 ml Maalox Plus oral suspension sugar-free | 500 ml GSL £3.90

ANTACIDS > MAGNESIUM

Magnesium trisilicate with magnesium carbonate and sodium bicarbonate

The properties listed below are those particular to the combination only. For the properties of the components please consider, sodium bicarbonate p. 544.

● **INDICATIONS AND DOSE**

Dyspepsia
▸ BY MOUTH
▸ Child 5–11 years: 5–10 mL 3 times a day, alternatively as required, dose to be made up with water
▸ Child 12–17 years: 10–20 mL 3 times a day, alternatively as required, dose to be made up with water

● **CONTRA-INDICATIONS** Hypophosphataemia · Severe renal failure
● **CAUTIONS** Heart failure · hypermagnesaemia · hypertension · metabolic alkalosis · respiratory alkalosis
● **INTERACTIONS** → Appendix 1 (antacids).
  Antacids should preferably not be taken at the same time as other drugs since they may impair absorption. Antacids may damage enteric coatings designed to prevent dissolution in the stomach.
● **SIDE-EFFECTS** Belching due to liberated carbon dioxide · diarrhoea
● **HEPATIC IMPAIRMENT** In patients with fluid retention avoid antacids containing large amounts of sodium. Avoid antacids containing magnesium salts in hepatic coma if there is a risk of renal failure.
● **RENAL IMPAIRMENT** Magnesium trisilicate and magnesium carbonate mixtures have high sodium content; avoid in patients with fluid retention.
● **PRESCRIBING AND DISPENSING INFORMATION** When prepared extemporaneously, the BP states Magnesium Trisilicate Mixture, BP consists of 5% each of magnesium trisilicate, light magnesium carbonate, and sodium bicarbonate in a suitable vehicle with a peppermint flavour.

● **MEDICINAL FORMS**
There can be variation in the licensing of different medicines containing the same drug.

Oral suspension
▸ Magnesium trisilicate with magnesium carbonate and sodium bicarbonate (Non-proprietary)
  Magnesium carbonate light 50 mg per 1 ml, Magnesium trisilicate 50 mg per 1 ml, Sodium bicarbonate 50 mg per 1 ml Magnesium trisilicate oral suspension | 200 ml GSL £1.50 DT price = £1.50

ANTIFOAMING DRUGS

Simeticone

(Activated dimeticone)

● **DRUG ACTION** Simeticone (activated dimeticone) is an antifoaming agent.

● **INDICATIONS AND DOSE**

DENTINOX®

Colic | Wind pains
▸ BY MOUTH
▸ Neonate: 2.5 mL, to be taken with or after each feed; may be added to bottle feed; maximum 6 doses per day.
▸ Child 1 month-1 year: 2.5 mL, to be taken with or after each feed; may be added to bottle feed; maximum 6 doses per day

INFACOL®

Colic | Wind pains
▸ BY MOUTH
▸ Neonate: 0.5–1 mL, to be taken before feeds.
▸ Child 1 month-1 year: 0.5–1 mL, to be taken before feeds

● **PRESCRIBING AND DISPENSING INFORMATION**
DENTINOX® The brand name Dentinox® is also used for other preparations including teething gel.
● **PATIENT AND CARER ADVICE**
INFACOL® Patients or carers should be given advice on use of the Infacol® dropper.
● **LESS SUITABLE FOR PRESCRIBING**
INFACOL® Infacol® is less suitable for prescribing (evidence of benefit in infantile colic uncertain).
DENTINOX® Dentinox® colic drops are less suitable for prescribing (evidence of benefit in infantile colic uncertain).

● **MEDICINAL FORMS**
There can be variation in the licensing of different medicines containing the same drug.

Oral suspension
▸ Infacol (Forest Laboratories UK Ltd)
  Simeticone 40 mg per 1 ml Infacol 40mg/ml oral suspension sugar-free | 50 ml GSL £2.71 DT price = £2.71

Oral drops
▸ Dentinox Infant (Dendron Ltd)
  Simeticone 8.4 mg per 1 ml Dentinox Infant colic drops | 100 ml GSL £1.73

Combinations available: *Simeticone with aluminium hydroxide and magnesium hydroxide,* above

Recommended regimens for _Helicobacter pylori_ eradication

Age range	Acid suppressant	Antibacterial		
		Amoxicillin	Clarithromycin	Metronidazole
Child 1–5 years	Omeprazole 1–2 mg/kg once daily (max. per dose 40 mg)	250 mg twice daily	7.5 mg/kg (max. 500 mg) twice daily	–
		125 mg 3 times a day	–	100 mg 3 times a day
		–	7.5 mg/kg (max. 500 mg) twice daily	100 mg twice daily
Child 6–11 years	Omeprazole 1–2 mg/kg once daily (max. per dose 40 mg)	500 mg twice daily	7.5 mg/kg (max. 500 mg) twice daily	–
		250 mg 3 times a day	–	200 mg 3 times a day
		–	7.5 mg/kg (max. 500 mg) twice daily	200 mg twice daily
Child 12–17 years	Omeprazole 40 mg once daily	1 g twice daily	500 mg twice daily	–
		500 mg 3 times a day	–	400 mg 3 times a day
		–	500 mg twice daily	400 mg twice daily

4.2 Gastric and duodenal ulceration

Peptic ulceration

Overview

Peptic ulceration commonly involves the stomach, duodenum, and lower oesophagus; after gastric surgery it involves the gastro-enterostomy stoma. Healing can be promoted by general measures, stopping smoking and taking antacids and by antisecretory drug treatment, but relapse is common when treatment ceases. Nearly all duodenal ulcers and most gastric ulcers not associated with NSAIDs are caused by _Helicobacter pylori_.

Helicobacter pylori infection

Eradication of _Helicobacter pylori_ reduces the recurrence of gastric and duodenal ulcers and the risk of rebleeding. The presence of _H. pylori_ should be confirmed before starting eradication treatment. If possible, the antibacterial sensitivity of the organism should be established at the time of endoscopy and biopsy. Acid inhibition combined with antibacterial treatment is highly effective in the eradication of _H. pylori_; reinfection is rare. Antibiotic-associated colitis is an uncommon risk.

Treatment to eradicate _H. pylori_ infection in children should be initiated under specialist supervision. One week triple-therapy regimens that comprise omeprazole p. 54, amoxicillin p. 320, and either clarithromycin p. 309 or metronidazole p. 313 are recommended, see table above. Resistance to clarithromycin or to metronidazole is much more common than to amoxicillin and can develop during treatment. A regimen containing amoxicillin and clarithromycin is therefore recommended for initial therapy and one containing amoxicillin and metronidazole is recommended for eradication failure or for a child who has been treated with a macrolide for other infections. There is usually no need to continue antisecretory treatment (with a proton pump inhibitor or H_2-receptor antagonist); however, if the ulcer is large, or complicated by haemorrhage or perforation then antisecretory treatment is continued for a further 3 weeks. Lansoprazole p. 53 may be considered if omeprazole is unsuitable. Treatment failure usually indicates antibacterial resistance or poor compliance.

Two-week triple-therapy regimens offer the possibility of higher eradication rates compared to one-week regimens, but adverse effects are common and poor compliance is likely to offset any possible gain.

Two-week dual-therapy regimens using a proton pump inhibitor and a single antibacterial produce low rates of _H. pylori_ eradication and are **not** recommended.

See under _NSAID-associated ulcers_ for the role of _H. pylori_ eradication therapy in children starting or taking NSAIDs.

Test for _Helicobacter pylori_

^{13}C-Urea breath test kits are available for confirming the presence of gastro-duodenal infection with _Helicobacter pylori_. The test involves collection of breath samples before and after ingestion of an oral solution of ^{13}C-urea; the samples are sent for analysis by an appropriate laboratory. The test should not be performed within 4 weeks of treatment with an antibacterial or within 2 weeks of treatment with an antisecretory drug. A specific ^{13}C-Urea breath test kit for children is available (_Helicobacter Test INFAI for children of the age_ 3–11 ®). However the appropriateness of testing for _H. pylori_ infection in children has not been established. Breath, saliva, faecal, and urine tests for _H. pylori_ are frequently unreliable in children; the most accurate method of diagnosis is endoscopy with biopsy.

NSAID-associated ulcers

Gastro-intestinal bleeding and ulceration can occur with NSAID use. Whenever possible, NSAIDs should be **withdrawn** if an ulcer occurs.

Children at high risk of developing gastro-intestinal complications with a NSAID include those with a history of peptic ulcer disease or serious upper gastro-intestinal complication, those taking other medicines that increase the risk of upper gastro-intestinal side-effects, or those with serious co-morbidity. In children at risk of ulceration, a proton pump inhibitor can be considered for protection against gastric and duodenal ulcers associated with non-selective NSAIDs; high dose ranitidine p. 50 is an alternative.

NSAID use and _H. pylori_ infection are independent risk factors for gastro-intestinal bleeding and ulceration. In children already taking a NSAID, eradication of _H. pylori_ is unlikely to reduce the risk of NSAID-induced bleeding or ulceration. However, in children about to start long-term NSAID treatment who are _H. pylori_ positive and have dyspepsia or a history of gastric or duodenal ulcer, eradication of _H. pylori_ may reduce the overall risk of ulceration.

If the NSAID can be _discontinued_ in a child who has developed an ulcer, a proton pump inhibitor usually produces the most rapid healing; alternatively the ulcer can be treated with an H_2-receptor antagonist.

If _NSAID treatment needs to continue_, the ulcer is treated with a proton pump inhibitor.

GASTROPROTECTIVE COMPLEXES AND CHELATORS

Chelates and complexes

Sucralfate

Sucralfate below is a complex of aluminium hydroxide and sulfated sucrose that appears to act by protecting the mucosa from acid-pepsin attack; it has minimal antacid properties.

Sucralfate

- **INDICATIONS AND DOSE**

Benign gastric ulceration | Benign duodenal ulceration
▸ BY MOUTH
- ▸ Child 1 month–1 year: 250 mg 4–6 times a day
- ▸ Child 2–11 years: 500 mg 4–6 times a day
- ▸ Child 12–14 years: 1 g 4–6 times a day
- ▸ Child 15–17 years: 2 g twice daily, dose to be taken on rising and at bedtime, alternatively 1 g 4 times a day for 4–6 weeks, or in resistant cases up to 12 weeks, dose to be taken 1 hour before meals and at bedtime; maximum 8 g per day

Prophylaxis of stress ulceration in child under intensive care
▸ BY MOUTH
- ▸ Child 1 month–1 year: 250 mg 4–6 times a day
- ▸ Child 2–11 years: 500 mg 4–6 times a day
- ▸ Child 12–14 years: 1 g 4–6 times a day
- ▸ Child 15–17 years: 1 g 6 times a day; maximum 8 g per day

- **UNLICENSED USE** Not licensed for use in children under 15 years. Tablets not licensed for prophylaxis of stress ulceration.
- **CAUTIONS** Patients under intensive care (**Important:** reports of bezoar formation)
  CAUTIONS, FURTHER INFORMATION
▸ Bezoar formation Following reports of bezoar formation associated with sucralfate, caution is advised in seriously ill patients, especially those receiving concomitant enteral feeds or those with predisposing conditions such as delayed gastric emptying.
- **INTERACTIONS** → Appendix 1 (sucralfate).
- **SIDE-EFFECTS**
▸ **Common or very common** Constipation
▸ **Uncommon** Back pain · bezoar formation · diarrhoea · dizziness · drowsiness · dry mouth · eadache · flatulence · gastric discomfort · indigestion · nausea · rash
- **PREGNANCY** No evidence of harm; absorption from gastro-intestinal tract negligible.
- **BREAST FEEDING** Amount probably too small to be harmful.
- **RENAL IMPAIRMENT** Use with caution; aluminium is absorbed and may accumulate.
- **DIRECTIONS FOR ADMINISTRATION** Administration of sucralfate and enteral feeds should be separated by 1 hour and for administration by *mouth*, sucralfate should be given 1 hour before meals. *Oral suspension* blocks fine-bore feeding tubes. Crushed *tablets* may be dispersed in water.
- **PRESCRIBING AND DISPENSING INFORMATION** Flavours of oral liquid formulations may include aniseed and caramel.

- **MEDICINAL FORMS** There can be variation in the licensing of different medicines containing the same drug. Forms available from special-order manufacturers include: tablet, oral suspension

Tablet
CAUTIONARY AND ADVISORY LABELS 5
▸ Sucralfate (Non-proprietary)
  Sucralfate 1 gram Sulcrate 1g tablets | 100 tablet no price available

H₂-RECEPTOR ANTAGONISTS

H₂-receptor antagonists

Overview

Histamine H_2-receptor antagonists heal *gastric and duodenal ulcers* by reducing gastric acid output as a result of histamine H_2-receptor blockade; they are also used to relieve symptoms of *dyspepsia* and *gastro-oesophageal reflux disease*. H_2-receptor antagonists should not normally be used for *Zollinger–Ellison syndrome* because proton pump inhibitors are more effective.

Maintenance treatment with low doses has largely been replaced in *Helicobacter pylori* positive children by eradication regimens.

H_2-receptor antagonist therapy can promote healing of *NSAID-associated ulcers*.

Treatment with a H_2-receptor antagonist has not been shown to be beneficial in haematemesis and melaena, but prophylactic use reduces the frequency of bleeding from *gastroduodenal erosions in hepatic coma*, and possibly in other conditions requiring intensive care. Treatment also reduces the risk of *acid aspiration* in obstetric patients at delivery (Mendelson's syndrome).

H_2-receptor antagonists are also used to reduce the degradation of pancreatic enzyme supplements in children with cystic fibrosis.

H₂-receptor antagonists

- **SIDE-EFFECTS**
▸ **Common or very common** Diarrhoea · dizziness · headache
▸ **Uncommon** Erythema multiforme · rash · toxic epidermal necrolysis
▸ **Rare** Arthralgia · blood disorders · bradycardia · cholestatic jaundice · confusion · depression · hallucinations · hepatitis · leucopenia · myalgia · pancytopenia · psychiatric reactions · thrombocytopenia
▸ **Frequency not known** Gynaecomastia · impotence
SIDE-EFFECTS, FURTHER INFORMATION
▸ Psychiatric reactions Psychiatric reactions, including confusion, depression, and hallucinations occur particularly in the very ill.

▸ above

Ranitidine

- **INDICATIONS AND DOSE**

Benign gastric ulceration | Duodenal ulceration
▸ BY MOUTH
- ▸ Neonate: 2 mg/kg 3 times a day (max. per dose 3 mg/kg 3 times a day), oral absorption is unreliable.
- ▸ Child 1–5 months: 1 mg/kg 3 times a day (max. per dose 3 mg/kg 3 times a day)
- ▸ Child 6 months–2 years: 2–4 mg/kg twice daily
- ▸ Child 3–11 years: 2–4 mg/kg twice daily (max. per dose 150 mg)
- ▸ Child 12–17 years: 150 mg twice daily, alternatively 300 mg once daily, dose to be taken at night

Prophylaxis of stress ulceration

▸ INITIALLY BY SLOW INTRAVENOUS INJECTION

▸ **Neonate:** 0.5–1 mg/kg every 6–8 hours.

▸ **Child 1 month–11 years:** 1 mg/kg every 6–8 hours (max. per dose 50 mg), may be given as an intermittent infusion at a rate of 25 mg/hour

▸ **Child 12–17 years:** 50 mg every 8 hours, dose to be diluted to 20 mL and given over at least 2 minutes, then (by mouth) 150 mg twice daily, may be given when oral feeding commences

Reflux oesophagitis and other conditions where gastric acid reduction is beneficial

▸ BY MOUTH

▸ **Neonate:** 2 mg/kg 3 times a day (max. per dose 3 mg/kg 3 times a day), oral absorption is unreliable.

▸ **Child 1–5 months:** 1 mg/kg 3 times a day (max. per dose 3 mg/kg 3 times a day)

▸ **Child 6 months–2 years:** 2–4 mg/kg twice daily

▸ **Child 3–11 years:** 2–4 mg/kg twice daily (max. per dose 150 mg); increased to up to 5 mg/kg twice daily (max. per dose 300 mg), dose increase for severe gastro-oesophageal disease

▸ **Child 12–17 years:** 150 mg twice daily, alternatively 300 mg once daily, dose to be taken at night, then increased if necessary to 300 mg twice daily for up to 12 weeks in moderate to severe gastro-oesophageal reflux disease, alternatively increased if necessary to 150 mg 4 times a day for up to 12 weeks in moderate to severe gastro-oesophageal reflux disease

▸ BY SLOW INTRAVENOUS INJECTION

▸ **Neonate:** 0.5–1 mg/kg every 6–8 hours.

▸ **Child:** 1 mg/kg every 6–8 hours (max. per dose 50 mg), may be given as an intermittent infusion at a rate of 25 mg/hour

● **UNLICENSED USE** *Oral* preparations not licensed for use in children under 3 years. *Injection* not licensed for use in children under 6 months.

● **INTERACTIONS** → Appendix 1 (histamine H_2-antagonists).

● **SIDE-EFFECTS**

▸ **Uncommon** Blurred vision

▸ **Frequency not known** Alopecia · interstitial nephritis · involuntary movement disorders · pancreatitis

● **PREGNANCY** Manufacturer advises avoid unless essential, but not known to be harmful.

● **BREAST FEEDING** Significant amount present in milk, but not known to be harmful.

● **RENAL IMPAIRMENT** Use half normal dose if estimated glomerular filtration rate less than 50 mL/minute/1.73 m².

● **DIRECTIONS FOR ADMINISTRATION**

▸ With intravenous use For *slow intravenous injection* dilute to a concentration of 2.5 mg/mL with Glucose 5% or Sodium Chloride 0.9%; give over at least 3 minutes.

● **PATIENT AND CARER ADVICE**

Medicines for Children leaflet: Ranitidine for acid reflux www.medicinesforchildren.org.uk/ranitidine-for-acid-reflux

In fat malabsorption syndrome, give oral doses 1–2 hours before food to enhance effects of pancreatic enzyme replacement.

● **EXCEPTIONS TO LEGAL CATEGORY** Ranitidine can be sold to the public for children over 16 years (provided packs do not contain more than 2 weeks' supply) for the short-term symptomatic relief of heartburn, dyspepsia, and hyperacidity, and for the prevention of these symptoms when associated with consumption of food or drink (max. single dose 75 mg, max. daily dose 300 mg).

● **MEDICINAL FORMS**
There can be variation in the licensing of different medicines containing the same drug. Forms available from special-order manufacturers include: oral suspension, oral solution, infusion

Tablet

▸ **Ranitidine (Non-proprietary)**
Ranitidine (as Ranitidine hydrochloride) 75 mg
Ranitidine (as Ranitidine hydrochloride) 150 mg Ranitidine 150mg tablets | 60 tablet P no price available DT price = £1.15 | 60 tablet PoM £2.50 DT price = £1.15
Ranitidine (as Ranitidine hydrochloride) 300 mg Ranitidine 300mg tablets | 30 tablet P no price available DT price = £1.17 | 30 tablet PoM £1.61 DT price = £1.17

▸ **Ranitil (Tillomed Laboratories Ltd)**
Ranitidine (as Ranitidine hydrochloride) 150 mg Ranitil 150mg tablets | 60 tablet PoM £18.13 DT price = £1.15
Ranitidine (as Ranitidine hydrochloride) 300 mg Ranitil 300mg tablets | 30 tablet PoM £17.64 DT price = £1.17

▸ **Zantac (Omega Pharma Ltd, GlaxoSmithKline UK Ltd)**
Ranitidine (as Ranitidine hydrochloride) 150 mg Zantac 150mg tablets | 60 tablet PoM £1.30 DT price = £1.15
Ranitidine (as Ranitidine hydrochloride) 300 mg Zantac 300mg tablets | 30 tablet PoM £1.30 DT price = £1.17

Effervescent tablet
CAUTIONARY AND ADVISORY LABELS 13
ELECTROLYTES: May contain Sodium

▸ **Ranitidine (Non-proprietary)**
Ranitidine (as Ranitidine hydrochloride) 150 mg Ranitidine 150mg effervescent tablets | 60 tablet PoM £35.00 DT price = £34.76
Ranitidine (as Ranitidine hydrochloride) 300 mg Ranitidine 300mg effervescent tablets | 30 tablet PoM £35.00 DT price = £34.76

Oral solution
EXCIPIENTS: May contain Alcohol

▸ **Ranitidine (Non-proprietary)**
Ranitidine (as Ranitidine hydrochloride) 15 mg per 1 ml Ranitidine 75mg/5ml oral solution sugar free sugar-free | 100 ml PoM £2.10–£2.88 sugar-free | 300 ml PoM £21.55 DT price = £6.45

▸ **Zantac (GlaxoSmithKline UK Ltd)**
Ranitidine (as Ranitidine hydrochloride) 15 mg per 1 ml Zantac 150mg/10ml syrup sugar-free | 300 ml PoM £20.76 DT price = £6.45

Solution for injection

▸ **Ranitidine (Non-proprietary)**
Ranitidine (as Ranitidine hydrochloride) 25 mg per 1 ml Ranitidine 50mg/2ml solution for injection ampoules | 5 ampoule PoM £2.69–£5.00

▸ **Zantac (GlaxoSmithKline UK Ltd)**
Ranitidine (as Ranitidine hydrochloride) 25 mg per 1 ml Zantac 50mg/2ml solution for injection ampoules | 5 ampoule PoM £2.82

PROTON PUMP INHIBITORS

Proton pump inhibitors

Overview

Omeprazole p. 54 is an effective short-term treatment for *gastric* and *duodenal ulcers*; it is also used in combination with antibacterials for the eradication of *Helicobacter pylori*. An initial short course of omeprazole is the treatment of choice in *gastro-oesophageal reflux disease* with severe symptoms; children with endoscopically confirmed *erosive, ulcerative, or stricturing oesophagitis* usually need to be maintained on omeprazole.

Omeprazole is also used for the prevention and treatment of NSAID-associated ulcers. In children who need to continue NSAID treatment after an ulcer has healed, the dose of omeprazole should not normally be reduced because asymptomatic ulcer deterioration may occur.

Omeprazole is effective in the treatment of the *Zollinger-Ellison syndrome* (including cases resistant to other treatment). It is also used to reduce the degradation of pancreatic enzyme supplements in children with cystic fibrosis.

Lansoprazole p. 53 is not licensed for use in children, but may be considered when the available formulations of omeprazole are unsuitable.

Esomeprazole below can be used for the management of gastro-oesophageal reflux disease when the available formulations of omeprazole and lansoprazole are unsuitable.

Proton pump inhibitors

- **DRUG ACTION** Proton pump inhibitors inhibit gastric acid secretion by blocking the hydrogen-potassium adenosine triphosphatase enzyme system (the 'proton pump') of the gastric parietal cell.

IMPORTANT SAFETY INFORMATION

MHRA ADVICE: PROTON PUMP INHIBITORS (PPIS): VERY LOW RISK OF SUBACUTE CUTANEOUS LUPUS ERYTHEMATOSUS (SEPTEMBER 2015)

Very infrequent cases of subacute cutaneous lupus erythematosus (SCLE) have been reported in patients taking PPIs. Drug-induced SCLE can occur weeks, months or even years after exposure to the drug.

If a patient treated with a PPI develops lesions—especially in sun-exposed areas of the skin—and it is accompanied by arthralgia:

- advise them to avoid exposing the skin to sunlight;
- consider SCLE as a possible diagnosis;
- consider discontinuing PPI treatment unless it is imperative for a serious acid-related condition; a patient who develops SCLE with a particular PPI may be at risk of the same reaction with another;
- in most cases, symptoms resolve on PPI withdrawal; topical or systemic steroids might be necessary for treatment of SCLE only if there are no signs of remission after a few weeks or months.

- **CAUTIONS** May increase the risk of gastro-intestinal infections (including *Clostridium difficile* infection) · patients at risk of osteoporosis

  CAUTIONS, FURTHER INFORMATION

- Risk of osteoporosis Patients at risk of osteoporosis should maintain an adequate intake of calcium and vitamin D, and if necessary, receive other preventative therapy.

- **SIDE-EFFECTS**
- Common or very common Abdominal pain · constipation · diarrhoea · flatulence · gastro-intestinal disturbances · headache · nausea · vomiting
- Uncommon Arthralgia · dizziness · dry mouth · fatigue · myalgia · paraesthesia · peripheral oedema · pruritus · rash · sleep disturbances
- Rare Alopecia · anaphylaxis · blood disorders · bronchospasm · confusion · depression · fever · gynaecomastia · hallucinations · hepatitis · hypersensitivity reactions · hypomagnesaemia (usually after 1 year of treatment, but sometimes after 3 months of treatment) · hyponatraemia · interstitial nephritis · jaundice · leucocytosis · leucopenia · pancytopenia · photosensitivity · Stevens-Johnson syndrome · stomatitis · sweating · taste disturbance · thrombocytopenia · toxic epidermal necrolysis · visual disturbances

  SIDE-EFFECTS, FURTHER INFORMATION

  Rebound acid hypersecretion and protracted dyspepsia may occur after stopping prolonged treatment with a proton pump inhibitor.

- **MONITORING REQUIREMENTS** Measurement of serum-magnesium concentrations should be considered before and during prolonged treatment with a proton pump inhibitor, especially when used with other drugs that cause hypomagnesaemia or with digoxin.

- **PRESCRIBING AND DISPENSING INFORMATION** A proton pump inhibitor should be prescribed for appropriate indications at the lowest effective dose for the shortest period; the need for long-term treatment should be reviewed periodically.

☞ above

Esomeprazole

- **INDICATIONS AND DOSE**

Gastro-oesophageal reflux disease (in the presence of erosive reflux oesophagitis)

- BY MOUTH
- Child 1-11 years (body-weight 10-19 kg): 10 mg once daily for 8 weeks
- Child 1-11 years (body-weight 20 kg and above): 10–20 mg once daily for 8 weeks
- Child 12-17 years: Initially 40 mg once daily for 4 weeks, continued for further 4 weeks if not fully healed or symptoms persist; maintenance 20 mg daily
- BY INTRAVENOUS INJECTION, OR BY INTRAVENOUS INFUSION
- Child 1-11 years (body-weight up to 20 kg): 10 mg once daily, injection to be given over at least 3 minutes
- Child 1-11 years (body-weight 20 kg and above): 10–20 mg once daily, injection to be given over at least 3 minutes
- Child 12-17 years: 40 mg daily, injection to be given over at least 3 minutes

Symptomatic treatment of gastro-oesophageal reflux disease (in the absence of oesophagitis)

- BY MOUTH
- Child 1-11 years (body-weight 10 kg and above): 10 mg once daily for up to 8 weeks
- Child 12-17 years: 20 mg once daily for up to 4 weeks
- BY INTRAVENOUS INJECTION, OR BY INTRAVENOUS INFUSION
- Child 1-11 years: 10 mg once daily, injection to be given over at least 3 minutes
- Child 12-17 years: 20 mg once daily, injection to be given over at least 3 minutes

- **UNLICENSED USE** Tablets and capsules not licensed for use in children 1–11 years.

- **INTERACTIONS** → Appendix 1 (proton pump inhibitors).

- **PREGNANCY** Manufacturer advises caution—no information available.

- **BREAST FEEDING** Manufacturer advises avoid—no information available.

- **HEPATIC IMPAIRMENT** 1–11 years max. 10 mg daily in severe impairment. 12–17 years max. 20 mg daily in severe impairment.

- **RENAL IMPAIRMENT** Manufacturer advises caution in severe renal insufficiency.

- **DIRECTIONS FOR ADMINISTRATION**
- With intravenous use For *intravenous infusion*, dilute reconstituted solution to a concentration not exceeding 800 micrograms/mL with Sodium Chloride 0.9%; give over 10–30 minutes.
- With oral use Do not chew or crush capsules; swallow whole or mix capsule contents in water and drink within 30 minutes. Do not crush or chew tablets; swallow whole or disperse in water and drink within 30 minutes. Disperse the contents of each sachet of gastro-resistant granules in approx. 15 mL water. Stir and leave to thicken for a few minutes; stir again before administration and use within 30 minutes; rinse container with 15 mL water to obtain full dose. For administration through a gastric tube, consult product literature.

- **PATIENT AND CARER ADVICE**
- With oral use Counselling on administration of gastro-resistant capsules, tablets, and granules advised.

● **MEDICINAL FORMS**
There can be variation in the licensing of different medicines containing the same drug. Forms available from special-order manufacturers include: oral suspension

Gastro-resistant tablet

▸ Esomeprazole (Non-proprietary)
Esomeprazole (as Esomeprazole magnesium trihydrate)
20 mg Esomeprazole 20mg gastro-resistant tablets | 28 tablet [PoM] £18.50 DT price = £3.31
Esomeprazole (as Esomeprazole magnesium trihydrate)
40 mg Esomeprazole 40mg gastro-resistant tablets | 28 tablet [PoM] £25.19 DT price = £4.18

▸ Nexium (AstraZeneca UK Ltd, Pfizer Consumer Healthcare Ltd)
Esomeprazole (as Esomeprazole magnesium trihydrate)
20 mg Nexium 20mg gastro-resistant tablets | 28 tablet [PoM] £18.50 DT price = £3.31
Esomeprazole (as Esomeprazole magnesium trihydrate)
40 mg Nexium 40mg gastro-resistant tablets | 28 tablet [PoM] £25.19 DT price = £4.18

Gastro-resistant capsule

▸ Esomeprazole (Non-proprietary)
Esomeprazole (as Esomeprazole magnesium dihydrate)
20 mg Esomeprazole 20mg gastro-resistant capsules | 28 capsule [PoM] £12.95 DT price = £3.40
Esomeprazole (as Esomeprazole magnesium dihydrate)
40 mg Esomeprazole 40mg gastro-resistant capsules | 28 capsule [PoM] £17.63 DT price = £3.96

▸ Emozul (Consilient Health Ltd)
Esomeprazole (as Esomeprazole magnesium dihydrate)
20 mg Emozul 20mg gastro-resistant capsules | 28 capsule [PoM] £3.40 DT price = £3.40
Esomeprazole (as Esomeprazole magnesium dihydrate)
40 mg Emozul 40mg gastro-resistant capsules | 28 capsule [PoM] £3.96 DT price = £3.96

Gastro-resistant granules
CAUTIONARY AND ADVISORY LABELS 25

▸ Nexium (AstraZeneca UK Ltd)
Esomeprazole (as Esomeprazole magnesium trihydrate)
10 mg Nexium 10mg gastro-resistant granules sachets | 28 sachet [PoM] £25.19 DT price = £25.19

Powder for solution for injection

▸ Esomeprazole (Non-proprietary)
Esomeprazole (as Esomeprazole sodium) 40 mg Esomeprazole 40mg powder for solution for injection vials | 1 vial [PoM] £3.07–£3.13 (Hospital only)

▸ Nexium (AstraZeneca UK Ltd)
Esomeprazole (as Esomeprazole sodium) 40 mg Nexium I.V 40mg powder for solution for injection vials | 1 vial [PoM] £4.25 (Hospital only)

◀ 52

Lansoprazole

● **INDICATIONS AND DOSE**

Benign gastric ulcer

▸ BY MOUTH

▸ Child (body-weight up to 30 kg): 0.5–1 mg/kg once daily (max. per dose 15 mg once daily), doses to be taken in the morning

▸ Child (body-weight 30 kg and above): 15–30 mg once daily, doses to be taken in the morning

Duodenal ulcer

▸ BY MOUTH

▸ Child (body-weight up to 30 kg): 0.5–1 mg/kg once daily (max. per dose 15 mg once daily), doses to be taken in the morning

▸ Child (body-weight 30 kg and above): 15–30 mg once daily, doses to be taken in the morning

NSAID-associated duodenal ulcer | NSAID-associated gastric ulcer

▸ BY MOUTH

▸ Child (body-weight up to 30 kg): 0.5–1 mg/kg once daily (max. per dose 15 mg once daily), doses to be taken in the morning

▸ Child (body-weight 30 kg and above): 15–30 mg once daily, doses to be taken in the morning

Gastro-oesophageal reflux disease

▸ BY MOUTH

▸ Child (body-weight up to 30 kg): 0.5–1 mg/kg once daily (max. per dose 15 mg once daily), doses to be taken in the morning

▸ Child (body-weight 30 kg and above): 15–30 mg once daily, doses to be taken in the morning

Acid-related dyspepsia

▸ BY MOUTH

▸ Child (body-weight up to 30 kg): 0.5–1 mg/kg once daily (max. per dose 15 mg once daily), doses to be taken in the morning

▸ Child (body-weight 30 kg and above): 15–30 mg once daily, doses to be taken in the morning

Fat malabsorption despite pancreatic enzyme replacement therapy in cystic fibrosis

▸ BY MOUTH

▸ Child (body-weight up to 30 kg): 0.5–1 mg/kg once daily (max. per dose 15 mg once daily), doses to be taken in the morning

▸ Child (body-weight 30 kg and above): 15–30 mg once daily, doses to be taken in the morning

● **UNLICENSED USE** Not licensed for use in children.

● **INTERACTIONS** → Appendix 1 (proton pump inhibitors).

● **SIDE-EFFECTS**

▸ **Very rare** Colitis · raised serum cholesterol · raised triglycerides

▸ **Frequency not known** Anorexia · glossitis · impotence · pancreatitis · petechiae · purpura · restlessness · tremor

● **PREGNANCY** Manufacturer advises avoid.

● **BREAST FEEDING** Avoid—present in milk in *animal* studies.

● **HEPATIC IMPAIRMENT** Use half normal dose in moderate to severe liver disease.

● **DIRECTIONS FOR ADMINISTRATION** Orodispersible tablets should be placed on the tongue, allowed to disperse and swallowed, or may be swallowed whole with a glass of water. Alternatively, tablets can be dispersed in a small amount of water and administered by an oral syringe or nasogastric tube.

● **PATIENT AND CARER ADVICE**
Medicines for Children leaflet: Lansoprazole for gastro-oesophageal reflux disease (GORD) and ulcers www.medicinesforchildren.org.uk/lansoprazole-for-gord-and-ulcers
Counselling on administration of orodispersible tablet advised.

● **MEDICINAL FORMS**
There can be variation in the licensing of different medicines containing the same drug. Forms available from special-order manufacturers include: oral suspension, oral solution

Orodispersible tablet
CAUTIONARY AND ADVISORY LABELS 5, 22
EXCIPIENTS: May contain Aspartame

▸ Lansoprazole (Non-proprietary)
Lansoprazole 15 mg Lansoprazole 15mg orodispersible tablets | 28 tablet [PoM] £3.99 DT price = £2.42
Lansoprazole 30 mg Lansoprazole 30mg orodispersible tablets | 28 tablet [PoM] £6.99 DT price = £4.18

▸ Zoton FasTab (Pfizer Ltd)
Lansoprazole 15 mg Zoton FasTab 15mg | 28 tablet [PoM] £2.99 DT price = £2.42
Lansoprazole 30 mg Zoton FasTab 30mg | 28 tablet [PoM] £5.50 DT price = £4.18

Gastro-resistant capsule
CAUTIONARY AND ADVISORY LABELS 5, 22, 25

▸ Lansoprazole (Non-proprietary)
Lansoprazole 15 mg Lansoprazole 15mg gastro-resistant capsules | 28 capsule [PoM] £12.92 DT price = £0.97
Lansoprazole 30 mg Lansoprazole 30mg gastro-resistant capsules | 28 capsule [PoM] £23.63 DT price = £1.37

Omeprazole

F 52

● INDICATIONS AND DOSE

Helicobacter pylori **eradication in combination with amoxicillin and clarithromycin; or in combination with amoxicillin and metronidazole; or in combination with clarithromycin and metronidazole**
▸ BY MOUTH

▸ Child 1–11 years: 1–2 mg/kg once daily (max. per dose 40 mg)
▸ Child 12–17 years: 40 mg once daily

Treatment of duodenal ulcers including those complicating NSAID therapy | Treatment of benign gastric ulcers including those complicating NSAID therapy
▸ BY MOUTH

▸ Neonate: 700 micrograms/kg once daily for 7–14 days, then increased if necessary to 1.4–2.8 mg/kg once daily.

▸ Child 1 month–1 year: 700 micrograms/kg once daily, increased if necessary to 3 mg/kg once daily (max. per dose 20 mg)
▸ Child 2–17 years (body-weight 10–19 kg): 10 mg once daily, increased if necessary to 20 mg once daily
▸ Child 2–17 years (body-weight 20 kg and above): 20 mg once daily, increased if necessary to 40 mg once daily
▸ BY INTRAVENOUS INJECTION, OR BY INTRAVENOUS INFUSION
▸ Child 1 month–11 years: Initially 500 micrograms/kg once daily (max. per dose 20 mg), increased if necessary to 2 mg/kg once daily (max. per dose 40 mg), injection to be given over 5 minutes
▸ Child 12–17 years: 40 mg once daily, injection to be given over 5 minutes

Zollinger–Ellison syndrome
▸ BY MOUTH

▸ Neonate: 700 micrograms/kg once daily for 7–14 days, then increased if necessary to 1.4–2.8 mg/kg once daily.

▸ Child 1 month–1 year: 700 micrograms/kg once daily, increased if necessary to 3 mg/kg once daily (max. per dose 20 mg)
▸ Child 2–17 years (body-weight 10–19 kg): 10 mg once daily, increased if necessary to 20 mg once daily
▸ Child 2–17 years (body-weight 20 kg and above): 20 mg once daily, increased if necessary to 40 mg once daily
▸ BY INTRAVENOUS INJECTION, OR BY INTRAVENOUS INFUSION
▸ Child 1 month–11 years: Initially 500 micrograms/kg once daily (max. per dose 20 mg), increased if necessary to 2 mg/kg once daily (max. per dose 40 mg), injection to be given over 5 minutes
▸ Child 12–17 years: 40 mg once daily, injection to be given over 5 minutes

Gastro-oesophageal reflux disease
▸ BY MOUTH

▸ Neonate: 700 micrograms/kg once daily for 7–14 days, then increased if necessary to 1.4–2.8 mg/kg once daily.

▸ Child 1 month–1 year: 700 micrograms/kg once daily, increased if necessary to 3 mg/kg once daily (max. per dose 20 mg)
▸ Child 2–17 years (body-weight 10–19 kg): 10 mg once daily, increased if necessary to 20 mg once daily, in severe ulcerating reflux oesophagitis, maximum 12 weeks at higher dose
▸ Child 2–17 years (body-weight 20 kg and above): 20 mg once daily, increased if necessary to 40 mg once daily, in severe ulcerating reflux oesophagitis, maximum 12 weeks at higher dose
▸ BY INTRAVENOUS INJECTION, OR BY INTRAVENOUS INFUSION
▸ Child 1 month–11 years: Initially 500 micrograms/kg once daily (max. per dose 20 mg), increased if necessary to

2 mg/kg once daily (max. per dose 40 mg), injection to be given over 5 minutes
▸ Child 12–17 years: 40 mg once daily, injection to be given over 5 minutes

Acid-related dyspepsia
▸ BY MOUTH

▸ Neonate: 700 micrograms/kg once daily for 7–14 days, then increased if necessary to 1.4–2.8 mg/kg once daily.

▸ Child 1 month–1 year: 700 micrograms/kg once daily, increased if necessary to 3 mg/kg once daily (max. per dose 20 mg)
▸ Child 2–17 years (initiated by a specialist) (body-weight 10–19 kg): 10 mg once daily, increased if necessary to 20 mg once daily
▸ Child 2–17 years (initiated by a specialist) (body-weight 20 kg and above): 20 mg once daily, increased if necessary to 40 mg once daily
▸ BY INTRAVENOUS INJECTION, OR BY INTRAVENOUS INFUSION
▸ Child 1 month–11 years: Initially 500 micrograms/kg once daily (max. per dose 20 mg), increased if necessary to 2 mg/kg once daily (max. per dose 40 mg), injection to be given over 5 minutes
▸ Child 12–17 years: 40 mg once daily, injection to be given over 5 minutes

Fat malabsorption despite pancreatic enzyme replacement therapy in cystic fibrosis
▸ BY MOUTH

▸ Neonate: 700 micrograms/kg once daily for 7–14 days, then increased if necessary to 1.4–2.8 mg/kg once daily.

▸ Child 1 month–1 year: 700 micrograms/kg once daily, increased if necessary to 3 mg/kg once daily (max. per dose 20 mg)
▸ Child 2–17 years (body-weight 10–19 kg): 10 mg once daily, increased if necessary to 20 mg once daily
▸ Child 2–17 years (body-weight 20 kg and above): 20 mg once daily, increased if necessary to 40 mg once daily
▸ BY INTRAVENOUS INJECTION, OR BY INTRAVENOUS INFUSION
▸ Child 1 month–11 years: Initially 500 micrograms/kg once daily (max. per dose 20 mg), increased if necessary to 2 mg/kg once daily (max. per dose 40 mg), injection to be given over 5 minutes
▸ Child 12–17 years: 40 mg once daily, injection to be given over 5 minutes

● UNLICENSED USE *Capsules and tablets* not licensed for use in children except for severe ulcerating reflux oesophagitis in children over 1 year. *Injection* not licensed for use in children under 12 years.

● INTERACTIONS → Appendix 1 (proton pump inhibitors).

● SIDE-EFFECTS Agitation · impotence

● PREGNANCY Not known to be harmful.

● BREAST FEEDING Present in milk but not known to be harmful.

● HEPATIC IMPAIRMENT No more than 700 micrograms/kg (max. 20 mg) once daily.

● DIRECTIONS FOR ADMINISTRATION For administration by *mouth*, swallow whole, or disperse *Losec MUPS*® tablets in water, *or* mix capsule contents or *Losec MUPS*® tablets with fruit juice or yoghurt. Preparations consisting of an e/c tablet within a capsule should **not** be opened.

For administration through an *enteral feeding tube*, use *Losec MUPS*® or the contents of a capsule containing omeprazole dispersed in a large volume of water, or in 10 mL Sodium Bicarbonate 8.4% (1 mmol Na⁺/mL). Allow to stand for 10 minutes before administration.

▸ With intravenous use For *intermittent intravenous infusion*, dilute reconstituted solution to a concentration of 400 micrograms/mL with Glucose 5% or Sodium Chloride 0.9%; give over 20–30 minutes.

- **PATIENT AND CARER ADVICE**
  Medicines for Children leaflet: Omeprazole for gastro-oesophageal reflux disease (GORD) www.medicinesforchildren.org.uk/omeprazole-for-gord
  ‣ With oral use Counselling on administration advised.
- **PROFESSION SPECIFIC INFORMATION**
  Dental practitioners' formulary
  Gastro-resistant omeprazole capsules may be prescribed.

- **MEDICINAL FORMS**
  There can be variation in the licensing of different medicines containing the same drug. Forms available from special-order manufacturers include: oral suspension, oral solution

Gastro-resistant tablet
CAUTIONARY AND ADVISORY LABELS 25
‣ Omeprazole (Non-proprietary)
Omeprazole 10 mg Omeprazole 10mg gastro-resistant tablets | 28 tablet PoM £18.91 DT price = £7.90
Omeprazole (as Omeprazole magnesium) 10 mg Omeprazole 10mg dispersible gastro-resistant tablets | 28 tablet PoM £8.94 DT price = £7.75
Omeprazole 20 mg Omeprazole 20mg gastro-resistant tablets | 28 tablet PoM £28.56 DT price = £5.87
Omeprazole (as Omeprazole magnesium) 20 mg Omeprazole 20mg dispersible gastro-resistant tablets | 28 tablet PoM £12.53 DT price = £11.60
Omeprazole 40 mg Omeprazole 40mg gastro-resistant tablets | 7 tablet PoM £15.00 DT price = £4.97
Omeprazole (as Omeprazole magnesium) 40 mg Omeprazole 40mg dispersible gastro-resistant tablets | 7 tablet PoM £6.78 DT price = £5.80
‣ Losec (AstraZeneca UK Ltd)
Omeprazole (as Omeprazole magnesium) 10 mg Losec MUPS 10mg gastro-resistant tablets | 28 tablet PoM £7.75 DT price = £7.75
Omeprazole (as Omeprazole magnesium) 20 mg Losec MUPS 20mg gastro-resistant tablets | 28 tablet PoM £11.60 DT price = £11.60
Omeprazole (as Omeprazole magnesium) 40 mg Losec MUPS 40mg gastro-resistant tablets | 7 tablet PoM £5.80 DT price = £5.80
‣ Mezzopram (Sandoz Ltd)
Omeprazole (as Omeprazole magnesium) 10 mg Mezzopram 10mg gastro-resistant tablets | 28 tablet PoM £6.58 DT price = £7.75
Omeprazole (as Omeprazole magnesium) 20 mg Mezzopram 20mg gastro-resistant tablets | 28 tablet PoM £9.86 DT price = £11.60
Omeprazole (as Omeprazole magnesium) 40 mg Mezzopram 40mg gastro-resistant tablets | 7 tablet PoM £4.93 DT price = £5.80

Gastro-resistant capsule
‣ Omeprazole (Non-proprietary)
Omeprazole 10 mg Omeprazole 10mg gastro-resistant capsules | 28 capsule PoM £9.30 DT price = £0.92
Omeprazole 20 mg Omeprazole 20mg gastro-resistant capsules | 28 capsule PoM £13.50 DT price = £0.92
Omeprazole 40 mg Omeprazole 40mg gastro-resistant capsules | 7 capsule PoM £6.96 DT price = £0.78 | 28 capsule PoM £21.65
‣ Losec (AstraZeneca UK Ltd)
Omeprazole 10 mg Losec 10mg gastro-resistant capsules | 28 capsule PoM £9.30 DT price = £0.92
Omeprazole 20 mg Losec 20mg gastro-resistant capsules | 28 capsule PoM £13.92 DT price = £0.92
Omeprazole 40 mg Losec 40mg gastro-resistant capsules | 7 capsule PoM £6.96 DT price = £0.78
‣ Mepradec (Discovery Pharmaceuticals)
Omeprazole 10 mg Mepradec 10mg gastro-resistant capsules | 28 capsule PoM £0.92 DT price = £0.92
Omeprazole 20 mg Mepradec 20mg gastro-resistant capsules | 28 capsule PoM £0.92 DT price = £0.92

Powder for solution for infusion
‣ Omeprazole (Non-proprietary)
Omeprazole (as Omeprazole sodium) 40 mg Omeprazole 40mg powder for solution for infusion vials | 5 vial PoM £32.45 (Hospital only) | 5 vial PoM £16.54

4.3 Gastro-oesophageal reflux disease

Gastro-oesophageal reflux disease

Management

Gastro-oesophageal reflux disease includes non-erosive gastro-oesophageal reflux and erosive oesophagitis. Uncomplicated gastro-oesophageal reflux is common in infancy and most symptoms, such as intermittent vomiting or repeated, effortless regurgitation, resolve without treatment between 12 and 18 months of age. Older children with gastro-oesophageal reflux disease may have heartburn, acid regurgitation and dysphagia. Oesophageal inflammation (oesophagitis), ulceration or stricture formation may develop in early childhood; gastro-oesophageal reflux disease may also be associated with chronic respiratory disorders including asthma.

Parents and carers of *neonates* and *infants* should be reassured that most symptoms of uncomplicated gastro-oesophageal reflux resolve without treatment. An increase in the frequency and a decrease in the volume of feeds may reduce symptoms. A feed thickener or pre-thickened formula feed can be used on the advice of a dietician. If necessary, a suitable alginate-containing preparation can be used instead of thickened feeds. A thickening agent should be tried for up to 2 weeks before considering other treatment.

Older children should be advised about life-style changes such as weight reduction if overweight, and the avoidance of alcohol and smoking. An alginate-containing antacid can be used to relieve symptoms.

Children who do not respond to these measures or who have problems such as respiratory disorders or suspected oesophagitis need to be referred to hospital. On the advice of a paediatrician, a **histamine H$_2$-receptor antagonist** can be used to relieve symptoms of gastro-oesophageal reflux disease, promote mucosal healing and permit reduction in antacid consumption. A **proton pump inhibitor** can be used for the treatment of moderate, non-erosive oesophagitis that is unresponsive to an H$_2$- receptor antagonist. Endoscopically confirmed *erosive, ulcerative,* or *stricturing* disease in children is usually treated with a proton pump inhibitor. Reassessment is necessary if symptoms persist despite 4–6 weeks of treatment; long-term use of an H$_2$-receptor antagonist or proton pump inhibitor should not be undertaken without full assessment of the underlying condition. For endoscopically confirmed *erosive, ulcerative,* or *stricturing* disease, the proton pump inhibitor usually needs to be maintained at the minimum effective dose.

Motility stimulants, such as erythromycin p. 310 may improve gastro-oesophageal sphincter contraction and accelerate gastric emptying. Evidence for the long-term efficacy of motility stimulants in the management of gastro-oesophageal reflux in children is unconvincing.

For advice on specialised formula feeds, see Enteral feeds.

Pregnancy

If dietary and lifestyle changes fail to control gastro-oesophageal reflux disease in pregnancy, an antacid or an alginate can be used. If this is ineffective, ranitidine p. 50 can be tried. Omeprazole p. 54 is reserved for women with severe or complicated reflux disease.

> **Drugs used for Gastro-oesophageal reflux disease not listed below** Esomeprazole, p. 52 · Lansoprazole, p. 53

Gastro-intestinal system

1

Sodium alginate with calcium carbonate and sodium bicarbonate

The properties listed below are those particular to the combination only. For the properties of the components please consider, alginic acid p. 46, sodium bicarbonate p. 544, calcium carbonate p. 552.

● **INDICATIONS AND DOSE**

Mild symptoms of gastro-oesophageal reflux disease
▸ BY MOUTH
▸ Child 6–11 years: 5–10 mL, to be taken after meals and at bedtime
▸ Child 12–17 years: 10–20 mL, to be taken after meals and at bedtime

● **PRESCRIBING AND DISPENSING INFORMATION** Flavours of oral liquid formulations may include aniseed or peppermint.

● **PATIENT AND CARER ADVICE**
Medicines for Children leaflet: Gaviscon for gastro-oesophageal reflux disease www.medicinesforchildren.org.uk/gaviscon-gastro-oesophageal-reflux-disease

● **MEDICINAL FORMS**
There can be variation in the licensing of different medicines containing the same drug.
Oral suspension
ELECTROLYTES: May contain Sodium
▸ **Sodium alginate with calcium carbonate and sodium bicarbonate** (Non-proprietary)
Calcium carbonate 16 mg per 1 ml, Sodium bicarbonate 26.7 mg per 1 ml, Sodium alginate 50 mg per 1 ml Alginate raft-forming oral suspension sugar free peppermint sugar-free | 500 ml GSL no price available DT price = £1.95
Alginate raft-forming oral suspension sugar free aniseed sugar-free | 500 ml GSL no price available DT price = £1.95
▸ Brands may include Acidex, Entrocalm Heartburn and Indigestion Relief, Gaviscon, Gaviscon Cool, Gaviscon Liquid Relief, Peptac

4.4 *Helicobacter pylori* diagnosis

DIAGNOSTIC AGENTS

Urea (13C)

● **INDICATIONS AND DOSE**

Diagnosis of gastro-duodenal *Helicobacter pylori* infection
▸ BY MOUTH
▸ Child: (consult product literature)

● **MEDICINAL FORMS**
There can be variation in the licensing of different medicines containing the same drug.
Tablet
▸ **Diabact UBT** (Seahorse Laboratories Ltd)
Urea [13-C] 50 mg diabact UBT 50mg tablets | 1 tablet PoM £21.25 | 10 tablet PoM no price available (Hospital only)
Soluble tablet
▸ **Pylobactell** (Torbet Laboratories Ltd)
Urea [13-C] 100 mg Pylobactell breath test kit | 1 kit PoM £20.75
Powder
▸ **Helicobacter Test INFAI** (INFAI UK Ltd)
Urea [13-C] 45 mg Helicobacter Test INFAI for children breath test kit sugar-free | 1 kit PoM £19.10
Urea [13-C] 75 mg Helicobacter Test INFAI breath test kit sugar-free | 1 kit PoM £21.70

5 Food allergy

Food allergy

Management

Allergy with classical symptoms of vomiting, colic and diarrhoea caused by specific foods such as cow's milk or shellfish should be managed by strict avoidance. The condition should be distinguished from symptoms of occasional food intolerance in those with irritable bowel syndrome. Sodium cromoglicate p. 157 may be helpful as an adjunct to dietary avoidance.

> **Other drugs used for Food allergy** Chlorphenamine maleate, p. 168

6 Gastro-intestinal smooth muscle spasm

Antispasmodics

Antimuscarinics

The intestinal smooth muscle relaxant properties of antimuscarinic and other antispasmodic drugs may be useful in *irritable bowel syndrome*.

Antimuscarinics (formerly termed 'anticholinergics') reduce intestinal motility. They are occasionally used for the management of *irritable bowel syndrome*. However, evidence of their value has not been established and response varies.

Antimuscarinics that are used for gastro-intestinal smooth muscle spasm includes the tertiary amine dicycloverine hydrochloride p. 57 and the quaternary ammonium compounds propantheline bromide p. 58 and hyoscine butylbromide p. 57. The quaternary ammonium compounds are less lipid soluble than atropine and are less likely to cross the blood-brain barrier; they are also less well absorbed from the gastro-intestinal tract.

Dicycloverine hydrochloride, may also have some direct action on smooth muscle. Hyoscine butylbromide is advocated as a gastro-intestinal antispasmodic, but it is poorly absorbed; the injection may be useful in endoscopy and radiology.

Other indications for antimuscarinic drugs include asthma and airways disease, motion sickness, urinary frequency and enuresis, mydriasis and cycloplegia, premedication, palliative care and as an antidote to organophosphorus poisoning.

Other antispasmodics

Alverine citrate p. 58, mebeverine hydrochloride p. 58, and peppermint oil p. 32 are believed to be direct relaxants of intestinal smooth muscle and may relieve pain in *irritable bowel syndrome*, and *primary dysmenorrhoea*. They have no serious adverse effects but, like all antispasmodics, should be avoided in paralytic ileus.

Motility stimulants

Domperidone is a dopamine receptor antagonist which stimulates gastric emptying and small intestinal transit, and enhances the strength of oesophageal sphincter contraction. The MHRA/CHM has issued restrictions on its use because domperidone is associated with a small increased risk of serious cardiac side effects.

A low dose of erythromycin p. 310 stimulates gastro-intestinal motility and may be used on the advice of a paediatric gastroenterologist to promote tolerance of enteral feeds; erythromycin may be less effective as a prokinetic drug in preterm neonates than in older children.

ANTIMUSCARINICS

Dicycloverine hydrochloride
▸ 457

(Dicyclomine hydrochloride)

- **INDICATIONS AND DOSE**

Symptomatic relief of gastro-intestinal disorders characterised by smooth muscle spasm
  ▸ BY MOUTH
  ▸ Child 6-23 months: 5–10 mg 3–4 times a day, dose to be taken 15 minutes before feeds
  ▸ Child 2-11 years: 10 mg 3 times a day
  ▸ Child 12-17 years: 10–20 mg 3 times a day

- **CONTRA-INDICATIONS** Child under 6 months
- **PREGNANCY** Not known to be harmful; manufacturer advises use only if essential.
- **BREAST FEEDING** Avoid—present in milk; apnoea reported in infant.
- **EXCEPTIONS TO LEGAL CATEGORY** Dicycloverine hydrochloride can be sold to the public provided that max. single dose is 10 mg and max. daily dose is 60 mg.
- **MEDICINAL FORMS**
  There can be variation in the licensing of different medicines containing the same drug.
  Tablet
  ▸ Dicycloverine hydrochloride (Non-proprietary)
  Dicycloverine hydrochloride 10 mg Dicycloverine 10mg tablets | 100 tablet [PoM] £190.80 DT price = £159.30
  Dicycloverine hydrochloride 20 mg Dicycloverine 20mg tablets | 84 tablet [PoM] £203.42 DT price = £169.86
  Oral solution
  ▸ Dicycloverine hydrochloride (Non-proprietary)
  Dicycloverine hydrochloride 2 mg per 1 ml Dicycloverine 10mg/5ml oral solution | 100 ml [PoM] no price available | 120 ml [PoM] £189.49 DT price = £158.25 | 300 ml [PoM] no price available

Dicycloverine hydrochloride with aluminium hydroxide, magnesium oxide and simeticone

The properties listed below are those particular to the combination only. For the properties of the components please consider, dicycloverine hydrochloride above, aluminium hydroxide p. 558, simeticone p. 48.

- **INDICATIONS AND DOSE**

Symptomatic relief of gastro-intestinal disorders characterised by smooth muscle spasm
  ▸ BY MOUTH
  ▸ Child 12-17 years: 10–20 mL every 4 hours as required

- **MEDICINAL FORMS**
  There can be variation in the licensing of different medicines containing the same drug.
  Oral suspension
  ▸ Kolanticon (Peckforton Pharmaceuticals Ltd)
  Dicycloverine hydrochloride 500 microgram per 1 ml, Simeticone 4 mg per 1 ml, Magnesium oxide light 20 mg per 1 ml, Aluminium hydroxide dried 40 mg per 1 ml Kolanticon gel sugar-free | 200 ml [P] £4.00 sugar-free | 500 ml [P] £6.00

Hyoscine butylbromide
▸ 457

- **INDICATIONS AND DOSE**

Symptomatic relief of gastro-intestinal or genito-urinary disorders characterised by smooth muscle spasm
  ▸ BY MOUTH
  ▸ Child 6-11 years: 10 mg 3 times a day
  ▸ Child 12-17 years: 20 mg 4 times a day

Acute spasm | Spasm in diagnostic procedures
  ▸ INITIALLY BY INTRAMUSCULAR INJECTION, OR BY SLOW INTRAVENOUS INJECTION
  ▸ Child 2-5 years: 5 mg, then (by intramuscular injection or by slow intravenous injection) 5 mg after 30 minutes if required, dose may be repeated more frequently in endoscopy; maximum 15 mg per day
  ▸ Child 6-11 years: 5–10 mg, then (by intramuscular injection or by intravenous injection) 5–10 mg after 30 minutes if required, dose may be repeated more frequently in endoscopy; maximum 30 mg per day
  ▸ Child 12-17 years: 20 mg, then (by intramuscular injection or by slow intravenous injection) 20 mg after 30 minutes if required, dose may be repeated more frequently in endoscopy; maximum 80 mg per day

Excessive respiratory secretions in palliative care
  ▸ BY MOUTH
  ▸ Child 1 month-1 year: 300–500 micrograms/kg 3–4 times a day (max. per dose 5 mg)
  ▸ Child 2-4 years: 5 mg 3–4 times a day
  ▸ Child 5-11 years: 10 mg 3–4 times a day
  ▸ Child 12-17 years: 10–20 mg 3–4 times a day
  ▸ BY INTRAMUSCULAR INJECTION, OR BY INTRAVENOUS INJECTION
  ▸ Child 1 month-4 years: 300–500 micrograms/kg 3–4 times a day (max. per dose 5 mg)
  ▸ Child 5-11 years: 5–10 mg 3–4 times a day
  ▸ Child 12-17 years: 10–20 mg 3–4 times a day

Bowel colic (in palliative care)
  ▸ BY MOUTH
  ▸ Child 1 month-1 year: 300–500 micrograms/kg 3–4 times a day (max. per dose 5 mg)
  ▸ Child 2-4 years: 5 mg 3–4 times a day
  ▸ Child 5-11 years: 10 mg 3–4 times a day
  ▸ Child 12-17 years: 10–20 mg 3–4 times a day
  ▸ BY INTRAMUSCULAR INJECTION, OR BY INTRAVENOUS INJECTION
  ▸ Child 1 month-4 years: 300–500 micrograms/kg 3–4 times a day (max. per dose 5 mg)
  ▸ Child 5-11 years: 5–10 mg 3–4 times a day
  ▸ Child 12-17 years: 10–20 mg 3–4 times a day

PHARMACOKINETICS
Administration by mouth is associated with poor absorption.

- **UNLICENSED USE** *Tablets* not licensed for use in children under 6 years. *Injection* not licensed for use in children (age range not specified by manufacturer).
- **PREGNANCY** Manufacturer advises avoid.
- **BREAST FEEDING** Amount too small to be harmful.
- **DIRECTIONS FOR ADMINISTRATION**
  ▸ With oral use For administration by *mouth*, injection solution may be used; content of ampoule may be stored in a refrigerator for up to 24 hours after opening.
  ▸ With intravenous use For *intravenous injection*, may be diluted with Glucose 5% or Sodium Chloride 0.9%; give over at least 1 minute.

- **MEDICINAL FORMS**
  There can be variation in the licensing of different medicines containing the same drug. Forms available from special-order manufacturers include: oral suspension, oral solution

Tablet
- ▸ Buscopan (Boehringer Ingelheim Ltd)
  Hyoscine butylbromide 10 mg Buscopan 10mg tablets | 56 tablet [PoM] £3.00 DT price = £3.00

Solution for injection
- ▸ Buscopan (Boehringer Ingelheim Ltd)
  Hyoscine butylbromide 20 mg per 1 ml Buscopan 20mg/1ml solution for injection ampoules | 10 ampoule [PoM] £2.92 DT price = £2.92

▸ 457

Propantheline bromide

- **INDICATIONS AND DOSE**

Symptomatic relief of gastro-intestinal disorders characterised by smooth muscle spasm
- ▸ BY MOUTH
- ▸ Child 1 month–11 years: 300 micrograms/kg 3–4 times a day (max. per dose 15 mg), dose to be taken at least one hour before food
- ▸ Child 12–17 years: 15 mg 3 times a day, dose to be taken at least one hour before food and 30 mg, dose to be taken at night; maximum 120 mg per day

- **UNLICENSED USE** *Tablets* not licensed for use in children under 12 years.
- **SIDE-EFFECTS** Facial flushing
- **PREGNANCY** Manufacturer advises avoid unless essential—no information available.
- **BREAST FEEDING** May suppress lactation.
- **HEPATIC IMPAIRMENT** Manufacturer advises caution.
- **RENAL IMPAIRMENT** Manufacturer advises caution.

- **MEDICINAL FORMS**
  There can be variation in the licensing of different medicines containing the same drug. Forms available from special-order manufacturers include: oral suspension, oral solution

Tablet
CAUTIONARY AND ADVISORY LABELS 23
- ▸ Propantheline bromide (Non-proprietary)
  Propantheline bromide 15 mg Propantheline bromide 15mg tablets | 100 tablet [PoM] no price available
- ▸ Pro-Banthine (ProStrakan Ltd)
  Propantheline bromide 15 mg Pro-Banthine 15mg tablets | 112 tablet [PoM] £20.74 DT price = £20.74

ANTISPASMODICS

Alverine citrate

24.2.2016

- **INDICATIONS AND DOSE**

Symptomatic relief of gastro-intestinal disorders characterised by smooth muscle spasm | Dysmenorrhoea
- ▸ BY MOUTH
- ▸ Child 12–17 years: 60–120 mg 1–3 times a day

- **CONTRA-INDICATIONS** Intestinal obstruction · paralytic ileus
- **SIDE-EFFECTS** Dizziness · dyspnoea · headache · hepatitis · jaundice (resolves with cessation) · nausea · pruritus · wheezing
- **PREGNANCY** Manufacturer advises avoid—limited information available
- **BREAST FEEDING** Manufacturer advises avoid—limited information available.

- **PATIENT AND CARER ADVICE**
  Driving and skilled tasks
  Dizziness may affect performance of skilled tasks (e.g. driving).

- **MEDICINAL FORMS**
  There can be variation in the licensing of different medicines containing the same drug.

Capsule
- ▸ Alverine citrate (Non-proprietary)
  Alverine citrate 60 mg Alverine 60mg capsules | 100 capsule [P] £19.49 DT price = £19.48
  Alverine citrate 120 mg Alverine 120mg capsules | 60 capsule [P] £23.30 DT price = £23.11
- ▸ Audmonal (Auden McKenzie (Pharma Division) Ltd)
  Alverine citrate 60 mg Audmonal 60mg capsules | 100 capsule [P] £14.80 DT price = £19.48
  Alverine citrate 120 mg Audmonal Forte 120mg capsules | 60 capsule [P] £17.75 DT price = £23.11
- ▸ Spasmonal (Meda Pharmaceuticals Ltd)
  Alverine citrate 60 mg Spasmonal 60mg capsules | 100 capsule [P] £16.45 DT price = £19.48
  Alverine citrate 120 mg Spasmonal Forte 120mg capsules | 60 capsule [P] £19.42 DT price = £23.11

Mebeverine hydrochloride

- **INDICATIONS AND DOSE**

Adjunct in gastro-intestinal disorders characterised by smooth muscle spasm
- ▸ BY MOUTH USING IMMEDIATE-RELEASE MEDICINES
- ▸ Child 3 years: 25 mg 3 times a day, dose preferably taken 20 minutes before meals
- ▸ Child 4–7 years: 50 mg 3 times a day, dose preferably taken 20 minutes before meals
- ▸ Child 8–9 years: 100 mg 3 times a day, dose preferably taken 20 minutes before meals
- ▸ Child 10–17 years: 135–150 mg 3 times a day, dose preferably taken 20 minutes before meals

Irritable bowel syndrome
- ▸ BY MOUTH USING MODIFIED-RELEASE MEDICINES
- ▸ Child 12–17 years: 200 mg twice daily

- **UNLICENSED USE** *Tablets and liquid* not licensed for use in children under 10 years. *Granules* not licensed for use in children under 12 years. *Modified-release capsules* not licensed for use in children under 18 years.
- **CONTRA-INDICATIONS** Paralytic ileus
- **SIDE-EFFECTS** Allergic reactions · angioedema · rash · urticaria
- **PREGNANCY** Not known to be harmful—manufacturers advise avoid.
- **BREAST FEEDING** Manufacturers advise avoid—no information available.
- **PATIENT AND CARER ADVICE**
  Medicines for Children leaflet: Mebeverine for intestinal spasm www.medicinesforchildren.org.uk/mebeverine-for-intestinal-spasms
  Patients or carers should be given advice on the timing of administration of mebeverine hydrochloride tablets and oral suspension.

- **MEDICINAL FORMS**
  There can be variation in the licensing of different medicines containing the same drug.

Tablet
- ▸ Mebeverine hydrochloride (Non-proprietary)
  Mebeverine hydrochloride 135 mg Mebeverine 135mg tablets | 15 tablet [PoM] £4.50 | 100 tablet [PoM] £20.00 DT price = £7.59
- ▸ Colofac (BGP Products Ltd)
  Mebeverine hydrochloride 135 mg Colofac 135mg tablets | 100 tablet [PoM] £9.02 DT price = £7.59

Modified-release capsule

CAUTIONARY AND ADVISORY LABELS 25

▸ **Colofac MR** (BGP Products Ltd)
Mebeverine hydrochloride 200 mg Colofac MR 200mg capsules | 60 capsule [PoM] £6.92 DT price = £6.92

Oral suspension

▸ **Mebeverine hydrochloride** (Non-proprietary)
Mebeverine hydrochloride (as Mebeverine pamoate) 10 mg per 1 ml Mebeverine 50mg/5ml oral suspension sugar free sugar-free | 300 ml [PoM] £163.43 DT price = £163.43

7 Liver disorders and related conditions

7.1 Biliary disorders

Biliary disorders

Drugs affecting biliary composition and flow

Bile acids (ursodeoxycholic acid p. 60, chenodeoxycholic acid below and cholic acid p. 60) may be used as dietary supplements in children with inborn errors of bile acid synthesis. Ursodeoxycholic acid is used to improve the flow of bile in children with cholestatic conditions such as familial intrahepatic cholestasis, biliary atresia in infants, cystic-fibrosis related liver disease, and cholestasis caused by total parenteral nutrition or following liver transplantation. Ursodeoxycholic acid may also relieve the severe itching associated with cholestasis.

In sclerosing cholangitis, ursodeoxycholic acid is used to lower liver enzyme and serum-bilirubin concentrations.

Ursodeoxycholic acid is also used in the treatment of intrahepatic cholestasis in pregnancy.

Smith-Lemli-Opitz syndrome

Chenodeoxycholic acid and ursodeoxycholic acid have been used with cholesterol in children with Smith-Lemli-Opitz syndrome. Chenodeoxycholic acid is also used in combination with cholic acid to treat bile acid synthesis defects. Chenodeoxycholic acid and cholesterol p. 61 are available from 'special-order' manufacturers or specialist importing companies.

Bile acid sequestrants

Colestyramine p. 120 is an anion-exchange resin that forms an insoluble complex with bile acids in the gastro-intestinal tract; it is used to relieve diarrhoea associated with surgical procedures such as ileal resection, or following radiation therapy. Colestyramine is also used in the treatment of familial hypercholesterolaemia, and to relieve pruritus in children with partial biliary obstruction. Colestyramine is not absorbed from the gastro-intestinal tract.

Pancreatin

Pancreatin p. 66, containing a mixture of protease, lipase and amylase in varying proportions, aids the digestion of starch, fat, and protein. Supplements of pancreatin are given by mouth to compensate for reduced or absent exocrine secretion in cystic fibrosis, and following pan- createctomy, total gastrectomy, or chronic pancreatitis.

The dose of pancreatin is adjusted according to size, number, and consistency of stools, and the nutritional status of the child; extra allowance will be needed if snacks are taken between meals.

Pancreatin preparations			
Preparation	Protease units	Amylase units	Lipase units
Creon® 10 000 capsule, e/c granules	600	8000	10 000
Creon® Micro e/c granules (per 100 mg)	200	3600	5000
Pancrex® granules (per gram)	300	4000	5000
Pancrex V® capsule, powder	430	9000	8000
Pancrex V '125'® capsule, powder	160	3300	2950
Pancrex V® e/c tablet	110	1700	1900
Pancrex V® Forte e/c tablet	330	5000	5600
Pancrex V® powder (per gram)	1400	30 000	25 000

Higher-strength pancreatin preparations Pancrease HL® and Nutrizym 22® have been associated with the development of large bowel strictures (fibrosing colonopathy) in children with cystic fibrosis aged between 2 and 13 years. The following is recommended:

- Pancrease HL®, Nutrizym 22® should not be used in children under 16 years with cystic fibrosis;
- the total dose of pancreatic enzyme supplements used in patients with cystic fibrosis should not usually exceed 10 000 units of lipase per kg body-weight daily;
- if a patient on any pancreatin preparation develops new abdominal symptoms (or any change in existing abdominal symptoms) the patient should be reviewed to exclude the possibility of colonic damage.

Possible risk factors are gender (boys at greater risk than girls), more severe cystic fibrosis, and concomitant use of laxatives. The peak age for developing fibrosing colonopathy is between 2 and 8 years.

Higher-strength pancreatin preparations			
Preparation	Protease units	Amylase units	Lipase units
Creon® 25 000 capsule, e/c pellets	1000	18 000	25 000
Creon® 40 000 capsule, e/c granules	1600	25 000	40 000
Nutrizym 22® capsule, e/c minitablets	1100	19 800	22 000
Pancrease HL® capsule, e/c minitablets	1250	22 500	25 000

In children with cystic fibrosis with persistent fat malabsorption despite optimal use of enzyme replacement, an H_2-receptor antagonist, or a proton pump inhibitor may improve fat digestion and absorption.

BILE ACIDS

Chenodeoxycholic acid

● **INDICATIONS AND DOSE**

Cerebrotendinous xanthomatosis
▸ BY MOUTH

▸ **Neonate:** 5 mg/kg 3 times a day.

▸ **Child:** 5 mg/kg 3 times a day

Defective synthesis of bile acid
▸ BY MOUTH

▸ **Neonate:** Initially 5 mg/kg 3 times a day, reduced to 2.5 mg/kg 3 times a day.

▸ **Child:** Initially 5 mg/kg 3 times a day, reduced to 2.5 mg/kg 3 times a day continued →

Smith-Lemli-Opitz syndrome
▸ BY MOUTH

▸ **Neonate:** 7 mg/kg once daily, alternatively 7 mg/kg daily in divided doses.

▸ **Child:** 7 mg/kg once daily, alternatively 7 mg/kg daily in divided doses

● **UNLICENSED USE** Not licensed.

● **CONTRA-INDICATIONS** Non-functioning gall bladder · radio-opaque stones

● **INTERACTIONS** → Appendix 1 (bile acids).

● **SIDE-EFFECTS**
▸ **Rare** Diarrhoea

● **PREGNANCY** Avoid—fetotoxicity reported in *animal* studies.

● **DIRECTIONS FOR ADMINISTRATION** For administration *by mouth*, add the contents of a 250 mg capsule to 25 mL of sodium bicarbonate solution 8.4% (1 mmol/mL) to produce a suspension containing chenodeoxycholic acid 10 mg/mL; use immediately after preparation, discard any remaining suspension.

● **MEDICINAL FORMS**
There can be variation in the licensing of different medicines containing the same drug. Forms available from special-order manufacturers include: tablet, capsule

Tablet
▸ **Chenodeoxycholic acid (Non-proprietary)**
Chenodeoxycholic acid 250 mg Chenodiol 250mg tablets | 100 tablet [PoM] no price available

Capsule
▸ **Chenodeoxycholic acid (Non-proprietary)**
Chenodeoxycholic acid 250 mg Xenbilox 250mg capsules | 100 capsule [PoM] no price available

▌ Cholic acid   21.3.2016

● **DRUG ACTION** Cholic acid is the predominant primary bile acid in humans, which can be used to provide a source of bile acid in patients with inborn deficiencies in bile acid synthesis.

● **INDICATIONS AND DOSE**

Inborn errors of primary bile acid synthesis (initiated by a specialist)
▸ BY MOUTH

▸ **Child (body-weight up to 10 kg):** 50 mg daily, then increased in steps of 50 mg daily in divided doses; usual dose 5–15 mg/kg daily in divided doses, dose to be given with food at the same time each day

▸ **Child (body-weight 10 kg and above):** Usual dose 5–15 mg/kg daily; increased in steps of 50 mg daily in divided doses if required, dose to be given with food at the same time each day; Usual maximum 500 mg/24 hours

● **INTERACTIONS** → Appendix 1 (bile acids).

● **SIDE-EFFECTS** Diarrhoea · gallstones (long term use) · pruritus

SIDE-EFFECTS, FURTHER INFORMATION
Patients presenting with pruritus and/or persistent diarrhoea should be investigated for potential overdose by a serum and/or urine bile acid assay.

● **PREGNANCY** Limited data available—not known to be harmful, manufacturer advises continue treatment. Manufacturer advises monitor patient parameters more frequently in pregnancy.

● **BREAST FEEDING** Present in milk but not known to be harmful.

● **HEPATIC IMPAIRMENT** Manufacturer advises monitor closely.

● **MONITORING REQUIREMENTS** Manufacturer advises monitor serum and/or urine bile-acid concentrations every 3 months for the first year, then every 6 months for three years, then annually; monitor liver function tests at the same or greater frequency.

● **DIRECTIONS FOR ADMINISTRATION** Manufacturer advises capsules may be opened and the content added to infant formula, juice, fruit compote, or yoghurt for administration.

● **PATIENT AND CARER ADVICE** Counselling advised on administration.

● **MEDICINAL FORMS**
There can be variation in the licensing of different medicines containing the same drug.

Capsule
CAUTIONARY AND ADVISORY LABELS 25
▸ Kolbam (Lucane Pharma Ltd) ▼
Cholic acid 50 mg Kolbam 50mg capsules | 90 capsule [PoM] £3,240.00
Cholic acid 250 mg Kolbam 250mg capsules | 90 capsule [PoM] £11,340.00
▸ Orphacol (Laboratoires CTRS) ▼
Cholic acid 50 mg Orphacol 50mg capsules | 30 capsule [PoM] £1,860.00 | 60 capsule [PoM] £3,720.00
Cholic acid 250 mg Orphacol 250mg capsules | 30 capsule [PoM] £6,630.00

▌ Ursodeoxycholic acid

● **INDICATIONS AND DOSE**

Cholestasis
▸ BY MOUTH

▸ **Neonate:** 5 mg/kg 3 times a day (max. per dose 10 mg/kg 3 times a day), adjusted according to response.

▸ **Child 1–23 months:** 5 mg/kg 3 times a day (max. per dose 10 mg/kg 3 times a day), adjusted according to response

Improvement of hepatic metabolism of essential fatty acids and bile flow, in children with cystic fibrosis
▸ BY MOUTH

▸ **Child:** 10–15 mg/kg twice daily, total daily dose may alternatively be given in 3 divided doses

Cholestasis associated with total parenteral nutrition
▸ BY MOUTH

▸ **Neonate:** 10 mg/kg 3 times a day.

▸ **Child:** 10 mg/kg 3 times a day

Sclerosing cholangitis
▸ BY MOUTH

▸ **Child:** 5–10 mg/kg 2–3 times a day (max. per dose 15 mg/kg 3 times a day), adjusted according to response

● **UNLICENSED USE** Not licensed for use in children for the treatment of cholestasis, sclerosing cholangitis, cholestasis associated with total parenteral nutrition or the improvement of hepatic metabolism of essential fatty acids and bile flow in cystic fibrosis.

● **CONTRA-INDICATIONS** Non-functioning gall bladder · radio-opaque stones

● **INTERACTIONS** → Appendix 1 (bile acids).

● **SIDE-EFFECTS**
▸ **Rare** Diarrhoea

● **PREGNANCY** No evidence of harm but manufacturer advises avoid.

● **BREAST FEEDING** Not known to be harmful but manufacturer advises avoid.

- **HEPATIC IMPAIRMENT** Avoid in chronic liver disease (but used in primary biliary cirrhosis).
- **PATIENT AND CARER ADVICE**
  Medicines for Children leaflet: Ursodeoxycholic acid for cholestasis and sclerosing cholangitis www.medicinesforchildren.org.uk/ursodeoxycholic-acid-for-cholestasis-and-sclerosing-cholangitis
  Patients should be given dietary advice (including avoidance of excessive cholesterol and calories).
- **MEDICINAL FORMS**
  There can be variation in the licensing of different medicines containing the same drug. Forms available from special-order manufacturers include: oral suspension, oral solution

Tablet
CAUTIONARY AND ADVISORY LABELS 21
▸ Ursodeoxycholic acid (Non-proprietary)
  Ursodeoxycholic acid 150 mg Ursodeoxycholic acid 150mg tablets | 60 tablet [PoM] £19.02 DT price = £19.02
  Ursodeoxycholic acid 300 mg Ursodeoxycholic acid 300mg tablets | 60 tablet [PoM] £47.63 DT price = £47.63
▸ Destolit (Norgine Pharmaceuticals Ltd)
  Ursodeoxycholic acid 150 mg Destolit 150mg tablets | 60 tablet [PoM] £18.39 DT price = £19.02
▸ Ursofalk (Dr. Falk Pharma UK Ltd)
  Ursodeoxycholic acid 500 mg Ursofalk 500mg tablets | 100 tablet [PoM] £80.00

Capsule
CAUTIONARY AND ADVISORY LABELS 21
▸ Ursodeoxycholic acid (Non-proprietary)
  Ursodeoxycholic acid 250 mg Ursodeoxycholic acid 250mg capsules | 60 capsule [PoM] £25.93 DT price = £25.29
▸ Ursofalk (Dr. Falk Pharma UK Ltd)
  Ursodeoxycholic acid 250 mg Ursofalk 250mg capsules | 60 capsule [PoM] £30.17 DT price = £25.29 | 100 capsule [PoM] £31.88

Oral suspension
CAUTIONARY AND ADVISORY LABELS 21
▸ Ursofalk (Dr. Falk Pharma UK Ltd)
  Ursodeoxycholic acid 50 mg per 1 ml Ursofalk 250mg/5ml oral suspension sugar-free | 250 ml [PoM] £26.98 DT price = £26.98

LIPIDS ⟩ STEROLS

Cholesterol

- **INDICATIONS AND DOSE**
  Smith-Lemli-Opitz syndrome
  ▸ BY MOUTH
  ▸ Neonate: 5–10 mg/kg 3–4 times a day.
  ▸ Child: 5–10 mg/kg 3–4 times a day, doses up to 15 mg/kg 4 times daily have been used

- **UNLICENSED USE** Not licensed.
- **CONTRA-INDICATIONS**
  CONTRA-INDICATIONS, FURTHER INFORMATION
  For contra-indications, consult product literature.
- **CAUTIONS**
  CAUTIONS, FURTHER INFORMATION
  For advice on cautions, consult product literature.
- **DIRECTIONS FOR ADMINISTRATION** Cholesterol powder can be mixed with a vegetable oil before administration.

- **MEDICINAL FORMS**
  There can be variation in the licensing of different medicines containing the same drug. Forms available from special-order manufacturers include: oral suspension, powder

7.2 Oesophageal varices

PITUITARY AND HYPOTHALAMIC HORMONES AND ANALOGUES ⟩ VASOPRESSIN AND ANALOGUES

Terlipressin acetate

- **INDICATIONS AND DOSE**
  GLYPRESSIN® INJECTION

  Adjunct in acute massive haemorrhage of gastro-intestinal tract or oesophageal varices (specialist use only)
  ▸ BY INTRAVENOUS INJECTION
  ▸ Child 12–17 years (body-weight up to 50 kg): Initially 2 mg every 4 hours until bleeding controlled, then reduced to 1 mg every 4 hours if required, maximum duration 48 hours
  ▸ Child 12–17 years (body-weight 50 kg and above): Initially 2 mg every 4 hours until bleeding controlled, reduced if not tolerated to 1 mg every 4 hours, maximum duration 48 hours

  VARIQUEL® INJECTION

  Adjunct in acute massive haemorrhage of gastro-intestinal tract or oesophageal varices (specialist use only)
  ▸ BY INTRAVENOUS INJECTION
  ▸ Child 12–17 years (body-weight up to 50 kg): Initially 1 mg, then 1 mg every 4–6 hours for up to 72 hours, to be administered over 1 minute
  ▸ Child 12–17 years (body-weight 50–69 kg): Initially 1.5 mg, then 1 mg every 4–6 hours for up to 72 hours, to be administered over 1 minute
  ▸ Child 12–17 years (body-weight 70 kg and above): Initially 2 mg, then 1 mg every 4–6 hours for up to 72 hours, to be administered over 1 minute

- **UNLICENSED USE** Unlicensed for use in children.
- **CAUTIONS** Arrhythmia · electrolyte and fluid disturbances · heart disease · history of QT-interval prolongation · respiratory disease · septic shock · uncontrolled hypertension · vascular disease
- **INTERACTIONS** Caution with concomitant use of drugs that prolong the QT-interval.
- **SIDE-EFFECTS**
  ▸ **Common or very common** Abdominal cramps · arrhythmia · bradycardia · diarrhoea · headache · hypertension · hypotension · pallor · peripheral ischaemia
  ▸ **Uncommon** Angina · bronchospasm · convulsions · hot flushes · hyponatraemia · intestinal ischaemia · myocardial infarction · nausea · pulmonary oedema · respiratory failure · tachycardia · vomiting
  ▸ **Rare** Dyspnoea
  ▸ **Very rare** Hyperglycaemia · stroke
  ▸ **Frequency not known** Heart failure · skin necrosis
- **PREGNANCY** Avoid unless benefits outweigh risk—uterine contractions and increased intra-uterine pressure in early pregnancy, and decreased uterine blood flow reported.
- **BREAST FEEDING** Avoid unless benefits outweigh risk—no information available.
- **RENAL IMPAIRMENT** Use with caution in chronic renal failure.

- **MEDICINAL FORMS**
  There can be variation in the licensing of different medicines containing the same drug.
  Solution for injection
  ▸ Glypressin (Ferring Pharmaceuticals Ltd)
  Terlipressin acetate 120 microgram per 1 ml Glypressin 1mg/8.5ml solution for injection ampoules | 5 ampoule [PoM] no price available
  ▸ Variquel (Sinclair IS Pharma Plc)
  Terlipressin acetate 200 microgram per 1 ml Variquel 1mg/5ml solution for injection vials | 5 vial [PoM] £89.98 (Hospital only)
  Powder and solvent for solution for injection
  ▸ Glypressin (Ferring Pharmaceuticals Ltd)
  Terlipressin acetate 1 mg Glypressin 1mg powder and solvent for solution for injection vials | 5 vial [PoM] £92.33
  ▸ Variquel (Sinclair IS Pharma Plc)
  Terlipressin acetate 1 mg Variquel 1mg powder and solvent for solution for injection vials | 5 vial [PoM] £89.48

Vasopressin

- **INDICATIONS AND DOSE**

  Adjunct in acute massive haemorrhage of gastrointestinal tract or oesophageal varices (specialist use only)
  ▸ BY CONTINUOUS INTRAVENOUS INFUSION
  ▸ **Child:** Initially 0.3 unit/kg (max. per dose 20 units), dose to be administered over 20–30 minutes, then 0.3 unit/kg/hour, adjusted according to response (max. per dose 1 unit/kg/hour), if bleeding stops, continue at same dose for 12 hours, then withdraw gradually over 24–48 hours; max. duration of treatment 72 hours, dose may alternatively be infused directly into the superior mesenteric artery

- **UNLICENSED USE** Not licensed for use in children.
- **CONTRA-INDICATIONS** Chronic nephritis (until reasonable blood nitrogen concentrations attained) · vascular disease (especially disease of coronary arteries) unless extreme caution
- **CAUTIONS** Asthma · avoid fluid overload · conditions which might be aggravated by water retention · epilepsy · heart failure · hypertension · migraine
- **SIDE-EFFECTS**
  ▸ Rare Gangrene
  ▸ Frequency not known Abdominal cramps · anaphylaxis · anginal attacks · belching · constriction of coronary arteries · desire to defaecate · fluid retention · headache · hypersensitivity reactions · myocardial ischaemia · nausea · pallor · peripheral ischaemia · sweating · tremor · vertigo · vomiting
- **PREGNANCY** Oxytocic effect in third trimester.
- **BREAST FEEDING** Not known to be harmful.
- **DIRECTIONS FOR ADMINISTRATION** For *intravenous infusion* (argipressin); dilute with Glucose 5% or Sodium Chloride 0.9% to a concentration of 0.2–1 unit/mL.

- **MEDICINAL FORMS**
  There can be variation in the licensing of different medicines containing the same drug.
  Solution for injection
  ▸ Vasopressin (Non-proprietary)
  Argipressin 20 unit per 1 ml Argipressin 20units/1ml solution for injection ampoules | 10 ampoule [PoM] £800.00 (Hospital only)

8 Obesity

Obesity

1.6.2016

Description of condition

Obesity is directly linked to many health problems including cardiovascular disease, type 2 diabetes, and obstructive sleep apnoea syndrome. It can also contribute to psychological and psychiatric morbidities.

In children and adolescents, body mass index (BMI) should be used as a practical estimation of body fat. However, it should be interpreted with caution as it is not a direct measure of adiposity. Assessing the BMI of children is more complicated than for adults because it changes as they grow and mature, with different growth patterns seen between boys and girls.

Public Health England advises that the British 1990 (UK90) growth reference charts should be used to determine the weight status of children. A child $\geq$ the 91st centile is classified as overweight, and as obese if $\geq$ the 98th centile. Waist circumference is not recommended as a routine measure, but should be used as an additional predictor for risk of developing other long-term health problems. Children who are overweight or obese and have significant comorbidities or complex needs should be considered for specialist referral.

Aims of treatment

Children who are overweight or obese and are no longer growing taller will ultimately need to lose weight and maintain weight loss to improve their BMI. However, preventing further weight gain while making lifestyle changes, may be an appropriate short-term aim.

Overview

[EvGr] The goals of management of obesity should be agreed together with the child and their parents or carers; parents or carers should be encouraged to take responsibility for lifestyle changes of their children. Referral to a specialist can be considered for children who are overweight or obese and have significant comorbidities or complex needs (e.g. learning disabilities). Children should be assessed for comorbidities such as hypertension, hyperinsulinaemia, dyslipidaemia, type 2 diabetes, psychosocial dysfunction, and exacerbation of conditions such as asthma. ⟨A⟩
[EvGr] An initial assessment should consider potential underlying causes (e.g. hypothyroidism) and a review of the appropriateness of current medications, which are known to cause weight gain, e.g. atypical antipsychotics, beta-adrenoceptor blocking drugs, insulin (when used in the treatment of type 2 diabetes), sodium valproate, and tricyclic antidepressants. ⟨A⟩

Lifestyle changes

[EvGr] Obese children should be encouraged to engage in a sustainable weight management programme which includes strategies to change behaviour, increase physical activity and improve diet and eating behaviour. These changes should be encouraged within the whole family. Any dietary changes should be age appropriate and consistent with healthy eating recommendations. Surgical intervention is not generally recommended in children or adolescents. ⟨A⟩

Drug treatment

EvGr Drug treatment is not generally recommended for children younger than 12 years, unless there are exceptional circumstances, such as if severe comorbidities are present. In children over 12 years, drug treatment is only recommended if physical comorbidities, such as orthopaedic problems or sleep apnoea, or severe psychological comorbidities are present. Drug treatment should **never** be used as the sole element of treatment and should be used as part of an overall weight management plan. Orlistat below [unlicensed use] is the only drug currently available in the UK that is recommended specifically for the treatment of obesity; it acts by reducing the absorption of dietary fat. Treatment should be started and monitored in a specialist paediatric setting by experienced multidisciplinary teams. An initial 6–12 month trial is recommended, with regular review to assess effectiveness, adverse effects and adherence. ⟨A⟩

EvGr Treatment may also be used to maintain weight loss rather than to continue to lose weight. A vitamin and mineral supplement may also be considered if there is concern about inadequate micronutrient intake, particularly for younger children who need vitamins and minerals for growth and development. ⟨A⟩

Useful Resources

Obesity: identification, assessment and management. Clinical Guideline 189. National Institute for Health and Care Excellence. November 2014.
www.nice.org.uk/guidance/cg189
Measuring and interpreting BMI in Children. Public Health England.
www.noo.org.uk/NOO_about_obesity/measurement/children

PERIPHERALLY ACTING ANTIOBESITY DRUGS ⟩
LIPASE INHIBITORS

Orlistat

- **DRUG ACTION** Orlistat, a lipase inhibitor, reduces the absorption of dietary fat.

- **INDICATIONS AND DOSE**

  Adjunct in obesity
  ▶ BY MOUTH
  ▶ Child 12–17 years (initiated by a specialist): 120 mg up to 3 times a day, dose to be taken immediately before, during, or up to 1 hour after each main meal, continue treatment beyond 12 weeks only under specialist supervision, if a meal is missed or contains no fat, the dose of orlistat should be omitted

- **UNLICENSED USE** Not licensed for use in children.

- **CONTRA-INDICATIONS** Cholestasis · chronic malabsorption syndrome

- **CAUTIONS** Chronic kidney disease · may impair absorption of fat-soluble vitamins · volume depletion

  CAUTIONS, FURTHER INFORMATION
  Vitamin supplementation (especially of vitamin D) may be considered if there is concern about deficiency of fat-soluble vitamins.

- **INTERACTIONS** → Appendix 1 (orlistat).
  ▶ **Multivitamins** If a multivitamin supplement is required, it should be taken at least 2 hours after orlistat dose or at bedtime.

- **SIDE-EFFECTS**
  ▶ **Common or very common** Abdominal distension (gastro-intestinal effects minimised by reduced fat intake) · abdominal pain (gastro-intestinal effects minimised by reduced fat intake) · anxiety · faecal incontinence · faecal urgency · flatulence · gingival disorders · headache · hypoglycaemia · liquid stools · malaise · menstrual

disturbances · oily leakage from rectum · oily stools · respiratory infections · tooth disorders · urinary tract infection
▶ **Frequency not known** Bullous eruptions · cholelithiasis · diverticulitis · hepatitis · hypothyroidism · oxalate nephropathy · rectal bleeding

- **PREGNANCY** Use with caution.

- **BREAST FEEDING** Avoid—no information available.

- **MEDICINAL FORMS**
  There can be variation in the licensing of different medicines containing the same drug.
  Capsule
  ▶ Orlistat (Non-proprietary)
  Orlistat 120 mg Orlistat 120mg capsules | 84 capsule PoM £30.05 DT price = £20.07
  ▶ Alli (GlaxoSmithKline Consumer Healthcare)
  Orlistat 60 mg Alli 60mg capsules | 42 capsule P £19.20 | 84 capsule P £29.10 | 120 capsule P £36.32
  ▶ Beacita (Actavis UK Ltd)
  Orlistat 120 mg Beacita 120mg capsules | 84 capsule PoM £31.63 DT price = £20.07
  ▶ Xenical (Roche Products Ltd)
  Orlistat 120 mg Xenical 120mg capsules | 84 capsule PoM £31.63 DT price = £20.07

9　Rectal and anal disorders

Rectal and anal disorders

Overview

In children with perianal soreness or pruritus ani, good toilet hygiene is essential; the use of alcohol-free 'wet-wipes' after each bowel motion, regular bathing and the avoidance of local irritants such as bath additives is recommended. Excoriated skin is best treated with a protective barrier emollient; in children over 1 month, hydrocortisone p. 411 ointment or cream or a compound rectal preparation may be used for a short period of time, up to a maximum of 7 days.

Pruritus ani caused by threadworm infection requires treatment with an anthelmintic. Topical application of **white soft paraffin** or other bland emollient may reduce anal irritation caused by threadworms.

Perianal erythema caused by streptococcal infection should be treated initially with an oral antibacterial such as phenoxymethylpenicillin p. 319 or erythromycin p. 310, while awaiting results of culture and sensitivity testing.

Perianal candidiasis (thrush) requires treatment with a topical antifungal preparation.

Proctitis associated with inflammatory bowel disease in children is treated with corticosteroids and aminosalicylates.

Soothing anal and rectal preparations

Haemorrhoids in children are rare, but may occur in infants with portal hypertension. Soothing rectal preparations containing mild astringents such as bismuth subgallate, zinc oxide, and hammamelis may provide symptomatic relief, but proprietary preparations which also contain lubricants, vasoconstrictors, or mild antiseptics may cause further perianal irritation.

Local anaesthetics may be used to relieve pain in children with anal fissures or pruritus ani, but local anaesthetics are absorbed through the rectal mucosa and may cause sensitisation of the anal skin. Excessive use of local anaesthetics may result in systemic effects. Preparations containing local anaesthetics should be used for no longer than 2–3 days.

Lidocaine hydrochloride ointment p. 780 may be applied before defaecation to relieve pain associated with anal fissure, but local anaesthetics can cause stinging initially and this may aggravate the child's fear of pain.

Other local anaesthetics such as tetracaine p. 635, cinchocaine (dibucaine), and pramocaine (pramoxine) may be included in rectal preparations, but these are more irritant than lidocaine hydrochloride.

Corticosteroids are often combined with local anaesthetics and soothing agents in topical preparations for haemorrhoids and proctitis. Topical preparations containing corticosteroids should not be used long-term or if infection (such as herpes simplex) is present.

Anal fissures

The management of anal fissures includes stool softening and the short-term use of a topical preparation containing a local anaesthetic. If these measures are inadequate, children with chronic anal fissures should be referred for specialist treatment in hospital. Topical glyceryl trinitrate 0.05% or 0.1% ointment p. 127, may be used in children to relax the anal sphincter, relieve pain and aid healing of anal fissures. Excessive application of topical nitrates causes side-effects such as headache, flushing, dizziness, and postural hypotension.

Before considering surgery, diltiazem hydrochloride 2% ointment may be used in children with chronic anal fissures resistant to topical nitrates.

Ointments containing glyceryl trinitrate in a range of strengths or diltiazem hydrochloride 2% are available as manufactured specials.

9.1 Haemorrhoids

CORTICOSTEROIDS

Benzyl benzoate with bismuth oxide, bismuth subgallate, hydrocortisone acetate, peru balsam and zinc oxide

● **INDICATIONS AND DOSE**

Haemorrhoids | Pruritus ani

▸ BY RECTUM USING OINTMENT

▸ Child 12-17 years: Apply twice daily for no longer than 7 days, to be applied morning and night, an additional dose should be applied after a bowel movement

▸ BY RECTUM USING SUPPOSITORIES

▸ Child 12-17 years: 1 suppository twice daily for no longer than 7 days, to be inserted night and morning, additional dose after a bowel movement

● **CAUTIONS** Local anaesthetic component can be absorbed through the rectal mucosa (avoid excessive application) · local anaesthetic component may cause sensitisation (use for short periods only—no longer than a few days)

● **PRESCRIBING AND DISPENSING INFORMATION** A proprietary brand *Anusol Plus HC*® (ointment and suppositories) is on sale to the public.

● **MEDICINAL FORMS**
There can be variation in the licensing of different medicines containing the same drug.
Suppository
▸ Benzyl benzoate with bismuth oxide, bismuth subgallate, hydrocortisone acetate, peru balsam and zinc oxide (Non-proprietary)
Hydrocortisone acetate 10 mg, Bismuth oxide 24 mg, Benzyl benzoate 33 mg, Peru Balsam 49 mg, Bismuth subgallate 59 mg, Zinc oxide 296 mg Anusol Soothing Relief suppositories | 12 suppository GSL £3.34
▸ Anusol-Hc (McNeil Products Ltd)
Hydrocortisone acetate 10 mg, Bismuth oxide 24 mg, Benzyl benzoate 33 mg, Peru Balsam 49 mg, Bismuth subgallate 59 mg, Zinc oxide 296 mg Anusol HC suppositories | 12 suppository PoM £1.74
Anusol Plus HC suppositories | 12 suppository P £3.03

Ointment

▸ Benzyl benzoate with bismuth oxide, bismuth subgallate, hydrocortisone acetate, peru balsam and zinc oxide (Non-proprietary)
Hydrocortisone acetate 2.5 mg per 1 gram, Bismuth oxide 8.75 mg per 1 gram, Benzyl benzoate 12.5 mg per 1 gram, Peru Balsam 18.75 mg per 1 gram, Bismuth subgallate 22.5 mg per 1 gram, Zinc oxide 107.5 mg per 1 gram Anusol Soothing Relief ointment | 15 gram GSL £3.34
▸ Anusol-Hc (McNeil Products Ltd)
Hydrocortisone acetate 2.5 mg per 1 gram, Bismuth oxide 8.75 mg per 1 gram, Benzyl benzoate 12.5 mg per 1 gram, Peru Balsam 18.75 mg per 1 gram, Bismuth subgallate 22.5 mg per 1 gram, Zinc oxide 107.5 mg per 1 gram Anusol Plus HC ointment | 15 gram P £3.03
Anusol HC ointment | 30 gram PoM £2.49

Benzyl benzoate with bismuth oxide, hydrocortisone acetate, peru balsam, pramocaine hydrochloride and zinc oxide

● **INDICATIONS AND DOSE**

Haemorrhoids | Pruritus ani

▸ BY RECTUM

▸ Child 12-17 years: Apply twice daily for no longer than 7 days, to be applied morning and night and after a bowel movement

● **CAUTIONS** Local anaesthetic component can be absorbed through the rectal mucosa (avoid excessive application) · local anaesthetic component may cause sensitisation (use for short periods only—no longer than a few days)

● **MEDICINAL FORMS**
There can be variation in the licensing of different medicines containing the same drug.
Cream
▸ Anugesic-Hc (Pfizer Ltd)
Hydrocortisone acetate 5 mg per 1 gram, Bismuth oxide 8.75 mg per 1 gram, Pramocaine hydrochloride 10 mg per 1 gram, Benzyl benzoate 12 mg per 1 gram, Peru Balsam 18.5 mg per 1 gram, Zinc oxide 123.5 mg per 1 gram Anugesic-HC cream | 30 gram PoM £3.71

Cinchocaine hydrochloride with fluocortolone caproate and fluocortolone pivalate

● **INDICATIONS AND DOSE**

Haemorrhoids | Pruritus ani

▸ BY RECTUM USING OINTMENT

▸ Child: Apply twice daily for 5–7 days, apply 3–4 times a day if required, on the first day of treatment, then apply once daily for a few days after symptoms have cleared

▸ BY RECTUM USING SUPPOSITORIES

▸ Child 12-17 years: Initially 1 suppository daily for 5–7 days, to be inserted after a bowel movement, then 1 suppository once daily on alternate days for 1 week

Haemorrhoids (severe cases) | Pruritus ani (severe cases)

▸ BY RECTUM USING SUPPOSITORIES

▸ Child 12-17 years: Initially 1 suppository 2–3 times a day for 5–7 days, then 1 suppository once daily on alternate days for 1 week

● **CAUTIONS** Local anaesthetic component can be absorbed through the rectal mucosa (avoid excessive application) · local anaesthetic component may cause sensitisation (use for short periods only—no longer than a few days)

● **MEDICINAL FORMS**
There can be variation in the licensing of medicines containing the same drug.

Suppository
▸ Ultraproct (Meadow Laboratories Ltd)
Fluocortolone pivalate 610 microgram, Fluocortolone caproate 630 microgram, Cinchocaine hydrochloride 1 mg Ultraproct suppositories | 12 suppository PoM £4.06

Ointment
▸ Ultraproct (Meadow Laboratories Ltd)
Fluocortolone pivalate 920 microgram per 1 gram, Fluocortolone caproate 950 microgram per 1 gram, Cinchocaine hydrochloride 5 mg per 1 gram Ultraproct ointment | 30 gram PoM £8.27

Cinchocaine with hydrocortisone

● **INDICATIONS AND DOSE**

PROCTOSEDYL® OINTMENT

Haemorrhoids | Pruritus ani
▸ TO THE SKIN, OR BY RECTUM
▸ Child: Apply twice daily, to be administered morning and night and after a bowel movement. Apply externally or by rectum. Do not use for longer than 7 days

PROCTOSEDYL® SUPPOSITORIES

Haemorrhoids | Pruritus ani
▸ BY RECTUM
▸ Child 12–17 years: 1 suppository, insert suppository night and morning and after a bowel movement. Do not use for longer than 7 days

UNIROID-HC® OINTMENT

Haemorrhoids | Pruritus ani
▸ TO THE SKIN, OR BY RECTUM
▸ Child 1 month–11 years (under medical advice only): Apply twice daily, and apply after a bowel movement, apply externally or by rectum, do not use for longer than 7 days
▸ Child 12–17 years: Apply twice daily, and apply after a bowel movement, apply externally or by rectum, do not use for longer than 7 days

UNIROID-HC® SUPPOSITORIES

Haemorrhoids | Pruritus ani
▸ BY RECTUM
▸ Child 12–17 years: 1 suppository, insert twice daily and after a bowel movement. Do not use for longer than 7 days

● **CAUTIONS** Local anaesthetic component can be absorbed through the rectal mucosa (avoid excessive application) · local anaesthetic component may cause sensitisation (use for short periods only—no longer than a few days)

● **MEDICINAL FORMS**
There can be variation in the licensing of different medicines containing the same drug.

Suppository
▸ Cinchocaine with hydrocortisone (Non-proprietary)
Cinchocaine hydrochloride 5 mg, Hydrocortisone 5 mg Cinchocaine 5mg / Hydrocortisone 5mg suppositories | 12 suppository PoM no price available
▸ Proctosedyl (Sanofi)
Cinchocaine hydrochloride 5 mg, Hydrocortisone 5 mg Proctosedyl suppositories | 12 suppository PoM £5.08
▸ Uniroid HC (Chemidex Pharma Ltd)
Cinchocaine hydrochloride 5 mg, Hydrocortisone 5 mg Uniroid HC suppositories | 12 suppository PoM £1.91

Ointment
▸ Cinchocaine with hydrocortisone (Non-proprietary)
Cinchocaine hydrochloride 5 mg per 1 gram, Hydrocortisone 5 mg per 1 gram Cinchocaine 0.5% / Hydrocortisone 0.5% ointment | 30 gram PoM no price available

▸ Proctosedyl (Sanofi)
Cinchocaine hydrochloride 5 mg per 1 gram, Hydrocortisone 5 mg per 1 gram Proctosedyl ointment | 30 gram PoM £10.34
▸ Uniroid HC (Chemidex Pharma Ltd)
Cinchocaine hydrochloride 5 mg per 1 gram, Hydrocortisone 5 mg per 1 gram Uniroid HC ointment | 30 gram PoM £4.23

Cinchocaine with prednisolone

● **INDICATIONS AND DOSE**

Haemorrhoids | Pruritus ani
▸ BY RECTUM USING OINTMENT
▸ Child: Apply twice daily for 5–7 days, apply 3–4 times a day on the first day if necessary, then apply once daily for a few days after symptoms have cleared
▸ BY RECTUM USING SUPPOSITORIES
▸ Child 12–17 years: 1 suppository daily for 5–7 days, to be inserted after a bowel movement

Haemorrhoids (severe cases) | Pruritus ani (severe cases)
▸ BY RECTUM USING SUPPOSITORIES
▸ Child 12–17 years: Initially 1 suppository 2–3 times a day, then 1 suppository daily for a total of 5–7 days, to be inserted after a bowel movement

● **CAUTIONS** Local anaesthetic component can be absorbed through the rectal mucosa (avoid excessive application) · local anaesthetic component may cause sensitisation (use for short periods only—no longer than a few days)

● **MEDICINAL FORMS**
There can be variation in the licensing of different medicines containing the same drug.

Suppository
▸ Scheriproct (Bayer Plc)
Cinchocaine hydrochloride 1 mg, Prednisolone hexanoate 1.3 mg Scheriproct suppositories | 12 suppository PoM £1.38 DT price = £1.38

Ointment
▸ Scheriproct (Bayer Plc)
Prednisolone hexanoate 1.9 mg per 1 gram, Cinchocaine hydrochloride 5 mg per 1 gram Scheriproct ointment | 30 gram PoM £2.94 DT price = £2.94

Hydrocortisone with lidocaine

● **INDICATIONS AND DOSE**

Haemorrhoids | Pruritus ani
▸ BY RECTUM USING AEROSOL SPRAY
▸ Child 2–13 years (under medical advice only): 1 spray up to 3 times a day, spray once over the affected area
▸ Child 14–17 years: 1 spray up to 3 times a day for no longer than 7 days without medical advice, spray once over the affected area
▸ BY RECTUM USING OINTMENT
▸ Child: Apply several times daily, for short term use only

● **CAUTIONS** Local anaesthetic component can be absorbed through the rectal mucosa (avoid excessive application) · local anaesthetic component may cause sensitisation (use for short periods only—no longer than a few days)

● **MEDICINAL FORMS**
There can be variation in the licensing of different medicines containing the same drug.

Ointment
▸ Hydrocortisone with lidocaine (Non-proprietary)
Hydrocortisone acetate 2.75 mg per 1 gram, Lidocaine 50 mg per 1 gram Lidocaine 5% / Hydrocortisone acetate 0.275% ointment | 20 gram PoM no price available DT price = £4.19
▸ Xyloproct (AstraZeneca UK Ltd)
Hydrocortisone acetate 2.75 mg per 1 gram, Lidocaine 50 mg per 1 gram Xyloproct 5%/0.275% ointment | 20 gram PoM £4.19 DT price = £4.19

Gastro-intestinal system

1

Spray

▸ **Germoloids HC** (Bayer Plc)
Hydrocortisone 2 mg per 1 gram, Lidocaine hydrochloride 10 mg per 1 gram Germoloids HC spray | 30 ml [GSL] £5.20
▸ **Perinal** (Dermal Laboratories Ltd)
Hydrocortisone 2 mg per 1 gram, Lidocaine hydrochloride 10 mg per 1 gram Perinal spray | 30 ml [P] £6.11

Hydrocortisone with pramocaine

● **INDICATIONS AND DOSE**

Pain and irritation associated with local, non-infected anal or perianal conditions

▸ BY RECTUM

▸ Child 12–17 years: 1 applicatorful 2–3 times a day and 1 applicatorful, after a bowel movement, do not use for longer than 7 days; maximum 4 applicatorfuls per day

● **CAUTIONS** Local anaesthetic component can be absorbed through the rectal mucosa (avoid excessive application) · local anaesthetic component may cause sensitisation (use for short periods only—no longer than a few days)

● **MEDICINAL FORMS**
There can be variation in the licensing of different medicines containing the same drug.

Foam

▸ **Proctofoam HC** (Meda Pharmaceuticals Ltd)
Hydrocortisone acetate 10 mg per 1 gram, Pramocaine hydrochloride 10 mg per 1 gram Proctofoam HC foam enema | 40 dose [PoM] £6.07 DT price = £6.07

10 Reduced exocrine secretions

PANCREATIC ENZYMES

Pancreatin

● **DRUG ACTION** Supplements of pancreatin are given to compensate for reduced or absent exocrine secretion. They assist the digestion of starch, fat, and protein.

● **INDICATIONS AND DOSE**

CREON® 10000

Pancreatic insufficiency

▸ BY MOUTH

▸ Child: Initially 1–2 capsules, dose to be taken with each meal either taken whole or contents mixed with acidic fluid or soft food (then swallowed immediately without chewing)

CREON® 25000

Pancreatic insufficiency

▸ BY MOUTH

▸ Child 2–17 years: Initially 1–2 capsules, dose to be taken with each meal either taken whole or contents mixed with acidic fluid or soft food (then swallowed immediately without chewing)

CREON® 40000

Pancreatic insufficiency

▸ BY MOUTH

▸ Child 2–17 years: Initially 1–2 capsules, dose to be taken with each meal either taken whole or contents mixed with acidic fluid or soft food (then swallowed immediately without chewing)

CREON® MICRO

Pancreatic insufficiency

▸ BY MOUTH

▸ Neonate: Initially 100 mg, to be given before each feed; granules can be mixed with a small amount of breast milk or formula feed and administered immediately (manufacturer recommends mixing with a small amount of apple juice before administration), granules should not be chewed before swallowing.

▸ Child: Initially 100 mg, to be taken before each feed or meal; granules can be mixed with a small amount of milk or soft food and administered immediately (manufacturer recommends mixing with acidic liquid or pureed fruit before administration), granules should not be chewed before swallowing

DOSE EQUIVALENCE AND CONVERSION
For *Creon®* Micro: 100 mg granules = one measured scoopful (scoop supplied with product).

NUTRIZYM 22® GASTRO-RESISTANT CAPSULES

Pancreatic insufficiency

▸ BY MOUTH

▸ Child 15–17 years: Initially 1–2 capsules, dose to be taken with meals and 1 capsule as required, dose to be taken with snacks, doses should be swallowed whole or contents taken with water or mixed with soft food (then swallowed immediately without chewing)

PANCREASE HL®

Pancreatic insufficiency

▸ BY MOUTH

▸ Child 15–17 years: Initially 1–2 capsules, dose to be taken during each meal and 1 capsule, to be taken with snacks, all doses either taken whole or contents mixed with slightly acidic liquid or soft food (then swallowed immediately without chewing)

PANCREX®

Pancreatic insufficiency

▸ BY MOUTH

▸ Child 2–17 years: 5–10 g, to be taken just before meals, washed down or mixed with milk or water

PANCREX® V

Pancreatic insufficiency

▸ BY MOUTH

▸ Child 1–11 months: 1–2 capsules, contents of capsule to be mixed with feeds

▸ Child 1–17 years: 2–6 capsules, dose to be taken with each meal either swallowed whole or sprinkled on food

PANCREX® V CAPSULES '125'

Pancreatic insufficiency

▸ BY MOUTH

▸ Neonate: 1–2 capsules, contents of capsule to be given in each feed (or mixed with feed and given by spoon).

PANCREX® V POWDER

Pancreatic insufficiency

▸ BY MOUTH

▸ Neonate: 250–500 mg, dose to be taken with each feed.

▸ Child: 0.5–2 g, to be taken before or with meals, washed down or mixed with milk or water

PANCREX® V TABLETS

Pancreatic insufficiency

▸ BY MOUTH

▸ Child 2–17 years: 5–15 tablets, to be taken before meals

PANCREX® V TABLETS FORTE

Pancreatic insufficiency

▸ BY MOUTH

▸ Child 2–17 years: 6–10 tablets, to be taken before meals

- **CONTRA-INDICATIONS**
  PANCREASE HL® Should not be used in children aged 15 years or less with cystic fibrosis
- **CAUTIONS** Can irritate the perioral skin and buccal mucosa if retained in the mouth · excessive doses can cause perianal irritation
- **INTERACTIONS** → Appendix 1 (pancreatin).
- **SIDE-EFFECTS** Abdominal discomfort · hyperuricaemia (associated with very high doses) · hyperuricosuria (associated with very high doses) · mucosal irritation · nausea · skin irritation · vomiting
- **PREGNANCY** Not known to be harmful.
- **DIRECTIONS FOR ADMINISTRATION** Enteric-coated preparations deliver a higher enzyme concentration in the duodenum (provided the capsule contents are swallowed whole without chewing). Since pancreatin is inactivated by heat, excessive heat should be avoided if preparations are mixed with liquids or food; the resulting mixtures should not be kept for more than one hour. Gastro-resistant granules should be mixed with milk, slightly acidic soft food or liquid such as apple juice, and then swallowed immediately without chewing. Any left-over food or liquid containing pancreatin should be discarded. Capsules containing enteric-coated granules can be opened and the granules administered in the same way. Pancreatin is inactivated by gastric acid therefore pancreatin preparations are best taken with food (or immediately before or after food).

  In children with cystic fibrosis with persistent fat malabsorption despite optimal use of enzyme replacement, an H_2-receptor antagonist or a proton pump inhibitor may improve fat digestion and absorption.
- **PRESCRIBING AND DISPENSING INFORMATION** Preparations may contain pork pancreatin—consult product literature.
- **HANDLING AND STORAGE** Hypersensitivity reactions occur occasionally and may affect those handling the powder.
- **PATIENT AND CARER ADVICE**
  Medicines for Children leaflet: Pancreatin for pancreatic insufficiency www.medicinesforchildren.org.uk/pancreatin-for-pancreatic-insufficiency

  Patients or carers should be given advice on administration.

  It is important to ensure adequate hydration at all times in patients receiving higher-strength pancreatin preparations.
- **MEDICINAL FORMS**
  There can be variation in the licensing of different medicines containing the same drug.
  Gastro-resistant tablet
  CAUTIONARY AND ADVISORY LABELS 5, 25
  ▸ Pancrex (Essential Pharmaceuticals Ltd)
  Protease 110 unit, Amylase 1700 unit, Lipase 1900 unit Pancrex V gastro-resistant tablets | 300 tablet ℗ £38.79
  Protease 330 unit, Amylase 5000 unit, Lipase 5600 unit Pancrex V Forte gastro-resistant tablets | 300 tablet ℗ £48.11
  Capsule
  ▸ Pancrex (Essential Pharmaceuticals Ltd)
  Protease 160 unit, Lipase 2950 unit, Amylase 3300 unit Pancrex V 125mg capsules | 300 capsule ℗ £42.07
  Protease 430 unit, Lipase 8000 unit, Amylase 9000 unit Pancrex V capsules | 300 capsule ℗ £53.20
  Gastro-resistant capsule
  ▸ Creon (BGP Products Ltd)
  Protease 600 unit, Amylase 8000 unit, Lipase 10000 unit Creon 10000 gastro-resistant capsules | 100 capsule ℗ £12.93
  Protease 1000 unit, Amylase 18000 unit, Lipase 25000 unit Creon 25000 gastro-resistant capsules | 100 capsule PoM £28.25
  Protease 1600 unit, Amylase 25000 unit, Lipase 40000 unit Creon 40000 gastro-resistant capsules | 100 capsule PoM £41.80

  ▸ Nutrizym (Merck Serono Ltd)
  Protease 1100 unit, Amylase 19800 unit, Lipase 22000 unit Nutrizym 22 gastro-resistant capsules | 100 capsule PoM £33.33
  ▸ Pancrease (Janssen-Cilag Ltd)
  Protease 1250 unit, Amylase 22500 unit, Lipase 25000 unit Pancrease HL gastro-resistant capsules | 100 capsule PoM £40.38
  Gastro-resistant granules
  CAUTIONARY AND ADVISORY LABELS 25
  ▸ Creon (BGP Products Ltd)
  Protease 200 unit, Amylase 3600 unit, Lipase 5000 unit Creon Micro Pancreatin 60.12mg gastro-resistant granules | 20 gram ℗ £31.50
  ▸ Pancrex (Essential Pharmaceuticals Ltd)
  Protease 300 unit, Amylase 4000 unit, Lipase 5000 unit Pancrex gastro-resistant granules | 300 gram ℗ £57.00
  Powder
  ▸ Pancrex (Essential Pharmaceuticals Ltd)
  Protease 1400 unit, Lipase 25000 unit, Amylase 30000 unit Pancrex V oral powder sugar-free | 300 gram ℗ £58.88

11   Stoma care

Stoma care

24.2.2016

Description of condition

A stoma is an artificial opening on the abdomen to divert flow of faeces or urine into an external pouch located outside of the body. This procedure may be temporary or permanent. Colostomy and ileostomy are the most common forms of stoma but a gastrostomy, jejunostomy, duodenostomy or caecostomy may also be performed. Understanding the type and extent of surgical intervention in each patient is crucial in managing the patient's pharmaceutical needs correctly.

Overview

Prescribing for patients with stoma calls for special care due to modifications in drug delivery, resulting in a higher risk of sub-optimal absorption. The following is a brief account of some of the main points to be borne in mind.

Enteric-coated and modified-release medicines are **unsuitable**, particularly in patients with an ileostomy, as there may not be sufficient release of active ingredient. Soluble tablets, liquids, capsules or uncoated tablets are more suitable due to their quicker dissolution. When a solid-dose form such as a capsule or a tablet is given, the contents of the ostomy bag should be checked for any remnants.

Preparations containing sorbitol as an excipient should be avoided, due to its laxative side effects.

Analgesics

Opioid analgesics may cause troublesome constipation in colostomy patients. When a non-opioid analgesic is required, paracetamol is usually suitable. Anti-inflammatory analgesics may cause gastric irritation and bleeding; faecal output should be monitored for traces of blood.

Antacids

The tendency to diarrhoea from magnesium salts or constipation from aluminium or calcium salts may be increased in patients with stoma.

Antisecretory drugs

The gastric acid secretion often increases stoma output. Proton pump inhibitors and somatostatin analogues (octreotide p. 434) are often used to reduce this risk.

Antidiarrhoeal drugs

Loperamide hydrochloride p. 44 and codeine phosphate p. 259 reduce intestinal motility and decrease water and

Gastro-intestinal system

1

sodium output from an ileostomy. Loperamide hydrochloride circulates through the enterohepatic circulation, which is disrupted in patients with a short bowel; high doses of loperamide hydrochloride may be required. Codeine phosphate can be added if response with loperamide hydrochloride alone is inadequate.

Digoxin

Children with a stoma are particularly susceptible to hypokalaemia. This predisposes children on digoxin p. 75 to digoxin toxicity; potassium supplements or a potassium-sparing diuretic may be advisable.

Diuretics

Diuretics should be used with caution in patients with an ileostomy or with urostomy as they may become excessively dehydrated and potassium depletion may easily occur. It is usually advisable to use a potassium-sparing diuretic.

Iron preparations

Iron preparations may cause loose stools and sore skin in these patients. If this is troublesome and if iron is definitely indicated, an intramuscular iron preparation should be used. Modified-release preparations should be avoided for the reasons given above.

Laxatives

Laxatives should be used in children with stoma only under specialist supervision; they should be prescribed with caution for those with an ileostomy as they may cause rapid and severe loss of water and electrolytes.

Colostomy patients may suffer from constipation and whenever possible it should be treated by increasing fluid intake or dietary fibre. If a laxative is required, it should generally be used for short periods only.

Care of stoma

Patients and their carers are usually given advice about the use of cleansing agents, protective creams, lotions, deodorants, or sealants whilst in hospital, either by the surgeon or by stoma care nurses. Voluntary organisations offer help and support to patients with stoma.

Chapter 2
Cardiovascular system

CONTENTS

1	**Arrhythmias**	page 69
2	**Bleeding disorders**	76
2.1	Coagulation factor deficiencies	77
2.2	Subarachnoid haemorrhage	80
3	**Blood clots**	81
3.1	Thromboembolism	81
4	**Blood pressure conditions**	90
4.1	Hypertension	90
	4.1a Hypertension associated with phaeochromocytoma	109
	4.1b Hypertensive crises	109

	4.1c Pulmonary hypertension	page 110
4.2	Hypotension and shock	112
5	**Heart failure**	116
6	**Hyperlipidaemia**	119
7	**Myocardial ischaemia**	125
7.1	Cardiac arrest	128
8	**Oedema**	130
9	**Patent ductus arteriosus**	134
10	**Vascular disease**	135

1   Arrhythmias

Arrhythmias

Overview

Management of an arrhythmia requires precise diagnosis of the type of arrhythmia; electrocardiography and referral to a paediatric cardiologist is essential; underlying causes such as heart failure require appropriate treatment.

Bradycardia

Adrenaline/epinephrine p. 128 is useful in the treatment of symptomatic bradycardia in an infant or child.

Supraventricular tachycardia

In supraventricular tachycardia adenosine p. 73 is given by rapid intravenous injection. If adenosine is ineffective, intravenous amiodarone hydrochloride p. 72, flecainide acetate p. 71, or a beta-blocker (such as esmolol hydrochloride p. 98) can be tried; verapamil hydrochloride p. 101 can also be considered in children over 1 year. Atenolol p. 97, sotalol hydrochloride p. 74 and flecainide acetate are used for the prophylaxis of paroxysmal supraventricular tachycardias.

The use of d.c. shock and vagal stimulation also have a role in the treatment of supraventricular tachycardia.

Syndromes associated with accessory conducting pathways

Amiodarone hydrochloride, flecainide acetate, or a beta-blocker is used to prevent recurrence of supraventricular tachycardia in infants and young children with these syndromes (e.g. Wolff-Parkinson-White syndrome).

Atrial flutter

In atrial flutter without structural heart defects, sinus rhythm is restored with d.c. shock or cardiac pacing; drug treatment is usually not necessary. Amiodarone hydrochloride is used in atrial flutter when structural heart defects are present or after heart surgery. Sotalol hydrochloride may also be considered.

Atrial fibrillation

Atrial fibrillation is very rare in children. To restore sinus rhythm d.c. shock is used; beta-blockers, alone or together with digoxin p. 75 may be useful for ventricular rate control.

Ectopic tachycardia

Intravenous amiodarone hydrochloride is used in conjunction with body cooling and synchronised pacing in postoperative junctional ectopic tachycardia. Oral amiodarone hydrochloride or flecainide acetate are used in congenital junctional ectopic tachycardia.

Amiodarone hydrochloride, flecainide acetate, or a beta-blocker are used in atrial ectopic tachycardia; amiodarone hydrochloride is preferred in those with poor ventricular function.

Ventricular tachycardia and ventricular fibrillation

Pulseless ventricular tachycardia or ventricular fibrillation require resuscitation, see Paediatric Advanced Life Support algorithm. Amiodarone hydrochloride is used in resuscitation for pulseless ventricular tachycardia or ventricular fibrillation unresponsive to d.c. shock; lidocaine hydrochloride p. 70 can be used as an alternative only if amiodarone hydrochloride is not available.

Amiodarone hydrochloride is also used in a haemodynamically stable child when drug treatment is required; lidocaine hydrochloride can be used as an alternative only if amiodarone hydrochloride is not available.

Torsade de pointes

Torsade de pointes is a form of ventricular tachycardia associated with long QT syndrome, which may be congenital or drug induced. Episodes may be self-limiting, but are frequently recurrent and can cause impairment or loss of consciousness. If not controlled, the arrhythmia can progress to ventricular fibrillation and sometimes death. Intravenous magnesium sulfate can be used to treat torsade de pointes (dose recommendations vary—consult local guidelines). Anti-arrhythmics can further prolong the QT interval, thus worsening the condition.

Drugs for arrhythmias

Anti-arrhythmic drugs can be classified clinically into those that act on supraventricular arrhythmias (e.g. verapamil hydrochloride), those that act on both supraventricular and ventricular arrhythmias (e.g. amiodarone hydrochloride), and those that act on ventricular arrhythmias (e.g. lidocaine hydrochloride).

Anti-arrhythmic drugs can also be classified according to their effects on the electrical behaviour of myocardial cells during activity (the Vaughan Williams classification) although this classification is of less clinical significance:

- Class I: membrane stabilising drugs (e.g. lidocaine, flecainide)
- Class II: beta-blockers
- Class III: amiodarone; sotalol (also Class II)
- Class IV: calcium-channel blockers (includes verapamil but not dihydropyridines)

The negative inotropic effects of anti-arrhythmic drugs tend to be additive. Therefore special care should be taken if two or more are used, especially if myocardial function is impaired. Most drugs that are effective in countering arrhythmias can also provoke them in some circumstances; moreover, hypokalaemia enhances the arrhythmogenic (pro-arrhythmic) effect of many drugs.

Adenosine is the treatment of choice for terminating supraventricular tachycardias, including those associated with accessory conducting pathways (e.g. Wolff-Parkinson-White syndrome). It is also used in the diagnosis of supraventricular arrhythmias. It is not negatively inotropic and does not cause significant hypotension. The injection should be administered by rapid intravenous injection into a central or large peripheral vein.

Amiodarone hydrochloride is useful in the management of both supraventricular and ventricular tachyarrhythmias. It can be given by intravenous infusion and by mouth, and causes little or no myocardial depression. Unlike oral amiodarone hydrochloride, intravenous amiodarone hydrochloride acts relatively rapidly. Intravenous amiodarone hydrochloride is also used in cardiopulmonary resuscitation for ventricular fibrillation or pulseless ventricular tachycardia unresponsive to d.c. shock.

Amiodarone hydrochloride has a very long half-life (extending to several weeks) and only needs to be given once daily (but high doses may cause nausea unless divided). Many weeks or months may be required to achieve steady state plasma-amiodarone concentration; this is particularly important when drug interactions are likely.

Beta-blockers act as anti-arrhythmic drugs principally by attenuating the effects of the sympathetic system on automaticity and conductivity within the heart. Sotalol hydrochloride has a role in the management of ventricular arrhythmias.

Oral administration of digoxin slows the ventricular rate in atrial fibrillation and in atrial flutter. However, intravenous infusion of digoxin is rarely effective for rapid control of ventricular rate.

Flecainide acetate is useful for the treatment of resistant re-entry supraventricular tachycardia, ventricular tachycardia, ventricular ectopic beats, arrhythmias associated with accessory conducting pathways (e.g. Wolff-Parkinson- White syndrome), and paroxysmal atrial fibrillation. Flecainide acetate crosses the placenta and can be used to control fetal supraventricular arrhythmias.

Lidocaine hydrochloride can be used in cardiopulmonary resuscitation in children with ventricular fibrillation or pulseless ventricular tachycardia unresponsive to d.c. shock, but only if amiodarone hydrochloride is not available. Doses may need to be reduced in children with persistently poor cardiac output and hepatic or renal failure.

Verapamil hydrochloride can cause severe haemodynamic compromise (refractory hypotension and cardiac arrest) when used for the acute treatment of arrhythmias in neonates and infants; it is contra-indicated in children under 1 year. It is also contra-indicated in those with congestive heart failure, syndromes associated with accessory conducting pathways (e.g. Wolff-Parkinson-White syndrome) and in most receiving concomitant beta-blockers. It can be useful in older children with supraventricular tachycardia.

Drugs used for Arrhythmias not listed below Atropine sulfate p. 764 · Metoprolol tartrate, p. 98 · Propranolol hydrochloride p. 96

ANTIARRHYTHMICS ⟩ CLASS IB

Lidocaine hydrochloride
(Lignocaine hydrochloride)

- **INDICATIONS AND DOSE**

Ventricular arrhythmias | Pulseless ventricular tachycardia | Ventricular fibrillation
▶ INITIALLY BY INTRAVENOUS INJECTION, OR BY INTRAOSSEOUS INJECTION

▶ Neonate: Initially 0.5–1 mg/kg, followed immediately by (by intravenous infusion) 0.6–3 mg/kg/hour, alternatively (by intravenous injection or by intraosseous injection) 0.5–1 mg/kg repeated at intervals of not less than 5 minutes if infusion is not immediately available following initial injection, until infusion can be initiated; maximum 3 mg/kg per course.

▶ Child 1 month-11 years: Initially 0.5–1 mg/kg, followed immediately by (by intravenous infusion) 0.6–3 mg/kg/hour, alternatively (by intravenous injection or by intraosseous injection) 0.5–1 mg/kg repeated at intervals of not less than 5 minutes if infusion is not immediately available following initial injection, until infusion can be initiated; maximum 3 mg/kg per course

▶ Child 12-17 years: Initially 50–100 mg, followed by (by intravenous infusion) 120 mg, dose to be given over 30 minutes, then (by intravenous infusion) 240 mg, dose to be given over 2 hours, then (by intravenous infusion) 60 mg/hour, reduce dose further if infusion is continued beyond 24 hours, if infusion not immediately available following initial injection, the initial injection dose may be repeated at intervals of not less than 5 minutes (to a maximum 300 mg dose in 1 hour) until infusion can be initiated

Neonatal seizures
▶ BY INTRAVENOUS INFUSION

▶ Neonate: Initially 2 mg/kg, dose to be given over 10 minutes, followed by 6 mg/kg/hour for 6 hours; reduced to 4 mg/kg/hour for 12 hours, then reduced to 2 mg/kg/hour for a further 12 hours, preterm neonates may require lower doses.

- **UNLICENSED USE** Not licensed for use in children under 1 year.
- **CONTRA-INDICATIONS** All grades of atrioventricular block · severe myocardial depression · sino-atrial disorders
- **CAUTIONS** Acute porphyria (consider infusion with glucose for its anti-porphyrinogenic effects) · congestive cardiac failure (consider lower dose) · post cardiac surgery (consider lower dose)
- **INTERACTIONS** → Appendix 1 (lidocaine).
- **SIDE-EFFECTS**
▶ **Common or very common** Bradycardia (may lead to cardiac arrest) · confusion · convulsions · dizziness (particularly if injection too rapid) · drowsiness (particularly if injection too rapid) · hypotension (may lead to cardiac arrest) · paraesthesia (particularly if injection too rapid) · respiratory depression
▶ **Rare** Anaphylaxis
- **PREGNANCY** Crosses the placenta but not known to be harmful in *animal* studies—use if benefit outweighs risk.
- **BREAST FEEDING** Present in milk but amount too small to be harmful.
- **HEPATIC IMPAIRMENT** Caution—increased risk of side-effects.
- **RENAL IMPAIRMENT** Possible accumulation of lidocaine and active metabolite; caution in severe impairment.

● **MONITORING REQUIREMENTS**
▶ Monitor ECG and have resuscitation facilities available.
● **DIRECTIONS FOR ADMINISTRATION** For *intravenous infusion*, dilute with Glucose 5% or Sodium Chloride 0.9%.

● **MEDICINAL FORMS**
There can be variation in the licensing of different medicines containing the same drug. Forms available from special-order manufacturers include: solution for injection
Solution for injection
▶ Lidocaine hydrochloride (Non-proprietary)
Lidocaine hydrochloride 5 mg per 1 ml Lidocaine 50mg/10ml (0.5%) solution for injection ampoules | 10 ampoule PoM £7.00
Lidocaine hydrochloride 10 mg per 1 ml Lidocaine 100mg/10ml (1%) solution for injection Mini-Plasco ampoules | 20 ampoule PoM £10.89
Lidocaine 100mg/10ml (1%) solution for injection ampoules | 10 ampoule PoM £4.50 DT price = £4.01
Lidocaine 100mg/10ml (1%) solution for injection Sure-Amp ampoules | 20 ampoule PoM £8.80
Lidocaine 200mg/20ml (1%) solution for injection vials | 10 vial PoM £18.00–£19.00
Lidocaine 200mg/20ml (1%) solution for injection ampoules | 10 ampoule PoM £7.00–£8.75 DT price = £8.75
Lidocaine 50mg/5ml (1%) solution for injection ampoules | 10 ampoule PoM £2.35–£3.10 DT price = £2.36
Lidocaine 20mg/2ml (1%) solution for injection ampoules | 10 ampoule PoM £3.50 DT price = £1.98
Lidocaine 50mg/5ml (1%) solution for injection Sure-Amp ampoules | 20 ampoule PoM £6.00
Lidocaine hydrochloride 20 mg per 1 ml Lidocaine 100mg/5ml (2%) solution for injection ampoules | 10 ampoule PoM £2.40–£3.80 DT price = £2.41
Lidocaine 400mg/20ml (2%) solution for injection vials | 10 vial PoM £18.50–£19.50
Lidocaine 200mg/10ml (2%) solution for injection Mini-Plasco ampoules | 20 ampoule PoM £14.52
Lidocaine 40mg/2ml (2%) solution for injection ampoules | 10 ampoule PoM £4.00 DT price = £2.11
Lidocaine 100mg/5ml (2%) solution for injection Sure-Amp ampoules | 20 ampoule PoM £6.00
Lidocaine 400mg/20ml (2%) solution for injection ampoules | 10 ampoule PoM £8.00–£9.00 DT price = £9.00

ANTIARRHYTHMICS > CLASS IC

Flecainide acetate

● **INDICATIONS AND DOSE**
Supraventricular arrhythmias
▶ BY MOUTH USING MODIFIED-RELEASE MEDICINES
▶ Child 12–17 years: 200 mg daily
Resistant re-entry supraventricular tachycardia | Ventricular ectopic beats or ventricular tachycardia | Arrhythmias associated with accessory conduction pathways (e.g. Wolff-Parkinson-White syndrome) | Paroxysmal atrial fibrillation
▶ BY MOUTH USING IMMEDIATE-RELEASE MEDICINES
▶ Neonate: 2 mg/kg 2–3 times a day, adjusted according to response, also adjust dose according to plasma-flecainide concentration.
▶ Child 1 month–11 years: 2 mg/kg 2–3 times a day, adjusted according to response, also adjust dose according to plasma-flecainide concentration,; maximum 8 mg/kg per day; maximum 300 mg per day
▶ Child 12–17 years: Initially 50–100 mg twice daily; increased if necessary up to 300 mg daily, maximum 400 mg daily for ventricular arrhythmias in heavily built children
▶ INITIALLY BY SLOW INTRAVENOUS INJECTION, OR BY INTRAVENOUS INFUSION
▶ Neonate: Initially 1–2 mg/kg, dose to be given over 10–30 minutes, followed by (by continuous intravenous infusion) 100–250 micrograms/kg/hour if required until arrhythmia controlled, transfer to oral treatment following intravenous treatment.

▶ Child 1 month–11 years: Initially 2 mg/kg, dose to be given over 10–30 minutes, followed by (by continuous intravenous infusion) 100–250 micrograms/kg/hour if required until arrhythmia controlled, maximum cumulative dose of 600 mg in the first 24 hours, transfer patient to oral treatment following intravenous treatment
▶ Child 12–17 years: Initially 2 mg/kg (max. per dose 150 mg), dose to be given over 10–30 minutes, followed by (by continuous intravenous infusion) 1.5 mg/kg/hour if required for 1 hour, then (by continuous intravenous infusion) reduced to 100–250 micrograms/kg/hour until arrhythmia controlled, maximum cumulative dose of 600 mg in the first 24 hours, transfer patient to oral treatment following intravenous treatment

DOSE EQUIVALENCE AND CONVERSION
Patients stabilised on 200 mg daily immediate-release flecainide may be transferred to modified-release medicines.

● **UNLICENSED USE** Not licensed for use in children under 12 years.

● **CONTRA-INDICATIONS** Abnormal left ventricular function · atrial conduction defects (unless pacing rescue available) · bundle branch block (unless pacing rescue available) · control of arrhythmias in acute situations (for modified-release forms only) · distal block (unless pacing rescue available) · haemodynamically significant valvular heart disease · heart failure · long-standing atrial fibrillation where conversion to sinus rhythm not attempted · second-degree or greater AV block (unless pacing rescue available) · sinus node dysfunction (unless pacing rescue available)

● **CAUTIONS** Atrial fibrillation following heart surgery · patients with pacemakers (especially those who may be pacemaker dependent because stimulation threshold may rise appreciably)

● **INTERACTIONS** → Appendix 1 (flecainide).

● **SIDE-EFFECTS**
▶ **Common or very common** Asthenia · dizziness · dyspnoea · fatigue · fever · oedema · pro-arrhythmic effects · visual disturbances
▶ **Rare** Amnesia · confusion · convulsions · depression · dyskinesia · hallucinations · peripheral neuropathy · pneumonitis
▶ **Frequency not known** Anaemia · anorexia · anxiety · ataxia · corneal deposits · drowsiness · flushing · gastrointestinal disturbances · headache · hepatic dysfunction · hypersensitivity reactions · hypoaesthesia · increased antinuclear antibodies · increased sweating · insomnia · leucopenia · paraesthesia · photosensitivity · rash · syncope · thrombocytopenia · tinnitus · tremor · urticaria · vertigo

● **PREGNANCY** Used in pregnancy to treat maternal and fetal arrhythmias in specialist centres; toxicity reported in *animal* studies; infant hyperbilirubinaemia also reported.

● **BREAST FEEDING** Significant amount present in milk but not known to be harmful.

● **HEPATIC IMPAIRMENT** Avoid or reduce dose in severe impairment. Monitor plasma-flecainide concentration.

● **RENAL IMPAIRMENT** Reduce dose by 25–50% if estimated glomerular filtration rate less than 35 mL/minute/1.73 m². Monitor plasma-flecainide concentration.

● **MONITORING REQUIREMENTS**
▶ Plasma-flecainide concentration for optimal response 200–800 micrograms/litre; blood sample should be taken immediately before next dose.
▶ With intravenous use ECG monitoring and resuscitation facilities must be available.

- **DIRECTIONS FOR ADMINISTRATION**
- ▸ With oral use For administration *by mouth*, milk, infant formula, and dairy products may reduce absorption of flecainide—separate doses from feeds. Liquid has a local anaesthetic effect and should be given at least 30 minutes before or after food. Do not store liquid in refrigerator as precipitation occurs.
- ▸ With intravenous use For *intravenous administration* give initial dose over 30 minutes in children with sustained ventricular tachycardia or cardiac failure. Dilute injection using Glucose 5%; concentrations of more than 300 micrograms/mL are unstable in chloride-containing solutions.

- **PATIENT AND CARER ADVICE**
  Medicines for Children leaflet: Flecainide for arrhythmias
  www.medicinesforchildren.org.uk/flecainide-for-arrhythmias

- **MEDICINAL FORMS**
  There can be variation in the licensing of different medicines containing the same drug. Forms available from special-order manufacturers include: oral suspension, oral solution

  Tablet
  - ▸ Flecainide acetate (Non-proprietary)
    Flecainide acetate 50 mg Flecainide 50mg tablets | 60 tablet PoM £19.50 DT price = £3.02
    Flecainide acetate 100 mg Flecainide 100mg tablets | 60 tablet PoM £29.00 DT price = £3.89
  - ▸ Tambocor (Meda Pharmaceuticals Ltd)
    Flecainide acetate 50 mg Tambocor 50mg tablets | 60 tablet PoM £11.57 DT price = £3.02
    Flecainide acetate 100 mg Tambocor 100mg tablets | 60 tablet PoM £16.53 DT price = £3.89

  Modified-release capsule
  CAUTIONARY AND ADVISORY LABELS 25
  - ▸ Tambocor XL (Meda Pharmaceuticals Ltd)
    Flecainide acetate 200 mg Tambocor XL 200mg capsules | 30 capsule PoM £14.77

  Solution for injection
  - ▸ Tambocor (Meda Pharmaceuticals Ltd)
    Flecainide acetate 10 mg per 1 ml Tambocor 150mg/15ml solution for injection ampoules | 5 ampoule PoM £21.99

ANTIARRHYTHMICS ⟩ CLASS III

▌Amiodarone hydrochloride

- **INDICATIONS AND DOSE**
  Supraventricular and ventricular arrhythmias (initiated in hospital or under specialist supervision)
  ▸ BY MOUTH

- ▸ Neonate: Initially 5–10 mg/kg twice daily for 7–10 days, then reduced to 5–10 mg/kg daily.

- ▸ Child 1 month–11 years: Initially 5–10 mg/kg twice daily (max. per dose 200 mg) for 7–10 days, then reduced to 5–10 mg/kg once daily; maximum 200 mg per day

- ▸ Child 12–17 years: 200 mg 3 times a day for 1 week, then 200 mg twice daily for 1 week, then usually 200mg daily adjusted according to response
  ▸ BY INTRAVENOUS INFUSION

- ▸ Neonate: Initially 5 mg/kg, then 5 mg/kg every 12–24 hours, dose to be given over 30 minutes.

- ▸ Child: Initially 5–10 mg/kg, dose to be given over 20 minutes to 2 hours, then (by continuous intravenous infusion) 300 micrograms/kg/hour, adjusted according to response; (by continuous intravenous infusion) increased if necessary up to 1.5 mg/kg/hour; maximum 1.2 g per day

Ventricular fibrillation or pulseless ventricular tachycardia refractory to defibrillation (for cardiopulmonary resuscitation)
▸ BY INTRAVENOUS INJECTION

- ▸ Neonate: 5 mg/kg, dose to be given over at least 3 minutes.

- ▸ Child: 5 mg/kg (max. per dose 300 mg), dose to be given over at least 3 minutes

- **UNLICENSED USE** Not licensed for use in children under 3 years.

- **CONTRA-INDICATIONS**
  GENERAL CONTRA-INDICATIONS
  Avoid in severe conduction disturbances (unless pacemaker fitted) · avoid in sinus node disease (unless pacemaker fitted) · avoid rapid loading after cardiac surgery · iodine sensitivity · sino-atrial heart block (except in cardiac arrest) · sinus bradycardia (except in cardiac arrest) · thyroid dysfunction
  SPECIFIC CONTRA-INDICATIONS
  - ▸ With intravenous use Avoid bolus injection in cardiomyopathy · avoid bolus injection in congestive heart failure · avoid in circulatory collapse · avoid in severe arterial hypotension · avoid in severe respiratory failure

- **CAUTIONS**
  GENERAL CAUTIONS
  Acute porphyrias p. 562 · conduction disturbances (in excessive dosage) · heart failure · hypokalaemia · severe bradycardia (in excessive dosage)
  SPECIFIC CAUTIONS
  - ▸ With intravenous use Avoid benzyl alcohol containing injections in neonates (in neonates) · moderate and transient fall in blood pressure (circulatory collapse precipitated by rapid administration or overdosage) · severe hepatocellular toxicity

- **INTERACTIONS** → Appendix 1 (amiodarone).
  Amiodarone has a long half-life; there is a potential for drug interactions to occur for several weeks (or even months) after treatment with it has been stopped. Use extreme caution or avoid concomitant use of drugs that prolong QT interval.

- **SIDE-EFFECTS**
  GENERAL SIDE-EFFECTS
  - ▸ **Common or very common** Bradycardia · hyperthyroidism · hypothyroidism · jaundice · nausea · persistent slate grey skin discoloration · phototoxicity · pulmonary toxicity (including pneumonitis and fibrosis) · raised serum transaminases (may require dose reduction or withdrawal if accompanied by acute liver disorders) · reversible corneal microdeposits (sometimes with night glare) · sleep disorders · taste disturbances · tremor · vomiting
  - ▸ **Uncommon** Conduction disturbances · onset or worsening of arrhythmia · peripheral myopathy (usually reversible on withdrawal) · peripheral neuropathy (usually reversible on withdrawal)
  - ▸ **Very rare** Alopecia · aplastic anaemia · ataxia · benign intracranial hypertension · bronchospasm (in patients with severe respiratory failure) · chronic liver disease · cirrhosis · epididymo-orchitis · exfoliative dermatitis · haemolytic anaemia · headache · hypersensitivity · impaired vision due to optic neuritis or optic neuropathy (including blindness) · impotence · rash · sinus arrest · thrombocytopenia · vasculitis · vertigo
  - ▸ **Frequency not known** Hot flushes · hypotension · respiratory distress syndrome · sweating
    SPECIFIC SIDE-EFFECTS
  - ▸ **Very rare**
  - ▸ With intravenous use Anaphylaxis on rapid injection

SIDE-EFFECTS, FURTHER INFORMATION

▸ Corneal microdeposits Most patients taking amiodarone develop corneal microdeposits (reversible on withdrawal of treatment); these rarely interfere with vision, but drivers may be dazzled by headlights at night. However, if vision is impaired or if optic neuritis or optic neuropathy occur, amiodarone must be stopped to prevent blindness and expert advice sought.

▸ Thyroid function Amiodarone contains iodine and can cause disorders of thyroid function; both hypothyroidism and hyperthyroidism can occur. Thyrotoxicosis may be very refractory, and amiodarone should usually be withdrawn at least temporarily to help achieve control; treatment with carbimazole may be required. Hypothyroidism can be treated with replacement therapy without withdrawing amiodarone if it is essential; careful supervision is required.

▸ Hepatotoxicity Amiodarone is also associated with hepatotoxicity and treatment should be discontinued if severe liver function abnormalities or clinical signs of liver disease develop.

▸ Pulmonary toxicity Pneumonitis should always be suspected if new or progressive shortness of breath or cough develops in a patient taking amiodarone.

▸ Peripheral neuropathy Fresh neurological symptoms should raise the possibility of peripheral neuropathy.

● **PREGNANCY** Possible risk of neonatal goitre; use only if no alternative.

● **BREAST FEEDING** Avoid; present in milk in significant amounts; theoretical risk of neonatal hypothyroidism from release of iodine.

● **MONITORING REQUIREMENTS**

▸ Thyroid function tests should be performed before treatment and then every 6 months. Clinical assessment of thyroid function alone is unreliable. Thyroxine (T4) may be raised in the absence of hyperthyroidism; therefore tri-iodothyronine (T3), T4, and thyroid-stimulating hormone (thyrotrophin, TSH) should all be measured. A raised T3 and T4 with a very low or undetectable TSH concentration suggests the development of thyrotoxicosis.

▸ Liver function tests required before treatment and then every 6 months.

▸ Serum potassium concentration should be measured before treatment.

▸ Chest x-ray required before treatment.

▸ Pulmonary function tests required before treatment.

▸ With intravenous use ECG monitoring and resuscitation facilities must be available. Monitor liver transaminases closely.

● **DIRECTIONS FOR ADMINISTRATION**

▸ With intravenous use Intravenous administration via central venous catheter recommended if repeated or continuous infusion required, as infusion via peripheral veins may cause pain and inflammation. For *intravenous infusion*, dilute to a concentration of not less than 600 micrograms/mL with Glucose 5%. Incompatible with Sodium Chloride infusion fluids; avoid equipment containing the plasticizer di-2-ethylhexphthalate (DEHP).

▸ With oral use For administration *by mouth*, tablets may be crushed and dispersed in water; injection solution should **not** be given orally (irritant).

● **PATIENT AND CARER ADVICE**

Because of the possibility of phototoxic reactions, patients should be advised to shield the skin from light during treatment and for several months after discontinuing amiodarone; a wide-spectrum sunscreen to protect against both long-wave ultraviolet and visible light should be used.

Medicines for Children leaflet: Amiodarone for abnormal heart rhythms www.medicinesforchildren.org.uk/amiodarone-for-abnormal-heart-rhythms

● **MEDICINAL FORMS**

There can be variation in the licensing of different medicines containing the same drug. Forms available from special-order manufacturers include: oral suspension, oral solution

Tablet

CAUTIONARY AND ADVISORY LABELS 11

▸ Amiodarone hydrochloride (Non-proprietary)

Amiodarone hydrochloride 100 mg Amiodarone 100mg tablets | 28 tablet [PoM] £4.25 DT price = £0.96

Amiodarone hydrochloride 200 mg Amiodarone 200mg tablets | 28 tablet [PoM] £7.80 DT price = £1.45

▸ Cordarone X (Sanofi)

Amiodarone hydrochloride 100 mg Cordarone X 100 tablets | 28 tablet [PoM] £4.28 DT price = £0.96

Amiodarone hydrochloride 200 mg Cordarone X 200 tablets | 28 tablet [PoM] £6.99 DT price = £1.45

Solution for injection

EXCIPIENTS: May contain Benzyl alcohol

▸ Amiodarone hydrochloride (Non-proprietary)

Amiodarone hydrochloride 30 mg per 1 ml Amiodarone 300mg/10ml solution for injection pre-filled syringes | 1 pre-filled disposable injection [PoM] £13.80

Amiodarone hydrochloride 50 mg per 1 ml Amiodarone 150mg/3ml concentrate for solution for injection ampoules | 10 ampoule [PoM] £15.00

▸ Cordarone X (Sanofi)

Amiodarone hydrochloride 50 mg per 1 ml Cordarone X 150mg/3ml solution for injection ampoules | 6 ampoule [PoM] £9.60

ANTIARRHYTHMICS ＞ OTHER

Adenosine

● **INDICATIONS AND DOSE**

Used in conjunction with radionuclide myocardial perfusion imaging in patients who cannot exercise adequately or for whom exercise is inappropriate

▸ BY INTRAVENOUS INFUSION

▸ Child: (consult product literature)

Termination of supraventricular tachycardias, including those associated with accessory conducting pathways (e.g. Wolff-Parkinson-White syndrome) | Diagnosis of supraventricular arrhythmias

▸ BY RAPID INTRAVENOUS INJECTION

▸ Neonate: Initially 150 micrograms/kg, then increased in steps of 50–100 micrograms/kg every 1–2 minutes (max. per dose 300 micrograms/kg) if required, dose to be repeated until tachycardia terminated or maximum single dose given.

▸ Child 1–11 months: Initially 150 micrograms/kg, then increased in steps of 50–100 micrograms/kg every 1–2 minutes (max. per dose 500 micrograms/kg) if required, dose to be repeated until tachycardia terminated or maximum single dose given

▸ Child 1–11 years: Initially 100 micrograms/kg, then increased in steps of 50–100 micrograms/kg every 1–2 minutes (max. per dose 12 mg) if required, dose to be repeated until tachycardia terminated or maximum single dose given

▸ Child 12–17 years: Initially 3 mg, followed by 6 mg after 1–2 minutes if required, followed by 12 mg after 1–2 minutes if required, in some children over 12 years 3 mg dose ineffective (e.g. if a small peripheral vein is used for administration) and higher initial dose sometimes used; however, those with *heart transplant* are **very sensitive** to the effects of adenosine, and should **not** receive higher initial doses

DOSE ADJUSTMENTS DUE TO INTERACTIONS

If essential to give with dipyridamole reduce adenosine dose to a quarter of the usual dose.

● **UNLICENSED USE** *Adenocor®* licensed for treatment of paroxysmal supraventricular tachycardia in children; not licensed for diagnosis in children; *Adenoscan*® not licensed in children.

- CONTRA-INDICATIONS Asthma · decompensated heart failure · long QT syndrome · second- or third-degree AV block and sick sinus syndrome (unless pacemaker fitted) · severe hypotension
- CAUTIONS Atrial fibrillation with accessory pathway (conduction down anomalous pathway may increase) · atrial flutter with accessory pathway (conduction down anomalous pathway may increase) · autonomic dysfunction · bundle branch block · first-degree AV block · heart transplant · left main coronary artery stenosis · left to right shunt · pericardial effusion · pericarditis · QT-interval prolongation · recent myocardial infarction · severe heart failure · stenotic carotid artery disease with cerebrovascular insufficiency · stenotic valvular heart disease · uncorrected hypovolaemia
- INTERACTIONS → Appendix 1 (adenosine); also possibility of interaction with drugs tending to impair myocardial conduction.
- SIDE-EFFECTS
  ▶ **Common or very common** Angina (discontinue) · apprehension · arrhythmia (discontinue if asystole or severe bradycardia occur) · AV block · dizziness · dyspnoea · flushing · headache · nausea · sinus pause
  ▶ **Uncommon** Blurred vision · hyperventilation · metallic taste · palpitation · sweating · weakness
  ▶ **Very rare** Bronchospasm · injection-site reactions · transient worsening of intracranial hypertension
  ▶ **Frequency not known** Cardiac arrest · convulsions · hypotension (discontinue if severe) · respiratory failure (discontinue) · syncope · vomiting
- PREGNANCY Large doses may produce fetal toxicity; manufacturer advises use only if potential benefit outweighs risk.
- BREAST FEEDING No information available—unlikely to be present in milk owing to short half-life.
- MONITORING REQUIREMENTS Monitor ECG and have resuscitation facilities available.
- DIRECTIONS FOR ADMINISTRATION For *rapid intravenous injection* give over 2 seconds into central or large peripheral vein followed by rapid Sodium Chloride 0.9% flush; injection solution may be diluted with Sodium Chloride 0.9% if required.

- MEDICINAL FORMS
  There can be variation in the licensing of different medicines containing the same drug. Forms available from special-order manufacturers include: solution for injection, infusion, solution for infusion

  Solution for injection
  ELECTROLYTES: May contain Sodium
  ▶ Adenosine (Non-proprietary)
  Adenosine 3 mg per 1 ml Adenosine 6mg/2ml solution for injection vials | 6 vial [PoM] £26.70–£29.24 (Hospital only)
  ▶ Adenocor (Sanofi)
  Adenosine 3 mg per 1 ml Adenocor 6mg/2ml solution for injection vials | 6 vial [PoM] £29.94 (Hospital only)

  Solution for infusion
  ELECTROLYTES: May contain Sodium
  ▶ Adenosine (Non-proprietary)
  Adenosine 3 mg per 1 ml Adenosine 30mg/10ml solution for infusion vials | 6 vial [PoM] £70.00–£85.57 (Hospital only)
  ▶ Adenoscan (Sanofi)
  Adenosine 3 mg per 1 ml Adenosine 30mg/10ml solution for infusion vials | 6 vial [PoM] £85.57

BETA-ADRENOCEPTOR BLOCKERS 〉
NON-SELECTIVE

☞ 95

Sotalol hydrochloride

- INDICATIONS AND DOSE
  Life-threatening arrhythmias including ventricular tachyarrhythmias
  ▶ BY MOUTH
  ▶ Child 12–17 years: Initially 80 mg once daily, alternatively initially 40 mg twice daily, then increased to 80–160 mg twice daily, dose to be increased gradually at intervals of 2–3 days; higher doses of 480–640 mg daily may be required for life-threatening ventricular arrhythmias (under specialist supervision)

  Ventricular arrhythmias, life-threatening ventricular tachyarrhythmia and supraventricular arrhythmias (initiated under specialist supervision)
  ▶ BY MOUTH
  ▶ Neonate: Initially 1 mg/kg twice daily, increased if necessary up to 4 mg/kg twice daily, dose to be increased at intervals of 3–4 days.

  Atrial flutter, ventricular arrhythmias, life-threatening ventricular tachyarrhythmia and supraventricular arrhythmias (initiated under specialist supervision)
  ▶ BY MOUTH
  ▶ Child 1 month–11 years: Initially 1 mg/kg twice daily, then increased if necessary up to 4 mg/kg twice daily (max. per dose 80 mg twice daily), dose to be increased at intervals of 2–3 days
  ▶ Child 12–17 years: Initially 80 mg once daily, alternatively initially 40 mg twice daily, increased to 80–160 mg twice daily, dose to be increased gradually at intervals of 2–3 days

- UNLICENSED USE Not licensed for use in children under 12 years.

> IMPORTANT SAFETY INFORMATION
> Sotalol may prolong the QT interval, and it occasionally causes life threatening ventricular arrhythmias (**important**: particular care is required to avoid hypokalaemia in patients taking sotalol—electrolyte disturbances, particularly hypokalaemia and hypomagnesaemia should be corrected before sotalol started and during use).
>   Reduce dose or discontinue if corrected QT interval exceeds 550 msec.

- CONTRA-INDICATIONS Long QT syndrome (congenital or acquired) · torsade de pointes
- CAUTIONS Diarrhoea (severe or prolonged)
- INTERACTIONS Extreme caution or avoid concomitant use of drugs that prolong QT interval.
- SIDE-EFFECTS Arrhythmogenic (pro-arrhythmic) effect (torsade de pointes—increased risk in females)
- BREAST FEEDING Water soluble beta-blockers such as sotalol are present in breast milk in greater amounts than other beta blockers.
- RENAL IMPAIRMENT Halve normal dose if estimated glomerular filtration rate 30–60 mL/minute/1.73 m^2; use one-quarter normal dose if estimated glomerular filtration rate 10–30 mL/minute/1.73 m^2. Avoid if estimated glomerular filtration rate less than 10 mL/minute/1.73 m^2.
- MONITORING REQUIREMENTS Measurement of corrected QT interval, and monitoring of ECG and electrolytes required; correct hypokalaemia, hypomagnesaemia, or other electrolyte disturbances.

- **DIRECTIONS FOR ADMINISTRATION** For administration *by mouth*, tablets may be crushed and dispersed in water.

- **MEDICINAL FORMS**
There can be variation in the licensing of different medicines containing the same drug. Forms available from special-order manufacturers include: oral suspension, oral solution
  Tablet
  CAUTIONARY AND ADVISORY LABELS 8
  ▸ Sotalol hydrochloride (Non-proprietary)
  Sotalol hydrochloride 40 mg Sotalol 40mg tablets |
  28 tablet [PoM] £3.00 DT price = £1.09
  Sotalol hydrochloride 80 mg Sotalol 80mg tablets |
  28 tablet [PoM] £3.75 DT price = £1.30 | 56 tablet [PoM] no price available
  Sotalol hydrochloride 160 mg Sotalol 160mg tablets |
  28 tablet [PoM] £6.25 DT price = £5.93
  ▸ Beta-Cardone (Focus Pharmaceuticals Ltd)
  Sotalol hydrochloride 200 mg Beta-Cardone 200mg tablets |
  28 tablet [PoM] £2.40 DT price = £2.40
  ▸ Sotacor (Bristol-Myers Squibb Pharmaceuticals Ltd)
  Sotalol hydrochloride 80 mg Sotacor 80mg tablets |
  30 tablet [PoM] £3.28

CARDIAC GLYCOSIDES

Cardiac glycosides

Digoxin-specific antibody

Serious cases of digoxin toxicity should be discussed with the National Poisons Information Service (see further information, under Emergency treatment of poisoning p. 786). Digoxin-specific antibody p. 795 fragments are indicated for the treatment of known or strongly suspected life-threatening digoxin toxicity associated with ventricular arrhythmias or bradyarrhythmias unresponsive to atropine sulfate p. 764 and when measures beyond the withdrawal of digoxin below and correction of any electrolyte abnormalities are considered necessary.

Digoxin

Digoxin is most useful in the treatment of supraventricular tachycardias, especially for controlling ventricular response in persistent atrial fibrillation. Digoxin has a limited role in children with chronic heart failure.

For the management of atrial fibrillation, the maintenance dose of digoxin is determined on the basis of the ventricular rate at rest, which should not be allowed to fall below an acceptable level for the child.

Digoxin is now rarely used for rapid control of heart rate, even with intravenous administration, response may take many hours; persistence of tachycardia is therefore not an indication for exceeding the recommended dose. The intramuscular route is **not** recommended.

In children with heart failure who are in sinus rhythm, a loading dose may not be required.

Unwanted effects depend both on the concentration of digoxin in the plasma and on the sensitivity of the conducting system or of the myocardium, which is often increased in heart disease. It can sometimes be difficult to distinguish between toxic effects and clinical deterioration because the symptoms of both are similar. The plasma-digoxin concentration alone cannot indicate toxicity reliably, but the likelihood of toxicity increases progressively through the range 1.5 to 3 micrograms/litre for digoxin. Renal function is very important in determining digoxin dosage.

Hypokalaemia predisposes the child to digitalis toxicity and should be avoided; it is managed by giving a potassium-sparing diuretic or, if necessary, potassium supplements.

If toxicity occurs, digoxin should be withdrawn; serious manifestations require urgent specialist management. Digoxin-specific antibody fragments are available for reversal of life-threatening overdosage.

Digoxin

- **DRUG ACTION** Digoxin is a cardiac glycoside that increases the force of myocardial contraction and reduces conductivity within the atrioventricular (AV) node.

- **INDICATIONS AND DOSE**
Supraventricular arrhythmias | Chronic heart failure
  ▸ BY MOUTH
  ▸ Neonate (body-weight up to 1.5 kg): Initially 25 micrograms/kg in 3 divided doses for 24 hours, then 4–6 micrograms/kg daily in 1–2 divided doses.
  ▸ Neonate (body-weight 1.5–2.5 kg): Initially 30 micrograms/kg in 3 divided doses for 24 hours, then 4–6 micrograms/kg daily in 1–2 divided doses.
  ▸ Neonate (body-weight 2.6 kg and above): Initially 45 micrograms/kg in 3 divided doses for 24 hours, then 10 micrograms/kg daily in 1–2 divided doses.
  ▸ Child 1 month–1 year: Initially 45 micrograms/kg in 3 divided doses for 24 hours, then 10 micrograms/kg daily in 1–2 divided doses
  ▸ Child 2–4 years: Initially 35 micrograms/kg in 3 divided doses for 24 hours, then 10 micrograms/kg daily in 1–2 divided doses
  ▸ Child 5–9 years: Initially 25 micrograms/kg in 3 divided doses (max. per dose 750 micrograms) for 24 hours, then 6 micrograms/kg daily in 1–2 divided doses; maximum 250 micrograms per day
  ▸ Child 10–17 years: Initially 0.75–1.5 mg in 3 divided doses for 24 hours, then 62.5–250 micrograms daily in 1–2 divided doses, higher doses may be necessary
  ▸ BY INTRAVENOUS INFUSION
  ▸ Neonate (body-weight up to 1.5 kg): Initially 20 micrograms/kg in 3 divided doses for 24 hours, then 4–6 micrograms/kg daily in 1–2 divided doses.
  ▸ Neonate (body-weight 1.5–2.5 kg): Initially 30 micrograms/kg in 3 divided doses for 24 hours, then 4–6 micrograms/kg daily in 1–2 divided doses.
  ▸ Neonate (body-weight 2.6 kg and above): Initially 35 micrograms/kg in 3 divided doses for 24 hours, then 10 micrograms/kg daily in 1–2 divided doses.
  ▸ Child 1 month–1 year: Initially 35 micrograms/kg in 3 divided doses for 24 hours, then 10 micrograms/kg daily in 1–2 divided doses
  ▸ Child 2–4 years: Initially 35 micrograms/kg in 3 divided doses for 24 hours, then 10 micrograms/kg daily in 1–2 divided doses
  ▸ Child 5–9 years: Initially 25 micrograms/kg in 3 divided doses (max. per dose 500 micrograms) for 24 hours, then 6 micrograms/kg daily in 1–2 divided doses; maximum 250 micrograms per day
  ▸ Child 10–17 years: Initially 0.5–1 mg in 3 divided doses for 24 hours, then 62.5–250 micrograms daily in 1–2 divided doses, higher doses may be necessary

  DOSE EQUIVALENCE AND CONVERSION
  Dose may need to be reduced if digoxin (or another cardiac glycoside) has been given in the preceding 2 weeks.
  When switching from intravenous to oral route may need to increase dose by 20–33% to maintain the same plasma-digoxin concentration.

- **UNLICENSED USE** Digoxin is licensed for use in heart failure and supraventricular arrhythmias.

- **CONTRA-INDICATIONS** Constrictive pericarditis (unless to control atrial fibrillation or improve systolic dysfunction—but use with caution) · hypertrophic cardiomyopathy (unless concomitant atrial fibrillation and heart failure—

but use with caution) · intermittent complete heart block · myocarditis · second degree AV block · supraventricular arrhythmias associated with accessory conducting pathways e.g. Wolff-Parkinson-White syndrome (although can be used in infancy) · ventricular tachycardia or fibrillation

- **CAUTIONS** Avoid hypercalcaemia (risk of digitalis toxicity) · avoid hypokalaemia (risk of digitalis toxicity) · avoid hypomagnesaemia (risk of digitalis toxicity) · avoid hypoxia (risk of digitalis toxicity) · severe respiratory disease · sick sinus syndrome · thyroid disease

- **INTERACTIONS** → Appendix 1 (cardiac glycosides).

- **SIDE-EFFECTS**
- **Common or very common** Arrhythmias · blurred vision · conduction disturbances · diarrhoea · dizziness · eosinophilia · nausea · rash · vomiting · yellow vision
- **Uncommon** Depression
- **Very rare** Anorexia · apathy · confusion · fatigue · gynaecomastia on long-term use · headache · intestinal ischaemia and necrosis · psychosis · thrombocytopenia · weakness

Overdose
If toxicity occurs, digoxin should be withdrawn; serious manifestations require urgent specialist management.

- **PREGNANCY** May need dosage adjustment.
- **BREAST FEEDING** Amount too small to be harmful.
- **RENAL IMPAIRMENT** Use half normal dose if estimated glomerular filtration rate is 10–50 mL/minute/1.73 m^2 and use a quarter normal dose if estimated glomerular filtration rate is less than 10 mL/minute/1.73 m^2. Monitor plasma-digoxin concentration in renal impairment.

- **MONITORING REQUIREMENTS**
- For plasma-digoxin concentration assay, blood should be taken at least 6 hours after a dose.
- Plasma-digoxin concentration should be maintained in the range 0.8–2 micrograms/litre.
- Monitor serum electrolytes and renal function. Toxicity increased by electrolyte disturbances.

- **DIRECTIONS FOR ADMINISTRATION**
- With intravenous use Avoid rapid intravenous administration (risk of hypertension and reduced coronary flow). For *intravenous infusion*, dilute with Sodium Chloride 0.9% or Glucose 5% to a max. concentration of 62.5 micrograms/mL; loading doses should be given over 30–60 minutes and maintenance dose over 10–20 minutes.
- With oral use For *oral* administration, oral solution must **not** be diluted.

- **PATIENT AND CARER ADVICE** Patient counselling is advised for digoxin elixir (use pipette).

- **MEDICINAL FORMS**
There can be variation in the licensing of different medicines containing the same drug. Forms available from special-order manufacturers include: oral suspension, oral solution, solution for injection

Tablet
- Digoxin (Non-proprietary)
  Digoxin 62.5 microgram Digoxin 62.5microgram tablets | 28 tablet [PoM] £9.99 DT price = £2.87 | 500 tablet [PoM] no price available
  Digoxin 125 microgram Digoxin 125microgram tablets | 28 tablet [PoM] £5.02 DT price = £3.02
  Digoxin 250 microgram Digoxin 250microgram tablets | 28 tablet [PoM] £5.09 DT price = £2.85 | 500 tablet [PoM] no price available
- Lanoxin (Aspen Pharma Trading Ltd)
  Digoxin 62.5 microgram Lanoxin PG 62.5microgram tablets | 500 tablet [PoM] £8.09
  Digoxin 125 microgram Lanoxin 125 tablets | 500 tablet [PoM] £8.09
  Digoxin 250 microgram Lanoxin 250microgram tablets | 500 tablet [PoM] £8.09

Oral solution
- Lanoxin (Aspen Pharma Trading Ltd)
  Digoxin 50 microgram per 1 ml Lanoxin PG 50micrograms/ml elixir | 60 ml [PoM] £5.35 DT price = £5.35

Solution for injection
EXCIPIENTS: May contain Alcohol, propylene glycol
- Digoxin (Non-proprietary)
  Digoxin 100 microgram per 1 ml Lanoxin Injection Pediatric 100micrograms/1ml solution for injection ampoules | 10 ampoule [PoM] no price available

Solution for infusion
- Digoxin (Non-proprietary)
  Digoxin 250 microgram per 1 ml Digoxin 500micrograms/2ml solution for infusion ampoules | 10 ampoule [PoM] £7.00
- Lanoxin (Aspen Pharma Trading Ltd)
  Digoxin 250 microgram per 1 ml Lanoxin 500micrograms/2ml solution for infusion ampoules | 5 ampoule [PoM] £3.30

2 Bleeding disorders

Antifibrinolytic drugs and haemostatics

Overview

Fibrin dissolution can be impaired by the administration of tranexamic acid below, which inhibits fibrinolysis. It can be used to prevent bleeding or treat bleeding associated with excessive fibrinolysis (e.g. in surgery, dental extraction, obstetric disorders, and traumatic hyphaema) and in the management of menorrhagia; it may also be used in hereditary angioedema, epistaxis, and thrombolytic overdose. Tranexamic acid can also be used in cardiac surgery to reduce blood loss and to reduce the need for use of blood products.

Desmopressin p. 403 is used in the management of mild to moderate haemophilia and von Willebrand's disease. It is also used for fibrinolytic response testing.

ANTIHAEMORRHAGICS > ANTIFIBRINOLYTICS

Tranexamic acid

- **INDICATIONS AND DOSE**
Inhibition of fibrinolysis
- BY MOUTH
- **Child:** 15–25 mg/kg 2–3 times a day (max. per dose 1.5 g)
- BY SLOW INTRAVENOUS INJECTION
- **Child:** 10 mg/kg 2–3 times a day (max. per dose 1 g), dose to be given over at least 10 minutes
- BY CONTINUOUS INTRAVENOUS INFUSION
- **Child:** 45 mg/kg, dose to be given over 24 hours

Menorrhagia
- BY MOUTH
- **Child 12-17 years:** 1 g 3 times a day for up to 4 days, to be initiated when menstruation has started; maximum 4 g per day

Hereditary angioedema
- BY MOUTH
- **Child:** 15–25 mg/kg 2–3 times a day (max. per dose 1.5 g), for short-term prophylaxis of hereditary angioedema, tranexamic acid is started several days before planned procedures which may trigger an acute attack of hereditary angioedema (e.g. dental work) and continued for 2–5 days afterwards
- BY SLOW INTRAVENOUS INJECTION
- **Child:** 10 mg/kg 2–3 times a day (max. per dose 1 g), dose to be given over at least 10 minutes

▸ BY CONTINUOUS INTRAVENOUS INFUSION
▸ Child: 45 mg/kg, dose to be given over 24 hours

Prevention of excessive bleeding after dental procedures (e.g. in haemophilia)

▸ BY INTRAVENOUS INJECTION
▸ Child 6–17 years: 10 mg/kg (max. per dose 1.5 g), dose to be given pre-operatively

▸ BY MOUTH
▸ Child 6–17 years: 15–25 mg/kg (max. per dose 1.5 g), dose to be given pre-operatively, then 15–25 mg/kg 2–3 times a day (max. per dose 1.5 g) for up to 8 days, dose to be given postoperatively

Prevention of excessive bleeding after dental procedures (e.g. in haemophilia) with mouthwash 5% solution (specialist use only)

▸ BY MOUTH
▸ Child 6–17 years: 5–10 mL 4 times a day for 2 days, rinse mouth with solution; the solution should not be swallowed

Reduction of blood loss during cardiac surgery

▸ BY SLOW INTRAVENOUS INJECTION, OR BY INTRAVENOUS INFUSION
▸ Child: (consult local protocol)

● **UNLICENSED USE** Not licensed for reduction of blood loss during cardiac surgery; injection not licensed for use in children under 1 year or for administration by intravenous infusion.

● **CONTRA-INDICATIONS** Fibrinolytic conditions following disseminated intravascular coagulation (unless predominant activation of fibrinolytic system with severe bleeding) · history of convulsions · thromboembolic disease

● **CAUTIONS** Irregular menstrual bleeding (establish cause before initiating therapy) · massive haematuria (avoid if risk of ureteric obstruction) · patients receiving oral contraceptives (increased risk of thrombosis)

CAUTIONS, FURTHER INFORMATION
▸ **Menorrhagia** Before initiating treatment for menorrhagia, exclude structural or histological causes or fibroids causing distortion of uterine cavity.

● **SIDE-EFFECTS**
▸ **Common or very common** Diarrhoea (reduce dose) · nausea · vomiting
▸ **Uncommon** Dermatitis
▸ **Rare** Impairment of colour vision (discontinue) · thromboembolic events · visual disturbances (discontinue)
▸ **Frequency not known** Convulsions (usually with high doses) · hypotension (on rapid intravenous injection) · malaise (on rapid intravenous injection)

● **PREGNANCY** No evidence of teratogenicity in *animal* studies; manufacturer advises use only if potential benefit outweighs risk—crosses the placenta.

● **BREAST FEEDING** Small amount present in milk—antifibrinolytic effect in infant unlikely.

● **RENAL IMPAIRMENT** Reduce dose in mild to moderate impairment. Avoid in severe impairment.

● **MONITORING REQUIREMENTS** Regular liver function tests in long-term treatment of hereditary angioedema.

● **DIRECTIONS FOR ADMINISTRATION** For *intravenous administration*, dilute with Glucose 5% *or* Sodium chloride 0.9%.

● **PATIENT AND CARER ADVICE**
Medicines for Children leaflet: Tranexamic acid for heavy bleeding during periods www.medicinesforchildren.org.uk/tranexamic-acid-for-heavy-bleeding-during-periods
Medicines for Children leaflet: Tranexamic acid for treatment for prevention of bleeding www.medicinesforchildren.org.uk/tranexamic-acid-for-treatment-or-prevention-of-bleeding

● **MEDICINAL FORMS**
There can be variation in the licensing of different medicines containing the same drug. Forms available from special-order manufacturers include: oral suspension, oral solution, mouthwash

Tablet
▸ Tranexamic acid (Non-proprietary)
 Tranexamic acid 500 mg Tranexamic acid 500mg tablets | 60 tablet [PoM] £18.87 DT price = £4.42
▸ Cyklokapron (Meda Pharmaceuticals Ltd)
 Tranexamic acid 500 mg Cyklokapron 500mg tablets | 60 tablet [PoM] £14.30 DT price = £4.42

Solution for injection
▸ Tranexamic acid (Non-proprietary)
 Tranexamic acid 100 mg per 1 ml Tranexamic acid 500mg/5ml solution for injection ampoules | 5 ampoule [PoM] £7.50 (Hospital only) | 10 ampoule [PoM] £15.47 (Hospital only)
▸ Cyklokapron (Pfizer Ltd)
 Tranexamic acid 100 mg per 1 ml Cyklokapron 500mg/5ml solution for injection ampoules | 10 ampoule [PoM] £15.47

2.1 Coagulation factor deficiencies

BLOOD AND RELATED PRODUCTS ⟩
COAGULATION PROTEINS

Dried prothrombin complex

(Human prothrombin complex)

● **INDICATIONS AND DOSE**

Treatment and peri-operative prophylaxis of haemorrhage in patients with congenital deficiency of factors II, VII, IX, or X if purified specific coagulation factors not available | Treatment and peri-operative prophylaxis of haemorrhage in patients with acquired deficiency of factors II, VII, IX, or X (e.g. during warfarin treatment)

▸ BY INTRAVENOUS INFUSION
▸ Child: (consult haematologist)

● **CONTRA-INDICATIONS** Angina · history of heparin induced thrombocytopenia · recent myocardial infarction (except in life-threatening haemorrhage following overdosage of oral anticoagulants, and before induction of fibrinolytic therapy)

● **CAUTIONS** Disseminated intravascular coagulation · history of myocardial infarction or coronary heart disease · postoperative use · risk of thrombosis · vaccination against hepatitis A and hepatitis B may be required

● **SIDE-EFFECTS**
▸ **Rare** Headache
▸ **Very rare** Anaphylaxis · antibody formation · hypersensitivity reactions · pyrexia
▸ **Frequency not known** Disseminated intravascular coagulation · nephrotic syndrome · thrombotic events

● **HEPATIC IMPAIRMENT** Monitor closely in hepatic impairment (risk of thromboembolic complications).

● **PRESCRIBING AND DISPENSING INFORMATION** Dried prothrombin complex is prepared from human plasma by a suitable fractionation technique, and contains factor IX, together with variable amounts of factors II, VII, and X.
  Available from CSL Behring (*Beriplix® P/N*), Octapharma (*Octaplex®*).

● **MEDICINAL FORMS**
There can be variation in the licensing of different medicines containing the same drug.
No licensed medicines identified.

Factor IX fraction, dried

- **INDICATIONS AND DOSE**

Treatment and prophylaxis of haemorrhage in congenital factor IX deficiency (haemophilia B)
  - ▸ BY INTRAVENOUS INJECTION, OR BY CONTINUOUS INTRAVENOUS INFUSION
  - ▸ Child: (consult haematologist)

- **CONTRA-INDICATIONS** Disseminated intravascular coagulation

- **CAUTIONS** Risk of thrombosis—principally with former low purity products · vaccination against hepatitis A and hepatitis B may be required (not necessary with recombinant preparation)

- **SIDE-EFFECTS** Allergic reactions · chills · dizziness · fever · gastro-intestinal disturbances · headache

- **PRESCRIBING AND DISPENSING INFORMATION** Dried factor IX fraction is prepared from human plasma by a suitable fractionation technique; it may also contain clotting factors II, VII, and X.

- **MEDICINAL FORMS**
There can be variation in the licensing of different medicines containing the same drug.
Powder and solvent for solution for injection
  - ▸ AlphaNine (Grifols UK Ltd)
    Factor IX high purity 1000 unit AlphaNine 1,000unit powder and solvent for solution for injection vials | 1 vial PoM £390.00
    Factor IX high purity 1500 unit AlphaNine 1,500unit powder and solvent for solution for injection vials | 1 vial PoM no price available
  - ▸ Haemonine (Biotest (UK) Ltd)
    Factor IX high purity 500 unit Haemonine 500unit powder and solvent for solution for injection vials | 1 vial PoM £255.00 (Hospital only)
    Factor IX high purity 1000 unit Haemonine 1,000unit powder and solvent for solution for injection vials | 1 vial PoM £510.00 (Hospital only)
  - ▸ Mononine (CSL Behring UK Ltd)
    Factor IX high purity 1000 unit Mononine 1,000unit powder and solvent for solution for injection vials | 1 vial PoM £478.43
  - ▸ Replenine-VF (Bio Products Laboratory Ltd)
    Factor IX high purity 500 unit Replenine-VF 500unit powder and solvent for solution for injection vials | 1 vial PoM £180.00 | 10 vial PoM no price available
    Factor IX high purity 1000 unit Replenine-VF 1,000unit powder and solvent for solution for injection vials | 1 vial PoM £360.00 | 10 vial PoM no price available

Powder and solvent for solution for infusion
  - ▸ BeneFIX (Pfizer Ltd)
    Nonacog alfa 250 unit BeneFIX 250unit powder and solvent for solution for infusion vials | 1 vial PoM £151.80 (Hospital only)
    Nonacog alfa 500 unit BeneFIX 500unit powder and solvent for solution for infusion vials | 1 vial PoM £303.60 (Hospital only)
    Nonacog alfa 1000 unit BeneFIX 1,000unit powder and solvent for solution for infusion vials | 1 vial PoM £607.20 (Hospital only)
    Nonacog alfa 2000 unit BeneFIX 2,000unit powder and solvent for solution for infusion vials | 1 vial PoM £1,214.40 (Hospital only)
    Nonacog alfa 3000 unit BeneFIX 3,000unit powder and solvent for solution for infusion vials | 1 vial PoM £1,821.60 (Hospital only)

Factor VIIa (recombinant)

(Eptacog alfa (activated))

- **INDICATIONS AND DOSE**

Treatment and prophylaxis of haemorrhage in patients with haemophilia A or B with inhibitors to factors VIII or IX, acquired haemophilia, factor VII deficiency, or Glanzmann's thrombasthenia
  - ▸ BY INTRAVENOUS INJECTION
  - ▸ Child: (consult haematologist)

- **CAUTIONS** Disseminated intravascular coagulation · risk of thrombosis

- **SIDE-EFFECTS**
  - ▸ **Very rare** Allergic reactions · cerebrovascular accident · coagulation disorders · fever · myocardial infarction · nausea · pain · rash · thrombotic events

- **MEDICINAL FORMS**
There can be variation in the licensing of different medicines containing the same drug.
Powder and solvent for solution for injection
  - ▸ NovoSeven (Novo Nordisk Ltd)
    Eptacog alfa activated 50000 unit NovoSeven 1mg (50,000units) powder and solvent for solution for injection pre-filled syringes | 1 pre-filled disposable injection PoM £525.20 (Hospital only)
    NovoSeven 1mg (50,000units) powder and solvent for solution for injection vials | 1 vial PoM £525.20 (Hospital only)
    Eptacog alfa activated 100000 unit NovoSeven 2mg (100,000units) powder and solvent for solution for injection vials | 1 vial PoM £1,050.40 (Hospital only)
    NovoSeven 2mg (100,000units) powder and solvent for solution for injection pre-filled syringes | 1 pre-filled disposable injection PoM £1,050.40 (Hospital only)
    Eptacog alfa activated 250000 unit NovoSeven 5mg (250,000units) powder and solvent for solution for injection pre-filled syringes | 1 pre-filled disposable injection PoM £2,626.00 (Hospital only)
    NovoSeven 5mg (250,000units) powder and solvent for solution for injection vials | 1 vial PoM £2,626.00 (Hospital only)
    Eptacog alfa activated 400000 unit NovoSeven 8mg (400,000units) powder and solvent for solution for injection vials | 1 vial PoM £4,201.60 (Hospital only)
    NovoSeven 8mg (400,000units) powder and solvent for solution for injection pre-filled syringes | 1 pre-filled disposable injection PoM £4,201.60 (Hospital only)

Factor VIII fraction, dried

(Human coagulation factor VIII, dried)

- **INDICATIONS AND DOSE**

Treatment and prophylaxis of haemorrhage in congenital factor VIII deficiency (haemophilia A), acquired factor VIII deficiency | Von Willebrand's disease
  - ▸ BY INTRAVENOUS INJECTION, OR BY INTRAVENOUS INFUSION, OR BY CONTINUOUS INTRAVENOUS INFUSION
  - ▸ Child: (consult haematologist)

- **CAUTIONS** Intravascular haemolysis after large or frequently repeated doses in patients with blood groups A, B, or AB—less likely with high potency concentrates · vaccination against hepatitis A and hepatitis B may be required (not necessary with recombinant preparation)

- **SIDE-EFFECTS** Anaphylaxis · angioedema · antibody formation · blurred vision · chills · coughing · dizziness · drowsiness · dyspnoea · fever · flushing · gastro-intestinal disturbances · headache · hypersensitivity reactions · hypotension · palpitation · paraesthesia · taste disturbances · urticaria

- **MONITORING REQUIREMENTS** Monitor for development of factor VIII inhibitors.

- **PRESCRIBING AND DISPENSING INFORMATION** Dried factor VIII fraction is prepared from human plasma by a suitable fractionation technique; it may also contain varying amounts of von Willebrand factor. *Optivate*®, *Fanhdi*®, and *Octanate*® are not indicated for use in von Willebrand's disease.

  Recombinant human coagulation factor VIII including octocog alfa, moroctocog alfa, and simoctocog alfa are not indicated for use in von Willebrand's disease.

- **MEDICINAL FORMS**
There can be variation in the licensing of different medicines containing the same drug.
Powder and solvent for solution for injection
  - ▸ Advate (Baxalta UK Ltd)
    Octocog alfa 250 unit Advate 250unit powder and solvent for solution for injection vials | 1 vial PoM no price available

Octocog alfa 500 unit Advate 500unit powder and solvent for solution for injection vials | 1 vial [PoM] no price available
Octocog alfa 1000 unit Advate 1,000unit powder and solvent for solution for injection vials | 1 vial [PoM] no price available
Octocog alfa 2000 unit Advate 2,000unit powder and solvent for solution for injection vials | 1 vial [PoM] no price available

▸ **Elocta** (Swedish Orphan Biovitrum Ltd) ▼
Efmoroctocog alfa 250 unit Elocta 250unit powder and solvent for solution for injection vials | 1 vial [PoM] no price available (Hospital only)
Efmoroctocog alfa 500 unit Elocta 500unit powder and solvent for solution for injection vials | 1 vial [PoM] no price available (Hospital only)
Efmoroctocog alfa 1000 unit Elocta 1,000unit powder and solvent for solution for injection vials | 1 vial [PoM] no price available (Hospital only)
Efmoroctocog alfa 1500 unit Elocta 1,500unit powder and solvent for solution for injection vials | 1 vial [PoM] no price available (Hospital only)
Efmoroctocog alfa 2000 unit Elocta 2,000unit powder and solvent for solution for injection vials | 1 vial [PoM] no price available (Hospital only)
Efmoroctocog alfa 3000 unit Elocta 3,000unit powder and solvent for solution for injection vials | 1 vial [PoM] no price available (Hospital only)

▸ **Fanhdi** (Grifols UK Ltd)
Factor VIII high purity 500 unit Fanhdi 500unit powder and solvent for solution for injection vials | 1 vial [PoM] £165.00 (Hospital only)
Factor VIII high purity 1000 unit Fanhdi 1,000unit powder and solvent for solution for injection vials | 1 vial [PoM] £330.00 (Hospital only)
Factor VIII high purity 1500 unit Fanhdi 1,500unit powder and solvent for solution for injection vials | 1 vial [PoM] £495.00

▸ **Haemoctin** (Biotest (UK) Ltd)
Factor VIII high purity 250 unit Haemoctin 250unit powder and solvent for solution for injection vials | 1 vial [PoM] £127.50 (Hospital only)
Factor VIII high purity 500 unit Haemoctin 500unit powder and solvent for solution for injection vials | 1 vial [PoM] £255.00 (Hospital only)
Factor VIII high purity 1000 unit Haemoctin 1,000unit powder and solvent for solution for injection vials | 1 vial [PoM] £510.00 (Hospital only)

▸ **Helixate NexGen** (CSL Behring UK Ltd)
Octocog alfa 250 unit Helixate NexGen 250unit powder and solvent for solution for injection vials | 1 vial [PoM] £118.57
Octocog alfa 500 unit Helixate NexGen 500unit powder and solvent for solution for injection vials | 1 vial [PoM] £237.15
Octocog alfa 1000 unit Helixate NexGen 1,000unit powder and solvent for solution for injection vials | 1 vial [PoM] £474.30
Octocog alfa 2000 unit Helixate NexGen 2,000unit powder and solvent for solution for injection vials | 1 vial [PoM] £948.60

▸ **Kogenate** (Bayer Plc)
Octocog alfa 250 unit Kogenate Bayer 250unit powder and solvent for solution for injection vials | 1 vial [PoM] £157.50
Octocog alfa 500 unit Kogenate Bayer 500unit powder and solvent for solution for injection vials | 1 vial [PoM] £315.00
Octocog alfa 1000 unit Kogenate Bayer 1,000unit powder and solvent for solution for injection vials | 1 vial [PoM] £630.00
Octocog alfa 2000 unit Kogenate Bayer 2,000unit powder and solvent for solution for injection vials | 1 vial [PoM] £1,260.00

▸ **Nuwiq** (Octapharma Ltd) ▼
Simoctocog alfa 250 unit Nuwiq 250unit powder and solvent for solution for injection vials | 1 vial [PoM] £190.00 (Hospital only)
Simoctocog alfa 500 unit Nuwiq 500unit powder and solvent for solution for injection vials | 1 vial [PoM] £380.00 (Hospital only)
Simoctocog alfa 1000 unit Nuwiq 1,000unit powder and solvent for solution for injection vials | 1 vial [PoM] £760.00 (Hospital only)
Simoctocog alfa 2000 unit Nuwiq 2,000unit powder and solvent for solution for injection vials | 1 vial [PoM] £1,520.00 (Hospital only)

Powder and solvent for solution for infusion
▸ **Advate** (Baxalta UK Ltd)
Octocog alfa 1500 unit Advate 1,500unit powder and solvent for solution for infusion vials | 1 vial [PoM] no price available
Octocog alfa 3000 unit Advate 3,000unit powder and solvent for solution for infusion vials | 1 vial [PoM] no price available
▸ **Kogenate** (Bayer Plc)
Octocog alfa 3000 unit Kogenate Bayer 3,000unit powder and solvent for solution for injection vials | 1 vial [PoM] £1,890.00

Factor XIII fraction, dried
(Human fibrin-stabilising factor, dried)

● **INDICATIONS AND DOSE**
Congenital factor XIII deficiency
▸ BY INTRAVENOUS INJECTION, OR BY INTRAVENOUS INFUSION
▸ Child: (consult haematologist)

● **CAUTIONS** Vaccination against hepatitis A and hepatitis B may be required

● **SIDE-EFFECTS**
▸ **Rare** Allergic reactions · fever

● **MEDICINAL FORMS**
There can be variation in the licensing of different medicines containing the same drug.
Powder and solvent for solution for injection
▸ **Fibrogammin P** (CSL Behring UK Ltd)
Factor XIII 250 unit Fibrogammin 250unit powder and solvent for solution for injection vials | 1 vial [PoM] £90.59
Factor XIII 1250 unit Fibrogammin 1,250unit powder and solvent for solution for injection vials | 1 vial [PoM] £452.95

Fibrinogen, dried
(Human fibrinogen)

● **INDICATIONS AND DOSE**
Treatment of haemorrhage in congenital hypofibrinogenaemia or afibrinogenaemia
▸ BY INTRAVENOUS INJECTION, OR BY INTRAVENOUS INFUSION
▸ Child: (consult haematologist)

● **CAUTIONS** Risk of thrombosis
● **SIDE-EFFECTS**
▸ **Rare** Allergic reactions · fever
▸ **Very rare** Myocardial infarction · pulmonary embolism · thromboembolic events

● **PREGNANCY** Manufacturer advises not known to be harmful—no information available.

● **BREAST FEEDING** Manufacturer advises avoid—no information available.

● **PRESCRIBING AND DISPENSING INFORMATION** Fibrinogen is prepared from human plasma.

● **MEDICINAL FORMS**
There can be variation in the licensing of different medicines containing the same drug.
Powder for solution for infusion
▸ **Riastap** (CSL Behring UK Ltd)
Fibrinogen 1 gram Riastap 1g powder for solution for infusion vials | 1 vial [PoM] £340.00

Protein C concentrate

● **INDICATIONS AND DOSE**
Congenital protein C deficiency
▸ BY INTRAVENOUS INJECTION
▸ Child: (consult haematologist)

● **CAUTIONS** Hypersensitivity to heparins · vaccination against hepatitis A and hepatitis B may be required
● **SIDE-EFFECTS**
▸ **Very rare** Bleeding · dizziness · fever · hypersensitivity reactions

● **PRESCRIBING AND DISPENSING INFORMATION** Protein C is prepared from human plasma.

2

Cardiovascular system

- **MEDICINAL FORMS**
  There can be variation in the licensing of different medicines containing the same drug.
  Powder and solvent for solution for injection
  - Ceprotin (Baxalta UK Ltd)
    Protein C 500 unit Ceprotin 500unit powder and solvent for solution for injection vials | 1 vial [PoM] no price available
    Protein C 1000 unit Ceprotin 1000unit powder and solvent for solution for injection vials | 1 vial [PoM] no price available

BLOOD AND RELATED PRODUCTS >
HAEMOSTATIC PRODUCTS

Factor VIII inhibitor bypassing fraction

- **INDICATIONS AND DOSE**
  Treatment and prophylaxis of haemorrhage in patients with congenital factor VIII deficiency (haemophilia A) and factor VIII inhibitors | Treatment of haemorrhage in non-haemophiliac patients with acquired factor VIII inhibitors
  - BY INTRAVENOUS INFUSION, OR BY INTRAVENOUS INJECTION
  - Child: (consult haematologist)

- **CONTRA-INDICATIONS** Disseminated intravascular coagulation
- **CAUTIONS** Vaccination against hepatitis A and hepatitis B may be required
- **SIDE-EFFECTS** Anaphylaxis · disseminated intravascular coagulation · flushing · hypersensitivity · hypotension · myocardial infarction · paraesthesia · pyrexia · rash · thrombosis · urticaria
- **PRESCRIBING AND DISPENSING INFORMATION** Preparations with factor VIII inhibitor bypassing activity are prepared from human plasma.

- **MEDICINAL FORMS**
  There can be variation in the licensing of different medicines containing the same drug.
  Powder and solvent for solution for injection
  - FEIBA Imuno (Baxalta UK Ltd)
    Factor VIII inhibitor bypassing fraction 500 unit FEIBA 500unit powder and solvent for solution for injection vials | 1 vial [PoM] no price available
  Powder and solvent for solution for infusion
  - FEIBA Imuno (Baxalta UK Ltd)
    Factor VIII inhibitor bypassing fraction 1000 unit FEIBA 1,000unit powder and solvent for solution for infusion vials | 1 vial [PoM] no price available

BLOOD AND RELATED PRODUCTS > PLASMA
PRODUCTS

Fresh frozen plasma

- **INDICATIONS AND DOSE**
  Replacement of coagulation factors or other plasma proteins where their concentration or functional activity is critically reduced
  - BY INTRAVENOUS INFUSION
  - Child: (consult haematologist)

- **CONTRA-INDICATIONS** Avoid use as a volume expander · IgA deficiency with confirmed antibodies to IgA
- **CAUTIONS** Cardiac decompensation · need for compatibility · pulmonary oedema · severe protein S deficiency (avoid products with low protein S activity e.g. *OctaplasLG*®) · vaccination against hepatitis A and hepatitis B may be required
- **SIDE-EFFECTS**
- **Common or very common** Nausea · pruritus · rash
- **Uncommon** Oedema · vomiting
- **Rare** Agitation · allergic reactions · bronchospasm · cardiorespiratory collapse · chills · fever · tachycardia
- **Very rare** Arrhythmia · hypertension · thromboembolism
- **PRESCRIBING AND DISPENSING INFORMATION** Fresh frozen plasma is prepared from the supernatant liquid obtained by centrifugation of one donation of whole blood.

  A preparation of solvent/detergent treated human plasma (frozen) from pooled donors is available from Octapharma (*OctaplasLG*®).

  Children under 16 years should only receive virucidally inactivated preparations of fresh frozen plasma, sourced from 'low prevalence BSE regions' such as the USA.

- **MEDICINAL FORMS**
  There can be variation in the licensing of different medicines containing the same drug.
  No licensed medicines identified.

2.2 Subarachnoid haemorrhage

CALCIUM-CHANNEL BLOCKERS

[F 99]

Nimodipine

- **DRUG ACTION** Nimodipine is a dihydropyridine calcium-channel blocker.

- **INDICATIONS AND DOSE**
  Treatment of vasospasm following subarachnoid haemorrhage (specialist use only)
  - BY INTRAVENOUS INFUSION
  - Child 1 month-11 years: Initially 15 micrograms/kg/hour (max. per dose 500 micrograms/hour), increased after 2 hours if no severe decrease in blood pressure; increased to 30 micrograms/kg/hour (max. per dose 2 mg/hour), continue for at least 5 days (max. 14 days), use initial dose of 7.5 micrograms/kg/hour if blood pressure unstable
  - Child 12-17 years (body-weight up to 70 kg): Initially 0.5 mg/hour, increased after 2 hours if no severe decrease in blood pressure; increased to 1-2 mg/hour, continue for at least 5 days (max. 14 days)
  - Child 12-17 years (body-weight 70 kg and above): Initially up to 1 mg/hour, use dose if blood pressure stable; increased after 2 hours if no severe decrease in blood pressure; increased to 1-2 mg/hour, continue for at least 5 days (max. 14 days)
  Prevention of vasospasm following subarachnoid haemorrhage
  - BY MOUTH
  - Child: 0.9-1.2 mg/kg 6 times a day (max. per dose 60 mg), started within 4 days of haemorrhage and continued for 21 days

- **UNLICENSED USE** Not licensed for use in children.
- **CONTRA-INDICATIONS** Acute porphyrias p. 562
- **CAUTIONS** Cerebral oedema · hypotension · severely raised intracranial pressure
- **INTERACTIONS** → Appendix 1 (calcium-channel blockers, alcohol (infusion only)).
  Avoid concomitant administration with other calcium-channel blockers, beta-blocker and nephrotoxic drugs.
- **SIDE-EFFECTS** Flushing · gastro-intestinal disorders · headache · hypotension · ileus · nausea · sweating and feeling of warmth · thrombocytopenia · variation in heart-rate
- **PREGNANCY** Manufacturer advises use only if potential benefit outweighs risk.

- **BREAST FEEDING** Manufacturer advises avoid—present in milk.
- **HEPATIC IMPAIRMENT**
  Monitoring
  Elimination reduced in cirrhosis—monitor blood pressure.
- **RENAL IMPAIRMENT**
  Monitoring
  ▸ With intravenous use Manufacturer advises monitor renal function closely in renal impairment.
- **DIRECTIONS FOR ADMINISTRATION** Avoid concomitant administration of nimodipine infusion and tablets.
  ▸ With oral use For administration *by mouth*, tablets may be crushed or halved but are light sensitive—administer immediately.
  ▸ With intravenous use For *continuous intravenous infusion*, administer undiluted *via* a Y-piece on a central venous catheter connected to a running infusion of Glucose 5%, or Sodium Chloride 0.9%; not to be added to an infusion container; incompatible with polyvinyl chloride giving sets or containers; protect infusion from light.
  ▸ With intravenous use Polyethylene, polypropylene, or glass apparatus should be used. PVC should be avoided.

- **MEDICINAL FORMS**
  There can be variation in the licensing of different medicines containing the same drug. Forms available from special-order manufacturers include: oral suspension
  Tablet
  ▸ Nimotop (Bayer Plc)
    Nimodipine 30 mg Nimotop 30mg tablets | 100 tablet PoM £40.00
  Solution for infusion
  ▸ Nimotop (Bayer Plc)
    Nimodipine 200 microgram per 1 ml Nimotop 0.02% solution for infusion 50ml vials | 5 vial PoM £68.00 (Hospital only)

3   Blood clots

ANTITHROMBOTIC DRUGS ▸ TISSUE
PLASMINOGEN ACTIVATORS

⌕ 126

▌ Urokinase

- **INDICATIONS AND DOSE**
  Occluded arteriovenous shunts, catheters, and indwelling central lines
  ▸ TO THE DEVICE AS A FLUSH

  ▸ **Neonate:** 5000–25 000 units, inject directly into occluded catheter or central line, dilute dose in sodium chloride 0.9% to fill catheter dead space **only**. Leave for 20–60 minutes then aspirate the lysate and flush with sodium chloride 0.9%.

  ▸ **Child:** 5000–25 000 units, inject directly into occluded catheter or central line, dilute dose in sodium chloride 0.9% to fill catheter dead space **only**. Leave for 20–60 minutes then aspirate the lysate and flush with sodium chloride 0.9%

- **CONTRA-INDICATIONS** Recent stroke
- **CAUTIONS** Atrial fibrillation · cavernous pulmonary disease · mitral valve defect · recent delivery · septic thrombotic disease · severe cerebrovascular disease
- **INTERACTIONS** Contra-indicated if concomitant treatment with oral anticoagulants or heparin.
- **BREAST FEEDING** Manufacturer advises avoid—no information available.
- **DIRECTIONS FOR ADMINISTRATION** May be diluted, after reconstitution, with Sodium Chloride 0.9%.

- **MEDICINAL FORMS**
  There can be variation in the licensing of different medicines containing the same drug.
  Powder for solution for injection
  ▸ Urokinase (Non-proprietary)
    Urokinase 10000 unit Urokinase 10,000unit powder for solution for injection vials | 1 vial PoM £33.79
    Urokinase 50000 unit Urokinase 50,000unit powder for solution for injection vials | 1 vial PoM £69.70
    Urokinase 100000 unit Urokinase 100,000unit powder for solution for injection vials | 1 vial PoM £106.17
    Urokinase 250000 unit Urokinase 250,000unit powder for solution for injection vials | 1 vial PoM £185.65
    Urokinase 500000 unit Urokinase 500,000unit powder for solution for injection vials | 1 vial PoM £365.00

3.1   Thromboembolism

Venous thromboembolism

Prophylaxis of venous thromboembolism

Low-dose heparin (unfractionated) p. 87 by subcutaneous injection is used to prevent thrombotic episodes in 'high-risk' patients; laboratory monitoring of APTT or anti-Factor Xa concentration is also required in prophylactic regimens in children. Low molecular weight heparins, aspirin (antiplatelet dose), and warfarin sodium p. 89 can also be used for prophylaxis.

Treatment of venous thromboembolism

For the initial treatment of thrombotic episodes heparin (unfractionated) is given as an intravenous loading dose, followed by continuous intravenous infusion (using an infusion pump) or by intermittent subcutaneous injection; the use of intermittent intravenous injection is no longer recommended. Alternatively, a low molecular weight heparin may be given for initial treatment. If an oral anticoagulant (usually warfarin sodium) is also required, it may be started at the same time as the heparin (the heparin needs to be continued for at least 5 days and until the INR has been in the therapeutic range for 2 consecutive days). Laboratory monitoring of coagulation activity, preferably on a daily basis, involves determination of the activated partial thromboplastin time (APTT) (for heparin (unfractionated) only) or of the anti-Factor Xa concentration (for low molecular weight heparins). Local guidelines on recommended APTT for neonates and children should be followed; monitoring of APTT should be discussed with a specialist prior to treatment for thrombotic episodes in neonates.

Management of venous thromboembolism in pregnancy

Heparins are used for the management of venous thromboembolism in pregnancy because they do not cross the placenta. Low molecular weight heparins are preferred because they have a lower risk of osteoporosis and of heparin-induced thrombocytopenia. Low molecular weight heparins are eliminated more rapidly in pregnancy, requiring alteration of the dosage regimen for drugs such as dalteparin sodium p. 86, enoxaparin sodium p. 86 and tinzaparin sodium p. 88; see also under individual drugs. Treatment should be stopped at the onset of labour and advice sought from a specialist on continuing therapy after birth.

Extracorporeal circuits

Heparin (unfractionated) is also used in the maintenance of extracorporeal circuits in cardiopulmonary bypass and haemodialysis.

2

Cardiovascular system

Haemorrhage

If haemorrhage occurs it is usually sufficient to withdraw unfractionated or low molecular weight heparin (unfractionated), but if rapid reversal of the effects of the heparin (unfractionated) is required, protamine sulfate p. 795 is a specific antidote (but only partially reverses the effects of low molecular weight heparin (unfractionated)).

Oral anticoagulants

Overview

The main use of anticoagulants is to prevent thrombus formation or extension of an existing thrombus in the slower-moving venous side of the circulation, where the thrombus consists of a fibrin web enmeshed with platelets and red cells.

Anticoagulants are of less use in preventing thrombus formation in arteries, for in faster-flowing vessels thrombi are composed mainly of platelets with little fibrin.

Oral anticoagulants antagonise the effects of vitamin K and take at least 48 to 72 hours for the anticoagulant effect to develop fully; if an immediate effect is required, unfractionated or low molecular weight heparin must be given concomitantly.

Uses

Warfarin sodium p. 89 is the drug of choice for the treatment of systemic thromboembolism in children (not neonates) after initial heparinisation. It may also be used occasionally for the treatment of intravascular or intracardiac thrombi. Warfarin sodium is used prophylactically in those with chronic atrial fibrillation, dilated cardiomyopathy, certain forms of reconstructive heart surgery, mechanical prosthetic heart valves, and some forms of hereditary thrombophilia (e.g. homozygous protein C deficiency).

Unfractionated or a low molecular weight heparin (see under Parenteral anticoagulants p. 83) is usually preferred for the prophylaxis of venous thromboembolism in children undergoing surgery; alternatively warfarin sodium can be continued in selected children currently taking warfarin sodium and who are at a high risk of thromboembolism (seek expert advice).

Dose

The base-line prothrombin time should be determined but the initial dose should not be delayed whilst awaiting the result.

An induction dose is usually given over 4 days. The subsequent maintenance dose depends on the prothrombin time, reported as INR (international normalised ratio) and should be taken at the same time each day.

Target INR

The following indications and target INRs for adults for warfarin take into account recommendations of the British Society for Haematology Guidelines on Oral Anticoagulation with warfarin—fourth edition. *Br J Haematol* 2011; **154**: 311–324:

An INR which is within 0.5 units of the target value is generally satisfactory; larger deviations require dosage adjustment. Target values (rather than ranges) are now recommended.

INR 2.5 for:

- treatment of deep-vein thrombosis or pulmonary embolism (including those associated with antiphospholipid syndrome or for recurrence in patients no longer receiving warfarin sodium)
- atrial fibrillation
- cardioversion—target INR should be achieved at least 3 weeks before cardioversion and anticoagulation should

continue for at least 4 weeks after the procedure (higher target values, such as an INR of 3, can be used for up to 4 weeks before the procedure to avoid cancellations due to low INR)

- dilated cardiomyopathy
- mitral stenosis or regurgitation in patients with either atrial fibrillation, a history of systemic embolism, a left atrial thrombus, or an enlarged left atrium
- bioprosthetic heart valves in the mitral position (treat for 3 months), or in patients with a history of systemic embolism (treat for at least 3 months), or with a left atrial thrombus at surgery (treat until clot resolves), or with other risk factors (e.g. atrial fibrillation or a low ventricular ejection fraction)
- acute arterial embolism requiring embolectomy (consider long-term treatment)
- myocardial infarction

INR 3.5 for:

- recurrent deep-vein thrombosis or pulmonary embolism in patients currently receiving anticoagulation and with an INR above 2;

Mechanical prosthetic heart valves:

- the recommended target INR depends on the type and location of the valve, and patient-related risk factors
- consider increasing the INR target or adding an antiplatelet drug, if an embolic event occurs whilst anticoagulated at the target INR.

Haemorrhage

The main adverse effect of all oral anticoagulants is haemorrhage. Checking the INR and omitting doses when appropriate is essential; if the anticoagulant is stopped but not reversed, the INR should be measured 2–3 days later to ensure that it is falling. The cause of an elevated INR should be investigated. The following recommendations (which take into account the recommendations of the British Society for Haematology Guidelines on Oral Anticoagulation with Warfarin—fourth edition. *Br J Haematol* 2011; **154**: 311–324) are based on the result of the INR and whether there is major or minor bleeding; the recommendations apply to adults taking warfarin:

- Major bleeding—stop warfarin sodium; give phytomenadione (vitamin K₁) p. 593 by slow intravenous injection; give dried prothrombin complex p. 77 (factors II, VII, IX, and X); if dried prothrombin complex unavailable, fresh frozen plasma can be given but is less effective; recombinant factor VIIa is not recommended for emergency anticoagulation reversal
- INR >8.0, minor bleeding—stop warfarin sodium; give phytomenadione (vitamin K₁) by slow intravenous injection; repeat dose of phytomenadione if INR still too high after 24 hours; restart warfarin sodium when INR <5.0
- INR >8.0, no bleeding—stop warfarin sodium; give phytomenadione (vitamin K₁) by mouth using the intravenous preparation orally [unlicensed use]; repeat dose of phytomenadione if INR still too high after 24 hours; restart warfarin sodium when INR <5.0
- INR 5.0–8.0, minor bleeding—stop warfarin sodium; give phytomenadione (vitamin K₁) by slow intravenous injection; restart warfarin sodium when INR <5.0
- INR 5.0–8.0, no bleeding—withhold 1 or 2 doses of warfarin sodium and reduce subsequent maintenance dose
- Unexpected bleeding at therapeutic levels—always investigate possibility of underlying cause e.g. unsuspected renal or gastro-intestinal tract pathology

Parenteral anticoagulants

Anticoagulants

Although thrombotic episodes are uncommon in childhood, anticoagulants may be required in children with congenital heart disease; in children undergoing haemodialysis; for preventing thrombosis in children requiring chemotherapy and following surgery; and for systemic venous thromboembolism secondary to inherited thrombophilias, systemic lupus erythematosus, or indwelling central venous catheters.

Heparin

Heparin initiates anticoagulation rapidly but has a short duration of action. It is now often referred to as being **standard** or heparin (unfractionated) p. 87 to distinguish it from the **low molecular weight heparins**, which have a longer duration of action. For children at high risk of bleeding, heparin (unfractionated) is more suitable than low molecular weight heparin because its effect can be terminated rapidly by stopping the infusion.

Heparins are used in both the treatment and prophylaxis of thromboembolic disease, mainly to prevent further clotting rather than to lyse existing clots—surgery or a thrombolytic drug may be necessary if a thrombus obstructs major vessels.

Low molecular weight heparins

Dalteparin sodium p. 86, enoxaparin sodium p. 86, and tinzaparin sodium p. 88 are low molecular weight heparins used for treatment and prophylaxis of thrombotic episodes in children. Their duration of action is longer than that of heparin (unfractionated) and in adults and older children *once-daily subcutaneous* dosage is sometimes possible; however, younger children require relatively higher doses (possibly due to larger volume of distribution, altered heparin pharmacokinetics, or lower plasma concentrations of antithrombin) and twice daily dosage is sometimes necessary. Low molecular weight heparins are convenient to use, especially in children with poor venous access.

Heparinoids

Danaparoid sodium p. 85 is a heparinoid that has a role in children who develop heparin-induced thrombocytopenia, providing they have no evidence of cross-reactivity.

Heparin flushes

The use of heparin flushes should be kept to a minimum. For maintaining patency of peripheral venous catheters, sodium chloride injection 0.9% is as effective as heparin flushes. The role of heparin flushes in maintaining patency of arterial and central venous catheters is unclear.

Epoprostenol

Epoprostenol (prostacyclin) p. 110 can be given to inhibit platelet aggregation during renal dialysis when heparins are unsuitable or contra-indicated. It is a potent vasodilator and therefore its side-effects include flushing, headache and hypotension.

> **Drugs used for Thromboembolism not listed below**
> Alteplase, p. 126 · Streptokinase, p. 126

Antiplatelet drugs

Antiplatelet drugs decrease platelet aggregation and inhibit thrombus formation in the arterial circulation, because in faster-flowing vessels, thrombi are composed mainly of platelets with little fibrin.

Aspirin below has limited use in children because it has been associated with Reye's syndrome. Aspirin-containing preparations should not be given to children and adolescents under 16 years, unless specifically indicated, such as for Kawasaki disease, for prophylaxis of clot formation after cardiac surgery, or for prophylaxis of stroke in children at high risk.

If aspirin causes dyspepsia, or if the child is at a high risk of gastro-intestinal bleeding, a proton pump inhibitor or a H_2-receptor antagonist can be added.

Dipyridamole p. 84 is also used as an antiplatelet drug to prevent clot formation after cardiac surgery and may be used with specialist advice for treatment of persistent coronary artery aneurysms in Kawasaki disease.

Kawasaki disease

Initial treatment is with high dose aspirin and a single dose of intravenous normal immunoglobulin; this combination has an additive anti-inflammatory effect resulting in faster resolution of fever and a decreased incidence of coronary artery complications. After the acute phase, when the patient is afebrile, aspirin is continued at a lower dose to prevent coronary artery abnormalities.

Aspirin
(Acetylsalicylic Acid)

● **INDICATIONS AND DOSE**
Antiplatelet | Prevention of thrombus formation after cardiac surgery
▸ BY MOUTH
▸ Neonate: 1–5 mg/kg once daily.
▸ Child 1 month–11 years: 1–5 mg/kg once daily (max. per dose 75 mg)
▸ Child 12–17 years: 75 mg once daily
Kawasaki disease
▸ BY MOUTH
▸ Neonate: Initially 8 mg/kg 4 times a day for 2 weeks *or* until afebrile, followed by 5 mg/kg once daily for 6–8 weeks, if no evidence of coronary lesions after 8 weeks, discontinue treatment or seek expert advice.
▸ Child 1 month–11 years: Initially 7.5–12.5 mg/kg 4 times a day for 2 weeks *or* until afebrile, then 2–5 mg/kg once daily for 6–8 weeks, if no evidence of coronary lesions after 8 weeks, discontinue treatment or seek expert advice

● **UNLICENSED USE** Not licensed for use in children under 16 years.
● **CONTRA-INDICATIONS** Active peptic ulceration · bleeding disorders (antiplatelet dose) · children under 16 years (risk of Reye's syndrome) · haemophilia · previous peptic ulceration (analgesic dose) · severe cardiac failure (analgesic dose)
CONTRA-INDICATIONS, FURTHER INFORMATION
▸ Reye's syndrome Owing to an association with Reye's syndrome, aspirin-containing preparations should not be given to children under 16 years, unless specifically indicated, e.g. for Kawasaki disease.

Cardiovascular system

- **CAUTIONS** Allergic disease · anaemia · asthma · dehydration · G6PD deficiency · preferably avoid during fever or viral infection in children (risk of Reye's syndrome) · previous peptic ulceration (but manufacturers may advise avoidance of low-dose aspirin in history of peptic ulceration) · thyrotoxicosis · uncontrolled hypertension
- **INTERACTIONS** → Appendix 1 (aspirin). Caution with concomitant use of drugs that increase risk of bleeding.
- **SIDE-EFFECTS** Blood disorders (with analgesic doses) · bronchospasm · confusion (with analgesic doses) · gastro-intestinal haemorrhage (occasionally major) · gastro-intestinal irritation (with slight asymptomatic blood loss at higher doses) · haemorrhage including subconjunctival haemorrhage (reported with antiplatelet doses) · increased bleeding time · skin reactions in hypersensitive patients · tinnitus (with analgesic doses)

Overdose
The main features of salicylate poisoning are hyperventilation, tinnitus, deafness, vasodilatation, and sweating. Coma is uncommon but indicates very severe poisoning.
For specific details on the management of poisoning, see *Aspirin*, under Emergency treatment of poisoning p. 786.

- **ALLERGY AND CROSS-SENSITIVITY** Aspirin is **contra-indicated** in history of hypersensitivity to aspirin or any other NSAID—which includes those in whom attacks of asthma, angioedema, urticaria, or rhinitis have been precipitated by aspirin or any other NSAID.
- **PREGNANCY** Use antiplatelet doses with caution during third trimester; impaired platelet function and risk of haemorrhage; delayed onset and increased duration of labour with increased blood loss; avoid analgesic doses if possible in last few weeks (low doses probably not harmful); high doses may be related to intra-uterine growth restriction, teratogenic effects, closure of fetal ductus arteriosus in utero and possibly persistent pulmonary hypertension of newborn; kernicterus may occur in jaundiced neonates.
- **BREAST FEEDING** Avoid—possible risk of Reye's syndrome; regular use of high doses could impair platelet function and reduce hypoprothrombinaemia in infant if neonatal vitamin K stores low.
- **HEPATIC IMPAIRMENT** Avoid in severe impairment—increased risk of gastro-intestinal bleeding.
- **RENAL IMPAIRMENT** Use with caution; avoid in severe impairment; sodium and water retention; deterioration in renal function; increased risk of gastro-intestinal bleeding.
- **PATIENT AND CARER ADVICE**
Medicines for Children leaflet: Aspirin for prevention of blood clots www.medicinesforchildren.org.uk/aspirin-prevention-blood-clots-0

- **MEDICINAL FORMS**
There can be variation in the licensing of different medicines containing the same drug. Forms available from special-order manufacturers include: capsule, oral suspension, oral solution,

Tablet
CAUTIONARY AND ADVISORY LABELS 21, 32
▸ **Aspirin (Non-proprietary)**
Aspirin 75 mg Aspirin 75mg tablets | 28 tablet PoM £1.13 DT price = £0.98
Aspirin 300 mg Aspirin 300mg tablets | 16 tablet GSL no price available | 32 tablet P £3.35 DT price = £3.35 | 32 tablet GSL £3.35 DT price = £3.35 | 100 tablet PoM £10.47

Dispersible tablet
CAUTIONARY AND ADVISORY LABELS 13, 21, 32
▸ **Aspirin (Non-proprietary)**
Aspirin 75 mg Aspirin 75mg dispersible tablets | 28 tablet GSL £1.04 DT price = £0.68 | 28 tablet P £0.75 DT price = £0.68 | 100 tablet P £0.64 DT price = £2.43 | 100 tablet GSL £1.27 DT price = £2.43 | 1000 tablet PoM £31.28
Aspirin 300 mg Aspirin 300mg dispersible tablets | 32 tablet PoM no price available DT price = £1.09 | 32 tablet P £1.12 DT price = £1.09 | 100 tablet PoM £4.28 DT price = £3.41 | 1000 tablet PoM £37.80

Gastro-resistant tablet
CAUTIONARY AND ADVISORY LABELS 5, 25, 32
▸ **Aspirin (Non-proprietary)**
Aspirin 75 mg Aspirin 75mg gastro-resistant tablets | 28 tablet GSL £0.80 DT price = £0.73 | 28 tablet P £0.80–£0.93 DT price = £0.73 | 56 tablet PoM no price available | 56 tablet P £1.93 | 56 tablet GSL £1.60
Aspirin 300 mg Aspirin 300mg gastro-resistant tablets | 100 tablet PoM £20.34 DT price = £20.34
▸ **Micropirin** (Dexcel-Pharma Ltd)
Aspirin 75 mg Micropirin 75mg gastro-resistant tablets | 28 tablet P £1.45 DT price = £0.73 | 56 tablet P £2.87
▸ **Nu-Seals** (Alliance Pharmaceuticals Ltd)
Aspirin 75 mg Nu-Seals 75 gastro-resistant tablets | 56 tablet P £3.12

Dipyridamole

- **INDICATIONS AND DOSE**

Kawasaki disease (initiated under specialist supervision)
▸ BY MOUTH USING IMMEDIATE-RELEASE MEDICINES
▸ Child 1 month–11 years: 1 mg/kg 3 times a day
Prevention of thrombus formation after cardiac surgery
▸ BY MOUTH USING IMMEDIATE-RELEASE MEDICINES
▸ Child 1 month–11 years: 2.5 mg/kg twice daily
▸ Child 12–17 years: 100–200 mg 3 times a day

- **UNLICENSED USE** Not licensed for use in children.
- **CAUTIONS** Aortic stenosis · coagulation disorders · heart failure · hypotension · left ventricular outflow obstruction · may exacerbate migraine · myasthenia gravis (risk of exacerbation)
- **INTERACTIONS** → Appendix 1 (dipyridamole). Caution with concomitant use of drugs that increase risk of bleeding.
- **SIDE-EFFECTS** Angioedema · dizziness · gastro-intestinal effects · hot flushes · hypersensitivity reactions · hypotension · increased bleeding after surgery · increased bleeding during surgery · myalgia · rash · severe bronchospasm · tachycardia · throbbing headache · thrombocytopenia · urticaria
- **PREGNANCY** Not known to be harmful.
- **BREAST FEEDING** Manufacturers advise use only if essential—small amount present in milk.
- **DIRECTIONS FOR ADMINISTRATION**
▸ With oral use Injection solution can be given orally.

- **MEDICINAL FORMS**
There can be variation in the licensing of different medicines containing the same drug. Forms available from special-order manufacturers include: oral suspension, oral solution

Tablet
CAUTIONARY AND ADVISORY LABELS 22
▸ **Dipyridamole (Non-proprietary)**
Dipyridamole 25 mg Dipyridamole 25mg tablets | 84 tablet PoM £9.40 DT price = £9.40
Dipyridamole 100 mg Dipyridamole 100mg tablets | 84 tablet PoM £12.50 DT price = £4.48
▸ **Persantin** (Boehringer Ingelheim Ltd)
Dipyridamole 100 mg Persantin 100mg tablets | 84 tablet PoM £6.30 DT price = £4.48

Oral suspension

▸ Dipyridamole (Non-proprietary)

Dipyridamole 10 mg per 1 ml Dipyridamole 50mg/5ml oral suspension sugar free sugar-free | 150 ml [PoM] £41.06 DT price = £41.06

Dipyridamole 40 mg per 1 ml Dipyridamole 200mg/5ml oral suspension sugar free sugar-free | 150 ml [PoM] £109.35–£131.22 DT price = £120.29

ANTITHROMBOTIC DRUGS › HEPARINOIDS

Danaparoid sodium

● **INDICATIONS AND DOSE**

Thromboembolic disease in patients with history of heparin-induced thrombocytopenia

▸ INITIALLY BY INTRAVENOUS INJECTION

▸ **Neonate:** Initially 30 units/kg, then (by continuous intravenous infusion) 1.2–2 units/kg/hour, infusion dose to be adjusted according to coagulation activity

▸ Child 1 month–15 years (body-weight up to 55 kg): Initially 30 units/kg (max. per dose 1250 units), then (by continuous intravenous infusion) 1.2–2 units/kg/hour, infusion dose to be adjusted according to coagulation activity

▸ Child 1 month–15 years (body-weight 55 kg and above): Initially 30 units/kg (max. per dose 2500 units), then (by continuous intravenous infusion) 1.2–2 units/kg/hour, infusion dose to be adjusted according to coagulation activity

▸ Child 16–17 years (body-weight up to 55 kg): Initially 1250 units, then (by continuous intravenous infusion) 400 units/hour for 2 hours, then (by continuous intravenous infusion) 300 units/hour for 2 hours, then (by continuous intravenous infusion) 200 units/hour for 5 days, infusion dose to be adjusted according to coagulation activity

▸ Child 16–17 years (body-weight 55–90 kg): Initially 2500 units, then (by continuous intravenous infusion) 400 units/hour for 2 hours, then (by continuous intravenous infusion) 300 units/hour for 2 hours, then (by continuous intravenous infusion) 200 units/hour for 5 days, infusion dose to be adjusted according to coagulation activity

▸ Child 16–17 years (body-weight 91 kg and above): Initially 3750 units, then (by continuous intravenous infusion) 400 units/hour for 2 hours, then (by continuous intravenous infusion) 300 units/hour for 2 hours, then (by continuous intravenous infusion) 200 units/hour for 5 days, infusion dose to be adjusted according to coagulation activity

● **UNLICENSED USE** Not licensed for use in children.

● **CONTRA-INDICATIONS** Active peptic ulcer (unless this is the reason for operation) · acute bacterial endocarditis · diabetic retinopathy · epidural anaesthesia (with treatment doses) · haemophilia and other haemorrhagic disorders · recent cerebral haemorrhage · severe hypertension · spinal anaesthesia (with treatment doses) · thrombocytopenia (unless patient has heparin-induced thrombocytopenia)

● **CAUTIONS** Antibodies to heparins (risk of antibody-induced thrombocytopenia) · body-weight over 90 kg · recent bleeding · risk of bleeding

● **INTERACTIONS** → Appendix 1 (danaparoid). Caution with concomitant use of drugs that increase risk of bleeding.

● **SIDE-EFFECTS** Bleeding · hypersensitivity reactions · rash

● **PREGNANCY** Manufacturer advises avoid—limited information available but not known to be harmful.

● **BREAST FEEDING** Amount probably too small to be harmful but manufacturer advises avoid.

● **HEPATIC IMPAIRMENT** Caution in moderate impairment (increased risk of bleeding). Avoid in severe impairment unless patient has heparin-induced thrombocytopenia and no alternative available.

● **RENAL IMPAIRMENT** Use with caution in moderate impairment. Avoid in severe impairment unless patient has heparin-induced thrombocytopenia and no alternative available. Increased risk of bleeding in renal impairment, monitor anti-Factor Xa activity.

● **MONITORING REQUIREMENTS** Monitor anti factor Xa activity in patients with body-weight over 90 kg.

● **DIRECTIONS FOR ADMINISTRATION** For *intravenous infusion*, dilute with Glucose 5% or Sodium Chloride 0.9%.

● **MEDICINAL FORMS**
There can be variation in the licensing of different medicines containing the same drug.

Solution for injection

▸ Organan (Aspen Pharma Trading Ltd)
Danaparoid sodium 1250 unit per 1 ml Organan 750units/0.6ml solution for injection ampoules | 10 ampoule [PoM] £266.73

ANTITHROMBOTIC DRUGS › HEPARINS

Heparins

● **CONTRA-INDICATIONS** Acute bacterial endocarditis · after major trauma · epidural anaesthesia with treatment doses · haemophilia and other haemorrhagic disorders · peptic ulcer · recent cerebral haemorrhage · recent surgery to eye · recent surgery to nervous system · severe hypertension · spinal anaesthesia with treatment doses · thrombocytopenia (including history of heparin-induced thrombocytopenia)

● **INTERACTIONS** → Appendix 1 (heparins).
Caution with concomitant use of drugs that increase risk of bleeding.

● **SIDE-EFFECTS**

▸ **Rare** Alopecia (on prolonged use) · anaphylaxis · angioedema · hyperkalaemia · hypersensitivity reactions · injection-site reactions · osteoporosis (risk lower with low molecular weight heparins) · priapism · rebound hyperlipidaemia (following unfractionated heparin withdrawal) · skin necrosis · urticaria

▸ **Frequency not known** Haemorrhage · thrombocytopenia

SIDE-EFFECTS, FURTHER INFORMATION

▸ Haemorrhage If haemorrhage occurs it is usually sufficient to withdraw unfractionated or low molecular weight heparin, but if rapid reversal of the effects of the heparin is required, protamine sulfate is a specific antidote (but only partially reverses the effects of low molecular weight heparins).

▸ Heparin-induced thrombocytopenia Clinically important heparin-induced thrombocytopenia is immune-mediated and does not usually develop until after 5–10 days; it can be complicated by thrombosis.

Signs of heparin-induced thrombocytopenia include a 30% reduction of platelet count, thrombosis, or skin allergy. If heparin-induced thrombocytopenia is strongly suspected or confirmed, the heparin should be **stopped** and an alternative anticoagulant, such as danaparoid, should be given. Ensure platelet counts return to normal range in those who require warfarin.

▸ Hyperkalaemia Inhibition of aldosterone secretion by unfractionated or low molecular weight heparin can result in hyperkalaemia; patients with diabetes mellitus, chronic renal failure, acidosis, raised plasma potassium or those taking potassium-sparing drugs seem to be more susceptible. The risk appears to increase with duration of therapy.

- **ALLERGY AND CROSS-SENSITIVITY** Hypersensitivity to unfractionated or low molecular weight heparin.
- **MONITORING REQUIREMENTS**
  - ▶ Heparin-induced thrombocytopenia Platelet counts should be measured just before treatment with unfractionated or low molecular weight heparin, and regular monitoring of platelet counts may be required if given for longer than 4 days. See the British Society for Haematology's Guidelines on the diagnosis and management of heparin-induced thrombocytopenia: second edition. *Br J Haematol* 2012; **159**: 528–540.
  - ▶ Hyperkalaemia Plasma-potassium concentration should be measured in patients at risk of hyperkalaemia before starting the heparin and monitored regularly thereafter, particularly if treatment is to be continued for longer than 7 days.

F 85

Dalteparin sodium

- **INDICATIONS AND DOSE**

Treatment of thrombotic episodes
  - ▶ BY SUBCUTANEOUS INJECTION
  - ▶ Neonate: 100 units/kg twice daily.
  - ▶ Child 1 month–11 years: 100 units/kg twice daily
  - ▶ Child 12–17 years: 200 units/kg once daily (max. per dose 18 000 units); reduced to 100 units/kg twice daily, dose reduced if increased risk of bleeding

Treatment of venous thromboembolism in pregnancy
  - ▶ BY SUBCUTANEOUS INJECTION
  - ▶ Child 12–17 years (body-weight up to 50 kg): 5000 units twice daily, use body-weight in early pregnancy to calculate the dose
  - ▶ Child 12–17 years (body-weight 50–69 kg): 6000 units twice daily, use body-weight in early pregnancy to calculate the dose
  - ▶ Child 12–17 years (body-weight 70–89 kg): 8000 units twice daily, use body-weight in early pregnancy to calculate the dose
  - ▶ Child 12–17 years (body-weight 90 kg and above): 10 000 units twice daily, use body-weight in early pregnancy to calculate the dose

Prophylaxis of thrombotic episodes.
  - ▶ BY SUBCUTANEOUS INJECTION
  - ▶ Neonate: 100 units/kg once daily.
  - ▶ Child 1 month–11 years: 100 units/kg once daily
  - ▶ Child 12–17 years: 2500–5000 units once daily

- **UNLICENSED USE** Not licensed for use in children.
- **PREGNANCY** Not known to be harmful, low molecular weight heparins do not cross the placenta. Multidose vial contains benzyl alcohol—manufacturer advises avoid.
- **BREAST FEEDING** Due to the relatively high molecular weight and inactivation in the gastro-intestinal tract, passage into breast-milk and absorption by the nursing infant are likely to be negligible, however manufacturers advise avoid.
- **HEPATIC IMPAIRMENT** Dose reduction may be required in severe impairment—risk of bleeding may be increased.
- **RENAL IMPAIRMENT** Risk of bleeding may be increased—dose reduction may be required. Use of unfractionated heparin may be preferable.
- **MONITORING REQUIREMENTS** Routine monitoring of anti-Factor Xa activity is not usually required during treatment with dalteparin, except in neonates; monitoring may also be necessary in severely ill children and those with renal or hepatic impairment.

- **MEDICINAL FORMS**
  There can be variation in the licensing of different medicines containing the same drug.

Solution for injection
EXCIPIENTS: May contain Benzyl alcohol
  - ▶ **Dalteparin sodium (Non-proprietary)**
    Dalteparin sodium 10000 unit per 1 ml Dalteparin sodium 10,000units/1ml solution for injection pre-filled syringes | 5 pre-filled disposable injection [PoM] no price available | 5 pre-filled disposable injection no price available
    Dalteparin sodium 12500 unit per 1 ml Dalteparin sodium 2,500units/0.2ml solution for injection pre-filled syringes | 10 pre-filled disposable injection [PoM] no price available
    Dalteparin sodium 25000 unit per 1 ml Dalteparin sodium 7,500units/0.3ml solution for injection pre-filled syringes | 10 pre-filled disposable injection [PoM] no price available
    Dalteparin sodium 12,500units/0.5ml solution for injection pre-filled syringes | 5 pre-filled disposable injection [PoM] no price available
    Dalteparin sodium 5,000units/0.2ml solution for injection pre-filled syringes | 10 pre-filled disposable injection [PoM] no price available
    Dalteparin sodium 15,000units/0.6ml solution for injection pre-filled syringes | 5 pre-filled disposable injection [PoM] no price available
    Dalteparin sodium 10,000units/0.4ml solution for injection pre-filled syringes | 5 pre-filled disposable injection [PoM] no price available
    Dalteparin sodium 18,000units/0.72ml solution for injection pre-filled syringes | 5 pre-filled disposable injection [PoM] no price available
  - ▶ **Fragmin** (Pfizer Ltd)
    Dalteparin sodium 2500 unit per 1 ml Fragmin 10,000units/4ml solution for injection ampoules | 10 ampoule [PoM] £51.22
    Dalteparin sodium 10000 unit per 1 ml Fragmin 10,000units/1ml solution for injection pre-filled syringes | 5 pre-filled disposable injection [PoM] £28.23
    Fragmin 10,000units/1ml solution for injection ampoules | 10 ampoule [PoM] £51.22
    Dalteparin sodium 12500 unit per 1 ml Fragmin 2,500units/0.2ml solution for injection pre-filled syringes | 10 pre-filled disposable injection [PoM] £18.58
    Dalteparin sodium 25000 unit per 1 ml Fragmin 18,000units/0.72ml solution for injection pre-filled syringes | 5 pre-filled disposable injection [PoM] £50.82
    Fragmin 15,000units/0.6ml solution for injection pre-filled syringes | 5 pre-filled disposable injection [PoM] £42.34
    Fragmin 5,000units/0.2ml solution for injection pre-filled syringes | 10 pre-filled disposable injection [PoM] £28.23
    Fragmin 12,500units/0.5ml solution for injection pre-filled syringes | 5 pre-filled disposable injection [PoM] £35.29
    Fragmin 7,500units/0.3ml solution for injection pre-filled syringes | 10 pre-filled disposable injection [PoM] £42.34
    Fragmin 100,000units/4ml solution for injection vials | 1 vial [PoM] £48.66
    Fragmin 10,000units/0.4ml solution for injection pre-filled syringes | 5 pre-filled disposable injection [PoM] £28.23

F 85

Enoxaparin sodium

- **INDICATIONS AND DOSE**

Treatment of thrombotic episodes
  - ▶ BY SUBCUTANEOUS INJECTION
  - ▶ Neonate: 1.5–2 mg/kg twice daily.
  - ▶ Child 1 month: 1.5 mg/kg twice daily
  - ▶ Child 2 months–17 years: 1 mg/kg twice daily

Treatment of venous thromboembolism in pregnancy
  - ▶ BY SUBCUTANEOUS INJECTION
  - ▶ Child 12–17 years (body-weight up to 50 kg): 40 mg twice daily, dose based on early pregnancy body-weight
  - ▶ Child 12–17 years (body-weight 50–69 kg): 60 mg twice daily, dose based on early pregnancy body-weight
  - ▶ Child 12–17 years (body-weight 70–89 kg): 80 mg twice daily, dose based on early pregnancy body-weight
  - ▶ Child 12–17 years (body-weight 90 kg and above): 100 mg twice daily, dose based on early pregnancy body-weight

Prophylaxis of thrombotic episodes
▸ BY SUBCUTANEOUS INJECTION

▸ Neonate: 750 micrograms/kg twice daily.

▸ Child 1 month: 750 micrograms/kg twice daily
▸ Child 2 months–17 years: 500 micrograms/kg twice daily; maximum 40 mg per day

DOSE EQUIVALENCE AND CONVERSION
1 mg equivalent to 100 units.

● **UNLICENSED USE** Not licensed for use in children.

● **PREGNANCY** Not known to be harmful, low molecular weight heparins do not cross the placenta. Multidose vial contains benzyl alcohol—avoid.

● **BREAST FEEDING** Due to the relatively high molecular weight of enoxaparin and inactivation in the gastrointestinal tract, passage into breast-milk and absorption by the nursing infant are likely to be negligible; however manufacturers advise avoid.

● **HEPATIC IMPAIRMENT** Reduce dose in severe impairment—risk of bleeding may be increased.

● **RENAL IMPAIRMENT** Risk of bleeding increased; reduce dose if estimated glomerular filtration rate less than 30 mL/minute/1.73 m^2—consult product literature for details. Use of unfractionated heparin may be preferable.

● **MONITORING REQUIREMENTS** Routine monitoring of anti-Factor Xa activity is not usually required during treatment with enoxaparin, except in neonates; monitoring may also be necessary in severely ill children and those with renal or hepatic impairment.

● **MEDICINAL FORMS**
There can be variation in the licensing of different medicines containing the same drug.
Solution for injection
EXCIPIENTS: May contain Benzyl alcohol
▸ Clexane (Sanofi)
Enoxaparin sodium 100 mg per 1 ml Clexane 60mg/0.6ml solution for injection pre-filled syringes | 10 pre-filled disposable injection [PoM] £39.26 DT price = £39.26
Clexane 300mg/3ml solution for injection multidose vials | 1 vial [PoM] £21.33
Clexane 80mg/0.8ml solution for injection pre-filled syringes | 10 pre-filled disposable injection [PoM] £55.13 DT price = £55.13
Clexane 40mg/0.4ml solution for injection pre-filled syringes | 10 pre-filled disposable injection [PoM] £30.27 DT price = £30.27
Clexane 100mg/1ml solution for injection pre-filled syringes | 10 pre-filled disposable injection [PoM] £72.30 DT price = £72.30
Clexane 20mg/0.2ml solution for injection pre-filled syringes | 10 pre-filled disposable injection [PoM] £20.86 DT price = £20.86
Enoxaparin sodium 150 mg per 1 ml Clexane Forte 120mg/0.8ml solution for injection pre-filled syringes | 10 pre-filled disposable injection [PoM] £87.93 DT price = £87.93
Clexane Forte 150mg/1ml solution for injection pre-filled syringes | 10 pre-filled disposable injection [PoM] £99.91 DT price = £99.91

◀ 85

Heparin (unfractionated)

● **INDICATIONS AND DOSE**
Prevention of clotting in extracorporeal circuits
▸ TO THE DEVICE AS A FLUSH
▸ Child: (consult product literature)
Maintenance of neonatal umbilical arterial catheter
▸ BY INTRAVENOUS INFUSION

▸ Neonate: 0.5 unit/hour.

Treatment of thrombotic episodes
▸ INITIALLY BY INTRAVENOUS INJECTION

▸ Neonate up to 35 weeks corrected gestational age: Initially 50 units/kg, then (by continuous intravenous infusion) 25 units/kg/hour, adjusted according to APTT.

▸ Neonate: Initially 75 units/kg, then (by continuous intravenous infusion) 25 units/kg/hour, adjusted according to APTT.

▸ Child 1–11 months: Initially 75 units/kg, then (by continuous intravenous infusion) 25 units/kg/hour, adjusted according to APTT

▸ Child 1–17 years: Initially 75 units/kg, then (by continuous intravenous infusion) 20 units/kg/hour, adjusted according to APTT
▸ BY SUBCUTANEOUS INJECTION
▸ Child: 250 units/kg twice daily, adjusted according to APTT

Prophylaxis of thrombotic episodes
▸ BY SUBCUTANEOUS INJECTION
▸ Child: 100 units/kg twice daily (max. per dose 5000 units), adjusted according to APTT

Maintenance of cardiac shunts and critical stents
▸ TO THE DEVICE AS A FLUSH
▸ Child: (consult local protocol)

● **UNLICENSED USE** Check product literature for licensed use in children.

● **PREGNANCY** Does not cross the placenta; maternal osteoporosis reported after prolonged use; multidose vials may contain benzyl alcohol—some manufacturers advise avoid.

● **BREAST FEEDING** Not excreted into milk due to high molecular weight.

● **HEPATIC IMPAIRMENT** Risk of bleeding increased—reduce dose or avoid in severe impairment (including oesophageal varices).

● **RENAL IMPAIRMENT** Risk of bleeding increased in severe impairment—dose may need to be reduced.

● **DIRECTIONS FOR ADMINISTRATION** For *continuous intravenous infusion*, dilute with Glucose 5% or Sodium chloride 0.9%.

▸ In neonates For *maintenance of neonatal umbilical arterial catheter*, dilute 50 units to a final volume of 50 mL with Sodium Chloride 0.45% or use ready-made bag containing 500 units in 500 mL Sodium Chloride 0.9%; infuse at 0.5 mL/hour. For *neonatal intensive care (treatment of thrombosis)*, dilute 1250 units/kg body-weight to a final volume of 50 mL with infusion fluid; an intravenous infusion rate of 1 mL/hour provides a dose of 25 units/kg/hour.

● **MEDICINAL FORMS**
There can be variation in the licensing of different medicines containing the same drug. Forms available from special-order manufacturers include: solution for injection, solution for infusion
Solution for injection
EXCIPIENTS: May contain Benzyl alcohol
▸ Heparin (unfractionated) (Non-proprietary)
Heparin sodium 1000 unit per 1 ml Heparin sodium 1,000units/1ml solution for injection ampoules | 10 ampoule [PoM] £14.85
Heparin sodium 5,000units/5ml solution for injection vials | 10 vial [PoM] £16.50–£37.41
Heparin sodium 20,000units/20ml solution for injection ampoules | 10 ampoule [PoM] £70.80–£70.88
Heparin sodium 5,000units/5ml solution for injection ampoules | 10 ampoule [PoM] £37.45–£37.47
Heparin sodium 10,000units/10ml solution for injection ampoules | 10 ampoule [PoM] £64.50–£64.59
Heparin sodium 5000 unit per 1 ml Heparin sodium 5,000units/1ml solution for injection ampoules | 10 ampoule [PoM] £29.04
Heparin sodium 25,000units/5ml solution for injection vials | 10 vial [PoM] £45.00–£84.60
Heparin sodium 25,000units/5ml solution for injection ampoules | 10 ampoule [PoM] £75.78
Heparin calcium 25000 unit per 1 ml Heparin calcium 5,000units/0.2ml solution for injection ampoules | 10 ampoule [PoM] £44.70

Heparin sodium 25000 unit per 1 ml Heparin sodium 25,000units/1ml solution for injection ampoules | 10 ampoule [PoM] £76.95
Heparin sodium 5,000units/0.2ml solution for injection ampoules | 10 ampoule [PoM] £37.35

Infusion
▸ Heparin (unfractionated) (Non-proprietary)
Heparin sodium 2 unit per 1 ml Heparin sodium 1,000units/500ml infusion Viaflex bags | 1 bag [PoM] no price available
Heparin sodium 2,000units/1,000ml infusion Viaflex bags | 1 bag [PoM] no price available
Heparin sodium 5 unit per 1 ml Heparin sodium 5,000units/1litre infusion Viaflex bags | 1 bag [PoM] no price available

Intravenous flush
EXCIPIENTS: May contain Benzyl alcohol
▸ Heparin (unfractionated) (Non-proprietary)
Heparin sodium 10 unit per 1 ml Heparin sodium 50units/5ml patency solution ampoules | 10 ampoule [PoM] £14.96
Heparin sodium 50units/5ml I.V. flush solution ampoules | 10 ampoule [PoM] £14.96
Heparin sodium 100 unit per 1 ml Heparin sodium 200units/2ml I.V. flush solution ampoules | 10 ampoule [PoM] £15.68
Heparin sodium 200units/2ml patency solution ampoules | 10 ampoule [PoM] £15.68

F 85

Tinzaparin sodium

● **INDICATIONS AND DOSE**
Treatment of thrombotic episodes
▸ BY SUBCUTANEOUS INJECTION
▸ Child 1 month: 275 units/kg once daily
▸ Child 2-11 months: 250 units/kg once daily
▸ Child 1-4 years: 240 units/kg once daily
▸ Child 5-9 years: 200 units/kg once daily
▸ Child 10-17 years: 175 units/kg once daily

Treatment of venous thromboembolism in pregnancy
▸ BY SUBCUTANEOUS INJECTION
▸ Child 12-17 years: 175 units/kg once daily, dose based on early pregnancy body-weight

Prophylaxis of thrombotic episodes
▸ BY SUBCUTANEOUS INJECTION
▸ Child: 50 units/kg once daily

● **UNLICENSED USE** Not licensed for use in children.

● **SIDE-EFFECTS**
▸ **Uncommon** Headache

● **PREGNANCY** Not known to be harmful, low molecular weight heparins do not cross the placenta. Vials contain benzyl alcohol—manufacturer advises avoid.

● **BREAST FEEDING** Due to the relatively high molecular weight of tinzaparin and inactivation in the gastro-intestinal tract, passage into breast-milk and absorption by the nursing infant are likely to be negligible; however manufacturer advise avoid.

● **RENAL IMPAIRMENT** Manufacturer advises caution if estimated glomerular filtration rate less than 30 mL/minute/1.73 m². Risk of bleeding may be increased. Unfractionated heparin may be preferable. In renal impairment monitoring of anti-Factor Xa may be required if estimated glomerular filtration rate less than 30 mL/minute/1.73 m².

● **MONITORING REQUIREMENTS** Routine monitoring of anti-Factor Xa activity is not usually required except in neonates; monitoring may also be necessary in severely ill children and those with renal or hepatic impairment.

● **MEDICINAL FORMS**
There can be variation in the licensing of different medicines containing the same drug.
Solution for injection
EXCIPIENTS: May contain Benzyl alcohol, sulfites
▸ Tinzaparin sodium (Non-proprietary)
Tinzaparin sodium 10000 unit per 1 ml Tinzaparin sodium 3,500units/0.35ml solution for injection pre-filled syringes | 10 pre-filled disposable injection [PoM] £27.71
Tinzaparin sodium 4,500units/0.45ml solution for injection pre-filled syringes | 10 pre-filled disposable injection [PoM] £35.63
Tinzaparin sodium 2,500units/0.25ml solution for injection pre-filled syringes | 10 pre-filled disposable injection [PoM] £19.80
Tinzaparin sodium 20,000units/2ml solution for injection vials | 10 vial [PoM] no price available
Tinzaparin sodium 20000 unit per 1 ml Tinzaparin sodium 40,000units/2ml solution for injection vials | 1 vial [PoM] no price available
Tinzaparin sodium 14,000units/0.7ml solution for injection pre-filled syringes | 2 pre-filled disposable injection [PoM] no price available | 6 pre-filled disposable injection [PoM] no price available
Tinzaparin sodium 10,000units/0.5ml solution for injection pre-filled syringes | 2 pre-filled disposable injection [PoM] no price available | 6 pre-filled disposable injection [PoM] no price available
Tinzaparin sodium 18,000units/0.9ml solution for injection pre-filled syringes | 2 pre-filled disposable injection [PoM] no price available | 6 pre-filled disposable injection [PoM] no price available

ANTITHROMBOTIC DRUGS ⟩ VITAMIN K ANTAGONISTS

Vitamin K antagonists

● **CONTRA-INDICATIONS** Avoid use within 48 hours postpartum · haemorrhagic stroke · significant bleeding

● **CAUTIONS** Bacterial endocarditis (use only if warfarin otherwise indicated) · conditions in which risk of bleeding is increased · history of gastrointestinal bleeding · peptic ulcer · postpartum (delay warfarin until risk of haemorrhage is low—usually 5–7 days after delivery) · recent ischaemic stroke · recent surgery · uncontrolled hypertension

● **INTERACTIONS** → Appendix 1 (coumarins, phenindione). Major changes in diet (especially involving salads and vegetables) and in alcohol consumption may affect warfarin control.
Caution if concomitant use of drugs that increase risk of bleeding. Avoid cranberry juice.

● **SIDE-EFFECTS** Alopecia · diarrhoea · haemorrhage · hepatic dysfunction · jaundice · nausea · pancreatitis · purpura · pyrexia · rash · skin necrosis (increased risk in patients with protein C or protein S deficiency) · vomiting · 'purple toes'

● **CONCEPTION AND CONTRACEPTION** Women of child-bearing age should be warned of the danger of teratogenicity.

● **PREGNANCY** Should not be given in the first trimester of pregnancy. Warfarin, acenocoumarol, and phenindione cross the placenta with risk of congenital malformations, and placental, fetal, or neonatal haemorrhage, especially during the last few weeks of pregnancy and at delivery. Therefore, if at all possible, they should be avoided in pregnancy, especially in the first and third trimesters (difficult decisions may have to be made, particularly in women with prosthetic heart valves, atrial fibrillation, or with a history of recurrent venous thrombosis or pulmonary embolism). Stopping these drugs before the sixth week of gestation may largely avoid the risk of fetal abnormality.

● **MONITORING REQUIREMENTS**
▸ The base-line prothrombin time should be determined but the initial dose should not be delayed whilst awaiting the result.
▸ It is essential that the INR be determined daily or on alternate days in early days of treatment, *then* at longer

intervals (depending on response), *then* up to every 12 weeks.

▸ Change in patient's clinical condition, particularly associated with liver disease, intercurrent illness, or drug administration, necessitates more frequent testing.

● **PATIENT AND CARER ADVICE** Anticoagulant treatment booklets should be issued to all patients or their carers; these booklets include advice for patients on anticoagulant treatment, an alert card to be carried by the patient at all times, and a section for recording of INR results and dosage information. In **England, Wales,** and **Northern Ireland,** they are available for purchase from:
Gorse Street, Chadderton
Oldham
OL9 9QH
Tel: 0845 610 1112

GP practices can obtain supplies through their Local Area Team stores. NHS Trusts can order supplies from www.nhsforms.co.uk or by emailing nhsforms@mmm.com.

In **Scotland,** treatment booklets and starter information packs can be obtained by emailing stockorders. dppas@theapsgroup.com or by fax on (0131) 6299 967

Electronic copies of the booklets and further advice are also available at www.npsa.nhs.uk/nrls/alerts-and-directives/alerts/anticoagulant.

▸ 88

Warfarin sodium

● **INDICATIONS AND DOSE**

Treatment and prophylaxis of thrombotic episodes (induction)
▸ BY MOUTH

▸ Neonate (initiated under specialist supervision): Initially 200 micrograms/kg for 1 dose on day 1, then reduced to 100 micrograms/kg once daily for the following 3 days, subsequent doses dependent on INR levels, induction dose may need to be altered according to condition (e.g. abnormal liver function tests, cardiac failure), concomitant interacting drugs, and if baseline INR above 1.3.

▸ Child: Initially 200 micrograms/kg (max. per dose 10 mg) for 1 dose on day 1, then reduced to 100 micrograms/kg once daily (max. per dose 5 mg) for the following 3 days, subsequent doses adjusted according to INR levels, induction dose may need to be altered according to condition (e.g. abnormal liver function tests, cardiac failure), concomitant interacting drugs, and if baseline INR above 1.3

Treatment and prophylaxis of thrombotic episodes following induction dose (if INR still below 1.4)
▸ BY MOUTH

▸ Neonate: 200 micrograms/kg once daily.

▸ Child: 200 micrograms/kg once daily (max. per dose 10 mg)

Treatment and prophylaxis of thrombotic episodes following induction dose (if INR above 3.0)
▸ BY MOUTH

▸ Neonate: 50 micrograms/kg once daily.

▸ Child: 50 micrograms/kg once daily (max. per dose 2.5 mg)

Treatment and prophylaxis of thrombotic episodes following induction dose (if INR above 3.5)
▸ BY MOUTH

▸ Neonate: Dose to be omitted.

▸ Child: Dose to be omitted

Treatment and prophylaxis of thrombotic episodes (usual maintenance)
▸ BY MOUTH

▸ Neonate: Maintenance 100–300 micrograms/kg once daily, doses up to 400 micrograms/kg once daily may be required especially if bottle fed, to be adjusted according to INR.

▸ Child: Maintenance 100–300 micrograms/kg once daily, doses up to 400 micrograms/kg once daily may be required especially if bottle fed, to be adjusted according to INR

● **UNLICENSED USE** Not licensed for use in children.

● **PREGNANCY** Babies of mothers taking warfarin at the time of delivery need to be offered immediate prophylaxis with intramuscular phytomenadione (vitamin K_1).

● **BREAST FEEDING** Not present in milk in significant amounts and appears safe. Risk of haemorrhage which is increased by vitamin K deficiency.

● **HEPATIC IMPAIRMENT** Avoid in severe impairment, especially if prothrombin time is already prolonged.

● **RENAL IMPAIRMENT** Use with caution in mild to moderate impairment. In severe renal impairment, monitor INR more frequently.

● **PRESCRIBING AND DISPENSING INFORMATION**
Dietary differences Infant formula is supplemented with vitamin K, which makes formula-fed infants resistant to warfarin; they may therefore need higher doses. In contrast breast milk contains low concentrations of vitamin K making breast-fed infants more sensitive to warfarin.

● **PATIENT AND CARER ADVICE** Anticoagulant card to be provided.
Medicines for Children leaflet: Warfarin for the treatment and prevention of thrombosis www.medicinesforchildren.org.uk/warfarin-treatment-and-prevention-thrombosis

● **MEDICINAL FORMS**
There can be variation in the licensing of different medicines containing the same drug. Forms available from special-order manufacturers include: capsule, oral suspension, oral solution

Tablet
CAUTIONARY AND ADVISORY LABELS 10
▸ **Warfarin sodium (Non-proprietary)**
  Warfarin sodium 500 microgram Warfarin 500microgram tablets | 28 tablet [PoM] £1.92 DT price = £1.54
  Warfarin sodium 1 mg Warfarin 1mg tablets | 28 tablet [PoM] £1.16 DT price = £0.76 | 500 tablet [PoM] £14.82
  Warfarin sodium 3 mg Warfarin 3mg tablets | 28 tablet [PoM] £1.20 DT price = £0.79 | 500 tablet [PoM] £15.71
  Warfarin sodium 4 mg Coumadin 4mg tablets | 100 tablet [PoM] no price available
  Warfarin sodium 5 mg Warfarin 5mg tablets | 28 tablet [PoM] £1.29 DT price = £0.82 | 500 tablet [PoM] no price available
▸ **Marevan (AMCo)**
  Warfarin sodium 1 mg Marevan 1mg tablets | 28 tablet [PoM] £0.31 DT price = £0.76
  Warfarin sodium 3 mg Marevan 3mg tablets | 28 tablet [PoM] £0.35 DT price = £0.79
  Warfarin sodium 5 mg Marevan 5mg tablets | 28 tablet [PoM] £0.47 DT price = £0.82

Oral suspension
CAUTIONARY AND ADVISORY LABELS 10
▸ **Warfarin sodium (Non-proprietary)**
  Warfarin sodium 1 mg per 1 ml Warfarin 1mg/ml oral suspension sugar free sugar-free | 150 ml [PoM] £108.00 DT price = £108.00

4 Blood pressure conditions
4.1 Hypertension

Hypertension

Overview

Hypertension in children and adolescents can have a substantial effect on long-term health. Possible causes of hypertension (e.g. congenital heart disease, renal disease and endocrine disorders) and the presence of any complications (e.g. left ventricular hypertrophy) should be established. Treatment should take account of contributory factors and any factors that increase the risk of cardiovascular complications.

Serious hypertension is rare in *neonates* but it can present with signs of congestive heart failure; the cause is often renal and can follow embolic arterial damage.

Children (or their parents or carers) should be given advice on lifestyle changes to reduce blood pressure or cardiovascular risk; these include weight reduction (in obese children), reduction of dietary salt, reduction of total and saturated fat, increasing exercise, increasing fruit and vegetable intake, and not smoking.

Indications for antihypertensive therapy in children include symptomatic hypertension, secondary hypertension, hypertensive target-organ damage, diabetes mellitus, persistent hypertension despite lifestyle measures, and pulmonary hypertension. The effect of antihypertensive treatment on growth and development is not known; treatment should be started only if benefits are clear.

Antihypertensive therapy should be initiated with a single drug at the lowest recommended dose; the dose can be increased until the target blood pressure is achieved. Once the highest recommended dose is reached, or sooner if the patient begins to experience side-effects, a second drug may be added if blood pressure is not controlled. If more than one drug is required, these should be given as separate products to allow dose adjustment of individual drugs, but fixed-dose combination products may be useful in adolescents if compliance is a problem.

Acceptable drug classes for use in children with hypertension include **ACE inhibitors, alpha-blockers, beta-blockers, calcium-channel blockers,** and **thiazide diuretics**. There is limited information on the use of **angiotensin-II receptor antagonists** in children. Diuretics and beta-blockers have a long history of safety and efficacy in children. The newer classes of antihypertensive drugs, including ACE inhibitors and calcium-channel blockers have been shown to be safe and effective in short-term studies in children. Refractory hypertension may require additional treatment with agents such as minoxidil p. 108 or clonidine hydrochloride p. 93.

Other measures to reduce cardiovascular risk

Aspirin p. 83 may be used to reduce the risk of cardiovascular events; however, concerns about an increased risk of bleeding and Reye's syndrome need to be considered.

A **statin** can be of benefit in older children who have a high risk of cardiovascular disease and have hypercholesterolaemia.

Hypertension in diabetes

Hypertension can occur in type 2 diabetes and treatment prevents both macrovascular and microvascular complications. ACE inhibitors should be considered in children with diabetes and microalbuminaemia or proteinuric renal disease. Beta-blockers are best avoided in children with, or at a high risk of developing, diabetes, especially when combined with a thiazide diuretic.

Hypertension in renal disease

ACE inhibitors may be considered in children with microalbuminuria or proteinuric renal disease. High doses of loop diuretics may be required. Specific cautions apply to the use of ACE inhibitors in renal impairment, but ACE inhibitors may be effective. Dihydropyridine calcium-channel blockers may be added.

Hypertension in pregnancy

High blood pressure in pregnancy may usually be due to pre-existing essential hypertension or to pre-eclampsia. Methyldopa is safe in pregnancy. Beta-blockers are effective and safe in the third trimester. Modified-release preparations of nifedipine p. 100 [unlicensed] are also used for hypertension in pregnancy. Intravenous administration of labetalol hydrochloride p. 95 can be used to control hypertensive crises; alternatively hydralazine hydrochloride p. 108 can be given by the intravenous route.

Hypertensive emergencies

Hypertensive emergencies in children may be accompanied by signs of hypertensive encephalopathy, including seizures. Controlled reduction in blood pressure over 72–96 hours is essential; rapid reduction can reduce perfusion leading to organ damage. Treatment should be initiated with intravenous drugs; once blood pressure is controlled, oral therapy can be started. It may be necessary to infuse fluids particularly during the first 12 hours to expand plasma volume should the blood pressure drop too rapidly.

Controlled reduction of blood pressure is achieved by intravenous administration of labetalol hydrochloride or sodium nitroprusside p. 109. Esmolol hydrochloride p. 98 is useful for short-term use and has a short duration of action. Nicardipine hydrochloride p. 100 can be administered as a continuous intravenous infusion for life-threatening hypertension in paediatric intensive care settings. In less severe cases, nifedipine capsules can be used.

Other antihypertensive drugs which can be given intravenously include hydralazine hydrochloride and clonidine hydrochloride.

Hypertension in acute nephritis occurs as a result of sodium and water retention; it should be treated with sodium and fluid restriction, and with furosemide p. 132; antihypertensive drugs may be added if necessary.

Also see advice on short-term management of hypertensive episodes in phaeochromocytoma.

Phaeochromocytoma

Long-term management of phaeochromocytoma involves surgery. However, surgery should not take place until there is adequate blockade of both alpha- and beta-adrenoceptors. Alpha-blockers are used in the short-term management of hypertensive episodes in phaeochromocytoma. Once alpha blockade is established, tachycardia can be controlled by the cautious addition of a beta-blocker; a cardioselective beta-blocker is preferred. There is no nationwide consensus on the optimal drug regimen or doses used for the management of phaeochromocytoma.

Phenoxybenzamine hydrochloride p. 109, a powerful alpha-blocker, is effective in the management of phaeochromocytoma but it has many side-effects.

Pulmonary hypertension

Only pulmonary *arterial* hypertension is currently suitable for drug treatment. Pulmonary arterial hypertension includes persistent pulmonary hypertension of the newborn, idiopathic pulmonary arterial hypertension in children, and pulmonary hypertension related to congenital heart disease and cardiac surgery.

Some types of pulmonary hypertension are treated with vasodilator antihypertensive therapy and oxygen. Diuretics may also have a role in children with right-sided heart failure.

Initial treatment of *persistent pulmonary hypertension of the newborn* involves the administration of **nitric oxide**; epoprostenol p. 110 can be used until nitric oxide is available. Oral sildenafil p. 111 may be helpful in less severe cases. Epoprostenol and sildenafil can cause profound systemic hypotension. In rare circumstances either tolazoline p. 112 or magnesium sulfate p. 556 can be given by intravenous infusion when nitric oxide and epoprostenol have failed.

Treatment of *idiopathic pulmonary arterial hypertension* is determined by acute vasodilator testing; drugs used for treatment include calcium-channel blockers (usuallynifedipine), long-term intravenous epoprostenol, nebulised iloprost p. 110, bosentan p. 111, or sildenafil. Anticoagulation (usually with warfarin sodium p. 89) may also be required to prevent secondary thrombosis.

Inhaled nitric oxide is a potent and selective pulmonary vasodilator. It acts on cyclic guanosine monophosphate (cGMP) resulting in smooth muscle relaxation. Inhaled nitric oxide is used in the treatment of persistent pulmonary hypertension of the newborn, and may also be useful in other forms of arterial pulmonary hypertension. Dependency can occur with high doses and prolonged use; to avoid rebound pulmonary hypertension the drug should be withdrawn gradually, often with the aid of sildenafil p. 111.

Excess nitric oxide can cause methaemoglobinaemia; therefore, methaemoglobin concentration should be measured regularly, particularly in neonates.

Nitric oxide increases the risk of haemorrhage by inhibiting platelet aggregation, but it does not usually cause bleeding.

Epoprostenol (prostacyclin) p. 110 is a prostaglandin and a potent vasodilator. It is used in the treatment of persistent pulmonary hypertension of the newborn, idiopathic pulmonary arterial hypertension, and in the acute phase following cardiac surgery. It is given by continuous 24-hour intravenous infusion.

Epoprostenol is a powerful inhibitor of platelet aggregation and there is a possible risk of haemorrhage. It is sometimes used as an antiplatelet in renal dialysis when heparins are unsuitable or contra-indicated. It can also cause serious systemic hypotension and, if withdrawn suddenly, can cause pulmonary hypertensive crisis.

Children on prolonged treatment can become tolerant to epoprostenol, and therefore require an increase in dose.

Iloprost p. 110 is a synthetic analogue of epoprostenol and is efficacious when nebulised in adults with pulmonary arterial hypertension, but experience in children is limited. It is more stable than epoprostenol and has a longer half-life.

Bosentan p. 111 is a dual endothelin receptor antagonist used orally in the treatment of pulmonary arterial hypertension. The concentration of endothelin, a potent vasoconstrictor, is raised in sustained pulmonary hypertension.

Sildenafil, a vasodilator developed for the treatment of erectile dysfunction, is also used for pulmonary arterial hypertension. It is used either alone or as an adjunct to other drugs.

Sildenafil is a selective phosphodiesterase type-5 inhibitor. Inhibition of this enzyme in the lungs enhances the vasodilatory effects of nitric oxide and promotes relaxation of vascular smooth muscle.

Sildenafil has also been used in pulmonary hypertension for weaning children off inhaled nitric oxide following cardiac surgery, and less successfully in idiopathic pulmonary arterial hypertension.

Tolazoline p. 112 is now rarely used to correct pulmonary artery vasospasm in pulmonary hypertension of the newborn as better alternatives are available. Tolazoline is an alpha-blocker and produces both pulmonary and systemic vasodilation.

Antihypertensive drugs

Vasodilator antihypertensive drugs

Vasodilators have a potent hypotensive effect, especially when used in combination with a beta-blocker and a thiazide. **Important:** see Hypertension (hypertensive emergencies) for a warning on the hazards of a very rapid fall in blood pressure.

Hydralazine hydrochloride p. 108 is given by mouth as an adjunct to other antihypertensives for the treatment of resistant hypertension but is rarely used; when used alone it causes tachycardia and fluid retention.

Sodium nitroprusside p. 109 is given by intravenous infusion to control severe hypertensive crisis when parenteral treatment is necessary. At low doses it reduces systemic vascular resistance and increases cardiac output; at high doses it can produce profound systemic hypotension— continuous blood pressure monitoring is therefore essential. Sodium nitroprusside may also be used to control paradoxical hypertension after surgery for coarctation of the aorta.

Minoxidil p. 108 should be reserved for the treatment of severe hypertension resistant to other drugs. Vasodilatation is accompanied by increased cardiac output and tachycardia and children develop fluid retention. For this reason the addition of a beta-blocker and a diuretic (usually furosemide p. 132, in high dosage) are mandatory. Hypertrichosis is troublesome and renders this drug unsuitable for females.

Prazosin p. 92 and doxazosin p. 458 have alpha-blocking and vasodilator properties.

Centrally acting antihypertensive drugs

Methyldopa, a centrally acting antihypertensive, is of little value in the management of refractory sustained hypertension in infants and children. On prolonged use it is associated with fluid retention (which may be alleviated by concomitant use of diuretics).

Methyldopa is also effective for the management of hypertension in pregnancy.

Clonidine hydrochloride p. 93 is also a centrally acting antihypertensive but has the disadvantage that sudden withdrawal may cause a hypertensive crisis. Clonidine hydrochloride is also used under specialist supervision for pain management, sedation, and opioid withdrawal, attention deficit hyperactivity disorder, and Tourette syndrome.

Adrenergic neurone blocking drugs

Adrenergic neurone blocking drugs prevent the release of noradrenaline from postganglionic adrenergic neurones. These drugs do not control supine blood pressure and may cause postural hypotension. For this reason they have largely fallen from use in adults and are rarely used in children.

Alpha-adrenoceptor blocking drugs

Doxazosin and prazosin have post-synaptic alpha-blocking and vasodilator properties and rarely cause tachycardia. They can, however, reduce blood pressure rapidly after the first dose and should be introduced with caution.

Alpha-blockers can be used with other antihypertensive drugs in the treatment of resistant hypertension.

2

Cardiovascular system

Drugs affecting the renin-angiotensin system

Angiotensin-converting enzyme inhibitors

Angiotensin-converting enzyme inhibitors (ACE inhibitors) inhibit the conversion of angiotensin I to angiotensin II. The main indications of ACE inhibitors in children are shown below. In infants and young children, captopril p. 103 is often considered first.

Initiation under specialist supervision

Treatment with ACE inhibitors should be initiated under specialist supervision and with careful clinical monitoring in children.

Heart failure

ACE inhibitors have a valuable role in all grades of heart failure, usually combined with a loop diuretic. Potassium supplements and potassium-sparing diuretics should be discontinued before introducing an ACE inhibitor because of the risk of hyperkalaemia. Profound first-dose hypotension can occur when ACE inhibitors are introduced to children with heart failure who are already taking a high dose of a loop diuretic. Temporary withdrawal of the loop diuretic reduces the risk, but can cause severe rebound pulmonary oedema.

Hypertension

ACE inhibitors may be considered for hypertension when thiazides and beta-blockers are contra-indicated, not tolerated, or fail to control blood pressure; they may be considered for hypertension in children with type 1 diabetes with nephropathy. ACE inhibitors can reduce blood pressure very rapidly in some patients particularly in those receiving diuretic therapy.

Diabetic nephropathy

ACE inhibitors also have a role in the management of diabetic nephropathy.

Renal effects

Renal function and electrolytes should be checked before starting ACE inhibitors (or increasing the dose) and monitored during treatment (more frequently if features mentioned below are present). Hyperkalaemia and other side-effects of ACE inhibitors are more common in children with impaired renal function and the dose may need to be reduced.

Concomitant treatment with NSAIDs increases the risk of renal damage, and potassium-sparing diuretics (or potassium-containing salt substitutes) increase the risk of hyperkalaemia.

In children with severe bilateral renal artery stenosis (or severe stenosis of the artery supplying a single functioning kidney), ACE inhibitors reduce or abolish glomerular filtration and are likely to cause severe and progressive renal failure. They are therefore contra-indicated in children known to have these forms of critical renovascular disease.

ACE inhibitor treatment is unlikely to have an adverse effect on overall renal function in children with severe unilateral renal artery stenosis and a normal contralateral kidney, but glomerular filtration is likely to be reduced (or even abolished) in the affected kidney and the long-term consequences are unknown.

ACE inhibitors are therefore best avoided in those with known or suspected renovascular disease, unless the blood pressure cannot be controlled by other drugs. If they are used in these circumstances renal function needs to be monitored.

ACE inhibitors should also be used with particular caution in children who may have undiagnosed and clinically silent renovascular disease. ACE inhibitors are useful for the management of hypertension and proteinuria in children with nephritis. They are thought to have a beneficial effect by reducing intra-glomerular hypertension and protecting the glomerular capillaries and membrane.

ACE inhibitors in combination with other drugs

Concomitant diuretics

ACE inhibitors can cause a very rapid fall in blood pressure in volume-depleted children; treatment should therefore be initiated with very low doses. In some children the diuretic dose may need to be reduced or the diuretic discontinued at least 24 hours beforehand (may not be possible in heart failure—risk of pulmonary oedema). If high-dose diuretic therapy cannot be stopped, close observation is recommended after administration of the first dose of ACE inhibitor, for at least 2 hours or until the blood pressure has stabilised.

Angiotensin-II receptor antagonists

Candesartan cilexetil p. 106, losartan potassium p. 107 and valsartan p. 107 are specific angiotensin-II receptor antagonists with many properties similar to those of the ACE inhibitors. However, unlike ACE inhibitors, they do not inhibit the breakdown of bradykinin and other kinins, and thus are less likely to cause the persistent dry cough which can complicate ACE inhibitor therapy. They are therefore a useful alternative for children who have to discontinue an ACE inhibitor because of persistent cough.

Candesartan cilexetil, losartan potassium or valsartan can be used as an alternative to an ACE inhibitor in the management of hypertension.

Renal effects

Angiotensin-II receptor antagonists should be used with caution in renal artery stenosis (see also Renal effects under ACE Inhibitors, above).

Neonates

The neonatal response to treatment with ACE inhibitors is very variable, and some neonates develop profound hypotension with even small doses; a test-dose should be used initially and increased cautiously. Adverse effects such as apnoea, seizures, renal failure, and severe unpredictable hypotension are very common in the first month of life and it is therefore recommended that ACE inhibitors are avoided whenever possible, particularly in preterm neonates.

> **Drugs used for Hypertension not listed below**
> Chlortalidone, p. 134 · Diazoxide p. 434

ALPHA-ADRENOCEPTOR BLOCKERS

| Prazosin

- **● INDICATIONS AND DOSE**
  Hypertension
  ► BY MOUTH
  ► Child 1 month-11 years: Initially 10–15 micrograms/kg 2–4 times a day, initial dose to be taken at bedtime, then increased to 500 micrograms/kg daily in divided doses, dose to be increased gradually; maximum 20 mg per day
  ► Child 12-17 years: Initially 500 micrograms 2–3 times a day for 3-7 days, initial dose to be taken at bedtime, then increased to 1 mg 2–3 times a day for a further 3–7 days, then increased if necessary up to 20 mg daily in divided doses, dose should be increased gradually

Congestive heart failure (rarely used)
▶ BY MOUTH
▶ Child 1 month–11 years: 5 micrograms/kg twice daily, initial dose to be taken at bedtime, then increased to 100 micrograms/kg daily in divided doses, doses should be increased gradually
▶ Child 12–17 years: 500 micrograms 2–4 times a day, initial dose to be taken at bedtime, then increased to 4 mg daily in divided doses; maintenance 4–20 mg daily in divided doses

● UNLICENSED USE Not licensed for use in children under 12 years.
● CONTRA-INDICATIONS History of micturition syncope · history of postural hypotension · not recommended for congestive heart failure due to mechanical obstruction (e.g. aortic stenosis)
● CAUTIONS Cataract surgery (risk of intra-operative floppy iris syndrome) · first dose hypotension
● INTERACTIONS → Appendix 1 (alpha-blockers).
● SIDE-EFFECTS
▶ Common or very common Blurred vision · depression · dizziness · drowsiness · dry mouth · dyspnoea · gastro-intestinal disturbances · headache · nasal congestion · nervousness · oedema · palpitations · syncope · urinary frequency · vertigo · weakness
▶ Uncommon Allergic reactions · arthralgia · epistaxis · eye disorders · impotence · insomnia · paraesthesia · pruritus · rash · sweating · tachycardia · tinnitus · urticaria
▶ Rare Alopecia · bradycardia · flushing · gynaecomastia · hallucinations · pancreatitis · priapism · urinary incontinence · vasculitis · worsening of narcolepsy
▶ Frequency not known Angioedema · asthenia · hypotension · postural hypotension
● PREGNANCY No evidence of teratogenicity; manufacturers advise use only when potential benefit outweighs risk.
● BREAST FEEDING Present in milk, amount probably too small to be harmful; manufacturer advises use with caution.
● HEPATIC IMPAIRMENT Start with low doses and adjust according to response.
● RENAL IMPAIRMENT Start with low doses in moderate to severe impairment; increase with caution.
● DIRECTIONS FOR ADMINISTRATION
▶ With oral use For administration *by mouth*, tablets may be dispersed in water.
● PATIENT AND CARER ADVICE
Driving and skilled tasks
May affect performance of skilled tasks e.g. driving.
First dose effect First dose may cause collapse due to hypotensive effect (therefore should be taken on retiring to bed).

● MEDICINAL FORMS
There can be variation in the licensing of different medicines containing the same drug. Forms available from special-order manufacturers include: tablet, oral suspension, oral solution
Tablet
▶ Prazosin (Non-proprietary)
Prazosin (as Prazosin hydrochloride) 2 mg Minipress 2mg tablets | 100 tablet [PoM] no price available
Prazosin (as Prazosin hydrochloride) 5 mg Minipress 5mg tablets | 100 tablet [PoM] no price available
▶ Hypovase (Pfizer Ltd)
Prazosin (as Prazosin hydrochloride) 500 microgram Hypovase 500microgram tablets | 60 tablet [PoM] £2.69 DT price = £2.69
Prazosin (as Prazosin hydrochloride) 1 mg Hypovase 1mg tablets | 60 tablet [PoM] £3.46 DT price = £3.46

ANTIHYPERTENSIVES, CENTRALLY ACTING

Clonidine hydrochloride

● INDICATIONS AND DOSE
Severe hypertension
▶ BY MOUTH
▶ Child 2–17 years: Initially 0.5–1 microgram/kg 3 times a day, then increased if necessary up to 25 micrograms/kg daily in divided doses, increase dose gradually; maximum 1.2 mg per day
▶ BY SLOW INTRAVENOUS INJECTION
▶ Child 2–17 years: 2–6 micrograms/kg (max. per dose 300 micrograms) for 1 dose

● UNLICENSED USE Not licensed for use in children.
● CONTRA-INDICATIONS Severe bradyarrhythmia secondary to second- or third-degree AV block or sick sinus syndrome
● CAUTIONS Cerebrovascular disease · constipation · heart failure · history of depression · mild to moderate bradyarrhythmia · polyneuropathy · Raynaud's syndrome or other occlusive peripheral vascular disease
● INTERACTIONS → Appendix 1 (clonidine).
● SIDE-EFFECTS
▶ Common or very common Constipation · depression · dizziness · drowsiness · dry mouth · headache · malaise · nausea · postural hypotension · salivary gland pain · sexual dysfunction · sleep disturbances · vomiting
▶ Uncommon Bradycardia · delusion · hallucination · paraesthesia · pruritus · rash · Raynaud's syndrome · urticaria
▶ Rare Alopecia · AV block · colonic pseudo-obstruction · decreased lacrimation · gynaecomastia · nasal dryness
▶ Frequency not known Bradyarrhythmia · confusion · fluid retention · hepatitis · impaired visual accommodation
● PREGNANCY May lower fetal heart rate. Avoid oral use unless potential benefit outweighs risk. Avoid using injection.
● BREAST FEEDING Avoid—present in milk.
● RENAL IMPAIRMENT Use with caution.
● TREATMENT CESSATION Must be withdrawn gradually to avoid hypertensive crisis.
● DIRECTIONS FOR ADMINISTRATION
▶ With intravenous use For *intravenous injection*, give over 10–15 minutes; compatible with Sodium Chloride 0.9% *or* Glucose 5%.
▶ With oral use For administration *by mouth*, tablets may be crushed and dissolved in water.
● PATIENT AND CARER ADVICE
Medicines for Children leaflet: Clonidine for Tourette's syndrome, ADHD and sleep-onset disorder www.medicinesforchildren.org.uk/clonidine-tourettes-syndrome-adhd-and-sleep-onset-disorder
Driving and skilled tasks
Drowsiness may affect performance of skilled tasks (e.g. driving); effects of alcohol may be enhanced.
● LESS SUITABLE FOR PRESCRIBING Clonidine is less suitable for prescribing.

● MEDICINAL FORMS
There can be variation in the licensing of different medicines containing the same drug. Forms available from special-order manufacturers include: oral suspension, oral solution, solution for injection
Tablet
CAUTIONARY AND ADVISORY LABELS 3, 8
▶ Clonidine hydrochloride (Non-proprietary)
Clonidine hydrochloride 25 microgram Clonidine 25microgram tablets | 112 tablet [PoM] £12.79 DT price = £6.15

▸ **Catapres** (Boehringer Ingelheim Ltd)
Clonidine hydrochloride 100 microgram Catapres 100microgram tablets | 100 tablet [PoM] £8.04 DT price = £8.04
▸ **Dixarit** (Boehringer Ingelheim Ltd)
Clonidine hydrochloride 25 microgram Dixarit 25microgram tablets | 112 tablet [PoM] £6.99 DT price = £6.15

Solution for injection
▸ **Catapres** (Boehringer Ingelheim Ltd)
Clonidine hydrochloride 150 microgram per 1 ml Catapres 150micrograms/1ml solution for injection ampoules | 5 ampoule [PoM] £2.09

BETA-ADRENOCEPTOR BLOCKERS

Beta-adrenoceptor blocking drugs

Overview

Beta-adrenoceptor blocking drugs (beta-blockers) block the beta-adrenoceptors in the heart, peripheral vasculature, bronchi, pancreas, and liver.

Many beta-blockers are available but experience in children is limited to the use of only a few.

Differences between beta-blockers may affect choice. The water-soluble beta-blockers, atenolol p. 97 and sotalol hydrochloride p. 74, are less likely to enter the brain and may therefore cause less sleep disturbance and nightmares. Water-soluble beta-blockers are excreted by the kidneys and dosage reduction is often necessary in renal impairment.

Some beta-blockers, such as atenolol, have an intrinsically longer duration of action and need to be given only once daily. Carvedilol p. 116 and labetalol hydrochloride p. 95 are beta-blockers which have, in addition, an arteriolar vasodilating action and thus lower peripheral resistance. Although carvedilol and labetalol hydrochloride possess both alpha- and beta-blocking properties, these drugs have no important advantages over other beta-blockers in the treatment of hypertension.

Beta-blockers slow the heart and can depress the myocardium; they are contra-indicated in children with second- or third-degree heart block.

Beta-blockers can precipitate asthma and should usually be avoided in children with a history of asthma or bronchospasm. If there is no alternative, a child with well-controlled asthma can be treated for a co-existing condition (e.g. arrhythmia) with a cardioselective beta-blocker, which should be initiated with caution at a low dose by a specialist and the child monitored closely for adverse effects. Atenolol and metoprolol tartrate p. 98 have less effect on the beta$_2$ (bronchial) receptors and are, therefore, relatively *cardioselective*, but they are not *cardiospecific*; they have a lesser effect on airways resistance but are not free of this side-effect.

Beta-blockers are also associated with fatigue, coldness of the extremities, and sleep disturbances with nightmares (may be less common with the water-soluble beta-blockers).

Beta-blockers can affect carbohydrate metabolism causing hypoglycaemia or hyperglycaemia in children with or without diabetes; they can also interfere with metabolic and autonomic responses to hypoglycaemia thereby masking symptoms such as tachycardia. However, beta-blockers are not contra-indicated in diabetes, although the cardioselective beta-blockers (e.g. atenolol and metoprolol tartrate) may be preferred. Beta-blockers should be avoided altogether in those with frequent episodes of hypoglycaemia.

Hypertension

Beta-blockers are effective for reducing blood pressure, but their mode of action is not understood; they reduce cardiac output, alter baroceptor reflex sensitivity, and block peripheral adrenoceptors. Some beta-blockers depress plasma renin secretion. It is possible that a central effect may also partly explain their mode of action. Blood pressure

can usually be controlled with relatively few side-effects. In general the dose of beta-blocker does not have to be high.

Labetalol hydrochloride may be given intravenously for *hypertensive emergencies* in children; however, care is needed to avoid dangerous hypotension or beta-blockade, particularly in neonates. Esmolol hydrochloride p. 98 is also used intravenously for the treatment of hypertension particularly in the peri-operative period.

Beta-blockers can be used to control the pulse rate in children with *phaeochromocytoma*. However, they should never be used alone as beta-blockade without concurrent alpha-blockade may lead to a hypertensive crisis; phenoxybenzamine hydrochloride p. 109 should always be used together with the beta-blocker.

Arrhythmias

In arrhythmias, beta-blockers act principally by attenuating the effects of the sympathetic system on automaticity and conductivity within the heart. They can be used alone or in conjunction with digoxin p. 75 to control the ventricular rate in *atrial fibrillation*. Beta-blockers are also useful in the management of *supraventricular tachycardias* and *ventricular tachycardias* particularly to prevent recurrence of the tachycardia.

Esmolol hydrochloride is a relatively cardioselective beta-blocker with a very short duration of action, used intravenously for the short-term treatment of supraventricular arrhythmias and sinus tachycardia, particularly in the peri-operative period.

Sotalol hydrochloride is a non-cardioselective beta-blocker with additional class III anti-arrhythmic activity. Atenololand sotalol hydrochloride suppress ventricular ectopic beats and non-sustained ventricular tachycardia. However, the pro-arrhythmic effects of sotalol hydrochloride, particularly in children with sick sinus syndrome, may prolong the QT interval and induce torsade de pointes.

Heart failure

Beta-blockers may produce benefit in heart failure by blocking sympathetic activity and the addition of a beta-blocker such as carvedilol to other treatment for heart failure may be beneficial. Treatment should be initiated by those experienced in the management of heart failure.

Thyrotoxicosis

Beta-blockers are used in the management of *thyrotoxicosis* including neonatal thyrotoxicosis; propranolol hydrochloride p. 96 can reverse clinical symptoms within 4 days. Beta-blockers are also used for the pre-operative preparation for thyroidectomy; the thyroid gland is rendered less vascular, thus facilitating surgery.

Other uses

In tetralogy of Fallot, esmolol hydrochloride or propranolol hydrochloride may be given intravenously in the initial management of *cyanotic spells*; propranolol hydrochloride is given by mouth for preventing cyanotic spells. If a severe cyanotic spell in a child with congenital heart disease persists despite optimal use of 100% oxygen, propranolol hydrochloride is given by intravenous infusion. If cyanosis is still present after 10 minutes, sodium bicarbonate p. 544 intravenous infusion is given in a dose to correct acidosis (or dose calculated according to arterial blood gas results); sodium bicarbonate 4.2% intravenous infusion is appropriate for a child under 1 year and sodium bicarbonate 8.4% intravenous infusion in children over 1 year. If blood-glucose concentration is less than 3 mmol/litre, glucose 10% intravenous infusion is given, followed by intravenous or intramuscular injection of morphine p. 265.

Beta-blockers are also used in the *prophylaxis of migraine*. Betaxolol p. 637, carteolol hydrochloride p. 637, levobunolol hydrochloride p. 637, and timolol maleate p. 638 are used topically in *glaucoma*.

Beta-adrenoceptor blockers (systemic) ⬛

- **CONTRA-INDICATIONS** Asthma · cardiogenic shock · hypotension · marked bradycardia · metabolic acidosis · phaeochromocytoma (apart from specific use with alpha-blockers) · second-degree AV block · severe peripheral arterial disease · sick sinus syndrome · third-degree AV block · uncontrolled heart failure

  CONTRA-INDICATIONS, FURTHER INFORMATION

  ▸ Bronchospasm Beta-blockers, including those considered to be cardioselective, should usually be avoided in patients with a history of asthma, bronchospasm or a history of obstructive airways disease. However, when there is no alternative, a cardioselective beta-blocker can be given to these patients with caution and under specialist supervision. In such cases the risk of inducing bronchospasm should be appreciated and appropriate precautions taken.

- **CAUTIONS** Diabetes · first-degree AV block · history of obstructive airways disease (introduce cautiously) · myasthenia gravis · portal hypertension (risk of deterioration in liver function) · psoriasis · symptoms of thyrotoxicosis may be masked

- **INTERACTIONS** → Appendix 1 (beta-blockers).

  ▸ **Verapamil and beta-blockers** Verapamil injection should not be given to patients recently treated with beta-blockers because of the risk of hypotension and asystole. The suggestion that when verapamil injection has been given first, an interval of 30 minutes before giving a beta-blocker is sufficient has not been confirmed.

  It may also be hazardous to give verapamil and a beta-blocker together by mouth (should only be contemplated if myocardial function well preserved).

  There is a risk of precipitating heart failure when beta-blockers and verapamil are used together in established ischaemic heart disease.

- **SIDE-EFFECTS**

  ▸ **Rare** Dry eyes (reversible on withdrawal) · rashes (reversible on withdrawal)

  ▸ **Frequency not known** Alopecia · bradycardia · bronchospasm · coldness of the extremities · conduction disorders · dizziness · dyspnoea · exacerbation of intermittent claudication · exacerbation of psoriasis · exacerbation of Raynaud's phenomenon · fatigue · gastro-intestinal disturbances · headache · heart failure · hyperglycaemia (in patients with or without diabetes) · hypoglycaemia (in patients with or without diabetes) · hypotension · paraesthesia · peripheral vasoconstriction · psychoses · purpura · sexual dysfunction · sleep disturbances (with nightmares) · symptoms of hypoglycaemia masked · thrombocytopenia · vertigo · visual disturbances

  SIDE-EFFECTS, FURTHER INFORMATION

  ▸ Bradycardia With administration by intravenous injection, excessive bradycardia can occur and may be countered with **intravenous injection** of atropine sulfate.

  Overdose

  Therapeutic overdosages with beta-blockers may cause lightheadedness, dizziness, and possibly syncope as a result of bradycardia and hypotension; heart failure may be precipitated or exacerbated. For details on the management of poisoning, see Beta-blockers, under Emergency treatment of poisoning p. 786.

- **ALLERGY AND CROSS-SENSITIVITY** Caution is advised in patients with a history of hypersensitivity—may increase sensitivity to allergens and result in more serious hypersensitivity response. Furthermore beta-adrenoceptor blockers may reduce response to adrenaline (epinephrine).

- **PREGNANCY** Beta-blockers may cause intra-uterine growth restriction, neonatal hypoglycaemia, and bradycardia; the risk is greater in severe hypertension.

- **BREAST FEEDING** With systemic use in the mother, infants should be monitored as there is a risk of possible toxicity due to beta-blockade. However, the amount of most beta-blockers present in milk is too small to affect infants.

- **MONITORING REQUIREMENTS** Monitor lung function (in patients with a history of obstructive airway disease).

- **TREATMENT CESSATION** Avoid abrupt withdrawal.

BETA-ADRENOCEPTOR BLOCKERS ⟩ ALPHA- AND BETA-ADRENOCEPTOR BLOCKERS

⬛ above

Labetalol hydrochloride

- ● **INDICATIONS AND DOSE**

  Hypertensive emergencies

  ▸ BY INTRAVENOUS INFUSION

  ▸ **Neonate:** Initially 0.5 mg/kg/hour (max. per dose 4 mg/kg/hour), dose to be adjusted according to response at intervals of at least 15 minutes.

  ▸ **Child 1 month–11 years:** Initially 0.5–1 mg/kg/hour (max. per dose 3 mg/kg/hour), dose to be adjusted according to response at intervals of at least 15 minutes

  ▸ **Child 12–17 years:** Initially 30–120 mg/hour, dose to be adjusted according to response at intervals of at least 15 minutes

  Hypertension

  ▸ BY MOUTH

  ▸ **Child 1 month–11 years:** 1–2 mg/kg 3–4 times a day

  ▸ **Child 12–17 years:** Initially 50–100 mg twice daily, dose to be increased if required at intervals of 3–14 days; usual dose 200–400 mg twice daily, higher doses to be given in 3–4 divided doses; maximum 2.4 g per day

  ▸ BY INTRAVENOUS INJECTION

  ▸ **Child 1 month–11 years:** 250–500 micrograms/kg (max. per dose 20 mg) for 1 dose

  ▸ **Child 12–17 years:** 50 mg, dose to be given over at least 1 minute, then 50 mg after 5 minutes if required; maximum 200 mg per course

- ● **UNLICENSED USE** Not licensed for use in children.

  > **IMPORTANT SAFETY INFORMATION**
  > ▸ With intravenous use
  > Consult local guidelines. In hypertensive encephalopathy reduce blood pressure to normotensive level over 24–48 hours (more rapid reduction may lead to cerebral infarction, blindness, and death). If child fitting, reduce blood pressure rapidly, but not to normal levels.

- ● **CAUTIONS** Liver damage

- ● **SIDE-EFFECTS**

  ▸ **Rare** Lichenoid rash

  ▸ **Frequency not known** Difficulty in micturition · epigastric pain · liver damage · nausea · postural hypotension · vomiting · weakness

- ● **PREGNANCY** The use of labetalol in maternal hypertension is not known to be harmful, except possibly in the first trimester. If labetalol is used close to delivery, infants should be monitored for signs of alpha-blockade (as well as beta-blockade).

- ● **BREAST FEEDING** Infants should be monitored as there is a risk of possible toxicity due to alpha-blockade (in addition to beta-blockade).

- **HEPATIC IMPAIRMENT** Avoid—severe hepatocellular injury reported.
- **RENAL IMPAIRMENT** Dose reduction may be required.
- **MONITORING REQUIREMENTS**
▸ Liver damage Severe hepatocellular damage reported after both short-term and long-term treatment. Appropriate laboratory testing needed at first symptom of liver dysfunction and if laboratory evidence of damage (or if jaundice) labetalol should be stopped and not restarted.
- **EFFECT ON LABORATORY TESTS** Interferes with laboratory tests for catecholamines.
- **DIRECTIONS FOR ADMINISTRATION**
▸ With intravenous use For *intravenous infusion*, dilute to a concentration of 1 mg/mL in Glucose 5% or Sodium Chloride and Glucose 5%; if fluid restricted may be given undiluted, preferably through a central venous catheter. Avoid upright position during and for 3 hours after intravenous administration.
▸ With oral use For administration *by mouth*, injection may be given orally with squash or juice.
- **PATIENT AND CARER ADVICE**
Medicines for Children leaflet: Labetalol hydrochloride for hypertension www.medicinesforchildren.org.uk/ labetalol-hydrochloride-for-hypertension

- **MEDICINAL FORMS**
There can be variation in the licensing of different medicines containing the same drug. Forms available from special-order manufacturers include: oral suspension, oral solution

Tablet
▸ CAUTIONARY AND ADVISORY LABELS 8, 21
▸ **Labetalol hydrochloride (Non-proprietary)**
Labetalol hydrochloride 100 mg Labetalol 100mg tablets |
56 tablet [PoM] £7.21 DT price = £5.81
Labetalol hydrochloride 200 mg Labetalol 200mg tablets |
56 tablet [PoM] £9.97 DT price = £8.83
Labetalol hydrochloride 400 mg Labetalol 400mg tablets |
56 tablet [PoM] £23.14 DT price = £23.14
▸ **Trandate** (Focus Pharmaceuticals Ltd)
Labetalol hydrochloride 50 mg Trandate 50mg tablets |
56 tablet [PoM] £3.79 DT price = £3.79
Labetalol hydrochloride 100 mg Trandate 100mg tablets |
56 tablet [PoM] £4.64 DT price = £5.81 | 250 tablet [PoM] £15.62
Labetalol hydrochloride 200 mg Trandate 200mg tablets |
56 tablet [PoM] £7.41 DT price = £8.83 | 250 tablet [PoM] £24.76
Labetalol hydrochloride 400 mg Trandate 400mg tablets |
56 tablet [PoM] £10.15 DT price = £23.14

Solution for injection
▸ Labetalol hydrochloride (Non-proprietary)
Labetalol hydrochloride 5 mg per 1 ml Labetalol 100mg/20ml solution for injection ampoules | 5 ampoule [PoM] £44.44–£53.33

BETA-ADRENOCEPTOR BLOCKERS ›
NON-SELECTIVE

F 95

Propranolol hydrochloride

- **INDICATIONS AND DOSE**

Hyperthyroidism with autonomic symptoms
▸ BY MOUTH

▸ **Neonate:** Initially 250–500 micrograms/kg every 6–8 hours, adjusted according to response.

▸ **Child:** Initially 250–500 micrograms/kg every 8 hours, adjusted according to response; increased if necessary up to 1 mg/kg every 8 hours (max. per dose 40 mg every 8 hours)
▸ BY INTRAVENOUS INJECTION

▸ **Neonate:** Initially 20–50 micrograms/kg every 6–8 hours, adjusted according to response, to be given over 10 minutes.

▸ **Child:** Initially 25–50 micrograms/kg every 6–8 hours (max. per dose 5 mg), adjusted according to response, to be given over 10 minutes

Thyrotoxicosis (adjunct)
▸ BY MOUTH

▸ **Neonate:** Initially 250–500 micrograms/kg every 6–8 hours, adjusted according to response.

▸ **Child:** Initially 250–500 micrograms/kg every 8 hours, adjusted according to response; increased if necessary up to 1 mg/kg every 8 hours (max. per dose 40 mg every 8 hours)
▸ BY INTRAVENOUS INJECTION

▸ **Neonate:** Initially 20–50 micrograms/kg every 6–8 hours, adjusted according to response, to be given over 10 minutes.

▸ **Child:** Initially 25–50 micrograms/kg every 6–8 hours (max. per dose 5 mg), adjusted according to response, to be given over 10 minutes

Thyrotoxic crisis
▸ BY MOUTH

▸ **Neonate:** Initially 250–500 micrograms/kg every 6–8 hours, adjusted according to response.

▸ **Child:** Initially 250–500 micrograms/kg every 8 hours, adjusted according to response; increased if necessary up to 1 mg/kg every 8 hours (max. per dose 40 mg every 8 hours)
▸ BY INTRAVENOUS INJECTION

▸ **Neonate:** Initially 20–50 micrograms/kg every 6–8 hours, adjusted according to response, to be given over 10 minutes.

▸ **Child:** Initially 25–50 micrograms/kg every 6–8 hours (max. per dose 5 mg), adjusted according to response, to be given over 10 minutes

Hypertension
▸ BY MOUTH

▸ **Neonate:** Initially 250 micrograms/kg 3 times a day, then increased if necessary up to 2 mg/kg 3 times a day.

▸ **Child 1 month-11 years:** Initially 0.25–1 mg/kg 3 times a day, then increased to 5 mg/kg daily in divided doses, dose should be increased at weekly intervals

▸ **Child 12-17 years:** Initially 80 mg twice daily, then increased if necessary up to 160–320 mg daily, dose should be increased at weekly intervals, slow-release preparations may be used for once daily administration

Migraine prophylaxis
▸ BY MOUTH

▸ **Child 2-11 years:** Initially 200–500 micrograms/kg twice daily; usual dose 10–20 mg twice daily (max. per dose 2 mg/kg twice daily)

▸ **Child 12-17 years:** Initially 20–40 mg twice daily; usual dose 40–80 mg twice daily (max. per dose 120 mg); maximum 4 mg/kg per day

Arrhythmias
▸ BY MOUTH

▸ **Neonate:** 250–500 micrograms/kg 3 times a day, adjusted according to response.

▸ **Child:** 250–500 micrograms/kg 3–4 times a day (max. per dose 1 mg/kg 4 times a day), adjusted according to response; maximum 160 mg per day
▸ BY SLOW INTRAVENOUS INJECTION

▸ **Neonate:** 20–50 micrograms/kg, then 20–50 micrograms/kg every 6–8 hours if required, eCG monitoring required.

▸ **Child:** 25–50 micrograms/kg, then 25–50 micrograms/kg every 6–8 hours if required, eCG monitoring required

Tetralogy of Fallot
▶ BY MOUTH

▸ **Neonate:** 0.25–1 mg/kg 2–3 times a day (max. per dose 2 mg/kg 3 times a day).

▸ **Child 1 month–11 years:** 0.25–1 mg/kg 3–4 times a day, maximum dose to be given in divided doses; maximum 5 mg/kg per day

▶ BY SLOW INTRAVENOUS INJECTION

▸ **Neonate:** Initially 15–20 micrograms/kg (max. per dose 100 micrograms/kg), then 15–20 micrograms/kg every 12 hours if required, eCG monitoring is required with administration.

▸ **Child 1 month–11 years:** Initially 15–20 micrograms/kg (max. per dose 100 micrograms/kg), higher doses are rarely necessary, then 15–20 micrograms/kg every 6–8 hours if required, eCG monitoring is required with administration

● **UNLICENSED USE** Not licensed for treatment of hypertension in children under 12 years.

● **SIDE-EFFECTS**

● **Rare** Dry eyes (reversible on withdrawal)

● **HEPATIC IMPAIRMENT** Reduce oral dose.

● **RENAL IMPAIRMENT** Manufacturer advises caution; dose reduction may be required.

● **DIRECTIONS FOR ADMINISTRATION** For *slow intravenous injection*, give over at least 3–5 minutes; rate of administration should not exceed 1 mg/minute. May be diluted with Sodium Chloride 0.9% or Glucose 5%. Incompatible with bicarbonate.

● **PRESCRIBING AND DISPENSING INFORMATION** Modified-release preparations can be used for once daily administration.

● **MEDICINAL FORMS**
There can be variation in the licensing of different medicines containing the same drug. Forms available from special-order manufacturers include: oral suspension, oral solution

Tablet
CAUTIONARY AND ADVISORY LABELS 8

▸ Propranolol hydrochloride (Non-proprietary)
Propranolol hydrochloride 10 mg Propranolol 10mg tablets | 28 tablet [PoM] £1.47 DT price = £0.85
Propranolol hydrochloride 40 mg Propranolol 40mg tablets | 28 tablet [PoM] £1.85 DT price = £0.89
Propranolol hydrochloride 80 mg Propranolol 80mg tablets | 28 tablet [PoM] no price available | 56 tablet [PoM] £9.33 DT price = £1.93
Propranolol hydrochloride 160 mg Propranolol 160mg tablets | 56 tablet [PoM] £6.23 DT price = £5.65

Modified-release capsule
CAUTIONARY AND ADVISORY LABELS 8, 25

▸ Propranolol hydrochloride (Non-proprietary)
Propranolol hydrochloride 80 mg Propranolol 80mg modified-release capsules | 28 capsule [PoM] £6.98 DT price = £4.95
Propranolol hydrochloride 160 mg Propranolol 160mg modified-release capsules | 28 capsule [PoM] £4.88 DT price = £5.13
▸ Bedranol SR (Almus Pharmaceuticals Ltd, Sandoz Ltd)
Propranolol hydrochloride 80 mg Bedranol SR 80mg capsules | 28 capsule [PoM] £4.16 DT price = £4.95
Propranolol hydrochloride 160 mg Bedranol SR 160mg capsules | 28 capsule [PoM] £5.09 DT price = £5.13
▸ Beta-Prograne (Actavis UK Ltd, Tillomed Laboratories Ltd, Teva UK Ltd)
Propranolol hydrochloride 160 mg Beta-Prograne 160mg modified-release capsules | 28 capsule [PoM] £6.11 DT price = £5.13
▸ Half Beta-Prograne (Tillomed Laboratories Ltd, Teva UK Ltd, Actavis UK Ltd)
Propranolol hydrochloride 80 mg Half Beta-Prograne 80mg modified-release capsules | 28 capsule [PoM] £4.95 DT price = £4.95

Oral solution
CAUTIONARY AND ADVISORY LABELS 8

▸ Propranolol hydrochloride (Non-proprietary)
Propranolol hydrochloride 1 mg per 1 ml Propranolol 5mg/5ml oral solution sugar free sugar-free | 150 ml [PoM] £15.50 DT price = £12.50
Propranolol hydrochloride 2 mg per 1 ml Propranolol 10mg/5ml oral solution sugar free sugar-free | 150 ml [PoM] £20.45 DT price = £16.45
Propranolol hydrochloride 8 mg per 1 ml Propranolol 40mg/5ml oral solution sugar free sugar-free | 150 ml [PoM] £31.50 DT price = £31.50
Propranolol hydrochloride 10 mg per 1 ml Propranolol 50mg/5ml oral solution sugar free sugar-free | 150 ml [PoM] £24.98 DT price = £19.98
▸ Syprol (Rosemont Pharmaceuticals Ltd)
Propranolol hydrochloride 1 mg per 1 ml Syprol 5mg/5ml oral solution sugar-free | 150 ml [PoM] £12.50 DT price = £12.50
Propranolol hydrochloride 2 mg per 1 ml Syprol 10mg/5ml oral solution sugar-free | 150 ml [PoM] £16.45 DT price = £16.45
Propranolol hydrochloride 8 mg per 1 ml Syprol 40mg/5ml oral solution sugar-free | 150 ml [PoM] £31.50 DT price = £31.50
Propranolol hydrochloride 10 mg per 1 ml Syprol 50mg/5ml oral solution sugar-free | 150 ml [PoM] £19.98 DT price = £19.98

BETA-ADRENOCEPTOR BLOCKERS ›
SELECTIVE

⬛ 95

Atenolol

● **INDICATIONS AND DOSE**
Hypertension
▶ BY MOUTH

▸ **Neonate:** 0.5–2 mg/kg once daily, dose may be given in 2 divided doses.

▸ **Child 1 month–11 years:** 0.5–2 mg/kg once daily, dose may be given in 2 divided doses, doses higher than 50 mg daily are rarely necessary

▸ **Child 12–17 years:** 25–50 mg once daily, dose may be given in 2 divided doses, higher doses are rarely necessary

Arrhythmias
▶ BY MOUTH

▸ **Neonate:** 0.5–2 mg/kg once daily, dose may be given in 2 divided doses.

▸ **Child 1 month–11 years:** 0.5–2 mg/kg once daily, dose may be given in 2 divided doses; maximum 100 mg per day

▸ **Child 12–17 years:** 50–100 mg once daily, dose may be given in 2 divided doses

● **UNLICENSED USE** Not licensed for use in children under 12 years.

● **BREAST FEEDING** Water soluble beta-blockers such as atenolol are present in breast milk in greater amounts than other beta blockers.

● **RENAL IMPAIRMENT** Initially use 50% of usual dose if estimated glomerular filtration rate 10–35 mL/minute/1.73 m^2; initially use 30–50% of usual dose if estimated glomerular filtration rate less than 10 mL/minute/1.73 m^2.

● **PATIENT AND CARER ADVICE**
Medicines for Children leaflet: Atenolol for hypertension
www.medicinesforchildren.org.uk/atenolol-hypertension-0

● MEDICINAL FORMS
There can be variation in the licensing of different medicines containing the same drug. Forms available from special-order manufacturers include: oral suspension, oral solution

Tablet
CAUTIONARY AND ADVISORY LABELS 8
▸ Atenolol (Non-proprietary)
Atenolol 25 mg Atenolol 25mg tablets | 28 tablet [PoM] £1.39 DT price = £0.70
Atenolol 50 mg Atenolol 50mg tablets | 28 tablet [PoM] £1.44 DT price = £0.77
Atenolol 100 mg Atenolol 100mg tablets | 28 tablet [PoM] £1.74 DT price = £0.73
▸ Tenormin (AstraZeneca UK Ltd)
Atenolol 50 mg Tenormin LS 50mg tablets | 28 tablet [PoM] £5.11 DT price = £0.77
Atenolol 100 mg Tenormin 100mg tablets | 28 tablet [PoM] £6.49 DT price = £0.73

Oral solution
▸ Atenolol (Non-proprietary)
Atenolol 5 mg per 1 ml Atenolol 25mg/5ml oral solution sugar free sugar-free | 300 ml [PoM] £6.72 DT price = £5.59

◤ 95

Esmolol hydrochloride

● INDICATIONS AND DOSE
Arrhythmias | Hypertensive emergencies
▸ INITIALLY BY INTRAVENOUS INJECTION
▸ Child: Loading dose 500 micrograms/kg, to be given over 1 minute, then (by intravenous infusion) maintenance 50 micrograms/kg/minute for 4 minutes (rate reduced if low blood pressure or low heart rate), if inadequate response, repeat loading dose and increase maintenance infusion, (by intravenous injection) loading dose 500 micrograms/kg, given over 1 minute, then (by intravenous infusion) maintenance 100 micrograms/kg/minute for 4 minutes, if response still inadequate, repeat loading dose and increase maintenance infusion, (by intravenous injection) loading dose 500 micrograms/kg, given over 1 minute, then (by intravenous infusion) maintenance 150 micrograms/kg/minute for 4 minutes, if response still inadequate, repeat loading dose and increase maintenance infusion, (by intravenous injection) loading dose 500 micrograms/kg, given over 1 minute, then (by intravenous infusion) maintenance 200 micrograms/kg/minute for 4 minutes, doses over 300 micrograms/kg/minute not recommended

Tetralogy of Fallot
▸ INITIALLY BY INTRAVENOUS INJECTION
▸ Neonate: Initially 600 micrograms/kg, dose to be given over 1–2 minutes, then (by intravenous infusion) 300–900 micrograms/kg/minute if required.

● UNLICENSED USE Not licensed for use in children.
● SIDE-EFFECTS Thrombophlebitis · venous irritation
● BREAST FEEDING Manufacturer advises avoidance.
● RENAL IMPAIRMENT Manufacturer advises caution.
● DIRECTIONS FOR ADMINISTRATION Give through a central venous catheter; incompatible with bicarbonate.

● MEDICINAL FORMS
There can be variation in the licensing of different medicines containing the same drug.
Solution for injection
▸ Brevibloc (Baxter Healthcare Ltd)
Esmolol hydrochloride 10 mg per 1 ml Brevibloc Premixed 100mg/10ml solution for injection vials | 5 vial [PoM] no price available

Solution for infusion
▸ Brevibloc (Baxter Healthcare Ltd)
Esmolol hydrochloride 10 mg per 1 ml Brevibloc Premixed 2.5g/250ml infusion bags | 1 bag [PoM] £89.69

◤ 95

Metoprolol tartrate

● INDICATIONS AND DOSE
Hypertension
▸ BY MOUTH USING IMMEDIATE-RELEASE MEDICINES
▸ Child 1 month–11 years: Initially 1 mg/kg twice daily, increased if necessary up to 8 mg/kg daily in 2–4 divided doses (max. per dose 400 mg)
▸ Child 12–17 years: Initially 50–100 mg daily, increased if necessary to 200 mg daily in 1–2 divided doses, high doses are rarely necessary; maximum 400 mg per day
▸ BY MOUTH USING MODIFIED-RELEASE MEDICINES
▸ Child 12–17 years: 200 mg once daily

Arrhythmias
▸ BY MOUTH USING IMMEDIATE-RELEASE MEDICINES
▸ Child 12–17 years: Usual dose 50 mg 2–3 times a day, then increased if necessary up to 300 mg daily in divided doses

● UNLICENSED USE Not licensed for use in children.
● HEPATIC IMPAIRMENT Reduce dose in severe impairment.

● MEDICINAL FORMS
There can be variation in the licensing of different medicines containing the same drug. Forms available from special-order manufacturers include: capsule, oral suspension, oral solution

Tablet
CAUTIONARY AND ADVISORY LABELS 8
▸ Metoprolol tartrate (Non-proprietary)
Metoprolol tartrate 50 mg Metoprolol 50mg tablets | 28 tablet [PoM] £3.00 DT price = £1.31 | 56 tablet [PoM] £3.52
Metoprolol tartrate 100 mg Metoprolol 100mg tablets | 28 tablet [PoM] £3.00 DT price = £1.50 | 56 tablet [PoM] £4.64
▸ Lopresor (Recordati Pharmaceuticals Ltd)
Metoprolol tartrate 50 mg Lopresor 50mg tablets | 56 tablet [PoM] £2.57
Metoprolol tartrate 100 mg Lopresor 100mg tablets | 56 tablet [PoM] £6.68

CALCIUM-CHANNEL BLOCKERS

Calcium-channel blockers

Overview

Calcium-channel blockers differ in their predilection for the various possible sites of action and, therefore, their therapeutic effects are disparate, with much greater variation than those of beta-blockers. There are important differences between verapamil hydrochloride p. 101, diltiazem hydrochloride p. 136, and the dihydropyridine calcium-channel blockers (amlodipine p. 99, nicardipine hydrochloride p. 100, nifedipine p. 100, and nimodipine p. 80). Verapamil hydrochloride and diltiazem hydrochloride should usually be **avoided** in heart failure because they may further depress cardiac function and cause clinically significant deterioration.

Verapamil hydrochloride is used for the treatment of hypertension and arrhythmias. However, it is no longer first-line treatment for arrhythmias in children because it has been associated with fatal collapse especially in infants under 1 year; adenosine p. 73 is now recommended for first-line use.

Verapamil hydrochloride is a highly negatively inotropic calcium channel-blocker and it reduces cardiac output, slows the heart rate, and may impair atrioventricular conduction. It may precipitate heart failure, exacerbate conduction disorders, and cause hypotension at high doses and should

not be used with beta-blockers. Constipation is the most common side-effect.

Nifedipine relaxes vascular smooth muscle and dilates coronary and peripheral arteries. It has more influence on vessels and less on the myocardium than does verapamil hydrochloride and unlike verapamil hydrochloride has no anti-arrhythmic activity. It rarely precipitates heart failure because any negative inotropic effect is offset by a reduction in left ventricular work. Short-acting formulations of nifedipine may be used if a modified-release preparation delivering the appropriate dose is not available or if a child is unable to swallow (a liquid preparation may be prepared using capsules). Nifedipine may also be used for the management of angina due to coronary artery disease in Kawasaki disease or progeria and in the management of Raynaud's syndrome.

Nicardipine hydrochloride has similar effects to those of nifedipine and may produce less reduction of myocardial contractility; it should only be used for the treatment of life-threatening hypertension in paediatric intensive care settings and in postoperative hypertension.

Amlodipine also resembles nifedipine and nicardipine hydrochloride in its effects and does not reduce myocardial contractility or produce clinical deterioration in heart failure. It has a longer duration of action and can be given once daily. Nifedipine and amlodipine are used for the treatment of hypertension. Side-effects associated with vasodilatation such as flushing and headache (which become less obtrusive after a few days), and ankle swelling (which may respond only partially to diuretics) are common.

Nimodipine is related to nifedipine but the smooth muscle relaxant effect preferentially acts on cerebral arteries. Its use is confined to prevention and treatment of vascular spasm following aneurysmal subarachnoid haemorrhage.

Diltiazem hydrochloride is a peripheral vasodilator and also has mild depressor effects on the myocardium. It is used in the treatment of Raynaud's syndrome.

Calcium-channel blockers

- **DRUG ACTION** Calcium-channel blockers (less correctly called 'calcium-antagonists') interfere with the inward displacement of calcium ions through the slow channels of active cell membranes. They influence the myocardial cells, the cells within the specialised conducting system of the heart, and the cells of vascular smooth muscle. Thus, myocardial contractility may be reduced, the formation and propagation of electrical impulses within the heart may be depressed, and coronary or systemic vascular tone may be diminished.

- **SIDE-EFFECTS**
Overdose
Features of calcium-channel blocker poisoning include nausea, vomiting, dizziness, agitation, confusion, and coma in severe poisoning. Metabolic acidosis and hyperglycaemia may occur.
For details on the management of poisoning, see Calcium-channel blockers, under Emergency treatment of poisoning p. 786.

- **TREATMENT CESSATION** There is some evidence that sudden withdrawal of calcium-channel blockers may be associated with an exacerbation of myocardial ischaemia.

---

above

Amlodipine

- **DRUG ACTION** Amlodipine is a dihydropyridine calcium-channel blocker.

- **INDICATIONS AND DOSE**
Hypertension
▸ BY MOUTH
  ▸ Child 1 month–11 years: Initially 100–200 micrograms/kg once daily; increased if necessary up to 400 micrograms/kg once daily, adjusted at intervals of 1–2 weeks; maximum 10 mg per day
  ▸ Child 12–17 years: Initially 5 mg once daily, then increased if necessary up to 10 mg once daily, adjusted at intervals of 1–2 weeks

DOSE EQUIVALENCE AND CONVERSION
Tablets from various suppliers may contain different salts (e.g. amlodipine besilate, amlodipine maleate, and amlodipine mesilate) but the strength is expressed in terms of amlodipine (base); tablets containing different salts are considered interchangeable.

- **UNLICENSED USE** Not licensed for use in children under 6 years.

- **CONTRA-INDICATIONS** Cardiogenic shock · significant aortic stenosis

- **INTERACTIONS** → Appendix 1 (calcium-channel blockers).

- **SIDE-EFFECTS**
▸ **Common or very common** Abdominal pain · dizziness · fatigue · flushing · headache · nausea · oedema · palpitation · sleep disturbances
▸ **Uncommon** Alopecia · arthralgia · asthenia · back pain · chest pain · dry mouth · dyspnoea · gastro-intestinal disturbances · gynaecomastia · hypotension · impotence · mood changes · muscle cramps · myalgia · paraesthesia · pruritus · purpura · rashes · rhinitis · skin discolouration · sweating · syncope · taste disturbances · tinnitus · tremor · urinary disturbances · visual disturbances · weight changes
▸ **Very rare** Angioedema · arrhythmias · cholestasis · coughing · gastritis · gingival hyperplasia · hepatitis · hyperglycaemia · jaundice · myocardial infarction · pancreatitis · peripheral neuropathy · tachycardia · thrombocytopenia · urticaria · vasculitis
▸ **Frequency not known** Erythema multiforme
Overdose
In overdose, the dihydropyridine calcium-channel blockers cause severe hypotension secondary to profound peripheral vasodilatation.

- **PREGNANCY** No information available—manufacturer advises avoid, but risk to fetus should be balanced against risk of uncontrolled maternal hypertension.

- **BREAST FEEDING** Manufacturer advises avoid—no information available.

- **HEPATIC IMPAIRMENT** May need dose reduction—half-life prolonged.

- **DIRECTIONS FOR ADMINISTRATION** Tablets may be dispersed in water.

- **PATIENT AND CARER ADVICE**
Medicines for Children leaflet: Amlodipine for hypertension www.medicinesforchildren.org.uk/amlodipine-for-hypertension

- **MEDICINAL FORMS**
There can be variation in the licensing of different medicines containing the same drug. Forms available from special-order manufacturers include: oral suspension, oral solution
Tablet
▸ Amlodipine (Non-proprietary)
  Amlodipine 5 mg Amlodipine 5mg tablets | 28 tablet PoM £9.42 DT price = £0.72
  Amlodipine 10 mg Amlodipine 10mg tablets | 28 tablet PoM £14.07 DT price = £0.77

▸ **Amlostin** (Discovery Pharmaceuticals)
  Amlodipine 5 mg Amlostin 5mg tablets | 28 tablet [PoM] £0.73 DT price = £0.72
  Amlodipine 10 mg Amlostin 10mg tablets | 28 tablet [PoM] £0.77 DT price = £0.77
▸ **Istin** (Pfizer Ltd)
  Amlodipine 5 mg Istin 5mg tablets | 28 tablet [PoM] £11.08 DT price = £0.72
  Amlodipine 10 mg Istin 10mg tablets | 28 tablet [PoM] £16.55 DT price = £0.77

Oral solution
▸ **Amlodipine** (Non-proprietary)
  Amlodipine 1 mg per 1 ml Amlodipine 5mg/5ml oral solution sugar free sugar-free | 150 ml [PoM] £77.82 DT price = £76.65
  Amlodipine 2 mg per 1 ml Amlodipine 10mg/5ml oral solution sugar free sugar-free | 150 ml [PoM] £118.89 DT price = £117.11

F 99

Nicardipine hydrochloride

● **DRUG ACTION** Nicardipine is a dihydropyridine calcium-channel blocker.

● **INDICATIONS AND DOSE**

Life-threatening hypertension (specialist use only) | Post-operative hypertension (specialist use only)
▸ BY CONTINUOUS INTRAVENOUS INFUSION
▸ **Neonate:** Initially 500 nanograms/kg/minute (max. per dose 5 micrograms/kg/minute), adjusted according to response; maintenance 1–4 micrograms/kg/minute.
▸ **Child:** Initially 500 nanograms/kg/minute (max. per dose 5 micrograms/kg/minute), adjusted according to response; maintenance 1–4 micrograms/kg/minute (max. per dose 250 micrograms/minute)

● **CONTRA-INDICATIONS** Acute porphyrias p. 562 · avoid within 8 days of myocardial infarction · cardiogenic shock · compensatory hypertension · significant or advanced aortic stenosis

● **CAUTIONS** Congestive heart failure · elevated intracranial pressure · increased risk of serious hypotension · portal hypertension · pulmonary oedema · significantly impaired left ventricular function · stroke

● **INTERACTIONS** → Appendix 1 (calcium-channel blockers).

● **SIDE-EFFECTS** Atrioventricular block · dizziness · flushing · headache · hypotension · nausea · palpitations · paralytic ileus · peripheral oedema · pulmonary oedema · tachycardia · thrombocytopenia · vomiting

SIDE-EFFECTS, FURTHER INFORMATION
▸ Hypotension and reflex tachycardia Systemic hypotension and reflex tachycardia with rapid reduction of blood pressure may occur—during intravenous use consider stopping infusion or decreasing dose by half.

Overdose
In overdose, the dihydropyridine calcium-channel blockers cause severe hypotension secondary to profound peripheral vasodilatation.

● **PREGNANCY** May inhibit labour. Not to be used in multiple pregnancy (twins or more) unless there is no other acceptable alternative. Toxicity in *animal* studies. Risk of severe maternal hypotension and fatal foetal hypoxia—avoid excessive decrease in blood pressure.

● **BREAST FEEDING** Manufacturer advises avoid—present in breast milk.

● **HEPATIC IMPAIRMENT** Half-life prolonged in severe impairment—consider using low initial dose. Use with caution in hepatic impairment—increased risk of serious hypotension.

● **RENAL IMPAIRMENT** Use with caution—increased risk of serious hypotension; consider using low initial dose.

● **MONITORING REQUIREMENTS** Monitor blood pressure and heart rate at least every 5 minutes during intravenous

infusion, and then until stable, and continue monitoring for at least 12 hours after end of infusion.

● **DIRECTIONS FOR ADMINISTRATION** Intravenous nicardipine should only be administered under the supervision of a specialist and in a hospital or intensive care setting in which patients can be closely monitored.
  For *continuous intravenous infusion*, dilute to a concentration of 100–200 micrograms/mL with Glucose 5% and give *via* volumetric infusion pump or syringe driver; protect from light; to minimise peripheral venous irritation, change site of infusion every 12 hours; risk of adsorption on to plastic in the presence of saline solutions; incompatible with bicarbonate or alkaline solutions—consult product literature.

● **MEDICINAL FORMS** There can be variation in the licensing of different medicines containing the same drug.

Solution for infusion
▸ **Nicardipine hydrochloride** (Non-proprietary)
  Nicardipine hydrochloride 1 mg per 1 ml Nicardipine 10mg/10ml solution for injection ampoules | 5 ampoule [PoM] £50.00
  Nicardipine hydrochloride 2.5 mg per 1 ml Cardene I.V. 25mg/10ml solution for infusion ampoules | 10 ampoule [PoM] no price available

F 99

Nifedipine

● **DRUG ACTION** Nifedipine is a dihydropyridine calcium-channel blocker.

● **INDICATIONS AND DOSE**

Hypertensive crisis | Acute angina in Kawasaki disease or progeria
▸ BY MOUTH USING IMMEDIATE-RELEASE MEDICINES
▸ **Child:** Initially 250–500 micrograms/kg (max. per dose 10 mg), then repeat once if necessary, may cause unpredictable and severe reduction of blood pressure—monitor closely following administration; if ineffective consider alternative treatment and seek specialist advice

Hypertension | Angina in Kawasaki disease or progeria
▸ BY MOUTH USING IMMEDIATE-RELEASE MEDICINES
▸ **Child 1 month–11 years:** 200–300 micrograms/kg 3 times a day, dose frequency depends on preparation used; maximum 3 mg/kg per day; maximum 90 mg per day
▸ **Child 12–17 years:** 5–20 mg 3 times a day, dose frequency depends on preparation used; maximum 90 mg per day

Raynaud's syndrome
▸ BY MOUTH USING IMMEDIATE-RELEASE MEDICINES
▸ **Child 2–17 years:** 2.5–10 mg 2–4 times a day, start with low doses at night and increase gradually to avoid postural hypotension, dose frequency depends on preparation used

Persistent hyperinsulinaemic hypoglycaemia
▸ BY MOUTH USING IMMEDIATE-RELEASE MEDICINES
▸ **Neonate:** 100–200 micrograms/kg 4 times a day (max. per dose 600 micrograms/kg).

DOSE EQUIVALENCE AND CONVERSION
ADALAT®
Adalat liquid gel capsules contain 5 mg nifedipine in 0.17 mL and 10 mg nifedipine in 0.34 mL.

● **UNLICENSED USE** Not licensed for use in children.

● **CONTRA-INDICATIONS** Cardiogenic shock · significant aortic stenosis

● **CAUTIONS** Diabetes mellitus · heart failure · poor cardiac reserve · severe hypotension · short-acting formulations are not recommended for angina or long-term management of hypertension; their use may be associated with large variations in blood pressure and reflex tachycardia · significantly impaired left ventricular function (heart failure deterioration observed)

● **INTERACTIONS** → Appendix 1 (calcium-channel blockers).

● **SIDE-EFFECTS**

▸ **Common or very common** Asthenia · dizziness · gastro-intestinal disturbance · headache · hypotension · lethargy · oedema · palpitation · vasodilatation

▸ **Uncommon** Angioedema · anxiety · chills · dyspnoea · dysuria · epistaxis · erectile dysfunction · hypersensitivity reactions · jaundice · joint swelling · migraine · myalgia · nasal congestion · nocturia · paraesthesia · polyuria · pruritus · rash · sleep disturbance · sweating · syncope · tachycardia · tremor · urticaria · vertigo · visual disturbance

▸ **Rare** Anorexia · gum hyperplasia · hyperglycaemia · male infertility · mood disturbances · photosensitivity reactions · purpura

▸ **Frequency not known** Agranulocytosis · anaphylaxis · dysphagia · gynaecomastia · intestinal obstruction · intestinal ulcer

Overdose

In overdose, the dihydropyridine calcium-channel blockers cause severe hypotension secondary to profound peripheral vasodilatation.

● **PREGNANCY** May inhibit labour; manufacturer advises avoid before week 20, but risk to fetus should be balanced against risk of uncontrolled maternal hypertension. Use only if other treatment options are not indicated or have failed.

● **BREAST FEEDING** Amount too small to be harmful but manufacturers advise avoid.

● **HEPATIC IMPAIRMENT** Dose reduction may be required in severe liver disease.

● **DIRECTIONS FOR ADMINISTRATION** For rapid effect in *hypertensive crisis*, bite capsules and swallow liquid or use liquid preparation if 5 mg or 10 mg dose inappropriate. If liquid unavailable, extract contents of capsule via a syringe and use immediately—cover syringe with foil to protect contents from light; capsule contents may be diluted with water if necessary.

● **PATIENT AND CARER ADVICE**

Medicines for Children leaflet: Nifedipine for high blood pressure www.medicinesforchildren.org.uk/nifedipine-for-high-blood-pressure

● **MEDICINAL FORMS**

There can be variation in the licensing of different medicines containing the same drug. Forms available from special-order manufacturers include: oral suspension, oral drops, ointment

Capsule

▸ Nifedipine (Non-proprietary)
Nifedipine 5 mg Nifedipine 5mg capsules | 84 capsule PoM £19.99 DT price = £16.21
Nifedipine 10 mg Nifedipine 10mg capsules | 84 capsule PoM £21.00 DT price = £11.36

▸ Adalat (Bayer Plc)
Nifedipine 5 mg Adalat 5mg capsules | 90 capsule PoM £5.73
Nifedipine 10 mg Adalat 10mg capsules | 90 capsule PoM £7.30

Oral drops

▸ Nifedipine (Non-proprietary)
Nifedipine 20 mg per 1 ml Nifedipin-ratiopharm 20mg/ml oral drops | 30 ml PoM no price available | 100 ml PoM no price available

⚑ 99

Verapamil hydrochloride

● **INDICATIONS AND DOSE**

Treatment of supraventricular arrhythmias

▸ BY SLOW INTRAVENOUS INJECTION

▸ Child 1–17 years (administered on expert advice): 100–300 micrograms/kg (max. per dose 5 mg) for 1 dose, to be given over 2–3 minutes (with ECG and

blood-pressure monitoring), dose can be repeated after 30 minutes if necessary

Hypertension

▸ BY MOUTH USING IMMEDIATE-RELEASE MEDICINES

▸ Child 12–23 months (administered on expert advice): 20 mg 2–3 times a day

▸ Child 2–17 years (administered on expert advice): 40–120 mg 2–3 times a day

Prophylaxis of supraventricular arrhythmias (administered on expert advice)

▸ BY MOUTH USING IMMEDIATE-RELEASE MEDICINES

▸ Child 12–23 months: 20 mg 2–3 times a day

▸ Child 2–17 years: 40–120 mg 2–3 times a day

● **CONTRA-INDICATIONS** Acute porphyrias p. 562 · atrial flutter or fibrillation associated with accessory conducting pathways (e.g. Wolff-Parkinson-White-syndrome) · bradycardia · cardiogenic shock · history of heart failure (even if controlled by therapy) · history of significantly impaired left ventricular function (even if controlled by therapy) · hypotension · second- and third-degree AV block · sick sinus syndrome · sino-atrial block

● **CAUTIONS** First-degree AV block

● **INTERACTIONS** → Appendix 1 (calcium-channel blockers).

▸ **Verapamil and beta-blockers** Verapamil injection should not be given to patients recently treated with beta-blockers because of the risk of hypotension and asystole. The suggestion that when verapamil injection has been given first, an interval of 30 minutes before giving a beta-blocker is sufficient has not been confirmed.

It may also be hazardous to give verapamil and a beta–blocker together by mouth (should only be contemplated if myocardial function well preserved).

● **SIDE-EFFECTS**

▸ **Common or very common** Constipation

▸ **Uncommon** Ankle oedema · dizziness · fatigue · flushing · headache · nausea · vomiting

▸ **Rare** Allergic reactions · angioedema · arthralgia · asystole · bradycardia · erythema · erythromelalgia · gingival hyperplasia after long-term treatment · gynaecomastia after long-term treatment · heart block · heart failure · hypersensitivity reactions involving reversibly raised liver function tests · hypotension · increased prolactin concentration · myalgia · paraesthesia · pruritus · Stevens-Johnson syndrome · urticaria

SIDE-EFFECTS, FURTHER INFORMATION

▸ Intravenous administration or high doses Hypotension, heart failure, bradycardia, heart block, and asystole are side-effects associated with intravenous administration or high doses.

Overdose

In overdose, verapamil has a profound cardiac depressant effect causing hypotension and arrhythmias, including complete heart block and asystole.

● **PREGNANCY** May reduce uterine blood flow with fetal hypoxia. Manufacturer advises avoid in first trimester unless absolutely necessary. May inhibit labour.

● **BREAST FEEDING** Amount too small to be harmful.

● **HEPATIC IMPAIRMENT** Oral dose may need to be reduced.

● **DIRECTIONS FOR ADMINISTRATION** For *intravenous injection*, may be diluted with Glucose 5% *or* Sodium Chloride 0.9%. Incompatible with solutions of pH greater than 6.

Cardiovascular system

2

● **MEDICINAL FORMS**
There can be variation in the licensing of different medicines containing the same drug. Forms available from special-order manufacturers include: oral suspension, oral solution

Tablet
▸ **Verapamil hydrochloride (Non-proprietary)**
Verapamil hydrochloride 40 mg Verapamil 40mg tablets | 84 tablet PoM £2.07 DT price = £1.65
Verapamil hydrochloride 80 mg Verapamil 80mg tablets | 84 tablet PoM £2.33 DT price = £1.90
Verapamil hydrochloride 120 mg Verapamil 120mg tablets | 28 tablet PoM £2.01 DT price = £1.47
Verapamil hydrochloride 160 mg Verapamil 160mg tablets | 56 tablet PoM £33.84 DT price = £28.20

Oral solution
▸ **Verapamil hydrochloride (Non-proprietary)**
Verapamil hydrochloride 8 mg per 1 ml Verapamil 40mg/5ml oral solution sugar free sugar-free | 150 ml PoM £39.00 DT price = £36.90
▸ **Zolvera** (Rosemont Pharmaceuticals Ltd)
Verapamil hydrochloride 8 mg per 1 ml Zolvera 40mg/5ml oral solution sugar-free | 150 ml PoM £36.90 DT price = £36.90

Solution for injection
▸ **Securon** (BGP Products Ltd)
Verapamil hydrochloride 2.5 mg per 1 ml Securon IV 5mg/2ml solution for injection ampoules | 5 ampoule PoM £5.41

DIURETICS ＞ THIAZIDES AND RELATED DIURETICS

Thiazides and related diuretics

● **CONTRA-INDICATIONS** Addison's disease · hypercalcaemia · hyponatraemia · refractory hypokalaemia · symptomatic hyperuricaemia
● **CAUTIONS** Diabetes · gout · hyperaldosteronism · malnourishment · nephrotic syndrome · systemic lupus erythematosus

CAUTIONS, FURTHER INFORMATION
▸ **Potassium loss** Hypokalaemia can occur with both thiazide and loop diuretics. The risk of hypokalaemia depends on the duration of action as well as the potency and is thus greater with thiazides than with an equipotent dose of a loop diuretic.

Hypokalaemia is particularly dangerous in children being treated with cardiac glycosides. In hepatic failure hypokalaemia caused by diuretics can precipitate encephalopathy.

The use of potassium-sparing diuretics avoids the need to take potassium supplements.
▸ **Existing conditions** Thiazides and related diuretics can exacerbate diabetes, gout, and systemic lupus erythematosus.

● **INTERACTIONS** → Appendix 1 (diuretics).
● **SIDE-EFFECTS**
▸ **Common or very common** Altered plasma-lipid concentrations · gout · hypercalcaemia · hyperglycaemia · hyperuricaemia · hypochloraemic alkalosis · hypokalaemia · hypomagnesaemia · hyponatraemia · metabolic and electrolyte disturbances · mild gastrointestinal disturbances · postural hypotension
▸ **Uncommon** Agranulocytosis · blood disorders · impotence · leucopenia · thrombocytopenia
▸ **Frequency not known** Cardiac arrhythmias · dizziness · headache · hypersensitivity reactions · intrahepatic cholestasis · pancreatitis · paraesthesia · photosensitivity · pneumonitis · pulmonary oedema · severe skin reactions · visual disturbances
● **PREGNANCY** Thiazides and related diuretics should not be used to treat gestational hypertension. They may cause neonatal thrombocytopenia, bone marrow suppression, jaundice, electrolyte disturbances, and hypoglycaemia; placental perfusion may also be reduced. Stimulation of labour, uterine inertia, and meconium staining have also been reported.

● **HEPATIC IMPAIRMENT** Caution in mild to moderate impairment. Avoid in severe liver disease. Hypokalaemia may precipitate coma in hepatic impairment, although hypokalaemia can be prevented by using a potassium-sparing diuretic.
● **RENAL IMPAIRMENT** Thiazides and related diuretics should be used with caution because they can further reduce renal function. They are ineffective if estimated glomerular filtration rate is less than 30 mL/minute/1.73 m^2 and should be avoided. Metolazone remains effective if estimated glomerular filtration rate is less than 30 mL/minute/1.73 m^2 but is associated with a risk of excessive diuresis. Electrolytes should be monitored in renal impairment.
● **MONITORING REQUIREMENTS** Electrolytes should be monitored, particularly with high doses and long-term use.

⌐ above

Bendroflumethiazide
(Bendrofluazide)

● **INDICATIONS AND DOSE**
Hypertension
▸ BY MOUTH
▸ Child 1 month-1 year: 50–100 micrograms/kg daily, adjusted according to response
▸ Child 2-11 years: Initially 50–400 micrograms/kg daily (max. per dose 10 mg), then maintenance 50–100 micrograms/kg daily, adjusted according to response; maximum 10 mg per day
▸ Child 12-17 years: 2.5 mg once daily, dose to be taken as a single dose in the morning, higher doses are rarely necessary

Oedema in heart failure, renal disease and hepatic disease | Pulmonary oedema
▸ BY MOUTH
▸ Child 1 month-1 year: 50–100 micrograms/kg daily, adjusted according to response
▸ Child 2-11 years: Initially 50–400 micrograms/kg daily (max. per dose 10 mg), then maintenance 50–100 micrograms/kg daily, adjusted according to response; maximum 10 mg per day
▸ Child 12-17 years: Initially 5–10 mg once daily or on alternate days, adjusted according to response, dose to be taken as a single dose in the morning; maximum 10 mg per day

● **BREAST FEEDING** The amount present in milk is too small to be harmful. Large doses may suppress lactation.

● **MEDICINAL FORMS**
There can be variation in the licensing of different medicines containing the same drug. Forms available from special-order manufacturers include: oral suspension, oral solution

Tablet
▸ **Bendroflumethiazide (Non-proprietary)**
Bendroflumethiazide 2.5 mg Bendroflumethiazide 2.5mg tablets | 28 tablet PoM £3.68 DT price = £0.67 | 500 tablet PoM £65.71
Bendroflumethiazide 5 mg Bendroflumethiazide 5mg tablets | 28 tablet PoM £7.36 DT price = £0.97 | 500 tablet PoM £73.60
▸ **Aprinox** (AMCo)
Bendroflumethiazide 2.5 mg Aprinox 2.5mg tablets | 500 tablet PoM £27.31
▸ **Neo-Naclex** (AMCo)
Bendroflumethiazide 2.5 mg Neo-Naclex 2.5mg tablets | 28 tablet PoM £0.33 DT price = £0.67

Chlorothiazide

📰 102

- **INDICATIONS AND DOSE**

Heart failure | Hypertension | Ascites
- BY MOUTH

- Neonate: 10–20 mg/kg twice daily.

- Child 1–5 months: 10–20 mg/kg twice daily
- Child 6 months–11 years: 10 mg/kg twice daily; maximum 1 g per day
- Child 12–17 years: 0.25–1 g once daily, alternatively 125–500 mg twice daily

Reduction of diazoxide-induced sodium and water retention in the management of chronic hypoglycaemia | Potentiating the glycaemic effect of diazoxide in the management of chronic hypoglycaemia
- BY MOUTH

- Child: 3–5 mg/kg twice daily

Nephrogenic and partial pituitary diabetes insipidus
- BY MOUTH

- Child: 10–20 mg/kg twice daily (max. per dose 500 mg)

- **UNLICENSED USE** Not licensed.
- **CAUTIONS** Neonate (theoretical risk of kernicterus if very jaundiced)
- **BREAST FEEDING** The amount present in milk is too small to be harmful. Large doses may suppress lactation.

- **MEDICINAL FORMS**
  There can be variation in the licensing of different medicines containing the same drug. Forms available from special-order manufacturers include: tablet, oral suspension, oral solution

  Tablet
  - Chlorothiazide (Non-proprietary)
    Chlorothiazide 250 mg Diuril 250mg tablets | 100 tablet PoM no price available

  Oral suspension
  - Chlorothiazide (Non-proprietary)
    Chlorothiazide 50 mg per 1 ml Diuril 250mg/5ml oral suspension | 237 ml PoM no price available

DRUGS ACTING ON THE RENIN-ANGIOTENSIN SYSTEM > ACE INHIBITORS

Angiotensin-converting enzyme inhibitors 🅟

- **CONTRA-INDICATIONS** Bilateral renovascular disease
- **CAUTIONS** Afro-Caribbean patients (may respond less well to ACE inhibitors) · concomitant diuretics · first dose hypotension (especially in patients taking high doses of diuretics, on a low-sodium diet, on dialysis, dehydrated, or with heart failure) · neonates (in neonates) · primary aldosteronism (patients may respond less well to ACE inhibitors) · the risk of agranulocytosis is possibly increased in collagen vascular disease (blood counts recommended) · use with care (or avoid) in those with a history of idiopathic or hereditary angioedema · use with care in patients with hypertrophic cardiomyopathy · use with care in patients with severe or symptomatic aortic stenosis (risk of hypotension)

  CAUTIONS, FURTHER INFORMATION
- Anaphylactoid reactions To prevent anaphylactoid reactions, ACE inhibitors should be avoided during dialysis with high-flux polyacrylonitrile membranes and during low-density lipoprotein apheresis with dextran sulfate; they should also be withheld before desensitisation with wasp or bee venom.

- **INTERACTIONS** → Appendix 1 (ACE inhibitors).

- **SIDE-EFFECTS**
- ▸ **Common or very common** Apnoea (in neonates) · renal failure (in neonates) · seizures (in neonates) · severe unpredictable hypotension (in neonates)
- ▸ **Frequency not known** Pruritus · abdominal pain · altered liver function tests · angioedema (onset may be delayed; higher incidence reported in Afro-Caribbean patients) · arthralgia · blood disorders · bronchospasm · cholestatic jaundice · constipation · diarrhoea · dizziness · dyspepsia · eosinophilia · fatigue · fever · fulminant hepatic necrosis · haemolytic anaemia · headache · hepatic failure · hepatitis · hyperkalaemia · hypoglycaemia · leucocytosis · leucopenia · malaise · myalgia · nausea · neutropenia · pancreatitis · paraesthesia · persistent dry cough · photosensitivity · positive antinuclear antibody · profound hypotension · raised erythrocyte sedimentation rate · rash · renal impairment · rhinitis · serositis · sinusitis · sore throat · taste disturbance · thrombocytopenia · urticaria · vasculitis · vomiting

  SIDE-EFFECTS, FURTHER INFORMATION
- ▸ Hepatic effects In light of reports of cholestatic jaundice, hepatitis, fulminant hepatic necrosis, and hepatic failure, ACE inhibitors should be discontinued if marked elevation of hepatic enzymes or jaundice occur.

- **ALLERGY AND CROSS-SENSITIVITY** ACE inhibitors are contra-indicated in patients with hypersensitivity to ACE inhibitors (including angioedema).
- **PREGNANCY** ACE inhibitors should be avoided in pregnancy unless essential. They may adversely affect fetal and neonatal blood pressure control and renal function; skull defects and oligohydramnios have also been reported.
- **BREAST FEEDING** Information on the use of ACE inhibitors in breast-feeding is limited.
- **RENAL IMPAIRMENT** Use with caution, starting with low dose, and adjust according to response. Hyperkalaemia and other side-effects of ACE inhibitors are more common in those with impaired renal function and the dose may need to be reduced.
- **MONITORING REQUIREMENTS** Renal function and electrolytes should be checked before starting ACE inhibitors (or increasing the dose) and monitored during treatment (more frequently if side effects mentioned are present).
- **DIRECTIONS FOR ADMINISTRATION** For hypertension the first dose should preferably be given at bedtime.

📰 above

Captopril

- **INDICATIONS AND DOSE**

Hypertension
- BY MOUTH

- Preterm neonate (initiated under specialist supervision): Test dose 10 micrograms/kg, monitor blood pressure carefully for 1–2 hours; usual dose 10–50 micrograms/kg 2–3 times a day, then increased if necessary up to 300 micrograms/kg daily in divided doses, ongoing doses should only be given if test dose tolerated.

- Neonate (initiated under specialist supervision): Test dose 10–50 micrograms/kg, monitor blood pressure carefully for 1–2 hours; usual dose 10–50 micrograms/kg 2–3 times a day, then increased if necessary up to 2 mg/kg daily in divided doses, ongoing doses should only be given if test dose tolerated.

- Child 1–11 months (initiated under specialist supervision): Test dose 100 micrograms/kg (max. per dose 6.25 mg), monitor blood pressure carefully for continued →

1–2 hours; usual dose 100–300 micrograms/kg 2–3 times a day, then increased if necessary up to 4 mg/kg daily in divided doses, ongoing doses should only be given if test dose tolerated
▸ **Child 1-11 years** (initiated under specialist supervision): Test dose 100 micrograms/kg (max. per dose 6.25 mg), monitor blood pressure carefully for 1–2 hours; usual dose 100–300 micrograms/kg 2–3 times a day, then increased if necessary up to 6 mg/kg daily in divided doses, ongoing doses should only be given if test dose tolerated
▸ **Child 12-17 years** (initiated under specialist supervision): Test dose 100 micrograms/kg, alternatively test dose 6.25 mg, monitor blood pressure carefully for 1–2 hours; usual dose 12.5–25 mg 2–3 times a day, then increased if necessary up to 150 mg daily in divided doses, ongoing doses should only be given if test dose tolerated

Heart failure
▸ BY MOUTH

▸ **Preterm neonate** (initiated under specialist supervision): Test dose 10 micrograms/kg, monitor blood pressure carefully for 1–2 hours; usual dose 10–50 micrograms/kg 2–3 times a day, then increased if necessary up to 300 micrograms/kg daily in divided doses, ongoing doses should only be given if test dose tolerated.

▸ **Neonate** (initiated under specialist supervision): Test dose 10–50 micrograms/kg, monitor blood pressure carefully for 1–2 hours; usual dose 10–50 micrograms/kg 2–3 times a day, then increased if necessary up to 2 mg/kg daily in divided doses, ongoing doses should only be given if test dose tolerated.

▸ **Child 1-11 months** (initiated under specialist supervision): Test dose 100 micrograms/kg (max. per dose 6.25 mg), monitor blood pressure carefully for 1–2 hours; usual dose 100–300 micrograms/kg 2–3 times a day, then increased if necessary up to 4 mg/kg daily in divided doses, ongoing doses should only be given if test dose tolerated

▸ **Child 1-11 years** (initiated under specialist supervision): Test dose 100 micrograms/kg (max. per dose 6.25 mg), monitor blood pressure carefully for 1–2 hours; usual dose 100–300 micrograms/kg 2–3 times a day, then increased if necessary up to 6 mg/kg daily in divided doses, ongoing doses should only be given if test dose tolerated

▸ **Child 12-17 years** (initiated under specialist supervision): Test dose 100 micrograms/kg, alternatively test dose 6.25 mg, monitor blood pressure carefully for 1–2 hours; usual dose 12.5–25 mg 2–3 times a day, then increased if necessary up to 150 mg daily in divided doses, ongoing doses should only be given if test dose tolerated

Proteinuria in nephritis (under expert supervision)
▸ BY MOUTH

▸ **Preterm neonate:** Test dose 10 micrograms/kg, monitor blood pressure carefully for 1–2 hours; usual dose 10–50 micrograms/kg 2–3 times a day, then increased if necessary up to 300 micrograms/kg daily in divided doses, ongoing doses should only be given if test dose tolerated.

▸ **Neonate:** Test dose 10–50 micrograms/kg, monitor blood pressure carefully for 1–2 hours; usual dose 10–50 micrograms/kg 2–3 times a day, then increased if necessary up to 2 mg/kg daily in divided doses, ongoing doses should only be given if test dose tolerated.

▸ **Child 1-11 months:** Test dose 100 micrograms/kg (max. per dose 6.25 mg), monitor blood pressure carefully for 1–2 hours; usual dose 100–300 micrograms/kg 2–3 times a day, then increased if necessary up to 4 mg/kg daily in divided doses, ongoing doses should only be given if test dose tolerated

▸ **Child 1-11 years:** Test dose 100 micrograms/kg (max. per dose 6.25 mg), monitor blood pressure carefully for 1–2 hours; usual dose 100–300 micrograms/kg 2–3 times a day, then increased if necessary up to 6 mg/kg daily in divided doses, ongoing doses should only be given if test dose tolerated

▸ **Child 12-17 years:** Test dose 100 micrograms/kg, alternatively test dose 6.25 mg, monitor blood pressure carefully for 1–2 hours; usual dose 12.5–25 mg 2–3 times a day, then increased if necessary up to 150 mg daily in divided doses, ongoing doses should only be given if test dose tolerated

Diabetic nephropathy in type 1 diabetes mellitus
▸ BY MOUTH

▸ **Child 12-17 years** (under expert supervision): Test dose 100 micrograms/kg, alternatively test dose 6.25 mg, monitor blood pressure carefully for 1– 2 hours; usual dose 12.5–25 mg 2–3 times a day, increased if necessary up to 100 mg daily in divided doses, ongoing doses should only be given if test dose tolerated

● **UNLICENSED USE** Not licensed for use in children under 18 years.

● **SIDE-EFFECTS**
▸ **Common or very common** Alopecia · dry mouth · dyspnoea · sleep disorder
▸ **Uncommon** Angina · arrhythmia · flushing · pallor · palpitation · Raynaud's syndrome · tachycardia
▸ **Rare** Anorexia · stomatitis
▸ **Very rare** Allergic alveolitis · blurred vision · cardiac arrest · cardiogenic shock · cerebrovascular events · confusion · depression · eosinophilic pneumonia · glossitis · gynaecomastia · hyponatraemia · impotence · peptic ulcer · photosensitivity · Stevens-Johnson syndrome · syncope

● **BREAST FEEDING** Avoid in first few weeks after delivery, particularly in preterm infants—risk of profound neonatal hypotension; can be used in mothers breast-feeding older infants if essential but monitor infant's blood pressure.

● **DIRECTIONS FOR ADMINISTRATION** Administer under close supervision. Give test dose whilst child supine. Tablets can be dispersed in water.

● **PATIENT AND CARER ADVICE**
Medicines for Children leaflet: Captopril for heart failure www.medicinesforchildren.org.uk/captopril-heart-failure-0

● **MEDICINAL FORMS**
There can be variation in the licensing of different medicines containing the same drug. Forms available from special-order manufacturers include: tablet, capsule, oral suspension, oral solution
Tablet
▸ Captopril (Non-proprietary)
Captopril 12.5 mg Captopril 12.5mg tablets | 56 tablet [PoM] £2.80 DT price = £2.44 | 100 tablet [PoM] £5.00
Captopril 25 mg Captopril 25mg tablets | 56 tablet [PoM] £4.52 DT price = £3.32 | 100 tablet [PoM] £8.07
Captopril 50 mg Captopril 50mg tablets | 56 tablet [PoM] £5.83 DT price = £2.47 | 100 tablet [PoM] £10.41
▸ Capoten (Bristol-Myers Squibb Pharmaceuticals Ltd)
Captopril 25 mg Capoten 25mg tablets | 28 tablet [PoM] £5.26

▸ Ecopace (AMCo)
Captopril 12.5 mg Ecopace 12.5mg tablets | 56 tablet PoM £0.48 DT price = £2.44
Captopril 25 mg Ecopace 25mg tablets | 56 tablet PoM £0.60 DT price = £3.32
Captopril 50 mg Ecopace 50mg tablets | 56 tablet PoM £0.72 DT price = £2.47

Oral solution
ELECTROLYTES: May contain Sodium
▸ Noyada (Martindale Pharmaceuticals Ltd)
Captopril 1 mg per 1 ml Noyada 5mg/5ml oral solution sugar-free | 100 ml PoM £98.21 DT price = £98.21
Captopril 5 mg per 1 ml Noyada 25mg/5ml oral solution sugar-free | 100 ml PoM £108.94 DT price = £108.94

⚑ 103

Enalapril maleate

● **INDICATIONS AND DOSE**

Hypertension
▸ BY MOUTH

▸ Neonate (under expert supervision): Initially 10 micrograms/kg once daily, monitor blood pressure carefully for 1–2 hours, increased if necessary up to 500 micrograms/kg daily in 1–3 divided doses, limited information.

▸ Child 1 month–11 years (under expert supervision): Initially 100 micrograms/kg once daily, monitor blood pressure carefully for 1–2 hours, then increased if necessary up to 1 mg/kg daily in 1–2 divided doses

▸ Child 12–17 years (under expert supervision) (body-weight up to 50 kg): Initially 2.5 mg once daily, monitor blood pressure carefully for 1–2 hours, maintenance 10–20 mg daily in 1–2 divided doses

▸ Child 12–17 years (under expert supervision) (body-weight 50 kg and above): Initially 2.5 mg once daily, monitor blood pressure carefully for 1–2 hours, maintenance 10–20 mg daily in 1–2 divided doses; maximum 40 mg per day

Heart failure
▸ BY MOUTH

▸ Neonate (under expert supervision): Initially 10 micrograms/kg once daily, monitor blood pressure carefully for 1–2 hours, increased if necessary up to 500 micrograms/kg daily in 1–3 divided doses, limited information.

▸ Child 1 month–11 years (under expert supervision): Initially 100 micrograms/kg once daily, monitor blood pressure carefully for 1–2 hours, then increased if necessary up to 1 mg/kg daily in 1–2 divided doses

▸ Child 12–17 years (under expert supervision) (body-weight up to 50 kg): Initially 2.5 mg once daily, monitor blood pressure carefully for 1–2 hours, maintenance 10–20 mg daily in 1–2 divided doses

▸ Child 12–17 years (under expert supervision) (body-weight 50 kg and above): Initially 2.5 mg once daily, monitor blood pressure carefully for 1–2 hours, maintenance 10–20 mg daily in 1–2 divided doses; maximum 40 mg per day

Proteinuria in nephritis (under expert supervision)
▸ BY MOUTH

▸ Neonate: Initially 10 micrograms/kg once daily, monitor blood pressure carefully for 1–2 hours, increased if necessary up to 500 micrograms/kg daily in 1–3 divided doses, limited information.

▸ Child 1 month–11 years: Initially 100 micrograms/kg once daily, monitor blood pressure carefully for 1–2 hours, then increased if necessary up to 1 mg/kg daily in 1–2 divided doses

▸ Child 12–17 years (body-weight up to 50 kg): Initially 2.5 mg once daily, monitor blood pressure carefully for 1–2 hours, maintenance 10–20 mg daily in 1–2 divided doses

▸ Child 12–17 years (body-weight 50 kg and above): Initially 2.5 mg once daily, monitor blood pressure carefully for 1–2 hours, maintenance 10–20 mg daily in 1–2 divided doses; maximum 40 mg per day

Diabetic nephropathy (under expert supervision)
▸ BY MOUTH

▸ Child 12–17 years (body-weight up to 50 kg): Initially 2.5 mg once daily, monitor blood pressure carefully for 1–2 hours; maintenance 10–20 mg daily in 1–2 divided doses

▸ Child 12–17 years (body-weight 50 kg and above): Initially 2.5 mg once daily, monitor blood pressure carefully for 1–2 hours; maintenance 10–20 mg daily in 1–2 divided doses; maximum 40 mg per day

● **UNLICENSED USE** Not licensed for use in children for congestive heart failure, proteinuria in nephritis or diabetic nephropathy; not licensed for use in children less than 20 kg for hypertension.

● **SIDE-EFFECTS**
▸ **Common or very common** Asthenia · blurred vision · depression · dyspnoea
▸ **Uncommon** Alopecia · anorexia · arrhythmias · confusion · drowsiness · dry mouth · flushing · hyponatraemia · ileus · impotence · insomnia · muscle cramps · nervousness · palpitation · peptic ulcer · sweating · tinnitus · vertigo
▸ **Rare** Abnormal dreams · allergic alveolitis · exfoliative dermatitis · glossitis · gynaecomastia · pemphigus · pulmonary infiltrates · Raynaud's syndrome · Stevens-Johnson syndrome · stomatitis · toxic epidermal necrolysis
▸ **Very rare** Gastro-intestinal angioedema

● **BREAST FEEDING** Avoid in first few weeks after delivery, particularly in preterm infants—risk of profound neonatal hypotension; can be used in mothers breast-feeding older infants if essential but monitor infant's blood pressure.

● **HEPATIC IMPAIRMENT** Enalapril is a prodrug and requires close monitoring in patients with hepatic impairment.

● **DIRECTIONS FOR ADMINISTRATION** Tablets may be crushed and suspended in water immediately before use.

● **PATIENT AND CARER ADVICE**
Medicines for Children leaflet: Enalapril for high blood pressure www.medicinesforchildren.org.uk/enalapril-for-high-blood-pressure

● **MEDICINAL FORMS**
There can be variation in the licensing of different medicines containing the same drug. Forms available from special-order manufacturers include: oral suspension, oral solution

Tablet
▸ Enalapril maleate (Non-proprietary)
Enalapril maleate 2.5 mg Enalapril 2.5mg tablets | 28 tablet PoM £3.60 DT price = £2.38
Enalapril maleate 5 mg Enalapril 5mg tablets | 28 tablet PoM £4.13 DT price = £0.87
Enalapril maleate 10 mg Enalapril 10mg tablets | 28 tablet PoM £5.64 DT price = £0.89
Enalapril maleate 20 mg Enalapril 20mg tablets | 28 tablet PoM £6.63 DT price = £1.42
▸ Innovace (Merck Sharp & Dohme Ltd)
Enalapril maleate 2.5 mg Innovace 2.5mg tablets | 28 tablet PoM £5.35 DT price = £2.38
Enalapril maleate 5 mg Innovace 5mg tablets | 28 tablet PoM £7.51 DT price = £0.87
Enalapril maleate 10 mg Innovace 10mg tablets | 28 tablet PoM £10.53 DT price = £0.89
Enalapril maleate 20 mg Innovace 20mg tablets | 28 tablet PoM £12.51 DT price = £1.42

Cardiovascular system

⬤ 103

Lisinopril

- **INDICATIONS AND DOSE**

Hypertension
- BY MOUTH
  - Child 6–11 years (under expert supervision): Initially 70 micrograms/kg once daily (max. per dose 5 mg), increased to up to 600 micrograms/kg once daily, alternatively increased to up to 40 mg once daily, dose to be increased in intervals of 1–2 weeks
  - Child 12–17 years (under expert supervision): Initially 5 mg once daily; usual maintenance 10–20 mg once daily; maximum 80 mg per day

Proteinuria in nephritis (under expert supervision)
- BY MOUTH
  - Child 6–11 years: Initially 70 micrograms/kg once daily (max. per dose 5 mg), increased to up to 600 micrograms/kg once daily, alternatively increased to up to 40 mg once daily, dose to be increased in intervals of 1–2 weeks
  - Child 12–17 years: Initially 5 mg once daily; usual maintenance 10–20 mg once daily; maximum 80 mg per day

Diabetic nephropathy (under expert supervision)
- BY MOUTH
  - Child 12–17 years: Initially 5 mg once daily; usual maintenance 10–20 mg once daily; maximum 80 mg per day

Heart failure (adjunct) (under close medical supervision)
- BY MOUTH
  - Child 12–17 years: Initially 2.5 mg once daily; increased in steps of up to 10 mg at least every 2 weeks; maximum 35 mg per day

- **UNLICENSED USE** Not licensed for use in children.
- **SIDE-EFFECTS**
- **Uncommon** Raynaud's syndrome · vertigo · asthenia · cerebrovascular accident · confusion · impotence · mood changes · palpitation · sleep disturbances · tachycardia
- **Rare** Alopecia · dry mouth · gynaecomastia · psoriasis
- **Very rare** Allergic alveolitis · pemphigus · profuse sweating · pulmonary infiltrates · Stevens-Johnson syndrome · toxic epidermal necrolysis
- **BREAST FEEDING** Not recommended; alternative treatment options, with better established safety information during breast-feeding, are available.
- **PATIENT AND CARER ADVICE**
  Medicines for Children leaflet: Lisinopril for high blood pressure www.medicinesforchildren.org.uk/lisinopril-for-high-blood-pressure

- **MEDICINAL FORMS**
  There can be variation in the licensing of different medicines containing the same drug. Forms available from special-order manufacturers include: oral suspension, oral solution
  Tablet
  - Lisinopril (Non-proprietary)
    Lisinopril 2.5 mg Lisinopril 2.5mg tablets | 28 tablet [PoM] £1.51 DT price = £0.72
    Lisinopril 5 mg Lisinopril 5mg tablets | 28 tablet [PoM] £7.80 DT price = £0.74
    Lisinopril 10 mg Lisinopril 10mg tablets | 28 tablet [PoM] £9.60 DT price = £0.76
    Lisinopril 20 mg Lisinopril 20mg tablets | 28 tablet [PoM] £10.90 DT price = £0.85
  - Zestril (AstraZeneca UK Ltd)
    Lisinopril 5 mg Zestril 5mg tablets | 28 tablet [PoM] £4.71 DT price = £0.74
    Lisinopril 10 mg Zestril 10mg tablets | 28 tablet [PoM] £7.38 DT price = £0.76
    Lisinopril 20 mg Zestril 20mg tablets | 28 tablet [PoM] £6.51 DT price = £0.85

Oral solution
- Lisinopril (Non-proprietary)
  Lisinopril 1 mg per 1 ml Lisinopril 5mg/5ml oral solution sugar free sugar-free | 150 ml [PoM] £154.11 DT price = £154.11

DRUGS ACTING ON THE RENIN-ANGIOTENSIN SYSTEM > ANGIOTENSIN II RECEPTOR ANTAGONISTS

Angiotensin II receptor antagonists

- **CAUTIONS** Afro-Caribbean patients—particularly those with left ventricular hypertrophy (may not benefit from an angiotensin-II receptor antagonist) · aortic or mitral valve stenosis · hypertrophic cardiomyopathy · patients with a history of angioedema · patients with primary aldosteronism (may not benefit from an angiotensin-II receptor antagonist) · renal artery stenosis
- **INTERACTIONS** → Appendix 1 (angiotensin-II receptor antagonists).
- **SIDE-EFFECTS** Hyperkalaemia · angioedema (may be delayed onset) · symptomatic hypotension including dizziness (particularly in children with hyponatraemia or intravascular volume depletion e.g. those taking high-dose diuretics)
- **PREGNANCY** Angiotensin-II receptor antagonists should be avoided in pregnancy unless essential. They may adversely affect fetal and neonatal blood pressure control and renal function; neonatal skull defects and oligohydramnios have also been reported.
- **BREAST FEEDING** Information on the use of angiotensin-II receptor antagonists in breast-feeding is limited. They are not recommended in breast-feeding and alternative treatment options, with better established safety information during breast-feeding, are available.
- **RENAL IMPAIRMENT** Use with caution, starting with low dose, and adjust according to response.
- **MONITORING REQUIREMENTS** Monitor plasma-potassium concentration, particularly in children with renal impairment.

⬤ above

Candesartan cilexetil

- **INDICATIONS AND DOSE**

Hypertension
- BY MOUTH
  - Child 6–17 years (under expert supervision) (body-weight up to 50 kg): Initially 4 mg once daily, adjusted according to response, lower dose may be used in intravascular volume depletion; maximum 8 mg per day
  - Child 6–17 years (under expert supervision) (body-weight 50 kg and above): Initially 4 mg once daily, adjusted according to response, lower dose may be used in intravascular volume depletion; maximum 16 mg per day

- **CONTRA-INDICATIONS** Cholestasis
- **SIDE-EFFECTS**
- **Common or very common** Cough · headache · rash · vertigo
- **Uncommon** Hyponatraemia
- **Very rare** Arthralgia · back pain · blood disorders · hepatitis · myalgia · nausea · pruritus · urticaria
- **HEPATIC IMPAIRMENT** Reduce initial dose in mild or moderate impairment. Avoid in severe hepatic impairment.
- **RENAL IMPAIRMENT** Reduce initial dose. Use with caution if estimated glomerular filtration rate is less than 30 mL/minute/1.73 m^2—no information available.

- **MEDICINAL FORMS**
  There can be variation in the licensing of different medicines containing the same drug. Forms available from special-order manufacturers include: oral suspension, oral solution

  Tablet
  - Candesartan cilexetil (Non-proprietary)
    Candesartan cilexetil 2 mg Candesartan 2mg tablets |
    7 tablet [PoM] £3.40 DT price = £1.02
    Candesartan cilexetil 4 mg Candesartan 4mg tablets |
    7 tablet [PoM] £3.88 DT price = £0.68 | 28 tablet [PoM] £9.78
    Candesartan cilexetil 8 mg Candesartan 8mg tablets |
    28 tablet [PoM] £9.89 DT price = £1.05
    Candesartan cilexetil 16 mg Candesartan 16mg tablets |
    28 tablet [PoM] £12.72 DT price = £1.26
    Candesartan cilexetil 32 mg Candesartan 32mg tablets |
    28 tablet [PoM] £16.13 DT price = £1.79
  - Amias (Takeda UK Ltd)
    Candesartan cilexetil 2 mg Amias 2mg tablets | 7 tablet [PoM]
    £3.58 DT price = £1.02
    Candesartan cilexetil 4 mg Amias 4mg tablets | 7 tablet [PoM]
    £3.88 DT price = £0.68 | 28 tablet [PoM] £9.78
    Candesartan cilexetil 8 mg Amias 8mg tablets | 28 tablet [PoM]
    £9.89 DT price = £1.05
    Candesartan cilexetil 16 mg Amias 16mg tablets | 28 tablet [PoM]
    £12.72 DT price = £1.26
    Candesartan cilexetil 32 mg Amias 32mg tablets | 28 tablet [PoM]
    £16.13 DT price = £1.79

⌐ 106

Losartan potassium

- **INDICATIONS AND DOSE**

Hypertension
- BY MOUTH
- Child 6–17 years (under expert supervision) (body-weight 20–49 kg): Initially 700 micrograms/kg once daily (max. per dose 25 mg), adjusted according to response to 50 mg daily, lower initial dose may be used in intravascular volume depletion; maximum 50 mg per day
- Child 6–17 years (under expert supervision) (body-weight 50 kg and above): Initially 50 mg once daily, adjusted according to response to 1.4 mg/kg once daily; maximum 100 mg per day

Hypertension with intravascular volume depletion
- BY MOUTH
- Child 6–17 years (under expert supervision) (body-weight 50 kg and above): Initially 25 mg once daily; adjusted according to response to 1.4 mg/kg once daily; maximum 100 mg per day

- **CAUTIONS** Severe heart failure
- **SIDE-EFFECTS**
- **Common or very common** Anaemia · malaise
- **Uncommon** Abdominal pain · angina · constipation · cough · diarrhoea · drowsiness · dyspnoea · headache · nausea · oedema · palpitation · pruritus · rash · sleep disorders · urticaria · vomiting
- **Rare** Atrial fibrillation · cerebrovascular accident · hepatitis · paraesthesia
- **Frequency not known** Arthralgia · depression · erectile dysfunction · Henoch-Schönlein purpura · hyponatraemia · myalgia · pancreatitis · photosensitivity · rhabdomyolysis · thrombocytopenia · tinnitus · vasculitis
- **HEPATIC IMPAIRMENT** Avoid—no information available.
- **RENAL IMPAIRMENT** Avoid if estimated glomerular filtration rate is less than 30 mL/minute/1.73 m²—no information available.
- **PRESCRIBING AND DISPENSING INFORMATION** Flavours of oral liquid formulations may include berry-citrus.

- **MEDICINAL FORMS**
  There can be variation in the licensing of different medicines containing the same drug. Forms available from special-order manufacturers include: oral suspension, oral solution

  Tablet
  - Losartan potassium (Non-proprietary)
    Losartan potassium 12.5 mg Losartan 12.5mg tablets |
    28 tablet [PoM] £30.00 DT price = £5.15
    Losartan potassium 25 mg Losartan 25mg tablets | 28 tablet [PoM]
    £16.17 DT price = £0.82
    Losartan potassium 50 mg Losartan 50mg tablets | 28 tablet [PoM]
    £12.80 DT price = £0.89
    Losartan potassium 100 mg Losartan 100mg tablets |
    28 tablet [PoM] £16.18 DT price = £1.05
  - Cozaar (Merck Sharp & Dohme Ltd)
    Losartan potassium 12.5 mg Cozaar 12.5mg tablets |
    28 tablet [PoM] £8.09 DT price = £5.15
    Losartan potassium 25 mg Cozaar 25mg tablets | 28 tablet [PoM]
    £16.18 DT price = £0.82
    Losartan potassium 50 mg Cozaar 50mg tablets | 28 tablet [PoM]
    £12.80 DT price = £0.89
    Losartan potassium 100 mg Cozaar 100mg tablets |
    28 tablet [PoM] £16.18 DT price = £1.05

  Oral suspension
  - Cozaar (Merck Sharp & Dohme Ltd)
    Losartan potassium 2.5 mg per 1 ml Cozaar 2.5mg/ml oral
    suspension sugar-free | 200 ml [PoM] £53.68

⌐ 106

Valsartan

- **INDICATIONS AND DOSE**

Hypertension
- BY MOUTH
- Child 6–17 years (under expert supervision) (body-weight 18–34 kg): Initially 40 mg once daily, adjusted according to response; maximum 80 mg per day
- Child 6–17 years (under expert supervision) (body-weight 35–79 kg): Initially 80 mg once daily, adjusted according to response; maximum 160 mg per day
- Child 6–17 years (under expert supervision) (body-weight 80 kg and above): Initially 80 mg once daily, adjusted according to response; maximum 320 mg per day

- **UNLICENSED USE** Capsules not licensed for use in children.
- **CONTRA-INDICATIONS** Biliary cirrhosis · cholestasis
- **SIDE-EFFECTS**
- **Uncommon** Abdominal pain · cough · diarrhoea · headache · malaise · nausea
- **Frequency not known** Anaemia · myalgia · neutropenia · pruritus · rash · renal failure · serum sickness · thrombocytopenia · vasculitis
- **HEPATIC IMPAIRMENT** Max. dose 80 mg daily in mild to moderate impairment. Avoid in severe hepatic impairment.
- **RENAL IMPAIRMENT** Avoid if estimated glomerular filtration rate is less than 30 mL/minute/1.73 m²—no information available.

- **MEDICINAL FORMS**
  There can be variation in the licensing of different medicines containing the same drug. Forms available from special-order manufacturers include: oral suspension, oral solution

  Tablet
  - Valsartan (Non-proprietary)
    Valsartan 40 mg Valsartan 40mg tablets | 7 tablet [PoM] £3.49 DT
    price = £2.66 | 28 tablet [PoM] no price available
    Valsartan 80 mg Valsartan 80mg tablets | 28 tablet [PoM] £13.69
    DT price = £13.69
    Valsartan 160 mg Valsartan 160mg tablets | 28 tablet [PoM] £14.69
    DT price = £14.69
    Valsartan 320 mg Valsartan 320mg tablets | 28 tablet [PoM] £20.23
    DT price = £14.32

2

Cardiovascular system

Capsule
‣ Valsartan (Non-proprietary)
Valsartan 40 mg Valsartan 40mg capsules | 28 capsule PoM
£13.97 DT price = £1.00
Valsartan 80 mg Valsartan 80mg capsules | 28 capsule PoM
£13.97 DT price = £1.06
Valsartan 160 mg Valsartan 160mg capsules | 28 capsule PoM
£18.41 DT price = £1.48

Oral solution
‣ Diovan (Novartis Pharmaceuticals UK Ltd)
Valsartan 3 mg per 1 ml Diovan 3mg/1ml oral solution |
160 ml PoM £7.20

VASODILATORS › VASODILATOR ANTIHYPERTENSIVES

Hydralazine hydrochloride

● **INDICATIONS AND DOSE**
Resistant hypertension (adjunct)
▶ BY MOUTH
‣ **Neonate:** 250–500 micrograms/kg every 8–12 hours, increased if necessary to 2–3 mg/kg every 8 hours.
‣ **Child 1 month–11 years:** 250–500 micrograms/kg every 8–12 hours, increased if necessary to 7.5 mg/kg daily; maximum 200 mg per day
‣ **Child 12–17 years:** 25 mg twice daily, increased to 50–100 mg twice daily
▶ BY SLOW INTRAVENOUS INJECTION
‣ **Neonate:** 100–500 micrograms/kg, dose may be repeated if necessary every 4–6 hours; maximum 3 mg/kg per day.
‣ **Child 1 month–11 years:** 100–500 micrograms/kg, dose may be repeated if necessary every 4–6 hours; maximum 3 mg/kg per day; maximum 60 mg per day
‣ **Child 12–17 years:** 5–10 mg, dose may be repeated if necessary every 4–6 hours
▶ BY CONTINUOUS INTRAVENOUS INFUSION
‣ **Neonate:** 12.5–50 micrograms/kg/hour, continuous intravenous infusion is the preferred route in cardiac patients; maximum 2 mg/kg per day.
‣ **Child 1 month–11 years:** 12.5–50 micrograms/kg/hour, continuous intravenous infusion is the preferred route in cardiac patients; maximum 3 mg/kg per day
‣ **Child 12–17 years:** 3–9 mg/hour, continuous intravenous infusion is the preferred route in cardiac patients; maximum 3 mg/kg per day

● **UNLICENSED USE** Not licensed for use in children.
● **CONTRA-INDICATIONS** Acute porphyrias p. 562 · cor pulmonale · high output heart failure · idiopathic systemic lupus erythematosus · myocardial insufficiency due to mechanical obstruction · severe tachycardia
● **CAUTIONS** Cerebrovascular disease · occasionally blood pressure reduction too rapid even with low parenteral doses
● **INTERACTIONS** → Appendix 1 (hydralazine).
● **SIDE-EFFECTS**
▶ **Rare** Rashes
▶ **Frequency not known** Abnormal liver function · agitation · anorexia · anxiety · arthralgia · blood disorders · dizziness · dyspnoea · fever · fluid retention · flushing · gastro-intestinal disturbances · haematuria · haemolytic anaemia · headache · hypotension · increased lacrimation · jaundice · leucopenia · myalgia · nasal congestion · palpitation · paraesthesia · peripheral neuritis · polyneuritis · proteinuria · raised plasma creatinine · systemic lupus erythematosus-like syndrome after long-term therapy (especially in slow acetylator individuals) · tachycardia · thrombocytopenia

● **SIDE-EFFECTS, FURTHER INFORMATION**
The incidence of side-effects is lower if the dose is kept low, but systemic lupus erythematosus should be suspected if there is unexplained weight loss, arthritis, or any other unexplained ill health.
● **PREGNANCY** Neonatal thrombocytopenia reported, but risk should be balanced against risk of uncontrolled maternal hypertension. Manufacturer advises avoid before third trimester.
● **BREAST FEEDING** Present in milk but not known to be harmful.
Monitor infant in breast-feeding.
● **HEPATIC IMPAIRMENT** Reduce dose.
● **RENAL IMPAIRMENT** Reduce dose if estimated glomerular filtration rate less than 30 mL/minute/1.73 m^2.
● **MONITORING REQUIREMENTS** Manufacturer advises test for antinuclear factor and for proteinuria every 6 months and check acetylator status before increasing dose, but evidence of clinical value unsatisfactory.
● **DIRECTIONS FOR ADMINISTRATION**
‣ **With oral use** For administration *by mouth*, diluted injection may be given orally.
‣ **With intravenous use** For *continuous intravenous infusion*, initially reconstitute 20 mg with 1 mL Water for Injections, then dilute with Sodium Chloride 0.9%. Incompatible with Glucose intravenous infusion. For *intravenous injection*, initially reconstitute 20 mg with 1 mL Water for Injections, then dilute to a concentration of 0.5–1 mg/mL with Sodium Chloride 0.9% and administer over 5–20 minutes.

● **MEDICINAL FORMS**
There can be variation in the licensing of different medicines containing the same drug. Forms available from special-order manufacturers include: oral suspension, oral solution
Tablet
EXCIPIENTS: May contain Gluten, propylene glycol
‣ Hydralazine hydrochloride (Non-proprietary)
Hydralazine hydrochloride 10 mg Apo-Hydralazine 10mg tablets | 100 tablet PoM no price available
Hydralazine hydrochloride 25 mg Hydralazine 25mg tablets | 56 tablet PoM £8.56 DT price = £7.71 | 84 tablet PoM £14.00
Hydralazine hydrochloride 50 mg Hydralazine 50mg tablets | 56 tablet PoM £15.74 DT price = £13.15
‣ Apresoline (AMCo)
Hydralazine hydrochloride 25 mg Apresoline 25mg tablets | 84 tablet PoM £3.38
Powder for solution for injection
‣ Hydralazine hydrochloride (Non-proprietary)
Hydralazine hydrochloride 20 mg Hydralazine 20mg powder for concentrate for solution for injection ampoules | 5 ampoule PoM £64.50
‣ Apresoline (AMCo)
Hydralazine hydrochloride 20 mg Apresoline 20mg powder for solution for injection ampoules | 5 ampoule PoM £11.09

Minoxidil

● **INDICATIONS AND DOSE**
Severe hypertension
▶ BY MOUTH
‣ **Child 1 month–11 years:** Initially 200 micrograms/kg daily in 1–2 divided doses, then increased in steps of 100–200 micrograms/kg, at intervals of at least 3 days; maximum 1 mg/kg per day
‣ **Child 12–17 years:** Initially 5 mg daily in 1–2 divided doses, then increased in steps of 5–10 mg daily, increased at intervals of at least 3 days, seldom necessary to exceed 50 mg daily; maximum 100 mg per day

● **CONTRA-INDICATIONS** Phaeochromocytoma
● **CAUTIONS** Acute porphyrias p. 562

- **INTERACTIONS** → Appendix 1 (vasodilator antihypertensives).
- **PREGNANCY** Avoid—possible toxicity including reduced placental perfusion. Neonatal hirsutism reported.
- **BREAST FEEDING** Present in milk but not known to be harmful.
- **RENAL IMPAIRMENT** Use with caution in significant impairment.

- **MEDICINAL FORMS**
  There can be variation in the licensing of different medicines containing the same drug.
  Tablet
  ▸ **Loniten** (Pfizer Ltd)
    Minoxidil 2.5 mg Loniten 2.5mg tablets | 60 tablet [PoM] £8.88 DT price = £8.88
    Minoxidil 5 mg Loniten 5mg tablets | 60 tablet [PoM] £15.83 DT price = £15.83
    Minoxidil 10 mg Loniten 10mg tablets | 60 tablet [PoM] £30.68 DT price = £30.68

4.1a Hypertension associated with phaeochromocytoma

VASODILATORS > PERIPHERAL VASODILATORS

Phenoxybenzamine hydrochloride

- **INDICATIONS AND DOSE**
  Hypertension in phaeochromocytoma
  ▸ BY MOUTH
  ▸ Child: 0.5–1 mg/kg twice daily, adjusted according to response

- **UNLICENSED USE** Not licensed for use in children.
- **CONTRA-INDICATIONS** History of cerebrovascular accident
- **CAUTIONS** Avoid contact with skin (risk of contact sensitisation) · avoid in Acute porphyrias p. 562 · carcinogenic in *animals* · cerebrovascular disease · congestive heart failure · severe ischaemic heart disease
- **SIDE-EFFECTS**
  ▸ **Rare** Gastro-intestinal disturbances
  ▸ **Frequency not known** Inhibition of ejaculation · lassitude · miosis · nasal congestion · postural hypotension (with dizziness and marked compensatory tachycardia)
- **PREGNANCY** Hypotension may occur in newborn.
- **BREAST FEEDING** May be present in milk.
- **RENAL IMPAIRMENT** Use with caution.
- **DIRECTIONS FOR ADMINISTRATION** For administration *by mouth*, capsules may be opened.
- **HANDLING AND STORAGE** Owing to risk of contact sensitisation healthcare professionals should avoid contamination of hands.

- **MEDICINAL FORMS**
  There can be variation in the licensing of different medicines containing the same drug. Forms available from special-order manufacturers include: oral suspension, oral solution
  Capsule
  ▸ **Phenoxybenzamine hydrochloride** (Non-proprietary)
    Phenoxybenzamine hydrochloride 10 mg Phenoxybenzamine 10mg capsules | 30 capsule [PoM] £97.38 DT price = £97.38

4.1b Hypertensive crises

Drugs used for Hypertensive crises not listed below
Esmolol hydrochloride p. 98 · Labetalol hydrochloride, p. 95

VASODILATORS > VASODILATOR ANTIHYPERTENSIVES

Sodium nitroprusside

- **INDICATIONS AND DOSE**
  Hypertensive emergencies
  ▸ BY CONTINUOUS INTRAVENOUS INFUSION
  ▸ Neonate: Initially 500 nanograms/kg/minute, then increased in steps of 200 nanograms/kg/minute (max. per dose 8 micrograms/kg/minute) as required, max. 4 micrograms/kg/minute if used for longer than 24 hours.
  ▸ Child: Initially 500 nanograms/kg/minute, then increased in steps of 200 nanograms/kg/minute (max. per dose 8 micrograms/kg/minute) as required, max. 4 micrograms/kg/minute if used for longer than 24 hours

- **UNLICENSED USE** Not licensed for use in the UK.
- **CONTRA-INDICATIONS** Compensatory hypertension · Leber's optic atrophy · severe vitamin B_{12} deficiency
- **CAUTIONS** Hyponatraemia · hypothermia · hypothyroidism · impaired cerebral circulation
- **INTERACTIONS** → Appendix 1 (sodium nitroprusside).
- **SIDE-EFFECTS** Abdominal pain · acute transient phlebitis · anxiety · dizziness · headache · nausea · palpitation · perspiration · reduced platelet count · retching · retrosternal discomfort
  SIDE-EFFECTS, FURTHER INFORMATION
  ▸ Side-effects associated with over rapid reduction in blood pressure: Headache, dizziness, nausea, retching, abdominal pain, perspiration, palpitation, anxiety, retrosternal discomfort—reduce infusion rate if any of these side-effects occur.
  Overdose
  Side-effects caused by excessive plasma concentration of the cyanide metabolite include tachycardia, sweating, hyperventilation, arrhythmias, marked metabolic acidosis (discontinue and give antidote, see cyanide in Emergency treatment of poisoning p. 786).
- **PREGNANCY** Avoid prolonged use—potential for accumulation of cyanide in fetus.
- **BREAST FEEDING** No information available. Caution advised due to thiocyanate metabolite.
- **HEPATIC IMPAIRMENT** Use with caution. Avoid in hepatic failure—cyanide or thiocyanate metabolites may accumulate.
- **RENAL IMPAIRMENT** Avoid prolonged use—cyanide or thiocyanate metabolites may accumulate.
- **MONITORING REQUIREMENTS** Monitor blood pressure (including intra-arterial blood pressure) and blood-cyanide concentration, and if treatment exceeds 3 days, also blood thiocyanate concentration.
- **TREATMENT CESSATION** Avoid sudden withdrawal—terminate infusion over 15–30 minutes.
- **DIRECTIONS FOR ADMINISTRATION** For *continuous intravenous infusion* in Glucose 5%, infuse *via* infusion device to allow precise control. For further details, consult product literature. Protect infusion from light.

Cardiovascular system

2

- **MEDICINAL FORMS**
  There can be variation in the licensing of different medicines containing the same drug.
  Powder and solvent for solution for infusion
  ‣ Sodium nitroprusside (Non-proprietary)
  Sodium nitroprusside dihydrate 50 mg Sodium nitroprusside 50mg powder and solvent for solution for infusion vials | 1 vial [PoM] no price available

4.1c Pulmonary hypertension

ANTITHROMBOTIC DRUGS › PROSTAGLANDINS, CARDIOVASCULAR

Epoprostenol

(Prostacyclin)

- **DRUG ACTION** Epoprostenol is a prostaglandin and a potent vasodilator. It is also a powerful inhibitor of platelet aggregation.

- **INDICATIONS AND DOSE**
  Persistent pulmonary hypertension of the newborn
  ‣ BY CONTINUOUS INTRAVENOUS INFUSION
  ‣ Neonate: Initially 2 nanograms/kg/minute (max. per dose 20 nanograms/kg/minute), adjusted according to response, rarely doses up to 40 nanograms/kg/minute are used.

  Idiopathic pulmonary arterial hypertension
  ‣ BY CONTINUOUS INTRAVENOUS INFUSION
  ‣ Child: Initially 2 nanograms/kg/minute, increased if necessary up to 40 nanograms/kg/minute
  PHARMACOKINETICS
  Short half-life of approximately 3 minutes, therefore it must be administered by continuous intravenous infusion.

- **UNLICENSED USE** Not licensed for use in children.
- **CONTRA-INDICATIONS** Pulmonary veno-occlusive disease · severe left ventricular dysfunction
- **CAUTIONS** Avoid abrupt withdrawal (risk of rebound pulmonary hypertension/pulmonary hypertensive crisis) · haemorrhagic diathesis
- **INTERACTIONS** Caution with concomitant use of drugs that increase risk of bleeding.
- **SIDE-EFFECTS**
  ‣ **Common or very common** Abdominal pain · anxiety · arthralgia · bleeding · bradycardia · chest pain · diarrhoea · flushing · headache · hypotension · jaw pain · nausea · sepsis · tachycardia · vomiting
  ‣ **Uncommon** Dry mouth · pulmonary oedema · sweating
  ‣ **Rare** Agitation · pallor
  ‣ **Frequency not known** Serious systemic hypotension
- **PREGNANCY** Manufacturer advises caution—no information available.
- **BREAST FEEDING** Manufacturer advises avoid—no information available.
- **MONITORING REQUIREMENTS**
  ‣ Anticoagulant monitoring required when given with anticoagulants.
  ‣ Monitor blood pressure.
- **TREATMENT CESSATION** Avoid abrupt withdrawal (risk of rebound pulmonary hypertension and pulmonary hypertensive crisis).
- **DIRECTIONS FOR ADMINISTRATION** Reconstitute using the glycine buffer diluent provided to make a concentrate (pH 10.5); filter the concentrate using the filter provided. The concentrate can be administered via a central venous

catheter, alternatively it may be diluted further either with the glycine buffer diluent *or* to a minimum concentration of 1.43 micrograms/mL with Sodium Chloride 0.9%. Solution stable for 12 hours at room temperature, although some units use for 24 hours and allow for loss of potency; solution stable for 24 hours if prepared in glycine buffer diluent only and administered via an ambulatory cold pouch system (to maintain solution at 2–8°C).
Neonatal intensive care, prepare a filtered concentrate of 10 micrograms/mL using the 500-microgram vial. *Neonate body-weight under 2 kg,* using the concentrate, dilute 150 micrograms/kg body-weight to a final volume of 50 mL with Sodium Chloride 0.9%; an intravenous infusion rate of 0.1 mL/hour provides a dose of 5 nanograms/kg/minute. *Neonate body-weight over 2 kg,* using the concentrate, dilute 60 micrograms/kg body-weight to a final volume of 50 mL with Sodium Chloride 0.9%; an intravenous infusion rate of 0.1 mL/hour provides a dose of 2 nanograms/kg/minute.

- **MEDICINAL FORMS**
  There can be variation in the licensing of different medicines containing the same drug.
  Powder for solution for infusion
  ‣ Veletri (Actelion Pharmaceuticals UK Ltd)
  Epoprostenol (as Epoprostenol sodium) 500 microgram Veletri 500microgram powder for solution for infusion vials | 1 vial [PoM] £24.44
  Epoprostenol (as Epoprostenol sodium) 1.5 mg Veletri 1.5mg powder for solution for infusion vials | 1 vial [PoM] £49.24
  Powder and solvent for solution for infusion
  ‣ Epoprostenol (Non-proprietary)
  Epoprostenol (as Epoprostenol sodium)
  500 microgram Epoprostenol 500microgram powder and solvent for solution for infusion vials | 1 vial [PoM] £22.22
  Epoprostenol (as Epoprostenol sodium) 1.5 mg Epoprostenol 1.5mg powder and solvent for solution for infusion vials | 1 vial [PoM] £49.24
  ‣ Flolan (GlaxoSmithKline UK Ltd)
  Epoprostenol (as Epoprostenol sodium) 500 microgram Flolan 500microgram powder and solvent for solution for infusion vials | 1 vial [PoM] £22.22
  Epoprostenol (as Epoprostenol sodium) 1.5 mg Flolan 1.5mg powder and solvent for solution for infusion vials | 1 vial [PoM] £44.76

Iloprost

- **INDICATIONS AND DOSE**
  Idiopathic or familial pulmonary arterial hypertension (initiated under specialist supervision)
  ‣ BY INHALATION OF NEBULISED SOLUTION
  ‣ Child 8–17 years: Initially 2.5 micrograms for 1 dose, increased to 5 micrograms for 1 dose, increased if tolerated to 5 micrograms 6–9 times a day, adjusted according to response; reduced if not tolerated to 2.5 micrograms 6–9 times a day, reduce to lower maintenance dose if high dose not tolerated

  Raynaud's syndrome
  ‣ BY INTRAVENOUS INFUSION
  ‣ Child 12–17 years: Initially 30 nanograms/kg/hour, increased to 60–120 nanograms/kg/hour daily for 3–5 days, dose to be given over 6 hours, dose increase should be performed gradually

- **UNLICENSED USE** Not licensed for use in children.
- **CONTRA-INDICATIONS** Conditions which increase risk of haemorrhage · congenital or acquired valvular defects of the myocardium · decompensated cardiac failure (unless under close medical supervision) · pulmonary veno-occlusive disease · severe arrhythmias · severe coronary heart disease

- **CAUTIONS**
  GENERAL CAUTIONS
  Hypotension (do not initiate if systolic blood pressure below 85 mmHg) · unstable pulmonary hypertension with advanced right heart failure
  SPECIFIC CAUTIONS
- When used by inhalation Acute pulmonary infection · severe asthma
- **INTERACTIONS** → Appendix 1 (iloprost).
- **SIDE-EFFECTS**
- Common or very common Chest pain · cough · diarrhoea · dyspnoea · haemorrhage · headache · hypotension · jaw pain · nausea · oral irritation · rash · throat pain · vomiting
- Frequency not known Bronchospasm · taste disturbance · thrombocytopenia · wheezing
- **PREGNANCY**
- When used by inhalation Use if potential benefit outweighs risk.
- **BREAST FEEDING**
- When used by inhalation Manufacturer advises avoid—no information available.
- **HEPATIC IMPAIRMENT** Dose may need to be halved in liver cirrhosis.
- When used by inhalation Initially 2.5 micrograms at intervals of 3–4 hours (max. 6 times daily), adjusted according to response (consult product literature).
- **DIRECTIONS FOR ADMINISTRATION**
- With intravenous use For *intravenous infusion* dilute to a concentration of 200 nanograms/mL with Glucose 5% or Sodium Chloride 0.9%; alternatively, may be diluted to a concentration of 2 micrograms/mL and given via syringe driver.
- When used by inhalation For *inhaled treatment*, to minimise accidental exposure use only with nebulisers listed in *Ventavis®* product literature in a well ventilated room.
- **PRESCRIBING AND DISPENSING INFORMATION**
- When used by inhalation Delivery characteristics of nebuliser devices may vary—only switch devices under medical supervision.
- With intravenous use Concentrate for infusion available on a named patient basis from Bayer Schering in 0.5 mL and 1 mL ampoules.

- **MEDICINAL FORMS**
  There can be variation in the licensing of different medicines containing the same drug. No intravenous preparations listed
  Nebuliser liquid
- Ventavis (Bayer Plc)
  Iloprost (as Iloprost trometamol) 10 microgram per 1 ml Ventavis 10micrograms/ml nebuliser solution 1ml ampoules | 30 ampoule PoM £400.19 | 168 ampoule PoM £2,241.08

ENDOTHELIN RECEPTOR ANTAGONISTS

Bosentan

- **INDICATIONS AND DOSE**
  Pulmonary arterial hypertension (initiated under specialist supervision)
- BY MOUTH
- Child 2–17 years (body-weight 10–20 kg): Initially 31.25 mg once daily for 4 weeks, then increased to 31.25 mg twice daily
- Child 2–17 years (body-weight 20–40 kg): Initially 31.25 mg twice daily for 4 weeks, then increased to 62.5 mg twice daily
- Child 12–17 years (body-weight 40 kg and above): Initially 62.5 mg twice daily for 4 weeks, then increased to 125 mg twice daily (max. per dose 250 mg)

- **CONTRA-INDICATIONS** Acute porphyrias p. 562

- **CAUTIONS** Not to be initiated if systemic systolic blood pressure is below 85 mmHg
- **INTERACTIONS** → Appendix 1 (bosentan).
- **SIDE-EFFECTS**
- Common or very common Anaemia · diarrhoea · flushing · gastro-oesophageal reflux · headache · hypotension · oedema · palpitation · syncope
- Uncommon Leucopenia · neutropenia · thrombocytopenia
- Rare Liver cirrhosis · liver failure
- **CONCEPTION AND CONTRACEPTION** Effective contraception required during administration (hormonal contraception not considered effective). Monthly pregnancy tests advised.
- **PREGNANCY** Avoid (teratogenic in *animal* studies).
- **BREAST FEEDING** Manufacturer advises avoid—no information available.
- **HEPATIC IMPAIRMENT** Avoid in moderate and severe impairment.
- **MONITORING REQUIREMENTS**
- Monitor haemoglobin before and during treatment (monthly for first 4 months, then 3-monthly).
- Monitor liver function before treatment, at monthly intervals during treatment, and 2 weeks after dose increase (reduce dose or suspend treatment if liver enzymes raised significantly)—discontinue if symptoms of liver impairment.
- **TREATMENT CESSATION** Avoid abrupt withdrawal—withdraw treatment gradually.
- **DIRECTIONS FOR ADMINISTRATION** Tablets may be cut, or suspended in water or non-acidic liquid. Suspension is stable at room-temperature (max. 25°C) for 24 hours.

- **MEDICINAL FORMS**
  There can be variation in the licensing of different medicines containing the same drug.
  Tablet
- Tracleer (Actelion Pharmaceuticals UK Ltd)
  Bosentan (as Bosentan monohydrate) 62.5 mg Tracleer 62.5mg tablets | 56 tablet PoM £1,510.21
  Bosentan (as Bosentan monohydrate) 125 mg Tracleer 125mg tablets | 56 tablet PoM £1,510.21

PHOSPHODIESTERASE TYPE-5 INHIBITORS

Sildenafil

- **INDICATIONS AND DOSE**
  Pulmonary arterial hypertension (initiated under specialist supervision)
- BY MOUTH
- Neonate: Initially 250–500 micrograms/kg every 4–8 hours, adjusted according to response, start with the lower dose and frequency, especially if used with other vasodilators; maximum 30 mg per day.
- Child 1–11 months: Initially 250–500 micrograms/kg every 4–8 hours, adjusted according to response, start with the lower dose and frequency, especially if used with other vasodilators; maximum 30 mg per day
- Child 1–17 years (body-weight up to 20 kg): 10 mg 3 times a day
- Child 1–17 years (body-weight 20 kg and above): 20 mg 3 times a day

- **UNLICENSED USE** Not licensed for use in children under 1 year.
- **CONTRA-INDICATIONS** Hereditary degenerative retinal disorders · history of non-arteritic anterior ischaemic optic neuropathy · recent history of stroke · sickle-cell anaemia
- **CAUTIONS** Active peptic ulceration · anatomical deformation of the penis · autonomic dysfunction ·

bleeding disorders · cardiovascular disease · hypotension (avoid if severe) · intravascular volume depletion · left ventricular outflow obstruction · ocular disorders · predisposition to priapism · pulmonary veno-occlusive disease

- **INTERACTIONS** → Appendix 1 (sildenafil). Initiate cautiously if child also on epoprostenol, iloprost, bosentan or nitric oxide.
- **SIDE-EFFECTS**
  ▶ **Common or very common** Abdominal distension · alopecia · anaemia · anxiety · back pain · bronchitis · cellulitis · cough · diarrhoea · dry mouth · dyspepsia · epistaxis · fever · flushing · gastritis · gastro-oesophageal reflux · haemorrhoids · headache · influenza-like symptoms · insomnia · limb pain · migraine · myalgia · nasal congestion · night sweats · oedema · painful red eyes · paraesthesia · photophobia · retinal haemorrhage · tremor · vertigo · visual disturbances
  ▶ **Uncommon** Gynaecomastia · haematuria · penile haemorrhage · priapism
  ▶ **Frequency not known** Non-arteritic anterior ischaemic optic neuropathy (discontinue if sudden visual impairment occurs) · rash · retinal vascular occlusion · sudden hearing loss (advise patient to seek medical help)
- **PREGNANCY** Use only if potential benefit outweighs risk—no evidence of harm in *animal* studies.
- **BREAST FEEDING** Manufacturer advises avoid—no information available.
- **HEPATIC IMPAIRMENT** Reduce dose if not tolerated in mild to moderate impairment. Manufacturer advises avoid in severe impairment.
- **RENAL IMPAIRMENT** Reduce dose if not tolerated
- **TREATMENT CESSATION** Avoid abrupt withdrawal.
- **PATIENT AND CARER ADVICE**
  Medicines for Children leaflet: Sildenafil for pulmonary hypertension www.medicinesforchildren.org.uk/sildenafil-for-pulmonary-hypertension
- **NATIONAL FUNDING/ACCESS DECISIONS**
  Scottish Medicines Consortium (SMC) Decisions
  The *Scottish Medicines Consortium* has advised (October 2012) that sildenafil (*Revatio*®) is accepted for restricted use within NHS Scotland for the treatment of pulmonary arterial hypertension in children aged 1–17 years; sildenafil should only be prescribed on the advice of specialists in the Scottish Pulmonary Vascular Unit or the Scottish Adult Congenital Cardiac Service.

- **MEDICINAL FORMS**
  There can be variation in the licensing of different medicines containing the same drug. Forms available from special-order manufacturers include: oral suspension, oral solution
  Tablet
  ▶ **Revatio** (Pfizer Ltd)
  Sildenafil (as Sildenafil citrate) 20 mg Revatio 20mg tablets | 90 tablet PoM £446.33
  Oral suspension
  ▶ **Revatio** (Pfizer Ltd)
  Sildenafil (as Sildenafil citrate) 10 mg per 1 ml Revatio 10mg/ml oral suspension sugar-free | 112 ml PoM £186.75

VASODILATORS ⟩ PERIPHERAL VASODILATORS

Tolazoline

- **DRUG ACTION** Tolazoline is an alpha-blocker and produces both pulmonary and systemic vasodilation.

- **INDICATIONS AND DOSE**
  Correction of pulmonary vasospasm in neonates
  ▶ INITIALLY BY INTRAVENOUS INJECTION
  ▶ Neonate: Initially 1 mg/kg, to be given over 2–5 minutes, followed by (by continuous intravenous infusion) maintenance 200 micrograms/kg/hour if required, careful blood pressure monitoring should be carried out, doses above 300 micrograms/kg/hour associated with cardiotoxicity and renal failure.

  ▶ BY ENDOTRACHEAL TUBE
  ▶ Neonate: 200 micrograms/kg.

- **UNLICENSED USE** Not licensed for use in children.
- **CONTRA-INDICATIONS** Peptic ulcer disease
- **CAUTIONS** Cardiotoxic accumulation may occur with continuous infusion (particularly in renal impairment) · mitral stenosis
- **INTERACTIONS** → Appendix 1 (alpha-blockers).
- **SIDE-EFFECTS** Blood dyscrasias · blotchy skin · cardiac arrhythmias · diarrhoea · epigastric pain · flushing · haematuria · haemorrhage (with high doses) · headache · marked hypertension (with high doses) · metabolic alkalosis · nausea · oliguria · renal failure (with high doses) · severe hypotension (with high doses) · shivering · sweating · tachycardia · thrombocytopenia · vomiting
- **RENAL IMPAIRMENT** Lower doses may be necessary. Accumulates in renal impairment. Risk of cardiotoxicity.
- **MONITORING REQUIREMENTS** Monitor blood pressure regularly for sustained systemic hypotension.
- **DIRECTIONS FOR ADMINISTRATION** For *continuous intravenous infusion*, dilute with Glucose 5% or Sodium Chloride 0.9%. Prepare a fresh solution every 24 hours. For *endotracheal administration*, dilute with 0.5–1 mL of Sodium Chloride 0.9%.

- **MEDICINAL FORMS**
  There can be variation in the licensing of different medicines containing the same drug. Forms available from special-order manufacturers include: solution for injection

4.2 Hypotension and shock

Sympathomimetics

Overview

The properties of sympathomimetics vary according to whether they act on alpha or on beta adrenergic receptors. Response to sympathomimetics can also vary considerably in children, particularly neonates. It is important to titrate the dose to the desired effect and to monitor the child closely.

Inotropic sympathomimetics

Dopamine hydrochloride p. 114 has a variable, unpredictable, and dose dependent impact on vascular tone. Low dose infusion normally causes vasodilatation, but there is little evidence that this is clinically beneficial; moderate doses increase myocardial contractility and cardiac output in older children, but in neonates moderate doses may cause a reduction in cardiac output. High doses cause vasoconstriction and increase vascular resistance, and should therefore be used with caution following cardiac surgery, or where there is co-existing neonatal pulmonary hypertension.

In neonates the response to inotropic sympathomimetics varies considerably, particularly in those born prematurely; careful dose titration and monitoring are necessary.

Isoprenaline injection is available from 'special-order' manufacturers or specialist importing companies.

Shock

Shock is a medical emergency associated with a high mortality. The underlying causes of shock such as haemorrhage, sepsis or myocardial insufficiency should be corrected. Additional treatment is dependent on the type of shock.

Septic shock is associated with severe hypovolaemia (due to vasodilation and capillary leak) which should be corrected with crystalloids or colloids. If hypotension persists despite volume replacement, dopamine hydrochloride should be started. For shock refractory to treatment with dopamine hydrochloride, if cardiac output is high and peripheral vascular resistance is low (warm shock), noradrenaline/norepinephrine p. 115 should be added *or* if cardiac output is low and peripheral vascular resistance is high (cold shock), adrenaline/epinephrine p. 128 should be added. Additionally, in cold shock, a vasodilator such as milrinone p. 118, glyceryl trinitrate p. 127, or sodium nitroprusside p. 109 (on specialist advice only) can be used to reduce vascular resistance.

If the shock is resistant to volume expansion and catecholamines, and there is suspected or proven adrenal insufficiency, low dose hydrocortisone p. 411 can be used. ACTH-stimulated plasma-cortisol concentration should be measured; however, hydrocortisone can be started without such information. Alternatively, if the child is resistant to catecholamines, and vascular resistance is low, vasopressin p. 62 can be added.

Neonatal septic shock can be complicated by the transition from fetal to neonatal circulation. Treatment to reverse right ventricular failure, by decreasing pulmonary artery pressures, is commonly needed in neonates with fluid-refractory shock and persistent pulmonary hypertension of the newborn. Rapid administration of fluid in neonates with patent ductus arteriosus may cause left-to-right shunting and congestive heart failure induced by ventricular overload.

In *cardiogenic shock*, the aim is to improve cardiac output and to reduce the afterload on the heart. If central venous pressure is low, cautious volume expansion with a colloid or crystalloid can be used. An inotrope such as adrenaline/epinephrine or dopamine hydrochloride should be given to increase cardiac output. Dobutamine below is a peripheral vasodilator and is an alternative if hypotension is not significant.

Milrinone has both inotropic and vasodilatory effects and can be used when vascular resistance is high. Alternatively, glyceryl trinitrate or sodium nitroprusside (on specialist advice only) can be used to reduce vasoconstriction.

Hypovolaemic shock should be treated with a crystalloid or colloid solution (or whole or reconstituted blood if source of hypovolaemia is haemorrhage) and further steps to improve cardiac output and decrease vascular resistance can be taken, as in cardiogenic shock.

The use of sympathomimetic inotropes and vasoconstrictors should preferably be confined to the intensive care setting and undertaken with invasive haemodynamic monitoring.

See also advice on the management of anaphylactic shock in Antihistamines, allergen immunotherapy and allergic emergencies p. 162.

Vasoconstrictor sympathomimetics

Vasoconstrictor sympathomimetics raise blood pressure transiently by acting on alpha-adrenergic receptors to constrict peripheral vessels. They are sometimes used as an emergency method of elevating blood pressure where other measures have failed.

The danger of vasoconstrictors is that although they raise blood pressure they also reduce perfusion of vital organs such as the kidney.

Ephedrine hydrochloride p. 114 is used to reverse hypotension caused by spinal and epidural anaesthesia.

Metaraminol p. 115 is used as a vasopressor during cardiopulmonary bypass.

Phenylephrine hydrochloride p. 116 causes peripheral vasoconstriction and increases arterial pressure.

Ephedrine hydrochloride, metaraminol and phenylephrine hydrochloride are rarely needed in children and should be used under specialist supervision.

Noradrenaline/norepinephrine is reserved for children with low systemic vascular resistance that is unresponsive to fluid resuscitation following septic shock, spinal shock, and anaphylaxis.

Adrenaline/epinephrine is mainly used for its inotropic action. Low doses (acting on beta receptors) cause systemic and pulmonary vasodilation, some increase in heart rate and stroke volume and also an increase in contractility; high doses act predominantly on alpha receptors causing intense systemic vasoconstriction.

SYMPATHOMIMETICS > INOTROPIC

Dobutamine

- **DRUG ACTION** Dobutamine is a cardiac stimulant which acts on beta$_1$ receptors in cardiac muscle, and increases contractility with little effect on rate.

- **INDICATIONS AND DOSE**

  Inotropic support in low cardiac output states, after cardiac surgery, cardiomyopathies, shock
  ▸ BY CONTINUOUS INTRAVENOUS INFUSION

  ▸ Neonate: Initially 5 micrograms/kg/minute, then adjusted according to response to 2–20 micrograms/kg/minute, doses as low as 0.5–1 microgram/kg/minute have been used.

  ▸ Child: Initially 5 micrograms/kg/minute, then adjusted according to response to 2–20 micrograms/kg/minute, doses as low as 0.5–1 microgram/kg/minute have been used

- **CONTRA-INDICATIONS** Phaeochromocytoma

- **CAUTIONS** Acute heart failure · acute myocardial infarction · arrhythmias · correct hypercapnia before starting and during treatment · correct hypovolaemia before starting and during treatment · correct hypoxia before starting and during treatment · correct metabolic acidosis before starting and during treatment · diabetes mellitus · extravasation may cause tissue necrosis · extreme caution or avoid in marked obstruction of cardiac ejection (such as idiopathic hypertrophic subaortic stenosis) · hyperthyroidism · ischaemic heart disease · occlusive vascular disease · severe hypotension · susceptibility to angle-closure glaucoma · tachycardia · tolerance may develop with continuous infusions longer than 72 hours

- **INTERACTIONS** → Appendix 1 (sympathomimetics).

- **SIDE-EFFECTS**
  ▸ **Rare** Psychosis
  ▸ **Very rare** Angle-closure glaucoma · AV block · bradycardia · cardiac arrest · coronary artery spasm · hypokalaemia · myocardial infarction · petechial bleeding
  ▸ **Frequency not known** Anxiety · arrhythmias · bronchospasm · cerebral haemorrhage · chest pain · dyspnoea · eosinophilia · fever · headache · hypertension (marked increase in systolic blood pressure indicates overdose) · hypotension · increased urinary urgency ·

myoclonic spasm · nausea · palpitation · paraesthesia · phlebitis · pruritus of scalp · pulmonary oedema · rash · reduced platelet aggregation (on prolonged use) · tachycardia · tremor · vomiting

- **PREGNANCY** No evidence of harm in *animal* studies—manufacturers advise use only if potential benefit outweighs risk.
- **BREAST FEEDING** Manufacturers advise avoid—no information available.
- **DIRECTIONS FOR ADMINISTRATION** Dobutamine injection should be diluted before use or given undiluted with syringe pump. Dobutamine concentrate for intravenous infusion should be diluted before use.

    For *continuous intravenous infusion*, using infusion pump, dilute to a concentration of 0.5–1 mg/mL (max. 5 mg/mL if fluid restricted) with Glucose 5% *or* Sodium Chloride 0.9%; infuse higher concentration solutions through central venous catheter only. Incompatible with bicarbonate and other strong alkaline solutions.

  ▸ In neonates *Neonatal intensive care*, dilute 30 mg/kg body-weight to a final volume of 50 mL with infusion fluid; an intravenous infusion rate of 0.5 mL/hour provides a dose of 5 micrograms/kg/minute; max. concentration of 5 mg/mL; infuse higher concentration solutions through central venous catheter only. Incompatible with bicarbonate and other strong alkaline solutions.

- **MEDICINAL FORMS**
  There can be variation in the licensing of different medicines containing the same drug.
  Solution for infusion
  EXCIPIENTS: May contain Sulfites
  ▸ **Dobutamine (Non-proprietary)**
    Dobutamine (as Dobutamine hydrochloride) 5 mg per 1 ml Dobutamine 250mg/50ml solution for infusion vials | 1 vial PoM £7.50
    Dobutamine (as Dobutamine hydrochloride) 12.5 mg per 1 ml Dobutamine 250mg/20ml concentrate for solution for infusion ampoules | 5 ampoule PoM £26.00–£26.25

Dopamine hydrochloride

- **DRUG ACTION** Dopamine is a cardiac stimulant which acts on beta$_1$ receptors in cardiac muscle, and increases contractility with little effect on rate.

- **INDICATIONS AND DOSE**

  To correct the haemodynamic imbalance due to acute hypotension, shock, cardiac failure, adjunct following cardiac surgery
  ▸ BY CONTINUOUS INTRAVENOUS INFUSION

  ▸ Neonate: Initially 3 micrograms/kg/minute (max. per dose 20 micrograms/kg/minute), adjusted according to response.

  ▸ Child: Initially 5 micrograms/kg/minute (max. per dose 20 micrograms/kg/minute), adjusted according to response

- **UNLICENSED USE** Not licensed for use in children under 12 years.
- **CONTRA-INDICATIONS** Phaeochromocytoma · tachyarrhythmia
- **CAUTIONS** Correct hypovolaemia · hyperthyroidism
- **INTERACTIONS** → Appendix 1 (sympathomimetics).
- **SIDE-EFFECTS**
  ▸ **Common or very common** Chest pain · dyspnoea · headache · hypotension · nausea · palpitation · tachycardia · vasoconstriction · vomiting
  ▸ **Uncommon** Bradycardia · gangrene · hypertension · mydriasis
  ▸ **Rare** Fatal ventricular arrhythmias

- **PREGNANCY** No evidence of harm in *animal* studies—manufacturer advises use only if potential benefit outweighs risk.
- **BREAST FEEDING** May suppress lactation—not known to be harmful.
- **DIRECTIONS FOR ADMINISTRATION** Dopamine concentrate for intravenous infusion to be diluted before use.

    For *continuous intravenous infusion*, dilute to a max. concentration of 3.2 mg/mL with Glucose 5% *or* Sodium Chloride 0.9%. Infuse higher concentrations through central venous catheter using a syringe pump to avoid extravasation and fluid overload. Incompatible with bicarbonate and other alkaline solutions.

  ▸ In neonates *Neonatal intensive care*, dilute 30 mg/kg body-weight to a final volume of 50 mL with infusion fluid; an intravenous infusion rate of 0.3 mL/hour provides a dose of 3 micrograms/kg/minute; max. concentration of 3.2 mg/mL; infuse higher concentrations through central venous catheter. Incompatible with bicarbonate and other alkaline solutions.

- **MEDICINAL FORMS**
  There can be variation in the licensing of different medicines containing the same drug. Forms available from special-order manufacturers include: solution for infusion
  Solution for infusion
  ▸ **Dopamine hydrochloride (Non-proprietary)**
    Dopamine hydrochloride 40 mg per 1 ml Dopamine 200mg/5ml solution for infusion ampoules | 5 ampoule PoM £19.42–£20.00 | 10 ampoule PoM £9.04
    Dopamine 200mg/5ml concentrate for solution for infusion ampoules | 10 ampoule PoM no price available
    Dopamine hydrochloride 160 mg per 1 ml Dopamine 800mg/5ml solution for infusion ampoules | 10 ampoule PoM £34.00

SYMPATHOMIMETICS ⟩ VASOCONSTRICTOR

Ephedrine hydrochloride

- **INDICATIONS AND DOSE**

  Reversal of hypotension from spinal or epidural anaesthesia
  ▸ BY SLOW INTRAVENOUS INJECTION
  ▸ Child 1-11 years: 500–750 micrograms/kg every 3–4 minutes, adjusted according to response, alternatively 17–25 mg/m^2 every 3–4 minutes, adjusted according to response, injection solution to contain ephedrine hydrochloride 3 mg/ml; maximum 30 mg per course
  ▸ Child 12-17 years: 3–7.5 mg every 3–4 minutes (max. per dose 9 mg), adjusted according to response, injection solution to contain ephedrine hydrochloride 3 mg/ml; maximum 30 mg per course

- **CAUTIONS** Diabetes mellitus · hypertension · hyperthyroidism · susceptibility to angle-closure glaucoma
- **INTERACTIONS** → Appendix 1 (sympathomimetics).
- **SIDE-EFFECTS**
  ▸ **Common or very common** Anginal pain · anorexia · anxiety · arrhythmias · changes in blood-glucose concentration · confusion · difficulty in micturition · dizziness · dyspnoea · flushing · headache · hypersalivation · insomnia · nausea · psychoses · restlessness · sweating · tachycardia · tremor · urine retention · vasoconstriction with hypertension · vasodilation with hypotension · vomiting
  ▸ **Very rare** Angle-closure glaucoma
  ▸ **Frequency not known** Bradycardia · Increased lacrimation (can have adverse effects on contact lens wear)

- **PREGNANCY** Increased fetal heart rate reported with parenteral ephedrine.
- **BREAST FEEDING** Present in milk; manufacturer advises avoid—irritability and disturbed sleep reported.

- **RENAL IMPAIRMENT** Use with caution.
- **DIRECTIONS FOR ADMINISTRATION** For *slow intravenous injection*, give via central venous catheter using a solution containing ephedrine hydrochloride 3 mg/ml.
- **MEDICINAL FORMS**
  There can be variation in the licensing of different medicines containing the same drug. Forms available from special-order manufacturers include: solution for injection
  Solution for injection
  ▸ Ephedrine hydrochloride (Non-proprietary)
  Ephedrine hydrochloride 3 mg per 1 ml Ephedrine 30mg/10ml solution for injection ampoules | 10 ampoule PoM £73.21
  Ephedrine 30mg/10ml solution for injection pre-filled syringes | 1 pre-filled disposable injection PoM £7.59–£9.50 | 12 pre-filled disposable injection PoM £114.00
  Ephedrine hydrochloride 30 mg per 1 ml Ephedrine 30mg/1ml solution for injection ampoules | 10 ampoule PoM £4.31–£4.74

Metaraminol

- **INDICATIONS AND DOSE**
  Acute hypotension
  ▸ BY INTRAVENOUS INFUSION
  ▸ Child 12–17 years: 15–100 mg, adjusted according to response
  Emergency treatment of acute hypotension
  ▸ INITIALLY BY INTRAVENOUS INJECTION
  ▸ Child 12–17 years: Initially 0.5–5 mg, then (by intravenous infusion) 15–100 mg, adjusted according to response
- **UNLICENSED USE** Not licensed for use in children.
- **CONTRA-INDICATIONS** Hypertension
- **CAUTIONS** Cirrhosis · coronary vascular thrombosis · diabetes mellitus · extravasation at injection site may cause necrosis · following myocardial infarction · hypercapnia · hyperthyroidism · hypoxia · mesenteric vascular thrombosis · peripheral vascular thrombosis · Prinzmetal's variant angina · susceptibility to angle-closure glaucoma · uncorrected hypovolaemia
  CAUTIONS, FURTHER INFORMATION
  ▸ Hypertensive response
  Metaraminol has a longer duration of action than noradrenaline, and an excessive vasopressor response may cause a prolonged rise in blood pressure.
- **INTERACTIONS** → Appendix 1 (sympathomimetics).
- **SIDE-EFFECTS** Angle-closure glaucoma · anorexia · anxiety · arrhythmias · bradycardia · confusion · dyspnoea · fatal ventricular arrhythmia reported in Laennec's cirrhosis · headache · hypertension · hypoxia · insomnia · nausea · palpitation · peripheral ischaemia · psychosis · tachycardia · tremor · urinary retention · vomiting · weakness
- **PREGNANCY** May reduce placental perfusion—manufacturer advises use only if potential benefit outweighs risk.
- **BREAST FEEDING** Manufacturer advises caution—no information available.
- **MONITORING REQUIREMENTS** Monitor blood pressure and rate of flow frequently.
- **DIRECTIONS FOR ADMINISTRATION** For *intravenous infusion*, dilute to a concentration of 30–200 micrograms/mL with Glucose 5% or Sodium Chloride 0.9% and give through a central venous catheter.

- **MEDICINAL FORMS**
  There can be variation in the licensing of different medicines containing the same drug. Forms available from special-order manufacturers include: solution for injection
  Solution for injection
  ▸ Metaraminol (Non-proprietary)
  Metaraminol (as Metaraminol tartrate) 10 mg per 1 ml Metaraminol 10mg/1ml solution for injection ampoules | 10 ampoule PoM £31.97

Noradrenaline/norepinephrine

- **INDICATIONS AND DOSE**
  Acute hypotension (septic shock) | Shock secondary to excessive vasodilation (as noradrenaline)
  ▸ BY CONTINUOUS INTRAVENOUS INFUSION
  ▸ Neonate: 20–100 nanograms/kg/minute (max. per dose 1 microgram/kg/minute), adjusted according to response.
  ▸ Child: 20–100 nanograms/kg/minute (max. per dose 1 microgram/kg/minute), adjusted according to response
  DOSE EQUIVALENCE AND CONVERSION
  1 mg of noradrenaline base is equivalent to 2 mg of noradrenaline acid tartrate. **Doses expressed as the base.**
- **UNLICENSED USE** Not licensed for use in children.
- **CONTRA-INDICATIONS** Hypertension
- **CAUTIONS** Coronary vascular thrombosis · diabetes mellitus · extravasation at injection site may cause necrosis · following myocardial infarction · hypercapnia · hyperthyroidism · hypoxia · mesenteric vascular thrombosis · peripheral vascular thrombosis · Prinzmetal's variant angina · susceptibility to angle-closure glaucoma · uncorrected hypovolaemia
- **INTERACTIONS** → Appendix 1 (sympathomimetics).
- **SIDE-EFFECTS** Angle-closure glaucoma · anorexia · anxiety · arrhythmias · bradycardia · confusion · dyspnoea · headache · hypertension · hypoxia · insomnia · nausea · palpitation · peripheral ischaemia · psychosis · tachycardia · tremor · urinary retention · vomiting · weakness
- **PREGNANCY** Avoid—may reduce placental perfusion.
- **MONITORING REQUIREMENTS** Monitor blood pressure and rate of flow frequently.
- **DIRECTIONS FOR ADMINISTRATION** For *continuous intravenous infusion*, dilute to a max. concentration of noradrenaline (base) 40 micrograms/mL (higher concentrations can be used if fluid-restricted) with Glucose 5% or Sodium Chloride and Glucose. Infuse through central venous catheter; discard if discoloured. Incompatible with bicarbonate or alkaline solutions.
  ▸ In neonates *Neonatal intensive care*, dilute 600 micrograms (base)/kg body-weight to a final volume of 50 mL with infusion fluid; an intravenous infusion rate of 0.1 mL/hour provides a dose of 20 nanograms(base)/kg/minute; infuse through central venous catheter; max. concentration of noradrenaline (base) 40 micrograms/mL (higher concentrations can be used if fluid-restricted). Discard if discoloured. Incompatible with bicarbonate or alkaline solutions.
- **PRESCRIBING AND DISPENSING INFORMATION** For a period of time, preparations on the UK market may be described as either noradrenaline base or noradrenaline acid tartrate; doses in the BNF are expressed as the base.

2

Cardiovascular system

- **MEDICINAL FORMS**
  There can be variation in the licensing of different medicines containing the same drug. Forms available from special-order manufacturers include: infusion, solution for infusion

  Solution for infusion
  ▶ Noradrenaline/norepinephrine (Non-proprietary)
  Noradrenaline (as Noradrenaline acid tartrate) 1 mg per 1 ml Noradrenaline (Norepinephrine) 4mg/4ml concentrate for solution for infusion ampoules | 10 ampoule [PoM] £44.00
  Noradrenaline (base) 8mg/8ml concentrate for solution for infusion ampoules | 10 ampoule [PoM] £116.00
  Noradrenaline (base) 2mg/2ml solution for infusion ampoules | 5 ampoule [PoM] £12.00 (Hospital only)
  Noradrenaline (base) 4mg/4ml solution for infusion ampoules | 5 ampoule [PoM] £22.00 (Hospital only)
  Noradrenaline (base) 4mg/4ml solution for infusion ampoules | 10 ampoule [PoM] £58.00
  Noradrenaline (Norepinephrine) 2mg/2ml concentrate for solution for Infusion ampoules | 5 ampoule [PoM] £11.00

Phenylephrine hydrochloride

- **INDICATIONS AND DOSE**

  Acute hypotension
  ▶ BY SUBCUTANEOUS INJECTION, OR BY INTRAMUSCULAR INJECTION
  ▶ Child 1–11 years: 100 micrograms/kg every 1–2 hours (max. per dose 5 mg) as required
  ▶ Child 12–17 years: Initially 2–5 mg (max. per dose 5 mg), followed by 1–10 mg, after at least 15 minutes if required
  ▶ BY SLOW INTRAVENOUS INJECTION
  ▶ Child 1–11 years: Initially 5–20 micrograms/kg (max. per dose 500 micrograms), repeated as necessary after at least 15 minutes
  ▶ Child 12–17 years: 100–500 micrograms, repeated as necessary after at least 15 minutes
  ▶ BY INTRAVENOUS INFUSION
  ▶ Child 1–15 years: Initially 100–500 nanograms/kg/minute, adjusted according to response
  ▶ Child 16–17 years: Initially up to 180 micrograms/minute, reduced to 30–60 micrograms/minute, adjusted according to response

- **UNLICENSED USE** Not licensed for use in children by intravenous infusion or injection.

- **CONTRA-INDICATIONS** Hypertension · severe hyperthyroidism

- **CAUTIONS** Coronary disease · coronary vascular thrombosis · diabetes · extravasation at injection site may cause necrosis · following myocardial infarction · hypercapnia · hyperthyroidism · hypoxia · mesenteric vascular thrombosis · peripheral vascular thrombosis · Prinzmetal's variant angina · susceptibility to angle-closure glaucoma · uncorrected hypovolaemia
  CAUTIONS, FURTHER INFORMATION
  ▶ Hypertensive response Phenylephrine has a longer duration of action than noradrenaline (norepinephrine), and an excessive vasopressor response may cause a prolonged rise in blood pressure.

- **INTERACTIONS** → Appendix 1 (sympathomimetics). Phenylephrine may interact with systemically administered monoamine-oxidase inhibitors.

- **SIDE-EFFECTS** Angle-closure glaucoma · anorexia · anxiety · arrhythmias · bradycardia (also reflex bradycardia) · confusion · dyspnoea · headache · hypertension · hypoxia · insomnia · nausea · palpitation · peripheral ischaemia · psychosis · tachycardia · tremor · urinary retention · vomiting · weakness

- **PREGNANCY** Avoid if possible; malformations reported following use in first trimester; fetal hypoxia and bradycardia reported in late pregnancy and labour.

- **MONITORING REQUIREMENTS**
  ▶ Contra-indicated in hypertension—monitor blood pressure and rate of flow frequently.

- **DIRECTIONS FOR ADMINISTRATION** For *intravenous injection*, dilute to a concentration of 1 mg/mL with Water for Injections and administer slowly. For *intravenous infusion*, dilute to a concentration of 20 micrograms/mL with Glucose 5% or Sodium Chloride 0.9% and administer as a continuous infusion via a central venous catheter using a controlled infusion device.

- **PRESCRIBING AND DISPENSING INFORMATION** Intravenous administration preferred when managing acute hypotension in children.

- **MEDICINAL FORMS**
  There can be variation in the licensing of different medicines containing the same drug. Forms available from special-order manufacturers include: solution for injection

  Solution for injection
  ▶ Phenylephrine hydrochloride (Non-proprietary)
  Phenylephrine (as Phenylephrine hydrochloride) 50 microgram per 1 ml Phenylephrine 500micrograms/10ml solution for injection pre-filled syringes | 1 pre-filled disposable injection [PoM] £15.00 | 10 pre-filled disposable injection [PoM] £150.00
  Phenylephrine hydrochloride 100 microgram per 1 ml Phenylephrine 1mg/10ml solution for injection ampoules | 10 ampoule [PoM] £40.00
  Phenylephrine hydrochloride 10 mg per 1 ml Phenylephrine 10mg/1ml solution for injection ampoules | 10 ampoule [PoM] £99.12

5 Heart failure

Drugs used for Heart failure not listed below
Bendroflumethiazide, p. 102 · Captopril, p. 103 · Chlorothiazide, p. 103 · Chlortalidone, p. 134 · Digoxin, p. 75 · Enalapril maleate, p. 105 · Glyceryl trinitrate, p. 127 · Lisinopril, p. 106 · Prazosin, p. 92

BETA-ADRENOCEPTOR BLOCKERS ❯
ALPHA- AND BETA-ADRENOCEPTOR BLOCKERS

☞ 95

Carvedilol

- **INDICATIONS AND DOSE**

  Adjunct in heart failure (limited information available)
  ▶ BY MOUTH
  ▶ Child 2–17 years: Initially 50 micrograms/kg twice daily (max. per dose 3.125 mg) for at least 2 weeks, then increased to 100 micrograms/kg twice daily for at least 2 weeks, then increased to 200 micrograms/kg twice daily, then increased if necessary up to 350 micrograms/kg twice daily (max. per dose 25 mg)

- **UNLICENSED USE** Not licensed for use in children under 18 years.

- **CONTRA-INDICATIONS** Acute or decompensated heart failure requiring intravenous inotropes

- **SIDE-EFFECTS** Allergic skin reactions · angina · AV block · changes in liver enzymes · depressed mood · disturbances of micturition · influenza-like symptoms · leucopenia · nasal stuffiness · postural hypotension · thrombocytopenia · wheezing

- **PREGNANCY** Information on the safety of carvedilol during pregnancy is lacking. If carvedilol is used close to delivery, infants should be monitored for signs of alpha-blockade (as well as beta-blockade).

- **BREAST FEEDING** Infants should be monitored as there is a risk of possible toxicity due to alpha-blockade (in addition to beta-blockade).
- **HEPATIC IMPAIRMENT** Avoid in hepatic impairment.
- **MONITORING REQUIREMENTS** Monitor renal function during dose titration in patients with heart failure who also have renal impairment, low blood pressure, ischaemic heart disease, or diffuse vascular disease.
- **PATIENT AND CARER ADVICE**
  Medicines for Children leaflet: Carvedilol for heart failure www.medicinesforchildren.org.uk/carvedilol-heart-failure-0

- **MEDICINAL FORMS**
  There can be variation in the licensing of different medicines containing the same drug. Forms available from special-order manufacturers include: oral suspension

  Tablet
  CAUTIONARY AND ADVISORY LABELS 8
  ▸ Carvedilol (Non-proprietary)
    Carvedilol 3.125 mg Carvedilol 3.125mg tablets | 28 tablet [PoM]
    £8.00 DT price = £0.89
    Carvedilol 6.25 mg Carvedilol 6.25mg tablets | 28 tablet [PoM]
    £8.99 DT price = £0.98
    Carvedilol 12.5 mg Carvedilol 12.5mg tablets | 28 tablet [PoM] £9.99
    DT price = £0.99
    Carvedilol 25 mg Carvedilol 25mg tablets | 28 tablet [PoM] £12.50
    DT price = £1.15

DIURETICS > POTASSIUM-SPARING DIURETICS > ALDOSTERONE ANTAGONISTS

Potassium canrenoate

- **INDICATIONS AND DOSE**
  Short-term diuresis for oedema in heart failure and in ascites
  ▸ BY INTRAVENOUS INJECTION, OR BY INTRAVENOUS INFUSION
  ▸ Neonate: 1–2 mg/kg twice daily.
  ▸ Child 1 month–11 years: 1–2 mg/kg twice daily
  ▸ Child 12–17 years: 1–2 mg/kg twice daily (max. per dose 200 mg)

  DOSE EQUIVALENCE AND CONVERSION
  To convert to equivalent oral spironolactone dose, multiply potassium canrenoate dose by 0.7.

- **UNLICENSED USE** Not licensed for use in the UK.
- **CONTRA-INDICATIONS** Hyperkalaemia · hyponatraemia
- **CAUTIONS** Acute porphyrias p. 562 · hypotension · potential metabolic products carcinogenic in *rodents*
- **INTERACTIONS** → Appendix 1 (diuretics).
- **SIDE-EFFECTS**
- **Common or very common** Ataxia · drowsiness · headache · hyperuricaemia · menstrual irregularities · pain at injection site on rapid administration
- **Uncommon** Eosinophilia · hyperkalaemia · thrombocytopenia
- **Rare** Agranulocytosis · alopecia · deepening of voice · erythema · hepatotoxicity · hoarseness · hypersensitivity reactions · osteomalacia · urticaria
- **Frequency not known** Gastro-intestinal disturbances · gynaecomastia · hirsutism · hypochloraemic acidosis · hyponatraemia · hypotension · mastalgia · transient confusion with high doses
- **PREGNANCY** Crosses placenta. Feminisation and undescended testes in male fetus in *animal* studies—manufacturer advises avoid.
- **BREAST FEEDING** Present in breast milk—manufacturer advises avoid.

- **RENAL IMPAIRMENT** Use with caution if estimated glomerular filtration rate 30–60 mL/minute/1.73 m². Avoid if estimated glomerular filtration rate less than 30 mL/minute/1.73 m². Monitor plasma-potassium concentration if estimated glomerular filtration rate 30–60 mL/minute/1.73 m².
- **MONITORING REQUIREMENTS** Monitor electrolytes (discontinue if hyperkalaemia occurs).
- **DIRECTIONS FOR ADMINISTRATION** Consult product literature. Intravenous injection to be given over at least 3 minutes.
- **PRESCRIBING AND DISPENSING INFORMATION** Potassium canrenoate injection is available from 'special-order' manufacturers or specialist importing companies.

- **MEDICINAL FORMS**
  There can be variation in the licensing of different medicines containing the same drug.
  Solution for injection
  ▸ Potassium canrenoate (Non-proprietary)
    Potassium canrenoate 20 mg per 1 ml Aldactone 200mg/10ml solution for injection ampoules | 10 ampoule [PoM] no price available

Spironolactone

- **INDICATIONS AND DOSE**
  Oedema in heart failure and in ascites | Nephrotic syndrome | Reduction of hypokalaemia induced by diuretics or amphotericin
  ▸ BY MOUTH
  ▸ Neonate: Initially 1–2 mg/kg daily in 1–2 divided doses; increased if necessary up to 7 mg/kg daily, in resistant ascites.
  ▸ Child 1 month–11 years: Initially 1–3 mg/kg daily in 1–2 divided doses; increased if necessary up to 9 mg/kg daily, in resistant ascites
  ▸ Child 12–17 years: Initially 50–100 mg daily in 1–2 divided doses; increased if necessary up to 9 mg/kg daily, in resistant ascites; maximum 400 mg per day

- **UNLICENSED USE** Not licensed for reduction of hypokalaemia induced by diuretics or amphotericin.
- **CONTRA-INDICATIONS** Addison's disease · anuria · hyperkalaemia
- **CAUTIONS** Acute porphyrias p. 562 · potential metabolic products carcinogenic in *rodents*
- **INTERACTIONS** → Appendix 1 (diuretics).
  Potassium supplements must **not** be given with potassium-sparing diuretics.
  Administration of a potassium-sparing diuretic to a patient receiving an ACE inhibitor or an angiotensin-II receptor antagonist can also cause severe hyperkalaemia.
- **SIDE-EFFECTS** Acute renal failure · agranulocytosis · alopecia · benign breast tumour · breast pain · changes in libido · confusion · dizziness · drowsiness · electrolyte disturbances · gastro-intestinal disturbances · gynaecomastia · hepatotoxicity · hyperkalaemia (discontinue) · hypertrichosis · hyperuricaemia · hyponatraemia · leg cramps · leucopenia · malaise · menstrual disturbances · rash · Stevens-Johnson syndrome · thrombocytopenia
- **PREGNANCY** Use only if potential benefit outweighs risk—feminisation of male fetus in *animal* studies.
- **BREAST FEEDING** Metabolites present in milk, but amount probably too small to be harmful.
- **RENAL IMPAIRMENT** Avoid in acute renal insufficiency or severe impairment. Monitor plasma-potassium concentration (high risk of hyperkalaemia in renal impairment).

- **MONITORING REQUIREMENTS** Monitor electrolytes—discontinue if hyperkalaemia occurs.
- **PATIENT AND CARER ADVICE**
  Medicines for Children leaflet: Spironolactone for heart failure www.medicinesforchildren.org.uk/spironolactone-for-heart-failure
- **MEDICINAL FORMS**
  There can be variation in the licensing of different medicines containing the same drug. Forms available from special-order manufacturers include: oral suspension, oral solution

Tablet

CAUTIONARY AND ADVISORY LABELS 21

▸ Spironolactone (Non-proprietary)
  Spironolactone 25 mg Spironolactone 25mg tablets | 28 tablet [PoM] £1.95 DT price = £1.23
  Spironolactone 50 mg Spironolactone 50mg tablets | 28 tablet [PoM] £6.00 DT price = £1.74
  Spironolactone 100 mg Spironolactone 100mg tablets | 28 tablet [PoM] £6.24 DT price = £2.04 | 30 tablet [PoM] no price available

▸ Aldactone (Pfizer Ltd)
  Spironolactone 25 mg Aldactone 25mg tablets | 100 tablet [PoM] £8.89
  Spironolactone 50 mg Aldactone 50mg tablets | 100 tablet [PoM] £17.78
  Spironolactone 100 mg Aldactone 100mg tablets | 28 tablet [PoM] £9.96 DT price = £2.04 | 100 tablet [PoM] £35.56

PHOSPHODIESTERASE TYPE-3 INHIBITORS

Enoximone

- **DRUG ACTION** Enoximone is a phosphodiesterase type-3 inhibitor that exerts most effect on the myocardium; it has positive inotropic properties and vasodilator activity.

- **INDICATIONS AND DOSE**

Congestive heart failure, low cardiac output following cardiac surgery
▸ INITIALLY BY SLOW INTRAVENOUS INJECTION

▸ **Neonate:** Loading dose 500 micrograms/kg, followed by (by continuous intravenous infusion) 5–20 micrograms/kg/minute, adjusted according to response, infusion to be given over 24 hours; maximum 24 mg/kg per day.

▸ **Child:** Loading dose 500 micrograms/kg, followed by (by continuous intravenous infusion) 5–20 micrograms/kg/minute, adjusted according to response, infusion dose to be given over 24 hours; maximum 24 mg/kg per day

- **UNLICENSED USE** Not licensed for use in children.
- **CAUTIONS** Heart failure associated with hypertrophic cardiomyopathy, stenotic or obstructive valvular disease or other outlet obstruction
- **INTERACTIONS** → Appendix 1 (phosphodiesterase type-3 inhibitors).
- **SIDE-EFFECTS** Chills · diarrhoea · ectopic beats · fever · headache · hypotension · insomnia · nausea · oliguria · supraventricular arrhythmias (more likely in patients with pre-existing arrhythmias) · upper and lower limb pain · urinary retention · ventricular tachycardia (more likely in patients with pre-existing arrhythmias) · vomiting
- **PREGNANCY** Manufacturer advises use only if potential benefit outweighs risk.
- **BREAST FEEDING** Manufacturer advises caution—no information available.
- **HEPATIC IMPAIRMENT** Dose reduction may be required.
- **RENAL IMPAIRMENT** Consider dose reduction.
- **MONITORING REQUIREMENTS** Monitor blood pressure, heart rate, ECG, central venous pressure, fluid and electrolyte status, renal function, platelet count and hepatic enzymes.
- **DIRECTIONS FOR ADMINISTRATION** Incompatible with glucose solutions. Use only plastic containers or syringes; crystal formation if glass used. Avoid extravasation.
  For *intravenous administration*, dilute to concentration of 2.5 mg/mL with Sodium Chloride 0.9% or Water for Injections; the initial loading dose should be given by slow intravenous injection over at least 15 minutes.
- **PRESCRIBING AND DISPENSING INFORMATION**
  Phosphodiesterase type-3 inhibitors possess positive inotropic and vasodilator activity and are useful in infants and children with low cardiac output especially after cardiac surgery. Phosphodiesterase type-3 inhibitors should be limited to short-term use because long-term oral administration has been associated with increased mortality in adults with congestive heart failure.
- **PATIENT AND CARER ADVICE**
  Medicines for Children leaflet: Enoximone for pulmonary hypertension www.medicinesforchildren.org.uk/enoximone-for-pulmonary-hypertension
- **MEDICINAL FORMS**
  There can be variation in the licensing of different medicines containing the same drug.
  Solution for injection
  EXCIPIENTS: May contain Alcohol, propylene glycol
  ▸ Perfan (Myogen GmbH)
    Enoximone 5 mg per 1 ml Perfan 100mg/20ml solution for injection ampoules | 10 ampoule [PoM] no price available (Hospital only)

Milrinone

- **DRUG ACTION** Milrinone is a phosphodiesterase type-3 inhibitor that exerts most effect on the myocardium; it has positive inotropic properties and vasodilator activity.

- **INDICATIONS AND DOSE**

Congestive heart failure, low cardiac output following cardiac surgery, shock
▸ INITIALLY BY INTRAVENOUS INFUSION

▸ **Neonate:** Initially 50–75 micrograms/kg, given over 30–60 minutes, reduce or omit initial dose if at risk of hypotension, then (by continuous intravenous infusion) 30–45 micrograms/kg/hour for 2–3 days (usually for 12 hours after cardiac surgery).

▸ **Child:** Initially 50–75 micrograms/kg, given over 30–60 minutes, reduce or omit initial dose if at risk of hypotension, then (by continuous intravenous infusion) 30–45 micrograms/kg/hour for 2–3 days (usually for 12 hours after cardiac surgery)

- **UNLICENSED USE** Not licensed for use in children under 18 years.
- **CONTRA-INDICATIONS** Severe hypovolaemia
- **CAUTIONS** Correct hypokalaemia · heart failure associated with hypertrophic cardiomyopathy, stenotic or obstructive valvular disease or other outlet obstruction
- **INTERACTIONS** → Appendix 1 (phosphodiesterase type-3 inhibitors).
- **SIDE-EFFECTS**
  ▸ **Common or very common** Ectopic beats · headache · hypotension · supraventricular arrhythmias (more likely in patients with pre-existing arrhythmias) · ventricular tachycardia
  ▸ **Uncommon** Chest pain · hypokalaemia · thrombocytopenia · tremor · ventricular fibrillation
  ▸ **Very rare** Anaphylaxis · bronchospasm · rash
- **PREGNANCY** Manufacturer advises use only if potential benefit outweighs risk.

- **BREAST FEEDING** Manufacturer advises avoid—no information available.
- **RENAL IMPAIRMENT** Use half to three-quarters normal dose and monitor response if estimated glomerular filtration rate less than 50 mL/minute/1.73 m^2.
- **MONITORING REQUIREMENTS**
▸ Monitor blood pressure, heart rate, ECG, central venous pressure, fluid and electrolyte status, renal function, platelet count and hepatic enzymes.
▸ Monitor renal function.
- **DIRECTIONS FOR ADMINISTRATION** Avoid extravasation. For *intravenous infusion* dilute with Glucose 5% or Sodium Chloride 0.9% *or* Sodium Chloride and Glucose intravenous infusion to a concentration of 200 micrograms/mL (higher concentrations of 400 micrograms/mL have been used). Loading dose may be given undiluted if fluid-restricted.
- **PRESCRIBING AND DISPENSING INFORMATION** Phosphodiesterase type-3 inhibitors possess positive inotropic and vasodilator activity and are useful in infants and children with low cardiac output especially after cardiac surgery. Phosphodiesterase type-3 inhibitors should be limited to short-term use because long-term oral administration has been associated with increased mortality in adults with congestive heart failure.

- **MEDICINAL FORMS**
There can be variation in the licensing of different medicines containing the same drug. Forms available from special-order manufacturers include: solution for infusion
Solution for injection
▸ Primacor (Sanofi)
Milrinone 1 mg per 1 ml Primacor 10mg/10ml solution for injection ampoules | 10 ampoule PoM £199.06

6 Hyperlipidaemia

Lipid-regulating drugs

Risk factors for cardiovascular disease

Atherosclerosis begins in childhood and raised serum cholesterol in children is associated with cardiovascular disease in adulthood. Lowering the cholesterol, without hindering growth and development in children and adolescents, should reduce the risk of cardiovascular disease in later life.

The risk factors for developing cardiovascular disease include raised serum cholesterol concentration, smoking, hypertension, impaired glucose tolerance, male sex, ethnicity, obesity, triglyceride concentration, chronic kidney disease, and a family history of cardiovascular disease. Heterozygous familial hypercholesterolaemia is the most common cause of raised serum cholesterol in children; homozygous familial hypercholesterolaemia is very rare and its specialised management is not covered in *BNF for Children*. Familial hypercholesterolaemia can lead to a greater risk of early coronary heart disease and should be managed by a specialist.

Secondary causes of hypercholesterolaemia should be addressed, these include obesity, diet, diabetes mellitus, hypothyroidism, nephrotic syndrome, obstructive biliary disease, glycogen storage disease, and drugs such as corticosteroids.

Management
The aim of management of hypercholesterolaemia is to reduce the risk of atherosclerosis while ensuring adequate growth and development. Children with hypercholesterolaemia (or their carers) should receive advice on appropriate lifestyle changes such as improved diet,

increased exercise, weight reduction, and not smoking; Hypertension p. 90 should also be managed appropriately. Drug therapy may also be necessary.

Hypothyroidism
Children with hypothyroidism should receive adequate thyroid replacement therapy before their requirement for lipid-regulating treatment is assessed because correction of hypothyroidism itself may resolve the lipid abnormality. Untreated hypothyroidism increases the risk of myositis with lipid regulating drugs.

Drug treatment in heterozygous familial hypercholesterolaemia
Lifestyle modifications alone are unlikely to lower cholesterol concentration adequately in heterozygous familial hypercholesterolaemia and drug treatment is often required. Lipid-regulating drugs should be considered by the age of 10 years. The decision to initiate drug treatment will depend on the child's age, the age of onset of coronary heart disease within the family, and the presence of other cardiovascular risk factors. In children with a family history of coronary heart disease in early adulthood, drug treatment before the age of 10 years, and a combination of lipid-regulating drugs may be necessary.

Drug treatment in secondary hypercholesterolaemia
If 6–12 months of dietary and other lifestyle interventions has failed to lower cholesterol concentration adequately, drug treatment may be indicated in children 10 years and older (rarely necessary in younger children) who are at a high risk of developing cardiovascular disease.

Choice of drugs
Experience in the use of lipid-regulating drugs in children is limited and they should be initiated on specialist advice.

Statins are more effective than other classes of drugs in lowering LDL-cholesterol but less effective than the fibrates in reducing triglycerides. Statins also increase concentrations of HDL-cholesterol. Statins reduce cardiovascular disease events and total mortality in adults, irrespective of the initial cholesterol concentration. They are the drugs of first choice in children and are generally well tolerated; atorvastatin p. 123 and simvastatin p. 125 are the preferred statins. Other lipid-regulating drugs can be used if statins are ineffective or are not tolerated.

Ezetimibe p. 121 can be used alone when statins are not tolerated, or in combination with a statin when a high dose statin fails to control cholesterol concentration adequately.

Bile acid sequestrants are also available but tolerability of and compliance with these drugs is poor, and their use is declining.

Fibrates may reduce the risk of coronary heart disease in those with low HDL-cholesterol or with raised triglycerides. Evidence for the use of a fibrate (bezafibrate p. 121 or fenofibrate p. 122) in children is limited; fibrates should be considered only if dietary intervention and treatment with a statin and a bile acid sequestrant is unsuccessful or contra-indicated.

In hypertriglyceridaemia which cannot be controlled by very strict diet, omega-3 fatty acid compounds can be considered.

2

Cardiovascular system

↰ above

LIPID MODIFYING DRUGS ›BILE ACID SEQUESTRANTS

Bile acid sequestrants

- **DRUG ACTION** Bile acid sequestrants act by binding bile acids, preventing their reabsorption; this promotes hepatic conversion of cholesterol into bile acids; the resultant increased LDL-receptor activity of liver cells increases the clearance of LDL-cholesterol from the plasma.

- **CAUTIONS** Interference with the absorption of fat-soluble vitamins (supplements of vitamins A, D, K, and folic acid may be required when treatment is prolonged).

- **SIDE-EFFECTS** Constipation · diarrhoea · gastro-intestinal discomfort · hypertriglyceridaemia (aggravation) · hypoprothrombinaemia associated with vitamin K deficiency · increased risk of bleeding · nausea · vomiting

- **PREGNANCY** Bile acid sequestrants should be used with caution as although the drugs are not absorbed, they may cause fat-soluble vitamin deficiency on prolonged use.

- **BREAST FEEDING** Bile acid sequestrants should be used with caution as although the drugs are not absorbed, they may cause fat-soluble vitamin deficiency on prolonged use.

- **MONITORING REQUIREMENTS** A child's growth and development should be monitored.

↰ above

Colestipol hydrochloride

- **INDICATIONS AND DOSE**
  Familial hypercholesterolaemia
  ▸ BY MOUTH
  ▸ Child 12–17 years: Initially 5 g 1–2 times a day, then increased in steps of 5 g every 1 month, total daily dose may be given in 1–2 divided doses or as a single dose if tolerated; maximum 30 g per day

- **UNLICENSED USE** Not licensed for use in children.

- **INTERACTIONS** → Appendix 1 (colestipol).

- **DIRECTIONS FOR ADMINISTRATION** The contents of each sachet should be mixed with at least 100 mL of water or other suitable liquid such as fruit juice or skimmed milk; alternatively it can be mixed with thin soups, cereals, yoghurt, or pulpy fruits ensuring at least 100 mL of liquid is provided.
  Other drugs should be taken at least 1 hour before or 4–6 hours after colestipol to reduce possible interference with absorption.

- **PATIENT AND CARER ADVICE** Patient counselling on administration is advised for colestipol hydrochloride granules (avoid other drugs at same time).

- **MEDICINAL FORMS**
  There can be variation in the licensing of different medicines containing the same drug.
  Tablet
  ▸ Colestipol hydrochloride (Non-proprietary)
  Colestipol hydrochloride 1 gram Colestid 1g tablets |
  120 tablet PoM no price available
  Granules
  CAUTIONARY AND ADVISORY LABELS 13
  ▸ Colestid (Pfizer Ltd)
  Colestipol hydrochloride 5 gram Colestid 5g granules sachets plain sugar-free | 30 sachet PoM £15.05
  Colestid Orange 5g granules sachets sugar-free | 30 sachet PoM £15.05

↰ above

Colestyramine
(Cholestyramine)

- **INDICATIONS AND DOSE**
  Familial hypercholesterolaemia
  ▸ BY MOUTH
  ▸ Child 6–11 years: Initially 4 g once daily, then increased to 4 g up to 3 times a day, adjusted according to response
  ▸ Child 12–17 years: Initially 4 g once daily, then increased in steps of 4 g every 1 week; increased to 12–24 g daily in 1–4 divided doses, adjusted according to response; maximum 36 g per day

  Pruritus associated with partial biliary obstruction and primary biliary cirrhosis
  ▸ BY MOUTH
  ▸ Child 1–11 months: 1 g once daily, adjusted according to response, total daily dose may alternatively be given in 2–4 divided doses; maximum 9 g per day
  ▸ Child 1–5 years: 2 g once daily, adjusted according to response, total daily dose may alternatively be given in 2–4 divided doses; maximum 18 g per day
  ▸ Child 6–11 years: 4 g once daily, adjusted according to response, total daily dose may alternatively be given in 2–4 divided doses; maximum 24 g per day
  ▸ Child 12–17 years: 4–8 g once daily, adjusted according to response, total daily dose may alternatively be given in 2–4 divided doses; maximum 36 g per day

  Diarrhoea associated with Crohn's disease, ileal resection, vagotomy, diabetic vagal neuropathy, and radiation
  ▸ BY MOUTH
  ▸ Child 1–11 months: 1 g once daily, adjusted according to response, total daily dose may alternatively be given in 2–4 divided doses, if no response within 3 days an alternative therapy should be initiated; maximum 9 g per day
  ▸ Child 1–5 years: 2 g once daily, adjusted according to response, total daily dose may alternatively be given in 2–4 divided doses, if no response within 3 days an alternative therapy should be initiated; maximum 18 g per day
  ▸ Child 6–11 years: 4 g once daily, adjusted according to response, total daily dose may alternatively be given in 2–4 divided doses, if no response within 3 days an alternative therapy should be initiated; maximum 24 g per day
  ▸ Child 12–17 years: 4–8 g once daily, adjusted according to response, total daily dose may alternatively be given in 2–4 divided doses, if no response within 3 days an alternative therapy should be initiated; maximum 36 g per day

- **UNLICENSED USE** Not licensed for use in children under 6 years to reduce cholesterol.

- **CONTRA-INDICATIONS** Complete biliary obstruction (not likely to be effective)

- **INTERACTIONS** → Appendix 1 (colestyramine).

- **SIDE-EFFECTS**
- **Rare** Intestinal obstruction
- **Frequency not known** Hyperchloraemic acidosis (on prolonged use)

- **DIRECTIONS FOR ADMINISTRATION** The contents of each sachet should be mixed with at least 150 mL of water or other suitable liquid such as fruit juice, skimmed milk, thin soups, and pulpy fruits with a high moisture content.
  Other drugs should be taken at least 1 hour before or 4–6 hours after colestyramine to reduce possible interference with absorption.

• **PATIENT AND CARER ADVICE** Patient counselling on administration is advised for colestyramine powder (avoid other drugs at same time).

• **MEDICINAL FORMS**
There can be variation in the licensing of different medicines containing the same drug. Forms available from special-order manufacturers include: oral suspension, oral solution
Powder
CAUTIONARY AND ADVISORY LABELS 13
EXCIPIENTS: May contain Aspartame, sucrose
▸ **Colestyramine (Non-proprietary)**
Colestyramine anhydrous 4 gram Colestyramine 4g oral powder sachets | 50 sachet [PoM] no price available
Colestyramine 4g oral powder sachets sugar free sugar-free | 50 sachet [PoM] £30.00–£32.78 DT price = £31.85
▸ **Questran** (Bristol-Myers Squibb Pharmaceuticals Ltd)
Colestyramine anhydrous 4 gram Questran 4g oral powder sachets | 50 sachet [PoM] £10.76
▸ **Questran Light** (Bristol-Myers Squibb Pharmaceuticals Ltd)
Colestyramine anhydrous 4 gram Questran Light 4g oral powder sachets sugar-free | 50 sachet [PoM] £16.15 DT price = £31.85

LIPID MODIFYING DRUGS > CHOLESTEROL ABSORPTION INHIBITORS

Ezetimibe

• **DRUG ACTION** Ezetimibe inhibits the intestinal absorption of cholesterol.

• **INDICATIONS AND DOSE**
Adjunct to dietary measures and statin treatment in primary hypercholesterolaemia | Adjunct to dietary measures and statin in homozygous familial hypercholesterolaemia | Primary hypercholesterolaemia (if statin inappropriate or not tolerated) | Adjunct to dietary measures in homozygous sitosterolaemia
▸ BY MOUTH
▸ Child 10–17 years: 10 mg daily

• **INTERACTIONS** → Appendix 1 (ezetimibe).
There is an increased risk of rhabdomyolysis if ezetimibe is used in combination with a statin.

• **SIDE-EFFECTS**
▸ **Common or very common** Fatigue · gastro-intestinal disturbances · headache · myalgia
▸ **Rare** Anaphylaxis · angioedema · arthralgia · hepatitis · hypersensitivity reactions · rash
▸ **Very rare** Cholecystitis · cholelithiasis · myopathy · pancreatitis · raised creatine kinase · rhabdomyolysis · thrombocytopenia

• **PREGNANCY** Manufacturer advises use only if potential benefit outweighs risk—no information available.

• **BREAST FEEDING** Manufacturer advises avoid—present in milk in *animal* studies.

• **HEPATIC IMPAIRMENT** Avoid in moderate and severe impairment—may accumulate.

• **MEDICINAL FORMS**
There can be variation in the licensing of different medicines containing the same drug.
Tablet
▸ **Ezetrol** (Merck Sharp & Dohme Ltd)
Ezetimibe 10 mg Ezetrol 10mg tablets | 28 tablet [PoM] £26.31 DT price = £26.31

Combinations available: *Simvastatin with ezetimibe*, p. 125

LIPID MODIFYING DRUGS > FIBRATES

Bezafibrate

• **DRUG ACTION** Fibrates act by decreasing serum triglycerides; they have variable effect on LDL-cholestrol.

• **INDICATIONS AND DOSE**
Hyperlipidaemia including familial hypercholesterolaemia (administered on expert advice)
▸ BY MOUTH USING IMMEDIATE-RELEASE MEDICINES
▸ Child 10–17 years: 200 mg once daily (max. per dose 200 mg 3 times a day), adjusted according to response

• **UNLICENSED USE** Not licensed for use in children.

• **CONTRA-INDICATIONS** Gall bladder disease · hypoalbuminaemia · nephrotic syndrome · photosensitivity to fibrates

• **CAUTIONS** Correct hypothyroidism before initiating treatment

• **INTERACTIONS** → Appendix 1 (fibrates).
Combination of a fibrate with a statin increases the risk of muscle effects (especially rhabdomyolysis) and should be used with caution.

• **SIDE-EFFECTS**
▸ **Common or very common** Abdominal distension · anorexia · diarrhoea · nausea
▸ **Uncommon** Alopecia · cholestasis · dizziness · erectile dysfunction · headache · myotoxicity (with myasthenia, myalgia, or very rarely rhabdomyolysis)—special risk in renal impairment · photosensitivity reactions · pruritus · rash · renal failure · urticaria
▸ **Rare** Pancreatitis · peripheral neuropathy
▸ **Very rare** Anaemia · gallstones · increased platelet count · interstitial lung disease · leucopenia · pancytopenia · Stevens-Johnson syndrome · thrombocytopenic purpura · toxic epidermal necrolysis

• **PREGNANCY** Manufacturers advise avoid—no information available.

• **BREAST FEEDING** Manufacturer advises avoid—no information available.

• **HEPATIC IMPAIRMENT** Avoid in severe liver disease.

• **RENAL IMPAIRMENT** Reduce dose if estimated glomerular filtration rate 15–60 mL/minute/1.73 m^2.
Myotoxicity Special care needed in patients with renal disease, as progressive increases in serum creatinine concentration or failure to follow dosage guidelines may result in myotoxicity (rhabdomyolysis); discontinue if myotoxicity suspected or creatine kinase concentration increases significantly.
Avoid if estimated glomerular filtration rate less than 15 mL/minute/1.73 m^2.

• **MONITORING REQUIREMENTS** Consider monitoring of liver function and creatine kinase when fibrates used in combination with a statin.

• **PRESCRIBING AND DISPENSING INFORMATION** Fibrates are mainly used in those whose serum-triglyceride concentration is greater than 10 mmol/litre or in those who cannot tolerate a statin (specialist use).

• **MEDICINAL FORMS**
There can be variation in the licensing of different medicines containing the same drug. Forms available from special-order manufacturers include: oral suspension
Tablet
CAUTIONARY AND ADVISORY LABELS 21
▸ **Bezafibrate (Non-proprietary)**
Bezafibrate 200 mg Bezafibrate 200mg tablets | 100 tablet [PoM] £8.50 DT price = £4.51
▸ **Bezalip** (Actavis UK Ltd)
Bezafibrate 200 mg Bezalip 200mg tablets | 100 tablet [PoM] £8.63 DT price = £4.51

Cardiovascular system

2

Fenofibrate

- **DRUG ACTION** Fibrates act by decreasing serum triglycerides; they have variable effect on LDL-cholestrol.

- **INDICATIONS AND DOSE**

  Hyperlipidaemias including familial hypercholesterolaemia (administered on expert advice)
  ▸ BY MOUTH USING CAPSULES
  ▸ Child 4-14 years: One 67 mg (micronised) capsule per 20 kg body-weight daily, maximum four 67 mg capsules daily, or max. three 67 mg capsules daily with concomitant statin
  ▸ Child 15-17 years: Initially 3 capsules daily, then increased if necessary to 4 capsules daily, max. 3 capsules daily with concomitant statin, dose relates to 67 mg (micronised) capsules

- **UNLICENSED USE** 200 mg and 267 mg capsules not licensed in children.
- **CONTRA-INDICATIONS** Gall bladder disease · pancreatitis (unless due to severe hypertriglyceridaemia) · photosensitivity to ketoprofen
- **CAUTIONS** Correct hypothyroidism before initiating treatment
- **INTERACTIONS** → Appendix 1 (fibrates).
  Combination of a fibrate with a statin increases the risk of muscle effects (especially rhabdomyolysis) and should be used with caution.
- **SIDE-EFFECTS**
  ▸ **Common or very common** Abdominal distension · anorexia · diarrhoea · nausea
  ▸ **Uncommon** Alopecia · cholestasis · dizziness · erectile dysfunction · headache · myotoxicity (with myasthenia, myalgia, or very rarely rhabdomyolysis)—special risk in renal impairment · pancreatitis · photosensitivity reactions · pruritus · pulmonary embolism · rash · renal failure · urticaria
  ▸ **Rare** Hepatitis · peripheral neuropathy
  ▸ **Very rare** Anaemia · gallstones · increased platelet count · interstitial lung disease · leucopenia · pancytopenia · Stevens-Johnson syndrome · thrombocytopenic purpura · toxic epidermal necrolysis
  ▸ **Frequency not known** Interstitial pneumopathies
- **PREGNANCY** Avoid—embryotoxicity in *animal* studies.
- **BREAST FEEDING** Manufacturers advise avoid—no information available.
- **HEPATIC IMPAIRMENT** Avoid.
- **RENAL IMPAIRMENT** Reduce dose if estimated glomerular filtration rate less than 60 mL/minute/1.73 m². Avoid if estimated glomerular filtration rate less than 15 mL/minute/1.73 m².
  Myotoxicity Special care needed in patients with renal disease, as progressive increases in serum creatinine concentration or failure to follow dosage guidelines may result in myotoxicity (rhabdomyolysis); discontinue if myotoxicity suspected or creatine kinase concentration increases significantly.
- **MONITORING REQUIREMENTS**
  ▸ Liver function tests recommended every 3 months for first year (discontinue treatment if significantly raised).
  ▸ Consider monitoring liver function and creatine kinase when fibrates used in combination with a statin.
- **PRESCRIBING AND DISPENSING INFORMATION** Fibrates are mainly used in those whose serum-triglyceride concentration is greater than 10 mmol/litre or in those who cannot tolerate a statin (specialist use).

- **MEDICINAL FORMS**
  There can be variation in the licensing of different medicines containing the same drug.
  Capsule
  CAUTIONARY AND ADVISORY LABELS 21
  ▸ Fenofibrate (Non-proprietary)
    Fenofibrate micronised 67 mg Fenofibrate micronised 67mg capsules | 90 capsule ‖PoM‖ £23.30 DT price = £22.37
    Fenofibrate micronised 200 mg Fenofibrate micronised 200mg capsules | 28 capsule ‖PoM‖ £21.75 DT price = £7.38
    Fenofibrate micronised 267 mg Fenofibrate micronised 267mg capsules | 28 capsule ‖PoM‖ £21.75 DT price = £4.33
  ▸ Lipantil Micro (BGP Products Ltd)
    Fenofibrate micronised 67 mg Lipantil Micro 67 capsules | 90 capsule ‖PoM‖ £23.30 DT price = £22.37
    Fenofibrate micronised 200 mg Lipantil Micro 200 capsules | 28 capsule ‖PoM‖ £14.23 DT price = £7.38
    Fenofibrate micronised 267 mg Lipantil Micro 267 capsules | 28 capsule ‖PoM‖ £21.75 DT price = £4.33

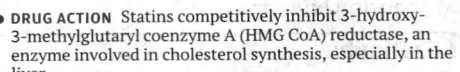 LIPID MODIFYING DRUGS ▸ STATINS

Statins

- **DRUG ACTION** Statins competitively inhibit 3-hydroxy-3-methylglutaryl coenzyme A (HMG CoA) reductase, an enzyme involved in cholesterol synthesis, especially in the liver.
- **CAUTIONS** High alcohol intake · history of liver disease · hypothyroidism · patients at increased risk of muscle toxicity, including myopathy or rhabdomyolysis (e.g. those with a personal or family history of muscular disorders, previous history of muscular toxicity and a high alcohol intake)
  CAUTIONS, FURTHER INFORMATION
  ▸ Muscle effects Muscle toxicity can occur with all statins, however the likelihood increases with higher doses and in certain patients (see below). Statins should be used with caution in patients at increased risk of muscle toxicity, including those with a personal or family history of muscular disorders, previous history of muscular toxicity, a high alcohol intake, renal impairment or hypothyroidism.
    In patients at increased risk of muscle effects, a statin should not usually be started if the baseline creatine kinase concentration is more than 5 times the upper limit of normal (some patients may present with an extremely elevated baseline creatine kinase concentration, for example because of a physical occupation or rigorous exercise—specialist advice should be sought regarding consideration of statin therapy in these patients).
  ▸ Hypothyroidism Hypothyroidism should be managed adequately before starting treatment with a statin.
- **INTERACTIONS** → Appendix 1 (statins).
  There is an increased incidence of myopathy if a statin is given with a fibrate (the combination of a statin and gemfibrozil should preferably be avoided), with lipid-lowering doses of nicotinic acid, with fusidic acid (risk of rhabdomyolysis—the combination of a statin and fusidic acid should be avoided; temporarily discontinue statin and restart 7 days after last fusidic acid dose), or with drugs that increase the plasma-statin concentration, such as macrolide antibiotics, imidazole and triazole antifungals, and ciclosporin; close monitoring of liver function and, if muscular symptoms occur, of creatine kinase is necessary.
- **SIDE-EFFECTS**
  ▸ **Rare** Hepatitis · jaundice
  ▸ **Very rare** Hepatic failure. · interstitial lung disease · lupus erythematosus-like reactions · pancreatitis
  ▸ **Frequency not known** Alopecia · altered liver function tests · amnesia · arthralgia · asthenia · depression · dizziness · fatigue · gastro-intestinal disturbances · headache · hyperglycaemia · hypersensitivity reactions · may be

associated with the development of diabetes mellitus (particularly in those already at risk of the condition) · myalgia · myopathy · myositis · paraesthesia · peripheral neuropathy · pruritus · rash · rhabdomyolysis · sexual dysfunction · sleep disturbance · thrombocytopenia · urticaria · visual disturbance

SIDE-EFFECTS, FURTHER INFORMATION
▸ **Muscle effects** The risk of myopathy, myositis, and rhabdomyolysis associated with statin use is rare. Although myalgia has been reported commonly in patients receiving statins, muscle toxicity truly attributable to statin use is rare. Muscle toxicity can occur with all statins, however the likelihood increases with higher doses.

If muscular symptoms or raised creatine kinase occur during treatment, other possible causes (e.g. rigorous physical activity, hypothyroidism, infection, recent trauma, and drug or alcohol addiction) should be excluded before statin therapy is implicated, particularly if statin treatment has previously been tolerated for more than 3 months. When a statin is suspected to be the cause of myopathy, and creatine kinase concentration is markedly elevated (more than 5 times upper limit of normal), or if muscular symptoms are severe, treatment should be discontinued. If symptoms resolve and creatine kinase concentrations return to normal, the statin should be reintroduced at a lower dose and the patient monitored closely; an alternative statin should be prescribed if unacceptable side-effects are experienced with a particular statin. Statins should not be discontinued in the event of small, asymptomatic elevations of creatine kinase. Routine monitoring of creatine kinase is unnecessary in asymptomatic patients.
▸ **Interstitial lung disease** If patients develop symptoms such as dyspnoea, cough, and weight loss, they should seek medical attention.

● **CONCEPTION AND CONTRACEPTION** Adequate contraception is required during treatment and for 1 month afterwards.

● **PREGNANCY** Statins should be avoided in pregnancy (discontinue 3 months before attempting to conceive) as congenital anomalies have been reported and the decreased synthesis of cholesterol possibly affects fetal development.

● **HEPATIC IMPAIRMENT** Statins should be used with caution in those with a history of liver disease. Avoid in active liver disease or when there are unexplained persistent elevations in serum transaminases.

● **MONITORING REQUIREMENTS**
▸ Before starting treatment with statins, at least one full lipid profile (non-fasting) should be measured, including total cholesterol, HDL-cholesterol, non-HDL-cholesterol (calculated as total cholesterol minus HDL-cholesterol), and triglyceride concentrations, thyroid-stimulating hormone, and renal function should also be assessed.
▸ **Liver function** There is little information available on a rational approach to liver-function monitoring; however, NICE suggests that liver enzymes should be measured before treatment, and repeated within 3 months and at 12 months of starting treatment, unless indicated at other times by signs or symptoms suggestive of hepatotoxicity (NICE clinical guideline 181 (July 2014). Lipid Modification—Cardiovascular risk assessment and the modification of blood lipids for the primary and secondary prevention of cardiovascular disease).
Those with serum transaminases that are raised, but less than 3 times the upper limit of the reference range, should **not** be routinely excluded from statin therapy. Those with serum transaminases of more than 3 times the upper limit of the reference range should discontinue statin therapy.

▸ **Creatine kinase** Creatine kinase concentration should be measured in children before treatment and if unexplained muscle pain occurs.

● **PATIENT AND CARER ADVICE** Advise patients to report promptly unexplained muscle pain, tenderness, or weakness.

◀ 122

Atorvastatin

● **INDICATIONS AND DOSE**

Hyperlipidaemia including familial hypercholesterolaemia
▸ BY MOUTH
 ▸ **Child 10–17 years:** Initially 10 mg once daily, then increased if necessary up to 20 mg once daily, dose to be adjusted at intervals of at least 4 weeks

Homozygous familial hypercholestrolaemia
▸ BY MOUTH
 ▸ **Child 10–17 years:** Initially 10 mg once daily, then increased if necessary up to 80 mg once daily, dose to be adjusted at intervals of at least 4 weeks

DOSE ADJUSTMENTS DUE TO INTERACTIONS
Reduced dose required (max. 10 mg daily) with concomitant ciclosporin, or tipranavir combined with ritonavir—seek specialist advice.

● **CAUTIONS** Haemorrhagic stroke

● **SIDE-EFFECTS**
▸ **Common or very common** Back pain · epistaxis · hyperglycaemia · nasopharyngitis · pharyngeolaryngeal pain
▸ **Uncommon** Anorexia · blurred vision · chest pain · hypoglycaemia · malaise · neck pain · peripheral oedema · pyrexia · tinnitus · weight gain
▸ **Rare** Cholestasis · Stevens-Johnson syndrome · toxic epidermal necrolysis
▸ **Very rare** Gynaecomastia · hearing loss

● **BREAST FEEDING** Manufacturer advises avoid—no information available.

● **PATIENT AND CARER ADVICE** Patient counselling is advised for atorvastatin tablets (muscle effects).
Medicines for Children leaflet: Atorvastatin for high cholesterol www.medicinesforchildren.org.uk/atorvastatin-high-cholesterol-0

● **MEDICINAL FORMS**
There can be variation in the licensing of different medicines containing the same drug. Forms available from special-order manufacturers include: oral suspension, oral solution
Tablet
▸ Atorvastatin (Non-proprietary)
  Atorvastatin (as Atorvastatin calcium trihydrate)
  10 mg Atorvastatin 10mg tablets | 28 tablet PoM £13.00 DT price = £0.95 | 90 tablet PoM £41.78
  Atorvastatin (as Atorvastatin calcium trihydrate)
  20 mg Atorvastatin 20mg tablets | 28 tablet PoM £24.64 DT price = £1.12 | 90 tablet PoM £79.20
  Atorvastatin (as Atorvastatin calcium trihydrate)
  30 mg Atorvastatin 30mg tablets | 28 tablet PoM £24.50 DT price = £24.50
  Atorvastatin (as Atorvastatin calcium trihydrate)
  40 mg Atorvastatin 40mg tablets | 28 tablet PoM £24.64 DT price = £1.28 | 90 tablet PoM £79.20
  Atorvastatin (as Atorvastatin calcium trihydrate)
  60 mg Atorvastatin 60mg tablets | 28 tablet PoM £28.00 DT price = £28.00
  Atorvastatin (as Atorvastatin calcium trihydrate)
  80 mg Atorvastatin 80mg tablets | 28 tablet PoM £28.21 DT price = £2.18 | 90 tablet PoM £90.67
▸ Lipitor (Pfizer Ltd)
  Atorvastatin (as Atorvastatin calcium trihydrate) 10 mg Lipitor 10mg tablets | 28 tablet PoM £13.00 DT price = £0.95
  Atorvastatin (as Atorvastatin calcium trihydrate) 20 mg Lipitor 20mg tablets | 28 tablet PoM £24.64 DT price = £1.12

Atorvastatin (as Atorvastatin calcium trihydrate) 40 mg Lipitor 40mg tablets | 28 tablet [PoM] £24.64 DT price = £1.28
Atorvastatin (as Atorvastatin calcium trihydrate) 80 mg Lipitor 80mg tablets | 28 tablet [PoM] £28.21 DT price = £2.18

Chewable tablet
CAUTIONARY AND ADVISORY LABELS 24
▶ Lipitor (Pfizer Ltd)
Atorvastatin (as Atorvastatin calcium trihydrate) 10 mg Lipitor 10mg chewable tablets sugar-free | 30 tablet [PoM] £13.80 DT price = £13.80
Atorvastatin (as Atorvastatin calcium trihydrate) 20 mg Lipitor 20mg chewable tablets sugar-free | 30 tablet [PoM] £26.40 DT price = £26.40

F 122

Fluvastatin

● **INDICATIONS AND DOSE**
Heterozygous familial hypercholesterolaemia
▶ INITIALLY BY MOUTH USING IMMEDIATE-RELEASE MEDICINES
▷ Child 9-17 years: Initially 20 mg daily, dose to be taken in the evening, then (by mouth) adjusted in steps of 20 mg daily (max. per dose 40 mg twice daily), adjusted at intervals of at least 6 weeks; maximum 80 mg per day
▶ BY MOUTH USING MODIFIED-RELEASE MEDICINES
▷ Child 9-17 years: 80 mg daily, dose form is not appropriate for initial dose titration

● SIDE-EFFECTS
▶ Very rare Vasculitis

● BREAST FEEDING Manufacturer advises avoid—no information available.

● RENAL IMPAIRMENT Manufacturer advises doses above 40 mg daily should be initiated with caution if estimated glomerular filtration rate less than 30 mL/minute/1.73 m^2.

● PATIENT AND CARER ADVICE Patient counselling is advised for fluvastatin tablets/capsules (muscle effects).

● MEDICINAL FORMS
There can be variation in the licensing of different medicines containing the same drug.
Modified-release tablet
CAUTIONARY AND ADVISORY LABELS 25
▶ Fluvastatin (Non-proprietary)
Fluvastatin (as Fluvastatin sodium) 80 mg Fluvastatin 80mg modified-release tablets | 28 tablet [PoM] no price available DT price = £19.20
▶ Dorisin XL (Aspire Pharma Ltd)
Fluvastatin (as Fluvastatin sodium) 80 mg Dorisin XL 80mg tablets | 28 tablet [PoM] £19.20 DT price = £19.20
▶ Lescol XL (Novartis Pharmaceuticals UK Ltd)
Fluvastatin (as Fluvastatin sodium) 80 mg Lescol XL 80mg tablets | 28 tablet [PoM] £19.20 DT price = £19.20
▶ Luvinsta XL (Actavis UK Ltd)
Fluvastatin (as Fluvastatin sodium) 80 mg Luvinsta XL 80mg tablets | 28 tablet [PoM] £19.20 DT price = £19.20
▶ Nandovar XL (Sandoz Ltd)
Fluvastatin (as Fluvastatin sodium) 80 mg Nandovar XL 80mg tablets | 28 tablet [PoM] £16.32 DT price = £19.20
▶ Pinmactil (Mylan Ltd)
Fluvastatin (as Fluvastatin sodium) 80 mg Pinmactil 80mg modified-release tablets | 28 tablet [PoM] £19.20 DT price = £19.20

Capsule
▶ Fluvastatin (Non-proprietary)
Fluvastatin (as Fluvastatin sodium) 20 mg Fluvastatin 20mg capsules | 28 capsule [PoM] £6.96 DT price = £2.16
Fluvastatin (as Fluvastatin sodium) 40 mg Fluvastatin 40mg capsules | 28 capsule [PoM] £7.42 DT price = £2.38
▶ Lescol (Novartis Pharmaceuticals UK Ltd)
Fluvastatin (as Fluvastatin sodium) 20 mg Lescol 20mg capsules | 28 capsule [PoM] £15.26 DT price = £2.16
Fluvastatin (as Fluvastatin sodium) 40 mg Lescol 40mg capsules | 28 capsule [PoM] £15.26 DT price = £2.38

F 122

Pravastatin sodium

● **INDICATIONS AND DOSE**
Hyperlipidaemia including familial hypercholesterolaemia
▶ BY MOUTH
▷ Child 8-13 years: 10 mg daily, then increased if necessary up to 20 mg daily, dose to be taken at night, dose to be adjusted at intervals of at least 4 weeks
▷ Child 14-17 years: 10 mg daily, then increased if necessary up to 40 mg daily, dose to be taken at night, dose to be adjusted at intervals of at least 4 weeks

● SIDE-EFFECTS
▶ Uncommon Abnormal urination · dysuria · nocturia · urinary frequency
▶ Very rare Fulminant hepatic necrosis

● BREAST FEEDING Manufacturer advises avoid—small amount of drug present in breast milk.

● RENAL IMPAIRMENT Start with lower doses in moderate to severe impairment.

● PATIENT AND CARER ADVICE Patient counselling is advised for pravastatin tablets (muscle effects).

● MEDICINAL FORMS
There can be variation in the licensing of different medicines containing the same drug. Forms available from special-order manufacturers include: oral suspension, oral solution, powder
Tablet
▶ Pravastatin sodium (Non-proprietary)
Pravastatin sodium 10 mg Pravastatin 10mg tablets | 28 tablet [PoM] £16.10 DT price = £0.91
Pravastatin sodium 20 mg Pravastatin 20mg tablets | 28 tablet [PoM] £29.60 DT price = £1.08
Pravastatin sodium 40 mg Pravastatin 40mg tablets | 28 tablet [PoM] £29.60 DT price = £1.37

F 122

Rosuvastatin

● **INDICATIONS AND DOSE**
Hyperlipidaemia including familial hypercholesterolaemia
▶ BY MOUTH
▷ Child 10-17 years: Initially 5 mg once daily, then increased if necessary up to 20 mg once daily, dose to be increased at intervals of at least 4 weeks, use lower max. dose in children with risk factors for myopathy or rhabdomyolysis (including personal or family history of muscular disorders or toxicity)

DOSE ADJUSTMENTS DUE TO INTERACTIONS
Reduced dose required with concomitant atazanavir, darunavir, ezetimibe, fibrate, itraconazole, lopinavir, or tipranavir—seek specialist advice.

● CAUTIONS Patients of Asian origin

● SIDE-EFFECTS
▶ Common or very common Proteinuria
▶ Very rare Gynaecomastia · haematuria
▶ Frequency not known Oedema · Stevens-Johnson syndrome

● BREAST FEEDING Manufacturer advises avoid—no information available.

● RENAL IMPAIRMENT Reduce dose if estimated glomerular filtration rate less than 60 mL/minute/1.73 m^2. Avoid if estimated glomerular filtration rate less than 30 mL/minute/1.73 m^2.

● PATIENT AND CARER ADVICE Patient counselling is advised for rosuvastatin tablets (muscle effects).

- **MEDICINAL FORMS**
There can be variation in the licensing of different medicines containing the same drug. Forms available from special-order manufacturers include: oral suspension

Tablet
- ▸ Crestor (AstraZeneca UK Ltd)
  Rosuvastatin (as Rosuvastatin calcium) 5 mg Crestor 5mg tablets | 28 tablet [PoM] £18.03 DT price = £18.03
  Rosuvastatin (as Rosuvastatin calcium) 10 mg Crestor 10mg tablets | 28 tablet [PoM] £18.03 DT price = £18.03
  Rosuvastatin (as Rosuvastatin calcium) 20 mg Crestor 20mg tablets | 28 tablet [PoM] £26.02 DT price = £26.02
  Rosuvastatin (as Rosuvastatin calcium) 40 mg Crestor 40mg tablets | 28 tablet [PoM] £29.69 DT price = £29.69

▸ 122

Simvastatin

- **INDICATIONS AND DOSE**

Hyperlipidaemia including familial hypercholesterolaemia
- ▸ BY MOUTH
- ▸ Child 5–9 years: Initially 10 mg once daily, then increased if necessary up to 20 mg once daily, dose to be taken at night, increased at intervals of at least 4 weeks
- ▸ Child 10-17 years: Initially 10 mg once daily, then increased if necessary up to 40 mg once daily, dose to be taken at night, increased at intervals of at least 4 weeks

DOSE ADJUSTMENTS DUE TO INTERACTIONS
Reduced dose required with concomitant amiodarone, bezafibrate, amlodipine, diltiazem, or verapamil—seek specialist advice.

- **UNLICENSED USE** Not licensed for use in children under 10 years.
- **SIDE-EFFECTS**
- ▸ **Rare** Anaemia
- ▸ **Frequency not known** Tendinopathy
- **BREAST FEEDING** Manufacturer advises avoid—no information available.
- **RENAL IMPAIRMENT** Doses above 10 mg daily should be used with caution if estimated glomerular filtration rate less than 30 mL/minute/1.73 m².
- **PATIENT AND CARER ADVICE** Patient counselling is advised for simvastatin tablets/oral suspension (muscle effects).

- **MEDICINAL FORMS**
There can be variation in the licensing of different medicines containing the same drug. Forms available from special-order manufacturers include: oral suspension, oral solution

Tablet
- ▸ Simvastatin (Non-proprietary)
  Simvastatin 10 mg Simvastatin 10mg tablets | 28 tablet [PoM] £18.00 DT price = £0.67
  Simvastatin 20 mg Simvastatin 20mg tablets | 28 tablet [PoM] £29.60 DT price = £0.77
  Simvastatin 40 mg Simvastatin 40mg tablets | 28 tablet [PoM] £29.60 DT price = £0.86
  Simvastatin 80 mg Simvastatin 80mg tablets | 28 tablet [PoM] £29.61 DT price = £1.71
- ▸ Simvador (Discovery Pharmaceuticals)
  Simvastatin 10 mg Simvador 10mg tablets | 28 tablet [PoM] £0.67 DT price = £0.67
  Simvastatin 20 mg Simvador 20mg tablets | 28 tablet [PoM] £0.77 DT price = £0.77
  Simvastatin 40 mg Simvador 40mg tablets | 28 tablet [PoM] £0.86 DT price = £0.86
  Simvastatin 80 mg Simvador 80mg tablets | 28 tablet [PoM] £1.71 DT price = £1.71
- ▸ Zocor (Merck Sharp & Dohme Ltd)
  Simvastatin 10 mg Zocor 10mg tablets | 28 tablet [PoM] £18.03 DT price = £0.67
  Simvastatin 20 mg Zocor 20mg tablets | 28 tablet [PoM] £29.69 DT price = £0.77

Simvastatin 40 mg Zocor 40mg tablets | 28 tablet [PoM] £29.69 DT price = £0.86
Simvastatin 80 mg Zocor 80mg tablets | 28 tablet [PoM] £29.69 DT price = £1.71

Oral suspension
EXCIPIENTS: May contain Propylene glycol
- ▸ Simvastatin (Non-proprietary)
  Simvastatin 4 mg per 1 ml Simvastatin 20mg/5ml oral suspension sugar free sugar-free | 150 ml [PoM] £119.40 DT price = £119.40
  Simvastatin 8 mg per 1 ml Simvastatin 40mg/5ml oral suspension sugar free sugar-free | 150 ml [PoM] £182.40 DT price = £182.40

Simvastatin with ezetimibe

The properties listed below are those particular to the combination only. For the properties of the components please consider, simvastatin above, ezetimibe p. 121.

- **INDICATIONS AND DOSE**

Homozygous familial hypercholesterolaemia, primary hypercholesterolaemia, and mixed hyperlipidaemia in patients over 10 years stabilised on the individual components in the same proportions, or for patients not adequately controlled by statin alone
- ▸ BY MOUTH
- ▸ Child (initiated by a specialist): (consult product literature)

- **MEDICINAL FORMS**
There can be variation in the licensing of different medicines containing the same drug.

Tablet
- ▸ Inegy (Merck Sharp & Dohme Ltd)
  Ezetimibe 10 mg, Simvastatin 20 mg Inegy 10mg/20mg tablets | 28 tablet [PoM] £33.42 DT price = £33.42
  Ezetimibe 10 mg, Simvastatin 40 mg Inegy 10mg/40mg tablets | 28 tablet [PoM] £38.98 DT price = £38.98
  Ezetimibe 10 mg, Simvastatin 80 mg Inegy 10mg/80mg tablets | 28 tablet [PoM] £41.21 DT price = £41.21

7 Myocardial ischaemia

ANTITHROMBOTIC DRUGS > TISSUE PLASMINOGEN ACTIVATORS

Fibrinolytic drugs

Overview

Alteplase p. 126, streptokinase p. 126 and urokinase p. 81 are used in children to dissolve intravascular thrombi and unblock occluded arteriovenous shunts, catheters, and indwelling central lines blocked with fibrin clots. Treatment should be started as soon as possible after a clot has formed and discontinued once a pulse in the affected limb is detected, or the shunt or catheter unblocked.

The safety and efficacy of treatment remains uncertain, especially in neonates. A fibrinolytic drug is probably only appropriate where arterial occlusion threatens ischaemic damage; an anticoagulant may stop the clot getting bigger. Alteplase is the preferred fibrinolytic in children and neonates; there is less risk of adverse effects including allergic reactions.

Fibrinolytics ▣

- **DRUG ACTION** Fibrinolytic drugs act as thrombolytics by activating plasminogen to form plasmin, which degrades fibrin and so breaks up thrombi.
- **CONTRA-INDICATIONS** Acute pancreatitis · aneurysm · arteriovenous malformation · bacterial endocarditis · bleeding diatheses · coagulation defects · neoplasm with risk of haemorrhage · pericarditis · recent haemorrhage · recent surgery (including dental extraction) · recent trauma · severe hypertension
- **CAUTIONS** Conditions with an increased risk of haemorrhage · hypertension · risk of bleeding (including that from venepuncture or invasive procedures)
- **INTERACTIONS** Caution with recent or concomitant use of drugs that increase the risk of bleeding.
- **SIDE-EFFECTS** Allergic reactions · anaphylaxis · back pain · bleeding · bleeding (usually limited to the site of injection, but can occur from other sites) · cerebral oedema (caused by reperfusion) · convulsions · fever · flushing · hypotension · intracerebral haemorrhage · nausea · pulmonary oedema (caused by reperfusion) · rash · uveitis · vomiting

  SIDE-EFFECTS, FURTHER INFORMATION
  ▸ **Bleeding** Serious bleeding calls for discontinuation of the thrombolytic and may require administration of coagulation factors and antifibrinolytic drugs (e.g. tranexamic acid). Rarely further embolism may occur (either due to clots that break away from the original thrombus or to cholesterol crystal emboli).
  ▸ **Hypotension** Hypotension can usually be controlled by elevating the patient's legs, or by reducing the rate of infusion or stopping it temporarily.
- **PREGNANCY** Thrombolytic drugs can possibly lead to premature separation of the placenta in the first 18 weeks of pregnancy. There is also a risk of maternal haemorrhage throughout pregnancy and post-partum, and also a theoretical risk of fetal haemorrhage throughout pregnancy.
- **HEPATIC IMPAIRMENT** Avoid in severe hepatic impairment as there is an increased risk of bleeding.

⌐ above

Alteplase

(rt-PA; Tissue-type plasminogen activator)

- **INDICATIONS AND DOSE**
  Intravascular thrombosis
  ▸ BY INTRAVENOUS INFUSION
  ▸ Neonate: 100–500 micrograms/kg/hour for 3–6 hours, use ultrasound assessment to monitor effect before considering a second course of treatment (consult local protocol).
  ▸ Child: 100–500 micrograms/kg/hour for 3–6 hours, use ultrasound assessment to monitor effect before considering a second course of treatment; maximum 100 mg per day

  ACTILYSE CATHFLO®
  Thrombolytic treatment of occluded central venous access devices (including those used for haemodialysis)
  ▸ BY INTRAVENOUS INJECTION
  ▸ Child: (consult product literature)

- **UNLICENSED USE** *Actilyse*® not licensed for use in children.
- **CONTRA-INDICATIONS** Oesophageal varices · recent delivery · recent ulcerative gastro-intestinal disease · stroke

- **INTERACTIONS** Contra-indicated if concomitant treatment with oral anticoagulants.
- **SIDE-EFFECTS** Risk of cerebral bleeding increased in acute stroke
- **ALLERGY AND CROSS-SENSITIVITY** Contra-indicated if history of hypersensitivity to gentamicin (residue from manufacturing process).
- **DIRECTIONS FOR ADMINISTRATION** For *intravenous infusion* (*Actilyse*®), dissolve in Water for Injections to a concentration of 1 mg/mL or 2 mg/mL and infuse intravenously; alternatively dilute further in Sodium Chloride 0.9% to a concentration of not less than 200 micrograms/mL; not to be diluted in Glucose.

- **MEDICINAL FORMS**
  There can be variation in the licensing of different medicines containing the same drug. Forms available from special-order manufacturers include: solution for injection
  Powder and solvent for solution for injection
  ▸ Actilyse (Boehringer Ingelheim Ltd)
    Alteplase 10 mg Actilyse 10mg powder and solvent for solution for injection vials | 1 vial PoM £144.00
    Alteplase 20 mg Actilyse 20mg powder and solvent for solution for injection vials | 1 vial PoM £216.00
  ▸ Actilyse Cathflo (Boehringer Ingelheim Ltd)
    Alteplase 2 mg Actilyse Cathflo 2mg powder and solvent for solution for injection vials | 5 vial PoM £225.00 (Hospital only)
  Powder and solvent for solution for infusion
  ▸ Actilyse (Boehringer Ingelheim Ltd)
    Alteplase 50 mg Actilyse 50mg powder and solvent for solution for infusion vials | 1 vial PoM £360.00

⌐ above

Streptokinase

- **INDICATIONS AND DOSE**
  Intravascular thrombosis
  ▸ INITIALLY BY INTRAVENOUS INFUSION
  ▸ Child 1 month–11 years: Initially 2500–4000 units/kg, dose to be given over 30 minutes, followed by (by continuous intravenous infusion) 500–1000 units/kg/hour for up to 3 days until reperfusion occurs
  ▸ Child 12–17 years: Initially 250 000 units, dose to be given over 30 minutes, followed by (by continuous intravenous infusion) 100 000 units/hour for up to 3 days until reperfusion occurs

- **UNLICENSED USE** Not licensed for use in children.
- **CONTRA-INDICATIONS** Avoid in children who have had streptococcal infection in the last 12 months
- **CAUTIONS** Atrial fibrillation · cavernous pulmonary disease · cerebrovascular disease · mitral valve defect · recent delivery or abortion · septic thrombotic disease
- **INTERACTIONS** Contra-indicated if concomitant treatment with oral anticoagulants.
- **SIDE-EFFECTS**
  ▸ **Rare** Guillain-Barré syndrome
- **ALLERGY AND CROSS-SENSITIVITY** Contra-indicated if previous allergic reaction to either streptokinase or anistreplase (no longer available). Prolonged persistence of antibodies to streptokinase and anistreplase (no longer available) can reduce the effectiveness of subsequent treatment; therefore, streptokinase should not be used again beyond 4 days of first administration of either streptokinase or anistreplase.
- **DIRECTIONS FOR ADMINISTRATION** For *intravenous infusion*, reconstitute with Sodium Chloride 0.9%, then dilute further with Glucose 5% or Sodium Chloride 0.9% after reconstitution. Monitor fibrinogen concentration closely; if fibrinogen concentration less than 1 g/litre, stop streptokinase infusion and start unfractionated heparin;

restart streptokinase once fibrinogen concentration reaches 1 g/litre.

● **MEDICINAL FORMS**
There can be variation in the licensing of different medicines containing the same drug.
Powder for solution for infusion
▸ Streptokinase (Non-proprietary)
Streptokinase 1.5 mega u Biofactor Streptokinase 1.5million unit powder for solution for infusion vials | 1 vial [PoM] £83.44
Streptokinase 250000 unit Biofactor Streptokinase 250,000unit powder for solution for infusion vials | 1 vial [PoM] £15.91
Streptokinase 750000 unit Biofactor Streptokinase 750,000unit powder for solution for infusion vials | 1 vial [PoM] £41.72

NITRATES

Nitrates

Overview

Nitrates are potent coronary vasodilators, but their principal benefit follows from a reduction in venous return which reduces left ventricular strain. Unwanted effects such as flushing, headache, and postural hypotension may limit therapy, especially if the child is unusually sensitive to the effects of nitrates or is hypovolaemic. Glyceryl trinitrate below is also used in extravasation.

Nitrates

● **CONTRA-INDICATIONS** Aortic stenosis · cardiac tamponade · constrictive pericarditis · hypertrophic cardiomyopathy · hypotensive conditions · hypovolaemia · marked anaemia · mitral stenosis · raised intracranial pressure due to cerebral haemorrhage · raised intracranial pressure due to head trauma · toxic pulmonary oedema

● **CAUTIONS** Heart failure due to obstruction · hypothermia · hypothyroidism · hypoxaemia · malnutrition · metal-containing transdermal systems should be removed before magnetic resonance imaging procedures, cardioversion, or diathermy · recent history of myocardial infarction · susceptibility to angle-closure glaucoma · tolerance · ventilation and perfusion abnormalities

CAUTIONS, FURTHER INFORMATION
▸ Tolerance Children receiving nitrates continuously throughout the day can develop tolerance (with reduced therapeutic effects). Reduction of blood-nitrate concentrations to low levels for 4 to 8 hours each day usually maintains effectiveness in such patients.

● **INTERACTIONS** → Appendix 1 (nitrates).

● **SIDE-EFFECTS**

GENERAL SIDE-EFFECTS
▸ **Common or very common** Dizziness · postural hypotension · tachycardia · throbbing headache
▸ **Uncommon** Flushing · heartburn · nausea · rash · syncope · temporary hypoxaemia · vomiting
▸ **Very rare** Angle-closure glaucoma
▸ **Frequency not known** Paradoxical bradycardia

SPECIFIC SIDE-EFFECTS
▸ With intravenous use Abdominal pain · apprehension · diaphoresis · muscle twitching · palpitation · prolonged administration has been associated with methaemoglobinaemia · restlessness · retrosternal discomfort · severe hypotension

SIDE-EFFECTS, FURTHER INFORMATION
▸ With intravenous use Specific side-effects following injection (particularly if given too rapidly) include severe hypotension, diaphoresis, apprehension, restlessness, muscle twitching, retrosternal discomfort, palpitation,

abdominal pain; prolonged administration has been associated with methaemoglobinaemia.

● **ALLERGY AND CROSS-SENSITIVITY** Contra-indicated in nitrate hypersensitivity.

● **BREAST FEEDING** No information available—manufacturers advise use only if potential benefit outweighs risk.

● **HEPATIC IMPAIRMENT** Caution in severe impairment.

● **RENAL IMPAIRMENT** Manufacturers advise use with caution in severe impairment.

● **MONITORING REQUIREMENTS** Monitor blood pressure and heart rate during intravenous infusion.

● **TREATMENT CESSATION** Avoid abrupt withdrawal.

⌐ above

Glyceryl trinitrate

● **INDICATIONS AND DOSE**

Hypertension during and after cardiac surgery | Heart failure after cardiac surgery | Coronary vasoconstriction in myocardial ischaemia | Vasoconstriction in shock
▸ BY CONTINUOUS INTRAVENOUS INFUSION

▸ Neonate: 0.2–0.5 microgram/kg/minute, adjusted according to response, maintenance 1–3 micrograms/kg/minute (max. per dose 10 micrograms/kg/minute).

▸ Child: Initially 0.2–0.5 microgram/kg/minute, adjusted according to response, maintenance 1–3 micrograms/kg/minute (max. per dose 10 micrograms/kg/minute); maximum 200 micrograms/minute

● **UNLICENSED USE** Not licensed for use in children.

● **PREGNANCY** Not known to be harmful.

● **DIRECTIONS FOR ADMINISTRATION**
▸ With intravenous use For *continuous intravenous infusion*, dilute to max. concentration of 400 micrograms/mL (but concentration of 1 mg/mL has been used via a central venous catheter) with Glucose 5% or Sodium Chloride 0.9%. *Neonatal intensive care*, dilute 3 mg/kg body-weight to a final volume of 50 mL with Glucose 5% or Sodium Chloride 0.9%; an intravenous infusion rate of 1 mL/hour provides a dose of 1 microgram/kg/minute; max. concentration of 400 micrograms/mL (but concentration of 1 mg/mL has been used via a central venous catheter).
▸ With intravenous use Glass or polyethylene apparatus is preferable; loss of potency will occur if PVC is used. Glyceryl trinitrate 1 mg/ml to be diluted before use or given undiluted with syringe pump. Glyceryl trinitrate 5 mg/ml to be diluted before use.

● **MEDICINAL FORMS**
There can be variation in the licensing of different medicines containing the same drug.
Solution for infusion
EXCIPIENTS: May contain Ethanol, propylene glycol
▸ Glyceryl trinitrate (Non-proprietary)
Glyceryl trinitrate 1 mg per 1 ml Glyceryl trinitrate 50mg/50ml solution for infusion vials | 1 vial [PoM] £15.90 | 25 vial [PoM] no price available
Glyceryl trinitrate 5 mg per 1 ml Glyceryl trinitrate 50mg/10ml solution for infusion ampoules | 5 ampoule [PoM] £64.90
Glyceryl trinitrate 25mg/5ml solution for infusion ampoules | 5 ampoule [PoM] £32.45
▸ Nitrocine (UCB Pharma Ltd)
Glyceryl trinitrate 1 mg per 1 ml Nitrocine 10mg/10ml solution for infusion ampoules | 10 ampoule [PoM] £58.75 (Hospital only)
▸ Nitronal (Merck Serono Ltd)
Glyceryl trinitrate 1 mg per 1 ml Nitronal 5mg/5ml solution for infusion ampoules | 10 ampoule [PoM] £18.04
Nitronal 50mg/50ml solution for infusion vials | 1 vial [PoM] £14.76

7.1 Cardiac arrest

Cardiopulmonary resuscitation

Overview

The algorithms for cardiopulmonary resuscitation (Life support algorithm (see inside back cover)) reflect the recommendations of the Resuscitation Council (UK); they cover paediatric basic life support, paediatric advanced life support, and newborn life support. The guidelines are available at www.resus.org.uk.

Paediatric advanced life support

Cardiopulmonary (cardiac) arrest in children is rare and frequently represents the terminal event of progressive shock or respiratory failure.

During cardiopulmonary arrest in children without intravenous access, the intraosseous route is chosen because it provides rapid and effective response; if circulatory access cannot be gained, the endotracheal tube can be used. When the endotracheal route is used ten times the intravenous dose should be used; the drug should be injected quickly down a narrow bore suction catheter beyond the tracheal end of the tube and then flushed in with 1 or 2 mL of sodium chloride 0.9%. The endotracheal route is useful for lipid-soluble drugs, including lidocaine hydrochloride p. 70, adrenaline/epinephrine below, atropine sulfate p. 764, and naloxone hydrochloride p. 796. Drugs that are not lipid-soluble (e.g. sodium bicarbonate p. 544 and calcium chloride p. 553) should **not** be administered by this route because they will injure the airways.

For the management of acute anaphylaxis, see allergic emergencies under Antihistamines, allergen immunotherapy and allergic emergencies p. 162..

SYMPATHOMIMETICS ⟩ VASOCONSTRICTOR

Adrenaline/epinephrine

● **DRUG ACTION** Acts on both alpha and beta receptors and increases both heart rate and contractility (beta$_1$ effects); it can cause peripheral vasodilation (a beta$_2$ effect) or vasoconstriction (an alpha effect).

● INDICATIONS AND DOSE

Acute hypotension
▶ BY CONTINUOUS INTRAVENOUS INFUSION
▶ Neonate: Initially 100 nanograms/kg/minute, adjusted according to response, higher doses up to 1.5 micrograms/kg/minute have been used in acute hypotension.
▶ Child: Initially 100 nanograms/kg/minute, adjusted according to response, higher doses up to 1.5 micrograms/kg/minute have been used in acute hypotension

Croup (when not effectively controlled with corticosteroid treatment)
▶ BY INHALATION OF NEBULISED SOLUTION
▶ Child 1 month–11 years: 400 micrograms/kg (max. per dose 5 mg), dose to be repeated after 30 minutes if necessary

PHARMACOKINETICS

The effects of nebulised adrenaline for the treatment of croup lasts for 2–3 hours.

Emergency treatment of acute anaphylaxis (under expert supervision) | Angioedema (if laryngeal oedema is present) (under expert supervision)
▶ BY INTRAMUSCULAR INJECTION
▶ Child 1 month–5 years: 150 micrograms, doses may be repeated several times if necessary at 5 minute intervals according to blood pressure, pulse, and respiratory function, suitable syringe to be used for measuring small volume; injected preferably into the anterolateral aspect of the middle third of the thigh
▶ Child 6–11 years: 300 micrograms, doses may be repeated several times if necessary at 5 minute intervals according to blood pressure, pulse, and respiratory function, to be injected preferably into the anterolateral aspect of the middle third of the thigh
▶ Child 12–17 years: 500 micrograms, to be injected preferably into the anterolateral aspect of the middle third of the thigh, doses may be repeated several times if necessary at 5 minute intervals according to blood pressure, pulse, and respiratory function, 300 micrograms (0.3 mL) to be administered if child small or prepubertal

Acute anaphylaxis when there is doubt as to the adequacy of the circulation (specialist use only) | Angioedema (if laryngeal oedema is present) (specialist use only)
▶ BY SLOW INTRAVENOUS INJECTION
▶ Child: 1 microgram/kg (max. per dose 50 micrograms), using dilute 1 in 10 000 adrenaline injection, dose to be repeated according to response, if multiple doses required, adrenaline should be given as a slow intravenous infusion stopping when a response has been obtained

EMERADE® 150 MICROGRAMS

Acute anaphylaxis (for self-administration)
▶ BY INTRAMUSCULAR INJECTION
▶ Child (body-weight up to 15 kg): 150 micrograms, then 150 micrograms after 5–15 minutes as required
▶ Child (body-weight 15–30 kg): 150 micrograms, then 150 micrograms after 5–15 minutes as required, on the basis of a dose of 10 micrograms/kg, 300 micrograms may be more appropriate for some children

EMERADE® 300 MICROGRAMS

Acute anaphylaxis (for self-administration)
▶ BY INTRAMUSCULAR INJECTION
▶ Child (body-weight 30 kg and above): 300 micrograms, then 300 micrograms after 5–15 minutes as required

EMERADE® 500 MICROGRAMS

Acute anaphylaxis (for self-administration for patients at risk of severe anaphylaxis)
▶ BY INTRAMUSCULAR INJECTION
▶ Child 12–17 years: 500 micrograms, then 500 micrograms after 5–15 minutes as required

EPIPEN® AUTO-INJECTOR 0.3MG

Acute anaphylaxis (for self-administration)
▶ BY INTRAMUSCULAR INJECTION
▶ Child (body-weight 30 kg and above): 300 micrograms, then 300 micrograms after 5–15 minutes as required

EPIPEN® JR AUTO-INJECTOR 0.15MG

Acute anaphylaxis (for self-administration)
▶ BY INTRAMUSCULAR INJECTION
▶ Child (body-weight up to 15 kg): 150 micrograms, then 150 micrograms after 5–15 minutes as required
▶ Child (body-weight 15–30 kg): 150 micrograms, then 150 micrograms after 5–15 minutes as required, on the basis of a dose of 10 micrograms/kg, 300 micrograms may be more appropriate for some children

JEXT® 150 MICROGRAMS

Acute anaphylaxis (for self-administration)
▸ BY INTRAMUSCULAR INJECTION
▸ **Child (body-weight up to 15 kg):** 150 micrograms, then 150 micrograms after 5–15 minutes as required
▸ **Child (body-weight 15-30 kg):** 150 micrograms, then 150 micrograms after 5–15 minutes as required, on the basis of a dose of 10 micrograms/kg, 300 micrograms may be more appropriate for some children

JEXT® 300 MICROGRAMS

Acute anaphylaxis (for self-administration)
▸ BY INTRAMUSCULAR INJECTION
▸ **Child (body-weight 30 kg and above):** 300 micrograms, then 300 micrograms after 5–15 minutes as required

● **UNLICENSED USE**
▸ With intramuscular use for acute anaphylaxis Auto-injectors delivering 150-microgram dose of adrenaline may not be licensed for use in children with body-weight under 15 kg.
▸ With intravenous use for acute hypotension Adrenaline 1 in 1000 (1 mg/mL) solution is not licensed for intravenous administration.

IMPORTANT SAFETY INFORMATION
SAFE PRACTICE
Intravenous route should be used with **extreme care** by specialists only.

● **CAUTIONS** Arrhythmias · cerebrovascular disease · cor pulmonale · diabetes mellitus · hypercalcaemia · hyperreflexia · hypertension · hyperthyroidism · hypokalaemia · ischaemic heart disease · obstructive cardiomyopathy · occlusive vascular disease · organic brain damage · phaeochromocytoma · prostate disorders · psychoneurosis · severe angina · susceptibility to angle-closure glaucoma

CAUTIONS, FURTHER INFORMATION
Cautions listed are only for non-life-threatening situations.

● **INTERACTIONS** → Appendix 1 (sympathomimetics)
Severe anaphylaxis in patients taking beta-blockers may not respond to adrenaline—consider bronchodilator therapy. Furthermore, adrenaline can cause severe hypertension and bradycardia in those taking non-cardioselective beta-blockers.

● **SIDE-EFFECTS** Angina · angle-closure glaucoma · anorexia · anxiety · arrhythmias · cold extremities · confusion · difficulty in micturition · dizziness · dry mouth · dyspnoea · headache · hyperglycaemia · hypersalivation · hypertension (risk of cerebral haemorrhage) · hypokalaemia · insomnia · metabolic acidosis · mydriasis · myocardial infarction · nausea · pallor · palpitation · psychosis · pulmonary oedema (on excessive dosage or extreme sensitivity) · restlessness · sweating · tachycardia · tissue necrosis at injection site · tissue necrosis of bowel · tissue necrosis of extremities · tissue necrosis of kidneys · tissue necrosis of liver · tremor · urinary retention · vomiting · weakness

● **PREGNANCY** May reduce placental perfusion and cause tachycardia, cardiac irregularities, and extrasystoles in fetus. Can delay second stage of labour. Manufacturers advise use only if benefit outweighs risk.

● **BREAST FEEDING** Present in milk but unlikely to be harmful as poor oral bioavailability.

● **RENAL IMPAIRMENT** Manufacturers advise use with caution in severe impairment.

● **MONITORING REQUIREMENTS** Monitor blood pressure and ECG.

● **DIRECTIONS FOR ADMINISTRATION**
▸ With intravenous use for acute hypotension For *continuous intravenous infusion*, dilute with Glucose 5% or Sodium Chloride 0.9% and give through a central venous catheter. Incompatible with bicarbonate and alkaline solutions. *Neonatal intensive care*, dilute 3 mg/kg body-weight to a final volume of 50 mL with infusion fluid; an intravenous infusion rate of 0.1 mL/hour provides a dose of 100 nanograms/kg/minute; infuse through a central venous catheter. Incompatible with bicarbonate and alkaline solutions. These infusions are usually made up with adrenaline 1 in 1000 (1 mg/mL) solution.
▸ When used by inhalation For nebulisation in croup, adrenaline 1 in 1000 solution may be diluted with sterile sodium chloride 0.9% solution.

● **PRESCRIBING AND DISPENSING INFORMATION** It is important, in acute anaphylaxis where intramuscular injection might still succeed, time should not be wasted seeking intravenous access.

Great vigilance is needed to ensure that the *correct strength* of adrenaline injection is used; anaphylactic shock kits need to make a *very clear distinction* between the 1 in 10 000 strength and the 1 in 1000 strength.

Patients with severe allergy should be instructed in the self-administration of adrenaline by intramuscular injection.

Packs for self-administration need to be **clearly labelled with instructions** on how to administer adrenaline (intramuscularly, preferably at the midpoint of the outer thigh, through light clothing if necessary) so that in the case of rapid collapse someone else is able to give it. It is important to ensure individuals at risk and their carers understand that:
● two injection devices should be carried at all times to treat symptoms until medical assistance is available; if, after the first injection, the individual does not start to feel better, the second injection should be given 5 to 15 minutes after the first;
● an ambulance should be called after every administration, even if symptoms improve;
● the individual should lie down with their legs raised (unless they have breathing difficulties, in which case they should sit up) and should not be left alone.

Adrenaline for administration by intramuscular injection is available in 'auto-injectors' (e.g. *Emerade®*, *EpiPen®*, or *Jext®*), pre-assembled syringes fitted with a needle suitable for very rapid administration (if necessary by a bystander or a healthcare provider if it is the only preparation available); injection technique is device specific.

To ensure patients receive the auto-injector device that they have been trained to use, prescribers should specify the brand to be dispensed.

● **PATIENT AND CARER ADVICE**
Individuals at considerable risk of anaphylaxis need to carry (or have available) adrenaline at all times and the patient, or their carers, need to be *instructed in advance* when and how to inject it.

JEXT® 300 MICROGRAMS 1.1 mL of the solution remains in the auto-injector device after use.

JEXT® 150 MICROGRAMS 1.25 mL of the solution remains in the auto-injector device after use.

EPIPEN® JR AUTO-INJECTOR 0.15MG 1.7 mL of the solution remains in the auto-injector device after use.

EPIPEN® AUTO-INJECTOR 0.3MG 1.7 mL of the solution remains in the auto-injector device after use.

EMERADE® 300 MICROGRAMS 0.2 mL of the solution remains in the auto-injector device after use.

EMERADE® 500 MICROGRAMS No solution remains in the auto-injector device after use.

EMERADE® 150 MICROGRAMS 0.35 mL of the solution remains in the auto-injector device after use.

Medicines for Children leaflet: Adrenaline auto-injector for anaphylaxis www.medicinesforchildren.org.uk/adrenaline-for-anapylaxis

- **EXCEPTIONS TO LEGAL CATEGORY** POM restriction does not apply to the intramuscular administration of up to 1 mg of adrenaline injection 1 in 1000 (1 mg/mL) for the emergency treatment of anaphylaxis.

- **MEDICINAL FORMS**
There can be variation in the licensing of different medicines containing the same drug. Forms available from special-order manufacturers include: solution for injection

Solution for injection
EXCIPIENTS: May contain Sulfites

▸ **Adrenaline/epinephrine (Non-proprietary)**
Adrenaline 100 microgram per 1 ml Adrenaline (base) 100micrograms/1ml (1 in 10,000) dilute solution for injection ampoules | 10 ampoule PoM £60.09
Adrenaline (base) 1mg/10ml (1 in 10,000) dilute solution for injection pre-filled syringes | 1 pre-filled disposable injection PoM £6.87
Adrenaline (base) 1mg/10ml (1 in 10,000) dilute solution for injection Minijet pre-filled syringes | 1 pre-filled disposable injection PoM £6.99
Adrenaline (as Adrenaline acid tartrate) 100 microgram per 1 ml Adrenaline (base) 1mg/10ml (1 in 10,000) dilute solution for injection ampoules | 1 ampoule PoM £43.53 | 10 ampoule PoM £69.65
Adrenaline (base) 500micrograms/5ml (1 in 10,000) dilute solution for injection ampoules | 10 ampoule PoM £64.02
Adrenaline 1 mg per 1 ml Adrenaline (base) for anaphylaxis 1mg/1ml (1 in 1,000) solution for injection pre-filled syringes | 1 pre-filled disposable injection PoM £10.40
Adrenaline (base) 1mg/1ml (1 in 1,000) solution for injection Minijet pre-filled syringes 21 gauge | 1 pre-filled disposable injection PoM £15.00
Adrenaline (base) 1mg/1ml (1 in 1,000) solution for injection pre-filled syringes | 1 pre-filled disposable injection PoM £10.40–£30.00
Adrenaline (base) 1mg/1ml (1 in 1,000) solution for injection Minijet pre-filled syringes 25 gauge | 1 pre-filled disposable injection PoM £13.90
Adrenaline (as Adrenaline acid tartrate) 1 mg per 1 ml Adrenaline (base) 5mg/5ml (1 in 1,000) solution for injection ampoules | 10 ampoule PoM £73.66
Adrenaline (base) 500micrograms/0.5ml (1 in 1,000) solution for injection ampoules | 10 ampoule PoM £58.08–£58.41 DT price = £58.25
Adrenaline (base) 1mg/1ml (1 in 1,000) solution for injection ampoules | 10 ampoule PoM £5.82 DT price = £5.81
▸ **Emerade** (Imed Systems Ltd)
Adrenaline 1 mg per 1 ml Emerade 300micrograms/0.3ml (1 in 1,000) solution for injection auto-injectors | 1 pre-filled disposable injection PoM £26.94 DT price = £26.45
Adrenaline (as Adrenaline acid tartrate) 1 mg per 1 ml Emerade 150micrograms/0.15ml (1 in 1,000) solution for injection auto-injectors | 1 pre-filled disposable injection PoM £26.94
Emerade 500micrograms/0.5ml (1 in 1,000) solution for injection auto-injectors | 1 pre-filled disposable injection PoM £28.74
▸ **EpiPen** (Meda Pharmaceuticals Ltd)
Adrenaline 500 microgram per 1 ml EpiPen Jr. 150micrograms/0.3ml (1 in 2,000) solution for injection auto-injectors | 1 pre-filled disposable injection PoM £26.45 | 2 pre-filled disposable injection PoM £52.90
Adrenaline 1 mg per 1 ml EpiPen 300micrograms/0.3ml (1 in 1,000) solution for injection auto-injectors | 1 pre-filled disposable injection PoM £26.45 DT price = £26.45 | 2 pre-filled disposable injection PoM £52.90
▸ **Jext** (ALK-Abello Ltd)
Adrenaline 1 mg per 1 ml Jext 300micrograms/0.3ml (1 in 1,000) solution for injection auto-injectors | 1 pre-filled disposable injection PoM £23.99 DT price = £26.45
Adrenaline (as Adrenaline acid tartrate) 1 mg per 1 ml Jext 150micrograms/0.15ml (1 in 1,000) solution for injection auto-injectors | 1 pre-filled disposable injection PoM £23.99

8 Oedema

Diuretics

Overview

Diuretics are used for a variety of conditions in children including pulmonary oedema (caused by conditions such as respiratory distress syndrome and bronchopulmonary dysplasia), congestive heart failure, and hypertension. Hypertension in children is often resistant to therapy and may require the use of several drugs in combination. Maintenance of fluid and electrolyte balance can be difficult in children on diuretics, particularly neonates whose renal function may be immature.

Loop diuretics are used for pulmonary oedema, congestive heart failure, and in renal disease.

Thiazides are used less commonly than loop diuretics but are often used in combination with loop diuretics or spironolactone p. 117 in the management of pulmonary oedema and, in lower doses, for hypertension associated with cardiac disease.

Aminophylline p. 158 **infusion** has been used with intravenous furosemide p. 132 to relieve fluid overload in critically ill children.

Heart failure

Heart failure is less common in children than in adults; it can occur as a result of congenital heart disease (e.g. septal defects), dilated cardiomyopathy, myocarditis, or cardiac surgery. Drug treatment of heart failure due to left ventricular systolic dysfunction is covered below; optimal management of heart failure with preserved left ventricular function has not been established.

Acute heart failure can occur after cardiac surgery or as a complication in severe acute infections with or without myocarditis. Therapy consists of volume loading, vasodilator or inotropic drugs.

Chronic heart failure is initially treated with a **loop diuretic**, usually furosemide supplemented with spironolactone, amiloride hydrochloride p. 133, or potassium chloride p. 561.

If diuresis with furosemide is insufficient, the addition of metolazone p. 134 or a **thiazide diuretic** can be considered. With metolazone the resulting diuresis can be profound and care is needed to avoid potentially dangerous electrolyte disturbance.

If diuretics are insufficient an ACE inhibitor, titrated to the maximum tolerated dose, can be used. **ACE inhibitors** are used for the treatment of all grades of heart failure in adults and can also be useful for children with heart failure. Addition of digoxin p. 75 can be considered in children who remain symptomatic despite treatment with a diuretic and an ACE inhibitor.

Some beta-blockers improve outcome in adults with heart failure, but data on beta-blockers in children are limited. Carvedilol p. 116 has vasodilatory properties and therefore (like ACE inhibitors) also lowers afterload.

In children receiving specialist cardiology care, the phosphodiesterase type-3 inhibitor enoximone p. 118 is sometimes used by mouth for its inotropic and vasodilator effects. Spironolactone is usually used as a potassium-sparing drug with a loop diuretic; in adults low doses of spironolactone are effective in the treatment of heart failure. Careful monitoring of serum potassium is necessary if spironolactone is used in combination with an ACE inhibitor.

Thiazides and related diuretics

Thiazides and related compounds are moderately potent diuretics; they inhibit sodium reabsorption at the beginning of the distal convoluted tubule. They are usually administered early in the day so that the diuresis does not interfere with sleep.

In the management of *hypertension* a low dose of a thiazide produces a maximal or near-maximal blood pressure lowering effect, with very little biochemical disturbance. Higher doses cause more marked changes in plasma potassium, sodium, uric acid, glucose, and lipids, with little advantage in blood pressure control. Thiazides also have a role in chronic heart failure.

Bendroflumethiazide p. 102 is licensed for use in children; chlorothiazide p. 103 is also used.

Chlortalidone p. 134, a thiazide-related compound, has a longer duration of action than the thiazides and may be given on alternate days in younger children.

Metolazone is particularly effective when combined with a loop diuretic (even in renal failure) and is most effective when given 30–60 minutes before furosemide profound diuresis can occur and the child should therefore be monitored carefully.

Loop diuretics

Loop diuretics inhibit reabsorption of sodium, potassium, and chloride from the ascending limb of the loop of Henlé in the renal tubule and are powerful diuretics.

Furosemide and bumetanide p. 132 are similar in activity; they produce dose-related diuresis. Furosemide is used extensively in children. It can be used for pulmonary oedema (e.g. in respiratory distress syndrome and bronchopulmonary dysplasia), congestive heart failure, and in renal disease.

Potassium-sparing diuretics and aldosterone antagonists

Spironolactone is the most commonly used potassium sparing diuretic in children; it is an aldosterone antagonist and enhances potassium retention and sodium excretion in the distal tubule. Spironolactone is combined with other diuretics to reduce urinary potassium loss. It is also used in nephrotic syndrome, the long-term management of Bartter's syndrome, and high doses can help to control ascites in babies with chronic neonatal hepatitis. The clinical value of spironolactone in the management of pulmonary oedema in preterm neonates with chronic lung disease is uncertain.

Potassium canrenoate p. 117 given intravenously, is an alternative aldosterone antagonist that may be useful if a potassium-sparing diuretic is required and the child is unable to take oral medication. It is metabolised to canrenone, which is also a metabolite of spironolactone.

Amiloride hydrochloride on its own is a weak diuretic. It causes retention of potassium and is therefore given with thiazide or loop diuretics as an alternative to giving potassium supplements.

A potassium-sparing diuretic such as spironolactone or amiloride hydrochloride may also be used in the management of amphotericin-induced hypokalaemia.

Potassium supplements must **not** be given with potassium-sparing diuretics. Administration of a potassium-sparing diuretic to a child receiving an ACE inhibitor or an angiotensin-II receptor antagonist can also cause severe hyperkalaemia.

Potassium-sparing diuretics with other diuretics

Although it is preferable to prescribe diuretics separately in children, the use of fixed combinations may be justified in older children if compliance is a problem. (Some preparations may not be licensed for use in children—consult product literature).

Other diuretics

Mannitol p. 133 is used to treat cerebral oedema, raised intraocular pressure, peripheral oedema, and acites.

The carbonic anhydrase inhibitor acetazolamide p. 638 is a weak diuretic although it is little used for its diuretic effect. Acetazolamide and eye drops of dorzolamide p. 639 and brinzolamide p. 639 inhibit the formation of aqueous humour and are used in glaucoma. Acetazolamide is also used in the treatment of epilepsy, and raised intracranial pressure.

Diuretics with potassium

Diuretics and potassium supplements should be prescribed separately.

DIURETICS ⟩ LOOP DIURETICS

Loop diuretics   🅖

- **DRUG ACTION** Loop diuretics inhibit reabsorption from the ascending limb of the loop of Henlé in the renal tubule and are powerful diuretics.
- **CONTRA-INDICATIONS** Anuria · renal failure due to nephrotoxic or hepatotoxic drugs · severe hypokalaemia · severe hyponatraemia
- **CAUTIONS** Can cause acute urinary retention in children with obstruction of urinary outflow · can exacerbate diabetes (but hyperglycaemia less likely than with thiazides) · can excacerbate gout · comatose and precomatose states associated with liver cirrhosis · hypotension should be corrected before initiation of treatment · hypovolaemia should be corrected before initiation of treatment

CAUTIONS, FURTHER INFORMATION

▸ Potassium loss Hypokalaemia can occur with both thiazide and loop diuretics. The risk of hypokalaemia depends on the duration of action as well as the potency and is thus greater with thiazides than with an equipotent dose of a loop diuretic.

Hypokalaemia is particularly dangerous in children being treated with cardiac glycosides. In hepatic failure hypokalaemia caused by diuretics can precipitate encephalopathy.

The use of potassium-sparing diuretics avoids the need to take potassium supplements.

▸ Urinary retention Loop diuretics can cause acute urinary retention in children with obstruction of urinary outflow, therefore adequate urinary output should be established before initiating treatment.

- **INTERACTIONS** → Appendix 1 (diuretics).
- **SIDE-EFFECTS**
- ▸ Very rare Hyperuricaemia
- ▸ **Frequency not known** Acute urinary retention · blood disorders · bone-marrow depression · deafness (usually with high doses and rapid intravenous administration, and in renal impairment) · electrolyte disturbances · hepatic encephalopathy · hyperglycaemia (less common than with thiazides) · hypersensitivity reactions · hypochloraemia · hypokalaemia · hypomagnesaemia · hyponatraemia · increased calcium excretion (nephrocalcinosis and nephrolithiasis reported with long-term use of furosemide in preterm infants) · leucopenia · metabolic alkalosis · mild gastro-intestinal disturbances · pancreatitis · photosensitivity · postural hypotension · rash · temporary increase in serum-cholesterol and triglyceride concentration · thrombocytopenia · tinnitus (usually with high doses and rapid intravenous administration, and in renal impairment) · visual disturbances
- **HEPATIC IMPAIRMENT** Hypokalaemia induced by loop diuretics may precipitate hepatic encephalopathy and coma—potassium-sparing diuretics can be used to prevent this.
- **RENAL IMPAIRMENT** High doses of loop diuretics may occasionally be needed in renal impairment. High doses or

rapid intravenous administration can cause tinnitus and deafness.

- **MONITORING REQUIREMENTS** Monitor electrolytes during treatment.

☞ 131

Bumetanide

- **INDICATIONS AND DOSE**

Oedema in heart failure, renal disease, and hepatic disease | Pulmonary oedema
- ▸ BY MOUTH
- ▸ Child 1 month–11 years: 15–50 micrograms/kg 1–4 times a day (max. per dose 2 mg); maximum 5 mg per day
- ▸ Child 12–17 years: Initially 1 mg to be taken in the morning, then 1 mg after 6–8 hours if required

Oedema in heart failure, renal disease, and hepatic disease (severe cases) | Pulmonary oedema (severe cases)
- ▸ BY MOUTH
- ▸ Child 12–17 years: Initially 5 mg daily, increased in steps of 5 mg every 12–24 hours, adjusted according to response

- **UNLICENSED USE** Not licensed for use in children under 12 years.
- **SIDE-EFFECTS** Breast pain · gynaecomastia · musculoskeletal pain (associated with high doses in renal failure)
- **PREGNANCY** Bumetanide should not be used to treat gestational hypertension because of the maternal hypovolaemia associated with this condition.
- **BREAST FEEDING** No information available. May inhibit lactation.

- **MEDICINAL FORMS**
There can be variation in the licensing of different medicines containing the same drug. Forms available from special-order manufacturers include: oral suspension
Tablet
- ▸ Bumetanide (Non-proprietary)
Bumetanide 1 mg Bumetanide 1mg tablets | 28 tablet [PoM] £3.00 DT price = £1.18
Bumetanide 5 mg Bumetanide 5mg tablets | 28 tablet [PoM] £7.00 DT price = £6.98
Oral solution
- ▸ Bumetanide (Non-proprietary)
Bumetanide 200 microgram per 1 ml Bumetanide 1mg/5ml oral solution sugar free sugar-free | 150 ml [PoM] £168.00 DT price = £168.00

☞ 131

Furosemide

(Frusemide)

- **INDICATIONS AND DOSE**

Oedema in heart failure, renal disease, and hepatic disease | Pulmonary oedema
- ▸ BY MOUTH
- ▸ Neonate: 0.5–2 mg/kg every 12–24 hours, alternatively 0.5–2 mg/kg every 24 hours, if corrected gestational age under 31 weeks.
- ▸ Child 1 month–11 years: 0.5–2 mg/kg 2–3 times a day, alternatively 0.5–2 mg/kg every 24 hours, if corrected gestational age of under 31 weeks, higher doses may be required in resistant oedema; maximum 80 mg per day; maximum 12 mg/kg per day
- ▸ Child 12–17 years: 20–40 mg daily; increased to 80–120 mg daily, in resistant oedema

- ▸ BY SLOW INTRAVENOUS INJECTION
- ▸ Neonate: 0.5–1 mg/kg every 12–24 hours, alternatively 0.5–1 mg/kg every 24 hours, if corrected gestational age under 31 weeks.
- ▸ Child 1 month–11 years: 0.5–1 mg/kg every 8 hours (max. per dose 40 mg every 8 hours) as required; maximum 6 mg/kg per day
- ▸ Child 12–17 years: 20–40 mg every 8 hours as required, higher doses may be required in resistant cases
- ▸ BY CONTINUOUS INTRAVENOUS INFUSION
- ▸ Child: 0.1–2 mg/kg/hour

Oedema in heart failure, renal disease, and hepatic disease following cardiac surgery | Pulmonary oedema following cardiac surgery
- ▸ BY CONTINUOUS INTRAVENOUS INFUSION
- ▸ Child: Initially 100 micrograms/kg/hour, dose to be doubled every 2 hours until urine output exceeds 1 mL/kg/hour

Oliguria
- ▸ BY MOUTH
- ▸ Child 12–17 years: Initially 250 mg daily, then increased in steps of 250 mg every 4–6 hours (max. per dose 2 g) if required
- ▸ BY INTRAVENOUS INFUSION
- ▸ Child 1 month–11 years: 2–5 mg/kg up to 4 times a day; maximum 1 g per day
- ▸ Child 12–17 years: Initially 250 mg, dose to be administered over 1 hour, increased to 500 mg, increased dose is given if satisfactory urine output not obtained; dose administered over 2 hours, then increased to 1 g, increased dose given if satisfactory response not obtained within subsequent hour; dose to be administered over 4 hours. If no response obtained dialysis probably required;, effective dose of up to 1 g given at a maximum rate of 4 mg/minute can be repeated every 24 hours

- **CAUTIONS** Effect may be prolonged in neonates (in neonates) · hepatorenal syndrome · hypoproteinaemia may reduce diuretic effect and increase risk of side-effects
- **SIDE-EFFECTS** Gout · intrahepatic cholestasis
- **PREGNANCY** Furosemide should not be used to treat gestational hypertension because of the maternal hypovolaemia associated with this condition.
- **BREAST FEEDING** Amount too small to be harmful. May inhibit lactation.

- **DIRECTIONS FOR ADMINISTRATION**
- ▸ With intravenous use For *intravenous injection*, give over 5–10 minutes at a usual rate of 100 micrograms/kg/minute (not exceeding 500 micrograms/kg/minute), max. 4 mg/minute; lower rate of infusion may be necessary in renal impairment. For *intravenous infusion*, dilute with Sodium Chloride 0.9% to a concentration of 1–2 mg/mL. Glucose solutions unsuitable (infusion pH must be above 5.5).
- ▸ With oral use For administration by *mouth*, tablets can be crushed and mixed with water or injection solution diluted and given by mouth. Risk of ototoxicity may be reduced by giving high oral doses in 2 or more divided doses.
- **PRESCRIBING AND DISPENSING INFORMATION**
- ▸ With oral use Some liquid preparations contain alcohol, caution especially in neonates.

- **MEDICINAL FORMS**
There can be variation in the licensing of different medicines containing the same drug. Forms available from special-order manufacturers include: oral suspension, oral solution
Tablet
- ▸ Furosemide (Non-proprietary)
Furosemide 20 mg Furosemide 20mg tablets | 28 tablet [PoM] £1.02 DT price = £0.73

Furosemide 40 mg Furosemide 40mg tablets | 28 tablet [PoM]
£1.03 DT price = £0.70 | 1000 tablet [PoM] £35.00
Furosemide 500 mg Furosemide 500mg tablets | 28 tablet [PoM]
£70.00 DT price = £37.09
▸ Diuresal (Ennogen Pharma Ltd)
Furosemide 500 mg Diuresal 500mg tablets | 28 tablet [PoM]
£44.80 DT price = £37.09

Oral solution
EXCIPIENTS: May contain Alcohol
▸ Furosemide (Non-proprietary)
Furosemide 4 mg per 1 ml Furosemide 20mg/5ml oral solution
sugar free sugar-free | 150 ml [PoM] £14.49 DT price = £14.49
Furosemide 8 mg per 1 ml Furosemide 40mg/5ml oral solution
sugar free sugar-free | 150 ml [PoM] £18.69 DT price = £18.69
Furosemide 10 mg per 1 ml Furosemide 50mg/5ml oral solution
sugar free sugar-free | 150 ml [PoM] £20.21 DT price = £20.21
▸ Frusol (Rosemont Pharmaceuticals Ltd)
Furosemide 4 mg per 1 ml Frusol 20mg/5ml oral solution sugar-free
| 150 ml [PoM] £12.07 DT price = £14.49
Furosemide 8 mg per 1 ml Frusol 40mg/5ml oral solution sugar-free
| 150 ml [PoM] £15.58 DT price = £18.69
Furosemide 10 mg per 1 ml Frusol 50mg/5ml oral solution sugar-
free | 150 ml [PoM] £16.84 DT price = £20.21

Solution for injection
▸ Furosemide (Non-proprietary)
Furosemide 10 mg per 1 ml Furosemide 250mg/25ml solution for
injection ampoules | 10 ampoule [PoM] £25.00–£40.00
Furosemide 50mg/5ml solution for injection ampoules |
10 ampoule [PoM] £4.50–£7.60
Furosemide 20mg/2ml solution for injection ampoules |
10 ampoule [PoM] £4.50
▸ Lasix (Sanofi)
Furosemide 10 mg per 1 ml Lasix 20mg/2ml solution for injection
ampoules | 5 ampoule [PoM] £3.74

DIURETICS > OSMOTIC DIURETICS

Mannitol

● **INDICATIONS AND DOSE**
Cerebral oedema
▸ BY INTRAVENOUS INFUSION
▸ Child 1 month–11 years: 0.25–1.5 g/kg, repeated if
necessary, to be administered over 30–60 minutes,
dose may be repeated 1–2 times after 4–8 hours
▸ Child 12–17 years: 0.25–2 g/kg, repeated if necessary, to
be administered over 30-60 minutes, dose may be
repeated 1–2 times after 4–8 hours
Peripheral oedema and ascites
▸ BY INTRAVENOUS INFUSION
▸ Child: 1–2 g/kg, to be given over 2–6 hours

● **UNLICENSED USE** Not licensed for use in children under
12 years.
● **CONTRA-INDICATIONS** Anuria · intracranial bleeding
(except during craniotomy) · severe cardiac failure · severe
dehydration · severe pulmonary oedema
● **CAUTIONS** Extravasation causes inflammation and
thrombophlebitis
● **INTERACTIONS** → Appendix 1 (mannitol).
● **SIDE-EFFECTS**
▸ **Uncommon** Electrolyte imbalance · fluid imbalance ·
hypotension · thrombophlebitis
▸ **Rare** Anaphylaxis · arrhythmia · blurred vision · chest pain
· chills · convulsions · cramp · dehydration · dizziness · dry
mouth · fever · focal osmotic nephrosis · headache ·
hypersensitivity reactions · hypertension · nausea · oedema
· pulmonary oedema · raised intracranial pressure · rhinitis
· skin necrosis · thirst · urinary retention · urticaria ·
vomiting
▸ **Very rare** Acute renal failure · congestive heart failure
● **PREGNANCY** Manufacturer advises avoid unless
essential— no information available.

● **BREAST FEEDING** Manufacturer advises avoid unless
essential—no information available.
● **RENAL IMPAIRMENT** Use with caution in severe
impairment.
● **PRE-TREATMENT SCREENING** Assess cardiac function
before treatment.
● **MONITORING REQUIREMENTS**
▸ Monitor fluid and electrolyte balance, serum osmolality,
and cardiac, pulmonary and renal function.
● **DIRECTIONS FOR ADMINISTRATION** Examine infusion for
crystals. If crystals present, dissolve by warming infusion
fluid (allow to cool to body temperature before
administration).
For mannitol 20%, an in-line filter is recommended
(15-micron filters have been used).

● **MEDICINAL FORMS**
There can be variation in the licensing of different medicines
containing the same drug. Forms available from special-order
manufacturers include: infusion, solution for infusion
Infusion
▸ Mannitol (Non-proprietary)
Mannitol 100 mg per 1 ml Mannitol 50g/500ml (10%) infusion Viaflo
bags | 1 bag [PoM] no price available | 20 bag [PoM] no price
available
Mannitol 50g/500ml (10%) infusion Viaflex bags | 1 bag [PoM] no
price available | 20 bag [PoM] no price available
Polyfusor K mannitol 10% infusion 500ml bottles | 1 bottle [PoM]
£4.46 | 12 bottle [PoM] no price available
Mannitol 150 mg per 1 ml Mannitol 75g/500ml (15%) infusion Viaflo
bags | 20 bag [PoM] no price available
Mannitol 200 mg per 1 ml Mannitol 100g/500ml (20%) infusion
Viaflex bags | 1 bag [PoM] no price available | 20 bag [PoM] no price
available
Polyfusor M mannitol 20% infusion 500ml bottles | 1 bottle [PoM]
£5.86 | 12 bottle [PoM] no price available
Mannitol 50g/250ml (20%) infusion Viaflex bags | 1 bag [PoM] no
price available | 30 bag [PoM] no price available
Mannitol 100g/500ml (20%) infusion Viaflo bags | 1 bag [PoM] no
price available | 20 bag [PoM] no price available

DIURETICS > POTASSIUM-SPARING DIURETICS

Amiloride hydrochloride

● **INDICATIONS AND DOSE**
**Adjunct to thiazide or loop diuretics for oedema in heart
failure, and hepatic disease (where potassium
conservation desirable)**
▸ BY MOUTH
▸ Neonate: 100–200 micrograms/kg twice daily.
▸ Child 1 month–11 years: 100–200 micrograms/kg twice
daily; maximum 20 mg per day
▸ Child 12–17 years: 5–10 mg twice daily

● **UNLICENSED USE** Not licensed for use in children.
● **CONTRA-INDICATIONS** Addison's disease · anuria ·
hyperkalaemia
● **CAUTIONS** Diabetes mellitus
● **INTERACTIONS** → Appendix 1 (diuretics).
● **SIDE-EFFECTS** Abdominal pain · agitation · alopecia ·
angina · anorexia · arrhythmias · arthralgia · confusion ·
constipation · cough · diarrhoea · dizziness · dry mouth ·
dyspepsia · dyspnoea · encephalopathy · flatulence · gastro-
intestinal bleeding · headache · hyperkalaemia · insomnia ·
jaundice · malaise · muscle cramp · nasal congestion ·
nausea · palpitation · paraesthesia · postural hypotension ·
pruritus · raised intra-ocular pressure · rash · sexual
dysfunction · thirst · tinnitus · tremor · urinary
disturbances · visual disturbance · vomiting · weakness
● **PREGNANCY** Not to be used to treat gestational
hypertension.

Cardiovascular system

- **BREAST FEEDING** Manufacturer advises avoid—no information available.
- **RENAL IMPAIRMENT** Manufacturers advise avoid in severe impairment. Monitor plasma-potassium concentration (high risk of hyperkalaemia in renal impairment).
- **MONITORING REQUIREMENTS** Monitor electrolytes.
- **MEDICINAL FORMS**
There can be variation in the licensing of different medicines containing the same drug. Forms available from special-order manufacturers include: oral suspension, oral solution

Tablet
▸ Amiloride hydrochloride (Non-proprietary)
Amiloride hydrochloride 5 mg Amiloride 5mg tablets | 28 tablet PoM £6.72 DT price = £4.31

Oral solution
EXCIPIENTS: May contain Propylene glycol
▸ Amiloride hydrochloride (Non-proprietary)
Amiloride hydrochloride 1 mg per 1 ml Amiloride 5mg/5ml oral solution sugar free sugar-free | 150 ml PoM no price available DT price = £37.35
▸ Amilamont (Rosemont Pharmaceuticals Ltd)
Amiloride hydrochloride 1 mg per 1 ml Amilamont 5mg/5ml oral solution sugar free sugar-free | 150 ml PoM £37.35 DT price = £37.35

DIURETICS ⟩ THIAZIDES AND RELATED DIURETICS

F 102

Chlortalidone

(Chlorthalidone)

- **INDICATIONS AND DOSE**

Ascites | Oedema in nephrotic syndrome
▸ BY MOUTH
▸ Child 5–11 years: 0.5–1 mg/kg every 48 hours (max. per dose 1.7 mg/kg every 48 hours), dose to be taken in the morning
▸ Child 12–17 years: Up to 50 mg daily

Hypertension
▸ BY MOUTH
▸ Child 5–11 years: 0.5–1 mg/kg every 48 hours (max. per dose 1.7 mg/kg every 48 hours), dose to be taken in the morning
▸ Child 12–17 years: 25 mg daily, dose to be taken in the morning, then increased if necessary to 50 mg daily

Stable heart failure
▸ BY MOUTH
▸ Child 5–11 years: 0.5–1 mg/kg every 48 hours (max. per dose 1.7 mg/kg every 48 hours), dose to be taken in the morning
▸ Child 12–17 years: 25–50 mg daily, dose to be taken in the morning, then increased if necessary to 100–200 mg daily, reduce to lowest effective dose for maintenance

- **SIDE-EFFECTS**
▸ Rare Jaundice
- **BREAST FEEDING** The amount present in milk is too small to be harmful. Large doses may suppress lactation.
- **MEDICINAL FORMS**
There can be variation in the licensing of different medicines containing the same drug. Forms available from special-order manufacturers include: oral suspension

Tablet
▸ Chlortalidone (Non-proprietary)
Chlortalidone 25 mg Chlortalidone 25mg tablets | 100 tablet PoM no price available
Chlortalidone 50 mg Chlortalidone 50mg tablets | 30 tablet PoM £88.00 DT price = £88.00

F 102

Metolazone

- **INDICATIONS AND DOSE**

Oedema resistant to loop diuretics in heart failure, renal disease and hepatic disease | Pulmonary oedema | Adjunct to loop diuretics to induce diuresis
▸ BY MOUTH
▸ Child 1 month–11 years: 100–200 micrograms/kg 1–2 times a day
▸ Child 12–17 years: 5–10 mg once daily, dose to be taken in the morning; increased if necessary to 5–10 mg twice daily, dose increased in resistant oedema

- **UNLICENSED USE** Not licensed for use in children.
- **CAUTIONS** Acute porphyrias p. 562
- **SIDE-EFFECTS** Chest pain · chills
- **BREAST FEEDING** The amount present in milk is too small to be harmful. Large doses may suppress lactation.
- **DIRECTIONS FOR ADMINISTRATION** Tablets may be crushed and mixed with water immediately before use.
- **MEDICINAL FORMS**
There can be variation in the licensing of different medicines containing the same drug. Forms available from special-order manufacturers include: tablet, oral suspension, oral solution

Tablet
▸ Metolazone (Non-proprietary)
Metolazone 2.5 mg Zaroxolyn 2.5mg tablets | 100 tablet PoM no price available
Metolazone 5 mg Zaroxolyn 5mg tablets | 50 tablet PoM no price available

9 Patent ductus arteriosus

Drugs affecting the ductus arteriosus

Drugs used for Patent ductus arteriosus not listed below
Ibuprofen p. 608 · Indometacin p. 611

Closure of the ductus arteriosus

Patent ductus arteriosus is a frequent problem in premature neonates with respiratory distress syndrome. Substantial left-to-right shunting through the ductus arteriosus may increase the risk of intraventricular haemorrhage, necrotising enterocolitis, bronchopulmonary dysplasia, and possibly death. Indometacin p. 611 or ibuprofen p. 608 can be used to close the ductus arteriosus. Indometacin has been used for many years and is effective but it reduces cerebral blood flow, and causes a transient fall in renal and gastro-intestinal blood flow. Ibuprofen may also be used; it has little effect on renal function (there may be a small reduction in sodium excretion) when used in doses for closure of the ductus arteriosus; gastro-intestinal problems are uncommon. If drug treatment fails to close the ductus arteriosus, surgery may be indicated.

Maintenance of patency

In the newborn with duct-dependent congenital heart disease it is often necessary to maintain the patency of the ductus arteriosus whilst awaiting surgery. Alprostadil p. 135 (prostaglandin E1) and dinoprostone p. 135 (prostaglandin E2) are potent vasodilators that are effective for maintaining the patency of the ductus arteriosus. They are usually given by continuous intravenous infusion, but oral dosing of dinoprostone is still used in some centres. During the infusion of a prostaglandin, the newborn requires careful monitoring of heart rate, blood pressure, respiratory rate, and core body temperature. In the event of complications such as apnoea, profound bradycardia, or severe hypotension, the infusion should be temporarily stopped and the complication dealt with; the infusion should be restarted at a lower dose. Recurrent or prolonged apnoea may require ventilatory support in order for the prostaglandin infusion to continue.

PROSTAGLANDIN ANALOGUES AND PROSTAMIDES > PROSTAGLANDINS

Alprostadil

- ● **INDICATIONS AND DOSE**
Maintaining patency of the ductus arteriosus
▶ BY CONTINUOUS INTRAVENOUS INFUSION

▶ Neonate: Initially 5 nanograms/kg/minute, adjusted according to response, adjusted in steps of 5 nanograms/kg/minute (max. per dose 100 nanograms/kg/minute), maximum dose associated with increased side-effects.

- ● **UNLICENSED USE** Alprostadil doses in BNFC may differ from those in product literature.
- ● **CONTRA-INDICATIONS** Avoid in hyaline membrane disease
- ● **CAUTIONS** History of haemorrhage
- ● **INTERACTIONS** → Appendix 1 (alprostadil).
- ● **SIDE-EFFECTS** Apnoea (particularly in neonates under 2 kg) · bradycardia · cardiac arrest · convulsions · cortical proliferation of long bones · diarrhoea · disseminated intravascular coagulation · fever · flushing · gastric-outlet obstruction · hypokalaemia · hypotension · oedema · tachycardia · weakening of the wall of the ductus arteriosus and pulmonary artery (following prolonged use)
- ● **MONITORING REQUIREMENTS**
▶ During the infusion of a prostaglandin, the newborn requires careful monitoring of heart rate, blood pressure, respiratory rate, and core body temperature.
▶ Monitor arterial pressure, respiratory rate, heart rate, temperature, and venous blood pressure in arm and leg; facilities for intubation and ventilation must be immediately available
- ● **DIRECTIONS FOR ADMINISTRATION** Dilute 150 micrograms/kg body-weight to a final volume of 50 mL with Glucose 5% or Sodium Chloride 0.9%; an intravenous infusion rate of 0.1 mL/hour provides a dose of 5 nanograms/kg/minute. Undiluted solution must not come into contact with the barrel of the plastic syringe; add the required volume of alprostadil to a volume of infusion fluid in the syringe and then make up to final volume.

- ● **MEDICINAL FORMS**
There can be variation in the licensing of different medicines containing the same drug.
Solution for infusion
▶ Prostin VR (Pfizer Ltd)
Alprostadil 500 microgram per 1 ml Prostin VR 500micrograms/1ml solution for infusion ampoules | 5 ampoule [PoM] £375.96 (Hospital only)

Dinoprostone

- ● **INDICATIONS AND DOSE**
Maintaining patency of the ductus arteriosus
▶ BY CONTINUOUS INTRAVENOUS INFUSION

▶ Neonate: Initially 5 nanograms/kg/minute, then increased in steps of 5 nanograms/kg/minute as required; increased to 20 nanograms/kg/minute, doses up to 100 nanogram/kg/minute have been used but are associated with increased side-effects.

▶ BY MOUTH

▶ Neonate: 20–25 micrograms/kg every 1–2 hours, then increased if necessary to 40–50 micrograms/kg every 1–2 hours, if treatment continues for more than 1 week gradually reduce the dose.

- ● **UNLICENSED USE** Not licensed for use in children.
- ● **CONTRA-INDICATIONS** Avoid in hyaline membrane disease
- ● **CAUTIONS** History of haemorrhage
- ● **INTERACTIONS** → Appendix 1 (prostaglandins).
- ● **SIDE-EFFECTS**
Cortical hyperostosis (prolonged use) · apnoea (particularly with high doses and in low birth-weight neonates) · bradycardia · bronchospasm · cardiac arrest · diarrhoea · erythema · flushing · gastric outlet obstruction (if used for longer than 5 days) · hypotension · local reactions · nausea · pyrexia · raised white blood cell count · respiratory depression (particularly with high doses and in low birth-weight neonates) · shivering · temporary pyrexia · vomiting
- ● **HEPATIC IMPAIRMENT** Manufacturers advise avoid.
- ● **RENAL IMPAIRMENT** Manufacturers advise avoid.
- ● **MONITORING REQUIREMENTS** Monitor arterial oxygenation, heart rate, temperature, and blood pressure in arm and leg; facilities for intubation and ventilation must be immediately available. During infusion of dinoprostone, the newborn requires careful monitoring of heart rate, blood pressure, respiratory rate and core body temperature.
- ● **DIRECTIONS FOR ADMINISTRATION**
▶ With intravenous use For *continuous intravenous infusion*, dilute to a concentration of 1 microgram/mL with Glucose 5% or Sodium Chloride 0.9%.
▶ With oral use in neonates For administration by *mouth*, injection solution can be given orally; dilute with water.

- ● **MEDICINAL FORMS**
There can be variation in the licensing of different medicines containing the same drug.
Solution for infusion
▶ Prostin E2 (Pfizer Ltd)
Dinoprostone 1 mg per 1 ml Prostin E2 750micrograms/0.75ml solution for infusion ampoules | 1 ampoule [PoM] £8.52 (Hospital only)
Dinoprostone 10 mg per 1 ml Prostin E2 5mg/0.5ml solution for infusion ampoules | 1 ampoule [PoM] £18.40 (Hospital only)

10 Vascular disease

Peripheral vascular disease

Classification and management

Raynaud's syndrome, a vasospastic peripheral vascular disease, consists of recurrent, long-lasting, and episodic vasospasm of the fingers and toes often associated with exposure to cold. Management includes avoidance of exposure to cold and stopping smoking (if appropriate).

More severe symptoms may require vasodilator treatment, which is most often successful in primary Raynaud's syndrome. Nifedipine p. 100 and diltiazem hydrochloride below are useful for reducing the frequency and severity of vasospastic attacks. In very severe cases, where digital infarction is likely, intravenous infusion of the prostacyclin analogue iloprost p. 110 may be helpful.

Vasodilator therapy is not established as being effective for *chilblains*.

CALCIUM-CHANNEL BLOCKERS

F 99

Diltiazem hydrochloride

● **INDICATIONS AND DOSE**
Raynaud's syndrome
▶ BY MOUTH
▶ Child 12-17 years: 30–60 mg 2–3 times a day

● **UNLICENSED USE** Not licensed for use in children.

● **CONTRA-INDICATIONS** Acute porphyrias p. 562 · cardiogenic shock · left ventricular failure with pulmonary congestion · second- or third-degree AV block (unless pacemaker fitted) · severe bradycardia · sick sinus syndrome · significant aortic stenosis

● **CAUTIONS** Bradycardia (avoid if severe) · first degree AV block · heart failure · prolonged PR interval · significantly impaired left ventricular function

● **INTERACTIONS** → Appendix 1 (calcium-channel blockers).

● **SIDE-EFFECTS**
▶ **Common or very common** Asthenia · AV block · bradycardia · dizziness · gastro-intestinal disturbances · headache · hot flushes · hypotension · malaise · oedema (notably of ankles) · palpitation · sino-atrial block
▶ **Rare** Erythema multiforme · exfoliative dermatitis · photosensitivity · rashes
▶ **Frequency not known** Depression · extrapyramidal symptoms · gum hyperplasia · gynaecomastia · hepatitis

Overdose
In overdose, diltiazem has a profound cardiac depressant effect causing hypotension and arrhythmias, including complete heart block and asystole.

● **PREGNANCY** Avoid.

● **BREAST FEEDING** Significant amount present in milk—no evidence of harm but avoid unless no safer alternative.

● **HEPATIC IMPAIRMENT** Reduce dose.

● **RENAL IMPAIRMENT** Start with smaller dose.

● **MEDICINAL FORMS**
There can be variation in the licensing of different medicines containing the same drug. Forms available from special-order manufacturers include: oral suspension, oral solution
Modified-release tablet
CAUTIONARY AND ADVISORY LABELS 25
▶ **Diltiazem hydrochloride (Non-proprietary)**
Diltiazem hydrochloride 60 mg Diltiazem 60mg modified-release tablets | 84 tablet PoM £41.87 DT price = £41.50 | 100 tablet PoM £49.40
Diltiazem hydrochloride 90 mg Diltiazem 90mg modified-release tablets | 56 tablet PoM no price available
Diltiazem hydrochloride 120 mg Diltiazem 120mg modified-release tablets | 56 tablet PoM no price available
▶ **Tildiem (Sanofi)**
Diltiazem hydrochloride 60 mg Tildiem 60mg modified-release tablets | 90 tablet PoM £7.96

Chapter 3
Respiratory system

CONTENTS

1	Airways disease, obstructive	page 138
2	Allergic conditions	162
2.1	Angioedema	174
3	Conditions affecting sputum viscosity	174
3.1	Cystic fibrosis	175

4	Cough and congestion	page 176
5	Respiratory depression, respiratory distress syndrome and apnoea	178
5.1	Neonatal apnoea	179

Respiratory system, drug delivery

Inhalation

This route delivers the drug directly to the airways; the dose required is smaller than when given by mouth and side-effects are reduced.

Children and their carers should be advised to follow manufacturers' instructions on the care and cleansing of inhaler devices.

Inhaler devices

A *pressurised metered-dose inhaler* is an effective method of drug administration in mild to moderate chronic asthma; to deliver the drug effectively, particularly in children under 12 years, a spacer device should also be used (see also NICE guidance). By the age of 3 years, a child can usually be taught to use a spacer device without a mask. As soon as a child is able to use the mouthpiece, then this is the preferred delivery system. When a pressurised metered-does inhaler with a spacer is unsuitable or inconvenient, a *dry-powder inhaler* or *breath-actuated inhaler* may be used instead if the child is able to use the device effectively.

Dry powder inhalers may be useful in children over 5 years, who are unwilling or unable to use a pressurised metered-dose inhaler with a spacer device; *breath-actuated inhalers* may be useful in older children if they are able to use the device effectively. The child or child's carer should be instructed carefully on the use of the inhaler. It is important to check that the inhaler is being used correctly; poor inhalation technique may be mistaken for a lack of response to the drug.

On changing from a pressurised metered-dose inhaler to a dry powder inhaler, the child may notice a lack of sensation in the mouth and throat previously associated with each actuation; coughing may occur more frequently following use of a dry-powder inhaler.

CFC-free metered-dose inhalers should be cleaned **weekly** according to the manufacturer's instructions.

Spacer devices

Spacer devices are particularly useful for infants, for children with poor inhalation technique, or for nocturnal asthma, because the device reduces the need for coordination between actuation of a pressurised metered-dose inhaler and inhalation. The spacer device reduces the velocity of the aerosol and subsequent impaction on the oropharynx and allows more time for evaporation of the propellant so that a larger proportion of the particles can be inhaled and deposited in the lungs. Smaller-volume spacers may be more manageable for pre-school children and infants. The spacer device used must be compatible with the prescribed metered-dose inhaler.

Use and care of spacer devices
The suitability of the spacer device should be carefully assessed; opening the one-way valve is dependent on the child's inspiratory flow. Some devices can be tipped to 45° to open the valve during inhaler actuation and inspiration to assist the child.

Inhalation from the spacer device should follow the actuation as soon as possible because the drug aerosol is very short-lived. The total dose (which may be more than a single puff) should be administered as single actuations (with tidal breathing for 10–20 seconds or 5 breaths for each actuation) for children with good inspiratory flow. Larger doses may be necessary for a child with acute bronchospasm.

The device should be cleansed once a month by washing in mild detergent and then allowed to dry in air without rinsing; the mouthpiece should be wiped clean of detergent before use. Some manufacturers recommend more frequent cleaning, but this should be avoided since any electrostatic charge may affect drug delivery. Spacer devices should be replaced every 6–12 months.

Nebulisers

Solutions for nebulisation for use in acute severe asthma are administered over 5–10 minutes from a nebuliser, usually driven by oxygen in hospital.

Children with a severe attack of asthma should preferably have oxygen during nebulisation since beta$_2$ agonists can increase arterial hypoxaemia.

A nebuliser converts a solution of a drug into an aerosol for inhalation. It is used to deliver higher doses of drug to the airways than is usual with standard inhalers. The main indications for use of a nebuliser are:

- to deliver a beta$_2$ agonist or ipratropium bromide p. 143 to a child with an *acute exacerbation* of asthma or of airways obstruction;
- to deliver *prophylactic medication* to a child unable to use other conventional devices;
- to deliver an antibacterial (such as colistimethate sodium p. 326 or tobramycin p. 294) to a child with chronic purulent infection (as in cystic fibrosis or bronchiectasis);
- to deliver budesonide p. 151 to a child with severe croup.

The proportion of a nebuliser solution that reaches the lungs depends on the type of nebuliser and although it can be as high as 30% it is more frequently close to 10% and sometimes below 10%. The remaining solution is left in the nebuliser as residual volume or it is deposited in the mouthpiece and tubing. The extent to which the nebulised solution is deposited in the airways or alveoli depends on particle size. Particles with a median diameter of 1–5 microns are deposited in the airways and are therefore appropriate for asthma whereas a particle size of 1–2 microns is needed for alveolar deposition. The type of

Respiratory system

3

nebuliser is therefore chosen according to the deposition required and according to the viscosity of the solution.

Nebulised bronchodilators are appropriate for children with chronic persistent asthma or those with severe acute asthma. In chronic asthma, nebulised bronchodilators should only be used to relieve persistent daily wheeze, however, with the development of spacers with facemasks, it is now unusual for a child to require long-term nebulised asthma therapy. The use of nebulisers in chronic persistent asthma should be considered only:

- after a review of the diagnosis and use of current inhaler devices;
- if the airflow obstruction is significantly reversible by bronchodilators without unacceptable side-effects;
- if the child does not benefit from use of conventional inhaler device, such as pressurised metered-dose inhaler plus spacer;
- if the child is complying with the prescribed dose and frequency of anti-inflammatory treatment including regular use of high-dose inhaled corticosteroid.

When a nebuliser is prescribed, the child or child's carer must:

- have clear instructions from a doctor, specialist nurse, physiotherapist, or pharmacist on the use of the nebuliser (and on peak-flow monitoring);
- be instructed not to treat acute attacks without also seeking medical help;
- have regular follow up with doctor or specialist nurse.

Jet nebulisers
Jet nebulisers are more widely used than ultrasonic nebulisers. Most jet nebulisers require an optimum flow rate of 6–8 litres/minute and in hospital can be driven by piped air or oxygen; in acute asthma the nebuliser should always be driven by oxygen. Domiciliary oxygen cylinders do not provide an adequate flow rate therefore an electrical compressor is required for domiciliary use.

Some jet nebulisers are able to increase drug output during inspiration and hence increase efficiency.

Safe practice
The Department of Health has reminded users of the need to use the correct grade of tubing when connecting a nebuliser to a medical gas supply or compressor.

Nebuliser diluent
Nebulisation may be carried out using an undiluted nebuliser solution or it may require dilution beforehand. The usual diluent is sterile sodium chloride 0.9% (physiological saline).

In England and Wales nebulisers and compressors are not available on the NHS (but they are free of VAT); some nebulisers (but not compressors) are available on form GP10A in Scotland (for details consult Scottish Drug Tariff).

Oral

Systemic side-effects occur more frequently when a drug is given orally rather than by inhalation. Oral corticosteroids, theophylline p. 159, and leukotriene receptor antagonists are sometimes required for the management of asthma. Oral administration of a beta$_2$ agonist is generally not recommended for children, but may be necessary in infants and young children who are unable or unwilling to use an inhaler device.

Parenteral

Drugs such as beta$_2$ agonists, corticosteroids, and aminophylline p. 158 can be given by injection in acute severe asthma when drug administration by nebulisation is inadequate or inappropriate; in these circumstances the child should generally be treated in a high dependency or intensive care unit.

Peak flow meters

Peak flow meters may be used to assess lung function in children over 5 years with asthma, but symptom monitoring is the most reliable assessment of asthma control. They are best used for short periods to assess the severity of asthma and to monitor response to treatment; continuous use of peak flow meters may detract from compliance with inhalers.

Peak flow charts should be issued to patients where appropriate, and are available to purchase from:

3M Security Print and Systems Limited. Gorse Street, Chadderton, Oldham, OL9 9QH. Tel: 0845 610 1112

GP practices can obtain supplies through their Area Team stores.

NHS Hospitals can order supplies from www.nhsforms.co.uk or by emailing nhsforms@mmm.com.

In Scotland, peak flow charts can be obtained by emailing stockorders.dppas@apsgroup.co.uk.

NICE technology appraisals (TAs)
Inhaler devices for children under 5 years with chronic asthma (August 2000) NICE TA10
A child's needs and likelihood of good compliance should govern the choice of inhaler and spacer device; only then should cost be considered.

- corticosteroid and bronchodilator therapy should be delivered by pressurised metered-dose inhaler and spacer device, with a facemask if necessary;
- if this is not effective, and depending on the child's condition, nebulised therapy may be considered and, in children over 3 years, a dry powder inhaler may also be considered.

www.nice.org.uk/TA10

Inhaler devices for children 5–15 years with chronic asthma (March 2002) NICE TA38
A child's needs, ability to develop and maintain effective technique, and likelihood of good compliance should govern the choice of inhaler and spacer device; only then should cost be considered.

- corticosteroid therapy should be routinely delivered by a pressurised metered-dose inhaler and spacer device;
- for other inhaled drugs, particularly bronchodilators, a wider range of devices should be considered;
- children and their carers should be trained in the use of the chosen device; suitability of the device should be reviewed at least annually. Inhaler technique and compliance should be monitored.

www.nice.org.uk/TA38

1 Airways disease, obstructive

Asthma

31.3.2016

Description of condition

Asthma is a common chronic inflammatory condition of the airways characterised by bronchoconstriction. The most frequent symptoms are cough, wheezing, chest tightness, and shortness of breath. The bronchoconstriction is usually reversible (either spontaneously or with the aid of medication) leading to intermittent symptoms, but in some patients with chronic asthma the inflammation may result in irreversible airway obstruction. Occasionally, asthma symptoms can get gradually or suddenly worse provoking an acute asthma attack that, if severe, may require hospitalisation.

Aims of treatment

In clinical practice, patients may choose to balance the aims of asthma management against the potential side-effects or inconvenience of taking medication necessary to achieve perfect control. Complete control of asthma is defined as no daytime symptoms, no night-time awakening due to asthma, no asthma attacks, no need for rescue medication, no limitations on activity including exercise, and normal lung function (in practical terms FEV_1 and/or peak flow > 80% predicted or best).

Lifestyle changes

EvGr Weight loss in overweight patients may lead to an improvement in asthma symptoms. Parents with asthma should be advised about the danger to themselves and to their children with asthma, of smoking, and be offered appropriate support to stop smoking. Breathing exercise programmes (including physiotherapist-taught methods) can be offered as an adjuvant to drug treatment in order to improve quality of life and reduce symptoms. A

Management of chronic asthma

EvGr A stepwise approach aims to stop symptoms quickly and to improve peak flow. Start at the step most appropriate to initial severity of asthma. The aim is to achieve early control and to maintain it by *stepping up* treatment as necessary and *stepping down* treatment when control is good. Before initiating a new drug consider whether diagnosis is correct, check compliance and inhaler technique, and eliminate trigger factors for acute attacks. A

Child over 5 years
Step 1—Mild intermittent asthma

▶ EvGr Start inhaled short-acting beta₂ agonist (such as salbutamol p. 146 or terbutaline sulfate p. 148) as required A

EvGr Children using more than one short-acting bronchodilator inhaler a month should have their asthma urgently assessed and action taken to improve poorly controlled asthma. Inhaled ipratropium bromide p. 143 also acts as a short-acting bronchodilator but inhaled short-acting beta₂ agonists are preferred.

Move to **step 2** if the child presents with any one of the following features; is using an inhaled beta₂ agonist three times a week or more, being symptomatic three times a week or more, experiencing night-time symptoms at least once a week, or has had an asthma attack in the last 2 years. A

Step 2—Regular preventer therapy

▶ EvGr Consider adding regular inhaled standard-dose corticosteroid (alternatives to inhaled corticosteroid are leukotriene receptor antagonists, theophylline p. 159, inhaled sodium cromoglicate p. 157, or inhaled nedocromil sodium p. 157, but are less effective) A

EvGr Start the inhaled corticosteroid at a dose appropriate to severity of disease and adjust to the lowest effective dose at which control of asthma is maintained. Inhaled corticosteroids (except ciclesonide p. 152) should be initially taken twice daily, however, the same total daily dose can be considered once a day if good control is established. A

Note, inhaled standard-dose corticosteroid
Child over 12 years: 200–800 micrograms/day beclometasone dipropionate p. 150 or equivalent
Child 5–12 years: 200–400 micrograms/day beclometasone dipropionate or equivalent

EvGr Beclometasone dipropionate and budesonide p. 151 are approximately equivalent in clinical practice although there may be variations with different drug delivery devices. Fluticasone p. 152 provides equal clinical activity to beclometasone dipropionate and budesonide at half the dosage. A

EvGr In children, administration of high doses of inhaled corticosteroids may be associated with systemic side-effects, including growth failure, reduced bone mineral density, and adrenal suppression, see individual drug monographs for monitoring information.

If asthma is not adequately controlled, move to **step 3**. A

Step 3—Initial add-on therapy

▶ EvGr Consider adding a regular inhaled long-acting beta₂ agonist (LABA) such as formoterol fumarate p. 144 or salmeterol p. 145 to be used in conjunction with an inhaled corticosteroid (see also CHM advice for formoterol fumarate and salmeterol) A

EvGr If the child is gaining some benefit from addition of a LABA but control is *inadequate* then continue the LABA and increase dose of inhaled corticosteroid to top end of inhaled standard-dose corticosteroid range. If there is *no response* to the LABA, discontinue and increase dose of inhaled corticosteroid. If control is still inadequate, start a trial of either a leukotriene receptor antagonist (montelukast p. 155, or zafirlukast p. 156 if over 12 years) or modified-release theophylline. A

Step 4—Persistent poor control
Consider the following options:

▶ EvGr Increase dose of inhaled corticosteroid (a spacer should be used), or A
▶ EvGr Add a leukotriene receptor antagonist, modified-release theophylline, or modified-release oral beta₂ agonist (caution in children already taking a LABA) A

Note, increased inhaled corticosteroid dose
Child over 12 years: up to 2000 micrograms/day beclometasone dipropionate or equivalent
Child 5–12 years: up to 800 micrograms/day beclometasone dipropionate or equivalent
EvGr Before proceeding to **step 5**, refer children with inadequately controlled asthma to specialist care. A

Step 5—Continuous or frequent use of oral corticosteroids

▶ EvGr Add regular oral corticosteroid (prednisolone p. 413, as single daily dose) at lowest dose to provide adequate control; continue high-dose inhaled corticosteroid (in exceptional cases, this may exceed licensed doses) A

Child under 5 years
Step 1—Mild intermittent asthma

▶ EvGr Inhaled short-acting beta₂ agonist (such as salbutamol or terbutaline sulfate) as required A

EvGr Children identified to be using more than one short-acting bronchodilator inhaler a month should have their asthma urgently assessed and action taken to improve poorly controlled asthma.

Move to **step 2** if the child presents with any one of the following features; is using an inhaled beta₂ agonist three times a week or more, being symptomatic three times a week or more, experiencing night-time symptoms at least once a week. A

Step 2—Regular preventer therapy

▶ EvGr Consider adding regular standard-dose inhaled corticosteroid A
▶ EvGr If child is unable to take an inhaled corticosteroid, a leukotriene receptor antagonist (such as montelukast) is an effective first-line preventer A

EvGr Start inhaled corticosteroid at a dose appropriate to severity of disease and adjust to the lowest effective dose at which control of asthma is maintained. A

Note, inhaled standard-dose corticosteroid
Child under 5 years: 200–400 micrograms/day beclometasone dipropionate or equivalent

EvGr Beclometasone dipropionate and budesonide are approximately equivalent in clinical practice although there may be variations with different drug delivery devices. Fluticasone provides equal clinical activity to beclometasone dipropionate and budesonide at half the dosage. ⟨A⟩

EvGr In children, administration of high doses of inhaled corticosteroids may be associated with systemic side-effects, including growth failure, reduced bone mineral density and adrenal suppression, see individual drug monographs for monitoring information.

If asthma is not adequately controlled, move to **step 3**. ⟨A⟩

Step 3—Initial add-on therapy

▸ EvGr In children 2–5 years, add a leukotriene receptor antagonist if not added during step 2. If a leukotriene receptor antagonist was added at step 2, reconsider addition of standard-dose inhaled corticosteroid. ⟨A⟩

▸ EvGr In children under 2 years, consider proceeding to **step 4** ⟨A⟩

Step 4—Persistent poor control

▸ EvGr Refer child to respiratory paediatrician ⟨A⟩

Stepping down

EvGr Once asthma is controlled, it is recommended to step down therapy and continue to regularly review the child. When deciding which drug to step down first and at what rate, the severity of asthma, the side-effects of treatment, duration on current dose, the beneficial effects achieved, and the child's preference, should be considered.

The child should be maintained at the lowest possible dose of inhaled corticosteroid. Reductions should be considered every three months, decreasing the dose by approximately 25–50% each time. Reduce the dose slowly as children deteriorate at different rates. ⟨A⟩

Management of acute asthma

Child over 2 years

The nature of treatment required for the management of acute asthma depends on the level of severity, described as follows:

Moderate acute asthma

- Able to talk in sentences
- Arterial oxygen saturation (SpO$_2$) $\geq$ 92%
- Peak flow $\geq$ 50% best or predicted
- Heart rate $\leq$ 140/minute in children aged 2–5 years; heart rate $\leq$ 125/minute in children over 5 years
- Respiratory rate $\leq$ 40/minute in children aged 2–5 years; respiratory rate $\leq$ 30/minute in children over 5 years

Severe acute asthma

- Can't complete sentences in one breath or too breathless to talk or feed
- SpO$_2$ < 92%
- Peak flow 33–50% best or predicted
- Heart rate > 140/minute in children aged 2–5 years; heart rate > 125/minute in children aged over 5 years
- Respiratory rate > 40/minute in children aged 2–5 years; respiratory rate > 30/minute in children aged over 5 years

Life-threatening acute asthma

Any one of the following in a child with severe asthma:

- SpO$_2$ < 92%
- Peak flow < 33% best or predicted
- Silent chest
- Cyanosis
- Poor respiratory effort
- Hypotension
- Exhaustion
- Confusion

EvGr Following initial assessment, supplementary high flow oxygen should be given to all children with life-threatening acute asthma or SpO$_2$ < 94% to achieve normal saturations of 94–98%. ⟨A⟩

EvGr First-line treatment for acute asthma is an inhaled short-acting beta$_2$ agonist (salbutamol p. 146 or terbutaline sulfate p. 148) given as soon as possible, ideally via a metered dose inhaler and spacer device in mild to moderate acute asthma. Children with severe or life-threatening acute asthma should be transferred to hospital urgently. ⟨A⟩

EvGr In all cases of acute asthma, children should be prescribed an adequate once daily dose of oral prednisolone p. 413. Treatment for up to 3 days is usually sufficient, but the length of course should be tailored to the number of days necessary to bring about recovery. Intravenous hydrocortisone p. 411 should be reserved for severely affected children who are unable to retain oral medication.

Nebulised ipratropium bromide p. 143 may be combined with beta$_2$ agonist treatment for children with severe or life-threatening acute asthma or in those with a poor initial response to beta$_2$ agonist therapy to provide greater bronchodilation. Consider adding magnesium sulfate p. 556 to nebulised salbutamol and ipratropium bromide in the first hour in children with a short duration of acute severe asthma symptoms presenting with an oxygen saturation less than 92%. ⟨A⟩

EvGr Children with continuing severe asthma despite frequent nebulised beta$_2$ agonists and ipratropium bromide plus oral corticosteroids, and those with life-threatening features, need urgent review by a specialist with a view to transfer to a high dependency unit or paediatric intensive care unit (PICU) to receive second-line intravenous therapies.

In a severe asthma attack where the child has not responded to initial inhaled therapy, early addition of a single bolus dose of intravenous salbutamol may be an option. Continuous intravenous infusion of salbutamol, administered under specialist supervision with continuous ECG and electrolyte monitoring, should be considered in patients with unreliable inhalation or severe refractory asthma. Aminophylline p. 158 may be considered in children with severe or life-threatening acute asthma unresponsive to maximal doses of bronchodilators and corticosteroids. Aminophylline is not recommended in children with mild to moderate acute asthma. Intravenous magnesium sulfate has been used for acute asthma [unlicensed use] although its place in management is not yet established. ⟨A⟩

Child under 2 years

EvGr Inhaled short-acting beta$_2$ agonists are the initial treatment of choice for acute asthma in children under 2 years. For mild to moderate acute asthma attacks, a metered-dose inhaler with a spacer and mask is the optimal drug delivery device. In a hospital setting, consider oral prednisolone daily for up to 3 days, early in the management of severe asthma attacks. For more severe symptoms, inhaled ipratropium bromide in combination with an inhaled beta$_2$ agonist is also an option. ⟨A⟩

Follow up in all cases

EvGr Episodes of acute asthma may be a failure of preventative therapy, review is required to prevent further episodes. A careful history should be taken to establish the reason for the asthma attack. Inhaler technique should be checked and regular treatment should be reviewed. Children and their carers should be given a written asthma action plan aimed at preventing relapse, optimising treatment, and preventing delay in seeking assistance in future attacks. It is essential that the child's GP practice is informed within 24 hours of discharge from the emergency department or hospital following an asthma attack. Children who have had a near-fatal asthma attack should be kept under specialist supervision indefinitely. A respiratory specialist should follow up all patients admitted with a severe asthma attack for at least one year after the admission. ⟨A⟩

Pregnancy and breast-feeding

EvGr Women with asthma should be closely monitored during pregnancy. It is particularly important that asthma should be well controlled during pregnancy; when this is achieved asthma has no important effects on pregnancy, labour, or on the fetus. Women planning to become pregnant should be counselled about the importance of taking their asthma medication regularly to maintain good control. Drugs for asthma should preferably be administered by inhalation to minimise exposure of the fetus. Short-acting beta$_2$ agonists, long-acting beta$_2$ agonists, oral and inhaled corticosteroids, sodium cromoglicate p. 157, nedocromil sodium p. 157, and oral and intravenous theophyllines can be used as normal during pregnancy. There is limited information on use of leukotriene receptor antagonists during pregnancy, however they may be used if potential benefit outweighs risk. Drugs for asthma, including corticosteroid tablets, can be used as normal and in-line with manufacturers' recommendations in breast-feeding. A

EvGr Severe acute attacks of asthma can have an adverse effect on pregnancy and should be treated promptly in hospital with conventional therapy, including nebulisation of a beta$_2$ agonist and oral or parenteral administration of a corticosteroid; prednisolone p. 413 is the preferred corticosteroid for oral administration since very little of the drug reaches the fetus. Oxygen should be given immediately to maintain arterial oxygen saturation of 94–98% and prevent maternal and fetal hypoxia. A

Useful Resources

British guideline on the management of asthma. British Thoracic Society and Scottish Intercollegiate Guidelines Network. Quick Reference Guide 141. October 2014. sign.ac.uk/pdf/QRG141.pdf

British guideline on the management of asthma. British Thoracic Society and Scottish Intercollegiate Guidelines Network. Full guidance - A national clinical guideline 141. October 2014.
sign.ac.uk/pdf/SIGN141.pdf

Bronchodilators

Beta$_2$ agonists

Selective beta$_2$ agonists produce bronchodilation. A short-acting beta$_2$ agonist is used for immediate relief of asthma symptoms while a long-acting beta$_2$ agonist is used in addition to an inhaled corticosteroid in children requiring prophylactic treatment.

The selective beta$_2$ agonists (selective beta$_2$-adrenoceptor agonists, selective beta$_2$ stimulants) such as salbutamol p. 146 or terbutaline sulfate p. 148 are the safest and most effective short-acting beta$_2$ agonists for the treatment of asthma.

Adrenaline/epinephrine p. 128 (which has both alpha-and beta-adrenoceptor agonist properties) is used in the emergency management of acute allergic and anaphylactic reactions, in angioedema, and in cardiopulmonary resuscitation; it is also used as a nebuliser solution to treat severe croup.

Short-acting beta$_2$ agonists

Mild to moderate symptoms of asthma respond rapidly to the inhalation of a selective short-acting beta$_2$ agonist such as salbutamol or terbutaline sulfate. If beta$_2$ agonist inhalation is needed more often than twice a week, or if night-time symptoms occur at least once a week, or if the patient has suffered an exacerbation in the last 2 years, then prophylactic treatment should be considered using a stepped approach.

A short-acting beta$_2$ agonist inhaled immediately before exertion reduces *exercise-induced asthma*; however, frequent exercise-induced asthma probably reflects poor overall control and calls for reassessment of asthma treatment.

Long-acting beta$_2$ agonists

Formoterol fumarate p. 144 (eformoterol) and salmeterol p. 145 are longer-acting beta$_2$ agonists which are administered by inhalation. They should be used for asthma only in children who regularly use an inhaled corticosteroid. They have a role in the long-term management of chronic asthma and can be useful in nocturnal asthma.

Salmeterol should not be used for the relief of an asthma attack; it has a slower onset of action than salbutamol or terbutaline sulfate. Formoterol fumarate is licensed for short-term symptom relief and for the prevention of exercise-induced bronchospasm; its speed of onset of action is similar to that of salbutamol.

Vilanterol is a long-acting beta$_2$ agonist available in a combination inhaler with fluticasone furoate.

Combination inhalers that contain a long-acting beta$_2$ agonist and a corticosteroid ensure that long-acting beta$_2$ agonists are not used without concomitant corticosteroids, but reduce the flexibility to adjust the dose of each component.

Oral

Oral preparations of beta$_2$ agonists may be used for children if an inhaler device cannot be used but inhaled beta$_2$ agonists are more effective and have fewer side-effects. A modified-release formulation of salbutamol may be of value in nocturnal asthma as an alternative to modified-release theophylline p. 159 preparations, but an inhaled long-acting beta$_2$ agonist is preferable.

Parenteral

Beta$_2$ agonists can be given intravenously in children with severe or life-threatening acute asthma. Chronic asthma unresponsive to stepwise treatment may benefit from continuous subcutaneous infusion of a beta$_2$ agonist, but this should be used only under the supervision of a respiratory specialist; the evidence of benefit is uncertain and it may be difficult to withdraw such treatment once started.

Antimuscarinic bronchodilators

Ipratropium bromide p. 143 by nebulisation can be added to other standard treatment in life-threatening acute asthma or if acute asthma fails to improve with standard therapy. Ipratropium bromide can be used to provide short-term relief in chronic asthma, but short-acting beta$_2$ agonists act more quickly and are preferred.

The aerosol inhalation of ipratropium bromide has a maximum effect 30–60 minutes after use; its duration of action is 3 to 6 hours.

Theophylline

Theophylline is a xanthine used as a bronchodilator in asthma. It may have an additive effect when used in conjunction with small doses of beta$_2$ agonists; the combination may increase the risk of side-effects, including hypokalaemia.

Theophylline is given by injection as aminophylline p. 158, a mixture of theophylline with ethylenediamine, which is 20 times more soluble than theophylline alone. Aminophylline injection is needed rarely for severe acute asthma.

Compound bronchodilator preparations

In general, children are best treated with single-ingredient preparations, such as a selective beta$_2$ agonist or ipratropium bromide, so that the dose of each drug can be adjusted. This flexibility is lost with compound bronchodilator preparations.

Croup

Management

Mild croup is largely self-limiting, but treatment with a single dose of a corticosteroid (e.g. dexamethasone p. 410) by mouth may be of benefit.

More severe croup (or mild croup that might cause complications) calls for hospital admission; a single dose of a corticosteroid (e.g. dexamethasone or prednisolone p. 413 by mouth) should be administered before transfer to hospital. In hospital, dexamethasone (by mouth or by injection) or budesonide p. 151 (by nebulisation) will often reduce symptoms; the dose may need to be repeated after 12 hours if necessary.

For severe croup not effectively controlled with corticosteroid treatment, nebulised adrenaline/epinephrine solution 1 in 1000 (1 mg/mL) p. 128 should be given with close clinical monitoring; the effects of nebulised adrenaline/epinephrine last 2–3 hours and the child needs to be monitored carefully for recurrence of the obstruction.

Oxygen

Overview

Oxygen should be regarded as a drug. It is prescribed for hypoxaemic patients to increase alveolar oxygen tension and decrease the work of breathing. The concentration of oxygen required depends on the condition being treated; administration of an inappropriate concentration of oxygen may have serious or even fatal consequences. High concentrations of oxygen can cause pulmonary epithelial damage (bronchopulmonary dysplasia), convulsions, and retinal damage, especially in preterm neonates.

Oxygen is probably the most common drug used in medical emergencies. It should be prescribed initially to achieve a normal or near-normal oxygen saturation. In most acutely ill children with an expected or known normal or low arterial carbon dioxide (P_aCO_2), oxygen saturation should be maintained above 92%; some clinicians may aim for a target of 94–98%. In some clinical situations, such as carbon monoxide poisoning, it is more appropriate to aim for the highest possible oxygen saturation until the child is stable. Hypercapnic respiratory failure is rare in children; in those children at risk, a lower oxygen saturation target of 88–92% is indicated.

High concentration oxygen therapy is safe in uncomplicated cases of conditions such as pneumonia, pulmonary thromboembolism, pulmonary fibrosis, shock, severe trauma, sepsis, or anaphylaxis. In such conditions low arterial oxygen (P_aO_2) is usually associated with low or normal arterial carbon dioxide (P_aCO_2), and therefore there is little risk of hypoventilation and carbon dioxide retention.

In severe acute asthma, the arterial carbon dioxide (P_aCO_2) is usually subnormal but as asthma deteriorates it may rise steeply (particularly in children). These patients usually require high concentrations of oxygen and if the arterial carbon dioxide (P_aCO_2) remains high despite other treatment, intermittent positive-pressure ventilation needs to be considered urgently.

Oxygen should not be given to neonates except under expert supervision. Particular care is required in preterm neonates because of the risk of hyperoxia.

Low concentration oxygen therapy (controlled oxygen therapy) is reserved for children at risk of hypercapnic respiratory failure, which is more likely in children with:

- advanced cystic fibrosis
- advanced non-cystic fibrosis bronchiectasis
- severe kyphoscoliosis or severe ankylosing spondylitis
- severe lung scarring caused by tuberculosis

- musculoskeletal disorders with respiratory weakness, especially if on home ventilation
- an overdose of opioids, benzodiazepines, or other drugs causing respiratory depression.

Until blood gases can be measured, initial oxygen should be given using a controlled concentration of 28% or less, titrated towards a target concentration of 88–92%. The aim is to provide the child with enough oxygen to achieve an acceptable arterial oxygen tension without worsening carbon dioxide retention and respiratory acidosis.

Domiciliary oxygen

Oxygen should only be prescribed for use in the home after careful evaluation in hospital by a respiratory care specialist. Carers and children who smoke should be advised of the risks of smoking when receiving oxygen, including the risk of fire. Smoking cessation therapy should be recommended before home oxygen prescription.

Long-term oxygen therapy

The aim of long-term oxygen therapy is to maintain oxygen saturation of at least 92%. Children (especially those with chronic neonatal lung disease) often require supplemental oxygen, either for 24-hours a day or during periods of sleep; many children are eventually weaned off long-term oxygen therapy as their condition improves.

Long-term oxygen therapy should be considered for children with conditions such as:

- bronchopulmonary dysplasia (chronic neonatal lung disease);
- congenital heart disease with pulmonary hypertension;
- pulmonary hypertension secondary to pulmonary disease;
- idiopathic pulmonary hypertension;
- sickle-cell disease with persistent nocturnal hypoxia;
- interstitial lung disease and obliterative bronchiolitis;
- cystic fibrosis;
- obstructive sleep apnoea syndrome;
- neuromuscular or skeletal disease requiring non-invasive ventilation;
- pulmonary malignancy or other terminal disease with disabling dyspnoea.

Increased respiratory depression is seldom a problem in children with stable respiratory failure treated with low concentrations of oxygen although it may occur during exacerbations; children and their carers should be warned to call for medical help if drowsiness or confusion occurs.

Short-burst oxygen therapy

Oxygen is occasionally prescribed for short-burst (intermittent) use for episodes of breathlessness.

Ambulatory oxygen therapy

Ambulatory oxygen is prescribed for children on long-term oxygen therapy who need to be away from home on a regular basis.

Oxygen therapy equipment

Under the NHS oxygen may be supplied as **oxygen cylinders**. Oxygen flow can be adjusted as the cylinders are equipped with an oxygen flow meter. Oxygen delivered from a cylinder should be passed through a humidifier if used for long periods.

Oxygen concentrators are more economical for children who require oxygen for long periods, and in England and Wales can be ordered on the NHS on a regional tendering basis. A concentrator is recommended for a child who requires oxygen for more than 8 hours a day (or 21 cylinders per month). Exceptionally, if a higher concentration of oxygen is required the output of 2 oxygen concentrators can be combined using a 'Y' connection.

A nasal cannula is usually preferred to a face mask for long-term oxygen therapy from an oxygen concentrator.

Nasal cannulas can, however, cause dermatitis and mucosal drying in sensitive individuals.

Giving oxygen by nasal cannula allows the child to talk, eat, and drink, but the concentration of oxygen is not controlled and the method may not be appropriate for acute respiratory failure. When oxygen is given through a nasal cannula at a rate of 1–2 litres/minute the inspiratory oxygen concentration is usually low, but it varies with ventilation and can be high if the patient is underventilating.

Arrangements for supplying oxygen

The following oxygen services may be ordered in England and Wales:

- emergency oxygen;
- short-burst (intermittent) oxygen therapy;
- long-term oxygen therapy;
- ambulatory oxygen.

The type of oxygen service (or combination of services) should be ordered on a Home Oxygen Order Form (HOOF); the amount of oxygen required (hours per day) and flow rate should be specified. The clinician will determine the appropriate equipment to be provided. Special needs or preferences should be specified on the HOOF.

The clinician should obtain the consent of the child or carers to pass on the child's details to the supplier, the fire brigade, and other relevant organisations. The supplier will contact the child or carer to make arrangements for delivery, installation, and maintenance of the equipment. The supplier will also train the child or carer to use the equipment.

The clinician should send the HOOF to the supplier who will continue to provide the service until a revised HOOF is received, or until notified that the child no longer requires the home oxygen service.

HOOF and further instructions are available at www.bprs.co.uk/oxygen.html.

- East of England, North East: BOC Medical: Tel: 0800 136 603 Fax: 0800 169 9989
- South West: Air Liquide: Tel: 0808 202 2229 Fax: 0191 497 4340
- London East, Midlands, North West:Air Liquide: Tel: 0500 823 773 Fax: 0800 781 4610
- Yorkshire and Humberside, West Midlands, Wales: Air Products: Tel: 0800 373 580 Fax: 0800 214 709
- South East Coast, South Central: Dolby Vivisol: Tel: 08443 814 402 Fax: 0800 781 4610

In **Scotland** refer the child for assessment by a paediatric respiratory consultant. If the need for a concentrator is confirmed the consultant will arrange for the provision of a concentrator through the Common Services Agency. Prescribers should complete a Scottish Home Oxygen Order Form (SHOOF) and email it to Health Facilities Scotland. Health Facilities Scotland will then liaise with their contractor to arrange the supply of oxygen. Further information can be obtained at www.dolbyvivisol.com/our-services/healthcare-professionals/home-oxygen-services-sco.aspx.

In **Northern Ireland** oxygen concentrators and cylinders should be prescribed on form HS21; oxygen concentrators are supplied by a local contractor. Prescriptions for oxygen cylinders and accessories can be dispensed by pharmacists contracted to provide domiciliary oxygen services.

ANTIMUSCARINICS

Antimuscarinics (inhaled) 9.2.2016

- **CAUTIONS** Bladder outflow obstruction · paradoxical bronchospasm · prostatic hyperplasia · susceptibility to angle-closure glaucoma
- **INTERACTIONS** → Appendix 1 (antimuscarinics). However, note that interactions do not *generally* apply to antimuscarinics used by inhalation.
- **SIDE-EFFECTS**
- **Common or very common** Constipation · cough · diarrhoea · dry mouth · gastro-intestinal motility disorder · headache · sinusitis
- **Uncommon** Angle-closure glaucoma · atrial fibrillation · blurred vision · dizziness · mydriasis · nasopharyngitis · nausea · palpitation · paradoxical bronchospasm · pharyngitis · rash · tachycardia · throat irritation · urinary retention
- **Rare** Dental caries

⚑ above

| Ipratropium bromide 24.2.2016

- **INDICATIONS AND DOSE**
Reversible airways obstruction
- BY INHALATION OF AEROSOL
- Child 1 month–5 years: 20 micrograms 3 times a day
- Child 6–11 years: 20–40 micrograms 3 times a day
- Child 12–17 years: 20–40 micrograms 3–4 times a day

Acute bronchospasm
- BY INHALATION OF NEBULISED SOLUTION
- Child 1 month–5 years: 125–250 micrograms as required; maximum 1 mg per day
- Child 6–11 years: 250 micrograms as required; maximum 1 mg per day
- Child 12–17 years: 500 micrograms as required, doses higher than max. can be given under medical supervision; maximum 2 mg per day

Severe or life-threatening acute asthma
- BY INHALATION OF NEBULISED SOLUTION
- Child 1 month–11 years: 250 micrograms every 20–30 minutes for the first 2 hours, then 250 micrograms every 4–6 hours as required
- Child 12–17 years: 500 micrograms every 4–6 hours as required

PHARMACOKINETICS
The maximal effect of inhaled ipratropium occurs 30–60 minutes after use; its duration of action is 3 to 6 hours and bronchodilation can usually be maintained with treatment 3 times a day.

- **UNLICENSED USE** EvGr The dose of ipratropium for severe or life-threatening acute asthma is unlicensed. ⚠
- **CAUTIONS** Cystic fibrosis
  CAUTIONS, FURTHER INFORMATION
- Glaucoma *Acute angle-closure glaucoma* has been reported with nebulised ipratropium, particularly when given with nebulised salbutamol (and possibly other beta₂ agonists); care needed to protect the patient's eyes from nebulised drug or from drug powder.
- **SIDE-EFFECTS**
- **Uncommon** Laryngospasm · pharyngeal oedema · stomatitis · vomiting
- **Rare** Ocular accommodation disorder
- **PREGNANCY** Manufacturer advises only use if potential benefit outweighs the risk.
- **BREAST FEEDING** No information available—manufacturer advises only use if potential benefit outweighs risk.

3

Respiratory system

- **DIRECTIONS FOR ADMINISTRATION** If dilution of ipratropium bromide nebuliser solution is necessary use only sterile sodium chloride 0.9%.
- **PATIENT AND CARER ADVICE** Patients or carers should be given advice on appropriate inhaler technique.
- **MEDICINAL FORMS**
  There can be variation in the licensing of different medicines containing the same drug.

Pressurised inhalation
- ▸ Ipratropium bromide (Non-proprietary)
  Ipratropium bromide 20 microgram per 1 dose Ipratropium bromide 20micrograms/dose inhaler CFC free | 200 dose PoM £5.00 DT price = £5.56
- ▸ Atrovent (Boehringer Ingelheim Ltd)
  Ipratropium bromide 20 microgram per 1 dose Atrovent 20micrograms/dose inhaler CFC free | 200 dose PoM £5.56 DT price = £5.56

Nebuliser liquid
- ▸ Ipratropium bromide (Non-proprietary)
  Ipratropium bromide 250 microgram per 1 ml Ipratropium bromide 500micrograms/2ml nebuliser liquid unit dose vials | 20 unit dose PoM £8.93 DT price = £2.95
  Ipratropium bromide 250micrograms/1ml nebuliser liquid unit dose vials | 20 unit dose PoM £4.52 DT price = £4.44
  Ipratropium 250micrograms/1ml nebuliser liquid Steri-Neb unit dose vials | 20 unit dose PoM £14.99 DT price = £4.44
  Ipratropium 500micrograms/2ml nebuliser liquid Steri-Neb unit dose vials | 20 unit dose PoM £15.99 DT price = £2.95
- ▸ Atrovent UDV (Boehringer Ingelheim Ltd)
  Ipratropium bromide 250 microgram per 1 ml Atrovent 500micrograms/2ml nebuliser liquid UDVs | 20 unit dose PoM £4.87 DT price = £2.95 | 60 unit dose PoM £14.59
  Atrovent 250micrograms/1ml nebuliser liquid UDVs | 20 unit dose PoM £4.14 DT price = £4.44 | 60 unit dose PoM £12.44
- ▸ Respontin (GlaxoSmithKline UK Ltd)
  Ipratropium bromide 250 microgram per 1 ml Respontin 250micrograms/1ml Nebules | 20 unit dose PoM £4.78 DT price = £4.44
  Respontin 500micrograms/2ml Nebules | 20 unit dose PoM £5.60 DT price = £2.95

BETA₂-ADRENOCEPTOR AGONISTS, SELECTIVE

Beta₂-adrenoceptor agonists, selective

12.2.2016

- **CONTRA-INDICATIONS** Severe pre-eclampsia
- **CAUTIONS** Arrhythmias · cardiovascular disease · diabetes (risk of hyperglycaemia and ketoacidosis, especially with intravenous use) · high doses of beta₂ agonists can be dangerous in some children · hypertension · hyperthyroidism · hypokalaemia · susceptibility to QT-interval prolongation

  CAUTIONS, FURTHER INFORMATION
  ▸ Hypokalaemia Potentially serious hypokalaemia may result from beta₂ agonist therapy. Particular caution is required in severe asthma, because this effect may be potentiated by concomitant treatment with theophylline and its derivatives, corticosteroids, diuretics, and by hypoxia.
- **INTERACTIONS** → Appendix 1 (sympathomimetics, beta₂). Hypokalaemia may be potentiated by concomitant treatment with theophylline and its derivatives, corticosteroids, and diuretics.
- **SIDE-EFFECTS** Angioedema · arrhythmias · behavioural disturbances · collapse · fine tremor (particularly in the hands) · headache · hyperglycaemia (especially when given intravenously) · hypersensitivity reactions · hypokalaemia (with high doses) · hypotension · ketoacidosis (especially when given intravenously) · muscle cramps · myocardial ischaemia · nervous tension · palpitation · paradoxical bronchospasm (occasionally severe) · peripheral vasodilation · rash · sleep disturbances · tachycardia · urticaria

- **PREGNANCY** Women planning to become pregnant should be counselled about the importance of taking their asthma medication regularly to maintain good control.
- **MONITORING REQUIREMENTS**
  ▸ In severe asthma, plasma-potassium concentration should be monitored (risk of hypokalaemia).
  ▸ In patients with diabetes, monitor blood glucose (risk of hyperglycaemia and ketoacidosis, especially when beta₂ agonist given intravenously).
- **PATIENT AND CARER ADVICE**
  ▸ When used by inhalation The **dose**, the frequency, and the maximum number of inhalations in 24 hours of the beta₂ agonist should be **stated explicitly** to the patient or their carer. The patient or their carer should be advised to seek medical advice when the prescribed dose of beta₂ agonist fails to provide the usual degree of symptomatic relief because this usually indicates a worsening of the asthma and the patient may require a prophylactic drug. Patients or their carers should be advised to follow manufacturers' instructions on the care and cleansing of inhaler devices.

BETA₂-ADRENOCEPTOR AGONISTS, SELECTIVE ⟩ LONG-ACTING

⟟ above

Formoterol fumarate

(Eformoterol fumarate)

- **INDICATIONS AND DOSE**

  Reversible airways obstruction in patients requiring long-term regular bronchodilator therapy | Nocturnal asthma in patients requiring long-term regular bronchodilator therapy | Prophylaxis of exercise-induced bronchospasm in patients requiring long-term regular bronchodilator therapy | Chronic asthma in patients who regularly use an inhaled corticosteroid
  ▸ BY INHALATION OF POWDER
  ▸ Child 6-11 years: 12 micrograms twice daily, a daily dose of 24 micrograms of formoterol should be sufficient for the majority of children, particularly for younger age-groups; higher doses should be used rarely, and only when control is not maintained on the lower dose
  ▸ Child 12-17 years: 12 micrograms twice daily, dose may be increased in more severe airway obstruction; increased to 24 micrograms twice daily, a daily dose of 24 micrograms of formoterol should be sufficient for the majority of children, particularly for younger age-groups; higher doses should be used rarely, and only when control is not maintained on the lower dose
  ▸ BY INHALATION OF AEROSOL
  ▸ Child 12-17 years: 12 micrograms twice daily, dose may be increased in more severe airway obstruction; increased to 24 micrograms twice daily, a daily dose of 24 micrograms of formoterol should be sufficient for the majority of children, particularly for younger age-groups; higher doses should be used rarely, and only when control is not maintained on the lower dose

  OXIS®

  Chronic asthma
  ▸ BY INHALATION OF POWDER
  ▸ Child 6-17 years: 6–12 micrograms 1–2 times a day (max. per dose 12 micrograms), occasionally doses up to the maximum daily may be needed, reassess treatment if additional doses required on more than 2 days a week; maximum 48 micrograms per day

  Relief of bronchospasm
  ▸ BY INHALATION OF POWDER
  ▸ Child 6-17 years: 6–12 micrograms

Prophylaxis of exercise-induced bronchospasm
▶ BY INHALATION OF POWDER
▶ Child 6–17 years: 6–12 micrograms, dose to be taken before exercise

PHARMACOKINETICS
At recommended inhaled doses, the duration of action of formoterol is about 12 hours.

IMPORTANT SAFETY INFORMATION
CHM ADVICE
To ensure safe use, the CHM has advised that for the management of chronic asthma, long-acting beta₂ agonist (formoterol) should:
- be added only if regular use of standard-dose inhaled corticosteroids has failed to control asthma adequately;
- not be initiated in patients with rapidly deteriorating asthma;
- be introduced at a low dose and the effect properly monitored before considering dose increase;
- be discontinued in the absence of benefit;
- not be used for the relief of exercise-induced asthma symptoms unless regular inhaled corticosteroids are also used;
- be reviewed as clinically appropriate: stepping down therapy should be considered when good long-term asthma control has been achieved.

● SIDE-EFFECTS
▶ **Very rare** QT-interval prolongation
▶ **Frequency not known** Dizziness · nausea · pruritus · taste disturbances

● PREGNANCY Inhaled drugs for asthma can be taken as normal during pregnancy.

● BREAST FEEDING Inhaled drugs for asthma can be taken as normal during breast-feeding.

● PATIENT AND CARER ADVICE Advise patients not to exceed prescribed dose, and to follow manufacturer's directions; if a previously effective dose of inhaled formoterol fails to provide adequate relief, a doctor's advice should be obtained as soon as possible. Patients should be advised to report any deterioration in symptoms following initiation of treatment with a long-acting beta₂ agonist. Patient or carer should be given advice on how to administer formoterol fumarate inhalers.

● MEDICINAL FORMS
There can be variation in the licensing of different medicines containing the same drug.
Pressurised inhalation
▶ Atimos Modulite (Chiesi Ltd)
Formoterol fumarate dihydrate 12 microgram per 1 dose Atimos Modulite 12micrograms/dose inhaler | 100 dose [PoM] £30.06 DT price = £30.06
Inhalation powder
▶ Easyhaler (formoterol) (Orion Pharma (UK) Ltd)
Formoterol fumarate dihydrate 12 microgram per 1 dose Formoterol Easyhaler 12micrograms/dose dry powder inhaler | 120 dose [PoM] £23.75 DT price = £23.75
▶ Foradil (Novartis Pharmaceuticals UK Ltd)
Formoterol fumarate dihydrate 12 microgram Foradil 12microgram inhalation powder capsules with device | 60 capsule [PoM] £28.06 DT price = £28.06
▶ Oxis Turbohaler (AstraZeneca UK Ltd)
Formoterol fumarate dihydrate 6 microgram per 1 dose Oxis 6 Turbohaler | 60 dose [PoM] £24.80 DT price = £24.80
Formoterol fumarate dihydrate 12 microgram per 1 dose Oxis 12 Turbohaler | 60 dose [PoM] £24.80 DT price = £24.80

Combinations available: *Budesonide with formoterol*, p. 152 · *Fluticasone with formoterol*, p. 153

◀ 144

⎮ Salmeterol

● INDICATIONS AND DOSE
Reversible airways obstruction in patients requiring long-term regular bronchodilator therapy | Nocturnal asthma in patients requiring long-term regular bronchodilator therapy | Prevention of exercise-induced bronchospasm in patients requiring long-term regular bronchodilator therapy | Chronic asthma only in patients who regularly use an inhaled corticosteroid (not for immediate relief of acute asthma)
▶ BY INHALATION OF AEROSOL, OR BY INHALATION OF POWDER
▶ Child 5–11 years: 50 micrograms twice daily
▶ Child 12–17 years: 50 micrograms twice daily, dose may be increased in more severe airway obstruction; increased to 100 micrograms twice daily

PHARMACOKINETICS
At recommended inhaled doses, the duration of action of salmeterol is about 12 hours.

● UNLICENSED USE *Neovent* ® not licensed for use in children under 12 years.

IMPORTANT SAFETY INFORMATION
CHM ADVICE
To ensure safe use, the CHM has advised that for the management of chronic asthma, long-acting beta₂ agonist (salmeterol) should:
- be added only if regular use of standard-dose inhaled corticosteroids has failed to control asthma adequately;
- not be initiated in patients with rapidly deteriorating asthma;
- be introduced at a low dose and the effect properly monitored before considering dose increase;
- be discontinued in the absence of benefit;
- not be used for the relief of exercise-induced asthma symptoms unless regular inhaled corticosteroids are also used;
- be reviewed as clinically appropriate: stepping down therapy should be considered when good long-term asthma control has been achieved.

● SIDE-EFFECTS Arthralgia · dizziness · nausea

● PREGNANCY Inhaled drugs for asthma can be taken as normal during pregnancy.

● BREAST FEEDING Inhaled drugs for asthma can be taken as normal during breast-feeding.

● PATIENT AND CARER ADVICE
Advise patients that salmeterol should **not** be used for relief of acute attacks, not to exceed prescribed dose, and to follow manufacturer's directions; if a previously effective dose of inhaled salmeterol fails to provide adequate relief, a doctor's advice should be obtained as soon as possible.
Patients should be advised to report any deterioration in symptoms following initiation of treatment with a long-acting beta₂ agonist.
Medicines for Children leaflet: Salmeterol inhaler for asthma prevention (prophylaxis) www.medicinesforchildren.org.uk/salmeterol-inhaler-for-asthma-prevention

● MEDICINAL FORMS
There can be variation in the licensing of different medicines containing the same drug.
Pressurised inhalation
▶ Salmeterol (Non-proprietary)
Salmeterol (as Salmeterol xinafoate) 25 microgram per 1 dose Salmeterol 25micrograms/dose inhaler CFC free | 120 dose [PoM] £29.26 DT price = £29.26

▸ **Neovent** (Kent Pharmaceuticals Ltd)
Salmeterol (as Salmeterol xinafoate) 25 microgram per 1 dose Neovent 25micrograms/dose inhaler CFC free | 120 dose [PoM] £29.26 DT price = £29.26

▸ **Serevent Evohaler** (GlaxoSmithKline UK Ltd)
Salmeterol (as Salmeterol xinafoate) 25 microgram per 1 dose Serevent 25micrograms/dose Evohaler | 120 dose [PoM] £29.26 DT price = £29.26

▸ **Vertine** (Teva UK Ltd)
Salmeterol (as Salmeterol xinafoate) 25 microgram per 1 dose Vertine 25micrograms/dose inhaler CFC free | 120 dose [PoM] £23.40 DT price = £29.26

Inhalation powder

▸ **Serevent Accuhaler** (GlaxoSmithKline UK Ltd)
Salmeterol (as Salmeterol xinafoate) 50 microgram per 1 dose Serevent 50micrograms/dose Accuhaler | 60 dose [PoM] £29.26 DT price = £29.26

Combinations available: *Fluticasone with salmeterol*, p. 153

BETA₂-ADRENOCEPTOR AGONISTS, SELECTIVE ⟩ SHORT-ACTING

▸ 144

Salbutamol

(Albuterol)

● **INDICATIONS AND DOSE**

Acute asthma

▸ BY INTRAVENOUS INJECTION

▸ **Child 1-23 months:** 5 micrograms/kg for 1 dose, dose to be administered over 5 minutes, reserve intravenous beta₂ agonists for those in whom inhaled therapy cannot be used reliably or there is no current effect

▸ **Child 2-17 years:** 15 micrograms/kg (max. per dose 250 micrograms) for 1 dose, dose to be administered over 5 minutes, reserve intravenous beta₂ agonists for those in whom inhaled therapy cannot be used reliably or there is no current effect

▸ BY CONTINUOUS INTRAVENOUS INFUSION

▸ **Child:** 1-2 micrograms/kg/minute, adjusted according to response and heart rate, increased if necessary up to 5 micrograms/kg/minute, doses above 2 micrograms/kg/minute should be given in an intensive care setting, reserve intravenous beta₂ agonists for those in whom inhaled therapy cannot be used reliably or there is no current effect

Moderate, severe, or life-threatening acute asthma

▸ BY INHALATION OF NEBULISED SOLUTION

▸ **Child 1 month-4 years:** 2.5 mg, repeat every 20-30 minutes or when required, give via oxygen-driven nebuliser if available

▸ **Child 5-11 years:** 2.5-5 mg, repeat every 20-30 minutes or when required, give via oxygen-driven nebuliser if available

▸ **Child 12-17 years:** 5 mg, repeat every 20-30 minutes or when required, give via oxygen-driven nebuliser if available

Moderate and severe acute asthma

▸ BY INHALATION OF AEROSOL

▸ **Child:** 2-10 puffs, each puff is to be inhaled separately, repeat every 10-20 minutes or when required, give via large volume spacer (and a close-fitting face mask in children under 3 years), each puff is equivalent to 100 micrograms

Exacerbation of reversible airways obstruction (including nocturnal asthma) | Prophylaxis of allergen- or exercise-induced bronchospasm

▸ BY INHALATION OF AEROSOL

▸ **Child:** 100-200 micrograms, up to 4 times a day for persistent symptoms

▸ BY MOUTH

▸ **Child 1 month-1 year:** 100 micrograms/kg 3-4 times a day (max. per dose 2 mg), inhalation route preferred over oral route

▸ **Child 2-5 years:** 1-2 mg 3-4 times a day, inhalation route preferred over oral route

▸ **Child 6-11 years:** 2 mg 3-4 times a day, inhalation route preferred over oral route

▸ **Child 12-17 years:** 2-4 mg 3-4 times a day, inhalation route preferred over oral route

Severe hyperkalaemia

▸ BY INTRAVENOUS INJECTION

▸ **Neonate:** 4 micrograms/kg, repeated if necessary, to be administered over 5 minutes.

▸ **Child:** 4 micrograms/kg, repeated if necessary, to be administered over 5 minutes

▸ BY INHALATION OF NEBULISED SOLUTION

▸ **Neonate:** 2.5-5 mg, repeated if necessary, intravenous injection route preferred over inhalation of nebulised solution.

▸ **Child:** 2.5-5 mg, repeated if necessary, intravenous injection route preferred over inhalation of nebulised solution

Chronic asthma

▸ BY MOUTH USING MODIFIED-RELEASE MEDICINES

▸ **Child 3-11 years:** 4 mg twice daily

▸ **Child 12-17 years:** 8 mg twice daily

ASMASAL CLICKHALER®

Acute bronchospasm

▸ BY INHALATION OF POWDER

▸ **Child 5-17 years:** 1-2 puffs, up to 4 times daily for persistent symptoms

Prophylaxis of allergen- or exercise-induced bronchospasm

▸ BY INHALATION OF POWDER

▸ **Child 5-17 years:** 1-2 puffs

EASYHALER® SALBUTAMOL

Acute bronchospasm

▸ BY INHALATION OF POWDER

▸ **Child 5-11 years:** 100-200 micrograms; maximum 800 micrograms per day

▸ **Child 12-17 years:** Initially 100-200 micrograms, increased if necessary to 400 micrograms; maximum 800 micrograms per day

Prophylaxis of allergen- or exercise-induced bronchospasm

▸ BY INHALATION OF POWDER

▸ **Child 5-11 years:** 100-200 micrograms

▸ **Child 12-17 years:** 200 micrograms

PULVINAL® SALBUTAMOL

Acute bronchospasm

▸ BY INHALATION OF POWDER

▸ **Child 5-17 years:** Initially 200 micrograms, up to 800 micrograms daily for persistent symptoms

Prophylaxis of allergen- or exercise-induced bronchospasm

▸ BY INHALATION OF POWDER

▸ **Child 5-17 years:** 200 micrograms

SALBULIN NOVOLIZER®

Acute bronchospasm

▸ BY INHALATION OF POWDER

▸ **Child 6-11 years:** 100-200 micrograms, up to 400 micrograms daily for persistent symptoms

▸ **Child 12-17 years:** Initially 100-200 micrograms, up to 800 micrograms daily for persistent symptoms

Prophylaxis of allergen- or exercise-induced bronchospasm
▸ BY INHALATION OF POWDER
▸ Child 6–11 years: 100–200 micrograms
▸ Child 12–17 years: 200 micrograms

VENTOLIN ACCUHALER®

Acute bronchospasm
▸ BY INHALATION OF POWDER
▸ Child 5–17 years: Initially 200 micrograms, up to 4 times daily for persistent symptoms

Prophylaxis of allergen- or exercise-induced bronchospasm
▸ BY INHALATION OF POWDER
▸ Child 5–17 years: 200 micrograms

PHARMACOKINETICS
At recommended inhaled doses, the duration of action of salbutamol is about 3 to 5 hours.

● **UNLICENSED USE** Not licensed for use in hyperkalaemia.
▸ With oral use Syrup and tablets not licensed for use in children under 2 years. Modified-release tablets not licensed for use in children under 3 years.
▸ With intravenous use or subcutaneous use Injection and solution for intravenous infusion not licensed for use in children under 12 years.
▸ With intravenous use Administration of undiluted salbutamol injection through a central venous catheter is not licensed.

● **SIDE-EFFECTS** Lactic acidosis (with high doses) · nausea

● **BREAST FEEDING** Inhaled drugs for asthma can be taken as normal during breast-feeding.

● **DIRECTIONS FOR ADMINISTRATION**
▸ With intravenous use For *continuous intravenous infusion*, dilute to a concentration of 200 micrograms/mL with Glucose 5% *or* Sodium Chloride 0.9%. If fluid-restricted, can be given undiluted through central venous catheter [unlicensed]. For *intravenous injection*, dilute to a concentration of 50 micrograms/mL with Glucose 5%, Sodium Chloride 0.9%, *or* Water for injections.
▸ When used by inhalation For *nebulisation*, dilute nebuliser solution with a suitable volume of sterile Sodium Chloride 0.9% solution according to nebuliser type and duration of administration; salbutamol and ipratropium bromide solutions are compatible and can be mixed for nebulisation.

● **PATIENT AND CARER ADVICE**
Medicines for Children leaflet: Salbutamol inhaler for asthma and wheeze www.medicinesforchildren.org.uk/salbutamol-inhaler-for-asthma-and-wheeze
▸ When used by inhalation *For inhalation by aerosol or dry powder*, advise patients and carers not to exceed prescribed dose and to follow manufacturer's directions; if a previously effective dose of inhaled salbutamol fails to provide at least 3 hours relief, a doctor's advice should be obtained as soon as possible. *For inhalation by nebuliser*, the dose given by nebuliser is substantially higher than that given by inhaler. Patients should therefore be warned that it is dangerous to exceed the prescribed dose and they should seek medical advice if they fail to respond to the usual dose of the respirator solution.

● **MEDICINAL FORMS**
There can be variation in the licensing of different medicines containing the same drug.

Tablet
▸ Salbutamol (Non-proprietary)
Salbutamol (as Salbutamol sulfate) 2 mg Salbutamol 2mg tablets | 28 tablet [PoM] £113.09 DT price = £104.95
Salbutamol (as Salbutamol sulfate) 4 mg Salbutamol 4mg tablets | 28 tablet [PoM] £115.76 DT price = £107.43

Oral solution
▸ Salbutamol (Non-proprietary)
Salbutamol (as Salbutamol sulfate) 400 microgram per 1 ml Salbutamol 2mg/5ml oral solution sugar free sugar-free | 150 ml [PoM] no price available DT price = £0.72
▸ Ventolin (GlaxoSmithKline UK Ltd)
Salbutamol (as Salbutamol sulfate) 400 microgram per 1 ml Ventolin 2mg/5ml syrup sugar-free | 150 ml [PoM] £0.72 DT price = £0.72

Solution for injection
▸ Ventolin (GlaxoSmithKline UK Ltd)
Salbutamol (as Salbutamol sulfate) 500 microgram per 1 ml Ventolin 500micrograms/1ml solution for injection ampoules | 5 ampoule [PoM] £1.91

Solution for infusion
▸ Ventolin (GlaxoSmithKline UK Ltd)
Salbutamol (as Salbutamol sulfate) 1 mg per 1 ml Ventolin 5mg/5ml solution for infusion ampoules | 10 ampoule [PoM] £24.81

Pressurised inhalation
▸ Salbutamol (Non-proprietary)
Salbutamol (as Salbutamol sulfate) 100 microgram per 1 dose Salbutamol 100micrograms/dose inhaler CFC free | 200 dose [PoM] £1.50 DT price = £1.50
▸ AirSalb (Sandoz Ltd)
Salbutamol (as Salbutamol sulfate) 100 microgram per 1 dose AirSalb 100micrograms/dose inhaler CFC free | 200 dose [PoM] £1.50 DT price = £1.50
▸ Airomir (Teva UK Ltd)
Salbutamol (as Salbutamol sulfate) 100 microgram per 1 dose Airomir 100micrograms/dose inhaler | 200 dose [PoM] £1.97 DT price = £1.50
▸ Airomir Autohaler (Teva UK Ltd)
Salbutamol (as Salbutamol sulfate) 100 microgram per 1 dose Airomir 100micrograms/dose Autohaler | 200 dose [PoM] £6.02 DT price = £6.30
▸ Asmavent (Kent Pharmaceuticals Ltd)
Salbutamol (as Salbutamol sulfate) 100 microgram per 1 dose Asmavent 100micrograms/dose inhaler CFC free | 200 dose [PoM] £1.50 DT price = £1.50
▸ Salamol (Teva UK Ltd)
Salbutamol (as Salbutamol sulfate) 100 microgram per 1 dose Salamol 100micrograms/dose inhaler CFC free | 200 dose [PoM] £1.46 DT price = £1.50
▸ Salamol Easi-Breathe (Teva UK Ltd)
Salbutamol (as Salbutamol sulfate) 100 microgram per 1 dose Salamol 100micrograms/dose Easi-Breathe inhaler | 200 dose [PoM] £6.30 DT price = £6.30
▸ Ventolin Evohaler (GlaxoSmithKline UK Ltd)
Salbutamol (as Salbutamol sulfate) 100 microgram per 1 dose Ventolin 100micrograms/dose Evohaler | 200 dose [PoM] £1.50 DT price = £1.50

Inhalation powder
▸ Easyhaler (salbutamol) (Orion Pharma (UK) Ltd)
Salbutamol 100 microgram per 1 dose Easyhaler Salbutamol sulfate 100micrograms/dose dry powder inhaler | 200 dose [PoM] £3.31 DT price = £3.31
Salbutamol 200 microgram per 1 dose Easyhaler Salbutamol sulfate 200micrograms/dose dry powder inhaler | 200 dose [PoM] £6.63 DT price = £6.63
▸ Salbulin Novolizer (Meda Pharmaceuticals Ltd)
Salbutamol (as Salbutamol sulfate) 100 microgram per 1 dose Salbulin Novolizer 100micrograms/dose inhalation powder | 200 dose [PoM] £4.95
Salbulin Novolizer 100micrograms/dose inhalation powder refill | 200 dose [PoM] £2.75
▸ Ventolin Accuhaler (GlaxoSmithKline UK Ltd)
Salbutamol 200 microgram per 1 dose Ventolin 200micrograms/dose Accuhaler | 60 dose [PoM] £3.00 DT price = £3.00

Nebuliser liquid
▸ Salbutamol (Non-proprietary)
Salbutamol (as Salbutamol sulfate) 1 mg per 1 ml Salbutamol 2.5mg/2.5ml nebuliser liquid unit dose vials | 20 unit dose [PoM] £7.00 DT price = £1.91
Salbutamol (as Salbutamol sulfate) 2 mg per 1 ml Salbutamol 5mg/2.5ml nebuliser liquid unit dose vials | 20 unit dose [PoM] £7.35 DT price = £3.82

‣ **Salamol Steri-Neb** (Teva UK Ltd)
  Salbutamol (as Salbutamol sulfate) 1 mg per 1 ml Salamol 2.5mg/2.5ml nebuliser liquid Steri-Neb unit dose vials | 20 unit dose [PoM] £1.91 DT price = £1.91
  Salbutamol (as Salbutamol sulfate) 2 mg per 1 ml Salamol 5mg/2.5ml nebuliser liquid Steri-Neb unit dose vials | 20 unit dose [PoM] £3.82 DT price = £3.82
‣ **Ventolin** (GlaxoSmithKline UK Ltd)
  Salbutamol (as Salbutamol sulfate) 5 mg per 1 ml Ventolin 5mg/ml respirator solution | 20 ml [PoM] £2.18 DT price = £2.18
‣ **Ventolin Nebules** (GlaxoSmithKline UK Ltd)
  Salbutamol (as Salbutamol sulfate) 1 mg per 1 ml Ventolin 2.5mg Nebules | 20 unit dose [PoM] £1.65 DT price = £1.91
  Salbutamol (as Salbutamol sulfate) 2 mg per 1 ml Ventolin 5mg Nebules | 20 unit dose [PoM] £2.78 DT price = £3.82

F 144

Terbutaline sulfate

● **INDICATIONS AND DOSE**

Acute asthma
‣ BY SUBCUTANEOUS INJECTION, OR BY SLOW INTRAVENOUS INJECTION
▸ Child 2-14 years: 10 micrograms/kg up to 4 times a day (max. per dose 300 micrograms), reserve intravenous beta$_2$ agonists for those in whom inhaled therapy cannot be used reliably or there is no current effect
▸ Child 15-17 years: 250–500 micrograms up to 4 times a day, reserve intravenous beta$_2$ agonists for those in whom inhaled therapy cannot be used reliably or there is no current effect
‣ BY CONTINUOUS INTRAVENOUS INFUSION
▸ Child: Loading dose 2–4 micrograms/kg, then 1–10 micrograms/kg/hour, dose to be adjusted according to response and heart rate, close monitoring is required for doses above 10 micrograms/kg/hour, reserve intravenous beta$_2$ agonists for those in whom inhaled therapy cannot be used reliably or there is no current effect

Moderate, severe, or life-threatening acute asthma
‣ BY INHALATION OF NEBULISED SOLUTION
▸ Child 1 month-4 years: 5 mg, repeat every 20–30 minutes or when required, give via oxygen-driven nebuliser if available
▸ Child 5-11 years: 5–10 mg, repeat every 20–30 minutes or when required, give via oxygen-driven nebuliser if available
▸ Child 12-17 years: 10 mg, repeat every 20–30 minutes or when required, give via oxygen-driven nebuliser if available

Exacerbation of reversible airways obstruction (including nocturnal asthma) | Prevention of exercise-induced bronchospasm
‣ BY INHALATION OF POWDER
▸ Child 5-17 years: 500 micrograms up to 4 times a day, for occasional use only
‣ BY MOUTH
▸ Child 1 month-6 years: 75 micrograms/kg 3 times a day (max. per dose 2.5 mg), administration by mouth is not recommended
▸ Child 7-14 years: 2.5 mg 2–3 times a day, administration by mouth is not recommended
▸ Child 15-17 years: Initially 2.5 mg 3 times a day, then increased if necessary to 5 mg 3 times a day, administration by mouth is not recommended

PHARMACOKINETICS
At recommended inhaled doses, the duration of action of terbutaline is about 3 to 5 hours.

● **UNLICENSED USE**
‣ With oral use Tablets not licensed for use in children under 7 years.
‣ With intravenous use or subcutaneous use Injection not licensed for use in children under 2 years.

● **SIDE-EFFECTS** Nausea

● **PREGNANCY** Inhaled drugs for asthma can be taken as normal during pregnancy.

● **BREAST FEEDING** Inhaled drugs for asthma can be taken as normal during breast-feeding.

● **DIRECTIONS FOR ADMINISTRATION**
‣ With intravenous use For *continuous intravenous infusion*, dilute to a concentration of 5 micrograms/mL with Glucose 5% or Sodium Chloride 0.9%; if fluid-restricted, dilute to a concentration of 100 micrograms/mL.
‣ When used by inhalation For *nebulisation*, dilute nebuliser solution with sterile Sodium Chloride 0.9% solution according to nebuliser type and duration of administration; terbutaline and ipratropium bromide solutions are compatible and may be mixed for nebulisation.

● **PATIENT AND CARER ADVICE**
‣ When used by inhalation For inhalation by dry powder, advise patients and carers not to exceed prescribed dose and to follow manufacturer's directions; if a previously effective dose of inhaled terbutaline fails to provide at least 3 hours relief, a doctor's advice should be obtained as soon as possible. For inhalation by nebuliser, the dose given by nebuliser is substantially higher than that given by inhaler. Patients should therefore be warned that it is dangerous to exceed the prescribed dose and they should seek medical advice if they fail to respond to the usual dose of the respirator solution.

● **MEDICINAL FORMS**
There can be variation in the licensing of different medicines containing the same drug. Forms available from special-order manufacturers include: solution for injection

Tablet
‣ **Bricanyl** (AstraZeneca UK Ltd)
  Terbutaline sulfate 5 mg Bricanyl 5mg tablets | 100 tablet [PoM] £4.91 DT price = £4.91

Oral solution
‣ **Bricanyl** (AstraZeneca UK Ltd)
  Terbutaline sulfate 300 microgram per 1 ml Bricanyl 1.5mg/5ml syrup sugar-free | 100 ml [PoM] £2.80 DT price = £2.80

Solution for injection
‣ **Bricanyl** (AstraZeneca UK Ltd)
  Terbutaline sulfate 500 microgram per 1 ml Bricanyl 2.5mg/5ml solution for injection ampoules | 10 ampoule [PoM] £16.74
  Bricanyl 500micrograms/1ml solution for injection ampoules | 5 ampoule [PoM] £2.16

Inhalation powder
‣ **Bricanyl Turbohaler** (AstraZeneca UK Ltd)
  Terbutaline sulfate 500 microgram per 1 dose Bricanyl 500micrograms/dose Turbohaler | 100 dose [PoM] £6.92 DT price = £6.92

Nebuliser liquid
‣ **Terbutaline sulfate** (Non-proprietary)
  Terbutaline sulfate 2.5 mg per 1 ml Terbutaline 5mg/2ml nebuliser liquid unit dose vials | 20 unit dose [PoM] £4.04 DT price = £4.04
‣ **Bricanyl Respules** (AstraZeneca UK Ltd)
  Terbutaline sulfate 2.5 mg per 1 ml Bricanyl 5mg/2ml Respules | 20 unit dose [PoM] £5.82 DT price = £4.04

CORTICOSTEROIDS

Airways disease, use of corticosteroids

Asthma

Inhaled corticosteroids

Corticosteroids are effective in the management of *asthma*; they reduce airway inflammation.

An inhaled corticosteroid is used regularly for prophylaxis of asthma when a child requires a beta$_2$ agonist more than twice a week, or if symptoms disturb sleep at least once a week, or if the child has suffered an exacerbation in the last 2 years requiring a systemic corticosteroid.

Current or previous smoking reduces the effectiveness of inhaled corticosteroids and higher doses may be necessary.

Corticosteroid inhalers must be used regularly for maximum benefit; alleviation of symptoms usually occurs 3 to 7 days after initiation but may take longer. Beclometasone dipropionate p. 150, budesonide p. 151, fluticasone p. 152, and mometasone furoate p. 154 appear to be equally effective. A spacer device should be used for administering inhaled corticosteroids in children under 15 years); a spacer device is also useful in children over 15 years, particularly if high doses are required.

In children 12–18 years using an inhaled corticosteroid and a long-acting beta$_2$ agonist for the prophylaxis of asthma, but who are poorly controlled, *Symbicort*® (budesonide with formoterol p. 152) may be used as a reliever (instead of a short-acting beta$_2$ agonist), in addition to its regular use for the prophylaxis of asthma [unlicensed]. *Symbicort*® can also be used in this way in children 12–18 years using an inhaled corticosteroid with a dose greater than 400 micrograms beclometasone dipropionate daily, but who are poorly controlled [unlicensed] (standard doses of other inhaled corticosteroids can be used). When starting this treatment, the total regular dose of inhaled corticosteroid should not be reduced. Children and their carers must be carefully instructed on the appropriate dose and management of exacerbations before initiating this treatment, preferably by a respiratory specialist. Children using budesonide with formoterol as a reliever once a day or more should have their treatment reviewed regularly. This management approach has not been investigated with combination inhalers containing other corticosteroids and long-acting beta$_2$ agonists.

High doses of inhaled corticosteroids can be prescribed for children who respond only partially to standard doses of an inhaled corticosteroid and a long-acting beta$_2$ agonist or to other long-acting bronchodilators. High doses should be continued only if there is clear benefit over the lower dose. The recommended maximum dose of an inhaled corticosteroid should not generally be exceeded; however, if a higher dose is required it should be initiated and supervised by a respiratory paediatrician. The use of high doses of an inhaled corticosteroid can minimise the requirement for an oral corticosteroid.

Oral corticosteroids

Systemic therapy may be required during periods of stress, such as during severe infections, or when airways obstruction or mucus prevent drug access to smaller airways.

An acute attack of asthma should be treated with a short course (3–5 days) of oral corticosteroid. The dose can usually be stopped abruptly but it should be reduced gradually in children under 12 years who have taken corticosteroids for more than 14 days. Tapering is not needed in children 12–18 years provided that the child receives an inhaled corticosteroid in an adequate dose (apart from those on maintenance oral corticosteroid treatment or where oral corticosteroids are required for 3 or more weeks).

In chronic continuing asthma, when the response to other drugs has been inadequate, longer term administration of an oral corticosteroid may be necessary; in such cases high doses of an inhaled corticosteroid should be continued to minimise oral corticosteroid requirements.

An oral corticosteroid should normally be taken as a single dose in the morning to reduce the disturbance to circadian cortisol secretion. Dosage should always be titrated to the lowest dose that controls symptoms. Some clinicians use alternate-day dosing of an oral corticosteroid.

Parenteral corticosteroids

Hydrocortisone injection p. 411 has a role in the emergency treatment of acute severe asthma.

Corticosteroids (inhaled)

- **INTERACTIONS** → Appendix 1 (corticosteroids). Interactions do not generally apply to corticosteroids used for inhalation unless specified.

- **SIDE-EFFECTS**
- ▸ **Very rare** Paradoxical bronchospasm
- ▸ **Frequency not known** Adrenal crisis (with prolonged high doses) · adrenal suppression (with prolonged high doses) · aggression · anxiety · behavioural changes · bruising · candidiasis of the mouth · candidiasis of the throat · cataracts · coma (with prolonged high doses) · Cushing's syndrome (with moon face, striae and acne) · depression · dysphonia · glaucoma (with prolonged high doses) · hoarseness · hyperactivity · hyperglycaemia (usually only with high doses) · irritability · reduced growth velocity · reduced mineral bone density (with long-term treatment of high doses) · side-effects applicable to systemic corticosteroids may also apply if absorption occurs following inhaled use · sleep disturbances · throat irritation

SIDE-EFFECTS, FURTHER INFORMATION

- ▸ Candidiasis The risk of oral candidiasis can be reduced by using a spacer device with the corticosteroid inhaler; rinsing the mouth with water after inhalation of a dose may also be helpful. An anti-fungal oral suspension or oral gel can be used to treat oral candidiasis without discontinuing corticosteroid therapy.

- ▸ Paradoxical bronchospasm The potential for paradoxical bronchospasm (calling for discontinuation and alternative therapy) should be borne in mind—mild bronchospasm may be prevented by inhalation of a short-acting beta$_2$ agonist beforehand (or by transfer from an aerosol inhalation to a dry powder inhalation).

- **PREGNANCY** Inhaled drugs for asthma can be taken as normal during pregnancy.

- **BREAST FEEDING** Inhaled corticosteroids for asthma can be taken as normal during breast-feeding.

- **MONITORING REQUIREMENTS** The height and weight of children receiving prolonged treatment with inhaled corticosteroids should be monitored annually; if growth is slowed, referral to a paediatrician should be considered.

- **NATIONAL FUNDING/ACCESS DECISIONS**

NICE technology appraisals (TAs)

- ▸ Inhaled corticosteroids for the treatment of chronic asthma in children under 12 years (November 2007) NICE TA131
For children under 12 years with chronic asthma in whom treatment with an inhaled corticosteroid is considered appropriate, the least costly product that is suitable for an individual child (taking into consideration NICE TAs 38 and 10), within its marketing authorisation, is recommended.

For children under 12 years with chronic asthma in whom treatment with an inhaled corticosteroid and a long-acting beta$_2$ agonist is considered appropriate, the following apply:

3

Respiratory system

- the use of a combination inhaler within its marketing authorisation is recommended as an option;
- the decision to use a combination inhaler or two agents in separate inhalers should be made on an individual basis, taking into consideration therapeutic need and the likelihood of treatment adherence;
- if a combination inhaler is chosen, then the least costly inhaler that is suitable for the individual child is recommended.

www.nice.org.uk/TA131

▸ **Inhaled corticosteroids for the treatment of chronic asthma in adults and children over 12 years (March 2008)** NICE TA138
For adults and children over 12 years with chronic asthma in whom treatment with an inhaled corticosteroid is considered appropriate, the least costly product that is suitable for an individual (taking into consideration NICE TAs 38 and 10), within its marketing authorisation is recommended.

For adults and children over 12 years with chronic asthma in whom treatment with an inhaled corticosteroid and a long-acting beta$_2$ agonist is considered appropriate, the following apply:

- the use of a combination inhaler within its marketing authorisation is recommended as an option;
- the decision to use a combination inhaler or two agents in separate inhalers should be made on an individual basis, taking into consideration therapeutic need, and the likelihood of treatment adherence;
- if a combination inhaler is chosen, then the least costly inhaler that is suitable for the individual is recommended.

www.nice.org.uk/TA138

▸ F 149

Beclometasone dipropionate

(Beclomethasone dipropionate)

● **INDICATIONS AND DOSE**
Prophylaxis of asthma
▸ BY INHALATION OF POWDER
▸ Child 5–11 years: 100–200 micrograms twice daily, dose to be adjusted as necessary
▸ Child 12–17 years: 200–400 micrograms twice daily; increased if necessary up to 800 micrograms twice daily, dose to be adjusted as necessary

ASMABEC CLICKHALER®
Prophylaxis of asthma
▸ BY INHALATION OF POWDER
▸ Child 6–11 years: 100–200 micrograms twice daily, dose to be adjusted as necessary
▸ Child 12–17 years: 100–400 micrograms twice daily (max. per dose 1 mg twice daily), dose to be adjusted as necessary

CLENIL MODULITE®
Prophylaxis of asthma
▸ BY INHALATION OF AEROSOL
▸ Child 2–11 years: 100–200 micrograms twice daily
▸ Child 12–17 years: 200–400 micrograms twice daily, adjusted according to response; increased if necessary up to 1 mg twice daily

QVAR® PREPARATIONS
Prophylaxis of asthma
▸ BY INHALATION OF AEROSOL
▸ Child 12–17 years: 50–200 micrograms twice daily; increased if necessary up to 400 micrograms twice daily

POTENCY
Qvar® has extra-fine particles, is more potent than traditional beclometasone dipropionate CFC-containing inhalers and is approximately twice as potent as *Clenil Modulite®*.

DOSE EQUIVALENCE AND CONVERSION
Dose adjustments may be required for some inhaler devices, see under individual preparations.

● **UNLICENSED USE** *Easyhaler® Beclometasone Dipropionate* is not licensed for use in children under 18 years. *Clenil Modulite®* -200 and -250 are not licensed for use in children under 12 years. *Qvar®* is not licensed for use in children under 12 years.

● **IMPORTANT SAFETY INFORMATION**
MHRA/CHM ADVICE (JULY 2008)
Beclometasone dipropionate CFC-free pressurised metered-dose inhalers (*Qvar®* and *Clenil Modulite®*) are **not** interchangeable and should be prescribed by brand name; *Qvar®* has extra-fine particles, is more potent than traditional beclometasone dipropionate CFC-containing inhalers, and is approximately twice as potent as *Clenil Modulite®*.

● **PRESCRIBING AND DISPENSING INFORMATION** The MHRA has advised (July 2008) that beclometasone dipropionate CFC-free inhalers should be prescribed by brand name.
CLENIL MODULITE® *Clenil Modulite®* is not interchangeable with other CFC-free beclometasone dipropionate inhalers.
QVAR® PREPARATIONS When switching a patient with well-controlled asthma from another corticosteroid inhaler, initially a 100-microgram metered dose of *Qvar®* should be prescribed for 200–250 micrograms of beclometasone dipropionate or budesonide and for 100 micrograms of fluticasone propionate. When switching a patient with poorly controlled asthma from another corticosteroid inhaler, initially a 100-microgram metered dose of *Qvar®* should be prescribed for 100 micrograms of beclometasone dipropionate, budesonide, or fluticasone propionate; the dose of *Qvar®* should be adjusted according to response.

● **PATIENT AND CARER ADVICE** Steroid card should be issued with high doses of inhaled beclometasone dipropionate. Medicines for Children leaflet: Beclometasone for asthma prevention (prophylaxis)
www.medicinesforchildren.org.uk/
beclometasone-inhaler-asthma-prevention-prophylaxis-0

● **PROFESSION SPECIFIC INFORMATION**
Dental practitioners' formulary
Clenil Modulite® 50 micrograms/metered inhalation may be prescribed.

● **MEDICINAL FORMS**
There can be variation in the licensing of different medicines containing the same drug.
Pressurised inhalation
CAUTIONARY AND ADVISORY LABELS 8, 10
▸ **Beclometasone dipropionate (Non-proprietary)**
Beclometasone dipropionate 50 microgram per 1 dose Beclometasone 50micrograms/dose inhaler CFC free | 200 dose [PoM] no price available
Beclometasone dipropionate 100 microgram per 1 dose Beclometasone 100micrograms/dose inhaler CFC free | 200 dose [PoM] £54.20
Beclometasone dipropionate 200 microgram per 1 dose Beclometasone 200micrograms/dose inhaler CFC free | 200 dose [PoM] no price available
▸ **Clenil Modulite** (Chiesi Ltd)
Beclometasone dipropionate 50 microgram per 1 dose Clenil Modulite 50micrograms/dose inhaler | 200 dose [PoM] £3.70
Beclometasone dipropionate 100 microgram per 1 dose Clenil Modulite 100micrograms/dose inhaler | 200 dose [PoM] £7.42
Beclometasone dipropionate 200 microgram per 1 dose Clenil Modulite 200micrograms/dose inhaler | 200 dose [PoM] £16.17
Beclometasone dipropionate 250 microgram per 1 dose Clenil Modulite 250micrograms/dose inhaler | 200 dose [PoM] £16.29

▸ **Qvar** (Teva UK Ltd)
Beclometasone dipropionate 50 microgram per 1 dose Qvar 50 inhaler | 200 dose PoM £7.87
Beclometasone dipropionate 100 microgram per 1 dose Qvar 100 inhaler | 200 dose PoM £17.21
▸ **Qvar Autohaler** (Teva UK Ltd)
Beclometasone dipropionate 50 microgram per 1 dose Qvar 50 Autohaler | 200 dose PoM £7.87 DT price = £7.87
Beclometasone dipropionate 100 microgram per 1 dose Qvar 100 Autohaler | 200 dose PoM £17.21 DT price = £17.21
▸ **Qvar Easi-Breathe** (Teva UK Ltd)
Beclometasone dipropionate 50 microgram per 1 dose Qvar 50micrograms/dose Easi-Breathe inhaler | 200 dose PoM £7.74 DT price = £7.87
Beclometasone dipropionate 100 microgram per 1 dose Qvar 100micrograms/dose Easi-Breathe inhaler | 200 dose PoM £16.95 DT price = £17.21

Inhalation powder
CAUTIONARY AND ADVISORY LABELS 8, 10
▸ **Asmabec Clickhaler** (Focus Pharmaceuticals Ltd)
Beclometasone dipropionate 100 microgram per 1 dose Asmabec 100 Clickhaler | 200 dose PoM £9.81
▸ **Easyhaler (beclometasone)** (Orion Pharma (UK) Ltd)
Beclometasone dipropionate 200 microgram per 1 dose Easyhaler Beclometasone 200micrograms/dose dry powder inhaler | 200 dose PoM £14.93

⬏ 149

Budesonide

● **INDICATIONS AND DOSE**
Bronchopulmonary dysplasia with spontaneous respiration
▸ BY INHALATION OF NEBULISED SUSPENSION
▸ **Neonate:** 500 micrograms twice daily.

▸ **Child 1–4 months:** 500 micrograms twice daily
Bronchopulmonary dysplasia with spontaneous respiration (severe symptoms)
▸ BY INHALATION OF NEBULISED SUSPENSION
▸ **Child 1–4 months (body-weight 2.5 kg and above):** 1 mg twice daily
Prophylaxis of mild to moderate asthma (in patients stabilised on twice daily dose)
▸ BY INHALATION OF POWDER
▸ **Child 6–11 years:** 200–400 micrograms once daily, dose to be given in the evening
▸ **Child 12–17 years:** 200–400 micrograms once daily (max. per dose 800 micrograms), dose to be given in the evening
Prophylaxis of asthma
▸ BY INHALATION OF POWDER
▸ **Child 6–11 years:** 100–400 micrograms twice daily, dose to be adjusted as necessary
▸ **Child 12–17 years:** 100–800 micrograms twice daily, dose to be adjusted as necessary
▸ BY INHALATION OF NEBULISED SUSPENSION
▸ **Child 6 months–11 years:** 125–500 micrograms twice daily, adjusted according to response; maximum 2 mg per day
▸ **Child 12–17 years:** Initially 0.25–1 mg twice daily, adjusted according to response, doses higher than recommended max. may be used in severe disease; maximum 2 mg per day
BUDELIN NOVOLIZER®
Prophylaxis of asthma
▸ BY INHALATION OF POWDER
▸ **Child 6–11 years:** 200–400 micrograms twice daily, dose is adjusted as necessary
▸ **Child 12–17 years:** 200–800 micrograms twice daily, dose is adjusted as necessary

Alternative in mild to moderate asthma, for patients previously stabilised on a twice daily dose
▸ BY INHALATION OF POWDER
▸ **Child 6–11 years:** 200–400 micrograms once daily, to be taken in the evening
▸ **Child 12–17 years:** 200–400 micrograms once daily (max. per dose 800 micrograms), to be taken in the evening
PULMICORT® RESPULES
Prophylaxis of asthma
▸ BY INHALATION OF NEBULISED SUSPENSION
▸ **Child 3 months–11 years:** Initially 0.5–1 mg twice daily, reduced to 250–500 micrograms twice daily
▸ **Child 12–17 years:** Initially 1–2 mg twice daily, reduced to 0.5–1 mg twice daily
Croup
▸ BY INHALATION OF NEBULISED SUSPENSION
▸ **Child:** 2 mg for 1 dose, alternatively 1 mg for 2 doses separated by a 30 minute interval, dose may be repeated every 12 hours until clinical improvement
PULMICORT® TURBOHALER
Prophylaxis of asthma
▸ BY INHALATION OF POWDER
▸ **Child 5–11 years:** 100–400 micrograms twice daily, dose to be adjusted as necessary
▸ **Child 12–17 years:** 100–800 micrograms twice daily, dose to be adjusted as necessary
Alternative in mild to moderate asthma, for patients previously stabilised on a twice daily dose
▸ BY INHALATION OF POWDER
▸ **Child 5–11 years:** 200–400 micrograms once daily, to be taken in the evening
▸ **Child 12–17 years:** 200–400 micrograms once daily (max. per dose 800 micrograms), to be taken in the evening
POTENCY
Dose adjustments may be required for some inhaler devices, see under individual preparations.

● **UNLICENSED USE** *Pulmicort® nebuliser solution* not licensed for use in children under 3 months; not licensed for use in bronchopulmonary dysplasia.

● **DIRECTIONS FOR ADMINISTRATION** Budesonide nebuliser suspension is not suitable for use in ultrasonic nebulisers.

● **PATIENT AND CARER ADVICE** With high doses, a steroid card should be supplied. Patients or carers should be given advice on how to administer budesonide dry powder inhaler and nebuliser suspension.
Medicines for Children leaflet: Budesonide inhaler for asthma prevention (prophylaxis) www.medicinesforchildren.org.uk/budesonide-inhaler-asthma-prevention-prophylaxis

BUDELIN NOVOLIZER® Patients or carers should be given advice on adminstration of *Budelin NovolizerA®*.

● **MEDICINAL FORMS**
There can be variation in the licensing of different medicines containing the same drug.
Inhalation powder
CAUTIONARY AND ADVISORY LABELS 8, 10
▸ **Budelin Novolizer** (Meda Pharmaceuticals Ltd)
Budesonide 200 microgram per 1 dose Budelin Novolizer 200micrograms/dose inhalation powder | 100 dose PoM £14.86
Budelin Novolizer 200micrograms/dose inhalation powder refill | 100 dose PoM £9.59
▸ **Easyhaler (budesonide)** (Orion Pharma (UK) Ltd)
Budesonide 100 microgram per 1 dose Easyhaler Budesonide 100micrograms/dose dry powder inhaler | 200 dose PoM £8.86 DT price = £11.84
Budesonide 200 microgram per 1 dose Easyhaler Budesonide 200micrograms/dose dry powder inhaler | 200 dose PoM £17.71
Budesonide 400 microgram per 1 dose Easyhaler Budesonide 400micrograms/dose dry powder inhaler | 100 dose PoM £17.71

▸ **Pulmicort Turbohaler** (AstraZeneca UK Ltd)
Budesonide 100 microgram per 1 dose Pulmicort 100 Turbohaler | 200 dose [PoM] £11.84 DT price = £11.84
Budesonide 200 microgram per 1 dose Pulmicort 200 Turbohaler | 100 dose [PoM] £11.84 DT price = £11.84
Budesonide 400 microgram per 1 dose Pulmicort 400 Turbohaler | 50 dose [PoM] £13.86 DT price = £13.86

Nebuliser liquid
CAUTIONARY AND ADVISORY LABELS 8, 10
▸ **Budesonide** (Non-proprietary)
Budesonide 250 microgram per 1 ml Budesonide 500micrograms/2ml nebuliser liquid unit dose vials | 20 unit dose [PoM] £63.00 DT price = £24.70
Budesonide 500 microgram per 1 ml Budesonide 1mg/2ml nebuliser liquid unit dose vials | 20 unit dose [PoM] £42.41 DT price = £34.62
▸ **Pulmicort Respules** (AstraZeneca UK Ltd)
Budesonide 250 microgram per 1 ml Pulmicort 0.5mg Respules | 20 unit dose [PoM] £26.42 DT price = £24.70
Budesonide 500 microgram per 1 ml Pulmicort 1mg Respules | 20 unit dose [PoM] £40.00 DT price = £34.62

Budesonide with formoterol

The properties listed below are those particular to the combination only. For the properties of the components please consider, budesonide p. 151, formoterol fumarate p. 144.

● INDICATIONS AND DOSE
SYMBICORT 100/6 TURBOHALER®
Asthma, maintenance therapy
▸ BY INHALATION OF POWDER
▸ Child 6-17 years: Initially 1–2 puffs twice daily; reduced to 1 puff daily, dose reduced only if control is maintained

Asthma, maintenance and reliever therapy
▸ BY INHALATION OF POWDER
▸ Child 12-17 years: Maintenance 2 puffs daily in 1–2 divided doses; 1 puff as required for relief of symptoms, increased if necessary up to 6 puffs as required; maximum 8 puffs per day

SYMBICORT 200/6 TURBOHALER®
Asthma, maintenance therapy
▸ BY INHALATION OF POWDER
▸ Child 12-17 years: Initially 1–2 puffs twice daily; reduced to 1 puff daily, dose reduced only if control is maintained

Asthma, maintenance and reliever therapy
▸ BY INHALATION OF POWDER
▸ Child 12-17 years: Maintenance 2 puffs daily in 1–2 divided doses, increased if necessary to 2 puffs twice daily; 1 puff as required for relief of symptoms, increased if necessary up to 6 puffs as required; maximum 8 puffs per day

SYMBICORT 400/12 TURBOHALER®
Asthma, maintenance therapy
▸ BY INHALATION OF POWDER
▸ Child 12-17 years: Initially 1 puff twice daily; reduced to 1 puff daily, dose reduced only if control is maintained

● UNLICENSED USE
SYMBICORT 100/6 TURBOHALER®
Symbicort® not licensed for use in children for asthma maintenance and reliever therapy.
SYMBICORT 200/6 TURBOHALER®
Symbicort® not licensed for use in children for asthma maintenance and reliever therapy.

● PATIENT AND CARER ADVICE With high doses, a steroid card should be supplied.

Patients counselling is advised for budesonide with formoterol dry powder inhalation (administration).

● MEDICINAL FORMS
There can be variation in the licensing of different medicines containing the same drug.
Inhalation powder
CAUTIONARY AND ADVISORY LABELS 8, 10 (high doses)
▸ **Symbicort Turbohaler** (AstraZeneca UK Ltd)
Formoterol fumarate dihydrate 6 microgram per 1 dose, Budesonide 100 microgram per 1 dose Symbicort 100/6 Turbohaler | 120 dose [PoM] £33.00 DT price = £33.00
Formoterol fumarate dihydrate 6 microgram per 1 dose, Budesonide 200 microgram per 1 dose Symbicort 200/6 Turbohaler | 120 dose [PoM] £38.00 DT price = £38.00
Formoterol fumarate dihydrate 12 microgram per 1 dose, Budesonide 400 microgram per 1 dose Symbicort 400/12 Turbohaler | 60 dose [PoM] £38.00 DT price = £38.00

▶ 149

Ciclesonide

● INDICATIONS AND DOSE
Prophylaxis of asthma
▸ BY INHALATION OF AEROSOL
▸ Child 12-17 years: 160 micrograms once daily; reduced to 80 micrograms daily, if control maintained

● SIDE-EFFECTS Nausea · taste disturbance

● PATIENT AND CARER ADVICE Patients or carers should be given advice on how to administer ciclesonide aerosol inhaler.

● MEDICINAL FORMS
There can be variation in the licensing of different medicines containing the same drug.
Pressurised inhalation
CAUTIONARY AND ADVISORY LABELS 8
▸ **Alvesco** (Takeda UK Ltd)
Ciclesonide 80 microgram per 1 dose Alvesco 80 inhaler | 120 dose [PoM] £32.83 DT price = £32.83
Ciclesonide 160 microgram per 1 dose Alvesco 160 inhaler | 60 dose [PoM] £19.31 DT price = £19.31 | 120 dose [PoM] £38.62 DT price = £38.62

▶ 149

Fluticasone

4.1.2016

● INDICATIONS AND DOSE
Prophylaxis of asthma
▸ BY INHALATION OF POWDER
▸ Child 5-15 years: Initially 50–100 micrograms twice daily (max. per dose 200 micrograms twice daily), dose to be adjusted as necessary
▸ Child 16-17 years: Initially 100–500 micrograms twice daily (max. per dose 1 mg twice daily), dose may be increased according to severity of asthma. Doses above 500 micrograms twice daily initiated by a specialist
▸ BY INHALATION OF AEROSOL
▸ Child 4-15 years: Initially 50–100 micrograms twice daily (max. per dose 200 micrograms twice daily), dose to be adjusted as necessary
▸ Child 16-17 years: Initially 100–500 micrograms twice daily (max. per dose 1 mg twice daily), dose may be increased according to severity of asthma. Doses above 500 micrograms twice daily initiated by a specialist
▸ BY INHALATION OF NEBULISED SUSPENSION
▸ Child 4-15 years: 1 mg twice daily
▸ Child 16-17 years: 0.5–2 mg twice daily

● SIDE-EFFECTS Arthralgia · dyspepsia

● DIRECTIONS FOR ADMINISTRATION Fluticasone nebuliser liquid may be diluted with sterile sodium chloride 0.9%. It is not suitable for use in ultrasonic nebulisers.

- **PATIENT AND CARER ADVICE** With high doses, a steroid card should be supplied.

   Patients or carers should be given advice on how to administer all fluticasone inhalations preparations. Medicines for Children leaflet: Fluticasone inhaler for asthma prevention (prophylaxis) www.medicinesforchildren.org.uk/fluticasone-inhaler-for-asthma-prevention

- **MEDICINAL FORMS**
   There can be variation in the licensing of different medicines containing the same drug.
   Pressurised inhalation
   CAUTIONARY AND ADVISORY LABELS 8, 10
   ▸ Flixotide Evohaler (GlaxoSmithKline UK Ltd)
   Fluticasone propionate 50 microgram per 1 dose Flixotide 50micrograms/dose Evohaler | 120 dose [PoM] £5.44 DT price = £5.44
   Fluticasone propionate 125 microgram per 1 dose Flixotide 125micrograms/dose Evohaler | 120 dose [PoM] £21.26 DT price = £21.26
   Fluticasone propionate 250 microgram per 1 dose Flixotide 250micrograms/dose Evohaler | 120 dose [PoM] £36.14 DT price = £36.14

   Inhalation powder
   CAUTIONARY AND ADVISORY LABELS 8, 10
   ▸ Flixotide Accuhaler (GlaxoSmithKline UK Ltd)
   Fluticasone propionate 50 microgram per 1 dose Flixotide 50micrograms/dose Accuhaler | 60 dose [PoM] £6.38 DT price = £6.38
   Fluticasone propionate 100 microgram per 1 dose Flixotide 100micrograms/dose Accuhaler | 60 dose [PoM] £8.93 DT price = £8.93
   Fluticasone propionate 250 microgram per 1 dose Flixotide 250micrograms/dose Accuhaler | 60 dose [PoM] £21.26 DT price = £21.26
   Fluticasone propionate 500 microgram per 1 dose Flixotide 500micrograms/dose Accuhaler | 60 dose [PoM] £36.14 DT price = £36.14

   Nebuliser liquid
   CAUTIONARY AND ADVISORY LABELS 8, 10
   ▸ Flixotide Nebule (GlaxoSmithKline UK Ltd)
   Fluticasone propionate 250 microgram per 1 ml Flixotide 0.5mg/2ml Nebules | 10 unit dose [PoM] £9.34
   Fluticasone propionate 1 mg per 1 ml Flixotide 2mg/2ml Nebules | 10 unit dose [PoM] £37.35

Fluticasone with formoterol

The properties listed below are those particular to the combination only. For the properties of the components please consider, fluticasone p. 152, formoterol fumarate p. 144.

- **INDICATIONS AND DOSE**
   FLUTIFORM® 50
   Prophylaxis of asthma
   ▸ BY INHALATION OF AEROSOL
   ▸ Child 12-17 years: 2 puffs twice daily
   FLUTIFORM® 125
   Prophylaxis of asthma
   ▸ BY INHALATION OF AEROSOL
   ▸ Child 12-17 years: 2 puffs twice daily

- **PATIENT AND CARER ADVICE** With high doses, a steroid card should be provided.

   Patients or carers should be given advice on how to administer fluticasone with formoterol aerosol inhalation.

- **MEDICINAL FORMS**
   There can be variation in the licensing of different medicines containing the same drug.
   Pressurised inhalation
   CAUTIONARY AND ADVISORY LABELS 8, 10 (high doses)
   ▸ Flutiform (Napp Pharmaceuticals Ltd)
   Formoterol fumarate dihydrate 5 microgram per 1 dose, Fluticasone propionate 50 microgram per 1 dose Flutiform

50micrograms/dose / 5micrograms/dose inhaler | 120 dose [PoM] £14.40 DT price = £14.40
Formoterol fumarate dihydrate 5 microgram per 1 dose, Fluticasone propionate 125 microgram per 1 dose Flutiform 125micrograms/dose / 5micrograms/dose inhaler | 120 dose [PoM] £28.00 DT price = £28.00

Fluticasone with salmeterol

The properties listed below are those particular to the combination only. For the properties of the components please consider, fluticasone p. 152, salmeterol p. 145.

- **INDICATIONS AND DOSE**
   SERETIDE 100 ACCUHALER®
   Prophylaxis of asthma
   ▸ BY INHALATION OF POWDER
   ▸ Child 5-17 years: 1 inhalation twice daily, reduced to 1 inhalation daily, use reduced dose only if control maintained

   SERETIDE 250 ACCUHALER®
   Prophylaxis of asthma
   ▸ BY INHALATION OF POWDER
   ▸ Child 12-17 years: 1 inhalation twice daily

   SERETIDE 500 ACCUHALER®
   Prophylaxis of asthma
   ▸ BY INHALATION OF POWDER
   ▸ Child 12-17 years: 1 inhalation twice daily

   SERETIDE 50 EVOHALER®
   Prophylaxis of asthma
   ▸ BY INHALATION OF AEROSOL
   ▸ Child 5-17 years: 2 puffs twice daily, reduced to 2 puffs once daily, use reduced dose only if control maintained

   SERETIDE 125 EVOHALER®
   Prophylaxis of asthma
   ▸ BY INHALATION OF AEROSOL
   ▸ Child 12-17 years: 2 puffs twice daily

   SERETIDE 250 EVOHALER®
   Prophylaxis of asthma
   ▸ BY INHALATION OF AEROSOL
   ▸ Child 12-17 years: 2 puffs twice daily

- **PATIENT AND CARER ADVICE** With preparations containing greater than 100 micrograms fluticasone, a steroid card should be provided.

   Patients or carers should be given advice on how to administer fluticasone with salmeterol dry powder inhalation and aerosol inhalation.

- **MEDICINAL FORMS**
   There can be variation in the licensing of different medicines containing the same drug.
   Pressurised inhalation
   CAUTIONARY AND ADVISORY LABELS 8, 10 (excluding Seretide 50 Evohaler®)
   ▸ Seretide Evohaler (GlaxoSmithKline UK Ltd)
   Salmeterol (as Salmeterol xinafoate) 25 microgram per 1 dose, Fluticasone propionate 50 microgram per 1 dose Seretide 50 Evohaler | 120 dose [PoM] £18.00 DT price = £18.00
   Salmeterol (as Salmeterol xinafoate) 25 microgram per 1 dose, Fluticasone propionate 125 microgram per 1 dose Seretide 125 Evohaler | 120 dose [PoM] £35.00 DT price = £35.00
   Salmeterol (as Salmeterol xinafoate) 25 microgram per 1 dose, Fluticasone propionate 250 microgram per 1 dose Seretide 250 Evohaler | 120 dose [PoM] £59.48 DT price = £59.48

Inhalation powder

CAUTIONARY AND ADVISORY LABELS 8, 10 (excluding Seretide 100 Accuhaler®)
- ▸ **Seretide Accuhaler** (GlaxoSmithKline UK Ltd)
  Salmeterol (as Salmeterol xinafoate) 50 microgram per 1 dose, Fluticasone propionate 100 microgram per 1 dose Seretide 100 Accuhaler | 60 dose [PoM] £18.00 DT price = £18.00
  Salmeterol (as Salmeterol xinafoate) 50 microgram per 1 dose, Fluticasone propionate 250 microgram per 1 dose Seretide 250 Accuhaler | 60 dose [PoM] £35.00 DT price = £35.00
  Salmeterol (as Salmeterol xinafoate) 50 microgram per 1 dose, Fluticasone propionate 500 microgram per 1 dose Seretide 500 Accuhaler | 60 dose [PoM] £40.92 DT price = £40.92

Fluticasone with vilanterol

The properties listed below are those particular to the combination only. For the properties of the components please consider, fluticasone p. 152.

- ● **INDICATIONS AND DOSE**
  RELVAR ELLIPTA® 184 MICROGRAMS/22 MICROGRAMS
  Prophylaxis of asthma
  - ▸ BY INHALATION OF POWDER
  - ▸ Child 12–17 years: 1 inhalation once daily
  RELVAR ELLIPTA® 92 MICROGRAMS/22 MICROGRAMS
  Prophylaxis of asthma
  - ▸ BY INHALATION OF POWDER
  - ▸ Child 12–17 years: 1 inhalation once daily
  DOSE EQUIVALENCE AND CONVERSION
  RELVAR ELLIPTA® 184 MICROGRAMS/22 MICROGRAMS
  1 inhalation (delivered dose) of fluticasone *furoate* 184 micrograms once daily is approximately equivalent to fluticasone *propionate* 500 micrograms twice daily.
  RELVAR ELLIPTA® 92 MICROGRAMS/22 MICROGRAMS
  1 inhalation (delivered dose) of fluticasone *furoate* 92 micrograms once daily is approximately equivalent to fluticasone *propionate* 250 micrograms twice daily.

- ● **SIDE-EFFECTS** Abdominal pain · back pain
- ● **PREGNANCY** Manufacturer advises use only if potential benefit outweighs risk.
- ● **BREAST FEEDING** Manufacturer advises avoid—no information available.
- ● **HEPATIC IMPAIRMENT** Max. dose fluticasone furoate 92 micrograms, vilanterol 22 micrograms.
  RELVAR ELLIPTA®
  184 MICROGRAMS/22 MICROGRAMS Avoid in moderate to severe impairment.
- ● **PATIENT AND CARER ADVICE** A steroid card should be provided.
  Patients or carers should be given advice on how to administer fluticasone with vilanterol powder for inhalation.

- ● **MEDICINAL FORMS**
  There can be variation in the licensing of different medicines containing the same drug.
  Inhalation powder
  CAUTIONARY AND ADVISORY LABELS 8, 10
  - ▸ **Relvar Ellipta** (GlaxoSmithKline UK Ltd) ▼
    Vilanterol 22 microgram per 1 dose, Fluticasone furoate 92 microgram per 1 dose Relvar Ellipta 92micrograms/dose / 22micrograms/dose dry powder inhaler | 30 dose [PoM] £22.00
    Vilanterol 22 microgram per 1 dose, Fluticasone furoate 184 microgram per 1 dose Relvar Ellipta 184micrograms/dose / 22micrograms/dose dry powder inhaler | 30 dose [PoM] £29.50

⌐ 149

Mometasone furoate

- ● **INDICATIONS AND DOSE**
  Prophylaxis of asthma
  - ▸ BY INHALATION OF POWDER
  - ▸ Child 12–17 years: Initially 400 micrograms daily in 1–2 divided doses, single dose to be inhaled in the evening, reduced to 200 micrograms once daily, if control maintained
  Prophylaxis of severe asthma
  - ▸ BY INHALATION OF POWDER
  - ▸ Child 12–17 years: Increased if necessary up to 400 micrograms twice daily

- ● **SIDE-EFFECTS**
- ▸ **Common or very common** Headache
- ▸ **Uncommon** Dyspepsia · palpitation · weight gain
- ● **PATIENT AND CARER ADVICE**
  Patients or carers should be given advice on how to administer mometasone by inhaler. With high doses, a steroid card should be supplied.
  Medicines for Children leaflet: Mometasone furoate inhaler for asthma prevention (prophylaxis) www.medicinesforchildren.org.uk/mometasone-furoate-inhaler-for-asthma-prevention-prophylaxis

- ● **NATIONAL FUNDING/ACCESS DECISIONS**
  Scottish Medicines Consortium (SMC) Decisions
  The *Scottish Medicines Consortium* has advised (November 2003) that *Asmanex*® is restricted for use following failure of first-line inhaled corticosteroids.

- ● **MEDICINAL FORMS**
  There can be variation in the licensing of different medicines containing the same drug.
  Inhalation powder
  CAUTIONARY AND ADVISORY LABELS 8, 10
  - ▸ **Asmanex Twisthaler** (Merck Sharp & Dohme Ltd)
    Mometasone furoate 200 microgram per 1 dose Asmanex 200micrograms/dose Twisthaler | 30 dose [PoM] £15.70 DT price = £15.70 | 60 dose [PoM] £23.54 DT price = £23.54
    Mometasone furoate 400 microgram per 1 dose Asmanex 400micrograms/dose Twisthaler | 30 dose [PoM] £21.78 DT price = £21.78 | 60 dose [PoM] £36.05 DT price = £36.05

DRUGS FOR RESPIRATORY DISEASES ⟩
MONOCLONAL ANTIBODIES

Omalizumab

- ● **INDICATIONS AND DOSE**
  Prophylaxis of severe persistent allergic asthma
  - ▸ BY SUBCUTANEOUS INJECTION
  - ▸ Child 6–17 years: Dose according to immunoglobulin E concentration and body-weight (consult product literature)
  Add-on therapy for chronic spontaneous urticaria in patients who have had an inadequate response to H_1 antihistamine treatment
  - ▸ BY SUBCUTANEOUS INJECTION
  - ▸ Child 12–17 years: 300 mg every 4 weeks

- ● **CAUTIONS** Autoimmune disease · susceptibility to helminth infection—discontinue if infection does not respond to anthelmintic
- ● **SIDE-EFFECTS**
- ▸ **Common or very common** Abdominal pain · arthralgia · headache · injection-site reactions · pyrexia · sinusitis · upper respiratory tract infection
- ▸ **Uncommon** Bronchospasm · cough · diarrhoea · dizziness · drowsiness · dyspepsia · flushing · influenza-like illness · malaise · nausea · paraesthesia · pharyngitis ·

photosensitivity · postural hypotension · pruritus · rash · syncope · urticaria · weight gain

▶ **Rare** Angioedema · antibody formation · laryngoedema · parasitic infection

▶ **Frequency not known** Alopecia · arterial thromboembolic events · Churg-Strauss syndrome · joint swelling · myalgia · serum sickness (including fever and lymphadenopathy) · thrombocytopenia

SIDE-EFFECTS, FURTHER INFORMATION

▶ Churg-Strauss syndrome Churg-Strauss syndrome has occurred rarely in patients given omalizumab; the reaction is usually associated with the reduction of oral corticosteroid therapy. Churg-Strauss syndrome can present as eosinophilia, vasculitic rash, cardiac complications, worsening pulmonary symptoms, or peripheral neuropathy.

▶ Hypersensitivity reactions Hypersensitivity reactions can also occur immediately following treatment with omalizumab or sometimes more than 24 hours after the first injection.

● **PREGNANCY** Manufacturer advises avoid unless essential—crosses the placenta.

● **BREAST FEEDING** Manufacturer advises avoid—present in milk in *animal* studies.

● **HEPATIC IMPAIRMENT** Manufacturer advises caution—no information available.

● **RENAL IMPAIRMENT** Manufacturer advises caution—no information available.

● **NATIONAL FUNDING/ACCESS DECISIONS**

NICE technology appraisals (TAs)

▶ **Omalizumab for severe persistent allergic asthma (April 2013)** NICE TA278

Omalizumab is recommended as an option for treating severe persistent confirmed allergic IgE-mediated asthma as an add-on to optimised standard therapy in patients aged 6 years and over:

● who need continuous or frequent treatment with oral corticosteroids (defined as 4 or more courses in the previous year), **and**

● only if the manufacturer makes omalizumab available with the discount agreed in the patient access scheme.

Optimised standard therapy is defined as a full trial of and, if tolerated, documented compliance with inhaled high-dose corticosteroids, long-acting beta$_2$ agonists, leukotriene receptor antagonists, theophyllines, oral corticosteroids, and smoking cessation if clinically appropriate.

Patients currently receiving omalizumab whose disease does not meet the criteria should be able to continue treatment until they and their clinician consider it appropriate to stop.

www.nice.org.uk/TA278

▶ **Omalizumab for previously treated chronic spontaneous urticaria (June 2015)** NICE TA339

Omalizumab is an option as add-on therapy for the treatment of severe chronic spontaneous urticaria in patients 12 years and over, only if:

● the severity of the condition is assessed objectively, for example, using a weekly urticaria activity score of 28 or more,

● the patient's condition has not responded to standard treatment with H$_1$-antihistamines and leukotriene receptor antagonists,

● omalizumab is stopped at or before the fourth dose if the condition has not responded,

● omalizumab is stopped at the end of a course of treatment (6 doses) if the condition has responded and is restarted only if the condition relapses,

● omalizumab is administered under the management of a secondary care specialist in dermatology, immunology or allergy,

● the manufacturer provides omalizumab with the discount agreed in the patient access scheme.

Patients currently receiving omalizumab whose disease does not meet the above criteria should have the option to continue treatment until they and their clinician consider it appropriate to stop.

www.nice.org.uk/TA339

Scottish Medicines Consortium (SMC) Decisions

The *Scottish Medicines Consortium* has advised (December 2014) that omalizumab (*Xolair*®) is accepted for restricted use within NHS Scotland for the treatment of chronic spontaneous urticaria in patients aged 12 years and over, who have had an inadequate response to combination therapy with H$_1$-antihistamines, leukotriene receptor antagonists and H$_2$-antihistamines, used according to current treatment guidelines.

● **MEDICINAL FORMS**

There can be variation in the licensing of different medicines containing the same drug.

Solution for injection

▶ Xolair (Novartis Pharmaceuticals UK Ltd)

Omalizumab 150 mg per 1 ml Xolair 150mg/1ml solution for injection pre-filled syringes | 1 pre-filled disposable injection PoM £256.15

Xolair 75mg/0.5ml solution for injection pre-filled syringes | 1 pre-filled disposable injection PoM £128.07

LEUKOTRIENE RECEPTOR ANTAGONISTS

Leukotriene receptor antagonists

The leukotriene receptor antagonists, montelukast below and zafirlukast p. 156, block the effects of cysteinyl leukotrienes in the airways; they can be used in children for the management of chronic asthma with an inhaled corticosteroid or as an alternative if an inhaled corticosteroid cannot be used.

Montelukast has not been shown to be more effective than a standard dose of inhaled corticosteroid, but the two drugs appear to have an additive effect. The leukotriene receptor antagonists may be of benefit in exercise- induced asthma and in those with concomitant rhinitis, but they are less effective in children with severe asthma who are also receiving high doses of other drugs.

There is some limited evidence to support the intermittent use of montelukast in children under 12 years with episodic wheeze associated with viral infections [unlicensed use]. Treatment is started at the onset of either asthma symptoms or of coryzal symptoms and continued for 7 days; there is no evidence to support this use in moderate or severe asthma.

Montelukast

● **INDICATIONS AND DOSE**

Prophylaxis of asthma

▶ BY MOUTH

▶ Child 6 months-5 years: 4 mg once daily, dose to be taken in the evening

▶ Child 6-14 years: 5 mg once daily, dose to be taken in the evening

▶ Child 15-17 years: 10 mg once daily, dose to be taken in the evening

Symptomatic relief of seasonal allergic rhinitis in patients with asthma.

▶ BY MOUTH

▶ Child 15-17 years: 10 mg once daily, dose to be taken in the evening

● **INTERACTIONS** → Appendix 1 (leukotriene receptor antagonists).

- **SIDE-EFFECTS**
- ▸ **Common or very common** Abdominal pain · headache · hyperkinesia (in young children) · thirst
- ▸ **Uncommon** Abnormal dreams · aggressive behaviour · agitation · anxiety · arthralgia · bruising · depression · dizziness · drowsiness · dry mouth · dyspepsia · epistaxis · hostility · hypoaesthesia · irritability · malaise · muscle cramps · myalgia · oedema · paraesthesia · psychomotor hyperactivity · restlessness · seizures · sleep disturbances · sleep-walking
- ▸ **Rare** Disturbance in attention · increased bleeding tendency · memory impairment · palpitation · tremor
- ▸ **Very rare** Churg-Strauss syndrome · disorientation · erythema multiforme · erythema nodosum · hallucinations · hepatic disorders · hepatic eosinophilic infiltration · suicidal behaviour · suicidal thoughts

SIDE-EFFECTS, FURTHER INFORMATION
Churg-Strauss syndrome has occurred very rarely in association with the use of montelukast; in many of the reported cases the reaction followed the reduction or withdrawal of oral corticosteroid therapy. Prescribers should be alert to the development of eosinophilia, vasculitic rash, worsening pulmonary symptoms, cardiac complications, or peripheral neuropathy.

- **PREGNANCY** Manufacturer advises avoid unless essential. There is limited evidence for the safe use of montelukast during pregnancy; however, it can be taken as normal in women who have shown a significant improvement in asthma not achievable with other drugs before becoming pregnant.
- **BREAST FEEDING** Manufacturer advises avoid unless essential.
- **DIRECTIONS FOR ADMINISTRATION**
- ▸ With oral use Granules may be swallowed or mixed with cold, soft food (not liquid) and taken immediately.
- **PRESCRIBING AND DISPENSING INFORMATION** Flavours of chewable tablet formulations may include cherry.
- **PATIENT AND CARER ADVICE** Patients or carers should be given advice on how to administer montelukast granules. Medicines for Children leaflet: Montelukast for asthma www.medicinesforchildren.org.uk/montelukast-for-asthma
- **NATIONAL FUNDING/ACCESS DECISIONS**
SINGULAIR® GRANULES

Scottish Medicines Consortium (SMC) Decisions
The *Scottish Medicines Consortium* has advised (June 2007) that *Singulair*® granules are restricted for use as an alternative to low-dose inhaled corticosteroids for children 2–14 years with mild persistent asthma who have not recently had serious asthma attacks that required oral corticosteroid use and who are not capable of using inhaled corticosteroids; *Singulair*® granules should be initiated by a specialist in paediatric asthma.

SINGULAIR® CHEWABLE TABLETS

Scottish Medicines Consortium (SMC) Decisions
The *Scottish Medicines Consortium* has advised (June 2007) that *Singulair*® chewable tablets are restricted for use as an alternative to low-dose inhaled corticosteroids for children 2–14 years with mild persistent asthma who have not recently had serious asthma attacks that required oral corticosteroid use and who are not capable of using inhaled corticosteroids; *Singulair*® chewable tablets should be initiated by a specialist in paediatric asthma.

- **MEDICINAL FORMS**
There can be variation in the licensing of different medicines containing the same drug.
Tablet
- ▸ Montelukast (Non-proprietary)
Montelukast (as Montelukast sodium) 10 mg Montelukast 10mg tablets | 28 tablet PoM £26.97 DT price = £1.54

- ▸ Singulair (Merck Sharp & Dohme Ltd)
Montelukast (as Montelukast sodium) 10 mg Singulair 10mg tablets | 28 tablet PoM £26.97 DT price = £1.54

Chewable tablet
CAUTIONARY AND ADVISORY LABELS 23, 24
EXCIPIENTS: May contain Aspartame
- ▸ Montelukast (Non-proprietary)
Montelukast (as Montelukast sodium) 4 mg Montelukast 4mg chewable tablets sugar free sugar-free | 28 tablet PoM £25.69 DT price = £1.35
Montelukast (as Montelukast sodium) 5 mg Montelukast 5mg chewable tablets sugar free sugar-free | 28 tablet PoM £25.69 DT price = £1.58
- ▸ Singulair (Merck Sharp & Dohme Ltd)
Montelukast (as Montelukast sodium) 4 mg Singulair Paediatric 4mg chewable tablets sugar-free | 28 tablet PoM £25.69 DT price = £1.35
Montelukast (as Montelukast sodium) 5 mg Singulair Paediatric 5mg chewable tablets sugar-free | 28 tablet PoM £25.69 DT price = £1.58

Granules
- ▸ Montelukast (Non-proprietary)
Montelukast (as Montelukast sodium) 4 mg Montelukast 4mg granules sachets sugar free sugar-free | 28 sachet PoM £24.41 DT price = £4.05
- ▸ Singulair (Merck Sharp & Dohme Ltd)
Montelukast (as Montelukast sodium) 4 mg Singulair Paediatric 4mg granules sachets sugar-free | 28 sachet PoM £25.69 DT price = £4.05

Zafirlukast

- **INDICATIONS AND DOSE**
Prophylaxis of asthma
- ▸ BY MOUTH
- ▸ Child 12–17 years: 20 mg twice daily

- **INTERACTIONS** → Appendix 1 (leukotriene receptor antagonists).
- **SIDE-EFFECTS**
- ▸ **Common or very common** Gastro-intestinal disturbances · headache · respiratory infections
- ▸ **Uncommon** Insomnia · malaise
- ▸ **Rare** Angioedema · arthralgia · bleeding disorders · hepatitis · hyperbilirubinaemia · hypersensitivity reactions · myalgia · skin reactions · thrombocytopenia
- ▸ **Very rare** Agranulocytosis · Churg-Strauss syndrome

SIDE-EFFECTS, FURTHER INFORMATION
- ▸ Hepatic disorder Patients or their carers should be told how to recognise development of liver disorder and advised to seek medical attention if symptoms or signs such as persistent nausea, vomiting, malaise, or jaundice develop.
Churg-Strauss syndrome has occurred very rarely in association with the use of zafirlukast; in many of the reported cases the reaction followed the reduction or withdrawal of oral corticosteroid therapy. Prescribers should be alert to the development of eosinophilia, vasculitic rash, worsening pulmonary symptoms, cardiac complications, or peripheral neuropathy.

- **PREGNANCY** Manufacturer advises use only if potential benefit outweighs risk. There is limited evidence for the safe use of zafirlukast during pregnancy; however, it can be taken as normal in women who have shown a significant improvement in asthma not achievable with other drugs before becoming pregnant.
- **BREAST FEEDING** Present in milk—manufacturer advises avoid.
- **HEPATIC IMPAIRMENT** Manufacturer advises avoid.
- **RENAL IMPAIRMENT** Manufacturer advises caution.
- **PATIENT AND CARER ADVICE**
Medicines for Children leaflet: Zafirlukast for asthma prevention (prophylaxis) www.medicinesforchildren.org.uk/zafirlukast-for-asthma-prevention

- **MEDICINAL FORMS**
  There can be variation in the licensing of different medicines containing the same drug.

  Tablet
  CAUTIONARY AND ADVISORY LABELS 23
  ▸ **Accolate** (AstraZeneca UK Ltd)
    Zafirlukast 20 mg Accolate 20mg tablets | 56 tablet [PoM] £17.75
    DT price = £17.75

MAST-CELL STABILISERS

Cromoglicate and related therapy

Overview

The mode of action of sodium cromoglicate below and nedocromil sodium below is not completely understood; they may be of value as *prophylaxis* in asthma with an allergic basis, but the evidence for benefit of sodium cromoglicate in children is contentious. Prophylaxis with sodium cromoglicate or nedocromil sodium is less effective than with inhaled corticosteroids.

Nedocromil sodium may be of some benefit in the prophylaxis of exercise-induced asthma.

Sodium cromoglicate and nedocromil sodium may also have a role in allergic conjunctivitis; sodium cromoglicate is used also in allergic rhinitis and allergy-related diarrhoea.

Nedocromil sodium

- **INDICATIONS AND DOSE**
  Prophylaxis of asthma
  ▸ BY INHALATION OF AEROSOL
  ▸ Child 5–17 years: Initially 4 mg 4 times a day, when control achieved may be possible to reduce to twice daily

  DOSE EQUIVALENCE AND CONVERSION
  2 puffs = 4 mg.

- **UNLICENSED USE** Not licensed for use in children under 6 years.

- **SIDE-EFFECTS**
- **Common or very common** Abdominal pain · dyspepsia · nausea · pharyngitis · vomiting
- **Rare** Taste disturbances
- **Frequency not known** Bronchospasm · cough · headache · paradoxical bronchospasm · throat irritation
  SIDE-EFFECTS, FURTHER INFORMATION
  ▸ Paradoxical bronchospasm If paradoxical bronchospasm occurs, a short-acting beta$_2$ agonist such as salbutamol or terbutaline should be used to control symptoms; treatment with nedocromil should be discontinued.

- **PREGNANCY** Inhaled drugs can be taken as normal during pregnancy.

- **BREAST FEEDING** Inhaled drugs can be taken as normal during breast-feeding.

- **TREATMENT CESSATION** Withdrawal should be done gradually over a period of one week—symptoms of asthma may recur.

- **PRESCRIBING AND DISPENSING INFORMATION** Flavours of inhalers may include mint.

- **PATIENT AND CARER ADVICE** Regular use is necessary. Patient counselling is advised for Nedocromil aerosol for inhalation (administration).

- **MEDICINAL FORMS**
  There can be variation in the licensing of different medicines containing the same drug.

  Pressurised inhalation
  CAUTIONARY AND ADVISORY LABELS 8
  ▸ **Tilade** (Sanofi)
    Nedocromil sodium 2 mg per 1 dose Tilade 2mg/dose inhaler CFC free | 112 dose [PoM] £39.94

Sodium cromoglicate

(Sodium cromoglycate)

- **INDICATIONS AND DOSE**
  Prophylaxis of asthma
  ▸ BY INHALATION OF AEROSOL
  ▸ Child 5–17 years: Initially 10 mg 4 times a day, additional dose may also be taken before exercise, increased if necessary to 10 mg 6–8 times a day; maintenance 5 mg 4 times a day, 5 mg is equivalent to 1 puff

  Food allergy (in conjunction with dietary restriction)
  ▸ BY MOUTH
  ▸ Child 2–13 years: Initially 100 mg 4 times a day for 2–3 weeks, then increased if necessary up to 40 mg/kg daily, then reduced according to response, to be taken before meals
  ▸ Child 14–17 years: Initially 200 mg 4 times a day for 2–3 weeks, then increased if necessary up to 40 mg/kg daily, then reduced according to response, to be taken before meals

- **CAUTIONS**
▸ When used by inhalation Discontinue if eosinophilic pneumonia occurs

- **SIDE-EFFECTS**
▸ When used by inhalation Bronchospasm · cough · eosinophilic pneumonia · headache · paradoxical bronchospasm · rhinitis · throat irritation
▸ With oral use Joint pain · occasional nausea · rashes
  SIDE-EFFECTS, FURTHER INFORMATION
▸ Paradoxical bronchospasm
▸ When used by inhalation If paradoxical bronchospasm occurs, a short-acting beta$_2$ agonist such as salbutamol or terbutaline should be used to control symptoms; treatment with sodium cromoglicate should be discontinued.

- **PREGNANCY** Not known to be harmful. Inhaled drugs can be taken as normal during pregnancy.

- **BREAST FEEDING** Unlikely to be present in milk. Inhaled drugs can be taken as normal during breast-feeding.

- **TREATMENT CESSATION**
▸ When used by inhalation Withdrawal of sodium cromoglicate should be done gradually over a period of one week—symptoms of asthma may recur.

- **DIRECTIONS FOR ADMINISTRATION**
▸ With oral use Capsules may be swallowed whole or the contents dissolved in hot water and diluted with cold water before taking.

- **PATIENT AND CARER ADVICE**
▸ With oral use Patient counselling is advised for sodium cromoglicate capsules (administration).
▸ When used by inhalation Patient counselling is advised for sodium cromoglicate pressurised inhalation (administration).

- **MEDICINAL FORMS**
  There can be variation in the licensing of different medicines containing the same drug. Forms available from special-order manufacturers include: oral solution,

Capsule
CAUTIONARY AND ADVISORY LABELS 22
▸ Nalcrom (Sanofi)
  Sodium cromoglicate 100 mg Nalcrom 100mg capsules |
  100 capsule [PoM] £41.14 DT price = £41.14

Pressurised inhalation
CAUTIONARY AND ADVISORY LABELS 8
▸ Intal (Sanofi)
  Sodium cromoglicate 5 mg per 1 dose Intal 5mg/dose inhaler CFC free | 112 dose [PoM] £18.33

XANTHINES

Aminophylline

- **INDICATIONS AND DOSE**

Severe acute asthma in patients not previously treated with theophylline
▸ BY SLOW INTRAVENOUS INJECTION
▸ Child: 5 mg/kg (max. per dose 500 mg), to be followed by intravenous infusion

Severe acute asthma
▸ BY INTRAVENOUS INFUSION
▸ Child 1 month–11 years: 1 mg/kg/hour, adjusted according to plasma-theophylline concentration
▸ Child 12-17 years: 500–700 micrograms/kg/hour, adjusted according to plasma-theophylline concentration

Chronic asthma
▸ BY MOUTH USING MODIFIED-RELEASE MEDICINES
▸ Child (body-weight 40 kg and above): Initially 225 mg twice daily for 1 week, then increased if necessary to 450 mg twice daily, adjusted according to plasma-theophylline concentration

DOSE ADJUSTMENTS DUE TO INTERACTIONS
Dose adjustment may be necessary if smoking started or stopped during treatment.

DOSES AT EXTREMES OF BODY-WEIGHT
To avoid excessive dosage in obese patients, dose should be calculated on the basis of ideal weight for height.

PHARMACOKINETICS
Aminophylline is a stable mixture or combination of theophylline and ethylenediamine; the ethylenediamine confers greater solubility in water.
Theophylline is metabolised in the liver. The plasma-theophylline concentration is increased in heart failure, hepatic impairment, and in viral infections. The plasma-theophylline concentration is decreased in smokers, and by alcohol consumption. Differences in the half-life of aminophylline are important because the toxic dose is close to the therapeutic dose.

- **UNLICENSED USE** Aminophylline injection not licensed for use in children under 6 months.
- **CAUTIONS** Arrhythmias following rapid intravenous injection · cardiac arrhythmias or other cardiac disease · epilepsy · fever · hypertension · hyperthyroidism · peptic ulcer · risk of hypokalaemia
- **INTERACTIONS** → Appendix 1 (aminophylline).
- **SIDE-EFFECTS** Arrhythmias (especially if given rapidly by intravenous injection) · CNS stimulation · convulsions (especially if given rapidly by intravenous injection) · diarrhoea · gastric irritation · headache · hypotension (especially if given rapidly by intravenous injection) · insomnia · nausea · palpitation · tachycardia · vomiting

SIDE-EFFECTS, FURTHER INFORMATION
▸ Hypokalaemia Potentially serious hypokalaemia may result from beta$_2$ agonist therapy. Particular caution is required in severe asthma, because this effect may be potentiated by concomitant treatment with theophylline and its derivatives, corticosteroids, and diuretics, and by hypoxia. Plasma-potassium concentration should therefore be monitored in severe asthma.

Overdose
Theophylline and related drugs are often prescribed as modified-release formulations and toxicity can therefore be delayed. They cause vomiting (which may be severe and intractable), agitation, restlessness, dilated pupils, sinus tachycardia, and hyperglycaemia. More serious effects are haematemesis, convulsions, and supraventricular and ventricular arrhythmias. Severe hypokalaemia may develop rapidly.
  For specific details on the management of poisoning, see *Theophylline*, under Emergency treatment of poisoning p. 791.

- **ALLERGY AND CROSS-SENSITIVITY** Allergy to ethylenediamine can cause urticaria, erythema, and exfoliative dermatitis.
- **PREGNANCY** Neonatal irritability and apnoea have been reported. Theophylline can be taken as normal during pregnancy as it is particularly important that asthma should be well controlled during pregnancy.
- **BREAST FEEDING** Present in milk—irritability in infant reported; modified-release preparations preferable. Theophylline can be taken as normal during breast-feeding.
- **HEPATIC IMPAIRMENT** Reduce dose.
- **MONITORING REQUIREMENTS**
▸ Aminophylline is monitored therapeutically in terms of plasma-theophylline concentrations.
▸ Measurement of plasma-theophylline concentration may be helpful and is **essential** if a loading dose of intravenous aminophylline is to be given to patients who are already taking theophylline, because serious side-effects such as convulsions and arrhythmias can occasionally precede other symptoms of toxicity.
▸ In most individuals, a plasma-theophylline concentration of 10–20 mg/litre (55–110 micromol/litre) is required for satisfactory bronchodilation, although a lower plasma-theophylline concentration of 5–15 mg/litre may be effective. Adverse effects can occur within the range 10–20 mg/litre and both the frequency and severity increase at concentrations above 20 mg/litre.
▸ If aminophylline is given intravenously, a blood sample should be taken 4–6 hours after starting treatment.
▸ With oral use Plasma-theophylline concentration is measured 5 days after starting oral treatment and at least 3 days after any dose adjustment. A blood sample should usually be taken 4–6 hours after an oral dose of a modified-release preparation (sampling times may vary—consult local guidelines).

- **DIRECTIONS FOR ADMINISTRATION**
▸ With intravenous use For *intravenous infusion*, dilute to a concentration of 1 mg/mL with Glucose 5% *or* Sodium Chloride 0.9%.
▸ With intravenous use For *intravenous injection*, give **very slowly** over at least 20 minutes (with close monitoring).
▸ With intramuscular use Aminophylline is too irritant for intramuscular use.

- **PRESCRIBING AND DISPENSING INFORMATION**
Patients taking oral theophylline or aminophylline should not normally receive a loading dose of intravenous aminophylline.
  Consider intravenous aminophylline for treatment of severe and life-threatening acute asthma only after consultation with senior medical staff.

Modified release The rate of absorption from modified-release preparations can vary between brands. If a prescription for a modified-release oral aminophylline preparation does not specify a brand name, the pharmacist should contact the prescriber and agree the brand to be dispensed. Additionally, it is essential that a patient discharged from hospital should be maintained on the brand on which that patient was stabilised as an in-patient.

- **MEDICINAL FORMS**
  There can be variation in the licensing of different medicines containing the same drug. Forms available from special-order manufacturers include: solution for infusion
  Modified-release tablet
  CAUTIONARY AND ADVISORY LABELS 25
  ‣ **Aminophylline** (Non-proprietary)
    Aminophylline hydrate 225 mg Aminophylline hydrate 225mg modified-release tablets | 56 tablet P no price available DT price = £2.40
  ‣ **Phyllocontin Continus** (Napp Pharmaceuticals Ltd)
    Aminophylline hydrate 225 mg Phyllocontin Continus 225mg tablets | 56 tablet P £2.40 DT price = £2.40
  Solution for injection
  ‣ **Aminophylline** (Non-proprietary)
    Aminophylline 25 mg per 1 ml Aminophylline 250mg/10ml solution for injection ampoules | 10 ampoule PoM £6.50 DT price = £6.50

Theophylline

- **INDICATIONS AND DOSE**
  NUELIN SA® 175MG TABLETS
  Chronic asthma
  ‣ BY MOUTH USING MODIFIED-RELEASE MEDICINES
  ‣ Child 6–11 years: 175 mg every 12 hours
  ‣ Child 12–17 years: 175–350 mg every 12 hours
  NUELIN SA® 250 TABLETS
  Chronic asthma
  ‣ BY MOUTH USING MODIFIED-RELEASE MEDICINES
  ‣ Child 6–11 years: 125–250 mg every 12 hours
  ‣ Child 12–17 years: 250–500 mg every 12 hours
  SLO-PHYLLIN®
  Chronic asthma
  ‣ BY MOUTH USING MODIFIED-RELEASE MEDICINES
  ‣ Child 6 months–1 year: 12 mg/kg every 12 hours (max. per dose 120 mg)
  ‣ Child 2–5 years: 60–120 mg every 12 hours
  ‣ Child 6–11 years: 125–250 mg every 12 hours
  ‣ Child 12–17 years: 250–500 mg every 12 hours
  UNIPHYLLIN CONTINUS®
  Chronic asthma
  ‣ BY MOUTH USING MODIFIED-RELEASE MEDICINES
  ‣ Child 2–11 years: 9 mg/kg every 12 hours (max. per dose 200 mg), dose may be increased in some children with chronic asthma; increased to 10–16 mg/kg every 12 hours (max. per dose 400 mg), may be appropriate to give larger evening or morning dose to achieve optimum therapeutic effect when symptoms most severe; in patients whose night or daytime symptoms persist despite other therapy, who are not currently receiving theophylline, total daily requirement may be added as single evening or morning dose
  ‣ Child 12–17 years: 200 mg every 12 hours, adjusted according to response to 400 mg every 12 hours, may be appropriate to give larger evening or morning dose to achieve optimum therapeutic effect when symptoms most severe; in patients whose night or daytime symptoms persist despite other therapy, who are not currently receiving theophylline, total daily

requirement may be added as single evening or morning dose

DOSE ADJUSTMENTS DUE TO INTERACTIONS
Dose adjustment may be necessary if smoking started or stopped during treatment.

PHARMACOKINETICS
Theophylline is metabolised in the liver. The plasma-theophylline concentration is increased in heart failure, hepatic impairment, and in viral infections. The plasma-theophylline concentration is decreased in smokers, and by alcohol consumption. Differences in the half-life of theophylline are important because the toxic dose is close to the therapeutic dose.

- **UNLICENSED USE**
  SLO-PHYLLIN® *Slo-phyllin®* capsules not licensed for use in children under 2 years.
- **CAUTIONS** Cardiac arrhythmias or other cardiac disease · epilepsy · fever · hypertension · hyperthyroidism · peptic ulcer · risk of hypokalaemia
- **INTERACTIONS** → Appendix 1 (theophylline).
- **SIDE-EFFECTS** Arrhythmias · CNS stimulation · convulsions · diarrhoea · gastric irritation · headache · insomnia · nausea · palpitation · tachycardia · vomiting
  SIDE-EFFECTS, FURTHER INFORMATION
  ‣ Hypokalaemia Potentially serious hypokalaemia may result from beta$_2$ agonist therapy. Particular caution is required in severe asthma, because this effect may be potentiated by concomitant treatment with theophylline and its derivatives, corticosteroids, and diuretics, and by hypoxia. Plasma-potassium concentration should therefore be monitored in severe asthma.
  Overdose
  Theophylline in overdose can cause vomiting (which may be severe and intractable), agitation, restlessness, dilated pupils, sinus tachycardia, and hyperglycaemia. More serious effects are haematemesis, convulsions, and supraventricular and ventricular arrhythmias. Severe hypokalaemia may develop rapidly.
     For details on the management of poisoning, see Theophylline, under Emergency treatment of poisoning p. 791.
- **PREGNANCY** Neonatal irritability and apnoea have been reported. Theophylline can be taken as normal during pregnancy as it is particularly important that asthma should be well controlled during pregnancy.
- **BREAST FEEDING** Present in milk—irritability in infant reported; modified-release preparations preferable. Theophylline can be taken as normal during breast-feeding.
- **HEPATIC IMPAIRMENT** Reduce dose.
- **MONITORING REQUIREMENTS**
  ‣ In most individuals, a plasma-theophylline concentration of 10–20 mg/litre (55–110 micromol/litre) is required for satisfactory bronchodilation, although a lower plasma-theophylline concentration of 5–15 mg/litre may be effective. Adverse effects can occur within the range 10–20 mg/litre and both the frequency and severity increase at concentrations above 20 mg/litre.
  ‣ Plasma-theophylline concentration is measured 5 days after starting oral treatment and at least 3 days after any dose adjustment. A blood sample should usually be taken 4–6 hours after an oral dose of a modified-release preparation (sampling times may vary—consult local guidelines).
- **DIRECTIONS FOR ADMINISTRATION**
  SLO-PHYLLIN® Contents of the capsule (enteric-coated granules) may be sprinkled on to a spoonful of soft food (e.g. yoghurt) and swallowed without chewing.

- **PRESCRIBING AND DISPENSING INFORMATION** The rate of absorption from modified-release preparations can vary between brands. If a prescription for a modified-release oral theophylline preparation does not specify a brand name, the pharmacist should contact the prescriber and agree the brand to be dispensed. Additionally, it is essential that a patient discharged from hospital should be maintained on the brand on which that patient was stabilised as an in-patient.

- **PATIENT AND CARER ADVICE**
SLO-PHYLLIN® Patient or carer should be given advice on how to administer theophylline modified release capsules.

- **MEDICINAL FORMS**
There can be variation in the licensing of different medicines containing the same drug.

Modified-release tablet
CAUTIONARY AND ADVISORY LABELS 21, 25
  - **Nuelin SA** (Meda Pharmaceuticals Ltd)
  Theophylline 175 mg Nuelin SA 175mg tablets | 60 tablet Ⓟ £6.38 DT price = £6.38
  Theophylline 250 mg Nuelin SA 250 tablets | 60 tablet Ⓟ £8.92 DT price = £8.92
  - **Uniphyllin Continus** (Napp Pharmaceuticals Ltd)
  Theophylline 200 mg Uniphyllin Continus 200mg tablets | 56 tablet Ⓟ £2.96
  Theophylline 300 mg Uniphyllin Continus 300mg tablets | 56 tablet Ⓟ £4.77
  Theophylline 400 mg Uniphyllin Continus 400mg tablets | 56 tablet Ⓟ £5.65 DT price = £5.65

Modified-release capsule
CAUTIONARY AND ADVISORY LABELS 25
  - **Slo-Phyllin** (Merck Serono Ltd)
  Theophylline 60 mg Slo-Phyllin 60mg capsules | 56 capsule Ⓟ £2.76 DT price = £2.76
  Theophylline 125 mg Slo-Phyllin 125mg capsules | 56 capsule Ⓟ £3.48 DT price = £3.48
  Theophylline 250 mg Slo-Phyllin 250mg capsules | 56 capsule Ⓟ £4.34 DT price = £4.34

Nebuliser solutions

- **HYPERTONIC SODIUM CHLORIDE SOLUTIONS**

- **INDICATIONS AND DOSE**
MUCOCLEAR® 3%

Mobilise lower respiratory tract secretions in mucous consolidation (e.g. cystic fibrosis) | Mild to moderate acute viral bronchiolitis in infants
  - BY INHALATION OF NEBULISED SOLUTION
  - Child: 4 mL 2–4 times a day, temporary irritation, such as coughing, hoarseness, or reversible bronchoconstriction may occur; an inhaled bronchodilator can be used before treatment with hypertonic sodium chloride to reduce the risk of these adverse effects

MucoClear 3% inhalation solution 4ml ampoules (Pari Medical Ltd) **Sodium chloride 30 mg per 1 ml** | 20 ampoule · NHS indicative price = £12.98 · Drug Tariff (Part IXa) | 60 ampoule · NHS indicative price = £27.00 · Drug Tariff (Part IXa)

- **INDICATIONS AND DOSE**
MUCOCLEAR® 6%

Mobilise lower respiratory tract secretions in mucous consolidation (e.g. cystic fibrosis)
  - BY INHALATION OF NEBULISED SOLUTION
  - Child: 4 mL twice daily, temporary irritation, such as coughing, hoarseness, or reversible bronchoconstriction may occur; an inhaled bronchodilator can be used before treatment with hypertonic sodium chloride to reduce the risk of these adverse effects

MucoClear 6% inhalation solution 4ml ampoules (Pari Medical Ltd) **Sodium chloride 60 mg per 1 ml** | 20 ampoule · NHS indicative price = £12.98 · Drug Tariff (Part IXa) | 60 ampoule · NHS indicative price = £27.00 · Drug Tariff (Part IXa)

- **INDICATIONS AND DOSE**
NEBUSAL®

Mobilise lower respiratory tract secretions in mucous consolidation (e.g. cystic fibrosis)
  - BY INHALATION OF NEBULISED SOLUTION
  - Child: 4 mL up to twice daily, temporary irritation, such as coughing, hoarseness, or reversible bronchoconstriction may occur; an inhaled bronchodilator can be used before treatment with hypertonic sodium chloride to reduce the risk of these adverse effects

Nebusal 7% inhalation solution 4ml vials (Forest Laboratories UK Ltd) **Sodium chloride 70 mg per 1 ml** | 60 vial · NHS indicative price = £27.00 · Drug Tariff (Part IXa)

Peak flow meters

- **LOW RANGE PEAK FLOW METERS**
MEDI® LOW RANGE
Range 40–420 litres/minute.
Compliant to standard EN ISO 23747:2007 except for scale range.

Medi peak flow meter low range (Medicareplus International Ltd) | 1 device · NHS indicative price = £6.50 · Drug Tariff (Part IXa) price = £6.50

MINI-WRIGHT® LOW RANGE
Range 30–400 litres/minute.
Compliant to standard EN ISO 23747:2007 except for scale range.

Mini-wright peak flow meter low range (Clement Clarke International Ltd) | 1 device · NHS indicative price = £6.50 · Drug Tariff (Part IXa) price = £7.14

POCKETPEAK® LOW RANGE
Range 50–400 litres/minute.
Compliant to standard EN ISO 23747:2007 except for scale range.

nSpire Pocket Peak peak flow meter low range (nSpire Health Ltd) | 1 device · NHS indicative price = £6.53 · Drug Tariff (Part IXa) price = £6.50

- **STANDARD RANGE PEAK FLOW METERS**
AIRZONE®
Range 60–720 litres/minute.
Conforms to standard EN ISO 23747:2007.

AirZone peak flow meter standard range (Clement Clarke International Ltd) | 1 device · NHS indicative price = £4.69 · Drug Tariff (Part IXa) price = £4.50

MEDI® STANDARD RANGE
Range 60–800 litres/minute.
Conforms to standard EN ISO 23747:2007.

Medi peak flow meter standard range (Medicareplus International Ltd) | 1 device · NHS indicative price = £4.50 · Drug Tariff (Part IXa) price = £4.50

MICROPEAK®
Range 60–900 litres/minute.
Conforms to standard EN ISO 23747:2007.

MicroPeak peak flow meter standard range (Micro Medical Ltd) | 1 device · NHS indicative price = £6.50 · Drug Tariff (Part IXa) price = £4.50

MINI-WRIGHT® STANDARD RANGE
Range 60–800 litres/minute.
Conforms to standard EN ISO 23747:2007.

Mini-Wright peak flow meter standard range (Clement Clarke International Ltd) | 1 device · NHS indicative price = £7.08 · Drug Tariff (Part IXa) price = £4.50

PIKO-1®
Range 15–999 litres/minute.
Conforms to standard EN ISO 23747:2007.

nSpire PiKo-1 peak flow meter standard range (nSpire Health Ltd) | 1 device · NHS indicative price = £9.50 · Drug Tariff (Part IXa) price = £4.50

PINNACLE®
Range 60–900 litres/minute.
Conforms to standard EN ISO 23747:2007.

Fyne Dynamics Pinnacle peak flow meter standard range (Fyne Dynamics Ltd) | 1 device · NHS indicative price = £6.50 · Drug Tariff (Part IXa) price = £4.50

POCKETPEAK® STANDARD RANGE
Range 60–800 litres/minute.
Conforms to standard EN ISO 23747:2007.

nSpire Pocket Peak peak flow meter standard range (nSpire Health Ltd) | 1 device · NHS indicative price = £6.53 · Drug Tariff (Part IXa) price = £4.50

VITALOGRAPH®
Range 50–800 litres/minute.
Conforms to standard EN ISO 23747:2007.

Vitalograph peak flow meter standard range (Vitalograph Ltd) | 1 device · NHS indicative price = £4.83 · Drug Tariff (Part IXa) price = £4.50

Spacers

● **SPACERS**

A2A SPACER®
For use with all pressurised (aerosol) inhalers.

A2A Spacer (Clement Clarke International Ltd) | 1 device · NHS indicative price = £4.15 · Drug Tariff (Part IXa)

A2A Spacer with medium mask (Clement Clarke International Ltd) | 1 device · NHS indicative price = £6.68 · Drug Tariff (Part IXa)

A2A Spacer with small mask (Clement Clarke International Ltd) | 1 device · NHS indicative price = £6.68 · Drug Tariff (Part IXa)

ABLE SPACER®
Small-volume device. For use with all pressurised (aerosol) inhalers.

Able Spacer (Clement Clarke International Ltd) | 1 device · NHS indicative price = £4.39 · Drug Tariff (Part IXa)

Able Spacer with medium mask (Clement Clarke International Ltd) | 1 device · NHS indicative price = £7.16 · Drug Tariff (Part IXa)

Able Spacer with small mask (Clement Clarke International Ltd) | 1 device · NHS indicative price = £7.16 · Drug Tariff (Part IXa)

AEROCHAMBER PLUS®
Medium-volume device. For use with all pressurised (aerosol) inhalers.

AeroChamber Plus (GlaxoSmithKline UK Ltd) | 1 device · NHS indicative price = £4.81 · Drug Tariff (Part IXa)

AeroChamber Plus with adult mask (GlaxoSmithKline UK Ltd) | 1 device · NHS indicative price = £8.02 · Drug Tariff (Part IXa)

AeroChamber Plus with child mask (GlaxoSmithKline UK Ltd) | 1 device · NHS indicative price = £8.02 · Drug Tariff (Part IXa)

AeroChamber Plus with infant mask (GlaxoSmithKline UK Ltd) | 1 device · NHS indicative price = £8.02 · Drug Tariff (Part IXa)

BABYHALER®
For paediatric use with *Flixotide®*, and *Ventolin®* inhalers.

● **PRESCRIBING AND DISPENSING INFORMATION**
Not available for NHS prescription.

Babyhaler (Allen & Hanburys Ltd) | 1 device · No NHS indicative price available · Drug Tariff (Part IXa)

HALERAID®
Device to place over pressurised (aerosol) inhalers to aid when strength in hands is impaired (e.g. in arthritis). For use with *Flixotide®*, *Seretide®*, *Serevent®*, and *Ventolin®* inhalers.

● **PRESCRIBING AND DISPENSING INFORMATION**
Not available for NHS prescription.

Haleraid-120 (Allen & Hanburys Ltd) | 1 device · No NHS indicative price available · Drug Tariff (Part IXa)

Haleraid-200 (Allen & Hanburys Ltd) | 1 device · No NHS indicative price available · Drug Tariff (Part IXa)

OPTICHAMBER®
For use with all pressurised (aerosol) inhalers.

OptiChamber (Respironics (UK) Ltd) | 1 device · NHS indicative price = £4.28 · Drug Tariff (Part IXa)

OPTICHAMBER® DIAMOND
For use with all pressurised (aerosol) inhalers.

OptiChamber Diamond (Respironics (UK) Ltd) | 1 device · NHS indicative price = £4.49 · Drug Tariff (Part IXa)

OptiChamber Diamond with large LiteTouch mask 5 years-adult (Respironics (UK) Ltd) | 1 device · NHS indicative price = £7.49 · Drug Tariff (Part IXa)

OptiChamber Diamond with medium LiteTouch mask 1-5 years (Respironics (UK) Ltd) | 1 device · NHS indicative price = £7.49 · Drug Tariff (Part IXa)

OptiChamber Diamond with small LiteTouch mask 0-18 months (Respironics (UK) Ltd) | 1 device · NHS indicative price = £7.49 · Drug Tariff (Part IXa)

POCKET CHAMBER®
Small volume device. For use with all pressurised (aerosol) inhalers.

Pocket Chamber (nSpire Health Ltd) | 1 device · NHS indicative price = £4.18 · Drug Tariff (Part IXa)

Pocket Chamber with adult mask (nSpire Health Ltd) | 1 device · NHS indicative price = £9.75 · Drug Tariff (Part IXa)

Pocket Chamber with child mask (nSpire Health Ltd) | 1 device · NHS indicative price = £9.75 · Drug Tariff (Part IXa)

Pocket Chamber with infant mask (nSpire Health Ltd) | 1 device · NHS indicative price = £9.75 · Drug Tariff (Part IXa)

Pocket Chamber with teenager mask (nSpire Health Ltd) | 1 device · NHS indicative price = £9.75 · Drug Tariff (Part IXa)

SPACE CHAMBER PLUS®
For use with all pressurised (aerosol) inhalers.

Space Chamber Plus (Medical Developments International Ltd) | 1 device · NHS indicative price = £4.26 · Drug Tariff (Part IXa)

Space Chamber Plus with large mask (Medical Developments International Ltd) | 1 device · NHS indicative price = £6.98 · Drug Tariff (Part IXa)

Space Chamber Plus with medium mask (Medical Developments International Ltd) | 1 device · NHS indicative price = £6.98 · Drug Tariff (Part IXa)

Space Chamber Plus with small mask (Medical Developments International Ltd) | 1 device · NHS indicative price = £6.98 · Drug Tariff (Part IXa)

VOLUMATIC®
Large-volume device. For use with *Clenil Modulite®*, *Flixotide®*, *Seretide®*, *Serevent®*, and *Ventolin®* inhalers.

Volumatic (GlaxoSmithKline UK Ltd) | 1 device · NHS indicative price = £3.81 · Drug Tariff (Part IXa)

Volumatic with paediatric mask (GlaxoSmithKline UK Ltd) | 1 device · NHS indicative price = £6.70 · Drug Tariff (Part IXa)

VORTEX®
Medium-volume device. For use with all pressurised (aerosol) inhalers.

Vortex Spacer (Pari Medical Ltd) | 1 device · NHS indicative price = £6.28 · Drug Tariff (Part IXa)

Vortex with child mask 0-2 years (Pari Medical Ltd) | 1 device · NHS indicative price = £7.99 · Drug Tariff (Part IXa)

Vortex with child mask 2 years+ (Pari Medical Ltd) | 1 device · NHS indicative price = £7.99 · Drug Tariff (Part IXa)

2 Allergic conditions

Antihistamines, allergen immunotherapy and allergic emergencies

Antihistamines

Antihistamines (histamine H_1-receptor antagonists) are classified as *sedating* or *non-sedating*, according to their relative potential for CNS depression. Antihistamines differ in their duration of action, incidence of drowsiness, and antimuscarinic effects; the response to an antihistamine may vary from child to child. Either a sedating or a non-sedating antihistamine may be used to treat an acute allergic reaction; for conditions with more persistent symptoms which require regular treatment, a non-sedating anti-histamine should be used to minimise the risk of sedation and psychomotor impairment associated with sedating antihistamines.

Oral antihistamines are used in the treatment of nasal allergies, particularly seasonal allergic rhinitis (hay fever), and may be of some value in vasomotor rhinitis; rhinorrhoea and sneezing is reduced, but antihistamines are usually less effective for nasal congestion. Antihistamines are used topically to treat allergic reactions in the eye and in the nose. Topical application of antihistamines to the skin is not recommended.

An oral antihistamine may be used to prevent urticaria, and for the treatment of acute urticarial rashes, pruritus, insect bites, and stings. Antihistamines are also used in the management of nausea and vomiting, of migraine, and the adjunctive management of anaphylaxis and angioedema.

The *non-sedating* antihistamine cetirizine hydrochloride p. 164 is safe and effective in children. Other non-sedating antihistamines that are used include acrivastine p. 163, bilastine p. 164, desloratadine p. 165 (an active metabolite of loratadine p. 166), fexofenadine hydrochloride p. 165 (an active metabolite of terfenadine), levocetirizine hydrochloride p. 166 (an isomer of cetirizine hydrochloride), loratadine, and mizolastine p. 167. Most non-sedating antihistamines are long-acting (usually 12–24 hours). There is little evidence that desloratadine or levocetirizine hydrochloride confer any additional benefit—they should be reserved for children who cannot tolerate other therapies.

Sedating antihistamines are occasionally useful when insomnia is associated with urticaria and pruritus. Most of the sedating antihistamines are relatively short-acting, but promethazine may be effective for up to 12 hours. Alimemazine tartrate p. 167 and **promethazine** have a more sedative effect than chlorphenamine maleate p. 168 and cyclizine p. 244. Chlorphenamine maleate is used as an adjunct to adrenaline/epinephrine p. 174 in the emergency treatment of anaphylaxis and angioedema.

Allergen immunotherapy

Immunotherapy using allergen vaccines containing house dust mite, animal dander (cat or dog), or extracts of grass and tree pollen can improve symptoms of asthma and allergic rhinoconjunctivitis in children. A vaccine containing extracts of wasp and bee venom is used to reduce the risk of severe anaphylaxis and systemic reactions in children with hypersensitivity to wasp and bee stings. An oral preparation of grass pollen extract (*Grazax*®) is also licensed for disease-modifying treatment of grass pollen-induced rhinitis and conjunctivitis. Children requiring immunotherapy must be referred to a hospital specialist for accurate diagnosis, assessment, and treatment.

Omalizumab p. 154 is a monoclonal antibody that binds to immunoglobulin E (IgE). It is licensed for use as additional therapy in children over 6 years with proven IgE-mediated sensitivity to inhaled allergens, whose severe persistent allergic asthma cannot be controlled adequately with high-dose inhaled corticosteroid together with a long-acting beta$_2$ agonist. Omalizumab should be initiated by physicians experienced in the treatment of severe persistent asthma. Omalizumab is also indicated as add-on therapy for the treatment of chronic spontaneous urticaria in patients who have had an inadequate response to H_1 antihistamine treatment.

Allergic emergencies

Anaphylaxis

Anaphylaxis is a severe, life-threatening, generalised or systemic hypersensitivity reaction. It is characterised by the rapid onset of respiratory and/or circulatory problems and is usually associated with skin and mucosal changes; prompt treatment is required. Children with pre-existing asthma, especially poorly controlled asthma, are at particular risk of life-threatening reactions. Insect stings are a recognised risk (in particular wasp and bee stings). Latex and certain foods, including eggs, fish, cows' milk protein, peanuts, sesame, shellfish, soy, and tree nuts may also precipitate anaphylaxis. Medicinal products particularly associated with anaphylaxis include blood products, vaccines, allergen immunotherapy preparations, antibacterials, aspirin p. 83 and other NSAIDs, and neuromuscular blocking drugs. In the case of drugs, anaphylaxis is more likely after parenteral administration; resuscitation facilities must always be available for injections associated with special risk. Refined arachis (peanut) oil, which may be present in some medicinal products, is unlikely to cause an allergic reaction—nevertheless it is wise to check the full formula of preparations which may contain allergens.

Treatment of anaphylaxis

Adrenaline/epinephrine provides physiological reversal of the immediate symptoms associated with hypersensitivity reactions such as *anaphylaxis* and *angioedema*.

First-line treatment includes:

- securing the airway, restoration of blood pressure (laying the child flat and raising the legs, or in the recovery position if unconscious or nauseous and at risk of vomiting);
- administering adrenaline/epinephrine by **intramuscular** injection; the dose should be repeated if necessary at 5-minute intervals according to blood pressure, pulse, and respiratory function;
- administering high-flow **oxygen** and **intravenous fluids**;
- administering an antihistamine, such as chlorphenamine maleate, by slow intravenous injection or intramuscular injection as adjunctive treatment given after adrenaline;
- Administering an intravenous corticosteroid such as hydrocortisone p. 411 (preferably as sodium succinate) is of secondary value in the initial management of anaphylaxis because the onset of action is delayed for several hours, but should be given to prevent further deterioration in severely affected children.

Continuing respiratory deterioration requires further treatment with **bronchodilators** including inhaled or intravenous salbutamol p. 146, inhaled ipratropium bromide p. 143, intravenous aminophylline p. 158, or intravenous magnesium sulfate p. 556 [unlicensed indication] (as for acute severe asthma); in addition to oxygen, assisted respiration and possibly emergency tracheotomy may be necessary.

When a child is so ill that there is doubt about the adequacy of the circulation, the initial injection of adrenaline/epinephrine may need to be given as a *dilute solution by the intravenous route*, or by the *intraosseous route* if venous access is difficult; for details see adrenaline/epinephrine.

On discharge, child should be considered for further treatment with an oral antihistamine and an oral corticosteroid for up to 3 days to reduce the risk of further reaction. The child, or carer, should be instructed to return to hospital if symptoms recur and to contact their general practitioner for follow-up.

Children who are suspected of having had an anaphylactic reaction should be referred to a specialist for specific allergy diagnosis. Avoidance of the allergen is the principal treatment; if appropriate, an adrenaline/epinephrine auto-injector should be given for self-administration or a replacement supplied.

Intramuscular adrenaline (epinephrine)
The *intramuscular route is the first choice route* for the administration of adrenaline/epinephrine p. 174) in the management of anaphylaxis. Adrenaline/epinephrine is best given as an intramuscular injection into the anterolateral aspect of the middle third of the thigh; it has a rapid onset of action after intramuscular administration and in the shocked patient its absorption from the intramuscular site is faster and more reliable than from the subcutaneous site.

Children with severe allergy, and their carers, should ideally be instructed in the self-administration of adrenaline/epinephrine by intramuscular injection (for details of self-administration.

Prompt injection of adrenaline/epinephrine is of paramount importance. The adrenaline/epinephrine doses recommended for the emergency treatment of anaphylaxis by appropriately trained healthcare professionals are based on the revised recommendations of the Working Group of the Resuscitation Council (UK).

Dose of intramuscular injection of adrenaline (epinephrine) for the emergency treatment of anaphylaxis by healthcare professionals

Age	Dose	Volume of adrenaline
▶ Child 1 month–5 years	150 micrograms	0.15 mL 1 in 1000 (1 mg/mL) adrenaline[1]
▶ Child 6–11 years	300 micrograms	0.3 mL 1 in 1000 (1 mg/mL) adrenaline
▶ Child 12–17 years	500 micrograms	0.5 mL 1 in 1000 (1 mg/mL) adrenaline[2]

These doses may be repeated several times if necessary at 5-minute intervals according to blood pressure, pulse and respiratory rate.

1. Use suitable syringe for measuring small volume

2. 300 micrograms (0.3 mL) if child is small or prepubertal

Intravenous adrenaline (epinephrine)
Intravenous adrenaline/epinephrine should be given only by those experienced in its use, in a setting where patients can be carefully monitored.

Where the child is severely ill and there is real doubt about adequacy of the circulation and absorption from the intramuscular injection site, adrenaline/epinephrine may be given by **slow** *intravenous injection*, repeated according to response; if multiple doses are required consider giving adrenaline by slow intravenous infusion.

It is also important that, where intramuscular injection might still succeed, time should not be wasted seeking intravenous access.

Adrenaline/epinephrine is also given by the intravenous route for *acute hypotension*.

Angioedema
Angioedema is dangerous if *laryngeal oedema* is present. In this circumstance adrenaline/epinephrine injection, oxygen, antihistamines and corticosteroids should be given as described under **Anaphylaxis**. Tracheal intubation may be necessary. In some children with laryngeal oedema,

adrenaline 1 in 1000 (1 mg/mL) solution may be given by nebuliser. However, nebulised adrenaline/epinephrine cannot be relied upon for a systemic effect—intramuscular adrenaline/epinephrine should be used.

Hereditary angioedema
The treatment of hereditary angioedema should be under specialist supervision. Unlike allergic angioedema, adrenaline/epinephrine, corticosteroids, and antihistamines should not be used for the treatment of acute attacks, including attacks involving laryngeal oedema, as they are ineffective and may delay appropriate treatment—intubation may be necessary. The administration of C1-esterase inhibitor p. 174 (in fresh frozen plasma or in partially purified form) can terminate acute attacks of *hereditary angioedema*; it can also be used for short-term prophylaxis before dental, medical, or surgical procedures. Tranexamic acid p. 76 is used for short-term or long-term prophylaxis of hereditary angioedema; short-term prophylaxis is started several days before planned procedures which may trigger an acute attack of hereditary angioedema (e.g. dental work) and continued for 2–5 days afterwards. Danazol [unlicensed indication] is best avoided in children because of its androgenic effects, but it can be used for short-term prophylaxis of hereditary angioedema.

ANTIHISTAMINES ⟩ NON-SEDATING

Acrivastine

- **INDICATIONS AND DOSE**

  Symptomatic relief of allergy such as hayfever, chronic idiopathic urticaria
  - ▶ BY MOUTH
  - ▶ Child 12–17 years: 8 mg 3 times a day

- **CONTRA-INDICATIONS** Avoid in Acute porphyrias p. 562 (some antihistamines are thought to be safe)

- **CAUTIONS** Epilepsy

- **INTERACTIONS** → Appendix 1 (antihistamines). Sedative antihistamine interactions apply to a lesser extent to the non-sedating antihistamines.

- **SIDE-EFFECTS**
  - ▶ **Uncommon** Antimuscarinic effects · gastro-intestinal disturbances · headache · psychomotor impairment
  - ▶ **Rare** Anaphylaxis · angioedema · arrhythmias · blood disorders · bronchospasm · confusion · convulsions · depression · dizziness · extrapyramidal effects · hypersensitivity reactions · hypotension · liver dysfunction · palpitation · photosensitivity reactions · rashes · sleep disturbances · tremor
  - ▶ **Frequency not known** Blurred vision · drowsiness · dry mouth · urinary retention

  SIDE-EFFECTS, FURTHER INFORMATION
  Non-sedating antihistamines such as acrivastine cause less sedation and psychomotor impairment than the older antihistamines because they penetrate the blood brain barrier only to a slight extent.

  If drowsiness occurs, it may diminish after a few days of treatment.

  Children are more susceptible to side-effects.

- **ALLERGY AND CROSS-SENSITIVITY** Contra-indicated if history of hypersensitivity to triprolidine.

- **PREGNANCY** Most manufacturers of antihistamines advise avoiding their use during pregnancy; however, there is no evidence of teratogenicity.

- **BREAST FEEDING** Most antihistamines are present in breast milk in varying amounts; although not known to be harmful, most manufacturers advise avoiding their use in mothers who are breast-feeding.

- **RENAL IMPAIRMENT** Avoid in severe impairment.

- **PATIENT AND CARER ADVICE**

Driving and skilled tasks

Although drowsiness is rare, nevertheless children and their carers should be advised that it can occur and may affect performance of skilled tasks (e.g. cycling or driving); alcohol should be avoided.

- **MEDICINAL FORMS**

There can be variation in the licensing of different medicines containing the same drug.

Capsule

▸ Benadryl Allergy Relief (McNeil Products Ltd)
  Acrivastine 8 mg Benadryl Allergy Relief 8mg capsules |
  24 capsule P £4.95

Bilastine

- **INDICATIONS AND DOSE**

Symptomatic relief of allergic rhinoconjunctivitis and urticaria

▸ BY MOUTH
▸ Child 12–17 years: 20 mg once daily

- **CONTRA-INDICATIONS** Avoid in Acute porphyrias p. 562 (some antihistamines are thought to be safe)
- **CAUTIONS** Epilepsy
- **INTERACTIONS** → Appendix 1 (antihistamines).
Sedative antihistamine interactions apply to a lesser extent to the non-sedating antihistamines.
- **SIDE-EFFECTS**
▸ **Common or very common** Headache · malaise
▸ **Uncommon** Abdominal pain · anxiety · diarrhoea · dizziness · dyspnoea · gastritis · increased appetite · insomnia · oral herpes · prolongation of the QT interval · pyrexia · thirst · tinnitus · vertigo · weight gain

SIDE-EFFECTS, FURTHER INFORMATION
Children are more susceptible to side-effects.
  Non-sedating antihistamines such as bilastine cause less sedation and psychomotor impairment than the older antihistamines because they penetrate the blood brain barrier only to a slight extent.

- **PREGNANCY** Avoid—limited information available. Most manufacturers of antihistamines advise avoiding their use during pregnancy; however, there is no evidence of teratogenicity.
- **BREAST FEEDING** Avoid—no information available. Most antihistamines are present in breast milk in varying amounts; although not known to be harmful, most manufacturers advise avoiding their use in mothers who are breast-feeding.
- **DIRECTIONS FOR ADMINISTRATION** Take tablet 1 hour before or 2 hours after food or fruit juice.
- **PATIENT AND CARER ADVICE** Patients or carers should be given advice on how to administer bilastine tablets.

Driving and skilled tasks

Although drowsiness is rare, nevertheless patients should be advised that it can occur and may affect performance of skilled tasks (e.g. cycling or driving); alcohol should be avoided.

- **MEDICINAL FORMS**

There can be variation in the licensing of different medicines containing the same drug.
No licensed medicines listed.

Cetirizine hydrochloride

- **INDICATIONS AND DOSE**

Symptomatic relief of allergy such as hay fever, chronic idiopathic urticaria, atopic dermatitis

▸ BY MOUTH
▸ Child 1 year: 250 micrograms/kg twice daily
▸ Child 2–5 years: 2.5 mg twice daily
▸ Child 6–11 years: 5 mg twice daily
▸ Child 12–17 years: 10 mg once daily

- **UNLICENSED USE** Not licensed for use in children under 2 years.
- **CONTRA-INDICATIONS** Avoid in Acute porphyrias p. 562 (some antihistamines are thought to be safe)
- **CAUTIONS** Epilepsy
- **INTERACTIONS** → Appendix 1 (antihistamines).
Sedative antihistamine interactions apply to a lesser extent to the non-sedating antihistamines.
- **SIDE-EFFECTS**
▸ **Uncommon** Antimuscarinic effects · blurred vision · dry mouth · gastro-intestinal disturbances · headache · psychomotor impairment · urinary retention
▸ **Rare** Anaphylaxis · angioedema · arrhythmias · blood disorders · bronchospasm · confusion · convulsions · depression · dizziness · extrapyramidal effects · hypersensitivity reactions · hypotension · liver dysfunction · palpitation · photosensitivity reactions · rashes · sleep disturbances · tremor
▸ **Frequency not known** Drowsiness

SIDE-EFFECTS, FURTHER INFORMATION
Non-sedating antihistamines such as cetirizine cause less sedation and psychomotor impairment than the older antihistamines because they penetrate the blood brain barrier only to a slight extent.
  If drowsiness occurs, it may diminish after a few days of treatment.
  Children are more susceptible to side-effects.

- **PREGNANCY** Most manufacturers of antihistamines advise avoiding their use during pregnancy; however, there is no evidence of teratogenicity.
- **BREAST FEEDING** Most antihistamines are present in breast milk in varying amounts; although not known to be harmful, most manufacturers advise avoiding their use in mothers who are breast-feeding.
- **RENAL IMPAIRMENT** Use half normal dose if estimated glomerular filtration rate 30–50 mL/minute/1.73 m^2. Use half normal dose and reduce dose frequency to alternate days if estimated glomerular filtration rate 10–30 mL/minute/1.73 m^2. Avoid if estimated glomerular filtration rate less than 10 mL/minute/1.73 m^2.
- **PATIENT AND CARER ADVICE**

Driving and skilled tasks

Although drowsiness is rare, nevertheless patients should be advised that it can occur and may affect performance of skilled tasks (e.g. cycling or driving); alcohol should be avoided.

Medicines for Children leaflet: Cetirizine hydrochloride for hay fever www.medicinesforchildren.org.uk/cetirizine-hay-fever-0

- **PROFESSION SPECIFIC INFORMATION**

Dental practitioners' formulary

Cetirizine Tablets 10 mg may be prescribed.
  Cetirizine Oral Solution 5 mg/5 mL may be prescribed.

- **MEDICINAL FORMS**
  There can be variation in the licensing of different medicines containing the same drug.
  Tablet
  ▸ Cetirizine hydrochloride (Non-proprietary)
    Cetirizine hydrochloride 10 mg Cetirizine 10mg tablets |
    7 tablet P £1.40 | 14 tablet GSL no price available |
    30 tablet PoM £1.26 DT price = £0.81 | 30 tablet P £8.29 DT price =
    £0.81 | 30 tablet GSL £0.89 DT price = £0.81
  ▸ Pollenshield (Actavis UK Ltd)
    Cetirizine hydrochloride 10 mg Pollenshield Hayfever 10mg tablets
    | 30 tablet P £2.17 DT price = £0.81
  ▸ Zirtek (UCB Pharma Ltd)
    Cetirizine hydrochloride 10 mg Zirtek Allergy 10mg tablets |
    21 tablet P £5.33 | 30 tablet P £8.12 DT price = £0.81
  Oral solution
  EXCIPIENTS: May contain Propylene glycol
  ▸ Cetirizine hydrochloride (Non-proprietary)
    Cetirizine hydrochloride 1 mg per 1 ml Cetirizine 1mg/ml oral
    solution sugar free sugar-free | 200 ml P no price available DT price
    = £1.58 sugar-free | 200 ml PoM £3.50 DT price = £1.58
  ▸ Benadryl Allergy (McNeil Products Ltd)
    Cetirizine hydrochloride 1 mg per 1 ml Benadryl Allergy Children's
    1mg/ml oral solution sugar-free | 100 ml P £3.21
    Benadryl Allergy 1mg/ml oral solution sugar-free | 100 ml P £3.15
  ▸ Zirtek (UCB Pharma Ltd)
    Cetirizine hydrochloride 1 mg per 1 ml Zirtek Allergy 1mg/ml oral
    solution sugar-free | 150 ml P £3.70 sugar-free | 200 ml P £9.77
    DT price = £1.58

Desloratadine

- **INDICATIONS AND DOSE**
  Symptomatic relief of allergy such as allergic rhinitis, urticaria, chronic idiopathic urticaria
  ▸ BY MOUTH
  ▸ Child 1–5 years: 1.25 mg once daily
  ▸ Child 6–11 years: 2.5 mg once daily
  ▸ Child 12–17 years: 5 mg once daily
  PHARMACOKINETICS
  Desloratadine is a metabolite of loratadine.

- **CAUTIONS** Acute porphyrias p. 562 · epilepsy
- **INTERACTIONS** → Appendix 1 (antihistamines).
  Sedative antihistamine interactions apply to a lesser extent to the non-sedating antihistamines.
- **SIDE-EFFECTS**
  ▸ **Uncommon** Antimuscarinic effects · blurred vision · dry mouth · gastro-intestinal disturbances · headache · psychomotor impairment · urinary retention
  ▸ **Rare** Anaphylaxis · angioedema · arrhythmias · blood disorders · bronchospasm · confusion · convulsions · depression · dizziness · extrapyramidal effects · hypersensitivity reactions · hypotension · liver dysfunction · myalgia · palpitation · photosensitivity reactions · rashes · sleep disturbances · tremor
  ▸ **Very rare** Hallucinations
  ▸ **Frequency not known** Drowsiness
  SIDE-EFFECTS, FURTHER INFORMATION
  Non-sedating antihistamines such as desloratadine cause less sedation and psychomotor impairment than the older antihistamines because they penetrate the blood brain barrier only to a slight extent.
  If drowsiness occurs, it may diminish after a few days of treatment.
  Children are more susceptible to side-effects.
- **ALLERGY AND CROSS-SENSITIVITY** Contra-indicated if history of hypersensitivity to loratadine.
- **PREGNANCY** Most manufacturers of antihistamines advise avoiding their use during pregnancy; however, there is no evidence of teratogenicity.

- **BREAST FEEDING** Most antihistamines are present in breast milk in varying amounts; although not known to be harmful, most manufacturers advise avoiding their use in mothers who are breast-feeding.
- **RENAL IMPAIRMENT** Use with caution in severe impairment.
- **PRESCRIBING AND DISPENSING INFORMATION** Flavours of oral liquid formulations may include bubblegum.
- **PATIENT AND CARER ADVICE**
  Driving and skilled tasks
  Although drowsiness is rare, nevertheless patients should be advised that it can occur and may affect performance of skilled tasks (e.g. cycling or driving); excess alcohol should be avoided.

- **MEDICINAL FORMS**
  There can be variation in the licensing of different medicines containing the same drug.
  Tablet
  ▸ Desloratadine (Non-proprietary)
    Desloratadine 5 mg Desloratadine 5mg tablets | 30 tablet PoM
    £6.77 DT price = £1.23
  ▸ Neoclarityn (Merck Sharp & Dohme Ltd)
    Desloratadine 5 mg Neoclarityn 5mg tablets | 30 tablet PoM £6.77
    DT price = £1.23
  Oral solution
  EXCIPIENTS: May contain Propylene glycol, sorbitol
  ▸ Desloratadine (Non-proprietary)
    Desloratadine 500 microgram per 1 ml Desloratadine 2.5mg/5ml
    oral solution sugar free sugar-free | 100 ml PoM no price available
    sugar-free | 150 ml PoM £8.00–£10.15 DT price = £10.15
  ▸ Neoclarityn (Merck Sharp & Dohme Ltd)
    Desloratadine 500 microgram per 1 ml Neoclarityn 2.5mg/5ml oral
    solution sugar-free | 100 ml PoM £6.77 sugar-free | 150 ml PoM
    £10.15 DT price = £10.15

Fexofenadine hydrochloride

- **INDICATIONS AND DOSE**
  Symptomatic relief of seasonal allergic rhinitis
  ▸ BY MOUTH
  ▸ Child 6–11 years: 30 mg twice daily
  ▸ Child 12–17 years: 120 mg once daily
  Symptomatic relief of chronic idiopathic urticaria
  ▸ BY MOUTH
  ▸ Child 12–17 years: 180 mg once daily
  PHARMACOKINETICS
  Fexofenadine is a metabolite of terfenadine.

- **CAUTIONS** Epilepsy
- **INTERACTIONS** → Appendix 1 (antihistamines).
  Sedative antihistamine interactions apply to a lesser extent to the non-sedating antihistamines.
- **SIDE-EFFECTS**
  ▸ **Uncommon** Antimuscarinic effects · blurred vision · dry mouth · gastro-intestinal disturbances · headache · psychomotor impairment · urinary retention
  ▸ **Rare** Anaphylaxis · angioedema · arrhythmias · blood disorders · bronchospasm · confusion · convulsions · depression · dizziness · extrapyramidal effects · hypersensitivity reactions · hypotension · liver dysfunction · palpitation · photosensitivity reactions · rashes · sleep disturbances · tremor
  ▸ **Frequency not known** Drowsiness
  SIDE-EFFECTS, FURTHER INFORMATION
  Non-sedating antihistamines such as fexofenadine cause less sedation and psychomotor impairment than the older antihistamines because they penetrate the blood brain barrier only to a slight extent.
  If drowsiness occurs, it may diminish after a few days of treatment.
  Children are more susceptible to side-effects.

Respiratory system

3

- **PREGNANCY** Most manufacturers of antihistamines advise avoiding their use during pregnancy; however, there is no evidence of teratogenicity.
- **BREAST FEEDING** Most antihistamines are present in breast milk in varying amounts; although not known to be harmful, most manufacturers advise avoiding their use in mothers who are breast-feeding.
- **PATIENT AND CARER ADVICE**
  Driving and skilled tasks
  Although drowsiness is rare, nevertheless patients should be advised that it can occur and may affect performance of skilled tasks (e.g. cycling or driving); alcohol should be avoided.
- **MEDICINAL FORMS**
  There can be variation in the licensing of different medicines containing the same drug. Forms available from special-order manufacturers include: oral suspension, oral solution
  Tablet
  CAUTIONARY AND ADVISORY LABELS 5
  ‣ Fexofenadine hydrochloride (Non-proprietary)
  Fexofenadine hydrochloride 120 mg Fexofenadine 120mg tablets | 30 tablet [PoM] £7.15 DT price = £2.28
  Fexofenadine hydrochloride 180 mg Fexofenadine 180mg tablets | 30 tablet [PoM] £9.65 DT price = £3.24
  ‣ Telfast (Sanofi)
  Fexofenadine hydrochloride 30 mg Telfast 30mg tablets | 60 tablet [PoM] £5.46 DT price = £5.46
  Fexofenadine hydrochloride 120 mg Telfast 120mg tablets | 30 tablet [PoM] £5.99 DT price = £2.28
  Fexofenadine hydrochloride 180 mg Telfast 180mg tablets | 30 tablet [PoM] £7.58 DT price = £3.24

Levocetirizine hydrochloride

- **INDICATIONS AND DOSE**
  Symptomatic relief of allergy such as hay fever, urticaria
  ‣ BY MOUTH
  ‣ Child 2–5 years: 1.25 mg twice daily
  ‣ Child 6–17 years: 5 mg once daily
  PHARMACOKINETICS
  Levocetirizine is an isomer of cetirizine.

- **UNLICENSED USE** Tablets not licensed for use in children under 6 years.
- **CONTRA-INDICATIONS** Avoid in Acute porphyrias p. 562 (some antihistamines are thought to be safe)
- **CAUTIONS** Epilepsy
- **INTERACTIONS** → Appendix 1 (antihistamines). Sedative antihistamine interactions apply to a lesser extent to the non-sedating antihistamines.
- **SIDE-EFFECTS**
  ‣ **Uncommon** Antimuscarinic effects · blurred vision · dry mouth · gastro-intestinal disturbances · headache · psychomotor impairment · urinary retention
  ‣ **Rare** Anaphylaxis · angioedema · arrhythmias · blood disorders · bronchospasm · confusion · convulsions · depression · dizziness · extrapyramidal effects · hypersensitivity reactions · hypotension · liver dysfunction · palpitation · photosensitivity reactions · rashes · sleep disturbances · tremor
  ‣ **Very rare** Weight gain
  ‣ **Frequency not known** Drowsiness
  SIDE-EFFECTS, FURTHER INFORMATION
  Non-sedating antihistamines such as levocetirizine cause less sedation and psychomotor impairment than the older antihistamines because they penetrate the blood brain barrier only to a slight extent.
  If drowsiness occurs, it may diminish after a few days of treatment.
  Children are more susceptible to side-effects.

- **PREGNANCY** Most manufacturers of antihistamines advise avoiding their use during pregnancy; however, there is no evidence of teratogenicity.
- **BREAST FEEDING** Most antihistamines are present in breast milk in varying amounts; although not known to be harmful, most manufacturers advise avoiding their use in mothers who are breast-feeding.
- **RENAL IMPAIRMENT** Reduce dose frequency to alternate days if estimated glomerular filtration rate 30–50 mL/minute/1.73 m^2. Reduce dose frequency to every 3 days if estimated glomerular filtration rate 10–30 mL/minute/1.73 m^2. Avoid if estimated glomerular filtration rate less than 10 mL/minute/1.73 m^2.
- **PATIENT AND CARER ADVICE**
  Driving and skilled tasks
  Although drowsiness is rare, nevertheless patients should be advised that it can occur and may affect performance of skilled tasks (e.g. cycling or driving); alcohol should be avoided.
- **MEDICINAL FORMS**
  There can be variation in the licensing of different medicines containing the same drug.
  Tablet
  ‣ Levocetirizine hydrochloride (Non-proprietary)
  Levocetirizine dihydrochloride 5 mg Levocetirizine 5mg tablets | 30 tablet [PoM] £4.39 DT price = £4.28
  ‣ Xyzal (UCB Pharma Ltd)
  Levocetirizine dihydrochloride 5 mg Xyzal 5mg tablets | 30 tablet [PoM] £4.39 DT price = £4.28
  Oral solution
  ‣ Xyzal (UCB Pharma Ltd)
  Levocetirizine dihydrochloride 500 microgram per 1 ml Xyzal 0.5mg/ml oral solution sugar-free | 200 ml [PoM] £6.00 DT price = £6.00

Loratadine

- **INDICATIONS AND DOSE**
  Symptomatic relief of allergy such as hay fever, chronic idiopathic urticaria
  ‣ BY MOUTH
  ‣ Child 2–11 years (body-weight up to 31 kg): 5 mg once daily
  ‣ Child 2–11 years (body-weight 31 kg and above): 10 mg once daily
  ‣ Child 12–17 years: 10 mg once daily

- **CAUTIONS** Acute porphyrias p. 562 · epilepsy
- **INTERACTIONS** → Appendix 1 (antihistamines). Sedative antihistamine interactions apply to a lesser extent to the non-sedating antihistamines. Interactions do not generally apply to antihistamines used for topical action (including inhalation).
- **SIDE-EFFECTS**
  ‣ **Uncommon** Antimuscarinic effects · blurred vision · dry mouth · gastro-intestinal disturbances · Headache · psychomotor impairment · urinary retention
  ‣ **Rare** Anaphylaxis · angioedema · arrhythmias · blood disorders · bronchospasm · confusion · convulsions · depression · dizziness · extrapyramidal effects · hypersensitivity reactions · hypotension · liver dysfunction · palpitation · photosensitivity reactions · rashes · sleep disturbances · tremor
  ‣ **Frequency not known** Drowsiness
  SIDE-EFFECTS, FURTHER INFORMATION
  Non-sedating antihistamines such as loratadine cause less sedation and psychomotor impairment than the older antihistamines because they penetrate the blood brain barrier only to a slight extent.
  If drowsiness occurs, it may diminish after a few days of treatment.
  Children are more susceptible to side-effects.

- **PREGNANCY** Most manufacturers of antihistamines advise avoiding their use during pregnancy; however, there is no evidence of teratogenicity.
- **BREAST FEEDING** Most antihistamines are present in breast milk in varying amounts; although not known to be harmful, most manufacturers advise avoiding their use in mothers who are breast-feeding.
- **HEPATIC IMPAIRMENT** Reduce dose frequency to alternate days in severe impairment.
- **PATIENT AND CARER ADVICE**
  Driving and skilled tasks
  Although drowsiness is rare, nevertheless patients and their carers should be advised that it can occur and may affect performance of skilled tasks (e.g. cycling or driving); alcohol should be avoided.
- **PROFESSION SPECIFIC INFORMATION**
  Dental practitioners' formulary
  Loratadine 10 mg tablets may be prescribed.
  Loratadine syrup 5 mg/5 mL may be prescribed.
- **MEDICINAL FORMS**
  There can be variation in the licensing of different medicines containing the same drug.
  Tablet
  ‣ **Loratadine (Non-proprietary)**
  Loratadine 10 mg Loratadine 10mg tablets | 14 tablet [GSL] no price available | 30 tablet [P] £8.20 DT price = £0.86
  ‣ **Clarityn (Loratadine)** (Bayer Plc)
  Loratadine 10 mg Clarityn Allergy 10mg tablets | 60 tablet [P] £8.85
  Oral solution
  EXCIPIENTS: May contain Propylene glycol
  ‣ **Loratadine (Non-proprietary)**
  Loratadine 1 mg per 1 ml Loratadine 5mg/5ml oral solution | 100 ml [P] £4.85 DT price = £1.80 | 100 ml [PoM] £2.63 DT price = £1.80 | 120 ml [P] £2.40–£2.47 | 120 ml [PoM] £2.40
  ‣ **Clarityn (Loratadine)** (Bayer Plc)
  Loratadine 1 mg per 1 ml Clarityn Allergy 5mg/5ml syrup | 70 ml [GSL] £2.43
  Oral lyophilisate
  ‣ **Clarityn (Loratadine)** (Bayer Plc)
  Loratadine 10 mg Clarityn Rapide Allergy 10mg tablets sugar-free | 10 tablet [GSL] £3.24

Mizolastine

- **INDICATIONS AND DOSE**
  Symptomatic relief of allergy such as hay fever, urticaria
  ‣ BY MOUTH
  ‣ Child 12–17 years: 10 mg once daily

- **CONTRA-INDICATIONS** Avoid in Acute porphyrias p. 562 (some antihistamines are thought to be safe) · cardiac disease · hypokalaemia · susceptibility to QT-interval prolongation
- **CAUTIONS** Epilepsy
- **INTERACTIONS** → Appendix 1 (antihistamines).
  Sedative antihistamine interactions apply to a lesser extent to the non-sedating antihistamines.
- **SIDE-EFFECTS**
  ‣ **Common or very common** Anxiety · asthenia · weight gain
  ‣ **Uncommon** Antimuscarinic effects · arthralgia · blurred vision · dry mouth · gastro-intestinal disturbances · headache · myalgia · psychomotor impairment · urinary retention
  ‣ **Rare** Anaphylaxis · angioedema · arrhythmias · blood disorders · bronchospasm · confusion · convulsions · depression · dizziness · extrapyramidal effects · hypersensitivity reactions · hypotension · liver dysfunction · palpitation · photosensitivity reactions · rashes · sleep disturbances · tremor
  ‣ **Frequency not known** Drowsiness

SIDE-EFFECTS, FURTHER INFORMATION
Non-sedating antihistamines such as mizolastine cause less sedation and psychomotor impairment than the older antihistamines because they penetrate the blood brain barrier only to a slight extent.
  If drowsiness occurs, it may diminish after a few days of treatment.
  Children are more susceptible to side-effects.

- **PREGNANCY** Most manufacturers of antihistamines advise avoiding their use during pregnancy; however, there is no evidence of teratogenicity.
- **BREAST FEEDING** Most antihistamines are present in breast milk in varying amounts; although not known to be harmful, most manufacturers advise avoiding their use in mothers who are breast-feeding.
- **HEPATIC IMPAIRMENT** Manufacturer advises avoid in significant impairment.
- **PATIENT AND CARER ADVICE**
  Driving and skilled tasks
  Although drowsiness is rare, nevertheless patients and their carers should be advised that it can occur and may affect performance of skilled tasks (e.g. cycling or driving); alcohol should be avoided.
- **MEDICINAL FORMS**
  There can be variation in the licensing of different medicines containing the same drug.
  Modified-release tablet
  CAUTIONARY AND ADVISORY LABELS 25
  ‣ **Mizollen** (Sanofi)
  Mizolastine 10 mg Mizollen 10mg modified-release tablets | 30 tablet [PoM] £6.92 DT price = £6.92

ANTIHISTAMINES ⟩ SEDATING

Alimemazine tartrate
(Trimeprazine tartrate)

- **INDICATIONS AND DOSE**
  Urticaria | Pruritus
  ‣ BY MOUTH
  ‣ Child 6 months–1 year (specialist use only): 250 micrograms/kg 3–4 times a day (max. per dose 2.5 mg)
  ‣ Child 2–4 years: 2.5 mg 3–4 times a day
  ‣ Child 5–11 years: 5 mg 3–4 times a day
  ‣ Child 12–17 years: 10 mg 2–3 times a day, in severe cases up to maximum daily dose has been used; maximum 100 mg per day
  Premedication to anaesthesia
  ‣ BY MOUTH
  ‣ Child 2–6 years: Up to 2 mg/kg, to be given 1–2 hours before operation

- **UNLICENSED USE** Not licensed for use in children under 2 years.
- **CONTRA-INDICATIONS** Children under 2 years except on specialist advice (safety of such use has not been established) · epilepsy · hepatic dysfunction · history of narrow angle glaucoma · hypothyroidism · many antihistamines should be avoided in Acute porphyrias p. 562 but alimemazine is thought to be safe · myasthenia gravis · neonate (with significant antimuscarinic activity) · phaeochromocytoma · renal dysfunction
- **CAUTIONS** Cardiovascular diseases (due to tachycardia-inducing and hypotensive effects of phenothiazines) · exposure to sunlight should be avoided during treatment with high doses · pyloroduodenal obstruction · urinary retention · volume depleted patients who are more susceptible to orthostatic hypotension
- **INTERACTIONS** → Appendix 1 (antihistamines).

- SIDE-EFFECTS
▸ **Rare** Anaphylaxis · angioedema · bronchospasm · hypersensitivity reactions
▸ **Frequency not known** Acute dystonia · agitation · agranulocytosis · akathisia · akinesia · angle-closure glaucoma · anti-muscarinic effects · arrhythmias (may be predisposed by hypokalaemia and cardiac disease)· blurred vision · contact sensitisation · convulsions · drowsiness · dry mouth · dyskinesia · gastro-intestinal disturbances · headache · hyperprolactinaemia · hypotension · insomnia · jaundice · leukopenia (on prolonged high dose) · nasal stuffiness · neuroleptic malignant syndrome · ocular changes · pallor · paradoxical excitement · parkinsonism · photosensitivity · postural hypotension (in volume depletion) · rashes · respiratory depression · rigidity · tardive dyskinesia (usually after prolonged high doses) · tremor · urinary retention

SIDE-EFFECTS, FURTHER INFORMATION
Patients on high dosage may develop photosensitivity and should avoid exposure to direct sunlight.
  Children are more susceptible to side-effects.
  Drowsiness is a significant side-effect with most of the older antihistamines although paradoxical stimulation may occur rarely in children, especially with high doses. Drowsiness may diminish after a few days of treatment and is considerably less of a problem with the newer antihistamines.

- PREGNANCY Most manufacturers of antihistamines advise avoiding their use during pregnancy; however, there is no evidence of teratogenicity. Use in the latter part of the third trimester may cause adverse effects in neonates such as irritability, paradoxical excitability, and tremor.

- BREAST FEEDING Most antihistamines are present in breast milk in varying amounts; although not known to be harmful, most manufacturers advise avoiding their use in mothers who are breast-feeding.

- HEPATIC IMPAIRMENT Avoid in severe liver disease— increased risk of coma.

- RENAL IMPAIRMENT Avoid.

- PATIENT AND CARER ADVICE
Driving and skilled tasks
Although drowsiness is rare, nevertheless children and their carers should be advised that it can occur and may affect performance of skilled tasks (e.g. cycling or driving); alcohol should be avoided.

- MEDICINAL FORMS
There can be variation in the licensing of different medicines containing the same drug. Forms available from special-order manufacturers include: oral solution
Tablet
CAUTIONARY AND ADVISORY LABELS 2
▸ **Alimemazine tartrate (Non-proprietary)**
Alimemazine tartrate 10 mg Alimemazine 10mg tablets | 25 tablet [PoM] no price available | 28 tablet [PoM] £67.81 DT price = £62.16
Oral solution
CAUTIONARY AND ADVISORY LABELS 2
▸ **Alimemazine tartrate (Non-proprietary)**
Alimemazine tartrate 1.5 mg per 1 ml Alimemazine 7.5mg/5ml oral solution | 100 ml [PoM] £124.74 DT price = £114.35
Alimemazine tartrate 6 mg per 1 ml Alimemazine 30mg/5ml oral solution | 100 ml [PoM] £180.00 DT price = £176.65

Chlorphenamine maleate
(Chlorpheniramine maleate)

- INDICATIONS AND DOSE
Symptomatic relief of allergy such as hay fever, urticaria, food allergy, drug reactions | Relief of itch associated with chickenpox
▸ BY MOUTH
▸ **Child 1–23 months:** 1 mg twice daily
▸ **Child 2–5 years:** 1 mg every 4–6 hours; maximum 6 mg per day
▸ **Child 6–11 years:** 2 mg every 4–6 hours; maximum 12 mg per day
▸ **Child 12–17 years:** 4 mg every 4–6 hours; maximum 24 mg per day
▸ BY INTRAMUSCULAR INJECTION, OR BY INTRAVENOUS INJECTION
▸ **Child 1–5 months:** 250 micrograms/kg (max. per dose 2.5 mg), repeated if necessary; maximum 4 doses per day
▸ **Child 6 months–5 years:** 2.5 mg, repeated if necessary; maximum 4 doses per day
▸ **Child 6–11 years:** 5 mg, repeated if necessary; maximum 4 doses per day
▸ **Child 12–17 years:** 10 mg, repeated if necessary; maximum 4 doses per day

Emergency treatment of anaphylactic reactions
▸ BY INTRAMUSCULAR INJECTION, OR BY INTRAVENOUS INJECTION
▸ **Child 1–5 months:** 250 micrograms/kg (max. per dose 2.5 mg), repeated if necessary; maximum 4 doses per day
▸ **Child 6 months–5 years:** 2.5 mg, repeated if necessary; maximum 4 doses per day
▸ **Child 6–11 years:** 5 mg, repeated if necessary; maximum 4 doses per day
▸ **Child 12–17 years:** 10 mg, repeated if necessary; maximum 4 doses per day

- UNLICENSED USE *Injection* not licensed for use in neonates. *Tablets* not licensed for use in children under 6 years. *Syrup* not licensed for use in children under 1 year.

> **IMPORTANT SAFETY INFORMATION**
> MHRA/CHM ADVICE (MARCH 2008 AND FEBRUARY 2009) OVER-THE-COUNTER COUGH AND COLD MEDICINES FOR CHILDREN
> Children under 6 years should not be given over-the-counter cough and cold medicines containing chlorphenamine.

- CONTRA-INDICATIONS Many antihistamines should be avoided in Acute porphyrias p. 562 but chlorphenamine is thought to be safe · neonate (due to significant antimuscarinic activity)

- CAUTIONS Epilepsy · pyloroduodenal obstruction · susceptibility to angle-closure glaucoma · urinary retention

- INTERACTIONS → Appendix 1 (antihistamines).

- SIDE-EFFECTS
GENERAL SIDE-EFFECTS
▸ **Common or very common** Blurred vision · dry mouth · gastro-intestinal disturbances · headache · psychomotor impairment · urinary retention
▸ **Rare** Anaphylaxis · angioedema · arrhythmias · bronchospasm · confusion · convulsions · depression · dizziness · extrapyramidal effects · hypersensitivity reactions · hypotension · liver dysfunction · palpitation · photosensitivity reactions · sleep disturbances · tremor
▸ **Frequency not known** Antimuscarinic effects · blood disorders · exfoliative dermatitis · rashes · tinnitus

SPECIFIC SIDE-EFFECTS
▸ With intramuscular or intravenous use CNS stimulation · irritant effects · transient hypotension

SIDE-EFFECTS, FURTHER INFORMATION
Children are more susceptible to side-effects.

Drowsiness is a significant side-effect with most of the older antihistamines although paradoxical stimulation may occur rarely in children, especially with high doses. Drowsiness may diminish after a few days of treatment and is considerably less of a problem with the newer antihistamines.

● **PREGNANCY** Most manufacturers of antihistamines advise avoiding their use during pregnancy; however, there is no evidence of teratogenicity. Use in the latter part of the third trimester may cause adverse effects in neonates such as irritability, paradoxical excitability, and tremor.

● **BREAST FEEDING** Most antihistamines are present in breast milk in varying amounts; although not known to be harmful, most manufacturers advise avoiding their use in mothers who are breast-feeding.

● **HEPATIC IMPAIRMENT** Avoid in severe liver disease—increased risk of coma.

● **DIRECTIONS FOR ADMINISTRATION** For *intravenous injection*, give over 1 minute; if small dose required, dilute with Sodium Chloride 0.9%.

● **PATIENT AND CARER ADVICE**
Driving and skilled tasks
Drowsiness may affect performance of skilled tasks (e.g. cycling or driving); sedating effects enhanced by alcohol.
Medicines for Children leaflet: Chlorphenamine maleate for allergy symptoms www.medicinesforchildren.org.uk/chlorphenamine-maleate-allergy-symptoms-0

● **PROFESSION SPECIFIC INFORMATION**
Dental practitioners' formulary
Chlorphenamine tablets may be prescribed.
Chlorphenamine oral solution may be prescribed.

● **EXCEPTIONS TO LEGAL CATEGORY**
▸ With intramuscular use or intravenous use Prescription only medicine restriction does not apply to chlorphenamine injection where administration is for saving life in emergency.

● **MEDICINAL FORMS**
There can be variation in the licensing of different medicines containing the same drug. Forms available from special-order manufacturers include: oral solution

Tablet
CAUTIONARY AND ADVISORY LABELS 2
▸ Chlorphenamine maleate (Non-proprietary)
Chlorphenamine maleate 4 mg Chlorphenamine 4mg tablets | 28 tablet [P] £1.08 DT price = £0.75 | 30 tablet [P] no price available
▸ Hayleve (Genesis Pharmaceuticals Ltd)
Chlorphenamine maleate 4 mg Hayleve 4mg tablets | 28 tablet [P] £0.84 DT price = £0.75
▸ Piriton (GlaxoSmithKline Consumer Healthcare)
Chlorphenamine maleate 4 mg Piriton 4mg tablets | 500 tablet [P] £4.06
Piriton Allergy 4mg tablets | 30 tablet [P] £2.06 | 60 tablet [P] £3.73
▸ Pollenase (chlorphenamine) (E M Pharma)
Chlorphenamine maleate 4 mg Pollenase Antihistamine 4mg tablets | 30 tablet [P] £1.20

Oral solution
CAUTIONARY AND ADVISORY LABELS 2
▸ Chlorphenamine maleate (Non-proprietary)
Chlorphenamine maleate 400 microgram per 1 ml Chlorphenamine 2mg/5ml oral solution sugar free | 150 ml [P] £2.62 DT price = £2.62
▸ Allerief (Orbis Consumer Products Ltd)
Chlorphenamine maleate 400 microgram per 1 ml Allerief 2mg/5ml oral solution sugar-free | 150 ml [P] £2.22 DT price = £2.62
▸ Piriton (GlaxoSmithKline Consumer Healthcare)
Chlorphenamine maleate 400 microgram per 1 ml Piriton 2mg/5ml syrup | 150 ml [P] £2.62 DT price = £2.62

Solution for injection
▸ Chlorphenamine maleate (Non-proprietary)
Chlorphenamine maleate 10 mg per 1 ml Chlorphenamine 10mg/1ml solution for injection ampoules | 5 ampoule [PoM] £22.48-£22.50 DT price = £22.50

Hydroxyzine hydrochloride
22.2.2016

● **DRUG ACTION** Hydroxyzine is a sedating antihistamine which exerts its actions by antagonising the effects of histamine.

● **INDICATIONS AND DOSE**
Pruritus
▸ BY MOUTH
▸ Child 6 months–5 years: 5–15 mg daily in divided doses, dose adjusted according to weight; maximum 2 mg/kg per day
▸ Child 6–17 years (body-weight up to 40 kg): Initially 15–25 mg daily in divided doses, dose increased as necessary, adjusted according to weight; maximum 2 mg/kg per day
▸ Child 6–17 years (body-weight 40 kg and above): Initially 15–25 mg daily in divided doses, increased if necessary to 50–100 mg daily in divided doses, dose adjusted according to weight

● **UNLICENSED USE** *Ucerax* ® preparations not licensed for use in children under 1 year.

> **IMPORTANT SAFETY INFORMATION**
> MHRA/CHM ADVICE: RISK OF QT-INTERVAL PROLONGATION AND TORSADE DE POINTES (APRIL 2015)
> Following concerns of heart rhythm abnormalities, the safety and efficacy of hydroxyzine has been reviewed by the European Medicines Agency. The review concludes that hydroxyzine is associated with a small risk of QT-interval prolongation and torsade de pointes; these events are most likely to occur in patients who have risk factors for QT prolongation, e.g. concomitant use of drugs that prolong the QT-interval, cardiovascular disease, family history of sudden cardiac death, significant electrolyte imbalance (low plasma-potassium or plasma-magnesium concentrations), or significant bradycardia.
> To minimise the risk of such adverse effects, the following dose restrictions have been made and new cautions and contra-indications added:
> ● Hydroxyzine is contra-indicated in patients with prolonged QT-interval or who have risk factors for QT-interval prolongation;
> ● Consider the risks of QT-interval prolongation and torsade de pointes before prescribing to patients taking drugs that lower heart rate or plasma-potassium concentration;
> ● In children with body-weight up to 40 kg, the maximum daily dose is 2 mg/kg;
> ● The lowest effective dose for the shortest period of time should be prescribed.

● **CONTRA-INDICATIONS** Acquired or congenital QT interval prolongation · avoid in Acute porphyrias p. 562 (some antihistamines are thought to be safe) · predisposition to QT interval prolongation

CONTRA-INDICATIONS, FURTHER INFORMATION
▸ QT interval prolongation Risk factors for QT interval prolongation include significant electrolyte imbalance, bradycardia, cardiovascular disease, and family history of sudden cardiac death.

● **CAUTIONS** Bladder outflow obstruction · breathing problems · cardiovascular disease · children · decreased gastrointestinal motility · dementia · epilepsy ·

Respiratory system

3

hypertension · hyperthyroidism · myasthenia gravis · pyloroduodenal obstruction · stenosing peptic ulcer · susceptibility to angle-closure glaucoma · urinary retention

CAUTIONS, FURTHER INFORMATION
Children have an increased susceptibility to side-effects, particularly CNS effects.

● INTERACTIONS → Appendix 1 (antihistamines).

● SIDE-EFFECTS
▸ **Common or very common** Dry mouth · fatigue · headache
▸ **Uncommon** Constipation · dizziness · insomnia · nausea
▸ **Rare** Blood disorders · bronchospasm · liver dysfunction · rashes
▸ **Frequency not known** Agitation · alopecia · anorexia · anxiety · blurred vision · coma · confusion · convulsions (with high doses) · depression · diarrhoea · drowsiness · dyskinesia (after stopping use) · extrapyramidal effects · flushing · hallucinations · hypotension · impotence · labrynthitis · menstrual disturbances · myalgia · palpitation · priapsim · psychomotor impairment · sleep disturbances · tachycardia · tinnitus · tremor (with high doses) · urinary retention · ventricular arrhythmias · vertigo · vomiting

SIDE-EFFECTS, FURTHER INFORMATION
Drowsiness is a significant side-effect with most of the older antihistamines although paradoxical stimulation may occur rarely, especially with high doses. Drowsiness may diminish after a few days of treatment and is considerably less of a problem with the newer antihistamines.

● ALLERGY AND CROSS-SENSITIVITY Manufacturer advises hydroxyzine should be avoided in patients with previous hypersensitivity to cetirizine or other piperazine derivatives, and aminophylline.

● PREGNANCY Manufacturers advise avoid—toxicity in *animal* studies with higher doses. Use in the latter part of the third trimester may cause irritability, paradoxical excitability, and tremor in the neonate.

● BREAST FEEDING Manufacturer advises avoid—expected to be present in milk but effect unknown.

● HEPATIC IMPAIRMENT Manufacturer advises reduce daily dose by one-third. Manufacturer advises avoid in severe liver disease—increased risk of coma.

● RENAL IMPAIRMENT Manufacturers advise reduce daily dose by half in moderate to severe renal impairment.

● EFFECT ON LABORATORY TESTS May interfere with methacholine test—manufacturer advises stop treatment 96 hours prior to test. May interfere with skin testing for allergy—manufacturer advises stop treatment one week prior to test.

● PATIENT AND CARER ADVICE
Driving and skilled tasks
Drowsiness may affect performance of skilled tasks (e.g. cycling or driving); sedating effects enhanced by alcohol.

● MEDICINAL FORMS
There can be variation in the licensing of different medicines containing the same drug. Forms available from special-order manufacturers include: oral suspension, oral solution
Tablet
CAUTIONARY AND ADVISORY LABELS 2
▸ **Atarax** (Alliance Pharmaceuticals Ltd)
Hydroxyzine hydrochloride 10 mg Atarax 10mg tablets | 84 tablet PoM £1.20 DT price = £1.20
Hydroxyzine hydrochloride 25 mg Atarax 25mg tablets | 28 tablet PoM £0.62 DT price = £0.62

Ketotifen

● INDICATIONS AND DOSE
Allergic rhinitis
▸ BY MOUTH
▸ Child 3–17 years: 1 mg twice daily

● CONTRA-INDICATIONS Avoid in Acute porphyrias p. 562 (some antihistamines are thought to be safe)

● CAUTIONS Epilepsy · pyloroduodenal obstruction · susceptibility to angle-closure glaucoma · urinary retention

● INTERACTIONS → Appendix 1 (antihistamines).
Sedative antihistamine interactions apply to a lesser extent to the non-sedating antihistamines.

● SIDE-EFFECTS
▸ **Common or very common** Irritability · nervousness
▸ **Uncommon** Cystitis
▸ **Rare** Weight gain
▸ **Very rare** Stevens-Johnson syndrome
▸ **Frequency not known** Anaphylaxis · angioedema · antimuscarinic effects · arrhythmias · blood disorders · blurred vision · bronchospasm · confusion · convulsions · depression · dizziness · dry mouth · extrapyramidal effects · gastro-intestinal disturbances · headache · hypersensitivity reactions · hypotension · liver dysfunction · palpitation · photosensitivity reactions · psychomotor impairment · rashes · sleep disturbances · tremor · urinary retention

SIDE-EFFECTS, FURTHER INFORMATION
Drowsiness is a significant side-effect with most of the older antihistamines although paradoxical stimulation may occur rarely, especially with high doses. Drowsiness may diminish after a few days of treatment and is considerably less of a problem with the newer antihistamines.

● PREGNANCY Most manufacturers of antihistamines advise avoiding their use during pregnancy; however, there is no evidence of teratogenicity. Use in the latter part of the third trimester may cause adverse effects in neonates such as irritability, paradoxical excitability, and tremor.

● BREAST FEEDING Most antihistamines are present in breast milk in varying amounts; although not known to be harmful, most manufacturers advise avoiding their use in mothers who are breast-feeding.

● HEPATIC IMPAIRMENT Avoid in severe liver disease—increased risk of coma.

● PATIENT AND CARER ADVICE
Driving and skilled tasks
Drowsiness may affect performance of skilled tasks (e.g. driving or cycling); sedating effects enhanced by alcohol.

● MEDICINAL FORMS
There can be variation in the licensing of different medicines containing the same drug.
Tablet
CAUTIONARY AND ADVISORY LABELS 2, 21
▸ **Zaditen** (CD Pharma AB)
Ketotifen (as Ketotifen fumarate) 1 mg Zaditen 1mg tablets | 60 tablet PoM £7.53
Oral solution
CAUTIONARY AND ADVISORY LABELS 2, 21
▸ **Zaditen** (CD Pharma AB)
Ketotifen (as Ketotifen fumarate) 200 microgram per 1 ml Zaditen 1mg/5ml elixir sugar-free | 300 ml PoM £8.91 DT price = £8.91

Promethazine hydrochloride

- **INDICATIONS AND DOSE**

Symptomatic relief of allergy such as hay fever and urticaria | Insomnia associated with urticaria and pruritus
▸ BY MOUTH
  - Child 2-4 years: 5 mg twice daily, alternatively 5–15 mg once daily, dose to be taken at night
  - Child 5-9 years: 5–10 mg twice daily, alternatively 10–25 mg once daily, dose to be taken at night
  - Child 10-17 years: 10–20 mg 2–3 times a day, alternatively 25 mg once daily, dose to be taken at night, increased if necessary to 25 mg twice daily

Sedation (short-term use)
▸ BY MOUTH
  - Child 2-4 years: 15–20 mg
  - Child 5-9 years: 20–25 mg
  - Child 10-17 years: 25–50 mg

Sedation in intensive care
▸ BY MOUTH, OR BY SLOW INTRAVENOUS INJECTION, OR BY DEEP INTRAMUSCULAR INJECTION
  - Child 1 month-11 years: 0.5–1 mg/kg 4 times a day (max. per dose 25 mg), adjusted according to response
  - Child 12-17 years: 25–50 mg 4 times a day, adjusted according to response

Nausea | Vomiting | Vertigo | Labyrinthine disorders | Motion sickness
▸ BY MOUTH
  - Child 2-4 years: 5 mg, to be taken at bedtime on night before travel, repeat following morning if necessary
  - Child 5-9 years: 10 mg, to be taken at bedtime on night before travel, repeat following morning if necessary
  - Child 10-17 years: 20–25 mg, to be taken at bedtime on night before travel, repeat following morning if necessary

- **UNLICENSED USE** Not licensed for use for sedation in children under 2 years.

> **IMPORTANT SAFETY INFORMATION**
> MHRA/CHM ADVICE (MARCH 2008 AND FEBRUARY 2009) OVER-THE-COUNTER COUGH AND COLD MEDICINES FOR CHILDREN
> Children under 6 years should not be given over-the-counter cough and cold medicines containing promethazine.

- **CONTRA-INDICATIONS** Many antihistamines should be avoided in Acute porphyrias p. 562 but promethazine is thought to be safe · neonate (due to significant antimuscarinic activity) · should not be given to children under 2 years, except on specialist advice, because the safety of such use has not been established
- **CAUTIONS**
  GENERAL CAUTIONS
  Epilepsy · pyloroduodenal obstruction · severe coronary artery disease · susceptibility to angle-closure glaucoma · urinary retention
  SPECIFIC CAUTIONS
▸ With intravenous use Avoid extravasation with intravenous injection
- **INTERACTIONS** → Appendix 1 (antihistamines).
- **SIDE-EFFECTS**
▸ **Rare** Anaphylaxis · angioedema · angle-closure glaucoma · arrhythmias · blood disorders · bronchospasm · confusion · convulsions · depression · dizziness · extrapyramidal effects · hypersensitivity reactions · hypotension · liver dysfunction · palpitation · photosensitivity reactions · rashes · sleep disturbances · tremor
▸ **Frequency not known** Antimuscarinic effects · blurred vision · drowsiness · dry mouth · gastro-intestinal

disturbances · headache · psychomotor impairment · restlessness · urinary retention
  SIDE-EFFECTS, FURTHER INFORMATION
  Children are more susceptible to side-effects.
    Drowsiness is a significant side-effect with most of the older antihistamines although paradoxical stimulation may occur rarely in children, especially with high doses. Drowsiness may diminish after a few days of treatment and is considerably less of a problem with the newer antihistamines.
- **PREGNANCY** Most manufacturers of antihistamines advise avoiding their use during pregnancy; however, there is no evidence of teratogenicity. Use in the latter part of the third trimester may cause adverse effects in neonates such as irritability, paradoxical excitability, and tremor.
- **BREAST FEEDING** Most antihistamines are present in breast milk in varying amounts; although not known to be harmful, most manufacturers advise avoiding their use in mothers who are breast-feeding.
- **HEPATIC IMPAIRMENT** Avoid in severe liver disease—increased risk of coma.
- **RENAL IMPAIRMENT** Use with caution.
- **PATIENT AND CARER ADVICE**
  Driving and skilled tasks
  Drowsiness may affect the performance of skilled tasks (e.g. cycling or driving); sedating effects enhanced by alcohol.
- **PROFESSION SPECIFIC INFORMATION**
  Dental practitioners' formulary
  Promethazine Hydrochloride Tablets 10 mg or 25 mg may be prescribed.
    Promethazine Hydrochloride Oral Solution (elixir) 5 mg/5 mL may be prescribed.
- **LESS SUITABLE FOR PRESCRIBING** Promethazine is less suitable for prescribing for sedation.
- **EXCEPTIONS TO LEGAL CATEGORY** Prescription only medicine restriction does not apply to promethazine hydrochloride injection where administration is for saving life in emergency.

- **MEDICINAL FORMS**
  There can be variation in the licensing of different medicines containing the same drug. Forms available from special-order manufacturers include: oral suspension, oral solution
  Tablet
  CAUTIONARY AND ADVISORY LABELS 2
  ▸ Promethazine hydrochloride (Non-proprietary)
    Promethazine hydrochloride 10 mg Promethazine hydrochloride 10mg tablets | 56 tablet PoM £3.30 DT price = £2.96
  ▸ Phenergan (Sanofi)
    Promethazine hydrochloride 10 mg Phenergan 10mg tablets | 56 tablet P £2.96 DT price = £2.96
    Promethazine hydrochloride 25 mg Phenergan 25mg tablets | 56 tablet P £4.65 DT price = £4.65
  Oral solution
  CAUTIONARY AND ADVISORY LABELS 2
  EXCIPIENTS: May contain Sulfites
  ELECTROLYTES: May contain Sodium
  ▸ Phenergan (Sanofi)
    Promethazine hydrochloride 1 mg per 1 ml Phenergan 5mg/5ml elixir sugar-free | 100 ml P £2.85 DT price = £2.85
  Solution for injection
  EXCIPIENTS: May contain Sulfites
  ▸ Phenergan (Sanofi)
    Promethazine hydrochloride 25 mg per 1 ml Phenergan 25mg/1ml solution for injection ampoules | 10 ampoule PoM £6.74

3

Respiratory system

Bee venom extract

- **INDICATIONS AND DOSE**

Hypersensitivity to bee venom
- ▶ BY SUBCUTANEOUS INJECTION
- ▶ Child: (consult product literature)

IMPORTANT SAFETY INFORMATION
DESENSITISING VACCINES
In view of concerns about the safety of desensitising vaccines, it is recommended that they are used by specialists and only for the following indications:
- seasonal allergic hay fever (caused by pollen) that has not responded to anti-allergic drugs;
- hypersensitivity to wasp and bee venoms.
Desensitising vaccines should generally be avoided or used with particular care in patients with asthma.

- **CONTRA-INDICATIONS** Children under 5 years · consult product literature
- **CAUTIONS** Consult product literature
- **INTERACTIONS** → Appendix 1 (bee venom extracts). Contra-indicated in patients taking beta-blockers (adrenaline may be ineffective in case of a hypersensitivity reaction).
- **SIDE-EFFECTS**
SIDE-EFFECTS, FURTHER INFORMATION
Consult product literature.
- ▶ Hypersensitivity reactions Hypersensitivity reactions to immunotherapy (especially to wasp and bee venom extracts) can be life-threatening; bronchospasm usually develops within 1 hour and anaphylaxis within 30 minutes of injection. Therefore, cardiopulmonary resuscitation must be immediately available and patients need to be monitored for at least 1 hour after injection. If symptoms or signs of hypersensitivity develop (e.g. rash, urticaria, bronchospasm, faintness), **even when mild**, the patient should be observed until these have **resolved completely**.
- **PREGNANCY** Avoid.
- **PRESCRIBING AND DISPENSING INFORMATION** Each set of allergen extracts usually contains vials for the administration of graded amounts of allergen to patients undergoing hyposensitisation. Maintenance sets containing vials at the highest strength are also available. Product literature must be consulted for details of allergens, vial strengths, and administration.
- **NATIONAL FUNDING/ACCESS DECISIONS**
NICE technology appraisals (TAs)
- ▶ *Pharmalgen*® for bee and wasp venom allergy (February 2012) NICE TA246
Pharmalgen® is an option for the treatment of IgE-mediated bee and wasp venom allergy in those who have had:
- a severe systemic reaction to bee or wasp venom;
- a moderate systemic reaction to bee or wasp venom and who have a raised baseline serum-tryptase concentration, a high risk of future stings, or anxiety about future stings.
Treatment with *Pharmalgen*® should be initiated and monitored in a specialist centre experienced in venom immunotherapy.
www.nice.org.uk/TA246

- **MEDICINAL FORMS**
There can be variation in the licensing of different medicines containing the same drug.
Powder and solvent for solution for injection
- ▶ Bee Venom (ALK-Abello Ltd)
Bee venom 1.2 microgram Pharmalgen Bee Venom 1.2microgram powder and solvent for solution for injection vials | 1 vial [PoM] no price available
Bee venom 12 microgram Pharmalgen Bee Venom 12microgram powder and solvent for solution for injection vials | 1 vial [PoM] no price available
Bee venom 120 microgram Pharmalgen Bee Venom maintenance set 120microgram powder and solvent for solution for injection vials | 1 vial [PoM] no price available | 4 vial [PoM] £150.00
Bee venom 120 nanogram Pharmalgen Bee Venom 120nanogram powder and solvent for solution for injection vials | 1 vial [PoM] no price available

Grass pollen extract

- **INDICATIONS AND DOSE**

Treatment of seasonal allergic hay fever due to grass pollen in patients who have failed to respond to anti-allergy drugs
- ▶ BY SUBCUTANEOUS INJECTION
- ▶ Child: (consult product literature)

Treatment of seasonal allergic hay fever due to grass pollen in patients who have failed to respond to anti-allergy drugs (initiated under specialist supervision)
- ▶ BY MOUTH
- ▶ Child 5-17 years: 1 tablet daily, treatment to be started at least 4 months before start of pollen season and continue for up to 3 years

IMPORTANT SAFETY INFORMATION
DESENSITISING VACCINES
In view of concerns about the safety of desensitising vaccines, it is recommended that they are used by specialists and only for the following indications:
- seasonal allergic hay fever (caused by pollen) that has not responded to anti-allergic drugs;
- hypersensitivity to wasp and bee venoms.
Desensitising vaccines should generally be avoided or used with particular care in patients with asthma.

- **CONTRA-INDICATIONS** Children under 5 years · consult product literature
- **CAUTIONS** Consult product literature
- **INTERACTIONS** Desensitising vaccines should be avoided in patients taking beta-blockers (adrenaline may be ineffective in case of a hypersensitivity reaction), or ACE inhibitors (risk of severe anaphylactoid reactions).
- **SIDE-EFFECTS**
SIDE-EFFECTS, FURTHER INFORMATION
Consult product literature.
- ▶ Hypersensitivity reactions Hypersensitivity reactions to immunotherapy can be life-threatening; bronchospasm usually develops within 1 hour and anaphylaxis within 30 minutes of injection. Therefore, cardiopulmonary resuscitation must be immediately available and patients need to be monitored for at least 1 hour after injection. If symptoms or signs of hypersensitivity develop (e.g. rash, urticaria, bronchospasm, faintness), **even when mild**, the patient should be observed until these have **resolved completely**.
- **PREGNANCY** Should be avoided in pregnant women— consult product literature.
- **MONITORING REQUIREMENTS** The first dose of grass pollen extract should be (*Grazax*®) should be taken under medical supervision and the patient should be monitored for 20–30 minutes.

- **DIRECTIONS FOR ADMINISTRATION** Oral lyophilisates should be placed under the tongue and allowed to disperse. Advise patient not to swallow for 1 minute, or eat or drink for 5 minutes after taking the tablet. The first should be taken under medical supervision and the patient should be monitored for 20–30 minutes.
- **PRESCRIBING AND DISPENSING INFORMATION** Each set of allergen extracts usually contains vials for the administration of graded amounts of allergen to patients undergoing hyposensitisation. Maintenance sets containing vials at the highest strength are also available. Product literature must be consulted for details of allergens, vial strengths, and administration.
- **PATIENT AND CARER ADVICE**
  - With oral use Patients or carers should be given advice on how to administer oral lyophilisates.
- **MEDICINAL FORMS**
  There can be variation in the licensing of different medicines containing the same drug.
  Oral lyophilisate
  - Grazax (ALK-Abello Ltd)
    Phleum pratense 75000 SQ-T Grazax 75,000 SQ-T oral lyophilisates sugar-free | 30 tablet [PoM] £80.12
  Suspension for injection
  - Pollinex Grasses + Rye (Allergy Therapeutics (UK) Ltd)
    Pollinex Grasses + Rye suspension for injection treatment and extension course vials | 4 vial [PoM] £450.00

Tree pollen extract

- **INDICATIONS AND DOSE**

Treatment of seasonal allergic hay fever due to tree pollen in patients who have failed to respond to anti-allergy drugs
  - BY SUBCUTANEOUS INJECTION
  - Child: (consult product literature)

> **IMPORTANT SAFETY INFORMATION**
> DESENSITISING VACCINES
> In view of concerns about the safety of desensitising vaccines, it is recommended that they are used by specialists and only for the following indications:
> - seasonal allergic hay fever (caused by pollen) that has not responded to anti-allergic drugs;
> - hypersensitivity to wasp and bee venoms.
> Desensitising vaccines should generally be avoided or used with particular care in patients with asthma.

- **CONTRA-INDICATIONS** Children under 5 years · consult product literature
- **CAUTIONS** Consult product literature
- **INTERACTIONS** Desensitising vaccines should be avoided in patients taking beta-blockers (adrenaline may be ineffective in case of a hypersensitivity reaction), or ACE inhibitors (risk of severe anaphylactoid reactions).
- **SIDE-EFFECTS**
  SIDE-EFFECTS, FURTHER INFORMATION
  Consult product literature.
  - Hypersensitivity reactions Hypersensitivity reactions to immunotherapy (especially to wasp and bee venom extracts) can be life-threatening; bronchospasm usually develops within 1 hour and anaphylaxis within 30 minutes of injection. Therefore, cardiopulmonary resuscitation must be immediately available and patients need to be monitored for at least 1 hour after injection. If symptoms or signs of hypersensitivity develop (e.g. rash, urticaria, bronchospasm, faintness), **even when mild**, the patient should be observed until these have **resolved completely**.

- **PREGNANCY** Should be avoided in pregnant women—consult product literature.
- **PRESCRIBING AND DISPENSING INFORMATION** Each set of allergen extracts usually contains vials for the administration of graded amounts of allergen to patients undergoing hyposensitisation. Maintenance sets containing vials at the highest strength are also available. Product literature must be consulted for details of allergens, vial strengths, and administration.

- **MEDICINAL FORMS**
  There can be variation in the licensing of different medicines containing the same drug.
  Suspension for injection
  - Pollinex Trees (Allergy Therapeutics (UK) Ltd)
    Pollinex Trees No 3 suspension for injection 1ml vials | 1 vial [PoM] no price available
    Pollinex Trees No 2 suspension for injection 1ml vials | 1 vial [PoM] no price available
    Pollinex Trees No 1 suspension for injection 1ml vials | 1 vial [PoM] no price available
  - Pollinex Trees (Allergy Therapeutics (UK) Ltd)
    Pollinex Trees suspension for injection treatment and extension course vials | 4 vial [PoM] £450.00

Wasp venom extract

- **INDICATIONS AND DOSE**

Hypersensitivity to wasp venom
  - BY SUBCUTANEOUS INJECTION
  - Child: (consult product literature)

> **IMPORTANT SAFETY INFORMATION**
> DESENSITISING VACCINES
> In view of concerns about the safety of desensitising vaccines, it is recommended that they are used by specialists and only for the following indications:
> - seasonal allergic hay fever (caused by pollen) that has not responded to anti-allergic drugs;
> - hypersensitivity to wasp and bee venoms.
> Desensitising vaccines should generally be avoided or used with particular care in patients with asthma.

- **CONTRA-INDICATIONS** Children under 5 years · consult product literature
- **CAUTIONS** Consult product literature
- **INTERACTIONS** → Appendix 1 (wasp venom extracts). Contra-indicated in patients taking beta-blockers (adrenaline may be ineffective in case of a hypersensitivity reaction).
- **SIDE-EFFECTS**
  SIDE-EFFECTS, FURTHER INFORMATION
  Consult product literature.
  - Hypersensitivity reactions Hypersensitivity reactions to immunotherapy (especially to wasp and bee venom extracts) can be life-threatening; bronchospasm usually develops within 1 hour and anaphylaxis within 30 minutes of injection. Therefore, cardiopulmonary resuscitation must be immediately available and patients need to be monitored for at least 1 hour after injection. If symptoms or signs of hypersensitivity develop (e.g. rash, urticaria, bronchospasm, faintness), **even when mild**, the patient should be observed until these have **resolved completely**.
- **PREGNANCY** Avoid.
- **PRESCRIBING AND DISPENSING INFORMATION** Each set of allergen extracts usually contains vials for the administration of graded amounts of allergen to patients undergoing hyposensitisation. Maintenance sets containing vials at the highest strength are also available. Product literature must be consulted for details of allergens, vial strengths, and administration.

- NATIONAL FUNDING/ACCESS DECISIONS

NICE technology appraisals (TAs)

▸ *Pharmalgen*® for bee and wasp venom allergy (February 2012) NICE TA246

Pharmalgen® is an option for the treatment of IgE-mediated bee and wasp venom allergy in those who have had:

- a severe systemic reaction to bee or wasp venom;
- a moderate systemic reaction to bee or wasp venom and who have a raised baseline serum-tryptase concentration, a high risk of future stings, or anxiety about future stings.

Treatment with *Pharmalgen*® should be initiated and monitored in a specialist centre experienced in venom immunotherapy.

www.nice.org.uk/TA246

- MEDICINAL FORMS

There can be variation in the licensing of different medicines containing the same drug.

Powder and solvent for solution for injection

▸ Wasp Venom (ALK-Abello Ltd)

Wasp venom 1.2 microgram Pharmalgen Wasp Venom 1.2microgram powder and solvent for solution for injection vials | 1 vial PoM no price available

Wasp venom 12 microgram Pharmalgen Wasp Venom 12microgram powder and solvent for solution for injection vials | 1 vial PoM no price available

Wasp venom 120 nanogram Pharmalgen Wasp Venom 120nanogram powder and solvent for solution for injection vials | 1 vial PoM no price available

Wasp venom 120 microgram Pharmalgen Wasp Venom maintenance set 120microgram vaccine powder and solvent for solution for injection vials | 1 vial PoM no price available | 4 vial PoM £150.00

2.1 Angioedema

Drugs used for Angioedema not listed below
Adrenaline/epinephrine p. 128

DRUGS USED IN HEREDITARY ANGIOEDEMA ›
COMPLEMENT REGULATORY PROTEINS

C1-esterase inhibitor

- INDICATIONS AND DOSE

BERINERT®

Acute attacks of hereditary angioedema (under expert supervision)

▸ BY SLOW INTRAVENOUS INJECTION, OR BY INTRAVENOUS INFUSION

▸ Child: 20 units/kg

Short-term prophylaxis of hereditary angioedema before dental, medical, or surgical procedures (under expert supervision)

▸ BY SLOW INTRAVENOUS INJECTION, OR BY INTRAVENOUS INFUSION

▸ Child: 15–30 units/kg (max. per dose 1000 units) for 1 dose, to be administered less than 6 hours before procedure

CINRYZE®

Acute attacks of hereditary angioedema (under expert supervision)

▸ BY SLOW INTRAVENOUS INJECTION

▸ Child 12-17 years: 1000 units for 1 dose, dose may be repeated if necessary

Short-term prophylaxis of hereditary angioedema before dental, medical, or surgical procedures (under expert supervision)

▸ BY SLOW INTRAVENOUS INJECTION

▸ Child 12-17 years: 1000 units for 1 dose, to be administered up to 24 hours before procedure

Long-term prophylaxis of severe, recurrent attacks of hereditary angioedema where oral prophylaxis is inadequate, or when oral prophylaxis is inadequate or not tolerated (under expert supervision)

▸ BY SLOW INTRAVENOUS INJECTION

▸ Child 12-17 years: 1000 units every 3–4 days, interval between doses to be adjusted according to response

- CAUTIONS Vaccination against hepatitis A and hepatitis B may be required

- SIDE-EFFECTS Fever · headache · thrombosis (with high doses)

- PREGNANCY Manufacturer advises avoid unless essential.

- DIRECTIONS FOR ADMINISTRATION

CINRYZE® ▸ With intravenous use For *slow intravenous injection*, reconstitute (with solvent provided) to a concentration of 100 units/mL; give at a rate of 1 mL/minute.

- PRESCRIBING AND DISPENSING INFORMATION C1-esterase inhibitor is prepared from human plasma.

- MEDICINAL FORMS

There can be variation in the licensing of different medicines containing the same drug.

Powder and solvent for solution for injection
ELECTROLYTES: May contain Sodium

▸ Berinert P (CSL Behring UK Ltd)

C1-esterase inhibitor 500 unit Berinert 500unit powder and solvent for solution for injection vials | 1 vial PoM £467.50

C1-esterase inhibitor 1500 unit Berinert 1,500unit powder and solvent for solution for injection vials | 1 vial PoM £1,402.50

▸ Cinryze (Shire Pharmaceuticals Ltd) ▾

C1-esterase inhibitor 500 unit Cinryze 500unit powder and solvent for solution for injection vials | 2 vial PoM £1,336.00

3 Conditions affecting sputum viscosity

Mucolytics for cystic fibrosis

Overview

Mucolytics, such as carbocisteine p. 175 are used to facilitate mucociliary clearance and expectoration by reducing sputum viscosity but evidence of efficacy is limited.

Dornase alfa p. 175 is used to reduce sputum viscosity in children with cystic fibrosis.

Nebulised hypertonic sodium chloride (3–7%) is used to mobilise lower respiratory tract secretions in mucus consolidation (e.g cystic fibrosis). Nebulised hypertonic sodium chloride solution (3%) is used for mild to moderate acute viral bronchiolitis in infants.

Mesna p. 515 (*Mistabron*®) is used in some children with cystic fibrosis when other mucolytics have failed to reduce sputum viscosity.

Acetylcysteine p. 797 has been used to treat meconium ileus in neonates and distal intestinal obstruction syndrome in children with cystic fibrosis, but evidence of efficacy is lacking. *Gastrografin*®, or a bowel cleansing preparation containing macrogols, is usually more effective.

Acetylcysteine may be used as a mucolytic to prevent further obstruction.

MUCOLYTICS

Carbocisteine

● INDICATIONS AND DOSE

Reduction of sputum viscosity
▸ BY MOUTH
- Child 2–4 years: 62.5–125 mg 4 times a day
- Child 5–11 years: 250 mg 3 times a day
- Child 12–17 years: Initially 2.25 g daily in divided doses, then reduced to 1.5 g daily in divided doses, as condition improves

- ● CONTRA-INDICATIONS Active peptic ulceration
- ● CAUTIONS History of peptic ulceration (may disrupt the gastric mucosal barrier)
- ● SIDE-EFFECTS
▸ **Rare** Gastro-intestinal bleeding
▸ **Frequency not known** Erythema multiforme · Stevens-Johnson syndrome
- ● PREGNANCY Manufacturer advises avoid in first trimester.
- ● BREAST FEEDING No information available.
- ● PRESCRIBING AND DISPENSING INFORMATION Flavours of oral liquid formulations may include cherry, raspberry, cinnamon, or rum.

- ● MEDICINAL FORMS
There can be variation in the licensing of different medicines containing the same drug.
Capsule
▸ Carbocisteine (Non-proprietary)
Carbocisteine 375 mg Carbocisteine 375mg capsules | 120 capsule PoM £18.98 DT price = £11.50
▸ Mucodyne (Sanofi)
Carbocisteine 375 mg Mucodyne 375mg capsules | 120 capsule PoM £18.98 DT price = £11.50
Oral solution
▸ Carbocisteine (Non-proprietary)
Carbocisteine 75 mg per 1 ml Carbocisteine 750mg/10ml oral solution 10ml sachets sugar free sugar-free | 15 sachet PoM £3.85 DT price = £3.85
▸ Mucodyne (Sanofi)
Carbocisteine 50 mg per 1 ml Mucodyne 250mg/5ml syrup | 300 ml PoM £8.39 DT price = £8.39

3.1 Cystic fibrosis

MUCOLYTICS

Dornase alfa

(Phosphorylated glycosylated recombinant human deoxyribonuclease 1 (rhDNase))

- ● DRUG ACTION Dornase alfa is a genetically engineered version of a naturally occurring human enzyme which cleaves extracellular deoxyribonucleic acid (DNA).

● INDICATIONS AND DOSE

Management of cystic fibrosis patients with a forced vital capacity (FVC) of greater than 40% of predicted to improve pulmonary function
▸ BY INHALATION OF NEBULISED SOLUTION
- Child 5–17 years: 2500 units once daily, administered by jet nebuliser

DOSE EQUIVALENCE AND CONVERSION
Dornase alfa 1000 units is equivalent to 1 mg

- ● SIDE-EFFECTS
▸ **Rare** Chest pain · conjunctivitis · dyspepsia · dysphonia · dyspnoea · laryngitis · pharyngitis · pyrexia · rash · rhinitis · urticaria

- ● PREGNANCY No evidence of teratogenicity; manufacturer advises use only if potential benefit outweighs risk.
- ● BREAST FEEDING Amount probably too small to be harmful—manufacturer advises caution.
- ● DIRECTIONS FOR ADMINISTRATION Dornase alfa is administered by inhalation using a jet nebuliser, usually once daily at least 1 hour before physiotherapy; however, alternate-day therapy may be as effective as daily treatment.
  For use undiluted with jet nebulisers only; ultrasonic nebulisers are unsuitable.
- ● PRESCRIBING AND DISPENSING INFORMATION Not all children benefit from treatment with dornase alfa; improvement occurs within 2 weeks, but in more severely affected children a trial of 6–12 weeks may be required.
- ● PATIENT AND CARER ADVICE
Medicines for Children leaflet: Dornase alfa for cystic fibrosis www.medicinesforchildren.org.uk/dornase-alfa-for-cystic-fibrosis

- ● MEDICINAL FORMS
There can be variation in the licensing of different medicines containing the same drug.
Nebuliser liquid
▸ Pulmozyme (Roche Products Ltd)
Dornase alfa 1 mg per 1 ml Pulmozyme 2.5mg nebuliser liquid 2.5ml ampoules | 30 ampoule PoM £496.43 DT price = £496.43

Ivacaftor

● INDICATIONS AND DOSE

Treatment of cystic fibrosis in patients who have a G551D mutation in the cystic fibrosis transmembrane conductance regulator (CFTR) gene (under expert supervision)
▸ BY MOUTH
- Child 6–17 years: 150 mg every 12 hours

DOSE ADJUSTMENTS DUE TO INTERACTIONS
Reduce dose to 150 mg twice a week with concomitant use of itraconazole, ketoconazole, posaconazole, voriconazole, telithromycin, and clarithromycin.
Reduce dose to 150 mg once daily with concomitant use of fluconazole and erythromycin.

- ● CONTRA-INDICATIONS Organ transplantation (no information available)
- ● INTERACTIONS → Appendix 1 (ivacaftor).
Avoid grapefruit and Seville oranges.
- ● SIDE-EFFECTS
▸ **Common or very common** Abdominal pain · diarrhoea · dizziness · ear discomfort · headache · nasal congestion · nasopharyngitis · oropharyngeal pain · pharyngeal oedema · rash · rhinitis · tinnitus · upper respiratory-tract infection
▸ **Uncommon** Gynaecomastia · vestibular disorder
- ● PREGNANCY Manufacturer advises use only if potential benefit outweighs risk—no information available.
- ● BREAST FEEDING Manufacturer advises use only if potential benefit outweighs risk—no information available.
- ● HEPATIC IMPAIRMENT Max. 150 mg once daily in moderate impairment; in severe impairment, manufacturer recommends use only if potential benefit outweighs risk—starting dose 150 mg on alternate days, dosing interval adjusted according to clinical response and tolerability.
- ● RENAL IMPAIRMENT Caution in severe impairment.
- ● PRE-TREATMENT SCREENING If the patient's genotype is unknown, a validated genotyping method should be performed to confirm the presence of the G551D mutation in at least one allele of the CFTR gene before starting treatment.

- **MONITORING REQUIREMENTS** Test liver function before treatment, every 3 months during the first year of treatment, then annually thereafter.
- **DIRECTIONS FOR ADMINISTRATION** Tablets should be taken with fat-containing food.
- **PRESCRIBING AND DISPENSING INFORMATION** Ivacaftor should be prescribed by a physician experienced in the treatment of cystic fibrosis.
- **PATIENT AND CARER ADVICE** Patients or carers should be given advice on how to administer ivacaftor tablets.

- **MEDICINAL FORMS**
  There can be variation in the licensing of different medicines containing the same drug.

  Tablet
  CAUTIONARY AND ADVISORY LABELS 25
  ‣ **Kalydeco** (Vertex Pharmaceuticals (UK) Ltd) ▼
  Ivacaftor 150 mg Kalydeco 150mg tablets | 56 tablet PoM £14,000.00

  Granules
  ‣ **Kalydeco** (Vertex Pharmaceuticals (UK) Ltd) ▼
  Ivacaftor 50 mg Kalydeco 50mg granules sachets sugar-free | 56 sachet PoM £14,000.00
  Ivacaftor 75 mg Kalydeco 75mg granules sachets sugar-free | 56 sachet PoM £14,000.00

4 Cough and congestion

Aromatic inhalations, cough preparations and systemic nasal decongestants

Aromatic inhalations

Inhalations containing volatile substances such as eucalyptus oil are traditionally used to relieve congestion and ease breathing. Although the vapour may contain little of the additive it encourages deliberate inspiration of warm moist air which is often comforting. Boiling water should not be used owing to the risk of scalding.

Strong aromatic decongestants (applied as rubs or to pillows) are not recommended for infants under the age of 3 months. Sodium chloride 0.9% solution given as nasal drops can be used to liquefy mucous secretions and relieve nasal congestion in infants and young children; administration before feeds may ease feeding difficulties caused by nasal congestion.

Cough preparations

Cough suppressants

Cough may be a symptom of an underlying disorder such as asthma, gastro-oesophageal reflux disease, or rhinitis, which should be addressed before prescribing cough suppressants. Cough may be associated with smoking or environmental pollutants. Cough can also result from bronchiectasis including that associated with cystic fibrosis; cough can also have a significant habit component. There is little evidence of any significant benefit from the use of cough suppressants in children with acute cough in ambulatory settings. Cough suppressants may cause sputum retention and this can be harmful in children with bronchiectasis.

The use of cough suppressants containing pholcodine below or similar opioid analgesics is not generally recommended in children and should be avoided in children under 6 years; the use of over-the-counter cough suppressants containing codeine phosphate p. 259 should be avoided in children under 12 years and in children of any age known to be CYP2D6 ultra-rapid metabolisers.

Sedating antihistamines are used as the cough suppressant component of many compound cough

preparations on sale to the public; all tend to cause drowsiness which may reflect their main mode of action.

Demulcent and expectorant cough preparations

Simple linctus and other demulcent cough preparations containing soothing substances, such as syrup or glycerol, may temporarily relieve a dry irritating cough. These preparations have the advantage of being harmless and inexpensive and sugar-free versions are available.

Expectorants are claimed to promote expulsion of bronchial secretions, but there is no evidence that any drug can specifically facilitate expectoration.

Compound cough preparations for children are on sale to the public but should not be used in children under 6 years; the rationale for some is dubious. Care should be taken to give the correct dose and to not use more than one preparation at a time.

MHRA/CHM advice (March 2008 and February 2009)

Children under 6 years should not be given over-the-counter cough and cold medicines containing the following ingredients:

- brompheniramine, chlorphenamine maleate p. 168, diphenhydramine, doxylamine, promethazine, or triprolidine (antihistamines);
- dextromethorphan or pholcodine (cough suppressants);
- guaifenesin or ipecacuanha (expectorants);
- phenylephrine hydrochloride p. 116, pseudoephedrine hydrochloride p. 649, ephedrine hydrochloride p. 649, oxymetazoline, or xylometazoline hydrochloride p. 650 (decongestants).

Over-the-counter cough and cold medicines can be considered for children aged 6–12 years after basic principles of best care have been tried, but treatment should be restricted to five days or less. Children should not be given more than 1 cough or cold preparation at a time because different brands may contain the same active ingredient; care should be taken to give the correct dose.

Systemic nasal decongestants

Nasal congestion in children due to allergic or vasomotor rhinitis should be treated with oral antihistamines, topical nasal preparations containing corticosteroids, or topical decongestants.

There is little evidence to support the use of systemic decongestants in children.

Pseudoephedrine hydrochloride has few sympathomimetic effects, and is commonly combined with other ingredients (including antihistamines) in preparations intended for the relief of cough and cold symptoms.

COUGH AND COLD PREPARATIONS ⟩ COUGH SUPPRESSANTS

▐ Pholcodine

- **INDICATIONS AND DOSE**
  Dry cough
  ‣ BY MOUTH USING LINCTUS
  ‣ Child 6–11 years: 2–5 mg 3–4 times a day
  ‣ Child 12–17 years: 5–10 mg 3–4 times a day

IMPORTANT SAFETY INFORMATION

MHRA/CHM ADVICE (MARCH 2008 AND FEBRUARY 2009) OVER-THE-COUNTER COUGH AND COLD MEDICINES FOR CHILDREN

Children under 6 years should not be given over-the-counter cough and cold medicines containing pholcodine (cough suppressant).

Over-the-counter cough and cold medicines can be considered for children aged 6–12 years after basic principles of best care have been tried, but treatment should be restricted to 5 days or less. Children should not be given more than 1 cough or cold preparation at a time because different brands may contain the same active ingredient; care should be taken to give the correct dose.

- **CONTRA-INDICATIONS** Bronchiectasis · bronchiolitis · chronic bronchitis · patients at risk of respiratory failure
- **CAUTIONS** Asthma · chronic cough · persistent cough · productive cough
- **INTERACTIONS** → Appendix 1 (pholcodine).
- **SIDE-EFFECTS** Confusion · constipation · dizziness · drowsiness · excitation · nausea · rash · sputum retention · vomiting
- **PREGNANCY** Manufacturer advises avoid unless potential benefit outweighs risk.
- **BREAST FEEDING** Manufacturer advises avoid unless potential benefit outweighs risk—no information available.
- **HEPATIC IMPAIRMENT** Avoid in hepatic impairment.
- **RENAL IMPAIRMENT** Use with caution in renal impairment. Avoid in severe renal impairment.
- **PRESCRIBING AND DISPENSING INFORMATION** Pholcodine is not generally recommended for children.
  Flavours of oral liquid formulations may include orange.
  When prepared extemporaneously, the BP states Pholcodine Linctus, BP consists of pholcodine 5 mg/5 mL in a suitable flavoured vehicle, containing citric acid monohydrate 1% and Pholcodine Linctus, Strong, BP consists of pholcodine 10 mg/5 mL in a suitable flavoured vehicle, containing citric acid monohydrate 2%

- **MEDICINAL FORMS**
There can be variation in the licensing of different medicines containing the same drug.
  Oral solution
  ▸ Pholcodine (Non-proprietary)
    Pholcodine 1 mg per 1 ml Pholcodine 5mg/5ml linctus | 200 ml Ⓟ £1.29 DT price = £1.29 Schedule 5 (CD Inv)
    Pholcodine 5mg/5ml linctus sugar free | 200 ml Ⓟ £1.31 DT price = £1.31 Schedule 5 (CD Inv) sugar-free | 2000 ml Ⓟ £13.10 Schedule 5 (CD Inv)
    Pholcodine 2 mg per 1 ml Pholcodine 10mg/5ml linctus strong sugar free | 2000 ml Ⓟ £10.88 DT price = £9.88 Schedule 5 (CD Inv)
    Pholcodine 10mg/5ml linctus strong | 200 ml Ⓟ £1.61 Schedule 5 (CD Inv)
  ▸ Galenphol (Thornton & Ross Ltd)
    Pholcodine 400 microgram per 1 ml Galenphol Paediatric 2mg/5ml linctus sugar-free | 2000 ml Ⓟ £4.50 DT price = £4.50 Schedule 5 (CD Inv)
    Pholcodine 1 mg per 1 ml Galenphol 5mg/5ml linctus sugar-free | 2000 ml Ⓟ £8.50 Schedule 5 (CD Inv)
    Pholcodine 2 mg per 1 ml Galenphol Strong 10mg/5ml linctus sugar-free | 2000 ml Ⓟ £9.88 DT price = £9.88 Schedule 5 (CD Inv)
  ▸ Pavacol-D (Alliance Pharmaceuticals Ltd)
    Pholcodine 1 mg per 1 ml Pavacol-D 5mg/5ml mixture sugar-free | 150 ml Ⓟ £1.69 Schedule 5 (CD Inv) sugar-free | 300 ml Ⓟ £2.55 Schedule 5 (CD Inv)

COUGH AND COLD PREPARATIONS ⟩ OTHER

Citric acid

(Formulated as Simple Linctus)

- **INDICATIONS AND DOSE**
Cough
▸ BY MOUTH
▸ Child 1 month–11 years: 5–10 mL 3–4 times a day, this dose is for Simple Linctus, Paediatric, BP (0.625%)
Cough
▸ BY MOUTH
▸ Child 12–17 years: 5 mL 3–4 times a day, this dose is for Simple Linctus, BP (2.5%)

- **PRESCRIBING AND DISPENSING INFORMATION** Flavours of oral liquid formulations may include anise.
  When prepared extemporaneously, the BP states Simple Linctus, Paediatric, BP consists of citric acid monohydrate 0.625% and Simple Linctus, BP consists of citric acid monohydrate 2.5%, both in a suitable vehicle with an anise flavour.

- **MEDICINAL FORMS**
There can be variation in the licensing of different medicines containing the same drug.
  Oral solution
  ▸ Citric acid (Non-proprietary)
    Citric acid monohydrate 6.25 mg per 1 ml Simple linctus paediatric sugar free sugar-free | 2000 ml GSL £12.50
    Simple linctus paediatric | 200 ml GSL £1.01 DT price = £1.01
    Citric acid monohydrate 25 mg per 1 ml Simple linctus sugar free sugar-free | 200 ml GSL £1.21 DT price = £0.89 sugar-free | 2000 ml GSL £8.40

MENTHOL AND DERIVATIVES

Eucalyptus with menthol

- **INDICATIONS AND DOSE**
Aromatic inhalation for relief of nasal congestion
▸ BY INHALATION
▸ Child: Add one teaspoonful to a pint of hot, **not** boiling, water and inhale the vapour

- **PRESCRIBING AND DISPENSING INFORMATION** When prepared extemporaneously, the BP states Menthol and Eucalyptus Inhalation, BP 1980 consists of racementhol or levomenthol 2 g, eucalyptus oil 10 mL, light magnesium carbonate 7 g, water to 100 mL.
  Not recommended (applied as a rub or to pillows) for infants under the age of 3 months.

- **PROFESSION SPECIFIC INFORMATION**
Dental practitioners' formulary
Menthol and Eucalyptus Inhalation BP, 1980 may be prescribed.

- **MEDICINAL FORMS**
There can be variation in the licensing of different medicines containing the same drug.
  Inhalation vapour
  ▸ Eucalyptus with menthol (Non-proprietary)
    Eucalyptus oil 100 microlitre per 1 ml, Menthol 20 mg per 1 ml, Magnesium carbonate light 70 mg per 1 ml Menthol and Eucalyptus inhalation | 100 ml GSL £1.34–£1.36 DT price = £1.35

RESINS

Benzoin tincture

(Friars' Balsam)

- **INDICATIONS AND DOSE**
Aromatic inhalation for relief of nasal congestion
▸ BY INHALATION
▸ Child: Add 5 mL to a pint of hot, **not** boiling, water and inhale the vapour; repeat after 4 hours if necessary

- **SIDE-EFFECTS** Allergic contact dermatitis
- **PRESCRIBING AND DISPENSING INFORMATION** Not recommended (applied as a rub or to pillows) for infants under 3 months.
  When prepared extemporaneously, the BP states Benzoin Tincture, Compound, BP consists of balsamic acids approx. 4.5%.

- **MEDICINAL FORMS**
There can be variation in the licensing of different medicines containing the same drug.
Liquid
CAUTIONARY AND ADVISORY LABELS 15
▸ **Benzoin tincture (Non-proprietary)**
Balsamic acids 16.5 mg per 1 ml Benzoin tincture | 500 ml GSL
£12.62–£22.78 DT price = £12.62

5 Respiratory depression, respiratory distress syndrome and apnoea

Respiratory stimulants

Respiratory stimulants

Respiratory stimulants (analeptic drugs), such as caffeine citrate p. 179, reduce the frequency of neonatal apnoea, and the need for mechanical ventilation during the first 7 days of treatment. They are typically used in the management of very preterm neonates, and continued until a corrected gestational age of 34 to 35 weeks is reached (or longer if necessary). They should only be given under **expert supervision** in hospital; it is important to rule out any underlying disorder, such as seizures, hypoglycaemia, or infection, causing respiratory exhaustion before starting treatment with a respiratory stimulant.

Pulmonary surfactants

Pulmonary surfactants derived from animal lungs, beractant below and poractant alfa below are used to prevent and treat respiratory distress syndrome (hyaline membrane disease) in neonates and preterm neonates. Prophylactic use of a pulmonary surfactant may reduce the need for mechanical ventilation and is more effective than 'rescue treatment' in preterm neonates of 29 weeks or less corrected gestational age. Pulmonary surfactants may also be of benefit in neonates with meconium aspiration syndrome or intrapartum streptococcal infection. Pulmonary immaturity with surfactant deficit is the commonest reason for respiratory failure in the neonate, especially in those of less than 30 weeks corrected gestational age. Betamethasone p. 409 given to the mother (at least 12 hours but preferably 48 hours) before delivery substantially enhances pulmonary maturity in the neonate.

PULMONARY SURFACTANTS

▌Beractant

- **INDICATIONS AND DOSE**
Treatment of respiratory distress syndrome in preterm neonates, birth-weight over 700 g (specialist use only)
▸ BY ENDOTRACHEAL TUBE

▸ Preterm neonate: 100 mg/kg, preferably administer within 8 hours of birth; dose may be repeated within 48 hours at intervals of at least 6 hours for up to 4 doses.

Prophylaxis of respiratory distress syndrome in preterm neonates (specialist use only)
▸ BY ENDOTRACHEAL TUBE

▸ Neonate up to 32 weeks corrected gestational age: 100 mg/kg, preferably administer within 15 minutes of birth; dose may be repeated within 48 hours at intervals of at least 6 hours for up to 4 doses.

- **DOSE EQUIVALENCE AND CONVERSION**
Phospholipid 100 mg/kg is equivalent to a volume of 4 mL/kg.

- **CAUTIONS** Consult product literature
- **SIDE-EFFECTS**
▸ **Rare** Bradycardia · decreased oxygen saturation · pulmonary haemorrhage
▸ **Frequency not known** Hyperoxia · intracranial haemorrhage · obstruction of the endotracheal tube by mucous secretions

- **MEDICINAL FORMS**
There can be variation in the licensing of different medicines containing the same drug.
Liquid
▸ **Survanta** (AbbVie Ltd)
Phospholipids (as Beractant) 25 mg per 1 ml Survanta 200mg/8ml endotracheopulmonary suspension bottles | 1 bottle PoM £306.43

▌Poractant alfa

- **INDICATIONS AND DOSE**
Treatment of respiratory distress syndrome in neonates, birth weight over 700 g (specialist use only)
▸ BY ENDOTRACHEAL TUBE

▸ Neonate: 100–200 mg/kg, then 100 mg/kg every 12 hours if required, maximum 300–400 mg/kg per course.

Prophylaxis of respiratory distress syndrome (specialist use only)
▸ BY ENDOTRACHEAL TUBE

▸ Neonate 24 weeks to 31 weeks corrected gestational age: 100–200 mg/kg, administer soon after birth, preferably within 15 minutes, then 100 mg/kg after 6–12 hours if required, then 100 mg/kg after 12 hours if required, and if neonate still intubated. Max 300–400 mg/kg per course.

- **CAUTIONS** Consult product literature
- **SIDE-EFFECTS**
▸ **Rare** Bradycardia · decreased oxygen saturation · hypotension · pulmonary haemorrhage
▸ **Frequency not known** Hyperoxia · intracranial haemorrhage · obstruction of the endotracheal tube by mucous secretions

- **MEDICINAL FORMS**
There can be variation in the licensing of different medicines containing the same drug.
Liquid
▸ **Curosurf** (Chiesi Ltd)
Phospholipids (as Poractant alfa) 80 mg per 1 ml Curosurf 240mg/3ml endotracheopulmonary suspension vials | 1 vial PoM £547.40 (Hospital only)
Curosurf 120mg/1.5ml endotracheopulmonary suspension vials | 1 vial PoM £281.64 (Hospital only)

5.1 Neonatal apnoea

XANTHINES

Caffeine citrate

24.2.2016

- **INDICATIONS AND DOSE**

Neonatal apnoea (specialist supervision in hospital)
▸ BY MOUTH, OR BY INTRAVENOUS INFUSION

▸ **Neonate:** Initially 20 mg/kg, administered over 30 minutes if given by intravenous infusion, then 5 mg/kg once daily, administered over 10 minutes if given by intravenous infusion, started 24 hours after initial dose; increased if necessary to 10 mg/kg daily.

DOSE EQUIVALENCE AND CONVERSION
Caffeine citrate 2 mg ≡ caffeine base 1 mg

PHARMACOKINETICS
Caffeine citrate is well absorbed when given orally.

- **UNLICENSED USE** EvGr Caffeine citrate loading doses in the BNF *for children* may differ to those in product literature. ◁E▷

IMPORTANT SAFETY INFORMATION

MHRA/CHM ADVICE: SAFE PRACTICE
From August 2013, all licensed preparations of caffeine are required to be labelled as caffeine citrate. To minimise the risk of dosing errors, **always state dose in terms of caffeine citrate when prescribing caffeine.** Some stock packaged as caffeine base.

- **CAUTIONS** Cardiovascular disease · gastro-oesophageal reflux · rhythm disorder · seizure disorders
- **INTERACTIONS** → Appendix 1 (caffeine citrate).
- **SIDE-EFFECTS**
▸ **Common or very common** Fluid and electrolyte imbalance · hyperglycaemia · hypertension · hypoglycaemia · irritability · restlessness · tachycardia
▸ **Frequency not known** Gastro-oesophageal reflux
- **HEPATIC IMPAIRMENT** Manufacturer advises caution with impaired hepatic function.
- **RENAL IMPAIRMENT** Reduced daily maintenance dose required—consult product literature. Manufacturer advises caution with impaired renal function—potential for accumulation of caffeine.
- **MONITORING REQUIREMENTS**
▸ EvGr The therapeutic range for plasma-caffeine concentration is usually 10–20 mg/litre (50–100 micromol/litre), but a concentration of 25–35 mg/litre (130–180 micromol/litre) may be required. Signs of toxicity only normally occur at concentrations greater than 50 mg/litre (260 micromol/litre). ◁D▷
▸ Monitor for recurrence of apnoea for 1 week after stopping treatment.
- **DIRECTIONS FOR ADMINISTRATION** Caffeine citrate injection may be administered *by mouth* or *by intravenous infusion.*
- **NATIONAL FUNDING/ACCESS DECISIONS**

Scottish Medicines Consortium (SMC) Decisions
The *Scottish Medicines Consortium* has advised (September 2013) that *Peyona®* is accepted for use within NHS Scotland for the treatment of primary apnoea of premature newborns only whilst *Peyona®* is available at the price agreed in the patient access scheme.

- **MEDICINAL FORMS**
There can be variation in the licensing of different medicines containing the same drug. Forms available from special-order manufacturers include: oral suspension, oral solution

Oral solution
▸ **Caffeine citrate (Non-proprietary)**
Caffeine citrate 10 mg per 1 ml Caffeine citrate 50mg/5ml oral solution | 5 ml PoM £24.41

Solution for injection
▸ **Caffeine citrate (Non-proprietary)**
Caffeine citrate 10 mg per 1 ml Caffeine citrate 10mg/1ml solution for injection ampoules | 10 ampoule PoM £48.82

Solution for infusion
▸ **Peyona** (Chiesi Ltd)
Caffeine citrate 20 mg per 1 ml Peyona 20mg/ml solution for infusion ampoules | 10 ampoule PoM £172.50 (Hospital only)

Chapter 4
Nervous system

CONTENTS

1	**Epilepsy and other seizure disorders**	page 180
1.1	Status epilepticus	208
2	**Mental health disorders**	212
2.1	Attention deficit hyperactivity disorder	212
2.2	Bipolar disorder and mania	217
2.3	Depression	221
2.4	Psychoses and schizophrenia	227
3	**Movement disorders**	240
3.1	Dystonias and other involuntary movements	240
4	**Nausea and labyrinth disorders**	243

5	**Pain**	page 252
5.1	Migraine	272
5.2	Neuropathic pain	275
6	**Sleep disorders**	275
6.1	Insomnia	275
7	**Substance dependence**	276
7.1	Nicotine dependence	277
7.2	Opioid dependence	279

1 Epilepsy and other seizure disorders

Epilepsy

Control of the epilepsies

The object of treatment is to prevent the occurrence of seizures by maintaining an effective dose of one or more antiepileptic drugs. Careful adjustment of doses is necessary, starting with low doses and increasing gradually until seizures are controlled or there are significant adverse effects.

When choosing an antiepileptic drug, the presenting epilepsy syndrome should first be considered. If the syndrome is not clear, the seizure type should determine the choice of treatment. Concomitant medication, co-morbidity, age, and sex should also be taken into account.

The frequency of administration is often determined by the plasma-drug half-life, and should be kept as low as possible to encourage better adherence. Most antiepileptics, when used in usual dosage, can be given twice daily. Lamotrigine p. 189, perampanel p. 193, phenobarbital p. 203 and phenytoin p. 193, which have long half-lives, can be given as a daily dose at bedtime. However, with large doses, some antiepileptics may need to be given three times daily to avoid adverse effects associated with high peak plasma-drug concentrations. Young children metabolise some antiepileptics more rapidly than adults and therefore may require more frequent doses and a higher amount per kilogram body-weight.

Management

When monotherapy with a first-line antiepileptic drug has failed, monotherapy with a second drug should be tried; the diagnosis should be checked before starting an alternative drug if the first drug showed lack of efficacy. The change from one antiepileptic drug to another should be cautious, slowly withdrawing the first drug only when the new regimen has been established. Combination therapy with two or more antiepileptic drugs may be necessary, but the concurrent use of antiepileptic drugs increases the risk of adverse effects and drug interactions. If combination therapy does not bring about worthwhile benefits, revert to the regimen (monotherapy or combination therapy) that provided the best balance between tolerability and efficacy. A single antiepileptic drug should be prescribed wherever possible and will achieve seizure control for the majority of children.

MHRA/CHM advice: Antiepileptic drugs: new advice on switching between different manufacturers' products for a particular drug (November 2013)

The CHM has reviewed spontaneous adverse reactions received by the MHRA and publications that reported potential harm arising from switching of antiepileptic drugs in patients previously stabilised on a branded product to a generic. The CHM concluded that reports of loss of seizure control and/or worsening of side-effects around the time of switching between products could be explained as chance associations, but that a causal role of switching could not be ruled out in all cases. The following guidance has been issued to help minimise risk:

- Different antiepileptic drugs vary considerably in their characteristics, which influences the risk of whether switching between different manufacturers' products of a particular drug may cause adverse effects or loss of seizure control;
- Antiepileptic drugs have been divided into three risk-based categories to help healthcare professionals decide whether it is necessary to maintain continuity of supply of a specific manufacturer's product. These categories are listed below;
- If it is felt desirable for a patient to be maintained on a specific manufacturer's product this should be prescribed either by specifying a brand name, or by using the generic drug name and name of the manufacturer (otherwise known as the Marketing Authorisation Holder);
- This advice relates only to antiepileptic drug use for treatment of epilepsy; it does not apply to their use in other indications (e.g. mood stabilisation, neuropathic pain);
- Please report on a Yellow Card any suspected adverse reactions to antiepileptic drugs;
- Dispensing pharmacists should ensure the continuity of supply of a particular product when the prescription specifies it. If the prescribed product is unavailable, it may be necessary to dispense a product from a different manufacturer to maintain continuity of treatment of that antiepileptic drug. Such cases should be discussed and agreed with both the prescriber and patient (or carer);
- Usual dispensing practice can be followed when a specific product is not stated.

Category 1

Phenytoin, carbamazepine p. 184, phenobarbital, primidone p. 204. For these drugs, doctors are advised to ensure that their patient is maintained on a specific manufacturer's product.

Category 2

Valproate, lamotrigine, perampanel, retigabine, rufinamide, clobazam p. 205, clonazepam p. 206, oxcarbazepine p. 192, eslicarbazepine acetate, zonisamide p. 202, topiramate p. 199. For these drugs, the need for continued supply of a particular manufacturer's product should be based on clinical judgement and consultation with the patient and/or carer taking into account factors such as seizure frequency and treatment history.

Category 3

Levetiracetam p. 191, lacosamide p. 188, tiagabine p. 199, gabapentin p. 187, pregabalin, ethosuximide p. 186, vigabatrin p. 201. For these drugs, it is usually unnecessary to ensure that patients are maintained on a specific manufacturer's product unless there are specific concerns such as patient anxiety, and risk of confusion or dosing errors Interactions.

Antiepileptic hypersensitivity syndrome

Antiepileptic hypersensitivity syndrome is a rare but potentially fatal syndrome associated with some antiepileptic drugs (carbamazepine, lacosamide, lamotrigine, oxcarbazepine, phenobarbital, phenytoin, primidone, and rufinamide p. 195); rarely cross-sensitivity occurs between some of these antiepileptic drugs. Some other antiepileptics (eslicarbazepine acetate, stiripentol p. 198, and zonisamide) have a theoretical risk. The symptoms usually start between 1 and 8 weeks of exposure; fever, rash, and lymphadenopathy are most commonly seen. Other warning signs include liver dysfunction, haematological, renal, and pulmonary abnormalities, vasculitis, and multi-organ failure. If signs or symptoms of hypersensitivity syndrome occur, the drug should be withdrawn immediately, the child should not be re-exposed, and expert advice should be sought.

Interactions

Interactions between antiepileptics are complex and may increase toxicity without a corresponding increase in antiepileptic effect. Interactions are usually caused by hepatic enzyme induction or inhibition; displacement from protein binding sites is not usually a problem. These interactions are highly variable and unpredictable.

Withdrawal

Antiepileptic drugs should be withdrawn under specialist supervision. Avoid abrupt withdrawal, particularly of barbiturates and benzodiazepines, because this can precipitate severe rebound seizures. Reduction in dosage should be gradual and, in the case of barbiturates, withdrawal of the drug may take months.

The decision to withdraw antiepileptic drugs from a seizure-free child, and its timing, is often difficult and depends on individual circumstances. Even in children who have been seizure-free for several years, there is a significant risk of seizure recurrence on drug withdrawal.

Drugs should be gradually withdrawn over at least 2–3 months by reducing the daily dose by 10–25% at intervals of 1–2 weeks. Benzodiazepines may need to be withdrawn over 6 months or longer.

In children receiving several antiepileptic drugs, only one drug should be withdrawn at a time.

Monitoring

Routine measurement of plasma concentrations of antiepileptic drugs is not usually justified, because the target concentration ranges are arbitrary and often vary between individuals. However, plasma-drug concentrations may be measured in children with worsening seizures, status epilepticus, suspected non-compliance, or suspected toxicity. Similarly, haematological and biochemical monitoring should not be undertaken unless clinically indicated.

Plasma concentration of some medications may change during pregnancy and monitoring may be required (see under *Pregnancy*).

Driving

Older children with epilepsy may drive a motor vehicle (but not a large goods or passenger carrying vehicle) provided that they have been seizure-free for one year or, if subject to attacks only while asleep, have established a 3-year period of asleep attacks without awake attacks. Those affected by drowsiness should not drive or operate machinery.

Guidance issued by the Drivers Medical Unit of the Driver and Vehicle Licensing Agency (DVLA) recommends that patients should be advised not to drive during medication changes or withdrawal of antiepileptic drugs, and for 6 months afterwards.

Patients who have had a first or single epileptic seizure must not drive for 6 months (5 years in the case of large goods or passenger carrying vehicles) after the event; driving may then be resumed, provided the patient has been assessed by a specialist as fit to drive because no abnormality was detected on investigation.

Pregnancy

Young women of child-bearing potential should discuss with a specialist the impact of both epilepsy, and its treatment, on the outcome of pregnancy.

There is an increased risk of teratogenicity associated with the use of antiepileptic drugs (especially if used during the first trimester and particularly if the patient takes two or more antiepileptic drugs). Valproate is associated with the highest risk of major and minor congenital malformations (in particular neural tube defects), and long-term developmental disorders. There is also an increased risk of teratogenicity with phenytoin, primidone, phenobarbital, lamotrigine, and carbamazepine. Topiramate carries an increased risk of cleft palate if taken in the first trimester of pregnancy. There is not enough evidence to establish the risk of teratogenicity with other antiepileptic drugs.

Prescribers should also consider carefully the choice of antiepileptic therapy in pre-pubescent girls who may later become pregnant. Young women of child-bearing potential who take antiepileptic drugs should be given advice about the need for an effective contraception method to avoid unplanned pregnancy. Some antiepileptic drugs can reduce the efficacy of hormonal contraceptives, and the efficacy of some antiepileptics may be affected by hormonal contraceptives.

Young women who want to become pregnant should be referred to a specialist for advice in advance of conception. For some women, the severity of seizure or the seizure type may not pose a serious threat, and drug withdrawal may be considered; therapy may be resumed after the first trimester. If treatment with antiepileptic drugs must continue throughout pregnancy, then monotherapy is preferable at the lowest effective dose.

Once an unplanned pregnancy is discovered it is usually too late for changes to be made to the treatment regimen; the risk of harm to the mother and fetus from convulsive seizures outweighs the risk of continued therapy. The likelihood of a woman who is taking antiepileptic drugs having a baby with no malformations is at least 90%, and it is important that women do not stop taking essential treatment because of concern over harm to the fetus. To reduce the risk of neural tube defects, folate supplementation is advised before conception and throughout the first trimester. In the case of sodium valproate p. 195 and valproic acid p. 200 an urgent

4

Nervous system

consultation is required to reconsider the benefits and risks of valproate therapy.

The concentration of antiepileptic drugs in the plasma can change during pregnancy. Doses of phenytoin, carbamazepine, and lamotrigine should be adjusted on the basis of plasma-drug concentration monitoring; the dose of other antiepileptic drugs should be monitored carefully during pregnancy and after birth, and adjustments made on a clinical basis. Plasma-drug concentration monitoring during pregnancy is also useful to check compliance. Additionally, in patients taking topiramate or levetiracetam, it is recommended that fetal growth should be monitored. Women who have seizures in the second half of pregnancy should be assessed for eclampsia before any change is made to antiepileptic treatment. Status epilepticus should be treated according to the standard protocol.

Routine injection of vitamin K at birth minimises the risk of neonatal haemorrhage associated with antiepileptics.

Withdrawal effects in the newborn may occur with some antiepileptic drugs, in particular benzodiazepines and phenobarbital, and can take several days to diminish.

Epilepsy and Pregnancy Register
All pregnant women with epilepsy, whether taking medication or not, should be encouraged to notify the UK Epilepsy and Pregnancy Register (Tel: 0800 389 1248).

Breast-feeding
Young women taking antiepileptic monotherapy should generally be encouraged to breast-feed; if a woman is on combination therapy or if there are other risk factors, such as premature birth, specialist advice should be sought.

All infants should be monitored for sedation, feeding difficulties, adequate weight gain, and developmental milestones. Infants should also be monitored for adverse effects associated with the antiepileptic drug particularly with newer antiepileptics, if the antiepileptic is readily transferred into breast-milk causing high infant serum-drug concentrations (e.g. ethosuximide, lamotrigine, primidone, and zonisamide), or if slower metabolism in the infant causes drugs to accumulate (e.g. phenobarbital and lamotrigine). Serum-drug concentration monitoring should be undertaken in breast-fed infants if suspected adverse reactions develop; if toxicity develops it may be necessary to introduce formula feeds to limit the infant's drug exposure, or to wean the infant off breast-milk altogether.

Primidone, phenobarbital, and the benzodiazepines are associated with an established risk of drowsiness in breast-fed babies and caution is required.

Withdrawal effects may occur in infants if a mother suddenly stops breast-feeding, particularly if she is taking phenobarbital, primidone, or lamotrigine.

Focal seizures with or without secondary generalisation

Carbamazepine p. 184 and lamotrigine p. 189 are the drugs of choice for focal seizures; levetiracetam p. 191, oxcarbazepine p. 192 and sodium valproate p. 195 can be considered if these are unsuitable. These drugs may also be used as adjunctive treatment. Other adjunctive options include clobazam p. 205, gabapentin p. 187, and topiramate p. 199. If adjunctive treatment is ineffective or not tolerated, a tertiary specialist should be consulted who may consider eslicarbazepine acetate, lacosamide p. 188, phenobarbital p. 203, phenytoin p. 193, pregabalin, tiagabine p. 199, vigabatrin p. 201, and zonisamide p. 202.

Generalised seizures

Tonic-clonic seizures
The drug of choice for newly diagnosed tonic-clonic seizures in children is sodium valproate (except in female patients, see *Valproate* below), or lamotrigine where sodium valproate is unsuitable (but may exacerbate myoclonic seizures). In

children with established epilepsy with generalised tonic-clonic seizures only, lamotrigine may be prescribed as the first-line choice. Carbamazepine or oxcarbazepine can also be considered but may exacerbate myoclonic or absence seizures. Clobazam, lamotrigine, levetiracetam, sodium valproate, or topiramate may be used as adjunctive treatment if monotherapy is ineffective or not tolerated.

Absence seizures
Ethosuximide p. 186 and sodium valproate (except in female patients, see *Valproate* below) are the drugs of choice for absence seizures and syndromes; lamotrigine can be used if these are unsuitable, ineffective or not tolerated. Sodium valproate should be used as the first choice if there is a high risk of generalised tonic-clonic seizures. A combination of any two of these drugs may be used if monotherapy is ineffective. Second-line therapy includes clobazam, clonazepam p. 206, levetiracetam, topiramate or zonisamide which may be considered by a tertiary specialist if adjunctive treatment fails. Carbamazepine, gabapentin, oxcarbazepine, phenytoin, pregabalin, tiagabine, and vigabatrin are not recommended in absence seizures or syndromes.

Myoclonic seizures
Myoclonic seizures (myoclonic jerks) occur in a variety of syndromes, and response to treatment varies considerably. Sodium valproate is the drug of choice (except in female patients, see *Valproate* below); consider levetiracetam or topiramate if sodium valproate is unsuitable (but consider the less favourable side-effect profile of topiramate). A combination of two of these drugs may be used if monotherapy is ineffective or poorly tolerated. Second-line therapy includes clobazam, clonazepam, piracetam or zonisamide which should be prescribed under the supervision of a tertiary specialist. Carbamazepine, gabapentin, oxcarbazepine, phenytoin, pregabalin, tiagabine, and vigabatrin are not recommended for the treatment of myoclonic seizures.

Tonic and atonic seizures
Tonic or atonic seizures are treated with sodium valproate (except in female patients, see *Valproate* below); lamotrigine can be considered as adjunctive treatment if sodium valproate is ineffective or not tolerated. If adjunctive treatment fails, a tertiary specialist should be consulted who may consider rufinamide p. 195 or topiramate. Carbamazepine, gabapentin, oxcarbazepine, pregabalin, tiagabine, and vigabatrin are not recommended in atonic or tonic seizures.

Epilepsy syndromes

Infantile spasms
Vigabatrin is the drug of choice for infantile spasms associated with tuberous sclerosis. Corticosteroids, such as prednisolone p. 413 or tetracosactide p. 441, are second-line options if vigabatrin is ineffective. In spasms of other causes, vigabatrin, prednisolone or tetracosactide can be considered as first-line options. A tertiary specialist should be consulted before treating infantile spasms.

Dravet syndrome
Sodium valproate (except in female patients, see *Valproate* below) or topiramate is the treatment of choice in Dravet syndrome. Clobazam or stiripentol p. 198 may be considered as adjunctive treatment. Carbamazepine, gabapentin, lamotrigine, oxcarbazepine, phenytoin, pregabalin, tiagabine, and vigabatrin should not be used as they may exacerbate myoclonic seizures. A tertiary specialist should be involved in decisions regarding treatment of Dravet syndrome.

Lennox-Gastaut syndrome
Sodium valproate is the first-line drug for treating Lennox-Gastaut syndrome (except in female patients, see *Valproate* below); lamotrigine can be used as adjunctive treatment if

sodium valproate is ineffective or not tolerated. Rufinamide and topiramate may be considered by tertiary epilepsy specialists. Carbamazepine, gabapentin, oxcarbazepine, pregabalin, tiagabine, and vigabatrin should not be used. Felbamate [unlicensed] may be used in tertiary specialist centres when all other treatment options have failed.

Landau-Kleffner syndrome
Always discuss with or refer to tertiary epilepsy specialists.

Neonatal seizures
Seizures can occur before delivery, but they are most common up to 24 hours after birth. Seizures in neonates occur as a result of biochemical disturbances, inborn errors of metabolism, hypoxic ischaemic encephalopathy, drug withdrawal, meningitis, stroke, cerebral haemorrhage or malformation, or severe jaundice (kernicterus).

Seizures caused by biochemical imbalance and those in neonates with inherited abnormal pyridoxine or biotin metabolism should be corrected by treating the underlying cause. Seizures caused by drug withdrawal following intra-uterine exposure are treated with a drug withdrawal regimen.

Phenobarbital can be used to manage neonatal seizures where there is a risk of recurrence; phenytoin is an alternative. Midazolam p. 210 and **rectal** paraldehyde p. 208 may also be useful in the management of acute neonatal seizures. Lidocaine hydrochloride p. 70 may be used if other treatments are unsuccessful; lidocaine hydrochloride should not be given to neonates who have received phenytoin infusion because of the risk of cardiac toxicity.

Antiepileptic drugs

Carbamazepine and related antiepileptics
Carbamazepine is a drug of choice for simple and complex focal seizures and is a first-line treatment option for generalised tonic-clonic seizures. It can be used as adjunctive treatment for focal seizures when monotherapy has been ineffective. It is essential to initiate carbamazepine therapy at a low dose and build this up slowly in small increments every 3–7 days. Carbamazepine may exacerbate tonic, atonic, myoclonic and absence seizures and is therefore not recommended if these seizures are present.

Oxcarbazepine is not recommended in tonic, atonic, absence or myoclonic seizures due to the risk of seizure exacerbation.

Ethosuximide
Ethosuximide is a first-line treatment option for absence seizures, and may be used as adjunctive treatment when monotherapy has failed.

Gabapentin
Gabapentin is used as adjunctive therapy for the treatment of focal seizures with or without secondary generalisation; it is licensed as monotherapy in children over 12 years. It is not recommended if tonic, atonic, absence or myoclonic seizures are present.

Lamotrigine
Lamotrigine is an antiepileptic drug recommended as a first-line treatment for focal seizures and primary and secondary generalised tonic-clonic seizures. It is also licensed as monotherapy for typical absence seizures in children (but efficacy may not be maintained in all children). It may be tried as an adjunctive treatment for atonic and tonic seizures if first-line treatment has failed [unlicensed]. Myoclonic seizures may be exacerbated by lamotrigine and it can cause serious rashes; dose recommendations should be adhered to closely.

Lamotrigine is used either as sole treatment or as an adjunct to treatment with other antiepileptic drugs. Valproate increases plasma-lamotrigine concentration, whereas the enzyme-inducing antiepileptics reduce it; care is therefore required in choosing the appropriate initial dose

and subsequent titration. When the potential for interaction is not known, treatment should be initiated with lower doses, such as those used with valproate.

Levetiracetam
Levetiracetam p. 191 is used for monotherapy and adjunctive treatment of focal seizures with or without secondary generalisation, and for adjunctive treatment of myoclonic seizures in children with juvenile myoclonic epilepsy and primary generalised tonic-clonic seizures. Levetiracetam may be prescribed alone and in combination for the treatment of myoclonic seizures, and under specialist supervision for absence seizures [both unlicensed].

Phenobarbital and primidone
Phenobarbital p. 203 is effective for tonic-clonic, focal seizures and neonatal seizures but may cause behavioural disturbances and hyperkinesia. It may be tried for atypical absence, atonic, and tonic seizures. For therapeutic purposes phenobarbital and *phenobarbital sodium* should be considered equivalent in effect. Rebound seizures may be a problem on withdrawal.

Primidone p. 204 is largely converted to phenobarbital and this is probably responsible for its antiepileptic action. It is used rarely in children. A low initial dose of primidone is essential.

Phenytoin
Phenytoin p. 193 is licensed for tonic-clonic and focal seizures but may exacerbate absence or myoclonic seizures and should be avoided if theses seizures are present. It has a narrow therapeutic index and the relationship between dose and plasma-drug concentration is non-linear; small dosage increases in some patients may produce large increases in plasma concentration with acute toxic side-effects. Similarly, a few missed doses or a small change in drug absorption may result in a marked change in plasma-drug concentration. Monitoring of plasma-drug concentration improves dosage adjustment.

When only parenteral administration is possible, fosphenytoin sodium p. 187, a pro-drug of phenytoin, may be convenient to give. Whereas phenytoin should be given intravenously only, fosphenytoin sodium may also be given by intramuscular injection.

Rufinamide
Rufinamide p. 195 is licensed for the adjunctive treatment of seizures in Lennox-Gastaut syndrome. It may be considered by a tertiary specialist for the treatment of refractory tonic or atonic seizures [unlicensed].

Topiramate
Topiramate p. 199 can be given alone or as adjunctive treatment in generalised tonic-clonic seizures or focal seizures. It can also be used for absence, tonic and atonic seizures under specialist supervision and as an option in myoclonic seizures [all unlicensed]. Topiramate is also licensed for prophylaxis of migraine.

Valproate
Valproate (as either sodium valproate p. 195 or valproic acid p. 200) is effective in controlling tonic-clonic seizures, particularly in primary generalised epilepsy. It is a drug of choice in primary generalised tonic-clonic seizures, focal seizures, generalised absences and myoclonic seizures, and can be tried in atypical absence seizures. It is recommended as a first-line option in atonic and tonic seizures. Valproate should generally be avoided in children under 2 years especially with other antiepileptics, but it may be required in infants with continuing epileptic tendency. Sodium valproate has widespread metabolic effects, and monitoring of liver function tests and full blood count is essential. Valproate should not be used in female children, in females of childbearing potential, and pregnant females, unless alternative treatments are ineffective or not tolerated, becuase of its high teratogenic potential; the benefits and

risks of valproate therapy should be carefully reconsidered at regular treatment reviews, see *Important safety information* in the sodium valproate and valproic acid drug monographs. Plasma-valproate concentrations are not a useful index of efficacy, therefore routine monitoring is unhelpful.

Zonisamide

Zonisamide p. 202 can be used as an adjunctive treatment for refractory focal seizures with or without secondary generalisation in children and adolescents aged 6 years and above. It can also be used under the supervision of a specialist for refractory absence and myoclonic seizures [unlicensed indications].

Benzodiazepines

Clobazam p. 205 may be used as adjunctive therapy in the treatment of generalised tonic-clonic and refractory focal seizures. It may be prescribed under the care of a specialist for refractory absence and myoclonic seizures. Clonazepam p. 206 may be prescribed by a specialist for refractory absence and myoclonic seizures, but its sedative side-effects may be prominent.

Other drugs

Acetazolamide p. 638, a carbonic anhydrase inhibitor, has a specific role in treating epilepsy associated with menstruation. Piracetam is used as adjunctive treatment for cortical myoclonus.

Status epilepticus

Convulsive status epilepticus

Immediate measures to manage status epilepticus include positioning the child to avoid injury, supporting respiration including the provision of oxygen, maintaining blood pressure, and the correction of any hypoglycaemia. Pyridoxine hydrochloride p. 585 should be administered if the status epilepticus is caused by pyridoxine deficiency.

Seizures lasting 5 minutes should be treated urgently with buccal midazolam p. 210 or intravenous lorazepam p. 209 (repeated once after 10 minutes if seizures recur or fail to respond). Intravenous diazepam p. 207 is effective but it carries a high risk of venous thrombophlebitis (reduced by using an emulsion formulation of diazepam injection). Patients should be monitored for respiratory depression and hypotension.

Important

If, after initial treatment with benzodiazepines, seizures recur or fail to respond 25 minutes after onset, phenytoin sodium should be used, or if the child is on regular phenytoin, give phenobarbital sodium intravenously over 5 minutes; the paediatric intensive care unit should be contacted. Paraldehyde p. 208 can be given after starting phenytoin infusion.

If these measures fail to control seizures 45 minutes after onset, anaesthesia with thiopental sodium p. 209 should be instituted with full intensive care support.

Phenytoin sodium can be given by intravenous infusion over 20 minutes, followed by the maintenance dosage if appropriate.

Paraldehyde given rectally causes little respiratory depression and is therefore useful where facilities for resuscitation are poor.

Non-convulsive status epilepticus

The urgency to treat non-convulsive status epilepticus depends on the severity of the child's condition. If there is incomplete loss of awareness, oral antiepileptic therapy should be continued or restarted. Children who fail to respond to oral antiepileptic therapy or have complete lack of awareness can be treated in the same way as for convulsive status epilepticus, although anaesthesia is rarely needed.

Febrile convulsions

Brief febrile convulsions need no specific treatment; antipyretic medication (e.g. paracetamol p. 254), is commonly used to reduce fever and prevent further convulsions but evidence to support this practice is lacking. *Prolonged febrile convulsions* (those lasting 5 minutes or longer), or *recurrent febrile convulsions* without recovery must be treated actively (as for convulsive status epilepticus).

Long-term anticonvulsant prophylaxis for febrile convulsions is rarely indicated.

ANTIEPILEPTICS

Carbamazepine

● INDICATIONS AND DOSE

Trigeminal neuralgia

▸ BY MOUTH USING IMMEDIATE-RELEASE MEDICINES

▸ Child 1 month–11 years: Initially 5 mg/kg once daily, dose to be taken at night, alternatively initially 2.5 mg/kg twice daily, then increased in steps of 2.5–5 mg/kg every 3–7 days as required; maintenance 5 mg/kg 2–3 times a day, increased if necessary up to 20 mg/kg daily

▸ Child 12–17 years: Initially 100–200 mg 1–2 times a day, then increased to 200–400 mg 2–3 times a day, increased if necessary up to 1.8 g daily, dose should be increased slowly

Prophylaxis of bipolar disorder

▸ BY MOUTH USING IMMEDIATE-RELEASE MEDICINES

▸ Child 1 month–11 years: Initially 5 mg/kg once daily, dose to be taken at night, alternatively initially 2.5 mg/kg twice daily, then increased in steps of 2.5–5 mg/kg every 3–7 days as required; maintenance 5 mg/kg 2–3 times a day, increased if necessary up to 20 mg/kg daily

▸ Child 12–17 years: Initially 100–200 mg 1–2 times a day, then increased to 200–400 mg 2–3 times a day, increased if necessary up to 1.8 g daily, dose should be increased slowly

Focal and generalised tonic-clonic seizures

▸ BY MOUTH USING IMMEDIATE-RELEASE MEDICINES

▸ Child 1 month–11 years: Initially 5 mg/kg once daily, dose to be taken at night, alternatively initially 2.5 mg/kg twice daily, then increased in steps of 2.5–5 mg/kg every 3–7 days as required; maintenance 5 mg/kg 2–3 times a day, increased if necessary up to 20 mg/kg daily

▸ Child 12–17 years: Initially 100–200 mg 1–2 times a day, then increased to 200–400 mg 2–3 times a day, increased if necessary up to 1.8 g daily, dose should be increased slowly

▸ BY RECTUM

▸ Child: Up to 250 mg up to 4 times a day, to be used for short-term use (max. 7 days) when oral therapy temporarily not possible, use approx. 25% more than the oral dose

DOSE EQUIVALENCE AND CONVERSION

Suppositories of 125 mg may be considered to be approximately equivalent in therapeutic effect to tablets of 100 mg but final adjustment should always depend on clinical response (plasma concentration monitoring recommended).

CARBAGEN® SR

Trigeminal neuralgia

▸ BY MOUTH

▸ Child 5–11 years: Initially 5 mg/kg daily in 1–2 divided doses, then increased in steps of 2.5–5 mg/kg every

3–7 days as required; maintenance 10–15 mg/kg daily in 1–2 divided doses, increased if necessary up to 20 mg/kg daily in 1–2 divided doses
▸ Child 12–17 years: Initially 100–400 mg daily in 1–2 divided doses, then increased to 400–1200 mg daily in 1–2 divided doses, increased if necessary up to 1.8 g daily in 1–2 divided doses, dose should be increased slowly

Focal and generalised tonic-clonic seizures | Prophylaxis of bipolar disorder
▸ BY MOUTH
▸ Child 5–11 years: Initially 5 mg/kg daily in 1–2 divided doses, then increased in steps of 2.5–5 mg/kg every 3–7 days as required, dose should be increased slowly; maintenance 10–15 mg/kg daily in 1–2 divided doses, increased if necessary up to 20 mg/kg daily in 1–2 divided doses
▸ Child 12–17 years: Initially 100–400 mg daily in 1–2 divided doses, then increased to 400–1200 mg daily in 1–2 divided doses, increased if necessary up to 1.8 g daily in 1–2 divided doses, dose should be increased slowly

TEGRETOL® PROLONGED RELEASE

Focal and generalised tonic-clonic seizures | Prophylaxis of bipolar disorder
▸ BY MOUTH
▸ Child 5–11 years: Initially 5 mg/kg daily in 2 divided doses, then increased in steps of 2.5–5 mg/kg every 3–7 days as required; maintenance 10–15 mg/kg daily in 2 divided doses, increased if necessary up to 20 mg/kg daily in 2 divided doses
▸ Child 12–17 years: Initially 100–400 mg daily in 2 divided doses, dose should be increased slowly; maintenance 400–1200 mg daily in 2 divided doses, increased if necessary up to 1.8 g daily in 2 divided doses

Trigeminal neuralgia
▸ BY MOUTH
▸ Child 5–11 years: Initially 5 mg/kg daily in 2 divided doses, then increased in steps of 2.5–5 mg/kg every 3–7 days as required; maintenance 10–15 mg/kg daily in 2 divided doses, increased if necessary up to 20 mg/kg daily in 2 divided doses
▸ Child 12–17 years: Initially 100–400 mg daily in 2 divided doses, dose should be increased slowly; maintenance 400–1200 mg daily in 2 divided doses, increased if necessary up to 1.8 g daily in 2 divided doses, dose should be increased slowly

● CONTRA-INDICATIONS Acute porphyrias p. 562 · AV conduction abnormalities (unless paced) · history of bone-marrow depression
● CAUTIONS Cardiac disease · history of haematological reactions to other drugs · may exacerbate absence and myoclonic seizures · skin reactions · susceptibility to angle-closure glaucoma
CAUTIONS, FURTHER INFORMATION
Consider vitamin D supplementation in patients who are immobilised for long periods or who have inadequate sun exposure or dietary intake of calcium.
▸ Blood, hepatic, or skin disorders Carbamazepine should be withdrawn immediately in cases of aggravated liver dysfunction or acute liver disease. Leucopenia that is severe, progressive, or associated with clinical symptoms requires withdrawal (if necessary under cover of a suitable alternative).
● INTERACTIONS → Appendix 1 (carbamazepine).
● SIDE-EFFECTS
▸ Common or very common Allergic skin reactions · aplastic anaemia · ataxia · blood disorders · blurring of vision · dermatitis · dizziness · drowsiness · dry mouth · eosinophilia · fatigue · haemolytic anaemia · headache ·

hyponatraemia (leading in rare cases to water intoxication) · leucopenia · nausea · oedema · thrombocytopenia · unsteadiness · urticaria · vomiting
▸ Uncommon Constipation · diarrhoea · involuntary movements (including nystagmus) · visual disturbances
▸ Rare Abdominal pain · aggression · agitation · anorexia · cardiac conduction disorders · confusion · delayed multi-organ hypersensitivity disorder · depression · dysarthria · hallucinations · hepatitis · hypertension · hypotension · jaundice · lymph node enlargement · muscle weakness · paraesthesia · peripheral neuropathy · restlessness · systemic lupus erythematosus · vanishing bile duct syndrome
▸ Very rare Arthralgia · muscle spasm · acne · alopecia · alterations in skin pigmentation · angle-closure glaucoma · aseptic meningitis · AV block with syncope · circulatory collapse · conjunctivitis · dyspnoea · exacerbation of coronary artery disease · galactorrhoea · gynaecomastia · hearing disorders · hepatic failure · hirsutism · hypercholesterolaemia · impaired male fertility · interstitial nephritis · muscle pain · neuroleptic malignant syndrome · osteomalacia · osteoporosis · pancreatitis · photosensitivity · pneumonia · pneumonitis · psychosis · pulmonary hypersensitivity · purpura · renal failure · sexual dysfunction · Stevens-Johnson syndrome · stomatitis · sweating · taste disturbance · thromboembolism · thrombophlebitis · toxic epidermal necrolysis · urinary frequency · urinary retention
▸ Frequency not known Suicidal ideation
SIDE-EFFECTS, FURTHER INFORMATION
Some side-effects (such as headache, ataxia, drowsiness, nausea, vomiting, blurring of vision, dizziness, unsteadiness, and allergic skin reactions) are dose-related, and may be dose-limiting. These side-effects are more common at the start of treatment. Children should be offered a modified-release preparation to reduce the risk of side-effects; altering the timing of medication may also be beneficial.

Overdose
For details on the management of poisoning, see Active elimination techniques, under Emergency treatment of poisoning p. 786.
● ALLERGY AND CROSS-SENSITIVITY Antiepileptic hypersensitivity syndrome associated with carbamazepine. See under Epilepsy p. 180 for more information. Caution—cross-sensitivity reported with oxcarbazepine and with phenytoin.
● PREGNANCY

Monitoring
Doses should be adjusted on the basis of plasma-drug concentration monitoring.
● BREAST FEEDING Amount probably too small to be harmful.
    Monitor infant for possible adverse reactions.
● HEPATIC IMPAIRMENT Metabolism impaired in advanced liver disease.
● RENAL IMPAIRMENT Use with caution.
● PRE-TREATMENT SCREENING Test for HLA-B*1502 allele in individuals of Han Chinese or Thai origin (avoid unless no alternative—risk of Stevens-Johnson syndrome in presence of HLA-B*1502 allele).
● MONITORING REQUIREMENTS
▸ Plasma concentration for optimum response 4–12 mg/litre (20–50 micromol/litre) measured after 1–2 weeks.
▸ Manufacturer recommends blood counts and hepatic and renal function tests (but evidence of practical value uncertain).
● TREATMENT CESSATION When stopping treatment with carbamazepine for bipolar disorder, reduce the dose gradually over a period of at least 4 weeks.

- **DIRECTIONS FOR ADMINISTRATION** Oral liquid has been used rectally—should be retained for at least 2 hours (but may have laxative effect).

  TEGRETOL® PROLONGED RELEASE *Tegretol® Prolonged Release* tablets can be halved but should not be chewed.

- **PRESCRIBING AND DISPENSING INFORMATION**
  Switching between formulations Different formulations of oral preparations may vary in bioavailability. Patients being treated for epilepsy should be maintained on a specific manufacturer's product.

- **PATIENT AND CARER ADVICE**
  Medicines for Children leaflet: Carbamazepine (oral) for preventing seizures www.medicinesforchildren.org.uk/carbamazepine-oral-preventing-seizures-0
  Blood, hepatic, or skin disorders Patients or their carers should be told how to recognise signs of blood, liver, or skin disorders, and advised to seek immediate medical attention if symptoms such as fever, rash, mouth ulcers, bruising, or bleeding develop.

- **PROFESSION SPECIFIC INFORMATION**
  Dental practitioners' formulary
  Carbamazepine Tablets may be prescribed.

- **MEDICINAL FORMS**
  There can be variation in the licensing of different medicines containing the same drug. Forms available from special-order manufacturers include: oral suspension, oral solution

  Tablet
  CAUTIONARY AND ADVISORY LABELS 3, 8
  ▸ **Carbamazepine (Non-proprietary)**
  Carbamazepine 100 mg Carbamazepine 100mg tablets |
  28 tablet [PoM] £6.75 | 84 tablet [PoM] no price available DT price = £2.07
  Carbamazepine 200 mg Carbamazepine 200mg tablets |
  28 tablet [PoM] £5.83 DT price = £5.26 | 84 tablet [PoM] no price available
  Carbamazepine 400 mg Carbamazepine 400mg tablets |
  28 tablet [PoM] no price available | 56 tablet [PoM] £6.15 DT price = £5.02
  ▸ **Carbagen (Mylan Ltd)**
  Carbamazepine 100 mg Carbagen 100mg tablets | 28 tablet [PoM] £5.74 | 56 tablet [PoM] no price available (Hospital only) |
  84 tablet [PoM] no price available DT price = £2.07 (Hospital only)
  Carbamazepine 200 mg Carbagen 200mg tablets | 28 tablet [PoM] £4.99 DT price = £5.26 | 56 tablet [PoM] no price available (Hospital only) | 84 tablet [PoM] no price available (Hospital only)
  Carbamazepine 400 mg Carbagen 400mg tablets | 28 tablet [PoM] £4.27 | 56 tablet [PoM] no price available DT price = £5.02 (Hospital only)
  ▸ **Tegretol (Novartis Pharmaceuticals UK Ltd)**
  Carbamazepine 100 mg Tegretol 100mg tablets | 84 tablet [PoM] £2.07 DT price = £2.07
  Carbamazepine 200 mg Tegretol 200mg tablets | 84 tablet [PoM] £3.83
  Carbamazepine 400 mg Tegretol 400mg tablets | 56 tablet [PoM] £5.02 DT price = £5.02

  Modified-release tablet
  CAUTIONARY AND ADVISORY LABELS 3, 8, 25
  ▸ **Carbagen SR (Mylan Ltd)**
  Carbamazepine 200 mg Carbagen SR 200mg tablets |
  56 tablet [PoM] £4.16 DT price = £5.20
  Carbamazepine 400 mg Carbagen SR 400mg tablets |
  56 tablet [PoM] £8.20 DT price = £10.24
  ▸ **Tegretol Retard (Novartis Pharmaceuticals UK Ltd)**
  Carbamazepine 200 mg Tegretol Prolonged Release 200mg tablets | 56 tablet [PoM] £5.20 DT price = £5.20
  Carbamazepine 400 mg Tegretol Prolonged Release 400mg tablets | 56 tablet [PoM] £10.24 DT price = £10.24

  Oral suspension
  CAUTIONARY AND ADVISORY LABELS 3, 8
  ▸ **Carbamazepine (Non-proprietary)**
  Carbamazepine 20 mg per 1 ml Carbamazepine 100mg/5ml oral suspension sugar free sugar-free | 300 ml [PoM] £7.13 DT price = £6.12

▸ **Tegretol (Novartis Pharmaceuticals UK Ltd)**
Carbamazepine 20 mg per 1 ml Tegretol 100mg/5ml liquid sugar-free | 300 ml [PoM] £6.12 DT price = £6.12

Suppository
CAUTIONARY AND ADVISORY LABELS 3, 8
▸ **Tegretol (Novartis Pharmaceuticals UK Ltd)**
Carbamazepine 125 mg Tegretol 125mg suppositories |
5 suppository [PoM] £8.03
Carbamazepine 250 mg Tegretol 250mg suppositories |
5 suppository [PoM] £10.71

Ethosuximide

- **INDICATIONS AND DOSE**

  Absence seizures | Atypical absence seizures (adjunct) | Myoclonic seizures
  ▸ BY MOUTH
  ▸ Child 1 month–5 years: Initially 5 mg/kg twice daily (max. per dose 125 mg), dose to be increased every 5–7 days; maintenance 10–20 mg/kg twice daily (max. per dose 500 mg), total daily dose may rarely be given in 3 divided doses
  ▸ Child 6–17 years: Initially 250 mg twice daily, then increased in steps of 250 mg every 5–7 days; usual dose 500–750 mg twice daily, increased if necessary up to 1 g twice daily

- **CAUTIONS** Avoid in Acute porphyrias p. 562

- **INTERACTIONS** → Appendix 1 (ethosuximide).

- **SIDE-EFFECTS**
  ▸ **Common or very common** Anorexia · abdominal pain · diarrhoea · gastro-intestinal disturbances · nausea · vomiting · weight loss
  ▸ **Uncommon** Aggression · ataxia · dizziness · drowsiness · euphoria · fatigue · headache · hiccup · impaired concentration · irritability
  ▸ **Rare** Depression · dyskinesia · gingival hypertrophy · increased libido · myopia · photophobia · psychosis · rash · sleep disturbances · tongue swelling · vaginal bleeding
  ▸ **Frequency not known** Agranulocytosis · aplastic anaemia · blood disorders · hyperactivity · increase in seizure frequency · leucopenia · pancytopenia · Stevens-Johnson syndrome · suicidal ideation · systemic lupus erythematosus

  SIDE-EFFECTS, FURTHER INFORMATION
  ▸ Blood disorders Blood counts required if features of infection.

- **PREGNANCY**
  Monitoring
  The dose should be monitored carefully during pregnancy and after birth, and adjustments made on a clinical basis.

- **BREAST FEEDING** Present in milk. Hyperexcitability and sedation reported.

- **HEPATIC IMPAIRMENT** Use with caution.

- **RENAL IMPAIRMENT** Use with caution.

- **PATIENT AND CARER ADVICE**
  Medicines for Children leaflet: Ethosuximide for preventing seizures www.medicinesforchildren.org.uk/ethosuximide-for-preventing-seizures
  Blood disorders Patients or their carers should be told how to recognise signs of blood disorders, and advised to seek immediate medical attention if symptoms such as fever, mouth ulcers, bruising, or bleeding develop.

- **MEDICINAL FORMS**
  There can be variation in the licensing of different medicines containing the same drug.

Capsule
CAUTIONARY AND ADVISORY LABELS 8
- Ethosuximide (Non-proprietary)
  Ethosuximide 250 mg Ethosuximide 250mg capsules | 56 capsule PoM £73.20 DT price = £73.20

Oral solution
CAUTIONARY AND ADVISORY LABELS 8
- Emeside (Essential Pharma Ltd)
  Ethosuximide 50 mg per 1 ml Emeside 250mg/5ml syrup | 200 ml PoM £6.60 DT price = £4.22
- Zarontin (Pfizer Ltd)
  Ethosuximide 50 mg per 1 ml Zarontin 250mg/5ml syrup | 200 ml PoM £4.22 DT price = £4.22

Fosphenytoin sodium

- **DRUG ACTION** Fosphenytoin is a pro-drug of phenytoin.

- **INDICATIONS AND DOSE**

Status epilepticus
▶ BY INTRAVENOUS INFUSION
▶ Child 5–17 years: Initially 20 mg(PE)/kg, dose to be administered at a rate of 2–3 mg(PE)/kg/minute, maximum 150 mg(PE)/minute, then 4–5 mg(PE)/kg daily in 1–4 divided doses, dose to be administered at a rate of 1–2 mg(PE)/kg/minute, maximum 100 mg (PE)/minute, dose to be adjusted according to response and trough plasma-phenytoin concentration

Prophylaxis or treatment of seizures associated with neurosurgery or head injury
▶ BY INTRAVENOUS INFUSION
▶ Child 5–17 years: Initially 10–15 mg(PE)/kg, then 4–5 mg(PE)/kg daily in 1–4 divided doses, dose to be administered at a rate of 1–2 mg(PE)/kg/minute, maximum 100 mg(PE)/minute, dose to be adjusted according to response and trough plasma-phenytoin concentration

Temporary substitution for oral phenytoin
▶ BY INTRAVENOUS INFUSION
▶ Child 5–17 years: Same dose and same dosing frequency as oral phenytoin therapy, intravenous infusion to be administered at a rate of 1–2 mg(PE)/kg/minute, maximum 100 mg(PE)/minute

DOSE EQUIVALENCE AND CONVERSION
Doses are expressed as phenytoin sodium equivalent (PE); fosphenytoin sodium 1.5 mg ≡ phenytoin sodium 1 mg.

- **UNLICENSED USE** Fosphenytoin sodium doses in BNFC may differ from those in product literature.

- **CONTRA-INDICATIONS** Acute porphyrias p. 562 · second-degree heart block · sino-atrial block · sinus bradycardia · Stokes-Adams syndrome · third-degree heart block

- **CAUTIONS** Heart failure · hypotension · injection solutions alkaline (irritant to tissues) · respiratory depression · resuscitation facilities must be available

- **INTERACTIONS** → Appendix 1 (fosphenytoin).

- **SIDE-EFFECTS**
- **Common or very common** Alterations in respiratory function · arrhythmias · asthenia · cardiovascular collapse · cardiovascular depression (particularly if injection too rapid) · chills · CNS depression (particularly if injection too rapid) · dry mouth · dysarthria · ecchymosis · euphoria · hypotension · incoordination · pruritus · respiratory arrest · taste disturbance · tinnitus · vasodilatation · visual disturbances

▶ **Uncommon** Decreased reflexes · hypoacusis · hypoaesthesia · increased reflexes · muscle spasm · muscle weakness · pain · stupor
▶ **Frequency not known** Confusion · extrapyramidal disorder · hyperglycaemia · purple glove syndrome · tonic seizures · twitching

SIDE-EFFECTS, FURTHER INFORMATION
▶ Cardiovascular reactions Intravenous infusion of fosphenytoin has been associated with severe cardiovascular reactions including asystole, ventricular fibrillation, and cardiac arrest. Hypotension, bradycardia, and heart block have also been reported. The following are recommended:
  - monitor heart rate, blood pressure, and respiratory function for duration of infusion;
  - observe patient for at least 30 minutes after infusion;
  - if hypotension occurs, reduce infusion rate or discontinue;
  - reduce dose or infusion in renal or hepatic impairment.

- **ALLERGY AND CROSS-SENSITIVITY** Cross-sensitivity reported with carbamazepine.

- **PREGNANCY** Changes in plasma-protein binding make interpretation of plasma-phenytoin concentrations difficult—monitor unbound fraction. The dose should be monitored carefully during pregnancy and after birth, and adjustments made on a clinical basis.

- **BREAST FEEDING** Small amounts present in milk, but not known to be harmful.

- **HEPATIC IMPAIRMENT** Consider 10–25% reduction in dose or infusion rate (except initial dose for status epilepticus).

- **RENAL IMPAIRMENT** Consider 10–25% reduction in dose or infusion rate (except initial dose for status epilepticus).

- **PRE-TREATMENT SCREENING** HLA-B* 1502 allele in individuals of Han Chinese or Thai origin—avoid unless essential (increased risk of Stevens-Johnson syndrome).

- **MONITORING REQUIREMENTS**
▶ Manufacturer recommends blood counts (but evidence of practical value uncertain).
▶ With intravenous use Monitor heart rate, blood pressure, ECG, and respiratory function for during infusion.

- **DIRECTIONS FOR ADMINISTRATION** For *intermittent intravenous infusion* (*Pro-Epanutin®*), give *in* Glucose 5% *or* Sodium chloride 0.9%; dilute to a concentration of 1.5–25 mg (phenytoin sodium equivalent (PE))/mL.

- **PRESCRIBING AND DISPENSING INFORMATION**
  Prescriptions for fosphenytoin sodium should state the dose in terms of phenytoin sodium equivalent (PE); fosphenytoin sodium 1.5 mg ≡ phenytoin sodium 1 mg.

- **MEDICINAL FORMS**
  There can be variation in the licensing of different medicines containing the same drug.

Solution for injection
ELECTROLYTES: May contain Phosphate
▶ Pro-Epanutin (Pfizer Ltd)
  Fosphenytoin sodium 75 mg per 1 ml Pro-Epanutin 750mg/10ml concentrate for solution for injection vials | 10 vial PoM £400.00 (Hospital only)

Gabapentin

- **INDICATIONS AND DOSE**

Adjunctive treatment of focal seizures with or without secondary generalisation
▶ BY MOUTH
▶ Child 2–5 years: 10 mg/kg once daily on day 1, then 10 mg/kg twice daily on day 2, then 10 mg/kg 3 times a day on day 3, then increased to 30–70 mg/kg daily in 3 divided doses, adjusted according to continued →

response, some children may not tolerate daily increments; longer intervals (up to weekly) may be more appropriate
- Child 6–11 years: 10 mg/kg once daily (max. per dose 300 mg) on day 1, then 10 mg/kg twice daily (max. per dose 300 mg) on day 2, then 10 mg/kg 3 times a day (max. per dose 300 mg) on day 3; usual dose 25–35 mg/kg daily in 3 divided doses, some children may not tolerate daily increments; longer intervals (up to weekly) may be more appropriate, daily dose maximum to be given in 3 divided doses; maximum 70 mg/kg per day
- Child 12–17 years: Initially 300 mg once daily on day 1, then 300 mg twice daily on day 2, then 300 mg 3 times a day on day 3, alternatively initially 300 mg 3 times a day on day 1, then increased in steps of 300 mg every 2–3 days in 3 divided doses, adjusted according to response; usual dose 0.9–3.6 g daily in 3 divided doses (max. per dose 1.6 g 3 times a day), some children may not tolerate daily increments; longer intervals (up to weekly) may be more appropriate

Monotherapy for focal seizures with or without secondary generalisation
▶ BY MOUTH
- Child 12–17 years: Initially 300 mg once daily on day 1, then 300 mg twice daily on day 2, then 300 mg 3 times a day on day 3, alternatively initially 300 mg 3 times a day on day 1, then increased in steps of 300 mg every 2–3 days in 3 divided doses, adjusted according to response; usual dose 0.9–3.6 g daily in 3 divided doses (max. per dose 1.6 g 3 times a day), some children may not tolerate daily increments; longer intervals (up to weekly) may be more appropriate

- **UNLICENSED USE** Not licensed for use in children under 6 years. Not licensed at doses over 50 mg/kg daily in children under 12 years.

> **IMPORTANT SAFETY INFORMATION**
> The levels of propylene glycol, acesulfame K and saccharin sodium may exceed the recommended WHO daily intake limits if high doses of gabapentin oral solution (Rosemont brand) are given to adolescents or adults with low body-weight (39–50 kg)—consult product literature.

- **CAUTIONS** Diabetes mellitus · high doses of oral solution in adolescents and adults with low body-weight · history of psychotic illness · mixed seizures (including absences)
- **INTERACTIONS** → Appendix 1 (gabapentin).
- **SIDE-EFFECTS**
▶ **Common or very common** Abdominal pain · abnormal reflexes · abnormal thoughts · acne · amnesia · anorexia · anxiety · arthralgia · ataxia · confusion · constipation · convulsions · cough · depression · diarrhoea · dizziness · drowsiness · dry mouth · dry throat · dyspepsia · dyspnoea · emotional lability · fever · flatulence · flu syndrome · gingivitis · headache · hostility · hypertension · impotence · increased appetite · insomnia · leucopenia · malaise · movement disorders · myalgia · nausea · nervousness · nystagmus · oedema · paraesthesia · pruritus · rash · rhinitis · speech disorder · tremor · twitching · vasodilatation · vertigo · visual disturbances · vomiting · weight gain
▶ **Uncommon** Palpitations
▶ **Frequency not known** Acute renal failure · alopecia · blood glucose fluctuations in patients with diabetes · breast hypertrophy · gynaecomastia · hallucinations · hepatitis · hypersensitivity syndrome · incontinence · pancreatitis · Stevens-Johnson syndrome · suicidal ideation · thrombocytopenia · tinnitus

- **PREGNANCY**
  Monitoring
  The dose should be monitored carefully during pregnancy and after birth, and adjustments made on a clinical basis.
- **BREAST FEEDING** Present in milk—manufacturer advises use only if potential benefit outweighs risk.
- **RENAL IMPAIRMENT** Reduce dose if estimated glomerular filtration rate less than 80 mL/minute/1.73 m^2; consult product literature.
- **EFFECT ON LABORATORY TESTS** False positive readings with some urinary protein tests.
- **DIRECTIONS FOR ADMINISTRATION** Capsules can be opened but the bitter taste is difficult to mask.
- **PATIENT AND CARER ADVICE**
  Medicines for Children leaflet: Gabapentin for preventing seizures www.medicinesforchildren.org.uk/gabapentin-for-preventing-seizures
- **MEDICINAL FORMS**
  There can be variation in the licensing of different medicines containing the same drug. Forms available from special-order manufacturers include: oral suspension, oral solution,

Tablet
CAUTIONARY AND ADVISORY LABELS 3, 5, 8
▶ Gabapentin (Non-proprietary)
  Gabapentin 600 mg Gabapentin 600mg tablets ┃ 100 tablet PoM £106.00 DT price = £7.62
  Gabapentin 800 mg Gabapentin 800mg tablets ┃ 100 tablet PoM £98.13 DT price = £25.93
▶ Neurontin (Pfizer Ltd)
  Gabapentin 600 mg Neurontin 600mg tablets ┃ 100 tablet PoM £84.80 DT price = £7.62
  Gabapentin 800 mg Neurontin 800mg tablets ┃ 100 tablet PoM £98.13 DT price = £25.93

Capsule
CAUTIONARY AND ADVISORY LABELS 3, 5, 8
▶ Gabapentin (Non-proprietary)
  Gabapentin 100 mg Gabapentin 100mg capsules ┃ 100 capsule PoM £22.00 DT price = £2.12
  Gabapentin 300 mg Gabapentin 300mg capsules ┃ 100 capsule PoM £42.40 DT price = £3.47
  Gabapentin 400 mg Gabapentin 400mg capsules ┃ 100 capsule PoM £49.06 DT price = £3.62
▶ Neurontin (Pfizer Ltd)
  Gabapentin 100 mg Neurontin 100mg capsules ┃ 100 capsule PoM £18.29 DT price = £2.12
  Gabapentin 300 mg Neurontin 300mg capsules ┃ 100 capsule PoM £42.40 DT price = £3.47
  Gabapentin 400 mg Neurontin 400mg capsules ┃ 100 capsule PoM £49.06 DT price = £3.62

Oral solution
CAUTIONARY AND ADVISORY LABELS 3, 5, 8
EXCIPIENTS: May contain Propylene glycol
ELECTROLYTES: May contain Potassium, sodium
▶ Gabapentin (Non-proprietary)
  Gabapentin 50 mg per 1 ml Neurontin 250mg/5ml oral solution ┃ 470 ml PoM no price available
  Gabapentin 50mg/ml oral solution sugar free sugar-free ┃ 150 ml PoM £69.00 DT price = £69.00

Lacosamide

- **INDICATIONS AND DOSE**

Adjunctive treatment of focal seizures with or without secondary generalisation
▶ BY MOUTH, OR BY INTRAVENOUS INFUSION
- Child 16–17 years: Initially 50 mg twice daily, infusion to be administered over 15–60 minutes (for up to 5 days), then increased, if tolerated, in steps of 50 mg twice daily, adjusted according to response, dose to be increased in weekly intervals; maintenance 100 mg twice daily (max. per dose 200 mg twice daily)

Adjunctive treatment of focal seizures with or without secondary generalisation (alternative loading dose regimen when it is necessary to rapidly attain therapeutic plasma concentrations) (under close medical supervision)

▶ BY MOUTH, OR BY INTRAVENOUS INFUSION

▶ **Child 16–17 years:** Loading dose 200 mg, infusion to be administered over 15–60 minutes (for up to 5 days), followed by maintenance 100 mg twice daily, to be given 12 hours after initial dose, then increased, if tolerated, in steps of 50 mg twice daily (max. per dose 200 mg twice daily), adjusted according to response, dose to be increased in weekly intervals

● CONTRA-INDICATIONS Second- or third-degree AV block

● CAUTIONS Conduction problems · risk of PR-interval prolongation · severe cardiac disease

● INTERACTIONS → Appendix 1 (lacosamide). Caution with concomitant use of drugs that prolong PR interval.

● SIDE-EFFECTS

▶ **Common or very common** Abnormal gait · blurred vision · cognitive disorder · constipation · depression · dizziness · drowsiness · fatigue · flatulence · headache · impaired coordination · nausea · nystagmus · pruritus · tremor · vomiting

▶ **Rare** Multi-organ hypersensitivity reaction

▶ **Frequency not known** Aggression · agitation · agranulocytosis · atrial fibrillation · atrial flutter · AV block · bradycardia · confusion · dry mouth · dysarthria · dyspepsia · euphoria · hypoesthesia · irritability · muscle spasm · PR-interval prolongation · psychosis · rash · suicidal ideation · tinnitus

● ALLERGY AND CROSS-SENSITIVITY Antiepileptic hypersensitivity syndrome associated with lacosamide. See under Epilepsy p. 180 for more information.

● PREGNANCY

Monitoring
The dose should be monitored carefully during pregnancy and after birth, and adjustments made on a clinical basis.

● BREAST FEEDING Manufacturer advises avoid—present in milk in *animal* studies.

● HEPATIC IMPAIRMENT Titrate with caution in mild to moderate impairment if co-existing renal impairment. Caution in severe impairment—no information available.

● RENAL IMPAIRMENT Loading dose regimen can be considered in mild to moderate impairment—titrate above 200 mg with caution. Titrate with caution in severe impairment, max. 250 mg daily.
   Consult product literature for loading dose if estimated glomerular filtration rate is less than 30 mL/minute/1.73 m².

● DIRECTIONS FOR ADMINISTRATION

▶ With intravenous use For *intravenous infusion*, give undiluted or dilute with Glucose 5% *or* Sodium Chloride 0.9%.

● PRESCRIBING AND DISPENSING INFORMATION Flavours of syrup may include strawberry.

● PATIENT AND CARER ADVICE
Medicines for Children leaflet: Lacosamide for preventing seizures www.medicinesforchildren.org.uk/lacosamide-for-preventing-seizures

● NATIONAL FUNDING/ACCESS DECISIONS

Scottish Medicines Consortium (SMC) Decisions
The *Scottish Medicines Consortium* has advised (January 2009) that lacosamide (*Vimpat* ®) is accepted for restricted use within NHS Scotland as adjunctive treatment for focal seizures with or without secondary generalisation in patients from 16 years. It is restricted for specialist use in refractory epilepsy.

● MEDICINAL FORMS
There can be variation in the licensing of different medicines containing the same drug.

Tablet
CAUTIONARY AND ADVISORY LABELS 8

▶ **Vimpat** (UCB Pharma Ltd)
Lacosamide 50 mg Vimpat 50mg tablets | 14 tablet [PoM] £10.81 DT price = £10.81
Lacosamide 100 mg Vimpat 100mg tablets | 14 tablet [PoM] £21.62 | 56 tablet [PoM] £86.50 DT price = £86.50
Lacosamide 150 mg Vimpat 150mg tablets | 14 tablet [PoM] £32.44 | 56 tablet [PoM] £129.74 DT price = £129.74
Lacosamide 200 mg Vimpat 200mg tablets | 56 tablet [PoM] £144.16 DT price = £144.16

Oral solution
CAUTIONARY AND ADVISORY LABELS 8
EXCIPIENTS: May contain Aspartame, propylene glycol
ELECTROLYTES: May contain Sodium

▶ **Vimpat** (UCB Pharma Ltd)
Lacosamide 10 mg per 1 ml Vimpat 10mg/ml syrup sugar-free | 200 ml [PoM] £25.74 DT price = £25.74

Solution for infusion
ELECTROLYTES: May contain Sodium

▶ **Vimpat** (UCB Pharma Ltd)
Lacosamide 10 mg per 1 ml Vimpat 200mg/20ml solution for infusion vials | 1 vial [PoM] £29.70

Lamotrigine

● INDICATIONS AND DOSE

Monotherapy of focal seizures | Monotherapy of primary and secondary generalised tonic-clonic seizures | Monotherapy of seizures associated with Lennox-Gastaut syndrome

▶ BY MOUTH

▶ **Child 12–17 years:** Initially 25 mg once daily for 14 days, then increased to 50 mg once daily for further 14 days, then increased in steps of up to 100 mg every 7–14 days; maintenance 100–200 mg daily in 1–2 divided doses; increased if necessary up to 500 mg daily, dose titration should be repeated if restarting after interval of more than 5 days

Monotherapy of typical absence seizures

▶ BY MOUTH

▶ **Child 2–11 years:** Initially 300 micrograms/kg daily in 1–2 divided doses, for 14 days, then 600 micrograms/kg daily in 1–2 divided doses, for further 14 days, then increased in steps of up to 600 micrograms/kg every 7–14 days; maintenance 1–10 mg/kg daily in 1–2 divided doses, increased if necessary up to 15 mg/kg daily, dose titration should be repeated if restarting after interval of more than 5 days

Adjunctive therapy of focal seizures with valproate | Adjunctive therapy of primary and secondary generalised tonic-clonic seizures with valproate | Adjunctive therapy of seizures associated with Lennox-Gastaut syndrome with valproate

▶ BY MOUTH

▶ **Child 2–11 years (body-weight up to 13 kg):** Initially 2 mg once daily on alternate days for first 14 days, then 300 micrograms/kg once daily for further 14 days, then increased in steps of up to 300 micrograms/kg every 7–14 days; maintenance 1–5 mg/kg daily in 1–2 divided doses, dose titration should be repeated if restarting after interval of more than 5 days; maximum 200 mg per day

▶ **Child 2–11 years (body-weight 13 kg and above):** Initially 150 micrograms/kg once daily for 14 days, then 300 micrograms/kg once daily for further 14 days, then increased in steps of up to 300 micrograms/kg every 7–14 days; maintenance 1–5 mg/kg daily in 1–2 divided doses, dose titration should be continued →

repeated if restarting after interval of more than 5 days; maximum 200 mg per day
- Child 12–17 years: Initially 25 mg once daily on alternate days for 14 days, then 25 mg once daily for further 14 days, then increased in steps of up to 50 mg every 7–14 days; maintenance 100–200 mg daily in 1–2 divided doses, dose titration should be repeated if restarting after interval of more than 5 days

Adjunctive therapy of focal seizures (with enzyme inducing drugs) without valproate | Adjunctive therapy of primary and secondary generalised tonic-clonic seizures (with enzyme inducing drugs) without valproate | Adjunctive therapy of seizures associated with Lennox-Gastaut syndromes (with enzyme inducing drugs) without valproate
- BY MOUTH
- Child 2–11 years: Initially 300 micrograms/kg twice daily for 14 days, then 600 micrograms/kg twice daily for further 14 days, then increased in steps of up to 1.2 mg/kg every 7–14 days; maintenance 5–15 mg/kg daily in 1–2 divided doses, dose titration should be repeated if restarting after interval of more than 5 days; maximum 400 mg per day
- Child 12–17 years: Initially 50 mg once daily for 14 days, then 50 mg twice daily for further 14 days, then increased in steps of up to 100 mg every 7–14 days; maintenance 200–400 mg daily in 2 divided doses, increased if necessary up to 700 mg daily, dose titration should be repeated if restarting after interval of more than 5 days

Adjunctive therapy of focal seizures (without enzyme inducing drugs) without valproate | Adjunctive therapy of primary and secondary generalised tonic-clonic seizures (without enzyme inducing drugs) without valproate | Adjunctive therapy of seizures associated with Lennox-Gastaut syndromes (without enzyme inducing drugs) without valproate
- BY MOUTH
- Child 2–11 years: Initially 300 micrograms/kg daily in 1–2 divided doses for 14 days, then 600 micrograms/kg daily in 1–2 divided doses for further 14 days, then increased in steps of up to 600 micrograms/kg every 7–14 days; maintenance 1–10 mg/kg daily in 1–2 divided doses, dose titration should be repeated if restarting after interval of more than 5 days; maximum 200 mg per day
- Child 12–17 years: Initially 25 mg once daily for 14 days, then increased to 50 mg once daily for further 14 days, then increased in steps of up to 100 mg every 7–14 days; maintenance 100–200 mg daily in 1–2 divided doses, dose titration should be repeated if restarting after interval of more than 5 days

---

IMPORTANT SAFETY INFORMATION

SAFE PRACTICE

Do not confuse the different combinations or indications.

- **CAUTIONS** Myoclonic seizures (may be exacerbated)
- **INTERACTIONS** → Appendix 1 (lamotrigine).
- **SIDE-EFFECTS**
- **Common or very common** Blurred vision · aggression · agitation · arthralgia · ataxia · back pain · diarrhoea · diplopia · dizziness · drowsiness · dry mouth · headache · insomnia · nausea · nystagmus · rash · tremor · vomiting
- **Rare** Conjunctivitis
- **Very rare** Anaemia · blood disorders · confusion · hallucination · hepatic failure · hypersensitivity syndrome · increase in seizure frequency · leucopenia · lupus erythematosus-like reactions · movement disorders · pancytopenia · thrombocytopenia · unsteadiness

- **Frequency not known** Aseptic meningitis · suicidal ideation

SIDE-EFFECTS, FURTHER INFORMATION
- Skin reactions Serious skin reactions including Stevens-Johnson syndrome and toxic epidermal necrolysis have developed (especially in children); most rashes occur in the first 8 weeks. Rash is sometimes associated with hypersensitivity syndrome and is more common in patients with history of allergy or rash from other antiepileptic drugs. Consider withdrawal if rash or signs of hypersensitivity syndrome develop. Factors associated with increased risk of serious skin reactions include concomitant use of valproate, initial lamotrigine dosing higher than recommended, and more rapid dose escalation than recommended.
- **ALLERGY AND CROSS-SENSITIVITY** Antiepileptic hypersensitivity syndrome associated with lamotrigine. See under Epilepsy p. 180 for more information.
- **PREGNANCY**

Monitoring
Doses should be adjusted on the basis of plasma-drug concentration monitoring.
- **BREAST FEEDING** Present in milk, but limited data suggest no harmful effect on infant.
- **HEPATIC IMPAIRMENT** Halve dose in moderate impairment. Quarter dose in severe impairment.
- **RENAL IMPAIRMENT** Consider reducing maintenance dose in significant impairment. Caution in renal failure; metabolite may accumulate.
- **TREATMENT CESSATION** Avoid abrupt withdrawal (taper off over 2 weeks or longer) unless serious skin reaction occurs.
- **PRESCRIBING AND DISPENSING INFORMATION** Patients being treated for epilepsy may need to be maintained on a specific manufacturer's branded or generic lamotrigine product.
Switching between formulations Care should be taken when switching between oral formulations in the treatment of epilepsy. The need for continued supply of a particular manufacturer's product should be based on clinical judgement and consultation with the patient or their carer, taking into account factors such as seizure frequency and treatment history.
- **PATIENT AND CARER ADVICE**
Medicines for Children leaflet: Lamotrigine for preventing seizures www.medicinesforchildren.org.uk/lamotrigine-for-preventing-seizures
Skin reactions Warn patients and carers to see their doctor immediately if rash or signs or symptoms of hypersensitivity syndrome develop.
Blood disorders Patients and their carers should be alert for symptoms and signs suggestive of bone-marrow failure, such as anaemia, bruising, or infection. Aplastic anaemia, bone-marrow depression, and pancytopenia have been associated rarely with lamotrigine.

- **MEDICINAL FORMS**
There can be variation in the licensing of different medicines containing the same drug. Forms available from special-order manufacturers include: oral suspension, oral solution

Tablet
CAUTIONARY AND ADVISORY LABELS 8
- Lamotrigine (Non-proprietary)
Lamotrigine 25 mg Lamotrigine 25mg tablets | 56 tablet [PoM] £20.41 DT price = £1.41
Lamotrigine 50 mg Lamotrigine 50mg tablets | 56 tablet [PoM] £9.00 DT price = £1.39
Lamotrigine 100 mg Lamotrigine 100mg tablets | 56 tablet [PoM] £5.87 DT price = £1.65
Lamotrigine 200 mg Lamotrigine 200mg tablets | 56 tablet [PoM] £12.00 DT price = £2.99
- Lamictal (GlaxoSmithKline UK Ltd)
Lamotrigine 25 mg Lamictal 25mg tablets | 56 tablet [PoM] £23.53 DT price = £1.41

Lamotrigine 50 mg Lamictal 50mg tablets | 56 tablet PoM £40.02
DT price = £1.39
Lamotrigine 100 mg Lamictal 100mg tablets | 56 tablet PoM
£69.04 DT price = £1.65
Lamotrigine 200 mg Lamictal 200mg tablets | 56 tablet PoM
£117.35 DT price = £2.99

Dispersible tablet

CAUTIONARY AND ADVISORY LABELS 8, 13

▸ Lamotrigine (Non-proprietary)
Lamotrigine 5 mg Lamotrigine 5mg dispersible tablets sugar free
sugar-free | 28 tablet PoM £15.00 DT price = £2.42
Lamotrigine 25 mg Lamotrigine 25mg dispersible tablets sugar free
sugar-free | 56 tablet PoM £20.41 DT price = £2.37
Lamotrigine 100 mg Lamotrigine 100mg dispersible tablets sugar
free sugar-free | 56 tablet PoM £6.98 DT price = £2.15

▸ Lamictal (GlaxoSmithKline UK Ltd)
Lamotrigine 2 mg Lamictal 2mg dispersible tablets sugar-free |
30 tablet PoM £12.54 DT price = £12.54
Lamotrigine 5 mg Lamictal 5mg dispersible tablets sugar-free |
28 tablet PoM £9.38 DT price = £2.42
Lamotrigine 25 mg Lamictal 25mg dispersible tablets sugar-free |
56 tablet PoM £23.53 DT price = £2.37
Lamotrigine 100 mg Lamictal 100mg dispersible tablets sugar-free
| 56 tablet PoM £69.04 DT price = £2.15

Levetiracetam

● INDICATIONS AND DOSE

Monotherapy of focal seizures with or without secondary generalisation

▸ BY MOUTH, OR BY INTRAVENOUS INFUSION

▸ **Child 16–17 years:** Initially 250 mg once daily for 1 week,
then increased to 250 mg twice daily, then increased in
steps of 250 mg twice daily (max. per dose 1.5 g twice
daily), adjusted according to response, dose to be
increased every 2 weeks

Adjunctive therapy of focal seizures with or without secondary generalisation

▸ BY MOUTH

▸ **Child 1–5 months:** Initially 7 mg/kg once daily, then
increased in steps of up to 7 mg/kg twice daily (max.
per dose 21 mg/kg twice daily), dose to be increased
every 2 weeks

▸ **Child 6 months–17 years (body-weight up to 50 kg):**
Initially 10 mg/kg once daily, then increased in steps of
up to 10 mg/kg twice daily (max. per dose 30 mg/kg
twice daily), dose to be increased every 2 weeks

▸ **Child 12–17 years (body-weight 50 kg and above):** Initially
250 mg twice daily, then increased in steps of 500 mg
twice daily (max. per dose 1.5 g twice daily), dose to be
increased every 2–4 weeks

▸ BY INTRAVENOUS INFUSION

▸ **Child 4–17 years (body-weight up to 50 kg):** Initially
10 mg/kg once daily, then increased in steps of up to
10 mg/kg twice daily (max. per dose 30 mg/kg twice
daily), dose to be increased every 2 weeks

▸ **Child 12–17 years (body-weight 50 kg and above):** Initially
250 mg twice daily, then increased in steps of 500 mg
twice daily (max. per dose 1.5 g twice daily), dose to be
increased every 2 weeks

Adjunctive therapy of myoclonic seizures and tonic-clonic seizures

▸ BY MOUTH, OR BY INTRAVENOUS INFUSION

▸ **Child 12–17 years (body-weight up to 50 kg):** Initially
10 mg/kg once daily, then increased in steps of up to
10 mg/kg twice daily (max. per dose 30 mg/kg twice
daily), dose to be increased every 2 weeks

▸ **Child 12–17 years (body-weight 50 kg and above):** Initially
250 mg twice daily, then increased in steps of 500 mg
twice daily (max. per dose 1.5 g twice daily), dose to be
increased every 2 weeks

● UNLICENSED USE

▸ With oral use *Granules* not licensed for use in children
under 6 years, for initial treatment in children with body-
weight less than 25 kg, or for the administration of doses
below 250 mg.

● INTERACTIONS → Appendix 1 (levetiracetam).

● SIDE-EFFECTS

▸ **Common or very common** Abdominal pain · aggression ·
anorexia · anxiety · ataxia · convulsion · cough · depression
· diarrhoea · dizziness · drowsiness · dyspepsia · headache ·
insomnia · irritability · malaise · nasopharyngitis · nausea ·
rash · tremor · vertigo · vomiting

▸ **Uncommon** Agitation · alopecia · amnesia · blurred vision ·
confusion · diplopia · eczema · impaired attention ·
leucopenia · myalgia · paraesthesia · pruritus · psychosis ·
suicidal ideation · thrombocytopenia · weight changes

▸ **Rare** Agranulocytosis · choreoathetosis · drug reaction
with eosinophilia and systemic symptoms (DRESS) ·
dyskinesia · erythema multiforme · hepatic failure ·
hyponatraemia · neutropenia · pancreatitis · pancytopenia ·
Stevens-Johnson syndrome · toxic epidermal necrolysis

▸ **Frequency not known** Completed suicide · pancytopenia

● PREGNANCY

Monitoring
The dose should be monitored carefully during pregnancy
and after birth, and adjustments made on a clinical basis.
It is recommended that the fetal growth should be
monitored.

● BREAST FEEDING Present in milk—manufacturer advises
avoid.

● HEPATIC IMPAIRMENT Halve dose in severe hepatic
impairment if estimated glomerular filtration rate less
than 60 mL/minute/1.73 m².

● RENAL IMPAIRMENT Reduce dose if estimated glomerular
filtration rate less than 80 mL/minute/1.73 m² (consult
product literature).

● DIRECTIONS FOR ADMINISTRATION

▸ With intravenous use For *intravenous infusion* (Keppra®),
dilute requisite dose with at least 100 mL Glucose 5% or
Sodium Chloride 0.9%; give over 15 minutes.

▸ With oral use For administration of *oral solution*, requisite
dose may be diluted in a glass of water.

● PRESCRIBING AND DISPENSING INFORMATION If switching
between oral therapy and intravenous therapy (for those
temporarily unable to take oral medication), the
intravenous dose should be the same as the established
oral dose.

● PATIENT AND CARER ADVICE
Medicines for Children leaflet: Levetiracetam for preventing
seizures www.medicinesforchildren.org.uk/levetiracetam-for-
preventing-seizures

● MEDICINAL FORMS
There can be variation in the licensing of different medicines
containing the same drug. Forms available from special-order
manufacturers include: oral suspension, oral solution

Tablet
CAUTIONARY AND ADVISORY LABELS 8

▸ Levetiracetam (Non-proprietary)
Levetiracetam 250 mg Levetiracetam 250mg tablets |
60 tablet PoM £28.01 DT price = £2.60
Levetiracetam 500 mg Levetiracetam 500mg tablets |
60 tablet PoM £49.32 DT price = £3.75
Levetiracetam 750 mg Levetiracetam 750mg tablets |
60 tablet PoM £84.02 DT price = £5.26
Levetiracetam 1 gram Levetiracetam 1g tablets | 60 tablet PoM
£95.34 DT price = £6.96

▸ Keppra (UCB Pharma Ltd)
Levetiracetam 250 mg Keppra 250mg tablets | 60 tablet PoM
£28.01 DT price = £2.60
Levetiracetam 500 mg Keppra 500mg tablets | 60 tablet PoM
£49.32 DT price = £3.75

Levetiracetam 750 mg Keppra 750mg tablets | 60 tablet PoM £84.02 DT price = £5.26
Levetiracetam 1 gram Keppra 1g tablets | 60 tablet PoM £95.34 DT price = £6.96
▸ **Matever** (Aspire Pharma Ltd)
Levetiracetam 250 mg Matever 250mg tablets | 60 tablet PoM £28.01 DT price = £2.60
Levetiracetam 500 mg Matever 500mg tablets | 60 tablet PoM £49.32 DT price = £3.75
Levetiracetam 750 mg Matever 750mg tablets | 60 tablet PoM £84.02 DT price = £5.26
Levetiracetam 1 gram Matever 1g tablets | 60 tablet PoM £95.34 DT price = £6.96

Granules
CAUTIONARY AND ADVISORY LABELS 8
▸ **Desitrend** (Desitin Pharma Ltd)
Levetiracetam 250 mg Desitrend 250mg granules sachets sugar-free | 60 sachet PoM £22.41
Levetiracetam 500 mg Desitrend 500mg granules sachet-free | 60 sachet PoM £39.46
Levetiracetam 1 gram Desitrend 1000mg granules sachets sugar-free | 60 sachet PoM £76.27

Oral solution
CAUTIONARY AND ADVISORY LABELS 8
▸ **Levetiracetam** (Non-proprietary)
Levetiracetam 100 mg per 1 ml Levetiracetam 100mg/ml oral solution sugar free sugar-free | 150 ml PoM £27.00–£33.48 sugar-free | 300 ml PoM £66.95 DT price = £6.88
▸ **Desitrend** (Desitin Pharma Ltd)
Levetiracetam 100 mg per 1 ml Desitrend 100mg/ml oral solution sugar-free | 300 ml PoM £15.90 DT price = £6.88
▸ **Keppra** (UCB Pharma Ltd)
Levetiracetam 100 mg per 1 ml Keppra 100mg/ml oral solution sugar-free | 150 ml PoM £33.48 sugar-free | 300 ml PoM £66.95 DT price = £6.88

Solution for infusion
ELECTROLYTES: May contain Sodium
▸ **Levetiracetam** (Non-proprietary)
Levetiracetam 100 mg per 1 ml Levetiracetam 500mg/5ml concentrate for solution for infusion vials | 1 vial PoM £127.31 | 10 vial PoM £114.57–£127.31
Levetiracetam 500mg/5ml solution for infusion vials | 10 vial £127.31
▸ **Desitrend** (Desitin Pharma Ltd)
Levetiracetam 100 mg per 1 ml Desitrend 500mg/5ml concentrate for solution for infusion ampoules | 10 ampoule PoM £127.31
▸ **Keppra** (UCB Pharma Ltd)
Levetiracetam 100 mg per 1 ml Keppra 500mg/5ml concentrate for solution for infusion vials | 10 vial PoM £127.31
▸ **Matever** (Aspire Pharma Ltd)
Levetiracetam 100 mg per 1 ml Matever 500mg/5ml concentrate for solution for infusion vials | 10 vial PoM £127.31

Oxcarbazepine

● **INDICATIONS AND DOSE**

Monotherapy for the treatment of focal seizures with or without secondary generalised tonic-clonic seizures
▸ BY MOUTH
▸ **Child 6-17 years:** Initially 4–5 mg/kg twice daily (max. per dose 300 mg), then increased in steps of up to 5 mg/kg twice daily, adjusted according to response, dose to be adjusted at weekly intervals; maximum 46 mg/kg per day

Adjunctive therapy for the treatment of focal seizures with or without secondary generalised tonic-clonic seizures
▸ BY MOUTH
▸ **Child 6-17 years:** Initially 4–5 mg/kg twice daily (max. per dose 300 mg), then increased in steps of up to 5 mg/kg twice daily, adjusted according to response, dose to be adjusted at weekly intervals; maintenance 15 mg/kg twice daily; maximum 46 mg/kg per day

DOSE ADJUSTMENTS DUE TO INTERACTIONS
In adjunctive therapy, the dose of concomitant antiepileptics may need to be reduced when using high doses of oxcarbazepine.

● **CAUTIONS** Avoid in Acute porphyrias p. 562 · cardiac conduction disorders · heart failure · hyponatraemia
● **INTERACTIONS** → Appendix 1 (oxcarbazepine).
● **SIDE-EFFECTS**
▸ **Common or very common** Abdominal pain · acne · agitation · alopecia · amnesia · asthenia · ataxia · confusion · constipation · depression · diarrhoea · diplopia · dizziness · drowsiness · headache · hyponatraemia · impaired concentration · nausea · nystagmus · rash · tremor · visual disorders · vomiting
▸ **Uncommon** Leucopenia · urticaria
▸ **Very rare** Arrhythmias · atrioventricular block · hepatitis · multi-organ hypersensitivity disorders · pancreatitis · Stevens-Johnson syndrome · systemic lupus erythematosus · thrombocytopenia · toxic epidermal necrolysis
▸ **Frequency not known** Aplastic anaemia · bone marrow depression · hypertension · hypothyroidism · neutropenia · osteoporotic bone disorders · pancytopenia · suicidal ideation
● **ALLERGY AND CROSS-SENSITIVITY** Caution in patients with hypersensitivity to carbamazepine. Antiepileptic hypersensitivity syndrome associated with oxcarbazepine. See under Epilepsy p. 180 for more information.
● **PREGNANCY**
Monitoring
The dose should be monitored carefully during pregnancy and after birth, and adjustments made on a clinical basis.
● **BREAST FEEDING** Amount probably too small to be harmful but manufacturer advises avoid.
● **HEPATIC IMPAIRMENT** Caution in severe impairment—no information available.
● **RENAL IMPAIRMENT** Halve initial dose if estimated glomerular filtration rate less than 30 mL/minute/1.73 m^2, increase according to response at intervals of at least 1 week.
● **PRE-TREATMENT SCREENING** Test for HLA-B*1502 allele in individuals of Han Chinese or Thai origin (avoid unless no alternative—risk of Stevens-Johnson syndrome in presence of HLA-B*1502 allele).
● **MONITORING REQUIREMENTS**
▸ Monitor plasma-sodium concentration in patients at risk of hyponatraemia.
▸ Monitor body-weight in patients with heart failure.
● **PRESCRIBING AND DISPENSING INFORMATION** Patients may need to be maintained on a specific manufacturer's branded or generic oxcarbazepine product.
Switching between formulations Care should be taken when switching between oral formulations. The need for continued supply of a particular manufacturer's product should be based on clinical judgement and consultation with the patient or their carer, taking into account factors such as seizure frequency and treatment history.
● **PATIENT AND CARER ADVICE**
Medicines for Children: Oxcarbazepine for preventing seizures www.medicinesforchildren.org.uk/oxcarbazepine-for-preventing-seizures
Blood, hepatic, or skin disorders Patients or their carers should be told how to recognise signs of blood, liver, or skin disorders, and advised to seek immediate medical attention if symptoms such as lethargy, confusion, muscular twitching, fever, rash, blistering, mouth ulcers, bruising, or bleeding develop.

● MEDICINAL FORMS
There can be variation in the licensing of different medicines containing the same drug. Forms available from special-order manufacturers include: oral suspension

Tablet
CAUTIONARY AND ADVISORY LABELS 3, 8
▸ Oxcarbazepine (Non-proprietary)
Oxcarbazepine 150 mg Oxcarbazepine 150mg tablets | 50 tablet PoM £11.14 DT price = £8.60
Oxcarbazepine 300 mg Oxcarbazepine 300mg tablets | 50 tablet PoM £22.61 DT price = £6.09
Oxcarbazepine 600 mg Oxcarbazepine 600mg tablets | 50 tablet PoM £45.19 DT price = £38.96
▸ Trileptal (Novartis Pharmaceuticals UK Ltd)
Oxcarbazepine 150 mg Trileptal 150mg tablets | 50 tablet PoM £12.24 DT price = £8.60
Oxcarbazepine 300 mg Trileptal 300mg tablets | 50 tablet PoM £24.48 DT price = £6.09
Oxcarbazepine 600 mg Trileptal 600mg tablets | 50 tablet PoM £48.96 DT price = £38.96

Oral suspension
CAUTIONARY AND ADVISORY LABELS 3, 8
EXCIPIENTS: May contain Propylene glycol
▸ Trileptal (Novartis Pharmaceuticals UK Ltd)
Oxcarbazepine 60 mg per 1 ml Trileptal 60mg/ml oral suspension sugar-free | 250 ml PoM £48.96

Perampanel

● INDICATIONS AND DOSE

Adjunctive treatment of focal seizures with or without secondary generalised seizures
▸ BY MOUTH
▸ Child 12–17 years: Initially 2 mg once daily, dose to be taken before bedtime, then increased, if tolerated, in steps of 2 mg at intervals of at least every 2 weeks, adjusted according to response; maintenance 4–8 mg once daily; maximum 12 mg per day

DOSE ADJUSTMENTS DUE TO INTERACTIONS
Titrate at intervals of at least 1 week with concomitant carbamazepine, fosphenytoin, oxcarbazepine, or phenytoin.

● INTERACTIONS → Appendix 1 (perampanel).

● SIDE-EFFECTS Aggression · anxiety · ataxia · back pain · blurred vision · changes in appetite · confusion · diplopia · dizziness · drowsiness · dysarthria · gait disturbance · irritability · malaise · nausea · suicidal behaviour · suicidal ideation · vertigo · weight increase

● PREGNANCY Manufacturer advises avoid.
The dose should be monitored carefully during pregnancy and after birth, and adjustments made on a clinical basis.

● BREAST FEEDING Avoid—present in milk in *animal* studies.

● HEPATIC IMPAIRMENT Increase at intervals of at least 2 weeks, up to max. 8 mg daily in mild or moderate impairment. Avoid in severe impairment.

● RENAL IMPAIRMENT Avoid in moderate or severe impairment.

● PRESCRIBING AND DISPENSING INFORMATION
Switching between formulations Care should be taken when switching between oral formulations. The need for continued supply of a particular manufacturer's product should be based on clinical judgement and consultation with the patient or their carer, taking into account factors such as seizure frequency and treatment history.
Patients may need to be maintained on a specific manufacturer's branded or generic perampanel product.

● MEDICINAL FORMS
There can be variation in the licensing of different medicines containing the same drug.

Tablet
CAUTIONARY AND ADVISORY LABELS 3, 8, 25
▸ Fycompa (Eisai Ltd) ▼
Perampanel 2 mg Fycompa 2mg tablets | 7 tablet PoM £35.00 | 28 tablet PoM £140.00
Perampanel 4 mg Fycompa 4mg tablets | 28 tablet PoM £140.00
Perampanel 6 mg Fycompa 6mg tablets | 28 tablet PoM £140.00
Perampanel 8 mg Fycompa 8mg tablets | 28 tablet PoM £140.00
Perampanel 10 mg Fycompa 10mg tablets | 28 tablet PoM £140.00
Perampanel 12 mg Fycompa 12mg tablets | 28 tablet PoM £140.00

Phenytoin

● INDICATIONS AND DOSE

Tonic-clonic seizures | Focal seizures | Prevention and treatment of seizures during or following neurosurgery or severe head injury
▸ BY MOUTH
▸ Child 1 month–11 years: Initially 1.5–2.5 mg/kg twice daily, then adjusted according to response to 2.5–5 mg/kg twice daily (max. per dose 7.5 mg/kg twice daily), dose also adjusted according to plasma-phenytoin concentration; maximum 300 mg per day
▸ Child 12–17 years: Initially 75–150 mg twice daily, then adjusted according to response to 150–200 mg twice daily (max. per dose 300 mg twice daily), dose also adjusted according to plasma-phenytoin concentration
▸ INITIALLY BY SLOW INTRAVENOUS INJECTION
▸ Neonate: Loading dose 18 mg/kg, dose to be administered over 20–30 minutes, then (by mouth) 2.5–5 mg/kg twice daily (max. per dose 7.5 mg/kg twice daily), adjusted according to response, dose also adjusted according to plasma-phenytoin concentration.

Status epilepticus | Acute symptomatic seizures associated with head trauma or neurosurgery
▸ INITIALLY BY SLOW INTRAVENOUS INJECTION, OR BY INTRAVENOUS INFUSION
▸ Neonate: Loading dose 20 mg/kg, then (by slow intravenous injection or by intravenous infusion) 2.5–5 mg/kg twice daily, to be given with blood pressure and ECG monitoring.
▸ Child 1 month–11 years: Loading dose 20 mg/kg, then (by slow intravenous injection or by intravenous infusion) 2.5–5 mg/kg twice daily, to be given with blood pressure and ECG monitoring
▸ Child 12–17 years: Loading dose 20 mg/kg, then (by intravenous infusion or by slow intravenous injection) up to 100 mg 3–4 times a day, to be given with blood pressure and ECG monitoring

DOSE EQUIVALENCE AND CONVERSION
Preparations containing phenytoin sodium are **not** bioequivalent to those containing phenytoin base (such as *Epanutin Infatabs*® and *Epanutin*® suspension); 100 mg of phenytoin sodium is approximately equivalent in therapeutic effect to 92 mg phenytoin base. The dose is the same for all phenytoin products when initiating therapy. However, if switching between these products the difference in phenytoin content may be clinically significant. Care is needed when making changes between formulations and plasma-phenytoin concentration monitoring is recommended.

● UNLICENSED USE
▸ With oral use Licensed for use in children (age range not specified by manufacturer).

- With intravenous use Phenytoin doses in BNF publications may differ from those in product literature.
- **CONTRA-INDICATIONS**
  GENERAL CONTRA-INDICATIONS
  Acute porphyrias p. 562
  SPECIFIC CONTRA-INDICATIONS
- With intravenous use Second- and third-degree heart block · sino-atrial block · sinus bradycardia · Stokes-Adams syndrome
- **CAUTIONS**
  GENERAL CAUTIONS
  Enteral feeding (interrupt feeding for 2 hours before and after dose; more frequent monitoring may be necessary)
  SPECIFIC CAUTIONS
- With intravenous use Heart failure · hypotension · injection solutions alkaline (irritant to tissues) · respiratory depression · resuscitation facilities must be available
  CAUTIONS, FURTHER INFORMATION
  Consider vitamin D supplementation in patients who are immobilised for long periods or who have inadequate sun exposure or dietary intake of calcium.
  Intramuscular phenytoin should not be used (absorption is slow and erratic).
- **INTERACTIONS** → Appendix 1 (phenytoin).
- **SIDE-EFFECTS**
  GENERAL SIDE-EFFECTS
- **Common or very common** Acne · anorexia · coarsening of facial appearance · constipation · dizziness · drowsiness · gingival hypertrophy and tenderness (maintain good oral hygiene) · headache · hirsutism · insomnia · nausea · paraesthesia · rash · transient nervousness · tremor · vomiting
- **Rare** Leucopenia · aplastic anaemia · blood disorders · dyskinesia · hepatotoxicity · lupus erythematosus · lymphadenopathy · megaloblastic anaemia · osteomalacia · peripheral neuropathy · polyarteritis nodosa · Stevens-Johnson syndrome · thrombocytopenia · toxic epidermal necrolysis
- **Frequency not known** Hypersensitivity syndrome · interstitial nephritis · pneumonitis · polyarthropathy · suicidal ideation
  SPECIFIC SIDE-EFFECTS
- **Common or very common**
- With intravenous use Alterations in respiratory function · arrhythmias · cardiovascular collapse · cardiovascular depression (particularly if injection too rapid) · CNS depression (particularly if injection too rapid) · hypotension · respiratory arrest
- **Frequency not known**
- With intravenous use Purple glove syndrome · tonic seizures
  SIDE-EFFECTS, FURTHER INFORMATION
- Hepatotoxicity Discontinue immediately and do not re-administer.
- Rash Discontinue; if mild re-introduce cautiously but discontinue immediately if recurrence.
- Use in adolescents Phenytoin may cause coarsening of the facial appearance, acne, hirsutism, and gingival hyperplasia and so may be particularly undesirable in adolescent patients.
- Bradycardia and hypotension
- With intravenous use Reduce rate of administration if bradycardia or hypotension occurs.
  Overdose
  Symptoms of phenytoin toxicity include nystagmus, diplopia, slurred speech, ataxia, confusion, and hyperglycaemia.
- **ALLERGY AND CROSS-SENSITIVITY** Cross-sensitivity reported with carbamazepine. Antiepileptic hypersensitivity syndrome associated with phenytoin. See under Epilepsy p. 180 for more information.

- **PREGNANCY** Changes in plasma-protein binding make interpretation of plasma-phenytoin concentrations difficult—monitor unbound fraction. Doses should be adjusted on the basis of plasma-drug concentration monitoring.
- **BREAST FEEDING** Small amounts present in milk, but not known to be harmful.
- **HEPATIC IMPAIRMENT** Reduce dose to avoid toxicity.
- **PRE-TREATMENT SCREENING** HLAB* 1502 allele in individuals of Han Chinese or Thai origin—avoid unless essential (increased risk of Stevens- Johnson syndrome).
- **MONITORING REQUIREMENTS**
- Therapeutic plasma-phenytoin concentrations reduced in first 3 months of life because of reduced protein binding.
- Trough plasma concentration for optimum response: neonate–3 months, 6–15 mg/litre (25–60 micromol/litre); child 3 months–18 years, 10–20 mg/litre (40–80 micromol/litre).
- Manufacturer recommends blood counts (but evidence of practical value uncertain).
- With intravenous use Monitor ECG and blood pressure.
- **DIRECTIONS FOR ADMINISTRATION**
- With intravenous use Before and after administration flush intravenous line with Sodium Chloride 0.9%. For *intravenous injection*, give into a large vein at rate not exceeding 1 mg/kg/minute (max. 50 mg/minute). For *intravenous infusion*, dilute to a concentration not exceeding 10 mg/mL with Sodium Chloride 0.9% and give into a large vein through an in-line filter (0.22–0.50 micron) at a rate not exceeding 1 mg/kg/minute (max. 50 mg/minute); complete administration within 1 hour of preparation.
- **PRESCRIBING AND DISPENSING INFORMATION**
  Switching between formulations Different formulations of oral preparations may vary in bioavailability. Patients being treated for epilepsy should be maintained on a specific manufacturer's product.
- **PATIENT AND CARER ADVICE**
  Medicines for Children leaflet: Phenytoin for preventing seizures www.medicinesforchildren.org.uk/phenytoin-for-preventing-seizures
  Blood or skin disorders Patients or their carers should be told how to recognise signs of blood or skin disorders, and advised to seek immediate medical attention if symptoms such as fever, rash, mouth ulcers, bruising, or bleeding develop. Leucopenia that is severe, progressive, or associated with clinical symptoms requires withdrawal (if necessary under cover of a suitable alternative).

- **MEDICINAL FORMS**
  There can be variation in the licensing of different medicines containing the same drug. Forms available from special-order manufacturers include: oral suspension, oral solution
  Tablet
  CAUTIONARY AND ADVISORY LABELS 8
- **Phenytoin (Non-proprietary)**
  Phenytoin sodium 100 mg Phenytoin sodium 100mg tablets | 28 tablet [PoM] £117.00 DT price = £26.75 | 100 tablet [PoM] no price available
  Chewable tablet
  CAUTIONARY AND ADVISORY LABELS 8, 24
- **Epanutin (Phenytoin)** (Pfizer Ltd)
  Phenytoin 50 mg Epanutin Infatabs 50mg chewable tablets | 200 tablet [PoM] £13.18
  Capsule
  CAUTIONARY AND ADVISORY LABELS 8
- **Phenytoin (Non-proprietary)**
  Phenytoin sodium 25 mg Phenytoin sodium 25mg capsules | 28 capsule [PoM] £15.74 DT price = £15.74
  Phenytoin sodium 50 mg Phenytoin sodium 50mg capsules | 28 capsule [PoM] £15.98 DT price = £15.98
  Phenytoin sodium 100 mg Phenytoin sodium 100mg capsules | 84 capsule [PoM] £68.76 DT price = £54.00

Phenytoin sodium 300 mg Phenytoin sodium 300mg capsules |
28 capsule [PoM] £57.38 DT price = £57.38

Oral suspension
CAUTIONARY AND ADVISORY LABELS 8
▸ Epanutin (Phenytoin) (Pfizer Ltd)
Phenytoin 6 mg per 1 ml Epanutin 30mg/5ml oral suspension |
500 ml [PoM] £4.27 DT price = £4.27

Solution for injection
EXCIPIENTS: May contain Alcohol, propylene glycol
ELECTROLYTES: May contain Sodium
▸ Phenytoin (Non-proprietary)
Phenytoin sodium 50 mg per 1 ml Phenytoin sodium 250mg/5ml
solution for injection ampoules | 5 ampoule [PoM] £15.50–£24.40 |
10 ampoule [PoM] no price available
▸ Epanutin (Phenytoin sodium) (Pfizer Ltd)
Phenytoin sodium 50 mg per 1 ml Epanutin Ready-Mixed
Parenteral 250mg/5ml solution for injection ampoules |
10 ampoule [PoM] £48.79

Rufinamide

● INDICATIONS AND DOSE
Adjunctive treatment of seizures in Lennox-Gastaut syndrome
▸ BY MOUTH
▸ Child 4–17 years (body-weight up to 30 kg): Initially
100 mg twice daily, then increased in steps of 100 mg
twice daily (max. per dose 500 mg twice daily), adjusted
according to response, dose to be increased at intervals
of not less than 2 days
▸ Child 4–17 years (body-weight 30–49 kg): Initially 200 mg
twice daily, then increased in steps of 200 mg twice
daily (max. per dose 900 mg twice daily), adjusted
according to response, dose to be increased at intervals
of not less than 2 days
▸ Child 4–17 years (body-weight 50–69 kg): Initially 200 mg
twice daily, then increased in steps of 200 mg twice
daily (max. per dose 1.2 g twice daily), adjusted
according to response, dose to be increased at intervals
of not less than 2 days
▸ Child 4–17 years (body-weight 70 kg and above): Initially
200 mg twice daily, then increased in steps of 200 mg
twice daily (max. per dose 1.6 g twice daily), adjusted
according to response, dose to be increased at intervals
of not less than 2 days

Adjunctive treatment of seizures in Lennox-Gastaut syndrome with valproate
▸ BY MOUTH
▸ Child 4–17 years (body-weight up to 30 kg): Initially
100 mg twice daily, then increased in steps of 100 mg
twice daily (max. per dose 300 mg twice daily), adjusted
according to response, dose to be increased at intervals
of not less than 2 days

● INTERACTIONS → Appendix 1 (rufinamide).

● SIDE-EFFECTS Abdominal pain · acne · anorexia · anxiety ·
back pain · blurred vision · constipation · diarrhoea ·
diplopia · dizziness · drowsiness · dyspepsia · epistaxis ·
fatigue · gait disturbances · headache · hyperactivity ·
hypersensitivity syndrome · impaired coordination ·
increase in seizure frequency · influenza-like symptoms ·
insomnia · nausea · nystagmus · oligomenorrhoea · rash ·
rhinitis · tremor · vomiting · weight loss

● ALLERGY AND CROSS-SENSITIVITY Antiepileptic
hypersensitivity syndrome associated with rufinamide. See
under Epilepsy p. 180 for more information.

● PREGNANCY
Monitoring
The dose should be monitored carefully during pregnancy
and after birth, and adjustments made on a clinical basis.

● BREAST FEEDING Manufacturer advises avoid—no
information available.

● HEPATIC IMPAIRMENT Caution and careful dose titration in
mild to moderate impairment. Avoid in severe
impairment.

● DIRECTIONS FOR ADMINISTRATION Tablets may be crushed
and given in half a glass of water.

● PRESCRIBING AND DISPENSING INFORMATION
Switching between formulations Care should be taken when
switching between oral formulations. The need for
continued supply of a particular manufacturer's product
should be based on clinical judgement and consultation
with the patient or their carer, taking into account factors
such as seizure frequency and treatment history.
  Patients may need to be maintained on a specific
manufacturer's branded or generic rufinamide product.

● PATIENT AND CARER ADVICE
Counselling on antiepileptic hypersensitivity syndrome is
advised.
Medicines for Children leaflet: Rufinamide for preventing
seizures www.medicinesforchildren.org.uk/rufinamide-for-
preventing-seizures

● NATIONAL FUNDING/ACCESS DECISIONS
Scottish Medicines Consortium (SMC) Decisions
The *Scottish Medicines Consortium* has advised (October
2008) that rufinamide (*Inovelon*®) is accepted for restricted
use within NHS Scotland as adjunctive therapy in the
treatment of seizures associated with Lennox-Gastaut
syndrome in patients 4 years and above. It is restricted for
use when alternative traditional antiepileptic drugs are
unsatisfactory.

● MEDICINAL FORMS
There can be variation in the licensing of different medicines
containing the same drug.
Tablet
CAUTIONARY AND ADVISORY LABELS 8, 21
▸ Inovelon (Eisai Ltd)
Rufinamide 100 mg Inovelon 100mg tablets | 10 tablet [PoM] £5.15
Rufinamide 200 mg Inovelon 200mg tablets | 60 tablet [PoM]
£61.77
Rufinamide 400 mg Inovelon 400mg tablets | 60 tablet [PoM]
£102.96

Oral suspension
CAUTIONARY AND ADVISORY LABELS 8, 21
EXCIPIENTS: May contain Propylene glycol
▸ Inovelon (Eisai Ltd)
Rufinamide 40 mg per 1 ml Inovelon 40mg/ml oral suspension
sugar-free | 460 ml [PoM] £94.71

Sodium valproate
9.6.2016

● INDICATIONS AND DOSE
All forms of epilepsy
▸ BY MOUTH USING IMMEDIATE-RELEASE MEDICINES
▸ Neonate: Initially 20 mg/kg once daily; maintenance
10 mg/kg twice daily.
▸ Child 1 month–11 years: Initially 10–15 mg/kg daily in
1–2 divided doses (max. per dose 600 mg);
maintenance 25–30 mg/kg daily in 2 divided doses,
doses up to 60 mg/kg daily in 2 divided doses may be
used in infantile spasms; monitor clinical chemistry
and haematological parameters if dose exceeds
40 mg/kg daily
▸ Child 12–17 years: Initially 600 mg daily in 1–2 divided
doses, increased in steps of 150–300 mg every 3 days;
maintenance 1–2 g daily in 2 divided doses; maximum
2.5 g per day continued →

4

Nervous system

▶ BY RECTUM

- ▶ **Neonate:** Initially 20 mg/kg once daily; maintenance 10 mg/kg twice daily.
- ▶ **Child 1 month–11 years:** Initially 10–15 mg/kg daily in 1–2 divided doses (max. per dose 600 mg); maintenance 25–30 mg/kg daily in 1–2 divided doses, doses up to 60 mg/kg daily in 2 divided doses may be used in infantile spasms; monitor clinical chemistry and haematological parameters if dose exceeds 40 mg/kg daily
- ▶ **Child 12–17 years:** Initially 600 mg daily in 1–2 divided doses, increased in steps of 150–300 mg every 3 days; maintenance 1–2 g daily in 2 divided doses; maximum 2.5 g per day

Initiation of valproate treatment

▶ INITIALLY BY INTRAVENOUS INJECTION

- ▶ **Neonate:** 10 mg/kg twice daily.
- ▶ **Child 1 month–11 years:** Initially 10 mg/kg, then (by intravenous infusion or by intravenous injection) increased to 20–40 mg/kg daily in 2–4 divided doses, alternatively (by continuous intravenous infusion) increased to 20–40 mg/kg daily, monitor clinical chemistry and haematological parameters if dose exceeds 40 mg/kg daily
- ▶ **Child 12–17 years:** Initially 10 mg/kg, followed by (by intravenous infusion or by intravenous injection) up to 2.5 g daily in 2–4 divided doses, alternatively (by continuous intravenous infusion) up to 2.5 g daily; (by intravenous injection or by intravenous infusion or by continuous intravenous infusion) usual dose 1–2 g daily, alternatively (by intravenous injection or by intravenous infusion or by continuous intravenous infusion) usual dose 20–30 mg/kg daily, intravenous injection to be administered over 3–5 minutes

Continuation of valproate treatment

▶ BY INTRAVENOUS INJECTION, OR BY INTRAVENOUS INFUSION, OR BY CONTINUOUS INTRAVENOUS INFUSION

- ▶ **Child:** If switching from oral therapy to intravenous therapy give the same dose as current oral daily dose, give over 3–5 minutes by intravenous injection *or* in 2–4 divided doses by intravenous infusion

EPILIM CHRONOSPHERE®

All forms of epilepsy

▶ BY MOUTH

- ▶ **Child:** Total daily dose to be given in 1–2 divided doses (consult product literature)

EPILIM CHRONO®

All forms of epilepsy

▶ BY MOUTH

- ▶ **Child (body-weight 20 kg and above):** Total daily dose to be given in 1–2 divided doses (consult product literature)

EPISENTA® CAPSULES

All forms of epilepsy

▶ BY MOUTH

- ▶ **Child:** Total daily dose to be given in 1–2 divided doses (consult product literature)

EPISENTA® GRANULES

All forms of epilepsy

▶ BY MOUTH

- ▶ **Child:** Total daily dose to be given in 1–2 divided doses (consult product literature)

EPIVAL®

All forms of epilepsy

▶ BY MOUTH

- ▶ **Child:** Total daily dose to be given in 1–2 divided doses (consult product literature)

IMPORTANT SAFETY INFORMATION

MHRA/CHM ADVICE: VALPROATE AND RISK OF ABNORMAL PREGNANCY OUTCOMES

Infants exposed to valproate in utero are at a high risk of serious developmental disorders (up to 30–40% risk) and congenital malformations (approx. 11% risk). Valproate should not be used in female children, females of childbearing potential or during pregnancy unless alternative treatments are ineffective or not tolerated.

- ● **CONTRA-INDICATIONS** Acute porphyrias p. 562 · known or suspected mitochondrial disorders (higher rate of acute liver failure and liver-related deaths) · personal or family history of severe hepatic dysfunction
- ● **CAUTIONS** Systemic lupus erythematosus

CAUTIONS, FURTHER INFORMATION

Consider vitamin D supplementation in patients that are immobilised for long periods or who have inadequate sun exposure or dietary intake of calcium.

- ▶ Liver toxicity Liver dysfunction (including fatal hepatic failure) has occurred in association with valproate (especially in children under 3 years and in those with metabolic or degenerative disorders, organic brain disease or severe seizure disorders associated with mental retardation) usually in first 6 months and usually involving multiple antiepileptic therapy. Raised liver enzymes during valproate treatment are usually transient but patients should be reassessed clinically and liver function (including prothrombin time) monitored until return to normal—discontinue if abnormally prolonged prothrombin time (particularly in association with other relevant abnormalities).
- ● **INTERACTIONS** → Appendix 1 (sodium valproate).
- ● **SIDE-EFFECTS**
- ▶ **Common or very common** Aggression · anaemia · confusion · convulsion · deafness · diarrhoea · extrapyramidal disorders · gastric irritation · haemorrhage · headache · hyponatraemia · memory impairment · menstrual disturbance · nausea · nystagmus · somnolence · stupor · thrombocytopenia · transient hair loss (regrowth may be curly) · tremor · weight gain
- ▶ **Uncommon** Angioedema · ataxia · coma · encephalopathy · increased alertness · lethargy · leucopenia · pancytopenia · paraesthesia · peripheral oedema · rash · reduced bone mineral density · syndrome of inappropriate secretion of antidiuretic hormone · vasculitis
- ▶ **Rare** Behavioural disturbance · blood disorders · bone marrow failure · drowsiness · drug rash with eosinophilia and systemic symptoms (DRESS) syndrome · enuresis · Fanconi's syndrome · hallucinations · hearing loss · hyperactivity · hyperammonaemia · hypothyroidism · learning disorders · male infertility · myelodysplastic syndrome · polycystic ovaries · Stevens-Johnson syndrome · systemic lupus erythematosus · toxic epidermal necrolysis
- ▶ **Very rare** Acne · gynaecomastia · hepatic dysfunction · hirsutism · increase in bleeding time · pancreatitis
- ▶ **Frequency not known** Hypersensitivity reactions · suicidal ideation

SIDE-EFFECTS, FURTHER INFORMATION

- ▶ Hepatic dysfunction Withdraw treatment immediately if persistent vomiting and abdominal pain, anorexia, jaundice, oedema, malaise, drowsiness, or loss of seizure control.

▸ Pancreatitis Discontinue treatment if symtoms of pancreatitis develop.

● **CONCEPTION AND CONTRACEPTION** Valproate is associated with teratogenic risks and should not be used in females of child-bearing potential unless there is no safer alternative—this should be fully considered and discussed before prescribing for females of child-bearing age. Exclude pregnancy before treatment—effective contraception advised in females of child-bearing potential. In females planning to become pregnant, all efforts should be made to switch to appropriate alternative treatment prior to conception.

● **PREGNANCY** Valproate is associated with the highest risk of major and minor congenital malformations (in particular neural tube defects), and long-term neurodevelopmental effects. Valproate should not be used during pregnancy unless there is no safer alternative and only after a careful discussion of the risks. If valproate is to be used during pregnancy, the lowest effective dose should be prescribed in divided doses or as modified-release tablets to avoid peaks in plasma-valproate concentrations; doses greater than 1 g daily are associated with an increased risk of teratogenicity. Neonatal bleeding (related to hypofibrinaemia) reported. Neonatal hepatotoxicity also reported.

Specialist prenatal monitoring should be instigated when valproate has been taken in pregnancy.

The dose should be monitored carefully during pregnancy and after birth, and adjustments made on a clinical basis.

● **BREAST FEEDING** Present in milk—risk of haematological disorders in breast-fed newborns and infants.

● **HEPATIC IMPAIRMENT** Avoid if possible—hepatotoxicity and hepatic failure may occasionally occur (usually in first 6 months). Avoid in active liver disease.

● **RENAL IMPAIRMENT** Reduce dose.

● **MONITORING REQUIREMENTS**
▸ Plasma-valproate concentrations are not a useful index of efficacy, therefore routine monitoring is unhelpful.
▸ Monitor liver function before therapy and during first 6 months especially in patients most at risk.
▸ Measure full blood count and ensure no undue potential for bleeding before starting and before surgery.

● **EFFECT ON LABORATORY TESTS** False-positive urine tests for ketones.

● **TREATMENT CESSATION** EvGr Avoid abrupt withdrawal; if treatment with valproate is stopped, reduce the dose gradually over at least 4 weeks. ⚠

● **DIRECTIONS FOR ADMINISTRATION**
▸ With intravenous use For *intravenous injection*, may be diluted in Glucose 5% *or* Sodium Chloride 0.9% and given over 3–5 minutes. For *intravenous infusion*, dilute injection solution with Glucose 5% *or* Sodium Chloride 0.9%.
▸ With rectal use For *rectal administration*, sodium valproate oral solution may be given rectally and retained for 15 minutes (may require dilution with water to prevent rapid expulsion).

EPIVAL® Tablets may be halved but not crushed or chewed.

EPISENTA® CAPSULES Contents of capsule may be mixed with soft food or drink that is cold or at room temperature, and swallowed immediately without chewing.

EPILIM® SYRUP May be diluted, preferably in Syrup BP; use within 14 days.

EPISENTA® GRANULES Granules may be mixed with soft food or drink that is cold or at room temperature, and swallowed immediately without chewing.

EPILIM CHRONOSPHERE® Granules may be mixed with soft food or drink that is cold or at room temperature, and swallowed immediately without chewing.

● **PRESCRIBING AND DISPENSING INFORMATION**
Switching between formulations Care should be taken when switching between oral formulations in the treatment of epilepsy. The need for continued supply of a particular manufacturer's product should be based on clinical judgement and consultation with the patient or their carer, taking into account factors such as seizure frequency and treatment history.

Patients being treated for epilepsy may need to be maintained on a specific manufacturer's branded or generic oral sodium valproate product.

EPILIM CHRONOSPHERE® Prescribe dose to the nearest whole 50-mg sachet.

● **PATIENT AND CARER ADVICE**
Risk of abnormal pregnancy outcomes A patient guide and card should be provided to all female patients.
Medicines for Children leaflet: Sodium valproate for preventing seizures www.medicinesforchildren.org.uk/sodium-valproate-for-preventing-seizures

Blood or hepatic disorders Patients or their carers should be told how to recognise signs and symptoms of blood or liver disorders and advised to seek immediate medical attention if symptoms develop.

Pancreatitis Patients or their carers should be told how to recognise signs and symptoms of pancreatitis and advised to seek immediate medical attention if symptoms such as abdominal pain, nausea, or vomiting develop.

MHRA advice: Valproate and risk of abnormal pregnancy outcomes Female patients and their carers should be counselled on the risk of valproate treatment during pregnancy. Ensure female patients are provided with relevant resources, to support their understanding of the risks. In particular the prescriber must ensure the patient understands:
● the risks associated with valproate during pregnancy;
● the need to use effective contraception;
● the need for regular review of treatment;
● the need to rapidly consult if she is planning a pregnancy or becomes pregnant

EPISENTA® CAPSULES Patients and carers should be counselled on the administration of capsules.

EPISENTA® GRANULES Patients and carers should be counselled on the administration of granules.

EPILIM CHRONOSPHERE® Patients and carers should be counselled on the administration of granules.

● **MEDICINAL FORMS**
There can be variation in the licensing of different medicines containing the same drug. Forms available from special-order manufacturers include: oral suspension, oral solution, suppository

Tablet
CAUTIONARY AND ADVISORY LABELS 8, 10, 21
▸ Epilim (Sanofi) ▼
   Sodium valproate 100 mg Epilim 100mg crushable tablets | 100 tablet PoM £5.60 DT price = £5.60

Modified-release tablet
CAUTIONARY AND ADVISORY LABELS 8, 10, 21, 25
▸ Epilim Chrono (Sanofi) ▼
   Sodium valproate 200 mg Epilim Chrono 200 tablets | 100 tablet PoM £11.65 DT price = £11.65
   Sodium valproate 300 mg Epilim Chrono 300 tablets | 100 tablet PoM £17.47 DT price = £17.47
   Sodium valproate 500 mg Epilim Chrono 500 tablets | 100 tablet PoM £29.10
▸ Epival CR (Chanelle Medical UK Ltd) ▼
   Sodium valproate 300 mg Epival CR 300mg tablets | 100 tablet PoM £12.13 DT price = £17.47
   Sodium valproate 500 mg Epival CR 500mg tablets | 100 tablet PoM £20.21

Gastro-resistant tablet
CAUTIONARY AND ADVISORY LABELS 5, 8, 10, 25
▶ **Sodium valproate (Non-proprietary)** ▼
Sodium valproate 200 mg Sodium valproate 200mg gastro-resistant tablets | 100 tablet PoM £7.70 DT price = £4.16
Sodium valproate 500 mg Sodium valproate 500mg gastro-resistant tablets | 100 tablet PoM £21.99 DT price = £7.98
▶ **Epilim (Sanofi)** ▼
Sodium valproate 200 mg Epilim 200 gastro-resistant tablets | 100 tablet PoM £7.70 DT price = £4.16
Sodium valproate 500 mg Epilim 500 gastro-resistant tablets | 100 tablet PoM £19.25 DT price = £7.98

Modified-release capsule
CAUTIONARY AND ADVISORY LABELS 8, 10, 21, 25
▶ **Episenta (Desitin Pharma Ltd)** ▼
Sodium valproate 150 mg Episenta 150mg modified-release capsules | 100 capsule PoM £7.00
Sodium valproate 300 mg Episenta 300mg modified-release capsules | 100 capsule PoM £13.00

Modified-release granules
CAUTIONARY AND ADVISORY LABELS 8, 10, 21, 25
▶ **Epilim Chronosphere MR (Sanofi)** ▼
Sodium valproate 50 mg Epilim Chronosphere MR 50mg granules sachets sugar-free | 30 sachet PoM £30.00
Sodium valproate 100 mg Epilim Chronosphere MR 100mg granules sachets sugar-free | 30 sachet PoM £30.00 DT price = £30.00
Sodium valproate 250 mg Epilim Chronosphere MR 250mg granules sachets sugar-free | 30 sachet PoM £30.00 DT price = £30.00
Sodium valproate 500 mg Epilim Chronosphere MR 500mg granules sachets sugar-free | 30 sachet PoM £30.00 DT price = £30.00
Sodium valproate 750 mg Epilim Chronosphere MR 750mg granules sachets sugar-free | 30 sachet PoM £30.00 DT price = £30.00
Sodium valproate 1 gram Epilim Chronosphere MR 1000mg granules sachets sugar-free | 30 sachet PoM £30.00 DT price = £30.00
▶ **Episenta (Desitin Pharma Ltd)** ▼
Sodium valproate 500 mg Episenta 500mg modified-release granules sachets sugar-free | 100 sachet PoM £21.00 DT price = £21.00
Sodium valproate 1 gram Episenta 1000mg modified-release granules sachets sugar-free | 100 sachet PoM £41.00 DT price = £41.00

Oral solution
CAUTIONARY AND ADVISORY LABELS 8, 10, 21
▶ **Sodium valproate (Non-proprietary)** ▼
Sodium valproate 40 mg per 1 ml Sodium valproate 200mg/5ml oral solution sugar free sugar-free | 300 ml PoM £4.77–£7.78 DT price = £4.30
▶ **Epilim (Sanofi)** ▼
Sodium valproate 40 mg per 1 ml Epilim 200mg/5ml liquid sugar-free | 300 ml PoM £7.78 DT price = £4.30
Epilim 200mg/5ml syrup | 300 ml PoM £9.33 DT price = £9.33

Solution for injection
▶ **Sodium valproate (Non-proprietary)** ▼
Sodium valproate 100 mg per 1 ml Sodium valproate 400mg/4ml solution for injection ampoules | 5 ampoule PoM £57.90
▶ **Episenta (Desitin Pharma Ltd)** ▼
Sodium valproate 100 mg per 1 ml Episenta 300mg/3ml solution for injection ampoules | 5 ampoule PoM £35.00

Powder and solvent for solution for injection
▶ **Sodium valproate (Non-proprietary)** ▼
Sodium valproate 400 mg Sodium valproate 400mg powder and solvent for solution for injection vials | 4 vial PoM £49.00
▶ **Epilim (Sanofi)** ▼
Sodium valproate 400 mg Epilim Intravenous 400mg powder and solvent for solution for injection vials | 1 vial PoM £13.32

Stiripentol

● **INDICATIONS AND DOSE**

Adjunctive therapy of refractory generalised tonic-clonic seizures in children with severe myoclonic epilepsy in infancy (Dravet Syndrome) in combination with clobazam and valproate (under expert supervision)
▶ BY MOUTH
▶ Child 3–17 years: Initially 10 mg/kg daily in 2–3 divided doses, increased to up to 50 mg/kg daily in 2–3 divided doses, titrated over minimum of 3 days

● **CONTRA-INDICATIONS** History of psychosis
● **INTERACTIONS** → Appendix 1 (stiripentol).
● **SIDE-EFFECTS**
▶ **Common or very common** Aggression · anorexia · ataxia · drowsiness · dystonia · hyperexcitability · hyperkinesia · hypotonia · irritability · nausea · neutropenia · sleep disorders · vomiting · weight loss
▶ **Uncommon** Fatigue · photosensitivity · rash · urticaria
● **ALLERGY AND CROSS-SENSITIVITY** Antiepileptic hypersensitivity syndrome theoretically associated with stiripentol. See under Epilepsy p. 180 for more information.
● **PREGNANCY**
Monitoring
The dose should be monitored carefully during pregnancy and after birth, and adjustments made on a clinical basis.
● **BREAST FEEDING** Present in milk in *animal* studies.
● **HEPATIC IMPAIRMENT** Avoid—no information available.
● **RENAL IMPAIRMENT** Avoid—no information available.
● **MONITORING REQUIREMENTS**
▶ Perform full blood count and liver function tests prior to initiating treatment and every 6 months thereafter.
▶ Monitor growth.
● **DIRECTIONS FOR ADMINISTRATION** Do not take with milk, dairy products, carbonated drinks, fruit juice, or with food or drinks that contains caffeine.
● **PATIENT AND CARER ADVICE**
Medicines for Children leaflet: Stiripentol for preventing seizures www.medicinesforchildren.org.uk/stiripentol-for-preventing-seizures

● **MEDICINAL FORMS**
There can be variation in the licensing of different medicines containing the same drug.

Capsule
CAUTIONARY AND ADVISORY LABELS 1, 8, 21
▶ **Diacomit (Alan Pharmaceuticals)**
Stiripentol 250 mg Diacomit 250mg capsules | 60 capsule PoM £284.00 DT price = £284.00
Stiripentol 500 mg Diacomit 500mg capsules | 60 capsule PoM £493.00

Powder
CAUTIONARY AND ADVISORY LABELS 1, 8, 13, 21
EXCIPIENTS: May contain Aspartame
▶ **Diacomit (Alan Pharmaceuticals)**
Stiripentol 250 mg Diacomit 250mg oral powder sachets | 60 sachet PoM £284.00
Stiripentol 500 mg Diacomit 500mg oral powder sachets | 60 sachet PoM £493.00

Tiagabine

● **INDICATIONS AND DOSE**

Adjunctive treatment for focal seizures with or without secondary generalisation that are not satisfactorily controlled by other antiepileptics (with enzyme-inducing drugs)

▸ BY MOUTH
  ▸ Child 12–17 years: Initially 5–10 mg daily in 1–2 divided doses, then increased in steps of 5–10 mg/24 hours every 1 week; maintenance 30–45 mg daily in 2–3 divided doses

Adjunctive treatment for focal seizures with or without secondary generalisation that are not satisfactorily controlled by other antiepileptics (without enzyme-inducing drugs)

▸ BY MOUTH
  ▸ Child 12–17 years: Initially 5–10 mg daily in 1–2 divided doses, then increased in steps of 5–10 mg/24 hours every 1 week; maintenance 15–30 mg daily in 2–3 divided doses

● **CAUTIONS** Avoid in Acute porphyrias p. 562

CAUTIONS, FURTHER INFORMATION
Tiagabine should be avoided in absence, myoclonic, tonic and atonic seizures due to risk of seizure exacerbation.

● **INTERACTIONS** → Appendix 1 (tiagabine).

● **SIDE-EFFECTS**
▸ **Common or very common** Diarrhoea · dizziness · emotional lability · impaired concentration · nervousness · speech impairment · tiredness · tremor
▸ **Rare** Bruising · confusion · depression · drowsiness · non-convulsive status epilepticus · psychosis · suicidal ideation · visual disturbances
▸ **Frequency not known** Leucopenia

● **PREGNANCY**

Monitoring
The dose should be monitored carefully during pregnancy and after birth, and adjustments made on a clinical basis.

● **HEPATIC IMPAIRMENT** In mild to moderate impairment reduce dose, prolong the dose interval, or both. Avoid in severe impairment.

● **PATIENT AND CARER ADVICE**

Medicines for Children leaflet: Tiagibine for preventing seizures www.medicinesforchildren.org.uk/tiagabine-for-preventing-seizures

Driving and skilled tasks
May impair performance of skilled tasks (e.g. driving).

● **MEDICINAL FORMS**
There can be variation in the licensing of different medicines containing the same drug. Forms available from special-order manufacturers include: oral suspension

Tablet

CAUTIONARY AND ADVISORY LABELS 21
▸ **Gabitril** (Teva UK Ltd)
  Tiagabine (as Tiagabine hydrochloride monohydrate)
  5 mg Gabitril 5mg tablets | 100 tablet [PoM] £52.04
  Tiagabine (as Tiagabine hydrochloride monohydrate)
  10 mg Gabitril 10mg tablets | 100 tablet [PoM] £104.09
  Tiagabine (as Tiagabine hydrochloride monohydrate)
  15 mg Gabitril 15mg tablets | 100 tablet [PoM] £156.13

Topiramate

● **INDICATIONS AND DOSE**

Monotherapy of generalised tonic-clonic seizures or focal seizures with or without secondary generalisation

▸ BY MOUTH
  ▸ Child 6–17 years: Initially 0.5–1 mg/kg once daily (max. per dose 25 mg) for 1 week, dose to be taken at night, then increased in steps of 250–500 micrograms/kg twice daily, dose to be increased by a maximum of 25 mg twice daily at intervals of 1–2 weeks; usual dose 50 mg twice daily (max. per dose 7.5 mg/kg twice daily), if child cannot tolerate titration regimens recommended above then smaller steps or longer interval between steps may be used; maximum 500 mg per day

Adjunctive treatment of generalised tonic-clonic seizures or focal seizures with or without secondary generalisation | Adjunctive treatment for seizures associated with Lennox-Gastaut syndrome

▸ BY MOUTH
  ▸ Child 2–17 years: Initially 1–3 mg/kg once daily (max. per dose 25 mg) for 1 week, dose to be taken at night, then increased in steps of 0.5–1.5 mg/kg twice daily, dose to be increased by a maximum of 25 mg twice daily at intervals of 1–2 weeks; usual dose 2.5–4.5 mg/kg twice daily (max. per dose 7.5 mg/kg twice daily), if child cannot tolerate recommended titration regimen then smaller steps or longer interval between steps may be used; maximum 400 mg per day

Migraine prophylaxis

▸ BY MOUTH
  ▸ Child 16–17 years: Initially 25 mg once daily for 1 week, dose to be taken at night, then increased in steps of 25 mg every 1 week; usual dose 50–100 mg daily in 2 divided doses, if child cannot tolerate recommended titration regimen then smaller steps or longer interval between steps may be used; maximum 200 mg per day

● **UNLICENSED USE** Not licensed for use in children for migraine prophylaxis.

● **CAUTIONS** Avoid in Acute porphyrias p. 562 · risk of metabolic acidosis · risk of nephrolithiasis—ensure adequate hydration (especially in strenuous activity or warm environment)

● **INTERACTIONS** → Appendix 1 (topiramate).

● **SIDE-EFFECTS**
▸ **Common or very common** Abdominal pain · aggression · agitation · alopecia · anaemia · anxiety · appetite changes · arthralgia · cognitive impairment · confusion · constipation · depression · diarrhoea · dizziness · drowsiness · dry mouth · dyspepsia · dyspnoea · epistaxis · gastritis · impaired attention · impaired coordination · irritability · malaise · mood changes · movement disorders · muscle spasm · muscular weakness · myalgia · nausea · nephrolithiasis · nystagmus · paraesthesia · pruritus · rash · seizures · sleep disturbance · speech disorder · taste disturbance · tinnitus · tremor · urinary disorders · visual disturbances · vomiting
▸ **Uncommon** Abdominal distension · altered sense of smell · blepharospasm · blood disorders · bradycardia · dry eye · flatulence · flushing · gingival bleeding · glossodynia · haematuria · halitosis · hearing loss · hypokalaemia · hypotension · increased lacrimation · influenza-like symptoms · leucopenia · metabolic acidosis · mydriasis · neutropenia · palpitation · pancreatitis · panic attack · peripheral neuropathy · photophobia · postural hypotension · psychosis · reduced sweating · salivation · sexual dysfunction · skin discoloration · suicidal ideation · thirst · thrombocytopenia · urinary calculus

▸ **Rare** Abnormal skin odour · calcinosis · hepatic failure · hepatitis · periorbital oedema · Raynaud's syndrome · Stevens-Johnson syndrome · unilateral blindness
▸ **Very rare** Angle-closure glaucoma
▸ **Frequency not known** Encephalopathy · hyperammonaemia · maculopathy · toxic epidermal necrolysis

SIDE-EFFECTS, FURTHER INFORMATION

▸ Acute myopia with secondary angle-closure glaucoma Topiramate has been associated with acute myopia with secondary angle-closure glaucoma, typically occurring within 1 month of starting treatment. Choroidal effusions resulting in anterior displacement of the lens and iris have also been reported. If raised intra-ocular pressure occurs:
seek specialist ophthalmological advice;
use appropriate measures to reduce intra-ocular pressure;
stop topiramate as rapidly as feasible

● **PREGNANCY** Increased risk of cleft palate if taken in the first trimester of pregnancy.
The dose should be monitored carefully during pregnancy and after birth, and adjustments made on a clinical basis.
It is recommended that the fetal growth should be monitored.

● **BREAST FEEDING** Manufacturer advises avoid—present in milk.

● **HEPATIC IMPAIRMENT** Use with caution in moderate to severe impairment—clearance may be reduced.

● **RENAL IMPAIRMENT** Half usual starting and maintenance dose if estimated glomerular filtration less than 70 mL/minute/1.73 m^2—reduced clearance and longer time to steady-state plasma concentration. Use with caution.

● **DIRECTIONS FOR ADMINISTRATION**
TOPAMAX® CAPSULES Swallow whole or sprinkle contents of capsule on soft food and swallow immediately without chewing.

● **PRESCRIBING AND DISPENSING INFORMATION**
Switching between formulations Care should be taken when switching between oral formulations in the treatment of epilepsy. The need for continued supply of a particular manufacturer's product should be based on clinical judgement and consultation with the patient or their carer, taking into account factors such as seizure frequency and treatment history.
Patients being treated for epilepsy may need to be maintained on a specific manufacturer's branded or generic topiramate product.

● **PATIENT AND CARER ADVICE**
Medicines for Children leaflet: Topiramate for preventing seizures www.medicinesforchildren.org.uk/topiramate-for-preventing-seizures

TOPAMAX® CAPSULES Patients or carers should be given advice on how to administer *Topamax*® capsules.

● **MEDICINAL FORMS**
There can be variation in the licensing of different medicines containing the same drug. Forms available from special-order manufacturers include: oral suspension, oral solution

Tablet
CAUTIONARY AND ADVISORY LABELS 3, 8
▸ **Topiramate (Non-proprietary)**
Topiramate 25 mg Topiramate 25mg tablets | 60 tablet [PoM] £7.62 DT price = £1.64
Topiramate 50 mg Topiramate 50mg tablets | 60 tablet [PoM] £12.83 DT price = £2.05
Topiramate 100 mg Topiramate 100mg tablets | 60 tablet [PoM] £57.60 DT price = £2.63
Topiramate 200 mg Topiramate 200mg tablets | 60 tablet [PoM] £111.50 DT price = £14.03
▸ **Topamax (Janssen-Cilag Ltd)**
Topiramate 25 mg Topamax 25mg tablets | 60 tablet [PoM] £19.29 DT price = £1.64

Topiramate 50 mg Topamax 50mg tablets | 60 tablet [PoM] £31.69 DT price = £2.05
Topiramate 100 mg Topamax 100mg tablets | 60 tablet [PoM] £56.76 DT price = £2.63
Topiramate 200 mg Topamax 200mg tablets | 60 tablet [PoM] £110.23 DT price = £14.03

Capsule
CAUTIONARY AND ADVISORY LABELS 3, 8
▸ **Topiramate (Non-proprietary)**
Topiramate 15 mg Topiramate 15mg capsules | 60 capsule [PoM] £28.11 DT price = £23.73
Topiramate 25 mg Topiramate 25mg capsules | 60 capsule [PoM] £25.95 DT price = £14.74
Topiramate 50 mg Topiramate 50mg capsules | 60 capsule [PoM] £62.81 DT price = £52.19
▸ **Topamax (Janssen-Cilag Ltd)**
Topiramate 15 mg Topamax 15mg sprinkle capsules | 60 capsule [PoM] £14.79 DT price = £23.73
Topiramate 25 mg Topamax 25mg sprinkle capsules | 60 capsule [PoM] £22.18 DT price = £14.74
Topiramate 50 mg Topamax 50mg sprinkle capsules | 60 capsule [PoM] £36.45 DT price = £52.19

❙ Valproic acid

9.6.2016

● **INDICATIONS AND DOSE**

CONVULEX®
Epilepsy
▸ BY MOUTH
▸ **Child 1 month-11 years:** Initially 10–15 mg/kg daily in 2–4 divided doses, max. 600 mg daily; usual maintenance 25–30 mg/kg daily in 2–4 divided doses, doses up to 60 mg/kg daily in 2–4 divided doses in infantile spasms; monitor clinical chemistry and haematological parameters if dose exceeds 40 mg/kg daily
▸ **Child 12-17 years:** Initially 600 mg daily in 2–4 divided doses, increased in steps of 150–300 mg every 3 days; usual maintenance 1–2 g daily in 2–4 divided doses, max. 2.5 g daily in 2–4 divided doses

DOSE EQUIVALENCE AND CONVERSION
Convulex® has a 1:1 dose relationship with products containing sodium valproate, but nevertheless care is needed if switching or making changes.

IMPORTANT SAFETY INFORMATION
MHRA/CHM ADVICE: VALPROATE AND RISK OF ABNORMAL PREGNANCY OUTCOMES
Infants exposed to valproate in utero are at a high risk of serious developmental disorders (up to 30–40% risk) and congenital malformations (approx. 11% risk). Valproate should not be used in female children, females of childbearing potential or during pregnancy unless alternative treatments are ineffective or not tolerated.

● **CONTRA-INDICATIONS** Acute porphyrias p. 562 · known or suspected mitochondrial disorders (higher rate of acute liver failure and liver-related deaths) · personal or family history of severe hepatic dysfunction

● **CAUTIONS** Systemic lupus erythematosus

CAUTIONS, FURTHER INFORMATION
Consider vitamin D supplementation in patients that are immobilised for long periods or who have inadequate sun exposure or dietary intake of calcium.
▸ Liver toxicity Liver dysfunction (including fatal hepatic failure) has occurred in association with valproate (especially in children under 3 years and in those with metabolic or degenerative disorders, organic brain disease or severe seizure disorders associated with mental retardation) usually in first 6 months and usually involving multiple antiepileptic therapy. Raised liver enzymes during valproate treatment are usually transient but

patients should be reassessed clinically and liver function (including prothrombin time) monitored until return to normal—discontinue if abnormally prolonged prothrombin time (particularly in association with other relevant abnormalities).

● INTERACTIONS → Appendix 1 (valproic acid).

● SIDE-EFFECTS

▸ **Common or very common** Diarrhoea · gastric irritation · hyperammonaemia · nausea · thrombocytopenia · transient hair loss (regrowth may be curly) · weight gain

▸ **Uncommon** Aggression · ataxia · behavioural disturbances · hyperactivity · increased alertness · tremor · vasculitis

▸ **Rare** Anaemia · blood disorders · confusion · drowsiness · hallucinations · hearing loss · hepatic dysfunction · lethargy · leucopenia · pancytopenia · rash · stupor

▸ **Very rare** Acne · coma · dementia · encephalopathy · enuresis · extrapyramidal symptoms · Fanconi's syndrome · gynaecomastia · hirsutism · hyponatraemia · increase in bleeding time · pancreatitis · peripheral oedema · reduced bone mineral density · Stevens-Johnson syndrome · suicidal ideation · toxic epidermal necrolysis

▸ **Frequency not known** Drug rash with eosinophilia and systemic symptoms (DRESS) syndrome · hypersensitivity reactions · male infertility · menstrual disturbances · syndrome of inappropriate secretion of antidiuretic hormone

SIDE-EFFECTS, FURTHER INFORMATION

▸ Hepatic dysfunction Withdraw treatment immediately if persistent vomiting and abdominal pain, anorexia, jaundice, oedema, malaise, drowsiness, or loss of seizure control.

▸ Pancreatitis Discontinue treatment if symptoms of pancreatitis develop.

● CONCEPTION AND CONTRACEPTION Valproate is associated with teratogenic risks and should not be used in females of child-bearing potential unless there is no safer alternative—this should be fully considered and discussed before prescribing for females of child-bearing age. Effective contraception advised in females of child-bearing potential. In females planning to become pregnant, all efforts should be made to switch to appropriate alternative treatment prior to conception.

● PREGNANCY Valproate is associated with the highest risk of major and minor congenital malformations (in particular neural tube defects), and long-term neurodevelopmental effects. Valproate should not be used during pregnancy unless there is no safer alternative and only after a careful discussion of the risks. If valproate is to be used during pregnancy, the lowest effective dose should be prescribed in divided doses to avoid peaks in plasma-valproate concentrations; doses greater than 1 g daily are associated with an increased risk of teratogenicity. Neonatal bleeding (related to hypofibrinaemia). Neonatal hepatotoxicity also reported.

Specialist prenatal monitoring should be instigated when valproate has been taken in pregnancy.

The dose should be monitored carefully during pregnancy and after birth, and adjustments made on a clinical basis.

● BREAST FEEDING Present in milk—risk of haematological disorders in breast-fed newborns and infants.

● HEPATIC IMPAIRMENT Avoid if possible—hepatotoxicity and hepatic failure may occasionally occur (usually in first 6 months). Avoid in active liver disease.

● RENAL IMPAIRMENT Reduce dose.

● MONITORING REQUIREMENTS

▸ Monitor closely if dose greater than 45 mg/kg daily.

▸ Monitor liver function before therapy and during first 6 months especially in patients most at risk.

▸ Measure full blood count and ensure no undue potential for bleeding before starting and before surgery.

● EFFECT ON LABORATORY TESTS False-positive urine tests for ketones.

● TREATMENT CESSATION EvGr Avoid abrupt withdrawal; if treatment with valproate is stopped, reduce the dose gradually over at least 4 weeks. ⟨A⟩

● PRESCRIBING AND DISPENSING INFORMATION

CONVULEX® Patients being treated for epilepsy may need to be maintained on a specific manufacturer's branded or generic oral valproic acid product.

● PATIENT AND CARER ADVICE

Risk of abnormal pregnancy outcomes A patient guide and card should be provided to all female patients.

Blood or hepatic disorders Patients or their carers should be told how to recognise signs and symptoms of blood or liver disorders and advised to seek immediate medical attention if symptoms develop.

Pancreatitis Patients or their carers should be told how to recognise signs and symptoms of pancreatitis and advised to seek immediate medical attention if symptoms such as abdominal pain, nausea, or vomiting develop.

MHRA advice: Valproate and risk of abnormal pregnancy outcomes Female patients and their carers should be counselled on the risk of valproate treatment during pregnancy. Ensure female patients are provided with relevant resources, to support their understanding of the risks. In particular the prescriber must ensure the patient understands:

● the risks associated with valproate during pregnancy;

● the need to use effective contraception;

● the need for regular review of treatment;

● the need to rapidly consult if she is planning a pregnancy or becomes pregnant

● MEDICINAL FORMS

There can be variation in the licensing of different medicines containing the same drug.

Gastro-resistant capsule

CAUTIONARY AND ADVISORY LABELS 8, 21, 25, 10

▸ Convulex (Pfizer Ltd) ▼

Valproic acid 150 mg Convulex 150mg gastro-resistant capsules | 100 capsule [PoM] £3.68

Valproic acid 300 mg Convulex 300mg gastro-resistant capsules | 100 capsule [PoM] £7.35

Valproic acid 500 mg Convulex 500mg gastro-resistant capsules | 100 capsule [PoM] £12.25

Vigabatrin

● INDICATIONS AND DOSE

Adjunctive treatment of focal seizures with or without secondary generalisation not satisfactorily controlled with other antiepileptics (under expert supervision)

▸ BY MOUTH

▸ **Neonate:** Initially 15–20 mg/kg twice daily, to be increased over 2–3 weeks to usual maintenance dose, usual maintenance 30–40 mg/kg twice daily (max. per dose 75 mg/kg).

▸ **Child 1-23 months:** Initially 15–20 mg/kg twice daily (max. per dose 250 mg), to be increased over 2–3 weeks to usual maintenance dose, usual maintenance 30–40 mg/kg twice daily (max. per dose 75 mg/kg)

▸ **Child 2-11 years:** Initially 15–20 mg/kg twice daily (max. per dose 250 mg), to be increased over 2–3 weeks to usual maintenance dose, usual maintenance 30–40 mg/kg twice daily (max. per dose 1.5 g)

▸ **Child 12-17 years:** Initially 250 mg twice daily, to be increased over 2–3 weeks to usual maintenance dose, usual maintenance 1–1.5 g twice daily continued →

▶ BY RECTUM
▶ Child 1–23 months: Initially 15–20 mg/kg twice daily (max. per dose 250 mg), to be increased over 2–3 weeks to usual maintenance dose, usual maintenance 30–40 mg/kg twice daily (max. per dose 75 mg/kg)
▶ Child 2–11 years: Initially 15–20 mg/kg twice daily (max. per dose 250 mg), to be increased over 2–3 weeks to usual maintenance dose, usual maintenance 30–40 mg/kg twice daily (max. per dose 1.5 g)
▶ Child 12–17 years: Initially 250 mg twice daily, to be increased over 2–3 weeks to usual maintenance dose, usual maintenance 1–1.5 g twice daily

Monotherapy in the management of infantile spasms in West's syndrome (under expert supervision)
▶ BY MOUTH
▶ Neonate: Initially 15–25 mg/kg twice daily, to be adjusted according to response over 7 days to usual maintenance dose; usual maintenance 40–50 mg/kg twice daily (max. per dose 75 mg/kg).
▶ Child 1 month–1 year: Initially 15–25 mg/kg twice daily, to be adjusted according to response over 7 days to usual maintenance dose; usual maintenance 40–50 mg/kg twice daily (max. per dose 75 mg/kg)

● UNLICENSED USE Granules not licensed for rectal use. Tablets not licensed to be crushed and dispersed in liquid. Vigabatrin doses in BNF publications may differ from those in product literature.
● CONTRA-INDICATIONS Visual field defects
● CAUTIONS History of behavioural problems · history of depression · history of psychosis
  CAUTIONS, FURTHER INFORMATION
  Vigabatrin may worsen absence, myoclonic, tonic and atonic seizures.
▶ Visual field defects Vigabatrin is associated with visual field defects. The onset of symptoms varies from 1 month to several years after starting. In most cases, visual field defects have persisted despite discontinuation, and further deterioration after discontinuation cannot be excluded. Product literature advises visual field testing before treatment and at 6-month intervals. Patients and their carers should be warned to report any new visual symptoms that develop and those with symptoms should be referred for an urgent ophthalmological opinion. Gradual withdrawal of vigabatrin should be considered.
● INTERACTIONS → Appendix 1 (vigabatrin).
● SIDE-EFFECTS
▶ Common or very common Abdominal pain · aggression · agitation · blurred vision · depression · diplopia · dizziness · drowsiness · excitation · fatigue · headache · impaired concentration · impaired memory · irritability · nausea · nervousness · nystagmus · oedema · paraesthesia · paranoia · speech disorder · tremor · visual field defects · vomiting · weight gain
▶ Uncommon Ataxia · mania · occasional increase in seizure frequency (especially if myoclonic) · psychosis · rash
▶ Rare Peripheral retinal neuropathy · retinal disorders · suicidal ideation
▶ Very rare Hepatitis · optic atrophy · optic neuritis
▶ Frequency not known Movement disorders in infantile spasms
  SIDE-EFFECTS, FURTHER INFORMATION
  Encephalopathic symptoms including marked sedation, stupor, and confusion with non-specific slow wave EEG can occur *rarely*—reduce dose or withdraw.
▶ Visual field defects About one-third of patients treated with vigabatrin have suffered visual field defects; counselling and **careful monitoring** for this side-effect are required.

● PREGNANCY
  Monitoring
  The dose should be monitored carefully during pregnancy and after birth, and adjustments made on a clinical basis.
● BREAST FEEDING Present in milk—manufacturer advises avoid.
● RENAL IMPAIRMENT Consider reduced dose or increased dose interval if estimated glomerular filtration rate less than 60 mL/minute/1.73 m².
● MONITORING REQUIREMENTS Closely monitor neurological function.
● DIRECTIONS FOR ADMINISTRATION
▶ With oral use The contents of a sachet should be dissolved in water or a soft drink immediately before taking. Tablets may be crushed and dispersed in liquid.
▶ With rectal use Dissolve contents of sachet in small amount of water and administer rectally [unlicensed use].
● PATIENT AND CARER ADVICE
  Patients and their carers should be warned to report any new visual symptoms that develop.
  Medicines for Children leaflet: Vigabatrin for preventing seizures www.medicinesforchildren.org.uk/vigabatrin-for-preventing-seizures

● MEDICINAL FORMS
  There can be variation in the licensing of different medicines containing the same drug. Forms available from special-order manufacturers include: oral solution

Tablet
CAUTIONARY AND ADVISORY LABELS 3, 8
▶ Sabril (Sanofi)
  Vigabatrin 500 mg Sabril 500mg tablets | 100 tablet [PoM] £44.41 DT price = £44.41

Powder
CAUTIONARY AND ADVISORY LABELS 3, 8, 13
▶ Sabril (Sanofi)
  Vigabatrin 500 mg Sabril 500mg oral powder sachets sugar-free | 50 sachet [PoM] £24.60 DT price = £24.60

Zonisamide

● INDICATIONS AND DOSE
Adjunctive treatment for refractory focal seizures with or without secondary generalisation
▶ BY MOUTH
▶ Child 6–17 years (body-weight 20–54 kg): Initially 1 mg/kg once daily for 7 days, then increased in steps of 1 mg/kg every 7 days, usual maintenance 6–8 mg/kg once daily (max. per dose 500 mg once daily), dose to be increased at 2-week intervals in patients who are **not** receiving concomitant carbamazepine, phenytoin, phenobarbital or other potent inducers of cytochrome P450 enzyme CYP3A4
▶ Child 6–17 years (body-weight 55 kg and above): Initially 1 mg/kg once daily for 7 days, then increased in steps of 1 mg/kg every 7 days, usual maintenance 300–500 mg once daily, dose to be increased at 2-week intervals in patients who are **not** receiving concomitant carbamazepine, phenytoin, phenobarbital or other potent inducers of cytochrome P450 enzyme CYP3A4

● CAUTIONS Low body-weight or poor appetite—monitor weight throughout treatment (fatal cases of weight loss reported in children) · metabolic acidosis—monitor serum bicarbonate concentration in children and those with other risk factors (consider dose reduction or discontinuation if metabolic acidosis develops) · risk factors for renal stone formation (particularly predisposition to nephrolithiasis)

CAUTIONS, FURTHER INFORMATION
Avoid overheating and ensure adequate hydration especially in children, during strenuous activity or if in warm environment (fatal cases of heat stroke reported in children).

- **INTERACTIONS** → Appendix 1 (zonisamide).
Caution with concomitant use of drugs that increase risk of nephrolithiasis.
Contra-indicated with use of drugs that increase risk of hyperthermia or metabolic acidosis.

- **SIDE-EFFECTS**
▸ **Common or very common** Abdominal pain · agitation · alopecia · anorexia · ataxia · confusion · constipation · depression · diarrhoea · diplopia · dizziness · drowsiness · ecchymosis · fatigue · impaired attention · impaired memory · insomnia · irritability · nausea · nystagmus · paraesthesia · peripheral oedema · pruritus · psychosis · pyrexia · rash (consider withdrawal) · speech disorder · tremor · weight loss
▸ **Uncommon** Aggression · cholecystitis · cholelithiasis · dyspepsia · hypokalaemia · pneumonia · seizures · suicidal ideation · urinary calculus · urinary tract infection · vomiting
▸ **Very rare** Amnesia · aspiration · blood disorders · coma · dyspnoea · hallucinations · heat stroke · hepatitis · hydronephrosis · impaired sweating · metabolic acidosis · myasthenic syndrome · neuroleptic malignant syndrome · pancreatitis · renal failure · renal tubular acidosis · rhabdomyolysis · Stevens-Johnson syndrome · toxic epidermal necrolysis

- **ALLERGY AND CROSS-SENSITIVITY** Contra-indicated in sulfonamide hypersensitivity.
Antiepileptic hypersensitivity syndrome theoretically associated with zonisamide. See under Epilepsy p. 180 for more information.

- **CONCEPTION AND CONTRACEPTION** Manufacturer advises women of childbearing potential should use adequate contraception during treatment and for 4 weeks after last dose.

- **PREGNANCY**
Monitoring
The dose should be monitored carefully during pregnancy and after birth, and adjustments made on a clinical basis.

- **BREAST FEEDING** Manufacturer advises avoid for 4 weeks after last dose.

- **HEPATIC IMPAIRMENT** Initially increase dose at 2-week intervals if mild or moderate impairment. Avoid in severe impairment.

- **RENAL IMPAIRMENT** Initially increase dose at 2-week intervals; discontinue if renal function deteriorates.

- **TREATMENT CESSATION** Avoid abrupt withdrawal (consult product literature for recommended withdrawal regimens in children).

- **PRESCRIBING AND DISPENSING INFORMATION**
Switching between formulations Care should be taken when switching between oral formulations. The need for continued supply of a particular manufacturer's product should be based on clinical judgement and consultation with the patient or their carer, taking into account factors such as seizure frequency and treatment history.
Patients may need to be maintained on a specific manufacturer's branded or generic zonisamide product.

- **PATIENT AND CARER ADVICE**
Children and their carers should be made aware of how to prevent and recognise overheating and dehydration.
Medicines for Children leaflet: Zonisamide for preventing seizures www.medicinesforchildren.org.uk/zonisamide-for-preventing-seizures

- **NATIONAL FUNDING/ACCESS DECISIONS**
Scottish Medicines Consortium (SMC) Decisions
The *Scottish Medicines Consortium* has advised (February 2014) that zonisamide (*Zonegran*®) is accepted for restricted use within NHS Scotland as adjunctive treatment of focal seizures, with or without secondary generalisation, in adolescents and children aged 6 years and above. It is restricted to use on advice from specialists in paediatric neurology or epilepsy.

- **MEDICINAL FORMS**
There can be variation in the licensing of different medicines containing the same drug. Forms available from special-order manufacturers include: oral suspension, oral solution
Capsule
CAUTIONARY AND ADVISORY LABELS 3, 8, 10
▸ Zonisamide (Non-proprietary)
Zonisamide 25 mg Zonisamide 25mg capsules | 14 capsule PoM £8.38–£9.26 DT price = £8.82
Zonisamide 50 mg Zonisamide 50mg capsule | 56 capsule PoM £47.04 DT price = £47.04
Zonisamide 50mg capsules | 56 capsule PoM £44.69–£49.40 DT price = £47.04
Zonisamide 100 mg Zonisamide 100mg capsules | 56 capsule PoM £59.58–£65.85 DT price = £62.72
Zonisamide 100mg capsule | 56 capsule PoM £62.72 DT price = £62.72
▸ Zonegran (Eisai Ltd)
Zonisamide 25 mg Zonegran 25mg capsules | 14 capsule PoM £8.82 DT price = £8.82
Zonisamide 50 mg Zonegran 50mg capsules | 56 capsule PoM £47.04 DT price = £47.04
Zonisamide 100 mg Zonegran 100mg capsules | 56 capsule PoM £62.72 DT price = £62.72

ANTIEPILEPTICS › BARBITURATES

Phenobarbital
(Phenobarbitone)

- **INDICATIONS AND DOSE**
All forms of epilepsy except typical absence seizures
▸ BY MOUTH
▸ **Child 1 month–11 years:** Initially 1–1.5 mg/kg twice daily, then increased in steps of 2 mg/kg daily as required; maintenance 2.5–4 mg/kg 1–2 times a day
▸ **Child 12–17 years:** 60–180 mg once daily
▸ INITIALLY BY SLOW INTRAVENOUS INJECTION

▸ **Neonate:** Initially 20 mg/kg, then (by slow intravenous injection or by mouth) 2.5–5 mg/kg once daily, adjusted according to response.

Status epilepticus
▸ BY SLOW INTRAVENOUS INJECTION

▸ **Neonate:** Initially 20 mg/kg, dose to be administered at a rate no faster than 1 mg/kg/minute, then 2.5–5 mg/kg 1–2 times a day.

▸ **Child 1 month–11 years:** Initially 20 mg/kg, dose to be administered at a rate no faster than 1 mg/kg/minute, then 2.5–5 mg/kg 1–2 times a day

▸ **Child 12–17 years:** Initially 20 mg/kg (max. per dose 1 g), dose to be administered at a rate no faster than 1 mg/kg/minute, then 300 mg twice daily

DOSE EQUIVALENCE AND CONVERSION
For therapeutic purposes phenobarbital and phenobarbital sodium may be considered equivalent in effect.

- **CAUTIONS** Avoid in Acute porphyrias p. 562 · children · debilitated · history of alcohol abuse · history of drug abuse · respiratory depression (avoid if severe)

CAUTIONS, FURTHER INFORMATION
Consider vitamin D supplementation in patients who are immobilised for long periods or who have inadequate sun exposure or dietary intake of calcium.

● INTERACTIONS → Appendix 1 (phenobarbital).

● SIDE-EFFECTS

▸ **Common or very common** Agranulocytosis · allergic skin reactions · ataxia · behavioural disturbances · cholestasis · depression · drowsiness · hallucinations · hepatitis · hyperactivity · hypotension · impaired cognition · impaired memory · irritability · lethargy · megaloblastic anaemia (may be treated with folic acid) · nystagmus · osteomalacia · respiratory depression · thrombocytopenia

▸ **Very rare** Antiepileptic Hypersensitivity Syndrome · Stevens-Johnson syndrome · suicidal ideation · toxic epidermal necrolysis

▸ **Frequency not known** Hyperkinesia

Overdose
For details on the management of poisoning, see Active elimination techniques, under Emergency treatment of poisoning p. 786.

● ALLERGY AND CROSS-SENSITIVITY Antiepileptic hypersensitivity syndrome associated with phenobarbital. See under Epilepsy p. 180 for more information.

● PREGNANCY

Monitoring
The dose should be monitored carefully during pregnancy and after birth, and adjustments made on a clinical basis.

● BREAST FEEDING Avoid if possible; drowsiness may occur.

● HEPATIC IMPAIRMENT May precipitate coma. Avoid in severe impairment.

● RENAL IMPAIRMENT Use with caution.

● MONITORING REQUIREMENTS

▸ Plasma-phenobarbital concentration for optimum response is 15–40 mg/litre (60–180 micromol/litre); however, monitoring the plasma-drug concentration is less useful than with other drugs because tolerance occurs.

● TREATMENT CESSATION Avoid abrupt withdrawal (dependence with prolonged use).

● DIRECTIONS FOR ADMINISTRATION

▸ With oral use For administration by *mouth*, tablets may be crushed.

▸ With intravenous use For *intravenous injection*, dilute to a concentration of 20 mg/mL with Water for Injections; give over 20 minutes (no faster than 1 mg/kg/minute).

● PRESCRIBING AND DISPENSING INFORMATION
Some hospitals supply **alcohol-free** formulations of varying phenobarbital strengths.
Switching between formulations Different formulations of oral preparations may vary in bioavailability. Patients should be maintained on a specific manufacturer's product.

● PATIENT AND CARER ADVICE
Medicines for Children leaflet: Phenobarbital for preventing seizures www.medicinesforchildren.org.uk/phenobarbital-for-preventing-seizures

● MEDICINAL FORMS
There can be variation in the licensing of different medicines containing the same drug. Forms available from special-order manufacturers include: tablet, capsule, oral suspension, oral solution

Tablet
CAUTIONARY AND ADVISORY LABELS 2, 8
▸ Phenobarbital (Non-proprietary)
Phenobarbital 15 mg Phenobarbital 15mg tablets | 28 tablet PoM £24.95 DT price = £22.14 CD3
Phenobarbital 30 mg Phenobarbital 30mg tablets | 28 tablet PoM £5.99 DT price = £0.79 CD3
Phenobarbital 60 mg Phenobarbital 60mg tablets | 28 tablet PoM £7.99 DT price = £6.07 CD3

Oral solution
CAUTIONARY AND ADVISORY LABELS 2, 8
▸ Phenobarbital (Non-proprietary)
Phenobarbital 3 mg per 1 ml Phenobarbital 15mg/5ml elixir | 500 ml PoM £83.00 DT price = £83.00 CD3

Solution for injection
EXCIPIENTS: May contain Propylene glycol
▸ Phenobarbital (Non-proprietary)
Phenobarbital sodium 15 mg per 1 ml Phenobarbital 15mg/1ml solution for injection ampoules | 10 ampoule PoM £19.68 CD3
Phenobarbital sodium 30 mg per 1 ml Phenobarbital 30mg/1ml solution for injection ampoules | 10 ampoule PoM £69.88–£76.87 CD3
Phenobarbital sodium 60 mg per 1 ml Phenobarbital 60mg/1ml solution for injection ampoules | 10 ampoule PoM £81.73 CD3
Phenobarbital sodium 200 mg per 1 ml Phenobarbital 200mg/1ml solution for injection ampoules | 10 ampoule PoM £60.57–£66.63 CD3

Primidone

● INDICATIONS AND DOSE
All forms of epilepsy except typical absence seizures
▸ BY MOUTH
▸ Child 1 month–1 year: Initially 125 mg daily, dose to be taken at bedtime, then increased in steps of 125 mg every 3 days, adjusted according to response; maintenance 125–250 mg twice daily
▸ Child 2–4 years: Initially 125 mg once daily, dose to be taken at bedtime, then increased in steps of 125 mg every 3 days, adjusted according to response; maintenance 250–375 mg twice daily
▸ Child 5–8 years: Initially 125 mg once daily, dose to be taken at bedtime, then increased in steps of 125 mg every 3 days, adjusted according to response; maintenance 375–500 mg twice daily
▸ Child 9–17 years: Initially 125 mg once daily, dose to be taken at bedtime, then increased in steps of 125 mg every 3 days, increased to 250 mg twice daily, then increased in steps of 250 mg every 3 days (max. per dose 750 mg twice daily), adjusted according to response

● CAUTIONS Avoid in acute porphyria · children · debilitated · history of alcohol abuse · history of drug abuse · respiratory depression (avoid if severe)

CAUTIONS, FURTHER INFORMATION
Consider vitamin D supplementation in patients who are immobilised for long periods or who have inadequate sun exposure or dietary intake of calcium.

● INTERACTIONS → Appendix 1 (primidone).

● SIDE-EFFECTS

▸ **Common or very common** Agranulocytosis · allergic skin reactions · ataxia · behavioural disturbances · cholestasis · depression · drowsiness · hallucinations · hepatitis · hyperactivity · hypotension · impaired cognition · impaired memory · irritability · lethargy · megaloblastic anaemia (may be treated with folic acid) · nausea · nystagmus · osteomalacia · respiratory depression · thrombocytopenia · visual disturbances

▸ **Uncommon** Dizziness · headache · vomiting

▸ **Rare** Arthralgia · lupus erythematosus · psychosis

▸ **Very rare** Antiepileptic Hypersensitivity Syndrome · Stevens-Johnson syndrome · suicidal ideation · toxic epidermal necrolysis

▸ **Frequency not known** Dupuytren's contracture

● ALLERGY AND CROSS-SENSITIVITY Antiepileptic hypersensitivity syndrome associated with primidone. See under Epilepsy p. 180 for more information.

- **PREGNANCY**
  Monitoring
  The dose should be monitored carefully during pregnancy and after birth, and adjustments made on a clinical basis.
- **HEPATIC IMPAIRMENT** Reduce dose. May precipitate coma.
- **RENAL IMPAIRMENT** Use with caution.
- **MONITORING REQUIREMENTS**
  ▸ Monitor plasma concentrations of derived phenobarbital; plasma concentration for optimum response is 15–40 mg/litre (60–180 micromol/litre).
- **TREATMENT CESSATION** Avoid abrupt withdrawal (dependence with prolonged use).
- **PRESCRIBING AND DISPENSING INFORMATION**
  Switching between formulations Different formulations of oral preparations may vary in bioavailability. Patients being treated for epilepsy should be maintained on a specific manufacturer's product.

- **MEDICINAL FORMS**
  There can be variation in the licensing of different medicines containing the same drug. Forms available from special-order manufacturers include: capsule, oral suspension
  Tablet
  CAUTIONARY AND ADVISORY LABELS 2, 8
  ▸ **Primidone (Non-proprietary)**
    Primidone 50 mg Primidone 50mg tablets | 100 tablet PoM £95.65–£112.37 DT price = £104.54
    Primidone 250 mg Primidone 250mg tablets | 90 tablet PoM no price available | 100 tablet PoM £99.65–£121.94 DT price = £112.59
  Oral suspension
  ▸ **Primidone (Non-proprietary)**
    Primidone 25 mg per 1 ml Liskantin Saft 125mg/5ml oral suspension | 250 ml PoM no price available

HYPNOTICS, SEDATIVES AND ANXIOLYTICS ›
BENZODIAZEPINES

Benzodiazepines 🔳

- **CONTRA-INDICATIONS** Acute pulmonary insufficiency · marked neuromuscular respiratory weakness · sleep apnoea syndrome · unstable myasthenia gravis
- **CAUTIONS** Avoid prolonged use (and abrupt withdrawal thereafter) · history of alcohol dependence or abuse · history of drug dependence or abuse · myasthenia gravis · respiratory disease
  CAUTIONS, FURTHER INFORMATION
  ▸ Paradoxical effects A paradoxical increase in hostility and aggression may be reported by patients taking benzodiazepines. The effects range from talkativeness and excitement to aggressive and antisocial acts. Adjustment of the dose (up or down) sometimes attenuates the impulses. Increased anxiety and perceptual disorders are other paradoxical effects.
- **INTERACTIONS** → Appendix 1 (anxiolytics and hypnotics).
- **SIDE-EFFECTS**
  Overdose
  Benzodiazepines taken alone cause drowsiness, ataxia, dysarthria, nystagmus, and occasionally respiratory depression, and coma. For details on the management of poisoning, see Benzodiazepines, under Emergency treatment of poisoning p. 786.
- **PREGNANCY** Risk of neonatal withdrawal symptoms when used during pregnancy. Avoid regular use and use only if there is a clear indication such as seizure control. High doses administered during late pregnancy or labour may cause neonatal hypothermia, hypotonia, and respiratory depression.
- **RENAL IMPAIRMENT** Increased cerebral sensitivity to benzodiazepines.

- **PATIENT AND CARER ADVICE**
  Driving and skilled tasks
  Drowsiness may persist the next day and affect performance of skilled tasks (e.g. driving); effects of alcohol enhanced.
  For information on 2015 legislation regarding driving whilst taking certain controlled drugs, including benzodiazepines, see *Drugs and driving* under Guidance on prescribing p. 1.

  ⏏ above

Clobazam

- **INDICATIONS AND DOSE**
  Adjunct in epilepsy
  ▸ BY MOUTH
  ▸ Child 1 month–5 years: Initially 125 micrograms/kg twice daily, dose to be increased if necessary every 5 days, maintenance 250 micrograms/kg twice daily (max. per dose 500 micrograms/kg twice daily); maximum 30 mg per day
  ▸ Child 6–17 years: Initially 5 mg daily, dose to be increased if necessary at intervals of 5 days, maintenance 0.3–1 mg/kg daily, daily doses of up to 30 mg may be given as a single dose at bedtime, higher doses should be divided; maximum 60 mg per day

  **Monotherapy for catamenial (menstruation) seizures (usually for 7–10 days each month, just before and during menstruation) (under expert supervision) |
  Cluster seizures**
  ▸ BY MOUTH
  ▸ Child 1 month–5 years: Initially 125 micrograms/kg twice daily, dose to be increased if necessary every 5 days, maintenance 250 micrograms/kg twice daily (max. per dose 500 micrograms/kg twice daily); maximum 30 mg per day
  ▸ Child 6–17 years: Initially 5 mg daily, dose to be increased if necessary at intervals of 5 days, maintenance 0.3–1 mg/kg daily, daily doses of up to 30 mg may be given as a single dose at bedtime, higher doses should be divided; maximum 60 mg per day

- **UNLICENSED USE** Not licensed for use in children under 6 years. Not licensed as monotherapy.
- **CONTRA-INDICATIONS** Hyperkinesis · obsessional states · phobic states · respiratory depression
- **CAUTIONS** Muscle weakness · organic brain changes · personality disorder (within the fearful group—dependent, avoidant, obsessive-compulsive) may increase risk of dependence
  CAUTIONS, FURTHER INFORMATION
  The effectiveness of clobazam may decrease significantly after weeks or months of continuous therapy.
- **SIDE-EFFECTS**
  ▸ **Common or very common** Amnesia · ataxia · confusion · dependence · drowsiness the next day · lightheadedness the next day · muscle weakness · paradoxical increase in aggression
  ▸ **Uncommon** Dizziness · dysarthria · gastro-intestinal disturbances · gynaecomastia · incontinence · salivation changes · tremor · visual disturbances
  ▸ **Rare** Apnoea · blood disorders · changes in libido · headache · hypotension · jaundice · respiratory depression · skin reactions · urinary retention · vertigo
  ▸ **Frequency not known** Delusions · excitement · hallucinations · irritability · psychosis · restlessness
- **BREAST FEEDING** Benzodiazepines are present in milk, and should be avoided if possible during breast-feeding.
  All infants should be monitored for sedation, feeding difficulties, adequate weight gain, and developmental milestones.

- **HEPATIC IMPAIRMENT** Start with smaller initial doses or reduce dose. Can precipitate coma. Avoid in severe impairment.
- **RENAL IMPAIRMENT** Start with small doses in severe impairment.
- **MONITORING REQUIREMENTS** Routine measurement of plasma concentrations of antiepileptic drugs is not usually justified, because the target concentration ranges are arbitrary and often vary between individuals. However, plasma drug concentrations may be measured in children with worsening seizures, status epilepticus, suspected noncompliance, or suspected toxicity. Similarly, haematological and biochemical monitoring should not be undertaken unless clinically indicated.
- **PRESCRIBING AND DISPENSING INFORMATION** Switching between formulations Care should be taken when switching between oral formulations in the treatment of epilepsy. The need for continued supply of a particular manufacturer's product should be based on clinical judgement and consultation with the patient or their carer, taking into account factors such as seizure frequency and treatment history.

  Patients being treated for epilepsy may need to be maintained on a specific manufacturer's branded or generic clobazam product.
- **PATIENT AND CARER ADVICE** Medicines for Children leaflet: Clobazam for preventing seizures www.medicinesforchildren.org.uk/clobazam-preventing-seizures-0
- **NATIONAL FUNDING/ACCESS DECISIONS** **NHS restrictions** Clobazam is not prescribable under the NHS except for epilepsy and endorsed 'SLS'.

- **MEDICINAL FORMS** There can be variation in the licensing of different medicines containing the same drug. Forms available from special-order manufacturers include: capsule, oral suspension

Tablet
CAUTIONARY AND ADVISORY LABELS 2, 19, 8
- ▶ Clobazam (Non-proprietary)
  Clobazam 10 mg Clobazam 10mg tablets | 30 tablet PoM £3.59 DT price = £3.29 CD4-1
- ▶ Frisium (Sanofi)
  Clobazam 10 mg Frisium 10mg tablets | 30 tablet PoM £2.51 DT price = £3.29 CD4-1

Oral suspension
CAUTIONARY AND ADVISORY LABELS 2, 19, 8
- ▶ Clobazam (Non-proprietary)
  Clobazam 1 mg per 1 ml Clobazam 5mg/5ml oral suspension sugar free sugar-free | 150 ml PoM £90.00 DT price = £90.00 CD4-1 sugar-free | 250 ml PoM £150.00 CD4-1
  Clobazam 2 mg per 1 ml Clobazam 10mg/5ml oral suspension sugar free sugar-free | 150 ml PoM £95.00–£97.50 DT price = £95.00 CD4-1 sugar-free | 250 ml PoM £162.50 CD4-1
- ▶ Perizam (Rosemont Pharmaceuticals Ltd)
  Clobazam 1 mg per 1 ml Perizam 1mg/ml oral suspension sugar-free | 150 ml PoM £90.00 DT price = £90.00 CD4-1
  Clobazam 2 mg per 1 ml Perizam 2mg/ml oral suspension sugar-free | 150 ml PoM £95.00 DT price = £95.00 CD4-1
- ▶ Tapclob (Martindale Pharmaceuticals Ltd)
  Clobazam 1 mg per 1 ml Tapclob 5mg/5ml oral suspension sugar-free | 150 ml PoM £90.00 DT price = £90.00 CD4-1 sugar-free | 250 ml PoM £150.00 CD4-1
  Clobazam 2 mg per 1 ml Tapclob 10mg/5ml oral suspension sugar-free | 150 ml PoM £95.00 DT price = £95.00 CD4-1 sugar-free | 250 ml PoM £158.34 CD4-1

▶ 205

Clonazepam

- **INDICATIONS AND DOSE**
All forms of epilepsy
- ▶ BY MOUTH
  - ▶ Child 1-11 months: Initially 250 micrograms once daily for 4 nights, dose to be increased over 2–4 weeks, usual dose 0.5–1 mg daily, dose to be taken at night; may be given in 3 divided doses if necessary
  - ▶ Child 1-4 years: Initially 250 micrograms once daily for 4 nights, dose to be increased over 2–4 weeks, usual dose 1–3 mg daily, dose to be taken at night; may be given in 3 divided doses if necessary
  - ▶ Child 5-11 years: Initially 500 micrograms once daily for 4 nights, dose to be increased over 2–4 weeks, usual dose 3–6 mg daily, dose to be taken at night; may be given in 3 divided doses if necessary
  - ▶ Child 12-17 years: Initially 1 mg once daily for 4 nights, dose to be increased over 2–4 weeks, usual dose 4–8 mg daily, dose usually taken at night; may be given in 3–4 divided doses if necessary

- **UNLICENSED USE** Clonazepam doses in BNFC may differ from those in product literature.
- **CONTRA-INDICATIONS** Coma · current alcohol abuse · current drug abuse · respiratory depression
- **CAUTIONS** Acute porphyrias p. 562 · airways obstruction · brain damage · cerebellar ataxia · depression · spinal ataxia · suicidal ideation
  CAUTIONS, FURTHER INFORMATION
  The effectiveness of clonazepam may decrease significantly after weeks or months of continuous therapy.
- **SIDE-EFFECTS**
- ▶ **Common or very common** Amnesia · bronchial hypersecretion in infants and small children · co-ordination disturbances · confusion · dependence · dizziness · drowsiness · fatigue · muscle hypotonia · nystagmus · poor concentration · restlessness · salivary hypersecretion in infants and small children · withdrawal symptoms
- ▶ **Rare** Aggression · anxiety · blood disorders · dysarthria · gastro-intestinal symptoms · headache · paradoxical effects · pruritus · respiratory depression · reversible hair loss · sexual dysfunction · skin pigmentation changes · urinary incontinence · urticaria · visual disturbances on long-term treatment
- ▶ **Very rare** Increase in seizure frequency
- **BREAST FEEDING** Present in milk, and should be avoided if possible during breast-feeding.
  All infants should be monitored for sedation, feeding difficulties, adequate weight gain, and developmental milestones.
- **HEPATIC IMPAIRMENT** Start with smaller initial doses or reduce dose. Can precipitate coma. Avoid in severe impairment.
- **RENAL IMPAIRMENT** Start with small doses in severe impairment.
- **MONITORING REQUIREMENTS** Routine measurement of plasma concentrations of antiepileptic drugs is not usually justified, because the target concentration ranges are arbitrary and often vary between individuals. However, plasma drug concentrations may be measured in children with worsening seizures, status epilepticus, suspected noncompliance, or suspected toxicity. Similarly, haematological and biochemical monitoring should not be undertaken unless clinically indicated.
- **PRESCRIBING AND DISPENSING INFORMATION** Switching between formulations Care should be taken when switching between oral formulations in the treatment of

epilepsy. The need for continued supply of a particular manufacturer's product should be based on clinical judgement and consultation with the patient or their carer, taking into account factors such as seizure frequency and treatment history.

Patients being treated for epilepsy may need to be maintained on a specific manufacturer's branded or generic oral clonazepam product.

● PATIENT AND CARER ADVICE
Medicines for Children leaflet: Clonazepam for preventing seizures www.medicinesforchildren.org.uk/clonazepam-preventing-seizures-0

● MEDICINAL FORMS
There can be variation in the licensing of different medicines containing the same drug. Forms available from special-order manufacturers include: orodispersible tablet, oral suspension, oral solution, oral drops

Tablet
CAUTIONARY AND ADVISORY LABELS 2, 8
▸ Clonazepam (Non-proprietary)
Clonazepam 500 microgram Clonazepam 500microgram tablets | 100 tablet [PoM] £30.11 DT price = £24.95 [CD4-1]
Clonazepam 2 mg Clonazepam 2mg tablets | 100 tablet [PoM] £33.41 DT price = £27.69 [CD4-1]

Oral solution
CAUTIONARY AND ADVISORY LABELS 2, 8
EXCIPIENTS: May contain Ethanol
▸ Clonazepam (Non-proprietary)
Clonazepam 100 microgram per 1 ml Clonazepam 500micrograms/5ml oral solution sugar free sugar-free | 150 ml [PoM] £83.40 DT price = £69.50 [CD4-1]
Clonazepam 400 microgram per 1 ml Clonazepam 2mg/5ml oral solution sugar free sugar-free | 150 ml [PoM] £108.36 DT price = £108.36 [CD4-1]

Oral drops
▸ Clonazepam (Non-proprietary)
Clonazepam 2.5 mg per 1 ml Rivotril 2.5mg/1ml drops sugar-free | 10 ml [PoM] no price available [CD4-1]

Oral lyophilisate
▸ Clonazepam (Non-proprietary)
Clonazepam 500 microgram Klonopin 0.5mg oral lyophilisates sugar-free | 60 tablet [PoM] no price available [CD4-1]

F 205

Diazepam

● INDICATIONS AND DOSE
Tetanus
▸ BY INTRAVENOUS INJECTION
▸ Child: 100–300 micrograms/kg every 1–4 hours
▸ BY INTRAVENOUS INFUSION, OR BY NASODUODENAL TUBE
▸ Child: 3–10 mg/kg, adjusted according to response, to be given over 24 hours

Muscle spasm in cerebral spasticity or in postoperative skeletal muscle spasm
▸ BY MOUTH
▸ Child 1–11 months: Initially 250 micrograms/kg twice daily
▸ Child 1–4 years: Initially 2.5 mg twice daily
▸ Child 5–11 years: Initially 5 mg twice daily
▸ Child 12–17 years: Initially 10 mg twice daily; maximum 40 mg per day

Status epilepticus | Febrile convulsions | Convulsions due to poisoning
▸ BY INTRAVENOUS INJECTION
▸ Neonate: 300–400 micrograms/kg, then 300–400 micrograms/kg after 10 minutes if required, to be given over 3–5 minutes.
▸ Child 1 month–11 years: 300–400 micrograms/kg (max. per dose 10 mg), then 300–400 micrograms/kg after 10 minutes if required, to be given over 3–5 minutes
▸ Child 12–17 years: 10 mg, then 10 mg after 10 minutes if required, to be given over 3–5 minutes

▸ BY RECTUM
▸ Neonate: 1.25–2.5 mg, then 1.25–2.5 mg after 10 minutes if required.
▸ Child 1 month–1 year: 5 mg, then 5 mg after 10 minutes if required
▸ Child 2–11 years: 5–10 mg, then 5–10 mg after 10 minutes if required
▸ Child 12–17 years: 10–20 mg, then 10–20 mg after 10 minutes if required

Life-threatening acute drug-induced dystonic reactions
▸ BY INTRAVENOUS INJECTION
▸ Child 1 month–11 years: 100 micrograms/kg, repeated if necessary, to be given over 3–5 minutes
▸ Child 12–17 years: 5–10 mg, repeated if necessary, to be given over 3–5 minutes

● UNLICENSED USE
▸ With rectal use *Diazepam Desitin*®, *Diazepam Rectubes*®, and *Stesolid Rectal Tubes*® not licensed for use in children under 1 year.

> **IMPORTANT SAFETY INFORMATION**
> ANAESTHESIA
> Benzodiazepines should only be administered for anaesthesia by, or under the direct supervision of, personnel experienced in their use, with adequate training in anaesthesia and airway management.

● CONTRA-INDICATIONS Avoid injections containing benzyl alcohol in neonates · CNS depression · compromised airway · hyperkinesis · obsessional states · phobic states · respiratory depression

● CAUTIONS
GENERAL CAUTIONS
Muscle weakness · organic brain changes · parenteral administration (close observation required until full recovery from sedation) · personality disorder (within the fearful group—dependent, avoidant, obsessive-compulsive) may increase risk of dependence
SPECIFIC CAUTIONS
▸ With intravenous use High risk of venous thrombophlebitis with intravenous use (reduced by using an emulsion formulation)
CAUTIONS, FURTHER INFORMATION
▸ Special precautions for intravenous injection
▸ With intravenous use When given intravenously facilities for reversing respiratory depression with mechanical ventilation must be immediately available.

● SIDE-EFFECTS
GENERAL SIDE-EFFECTS
▸ **Common or very common** Amnesia · ataxia · confusion · dependence · drowsiness the next day · lightheadedness the next day · muscle weakness · paradoxical increase in aggression
▸ **Uncommon** Dizziness · dysarthria · gastro-intestinal disturbances · gynaecomastia · incontinence · salivation changes · tremor · visual disturbances
▸ **Rare** Apnoea · blood disorders · changes in libido · headache · hypotension · jaundice · respiratory depression · skin reactions · urinary retention · vertigo
▸ **Frequency not known** Delusions · excitement · hallucinations · hypotonia (when used for muscle spasm) · irritability · marked respiratory depression, particularly with high dose (facilities for its treatment are essential) · psychosis · restlessness
SPECIFIC SIDE-EFFECTS
▸ With intravenous use Pain · thrombophlebitis

● PREGNANCY Women who have seizures in the second half of pregnancy should be assessed for eclampsia before any change is made to antiepileptic treatment. Status epilepticus should be treated according to the standard protocol.

Epilepsy and Pregnancy Register All pregnant women with epilepsy, whether taking medication or not, should be encouraged to notify the UK Epilepsy and Pregnancy Register (Tel: 0800 389 1248).

● BREAST FEEDING Present in milk, and should be avoided if possible during breast-feeding.

● HEPATIC IMPAIRMENT Start with smaller initial doses or reduce dose. Can precipitate coma. If treatment is necessary, benzodiazepines with shorter half lives are safer, such as temazepam or oxazepam.
Avoid in severe impairment.

● RENAL IMPAIRMENT Start with small doses in severe impairment.

● DIRECTIONS FOR ADMINISTRATION
▸ With intravenous use For *continuous intravenous infusion* of diazepam emulsion, dilute to a concentration of max. 400 micrograms/mL with Glucose 5% or 10%; max. 6 hours between addition and completion of infusion. For *continuous intravenous infusion* of diazepam solution, dilute to a concentration of max. 50 micrograms/mL with Glucose 5% or Sodium Chloride 0.9%.
▸ With intravenous use Diazepam is adsorbed by plastics of infusion bags and giving sets. Emulsion formulation preferred for intravenous injection.

● PATIENT AND CARER ADVICE

Driving and skilled tasks
May impair judgement and increase reaction time, and so affect ability to drive or perform skilled tasks; they increase the effects of alcohol. Moreover the hangover effects of a night dose may impair performance on the following day.

Patients given sedatives and analgesics during minor outpatient procedures should be very carefully warned about the risks of undertaking skilled tasks (e.g. driving) afterwards. For intravenous benzodiazepines the risk extends to **at least 24 hours** after administration. Responsible persons should be available to take patients home afterwards. The dangers of taking **alcohol** should be emphasised.

Medicines for Children leaflet: Diazepam (rectal) for stopping seizures www.medicinesforchildren.org.uk/diazepam-rectal-stopping-seizures-0

Medicines for Children leaflet: Diazepam for muscle spasm www.medicinesforchildren.org.uk/diazepam-for-muscle-spasm

● PROFESSION SPECIFIC INFORMATION

Dental practitioners' formulary
Diazepam Tablets may be prescribed.
Diazepam Oral Solution 2 mg/5 mL may be prescribed.

● MEDICINAL FORMS
There can be variation in the licensing of different medicines containing the same drug. Forms available from special-order manufacturers include: oral suspension, oral solution, suppository

Tablet
CAUTIONARY AND ADVISORY LABELS 2, 19
▸ Diazepam (Non-proprietary)
Diazepam 2 mg Diazepam 2mg tablets | 28 tablet [PoM] £3.80 DT price = £0.76 [CD4-1] | 1000 tablet [PoM] £135.71 [CD4-1]
Diazepam 5 mg Diazepam 5mg tablets | 28 tablet [PoM] £6.80 DT price = £0.79 [CD4-1] | 1000 tablet [PoM] £242.85 [CD4-1]
Diazepam 10 mg Diazepam 10mg tablets | 28 tablet [PoM] £9.80 DT price = £0.91 [CD4-1] | 500 tablet [PoM] £175.00 [CD4-1]

Oral suspension
▸ Diazepam (Non-proprietary)
Diazepam 400 microgram per 1 ml Diazepam 2mg/5ml oral suspension | 100 ml [PoM] £31.75 [CD4-1]
Diazepam 1 mg per 1 ml Diazepam 5mg/5ml oral suspension | 100 ml [PoM] £55.00 [CD4-1]

Oral solution
CAUTIONARY AND ADVISORY LABELS 2, 19
▸ Diazepam (Non-proprietary)
Diazepam 400 microgram per 1 ml Diazepam 2mg/5ml oral solution sugar free sugar-free | 100 ml [PoM] £40.49 DT price = £31.75 [CD4-1]

Solution for injection
EXCIPIENTS: May contain Benzyl alcohol, ethanol, propylene glycol
▸ Diazepam (Non-proprietary)
Diazepam 5 mg per 1 ml Diazepam 10mg/2ml solution for injection ampoules | 10 ampoule [PoM] £4.00–£5.50 DT price = £5.50 [CD4-1]

Emulsion for injection
▸ Diazemuls (Actavis UK Ltd)
Diazepam 5 mg per 1 ml Diazemuls 10mg/2ml emulsion for injection ampoules | 10 ampoule [PoM] £9.05 [CD4-1]

Enema
CAUTIONARY AND ADVISORY LABELS 2, 19
▸ Diazepam (Non-proprietary)
Diazepam 2 mg per 1 ml Diazepam 5mg RecTubes | 5 tube [PoM] £5.85 DT price = £5.85 [CD4-1]
Diazepam 2.5mg/1.25ml rectal solution tube | 5 tube [PoM] no price available [CD4-1]
Diazepam 2.5mg RecTubes | 5 tube [PoM] £5.65 [CD4-1]
Diazepam 5mg/2.5ml rectal solution tube | 5 tube [PoM] £6.30 DT price = £5.85 [CD4-1]
Diazepam 4 mg per 1 ml Diazepam 10mg RecTubes | 5 tube [PoM] £7.35 DT price = £7.35 [CD4-1]
Diazepam 10mg/2.5ml rectal solution tube | 5 tube [PoM] £8.00 DT price = £7.35 [CD4-1]
▸ Stesolid (Actavis UK Ltd)
Diazepam 2 mg per 1 ml Stesolid 5mg rectal tube | 5 tube [PoM] £6.89 DT price = £5.85 [CD4-1]
Diazepam 4 mg per 1 ml Stesolid 10mg rectal tube | 5 tube [PoM] £8.78 DT price = £7.35 [CD4-1]

1.1   Status epilepticus

> **Drugs used for Status epilepticus not listed below**
> Diazepam p. 207 · Fosphenytoin sodium p. 187 · Phenobarbital p. 203 · Phenytoin p. 193

ANTIEPILEPTICS

Paraldehyde

● INDICATIONS AND DOSE

Status epilepticus
▸ BY RECTUM

▸ Neonate: 0.8 mL/kilogram for 1 dose, the dose is based on the use of a premixed solution of paraldehyde in olive oil in equal volumes

▸ Child: 0.8 mL/kilogram (max. per dose 20 mL) for 1 dose, the dose is based on the use of a premixed solution of paraldehyde in olive oil in equal volumes

● UNLICENSED USE Not licensed for use in children as an enema.

● CONTRA-INDICATIONS Gastric disorders · rectal administration in colitis

● CAUTIONS Bronchopulmonary disease

● INTERACTIONS → Appendix 1 (paraldehyde).

● SIDE-EFFECTS Rash

● PREGNANCY Avoid unless essential—crosses placenta.

● BREAST FEEDING Avoid unless essential—present in milk.

● HEPATIC IMPAIRMENT Use with caution.

● PATIENT AND CARER ADVICE
Medicines for Children leaflet: Paraldehyde for seizures www.medicinesforchildren.org.uk/paraldehyde-for-seizures

● MEDICINAL FORMS
There can be variation in the licensing of different medicines containing the same drug. Forms available from special-order manufacturers include: enema

ANTIEPILEPTICS > BARBITURATES

Thiopental sodium

(Thiopentone sodium)

- **INDICATIONS AND DOSE**

Prolonged status epilepticus
▸ INITIALLY BY SLOW INTRAVENOUS INJECTION

- Neonate: Initially up to 2 mg/kg, then (by continuous intravenous infusion) up to 8 mg/kg/hour, adjusted according to response.
- Child: Initially up to 4 mg/kg, then (by continuous intravenous infusion) up to 8 mg/kg/hour, adjusted according to response

Induction of anaesthesia
▸ BY SLOW INTRAVENOUS INJECTION

- Neonate: Initially up to 2 mg/kg, then 1 mg/kg, repeated if necessary; maximum 4 mg/kg per course.
- Child: Initially up to 4 mg/kg, then 1 mg/kg, repeated if necessary; maximum 7 mg/kg per course

- **UNLICENSED USE** Not licensed for use in status epilepticus. Not licensed for use by intravenous infusion.

IMPORTANT SAFETY INFORMATION
Thiopental sodium should only be administered by, or under the direct supervision of, personnel experienced in its use, with adequate training in anaesthesia and airway management, and when resuscitation equipment is available.

- **CONTRA-INDICATIONS** Acute porphyrias p. 562 · myotonic dystrophy
- **CAUTIONS** Acute circulatory failure (shock) · avoid intra-arterial injection · cardiovascular disease · fixed cardiac output · hypovolaemia · reconstituted solution is highly alkaline (extravasation causes tissue necrosis and severe pain)
- **INTERACTIONS** → Appendix 1 (anaesthetics, general).
- **SIDE-EFFECTS** Arrhythmias · cough · headache · hypersensitivity reactions · hypotension · laryngeal spasm · myocardial depression · rash · sneezing
- **PREGNANCY** May depress neonatal respiration when used during delivery.
- **BREAST FEEDING** Breast-feeding can be resumed as soon as mother has recovered sufficiently from anaesthesia.
- **HEPATIC IMPAIRMENT** Use with caution—reduce dose.
- **RENAL IMPAIRMENT** Caution in severe impairment.
- **DIRECTIONS FOR ADMINISTRATION** For *intravenous injection*, reconstitute 500-mg vial with 20 mL Water for Injections to give 25 mg/mL solution; give over at least 10–15 seconds; for *intravenous infusion* reconstituted solution may be further diluted with Sodium Chloride 0.9%.
- **PATIENT AND CARER ADVICE**

Driving and skilled tasks
Patients given sedatives and analgesics during minor outpatient procedures should be very carefully warned about the risk of driving or undertaking skilled tasks afterwards. For a short general anaesthetic the risk extends to **at least 24 hours** after administration. Responsible persons should be available to take patients home. The dangers of taking **alcohol** should also be emphasised.

- **MEDICINAL FORMS**
There can be variation in the licensing of different medicines containing the same drug. Forms available from special-order manufacturers include: solution for injection

Powder for solution for injection
▸ Thiopental sodium (Non-proprietary)
   Thiopental sodium 500 mg Thiopental 500mg powder for solution for injection vials | 25 vial [PoM] £172.50

HYPNOTICS, SEDATIVES AND ANXIOLYTICS > BENZODIAZEPINES

◣ 205

Lorazepam

- **INDICATIONS AND DOSE**

Premedication
▸ BY MOUTH

- Child 1 month–11 years: 50–100 micrograms/kg (max. per dose 4 mg), to be given at least 1 hour before procedure, same dose may be given the night before procedure in addition to, or to replace, dose before procedure
- Child 12–17 years: 1–4 mg, to be given at least 1 hour before procedure, same dose may be given the night before procedure in addition to, or to replace, dose before procedure

▸ BY INTRAVENOUS INJECTION

- Child: 50–100 micrograms/kg (max. per dose 4 mg), to be administered 30–45 minutes before procedure

Status epilepticus | Febrile convulsions | Convulsions caused by poisoning
▸ BY SLOW INTRAVENOUS INJECTION

- Neonate: 100 micrograms/kg for 1 dose, then 100 micrograms/kg after 10 minutes if required for 1 dose, to be administered into a large vein.
- Child 1 month–11 years: 100 micrograms/kg (max. per dose 4 mg) for 1 dose, then 100 micrograms/kg after 10 minutes (max. per dose 4 mg) if required for 1 dose, to be administered into a large vein
- Child 12–17 years: 4 mg for 1 dose, then 4 mg after 10 minutes if required for 1 dose, to be administered into a large vein

- **UNLICENSED USE** Not licensed for use in febrile convulsions. Not licensed for use in convulsions caused by poisoning.
▸ With intravenous use Not licensed for use as intravenous premedication in children under 12 years.
▸ With oral use Not licensed for use as oral premedication in children under 5 years.

IMPORTANT SAFETY INFORMATION
ANAESTHESIA
Benzodiazepines should only be administered for anaesthesia by, or under the direct supervision of, personnel experienced in their use, with adequate training in anaesthesia and airway management.

- **CONTRA-INDICATIONS** Avoid injections containing benzyl alcohol in neonates · CNS depression · compromised airway · hyperkinesis · obsessional states · phobic states · respiratory depression
- **CAUTIONS** Personality disorder (within the fearful group—dependent, avoidant, obsessive-compulsive) may increase risk of dependence · muscle weakness · organic brain changes · parenteral administration

CAUTIONS, FURTHER INFORMATION
▸ Paradoxical effects A paradoxical increase in hostility and aggression may be reported by patients taking benzodiazepines. The effects range from talkativeness and excitement to aggressive and antisocial acts. Adjustment

of the dose (up or down) sometimes attenuates the impulses. Increased anxiety and perceptual disorders are other paradoxical effects.

- Special precautions for parenteral administration
- With intramuscular use or intravenous use When given parenterally, facilities for managing respiratory depression with mechanical ventilation must be available. Close observation required until full recovery from sedation.

● SIDE-EFFECTS
- **Common or very common** Amnesia · ataxia · confusion · dependence · drowsiness the next day · lightheadedness the next day · muscle weakness · paradoxical increase in aggression
- **Uncommon** Dizziness · dysarthria · gastro-intestinal disturbances · gynaecomastia · incontinence · salivation changes · tremor · visual disturbances
- **Rare** Apnoea · blood disorders · changes in libido · headache · hypotension · jaundice · respiratory depression · skin reactions · urinary retention · vertigo
- **Frequency not known** Delusions · excitement · hallucinations · irritability · marked respiratory depression, particularly with high dose and intravenous use (facilities for its treatment are essential) · pain (on intravenous injection) · psychosis · restlessness · thrombophlebitis (on intravenous injection)

● BREAST FEEDING Benzodiazepines are present in milk, and should be avoided if possible during breast-feeding.

● HEPATIC IMPAIRMENT Start with smaller initial doses or reduce dose. Can precipitate coma. Avoid in severe impairment.

● RENAL IMPAIRMENT Start with small doses in severe impairment.

● DIRECTIONS FOR ADMINISTRATION
- With intravenous use For *intravenous injection*, dilute with an equal volume of Sodium Chloride 0.9% (for neonates, dilute injection solution to a concentration of 100 micrograms/mL). Give over 3–5 minutes; max. rate 50 micrograms/kg over 3 minutes.

● PATIENT AND CARER ADVICE
Driving and skilled tasks
May impair judgement and increase reaction time, and so affect ability to drive or operate machinery; they increase the effects of alcohol. Moreover the hangover effects of a night dose may impair driving on the following day.

Patients given sedatives and analgesics during minor outpatient procedures should be very carefully warned about the risks of undertaking skilled tasks (e.g. driving) afterwards. For intravenous benzodiazepines the risk extends to **at least 24 hours** after administration. Responsible persons should be available to take patients home afterwards. The dangers of taking **alcohol** should be emphasised.

● MEDICINAL FORMS
There can be variation in the licensing of different medicines containing the same drug. Forms available from special-order manufacturers include: oral suspension, oral solution, solution for injection

Tablet
CAUTIONARY AND ADVISORY LABELS 2, 19
- Lorazepam (Non-proprietary)
  Lorazepam 1 mg Lorazepam 1mg tablets | 28 tablet [PoM] £12.21
  DT price = £2.02 [CD4-1] | 30 tablet [PoM] no price available [CD4-1]
  Lorazepam 2.5 mg Lorazepam 2.5mg tablets | 28 tablet [PoM]
  £12.50 DT price = £2.90 [CD4-1] | 30 tablet [PoM] no price available [CD4-1]

Solution for injection
EXCIPIENTS: May contain Benzyl alcohol, propylene glycol
- Ativan (Pfizer Ltd)
  Lorazepam 4 mg per 1 ml Ativan 4mg/1ml solution for injection ampoules | 10 ampoule [PoM] £3.54 [CD4-1]

☞ 205

Midazolam

● INDICATIONS AND DOSE
Status epilepticus | Febrile convulsions
▸ BY BUCCAL ADMINISTRATION

- Neonate: 300 micrograms/kg, then 300 micrograms/kg after 10 minutes if required.
- Child 1–2 months: 300 micrograms/kg (max. per dose 2.5 mg), then 300 micrograms/kg after 10 minutes (max. per dose 2.5 mg) if required
- Child 3–11 months: 2.5 mg, then 2.5 mg after 10 minutes if required
- Child 1–4 years: 5 mg, then 5 mg after 10 minutes if required
- Child 5–9 years: 7.5 mg, then 7.5 mg after 10 minutes if required
- Child 10–17 years: 10 mg, then 10 mg after 10 minutes if required

▸ INITIALLY BY INTRAVENOUS INJECTION

- Neonate: Initially 150–200 micrograms/kg, followed by (by continuous intravenous infusion) 60 micrograms/kg/hour, (by continuous intravenous infusion) increased in steps of 60 micrograms/kg/hour every 15 minutes (max. per dose 300 micrograms/kg/hour) until seizure controlled.
- Child: Initially 150–200 micrograms/kg, followed by (by continuous intravenous infusion) 60 micrograms/kg/hour, (by continuous intravenous infusion) increased in steps of 60 micrograms/kg/hour every 15 minutes (max. per dose 300 micrograms/kg/hour) until seizure controlled

Conscious sedation for procedures
▸ BY MOUTH
- Child: 500 micrograms/kg (max. per dose 20 mg), to be administered 30–60 minutes before procedure
▸ BY BUCCAL ADMINISTRATION
- Child 6 months–9 years: 200–300 micrograms/kg (max. per dose 5 mg)
- Child 10–17 years (body-weight up to 70 kg): 6–7 mg
- Child 10–17 years (body-weight 70 kg and above): 6–7 mg (max. per dose 8 mg)
▸ BY RECTUM
- Child 6 months–11 years: 300–500 micrograms/kg, to be administered 15–30 minutes before procedure
▸ BY INTRAVENOUS INJECTION
- Child 1 month–5 years: Initially 25–50 micrograms/kg, to be administered over 2–3 minutes, 5–10 minutes before procedure, dose can be increased if necessary in small steps to maximum total dose per course; maximum 6 mg per course
- Child 6–11 years: Initially 25–50 micrograms/kg, to be administered over 2–3 minutes, 5–10 minutes before procedure, dose can be increased if necessary in small steps to maximum total dose per course; maximum 10 mg per course
- Child 12–17 years: Initially 25–50 micrograms/kg, to be administered over 2–3 minutes, 5–10 minutes before procedure, dose can be increased if necessary in small steps to maximum total dose per course; maximum 7.5 mg per course

Premedication
▸ BY MOUTH
- Child: 500 micrograms/kg (max. per dose 20 mg), to be taken 15–30 minutes before the procedure
▸ BY RECTUM
- Child 6 months–11 years: 300–500 micrograms/kg, to be administered 15–30 minutes before induction

Induction of anaesthesia (but rarely used)

▸ BY SLOW INTRAVENOUS INJECTION

▸ **Child 7–17 years:** Initially 150 micrograms/kg (max. per dose 7.5 mg), dose to be given in steps of 50 micrograms/kg (max. 2.5 mg) over 2–5 minutes; wait for 2–5 minutes before subsequent dosing, then 50 micrograms/kg every 2 minutes (max. per dose 2.5 mg) if required; maximum 500 micrograms/kg per course; maximum 25 mg per course

Sedation of patient receiving intensive care

▸ INITIALLY BY SLOW INTRAVENOUS INJECTION

▸ **Child 6 months–11 years:** Initially 50–200 micrograms/kg, to be administered over at least 3 minutes, followed by (by continuous intravenous infusion) 30–120 micrograms/kg/hour, adjusted according to response, initial dose may not be required and lower maintenance doses needed if opioid analgesics also used; reduce dose (or reduce or omit initial dose) in hypovolaemia, vasoconstriction, or hypothermia

▸ **Child 12–17 years:** Initially 30–300 micrograms/kg, dose to be given in steps of 1–2.5 mg every 2 minutes, followed by (by continuous intravenous infusion) 30–200 micrograms/kg/hour, adjusted according to response, initial dose may not be required and lower maintenance doses needed if opioid analgesics also used; reduce dose (or reduce or omit initial dose) in hypovolaemia, vasoconstriction, or hypothermia

▸ BY CONTINUOUS INTRAVENOUS INFUSION

▸ **Neonate up to 32 weeks corrected gestational age:** 60 micrograms/kg/hour for 24 hours, then reduced to 30 micrograms/kg/hour, adjusted according to response for maximum treatment duration of 4 days.

▸ **Neonate 32 weeks corrected gestational age and above:** 60 micrograms/kg/hour, adjusted according to response for maximum treatment duration of 4 days.

▸ **Child 1–5 months:** 60 micrograms/kg/hour, adjusted according to response

● **UNLICENSED USE** Oromucosal solution not licensed for use in children under 3 months. Unlicensed oromucosal formulations are also available and may have different doses—refer to product literature.

Injection not licensed for use in status epilepticus or febrile convulsions.

Not licensed for use in children under 6 months for premedication and conscious sedation. Not licensed for use by buccal administration for conscious sedation.

Not licensed for use by mouth.

IMPORTANT SAFETY INFORMATION

ANAESTHESIA

Benzodiazepines should only be administered for anaesthesia by, or under the direct supervision of, personnel experienced in their use, with adequate training in anaesthesia and airway management.

PRESCRIBING OF MIDAZOLAM IN PALLIATIVE CARE

The use of high-strength midazolam (5 mg/mL in 2 mL and 10 mL ampoules, or 2 mg/mL in 5 mL ampoules) should be considered in palliative care and other situations where a higher strength may be more appropriate to administer the prescribed dose, and where the risk of overdosage has been assessed. It is advised that flumazenil is available when midazolam is used, to reverse the effects if necessary.

● **CONTRA-INDICATIONS** CNS depression · compromised airway · severe respiratory depression

● **CAUTIONS** Cardiac disease · children (particularly if cardiovascular impairment) · concentration of midazolam in children under 15 kg not to exceed 1 mg/mL · debilitated patients (reduce dose) · hypothermia · hypovolaemia (risk of severe hypotension) · neonates · risk of airways obstruction and hypoventilation in children under 6 months (monitor respiratory rate and oxygen saturation) · vasoconstriction

CAUTIONS, FURTHER INFORMATION

▸ **Recovery when used for sedation** Midazolam has a fast onset of action, recovery is faster than for other benzodiazepines such as diazepam, but may be significantly longer in patients with a low cardiac output, or after repeated dosing.

● **SIDE-EFFECTS** Amnesia · anaphylaxis · ataxia · blood disorders · bronchospasm · cardiac arrest · confusion · convulsions (more common in neonates) · depression of consciousness · dizziness · drowsiness · dry mouth · dysarthria · euphoria · fatigue · gastro-intestinal disturbances · hallucinations · headache · heart rate changes · hiccups · hypotension · incontinence · increased appetite · injection-site reactions · involuntary movements · jaundice · laryngospasm · muscle weakness · paradoxical aggression · paradoxical excitement · respiratory arrest (particularly with high doses or on rapid injection) · respiratory depression (may be severe with sedative and peri-operative use—facilities for its treatment are essential) · respiratory depression (particularly with high doses or on rapid injection) · restlessness (with sedative and peri-operative use) · salivation changes · severe disinhibition (with sedative and peri-operative use) · skin reactions · thrombosis · urinary retention · vertigo · visual disturbances

SIDE-EFFECTS, FURTHER INFORMATION

▸ **Sedation** Midazolam is associated with profound sedation when high doses are given or when it is used with certain other drugs. Midazolam is not recommended for prolonged sedation in neonates; drug accumulation is likely to occur.

Overdose

There have been reports of overdosage when high strength midazolam has been used for conscious sedation. The use of high-strength midazolam (5 mg/mL in 2 mL and 10 mL ampoules, or 2 mg/mL in 5 mL ampoules) should be restricted to general anaesthesia, intensive care, palliative care, or other situations where the risk has been assessed. It is advised that flumazenil is available when midazolam is used, to reverse the effects if necessary.

● **BREAST FEEDING** Small amount present in milk—avoid breast-feeding for 24 hours after administration (although amount probably too small to be harmful after single doses).

● **HEPATIC IMPAIRMENT** Use with caution particularly in sedative doses; can precipitate coma. For status epilepticus and febrile convulsions: use with caution in mild to moderate impairment; avoid in severe impairment.

● **RENAL IMPAIRMENT** Use with caution in chronic renal failure.

● **DIRECTIONS FOR ADMINISTRATION**

▸ **With intravenous use** For *intravenous infusion* (*Hypnovel®*), give continuously *in* Glucose 5% *or* Sodium chloride 0.9%. For *intravenous injection* in status epilepticus and febrile convulsions, dilute with Glucose 5% *or* Sodium Chloride 0.9%; rapid intravenous injection (less than 2 minutes) may cause seizure-like myoclonus in preterm neonate. For neonate and children under 15 kg dilute to a max. concentration of 1 mg/mL. *Neonatal intensive care*, dilute 15 mg/kg body-weight to a final volume of 50 mL with infusion fluid; an intravenous infusion rate of 0.1 mL/hour provides a dose of 30 micrograms/kg/hour.

▸ **With oral use** For administration *by mouth* for sedation and premedication, injection solution may be diluted with apple or black currant juice, chocolate sauce, or cola.

4

Nervous System

● PATIENT AND CARER ADVICE

Patients or carers should be given advice on how to administer midazolam oromucosal solution.

Patients given sedatives and analgesics during minor outpatient procedures should be very carefully warned about the risks of undertaking skilled tasks (e.g. driving) afterwards. For intravenous benzodiazepines the risk extends to **at least 24 hours** after administration. Responsible persons should be available to take patients home afterwards. The dangers of taking **alcohol** should be emphasised.

Medicines for Children leaflet: Midazolam for stopping seizures www.medicinesforchildren.org.uk/midazolam-for-stopping-seizures

● MEDICINAL FORMS

There can be variation in the licensing of different medicines containing the same drug. Forms available from special-order manufacturers include: tablet, oral suspension, oral solution, oromucosal solution, solution for injection, infusion, solution for infusion

Tablet

▸ Midazolam (Non-proprietary)
Midazolam maleate 7.5 mg Dormicum 7.5mg tablets |
30 tablet PoM no price available CD3
Midazolam maleate 15 mg Dormicum 15mg tablets |
30 tablet PoM no price available CD3

Oral solution

▸ Midazolam (Non-proprietary)
Midazolam (as Midazolam hydrochloride) 2 mg per
1 ml Midazolam 2mg/ml oral solution sugar free sugar-free |
118 ml PoM no price available CD3

Oromucosal solution

CAUTIONARY AND ADVISORY LABELS 2

▸ Buccolam (Shire Pharmaceuticals Ltd)
Midazolam (as Midazolam hydrochloride) 5 mg per
1 ml Buccolam 7.5mg/1.5ml oromucosal solution pre-filled oral
syringes | 4 unit dose PoM £89.00 CD3 sugar-free | 4 unit
dose PoM £89.00 DT price = £89.00 CD3
Buccolam 10mg/2ml oromucosal solution pre-filled oral syringes |
4 unit dose PoM £91.50 CD3 sugar-free | 4 unit dose PoM £91.50
DT price = £91.50 CD3
Buccolam 5mg/1ml oromucosal solution pre-filled oral syringes sugar-
free | 4 unit dose PoM £85.50 DT price = £85.50 CD3 | 4 unit
dose PoM £85.50 CD3
Buccolam 2.5mg/0.5ml oromucosal solution pre-filled oral syringes |
4 unit dose PoM £82.00 CD3 sugar-free | 4 unit dose PoM £82.00
DT price = £82.00 CD3

Solution for injection

▸ Midazolam (Non-proprietary)
Midazolam (as Midazolam hydrochloride) 1 mg per
1 ml Midazolam 5mg/5ml solution for injection ampoules |
10 ampoule PoM £6.00 CD3
Midazolam 2mg/2ml solution for injection ampoules |
10 ampoule PoM £5.00 CD3
Midazolam (as Midazolam hydrochloride) 2 mg per
1 ml Midazolam 10mg/5ml solution for injection ampoules |
10 ampoule PoM £9.80 CD3 | 10 ampoule PoM no price available
(Hospital only) CD3
Midazolam (as Midazolam hydrochloride) 5 mg per
1 ml Midazolam 50mg/10ml solution for injection ampoules |
10 ampoule PoM £78.00 CD3
Midazolam 10mg/2ml solution for injection ampoules |
10 ampoule PoM £7.97 DT price = £6.90 CD3
▸ Hypnovel (Roche Products Ltd)
Midazolam (as Midazolam hydrochloride) 5 mg per 1 ml Hypnovel
10mg/2ml solution for injection | 10 ampoule PoM £7.11
DT price = £6.90 CD3

Solution for infusion

▸ Midazolam (Non-proprietary)
Midazolam (as Midazolam hydrochloride) 1 mg per
1 ml Midazolam 50mg/50ml solution for infusion vials | 1 vial PoM
£9.56–£11.00 CD3
Midazolam (as Midazolam hydrochloride) 2 mg per
1 ml Midazolam 100mg/50ml solution for infusion vials | 1 vial PoM
£9.05–£12.50 CD3

2 Mental health disorders

2.1 Attention deficit hyperactivity disorder

Attention deficit hyperactivity disorder

Management

CNS stimulants should be prescribed for children with severe and persistent symptoms of *attention deficit hyperactivity disorder* (ADHD), when the diagnosis has been confirmed by a specialist; children with moderate symptoms of ADHD can be treated with CNS stimulants when psychological interventions have been unsuccessful or are unavailable. Prescribing of CNS stimulants may be continued by general practitioners, under a shared-care arrangement. Treatment of ADHD often needs to be continued into adolescence, and may need to be continued into adulthood.

Drug treatment of ADHD should be part of a comprehensive treatment programme. The choice of medication should take into consideration co-morbid conditions (such as tic disorders, Tourette syndrome, and epilepsy), the adverse effect profile, potential for drug misuse, tolerance and dependance; and preferences of the child and carers. Methylphenidate hydrochloride p. 213 and atomoxetine, below, are used for the management of ADHD; dexamfetamine sulfate p. 215 and lisdexamfetamine mesilate p. 216 are an alternative in children who do not respond to these drugs. Guanfacine p. 217, a non-stimulant alpha$_2$-adrenoceptor agonist, can be used in children for whom stimulants are not suitable, not tolerated, or ineffective. Therapeutic response to guanfacine should be evaluated every 3 months for the first year and then at least yearly, when prescribed for extended periods.

The need to continue drug treatment for ADHD should be reviewed at least annually. This may involve suspending treatment.

A tricyclic antidepressant such as imipramine hydrochloride p. 226 is sometimes used in the treatment of ADHD; it should not be prescribed concomitantly with a CNS stimulant.

CNS STIMULANTS 〉 CENTRALLY ACTING SYMPATHOMIMETICS

Atomoxetine

● INDICATIONS AND DOSE

Attention deficit hyperactivity disorder (initiated by a specialist)

▸ BY MOUTH

▸ Child 6–17 years (body-weight up to 70 kg): Initially 500 micrograms/kg daily for 7 days, dose is increased according to response; maintenance 1.2 mg/kg daily, total daily dose may be given either as a single dose in the morning or in 2 divided doses with last dose no later than early evening, high daily doses to be given under the direction of a specialist; maximum 1.8 mg/kg per day; maximum 120 mg per day

▸ Child 6–17 years (body-weight 70 kg and above): Initially 40 mg daily for 7 days, dose is increased according to response; maintenance 80 mg daily, total daily dose may be given either as a single dose in the morning or in 2 divided doses with last dose no later than early evening, high daily doses to be given under the direction of a specialist; maximum 120 mg per day

- **UNLICENSED USE** Doses above 100 mg daily not licensed. Atomoxetine doses in BNF may differ from those in product literature.
- **CONTRA-INDICATIONS** Phaeochromocytoma · severe cardiovascular disease · severe cerebrovascular disease
- **CAUTIONS** QT-interval prolongation · aggressive behaviour · cardiovascular disease · cerebrovascular disease · emotional lability · history of seizures · hostility · hypertension · mania · psychosis · structural cardiac abnormalities · susceptibility to angle-closure glaucoma · tachycardia
- **INTERACTIONS** → Appendix 1 (atomoxetine). Avoid concomitant use of drugs that prolong QT interval.
- **SIDE-EFFECTS**
  - **Common or very common** Abdominal pain · anorexia · anxiety · chills · constipation · depression · dermatitis · dizziness · drowsiness · dry mouth · dyspepsia · flatulence · flushing · headache · increased blood pressure · irritability · lethargy · malaise · mydriasis · nausea · palpitation · paraesthesia · prostatitis · rash · sexual dysfunction · sleep disturbances · sweating · tachycardia · taste disturbances · tremor · urinary dysfunction · vomiting
  - **Uncommon** Aggression · cold extremities · emotional lability · hostility · hypoaesthesia · menstrual disturbances · muscle spasms · pruritus · psychosis · QT-interval prolongation · suicidal ideation · syncope · tics
  - **Rare** Raynaud's phenomenon · seizures
  - **Very rare** Angle-closure glaucoma · hepatic disorders
- **PREGNANCY** Manufacturer advises avoid unless potential benefit outweighs risk.
- **BREAST FEEDING** Avoid-present in milk in *animal* studies.
- **HEPATIC IMPAIRMENT** Halve dose in moderate impairment. Quarter dose in severe impairment.
- **MONITORING REQUIREMENTS**
  - Monitor for appearance or worsening of anxiety, depression or tics.
  - Pulse, blood pressure, psychiatric symptoms, appetite, weight and height should be recorded at initiation of therapy, following each dose adjustment, and at least every 6 months thereafter.
- **PATIENT AND CARER ADVICE**
  Medicines for Children leaflet: Atomoxetine for attention deficit hyperactivity disorder (ADHD) www.medicinesforchildren.org.uk/atomoxetine-attention-deficit-hyperactivity-disorder-adhd

  Suicidal ideation Following reports of suicidal thoughts and behaviour, patients and their carers should be informed about the risk and told to report clinical worsening, suicidal thoughts or behaviour, irritability, agitation, or depression.

  Hepatic impairment Following rare reports of hepatic disorders, patients and carers should be advised of the risk and be told how to recognise symptoms; prompt medical attention should be sought in case of abdominal pain, unexplained nausea, malaise, darkening of the urine, or jaundice.
- **NATIONAL FUNDING/ACCESS DECISIONS**
  NICE technology appraisals (TAs)
  - Methylphenidate, atomoxetine and dexamfetamine for attention deficit hyperactivity disorder (ADHD) (March 2006) NICE TA98
  Atomoxetine is recommended, within its licensed indications, as an option for the management of ADHD in children and adolescents.
  www.nice.org.uk/TA98

- **MEDICINAL FORMS**
  There can be variation in the licensing of different medicines containing the same drug. Forms available from special-order manufacturers include: oral suspension, oral solution

Capsule
CAUTIONARY AND ADVISORY LABELS 3
- **Strattera** (Eli Lilly and Company Ltd)
  Atomoxetine (as Atomoxetine hydrochloride) 10 mg Strattera 10mg capsules | 7 capsule [PoM] £13.28 | 28 capsule [PoM] £53.09 DT price = £53.09
  Atomoxetine (as Atomoxetine hydrochloride) 18 mg Strattera 18mg capsules | 7 capsule [PoM] £13.28 | 28 capsule [PoM] £53.09 DT price = £53.09
  Atomoxetine (as Atomoxetine hydrochloride) 25 mg Strattera 25mg capsules | 7 capsule [PoM] £13.28 | 28 capsule [PoM] £53.09 DT price = £53.09
  Atomoxetine (as Atomoxetine hydrochloride) 40 mg Strattera 40mg capsules | 7 capsule [PoM] £13.28 | 28 capsule [PoM] £53.09 DT price = £53.09
  Atomoxetine (as Atomoxetine hydrochloride) 60 mg Strattera 60mg capsules | 28 capsule [PoM] £53.09 DT price = £53.09
  Atomoxetine (as Atomoxetine hydrochloride) 80 mg Strattera 80mg capsules | 28 capsule [PoM] £70.79 DT price = £70.79
  Atomoxetine (as Atomoxetine hydrochloride) 100 mg Strattera 100mg capsules | 28 capsule [PoM] £70.79 DT price = £70.79

Oral solution
CAUTIONARY AND ADVISORY LABELS 3
- **Strattera** (Eli Lilly and Company Ltd)
  Atomoxetine (as Atomoxetine hydrochloride) 4 mg per 1 ml Strattera 4mg/1ml oral solution sugar-free | 300 ml [PoM] £85.00 DT price = £85.00

Methylphenidate hydrochloride

- **INDICATIONS AND DOSE**
  Attention deficit hyperactivity disorder (initiated under specialist supervision)
  - BY MOUTH USING IMMEDIATE-RELEASE MEDICINES
  - Child 4–5 years: Initially 2.5 mg twice daily, increased in steps of 2.5 mg daily if required, at weekly intervals, increased if necessary up to 1.4 mg/kg daily in 2–3 divided doses, discontinue if no response after 1 month, if effect wears off in evening (with rebound hyperactivity) a dose at bedtime may be appropriate (establish need with trial bedtime dose). Treatment may be started using a modified-release preparation
  - Child 6–17 years: Initially 5 mg 1–2 times a day, increased in steps of 5–10 mg daily if required, at weekly intervals, increased if necessary up to 60 mg daily in 2–3 divided doses, increased if necessary up to 2.1 mg/kg daily in 2–3 divided doses, the licensed maximum dose is 60 mg daily in 2–3 doses, higher dose (up to a maximum of 90 mg daily) under the direction of a specialist, discontinue if no response after 1 month, if effect wears off in evening (with rebound hyperactivity) a dose at bedtime may be appropriate (establish need with trial bedtime dose). Treatment may be started using a modified-release preparation

CONCERTA® XL

Attention deficit hyperactivity disorder
- BY MOUTH
- Child 6–17 years: Initially 18 mg once daily, dose to be taken in the morning, increased in steps of 18 mg every 1 week, adjusted according to response; increased if necessary up to 2.1 mg/kg daily, licensed max. dose is 54 mg once daily, to be increased to higher dose only under direction of specialist; discontinue if no response after 1 month; maximum 108 mg per day

DOSE EQUIVALENCE AND CONVERSION
Total daily dose of 15 mg of standard-release formulation is considered equivalent to *Concerta*® XL 18 mg once daily. continued →

EQUASYM® XL

Attention deficit hyperactivity disorder

▶ BY MOUTH

▶ **Child 6-17 years:** Initially 10 mg once daily, dose to be taken in the morning before breakfast; increased gradually at weekly intervals if necessary; increased if necessary up to 2.1 mg/kg daily, licensed max. dose is 60 mg daily, to be increased to higher dose only under direction of specialist; discontinue if no response after 1 month; maximum 90 mg per day

MEDIKINET® XL

Attention deficit hyperactivity disorder

▶ BY MOUTH

▶ **Child 6-17 years:** Initially 10 mg once daily, dose to be taken in the morning with breakfast; adjusted at weekly intervals according to response; increased if necessary up to 2.1 mg/kg daily, licensed max. dose is 60 mg daily, to be increased to higher dose only under direction of specialist; discontinue if no response after 1 month; maximum 90 mg per day

● **UNLICENSED USE** Doses over 60 mg daily not licensed; doses of *Concerta XL* over 54 mg daily not licensed. Not licensed for use in children under 6 years.

● **CONTRA-INDICATIONS** Anorexia nervosa · arrhythmias · cardiomyopathy · cardiovascular disease · cerebrovascular disorders · heart failure · hyperthyroidism · phaeochromocytoma · psychosis · severe depression · severe hypertension · structural cardiac abnormalities · suicidal ideation · uncontrolled bipolar disorder · vasculitis

● **CAUTIONS** Agitation · alcohol dependence · anxiety · drug dependence · epilepsy (discontinue if increased seizure frequency) · family history of Tourette syndrome · susceptibility to angle-closure glaucoma · tics

CONCERTA® XL Dysphagia (dose form not appropriate) · restricted gastro-intestinal lumen (dose form not appropriate)

● **INTERACTIONS** → Appendix 1 (sympathomimetics).

● **SIDE-EFFECTS**

▶ **Common or very common** Abdominal pain · aggression · alopecia · anorexia · arrhythmias · arthralgia · asthenia · changes in blood pressure · cough · depression · diarrhoea · dizziness · drowsiness · dry mouth · dyspepsia · fever · growth restriction · headache · insomnia · irritability · movement disorders · nasopharyngitis · nausea · nervousness · palpitation · pruritus · rash · reduced weight gain · tachycardia · tics · vomiting

▶ **Uncommon** Abnormal dreams · confusion · constipation · dyspnoea · epistaxis · haematuria · muscle cramps · suicidal ideation · urinary frequency

▶ **Rare** Angina · sweating · visual disturbances;

▶ **Very rare** Angle-closure glaucoma · blood disorders · cerebral arteritis · dependence · erythema multiforme · exfoliative dermatitis · hepatic dysfunction · leucopenia · myocardial infarction · neuroleptic malignant syndrome · psychosis · seizures · thrombocytopenia · tolerance · Tourette syndrome

▶ **Frequency not known** Bradycardia · convulsions · supraventricular tachycardia

● **PREGNANCY** Limited experience—avoid unless potential benefit outweighs risk.

● **BREAST FEEDING** Limited information available—avoid.

● **MONITORING REQUIREMENTS**

▶ Monitor for psychiatric illness.

▶ Pulse, blood pressure, psychiatric symptoms, appetite, weight and height should be recorded at initiation of therapy, following each dose adjustment, and at least every 6 months thereafter.

● **TREATMENT CESSATION** Avoid abrupt withdrawal.

● **DIRECTIONS FOR ADMINISTRATION**

MEDIKINET® XL Contents of capsule can be sprinkled on a tablespoon of apple sauce or yoghurt (then swallowed immediately without chewing).

EQUASYM® XL Contents of capsule can be sprinkled on a tablespoon of apple sauce (then swallowed immediately without chewing).

● **PRESCRIBING AND DISPENSING INFORMATION** Different versions of modified-release preparations may not have the same clinical effect. To avoid confusion between these different formulations of methylphenidate, prescribers should specify the brand to be dispensed.

CONCERTA® XL Consists of an immediate-release component (22% of the dose) and a modified-release component (78% of the dose).

MEDIKINET® XL Consists of an immediate-release component (50% of the dose) and a modified-release component (50% of the dose).

EQUASYM® XL Consists of an immediate-release component (30% of the dose) and a modified-release component (70% of the dose).

● **PATIENT AND CARER ADVICE**

Driving and skilled tasks

Drugs and Driving Prescribers and other healthcare professionals should advise patients if treatment is likely to affect their ability to perform skilled tasks (e.g. driving). This applies especially to drugs with sedative effects; patients should be warned that these effects are increased by alcohol. General information about a patient's fitness to drive is available from the Driver and Vehicle Licensing Agency at www.dvla.gov.uk.

2015 legislation regarding driving whilst taking certain drugs, may also apply to methylphenidate, see *Drugs and driving* under Guidance on prescribing p. 1.

CONCERTA® XL Tablet membrane may pass through gastro-intestinal tract unchanged.

● **NATIONAL FUNDING/ACCESS DECISIONS**

NICE technology appraisals (TAs)

▶ **Methylphenidate, atomoxetine and dexamfetamine for attention deficit hyperactivity disorder (ADHD) (March 2006)** NICE TA98
Methylphenidate is recommended, within its licensed indications, as an option for the management of ADHD in children and adolescents.
www.nice.org.uk/TA98

● **MEDICINAL FORMS**
There can be variation in the licensing of different medicines containing the same drug. Forms available from special-order manufacturers include: oral suspension, oral solution

Tablet

▶ Methylphenidate hydrochloride (Non-proprietary)
Methylphenidate hydrochloride 5 mg Methylphenidate 5mg tablets | 30 tablet PoM £3.44 DT price = £3.03 CD2
Methylphenidate hydrochloride 10 mg Methylphenidate 10mg tablets | 30 tablet PoM £7.17 DT price = £5.49 CD2
Methylphenidate hydrochloride 20 mg Methylphenidate 20mg tablets | 30 tablet PoM £11.12 DT price = £10.92 CD2

▶ Medikinet (Flynn Pharma Ltd)
Methylphenidate hydrochloride 5 mg Medikinet 5mg tablets | 30 tablet PoM £3.03 DT price = £3.03 CD2
Methylphenidate hydrochloride 10 mg Medikinet 10mg tablets | 30 tablet PoM £5.49 DT price = £5.49 CD2
Methylphenidate hydrochloride 20 mg Medikinet 20mg tablets | 30 tablet PoM £10.92 DT price = £10.92 CD2

▶ Ritalin (Novartis Pharmaceuticals UK Ltd)
Methylphenidate hydrochloride 10 mg Ritalin 10mg tablets | 30 tablet PoM £6.68 DT price = £5.49 CD2

▶ Tranquilyn (Genesis Pharmaceuticals Ltd)
Methylphenidate hydrochloride 5 mg Tranquilyn 5mg tablets | 30 tablet PoM £3.03 DT price = £3.03 CD2
Methylphenidate hydrochloride 10 mg Tranquilyn 10mg tablets | 30 tablet PoM £5.49 DT price = £5.49 CD2

Methylphenidate hydrochloride 20 mg Tranquilyn 20mg tablets |
30 tablet [PoM] £10.92 DT price = £10.92 [CD2]

Modified-release tablet

CAUTIONARY AND ADVISORY LABELS 25
▸ Concerta XL (Janssen-Cilag Ltd)

Methylphenidate hydrochloride 18 mg Concerta XL 18mg tablets |
30 tablet [PoM] £31.19 DT price = £31.19 [CD2]
Methylphenidate hydrochloride 27 mg Concerta XL 27mg tablets |
30 tablet [PoM] £36.81 DT price = £36.81 [CD2]
Methylphenidate hydrochloride 36 mg Concerta XL 36mg tablets
| 30 tablet [PoM] £42.45 DT price = £42.45 [CD2]
Methylphenidate hydrochloride 54 mg Concerta XL 54mg tablets
| 30 tablet [PoM] £73.62 DT price = £60.48 [CD2]

Modified-release capsule

CAUTIONARY AND ADVISORY LABELS 25
▸ Equasym XL (Shire Pharmaceuticals Ltd)

Methylphenidate hydrochloride 10 mg Equasym XL 10mg capsules
| 30 capsule [PoM] £25.00 DT price = £25.00 [CD2]
Methylphenidate hydrochloride 20 mg Equasym XL 20mg capsules
| 30 capsule [PoM] £30.00 DT price = £30.00 [CD2]
Methylphenidate hydrochloride 30 mg Equasym XL 30mg capsules
| 30 capsule [PoM] £35.00 DT price = £35.00 [CD2]
▸ Medikinet XL (Flynn Pharma Ltd)

Methylphenidate hydrochloride 5 mg Medikinet XL 5mg capsules
| 30 capsule [PoM] £24.04 [CD2]
Methylphenidate hydrochloride 10 mg Medikinet XL 10mg
capsules | 30 capsule [PoM] £24.04 DT price = £25.00 [CD2]
Methylphenidate hydrochloride 20 mg Medikinet XL 20mg
capsules | 30 capsule [PoM] £28.86 DT price = £30.00 [CD2]
Methylphenidate hydrochloride 30 mg Medikinet XL 30mg
capsules | 30 capsule [PoM] £33.66 DT price = £35.00 [CD2]
Methylphenidate hydrochloride 40 mg Medikinet XL 40mg
capsules | 30 capsule [PoM] £57.72 DT price = £57.72 [CD2]
Methylphenidate hydrochloride 50 mg Medikinet XL 50mg
capsules | 30 capsule [PoM] £62.52 [CD2]
Methylphenidate hydrochloride 60 mg Medikinet XL 60mg
capsules | 30 capsule [PoM] £67.32 [CD2]

CNS STIMULANTS ⟩ CENTRALLY ACTING SYMPATHOMIMETICS ⟩ AMFETAMINES

Dexamfetamine sulfate

(Dexamphetamine sulfate)

● **INDICATIONS AND DOSE**

Refractory attention deficit hyperactivity disorder (initiated under specialist supervision)
▸ BY MOUTH
▸ Child 6–17 years: Initially 2.5 mg 2–3 times a day,
  increased in steps of 5 mg once weekly if required,
  increased if necessary up to 1 mg/kg daily,
  maintenance dose to be given in 2–4 divided doses, up
  to 20 mg daily (40 mg daily has been required in some
  children)

● **CONTRA-INDICATIONS** Agitated states · cardiovascular
disease · history of alcohol abuse · history of drug abuse ·
hyperexcitability · hyperthyroidism · moderate
hypertension · severe hypertension · structural cardiac
abnormalities

● **CAUTIONS** Anorexia · bipolar disorder · history of epilepsy
(discontinue if seizures occur) · mild hypertension ·
psychosis · susceptibility to angle-closure glaucoma · tics ·
Tourette syndrome

CAUTIONS, FURTHER INFORMATION
▸ Tics and Tourette syndrome Discontinue use if tics occur.
▸ Growth restriction in children Monitor height and weight as
growth restriction may occur during prolonged therapy
(drug-free periods may allow catch-up in growth but
withdraw slowly to avoid inducing depression or renewed
hyperactivity).

● **INTERACTIONS** → Appendix 1 (sympathomimetics).

● **SIDE-EFFECTS**
▸ **Common or very common** Abdominal cramps · acidosis ·
aggression · alopecia · anhedonia · anorexia · anxiety ·
ataxia · cardiomyopathy · cardiovascular collapse · cerebral
vasculitis · chest pain · confusion · depression · diarrhoea ·
dizziness · dry mouth · dysphoria · euphoria · growth
restriction in children · headache · hyperactivity ·
hyperpyrexia · hyperreflexia · hypertension · hypotension ·
impaired concentration · irritability · ischaemic colitis ·
malaise · mydriasis · myocardial infarction · nausea ·
nervousness · neuroleptic malignant syndrome · obsessive-
compulsive behaviour · palpitations · panic attack ·
paranoia · psychosis · rash · renal impairment · restlessness
· rhabdomyolysis · seizures · sexual dysfunction · sleep
disturbances · stroke · sweating · tachycardia · taste
disturbance · Tourette syndrome (in predisposed
individuals) · tremor · urticaria · visual disturbances ·
weight loss
▸ **Very rare** Angle-closure glaucoma
▸ **Frequency not known** Choreoathetoid movements (in
predisposed individuals) · dyskinesia (in predisposed
individuals) · increased appetite · tics (in predisposed
individuals)

Overdose
Amfetamines cause wakefulness, excessive activity,
paranoia, hallucinations, and hypertension followed by
exhaustion, convulsions, hyperthermia, and coma. See
Stimulants under Emergency treatment of poisoning
p. 786.

● **PREGNANCY** Avoid (retrospective evidence of uncertain
significance suggesting possible embryotoxicity).

● **BREAST FEEDING** Significant amount in milk—avoid.

● **RENAL IMPAIRMENT** Use with caution.

● **MONITORING REQUIREMENTS**
▸ Monitor growth in children.
▸ Monitor for aggressive behaviour or hostility during initial
treatment.
▸ Pulse, blood pressure, psychiatric symptoms, appetite,
weight and height should be recorded at initiation of
therapy, following each dose adjustment, and at least
every 6 months thereafter.

● **TREATMENT CESSATION** Avoid abrupt withdrawal.

● **DIRECTIONS FOR ADMINISTRATION**
▸ With oral use Tablets can be halved.

● **PRESCRIBING AND DISPENSING INFORMATION** Data on
safety and efficacy of long-term use not complete.

● **PATIENT AND CARER ADVICE**

Driving and skilled tasks
Drugs and Driving Prescribers and other healthcare
professionals should advise patients if treatment is likely
to affect their ability to perform skilled tasks (e.g. driving).
This applies especially to drugs with sedative effects;
patients should be warned that these effects are increased
by alcohol. General information about a patient's fitness to
drive is available from the Driver and Vehicle Licensing
Agency at www.dvla.gov.uk.

For information on 2015 legislation regarding driving
whilst taking certain controlled drugs, including
amfetamines, see *Drugs and driving* under Guidance on
prescribing p. 1.

● **NATIONAL FUNDING/ACCESS DECISIONS**

NICE technology appraisals (TAs)
▸ Methylphenidate, atomoxetine and dexamfetamine for
attention deficit hyperactivity disorder (ADHD) (March 2006)
NICE TA98
Dexamfetamine is recommended, within its licensed
indications, as an option for the management of ADHD in
children and adolescents.
www.nice.org.uk/TA98

● **MEDICINAL FORMS**
There can be variation in the licensing of different medicines containing the same drug. Forms available from special-order manufacturers include: oral suspension, oral solution

Tablet
▸ **Dexamfetamine sulfate (Non-proprietary)**
Dexamfetamine sulfate 5 mg Dexamfetamine 5mg tablets |
28 tablet [PoM] £24.75 DT price = £24.75 [CD2]
▸ **Amfexa** (Flynn Pharma Ltd)
Dexamfetamine sulfate 5 mg Amfexa 5mg tablets | 30 tablet [PoM]
£19.89 [CD2]

Oral solution
▸ **Dexamfetamine sulfate (Non-proprietary)**
Dexamfetamine sulfate 1 mg per 1 ml Dexamfetamine 5mg/5ml
oral solution sugar free sugar-free | 150 ml [PoM] £29.44–£34.35 [CD2]
sugar-free | 500 ml [PoM] £114.49 DT price = £114.49 [CD2]

Lisdexamfetamine mesilate

● **DRUG ACTION** Lisdexamfetamine is a prodrug of dexamfetamine.

● **INDICATIONS AND DOSE**

Attention deficit hyperactivity disorder refractory to methylphenidate (initiated by a specialist)
▸ BY MOUTH
▸ **Child 6–17 years:** Initially 30 mg once daily, increased in steps of 20 mg every 1 week if required, dose to be taken in the morning, discontinue if response insufficient after 1 month; maximum 70 mg per day

● **CONTRA-INDICATIONS** Advanced arteriosclerosis · agitated states · hyperexcitability · hyperthyroidism · moderate hypertension · severe hypertension · symptomatic cardiovascular disease
● **CAUTIONS** Anorexia · bipolar disorder · history of alcohol abuse · history of cardiac abnormalities · history of cardiovascular disease · history of drug abuse · may lower seizure threshold (discontinue if seizures occur) · psychosis · susceptibility to angle-closure glaucoma · tics · Tourette syndrome
CAUTIONS, FURTHER INFORMATION
▸ **Tics and Tourette syndrome** Discontinue use if tics occur.
▸ **Growth restriction in children** Monitor height and weight as growth restriction may occur during prolonged therapy (drug-free periods may allow catch-up in growth but withdraw slowly to avoid inducing depression or renewed hyperactivity).
● **INTERACTIONS** → Appendix 1 (sympathomimetics).
● **SIDE-EFFECTS**
▸ **Common or very common** Abdominal cramps · aggression · decreased appetite · diarrhoea · dizziness · drowsiness · dry mouth · dyspnoea · growth restriction in children · headache · labile mood · malaise · mydriasis · nausea · pyrexia · sleep disturbances · tics · vomiting · weight loss
▸ **Uncommon** Anorexia · anxiety · depression · dermatillomania · dysphoria · hallucination · hypertension · logorrhoea · mania · palpitation · paranoia · rash · restlessness · sexual dysfunction · sweating · tachycardia · tremor · visual disturbances
▸ **Very rare** Angle-closure glaucoma
▸ **Frequency not known** Cardiomyopathy · choreoathetoid movements (in predisposed individuals) · dyskinesia (in predisposed individuals) · euphoria · seizures · Tourette syndrome (in predisposed individuals)
Overdose
Amfetamines cause wakefulness, excessive activity, paranoia, hallucinations, and hypertension followed by exhaustion, convulsions, hyperthermia, and coma. See Stimulants under Emergency treatment of poisoning p. 786.

● **PREGNANCY** Manufacturer advises use only if potential benefit outweighs risk.
● **BREAST FEEDING** Manufacturer advises avoid—present in human milk.
● **RENAL IMPAIRMENT** Max. dose 50 mg daily in severe impairment.
● **MONITORING REQUIREMENTS**
▸ Monitor for aggressive behaviour or hostility during initial treatment.
▸ Monitor growth in children.
▸ Pulse, blood pressure, psychiatric symptoms, appetite, weight and height should be recorded at initiation of therapy, following each dose adjustment, and at least every 6 months thereafter.
● **TREATMENT CESSATION** Avoid abrupt withdrawal.
● **DIRECTIONS FOR ADMINISTRATION** Swallow whole or mix contents of capsule in yoghurt or a glass of water or orange juice; contents should be dispersed completely and consumed immediately.
● **PATIENT AND CARER ADVICE**
Patients and carers should be counselled on the administration of capsules.
Driving and skilled tasks
Drugs and Driving Prescribers and other healthcare professionals should advise patients if treatment is likely to affect their ability to perform skilled tasks (e.g. driving). This applies especially to drugs with sedative effects; patients should be warned that these effects are increased by alcohol. General information about a patient's fitness to drive is available from the Driver and Vehicle Licensing Agency at www.dvla.gov.uk.
For information on 2015 legislation regarding driving whilst taking certain controlled drugs, including amfetamines, see *Drugs and driving* under Guidance on prescribing p. 1.

● **MEDICINAL FORMS**
There can be variation in the licensing of different medicines containing the same drug.
Capsule
CAUTIONARY AND ADVISORY LABELS 3, 25
▸ **Elvanse** (Shire Pharmaceuticals Ltd) ▼
Lisdexamfetamine dimesylate 20 mg Elvanse 20mg capsules |
28 capsule [PoM] £54.62 [CD2]
Lisdexamfetamine dimesylate 30 mg Elvanse Adult 30mg capsules
| 28 capsule [PoM] £58.24 DT price = £58.24 [CD2]
Elvanse 30mg capsules | 28 capsule [PoM] £58.24 DT price =
£58.24 [CD2]
Lisdexamfetamine dimesylate 40 mg Elvanse 40mg capsules |
28 capsule [PoM] £62.82 [CD2]
Lisdexamfetamine dimesylate 50 mg Elvanse Adult 50mg capsules
| 28 capsule [PoM] £68.60 DT price = £68.60 [CD2]
Elvanse 50mg capsules | 28 capsule [PoM] £68.60 DT price =
£68.60 [CD2]
Lisdexamfetamine dimesylate 60 mg Elvanse 60mg capsules |
28 capsule [PoM] £75.18 [CD2]
Lisdexamfetamine dimesylate 70 mg Elvanse 70mg capsules |
28 capsule [PoM] £83.16 DT price = £83.16 [CD2]
Elvanse Adult 70mg capsules | 28 capsule [PoM] £83.16 DT price =
£83.16 [CD2]

SYMPATHOMIMETICS ⟩ ALPHA$_2$-ADRENOCEPTOR AGONISTS

Guanfacine

26.5.2016

- **INDICATIONS AND DOSE**

Attention deficit hyperactivity disorder in children for whom stimulants are not suitable, not tolerated or ineffective (initiated under specialist supervision)

▶ BY MOUTH

▶ Child 6–12 years (body-weight 25 kg and above): Initially 1 mg once daily; adjusted in steps of 1 mg every week if necessary and if tolerated; maintenance 0.05–0.12 mg/kg once daily (max. per dose 4 mg), for optimal weight-adjusted dose titrations, consult product literature

▶ Child 13–17 years (body-weight 34–41.4 kg): Initially 1 mg once daily; adjusted in steps of 1 mg every week if necessary and if tolerated; maintenance 0.05–0.12 mg/kg once daily (max. per dose 4 mg), for optimal weight-adjusted dose titrations, consult product literature

▶ Child 13–17 years (body-weight 41.5–49.4 kg): Initially 1 mg once daily; adjusted in steps of 1 mg every week if necessary and if tolerated; maintenance 0.05–0.12 mg/kg once daily (max. per dose 5 mg), for optimal weight-adjusted dose titrations, consult product literature

▶ Child 13–17 years (body-weight 49.5–58.4 kg): Initially 1 mg once daily; adjusted in steps of 1 mg every week if necessary and if tolerated; maintenance 0.05–0.12 mg/kg once daily (max. per dose 6 mg), for optimal weight-adjusted dose titrations, consult product literature

▶ Child 13–17 years (body-weight 58.5 kg and above): Initially 1 mg once daily; adjusted in steps of 1 mg every week if necessary and if tolerated; maintenance 0.05–0.12 mg/kg once daily (max. per dose 7 mg), for optimal weight-adjusted dose titrations, consult product literature

- **CAUTIONS** Bradycardia (risk of torsade de pointes) · heart block (risk of torsade de pointes) · history of cardiovascular disease · history of QT-interval prolongation · hypokalaemia (risk of torsade de pointes)

- **INTERACTIONS** → Appendix 1 (guanfacine). Caution with concomitant use of drugs that prolong QT-interval.

- **SIDE-EFFECTS**

▶ **Common or very common** Abdominal pain · anxiety · bradycardia · constipation · decreased appetite · depression · diarrhoea · dizziness · dry mouth · enuresis · headache · hypotension · irritability · malaise · mood lability · nausea · rash · sleep disturbance · somnolence · vomiting · weight increase

▶ **Uncommon** Agitation · chest pain · convulsion · dyspepsia · first-degree AV block · hallucination · pallor · pollakiuria · pruritus · sinus arrhythmia · syncope · tachycardia

▶ **Rare** Hypertension

▶ **Frequency not known** Suicidal ideation

SIDE-EFFECTS, FURTHER INFORMATION

▶ Somnolence and sedation Somnolence and sedation may occur, predominantly during the first 2-3 weeks of treatment and with dose increases; manufacturer advises to consider dose reduction or discontinuation of treatment if symptoms are clinically significant or persistent.

Overdose

Features may include hypotension, initial hypertension, bradycardia, lethargy, and respiratory depression. Manufacturer advises that patients who develop lethargy should be observed for development of more serious toxicity for up to 24 hours.

- **CONCEPTION AND CONTRACEPTION** Manufacturer recommends effective contraception in females of childbearing potential.

- **PREGNANCY** Manufacturer advises avoid—toxicity in *animal* studies.

- **BREAST FEEDING** Manufacturer advises avoid—present in milk in *animal* studies.

- **HEPATIC IMPAIRMENT** Manufacturer advises consider dose reduction.

- **RENAL IMPAIRMENT** Manufacturer advises consider dose reduction in severe impairment and end-stage renal disease.

- **MONITORING REQUIREMENTS**

▶ Manufacturer advises to conduct a baseline evaluation to identify patients at risk of somnolence, sedation, hypotension, bradycardia, QT-prolongation, and arrhythmia; this should include assessment of cardiovascular status. Monitor for signs of these adverse effects weekly during dose titration and then every 3 months during the first year of treatment, and every 6 months thereafter. Monitor BMI prior to treatment and then every 3 months for the first year of treatment, and every 6 months thereafter. More frequent monitoring is advised following dose adjustments.

▶ Monitor blood pressure and pulse during dose downward titration and following discontinuation of treatment.

- **TREATMENT CESSATION** Manufacturer advises avoid abrupt withdrawal; consider dose tapering to minimise potential withdrawal effects.

- **DIRECTIONS FOR ADMINISTRATION** Manufacturer advises avoid administration with high fat meals (may increase absorption).

- **PATIENT AND CARER ADVICE**
Patients or carers should be counselled on administration of guanfacine modified-release tablets.

Missed doses

Manufacturer advises that patients and carers should inform their prescriber if more than one dose is missed; consider dose re-titration.

Driving and skilled tasks

Manufacturer advises patients and carers should be counselled about the effects on driving and performance of skilled tasks—increased risk of dizziness and syncope.

- **MEDICINAL FORMS**
There can be variation in the licensing of different medicines containing the same drug.

Modified-release tablet

CAUTIONARY AND ADVISORY LABELS 25, 2

▶ Intuniv (Shire Pharmaceuticals Ltd) ▼

Guanfacine (as Guanfacine hydrochloride) 1 mg Intuniv 1mg modified-release tablets | 28 tablet [PoM] £56.00

Guanfacine (as Guanfacine hydrochloride) 2 mg Intuniv 2mg modified-release tablets | 28 tablet [PoM] £58.52

Guanfacine (as Guanfacine hydrochloride) 3 mg Intuniv 3mg modified-release tablets | 28 tablet [PoM] £65.52

Guanfacine (as Guanfacine hydrochloride) 4 mg Intuniv 4mg modified-release tablets | 28 tablet [PoM] £76.16

2.2 Bipolar disorder and mania

Drugs for mania and hypomania

Antimanic drugs are used to control acute attacks and to prevent recurrence of episodes of mania or hypomania. Long-term treatment of bipolar disorder should continue for at least two years from the last manic episode and up to five years if the patient has risk factors for relapse.

An antidepressant drug may also be required for the treatment of co-existing depression, but should be avoided in patients with rapid-cycling bipolar disorder, a recent history of hypomania, or with rapid mood fluctuations.

Benzodiazepines
Use of benzodiazepines may be helpful in the initial stages of treatment for behavioural disturbance or agitation; they should not be used for long periods because of the risk of dependence.

Antipsychotic drugs
Antipsychotic drugs (normally olanzapine p. 236, quetiapine p. 238, or risperidone p. 239) are useful in acute episodes of mania and hypomania; if the response to antipsychotic drugs is inadequate, lithium or valproate may be added. An antipsychotic drug may be used concomitantly with lithium or valproate in the initial treatment of severe acute mania.

Atypical antipsychotics are the treatment of choice for the long-term management of bipolar disorder in children and adolescents; if the patient has frequent relapses or continuing functional impairment, consider concomitant therapy with lithium or valproate. An atypical antipsychotic that causes less weight gain and does not increase prolactin levels is preferred.

When discontinuing antipsychotics, the dose should be reduced gradually over at least 4 weeks if the child is continuing on other antimanic drugs; if the child is not continuing on other antimanic drugs, or has a history of manic relapse, a withdrawal period of up to 3 months is required.

Carbamazepine
Carbamazepine p. 184 may be used under specialist supervision for the prophylaxis of bipolar disorder (manic-depressive disorder) in children unresponsive to a combination of other prophylactic drugs; it is used in patients with rapid-cycling manic-depressive illness (4 or more affective episodes per year). The dose of carbamazepine should not normally be increased if an acute episode of mania occurs.

Valproate
Valproic acid (as the semisodium salt) is licensed in adults for the treatment of manic episodes associated with bipolar disorder. Sodium valproate is unlicensed for the treatment of bipolar disorder. Valproate (valproic acid and sodium valproate) can also be used for the prophylaxis of bipolar disorder [unlicensed use]. It must be started and supervised by a specialist experienced in managing bipolar disorder.

Valproate (valproic acid and sodium valproate) should not be used in female children, in females of childbearing potential and pregnant females, unless alternative treatments are ineffective or not tolerated, because of its high teratogenic potential; the benefits and risks of valproate therapy should be carefully reconsidered at regular treatment reviews. In patients with frequent relapse or continuing functional impairment, consider switching therapy to lithium or an atypical antipsychotic, or adding lithium or an atypical antipsychotic to valproate. If a patient taking valproate experiences an acute episode of mania that is not ameliorated by increasing the valproate dose, consider concomitant therapy with olanzapine, quetiapine, or risperidone.

Lithium
Lithium salts are used in the prophylaxis and treatment of mania, in the prophylaxis of bipolar disorder (manic-depressive disorder), and bipolar depression, and as concomitant therapy with antidepressant medication in children who have had an incomplete response to treatment for acute depression in bipolar disorder [unlicensed

indication]. It is also used for the treatment of aggressive or self-harming behaviour [unlicensed indication].

The decision to give prophylactic lithium requires specialist advice, and must be based on careful consideration of the likelihood of recurrence in the individual child, and the benefit of treatment weighed against the risks. The full prophylactic effect of lithium may not occur for six to twelve months after the initiation of therapy. An atypical antipsychotic or valproate (given alone or as adjunctive therapy with lithium) are alternative prophylactic treatments in patients who experience frequent relapses or continued functional impairment.

> **Drugs used for Bipolar disorder and mania not listed below** Aripiprazole, p. 234 · Perphenazine, p. 232

ANTIPSYCHOTICS > LITHIUM SALTS

Lithium salts

- **CONTRA-INDICATIONS** Addison's disease · cardiac insufficiency · dehydration · family history of Brugada syndrome · low sodium diets · personal history of Brugada syndrome · rhythm disorder · untreated hypothyroidism
- **CAUTIONS** Avoid abrupt withdrawal · cardiac disease · concurrent ECT (may lower seizure threshold) · diuretic treatment (risk of toxicity) · epilepsy (may lower seizure threshold) · myasthenia gravis · psoriasis (risk of exacerbation) · QT interval prolongation · review dose as necessary in diarrhoea · review dose as necessary in intercurrent infection (especially if sweating profusely) · review dose as necessary in vomiting · surgery

CAUTIONS, FURTHER INFORMATION
▸ Long-term use Long-term use of lithium has been associated with thyroid disorders and mild cognitive and memory impairment. Long-term treatment should therefore be undertaken only with careful assessment of risk and benefit, and with monitoring of thyroid function every 6 months (more often if there is evidence of deterioration).

The need for continued therapy should be assessed regularly and patients should be maintained on lithium after 3–5 years only if benefit persists.

- **INTERACTIONS** → Appendix 1 (lithium).
Caution with concomitant use of drugs and any therapy that may lower seizure threshold.
Caution with concomitant use of drugs that prolong the QT interval.
Lithium toxicity is made worse by sodium depletion, therefore concurrent use of diuretics (particularly thiazides) is hazardous and should be avoided.
- **SIDE-EFFECTS**
▸ **Very rare** Nystagmus
▸ **Frequency not known** Acneiform eruptions · alopecia · anorexia · arrhythmia · arthralgia · AV block · benign intracranial hypertension · bradycardia · cardiomyopathy · cognitive impairment · dry mouth · dysgeusia · ECG changes · electrolyte imbalance · encephalopathy · euthyroid goitre · extrapyramidal side-effects · fine tremor · gastritis · gastro-intestinal disturbances · hallucinations · hyperparathyroidism · hypersalivation · hyperthyroidism · hypothyroidism · kidney changes · leucocytosis · malaise · memory loss · myalgia · myasthenia gravis · nephrogenic diabetes insipidus · nephrotic syndrome · oedema · other skin disorders · parathyroid adenoma · peripheral neuropathy · polydipsia · psoriasis exacerbation · QT interval prolongation · Raynaud's phenomena · renal impairment · sexual dysfunction · sinus node dysfunction · speech disorder · thyroid changes · vertigo · weight changes

Overdose
Signs of intoxication require withdrawal of treatment and include increasing gastro-intestinal disturbances (vomiting, diarrhoea), visual disturbances, polyuria, muscle weakness, fine tremor increasing to coarse tremor, CNS disturbances (confusion and drowsiness increasing to lack of coordination, restlessness, stupor); abnormal reflexes, myoclonus, incontinence, hypernatraemia. With severe overdosage seizures, cardiac arrhythmias (including sino-atrial block, bradycardia and first-degree heart block), blood pressure changes, circulatory failure, renal failure, coma and sudden death reported.

For details on the management of poisoning, see Lithium, under Emergency treatment of poisoning p. 786.

- **CONCEPTION AND CONTRACEPTION** Manufacturer advises effective contraception during treatment for women of child bearing potential.

- **PREGNANCY** Dose requirements increased during the second and third trimesters (but on delivery return abruptly to normal). Avoid if possible, particularly in the first trimester (risk of teratogenicity, including cardiac abnormalities).
  Close monitoring of serum-lithium concentration advised in pregnancy (risk of toxicity in neonate).

- **BREAST FEEDING** Present in milk and risk of toxicity in infant—avoid.

- **RENAL IMPAIRMENT** Caution in mild to moderate impairment. Avoid in severe impairment. In renal impairment monitor serum-lithium concentration closely and adjust dose accordingly.

- **MONITORING REQUIREMENTS**
  - Serum concentrations Lithium salts have a narrow therapeutic/toxic ratio and should therefore not be prescribed unless facilities for monitoring serum-lithium concentrations are available.
  Samples should be taken 12 hours after the dose to achieve a serum-lithium concentration of 0.4–1 mmol/litre (lower end of the range for maintenance therapy).
  A target serum-lithium concentration of 0.8–1 mmol/litre is recommended for acute episodes of mania, and for patients who have previously relapsed or have sub-syndromal symptoms. It is important to determine the optimum range for each individual patient.
  Routine serum-lithium monitoring should be performed weekly after initiation and after each dose change until concentrations are stable, then every 3 months thereafter. Additional serum-lithium measurements should be made if a patient develops significant intercurrent disease or if there is a significant change in a patient's sodium or fluid intake.
  - Renal function should be monitored at baseline and every 6 months thereafter (more often if there is evidence of deterioration or if the patient has other risk factors, such as starting ACE inhibitors, NSAIDs, or diuretics).
  - Assess cardiac and thyroid function before initiating, and thereafter every 6 months on stabilised regimens.

- **TREATMENT CESSATION** While there is no clear evidence of withdrawal or rebound psychosis, abrupt discontinuation of lithium increases the risk of relapse. If lithium is to be discontinued, the dose should be reduced gradually over a period of at least 4 weeks (preferably over a period of up to 3 months). Patients and their carers should be warned of the risk of relapse if lithium is discontinued abruptly. If lithium is stopped or is to be discontinued abruptly, consider changing therapy to an atypical antipsychotic or valproate.

- **PATIENT AND CARER ADVICE**
  Patients should be advised to report signs and symptoms of lithium toxicity, hypothyroidism, renal dysfunction (including polyuria and polydipsia), and benign intracranial hypertension (persistent headache and visual disturbance).
  Maintain adequate fluid intake and avoid dietary changes which reduce or increase sodium intake.
  Driving and skilled tasks May impair performance of skilled tasks (e.g. driving, operating machinery).
  Lithium treatment packs A lithium treatment pack should be given to patients on initiation of treatment with lithium. The pack consists of a patient information booklet, lithium alert card, and a record book for tracking serum-lithium concentration. Packs may be purchased from
  3M
  0845 610 1112
  nhsforms@mmm.uk.com

F 218

Lithium carbonate

- **INDICATIONS AND DOSE**

Treatment and prophylaxis of mania | Treatment and prophylaxis of bipolar disorder | Treatment and prophylaxis of recurrent depression | Treatment and prophylaxis of aggressive or self-harming behaviour
▸ BY MOUTH
- Child 12–17 years: Dose adjusted to achieve a serum-lithium concentration of 0.4–1 mmol/litre 12 hours after a dose on days 4–7 of treatment, then every week until dosage has remained constant for 4 weeks and every 3 months thereafter, doses are initially divided throughout the day, but once daily administration is preferred when serum-lithium concentration stabilised

CAMCOLIT® IMMEDIATE-RELEASE TABLET

Treatment of mania | Treatment of bipolar disorder | Treatment of recurrent depression | Treatment of aggressive or self-harming behaviour
▸ BY MOUTH
- Child 12-17 years: Initially 1–1.5 g daily, dose adjusted to achieve a serum-lithium concentration of 0.4–1 mmol/litre 12 hours after a dose on days 4–7 of treatment, then every week until dosage has remained constant for 4 weeks and every 3 months thereafter, doses are initially divided throughout the day, but once daily administration is preferred when serum-lithium concentration stabilised

Prophylaxis of mania | Prophylaxis of bipolar disorder | Prophylaxis of recurrent depression | Prophylaxis of aggressive or self-harming behaviour
▸ BY MOUTH
- Child 12-17 years: Initially 300–400 mg daily, dose adjusted to achieve a serum-lithium concentration of 0.4–1 mmol/litre 12 hours after a dose on days 4–7 of treatment, then every week until dosage has remained constant for 4 weeks and every 3 months thereafter, doses are initially divided throughout the day, but once daily administration is preferred when serum-lithium concentration stabilised

CAMCOLIT® MODIFIED-RELEASE TABLET

Treatment of mania | Treatment of bipolar disorder | Treatment of recurrent depression | Treatment of aggressive or self-harming behaviour
▸ BY MOUTH
- Child 12-17 years: Initially 1–1.5 g daily, dose adjusted to achieve a serum-lithium concentration of 0.4–1 mmol/litre 12 hours after a dose on days 4–7 of treatment, then every week until dosage has remained constant for 4 weeks and every 3 months thereafter, doses are initially divided throughout the day, but once daily administration is preferred when serum-lithium concentration stabilised continued →

4 Nervous system

☞ 218

Prophylaxis of mania | Prophylaxis of bipolar disorder | Prophylaxis of recurrent depression | Prophylaxis of aggressive or self-harming behaviour

▸ BY MOUTH
▸ Child 12-17 years: Initially 300–400 mg daily, dose adjusted to achieve a serum-lithium concentration of 0.4–1 mmol/litre 12 hours after a dose on days 4–7 of treatment, then every week until dosage has remained constant for 4 weeks and every 3 months thereafter, doses are initially divided throughout the day, but once daily administration is preferred when serum-lithium concentration stabilised

LISKONUM®

Treatment of mania | Treatment of bipolar disorder | Treatment of recurrent depression | Treatment of aggressive or self-harming behaviour

▸ BY MOUTH
▸ Child 12-17 years: Initially 225–675 mg twice daily, dose adjusted to achieve a serum-lithium concentration of 0.4–1 mmol/litre 12 hours after a dose on days 4–7 of treatment, then every week until dosage has remained constant for 4 weeks and every 3 months thereafter, doses are initially divided throughout the day, but once daily administration is preferred when serum-lithium concentration stabilised

Prophylaxis of mania | Prophylaxis of bipolar disorder | Prophylaxis of recurrent depression | Prophylaxis of aggressive or self-harming behaviour

▸ BY MOUTH
▸ Child 12-17 years: Initially 225–450 mg twice daily, dose adjusted to achieve a serum-lithium concentration of 0.4–1 mmol/litre 12 hours after a dose on days 4–7 of treatment, then every week until dosage has remained constant for 4 weeks and every 3 months thereafter, doses are initially divided throughout the day, but once daily administration is preferred when serum-lithium concentration stabilised

DOSE EQUIVALENCE AND CONVERSION

Preparations vary widely in bioavailability; changing the preparation requires the same precautions as initiation of treatment.

● UNLICENSED USE Not licensed for aggressive or self-harming behaviour. Not licensed for concomitant therapy with antidepressant medication in children who have had an incomplete response to treatment for acute depression in bipolar disorder.
Camcolit® brand not licensed for use in children.

● MEDICINAL FORMS
There can be variation in the licensing of different medicines containing the same drug. Forms available from special-order manufacturers include: oral suspension

Tablet
CAUTIONARY AND ADVISORY LABELS 10
▸ Lithium carbonate (Non-proprietary)
 Lithium carbonate 250 mg Lithium carbonate 250mg tablets | 100 tablet PoM £48.18 DT price = £48.18

Modified-release tablet
CAUTIONARY AND ADVISORY LABELS 10, 25
▸ Lithium carbonate (Non-proprietary)
 Lithium carbonate 400 mg Lithium carbonate 400mg modified-release tablets | 100 tablet PoM no price available DT price = £4.02
▸ Camcolit (Essential Pharma Ltd)
 Lithium carbonate 400 mg Camcolit 400 modified-release tablets | 100 tablet PoM £48.18 DT price = £4.02
▸ Liskonum (GlaxoSmithKline UK Ltd)
 Lithium carbonate 450 mg Liskonum 450mg modified-release tablets | 60 tablet PoM £2.88 DT price = £2.88
▸ Priadel (lithium carbonate) (Sanofi)
 Lithium carbonate 200 mg Priadel 200mg modified-release tablets | 100 tablet PoM £2.76 DT price = £2.76
 Lithium carbonate 400 mg Priadel 400mg modified-release tablets | 100 tablet PoM £4.02 DT price = £4.02

Lithium citrate

○ INDICATIONS AND DOSE

Treatment and prophylaxis of mania | Treatment and prophylaxis of bipolar disorder | Treatment and prophylaxis of recurrent depression | Treatment and prophylaxis of aggressive or self-harming behaviour

▸ BY MOUTH
▸ Child: Dose adjusted to achieve a serum-lithium concentration of 0.4–1 mmol/litre 12 hours after a dose on days 4–7 of treatment, then every week until dosage has remained constant for 4 weeks and every 3 months thereafter; doses are initially divided throughout the day, but once daily administration is preferred when serum-lithium concentration stabilised

DOSE EQUIVALENCE AND CONVERSION

Preparations vary widely in bioavailability; changing the preparation requires the same precautions as initiation of treatment.

LI-LIQUID®

Treatment and prophylaxis of mania | Treatment and prophylaxis of bipolar disorder | Treatment and prophylaxis of recurrent depression | Treatment and prophylaxis of aggressive or self-harming behaviour

▸ BY MOUTH
▸ Child: Dose adjusted to achieve a serum-lithium concentration of 0.4–1 mmol/litre 12 hours after a dose on days 4–7 of treatment, then every week until dosage has remained constant for 4 weeks and every 3 months thereafter, doses are initially divided throughout the day, but once daily administration is preferred when serum-lithium concentration stabilised

DOSE EQUIVALENCE AND CONVERSION

For *Li-Liquid®*: Lithium citrate tetrahydrate 509 mg is equivalent to lithium carbonate 200 mg.
Preparations vary widely in bioavailability; changing the preparation requires the same precautions as initiation of treatment.

PRIADEL® LIQUID

Treatment and prophylaxis of mania | Treatment and prophylaxis of bipolar disorder | Treatment and prophylaxis of recurrent depression | Treatment and prophylaxis of aggressive or self-harming behaviour

▸ BY MOUTH
▸ Child: Dose adjusted to achieve a serum-lithium concentration of 0.4–1 mmol/litre 12 hours after a dose on days 4–7 of treatment, then every week until dosage has remained constant for 4 weeks and every 3 months thereafter, doses are initially divided throughout the day, but once daily administration is preferred when serum-lithium concentration stabilised

DOSE EQUIVALENCE AND CONVERSION

For *Priadel®* liquid: Lithium citrate tetrahydrate 520 mg is equivalent to lithium carbonate 204 mg.
Preparations vary widely in bioavailability; changing the preparation requires the same precautions as initiation of treatment.

● UNLICENSED USE Not licensed for use in children.

● MEDICINAL FORMS
There can be variation in the licensing of different medicines containing the same drug.

Oral solution
CAUTIONARY AND ADVISORY LABELS 10
▸ Lithium citrate (Non-proprietary)
 Lithium citrate 101.8 mg per 1 ml Lithium citrate 509mg/5ml oral solution | 150 ml PoM no price available
 Lithium citrate 104 mg per 1 ml Lithium citrate 520mg/5ml oral solution sugar free sugar-free | 150 ml PoM no price available

Lithium citrate 203.6 mg per 1 ml Lithium citrate 1.018g/5ml oral
solution | 150 ml PoM no price available

▸ **Li-Liquid** (Rosemont Pharmaceuticals Ltd)
Lithium citrate 101.8 mg per 1 ml Li-Liquid 509mg/5ml oral
solution | 150 ml PoM £5.79
Lithium citrate 203.6 mg per 1 ml Li-Liquid 1.018g/5ml oral
solution | 150 ml PoM £11.58

▸ **Priadel (lithium citrate)** (Sanofi)
Lithium citrate 104 mg per 1 ml Priadel 520mg/5ml liquid sugar-
free | 150 ml PoM £6.73

2.3 Depression

Antidepressant drugs

Overview

Depression in children should be managed by an appropriate
specialist and treatment should involve psychological
therapy.

Choice

The major classes of antidepressant drugs include the
tricyclics and related antidepressant drugs, the selective
serotonin re-uptake inhibitors (SSRIs), and the monoamine
oxidase inhibitors (MAOIs).

Antidepressant drugs should not be used routinely in mild
depression, and psychological therapy should be considered
initially; however, a trial of antidepressant therapy may be
considered in cases refractory to psychological treatments or
in those associated with psychosocial or medical problems.
Drug treatment of mild depression may also be considered in
children with a history of moderate or severe depression.

Choice of antidepressant drug should be based on the
individual child's requirements, including the presence of
concomitant disease, existing therapy, suicide risk, and
previous response to antidepressant therapy.

When drug treatment of depression is considered
necessary in children, the SSRIs should be considered first-
line treatment; following a safety and efficacy review,
fluoxetine p. 223 is licensed to treat depression in children.

Tricyclic antidepressant drugs should be avoided for the
treatment of depression in children.

St John's wort (*Hypericum perforatum*) is a popular herbal
remedy on sale to the public for treating mild depression in
adults. It should not be used for the treatment of depression
in children because St John's wort can induce drug
metabolising enzymes and a number of important
interactions with conventional drugs, including
conventional antidepressants, have been identified.
Furthermore, the amount of active ingredient varies between
different preparations of St John's wort and switching from
one to another can change the degree of enzyme induction.
If a child stops taking St John's wort, the concentration of
interacting drugs may increase, leading to toxicity.

Management

Children should be reviewed every 1–2 weeks at the start of
antidepressant treatment. Treatment should be continued
for at least 4 weeks before considering whether to switch
antidepressant due to lack of efficacy. In cases of partial
response, continue for a further 2–4 weeks. Following
remission, antidepressant treatment should be continued at
the same dose for at least 6 months. Children with a history
of recurrent depression should continue treatment for at
least 2 years.

Hyponatraemia and antidepressant therapy

Hyponatraemia (possibly due to inappropriate secretion of
antidiuretic hormone) has been associated with all types of
antidepressants; however, it has been reported more
frequently with SSRIs than with other antidepressant drugs.
Hyponatraemia should be considered in all children who

develop drowsiness, confusion, or convulsions while taking
an antidepressant.

Suicidal behaviour and antidepressant therapy

The use of antidepressant drugs has been linked with
suicidal thoughts and behaviour. Where necessary, children
should be monitored for suicidal behaviour, self-harm, and
hostility, particularly at the beginning of treatment or if the
dose is changed.

Serotonin syndrome

Serotonin syndrome or serotonin toxicity is a relatively
uncommon adverse drug reaction caused by excessive
central and peripheral serotonergic activity. Onset of
symptoms, which range from mild to life-threatening, can
occur within hours or days following the initiation, dose
escalation, or overdose of a serotonergic drug, the addition
of a new serotonergic drug, or the replacement of one
serotonergic drug by another without allowing a long
enough washout period in-between, particularly when the
first drug is an irreversible MAOI or a drug with a long
halflife. Severe toxicity, which is a medical emergency,
usually occurs with a combination of serotonergic drugs, one
of which is generally an MAOI.

The characteristic symptoms of serotonin syndrome fall
into 3 main areas, although features from each group may
not be seen in all patients—neuromuscular hyperactivity
(such as tremor, hyperreflexia, clonus, myoclonus, rigidity),
autonomic dysfunction (tachycardia, blood pressure
changes, hyperthermia, diaphoresis, shivering, diarrhoea),
and altered mental state (agitation, confusion, mania).

Treatment consists of withdrawal of the serotonergic
medication and supportive care; specialist advice should be
sought.

**Important safety information: Depressive illness in children
and adolescents**

The balance of risks and benefits for the treatment of
depressive illness in individuals under 18 years is considered
unfavourable for the SSRIs citalopram, escitalopram,
paroxetine, and sertraline, and for mirtazapine and
venlafaxine. Clinical trials have failed to show efficacy and
have shown an increase in harmful outcomes. However, it is
recognised that specialists may sometimes decide to use
these drugs in response to individual clinical need; children
and adolescents should be monitored carefully for suicidal
behaviour, self-harm or hostility, particularly at the
beginning of treatment. Only fluoxetine has been shown in
clinical trials to be effective for treating depressive illness in
children and adolescents. However, it is possible that, in
common with the other SSRIs, it is associated with a small
risk of self-harm and suicidal thoughts. Overall, the balance
of risks and benefits for fluoxetine in the treatment of
depressive illness in individuals under 18 years is considered
favourable, but children and adolescents must be carefully
monitored as above.

Anxiety

Management of *acute anxiety* in children with drug treatment
is contentious. For *chronic anxiety* (of longer than 4 weeks'
duration), it may be appropriate to use an antidepressant
drug before a benzodiazepine.

Tricyclic antidepressants are not effective for treating
depression in children.

Some tricyclic antidepressant drugs may have a role in
some forms of *neuralgia*, and in *nocturnal enuresis* in
children.

Dosage

It is important to use doses that are sufficiently high for
effective treatment but not so high as to cause toxic effects.
Low doses should be used for initial treatment.

In most children the long half-life of tricyclic
antidepressant drugs allows **once-daily** administration,

usually at night; the use of modified-release preparations is therefore unnecessary.

> **Drugs used for Depression not listed below** Lithium carbonate, p. 219 · Lithium citrate, p. 220

ANTIDEPRESSANTS > SELECTIVE SEROTONIN RE-UPTAKE INHIBITORS

Selective serotonin re-uptake inhibitors

- **DRUG ACTION** Selectively inhibit the re-uptake of serotonin (5-hydroxytryptamine, 5-HT).
- **CONTRA-INDICATIONS** Poorly controlled epilepsy · SSRIs should not be used if the patient enters a manic phase.
- **CAUTIONS** Cardiac disease · concurrent electroconvulsive therapy · diabetes mellitus · epilepsy (discontinue if convulsions develop) · history of bleeding disorders (especially gastro-intestinal bleeding) · history of mania · susceptibility to angle-closure glaucoma
- **INTERACTIONS** → Appendix 1 (antidepressants, SSRI). Caution with other drugs that increase the risk of bleeding.
- **SIDE-EFFECTS**
- ▶ **Common or very common** Abdominal pain (dose-related) · constipation (dose-related) · diarrhoea (dose-related) · dyspepsia (dose-related) · gastro-intestinal effects (dose-related) · nausea (dose-related) · vomiting (dose-related)
- ▶ **Uncommon** Serotonin syndrome
- ▶ **Very rare** Angle-closure glaucoma
- ▶ **Frequency not known** Anaphylaxis · angioedema · anorexia with weight loss · anxiety · arthralgia · asthenia · bleeding disorders · convulsions · dizziness · drowsiness · dry mouth · dyskinesias · ecchymoses · galactorrhoea · hallucinations · headache · hypersensitivity reactions · hypomania · hyponatraemia · increased appetite · insomnia · mania · movement disorders · myalgia · nervousness · photosensitivity · purpura · rash · sexual dysfunction · suicidal behaviour · sweating · tremor · urinary retention · urticaria · visual disturbances · weight gain
  SIDE-EFFECTS, FURTHER INFORMATION
- ▶ **Hypersensitivity reactions** If hypersensitivity reactions (including rash) occur, consider discontinuation—may be sign of impending serious systemic reaction, possibly associated with vasculitis.

Overdose
Symptoms of poisoning by selective serotonin re-uptake inhibitors include nausea, vomiting, agitation, tremor, nystagmus, drowsiness, and sinus tachycardia; convulsions may occur. Rarely, severe poisoning results in the serotonin syndrome, with marked neuropsychiatric effects, neuromuscular hyperactivity, and autonomic instability; hyperthermia, rhabdomyolysis, renal failure, and coagulopathies may develop.

For details on the management of poisoning, see Selective serotonin re-uptake inhibitors, under Emergency treatment of poisoning p. 786.

- **PREGNANCY** Manufacturers advise avoid during pregnancy unless the potential benefit outweighs the risk. There is a small increased risk of congenital heart defects when taken during early pregnancy. If used during the third trimester there is a risk of neonatal withdrawal symptoms, and persistent pulmonary hypertension in the newborn has been reported.
- **TREATMENT CESSATION** Gastro-intestinal disturbances, headache, anxiety, dizziness, paraesthesia, electric shock sensation in the head, neck, and spine, tinnitus, sleep disturbances, fatigue, influenza-like symptoms, and sweating are the most common features of abrupt

withdrawal of an SSRI or marked reduction of the dose; palpitation and visual disturbances can occur less commonly. The dose should be tapered over at least a few weeks to avoid these effects. For some patients, it may be necessary to withdraw treatment over a longer period; consider obtaining specialist advice if symptoms persist.

Withdrawal effects may occur within 5 days of stopping treatment with antidepressant drugs; they are usually mild and self-limiting, but in some cases may be severe. The risk of withdrawal symptoms is increased if the antidepressant is stopped suddenly after regular administration for 8 weeks or more. The dose should preferably be reduced gradually over about 4 weeks, or longer if withdrawal symptoms emerge (6 months in patients who have been on long-term maintenance treatment).

- **PATIENT AND CARER ADVICE**
  Driving and skilled tasks
  May also impair performance of skilled tasks (e.g. driving, operating machinery).

> ◤ above

Citalopram

- **INDICATIONS AND DOSE**
  Major depression
  ▶ BY MOUTH USING TABLETS
  ▶ Child 12–17 years: Initially 10 mg once daily, increased if necessary to 20 mg once daily, dose to be increased over 2–4 weeks; maximum 40 mg per day
  ▶ BY MOUTH USING ORAL DROPS
  ▶ Child 12–17 years: Initially 8 mg once daily, increased if necessary to 16 mg once daily, dose to be increased over 2–4 weeks; maximum 32 mg per day

  DOSE EQUIVALENCE AND CONVERSION
  4 oral drops (8 mg) is equivalent in therapeutic effect to 10 mg tablet.

- **UNLICENSED USE** Not licensed for use in children.
- **CONTRA-INDICATIONS** QT-interval prolongation
- **CAUTIONS** Susceptibility to QT-interval prolongation
- **INTERACTIONS** Avoid concomitant administration of drugs that prolong QT interval.
- **SIDE-EFFECTS** Taste disturbance · abnormal dreams · aggression · amnesia · bradycardia · confusion · coughing · euphoria · haemorrhage · hepatitis · hypokalaemia · impaired concentration · increased salivation · malaise · micturition disorders · migraine · mydriasis · oedema · palpitation · paraesthesia · polyuria · postural hypotension · pruritus · QT-interval prolongation · rhinitis · tachycardia · tinnitus · yawning
- **BREAST FEEDING** Present in milk—use with caution.
- **HEPATIC IMPAIRMENT** Use doses at lower end of range; for *tablets* up to maximum 20 mg; for *oral solution* up to maximum 16 mg.
- **RENAL IMPAIRMENT** No information available for estimated glomerular filtration rate less than 20 mL/minute/1.73 m^2.
- **DIRECTIONS FOR ADMINISTRATION** *Cipramil*® oral drops should be mixed with water, orange juice, or apple juice before taking.
- **PATIENT AND CARER ADVICE**
  Counselling on administration of oral drops is advised.
  Driving and skilled tasks
  Patients should be advised of the effects of citalopram on driving and skilled tasks.

- **MEDICINAL FORMS**
There can be variation in the licensing of different medicines containing the same drug.

Tablet
▸ Citalopram (Non-proprietary)
Citalopram (as Citalopram hydrobromide) 10 mg Citalopram 10mg tablets | 28 tablet PoM £8.90 DT price = £0.77
Citalopram (as Citalopram hydrobromide) 20 mg Citalopram 20mg tablets | 28 tablet PoM £15.99 DT price = £0.82
Citalopram (as Citalopram hydrobromide) 40 mg Citalopram 40mg tablets | 28 tablet PoM £27.00 DT price = £0.96
▸ Cipramil (Lundbeck Ltd)
Citalopram (as Citalopram hydrobromide) 20 mg Cipramil 20mg tablets | 28 tablet PoM £8.95 DT price = £0.82

Oral drops
EXCIPIENTS: May contain Alcohol
▸ Citalopram (Non-proprietary)
Citalopram (as Citalopram hydrochloride) 40 mg per 1 ml Citalopram 40mg/ml oral drops sugar free sugar-free | 15 ml PoM £20.16 DT price = £5.17
▸ Cipramil (Lundbeck Ltd)
Citalopram (as Citalopram hydrochloride) 40 mg per 1 ml Cipramil 40mg/ml drops sugar-free | 15 ml PoM £10.08 DT price = £5.17

▶ 222

Fluoxetine

- **INDICATIONS AND DOSE**

Major depression
▸ BY MOUTH
▸ Child 8–17 years: Initially 10 mg daily, increased if necessary up to 20 mg daily, dose to be increased after 1–2 weeks of initial dose, daily dose may be administered as a single or divided dose

PHARMACOKINETICS
Consider the long half-life of fluoxetine when adjusting dosage (or in overdosage).

- **SIDE-EFFECTS** Alopecia · changes in blood sugar · chills · confusion · dysphagia · dyspnoea · euphoria · flushing · haemorrhage · hepatitis · hypotension · impaired concentration · malaise · neuroleptic malignant syndrome-like event · palpitation · pharyngitis · priapism · pulmonary fibrosis · pulmonary inflammation · sleep disturbances · taste disturbance · toxic epidermal necrolysis · urinary frequency · vasodilatation · yawning
- **BREAST FEEDING** Present in milk—avoid.
- **HEPATIC IMPAIRMENT** Reduce dose or increase dose interval.
- **DIRECTIONS FOR ADMINISTRATION** Dispersible tablets can be dispersed in water for administration or swallowed whole with plenty of water.
- **PATIENT AND CARER ADVICE**
Patients and carers should be counselled on the administration of dispersible tablets.

Driving and skilled tasks
Patients should be counselled about the effects on driving and skilled tasks.

Medicines for Children leaflet: Fluoxetine for depression, obsessive compulsive disorder and bulimia nervosa www.medicinesforchildren.org.uk/fluoxetine-depression-obsessive-compulsive-disorder-and-bulimia-nervosa

- **MEDICINAL FORMS**
There can be variation in the licensing of different medicines containing the same drug. Forms available from special-order manufacturers include: tablet, oral suspension, oral solution

Dispersible tablet
CAUTIONARY AND ADVISORY LABELS 10
▸ Olena (AMCo)
Fluoxetine (as Fluoxetine hydrochloride) 20 mg Olena 20mg dispersible tablets sugar-free | 28 tablet PoM £3.44 DT price = £3.44

Capsule
▸ Fluoxetine (Non-proprietary)
Fluoxetine (as Fluoxetine hydrochloride) 10 mg Fluoxetine 10mg capsules | 30 capsule PoM £55.00
Fluoxetine (as Fluoxetine hydrochloride) 20 mg Fluoxetine 20mg capsules | 30 capsule PoM £20.00 DT price = £0.92
Fluoxetine (as Fluoxetine hydrochloride) 60 mg Fluoxetine 60mg capsules | 30 capsule PoM £144.00 DT price = £11.26
▸ Oxactin (Discovery Pharmaceuticals)
Fluoxetine (as Fluoxetine hydrochloride) 20 mg Oxactin 20mg capsules | 30 capsule PoM £0.91 DT price = £0.92
▸ Prozac (Eli Lilly and Company Ltd)
Fluoxetine (as Fluoxetine hydrochloride) 20 mg Prozac 20mg capsules | 30 capsule PoM £1.50 DT price = £0.92

Oral solution
▸ Fluoxetine (Non-proprietary)
Fluoxetine (as Fluoxetine hydrochloride) 4 mg per 1 ml Fluoxetine 20mg/5ml oral solution | 70 ml PoM £12.75 DT price = £2.86
Fluoxetine 20mg/5ml oral solution sugar free sugar-free | 70 ml PoM £5.56
▸ Prozac (Eli Lilly and Company Ltd)
Fluoxetine (as Fluoxetine hydrochloride) 4 mg per 1 ml Prozac 20mg/5ml liquid | 70 ml PoM £11.12 DT price = £2.86
▸ Prozep (Chemidex Pharma Ltd)
Fluoxetine (as Fluoxetine hydrochloride) 4 mg per 1 ml Prozep 20mg/5ml oral solution sugar-free | 70 ml £12.95

▶ 222

Fluvoxamine maleate

- **INDICATIONS AND DOSE**

Obsessive-compulsive disorder
▸ BY MOUTH
▸ Child 8–17 years: Initially 25 mg daily, then increased in steps of 25 mg every 4–7 days (max. per dose 100 mg twice daily) if required, dose to be increased according to response, doses above 50 mg should be given in 2 divided doses, if no improvement in obsessive-compulsive disorder within 10 weeks, treatment should be reconsidered

- **SIDE-EFFECTS**
▸ **Common or very common** Malaise · palpitation · tachycardia
▸ **Uncommon** Ataxia · confusion · ppstural hypotension
▸ **Rare** Abnormal liver function, usually symptomatic (discontinue treatment)
▸ **Frequency not known** Neuroleptic malignant syndrome-like event · paraesthesia · taste disturbance
- **BREAST FEEDING** Present in milk—avoid.
- **HEPATIC IMPAIRMENT** Start with low dose.
- **RENAL IMPAIRMENT** Start with low dose.
- **PATIENT AND CARER ADVICE**

Driving and skilled tasks
Patients should be counselled about the effects on driving and skilled tasks.

- **MEDICINAL FORMS**
There can be variation in the licensing of different medicines containing the same drug. Forms available from special-order manufacturers include: oral suspension

Tablet
▸ Fluvoxamine maleate (Non-proprietary)
Fluvoxamine maleate 50 mg Fluvoxamine 50mg tablets | 60 tablet PoM £29.99 DT price = £25.57
Fluvoxamine maleate 100 mg Fluvoxamine 100mg tablets | 30 tablet PoM £29.99 DT price = £25.57
▸ Faverin (BGP Products Ltd)
Fluvoxamine maleate 50 mg Faverin 50mg tablets | 60 tablet PoM £17.10 DT price = £25.57
Fluvoxamine maleate 100 mg Faverin 100mg tablets | 30 tablet PoM £17.10 DT price = £25.57

4

Nervous system

F 222

Sertraline

- **INDICATIONS AND DOSE**

Obsessive-compulsive disorder
- BY MOUTH
  - Child 6–11 years: Initially 25 mg daily for 1 week, then increased to 50 mg daily, then increased in steps of 50 mg at intervals of at least 1 week if required; maximum 200 mg per day
  - Child 12–17 years: Initially 50 mg daily, then increased in steps of 50 mg at intervals of at least 1 week if required; maximum 200 mg per day

Major depression
- BY MOUTH
  - Child 12–17 years: Initially 50 mg once daily, then increased in steps of 50 mg at intervals of at least 1 week if required; maximum 200 mg per day

- **UNLICENSED USE** Not licensed for use in children for depression.
- **SIDE-EFFECTS** Aggression · amnesia · bronchospasm · hepatitis · hypercholesterolaemia · hyperprolactinaemia · hypertension · hypoglycaemia · hypothyroidism · jaundice · leucopenia · liver failure · menstrual irregularities · palpitation · pancreatitis · paraesthesia · postural hypotension · stomatitis · tachycardia · tinnitus · urinary incontinence
- **BREAST FEEDING** Not known to be harmful but consider discontinuing breast-feeding.
- **HEPATIC IMPAIRMENT** Reduce dose or increase dose interval in mild or moderate impairment. Avoid in severe impairment.
- **RENAL IMPAIRMENT** Use with caution.
- **PATIENT AND CARER ADVICE**

Driving and skilled tasks
Patients should be counselled on the effects on driving and skilled tasks.
Medicines for Children leaflet: Sertraline for OCD (obsessive compulsive disorder) and depression www.medicinesforchildren. org.uk/sertraline-for-ocd-obsessive-compulsive-disorder-and-depression

- **MEDICINAL FORMS**
There can be variation in the licensing of different medicines containing the same drug. Forms available from special-order manufacturers include: oral suspension

Tablet
- Sertraline (Non-proprietary)
  Sertraline (as Sertraline hydrochloride) 50 mg   Sertraline 50mg tablets | 28 tablet [PoM]   £19.25 DT price = £1.28
  Sertraline (as Sertraline hydrochloride) 100 mg   Sertraline 100mg tablets | 28 tablet [PoM]   £29.09 DT price = £1.39
- Lustral (Pfizer Ltd)
  Sertraline (as Sertraline hydrochloride) 50 mg   Lustral 50mg tablets | 28 tablet [PoM]   £17.82 DT price = £1.28
  Sertraline (as Sertraline hydrochloride) 100 mg   Lustral 100mg tablets | 28 tablet [PoM]   £29.16 DT price = £1.39

ANTIDEPRESSANTS › TRICYCLIC ANTIDEPRESSANTS

Amitriptyline hydrochloride

- **INDICATIONS AND DOSE**

Depressive illness (but not recommended)
- BY MOUTH
  - Child 16–17 years: Initially 10–25 mg 3 times a day, alternatively initially 30–75 mg once daily, dose to be taken at bedtime, increased if necessary to 150–200 mg daily, dose to be increased gradually

Neuropathic pain
- BY MOUTH
  - Child 2–11 years: Initially 200–500 micrograms/kg once daily (max. per dose 10 mg), dose to be taken at night, increased if necessary up to 1 mg/kg twice daily, to be given on specialist advice
  - Child 12–17 years: Initially 10 mg once daily, increased if necessary to 75 mg once daily, dose to be taken at night, dose to be increased gradually, higher doses to be given on specialist advice

- **UNLICENSED USE** Not licensed for use in neuropathic pain.
- **CONTRA-INDICATIONS** Acute porphyrias p. 562 · arrhythmias · during manic phase of bipolar disorder · heart block
- **CAUTIONS** Cardiovascular disease · chronic constipation · diabetes · epilepsy · history of bipolar disorder · history of psychosis · hyperthyroidism (risk of arrhythmias) · patients with a significant risk of suicide · phaeochromocytoma (risk of arrhythmias) · susceptibility to angle-closure glaucoma · urinary retention

CAUTIONS, FURTHER INFORMATION
Treatment should be stopped if the patient enters a manic phase.

- **INTERACTIONS** → Appendix 1 (Antidepressants, tricyclic).
- **SIDE-EFFECTS**
- **Common or very common** Abdominal pain · fatigue · hypertension · mydriasis · oedema · palpitation · restlessness · stomatitis
- **Rare** Dysarthria · extrapyramidal symptoms · paralytic ileus · tremor
- **Very rare** Neuroleptic malignant syndrome · precipitation of angle-closure glaucoma
- **Frequency not known** Agitation · alopecia · anorexia · anxiety · arrhythmia · blurred vision · breast enlargement · changes in blood sugar · chills (on withdrawal) · confusion · constipation · convulsions · delusions · dizziness · drowsiness · dry mouth · ECG changes · galactorrhoea · gynaecomastia · haematological reactions · hallucinations · headache (on withdrawal) · heart block · hepatic reactions · hypomania · hyponatraemia · increased appetite · increased intra-ocular pressure · influenza-like symptoms (on withdrawal) · Insomnia (on withdrawal) · irritability · mania · movement disorders (on withdrawal) · myalgia (on withdrawal) · nausea · nausea (on withdrawal) · paraesthesia · photosensitivity · postural hypotension · pruritus · rash · sexual dysfunction · sleep disturbances · sudden death of patients with cardiac disease · suicidal behaviour · sweating · sweating (on withdrawal) · tachycardia · taste disturbance · tinnitus · urinary retention · urticaria · vivid dreams (on withdrawal) · vomiting · weight gain · weight loss

Overdose
Overdosage with amitriptyline is associated with a relatively high rate of fatality. Symptoms of overdosage may include dry mouth, coma of varying degree, hypotension, hypothermia, hyperreflexia, extensor plantar responses, convulsions, respiratory failure, cardiac conduction defects, and arrhythmias. Dilated pupils and urinary retention also occur. For details on the management of poisoning, see Tricyclic and related antidepressants, under Emergency treatment of poisoning p. 786.

- **PREGNANCY** Use only if potential benefit outweighs risk.
- **BREAST FEEDING** The amount secreted into breast milk is too small to be harmful.
- **HEPATIC IMPAIRMENT** Sedative effects are increased in hepatic impairment. Avoid in severe liver disease.
- **TREATMENT CESSATION** Withdrawal effects may occur within 5 days of stopping treatment with antidepressant

drugs; they are usually mild and self-limiting, but in some cases may be severe. The risk of withdrawal symptoms is increased if the antidepressant is stopped suddenly after regular administration for 8 weeks or more. The dose should preferably be reduced gradually over about 4 weeks, or longer if withdrawal symptoms emerge (6 months in patients who have been on long-term maintenance treatment). If possible tricyclic and related antidepressants should be withdrawn slowly.

● **PRESCRIBING AND DISPENSING INFORMATION** Limited quantities of tricyclic antidepressants should be prescribed at any one time because their cardiovascular and epileptogenic effects are dangerous in overdosage.

● **PATIENT AND CARER ADVICE**

Driving and skilled tasks
Drowsiness may affect the performance of skilled tasks (e.g. driving).
      Effects of alcohol enhanced.

Medicines for Children leaflet: Amitriptyline for neuropathic pain www.medicinesforchildren.org.uk/amitriptyline-for-neuropathic-pain

● **MEDICINAL FORMS**
There can be variation in the licensing of different medicines containing the same drug. Forms available from special-order manufacturers include: oral suspension, oral solution

Tablet
CAUTIONARY AND ADVISORY LABELS 2
▸ **Amitriptyline hydrochloride (Non-proprietary)**
  Amitriptyline hydrochloride 10 mg Amitriptyline 10mg tablets |
  28 tablet [PoM] £1.23 DT price = £0.76
  Amitriptyline hydrochloride 25 mg Amitriptyline 25mg tablets |
  28 tablet [PoM] £1.13 DT price = £0.78
  Amitriptyline hydrochloride 50 mg Amitriptyline 50mg tablets |
  28 tablet [PoM] £3.60 DT price = £0.92

Oral solution
CAUTIONARY AND ADVISORY LABELS 2
▸ **Amitriptyline hydrochloride (Non-proprietary)**
  Amitriptyline hydrochloride 2 mg per 1 ml Amitriptyline 10mg/5ml
  oral solution sugar free sugar-free | 150 ml [PoM] £22.60-£129.25
  Amitriptyline hydrochloride 5 mg per 1 ml Amitriptyline 25mg/5ml
  oral solution sugar free sugar-free | 150 ml [PoM] £18.00 DT price =
  £18.00
  Amitriptyline hydrochloride 10 mg per 1 ml Amitriptyline
  50mg/5ml oral solution sugar free sugar-free | 150 ml [PoM] £19.20
  DT price = £19.20

Doxepin

● **INDICATIONS AND DOSE**

Depressive illness (particularly where sedation is required)
▸ BY MOUTH
▸ **Child 12-17 years:** Initially 75 mg daily in divided doses, alternatively 75 mg once daily, adjusted according to response, dose to taken at bedtime; maintenance 25–300 mg daily, doses above 100 mg given in 3 divided doses

● **CONTRA-INDICATIONS** Acute porphyrias p. 562 · arrhythmias · during manic phase of bipolar disorder · heart block

● **CAUTIONS** Cardiovascular disease · chronic constipation · diabetes · epilepsy · history of bipolar disorder · history of psychosis · hyperthyroidism (risk of arrhythmias) · patients with significant risk of suicide · phaeochromocytoma (risk of arrhythmias) · susceptibility to angle-closure glaucoma · urinary retention

CAUTIONS, FURTHER INFORMATION
Treatment should be stopped if the patient enters a manic phase.

● **INTERACTIONS** → Appendix 1 (antidepressants, tricyclic).

● **SIDE-EFFECTS**
▸ **Common or very common** Agitation · anxiety · confusion · dizziness · drowsiness · irritability · paraesthesia · sleep disturbances
▸ **Rare** Dysarthria · extrapyramidal symptoms · paralytic ileus · tremor
▸ **Very rare** Neuroleptic malignant syndrome · precipitation of angle-closure glaucoma
▸ **Frequency not known** Abdominal pain · alopecia · anorexia · arrhythmia · blurred vision · breast enlargement · changes in blood sugar · constipation · convulsions · delusions · diarrhoea · dry mouth · flushing · galactorrhoea · gynaecomastia · haematological reactions · hallucinations · headache (on withdrawal) · heart block · hepatic reactions · hypomania · hyponatraemia · increased appetite · influenza-like symptoms (on withdrawal) · insomnia (on withdrawal) · mania · movement disorders (on withdrawal) · myalgia (on withdrawal) · nausea · nausea (on withdrawal) · oedema · photosensitivity · pruritus · rash · sexual dysfunction · stomatitis · sudden death of patients with cardiac disease · suicidal behaviour · sweating · sweating (on withdrawal) · taste disturbance · tinnitus · urinary retention · urticaria · vivid dreams (on withdrawal) · vomiting · weight gain · weight loss

SIDE-EFFECTS, FURTHER INFORMATION
The patient should be encouraged to persist with treatment as some tolerance to these side-effects seems to develop. They are reduced if low doses are given initially and then gradually increased, but this must be balanced against the need to obtain a full therapeutic effect as soon as possible.

Overdose Tricyclic and related antidepressants cause dry mouth, coma of varying degree, hypotension, hypothermia, hyperreflexia, extensor plantar responses, convulsions, respiratory failure, cardiac conduction defects, and arrhythmias. Dilated pupils and urinary retention also occur. For details on the management of poisoning see Tricyclic and related antidepressants under Emergency treatment of poisoning p. 786.

● **PREGNANCY** Use with caution—limited information available.

● **BREAST FEEDING** The amount secreted into breast milk is too small to be harmful. Accumulation of metabolite may cause sedation and respiratory depression in neonate.

● **HEPATIC IMPAIRMENT** Sedative effects are increased in hepatic impairment. Avoid in severe liver disease.

● **RENAL IMPAIRMENT** Use with caution.

● **TREATMENT CESSATION** Withdrawal effects may occur within 5 days of stopping treatment with antidepressant drugs; they are usually mild and self-limiting, but in some cases may be severe. The risk of withdrawal symptoms is increased if the antidepressant is stopped suddenly after regular administration for 8 weeks or more. The dose should preferably be reduced gradually over about 4 weeks, or longer if withdrawal symptoms emerge (6 months in patients who have been on long-term maintenance treatment). If possible tricyclic and related antidepressants should be withdrawn slowly.

● **PRESCRIBING AND DISPENSING INFORMATION** Limited quantities of tricyclic antidepressants should be prescribed at any one time because their cardiovascular and epileptogenic effects are dangerous in overdosage.

● **PATIENT AND CARER ADVICE**

Driving and skilled tasks
Drowsiness may affect performance of skilled tasks (e.g. driving).
      Effects of alcohol enhanced.

● **MEDICINAL FORMS**
There can be variation in the licensing of different medicines containing the same drug. Forms available from special-order manufacturers include: capsule, oral suspension, oral solution
Capsule
CAUTIONARY AND ADVISORY LABELS 2
▸ Doxepin (Non-proprietary)
Doxepin (as Doxepin hydrochloride) 25 mg Doxepin 25mg capsules
| 28 capsule PoM £48.00–£97.00 DT price = £97.00
Doxepin (as Doxepin hydrochloride) 50 mg Doxepin 50mg capsules
| 28 capsule PoM £84.00–£154.00 DT price = £154.00

Imipramine hydrochloride

● **INDICATIONS AND DOSE**
Nocturnal enuresis
▸ BY MOUTH
▸ Child 6-7 years: 25 mg once daily, to be taken at bedtime, initial period of treatment (including gradual withdrawal) 3 months—full physical examination before further course
▸ Child 8-10 years: 25–50 mg once daily, to be taken at bedtime, initial period of treatment (including gradual withdrawal) 3 months—full physical examination before further course
▸ Child 11-17 years: 50–75 mg once daily, to be taken at bedtime, initial period of treatment (including gradual withdrawal) 3 months—full physical examination before further course

Attention deficit hyperactivity disorder (under expert supervision)
▸ BY MOUTH
▸ Child 6-17 years: 10–30 mg twice daily

● **UNLICENSED USE** Not licensed for use for attention deficit hyperactivity disorder.
● **CONTRA-INDICATIONS** Acute porphyrias p. 562 · arrhythmia · during the manic phase of bipolar disorder · heart block
● **CAUTIONS** Cardiovascular disease · chronic constipation · diabetes · epilepsy · history of bipolar disorder · history of psychosis · hyperthyroidism (risk of arrhythmias) · patients with a significant risk of suicide · phaeochromocytoma (risk of arrhythmias) · susceptibility to angle-closure glaucoma · urinary retention
CAUTIONS, FURTHER INFORMATION
Treatment should be stopped if the patient enters a manic phase.
● **INTERACTIONS** → Appendix 1 (antidepressants tricyclic).
● **SIDE-EFFECTS**
▸ **Common or very common** Fatigue · flushing · headache · palpitation · restlessness
▸ **Rare** Extrapyramidal symptoms · paralytic ileus
▸ **Very rare** Abdominal pain · aggression · allergic alveolitis · cardiac decompensation · diarrhoea · hypertension · mydriasis · myoclonus · neuroleptic malignant syndrome · oedema · peripheral vasospasm · precipitation of angle-closure glaucoma · stomatitis
▸ **Frequency not known** Agitation · alopecia · anorexia · anxiety · arrhythmia · blurred vision · breast enlargement · changes in blood sugar · chills (on withdrawal) · confusion · constipation · convulsions · delusions · dizziness · drowsiness · dry mouth · dysarthria · ECG changes · galactorrhoea · gynaecomastia · haematologial reactions · hallucinations · headache (on withdrawal) · heart block · hepatic reactions · hypomania · hyponatraemia · increased appetite · influenza-like symptoms (on withdrawal) · insomnia (on withdrawal) · irritability · mania · movement disorders (on withdrawal) · myalgia (on withdrawal) · nausea · nausea (on withdrawal) · paraesthesia · photosensitivity · postural hypotension · pruritus · rash ·

sexual dysfunction · sleep disturbances · sudden death of patients with cardiac disease · suicidal behaviour · sweating · sweating (on withdrawal) · tachycardia · taste disturbance · tinnitus · tremor · urinary retention · urticaria · vivid dreams (on withdrawal) · vomiting · weight gain · weight loss

Overdose
Tricyclic and related antidepressants cause dry mouth, coma of varying degree, hypotension, hypothermia, hyperreflexia, extensor plantar responses, convulsions, respiratory failure, cardiac conduction defects, and arrhythmias. Dilated pupils and urinary retention also occur. For details on the management of poisoning see Tricyclic and related antidepressants under Emergency treatment of poisoning p. 786.

● **PREGNANCY** Colic, tachycardia, dyspnoea, irritability, muscle spasms, respiratory depression and withdrawal symptoms reported in neonates when used in the third trimester.
● **BREAST FEEDING** The amount secreted into breast milk is too small to be harmful.
● **HEPATIC IMPAIRMENT** Sedative effects are increased in hepatic impairment. Avoid in severe liver disease.
● **RENAL IMPAIRMENT** Use with caution in severe impairment.
● **TREATMENT CESSATION** Withdrawal effects may occur within 5 days of stopping treatment with antidepressant drugs; they are usually mild and self-limiting, but in some cases may be severe. The risk of withdrawal symptoms is increased if the antidepressant is stopped suddenly after regular administration for 8 weeks or more. The dose should preferably be reduced gradually over about 4 weeks, or longer if withdrawal symptoms emerge (6 months in patients who have been on long-term maintenance treatment). If possible tricyclic antidepressants should be withdrawn slowly.
● **PRESCRIBING AND DISPENSING INFORMATION** Limited quantities of tricyclic antidepressants should be prescribed at any one time because their cardiovascular and epileptogenic effects are dangerous in overdosage.
● **PATIENT AND CARER ADVICE**
Medicines for Children leaflet: Imipramine www.medicinesforchildren.org.uk/imipramine
Driving and skilled tasks
Drowsiness may affect the performance of skilled tasks (e.g. driving).
Effects of alcohol enhanced.

● **MEDICINAL FORMS**
There can be variation in the licensing of different medicines containing the same drug. Forms available from special-order manufacturers include: oral suspension, oral solution
Tablet
CAUTIONARY AND ADVISORY LABELS 2
▸ Imipramine hydrochloride (Non-proprietary)
Imipramine hydrochloride 10 mg Imipramine 10mg tablets |
28 tablet PoM £1.17 DT price = £1.05
Imipramine hydrochloride 25 mg Imipramine 25mg tablets |
28 tablet PoM £1.16 DT price = £1.05
Oral solution
CAUTIONARY AND ADVISORY LABELS 2
▸ Imipramine hydrochloride (Non-proprietary)
Imipramine hydrochloride 5 mg per 1 ml Imipramine 25mg/5ml oral solution sugar free sugar-free | 150 ml PoM £39.31

Nortriptyline

- **INDICATIONS AND DOSE**
Depressive illness
  ▶ BY MOUTH
  ▸ **Child 12-17 years:** To be initiated at a low dose, then increased if necessary to 30–50 mg daily in divided doses, alternatively increased if necessary to 30–50 mg once daily; maximum 150 mg per day

- **CONTRA-INDICATIONS** Acute porphyrias p. 562 · arrhythmias · during the manic phase of bipolar disorder · heart block
- **CAUTIONS** Cardiovascular disease · chronic constipation · diabetes · epilepsy · history of bipolar disorder · history of psychosis · hyperthyroidism (risk of arrhythmias) · patients with a significant risk of suicide · phaeochromocytoma (risk of arrhythmias) · susceptibility to angle-closure glaucoma · urinary retention
  CAUTIONS, FURTHER INFORMATION
  Treatment should be stopped if the patient enters a manic phase.
- **INTERACTIONS** → Appendix 1 (antidepressants, tricyclic).
- **SIDE-EFFECTS**
  ▶ **Common or very common** Fatigue · hypertension · mydriasis · restlessness
  ▶ **Rare** Extrapyramidal symptoms · paralytic ileus
  ▶ **Very rare** Neuroleptic malignant syndrome · precipitation of angle-closure glaucoma
  ▶ **Frequency not known** Abdominal pain · agitation · alopecia · anorexia · anxiety · arrhythmia · blurred vision · breast enlargement · changes in blood sugar · chills (on withdrawal) · confusion · constipation · convulsions · delusions · diarrhoea · dizziness · drowsiness · dry mouth · dysarthria · ECG changes · flushing · galactorrhoea · gynaecomastia · haematological reactions · hallucinations · headache (on withdrawal) · heart block · hepatic reactions · hypomania · hyponatraemia · increased appetite · influenza-like symptoms (on withdrawal) · insomnia (on withdrawal) · irritability · mania · movement disorders (on withdrawal) · myalgia (on withdrawal) · nausea · nausea (on withdrawal) · oedema · paraesthesia · photosensitivity · postural hypotension · pruritus · rash · sexual dysfunction · sleep disturbances · stomatitis · sudden death of patients with cardiac disease · suicidal behaviour · sweating · sweating (on withdrawal) · tachycardia · taste disturbance · tinnitus · tremor · urinary retention · urticaria · vivid dreams (on withdrawal) · vomiting · weight gain · weight loss

Overdose
Tricyclic and related antidepressants cause dry mouth, coma of varying degree, hypotension, hypothermia, hyperreflexia, extensor plantar responses, convulsions, respiratory failure, cardiac conduction defects, and arrhythmias. Dilated pupils and urinary retention also occur. For details on the management of poisoning see Tricyclic and related antidepressants under Emergency treatment of poisoning p. 786.

- **PREGNANCY** Use only if potential benefit outweighs risk.
- **BREAST FEEDING** The amount secreted into breast milk is too small to be harmful.
- **HEPATIC IMPAIRMENT** Sedative effects are increased in hepatic impairment. Avoid in severe liver disease.
- **MONITORING REQUIREMENTS**
  ▶ Manufacturer advises plasma-nortriptyline concentration monitoring if dose above 100 mg daily, but evidence of practical value uncertain.
- **TREATMENT CESSATION** Withdrawal effects may occur within 5 days of stopping treatment with antidepressant drugs; they are usually mild and self-limiting, but in some cases may be severe. The risk of withdrawal symptoms is increased if the antidepressant is stopped suddenly after regular administration for 8 weeks or more. The dose should preferably be reduced gradually over about 4 weeks, or longer if withdrawal symptoms emerge (6 months in patients who have been on long-term maintenance treatment). If possible tricyclic and related antidepressants should be withdrawn slowly.
- **PRESCRIBING AND DISPENSING INFORMATION** Limited quantities of tricyclic antidepressants should be prescribed at any one time because their cardiovascular and epileptogenic effects are dangerous in overdosage.
- **PATIENT AND CARER ADVICE** Drowsiness may affect the performance of skilled tasks (e.g. driving). Effects of alcohol enhanced.
- **MEDICINAL FORMS**
  There can be variation in the licensing of different medicines containing the same drug. Forms available from special-order manufacturers include: oral suspension, oral solution
  Tablet
  CAUTIONARY AND ADVISORY LABELS 2
  ▸ Nortriptyline (Non-proprietary)
  Nortriptyline (as Nortriptyline hydrochloride) 10 mg Nortriptyline 10mg tablets | 100 tablet [PoM] £34.51-£68.41 DT price = £56.76
  Nortriptyline (as Nortriptyline hydrochloride) 25 mg Nortriptyline 25mg tablets | 100 tablet [PoM] £56.11-£111.06 DT price = £64.57

2.4 Psychoses and schizophrenia

Psychoses and related disorders

Advice on doses of antipsychotic drugs above BNF for Children upper limit

- Consider alternative approaches including adjuvant therapy.
- Bear in mind risk factors, including obesity. Consider potential for drug interactions—see interactions: Appendix 1 (antipsychotics).
- Carry out ECG to exclude untoward abnormalities such as prolonged QT interval; repeat ECG periodically **and** reduce dose if prolonged QT interval or other adverse abnormality develops.
- Increase dose slowly and not more often than once weekly.
- Carry out regular pulse, blood pressure, and temperature checks; ensure that patient maintains adequate fluid intake.
- Consider high-dose therapy to be for limited period and review regularly; abandon if no improvement after 3 months (return to standard dosage).

Important: When prescribing an antipsychotic for administration on an emergency basis, the intramuscular dose should be **lower** than the corresponding oral dose (owing to absence of first-pass effect), particularly if the child is very active (increased blood flow to muscle considerably increases the rate of absorption). The prescription should specify the dose for **each route** and should not imply that the same dose can be given by mouth or by intramuscular injection. The dose of antipsychotic for emergency use should be reviewed at least **daily**.

Antipsychotic drugs

There is little information on the efficacy and safety of antipsychotic drugs in children and adolescents and much of the information available has been extrapolated from adult data; in particular, little is known about the long-term effects of antipsychotic drugs on the developing nervous system. Antipsychotic drugs should be initiated and managed under the close supervision of an appropriate specialist.

4

Nervous system

Antipsychotic drugs are also known as 'neuroleptics' and (misleadingly) as 'major tranquillisers'.

In the short term they are used to calm disturbed children whatever the underlying psychopathology, which may be schizophrenia, brain damage, mania, toxic delirium, or agitated depression. Antipsychotic drugs are used to alleviate severe anxiety but this too should be a short-term measure.

Schizophrenia

The aim of treatment is to alleviate the suffering of the child (and carer) and to improve social and cognitive functioning. Many children require life-long treatment with antipsychotic medication. Antipsychotic drugs relieve positive psychotic symptoms such as thought disorder, hallucinations, and delusions, and prevent relapse; they are usually less effective on negative symptoms such as apathy and social withdrawal. In many patients, negative symptoms persist between episodes of treated positive symptoms, but earlier treatment of psychotic illness may protect against the development of negative symptoms over time. Children with acute schizophrenia generally respond better than those with chronic symptoms.

Long-term treatment of a child with a definitive diagnosis of schizophrenia is usually required after the first episode of illness in order to prevent relapses. Doses that are effective in acute episodes should generally be continued as prophylaxis.

First-generation antipsychotic drugs

The first-generation antipsychotic drugs act predominantly by blocking dopamine D_2 receptors in the brain. First-generation antipsychotic drugs are not selective for any of the four dopamine pathways in the brain and so can cause a range of side-effects, particularly extrapyramidal symptoms and elevated prolactin. The **phenothiazine** derivatives can be divided into 3 main groups:

- *Group* 1: chlorpromazine hydrochloride p. 230, levomepromazine p. 251, and promazine hydrochloride, generally characterised by pronounced sedative effects and moderate antimuscarinic and extrapyramidal side-effects.
- *Group* 2: pericyazine p. 232, generally characterised by moderate sedative effects, but fewer extrapyramidal side-effects than groups 1 or 3.
- *Group* 3: perphenazine p. 232, prochlorperazine p. 252, and trifluoperazine p. 233, generally characterised by fewer sedative and antimuscarinic effects, but more pronounced extrapyramidal side-effects than groups 1 and 2.

Butyrophenones (e.g. haloperidol p. 231) resemble the group 3 phenothiazines in their clinical properties. **Diphenylbutylpiperidines** (pimozide p. 232) and the **substituted benzamides** (sulpiride p. 233) have reduced sedative, antimuscarinic, and extrapyramidal effects.

Second-generation antipsychotic drugs

The second-generation antipsychotic drugs (also referred to as atypical antipsychotic drugs) act on a range of receptors in comparison to first-generation antipsychotic drugs and have more distinct clinical profiles, particularly with regard to side-effects.

Side effects of antipsychotic drugs

Side-effects caused by antipsychotic drugs are common and contribute significantly to non-adherence to therapy.

Extrapyramidal symptoms occur most frequently with the piperazine phenothiazines (fluphenazine, perphenazine, prochlorperazine, and trifluoperazine), the butyrophenones (benperidol and haloperidol), and the first-generation depot preparations. They are easy to recognise but cannot be predicted accurately because they depend on the dose, the type of drug, and on individual susceptibility.

Extrapyramidal symptoms consist of:

- *parkinsonian symptoms* (including tremor), which may appear gradually;
- *dystonia* (abnormal face and body movements) and dyskinesia, which occur more commonly in children or young adults and appear after only a few doses;
- *akathisia* (restlessness), which characteristically occurs after large initial doses and may resemble an exacerbation of the condition being treated;
- *tardive dyskinesia* (rhythmic, involuntary movements of tongue, face, and jaw), which usually develops on long-term therapy or with high dosage, but it may develop on short-term treatment with low doses—short-lived tardive dyskinesia may occur after withdrawal of the drug.

Parkinsonian symptoms remit if the drug is withdrawn and may be suppressed by the administration of antimuscarinic drugs. However, routine administration of such drugs is not justified because not all patients are affected and they may unmask or worsen tardive dyskinesia.

Tardive dyskinesia is the most serious manifestation of extrapyramidal symptoms; it is of particular concern because it may be irreversible on withdrawing therapy and treatment is usually ineffective. In children, tardive dyskinesia is more likely to occur when the antipsychotic drug is withdrawn. However, some manufacturers suggest that drug withdrawal at the earliest signs of tardive dyskinesia (fine vermicular movements of the tongue) may halt its full development. Tardive dyskinesia occurs fairly frequently and treatment must be carefully and regularly reviewed.

Hyperprolactinaemia

Most antipsychotic drugs, both first- and second-generation, increase prolactin concentration to some extent because dopamine inhibits prolactin release. Aripiprazole reduces prolactin because it is a dopamine-receptor partial agonist. Risperidone, amisulpride, and first-generation antipsychotic drugs are most likely to cause symptomatic hyperprolactinaemia. The clinical symptoms of hyperprolactinaemia include sexual dysfunction, reduced bone mineral density, menstrual disturbances, breast enlargement, and galactorrhoea.

Sexual dysfunction

Sexual dysfunction is one of the main causes of non-adherence to antipsychotic medication; physical illness, psychiatric illness, and substance misuse are contributing factors. Antipsychotic-induced sexual dysfunction is caused by more than one mechanism. Reduced dopamine transmission and hyperprolactinaemia decrease libido; antimuscarinic effects can cause disorders of arousal; and alpha$_1$-adrenoceptor antagonists are associated with erection and ejaculation problems in men. Risperidone and haloperidol commonly cause sexual dysfunction. If sexual dysfunction is thought to be antipsychotic-induced, dose reduction or switching medication should be considered.

Cardiovascular side-effects

Antipsychotic drugs have been associated with cardiovascular side-effects such as tachycardia, arrhythmias, and hypotension. QT-interval prolongation is a particular concern with pimozide and haloperidol. There is also a higher probability of QT-interval prolongation in patients using any intravenous antipsychotic drug, or any antipsychotic drug or combination of antipsychotic drugs with doses exceeding the recommended maximum. Cases of sudden death have occurred.

Hyperglycaemia

Hyperglycaemia and sometimes diabetes can occur with antipsychotic drugs, particularly clozapine, olanzapine, quetiapine, and risperidone. All antipsychotic drugs may cause weight gain, but the risk and extent varies. Clozapine and olanzapine commonly cause weight gain.

Hypotension and interference with temperature regulation
Hypotension and interference with temperature regulation are dose-related side-effects. Clozapine, chlorpromazine, and quetiapine can cause postural hypotension (especially during initial dose titration) which may be associated with syncope or reflex tachycardia in some children.

Neuroleptic malignant syndrome
Neuroleptic malignant syndrome (hyperthermia, fluctuating level of consciousness, muscle rigidity, and autonomic dysfunction with pallor, tachycardia, labile blood pressure, sweating, and urinary incontinence) is a rare but potentially fatal side-effect of all antipsychotic drugs. Discontinuation of the antipsychotic drug is essential because there is no proven effective treatment, but bromocriptine and dantrolene have been used. The syndrome, which usually lasts for 5–7 days after drug discontinuation, may be unduly prolonged if depot preparations have been used.

Blood dyscrasias
Perform blood counts if unexplained infection or fever develops.

Choice
The antipsychotic drugs most commonly used in children are haloperidol p. 231, risperidone p. 239, and olanzapine p. 236. There is little meaningful difference in efficacy between each of the antipsychotic drugs (other than clozapine p. 235), and response and tolerability to each antipsychotic drug varies. There is no first-line antipsychotic drug which is suitable for all children. Choice of antipsychotic medication is influenced by the child's medication history, the degree of sedation required (although tolerance to this usually develops), and consideration of individual patient factors such as risk of extrapyramidal side-effects, weight gain, impaired glucose tolerance, QT-interval prolongation, or the presence of negative symptoms.

Negative symptoms
Second generation antipsychotic drugs may be better at treating the negative symptoms of schizophrenia.

Extrapyramidal side-effects
Second-generation antipsychotic drugs may be prescribed if extrapyramidal side-effects are a particular concern. Of these, aripiprazole p. 234, clozapine, olanzapine, and quetiapine p. 238 are least likely to cause extrapyramidal side-effects. Although amisulpride p. 234 is a dopamine-receptor antagonist, extrapyramidal side-effects are less common than with the first-generation antipsychotic drugs because amisulpride selectively blocks mesolimbic dopamine receptors, and extrapyramidal symptoms are caused by blockade of the striatal dopamine pathway.

QT interval
Aripiprazole has negligible effect on the QT interval. Other antipsychotic drugs with a reduced tendency to prolong QT interval include amisulpride, clozapine, olanzapine, perphenazine p. 232, risperidone, and sulpiride p. 233.

Diabetes
Schizophrenia is associated with insulin resistance and diabetes; the risk of diabetes is increased in children with schizophrenia who take antipsychotic drugs. First-generation antipsychotic drugs are less likely to cause diabetes than second-generation antipsychotic drugs, and of the first-generation antipsychotic drugs, haloperidol has the lowest risk. Amisulpride and aripiprazole have the lowest risk of diabetes of the second-generation antipsychotic drugs. Amisulpride, aripiprazole, haloperidol, sulpiride, and trifluoperazine p. 233 are least likely to cause weight gain.

Sexual dysfunction and prolactin
The antipsychotic drugs with the lowest risk of sexual dysfunction are aripiprazole and quetiapine. Olanzapine may be considered if sexual dysfunction is judged to be secondary to hyperprolactinaemia. Hyperprolactinaemia is usually not clinically significant with aripiprazole, clozapine, olanzapine, and quetiapine treatment. When changing from other antipsychotic drugs, a reduction in prolactin concentration may increase fertility.

Children should receive an antipsychotic drug for 4–6 weeks before it is deemed ineffective. Prescribing more than one antipsychotic drug at a time should be avoided except in exceptional circumstances (e.g. clozapine augmentation or when changing medication during titration) because of the increased risk of adverse effects such as extrapyramidal symptoms, QT-interval prolongation, and sudden cardiac death.

Clozapine is used for the treatment of schizophrenia in children unresponsive to, or intolerant of, other antipsychotic drugs. Clozapine should be introduced if schizophrenia is not controlled despite the sequential use of two or more antipsychotic drugs (one of which should be a second-generation antipsychotic drug), each for at least 6–8 weeks. If symptoms do not respond adequately to an optimised dose of clozapine, plasma-clozapine concentration should be checked before adding a second antipsychotic drug to augment clozapine; allow 8–10 weeks' treatment to assess response. Children must be registered with a clozapine patient monitoring service.

Monitoring
Full blood count, urea and electrolytes, and liver function test monitoring is required at the start of therapy with antipsychotic drugs, and then annually thereafter.

Blood lipids and weight should be measured at baseline, at 3 months (weight should be measured at frequent intervals during the first 3 months), and then yearly.

Fasting blood glucose should be measured at baseline, at 4–6 months, and then yearly.

Before initiating antipsychotic drugs, an ECG may be required, particularly if physical examination identifies cardiovascular risk factors, if there is a personal history of cardiovascular disease, or if the child is being admitted as an inpatient.

Blood pressure monitoring is advised before starting therapy and frequently during dose titration of antipsychotic drugs.

Other uses
Nausea and vomiting, choreas, motor tics, and intractable hiccup.

Equivalent doses of oral antipsychotics
These equivalences are intended **only** as an approximate guide; individual dosage instructions should **also** be checked; children should be carefully monitored after **any** change in medication. Equivalent daily dose of antipsychotic drug:

- Chlorpromazine 100 mg
- Clozapine 50 mg
- Haloperidol 2–3 mg
- Pimozide 2 mg
- Risperidone 0.5–1 mg
- Sulpiride 200 mg
- Trifluoperazine 5 mg

Important:These equivalences must **not** be extrapolated beyond the maximum dose for the drug. Higher doses require careful titration in specialist units and the equivalences shown here may not be appropriate.

Dosage
After an initial period of stabilisation, the total daily oral dose of antipsychotic drugs can be given as a single dose in most children.

Antipsychotic depot injections

There is limited information on the use of antipsychotic depot injections in children and use should be restricted to specialist centres.

ANTIPSYCHOTICS

Antipsychotic drugs

- **CAUTIONS** Blood dyscrasias · cardiovascular disease · conditions predisposing to seizures · depression · epilepsy · history of jaundice · myasthenia gravis · photosensitisation (may occur with higher dosages) · severe respiratory disease · susceptibility to angle-closure glaucoma
  CAUTIONS, FURTHER INFORMATION
- ▸ Cardiovascular disease An ECG may be required, particularly if physical examination identifies cardiovascular risk factors, personal history of cardiovascular disease, or if the patient is being admitted as an inpatient.
- **INTERACTIONS** → Appendix 1 (antipsychotics). Increased risk of toxicity with myelosuppressive drugs.
- **SIDE-EFFECTS**
- ▸ **Rare** Neuroleptic malignant syndrome—discontinue (potentially fatal)
- ▸ **Very rare** Precipitation of angle-closure glaucoma
- ▸ **Frequency not known** Agitation · agranulocytosis · akathisia · antimuscarinic symptoms · apathy · blood dyscrasias · blurred vision · cardiovascular side-effects · confusion · constipation · contact sensitisation · convulsions · corneal and lens opacities · diabetes · difficulty with micturition · dizziness · drowsiness · dry mouth · dystonia · excitement · extrapyramidal symptoms · gastro-intestinal disturbances · headache · hyperglycaemia · hyperprolactinemia · hypotension (dose related) · insomnia · interference with temperature regulation (dose related) · jaundice (including cholestatic) · leucopenia · nasal congestion · parkinsonian symptoms · photosensitisation · purplish pigmentation of the conjunctiva · purplish pigmentation of the cornea · purplish pigmentation of the retina · purplish pigmentation of the skin · rashes · sexual dysfunction · tardive dyskinesia · venous thromboembolism · weight gain

Overdose
Phenothiazines cause less depression of consciousness and respiration than other sedatives. Hypotension, hypothermia, sinus tachycardia, and arrhythmias may complicate poisoning. For details on the management of poisoning see Antipsychotics under Emergency treatment of poisoning p. 786.

- **PREGNANCY** Extrapyramidal effects and withdrawal syndrome have been reported occasionally in the neonate when antipsychotic drugs are taken during the third trimester of pregnancy. Following maternal use of antipsychotic drugs in the third trimester, neonates should be monitored for symptoms including agitation, hypertonia, hypotonia, tremor, drowsiness, feeding problems, and respiratory distress.

- **BREAST FEEDING** There is limited information available on the short- and long-term effects of antipsychotic drugs on the breast-fed infant. *Animal studies* indicate possible adverse effects of antipsychotic medicines on the developing nervous system. Chronic treatment with antipsychotic drugs whilst breast-feeding should be avoided unless absolutely necessary. Phenothiazine derivatives are sometimes used in breast-feeding women for short-term treatment of nausea and vomiting.

- **MONITORING REQUIREMENTS**
- ▸ Regular clinical monitoring of endocrine function should be considered when children are taking an antipsychotic drug known to increase prolactin levels; this includes measuring weight and height, assessing sexual maturation, and monitoring menstrual function.
- ▸ It is advisable to monitor prolactin concentration at the start of therapy, at 6 months, and then yearly. Patients taking antipsychotic drugs not normally associated with symptomatic hyperprolactinaemia should be considered

for prolactin monitoring if they show symptoms of hyperprolactinaemia (such as breast enlargement and galactorrhoea).
- ▸ Patients with schizophrenia should have physical health monitoring (including cardiovascular disease risk assessment) at least once per year.

- **TREATMENT CESSATION** There is a high risk of relapse if medication is stopped after 1–2 years. Withdrawal of antipsychotic drugs after long-term therapy should always be gradual and closely monitored to avoid the risk of acute withdrawal syndromes or rapid relapse. Patients should be monitored for 2 years after withdrawal of antipsychotic medication for signs and symptoms of relapse.

- **PATIENT AND CARER ADVICE**
  As photosensitisation may occur with higher dosages, patients should avoid direct sunlight.

  Driving and skilled tasks
  Drowsiness may affect performance of skilled tasks (e.g. driving or operating machinery), especially at start of treatment; effects of alcohol are enhanced.

ANTIPSYCHOTICS > FIRST-GENERATION

▸ above

Chlorpromazine hydrochloride

- **INDICATIONS AND DOSE**

Childhood schizophrenia and other psychoses (under expert supervision)
- ▸ BY MOUTH
- ▸ Child 1–5 years: 500 micrograms/kg every 4–6 hours, adjusted according to response; maximum 40 mg per day
- ▸ Child 6–11 years: 10 mg 3 times a day, adjusted according to response; maximum 75 mg per day
- ▸ Child 12–17 years: Initially 25 mg 3 times a day, adjusted according to response, alternatively initially 75 mg once daily, adjusted according to response, dose to be taken at night; maintenance 75–300 mg daily, increased if necessary up to 1 g daily

Relief of acute symptoms of psychoses (under expert supervision)
- ▸ BY DEEP INTRAMUSCULAR INJECTION
- ▸ Child 1–5 years: 500 micrograms/kg every 6–8 hours; maximum 40 mg per day
- ▸ Child 6–11 years: 500 micrograms/kg every 6–8 hours; maximum 75 mg per day
- ▸ Child 12–17 years: 25–50 mg every 6–8 hours

Nausea and vomiting of terminal illness (where other drugs have failed or are not available)
- ▸ BY MOUTH
- ▸ Child 1–5 years: 500 micrograms/kg every 4–6 hours; maximum 40 mg per day
- ▸ Child 6–11 years: 500 micrograms/kg every 4–6 hours; maximum 75 mg per day
- ▸ Child 12–17 years: 10–25 mg every 4–6 hours
- ▸ BY DEEP INTRAMUSCULAR INJECTION
- ▸ Child 1–5 years: 500 micrograms/kg every 6–8 hours; maximum 40 mg per day
- ▸ Child 6–11 years: 500 micrograms/kg every 6–8 hours; maximum 75 mg per day
- ▸ Child 12–17 years: Initially 25 mg, then 25–50 mg every 3–4 hours until vomiting stops

DOSE ADJUSTMENTS DUE TO INTERACTIONS
Dose adjustment may be necessary if smoking started or stopped during treatment.

DOSE EQUIVALENCE AND CONVERSION
For equivalent therapeutic effect 20–25 mg chlorpromazine hydrochloride *by intramuscular injection* ≡ 40–50 mg of chlorpromazine base or hydrochloride given *by mouth*.

- **CONTRA-INDICATIONS** CNS depression · comatose states · hypothyroidism · phaeochromocytoma
- **CAUTIONS** Diabetes
- **SIDE-EFFECTS**

  SIDE-EFFECTS, FURTHER INFORMATION
  ▸ Acute dystonic reactions Phenothiazines can induce acute dystonic reactions such as facial and skeletal muscle spasms and oculogyric crises; children (especially girls, young women, and those under 10 kg) are particularly susceptible.
- **HEPATIC IMPAIRMENT** Can precipitate coma; phenothiazines are hepatotoxic.
- **RENAL IMPAIRMENT** Start with small doses in severe renal impairment because of increased cerebral sensitivity.
- **MONITORING REQUIREMENTS**
  ▸ With intramuscular use Patients should remain supine, with blood pressure monitoring for 30 minutes after intramuscular injection.
- **HANDLING AND STORAGE** Owing to the risk of contact sensitisation, pharmacists, nurses, and other health workers should avoid direct contact with chlorpromazine; tablets should not be crushed and solutions should be handled with care.

- **MEDICINAL FORMS**
  There can be variation in the licensing of different medicines containing the same drug. Forms available from special-order manufacturers include: tablet, capsule, oral suspension, oral solution
  Tablet
  CAUTIONARY AND ADVISORY LABELS 2, 11
  ▸ Chlorpromazine hydrochloride (Non-proprietary)
    Chlorpromazine hydrochloride 25 mg Chlorpromazine 25mg tablets | 28 tablet [PoM] £4.92 DT price = £1.84
    Chlorpromazine hydrochloride 50 mg Chlorpromazine 50mg tablets | 28 tablet [PoM] £5.28 DT price = £1.73
    Chlorpromazine hydrochloride 100 mg Chlorpromazine 100mg tablets | 28 tablet [PoM] £5.70 DT price = £1.85
  Oral solution
  CAUTIONARY AND ADVISORY LABELS 2, 11
  ▸ Chlorpromazine hydrochloride (Non-proprietary)
    Chlorpromazine hydrochloride 5 mg per 1 ml Chlorpromazine 25mg/5ml syrup | 150 ml [PoM] £2.35 DT price = £2.35
    Chlorpromazine 25mg/5ml oral solution sugar free sugar-free | 150 ml [PoM] £2.35
    Chlorpromazine 25mg/5ml oral solution | 150 ml [PoM] £2.35 DT price = £2.35
    Chlorpromazine hydrochloride 20 mg per 1 ml Chlorpromazine 100mg/5ml oral solution | 150 ml [PoM] £5.50 DT price = £5.50
  Solution for injection
  ▸ Largactil (Sanofi)
    Chlorpromazine hydrochloride 25 mg per 1 ml Largactil 50mg/2ml solution for injection ampoules | 10 ampoule [PoM] £7.51

◀ 230

▌Haloperidol

- **INDICATIONS AND DOSE**
  Schizophrenia (under expert supervision)
  ▸ BY MOUTH
  ▸ Child 3–12 years: Initially 500 micrograms daily in 2–3 divided doses; usual dose 1–4 mg daily in 2–3 divided doses; daily maximum to be given in 2–3 divided doses; maximum 6 mg per day
  ▸ Child 13–17 years: Initially 500 micrograms daily in 2–3 divided doses; usual dose 1–6 mg daily in 2–3 divided doses; daily maximum to be given in 2–3 divided doses; maximum 10 mg per day

Childhood behavioural disorders, especially when associated with hyperactivity and aggression (under expert supervision) | Gilles de la Tourette syndrome (under expert supervision)
▸ BY MOUTH
▸ Child 3–12 years: Initially 250 micrograms daily in 2–3 divided doses; usual dose 0.5–3 mg daily in 2–3 divided doses; daily maximum to be given in 2–3 divided doses; maximum 3 mg per day
▸ Child 13–17 years: Initially 250 micrograms daily in 2–3 divided doses; usual dose 2–6 mg daily in 2–3 divided doses; daily maximum to be given in 2–3 divided doses; maximum 6 mg per day

Nausea and vomiting in palliative care
▸ BY MOUTH
▸ Child 12–17 years: 1.5 mg once daily, dose to be taken at night, increased if necessary to 1.5 mg twice daily (max. per dose 5 mg twice daily)
▸ BY CONTINUOUS INTRAVENOUS INFUSION, OR BY CONTINUOUS SUBCUTANEOUS INFUSION
▸ Child 1 month–11 years: 25–85 micrograms/kg, to be administered over 24 hours
▸ Child 12–17 years: 1.5–5 mg, to be administered over 24 hours

Restlessness and confusion in palliative care
▸ BY MOUTH
▸ Child 1–17 years: 10–20 micrograms/kg every 8–12 hours

DOSE ADJUSTMENTS DUE TO INTERACTIONS
Dose adjustment may be necessary if smoking started or stopped during treatment.

- **UNLICENSED USE** Not licensed for use in children for nausea and vomiting in palliative care.
- **CONTRA-INDICATIONS** Bradycardia · CNS depression · comatose states · lesions of the basal ganglia · phaeochromocytoma · QT-interval prolongation
- **CAUTIONS** Hypocalcaemia · hypokalaemia · hypomagnesaemia · metabolic disturbances · subarachnoid haemorrhage
- **INTERACTIONS** Avoid concomitant administration of drugs that prolong QT interval.
- **SIDE-EFFECTS**
  ▸ **Common or very common** Depression · weight loss
  ▸ **Uncommon** Dyspnoea · oedema
  ▸ **Rare** Bronchospasm · hypoglycaemia · inappropriate antidiuretic hormone secretion
  ▸ **Frequency not known** Stevens-Johnson syndrome · toxic epidermal necrolysis
  SIDE-EFFECTS, FURTHER INFORMATION
  Less sedating and fewer antimuscarinic or hypotensive symptoms.
- **PREGNANCY** Avoid unless benefits outweigh risks.
- **HEPATIC IMPAIRMENT** Can precipitate coma.
- **RENAL IMPAIRMENT** Start with small doses in severe renal impairment because of increased cerebral sensitivity.
- **MONITORING REQUIREMENTS** Baseline ECG required before treatment—assess need for further ECGs during treatment on an individual basis.

- **MEDICINAL FORMS**
  There can be variation in the licensing of different medicines containing the same drug. Forms available from special-order manufacturers include: oral suspension, oral solution
  Tablet
  CAUTIONARY AND ADVISORY LABELS 2
  ▸ Haloperidol (Non-proprietary)
    Haloperidol 500 microgram Haloperidol 500microgram tablets | 28 tablet [PoM] £1.10–£20.05
    Haloperidol 1.5 mg Haloperidol 1.5mg tablets | 28 tablet [PoM] £5.99 DT price = £2.12

Haloperidol 5 mg Haloperidol 5mg tablets | 28 tablet [PoM] £3.80 DT price = £3.06
Haloperidol 10 mg Haloperidol 10mg tablets | 28 tablet [PoM] £12.99 DT price = £12.87
Haloperidol 20 mg Haloperidol 20mg tablets | 28 tablet [PoM] £21.97–£22.00 DT price = £21.98

Capsule
CAUTIONARY AND ADVISORY LABELS 2
▸ Serenace (Teva UK Ltd)
Haloperidol 500 microgram Serenace 500microgram capsules | 30 capsule [PoM] £1.18 DT price = £1.18

Oral solution
CAUTIONARY AND ADVISORY LABELS 2
▸ Haloperidol (Non-proprietary)
Haloperidol 1 mg per 1 ml Haloperidol 5mg/5ml oral solution sugar free sugar-free | 100 ml [PoM] £35.99 DT price = £6.45 sugar-free | 500 ml [PoM] £32.20
Haloperidol 2 mg per 1 ml Haloperidol 10mg/5ml oral solution sugar free sugar-free | 100 ml [PoM] £46.75 DT price = £7.10 sugar-free | 500 ml [PoM] £35.50
▸ Haldol (Janssen-Cilag Ltd)
Haloperidol 2 mg per 1 ml Haldol 2mg/ml oral solution sugar-free | 100 ml [PoM] £4.45 DT price = £7.10

Solution for injection
▸ Haloperidol (Non-proprietary)
Haloperidol 5 mg per 1 ml Haloperidol 5mg/1ml solution for injection ampoules | 10 ampoule [PoM] £35.00

F 230

Pericyazine

(Periciazine)

● INDICATIONS AND DOSE
Schizophrenia (under expert supervision) | Psychoses (severe mental or behavioural disorders only) (under expert supervision)
▸ BY MOUTH
▸ **Child 1–11 years:** Initially 500 micrograms daily for 10-kg child, increased by 1 mg for each additional 5 kg; dose may be gradually increased according to response but maintenance should not exceed twice initial dose; maximum 10 mg per day
▸ **Child 12–17 years:** Initially 25 mg 3 times a day, increased in steps of 25 mg every 1 week, adjusted according to response, increased if necessary up to 100 mg 3 times a day, total daily dose may alternatively be given in 2 divided doses

● UNLICENSED USE Tablets not licensed for use in children.
● CONTRA-INDICATIONS CNS depression · comatose states · phaeochromocytoma
● SIDE-EFFECTS
▸ **Common or very common** Hypotension (when treatment initiated)
▸ **Frequency not known** Respiratory depression
SIDE-EFFECTS, FURTHER INFORMATION
More sedating.
● HEPATIC IMPAIRMENT Can precipitate coma; phenothiazines are hepatotoxic.
● RENAL IMPAIRMENT Avoid in renal impairment.

● MEDICINAL FORMS
There can be variation in the licensing of different medicines containing the same drug. Forms available from special-order manufacturers include: oral suspension, oral solution

Tablet
CAUTIONARY AND ADVISORY LABELS 2
▸ Pericyazine (Non-proprietary)
Pericyazine 2.5 mg Pericyazine 2.5mg tablets | 84 tablet [PoM] £16.95 DT price = £16.23
Pericyazine 10 mg Pericyazine 10mg tablets | 84 tablet [PoM] £40.94 DT price = £40.47

Oral solution
CAUTIONARY AND ADVISORY LABELS 2
▸ Pericyazine (Non-proprietary)
Pericyazine 2 mg per 1 ml Pericyazine 10mg/5ml oral solution | 100 ml [PoM] £46.00–£46.01 DT price = £46.01

F 230

Perphenazine

● INDICATIONS AND DOSE
Schizophrenia and other psychoses | Mania | Short-term adjunctive management of anxiety | Severe psychomotor agitation, excitement, and violent or dangerously impulsive behaviour | Severe nausea and vomiting unresponsive to other anti-emetics
▸ BY MOUTH
▸ **Child 14–17 years (under close medical supervision):** Initially 4 mg 3 times a day, adjusted according to response; maximum 24 mg per day

● CONTRA-INDICATIONS CNS depression · comatose states · phaeochromocytoma
● CAUTIONS Hypothyroidism
● SIDE-EFFECTS
▸ **Rare** Systemic lupus erythematosus
▸ **Frequency not known** Dystonic reactions
SIDE-EFFECTS, FURTHER INFORMATION
Less sedating.
▸ **Acute dystonic reactions** Phenothiazines can all induce acute dystonic reactions such as facial and skeletal muscle spasms and oculogyric crises; children (especially girls, young women, and those under 10 kg) are particularly susceptible.
● HEPATIC IMPAIRMENT Can precipitate coma; phenothiazines are hepatotoxic.
● RENAL IMPAIRMENT Start with small doses in severe renal impairment because of increased cerebral sensitivity.

● MEDICINAL FORMS
There can be variation in the licensing of different medicines containing the same drug. Forms available from special-order manufacturers include: tablet, oral suspension

F 230

Pimozide

● INDICATIONS AND DOSE
Schizophrenia
▸ BY MOUTH
▸ **Child 12–17 years (under expert supervision):** Initially 1 mg daily, adjusted according to response, then increased in steps of 2–4 mg at intervals of not less than 1 week; usual dose 2–20 mg daily
Tourette syndrome (under expert supervision)
▸ BY MOUTH
▸ **Child 2–11 years:** 1–4 mg daily
▸ **Child 12–17 years:** 2–10 mg daily

● UNLICENSED USE Not licensed for use in Tourette syndrome.
● CONTRA-INDICATIONS CNS depression · comatose states · history of arrhythmias · history or family history of congenital QT prolongation · phaeochromocytoma
● SIDE-EFFECTS
▸ **Rare** Hyponatraemia
▸ **Frequency not known** Glycosuria · serious arrhythmias · venous thromboembolism
SIDE-EFFECTS, FURTHER INFORMATION
Less sedating.
● HEPATIC IMPAIRMENT Can precipitate coma.

- **RENAL IMPAIRMENT** Start with small doses in severe renal impairment because of increased cerebral sensitivity.
- **MONITORING REQUIREMENTS**
  - ECG monitoring Following reports of sudden unexplained death, an ECG is recommended before treatment. It is also recommended that patients taking pimozide should have an annual ECG (if the QT interval is prolonged, treatment should be reviewed and either withdrawn or dose reduced under close supervision) and that pimozide should not be given with other antipsychotic drugs (including depot preparations), tricyclic antidepressants or other drugs which prolong the QT interval, such as certain antimalarials, antiarrhythmic drugs and certain antihistamines and should not be given with drugs which cause electrolyte disturbances (especially diuretics).

- **MEDICINAL FORMS**
  There can be variation in the licensing of different medicines containing the same drug. Forms available from special-order manufacturers include: oral suspension
  Tablet
  CAUTIONARY AND ADVISORY LABELS 2
  - Pimozide (Non-proprietary)
    Pimozide 1 mg Orap 1mg tablets | 100 tablet PoM no price available
    Pimozide 4 mg Pimozide 4mg tablets | 100 tablet PoM no price available
  - Orap (Eumedica Pharmaceuticals)
    Pimozide 4 mg Orap 4mg tablets | 100 tablet PoM £40.31

⌐ 230

Sulpiride

- **INDICATIONS AND DOSE**
Schizophrenia with predominantly negative symptoms
  - BY MOUTH
    - Child 14–17 years (under expert supervision): 200–400 mg twice daily; maximum 800 mg per day
Schizophrenia with mainly positive symptoms
  - BY MOUTH
    - Child 14–17 years (under expert supervision): 200–400 mg twice daily; maximum 2.4 g per day
Tourette syndrome (under expert supervision)
  - BY MOUTH
    - Child 2–11 years: 50–400 mg twice daily
    - Child 12–17 years: 100–400 mg twice daily

- **UNLICENSED USE** Not licensed for use in Tourette syndrome.
- **CONTRA-INDICATIONS** CNS depression · comatose states · phaeochromocytoma
- **CAUTIONS** Aggressive patients (even low doses may aggravate symptoms) · agitated patients (even low doses may aggravate symptoms) · excited patients (even low doses may aggravate symptoms)
- **SIDE-EFFECTS** Hepatitis · venous thromboembolism
- **HEPATIC IMPAIRMENT** Can precipitate coma.
- **RENAL IMPAIRMENT** Start with small doses in severe renal impairment because of increased cerebral sensitivity.
- **MONITORING REQUIREMENTS** Sulpiride does not affect blood pressure to the same extent as other antipsychotic drugs and so blood pressure monitoring is not mandatory for this drug.
- **PRESCRIBING AND DISPENSING INFORMATION** Flavours of oral liquid formulations may include lemon and aniseed.
- **PATIENT AND CARER ADVICE**
  Medicines for Children leaflet: Sulpiride for schizophrenia and Tourette's syndrome www.medicinesforchildren.org.uk/sulpiride-for-schizophrenia-and-tourettes-syndrome

- **MEDICINAL FORMS**
  There can be variation in the licensing of different medicines containing the same drug. Forms available from special-order manufacturers include: oral suspension, oral solution
  Tablet
  CAUTIONARY AND ADVISORY LABELS 2
  - Sulpiride (Non-proprietary)
    Sulpiride 200 mg Sulpiride 200mg tablets | 30 tablet PoM £7.84 DT price = £3.96
    Sulpiride 400 mg Sulpiride 400mg tablets | 30 tablet PoM £18.80 DT price = £18.80
  - Dolmatil (Sanofi)
    Sulpiride 200 mg Dolmatil 200mg tablets | 100 tablet PoM £6.00
    Sulpiride 400 mg Dolmatil 400mg tablets | 100 tablet PoM £19.00
  Oral solution
  CAUTIONARY AND ADVISORY LABELS 2
  - Sulpiride (Non-proprietary)
    Sulpiride 40 mg per 1 ml Sulpiride 200mg/5ml oral solution sugar free sugar-free | 150 ml PoM £27.00 DT price = £25.38
  - Sulpor (Rosemont Pharmaceuticals Ltd)
    Sulpiride 40 mg per 1 ml Sulpor 200mg/5ml oral solution sugar-free | 150 ml PoM £25.38 DT price = £25.38

⌐ 230

Trifluoperazine

- **INDICATIONS AND DOSE**
Schizophrenia and other psychoses | Short-term adjunctive management of psychomotor agitation, excitement, and violent or dangerously impulsive behaviour
  - BY MOUTH
    - Child 12–17 years (under expert supervision): Initially 5 mg twice daily, increased by 5 mg daily after 1 week, then at intervals of 3 days, according to response
Short-term adjunctive management of severe anxiety
  - BY MOUTH
    - Child 3–5 years (under expert supervision): Up to 500 micrograms twice daily
    - Child 6–11 years (under expert supervision): Up to 2 mg twice daily
    - Child 12–17 years (under expert supervision): 1–2 mg twice daily, increased if necessary to 3 mg twice daily
Severe nausea and vomiting unresponsive to other antiemetics
  - BY MOUTH
    - Child 3–5 years: Up to 500 micrograms twice daily
    - Child 6–11 years: Up to 2 mg twice daily
    - Child 12–17 years: 1–2 mg twice daily (max. per dose 3 mg twice daily)

- **CONTRA-INDICATIONS** CNS depression · comatose states · phaeochromocytoma
- **SIDE-EFFECTS** Anorexia · dystonic reactions · muscle weakness
  SIDE-EFFECTS, FURTHER INFORMATION
  Extrapyramidal symptoms are more frequent, especially at doses exceeding 6 mg daily.
  Phenothiazines can all induce acute dystonic reactions such as facial and skeletal muscle spasms and oculogyric crises; children (especially girls, young women, and those under 10 kg) are particularly susceptible.
- **HEPATIC IMPAIRMENT** Can precipitate coma; phenothiazines are hepatotoxic.
- **RENAL IMPAIRMENT** Start with small doses in severe renal impairment because of increased cerebral sensitivity.
- **MONITORING REQUIREMENTS** Trifluoperazine does not affect blood pressure to the same extent as other antipsychotic drugs and so blood pressure monitoring is not mandatory for this drug.

● MEDICINAL FORMS
There can be variation in the licensing of different medicines containing the same drug.

Tablet
CAUTIONARY AND ADVISORY LABELS 2
▸ **Trifluoperazine (Non-proprietary)**
Trifluoperazine (as Trifluoperazine hydrochloride) 1 mg Stelazine 1mg tablets | 50 tablet [PoM] no price available
Trifluoperazine 1mg tablets | 112 tablet [PoM] £54.00 DT price = £54.00
Trifluoperazine (as Trifluoperazine hydrochloride) 5 mg Stelazine 5mg tablets | 50 tablet [PoM] no price available
Trifluoperazine 5mg tablets | 112 tablet [PoM] £123.20 DT price = £123.20

Oral solution
CAUTIONARY AND ADVISORY LABELS 2
▸ **Trifluoperazine (Non-proprietary)**
Trifluoperazine (as Trifluoperazine hydrochloride)
200 microgram per 1 ml Trifluoperazine 1mg/5ml oral solution sugar free sugar-free | 200 ml [PoM] £102.53 DT price = £102.53
Trifluoperazine (as Trifluoperazine hydrochloride) 1 mg per 1 ml Trifluoperazine 5mg/5ml oral solution sugar free sugar-free | 150 ml [PoM] £25.50 DT price = £25.50

ANTIPSYCHOTICS ⟩ SECOND-GENERATION

☞ 230

Amisulpride

● DRUG ACTION Amisulpride is a selective dopamine receptor antagonist with high affinity for mesolimbic D_2 and D_3 receptors.

● **INDICATIONS AND DOSE**
Acute psychotic episode in schizophrenia
▸ BY MOUTH
▸ Child 15–17 years (under expert supervision): 200–400 mg twice daily, adjusted according to response; maximum 1.2 g per day

Schizophrenia with predominantly negative symptoms
▸ BY MOUTH
▸ Child 15–17 years (under expert supervision): 50–300 mg daily

● UNLICENSED USE Not licensed for use in children under 18 years.

● CONTRA-INDICATIONS CNS depression · comatose states · phaeochromocytoma · pre-pubertal children · prolactin-dependent tumours

● SIDE-EFFECTS
▸ **Common or very common** Anxiety
▸ **Uncommon** Bradycardia

● PREGNANCY Avoid.

● BREAST FEEDING Avoid—no information available.

● RENAL IMPAIRMENT Halve dose if estimated glomerular filtration rate 30–60 mL/minute/1.73 m². Use one-third dose if estimated glomerular filtration rate 10–30 mL/minute/1.73 m². No information available if estimated glomerular filtration rate less than 10 mL/minute/1.73 m².

● MONITORING REQUIREMENTS Amisulpride does not affect blood pressure to the same extent as other antipsychotic drugs and so blood pressure monitoring is not mandatory for this drug.

● PRESCRIBING AND DISPENSING INFORMATION Flavours of oral liquid formulations may include caramel.

● MEDICINAL FORMS
There can be variation in the licensing of different medicines containing the same drug. Forms available from special-order manufacturers include: oral suspension, oral solution

Tablet
CAUTIONARY AND ADVISORY LABELS 2
▸ **Amisulpride (Non-proprietary)**
Amisulpride 50 mg Amisulpride 50mg tablets | 60 tablet [PoM] £27.00 DT price = £2.73
Amisulpride 100 mg Amisulpride 100mg tablets | 60 tablet [PoM] £51.27 DT price = £4.08
Amisulpride 200 mg Amisulpride 200mg tablets | 60 tablet [PoM] £66.00 DT price = £7.22
Amisulpride 400 mg Amisulpride 400mg tablets | 60 tablet [PoM] £132.00 DT price = £35.20
▸ **Solian** (Sanofi)
Amisulpride 50 mg Solian 50 tablets | 60 tablet [PoM] £22.76 DT price = £2.73
Amisulpride 100 mg Solian 100 tablets | 60 tablet [PoM] £35.29 DT price = £4.08
Amisulpride 200 mg Solian 200 tablets | 60 tablet [PoM] £58.99 DT price = £7.22
Amisulpride 400 mg Solian 400 tablets | 60 tablet [PoM] £117.97 DT price = £35.20

Oral solution
CAUTIONARY AND ADVISORY LABELS 2
▸ **Amisulpride (Non-proprietary)**
Amisulpride 100 mg per 1 ml Amisulpride 100mg/ml oral solution sugar free sugar-free | 60 ml [PoM] £36.00 DT price = £35.68
▸ **Solian** (Sanofi)
Amisulpride 100 mg per 1 ml Solian 100mg/ml oral solution sugar-free | 60 ml [PoM] £33.76 DT price = £35.68

☞ 230

Aripiprazole

● DRUG ACTION Aripiprazole is a dopamine D_2 partial agonist with weak 5-HT_{1a} partial agonism and 5-HT_{2A} receptor antagonism.

● **INDICATIONS AND DOSE**
Schizophrenia
▸ BY MOUTH
▸ Child 15–17 years (under expert supervision): Initially 2 mg once daily for 2 days, increased to 5 mg once daily for 2 days, then increased to 10 mg once daily, then increased in steps of 5 mg if required, for dose adjustments due to concomitant use of interacting drugs—consult product literature; maximum 30 mg per day

Treatment of mania (under expert supervision)
▸ BY MOUTH
▸ Child 13–17 years: Initially 2 mg once daily for 2 days, increased to 5 mg once daily for 2 days, then increased to 10 mg once daily, increased in steps of 5 mg if required, maximum duration of treatment 12 weeks, for dose adjustments due to concomitant use of interacting drugs—consult product literature, doses above 10 mg daily should only be used in exceptional cases; maximum 30 mg per day

● CONTRA-INDICATIONS CNS depression · comatose state · phaeochromocytoma

● CAUTIONS Cerebrovascular disease

● SIDE-EFFECTS
▸ **Common or very common** Anxiety · hypersalivation · malaise
▸ **Uncommon** Depression · dry mouth
▸ **Frequency not known** Alopecia · anorexia · bradycardia · hepatitis · hyponatraemia · infection · laryngospasm · myalgia · oedema · oropharyngeal spasm · pancreatitis · pathological gambling · respiratory disorders · rhabdomyolysis · suicidal ideation · sweating · urinary disorders

SIDE-EFFECTS, FURTHER INFORMATION

▸ With oral use Increased incidence of side-effects associated with doses of 30 mg daily; doses above 10 mg daily should only be used in exceptional cases and with close clinical monitoring.

● **PREGNANCY** Use only if potential benefit outweighs risk.

● **BREAST FEEDING** Manufacturer advises avoid—present in milk.

● **HEPATIC IMPAIRMENT** Use with caution in severe impairment.

● **MONITORING REQUIREMENTS** Aripiprazole does not affect blood pressure to the same extent as other antipsychotic drugs and so blood pressure monitoring is not mandatory for this drug.

● **DIRECTIONS FOR ADMINISTRATION** Orodispersible tablets should be placed on the tongue and allowed to dissolve, or be dispersed in water and swallowed.

● **PATIENT AND CARER ADVICE**
Patients or carers should be given advice on how to administer aripiprazole orodispersible tablets.

Medicines for Children leaflet: Aripiprazole for schizophrenia, bipolar disorder and movement disorders www. medicinesforchildren.org.uk/aripiprazole-schizophrenia-bipolar-disorder-and-movement-disorders

● **NATIONAL FUNDING/ACCESS DECISIONS**

NICE technology appraisals (TAs)

▸ Aripiprazole for the treatment of schizophrenia in people aged 15 to 17 years (January 2011) NICE TA213
Aripiprazole is recommended as an option for the treatment of schizophrenia in adolescents aged 15 to 17 years who have not responded adequately to, or who are intolerant of, risperidone, or for whom risperidone is contra-indicated.
www.nice.org.uk/ta213

▸ Aripiprazole for the treatment of moderate to severe manic episodes in adolescents with bipolar I disorder (July 2013) NICE TA292
Aripiprazole is recommended as an option for the treatment of moderate to severe manic episodes for up to 12 weeks in adolescents aged over 13 years with bipolar I disorder.
www.nice.org.uk/ta292

ABILIFY® ORAL SOLUTION

Scottish Medicines Consortium (SMC) Decisions
The *Scottish Medicines Consortium*, has advised (August 2013) that oral aripiprazole (*Abilify®*) is accepted for restricted use within NHS Scotland for the treatment of moderate to severe manic episodes in Bipolar I Disorder in adolescents aged 13 years and older for a period of up to 12 weeks. It is restricted to initiation and management under the supervision of a child/adolescent psychiatrist.

● **MEDICINAL FORMS**
There can be variation in the licensing of different medicines containing the same drug. Forms available from special-order manufacturers include: oral solution

Tablet
CAUTIONARY AND ADVISORY LABELS 2
▸ **Aripiprazole (Non-proprietary)**
Aripiprazole 5 mg Aripiprazole 5mg tablets | 28 tablet PoM £96.04 DT price = £5.79
Aripiprazole 10 mg Aripiprazole 10mg tablets | 28 tablet PoM £96.04 DT price = £5.79
Aripiprazole 15 mg Aripiprazole 15mg tablets | 28 tablet PoM £96.04 DT price = £5.72
Aripiprazole 30 mg Aripiprazole 30mg tablets | 28 tablet PoM £192.08 DT price = £103.07
▸ **Abilify** (Otsuka Pharmaceuticals (U.K.) Ltd)
Aripiprazole 5 mg Abilify 5mg tablets | 28 tablet PoM £96.04 DT price = £5.79
Aripiprazole 10 mg Abilify 10mg tablets | 28 tablet PoM £96.04 DT price = £5.79

Aripiprazole 15 mg Abilify 15mg tablets | 28 tablet PoM £96.04 DT price = £5.72
Aripiprazole 30 mg Abilify 30mg tablets | 28 tablet PoM £192.08 DT price = £103.07

Orodispersible tablet
CAUTIONARY AND ADVISORY LABELS 2
EXCIPIENTS: May contain Aspartame
▸ **Aripiprazole (Non-proprietary)**
Aripiprazole 10 mg Aripiprazole 10mg orodispersible tablets sugar free sugar-free | 28 tablet PoM £91.24 DT price = £87.05
Aripiprazole 15 mg Aripiprazole 15mg orodispersible tablets sugar free sugar-free | 28 tablet PoM £91.24 DT price = £87.05
▸ **Abilify** (Otsuka Pharmaceuticals (U.K.) Ltd)
Aripiprazole 10 mg Abilify 10mg orodispersible tablets sugar-free | 28 tablet PoM £96.04 DT price = £87.05
Aripiprazole 15 mg Abilify 15mg orodispersible tablets sugar-free | 28 tablet PoM £96.04 DT price = £87.05

Oral solution
CAUTIONARY AND ADVISORY LABELS 2
▸ **Aripiprazole (Non-proprietary)**
Aripiprazole 1 mg per 1 ml Aripiprazole 1mg/ml oral solution | 150 ml PoM no price available DT price = £102.90
▸ **Abilify** (Otsuka Pharmaceuticals (U.K.) Ltd)
Aripiprazole 1 mg per 1 ml Abilify 1mg/ml oral solution | 150 ml PoM £102.90 DT price = £102.90

⬏ 230

Clozapine

● **DRUG ACTION** Clozapine is a dopamine D_1, dopamine D_2, 5-HT_{2A}, alpha$_1$-adrenoceptor, and muscarinic-receptor antagonist.

● **INDICATIONS AND DOSE**

Schizophrenia in patients unresponsive to, or intolerant of, conventional antipsychotic drugs
▸ BY MOUTH
▸ Child 12–17 years (under expert supervision): 12.5 mg 1–2 times a day for day 1, then 25–50 mg for day 2, then increased, if tolerated, in steps of 25–50 mg daily, dose to be increased gradually over 14–21 days, increased to up to 300 mg daily in divided doses, larger dose to be taken at night, up to 200 mg daily may be taken as a single dose at bedtime; increased in steps of 50–100 mg 1–2 times a week if required, it is preferable to increase once a week; usual dose 200–450 mg daily, max. 900 mg per day, if restarting after interval of more than 48 hours, 12.5 mg once or twice on first day (but may be feasible to increase more quickly than on initiation)—extreme caution in case of previous respiratory or cardiac arrest with initial dosing

DOSE ADJUSTMENTS DUE TO INTERACTIONS
Dose adjustment may be necessary if smoking started or stopped during treatment.

● **UNLICENSED USE** Not licensed for use in children under 16 years.

● **CONTRA-INDICATIONS** Alcoholic and toxic psychoses · bone-marrow disorders · coma · drug intoxication · history of agranulocytosis · history of circulatory collapse · history of neutropenia · paralytic ileus · severe cardiac disorders (e.g. myocarditis) · severe CNS depression · uncontrolled epilepsy

● **CAUTIONS** Susceptibility to angle-closure glaucoma · taper off other antipsychotics before starting
CAUTIONS, FURTHER INFORMATION
▸ Agranulocytosis Neutropenia and potentially fatal agranulocytosis reported. Leucocyte and differential blood counts must be normal before starting; monitor counts every week for 18 weeks then at least every 2 weeks and if clozapine continued and blood count stable after 1 year at least every 4 weeks (and 4 weeks after discontinuation); if leucocyte count below 3000 /mm^3 or if absolute neutrophil count below 1500 /mm^3 discontinue permanently and refer

to haematologist. Patients who have a low white blood cell count because of benign ethnic neutropenia may be started on clozapine with the agreement of a haematologist. Avoid drugs which depress leucopoiesis; patients should report immediately symptoms of infection, especially influenza-like illness.

▸ **Myocarditis and cardiomyopathy** Fatal myocarditis (most commonly in first 2 months) and cardiomyopathy reported.

Perform physical examination and take full medical history before starting

Specialist examination required if cardiac abnormalities or history of heart disease found—clozapine initiated only in absence of severe heart disease and if benefit outweighs risk

Persistent tachycardia especially in first 2 months should prompt observation for other indicators for myocarditis or cardiomyopathy

If myocarditis or cardiomyopathy suspected clozapine should be stopped and patient evaluated urgently by cardiologist

Discontinue permanently in clozapine-induced myocarditis or cardiomyopathy

▸ **Intestinal obstruction** Impairment of intestinal peristalsis, including constipation, intestinal obstruction, faecal impaction, and paralytic ileus, (including fatal cases) reported. Clozapine should be used with caution in patients receiving drugs that may cause constipation (e.g. antimuscarinic drugs) or in those with a history of colonic disease or lower abdominal surgery. It is essential that constipation is recognised and actively treated.

● **INTERACTIONS** Avoid concomitant use of clozapine with drugs that have a substantial potential for causing agranulocytosis.

● **SIDE-EFFECTS**

▸ **Common or very common** Anorexia · constipation · hypersalivation · malaise · speech disorders · urinary incontinence

▸ **Uncommon** Agranulocytosis

▸ **Rare** Circulatory collapse · dysphagia · hepatitis · myocarditis · pancreatitis · pericarditis · pneumonia · pulmonary aspiration

▸ **Very rare** Cardiomyopathy · hypercholesterolaemia · hypertriglyceridaemia · interstitial nephritis · intestinal obstruction (including fatal cases) · myocardial infarction · obsessive compulsive disorder · parotid gland enlargement · respiratory depression

▸ **Frequency not known** Hepatic disorders · hepatic failure · muscle disorders · renal failure

SIDE-EFFECTS, FURTHER INFORMATION

▸ **Hypersalivation** Hypersalivation associated with clozapine therapy can be treated with hyoscine hydrobromide [unlicensed indication], provided that the patient is not at particular risk from the additive antimuscarinic side-effects of hyoscine and clozapine.

● **PREGNANCY** Use with caution.

● **BREAST FEEDING** Avoid.

● **HEPATIC IMPAIRMENT** Avoid in symptomatic liver disease. Avoid in progressive liver disease. Avoid in hepatic failure. Monitor hepatic function regularly.

● **RENAL IMPAIRMENT** Avoid in severe impairment.

● **MONITORING REQUIREMENTS**

▸ Monitor leucocyte and differential blood counts. Clozapine requires differential white blood cell monitoring weekly for 18 weeks, then fortnightly for up to one year, and then monthly as part of the clozapine patient monitoring service.

▸ Close medical supervision during initiation (risk of collapse because of hypotension and convulsions).

▸ Blood lipids and weight should be measured at baseline, at 3 months (weight should be measured at frequent intervals

during the first 3 months), and then yearly with antipsychotics. Patients taking clozapine require more frequent monitoring of these parameters: every 3 months for the first year, then yearly.

▸ Fasting blood glucose should be measured at baseline, at 4–6 months, and then yearly. Patients taking clozapine should have fasting blood glucose tested at baseline, after one months' treatment, then every 4–6 months.

▸ Patient, prescriber, and supplying pharmacist must be registered with the appropriate Patient Monitoring Service—it takes several days to do this.

● **TREATMENT CESSATION** On planned withdrawal reduce dose over 1–2 weeks to avoid risk of rebound psychosis. If abrupt withdrawal necessary observe patient carefully.

● **DIRECTIONS FOR ADMINISTRATION** Shake oral suspension well for 90 seconds when dispensing or if visibly settled and stand for 24 hours before use; otherwise shake well for 10 seconds before use. May be diluted with water.

● **PRESCRIBING AND DISPENSING INFORMATION** Clozapine has been used for psychosis in Parkinson's disease in children aged 16 years and over.

● **PATIENT AND CARER ADVICE** Patients or carers should be given advice on how to administer clozapine oral suspension.

● **MEDICINAL FORMS**
There can be variation in the licensing of different medicines containing the same drug. Forms available from special-order manufacturers include: oral suspension, oral solution

Tablet
CAUTIONARY AND ADVISORY LABELS 2, 10
▸ **Clozaril** (Novartis Pharmaceuticals UK Ltd)
Clozapine 25 mg Clozaril 25mg tablets | 28 tablet [PoM] £2.95 | 84 tablet [PoM] £6.30 (Hospital only) | 100 tablet [PoM] £7.50 (Hospital only)
Clozapine 100 mg Clozaril 100mg tablets | 28 tablet [PoM] £11.76 | 84 tablet [PoM] £25.21 (Hospital only) | 100 tablet [PoM] £30.01 (Hospital only)
▸ **Denzapine** (Britannia Pharmaceuticals Ltd)
Clozapine 25 mg Denzapine 25mg tablets | 84 tablet [PoM] £16.64 | 100 tablet [PoM] £19.80
Clozapine 100 mg Denzapine 100mg tablets | 84 tablet [PoM] £66.53 | 100 tablet [PoM] £79.20
▸ **Zaponex** (Teva UK Ltd)
Clozapine 25 mg Zaponex 25mg tablets | 84 tablet [PoM] £8.28 | 500 tablet [PoM] £48.39
Clozapine 100 mg Zaponex 100mg tablets | 84 tablet [PoM] £33.88 | 500 tablet [PoM] £196.43

Oral suspension
CAUTIONARY AND ADVISORY LABELS 2, 10
▸ **Denzapine** (Britannia Pharmaceuticals Ltd)
Clozapine 50 mg per 1 ml Denzapine 50mg/ml oral suspension sugar-free | 100 ml [PoM] £39.60

F 230

Olanzapine

● **DRUG ACTION** Olanzapine is a dopamine D_1, D_2, D_4, 5-HT_2, histamine- 1-, and muscarinic-receptor antagonist.

● **INDICATIONS AND DOSE**

Schizophrenia | Combination therapy for mania
▸ BY MOUTH
▸ **Child 12–17 years** (under expert supervision): Initially 5–10 mg daily, adjusted according to response, usual dose 5–20 mg daily, doses greater than 10 mg daily only after reassessment, when one or more factors present that might result in slower metabolism (e.g. female gender, non-smoker) consider lower initial dose and more gradual dose increase; maximum 20 mg per day

Monotherapy for mania
▶ BY MOUTH
▶ Child 12–17 years (under expert supervision): 15 mg daily, adjusted according to response, usual dose 5–20 mg daily, doses greater than 15 mg daily only after reassessment, when one or more factors present that might result in slower metabolism (e.g. female gender, non-smoker) consider lower initial dose and more gradual dose increase; maximum 20 mg per day

DOSE ADJUSTMENTS DUE TO INTERACTIONS
Dose adjustment may be necessary if smoking started or stopped during treatment.

● **UNLICENSED USE** Not licensed for use in children.
● **CAUTIONS** Bone-marrow depression · diabetes mellitus (risk of exacerbation or ketoacidosis) · hypereosinophilic disorders · low leucocyte count · low neutrophil count · myeloproliferative disease · paralytic ileus
● **SIDE-EFFECTS**
▶ **Common or very common** Arthralgia · hypercholesterolaemia · hypertriglyceridaemia · increased appetite · malaise · oedema
▶ **Uncommon** Alopecia · amnesia · bradycardia · epistaxis
▶ **Rare** Hepatitis · pancreatitis · rhabdomyolysis
● **PREGNANCY** Use only if potential benefit outweighs risk; neonatal lethargy, tremor, and hypertonia reported when used in third trimester.
● **BREAST FEEDING** Avoid—present in milk.
● **HEPATIC IMPAIRMENT** Consider initial dose of 5 mg daily.
● **RENAL IMPAIRMENT** Consider initial dose of 5 mg daily.
● **MONITORING REQUIREMENTS**
▶ Blood lipids and weight should be measured at baseline, at 3 months (weight should be measured at frequent intervals during the first 3 months), and then yearly with antipsychotic drugs. Patients taking olanzapine require more frequent monitoring of these parameters: every 3 months for the first year, then yearly.
▶ Fasting blood glucose should be measured at baseline, at 4–6 months, and then yearly. Patients taking olanzapine should have fasting blood glucose tested at baseline, after one months' treatment, then every 4–6 months.
● **DIRECTIONS FOR ADMINISTRATION** Olanzapine orodispersible tablet may be placed on the tongue and allowed to dissolve, or dispersed in water, orange juice, apple juice, milk, or coffee.
● **PATIENT AND CARER ADVICE**
Patients or carers should be given advice on how to administer orodispersible tablets.

Medicines for Children leaflet: Olanzapine for schizophrenia, bipolar disorder, mania and agitation www.medicinesforchildren. org.uk/olanzapine-schizophrenia-bipolar-disorder-mania-and-agitation

● **MEDICINAL FORMS**
There can be variation in the licensing of different medicines containing the same drug. Forms available from special-order manufacturers include: oral suspension, oral solution

Tablet
CAUTIONARY AND ADVISORY LABELS 2
▶ Olanzapine (Non-proprietary)
Olanzapine 2.5 mg Olanzapine 2.5mg tablets | 28 tablet PoM £21.85 DT price = £0.86
Olanzapine 5 mg Olanzapine 5mg tablets | 28 tablet PoM £43.70 DT price = £0.94
Olanzapine 7.5 mg Olanzapine 7.5mg tablets | 28 tablet PoM £65.55 DT price = £1.11 | 56 tablet PoM £131.10
Olanzapine 10 mg Olanzapine 10mg tablets | 28 tablet PoM £87.40 DT price = £1.13
Olanzapine 15 mg Olanzapine 15mg tablets | 28 tablet PoM £119.18 DT price = £1.31
Olanzapine 20 mg Olanzapine 20mg tablets | 28 tablet PoM £158.90 DT price = £1.53

▶ Zalasta (Consilient Health Ltd)
Olanzapine 2.5 mg Zalasta 2.5mg tablets | 28 tablet PoM £18.57 DT price = £0.86
Olanzapine 5 mg Zalasta 5mg tablets | 28 tablet PoM £37.14 DT price = £0.94
Olanzapine 7.5 mg Zalasta 7.5mg tablets | 56 tablet PoM £111.43
Olanzapine 10 mg Zalasta 10mg tablets | 28 tablet PoM £74.29 DT price = £1.13
Olanzapine 15 mg Zalasta 15mg tablets | 28 tablet PoM £101.30 DT price = £1.31
Olanzapine 20 mg Zalasta 20mg tablets | 28 tablet PoM £135.06 DT price = £1.53
▶ Zyprexa (Eli Lilly and Company Ltd)
Olanzapine 2.5 mg Zyprexa 2.5mg tablets | 28 tablet PoM £21.85 DT price = £0.86
Olanzapine 5 mg Zyprexa 5mg tablets | 28 tablet PoM £43.70 DT price = £0.94
Olanzapine 7.5 mg Zyprexa 7.5mg tablets | 56 tablet PoM £131.10
Olanzapine 10 mg Zyprexa 10mg tablets | 28 tablet PoM £87.40 DT price = £1.13
Olanzapine 15 mg Zyprexa 15mg tablets | 28 tablet PoM £119.18 DT price = £1.31
Olanzapine 20 mg Zyprexa 20mg tablets | 28 tablet PoM £158.90 DT price = £1.53

Orodispersible tablet
CAUTIONARY AND ADVISORY LABELS 2
EXCIPIENTS: May contain Aspartame
▶ Olanzapine (Non-proprietary)
Olanzapine 5 mg Olanzapine 5mg orodispersible tablets sugar free sugar-free | 28 tablet PoM £40.86 DT price = £1.79
Olanzapine 5mg orodispersible tablets | 28 tablet PoM £4.99 DT price = £2.54
Olanzapine 10 mg Olanzapine 10mg orodispersible tablets | 28 tablet PoM £5.99 DT price = £2.81
Olanzapine 10mg orodispersible tablets sugar free sugar-free | 28 tablet PoM £74.29 DT price = £2.41
Olanzapine 15 mg Olanzapine 15mg orodispersible tablets sugar free sugar-free | 28 tablet PoM £111.44 DT price = £2.99
Olanzapine 15mg orodispersible tablets | 28 tablet PoM £6.99 DT price = £3.20
Olanzapine 20 mg Olanzapine 20mg orodispersible tablets sugar free sugar-free | 28 tablet PoM £148.57 DT price = £4.46
Olanzapine 20mg orodispersible tablets | 28 tablet PoM £7.99 DT price = £4.32
▶ Arkolamyl (Mylan Ltd)
Olanzapine 5 mg Arkolamyl 5mg orodispersible tablets sugar-free | 28 tablet PoM £48.07 DT price = £1.79
Olanzapine 10 mg Arkolamyl 10mg orodispersible tablets sugar-free | 28 tablet PoM £87.40 DT price = £2.41
Olanzapine 15 mg Arkolamyl 15mg orodispersible tablets sugar-free | 28 tablet PoM £131.10 DT price = £2.99
Olanzapine 20 mg Arkolamyl 20mg orodispersible tablets sugar-free | 28 tablet PoM £174.79 DT price = £4.46
▶ Zalasta (Consilient Health Ltd)
Olanzapine 5 mg Zalasta 5mg orodispersible tablets sugar-free | 28 tablet PoM £40.85 DT price = £1.79
Olanzapine 10 mg Zalasta 10mg orodispersible tablets sugar-free | 28 tablet PoM £74.29 DT price = £2.41
Olanzapine 15 mg Zalasta 15mg orodispersible tablets sugar-free | 28 tablet PoM £111.43 DT price = £2.99
Olanzapine 20 mg Zalasta 20mg orodispersible tablets sugar-free | 28 tablet PoM £148.57 DT price = £4.46

Oral lyophilisate
▶ Zyprexa Velotabs (Eli Lilly and Company Ltd)
Olanzapine 5 mg Zyprexa 5mg Velotabs sugar-free | 28 tablet PoM £48.07 DT price = £48.07
Olanzapine 10 mg Zyprexa 10mg Velotabs sugar-free | 28 tablet PoM £87.40 DT price = £87.40
Olanzapine 15 mg Zyprexa 15mg Velotabs sugar-free | 28 tablet PoM £131.10 DT price = £131.10
Olanzapine 20 mg Zyprexa 20mg Velotabs sugar-free | 28 tablet PoM £174.79 DT price = £174.79

Nervous system

4

Quetiapine

F 230

- **DRUG ACTION** Quetiapine is a dopamine D_1, dopamine D_2, 5-HT_2, alpha$_1$-adrenoceptor, and histamine-1 receptor antagonist.

- **INDICATIONS AND DOSE**

Schizophrenia
▶ BY MOUTH USING IMMEDIATE-RELEASE MEDICINES
▶ Child 12–17 years (under expert supervision): Initially 25 mg twice daily, adjusted according to response. adjusted in steps of 25–50 mg; maximum 750 mg per day
▶ BY MOUTH USING MODIFIED-RELEASE MEDICINES
▶ Child 12–17 years (under expert supervision): Initially 50 mg once daily, adjusted according to response. adjusted in steps of 50 mg daily, usual dose 400–800 mg once daily; maximum 800 mg per day

Treatment of mania in bipolar disorder
▶ BY MOUTH USING IMMEDIATE-RELEASE MEDICINES
▶ Child 12–17 years (under expert supervision): 25 mg twice daily for day 1, then 50 mg twice daily for day 2, then 100 mg twice daily for day 3, then 150 mg twice daily for day 4, then 200 mg twice daily for day 5, then adjusted in steps of up to 100 mg daily, adjusted according to response, usual dose 400–600 mg daily in 2 divided doses

DOSE EQUIVALENCE AND CONVERSION
Patients can be switched from immediate-release to modified-release tablets at the equivalent daily dose; to maintain clinical response, dose titration may be required.

- **UNLICENSED USE** Not licensed for use in children.

- **CAUTIONS** Cerebrovascular disease · patients at risk of aspiration pneumonia · treatment of depression in patients under 25 years (increased risk of suicide)

- **SIDE-EFFECTS**
▶ **Common or very common** Asthenia · dysarthria · dyspnoea · elevated plasma-cholesterol concentrations · elevated plasma-triglyceride concentrations · increased appetite · irritability · peripheral oedema · sleep disorders
▶ **Uncommon** Hyponatraemia · hypothyroidism · restless legs syndrome · rhinitis
▶ **Rare** Hepatitis · pancreatitis
▶ **Very rare** Angioedema · inappropriate secretion of antidiuretic hormone · rhabdomyolysis · Stevens-Johnson syndrome
▶ **Frequency not known** Suicidal behaviour (particularly on initiation) · toxic epidermal necrolysis

- **PREGNANCY** Use only if potential benefit outweighs risk.

- **BREAST FEEDING** Manufacturer advises avoid.

- **HEPATIC IMPAIRMENT** For *immediate-release tablets*, initially 25 mg daily, increased daily in steps of 25–50 mg. For *modified-release tablets*, initially 50 mg daily, increased daily in steps of 50 mg.

- **MEDICINAL FORMS**
There can be variation in the licensing of different medicines containing the same drug. Forms available from special-order manufacturers include: oral suspension, oral solution

Tablet
CAUTIONARY AND ADVISORY LABELS 2
▶ Quetiapine (Non-proprietary)
Quetiapine (as Quetiapine fumarate) **25 mg** Quetiapine 25mg tablets | 60 tablet PoM £38.05 DT price = £1.11
Quetiapine (as Quetiapine fumarate) **100 mg** Quetiapine 100mg tablets | 60 tablet PoM £107.45 DT price = £1.79
Quetiapine (as Quetiapine fumarate) **150 mg** Quetiapine 150mg tablets | 60 tablet PoM £107.45 DT price = £2.27
Quetiapine (as Quetiapine fumarate) **200 mg** Quetiapine 200mg tablets | 60 tablet PoM £107.45 DT price = £2.50

Quetiapine (as Quetiapine fumarate) **300 mg** Quetiapine 300mg tablets | 60 tablet PoM £170.00 DT price = £3.20
▶ Seroquel (AstraZeneca UK Ltd)
Quetiapine (as Quetiapine fumarate) **25 mg** Seroquel 25mg tablets | 60 tablet PoM £40.50 DT price = £1.11
Quetiapine (as Quetiapine fumarate) **100 mg** Seroquel 100mg tablets | 60 tablet PoM £113.10 DT price = £1.79
Quetiapine (as Quetiapine fumarate) **200 mg** Seroquel 200mg tablets | 60 tablet PoM £113.10 DT price = £2.50
Quetiapine (as Quetiapine fumarate) **300 mg** Seroquel 300mg tablets | 60 tablet PoM £170.00 DT price = £3.20

Modified-release tablet
CAUTIONARY AND ADVISORY LABELS 2, 23, 25
▶ Atrolak XL (Accord Healthcare Ltd)
Quetiapine (as Quetiapine fumarate) **50 mg** Atrolak XL 50mg tablets | 60 tablet PoM £67.65 DT price = £67.66
Quetiapine (as Quetiapine fumarate) **200 mg** Atrolak XL 200mg tablets | 60 tablet PoM £113.09 DT price = £113.10
Quetiapine (as Quetiapine fumarate) **300 mg** Atrolak XL 300mg tablets | 60 tablet PoM £169.99 DT price = £170.00
Quetiapine (as Quetiapine fumarate) **400 mg** Atrolak XL 400mg tablets | 60 tablet PoM £226.19 DT price = £226.20
▶ Biquelle XL (Aspire Pharma Ltd)
Quetiapine (as Quetiapine fumarate) **50 mg** Biquelle XL 50mg tablets | 60 tablet PoM £29.45 DT price = £67.66
Quetiapine (as Quetiapine fumarate) **150 mg** Biquelle XL 150mg tablets | 60 tablet PoM £49.45 DT price = £113.10
Quetiapine (as Quetiapine fumarate) **200 mg** Biquelle XL 200mg tablets | 60 tablet PoM £49.45 DT price = £113.10
Quetiapine (as Quetiapine fumarate) **300 mg** Biquelle XL 300mg tablets | 60 tablet PoM £74.45 DT price = £170.00
Quetiapine (as Quetiapine fumarate) **400 mg** Biquelle XL 400mg tablets | 60 tablet PoM £98.95 DT price = £226.20
▶ Ebesque XL (DB Ashbourne Ltd)
Quetiapine (as Quetiapine fumarate) **50 mg** Ebesque XL 50mg tablets | 60 tablet PoM £31.80 DT price = £67.66
Quetiapine (as Quetiapine fumarate) **200 mg** Ebesque XL 200mg tablets | 60 tablet PoM £53.16 DT price = £113.10
Quetiapine (as Quetiapine fumarate) **300 mg** Ebesque XL 300mg tablets | 60 tablet PoM £79.90 DT price = £170.00
Quetiapine (as Quetiapine fumarate) **400 mg** Ebesque XL 400mg tablets | 60 tablet PoM £106.31 DT price = £226.20
▶ Mintreleq XL (CEB Pharma Ltd)
Quetiapine (as Quetiapine fumarate) **50 mg** Mintreleq XL 50mg tablets | 60 tablet PoM £29.45 DT price = £67.66
Quetiapine (as Quetiapine fumarate) **150 mg** Mintreleq XL 150mg tablets | 60 tablet PoM £49.45 DT price = £113.10
Quetiapine (as Quetiapine fumarate) **200 mg** Mintreleq XL 200mg tablets | 60 tablet PoM £49.45 DT price = £113.10
Quetiapine (as Quetiapine fumarate) **300 mg** Mintreleq XL 300mg tablets | 60 tablet PoM £74.45 DT price = £170.00
Quetiapine (as Quetiapine fumarate) **400 mg** Mintreleq XL 400mg tablets | 60 tablet PoM £98.95 DT price = £226.20
▶ Psyquet XL (Sandoz Ltd)
Quetiapine (as Quetiapine fumarate) **50 mg** Psyquet XL 50mg tablets | 60 tablet PoM £27.97 DT price = £67.66
Quetiapine (as Quetiapine fumarate) **150 mg** Psyquet XL 150mg tablets | 60 tablet PoM £46.97 DT price = £113.10
Quetiapine (as Quetiapine fumarate) **200 mg** Psyquet XL 200mg tablets | 60 tablet PoM £46.97 DT price = £113.10
Quetiapine (as Quetiapine fumarate) **300 mg** Psyquet XL 300mg tablets | 60 tablet PoM £70.72 DT price = £170.00
Quetiapine (as Quetiapine fumarate) **400 mg** Psyquet XL 400mg tablets | 60 tablet PoM £93.99 DT price = £226.20
▶ Seroquel XL (AstraZeneca UK Ltd)
Quetiapine (as Quetiapine fumarate) **50 mg** Seroquel XL 50mg tablets | 60 tablet PoM £67.66 DT price = £67.66
Quetiapine (as Quetiapine fumarate) **150 mg** Seroquel XL 150mg tablets | 60 tablet PoM £113.10 DT price = £113.10
Quetiapine (as Quetiapine fumarate) **200 mg** Seroquel XL 200mg tablets | 60 tablet PoM £113.10 DT price = £113.10
Quetiapine (as Quetiapine fumarate) **300 mg** Seroquel XL 300mg tablets | 60 tablet PoM £170.00 DT price = £170.00
Quetiapine (as Quetiapine fumarate) **400 mg** Seroquel XL 400mg tablets | 60 tablet PoM £226.20 DT price = £226.20
▶ Sondate XL (Teva UK Ltd)
Quetiapine (as Quetiapine fumarate) **50 mg** Sondate XL 50mg tablets | 60 tablet PoM £25.16 DT price = £67.66
Quetiapine (as Quetiapine fumarate) **150 mg** Sondate XL 150mg tablets | 60 tablet PoM £46.95 DT price = £113.10

Quetiapine (as Quetiapine fumarate) 200 mg Sondate XL 200mg
tablets | 60 tablet [PoM] £42.26 DT price = £113.10

Quetiapine (as Quetiapine fumarate) 300 mg Sondate XL 300mg
tablets | 60 tablet [PoM] £63.64 DT price = £170.00

Quetiapine (as Quetiapine fumarate) 400 mg Sondate XL 400mg
tablets | 60 tablet [PoM] £84.58 DT price = £226.20

▸ **Tenprolide XL** (Actavis UK Ltd)

Quetiapine (as Quetiapine fumarate) 50 mg Tenprolide XL 50mg
tablets | 60 tablet [PoM] £67.66 DT price = £67.66

Quetiapine (as Quetiapine fumarate) 200 mg Tenprolide XL
200mg tablets | 60 tablet [PoM] £113.10 DT price = £113.10

Quetiapine (as Quetiapine fumarate) 300 mg Tenprolide XL
300mg tablets | 60 tablet [PoM] £170.00 DT price = £170.00

Quetiapine (as Quetiapine fumarate) 400 mg Tenprolide XL
400mg tablets | 60 tablet [PoM] £226.20 DT price = £226.20

▸ **Zaluron XL** (Fontus Health Ltd)

Quetiapine (as Quetiapine fumarate) 50 mg Zaluron XL 50mg
tablets | 60 tablet [PoM] £27.96 DT price = £67.66

Quetiapine (as Quetiapine fumarate) 150 mg Zaluron XL 150mg
tablets | 60 tablet [PoM] £46.96 DT price = £113.10

Quetiapine (as Quetiapine fumarate) 200 mg Zaluron XL 200mg
tablets | 60 tablet [PoM] £46.96 DT price = £113.10

Quetiapine (as Quetiapine fumarate) 300 mg Zaluron XL 300mg
tablets | 60 tablet [PoM] £70.71 DT price = £170.00

Quetiapine (as Quetiapine fumarate) 400 mg Zaluron XL 400mg
tablets | 60 tablet [PoM] £93.98 DT price = £226.20

📑 230

Risperidone

● **DRUG ACTION** Risperidone is a dopamine D_2, 5-HT_{2A},
alpha$_1$-adrenoceptor, and histamine-1 receptor
antagonist.

● **INDICATIONS AND DOSE**

Acute and chronic psychosis

▸ BY MOUTH

▸ Child 12–17 years (under expert supervision): 2 mg daily in
1–2 divided doses for day 1, then 4 mg daily in
1–2 divided doses for day 2, slower titration is
appropriate in some patients; usual dose 4–6 mg daily,
doses above 10 mg daily only if benefit considered to
outweigh risk; maximum 16 mg per day

**Short-term monotherapy of mania in bipolar disorder
(under expert supervision)**

▸ BY MOUTH

▸ Child 12–17 years: Initially 500 micrograms once daily,
then adjusted in steps of 0.5–1 mg daily, adjusted
according to response; usual dose 2.5 mg daily in
1–2 divided doses; maximum 6 mg per day

**Short-term treatment (up to 6 weeks) of persistent
aggression in conduct disorder (under expert
supervision)**

▸ BY MOUTH

▸ Child 5–17 years (body-weight up to 50 kg): Initially
250 micrograms once daily, then increased in steps of
250 micrograms once daily on alternate days, adjusted
according to response; usual dose 500 micrograms
once daily; maximum 750 micrograms per day

▸ Child 5–17 years (body-weight 50 kg and above): Initially
500 micrograms once daily, then increased in steps of
500 micrograms once daily on alternate days, adjusted
according to response; usual dose 1 mg once daily;
maximum 1.5 mg per day

**Short-term treatment of severe aggression in autism
(under expert supervision)**

▸ BY MOUTH

▸ Child 5–17 years (body-weight 15–20 kg): Initially
250 micrograms daily for at least 4 days, then increased
if necessary to 500 micrograms daily, then increased in
steps of 250 micrograms daily, dose to be increased at
intervals of 2 weeks, review effectiveness and any side-
effects after 3–4 weeks; stop if no response at 6 weeks;
maximum 1 mg per day

▸ Child 5–17 years (body-weight 20–45 kg): Initially
500 micrograms daily for at least 4 days, then increased
if necessary to 1 mg daily, then increased in steps of
500 micrograms daily, dose to be increased at intervals
of 2 weeks, review effectiveness and any side-effects
after 3–4 weeks; stop if no response at 6 weeks;
maximum 2.5 mg per day

▸ Child 5–17 years (body-weight 45 kg and above): Initially
500 micrograms daily for at least 4 days, then increased
if necessary to 1 mg daily, then increased in steps of
500 micrograms daily, dose to be increased at intervals
of 2 weeks, review effectiveness and any side-effects
after 3–4 weeks; stop if no response at 6 weeks;
maximum 3 mg per day

● **UNLICENSED USE** Not licensed for use in children for
psychosis, mania, or autism.

● **CAUTIONS** Avoid in Acute porphyrias p. 562 · cataract
surgery (risk of intra-operative floppy iris syndrome) ·
dehydration · family history of sudden cardiac death
(perform ECG) · prolactin-dependent tumours

● **SIDE-EFFECTS**

▸ **Common or very common** Anxiety · appetite changes ·
arthralgia · depression · epistaxis · hypertension · infection
· malaise · myalgia · oedema · respiratory disorders · sleep
disorders · toothache · urinary disorders

▸ **Uncommon** Alopecia · elevated plasma-cholesterol
concentrations · elevated plasma-triglyceride
concentrations · hypoaesthesia · paraesthesia · taste
disturbances · tinnitus · visual disorders

▸ **Rare** Inappropriate antidiuretic hormone secretion ·
intestinal obstruction · intra-operative floppy iris
syndrome · pancreatitis · pulmonary embolism ·
rhabdomyolysis

● **PREGNANCY** Use only if potential benefit outweighs risk.

● **BREAST FEEDING** Use only if potential benefit outweighs
risk—small amount present in milk.

● **HEPATIC IMPAIRMENT**

▸ With oral use Initial and subsequent oral doses should be
halved.

● **RENAL IMPAIRMENT** Initial and subsequent oral doses
should be halved.

● **DIRECTIONS FOR ADMINISTRATION**

▸ With oral use Orodispersible tablets should be placed on the
tongue, allowed to dissolve and swallowed. Oral liquid may
be diluted with any non-alcoholic drink, except tea.

● **PATIENT AND CARER ADVICE**
Medicines for Children leaflet: Risperidone for psychological
disorders www.medicinesforchildren.org.uk/risperidone-for-
psychological-disorders

▸ With oral use Patients or carers should be given advice on
how to administer risperidone orodispersible tablets and
oral liquid (counselling on use of dose syringe advised).

● **MEDICINAL FORMS**
There can be variation in the licensing of different medicines
containing the same drug. Forms available from special-order
manufacturers include: oral solution

Tablet

CAUTIONARY AND ADVISORY LABELS 2

▸ Risperidone (Non-proprietary)

Risperidone 500 microgram Risperidone 500microgram tablets |
20 tablet [PoM] £6.18 DT price = £0.82

Risperidone 1 mg Risperidone 1mg tablets | 20 tablet [PoM] £1.02
DT price = £0.81 | 60 tablet [PoM] £25.07

Risperidone 2 mg Risperidone 2mg tablets | 60 tablet [PoM] £60.10
DT price = £1.37

Risperidone 3 mg Risperidone 3mg tablets | 60 tablet [PoM] £88.38
DT price = £1.67

Risperidone 4 mg Risperidone 4mg tablets | 60 tablet [PoM]
£116.67 DT price = £1.94

Risperidone 6 mg Risperidone 6mg tablets | 28 tablet [PoM] £82.50
DT price = £3.86 | 60 tablet [PoM] no price available

▸ **Risperdal** (Janssen-Cilag Ltd)
Risperdal 500 microgram Risperdal 500microgram tablets | 20 tablet [PoM] £5.08 DT price = £0.82
Risperdal 1 mg Risperdal 1mg tablets | 20 tablet [PoM] £8.36 DT price = £0.81 | 60 tablet [PoM] £17.56
Risperdal 2 mg Risperdal 2mg tablets | 60 tablet [PoM] £34.62 DT price = £1.37
Risperdal 3 mg Risperdal 3mg tablets | 60 tablet [PoM] £50.91 DT price = £1.67
Risperdal 4 mg Risperdal 4mg tablets | 60 tablet [PoM] £67.20 DT price = £1.94
Risperdal 6 mg Risperdal 6mg tablets | 28 tablet [PoM] £67.88 DT price = £3.86

Orodispersible tablet
CAUTIONARY AND ADVISORY LABELS 2
EXCIPIENTS: May contain Aspartame
▸ **Risperidone** (Non-proprietary)
Risperidone 500 microgram Risperidone 500microgram orodispersible tablets sugar free sugar-free | 28 tablet [PoM] £23.88 DT price = £23.86
Risperidone 1 mg Risperidone 1mg orodispersible tablets sugar free sugar-free | 28 tablet [PoM] £21.09 DT price = £21.07
Risperidone 2 mg Risperidone 2mg orodispersible tablets sugar free sugar-free | 28 tablet [PoM] £38.79 DT price = £38.77
Risperidone 3 mg Risperidone 3mg orodispersible tablets sugar free sugar-free | 28 tablet [PoM] £33.50 DT price = £33.50
Risperidone 4 mg Risperidone 4mg orodispersible tablets sugar free sugar-free | 28 tablet [PoM] £37.95 DT price = £37.95
▸ **Risperdal Quicklet** (Janssen-Cilag Ltd)
Risperidone 500 microgram Risperdal Quicklet 500microgram orodispersible tablets sugar-free | 28 tablet [PoM] £8.23 DT price = £23.86
Risperidone 1 mg Risperdal Quicklet 1mg orodispersible tablets sugar-free | 28 tablet [PoM] £13.86 DT price = £21.07
Risperidone 2 mg Risperdal Quicklet 2mg orodispersible tablets sugar-free | 28 tablet [PoM] £26.12 DT price = £38.77
Risperidone 3 mg Risperdal Quicklet 3mg orodispersible tablets sugar-free | 28 tablet [PoM] £28.99 DT price = £33.50
Risperidone 4 mg Risperdal Quicklet 4mg orodispersible tablets sugar-free | 28 tablet [PoM] £37.34 DT price = £37.95

Oral solution
CAUTIONARY AND ADVISORY LABELS 2
▸ **Risperidone** (Non-proprietary)
Risperidone 1 mg per 1 ml Risperidone 1mg/ml oral solution sugar free sugar-free | 100 ml [PoM] £61.15 DT price = £4.49
▸ **Risperdal** (Janssen-Cilag Ltd)
Risperdal 1 mg per 1 ml Risperdal 1mg/ml oral solution sugar-free | 100 ml [PoM] £37.01 DT price = £4.49

3 Movement disorders

3.1 Dystonias and other involuntary movements

Dystonias and related disorders

Dystonias

Dystonias may result from conditions such as cerebral palsy or may be related to a deficiency of the neurotransmitter dopamine as in Segawa syndrome.

Dopaminergic drugs used in dystonias

Levodopa, the amino-acid precursor of dopamine, acts by replenishing depleted striatal dopamine. It is given with an extracerebral **dopa-decarboxylase inhibitor**, which reduces the peripheral conversion of levodopa to dopamine, thereby limiting side-effects such as nausea, vomiting, and cardiovascular effects; additionally, effective brain-dopamine concentrations are achieved with lower doses of levodopa. The extracerebral dopa-decarboxylase inhibitor most commonly used in children is carbidopa (in co-careldopa p. 242).

Levodopa therapy should be initiated at a low dose and increased in small steps; the final dose should be as low as possible. Intervals between doses should be chosen to suit the needs of the individual child.

In severe dystonias related to cerebral palsy, improvement can be expected within 2 weeks. Children with Segawa syndrome are particularly sensitive to levodopa; they may even become symptom free on small doses. Levodopa also has a role in treating metabolic disorders such as defects in tetrahydrobiopterin synthesis and dihydrobiopterin reductase deficiency. Tetrahydrobiopterin may have a role in metabolic disorders.

Children may experience nausea within 2 hours of taking a dose; nausea and vomiting with co-careldopa is rarely dose-limiting.

In dystonic cerebral palsy, treatment with larger doses of levodopa is associated with the development of potentially troublesome motor complications (including response fluctuations and dyskinesias). Response fluctuations are characterised by large variations in motor performance, with normal function during the 'on' period, and weakness and restricted mobility during the 'off' period.

Antimuscarinic drugs used in dystonias

The antimuscarinic drugs procyclidine hydrochloride p. 241 and trihexyphenidyl hydrochloride p. 241 reduce the symptoms of dystonias, including those induced by antipsychotic drugs; there is no justification for giving them routinely in the absence of dystonic symptoms. Tardive dyskinesia is not improved by antimuscarinic drugs and may be made worse.

There are no important differences between the antimuscarinic drugs, but some children tolerate one better than another.

Procyclidine hydrochloride can be given parenterally and is effective emergency treatment for acute drug-induced dystonic reactions.

If treatment with an antimuscarinic is ineffective, intravenous diazepam p. 207 can be given for life-threatening acute drug-induced dystonic reactions.

Drugs used in essential tremor, chorea, tics, and related disorders

Haloperidol p. 231 can also improve motor tics and symptoms of Tourette syndrome and related choreas. Other treatments for Tourette syndrome include pimozide p. 232 [unlicensed indication] (**important**: ECG monitoring required), and sulpiride p. 233 [unlicensed indication].

Propranolol hydrochloride p. 96 or another beta-adrenoceptor blocking drug may be useful in treating essential tremor or tremor associated with anxiety or thyrotoxicosis.

Botulinum toxin type A p. 243 should be used under specialist supervision. Treatment with botulinum toxin type A can be considered after an acquired non-progressive brain injury if rapid-onset spasticity causes postural or functional difficulties, and in children with spasticity in whom focal dystonia causes postural or functional difficulties or pain.

> **Drugs used for Dystonias and other involuntary movements not listed below** Trifluoperazine, p. 233

ANTIMUSCARINICS

Procyclidine hydrochloride

- **DRUG ACTION** Procyclidine exerts its antiparkinsonian action by reducing the effects of the relative central cholinergic excess that occurs as a result of dopamine deficiency.

- **INDICATIONS AND DOSE**

Acute dystonia
- ▸ BY INTRAMUSCULAR INJECTION, OR BY INTRAVENOUS INJECTION
- ▸ Child 1 month-1 year: 0.5–2 mg for 1 dose, dose usually effective in 5–10 minutes but may need 30 minutes for relief
- ▸ Child 2-9 years: 2–5 mg for 1 dose, dose usually effective in 5–10 minutes but may need 30 minutes for relief
- ▸ Child 10-17 years: 5–10 mg, occasionally, more than 10 mg, dose usually effective in 5–10 minutes but may need 30 minutes for relief

Dystonia
- ▸ BY MOUTH
- ▸ Child 7-11 years: 1.25 mg 3 times a day
- ▸ Child 12-17 years: 2.5 mg 3 times a day

- **UNLICENSED USE** Not licensed for use in children.

- **CONTRA-INDICATIONS** Gastro-intestinal obstruction · myasthenia gravis

- **CAUTIONS** Cardiovascular disease · hypertension · liable to abuse · psychotic disorders · pyrexia · those susceptible to angle-closure glaucoma

- **INTERACTIONS** → Appendix 1 (antimuscarinics). Many drugs have antimuscarinic effects; concomitant use of two or more such drugs can increase side-effects such as dry mouth, urine retention, and constipation.

- **SIDE-EFFECTS** Angle-closure glaucoma · anxiety · blurred vision · confusion · constipation · dizziness · dry mouth · euphoria · gingivitis · hallucinations · impaired memory · nausea · rash · restlessness · tachycardia · urinary retention · vomiting

- **PREGNANCY** Use only if potential benefit outweighs risk.

- **BREAST FEEDING** No information available.

- **HEPATIC IMPAIRMENT** Use with caution.

- **RENAL IMPAIRMENT** Use with caution.

- **TREATMENT CESSATION** Avoid abrupt withdrawal in patients taking long-term treatment.

- **PATIENT AND CARER ADVICE**

Driving and skilled tasks
May affect performance of skilled tasks (e.g. driving).

- **MEDICINAL FORMS**
There can be variation in the licensing of different medicines containing the same drug. Forms available from special-order manufacturers include: oral suspension, oral solution

Tablet
- ▸ Procyclidine hydrochloride (Non-proprietary)
  Procyclidine hydrochloride 5 mg Procyclidine 5mg tablets | 28 tablet [PoM] £17.25 DT price = £11.97 | 100 tablet [PoM] £50.00 | 500 tablet [PoM] £255.00
- ▸ Kemadrin (Aspen Pharma Trading Ltd)
  Procyclidine hydrochloride 5 mg Kemadrin 5mg tablets | 100 tablet [PoM] £4.72 | 500 tablet [PoM] £23.62

Oral solution
- ▸ Procyclidine hydrochloride (Non-proprietary)
  Procyclidine hydrochloride 500 microgram per 1 ml Procyclidine 2.5mg/5ml oral solution sugar free sugar-free | 150 ml [PoM] £6.22 DT price = £4.22
  Procyclidine hydrochloride 1 mg per 1 ml Procyclidine 5mg/5ml oral solution sugar free sugar-free | 150 ml [PoM] £11.54 DT price = £7.54

- ▸ Arpicolin (Rosemont Pharmaceuticals Ltd)
  Procyclidine hydrochloride 500 microgram per 1 ml Arpicolin 2.5mg/5ml oral solution sugar-free | 150 ml [PoM] £4.22 DT price = £4.22
  Procyclidine hydrochloride 1 mg per 1 ml Arpicolin 5mg/5ml oral solution sugar-free | 150 ml [PoM] £7.54 DT price = £7.54

Solution for injection
- ▸ Procyclidine hydrochloride (Non-proprietary)
  Procyclidine hydrochloride 5 mg per 1 ml Procyclidine 10mg/2ml solution for injection ampoules | 5 ampoule [PoM] £60.00–£78.75 DT price = £72.18

Trihexyphenidyl hydrochloride

(Benzhexol hydrochloride)

- **DRUG ACTION** Trihexyphenidyl exerts its effects by reducing the effects of the relative central cholinergic excess that occurs as a result of dopamine deficiency.

- **INDICATIONS AND DOSE**

Dystonia
- ▸ BY MOUTH
- ▸ Child 3 months-17 years: Initially 1–2 mg daily in 1–2 divided doses, then increased in steps of 1 mg every 3–7 days, dose to be adjusted according to response and side-effects; maximum 2 mg/kg per day

- **UNLICENSED USE** Not licensed for use in children.

- **CONTRA-INDICATIONS** Gastro-intestinal obstruction · myasthenia gravis

- **CAUTIONS** Cardiovascular disease · hypertension · liable to abuse · psychotic disorders · pyrexia · those susceptible to angle-closure glaucoma

- **INTERACTIONS** → Appendix 1 (antimuscarinics). Many drugs have antimuscarinic effects; concomitant use of two or more such drugs can increase side-effects such as dry mouth, urine retention, and constipation.

- **SIDE-EFFECTS**
- ▸ Very rare Angle-closure glaucoma
- ▸ Frequency not known Anxiety · blurred vision · confusion · constipation · dizziness · dry mouth · euphoria · hallucinations · impaired memory · nausea · rash · restlessness · tachycardia · urinary retention · vomiting

- **PREGNANCY** Use only if potential benefit outweighs risk.

- **BREAST FEEDING** Avoid.

- **HEPATIC IMPAIRMENT** Use with caution.

- **RENAL IMPAIRMENT** Use with caution.

- **TREATMENT CESSATION** Avoid abrupt withdrawal in patients taking long-term treatment.

- **DIRECTIONS FOR ADMINISTRATION** Tablets should be taken with or after food.

- **PATIENT AND CARER ADVICE**

Driving and skilled tasks
May affect performance of skilled tasks (e.g. driving). Medicines for Children leaflet: Trihexyphenidyl hydrochloride for dystonia www.medicinesforchildren.org.uk/trihexyphenidyl-hydrochloride-for-dystonia

- **MEDICINAL FORMS**
There can be variation in the licensing of different medicines containing the same drug. Forms available from special-order manufacturers include: oral suspension, oral solution

Tablet
- ▸ Trihexyphenidyl hydrochloride (Non-proprietary)
  Trihexyphenidyl hydrochloride 2 mg Trihexyphenidyl 2mg tablets | 84 tablet [PoM] £11.80 DT price = £5.51
  Trihexyphenidyl hydrochloride 5 mg Trihexyphenidyl 5mg tablets | 84 tablet [PoM] £17.91 DT price = £17.91

4

Nervous system

Oral solution

EXCIPIENTS: May contain Propylene glycol

▸ **Trihexyphenidyl hydrochloride (Non-proprietary)**
Trihexyphenidyl hydrochloride 1 mg per 1 ml Trihexyphenidyl 5mg/5ml oral solution | 200 ml [PoM] £20.00–£24.00 DT price = £20.00

DOPAMINERGIC DRUGS ❯ DOPAMINE PRECURSORS

Co-careldopa

- **INDICATIONS AND DOSE**

Dopamine-sensitive dystonias including Segawa syndrome and dystonias related to cerebral palsy (dose expressed as levodopa)

▸ BY MOUTH

▸ Child 3 months-17 years: Initially 250 micrograms/kg 2–3 times a day, dose to be increased according to response every 2–3 days, increased if necessary up to 1 mg/kg 3 times a day, preparation containing 1:4 ratio of carbidopa:levodopa is to be used

Treatment of defects in tetrahydrobiopterin synthesis and dihydrobiopterin reductase deficiency (dose expressed as levodopa)

▸ BY MOUTH

▸ Neonate: Initially 250–500 micrograms/kg 4 times a day, dose to be increased every 4–5 days according to response, a preparation containing 1:4 carbidopa: levodopa to be administered; maintenance 2.5–3 mg/kg 4 times a day, at higher doses consider preparation containing 1:10 carbidopa:levodopa, review regularly (every 3–6 months).

▸ Child: Initially 250–500 micrograms/kg 4 times a day, dose to be increased every 4–5 days according to response, a preparation containing 1:4 carbidopa: levodopa to be administered; maintenance 2.5–3 mg/kg 4 times a day, at higher doses consider preparation containing 1:10 carbidopa:levodopa, review regularly (every 3–6 months in early childhood)

DOSE EQUIVALENCE AND CONVERSION

The proportions are expressed in the form x/y where x and y are the strengths in milligrams of carbidopa and levodopa respectively.
2 tablets *Sinemet*® 12.5 mg/50 mg is equivalent to 1 tablet *Sinemet*® Plus 25 mg/100 mg.

- **UNLICENSED USE** Not licensed for use in children.

- **CAUTIONS** Cardiovascular disease · diabetes mellitus · history of myocardial infarction with residual arrhythmia · history of peptic ulcer · history of skin melanoma (risk of activation) · osteomalacia · psychiatric illness (avoid if severe and discontinue if deterioration) · pulmonary disease · susceptibility to angle-closure glaucoma

- **INTERACTIONS** → Appendix 1 (co-careldopa, levodopa).

- **SIDE-EFFECTS**

▸ **Common or very common** Agitation · anorexia · arrhythmias · dizziness · insomnia · nausea · postural hypotension · reddish discoloration of urine and other body fluids · tachycardia · vomiting

▸ **Rare** Abnormal involuntary movements (may be dose-limiting) · Henoch-Schönlein purpura · hypersensitivity · labile hypertension · psychiatric symptoms (including hypomania, may be dose-limiting)

▸ **Very rare** Angle-closure glaucoma

▸ **Frequency not known** Depression · drowsiness · flushing · gastro-intestinal bleeding · headache · liver enzyme changes · peripheral neuropathy · pruritus · rash · sweating · syndrome resembling neuroleptic malignant syndrome (on withdrawal) · taste disturbance

- **PREGNANCY** Use with caution—toxicity has occurred in *animal* studies.

- **BREAST FEEDING** May suppress lactation; present in milk—avoid.

- **MONITORING REQUIREMENTS** In prolonged therapy, psychiatric, hepatic, haematological, renal, and cardiovascular monitoring is advisable; warn patients to resume normal activities gradually.

- **EFFECT ON LABORATORY TESTS** False positive tests for urinary ketones have been reported.

- **TREATMENT CESSATION** Avoid abrupt withdrawal.

- **PRESCRIBING AND DISPENSING INFORMATION** Co-careldopa is a mixture of carbidopa and levodopa; the proportions are expressed in the form x/y where x and y are the strengths in milligrams of carbidopa and levodopa respectively.

- **PATIENT AND CARER ADVICE**

Driving and skilled tasks
Sudden onset of sleep Excessive daytime sleepiness and sudden onset of sleep can occur with co-careldopa.

Patients starting treatment with these drugs should be warned of the risk and of the need to exercise caution when driving or operating machinery. Those who have experienced excessive sedation or sudden onset of sleep should refrain from driving or operating machines until these effects have stopped occurring.

Management of excessive daytime sleepiness should focus on the identification of an underlying cause, such as depression or concomitant medication. Patients should be counselled on improving sleep behaviour.

Warn patients to resume normal activity gradually.

- **MEDICINAL FORMS**
There can be variation in the licensing of different medicines containing the same drug. Forms available from special-order manufacturers include: oral suspension, oral solution

Tablet

CAUTIONARY AND ADVISORY LABELS 10, 14

▸ **Co-careldopa (Non-proprietary)**
Carbidopa (as Carbidopa monohydrate) 10 mg, Levodopa 100 mg Co-careldopa 10mg/100mg tablets | 100 tablet [PoM] £9.38 DT price = £8.68

Carbidopa (as Carbidopa monohydrate) 25 mg, Levodopa 100 mg Co-careldopa 25mg/100mg tablets | 100 tablet [PoM] £26.99 DT price = £14.39

Carbidopa (as Carbidopa monohydrate) 25 mg, Levodopa 250 mg Co-careldopa 25mg/250mg tablets | 100 tablet [PoM] £35.00 DT price = £34.98

▸ **Sinemet** (Merck Sharp & Dohme Ltd)
Carbidopa (as Carbidopa monohydrate) 12.5 mg, Levodopa 50 mg Sinemet 12.5mg/50mg tablets | 90 tablet [PoM] £6.28 DT price = £6.28

Carbidopa (as Carbidopa monohydrate) 10 mg, Levodopa 100 mg Sinemet 10mg/100mg tablets | 100 tablet [PoM] £7.30 DT price = £8.68

Carbidopa (as Carbidopa monohydrate) 25 mg, Levodopa 250 mg Sinemet 25mg/250mg tablets | 100 tablet [PoM] £18.29 DT price = £34.98

▸ **Sinemet Plus** (Merck Sharp & Dohme Ltd)
Carbidopa (as Carbidopa monohydrate) 25 mg, Levodopa 100 mg Sinemet Plus 25mg/100mg tablets | 100 tablet [PoM] £12.88 DT price = £14.39

4

Nervous system

MUSCLE RELAXANTS > PERIPHERALLY ACTING > NEUROTOXINS (BOTULINUM TOXINS)

Botulinum toxin type A

- **INDICATIONS AND DOSE**

Dynamic equinus foot deformity caused by spasticity in ambulant paediatric cerebral palsy
▸ **Child 2–17 years:** (consult product literature)

DOSE EQUIVALENCE AND CONVERSION
Important: information is specific to each individual preparation.

- **CONTRA-INDICATIONS** Generalised disorders of muscle activity · infection at injection site · myasthenia gravis
- **CAUTIONS** Atrophy in target muscle · chronic respiratory disorder · excessive weakness in target muscle · history of aspiration · history of dysphagia · inflammation in target muscle · neurological disorders · neuromuscular disorders · off-label use (fatal adverse events reported)

  CAUTIONS, FURTHER INFORMATION
  Neuromuscular or neurological disorders can lead to increased sensitivity and exaggerated muscle weakness including dysphagia and respiratory compromise.

- **SIDE-EFFECTS**
▸ **Common or very common** Abnormal gait · drowsiness · excessive doses may paralyse distant muscles · increased electrophysiologic jitter in some distant muscles · influenza-like symptoms · malaise · misplaced injections may paralyse nearby muscle groups · myalgia · pain in extremities · paraesthesia · urinary incontinence
▸ **Rare** Anaphylaxis · antibody formation (substantial deterioration in response) · arrhythmias · hypersensitivity reactions · myocardial infarction · pruritus · rash · seizures
▸ **Very rare** Aspiration · dysphagia · dysphonia · exaggerated muscle weakness · respiratory disorders

- **CONCEPTION AND CONTRACEPTION** Avoid in women of child-bearing age unless using effective contraception.
- **PREGNANCY** Avoid unless essential—toxicity in *animal* studies (manufacturer of *Botox*® advise avoid).
- **BREAST FEEDING** Low risk of systemic absorption but avoid unless essential.
- **PRESCRIBING AND DISPENSING INFORMATION** Preparations are not interchangeable.
- **PATIENT AND CARER ADVICE**
Patients and carers should be warned of the signs and symptoms of toxin spread, such as muscle weakness and breathing difficulties; they should be advised to seek immediate medical attention if swallowing, speech or breathing difficulties occur.
Medicines for Children leaflet: Botulinum toxin for muscle spasticity www.medicinesforchildren.org.uk/botulinum-toxin-muscle-spasticity-0

- **MEDICINAL FORMS**
There can be variation in the licensing of different medicines containing the same drug.
  Powder for solution for injection
  ▸ Azzalure (Galderma (UK) Ltd)
    Botulinum toxin type A 125 unit Azzalure 125unit powder for solution for injection vials | 1 vial PoM £64.00 | 2 vial PoM £128.00
  ▸ Bocouture (Merz Pharma UK Ltd)
    Botulinum toxin type A 50 unit Bocouture 50unit powder for solution for injection vials | 1 vial PoM £72.00
  ▸ Botox (Allergan Ltd)
    Botulinum toxin type A 50 unit Botox 50unit powder for solution for injection vials | 1 vial PoM £77.50
    Botulinum toxin type A 100 unit Botox 100unit powder for solution for injection vials | 1 vial PoM £138.20
    Botulinum toxin type A 200 unit Botox 200unit powder for solution for injection vials | 1 vial PoM £276.40

▸ Dysport (Ipsen Ltd)
  Botulinum toxin type A 300 unit Dysport 300unit powder for solution for injection vials | 1 vial PoM £92.40
  Botulinum toxin type A 500 unit Dysport 500unit powder for solution for injection vials | 2 vial PoM £308.00
▸ Xeomin (Merz Pharma UK Ltd)
  Botulinum toxin type A 50 unit Xeomin 50unit powder for solution for injection vials | 1 vial PoM £72.00
  Botulinum toxin type A 100 unit Xeomin 100unit powder for solution for injection vials | 1 vial PoM £129.90

4 Nausea and labyrinth disorders

Nausea and labyrinth disorders

Drug treatment

Antiemetics should be prescribed only when the cause of vomiting is known because otherwise they may delay diagnosis, particularly in children. Antiemetics are unnecessary and sometimes harmful when the cause can be treated, such as in diabetic ketoacidosis, or in digoxin p. 75 or antiepileptic overdose.

If antiemetic drug treatment is indicated, the drug is chosen according to the aetiology of vomiting.

Antihistamines are effective against nausea and vomiting resulting from many underlying conditions. There is no evidence that any one antihistamine is superior to another but their duration of action and incidence of adverse effects (drowsiness and antimuscarinic effects) differ.

The **phenothiazines** are dopamine antagonists and act centrally by blocking the chemoreceptor trigger zone. They are of considerable value for the prophylaxis and treatment of nausea and vomiting associated with diffuse neoplastic disease, radiation sickness, and the emesis caused by drugs such as opioids, general anaesthetics, and cytotoxics. Prochlorperazine p. 252, perphenazine p. 232, and trifluoperazine p. 233 are less sedating than chlorpromazine hydrochloride p. 230; severe dystonic reactions sometimes occur with phenothiazines. Some phenothiazines are available as rectal suppositories, which can be useful in children with persistent vomiting or with severe nausea; for children over 12 years prochlorperazine can also be administered as a buccal tablet which is placed between the upper lip and the gum.

Other antipsychotic drugs including haloperidol p. 231 and levomepromazine p. 251 are used for the relief of nausea in palliative care.

Metoclopramide hydrochloride p. 246 is an effective antiemetic and its activity closely resembles that of the phenothiazines. Metoclopramide hydrochloride also acts directly on the gastro-intestinal tract and it may be superior to the phenothiazines for emesis associated with gastroduodenal, hepatic, and biliary disease. Due to the risk of neurological side-effects, metoclopramide hydrochloride should only be used in children as second line therapy in postoperative and cytotoxic induced nausea and vomiting.

Domperidone p. 245 acts at the chemoreceptor trigger zone; it has the advantage over metoclopramide hydrochloride and the phenothiazines of being less likely to cause central effects such as sedation and dystonic reactions because it does not readily cross the blood-brain barrier.

Granisetron p. 247 and ondansetron p. 248 are specific $5HT_3$-receptor antagonists which block $5HT_3$ receptors in the gastro-intestinal tract and in the CNS. They are of value in the management of nausea and vomiting in children receiving cytotoxics and in postoperative nausea and vomiting.

Nabilone p. 245 is a synthetic cannabinoid with antiemetic properties. It may be used for nausea and vomiting caused by

4

Nervous system

cytotoxic chemotherapy that is unresponsive to conventional antiemetics.

Dexamethasone has antiemetic effects. Dexamethasone may also have a role in cytotoxic-induced nausea and vomiting.

Vomiting during pregnancy

Nausea in the first trimester of pregnancy is generally mild and does not require drug therapy. On rare occasions if vomiting is severe, short-term treatment with an antihistamine, such as **promethazine**, may be required. Prochlorperazine or metoclopramide hydrochloride are alternatives. If symptoms do not settle in 24 to 48 hours then specialist opinion should be sought. Hyperemesis gravidarum is a more serious condition, which requires regular antiemetic therapy, intravenous fluid and electrolyte replacement and sometimes nutritional support. Supplementation with thiamine p. 586 must be considered in order to reduce the risk of Wernicke's encephalopathy.

Postoperative nausea and vomiting

The incidence of postoperative nausea and vomiting depends on many factors including the anaesthetic used, and the type and duration of surgery. Other risk factors include female sex, non-smokers, a history of postoperative nausea and vomiting or motion sickness, and intraoperative and postoperative use of opioids. Therapy to prevent postoperative nausea and vomiting should be based on the assessed risk. Drugs used include **5HT$_3$-receptor antagonists**, droperidol p. 251, dexamethasone, some **phenothiazines** (e.g. prochlorperazine), and **antihistamines** (e.g. cyclizine below). A combination of two or more antiemetic drugs that have different mechanisms of action is often indicated in those at high risk of postoperative nausea and vomiting or where postoperative vomiting presents a particular danger (e.g. in some types of surgery). When a prophylactic antiemetic drug has failed, postoperative nausea and vomiting should be treated with one or more drugs from a different class.

Opioid-induced nausea and vomiting

Cyclizine, ondansetron, and prochlorperazine are used to relieve opioid-induced nausea and vomiting; ondansetron has the advantage of not producing sedation.

Motion sickness

Antiemetics should be given to prevent motion sickness rather than after nausea or vomiting develop. The most effective drug for the prevention of motion sickness is hyoscine hydrobromide p. 250. For children over 10 years old, a transdermal hyoscine patch provides prolonged activity but it needs to be applied several hours before travelling. The sedating antihistamines are slightly less effective against motion sickness, but are generally better tolerated than hyoscine. If a sedative effect is desired **promethazine** is useful, but generally a slightly less sedating antihistamine such as cyclizine or cinnarizine p. 249 is preferred. Domperidone, metoclopramide hydrochloride, 5HT$_3$-receptor antagonists, and the phenothiazines (except the antihistamine phenothiazine promethazine) are **ineffective** in motion sickness.

Other vestibular disorders

Management of vestibular diseases is aimed at treating the underlying cause as well as treating symptoms of the balance disturbance and associated nausea and vomiting. **Antihistamines** (such as cinnarizine), and **phenothiazines** (such as prochlorperazine) are effective for prophylaxis and treatment of nausea and vertigo resulting from vestibular disorders; however, when nausea and vertigo are associated with middle ear surgery, treatment can be difficult.

Cytotoxic chemotherapy, palliative care, and migraine

Antiemetics have a role in the management of nausea and vomiting induced by cytotoxic chemotherapy, in palliative care, and associated with migraine.

> **Drugs used for Nausea and labyrinth disorders not listed below** Promethazine hydrochloride, p. 171

ANTIEMETICS AND ANTINAUSEANTS ›
ANTIHISTAMINES

Cyclizine

- **INDICATIONS AND DOSE**

Nausea and vomiting of known cause | Nausea and vomiting associated with vestibular disorders and palliative care
- ▸ BY MOUTH, OR BY INTRAVENOUS INJECTION
- ▸ Child 1 month–5 years: 0.5–1 mg/kg up to 3 times a day (max. per dose 25 mg), intravenous injection to be given over 3–5 minutes, for motion sickness, take 1–2 hours before departure
- ▸ Child 6–11 years: 25 mg up to 3 times a day, intravenous injection to be given over 3–5 minutes, for motion sickness, take 1–2 hours before departure
- ▸ Child 12–17 years: 50 mg up to 3 times a day, intravenous injection to be given over 3–5 minutes, for motion sickness, take 1–2 hours before departure
- ▸ BY RECTUM
- ▸ Child 2–5 years: 12.5 mg up to 3 times a day
- ▸ Child 6–11 years: 25 mg up to 3 times a day
- ▸ Child 12–17 years: 50 mg up to 3 times a day
- ▸ BY CONTINUOUS INTRAVENOUS INFUSION, OR BY SUBCUTANEOUS INFUSION
- ▸ Child 1–23 months: 3 mg/kg, dose to be given over 24 hours
- ▸ Child 2–5 years: 50 mg, dose to be given over 24 hours
- ▸ Child 6–11 years: 75 mg, dose to be given over 24 hours
- ▸ Child 12–17 years: 150 mg, dose to be given over 24 hours

- **UNLICENSED USE** Tablets not licensed for use in children under 6 years. Injection not licensed for use in children.
- **CONTRA-INDICATIONS** Avoid in Acute porphyrias p. 562 (some antihistamines are thought to be safe) · neonate (due to significant antimuscarinic activity)
- **CAUTIONS** Epilepsy · glaucoma · may counteract haemodynamic benefits of opioids · neuromuscular disorders—increased risk of transient paralysis with intravenous use · pyloroduodenal obstruction · severe heart failure—may cause fall in cardiac output and associated increase in heart rate, mean arterial pressure and pulmonary wedge pressure · urinary retention
- **INTERACTIONS** → Appendix 1 (antihistamines).
- **SIDE-EFFECTS**
  GENERAL SIDE-EFFECTS
- ▸ **Common or very common** Drowsiness
- ▸ **Rare** Anaphylaxis · angioedema · angle-closure glaucoma · arrhythmias · blood disorders · bronchospasm · confusion · convulsions · depression · dizziness · extrapyramidal effects · hypersensitivity reactions · hypotension · liver dysfunction · palpitation · paradoxical stimulation (especially with high doses in children) · photosensitivity reactions · rashes · sleep disturbances · tremor
- ▸ **Frequency not known** Antimuscarinic effects · blurred vision · dry mouth · gastro-intestinal disturbances · hallucinations · headache · hypertension · movement disorders · oculogyric crisis · paraesthesia · psychomotor

impairment · tachycardia · transient speech disorders · twitching · urinary retention

SPECIFIC SIDE-EFFECTS

▶ **Rare**
▶ **With intravenous use** Transient paralysis
▶ **Frequency not known**
▶ **With subcutaneous use** Local irritation

SIDE-EFFECTS, FURTHER INFORMATION
Children are more susceptible to side-effects.

Drowsiness is a significant side-effect with most of the older antihistamines although paradoxical stimulation may occur rarely in children, especially with high doses. Drowsiness may diminish after a few days of treatment and is considerably less of a problem with the newer antihistamines.

● **PREGNANCY** Manufacturer advises avoid; however, there is no evidence of teratogenicity. The use of sedating antihistamines in the latter part of the third trimester may cause adverse effects in neonates such as irritability, paradoxical excitability, and tremor.

● **BREAST FEEDING** No information available. Most antihistamines are present in breast milk in varying amounts; although not known to be harmful, most manufacturers advise avoiding their use in mothers who are breast-feeding.

● **HEPATIC IMPAIRMENT** Avoid in severe liver disease—increased risk of coma.

● **DIRECTIONS FOR ADMINISTRATION** For administration *by mouth*, tablets may be crushed.
Mixing and compatibility for the use of syringe drivers in palliative care Cyclizine may precipitate at concentrations above 10 mg/mL or in the presence of sodium chloride 0.9% *or* as the concentration of diamorphine relative to cyclizine increases; mixtures of diamorphine and cyclizine are also likely to precipitate after 24 hours.

● **PATIENT AND CARER ADVICE**
Driving and skilled tasks
Drowsiness may affect performance of skilled tasks (e.g. cycling, driving); effects of alcohol enhanced.

● **MEDICINAL FORMS**
There can be variation in the licensing of different medicines containing the same drug. Forms available from special-order manufacturers include: oral suspension, oral solution, suppository
Tablet
CAUTIONARY AND ADVISORY LABELS 2
▶ Cyclizine (Non-proprietary)
  Cyclizine hydrochloride 50 mg Cyclizine 50mg tablets | 100 tablet P £15.62 DT price = £7.94
Solution for injection
▶ Cyclizine (Non-proprietary)
  Cyclizine lactate 50 mg per 1 ml Cyclizine 50mg/1ml solution for injection ampoules | 5 ampoule PoM £13.54 DT price = £13.54

ANTIEMETICS AND ANTINAUSEANTS ›
CANNIBINOIDS

Nabilone

● **INDICATIONS AND DOSE**
Nausea and vomiting caused by cytotoxic chemotherapy, unresponsive to conventional antiemetics (preferably in hospital setting) (under close medical supervision)
▶ BY MOUTH
▶ Child: (consult local protocol)

● **UNLICENSED USE** Not licensed for use in children.

● **CAUTIONS** Adverse effects on mental state can persist for 48–72 hours after stopping · heart disease · history of psychiatric disorder · hypertension

● **SIDE-EFFECTS**
▶ **Common or very common** Ataxia · concentration difficulties · drowsiness · dry mouth · dysphoria · euphoria · headache · hypotension · nausea · sleep disturbance · vertigo · visual disturbance
▶ **Frequency not known** Abdominal pain · confusion · decreased appetite · decreased coordination · depression · disorientation · hallucinations · psychosis · tachycardia · tremors

SIDE-EFFECTS, FURTHER INFORMATION
Drowsiness and dizziness occur frequently with standard doses.

● **PREGNANCY** Avoid unless essential.

● **BREAST FEEDING** Avoid—no information available.

● **HEPATIC IMPAIRMENT** Avoid in severe impairment.

● **PATIENT AND CARER ADVICE**
Driving and skilled tasks
Drowsiness may affect performance of skilled tasks (e.g. driving).

Effects of alcohol enhanced.

For information on 2015 legislation regarding driving whilst taking certain controlled drugs, including nabilone, see *Drugs and skilled tasks* under Guidance on prescribing p. 1.
Behavioural effects Patients should be made aware of possible changes of mood and other adverse behavioural effects.

● **MEDICINAL FORMS**
There can be variation in the licensing of different medicines containing the same drug. Forms available from special-order manufacturers include: capsule
Capsule
CAUTIONARY AND ADVISORY LABELS 2
▶ Nabilone (Non-proprietary)
  Nabilone 1 mg Nabilone 1mg capsules | 20 capsule PoM £196.00 CD2

ANTIEMETICS AND ANTINAUSEANTS ›
DOPAMINE RECEPTOR ANTAGONISTS

Domperidone

● **INDICATIONS AND DOSE**
Relief of nausea and vomiting
▶ BY MOUTH
▶ Child (body-weight up to 35 kg): 250 micrograms/kg up to 3 times a day; maximum 750 micrograms/kg per day
▶ Child 12–17 years (body-weight 35 kg and above): 10 mg up to 3 times a day; maximum 30 mg per day

Gastro-oesophageal reflux disease (but efficacy not proven)
▶ BY MOUTH
▶ Neonate: 250 micrograms/kg 3 times a day, dose can be increased if response inadequate, increased if necessary up to 400 micrograms/kg 3 times a day, interrupt treatment occasionally to assess recurrence—consider restarting if symptoms recur, discontinue if response inadequate at higher dose.
▶ Child: 250 micrograms/kg 3 times a day (max. per dose 10 mg), dose can be increased if response inadequate, increased if necessary up to 400 micrograms/kg 3 times a day (max. per dose 20 mg), interrupt treatment occasionally to assess recurrence—consider restarting if symptoms recur, discontinue if response inadequate at higher dose

4

Nervous system

- **UNLICENSED USE** Not licensed for use in children for gastro-oesophageal reflux disease.

IMPORTANT SAFETY INFORMATION

MHRA/CHM ADVICE—DOMPERIDONE: RISK OF CARDIAC SIDE-EFFECTS—RESTRICTED INDICATION, NEW CONTRA-INDICATIONS, REDUCED DOSE AND DURATION OF USE

The benefits and risks of domperidone have been reviewed. As domperidone is associated with a small increased risk of serious cardiac side-effects, the following restrictions to indication, dose and duration of treatment have been made, and new contra-indications added:

- Domperidone should only be used for the relief of the symptoms of nausea and vomiting;
- Domperidone should be used at the lowest effective dose for the shortest possible duration (max. treatment duration should not normally exceed 1 week);
- Domperidone is contra-indicated for use in conditions where cardiac conduction is, or could be impaired, or where there is underlying cardiac disease, when administered concomitantly with drugs that prolong the QT interval or potent CYP3A4 inhibitors, and in severe hepatic impairment;
- The recommended dose in adults and adolescents over 12 years and over 35 kg is 10 mg up to 3 times daily;
- The recommended dose in children under 35 kg is 250 micrograms/kg up to 3 times daily;
- Oral liquid formulations should be given via an appropriately designed, graduated oral syringe to ensure dose accuracy.

This advice does not apply to unlicensed uses of domperidone (e.g. palliative care).

- **CONTRA-INDICATIONS** Cardiac disease · gastro-intestinal haemorrhage · mechanical obstruction · mechanical perforation · predisposition to cardiac conduction disorders · prolactinoma
- **CAUTIONS** Children · if there are cardiac concerns, obtain ECG before and during treatment
- **INTERACTIONS** → Appendix 1 (domperidone). Contra-indicated with concomitant use of drugs that prolong the QT interval. Contra-indicated with concomitant use of potent CYP3A4 inhibitors.
- **SIDE-EFFECTS**
  - **Common or very common** Drowsiness · dry mouth · malaise
  - **Uncommon** Anxiety · breast pain · decreased libido · diarrhoea · galactorrhoea · headache · pruritus · rash
  - **Frequency not known** Agitation · amenorrhoea · convulsions · extrapyramidal disorders · gynaecomastia · nervousness · oculogyric crisis · QT-interval prolongation · sudden cardiac death · urinary retention · ventricular arrhythmias
- **PREGNANCY** Use only if potential benefit outweighs risk.
- **BREAST FEEDING** Amount too small to be harmful.
- **HEPATIC IMPAIRMENT** Avoid in moderate or severe impairment.
- **RENAL IMPAIRMENT** Reduce frequency.
- **PATIENT AND CARER ADVICE**
  Medicines for Children leaflet: Domperidone for gastro-oesophageal reflux www.medicinesforchildren.org.uk/domperidone-for-gastro-oesophageal-reflux
  Arrhythmia Patients and their carers should be told how to recognise signs of arrhythmia and advised to seek medical attention if symptoms such as palpitation or syncope develop.

- **MEDICINAL FORMS**
  There can be variation in the licensing of different medicines containing the same drug. Forms available from special-order manufacturers include: oral suspension

Tablet

CAUTIONARY AND ADVISORY LABELS 22
- ▶ **Domperidone (Non-proprietary)** ▼
  Domperidone (as Domperidone maleate) 10 mg Domperidone 10mg tablets | 30 tablet [PoM] £2.71 DT price = £1.19 | 100 tablet [PoM] £9.04 DT price = £3.97
- ▶ **Motilium (Zentiva)** ▼
  Domperidone (as Domperidone maleate) 10 mg Motilium 10mg tablets | 30 tablet [PoM] £2.71 DT price = £1.19 | 100 tablet [PoM] £9.04 DT price = £3.97

Oral suspension

CAUTIONARY AND ADVISORY LABELS 22
- ▶ **Domperidone (Non-proprietary)** ▼
  Domperidone 1 mg per 1 ml Domperidone 5mg/5ml oral suspension sugar free sugar-free | 200 ml [PoM] £13.43 DT price = £13.43

Metoclopramide hydrochloride

- **INDICATIONS AND DOSE**

Second-line option for treatment of established postoperative nausea and vomiting | Prevention of delayed chemotherapy-induced nausea and vomiting
- ▶ BY MOUTH, OR BY INTRAMUSCULAR INJECTION, OR BY INTRAVENOUS INJECTION
- ▶ **Child:** 100–150 micrograms/kg up to 3 times a day (max. per dose 10 mg), when administered by slow intravenous injection, to be given over at least 3 minutes

- **UNLICENSED USE** *Maxolon* ® tablets not licensed for use in children.

IMPORTANT SAFETY INFORMATION

MHRA/CHM ADVICE—METOCLOPRAMIDE: RISK OF NEUROLOGICAL ADVERSE EFFECTS—RESTRICTED DOSE AND DURATION OF USE (AUGUST 2013)

The benefits and risks of metoclopramide have been reviewed by the European Medicines Agency's Committee on Medicinal Products for Human Use, which concluded that the risk of neurological effects such as extrapyramidal disorders and tardive dyskinesia outweigh the benefits in long-term or high-dose treatment. To help minimise the risk of potentially serious neurological adverse effects, the following restrictions to indications, dose and duration of use have been made:

- In children aged 1–18 years, metoclopramide should only be used as a second-line option for prevention of delayed chemotherapy-induced nausea and vomiting and for treatment of established postoperative nausea and vomiting;
- Use of metoclopramide is contra-indicated in children aged under 1 year;
- Metoclopramide should only be prescribed for short-term use (up to 5 days);
- Recommended dose is 100–150 micrograms/kg (max. 10 mg), repeated up to 3 times daily;
- Intravenous doses should be administered as a slow bolus over at least 3 minutes;
- Oral liquid formulations should be given via an appropriately designed, graduated oral syringe to ensure dose accuracy.

This advice does not apply to unlicensed uses of metoclopramide (e.g. palliative care).

- **CONTRA-INDICATIONS** 3–4 days after gastrointestinal surgery · gastro-intestinal haemorrhage · gastro-intestinal obstruction · gastro-intestinal perforation · phaeochromocytoma

- **CAUTIONS** Asthma · atopic allergy · bradycardia · cardiac conduction disturbances · epilepsy · may mask underlying disorders such as cerebral irritation · uncorrected electrolyte imbalance
- **INTERACTIONS** → Appendix 1 (metoclopramide). Caution with concomitant use of other drugs affecting cardiac conduction.
- **SIDE-EFFECTS**
  GENERAL SIDE-EFFECTS
  ▸ **Common or very common** Extrapyramidal effects · galactorrhoea · gynaecomastia · hyperprolactinaemia · menstrual changes
  ▸ **Very rare** Depression · methaemoglobinaemia (more severe in G6PD deficiency) · neuroleptic malignant syndrome
  ▸ **Frequency not known** Anxiety · confusion · diarrhoea · dizziness · drowsiness · dyspnoea · hypotension · oedema · pruritus · rash · restlessness · tardive dyskinesia on prolonged administration · tremor · urticaria · visual disturbances
  SPECIFIC SIDE-EFFECTS
  ▸ **Very rare**
  ▸ **With intravenous use** Cardiac conduction abnormalities
  SIDE-EFFECTS, FURTHER INFORMATION
  ▸ **Acute dystonic reactions** Metoclopramide can induce acute dystonic reactions such as facial and skeletal muscle spasms and oculogyric crises; children (especially girls, young women, and those under 10 kg) are particularly susceptible. With metoclopramide, dystonic effects usually occur shortly after starting treatment and subside within 24 hours of stopping it. An antimuscarinic drug such as procyclidine is used to abort dystonic attacks.
- **PREGNANCY** Not known to be harmful.
- **BREAST FEEDING** Small amount present in milk; avoid.
- **HEPATIC IMPAIRMENT** Reduce dose.
- **RENAL IMPAIRMENT** Avoid or use small dose in severe impairment; increased risk of extrapyramidal reactions.
- **DIRECTIONS FOR ADMINISTRATION** Oral liquid preparation to be given via a graduated oral dosing syringe.
- **PATIENT AND CARER ADVICE** Counselling on use of pipette advised with oral solution.

- **MEDICINAL FORMS**
  There can be variation in the licensing of different medicines containing the same drug. Forms available from special-order manufacturers include: oral solution
  Tablet
  ▸ Metoclopramide hydrochloride (Non-proprietary)
  Metoclopramide hydrochloride 10 mg Metoclopramide 10mg tablets | 28 tablet PoM £1.23 DT price = £0.75
  ▸ Maxolon (AMCo)
  Metoclopramide hydrochloride 10 mg Maxolon 10mg tablets | 84 tablet PoM £5.24
  Oral solution
  ▸ Metoclopramide hydrochloride (Non-proprietary)
  Metoclopramide hydrochloride 1 mg per 1 ml Metoclopramide 5mg/5ml oral solution sugar free sugar-free | 150 ml PoM £19.77 DT price = £19.77
  Solution for injection
  ▸ Metoclopramide hydrochloride (Non-proprietary)
  Metoclopramide hydrochloride 5 mg per 1 ml Metoclopramide 10mg/2ml solution for injection ampoules | 5 ampoule PoM £1.31 | 10 ampoule PoM £3.50 DT price = £3.18
  ▸ Maxolon (AMCo)
  Metoclopramide hydrochloride 5 mg per 1 ml Maxolon 10mg/2ml solution for injection ampoules | 12 ampoule PoM £3.21

ANTIEMETICS AND ANTINAUSEANTS 〉
SEROTONIN (5HT3) RECEPTOR ANTAGONISTS

Granisetron

- **DRUG ACTION** Granisetron is a specific $5HT_3$-receptor antagonist which blocks $5HT_3$ receptors in the gastrointestinal tract and in the CNS.

- **INDICATIONS AND DOSE**
  Management of nausea and vomiting induced by cytotoxic chemotherapy
  ▸ BY MOUTH
  ▸ Child 12–17 years: 1–2 mg, to be taken within 1 hour before start of treatment, then 2 mg daily in 1–2 divided doses for up to 1 week following chemotherapy
  ▸ BY INTRAVENOUS INFUSION
  ▸ Child 2–17 years: 10–40 micrograms/kg (max. per dose 3 mg), repeated if necessary, to be given before start of chemotherapy, for treatment, dose may be repeated within 24 hours if necessary, not less than 10 minutes after initial dose; maximum 2 doses per day

- **UNLICENSED USE** Tablets not licensed in children (age range not specified by manufacturer).
- **CAUTIONS** Subacute intestinal obstruction · susceptibility to QT-interval prolongation (including electrolyte disturbances)
- **INTERACTIONS** → Appendix 1 ($5HT_3$-receptor Antagonists). Caution with concomitant use of drugs that prolong QT interval.
- **SIDE-EFFECTS**
  ▸ **Common or very common** Constipation · diarrhoea · headache · insomnia
  ▸ **Uncommon** Extrapyramidal reactions · QT-interval prolongation · rash
- **PREGNANCY** Manufacturer advises avoid.
- **BREAST FEEDING** Avoid—no information available.
- **HEPATIC IMPAIRMENT** Manufacturer advises use with caution.
- **DIRECTIONS FOR ADMINISTRATION**
  ▸ **With intravenous use** For *intravenous infusion*, dilute up to 3 mL of granisetron injection in Glucose 5% or Sodium Chloride 0.9% to a total volume of 10–30 mL; give over 5 minutes.

- **MEDICINAL FORMS**
  There can be variation in the licensing of different medicines containing the same drug.
  Tablet
  ▸ Granisetron (Non-proprietary)
  Granisetron (as Granisetron hydrochloride) 1 mg Granisetron 1mg tablets | 10 tablet PoM £51.20 DT price = £33.99
  Granisetron (as Granisetron hydrochloride) 2 mg Granisetron 2mg tablets | 5 tablet PoM no price available DT price = £52.39
  ▸ Kytril (Roche Products Ltd)
  Granisetron (as Granisetron hydrochloride) 1 mg Kytril 1mg tablets | 10 tablet PoM £52.39 DT price = £33.99
  Granisetron (as Granisetron hydrochloride) 2 mg Kytril 2mg tablets | 5 tablet PoM £52.39 DT price = £52.39
  Solution for injection
  ▸ Granisetron (Non-proprietary)
  Granisetron (as Granisetron hydrochloride) 1 mg per 1 ml Granisetron 3mg/3ml concentrate for solution for injection ampoules | 5 ampoule PoM £24.00
  Granisetron 1mg/1ml concentrate for solution for injection ampoules | 5 ampoule PoM £8.00

4

Nervous system

Nervous system

4

Ondansetron

- **DRUG ACTION** Ondansetron is a specific $5HT_3$-receptor antagonist which blocks $5HT_3$ receptors in the gastro-intestinal tract and in the CNS.

- **INDICATIONS AND DOSE**

Prevention of postoperative nausea and vomiting
- ▸ BY SLOW INTRAVENOUS INJECTION
- ▸ Child: 100 micrograms/kg (max. per dose 4 mg) for 1 dose, dose to be given over at least 30 seconds before, during, or after induction of anaesthesia

Treatment of postoperative nausea and vomiting
- ▸ BY SLOW INTRAVENOUS INJECTION
- ▸ Child: 100 micrograms/kg (max. per dose 4 mg) for 1 dose, dose to be given over at least 30 seconds

Prevention and treatment of chemotherapy- and radiotherapy-induced nausea and vomiting—initial dose
- ▸ BY INTRAVENOUS INFUSION
- ▸ Child 6 months–17 years (body surface area up to 1.3 m²): 5 mg/m² for 1 dose then give orally, alternatively 150 micrograms/kg (max. per dose 8 mg), dose to be administered immediately before chemotherapy, then 150 micrograms/kg every 4 hours (max. per dose 8 mg) for 2 further doses then give orally; maximum 32 mg per day
- ▸ Child 6 months–17 years (body surface area 1.3 m² and above): 8 mg for 1 dose then give orally, alternatively 150 micrograms/kg (max. per dose 8 mg), dose to be administered immediately before chemotherapy, then 150 micrograms/kg every 4 hours (max. per dose 8 mg) for 2 further doses then give orally, intravenous infusion to be administered over at least 15 minutes; maximum 32 mg per day

Prevention and treatment of chemotherapy- and radiotherapy-induced nausea and vomiting— (follow-on dose based on body surface area)
- ▸ BY MOUTH
- ▸ Child 6 months–17 years (body surface area up to 0.6 m²): 2 mg every 12 hours for up to 5 days (dose can be started 12 hours after intravenous administration); maximum 32 mg per day
- ▸ Child 6 months–17 years (body surface area 0.6–1.2 m²): 4 mg every 12 hours for up to 5 days (dose can be started 12 hours after intravenous administration); maximum 32 mg per day
- ▸ Child 6 months–17 years (body surface area 1.3 m² and above): 8 mg every 12 hours for up to 5 days (dose can be started 12 hours after intravenous administration); maximum 32 mg per day

Prevention and treatment of chemotherapy- and radiotherapy-induced nausea and vomiting—(follow-on dose based on body-weight)
- ▸ BY MOUTH
- ▸ Child 6 months–17 years (body-weight up to 10.1 kg): 2 mg every 12 hours for up to 5 days (dose can be started 12 hours after intravenous administration); maximum 32 mg per day
- ▸ Child 6 months–17 years (body-weight 10.1–40 kg): 4 mg every 12 hours for up to 5 days (dose can be started 12 hours after intravenous administration); maximum 32 mg per day
- ▸ Child 6 months–17 years (body-weight 41 kg and above): 8 mg every 12 hours for up to 5 days (dose can be started 12 hours after intravenous administration); maximum 32 mg per day

- **UNLICENSED USE** Not licensed for radiotherapy-induced nausea and vomiting in children.
- **CONTRA-INDICATIONS** Congenital long QT syndrome

- **CAUTIONS** Adenotonsillar surgery · subacute intestinal obstruction · susceptibility to QT-interval prolongation (including electrolyte disturbances)

- **INTERACTIONS** → Appendix 1 ($5HT_3$-receptor Antagonists). Caution with concomitant use of drugs that prolong QT interval.

- **SIDE-EFFECTS**
GENERAL SIDE-EFFECTS
- ▸ **Common or very common** Constipation · flushing · headache · injection site-reactions
- ▸ **Uncommon** Arrhythmias · bradycardia · chest pain · hiccups · hypotension · movement disorders · seizures
SPECIFIC SIDE-EFFECTS
- ▸ **Rare**
- ▸ With intravenous use Dizziness · transient visual disturbances
- ▸ **Very rare**
- ▸ With intravenous use Transient blindness

- **PREGNANCY** No information available; avoid unless potential benefit outweighs risk.

- **BREAST FEEDING** Present in milk in *animal* studies—avoid.

- **HEPATIC IMPAIRMENT** Reduce dose in moderate or severe impairment.

- **DIRECTIONS FOR ADMINISTRATION**
- ▸ With intravenous use For *intravenous infusion*, dilute to a concentration of 320–640 micrograms/mL with Glucose 5% or Sodium Chloride 0.9%; give over at least 15 minutes.
- ▸ With oral use Orodispersible films and lyophilisates should be placed on the tongue, allowed to disperse and swallowed.

- **PRESCRIBING AND DISPENSING INFORMATION** Flavours of oral liquid formulations may include strawberry.

- **PATIENT AND CARER ADVICE** Patients or carers should be given advice on how to administer orodispersible films and lyophilisates.

- **MEDICINAL FORMS**
There can be variation in the licensing of different medicines containing the same drug. Forms available from special-order manufacturers include: oral suspension, oral solution

Tablet
- ▸ **Ondansetron** (Non-proprietary)
  Ondansetron (as Ondansetron hydrochloride) 4 mg Ondansetron 4mg tablets | 10 tablet [PoM] £25.46 DT price = £1.22 | 30 tablet [PoM] £76.38
  Ondansetron (as Ondansetron hydrochloride) 8 mg Ondansetron 8mg tablets | 10 tablet [PoM] £47.99 DT price = £2.34
- ▸ **Ondemet** (Alliance Pharmaceuticals Ltd)
  Ondansetron (as Ondansetron hydrochloride) 4 mg Ondemet 4mg tablets | 30 tablet [PoM] £81.15
  Ondansetron (as Ondansetron hydrochloride) 8 mg Ondemet 8mg tablets | 10 tablet [PoM] £54.36 DT price = £2.34 (Hospital only)
- ▸ **Zofran** (Novartis Pharmaceuticals UK Ltd)
  Ondansetron (as Ondansetron hydrochloride) 4 mg Zofran 4mg tablets | 30 tablet [PoM] £107.91
  Ondansetron (as Ondansetron hydrochloride) 8 mg Zofran 8mg tablets | 10 tablet [PoM] £71.94 DT price = £2.34

Orodispersible tablet
- ▸ **Ondansetron** (Non-proprietary)
  Ondansetron 4 mg Ondansetron 4mg orodispersible tablets | 10 tablet [PoM] £43.46 DT price = £43.09
  Ondansetron 8 mg Ondansetron 8mg orodispersible tablets | 10 tablet [PoM] £85.43 DT price = £85.43

Orodispersible film
- ▸ **Setofilm** (Norgine Pharmaceuticals Ltd)
  Ondansetron 4 mg Setofilm 4mg orodispersible films sugar-free | 10 film [PoM] £28.50
  Ondansetron 8 mg Setofilm 8mg orodispersible films sugar-free | 10 film [PoM] £57.00

Oral solution
- ▸ **Ondansetron** (Non-proprietary)
  Ondansetron (as Ondansetron hydrochloride) 800 microgram per 1 ml Ondansetron 4mg/5ml oral solution sugar free sugar-free | 50 ml [PoM] £38.08 DT price = £38.02

▸ **Demorem** (Kappin Ltd)
　**Ondansetron (as Ondansetron hydrochloride) 800 microgram
　per 1 ml** Demorem 4mg/5ml oral solution sugar-free | 50 ml PoM
　£38.19 DT price = £38.02
▸ **Zofran** (Novartis Pharmaceuticals UK Ltd)
　**Ondansetron (as Ondansetron hydrochloride) 800 microgram
　per 1 ml** Zofran 4mg/5ml syrup sugar-free | 50 ml PoM　£35.97 DT
　price = £38.02

Oral lyophilisate
EXCIPIENTS: May contain Aspartame
▸ **Zofran Melt** (Novartis Pharmaceuticals UK Ltd)
　Ondansetron 4 mg Zofran Melt 4mg oral lyophilisates sugar-free |
　10 tablet PoM £35.97 DT price = £35.97
　Ondansetron 8 mg Zofran Melt 8mg oral lyophilisates sugar-free |
　10 tablet PoM £71.94 DT price = £71.94

Solution for injection
▸ **Ondansetron** (Non-proprietary)
　**Ondansetron (as Ondansetron hydrochloride) 2 mg per
　1 ml** Ondansetron 8mg/4ml solution for injection ampoules |
　5 ampoule PoM £58.45
　Ondansetron 4mg/2ml solution for injection ampoules |
　5 ampoule PoM £28.47 | 10 ampoule PoM £7.50
▸ **Zofran Flexi-amp** (Novartis Pharmaceuticals UK Ltd)
　**Ondansetron (as Ondansetron hydrochloride) 2 mg per
　1 ml** Zofran Flexi-amp 8mg/4ml solution for injection |
　5 ampoule PoM £59.95
　Zofran Flexi-amp 4mg/2ml solution for injection | 5 ampoule PoM
　£29.97

ANTIHISTAMINES ＞ SEDATING

Cinnarizine

● **INDICATIONS AND DOSE**
**Relief of symptoms of vestibular disorders, such as
vertigo, tinnitus, nausea, and vomiting in Ménière's
disease**
▸ BY MOUTH
▸ **Child 5–11 years:** 15 mg 3 times a day
▸ **Child 12–17 years:** 30 mg 3 times a day
Motion sickness
▸ BY MOUTH
▸ **Child 5–11 years:** Initially 15 mg, dose to be taken
　2 hours before travel, then 7.5 mg every 8 hours if
　required, dose to be taken during journey
▸ **Child 12–17 years:** Initially 30 mg, dose to be taken
　2 hours before travel, then 15 mg every 8 hours if
　required, dose to be taken during journey

● **CONTRA-INDICATIONS** Avoid in Acute porphyrias p. 562
(some antihistamines are thought to be safe) · neonate
(due to significant antimuscarinic activity)
● **CAUTIONS** Epilepsy · glaucoma · pyloroduodenal
obstruction · urinary retention
● **SIDE-EFFECTS**
▸ **Common or very common** Drowsiness
▸ **Rare** Anaphylaxis · angioedema · angle-closure glaucoma ·
arrhythmias · blood disorders · bronchospasm · confusion ·
convulsions · depression · dizziness · extrapyramidal
effects · hypersensitivity reactions · hypotension · lichen
planus · liver dysfunction · lupus-like skin reactions ·
palpitation · paradoxical stimulation (especially with high
doses in children) · photosensitivity reactions · rashes ·
sleep disturbances · sweating · tremor · weight gain
▸ **Frequency not known** Antimuscarinic effects · blurred
vision · dry mouth · gastro-intestinal disturbances ·
headache · psychomotor impairment · urinary retention
SIDE-EFFECTS, FURTHER INFORMATION
Children are more susceptible to side-effects.
　Drowsiness is a significant side-effect with most of the
older antihistamines although paradoxical stimulation
may occur rarely in children, especially with high doses.
Drowsiness may diminish after a few days of treatment and

is considerably less of a problem with the newer
antihistamines.
● **PREGNANCY** Manufacturer advises avoid; however, there
is no evidence of teratogenicity. The use of sedating
antihistamines in the latter part of the third trimester may
cause adverse effects in neonates such as irritability,
paradoxical excitability, and tremor.
● **BREAST FEEDING** Most antihistamines are present in
breast milk in varying amounts; although not known to be
harmful, most manufacturers advise avoiding their use in
mothers who are breast-feeding.
● **HEPATIC IMPAIRMENT** Avoid in severe liver disease—
increased risk of coma.
● **RENAL IMPAIRMENT** Use with caution—no information
available.
● **PATIENT AND CARER ADVICE**
Driving and skilled tasks
Drowsiness may affect performance of skilled tasks (e.g.
cycling, driving); sedating effects enhanced by alcohol.

● **MEDICINAL FORMS**
There can be variation in the licensing of different medicines
containing the same drug. Forms available from special-order
manufacturers include: oral suspension
Tablet
CAUTIONARY AND ADVISORY LABELS 2
▸ **Cinnarizine** (Non-proprietary)
　Cinnarizine 15 mg Boots Motion Sickness15mg tablets |
　15 tablet P no price available
　Cinnarizine 15mg tablets | 84 tablet P £15.40 DT price = £5.31
▸ **Mylan** (Mylan Ltd)
　Cinnarizine 15 mg Mylan Travel Sickness 15mg tablets |
　15 tablet P £2.50
▸ **Stugeron** (McNeil Products Ltd, Janssen-Cilag Ltd)
　Cinnarizine 15 mg Stugeron 15mg tablets | 15 tablet P £1.84 |
　100 tablet P £4.18

Promethazine teoclate

● **INDICATIONS AND DOSE**
Nausea | Vomiting | Labyrinthine disorders
▸ BY MOUTH
▸ **Child 5–9 years:** 12.5–37.5 mg daily
▸ **Child 10–17 years:** 25–75 mg daily; maximum 100 mg
　per day
**Motion sickness prevention (acts longer than
promethazine hydrochloride)**
▸ BY MOUTH
▸ **Child 5–9 years:** 12.5 mg once daily, dose to be taken at
　bedtime on night before travel or 1–2 hours before
　travel
▸ **Child 10–17 years:** 25 mg once daily, dose to be taken at
　bedtime on night before travel or 1–2 hours before
　travel
**Motion sickness treatment (acts longer than
promethazine hydrochloride)**
▸ BY MOUTH
▸ **Child 5–9 years:** 12.5 mg, dose to be taken at onset of
　motion sickness, then 12.5 mg daily for 2 days, dose to
　be taken at bedtime
▸ **Child 10–17 years:** 25 mg, dose to be taken at onset of
　motion sickness, then 25 mg once daily for 2 days, dose
　to be taken at bedtime

IMPORTANT SAFETY INFORMATION
MHRA/CHM ADVICE (MARCH 2008 AND FEBRUARY 2009) OVER-
THE-COUNTER COUGH AND COLD MEDICINES FOR CHILDREN
Children under 6 years should not be given over-the-
counter cough and cold medicines containing
promethazine.

4

Nervous system

- CAUTIONS Acute porphyrias p. 562 · asthma · bronchiectasis · bronchitis · epilepsy · pyloroduodenal obstruction · Reye's syndrome · severe coronary artery disease · susceptibility to angle-closure glaucoma · urinary retention
- INTERACTIONS → Appendix 1 (antihistamines).
- SIDE-EFFECTS
- **Rare** Anaphylaxis · angioedema · angle-closure glaucoma · arrhythmias · blood disorders · bronchospasm · confusion · convulsions · depression · dizziness · extrapyramidal effects · hypersensitivity reactions · hypotension · liver dysfunction · palpitation · photosensitivity reactions · rashes · sleep disturbances · tremor
- **Frequency not known** Antimuscarinic effects · blurred vision · drowsiness · dry mouth · gastro-intestinal disturbances · headache · psychomotor impairment · restlessness · urinary retention

  SIDE-EFFECTS, FURTHER INFORMATION
  Children are more susceptible to side-effects.
  Drowsiness is a significant side-effect with most of the older antihistamines although paradoxical stimulation may occur rarely in children, especially with high doses. Drowsiness may diminish after a few days of treatment and is considerably less of a problem with the newer antihistamines.
- PREGNANCY Most manufacturers of antihistamines advise avoiding their use during pregnancy; however, there is no evidence of teratogenicity. Use in the latter part of the third trimester may cause adverse effects in neonates such as irritability, paradoxical excitability, and tremor.
- BREAST FEEDING Most antihistamines are present in breast milk in varying amounts; although not known to be harmful, most manufacturers advise avoiding their use in mothers who are breast-feeding.
- HEPATIC IMPAIRMENT Avoid in severe liver disease—increased risk of coma.
- RENAL IMPAIRMENT Use with caution.
- PATIENT AND CARER ADVICE
  Driving and skilled tasks
  Drowsiness may affect performance of skilled tasks (e.g. cycling or driving); sedating effects enhanced by alcohol.

- MEDICINAL FORMS
  There can be variation in the licensing of different medicines containing the same drug.
  Tablet
  CAUTIONARY AND ADVISORY LABELS 2
- **Avomine** (Manx Healthcare Ltd)
  Promethazine teoclate 25 mg Avomine 25mg tablets |
  10 tablet Ⓟ £1.13 | 28 tablet Ⓟ £3.13 DT price = £3.13

ANTIMUSCARINICS

F 457

Hyoscine hydrobromide
(Scopolamine hydrobromide)

- INDICATIONS AND DOSE
  Motion sickness
- BY MOUTH
- Child 4–9 years: 75–150 micrograms, dose to be taken up to 30 minutes before the start of journey, then 75–150 micrograms every 6 hours if required; maximum 450 micrograms per day
- Child 10–17 years: 150–300 micrograms, dose to be taken up to 30 minutes before the start of journey, then 150–300 micrograms every 6 hours if required; maximum 900 micrograms per day

- BY TRANSDERMAL APPLICATION
- Child 10–17 years: Apply 1 patch, apply behind ear 5–6 hours before journey, then apply 1 patch after 72 hours if required, remove old patch and site replacement patch behind the other ear

Hypersalivation associated with clozapine therapy
- BY MOUTH
- Child 12–17 years: 300 micrograms up to 3 times a day; maximum 900 micrograms per day

Excessive respiratory secretions
- BY MOUTH, OR BY SUBLINGUAL ADMINISTRATION
- Child 2–11 years: 10 micrograms/kg 4 times a day (max. per dose 300 micrograms)
- Child 12–17 years: 300 micrograms 4 times a day
- BY TRANSDERMAL APPLICATION
- Child 1 month–2 years: 250 micrograms every 72 hours, dose equates to a quarter patch
- Child 3–9 years: 500 micrograms every 72 hours, dose equates to a half patch
- Child 10–17 years: 1 mg every 72 hours, dose equates to one patch

Excessive respiratory secretion (in palliative care)
- BY SUBCUTANEOUS INJECTION, OR BY INTRAVENOUS INJECTION
- Child: 10 micrograms/kg every 4–8 hours (max. per dose 600 micrograms)
- BY CONTINUOUS SUBCUTANEOUS INFUSION, OR BY INTRAVENOUS INFUSION
- Child: 40–60 micrograms/kg over 24 hours

Bowel colic pain in palliative care
- BY MOUTH USING SUBLINGUAL TABLETS
- Child: 10 micrograms/kg 3 times a day (max. per dose 300 micrograms), as *Kwells* ®.

Premedication
- BY SUBCUTANEOUS INJECTION, OR BY INTRAMUSCULAR INJECTION
- Child 1–11 years: 15 micrograms/kg (max. per dose 600 micrograms), to be administered 30–60 minutes before induction of anaesthesia
- Child 12–17 years: 200–600 micrograms, to be administered 30–60 minutes before induction of anaesthesia
- BY INTRAVENOUS INJECTION
- Child 1–11 years: 15 micrograms/kg (max. per dose 600 micrograms), to be administered immediately before induction of anaesthesia
- Child 12–17 years: 200–600 micrograms, to be administered immediately before induction of anaesthesia

- UNLICENSED USE Not licensed for use in excessive respiratory secretions or hypersalivation associated with clozapine therapy.

IMPORTANT SAFETY INFORMATION
Antimuscarininc drugs used for premedication to general anaesthesia should only be administered by, or under the direct supervision of, personnel experienced in their use.

- CAUTIONS Epilepsy
  CAUTIONS, FURTHER INFORMATION
- Anticholinergic syndrome
- With systemic use In some children hyoscine may cause the central anticholinergic syndrome (excitement, ataxia, hallucinations, behavioural abnormalities, and drowsiness).
- PREGNANCY Use only if potential benefit outweighs risk. Injection may depress neonatal respiration.
- BREAST FEEDING Amount too small to be harmful.
- HEPATIC IMPAIRMENT Use with caution.

- **RENAL IMPAIRMENT** Use with caution.
- **DIRECTIONS FOR ADMINISTRATION**
  ‣ With transdermal use *Patch* applied to hairless area of skin behind ear; if less than whole patch required **either** cut with scissors along full thickness ensuring membrane is not peeled away **or** cover portion to prevent contact with skin.
  ‣ With oral use For administration by *mouth*, injection solution may be given orally.
- **PRESCRIBING AND DISPENSING INFORMATION** Flavours of chewable tablet formulations may include raspberry.
- **PATIENT AND CARER ADVICE**
  ‣ With transdermal use Explain accompanying instructions to patient and in particular emphasise advice to wash hands after handling and to wash application site after removing, and to use one patch at a time.

  Driving and skilled tasks
  ‣ With transdermal use Drowsiness may persist for up to 24 hours or longer after removal of patch; effects of alcohol enhanced.

- **MEDICINAL FORMS**
  There can be variation in the licensing of different medicines containing the same drug. Forms available from special-order manufacturers include: oral suspension, oral solution
  Tablet
  CAUTIONARY AND ADVISORY LABELS 2
  ‣ **Hyoscine hydrobromide** (Non-proprietary)
  Hyoscine hydrobromide 300 microgram Hyoscine hydrobromide 300microgram tablets | 12 tablet Ⓟ no price available DT price = £1.67
  ‣ **Kwells** (Bayer Plc)
  Hyoscine hydrobromide 150 microgram Kwells Kids 150microgram tablets | 12 tablet Ⓟ £1.67 DT price = £1.67
  Hyoscine hydrobromide 300 microgram Kwells 300microgram tablets | 12 tablet Ⓟ £1.67 DT price = £1.67
  Chewable tablet
  CAUTIONARY AND ADVISORY LABELS 2, 24
  ‣ **Joy-Rides** (Forest Laboratories UK Ltd)
  Hyoscine hydrobromide 150 microgram Joy-rides 150microgram chewable tablets sugar-free | 12 tablet Ⓟ £1.55
  Solution for injection
  ‣ **Hyoscine hydrobromide** (Non-proprietary)
  Hyoscine hydrobromide 400 microgram per 1 ml Hyoscine hydrobromide 400micrograms/1ml solution for injection ampoules | 10 ampoule ⓅoⓂ £25.00-£43.84 DT price = £42.85
  Hyoscine hydrobromide 600 microgram per 1 ml Hyoscine hydrobromide 600micrograms/1ml solution for injection ampoules | 10 ampoule ⓅoⓂ £46.70 DT price = £45.64
  Transdermal patch
  CAUTIONARY AND ADVISORY LABELS 19
  ‣ **Scopoderm** (Novartis Consumer Health UK Ltd)
  Hyoscine 1 mg per 72 hour Scopoderm 1.5mg patches | 2 patch Ⓟ £4.52 DT price = £4.52

ANTIPSYCHOTICS ＞ FIRST-GENERATION

⟋ 230

Droperidol

- **DRUG ACTION** Droperidol is a butyrophenone, structurally related to haloperidol, which blocks dopamine receptors in the chemoreceptor trigger zone.

- **INDICATIONS AND DOSE**

  Prevention and treatment of postoperative nausea and vomiting
  ‣ BY INTRAVENOUS INJECTION
  ‣ Child 2-17 years: 20–50 micrograms/kg (max. per dose 1.25 mg), dose to be given 30 minutes before end of surgery, then 20–50 micrograms/kg every 6 hours (max. per dose 1.25 mg) if required

- **CONTRA-INDICATIONS** Bradycardia · CNS depression · comatose states · hypokalaemia · hypomagnesaemia · phaeochromocytoma · QT-interval prolongation
- **CAUTIONS** Chronic obstructive pulmonary disease · electrolyte disturbances · history of alcohol abuse · respiratory failure
- **INTERACTIONS** → Appendix 1 (droperidol).
  Avoid concomitant administration of drugs that prolong QT interval.
- **SIDE-EFFECTS** Anxiety · cardiac arrest · hallucinations · inappropriate antidiuretic hormone secretion
- **BREAST FEEDING** Limited information available—avoid repeated administration.
- **HEPATIC IMPAIRMENT** In postoperative nausea and vomiting, max. 625 micrograms repeated every 6 hours as required.
- **RENAL IMPAIRMENT** In postoperative nausea and vomiting, max. 625 micrograms repeated every 6 hours as required.
- **MONITORING REQUIREMENTS** Continuous pulse oximetry required if risk of ventricular arrhythmia—continue for 30 minutes following administration.

- **MEDICINAL FORMS**
  There can be variation in the licensing of different medicines containing the same drug.
  Solution for injection
  ‣ **Xomolix** (ProStrakan Ltd)
  Droperidol 2.5 mg per 1 ml Xomolix 2.5mg/1ml solution for injection ampoules | 10 ampoule ⓅoⓂ £39.40

⟋ 230

Levomepromazine

(Methotrimeprazine)

- **INDICATIONS AND DOSE**

  Restlessness and confusion in palliative care
  ‣ BY CONTINUOUS SUBCUTANEOUS INFUSION
  ‣ Child 1-11 years: 0.35–3 mg/kg, to be administered over 24 hours
  ‣ Child 12-17 years: 12.5–200 mg, to be administered over 24 hours

  Nausea and vomiting in palliative care
  ‣ BY CONTINUOUS INTRAVENOUS INFUSION, OR BY SUBCUTANEOUS INFUSION
  ‣ Child 1 month-11 years: 100–400 micrograms/kg, to be administered over 24 hours
  ‣ Child 12-17 years: 5–25 mg, to be administered over 24 hours

- **CONTRA-INDICATIONS** CNS depression · comatose states · phaeochromocytoma
- **CAUTIONS** Diabetes · patients receiving large initial doses should remain supine
- **SIDE-EFFECTS** Raised erythrocyte sedimentation rate
- **HEPATIC IMPAIRMENT** Can precipitate coma; phenothiazines are hepatotoxic.
- **RENAL IMPAIRMENT** Start with small doses in severe renal impairment because of increased cerebral sensitivity.
- **DIRECTIONS FOR ADMINISTRATION**
  ‣ With subcutaneous use For administration by *subcutaneous infusion* dilute with a suitable volume of Sodium Chloride 0.9%.

4

Nervous system

Nervous system

4

● **MEDICINAL FORMS**
There can be variation in the licensing of different medicines containing the same drug.

Solution for injection

▸ Levomepromazine (Non-proprietary)
Levomepromazine hydrochloride 25 mg per 1 ml Levomepromazine 25mg/1ml solution for injection ampoules | 10 ampoule [PoM] £20.13 DT price = £20.13

▸ Nozinan (Sanofi)
Levomepromazine hydrochloride 25 mg per 1 ml Nozinan 25mg/1ml solution for injection ampoules | 10 ampoule [PoM] £20.13 DT price = £20.13

F 230

Prochlorperazine

● **INDICATIONS AND DOSE**

Prevention and treatment of nausea and vomiting

▸ BY MOUTH
‣ Child 1–11 years (body-weight 10 kg and above): 250 micrograms/kg 2–3 times a day

‣ Child 12–17 years: 5–10 mg up to 3 times a day if required

▸ BY INTRAMUSCULAR INJECTION
‣ Child 2-4 years: 1.25–2.5 mg up to 3 times a day if required

‣ Child 5–11 years: 5–6.25 mg up to 3 times a day if required

‣ Child 12–17 years: 12.5 mg up to 3 times a day if required

Nausea and vomiting in previously diagnosed migraine

▸ BY MOUTH USING BUCCAL TABLET
‣ Child 12–17 years: 3–6 mg twice daily, tablets to be placed high between upper lip and gum and left to dissolve

DOSE EQUIVALENCE AND CONVERSION
Doses are expressed as prochlorperazine maleate or mesilate; 1 mg prochlorperazine maleate ≡ 1 mg prochlorperazine mesilate.

● **UNLICENSED USE**
▸ With intramuscular use Injection not licensed for use in children.
▸ With buccal use Buccal tablets not licensed for use in children.

● **CONTRA-INDICATIONS** Avoid oral route in child under 10 kg · children (in psychotic disorders) · CNS depression · comatose states · phaeochromocytoma

● **CAUTIONS** Hypotension (more likely after intramuscular injection)

● **SIDE-EFFECTS** Dystonic reactions · respiratory depression may occur in susceptible patients

SIDE-EFFECTS, FURTHER INFORMATION
▸ Acute dystonic reactions Phenothiazines can all induce acute dystonic reactions such as facial and skeletal muscle spasms and oculogyric crises; children (especially girls, young women, and those under 10 kg) are particularly susceptible.

● **HEPATIC IMPAIRMENT** Can precipitate coma; phenothiazines are hepatotoxic.

● **RENAL IMPAIRMENT** Start with small doses in severe renal impairment because of increased cerebral sensitivity.

● **DIRECTIONS FOR ADMINISTRATION**
▸ With buccal use Buccal tablets are placed high between upper lip and gum and left to dissolve.

● **PATIENT AND CARER ADVICE**
▸ With buccal use Patients or carers should be given advice on how to administer prochlorperazine buccal tablets.

● **MEDICINAL FORMS**
There can be variation in the licensing of different medicines containing the same drug.

Tablet
CAUTIONARY AND ADVISORY LABELS 2

▸ Prochlorperazine (Non-proprietary)
Prochlorperazine maleate 5 mg Prochlorperazine 5mg tablets | 28 tablet [PoM] £2.75 DT price = £0.93 | 84 tablet [PoM] £5.95

▸ Stemetil (Sanofi)
Prochlorperazine maleate 5 mg Stemetil 5mg tablets | 28 tablet [PoM] £1.98 DT price = £0.93 | 84 tablet [PoM] £5.94

Buccal tablet
CAUTIONARY AND ADVISORY LABELS 2

▸ Prochlorperazine (Non-proprietary)
Prochlorperazine maleate 3 mg Prochlorperazine 3mg buccal tablets | 50 tablet [PoM] £35.94–£43.13 DT price = £41.68

▸ Buccastem (Alliance Pharmaceuticals Ltd)
Prochlorperazine maleate 3 mg Buccastem M 3mg tablets | 8 tablet [P] £3.66

Oral solution
CAUTIONARY AND ADVISORY LABELS 2

▸ Stemetil (Sanofi)
Prochlorperazine mesilate 1 mg per 1 ml Stemetil 5mg/5ml syrup | 100 ml [PoM] £3.34 DT price = £3.34

Solution for injection

▸ Prochlorperazine (Non-proprietary)
Prochlorperazine mesilate 12.5 mg per 1 ml Prochlorperazine 12.5mg/1ml solution for injection ampoules | 10 ampoule [PoM] no price available DT price = £5.23

▸ Stemetil (Sanofi)
Prochlorperazine mesilate 12.5 mg per 1 ml Stemetil 12.5mg/1ml solution for injection ampoules | 10 ampoule [PoM] £5.23 DT price = £5.23

5 Pain

Analgesics

Drugs used for pain

The non-opioid drugs, paracetamol p. 254 and ibuprofen p. 608 (and other NSAIDs), are particularly suitable for pain in musculoskeletal conditions, whereas the opioid analgesics are more suitable for moderate to severe pain, particularly of visceral origin.

Pain in sickle-cell disease

The pain of mild sickle-cell crises is managed with paracetamol, an NSAID, codeine phosphate p. 259, or dihydrocodeine tartrate p. 262. Severe crises may require the use of morphine p. 265 or diamorphine hydrochloride p. 261; concomitant use of an NSAID may potentiate analgesia and allow lower doses of the opioid to be used. A mixture of nitrous oxide and oxygen (*Entonox*®, *Equanox*®) may also be used.

Dental and orofacial pain

Analgesics should be used judiciously in dental care as a **temporary** measure until the cause of the pain has been dealt with.

Dental pain of inflammatory origin, such as that associated with pulpitis, apical infection, localised osteitis or pericoronitis is usually best managed by treating the infection, providing drainage, restorative procedures, and other local measures. Analgesics provide temporary relief of pain (usually for about 1 to 7 days) until the causative factors have been brought under control. In the case of pulpitis, intra-osseous infection or abscess, reliance on analgesics alone is usually inappropriate.

Similarly the pain and discomfort associated with acute problems of the oral mucosa (e.g. acute herpetic gingivostomatitis, erythema multiforme) may be relieved by benzydamine hydrochloride p. 660 or topical anaesthetics until the cause of the mucosal disorder has been dealt with.

However, where a child is febrile, the antipyretic action of paracetamol or ibuprofen is often helpful.

The *choice* of an analgesic for dental purposes should be based on its suitability for the child. Most dental pain is relieved effectively by non-steroidal anti-inflammatory drugs (NSAIDs) e.g. ibuprofen. Paracetamol has analgesic and antipyretic effects but no anti-inflammatory effect.

Opioid analgesics such as dihydrocodeine tartrate act on the central nervous system and are traditionally used for *moderate to severe pain*. However, opioid analgesics are relatively ineffective in dental pain and their side-effects can be unpleasant.

Combining a non-opioid with an opioid analgesic can provide greater relief of pain than either analgesic given alone. However, this applies only when an adequate dose of each analgesic is used. Most combination analgesic preparations have not been shown to provide greater relief of pain than an adequate dose of the non-opioid component given alone. Moreover, combination preparations have the disadvantage of an increased number of side-effects.

Any analgesic given before a dental procedure should have a low risk of increasing postoperative bleeding. In the case of pain after the dental procedure, taking an analgesic before the effect of the local anaesthetic has worn off can improve control. Postoperative analgesia with ibuprofen is usually continued for about 24 to 72 hours.

Dysmenorrhoea
Paracetamol or a NSAID will generally provide adequate relief of pain from dysmenorrhoea. Alternatively use of a combined hormonal contraceptive in adolescent girls may prevent the pain.

Non-opioid analgesics and compound analgesic preparations

Paracetamol has analgesic and antipyretic properties but no demonstrable anti-inflammatory activity; unlike opioid analgesics, it does not cause respiratory depression and is less irritant to the stomach than the NSAIDs. **Overdosage** with paracetamol is particularly dangerous as it may cause hepatic damage which is sometimes not apparent for 4 to 6 days.

Non-steroidal anti-inflammatory analgesics (NSAIDs) are particularly useful for the treatment of children with chronic disease accompanied by pain and inflammation. Some of them are also used in the short-term treatment of mild to moderate pain including transient musculoskeletal pain but paracetamol is now often preferred. They are also suitable for the relief of pain in *dysmenorrhoea* and to treat pain caused by *secondary bone tumours*, many of which produce lysis of bone and release prostaglandins. Due to an association with Reye's syndrome, aspirin p. 83 should be avoided in children under 16 years except in Kawasaki disease or for its antiplatelet action. Several NSAIDs are also used for postoperative analgesia.

Compound analgesic preparations
Compound analgesic preparations that contain a simple analgesic (such as paracetamol) with an opioid component reduce the scope for effective titration of the individual components in the management of pain of varying intensity.

Compound analgesic preparations containing paracetamol with a *low dose* of an opioid analgesic (e.g. 8 mg of codeine phosphate per compound tablet) may be used in older children but the advantages have not been substantiated. The low dose of the opioid may be enough to cause opioid side-effects (in particular, constipation) and can complicate the treatment of **overdosage** yet may not provide significant additional relief of pain.

A *full dose* of the opioid component (e.g. 60 mg codeine phosphate) in compound analgesic preparations effectively augments the analgesic activity but is associated with the full range of opioid side-effects (including nausea, vomiting, severe constipation, drowsiness, respiratory depression, and risk of dependence on long-term administration).

In general, when assessing pain, it is necessary to weigh up carefully whether there is a need for a non-opioid and an opioid analgesic to be taken simultaneously.

Opioid analgesics

Opioid analgesics are usually used to relieve moderate to severe pain particularly of visceral origin. Repeated administration may cause tolerance, but this is no deterrent in the control of pain in terminal illness. Regular use of a potent opioid may be appropriate for certain cases of chronic non-malignant pain; treatment should be supervised by a specialist and the child should be assessed at regular intervals.

Strong opioids
Morphine remains the most valuable opioid analgesic for severe pain although it frequently causes nausea and vomiting. It is the standard against which other opioid analgesics are compared. In addition to relief of pain, morphine also confers a state of euphoria and mental detachment.

Morphine is the opioid of choice for the oral treatment of *severe pain in palliative care*. It is given regularly every 4 hours (or every 12 or 24 hours as modified-release preparations).

Buprenorphine p. 257 has both opioid agonist and antagonist properties and may precipitate withdrawal symptoms, including pain, in children dependent on other opioids. It has abuse potential and may itself cause dependence. It has a much longer duration of action than morphine and sublingually is an effective analgesic for 6 to 8 hours. Unlike most opioid analgesics, the effects of buprenorphine are only partially reversed by naloxone hydrochloride p. 796. It is rarely used in children.

Diamorphine hydrochloride (heroin) p. 261 is a powerful opioid analgesic. It may cause less nausea and hypotension than morphine p. 265. In *palliative care* the greater solubility of diamorphine hydrochloride allows effective doses to be injected in smaller volumes and this is important in the emaciated child. Diamorphine hydrochloride is sometimes given by the intranasal route to treat acute pain in children and is available as a nasal spray; intranasal administration of diamorphine injection has been used [unlicensed].

Alfentanil p. 772, fentanyl p. 262 and remifentanil p. 772 are used by injection for intra-operative analgesia. Fentanyl is available in a transdermal drug delivery system as a self-adhesive patch which is changed every 72 hours.

Methadone hydrochloride p. 279 is less sedating than morphine and acts for longer periods. In prolonged use, methadone hydrochloride should not be administered more often than twice daily to avoid the risk of accumulation and opioid overdosage. Methadone hydrochloride may be used instead of morphine when excitation (or exacerbation of pain) occurs with morphine. Methadone hydrochloride may also be used to treat children with neonatal abstinence syndrome.

Papaveretum p. 269 should not be used in children; morphine is easier to prescribe and less prone to error with regard to the strength and dose.

Pethidine hydrochloride p. 269 produces prompt but short-lasting analgesia; it is less constipating than morphine, but even in high doses is a less potent analgesic. Its use in children is not recommended. Pethidine hydrochloride is used for analgesia in labour; however, other opioids, such as morphine or diamorphine hydrochloride, are often preferred for obstetric pain.

Tramadol hydrochloride p. 270 is used in older children and produces analgesia by two mechanisms: an opioid effect and an enhancement of serotonergic and adrenergic pathways. It has fewer of the typical opioid side-effects (notably, less respiratory depression, less constipation and less addiction potential); psychiatric reactions have been reported.

Weak opioids
Codeine phosphate p. 259 can be used for the relief of short-term acute moderate pain in children older than 12 years where other painkillers such as paracetamol below or ibuprofen p. 608 have proved ineffective.

Dihydrocodeine tartrate p. 262 has an analgesic efficacy similar to that of codeine phosphate.

Postoperative analgesia
A combination of opioid and non-opioid analgesics is used to treat postoperative pain. The use of intra-operative opioids affects the prescribing of postoperative analgesics. A postoperative opioid analgesic should be given with care since it may potentiate any residual respiratory depression.

Morphine is used most widely. Tramadol hydrochloride is not as effective in severe pain as other opioid analgesics. Buprenorphine p. 257 may antagonise the analgesic effect of previously administered opioids and is generally not recommended. Pethidine hydrochloride is generally not recommended for postoperative pain because it is metabolised to norpethidine which may accumulate, particularly in neonates and in renal impairment; norpethidine stimulates the central nervous system and may cause convulsions.

Opioids are also given epidurally [unlicensed route] in the postoperative period but are associated with side-effects such as pruritus, urinary retention, nausea and vomiting; respiratory depression can be delayed, particularly with morphine.

Patient-controlled analgesia (PCA) and nurse-controlled analgesia (NCA) can be used to relieve postoperative pain—consult hospital protocols.

Pain management and opioid dependence
Although caution is necessary, patients who are dependent on opioids or have a history of drug dependence may be treated with opioid analgesics when there is a clinical need. Treatment with opioid analgesics in this patient group should normally be carried out with the advice of specialists. However, doctors do not require a special licence to prescribe opioid analgesics to patients with opioid dependence for relief of pain due to organic disease or injury.

> **Drugs used for Pain not listed below** Diclofenac potassium, p. 605 · Mefenamic acid, p. 612

ANALGESICS > NON-OPIOID

Paracetamol
5.5.2016
(Acetaminophen)

● **INDICATIONS AND DOSE**

Pain | Pyrexia with discomfort
▸ BY MOUTH

▸ Neonate 28 weeks to 32 weeks corrected gestational age: 20 mg/kg for 1 dose, then 10–15 mg/kg every 8–12 hours as required, maximum daily dose to be given in divided doses; maximum 30 mg/kg per day.

▸ Neonate 32 weeks corrected gestational age and above: 20 mg/kg for 1 dose, then 10–15 mg/kg every 6–8 hours as required, maximum daily dose to be given in divided doses; maximum 60 mg/kg per day.

▸ Child 1–2 months: 30–60 mg every 8 hours as required, maximum daily dose to be given in divided doses; maximum 60 mg/kg per day

▸ Child 3–5 months: 60 mg every 4–6 hours; maximum 4 doses per day

▸ Child 6 months–1 year: 120 mg every 4–6 hours; maximum 4 doses per day

▸ Child 2–3 years: 180 mg every 4–6 hours; maximum 4 doses per day

▸ Child 4–5 years: 240 mg every 4–6 hours; maximum 4 doses per day

▸ Child 6–7 years: 240–250 mg every 4–6 hours; maximum 4 doses per day

▸ Child 8–9 years: 360–375 mg every 4–6 hours; maximum 4 doses per day

▸ Child 10–11 years: 480–500 mg every 4–6 hours; maximum 4 doses per day

▸ Child 12–15 years: 480–750 mg every 4–6 hours; maximum 4 doses per day

▸ Child 16–17 years: 0.5–1 g every 4–6 hours; maximum 4 doses per day

▸ BY RECTUM

▸ Neonate 28 weeks to 32 weeks corrected gestational age: 20 mg/kg for 1 dose, then 10–15 mg/kg every 12 hours as required, maximum daily dose to be given in divided doses; maximum 30 mg/kg per day.

▸ Neonate 32 weeks corrected gestational age and above: 30 mg/kg for 1 dose, then 15–20 mg/kg every 8 hours as required, maximum daily dose to be given in divided doses; maximum 60 mg/kg per day.

▸ Child 1–2 months: 30–60 mg every 8 hours as required, maximum daily dose to be given in divided doses; maximum 60 mg/kg per day

▸ Child 3–11 months: 60–125 mg every 4–6 hours as required; maximum 4 doses per day

▸ Child 1–4 years: 125–250 mg every 4–6 hours as required; maximum 4 doses per day

▸ Child 5–11 years: 250–500 mg every 4–6 hours as required; maximum 4 doses per day

▸ Child 12–17 years: 500 mg every 4–6 hours
▸ BY INTRAVENOUS INFUSION

▸ Neonate 32 weeks corrected gestational age and above: 7.5 mg/kg every 8 hours, dose to be administered over 15 minutes.

▸ Neonate: 10 mg/kg every 4–6 hours, dose to be administered over 15 minutes; maximum 30 mg/kg per day.

▸ Child (body-weight up to 10 kg): 10 mg/kg every 4–6 hours, dose to be administered over 15 minutes; maximum 30 mg/kg per day

▸ Child (body-weight 10–50 kg): 15 mg/kg every 4–6 hours, dose to be administered over 15 minutes; maximum 60 mg/kg per day

▸ Child (body-weight 50 kg and above): 1 g every 4–6 hours, dose to be administered over 15 minutes; maximum 4 g per day

Pain in children with risk factors for hepatotoxicity | Pyrexia with discomfort in children with risk factors for hepatotoxicity
▸ BY INTRAVENOUS INFUSION

▸ Neonate 32 weeks corrected gestational age and above: 7.5 mg/kg every 8 hours, dose to be administered over 15 minutes.

▸ Neonate: 10 mg/kg every 4–6 hours, dose to be administered over 15 minutes; maximum 30 mg/kg per day.

▸ Child (body-weight up to 10 kg): 10 mg/kg every 4–6 hours, dose to be administered over 15 minutes; maximum 30 mg/kg per day

▸ Child (body-weight 10–50 kg): 15 mg/kg every 4–6 hours, dose to be administered over 15 minutes; maximum 60 mg/kg per day

‣ Child (body-weight 50 kg and above): 1 g every 4–6 hours, dose to be administered over 15 minutes; maximum 3 g per day

Post-operative pain

▸ BY MOUTH

‣ Child 1 month–5 years: 20–30 mg/kg for 1 dose, then 15–20 mg/kg every 4–6 hours, maximum daily dose to be given in divided doses; maximum 75 mg/kg per day

‣ Child 6–11 years: 20–30 mg/kg (max. per dose 1 g) for 1 dose, then 15–20 mg/kg every 4–6 hours, maximum daily dose to be given in divided doses; maximum 75 mg/kg per day; maximum 4 g per day

‣ Child 12–17 years: 1 g every 4–6 hours; maximum 4 doses per day

▸ BY RECTUM

‣ Child 1–2 months: 30 mg/kg for 1 dose, then 15–20 mg/kg every 4–6 hours, maximum daily dose to be given in divided doses; maximum 75 mg/kg per day

‣ Child 3 months–5 years: 30–40 mg/kg for 1 dose, then 15–20 mg/kg every 4–6 hours, maximum daily dose to be given in divided doses; maximum 75 mg/kg per day

‣ Child 6–11 years: 30–40 mg/kg (max. per dose 1 g) for 1 dose, then 15–20 mg/kg every 4–6 hours, maximum daily dose to be given in divided doses; maximum 75 mg/kg per day; maximum 4 g per day

‣ Child 12–17 years: 1 g every 4–6 hours; maximum 4 doses per day

Post-immunisation pyrexia in infants

▸ BY MOUTH

‣ Child 2–3 months: 60 mg for 1 dose, then 60 mg after 4–6 hours if required, (dose can be repeated twice for meningococcal B vaccine)

‣ Child 4 months: 60 mg for 1 dose, then 60 mg after 4–6 hours; maximum 4 doses per day

PANADOL OA®

Mild to moderate pain | Pyrexia

▸ BY MOUTH

‣ Child 12–17 years: 1 g up to 4 times a day, dose not to be taken more often than every 4 hours

● **UNLICENSED USE** Paracetamol oral suspension 500 mg/5 mL not licensed for use in children under 16 years. Not licensed for use in children under 2 months by mouth; under 3 months by rectum. [EvGr] Second further dose for post-immunisation pyrexia in infants 2–3 months for meningococcal B vaccine not licensed. ⟨E⟩ Intravenous infusion not licensed in preterm neonates. Intravenous infusion dose not licensed in children and neonates with body-weight under 10 kg.

● **CAUTIONS** Before administering, check when paracetamol last administered and cumulative paracetamol dose over previous 24 hours · body-weight under 50 kg · chronic alcohol consumption · chronic dehydration · chronic malnutrition · hepatocellular insufficiency · long-term use (especially in those who are malnourished)

CAUTIONS, FURTHER INFORMATION

[EvGr] Some patients may be at increased risk of experiencing toxicity at therapeutic doses, particularly those with a body-weight under 50 kg and those with risk factors for hepatotoxicity. Clinical judgement should be used to adjust the dose of oral and intravenous paracetamol in these patients. ⟨E⟩

[EvGr] Co-administration of enzyme-inducing antiepileptic medications may increase toxicity; doses should be reduced. ⟨E⟩

● **INTERACTIONS** → Appendix 1 (paracetamol).

● **SIDE-EFFECTS**

GENERAL SIDE-EFFECTS

▸ **Rare** Acute generalised exanthematous pustulosis · malaise · skin reactions · Stevens-Johnson syndrome · toxic epidermal necrolysis

▸ **Frequency not known** Blood disorders · leucopenia · neutropenia · thrombocytopenia

SPECIFIC SIDE-EFFECTS

▸ **Rare**

▸ With intravenous use Flushing · tachycardia

▸ **Frequency not known**

▸ With intravenous use Hypotension

Overdose

Important: liver damage and less frequently renal damage can occur following overdose.

Nausea and vomiting, the only early features of poisoning, usually settle within 24 hours. Persistence beyond this time, often associated with the onset of right subcostal pain and tenderness, usually indicates development of hepatic necrosis.

For specific details on the management of poisoning, see Paracetamol, under Emergency treatment of poisoning p. 786

● **PREGNANCY** Not known to be harmful.

● **BREAST FEEDING** Amount too small to be harmful.

● **HEPATIC IMPAIRMENT** Dose-related toxicity—avoid large doses.

● **RENAL IMPAIRMENT** Increase infusion dose interval to every 6 hours if estimated glomerular filtration rate less than 30 mL/minute/1.73 m^2.

● **DIRECTIONS FOR ADMINISTRATION**

▸ With intravenous use For *intravenous infusion* (*Perfalgan®*), give in Glucose 5% *or* Sodium Chloride 0.9%; dilute to a concentration of not less than 1 mg/mL and use within an hour; may also be given undiluted. For children under 33 kg, use 50 mL-vial.

● **PRESCRIBING AND DISPENSING INFORMATION** BP directs that when Paediatric Paracetamol Oral Suspension or Paediatric Paracetamol Mixture is prescribed Paracetamol Oral Suspension 120 mg/5 mL should be dispensed.

● **PATIENT AND CARER ADVICE**

Medicines for Children leaflet: Paracetamol for mild-to-moderate pain www.medicinesforchildren.org.uk/paracetamol-for-mildtomoderate-pain

● **PROFESSION SPECIFIC INFORMATION**

Dental practitioners' formulary

Paracetamol Tablets may be prescribed.

Paracetamol Soluble Tablets 500 mg may be prescribed.

Paracetamol Oral Suspension may be prescribed.

● **EXCEPTIONS TO LEGAL CATEGORY** Paracetamol capsules or tablets can be sold to the public provided packs contain no more than 32 capsules or tablets; pharmacists can sell multiple packs up to a total quantity of 100 capsules or tablets in justifiable circumstances.

● **MEDICINAL FORMS**

There can be variation in the licensing of different medicines containing the same drug. Forms available from special-order manufacturers include: oral suspension, oral solution, suppository

Tablet

CAUTIONARY AND ADVISORY LABELS 29 (does not apply to 1 g tablet), 30

▸ **Paracetamol (Non-proprietary)**

Paracetamol 500 mg Paracetamol 500mg caplets | 32 tablet [P] £0.38 DT price = £0.74 | 100 tablet [PoM] £3.18 DT price = £2.31

Paracetamol 500mg tablets | 32 tablet [P] £1.24 DT price = £0.74 | 100 tablet [PoM] £3.18 DT price = £2.31 | 1000 tablet [PoM] £25.63 | 5000 tablet [PoM] no price available

▸ **Mandanol** (M & A Pharmachem Ltd)

Paracetamol 500 mg Mandanol 500mg caplets | 32 tablet [P] £0.20 DT price = £0.74

Mandanol 500mg tablets | 100 tablet [PoM] £0.33 DT price = £2.31

4

Nervous system

▸ **Panadol** (GlaxoSmithKline Consumer Healthcare)
Paracetamol 500 mg Panadol Advance 500mg tablets |
32 tablet Ⓟ £1.74 DT price = £0.74

Effervescent tablet
CAUTIONARY AND ADVISORY LABELS 29, 30
▸ **Paracetamol (Non-proprietary)**
Paracetamol 500 mg Paracetamol 500mg soluble tablets |
60 tablet Ⓟ no price available | 60 tablet PoM £5.00 |
100 tablet PoM £8.33 DT price = £7.54 | 100 tablet Ⓟ no price
available DT price = £7.54

Soluble tablet
CAUTIONARY AND ADVISORY LABELS 13, 29, 30
▸ **Paracetamol (Non-proprietary)**
Paracetamol 120 mg Paracetamol 120mg soluble tablets sugar free
sugar-free | 16 tablet GSL no price available
▸ Brands may include Disprol

Orodispersible tablet
CAUTIONARY AND ADVISORY LABELS 30
▸ **Calpol Fastmelts** (McNeil Products Ltd)
Paracetamol 250 mg Calpol Six Plus Fastmelts 250mg tablets sugar-
free | 12 tablet £2.28 sugar-free | 24 tablet Ⓟ £3.59

Capsule
CAUTIONARY AND ADVISORY LABELS 29, 30
▸ **Paracetamol (Non-proprietary)**
Paracetamol 500 mg Paracetamol 500mg capsules | 16 capsule Ⓟ
£0.55 | 32 capsule Ⓟ £1.21 DT price = £1.00 | 100 capsule PoM
£8.20 DT price = £3.13

Oral suspension
CAUTIONARY AND ADVISORY LABELS 30
▸ **Paracetamol (Non-proprietary)**
Paracetamol 24 mg per 1 ml Paracetamol 120mg/5ml oral
suspension paediatric | 100 ml Ⓟ £0.72 | 500 ml Ⓟ £3.14 DT price
= £3.12
Paracetamol 120mg/5ml oral suspension paediatric sugar free sugar-
free | 100 ml Ⓟ £2.40 DT price = £1.23 sugar-free | 200 ml Ⓟ £2.72
sugar-free | 500 ml Ⓟ £6.80 sugar-free | 1000 ml Ⓟ £13.60
Paracetamol 50 mg per 1 ml Paracetamol 250mg/5ml oral
suspension | 100 ml Ⓟ £1.25 DT price = £1.13 | 500 ml Ⓟ £6.25
Paracetamol 250mg/5ml oral suspension sugar free sugar-free |
100 ml Ⓟ £2.75 sugar-free | 200 ml Ⓟ £1.99 DT price = £1.97
sugar-free | 500 ml Ⓟ £8.25 sugar-free | 1000 ml Ⓟ £16.50
Paracetamol 100 mg per 1 ml Paracetamol 500mg/5ml oral
suspension sugar free sugar-free | 150 ml PoM £24.00 DT price =
£24.00
▸ **Calpol** (McNeil Products Ltd)
Paracetamol 24 mg per 1 ml Calpol Infant 120mg/5ml oral
suspension | 200 ml Ⓟ £3.35
Calpol Infant 120mg/5ml oral suspension sugar free sugar-free |
200 ml Ⓟ £3.35
Paracetamol 50 mg per 1 ml Calpol Six Plus 250mg/5ml oral
suspension | 200 ml Ⓟ £3.88
Calpol Six Plus 250mg/5ml oral suspension sugar free sugar-free |
100 ml Ⓟ £2.40 sugar-free | 200 ml Ⓟ £3.88 DT price = £1.97
▸ **Mandanol** (M & A Pharmachem Ltd)
Paracetamol 24 mg per 1 ml Mandanol Infant paracetamol
120mg/5ml oral suspension sugar-free | 200 ml Ⓟ £1.05
Paracetamol 50 mg per 1 ml Mandanol 6+ paracetamol 250mg/5ml
oral suspension sugar-free | 100 ml Ⓟ £0.90 sugar-free | 200 ml Ⓟ
£1.10 DT price = £1.97

Oral solution
CAUTIONARY AND ADVISORY LABELS 30
▸ **Paracetamol (Non-proprietary)**
Paracetamol 24 mg per 1 ml Paracetamol 120mg/5ml oral solution
paediatric sugar free sugar-free | 500 ml Ⓟ £2.86 DT price = £2.86
sugar-free | 2000 ml Ⓟ £27.20
Paracetamol 100 mg per 1 ml Paracetamol 500mg/5ml oral
solution sugar free sugar-free | 200 ml PoM £18.00

Solution for infusion
▸ **Paracetamol (Non-proprietary)**
Paracetamol 10 mg per 1 ml Paracetamol 500mg/50ml solution for
infusion vials | 10 vial PoM £11.00
Paracetamol 1g/100ml solution for infusion vials | 10 vial PoM
£12.00
▸ **Perfalgan** (Bristol-Myers Squibb Pharmaceuticals Ltd)
Paracetamol 10 mg per 1 ml Perfalgan 1g/100ml solution for
infusion vials | 12 vial PoM £14.96
Perfalgan 500mg/50ml solution for infusion | 12 vial PoM
£13.60

Suppository
CAUTIONARY AND ADVISORY LABELS 30
▸ **Paracetamol (Non-proprietary)**
Paracetamol 80 mg Paracetamol 80mg suppositories |
10 suppository Ⓟ £10.00
Paracetamol 120 mg Paracetamol 120mg suppositories |
10 suppository Ⓟ £11.26 DT price = £11.26
Paracetamol 125 mg Paracetamol 125mg suppositories |
10 suppository Ⓟ £15.00 DT price = £13.80
Paracetamol 240 mg Paracetamol 240mg suppositories |
10 suppository Ⓟ £22.01 DT price = £22.01
Paracetamol 250 mg Paracetamol 250mg suppositories |
10 suppository Ⓟ £15.00 DT price = £27.60
Paracetamol 500 mg Paracetamol 500mg suppositories |
10 suppository Ⓟ £36.50 DT price = £36.50
Paracetamol 1 gram Paracetamol 1g suppositories |
10 suppository Ⓟ no price available | 12 suppository Ⓟ no price
available
▸ **Alvedon** (Intrapharm Laboratories Ltd)
Paracetamol 60 mg Alvedon 60mg suppositories |
10 suppository Ⓟ £11.95 DT price = £11.95
Paracetamol 125 mg Alvedon 125mg suppositories |
10 suppository Ⓟ £13.80 DT price = £13.80
Paracetamol 250 mg Alvedon 250mg suppositories |
10 suppository Ⓟ £27.60 DT price = £27.60

❙ Paracetamol with tramadol

The properties listed below are those particular to the
combination only. For the properties of the components
please consider, paracetamol p. 254, tramadol hydrochloride
p. 270.

● **INDICATIONS AND DOSE**
Moderate to severe pain
▸ BY MOUTH
▸ Child 12–17 years: 2 tablets up to every 6 hours;
maximum 8 tablets per day

● **MEDICINAL FORMS**
There can be variation in the licensing of different medicines
containing the same drug.

Tablet
CAUTIONARY AND ADVISORY LABELS 2, 25, 29, 30
▸ **Paracetamol with tramadol (Non-proprietary)**
Tramadol hydrochloride 37.5 mg, Paracetamol 325 mg Tramadol
37.5mg / Paracetamol 325mg tablets | 60 tablet PoM £9.68 DT price
= £9.22 CD3
▸ **Tramacet** (Grunenthal Ltd)
Tramadol hydrochloride 37.5 mg, Paracetamol 325 mg Tramacet
37.5mg/325mg tablets | 60 tablet PoM £9.68 DT price = £9.22 CD3

Effervescent tablet
CAUTIONARY AND ADVISORY LABELS 2, 13, 29, 30
ELECTROLYTES: May contain Sodium
▸ **Tramacet** (Grunenthal Ltd)
Tramadol hydrochloride 37.5 mg, Paracetamol 325 mg Tramacet
37.5mg/325mg effervescent tablets sugar-free | 60 tablet PoM £9.68
DT price = £9.68 CD3

ANALGESICS ❭ OPIOIDS

Opioids

● **CONTRA-INDICATIONS** Acute respiratory depression ·
comatose patients · head injury (opioid analgesics interfere
with pupillary responses vital for neurological assessment)
· raised intracranial pressure (opioid analgesics interfere
with pupillary responses vital for neurological assessment)
· risk of paralytic ileus
● **CAUTIONS** Adrenocortical insufficiency (reduced dose is
recommended) · asthma (avoid during an acute attack) ·
convulsive disorders · diseases of the biliary tract ·
hypotension · hypothyroidism (reduced dose is
recommended) · impaired respiratory function (avoid in
chronic obstructive pulmonary disease) · inflammatory

bowel disorders · myasthenia gravis · obstructive bowel disorders · shock

CAUTIONS, FURTHER INFORMATION

▶ **Dependence** Repeated use of opioid analgesics is associated with the development of psychological and physical dependence; although this is rarely a problem with therapeutic use, caution is advised if prescribing for patients with a history of drug dependence.

▶ **Palliative care** In the control of pain in terminal illness, the cautions listed should not necessarily be a deterrent to the use of opioid analgesics.

● INTERACTIONS → Appendix 1 (opioid analgesics).

● SIDE-EFFECTS

▶ **Common or very common** Biliary spasm · bradycardia · confusion · constipation · dependence · difficulty with micturition · dizziness · drowsiness · dry mouth · dysphoria · euphoria · flushing · hallucinations · headache · hypotension (larger doses) · miosis · mood changes · muscle rigidity (larger doses) · nausea (particularly in initial stages) · oedema · palpitation · postural hypotension · pruritus · rash · respiratory depression (larger doses) · sexual dysfunction · sleep disturbances · sweating · tachycardia · ureteric spasm · urinary retention · urticaria · vertigo · visual disturbances · vomiting (particularly in initial stages)

▶ **Frequency not known** Adrenal insufficiency (long-term use) · hyperalgesia (long-term use) · hypogonadism (long-term use)

SIDE-EFFECTS, FURTHER INFORMATION

▶ **Hypogonadism and adrenal insufficiency** Long-term use of opioid analgesics can cause hypogonadism and adrenal insufficiency in both males and females. This is thought to be dose related and can lead to amenorrhoea, reduced libido, infertility, depression, and erectile dysfunction.

▶ **Hyperalgesia** Long-term use of opioid analgesics has also been associated with a state of abnormal pain sensitivity (hyperalgesia). Pain associated with hyperalgesia is usually distinct from pain associated with disease progression or breakthrough pain, and is often more diffuse and less defined. Treatment of hyperalgesia involves reducing the dose of opioid medication or switching therapy; cases of suspected hyperalgesia should be referred to a specialist pain team.

▶ **Respiratory depression** Respiratory depression is a major concern with opioid analgesics; neonates (particularly if pre-term) may be more susceptible. It may be treated by artificial ventilation or be reversed by naloxone.

▶ **Dependence and withdrawal** Psychological dependence rarely occurs when opioids are used therapeutically (e.g. for pain relief) but tolerance can develop during long-term treatment.

Overdose
Opioids (narcotic analgesics) cause coma, respiratory depression, and pinpoint pupils. For details on the management of poisoning, see Opioids, under Emergency treatment of poisoning p. 786 and consider the specific antidote, naloxone hydrochloride p. 796.

● PREGNANCY Respiratory depression and withdrawal symptoms can occur in the neonate if opioid analgesics are used during delivery; also gastric stasis and inhalation pneumonia has been reported in the mother if opioid analgesics are used during labour.

● HEPATIC IMPAIRMENT Avoid use or reduce dose; may precipitate coma in patients with hepatic impairment.

● TREATMENT CESSATION Avoid abrupt withdrawal after long-term treatment; they should be withdrawn gradually to avoid abstinence symptoms.

● PATIENT AND CARER ADVICE

Driving and skilled tasks
Drowsiness may affect performance of skilled tasks (e.g. driving); effects of alcohol enhanced. Driving at the start of therapy with opioid analgesics, and following dose changes, should be avoided.

For information on 2015 legislation regarding driving whilst taking certain controlled drugs, including opioids, see *Drugs and driving* under Guidance on prescribing p. 1.

☞ 256

Buprenorphine

● DRUG ACTION Buprenorphine is an opioid-receptor partial agonist (it has opioid agonist and antagonist properties).

● INDICATIONS AND DOSE

Moderate to severe pain
▶ BY SUBLINGUAL ADMINISTRATION
▶ Child (body-weight 16–25 kg): 100 micrograms every 6–8 hours
▶ Child (body-weight 25–37.5 kg): 100–200 micrograms every 6–8 hours
▶ Child (body-weight 37.5–50 kg): 200–300 micrograms every 6–8 hours
▶ Child (body-weight 50 kg and above): 200–400 micrograms every 6–8 hours
▶ BY INTRAMUSCULAR INJECTION, OR BY SLOW INTRAVENOUS INJECTION
▶ Child 6 months–11 years: 3–6 micrograms/kg every 6–8 hours (max. per dose 9 micrograms/kg)
▶ Child 12–17 years: 300–600 micrograms every 6–8 hours

● UNLICENSED USE
▶ With oral use Sublingual tablets not licensed for use in children under 6 years.
▶ With intramuscular use or intravenous use Injection not licensed for use in children under 6 months.

● CAUTIONS Impaired consciousness

● INTERACTIONS Caution with concomitant use of hepatotoxic drugs.

● SIDE-EFFECTS

▶ **Common or very common** Abdominal pain · agitation · anorexia · anxiety · asthenia · diarrhoea · dyspepsia · dyspnoea · fatigue · mild withdrawal symptoms in patients dependent on opioids · paraesthesia · vasodilatation

▶ **Uncommon** Cough · depersonalisation · dry eye · dry skin · dysarthria · flatulence · hypertension · hypoaesthesia · hypoxia · impaired memory · influenza-like symptoms · muscle cramp · myalgia · pyrexia · restlessness · rhinitis · rigors · syncope · taste disturbance · tinnitus · tremor · wheezing

▶ **Rare** Diverticulitis · dysphagia · impaired concentration · paralytic ileus · psychosis

▶ **Very rare** Hiccups · hyperventilation · muscle fasciculation · retching

▶ **Frequency not known** Hepatic necrosis · hepatitis

Overdose
The effects of buprenorphine are only partially reversed by naloxone.

● BREAST FEEDING Present in low levels in breast milk. Neonates should be monitored for drowsiness, adequate weight gain, and developmental milestones.

● RENAL IMPAIRMENT Avoid use or reduce dose; opioid effects increased and prolonged and increased cerebral sensitivity occurs.

● PRE-TREATMENT SCREENING Documentation of viral hepatitis status is recommended before commencing therapy for opioid dependence.

● MONITORING REQUIREMENTS Monitor liver function; when used in opioid dependence baseline liver function test is recommended before commencing therapy, and regular liver function tests should be performed throughout treatment.

- **DIRECTIONS FOR ADMINISTRATION**
- ▶ With sublingual use For administration by *mouth*, tablets may be halved.

- **MEDICINAL FORMS**
There can be variation in the licensing of different medicines containing the same drug.
Sublingual tablet
CAUTIONARY AND ADVISORY LABELS 2, 26
  ▶ **Buprenorphine (Non-proprietary)**
  Buprenorphine (as Buprenorphine hydrochloride)
  200 microgram Buprenorphine 200microgram sublingual tablets sugar free sugar-free | 50 tablet PoM £6.05 DT price = £5.04 CD3
  Buprenorphine (as Buprenorphine hydrochloride)
  400 microgram Buprenorphine 400microgram sublingual tablets sugar free sugar-free | 7 tablet PoM £1.60 DT price = £1.60 CD3
  ▶ **Temgesic** (RB Pharmaceuticals Ltd)
  Buprenorphine (as Buprenorphine hydrochloride)
  200 microgram Temgesic 200microgram sublingual tablets sugar-free | 50 tablet PoM £5.04 DT price = £5.04 CD3
  Buprenorphine (as Buprenorphine hydrochloride)
  400 microgram Temgesic 400microgram sublingual tablets sugar-free | 50 tablet PoM £10.07 DT price = £10.07 CD3
  ▶ **Tephine** (Sandoz Ltd)
  Buprenorphine (as Buprenorphine hydrochloride)
  200 microgram Tephine 200microgram sublingual tablets sugar-free | 50 tablet PoM £4.27 DT price = £5.04 CD3
  Buprenorphine (as Buprenorphine hydrochloride)
  400 microgram Tephine 400microgram sublingual tablets sugar-free | 50 tablet PoM £8.54 DT price = £10.07 CD3
Solution for injection
  ▶ **Temgesic** (RB Pharmaceuticals Ltd)
  Buprenorphine (as Buprenorphine hydrochloride)
  300 microgram per 1 ml Temgesic 300micrograms/1ml solution for injection ampoules | 5 ampoule PoM £2.46 CD3

F 256

Co-codamol

- **INDICATIONS AND DOSE**

Short-term treatment of acute moderate pain (using co-codamol 8/500 preparations only)
  ▶ BY MOUTH
  ▶ **Child 12–17 years:** 8/500–16/1000 mg every 6 hours as required for maximum 3 days; maximum 64/4000 mg per day

Short-term treatment of acute moderate pain (using co-codamol 15/500 preparations only)
  ▶ BY MOUTH
  ▶ **Child 12–17 years:** 15/500–30/1000 mg every 6 hours as required for maximum 3 days; maximum 120/4000 mg per day

Short-term treatment of acute moderate pain (using co-codamol 30/500 preparations only)
  ▶ BY MOUTH
  ▶ **Child 12–17 years:** 30/500–60/1000 mg every 6 hours as required for maximum 3 days; maximum 240/4000 mg per day

KAPAKE® 15/500

Short-term treatment of acute pain
  ▶ BY MOUTH
  ▶ **Child 12–15 years:** 1 tablet every 6 hours as required for maximum 3 days; maximum 4 tablets per day

  ▶ **Child 16–17 years:** 2 tablets every 6 hours as required for maximum 3 days; maximum 8 tablets per day

> **IMPORTANT SAFETY INFORMATION**
> See codeine phosphate p. 259 for MHRA/CHM advice for restrictions on the use of codeine as an analgesic in children.

- **CONTRA-INDICATIONS** Acute ulcerative colitis · antibiotic-associated colitis · children who undergo the removal of tonsils or adenoids for the treatment of obstructive sleep apnoea · conditions where abdominal distention develops · conditions where inhibition of peristalsis should be avoided · known ultra-rapid codeine metabolisers
- **CAUTIONS** Acute abdomen · alcohol dependence · avoid abrupt withdrawal after long-term treatment · cardiac arrhythmias · chronic alcoholism · chronic dehydration · chronic malnutrition · convulsive disorders · gallstones · hepatocellular insufficiency
CAUTIONS, FURTHER INFORMATION
  ▶ Variation in metabolism The capacity to metabolise codeine to morphine can vary considerably between individuals; there is a marked increase in morphine toxicity in patients who are ultra-rapid codeine metabolisers (CYP2D6 ultra-rapid metabolisers) and a reduced therapeutic effect in poor codeine metabolisers.
- **INTERACTIONS** → Appendix 1 (paracetamol).
- **SIDE-EFFECTS** Abdominal pain · anorexia · blood disorders · depression (with larger doses) · hypothermia · leucopenia · malaise · muscle fasciculation · neutropenia · pancreatitis · seizures · thrombocytopenia
Overdose
Important: liver damage (and less frequently renal damage) following overdosage with paracetamol.
- **BREAST FEEDING** Avoid—although amount of codeine usually too small to be harmful, mothers vary considerably in their capacity to metabolise codeine—risk of morphine overdose in infant.
- **HEPATIC IMPAIRMENT** Dose-related toxicity with paracetamol—avoid large doses.
- **RENAL IMPAIRMENT** Reduce dose or avoid codeine; increased and prolonged effect; increased cerebral sensitivity.
- **PRESCRIBING AND DISPENSING INFORMATION** Co-codamol is a mixture of codeine phosphate and paracetamol; the proportions are expressed in the form x/y, where x and y are the strengths in milligrams of codeine phosphate and paracetamol respectively.
  When co-codamol tablets, dispersible (or effervescent) tablets, or capsules are prescribed and **no strength is stated**, tablets, dispersible (or effervescent) tablets, or capsules, respectively, containing codeine phosphate 8 mg and paracetamol 500 mg should be dispensed.
  The Drug Tariff allows tablets of co-codamol labelled 'dispersible' to be dispensed against an order for 'effervescent' and *vice versa*.
- **LESS SUITABLE FOR PRESCRIBING** Co-codamol is less suitable for prescribing.
- **EXCEPTIONS TO LEGAL CATEGORY** Co-codamol 8/500 can be sold to the public in certain circumstances; for exemptions see *Medicines, Ethics and Practice*, London, Pharmaceutical Press (always consult latest edition).

- **MEDICINAL FORMS**
There can be variation in the licensing of different medicines containing the same drug. Forms available from special-order manufacturers include: oral suspension, oral solution

Tablet
CAUTIONARY AND ADVISORY LABELS 2 (does not apply to the 8/500 tablet), 29, 30

► **Co-codamol** (Non-proprietary)
Codeine phosphate 8 mg, Paracetamol 500 mg Co-codamol 8mg/500mg tablets | 32 tablet P £1.02 Schedule 5 (CD Inv) | 100 tablet PoM £3.93 DT price = £3.07 Schedule 5 (CD Inv) | 500 tablet PoM £17.00 Schedule 5 (CD Inv) | 1000 tablet PoM £34.00 Schedule 5 (CD Inv)
Co-codamol 8mg/500mg caplets | 32 tablet P £1.20 Schedule 5 (CD Inv)

Codeine phosphate 15 mg, Paracetamol 500 mg Co-codamol 15mg/500mg tablets | 100 tablet PoM £15.00 DT price = £9.58 Schedule 5 (CD Inv)

Codeine phosphate 30 mg, Paracetamol 500 mg Co-codamol 30mg/500mg tablets | 100 tablet PoM £9.00 DT price = £4.17 Schedule 5 (CD Inv)
Co-codamol 30mg/500mg tablets | 30 tablet PoM £2.45 DT price = £1.25 Schedule 5 (CD Inv) | 100 tablet PoM £11.00 DT price = £4.17 Schedule 5 (CD Inv)

► **Codipar** (AMCo)
Codeine phosphate 15 mg, Paracetamol 500 mg Codipar 15mg/500mg tablets | 100 tablet PoM £8.25 DT price = £9.58 Schedule 5 (CD Inv)

► **Kapake** (Galen Ltd)
Codeine phosphate 30 mg, Paracetamol 500 mg Kapake 30mg/500mg tablets | 100 tablet PoM £6.04 DT price = £4.17 Schedule 5 (CD Inv)

► **Migraleve Yellow** (McNeil Products Ltd)
Codeine phosphate 8 mg, Paracetamol 500 mg Migraleve Yellow tablets | 16 tablet PoM no price available Schedule 5 (CD Inv)

► **Solpadol** (Sanofi)
Codeine phosphate 30 mg, Paracetamol 500 mg Solpadol 30mg/500mg caplets | 30 tablet PoM £2.02 DT price = £1.25 Schedule 5 (CD Inv) | 100 tablet PoM £6.74 DT price = £4.17 Schedule 5 (CD Inv)

► **Zapain** (AMCo)
Codeine phosphate 30 mg, Paracetamol 500 mg Zapain 30mg/500mg tablets | 100 tablet PoM £3.03 DT price = £4.17 Schedule 5 (CD Inv)

Effervescent tablet
CAUTIONARY AND ADVISORY LABELS 2 (does not apply to the 8/500 tablet), 13, 29, 30
EXCIPIENTS: May contain Aspartame
ELECTROLYTES: May contain Sodium

► **Co-codamol** (Non-proprietary)
Codeine phosphate 8 mg, Paracetamol 500 mg Co-codamol 8mg/500mg effervescent tablets | 32 tablet P £2.24 DT price = £2.25 Schedule 5 (CD Inv) | 100 tablet PoM £12.97 DT price = £7.03 Schedule 5 (CD Inv)

Codeine phosphate 30 mg, Paracetamol 500 mg Co-codamol 30mg/500mg effervescent tablets | 32 tablet PoM £5.40 DT price = £2.58 Schedule 5 (CD Inv) | 100 tablet PoM £19.20 DT price = £8.06 Schedule 5 (CD Inv)

► **Codipar** (AMCo)
Codeine phosphate 15 mg, Paracetamol 500 mg Codipar 15mg/500mg effervescent tablets sugar-free | 100 tablet PoM £8.25 DT price = £8.25 Schedule 5 (CD Inv)

► **Paracodol** (Bayer Plc)
Codeine phosphate 8 mg, Paracetamol 500 mg Paracodol 8mg/500mg effervescent tablets | 32 tablet P no price available DT price = £2.25 Schedule 5 (CD Inv)

► **Solpadol** (Sanofi)
Codeine phosphate 30 mg, Paracetamol 500 mg Solpadol 30mg/500mg effervescent tablets | 32 tablet PoM £2.59 DT price = £2.58 Schedule 5 (CD Inv) | 100 tablet PoM £8.90 DT price = £8.06 Schedule 5 (CD Inv)

► **Tylex** (UCB Pharma Ltd)
Codeine phosphate 30 mg, Paracetamol 500 mg Tylex 30mg/500mg effervescent tablets | 100 tablet PoM £9.06 DT price = £8.06 Schedule 5 (CD Inv)

Capsule
CAUTIONARY AND ADVISORY LABELS 2 (does not apply to the 8/500 capsule), 29, 30
EXCIPIENTS: May contain Sulfites

► **Co-codamol** (Non-proprietary)
Codeine phosphate 8 mg, Paracetamol 500 mg Co-codamol 8mg/500mg capsules | 100 capsule PoM £14.48 DT price = £12.63 Schedule 5 (CD Inv)

Codeine phosphate 30 mg, Paracetamol 500 mg Co-codamol 30mg/500mg capsules | 100 capsule PoM £15.00 DT price = £3.04 Schedule 5 (CD Inv)

► **Codipar** (AMCo)
Codeine phosphate 15 mg, Paracetamol 500 mg Codipar 15mg/500mg capsules | 100 capsule PoM £7.25 DT price = £7.25 Schedule 5 (CD Inv)

► **Kapake** (Galen Ltd)
Codeine phosphate 30 mg, Paracetamol 500 mg Kapake 30mg/500mg capsules | 100 capsule PoM £6.04 DT price = £3.04 Schedule 5 (CD Inv)

► **Paracodol** (Bayer Plc)
Codeine phosphate 8 mg, Paracetamol 500 mg Paracodol 8mg/500mg capsules | 20 capsule P £1.71 Schedule 5 (CD Inv) | 32 capsule P £2.69 DT price = £4.04 Schedule 5 (CD Inv)

► **Solpadol** (Sanofi)
Codeine phosphate 30 mg, Paracetamol 500 mg Solpadol 30mg/500mg capsules | 100 capsule PoM £6.74 DT price = £3.04 Schedule 5 (CD Inv)

► **Tylex** (UCB Pharma Ltd)
Codeine phosphate 30 mg, Paracetamol 500 mg Tylex 30mg/500mg capsules | 100 capsule PoM £7.93 DT price = £3.04 Schedule 5 (CD Inv)

► **Zapain** (AMCo)
Codeine phosphate 30 mg, Paracetamol 500 mg Zapain 30mg/500mg capsules | 100 capsule PoM £3.85 DT price = £3.04 Schedule 5 (CD Inv)

F 256

Codeine phosphate

- **INDICATIONS AND DOSE**

Acute diarrhoea
► BY MOUTH
► Child 12–17 years: 30 mg 3–4 times a day; usual dose 15–60 mg 3–4 times a day

Short-term treatment of acute moderate pain
► BY MOUTH, OR BY INTRAMUSCULAR INJECTION
► Child 12–17 years: 30–60 mg every 6 hours if required for maximum 3 days; maximum 240 mg per day

---

IMPORTANT SAFETY INFORMATION

MHRA/CHM ADVICE (JULY 2013) CODEINE FOR ANALGESIA: RESTRICTED USE IN CHILDREN DUE TO REPORTS OF MORPHINE TOXICITY

Codeine should only be used to relieve acute moderate pain in children older than 12 years and only if it cannot be relieved by other painkillers such as paracetamol or ibuprofen alone. A significant risk of serious and life-threatening adverse reactions has been identified in children with obstructive sleep apnoea who received codeine after tonsillectomy or adenoidectomy:

- in children aged 12–18 years, the maximum daily dose of codeine should not exceed 240 mg. Doses may be taken up to four times a day at intervals of no less than 6 hours. The lowest effective dose should be used and duration of treatment should be limited to 3 days
- codeine is contra-indicated in all children (under 18 years) who undergo the removal of tonsils or adenoids for the treatment of obstructive sleep apnoea
- codeine is not recommended for use in children whose breathing may be compromised, including those with neuromuscular disorders, severe cardiac or respiratory conditions, respiratory infections, multiple trauma or extensive surgical procedures
- codeine is contra-indicated in patients of any age who are known to be ultra-rapid metabolisers of codeine (CYP2D6 ultra-rapid metabolisers)

- codeine should not be used in breast-feeding mothers because it can pass to the baby through breast milk
- parents and carers should be advised on how to recognise signs and symptoms of morphine toxicity, and to stop treatment and seek medical attention if signs or symptoms of toxicity occur (including reduced consciousness, lack of appetite, somnolence, constipation, respiratory depression, 'pin-point' pupils, nausea, vomiting)

MHRA/CHM ADVICE (APRIL 2015) CODEINE FOR COUGH AND COLD: RESTRICTED USE IN CHILDREN

Do not use codeine in children under 12 years as it is associated with a risk of respiratory side effects. Codeine is not recommended for adolescents (12–18 years) who have problems with breathing. When prescribing or dispensing codeine-containing medicines for cough and cold, consider that codeine is contra-indicated in:

- children younger than 12 years old
- patients of any age known to be CYP2D6 ultra-rapid metabolisers
- breastfeeding mothers

- **CONTRA-INDICATIONS** Acute ulcerative colitis · antibiotic-associated colitis · children under 18 years who undergo the removal of tonsils or adenoids for the treatment of obstructive sleep apnoea · conditions where abdominal distension develops · conditions where inhibition of peristalsis should be avoided · known ultra-rapid codeine metabolisers
- **CAUTIONS** Acute abdomen · cardiac arrhythmias · gallstones · not recommended for adolescents aged 12–18 years with breathing problems

  CAUTIONS, FURTHER INFORMATION
- Variation in metabolism The capacity to metabolise codeine to morphine can vary considerably between individuals; there is a marked increase in morphine toxicity in patients who are ultra-rapid codeine metabolisers (CYP2D6 ultra-rapid metabolisers) and a reduced therapeutic effect in poor codeine metabolisers.
- **SIDE-EFFECTS** Abdominal pain · anorexia · antidiuretic effect · hypothermia · malaise · muscle fasciculation · pancreatitis · seizures
- **BREAST FEEDING** Avoid—although amount usually too small to be harmful, mothers vary considerably in their capacity to metabolise codeine—risk of morphine overdose in infant.
- **RENAL IMPAIRMENT** Avoid use or reduce dose; opioid effects increased and prolonged, and increased cerebral sensitivity occurs.
- **PRESCRIBING AND DISPENSING INFORMATION** BP directs that when Diabetic Codeine Linctus is prescribed, Codeine Linctus formulated with a vehicle appropriate for administration to diabetics, whether or not labelled 'Diabetic Codeine Linctus', shall be dispensed or supplied.
- **PATIENT AND CARER ADVICE** Medicines for Children leaflet: Codeine phosphate for pain www.medicinesforchildren.org.uk/codeine-phosphate-pain-0
- **MEDICINAL FORMS** There can be variation in the licensing of different medicines containing the same drug. Forms available from special-order manufacturers include: oral suspension, oral solution, solution for injection

  Tablet
  CAUTIONARY AND ADVISORY LABELS 2
  ▸ Codeine phosphate (Non-proprietary)
    Codeine phosphate 15 mg Codeine 15mg tablets | 28 tablet [PoM] £1.90 DT price = £0.94 Schedule 5 (CD Inv) | 30 tablet [PoM] no price available Schedule 5 (CD Inv) | 100 tablet [PoM] £6.60 DT price = £3.36 Schedule 5 (CD Inv) | 500 tablet [PoM] no price available Schedule 5 (CD Inv)

    Codeine phosphate 30 mg Codeine 30mg tablets | 28 tablet [PoM] £2.50 DT price = £1.10 Schedule 5 (CD Inv) | 30 tablet [PoM] no price available Schedule 5 (CD Inv) | 100 tablet [PoM] £5.68 DT price = £3.93 Schedule 5 (CD Inv) | 500 tablet [PoM] no price available Schedule 5 (CD Inv)

    Codeine phosphate 60 mg Codeine 60mg tablets | 28 tablet [PoM] £5.95 DT price = £1.84 Schedule 5 (CD Inv)

  Oral solution
  CAUTIONARY AND ADVISORY LABELS 2
  ▸ Codeine phosphate (Non-proprietary)
    Codeine phosphate 3 mg per 1 ml Codeine 15mg/5ml linctus sugar free sugar-free | 200 ml [P] £1.87 DT price = £1.63 Schedule 5 (CD Inv) sugar-free | 2000 ml [P] £16.30 Schedule 5 (CD Inv) Codeine 15mg/5ml linctus | 200 ml [P] £1.84 DT price = £1.84 Schedule 5 (CD Inv) | 2000 ml [P] no price available Schedule 5 (CD Inv)
    Codeine phosphate 5 mg per 1 ml Codeine 25mg/5ml oral solution | 500 ml [PoM] £6.46 DT price = £6.46 Schedule 5 (CD Inv)
  ▸ Galcodine (Thornton & Ross Ltd)
    Codeine phosphate 3 mg per 1 ml Galcodine 15mg/5ml linctus sugar-free | 2000 ml [P] £9.90 Schedule 5 (CD Inv)

  Solution for injection
  ▸ Codeine phosphate (Non-proprietary)
    Codeine phosphate 60 mg per 1 ml Codeine 60mg/1ml solution for injection ampoules | 10 ampoule [PoM] £23.70–£25.70 [CD2]

⟍ 256

Co-dydramol

- **INDICATIONS AND DOSE**

  Mild to moderate pain (using co-dydramol 10/500 preparations only)
  ▸ BY MOUTH
  ▸ Child 12–17 years: 10/500–20/1000 mg every 4–6 hours as required; maximum 80/4000 mg per day

  Severe pain (using co-dydramol 20/500 preparations only)
  ▸ BY MOUTH
  ▸ Child 12–17 years: 20/500–40/1000 mg every 4–6 hours as required; maximum 160/4000 mg per day

  Severe pain (using co-dydramol 30/500 preparations only)
  ▸ BY MOUTH
  ▸ Child 12–17 years: 30/500–60/1000 mg every 4–6 hours as required; maximum 240/4000 mg per day

  DOSE EQUIVALENCE AND CONVERSION
  A mixture of dihydrocodeine tartrate and paracetamol; the proportions are expressed in the form x/y, where x and y are the strengths in milligrams of dihydrocodeine and paracetamol respectively.

- **CAUTIONS** Alcohol dependence · before administering, check when paracetamol last administered and cumulative paracetamol dose over previous 24 hours · chronic alcoholism · chronic dehydration · chronic malnutrition · hepatocellular insufficiency · pancreatitis · severe cor pulmonale
- **INTERACTIONS** → Appendix 1 (paracetamol).
- **SIDE-EFFECTS** Abdominal pain · acute generalised exanthematous pustulosis · blood disorders · leucopenia · malaise · neutropenia · pancreatitis · paraesthesia · paralytic ileus · skin reactions · Stevens-Johnson syndrome · thrombocytopenia · toxic epidermal necrolysis

  Overdose
  Important: liver damage (and less frequently renal damage) following overdosage with paracetamol.
- **BREAST FEEDING** Amount of dihydrocodeine too small to be harmful but use only if potential benefit outweighs risk.
- **HEPATIC IMPAIRMENT** Dose-related toxicity with paracetamol—avoid large doses.
- **RENAL IMPAIRMENT** Reduce dose or avoid dihydrocodeine; increased and prolonged effect; increased cerebral sensitivity.

- **PRESCRIBING AND DISPENSING INFORMATION** When co-dydramol tablets are prescribed and **no strength is stated**, tablets containing dihydrocodeine tartrate 10 mg and paracetamol 500 mg should be dispensed.
- **LESS SUITABLE FOR PRESCRIBING** Co-dydramol is less suitable for prescribing.

- **MEDICINAL FORMS**
  There can be variation in the licensing of different medicines containing the same drug. Forms available from special-order manufacturers include: oral suspension, oral solution
  Tablet
  CAUTIONARY AND ADVISORY LABELS 2 (does not apply to the 10/500 tablet), 29, 30
  ‣ Co-dydramol (Non-proprietary)
  Dihydrocodeine tartrate 10 mg, Paracetamol 500 mg Co-dydramol 10mg/500mg tablets | 30 tablet [PoM] £3.30 DT price = £0.89 Schedule 5 (CD Inv) | 100 tablet [PoM] £11.00 DT price = £2.97 Schedule 5 (CD Inv) | 500 tablet [PoM] £16.35 Schedule 5 (CD Inv)

Diamorphine hydrochloride
(Heroin hydrochloride)

⚑ 256

10.6.2016

- **INDICATIONS AND DOSE**
Acute or chronic pain
  ‣ BY MOUTH
  ‣ Child 1 month–11 years: 100–200 micrograms/kg every 4 hours (max. per dose 10 mg), adjusted according to response
  ‣ Child 12–17 years: 5–10 mg every 4 hours, adjusted according to response
  ‣ BY CONTINUOUS INTRAVENOUS INFUSION
  ‣ Child 1 month–11 years: 12.5–25 micrograms/kg/hour, adjusted according to response
  ‣ BY INTRAVENOUS INJECTION
  ‣ Child 1-2 months: 20 micrograms/kg every 6 hours, adjusted according to response
  ‣ Child 3-5 months: 25–50 micrograms/kg every 6 hours, adjusted according to response
  ‣ Child 6-11 months: 75 micrograms/kg every 4 hours, adjusted according to response
  ‣ Child 1-11 years: 75–100 micrograms/kg every 4 hours (max. per dose 5 mg), adjusted according to response
  ‣ Child 12-17 years: 2.5–5 mg every 4 hours, adjusted according to response
  ‣ BY INTRAMUSCULAR INJECTION, OR BY SUBCUTANEOUS INJECTION
  ‣ Child 12-17 years: 5 mg every 4 hours, adjusted according to response

Acute or chronic pain in ventilated neonates
  ‣ INITIALLY BY INTRAVENOUS INJECTION
  ‣ Neonate: Initially 50 micrograms/kg, dose to be administered over 30 minutes, followed by (by continuous intravenous infusion) 15 micrograms/kg/hour, adjusted according to response.

Acute or chronic pain in non-ventilated neonates
  ‣ BY CONTINUOUS INTRAVENOUS INFUSION
  ‣ Neonate: 2.5–7 micrograms/kg/hour, adjusted according to response.

Acute severe nociceptive pain in an emergency setting (specialist supervision in hospital)
  ‣ BY INTRANASAL ADMINISTRATION
  ‣ Child 2-15 years (body-weight 12-17 kg): 1.44 mg for 1 dose, spray into alternate nostrils
  ‣ Child 2-15 years (body-weight 18-23 kg): 2.16 mg for 1 dose, spray into alternate nostrils
  ‣ Child 2-15 years (body-weight 24-29 kg): 2.88 mg for 1 dose, spray into alternate nostrils
  ‣ Child 2-15 years (body-weight 30-39 kg): 3.2 mg for 1 dose, spray into alternate nostrils
  ‣ Child 2-15 years (body-weight 40-50 kg): 4.8 mg for 1 dose, spray into alternate nostrils

- **CONTRA-INDICATIONS** Delayed gastric emptying · phaeochromocytoma
- **CAUTIONS** CNS depression · severe cor pulmonale · severe diarrhoea · toxic psychosis
- **SIDE-EFFECTS** Anorexia · asthenia · myocardial infarction · raised intracranial pressure · syncope · taste disturbance
- **BREAST FEEDING** Therapeutic doses unlikely to affect infant; withdrawal symptoms in infants of dependent mothers; breast-feeding not best method of treating dependence in offspring.
- **RENAL IMPAIRMENT** Avoid use or reduce dose; opioid effects increased and prolonged and increased cerebral sensitivity occurs.
- **DIRECTIONS FOR ADMINISTRATION**
  ‣ With intravenous use For *intravenous infusion*, dilute in Glucose 5% or Sodium Chloride 0.9%; Glucose 5% is preferable as an infusion fluid.
  ‣ With intranasal use Manufacturer advises spray should be directed at the nasal side wall whilst the patient is in a semi-recumbent position.
- **PRESCRIBING AND DISPENSING INFORMATION** Intranasal administration of diamorphine hydrochloride injection has been used [unlicensed]—no dose recommendation.

- **MEDICINAL FORMS**
  There can be variation in the licensing of different medicines containing the same drug. Forms available from special-order manufacturers include: capsule, oral solution, solution for injection, powder for solution for injection
  Tablet
  CAUTIONARY AND ADVISORY LABELS 2
  ‣ Diamorphine hydrochloride (Non-proprietary)
  Diamorphine hydrochloride 10 mg Diamorphine 10mg tablets | 100 tablet [PoM] £27.67–£27.82 DT price = £27.75 [CD2]
  Powder for solution for injection
  ‣ Diamorphine hydrochloride (Non-proprietary)
  Diamorphine hydrochloride 5 mg Diamorphine 5mg powder for solution for injection vials | 5 vial [PoM] £15.00 [CD2] Diamorphine 5mg powder for solution for injection ampoules | 5 ampoule [PoM] £11.36 DT price = £11.36 [CD2]
  Diamorphine hydrochloride 10 mg Diamorphine 10mg powder for solution for injection ampoules | 5 ampoule [PoM] £15.10 DT price = £13.61 [CD2] Diamorphine 10mg powder for solution for injection vials | 5 vial [PoM] £19.00 [CD2]
  Diamorphine hydrochloride 30 mg Diamorphine 30mg powder for solution for injection ampoules | 5 ampoule [PoM] £14.79 DT price = £13.33 [CD2] Diamorphine 30mg powder for solution for injection vials | 5 vial [PoM] £21.00 [CD2]
  Diamorphine hydrochloride 100 mg Diamorphine 100mg powder for solution for injection vials | 5 vial [PoM] £54.00 [CD2] Diamorphine 100mg powder for solution for injection ampoules | 5 ampoule [PoM] £42.39 DT price = £42.39 [CD2]
  Diamorphine hydrochloride 500 mg Diamorphine 500mg powder for solution for injection vials | 5 vial [PoM] £190.00–£235.00 DT price = £209.00 [CD2] Diamorphine 500mg powder for solution for injection ampoules | 5 ampoule [PoM] £187.70 DT price = £187.70 [CD2]
  Spray
  EXCIPIENTS: May contain Benzalkonium chloride, disodium edetate
  ‣ Ayendi (Wockhardt UK Ltd)
  Diamorphine (as Diamorphine hydrochloride) 720 microgram per 1 dose Ayendi 720micrograms/actuation nasal spray | 68 dose [PoM] £107.90 (Hospital only) [CD2] | 160 dose [PoM] £112.50 (Hospital only) [CD2]
  Diamorphine (as Diamorphine hydrochloride) 1.6 mg per 1 dose Ayendi 1600micrograms/actuation nasal spray | 68 dose [PoM] £113.52 (Hospital only) [CD2] | 160 dose [PoM] £123.75 (Hospital only) [CD2]

4

Nervous system

F 256

Dihydrocodeine tartrate

F 256

Fentanyl

● INDICATIONS AND DOSE

Moderate to severe pain

▶ BY MOUTH USING IMMEDIATE-RELEASE MEDICINES

- ▸ Child 1–3 years: 500 micrograms/kg every 4–6 hours
- ▸ Child 4–11 years: 0.5–1 mg/kg every 4–6 hours (max. per dose 30 mg)
- ▸ Child 12–17 years: 30 mg every 4–6 hours

▶ BY INTRAMUSCULAR INJECTION, OR BY SUBCUTANEOUS INJECTION

- ▸ Child 1–3 years: 500 micrograms/kg every 4–6 hours
- ▸ Child 4–11 years: 0.5–1 mg/kg every 4–6 hours (max. per dose 30 mg)
- ▸ Child 12–17 years: 30 mg every 4–6 hours (max. per dose 50 mg)

Chronic severe pain

▶ BY MOUTH USING MODIFIED-RELEASE MEDICINES

- ▸ Child 12–17 years: 60–120 mg every 12 hours

DF118 FORTE®

Severe pain

▶ BY MOUTH

- ▸ Child 12–17 years: 40–80 mg 3 times a day; maximum 240 mg per day

- ● UNLICENSED USE Most preparations not licensed for use in children under 4 years.
- ● CAUTIONS Pancreatitis · severe cor pulmonale
- ● SIDE-EFFECTS Abdominal pain · diarrhoea · paraesthesia · paralytic ileus · seizures
- ● BREAST FEEDING Use only if potential benefit outweighs risk.
- ● RENAL IMPAIRMENT Avoid use or reduce dose; opioid effects increased and prolonged and increased cerebral sensitivity occurs.
- ● PROFESSION SPECIFIC INFORMATION

Dental practitioners' formulary

Dihydrocodeine tablets 30 mg may be prescribed.

- ● MEDICINAL FORMS
There can be variation in the licensing of different medicines containing the same drug. Forms available from special-order manufacturers include: oral suspension, oral solution

Tablet

CAUTIONARY AND ADVISORY LABELS 2

- ▸ Dihydrocodeine tartrate (Non-proprietary)
 Dihydrocodeine tartrate 30 mg Dihydrocodeine 30mg tablets | 28 tablet [PoM] £1.75 DT price = £1.20 Schedule 5 (CD Inv) | 30 tablet [PoM] £1.56 Schedule 5 (CD Inv) | 100 tablet [PoM] £6.81 DT price = £4.29 Schedule 5 (CD Inv) | 500 tablet [PoM] £23.75 Schedule 5 (CD Inv)
- ▸ DF 118 (Martindale Pharmaceuticals Ltd)
 Dihydrocodeine tartrate 40 mg DF 118 Forte 40mg tablets | 100 tablet [PoM] £9.78 DT price = £9.78 Schedule 5 (CD Inv)

Modified-release tablet

CAUTIONARY AND ADVISORY LABELS 2, 25

- ▸ DHC Continus (Napp Pharmaceuticals Ltd)
 Dihydrocodeine tartrate 60 mg DHC Continus 60mg tablets | 56 tablet [PoM] £5.20 DT price = £5.20 Schedule 5 (CD Inv)
 Dihydrocodeine tartrate 90 mg DHC Continus 90mg tablets | 56 tablet [PoM] £8.66 DT price = £8.66 Schedule 5 (CD Inv)
 Dihydrocodeine tartrate 120 mg DHC Continus 120mg tablets | 56 tablet [PoM] £10.95 DT price = £10.95 Schedule 5 (CD Inv)

Oral solution

CAUTIONARY AND ADVISORY LABELS 2

- ▸ Dihydrocodeine tartrate (Non-proprietary)
 Dihydrocodeine tartrate 2 mg per 1 ml Dihydrocodeine 10mg/5ml oral solution | 150 ml [PoM] £7.16 DT price = £7.12 Schedule 5 (CD Inv)

Solution for injection

- ▸ Dihydrocodeine tartrate (Non-proprietary)
 Dihydrocodeine tartrate 50 mg per 1 ml Dihydrocodeine 50mg/1ml solution for injection ampoules | 10 ampoule [PoM] £91.14 DT price = £91.14 [CD2]

● INDICATIONS AND DOSE

Chronic intractable pain not currently treated with a strong opioid analgesic

▶ BY TRANSDERMAL APPLICATION

- ▸ Child 16–17 years: Initially 12 micrograms/hour every 72 hours, alternatively initially 25 micrograms/hour every 72 hours, when starting, evaluation of the analgesic effect should not be made before the system has been worn for 24 hours (to allow for the gradual increase in plasma-fentanyl concentration)—previous analgesic therapy should be phased out gradually from time of first patch application, dose should be adjusted at 48–72 hour intervals in steps of 12–25 micrograms/hour if necessary, more than one patch may be used at a time (but applied at the same time to avoid confusion)—consider additional or alternative analgesic therapy if dose required exceeds 300 micrograms/hour (important: it takes 17 hours or more for the plasma-fentanyl concentration to decrease by 50%— replacement opioid therapy should be initiated at a low dose and increased gradually)

Chronic intractable pain currently treated with a strong opioid analgesic

▶ BY TRANSDERMAL APPLICATION

- ▸ Child 2–17 years: Initial dose based on previous 24-hour opioid requirement (consult product literature), for evaluating analgesic efficacy and dose increments, see under *Chronic intractable pain not currently treated with a strong opioid analgesic*, for conversion from long term oral morphine to transdermal fentanyl, see *Pain management with opioids* p. 18.

Spontaneous respiration: analgesia and enhancement of anaesthesia, during operation

▶ BY INTRAVENOUS INJECTION

- ▸ Child 1 month–11 years: Initially 1–3 micrograms/kg, then 1 microgram/kg as required, dose to be administered over at least 30 seconds
- ▸ Child 12–17 years: Initially 50–100 micrograms (max. per dose 200 micrograms), dose maximum on specialist advice, then 25–50 micrograms as required, dose to be administered over at least 30 seconds

Assisted ventilation: analgesia and enhancement of anaesthesia during operation

▶ BY INTRAVENOUS INJECTION

- ▸ Neonate: Initially 1–5 micrograms/kg, then 1–3 micrograms/kg as required, dose to be administered over at least 30 seconds.
- ▸ Child 1 month–11 years: Initially 1–5 micrograms/kg, then 1–3 micrograms/kg as required, dose to be administered over at least 30 seconds
- ▸ Child 12–17 years: Initially 1–5 micrograms/kg, then 50–200 micrograms as required, dose to be administered over at least 30 seconds

Assisted ventilation: analgesia and respiratory depression in intensive care

▶ INITIALLY BY INTRAVENOUS INJECTION

- ▸ Neonate: Initially 1–5 micrograms/kg, then (by intravenous infusion) 1.5 micrograms/kg/hour, adjusted according to response
- ▸ Child: Initially 1–5 micrograms/kg, then (by intravenous infusion) 1–6 micrograms/kg/hour, adjusted according to response

Breakthrough pain in patients receiving opioid therapy for chronic cancer pain

▶ BY BUCCAL ADMINISTRATION USING LOZENGES
▶ Child 16–17 years: Initially 200 micrograms, dose to be given over 15 minutes, then 200 micrograms after 15 minutes if required, no more than 2 dose units for each pain episode; if adequate pain relief not achieved with 1 dose unit for consecutive breakthrough pain episodes, increase the strength of the dose unit until adequate pain relief achieved with 4 lozenges or less daily, if more than 4 episodes of breakthrough pain each day, adjust background analgesia

DOSE EQUIVALENCE AND CONVERSION
Fentanyl preparations for the treatment of breakthrough pain are not interchangeable; if patients are switched from another fentanyl-containing preparation, a new dose titration is required.

DOSES AT EXTREMES OF BODY-WEIGHT
To avoid excessive dosage in obese patients, weight-based doses may need to be calculated on the basis of ideal bodyweight.

● UNLICENSED USE
▶ With intravenous use Not licensed for use in children under 2 years; infusion not licensed for use in children under 12 years.

● CAUTIONS Cerebral tumour · diabetes mellitus (with *Actiq*® lozenges) · impaired consciousness
CAUTIONS, FURTHER INFORMATION
▶ With transdermal use Transdermal fentanyl patches are not suitable for acute pain or in those patients whose analgesic requirements are changing rapidly because the long time to steady state prevents rapid titration of the dose. Risk of fatal respiratory depression, particularly in patients not previously treated with a strong opioid analgesic; manufacturer recommends use only in opioid tolerant patients.
▶ With intravenous use Repeated intra-operative doses should be given with care since the resulting respiratory depression can persist postoperatively and occasionally it may become apparent for the first time postoperatively when monitoring of the patient might be less intensive.

● SIDE-EFFECTS
GENERAL SIDE-EFFECTS
▶ **Common or very common** Abdominal pain · aesthenia · anorexia · anxiety · appetite changes · application-site reactions · diarrhoea · dyspepsia · dyspnoea · gastro-oesophageal reflux disease · hypertension · myoclonus · paraesthesia · pharyngitis · rhinitis · stomatitis · tremor · vasodilation
▶ **Uncommon** Amnesia · arthralgia · blood disorders · chills · depressed level of consciousness · dysgeusia · flatulence · hypoventilation · ileus · impaired concentration · impaired coordination · loss of consciousness · malaise · parosmia · pyrexia · seizures · speech disorder · thirst · thrombocytopenia
▶ **Rare** Hiccups
▶ **Very rare** Apnoea · arrhythmia · ataxia · bladder pain · delusions · haemoptysis
SPECIFIC SIDE-EFFECTS
▶ **Common or very common**
▶ With intravenous use Myoclonic movements
▶ **Uncommon**
▶ With intravenous use Laryngospasm
▶ **Rare**
▶ With intravenous use Asystole · insomnia
SIDE-EFFECTS, FURTHER INFORMATION
▶ Fever or external heat Monitor patients using patches for increased side-effects if fever present (increased absorption possible); avoid exposing application site to

external heat, for example a hot bath or sauna (may also increase absorption).
▶ Muscle rigidity Intravenous administration of fentanyl can cause muscle rigidity, particularly of the chest wall or jaw; this can be managed by the use of neuromuscular blocking drugs.

● BREAST FEEDING Monitor infant for opioid-induced side-effects.

● RENAL IMPAIRMENT Avoid use or reduce dose; opioid effects increased and prolonged and increased cerebral sensitivity occurs.

● DIRECTIONS FOR ADMINISTRATION
▶ With transdermal use For *patches*, apply to dry, non-irritated, non-irradiated, non-hairy skin on torso or upper arm, removing after 72 hours and siting replacement patch on a different area (avoid using the same area for several days).
▶ With intravenous use For *intravenous infusion*, injection solution may be diluted in Glucose 5% or Sodium Chloride 0.9%.
▶ With buccal use Patients should be advised to place the lozenge in the mouth against the cheek and move it around the mouth using the applicator; each lozenge should be sucked over a 15 minute period. In patients with a dry mouth, water may be used to moisten the buccal mucosa. Patients with diabetes should be advised each lozenge contains approximately 2 g glucose.

● PRESCRIBING AND DISPENSING INFORMATION
▶ With transdermal use Prescriptions for fentanyl patches can be written to show the strength in terms of the release rate and it is acceptable to write *'Fentanyl 25 patches'* to prescribe patches that release fentanyl 25 micrograms per hour. The dosage should be expressed in terms of the interval between applying a patch and replacing it with a new one, e.g. *'one patch to be applied every 72 hours'*. The total quantity of patches to be supplied should be written in words and figures.

● PATIENT AND CARER ADVICE
Medicines for Children leaflet: Fentanyl lozenges for pain www.medicinesforchildren.org.uk/fentanyl-lozenges-for-pain
Medicines for Children leaflet: Fentanyl patches for pain www.medicinesforchildren.org.uk/fentanyl-patches-for-pain
▶ With transdermal use Patients and carers should be informed about safe use, including correct administration and disposal, strict adherence to dosage instructions, and the symptoms and signs of opioid overdosage. Patches should be removed immediately in case of breathing difficulties, marked drowsiness, confusion, dizziness, or impaired speech, and patients and carers should seek prompt medical attention.

● MEDICINAL FORMS
There can be variation in the licensing of different medicines containing the same drug. Forms available from special-order manufacturers include: solution for injection, infusion, solution for infusion

Lozenge
CAUTIONARY AND ADVISORY LABELS 2
EXCIPIENTS: May contain Propylene glycol
▶ Actiq (Teva UK Ltd)
Fentanyl (as Fentanyl citrate) 200 microgram Actiq 200microgram lozenges with integral oromucosal applicator |
3 lozenge PoM £21.05 CD2 | 30 lozenge PoM £210.41 CD2
Fentanyl (as Fentanyl citrate) 400 microgram Actiq 400microgram lozenges with integral oromucosal applicator |
3 lozenge PoM £21.05 CD2 | 30 lozenge PoM £210.41 CD2
Fentanyl (as Fentanyl citrate) 600 microgram Actiq 600microgram lozenges with integral oromucosal applicator |
3 lozenge PoM £21.05 CD2 | 30 lozenge PoM £210.41 CD2
Fentanyl (as Fentanyl citrate) 800 microgram Actiq 800microgram lozenges with integral oromucosal applicator |
3 lozenge PoM £21.05 CD2 | 30 lozenge PoM £210.41 CD2

Fentanyl (as Fentanyl citrate) **1.2 mg** Actiq 1.2mg lozenges with integral oromucosal applicator | 3 lozenge [PoM] £21.05 [CD2] | 30 lozenge [PoM] £210.41 [CD2]

Fentanyl (as Fentanyl citrate) **1.6 mg** Actiq 1.6mg lozenges with integral oromucosal applicator | 3 lozenge [PoM] £21.05 [CD2] | 30 lozenge [PoM] £210.41 [CD2]

Solution for injection

▸ **Fentanyl** (Non-proprietary)

Fentanyl (as Fentanyl citrate) 50 microgram per 1 ml Fentanyl 100micrograms/2ml solution for injection ampoules | 10 ampoule [PoM] £13.95 [CD2]

Fentanyl 500micrograms/10ml solution for injection ampoules | 10 ampoule [PoM] £12.50 [CD2]

▸ **Sublimaze** (Janssen-Cilag Ltd)

Fentanyl (as Fentanyl citrate) 50 microgram per 1 ml Sublimaze 500micrograms/10ml solution for injection ampoules | 5 ampoule [PoM] £6.53 [CD2]

Solution for infusion

▸ **Fentanyl** (Non-proprietary)

Fentanyl (as Fentanyl citrate) 50 microgram per 1 ml Fentanyl 2.5mg/50ml solution for infusion vials | 1 vial [PoM] £5.00 [CD2]

Transdermal patch

CAUTIONARY AND ADVISORY LABELS 2

▸ **Fentanyl** (Non-proprietary)

Fentanyl 12 microgram per 1 hour Fentanyl 12micrograms/hour transdermal patches | 5 patch [PoM] £12.59 DT price = £12.59 [CD2]

Fentanyl 25 microgram per 1 hour Fentanyl 25micrograms/hour transdermal patches | 5 patch [PoM] £17.99 DT price = £17.99 [CD2]

Fentanyl 50 microgram per 1 hour Fentanyl 50micrograms/hour transdermal patches | 5 patch [PoM] £35.91 DT price = £33.66 [CD2]

Fentanyl 75 microgram per 1 hour Fentanyl 75micrograms/hour transdermal patches | 5 patch [PoM] £50.12 DT price = £46.99 [CD2]

Fentanyl 100 microgram per 1 hour Fentanyl 100micrograms/hour transdermal patches | 5 patch [PoM] £61.72 DT price = £57.86 [CD2]

▸ **Durogesic DTrans** (Janssen-Cilag Ltd)

Fentanyl 12 microgram per 1 hour Durogesic DTrans 12micrograms transdermal patches | 5 patch [PoM] £12.59 DT price = £12.59 [CD2]

Fentanyl 25 microgram per 1 hour Durogesic DTrans 25micrograms transdermal patches | 5 patch [PoM] £17.99 DT price = £17.99 [CD2]

Fentanyl 50 microgram per 1 hour Durogesic DTrans 50micrograms transdermal patches | 5 patch [PoM] £33.66 DT price = £33.66 [CD2]

Fentanyl 75 microgram per 1 hour Durogesic DTrans 75micrograms transdermal patches | 5 patch [PoM] £46.99 DT price = £46.99 [CD2]

Fentanyl 100 microgram per 1 hour Durogesic DTrans 100micrograms transdermal patches | 5 patch [PoM] £57.86 DT price = £57.86 [CD2]

▸ **Fencino** (DB Ashbourne Ltd)

Fentanyl 12 microgram per 1 hour Fencino 12micrograms/hour transdermal patches | 5 patch [PoM] £8.46 DT price = £12.59 [CD2]

Fentanyl 25 microgram per 1 hour Fencino 25micrograms/hour transdermal patches | 5 patch [PoM] £12.10 DT price = £17.99 [CD2]

Fentanyl 50 microgram per 1 hour Fencino 50micrograms/hour transdermal patches | 5 patch [PoM] £22.62 DT price = £33.66 [CD2]

Fentanyl 75 microgram per 1 hour Fencino 75micrograms/hour transdermal patches | 5 patch [PoM] £31.54 DT price = £46.99 [CD2]

Fentanyl 100 microgram per 1 hour Fencino 100micrograms/hour transdermal patches | 5 patch [PoM] £38.88 DT price = £57.86 [CD2]

▸ **Fentalis** (Sandoz Ltd)

Fentanyl 25 microgram per 1 hour Fentalis Reservoir 25micrograms/hour transdermal patches | 5 patch [PoM] £22.89 DT price = £17.99 [CD2]

Fentanyl 50 microgram per 1 hour Fentalis Reservoir 50micrograms/hour transdermal patches | 5 patch [PoM] £42.77 DT price = £33.66 [CD2]

Fentanyl 75 microgram per 1 hour Fentalis Reservoir 75micrograms/hour transdermal patches | 5 patch [PoM] £59.62 DT price = £46.99 [CD2]

Fentanyl 100 microgram per 1 hour Fentalis Reservoir 100micrograms/hour transdermal patches | 5 patch [PoM] £73.49 DT price = £57.86 [CD2]

▸ **Matrifen** (Teva UK Ltd)

Fentanyl 12 microgram per 1 hour Matrifen 12micrograms/hour transdermal patches | 5 patch [PoM] £7.52 DT price = £12.59 [CD2]

Fentanyl 25 microgram per 1 hour Matrifen 25micrograms/hour transdermal patches | 5 patch [PoM] £10.76 DT price = £17.99 [CD2]

Fentanyl 50 microgram per 1 hour Matrifen 50micrograms/hour transdermal patches | 5 patch [PoM] £20.12 DT price = £33.66 [CD2]

Fentanyl 75 microgram per 1 hour Matrifen 75micrograms/hour transdermal patches | 5 patch [PoM] £28.06 DT price = £46.99 [CD2]

Fentanyl 100 microgram per 1 hour Matrifen 100micrograms/hour transdermal patches | 5 patch [PoM] £34.59 DT price = £57.86 [CD2]

▸ **Mezolar Matrix** (Sandoz Ltd)

Fentanyl 12 microgram per 1 hour Mezolar Matrix 12micrograms/hour transdermal patches | 5 patch [PoM] £7.53 DT price = £12.59 [CD2]

Fentanyl 25 microgram per 1 hour Mezolar Matrix 25micrograms/hour transdermal patches | 5 patch [PoM] £10.77 DT price = £17.99 [CD2]

Fentanyl 37.5 microgram per 1 hour Mezolar Matrix 37.5micrograms/hour transdermal patches | 5 patch [PoM] £15.46 [CD2]

Fentanyl 50 microgram per 1 hour Mezolar Matrix 50micrograms/hour transdermal patches | 5 patch [PoM] £20.13 DT price = £33.66 [CD2]

Fentanyl 75 microgram per 1 hour Mezolar Matrix 75micrograms/hour transdermal patches | 5 patch [PoM] £28.07 DT price = £46.99 [CD2]

Fentanyl 100 microgram per 1 hour Mezolar Matrix 100micrograms/hour transdermal patches | 5 patch [PoM] £34.60 DT price = £57.86 [CD2]

▸ **Mylafent** (Mylan Ltd)

Fentanyl 12 microgram per 1 hour Mylafent 12micrograms/hour transdermal patches | 5 patch [PoM] £7.53 DT price = £12.59 [CD2]

Fentanyl 25 microgram per 1 hour Mylafent 25micrograms/hour transdermal patches | 5 patch [PoM] £10.77 DT price = £17.99 [CD2]

Fentanyl 50 microgram per 1 hour Mylafent 50micrograms/hour transdermal patches | 5 patch [PoM] £20.13 DT price = £33.66 [CD2]

Fentanyl 75 microgram per 1 hour Mylafent 75micrograms/hour transdermal patches | 5 patch [PoM] £28.07 DT price = £46.99 [CD2]

Fentanyl 100 microgram per 1 hour Mylafent 100micrograms/hour transdermal patches | 5 patch [PoM] £34.60 DT price = £57.86 [CD2]

▸ **Opiodur** (Pfizer Ltd)

Fentanyl 12 microgram per 1 hour Opiodur 12micrograms/hour transdermal patches | 5 patch [PoM] £8.48 DT price = £12.59 [CD2]

Fentanyl 25 microgram per 1 hour Opiodur 25micrograms/hour transdermal patches | 5 patch [PoM] £12.12 DT price = £17.99 [CD2]

Fentanyl 50 microgram per 1 hour Opiodur 50micrograms/hour transdermal patches | 5 patch [PoM] £22.64 DT price = £33.66 [CD2]

Fentanyl 75 microgram per 1 hour Opiodur 75micrograms/hour transdermal patches | 5 patch [PoM] £31.56 DT price = £46.99 [CD2]

Fentanyl 100 microgram per 1 hour Opiodur 100micrograms/hour transdermal patches | 5 patch [PoM] £38.90 DT price = £57.86 [CD2]

▸ **Osmanil** (Zentiva)

Fentanyl 12 microgram per 1 hour Osmanil 12micrograms/hour transdermal patches | 5 patch [PoM] £18.11 DT price = £12.59 [CD2]

Fentanyl 25 microgram per 1 hour Osmanil 25micrograms/hour transdermal patches | 5 patch [PoM] £26.94 DT price = £17.99 [CD2]

Fentanyl 50 microgram per 1 hour Osmanil 50micrograms/hour transdermal patches | 5 patch [PoM] £50.32 DT price = £33.66 [CD2]

Fentanyl 75 microgram per 1 hour Osmanil 75micrograms/hour transdermal patches | 5 patch [PoM] £70.15 DT price = £46.99 [CD2]

Fentanyl 100 microgram per 1 hour Osmanil 100micrograms/hour transdermal patches | 5 patch [PoM] £86.46 DT price = £57.86 [CD2]

▸ **Tilofyl** (Tillomed Laboratories Ltd)

Fentanyl 25 microgram per 1 hour Tilofyl 25micrograms/hour transdermal patches | 5 patch [PoM] £27.00 DT price = £17.99 [CD2]

Fentanyl 50 microgram per 1 hour Tilofyl 50micrograms/hour transdermal patches | 5 patch [PoM] £51.00 DT price = £33.66 [CD2]

Fentanyl 75 microgram per 1 hour Tilofyl 75micrograms/hour transdermal patches | 5 patch [PoM] £71.00 DT price = £46.99 [CD2]

Fentanyl 100 microgram per 1 hour Tilofyl 100micrograms/hour transdermal patches | 5 patch [PoM] £88.00 DT price = £57.86 [CD2]

▸ **Victanyl** (Actavis UK Ltd)

Fentanyl 12 microgram per 1 hour Victanyl 12micrograms/hour transdermal patches | 5 patch [PoM] £12.58 DT price = £12.59 [CD2]

Fentanyl 25 microgram per 1 hour Victanyl 25micrograms/hour transdermal patches | 5 patch [PoM] £25.89 DT price = £17.99 [CD2]

Fentanyl 50 microgram per 1 hour Victanyl 50micrograms/hour transdermal patches | 5 patch [PoM] £48.36 DT price = £33.66 [CD2]

Fentanyl 75 microgram per 1 hour Victanyl 75micrograms/hour transdermal patches | 5 patch [PoM] £67.41 DT price = £46.99 [CD2]

Fentanyl 100 microgram per 1 hour Victanyl 100micrograms/hour transdermal patches | 5 patch [PoM] £83.09 DT price = £57.86 [CD2]

▸ **Yemex** (Sandoz Ltd)

Fentanyl 12 microgram per 1 hour Yemex 12micrograms/hour transdermal patches | 5 patch [PoM] £12.59 DT price = £12.59 [CD2]

Fentanyl 25 microgram per 1 hour Yemex 25micrograms/hour transdermal patches | 5 patch [PoM] £17.99 DT price = £17.99 [CD2]

Fentanyl 50 microgram per 1 hour Yemex 50micrograms/hour transdermal patches | 5 patch [PoM] £33.66 DT price = £33.66 [CD2]
Fentanyl 75 microgram per 1 hour Yemex 75micrograms/hour transdermal patches | 5 patch [PoM] £46.99 DT price = £46.99 [CD2]
Fentanyl 100 microgram per 1 hour Yemex 100micrograms/hour transdermal patches | 5 patch [PoM] £57.86 DT price = £57.86 [CD2]

☞ 256

Hydromorphone hydrochloride

- ● **INDICATIONS AND DOSE**
Severe pain in cancer
  - ▸ BY MOUTH USING IMMEDIATE-RELEASE MEDICINES
  - ▸ Child 12–17 years: 1.3 mg every 4 hours, dose to be increased if necessary according to severity of pain
  - ▸ BY MOUTH USING MODIFIED-RELEASE MEDICINES
  - ▸ Child 12–17 years: 4 mg every 12 hours, dose to be increased if necessary according to severity of pain

- ● **CONTRA-INDICATIONS** Acute abdomen
- ● **CAUTIONS** Pancreatitis · toxic psychosis
- ● **SIDE-EFFECTS**
  - ▸ **Common or very common** Abdominal pain · anorexia · anxiety
  - ▸ **Uncommon** Agitation · diarrhoea · dysgeusia · dyskinesia · myoclonus · paraesthesia · paralytic ileus · peripheral oedema · seizures · tremor
- ● **BREAST FEEDING** Avoid—no information available.
- ● **RENAL IMPAIRMENT** Avoid use or reduce dose; opioid effects increased and prolonged and increased cerebral sensitivity occurs.
- ● **DIRECTIONS FOR ADMINISTRATION** For *immediate-release* capsules, swallow whole capsule or sprinkle contents on soft food. For *modified-release* capsules, swallow whole or open capsule and sprinkle contents on soft cold food (swallow the pellets within the capsule whole; do not crush or chew).
- ● **PATIENT AND CARER ADVICE** Patients or carers should be given advice on how to administer hydromorphone hydrochloride capsules and modified-release capsules.

- ● **MEDICINAL FORMS**
There can be variation in the licensing of different medicines containing the same drug. Forms available from special-order manufacturers include: oral solution
Capsule
CAUTIONARY AND ADVISORY LABELS 2
  - ▸ Palladone (Napp Pharmaceuticals Ltd)
Hydromorphone hydrochloride 1.3 mg Palladone 1.3mg capsules | 56 capsule [PoM] £8.82 [CD2]
Hydromorphone hydrochloride 2.6 mg Palladone 2.6mg capsules | 56 capsule [PoM] £17.64 [CD2]
Modified-release capsule
CAUTIONARY AND ADVISORY LABELS 2
  - ▸ Palladone SR (Napp Pharmaceuticals Ltd)
Hydromorphone hydrochloride 2 mg Palladone SR 2mg capsules | 56 capsule [PoM] £20.98 [CD2]
Hydromorphone hydrochloride 4 mg Palladone SR 4mg capsules | 56 capsule [PoM] £28.75 [CD2]
Hydromorphone hydrochloride 8 mg Palladone SR 8mg capsules | 56 capsule [PoM] £56.08 [CD2]
Hydromorphone hydrochloride 16 mg Palladone SR 16mg capsules | 56 capsule [PoM] £106.53 [CD2]
Hydromorphone hydrochloride 24 mg Palladone SR 24mg capsules | 56 capsule [PoM] £159.82 [CD2]

☞ 256

Morphine

- ● **INDICATIONS AND DOSE**
Pain
  - ▸ BY SUBCUTANEOUS INJECTION
  - ▸ Neonate: Initially 100 micrograms/kg every 6 hours, adjusted according to response.
  - ▸ Child 1–5 months: Initially 100–200 micrograms/kg every 6 hours, adjusted according to response
  - ▸ Child 6 months–1 year: Initially 100–200 micrograms/kg every 4 hours, adjusted according to response
  - ▸ Child 2–11 years: Initially 200 micrograms/kg every 4 hours, adjusted according to response
  - ▸ Child 12–17 years: Initially 2.5–10 mg every 4 hours, adjusted according to response
  - ▸ INITIALLY BY INTRAVENOUS INJECTION
  - ▸ Neonate: 50 micrograms/kg every 6 hours, adjusted according to response, dose to be administered over at least 5 minutes, alternatively (by intravenous injection) initially 50 micrograms/kg, dose to be administered over at least 5 minutes, followed by (by continuous intravenous infusion) 5–20 micrograms/kg/hour, adjusted according to response
  - ▸ Child 1–5 months: 100 micrograms/kg every 6 hours, adjusted according to response, dose to be administered over at least 5 minutes, alternatively (by intravenous injection) initially 100 micrograms/kg, dose to be administered over at least 5 minutes, followed by (by continuous intravenous infusion) 10–30 micrograms/kg/hour, adjusted according to response
  - ▸ Child 6 months–11 years: 100 micrograms/kg every 4 hours, adjusted according to response, dose to be administered over at least 5 minutes, alternatively (by intravenous injection) initially 100 micrograms/kg, dose to be administered over at least 5 minutes, followed by (by continuous intravenous infusion) 20–30 micrograms/kg/hour, adjusted according to response
  - ▸ Child 12–17 years: 5 mg every 4 hours, adjusted according to response, dose to be administered over at least 5 minutes, alternatively (by intravenous injection) initially 5 mg, dose to be administered over at least 5 minutes, followed by (by continuous intravenous infusion) 20–30 micrograms/kg/hour, adjusted according to response
  - ▸ BY MOUTH, OR BY RECTUM
  - ▸ Child 1–2 months: Initially 50–100 micrograms/kg every 4 hours, adjusted according to response
  - ▸ Child 3–5 months: 100–150 micrograms/kg every 4 hours, adjusted according to response
  - ▸ Child 6–11 months: 200 micrograms/kg every 4 hours, adjusted according to response
  - ▸ Child 1 year: Initially 200–300 micrograms/kg every 4 hours, adjusted according to response
  - ▸ Child 2–11 years: Initially 200–300 micrograms/kg every 4 hours (max. per dose 10 mg), adjusted according to response
  - ▸ Child 12–17 years: Initially 5–10 mg every 4 hours, adjusted according to response
  - ▸ BY CONTINUOUS SUBCUTANEOUS INFUSION
  - ▸ Child 1–2 months: 10 micrograms/kg/hour, adjusted according to response
  - ▸ Child 3 months–17 years: 20 micrograms/kg/hour, adjusted according to response

continued →

4

Nervous system

Nervous system

4

Pain (with modified-release 12-hourly preparations)
▸ BY MOUTH USING MODIFIED-RELEASE MEDICINES
▸ Child: Every 12 hours, dose adjusted according to daily morphine requirements, dosage requirements should be reviewed if the brand is altered

Pain (with modified-release 24-hourly preparations)
▸ BY MOUTH USING MODIFIED-RELEASE MEDICINES
▸ Child: Every 24 hours, dose adjusted according to daily morphine requirements, dosage requirements should be reviewed if the brand is altered

Neonatal opioid withdrawal (under expert supervision)
▸ BY MOUTH

▸ Neonate: Initially 40 micrograms/kg every 4 hours until symptoms controlled, dose to be increased if necessary; reduce frequency gradually over 6–10 days, stop when 40 micrograms/kg once daily achieved, dose may vary—consult local guidelines.

Persistent cyanosis in congenital heart disease when blood glucose less than 3 mmol/litre (following glucose)
▸ BY INTRAVENOUS INJECTION, OR BY INTRAMUSCULAR INJECTION
▸ Child: 100 micrograms/kg

DOSE EQUIVALENCE AND CONVERSION
The doses stated refer equally to morphine hydrochloride and sulfate.

● **UNLICENSED USE**
▸ With oral use *Oramorph*® solution and *MXL*® capsules not licensed for use in children under 1 year. *Sevredol*® tablets not licensed for use in children under 3 years. *Oramorph*® unit dose vials and *Filnarine*® SR tablets not licensed for use in children under 6 years. *MST Continus*® preparations licensed to treat children with cancer pain (age-range not specified by manufacturer).
▸ With rectal use Suppositories are not licensed for use in children.

● **CONTRA-INDICATIONS** Acute abdomen · delayed gastric emptying · heart failure secondary to chronic lung disease · phaeochromocytoma

● **CAUTIONS** Cardiac arrhythmias · pancreatitis · severe cor pulmonale

● **SIDE-EFFECTS** Abdominal pain · agitation · amenorrhoea · anorexia · asthenia · bronchospasm · delirium · disorientation · dyspepsia · exacerbation of pancreatitis · excitation · hypertension · hypothermia · inhibition of cough reflex · malaise · muscle fasciculation · myoclonus · nystagmus · paraesthesia · paralytic ileus · raised intracranial pressure · restlessness · rhabdomyolysis · seizures · syncope · taste disturbance

● **BREAST FEEDING** Therapeutic doses unlikely to affect infant.

● **RENAL IMPAIRMENT** Avoid use or reduce dose; opioid effects increased and prolonged; increased cerebral sensitivity.

● **DIRECTIONS FOR ADMINISTRATION**
▸ With intravenous use For *continuous intravenous infusion*, dilute with Glucose 5% or 10% or Sodium Chloride 0.9%.
▸ With intravenous use in neonates *Neonatal intensive care*, dilute 2.5 mg/kg body-weight to a final volume of 50 mL with infusion fluid; an intravenous infusion rate of 0.1 mL/hour provides a dose of 5 micrograms/kg/hour.
▸ With oral use For *modified release capsules*—swallow whole or open capsule and sprinkle contents on soft food.

● **PRESCRIBING AND DISPENSING INFORMATION** Modified-release preparations are available as 12-hourly or 24-hourly formulations; prescribers must ensure that the correct preparation is prescribed. Preparations that should be given 12-hourly include *Filnarine*® SR, *MST Continus*®,

Morphgesic® SR and *Zomorph*®. Preparations that should be given 24-hourly include *MXL*®.
Prescriptions must specify the 'form'.
▸ With oral use Do not confuse modified-release 12-hourly preparations with 24-hourly preparations.
▸ With rectal use Both the strength of the suppositories and the morphine salt contained in them must be specified by the prescriber.

● **PATIENT AND CARER ADVICE**
Medicines for Children leaflet: Morphine for pain
www.medicinesforchildren.org.uk/morphine-for-pain
▸ With oral use Patients or carers should be given advice on how to administer morphine modified-release capsules.

● **EXCEPTIONS TO LEGAL CATEGORY**
Morphine Oral Solutions Prescription-only medicines or schedule 2 controlled drug. The proportion of morphine hydrochloride may be altered when specified by the prescriber; if above 13 mg per 5 mL the solution becomes a schedule 2 controlled drug. It is usual to adjust the strength so that the dose volume is 5 or 10 mL.
Oral solutions of morphine can be prescribed by writing the formula:
Morphine hydrochloride 5 mg
Chloroform water to 5 mL

● **MEDICINAL FORMS**
There can be variation in the licensing of different medicines containing the same drug. Forms available from special-order manufacturers include: capsule, oral solution, solution for injection, infusion, solution for infusion, suppository

Tablet
CAUTIONARY AND ADVISORY LABELS 2
▸ Sevredol (Napp Pharmaceuticals Ltd)
Morphine sulfate 10 mg Sevredol 10mg tablets | 56 tablet [PoM]
£5.31 DT price = £5.31 [CD2]
Morphine sulfate 20 mg Sevredol 20mg tablets | 56 tablet [PoM]
£10.61 DT price = £10.61 [CD2]
Morphine sulfate 50 mg Sevredol 50mg tablets | 56 tablet [PoM]
£28.02 DT price = £28.02 [CD2]

Modified-release tablet
CAUTIONARY AND ADVISORY LABELS 2, 25
▸ MST Continus (Napp Pharmaceuticals Ltd)
Morphine sulfate 5 mg MST Continus 5mg tablets | 60 tablet [PoM]
£3.29 DT price = £3.29 [CD2]
Morphine sulfate 10 mg MST Continus 10mg tablets | 60 tablet [PoM] £5.20 DT price = £5.20 [CD2]
Morphine sulfate 15 mg MST Continus 15mg tablets | 60 tablet [PoM] £9.10 DT price = £9.10 [CD2]
Morphine sulfate 30 mg MST Continus 30mg tablets | 60 tablet [PoM] £12.47 DT price = £12.47 [CD2]
Morphine sulfate 60 mg MST Continus 60mg tablets | 60 tablet [PoM] £24.32 DT price = £24.32 [CD2]
Morphine sulfate 100 mg MST Continus 100mg tablets | 60 tablet [PoM] £38.50 DT price = £38.50 [CD2]
Morphine sulfate 200 mg MST Continus 200mg tablets | 60 tablet [PoM] £81.34 DT price = £81.34 [CD2]
▸ Morphgesic SR (AMCo)
Morphine sulfate 10 mg Morphgesic SR 10mg tablets | 60 tablet [PoM] £3.85 DT price = £5.20 [CD2]
Morphine sulfate 30 mg Morphgesic SR 30mg tablets | 60 tablet [PoM] £9.24 DT price = £12.47 [CD2]
Morphine sulfate 60 mg Morphgesic SR 60mg tablets | 60 tablet [PoM] £18.04 DT price = £24.32 [CD2]
Morphine sulfate 100 mg Morphgesic SR 100mg tablets | 60 tablet [PoM] £28.54 DT price = £38.50 [CD2]

Modified-release capsule
CAUTIONARY AND ADVISORY LABELS 2
▸ MXL (Napp Pharmaceuticals Ltd)
Morphine sulfate 30 mg MXL 30mg capsules | 28 capsule [PoM]
£10.91 [CD2]
Morphine sulfate 60 mg MXL 60mg capsules | 28 capsule [PoM]
£14.95 [CD2]
Morphine sulfate 90 mg MXL 90mg capsules | 28 capsule [PoM]
£22.04 [CD2]
Morphine sulfate 120 mg MXL 120mg capsules | 28 capsule [PoM]
£29.15 [CD2]

Morphine sulfate 150 mg MXL 150mg capsules | 28 capsule [PoM] £36.43 [CD2]

Morphine sulfate 200 mg MXL 200mg capsules | 28 capsule [PoM] £46.15 [CD2]

▶ Zomorph (ProStrakan Ltd)

Morphine sulfate 10 mg Zomorph 10mg modified-release capsules | 60 capsule [PoM] £3.47 DT price = £3.47 [CD2]

Morphine sulfate 30 mg Zomorph 30mg modified-release capsules | 60 capsule [PoM] £8.30 DT price = £8.30 [CD2]

Morphine sulfate 60 mg Zomorph 60mg modified-release capsules | 60 capsule [PoM] £16.20 DT price = £16.20 [CD2]

Morphine sulfate 100 mg Zomorph 100mg modified-release capsules | 60 capsule [PoM] £21.80 [CD2]

Morphine sulfate 200 mg Zomorph 200mg modified-release capsules | 60 capsule [PoM] £43.60 DT price = £43.60 [CD2]

Modified-release granules

CAUTIONARY AND ADVISORY LABELS 2, 13

▶ MST Continus (Napp Pharmaceuticals Ltd)

Morphine sulfate 20 mg MST Continus Suspension 20mg granules sachets sugar-free | 30 sachet [PoM] £24.58 [CD2]

Morphine sulfate 30 mg MST Continus Suspension 30mg granules sachets sugar-free | 30 sachet [PoM] £25.54 [CD2]

Morphine sulfate 60 mg MST Continus Suspension 60mg granules sachets sugar-free | 30 sachet [PoM] £51.09 [CD2]

Morphine sulfate 100 mg MST Continus Suspension 100mg granules sachets sugar-free | 30 sachet [PoM] £85.15 [CD2]

Morphine sulfate 200 mg MST Continus Suspension 200mg granules sachets sugar-free | 30 sachet [PoM] £170.30 [CD2]

Oral solution

CAUTIONARY AND ADVISORY LABELS 2

▶ Morphine (Non-proprietary)

Morphine sulfate 2 mg per 1 ml Morphine sulfate 10mg/5ml oral solution unit dose vials sugar-free | 1 unit dose [PoM] no price available Schedule 5 (CD Inv)
Morphine sulfate 10mg/5ml oral solution | 100 ml [PoM] £1.82 Schedule 5 (CD Inv) | 300 ml [PoM] £5.45 DT price = £5.45 Schedule 5 (CD Inv) | 500 ml [PoM] £9.08 Schedule 5 (CD Inv)

▶ Oramorph (Boehringer Ingelheim Ltd)

Morphine sulfate 2 mg per 1 ml Oramorph 10mg/5ml oral solution | 100 ml [PoM] £1.89 Schedule 5 (CD Inv) | 300 ml [PoM] £5.45 DT price = £5.45 Schedule 5 (CD Inv) | 500 ml [PoM] £8.50 Schedule 5 (CD Inv)

Morphine sulfate 20 mg per 1 ml Oramorph 20mg/ml concentrated oral solution sugar-free | 30 ml [PoM] £4.98 [CD2] sugar-free | 120 ml [PoM] £19.50 DT price = £19.50 [CD2]

Solution for injection

▶ Morphine (Non-proprietary)

Morphine sulfate 1 mg per 1 ml Morphine sulfate 5mg/5ml solution for injection ampoules | 10 ampoule [PoM] £35.90 [CD2]
Morphine sulfate 1mg/1ml solution for injection ampoules | 10 ampoule [PoM] £26.10 [CD2]
Morphine sulfate 10mg/10ml solution for injection ampoules | 10 ampoule [PoM] £30.00-£38.00 [CD2]

Morphine sulfate 10 mg per 1 ml Morphine sulfate 10mg/1ml solution for injection ampoules | 10 ampoule [PoM] £9.36 DT price = £9.36 [CD2]

Morphine sulfate 15 mg per 1 ml Morphine sulfate 15mg/1ml solution for injection ampoules | 10 ampoule [PoM] £8.95 DT price = £8.95 [CD2]

Morphine sulfate 20 mg per 1 ml Morphine sulfate 20mg/1ml solution for injection ampoules | 10 ampoule [PoM] £51.69 [CD2]

Morphine sulfate 30 mg per 1 ml Morphine sulfate 30mg/1ml solution for injection ampoules | 10 ampoule [PoM] £9.04 DT price = £8.84 [CD2]
Morphine sulfate 60mg/2ml solution for injection ampoules | 5 ampoule [PoM] £10.07 [CD2]

Solution for infusion

▶ Morphine (Non-proprietary)

Morphine sulfate 1 mg per 1 ml Morphine sulfate 50mg/50ml solution for infusion vials | 1 vial [PoM] £5.25-£5.78 [CD2] | 10 vial [PoM] £28.90 [CD2]

Morphine sulfate 2 mg per 1 ml Morphine sulfate 100mg/50ml solution for injection vials | 1 vial [PoM] £6.48 [CD2] | 10 vial [PoM] £57.60 [CD2]

Suppository

CAUTIONARY AND ADVISORY LABELS 2

▶ Morphine (Non-proprietary)

Morphine sulfate 10 mg Morphine sulfate 10mg suppositories | 12 suppository [PoM] £18.34 [CD2]

Morphine sulfate 15 mg Morphine sulfate 15mg suppositories | 12 suppository [PoM] £16.48 DT price = £16.48 [CD2]

Morphine sulfate 30 mg Morphine sulfate 30mg suppositories | 12 suppository [PoM] £18.60 DT price = £18.60 [CD2]

Morphine with cyclizine

The properties listed below are those particular to the combination only. For the properties of the components please consider, morphine p. 265, cyclizine p. 244.

● **INDICATIONS AND DOSE**

CYCLIMORPH-10®

Moderate to severe pain (short-term use only)

▶ BY SUBCUTANEOUS INJECTION, OR BY INTRAMUSCULAR INJECTION, OR BY INTRAVENOUS INJECTION

▶ **Child 12-17 years:** 1 mL, do not repeat dose more often than every 4 hours; maximum 3 doses per day

CYCLIMORPH-15®

Moderate to severe pain (short-term use only)

▶ BY SUBCUTANEOUS INJECTION, OR BY INTRAMUSCULAR INJECTION, OR BY INTRAVENOUS INJECTION

▶ **Child 12-17 years:** 1 mL, do not repeat dose more often than every 4 hours; maximum 3 doses per day

● **CAUTIONS** Myocardial infarction (cyclizine may aggravate severe heart failure and counteract the haemodynamic benefits of opioids) · not recommended in palliative care

● **MEDICINAL FORMS**
There can be variation in the licensing of different medicines containing the same drug.

Solution for injection

▶ Cyclimorph (AMCo)

Morphine tartrate 15 mg per 1 ml, Cyclizine tartrate 50 mg per 1 ml Cyclimorph 15 solution for injection 1ml ampoules | 5 ampoule [PoM] £9.12 [CD2]

Morphine tartrate 10 mg per 1 ml, Cyclizine tartrate 50 mg per 1 ml Cyclimorph 10 solution for injection 1ml ampoules | 5 ampoule [PoM] £8.77 [CD2]

⚑ 256

Oxycodone hydrochloride

● **INDICATIONS AND DOSE**

Moderate to severe pain in palliative care

▶ BY MOUTH USING IMMEDIATE-RELEASE MEDICINES

▶ **Child 1 month-11 years:** Initially 200 micrograms/kg every 4–6 hours (max. per dose 5 mg), dose to be increased if necessary according to severity of pain

▶ **Child 12-17 years:** Initially 5 mg every 4–6 hours, dose to be increased if necessary according to severity of pain

▶ BY MOUTH USING MODIFIED-RELEASE MEDICINES

▶ **Child 8-11 years:** Initially 5 mg every 12 hours, dose to be increased if necessary according to severity of pain

▶ **Child 12-17 years:** Initially 10 mg every 12 hours, dose to be increased if necessary according to severity of pain

DOSE EQUIVALENCE AND CONVERSION
2 mg oral oxycodone is approximately equivalent to 1 mg parenteral oxycodone.

● **UNLICENSED USE** Oral solution, *Oxynorm*®, *Longtec*®, and *Oxycontin*® not licensed for use in children. Capsules and *Dolcodon*® *PR* not licensed for use in children under 12 years.

● **CONTRA-INDICATIONS** Acute abdomen · chronic constipation · cor pulmonale · delayed gastric emptying

● **CAUTIONS** Pancreatitis · toxic psychosis

● **SIDE-EFFECTS**

▶ Common or very common Abdominal pain · anorexia · anxiety · asthenia · bronchospasm · chills · diarrhoea · dyspepsia · dyspnoea · impaired cough reflex

▶ **Uncommon** Agitation · amenorrhoea · amnesia · belching · cholestasis · dehydration · disorientation · dry skin · dysphagia · flatulence · gastritis · hiccups · hypoaesthesia · hypotonia · malaise · muscle fasciculation · paraesthesia · paralytic ileus · pyrexia · restlessness · seizures · speech disorder · supraventricular tachycardia · syncope · taste disturbance · thirst · tremor · vasodilatation

● **BREAST FEEDING** Present in milk—avoid.

● **HEPATIC IMPAIRMENT** Max. initial dose 2.5 mg every 6 hours in patients not currently treated with an opioid with mild impairment. Avoid in moderate to severe impairment.

● **RENAL IMPAIRMENT** Max. initial dose 2.5 mg every 6 hours in patients not currently treated with an opioid with mild to moderate impairment. Opioid effects increased and prolonged and increased cerebral sensitivity occurs.
Avoid if estimated glomerular filtration rate less than 10 mL/minute/1.73 m^2.

● **MEDICINAL FORMS**
There can be variation in the licensing of different medicines containing the same drug. Forms available from special-order manufacturers include: oral solution

Modified-release tablet
CAUTIONARY AND ADVISORY LABELS 2, 25
▶ Abtard (DB Ashbourne Ltd)
Oxycodone hydrochloride 5 mg Abtard 5mg modified-release tablets | 28 tablet PoM £6.26 DT price = £12.52 CD2
Oxycodone hydrochloride 10 mg Abtard 10mg modified-release tablets | 56 tablet PoM £12.52 DT price = £25.04 CD2
Oxycodone hydrochloride 15 mg Abtard 15mg modified-release tablets | 56 tablet PoM £19.06 DT price = £38.12 CD2
Oxycodone hydrochloride 20 mg Abtard 20mg modified-release tablets | 56 tablet PoM £25.04 DT price = £50.08 CD2
Oxycodone hydrochloride 30 mg Abtard 30mg modified-release tablets | 56 tablet PoM £38.11 DT price = £76.23 CD2
Oxycodone hydrochloride 40 mg Abtard 40mg modified-release tablets | 56 tablet PoM £50.09 DT price = £100.19 CD2
Oxycodone hydrochloride 60 mg Abtard 60mg modified-release tablets | 56 tablet PoM £76.24 DT price = £152.49 CD2
Oxycodone hydrochloride 80 mg Abtard 80mg modified-release tablets | 56 tablet PoM £100.19 DT price = £200.39 CD2
▶ Carexil (Sandoz Ltd)
Oxycodone hydrochloride 5 mg Carexil 5mg modified-release tablets | 28 tablet PoM £6.26 DT price = £12.52 CD2
Oxycodone hydrochloride 10 mg Carexil 10mg modified-release tablets | 56 tablet PoM £12.52 DT price = £25.04 CD2
Oxycodone hydrochloride 20 mg Carexil 20mg modified-release tablets | 56 tablet PoM £25.04 DT price = £50.08 CD2
Oxycodone hydrochloride 40 mg Carexil 40mg modified-release tablets | 56 tablet PoM £60.11 DT price = £100.19 CD2
Oxycodone hydrochloride 80 mg Carexil 80mg modified-release tablets | 56 tablet PoM £120.23 DT price = £200.39 CD2
▶ Longtec (Qdem Pharmaceuticals Ltd)
Oxycodone hydrochloride 5 mg Longtec 5mg modified-release tablets | 28 tablet PoM £6.26 DT price = £12.52 CD2
Oxycodone hydrochloride 10 mg Longtec 10mg modified-release tablets | 56 tablet PoM £12.52 DT price = £25.04 CD2
Oxycodone hydrochloride 15 mg Longtec 15mg modified-release tablets | 56 tablet PoM £19.06 DT price = £38.12 CD2
Oxycodone hydrochloride 20 mg Longtec 20mg modified-release tablets | 56 tablet PoM £25.04 DT price = £50.08 CD2
Oxycodone hydrochloride 30 mg Longtec 30mg modified-release tablets | 56 tablet PoM £38.11 DT price = £76.23 CD2
Oxycodone hydrochloride 40 mg Longtec 40mg modified-release tablets | 56 tablet PoM £50.09 DT price = £100.19 CD2
Oxycodone hydrochloride 60 mg Longtec 60mg modified-release tablets | 56 tablet PoM £76.24 DT price = £152.49 CD2
Oxycodone hydrochloride 80 mg Longtec 80mg modified-release tablets | 56 tablet PoM £100.19 DT price = £200.39 CD2
Oxycodone hydrochloride 120 mg Longtec 120mg modified-release tablets | 56 tablet PoM £152.51 DT price = £305.02 CD2
▶ Oxeltra (Wockhardt UK Ltd)
Oxycodone hydrochloride 5 mg Oxeltra 5mg modified-release tablets | 28 tablet PoM £11.27 DT price = £12.52 CD2
Oxycodone hydrochloride 10 mg Oxeltra 10mg modified-release tablets | 56 tablet PoM £22.54 DT price = £25.04 CD2

Oxycodone hydrochloride 15 mg Oxeltra 15mg modified-release tablets | 56 tablet PoM £34.31 DT price = £38.12 CD2
Oxycodone hydrochloride 20 mg Oxeltra 20mg modified-release tablets | 56 tablet PoM £45.07 DT price = £50.08 CD2
Oxycodone hydrochloride 30 mg Oxeltra 30mg modified-release tablets | 56 tablet PoM £68.61 DT price = £76.23 CD2
Oxycodone hydrochloride 40 mg Oxeltra 40mg modified-release tablets | 56 tablet PoM £90.17 DT price = £100.19 CD2
Oxycodone hydrochloride 60 mg Oxeltra 60mg modified-release tablets | 56 tablet PoM £137.24 DT price = £152.49 CD2
Oxycodone hydrochloride 80 mg Oxeltra 80mg modified-release tablets | 56 tablet PoM £180.35 DT price = £200.39 CD2
▶ OxyContin (Napp Pharmaceuticals Ltd)
Oxycodone hydrochloride 5 mg OxyContin 5mg modified-release tablets | 28 tablet PoM £12.52 DT price = £12.52 CD2
Oxycodone hydrochloride 10 mg OxyContin 10mg modified-release tablets | 56 tablet PoM £25.04 DT price = £25.04 CD2
Oxycodone hydrochloride 15 mg OxyContin 15mg modified-release tablets | 56 tablet PoM £38.12 DT price = £38.12 CD2
Oxycodone hydrochloride 20 mg OxyContin 20mg modified-release tablets | 56 tablet PoM £50.08 DT price = £50.08 CD2
Oxycodone hydrochloride 30 mg OxyContin 30mg modified-release tablets | 56 tablet PoM £76.23 DT price = £76.23 CD2
Oxycodone hydrochloride 40 mg OxyContin 40mg modified-release tablets | 56 tablet PoM £100.19 DT price = £100.19 CD2
Oxycodone hydrochloride 60 mg OxyContin 60mg modified-release tablets | 56 tablet PoM £152.49 DT price = £152.49 CD2
Oxycodone hydrochloride 80 mg OxyContin 80mg modified-release tablets | 56 tablet PoM £200.39 DT price = £200.39 CD2
Oxycodone hydrochloride 120 mg OxyContin 120mg modified-release tablets | 56 tablet PoM £305.02 DT price = £305.02 CD2
▶ Oxylan (Chanelle Medical UK Ltd)
Oxycodone hydrochloride 5 mg Oxylan 5mg modified-release tablets | 28 tablet PoM £12.50 DT price = £12.52 CD2
Oxycodone hydrochloride 10 mg Oxylan 10mg modified-release tablets | 56 tablet PoM £24.99 DT price = £25.04 CD2
Oxycodone hydrochloride 20 mg Oxylan 20mg modified-release tablets | 56 tablet PoM £49.98 DT price = £50.08 CD2
Oxycodone hydrochloride 40 mg Oxylan 40mg modified-release tablets | 56 tablet PoM £99.98 DT price = £100.19 CD2
Oxycodone hydrochloride 80 mg Oxylan 80mg modified-release tablets | 56 tablet PoM £199.97 DT price = £200.39 CD2
▶ Reltebon (Actavis UK Ltd)
Oxycodone hydrochloride 5 mg Reltebon 5mg modified-release tablets | 28 tablet PoM £6.26 DT price = £12.52 CD2
Oxycodone hydrochloride 10 mg Reltebon 10mg modified-release tablets | 56 tablet PoM £12.52 DT price = £25.04 CD2
Oxycodone hydrochloride 15 mg Reltebon 15mg modified-release tablets | 56 tablet PoM £19.06 DT price = £38.12 CD2
Oxycodone hydrochloride 20 mg Reltebon 20mg modified-release tablets | 56 tablet PoM £25.04 DT price = £50.08 CD2
Oxycodone hydrochloride 30 mg Reltebon 30mg modified-release tablets | 56 tablet PoM £38.11 DT price = £76.23 CD2
Oxycodone hydrochloride 40 mg Reltebon 40mg modified-release tablets | 56 tablet PoM £50.09 DT price = £100.19 CD2
Oxycodone hydrochloride 60 mg Reltebon 60mg modified-release tablets | 56 tablet PoM £76.24 DT price = £152.49 CD2
Oxycodone hydrochloride 80 mg Reltebon 80mg modified-release tablets | 56 tablet PoM £100.19 DT price = £200.39 CD2
▶ Zomestine (Accord Healthcare Ltd)
Oxycodone hydrochloride 5 mg Zomestine 5mg modified-release tablets | 28 tablet PoM £5.01 DT price = £12.52 CD2
Oxycodone hydrochloride 10 mg Zomestine 10mg modified-release tablets | 56 tablet PoM £10.02 DT price = £25.04 CD2
Oxycodone hydrochloride 20 mg Zomestine 20mg modified-release tablets | 56 tablet PoM £20.03 DT price = £50.08 CD2
Oxycodone hydrochloride 40 mg Zomestine 40mg modified-release tablets | 56 tablet PoM £40.08 DT price = £100.19 CD2
Oxycodone hydrochloride 80 mg Zomestine 80mg modified-release tablets | 56 tablet PoM £80.16 DT price = £200.39 CD2

Capsule
CAUTIONARY AND ADVISORY LABELS 2
▶ Lynlor (Actavis UK Ltd)
Oxycodone hydrochloride 5 mg Lynlor 5mg capsules | 56 capsule PoM £6.86 DT price = £11.43 CD2
Oxycodone hydrochloride 10 mg Lynlor 10mg capsules | 56 capsule PoM £13.72 DT price = £22.86 CD2
Oxycodone hydrochloride 20 mg Lynlor 20mg capsules | 56 capsule PoM £27.43 DT price = £45.71 CD2

▸ **OxyNorm** (Napp Pharmaceuticals Ltd)
Oxycodone hydrochloride 5 mg OxyNorm 5mg capsules | 56 capsule [PoM] £11.43 DT price = £11.43 [CD2]
Oxycodone hydrochloride 10 mg OxyNorm 10mg capsules | 56 capsule [PoM] £22.86 DT price = £22.86 [CD2]
Oxycodone hydrochloride 20 mg OxyNorm 20mg capsules | 56 capsule [PoM] £45.71 DT price = £45.71 [CD2]

▸ **Shortec** (Qdem Pharmaceuticals Ltd)
Oxycodone hydrochloride 5 mg Shortec 5mg capsules | 56 capsule [PoM] £6.86 DT price = £11.43 [CD2]
Oxycodone hydrochloride 10 mg Shortec 10mg capsules | 56 capsule [PoM] £13.72 DT price = £22.86 [CD2]
Oxycodone hydrochloride 20 mg Shortec 20mg capsules | 56 capsule [PoM] £27.43 DT price = £45.71 [CD2]

Oral solution
CAUTIONARY AND ADVISORY LABELS 2
▸ **Oxycodone hydrochloride (Non-proprietary)**
Oxycodone hydrochloride 1 mg per 1 ml Oxycodone 5mg/5ml oral solution sugar free sugar-free | 250 ml [PoM] £9.71 DT price = £9.71 [CD2]
Oxycodone hydrochloride 10 mg per 1 ml Oxycodone 10mg/ml oral solution sugar free sugar-free | 120 ml [PoM] £46.63 DT price = £46.63 [CD2]

▸ **OxyNorm** (Napp Pharmaceuticals Ltd)
Oxycodone hydrochloride 1 mg per 1 ml OxyNorm liquid 5mg/5ml oral solution sugar-free | 250 ml [PoM] £9.71 DT price = £9.71 [CD2]
Oxycodone hydrochloride 10 mg per 1 ml OxyNorm 10mg/ml concentrate oral solution sugar-free | 120 ml [PoM] £46.63 DT price = £46.63 [CD2]

Solution for injection
▸ **Oxycodone hydrochloride (Non-proprietary)**
Oxycodone hydrochloride 10 mg per 1 ml Oxycodone 20mg/2ml solution for injection ampoules | 5 ampoule [PoM] £16.00 DT price = £16.00 [CD2]
Oxycodone 10mg/1ml solution for injection ampoules | 5 ampoule [PoM] £8.00 DT price = £8.00 [CD2]
Oxycodone hydrochloride 50 mg per 1 ml Oxycodone 50mg/1ml solution for injection ampoules | 5 ampoule [PoM] £70.10 DT price = £70.10 [CD2]

▸ **OxyNorm** (Napp Pharmaceuticals Ltd)
Oxycodone hydrochloride 10 mg per 1 ml OxyNorm 10mg/1ml solution for injection ampoules | 5 ampoule [PoM] £8.00 DT price = £8.00 [CD2]
OxyNorm 20mg/2ml solution for injection ampoules | 5 ampoule [PoM] £16.00 DT price = £16.00 [CD2]
Oxycodone hydrochloride 50 mg per 1 ml OxyNorm 50mg/1ml solution for injection ampoules | 5 ampoule [PoM] £70.10 DT price = £70.10 [CD2]

⚑ 256

Papaveretum

● **INDICATIONS AND DOSE**
Postoperative analgesia | Severe chronic pain
▸ BY SUBCUTANEOUS INJECTION, OR BY INTRAMUSCULAR INJECTION
▸ Neonate: 115 micrograms/kg every 4 hours if required.
▸ Child 1–11 months: 154 micrograms/kg every 4 hours if required
▸ Child 1–5 years: 1.93–3.85 mg every 4 hours if required
▸ Child 6–11 years: 3.85–7.7 mg every 4 hours if required
▸ Child 12–17 years: 7.7–15.4 mg every 4 hours if required
▸ BY INTRAVENOUS INJECTION
▸ Child: Use 25 to 50% of the corresponding subcutaneous/intramuscular dose

Premedication
▸ BY SUBCUTANEOUS INJECTION, OR BY INTRAMUSCULAR INJECTION
▸ Neonate: 115 micrograms/kg every 4 hours if required.
▸ Child 1–11 months: 154 micrograms/kg every 4 hours if required
▸ Child 1–5 years: 1.93–3.85 mg every 4 hours if required
▸ Child 6–11 years: 3.85–7.7 mg every 4 hours if required
▸ Child 12–17 years: 7.7–15.4 mg every 4 hours if required

▸ BY INTRAVENOUS INJECTION
▸ Child: Use 25 to 50% of the corresponding subcutaneous/intramuscular dose

> **IMPORTANT SAFETY INFORMATION**
> Do **not** confuse with papaverine.

● **CONTRA-INDICATIONS** Heart failure secondary to chronic lung disease · phaeochromocytoma
● **CAUTIONS** Supraventricular tachycardia
● **SIDE-EFFECTS** Hypothermia
● **BREAST FEEDING** Therapeutic doses unlikely to affect infant.
● **RENAL IMPAIRMENT** Avoid use or reduce dose; opioid effects increased and prolonged and increased cerebral sensitivity occurs.
● **PRESCRIBING AND DISPENSING INFORMATION** The name *Omnopon*® was formerly used for papaveretum preparations.
  Papaveretum is a mixture of 253 parts of morphine hydrochloride, 23 parts of papaverine hydrochloride and 20 parts of codeine hydrochloride.
● **LESS SUITABLE FOR PRESCRIBING** Papaveretum is less suitable for prescribing.

● **MEDICINAL FORMS**
There can be variation in the licensing of different medicines containing the same drug. Forms available from special-order manufacturers include: solution for injection
Solution for injection
▸ **Papaveretum (Non-proprietary)**
Papaveretum 15.4 mg per 1 ml Papaveretum 15.4mg/1ml solution for injection ampoules | 10 ampoule [PoM] £48.96 [CD2]

⚑ 256

Pethidine hydrochloride
(Meperidine)

● **INDICATIONS AND DOSE**
Obstetric analgesia
▸ BY SUBCUTANEOUS INJECTION, OR BY INTRAMUSCULAR INJECTION
▸ Child 12–17 years: 1 mg/kg (max. per dose 100 mg), then 1 mg/kg after 1–3 hours if required; maximum 400 mg per day

● **CONTRA-INDICATIONS** Phaeochromocytoma
● **CAUTIONS** Accumulation of metabolites may result in neurotoxicity · cardiac arrhythmias · not suitable for severe continuing pain · severe cor pulmonale
● **SIDE-EFFECTS** Hypothermia · restlessness · tremor
Overdose
Convulsions reported in overdosage.
● **BREAST FEEDING** Present in milk but not known to be harmful.
● **RENAL IMPAIRMENT** Avoid use or reduce dose; opioid effects increased and prolonged and increased cerebral sensitivity occurs.

● **MEDICINAL FORMS**
There can be variation in the licensing of different medicines containing the same drug. Forms available from special-order manufacturers include: solution for injection
Solution for injection
▸ **Pethidine hydrochloride (Non-proprietary)**
Pethidine hydrochloride 10 mg per 1 ml Pethidine 50mg/5ml solution for injection ampoules | 10 ampoule [PoM] £52.91 [CD2]
Pethidine hydrochloride 50 mg per 1 ml Pethidine 50mg/1ml solution for injection ampoules | 10 ampoule [PoM] £4.97 DT price = £4.97 [CD2]
Pethidine 100mg/2ml solution for injection ampoules | 10 ampoule [PoM] £4.66 DT price = £4.66 [CD2]

☞ 256

Tramadol hydrochloride

- **INDICATIONS AND DOSE**

Moderate to severe pain
▸ BY INTRAMUSCULAR INJECTION, OR BY INTRAVENOUS INJECTION, OR BY INTRAVENOUS INFUSION
  ▸ Child 12–17 years: 50–100 mg every 4–6 hours, intravenous injection to be given over 2–3 minutes

Moderate to severe acute pain
▸ BY MOUTH USING IMMEDIATE-RELEASE MEDICINES
  ▸ Child 12–17 years: Initially 100 mg, then 50–100 mg every 4–6 hours; usual maximum 400 mg per day

Moderate to severe chronic pain
▸ BY MOUTH USING IMMEDIATE-RELEASE MEDICINES
  ▸ Child 12–17 years: Initially 50 mg, then adjusted according to response; usual maximum 400 mg per day

Postoperative pain
▸ BY INTRAVENOUS INJECTION
  ▸ Child 12–17 years: Initially 100 mg, then 50 mg every 10–20 minutes if required up to total maximum 250 mg (including initial dose) in first hour, then 50–100 mg every 4–6 hours, intravenous injection to be given over 2–3 minutes; maximum 600 mg per day

Moderate to severe pain (with modified-release 12-hourly preparations)
▸ BY MOUTH USING MODIFIED-RELEASE MEDICINES
  ▸ Child 12–17 years: 50–100 mg twice daily, increased if necessary to 150–200 mg twice daily, doses exceeding the usual maximum not generally required; Usual maximum 400 micrograms/24 hours

Moderate to severe pain (with modified-release 24-hourly preparations)
▸ BY MOUTH USING MODIFIED-RELEASE MEDICINES
  ▸ Child 12–17 years: Initially 100–150 mg once daily, increased if necessary up to 400 mg once daily; Usual maximum 400 mg/24 hours

ZYDOL® XL

Moderate to severe pain
▸ BY MOUTH USING MODIFIED-RELEASE TABLETS
  ▸ Child 12–17 years: Initially 150 mg once daily, increased if necessary up to 400 mg once daily

- **CONTRA-INDICATIONS** Acute intoxication with alcohol · acute intoxication with analgesics · acute intoxication with hypnotics · acute intoxication with opioids · not suitable for narcotic withdrawal treatment · uncontrolled epilepsy

- **CAUTIONS** Excessive bronchial secretions · history of epilepsy—use tramadol only if compelling reasons · impaired consciousness · not suitable as a substitute in opioid-dependent patients · not suitable in some types of general anaesthesia · susceptibility to seizures—use tramadol only if compelling reasons
  CAUTIONS, FURTHER INFORMATION
  General anaesthesia Not recommended for analgesia during potentially light planes of general anaesthesia (possibly increased intra-operative recall reported).

- **SIDE-EFFECTS**
▸ **Common or very common** Malaise
▸ **Uncommon** Diarrhoea · flatulence · gastritis · retching
▸ **Rare** Abnormal coordination · anorexia · anxiety · bronchospasm · changes in appetite · delirium · dyspnoea · hypertension · muscle weakness · nightmares · paraesthesia · seizures · syncope · tremor · wheezing
▸ **Frequency not known** Blood disorders · hypoglycaemia · speech disorders

- **PREGNANCY** Embryotoxic in *animal* studies—manufacturers advise avoid.

- **BREAST FEEDING** Amount probably too small to be harmful, but manufacturer advises avoid.

- **HEPATIC IMPAIRMENT** Caution (avoid for *oral drops*) in severe impairment.

- **RENAL IMPAIRMENT** Avoid use or reduce dose; opioid effects increased and prolonged and increased cerebral sensitivity occurs. Caution (avoid for *oral drops*) in severe impairment.

- **DIRECTIONS FOR ADMINISTRATION** Tramadol hydrochloride *orodispersible tablets* should be sucked and then swallowed. May also be dispersed in water. Some tramadol hydrochloride modified-release capsule preparations may be opened and the contents swallowed immediately without chewing—check individual preparations.
  For *intravenous infusion*, dilute in Glucose 5% or Sodium Chloride 0.9%.

- **PRESCRIBING AND DISPENSING INFORMATION** Modified-release preparations are available as 12-hourly or 24-hourly formulations. Non-proprietary preparations of modified-release tramadol may be available as either 12-hourly or 24-hourly formulations; prescribers and dispensers must ensure that the correct formulation is prescribed and dispensed. Branded preparations that should be given 12-hourly include *Invodol® SR, Mabron®, Maneo®, Marol®, Maxitram® SR, Oldaram®, Tilodol® SR, Tramquel® SR, Tramulief® SR, Zamadol® SR, Zeridame® SR* and *Zydol SR®*. Preparations that should be given 24-hourly include *Tradorec XL®, Zamadol® 24hr*, and *Zydol XL®*.

- **PATIENT AND CARER ADVICE**
  Patients or carers should be given advice on how to administer tramadol hydochloride orodispersible tablets.
  Medicines for Children leaflet: Tramadol for pain
  www.medicinesforchildren.org.uk/tramadol-for-pain

- **MEDICINAL FORMS**
  There can be variation in the licensing of different medicines containing the same drug. Forms available from special-order manufacturers include: oral suspension

Soluble tablet
CAUTIONARY AND ADVISORY LABELS 2, 13
▸ Zydol (Grunenthal Ltd)
  Tramadol hydrochloride 50 mg Zydol 50mg soluble tablets sugar-free | 20 tablet [PoM] £2.79 [CD3] sugar-free | 100 tablet [PoM] £13.33 DT price = £13.33 [CD3]

Orodispersible tablet
CAUTIONARY AND ADVISORY LABELS 2
▸ Tramadol hydrochloride (Non-proprietary)
  Tramadol hydrochloride 50 mg Tramadol 50mg orodispersible tablets sugar free sugar-free | 60 tablet [PoM] no price available [CD3]
▸ Zamadol Melt (Meda Pharmaceuticals Ltd)
  Tramadol hydrochloride 50 mg Zamadol Melt 50mg tablets sugar-free | 60 tablet [PoM] £7.12 [CD3]

Modified-release tablet
CAUTIONARY AND ADVISORY LABELS 2, 25
▸ Tramadol hydrochloride (Non-proprietary)
  Tramadol hydrochloride 50 mg Tramadol 50mg modified-release tablets | 60 tablet [PoM] no price available DT price = £4.60 [CD3]
  Tramadol hydrochloride 100 mg Tramadol 100mg modified-release tablets | 60 tablet [PoM] £44.80 [CD3]
  Tramadol hydrochloride 150 mg Tramadol 150mg modified-release tablets | 60 tablet [PoM] £57.85 [CD3]
  Tramadol hydrochloride 200 mg Tramadol 200mg modified-release tablets | 30 tablet [PoM] no price available [CD3] | 60 tablet [PoM] £69.60 [CD3]
  Tramadol hydrochloride 300 mg Tramadol 300mg modified-release tablets | 30 tablet [PoM] no price available [CD3]
  Tramadol hydrochloride 400 mg Tramadol 400mg modified-release tablets | 28 tablet [PoM] no price available [CD3] | 30 tablet [PoM] no price available [CD3]
▸ Invodol SR (Ennogen Healthcare Ltd)
  Tramadol hydrochloride 100 mg Invodol SR 100mg tablets | 60 tablet [PoM] £14.61 [CD3]
  Tramadol hydrochloride 150 mg Invodol SR 150mg tablets | 60 tablet [PoM] £21.91 [CD3]

Tramadol hydrochloride 200 mg Invodol SR 200mg tablets |
60 tablet [PoM] £29.22 [CD3]

▸ **Mabron** (Morningside Healthcare Ltd)
Tramadol hydrochloride 100 mg Mabron 100mg modified-release
tablets | 60 tablet [PoM] £18.26 [CD3]
Tramadol hydrochloride 150 mg Mabron 150mg modified-release
tablets | 60 tablet [PoM] £27.39 [CD3]
Tramadol hydrochloride 200 mg Mabron 200mg modified-release
tablets | 60 tablet [PoM] £36.52 [CD3]

▸ **Maneo** (Mylan Ltd)
Tramadol hydrochloride 100 mg Maneo 100mg modified-release
tablets | 60 tablet [PoM] £6.95 [CD3]
Tramadol hydrochloride 150 mg Maneo 150mg modified-release
tablets | 60 tablet [PoM] £10.40 [CD3]
Tramadol hydrochloride 200 mg Maneo 200mg modified-release
tablets | 60 tablet [PoM] £14.20 [CD3]

▸ **Marol** (Teva UK Ltd)
Tramadol hydrochloride 100 mg Marol 100mg modified-release
tablets | 60 tablet [PoM] £6.94 [CD3]
Tramadol hydrochloride 150 mg Marol 150mg modified-release
tablets | 60 tablet [PoM] £10.39 [CD3]
Tramadol hydrochloride 200 mg Marol 200mg modified-release
tablets | 60 tablet [PoM] £14.19 [CD3]

▸ **Oldaram** (Ranbaxy (UK) Ltd)
Tramadol hydrochloride 100 mg Oldaram 100mg modified-release
tablets | 60 tablet [PoM] £18.80 [CD3]
Tramadol hydrochloride 150 mg Oldaram 150mg modified-release
tablets | 60 tablet [PoM] £28.21 [CD3]
Tramadol hydrochloride 200 mg Oldaram 200mg modified-release
tablets | 60 tablet [PoM] £37.62 [CD3]

▸ **Tilodol SR** (Sandoz Ltd)
Tramadol hydrochloride 100 mg Tilodol SR 100mg tablets |
60 tablet [PoM] £15.52 [CD3]
Tramadol hydrochloride 150 mg Tilodol SR 150mg tablets |
60 tablet [PoM] £23.28 [CD3]
Tramadol hydrochloride 200 mg Tilodol SR 200mg tablets |
60 tablet [PoM] £31.04 [CD3]

▸ **Tradorec XL** (Paladin Labs Europe Ltd)
Tramadol hydrochloride 100 mg Tradorec XL 100mg tablets |
30 tablet [PoM] £14.10 [CD3]
Tramadol hydrochloride 200 mg Tradorec XL 200mg tablets |
30 tablet [PoM] £14.98 [CD3]
Tramadol hydrochloride 300 mg Tradorec XL 300mg tablets |
30 tablet [PoM] £22.47 [CD3]

▸ **Tramulief SR** (AMCo)
Tramadol hydrochloride 100 mg Tramulief SR 100mg tablets |
60 tablet [PoM] £6.98 [CD3]
Tramadol hydrochloride 150 mg Tramulief SR 150mg tablets |
60 tablet [PoM] £10.48 [CD3]
Tramadol hydrochloride 200 mg Tramulief SR 200mg tablets |
60 tablet [PoM] £14.28 [CD3]

▸ **Zamadol 24hr** (Meda Pharmaceuticals Ltd)
Tramadol hydrochloride 150 mg Zamadol 24hr 150mg modified-
release tablets | 28 tablet [PoM] £10.70 [CD3]
Tramadol hydrochloride 200 mg Zamadol 24hr 200mg modified-
release tablets | 28 tablet [PoM] £14.26 [CD3]
Tramadol hydrochloride 300 mg Zamadol 24hr 300mg modified-
release tablets | 28 tablet [PoM] £21.39 [CD3]
Tramadol hydrochloride 400 mg Zamadol 24hr 400mg modified-
release tablets | 28 tablet [PoM] £28.51 [CD3]

▸ **Zeridame SR** (Actavis UK Ltd)
Tramadol hydrochloride 100 mg Zeridame SR 100mg tablets |
60 tablet [PoM] £17.21 [CD3]
Tramadol hydrochloride 150 mg Zeridame SR 150mg tablets |
60 tablet [PoM] £25.82 [CD3]
Tramadol hydrochloride 200 mg Zeridame SR 200mg tablets |
60 tablet [PoM] £34.43 [CD3]

▸ **Zydol SR** (Grunenthal Ltd)
Tramadol hydrochloride 50 mg Zydol SR 50mg tablets |
60 tablet [PoM] £4.60 DT price = £4.60 [CD3]
Tramadol hydrochloride 100 mg Zydol SR 100mg tablets |
60 tablet [PoM] £18.26 [CD3]
Tramadol hydrochloride 150 mg Zydol SR 150mg tablets |
60 tablet [PoM] £27.39 [CD3]
Tramadol hydrochloride 200 mg Zydol SR 200mg tablets |
60 tablet [PoM] £36.52 [CD3]

▸ **Zydol XL** (Grunenthal Ltd)
Tramadol hydrochloride 150 mg Zydol XL 150mg tablets |
30 tablet [PoM] £12.18 [CD3]

Tramadol hydrochloride 200 mg Zydol XL 200mg tablets |
30 tablet [PoM] £17.98 [CD3]
Tramadol hydrochloride 300 mg Zydol XL 300mg tablets |
30 tablet [PoM] £24.94 [CD3]
Tramadol hydrochloride 400 mg Zydol XL 400mg tablets |
30 tablet [PoM] £32.47 [CD3]

Capsule
CAUTIONARY AND ADVISORY LABELS 2
▸ **Tramadol hydrochloride (Non-proprietary)**
Tramadol hydrochloride 50 mg Tramadol 50mg capsules |
30 capsule [PoM] £4.71 DT price = £0.89 [CD3] | 100 capsule [PoM]
£14.40 DT price = £2.97 [CD3]
▸ **Zamadol** (Meda Pharmaceuticals Ltd)
Tramadol hydrochloride 50 mg Zamadol 50mg capsules |
100 capsule [PoM] £8.00 DT price = £2.97 [CD3]
▸ **Zydol** (Grunenthal Ltd)
Tramadol hydrochloride 50 mg Zydol 50mg capsules |
30 capsule [PoM] £2.29 DT price = £0.89 [CD3] | 100 capsule [PoM]
£7.63 DT price = £2.97 [CD3]

Modified-release capsule
CAUTIONARY AND ADVISORY LABELS 2, 25
▸ **Tramadol hydrochloride (Non-proprietary)**
Tramadol hydrochloride 50 mg Tramadol 50mg modified-release
capsules | 60 capsule [PoM] £7.75 DT price = £7.24 [CD3]
Tramadol hydrochloride 100 mg Tramadol 100mg modified-release
capsules | 60 capsule [PoM] £15.43 DT price = £14.47 [CD3]
Tramadol hydrochloride 150 mg Tramadol 150mg modified-release
capsules | 60 capsule [PoM] £23.35 DT price = £21.71 [CD3]
Tramadol hydrochloride 200 mg Tramadol 200mg modified-release
capsules | 60 capsule [PoM] £31.22 DT price = £28.93 [CD3]
▸ **Maxitram SR** (Chiesi Ltd)
Tramadol hydrochloride 50 mg Maxitram SR 50mg capsules |
60 capsule [PoM] £4.55 DT price = £7.24 [CD3]
Tramadol hydrochloride 100 mg Maxitram SR 100mg capsules |
60 capsule [PoM] £12.14 DT price = £14.47 [CD3]
Tramadol hydrochloride 150 mg Maxitram SR 150mg capsules |
60 capsule [PoM] £18.21 DT price = £21.71 [CD3]
Tramadol hydrochloride 200 mg Maxitram SR 200mg capsules |
60 capsule [PoM] £24.28 DT price = £28.93 [CD3]
▸ **Tramquel SR** (Beechmere Pharmaceuticals Ltd)
Tramadol hydrochloride 50 mg Tramquel SR 50mg capsules |
60 capsule [PoM] £7.24 DT price = £7.24 [CD3]
Tramadol hydrochloride 100 mg Tramquel 100mg capsules |
60 capsule [PoM] £14.47 DT price = £14.47 [CD3]
Tramadol hydrochloride 150 mg Tramquel SR 150mg capsules |
60 capsule [PoM] £21.71 DT price = £21.71 [CD3]
Tramadol hydrochloride 200 mg Tramquel SR 200mg capsules |
60 capsule [PoM] £28.93 DT price = £28.93 [CD3]
▸ **Zamadol SR** (Meda Pharmaceuticals Ltd)
Tramadol hydrochloride 50 mg Zamadol SR 50mg capsules |
60 capsule [PoM] £7.24 DT price = £7.24 [CD3]
Tramadol hydrochloride 100 mg Zamadol SR 100mg capsules |
60 capsule [PoM] £14.47 DT price = £14.47 [CD3]
Tramadol hydrochloride 150 mg Zamadol SR 150mg capsules |
60 capsule [PoM] £21.71 DT price = £21.71 [CD3]
Tramadol hydrochloride 200 mg Zamadol SR 200mg capsules |
60 capsule [PoM] £28.93 DT price = £28.93 [CD3]

Oral drops
CAUTIONARY AND ADVISORY LABELS 2, 13
▸ **Tramadol hydrochloride (Non-proprietary)**
Tramadol (as Tramadol hydrochloride) 100 mg per 1 ml Tramadol
100mg/ml oral drops | 10 ml [PoM] £3.50 DT price = £3.50 [CD3]

Solution for injection
▸ **Tramadol hydrochloride (Non-proprietary)**
Tramadol hydrochloride 50 mg per 1 ml Tramadol 100mg/2ml
solution for injection ampoules | 5 ampoule [PoM] £4.90-£4.92 [CD3]
| 10 ampoule [PoM] £10.00 [CD3]
▸ **Zamadol** (Meda Pharmaceuticals Ltd)
Tramadol hydrochloride 50 mg per 1 ml Zamadol 100mg/2ml
solution for injection ampoules | 5 ampoule [PoM] £5.49 [CD3]
▸ **Zydol** (Grunenthal Ltd)
Tramadol hydrochloride 50 mg per 1 ml Zydol 100mg/2ml solution
for injection ampoules | 5 ampoule [PoM] £4.00 [CD3]

Combinations available: *Paracetamol with tramadol,* p. 256

5.1 Migraine

Migraine

Treatment of acute migraine

Treatment of a migraine attack should be guided by response to previous treatment and the severity of the attacks. A simple analgesic such as paracetamol p. 254 (preferably in a soluble or dispersible form) or an NSAID, usually ibuprofen p. 608, is often effective; concomitant antiemetic treatment may be required. If treatment with an analgesic is inadequate, an attack may be treated with a specific antimigraine compound such as the 5HT$_1$- receptor agonist sumatriptan p. 273. **Ergot alkaloids** are associated with many side-effects and should be avoided.

Excessive use of acute treatments for migraine (opioid and non-opioid analgesics, 5HT$_1$-receptor agonists, and ergotamine) is associated with medication-overuse headache (analgesic-induced headache); therefore, increasing consumption of these medicines needs careful management.

5HT$_1$-receptor agonists

5HT$_1$-receptor agonists are used in the treatment of acute migraine attacks; treatment of children should be initiated by a specialist. A 5HT$_1$-receptor agonist may be used during the established headache phase of an attack and is the preferred treatment in those who fail to respond to conventional analgesics. 5HT$_1$-receptor agonists are **not** indicated for the treatment of hemiplegic, basilar, or opthalmoplegic migraine.

If a child does not respond to one 5HT$_1$-receptor agonist, an alternative 5HT$_1$-receptor agonist should be tried. For children who have prolonged attacks that frequently recur despite treatment with a 5HT$_1$-receptor agonist, combination therapy with an NSAID such as naproxen p. 614 can be considered. Sumatriptan and zolmitriptan p. 274 are used for migraine in children. They may also be of value in cluster headache.

Antiemetics

Antiemetics, including domperidone p. 245, phenothiazines, and antihistamines, relieve the nausea associated with migraine attacks. Antiemetics may be given by intramuscular injection or rectally if vomiting is a problem. Domperidone has the added advantage of promoting gastric emptying and normal peristalsis; a single dose should be given at the onset of symptoms.

Prophylaxis of migraine

Where migraine attacks are frequent, possible provoking factors such as stress should be sought; combined oral contraceptives may also provoke migraine. Preventive treatment should be considered if migraine attacks interfere with school and social life, particularly for children who:

- suffer at least two attacks a month;
- suffer an increasing frequency of headaches;
- suffer significant disability despite suitable treatment for migraine attacks;
- cannot take suitable treatment for migraine attacks.

In children it is often possible to stop prophylaxis after a period of treatment.

Propranolol hydrochloride p. 96 may be effective in preventing migraine in children but it is contra-indicated in those with asthma. Side-effects such as depression and postural hypotension can further limit its use.

Pizotifen below, an antihistamine and a serotonin-receptor antagonist, may also be used but its efficacy in children has not been clearly established. Common side-effects include drowsiness and weight gain.

Topiramate is licensed for migraine prophylaxis.

Cluster headache and the trigeminal autonomic cephalalgias

Cluster headache rarely responds to standard analgesics. Sumatriptan given by subcutaneous injection is the drug of choice for the treatment of cluster headache. If an injection is unsuitable, sumatriptan nasal spray or zolmitriptan nasal spray may be used. Treatment should be initiated by a specialist. Alternatively, 100% oxygen at a rate of 10–15 litres/minute for 10–20 minutes is useful in aborting an attack.

The other trigeminal autonomic cephalalgias, paroxysmal hemicrania (sensitive to indometacin p. 611), and short-lasting unilateral neuralgiform headache attacks with conjunctival injection and tearing, are seen rarely and are best managed by a specialist.

ANTIHISTAMINES ⟩ SEDATING

Paracetamol with buclizine hydrochloride and codeine phosphate

The properties listed below are those particular to the combination only. For the properties of the components please consider, paracetamol p. 254, codeine phosphate p. 259.

● **INDICATIONS AND DOSE**

MIGRALEVE®

Acute migraine
▸ BY MOUTH
▸ Child 12–14 years: Initially 1 tablet, (pink tablet) to be taken at onset of attack, or if it is imminent, followed by 1 tablet every 4 hours if required, (yellow tablet) to be taken following initial dose; maximum 1 pink and 3 yellow tablets in 24 hours
▸ Child 15–17 years: Initially 2 tablets, (pink tablet) to be taken at onset of attack or if it is imminent, followed by 2 tablets every 4 hours if required, (yellow tablets) to be taken following initial dose; maximum 2 pink and 6 yellow tablets in 24 hours

● **LESS SUITABLE FOR PRESCRIBING**
MIGRALEVE® *Migraleve®* is less suitable for prescribing.

● **MEDICINAL FORMS**
There can be variation in the licensing of different medicines containing the same drug.
Tablet
CAUTIONARY AND ADVISORY LABELS 2, 17, 30
▸ Migraleve Pink (McNeil Products Ltd)
Buclizine hydrochloride 6.25 mg, Codeine phosphate 8 mg, Paracetamol 500 mg Migraleve Pink tablets | 32 tablet [PoM] no price available Schedule 5 (CD Inv) | 48 tablet [PoM] £3.97 Schedule 5 (CD Inv)
▸ Migraleve (McNeil Products Ltd)
Migraleve tablets | 48 tablet [PoM] £3.64 Schedule 5 (CD Inv)

Pizotifen

● **INDICATIONS AND DOSE**
Prophylaxis of migraine
▸ BY MOUTH
▸ Child 5–17 years: Initially 500 micrograms once daily, dose to be taken at night, then increased to up to 1.5 mg daily in divided doses, dose to be increased gradually, max. single dose (at night) 1 mg

● **UNLICENSED USE** 1.5 mg tablets not licensed for use in children.

- **CAUTIONS** Avoid abrupt withdrawal · history of epilepsy · susceptibility to angle-closure glaucoma · urinary retention
- **INTERACTIONS** → Appendix 1 (pizotifen).
- **SIDE-EFFECTS**
  - **Common or very common** Dizziness · drowsiness · dry mouth · increased appetite · nausea · weight gain
  - **Uncommon** Constipation
  - **Rare** Aggression · anxiety · arthralgia · depression · hallucination · insomnia · myalgia · paraesthesia
  - **Very rare** Seizures
  - **Frequency not known** Hepatitis · jaundice · muscle cramps
- **PREGNANCY** Avoid unless potential benefit outweighs risk.
- **BREAST FEEDING** Amount probably too small to be harmful, but manufacturer advises avoid.
- **HEPATIC IMPAIRMENT** Use with caution.
- **RENAL IMPAIRMENT** Use with caution.
- **PATIENT AND CARER ADVICE**
  Medicines for Children leaflet: Pizotifen to prevent migraine headaches www.medicinesforchildren.org.uk/pizotifen-to-prevent-migraine-headaches
  Driving and skilled tasks
  Drowsiness may affect performance of skilled tasks (e.g. driving); effects of alcohol enhanced.
- **MEDICINAL FORMS**
  There can be variation in the licensing of different medicines containing the same drug. Forms available from special-order manufacturers include: oral suspension, oral solution
  Tablet
  CAUTIONARY AND ADVISORY LABELS 2
  - Pizotifen (Non-proprietary)
    Pizotifen (as Pizotifen hydrogen malate)
    500 microgram Pizotifen 500microgram tablets | 28 tablet [PoM] £9.56 DT price = £3.56
    Pizotifen (as Pizotifen hydrogen malate) 1.5 mg Pizotifen 1.5mg tablets | 28 tablet [PoM] £14.74 DT price = £3.70

TRIPTANS

Sumatriptan

- **INDICATIONS AND DOSE**
  Treatment of acute migraine
  - BY MOUTH
  - Child 6–9 years: Initially 25 mg for 1 dose, followed by 25 mg after at least 2 hours if required, to be taken only if migraine recurs (patient not responding to initial dose should not take second dose for same attack)
  - Child 10–11 years: Initially 50 mg for 1 dose, followed by 50 mg after at least 2 hours, to be taken only if migraine recurs (patient not responding to initial dose should not take second dose for same attack)
  - Child 12–17 years: Initially 50–100 mg for 1 dose, followed by 50–100 mg after at least 2 hours if required, to be taken only if migraine recurs (patient not responding to initial dose should not take second dose for same attack)
  - BY SUBCUTANEOUS INJECTION
  - Child 10–17 years: Initially 6 mg for 1 dose, followed by 6 mg after at least 1 hour if required, to be taken only if migraine recurs (patient not responding to initial dose should not take second dose for same attack), dose to be administered using an auto-injector; maximum 12 mg per day
  - BY INTRANASAL ADMINISTRATION
  - Child 12–17 years: Initially 10–20 mg for 1 dose, followed by 10–20 mg after at least 2 hours if required, to be taken only if migraine recurs (patient not responding to initial dose should not take second dose for same attack); maximum 40 mg per day

Treatment of acute cluster headache
  - BY SUBCUTANEOUS INJECTION
  - Child 10–17 years (under expert supervision): Initially 6 mg for 1 dose, followed by 6 mg after at least 1 hour if required, to be taken only if headache recurs (patient not responding to initial dose should not take second dose for same attack), dose to be administered using auto-injector; maximum 12 mg per day
  - BY INTRANASAL ADMINISTRATION
  - Child 12–17 years (under expert supervision): Initially 10–20 mg for 1 dose, followed by 10–20 mg after at least 2 hours if required, to be taken only if headache recurs (patient not responding to initial dose should not take second dose for same attack); maximum 40 mg per day

- **UNLICENSED USE** Tablets and injection not licensed for use in children. Intranasal dose for migraine not licensed. Not licensed for treating cluster headache in children.
- **CONTRA-INDICATIONS** Coronary vasospasm · ischaemic heart disease · mild uncontrolled hypertension · moderate and severe hypertension · peripheral vascular disease · previous cerebrovascular accident · previous myocardial infarction · previous transient ischaemic attack · Prinzmetal's angina
- **CAUTIONS** Conditions which predispose to coronary artery disease · history of seizures · mild, controlled hypertension · pre-existing cardiac disease · risk factors for seizures
- **INTERACTIONS** → Appendix 1 ($5HT_1$ agonists).
- **SIDE-EFFECTS**
  GENERAL SIDE-EFFECTS
  - **Common or very common** Dizziness · drowsiness · dyspnoea · fatigue · flushing · myalgia · nausea · sensory disturbances · transient increase in blood pressure · vomiting · weakness
  - **Frequency not known** Arrhythmias · angina · anxiety · arthralgia · bradycardia · diarrhoea · dystonia · hypersensitivity reactions · hypotension · ischaemic colitis · myocardial infarction · neck stiffness · nystagmus · palpitation · Raynaud's syndrome · seizures · sweating · tachycardia · transient ischaemic ECG changes · tremor · visual disturbances
  SPECIFIC SIDE-EFFECTS
  - **Common or very common**
  - **With intranasal use** Dysgeusia · epistaxis
  SIDE-EFFECTS, FURTHER INFORMATION
  Sensations of tingling, heat, heaviness, pressure, or tightness of any part of the body may occur (including throat and chest—discontinue if intense, may be due to coronary vasoconstriction or to anaphylaxis).
- **ALLERGY AND CROSS-SENSITIVITY** Caution in patients with sensitivity to sulfonamides.
- **PREGNANCY** There is limited experience of using $5HT_1$-receptor agonists during pregnancy; manufacturers advise that they should be avoided unless the potential benefit outweighs the risk.
- **BREAST FEEDING** Present in milk but amount probably too small to be harmful; withhold breast-feeding for 12 hours after treatment.
- **HEPATIC IMPAIRMENT** Reduce dose of oral therapy. Avoid in severe impairment.
- **RENAL IMPAIRMENT** Use with caution.
- **PATIENT AND CARER ADVICE**
  Driving and skilled tasks
  Drowsiness may affect performance of skilled tasks (e.g. driving).

- **MEDICINAL FORMS**
There can be variation in the licensing of different medicines containing the same drug.

Tablet

CAUTIONARY AND ADVISORY LABELS 3, 10

▶ Sumatriptan (Non-proprietary)

Sumatriptan (as Sumatriptan succinate) 50 mg Sumatriptan 50mg tablets | 6 tablet [PoM] £22.56 DT price = £1.20

Sumatriptan (as Sumatriptan succinate) 100 mg Sumatriptan 100mg tablets | 6 tablet [PoM] £36.47 DT price = £1.47

▶ Imigran (GlaxoSmithKline UK Ltd, Forest Laboratories UK Ltd)

Sumatriptan (as Sumatriptan succinate) 50 mg Imigran Radis 50mg tablets | 6 tablet [PoM] £23.90 DT price = £1.20

Imigran 50mg tablets | 6 tablet [PoM] £31.85 DT price = £1.20

Imigran Recovery 50mg tablets | 2 tablet [P] £4.76

Sumatriptan (as Sumatriptan succinate) 100 mg Imigran 100mg tablets | 6 tablet [PoM] £51.48 DT price = £1.47

Imigran Radis 100mg tablets | 6 tablet [PoM] £42.90 DT price = £1.47

▶ Migraitan (Bristol Laboratories Ltd)

Sumatriptan (as Sumatriptan succinate) 50 mg Migraitan 50mg tablets | 2 tablet [P] £4.24

Solution for injection

CAUTIONARY AND ADVISORY LABELS 3, 10

▶ Sumatriptan (Non-proprietary)

Sumatriptan (as Sumatriptan succinate) 12 mg per 1 ml Sumatriptan 6mg/0.5ml solution for injection pre-filled pen | 2 pre-filled disposable injection [PoM] £39.50 DT price = £39.50

▶ Imigran Subject (GlaxoSmithKline UK Ltd)

Sumatriptan (as Sumatriptan succinate) 12 mg per 1 ml Imigran Subject 6mg/0.5ml solution for injection syringe refill pack | 2 pre-filled disposable injection [PoM] £40.41 DT price = £40.41

Imigran Subject 6mg/0.5ml solution for injection pre-filled syringes with device | 2 pre-filled disposable injection [PoM] £42.47 DT price = £42.47

Spray

CAUTIONARY AND ADVISORY LABELS 3, 10

▶ Imigran (GlaxoSmithKline UK Ltd)

Sumatriptan 100 mg per 1 ml Imigran 10mg nasal spray | 2 unit dose [PoM] £11.80 DT price = £11.80

Sumatriptan 200 mg per 1 ml Imigran 20mg nasal spray | 2 unit dose [PoM] £14.16 | 6 unit dose [PoM] £35.39 DT price = £35.39

Zolmitriptan

- **INDICATIONS AND DOSE**

Treatment of acute migraine

▶ BY MOUTH

▶ Child 12–17 years: 2.5 mg, followed by 2.5 mg after at least 2 hours if required, dose to be taken only if migraine recurs, if response unsatisfactory after 3 attacks consider increasing dose to 5 mg or switching to alternative treatment; maximum 10 mg per day

▶ BY INTRANASAL ADMINISTRATION

▶ Child 12–17 years: 5 mg, dose to be administered as soon as possible after onset into one nostril only, followed by 5 mg after at least 2 hours if required, dose to be administered only if migraine recurs; maximum 10 mg per day

Treatment of acute cluster headache

▶ BY INTRANASAL ADMINISTRATION

▶ Child 12–17 years: 5 mg, dose to be administered as soon as possible after onset into one nostril only, followed by 5 mg after at least 2 hours if required, dose to be administered only if migraine recurs; maximum 10 mg per day

DOSE ADJUSTMENTS DUE TO INTERACTIONS

Max. 5 mg in 24 hours with concomitant cimetidine, fluvoxamine, moclobemide, or quinolone antibiotics.

DOSE EQUIVALENCE AND CONVERSION

1 spray of Zomig® nasal spray = 5 mg zolmitriptan.

- **UNLICENSED USE** Not licensed for use in children.
- **CONTRA-INDICATIONS** Arrhythmias associated with accessory cardiac conduction pathways · ischaemic heart disease · previous cerebrovascular accident · transient ischaemic attack · uncontrolled hypertension · vasospasm · Wolff-Parkinson-White syndrome

- **CAUTIONS** Should not be taken within 24 hours of any other 5HT₁-receptor agonist

- **INTERACTIONS** → Appendix 1 (5HT₁ agonists).

- **SIDE-EFFECTS**

GENERAL SIDE-EFFECTS

▶ **Common or very common** Abdominal pain · drowsiness · dry mouth · dysphagia · headache · muscle weakness · myalgia · palpitation · paraesthesia

▶ **Uncommon** Polyuria · tachycardia · transient increase in blood pressure

▶ **Rare** Urticaria

▶ **Very rare** Angina · gastro-intestinal infarction · ischaemic colitis · myocardial infarction · splenic infarction

▶ **Frequency not known** Asthenia · dizziness

SPECIFIC SIDE-EFFECTS

▶ With intranasal use Epistaxis · taste disturbance

SIDE-EFFECTS, FURTHER INFORMATION

Sensations of tingling, heat, heaviness, pressure, or tightness of any part of the body may occur (including throat and chest—discontinue if intense, may be due to coronary vasoconstriction or to anaphylaxis).

- **PREGNANCY** There is limited experience of using 5HT₁-receptor agonists during pregnancy; manufacturers advise that they should be avoided unless the potential benefit outweighs the risk.

- **BREAST FEEDING** Use with caution—present in milk in *animal* studies.

- **HEPATIC IMPAIRMENT** Max. 5 mg in 24 hours in moderate or severe impairment.

- **DIRECTIONS FOR ADMINISTRATION** Zolmitriptan orodispersible tablets should be placed on the tongue, allowed to disperse and swallowed.

- **PATIENT AND CARER ADVICE** Patients or carers should be given advice on how to administer zolmitriptan orodispersible tablets.

- **MEDICINAL FORMS**
There can be variation in the licensing of different medicines containing the same drug.

Tablet

▶ Zolmitriptan (Non-proprietary)

Zolmitriptan 2.5 mg Zolmitriptan 2.5mg tablets | 6 tablet [PoM] £16.20 DT price = £1.55 | 12 tablet [PoM] £3.42

Zolmitriptan 5 mg Zolmitriptan 5mg tablets | 6 tablet [PoM] £3.60 | 12 tablet [PoM] £7.20

▶ Zomig (AstraZeneca UK Ltd)

Zolmitriptan 2.5 mg Zomig 2.5mg tablets | 6 tablet [PoM] £23.94 DT price = £1.55

Orodispersible tablet

EXCIPIENTS: May contain Aspartame

▶ Zolmitriptan (Non-proprietary)

Zolmitriptan 2.5 mg Zolmitriptan 2.5mg orodispersible tablets sugar free sugar-free | 6 tablet [PoM] £1.58 DT price = £1.43

Zolmitriptan 5 mg Zolmitriptan 5mg orodispersible tablets sugar free sugar-free | 6 tablet [PoM] £11.49 DT price = £11.11

▶ Zomig Rapimelt (AstraZeneca UK Ltd)

Zolmitriptan 2.5 mg Zomig Rapimelt 2.5mg orodispersible tablets sugar-free | 6 tablet [PoM] £23.99 DT price = £1.43

Zolmitriptan 5 mg Zomig Rapimelt 5mg orodispersible tablets sugar-free | 6 tablet [PoM] £23.94 DT price = £11.11

Spray

▶ Zomig (AstraZeneca UK Ltd)

Zolmitriptan 50 mg per 1 ml Zomig 5mg/0.1ml nasal spray 0.1ml unit dose | 6 unit dose [PoM] £36.50 DT price = £36.50

5.2 Neuropathic pain

Neuropathic pain

Overview and management

Neuropathic pain, which occurs as a result of damage to neural tissue, includes *compression neuropathies, peripheral neuropathies* (e.g. due to Diabetes, HIV infection, chemotherapy), *trauma, idiopathic neuropathy, central pain* (e.g. pain following spinal cord injury and syringomyelia), *postherpetic neuralgia*, and *phantom limb pain*. The pain may occur in an area of sensory deficit and may be described as burning, shooting or scalding; it may be accompanied by pain that is evoked by a nonnoxious stimulus (allodynia).

Children with chronic neuropathic pain require multidisciplinary management, which may include physiotherapy and psychological support. Neuropathic pain is generally managed with a **tricyclic antidepressant** such as amitriptyline hydrochloride p. 224 or **antiepileptic drugs** such as carbamazepine p. 184. Children with localised pain may benefit from **topical local anaesthetic** preparations, particularly while awaiting specialist review. Neuropathic pain may respond only partially to **opioid analgesics**. A corticosteroid may help to relieve pressure in compression neuropathy and thereby reduce pain.

Chronic facial pain

Chronic oral and facial pain including *persistent idiopathic facial pain* (also termed 'atypical facial pain') and *temporomandibular dysfunction* (previously termed temporomandibular joint pain dysfunction syndrome) may call for prolonged use of analgesics or for other drugs. **Tricyclic antidepressants** may be useful for facial pain [unlicensed indication], but are not on the Dental Practitioners' List. Disorders of this type require specialist referral and psychological support to accompany drug treatment. Children on long-term therapy need to be monitored both for progress and for side-effects.

6 Sleep disorders
6.1 Insomnia

Hypnotics and anxiolytics

Overview

Most anxiolytics ('sedatives') will induce sleep when given at night and most hypnotics will sedate when given during the day. Hypnotics and anxiolytics should be reserved for short courses to alleviate acute conditions after causal factors have been established.

The role of drug therapy in the management of anxiety disorders in children and adolescents is uncertain; drug therapy should be initiated only by specialists after psychosocial interventions have failed. Benzodiazepines and tricyclic antidepressants have been used but adverse effects may be problematic.

Hypnotics

The prescribing of hypnotics to children, except for occasional use such as for sedation for procedures is not justified. There is a risk of habituation with prolonged use. Problems settling children at night should be managed with behavioural therapy.

Dental procedures

Some anxious children may benefit from the use of a hypnotic the night before a dental appointment.

Chloral and derivatives

Chloral hydrate below and derivatives were formerly popular hypnotics for children. Chloral hydrate is now mainly used for sedation during diagnostic procedures.

Antihistamines

Some **antihistamines** such as promethazine hydrochloride p. 171 are used for occasional insomnia in adults; their prolonged duration of action can often cause drowsiness the following day. The sedative effect of antihistamines may diminish after a few days of continued treatment; antihistamines are associated with headache, psychomotor impairment and antimuscarinic effects. The use of hypnotics in children is not usually justified.

Melatonin

Melatonin p. 276 is a pineal hormone that may affect sleep pattern. Clinical experience suggests that when appropriate behavioural sleep interventions fail, melatonin may be of value for treating sleep onset insomnia and delayed sleep phase syndrome in children with conditions such as visual impairment, cerebral palsy, attention deficit hyperactivity disorder, autism, and learning difficulties. It is also sometimes used before magnetic resonance imaging (MRI), computed tomography (CT), or EEG investigations. Little is known about its long-term effects in children, and there is uncertainty as to the effect on other circadian rhythms including endocrine or reproductive hormone secretion. The need to continue melatonin therapy should be reviewed every 6 months.

Anxiolytics

Anxiolytic treatment should be used in children only to relieve acute anxiety (and related insomnia) caused by fear (e.g. before surgery). Anxiolytic treatment should be limited to the lowest possible dose for the shortest possible time.

Buspirone

Buspirone hydrochloride is thought to act at specific serotonin ($5HT_{1A}$) receptors; safety and efficacy in children have yet to be determined.

HYPNOTICS, SEDATIVES AND ANXIOLYTICS >
NON-BENZODIAZEPINE

Chloral hydrate

● **INDICATIONS AND DOSE**

Sedation for painless procedures
▸ BY MOUTH, OR BY RECTUM

▸ Neonate: 30–50 mg/kg, to be given 45–60 minutes before procedure, doses up to 100 mg/kg may be used with respiratory monitoring, administration by rectum only if oral route not available.

▸ Child 1 month–11 years: 30–50 mg/kg (max. per dose 1 g), to be given 45–60 minutes before procedure, administration by rectum only if oral route not available, increased if necessary up to 100 mg/kg (max. per dose 2 g)

▸ Child 12–17 years: 1–2 g, to be given 45–60 minutes before procedure, administration by rectum only if oral route not available

Insomnia (short-term use), using chloral hydrate 143.3 mg/5 ml oral solution
▸ BY MOUTH USING ORAL SOLUTION

▸ Child 2–11 years: 1–1.75 mL/kilogram, alternatively 30–50 mg/kg once daily, dose to be taken with water or milk at bedtime; maximum 35 mL per day; maximum 1 g per day

▸ Child 12–17 years: 15–30 mL, alternatively 430–860 mg once daily, dose to be taken with water or continued →

4

Nervous system

milk at bedtime; maximum 70 mL per day; maximum 2 g per day

Insomnia (short-term use), using chloral betaine 707 mg (≡ 414 mg chloral hydrate) tablets

▶ BY MOUTH USING TABLETS

▶ Child 12–17 years: 1–2 tablets, alternatively 414–828 mg once daily, dose to be taken with water or milk at bedtime; maximum 4 tablets per day; maximum 2 g per day

● UNLICENSED USE Not licensed for sedation for painless procedures.

● CONTRA-INDICATIONS Acute porphyrias p. 562 · gastritis · severe cardiac disease

● CAUTIONS Avoid contact with mucous membranes · avoid contact with skin · avoid prolonged use (and abrupt withdrawal thereafter) · reduce dose in debilitated

● INTERACTIONS → Appendix 1 (anxiolytics and hypnotics).

● SIDE-EFFECTS Abdominal distention · delirium (especially on abrupt withdrawal) · dependence · excitement · flatulence · gastric irritation · headache · ketonuria · nausea · rash · tolerance · vomiting

● PREGNANCY Avoid.

● BREAST FEEDING Risk of sedation in infant—avoid.

● HEPATIC IMPAIRMENT Reduce dose in mild to moderate impairment. Can precipitate coma. Avoid in severe impairment.

● RENAL IMPAIRMENT Avoid in severe impairment.

● DIRECTIONS FOR ADMINISTRATION

▶ With oral use For administration *by mouth* dilute liquid with plenty of water or juice to mask unpleasant taste.

● PRESCRIBING AND DISPENSING INFORMATION Flavours of oral liquid formulations may include black currant.

When prepared extemporaneously, the BP states Chloral Mixture, BP 2000 consists of chloral hydrate 500 mg/5 mL in a suitable vehicle.

● PATIENT AND CARER ADVICE

Driving and skilled tasks

Drowsiness may persist the next day and affect performance of skilled tasks (e.g. driving); effects of alcohol enhanced.

● MEDICINAL FORMS

There can be variation in the licensing of different medicines containing the same drug. Forms available from special-order manufacturers include: oral suspension, oral solution, suppository, enema

Tablet

CAUTIONARY AND ADVISORY LABELS 19, 27

▶ Chloral hydrate (Non-proprietary)

Cloral betaine 707 mg Cloral betaine 707mg tablets | 30 tablet PoM £68.00–£138.59 DT price = £138.59

Oral solution

CAUTIONARY AND ADVISORY LABELS 1 (paediatric solution only), 19 (solution other than paediatric only), 27

▶ Chloral hydrate (Non-proprietary)

Chloral hydrate 28.66 mg per 1 ml Chloral hydrate 143.3mg/5ml oral solution BP | 150 ml PoM £120.00–£244.26 DT price = £244.26

Melatonin

● INDICATIONS AND DOSE

Sleep onset insomnia (initiated under specialist supervision) | Delayed sleep phase syndrome (initiated under specialist supervision)

▶ BY MOUTH USING MODIFIED-RELEASE TABLETS

▶ Child: Initially 2–3 mg daily for 1–2 weeks, then increased if necessary to 4–6 mg daily, dose to be taken before bedtime; maximum 10 mg per day

● UNLICENSED USE Not licensed for use in children.

● CAUTIONS Autoimmune disease (manufacturer advises avoid—no information available)

● INTERACTIONS → Appendix 1 (melatonin).

● SIDE-EFFECTS

▶ Uncommon Abdominal pain · abnormal dreams · anxiety · chest pain · dizziness · dry mouth · dry skin · dyspepsia · glycosuria · headache · hypertension · irritability · malaise · mouth ulceration · nausea · nervousness · proteinuria · pruritus · rash · restlessness · weight gain

▶ Rare Aggression · arthritis · electrolyte disturbances · flatulence · gastritis · haematuria · halitosis · hot flushes · hypersalivation · hypertriglyceridaemia · impaired memory · increased libido · lacrimation · leucopenia · mood changes · muscle spasm · nail disorder · palpitation · paraesthesia · polyuria · priapism · prostatitis · restless legs syndrome · syncope · thirst · thrombocytopenia · visual disturbances · vomiting

▶ Frequency not known Galactorrhoea · mouth oedema · tongue oedema

● PREGNANCY No information available—avoid.

● BREAST FEEDING Present in milk—avoid.

● HEPATIC IMPAIRMENT Clearance reduced—avoid.

● RENAL IMPAIRMENT No information available—use with caution.

● PRESCRIBING AND DISPENSING INFORMATION Treatment with melatonin should be initiated and supervised by a specialist, but may be continued by general practitioners under a shared-care arrangement. The need to continue melatonin therapy should be reviewed every 6 months.

Melatonin is available as a modified-release tablet (*Circadin*®) and also as unlicensed formulations. *Circadin*® is licensed for the short-term treatment of primary insomnia in adults over 55 years. Unlicensed immediate-release preparations are available; the manufacturer should be specified in the shared-care guideline because of variability in clinical effect of unlicensed formulations.

● PATIENT AND CARER ADVICE

Medicines for Children leaflet: Melatonin for sleep problems www.medicinesforchildren.org.uk/melatonin-for-sleep-disorders

● MEDICINAL FORMS

There can be variation in the licensing of different medicines containing the same drug.

Modified-release tablet

CAUTIONARY AND ADVISORY LABELS 2, 21, 25

▶ Melatonin (Non-proprietary)

Melatonin 3 mg Melatonin 3mg modified-release tablets | 120 tablet PoM no price available

▶ Circadin (Flynn Pharma Ltd)

Melatonin 2 mg Circadin 2mg modified-release tablets | 30 tablet PoM £15.39 DT price = £15.39

7 Substance dependence

Substance dependence

Guidance on treatment of drug misuse

Treatment of alcohol or opioid dependence in children requires specialist management. The UK health departments have produced guidance on the treatment of drug misuse in the UK. *Drug Misuse and Dependence: UK Guidelines on Clinical Management* (2007) is available at www.nta.nhs.uk/uploads/clinical_guidelines_2007.pdf.

Nicotine dependence

Smoking cessation interventions are a cost-effective way of reducing ill health and prolonging life. Smokers should be advised to stop and offered help with follow-up when appropriate. If possible, smokers should have access to smoking cessation services for behavioural support.

Therapy to aid smoking cessation is chosen according to the smoker's likely adherence, availability of counselling and support, previous experience of smoking-cessation aids, contra-indications and adverse effects of the preparations, and the smoker's preferences. **Nicotine replacement therapy** is an effective aid to smoking cessation. The use of nicotine below replacement therapy in an individual who is already accustomed to nicotine introduces few new risks and it is widely accepted that there are no circumstances in which it is safer to smoke than to use nicotine replacement therapy.

Some individuals benefit from having more than one type of nicotine replacement therapy prescribed, such as a combination of transdermal and oral preparations.

Concomitant medication
Cigarette smoking increases the metabolism of some medicines by stimulating the hepatic enzyme CYP1A2. When smoking is discontinued, the dose of these drugs, in particular theophylline p. 159, and some antipsychotics (including clozapine p. 235, olanzapine p. 236, chlorpromazine hydrochloride p. 230, and haloperidol p. 231, may need to be reduced. Regular monitoring for adverse effects is advised.

Nicotine replacement therapy
Nicotine replacement therapy can be used in place of cigarettes after abrupt cessation of smoking, or alternatively to reduce the amount of cigarettes used in advance of making a quit attempt. Nicotine replacement therapy can also be used to minimise passive smoking, and to treat cravings and reduce compensatory smoking after enforced abstinence in smoke-free environments. Smokers who find it difficult to achieve abstinence should consult a healthcare professional for advice.

Choice
Nicotine patches are a prolonged-release formulation and are applied for 16 hours (with the patch removed overnight) or for 24 hours. If the individual experiences strong cravings for cigarettes on waking, a 24-hour patch may be more suitable. Immediate-release nicotine preparations (gum, lozenges, sublingual tablets, inhalator, nasal spray, and oral spray) are used whenever the urge to smoke occurs or to prevent cravings.

The choice of nicotine replacement preparation depends largely on patient preference, and should take into account what preparations, if any, have been tried before. Patients with a high level of nicotine dependence, or who have failed with nicotine replacement therapy previously, may benefit from using a combination of an immediate-release preparation and patches to achieve abstinence.

Side-effects of specific nicotine preparations
Mild local reactions at the beginning of treatment are common because of the irritant effect of nicotine. Oral preparations and *inhalation cartridges* can cause irritation of the throat, *gum*, *lozenges*, and *oral spray* can cause increased salivation, and *patches* can cause minor skin irritation. The *nasal spray* commonly causes coughing, nasal irritation, epistaxis, sneezing, and watery eyes; the *oral spray* can cause watery eyes and blurred vision.

Gastro-intestinal disturbances are common and may be caused by swallowed nicotine. Nausea, vomiting, dyspepsia, and hiccup occur most frequently. Ulcerative stomatitis has also been reported. Dry mouth is a common side-effect of *lozenges*, *patches*, *oral spray*, and *sublingual tablets*. *Lozenges* cause diarrhoea, constipation, dysphagia, oesophagitis, gastritis, mouth ulcers, bloating, flatulence, and less commonly, taste disturbance, thirst, gingival bleeding, and halitosis. The *oral spray* may also cause abdominal pain, flatulence, and taste disturbance.

Palpitations may occur with nicotine replacement therapy and rarely *patches* and *oral spray* can cause arrhythmia. *Patches*, *lozenges*, and *oral spray* can cause chest pain. The *inhalator* can very rarely cause reversible atrial fibrillation.

Paraesthesia is a common side-effect of *oral spray*. Abnormal dreams can occur with *patches*; removal of the patch before bed may help. *Lozenges* and *oral spray* may cause rash and hot flushes. Sweating and myalgia can occur with *patches* and *oral spray*; the *patches* can also cause arthralgia.

Neonatal abstinence syndrome
Neonatal abstinence syndrome occurs at birth as a result of intra-uterine exposure to opioids or high-dose benzodiazepines. Treatment is usually initiated if:

- feeding becomes a problem and tube feeding is required;
- there is profuse vomiting or watery diarrhoea;
- the baby remains very unsettled after two consecutive feeds despite gentle swaddling and the use of a pacifier.

Treatment involves weaning the baby from the drug on which it is dependent. Morphine p. 265 or methadone hydrochloride p. 279 can be used in babies of mothers who have been taking opioids. Morphine is widely used because the dose can be easily adjusted, but methadone hydrochloride may provide smoother control of symptoms. Weaning babies from opioids usually takes 7–10 days.

Weaning babies from benzodiazepines that have a long half-life is difficult to manage; chlorpromazine hydrochloride may be used in these situations but excessive sedation may occur. For babies who are dependent on barbiturates, phenobarbital p. 203 may be tried, although it does not control gastro-intestinal symptoms.

7.1 Nicotine dependence

NICOTINIC RECEPTOR AGONISTS

▌ Nicotine

> ● **INDICATIONS AND DOSE**
>
> **Nicotine replacement therapy in individuals who smoke fewer than 20 cigarettes each day**
> ▸ BY MOUTH USING CHEWING GUM
> ▸ Child 12–17 years: 2 mg as required, chew 1 piece of gum when the urge to smoke occurs or to prevent cravings, if attempting smoking cessation, treatment should continue for 3 months before reducing the dose
> ▸ BY SUBLINGUAL ADMINISTRATION USING SUBLINGUAL TABLETS
> ▸ Child 12–17 years: 1 tablet every 1 hour, increased to 2 tablets every 1 hour if required, if attempting smoking cessation, treatment should continue for up to 3 months before reducing the dose; maximum 40 tablets per day
>
> **Nicotine replacement therapy in individuals who smoke more than 20 cigarettes each day or who require more than 15 pieces of 2-mg strength gum each day**
> ▸ BY MOUTH USING CHEWING GUM
> ▸ Child 12–17 years: 4 mg as required, chew 1 piece of gum when the urge to smoke occurs or to prevent cravings, individuals should not exceed 15 pieces of 4-mg strength gum daily, if attempting smoking cessation, treatment should continue for 3 months before reducing the dose
>
> **Nicotine replacement therapy in individuals who smoke more than 20 cigarettes each day**
> ▸ BY SUBLINGUAL ADMINISTRATION USING SUBLINGUAL TABLETS
> ▸ Child 12–17 years: 2 tablets every 1 hour, if attempting smoking cessation, treatment should continued →

continue for up to 3 months before reducing the dose; maximum 40 tablets per day

Nicotine replacement therapy

▸ BY INHALATION USING INHALATOR

▸ **Child 12–17 years:** As required, the cartridges can be used when the urge to smoke occurs or to prevent cravings, individuals should not exceed 12 cartridges of the 10-mg strength daily, or 6 cartridges of the 15-mg strength daily

▸ BY MOUTH USING LOZENGES

▸ **Child 12–17 years:** 1 lozenge every 1–2 hours as required, one lozenge should be used when the urge to smoke occurs, individuals who smoke less than 20 cigarettes each day should usually use the lower-strength lozenges; individuals who smoke more than 20 cigarettes each day and those who fail to stop smoking with the low-strength lozenges should use the higher-strength lozenges; If attempting smoking cessation, treatment should continue for 6–12 weeks before attempting a reduction in dose; maximum 15 lozenges per day

▸ BY MOUTH USING OROMUCOSAL SPRAY

▸ **Child 12–17 years:** 1–2 sprays as required, individuals can spray in the mouth when the urge to smoke occurs or to prevent cravings, individuals should not exceed 2 sprays per episode (up to 4 sprays every hour); maximum 64 sprays per day

▸ BY INTRANASAL ADMINISTRATION USING NASAL SPRAY

▸ **Child 12–17 years:** 1 spray as required, individuals can spray into each nostril when the urge to smoke occurs, up to twice every hour for 16 hours daily, if attempting smoking cessation, treatment should continue for 8 weeks before reducing the dose; maximum 64 sprays per day

▸ BY TRANSDERMAL APPLICATION USING PATCHES

▸ **Child 12–17 years:** Individuals who smoke more than 10 cigarettes daily should apply a high-strength patch daily for 6–8 weeks, followed by the medium-strength patch for 2 weeks, and then the low-strength patch for the final 2 weeks; individuals who smoke fewer than 10 cigarettes daily can usually start with the medium-strength patch for 6–8 weeks, followed by the low-strength patch for 2–4 weeks; a slower titration schedule can be used in individuals who are not ready to quit but want to reduce cigarette consumption before a quit attempt; if abstinence is not achieved, or if withdrawal symptoms are experienced, the strength of the patch used should be maintained or increased until the patient is stabilised; individuals using the high-strength patch who experience excessive side-effects, that do not resolve within a few days, should change to a medium-strength patch for the remainder of the initial period and then use the low-strength patch for 2–4 weeks

● UNLICENSED USE All preparations are licensed for adults and children over 12 years (with the exception of *Nicotinell*® lozenges which are licensed for children under 18 years only when recommended by a doctor).

● CAUTIONS

GENERAL CAUTIONS

Diabetes mellitus—blood-glucose concentration should be monitored closely when initiating treatment · haemodynamically unstable patients hospitalised with cerebrovascular accident · haemodynamically unstable patients hospitalised with myocardial infarction · haemodynamically unstable patients hospitalised with severe arrhythmias · phaeochromocytoma · uncontrolled hyperthyroidism

SPECIFIC CAUTIONS

▸ When used by inhalation Bronchospastic disease · chronic throat disease · obstructive lung disease

▸ With intranasal use Bronchial asthma (may exacerbate)

▸ With oral use Gastritis (can be aggravated by swallowed nicotine) · oesophagitis (can be aggravated by swallowed nicotine) · peptic ulcers (can be aggravated by swallowed nicotine)

▸ With oral (topical) use *gum* may also stick to and damage dentures

▸ With transdermal use *patches* should not be placed on broken skin · patients with skin disorders

CAUTIONS, FURTHER INFORMATION

Most warnings for nicotine replacement therapy also apply to continued cigarette smoking, but the risk of continued smoking outweighs any risks of using nicotine preparations.

Specific cautions for individual preparations are usually related to the local effect of nicotine.

● INTERACTIONS → Appendix 1 (nicotine).

● SIDE-EFFECTS

▸ **Common or very common** Bloating · blurred vision · constipation · coughing · diarrhoea · dry mouth · dyspepsia · dysphagia · epistaxis · flatulence · gastritis · gastro-intestinal disturbances (may be caused by swallowed nicotine) · hiccup · increased salivation · irritation of the throat · mild local reactions at the beginning of treatment are common because of the irritant effect of nicotine · minor skin irritation · mouth ulcers · nasal irritation · nausea · oesophagitis · paraesthesia · sneezing · vomiting · watery eyes

▸ **Uncommon** Gingival bleeding · halitosis · thirst

▸ **Rare** Arrhythmia

▸ **Very rare** Reversible atrial fibrillation

▸ **Frequency not known** Abdominal pain · abnormal dreams (may occur with patches, removal of the patch before bed may help) · arthralgia · chest pain · flatulence · hot flushes · myalgia · palpitations · rash · sweating · taste disturbance · ulcerative stomatitis

SIDE-EFFECTS, FURTHER INFORMATION

Side-effects listed have been reported with use of various nicotine replacement therapy preparations. See *Nicotine replacement therapy*, under Substance dependence p. 276 for further details on individual preparations.

▸ Nicotine withdrawal Some systemic effects occur on initiation of therapy, particularly if the patient is using high-strength preparations; however, the patient may confuse side-effects of the nicotine-replacement preparation with nicotine withdrawal symptoms.

Common symptoms of nicotine withdrawal include malaise, headache, dizziness, sleep disturbance, coughing, influenza–like symptoms, depression, irritability, increased appetite, weight gain, restlessness, anxiety, drowsiness, aphthous ulcers, decreased heart rate, and impaired concentration.

● PREGNANCY The use of nicotine replacement therapy in pregnancy is preferable to the continuation of smoking, but should be used only if smoking cessation without nicotine replacement fails. Intermittent therapy is preferable to patches but avoid liquorice-flavoured nicotine products. Patches are useful, however, if the patient is experiencing pregnancy-related nausea and vomiting. If patches are used, they should be removed before bed.

● BREAST FEEDING Nicotine is present in milk; however, the amount to which the infant is exposed is small and less hazardous than second-hand smoke. Intermittent therapy is preferred.

● HEPATIC IMPAIRMENT Use with caution in moderate to severe hepatic impairment.

● RENAL IMPAIRMENT Use with caution in severe renal impairment.

● DIRECTIONS FOR ADMINISTRATION Acidic beverages, such as coffee or fruit juice, may decrease the absorption of nicotine through the buccal mucosa and should be avoided for 15 minutes before the use of oral nicotine replacement therapy.

Administration by transdermal patch Patches should be applied on waking to dry, non-hairy skin on the hip, trunk, or upper arm and held in position for 10–20 seconds to ensure adhesion; place next patch on a different area and avoid using the same site for several days.

Administration by nasal spray Initially 1 spray should be used in both nostrils but when withdrawing from therapy, the dose can be gradually reduced to 1 spray in 1 nostril.

Administration by oral spray The oral spray should be released into the mouth, holding the spray as close to the mouth as possible and avoiding the lips. The patient should not inhale while spraying and avoid swallowing for a few seconds after use. If using the oral spray for the first time, or if unit not used for 2 or more days, prime the unit before administration.

Administration by sublingual tablet Each tablet should be placed under the tongue and allowed to dissolve.

Administration by lozenge Slowly allow each lozenge to dissolve in the mouth; periodically move the lozenge from one side of the mouth to the other. Lozenges last for 10–30 minutes, depending on their size.

Administration by inhalation Insert the cartridge into the device and draw in air through the mouthpiece; each session can last for approximately 5 minutes. The amount of nicotine from 1 puff of the cartridge is less than that from a cigarette, therefore it is necessary to inhale more often than when smoking a cigarette. A single 10 mg cartridge lasts for approximately 20 minutes of intense use; a single 15 mg cartridge lasts for approximately 40 minutes of intense use.

Administration by medicated chewing gum Chew the gum until the taste becomes strong, then rest it between the cheek and gum; when the taste starts to fade, repeat this process. One piece of gum lasts for approximately 30 minutes.

- **PRESCRIBING AND DISPENSING INFORMATION** Flavours of chewing gum and lozenges may include mint, freshfruit, freshmint, icy white, or cherry.

- **PATIENT AND CARER ADVICE** Patient or carers should be given advice on how to administer nicotine chewing gum, inhalators, lozenges, sublingual tablets, oral spray, nasal spray and patches.

- **MEDICINAL FORMS**
There can be variation in the licensing of different medicines containing the same drug.

Sublingual tablet
CAUTIONARY AND ADVISORY LABELS 26
▸ Nicotine (Non-proprietary)
　Nicotine (as Nicotine cyclodextrin complex) 2 mg sublingual tablets sugar-free | 100 tablet GSL no price available DT price = £13.12
▸ Brands may include Nicorette Microtab

Lozenge
EXCIPIENTS: May contain Aspartame
ELECTROLYTES: May contain Sodium
▸ Nicotine (Non-proprietary)
　Nicotine (as Nicotine bitartrate) 1 mg lozenges sugar-free | 96 lozenge GSL no price available DT price = £9.12
　Nicotine (as Nicotine bitartrate) 2 mg lozenges sugar-free | 96 lozenge GSL no price available
▸ Brands may include NiQuitin, Nicorette, Nicotinell

Medicated chewing-gum
▸ Nicotine (Non-proprietary)
　Nicotine 2 mg medicated chewing gum sugar-free | GSL no price available
　Nicotine 4 mg medicated chewing gum sugar-free | GSL no price available
▸ Brands may include NiQuitin, Nicorette, Nicorette Icy White, Nicotinell

Inhalation vapour
▸ Nicotine (Non-proprietary)
　Nicotine 15 mg Inhalator | 4 cartridge GSL no price available DT price = £4.27 | 20 cartridge GSL no price available DT price = £15.11
▸ Brands may include Nicorette

Transdermal patch
▸ Nicotine (Non-proprietary)
　Nicotine 7 mg per 24 hour transdermal patches | 7 patch GSL no price available
　Nicotine 10 mg per 16 hour patches | 7 patch GSL no price available DT price = £10.37
　Nicotine 14 mg per 24 hour transdermal patches | 7 patch GSL no price available
　Nicotine 15 mg per 16 hour patches | 7 patch GSL no price available DT price = £10.37
　Nicotine 21 mg per 24 hour transdermal patches | 7 patch GSL no price available DT price = £9.97
　Nicotine 25 mg per 16 hour patches | 7 patch GSL no price available DT price = £10.37
▸ Brands may include NiQuitin, NiQuitin Clear, Nicorette invisi, Nicotinell TTS

Spray
EXCIPIENTS: May contain Ethanol
▸ Nicotine (Non-proprietary)
　Nicotine 500 microgram per 1 actuation 10mg/ml nasal spray | 10 ml GSL no price available DT price = £13.80
▸ Brands may include Nicorette, Nicorette QuickMist

7.2　Opioid dependence

OPIOIDS

F 256

Methadone hydrochloride

- ● **INDICATIONS AND DOSE**

Neonatal opioid withdrawal
▸ BY MOUTH

▸ **Neonate:** Initially 100 micrograms/kg, then increased in steps of 50 micrograms/kg every 6 hours until symptoms are controlled, doses may vary, consult local guidelines, for maintenance, total daily dose that controls symptoms to be given in 2 divided doses.

- ● **UNLICENSED USE** Not licensed for use in children.

IMPORTANT SAFETY INFORMATION
Methadone oral solution 1 mg/mL is 2½ times the strength of Methadone Linctus (2 mg/5mL). Many preparations of Methadone oral solution are licensed for opioid drug addiction only but some are also licensed for analgesia in severe pain.

- ● **CONTRA-INDICATIONS** Phaeochromocytoma

- ● **CAUTIONS** Family history of sudden death (ECG monitoring recommended) · history of cardiac conduction abnormalities

CAUTIONS, FURTHER INFORMATION
▸ QT-interval prolongation Patients with the following risk factors for QT-interval prolongation should be carefully monitored while taking methadone: heart or liver disease, electrolyte abnormalities, or concomitant treatment with drugs that can prolong QT interval; patients requiring more than 100 mg daily should also be monitored.

- ● **SIDE-EFFECTS** Dry eyes · dysmenorrhoea · hyperprolactinaemia · hypothermia · QT-interval prolongation · raised intracranial pressure · restlessness · torsade de pointes

SIDE-EFFECTS, FURTHER INFORMATION
Methadone is a long-acting opioid therefore effects may be cumulative.

4

Nervous system

Methadone, even in low doses is a **special hazard** for children; non-dependent adults are also at risk of toxicity; dependent adults are at risk if tolerance is incorrectly assessed during induction.

Overdose

Methadone has a very long duration of action; patients may need to be monitored for long periods following large overdoses.

- **BREAST FEEDING** Withdrawal symptoms in infant; breast-feeding permissible during maintenance but dose should be as low as possible and infant monitored to avoid sedation (high doses of methadone carry an increased risk of sedation and respiratory depression in the neonate).

- **RENAL IMPAIRMENT** Avoid use or reduce dose; opioid effects increased and prolonged and increased cerebral sensitivity occurs.

- **TREATMENT CESSATION** Avoid abrupt withdrawal. When used for neonatal opioid withdrawal, reduce dose over 7–10 days.

- **DIRECTIONS FOR ADMINISTRATION** Syrup preserved with hydroxybenzoate (parabens) esters may be incompatible with methadone hydrochloride.

- **PRESCRIBING AND DISPENSING INFORMATION** Flavours of oral liquid formulations may include tolu.

- **MEDICINAL FORMS**
  There can be variation in the licensing of different medicines containing the same drug.

Oral solution
CAUTIONARY AND ADVISORY LABELS 2
- ▸ **Methadone hydrochloride (Non-proprietary)**
  Methadone hydrochloride 1 mg per 1 ml Methadone 1mg/ml oral solution | 100 ml [PoM] £1.10–£1.23 DT price = £1.11 [CD2] | 500 ml [PoM] £6.18 DT price = £5.55 [CD2] | 2500 ml [PoM] £27.50–£32.10 [CD2]
  Methadone 1mg/ml oral solution sugar free sugar-free | 50 ml [PoM] £1.04 DT price = £1.04 [CD2] sugar-free | 100 ml [PoM] £2.08 DT price = £2.08 [CD2] sugar-free | 500 ml [PoM] £6.30 DT price = £6.30 [CD2] sugar-free | 2500 ml [PoM] £31.50–£32.50 [CD2]
- ▸ **Metharose** (Rosemont Pharmaceuticals Ltd)
  Methadone hydrochloride 1 mg per 1 ml Metharose 1mg/ml oral solution sugar free sugar-free | 500 ml [PoM] £6.82 DT price = £6.30 [CD2]
- ▸ **Physeptone** (Martindale Pharmaceuticals Ltd)
  Methadone hydrochloride 1 mg per 1 ml Physeptone 1mg/ml mixture | 100 ml [PoM] £1.08 DT price = £1.11 [CD2] | 500 ml [PoM] £5.46 DT price = £5.55 [CD2] | 2500 ml [PoM] £27.29 [CD2]
  Physeptone 1mg/ml mixture sugar free sugar-free | 100 ml [PoM] £1.08 DT price = £2.08 [CD2] sugar-free | 500 ml [PoM] £5.46 DT price = £6.30 [CD2] sugar-free | 2500 ml [PoM] £27.29 [CD2]

Chapter 5
Infection

CONTENTS

1	**Amoebic infection**	page 281
2	**Bacterial infection**	281
2.1	Anthrax	339
2.2	Lyme disease	339
2.3	Methicillin-resistant staphylococcus aureus	339
2.4	Tuberculosis	340
2.5	Urinary tract infections	347
3	**Fungal infection**	348
3.1	Pneumocystis pneumonia	357
4	**Helminth infection**	359
5	**Protozoal infection**	362
5.1	Leishmaniasis	363

5.2	Malaria	page 363
5.3	Toxoplasmosis	377
6	**Viral infection**	377
6.1	Hepatitis	377
6.2	Hepatitis infections	378
	6.2a Chronic hepatitis C	378
6.3	Herpesvirus infections	380
	6.3a Cytomegalovirus infections	383
6.4	HIV infection	385
6.5	Influenza	399
6.6	Respiratory syncytial virus	402

1 Amoebic infection

Drugs used for Amoebic infection not listed below
Metronidazole, p. 313 · Tinidazole, p. 315

ANTIPROTOZOALS

Diloxanide furoate

● **INDICATIONS AND DOSE**

Chronic amoebiasis | Acute amoebiasis as adjunct to metronidazole or tinidazole
▸ BY MOUTH
▸ Child 1 month–11 years: 6.6 mg/kg 3 times a day for 10 days
▸ Child 12–17 years: 500 mg 3 times a day for 10 days

● **UNLICENSED USE** Not licensed for use in children under 25 kg body-weight.

● **SIDE-EFFECTS** Flatulence · pruritus · urticaria · vomiting

● **PREGNANCY** Manufacturer advises avoid—no information available.

● **BREAST FEEDING** Manufacturer advises avoid.

● **MEDICINAL FORMS**
There can be variation in the licensing of different medicines containing the same drug. Forms available from special-order manufacturers include: oral suspension, oral solution

Tablet
CAUTIONARY AND ADVISORY LABELS 9
▸ Diloxanide furoate (Non-proprietary)
Diloxanide furoate **500 mg** Diloxanide 500mg tablets |
30 tablet PoM £93.50

2 Bacterial infection

Antibacterials, principles of therapy

Choice of a suitable drug

Before selecting an antibacterial the clinician must first consider two factors— the patient and the known or likely causative organism. Factors related to the patient which must be considered include history of allergy, renal and hepatic function, susceptibility to infection (i.e. whether immunocompromised), ability to tolerate drugs by mouth, severity of illness, ethnic origin, age, whether taking other medication and, if female, whether pregnant, breast-feeding or taking an oral contraceptive.

The known or likely organism and its antibacterial sensitivity, in association with the above factors, will suggest one or more antibacterials, the final choice depending on the microbiological, pharmacological, and toxicological properties.

The principles involved in selection of an antibacterial must allow for a number of variables including changing renal and hepatic function, increasing bacterial resistance, and information on side-effects. Duration of therapy, dosage, and route of administration depend on site, type and severity of infection and response.

Antibacterial policies

Local policies often limit the antibacterials that may be used to achieve reasonable economy consistent with adequate cover, and to reduce the development of resistant organisms. A policy may indicate a range of drugs for general use, and permit other drugs only on the advice of the microbiologist or paediatric infectious diseases specialist.

Before starting therapy

The following precepts should be considered before starting:
● Viral infections should not be treated with antibacterials. However, antibacterials may be used to treat secondary bacterial infection (e.g. bacterial pneumonia secondary to influenza);
● Samples should be taken for culture and sensitivity testing; 'blind' antibacterial prescribing for unexplained

pyrexia usually leads to further difficulty in establishing the diagnosis;

- Knowledge of **prevalent organisms** and their current sensitivity is of great help in choosing an antibacterial before bacteriological confirmation is available. Generally, narrow-spectrum antibacterials are preferred to broad-spectrum antibacterials unless there is a clear clinical indication (e.g. life-threatening sepsis);
- The **dose** of an antibacterial varies according to a number of factors including age, weight, hepatic function, renal function, and severity of infection. The prescribing of the so-called 'standard' dose in serious infections may result in failure of treatment or even death of the patient; therefore it is important to prescribe a dose appropriate to the condition. An inadequate dose may also increase the likelihood of antibacterial resistance. On the other hand, for an antibacterial with a narrow margin between the toxic and therapeutic dose (e.g. an aminoglycoside) it is also important to avoid an excessive dose and the concentration of the drug in the plasma may need to be monitored;
- The **route** of administration of an antibacterial often depends on the severity of the infection. Life-threatening infections often require intravenous therapy. Antibacterials that are well absorbed may be given by mouth even for some serious infections. Parenteral administration is also appropriate when the oral route cannot be used (e.g. because of vomiting) or if absorption is inadequate (e.g. in neonates and young children). Whenever possible, painful intramuscular injections should be avoided in children;
- **Duration** of therapy depends on the nature of the infection and the response to treatment. Courses should not be unduly prolonged because they encourage resistance, they may lead to side-effects and they are costly. However, in certain infections such as tuberculosis or osteomyelitis it may be necessary to treat for prolonged periods. Conversely a single dose of an antibacterial may cure uncomplicated urinary-tract infections. The prescription for an antibacterial should specify the duration of treatment or the date when treatment is to be reviewed.

Superinfection

In general, broad-spectrum antibacterial drugs such as the cephalosporins are more likely to be associated with adverse reactions related to the selection of resistant organisms e.g. *fungal infections* or *antibiotic-associated colitis* (pseudomembranous colitis); other problems associated with superinfection include vaginitis and pruritus ani.

Therapy

When the pathogen has been isolated treatment may be changed to a more appropriate antibacterial if necessary. If no bacterium is cultured the antibacterial can be continued or stopped on clinical grounds.

Switching from parenteral to oral treatment

The ongoing parenteral administration of an antibacterial should be reviewed regularly. In older children it may be possible to switch to an oral antibacterial; in neonates and infants this should be done more cautiously because of the relatively high incidence of bacteraemia and the possibility of variable oral absorption.

Prophylaxis

In most situations, only a short course of prophylactic antibacterial is needed. Longer-term antibacterial prophylaxis is appropriate in specific indications such as vesico-ureteric reflux.

Notifiable diseases

Doctors must notify the Proper Officer of the local authority (usually the consultant in communicable disease control) when attending a patient suspected of suffering from any of the diseases listed below; a form is available from the Proper Officer.

- Anthrax
- Botulism
- Brucellosis
- Cholera
- Diarrhoea (infectious bloody)
- Diphtheria
- Encephalitis, acute
- Food poisoning
- Haemolytic uraemic syndrome
- Haemorrhagic fever (viral)
- Hepatitis, viral
- Legionnaires' disease
- Leprosy
- Malaria
- Measles
- Meningitis
- Meningococcal septicaemia
- Mumps
- Paratyphoid fever
- Plague
- Poliomyelitis, acute
- Rabies
- Rubella
- SARS
- Scarlet fever
- Smallpox
- Streptococcal disease (Group A, invasive)
- Tetanus
- Tuberculosis
- Typhoid fever
- Typhus
- Whooping cough
- Yellow fever

Note It is good practice for doctors to also inform the consultant in communicable disease control of instances of other infections (e.g. psittacosis) where there could be a public health risk.

Antibacterials, use for prophylaxis

Prevention of recurrence of rheumatic fever

- Phenoxymethylpenicillin p. 319 by mouth *or* erythromycin p. 310 by mouth.

Prevention of secondary case of invasive group A streptococcal infection

- Phenoxymethylpenicillin by mouth.

   If child penicillin allergic, *either* erythromycin by mouth or azithromycin p. 308 by mouth [unlicensed indication].

   For details of those who should receive chemoprophylaxis contact a consultant in communicable disease control (or a consultant in infectious diseases or the local Public Health England Laboratory).

Prevention of secondary case of meningococcal meningitis

- Ciprofloxacin p. 328 by mouth [unlicensed indication] *or* rifampicin p. 342 by mouth *or* ceftriaxone p. 302 by intramuscular injection [unlicensed indication].

   For details of those who should receive chemoprophylaxis contact a consultant in communicable disease control (or a consultant in infectious diseases or the local Public Health

England laboratory). Unless there has been direct exposure of the mouth or nose to infectious droplets from a patient with meningococcal disease who has received less than 24 hours of antibacterial treatment, healthcare workers do not generally require chemoprophylaxis.

Prevention of secondary case of *Haemophilus influenzae* type b disease

- Rifampicin by mouth *or* (if rifampicin cannot be used) ceftriaxone by intramuscular injection, or by intravenous injection, or by intravenous infusion [unlicensed indication].

    For details of those who should receive chemoprophylaxis contact a consultant in communicable disease control (or a consultant in infectious diseases or the local Public Health England laboratory). Unless there has been direct exposure of the mouth or nose to infectious droplets from a patient with meningococcal disease who has received less than 24 hours of antibacterial treatment, healthcare workers do not generally require chemoprophylaxis.

    Within 4 weeks of illness onset in an index case with confirmed or suspected invasive *Haemophilus influenzae* type b disease, give antibacterial prophylaxis to all household contacts if there is a vulnerable individual in the household. Also, give antibacterial prophylaxis to the index case if they are in contact with vulnerable household contacts or if they are under 10 years of age. Vulnerable individuals include the immunocompromised, those with asplenia, or children under 10 years of age. If there are 2 or more cases of invasive *Haemophilus influenzae* type b disease within 120 days in a pre-school or primary school, antibacterial prophylaxis should also be given to all room contacts (including staff). Also see immunisation against *Haemophilus influenzae* type b disease.

Prevention of secondary case of diphtheria in non-immune patient

- Erythromycin (*or* another macrolide e.g. azithromycin *or* clarithromycin p. 309) by mouth.

    Treat for further 10 days if nasopharyngeal swabs positive after first 7 days' treatment.

Prevention of pertussis

- Clarithromycin (*or* azithromycin *or* erythromycin) by mouth.

    Within 3 weeks of onset of cough in the index case, give antibacterial prophylaxis to all close contacts if amongst them there is at least one unimmunised or partially immunised child under 1 year of age, *or* if there is at least one individual who has not received a pertussis-containing vaccine more than 1 week and less than 5 years ago (so long as that individual lives or works with children under 4 months of age, is pregnant at over 32 weeks gestation, or is a healthcare worker who works with children under 1 year of age or with pregnant women).

Prevention of pneumococcal infection in asplenia or in patients with sickle-cell disease

- Phenoxymethylpenicillin by mouth.

    If cover also needed for *H. influenzae* in child give amoxicillin p. 320 instead.

    If penicillin-allergic, erythromycin by mouth.

    Antibacterial prophylaxis is not fully reliable. Antibacterial prophylaxis may be discontinued in children over 5 years of age with sickle-cell disease who have received pneumococcal immunisation and who do not have a history of severe pneumococcal infection.

Prevention of *Staphylococcus aureus* lung infection in cystic fibrosis

- *Primary prevention*, flucloxacillin p. 325 by mouth.
- *Secondary prevention*, flucloxacillin by mouth.

Prevention of tuberculosis in susceptible close contacts or those who have become tuberculin positive

- Isoniazid p. 345 for 6 months *or* isoniazid + rifampicin for 3 months *or* (if isoniazid-resistant tuberculosis) rifampicin for 6 months.

    For details of those who should receive chemoprophylaxis contact the lead clinician for local tuberculosis services (or a consultant in communicable disease control).

Prevention of urinary-tract infection

- Trimethoprim p. 338 by mouth *or* nitrofurantoin p. 347 by mouth.

    Antibacterial prophylaxis can be considered for recurrent infection, significant urinary-tract anomalies, or significant kidney damage.

Prevention of infection from animal and human bites

- Co-amoxiclav p. 323 alone (*or* clindamycin p. 307 if penicillin-allergic).

    Cleanse wound thoroughly. For tetanus-prone wound, give human tetanus immunoglobulin p. 729 (with a tetanus-containing vaccine if necessary, according to immunisation history and risk of infection).

    Consider rabies prophylaxis for bites from animals in endemic countries. Assess risk of blood-borne viruses (including HIV, hepatitis B and C) and give appropriate prophylaxis to prevent viral spread. Antibacterial prophylaxis recommended for wounds less than 48–72 hours old when the risk of infection is high (e.g. bites from humans or cats; bites to the hand, foot, face, or genital area; bites involving oedema, crush or puncture injury, or other moderate to severe injury; wounds that cannot be debrided adequately; patients with diabetes mellitus, cirrhosis, asplenia, prosthetic joints or valves, or those who are immunocompromised). Give antibacterial prophylaxis for up to 5 days.

Prevention of infection in gastro-intestinal procedures

Operations on stomach or oesophagus

- Single dose of i/v gentamicin p. 293 *or* i/v cefuroxime p. 300 *or* i/v co-amoxiclav (additional intra-operative or postoperative doses may be given for prolonged procedures or if there is major blood loss).

    Intravenous antibacterial prophylaxis should be given up to 30 minutes before the procedure.

    Add i/v teicoplanin p. 305 (*or* vancomycin p. 305) if high risk of meticillin-resistant *Staphylococcus aureus*.

Open biliary surgery

- Single dose of i/v cefuroxime + i/v metronidazole p. 313 *or* i/v gentamicin + i/v metronidazole *or* i/v co-amoxiclav alone (additional intra-operative or postoperative doses may be given for prolonged procedures or if there is major blood loss).

    Intravenous antibacterial prophylaxis should be given up to 30 minutes before the procedure.

    Where i/v metronidazole is suggested, it may alternatively be given by suppository but to allow adequate absorption, it should be given 2 hours before surgery.

    Add i/v teicoplanin (*or* vancomycin) if high risk of meticillin-resistant *Staphylococcus aureus*.

Resections of colon and rectum, and resections in inflammatory bowel disease, and appendicectomy

- Single dose of i/v gentamicin + i/v metronidazole *or* i/v cefuroxime + i/v metronidazole *or* i/v co-amoxiclav alone (additional intra-operative or postoperative doses may be given for prolonged procedures or if there is major blood loss).

Intravenous antibacterial prophylaxis should be given up to 30 minutes before the procedure.

Where i/v metronidazole p. 313 is suggested, it may alternatively be given by suppository but to allow adequate absorption, it should be given 2 hours before surgery.

Add i/v teicoplanin p. 305 (*or* vancomycin p. 305) if high risk of meticillin-resistant *Staphylococcus aureus*.

Endoscopic retrograde cholangiopancreatography

- Single dose of i/v gentamicin p. 293 *or* oral *or* i/v ciprofloxacin p. 328.

Intravenous antibacterial prophylaxis should be given up to 30 minutes before the procedure.

Prophylaxis recommended if pancreatic pseudocyst, immunocompromised, history of liver transplantation, or risk of incomplete biliary drainage. For biliary complications following liver transplantation, add i/v amoxicillin p. 320 or i/v teicoplanin (*or* vancomycin).

Percutaneous endoscopic gastrostomy or jejunostomy

- Single dose of i/v co-amoxiclav p. 323 or i/v cefuroxime p. 300.

Intravenous antibacterial prophylaxis should be given up to 30 minutes before the procedure.

Use single dose of i/v teicoplanin (*or* vancomycin) if history of allergy to penicillins or cephalosporins, or if high risk of meticillin-resistant *Staphylococcus aureus*.

Prevention of infection in orthopaedic surgery
Closed fractures

- Single dose of i/v cefuroxime *or* i/v flucloxacillin p. 325 (additional intra-operative or postoperative doses may be given for prolonged procedures or if there is major blood loss).

Intravenous antibacterial prophylaxis should be given up to 30 minutes before the procedure.

If history of allergy to penicillins or to cephalosporins or if high risk of meticillin-resistant *Staphylococcus aureus*, use single dose of i/v teicoplanin (*or* vancomycin) (additional intra-operative or postoperative doses may be given for prolonged procedures or if there is major blood loss).

Open fractures

- Use i/v co-amoxiclav alone *or* i/v cefuroxime + i/v metronidazole (*or* i/v clindamycin p. 307 alone if history of allergy to penicillins or to cephalosporins).

Add i/v teicoplanin (*or* vancomycin) if high risk of meticillin-resistant *Staphylococcus aureus*. Start prophylaxis within 3 hours of injury and continue until soft tissue closure (max. 72 hours).

At first debridement also use a single dose of i/v cefuroxime + i/v metronidazole + i/v gentamicin *or* i/v co-amoxiclav + i/v gentamicin (*or* i/v clindamycin + i/v gentamicin if history of allergy to penicillins or to cephalosporins).

At time of skeletal stabilisation and definitive soft tissue closure use a single dose of i/v gentamicin and i/v teicoplanin (*or* vancomycin) (intravenous antibacterial prophylaxis should be given up to 30 minutes before the procedure.

High lower-limb amputation

- Use i/v co-amoxiclav alone *or* i/v cefuroxime + i/v metronidazole.

Intravenous antibacterial prophylaxis should be given up to 30 minutes before the procedure.

Continue antibacterial prophylaxis for at least 2 doses after procedure (max. duration of prophylaxis 5 days). If history of allergy to penicillin or to cephalosporins, or if high risk of meticillin-resistant *Staphylococcus aureus*, use i/v teicoplanin (*or* vancomycin) + i/v gentamicin + i/v metronidazole.

Where i/v metronidazole is suggested, it may alternatively be given by suppository but to allow adequate absorption, it should be given 2 hours before surgery.

Prevention of infection in obstetric surgery
Termination of pregnancy

- Single dose of oral metronidazole (additional intra-operative or postoperative doses may be given for prolonged procedures or if there is major blood loss).

If genital chlamydial infection cannot be ruled out, give doxycycline p. 332 postoperatively.

Prevention of endocarditis

NICE guidance: Antimicrobial prophylaxis against infective endocarditis in adults and children undergoing interventional procedures (March 2008)

- Antibacterial prophylaxis and chlorhexidine mouthwash are **not** recommended for the prevention of endocarditis in patients undergoing dental procedures.

Antibacterial prophylaxis is **not** recommended for the prevention of endocarditis in patients undergoing procedures of the:

▸ upper and lower respiratory tract (including ear, nose, and throat procedures and bronchoscopy);

▸ genito-urinary tract (including urological, gynaecological, and obstetric procedures);

▸ upper and lower gastro-intestinal tract.

While these procedures can cause bacteraemia, there is no clear association with the development of infective endocarditis. Prophylaxis may expose patients to the adverse effects of antimicrobials when the evidence of benefit has not been proven.

Any infection in patients at risk of endocarditis should be investigated promptly and treated appropriately to reduce the risk of endocarditis.

If patients at risk of endocarditis are undergoing a gastro-intestinal or genito-urinary tract procedure at a site where infection is suspected, they should receive appropriate antibacterial therapy that includes cover against organisms that cause endocarditis.

Patients at risk of endocarditis should be:

▸ advised to maintain good oral hygiene;

▸ told how to recognise signs of infective endocarditis, and advised when to seek expert advice.

Patients at risk of endocarditis include those with valve replacement, acquired valvular heart disease with stenosis or regurgitation, structural congenital heart disease (including surgically corrected or palliated structural conditions, but excluding isolated atrial septal defect, fully repaired ventricular septal defect, fully repaired patent ductus arteriosus, and closure devices considered to be endothelialised), hypertrophic cardiomyopathy, or a previous episode of infective endocarditis.

Dermatological procedures

Advice of a Working Party of the British Society for Antimicrobial Chemotherapy is that patients who undergo dermatological procedures do not require antibacterial prophylaxis against endocarditis.

The British Association of Dermatologists Therapy Guidelines and Audit Subcommittee advise that such dermatological procedures include skin biopsies and excision of moles or of malignant lesions.

Joint prostheses and dental treatment

Advice of a Working Party of the British Society for Antimicrobial Chemotherapy is that patients with prosthetic joint implants (including total hip replacements) do not require antibacterial prophylaxis for dental treatment. The Working Party considers that it is unacceptable to expose patients to the adverse effects of antibacterials when there is no evidence that such prophylaxis is of any benefit, but that those who develop any intercurrent infection require prompt treatment with antibacterials to which the infecting organisms are sensitive.

The Working Party has commented that joint infections have rarely been shown to follow dental procedures and are even more rarely caused by oral streptococci.

Immunosuppression and indwelling intraperitoneal catheters

Advice of a Working Party of the British Society for Antimicrobial Chemotherapy is that patients who are immunosuppressed (including transplant patients) and patients with indwelling intraperitoneal catheters do not require antibacterial prophylaxis for dental treatment provided there is no other indication for prophylaxis.

The Working Party has commented that there is little evidence that dental treatment is followed by infection in immunosuppressed and immunodeficient patients nor is there evidence that dental treatment is followed by infection in patients with indwelling intraperitoneal catheters.

Blood infections, bacterial

Antibacterial therapy for septicaemia: community-acquired

* *Child 1 month*–18 *years*, aminoglycoside + amoxicillin p. 320 (*or* ampicillin p. 321) *or* cefotaxime p. 301 (*or* ceftriaxone p. 302) alone
▸ If pseudomonas or resistant micro-organisms suspected, use a broad-spectrum antipseudomonal beta-lactam antibacterial.
▸ If anaerobic infection suspected, add metronidazole p. 313.
▸ If Gram-positive infection suspected, add flucloxacillin p. 325 *or* vancomycin p. 305 (*or* teicoplanin p. 305).
▸ *Suggested duration of treatment* at least 5 days.

Antibacterial therapy for septicaemia: hospital-acquired

* *Child 1 month*–18 *years*, a broad-spectrum antipseudomonal beta-lactam antibacterial (e.g. piperacillin with tazobactam p. 317, ticarcillin with clavulanic acid p. 318, imipenem with cilastatin p. 295, *or* meropenem p. 296)
▸ If pseudomonas suspected, or if multiple-resistant organisms suspected, or if severe sepsis, add aminoglycoside.
▸ If meticillin-resistant *Staphylococcus aureus* suspected, add vancomycin (*or* teicoplanin).
▸ If anaerobic infection suspected, add metronidazole to a broad-spectrum cephalosporin.
▸ *Suggested duration of treatment* at least 5 days.

Septicaemia related to vascular catheter

* Vancomycin (*or* teicoplanin)
▸ If Gram-negative sepsis suspected, especially in the immunocompromised, add a broad-spectrum antipseudomonal beta-lactam.

▸ Consider removing vascular catheter, particularly if infection caused by *Staphylococcus aureus*, pseudomonas, or *Candida* species.

Meningococcal septicaemia

If meningococcal disease suspected, a single dose of benzylpenicillin sodium p. 318 should be given before urgent transfer to hospital, so long as this does not delay the transfer; cefotaxime may be an alternative in penicillin allergy; chloramphenicol p. 334 may be used if history of immediate hypersensitivity reaction to penicillin or to cephalosporins.

* Benzylpenicillin sodium or cefotaxime (*or* ceftriaxone)
* *If history of immediate hypersensitivity reaction to penicillin or to cephalosporins,* chloramphenicol
▸ To eliminate nasopharyngeal carriage, ciprofloxacin p. 328, *or* rifampicin p. 342, or ceftriaxone may be used.

Antibacterial therapy for septicaemia in neonates

* *Neonate less than* 72 *hours old*, benzylpenicillin sodium + gentamicin p. 293
▸ If Gram-negative septicaemia suspected, use benzylpenicillin sodium + gentamicin + cefotaxime; stop benzylpenicillin sodium if Gram-negative infection confirmed.
▸ *Suggested duration of treatment* usually 7 days.
* *Neonate more than* 72 *hours old*, flucloxacillin + gentamicin *or* amoxicillin (*or* ampicillin) + cefotaxime
▸ *Suggested duration of treatment* usually 7 days.

Cardiovascular system infections, bacterial

Antibacterial therapy for endocarditis: initial 'blind' therapy

* Flucloxacillin p. 325 (*or* benzylpenicillin sodium p. 318 if symptoms less severe) + gentamicin p. 293
* *If cardiac prostheses present, or if penicillin-allergic, or if meticillin-resistant Staphylococcus aureus suspected,* vancomycin p. 305 + rifampicin p. 342 + gentamicin

Antibacterial therapy for endocarditis caused by staphylococci

* Flucloxacillin
▸ Add rifampicin for at least 2 weeks in prosthetic valve endocarditis
▸ *Suggested duration of treatment* at least 4 weeks (at least 6 weeks for prosthetic valve endocarditis)
* *If penicillin-allergic or if meticillin-resistant Staphylococcus aureus,* vancomycin + rifampicin
▸ *Suggested duration of treatment* at least 4 weeks (at least 6 weeks for prosthetic valve endocarditis)

Antibacterial therapy for native-valve endocarditis caused by fully-sensitive streptococci (e.g. viridans streptococci)

* Benzylpenicillin sodium
▸ *Suggested duration of treatment* 4 weeks
* *Alternative if a large vegetation, intracardial abscess, or infected emboli are absent,* benzylpenicillin sodium + gentamicin
▸ *Suggested duration of treatment* 2 weeks
* *If penicillin-allergic,* vancomycin
▸ *Suggested duration of treatment* 4 weeks

Antibacterial therapy for native-valve endocarditis caused by less-sensitive streptococci

- Benzylpenicillin sodium + gentamicin
- *Suggested duration of treatment* 4–6 weeks (stop gentamicin after 2 weeks for micro-organisms moderately sensitive to penicillin)
- *If aminoglycoside cannot be used and if streptococci moderately sensitive to penicillin*, benzylpenicillin sodium
- *Suggested duration of treatment* 4 weeks
- *If penicillin-allergic or highly penicillin-resistant*, vancomycin (*or* teicoplanin p. 305) + gentamicin
- *Suggested duration of treatment* 4–6 weeks (stop gentamicin after 2 weeks for micro-organisms moderately sensitive to penicillin)

Antibacterial therapy for prosthetic valve endocarditis caused by streptococci

- Benzylpenicillin sodium + gentamicin
- *Suggested duration of treatment* at least 6 weeks (stop gentamicin after 2 weeks if micro-organisms fully sensitive to penicillin)
- *If penicillin-allergic or highly penicillin-resistant*, vancomycin (*or* teicoplanin) + gentamicin
- *Suggested duration of treatment* at least 6 weeks (stop gentamicin after 2 weeks if micro-organisms fully sensitive to penicillin)

Antibacterial therapy for endocarditis caused by enterococci (e.g. *Enterococcus faecalis*)

- Amoxicillin p. 320 (*or* ampicillin p. 321) + gentamicin
- If gentamicin-resistant, substitute gentamicin with streptomycin p. 293
- *Suggested duration of treatment* at least 4 weeks (at least 6 weeks for prosthetic valve endocarditis)
- *If penicillin-allergic or penicillin-resistant*, vancomycin (*or* teicoplanin) + gentamicin
- If gentamicin-resistant, substitute gentamicin with streptomycin
- *Suggested duration of treatment* at least 4 weeks (at least 6 weeks for prosthetic valve endocarditis)

Antibacterial therapy for endocarditis caused by *Haemophilus*, *Actinobacillus*, *Cardiobacterium*, *Eikenella*, and *Kingella* species ('HACEK' micro-organisms)

- Amoxicillin (*or* ampicillin) + gentamicin
- *Suggested duration of treatment* 4 weeks (6 weeks for prosthetic valve endocarditis); stop gentamicin after 2 weeks
- *If amoxicillin-resistant*, ceftriaxone p. 302 + gentamicin
- *Suggested duration of treatment* 4 weeks (6 weeks for prosthetic valve endocarditis); stop gentamicin after 2 weeks

Central nervous system infections, bacterial

Antibacterial therapy for meningitis: initial empirical therapy

- Transfer patient to hospital urgently.
- If *meningococcal disease* (meningitis with non-blanching rash or meningococcal septicaemia) suspected, benzylpenicillin sodium p. 318 should be given before transfer to hospital, so long as this does not delay the transfer. If a patient with suspected bacterial meningitis without non-blanching rash cannot be transferred to hospital urgently, benzylpenicillin sodium should be given before the transfer. Cefotaxime p. 301 may be an alternative in penicillin allergy; chloramphenicol p. 334 may be used if history of immediate hypersensitivity reaction to penicillin or to cephalosporins.
- In hospital, consider adjunctive treatment with dexamethasone p. 410, preferably starting before or with first dose of antibacterial, but no later than 12 hours after starting antibacterial; avoid dexamethasone in septic shock, meningococcal septicaemia, or if immunocompromised, or in meningitis following surgery.

In hospital, if aetiology unknown

- *Neonate and child 1–3 months*, cefotaxime (*or* ceftriaxone p. 302) + amoxicillin p. 320 (*or* ampicillin p. 321)
- Consider adding vancomycin p. 305 if prolonged or multiple use of other antibacterials in the last 3 months, or if travelled, in the last 3 months, to areas outside the UK with highly penicillin- and cephalosporin-resistant pneumococci
- *Suggested duration of treatment* at least 14 days
- *Child 3 months–18 years* cefotaxime (*or* ceftriaxone)
- Consider adding vancomycin if prolonged or multiple use of other antibacterials in the last 3 months, or if travelled, in the last 3 months, to areas outside the UK with highly penicillin- and cephalosporin-resistant pneumococci
- *Suggested duration of treatment* at least 10 days

Antibacterial therapy for meningitis caused by group B streptococcus

- Benzylpenicillin sodium + gentamicin p. 293 *or* cefotaxime (*or* ceftriaxone) alone
- *Suggested duration of treatment* at least 14 days; stop gentamicin after 5 days

Antibacterial therapy for meningitis caused by meningococci

- Benzylpenicillin sodium *or* cefotaxime (*or* ceftriaxone)
- *Suggested duration of treatment* 7 days.
- *If history of immediate hypersensitivity reaction to penicillin or to cephalosporins*, chloramphenicol
- *Suggested duration of treatment* 7 days.

Antibacterial therapy for meningitis caused by pneumococci

- Cefotaxime (*or* ceftriaxone)
- Consider adjunctive treatment with dexamethasone, preferably starting before or with first dose of antibacterial, but no later than 12 hours after starting antibacterial (may reduce penetration of vancomycin into cerebrospinal fluid).
- If micro-organism penicillin-sensitive, replace cefotaxime with benzylpenicillin sodium.
- If micro-organism highly penicillin- and cephalosporin-resistant, add vancomycin and if necessary rifampicin p. 342.
- *Suggested duration of antibacterial treatment* 14 days.

Antibacterial therapy for meningitis caused by *Haemophilus influenzae*

- Cefotaxime (*or* ceftriaxone)
- Consider adjunctive treatment with dexamethasone, preferably starting before or with first dose of antibacterial, but no later than 12 hours after starting antibacterial.
- *Suggested duration of antibacterial treatment* 10 days.

- For *H. influenzae* type b give rifampicin for 4 days before hospital discharge to those under 10 years of age or to those in contact with vulnerable household contacts
- *If history of immediate hypersensitivity reaction to penicillin or to cephalosporins, or if micro-organism resistant to* cefotaxime, chloramphenicol
- Consider adjunctive treatment with dexamethasone, preferably starting before or with first dose of antibacterial, but no later than 12 hours after starting antibacterial.
- *Suggested duration of antibacterial treatment* 10 days.
- For *H. influenzae* type b give rifampicin for 4 days before hospital discharge to those under 10 years of age or to those in contact with vulnerable household contacts

Antibacterial therapy for meningitis caused by Listeria

- Amoxicillin (*or* ampicillin) + gentamicin
- *Suggested duration of treatment* 21 days.
- Consider stopping gentamicin after 7 days
- *If history of immediate hypersensitivity reaction to penicillin*, co-trimoxazole p. 330
- *Suggested duration of treatment* 21 days.

Ear infections, bacterial

Antibacterial therapy for otitis externa

For topical treatments, consider *Otitis externa*, under Ear p. 643.

Consider systemic antibacterial if spreading cellulitis or patient systemically unwell.

- Flucloxacillin p. 325
- *If penicillin-allergic*, clarithromycin p. 309 (*or* azithromycin p. 308 *or* erythromycin p. 310)
- *If pseudomonas suspected*, ciprofloxacin p. 328 (*or an* aminoglycoside)

Antibacterial therapy for otitis media

Many infections caused by viruses. Most uncomplicated cases resolve without antibacterial treatment. In children without systemic features, antibacterial treatment may be started after 72 hours if no improvement. Consider earlier treatment if deterioration, if systemically unwell, if at high risk of serious complications (e.g. in immunosuppression, cystic fibrosis), if mastoiditis present, or in children under 2 years of age with bilateral otitis media.

- Amoxicillin p. 320 (*or* ampicillin p. 321)
- Consider co-amoxiclav p. 323 if no improvement after 48 hours.
- In severe infection, initial parenteral therapy with co-amoxiclav or cefuroxime p. 300.
- *Suggested duration of treatment* 5 days (longer if severely ill).
- *If penicillin-allergic*, clarithromycin (*or* azithromycin *or* erythromycin)
- *Suggested duration of treatment* 5 days (longer if severely ill)

Eye infections, bacterial

Antibacterial therapy for purulent conjunctivitis

- Chloramphenicol eye drops p. 631.

Antibacterial therapy for congenital chlamydial conjuctivitis

- Erythromycin p. 310 (by mouth)
- *Suggested duration of treatment* 14 days

Antibacterial therapy for congenital gonococcal conjunctivitis

- Cefotaxime p. 301 (*or* ceftriaxone p. 302)
- *Suggested duration of treatment* single dose.

Gastro-intestinal system infections, bacterial

Antibacterial therapy for gastro-enteritis

Frequently self-limiting and may not be bacterial.

- Antibacterial not usually indicated.

Antibacterial therapy for campylobacter enteritis

Frequently self-limiting; treat if immunocompromised or if severe infection.

- Clarithromycin p. 309 (*or* azithromycin p. 308 *or* erythromycin p. 310)
- *Alternative*, ciprofloxacin p. 328
- Strains with decreased sensitivity to ciprofloxacin isolated frequently

Antibacterial therapy for salmonella (non-typhoid)

Treat invasive or severe infection. Do not treat less severe infection unless there is a risk of developing invasive infection (e.g. immunocompromised children, those with haemoglobinopathy, or children under 6 months of age).

- Ciprofloxacin *or* cefotaxime p. 301

Antibacterial therapy for shigellosis

Antibacterial not indicated for mild cases.

- Azithromycin *or* ciprofloxacin
- *Alternatives if micro-organism sensitive*, amoxicillin p. 320 *or* trimethoprim p. 338

Antibacterial therapy for typhoid fever

Infections from Middle-East, South Asia, and South-East Asia may be multiple-antibacterial-resistant and sensitivity should be tested.

- Cefotaxime (*or* ceftriaxone p. 302)
- azithromycin may be an alternative in mild or moderate disease caused by multiple-antibacterial-resistant micro-organisms
- *Alternative if micro-organism sensitive*, ciprofloxacin *or* chloramphenicol p. 334

Antibacterial therapy for *Clostridium difficile* infection

- *For first episode of mild to moderate infection*, oral metronidazole p. 313
- *Suggested duration of treatment* 10–14 days
- *For second or subsequent episode of infection, for severe infection, for infection not responding to metronidazole, or in children intolerant of metronidazole*, oral vancomycin p. 305
- *Suggested duration of treatment* 10–14 days
- *For infection not responding to vancomycin, or for life-threatening infection, or in patients with ileus*, oral vancomycin + i/v metronidazole
- *Suggested duration of treatment* 10–14 days

Antibacterial therapy for peritonitis

- A cephalosporin + metronidazole *or* amoxicillin + gentamicin p. 293 + metronidazole *or* piperacillin with tazobactam p. 317 alone

Antibacterial therapy for peritonitis: peritoneal dialysis-associated

- Vancomycin (*or* teicoplanin p. 305) + ceftazidime p. 301 added to dialysis fluid *or* vancomycin added to dialysis fluid + ciprofloxacin by mouth
▸ *Suggested duration of treatment* 14 days or longer

Antibacterial therapy for necrotising enterocolitis in neonates

- Benzylpenicillin sodium p. 318 + gentamicin + metronidazole *or* amoxicillin (*or* ampicillin p. 321) + gentamicin + metronidazole *or* amoxicillin (*or* ampicillin) + cefotaxime + metronidazole

Genital system infections, bacterial

Antibacterial therapy for uncomplicated genital chlamydial infection, non-gonococcal urethritis, and non-specific genital infection

Contact tracing recommended.

- *Child under 12 years*, erythromycin p. 310
▸ *Suggested duration of treatment* 14 days
- *Child 12–18 years*, azithromycin p. 308 as a single dose *or* doxycycline p. 332 for 7 days
- *Alternatively*, erythromycin for 14 days

Antibacterial therapy for gonorrhoea: uncomplicated

Contact tracing recommended. Consider chlamydia co-infection. Choice of antibacterial depends on locality where infection acquired.

- *Child under 12 years*, single-dose of ceftriaxone p. 302
- *Child 12–18 years,* single-dose of cefixime p. 300
▸ *Alternatively, if micro-organism sensitive*, single-dose of ciprofloxacin p. 328
- *Child 12–18 years with pharyngeal infection*, single-dose of ceftriaxone

Antibacterial therapy for pelvic inflammatory disease

Contact tracing recommended.

- *Child 2–12 years*, erythromycin + metronidazole p. 313 + single-dose of i/m ceftriaxone
▸ *Suggested duration of treatment* 14 days (except i/m ceftriaxone)
- *Child 12–18 years*, doxycycline + metronidazole + single-dose of i/m ceftriaxone
▸ If severely ill, seek specialist advice.
▸ *Suggested duration of treatment* 14 days (except i/m ceftriaxone)

Antibacterial therapy for syphilis

Contact tracing recommended.

- *Child under 12 years*, benzylpenicillin sodium *or* procaine benzylpenicillin [unlicensed]
▸ *Suggested duration of treatment* 10 days

Early syphilis (infection of less than 2 years)

- *Child 12–18 years*, benzathine benzylpenicillin [unlicensed]

▸ *Suggested duration of treatment* single-dose (repeat dose after 7 days for females in the third trimester of pregnancy)
- *Alternatively*, doxycycline or erythromycin
▸ *Suggested duration of treatment* 14 days

Late latent syphilis (asymptomatic infection of more than 2 years)

- *Child 12–18 years*, benzathine benzylpenicillin [unlicensed].
▸ *Suggested duration of treatment* once weekly for 2 weeks
- *Alternatively*, doxycycline
▸ *Suggested duration of treatment* 28 days

Asymptomatic contacts of patients with infectious syphilis

- *Child 12–18 years*, doxycycline
▸ *Suggested duration of treatment* 14 days

Antibacterial therapy for neonatal congenital syphilis

- Benzylpenicillin sodium
▸ Also consider treating neonates with suspected congenital syphilis whose mothers were treated inadequately for syphilis, or whose mothers were treated for syphilis in the 4 weeks before delivery, or whose mothers were treated with non-penicillin antibacterials for syphilis.
▸ *Suggested duration of treatment* 10 days.

Musculoskeletal system infections, bacterial

Antibacterial therapy for osteomyelitis

Seek specialist advice if chronic infection or prostheses present.

- Flucloxacillin p. 325
▸ Consider adding fusidic acid p. 336 or rifampicin p. 342 for initial 2 weeks.
▸ *Suggested duration of treatment* 6 weeks for acute infection
- *If penicillin-allergic*, clindamycin p. 307
▸ Consider adding fusidic acid or rifampicin for initial 2 weeks.
▸ *Suggested duration of treatment* 6 weeks for acute infection
- *If meticillin-resistant Staphylococcus aureus suspected*, vancomycin p. 305 (*or* teicoplanin p. 305)
▸ Consider adding fusidic acid or rifampicin for initial 2 weeks.
▸ *Suggested duration of treatment* 6 weeks for acute infection

Antibacterial therapy for septic arthritis

Seek specialist advice if prostheses present.

- Flucloxacillin
▸ *Suggested duration of treatment* 4–6 weeks (longer if infection complicated).
- *If penicillin-allergic*, clindamycin
▸ *Suggested duration of treatment* 4–6 weeks (longer if infection complicated).
- *If meticillin-resistant Staphylococcus aureus suspected*, vancomycin (*or* teicoplanin)
▸ *Suggested duration of treatment* 4–6 weeks (longer if infection complicated).
- *If gonococcal arthritis or Gram-negative infection suspected*, cefotaxime p. 301 (*or* ceftriaxone p. 302)
▸ *Suggested duration of treatment* 4–6 weeks (longer if infection complicated; treat gonococcal infection for 2 weeks).

Nose infections, bacterial

Antibacterial therapy for sinusitis

Antibacterial should usually be used only for persistent symptoms and purulent discharge lasting at least 7 days or if severe symptoms. Also, consider antibacterial for those at high risk of serious complications (e.g. in immunosuppression, cystic fibrosis).

- Amoxicillin p. 320 (*or* ampicillin p. 321) or clarithromycin p. 309 (*or* azithromycin p. 308 *or* erythromycin p. 310)
- ‣ *Suggested duration of treatment* 7 days.
- ‣ Consider oral co-amoxiclav p. 323 if no improvement after 48 hours.
- ‣ In severe infection, initial parenteral therapy with co-amoxiclav or cefuroxime p. 300 may be required.

Oral bacterial infections

Antibacterial drugs

Antibacterial drugs should only be prescribed for the *treatment* of oral infections on the basis of defined need. They may be used in conjunction with (but not as an alternative to) other appropriate measures, such as providing drainage or extracting a tooth.

The 'blind' prescribing of an antibacterial for unexplained pyrexia, cervical lymphadenopathy, or facial swelling can lead to difficulty in establishing the diagnosis. In severe oral infections, a sample should always be taken for bacteriology.

Oral infections which may require antibacterial treatment include acute periapical or periodontal abscess, cellulitis, acutely created oral-antral communication (and acute sinusitis), severe pericoronitis, localised osteitis, acute necrotising ulcerative gingivitis, and destructive forms of chronic periodontal disease. Most of these infections are readily resolved by the early establishment of drainage and removal of the cause (typically an infected necrotic pulp). Antibacterials may be required if treatment has to be delayed, in immunocompromised patients, or in those with conditions such as diabetes. Certain rarer infections including bacterial sialadenitis, osteomyelitis, actinomycosis, and infections involving fascial spaces such as Ludwig's angina, require antibiotics and specialist hospital care.

Antibacterial drugs may also be useful after dental surgery in some cases of spreading infection. Infection may spread to involve local lymph nodes, to fascial spaces (where it can cause airway obstruction), or into the bloodstream (where it can lead to cavernous sinus thrombosis and other serious complications). Extension of an infection can also lead to maxillary sinusitis; osteomyelitis is a complication, which usually arises when host resistance is reduced.

If the oral infection fails to respond to antibacterial treatment within 48 hours the antibacterial should be changed, preferably on the basis of bacteriological investigation. Failure to respond may also suggest an incorrect diagnosis, lack of essential additional measures (such as drainage), poor host resistance, or poor patient compliance.

Combination of a penicillin (or a macrolide) with metronidazole p. 313 may sometimes be helpful for the treatment of severe oral infections or oral infections.

Penicillins

Phenoxymethylpenicillin p. 319 is effective for dentoalveolar abscess.

Broad-spectrum penicillins

Amoxicillin p. 320 is as effective as phenoxymethylpenicillin but is better absorbed; however, it may encourage emergence of resistant organisms.

Like phenoxymethylpenicillin, amoxicillin is ineffective against bacteria that produce beta-lactamases.

Co-amoxiclav p. 323 is active against beta-lactamase-producing bacteria that are resistant to amoxicillin. Co-amoxiclav may be used for severe dental infection with spreading cellulitis or dental infection not responding to first-line antibacterial treatment.

Cephalosporins

The cephalosporins offer little advantage over the penicillins in dental infections, often being less active against anaerobes. Infections due to oral streptococci (often termed viridans streptococci) which become resistant to penicillin are usually also resistant to cephalosporins. This is of importance in the case of patients who have had rheumatic fever and are on long-term penicillin therapy. Cefalexin p. 298 and cefradine p. 299 have been used in the treatment of oral infections.

Tetracyclines

In children over 12 years of age, tetracyclines can be effective against oral anaerobes but the development of resistance (especially by oral streptococci) has reduced their usefulness for the treatment of acute oral infections; they may still have a role in the treatment of destructive (refractory) forms of periodontal disease. Doxycycline p. 332 has a longer duration of action than tetracycline p. 334 or oxytetracycline p. 334 and need only be given once daily; it is reported to be more active against anaerobes than some other tetracyclines.

Doxycycline may have a role in the treatment of recurrent aphthous ulceration, or as an adjunct to gingival scaling and root planing for periodontitis.

Macrolides

The macrolides are an alternative for oral infections in penicillin-allergic patients or where a beta-lactamase producing organism is involved. However, many organisms are now resistant to macrolides or rapidly develop resistance; their use should therefore be limited to short courses.

Clindamycin

Clindamycin p. 307 should not be used routinely for the treatment of oral infections because it may be no more effective than penicillins against anaerobes and there may be cross-resistance with erythromycin p. 310-resistant bacteria. Clindamycin can be used for the treatment of dentoalveolar abscess that has not responded to penicillin or to metronidazole.

Metronidazole and tinidazole

Metronidazole is an alternative to a penicillin for the treatment of many oral infections where the patient is allergic to penicillin or the infection is due to beta-lactamase-producing anaerobes. It is the drug of first choice for the treatment of acute necrotising ulcerative gingivitis (Vincent's infection) and pericoronitis; amoxicillin is a suitable alternative. For these purposes metronidazole for 3 days is sufficient, but the duration of treatment may need to be longer in pericoronitis. Tinidazole p. 315 is licensed for the treatment of acute ulcerative gingivitis.

5

Infection

Respiratory system infections, bacterial

Antibacterial therapy for *Haemophilus influenzae* epiglottitis

- Cefotaxime p. 301 (*or* ceftriaxone p. 302)
- *If history of immediate hypersensitivity reaction to penicillin or to cephalosporins*, chloramphenicol p. 334

Antibacterial therapy for pneumonia: community-acquired

Children under 2 years with mild symptoms of lower respiratory tract infection (particularly those vaccinated with pneumococcal polysaccharide conjugate vaccine (adsorbed) and haemophilus type b conjugate vaccine) are unlikely to have pneumonia; antibacterial treatment may be considered if symptoms persist.

- *Neonate*, benzylpenicillin sodium p. 318 + gentamicin p. 293
- *Child* 1 *month*–18 *years*, amoxicillin p. 320 (*or* ampicillin p. 321) by mouth
- Pneumococci with decreased penicillin sensitivity have been isolated in the UK, but are not common.
- If no response to treatment, add clarithromycin p. 309 (*or* azithromycin p. 308 *or* erythromycin p. 310)
- If staphylococci suspected (e.g. in influenza or measles), give by mouth amoxicillin + flucloxacillin p. 325 *or* co-amoxiclav p. 323 alone
- If septicaemia, complicated pneumonia, or if oral administration not possible, initiate treatment with i/v amoxicillin *or* i/v co-amoxiclav *or* i/v cefuroxime p. 300 *or* i/v cefotaxime (*or* ceftriaxone)
- *Suggested duration of treatment* 7 days (may extend treatment to 14 days in some cases e.g. if staphylococci suspected)
- *Child* 1 *month*–18 *years, if penicillin-allergic*, clarithromycin (*or* azithromycin *or* erythromycin)
- *Suggested duration of treatment* 7 days (may extend treatment to 14 days in some cases e.g. if staphylococci suspected)

Antibacterial therapy for pneumonia possibly caused by atypical pathogens

- Clarithromycin (*or* azithromycin *or* erythromycin)
- *Suggested duration of treatment* 10–14 days
- *Alternative for chlamydial or mycoplasma infections in children over* 12 *years*, doxycycline p. 332
- *Suggested duration of treatment* 10–14 days

Antibacterial therapy for pneumonia: hospital-acquired

- *Early-onset infection* (less than 5 days after admission to hospital), treat as for severe community-acquired pneumonia of unknown aetiology; if life-threatening infection, or if recent history of antibacterial treatment, or if resistant organisms suspected, treat as for late-onset hospital-acquired pneumonia
- *Late-onset infection* (more than 5 days after admission to hospital), an antipseudomonal penicillin (e.g. piperacillin with tazobactam p. 317) *or* another antipseudomonal beta-lactam
- If meticillin-resistant *Staphylococcus aureus* suspected, add vancomycin p. 305.
- If severe illness caused by *Pseudomonas aeruginosa*, add an aminoglycoside.
- *Suggested duration of treatment* 7 days (longer if *Pseudomonas aeruginosa* confirmed)

Antibacterial therapy for staphylococcal lung infection in cystic fibrosis

- Flucloxacillin
- If child already taking flucloxacillin prophylaxis or if severe exacerbation, add fusidic acid p. 336 or rifampicin p. 342; use flucloxacillin at treatment dose
- *If penicillin-allergic*, clarithromycin (*or* azithromycin *or* erythromycin) or clindamycin p. 307
- Use clarithromycin only if micro-organism sensitive

Antibacterial therapy for *Haemophilus influenzae* lung infection in cystic fibrosis

- Amoxicillin *or* a broad-spectrum cephalosporin
- In severe exacerbation use a third-generation cephalosporin (e.g. cefotaxime)

Antibacterial therapy for pseudomonal lung infection in cystic fibrosis

- Ciprofloxacin p. 328 + *nebulised* colistimethate sodium p. 326
- *For severe exacerbation*, an antipseudomonal beta-lactam antibacterial + parenteral tobramycin p. 294

Skin infections, bacterial

Antibacterial therapy for impetigo: small areas of skin infected

Seek local microbiology advice before using topical treatment in hospital.

- Topical fusidic acid p. 336
- *Suggested duration of treatment* 7 days is usually adequate (max. 10 days).
- *Alternatively, if meticillin-resistant Staphylococcus aureus*, topical mupirocin p. 650
- *Suggested duration of treatment* 7 days is usually adequate (max. 10 days).

Impetigo: widespread infection

- Oral flucloxacillin p. 325
- If streptococci suspected in severe infection, add phenoxymethylpenicillin p. 319
- *Suggested duration of treatment* 7 days.
- *If penicillin-allergic*, oral clarithromycin p. 309 (*or* azithromycin p. 308 *or* erythromycin p. 310)
- *Suggested duration of treatment* 7 days.

Antibacterial therapy for erysipelas

- Phenoxymethylpenicillin *or* benzylpenicillin sodium p. 318
- If severe infection, replace phenoxymethylpenicillin or benzylpenicillin sodium with high-dose flucloxacillin
- *Suggested duration of treatment* at least 7 days
- *If penicillin-allergic*, clindamycin p. 307 or clarithromycin (*or* azithromycin *or* erythromycin)
- *Suggested duration of treatment* at least 7 days.

Antibacterial therapy for cellulitis

- Flucloxacillin (high dose)
- If streptococcal infection confirmed, replace flucloxacillin with phenoxymethylpenicillin or benzylpenicillin sodium
- If Gram-negative bacteria or anaerobes suspected (e.g. facial infection, orbital infection, or infection caused by animal or human bites), use broad-spectrum antibacterials; if periumbilical cellulitis, use flucloxacillin + gentamicin p. 293

- *If penicillin-allergic*, clindamycin *or* clarithromycin (*or* azithromycin *or* erythromycin)
- ▸ If Gram-negative bacteria suspected, use broad-spectrum antibacterials.

Antibacterial therapy for staphylococcal scalded skin syndrome

- Flucloxacillin
- ▸ *Suggested duration of treatment* 7–10 days.
- *If penicillin-allergic*, clarithromycin (*or* azithromycin *or* erythromycin)
- ▸ *Suggested duration of treatment* 7–10 days.

Antibacterial therapy for animal and human bites

Cleanse wound thoroughly. For tetanus-prone wound, give human tetanus immunoglobulin p. 729 (with a tetanus-containing vaccine if necessary, according to immunisation history and risk of infection). Consider rabies prophylaxis for bites from animals in endemic countries; assess risk of blood-borne viruses (including HIV, hepatitis B and C) and give appropriate prophylaxis to prevent viral spread.

- Co-amoxiclav p. 323
- *If penicillin-allergic*, clindamycin

Antibacterial therapy for surgical wound infection

- Flucloxacillin *or* co-amoxiclav

Antibacterial therapy for paronychia or 'septic spots' in neonate

- Flucloxacillin
- ▸ If systemically unwell, add an aminoglycoside.

ANTIBACTERIALS ⟩ AMINOGLYCOSIDES

Aminoglycosides

Overview

These include amikacin p. 292, gentamicin p. 293, neomycin sulfate p. 645, streptomycin p. 293, and tobramycin p. 294. All are bactericidal and active against some Gram-positive and many Gram-negative organisms. Amikacin, gentamicin, and tobramycin are also active against *Pseudomonas aeruginosa*; streptomycin is active against *Mycobacterium tuberculosis* and is now almost entirely reserved for tuberculosis.

The aminoglycosides are not absorbed from the gut (although there is a risk of absorption in inflammatory bowel disease and liver failure) and must therefore be given by injection for systemic infections.

Gentamicin is the aminoglycoside of choice in the UK and is used widely for the treatment of serious infections. It has a broad spectrum but is inactive against anaerobes and has poor activity against haemolytic streptococci and pneumococci. When used for the 'blind' therapy of undiagnosed serious infections it is usually given in conjunction with a penicillin or metronidazole p. 313 (or both). Gentamicin is used together with another antibiotic for the treatment of endocarditis. Streptomycin may be used as an alternative in gentamicin-resistant enterococcal endocarditis.

Loading and maintenance doses of gentamicin may be calculated on the basis of the patient's weight and renal function (e.g. using a nomogram); adjustments are then made according to serum-gentamicin concentrations. High doses are occasionally indicated for serious infections, especially in the neonate, in the patient with cystic fibrosis, or in the immunocompromised patient. Whenever possible treatment should not exceed 7 days.

Amikacin is more stable than gentamicin to enzyme inactivation. Amikacin is used in the treatment of serious infections caused by gentamicin-resistant Gram-negative bacilli.

Tobramycin has similar activity to gentamicin. It is slightly more active against *Ps. aeruginosa* but shows less activity against certain other Gram-negative bacteria..

Neomycin sulfate is too toxic for parenteral administration and can only be used for infections of the skin or mucous membranes or to reduce the bacterial population of the colon prior to bowel surgery or in hepatic failure. Oral administration may lead to malabsorption. Small amounts of neomycin sulfate may be absorbed from the gut in patients with hepatic failure and, as these patients may also be uraemic, cumulation may occur with resultant ototoxicity.

Cystic fibrosis

A higher dose of parenteral aminoglycoside is often required in children with cystic fibrosis because renal clearance of the aminoglycoside is increased. Aminoglycosides have a role in the treatment of pseudomonal lung infections in cystic fibrosis. Tobramycin can be administered by nebuliser or by inhalation of powder on a cyclical basis (28 days of tobramycin followed by a 28-day tobramycin-free interval) for the treatment of chronic pulmonary *Ps. aeruginosa* infection in cystic fibrosis; however, resistance may develop and some patients do not respond to treatment.

Once daily dosage

Once daily administration of aminoglycosides is more convenient, provides adequate serum concentrations, and has largely superseded *multiple- daily dose regimens* (given in 2–3 divided doses during the 24 hours). Local guidelines on dosage and serum concentrations should be consulted. A once-daily, high-dose regimen of an aminoglycoside should be avoided in children with endocarditis or burns of more than 20% of the total body surface area. There is insufficient evidence to recommend a once daily, high-dose regimen of an aminoglycoside in pregnancy.

Serum concentrations

Serum concentration monitoring avoids both excessive and subtherapeutic concentrations thus preventing toxicity and ensuring efficacy. Serum-aminoglycoside concentrations should be monitored in patients receiving parenteral aminoglycosides and **must** be determined in obesity, and in cystic fibrois, or if high doses are being given, or if there is renal impairment.

Neonates

▸ In neonates As aminoglycosides are eliminated principally via the kidney, neonatal treatment must reflect the changes in glomerular filtration that occur with increasing gestational and postnatal age. The *extended interval dose regimen* is used in neonates, and serum-aminoglycoside concentrations **must** be measured. In patients on single daily dose regimens it may become necessary to prolong the dose interval to more than 24 hours if the trough concentration is high.

Aminoglycosides (by injection)

- **CONTRA-INDICATIONS** Myasthenia gravis (aminoglycosides may impair neuromuscular transmission)
- **CAUTIONS** Care must be taken with dosage (the main side-effects of the aminoglycosides are dose-related) · conditions characterised by muscular weakness (aminoglycosides may impair neuromuscular transmission) · if possible, dehydration should be corrected before starting an aminoglycoside · whenever possible, parenteral treatment should not exceed 7 days

- **INTERACTIONS** → Appendix 1 (aminoglycosides). If possible, aminoglycosides should not be given with potentially ototoxic drugs (e.g. cisplatin). Administration of an aminoglycoside and of an ototoxic diuretic (e.g. furosemide) should be separated by as long a period as practicable.

- **SIDE-EFFECTS**
- **Rare** Antibiotic-associated colitis · electrolyte disturbances · hypocalcaemia · hypokalaemia · hypomagnesaemia on prolonged therapy · nausea · peripheral neuropathy · stomatitis · vomiting
- **Very rare** Blood disorders · CNS effects · convulsions · encephalopathy · headache
- **Frequency not known** Auditory damage · impaired neuromuscular transmission · irreversible ototoxicity · nephrotoxicity · transient myasthenic syndrome in patients with normal neuromuscular function with large doses given during surgery · vestibular damage

SIDE-EFFECTS, FURTHER INFORMATION
- Nephrotoxicity Occurs most commonly in children with renal failure.

- **PREGNANCY** There is a risk of auditory or vestibular nerve damage in the infant when aminoglycosides are used in the second and third trimesters of pregnancy. The risk is greatest with streptomycin. The risk is probably very small with gentamicin and tobramycin, but their use should be avoided unless essential.
    If given during pregnancy, serum-aminoglycoside concentration monitoring is essential.

- **RENAL IMPAIRMENT** If there is impairment of renal function, the interval between doses must be increased; if the renal impairment is severe, the dose itself should be reduced as well. Excretion of aminoglycosides is principally via the kidney and accumulation occurs in renal impairment.
    A once-daily, high-dose regimen of an aminoglycoside should be avoided in children over 1 month of age with a creatinine clearance less than 20 mL/minute/1.73 m^2.
    Ototoxicity and nephrotoxicity occur commonly in patients with renal failure. Serum-aminoglycoside concentrations **must** be monitored in patients with renal impairment; earlier and more frequent measurement of aminoglycoside concentration may be required.

- **MONITORING REQUIREMENTS**
- Serum concentrations Serum concentration monitoring avoids both excessive and subtherapeutic concentrations thus preventing toxicity and ensuring efficacy. Serum-aminoglycoside concentrations should be measured in all patients receiving parenteral aminoglycosides and **must** be determined in obesity, if high doses are being given and in cystic fibrosis.
- In neonates Serum aminoglycoside concentrations **must** be determined in neonates.
    In children with normal renal function, aminoglycoside concentrations should be measured after 3 or 4 doses of a multiple daily dose regimen.
    Blood samples should be taken just before the next dose is administered ('trough' concentration). If the pre-dose ('trough') concentration is high, the interval between doses must be increased. For multiple daily dose regimens, blood samples should also be taken approximately 1 hour after intramuscular or intravenous administration ('peak' concentration). If the post-dose ('peak') concentration is high, the dose must be decreased.
- Renal function should be assessed before starting an aminoglycoside and during treatment.
- Auditory and vestibular function should also be monitored during treatment.

⌐ 291

Amikacin

- **INDICATIONS AND DOSE**

Serious Gram-negative infections resistant to gentamicin (multiple daily dose regimen)
- BY SLOW INTRAVENOUS INJECTION
- Child 1 month–11 years: 7.5 mg/kg every 12 hours, to be administered over 3–5 minutes
- Child 12–17 years: 7.5 mg/kg every 12 hours; increased to 7.5 mg/kg every 8 hours (max. per dose 500 mg every 8 hours) for up to 10 days, higher dose to be used in severe infection, to be administered over 3–5 minutes; maximum 15 g per course

Serious Gram-negative infections resistant to gentamicin (once daily regimen)
- BY INTRAVENOUS INFUSION, OR BY INTRAVENOUS INJECTION
- Child: Initially 15 mg/kg adjusted according to plasma-concentration monitoring, not to be used for endocarditis or meningitis, dose to be adjusted according to serum-amikacin concentration, intravenous injection to be administered over 3–5 minutes

Neonatal sepsis (extended interval dose regimen)
- BY SLOW INTRAVENOUS INJECTION, OR BY INTRAVENOUS INFUSION
- Neonate: 15 mg/kg every 24 hours, intravenous injection to be administered over 3–5 minutes.

Neonatal sepsis (multiple daily dose regimen)
- BY INTRAMUSCULAR INJECTION, OR BY SLOW INTRAVENOUS INJECTION, OR BY INTRAVENOUS INFUSION
- Neonate: Loading dose 10 mg/kg, then 7.5 mg/kg every 12 hours, intravenous injection to be administered over 3–5 minutes.

Pseudomonal lung infection in cystic fibrosis
- BY SLOW INTRAVENOUS INJECTION, OR BY INTRAVENOUS INFUSION
- Child: 10 mg/kg every 8 hours (max. per dose 500 mg every 8 hours), intravenous injection to be administered over 3–5 minutes

DOSES AT EXTREMES OF BODY-WEIGHT
To avoid excessive dosage in obese patients, use ideal weight for height to calculate dose and monitor serum-amikacin concentration closely

- **UNLICENSED USE** Dose for cystic fibrosis not licensed.
- **SIDE-EFFECTS**
- **Uncommon** Rash
- **MONITORING REQUIREMENTS**
- *Multiple daily dose regimen*: one-hour ('peak') serum concentration should not exceed 30 mg/litre; pre-dose ('trough') concentration should be less than 10 mg/litre.
- With intravenous use *Once daily dose regimen*: pre-dose ('trough') concentration should be less than 5 mg/litre.
- **DIRECTIONS FOR ADMINISTRATION** For *intravenous infusion*, dilute with Glucose 5% or Sodium Chloride 0.9%; give over 30–60 minutes.
- **PRESCRIBING AND DISPENSING INFORMATION** Local guidelines may vary in the dosing advice provided.

- **MEDICINAL FORMS**
There can be variation in the licensing of different medicines containing the same drug.
Solution for injection
- Amikacin (Non-proprietary)
    Amikacin (as Amikacin sulfate) 250 mg per 1 ml Amikacin 500mg/2ml solution for injection vials | 5 vial PoM £60.00
- Amikin (Bristol-Myers Squibb Pharmaceuticals Ltd)
    Amikacin (as Amikacin sulfate) 50 mg per 1 ml Amikin 100mg/2ml solution for injection vials | 5 vial PoM £10.33

Gentamicin

▶ 291

- **INDICATIONS AND DOSE**

Septicaemia | Meningitis and other CNS infections | Biliary-tract infection | Acute pyelonephritis | Endocarditis | Pneumonia in hospital patients | Adjunct in listerial meningitis
▶ BY INTRAVENOUS INFUSION
- Child: Initially 7 mg/kg, to be given in a once daily regimen (not suitable for endocarditis or meningitis), subsequent doses adjusted according to serum-gentamicin concentration
▶ BY INTRAMUSCULAR INJECTION, OR BY SLOW INTRAVENOUS INJECTION
- Child 1 month–11 years: 2.5 mg/kg every 8 hours, to be given in a multiple daily dose regimen, intravenous injection to be administered over at least 3 minutes
- Child 12–17 years: 2 mg/kg every 8 hours, to be given in a multiple daily dose regimen, intravenous injection to be administered over at least 3 minutes

Neonatal sepsis
▶ BY SLOW INTRAVENOUS INJECTION, OR BY INTRAVENOUS INFUSION
- Neonate up to 7 days: 5 mg/kg every 36 hours, to be given in an extended interval dose regimen.

- Neonate 7 days to 28 days: 5 mg/kg every 24 hours, to be given in an extended interval dose regimen.

Pseudomonal lung infection in cystic fibrosis
▶ BY SLOW INTRAVENOUS INJECTION, OR BY INTRAVENOUS INFUSION
- Child: 3 mg/kg every 8 hours, to be given in a multiple daily dose regimen, intravenous injection to be administered over at least 3 minutes

Bacterial ventriculitis and CNS infection (supplement to systemic therapy) (administered on expert advice)
▶ BY INTRATHECAL INJECTION, OR BY INTRAVENTRICULAR INJECTION
- Neonate: (consult local protocol).
- Child: Initially 1 mg daily, then increased if necessary to 5 mg daily, seek specialist advice

DOSES AT EXTREMES OF BODY-WEIGHT
To avoid excessive dosage in obese patients, use ideal weight for height to calculate dose and monitor serum-gentamicin concentration closely.

- **SIDE-EFFECTS**
▶ **Uncommon** Rash
- **MONITORING REQUIREMENTS**
▶ With intravenous use in neonates Extended interval dose regimen in neonates: pre-dose ('trough') concentration should be less than 2 mg/litre (less than 1 mg/litre if more than 3 doses administered); consider monitoring one hour ('peak') concentration in neonates with poor response to treatment, with oedema, with Gram-negative infection, or with birth-weight greater than 4.5 kg (consider increasing dose if 'peak' concentration less than 8 mg/litre in severe sepsis).
▶ With intravenous use Once daily dose regimen: pre-dose ('trough') concentration should be less than 1 mg/litre.
▶ With intramuscular use or intravenous use Multiple daily dose regimen: one hour ('peak') serum concentration should be 5–10 mg/litre; pre-dose ('trough') concentration should be less than 2 mg/litre.
Multiple daily dose regimen for endocarditis: one hour ('peak') serum concentration should be 3–5 mg/litre; pre-dose ('trough') concentration should be less than 1 mg/litre. Serum-gentamicin concentration should be determined twice each week (more often in renal impairment).

Multiple daily dose regimen for cystic fibrosis: one hour ('peak') serum concentration should be 8–12 mg/litre; pre-dose ('trough') concentration should be less than 2 mg/litre.
▶ With intrathecal use or intraventricular use Intrathecal/intraventricular injection: cerebrospinal fluid concentration should not exceed 10 mg/litre.
- **DIRECTIONS FOR ADMINISTRATION**
▶ With intrathecal use or intraventricular use For *intrathecal* or *intraventricular* injection, use preservative-free intrathecal preparations only.
▶ With intravenous use For *intravenous infusion*, dilute in Glucose 5% or Sodium Chloride 0.9%; give over 30 minutes.
- **PRESCRIBING AND DISPENSING INFORMATION** Local guidelines may vary in the dosing advice provided.
▶ With intrathecal use Only preservative-free intrathecal preparation should be used.

- **MEDICINAL FORMS**
There can be variation in the licensing of different medicines containing the same drug.
Solution for injection
▶ **Gentamicin (Non-proprietary)**
  Gentamicin (as Gentamicin sulfate) 5 mg per 1 ml Gentamicin Intrathecal 5mg/1ml solution for injection ampoules | 5 ampoule PoM £22.50 (Hospital only)
  Gentamicin (as Gentamicin sulfate) 10 mg per 1 ml Gentamicin 20mg/2ml solution for injection ampoules | 5 ampoule PoM £11.25 Gentamicin Paediatric 20mg/2ml solution for injection vials | 5 vial PoM £11.25
  Gentamicin (as Gentamicin sulfate) 40 mg per 1 ml Gentamicin 80mg/2ml solution for injection vials | 5 vial PoM £20.00 Gentamicin 80mg/2ml solution for injection ampoules | 5 ampoule PoM £6.88 | 10 ampoule PoM £10.00
▶ **Cidomycin (Sanofi)**
  Gentamicin (as Gentamicin sulfate) 40 mg per 1 ml Cidomycin Adult Injectable 80mg/2ml solution for injection vials | 5 vial PoM £6.88
  Cidomycin Adult Injectable 80mg/2ml solution for injection ampoules | 5 ampoule PoM £6.88
Infusion
▶ **Gentamicin (Non-proprietary)**
  Gentamicin (as Gentamicin sulfate) 1 mg per 1 ml Gentamicin 80mg/80ml infusion bags | 20 bag PoM £39.00
  Gentamicin (as Gentamicin sulfate) 3 mg per 1 ml Gentamicin 240mg/80ml infusion bags | 20 bag PoM £119.00 Gentamicin 360mg/120ml infusion bags | 20 bag PoM £169.00

▶ 291

Streptomycin

- **INDICATIONS AND DOSE**

Tuberculosis, resistant to other treatment, in combination with other drugs
▶ BY DEEP INTRAMUSCULAR INJECTION
- Child: 15 mg/kg once daily (max. per dose 1 g)

Adjunct to doxycycline in brucellosis (administered on expert advice)
▶ BY DEEP INTRAMUSCULAR INJECTION
- Child: 5–10 mg/kg every 6 hours, total daily dose may alternatively be given in 2–3 divided doses

- **UNLICENSED USE** Not licensed for use in children.

IMPORTANT SAFETY INFORMATION
Side-effects increase after a cumulative dose of 100 g, which should only be exceeded in exceptional circumstances.

- **SIDE-EFFECTS**
▶ **Common or very common** Rash
▶ **Frequency not known** Hypersensitivity reactions · paraesthesia of mouth
- **RENAL IMPAIRMENT** Should preferably be avoided. If essential, use with great care and consider dose reduction.

- MONITORING REQUIREMENTS
► One-hour ('peak') concentration should be 15–40 mg/litre; pre-dose ('trough') concentration should be less than 5 mg/litre (less than 1 mg/litre in renal impairment).

- MEDICINAL FORMS
There can be variation in the licensing of different medicines containing the same drug. Forms available from special-order manufacturers include: powder for solution for injection

F 291

Tobramycin

- INDICATIONS AND DOSE

Chronic *Pseudomonas aeruginosa* infection in patients with cystic fibrosis

► BY INHALATION OF NEBULISED SOLUTION

► Child 6–17 years: 300 mg every 12 hours for 28 days, subsequent courses repeated after 28-day interval without tobramycin nebuliser solution

► BY INHALATION OF POWDER

► Child 6–17 years: 112 mg every 12 hours for 28 days, subsequent courses repeated after 28-day interval without tobramycin inhalation powder

Pseudomonal lung infection in cystic fibrosis

► BY SLOW INTRAVENOUS INJECTION

► Child: 8–10 mg/kg daily in 3 divided doses, to be given as a multiple daily dose regimen over 3–5 minutes

► BY INTRAVENOUS INFUSION

► Child: Initially 10 mg/kg once daily (max. per dose 660 mg), to be given over 30 minutes, subsequent doses adjusted according to serum-tobramycin concentration

Septicaemia | Meningitis and other CNS infections | Biliary-tract infection | Acute pyelonephritis | Pneumonia in hospital patients

► BY SLOW INTRAVENOUS INJECTION

► Child 1 month–11 years: 2–2.5 mg/kg every 8 hours, to be given as a multiple daily dose regimen over 3–5 minutes

► Child 12–17 years: 1 mg/kg every 8 hours, to be given as a multiple daily dose regimen over 3–5 minutes; increased if necessary up to 5 mg/kg daily in 3–4 divided doses, to be given in severe infections as a multiple daily dose regimen over 3–5 minutes, dose to be reduced back to 3 mg/kg as soon as clinically indicated

► BY INTRAVENOUS INFUSION

► Child: Initially 7 mg/kg, to be given as a once daily dose regimen, subsequent doses adjusted according to serum-tobramycin concentration

Neonatal sepsis

► BY INTRAVENOUS INJECTION, OR BY INTRAVENOUS INFUSION

► Neonate up to 32 weeks corrected gestational age: 4–5 mg/kg every 36 hours, to be given as an extended interval dose regimen, intravenous injection to be given over 3–5 minutes.

► Neonate 32 weeks corrected gestational age and above: 4–5 mg/kg every 24 hours, to be given as an extended interval dose regimen, intravenous injection to be given over 3–5 minutes.

► BY SLOW INTRAVENOUS INJECTION, OR BY INTRAVENOUS INFUSION

► Neonate up to 7 days: 2 mg/kg every 12 hours, to be given as a multiple daily dose regimen, intravenous injection to be given over 3–5 minutes.

► Neonate 7 days to 28 days: 2–2.5 mg/kg every 8 hours, to be given as a multiple daily dose regimen, intravenous injection to be given over 3–5 minutes.

- DOSES AT EXTREMES OF BODY-WEIGHT
► With intravenous use To avoid excessive dosage in obese patients, use ideal weight for height to calculate parenteral dose and monitor serum-tobramycin concentration closely.

- CAUTIONS
► When used by inhalation Severe haemoptysis—risk of further haemorrhage

- SIDE-EFFECTS
► **Uncommon**
► With intravenous use Rash
► **Frequency not known**
► When used by inhalation Bronchospasm · cough (more frequent by inhalation of powder) · dysphonia · epistaxis · haemoptysis · laryngitis · mouth ulcers · pharyngitis · salivary hypersecretion · taste disturbances

- MONITORING REQUIREMENTS
► With intravenous use in neonates *Extended interval dose regimen in neonates*: pre-dose ('trough') concentration should be less than 2 mg/litre.
► With intravenous use *Once daily dose regimen*: pre-dose ('trough') concentration should be less than 1 mg/litre. *Multiple daily dose regimen*: one-hour ('peak') serum concentration should not exceed 10 mg/litre (8–12 mg/litre in cystic fibrosis); pre-dose ('trough') concentration should be less than 2 mg/litre.
► When used by inhalation Measure lung function before and after initial dose of tobramycin and monitor for bronchospasm; if bronchospasm occurs in a patient not using a bronchodilator, repeat test using bronchodilator. Monitor renal function before treatment and then annually.

- DIRECTIONS FOR ADMINISTRATION
► With intravenous use For *intravenous infusion*, dilute with Glucose 5% or Sodium Chloride 0.9%; give over 20–60 minutes.
► When used by inhalation Other inhaled drugs should be administered before tobramycin.

- PRESCRIBING AND DISPENSING INFORMATION
► With intravenous use or when used by inhalation Local guidelines may vary in dosing advice provided.

- PATIENT AND CARER ADVICE
► When used by inhalation Patient counselling is advised for Tobramycin dry powder for inhalation (administration).

- NATIONAL FUNDING/ACCESS DECISIONS
► **NICE technology appraisals (TAs)**
► **Tobramycin by dry powder inhalation for pseudomonal lung infection in cystic fibrosis (March 2013) NICE TA276**
► When used by inhalation Tobramycin dry powder for inhalation is recommended for chronic pulmonary infection caused by *Pseudomonas aeruginosa* in patients with cystic fibrosis only if there is an inadequate response to colistimethate sodium, or if colistimethate sodium cannot be used because of contra-indications or intolerance. The manufacturer must provide tobramycin dry powder for inhalation at the discount agreed as part of the patient access scheme to primary, secondary and tertiary care in the NHS. Patients currently receiving tobramycin dry powder for inhalation can continue treatment until they and their clinician consider it appropriate to stop.
www.nice.org.uk/TA276

- MEDICINAL FORMS
There can be variation in the licensing of different medicines containing the same drug. Forms available from special-order manufacturers include: oral solution

Solution for injection
► Tobramycin (Non-proprietary)
Tobramycin (as Tobramycin sulfate) 40 mg per 1 ml Tobramycin 40mg/1ml solution for injection vials | 10 vial PoM £37.00 | 10 vial PoM £37.00 (Hospital only)

Tobramycin 80mg/2ml solution for injection vials | 5 vial PoM £20.80 | 10 vial PoM £37.72 | 10 vial PoM £47.00 (Hospital only) Tobramycin 240mg/6ml solution for injection vials | 1 vial PoM £19.20
‣ **Nebcin** (Flynn Pharma Ltd)
Tobramycin (as Tobramycin sulfate) 40 mg per 1 ml Nebcin 80mg/2ml solution for injection vials | 1 vial PoM £5.37

Inhalation powder
‣ **Tobi Podhaler** (Novartis Pharmaceuticals UK Ltd)
Tobramycin 28 mg Tobi Podhaler 28mg inhalation powder capsules with device | 56 capsule PoM £447.50 | 224 capsule PoM £1,790.00

Nebuliser liquid
‣ **Bramitob** (Chiesi Ltd)
Tobramycin 75 mg per 1 ml Bramitob 300mg/4ml nebuliser solution 4ml ampoules | 56 ampoule PoM £1,187.00
‣ **TOBI** (Novartis Pharmaceuticals UK Ltd)
Tobramycin 60 mg per 1 ml Tobi 300mg/5ml nebuliser solution 5ml ampoules | 56 ampoule PoM £1,305.92 DT price = £1,305.92
‣ **Tymbrineb** (Teva UK Ltd)
Tobramycin 60 mg per 1 ml Tymbrineb 300mg/5ml nebuliser solution 5ml ampoules | 56 ampoule PoM £1,127.84 DT price = £1,305.92

ANTIBACTERIALS > CARBAPENEMS

Carbapenems

Overview
The carbapenems are beta-lactam antibacterials with a broad-spectrum of activity which includes many Gram-positive and Gram-negative bacteria, and anaerobes; **imipenem** (imipenem with cilastatin below) and meropenem p. 296 have good activity against *Pseudomonas aeruginosa*. The carbapenems are not active against meticillin-resistant *Staphylococcus aureus* and *Enterococcus faecium*.

Imipenem (imipenem with cilastatin) and meropenem are used for the treatment of severe hospital-acquired infections and polymicrobial infections caused by multiple-antibacterial resistant organisms (including septicaemia, hospital-acquired pneumonia, intra-abdominal infections, skin and soft-tissue infections, and complicated urinary-tract infections).

Ertapenem below is licensed for treating abdominal and gynaecological infections and for community-acquired pneumonia, but it is not active against atypical respiratory pathogens and it has limited activity against penicillin-resistant pneumococci. Unlike the other carbapenems, ertapenem is not active against *Pseudomonas* or against *Acinetobacter spp*.

Imipenem is partially inactivated in the kidney by enzymatic activity and is therefore administered in combination with **cilastatin** (imipenem with cilastatin), a specific enzyme inhibitor, which blocks its renal metabolism. Meropenem and ertapenem are stable to the renal enzyme which inactivates imipenem and therefore can be given without cilastatin.

Side-effects of imipenem with cilastatin are similar to those of other beta-lactam antibiotics. Meropenem has less seizure-inducing potential and can be used to treat central nervous system infection.

Ertapenem

● **INDICATIONS AND DOSE**
Abdominal infections | Acute gynaecological infections | Community-acquired pneumonia
‣ BY INTRAVENOUS INFUSION
▸ **Child 3 months–12 years:** 15 mg/kg every 12 hours; maximum 1 g per day
▸ **Child 13–17 years:** 1 g once daily

Diabetic foot infections of the skin and soft-tissue
‣ BY INTRAVENOUS INFUSION
▸ **Child 13–17 years:** 1 g once daily

● **CAUTIONS** CNS disorders—risk of seizures
● **INTERACTIONS** → Appendix 1 (ertapenem).
● **SIDE-EFFECTS**
▸ **Common or very common** Diarrhoea · headache · injection-site reactions · nausea · pruritus · raised platelet count · rash (also reported with eosinophilia and systemic symptoms) · vomiting
▸ **Uncommon** Abdominal pain · anorexia · antibiotic-associated colitis · asthenia · bradycardia · chest pain · confusion · constipation · dizziness · dry mouth · dyspepsia · dyspnoea · hypotension · melaena · oedema · petechiae · pharyngeal discomfort · raised glucose · seizures · sleep disturbances · taste disturbances
▸ **Rare** Agitation · anxiety · arrhythmia · blood disorders · cholecystitis · cough · depression · dysphagia · electrolyte disturbances · haemorrhage · hypoglycaemia · increase in blood pressure · jaundice · liver disorder · muscle cramp · nasal congestion · neutropenia · pelvic peritonitis · renal impairment · scleral disorder · syncope · thrombocytopenia · tremor · wheezing
▸ **Frequency not known** Dyskinesia · hallucinations · muscular weakness

● **ALLERGY AND CROSS-SENSITIVITY** Avoid if history of **immediate hypersensitivity** reaction to beta-lactam antibacterials.
Use with caution in patients with sensitivity to beta-lactam antibacterials.
● **PREGNANCY** Manufacturer advises avoid unless potential benefit outweighs risk.
● **BREAST FEEDING** Present in milk—manufacturer advises avoid.
● **RENAL IMPAIRMENT** Use with caution (risk of seizures); avoid if estimated glomerular filtration rate less than 30 mL/minute/1.73 m^2.
● **DIRECTIONS FOR ADMINISTRATION** For *intravenous infusion* (*Invanz*®), give intermittently *in* Sodium chloride 0.9%. Reconstitute 1 g with 10 mL Water for injections *or* Sodium chloride 0.9%; dilute requisite dose in infusion fluid to a final concentration not exceeding 20 mg/mL; give over 30 minutes; incompatible with glucose solutions.

● **MEDICINAL FORMS**
There can be variation in the licensing of different medicines containing the same drug.
Powder for solution for infusion
ELECTROLYTES: May contain Sodium
‣ **Invanz** (Merck Sharp & Dohme Ltd)
Ertapenem (as Ertapenem sodium) 1 gram Invanz 1g powder for solution for infusion vials | 1 vial PoM £31.65

Imipenem with cilastatin

● **INDICATIONS AND DOSE**
Aerobic and anaerobic Gram-positive and Gram-negative infections (not indicated for CNS infections) | Hospital-acquired septicaemia
‣ BY INTRAVENOUS INFUSION
▸ **Neonate up to 7 days:** 20 mg/kg every 12 hours.
▸ **Neonate 7 days to 20 days:** 20 mg/kg every 8 hours.
▸ **Neonate 21 days to 28 days:** 20 mg/kg every 6 hours.
▸ **Child 1–2 months:** 20 mg/kg every 6 hours
▸ **Child 3 months–17 years:** 15 mg/kg every 6 hours (max. per dose 500 mg) continued →

Infection caused by *Pseudomonas* or other less sensitive organisms | Empirical treatment of infection in febrile patients with neutropenia | Life-threatening infection

▸ BY INTRAVENOUS INFUSION
  ▸ Child 3 months–17 years: 25 mg/kg every 6 hours (max. per dose 1 g)

Cystic fibrosis

▸ BY INTRAVENOUS INFUSION
  ▸ Child: 25 mg/kg every 6 hours (max. per dose 1 g)

DOSE EQUIVALENCE AND CONVERSION
Dose expressed in terms of imipenem.

● **UNLICENSED USE** Not licensed for use in children under 1 year; not licensed for use in children with renal impairment.

● **CAUTIONS** CNS disorders · epilepsy

● **INTERACTIONS** → Appendix 1 (imipenem with cilastatin).

● **SIDE-EFFECTS**
▸ **Common or very common** Diarrhoea · eosinophilia · nausea (may reduce rate of infusion) · rash · vomiting
▸ **Uncommon** Confusion · dizziness · drowsiness · hallucinations · hypotension · leucopenia · myoclonic activity · seizures · thrombocytopenia · thrombocytosis
▸ **Rare** Acute renal failure · anaphylactic reactions · antibiotic-associated colitis · encephalopathy · hearing loss · hepatitis · paraesthesia · polyuria · Stevens-Johnson syndrome · taste disturbances · tooth, tongue or urine discoloration · toxic epidermal necrolysis · tremor
▸ **Very rare** Abdominal pain · aggravation of myasthenia gravis · asthenia · cyanosis · dyspnoea · flushing · glossitis · haemolytic anaemia · headache · heartburn · hyperhidrosis · hypersalivation · hyperventilation · palpitation · polyarthralgia · tachycardia · tinnitus
▸ **Frequency not known** Neurotoxicity (at high dose, renal failure, CNS disease)

● **ALLERGY AND CROSS-SENSITIVITY** Avoid if history of **immediate hypersensitivity** reaction to beta-lactam antibacterials.
    Use with caution in patients with sensitivity to beta-lactam antibacterials.

● **PREGNANCY** Manufacturer advises avoid unless potential benefit outweighs risk (toxicity in *animal* studies).

● **BREAST FEEDING** Present in milk but unlikely to be absorbed.

● **RENAL IMPAIRMENT** Reduce dose if estimated glomerular filtration rate less than 70 mL/minute/1.73 m^2, risk of CNS side-effects.

● **EFFECT ON LABORATORY TESTS** Positive Coombs' test.

● **DIRECTIONS FOR ADMINISTRATION** For *intravenous infusion* dilute to a concentration of 5 mg (as imipenem)/mL in Sodium chloride 0.9%; give up to 500 mg (as imipenem) over 20–30 minutes, give dose greater than 500 mg (as imipenem) over 40–60 minutes.

● **MEDICINAL FORMS**
There can be variation in the licensing of different medicines containing the same drug.
Powder for solution for infusion
ELECTROLYTES: May contain Sodium
▸ **Imipenem with cilastatin** (Non-proprietary)
  Cilastatin (as Cilastatin sodium) 500 mg, Imipenem (as Imipenem monohydrate) 500 mg Imipenem 500mg / Cilastatin 500mg powder for solution for infusion vials | 1 vial [PoM] £12.00 (Hospital only) | 5 vial [PoM] £60.00 (Hospital only) | 10 vial [PoM] £75.45-£120.00
▸ **Primaxin I.V.** (Merck Sharp & Dohme Ltd)
  Cilastatin (as Cilastatin sodium) 500 mg, Imipenem (as Imipenem monohydrate) 500 mg Primaxin IV 500mg powder for solution for infusion vials | 1 vial [PoM] £12.00

Meropenem

● **INDICATIONS AND DOSE**
Aerobic and anaerobic Gram-positive and Gram-negative infections | Hospital-acquired septicaemia
▸ BY INTRAVENOUS INFUSION, OR BY INTRAVENOUS INJECTION
  ▸ Neonate up to 7 days: 20 mg/kg every 12 hours.
  ▸ Neonate 7 days to 28 days: 20 mg/kg every 8 hours.
  ▸ Child 1 month–11 years (body-weight up to 50 kg): 10–20 mg/kg every 8 hours
  ▸ Child 1 month–11 years (body-weight 50 kg and above): 0.5–1 g every 8 hours
  ▸ Child 12–17 years: 0.5–1 g every 8 hours

Severe aerobic and anaerobic Gram-positive and Gram-negative infections
▸ BY INTRAVENOUS INFUSION, OR BY INTRAVENOUS INJECTION
  ▸ Neonate up to 7 days: 40 mg/kg every 12 hours.
  ▸ Neonate 7 days to 28 days: 40 mg/kg every 8 hours.

Exacerbations of chronic lower respiratory-tract infection in cystic fibrosis
▸ BY INTRAVENOUS INFUSION
  ▸ Child 1 month–11 years (body-weight up to 50 kg): 40 mg/kg every 8 hours
  ▸ Child 1 month–11 years (body-weight 50 kg and above): 2 g every 8 hours
  ▸ Child 12–17 years: 2 g every 8 hours

Meningitis
▸ BY INTRAVENOUS INFUSION
  ▸ Neonate up to 7 days: 40 mg/kg every 12 hours.
  ▸ Neonate 7 days to 28 days: 40 mg/kg every 8 hours.
  ▸ Child 1 month–11 years (body-weight up to 50 kg): 40 mg/kg every 8 hours
  ▸ Child 1 month–11 years (body-weight 50 kg and above): 2 g every 8 hours
  ▸ Child 12–17 years: 2 g every 8 hours

● **UNLICENSED USE** Not licensed for use in children under 3 months.

● **INTERACTIONS** → Appendix 1 (meropenem).

● **SIDE-EFFECTS**
▸ **Common or very common** Abdominal pain · diarrhoea · disturbances in liver function tests · headache · nausea · pruritus · rash · thrombocythaemia · vomiting
▸ **Uncommon** Eosinophilia · leucopenia · paraesthesia · thrombocytopenia
▸ **Rare** Convulsions
▸ **Frequency not known** Antibiotic-associated colitis · haemolytic anaemia · Stevens-Johnson syndrome · toxic epidermal necrolysis

● **ALLERGY AND CROSS-SENSITIVITY** Avoid if history of **immediate hypersensitivity** reaction to beta-lactam antibacterials.
    Use with caution in patients with sensitivity to beta-lactam antibacterials.

● **PREGNANCY** Use only if potential benefit outweighs risk—no information available.

● **BREAST FEEDING** Unlikely to be absorbed (however, manufacturer advises avoid).

● **HEPATIC IMPAIRMENT**
Monitoring
Monitor liver function in hepatic impairment.

- **RENAL IMPAIRMENT** Use normal dose every 12 hours if estimated glomerular filtration rate 26–50 mL/minute/1.73 m². Use half normal dose every 12 hours if estimated glomerular filtration rate 10–25 mL/minute/1.73 m². Use half normal dose every 24 hours if estimated glomerular filtration rate less than 10 mL/minute/1.73 m².

- **EFFECT ON LABORATORY TESTS** Positive Coombs' test.

- **DIRECTIONS FOR ADMINISTRATION** *Intravenous injection* to be administered over 5 minutes.
  Displacement value may be significant when reconstituting injection, consult local guidelines. For *intravenous infusion*, dilute reconstituted solution further to a concentration of 1–20 mg/mL *in* Glucose 5% *or* Sodium Chloride 0.9%; give over 15–30 minutes.

- **MEDICINAL FORMS**
  There can be variation in the licensing of different medicines containing the same drug.
  Powder for solution for injection
  ELECTROLYTES: May contain Sodium
  ▸ **Meropenem (Non-proprietary)**
  Meropenem (as Meropenem trihydrate) 500 mg Meropenem 500mg powder for solution for injection vials | 10 vial PoM £76.90–£90.00
  Meropenem (as Meropenem trihydrate) 1 gram Meropenem 1g powder for solution for injection vials | 10 vial PoM £153.50–£206.28 | 10 vial PoM £171.90–£206.28 (Hospital only)
  ▸ **Meronem** (AstraZeneca UK Ltd)
  Meropenem (as Meropenem trihydrate) 500 mg Meronem 500mg powder for solution for injection vials | 10 vial PoM £103.14
  Meropenem (as Meropenem trihydrate) 1 gram Meronem 1g powder for solution for injection vials | 10 vial PoM £206.28

ANTIBACTERIALS ⟩ CEPHALOSPORINS

Cephalosporins

Overview

The cephalosporins are broad-spectrum antibiotics which are used for the treatment of septicaemia, pneumonia, meningitis, biliary-tract infections, peritonitis, and urinary-tract infections. The pharmacology of the cephalosporins is similar to that of the penicillins, excretion being principally renal. Cephalosporins penetrate the cerebrospinal fluid poorly unless the meninges are inflamed; cefotaxime p. 301 and ceftriaxone p. 302 are suitable cephalosporins for infections of the CNS (e.g meningitis).

The principal side-effect of the cephalosporins is hypersensitivity and about 0.5–6.5% of penicillin-sensitive patients will also be allergic to the cephalosporins. If a cephalosporin is essential in patients with a history of immediate hypersensitivity to penicillin, because a suitable alternative antibacterial is not available, then cefixime p. 300, cefotaxime, ceftazidime p. 301, ceftriaxone, or cefuroxime p. 300 can be used with caution; cefaclor p. 299, cefadroxil p. 298, cefalexin p. 298, and cefradine p. 299 should be avoided.

The orally active 'first generation' cephalosporins, cefalexin, cefradine, and cefadroxil and the 'second generation' cephalosporin, cefaclor have a similar antimicrobial spectrum. They are useful for urinary-tract infections which do not respond to other drugs or which occur in pregnancy, respiratory-tract infections, otitis media, sinusitis, and skin and soft-tissue infections. Cefaclor has good activity against *H. influenzae*. Cefadroxil has a long duration of action and can be given twice daily; it has poor activity against *H. influenzae*. **Cefuroxime axetil**, an ester of the 'second generation' cephalosporin cefuroxime, has the same antibacterial spectrum as the parent compound; it is poorly absorbed and needs to be given with food to maximise absorption.

Cefixime is an orally active 'third generation' cephalosporin. It has a longer duration of action than the other cephalosporins that are active by mouth. It is only licensed for acute infections.

Cefuroxime is a 'second generation' cephalosporin that is less susceptible than the earlier cephalosporins to inactivation by beta-lactamases. It is, therefore, active against certain bacteria which are resistant to the other drugs and has greater activity against *Haemophilus influenzae*.

Cefotaxime, ceftazidime and ceftriaxone are 'third generation' cephalosporins with greater activity than the 'second generation' cephalosporins against certain Gram-negative bacteria. However, they are less active than cefuroxime against Gram-positive bacteria, most notably *Staphylococcus aureus*. Their broad antibacterial spectrum may encourage superinfection with resistant bacteria or fungi.

Ceftazidime has good activity against pseudomonas. It is also active against other Gram-negative bacteria.

Ceftriaxone has a longer half-life and therefore needs to be given only once daily. Indications include serious infections such as septicaemia, pneumonia, and meningitis. The calcium salt of ceftriaxone forms a precipitate in the gall bladder which may rarely cause symptoms but these usually resolve when the antibacterial is stopped. In neonates, ceftriaxone may displace bilirubin from plasma-albumin and should be avoided in neonates with unconjugated hyperbilirubinaemia, hypoalbuminaemia, acidosis or impaired bilirubin binding.

Cephalosporins

- **INTERACTIONS** → Appendix 1 (cephalosporins).

- **SIDE-EFFECTS**
  ▸ **Rare** Antibiotic-associated colitis
  ▸ **Frequency not known** Abdominal discomfort · agranulocytosis · allergic reactions · anaphylaxis · aplastic anaemia · blood disorders · confusion · diarrhoea · disturbances in liver enzymes · dizziness · eosinophilia · haemolytic anaemia · hallucinations · headache · hyperactivity · hypertonia · leucopenia · nausea · nervousness · pruritus · rashes · reversible interstitial nephritis · serum sickness-like reactions with rashes, fever and arthralgia · sleep disturbances · Stevens-Johnson syndrome · thrombocytopenia · toxic epidermal necrolysis · transient cholestatic jaundice · transient hepatitis · urticaria · vomiting

  SIDE-EFFECTS, FURTHER INFORMATION
  ▸ Antibiotic-associated colitis Antibiotic-associated colitis may occur more commonly with second- and third-generation cephalosporins.

- **ALLERGY AND CROSS-SENSITIVITY** Contra-indicated in patients with cephalosporin hypersensitivity.
  ▸ Cross-sensitivity with other beta-lactam antibacterials About 0.5–6.5% of penicillin-sensitive patients will also be allergic to the cephalosporins. Patients with a history of **immediate hypersensitivity** to penicillin and other beta-lactams should not receive a cephalosporin. Cephalosporins should be used with caution in patients with sensitivity to penicillin and other beta-lactams.

- **EFFECT ON LABORATORY TESTS** False positive urinary glucose (if tested for reducing substances). False positive Coombs' test.

ANTIBACTERIALS > CEPHALOSPORINS, FIRST-GENERATION

F 297

Cefadroxil

● **INDICATIONS AND DOSE**

Susceptible infections due to sensitive Gram-positive and Gram-negative bacteria

▶ BY MOUTH

▶ Child 6-17 years (body-weight up to 40 kg): 0.5 g twice daily

▶ Child 6-17 years (body-weight 40 kg and above): 0.5–1 g twice daily

Skin infections | Soft-tissue infections | Uncomplicated urinary-tract infections

▶ BY MOUTH

▶ Child 6-17 years (body-weight 40 kg and above): 1 g once daily

● **PREGNANCY** Not known to be harmful.

● **BREAST FEEDING** Present in milk in low concentration, but appropriate to use.

● **RENAL IMPAIRMENT** Reduce dose if estimated glomerular filtration rate less than 50 mL/minute/1.73 m^2.

● **MEDICINAL FORMS**
There can be variation in the licensing of different medicines containing the same drug.

Capsule
CAUTIONARY AND ADVISORY LABELS 9
▶ Cefadroxil (Non-proprietary)
Cefadroxil (as Cefadroxil monohydrate) 500 mg Cefadroxil 500mg capsules | 20 capsule PoM £22.38 DT price = £22.38 | 100 capsule PoM £111.90

F 297

Cefalexin

(Cephalexin)

● **INDICATIONS AND DOSE**

Susceptible infections due to sensitive Gram-positive and Gram-negative bacteria

▶ BY MOUTH

▶ Neonate up to 7 days: 25 mg/kg twice daily (max. per dose 125 mg).

▶ Neonate 7 days to 20 days: 25 mg/kg 3 times a day (max. per dose 125 mg).

▶ Neonate 21 days to 28 days: 25 mg/kg 4 times a day (max. per dose 125 mg).

▶ Child 1-11 months: 12.5 mg/kg twice daily, alternatively 125 mg twice daily

▶ Child 1-4 years: 12.5 mg/kg twice daily, alternatively 125 mg 3 times a day

▶ Child 5-11 years: 12.5 mg/kg twice daily, alternatively 250 mg 3 times a day

▶ Child 12-17 years: 500 mg 2–3 times a day

Serious susceptible infections due to sensitive Gram-positive and Gram-negative bacteria

▶ BY MOUTH

▶ Child 1 month-11 years: 25 mg/kg 2–4 times a day (max. per dose 1 g 4 times a day)

▶ Child 12-17 years: 1–1.5 g 3–4 times a day

Prophylaxis of recurrent urinary-tract infection

▶ BY MOUTH

▶ Child: 12.5 mg/kg once daily (max. per dose 125 mg), dose to be taken at night

● **PREGNANCY** Not known to be harmful.

● **BREAST FEEDING** Present in milk in low concentration, but appropriate to use.

● **RENAL IMPAIRMENT** Reduce dose in moderate impairment.

● **PATIENT AND CARER ADVICE**
Medicines for Children leaflet: Cefalexin for bacterial infections www.medicinesforchildren.org.uk/cefalexin-bacterial-infections-0

● **PROFESSION SPECIFIC INFORMATION**

Dental practitioners' formulary
Cefalexin Capsules may be prescribed. Cefalexin Tablets may be prescribed. Cefalexin Oral Suspension may be prescribed.

● **MEDICINAL FORMS**
There can be variation in the licensing of different medicines containing the same drug.

Tablet
CAUTIONARY AND ADVISORY LABELS 9
▶ Cefalexin (Non-proprietary)
Cefalexin 250 mg Cefalexin 250mg tablets | 28 tablet PoM £5.02 DT price = £1.95 | 100 tablet PoM £4.93
Cefalexin 500 mg Cefalexin 500mg tablets | 21 tablet PoM £5.88 DT price = £1.98
▶ Ceporex (Co-Pharma Ltd)
Cefalexin 250 mg Ceporex 250mg tablets | 28 tablet PoM £4.02 DT price = £1.95 | 100 tablet PoM £13.74
Cefalexin 500 mg Ceporex 500mg tablets | 28 tablet PoM £7.85 | 100 tablet PoM £26.90
▶ Keflex (Flynn Pharma Ltd)
Cefalexin 250 mg Keflex 250mg tablets | 28 tablet PoM £1.60 DT price = £1.95
Cefalexin 500 mg Keflex 500mg tablets | 21 tablet PoM £2.08 DT price = £1.98

Capsule
CAUTIONARY AND ADVISORY LABELS 9
▶ Cefalexin (Non-proprietary)
Cefalexin 250 mg Cefalexin 250mg capsules | 28 capsule £4.01 DT price = £1.22 | 100 capsule PoM £5.01
Cefalexin 500 mg Cefalexin 500mg capsules | 21 capsule PoM £5.88 DT price = £1.40 | 100 capsule PoM £9.43
▶ Ceporex (Co-Pharma Ltd)
Cefalexin 250 mg Ceporex 250mg capsules | 28 capsule PoM £4.02 DT price = £1.22 | 100 capsule PoM £13.74
Cefalexin 500 mg Ceporex 500mg capsules | 28 capsule PoM £7.85 | 100 capsule PoM £26.90
▶ Keflex (Flynn Pharma Ltd)
Cefalexin 250 mg Keflex 250mg capsules | 28 capsule PoM £1.46 DT price = £1.22
Cefalexin 500 mg Keflex 500mg capsules | 21 capsule PoM £1.98 DT price = £1.40

Oral suspension
CAUTIONARY AND ADVISORY LABELS 9
▶ Cefalexin (Non-proprietary)
Cefalexin 25 mg per 1 ml Cefalexin 125mg/5ml oral suspension sugar free sugar-free | 100 ml PoM no price available
Cefalexin 125mg/5ml oral suspension | 100 ml PoM £4.90 DT price = £2.03
Cefalexin 50 mg per 1 ml Cefalexin 250mg/5ml oral suspension sugar free sugar-free | 100 ml PoM no price available
Cefalexin 250mg/5ml oral suspension | 100 ml PoM £5.25 DT price = £1.75
Cefalexin 100 mg per 1 ml Cefalexin 500mg/5ml oral suspension | 100 ml PoM no price available
▶ Ceporex (Co-Pharma Ltd)
Cefalexin 25 mg per 1 ml Ceporex 125mg/5ml syrup | 100 ml PoM £1.43 DT price = £2.03
Cefalexin 50 mg per 1 ml Ceporex 250mg/5ml syrup | 100 ml PoM £2.87 DT price = £1.75
Cefalexin 100 mg per 1 ml Ceporex 500mg/5ml syrup | 100 ml PoM £5.57
▶ Keflex (Flynn Pharma Ltd)
Cefalexin 25 mg per 1 ml Keflex 125mg/5ml oral suspension | 100 ml PoM £0.84 DT price = £2.03
Cefalexin 50 mg per 1 ml Keflex 250mg/5ml oral suspension | 100 ml PoM £1.40 DT price = £1.75

Cefradine

F 297

(Cephradine)

- **INDICATIONS AND DOSE**

Susceptible infections due to sensitive Gram-positive and Gram-negative bacteria | Surgical prophylaxis
▸ BY MOUTH
- Child 7–11 years: 25–50 mg/kg daily in 2–4 divided doses
- Child 12–17 years: 250–500 mg 4 times a day, alternatively 0.5–1 g twice daily; increased if necessary up to 1 g 4 times a day, increased dose may be used in severe infections

Prevention of *Staphylococcus aureus* lung infection in cystic fibrosis
▸ BY MOUTH
- Child 7–17 years: 2 g twice daily

- **UNLICENSED USE** Not licensed for use in children for prevention of *Staphylococcus aureus* lung infection in cystic fibrosis.
- **PREGNANCY** Not known to be harmful.
- **BREAST FEEDING** Present in milk in low concentration, but appropriate to use.
- **RENAL IMPAIRMENT** Reduce dose if estimated glomerular filtration rate less than 20 mL/minute/1.73 m^2.
- **PROFESSION SPECIFIC INFORMATION**

Dental practitioners' formulary
Cefradine Capsules may be prescribed.

- **MEDICINAL FORMS**
There can be variation in the licensing of different medicines containing the same drug.

Capsule
CAUTIONARY AND ADVISORY LABELS 9
▸ Cefradine (Non-proprietary)
  Cefradine 250 mg Cefradine 250mg capsules | 20 capsule [PoM]
  £6.00 DT price = £1.83 | 100 capsule [PoM] no price available
  Cefradine 500 mg Cefradine 500mg capsules | 20 capsule [PoM]
  £8.75 DT price = £2.70 | 100 capsule [PoM] no price available
▸ Nicef (Co-Pharma Ltd)
  Cefradine 250 mg Nicef 250mg capsules | 20 capsule [PoM] £3.55
  DT price = £1.83 | 100 capsule [PoM] £9.39
  Cefradine 500 mg Nicef 500mg capsules | 20 capsule [PoM] £5.58
  DT price = £2.70 | 100 capsule [PoM] £33.72

ANTIBACTERIALS > CEPHALOSPORINS, SECOND-GENERATION

Cefaclor

F 297

- **INDICATIONS AND DOSE**

Susceptible infections due to sensitive Gram-positive and Gram-negative bacteria
▸ BY MOUTH USING IMMEDIATE-RELEASE MEDICINES
- Child 1–11 months: 20 mg/kg daily in 3 divided doses, alternatively 62.5 mg 3 times a day
- Child 1–4 years: 20 mg/kg daily in 3 divided doses, alternatively 125 mg 3 times a day
- Child 5–11 years: 20 mg/kg daily in 3 divided doses, usual max. 1 g daily, alternatively 250 mg 3 times a day
- Child 12–17 years: 250 mg 3 times a day; maximum 4 g per day
▸ BY MOUTH USING MODIFIED-RELEASE MEDICINES
- Child 12–17 years: 375 mg every 12 hours, dose to be taken with food

Severe susceptible infections due to sensitive Gram-positive and Gram-negative bacteria
▸ BY MOUTH USING IMMEDIATE-RELEASE MEDICINES
- Child 1–11 months: 40 mg/kg daily in 3 divided doses, usual max. 1 g daily, alternatively 125 mg 3 times a day
- Child 1–4 years: 40 mg/kg daily in 3 divided doses, usual max. 1 g daily, alternatively 250 mg 3 times a day
- Child 5–11 years: 40 mg/kg daily in 3 divided doses, usual max. 1 g daily
- Child 12–17 years: 500 mg 3 times a day; maximum 4 g per day

Pneumonia
▸ BY MOUTH USING MODIFIED-RELEASE TABLETS
- Child 12–17 years: 750 mg every 12 hours, dose to be taken with food

Lower urinary-tract infections
▸ BY MOUTH USING MODIFIED-RELEASE MEDICINES
- Child 12–17 years: 375 mg every 12 hours, dose to be taken with food

Asymptomatic carriage of *Haemophilus influenzae* or mild exacerbations in cystic fibrosis
▸ BY MOUTH USING IMMEDIATE-RELEASE MEDICINES
- Child 1–11 months: 125 mg every 8 hours
- Child 1–6 years: 250 mg 3 times a day
- Child 7–17 years: 500 mg 3 times a day

- **SIDE-EFFECTS**
SIDE-EFFECTS, FURTHER INFORMATION
▸ Skin reactions Cefaclor is associated with protracted skin reactions, especially in children.

- **PREGNANCY** Not known to be harmful.
- **BREAST FEEDING** Present in milk in low concentration, but appropriate to use.
- **RENAL IMPAIRMENT** No dose adjustment required. Manufacturer advises caution.

- **MEDICINAL FORMS**
There can be variation in the licensing of different medicines containing the same drug.

Modified-release tablet
CAUTIONARY AND ADVISORY LABELS 9, 21, 25
▸ Distaclor MR (Flynn Pharma Ltd)
  Cefaclor (as Cefaclor monohydrate) 375 mg Distaclor MR 375mg
  tablets | 14 tablet [PoM] £9.10 DT price = £9.10

Capsule
CAUTIONARY AND ADVISORY LABELS 9
▸ Cefaclor (Non-proprietary)
  Cefaclor (as Cefaclor monohydrate) 250 mg Cefaclor 250mg
  capsules | 21 capsule [PoM] no price available DT price = £6.80
  Cefaclor (as Cefaclor monohydrate) 500 mg Cefaclor 500mg
  capsules | 50 capsule [PoM] no price available
▸ Distaclor (Flynn Pharma Ltd)
  Cefaclor (as Cefaclor monohydrate) 500 mg Distaclor 500mg
  capsules | 21 capsule [PoM] £7.50 DT price = £7.50
▸ Keftid (Co-Pharma Ltd)
  Cefaclor (as Cefaclor monohydrate) 250 mg Keftid 250mg capsules
  | 21 capsule [PoM] £6.80 DT price = £6.80
  Cefaclor (as Cefaclor monohydrate) 500 mg Keftid 500mg
  capsules | 50 capsule [PoM] £31.99

Oral suspension
CAUTIONARY AND ADVISORY LABELS 9
▸ Cefaclor (Non-proprietary)
  Cefaclor (as Cefaclor monohydrate) 25 mg per 1 ml Cefaclor
  125mg/5ml oral suspension sugar free sugar-free | 100 ml [PoM]
  £5.16 DT price = £5.16
  Cefaclor 125mg/5ml oral suspension | 100 ml [PoM] no price
  available
  Cefaclor (as Cefaclor monohydrate) 50 mg per 1 ml Cefaclor
  250mg/5ml oral suspension | 100 ml [PoM] no price available
▸ Distaclor (Flynn Pharma Ltd)
  Cefaclor (as Cefaclor monohydrate) 25 mg per 1 ml Distaclor
  125mg/5ml oral suspension | 100 ml [PoM] £4.13
  Cefaclor (as Cefaclor monohydrate) 50 mg per 1 ml Distaclor
  250mg/5ml oral suspension | 100 ml [PoM] £8.26

5

Infection

5

Infection

► **Keftid** (Co-Pharma Ltd)
Cefaclor (as Cefaclor monohydrate) 25 mg per 1 ml Keftid 125mg/5ml oral suspension sugar-free | 100 ml [PoM] £5.16 DT price = £5.16
Cefaclor (as Cefaclor monohydrate) 50 mg per 1 ml Keftid 250mg/5ml oral suspension sugar-free | 100 ml [PoM] £10.32 DT price = £10.32

F 297

Cefuroxime

● **INDICATIONS AND DOSE**

Susceptible infections due to Gram-positive and Gram-negative bacteria
► BY MOUTH
► Child 3 months–1 year: 10 mg/kg twice daily (max. per dose 125 mg)
► Child 2–11 years: 15 mg/kg twice daily (max. per dose 250 mg)
► Child 12–17 years: 250 mg twice daily, dose may be doubled in severe lower respiratory-tract infections or if pneumonia is suspected
► BY INTRAVENOUS INFUSION, OR BY INTRAVENOUS INJECTION
► Neonate up to 7 days: 25 mg/kg every 12 hours, increased if necessary to 50 mg/kg every 12 hours, increased dose used in severe infection.
► Neonate 7 days to 20 days: 25 mg/kg every 8 hours, increased if necessary to 50 mg/kg every 8 hours, increased dose used in severe infection.
► Neonate 21 days to 28 days: 25 mg/kg every 6 hours, increased if necessary to 50 mg/kg every 6 hours, increased dose used in severe infection.
► BY INTRAVENOUS INFUSION, OR BY INTRAVENOUS INJECTION, OR BY INTRAMUSCULAR INJECTION
► Child: 20 mg/kg every 8 hours (max. per dose 750 mg); increased to 50–60 mg/kg every 6–8 hours (max. per dose 1.5 g), increased dose used for severe infection and cystic fibrosis

Lyme disease
► BY MOUTH
► Child 3 months–11 years: 15 mg/kg twice daily (max. per dose 500 mg) for 14–21 days (for 28 days in Lyme arthritis)
► Child 12–17 years: 500 mg twice daily for 14–21 days (for 28 days in Lyme arthritis)

Lower urinary-tract infection
► BY MOUTH
► Child 12–17 years: 125 mg twice daily

Surgical prophylaxis
► INITIALLY BY INTRAVENOUS INJECTION
► Child: 50 mg/kg (max. per dose 1.5 g), to be administered up to 30 minutes before the procedure, then (by intravenous injection or by intramuscular injection) 30 mg/kg every 8 hours (max. per dose 750 mg) if required for up to 3 doses (for high-risk procedures)

● **UNLICENSED USE**
► With oral use Not licensed for treatment of Lyme disease in children under 12 years. Duration of treatment in Lyme disease is unlicensed.
● **PREGNANCY** Not known to be harmful.
● **BREAST FEEDING** Present in milk in low concentration, but appropriate to use.
● **RENAL IMPAIRMENT** Reduce parenteral dose if estimated glomerular filtration rate less than 20 mL/minute/1.73 m^2.
● **DIRECTIONS FOR ADMINISTRATION** Single doses over 750 mg should be administered by the intravenous route only.

► With intravenous use Displacement value may be significant when reconstituting injection, consult local guidelines. For intermittent intravenous infusion, dilute reconstituted solution further in glucose 5% or sodium chloride 0.9%; give over 30 minutes.

● **MEDICINAL FORMS**
There can be variation in the licensing of different medicines containing the same drug. Forms available from special-order manufacturers include: solution for injection, infusion

Tablet
CAUTIONARY AND ADVISORY LABELS 9, 21, 25
► **Cefuroxime** (Non-proprietary)
Cefuroxime (as Cefuroxime axetil) 250 mg Cefuroxime 250mg tablets | 14 tablet [PoM] £17.72 DT price = £17.72
► **Zinnat** (GlaxoSmithKline UK Ltd)
Cefuroxime (as Cefuroxime axetil) 125 mg Zinnat 125mg tablets | 14 tablet [PoM] £4.56 DT price = £4.56
Cefuroxime (as Cefuroxime axetil) 250 mg Zinnat 250mg tablets | 14 tablet [PoM] £9.11 DT price = £17.72

Oral suspension
CAUTIONARY AND ADVISORY LABELS 9, 21
EXCIPIENTS: May contain Aspartame, sucrose
► **Zinnat** (GlaxoSmithKline UK Ltd)
Cefuroxime (as Cefuroxime axetil) 25 mg per 1 ml Zinnat 125mg/5ml oral suspension | 70 ml [PoM] £5.20

Powder for injection
ELECTROLYTES: May contain Sodium
► **Cefuroxime** (Non-proprietary)
Cefuroxime (as Cefuroxime sodium) 250 mg Cefuroxime 250mg powder for injection vials | 10 vial [PoM] £9.25
Cefuroxime (as Cefuroxime sodium) 750 mg Cefuroxime 750mg powder for injection vials | 1 vial [PoM] £2.52 | 10 vial [PoM] £25.20
Cefuroxime (as Cefuroxime sodium) 1.5 gram Cefuroxime 1.5g powder for injection vials | 1 vial [PoM] £5.05 | 10 vial [PoM] £50.50
► **Zinacef** (GlaxoSmithKline UK Ltd)
Cefuroxime (as Cefuroxime sodium) 250 mg Zinacef 250mg powder for injection vials | 5 vial [PoM] £4.70
Cefuroxime (as Cefuroxime sodium) 750 mg Zinacef 750mg powder for injection vials | 5 vial [PoM] £11.72 (Hospital only)
Cefuroxime (as Cefuroxime sodium) 1.5 gram Zinacef 1.5g powder for injection vials | 1 vial [PoM] £4.70

ANTIBACTERIALS 〉 CEPHALOSPORINS, THIRD-GENERATION

F 297

Cefixime

● **INDICATIONS AND DOSE**

Acute infections due to sensitive Gram-positive and Gram-negative bacteria
► BY MOUTH
► Child 6–11 months: 75 mg daily
► Child 1–4 years: 100 mg daily
► Child 5–9 years: 200 mg daily
► Child 10–17 years: 200–400 mg daily, alternatively 100–200 mg twice daily

Uncomplicated gonorrhoea
► BY MOUTH
► Child 12–17 years: 400 mg for 1 dose

● **UNLICENSED USE** Use of cefixime for uncomplicated gonorrhoea is an unlicensed indication.
● **PREGNANCY** Not known to be harmful.
● **BREAST FEEDING** Manufacturer advises avoid unless essential—no information available.
● **RENAL IMPAIRMENT** Reduce dose if estimated glomerular filtration rate less than 20 mL/minute/1.73 m^2.

- **MEDICINAL FORMS**
There can be variation in the licensing of different medicines containing the same drug.

Tablet
CAUTIONARY AND ADVISORY LABELS 9
▶ **Suprax** (Sanofi)
Cefixime 200 mg Suprax 200mg tablets | 7 tablet [PoM] £13.23 DT price = £13.23

F 297

Cefotaxime

- **INDICATIONS AND DOSE**

Uncomplicated gonorrhoea
▶ BY INTRAMUSCULAR INJECTION
▷ Child 12–17 years: 500 mg for 1 dose

Severe exacerbations of *Haemophilus influenzae* infection in cystic fibrosis
▶ BY INTRAVENOUS INJECTION, OR BY INTRAVENOUS INFUSION
▷ Child: 50 mg/kg every 6–8 hours; maximum 12 g per day

Congenital gonococcal conjunctivitis
▶ BY INTRAMUSCULAR INJECTION
▷ Neonate: 100 mg/kg (max. per dose 1 g) for 1 dose.

Infections due to sensitive Gram-positive and Gram-negative bacteria | Surgical prophylaxis | Haemophilus epiglottitis
▶ BY INTRAMUSCULAR INJECTION, OR BY INTRAVENOUS INJECTION, OR BY INTRAVENOUS INFUSION
▷ Neonate up to 7 days: 25 mg/kg every 12 hours.
▷ Neonate 7 days to 20 days: 25 mg/kg every 8 hours.
▷ Neonate 21 days to 28 days: 25 mg/kg every 6–8 hours.
▷ Child: 50 mg/kg every 8–12 hours

Severe susceptible infections due to sensitive Gram-positive and Gram-negative bacteria | Meningitis
▶ BY INTRAMUSCULAR INJECTION, OR BY INTRAVENOUS INJECTION, OR BY INTRAVENOUS INFUSION
▷ Neonate up to 7 days: 50 mg/kg every 12 hours.
▷ Neonate 7 days to 20 days: 50 mg/kg every 8 hours.
▷ Neonate 21 days to 28 days: 50 mg/kg every 6–8 hours.
▷ Child: 50 mg/kg every 6 hours; maximum 12 g per day

Emergency treatment of suspected bacterial meningitis or meningococcal disease, before urgent transfer to hospital, in patients who cannot be given benzylpenicillin (e.g. because of an allergy)
▶ BY INTRAVENOUS INJECTION, OR BY INTRAMUSCULAR INJECTION
▷ Child 1 month–11 years: 50 mg/kg for 1 dose
▷ Child 12–17 years: 1 g for 1 dose

- **SIDE-EFFECTS**
▶ **Rare** Arrhythmias (following rapid injection)

- **PREGNANCY** Not known to be harmful.

- **BREAST FEEDING** Present in milk in low concentration, but appropriate to use.

- **RENAL IMPAIRMENT** Usual initial dose, then use half normal dose if estimated glomerular filtration rate less than 5 mL/minute/1.73 m^2.

- **DIRECTIONS FOR ADMINISTRATION**
▶ With intravenous use Displacement value may be significant, consult local guidelines. For intermittent *intravenous infusion* dilute in glucose 5% *or* sodium chloride 0.9%; administer over 20–60 minutes; incompatible with alkaline solutions.

- **MEDICINAL FORMS**
There can be variation in the licensing of different medicines containing the same drug.

Powder for solution for injection
▶ **Cefotaxime** (Non-proprietary)
Cefotaxime (as Cefotaxime sodium) 500 mg Cefotaxime 500mg powder for solution for injection vials | 1 vial [PoM] £1.50 | 10 vial [PoM] £25.50–£30.00
Cefotaxime (as Cefotaxime sodium) 1 gram Cefotaxime 1g powder for solution for injection vials | 1 vial [PoM] £3.00 | 10 vial [PoM] £35.00
Cefotaxime (as Cefotaxime sodium) 2 gram Cefotaxime 2g powder for solution for injection vials | 1 vial [PoM] £8.00 | 10 vial [PoM] £37.50

F 297

Ceftazidime

- **INDICATIONS AND DOSE**

Pseudomonal lung infection in cystic fibrosis
▶ BY INTRAVENOUS INFUSION, OR BY INTRAVENOUS INJECTION, OR BY DEEP INTRAMUSCULAR INJECTION
▷ Child: 50 mg/kg every 8 hours; maximum 9 g per day

Febrile neutropenia
▶ BY INTRAVENOUS INFUSION, OR BY INTRAVENOUS INJECTION
▷ Child: 50 mg/kg every 8 hours; maximum 6 g per day

Meningitis
▶ BY INTRAVENOUS INJECTION, OR BY INTRAVENOUS INFUSION
▷ Neonate up to 7 days: 50 mg/kg every 24 hours.
▷ Neonate 7 days to 20 days: 50 mg/kg every 12 hours.
▷ Neonate 21 days to 28 days: 50 mg/kg every 8 hours.
▷ Child: 50 mg/kg every 8 hours; maximum 6 g per day

Susceptible infections due to sensitive Gram-positive and Gram-negative bacteria
▶ BY INTRAVENOUS INJECTION, OR BY INTRAVENOUS INFUSION
▷ Neonate up to 7 days: 25 mg/kg every 24 hours.
▷ Neonate 7 days to 20 days: 25 mg/kg every 12 hours.
▷ Neonate 21 days to 28 days: 25 mg/kg every 8 hours.
▷ Child: 25 mg/kg every 8 hours; maximum 6 g per day

Severe susceptible infections due to sensitive Gram-positive and Gram-negative bacteria
▶ BY INTRAVENOUS INJECTION, OR BY INTRAVENOUS INFUSION
▷ Neonate up to 7 days: 50 mg/kg every 24 hours.
▷ Neonate 7 days to 20 days: 50 mg/kg every 12 hours.
▷ Neonate 21 days to 28 days: 50 mg/kg every 8 hours.
▷ Child: 50 mg/kg every 8 hours; maximum 6 g per day

Chronic *Burkholderia cepacia* infection in cystic fibrosis
▶ BY INHALATION OF NEBULISED SOLUTION
▷ Child: 1 g twice daily

- **UNLICENSED USE**
▶ When used by inhalation Nebulised route unlicensed.

- **SIDE-EFFECTS** Paraesthesia · taste disturbances

- **PREGNANCY** Not known to be harmful.

- **BREAST FEEDING** Present in milk in low concentration, but appropriate to use.

- **HEPATIC IMPAIRMENT** Manufacturer advises caution in severe impairment.

- **RENAL IMPAIRMENT** Reduce dose if estimated glomerular filtration rate less than 50 mL/minute/1.73 m^2—consult product literature.

- **DIRECTIONS FOR ADMINISTRATION** Intramuscular administration used when intravenous administration not possible; single doses over 1 g by intravenous route only.

▸ **With intravenous use** Displacement value may be significant, consult local guidelines. For intermittent intravenous infusion dilute reconstituted solution further to a concentration of not more than 40 mg/mL in Glucose 5% or Glucose 10% or Sodium chloride 0.9%; give over 20–30 minutes.

▸ **When used by inhalation** For nebulisation, dissolve dose in 3 mL of water for injection.

● **MEDICINAL FORMS**
There can be variation in the licensing of different medicines containing the same drug. Forms available from special-order manufacturers include: infusion, solution for infusion

Powder for solution for injection
ELECTROLYTES: May contain Sodium

▸ Ceftazidime (Non-proprietary)
Ceftazidime (as Ceftazidime pentahydrate) 500 mg Ceftazidime 500mg powder for solution for injection vials | 1 vial PoM £4.70
Ceftazidime (as Ceftazidime pentahydrate) 1 gram Ceftazidime 1g powder for solution for injection vials | 1 vial PoM £11.40 | 5 vial PoM £39.55 | 10 vial PoM £13.90
Ceftazidime (as Ceftazidime pentahydrate) 2 gram Ceftazidime 2g powder for solution for injection vials | 1 vial PoM £22.10 | 5 vial PoM £79.15 | 10 vial PoM £27.70

▸ Fortum (GlaxoSmithKline UK Ltd)
Ceftazidime (as Ceftazidime pentahydrate) 500 mg Fortum 500mg powder for solution for injection vials | 1 vial PoM £4.40 (Hospital only)
Ceftazidime (as Ceftazidime pentahydrate) 1 gram Fortum 1g powder for solution for injection vials | 1 vial PoM £8.79 (Hospital only)
Ceftazidime (as Ceftazidime pentahydrate) 2 gram Fortum 2g powder for solution for injection vials | 1 vial PoM £17.59 (Hospital only)
Ceftazidime (as Ceftazidime pentahydrate) 3 gram Fortum 3g powder for solution for injection vials | 1 vial PoM £25.76 (Hospital only)

F 297

Ceftriaxone

15.6.2016

● **INDICATIONS AND DOSE**

Community-acquired pneumonia | Hospital-acquired pneumonia | Intra-abdominal infections | Complicated urinary-tract infections
▸ BY INTRAVENOUS INFUSION

▸ Neonate up to 15 days: 20–50 mg/kg once daily, doses at the higher end of the recommended range used in severe cases.

▸ Neonate 15 days to 28 days: 50–80 mg/kg once daily, doses at the higher end of the recommended range used in severe cases.

▸ Child 1 month–11 years (body-weight up to 50 kg): 50–80 mg/kg once daily, doses at the higher end of the recommended range used in severe cases; maximum 4 g per day

▸ Child 9–11 years (body-weight 50 kg and above): 1–2 g once daily, 2 g dose to be used for hospital-acquired pneumonia and severe cases

▸ Child 12–17 years: 1–2 g once daily, 2 g dose to be used for hospital-acquired pneumonia and severe cases
▸ BY INTRAVENOUS INJECTION

▸ Child 9–11 years (body-weight 50 kg and above): 1–2 g once daily, 2 g dose to be used for hospital-acquired pneumonia and severe cases

▸ Child 12–17 years: 1–2 g once daily, 2 g dose to be used for hospital-acquired pneumonia and severe cases
▸ BY DEEP INTRAMUSCULAR INJECTION

▸ Child 1 month–11 years (body-weight up to 50 kg): 50–80 mg/kg once daily, doses at the higher end of the recommended range used in severe cases; maximum 4 g per day

▸ Child 9–11 years (body-weight 50 kg and above): 1–2 g once daily, 2 g dose to be used for hospital-acquired pneumonia and severe cases

▸ Child 12–17 years: 1–2 g once daily, 2 g dose to be used for hospital-acquired pneumonia and severe cases

Complicated skin and soft tissue infections | Infections of bones and joints
▸ BY INTRAVENOUS INFUSION

▸ Neonate up to 15 days: 20–50 mg/kg once daily, doses at the higher end of the recommended range used in severe cases.

▸ Neonate 15 days to 28 days: 50–100 mg/kg once daily, doses at the higher end of the recommended range used in severe cases.

▸ Child 1 month–11 years (body-weight up to 50 kg): 50–100 mg/kg once daily, doses at the higher end of the recommended range used in severe cases; maximum 4 g per day

▸ Child 9–11 years (body-weight 50 kg and above): 2 g once daily

▸ Child 12–17 years: 2 g once daily
▸ BY INTRAVENOUS INJECTION

▸ Child 9–11 years (body-weight 50 kg and above): 2 g once daily

▸ Child 12–17 years: 2 g once daily
▸ BY DEEP INTRAMUSCULAR INJECTION

▸ Child 1 month–11 years (body-weight up to 50 kg): 50–100 mg/kg once daily, doses at the higher end of the recommended range used in severe cases; maximum 4 g per day

▸ Child 9–11 years (body-weight 50 kg and above): 2 g once daily

▸ Child 12–17 years: 2 g once daily

Suspected bacterial infection in neutropenic patients
▸ BY INTRAVENOUS INFUSION

▸ Neonate up to 15 days: 20–50 mg/kg once daily, doses at the higher end of the recommended range used in severe cases.

▸ Neonate 15 days to 28 days: 50–100 mg/kg once daily, doses at the higher end of the recommended range used in severe cases.

▸ Child 1 month–11 years (body-weight up to 50 kg): 50–100 mg/kg once daily, doses at the higher end of the recommended range used in severe cases; maximum 4 g per day

▸ Child 9–11 years (body-weight 50 kg and above): 2–4 g once daily, doses at the higher end of the recommended range used in severe cases

▸ Child 12–17 years: 2–4 g once daily, doses at the higher end of the recommended range used in severe cases
▸ BY INTRAVENOUS INJECTION

▸ Child 9–11 years (body-weight 50 kg and above): 2–4 g once daily, doses at the higher end of the recommended range used in severe cases

▸ Child 12–17 years: 2–4 g once daily, doses at the higher end of the recommended range used in severe cases
▸ BY DEEP INTRAMUSCULAR INJECTION

▸ Child 1 month–11 years (body-weight up to 50 kg): 50–100 mg/kg once daily, doses at the higher end of the recommended range used in severe cases; maximum 4 g per day

▸ Child 9–11 years (body-weight 50 kg and above): 2–4 g once daily, doses at the higher end of the recommended range used in severe cases

▸ Child 12–17 years: 2–4 g once daily, doses at the higher end of the recommended range used in severe cases

Bacterial meningitis | Bacterial endocarditis

▶ BY INTRAVENOUS INFUSION

▸ Neonate up to 15 days: 50 mg/kg once daily.

▸ Neonate 15 days to 28 days: 80–100 mg/kg once daily, 100 mg/kg once daily dose should be used for bacterial endocarditis.

▸ Child 1 month–11 years (body-weight up to 50 kg): 80–100 mg/kg once daily, 100 mg/kg once daily dose should be used for bacterial endocarditis; maximum 4 g per day

▸ Child 9–11 years (body-weight 50 kg and above): 2–4 g once daily, doses at the higher end of the recommended range used in severe cases

▸ Child 12–17 years: 2–4 g once daily, doses at the higher end of the recommended range used in severe cases

▶ BY INTRAVENOUS INJECTION

▸ Child 9–11 years (body-weight 50 kg and above): 2–4 g once daily, doses at the higher end of the recommended range used in severe cases

▸ Child 12–17 years: 2–4 g once daily, doses at the higher end of the recommended range used in severe cases

▶ BY DEEP INTRAMUSCULAR INJECTION

▸ Child 1 month–11 years (body-weight up to 50 kg): 80–100 mg/kg once daily, 100 mg/kg once daily dose should be used for bacterial endocarditis; maximum 4 g per day

▸ Child 9–11 years (body-weight 50 kg and above): 2–4 g once daily, doses at the higher end of the recommended range used in severe cases

▸ Child 12–17 years: 2–4 g once daily, doses at the higher end of the recommended range used in severe cases

Surgical prophylaxis

▶ BY INTRAVENOUS INFUSION

▸ Neonate up to 15 days: 20–50 mg/kg for 1 dose, dose to be administered 30–90 minutes before procedure.

▸ Neonate 15 days to 28 days: 50–80 mg/kg for 1 dose, dose to be administered 30–90 minutes before procedure.

▸ Child 1 month–11 years (body-weight up to 50 kg): 50–80 mg/kg for 1 dose, dose to be administered 30–90 minutes before procedure; maximum 4 g per day

▸ Child 9–11 years (body-weight 50 kg and above): 2 g for 1 dose, dose to be administered 30–90 minutes before procedure

▸ Child 12–17 years: 2 g for 1 dose, dose to be administered 30–90 minutes before procedure

▶ BY INTRAVENOUS INJECTION

▸ Child 9–11 years (body-weight 50 kg and above): 2 g for 1 dose, dose to be administered 30–90 minutes before procedure

▸ Child 12–17 years: 2 g for 1 dose, dose to be administered 30–90 minutes before procedure

▶ BY DEEP INTRAMUSCULAR INJECTION

▸ Child 1 month–11 years (body-weight up to 50 kg): 50–80 mg/kg for 1 dose, dose to be administered 30–90 minutes before procedure; maximum 4 g per day

▸ Child 9–11 years (body-weight 50 kg and above): 2 g for 1 dose, dose to be administered 30–90 minutes before procedure

▸ Child 12–17 years: 2 g for 1 dose, dose to be administered 30–90 minutes before procedure

Uncomplicated gonorrhoea | Pelvic inflammatory disease

▶ BY DEEP INTRAMUSCULAR INJECTION

▸ Child 1 month–11 years (body-weight up to 45 kg): 125 mg for 1 dose

▸ Child 9–11 years (body-weight 45 kg and above): 250 mg for 1 dose

▸ Child 12–17 years: 500 mg for 1 dose

Syphilis

▶ BY INTRAVENOUS INFUSION

▸ Neonate up to 15 days: 50 mg/kg once daily for 10–14 days.

▸ Neonate 15 days to 28 days: 75–100 mg/kg once daily for 10–14 days.

▸ Child 1 month–11 years (body-weight up to 50 kg): 75–100 mg/kg once daily for 10–14 days; maximum 4 g per day

▸ Child 9–11 years (body-weight 50 kg and above): 0.5–1 g once daily for 10–14 days, dose can be increased to 2 g once daily for neurosyphilis

▸ Child 12–17 years: 0.5–1 g once daily for 10–14 days, dose can be increased to 2 g once daily for neurosyphilis

▶ BY INTRAVENOUS INJECTION

▸ Child 9–11 years (body-weight 50 kg and above): 0.5–1 g once daily for 10–14 days, dose can be increased to 2 g once daily for neurosyphilis

▸ Child 12–17 years: 0.5–1 g once daily for 10–14 days, dose can be increased to 2 g once daily for neurosyphilis

▶ BY DEEP INTRAMUSCULAR INJECTION

▸ Child 1 month–11 years (body-weight up to 50 kg): 75–100 mg/kg once daily for 10–14 days; maximum 4 g per day

▸ Child 9–11 years (body-weight 50 kg and above): 0.5–1 g once daily for 10–14 days, dose can be increased to 2 g once daily for neurosyphilis

▸ Child 12–17 years: 0.5–1 g once daily for 10–14 days, dose can be increased to 2 g once daily for neurosyphilis

Disseminated Lyme borreliosis (early [Stage II] and late [Stage III]

▶ BY INTRAVENOUS INFUSION

▸ Neonate 15 days to 28 days: 50–80 mg/kg once daily for 14–21 days, the recommended treatment durations vary and national or local guidelines should be taken into consideration.

▸ Child 1 month–11 years (body-weight up to 50 kg): 50–80 mg/kg once daily for 14–21 days, the recommended treatment durations vary and national or local guidelines should be taken into consideration; maximum 4 g per day

▸ Child 9–11 years (body-weight 50 kg and above): 2 g once daily for 14–21 days, the recommended treatment durations vary and national or local guidelines should be taken into consideration

▸ Child 12–17 years: 2 g once daily for 14–21 days, the recommended treatment durations vary and national or local guidelines should be taken into consideration

▶ BY INTRAVENOUS INJECTION

▸ Child 9–11 years (body-weight 50 kg and above): 2 g once daily for 14–21 days, the recommended treatment durations vary and national or local guidelines should be taken into consideration

▸ Child 12–17 years: 2 g once daily for 14–21 days, the recommended treatment durations vary and national or local guidelines should be taken into consideration

▶ BY DEEP INTRAMUSCULAR INJECTION

▸ Child 1 month–11 years (body-weight up to 50 kg): 50–80 mg/kg once daily for 14–21 days, the recommended treatment durations vary and national or local guidelines should be taken into consideration; maximum 4 g per day

▸ Child 9–11 years (body-weight 50 kg and above): 2 g once daily for 14–21 days, the recommended treatment durations vary and national or local guidelines should be taken into consideration continued →

- Child 12–17 years: 2 g once daily for 14–21 days, the recommended treatment durations vary and national or local guidelines should be taken into consideration

Congenital gonococcal conjunctivitis

▶ BY DEEP INTRAMUSCULAR INJECTION, OR BY INTRAVENOUS INFUSION

- Neonate: 25–50 mg/kg (max. per dose 125 mg) for 1 dose, intravenous infusion to be administered over 60 minutes.

Prevention of secondary case of meningococcal meningitis

▶ BY INTRAMUSCULAR INJECTION

- Child 1 month–11 years: 125 mg for 1 dose
- Child 12–17 years: 250 mg for 1 dose

Prevention of secondary case of *Haemophilus influenzae* type b disease

▶ BY INTRAVENOUS INFUSION

- Child 1 month–11 years: 50 mg/kg daily (max. per dose 1 g) for 2 days

▶ BY INTRAMUSCULAR INJECTION, OR BY INTRAVENOUS INJECTION

- Child 12–17 years: 1 g daily for 2 days

Acute otitis media

▶ BY INTRAMUSCULAR INJECTION

- Child 1 month–11 years (body-weight up to 50 kg): 50 mg/kg for 1 dose, dose can be given for 3 days if severely ill or previous therapy failed
- Child 9-11 years (body-weight 50 kg and above): 1–2 g for 1 dose, dose can be given for 3 days if severely ill or previous therapy failed
- Child 12–17 years: 1–2 g for 1 dose, dose can be given for 3 days if severely ill or previous therapy failed

● **UNLICENSED USE** EvGr Not licensed for prophylaxis of *Haemophilus influenzae* type b disease. ⟨E⟩ Not licensed for prophylaxis of meningococcal meningitis.
  EvGr Not licensed for congenital gonococcal conjunctivitis. ⟨E⟩
  EvGr Not licensed for use in children under 12 years of age for uncomplicated gonorrhoea. ⟨E⟩
  EvGr Not licensed for use in children for pelvic inflammatory disease. ⟨E⟩

● **CONTRA-INDICATIONS** Concomitant treatment with intravenous calcium (including total parenteral nutrition containing calcium) in neonates over 41 weeks corrected gestational age—risk of precipitation in urine and lungs · neonates less than 41 weeks corrected gestational age · neonates over 41 weeks corrected gestational age with jaundice, hypoalbuminaemia, acidosis, unconjugated hyperbilirubinaemia, or impaired bilirubin binding

● **CAUTIONS** History of hypercalciuria · history of kidney stones · use with caution in neonates

● **SIDE-EFFECTS**

▶ **Common or very common** Calcium ceftriaxone precipitates in gall bladder—consider discontinuation if symptomatic · calcium ceftriaxone precipitates in urine (particularly in very young, dehydrated or those who are immobilised)—consider discontinuation if symptomatic

▶ **Rare** Pancreatitis · prolongation of prothrombin time

● **PREGNANCY** Not known to be harmful.

● **BREAST FEEDING** Present in milk in low concentration, but appropriate to use.

● **HEPATIC IMPAIRMENT** Reduce dose if both hepatic and severe renal impairment. Monitor plasma concentration if both hepatic and severe renal impairment.

● **RENAL IMPAIRMENT** Max. 50 mg/kg daily (max. 2 g daily) in severe renal impairment. Use with caution in renal failure. Monitor plasma concentration if both hepatic and severe renal impairment.

● **DIRECTIONS FOR ADMINISTRATION**

▶ With intravenous use For *intravenous infusion* (preferred route), dilute reconstituted solution with Glucose 5% (or 10% in neonates) *or* Sodium Chloride 0.9%; give over at least 30 minutes (60 minutes in neonates—may displace bilirubin from serum albumin). Not to be given simultaneously with parenteral nutrition or infusion fluids containing calcium, even by different infusion lines; in children, may be infused sequentially with infusion fluids containing calcium if flush with sodium chloride 0.9% between infusions or give infusions by different infusion lines at different sites. Displacement value may be significant, consult local guidelines.
  For *intravenous injection*, give over 5 minutes; intravenous doses of 50 mg/kg or more in children under 12 years should be given by infusion.

▶ With intramuscular use or intravenous use Twice daily dosing may be considered for doses greater than 2 g daily.

▶ With intramuscular use For *intramuscular injection*, may be mixed with 1% Lidocaine Hydrochloride Injection to reduce pain at intramuscular injection site. Intramuscular injection should only be considered when the intravenous route is not possible or less appropriate. If administered by intramuscular injection, the lower end of the dose range should be used for the shortest time possible; volume depends on the age and size of the child, but doses over 1 g must be divided between more than one site. The maximum intramuscular dose is 2 g, doses greater than 2 g must be given by intravenous infusion or intravenous injection (see above). Displacement value may be significant, consult local guidelines.

● **MEDICINAL FORMS**
There can be variation in the licensing of different medicines containing the same drug. Forms available from special-order manufacturers include: infusion

Powder for solution for injection
ELECTROLYTES: May contain Sodium

▶ Ceftriaxone (Non-proprietary)
  Ceftriaxone (as Ceftriaxone sodium) 250 mg Ceftriaxone 250mg powder for solution for injection vials | 1 vial PoM £1.80–£2.30 DT price = £2.40
  Ceftriaxone (as Ceftriaxone sodium) 1 gram Ceftriaxone 1g powder for solution for injection vials | 1 vial PoM no price available DT price = £9.58 | 5 vial PoM £45.75 | 10 vial PoM £11.00
  Ceftriaxone (as Ceftriaxone sodium) 2 gram Ceftriaxone 2g powder for solution for injection vials | 1 vial PoM £18.00 DT price = £19.18 | 10 vial PoM £21.00

▶ Rocephin (Roche Products Ltd)
  Ceftriaxone (as Ceftriaxone sodium) 250 mg Rocephin 250mg powder for solution for injection vials | 1 vial PoM £2.40 DT price = £2.40
  Ceftriaxone (as Ceftriaxone sodium) 1 gram Rocephin 1g powder for solution for injection vials | 1 vial PoM £9.58 DT price = £9.58
  Ceftriaxone (as Ceftriaxone sodium) 2 gram Rocephin 2g powder for solution for injection vials | 1 vial PoM £19.18 DT price = £19.18

ANTIBACTERIALS > GLYCOPEPTIDE
ANTIBACTERIALS

Teicoplanin

- **DRUG ACTION** The glycopeptide antibiotic teicoplanin has bactericidal activity against aerobic and anaerobic Gram-positive bacteria including multi-resistant staphylococci. However, there are reports of *Staphylococcus aureus* with reduced susceptibility to glycopeptides and increasing reports of glycopeptide-resistant enterococci. Teicoplanin is similar to vancomycin, but has a significantly longer duration of action, allowing once daily administration after the loading dose.

- **INDICATIONS AND DOSE**
Surgical prophylaxis
  ▸ BY INTRAVENOUS INJECTION
  ▸ Child: (consult local protocol)
Potentially serious Gram-positive infections including endocarditis, and serious infections due to *Staphylococcus aureus*
  ▸ INITIALLY BY INTRAVENOUS INJECTION, OR BY INTRAVENOUS INFUSION
  ▸ Neonate: Initially 16 mg/kg for 1 dose, followed by (by intravenous infusion) 8 mg/kg once daily, subsequent dose to be administered 24 hours after initial dose.
  ▸ Child: Initially 10 mg/kg every 12 hours (max. per dose 400 mg) for 3 doses, then (by intravenous injection or by intravenous infusion or by intramuscular injection) 6 mg/kg once daily (max. per dose 400 mg), (After initial 3 doses subsequent doses can be given by intramuscular route, if necessary, although, intravenous route is preferable)
Severe Gram-positive infections (including burns, septicaemia, septic arthritis and osteomyelitis)
  ▸ BY INTRAVENOUS INJECTION, OR BY INTRAVENOUS INFUSION
  ▸ Child: Initially 10 mg/kg every 12 hours for 3 doses, then 10 mg/kg once daily
PHARMACOKINETICS
Teicoplanin should **not** be given by mouth for systemic infections because it is not absorbed significantly.

- **UNLICENSED USE** Not licensed for surgical prophylaxis.
- **INTERACTIONS** → Appendix 1 (teicoplanin).
If other nephrotoxic or neurotoxic drugs given, monitor renal and auditory function on prolonged administration.
- **SIDE-EFFECTS**
▸ **Common or very common** Pruritus · rash
▸ **Uncommon** Bronchospasm · diarrhoea · dizziness · eosinophilia · fever · headache · leucopenia · mild hearing loss · nausea · thrombocytopenia · thrombophlebitis · tinnitus · vestibular disorders · vomiting
▸ **Frequency not known** Exfoliative dermatitis · nephrotoxicity · renal failure · Stevens-Johnson syndrome · toxic epidermal necrolysis
SIDE-EFFECTS, FURTHER INFORMATION
▸ Nephrotoxicity Teicoplanin is associated with a lower incidence of nephrotoxicity than vancomycin.
- **ALLERGY AND CROSS-SENSITIVITY** Caution if history of vancomycin sensitivity.
- **PREGNANCY** Manufacturer advises use only if potential benefit outweighs risk.
- **BREAST FEEDING** No information available.
- **RENAL IMPAIRMENT** Use normal dose regimen on days 1–4, then use normal maintenance dose every 48 hours if estimated glomerular filtration rate 30–80 mL/minute/1.73 m² and use normal maintenance dose every 72 hours if estimated glomerular filtration rate less than 30 mL/minute/1.73 m². Plasma-teicoplanin

concentration should be monitored during parenteral maintenance treatment. Also monitor renal and auditory function during prolonged treatment in renal impairment.
- **MONITORING REQUIREMENTS**
▸ With intramuscular use or intravenous use Plasma-teicoplanin concentration is not measured routinely because a relationship between plasma concentration and toxicity has not been established. However, the plasma-teicoplanin concentration can be used to optimise parenteral treatment in severe sepsis or burns, deep-seated staphylococcal infection (including bone and joint infection), endocarditis, and in intravenous drug abusers. Pre-dose ('trough') concentrations should be greater than 15 mg/litre (greater than 20 mg/litre in endocarditis or deep-seated infection such as bone and joint infection), but less than 60 mg/litre.
▸ Blood counts and liver and kidney function tests required.
- **DIRECTIONS FOR ADMINISTRATION**
▸ With intravenous use For intermittent intravenous infusion, dilute reconstituted solution further in sodium chloride 0.9% *or* glucose 5%; give over 30 minutes. Intermittent intravenous infusion preferred in neonates.

- **MEDICINAL FORMS**
There can be variation in the licensing of different medicines containing the same drug. Forms available from special-order manufacturers include: solution for injection
Powder and solvent for solution for injection
ELECTROLYTES: May contain Sodium
  ▸ Targocid (Sanofi) ▼
  Teicoplanin 200 mg Targocid 200mg powder and solvent for solution for injection vials | 1 vial PoM £3.93
  Teicoplanin 400 mg Targocid 400mg powder and solvent for solution for injection vials | 1 vial PoM £7.32

Vancomycin

- **DRUG ACTION** The glycopeptide antibiotic vancomycin has bactericidal activity against aerobic and anaerobic Gram-positive bacteria including multi-resistant staphylococci. However, there are reports of *Staphylococcus aureus* with reduced susceptibility to glycopeptides. There are increasing reports of glycopeptide-resistant enterococci. Penetration into cerebrospinal fluid is poor.

- **INDICATIONS AND DOSE**
***Clostridium difficile* infection**
  ▸ BY MOUTH
  ▸ Child 1 month-4 years: 5 mg/kg 4 times a day for 10–14 days, dose may be increased if infection fails to respond or is life-threatening, increased if necessary up to 10 mg/kg 4 times a day
  ▸ Child 5-11 years: 62.5 mg 4 times a day for 10–14 days, dose may be increased if infection fails to respond or is life-threatening, increased if necessary up to 250 mg 4 times a day
  ▸ Child 12-17 years: 125 mg 4 times a day for 10–14 days, dose may be increased if infection fails to respond or is life-threatening, increased if necessary up to 500 mg 4 times a day
Infections due to Gram-positive bacteria including endocarditis, osteomyelitis, septicaemia and soft-tissue infections
  ▸ BY INTRAVENOUS INFUSION
  ▸ Neonate up to 29 weeks corrected gestational age: 15 mg/kg every 24 hours adjusted according to plasma-concentration monitoring.
  ▸ Neonate 29 weeks to 35 weeks corrected gestational age: 15 mg/kg every 12 hours adjusted according to plasma-concentration monitoring.

continued →

▸ Neonate 35 weeks corrected gestational age and above: 15 mg/kg every 8 hours adjusted according to plasma-concentration monitoring.

▸ Child: 15 mg/kg every 8 hours adjusted according to plasma-concentration monitoring; maximum 2 g per day

Surgical prophylaxis (when high risk of MRSA)
▸ BY INTRAVENOUS INFUSION
▸ Child: (consult local protocol)

CNS infection e.g. ventriculitis (administered on expert advice)
▸ BY INTRAVENTRICULAR ADMINISTRATION
▸ Neonate: 10 mg every 24 hours.

▸ Child: 10 mg every 24 hours, for all children reduce to 5 mg daily if ventricular size reduced or increase to 15–20 mg once daily if ventricular size increased, adjust dose according to CSF concentration after 3–4 days; aim for pre-dose ('trough') concentration less than 10 mg/litre. If CSF not draining free reduce dose frequency to once every 2–3 days

Peritonitis associated with peritoneal dialysis
▸ BY INTRAPERITONEAL ADMINISTRATION
▸ Child: Add to each bag of dialysis fluid to achieve a concentration of 20–25 mg/litre

Eradication of meticillin-resistant *Staphylococcus aureus* from the respiratory tract in cystic fibrosis
▸ BY INHALATION OF NEBULISED SOLUTION
▸ Child: 4 mg/kg twice daily (max. per dose 250 mg) for 5 days, alternatively 4 mg/kg 4 times a day (max. per dose 250 mg) for 5 days

PHARMACOKINETICS
Vancomycin should **not** be given by mouth for systemic infections because it is not absorbed significantly.

● UNLICENSED USE Vancomycin doses in BNF publications may differ from those in product literature. Use of vancomycin (added to dialysis fluid) for the treatment of peritonitis associated with peritoneal dialysis is an unlicensed route.
Not licensed for intraventricular use or inhalation.
Not licensed for use by the *intrathecal* route for the treatment of meningitis.

> **IMPORTANT SAFETY INFORMATION**
> SAFE PRACTICE
> For intraventricular administration, seek specialist advice.

● CAUTIONS
GENERAL CAUTIONS
Avoid if history of deafness
SPECIFIC CAUTIONS
▸ With oral use Systemic absorption may follow oral administration especially in inflammatory bowel disorders or following multiple doses

● INTERACTIONS → Appendix 1 (vancomycin).

● SIDE-EFFECTS
▸ Common or very common
▸ With intravenous use Blood disorders, including neutropenia (usually after 1 week or high cumulative dose) · interstitial nephritis · nephrotoxicity · ototoxicity (discontinue if tinnitus occurs) · renal failure
▸ Rare
▸ With intravenous use Agranulocytosis · thrombocytopenia
▸ Frequency not known
▸ With intravenous use Anaphylaxis · cardiac arrest on rapid infusion · chills · dyspnoea · eosinophilia · exfoliative dermatitis · fever · flushing of the upper body ('red man' syndrome) · nausea · pain and muscle spasm of back and chest · phlebitis (irritant to tissue) · pruritus · rashes ·

severe hypotension on rapid infusion · shock on rapid infusion · Stevens-Johnson syndrome · toxic epidermal necrolysis · urticaria · vasculitis · wheezing

SIDE-EFFECTS, FURTHER INFORMATION
▸ Nephrotoxicity Vancomycin is associated with a higher incidence of nephrotoxicity than teicoplanin.

● ALLERGY AND CROSS-SENSITIVITY Caution if teicoplanin sensitivity.

● PREGNANCY Manufacturer advises use only if potential benefit outweighs risk.
Plasma-vancomycin concentration monitoring essential to reduce risk of fetal toxicity.

● BREAST FEEDING Present in milk—significant absorption following oral administration unlikely.

● RENAL IMPAIRMENT Reduce dose. In renal impairment monitor plasma-vancomycin concentration and renal function regularly. Also monitor auditory function.

● MONITORING REQUIREMENTS
▸ All patients require plasma-vancomycin measurement (after 3 or 4 doses if renal function normal, earlier if renal impairment).
▸ All patients require blood counts, urinalysis, and renal function tests.
▸ With intravenous use Pre-dose ('trough') concentration should be 10–15 mg/litre (15–20 mg/litre for less sensitive strains of meticillin-resistant *Staphylococcus aureus*).
▸ With intraventricular use Aim for pre-dose ('trough') concentration less than 10 mg/litre.
▸ When used by inhalation Measure lung function before and after initial dose of vancomycin and monitor for bronchospasm.

● DIRECTIONS FOR ADMINISTRATION
▸ With intravenous use Avoid rapid infusion (risk of anaphylactoid reactions) and rotate infusion sites. Displacement value may be significant, consult product literature and local guidelines. For intermittent intravenous infusion, the reconstituted preparation should be further diluted in sodium chloride 0.9% *or* glucose 5% to a concentration of up to 5 mg/mL; give over at least 60 minutes (rate not to exceed 10 mg/minute for doses over 500 mg); use continuous infusion only if intermittent not available (limited evidence); 10 mg/mL can be used if infused via a central venous line over at least 1 hour.
▸ With oral use Injection can be used to prepare solution for oral administration; flavouring syrups may be added to the solution at the time of administration.
▸ When used by inhalation *For nebulisation* administer required dose in 4 mL of sodium chloride 0.9% (or water for injections). Administer inhaled bronchodilator before vancomycin.

● MEDICINAL FORMS
There can be variation in the licensing of different medicines containing the same drug. Forms available from special-order manufacturers include: oral suspension, oral solution, pastille, solution for injection, infusion

Capsule
CAUTIONARY AND ADVISORY LABELS 9
▸ Vancomycin (Non-proprietary)
Vancomycin (as Vancomycin hydrochloride) 125 mg Vancomycin 125mg capsules | 28 capsule [PoM] £132.47 DT price = £132.47
Vancomycin (as Vancomycin hydrochloride) 250 mg Vancomycin 250mg capsules | 28 capsule [PoM] £140.08 DT price = £140.08
▸ Vancocin Matrigel (Flynn Pharma Ltd)
Vancomycin (as Vancomycin hydrochloride) 125 mg Vancocin Matrigel 125mg capsules | 28 capsule [PoM] £88.31 DT price = £132.47

Powder for solution for infusion

▶ Vancomycin (Non-proprietary)

Vancomycin (as Vancomycin hydrochloride) 500 mg Vancomycin 500mg powder for solution for infusion vials | 1 vial [PoM] £7.25 (Hospital only) | 1 vial [PoM] £7.25
Vancomycin 500mg powder for concentrate for solution for infusion vials | 1 vial [PoM] £8.50
Vancomycin (as Vancomycin hydrochloride) 1 gram Vancomycin 1g powder for solution for infusion vials | 1 vial [PoM] £14.50 (Hospital only) | 1 vial [PoM] £17.25
Vancomycin 1g powder for concentrate for solution for infusion vials | 1 vial [PoM] £17.25

▶ Vancocin (Flynn Pharma Ltd)

Vancomycin (as Vancomycin hydrochloride) 500 mg Vancocin 500mg powder for solution for infusion vials | 1 vial [PoM] £6.25
Vancomycin (as Vancomycin hydrochloride) 1 gram Vancocin 1g powder for solution for infusion vials | 1 vial [PoM] £12.50

ANTIBACTERIALS > LINCOSAMIDES

Clindamycin

● **DRUG ACTION**
▶ With systemic use Clindamycin is active against Gram-positive cocci, including streptococci and penicillin-resistant staphylococci, and also against many anaerobes, especially *Bacteroides fragilis*. It is well concentrated in bone and excreted in bile and urine.

● **INDICATIONS AND DOSE**

Staphylococcal bone and joint infections such as osteomyelitis | Peritonitis | Intra-abdominal sepsis | Meticillin-resistant *Staphylococcus aureus* (MRSA) in bronchiectasis, bone and joint infections, and skin and soft-tissue infections | Erysipelas or cellulitis in penicillin-allergic patients (alternative to macrolides)
▶ BY MOUTH

▶ Neonate up to 14 days: 3–6 mg/kg 3 times a day.

▶ Neonate 14 days to 28 days: 3–6 mg/kg 4 times a day.

▶ Child: 3–6 mg/kg 4 times a day (max. per dose 450 mg)
▶ BY DEEP INTRAMUSCULAR INJECTION, OR BY INTRAVENOUS INFUSION

▶ Child: 3.75–6.25 mg/kg 4 times a day; increased if necessary up to 10 mg/kg 4 times a day (max. per dose 1.2 g), increased dose used for severe infections, total daily dose may alternatively be given in 3 divided doses, single doses above 600 mg to be administered by intravenous infusion only, single doses by intravenous infusion not to exceed 1.2 g

Staphylococcal lung infection in cystic fibrosis
▶ BY MOUTH

▶ Child: 5–7 mg/kg 4 times a day (max. per dose 600 mg)

Treatment of falciparum malaria (to be given with or following quinine)
▶ BY MOUTH

▶ Child: 7–13 mg/kg every 8 hours (max. per dose 450 mg) for 7 days

● **UNLICENSED USE** Not licensed for treatment of falciparum malaria.

● **CONTRA-INDICATIONS** Avoid injections containing benzyl alcohol in neonates · diarrhoeal states

● **CAUTIONS** Avoid in Acute porphyrias p. 562

● **INTERACTIONS** → Appendix 1 (clindamycin).

● **SIDE-EFFECTS**
▶ With intramuscular use Abscess · induration · pain
▶ With intravenous use Thrombophlebitis
▶ With systemic use Abdominal discomfort · anaphylactoid reactions · antibiotic-associated colitis · diarrhoea (discontinue treatment) · eosinophilia · exfoliative dermatitis · jaundice · leucopenia · nausea · oesophageal ulcers · oesophagitis · polyarthritis · pruritus · rash ·

Stevens-Johnson syndrome · taste disturbances · thrombocytopenia · toxic epidermal necrolysis · urticaria · vesiculobullous dermatitis · vomiting

SIDE-EFFECTS, FURTHER INFORMATION
▶ Antibiotic-associated colitis Clindamycin has been associated with antibiotic-associated colitis, which may be fatal. Although antibiotic-associated colitis can occur with most antibacterials, it occurs more frequently with clindamycin. Patients should therefore discontinue treatment immediately if diarrhoea develops.

● **PREGNANCY** Not known to be harmful.

● **BREAST FEEDING** Amount probably too small to be harmful but bloody diarrhoea reported in 1 infant.

● **MONITORING REQUIREMENTS**
▶ Monitor liver and renal function if treatment exceeds 10 days.
▶ Monitor liver and renal function in neonates and infants.

● **DIRECTIONS FOR ADMINISTRATION**
▶ With intravenous use Avoid rapid intravenous administration.
▶ With intravenous use For *intravenous infusion*, dilute to a concentration of not more than 18 mg/mL with Glucose 5% or Sodium Chloride 0.9%; give over 10–60 minutes at a max. rate of 20 mg/kg/hour.

● **PATIENT AND CARER ADVICE** Capsules should be swallowed with a glass of water. Patients and their carers should be advised to discontinue immediately and contact doctor if diarrhoea develops.

● **PROFESSION SPECIFIC INFORMATION**
Dental practitioners' formulary
Clindamycin capsules may be prescribed.

● **MEDICINAL FORMS**
There can be variation in the licensing of different medicines containing the same drug. Forms available from special-order manufacturers include: oral suspension, oral solution

Capsule
CAUTIONARY AND ADVISORY LABELS 9, 27
▶ Clindamycin (Non-proprietary)

Clindamycin (as Clindamycin hydrochloride) 150 mg Clindamycin 150mg capsules | 24 capsule [PoM] £48.00 DT price = £12.00 | 100 capsule [PoM] £60.00
Clindamycin (as Clindamycin hydrochloride) 300 mg Clindamycin 300mg capsules | 30 capsule [PoM] £38.96 DT price = £37.46

▶ Dalacin C (Pfizer Ltd)

Clindamycin (as Clindamycin hydrochloride) 75 mg Dalacin C 75mg capsules | 24 capsule [PoM] £7.45 DT price = £7.45
Clindamycin (as Clindamycin hydrochloride) 150 mg Dalacin C 150mg capsules | 24 capsule [PoM] £13.72 DT price = £12.00 | 100 capsule [PoM] £55.08

Solution for injection
EXCIPIENTS: May contain Benzyl alcohol
▶ Clindamycin (Non-proprietary)

Clindamycin (as Clindamycin phosphate) 150 mg per 1 ml Clindamycin 600mg/4ml solution for injection ampoules | 5 ampoule [PoM] £61.75
Clindamycin 300mg/2ml solution for injection ampoules | 5 ampoule [PoM] £28.50–£31.01

▶ Dalacin C (Pfizer Ltd)

Clindamycin (as Clindamycin phosphate) 150 mg per 1 ml Dalacin C Phosphate 300mg/2ml solution for injection ampoules | 5 ampoule [PoM] £31.01
Dalacin C Phosphate 600mg/4ml solution for injection ampoules | 5 ampoule [PoM] £61.75

ANTIBACTERIALS > MACROLIDES

Macrolides

Overview

The macrolides have an antibacterial spectrum that is similar but not identical to that of penicillin; they are thus an alternative in penicillin-allergic patients. They are active against many-penicillin-resistant staphylococci, but some are now also resistant to the macrolides.

Indications for the macrolides include campylobacter enteritis, respiratory infections (including pneumonia, whooping cough, Legionella, chlamydia, and mycoplasma infection), and skin infections.

Erythromycin p. 310 is also used in the treatment of early syphilis, uncomplicated genital chlamydial infection, and non-gonococcal urethritis. Erythromycin has poor activity against *Haemophilus influenzae*. Erythromycin causes nausea, vomiting, and diarrhoea in some patients; in mild to moderate infections this can be avoided by giving a lower dose or the total dose in 4 divided doses, but if a more serious infection, such as Legionella pneumonia, is suspected higher doses are needed.

Azithromycin below is a macrolide with slightly less activity than erythromycin against Gram-positive bacteria, but enhanced activity against some Gram-negative organisms including *H. influenzae*. Plasma concentrations are very low, but tissue concentrations are much higher. It has a long tissue half-life and once daily dosage is recommended. Azithromycin is also used in the treatment of uncomplicated genital chlamydial infection, non-gonococcal urethritis, typhoid [unlicensed indication], and trachoma [unlicensed indication].

Clarithromycin p. 309 is an erythromycin derivative with slightly greater activity than the parent compound. Tissue concentrations are higher than with erythromycin. It is given twice daily. Clarithromycin is also used in regimens for *Helicobacter pylori* eradication.

Erythromycin, azithromycin, and clarithromycin have a role in the treatment of Lyme disease p. 339.

Spiramycin is also a macrolide which is used for the treatment of toxoplasmosis.

Macrolides ⊝

- ● CAUTIONS
- ▸ With intravenous use Electrolyte disturbances (predisposition to QT interval prolongation) · may aggravate myasthenia gravis · predisposition to QT interval prolongation
- ▸ With oral use Electrolyte disturbances (predisposition to QT interval prolongation) · may aggravate myasthenia gravis · predisposition to QT interval prolongation
- ● SIDE-EFFECTS
- ▸ Common or very common
- ▸ With intravenous use Abdominal discomfort · diarrhoea · nausea · vomiting
- ▸ With oral use Abdominal discomfort · diarrhoea · nausea · vomiting
- ▸ Uncommon
- ▸ With intravenous use Cholestatic jaundice · hepatotoxicity · rash
- ▸ With oral use Cholestatic jaundice · hepatotoxicity · rash
- ▸ Rare
- ▸ With intravenous use Antibiotic-associated colitis · arrhythmias · pancreatitis · QT interval prolongation · Stevens-Johnson syndrome · toxic epidermal necrolysis
- ▸ With oral use Antibiotic-associated colitis · arrhythmias · pancreatitis · QT interval prolongation · Stevens-Johnson syndrome · toxic epidermal necrolysis
- ▸ Frequency not known
- ▸ With intravenous use Local tenderness · phlebitis · reversible hearing loss (sometimes with tinnitus) can occur after large doses
- ▸ With oral use Reversible hearing loss (sometimes with tinnitus) can occur after large doses

SIDE-EFFECTS, FURTHER INFORMATION
- ▸ With intravenous use or oral use Gastro-intestinal side-effects are mild and less frequent with azithromycin and clarithromycin than with erythromycin.

▶ above

Azithromycin

- ● INDICATIONS AND DOSE

Prevention of secondary case of invasive group A streptococcal infection in patients who are allergic to penicillin
- ▸ BY MOUTH
- ▸ Child 6 months–11 years: 12 mg/kg once daily (max. per dose 500 mg) for 5 days
- ▸ Child 12–17 years: 500 mg once daily for 5 days

Respiratory-tract infections, otitis media, skin and soft-tissue infections
- ▸ BY MOUTH
- ▸ Child 6 months–17 years: 10 mg/kg once daily (max. per dose 500 mg) for 3 days
- ▸ Child 6 months–17 years (body-weight 15–25 kg): 200 mg once daily for 3 days
- ▸ Child 6 months–17 years (body-weight 26–35 kg): 300 mg once daily for 3 days
- ▸ Child 6 months–17 years (body-weight 36–45 kg): 400 mg once daily for 3 days
- ▸ Child 6 months–17 years (body-weight 46 kg and above): 500 mg once daily for 3 days

Infection in cystic fibrosis
- ▸ BY MOUTH
- ▸ Child 6 months–17 years: 10 mg/kg once daily (max. per dose 500 mg) for 3 days, repeated after 1 week to complete course, treatment may be repeated as necessary

Chronic *Pseudomonas aeruginosa* infection in cystic fibrosis
- ▸ BY MOUTH
- ▸ Child 6–17 years (body-weight 25–40 kg): 250 mg 3 times a week
- ▸ Child 6–17 years (body-weight 41 kg and above): 500 mg 3 times a week

Uncomplicated genital chlamydial infections | Non-gonococcal urethritis
- ▸ BY MOUTH
- ▸ Child 12–17 years: 1 g for 1 dose

Lyme disease (under expert supervision)
- ▸ BY MOUTH
- ▸ Child 6 months–17 years: 10 mg/kg once daily (max. per dose 500 mg) for 7–10 days

Mild to moderate typhoid due to multiple-antibacterial resistant organisms
- ▸ BY MOUTH
- ▸ Child 6 months–17 years: 10 mg/kg once daily (max. per dose 500 mg) for 7 days

- ● UNLICENSED USE Not licensed for typhoid fever, Lyme disease, chronic *Pseudomonas aeruginosa* infection in cystic fibrosis, or prophylaxis of group A streptococcal infection.

- ● INTERACTIONS → Appendix 1 (macrolides).
Caution with concomitant use of drugs that prolong the QT interval.

- SIDE-EFFECTS
- ▶ **Common or very common** Anorexia · arthralgia · disturbances in taste · disturbances in vision · dizziness · dyspepsia · flatulence · headache · malaise · paraesthesia · reversible hearing loss (sometimes with tinnitus) after long-term therapy
- ▶ **Uncommon**
- ▶ With oral use Anxiety · chest pain · constipation · gastritis · hypoaesthesia · leucopenia · oedema · photosensitivity · sleep disturbances
- ▶ **Rare** Agitation
- ▶ **Frequency not known** Acute renal failure · convulsions · haemolytic anaemia · interstitial nephritis · smell disturbances · syncope · thrombocytopenia · tongue discoloration

- **PREGNANCY** Manufacturers advise use only if adequate alternatives not available.

- **BREAST FEEDING** Present in milk; use only if no suitable alternatives.

- **HEPATIC IMPAIRMENT** Manufacturers advise avoid in severe liver disease—no information available.

- **RENAL IMPAIRMENT** Use with caution if estimated glomerular filtration rate less than 10 mL/minute/1.73 m^2.

- **PRESCRIBING AND DISPENSING INFORMATION** Flavours of oral liquid formulations may include cherry or banana.

- PATIENT AND CARER ADVICE
  Medicines for Children leaflet: Azithromycin for bacterial infections www.medicinesforchildren.org.uk/azithromycin-bacterial-infections-0

- PROFESSION SPECIFIC INFORMATION
  Dental practitioners' formulary
  Azithromycin Capsules may be prescribed. Azithromycin Tablets may be prescribed. Azithromycin Oral Suspension 200 mg/5 mL may be prescribed.

- **EXCEPTIONS TO LEGAL CATEGORY** Azithromycin tablets can be sold to the public for the treatment of confirmed, asymptomatic *Chlamydia trachomatis* genital infection in those over 16 years of age, and for the epidemiological treatment of their sexual partners, subject to maximum single dose of 1 g, maximum daily dose 1 g, and a pack size of 1 g.

- MEDICINAL FORMS
  There can be variation in the licensing of different medicines containing the same drug. Forms available from special-order manufacturers include: oral suspension

Tablet
CAUTIONARY AND ADVISORY LABELS 5, 9
- ▶ Azithromycin (Non-proprietary)
  Azithromycin 250 mg Azithromycin 250mg tablets | 4 tablet [PoM] £10.11 DT price = £1.38 | 6 tablet [PoM] £14.46
  Azithromycin 500 mg Azithromycin 500mg tablets | 3 tablet [PoM] £9.80 DT price = £1.34

Capsule
CAUTIONARY AND ADVISORY LABELS 5, 9, 23
- ▶ Azithromycin (Non-proprietary)
  Azithromycin (as Azithromycin dihydrate) 250 mg Azithromycin 250mg capsules | 4 capsule [PoM] £10.10 | 6 capsule [PoM] £15.15 DT price = £15.13
- ▶ Zithromax (Pfizer Ltd)
  Azithromycin (as Azithromycin dihydrate) 250 mg Zithromax 250mg capsules | 4 capsule [PoM] £7.16 | 6 capsule [PoM] £10.74 DT price = £15.13

Oral suspension
CAUTIONARY AND ADVISORY LABELS 5, 9
- ▶ Azithromycin (Non-proprietary)
  Azithromycin 40 mg per 1 ml Azithromycin 200mg/5ml oral suspension | 15 ml [PoM] £6.18 DT price = £4.06 | 30 ml [PoM] £11.04 DT price = £11.04
- ▶ Zithromax (Pfizer Ltd)
  Azithromycin 40 mg per 1 ml Zithromax 200mg/5ml oral suspension | 15 ml [PoM] £4.06 DT price = £4.06 | 22.5 ml [PoM] £6.10 DT price = £6.10 | 30 ml [PoM] £11.04 DT price = £11.04

F 308

Clarithromycin

- INDICATIONS AND DOSE
  Respiratory-tract infections | Mild to moderate skin and soft-tissue infections | Otitis media
  - ▶ BY MOUTH USING IMMEDIATE-RELEASE MEDICINES
  - ▶ Neonate: 7.5 mg/kg twice daily.
  - ▶ Child 1 month–11 years (body-weight up to 8 kg): 7.5 mg/kg twice daily
  - ▶ Child 1 month–11 years (body-weight 8–11 kg): 62.5 mg twice daily
  - ▶ Child 1 month–11 years (body-weight 12–19 kg): 125 mg twice daily
  - ▶ Child 1 month–11 years (body-weight 20–29 kg): 187.5 mg twice daily
  - ▶ Child 1 month–11 years (body-weight 30–40 kg): 250 mg twice daily
  - ▶ Child 12–17 years: 250 mg twice daily usually for 7–14 days, increased to 500 mg twice daily, if required in severe infections (e.g. pneumonia)
  - ▶ BY MOUTH USING MODIFIED-RELEASE MEDICINES
  - ▶ Child 12–17 years: 500 mg once daily usually for 7–14 days, increased to 1 g once daily, if required in severe infections (e.g. pneumonia)
  - ▶ BY INTRAVENOUS INFUSION
  - ▶ Child 1 month–11 years: 7.5 mg/kg every 12 hours (max. per dose 500 mg every 12 hours) maximum duration 5 days, switch to oral route when appropriate, to be administered into a large proximal vein
  - ▶ Child 12–17 years: 500 mg every 12 hours maximum duration 5 days, switch to oral route when appropriate, to be administered into a large proximal vein

  Lyme disease
  - ▶ BY MOUTH
  - ▶ Child 1 month–11 years: 7.5 mg/kg twice daily (max. per dose 500 mg) for 14–21 days
  - ▶ Child 12–17 years: 500 mg twice daily for 14–21 days

  Prevention of pertussis
  - ▶ BY MOUTH
  - ▶ Neonate: 7.5 mg/kg twice daily for 7 days.
  - ▶ Child 1 month–11 years (body-weight up to 8 kg): 7.5 mg/kg twice daily for 7 days
  - ▶ Child 1 month–11 years (body-weight 8–11 kg): 62.5 mg twice daily for 7 days
  - ▶ Child 1 month–11 years (body-weight 12–19 kg): 125 mg twice daily for 7 days
  - ▶ Child 1 month–11 years (body-weight 20–29 kg): 187.5 mg twice daily for 7 days
  - ▶ Child 1 month–11 years (body-weight 30–40 kg): 250 mg twice daily for 7 days
  - ▶ Child 12–17 years: 500 mg twice daily for 7 days

  ***Helicobacter pylori* eradication in combination with omeprazole, and amoxicillin or metronidazole**
  - ▶ BY MOUTH
  - ▶ Child 1–5 years: 7.5 mg/kg twice daily (max. per dose 500 mg)
  - ▶ Child 6–11 years: 7.5 mg/kg twice daily (max. per dose 500 mg)
  - ▶ Child 12–17 years: 500 mg twice daily

- UNLICENSED USE
  - ▶ With oral use Tablets not licensed for use in children under 12 years; oral suspension not licensed for use in infants under 6 months.
  - ▶ With intravenous use Intravenous infusion not licensed for use in children under 12 years.

- INTERACTIONS → Appendix 1 (macrolides).
  Caution with concomitant use of drugs that prolong the QT interval.

Infection

5

- **SIDE-EFFECTS**
- ▸ **Common or very common** Dyspepsia · headache · hyperhidrosis · insomnia · taste disturbances
- ▸ **Uncommon** Anorexia · anxiety · blood disorders · chest pain · constipation · dizziness · dry mouth · flatulence · gastritis · glossitis · hepatic dysfunction including jaundice · leucopenia · malaise · myalgia · stomatitis · tinnitus · tremor
- ▸ **Frequency not known** Abnormal dreams · confusion · convulsions · depression · hypoglycaemia · interstitial nephritis · myopathy · paraesthesia · psychotic disorders · renal failure · smell disturbances · tongue discoloration · tooth discoloration
- **PREGNANCY** Manufacturer advises avoid, particularly in the first trimester, unless potential benefit outweighs risk.
- **BREAST FEEDING** Manufacturer advises avoid unless potential benefit outweighs risk—present in milk.
- **HEPATIC IMPAIRMENT** Avoid in severe impairment if renal impairment also present.
- **RENAL IMPAIRMENT** Use half normal dose if estimated glomerular filtration rate less than 30 mL/minute/1.73 m^2, max. duration 14 days. Avoid if severe hepatic impairment also present.
- ▸ With oral use Avoid *Klaricid XL* ® or clarithromyin m/r preparations if estimated glomerular filtration rate less than 30 mL/minute/1.73 m^2.
- **DIRECTIONS FOR ADMINISTRATION**
- ▸ With intravenous use For intermittent intravenous infusion dilute reconstituted solution further in Glucose 5% *or* Sodium chloride 0.9% to a concentration of 2 mg/mL; give into large proximal vein over 60 minutes.
- **PATIENT AND CARER ADVICE**
  Medicines for Children leaflet: Clarithromycin for bacterial infections www.medicinesforchildren.org.uk/clarithromycin-bacterial-infections
- **PROFESSION SPECIFIC INFORMATION**
  Dental practitioners' formulary
  Clarithromycin Tablets may be prescribed. Clarithromycin Oral Suspension may be prescribed.

- **MEDICINAL FORMS**
  There can be variation in the licensing of different medicines containing the same drug. Forms available from special-order manufacturers include: infusion
  Tablet
  CAUTIONARY AND ADVISORY LABELS 9
  ▸ **Clarithromycin (Non-proprietary)**
  Clarithromycin 250 mg Clarithromycin 250mg tablets | 14 tablet ᴾᴼᴹ £10.50 DT price = £1.40
  Clarithromycin 500 mg Clarithromycin 500mg tablets | 14 tablet ᴾᴼᴹ £21.50 DT price = £2.35
  Modified-release tablet
  CAUTIONARY AND ADVISORY LABELS 9, 21, 25
  ▸ **Clarie XL** (Teva UK Ltd)
  Clarithromycin 500 mg Clarie XL 500mg tablets | 7 tablet ᴾᴼᴹ £6.72 DT price = £6.72 | 14 tablet ᴾᴼᴹ £13.23
  ▸ **Klaricid XL** (BGP Products Ltd)
  Clarithromycin 500 mg Klaricid XL 500mg tablets | 7 tablet ᴾᴼᴹ £6.72 DT price = £6.72 | 14 tablet ᴾᴼᴹ £13.23
  Granules
  CAUTIONARY AND ADVISORY LABELS 9, 13
  ▸ **Klaricid** (BGP Products Ltd)
  Clarithromycin 250 mg Klaricid Adult 250mg granules sachets | 14 sachet ᴾᴼᴹ £11.68
  Oral suspension
  CAUTIONARY AND ADVISORY LABELS 9
  ▸ **Clarithromycin (Non-proprietary)**
  Clarithromycin 25 mg per 1 ml Clarithromycin 125mg/5ml oral suspension | 70 ml ᴾᴼᴹ £11.99 DT price = £3.87
  Clarithromycin 50 mg per 1 ml Clarithromycin 250mg/5ml oral suspension | 70 ml ᴾᴼᴹ £21.75 DT price = £5.74

- ▸ **Klaricid** (BGP Products Ltd)
  Clarithromycin 25 mg per 1 ml Klaricid Paediatric 125mg/5ml oral suspension | 70 ml ᴾᴼᴹ £5.26 DT price = £3.87 | 100 ml ᴾᴼᴹ £9.04
  Clarithromycin 50 mg per 1 ml Klaricid Paediatric 250mg/5ml oral suspension | 70 ml ᴾᴼᴹ £10.51 DT price = £5.74
  Powder for solution for infusion
  ELECTROLYTES: May contain Sodium
  ▸ **Clarithromycin (Non-proprietary)**
  Clarithromycin 500 mg Clarithromycin 500mg powder for solution for infusion vials | 1 vial ᴾᴼᴹ £11.25 DT price = £9.45
  Clarithromycin 500mg powder for concentrate for solution for infusion vials | 1 vial ᴾᴼᴹ £8.98 DT price = £9.45
  ▸ **Klaricid** (BGP Products Ltd)
  Clarithromycin 500 mg Klaricid IV 500mg powder for solution for infusion vials | 1 vial ᴾᴼᴹ £9.45 DT price = £9.45

ꜰ 308

Erythromycin

- **INDICATIONS AND DOSE**

Susceptible infections in patients with penicillin hypersensitivity (e.g. respiratory-tract infections (including Legionella infection), skin and oral infections, and campylobacter enteritis)
- ▸ BY MOUTH
- ▸ Neonate: 12.5 mg/kg every 6 hours.

- ▸ Child 1 month–1 year: 125 mg 4 times a day, total daily dose may alternatively be given in two divided doses, increased to 250 mg 4 times a day, dose increase may be used in severe infections
- ▸ Child 2–7 years: 250 mg 4 times a day, total daily dose may alternatively be given in two divided doses, increased to 500 mg 4 times a day, dose increase may be used in severe infections
- ▸ Child 8–17 years: 250–500 mg 4 times a day, total daily dose may alternatively be given in two divided doses, increased to 500–1000 mg 4 times a day, dose increase may be used in severe infections
- ▸ BY INTRAVENOUS INFUSION
- ▸ Neonate: 10–12.5 mg/kg every 6 hours.
- ▸ Child: 12.5 mg/kg every 6 hours (max. per dose 1 g)

Lyme disease (under expert supervision)
- ▸ BY MOUTH
- ▸ Child: 12.5 mg/kg 4 times a day (max. per dose 500 mg) for 14–21 days

Chlamydial ophthalmia
- ▸ BY MOUTH
- ▸ Neonate: 12.5 mg/kg every 6 hours.

- ▸ Child 1 month–1 year: 125 mg 4 times a day, increased to 250 mg every 6 hours, dose increase for severe infections, total daily dose may alternatively be given in two divided doses
- ▸ Child 2–7 years: 250 mg 4 times a day, increased to 500 mg every 6 hours, dose increase for severe infections, total daily dose may alternatively be given in two divided doses
- ▸ Child 8–17 years: 250–500 mg 4 times a day, increased to 500–1000 mg every 6 hours, dose increase for severe infections, total daily dose may alternatively be given in two divided doses
- ▸ BY INTRAVENOUS INFUSION
- ▸ Neonate: 10–12.5 mg/kg every 6 hours.
- ▸ Child: 12.5 mg/kg every 6 hours (max. per dose 1 g)

Early syphilis
- ▸ BY MOUTH
- ▸ Child 12–17 years: 500 mg 4 times a day for 14 days

Uncomplicated genital chlamydia | Non-gonococcal urethritis
▶ BY MOUTH
▶ Child 1 month–1 year: 12.5 mg/kg 4 times a day for 14 days
▶ Child 2–11 years: 250 mg twice daily for 14 days
▶ Child 12–17 years: 500 mg twice daily for 14 days

Pelvic inflammatory disease
▶ BY MOUTH
▶ Child 1 month–1 year: 12.5 mg/kg 4 times a day for 14 days
▶ Child 2–11 years: 250 mg twice daily for 14 days
▶ Child 12–17 years: 500 mg twice daily for 14 days

Prevention and treatment of pertussis
▶ BY MOUTH
▶ Neonate: 12.5 mg/kg every 6 hours.
▶ Child 1 month–1 year: 125 mg 4 times a day, total daily dose may alternatively be given in two divided doses, increased to 250 mg 4 times a day, dose increase may be used in severe infections
▶ Child 2–7 years: 250 mg 4 times a day, total daily dose may alternatively be given in two divided doses, increased to 500 mg 4 times a day, dose increase may be used in severe infections
▶ Child 8–17 years: 250–500 mg 4 times a day, total daily dose may alternatively be given in two divided doses, increased to 500–1000 mg 4 times a day, dose increase may be used in severe infections
▶ BY INTRAVENOUS INFUSION
▶ Neonate: 10–12.5 mg/kg every 6 hours.
▶ Child: 12.5 mg/kg every 6 hours (max. per dose 1 g)

Prevention of secondary case of diphtheria in non-immune patient
▶ BY MOUTH
▶ Child 1 month–1 year: 125 mg every 6 hours for 7 days, treat for further 10 days if nasopharyngeal swabs positive after first 7 days' treatment
▶ Child 2–7 years: 250 mg every 6 hours for 7 days, treat for further 10 days if nasopharyngeal swabs positive after first 7 days' treatment
▶ Child 8–17 years: 500 mg every 6 hours for 7 days, treat for further 10 days if nasopharyngeal swabs positive after first 7 days' treatment

Prevention of secondary case of invasive group A streptococcal infection in penicillin allergic patients
▶ BY MOUTH
▶ Child 1 month–1 year: 125 mg every 6 hours for 10 days
▶ Child 2–7 years: 250 mg every 6 hours for 10 days
▶ Child 8–17 years: 250–500 mg every 6 hours for 10 days

Prevention of pneumococcal infection in asplenia or in patients with sickle-cell disease (if penicillin-allergic)
▶ BY MOUTH
▶ Child 1 month–1 year: 125 mg twice daily, antibiotic prophylaxis is not fully reliable
▶ Child 2–7 years: 250 mg twice daily, antibiotic prophylaxis is not fully reliable. It may be discontinued in those over 5 years of age with sickle-cell disease who have received pneumococcal immunisation and who do not have a history of severe pneumococcal infection
▶ Child 8–17 years: 500 mg twice daily, antibiotic prophylaxis is not fully reliable. It may be discontinued in those with sickle-cell disease who have received pneumococcal immunisation and who do not have a history of severe pneumococcal infection

Prevention of recurrence of rheumatic fever
▶ BY MOUTH
▶ Child 1 month–1 year: 125 mg twice daily
▶ Child 2–17 years: 250 mg twice daily

Acne
▶ BY MOUTH
▶ Child 1–23 months: 250 mg once daily, alternatively 125 mg twice daily
▶ Child 12–17 years: 500 mg twice daily

Gastro-intestinal stasis
▶ BY MOUTH
▶ Neonate: 3 mg/kg 4 times a day.
▶ Child: 3 mg/kg 4 times a day
▶ BY INTRAVENOUS INFUSION
▶ Neonate: 3 mg/kg 4 times a day.
▶ Child 1–11 months: 3 mg/kg 4 times a day

● UNLICENSED USE Not licensed for use in gastro-intestinal stasis.
● CAUTIONS Avoid in Acute porphyrias p. 562 · neonate under 2 weeks (risk of hypertrophic pyloric stenosis)
● INTERACTIONS → See Appendix 1 (macrolides). Caution with concomitant use of drugs that prolong the QT interval.
● PREGNANCY Not known to be harmful.
● BREAST FEEDING Only small amounts in milk—not known to be harmful.
● HEPATIC IMPAIRMENT May cause idiosyncratic hepatotoxicity.
● RENAL IMPAIRMENT Reduce dose in severe renal impairment (ototoxicity).
● DIRECTIONS FOR ADMINISTRATION
▶ With intravenous use Dilute reconstituted solution further in glucose 5% (neutralised with Sodium bicarbonate) or sodium chloride 0.9% to a concentration of 1–5 mg/mL; give over 20–60 minutes. Concentration of up to 10 mg/mL may be used in fluid-restriction if administered via a central venous catheter.
● PRESCRIBING AND DISPENSING INFORMATION Flavours of oral liquid formulations may include banana.
● PATIENT AND CARER ADVICE
Medicines for Children leaflet: Erythromycin for bacterial infections www.medicinesforchildren.org.uk/erythromycin-for-bacterial-infections
● PROFESSION SPECIFIC INFORMATION
Dental practitioners' formulary
▶ With oral use Erythromycin tablets e/c may be prescribed. Erythromycin ethyl succinate oral suspension may be prescribed. Erythromycin stearate tablets may be prescribed. Erythromycin ethyl succinate tablets may be prescribed.

● MEDICINAL FORMS
There can be variation in the licensing of different medicines containing the same drug.

Tablet
CAUTIONARY AND ADVISORY LABELS 9
▶ Erythromycin (Non-proprietary)
Erythromycin (as Erythromycin ethyl succinate) 500 mg Erythromycin ethyl succinate 500mg tablets | 28 tablet PoM £15.95–£19.50 DT price = £10.78
▶ Erythrocin (AMCo)
Erythromycin (as Erythromycin stearate) 250 mg Erythrocin 250 tablets | 100 tablet PoM £18.20 DT price = £18.20
Erythromycin (as Erythromycin stearate) 500 mg Erythrocin 500 tablets | 100 tablet PoM £36.40 DT price = £36.40
▶ Erythrolar (Ennogen Pharma Ltd)
Erythromycin (as Erythromycin stearate) 250 mg Erythrolar 250mg tablets | 100 tablet PoM £22.80 DT price = £18.20
Erythromycin (as Erythromycin stearate) 500 mg Erythrolar 500mg tablets | 100 tablet PoM £45.60 DT price = £36.40
▶ Erythroped A (AMCo)
Erythromycin (as Erythromycin ethyl succinate) 500 mg Erythroped A 500mg tablets | 28 tablet PoM £10.78 DT price = £10.78

5

Infection

Gastro-resistant tablet

CAUTIONARY AND ADVISORY LABELS 5, 9, 25

▸ **Erythromycin (Non-proprietary)**

Erythromycin 250 mg Erythromycin 250mg gastro-resistant tablets | 28 tablet [PoM] £3.00 DT price = £1.44 | 500 tablet [PoM] £28.57

Gastro-resistant capsule

CAUTIONARY AND ADVISORY LABELS 5, 9, 25

▸ **Erythromycin (Non-proprietary)**

Erythromycin 250 mg Erythromycin 250mg gastro-resistant capsules | 28 capsule [PoM] no price available DT price = £5.61 | 30 capsule [PoM] no price available

▸ **Erymax** (Teva UK Ltd)

Erythromycin 250 mg Erymax 250mg gastro-resistant capsules | 28 capsule [PoM] £5.61 DT price = £5.61 | 112 capsule [PoM] £22.44

▸ **Tiloryth** (Tillomed Laboratories Ltd)

Erythromycin 250 mg Tiloryth 250mg gastro-resistant capsules | 30 capsule [PoM] £5.65 | 100 capsule [PoM] £18.66

Oral suspension

CAUTIONARY AND ADVISORY LABELS 9

▸ **Erythromycin (Non-proprietary)**

Erythromycin (as Erythromycin ethyl succinate) 25 mg per 1 ml Erythromycin ethyl succinate 125mg/5ml oral suspension | 100 ml [PoM] £4.05 DT price = £4.04
Erythromycin ethyl succinate 125mg/5ml oral suspension sugar free sugar-free | 100 ml [PoM] £4.05 DT price = £3.31

Erythromycin (as Erythromycin ethyl succinate) 50 mg per 1 ml Erythromycin ethyl succinate 250mg/5ml oral suspension | 100 ml [PoM] £6.38 DT price = £6.36
Erythromycin ethyl succinate 250mg/5ml oral suspension sugar free sugar-free | 100 ml [PoM] £7.99 DT price = £4.76

Erythromycin (as Erythromycin ethyl succinate) 100 mg per 1 ml Erythromycin ethyl succinate 500mg/5ml oral suspension | 100 ml [PoM] £11.24 DT price = £11.24
Erythromycin ethyl succinate 500mg/5ml oral suspension sugar free sugar-free | 100 ml [PoM] no price available DT price = £12.99

▸ **Erythroped** (AMCo)

Erythromycin (as Erythromycin ethyl succinate) 25 mg per 1 ml Erythroped PI SF 125mg/5ml oral suspension sugar-free | 140 ml [PoM] £3.06

Erythromycin (as Erythromycin ethyl succinate) 50 mg per 1 ml Erythroped SF 250mg/5ml oral suspension sugar-free | 140 ml [PoM] £5.95

Erythromycin (as Erythromycin ethyl succinate) 100 mg per 1 ml Erythroped Forte SF 500mg/5ml oral suspension sugar-free | 140 ml [PoM] £10.56

Powder for solution for infusion

▸ **Erythromycin (Non-proprietary)**

Erythromycin (as Erythromycin lactobionate)

1 gram Erythromycin 1g powder for solution for infusion vials | 1 vial [PoM] £22.92

| Telithromycin

● **DRUG ACTION** The ketolide telithromycin is a derivative of erythromycin. The antibacterial spectrum of telithromycin is similar to that of macrolides and it is also active against penicillin- and erythromycin-resistant *Streptococcus pneumoniae*.

● **INDICATIONS AND DOSE**

Treatment of beta-haemolytic streptococcal pharyngitis if caused by organisms resistant to beta-lactam antibacterials and other macrolides, or if conventional treatment is contra-indicated | Treatment of beta-haemolytic streptococcal tonsillitis if caused by organisms resistant to beta-lactam antibacterials and other macrolides, or if conventional treatment is contra-indicated

▸ BY MOUTH

▸ Child 12-17 years: 800 mg once daily for 5 days

● **CONTRA-INDICATIONS** Congenital history of QT interval prolongation (if not excluded by ECG) · family history of QT interval prolongation (if not excluded by ECG) · history of telithromycin-associated hepatitis · history of

telithromycin-associated jaundice · myasthenia gravis · prolongation of QT interval

● **CAUTIONS** Avoid in Acute porphyrias p. 562 · bradycardia—risk of QT interval prolongation · coronary heart disease—risk of QT interval prolongation · hypokalaemia—risk of QT interval prolongation · hypomagnesaemia—risk of QT interval prolongation · ventricular arrhythmias—risk of QT interval prolongation

● **INTERACTIONS** → Appendix 1 (telithromycin). Caution with concomitant use of drugs that prolong the QT interval.

● **SIDE-EFFECTS**

▸ **Common or very common** Abdominal pain · diarrhoea · dizziness · flatulence · headache · nausea · taste disturbances · vomiting

▸ **Uncommon** Anorexia · blurred vision · constipation · drowsiness · eosinophilia · flushing · hepatitis · insomnia · nervousness · palpitations · pruritus · rash · stomatitis · urticaria

▸ **Rare** Arrhythmias · cholestatic jaundice · diplopia · hypotension · paraesthesia · transient loss of consciousness

▸ **Very rare** Altered sense of smell · antibiotic-associated colitis · erythema multiforme · muscle cramp

▸ **Frequency not known** Arthralgia · confusion · hallucinations · pancreatitis

● **PREGNANCY** Toxicity in *animal* studies—manufacturer advises use only if potential benefit outweighs risk.

● **BREAST FEEDING** Manufacturer advises avoid—present in milk in *animal* studies.

● **HEPATIC IMPAIRMENT** Manufacturer advises caution.

● **RENAL IMPAIRMENT** Manufacturer advises avoid if possible if eGFR less than 30 mL/minute/1.73 m^2—if no alternative, use alternating daily doses of 800 mg and 400 mg, starting with 800 mg dose.

● **PATIENT AND CARER ADVICE**

Driving and skilled tasks
Visual disturbances or transient loss of consciousness may affect performance of skilled tasks (e.g. driving); effects may occur after the first dose. Administration at bedtime may reduce these side-effects. Patients should be advised not to drive or operate machinery if affected.

Hepatic disorders Counselling on hepatic disorders is advised. Patients should be told how to recognise signs of liver disorder, and advised to discontinue treatment and seek prompt medical attention if symptoms such as anorexia, nausea, vomiting, abdominal pain, jaundice, or dark urine develop.

● **MEDICINAL FORMS**
There can be variation in the licensing of different medicines containing the same drug.
No licensed medicines listed.

ANTIBACTERIALS > MONOBACTAMS

Aztreonam

- **DRUG ACTION** Aztreonam is a monocyclic beta-lactam ('monobactam') antibiotic with an antibacterial spectrum limited to Gram-negative aerobic bacteria including *Pseudomonas aeruginosa, Neisseria meningitidis,* and *Haemophilus influenzae*; it should not be used alone for 'blind' treatment since it is not active against Gram-positive organisms. Aztreonam is also effective against *Neisseria gonorrhoeae* (but not against concurrent chlamydial infection).

- **INDICATIONS AND DOSE**

Gram-negative infections including *Pseudomonas aeruginosa, Haemophilus influenzae,* and *Neisseria meningitidis*
  ▸ BY INTRAVENOUS INJECTION, OR BY INTRAVENOUS INFUSION
  ▸ Neonate up to 7 days: 30 mg/kg every 12 hours.
  ▸ Neonate 7 days to 28 days: 30 mg/kg every 6–8 hours.
  ▸ Child 1 month–11 years: 30 mg/kg every 6–8 hours
  ▸ Child 12–17 years: 1 g every 8 hours, alternatively 2 g every 12 hours

Severe gram-negative infections including *Pseudomonas aeruginosa, Haemophilus influenzae, Neisseria meningitidis,* and lung infections in cystic fibrosis
  ▸ BY INTRAVENOUS INFUSION, OR BY INTRAVENOUS INJECTION
  ▸ Child 2–11 years: 50 mg/kg every 6–8 hours (max. per dose 2 g 4 times a day)
  ▸ Child 12–17 years: 2 g every 6–8 hours

Chronic pulmonary *Pseudomonas aeruginosa* infection in patients with cystic fibrosis
  ▸ BY INHALATION OF NEBULISED SOLUTION
  ▸ Child 6–17 years: 75 mg 3 times a day for 28 days, doses to be administered at least 4 hours apart, subsequent courses repeated after 28-day interval without aztreonam nebuliser solution

- **UNLICENSED USE**
  ▸ With systemic use Injection not licensed for use in children under 7 days.

- **CAUTIONS**
  ▸ When used by inhalation Haemoptysis— risk of further haemorrhage

- **INTERACTIONS** → Appendix 1 (aztreonam).

- **SIDE-EFFECTS**
  GENERAL SIDE-EFFECTS
  Bronchospasm · rash
  SPECIFIC SIDE-EFFECTS
  ▸ Rare
  ▸ With systemic use Antibiotic-associated colitis · asthenia · blood disorders · breast tenderness · chest pain · confusion · diplopia · dizziness · dyspnoea · gastro-intestinal bleeding · halitosis · headache · hepatitis · hypotension · insomnia · jaundice · myalgia · neutropenia · paraesthesia · seizures · thrombocytopenia · tinnitus
  ▸ Frequency not known
  ▸ When used by inhalation Arthralgia · cough · haemoptysis · pharyngolaryngeal pain · pyrexia · rhinorrhoea · wheezing
  ▸ With systemic use Abdominal pain · diarrhoea · erythema multiforme · flushing · mouth ulcers · nausea · taste disturbances · toxic epidermal necrolysis · vomiting

- **ALLERGY AND CROSS-SENSITIVITY** Contra-indicated in aztreonam hypersensitivity.
  Use with caution in patients with hypersensitivity to other beta-lactam antibiotics (although aztreonam may be less likely than other beta-lactams to cause hypersensitivity in penicillin-sensitive patients).

- **PREGNANCY**
  ▸ With systemic use No information available; manufacturer of injection advises avoid.
  ▸ When used by inhalation No information available; manufacturer of powder for nebuliser solution advises avoid unless essential.

- **BREAST FEEDING** Amount in milk probably too small to be harmful.

- **HEPATIC IMPAIRMENT**
  ▸ With systemic use Use injection with caution. Monitor liver function.

- **RENAL IMPAIRMENT**
  ▸ With systemic use If estimated glomerular filtration rate 10–30 mL/minute/1.73 m^2, usual initial dose of injection, then half normal dose. If estimated glomerular filtration rate less than 10 mL/minute/1.73 m^2, usual initial dose of injection, then one-quarter normal dose.

- **MONITORING REQUIREMENTS**
  ▸ When used by inhalation Measure lung function before and after initial dose of aztreonam and monitor for bronchospasm.

- **DIRECTIONS FOR ADMINISTRATION** For *intravenous injection*, give over 3–5 minutes.
  ▸ With intravenous use Displacement value of injection may be significant, consult local guidelines. For intermittent intravenous infusion, dilute reconstituted solution further in Glucose 5% *or* Sodium chloride 0.9% to a concentration of less than 20 mg/mL; to be given over 20–60 minutes.
  ▸ When used by inhalation Other inhaled drugs should be administered before aztreonam; a bronchodilator should be administered before each dose.

- **NATIONAL FUNDING/ACCESS DECISIONS**
  Scottish Medicines Consortium (SMC) Decisions
  The *Scottish Medicines Consortium* has advised (December 2014) that aztreonam powder for nebuliser solution (*Cayston* ®) is accepted for restricted use within NHS Scotland when inhaled colistimethate sodium and inhaled tobramycin are not tolerated or are not providing satisfactory therapeutic benefit (measured as ≥2% decline in forced expiratory volume in 1 second).

- **MEDICINAL FORMS**
  There can be variation in the licensing of different medicines containing the same drug.
  Powder for solution for injection
  ▸ Azactam (Bristol-Myers Squibb Pharmaceuticals Ltd)
    Aztreonam 1 gram Azactam 1g powder for solution for injection vials
    | 1 vial PoM £9.40 (Hospital only)
    Aztreonam 2 gram Azactam 2g powder for solution for injection vials
    | 1 vial PoM £18.82 (Hospital only)
  Powder and solvent for nebuliser solution
  ▸ Cayston (Gilead Sciences International Ltd)
    Aztreonam (as Aztreonam lysine) 75 mg Cayston 75mg powder and solvent for nebuliser solution vials with Altera Nebuliser Handset
    | 84 vial PoM £2,181.53

ANTIBACTERIALS > NITROIMIDAZOLE DERIVATIVES

Metronidazole

- **DRUG ACTION** Metronidazole is an antimicrobial drug with high activity against anaerobic bacteria and protozoa.

- **INDICATIONS AND DOSE**
  Anaerobic infections
  ▸ BY MOUTH
  ▸ Child 1 month: 7.5 mg/kg every 12 hours usually treated for 7 days (for 10–14 days in *Clostridium difficile* infection) continued →

- Child 2 months–11 years: 7.5 mg/kg every 8 hours (max. per dose 400 mg) usually treated for 7 days (for 10–14 days in *Clostridium difficile* infection)
- Child 12–17 years: 400 mg every 8 hours usually treated for 7 days (for 10–14 days in *Clostridium difficile* infection)
▶ BY RECTUM
- Child 1–11 months: 125 mg 3 times a day for 3 days, then 125 mg twice daily, for usual total treatment duration of 7 days
- Child 1–4 years: 250 mg 3 times a day for 3 days, then 250 mg twice daily, for usual total treatment duration of 7 days
- Child 5–9 years: 500 mg 3 times a day for 3 days, then 500 mg twice daily, for usual total treatment duration of 7 days
- Child 10–17 years: 1 g 3 times a day for 3 days, then 1 g twice daily, for usual total treatment duration of 7 days
▶ BY INTRAVENOUS INFUSION
- Neonate up to 26 weeks corrected gestational age: Loading dose 15 mg/kg, followed by 7.5 mg/kg after 24 hours, then 7.5 mg/kg daily usually treated for a total duration of 7 days (for 10–14 days in *Clostridium difficile* infection).
- Neonate 26 weeks to 34 weeks corrected gestational age: Loading dose 15 mg/kg, followed by 7.5 mg/kg after 12 hours, then 7.5 mg/kg every 12 hours usually treated for a total duration of 7 days (for 10–14 days in *Clostridium difficile* infection).
- Neonate 34 weeks corrected gestational age and above: Loading dose 15 mg/kg, followed by 7.5 mg/kg after 8 hours, then 7.5 mg/kg every 8 hours usually treated for a total duration of 7 days (for 10–14 days in *Clostridium difficile* infection).
- Child 1 month: Loading dose 15 mg/kg, followed by 7.5 mg/kg after 8 hours, then 7.5 mg/kg every 8 hours usually treated for a total duration of 7 days (for 10–14 days in *Clostridium difficile* infection)
- Child 2 months–17 years: 7.5 mg/kg every 8 hours (max. per dose 500 mg) usually treated for 7 days (for 10–14 days in *Clostridium difficile* infection)

Helicobacter pylori eradication; in combination with clarithromycin and omeprazole
▶ BY MOUTH
- Child 1–5 years: 100 mg twice daily
- Child 6–11 years: 200 mg twice daily
- Child 12–17 years: 400 mg twice daily

Helicobacter pylori eradication; in combination with amoxicillin and omeprazole
▶ BY MOUTH
- Child 1–5 years: 100 mg 3 times a day
- Child 6–11 years: 200 mg 3 times a day
- Child 12–17 years: 400 mg 3 times a day

Fistulating Crohn's disease
▶ BY MOUTH
- Child: 7.5 mg/kg 3 times a day usually given for 1 month but should not be used for longer than 3 months because of concerns about peripheral neuropathy

Pelvic inflammatory disease
▶ BY MOUTH
- Child 12–17 years: 400 mg twice daily for 14 days

Acute ulcerative gingivitis
▶ BY MOUTH
- Child 1–2 years: 50 mg every 8 hours for 3 days
- Child 3–6 years: 100 mg every 12 hours for 3 days
- Child 7–9 years: 100 mg every 8 hours for 3 days
- Child 10–17 years: 200–250 mg every 8 hours for 3 days

Acute oral infections
▶ BY MOUTH
- Child 1–2 years: 50 mg every 8 hours for 3–7 days
- Child 3–6 years: 100 mg every 12 hours for 3–7 days
- Child 7–9 years: 100 mg every 8 hours for 3–7 days
- Child 10–17 years: 200–250 mg every 8 hours for 3–7 days

Surgical prophylaxis
▶ BY MOUTH
- Child 1 month–11 years: 30 mg/kg (max. per dose 500 mg), to be administered 2 hours before surgery
- Child 12–17 years: 400–500 mg, to be administered 2 hours before surgery, then 400–500 mg every 8 hours if required for up to 3 doses (in high-risk procedures)
▶ BY RECTUM
- Child 5–9 years: 500 mg, to be administered 2 hours before surgery, then 500 mg every 8 hours if required for up to 3 doses (in high-risk procedures)
- Child 10–17 years: 1 g, to be administered 2 hours before surgery, then 1 g every 8 hours if required for up to 3 doses (in high-risk procedures)
▶ BY INTRAVENOUS INFUSION
- Neonate up to 40 weeks corrected gestational age: 10 mg/kg, to be administered up to 30 minutes before the procedure.
- Neonate 40 weeks corrected gestational age and above: 20–30 mg/kg, to be administered up to 30 minutes before the procedure.
- Child 1 month–11 years: 30 mg/kg (max. per dose 500 mg), to be administered up to 30 minutes before the procedure
- Child 12–17 years: 500 mg, to be administered up to 30 minutes before the procedure, then 500 mg every 8 hours if required for up to 3 further doses (in high-risk procedures)

Invasive intestinal amoebiasis | Extra-intestinal amoebiasis (including liver abscess)
▶ BY MOUTH
- Child 1–2 years: 200 mg 3 times a day for 5 days in intestinal infection (for 5–10 days in extra-intestinal infection)
- Child 3–6 years: 200 mg 4 times a day for 5 days in intestinal infection (for 5–10 days in extra-intestinal infection)
- Child 7–9 years: 400 mg 3 times a day for 5 days in intestinal infection (for 5–10 days in extra-intestinal infection)
- Child 10–17 years: 800 mg 3 times a day for 5 days in intestinal infection (for 5–10 days in extra-intestinal infection)

Urogenital trichomoniasis
▶ BY MOUTH
- Child 1–2 years: 50 mg 3 times a day for 7 days
- Child 3–6 years: 100 mg twice daily for 7 days
- Child 7–9 years: 100 mg 3 times a day for 7 days
- Child 10–17 years: 200 mg 3 times a day for 7 days, alternatively 400–500 mg twice daily for 5–7 days, alternatively 2 g for 1 dose

Giardiasis
▶ BY MOUTH
- Child 1–2 years: 500 mg once daily for 3 days
- Child 3–6 years: 600–800 mg once daily for 3 days
- Child 7–9 years: 1 g once daily for 3 days
- Child 10–17 years: 2 g once daily for 3 days, alternatively 400 mg 3 times a day for 5 days, alternatively 500 mg twice daily for 7–10 days

Established case of tetanus
▶ BY INTRAVENOUS INFUSION
- Child: (consult product literature)

- **INTERACTIONS** → Appendix 1 (metronidazole). Caution—disulfiram-like reaction with alcohol.
- **SIDE-EFFECTS**
  ► **Very rare** Arthralgia · ataxia · darkening of urine · dizziness · drowsiness · erythema multiforme · headache · hepatitis · jaundice · leucopenia (on prolonged or intensive therapy) · myalgia · pancreatitis · pancytopenia · peripheral neuropathy (on prolonged or intensive therapy) · pruritus · psychotic disorders · rash · thrombocytopenia · transient epileptiform seizures (on prolonged or intensive therapy) · visual disturbances
  ► **Frequency not known** Anorexia · aseptic meningitis · furred tongue · gastro-intestinal disturbances · nausea · optic neuropathy · oral mucositis · taste disturbances · vomiting
- **PREGNANCY** Manufacturer advises avoidance of high-dose regimens; use only if potential benefit outweighs risk.
- **BREAST FEEDING** Significant amount in milk; manufacturer advises avoid large single doses though otherwise compatible; may give milk a bitter taste.
- **HEPATIC IMPAIRMENT** In severe liver disease reduce total daily dose to one-third, and give once daily.
  ► With systemic use Use with caution in hepatic encephalopathy.
- **MONITORING REQUIREMENTS** Clinical and laboratory monitoring advised if treatment exceeds 10 days.
- **DIRECTIONS FOR ADMINISTRATION** For *intravenous infusion*, give over 20–30 minutes.
- **PRESCRIBING AND DISPENSING INFORMATION** Metronidazole is well absorbed orally and the intravenous route is normally reserved for severe infections. Metronidazole by the rectal route is an effective alternative to the intravenous route when oral administration is not possible.
- **PATIENT AND CARER ADVICE** Medicines for Children leaflet: Metronidazole for bacterial infections www.medicinesforchildren.org.uk/metronidazole-for-bacterial-infections
- **PROFESSION SPECIFIC INFORMATION**
  Dental practitioners' formulary
  ► With oral use Metronidazole Tablets may be prescribed. Metronidazole Oral Suspension may be prescribed.

- **MEDICINAL FORMS**
  There can be variation in the licensing of different medicines containing the same drug. Forms available from special-order manufacturers include: oral suspension, oral solution
  Tablet
  CAUTIONARY AND ADVISORY LABELS 4, 9, 21, 25, 27
  ► **Metronidazole (Non-proprietary)**
  Metronidazole 200 mg Metronidazole 200mg tablets | 21 tablet PoM £11.66 DT price = £1.40 | 250 tablet PoM £19.69
  Metronidazole 400 mg Metronidazole 400mg tablets | 21 tablet PoM £7.95 DT price = £1.03
  Metronidazole 500 mg Metronidazole 500mg tablets | 21 tablet PoM £37.82 DT price = £37.82
  ► **Flagyl** (Zentiva)
  Metronidazole 200 mg Flagyl 200mg tablets | 21 tablet PoM £4.49 DT price = £1.40
  Metronidazole 400 mg Flagyl 400mg tablets | 14 tablet PoM £6.34
  Oral suspension
  CAUTIONARY AND ADVISORY LABELS 4, 9
  ► **Metronidazole (Non-proprietary)**
  Metronidazole (as Metronidazole benzoate) 40 mg per 1 ml Metronidazole 200mg/5ml oral suspension | 100 ml PoM £32.93 DT price = £32.93
  Infusion
  ELECTROLYTES: May contain Sodium
  ► **Metronidazole (Non-proprietary)**
  Metronidazole 5 mg per 1 ml Metronidazole 500mg/100ml infusion 100ml bags | 20 bag PoM £62.00
  Metronidazole 500mg/100ml infusion 100ml Macoflex bags | 1 bag PoM no price available | 60 bag PoM no price available

Suppository
CAUTIONARY AND ADVISORY LABELS 4, 9
► **Flagyl** (Zentiva)
Metronidazole 500 mg Flagyl 500mg suppositories | 10 suppository PoM £15.18
Metronidazole 1 gram Flagyl 1g suppositories | 10 suppository PoM £23.06

Tinidazole

- **DRUG ACTION** Tinidazole is an antimicrobial drug with high activity against anaerobic bacteria and protozoa; it has a longer duration of action than metronidazole.

- **INDICATIONS AND DOSE**
  Intestinal amoebiasis
  ► BY MOUTH
  ► Child 1 month–11 years: 50–60 mg/kg once daily (max. per dose 2 g) for 3 days
  ► Child 12–17 years: 2 g once daily for 2–3 days
  Amoebic involvement of liver
  ► BY MOUTH
  ► Child 1 month–11 years: 50–60 mg/kg once daily (max. per dose 2 g) for 5 days
  ► Child 12–17 years: 1.5–2 g once daily for 3–6 days
  Urogenital trichomoniasis | Giardiasis
  ► BY MOUTH
  ► Child 1 month–11 years: 50–75 mg/kg (max. per dose 2 g) for 1 single dose, dose may be repeated once if necessary
  ► Child 12–17 years: 2 g for 1 single dose, dose may be repeated once if necessary

- **CAUTIONS** Avoid in Acute porphyrias p. 562
- **INTERACTIONS** → Appendix 1 (tinidazole). Caution—disulfiram-like reaction with alcohol.
- **SIDE-EFFECTS**
  ► **Common or very common** Anorexia · furred tongue · gastro-intestinal disturbances · nausea · oral mucositis · taste disturbances · vomiting
  ► **Very rare** Arthralgia · ataxia · darkening of urine · dizziness · drowsiness · erythema multiforme · headache · hepatitis · jaundice · leucopenia (on prolonged or intensive therapy) · myalgia · pancreatitis · pancytopenia · peripheral neuropathy (on prolonged or intensive therapy) · pruritus · psychotic disorders · rash · thrombocytopenia · transient epileptiform seizures (on prolonged or intensive therapy) · visual disturbances
  ► **Frequency not known** Aseptic meningitis · optic neuropathy
- **PREGNANCY** Manufacturer advises avoid in first trimester.
- **BREAST FEEDING** Present in milk—manufacturer advises avoid breast-feeding during and for 3 days after stopping treatment.
- **MONITORING REQUIREMENTS** Clinical and laboratory monitoring advised if treatment exceeds 10 days.

- **MEDICINAL FORMS**
  There can be variation in the licensing of different medicines containing the same drug.
  Tablet
  CAUTIONARY AND ADVISORY LABELS 4, 9, 21, 25
  ► **Fasigyn** (Pfizer Ltd)
  Tinidazole 500 mg Fasigyn 500mg tablets | 16 tablet PoM £11.04 DT price = £11.04

5

Infection

Penicillins

Benzylpenicillin and phenoxymethylpenicillin

Benzylpenicillin sodium p. 318 (Penicillin G) remains an important and useful antibiotic but is inactivated by bacterial beta-lactamases. It is effective for many streptococcal (including pneumococcal), gonococcal, and meningococcal infections and also for anthrax, diphtheria, gas-gangrene, leptospirosis, and treatment of Lyme disease in children. It is also used in combination with gentamicin p. 293 for the empirical treatment of sepsis in neonates less than 48 hours old. Pneumococci, meningococci, and gonococci which have decreased sensitivity to penicillin have been isolated; benzylpenicillin sodium **is no longer the drug of first choice for pneumococcal meningitis**. Although benzylpenicillin sodium is effective in the treatment of tetanus, metronidazole p. 313 is preferred. Benzylpenicillin sodium is inactivated by gastric acid and absorption from the gastro-intestinal tract is low; therefore it must be given by injection.

Benzathine benzylpenicillin or **procaine benzylpenicillin** are used in the treatment of syphilis.

Phenoxymethylpenicillin p. 319 (Penicillin V) has a similar antibacterial spectrum to benzylpenicillin sodium, but is less active. It is gastric acid-stable, so is suitable for oral administration. It should not be used for serious infections because absorption can be unpredictable and plasma concentrations variable. It is indicated principally for respiratory-tract infections in children, for streptococcal tonsillitis, and for continuing treatment after one or more injections of benzylpenicillin sodium when clinical response has begun. It should not be used for meningococcal or gonococcal infections. Phenoxymethylpenicillin is used for prophylaxis against streptococcal infections following rheumatic fever and against pneumococcal infections following splenectomy or in sickle cell disease.

Penicillinase-resistant penicillins

Most staphylococci are now resistant to benzylpenicillin sodium because they produce penicillinases. Flucloxacillin p. 325, however, is not inactivated by these enzymes and is thus effective in infections caused by penicillin-resistant staphylococci, which is the main indication for its use. Flucloxacillin is acid-stable and can, therefore, be given by mouth as well as by injection. Flucloxacillin is well absorbed from the gut.

Broad-spectrum penicillins

Ampicillin p. 321 is active against certain Gram-positive and Gram-negative organisms but is inactivated by penicillinases including those produced by *Staphylococcus aureus* and by common Gram-negative bacilli such as *Escherichia coli*. Ampicillin is also active against *Listeria* spp. and enterococci. Almost all staphylococci, approx. 60% of *E. coli* strains and approx. 20% of *Haemophilus influenzae* strains are now resistant. The likelihood of resistance should therefore be considered before using ampicillin for the 'blind' treatment of infections; in particular, it should not be used for hospital patients without checking sensitivity.

Ampicillin can be given by mouth, but less than half the dose is absorbed and absorption is further decreased by the presence of food in the gut. Ampicillin is well excreted in the bile and urine.

Amoxicillin p. 320 is a derivative of ampicillin and has a similar antibacterial spectrum. It is better absorbed than ampicillin when given by mouth, producing higher plasma and tissue concentrations; unlike ampicillin, absorption is not affected by the presence of food in the stomach.

Amoxicillin or ampicillin are principally indicated for the treatment of community-acquired pneumonia and middle ear infections, both of which may be due to *Streptococcus pneumoniae* and *H. influenzae*, and for urinary-tract infections. They are also used in the treatment of endocarditis and listerial meningitis. Amoxicillin may also be used for the treatment of Lyme disease [not licensed].

Maculopapular rashes occur commonly with ampicillin (and amoxicillin) but are not usually related to true penicillin allergy. They often occur in children with glandular fever; broad-spectrum penicillins should not therefore be used for 'blind' treatment of a sore throat. The risk of rash is also increased in children with acute or chronic lymphocytic leukaemia or in cytomegalovirus infection.

Co-amoxiclav p. 323 consists of amoxicillin with the beta-lactamase inhibitor clavulanic acid. Clavulanic acid itself has no significant antibacterial activity but, by inactivating beta-lactamases, it makes the combination active against beta-lactamase-producing bacteria that are resistant to amoxicillin. These include resistant strains of *Staph. aureus*, *E. coli*, and *H. influenzae*, as well as many *Bacteroides* and *Klebsiella* spp. Co-amoxiclav should be reserved for infections likely, or known, to be caused by amoxicillin-resistant beta-lactamase-producing strains.

A combination of ampicillin with flucloxacillin (as co-fluampicil p. 322) is available to treat infections involving either streptococci or staphylococci (e.g. cellulitis).

Antipseudomonal penicillins

Piperacillin, a ureidopenicillin, is only available in combination with the beta-lactamase inhibitor tazobactam. **Ticarcillin**, a carboxypenicillin, is only available in combination with the beta-lactamase inhibitor clavulanic acid. Both preparations have a broad spectrum of activity against a range of Gram-positive and Gram-negative bacteria, and anaerobes. Piperacillin with tazobactam p. 317 has activity against a wider range of Gram-negative organisms than ticarcillin with clavulanic acid p. 318 and it is more active against *Pseudomonas aeruginosa*. These antibacterials are not active against MRSA. They are used in the treatment of septicaemia, hospital-acquired pneumonia, and complicated infections involving the urinary-tract, skin and soft tissue, or intra-abdomen. They may be used for the empirical treatment of septicaemia in immunocompromised children but otherwise should generally be reserved for serious infections resistant to other antibacterials. For severe pseudomonas infections these antipseudomonal penicillins can be given with an aminoglycoside (e.g. gentamicin) since they have a synergistic effect.

Piperacillin with tazobactam is used in cystic fibrosis for the treatment of *Ps. aeruginosa* colonisation when ciprofloxacin p. 328 and nebulised colistimethate sodium p. 326 have been ineffective; it can also be used in infective exacerbations, when it is combined with an aminoglycoside.

Mecillinams

Pivmecillinam hydrochloride p. 324 has significant activity against many Gram-negative bacteria including *Escherichia coli*, klebsiella, enterobacter, and salmonellae. It is not active against *Pseudomonas aeruginosa* or enterococci. Pivmecillinam hydrochloride is hydrolysed to mecillinam, which is the active drug.

Penicillins ⊖

- **DRUG ACTION** The penicillins are bactericidal and act by interfering with bacterial cell wall synthesis. They diffuse well into body tissues and fluids, but penetration into the cerebrospinal fluid is poor except when the meninges are inflamed. They are excreted in the urine in therapeutic concentrations.
- **CAUTIONS** History of allergy
- **INTERACTIONS** → Appendix 1 (penicillins).

- **SIDE-EFFECTS**
- ▶ **Common or very common** Anaphylaxis · angioedema · diarrhoea · fever · hypersensitivity reactions · joint pains · rashes · serum sickness-like reaction · urticaria
- ▶ **Rare** Cerebral irritation · CNS toxicity (including convulsions) · coagulation disorders · encephalopathy · haemolytic anaemia · interstitial nephritis · leucopenia · thrombocytopenia
- ▶ **Frequency not known** Antibiotic-associated colitis

SIDE-EFFECTS, FURTHER INFORMATION
- ▶ CNS toxicity A rare but serious toxic effect of the penicillins is encephalopathy due to cerebral irritation. This may result from excessively high doses or in patients with severe renal failure. The penicillins should **not** be given by intrathecal injection because they can cause encephalopathy which may be fatal.
- ▶ Diarrhoea Diarrhoea frequently occurs during oral penicillin therapy. It is most common with broad-spectrum penicillins, which can also cause antibiotic-associated colitis.
- **ALLERGY AND CROSS-SENSITIVITY** The most important side-effect of the penicillins is hypersensitivity which causes rashes and anaphylaxis and can be fatal. Allergic reactions to penicillins occur in 1–10% of exposed individuals; anaphylactic reactions occur in fewer than 0.05% of treated patients. Patients with a history of atopic allergy (e.g. asthma, eczema, hay fever) are at a higher risk of anaphylactic reactions to penicillins. Individuals with a history of anaphylaxis, urticaria, or rash immediately after penicillin administration are at risk of immediate hypersensitivity to a penicillin; these individuals should not receive a penicillin. Individuals with a history of a minor rash (i.e. non-confluent, non-pruritic rash restricted to a small area of the body) or a rash that occurs more than 72 hours after penicillin administration are probably not allergic to penicillin and in these individuals a penicillin should not be withheld unnecessarily for serious infections; the possibility of an allergic reaction should, however, be borne in mind. Other beta-lactam antibiotics (including cephalosporins) can be used in these patients.

    Patients who are allergic to one penicillin will be allergic to all because the hypersensitivity is related to the basic penicillin structure. Patients with a history of immediate hypersensitivity to penicillins may also react to the cephalosporins and other beta-lactam antibiotics, they should not receive these antibiotics. If a penicillin (or another beta-lactam antibiotic) is essential in an individual with immediate hypersensitivity to penicillin then specialist advice should be sought on hypersensitivity testing or using a beta-lactam antibiotic with a different structure to the penicillin that caused the hypersensitivity.

ANTIBACTERIALS ⟩ PENICILLINS, ANTIPSEUDOMONAL WITH BETA-LACTAMASE INHIBITOR

📄 316

Piperacillin with tazobactam

- **INDICATIONS AND DOSE**

Hospital-acquired pneumonia | Septicaemia | Complicated infections involving the urinary-tract | Complicated infections involving the skin | Complicated infections involving the soft-tissues
- ▶ BY INTRAVENOUS INFUSION
- ▶ **Neonate:** 90 mg/kg every 8 hours.
- ▶ **Child 1 month–11 years:** 90 mg/kg every 6–8 hours (max. per dose 4.5 g every 6 hours)
- ▶ **Child 12–17 years:** 4.5 g every 8 hours; increased if necessary to 4.5 g every 6 hours, increased frequency may be used for severe infections

Complicated intra-abdominal infections
- ▶ BY INTRAVENOUS INFUSION
- ▶ **Child 2–11 years:** 112.5 mg/kg every 8 hours (max. per dose 4.5 g)
- ▶ **Child 12–17 years:** 4.5 g every 8 hours; increased if necessary to 4.5 g every 6 hours, increased frequency may be used for severe infections

Infections in neutropenic patients
- ▶ BY INTRAVENOUS INFUSION
- ▶ **Child:** 90 mg/kg every 6 hours (max. per dose 4.5 g)

- **UNLICENSED USE** Not licensed for use in children under 12 years (except for children 2–12 years with neutropenia and complicated intra-abdominal infections).
- **CAUTIONS** High doses may lead to hypernatraemia (owing to sodium content of preparations)
- **SIDE-EFFECTS**
- ▶ **Common or very common** Nausea · vomiting
- ▶ **Uncommon** Constipation · dyspepsia · headache · hypotension · injection-site reactions · insomnia · jaundice · stomatitis
- ▶ **Rare** Abdominal pain · eosinophilia · hepatitis
- ▶ **Very rare** Hypoglycaemia · hypokalaemia · pancytopenia · Steven-Johnson syndrome · toxic epidermal necrolysis
- **PREGNANCY** Manufacturers advise use only if potential benefit outweighs risk.
- **BREAST FEEDING** Trace amount in milk, but appropriate to use.
- **RENAL IMPAIRMENT** *Child under 12 years* 78.75 mg/kg (max. 4.5 g) every 8 hours if estimated glomerular filtration rate less than 50 mL/minute/1.73 m^2. *Child 12–18 years* max. 4.5 g every 8 hours if estimated glomerular filtration rate 20–40 mL/minute/1.73 m^2; max. 4.5 g every 12 hours if estimated glomerular filtration rate less than 20 mL/minute/1.73 m^2.
- **EFFECT ON LABORATORY TESTS** False-positive urinary glucose (if tested for reducing substances).
- **DIRECTIONS FOR ADMINISTRATION**
- ▶ With intravenous use Displacement value may be significant when reconstituting injection, consult local guidelines. For *intravenous infusion*, dilute reconstituted solution to a concentration of 15–90 mg/mL with Glucose 5% *or* Sodium Chloride 0.9%; give over 30 minutes.
- **PRESCRIBING AND DISPENSING INFORMATION** Dose expressed as a combination of piperacillin and tazobactam (both as sodium salts) in a ratio of 8:1.
- **MEDICINAL FORMS**
There can be variation in the licensing of different medicines containing the same drug. Forms available from special-order manufacturers include: infusion
Powder for solution for injection
ELECTROLYTES: May contain Sodium
- ▶ **Piperacillin with tazobactam (Non-proprietary)**
Tazobactam (as Tazobactam sodium) 250 mg, Piperacillin (as Piperacillin sodium) 2 gram Piperacillin 2g / Tazobactam 250mg powder for solution for injection vials | 1 vial PoM £7.96 DT price = £7.91 (Hospital only) | 1 vial PoM £6.50-£7.91 DT price = £7.91 | 10 vial PoM £10.31-£60.80
Tazobactam (as Tazobactam sodium) 500 mg, Piperacillin (as Piperacillin sodium) 4 gram Piperacillin 4g / Tazobactam 500mg powder for solution for injection vials | 1 vial PoM £15.77-£15.79 (Hospital only) | 1 vial PoM £12.90
- ▶ **Tazocin (Pfizer Ltd)**
Tazobactam (as Tazobactam sodium) 250 mg, Piperacillin (as Piperacillin sodium) 2 gram Tazocin 2.25g powder for solution for injection vials | 1 vial PoM £7.65 DT price = £7.91
Tazobactam (as Tazobactam sodium) 500 mg, Piperacillin (as Piperacillin sodium) 4 gram Tazocin 4.5g powder for solution for injection vials | 1 vial PoM £15.17 (Hospital only)

5

Infection

Ticarcillin with clavulanic acid

☞ 316

● INDICATIONS AND DOSE

Infections due to *Pseudomonas* and *Proteus* spp.

▸ BY INTRAVENOUS INFUSION

▸ Preterm neonate (body-weight up to 2 kg): 80 mg/kg every 12 hours.

▸ Preterm neonate (body-weight 2 kg and above): 80 mg/kg every 8 hours; increased if necessary to 80 mg/kg every 6 hours, increased frequency used for more severe infections.

▸ Neonate: 80 mg/kg every 8 hours; increased if necessary to 80 mg/kg every 6 hours, increased frequency used for more severe infections.

▸ Child (body-weight up to 40 kg): 80 mg/kg every 8 hours; increased if necessary to 80 mg/kg every 6 hours, increased frequency used for more severe infections

▸ Child (body-weight 40 kg and above): 3.2 g every 6–8 hours; increased if necessary to 3.2 g every 4 hours, increased frequency used for more severe infections

● **CAUTIONS** High doses may lead to hypernatraemia (owing to sodium content of preparations)

CAUTIONS, FURTHER INFORMATION

▸ Cholestatic jaundice Cholestatic jaundice is possibly associated with clavulanic acid. An epidemiological study has shown that the risk of acute liver toxicity was about 6 times greater with co-amoxiclav (amoxicillin, clavulanic acid) than with amoxicillin. Cholestatic jaundice is more common in patients above the age of 65 years and in men; these reactions have only rarely been reported in children. Jaundice is usually self-limiting and very rarely fatal. The duration of treatment should be appropriate to the indication and should not usually exceed 14 days.

● **SIDE-EFFECTS** Eosinophilia · haemorrhagic cystitis (more frequent in children) · hypokalaemia · injection-site reactions · nausea · Stevens-Johnson syndrome · toxic epidermal necrolysis · vomiting

● **PREGNANCY** Not known to be harmful.

● **BREAST FEEDING** Trace amounts in milk, but appropriate to use.

● **HEPATIC IMPAIRMENT** Manufacturer advises caution in severe impairment.

● **RENAL IMPAIRMENT**

▸ In neonates Reduce dose if estimated glomerular filtration rate less than 60 mL/minute/1.73 m^2.
Child 1 month–18 years: use normal dose every 8 hours if estimated glomerular filtration rate 30–60 mL/minute/1.73 m^2; use half normal dose every 8 hours if estimated glomerular filtration rate 10–30 mL/minute/1.73 m^2; use half normal dose every 12 hours if estimated glomerular filtration rate less than 10 mL/minute/1.73 m^2. Accumulation of electrolytes contained in preparation can occur in patients with renal failure.

● **EFFECT ON LABORATORY TESTS** False-positive urinary glucose (if tested for reducing substances).

● **DIRECTIONS FOR ADMINISTRATION** Displacement value may be important, consult local guidelines. For intermittent infusion, dilute reconstituted solution further to a concentration of 16–32 mg/mL with glucose 5%; infuse over 30–40 minutes.

● **PRESCRIBING AND DISPENSING INFORMATION** Dose is expressed as a combination of ticarcillin (as sodium salt) and clavulanic acid (as potassium salt) in a ratio of 15:1.

● **MEDICINAL FORMS**
There can be variation in the licensing of different medicines containing the same drug.
Powder for solution for infusion
ELECTROLYTES: May contain Potassium, sodium
▸ Timentin (GlaxoSmithKline UK Ltd)
Clavulanic acid (as Potassium clavulanate) 200 mg, Ticarcillin (as Ticarcillin sodium) 3 gram Timentin 3.2g powder for solution for infusion vials | 4 vial [PoM] £21.32

ANTIBACTERIALS ⟩ PENICILLINS, BETA-LACTAMASE SENSITIVE

☞ 316

Benzylpenicillin sodium

(Penicillin G)

● **INDICATIONS AND DOSE**

Mild to moderate susceptible infections | Throat infections | Otitis media | Cellulitis | Pneumonia

▸ BY INTRAMUSCULAR INJECTION, OR BY SLOW INTRAVENOUS INJECTION, OR BY INTRAVENOUS INFUSION

▸ Neonate up to 7 days: 25 mg/kg every 12 hours; increased if necessary to 25 mg/kg every 8 hours, intravenous route recommended in neonates.

▸ Neonate 7 days to 28 days: 25 mg/kg every 8 hours; increased if necessary to 50 mg/kg every 8 hours in severe infection, intravenous route recommended in neonates.

▸ Child: 25 mg/kg every 6 hours; increased if necessary to 50 mg/kg every 4–6 hours (max. per dose 2.4 g every 4 hours) in severe infection, intravenous route recommended in infants

Endocarditis (in combination with other antibacterial if necessary)

▸ BY SLOW INTRAVENOUS INJECTION, OR BY INTRAVENOUS INFUSION

▸ Child: 25 mg/kg every 4 hours; increased if necessary to 50 mg/kg every 4 hours (max. per dose 2.4 g every 4 hours)

Meningitis | Meningococcal disease

▸ BY INTRAVENOUS INFUSION

▸ Neonate up to 7 days: 50 mg/kg every 12 hours.

▸ Neonate 7 days to 28 days: 50 mg/kg every 8 hours.

▸ Child: 50 mg/kg every 4–6 hours (max. per dose 2.4 g every 4 hours)

Suspected meningococcal disease (meningitis with non-blanching rash or meningococcal septicaemia) prior to urgent transfer to hospital

▸ BY INTRAVENOUS INJECTION, OR BY INTRAMUSCULAR INJECTION

▸ Child 1–11 months: 300 mg, administer as single dose prior to urgent transfer to hospital so long as does not delay transfer

▸ Child 1–9 years: 600 mg, administer as single dose prior to urgent transfer to hospital so long as does not delay transfer

▸ Child 10–17 years: 1.2 g, administer as single dose prior to urgent transfer to hospital so long as does not delay transfer

Suspected bacterial meningitis without non-blanching rash where patient cannot be transferred to hospital urgently

▸ BY INTRAVENOUS INJECTION, OR BY INTRAMUSCULAR INJECTION

▸ Child 1–11 months: 300 mg, administer as single dose prior to transfer to hospital

▸ Child 1–9 years: 600 mg, administer as single dose prior to transfer to hospital

▸ Child 10–17 years: 1.2 g, administer as single dose prior to transfer to hospital

Neonatal sepsis

▸ BY INTRAMUSCULAR INJECTION, OR BY SLOW INTRAVENOUS INJECTION, OR BY INTRAVENOUS INFUSION

▸ Neonate up to 7 days: 25 mg/kg every 12 hours; increased if necessary to 25 mg/kg every 8 hours, intravenous route recommended in neonates.

▸ Neonate 7 days to 28 days: 25 mg/kg every 8 hours; increased if necessary to 50 mg/kg every 8 hours in severe infection, intravenous route recommended in neonates.

IMPORTANT SAFETY INFORMATION
Intrathecal injection of benzylpenicillin is **not** recommended.

● CAUTIONS Accumulation of sodium from injection can occur with high doses

● PREGNANCY Not known to be harmful.

● BREAST FEEDING Trace amounts in milk, but appropriate to use.

● RENAL IMPAIRMENT Estimated glomerular filtration rate 10–50 mL/minute/1.73 m^2, use normal dose every 8–12 hours. Estimated glomerular filtration rate less than 10 mL/minute/1.73 m^2 use normal dose every 12 hours. Accumulation of sodium from injection can occur in renal failure.

High doses may cause neurotoxicity, including cerebral irritation, convulsions, or coma.

● EFFECT ON LABORATORY TESTS False-positive urinary glucose (if tested for reducing substances).

● DIRECTIONS FOR ADMINISTRATION

▸ With intravenous use Intravenous route recommended in neonates and infants. For *intravenous infusion*, dilute with Glucose 5% *or* Sodium Chloride 0.9%; give over 15–30 minutes. Longer administration time is particularly important when using doses of 50 mg/kg (or greater) to avoid CNS toxicity.

● MEDICINAL FORMS
There can be variation in the licensing of different medicines containing the same drug. Forms available from special-order manufacturers include: infusion

Powder for solution for injection
ELECTROLYTES: May contain Sodium

▸ Benzylpenicillin sodium (Non-proprietary)
Benzylpenicillin sodium 600 mg Benzylpenicillin 600mg powder for solution for injection vials | 2 vial [PoM] £4.67 DT price = £4.67 | 25 vial [PoM] £58.37–£58.38
Benzylpenicillin sodium 1.2 gram Benzylpenicillin 1.2g powder for solution for injection vials | 25 vial [PoM] £78.64 DT price = £78.64

[▶ 316]

Phenoxymethylpenicillin

(Penicillin V)

● INDICATIONS AND DOSE

Oral infections | Tonsillitis | Otitis media | Erysipelas | Cellulitis

▸ BY MOUTH

▸ Child 1–11 months: 62.5 mg 4 times a day; increased if necessary up to 12.5 mg/kg 4 times a day

▸ Child 1–5 years: 125 mg 4 times a day; increased if necessary up to 12.5 mg/kg 4 times a day

▸ Child 6–11 years: 250 mg 4 times a day; increased if necessary up to 12.5 mg/kg 4 times a day

▸ Child 12–17 years: 500 mg 4 times a day; increased if necessary up to 1 g 4 times a day

Prevention of recurrence of rheumatic fever

▸ BY MOUTH

▸ Child 1 month–5 years: 125 mg twice daily

▸ Child 6–17 years: 250 mg twice daily

Prevention of secondary case of invasive group A streptococcal infection

▸ BY MOUTH

▸ Neonate: 12.5 mg/kg every 6 hours (max. per dose 62.5 mg) for 10 days.

▸ Child 1–11 months: 62.5 mg every 6 hours for 10 days

▸ Child 1–5 years: 125 mg every 6 hours for 10 days

▸ Child 6–11 years: 250 mg every 6 hours for 10 days

▸ Child 12–17 years: 250–500 mg every 6 hours for 10 days

Prevention of pneumococcal infection in asplenia or in patients with sickle-cell disease

▸ BY MOUTH

▸ Child 1–11 months: 62.5 mg twice daily

▸ Child 1–4 years: 125 mg twice daily

▸ Child 5–17 years: 250 mg twice daily

● PREGNANCY Not known to be harmful.

● BREAST FEEDING Trace amounts in milk, but appropriate to use.

● EFFECT ON LABORATORY TESTS False-positive urinary glucose (if tested for reducing substances).

● PATIENT AND CARER ADVICE
Medicines for Children leaflet: Penicillin V for bacterial infections www.medicinesforchildren.org.uk/penicillin-v-for-bacterial-infections
Medicines for Children leaflet: Penicillin V for prevention of pneumococcal infection www.medicinesforchildren.org.uk/penicillin-v-for-prevention-of-pneumococcal-infection

● PROFESSION SPECIFIC INFORMATION
Dental practitioners' formulary
Phenoxymethylpenicillin Tablets may be prescribed.
Phenoxymethylpenicillin Oral Solution may be prescribed.

● MEDICINAL FORMS
There can be variation in the licensing of different medicines containing the same drug.

Tablet
CAUTIONARY AND ADVISORY LABELS 9, 23

▸ Phenoxymethylpenicillin (Non-proprietary)
Phenoxymethylpenicillin (as Phenoxymethylpenicillin potassium) 250 mg Phenoxymethylpenicillin 250mg tablets | 28 tablet [PoM] £5.00 DT price = £0.91

Oral solution
CAUTIONARY AND ADVISORY LABELS 9, 23

▸ Phenoxymethylpenicillin (Non-proprietary)
Phenoxymethylpenicillin (as Phenoxymethylpenicillin potassium) 25 mg per 1 ml Phenoxymethylpenicillin 125mg/5ml oral solution | 100 ml [PoM] £80.00 DT price = £14.73
Phenoxymethylpenicillin 125mg/5ml oral solution sugar free sugar-free | 100 ml [PoM] £25.00 DT price = £16.02
Phenoxymethylpenicillin (as Phenoxymethylpenicillin potassium) 50 mg per 1 ml Phenoxymethylpenicillin 250mg/5ml oral solution | 100 ml [PoM] £80.00 DT price = £14.66
Phenoxymethylpenicillin 250mg/5ml oral solution sugar free sugar-free | 100 ml [PoM] £35.00 DT price = £16.02

5

Infection

F 316

Amoxicillin

(Amoxycillin)

● **INDICATIONS AND DOSE**

Susceptible infections (including urinary-tract infections, otitis media, sinusitis, uncomplicated community acquired pneumonia, salmonellosis, oral infections)

▶ BY MOUTH

▸ Neonate 7 days to 28 days: 30 mg/kg 3 times a day (max. per dose 125 mg).

▸ Child 1-11 months: 125 mg 3 times a day; increased if necessary up to 30 mg/kg 3 times a day

▸ Child 1-4 years: 250 mg 3 times a day; increased if necessary up to 30 mg/kg 3 times a day

▸ Child 5-11 years: 500 mg 3 times a day; increased if necessary up to 30 mg/kg 3 times a day (max. per dose 1 g)

▸ Child 12-17 years: 500 mg 3 times a day; increased if necessary up to 1 g 3 times a day, use increased dose in severe infections

▶ BY INTRAVENOUS INJECTION, OR BY INTRAVENOUS INFUSION

▸ Neonate up to 7 days: 30 mg/kg every 12 hours, increased if necessary to 60 mg/kg every 12 hours, increased dose used in severe infection, community-acquired pneumonia or salmonellosis.

▸ Neonate 7 days to 28 days: 30 mg/kg every 8 hours, increased if necessary to 60 mg/kg every 8 hours, increased dose used in severe infection, community-acquired pneumonia or salmonellosis.

▸ Child: 20–30 mg/kg every 8 hours (max. per dose 500 mg), increased if necessary to 40–60 mg/kg every 8 hours (max. per dose 1 g every 8 hours), increased dose used in severe infection

Cystic fibrosis (treatment of asymptomatic *Haemophilus influenzae* carriage or mild exacerbation)

▶ BY MOUTH

▸ Neonate 7 days to 28 days: 30 mg/kg 3 times a day (max. per dose 125 mg).

▸ Child 1-11 months: 125 mg 3 times a day; increased if necessary up to 30 mg/kg 3 times a day

▸ Child 1-4 years: 250 mg 3 times a day; increased if necessary up to 30 mg/kg 3 times a day

▸ Child 5-11 years: 500 mg 3 times a day; increased if necessary up to 30 mg/kg 3 times a day (max. per dose 1 g)

▸ Child 12-17 years: 500 mg 3 times a day; increased if necessary up to 1 g 3 times a day, use increased dose in severe infections

▶ BY INTRAVENOUS INJECTION, OR BY INTRAVENOUS INFUSION

▸ Neonate up to 7 days: 30 mg/kg every 12 hours, increased if necessary to 60 mg/kg every 12 hours, increased dose used in severe infection.

▸ Neonate 7 days to 28 days: 30 mg/kg every 8 hours, increased if necessary to 60 mg/kg every 8 hours, increased dose used in severe infection.

▸ Child: 20–30 mg/kg every 8 hours (max. per dose 500 mg), increased if necessary to 40–60 mg/kg every 8 hours (max. per dose 1 g every 8 hours), increased dose used in severe infection

Lyme disease (under expert supervision)

▶ BY MOUTH

▸ Neonate 7 days to 28 days: 30 mg/kg 3 times a day (max. per dose 125 mg 3 times a day) usual duration 2–4 weeks.

▸ Child 1-11 months: 125 mg 3 times a day; increased if necessary up to 30 mg/kg 3 times a day usual duration 2–4 weeks

▸ Child 1-4 years: 250 mg 3 times a day; increased if necessary up to 30 mg/kg 3 times a day usual duration 2–4 weeks

▸ Child 5-17 years: 500 mg 3 times a day for 14–21 days (for 28 days in Lyme arthritis)

Anthrax (treatment and post-exposure prophylaxis)

▶ BY MOUTH

▸ Child (body-weight up to 20 kg): 80 mg/kg daily in 3 divided doses

▸ Child (body-weight 20 kg and above): 500 mg 3 times a day

Listerial meningitis (in combination with another antibiotic)

▶ BY INTRAVENOUS INFUSION

▸ Neonate up to 7 days: 50–100 mg/kg every 12 hours.

▸ Neonate 7 days to 28 days: 50–100 mg/kg every 8 hours.

▸ Child: 50 mg/kg every 4–6 hours (max. per dose 2 g every 4 hours)

Group B streptococcal infection | Enterococcal endocarditis (in combination with another antibiotic)

▶ BY INTRAVENOUS INFUSION

▸ Neonate up to 7 days: 50 mg/kg every 12 hours.

▸ Neonate 7 days to 28 days: 50 mg/kg every 8 hours.

▸ Child: 50 mg/kg every 4–6 hours (max. per dose 2 g every 4 hours)

Prevention of pneumococcal infection in asplenia or in patients with sickle-cell disease—if cover also needed for *Haemophilus influenzae*

▶ BY MOUTH

▸ Child 1 month-4 years: 125 mg twice daily

▸ Child 5-11 years: 250 mg twice daily

▸ Child 12-17 years: 500 mg twice daily

***Helicobacter pylori* eradication in combination with clarithromycin and omeprazole**

▶ BY MOUTH

▸ Child 1-5 years: 250 mg twice daily

▸ Child 6-11 years: 500 mg twice daily

▸ Child 12-17 years: 1 g twice daily

***Helicobacter pylori* eradication in combination with metronidazole and omeprazole**

▶ BY MOUTH

▸ Child 1-5 years: 125 mg 3 times a day

▸ Child 6-11 years: 250 mg 3 times a day

▸ Child 12-17 years: 500 mg 3 times a day

● **UNLICENSED USE** Amoxicillin doses in BNF Publications may differ from those in product literature.

● **CAUTIONS**

GENERAL CAUTIONS

Acute lymphocytic leukaemia (increased risk of erythematous rashes) · chronic lymphocytic leukaemia (increased risk of erythematous rashes) · cytomegalovirus infection (increased risk of erythematous rashes) · glandular fever (erythematous rashes common) · maintain adequate hydration with high doses (particularly during parenteral therapy)

SPECIFIC CAUTIONS

▸ With intravenous use Accumulation of sodium can occur with high parenteral doses

- **SIDE-EFFECTS**
- **Common or very common** Nausea · vomiting
  SIDE-EFFECTS, FURTHER INFORMATION
- **Rash** If rash occurs, discontinue treatment.
- **PREGNANCY** Not known to be harmful.
- **BREAST FEEDING** Trace amount in milk, but appropriate to use.
- **RENAL IMPAIRMENT** Reduce dose in severe impairment; rashes more common. Risk of crystalluria with high doses (particularly during parenteral therapy).
- With intravenous use Accumulation of sodium from injection can occur in patients with renal failure.
- **DIRECTIONS FOR ADMINISTRATION**
- With intravenous use Displacement value may be significant when reconstituting injection, consult local guidelines. Dilute intravenous injection to a concentration of 50 mg/mL (100 mg/mL for neonates). May be further diluted with Glucose 5% or Glucose 10% or Sodium chloride 0.9% or 0.45% for intravenous infusion. Give intravenous infusion over 30 minutes when using doses over 30 mg/kg.
- **PRESCRIBING AND DISPENSING INFORMATION** Flavours of oral liquid formulations and sachets may include peach, strawberry, or lemon.
- **PATIENT AND CARER ADVICE**
  Patient counselling is advised for Amoxicillin (*Amoxil*®) paediatric suspension (use of pipette).

  Medicines for Children leaflet: Amoxicillin for bacterial infections www.medicinesforchildren.org.uk/amoxicillin-bacterial-infections-0
- **PROFESSION SPECIFIC INFORMATION**
  Dental practitioners' formulary
  Amoxicillin capsules may be prescribed. Amoxicillin sachets may be prescribed as Amoxicillin Oral Powder. Amoxicillin Oral Suspension may be prescribed.

- **MEDICINAL FORMS**
  There can be variation in the licensing of different medicines containing the same drug.
  Capsule
  CAUTIONARY AND ADVISORY LABELS 9
  - Amoxicillin (Non-proprietary)
    Amoxicillin (as Amoxicillin trihydrate) 250 mg Amoxicillin 250mg capsules | 15 capsule [PoM] £5.00 DT price = £0.73 | 21 capsule [PoM] £5.00 DT price = £1.02 | 500 capsule [PoM] £120.00
    Amoxicillin (as Amoxicillin trihydrate) 500 mg Amoxicillin 500mg capsules | 15 capsule [PoM] £7.50 DT price = £0.91 | 21 capsule [PoM] £15.00 DT price = £1.27 | 100 capsule [PoM] £75.00
  - Amoxil (GlaxoSmithKline UK Ltd)
    Amoxicillin (as Amoxicillin trihydrate) 250 mg Amoxil 250mg capsules | 21 capsule [PoM] £3.38 DT price = £1.02
    Amoxicillin (as Amoxicillin trihydrate) 500 mg Amoxil 500mg capsules | 21 capsule [PoM] £6.77 DT price = £1.27
  Oral suspension
  CAUTIONARY AND ADVISORY LABELS 9
  EXCIPIENTS: May contain Sucrose
  - Amoxicillin (Non-proprietary)
    Amoxicillin (as Amoxicillin trihydrate) 25 mg per 1 ml Amoxicillin 125mg/5ml oral suspension sugar free sugar-free | 100 ml [PoM] £25.00 DT price = £1.02
    Amoxicillin 125mg/5ml oral suspension | 100 ml [PoM] £25.00 DT price = £0.97
    Amoxicillin (as Amoxicillin trihydrate) 50 mg per 1 ml Amoxicillin 250mg/5ml oral suspension sugar free sugar-free | 100 ml [PoM] £35.00 DT price = £1.18
    Amoxicillin 250mg/5ml oral suspension | 100 ml [PoM] £35.00 DT price = £1.15
  - Amoxil (GlaxoSmithKline UK Ltd)
    Amoxicillin (as Amoxicillin trihydrate) 100 mg per 1 ml Amoxil 125mg/1.25ml paediatric oral suspension | 20 ml [PoM] £3.18 DT price = £3.18

Powder for solution for injection
ELECTROLYTES: May contain Sodium
- Amoxicillin (Non-proprietary)
  Amoxicillin (as Amoxicillin sodium) 250 mg Amoxicillin 250mg powder for solution for injection vials | 10 vial [PoM] £4.65–£4.80
  Amoxicillin (as Amoxicillin sodium) 500 mg Amoxicillin 500mg powder for solution for injection vials | 10 vial [PoM] £8.55–£9.60 DT price = £5.48
  Amoxicillin (as Amoxicillin sodium) 1 gram Amoxicillin 1g powder for solution for injection vials | 1 vial [PoM] £1.92 | 10 vial [PoM] £16.50 DT price = £10.96
- Amoxil (GlaxoSmithKline UK Ltd)
  Amoxicillin (as Amoxicillin sodium) 500 mg Amoxil 500mg powder for solution for injection | 10 vial [PoM] £5.48 DT price = £5.48
  Amoxicillin (as Amoxicillin sodium) 1 gram Amoxil 1g powder for solution for injection | 10 vial [PoM] £10.96 DT price = £10.96

Powder
CAUTIONARY AND ADVISORY LABELS 9, 13
- Amoxicillin (Non-proprietary)
  Amoxicillin (as Amoxicillin trihydrate) 3 gram Amoxicillin 3g oral powder sachets sugar free sugar-free | 2 sachet [PoM] £15.00 DT price = £9.98
- Amoxil (GlaxoSmithKline UK Ltd)
  Amoxicillin (as Amoxicillin trihydrate) 3 gram Amoxil 3g oral powder sachets sucrose free sugar-free | 2 sachet [PoM] £2.99 DT price = £9.98

⮞ 316

Ampicillin

- **INDICATIONS AND DOSE**

Susceptible infections (including bronchitis, urinary-tract infections, otitis media, sinusitis, uncomplicated community-acquired pneumonia, salmonellosis)
▸ BY MOUTH

- Neonate 7 days to 20 days: 30 mg/kg 3 times a day (max. per dose 125 mg).
- Neonate 21 days to 28 days: 30 mg/kg 4 times a day (max. per dose 125 mg).
- Child 1–11 months: 125 mg 4 times a day; increased if necessary up to 30 mg/kg 4 times a day
- Child 1–4 years: 250 mg 4 times a day; increased if necessary up to 30 mg/kg 4 times a day
- Child 5–11 years: 500 mg 4 times a day; increased if necessary up to 30 mg/kg 4 times a day (max. per dose 1 g)
- Child 12–17 years: 500 mg 4 times a day; increased if necessary to 1 g 4 times a day, use increased dose in severe infection
▸ BY INTRAVENOUS INJECTION, OR BY INTRAVENOUS INFUSION

- Neonate up to 7 days: 30 mg/kg every 12 hours, increased if necessary to 60 mg/kg every 12 hours, increased dose used in severe infection, community-acquired pneumonia or salmonellosis.
- Neonate 7 days to 20 days: 30 mg/kg every 8 hours, increased if necessary to 60 mg/kg every 8 hours, increased dose used in severe infection, community-acquired pneumonia or salmonellosis.
- Neonate 21 days to 28 days: 30 mg/kg every 6 hours, increased if necessary to 60 mg/kg every 6 hours, increased dose used in severe infection, community-acquired pneumonia or salmonellosis.
- Child: 25 mg/kg every 6 hours (max. per dose 500 mg every 6 hours), increased if necessary to 50 mg/kg every 6 hours (max. per dose 1 g every 6 hours), increased dose used in severe infection

continued →

5

Infection

5

Infection

Group B streptococcal infection | Enterococcal endocarditis (in combination with another antibacterial)
▸ BY INTRAVENOUS INFUSION

▸ Neonate up to 7 days: 50 mg/kg every 12 hours.

▸ Neonate 7 days to 20 days: 50 mg/kg every 8 hours.

▸ Neonate 21 days to 28 days: 50 mg/kg every 6 hours.

▸ Child: 50 mg/kg every 4–6 hours (max. per dose 2 g every 4 hours)

Listerial meningitis
▸ BY INTRAVENOUS INFUSION

▸ Neonate up to 7 days: 100 mg/kg every 12 hours.

▸ Neonate 7 days to 20 days: 100 mg/kg every 8 hours.

▸ Neonate 21 days to 28 days: 100 mg/kg every 6 hours.

▸ Child: 50 mg/kg every 4–6 hours (max. per dose 2 g every 4 hours)

● **CAUTIONS**
GENERAL CAUTIONS
Acute lymphocytic leukaemia (increased risk of erythematous rashes) · chronic lymphocytic leukaemia (increased risk of erythematous rashes) · cytomegalovirus infection (increased risk of erythematous rashes) · glandular fever (erythematous rashes common)
SPECIFIC CAUTIONS
▸ With intravenous use Accumulation of electrolytes contained in parenteral preparations can occur with high doses

● **SIDE-EFFECTS**
▸ Common or very common Nausea · vomiting
SIDE-EFFECTS, FURTHER INFORMATION
▸ Rash If rash occurs, discontinue treatment.

● **PREGNANCY** Not known to be harmful.

● **BREAST FEEDING** Trace amounts in milk, but appropriate to use.

● **RENAL IMPAIRMENT** If estimated glomerular filtration rate less than 10 mL/minute/1.73 m^2 reduce dose or frequency; rashes more common.
▸ With intravenous use Accumulation of electrolytes contained in parenteral preparations can occur in patients with renal failure.

● **DIRECTIONS FOR ADMINISTRATION**
▸ With oral use Administer at least 30 minutes before food.
▸ With intravenous use Displacement value may be significant when reconstituting injection, consult local guidelines. Dilute intravenous injection to a concentration of 50–100 mg/mL. May be further diluted with glucose 5% or 10% or sodium chloride 0.9% or 0.45% for infusion. Give over 30 minutes when using doses of greater than 50 mg/kg to avoid CNS toxicity including convulsions.

● **PATIENT AND CARER ADVICE**
Medicines for Children leaflet: Ampicillin for bacterial infection www.medicinesforchildren.org.uk/ampicillin-bacterial-infection

● **MEDICINAL FORMS**
There can be variation in the licensing of different medicines containing the same drug.
Capsule
CAUTIONARY AND ADVISORY LABELS 9, 23
▸ **Ampicillin** (Non-proprietary)
Ampicillin 250 mg Ampicillin 250mg capsules | 28 capsule [PoM] £25.00 DT price = £5.48
Ampicillin 500 mg Ampicillin 500mg capsules | 28 capsule [PoM] £35.00 DT price = £29.92
▸ **Penbritin** (Chemidex Pharma Ltd)
Ampicillin 250 mg Penbritin 250mg capsules | 28 capsule [PoM] £2.10 DT price = £5.48
Ampicillin 500 mg Penbritin 500mg capsules | 28 capsule [PoM] £5.28 DT price = £29.92

Oral suspension
CAUTIONARY AND ADVISORY LABELS 9, 23
▸ **Ampicillin** (Non-proprietary)
Ampicillin 25 mg per 1 ml Ampicillin 125mg/5ml oral suspension | 100 ml [PoM] £29.86 DT price = £29.86
Ampicillin 50 mg per 1 ml Ampicillin 250mg/5ml oral suspension | 100 ml [PoM] £38.86 DT price = £38.86
Powder for solution for injection
▸ **Ampicillin** (Non-proprietary)
Ampicillin (as Ampicillin sodium) 500 mg Ampicillin 500mg powder for solution for injection vials | 10 vial [PoM] £78.30 DT price = £78.30

▸ 316

Co-fluampicil

● **INDICATIONS AND DOSE**
Mixed infections involving beta-lactamase-producing staphylococci
▸ BY MOUTH

▸ Child 1 month–9 years: 125/125 mg every 6 hours

▸ Child 10–17 years: 250/250 mg every 6 hours

▸ BY INTRAMUSCULAR INJECTION, OR BY SLOW INTRAVENOUS INJECTION, OR BY INTRAVENOUS INFUSION

▸ Child 1 month–1 year: 62.5/62.5 mg every 6 hours

▸ Child 2–9 years: 125/125 mg every 6 hours

▸ Child 10–17 years: 250/250 mg every 6 hours

Severe mixed infections involving beta-lactamase-producing staphylococci
▸ BY MOUTH

▸ Child 1 month–9 years: 250/250 mg every 6 hours

▸ Child 10–17 years: 500/500 mg every 6 hours

▸ BY INTRAMUSCULAR INJECTION, OR BY SLOW INTRAVENOUS INJECTION, OR BY INTRAVENOUS INFUSION

▸ Child 1 month–1 year: 125/125 mg every 6 hours

▸ Child 2–9 years: 250/250 mg every 6 hours

▸ Child 10–17 years: 500/500 mg every 6 hours

IMPORTANT SAFETY INFORMATION
HEPATIC DISORDERS
Cholestatic jaundice and hepatitis may occur very rarely, up to two months after treatment with flucloxacillin has been stopped. Administration for more than 2 weeks and increasing age are risk factors. Healthcare professionals are reminded that:
● flucloxacillin should not be used in patients with a history of hepatic dysfunction associated with flucloxacillin;
● flucloxacillin should be used with caution in patients with hepatic impairment;
● careful enquiry should be made about hypersensitivity reactions to beta-lactam antibacterials.

● **CAUTIONS**
GENERAL CAUTIONS
Acute lymphocytic leukaemia (increased risk of erythematous rashes) · chronic lymphocytic leukaemia (increased risk of erythematous rashes) · cytomegalovirus infection (increased risk of erythematous rashes) · glandular fever (erythematous rashes common)
SPECIFIC CAUTIONS
▸ With intravenous use Accumulation of electrolytes contained in parenteral preparations can occur with high doses · risk of kernicterus in jaundiced neonates when high doses given parenterally

● **SIDE-EFFECTS**
▸ Common or very common Gastro-intestinal disturbances · nausea · vomiting
▸ Very rare Cholestatic jaundice · hepatitis
SIDE-EFFECTS, FURTHER INFORMATION
▸ Rash If rash occurs, discontinue treatment.

- **PREGNANCY** Not known to be harmful.
- **BREAST FEEDING** Trace amount in milk, but appropriate to use.
- **HEPATIC IMPAIRMENT** Use with caution.
- **RENAL IMPAIRMENT** Reduce dose or frequency if estimated glomerular filtration rate less than 10 mL/minute/1.73 m²; rashes more common.
- With intravenous use Accumulation of electrolytes contained in parenteral preparations can occur in patients with renal failure.
- **EFFECT ON LABORATORY TESTS** False-positive urinary glucose (if tested for reducing substances).
- **PRESCRIBING AND DISPENSING INFORMATION** Dose expressed as a combination of equal parts by mass of flucloxacillin and ampicillin.

- **MEDICINAL FORMS**
  There can be variation in the licensing of different medicines containing the same drug.
  Capsule
  CAUTIONARY AND ADVISORY LABELS 9, 22
  - Co-fluampicil (Non-proprietary)
    Ampicillin (as Ampicillin trihydrate) 250 mg, Flucloxacillin (as Flucloxacillin sodium) 250 mg Co-fluampicil 250mg/250mg capsules | 28 capsule [PoM] £10.31 DT price = £2.21 | 100 capsule [PoM] £13.41–£42.99
  Oral suspension
  CAUTIONARY AND ADVISORY LABELS 9, 22
  - Co-fluampicil (Non-proprietary)
    Ampicillin (as Ampicillin trihydrate) 25 mg per 1 ml, Flucloxacillin (as Flucloxacillin magnesium) 25 mg per 1 ml Co-fluampicil 125mg/125mg/5ml oral suspension | 100 ml [PoM] £23.93 DT price = £23.93
  Powder for solution for injection
  ELECTROLYTES: May contain Sodium
  - Co-fluampicil (Non-proprietary)
    Ampicillin (as Ampicillin sodium) 250 mg, Flucloxacillin (as Flucloxacillin sodium) 250 mg Co-fluampicil 250mg/250mg powder for solution for injection vials | 10 vial [PoM] £13.33

ANTIBACTERIALS > **PENICILLINS, BROAD-SPECTRUM WITH BETA-LACTAMASE INHIBITOR**

⮞ 316

Co-amoxiclav

- **INDICATIONS AND DOSE**
  Infections due to beta-lactamase-producing strains (where amoxicillin alone not appropriate), including respiratory tract infections, bone and joint infections, genito-urinary and abdominal infections, cellulitis and animal bites
  ▸ BY MOUTH USING TABLETS
  - Child 12–17 years: 250/125 mg every 8 hours; increased to 500/125 mg every 8 hours, increased dose used for severe infection
  ▸ BY INTRAVENOUS INJECTION, OR BY INTRAVENOUS INFUSION
  - Neonate: 30 mg/kg every 12 hours.
  - Child 1–2 months: 30 mg/kg every 12 hours
  - Child 3 months–17 years: 30 mg/kg every 8 hours (max. per dose 1.2 g every 8 hours)
  Infections due to beta-lactamase-producing strains (where amoxicillin alone not appropriate) including respiratory-tract infections, bone and joint infections, genito-urinary and abdominal infections, cellulitis, animal bites (doses for 125/31 suspension)
  ▸ BY MOUTH USING ORAL SUSPENSION
  - Neonate: 0.25 mL/kilogram 3 times a day.
  - Child 1–11 months: 0.25 mL/kilogram 3 times a day, dose doubled in severe infection

- Child 1–5 years: 0.25 mL/kilogram 3 times a day, alternatively 5 mL 3 times a day, dose doubled in severe infection

  Infections due to beta-lactamase-producing strains (where amoxicillin alone not appropriate) including respiratory-tract infections, bone and joint infections, genito-urinary and abdominal infections, cellulitis, animal bites (doses for 250/62 suspension)
  ▸ BY MOUTH USING ORAL SUSPENSION
  - Child 6–11 years: 0.15 mL/kilogram 3 times a day, alternatively 5 mL 3 times a day, dose doubled in severe infection

  Infections due to beta-lactamase-producing strains (where amoxicillin alone not appropriate) including respiratory-tract infections, bone and joint infections, genito-urinary and abdominal infections, cellulitis, animal bites (doses for 400/57 suspension)
  ▸ BY MOUTH USING ORAL SUSPENSION
  - Child 2 months–1 year: 0.15 mL/kilogram twice daily, doubled in severe infection
  - Child 2–6 years (body-weight 13–21 kg): 2.5 mL twice daily, doubled in severe infection
  - Child 7–12 years (body-weight 22–40 kg): 5 mL twice daily, doubled in severe infection
  - Child 12–17 years (body-weight 41 kg and above): 10 mL twice daily; increased if necessary to 10 mL 3 times a day, increased frequency to be used in severe infection

  Severe dental infection with spreading cellulitis | Dental infection not responding to first-line antibacterial
  ▸ BY MOUTH USING TABLETS
  - Child 12–17 years: 250/125 mg every 8 hours for 5 days

  DOSE EQUIVALENCE AND CONVERSION
  Doses are expressed as co-amoxiclav.
  A mixture of amoxicillin (as the trihydrate or as the sodium salt) and clavulanic acid (as potassium clavulanate); the proportions are expressed in the form x/y where x and y are the strengths in milligrams of amoxicillin and clavulanic acid respectively.

- **CONTRA-INDICATIONS** History of co-amoxiclav-associated jaundice or hepatic dysfunction · history of penicillin-associated jaundice or hepatic dysfunction
- **CAUTIONS**
  GENERAL CAUTIONS
  Acute lymphocytic leukaemia (increased risk of erythematous rashes) · chronic lymphocytic leukaemia (increased risk of erythematous rashes) · cytomegalovirus infection (increased risk of erythematous rashes) · glandular fever (erythematous rashes common) · maintain adequate hydration with high doses (particularly during parental therapy)
  SPECIFIC CAUTIONS
  - With intravenous use Accumulation of electrolytes contained in parenteral preparations can occur with high doses
  CAUTIONS, FURTHER INFORMATION
  - Cholestatic jaundice Cholestatic jaundice can occur either during or shortly after the use of co-amoxiclav. An epidemiological study has shown that the risk of acute liver toxicity was about 6 times greater with co-amoxiclav than with amoxicillin. Cholestatic jaundice is more common in patients above the age of 65 years and in men; these reactions have only rarely been reported in children. Jaundice is usually self-limiting and very rarely fatal. The duration of treatment should be appropriate to the indication and should not usually exceed 14 days.
- **SIDE-EFFECTS**
  GENERAL SIDE-EFFECTS
  - **Common or very common** Cholestatic jaundice · hepatitis · nausea · vomiting
  - **Rare** Dizziness · headache · prolongation of bleeding time

Infection

5

▶ **Frequency not known** Exfoliative dermatitis · Steven-Johnson syndrome · toxic epidermal necrolysis · vasculitis
SPECIFIC SIDE-EFFECTS
▶ **Rare**
▶ With intravenous use Phlebitis at injection site
▶ With oral use Superficial staining of teeth with suspension
SIDE-EFFECTS, FURTHER INFORMATION
▶ Rash If rash occurs, discontinue treatment.
● **PREGNANCY** Not known to be harmful.
● **BREAST FEEDING** Trace amount in milk, but appropriate to use.
● **HEPATIC IMPAIRMENT** Monitor liver function in liver disease.
● **RENAL IMPAIRMENT**
▶ With oral use Co-amoxiclav 125/31 suspension, 250/62 suspension, 250/125 tablets, or 500/125 tablets : use normal dose every 12 hours if estimated glomerular filtration rate 10–30 mL/minute/1.73 m^2. Use the normal dose recommended for mild or moderate infections every 12 hours if estimated glomerular filtration rate less than 10 mL/minute/1.73 m^2. Co-amoxiclav 400/57 suspension : avoid if estimated glomerular filtration rate less than 30 mL/minute/1.73 m^2.
▶ With intravenous use Co-amoxiclav injection : use normal initial dose and then use half normal dose every 12 hours if estimated glomerular filtration rate 10–30 mL/minute/1.73 m^2; use normal initial dose and then use half normal dose every 24 hours if estimated glomerular filtration rate less than 10 mL/minute/1.73 m^2. Risk of crystalluria with high doses (particularly during parenteral therapy). Accumulation of electrolytes contained in parenteral preparations can occur in patients with renal failure.
● **DIRECTIONS FOR ADMINISTRATION**
▶ With intravenous use For intravenous infusion, dilute reconstituted solution to a concentration of 10 mg/mL with Sodium Chloride 0.9%; give intermittently over 30–40 minutes. For intravenous injection, administer over 3–4 minutes.
● **PRESCRIBING AND DISPENSING INFORMATION** Doses are expressed as co-amoxiclav: a mixture of amoxicillin (as the trihydrate or as the sodium salt) and clavulanic acid (as potassium clavulanate); the proportions are expressed in the form x/y where x and y are the strengths in milligrams of amoxicillin and clavulanic acid respectively.
▶ With oral use Flavours of oral liquid formulations may include raspberry and orange.
● **PATIENT AND CARER ADVICE**
Medicines for Children leaflet: Co-amoxiclav for bacterial infections www.medicinesforchildren.org.uk/co-amoxiclav-bacterial-infections-0
● **PROFESSION SPECIFIC INFORMATION**
Dental practitioners' formulary
Co-amoxiclav 250/125 Tablets may be prescribed. Co-amoxiclav 125/31 Suspension may be prescribed. Co-amoxiclav 250/62 Suspension may be prescribed.

● **MEDICINAL FORMS**
There can be variation in the licensing of different medicines containing the same drug. Forms available from special-order manufacturers include: infusion

Tablet
CAUTIONARY AND ADVISORY LABELS 9
▶ Co-amoxiclav (Non-proprietary)
Clavulanic acid (as Potassium clavulanate) 125 mg, Amoxicillin (as Amoxicillin trihydrate) 250 mg Co-amoxiclav 250mg/125mg tablets | 21 tablet PoM £7.00 DT price = £2.42 | 100 tablet PoM no price available
Clavulanic acid (as Potassium clavulanate) 125 mg, Amoxicillin (as Amoxicillin trihydrate) 500 mg Co-amoxiclav 500mg/125mg tablets | 21 tablet PoM £15.00 DT price = £2.38

Clavulanic acid (as Potassium clavulanate) 125 mg, Amoxicillin (as Amoxicillin trihydrate) 875 mg Co-amoxiclav 875mg/125mg tablets | 14 tablet PoM £18.00 DT price = £8.60
▶ Augmentin (GlaxoSmithKline UK Ltd)
Clavulanic acid (as Potassium clavulanate) 125 mg, Amoxicillin (as Amoxicillin trihydrate) 250 mg Augmentin 375mg tablets | 21 tablet PoM £5.03 DT price = £2.42
Clavulanic acid (as Potassium clavulanate) 125 mg, Amoxicillin (as Amoxicillin trihydrate) 500 mg Augmentin 625mg tablets | 21 tablet PoM £9.60 DT price = £2.38

Oral suspension
CAUTIONARY AND ADVISORY LABELS 9
EXCIPIENTS: May contain Aspartame
▶ Co-amoxiclav (Non-proprietary)
Clavulanic acid (as Potassium clavulanate) 6.25 mg per 1 ml, Amoxicillin (as Amoxicillin trihydrate) 25 mg per 1 ml Co-amoxiclav 125mg/31mg/5ml oral suspension | 100 ml PoM £5.00 DT price = £5.00
Co-amoxiclav 125mg/31mg/5ml oral suspension sugar free sugar-free | 100 ml PoM £25.00 DT price = £1.79
Clavulanic acid (as Potassium clavulanate) 12.5 mg per 1 ml, Amoxicillin (as Amoxicillin trihydrate) 50 mg per 1 ml Co-amoxiclav 250mg/62mg/5ml oral suspension | 100 ml PoM £5.00 DT price = £5.00
Co-amoxiclav 250mg/62mg/5ml oral suspension sugar free sugar-free | 100 ml PoM £35.00 DT price = £1.62
Clavulanic acid (as Potassium clavulanate) 11.4 mg per 1 ml, Amoxicillin (as Amoxicillin trihydrate) 80 mg per 1 ml Co-amoxiclav 400mg/57mg/5ml oral suspension sugar free sugar-free | 35 ml PoM £4.13 DT price = £4.13 sugar-free | 70 ml PoM £6.97 DT price = £5.79
▶ Augmentin (GlaxoSmithKline UK Ltd)
Clavulanic acid (as Potassium clavulanate) 6.25 mg per 1 ml, Amoxicillin (as Amoxicillin trihydrate) 25 mg per 1 ml Augmentin 125/31 SF oral suspension sugar-free | 100 ml PoM £3.54 DT price = £1.79
Clavulanic acid (as Potassium clavulanate) 12.5 mg per 1 ml, Amoxicillin (as Amoxicillin trihydrate) 50 mg per 1 ml Augmentin 250/62 SF oral suspension sugar-free | 100 ml PoM £3.60 DT price = £1.62
▶ Augmentin-Duo (GlaxoSmithKline UK Ltd)
Clavulanic acid (as Potassium clavulanate) 11.4 mg per 1 ml, Amoxicillin (as Amoxicillin trihydrate) 80 mg per 1 ml Augmentin-Duo 400/57 oral suspension sugar-free | 35 ml PoM £4.13 sugar-free | 70 ml PoM £5.79 DT price = £5.79

Powder for solution for injection
ELECTROLYTES: May contain Potassium, sodium
▶ Co-amoxiclav (Non-proprietary)
Clavulanic acid (as Potassium clavulanate) 100 mg, Amoxicillin (as Amoxicillin sodium) 500 mg Co-amoxiclav 500mg/100mg powder for solution for injection vials | 10 vial PoM £11.39–£14.90
Clavulanic acid (as Potassium clavulanate) 200 mg, Amoxicillin (as Amoxicillin sodium) 1000 mg Co-amoxiclav 1000mg/200mg powder for solution for injection vials | 10 vial PoM £29.70
▶ Augmentin Intravenous (GlaxoSmithKline UK Ltd)
Clavulanic acid (as Potassium clavulanate) 100 mg, Amoxicillin (as Amoxicillin sodium) 500 mg Augmentin Intravenous 600mg powder for solution for injection vials | 10 vial PoM £10.60
Clavulanic acid (as Potassium clavulanate) 200 mg, Amoxicillin (as Amoxicillin sodium) 1000 mg Augmentin Intravenous 1.2g powder for solution for injection vials | 10 vial PoM £10.60

ANTIBACTERIALS 〉 PENICILLINS, MECILLINAM-TYPE

�F 316

Pivmecillinam hydrochloride

● **INDICATIONS AND DOSE**
Acute uncomplicated cystitis
▶ BY MOUTH
▶ Child (body-weight 40 kg and above): Initially 400 mg for 1 dose, then 200 mg every 8 hours for 3 days
Chronic or recurrent bacteriuria
▶ BY MOUTH
▶ Child (body-weight 40 kg and above): 400 mg every 6–8 hours

Urinary-tract infections
- ▸ BY MOUTH
- ▸ Child (body-weight up to 40 kg): 5–10 mg/kg every 6 hours, alternatively 20–40 mg/kg daily in 3 divided doses

- **UNLICENSED USE** Not licensed for use in children under 3 months.
- **CONTRA-INDICATIONS** Carnitine deficiency · gastro-intestinal obstruction · infants under 3 months · oesophageal strictures
- **CAUTIONS** Avoid in Acute porphyrias p. 562
- **SIDE-EFFECTS**
- ▸ **Common or very common** Abdominal pain · dizziness · headache · nausea · vomiting
- ▸ **Frequency not known** Mouth ulcers · oesophagitis · reduced serum and total body carnitine (especially with long-term or repeated use)
- **PREGNANCY** Not known to be harmful, but manufacturer advises avoid.
- **BREAST FEEDING** Trace amount in milk, but appropriate to use.
- **MONITORING REQUIREMENTS** Liver and renal function tests required in long-term use.
- **EFFECT ON LABORATORY TESTS** False-positive urinary glucose (if tested for reducing substances).
- **DIRECTIONS FOR ADMINISTRATION** Tablets should be swallowed whole with plenty of fluid during meals while sitting or standing.
- **PATIENT AND CARER ADVICE** Patient counselling is advised on administration of pivmecillinam hydrochloride tablets (posture).

- **MEDICINAL FORMS**
  There can be variation in the licensing of different medicines containing the same drug. Forms available from special-order manufacturers include: oral suspension
  Tablet
  CAUTIONARY AND ADVISORY LABELS 9, 21, 27
  - ▸ Selexid (LEO Pharma)
    Pivmecillinam hydrochloride 200 mg Selexid 200mg tablets | 10 tablet [PoM] £4.50 DT price = £4.50

ANTIBACTERIALS > PENICILLINS, PENICILLINASE-RESISTANT

ⓕ 316

Flucloxacillin

- **INDICATIONS AND DOSE**
  Infections due to beta-lactamase-producing staphylococci including otitis externa | Adjunct in pneumonia | Adjunct in impetigo | Adjunct in cellulitis
  - ▸ BY MOUTH
  - ▸ Neonate up to 7 days: 25 mg/kg twice daily.
  - ▸ Neonate 7 days to 20 days: 25 mg/kg 3 times a day.
  - ▸ Neonate 21 days to 28 days: 25 mg/kg 4 times a day.
  - ▸ Child 1 month–1 year: 62.5–125 mg 4 times a day
  - ▸ Child 2–9 years: 125–250 mg 4 times a day
  - ▸ Child 10–17 years: 250–500 mg 4 times a day
  - ▸ BY INTRAMUSCULAR INJECTION
  - ▸ Child: 12.5–25 mg/kg every 6 hours (max. per dose 500 mg every 6 hours)
  - ▸ BY SLOW INTRAVENOUS INJECTION, OR BY INTRAVENOUS INFUSION
  - ▸ Neonate up to 7 days: 25 mg/kg every 12 hours.
  - ▸ Neonate 7 days to 20 days: 25 mg/kg every 8 hours.

- ▸ Neonate 21 days to 28 days: 25 mg/kg every 6 hours.
- ▸ Child: 12.5–25 mg/kg every 6 hours (max. per dose 1 g every 6 hours)

Severe infections due to beta-lactamase-producing staphylococci including otitis externa | Adjunct in pneumonia (severe infection) | Adjunct in impetigo (severe infection) | Adjunct in cellulitis (severe infection)
- ▸ BY SLOW INTRAVENOUS INJECTION, OR BY INTRAVENOUS INFUSION
- ▸ Neonate up to 7 days: 50 mg/kg every 12 hours.
- ▸ Neonate 7 days to 20 days: 50 mg/kg every 8 hours.
- ▸ Neonate 21 days to 28 days: 50 mg/kg every 6 hours.
- ▸ Child: 25–50 mg/kg every 6 hours (max. per dose 2 g every 6 hours)

Endocarditis (in combination with other antibacterial if necessary)
- ▸ BY SLOW INTRAVENOUS INJECTION, OR BY INTRAVENOUS INFUSION
- ▸ Child: 50 mg/kg every 6 hours (max. per dose 2 g every 6 hours)

Osteomyelitis
- ▸ BY SLOW INTRAVENOUS INJECTION, OR BY INTRAVENOUS INFUSION
- ▸ Neonate up to 7 days: 50–100 mg/kg every 12 hours.
- ▸ Neonate 7 days to 20 days: 50–100 mg/kg every 8 hours.
- ▸ Neonate 21 days to 28 days: 50–100 mg/kg every 6 hours.
- ▸ Child: 50 mg/kg every 6 hours (max. per dose 2 g every 6 hours)

Cerebral abscess | Staphylococcal meningitis
- ▸ BY SLOW INTRAVENOUS INJECTION, OR BY INTRAVENOUS INFUSION
- ▸ Neonate up to 7 days: 50–100 mg/kg every 12 hours.
- ▸ Neonate 7 days to 20 days: 50–100 mg/kg every 8 hours.
- ▸ Neonate 21 days to 28 days: 50–100 mg/kg every 6 hours.
- ▸ Child: 50 mg/kg every 6 hours (max. per dose 2 g every 6 hours)

Staphylococcal lung infection in cystic fibrosis
- ▸ BY MOUTH
- ▸ Child: 25 mg/kg 4 times a day (max. per dose 1 g), alternatively 100 mg/kg daily in 3 divided doses; maximum 4 g per day
- ▸ BY SLOW INTRAVENOUS INJECTION, OR BY INTRAVENOUS INFUSION
- ▸ Child: 50 mg/kg every 6 hours (max. per dose 2 g every 6 hours)

Prevention of *Staphylococcus aureus* lung infection in cystic fibrosis—primary prevention
- ▸ BY MOUTH
- ▸ Neonate: 125 mg twice daily.
- ▸ Child 1 month–3 years: 125 mg twice daily

Prevention of *Staphylococcus aureus* lung infection in cystic fibrosis—secondary prevention
- ▸ BY MOUTH
- ▸ Child: 50 mg/kg twice daily (max. per dose 1 g twice daily)

IMPORTANT SAFETY INFORMATION
HEPATIC DISORDERS
Cholestatic jaundice and hepatitis may occur very rarely, up to two months after treatment with flucloxacillin has been stopped. Administration for more than 2 weeks and increasing age are risk factors. Healthcare professionals are reminded that:

- fluxloxacillin should not be used in patients with a history of hepatic dysfunction associated with flucloxacillin
- flucloxacillin should be used with caution in patients with hepatic impairment
- careful enquiry should be made about hypersensitivity reactions to beta-lactam antibacterials

- **CAUTIONS**
  ‣ With intravenous use Accumulation of electrolytes can occur with high doses · risk of kernicterus in jaundiced neonates when high doses given parenterally
- **SIDE-EFFECTS**
  ‣ **Common or very common** Gastrointestinal disturbances
  ‣ **Very rare** Cholestatic jaundice · hepatitis
- **PREGNANCY** Not known to be harmful.
- **BREAST FEEDING** Trace amounts in milk, but appropriate to use.
- **HEPATIC IMPAIRMENT** Use with caution.
- **RENAL IMPAIRMENT** Use normal dose every 8 hours if estimated glomerular filtration rate less than 10 mL/minute/1.73 m^2.
  ‣ With intravenous use Accumulation of electrolytes can occur in patients with renal failure.
- **EFFECT ON LABORATORY TESTS** False-positive urinary glucose (if tested for reducing substances).
- **DIRECTIONS FOR ADMINISTRATION**
  ‣ With intravenous use For *intravenous infusion*, dilute reconstituted solution *in* Glucose 5% *or* Sodium Chloride 0.9% and give intermittently over 30–60 minutes.
- **PATIENT AND CARER ADVICE**
  Medicines for Children leaflet: Flucloxacillin for bacterial infections www.medicinesforchildren.org.uk/flucloxacillin-for-bacterial-infections

- **MEDICINAL FORMS**
  There can be variation in the licensing of different medicines containing the same drug. Forms available from special-order manufacturers include: infusion
  Capsule
  CAUTIONARY AND ADVISORY LABELS 9, 23
  ‣ Flucloxacillin (Non-proprietary)
  Flucloxacillin (as Flucloxacillin sodium) 250 mg Flucloxacillin 250mg capsules | 20 capsule [PoM] £3.58 | 28 capsule [PoM] £5.00 DT price = £1.29 | 100 capsule [PoM] £17.80 | 500 capsule [PoM] £52.14
  Flucloxacillin (as Flucloxacillin sodium) 500 mg Flucloxacillin 500mg capsules | 20 capsule [PoM] £7.50 | 28 capsule [PoM] £10.50 DT price = £2.19 | 100 capsule [PoM] £37.50
  Oral solution
  CAUTIONARY AND ADVISORY LABELS 9, 23
  ‣ Flucloxacillin (Non-proprietary)
  Flucloxacillin (as Flucloxacillin sodium) 25 mg per 1 ml Flucloxacillin 125mg/5ml oral solution | 100 ml [PoM] £21.87 DT price = £5.10
  Flucloxacillin 125mg/5ml oral solution sugar free sugar-free | 100 ml [PoM] £31.41 DT price = £22.58
  Flucloxacillin (as Flucloxacillin sodium) 50 mg per 1 ml Flucloxacillin 250mg/5ml oral solution sugar free sugar-free | 100 ml [PoM] £38.94 DT price = £27.23
  Flucloxacillin 250mg/5ml oral solution | 100 ml [PoM] £28.72 DT price = £26.04
  Powder for solution for injection
  ‣ Flucloxacillin (Non-proprietary)
  Flucloxacillin (as Flucloxacillin sodium) 250 mg Flucloxacillin 250mg powder for solution for injection vials | 10 vial [PoM] £10.43–£12.25
  Flucloxacillin (as Flucloxacillin sodium) 500 mg Flucloxacillin 500mg powder for solution for injection vials | 10 vial [PoM] £20.85–£24.50
  Flucloxacillin (as Flucloxacillin sodium) 1 gram Flucloxacillin 1g powder for solution for injection vials | 10 vial [PoM] £41.75–£49.00

ANTIBACTERIALS ⟩ POLYMYXINS

Colistimethate sodium
(Colistin sulfomethate sodium)

- **DRUG ACTION** The polymyxin antibiotic, **colistimethate sodium** (colistin sulfomethate sodium), is active against Gram-negative organisms including *Pseudomonas aeruginosa*, *Acinetobacter baumanii*, and *Klebsiella pneumoniae*. It is not absorbed by mouth and thus needs to be given by injection for a systemic effect.

- **INDICATIONS AND DOSE**
  Gram-negative infections resistant to other antibacterials, including those caused by *Pseudomonas aeruginosa*, *Acinetobacter baumanii* and *Klebsiella pneumoniae*
  ‣ BY SLOW INTRAVENOUS INJECTION, OR BY INTRAVENOUS INFUSION
  ‣ Child (body-weight up to 60 kg): 50 000–75 000 units/kg daily in 3 divided doses, to be administered into a totally implantable venous access device when giving via slow intravenous injection
  ‣ Child (body-weight 60 kg and above): 1–2 million units 3 times a day, to be administered into a totally implantable venous access device when giving via slow intravenous injection; maximum 6 million units per day

  Adjunct to standard antibacterial therapy for *Pseudomonas aeruginosa* infection in cystic fibrosis
  ‣ BY INHALATION OF NEBULISED SOLUTION
  ‣ Child 1 month-1 year: 0.5–1 million units twice daily, adjusted according to response, increased to 2 million units 3 times daily for subsequent respiratory isolates of *Pseudomonas aeruginosa*
  ‣ Child 2-17 years: 1–2 million units twice daily, adjusted according to response, increased to 2 million units 3 times daily for subsequent respiratory isolates of *Pseudomonas aeruginosa*

  PROMIXIN®
  Gram-negative infections resistant to other antibacterials, including those caused by *Pseudomonas aeruginosa*, *Acinetobacter baumanii* , *Klebsiella pneumoniae*
  ‣ BY SLOW INTRAVENOUS INJECTION, OR BY INTRAVENOUS INFUSION
  ‣ Child (body-weight up to 40 kg): 75 000–150 000 units/kg daily in 3 divided doses, to be administered into a totally implantable venous access device when giving via slow intravenous injection
  ‣ Child (body-weight 40 kg and above): 9 million units daily in 2–3 divided doses, to be administered into a totally implantable venous access device when giving via slow intravenous injection

  PROMIXIN®
  Management of chronic pulmonary infections due to *Pseudomonas aeruginosa* in patients with cystic fibrosis
  ‣ BY INHALATION OF NEBULISED SOLUTION
  ‣ Child 1 month-1 year: 0.5–1 million units twice daily, for specific advice on administration using nebulisers—consult product literature; maximum 2 million units per day
  ‣ Child 2-17 years: 1–2 million units 2–3 times a day, for specific advice on administration using nebulisers—consult product literature; maximum 6 million units per day

- **CONTRA-INDICATIONS** Myasthenia gravis

● **CAUTIONS**

GENERAL CAUTIONS
Acute porphyrias p. 562
SPECIFIC CAUTIONS
‣ When used by inhalation Severe haemoptysis—risk of further haemorrhage

● **INTERACTIONS** → Appendix 1 (polymyxins).

● **SIDE-EFFECTS**
‣ **Common or very common**
‣ When used by inhalation Bronchospasm · cough · dysphonia · nausea · sore mouth · Sore throat · taste disturbances · vomiting
‣ **Uncommon**
‣ When used by inhalation Hypersalivation · thirst
‣ **Rare**
‣ With intravenous use Vasomotor instability
‣ **Frequency not known**
‣ With intravenous use Apnoea · confusion · headache · muscle weakness · nephrotoxicity · neurotoxicity reported especially with excessive doses · perioral paraesthesia · peripheral paraesthesia · psychosis · rash · slurred speech · vertigo · visual disturbances

SIDE-EFFECTS, FURTHER INFORMATION
‣ Dose-related side-effects The major adverse effects are dose-related neurotoxicity and nephrotoxicity.

● **PREGNANCY**
‣ When used by inhalation Clinical use suggests probably safe.
‣ With intravenous use Use only if potential benefit outweighs risk.

● **BREAST FEEDING** Present in milk but poorly absorbed from gut; manufacturers advise avoid (or use only if potential benefit outweighs risk).

● **RENAL IMPAIRMENT**
‣ With intravenous use Reduce dose.
‣ With intravenous use In renal impairment, monitor plasma colistimethate sodium concentration during parenteral treatment—consult product literature. Recommended 'peak' plasma colistimethate sodium concentration (approx. 1 hour after intravenous injection or infusion) 5–15 mg/litre; pre-dose ('trough') concentration 2–6 mg/litre.

● **MONITORING REQUIREMENTS**
‣ With intravenous use Monitor renal function.
‣ When used by inhalation Measure lung function before and after initial dose of colistimethate sodium and monitor for bronchospasm; if bronchospasm occurs in a patient not using a bronchodilator, repeat test using a bronchodilator before the dose of colistimethate sodium.

● **DIRECTIONS FOR ADMINISTRATION**
‣ When used by inhalation Other inhaled drugs should be administered before colistimethate sodium. For *nebulisation* administer required dose in 2–4 mL of sodium chloride 0.9% (or water for injections) or a 1:1 mixture of sodium chloride 0.9% and water for injection.
‣ With intravenous use For *intravenous infusion*, dilute to a concentration of 40 000 units/mL with Sodium Chloride 0.9%; give over 30 minutes. For *slow intravenous injection* into a totally implantable venous access device, dilute to a concentration of 90 000 units/mL with Sodium Chloride 0.9% for child under 12 years (200 000 units/mL for child over 12 years).

COLOMYCIN® Colomycin® Injection may be used for nebulisation; administer required dose in 2–4 mL of sodium chloride 0.9%, (or water for injections) or a 1:1 mixture of sodium chloride 0.9% and water for injection.

● **PRESCRIBING AND DISPENSING INFORMATION**
Colistimethate sodium is included in some preparations for topical application.

● **PATIENT AND CARER ADVICE**
‣ When used by inhalation Patient should be advised to rinse mouth with water after each dose of dry powder inhalation.

● **NATIONAL FUNDING/ACCESS DECISIONS**
NICE technology appraisals (TAs)
‣ **Colistimethate sodium by dry powder inhalation for pseudomonal lung infection in cystic fibrosis (March 2013)**
NICE TA276
Colistimethate sodium dry powder for inhalation is recommended for chronic pulmonary infection caused by *Pseudomonas aeruginosa* in patients with cystic fibrosis who would benefit from continued treatment, but do not tolerate the drug in its nebulised form. The manufacturer must provide colistimethate sodium dry powder for inhalation at the discount agreed as part of the patient access scheme to primary, secondary and tertiary care in the NHS. Patients currently receiving colistimethate sodium dry powder for inhalation can continue treatment until they and their clinician consider it appropriate to stop.
www.nice.org.uk/TA276

● **MEDICINAL FORMS**
There can be variation in the licensing of different medicines containing the same drug.
Powder for solution for injection
ELECTROLYTES: May contain Sodium
‣ Colistimethate sodium (Non-proprietary)
 Colistimethate sodium 1000000 unit Colistimethate 1million unit powder for solution for injection vials | 10 vial [PoM] £18.00 | 10 vial [PoM] £16.79 (Hospital only)
‣ Colomycin (Forest Laboratories UK Ltd)
 Colistimethate sodium 1000000 unit Colomycin 1million unit powder for solution for injection vials | 10 vial [PoM] £18.00
 Colistimethate sodium 2000000 unit Colomycin 2million unit powder for solution for injection vials | 10 vial [PoM] £32.40
‣ Promixin (Profile Pharma Ltd)
 Colistimethate sodium 1000000 unit Promixin 1million unit powder for solution for injection vials | 10 vial [PoM] £30.00 (Hospital only)

Powder for nebuliser solution
‣ Promixin (Profile Pharma Ltd)
 Colistimethate sodium 1000000 unit Promixin 1million unit powder for nebuliser solution unit dose vials | 30 unit dose [PoM] £168.00

ANTIBACTERIALS ⟩ QUINOLONES

Quinolones

Overview

Ciprofloxacin p. 328 is active against both Gram-positive and Gram-negative bacteria. It is particularly active against Gram-negative bacteria, including salmonella, shigella, campylobacter, neisseria, and pseudomonas. Ciprofloxacin has only moderate activity against Gram-positive bacteria such as *Streptococcus pneumoniae* and *Enterococcus faecalis*; it should not be used for pneumococcal pneumonia. It is active against chlamydia and some mycobacteria. Most anaerobic organisms are not susceptible. Ciprofloxacin is licensed in children over 1 year of age for pseudomonal infections in cystic fibrosis, for complicated urinary-tract infections, and for treatment and prophylaxis of inhalation anthrax. When the benefits of treatment outweigh the risks, ciprofloxacin is licensed in children over 1 year of age for severe infections of the respiratory tract and of the gastro-intestinal system (including typhoid fever). It is also used in the treatment of septicaemia caused by multi-resistant organisms (usually hospital acquired) and gonorrhoea (although resistance is increasing). Ciprofloxacin is also used in the prophylaxis of meningococcal disease.

Nalidixic acid p. 329 may be used in uncomplicated urinary-tract infections that are resistant to other antibiotics in children over 3 months of age.

Many staphylococci are resistant to quinolones and their use should be avoided in MRSA infections.

Ofloxacin eye drops p. 631 are used in ophthalmic infections.

There is much less experience of the other quinolones in children; expert advice should be sought.

Quinolones

> **IMPORTANT SAFETY INFORMATION**
> The CSM has warned that quinolones may induce **convulsions** in patients with or without a history of convulsions; taking NSAIDs at the same time may also induce them.
>
> TENDON DAMAGE
> Tendon damage (including rupture) has been reported rarely in patients receiving quinolones. Tendon rupture may occur within 48 hours of starting treatment; cases have also been reported several months after stopping a quinolone. Healthcare professionals are reminded that:
> - quinolones are contra-indicated in patients with a history of tendon disorders related to quinolone use;
> - the risk of tendon damage is increased by the concomitant use of corticosteroids;
> - if tendinitis is suspected, the quinolone should be discontinued immediately.

- **CONTRA-INDICATIONS** History of tendon disorders related to quinolone use
- **CAUTIONS** Can prolong the QT interval · children or adolescents (arthropathy has developed in weight-bearing joints in young *animals*) · conditions that predispose to seizures · exposure to excessive sunlight should be avoided (discontinue if photosensitivity occurs) · G6PD deficiency · history of epilepsy · myasthenia gravis (risk of exacerbation)

  CAUTIONS, FURTHER INFORMATION
  Quinolones cause arthropathy in the weight-bearing joints of immature *animals* and are therefore generally not recommended in children and growing adolescents. However, the significance of this effect in humans is uncertain and in some specific circumstances short-term use of either ciprofloxacin or nalidixic acid may be justified in children.
- **INTERACTIONS** → Appendix 1 (quinolones).
- **SIDE-EFFECTS**
- ▶ **Common or very common** Diarrhoea · dizziness · headache · nausea · vomiting
- ▶ **Uncommon** Abdominal pain · anorexia · anxiety · arthralgia · asthenia · blood disorders · confusion · depression · disturbances in taste · disturbances in vision · dyspepsia · eosinophilia · hallucinations · leucopenia · myalgia · rash · sleep disturbances · thrombocytopenia · tremor
- ▶ **Rare** Antibiotic-associated colitis · convulsions · disturbances in hearing · disturbances in smell · dyspnoea · hepatic dysfunction · hepatitis · hypotension · interstitial nephritis · jaundice · photosensitivity · psychoses · renal failure · symptoms of peripheral neuropathy (sometimes irreversible) · tendon damage · tendon inflammation · vasculitis
- ▶ **Very rare** Stevens-Johnson syndrome · toxic epidermal necrolysis

  SIDE-EFFECTS, FURTHER INFORMATION
  The drug should be **discontinued** if psychiatric, neurological, or hypersensitivity reactions (including severe rash) occur.

- **ALLERGY AND CROSS-SENSITIVITY** Use of quinolones contra-indicated in quinolone hypersensitivity.
- **PREGNANCY** Avoid in pregnancy—shown to cause arthropathy in *animal* studies; safer alternatives are available.

◤ above

Ciprofloxacin

- **INDICATIONS AND DOSE**

Fistulating Crohn's disease
▶ BY MOUTH
- ▶ Child: 5 mg/kg twice daily

Severe respiratory-tract infections, gastro-intestinal infection
▶ BY MOUTH
- ▶ Neonate: 15 mg/kg twice daily.
- ▶ Child: 20 mg/kg twice daily (max. per dose 750 mg)
▶ BY INTRAVENOUS INFUSION
- ▶ Neonate: 10 mg/kg every 12 hours, to be given over 60 minutes.
- ▶ Child: 10 mg/kg every 8 hours (max. per dose 400 mg), to be given over 60 minutes

Pseudomonal lower respiratory-tract infection in cystic fibrosis
▶ BY MOUTH
- ▶ Child: 20 mg/kg twice daily (max. per dose 750 mg)
▶ BY INTRAVENOUS INFUSION
- ▶ Child: 10 mg/kg every 8 hours (max. per dose 400 mg), to be given over 60 minutes

Complicated urinary-tract infections
▶ BY MOUTH
- ▶ Neonate: 10 mg/kg twice daily.
- ▶ Child: 10 mg/kg twice daily, dose to be doubled in severe infection (max. 750 mg twice daily)
▶ BY INTRAVENOUS INFUSION
- ▶ Neonate: 6 mg/kg every 12 hours, to be given over 60 minutes.
- ▶ Child: 6 mg/kg every 8 hours; increased to 10 mg/kg every 8 hours (max. per dose 400 mg), in severe infection

Gonorrhoea
▶ BY MOUTH
- ▶ Child 12-17 years: 500 mg for 1 dose

Anthrax (treatment and post-exposure prophylaxis)
▶ BY MOUTH
- ▶ Child: 15 mg/kg twice daily (max. per dose 500 mg)
▶ BY INTRAVENOUS INFUSION
- ▶ Child: 10 mg/kg every 12 hours (max. per dose 400 mg)

Prevention of secondary case of meningococcal meningitis
▶ BY MOUTH
- ▶ Neonate: 30 mg/kg (max. per dose 125 mg) for 1 dose.
- ▶ Child 1 month-4 years: 30 mg/kg (max. per dose 125 mg) for 1 dose
- ▶ Child 5-11 years: 250 mg for 1 dose
- ▶ Child 12-17 years: 500 mg for 1 dose

- **UNLICENSED USE** Not licensed for use in children under 1 year of age. Licensed for use in children over 1 year for complicated urinary-tract infections, for pseudomonal lower respiratory-tract infections in cystic fibrosis, for prophylaxis and treatment of inhalational anthrax. Licensed for use in children over 1 year for other infections where the benefit is considered to outweigh the potential risks. Not licensed for use in children for gastro-intestinal anthrax. Not licensed for use in children for prophylaxis of meningococcal meningitis.

- **CAUTIONS** Acute myocardial infarction (risk factor for QT interval prolongation) · avoid excessive alkalinity of urine (risk of crystalluria) · bradycardia (risk factor for QT interval prolongation) · congenital long QT syndrome (risk factor for QT interval prolongation) · electrolyte disturbances (risk factor for QT interval prolongation) · ensure adequate fluid intake (risk of crystalluria) · heart failure with reduced left ventricular ejection fraction (risk factor for QT interval prolongation) · history of symptomatic arrhythmias (risk factor for QT interval prolongation)

- **INTERACTIONS** Caution if concomitant use with other drugs known to prolong the QT interval.

- **SIDE-EFFECTS**
  - ▶ **Common or very common**
  - ▶ With intravenous use Flatulence · pain at injection site · phlebitis at injection site
  - ▶ With oral use Flatulence
  - ▶ **Rare** Abnormal dreams · chest pain · dysphagia · dyspnoea · erythema nodosum · hot flushes · hyperglycaemia · hypoglycaemia · oedema · pancreatitis · sweating · syncope · tachycardia
  - ▶ **Very rare** Intracranial hypertension · movement disorders · tenosynovitis · tinnitus · vasculitis
  - ▶ **Frequency not known** Peripheral neuropathy · polyneuropathy

- **PREGNANCY** A single dose of ciprofloxacin may be used for the prevention of a secondary case of meningococcal meningitis.

- **BREAST FEEDING** Amount too small to be harmful but manufacturer advises avoid.

- **RENAL IMPAIRMENT** Reduce dose if estimated glomerular filtration rate less than 30 mL/minute/1.73 m²—consult product literature.

- **PRESCRIBING AND DISPENSING INFORMATION** Flavours of oral liquid formulations may include strawberry.

- **PATIENT AND CARER ADVICE**
  Driving and skilled tasks
  May impair performance of skilled tasks (e.g. driving); effects enhanced by alcohol.
  Medicines for Children leaflet: Ciprofloxacin for bacterial infections www.medicinesforchildren.org.uk/ciprofloxacin-bacterial-infections-0

- **MEDICINAL FORMS**
  There can be variation in the licensing of different medicines containing the same drug. Forms available from special-order manufacturers include: oral suspension

Tablet
CAUTIONARY AND ADVISORY LABELS 7, 9, 25
- ▶ Ciprofloxacin (Non-proprietary)
  Ciprofloxacin (as Ciprofloxacin hydrochloride)
  100 mg Ciprofloxacin 100mg tablets | 6 tablet [PoM] £4.50 DT price = £1.86
  Ciprofloxacin (as Ciprofloxacin hydrochloride)
  250 mg Ciprofloxacin 250mg tablets | 10 tablet [PoM] £7.25 DT price = £0.75 | 20 tablet [PoM] £11.20 | 100 tablet [PoM] no price available
  Ciprofloxacin (as Ciprofloxacin hydrochloride)
  500 mg Ciprofloxacin 500mg tablets | 10 tablet [PoM] £14.00 DT price = £0.92 | 20 tablet [PoM] £21.23 | 100 tablet [PoM] no price available
  Ciprofloxacin (as Ciprofloxacin hydrochloride)
  750 mg Ciprofloxacin 750mg tablets | 10 tablet [PoM] £20.00 DT price = £8.00 | 20 tablet [PoM] no price available
- ▶ Ciproxin (Bayer Plc)
  Ciprofloxacin (as Ciprofloxacin hydrochloride) 250 mg Ciproxin 250mg tablets | 10 tablet [PoM] £6.59 DT price = £0.75
  Ciprofloxacin (as Ciprofloxacin hydrochloride) 500 mg Ciproxin 500mg tablets | 10 tablet [PoM] £12.49 DT price = £0.92
  Ciprofloxacin (as Ciprofloxacin hydrochloride) 750 mg Ciproxin 750mg tablets | 10 tablet [PoM] £17.78 DT price = £8.00

Oral suspension
CAUTIONARY AND ADVISORY LABELS 7, 9, 25
- ▶ Ciproxin (Bayer Plc)
  Ciprofloxacin 50 mg per 1 ml Ciproxin 250mg/5ml oral suspension | 100 ml [PoM] £19.80 DT price = £19.80

Infusion
- ▶ Ciprofloxacin (Non-proprietary)
  Ciprofloxacin (as Ciprofloxacin lactate) 2 mg per 1 ml Ciprofloxacin 200mg/100ml infusion bags | 10 bag [PoM] £100.00
  Ciprofloxacin 400mg/200ml infusion bags | 10 bag [PoM] £200.00 | 15 bag [PoM] £64.35

Solution for infusion
ELECTROLYTES: May contain Sodium
- ▶ Ciprofloxacin (Non-proprietary)
  Ciprofloxacin (as Ciprofloxacin lactate) 2 mg per 1 ml Ciprofloxacin 200mg/100ml solution for infusion vials | 1 vial [PoM] £14.45
  Ciprofloxacin 400mg/200ml solution for infusion vials | 1 vial [PoM] £19.79 (Hospital only) | 1 vial [PoM] £19.59
  Ciprofloxacin 100mg/50ml solution for infusion vials | 1 vial [PoM] £7.57
- ▶ Ciproxin (Bayer Plc)
  Ciprofloxacin (as Ciprofloxacin lactate) 2 mg per 1 ml Ciproxin Infusion 100mg/50ml solution for infusion bottles | 1 bottle [PoM] £7.61 (Hospital only)
  Ciproxin Infusion 400mg/200ml solution for infusion bottles | 5 bottle [PoM] £114.23 (Hospital only)
  Ciproxin Infusion 200mg/100ml solution for infusion bottles | 5 bottle [PoM] £75.06 (Hospital only)

F 328

Nalidixic acid

- **INDICATIONS AND DOSE**

  Treatment of urinary tract infection resistant to other antibiotics
  - ▶ BY MOUTH
    - ▶ Child 3 months–11 years: 12.5 mg/kg 4 times a day for 7 days, then reduced to 7.5 mg/kg 4 times a day for prolonged therapy in chronic infections
    - ▶ Child 12–17 years: 900 mg 4 times a day for 7 days, then reduced to 600 mg 4 times a day for prolonged therapy in chronic infections

  Prophylaxis of urinary tract infections resistant to other antibiotics
  - ▶ BY MOUTH
    - ▶ Child 3 months–11 years: 15 mg/kg twice daily

- **UNLICENSED USE** Not licensed for use in children under 3 months of age.

- **CAUTIONS** Acute myocardial infarction (risk factor for QT interval prolongation) · avoid in Acute porphyrias p. 562 · bradycardia (risk factor for QT interval prolongation) · congenital long QT syndrome (risk factor for QT interval prolongation) · electrolyte disturbances (risk factor for QT interval prolongation) · heart failure with reduced left ventricular ejection fraction (risk factor for QT interval prolongation) · history of symptomatic arrhythmias (risk factor for QT interval prolongation)

- **INTERACTIONS** Caution if concomitant use with other drugs known to prolong the QT interval.

- **SIDE-EFFECTS** Cranial nerve palsy · increased intracranial pressure · metabolic acidosis · peripheral neuropathy · toxic psychosis

- **BREAST FEEDING** Risk to infant very small but one case of haemolytic anaemia reported.

- **HEPATIC IMPAIRMENT** Manufacturer advises caution in liver disease.

- **RENAL IMPAIRMENT** Use with caution; avoid if estimated glomerular filtration rate less than 20 mL/minute/1.73 m².

- **MONITORING REQUIREMENTS** Monitor blood counts, renal and liver function if treatment exceeds 2 weeks.

Infection

5

- **EFFECT ON LABORATORY TESTS** False positive urinary glucose (if tested for reducing substances).
- **PRESCRIBING AND DISPENSING INFORMATION** Flavours of oral liquid formulations may include raspberry and strawberry.
- **MEDICINAL FORMS**
  There can be variation in the licensing of different medicines containing the same drug.
  No licensed medicines listed.

ANTIBACTERIALS > SULFONAMIDES

Co-trimoxazole

- **DRUG ACTION** Sulfamethoxazole and trimethoprim are used in combination (as **co-trimoxazole**) because of their synergistic activity (the importance of the sulfonamides has decreased as a result of increasing bacterial resistance and their replacement by antibacterials which are generally more active and less toxic).

- **INDICATIONS AND DOSE**
  Treatment of susceptible infections
  ▸ BY MOUTH
  ▸ Child 6 weeks-5 months: 120 mg twice daily, alternatively 24 mg/kg twice daily
  ▸ Child 6 months-5 years: 240 mg twice daily, alternatively 24 mg/kg twice daily
  ▸ Child 6-11 years: 480 mg twice daily, alternatively 24 mg/kg twice daily
  ▸ Child 12-17 years: 960 mg twice daily
  ▸ BY INTRAVENOUS INFUSION
  ▸ Child 6 weeks-17 years: 18 mg/kg every 12 hours; increased to 27 mg/kg every 12 hours (max. per dose 1.44 g), increased dose used in severe infection

  Treatment of *Pneumocystis jirovecii* (*Pneumocystis carinii*) infections (undertaken where facilities for appropriate monitoring available--consult microbiologist and product literature)
  ▸ BY MOUTH, OR BY INTRAVENOUS INFUSION
  ▸ Child: 120 mg/kg daily in 2-4 divided doses for 14-21 days, oral route preferred for children

  Prophylaxis of *Pneumocystis jirovecii* (*Pneumocystis carinii*) infections
  ▸ BY MOUTH
  ▸ Child: 450 mg/m^2 twice daily (max. per dose 960 mg twice daily) for 3 days of the week (either consecutively or on alternate days), dose regimens may vary, consult local guidelines

  DOSE EQUIVALENCE AND CONVERSION
  480 mg of co-trimoxazole consists of sulfamethoxazole 400 mg and trimethoprim 80 mg.

- **UNLICENSED USE** Not licensed for *Burkholderia cepacia* infections in cystic fibrosis. Not licensed for *Stenotrophomonas maltophilia* infections. Not licensed for use in children under 6 weeks.

  IMPORTANT SAFETY INFORMATION
  RESTRICTIONS ON THE USE OF CO-TRIMOXAZOLE
  Co-trimoxazole is the drug of choice in the prophylaxis and treatment of *Pneumocystis jirovecii* (*Pneumocystis carinii*) pneumonia; it is also indicated for nocardiasis, *Stenotrophomonas maltophilia* infection [unlicensed indication], and toxoplasmosis. It should only be considered for use in acute exacerbations of chronic bronchitis and infections of the urinary tract when there is bacteriological evidence of sensitivity to co-trimoxazole and good reason to prefer this combination to a single antibacterial; similarly it should only be used in acute otitis media in children when there is good reason to prefer it. Co-trimoxazole is also used for the

treatment of infections caused by *Burkholderia cepacia* in cystic fibrosis [unlicensed indication].

- **CONTRA-INDICATIONS** Acute porphyrias p. 562
- **CAUTIONS** Asthma · avoid in blood disorders (unless under specialist supervision) · avoid in infants under 6 weeks (except for treatment or prophylaxis of pneumocystis pneumonia) because of the risk of kernicterus · G6PD deficiency (risk of haemolytic anaemia) · maintain adequate fluid intake · predisposition to folate deficiency
- **INTERACTIONS** → Appendix 1 (trimethoprim, sulfamethoxazole).
- **SIDE-EFFECTS**
  ▸ **Common or very common** Diarrhoea · headache · hyperkalaemia · nausea · rash
  ▸ **Uncommon** Vomiting
  ▸ **Rare** Agranulocytosis · bone marrow depression
  ▸ **Very rare** Anorexia · antibiotic-associated colitis · arthralgia · aseptic meningitis · ataxia · blood disorders · convulsions · cough · depression · eosinophilia · glossitis · hallucinations · hepatic necrosis · hypoglycaemia · hyponatraemia · interstitial nephritis · jaundice · leucopenia · liver damage · megaloblastic anaemia · myalgia · myocarditis · pancreatitis · peripheral neuropathy · photosensitivity · pulmonary infiltrates · renal disorders · shortness of breath · Stevens-Johnson syndrome · stomatitis · systemic lupus erythematosus · thrombocytopenia · tinnitus · toxic epidermal necrolysis · uveitis · vasculitis · vertigo
  ▸ **Frequency not known** Rhabdomyolysis reported in HIV-infected patients
  SIDE-EFFECTS, FURTHER INFORMATION
  ▸ Blood disorders or rash Co-trimoxazole is associated with rare but serious side effects. Discontinue immediately if blood disorders (including leucopenia, thrombocytopenia, megaloblastic anaemia, eosinophilia) or rash (including Stevens-Johnson syndrome, toxic epidermal necrolysis, photosensitivity) develop.
- **PREGNANCY** Teratogenic risk in first trimester (trimethoprim a folate antagonist). Neonatal haemolysis and methaemoglobinaemia in third trimester; fear of increased risk of kernicterus in neonates appears to be unfounded.
- **BREAST FEEDING** Small risk of kernicterus in jaundiced infants and of haemolysis in G6PD-deficient infants (due to sulfamethoxazole).
- **HEPATIC IMPAIRMENT** Manufacturer advises avoid in severe liver disease.
- **RENAL IMPAIRMENT** Use half normal dose if estimated glomerular filtration rate 15-30 mL/minute/1.73 m^2. Avoid if estimated glomerular filtration rate less than 15 mL/minute/1.73 m^2 and if plasma-sulfamethoxazole concentration cannot be monitored. Plasma concentration monitoring may be required in patients with moderate to severe renal impairment; seek expert advice.
- **MONITORING REQUIREMENTS**
  ▸ Plasma concentration monitoring may be required with high doses; seek expert advice.
  ▸ Monitor blood counts on prolonged treatment.
- **DIRECTIONS FOR ADMINISTRATION**
  ▸ With intravenous use For intermittent *intravenous infusion*, may be further diluted in glucose 5% and 10% or sodium chloride 0.9%. Dilute contents of 1 ampoule (5 mL) to 125 mL, 2 ampoules (10 mL) to 250 mL or 3 ampoules (15 mL) to 500 mL; suggested duration of infusion 60-90 minutes (but may be adjusted according to fluid requirements); if fluid restriction necessary, 1 ampoule (5 mL) may be diluted with 75 mL glucose 5% and the required dose infused over max. 60 minutes; check container for haze or precipitant during administration. In

severe fluid restriction may be given undiluted via a central venous line.

- **PRESCRIBING AND DISPENSING INFORMATION** Co-trimoxazole is a mixture of trimethoprim and sulfamethoxazole (sulphamethoxazole) in the proportions of 1 part to 5 parts.
- With oral use Flavours of oral liquid formulations may include banana, or vanilla.

- **MEDICINAL FORMS**
  There can be variation in the licensing of different medicines containing the same drug.

Tablet

CAUTIONARY AND ADVISORY LABELS 9
- Co-trimoxazole (Non-proprietary)
  Trimethoprim 80 mg, Sulfamethoxazole 400 mg Co-trimoxazole 80mg/400mg tablets | 28 tablet PoM £23.00 DT price = £2.50 | 100 tablet PoM £9.89–£10.91
  Trimethoprim 160 mg, Sulfamethoxazole 800 mg Co-trimoxazole 160mg/800mg tablets | 100 tablet PoM £23.40–£23.46 DT price = £23.46

Oral suspension

CAUTIONARY AND ADVISORY LABELS 9
- Co-trimoxazole (Non-proprietary)
  Trimethoprim 8 mg per 1 ml, Sulfamethoxazole 40 mg per 1 ml Co-trimoxazole 40mg/200mg/5ml oral suspension sugar free sugar-free | 100 ml PoM £9.95
  Trimethoprim 16 mg per 1 ml, Sulfamethoxazole 80 mg per 1 ml Co-trimoxazole 80mg/400mg/5ml oral suspension | 100 ml PoM £10.95

Solution for infusion

EXCIPIENTS: May contain Alcohol, propylene glycol, sulfites
ELECTROLYTES: May contain Sodium
- Co-trimoxazole (Non-proprietary)
  Trimethoprim 16 mg per 1 ml, Sulfamethoxazole 80 mg per 1 ml Co-trimoxazole 80mg/400mg/5ml solution for infusion ampoules | 10 ampoule PoM £35.00
- Septrin (Aspen Pharma Trading Ltd)
  Trimethoprim 16 mg per 1 ml, Sulfamethoxazole 80 mg per 1 ml Septrin for Infusion 80mg/400mg/5ml solution for infusion ampoules | 10 ampoule PoM £17.76

Sulfadiazine

(Sulphadiazine)

- **DRUG ACTION** Sulfadiazine is a short-acting sulphonamide with bacteriostatic activity against a broad spectrum of organisms. The importance of the sulfonamides has decreased as a result of increasing bacterial resistance and their replacement by antibacterials which are generally more active and less toxic.

- **INDICATIONS AND DOSE**

Toxoplasmosis in pregnancy (in combination with pyrimethamine and folinic acid)
- BY MOUTH
- Child 12–17 years: 1 g 3 times a day until delivery

Congenital toxoplasmosis (in combination with pyrimethamine and folinic acid)
- BY MOUTH
- Neonate: 50 mg/kg twice daily for 12 months.

- **UNLICENSED USE** Not licensed for use in toxoplasmosis.
- **CONTRA-INDICATIONS** Acute porphyrias p. 562
- **CAUTIONS** Asthma · avoid in blood disorders (unless under specialist supervision) · avoid in infants under 6 weeks (except for treatment or prophylaxis of *pneumocystis pneumonia*) because of the risk of kernicterus · G6PD deficiency (risk of haemolytic anaemia) · maintain adequate fluid intake · predisposition to folate deficiency
- **INTERACTIONS** → Appendix 1 (sulfonamides).

- **SIDE-EFFECTS**
- **Common or very common** Diarrhoea · headache · hyperkalaemia · nausea · rash
- **Uncommon** Vomiting
- **Rare** Agranulocytosis · bone marrow depression
- **Very rare** Anorexia · antibiotic-associated colitis · arthralgia · aseptic meningitis · ataxia · blood disorders · convulsions · cough · depression · eosinophilia · glossitis · hallucinations · hepatic necrosis · hypoglycaemia · hyponatraemia · interstitial nephritis · jaundice · leucopenia · liver damage · megaloblastic anaemia · myalgia · myocarditis · pancreatitis · peripheral neuropathy · photosensitivity · pulmonary infiltrates · renal disorders · shortness of breath · Stevens-Johnson syndrome · stomatitis · systemic lupus erythematosus · thrombocytopenia · tinnitus · toxic epidermal necrolysis · uveitis · vasculitis · vertigo
- **Frequency not known** Benign intracranial hypertension · hypothyroidism · optic neuropathy · rhabdomyolysis reported in HIV-infected patients

SIDE-EFFECTS, FURTHER INFORMATION
- Blood disorders or rash Discontinue immediately if blood disorders (including leucopenia, thrombocytopenia, megaloblastic anaemia, eosinophilia) or rash (including Stevens-Johnson syndrome, toxic epidermal necrolysis, photosensitivity) develop.

- **PREGNANCY** Risk of neonatal haemolysis and methaemoglobinaemia in third trimester; fear of increased risk of kernicterus in neonates appears to be unfounded.
- **BREAST FEEDING** Small risk of kernicterus in jaundiced infants and of haemolysis in G6PD-deficient infants.
- **HEPATIC IMPAIRMENT** Use with caution in mild to moderate impairment; avoid in severe impairment.
- **RENAL IMPAIRMENT** Use with caution in mild to moderate impairment; avoid in severe impairment; high risk of crystalluria.
- **MONITORING REQUIREMENTS** Monitor blood counts on prolonged treatment.

- **MEDICINAL FORMS**
  There can be variation in the licensing of different medicines containing the same drug. Forms available from special-order manufacturers include: oral suspension

Tablet

CAUTIONARY AND ADVISORY LABELS 9, 27
- Sulfadiazine (Non-proprietary)
  Sulfadiazine 500 mg Sulfadiazine 500mg tablets | 56 tablet PoM £85.55 DT price = £81.99

ANTIBACTERIALS › TETRACYCLINES AND RELATED DRUGS

Tetracyclines

Overview

The tetracyclines are broad-spectrum antibiotics whose value has decreased owing to increasing bacterial resistance. In children over 12 years of age they are useful for infections caused by chlamydia (trachoma, psittacosis, salpingitis, urethritis, and lymphogranuloma venereum), rickettsia (including Q-fever), brucella (doxycycline p. 332 with either streptomycin p. 293 or rifampicin p. 342), and the spirochaete, *Borrelia burgdorferi* (See Lyme disease). They are also used in respiratory and genital mycoplasma infections, in acne, in destructive (refractory) periodontal disease, in exacerbations of chronic respiratory diseases (because of their activity against *Haemophilus influenzae*), and for leptospirosis in penicillin hypersensitivity (as an alternative to erythromycin p. 310).

Microbiologically, there is little to choose between the various tetracyclines, the only exception being minocycline

5

Infection

p. 333 which has a broader spectrum; it is active against *Neisseria meningitidis* and has been used for meningococcal prophylaxis but is no longer recommended because of side-effects including dizziness and vertigo. Compared to other tetracyclines, minocycline is associated with a greater risk of lupus-erythematosus-like syndrome. Minocycline sometimes causes irreversible pigmentation.

Tetracyclines have a role in the management of meticillin-resistant *Staphylococcus aureus* (MRSA) infections.

Tetracyclines

- **CONTRA-INDICATIONS** Children under 12 years (deposition in growing bone and teeth, by binding to calcium, causes staining and occasionally dental hypoplasia)
- **CAUTIONS** Myasthenia gravis (muscle weakness may be increased) · systemic lupus erythematosus (may be exacerbated)
- **INTERACTIONS** → Appendix 1 (tetracyclines). Antacids, and aluminium, calcium, iron, magnesium and zinc salts decrease the absorption of tetracyclines. Use with caution in those receiving potentially hepatotoxic drugs.
- **SIDE-EFFECTS**
  - **Rare** Anaphylaxis · angioedema · blood disorders · exfoliative dermatitis · hepatotoxicity · hypersensitivity reactions · pancreatitis · pericarditis · photosensitivity (particularly with demeclocycline) · rash · Stevens-Johnson syndrome · urticaria
  - **Frequency not known** Antibiotic-associated colitis · benign intracranial hypertension · bulging fontanelles (in infants) · diarrhoea · dysphagia · headache · nausea · oesophageal irritation · visual disturbances · vomiting

  SIDE-EFFECTS, FURTHER INFORMATION
  - Benign intracranial hypertension Headache and visual disturbances may indicate benign intracranial hypertension (discontinue treatment).
- **PREGNANCY** Should **not** be given to pregnant women; effects on skeletal development have been documented in the first trimester in *animal* studies. Administration during the second or third trimester may cause discoloration of the child's teeth, and maternal hepatotoxicity has been reported with large parenteral doses.
- **BREAST FEEDING** Should **not** be given to women who are breast-feeding (although absorption and therefore discoloration of teeth in the infant is probably usually prevented by chelation with calcium in milk).
- **HEPATIC IMPAIRMENT** Should be avoided or used with caution in patients with hepatic impairment.

▶ above

Demeclocycline hydrochloride

- **INDICATIONS AND DOSE**
Susceptible infections (e.g. chlamydia, rickettsia and mycoplasma)
- ▸ BY MOUTH
- ▸ Child 12-17 years: 150 mg 4 times a day, alternatively 300 mg twice daily

- **CAUTIONS** Photosensitivity more common than with other tetracyclines
- **INTERACTIONS** Milk reduces absorption.
- **SIDE-EFFECTS** Acute renal failure · reversible nephrogenic diabetes insipidus
- **HEPATIC IMPAIRMENT** Max. 1 g daily in divided doses.
- **RENAL IMPAIRMENT** May exacerbate renal failure and should **not** be given to patients with renal impairment.

- **PATIENT AND CARER ADVICE** Patients should be advised to avoid exposure to sunlight or sun lamps.

- **MEDICINAL FORMS**
There can be variation in the licensing of different medicines containing the same drug. Forms available from special-order manufacturers include: oral suspension, oral solution
Tablet
- ▸ **Demeclocycline hydrochloride (Non-proprietary)**
  Demeclocycline hydrochloride 150 mg Demeclocycline 150mg tablets | 100 tablet PoM no price available
Capsule
CAUTIONARY AND ADVISORY LABELS 7, 9, 11, 23
- ▸ **Demeclocycline hydrochloride (Non-proprietary)**
  Demeclocycline hydrochloride 150 mg Demeclocycline 150mg capsules | 28 capsule PoM £160.89 DT price = £160.89

▶ above

Doxycycline

- **INDICATIONS AND DOSE**
Susceptible infections (e.g. chlamydia, rickettsia and mycoplasma)
- ▸ BY MOUTH USING IMMEDIATE-RELEASE MEDICINES
- ▸ Child 12-17 years: Initially 200 mg daily for 1 dose, then maintenance 100 mg once daily

Severe infections (including refractory urinary-tract infections)
- ▸ BY MOUTH USING IMMEDIATE-RELEASE MEDICINES
- ▸ Child 12-17 years: 200 mg daily

Acne
- ▸ BY MOUTH USING IMMEDIATE-RELEASE MEDICINES
- ▸ Child 12-17 years: 100 mg once daily

Early syphilis
- ▸ BY MOUTH USING IMMEDIATE-RELEASE MEDICINES
- ▸ Child 12-17 years: 100 mg twice daily for 14 days

Late latent syphilis
- ▸ BY MOUTH USING IMMEDIATE-RELEASE MEDICINES
- ▸ Child 12-17 years: 100 mg twice daily for 28 days

Uncomplicated genital chlamydia | Non-gonococcal urethritis
- ▸ BY MOUTH USING IMMEDIATE-RELEASE MEDICINES
- ▸ Child 12-17 years: 100 mg twice daily for 7 days

Pelvic inflammatory disease
- ▸ BY MOUTH USING IMMEDIATE-RELEASE MEDICINES
- ▸ Child 12-17 years: 100 mg twice daily for 14 days

Lyme disease (under expert supervision)
- ▸ BY MOUTH USING IMMEDIATE-RELEASE MEDICINES
- ▸ Child 12-17 years: 100 mg twice daily for 10–14 days (for 28 days in Lyme arthritis)

Anthrax (treatment or post-exposure prophylaxis)
- ▸ BY MOUTH USING IMMEDIATE-RELEASE MEDICINES
- ▸ Child 1 month-11 years: 2.5 mg/kg twice daily (max. per dose 100 mg twice daily), only to be used in children under 12 years if alternative antibacterial cannot be given
- ▸ Child 12-17 years: 100 mg twice daily

Prophylaxis of malaria
- ▸ BY MOUTH USING IMMEDIATE-RELEASE MEDICINES
- ▸ Child 12-17 years: 100 mg once daily, to be started 1–2 days before entering endemic area and continued for 4 weeks after leaving, can be used for up to 2 years

Adjunct to quinine in treatment of *Plasmodium falciparum* malaria
- ▸ BY MOUTH USING IMMEDIATE-RELEASE MEDICINES
- ▸ Child 12-17 years: 200 mg daily for 7 days

Periodontitis (as an adjunct to gingival scaling and root planing)
- ▸ BY MOUTH USING IMMEDIATE-RELEASE MEDICINES
- ▸ Child 12-17 years: 20 mg twice daily for 3 months

- **UNLICENSED USE** Not licensed for use in children under 12 years. Doxycycline doses in BNF Publications may differ from those in product literature. Not licensed for severe recurrent aphthous ulceration. Not licensed for malaria prophylaxis during pregnancy. Not licensed for treatment or post-exposure prophylaxis of anthrax.
- **CAUTIONS** Alcohol dependence
- **INTERACTIONS** The metabolism of doxycycline may be influenced by antiepileptics.
- **SIDE-EFFECTS** Anorexia · anxiety · dry mouth · flushing · fungal superinfection (when used for periodontitis) · tinnitus
- **PREGNANCY** When travel to malarious areas is unavoidable during pregnancy, doxycycline can be used for malaria prophylaxis if other regimens are unsuitable, and if the entire course of doxycycline can be completed before 15 weeks' gestation.
- **RENAL IMPAIRMENT** Use with caution (avoid excessive doses).
- **MONITORING REQUIREMENTS** When used for periodontitis, monitor for superficial fungal infection, particularly if predisposition to oral candidiasis.
- **DIRECTIONS FOR ADMINISTRATION** Capsules and Tablets should be swallowed whole with plenty of fluid, while sitting or standing. Capsules should be taken during meals.
- **PATIENT AND CARER ADVICE** Counselling on administration advised (posture).
  Photosensitivity Patients should be advised to avoid exposure to sunlight or sun lamps.
- **PROFESSION SPECIFIC INFORMATION**

  Dental practitioners' formulary
  Doxycycline Capsules 100 mg may be prescribed. Dispersible tablets may be prescribed as Dispersible Doxycycline Tablets. Tablets may be prescribed as Doxycycline Tablets 20 mg.

- **MEDICINAL FORMS**
  There can be variation in the licensing of different medicines containing the same drug. Forms available from special-order manufacturers include: oral suspension, oral solution

Tablet
CAUTIONARY AND ADVISORY LABELS 6, 11, 27
- Periostat (Alliance Pharmaceuticals Ltd)
  Doxycycline (as Doxycycline hyclate) 20 mg Periostat 20mg tablets | 56 tablet [PoM] £17.30 DT price = £17.30

Dispersible tablet
CAUTIONARY AND ADVISORY LABELS 6, 9, 11, 13
- Vibramycin-D (Pfizer Ltd)
  Doxycycline (as Doxycycline monohydrate) 100 mg Vibramycin-D 100mg dispersible tablets sugar-free | 8 tablet [PoM] £4.91 DT price = £4.91

Capsule
CAUTIONARY AND ADVISORY LABELS 6, 9, 11, 27
- Doxycycline (Non-proprietary)
  Doxycycline (as Doxycycline hyclate) 50 mg Doxycycline 50mg capsules | 28 capsule [PoM] £4.00 DT price = £1.30
  Doxycycline (as Doxycycline hyclate) 100 mg Doxycycline 100mg capsules | 8 capsule [PoM] £3.00 DT price = £0.88 | 50 capsule [PoM] £19.00
- Vibrox (Kent Pharmaceuticals Ltd)
  Doxycycline (as Doxycycline hyclate) 100 mg Vibrox 100mg capsules | 8 capsule [PoM] £3.97 DT price = £0.88 | 14 capsule [PoM] £4.48 | 50 capsule [PoM] £10.65

F 332

Lymecycline

- **INDICATIONS AND DOSE**

Susceptible infections (e.g. chlamydia, rickettsia and mycoplasma)
- ▶ BY MOUTH
- ▸ Child 12–17 years: 408 mg twice daily, increased to 1.224–1.632 g daily, (in severe infection)

Acne
- ▶ BY MOUTH
- ▸ Child 12–17 years: 408 mg daily for at least 8 weeks

- **RENAL IMPAIRMENT** May exacerbate renal failure and should **not** be given to patients with renal impairment.

- **MEDICINAL FORMS**
  There can be variation in the licensing of different medicines containing the same drug.
  Capsule
  CAUTIONARY AND ADVISORY LABELS 6, 9
  - Lymecycline (Non-proprietary)
    Lymecycline 408 mg Lymecycline 408mg capsules | 28 capsule [PoM] £8.11 DT price = £7.23 | 56 capsule [PoM] £16.22
  - Tetralysal (Galderma (UK) Ltd)
    Lymecycline 408 mg Tetralysal 300 capsules | 28 capsule [PoM] £6.95 DT price = £7.23 | 56 capsule [PoM] £11.53

F 332

Minocycline

- **INDICATIONS AND DOSE**

Susceptible infections (e.g. chlamydia, rickettsia and mycoplasma)
- ▶ BY MOUTH USING IMMEDIATE-RELEASE MEDICINES
- ▸ Child 12–17 years: 100 mg twice daily

Acne
- ▶ BY MOUTH USING IMMEDIATE-RELEASE MEDICINES
- ▸ Child 12–17 years: 100 mg once daily, alternatively 50 mg twice daily
- ▶ BY MOUTH USING MODIFIED-RELEASE MEDICINES
- ▸ Child 12–17 years: 100 mg daily

- **CAUTIONS** Systemic lupus erythematosus
- **SIDE-EFFECTS**
- ▶ **Rare** Acute renal failure · alopecia · anorexia · hyperaesthesia · impaired hearing · paraesthesia · pigmentation (sometimes irreversible) · tinnitus
- ▶ **Very rare** Discoloration of conjunctiva · discoloration of sweat · discoloration of tears · systemic lupus erythematosus
- ▶ **Frequency not known** Dizziness (more common in women) · vertigo (more common in women)
- **RENAL IMPAIRMENT** Use with caution (avoid excessive doses).
- **MONITORING REQUIREMENTS** If treatment continued for longer than 6 months, monitor every 3 months for hepatotoxicity, pigmentation and for systemic lupus erythematosus—discontinue if these develop or if pre-existing systemic lupus erythematosus worsens.
- **DIRECTIONS FOR ADMINISTRATION** Tablets or capsules should be swallowed whole with plenty of fluid while sitting or standing.
- **PATIENT AND CARER ADVICE** Counselling on administration advised (posture).
- **LESS SUITABLE FOR PRESCRIBING** Less suitable for prescribing (compared with other tetracyclines, minocycline is associated with a greater risk of lupus-erythematosus-like syndrome; it sometimes causes irreversible pigmentation).

5

Infection

Infection

5

- **MEDICINAL FORMS**
There can be variation in the licensing of different medicines containing the same drug. Forms available from special-order manufacturers include: oral suspension, oral solution

Tablet
CAUTIONARY AND ADVISORY LABELS 6, 9
▸ Minocycline (Non-proprietary)
Minocycline (as Minocycline hydrochloride) 50 mg Minocycline 50mg tablets | 28 tablet PoM £8.50 DT price = £6.19
Minocycline (as Minocycline hydrochloride) 100 mg Minocycline 100mg tablets | 28 tablet PoM £14.50 DT price = £14.01

Capsule
CAUTIONARY AND ADVISORY LABELS 6, 9
▸ Aknemin (Almirall Ltd)
Minocycline (as Minocycline hydrochloride) 50 mg Aknemin 50 capsules | 56 capsule PoM £15.27 DT price = £15.27
Minocycline (as Minocycline hydrochloride) 100 mg Aknemin 100mg capsules | 28 capsule PoM £13.09 DT price = £13.09

Modified-release capsule
CAUTIONARY AND ADVISORY LABELS 6, 25
▸ Minocycline (Non-proprietary)
Minocycline (as Minocycline hydrochloride) 100 mg Minocycline 100mg modified-release capsules | 56 capsule PoM £24.00 DT price = £20.08
▸ Acnamino MR (Almus Pharmaceuticals Ltd, Dexcel-Pharma Ltd)
Minocycline (as Minocycline hydrochloride) 100 mg Acnamino MR 100mg capsules | 56 capsule PoM £21.14 DT price = £20.08
▸ Minocin MR (Meda Pharmaceuticals Ltd)
Minocycline (as Minocycline hydrochloride) 100 mg Minocin MR 100mg capsules | 56 capsule PoM £20.08 DT price = £20.08

▶ 332

Oxytetracycline

- **INDICATIONS AND DOSE**

Susceptible infections (e.g. chlamydia, rickettsia and mycoplasma)
▸ BY MOUTH
▹ Child 12–17 years: 250–500 mg 4 times a day

Acne
▸ BY MOUTH
▹ Child 12–17 years: 500 mg twice daily for at least 3 months, if there is no improvement after the first 3 months another oral antibacterial should be used, maximum improvement usually occurs after 4 to 6 months but in more severe cases treatment may need to be continued for 2 years or longer

- **INTERACTIONS** Milk reduces absorption.
- **RENAL IMPAIRMENT** May exacerbate renal failure and should **not** be given to patients with renal impairment.
- **PROFESSION SPECIFIC INFORMATION**

Dental practitioners' formulary
Oxytetracycline Tablets may be prescribed.

- **MEDICINAL FORMS**
There can be variation in the licensing of different medicines containing the same drug. Forms available from special-order manufacturers include: oral suspension

Tablet
CAUTIONARY AND ADVISORY LABELS 7, 9, 23
▸ Oxytetracycline (Non-proprietary)
Oxytetracycline (as Oxytetracycline dihydrate) 250 mg Oxytetracycline 250mg tablets | 28 tablet PoM £12.50 DT price = £0.91 | 1000 tablet PoM no price available

Tetracycline

▶ 332

- **INDICATIONS AND DOSE**

Susceptible infections (e.g. chlamydia, rickettsia, mycoplasma)
▸ BY MOUTH
▹ Child 12–17 years: 250 mg 4 times a day, increased if necessary to 500 mg 3–4 times a day, increased dose used in severe infections

Acne
▸ BY MOUTH
▹ Child 12–17 years: 500 mg twice daily for at least 3 months, if there is no improvement after the first 3 months another oral antibacterial should be used, maximum improvement usually occurs after 4 to 6 months but in more severe cases treatment may need to be continued for 2 years or longer

Non-gonococcal urethritis
▸ BY MOUTH
▹ Child 12–17 years: 500 mg 4 times a day for 7–14 days (21 days if failure or relapse after first course)

- **INTERACTIONS** Milk reduces absorption.
- **SIDE-EFFECTS** Acute renal failure · skin discoloration
- **HEPATIC IMPAIRMENT** Max. 1 g daily in divided doses.
- **RENAL IMPAIRMENT** May exacerbate renal failure and should **not** be given to patients with renal impairment.
- **DIRECTIONS FOR ADMINISTRATION** Tablets should be swallowed whole with plenty of fluid while sitting or standing.
- **PATIENT AND CARER ADVICE** Counselling on administration advised.
- **PROFESSION SPECIFIC INFORMATION**

Dental practitioners' formulary
Tetracycline Tablets may be prescribed.

- **MEDICINAL FORMS**
There can be variation in the licensing of different medicines containing the same drug. Forms available from special-order manufacturers include: capsule, oral solution

Tablet
CAUTIONARY AND ADVISORY LABELS 7, 9, 23
▸ Tetracycline (Non-proprietary)
Tetracycline hydrochloride 250 mg Tetracycline 250mg tablets | 28 tablet PoM £25.65 DT price = £2.04

ANTIBACTERIALS > OTHER

Chloramphenicol

- **DRUG ACTION** Chloramphenicol is a potent broad-spectrum antibiotic.

- **INDICATIONS AND DOSE**

Life threatening infections particularly those caused by Haemophilus infuenzae | Typhoid fever
▸ BY MOUTH, OR BY INTRAVENOUS INJECTION, OR BY INTRAVENOUS INFUSION
▹ Child: 12.5 mg/kg every 6 hours, dose may be doubled in severe infections such as septicaemia, meningitis and epiglottitis providing plasma-chloramphenicol concentrations are measured and high doses reduced as soon as indicated
▸ BY INTRAVENOUS INJECTION

▹ Neonate up to 14 days: 12.5 mg/kg twice daily, doses should be checked carefully as overdosage can be fatal.

▹ Neonate 14 days to 28 days: 12.5 mg/kg 2–4 times a day, doses should be checked carefully as overdosage can be fatal.

Cystic fibrosis for the treatment of respiratory *Burkholderia cepacia* infection resistant to other antibacterials
‣ BY MOUTH, OR BY INTRAVENOUS INFUSION, OR BY INTRAVENOUS INJECTION
  ‣ Child: (consult product literature)

- **CONTRA-INDICATIONS** Acute porphyrias p. 562
- **CAUTIONS** Avoid repeated courses and prolonged treatment
- **INTERACTIONS** → Appendix 1 (chloramphenicol).
- **SIDE-EFFECTS** Blood disorders · depression · diarrhoea · dry mouth · erythema multiforme · glossitis · headache · nausea · nocturnal haemoglobinuria · optic neuritis · peripheral neuritis · reversible and irreversible aplastic anaemia · (with reports of resulting leukaemia) · stomatitis · urticaria · vomiting

  SIDE-EFFECTS, FURTHER INFORMATION
  ‣ With intravenous use in neonates Grey syndrome (abdominal distension, pallid cyanosis, circulatory collapse) may follow excessive doses in neonates with immature hepatic metabolism.
  ‣ With intravenous use or oral use Associated with serious haematological side-effects when given systemically and should therefore be reserved for the treatment of life-threatening infections.
- **PREGNANCY** Manufacturer advises avoid; neonatal 'grey-baby syndrome' if used in third trimester.
- **BREAST FEEDING** Manufacturer advises avoid; use another antibiotic; may cause bone-marrow toxicity in infant; concentration in milk usually insufficient to cause 'grey syndrome'.
- **HEPATIC IMPAIRMENT** Avoid if possible—increased risk of bone-marrow depression. Reduce dose and monitor plasma-chloramphenicol concentration in hepatic impairment.
- **RENAL IMPAIRMENT** Avoid in severe renal impairment unless no alternative; dose-related depression of haematopoiesis.
- **MONITORING REQUIREMENTS**
  ‣ Plasma concentration monitoring preferred in those under 4 years of age.
  ‣ Recommended peak plasma concentration (approx. 2 hours after administration by mouth, intravenous injection or infusion) 10–25 mg/litre; pre-dose ('trough') concentration should not exceed 15 mg/litre. Blood counts required before and periodically during treatment.
  ‣ In neonates use Plasma concentration monitoring required in neonates. Grey baby syndrome may follow excessive doses in neonates with immature hepatic metabolism.
- **DIRECTIONS FOR ADMINISTRATION**
  ‣ With intravenous use Displacement value may be significant for injection, consult local guidelines. For intermittent intravenous use, dilute reconstituted solution further in glucose 5% or sodium chloride 0.9%.

- **MEDICINAL FORMS**
  There can be variation in the licensing of different medicines containing the same drug.
  Capsule
  ‣ Chloramphenicol (Non-proprietary)
    Chloramphenicol 250 mg Chloramphenicol 250mg capsules | 60 capsule PoM £377.00 DT price = £377.00
  Powder for solution for injection
  ELECTROLYTES: May contain Sodium
  ‣ Kemicetine (Pfizer Ltd)
    Chloramphenicol (as Chloramphenicol sodium succinate)
    1 gram Kemicetine 1g powder for solution for injection vials | 1 vial PoM £1.39

Fosfomycin

- **DRUG ACTION** Fosfomycin, a phosphonic acid antibacterial, is active against a range of Gram-positive and Gram-negative bacteria including *Staphylococcus aureus* and Enterobacteriaceae.

- **INDICATIONS AND DOSE**

  Osteomyelitis when first-line treatments are inappropriate or ineffective | Hospital-acquired lower respiratory-tract infections when first-line treatments are inappropriate or ineffective
  ‣ BY INTRAVENOUS INFUSION

  ‣ Neonate up to 40 weeks corrected gestational age: 100 mg/kg daily in 2 divided doses.

  ‣ Neonate 40 weeks to 44 weeks corrected gestational age: 200 mg/kg daily in 3 divided doses.

  ‣ Child 1–11 months (body-weight up to 10 kg): 200–300 mg/kg daily in 3 divided doses, consider using the high-dose regimen in severe infection, particularly when suspected or known to be caused by less sensitive organisms
  ‣ Child 1–11 years (body-weight 10-39 kg): 200–400 mg/kg daily in 3–4 divided doses, consider using the high-dose regimen in severe infection, particularly when suspected or known to be caused by less sensitive organisms
  ‣ Child 12-17 years (body-weight 40 kg and above): 12–24 g daily in 2–3 divided doses (max. per dose 8 g), use the high-dose regimen in severe infection, particularly when suspected or known to be caused by less sensitive organisms

  Complicated urinary-tract infections when first-line treatment ineffective or inappropriate
  ‣ BY INTRAVENOUS INFUSION

  ‣ Neonate up to 40 weeks corrected gestational age: 100 mg/kg daily in 2 divided doses.

  ‣ Neonate 40 weeks to 44 weeks corrected gestational age: 200 mg/kg daily in 3 divided doses.

  ‣ Child 1–11 months (body-weight up to 10 kg): 200–300 mg/kg daily in 3 divided doses, consider using the high-dose regimen in severe infection, particularly when suspected or known to be caused by less sensitive organisms
  ‣ Child 1–11 years (body-weight 10-39 kg): 200–400 mg/kg daily in 3–4 divided doses, consider using the high-dose regimen in severe infection, particularly when suspected or known to be caused by less sensitive organisms
  ‣ Child 12-17 years (body-weight 40 kg and above): 12–16 g daily in 2–3 divided doses (max. per dose 8 g), use the high-dose regimen in severe infection, particularly when suspected or known to be caused by less sensitive organisms

  Bacterial meningitis when first-line treatment ineffective or inappropriate
  ‣ BY INTRAVENOUS INFUSION

  ‣ Neonate up to 40 weeks corrected gestational age: 100 mg/kg daily in 2 divided doses.

  ‣ Neonate 40 weeks to 44 weeks corrected gestational age: 200 mg/kg daily in 3 divided doses.

  ‣ Child 1–11 months (body-weight up to 10 kg): 200–300 mg/kg daily in 3 divided doses, consider using the high-dose regimen in severe infection, particularly when suspected or known to be caused by less sensitive organisms
  ‣ Child 1–11 years (body-weight 10-39 kg): 200–400 mg/kg daily in 3–4 divided doses, consider using continued →

5

Infection

the high-dose regimen in severe infection, particularly when suspected or known to be caused by less sensitive organisms

▸ Child 12-17 years (body-weight 40 kg and above): 16–24 g daily in 3–4 divided doses (max. per dose 8 g), use the high-dose regimen in severe infection suspected or known to be caused by less sensitive organisms

● CAUTIONS Cardiac insufficiency · hyperaldosteronism · hypernatraemia · hypertension · pulmonary oedema

● INTERACTIONS → Appendix 1 (fosfomycin).

● SIDE-EFFECTS

GENERAL SIDE-EFFECTS

▸ **Common or very common** Gastro-intestinal disturbances · rash

▸ **Uncommon** Diarrhoea · nausea · vomiting

▸ **Frequency not known** Abdominal pain

SPECIFIC SIDE-EFFECTS

▸ **Uncommon** Decreased appetite · dyspnoea · fatigue · headache · hypernatraemia · hypokalaemia · taste disturbances · vertigo

▸ **Rare** Aplastic anaemia · blood disorders · eosinophilia

▸ **Very rare** Fatty liver · visual impairment

▸ **Frequency not known** Antibiotic-associated colitis · bronchospasm · confusion · hepatitis · jaundice · tachycardia

● PREGNANCY Manufacturer advises use only if potential benefit outweighs risk.

● BREAST FEEDING Manufacturer advises use only if potential benefit outweighs risk—present in milk.

● RENAL IMPAIRMENT Age under 12 years (body-weight under 40 kg)—no information available. Age 12–17 years (body-weight over 40 kg)—use with caution if estimated glomerular filtration rate 40–80 mL/minute/1.73 m^2, and consult product literature for dose if estimated glomerular filtration rate less than 40 mL/minute/1.73 m^2.

● MONITORING REQUIREMENTS

▸ Monitor electrolytes and fluid balance.

● DIRECTIONS FOR ADMINISTRATION Displacement value may be significant when reconstituting injection, consult local guidelines. Reconstitute each 2-g vial with 50 mL Glucose 5% or Glucose 10% or Water for Injections; do not exceed infusion rate of 133 mg/minute.

● PRESCRIBING AND DISPENSING INFORMATION Doses expressed as fosfomycin base.

● NATIONAL FUNDING/ACCESS DECISIONS

Scottish Medicines Consortium (SMC) Decisions
The *Scottish Medicines Consortium* has advised (February 2015) that Fosfomycin (*Fomicyt* ®) is accepted for restricted use within NHS Scotland; initiation should be restricted to microbiologists or infectious disease specialists.

● MEDICINAL FORMS
There can be variation in the licensing of different medicines containing the same drug.

Powder for solution for infusion
ELECTROLYTES: May contain Sodium
▸ Fomicyt (Nordic Pharma Ltd)
Fosfomycin (as Fosfomycin sodium) 2 gram Fomicyt 2g powder for solution for infusion vials | 10 vial PoM £150.00
Fosfomycin (as Fosfomycin sodium) 4 gram Fomicyt 4g powder for solution for infusion vials | 10 vial PoM £300.00

Fusidic acid

● DRUG ACTION Fusidic acid and its salts are narrow-spectrum antibiotics used for staphylococcal infections.

● INDICATIONS AND DOSE

Staphylococcal skin infection
▸ TO THE SKIN
▸ Child: Apply 3–4 times a day usually for 7 days
▸ BY MOUTH USING TABLETS
▸ Child 12-17 years: 250 mg every 12 hours for 5-10 days

Penicillin-resistant staphylococcal infection including osteomyelitis | Staphylococcal endocarditis in combination with other antibacterials
▸ BY MOUTH USING ORAL SUSPENSION
▸ Neonate: 15 mg/kg 3 times a day.

▸ Child 1-11 months: 15 mg/kg 3 times a day
▸ Child 1-4 years: 250 mg 3 times a day
▸ Child 5-11 years: 500 mg 3 times a day
▸ Child 12-17 years: 750 mg 3 times a day
▸ BY MOUTH USING TABLETS
▸ Child 12-17 years: 500 mg every 8 hours, increased to 1 g every 8 hours, increased dose can be used for severe infections

DOSE EQUIVALENCE AND CONVERSION
▸ With oral use Fusidic acid is incompletely absorbed and doses recommended for suspension are proportionally higher than those for sodium fusidate tablets.

● CAUTIONS
▸ With topical use Avoid contact of cream or ointment with eyes
CAUTIONS, FURTHER INFORMATION
▸ Avoiding resistance
▸ With topical use To avoid the development of resistance, fusidic acid should not be used for longer than 10 days and local microbiology advice should be sought before using it in hospital.

● INTERACTIONS → Appendix 1 (fusidic acid).

● SIDE-EFFECTS
▸ **Common or very common**
▸ With oral use Abdominal pain · diarrhoea · dizziness · drowsiness · dyspepsia · nausea · vomiting
▸ **Uncommon**
▸ With oral use Anorexia · headache · malaise · pruritus · rash
▸ **Rare**
▸ With topical use Hypersensitivity reactions
▸ **Frequency not known**
▸ With oral use Acute renal failure (usually with jaundice) · blood disorders · reversible jaundice especially after high dosage (withdraw therapy if persistent)

● PREGNANCY
▸ With oral use Not known to be harmful; manufacturer advises use only if potential benefit outweighs risk.

● BREAST FEEDING
▸ With oral use Present in milk—manufacturer advises caution.

● HEPATIC IMPAIRMENT
▸ With oral use Impaired biliary excretion; possibly increased risk of hepatotoxicity; avoid or reduce dose. Elimination may be reduced in hepatic impairment or biliary disease or biliary obstruction. Monitor liver function in hepatic impairment.

● MONITORING REQUIREMENTS
▸ With oral use Monitor liver function with high doses or on prolonged therapy.

● PRESCRIBING AND DISPENSING INFORMATION
▸ With oral use Flavours of oral liquid formulations may include banana and orange.

- **PROFESSION SPECIFIC INFORMATION**
  Dental practitioners' formulary
- ▸ With topical use May be prescribed as Sodium Fusidate ointment.

- **MEDICINAL FORMS**
  There can be variation in the licensing of different medicines containing the same drug.

Tablet
CAUTIONARY AND ADVISORY LABELS 9
- ▸ Fucidin (Sodium fusidate) (LEO Pharma)
  Sodium fusidate 250 mg Fucidin 250mg tablets | 10 tablet [PoM]
  £6.02 DT price = £6.02 | 100 tablet [PoM] £54.99

Oral suspension
CAUTIONARY AND ADVISORY LABELS 9, 21
- ▸ Fucidin (Fusidic acid) (LEO Pharma)
  Fusidic acid 50 mg per 1 ml Fucidin 250mg/5ml oral suspension | 50 ml [PoM] £6.73

Cream
EXCIPIENTS: May contain Butylated hydroxyanisole, cetostearyl alcohol (including cetyl and stearyl alcohol)
- ▸ Fusidic acid (Non-proprietary)
  Fusidic acid 20 mg per 1 gram Fusidic acid 2% cream | 15 gram [PoM] £1.92 DT price = £1.92 | 30 gram [PoM] £3.59 DT price = £3.59
- ▸ Fucidin (Fusidic acid) (LEO Pharma)
  Fusidic acid 20 mg per 1 gram Fucidin 20mg/g cream | 15 gram [PoM] £1.92 DT price = £1.92 | 30 gram [PoM] £3.59 DT price = £3.59

Ointment
EXCIPIENTS: May contain Cetostearyl alcohol (including cetyl and stearyl alcohol), wool fat and related substances including lanolin
- ▸ Fucidin (Sodium fusidate) (LEO Pharma)
  Sodium fusidate 20 mg per 1 gram Fucidin 20mg/g ointment | 15 gram [PoM] £2.68 DT price = £2.68 | 30 gram [PoM] £4.55 DT price = £4.55

Linezolid

- **DRUG ACTION** Linezolid, an oxazolidinone antibacterial, is active against Gram-positive bacteria including meticillin-resistant *Staphylococcus aureus* (MRSA), and glycopeptide-resistant enterococci. Resistance to linezolid can develop with prolonged treatment or if the dose is less than that recommended. Linezolid is **not** active against common Gram-negative organisms; it must be given in combination with other antibacterials for mixed infections that also involve Gram-negative organisms.

- **INDICATIONS AND DOSE**
  Pneumonia (when other antibacterials e.g. a glycopeptide, such as vancomycin, cannot be used) (initiated under specialist supervision) | Complicated skin and soft-tissue infections caused by Gram-positive bacteria, when other antibacterials cannot be used (initiated under specialist supervision)
  - ▸ BY MOUTH, OR BY INTRAVENOUS INFUSION
  - ▸ Neonate up to 7 days: 10 mg/kg every 12 hours, increased if necessary to 10 mg/kg every 8 hours, increased dose can be used if poor response.
  - ▸ Neonate 7 days to 28 days: 10 mg/kg every 8 hours.
  - ▸ Child 1 month-11 years: 10 mg/kg every 8 hours (max. per dose 600 mg)
  - ▸ Child 12-17 years: 600 mg every 12 hours

- **UNLICENSED USE** Not licensed for use in children.

IMPORTANT SAFETY INFORMATION
CHM ADVICE (OPTIC NEUROPATHY)
Severe optic neuropathy may occur rarely, particularly if linezolid is used for longer than 28 days. The CHM recommends that:

- patients should be warned to report symptoms of visual impairment (including blurred vision, visual field defect, changes in visual acuity and colour vision) immediately;
- patients experiencing new visual symptoms (regardless of treatment duration) should be evaluated promptly, and referred to an ophthalmologist if necessary;
- visual function should be monitored regularly if treatment is required for longer than 28 days.

BLOOD DISORDERS
Haemopoietic disorders (including thrombocytopenia, anaemia, leucopenia, and pancytopenia) have been reported in patients receiving linezolid. It is recommended that full blood counts are monitored weekly. Close monitoring is recommended in patients who:

- receive treatment for more than 10–14 days;
- have pre-existing myelosuppression;
- are receiving drugs that may have adverse effects on haemoglobin, blood counts, or platelet function;
- have severe renal impairment.

If significant myelosuppression occurs, treatment should be stopped unless it is considered essential, in which case intensive monitoring of blood counts and appropriate management should be implemented.

- **CAUTIONS** Acute confusional states · bipolar depression · carcinoid tumour · phaeochromocytoma · schizophrenia · thyrotoxicosis · uncontrolled hypertension
  CAUTIONS, FURTHER INFORMATION
- ▸ Close observation Unless close observation and blood pressure monitoring possible, linezolid should be avoided in uncontrolled hypertension, phaeochromocytoma, carcinoid tumour, thyrotoxicosis, bipolar depression, schizophrenia, or acute confusional states.

- **INTERACTIONS** → Appendix 1 (MAOIs).
- ▸ Monoamine oxidase inhibition Linezolid is a reversible, non-selective monoamine oxidase inhibitor (MAOI). Patients should avoid consuming large amounts of tyramine-rich foods (such as mature cheese, yeast extracts, undistilled alcoholic beverages, and fermented soya bean products). In addition, linezolid should not be given with another MAOI or within 2 weeks of stopping another MAOI. Unless close observation and blood-pressure monitoring is possible, avoid in those receiving SSRIs, 5HT$_1$ agonists ('triptans'), tricyclic antidepressants, sympathomimetics, dopaminergics, buspirone, pethidine and possibly other opioid analgesics.

- **SIDE-EFFECTS**
  GENERAL SIDE-EFFECTS
- ▸ Common or very common Diarrhoea · eosinophilia · headache · nausea · taste disturbances · vomiting
- ▸ Uncommon Abdominal pain · blurred vision · constipation · diaphoresis · dizziness · dry mouth · dyspepsia · electrolyte disturbances · fatigue · fever · gastritis · glossitis · hypertension · hypoaesthesia · insomnia · leucopenia · pancreatitis · paraesthesia · polyuria · pruritus · rash · stomatitis · thirst · thrombocytopenia · tinnitus · tongue discoloration
- ▸ Rare Renal failure · tachycardia · transient ischaemic attacks
- ▸ Frequency not known Anaemia · antibiotic-associated colitis · convulsions · hyponatraemia · lactic acidosis · optic neuropathy reported on prolonged therapy · pancytopenia · peripheral neuropathy reported on prolonged therapy · Stevens-Johnson syndrome · tooth discoloration · toxic epidermal necrolysis
  SPECIFIC SIDE-EFFECTS
- ▸ Uncommon
- ▸ With intravenous use Injection-site reactions

- PREGNANCY Manufacturer advises use only if potential benefit outweighs risk—no information available.
- BREAST FEEDING Manufacturer advises avoid—present in milk in *animal* studies.
- HEPATIC IMPAIRMENT No dose adjustment necessary but in severe hepatic impairment use only if potential benefit outweighs risk.
- RENAL IMPAIRMENT No dose adjustment necessary but metabolites may accumulate if estimated glomerular filtration rate less than 30 mL/minute/1.73 m^2.
- MONITORING REQUIREMENTS Monitor full blood count (including platelet count) weekly.
- DIRECTIONS FOR ADMINISTRATION
  - With intravenous use Infusion to be administered over 30–120 minutes.
- PRESCRIBING AND DISPENSING INFORMATION Flavours of oral liquid formulations may contain orange.
  There is limited information on use in children and expert advice should be sought.
- PATIENT AND CARER ADVICE Patients should be advised to read the patient information leaflet given with linezolid.

- MEDICINAL FORMS
  There can be variation in the licensing of different medicines containing the same drug.
  Tablet
  CAUTIONARY AND ADVISORY LABELS 9, 10
  - Linezolid (Non-proprietary)
    Linezolid 600 mg Linezolid 600mg tablets | 10 tablet PoM £228.86–£445.00
  - Zyvox (Pfizer Ltd)
    Linezolid 600 mg Zyvox 600mg tablets | 10 tablet PoM £445.00
  Oral suspension
  CAUTIONARY AND ADVISORY LABELS 9, 10
  EXCIPIENTS: May contain Aspartame
  - Zyvox (Pfizer Ltd)
    Linezolid 20 mg per 1 ml Zyvox 100mg/5ml granules for oral suspension | 150 ml PoM £222.50
  Infusion
  EXCIPIENTS: May contain Glucose
  ELECTROLYTES: May contain Sodium
  - Linezolid (Non-proprietary)
    Linezolid 2 mg per 1 ml Linezolid 600mg/300ml infusion bags | 10 bag PoM £445.00 (Hospital only)
  - Zyvox (Pfizer Ltd)
    Linezolid 2 mg per 1 ml Zyvox 600mg/300ml infusion bags | 10 bag PoM £445.00

Trimethoprim

- **INDICATIONS AND DOSE**

Urinary-tract infections | Respiratory tract infections
- BY MOUTH
  - Neonate: Initially 3 mg/kg for 1 dose, then 1–2 mg/kg twice daily.
  - Child 4–5 weeks: 4 mg/kg twice daily (max. per dose 200 mg)
  - Child 6 weeks–5 months: 4 mg/kg twice daily (max. per dose 200 mg), alternatively 25 mg twice daily
  - Child 6 months–5 years: 4 mg/kg twice daily (max. per dose 200 mg), alternatively 50 mg twice daily
  - Child 6–11 years: 4 mg/kg twice daily (max. per dose 200 mg), alternatively 100 mg twice daily
  - Child 12–17 years: 200 mg twice daily

Prophylaxis of urinary-tract infection (considered for recurrent infection, significant urinary-tract anomalies, or significant kidney damage)
- BY MOUTH
  - Neonate: 2 mg/kg once daily, dose to be taken at night.
  - Child 4–5 weeks: 2 mg/kg once daily (max. per dose 100 mg), dose to be taken at night
  - Child 6 weeks–5 months: 2 mg/kg once daily (max. per dose 100 mg), dose to be taken at night, alternatively 12.5 mg once daily, dose to be taken at night
  - Child 6 months–5 years: 2 mg/kg once daily (max. per dose 100 mg), dose to be taken at night, alternatively 25 mg once daily, dose to be taken at night
  - Child 6–11 years: 2 mg/kg once daily (max. per dose 100 mg), dose to be taken at night, alternatively 50 mg once daily, dose to be taken at night
  - Child 12–17 years: 100 mg once daily, dose to be taken at night

Treatment of mild to moderate *Pneumocystis jirovecii* (*Pneumocystis carinii*) pneumonia in patients who cannot tolerate co-trimoxazole (in combination with dapsone)
- BY MOUTH
  - Child: 5 mg/kg every 6–8 hours

Shigellosis | Invasive salmonella infection
- BY MOUTH
  - Child: (consult product literature)

- UNLICENSED USE Not licensed for treatment of pneumocystis pneumonia.
  Not licensed for use in children under 6 weeks.
- CONTRA-INDICATIONS Blood dyscrasias
- CAUTIONS Acute porphyrias p. 562 · neonates (specialist supervision required) · predisposition to folate deficiency
- INTERACTIONS → Appendix 1 (trimethoprim).
- SIDE-EFFECTS
  - Rare Allergic reactions · anaphylaxis · angioedema · erythema multiforme · photosensitivity · toxic epidermal necrolysis
  - Frequency not known Aseptic meningitis · depression of haematopoiesis · gastro-intestinal disturbances · hyperkalaemia · nausea · pruritus · rashes · vomiting
  SIDE-EFFECTS, FURTHER INFORMATION
  Trimethoprim has side-effects similar to co-trimoxazole but they are less severe and occur less frequently.
- PREGNANCY Teratogenic risk in first trimester (folate antagonist). Manufacturers advise avoid during pregnancy.
- BREAST FEEDING Present in milk—short-term use not known to be harmful.
- RENAL IMPAIRMENT Use half normal dose after 3 days if estimated glomerular filtration rate 15–30 mL/minute/1.73 m^2. Use half normal dose if estimated glomerular filtration rate less than 15 mL/minute/1.73 m^2. Monitor plasma-trimethoprim concentration if estimated glomerular filtration rate less than 10 mL/minute/1.73 m^2.
- MONITORING REQUIREMENTS Manufacturer recommends blood counts on long-term therapy (but evidence of practical value unsatisfactory).
- PATIENT AND CARER ADVICE
  Medicines for Children leaflet: Trimethoprim for bacterial infections www.medicinesforchildren.org.uk/trimethoprim-for-bacterial-infections
  Blood disorders On long-term treatment, patients and their carers should be told how to recognise signs of blood disorders and advised to seek immediate medical attention if symptoms such as fever, sore throat, rash, mouth ulcers, purpura, bruising or bleeding develop.

● MEDICINAL FORMS
There can be variation in the licensing of different medicines containing the same drug. Forms available from special-order manufacturers include: oral suspension, oral solution

Tablet
CAUTIONARY AND ADVISORY LABELS 9
▸ **Trimethoprim (Non-proprietary)**
   Trimethoprim 100 mg Trimethoprim 100mg tablets |
   28 tablet [PoM] £9.99 DT price = £1.68
   Trimethoprim 200 mg Trimethoprim 200mg tablets | 6 tablet [PoM]
   £2.15 DT price = £1.03 | 14 tablet [PoM] £9.99 DT price = £2.40

Oral suspension
CAUTIONARY AND ADVISORY LABELS 9
▸ **Trimethoprim (Non-proprietary)**
   Trimethoprim 10 mg per 1 ml Trimethoprim 50mg/5ml oral
   suspension sugar free sugar-free | 100 ml [PoM] £15.00 DT price =
   £1.72
▸ **Monotrim** (Chemidex Pharma Ltd)
   Trimethoprim 10 mg per 1 ml Monotrim 50mg/5ml oral suspension
   sugar-free | 100 ml [PoM] £1.77 DT price = £1.72

2.1 ANTHRAX

Anthrax

Treatment and post-exposure prophylaxis

Inhalation or *gastro-intestinal anthrax* should be treated initially with either ciprofloxacin p. 328 or, in patients over 12 years, doxycycline p. 332 [unlicensed indication] combined with one or two other antibacterials (such as amoxicillin p. 320, benzylpenicillin sodium p. 318, chloramphenicol p. 334, clarithromycin p. 309, clindamycin p. 307, imipenem with cilastatin p. 295, rifampicin p. 342 [unlicensed indication], and vancomycin p. 305). When the condition improves and the sensitivity of the *Bacillus anthracis* strain is known, treatment may be switched to a single antibacterial. Treatment should continue for 60 days because germination may be delayed.

Cutaneous anthrax should be treated with either ciprofloxacin [unlicensed indication] or doxycycline [unlicensed indication] for 7 days. Treatment may be switched to amoxicillin if the infecting strain is susceptible. Treatment may need to be extended to 60 days if exposure is due to aerosol. A combination of antibacterials for 14 days is recommended for cutaneous anthrax with systemic features, extensive oedema, or lesions of the head or neck.

Ciprofloxacin or doxycycline may be given for *post-exposure prophylaxis*. If exposure is confirmed, antibacterial prophylaxis should continue for 60 days. Antibacterial prophylaxis may be switched to amoxicillin after 10–14 days if the strain of *B. anthracis* is susceptible. Vaccination against anthrax may allow the duration of antibacterial prophylaxis to be shortened.

2.2 Lyme disease

Lyme disease

Treatment

Lyme disease should generally be treated by those experienced in its management. Amoxicillin p. 320 [unlicensed indication], cefuroxime p. 300 (as cefuroxime axetil) or doxycycline p. 332 are the antibacterials of choice for *early Lyme disease* or *Lyme arthritis* but doxycycline should only be used in children over 12 years of age. If these antibacterials are contra-indicated, a **macrolide** (e.g. clarithromycin p. 309) can be used for early Lyme disease.

Intravenous administration of ceftriaxone p. 302, cefotaxime p. 301, or benzylpenicillin sodium p. 318 is recommended for Lyme disease associated with cardiac or neurological complications. The duration of treatment is usually 2–4 weeks; Lyme arthritis may require further treatment.

2.3 Methicillin-resistant staphylococcus aureus

MRSA

Management

Infection from *Staphylococcus aureus* strains resistant to meticillin [now discontinued] (meticillin-resistant *Staph. aureus*, MRSA) and to flucloxacillin p. 325 can be difficult to manage. Treatment is guided by the sensitivity of the infecting strain.

Rifampicin p. 342 or fusidic acid p. 336 should **not** be used alone because resistance may develop rapidly. Clindamycin p. 307 alone or a combination of rifampicin and fusidic acid can be used for *skin* and *soft-tissue infections* caused by MRSA; a **tetracycline** is an alternative in children over 12 years of age. A **glycopeptide** (e.g. vancomycin p. 305) can be used for severe skin and soft-tissue infections associated with MRSA. A combination of a glycopeptide and fusidic acid or a glycopeptide and rifampicin can be considered for skin and soft-tissue infections that have failed to respond to a single antibacterial. Linezolid p. 337 should be reserved for skin and soft-tissue infections that have not responded to other antibacterials or for children who cannot tolerate other antibacterials.

A **glycopeptide** can be used for *pneumonia* associated with MRSA. Linezolid should be reserved for hospital-acquired pneumonia that has not responded to other antibacterials or for children who cannot tolerate other antibacterials.

Trimethoprim p. 338 or nitrofurantoin p. 347 can be used for *urinary-tract infections* caused by MRSA; a **tetracycline** is an alternative in children over 12 years of age. A **glycopeptide** can be used for urinary-tract infections that are severe or resistant to other antibacterials.

A **glycopeptide** can be used for septicaemia associated with MRSA.

See the management of endocarditis, osteomyelitis, or septic arthritis associated with MRSA.

Prophylaxis with vancomycin or teicoplanin p. 305 (alone or in combination with another antibacterial active against other pathogens) is appropriate for patients undergoing surgery if:

- there is a history of MRSA colonisation or infection without documented eradication;
- there is a risk that the patient's MRSA carriage has recurred;
- the patient comes from an area with a high prevalence of MRSA.

It is important that hospitals have infection control guidelines to minimise MRSA transmission, including policies on isolation and treatment of MRSA carriers and on hand hygiene. See eradication of nasal carriage of MRSA in Nose p. 648.

5

Infection

2.4 Tuberculosis

Tuberculosis

Treatment phases, overview

Tuberculosis is treated in two phases—an *initial phase* using 4 drugs and a *continuation phase* using 2 drugs in fully sensitive cases. Treatment requires specialised knowledge and supervision, particularly where the disease involves resistant organisms or non-respiratory organs.

There are two regimens recommended for the treatment of tuberculosis in the UK; variations occur in other countries. Either the unsupervised regimen or the supervised regimen should be used; the two regimens should **not** be used concurrently. Compliance with therapy is a major determinant of its success. Treatment needs to be carefully monitored in families in whom concordance may be problematic.

Initial phase

The concurrent use of 4 drugs during the initial phase is designed to reduce the bacterial population as rapidly as possible and to prevent the emergence of drug-resistant bacteria. The drugs are best given as combination preparations, provided the respective dose of each drug is appropriate, unless the child is unable to swallow the tablets or one of the components cannot be given because of resistance or intolerance. The treatment of choice for the initial phase is the daily use of isoniazid p. 345, rifampicin p. 342, pyrazinamide p. 346 and ethambutol hydrochloride p. 345. Treatment should be started without waiting for culture results if clinical features or histology results are consistent with tuberculosis; treatment should be continued even if initial culture results are negative. The initial phase drugs should be continued for 2 months. Where a positive culture for *M. tuberculosis* has been obtained, but susceptibility results are not available after 2 months, treatment with rifampicin, isoniazid, pyrazinamide and ethambutol hydrochloride should be continued until full susceptibility is confirmed, even if this is for longer than 2 months.

Streptomycin p. 293 is rarely used in the UK although it may be used in the initial phase of treatment if resistance to isoniazid has been established before therapy is commenced and ethambutol hydrochloride is contra-indicated.

Continuation phase

After the initial phase, treatment is continued for a further 4 months with isoniazid and rifampicin (preferably given as a combination preparation). Longer treatment is necessary for meningitis, direct spinal cord involvement, and for resistant organisms which may also require modification of the regimen.

Unsupervised treatment

The following regimen should be used for those who are likely to take antituberculous drugs reliably **without supervision** by a healthcare worker. Children and families who are unlikely to comply with daily administration of antituberculous drugs should be treated with the regimen described under Supervised Treatment.

Pregnancy and breast-feeding

The standard unsupervised 6-month treatment regimen may be used during pregnancy. Streptomycin should not be given in pregnancy.

The standard unsupervised 6-month treatment regimen may be used during breast-feeding.

Neonates

Congenital tuberculosis is acquired from maternal extrapulmonary sites at birth, particularly the genital tract; if infection is suspected, the baby will require treatment with isoniazid, rifampicin, pyrazinamide, and ethambutol hydrochloride. Isoniazid, rifampicin, pyrazinamide, and ethambutol hydrochloride are used for 2 months during the initial phase of treatment. After the initial phase, treatment is continued for a further 4 months with isoniazid and rifampicin.

Supervised treatment

Drug administration needs to be **fully supervised** by a healthcare worker (directly observed therapy, DOT) in children or families who cannot comply reliably with the treatment regimen. These patients are given isoniazid, rifampicin, pyrazinamide and ethambutol hydrochloride (or streptomycin) 3 times a week under supervision for the first 2 months followed by isoniazid and rifampicin 3 times a week for a further 4 months.

Immunocompromised patients

Multi-resistant *Mycobacterium tuberculosis* may be present in immunocompromised children. The organism should always be cultured to confirm its type and drug sensitivity. Confirmed *M. tuberculosis* infection sensitive to first-line drugs should be treated with a standard 6-month regimen; after completing treatment, children should be closely monitored. The regimen may need to be modified if infection is caused by resistant organisms, and specialist advice is needed.

Specialist advice should be sought about tuberculosis treatment or chemoprophylaxis in a HIV-positive individual; care is required in choosing the regimen and in avoiding potentially serious interactions. Starting antiretroviral treatment in the first 2 months of antituberculosis treatment increases the risk of immune reconstitution syndrome.

Infection may also be caused by other mycobacteria e.g. *M. avium*complex in which case specialist advice on management is needed.

Corticosteroids

A corticosteroid should be given (in addition to antituberculosis therapy) for meningeal or pericardial tuberculosis.

Prevention of tuberculosis

Chemoprophylaxis may be required in children who are close contacts of a case of smear-positive pulmonary tuberculosis and who are severely immunosuppressed (including congenital immunodeficiencies, cytotoxic or immunosuppressive therapy) and in those who have evidence of latent tuberculosis and require treatment with immunosuppressants; expert advice should be sought.

Chemoprophylaxis involves use of either isoniazid alone for 6 months or of isoniazid and rifampicin for 3 months.

See prevention of tuberculosis in susceptible close contacts or those who have become tuberculin-positive. See advice on immunisation against tuberculosis and tuberculin testing.

Treatment failure

Major causes of treatment failure are incorrect prescribing by the physician and inadequate compliance by the child or their carer. Monthly tablet counts and urine examination (rifampicin imparts an orange-red coloration) may be useful indicators of compliance with treatment. Avoid both excessive and inadequate dosage. Treatment should be specialised by a specialist paediatrician.

Recommended dosage for standard unsupervised 6-month treatment

Isoniazid	Child: 10 mg/kg once daily (max. per dose 300 mg) for 6 months (initial and continuation phases)
Rifampicin	Child: ▸ body-weight up to 50 kg: 15 mg/kg once daily for 6 months (initial and continuation phases); maximum 450 mg per day; ▸ body-weight 50 kg and above: 15 mg/kg once daily for 6 months (initial and continuation phases); maximum 600 mg per day
Pyrazinamide	Child: ▸ body-weight up to 50 kg: 35 mg/kg once daily for 2 months (initial phase); maximum 1.5 g per day; ▸ body-weight 50 kg and above: 35 mg/kg once daily for 2 months (initial phase); maximum 2 g per day
Ethambutol hydrochloride	Child: 20 mg/kg once daily for 2 months (initial phase)

In general, doses should be rounded up to facilitate administration of suitable volumes of liquid or an appropriate strength of tablet. The exception is ethambutol hydrochloride due to the risk of toxicity. Doses may also need to be recalculated to allow for weight gain in younger children. The fixed-dose combination preparations (*Rifater*®, *Rifinah*®) are unlicensed for use in children. Consideration may be given to use of these preparations in older children, provided the respective dose of each drug is appropriate for the weight of the child.

Recommended dosage for intermittent supervised 6-month treatment

Isoniazid	Child: 15 mg/kg 3 times a week (max. per dose 900 mg) for 6 months (initial and continuation phases)
Rifampicin	Child: 15 mg/kg 3 times a week (max. per dose 900 mg) for 6 months (initial and continuation phases)
Pyrazinamide	Child: ▸ body-weight up to 50 kg: 50 mg/kg 3 times a week (max. per dose 2 g 3 times a week) for 2 months (initial phase); ▸ body-weight 50 kg and above: 50 mg/kg 3 times a week (max. per dose 2.5 g 3 times a week) for 2 months (initial phase)
Ethambutol hydrochloride	Child: 30 mg/kg 3 times a week for 2 months (initial phase)

In general, doses should be rounded up to facilitate administration of suitable volumes of liquid or an appropriate strength of tablet. The exception is ethambutol hydrochloride due to the risk of toxicity. Doses may also need to be recalculated to allow for weight gain in younger children. The fixed-dose combination preparations (*Rifater*®, *Rifinah*®) are unlicensed for use in children. Consideration may be given to use of these preparations in older children, provided the respective dose of each drug is appropriate for the weight of the child.

Antituberculosis drugs

Isoniazid is cheap and highly effective. Like rifampicin it should always be included in any antituberculous regimen unless there is a specific contra-indication.

Rifampicin, a rifamycin, is a key component of any antituberculous regimen. Like isoniazid it should always be included unless there is a specific contra-indication.

During the first two months ('initial phase') of rifampicin administration transient disturbance of liver function with elevated serum transaminases is common but generally does not require interruption of treatment. Occasionally more serious liver toxicity requires a change of treatment particularly in those with pre-existing liver disease.

On intermittent treatment six toxicity syndromes have been recognised—influenza-like, abdominal, and respiratory symptoms, shock, renal failure, and thrombocytopenic purpura—and can occur in 20 to 30% of patients.

Rifabutin below is licensed in adults for the *treatment* of non-tuberculous mycobacterial disease and pulmonary tuberculosis. There is limited experience in children.

Pyrazinamide is a bactericidal drug only active against intracellular dividing forms of *Mycobacterium tuberculosis*; it exerts its main effect only in the first two or three months. It is particularly useful in tuberculous meningitis because of good meningeal penetration. It is not active against *M. bovis*.

Ethambutol hydrochloride p. 345 is included in a treatment regimen if isoniazid p. 345 resistance is suspected; it can be omitted if the risk of resistance is low.

Streptomycin p. 293 [unlicensed] is now rarely used in the UK except for resistant organisms.

Drug-resistant tuberculosis should be treated by a specialist paediatrician with experience in such cases, and where appropriate facilities for infection-control exist. Second-line drugs available for infections caused by resistant organisms, or when first-line drugs cause unacceptable side-effects, include amikacin p. 292, capreomycin, cycloserine p. 344, newer macrolides (e.g. azithromycin p. 308 and clarithromycin p. 309), quinolones (e.g. moxifloxacin p. 631) and protionamide (prothionamide; no longer on UK market). Availability of suitable formulations may limit choice in children.

ANTIMYCOBACTERIALS ﹥ RIFAMYCINS

▌ Rifabutin

● **INDICATIONS AND DOSE**

Prophylaxis of *Mycobacterium avium* complex infections in immunosuppressed patients with low CD4 count

▸ BY MOUTH
▸ Child 1 month–11 years: 5 mg/kg once daily (max. per dose 300 mg), also consult product literature
▸ Child 12–17 years: 300 mg once daily, also consult product literature

Treatment of non-tuberculous mycobacterial disease, in combination with other drugs

▸ BY MOUTH
▸ Child 1 month–11 years: 5 mg/kg once daily for up to 6 months after cultures negative
▸ Child 12–17 years: 450–600 mg once daily for up to 6 months after cultures negative

Treatment of pulmonary tuberculosis, in combination with other drugs

▸ BY MOUTH
▸ Child 12–17 years: 150–450 mg once daily for at least 6 months

● **UNLICENSED USE** Not licensed for use in children.
● **CAUTIONS** Acute porphyrias p. 562 · discolours soft contact lenses
● **INTERACTIONS** → Appendix 1 (rifamycins).
● **SIDE-EFFECTS**
● **Common or very common** Anaemia · blood disorders · leucopenia · myalgia · nausea · pyrexia · rash · thrombocytopenia

▸ **Uncommon** Arthralgia · body secretions coloured orange-red · bronchospasm · corneal deposits · eosinophilia · hypersensitivity reactions · jaundice · raised liver enzymes · saliva coloured orange-red · skin coloured orange-red · urine coloured orange-red · uveitis (especially following high doses or concomitant use with drugs that increase plasma concentration) · vomiting

▸ **Rare** Haemolysis

▸ **Frequency not known** Chest pain · dyspnoea · hepatitis · influenza-like symptoms

SIDE-EFFECTS, FURTHER INFORMATION
Discontinue permanently if serious side-effects develop.

● **ALLERGY AND CROSS-SENSITIVITY** Contra-indicated in patients with rifamycin hypersensitivity.

● **CONCEPTION AND CONTRACEPTION**
Important Rifabutin induces hepatic enzymes and the effectiveness of hormonal contraceptives is reduced; alternative family planning advice should be offered.

● **PREGNANCY** Manufacturer advises avoid—no information available.

● **BREAST FEEDING** Manufacturer advises avoid—no information available.

● **HEPATIC IMPAIRMENT** Reduce dose in severe impairment. In patients with pre-existing liver disease or hepatic impairment monitor liver function regularly and particularly frequently in the first 2 months; blood counts should also be monitored in these patients.

● **RENAL IMPAIRMENT** Use half normal dose if estimated glomerular filtration rate less than 30 mL/minute/1.73 m².

● **MONITORING REQUIREMENTS**
▸ *Renal function* should be checked before treatment.
▸ *Hepatic function* should be checked before treatment. If there is no evidence of liver disease (and pre-treatment liver function is normal), further checks are only necessary if the patient develops fever, malaise, vomiting, jaundice or unexplained deterioration during treatment. However, hepatic function should be monitored on prolonged therapy.
▸ Blood counts should be monitored on prolonged therapy.

● **PRESCRIBING AND DISPENSING INFORMATION** If treatment interruption occurs, re-introduce with low dosage and increase gradually.

● **PATIENT AND CARER ADVICE**
Soft contact lenses Patients or their carers should be advised that rifabutin discolours soft contact lenses.
Hepatic disorders Patients or their carers should be told how to recognise signs of liver disorder, and advised to discontinue treatment and seek immediate medical attention if symptoms such as persistent nausea, vomiting, malaise or jaundice develop.

● **MEDICINAL FORMS**
There can be variation in the licensing of different medicines containing the same drug. Forms available from special-order manufacturers include: oral suspension, oral solution

Capsule
CAUTIONARY AND ADVISORY LABELS 8, 14
▸ Mycobutin (Pfizer Ltd)
Rifabutin 150 mg Mycobutin 150mg capsules | 30 capsule [PoM]
£90.38

Rifampicin

● **INDICATIONS AND DOSE**

Brucellosis in combination with other antibacterials | Legionnaires disease in combination with other antibacterials | Serious staphylococcal infections in combination with other antibacterials
▸ BY MOUTH, OR BY INTRAVENOUS INFUSION
▸ Neonate: 5–10 mg/kg twice daily.
▸ Child 1–11 months: 5–10 mg/kg twice daily
▸ Child 1–17 years: 10 mg/kg twice daily (max. per dose 600 mg)

Tuberculosis, in combination with other drugs (intermittent supervised 6-month treatment) (under expert supervision)
▸ BY MOUTH
▸ Child: 15 mg/kg 3 times a week (max. per dose 900 mg) for 6 months (initial and continuation phases)

Tuberculosis, in combination with other drugs (standard unsupervised 6-month treatment)
▸ BY MOUTH
▸ Child (body-weight up to 50 kg): 15 mg/kg once daily for 6 months (initial and continuation phases); maximum 450 mg per day
▸ Child (body-weight 50 kg and above): 15 mg/kg once daily for 6 months (initial and continuation phases); maximum 600 mg per day

Congenital tuberculosis
▸ BY MOUTH
▸ Neonate: 15 mg/kg once daily for 6 months (initial and continuation phases).

Prevention of tuberculosis in susceptible close contacts or those who have become tuberculin positive, in combination with isoniazid
▸ BY MOUTH
▸ Child 1 month–11 years (body-weight up to 50 kg): 15 mg/kg daily for 3 months; maximum 450 mg per day
▸ Child 1 month–11 years (body-weight 50 kg and above): 15 mg/kg daily for 3 months; maximum 600 mg per day
▸ Child 12–17 years (body-weight up to 50 kg): 450 mg daily for 3 months
▸ Child 12–17 years (body-weight 50 kg and above): 600 mg daily for 3 months

Prevention of tuberculosis in susceptible close contacts or those who have become tuberculin positive, who are isoniazid-resistant
▸ BY MOUTH
▸ Child 1 month–11 years (body-weight up to 50 kg): 15 mg/kg daily for 6 months; maximum 450 mg per day
▸ Child 1 month–11 years (body-weight 50 kg and above): 15 mg/kg daily for 6 months; maximum 600 mg per day
▸ Child 12–17 years (body-weight up to 50 kg): 450 mg daily for 6 months
▸ Child 12–17 years (body-weight 50 kg and above): 600 mg daily for 6 months

Prevention of secondary case of *Haemophilus influenzae* type b disease
▸ BY MOUTH
▸ Child 1–2 months: 10 mg/kg once daily for 4 days
▸ Child 3 months–11 years: 20 mg/kg once daily (max. per dose 600 mg) for 4 days
▸ Child 12–17 years: 600 mg once daily for 4 days

Prevention of secondary case of meningococcal meningitis
▶ BY MOUTH
▸ Neonate: 5 mg/kg every 12 hours for 2 days.

▸ Child 1–11 months: 5 mg/kg every 12 hours for 2 days
▸ Child 1–11 years: 10 mg/kg every 12 hours (max. per dose 600 mg), for 2 days
▸ Child 12–17 years: 600 mg every 12 hours for 2 days

Pruritus due to cholestasis
▶ BY MOUTH
▸ Child: 5–10 mg/kg once daily (max. per dose 600 mg)

● **UNLICENSED USE** Not licensed for use in children for pruritus due to cholestasis.

● **CONTRA-INDICATIONS** Acute porphyrias p. 562 · jaundice

● **CAUTIONS** Discolours soft contact lenses

● **INTERACTIONS** → Appendix 1 (rifamycins). Rifampicin induces hepatic enzymes which accelerate the metabolism of several drugs including oestrogens, corticosteroids, phenytoin, sulfonylureas, and anticoagulants.

● **SIDE-EFFECTS**
GENERAL SIDE-EFFECTS
Acute renal failure · adrenal insufficiency · alterations of liver function · anorexia · antibiotic-associated colitis · body secretions coloured orange-red · collapse and shock · diarrhoea · disseminated intravascular coagulation · drowsiness · eosinophilia · exfoliative dermatitis · flushing · gastro-intestinal symptoms · haemolytic anaemia · headache · influenza-like symptoms (with chills, fever, dizziness, bone pain) · jaundice · leucopenia · menstrual disturbances · muscular weakness · myopathy · nausea · oedema · pemphigoid reactions · psychoses · rashes · respiratory symptoms · saliva coloured orange-red · shortness of breath · Stevens-Johnson syndrome · thrombocytopenic purpura · toxic epidermal necrolysis · urine coloured orange-red · urticaria · vomiting

SPECIFIC SIDE-EFFECTS
▸ With intravenous use Thrombophlebitis reported if infusion used for prolonged period

SIDE-EFFECTS, FURTHER INFORMATION
Discontinue permanently if serious side-effects develop.
▸ Intermittent therapy Side-effects that mainly occur with intermittent therapy include influenza-like symptoms (with chills, fever, dizziness, bone pain), respiratory symptoms (including shortness of breath), collapse and shock, haemolytic anaemia, thrombocytopenic purpura, disseminated intravascular coagulation, and acute renal failure

● **ALLERGY AND CROSS-SENSITIVITY** Contra-indicated in patients with rifamycin hypersensitivity.

● **CONCEPTION AND CONTRACEPTION** Important Effectiveness of hormonal contraceptives is reduced and alternative family planning advice should be offered.

● **PREGNANCY** Manufacturers advise very high doses teratogenic in *animal* studies in first trimester; risk of neonatal bleeding may be increased in third trimester.

● **BREAST FEEDING** Amount too small to be harmful.

● **HEPATIC IMPAIRMENT** Avoid or do not exceed 8 mg/kg daily. Impaired elimination. In patients with pre-existing liver disease or hepatic impairment, monitor liver function regularly and particularly frequently in the first 2 months; blood counts should also be monitored in these patients.

● **RENAL IMPAIRMENT** Use with caution if doses above 10 mg/kg daily.

● **MONITORING REQUIREMENTS**
▸ *Renal function* should be checked before treatment.
▸ *Hepatic function* should be checked before treatment. If there is no evidence of liver disease (and pre-treatment liver function is normal), further checks are only necessary if the patient develops fever, malaise, vomiting, jaundice or unexplained deterioration during treatment. However, liver function should be monitored on prolonged therapy.
▸ Blood counts should be monitored in patients on prolonged therapy.

● **DIRECTIONS FOR ADMINISTRATION**
▸ With intravenous use Displacement value may be significant, consult local reconstitution guidelines; reconstitute with solvent provided. May be further diluted with Glucose 5% or Sodium chloride 0.9% to a final concentration of 1.2 mg/mL. Infuse over 2–3 hours.

● **PRESCRIBING AND DISPENSING INFORMATION** If treatment interruption occurs, re-introduce with low dosage and increase gradually.
▸ With oral use In general, doses should be rounded up to facilitate administration of suitable volumes of liquid or an appropriate strength of tablet. Doses may also need to be recalculated to allow for weight gain in younger children. Flavours of syrup may include raspberry.

● **PATIENT AND CARER ADVICE**
Medicines for Children leaflet: Rifampicin for meningococcal prophylaxis www.medicinesforchildren.org.uk/rifampicin-for-meningococcal-prophylaxis
Medicines for Children leaflet: Rifampicin for the treatment of tuberculosis www.medicinesforchildren.org.uk/rifampicin-for-treatment-of-tuberculosis
Soft contact lenses Patients or their carers should be advised that rifampicin discolours soft contact lenses.
Hepatic disorders Patients or their carers should be told how to recognise signs of liver disorder, and advised to discontinue treatment and seek immediate medical attention if symptoms such as persistent nausea, vomiting, malaise or jaundice develop.

● **MEDICINAL FORMS**
There can be variation in the licensing of different medicines containing the same drug. Forms available from special-order manufacturers include: oral suspension, oral solution

Capsule
CAUTIONARY AND ADVISORY LABELS 8, 14, 23
▸ **Rifampicin (Non-proprietary)**
  Rifampicin 150 mg Rifampicin 150mg capsules | 100 capsule [PoM] £44.84 DT price = £38.48
  Rifampicin 300 mg Rifampicin 300mg capsules | 100 capsule [PoM] £103.25 DT price = £87.77
▸ **Rifadin (Sanofi)**
  Rifampicin 150 mg Rifadin 150mg capsules | 100 capsule [PoM] £18.32 DT price = £38.48
  Rifampicin 300 mg Rifadin 300mg capsules | 100 capsule [PoM] £36.63 DT price = £87.77
▸ **Rimactane (Sandoz Ltd)**
  Rifampicin 300 mg Rimactane 300mg capsules | 60 capsule [PoM] £25.92

Oral suspension
CAUTIONARY AND ADVISORY LABELS 8, 14, 23
EXCIPIENTS: May contain Sucrose
▸ **Rifadin (Sanofi)**
  Rifampicin 20 mg per 1 ml Rifadin 100mg/5ml syrup | 120 ml [PoM] £4.27

Powder and solvent for solution for injection
▸ **Rifampicin (Non-proprietary)**
  Rifampicin 300 mg RIFA parenteral 300mg powder and solvent for solution for injection vials | 1 vial [PoM] no price available

Powder and solvent for solution for infusion
ELECTROLYTES: May contain Sodium
▸ **Rifadin (Sanofi)**
  Rifampicin 600 mg Rifadin 600mg powder and solvent for solution for infusion vials | 1 vial [PoM] £9.20

5

Infection

Rifampicin with isoniazid

The properties listed below are those particular to the combination only. For the properties of the components please consider, rifampicin p. 342, isoniazid p. 345.

● **INDICATIONS AND DOSE**
Treatment of tuberculosis (continuation phase)
▶ BY MOUTH
▶ Child: Although not licensed in children, consideration may be given to use of *Rifinah* ® in older children, provided the respective dose of each drug is appropriate for the weight of the child (consult local protocol).
DOSE EQUIVALENCE AND CONVERSION
Rifinah ® Tablets contain rifampicin and isoniazid; the proportions are expressed in the form x/y where x and y are the strengths in milligrams of rifampicin and isoniazid respectively.
Each *Rifinah* ® 150/100 Tablet contains rifampicin 150 mg and isoniazid 100 mg.
Each *Rifinah* ® 300/150 Tablet contains rifampicin 300 mg and isoniazid 150 mg.

● **UNLICENSED USE** Not licensed for use in children.

● **PATIENT AND CARER ADVICE**
Medicines for Children leaflet: Isoniazid and rifampicin combination for latent tuberculosis
www.medicinesforchildren.org.uk/
isoniazid-and-rifampicin-combination-latent-tuberculosis

● **MEDICINAL FORMS**
There can be variation in the licensing of different medicines containing the same drug.
Tablet
CAUTIONARY AND ADVISORY LABELS 8, 14, 23
▶ Rifinah (Sanofi)
Isoniazid 100 mg, Rifampicin 150 mg Rifinah 150mg/100mg tablets | 84 tablet PoM £19.09
Isoniazid 150 mg, Rifampicin 300 mg Rifinah 300mg/150mg tablets | 56 tablet PoM £25.22

Rifampicin with isoniazid and pyrazinamide

The properties listed below are those particular to the combination only. For the properties of the components please consider, rifampicin p. 342, isoniazid p. 345, pyrazinamide p. 346.

● **INDICATIONS AND DOSE**
Initial treatment of tuberculosis (in combination with ethambutol)
▶ Child: Although not licensed in children, consideration may be given to use of *Rifater* ® in older children, provided the respective dose of each drug is appropriate for the weight of the child (consult local protocol).
DOSE EQUIVALENCE AND CONVERSION
Tablet quantities refer to the number of *Rifater* ® Tablets which should be taken. Each *Rifater* ® Tablet contains isoniazid 50 mg, pyrazinamide 300 mg and rifampicin 120 mg.

● **UNLICENSED USE** Not licensed for use in children.

● **MEDICINAL FORMS**
There can be variation in the licensing of different medicines containing the same drug.
Tablet
CAUTIONARY AND ADVISORY LABELS 8, 14, 22
▶ Rifater (Sanofi)
Isoniazid 50 mg, Rifampicin 120 mg, Pyrazinamide 300 mg Rifater tablets | 100 tablet PoM £26.34

ANTIMYCOBACTERIALS 〉 OTHER

Cycloserine

● **INDICATIONS AND DOSE**
Tuberculosis resistant to first-line drugs, in combination with other drugs
▶ BY MOUTH
▶ Child 2–11 years: Initially 5 mg/kg twice daily (max. per dose 250 mg), then increased if necessary up to 10 mg/kg twice daily (max. per dose 500 mg), dose to be increased according to blood concentration and response
▶ Child 12–17 years: Initially 250 mg every 12 hours for 2 weeks, then increased if necessary up to 500 mg every 12 hours, dose to be increased according to blood concentration and response
PHARMACOKINETICS
Cycloserine penetrates the CNS.

● **UNLICENSED USE** Licensed for use in children (age range not specified by manufacturer).

● **CONTRA-INDICATIONS** Alcohol dependence · depression · epilepsy · psychotic states · severe anxiety

● **INTERACTIONS** → Appendix 1 (cycloserine).

● **SIDE-EFFECTS** Allergic dermatitis · changes in liver function tests · confusion · convulsions · depression · dizziness · drowsiness · headache · heart failure at high doses · megaloblastic anaemia · psychosis · rashes · tremor · vertigo
SIDE-EFFECTS, FURTHER INFORMATION
▶ CNS toxicity Discontinue or reduce dose if symptoms of CNS toxicity occur.
▶ Rashes or allergic dermatitis Discontinue or reduce dose if rashes or allergic dermatitis develops.

● **PREGNANCY** Manufacturer advises use only if potential benefit outweighs risk—crosses the placenta.

● **BREAST FEEDING** Present in milk—amount too small to be harmful.

● **RENAL IMPAIRMENT** Increase interval between doses if creatinine clearance less than 50 mL/minute/1.73 m². Monitor blood-cycloserine concentration if creatinine clearance less than 50 mL/minute/1.73 m².

● **MONITORING REQUIREMENTS**
▶ Blood concentration should not exceed a peak concentration of 30 mg/litre (measured 3–4 hours after the dose).
▶ Monitor haematological, renal, and hepatic function.

● **MEDICINAL FORMS**
There can be variation in the licensing of different medicines containing the same drug.
Capsule
CAUTIONARY AND ADVISORY LABELS 2, 8
▶ Cycloserine (Non-proprietary)
Cycloserine 250 mg Cycloserine 250mg capsules | 100 capsule PoM £402.63 DT price = £402.63

Ethambutol hydrochloride

- **INDICATIONS AND DOSE**

Tuberculosis, in combination with other drugs (standard unsupervised 6-month treatment)
▶ BY MOUTH
  ▶ Child: 20 mg/kg once daily for 2 months (initial phase)

Tuberculosis, in combination with other drugs (intermittent supervised 6-month treatment) (under expert supervision)
▶ BY MOUTH
  ▶ Child: 30 mg/kg 3 times a week for 2 months (initial phase)

Congenital tuberculosis, in combination with other drugs
▶ BY MOUTH
  ▶ Neonate: 20 mg/kg once daily for 2 months (initial phase).

- **CONTRA-INDICATIONS** Optic neuritis · poor vision
- **CAUTIONS** Young children

  CAUTIONS, FURTHER INFORMATION
▶ Understanding warnings Patients who cannot understand warnings about visual side-effects should, if possible, be given an alternative drug. In particular, ethambutol should be used with caution in children until they are at least 5 years old and capable of reporting symptomatic visual changes accurately.

- **INTERACTIONS** → Appendix 1 (ethambutol).
- **SIDE-EFFECTS**
▶ **Rare** Pruritus · rash · thrombocytopenia · urticaria
▶ **Frequency not known** Colour blindness · loss of visual acuity · optic neuritis · peripheral neuritis · red/green colour blindness · restriction of visual fields · visual disturbances

  SIDE-EFFECTS, FURTHER INFORMATION
▶ Ocular toxicity Ocular toxicity is more common where excessive dosage is used or if the patient's renal function is impaired. Early discontinuation of the drug is almost always followed by recovery of eyesight.

- **PREGNANCY** Not known to be harmful.
- **BREAST FEEDING** Amount too small to be harmful.
- **RENAL IMPAIRMENT** If creatinine clearance less than 30 mL/minute/1.73 m², use 15–25 mg/kg (max. 2.5 g) 3 times a week. Risk of optic nerve damage. Should preferably be avoided in patients with renal impairment. If creatinine clearance less than 30 mL/minute/1.73 m², monitor plasma-ethambutol concentration.
- **MONITORING REQUIREMENTS**
▶ 'Peak' concentration (2–2.5 hours after dose) should be 2–6 mg/litre (7–22 micromol/litre); 'trough' (pre-dose) concentration should be less than 1 mg/litre (4 micromol/litre).
▶ Renal function should be checked before treatment.
▶ Visual acuity should be tested by Snellen chart before treatment with ethambutol.
▶ In young children, routine ophthalmological monitoring recommended.
- **PATIENT AND CARER ADVICE**
  Medicines for Children leaflet: Ethambutol for the treatment of tuberculosis www.medicinesforchildren.org.uk/ethambutol-for-the-treatment-of-tuberculosis
  Ocular toxicity The earliest features of ocular toxicity are subjective and patients should be advised to discontinue therapy immediately if they develop deterioration in vision and promptly seek further advice.

- **MEDICINAL FORMS**
  There can be variation in the licensing of different medicines containing the same drug. Forms available from special-order manufacturers include: oral suspension, oral solution

  Tablet
  CAUTIONARY AND ADVISORY LABELS 8
  ▶ Ethambutol hydrochloride (Non-proprietary)
  Ethambutol hydrochloride 100 mg Ethambutol 100mg tablets | 56 tablet PoM £11.51 DT price = £11.51
  Ethambutol hydrochloride 400 mg Ethambutol 400mg tablets | 56 tablet PoM £42.74 DT price = £42.74

  Solution for infusion
  ▶ Ethambutol hydrochloride (Non-proprietary)
  Ethambutol hydrochloride 100 mg per 1 ml EMB-Fatol 1g/10ml concentrate for solution for infusion vials | 10 vial PoM no price available

Isoniazid

- **INDICATIONS AND DOSE**

Tuberculosis, in combination with other drugs (standard unsupervised 6-month treatment)
▶ BY MOUTH, OR BY INTRAMUSCULAR INJECTION, OR BY INTRAVENOUS INJECTION
  ▶ Child: 10 mg/kg once daily (max. per dose 300 mg) for 6 months (initial and continuation phases)

Tuberculosis, in combination with other drugs (intermittent supervised 6-month treatment) (under expert supervision)
▶ BY MOUTH, OR BY INTRAMUSCULAR INJECTION, OR BY INTRAVENOUS INJECTION
  ▶ Child: 15 mg/kg 3 times a week (max. per dose 900 mg) for 6 months (initial and continuation phases)

Congenital tuberculosis, in combination with other drugs
▶ BY MOUTH, OR BY INTRAMUSCULAR INJECTION, OR BY INTRAVENOUS INJECTION
  ▶ Neonate: 10 mg/kg daily for 6 months (initial and continuation phases).

Prevention of tuberculosis in susceptible close contacts or those who have become tuberculin positive
▶ BY MOUTH, OR BY INTRAMUSCULAR INJECTION, OR BY INTRAVENOUS INJECTION
  ▶ Neonate: 10 mg/kg daily for 6 months.
  ▶ Child 1 month–11 years: 10 mg/kg daily (max. per dose 300 mg) for 6 months, alternatively 10 mg/kg daily (max. per dose 300 mg) for 3 months, to be taken in combination with rifampicin
  ▶ Child 12–17 years: 300 mg daily for 6 months, alternatively 300 mg daily for 3 months, to be taken in combination with rifampicin

- **CONTRA-INDICATIONS** Drug-induced liver disease
- **CAUTIONS** Acute porphyrias p. 562 · alcohol dependence · diabetes mellitus · epilepsy · history of psychosis · HIV infection · malnutrition · slow acetylator status (increased risk of side-effects)

  CAUTIONS, FURTHER INFORMATION
▶ Peripheral neuropathy Peripheral neuropathy is more likely to occur where there are pre-existing risk factors such as diabetes, alcohol dependence, chronic renal failure, pregnancy, malnutrition and HIV infection. In patients at increased risk of peripheral neuropathy, pyridoxine hydrochloride p. 585 should be given prophylactically from the start of treatment.

- **INTERACTIONS** → Appendix 1 (isoniazid).
  When used with tyramine or histamine rich foods, tachycardia, palpitation, hypotension, flushing, headache, dizziness, and sweating reported.

- **SIDE-EFFECTS**
▶ **Common or very common** Peripheral neuropathy
▶ **Rare** Hepatitis · psychotic episodes
▶ **Frequency not known** Agranulocytosis · aplastic anaemia · blood disorders · constipation · convulsions · difficulty with micturition · dry mouth · fever · gynaecomastia · haemolytic anaemia · hearing loss (in patients with end-stage renal impairment) · hyperglycaemia · hyperreflexia · hypersensitivity reactions · interstitial pneumonitis · nausea · optic neuritis · pancreatitis · pellagra · peripheral neuritis with high doses · purpura · Stevens-Johnson syndrome · systemic lupus erythematosus-like syndrome · tinnitus (in patients with end-stage renal impairment) · vertigo · vomiting

- **PREGNANCY** Not known to be harmful; prophylactic pyridoxine recommended.

- **BREAST FEEDING** Theoretical risk of convulsions and neuropathy; prophylactic pyridoxine advisable in mother. In breast-feeding, monitor infant for possible toxicity.

- **HEPATIC IMPAIRMENT** Use with caution. In patients with pre-existing liver disease or hepatic impairment monitor liver function regularly and particularly frequently in the first 2 months.

- **RENAL IMPAIRMENT** Risk of ototoxicity and peripheral neuropathy; prophylactic pyridoxine hydrochloride p. 585 recommended.

- **MONITORING REQUIREMENTS**
▶ *Renal function* should be checked before treatment.
▶ *Hepatic function* should be checked before treatment. If there is no evidence of liver disease (and pre-treatment liver function is normal), further checks are only necessary if the patient develops fever, malaise, vomiting, jaundice or unexplained deterioration during treatment.

- **PRESCRIBING AND DISPENSING INFORMATION**
Doses may need to be recalculated to allow for weight gain in younger children.
▶ With oral use In general, doses should be rounded up to facilitate administration of suitable volumes of liquid or an appropriate strength of tablet.

- **PATIENT AND CARER ADVICE**
Medicines for Children leaflet: Isoniazid for latent tuberculosis www.medicinesforchildren.org.uk/isoniazid-for-latent-tuberculosis
Medicines for Children leaflet: Isoniazid for treatment of tuberculosis www.medicinesforchildren.org.uk/isoniazid-for-the-treatment-of-tuberculosis
Hepatic disorders Patients or their carers should be told how to recognise signs of liver disorder, and advised to discontinue treatment and seek immediate medical attention if symptoms such as persistent nausea, vomiting, malaise or jaundice develop.

- **MEDICINAL FORMS**
There can be variation in the licensing of different medicines containing the same drug. Forms available from special-order manufacturers include: oral suspension, oral solution

Tablet
CAUTIONARY AND ADVISORY LABELS 8, 22
▶ **Isoniazid (Non-proprietary)**
Isoniazid 50 mg Isoniazid 50mg tablets | 56 tablet [PoM] £19.24 DT price = £19.24
Isoniazid 100 mg Isoniazid 100mg tablets | 28 tablet [PoM] £19.24 DT price = £19.24
Isoniazid 300 mg Isoniazid 300mg tablets | 30 tablet [PoM] no price available

Solution for injection
▶ **Isoniazid (Non-proprietary)**
Isoniazid 20 mg per 1 ml Tebesium-S 100mg/5ml solution for injection ampoules | 12 ampoule [PoM] no price available
Isoniazid 25 mg per 1 ml Isoniazid 50mg/2ml solution for injection ampoules | 10 ampoule [PoM] £299.16

Combinations available: *Rifampicin with isoniazid*, p. 344 · *Rifampicin with isoniazid and pyrazinamide*, p. 344

Pyrazinamide

- **INDICATIONS AND DOSE**

Tuberculosis, in combination with other drugs (standard unsupervised 6-month treatment)
▶ BY MOUTH
▷ Child (body-weight up to 50 kg): 35 mg/kg once daily for 2 months (initial phase); maximum 1.5 g per day
▷ Child (body-weight 50 kg and above): 35 mg/kg once daily for 2 months (initial phase); maximum 2 g per day

Tuberculosis, in combination with other drugs (intermittent supervised 6-month treatment) (under expert supervision)
▶ BY MOUTH
▷ Child (body-weight up to 50 kg): 50 mg/kg 3 times a week (max. per dose 2 g 3 times a week) for 2 months (initial phase)
▷ Child (body-weight 50 kg and above): 50 mg/kg 3 times a week (max. per dose 2.5 g 3 times a week) for 2 months (initial phase)

Congenital tuberculosis, in combination with other drugs
▶ BY MOUTH
▷ Neonate: 35 mg/kg once daily for 2 months (initial phase).

- **CAUTIONS** Diabetes
- **INTERACTIONS** → Appendix 1 (pyrazinamide).
- **SIDE-EFFECTS** Anorexia · arthralgia · dysuria · fever · hepatomegaly · hepatotoxicity · jaundice · liver failure · nausea · photosensitivity · rash · sideroblastic anaemia · splenomegaly · thrombocytopenia · vomiting
- **PREGNANCY** Manufacturer advises use only if potential benefit outweighs risk.
- **BREAST FEEDING** Amount too small to be harmful.
- **HEPATIC IMPAIRMENT** Idiosyncratic hepatotoxicity more common; avoid in severe hepatic impairment. In patients with pre-existing liver disease or hepatic impairment monitor liver function regularly and particularly frequently in the first 2 months.
- **RENAL IMPAIRMENT** If estimated glomerular filtration rate less than 30 mL/minute/1.73 m^2, use 25–30 mg/kg 3 times a week.
- **MONITORING REQUIREMENTS**
▶ *Renal function* should be checked before treatment.
▶ *Hepatic function* should be checked before treatment. If there is no evidence of liver disease (and pre-treatment liver function is normal), further checks are only necessary if the patient develops fever, malaise, vomiting, jaundice or unexplained deterioration during treatment.
- **PRESCRIBING AND DISPENSING INFORMATION** In general, doses should be rounded up to facilitate administration of suitable volumes of liquid or an appropriate strength of tablet. Doses may also need to be recalculated to allow for weight gain in younger children.
- **PATIENT AND CARER ADVICE**
Medicines for Children leaflet: Pyrazinamide for treatment of tuberculosis www.medicinesforchildren.org.uk/pyrazinamide-for-tuberculosis
Hepatic disorders Patients or their carers should be told how to recognise signs of liver disorder, and advised to discontinue treatment and seek immediate medical attention if symptoms such as persistent nausea, vomiting, malaise or jaundice develop.

● MEDICINAL FORMS

There can be variation in the licensing of different medicines containing the same drug. Forms available from special-order manufacturers include: oral suspension, oral solution

Tablet

CAUTIONARY AND ADVISORY LABELS 8

▸ Pyrazinamide (Non-proprietary)

Pyrazinamide 500 mg Pyrazinamide 500mg tablets |
30 tablet ꞎPoMꞏ £31.35–£38.34 | 50 tablet ꞎPoMꞏ £52.25

▸ Zinamide (Thornton & Ross Ltd)

Pyrazinamide 500 mg Zinamide 500mg tablets | 30 tablet ꞎPoMꞏ
£31.35

Combinations available: **Rifampicin with isoniazid and pyrazinamide**, p. 344

2.5 Urinary tract infections

Urinary-tract infections

Overview

Urinary-tract infection is more common in adolescent girls than in boys; when it occurs in adolescent boys there is frequently an underlying abnormality of the renal tract. Recurrent episodes of infection are an indication for radiological investigation especially in children in whom untreated pyelonephritis may lead to permanent kidney damage.

Escherichia coli is the most common cause of urinary-tract infection; *Staphylococcus saprophyticus* is also common in sexually active young women. Less common causes include *Proteus* and *Klebsiella* spp. *Pseudomonas aeruginosa* infections usually occur in the hospital setting and may be associated with functional or anatomical abnormalities of the renal tract. *Staphylococcus epidermidis* and *Enterococcus faecalis* infection may complicate catheterisation or instrumentation.

A specimen of urine should be collected for culture and sensitivity testing before starting antibacterial therapy;

- in children under 3 years of age;
- in children with suspected upper urinary-tract infection, complicated infection, or recurrent infection;
- if resistant organisms are suspected;
- if urine dipstick testing gives a single positive result for leucocyte esterase or nitrite;
- if clinical symptoms are not consistent with results of dipstick testing;
- in pregnant women.

Treatment should not be delayed while waiting for results. The antibacterial chosen should reflect current local bacterial sensitivity to antibacterials.

Antibacterial therapy for urinary-tract infections

Urinary-tract infections in children require prompt antibacterial treatment to minimise the risk of renal scarring.

Children under 3 months of age should be transferred to hospital and treated initially with intravenous antibacterials such as amoxicillin p. 320 (*or* ampicillin p. 321) with gentamicin p. 293, or a cephalosporin (such as cefotaxime p. 301) alone, until the infection responds; full doses of oral antibacterials are then given for a further period.

Children over 3 months of age with uncomplicated lower urinary-tract infection, can be treated with trimethoprim p. 338 or nitrofurantoin below. *Suggested duration of treatment* 3 days. Re-assess child if they remain unwell 24–48 hours after initial assessment.

Alternatively, *children over 3 months of age, with uncomplicated lower urinary-tract infection*, may be treated with amoxicillin (*or* ampicillin) *or* oral first generation cephalosporin (e.g. cefalexin p. 298). Use amoxicillin only if

micro-organism sensitive. *Suggested duration of treatment* 3 days. Re-assess child if unwell 24–48 hours after initial assessment.

Acute pyelonephritis in children over 3 months of age can be treated with a first generation cephalosporin or co-amoxiclav p. 323 for 7–10 days.

If the patient is severely ill, then the infection is best treated initially by intravenous injection of a broad-spectrum antibacterial such as cefotaxime or co-amoxiclav; gentamicin is an alternative.

Resistant infections

Widespread bacterial resistance to ampicillin, amoxicillin, and trimethoprim has been reported. Alternatives for resistant organisms include co-amoxiclav (amoxicillin with clavulanic acid), an oral cephalosporin, pivmecillinam hydrochloride p. 324, or a quinolone.

Antibacterial prophylaxis

Recurrent episodes of infection are an indication for imaging tests. *Antibacterial prophylaxis* with low doses of trimethoprim or nitrofurantoin may be considered for children with recurrent infection, significant urinary-tract anomalies, or significant kidney damage. Nitrofurantoin is contra-indicated in children under 3 months of age because of the theoretical possibility of haemolytic anaemia.

Pregnancy

Urinary-tract infection in *pregnancy* may be asymptomatic and requires prompt treatment to prevent progression to acute pyelonephritis. Penicillins and cephalosporins are suitable for treating urinary-tract infection during pregnancy. Nitrofurantoin may also be used but it should be avoided at term. Sulfonamides, quinolones, and tetracyclines should be avoided during pregnancy; trimethoprim should also preferably be avoided particularly in the first trimester.

Renal impairment

In *renal failure* antibacterials normally excreted by the kidney accumulate with resultant toxicity unless the dose is reduced. This applies especially to the aminoglycosides which should be used with great caution; tetracyclines, methenamine hippurate, and nitrofurantoin should be avoided altogether.

ANTIBACTERIALS ⟩ OTHER

Nitrofurantoin

● INDICATIONS AND DOSE

Acute uncomplicated urinary-tract infections

▸ BY MOUTH USING IMMEDIATE-RELEASE MEDICINES

▸ Child 3 months–11 years: 750 micrograms/kg 4 times a day for 3–7 days

▸ Child 12–17 years: 50 mg 4 times a day for 3–7 days

▸ BY MOUTH USING MODIFIED-RELEASE MEDICINES

▸ Child 12–17 years: 100 mg twice daily, dose to be taken with food

Severe chronic recurrent urinary-tract infections

▸ BY MOUTH USING IMMEDIATE-RELEASE MEDICINES

▸ Child 12–17 years: 100 mg 4 times a day for 3–7 days

Prophylaxis of urinary-tract infection (considered for recurrent infection, significant urinary-tract anomalies, or significant kidney damage)

▸ BY MOUTH USING IMMEDIATE-RELEASE MEDICINES

▸ Child 3 months–11 years: 1 mg/kg once daily, dose to be taken at night

▸ Child 12–17 years: 50–100 mg once daily, dose to be taken at night continued →

Genito-urinary surgical prophylaxis
▶ BY MOUTH USING MODIFIED-RELEASE MEDICINES
▶ Child 12-17 years: 100 mg twice daily on day of procedure and for 3 days after

● CONTRA-INDICATIONS Acute porphyrias p. 562 · G6PD deficiency · infants less than 3 months old
● CAUTIONS Anaemia · diabetes mellitus · electrolyte imbalance · folate deficiency · pulmonary disease · susceptibility to peripheral neuropathy · urine may be coloured yellow or brown · vitamin B deficiency
● INTERACTIONS → Appendix 1 (nitrofurantoin).
● SIDE-EFFECTS
▶ Rare Agranulocytosis · aplastic anaemia · arthralgia · benign intracranial hypertension · blood disorders · cholestatic jaundice · erythema multiforme · exfoliative dermatitis · hepatitis · pancreatitis · thrombocytopenia · transient alopecia
▶ Frequency not known Acute pulmonary reactions · anaphylaxis · angioedema · anorexia · chronic pulmonary reactions (pulmonary fibrosis reported) · possible association with lupus erythematosus-like syndrome) · diarrhoea · hypersensitivity reactions · nausea · peripheral neuropathy · pruritus · rash · sialadenitis · urticaria · vomiting
● PREGNANCY Avoid at term—may produce neonatal haemolysis.
● BREAST FEEDING Avoid; only small amounts in milk but enough to produce haemolysis in G6PD-deficient infants.
● HEPATIC IMPAIRMENT Use with caution; cholestatic jaundice and chronic active hepatitis reported.
● RENAL IMPAIRMENT Risk of peripheral neuropathy; antibacterial efficacy depends on renal secretion of the drug into urinary tract. Avoid if estimated glomerular filtration rate less than 45 mL/minute/1.73 m^2; may be used with caution if estimated glomerular filtration rate 30–44 mL/minute/1.73 m^2 as a short-course only (3 to 7 days), to treat uncomplicated lower urinary-tract infection caused by suspected or proven multidrug resistant bacteria and only if potential benefit outweighs risk.
● MONITORING REQUIREMENTS On long-term therapy, monitor liver function and monitor for pulmonary symptoms (discontinue if deterioration in lung function).
● EFFECT ON LABORATORY TESTS False positive urinary glucose (if tested for reducing substances).
● PATIENT AND CARER ADVICE Medicines for Children leaflet: Nitrofurantoin for urinary tract infections www.medicinesforchildren.org.uk/nitrofurantoin-for-urinary-tract-infections
● MEDICINAL FORMS There can be variation in the licensing of different medicines containing the same drug. Forms available from special-order manufacturers include: oral suspension, oral solution

Tablet
CAUTIONARY AND ADVISORY LABELS 9, 14, 21
▶ Nitrofurantoin (Non-proprietary)
Nitrofurantoin 50 mg Nitrofurantoin 50mg tablets | 28 tablet PoM £35.00 DT price = £7.42 | 100 tablet PoM £111.89
Nitrofurantoin 100 mg Nitrofurantoin 100mg tablets | 28 tablet PoM £13.28 DT price = £2.60 | 100 tablet PoM £45.00
▶ Genfura (Genesis Pharmaceuticals Ltd)
Nitrofurantoin 50 mg Genfura 50mg tablets | 28 tablet PoM £14.40 DT price = £7.42
Nitrofurantoin 100 mg Genfura 100mg tablets | 28 tablet PoM £10.62 DT price = £2.60 | 100 tablet PoM £37.92

Capsule
CAUTIONARY AND ADVISORY LABELS 9, 14, 21
▶ Nitrofurantoin (Non-proprietary)
Nitrofurantoin 50 mg Nitrofurantoin 50mg capsules | 30 capsule PoM £15.42 DT price = £15.42

Nitrofurantoin 100 mg Nitrofurantoin 100mg capsules | 30 capsule PoM £10.42 DT price = £10.42

Modified-release capsule
CAUTIONARY AND ADVISORY LABELS 9, 14, 21, 25
▶ Macrobid (AMCo)
Nitrofurantoin 100 mg Macrobid 100mg modified-release capsules | 14 capsule PoM £9.50 DT price = £9.50

Oral suspension
CAUTIONARY AND ADVISORY LABELS 9, 14, 21
▶ Nitrofurantoin (Non-proprietary)
Nitrofurantoin 5 mg per 1 ml Nitrofurantoin 25mg/5ml oral suspension sugar free sugar-free | 300 ml PoM £446.95 DT price = £446.95

3   Fungal infection

Antifungals, systemic use

Common fungal infections

The systemic treatment of common fungal infections is outlined below; specialist treatment is required in most forms of systemic or disseminated fungal infections. Local treatment is suitable for a number of fungal infections (genital, bladder, eye, ear, oropharynx, and skin).

Aspergillosis

Aspergillosis most commonly affects the respiratory tract but in severely immunocompromised patients, invasive forms can affect the heart, brain, and skin. Voriconazole p. 355 is the treatment of choice for aspergillosis; liposomal amphotericin p. 351 is an alternative first-line treatment when voriconazole cannot be used. Caspofungin p. 350 or itraconazole p. 353 can be used in patients who are refractory to, or intolerant of voriconazole and liposomal amphotericin. Itraconazole is also used for the treatment of chronic pulmonary aspergillosis or as an adjunct in the treatment of allergic bronchopulmonary aspergillosis [unlicensed indication].

Candidiasis

Many superficial candidal infections, including infections of the skin, are treated locally. Systemic antifungal treatment is required in widespread or intractable infection. Vaginal candidiasis can be treated with locally acting antifungals; alternatively, fluconazole p. 352 can be given by mouth.

Oropharyngeal candidiasis generally responds to topical therapy. Fluconazole is given by mouth for unresponsive infections; it is reliably absorbed and is effective. Itraconazole may be used for infections that do not respond to fluconazole. Topical therapy may not be adequate in immunocompromised children and an oral triazole antifungal is preferred.

For *invasive or disseminated candidiasis*, either amphotericin by intravenous infusion or an **echinocandin** can be used. Fluconazole is an alternative for *Candida albicans* infection in clinically stable children who have not received an azole antifungal recently. Amphotericin should be considered for the initial treatment of CNS candidiasis. Voriconazole can be used for infections caused by fluconazole-resistant *Candida* spp. when oral therapy is required, or in children intolerant of amphotericin or an echinocandin. In refractory cases, flucytosine p. 356 can be used with intravenous amphotericin.

Cryptococcosis

Cryptococcosis is uncommon but infection in the immunocompromised, especially in HIV-positive patients, can be life-threatening; cryptococcal meningitis is the most common form of fungal meningitis. The treatment of choice in cryptococcal meningitis is amphotericin by intravenous infusion and flucytosine by intravenous infusion for 2 weeks, followed by fluconazole by mouth for 8 weeks or until cultures are negative. In cryptococcosis, fluconazole is sometimes given alone as an alternative in HIV-positive patients with mild, localised infections or in those who cannot tolerate amphotericin. Following successful treatment, fluconazole can be used for prophylaxis against relapse until immunity recovers.

Histoplasmosis

Histoplasmosis is rare in temperate climates; it can be life-threatening, particularly in HIV-infected persons. Itraconazole can be used for the treatment of immunocompetent patients with indolent non-meningeal infection, including chronic pulmonary histoplasmosis. Amphotericin by intravenous infusion is used for the initial treatment of fulminant or severe infections, followed by a course of itraconazole by mouth. Following successful treatment, itraconazole can be used for prophylaxis against relapse until immunity recovers.

Skin and nail infections

Mild localised fungal infections of the skin (including tinea corporis, tinea cruris, and tinea pedis) respond to topical therapy. Systemic therapy is appropriate if topical therapy fails, if many areas are affected, or if the site of infection is difficult to treat such as in infections of the nails (onychomycosis) and of the scalp (tinea capitis).

Oral imidazole or triazole antifungals (particularly itraconazole) and terbinafine p. 680 are used more frequently than griseofulvin p. 357 because they have a broader spectrum of activity and require a shorter duration of treatment.

Tinea capitis is treated systemically; additional topical application of an antifungal may reduce transmission. Griseofulvin is used for tinea capitis in adults and children; it is effective against infections caused by *Trichophyton tonsurans* and *Microsporum* spp. Terbinafine is used for tinea capitis caused by *T. tonsurans* [unlicensed indication]. The role of terbinafine in the management of *Microsporum* infections is uncertain. Fluconazole or itraconazole are alternatives in the treatment of tinea capitis caused by *T. tonsurans* or *Microsporum* spp. [both unlicensed indications].

Pityriasis versicolor may be treated with itraconazole by mouth if topical therapy is ineffective; fluconazole by mouth is an alternative. Oral terbinafine is **not** effective for pityriasis versicolor.

Antifungal treatment may not be necessary in asymptomatic patients with tinea infection of the nails. If treatment is necessary, a systemic antifungal is more effective than topical therapy. Terbinafine and itraconazole have largely replaced griseofulvin for the systemic treatment of *onychomycosis*, particularly of the toenail; they should be used under specialist advice in children. Although terbinafine is not licensed for use in children, it is considered to be the drug of choice for onychomycosis. Itraconazole can be administered as intermittent 'pulse' therapy. Topical antifungals also have a role in the treatment of onychomycosis.

Immunocompromised children

Immunocompromised children are at particular risk of fungal infections and may receive antifungal drugs prophylactically; oral triazole antifungals are the drugs of choice for prophylaxis. Fluconazole is more reliably absorbed than itraconazole, but fluconazole is not effective against *Aspergillus* spp. Itraconazole is preferred in patients at risk of invasive aspergillosis. Micafungin p. 350 can be used for prophylaxis of candidiasis in patients undergoing haematopoietic stem cell transplantation when fluconazole or itraconazole cannot be used.

Amphotericin by intravenous infusion or caspofungin is used for the empirical *treatment* of serious fungal infections in immunocompromised children; caspofungin is not effective against fungal infections of the CNS.

Triazole antifungals

Triazole antifungal drugs have a role in the prevention and systemic treatment of fungal infections.

Fluconazole is very well absorbed after oral administration. It also achieves good penetration into the cerebrospinal fluid to treat fungal meningitis. Fluconazole is excreted largely unchanged in the urine and can be used to treat candiduria.

Itraconazole is active against a wide range of dermatophytes. There is limited information available on use in children. Itraconazole capsules require an acid environment in the stomach for optimal absorption. Itraconazole has been associated with liver damage and should be avoided or used with caution in patients with liver disease; fluconazole is less frequently associated with hepatotoxicity.

Voriconazole is a broad-spectrum antifungal drug which is licensed in adults for use in life-threatening infections.

Imidazole antifungals

The imidazole antifungals include clotrimazole p. 481, p. 678, econazole nitrate p. 481, p. 678, ketoconazole p. 414, p. 678, and tioconazole p. 679. They are used for the local treatment of vaginal candidiasis and for dermatophyte infections. Miconazole p. 663 can be used locally for oral infections; it is also effective in intestinal infections. Systemic absorption may follow use of miconazole oral gel and may result in significant drug interactions.

Polyene antifungals

The polyene antifungals include amphotericin and nystatin p. 663; neither drug is absorbed when given by mouth. Nystatin p. 663 is used for oral, oropharyngeal, and perioral infections by local application in the mouth. Nystatin is also used for *Candida albicans* infection of the skin.

Amphotericin p. 351 by intravenous infusion is used for the treatment of systemic fungal infections and is active against most fungi and yeasts. It is highly protein bound and penetrates poorly into body fluids and tissues. When given parenterally amphotericin is toxic and side-effects are common. Lipid formulations of amphotericin (*Abelcet*® and *AmBisome*®) are significantly less toxic and are recommended when the conventional formulation of amphotericin is contra-indicated because of toxicity, especially nephrotoxicity or when response to conventional amphotericin is inadequate; lipid formulations are more expensive.

Echinocandin antifungals

The echinocandin antifungals include caspofungin p. 350 and micafungin p. 350. They are only active against *Aspergillus* spp. and *Candida* spp.; however, micafungin is not used for the treatment of aspergillosis. Echinocandins are not effective against fungal infections of the CNS. Echinocandin antifungals have a role in the prevention and systemic treatment of fungal infections.

Other antifungals

Flucytosine p. 356 is used with amphotericin in a synergistic combination. Bone marrow depression can occur which limits its use, particularly in HIV-positive patients; weekly blood counts are necessary during prolonged therapy. Resistance to flucytosine can develop during therapy and sensitivity testing is essential before and during treatment. Flucytosine has a role in the treatment of systemic candidiasis and cryptococcal meningitis.

Griseofulvin p. 357 is effective for widespread or intractable dermatophyte infections but has been superseded by newer antifungals, particularly for nail infections. Griseofulvin is used in the treatment of tinea capitis. It is the drug of choice for trichophyton infections in

5

Infection

children. Duration of therapy is dependent on the site of the infection and may extend to a number of months.

Terbinafine p. 680 is the drug of choice for fungal nail infections and is also used for ringworm infections where oral treatment is considered appropriate.

ANTIFUNGALS > ECHINOCANDIN ANTIFUNGALS

Caspofungin

- **INDICATIONS AND DOSE**

Invasive aspergillosis | Invasive candidiasis | Empirical treatment of systemic fungal infections in patients with neutropenia
  - ► BY INTRAVENOUS INFUSION
  - ► Neonate: 25 mg/m^2 once daily.
  - ► Child 1–2 months: 25 mg/m^2 once daily
  - ► Child 3–11 months: 50 mg/m^2 once daily
  - ► Child 1–17 years: 70 mg/m^2 once daily (max. per dose 70 mg) for 1 day, then 50 mg/m^2 once daily (max. per dose 70 mg); increased to 70 mg/m^2 once daily (max. per dose 70 mg), dose may be increased if lower dose tolerated but inadequate response

- **INTERACTIONS** → Appendix 1 (caspofungin).
- **SIDE-EFFECTS**
  - ► **Common or very common** Arthralgia · diarrhoea · dyspnoea · flushing · headache · hypokalaemia · hypomagnesaemia · hypotension · injection-site reactions · nausea · pruritus · rash · sweating · tachycardia · vomiting
  - ► **Uncommon** Abdominal pain · anaemia · anorexia · anxiety · arrhythmia · ascites · blurred vision · bronchospasm · chest pain · cholestasis · constipation · cough · disorientation · dizziness · dry mouth · dyspepsia · dysphagia · erythema multiforme · fatigue · flatulence · heart failure · hepatic dysfunction · hyperglycaemia · hypertension · hypoaesthesia · hypocalcaemia · leucopenia · metabolic acidosis · muscular weakness · myalgia · palpitation · paraesthesia · renal failure · sleep disturbances · taste disturbances · thrombocytopenia · thrombophlebitis · tremor
  - ► **Frequency not known** Acute respiratory distress syndrome · anaphylaxis · hypercalcaemia
- **PREGNANCY** Manufacturer advises avoid unless essential—toxicity in *animal* studies.
- **BREAST FEEDING** Present in milk in *animal* studies—manufacturer advises avoid.
- **HEPATIC IMPAIRMENT** Usual initial dose, then use 70% of normal maintenance dose in moderate impairment. No information available for severe impairment.
- **DIRECTIONS FOR ADMINISTRATION** For *intravenous infusion* (*Candidas*®), allow vial to reach room temperature; initially reconstitute 50 mg with 10.5 mL Water for Injections to produce a 5.2 mg/mL solution, or reconstitute 70 mg with 10.5 mL Water for Injections to produce a 7.2 mg/mL solution; mix gently to dissolve; dilute requisite dose to a final concentration not exceeding 500 micrograms/mL with Sodium Chloride 0.9%; give over 60 minutes; incompatible with glucose solutions.

- **MEDICINAL FORMS**
  There can be variation in the licensing of different medicines containing the same drug.

  Powder for solution for infusion
  - ► Cancidas (Merck Sharp & Dohme Ltd)
    Caspofungin (as Caspofungin acetate) 50 mg Cancidas 50mg powder for solution for infusion vials | 1 vial [PoM] £327.67
    Caspofungin (as Caspofungin acetate) 70 mg Cancidas 70mg powder for solution for infusion vials | 1 vial [PoM] £416.78

Micafungin

- **INDICATIONS AND DOSE**

Invasive candidiasis
  - ► BY INTRAVENOUS INFUSION
  - ► Neonate (administered on expert advice): 2 mg/kg once daily for at least 14 days; increased if necessary to 4 mg/kg once daily, increase dose if response inadequate.
  - ► Child (body-weight up to 40 kg): 2 mg/kg once daily for at least 14 days; increased if necessary to 4 mg/kg once daily, increase dose if response inadequate
  - ► Child (body-weight 40 kg and above): 100 mg once daily for at least 14 days; increased if necessary to 200 mg once daily, increase dose if response inadequate

Oesophageal candidiasis
  - ► BY INTRAVENOUS INFUSION
  - ► Child 16–17 years (body-weight up to 40 kg): 3 mg/kg once daily
  - ► Child 16–17 years (body-weight 40 kg and above): 150 mg once daily

Prophylaxis of candidiasis in patients undergoing bone-marrow transplantation or who are expected to become neutropenic for over 10 days
  - ► BY INTRAVENOUS INFUSION
  - ► Neonate: 1 mg/kg once daily continue for at least 7 days after neutrophil count is in desirable range.
  - ► Child (body-weight up to 40 kg): 1 mg/kg once daily continue for at least 7 days after neutrophil count is in desirable range
  - ► Child (body-weight 40 kg and above): 50 mg once daily continue for at least 7 days after neutrophil count is in desirable range

- **INTERACTIONS** → Appendix 1 (micafungin).
  Caution with concomitant use of other hepatotoxic drugs.
- **SIDE-EFFECTS**
  - ► **Common or very common** Abdominal pain · anaemia · blood pressure changes · diarrhoea · fever · headache · hepatomegaly · hypocalcaemia · hypokalaemia · hypomagnesaemia · leucopenia · nausea · phlebitis · rash · renal failure · tachycardia · thrombocytopenia · vomiting
  - ► **Uncommon** Anorexia · anxiety · bradycardia · cholestasis · confusion · constipation · dizziness · dyspepsia · dyspnoea · eosinophilia · flushing · hepatitis · hyperhidrosis · hyperkalaemia · hyponatraemia · hypophosphataemia · palpitation · pancytopenia · pruritus · sleep disturbances · tachycardia · taste disturbances · tremor
  - ► **Rare** Haemolytic anaemia
  - ► **Frequency not known** Disseminated intravascular coagulation · hepatotoxicity (potentially life-threatening; more common in children under 1 year) · Stevens-Johnson syndrome · toxic epidermal necrolysis
- **PREGNANCY** Manufacturer advises avoid unless essential—toxicity in *animal* studies.
- **BREAST FEEDING** Manufacturer advises use only if potential benefit outweighs risk—present in milk in *animal* studies.
- **HEPATIC IMPAIRMENT** Use with caution in mild to moderate impairment. Avoid in severe impairment.
- **RENAL IMPAIRMENT** Use with caution; renal function may deteriorate.
- **MONITORING REQUIREMENTS**
  - ► Monitor renal function.
  - ► Monitor liver function—discontinue if significant and persistent abnormalities in liver function tests develop.
- **DIRECTIONS FOR ADMINISTRATION** For *intravenous infusion* reconstitute each vial with 5 mL Glucose 5% *or* Sodium Chloride 0.9%; gently rotate vial, without shaking, to

dissolve; dilute requisite dose to a concentration of 0.5–2 mg/mL with Glucose 5% *or* Sodium Chloride 0.9%; protect infusion from light; give over 60 minutes.

● MEDICINAL FORMS
There can be variation in the licensing of different medicines containing the same drug.
Powder for solution for infusion
▸ Mycamine (Astellas Pharma Ltd)
Micafungin (as Micafungin sodium) 50 mg Mycamine 50mg powder for solution for infusion vials | 1 vial PoM £196.08
Micafungin (as Micafungin sodium) 100 mg Mycamine 100mg powder for solution for infusion vials | 1 vial PoM £341.00

ANTIFUNGALS ⟩ POLYENE ANTIFUNGALS

Amphotericin

(Amphotericin B)

● INDICATIONS AND DOSE
ABELCET®

Severe invasive candidiasis | Severe systemic fungal infections in patients not responding to conventional amphotericin or to other antifungal drugs or where toxicity or renal impairment precludes conventional amphotericin, including invasive aspergillosis, cryptococcal meningitis and disseminated cryptococcosis in HIV patients
▸ BY INTRAVENOUS INFUSION
▸ Child: Test dose 100 micrograms/kg (max. per dose 1 mg), then 5 mg/kg once daily

AMBISOME®

Severe systemic or deep mycoses where toxicity (particularly nephrotoxicity) precludes use of conventional amphotericin | Suspected or proven infection in febrile neutropenic patients unresponsive to broad-spectrum antibacterials
▸ BY INTRAVENOUS INFUSION
▸ Neonate: 1 mg/kg once daily, increased if necessary to 3 mg/kg once daily; maximum 5 mg/kg per day.
▸ Child: Test dose 100 micrograms/kg (max. per dose 1 mg), to be given over 10 minutes, then 3 mg/kg once daily; maximum 5 mg/kg per day

Visceral leishmaniasis (unresponsive to the antimonial alone)
▸ BY INTRAVENOUS INFUSION
▸ Child: 1–3 mg/kg daily for 10–21 days to a cumulative dose of 21–30 mg/kg, alternatively 3 mg/kg for 5 consecutive days, followed by 3 mg/kg after 6 days for 1 dose

FUNGIZONE®

Systemic fungal infections
▸ BY INTRAVENOUS INFUSION
▸ Neonate: 1 mg/kg once daily, increased if necessary to 1.5 mg/kg daily for 7 days, then reduced to 1–1.5 mg/kg once daily on alternate days if required.
▸ Child: Test dose 100 micrograms/kg (max. per dose 1 mg), included as part of first dose of 250 micrograms/kg daily, then increased if tolerated to 1 mg/kg daily, dose is gradually increased over 2–4 days; in severe infection max. 1.5 mg/kg daily or on alternate days. Prolonged treatment usually necessary; if interrupted for longer than 7 days recommence at 250 micrograms/kg daily and increase gradually

● UNLICENSED USE
AMBISOME® *Ambisome*® not licensed for use in children under 1 month.

FUNGIZONE® Intravenous conventional formulation amphotericin (*Fungizone*®) is licensed for use in children (age range not specified by manufacturer).

● CAUTIONS Avoid rapid infusion (risk of arrhythmias) · when given parenterally, toxicity common (close supervision necessary and close observation required for at least 30 minutes after test dose)
CAUTIONS, FURTHER INFORMATION
▸ Anaphylaxis Anaphylaxis can occur with any intravenous amphotericin product and a test dose is advisable before the first infusion in children over 1 month of age; the patient should be carefully observed for at least 30 minutes after the test dose. Prophylactic antipyretics or hydrocortisone should only be used in patients who have previously experienced acute adverse reactions (in whom continued treatment with amphotericin is essential).

● INTERACTIONS → Appendix 1 (amphotericin). Caution—corticosteroids (avoid except to control reactions).

● SIDE-EFFECTS
▸ Common or very common Abdominal pain · abnormal liver function (discontinue treatment) · anaemia · arrhythmias · blood disorders · blood pressure changes · cardiovascular effects · chest pain · diarrhoea · disturbances in renal function · dyspnoea · electrolyte disturbances · febrile reactions · headache · hypokalaemia · hypomagnesaemia · nausea · rash · renal tubular acidosis · thrombocytopenia · vomiting
▸ Uncommon Anaphylactoid reactions · bronchospasm · convulsions · diplopia · encephalopathy · hearing loss · neurological disorders · peripheral neuropathy · tremor
▸ Frequency not known Anorexia · arthralgia · myalgia · Stevens-Johnson syndrome · toxic epidermal necrolysis

● PREGNANCY Not known to be harmful but manufacturers advise avoid unless potential benefit outweighs risk.

● BREAST FEEDING No information available.

● RENAL IMPAIRMENT Use only if no alternative; nephrotoxicity may be reduced with use of lipid formulation.

● MONITORING REQUIREMENTS Hepatic and renal function tests, blood counts, and plasma electrolyte (including plasma-potassium and magnesium concentration) monitoring required.

● DIRECTIONS FOR ADMINISTRATION
ABELCET® Amphotericin (lipid complex)
For *intravenous infusion*, allow suspension to reach room temperature, shake gently to ensure no yellow settlement, withdraw requisite dose (using 17–19 gauge needle) into one or more 20-mL syringes; replace needle on syringe with a 5-micron filter needle provided (fresh needle for each syringe) and dilute in Glucose 5% to a concentration of 2 mg/mL; preferably give *via* an infusion pump at a rate of 2.5 mg/kg/hour (initial test dose given over 15 minutes); an in-line filter (pore size no less than 15 micron) may be used; do not use sodium chloride or other electrolyte solutions—flush existing intravenous line with Glucose 5% or use separate line.

AMBISOME® Amphotericin (liposomal)
For *intravenous infusion,* reconstitute each vial with 12 mL Water for Injections and shake vigorously to produce a preparation containing 4 mg/mL; withdraw requisite dose from vial and introduce into Glucose 5% or 10% through the 5-micron filter provided, to produce a final concentration of 0.2–2 mg/mL; infuse over 30–60 minutes, or if non-anaphylactic infusion-related reactions occur infuse over 2 hours (initial test dose given over 10 minutes); an in-line filter (pore size no less than 1 micron) may be used; incompatible with sodium chloride solutions—flush existing intravenous line with Glucose 5% or 10%, or use separate line.

5

Infection

FUNGIZONE® **Amphotericin (as sodium deoxycholate complex)**

For *intravenous infusion*, reconstitute each vial with 10 mL Water for Injections and shake immediately to produce a 5 mg/mL colloidal solution; dilute further in Glucose 5% to a concentration of 100 micrograms/mL (in fluid-restricted children, up to 400 micrograms/mL given via a central line); pH of glucose solution must not be below 4.2 (check each container—consult product literature for details of buffer); infuse over 4–6 hours, or if tolerated over a minimum of 2 hours (initial test dose given over 20–30 minutes); begin infusion immediately after dilution and protect from light; incompatible with Sodium Chloride solutions—flush existing intravenous line with Glucose 5% or use separate line; an in-line filter (pore size no less than 1 micron) may be used.

- **PRESCRIBING AND DISPENSING INFORMATION** Different preparations of intravenous amphotericin vary in their pharmacodynamics, pharmacokinetics, dosage, and administration; these preparations should **not** be considered interchangeable. To avoid confusion, prescribers should specify the brand to be dispensed.

- **MEDICINAL FORMS**
There can be variation in the licensing of different medicines containing the same drug.
Powder for solution for infusion
EXCIPIENTS: May contain Sucrose
ELECTROLYTES: May contain Sodium
  - AmBisome (Gilead Sciences International Ltd)
    Amphotericin B liposomal 50 mg AmBisome 50mg powder for solution for infusion vials | 10 vial [PoM] £821.87
  - Fungizone (Bristol-Myers Squibb Pharmaceuticals Ltd)
    Amphotericin B 50 mg Fungizone Intravenous 50mg powder for solution for infusion vials | 1 vial [PoM] £3.88
Suspension for infusion
ELECTROLYTES: May contain Sodium
  - Abelcet (Teva UK Ltd)
    Amphotericin B (as Amphotericin B phospholipid complex) 5 mg per 1 ml Abelcet 100mg/20ml concentrate for suspension for infusion vials | 10 vial [PoM] £775.04 (Hospital only)

ANTIFUNGALS > TRIAZOLE ANTIFUNGALS

Fluconazole

- **INDICATIONS AND DOSE**
Candidal balanitis
  - BY MOUTH
  - Child 16–17 years: 150 mg for 1 dose
Vaginal candidiasis
  - BY MOUTH
  - Child 1 month–15 years: 150 mg for 1 dose, for use in patients who are post-puberty
  - Child 16–17 years: 150 mg for 1 dose
Vulvovaginal candidiasis (recurrent)
  - BY MOUTH
  - Child: Initially 150 mg every 72 hours for 3 doses, then 150 mg once weekly for 6 months, for use in patients who are post-puberty
Mucosal candidiasis (except genital)
  - BY MOUTH, OR BY INTRAVENOUS INFUSION
  - Neonate up to 14 days: 3–6 mg/kg, dose to be given on first day, then 3 mg/kg every 72 hours.
  - Neonate 14 days to 28 days: 3–6 mg/kg, dose to be given on first day, then 3 mg/kg every 48 hours.
  - Child 1 month–11 years: 3–6 mg/kg, dose to be given on first day, then 3 mg/kg daily (max. per dose 100 mg) for 7–14 days in oropharyngeal candidiasis (max. 14 days except in severely immunocompromised patients); for 14–30 days in other mucosal infections (e.g.

oesophagitis, candiduria, non-invasive bronchopulmonary infections)
  - Child 12–17 years: 50 mg daily for 7–14 days in oropharyngeal candidiasis (max. 14 days except in severely immunocompromised patients); for 14–30 days in other mucosal infections (e.g. oesophagitis, candiduria, non-invasive bronchopulmonary infections); increased to 100 mg daily, increased dose only for unusually difficult infections
Tinea capitis
  - BY MOUTH
  - Child 1–17 years: 6 mg/kg daily (max. per dose 300 mg) for 2–4 weeks
Tinea pedis, corporis, cruris, pityriasis versicolor | Dermal candidiasis
  - BY MOUTH
  - Child: 3 mg/kg daily (max. per dose 50 mg) for 2–4 weeks (for up to 6 weeks in tinea pedis); max. duration of treatment 6 weeks
Invasive candidal infections (including candidaemia and disseminated candidiasis) and cryptococcal infections (including meningitis)
  - BY MOUTH, OR BY INTRAVENOUS INFUSION
  - Neonate up to 14 days: 6–12 mg/kg every 72 hours, treatment continued according to response (at least 8 weeks for cryptococcal meningitis).
  - Neonate 14 days to 28 days: 6–12 mg/kg every 48 hours, treatment continued according to response (at least 8 weeks for cryptococcal meningitis).
  - Child: 6–12 mg/kg daily (max. per dose 800 mg), treatment continued according to response (at least 8 weeks for cryptococcal meningitis)
Prevention of fungal infections in immunocompromised patients
  - BY MOUTH, OR BY INTRAVENOUS INFUSION
  - Neonate up to 14 days: 3–12 mg/kg every 72 hours, dose given according to extent and duration of neutropenia.
  - Neonate 14 days to 28 days: 3–12 mg/kg every 48 hours, dose given according to extent and duration of neutropenia.
  - Child: 3–12 mg/kg daily (max. per dose 400 mg), commence treatment before anticipated onset of neutropenia and continue for 7 days after neutrophil count in desirable range, dose given according to extent and duration of neutropenia
Prevention of fungal infections in immunocompromised patients (for patients with high risk of systemic infections e.g. following bone-marrow transplantation)
  - BY MOUTH, OR BY INTRAVENOUS INFUSION
  - Child: 12 mg/kg daily (max. per dose 400 mg), commence treatment before anticipated onset of neutropenia and continue for 7 days after neutrophil count in desirable range
Prevention of relapse of cryptococcal meningitis in HIV-infected patients after completion of primary therapy
  - BY MOUTH, OR BY INTRAVENOUS INFUSION
  - Child: 6 mg/kg daily (max. per dose 200 mg)

- **UNLICENSED USE** Not licensed for tinea infections in children, or for vaginal candidiasis in girls under 16 years, or for prevention of relapse of cryptococcal meningitis after completion of primary therapy in children with HIV.
- **CONTRA-INDICATIONS** Acute porphyrias p. 562
- **CAUTIONS** Susceptibility to QT interval prolongation
- **INTERACTIONS** → Appendix 1 (antifungals, triazole); in general, fluconazole interactions in Appendix 1 relate to multiple-dose treatment.

Caution with concomitant use of hepatotoxic drugs.

- **SIDE-EFFECTS**
- ▶ **Common or very common** Abdominal discomfort · diarrhoea · flatulence · headache · nausea · rash
- ▶ **Uncommon** Alopecia · anaphylaxis · angioedema · dizziness · dyspepsia · hepatic disorders · hyperlipidaemia · pruritus · seizures · Stevens-Johnson syndrome · taste disturbance · toxic epidermal necrolysis · vomiting
- ▶ **Frequency not known** Hypokalaemia · leucopenia · thrombocytopenia

  SIDE-EFFECTS, FURTHER INFORMATION
  If rash occurs, discontinue treatment (or monitor closely if infection invasive or systemic); severe cutaneous reactions are more likely in patients with AIDS.

- **PREGNANCY** Manufacturer advises avoid—multiple congenital abnormalities reported with long-term high doses.
- **BREAST FEEDING** Present in milk but amount probably too small to be harmful.
- **HEPATIC IMPAIRMENT** Toxicity with related drugs.
- **RENAL IMPAIRMENT** Usual initial dose then halve subsequent doses if estimated glomerular filtration rate less than 50 mL/minute/1.73 m^2.
- **MONITORING REQUIREMENTS** Monitor liver function with high doses or extended courses—discontinue if signs or symptoms of hepatic disease (risk of hepatic necrosis).
- **DIRECTIONS FOR ADMINISTRATION**
- ▶ With intravenous use For *intravenous infusion*, give over 10–30 minutes; do not exceed an infusion rate of 5–10 mL/minute.
- **PRESCRIBING AND DISPENSING INFORMATION** Flavours of oral liquid formulations may include orange.
- **PROFESSION SPECIFIC INFORMATION**

  Dental practitioners' formulary
  Fluconazole Capsules 50 mg may be prescribed.
  Fluconazole Oral Suspension 50 mg/5 mL may be prescribed.

- **EXCEPTIONS TO LEGAL CATEGORY** Fluconazole capsules can be sold to the public for vaginal candidiasis and associated candidal balanitis in those aged 16–60 years, in a container or packaging containing not more than 150 mg and labelled to show a max. dose of 150 mg.

- **MEDICINAL FORMS**
  There can be variation in the licensing of different medicines containing the same drug.

  Capsule
  CAUTIONARY AND ADVISORY LABELS 9 (50 mg and 200 mg strengths only)
- ▶ Fluconazole (Non-proprietary)
  Fluconazole 50 mg Fluconazole 50mg capsules | 7 capsule [PoM] £5.00 DT price = £0.86
  Fluconazole 150 mg Fluconazole 150mg capsules | 1 capsule [PoM] £8.50 DT price = £0.81 | 1 capsule [P] no price available DT price = £0.81
  Fluconazole 200 mg Fluconazole 200mg capsules | 7 capsule [PoM] £12.50 DT price = £6.05
- ▶ Canesten (fluconazole) (Bayer Plc)
  Fluconazole 150 mg Canesten 150mg capsules | 1 capsule [P] £6.33 DT price = £0.81
- ▶ Diflucan (Pfizer Ltd)
  Fluconazole 50 mg Diflucan 50mg capsules | 7 capsule [PoM] £16.61 DT price = £0.86
  Fluconazole 150 mg Diflucan 150mg capsules | 1 capsule [PoM] £7.12 DT price = £0.81
  Fluconazole 200 mg Diflucan 200mg capsules | 7 capsule [PoM] £66.42 DT price = £6.05

  Oral suspension
  CAUTIONARY AND ADVISORY LABELS 9
- ▶ Fluconazole (Non-proprietary)
  Fluconazole 10 mg per 1 ml Fluconazole 50mg/5ml oral suspension | 35 ml [PoM] £20.51 DT price = £20.51

- ▶ Diflucan (Pfizer Ltd)
  Fluconazole 10 mg per 1 ml Diflucan 50mg/5ml oral suspension | 35 ml [PoM] £16.61 DT price = £20.51
  Fluconazole 40 mg per 1 ml Diflucan 200mg/5ml oral suspension | 35 ml [PoM] £66.42 DT price = £66.42

  Solution for infusion
  ELECTROLYTES: May contain Sodium
- ▶ Fluconazole (Non-proprietary)
  Fluconazole 2 mg per 1 ml Fluconazole 100mg/50ml solution for infusion bottles | 5 bottle [PoM] £12.60
  Fluconazole 200mg/100ml solution for infusion vials | 1 vial [PoM] £29.28
  Fluconazole 50mg/25ml solution for infusion vials | 1 vial [PoM] £7.31-£7.32
- ▶ Diflucan (Pfizer Ltd)
  Fluconazole 2 mg per 1 ml Diflucan 200mg/100ml solution for infusion vials | 1 vial [PoM] £29.28

Itraconazole

- **INDICATIONS AND DOSE**

Oropharyngeal candidiasis
- ▶ BY MOUTH
- ▶ Child 1 month–11 years: 3–5 mg/kg once daily for 15 days; maximum 100 mg per day
- ▶ Child 12–17 years: 100 mg once daily for 15 days

Oropharyngeal candidiasis in patients with AIDS or neutropenia
- ▶ BY MOUTH
- ▶ Child 1 month–11 years: 3–5 mg/kg once daily for 15 days; maximum 200 mg per day
- ▶ Child 12–17 years: 200 mg once daily for 15 days

Systemic candidiasis where other antifungal drugs inappropriate or ineffective
- ▶ BY MOUTH
- ▶ Child: 5 mg/kg once daily (max. per dose 200 mg), dose increased in invasive or disseminated disease and in cryptococcal meningitis, increased to 5 mg/kg twice daily (max. per dose 200 mg)
- ▶ BY INTRAVENOUS INFUSION
- ▶ Child: 2.5 mg/kg every 12 hours (max. per dose 200 mg) for 2 days, then 2.5 mg/kg once daily (max. per dose 200 mg) for max. 12 days

Pityriasis versicolor
- ▶ BY MOUTH
- ▶ Child 1 month–11 years: 3–5 mg/kg once daily (max. per dose 200 mg) for 7 days
- ▶ Child 12–17 years: 200 mg once daily for 7 days

Tinea pedis | Tinea manuum
- ▶ BY MOUTH
- ▶ Child 1 month–11 years: 3–5 mg/kg once daily (max. per dose 100 mg) for 30 days
- ▶ Child 12–17 years: 100 mg once daily for 30 days, alternatively 200 mg twice daily for 7 days

Tinea corporis | Tinea cruris
- ▶ BY MOUTH
- ▶ Child 1 month–11 years: 3–5 mg/kg once daily (max. per dose 100 mg) for 15 days
- ▶ Child 12–17 years: 100 mg once daily for 15 days, alternatively 200 mg once daily for 7 days

Tinea capitis
- ▶ BY MOUTH
- ▶ Child 1–17 years: 3–5 mg/kg once daily (max. per dose 200 mg) for 2–6 weeks

Onychomycosis
- ▶ BY MOUTH
- ▶ Child 1–11 years: 5 mg/kg daily (max. per dose 200 mg) for 7 days, subsequent courses repeated after 21-day intervals; fingernails 2 courses, toenails 3 courses
- ▶ Child 12–17 years: 200 mg once daily for 3 months, alternatively 200 mg twice daily for 7 days, continued →

subsequent courses repeated after 21-day intervals; fingernails 2 courses, toenails 3 courses

Systemic aspergillosis where other antifungal drugs inappropriate or ineffective

▶ BY INTRAVENOUS INFUSION
▹ Child: 2.5 mg/kg every 12 hours (max. per dose 200 mg) for 2 days, then 2.5 mg/kg once daily (max. per dose 200 mg) for max. 12 days
▶ BY MOUTH
▹ Child: 5 mg/kg once daily (max. per dose 200 mg), increased to 5 mg/kg twice daily (max. per dose 200 mg), dose increased in invasive or disseminated disease and in cryptococcal meningitis

Histoplasmosis

▶ BY MOUTH
▹ Child: 5 mg/kg 1–2 times a day (max. per dose 200 mg)

Systemic cryptococcosis including cryptococcal meningitis where other antifungal drugs inappropriate or ineffective

▶ BY MOUTH
▹ Child: 5 mg/kg once daily (max. per dose 200 mg), dose increased in invasive or disseminated disease and in cryptococcal meningitis, increased to 5 mg/kg twice daily (max. per dose 200 mg)
▶ BY INTRAVENOUS INFUSION
▹ Child: 2.5 mg/kg every 12 hours (max. per dose 200 mg) for 2 days, then 2.5 mg/kg once daily (max. per dose 200 mg) for max. 12 days

Maintenance in HIV-infected patients to prevent relapse of underlying fungal infection and prophylaxis in neutropenia when standard therapy inappropriate

▶ BY MOUTH
▹ Child: 5 mg/kg once daily (max. per dose 200 mg), then increased to 5 mg/kg twice daily (max. per dose 200 mg), dose increased only if low plasma-itraconazole concentration

Prophylaxis of deep fungal infections (when standard therapy inappropriate) in patients with haematological malignancy or undergoing bone-marrow transplantation who are expected to become neutropenic

▶ BY MOUTH USING ORAL SOLUTION
▹ Child: 2.5 mg/kg twice daily, to be started before transplantation or before chemotherapy (taking care to avoid interaction with cytotoxic drugs) and continued until neutrophil count recovers, safety and efficacy not established

● UNLICENSED USE Not licensed for use in children (age range not specified by manufacturer).

IMPORTANT SAFETY INFORMATION

HEART FAILURE

Following reports of heart failure, caution is advised when prescribing itraconazole to patients at high risk of heart failure. Those at risk include:
● patients receiving high doses and longer treatment courses;
● older adults and those with cardiac disease;
● patients with chronic lung disease (including chronic obstructive pulmonary disease) associated with pulmonary hypertension;
● patients receiving treatment with negative inotropic drugs, e.g. calcium channel blockers.
Itraconazole should be avoided in patients with ventricular dysfunction or a history of heart failure unless the infection is serious.

● CONTRA-INDICATIONS Acute porphyrias p. 562
● CAUTIONS Active liver disease · history of hepatotoxicity with other drugs · susceptibility to congestive heart failure
● INTERACTIONS → Appendix 1 (antifungals, triazole).

● SIDE-EFFECTS

GENERAL SIDE-EFFECTS
▶ **Common or very common** Abdominal pain · blood pressure changes · cough · diarrhoea · dyspnoea · headache · hepatitis · hypokalaemia · nausea · rash · taste disturbances · vomiting
▶ **Uncommon** Constipation · dizziness · dyspepsia · flatulence · menstrual disorder · myalgia · oedema · peripheral neuropathy (discontinue treatment)
▶ **Rare** Alopecia · deafness · erectile dysfunction · heart failure · hypertriglyceridaemia · leucopenia · pancreatitis · photosensitivity · Stevens-Johnson syndrome · tinnitus · toxic epidermal necrolysis · urinary frequency · visual disturbances
▶ **Frequency not known** Arthralgia · confusion · drowsiness · hepatotoxicity · renal impairment · thrombocytopenia · tremor

SPECIFIC SIDE-EFFECTS
▶ With intravenous use Hyperglycaemia

SIDE-EFFECTS, FURTHER INFORMATION
▶ Hepatotoxicity Potentially life-threatening hepatotoxicity reported very rarely—discontinue if signs of hepatitis develop.

● CONCEPTION AND CONTRACEPTION Ensure effective contraception during treatment and until the next menstrual period following end of treatment.

● PREGNANCY Manufacturer advises use only in life-threatening situations (toxicity at high doses in *animal* studies).

● BREAST FEEDING Small amounts present in milk—may accumulate; manufacturer advises avoid.

● HEPATIC IMPAIRMENT Dose reduction may be necessary. Use only if potential benefit outweighs risk of hepatotoxicity.

● RENAL IMPAIRMENT Risk of congestive heart failure.
▶ With oral use Bioavailability of oral formulations possibly reduced.
▶ With intravenous use Use intravenous infusion with caution if estimated glomerular filtration rate 30–80 mL/minute/1.73 m^2 (monitor renal function); avoid intravenous infusion if estimated golmerular filtration rate less than 30 mL/minute/1.73 m^2.

● MONITORING REQUIREMENTS
▶ Absorption reduced in AIDS and neutropenia (monitor plasma-itraconazole concentration and increase dose if necessary).
▶ Monitor liver function if treatment continues for longer than one month, if receiving other hepatotoxic drugs, if history of hepatotoxicity with other drugs, or in hepatic impairment.

● DIRECTIONS FOR ADMINISTRATION
▶ With intravenous use For *intravenous infusion*, dilute 250 mg with 50 mL Sodium Chloride 0.9% and give requisite dose through an in-line filter (0.2 micron) over 60 minutes.
▶ With oral use For *oral liquid*, do not take with food; swish around mouth and swallow, do not rinse afterwards.

● PRESCRIBING AND DISPENSING INFORMATION Flavours of oral liquid formulations may include cherry.

● PATIENT AND CARER ADVICE Patients should be told how to recognise signs of liver disorder and advised to seek prompt medical attention if symptoms such as anorexia, nausea, vomiting, fatigue, abdominal pain or dark urine develop.
▶ With oral use Patients or carers should be given advice on how to administer itraconazole oral liquid.

- **MEDICINAL FORMS**
There can be variation in the licensing of different medicines containing the same drug. Forms available from special-order manufacturers include: oral suspension, oral solution

Capsule

CAUTIONARY AND ADVISORY LABELS 5, 9, 21, 25
▸ Itraconazole (Non-proprietary)
Itraconazole 100 mg Itraconazole 100mg capsules |
15 capsule [PoM] £21.50 DT price = £3.64 | 60 capsule [PoM] £56.21
Itraconazole 100mg Capsules | 15 capsule [PoM] £4.04 DT price = £3.64
▸ Sporanox (Janssen-Cilag Ltd)
Itraconazole 100 mg Sporanox-Pulse 100mg capsules |
28 capsule [PoM] £25.72
Sporanox 100mg capsules | 4 capsule [PoM] £3.67 | 15 capsule [PoM] £13.77 DT price = £3.64 | 60 capsule [PoM] £55.10

Oral solution

CAUTIONARY AND ADVISORY LABELS 9, 23
▸ Itraconazole (Non-proprietary)
Itraconazole 10 mg per 1 ml Itraconazole 50mg/5ml oral solution sugar free sugar-free | 150 ml [PoM] £58.34 DT price = £58.34
▸ Sporanox (Janssen-Cilag Ltd)
Itraconazole 10 mg per 1 ml Sporanox 50mg/5ml oral solution sugar-free | 150 ml [PoM] £58.34 DT price = £58.34

Solution for infusion

EXCIPIENTS: May contain Propylene glycol
▸ Sporanox (Janssen-Cilag Ltd)
Itraconazole 10 mg per 1 ml Sporanox I.V. 250mg/25ml solution for infusion ampoules and diluent | 1 ampoule [PoM] £79.71

Voriconazole

- **INDICATIONS AND DOSE**

Invasive aspergillosis | Serious infections caused by *Scedosporium* **spp.,** *Fusarium* **spp., or invasive fluconazole-resistant** *Candida* **spp. (including** *C. krusei***)**
▸ BY MOUTH
▸ Child 2–11 years: Treatment should be initiated with intravenous regimen, and oral regimen should be considered only after there is a significant clinical improvement; maintenance 9 mg/kg every 12 hours, adjusted in steps of 1 mg/kg and increased if necessary up to 350 mg every 12 hours, then adjusted in steps of 50 mg as required
▸ Child 12–14 years (body-weight up to 50 kg): Treatment should be initiated with intravenous regimen, and oral regimen should be considered only after there is a significant clinical improvement; maintenance 9 mg/kg every 12 hours, adjusted in steps of 1 mg/kg and increased if necessary up to 350 mg every 12 hours, then adjusted in steps of 50 mg as required
▸ Child 12–14 years (body-weight 50 kg and above): Initially 400 mg every 12 hours for 2 doses, then 200 mg every 12 hours, increased if necessary to 300 mg every 12 hours
▸ Child 15–17 years (body-weight up to 40 kg): Initially 200 mg every 12 hours for 2 doses, then 100 mg every 12 hours, increased if necessary to 150 mg every 12 hours
▸ Child 15–17 years (body-weight 40 kg and above): Initially 400 mg every 12 hours for 2 doses, then 200 mg every 12 hours, increased if necessary to 300 mg every 12 hours
▸ BY INTRAVENOUS INFUSION
▸ Child 2–11 years: Initially 9 mg/kg every 12 hours for 2 doses, then 8 mg/kg every 12 hours; adjusted in steps of 1 mg/kg as required; for max. 6 months
▸ Child 12–14 years (body-weight up to 50 kg): Initially 9 mg/kg every 12 hours for 2 doses, then 8 mg/kg every 12 hours; adjusted in steps of 1 mg/kg as required; for max. 6 months
▸ Child 12–14 years (body-weight 50 kg and above): Initially 6 mg/kg every 12 hours for 2 doses, then 4 mg/kg every

12 hours; reduced if not tolerated to 3 mg/kg every 12 hours; for max. 6 months
▸ Child 15–17 years: Initially 6 mg/kg every 12 hours for 2 doses, then 4 mg/kg every 12 hours; reduced if not tolerated to 3 mg/kg every 12 hours; for max. 6 months

- **CONTRA-INDICATIONS** Acute porphyrias p. 562
- **CAUTIONS** Avoid exposure to sunlight · bradycardia · cardiomyopathy · electrolyte disturbances · history of QT interval prolongation · patients at risk of pancreatitis · symptomatic arrhythmias
- **INTERACTIONS** → Appendix 1 (antifungals, triazole). Caution with concomitant use with other drugs that prolong QT interval.
- **SIDE-EFFECTS**

GENERAL SIDE-EFFECTS
▸ **Common or very common** Abdominal pain · acute renal failure · agitation · alopecia · altered perception · anaemia · anxiety · asthenia · blood disorders · blurred vision · cheilitis · chest pain · confusion · depression · diarrhoea · dizziness · haematuria · hallucinations · headache · hypoglycaemia · hypokalaemia · hypotension · influenza-like symptoms · jaundice · leucopenia · nausea · oedema · pancytopenia · paraesthesia · photophobia · photosensitivity · pruritus · rash · respiratory distress syndrome · sinusitis · thrombocytopenia · tremor · visual disturbances · vomiting
▸ **Uncommon** Adrenocortical insufficiency · arrhythmias · arthritis · ataxia · blepharitis · cholecystitis · constipation · duodenitis · dyspepsia · flushing · fulminant hepatic failure · gingivitis · glossitis · hepatitis · hypersensitivity reactions · hypoaesthesia · hyponatraemia · nystagmus · optic neuritis · pancreatitis · psoriasis · QT interval prolongation · raised serum cholesterol · scleritis · Stevens-Johnson syndrome · syncope
▸ **Rare** Convulsions · discoid lupus erythematosus · extrapyramidal effects · hearing disturbances · hyperthyroidism · hypertonia · hypothyroidism · insomnia · optic atrophy · pseudomembranous colitis · pseudoporphyria · retinal haemorrhage · taste disturbances (more common with oral suspension) · tinnitus · toxic epidermal necrolysis
▸ **Frequency not known** On long term treatment, squamous cell carcinoma of skin (particularly in presence of phototoxicity) · periostitis (particularly in transplant patients)

SPECIFIC SIDE-EFFECTS
▸ **Common or very common**
▸ **With intravenous use** Injection-site reactions

SIDE-EFFECTS, FURTHER INFORMATION
▸ **Hepatotoxicity** Hepatitis, cholestasis, and fulminant hepatic failure usually occur in the first 10 days; risk of hepatotoxicity increased in patients with haematological malignancy. Consider treatment discontinuation if severe abnormalities in liver function tests.
▸ **Phototoxicity** Phototoxicity occurs commonly. If phototoxicity occurs, consider treatment discontinuation; if treatment is continued, monitor for pre-malignant skin lesions and squamous cell carcinoma, and discontinue treatment if they occur.

- **CONCEPTION AND CONTRACEPTION** Effective contraception required during treatment.
- **PREGNANCY** Toxicity in *animal* studies—manufacturer advises avoid unless potential benefit outweighs risk.
- **BREAST FEEDING** Manufacturer advises avoid—no information available.
- **HEPATIC IMPAIRMENT**
Child 12–17 years In mild to moderate hepatic cirrhosis use usual initial dose then halve subsequent doses. No information available for severe hepatic cirrhosis—

5

Infection

manufacturer advises use only if potential benefit outweighs risk.

- **RENAL IMPAIRMENT**
  Child 2-12 years No information available.
  Child 12-17 years Intravenous vehicle may accumulate if estimated glomerular filtration rate less than 50 mL/minute/1.73 m² —use intravenous infusion only if potential benefit outweighs risk, and monitor renal function; alternatively, use tablets or oral suspension (no dose adjustment required).

- **MONITORING REQUIREMENTS**
  - Monitor renal function.
  - Monitor liver function before starting treatment, then at least weekly for 1 month, and then monthly during treatment.

- **DIRECTIONS FOR ADMINISTRATION**
  - With intravenous use For *intravenous infusion*, reconstitute each 200 mg with 19 mL Water for Injections or Sodium Chloride 0.9% to produce a 10 mg/mL solution; dilute dose to concentration of 0.5–5 mg/mL with Glucose 5% or Sodium Chloride 0.9% and give intermittently at a rate not exceeding 3 mg/kg/hour.

- **PRESCRIBING AND DISPENSING INFORMATION** Flavours of oral liquid formulations may include orange.

- **PATIENT AND CARER ADVICE** Patients and their carers should be advised to keep the alert card with them at all times.

  Patients and their carers should be told how to recognise symptoms of liver disorder, and advised to seek immediate medical attention if symptoms such as persistent nausea, vomiting, malaise or jaundice develop.

  Patients and their carers should be advised that patients should avoid intense or prolonged exposure to direct sunlight, and to avoid the use of sunbeds. In sunlight, patients should cover sun-exposed areas of skin and use a sunscreen with a high sun protection factor. Patients should seek medical attention if they experience sunburn or a severe skin reaction following exposure to light or sun.

- **MEDICINAL FORMS**
  There can be variation in the licensing of different medicines containing the same drug.

  Tablet
  CAUTIONARY AND ADVISORY LABELS 9, 11, 23
  - VFEND (Pfizer Ltd)
    Voriconazole 50 mg VFEND 50mg tablets | 28 tablet PoM £275.68
    Voriconazole 200 mg VFEND 200mg tablets | 28 tablet PoM £1,102.74

  Oral suspension
  CAUTIONARY AND ADVISORY LABELS 9, 11, 23
  - VFEND (Pfizer Ltd)
    Voriconazole 40 mg per 1 ml VFEND 40mg/ml oral suspension | 75 ml PoM £551.37

  Powder for solution for infusion
  EXCIPIENTS: May contain Sulfobutylether beta cyclodextrin sodium
  ELECTROLYTES: May contain Sodium
  - VFEND (Pfizer Ltd)
    Voriconazole 200 mg VFEND 200mg powder for solution for infusion vials | 1 vial PoM £77.14 (Hospital only)

  Powder and solvent for solution for infusion
  EXCIPIENTS: May contain Sulfobutylether beta cyclodextrin sodium
  ELECTROLYTES: May contain Sodium
  - VFEND (Pfizer Ltd)
    Voriconazole 200 mg VFEND 200mg powder and solvent for solution for infusion vials | 1 vial PoM £77.14 (Hospital only)

ANTIFUNGALS 〉 OTHER

Flucytosine

- **INDICATIONS AND DOSE**

  Systemic yeast and fungal infections | Adjunct to amphotericin in severe systemic candidiasis and in other severe or long-standing infections
  ▸ BY INTRAVENOUS INFUSION, OR BY MOUTH
  - Neonate: 50 mg/kg every 12 hours.

  - Child: Usual dose 50 mg/kg every 6 hours usually for not more than 7 days, alternatively 25–37.5 mg/kg every 6 hours usually for not more than 7 days, lower dose may be sufficient for sensitive organisms

  Cryptococcal meningitis (adjunct to amphotericin)
  ▸ BY INTRAVENOUS INFUSION, OR BY MOUTH
  - Neonate: 50 mg/kg every 12 hours.

  - Child: 25 mg/kg every 6 hours for 2 weeks

- **UNLICENSED USE** Tablets not licensed.

- **CAUTIONS** Blood disorders

- **INTERACTIONS** → Appendix 1 (flucytosine).

- **SIDE-EFFECTS**
  - **Common or very common** Diarrhoea · nausea · rashes · vomiting
  - **Uncommon** Alterations in liver function tests · cardiotoxicity · confusion · convulsions · hallucinations · headache · sedation · toxic epidermal necrolysis · vertigo
  - **Frequency not known** Aplastic anaemia · blood disorders · hepatic necrosis · hepatitis · leucopenia · thrombocytopenia

- **PREGNANCY** Teratogenic in *animal* studies; manufacturer advises use only if potential benefit outweighs risk.

- **BREAST FEEDING** Manufacturer advises avoid.

- **RENAL IMPAIRMENT** Use normal dose every 12 hours if creatinine clearance 20–40 mL/minute; use normal dose every 24 hours if creatinine clearance 10–20 mL/minute; use initial normal dose if creatinine clearance less than 10 mL/minute and then adjust dose according to plasma-flucytosine concentration. In renal impairment liver- and kidney-function tests and blood counts required weekly.

- **MONITORING REQUIREMENTS**
  - For plasma concentration monitoring, blood should be taken shortly before starting the next infusion; plasma concentration for optimum response 25–50 mg/litre (200–400 micromol/litre)—should not be allowed to exceed 80 mg/litre (620 micromol/litre).
  - Liver- and kidney-function tests and blood counts required (weekly in blood disorders).

- **DIRECTIONS FOR ADMINISTRATION** For *intravenous infusion*, give over 20–40 minutes.

- **MEDICINAL FORMS**
  There can be variation in the licensing of different medicines containing the same drug. Forms available from special-order manufacturers include: oral solution

  Solution for infusion
  ELECTROLYTES: May contain Sodium
  - Ancotil (Meda Pharmaceuticals Ltd)
    Flucytosine 10 mg per 1 ml Ancotil 2.5g/250ml solution for infusion bottles | 5 bottle PoM £151.67 (Hospital only)

Griseofulvin

- **INDICATIONS AND DOSE**

Dermatophyte infections of the skin, scalp, hair and nails where topical therapy has failed or is inappropriate
▶ BY MOUTH
- Child 1 month–11 years: Usual dose 10 mg/kg daily (max. per dose 500 mg), increased if necessary to 20 mg/kg daily (max. per dose 1 g) for severe infections; reduce dose when response occurs, daily dose may be taken once daily or in divided doses
- Child 12–17 years: 500 mg daily, increased if necessary to 1 g daily for severe infections; reduce dose when response occurs, daily dose may be taken once daily or in divided doses

Tinea capitis caused by *Trichophyton tonsurans*
▶ BY MOUTH
- Child 1 month–11 years: 15–20 mg/kg once daily (max. per dose 1 g), alternatively 15–20 mg/kg daily (max. per dose 1 g) in divided doses
- Child 12–17 years: 1 g once daily, alternatively 1 g daily in divided doses

- **UNLICENSED USE** Licensed for use in children (age range not specified by manufacturer).

- **CONTRA-INDICATIONS**
▶ With oral use Acute porphyrias p. 562 · systemic lupus erythematosus (risk of exacerbation)

- **INTERACTIONS** → Appendix 1 (griseofulvin).

- **SIDE-EFFECTS**
▶ **Rare** Erythema multiforme · toxic epidermal necrolysis
▶ **Very rare** Headache
▶ **Frequency not known** Abdominal pain · agitation · confusion · depression · diarrhoea · dizziness · dyspepsia · fatigue · glossitis · hepatotoxicity · impaired coordination · impaired hearing · leucopenia · menstrual disturbances · nausea · peripheral neuropathy · photosensitivity · rash · renal failure · sleep disturbances · systemic lupus erythematosus · taste disturbances · vomiting

- **CONCEPTION AND CONTRACEPTION** Effective contraception required during and for at least 1 month after administration to women (important: effectiveness of oral contraceptives may be reduced, additional contraceptive precautions e.g. barrier method, required). Men should avoid fathering a child during and for at least 6 months after administration

- **PREGNANCY** Avoid (fetotoxicity and teratogenicity in *animals*).

- **BREAST FEEDING** Avoid—no information available.

- **HEPATIC IMPAIRMENT** Avoid in severe liver disease.

- **PATIENT AND CARER ADVICE**
Driving and skilled tasks
▶ With oral use May impair performance of skilled tasks (e.g. driving); effects of alcohol enhanced.
Medicines for Children leaflet: Griseofulvin for fungal infections www.medicinesforchildren.org.uk/griseofulvin-for-fungal-infections

- **MEDICINAL FORMS**
There can be variation in the licensing of different medicines containing the same drug. Forms available from special-order manufacturers include: oral suspension

Tablet
CAUTIONARY AND ADVISORY LABELS 9, 21
▶ Griseofulvin (Non-proprietary)
Griseofulvin 125 mg Griseofulvin 125mg tablets | 100 tablet PoM £96.67 DT price = £96.67
Griseofulvin 500 mg Griseofulvin 500mg tablets | 90 tablet PoM £99.00 | 100 tablet PoM £90.34 DT price = £100.17

3.1 Pneumocystis pneumonia

Pneumocystis pneumonia

Overview

Pneumonia caused by *Pneumocystis jirovecii* (*Pneumocystis carinii*) occurs in immunosuppressed patients; it is a common cause of pneumonia in AIDS. Pneumocystis pneumonia should generally be treated by those experienced in its management. Blood gas measurement is used to assess disease severity.

Treatment

The recommended duration of treatment is generally 14–21 days.

Mild to moderate disease
Co-trimoxazole p. 330 in high dosage is the drug of choice for the treatment of mild to moderate pneumocystis pneumonia.

Atovaquone p. 358 or a combination of dapsone p. 358 with trimethoprim p. 338 is given by mouth for the treatment of mild to moderate disease [unlicensed indication] in children who cannot tolerate co-trimoxazole.

A combination of clindamycin p. 307 and primaquine p. 374 may be used in the treatment of mild to moderate disease [unlicensed indication]; this combination is associated with considerable toxicity.

Severe disease
Co-trimoxazole in high dosage, given by mouth or by intravenous infusion, is the drug of choice for the treatment of severe pneumocystis pneumonia. Pentamidine isetionate p. 358 given by intravenous infusion is an alternative for children who cannot tolerate co-trimoxazole, or who have not responded to it. Pentamidine isetionate is a potentially toxic drug that can cause severe hypotension during or immediately after infusion. If there is clinical improvement after 7–10 days of intravenous therapy with pentamidine isetionate, patients can be switched to oral treatment (e.g. atovaquone) to complete 21 days treatment.

Corticosteroid treatment can be lifesaving in those with severe pneumocystis pneumonia.

Adjunctive therapy
In moderate to severe pneumocystis infections associated with HIV infection, prednisolone p. 413 is given by mouth for 5 days (alternatively, hydrocortisone p. 411 may be given parenterally); the dose is then reduced over the next 16 days and then stopped. Corticosteroid treatment should ideally be started at the same time as the anti-pneumocystis therapy and certainly no later than 24–72 hours afterwards. The corticosteroid should be withdrawn before anti-pneumocystis treatment is complete.

Prophylaxis

Prophylaxis against pneumocystis pneumonia should be given to all children with a history of this infection, and to all HIV-infected infants aged 1 month–1 year. Prophylaxis against pneumocystis pneumonia should also be considered for severely immunocompromised children. Prophylaxis should continue until immunity recovers sufficiently. It should not be discontinued if the child has oral candidiasis, continues to lose weight, or is receiving cytotoxic therapy or long-term immunosuppressant therapy.

Prophylaxis should also be given to infants aged 1 month–1 year who are suspected to be HIV-positive, *or* whose mothers had a viral load greater than 1000 HIV RNA copies/mL between 36 weeks' gestation and delivery; prophylaxis should be continued until HIV infection is excluded or until immunity recovers.

5

Infection

5

Infection

Co-trimoxazole by mouth is the drug of choice for prophylaxis against pneumocystis pneumonia. Co-trimoxazole may be used in infants born to mothers with a high risk of transmission of infection.

Inhaled pentamidine isetionate is better tolerated than parenteral pentamidine isetionate. Intermittent inhalation of pentamidine isetionate is used for prophylaxis against pneumocystis pneumonia in children unable to tolerate co-trimoxazole. It is effective but children may be prone to extrapulmonary infection. Alternatively, dapsone can be used.

ANTIPROTOZOALS

Atovaquone

● **INDICATIONS AND DOSE**
Treatment of mild to moderate *Pneumocystis jirovecii* (*Pneumocystis carinii*) pneumonia in patients intolerant of co-trimoxazole
▸ BY MOUTH
▸ Child 1–2 months: 15–20 mg/kg twice daily for 14–21 days, dose to be taken with food, particularly high fat food
▸ Child 3 months–1 year: 22.5 mg/kg twice daily for 14–21 days, dose to be taken with food, particularly high fat food
▸ Child 2–17 years: 15–20 mg/kg twice daily (max. per dose 750 mg) for 14–21 days, dose to be taken with food, particularly high fat food

● **UNLICENSED USE** Not licensed for use in children.
● **CAUTIONS** Other causes of pulmonary disease should be sought and treated · initial diarrhoea and difficulty in taking with food may reduce absorption (and require alternative therapy)
● **INTERACTIONS** → Appendix 1 (atovaquone).
● **SIDE-EFFECTS** Anaemia · diarrhoea · fever · headache · hyponatraemia · insomnia · nausea · neutropenia · pruritus · rash · Stevens-Johnson syndrome · vomiting
● **PREGNANCY** Manufacturer advises avoid unless potential benefit outweighs risk—no information available.
● **BREAST FEEDING** Manufacturer advises avoid.
● **HEPATIC IMPAIRMENT** Manufacturer advises caution. Monitor more closely in hepatic impairment.
● **RENAL IMPAIRMENT** Manufacturer advises caution. Monitor more closely in renal impairment.
● **PRESCRIBING AND DISPENSING INFORMATION** Flavours of oral liquid formulations may include tutti-frutti.
● **MEDICINAL FORMS**
There can be variation in the licensing of different medicines containing the same drug.
Oral suspension
CAUTIONARY AND ADVISORY LABELS 21
▸ Wellvone (GlaxoSmithKline UK Ltd)
Atovaquone 150 mg per 1 ml Wellvone 750mg/5ml oral suspension sugar-free | 226 ml [PoM] £486.37

Dapsone

● **INDICATIONS AND DOSE**
Treatment of mild to moderate *Pneumocystis jirovecii* (*Pneumocystis carinii*) pneumonia (in combination with trimethoprim)
▸ BY MOUTH
▸ Child 1 month–11 years: 2 mg/kg once daily (max. per dose 100 mg)
▸ Child 12–17 years: 100 mg once daily

Prophylaxis of *Pneumocystis jirovecii* (*Pneumocystis carinii*) pneumonia
▸ BY MOUTH
▸ Child: 2 mg/kg once daily (max. per dose 100 mg)

● **UNLICENSED USE** Not licensed for treatment of pneumocystis (*P. jirovecii*) pneumonia. Monotherapy not licensed for children for prophylaxis of *P. jirovecii* pneumonia.
● **CAUTIONS** Anaemia (treat severe anaemia before starting) · avoid in Acute porphyrias p. 562 · cardiac disease · G6PD deficiency · pulmonary disease · susceptibility to haemolysis
● **INTERACTIONS** → Appendix 1 (dapsone).
● **SIDE-EFFECTS**
▸ **Rare** Stevens-Johnson syndrome · toxic epidermal necrolysis
▸ **Frequency not known** Agranulocytosis · allergic dermatitis · anorexia · dapsone syndrome · haemolysis · headache · hepatitis · insomnia · methaemoglobinaemia · nausea · neuropathy · psychosis · tachycardia · vomiting
SIDE-EFFECTS, FURTHER INFORMATION
▸ **Dapsone syndrome** If dapsone syndrome occurs (rash with fever and eosinophilia)—discontinue immediately (may progress to exfoliative dermatitis, hepatitis, hypoalbuminaemia, psychosis and death).
● **PREGNANCY** Folic acid p. 533 (higher dose) should be given to mother throughout pregnancy; neonatal haemolysis and methaemoglobinaemia reported in third trimester.
● **BREAST FEEDING** Haemolytic anaemia; although significant amount in milk, risk to infant very small unless infant is G6PD deficient.
● **PATIENT AND CARER ADVICE**
Blood disorders On long-term treatment, patients and their carers should be told how to recognise signs of blood disorders and advised to seek immediate medical attention if symptoms such as fever, sore throat, rash, mouth ulcers, purpura, bruising or bleeding develop.
● **MEDICINAL FORMS**
There can be variation in the licensing of different medicines containing the same drug. Forms available from special-order manufacturers include: oral suspension, oral solution
Tablet
CAUTIONARY AND ADVISORY LABELS 8
▸ Dapsone (Non-proprietary)
Dapsone 50 mg Dapsone 50mg tablets | 28 tablet [PoM] £64.77 DT price = £21.12
Dapsone 100 mg Dapsone 100mg tablets | 28 tablet [PoM] £117.80 DT price = £104.60

Pentamidine isetionate

● **INDICATIONS AND DOSE**
Treatment of *Pneumocystis jirovecii* (*Pneumocystis carinii*) pneumonia (specialist use only)
▸ BY INTRAVENOUS INFUSION
▸ Child: 4 mg/kg once daily for at least 7–10 days
Prophylaxis of *Pneumocystis jirovecii* (*Pneumocystis carinii*) pneumonia (specialist use only)
▸ BY INHALATION OF NEBULISED SOLUTION
▸ Child 5–17 years: 300 mg every 4 weeks, alternatively 150 mg every 2 weeks, using suitable equipment—consult product literature
Visceral leishmaniasis (specialist use only)
▸ BY DEEP INTRAMUSCULAR INJECTION
▸ Child 1–17 years: 3–4 mg/kg once daily on alternate days, maximum total of 10 injections, course may be repeated if necessary

Cutaneous leishmaniasis (specialist use only)
▶ BY DEEP INTRAMUSCULAR INJECTION
▶ Child 1-17 years: 3–4 mg/kg 1–2 times a week until condition resolves

Trypanosomiasis (specialist use only)
▶ BY DEEP INTRAMUSCULAR INJECTION, OR BY INTRAVENOUS INFUSION
▶ Child 1-17 years: 4 mg/kg once daily or on alternate days for a total of 7–10 injections

- **UNLICENSED USE** Not licensed for prevention of pneumocystis pneumonia in children.

- **CAUTIONS** Anaemia · bradycardia · coronary heart disease · history of ventricular arrhythmias · hyperglycaemia · hypertension · hypoglycaemia · hypokalaemia · hypomagnesaemia · hypotension · leucopenia · risk of severe hypotension following administration · thrombocytopenia

- **INTERACTIONS** → Appendix 1 (pentamidine isetionate). Caution with concomitant use of other drugs that prolong the QT interval.

- **SIDE-EFFECTS**
  GENERAL SIDE-EFFECTS
  Abnormal liver-function tests · acute renal failure · anaemia · arrhythmias (can be severe and sometimes fatal) · azotaemia · dizziness · flushing · hyperglycaemia · hyperkalaemia · hypocalcaemia · hypoglycaemia (can be severe and sometimes fatal) · hypotension (can be severe and sometimes fatal) · leucopenia · nausea · pancreatitis (can be severe and sometimes fatal) · rash · Stevens-Johnson syndrome · syncope · taste disturbances · thrombocytopenia · vomiting

  SPECIFIC SIDE-EFFECTS
  ▶ When used by inhalation Bronchoconstriction (may be prevented by prior use of bronchodilators) · cough · shortness of breath
  ▶ With intramuscular use Injection site reactions (muscle necrosis, discomfort, pain, induration, abscess formation)
  ▶ With intravenous use Injection site reactions (muscle necrosis, discomfort, pain, induration, abscess formation)

- **PREGNANCY** Manufacturer advises avoid unless essential.

- **BREAST FEEDING** Manufacturer advises avoid unless essential—no information available.

- **HEPATIC IMPAIRMENT** Manufacturer advises caution.

- **RENAL IMPAIRMENT** Reduce intravenous dose for pneumocystis pneumonia if creatinine clearance less than 10 mL/minute: in life-threatening infection, use 4 mg/kg once daily for 7–10 days, then 4 mg/kg on alternate days to complete course of at least 14 doses; in less severe infection, use 4 mg/kg on alternate days for at least 14 doses.

- **MONITORING REQUIREMENTS**
  ▶ Monitor blood pressure before starting treatment, during administration, and at regular intervals, until treatment concluded.
  ▶ Carry out laboratory monitoring according to product literature.

- **DIRECTIONS FOR ADMINISTRATION** Patient should be lying down when receiving drug parenterally. Direct intravenous injection should be avoided whenever possible and **never** given rapidly; intramuscular injections should be deep and preferably given into the buttock. For intravenous infusion, reconstitute 300 mg with 3–5 mL Water for Injections (displacement value may be significant), then dilute required dose with 50–250 mL Glucose 5% or Sodium Chloride 0.9%; give over at least 60 minutes.
  Powder for injection (dissolved in water for injection) may be used for nebulisation.

- **HANDLING AND STORAGE** Pentamidine isetionate is toxic and personnel should be adequately protected during handling and administration—consult product literature.

- **MEDICINAL FORMS**
  There can be variation in the licensing of different medicines containing the same drug.

  Powder for solution for injection
  ▶ Pentacarinat (Sanofi)
  Pentamidine isetionate 300 mg Pentacarinat 300mg powder for solution for injection vials | 5 vial [PoM] £158.86

4 Helminth infection

Helminth infections

Specialist centres

Advice on prophylaxis and treatment of helminth infections is available from the following specialist centres:

Birmingham	(0121) 424 0357
Scotland	Contact local Infectious Diseases Unit
Liverpool	(0151) 705 3100
London	0845 155 5000 (treatment)

Drugs for threadworms

Anthelmintics are effective in threadworm (pinworms, Enterobius vermicularis) infections, but their use needs to be combined with hygienic measures to break the cycle of auto-infection. All members of the family require treatment.

Adult threadworms do not live for longer than 6 weeks and for development of fresh worms, ova must be swallowed and exposed to the action of digestive juices in the upper intestinal tract. Direct multiplication of worms does not take place in the large bowel. Adult female worms lay ova on the perianal skin which causes pruritus; scratching the area then leads to ova being transmitted on fingers to the mouth, often via food eaten with unwashed hands. Washing hands and scrubbing nails before each meal and after each visit to the toilet is essential. A bath taken immediately after rising will remove ova laid during the night.

Mebendazole p. 361 is the drug of choice for treating threadworm infection in patients of all ages over 6 months. It is given as a single dose; as reinfection is very common, a second dose may be given after 2 weeks.

Ascaricides (common roundworm infections)

Mebendazole is effective against Ascaris lumbricoides and is generally considered to be the drug of choice.

Levamisole p. 361 [unlicensed] (available from 'special-order' manufacturers or specialist importing companies) is an alternative when mebendazole cannot be used. It is very well tolerated.

Drugs for tapeworm infections

Taenicides
Niclosamide [unlicensed] (available from 'special-order' manufacturers or specialist importing companies) is the most widely used drug for tapeworm infections and side-effects are limited to occasional gastro-intestinal upset, lightheadedness, and pruritus; it is not effective against larval worms. Fears of developing cysticercosis in Taenia solium infections have proved unfounded. All the same, an antiemetic can be given before treatment and a laxative can be given 2 hours after niclosamide.

Praziquantel p. 362 [unlicensed] (available from 'special-order' manufacturers or specialist importing companies) is as effective as niclosamide.

Hydatid disease

Cysts caused by Echinococcus granulosus grow slowly and asymptomatic patients do not always require treatment.

Surgical treatment remains the method of choice in many situations. Albendazole below [unlicensed] (available from 'special-order' manufacturers or specialist importing companies) is used in conjunction with surgery to reduce the risk of recurrence or as primary treatment in inoperable cases. Alveolar echinococcosis due to *E. multilocularis* is usually fatal if untreated. Surgical removal with albendazole cover is the treatment of choice, but where effective surgery is impossible, repeated cycles of albendazole (for a year or more) may help. Careful monitoring of liver function is particularly important during drug treatment.

Drugs for hookworms

Hookworms (ancylostomiasis, necatoriasis) live in the upper small intestine and draw blood from the point of their attachment to their host. An iron-deficiency anaemia may occur and, if present, effective treatment of the infection requires not only expulsion of the worms but treatment of the anaemia.

Mebendazole has a useful broad-spectrum activity, and is effective against hookworms. Albendazole [unlicensed] (available from 'special-order' manufacturers or specialist importing companies) is an alternative. Levamisole is also is also effective in children.

Schistosomicides (bilharziasis)

Adult *Schistosoma haematobium* worms live in the genitourinary veins and adult *S. mansoni* in those of the colon and mesentery.*S. japonicum* is more widely distributed in veins of the alimentary tract and portal system.

Praziquantel [unlicensed] is available from Merck Serono (*Cysticide®*) and is effective against all human schistosomes. No serious adverse effects have been reported. Of all the available schistosomicides, it has the most attractive combination of effectiveness, broad-spectrum activity, and low toxicity.

Filaricides

Diethylcarbamazine [unlicensed] (available from 'special-order' manufacturers or specialist importing companies) is effective against microfilariae and adults of *Loa loa*, *Wuchereria bancrofti*, and *Brugia malayi*. To minimise reactions, treatment in adults and children over 1 month, is commenced with a dose of diethylcarbamazine citrate on the first day and increased gradually over 3 days. Length of treatment varies according to infection type, and usually gives a radical cure for these infections. Close medical supervision is necessary particularly in the early phase of treatment.

In heavy infections there may be a febrile reaction, and in heavy *Loa loa* infection there is a small risk of encephalopathy. In such cases specialist advice should be sought, and treatment must be given under careful in-patient supervision and stopped at the first sign of cerebral involvement.

Ivermectin p. 361 [unlicensed] (available from 'special-order' manufacturers or specialist importing companies) is very effective in *onchocerciasis* and it is now the drug of choice; reactions are usually slight. Diethylcarbamazine or suramin should no longer be used for *onchocerciasis* because of their toxicity.

Drugs for cutaneous larva migrans (creeping eruption)

Dog and cat hookworm larvae may enter human skin where they produce slowly extending itching tracks usually on the foot. Single tracks can be treated with topical tiabendazole (no commercial preparation available). Multiple infections respond to ivermectin, albendazole or **tiabendazole** (thiabendazole) by mouth [all unlicensed] (available from 'special-order' manufacturers or specialist importing companies).

Drugs for strongyloidiasis

Adult *Strongyloides stercoralis* live in the gut and produce larvae which penetrate the gut wall and invade the tissues, setting up a cycle of auto-infection. Ivermectin [unlicensed] (available from 'special-order' manufacturers or specialist importing companies) is the treatment of choice for chronic *Strongyloides* infection in adults and children over 5 years. Albendazole [unlicensed] (available from 'special order' manufacturers or specialist importing companies) is an alternative given to adults and children over 2 years.

ANTHELMINTICS

▌Albendazole

● **INDICATIONS AND DOSE**

Chronic *Strongyloides* infection

▸ BY MOUTH

▸ Child 2–17 years: 400 mg twice daily for 3 days, dose may be repeated after 3 weeks if necessary

Hydatid disease, in conjunction with surgery to reduce the risk of recurrence or as primary treatment in inoperable cases

▸ BY MOUTH

▸ Child 2–17 years: 7.5 mg/kg twice daily (max. per dose 400 mg twice daily) for 28 days followed by 14-day break, repeated for up to 2–3 cycles

Hookworm infections

▸ BY MOUTH

▸ Child 2–17 years: 400 mg for 1 dose

● **UNLICENSED USE** Albendazole is an unlicensed drug.

● **INTERACTIONS** → Appendix 1 (albendazole).

● **MEDICINAL FORMS**
There can be variation in the licensing of different medicines containing the same drug. Forms available from special-order manufacturers include: tablet, chewable tablet, oral suspension

Tablet
CAUTIONARY AND ADVISORY LABELS 9

▸ Albendazole (Non-proprietary)
  Albendazole 400 mg Eskazole 400mg tablets | 60 tablet ᴘᴏᴹ no price available

Chewable tablet
CAUTIONARY AND ADVISORY LABELS 9

▸ Albendazole (Non-proprietary)
  Albendazole 200 mg Zentel 200mg chewable tablets | 6 tablet ᴘᴏᴹ no price available
  Albendazole 400 mg Zentel 400mg chewable tablets | 1 tablet ᴘᴏᴹ no price available | 3 tablet ᴘᴏᴹ no price available

▌Diethylcarbamazine

● **INDICATIONS AND DOSE**

***Wuchereria bancrofti* infections | *Brugia malayi* infections**

▸ BY MOUTH

▸ Child 1 month–9 years: Initially 1 mg/kg daily in divided doses on the first day, then increased to 3 mg/kg daily in divided doses, dose to be increased gradually over 3 days

▸ Child 10–17 years: Initially 1 mg/kg daily in divided doses on the first day, then increased to 6 mg/kg daily in divided doses, dose to be increased gradually over 3 days

***Loa loa* infections**

▸ BY MOUTH

▸ Child 1 month–9 years: Initially 1 mg/kg daily in divided doses on the first day, then increased to 3 mg/kg daily in divided doses, dose to be increased gradually over 3 days

▸ **Child 10-17 years:** Initially 1 mg/kg daily in divided doses on the first day, then increased to 6 mg/kg daily in divided doses, dose to be increased gradually over 3 days

● UNLICENSED USE Diethylcarbamazine is an unlicensed drug.

● INTERACTIONS → Appendix 1 (diethylcarbamazine).

● MEDICINAL FORMS
There can be variation in the licensing of different medicines containing the same drug.
No licensed medicines listed.

Ivermectin

● INDICATIONS AND DOSE
Chronic *Strongyloides* infection
▸ BY MOUTH
▸ **Child 5-17 years:** 200 micrograms/kg daily for 2 days
Onchocerciasis
▸ BY MOUTH
▸ **Child 5-17 years:** 150 micrograms/kg for 1 dose, retreatment at intervals of 6 to 12 months may be required depending on symptoms
Scabies, in combination with topical drugs, for the treatment of hyperkeratotic (crusted or 'Norwegian') scabies that does not respond to topical treatment alone
▸ BY MOUTH
▸ **Child:** (consult product literature)

● UNLICENSED USE Ivermectin is an unlicensed drug.
● INTERACTIONS → Appendix 1 (ivermectin).
● SIDE-EFFECTS Aggravation of itching · aggravation of rash

● MEDICINAL FORMS
There can be variation in the licensing of different medicines containing the same drug. Forms available from special-order manufacturers include: tablet
Tablet
▸ Ivermectin (Non-proprietary)
Ivermectin 3 mg Stromectol 3mg tablets | 4 tablet PoM no price available | 20 tablet PoM no price available

Levamisole

● INDICATIONS AND DOSE
Roundworm infections
▸ BY MOUTH
▸ **Child:** 2.5-3 mg/kg (max. per dose 150 mg) for 1 dose
Hookworm infections
▸ BY MOUTH
▸ **Child:** 2.5 mg/kg (max. per dose 150 mg) for 1 dose, dose to be repeated after 7 days if severe
Nephrotic syndrome (initiated under specialist supervision)
▸ BY MOUTH
▸ **Child:** 2.5 mg/kg once daily on alternate days (max. per dose 150 mg)

● UNLICENSED USE Not licensed.
● CONTRA-INDICATIONS Blood disorders
● CAUTIONS Epilepsy · juvenile idiopathic arthritis · Sjögren's syndrome
● INTERACTIONS → Appendix 1 (levamisole).
● SIDE-EFFECTS Arthralgia (on *prolonged treatment*) · blood disorders (on *prolonged treatment*) · convulsions (on *prolonged treatment*) · diarrhoea · dizziness · headache · influenza-like syndrome (on *prolonged treatment*) · insomnia (on *prolonged treatment*) · myalgia (on *prolonged*

treatment) · nausea · rash (on *prolonged treatment*) · taste disturbances (on *prolonged treatment*) · vasculitis (on *prolonged treatment*) · vomiting

● PREGNANCY Embryotoxic in *animal* studies, avoid if possible.
● BREAST FEEDING No information available.
● HEPATIC IMPAIRMENT Use with caution—dose adjustment may be necessary.
● PATIENT AND CARER ADVICE
Medicines for Children leaflet: Levamisole for nephrotic syndrome www.medicinesforchildren.org.uk/levamisole-for-nephrotic-syndrome

● MEDICINAL FORMS
There can be variation in the licensing of different medicines containing the same drug. Forms available from special-order manufacturers include: tablet
Tablet
CAUTIONARY AND ADVISORY LABELS 4
▸ Ergamisol (Imported (Belgium))
Levamisole (as Levamisole hydrochloride) 50 mg Ergamisol 50mg tablets | 20 tablet PoM no price available

Mebendazole

● INDICATIONS AND DOSE
Threadworm infections
▸ BY MOUTH
▸ **Child 6 months-17 years:** 100 mg for 1 dose, if reinfection occurs, second dose may be needed after 2 weeks
Whipworm infections | Hookworm infections
▸ BY MOUTH
▸ **Child 1-17 years:** 100 mg twice daily for 3 days
Roundworm infections
▸ BY MOUTH
▸ **Child 1 year:** 100 mg twice daily for 3 days
▸ **Child 2-17 years:** 100 mg twice daily for 3 days, alternatively 500 mg for 1 dose

● UNLICENSED USE Not licensed for use in children under 2 years. Treatment of roundworm infections with mebendazole 500 mg as a single dose is an unlicensed dose.
● INTERACTIONS → Appendix 1 (mebendazole).
● SIDE-EFFECTS
▸ **Common or very common** Abdominal pain
▸ **Uncommon** Diarrhoea · flatulence
▸ **Rare** Alopecia · convulsions · dizziness · hepatitis · neutropenia · rash · Stevens- Johnson syndrome · toxic epidermal necrolysis · urticaria
● PREGNANCY Manufacturer advises avoid—toxicity in *animal* studies.
● BREAST FEEDING Amount present in milk too small to be harmful but manufacturer advises avoid.
● PRESCRIBING AND DISPENSING INFORMATION Flavours of oral liquid formulations may include banana.
● PATIENT AND CARER ADVICE
Medicines for Children leaflet: Mebendazole for worm infections www.medicinesforchildren.org.uk/mebendazole-for-worm-infections
● EXCEPTIONS TO LEGAL CATEGORY Mebendazole tablets can be sold to the public if supplied for oral use in the treatment of enterobiasis in adults and children over 2 years provided its container or package is labelled to show a max. single dose of 100 mg and it is supplied in a container or package containing not more than 800 mg.

● MEDICINAL FORMS
There can be variation in the licensing of different medicines
containing the same drug.
Chewable tablet
▶ Ovex (McNeil Products Ltd)
Mebendazole 100 mg Ovex 100mg chewable tablets sugar-free |
1 tablet [P] £2.03 sugar-free | 4 tablet [P] £4.74
▶ Vermox (Janssen-Cilag Ltd)
Mebendazole 100 mg Vermox 100mg chewable tablets sugar-free |
6 tablet [PoM] £1.34 DT price = £1.34
Oral suspension
▶ Ovex (McNeil Products Ltd)
Mebendazole 20 mg per 1 ml Ovex 100mg/5ml oral suspension |
30 ml [P] £6.03 DT price = £1.55
▶ Vermox (Janssen-Cilag Ltd)
Mebendazole 20 mg per 1 ml Vermox 100mg/5ml oral suspension
| 30 ml [PoM] £1.55 DT price = £1.55

Praziquantel

● **INDICATIONS AND DOSE**
Tapeworm infections (*Taenia solium*)
▶ BY MOUTH
▶ Child 4–17 years: 5–10 mg/kg for 1 dose, to be taken
after a light breakfast
Tapeworm infections (*Hymenolepis nana*)
▶ BY MOUTH
▶ Child 4–17 years: 25 mg/kg for 1 dose, to be taken after a
light breakfast
**_Schistosoma haematobium_ worm infections | _Schistosoma
mansoni_ worm infections**
▶ BY MOUTH
▶ Child 4–17 years: 20 mg/kg, followed by 20 mg/kg after
4–6 hours
Schistosoma japonicum worm infections
▶ BY MOUTH
▶ Child 4–17 years: 20 mg/kg 3 times a day for 1 day

● UNLICENSED USE Praziquantel is an unlicensed drug.

● INTERACTIONS → Appendix 1 (praziquantel).

● MEDICINAL FORMS
There can be variation in the licensing of different medicines
containing the same drug. Forms available from special-order
manufacturers include: tablet
Tablet
▶ Praziquantel (Non-proprietary)
Praziquantel 150 mg Cesol 150mg tablets | 6 tablet [PoM] no price
available
Praziquantel 600 mg Biltricide 600mg tablets | 6 tablet [PoM] no
price available
▶ Cysticide (Imported (Germany))
Praziquantel 500 mg Cysticide 500mg tablets | 90 tablet [PoM] no
price available

5 Protozoal infection

Antiprotozoal drugs

Amoebicides

Metronidazole p. 313 is the drug of choice for *acute invasive
amoebic dysentery* since it is very effective against vegetative
forms of *Entamoeba histolytica* in ulcers. Tinidazole p. 315 is
also effective. Metronidazole and tinidazole are also active
against amoebae which may have migrated to the liver.
Treatment with metronidazole (or tinidazole) is followed by
a 10-day course of diloxanide furoate p. 281.

Diloxanide furoate is the drug of choice for asymptomatic
patients with *E. histolytica* cysts in the faeces; metronidazole
and tinidazole are relatively ineffective. Diloxanide furoate is

relatively free from toxic effects and the usual course is of
10 days, given alone for chronic infections or following
metronidazole or tinidazole treatment.

For *amoebic abscesses* of the liver metronidazole is
effective; tinidazole is an alternative. Aspiration of the
abscess is indicated where it is suspected that it may rupture
or where there is no improvement after 72 hours of
metronidazole; the aspiration may need to be repeated.
Aspiration aids penetration of metronidazole and, for
abscesses with large volumes of pus, if carried out in
conjunction with drug therapy, may reduce the period of
disability.

Diloxanide furoate is not effective against hepatic
amoebiasis, but a 10-day course should be given at the
completion of metronidazole or tinidazole treatment to
destroy any amoebae in the gut.

Trichomonacides

Metronidazole is the treatment of choice for *Trichomonas
vaginalis* infection. Contact tracing is recommended and
sexual contacts should be treated simultaneously. If
metronidazole is ineffective, tinidazole may be tried.

Antigiardial drugs

Metronidazole is the treatment of choice for *Giardia lamblia*
infections. Tinidazole may be used as an alternative to
metronidazole.

Leishmaniacides

Cutaneous leishmaniasis frequently heals spontaneously but
if skin lesions are extensive or unsightly, treatment is
indicated, as it is in visceral leishmaniasis (kala-azar).
Leishmaniasis should be treated under specialist
supervision.

Sodium stibogluconate p. 363, an organic pentavalent
antimony compound, is used for visceral leishmaniasis. The
dosage varies with different geographical regions and expert
advice should be obtained. Skin lesions can also be treated
with sodium stibogluconate.

Amphotericin p. 351 is used with or after an antimony
compound for visceral leishmaniasis unresponsive to the
antimonial alone; side-effects may be reduced by using
liposomal amphotericin (*AmBisome®*). *Abelcet®*, a lipid
formulation of amphotericin is also likely to be effective but
less information is available.

Pentamidine isetionate p. 358 (pentamidine isethionate)
has been used in antimony-resistant visceral leishmaniasis,
but although the initial response is often good, the relapse
rate is high; it is associated with serious side-effects. Other
treatments include paromomycin [unlicensed] (available
from 'special-order' manufacturers or specialist importing
companies).

Trypanocides

The prophylaxis and treatment of trypanosomiasis is difficult
and differs according to the strain of organism. Expert advice
should therefore be obtained.

Drugs for toxoplasmosis

Most infections caused by *Toxoplasma gondii* are self-
limiting, and treatment is not necessary. Exceptions are
patients with eye involvement (toxoplasma
choroidoretinitis), and those who are immunosuppressed.
Toxoplasmic encephalitis is a common complication of
AIDS. The treatment of choice is a combination of
pyrimethamine p. 375 and sulfadiazine p. 331, given for
several weeks (expert advice **essential**). Pyrimethamine is a
folate antagonist, and adverse reactions to this combination
are relatively common (folinic acid supplements and weekly
blood counts needed). Alternative regimens use
combinations of pyrimethamine with clindamycin p. 307 or
clarithromycin p. 309 or azithromycin p. 308. Long-term

secondary prophylaxis is required after treatment of toxoplasmosis in immunocompromised patients; prophylaxis should continue until immunity recovers.

If toxoplasmosis is acquired in pregnancy, transplacental infection may lead to severe disease in the fetus; specialist advice should be sought on management. Spiramycin [unlicensed] (available from 'special-order' manufacturers or specialist importing companies) may reduce the risk of transmission of maternal infection to the fetus. When there is evidence of placental or fetal infection, pyrimethamine may be given with sulfadiazine and folinic acid p. 515 after the first trimester.

In neonates without signs of toxoplasmosis, but born to mothers known to have become infected, spiramycin is given while awaiting laboratory results. If toxoplasmosis is confirmed in the infant, pyrimethamine and sulfadiazine are given for 12 months, together with folinic acid.

5.1 Leishmaniasis

ANTIPROTOZOALS

Sodium stibogluconate

● **INDICATIONS AND DOSE**
Visceral leishmaniasis (specialist use only)
▶ BY INTRAVENOUS INJECTION, OR BY INTRAMUSCULAR INJECTION
▶ Child: 20 mg/kg daily for at least 20 days

● **UNLICENSED USE** Licensed for use in children (age range not specified by manufacturer).

● **CAUTIONS** Heart disease (withdraw if conduction disturbances occur) · mucocutaneous disease · predisposition to QT interval prolongation · treat intercurrent infection (e.g. pneumonia)

CAUTIONS, FURTHER INFORMATION
▶ Mucocutaneous disease Successful treatment of mucocutaneous leishmaniasis may induce severe inflammation around the lesions (may be life-threatening if pharyngeal or tracheal involvement)—may require corticosteroid.

● **INTERACTIONS** → Appendix 1 (sodium stibogluconate). Caution with concomitant use of drugs that prolong QT interval.

● **SIDE-EFFECTS**
▶ **Rare** Bleeding from gums · bleeding from nose · fever · flushing · jaundice · rash · substernal pain · sweating · vertigo
▶ **Frequency not known** Abdominal pain · anaphylaxis · anorexia · arthralgia · coughing · diarrhoea · ECG changes · headache · lethargy · myalgia · nausea · pain on intramuscular injection · pain on intravenous administration · pancreatitis · thrombosis on intravenous administration · vomiting

● **PREGNANCY** Manufacturer advises use only if potential benefit outweighs risk.

● **BREAST FEEDING** Amount probably too small to be harmful.

● **HEPATIC IMPAIRMENT** Use with caution.

● **RENAL IMPAIRMENT** Avoid in significant impairment.

● **MONITORING REQUIREMENTS** Monitor ECG before and during treatment.

● **DIRECTIONS FOR ADMINISTRATION** Intravenous injections must be given slowly over 5 minutes (to reduce risk of local thrombosis) and stopped if coughing or substernal pain occur. Injection should be filtered immediately before administration using a filter of 5 microns or less.

● **MEDICINAL FORMS**
There can be variation in the licensing of different medicines containing the same drug.
Solution for injection
▶ Pentostam (GlaxoSmithKline UK Ltd)
Antimony pentavalent (as Sodium stibogluconate) 100 mg per 1 ml Pentostam 10g/100ml solution for injection vials | 1 vial [PoM] £66.43

5.2 Malaria

Antimalarials

Artemether with lumefantrine

Artemether with lumefantrine p. 370 is licensed for the *treatment of acute non-complicated falciparum malaria*.

Chloroquine

Chloroquine p. 372 is used for the *prophylaxis of malaria* in areas of the world where the *risk of chloroquine-resistant falciparum malaria is still low*. It is also used with proguanil hydrochloride p. 375 when chloroquine-resistant falciparum malaria is present but this regimen may not give optimal protection (see Recommended regimens for prophylaxis against malaria p. 366).

Chloroquine is **no longer recommended** for the *treatment of falciparum malaria* owing to widespread resistance, nor is it recommended if the infective species is *not known* or if the infection is *mixed*; in these cases treatment should be with quinine p. 376, *Malarone*®, or *Riamet*®. It is still recommended for the *treatment of non-falciparum malaria*.

Mefloquine

Mefloquine p. 373 is used for the *prophylaxis of malaria* in areas of the world where there is a *high risk of chloroquine resistant falciparum malaria* (for details, see Recommended regimens for prophylaxis against malaria p. 366).

Mefloquine is now rarely used for the *treatment of falciparum malaria* because of increased resistance. It is rarely used for the *treatment of non-falciparum malaria* because better tolerated alternatives are available. Mefloquine should not be used for treatment if it has been used for prophylaxis.

Piperaquine with artenimol

Artenimol with piperaquine phosphate p. 371 is not recommended for the first-line treatment of acute uncomplicated falciparum malaria because there is limited experience of its use in travellers who usually reside in areas where malaria is not endemic. Piperaquine has a long half-life.

Primaquine

Primaquine p. 374 is used to eliminate the liver stages of *P. vivax* or *P. ovale* following chloroquine treatment.

Proguanil

Proguanil hydrochloride is used (usually *with chloroquine*, but occasionally *alone*) for the *prophylaxis of malaria*, (for details, see Recommended regimens for prophylaxis against malaria p. 366).

Proguanil hydrochloride used alone is not suitable for the *treatment of malaria*; however, *Malarone*® (a combination of atovaquone with proguanil hydrochloride p. 371) is licensed for the treatment of acute uncomplicated falciparum malaria. *Malarone*® is also used for the *prophylaxis of falciparum malaria* in areas of *widespread mefloquine or chloroquine resistance*. *Malarone*® is also used as an alternative to mefloquine or doxycycline p. 332. *Malarone*® is particularly suitable for short trips to highly chloroquine-resistant areas because it needs to be taken only for 7 days after leaving an endemic area.

Pyrimethamine

Pyrimethamine p. 375 should not be used alone, but is used with sulfadoxine.

Pyrimethamine with sulfadoxine p. 375 is not recommended for the *prophylaxis of malaria*, but can be used in the *treatment of falciparum malaria with (or following) quinine*.

Quinine

Quinine is not suitable for the *prophylaxis of malaria*.

Quinine is used for the *treatment of falciparum malaria* or if the infective species is *not known* or if the infection is mixed (for details see Malaria, treatment p. 365).

Tetracyclines

Doxycycline is used in adults and children over 12 years for the *prophylaxis of malaria* in areas of *widespread mefloquine* or *chloroquine resistance*. Doxycycline is also used as an alternative to mefloquine or *Malarone*® (for details, see Recommended regimens for prophylaxis against malaria p. 366).

Malaria, prophylaxis

Prophylaxis against malaria

The recommendations on prophylaxis reflect guidelines agreed by UK malaria specialists; the advice is aimed at residents of the UK who travel to endemic areas. The choice of drug for a particular individual should take into account:

- risk of exposure to malaria
- extent of drug resistance
- efficacy of the recommended drugs
- side-effects of the drugs
- patient-related factors (e.g. age, pregnancy, renal or hepatic impairment, compliance with prophylactic regimen)

Prophylactic doses are based on guidelines agreed by UK malaria experts and may differ from advice in product literature. **Weight is a better guide than age**. If in doubt obtain advice from specialist centre (see under Malaria, treatment p. 365).

Protection against bites

Prophylaxis is not absolute, and breakthrough infection can occur with any of the drugs recommended. Personal protection against being bitten is very important. Mosquito nets impregnated with permethrin provide the most effective barrier protection against insects (infants should sleep with a mosquito net not stretched over the cot or baby carrier); mats and vaporised insecticides are also useful. Diethyltoluamide (DEET) 20–50% in lotions, sprays, or roll-on formulations is safe and effective when applied to the skin of adults and children over 2 months of age. It can also be used during pregnancy and breast-feeding. The duration of protection varies according to the concentration of DEET and is longest for DEET 50%. When sunscreen is also required, DEET should be applied after the sunscreen. DEET reduces the SPF of sunscreen, so a sunscreen of SPF 30-50 should be applied. Long sleeves and trousers worn after dusk also provide protection against bites.

Length of prophylaxis

In order to determine tolerance and to establish habit, prophylaxis should generally be started one week (2–3 weeks in the case of mefloquine p. 373) before travel into an endemic area; *Malarone*® or doxycycline p. 332 prophylaxis should be started 1–2 days before travel. Prophylaxis should be continued for **4 weeks after leaving** (except for *Malarone*® prophylaxis which should be stopped 1 week after

leaving). For extensive journeys across different regions, the traveller must be protected in all areas of risk.

In those requiring long-term prophylaxis, chloroquine p. 372 and proguanil hydrochloride p. 375 may be used for periods of over 5 years. Mefloquine is licensed for up to 1 year (although, if it is tolerated in the short term, there is no evidence of harm when it is used for up to 3 years). Doxycycline can be used for up to 2 years. *Malarone*® can be used for up to 1 year. Prophylaxis with mefloquine, doxycycline, or *Malarone*® may be considered for longer durations if it is justified by the risk of exposure to malaria. Specialist advice should be sought for long-term prophylaxis.

Return from malarial region

It is important to be aware that **any illness** that occurs within 1 year and **especially within 3 months of return might be malaria** even if all recommended precautions against malaria were taken. Travellers should be **warned** of this and told that if they develop any illness **particularly within 3 months** of their return they should go **immediately** to a doctor and specifically mention their exposure to malaria.

Epilepsy

Both chloroquine and mefloquine are unsuitable for malaria prophylaxis in individuals with a history of epilepsy. In areas *without chloroquine resistance* proguanil alone is recommended; in areas *with chloroquine resistance*, doxycycline or *Malarone*® may be considered.

Asplenia

Asplenic individuals (or those with severe splenic dysfunction) are at particular risk of severe malaria. If travel to malarious areas is unavoidable, rigorous precautions are required against contracting the disease.

Renal impairment

Avoidance (or dosage reduction) of proguanil hydrochloride is recommended since it is excreted by the kidneys. *Malarone*® should not be used for prophylaxis in patients with estimated glomerular filtration rate less than 30 mL/minute/1.73m². Chloroquine is only partially excreted by the kidneys and reduction of the dose for prophylaxis is not required except in severe impairment. Mefloquine is considered to be appropriate to use in renal impairment and does not require dosage reduction. Doxycycline is also considered to be appropriate.

Pregnancy

Travel to malarious areas should be avoided during pregnancy; if travel is unavoidable, effective prophylaxis must be used. Chloroquine and proguanil hydrochloride can be given in the usual doses during pregnancy, but these drugs are not appropriate for most areas because their effectiveness has declined, particularly in Sub-Saharan Africa; in the case of proguanil hydrochloride, folic acid p. 533 (in doses greater than standard pregnancy prophylaxis) should be given for at least the first trimester. The centres listed (see Malaria, treatment p. 365) should be consulted for advice on prophylaxis in chloroquine-resistant areas. Although the manufacturer advises that mefloquine should not be used during pregnancy, particularly in the first trimester, unless the potential benefit outweighs the risk, studies of mefloquine in pregnancy (including use in the first trimester) indicate that it can be considered for travel to chloroquine-resistant areas. Doxycycline is contra-indicated during pregnancy; however, it can be used for malaria prophylaxis if other regimens are unsuitable, and if the entire course of doxycycline can be completed before 15 weeks' gestation [unlicensed]. *Malarone*® should be avoided during pregnancy, however, it can be considered during the second and third trimesters if there is no suitable alternative.

5

Infection

Breast-feeding

Prophylaxis is required in **breast-fed infants**; although antimalarials are present in milk, the amounts are too variable to give reliable protection.

Anticoagulants

Travellers taking warfarin sodium p. 89 should begin chemoprophylaxis 2–3 weeks before departure. The INR should be stable before departure. It should be measured before starting chemoprophylaxis, 7 days after starting, and after completing the course. For prolonged stays, the INR should be checked at regular intervals.

Standby treatment

Children and their carers visiting remote, malarious areas for prolonged periods should carry standby treatment if they are likely to be more than 24 hours away from medical care. Self-medication should be **avoided** if medical help is accessible.

In order to avoid excessive self-medication, the traveller should be provided with **written instructions** that urgent medical attention should be sought if fever (38°C or more) develops 7 days (or more) after arriving in a malarious area and that self-treatment is indicated if medical help is not available within 24 hours of fever onset.

In view of the continuing emergence of resistant strains and of the different regimens required for different areas expert advice should be sought on the best treatment course for an individual traveller. A drug used for chemoprophylaxis should not be considered for standby treatment for the same traveller.

Specific recommendations

Where a journey requires two regimens, the regimen for the higher risk area should be used for the whole journey. Those travelling to remote or little-visited areas may require expert advice. See also *Recommended regimens for prophylaxis against malaria* .

Important

Settled immigrants (or long-term visitors) to the UK may be unaware that **any immunity they may have acquired while living in malarious areas is lost rapidly** after migration to the UK, or that any non-malarious areas where they lived previously **may now be malarious**.

Malaria, treatment

Advice for healthcare professionals

A number of specialist centres are able to provide advice on specific problems.

PHE (Public Health England) Malaria Reference Laboratory (020) 7637 0248 (fax) (prophylaxis only) www.malaria-reference.co.uk

National Travel Health Network and Centre 0845 602 6712

Travel Medicine Team, Health Protection Scotland (registered users of Travax only) www.travax.nhs.uk (for registered users of the NHS Travax website only) (0141) 300 1100 (weekdays 2–4 p.m. only)

Birmingham (0121) 424 2358

Liverpool (0151) 705 3100

London 0845 155 5000 (treatment)

Oxford (01865) 225 430

Advice for travellers

Hospital for Tropical Diseases Travel Healthline (020) 7950 7799 www.fitfortravel.nhs.uk

WHO advice on international travel and health www.who.int/ith

National Travel Health Network and Centre (NaTHNaC) www.nathnac.org/travel/index.htm

Treatment

Recommendations on the prophylaxis and treatment of malaria reflect guidelines agreed by UK malaria specialists. Choice will depend on the age of the child.

If the infective species is **not known**, or if the infection is **mixed**, initial treatment should be as for *falciparum malaria* with quinine p. 376, *Malarone*® (atovaquone with proguanil hydrochloride p. 371), or *Riamet*® (artemether with lumefantrine p. 370). Falciparum malaria can progress rapidly in unprotected individuals and antimalarial treatment should be considered in those with features of severe malaria and possible exposure, even if the initial blood tests for the organism are negative.

Falciparum malaria (treatment)

Falciparum malaria (malignant malaria) is caused by *Plasmodium falciparum*. In most parts of the world *P. falciparum* is now resistant to chloroquine p. 372 which should not therefore be given for treatment. Quinine, *Malarone*® (atovaquone with proguanil hydrochloride), or *Riamet*® (artemether with lumefantrine) can be given by mouth if the child can swallow and retain tablets and there are no serious manifestations (e.g. impaired consciousness); quinine should be given by intravenous infusion if the child is seriously ill or unable to take tablets. Mefloquine p. 373 is now rarely used for treatment because of concerns about resistance.

Oral quinine is well tolerated by children although the salts are bitter. Quinine is given by mouth together with or followed by clindamycin p. 307 [unlicensed indication] or, in children over 12 doxycycline p. 332.

If the parasite is likely to be sensitive, pyrimethamine with sulfadoxine p. 375 as a single dose [unlicensed] may be given (instead of either clindamycin or doxycycline) together with, or after, a course of quinine.

Alternatively, *Malarone*®, or *Riamet*® may be given instead of quinine. It is not necessary to give clindamycin, doxycycline, or pyrimethamine with sulfadoxine after *Malarone*® or *Riamet*® treatment.

If the child is seriously ill or unable to swallow tablets, or if more than 2% of red blood cell are parasitized, quinine should be given by *intravenous infusion* [unlicensed] (until patient can swallow tablets to complete the 7-day course *together with* or *followed by either* doxycycline in children over 12 years, or clindamycin).

Specialist advice should be sought in difficult cases (e.g. very high parasite count, deterioration on optimal doses of quinine, infection acquired in quinine-resistant areas of south east Asia) because intravenous **artesunate** may be available for 'named-patient' use.

Pregnancy

Falciparum malaria is particularly dangerous in pregnancy, especially in the last trimester. The treatment doses of oral and intravenous quinine (including the loading dose) can safely be given in pregnancy. Clindamycin [unlicensed indication] should be given for 7 days with or after quinine. Doxycycline should be avoided in pregnancy (affects teeth and skeletal development in fetus); pyrimethamine with sulfadoxine, Malarone®, and Riamet® are also best avoided until more information is available. Specialist advice should be sought in difficult cases (e.g. very high parasite count, deterioration on optimal doses of quinine, infection acquired in quinine-resistant areas of south east Asia) because intravenous artesunate may be available for 'named patient' use.

Non-falciparum malaria (treatment)

Non-falciparum malaria is usually caused by *Plasmodium vivax* and less commonly by *P. ovale* and *P. malariae*. *P. knowlesi* is also present in the Asia-Pacific region. Chloroquine is the drug of choice for the treatment of non-falciparum malaria (but chloroquine-resistant *P. vivax* has been reported in the Indonesian archipelago, the Malay

Key to recommended regimens for prophylaxis against malaria

Codes for regimens	Details of regimens for prophylaxis against malaria
1	Chemoprophylaxis not recommended, but avoid mosquito bites and consider malaria if fever presents
2	Chloroquine only
3	Chloroquine with proguanil
4	Atovaquone with proguanil hydrochloride or doxycycline or mefloquine
5	Atovaquone with proguanil hydrochloride or doxycycline

Specific recommendations

Country	Comments on risk of malaria and regional or seasonal variation	Codes for regimens
Afghanistan	Risk below 2000 m from May–November	3
	Low risk below 2000 m from December–April	1
Algeria	Very low risk in Illizi department only	1
Andaman and Nicobar Islands (India)	Risk present	1
Angola	High risk	4
Argentina	Low risk in low altitude areas of Salta provinces bordering Bolivia and in Chaco, Corrientes, and Misiones provinces close to border with Paraguay and Brazil	2
	No risk in Iguaçu Falls and areas other than those above	1
Armenia	No risk	1
Azerbaijan	Low to no risk	1
Bangladesh	High risk in Chittagong Hill Tract districts (but not Chittagong city)	4
	Low to no risk in Chittagong city and other areas, except Chittagong Hill Tract districts	1
Belize	Low risk in rural areas	2
	No risk in Belize district (including Belize city and islands)	1
Benin	High risk	4
Bhutan	Risk in southern belt districts, along border with India: Chukha, Geyleg-phug, Samchi, Samdrup Jonkhar, and Shemgang	3
	Low to no risk in areas other than those above	1
Bolivia	High risk in Amazon basin	4
	Risk in rural areas below 2500 m (other than above)	2
	No risk above 2500 m	1
Botswana	High risk from November–June in northern half, including Okavango Delta area	4
	Low risk from July–October in northern half; low to no risk all year in southern half	1
Brazil	Risk in Amazon basin, including city of Manaus	4
	Very low risk in areas other than those above, and no risk in Iguaçu Falls	1
Brunei Darussalam	Very low risk	1
Burkina Faso	High risk	4
Burundi	High risk	4
Cambodia	High risk, with widespread chloroquine and mefloquine resistance, in western provinces bordering Thailand	5
	High risk in areas other than those above and below	4
	Very low risk in Angkor Wat and Lake Tonle Sap, including Siem Reap; no risk in Phnom Penh	1
Cameroon	High risk	4
Cape Verde	Very low risk on island of Santiago (Sao Tiago) and Boa Vista	1
Central African Republic	High risk	4
Chad	High risk	4
China	High risk in Yunnan and Hainan provinces	4
	Very low risk in areas other than those above and below	1
	No risk in Hong Kong	–
Colombia	High risk in rural areas below 1600 m	4
	Low to no risk above 1600 m and in Cartagena	1
Comoros	High risk	4

Country	Comments on risk of malaria and regional or seasonal variation	Codes for regimens
Congo	High risk	4
Costa Rica	Risk in Limon province (but not city of Limon)	2
	Very low risk in areas other than those above	1
Cote d'Ivoire (Ivory Coast)	High risk	4
Democratic Republic of the Congo	High risk	4
Djibouti	High risk	4
Dominican Republic	Risk in all areas except cities of Santiago and Santo Domingo	2
	Cities of Santiago and Santo Domingo	1
East Timor (Timor-Leste)	High risk	4
Ecuador	Risk in areas below 1500 m including coastal provinces and Amazon basin (no risk in Galapagos islands or city of Guayaquil)	4
Egypt	No risk	1
El Salvador	Low risk in rural areas of Santa Ana, Ahuachapán, and La Unión provinces in western part of country; low to no risk in other areas	1
Equatorial Guinea	High risk	4
Eritrea	High risk below 2200 m	4
Ethiopia	High risk below 2000 m	4
French Guiana	High risk (particularly in border areas) except city of Cayenne or Devil's Island (Ile du Diable)	4
	No risk in city of Cayenne or Devil's Island (Ile du Diable)	1
Gabon	High risk	4
Gambia	High risk	4
Georgia	Very low risk in rural south east from June–October	1
Ghana	High risk	4
Guatemala	Low risk below 1500 m	2
	No risk in Guatemala City, Antigua, or Lake Atitlan	-
Guinea	High risk	4
Guinea-Bissau	High risk	4
Guyana	High risk in all interior regions	4
	Very low risk in Georgetown and coastal region	1
Haiti	Risk present	2
Honduras	Risk below 1000 m and in Roatán and other Bay Islands (no risk in San Pedro Sula or Tegucigalpa)	2
India	High risk in states of Assam and Orissa, districts of East Godavari, Srikakulam, Vishakhapatnam, and Vizianagaram in the state of Andhra Pradesh, and districts of Balaghat, Dindori, Mandla, and Seoni in the state of Madhya Pradesh	4
	Risk in areas other than those above or below (including Goa, Andaman and Nicobar islands)	1
	No risk in Lakshadweep islands	-
Indonesia	High risk in Lombok and Irian Jaya (Papua)	4
	Risk in areas other than those above or below	3
	Very low risk in Bali, and cities on islands of Java and Sumatra	1
	No risk in city of Jakarta	-
Indonesia (Borneo)	High risk	4
Iran	Risk from March–November in rural south eastern provinces and in north, along Azerbaijan border in Ardabil, and near Turkmenistan border in North Khorasan	3
	Low to no risk in areas other than those above	1
Iraq	Very low risk from May–November in rural northern area below 1500 m	1
Kenya	High risk below 2500 m (except city of Nairobi)	4
	Very low risk in the highlands above 2500 m and in city of Nairobi	1
Kyrgyzstan	Very low risk from June–October in southwest areas bordering Tajikistan and Uzbekistan	1

5

Infection

Key to recommended regimens for prophylaxis against malaria

Codes for regimens	Details of regimens for prophylaxis against malaria
1	Chemoprophylaxis not recommended, but avoid mosquito bites and consider malaria if fever presents
2	Chloroquine only
3	Chloroquine with proguanil
4	Atovaquone with proguanil hydrochloride or doxycycline or mefloquine
5	Atovaquone with proguanil hydrochloride or doxycycline

Specific recommendations

Country	Comments on risk of malaria and regional or seasonal variation	Codes for regimens
Laos	High risk along the border with Myanmar in the provinces of Bokeo and Louang Namtha, and along the border with Thailand in the province of Champasak and Saravan	5
	High risk in areas other than those above or below	4
	Low to no risk in city of Vientiane	1
Liberia	High risk	4
Libya	No risk	1
Madagascar	High risk	4
Malawi	High risk	4
Malaysia	Risk in inland forested areas of peninsular Malaysia	4
	Very low risk in rest of peninsular Malaysia, including Cameron Highlands and city of Kuala Lumpur	1
Malaysia (Borneo)	High risk in inland areas of eastern Sabah and in inland, forested areas of Sarawak	4
	Very low risk in areas other than those above, including coastal areas of Sabah and Sarawak	1
Mali	High risk	4
Mauritania	High risk all year in southern provinces, and from July-October in the northern provinces	4
	Low risk from November-June in the northern provinces	1
Mauritius	No risk	1
Mayotte	Risk present	4
Mexico	Low risk in Oaxaca and Chiapas	2
	Very low risk in areas other than those above	1
Mozambique	High risk	4
Myanmar	High risk (but not in cities of Mandalay and Yangon)	5
	No risk in cities of Mandalay and Yangon	1
Namibia	High risk all year in regions of Caprivi Strip, Kavango, and Kunene river, and from November-June in northern third of country	4
	Low to no risk in areas other than those above; low risk from July-October in northern third of country	1
Nepal	Risk below 1500 m, particularly in Terai district	3
	No risk in city of Kathmandu and on typical Himalayan treks	1
Nicaragua	Low risk (except Managua)	2
	Very low risk in Managua	1
Niger	High risk	4
Nigeria	High risk	4
North Korea	Very low risk in some southern areas	1
Pakistan	Risk below 2000 m	3
	Low to no risk above 2000 m	1
Panama	Risk east of Canal Zone	3
	Low risk west of Canal Zone	2
	No risk in Panama City or Canal Zone itself	1
Papua New Guinea	High risk below 1800 m	4
	Low to no risk above 1800 m	1

Country	Comments on risk of malaria and regional or seasonal variation	Codes for regimens
Paraguay	Low risk in departments of Alto Paraná and Caaguazú	2
	Very low risk in areas other than those above	1
Peru	High risk in Amazon basin along border with Brazil, particularly in Loreto province	4
	Risk in rural areas below 2000 m (other than those above and below) including in Amazon basin along border with Bolivia	2
	No risk in city of Lima and coastal region south of Chiclayo	1
Philippines	Risk in rural areas below 600 m and on islands of Luzon, Mindanao, Mindoro, and Palawan	3
	No risk in cities or on islands of Boracay, Bohol, Catanduanes, Cebu, or Leyte	1
Rwanda	High risk	4
São Tomé and Principe	High risk	4
Saudi Arabia	Risk in south-western provinces along border with Yemen, including below 2000 m in Asir province	3
	No risk in cities of Jeddah, Makkah (Mecca), Medina, Riyadh, or Ta'if, or above 2000 m in Asir province	1
Senegal	High risk	4
Sierra Leone	High risk	4
Solomon Islands	High risk	4
Somalia	High risk	4
South Africa	Moderate risk from September–May in low altitude areas of Mpumalanga and Limpopo, which border Mozambique and Zimbabwe (including Kruger National Park)	4
	Low risk in north-east KwaZulu-Natal	1
	Low risk in areas bordering those above	1
South Korea	Very low risk in northern areas, in Gangwon-do and Gyeonggi-do provinces, and Incheon city (towards Demilitarized Zone)	1
South Sudan	High risk	4
Sri Lanka	Low risk north of Vavuniya	1
	Very low risk in areas other than those above and below	1
	No risk in Colombo or Kandy	-
Sudan	High risk in central and southern areas; risk also present in rest of country (except Khartoum)	4
	Very low risk in Khartoum	1
Suriname	High risk (except coastal districts or city of Paramaribo)	4
	Very low risk in coastal districts; no risk in city of Paramaribo	1
Swaziland	High risk in northern and eastern regions bordering Mozambique and South Africa, including all of Lubombo district and Big Bend, Mhlume, Simunye, and Tshaneni regions	4
	Very low risk in the areas other than those above	1
Syria	Very low risk in small, remote foci of El Hasakah	1
Tajikistan	Risk below 2000 m from June–October	3
	Low risk below 2000 m from November–May	1
Tanzania	High risk below 1800 m; risk also in Zanzibar	4
Thailand	High risk, with chloroquine and mefloquine resistance, in rural forested borders with Cambodia, Laos, and Myanmar	5
	Very low risk in areas other than those above, including Kanchanaburi (Kwai Bridge); no risk in cities of Bangkok, Chiang Mai, Chiang Rai, Koh Phangan, Koh Samui, and Pattaya	1
Togo	High risk	4
Turkey	Low risk from May–October along the border plain with Syria, around Adana and east of Adana	2
	Very low risk from November–April along the border plain with Syria, around Adana and east of Adana; very low risk all year in rest of country	1
Uganda	High risk	4
Uzbekistan	Very low risk in extreme south-east	1
Vanuatu	Risk present	4

5

Infection

5

Infection

Key to recommended regimens for prophylaxis against malaria

Codes for regimens	Details of regimens for prophylaxis against malaria
1	Chemoprophylaxis not recommended, but avoid mosquito bites and consider malaria if fever presents
2	Chloroquine only
3	Chloroquine with proguanil
4	Atovaquone with proguanil hydrochloride or doxycycline or mefloquine
5	Atovaquone with proguanil hydrochloride or doxycycline

Specific recommendations

Country	Comments on risk of malaria and regional or seasonal variation	Codes for regimens
Venezuela	High risk in all areas south of, and including, the Orinoco river and Angel Falls	4
	Risk in rural areas of Apure, Monagas, Sucre, and Zulia states	3
	No risk in city of Caracas or on Margarita Island	1
Vietnam	Risk in rural areas, and in southern provinces of Tay Ninh, Lam Dong, Dac Lac, Gia Lai, and Kon Tum	5
	Very low risk in Mekong river delta until border area with Cambodia; no risk in large cities (including Ho Chi Minh (Saigon) and Hanoi), Red river delta, and coastal areas north of Nha Trang and Phu Quoc Island	1
Western Sahara	No risk	1
Yemen	Risk below 2000 m	3
	Very low risk on Socrota Island; no risk above 2000 m, including Sana'a city	1
Zambia	High risk	4
Zimbabwe	High risk all year in Zambezi valley, and from November–June in areas below 1200 m	4
	Low risk from July–October in areas below 1200 m; very low risk all year in Harare and Bulawayo	1

Peninsula, including Myanmar, and eastward to Southern Vietnam).

For the treatment of chloroquine-resistant non-falciparum malaria, *Malarone*® [unlicensed indication], quinine, or *Riamet*® [unlicensed indication] can be used; as with chloroquine, primaquine p. 374 should be given for radical cure.

Chloroquine alone is adequate for *P. malariae* and *P. knowlesi* infections but in the case of *P. vivax* and *P. ovale*, a *radical cure* (to destroy parasites in the liver and thus prevent relapses) is required. This is achieved with primaquine [unlicensed] given after chloroquine.

For a radical cure, primaquine [unlicensed] is then given to children over 6 months of age; specialist advice should be sought for children under 6 months of age.

Parenteral
If the child is unable to take oral therapy, quinine can be given by intravenous infusion, changed to oral chloroquine as soon as the patient's condition permits.

Pregnancy
Treatment doses of chloroquine can be given for non-falciparum malaria. In the case of *P.vivax* or *P.ovale*, however, the radical cure with primaquine should be **postponed** until the pregnancy is over; instead chloroquine should be continued, given weekly, during the pregnancy.

ANTIPROTOZOALS ⟩ ANTIMALARIALS

Artemether with lumefantrine

- **INDICATIONS AND DOSE**
  Treatment of acute uncomplicated falciparum malaria | Treatment of chloroquine-resistant non-falciparum malaria
  ▸ BY MOUTH
  ▸ Child (body-weight 5–14 kg): Initially 1 tablet, followed by 1 tablet for 5 doses each given at 8, 24, 36, 48, and 60 hours (total 6 tablets over 60 hours)
  ▸ Child (body-weight 15–24 kg): Initially 2 tablets, followed by 2 tablets for 5 doses each given at 8, 24, 36, 48, and 60 hours (total 12 tablets over 60 hours)
  ▸ Child (body-weight 25–34 kg): Initially 3 tablets, followed by 3 tablets for 5 doses each given at 8, 24, 36, 48, and 60 hours (total 18 tablets over 60 hours)
  ▸ Child 12–17 years (body-weight 35 kg and above): Initially 4 tablets, followed by 4 tablets for 5 doses each given at 8, 24, 36, 48, and 60 hours (total 24 tablets over 60 hours)

- **UNLICENSED USE** Use in treatment of non-falciparum malaria is an unlicensed indication.

- **CONTRA-INDICATIONS** Family history of congenital QT interval prolongation · family history of sudden death · history of arrhythmias · history of clinically relevant bradycardia · history of congestive heart failure accompanied by reduced left ventricular ejection fraction

- **CAUTIONS** Avoid in Acute porphyrias p. 562 · electrolyte disturbances

- **INTERACTIONS** → Appendix 1 (artemether with lumefantrine).
  Caution if concomitant use with other drugs known to cause QT-interval prolongation.

- **SIDE-EFFECTS**
- ▶ **Common or very common** Abdominal pain · anorexia · arthralgia · asthenia · cough · diarrhoea · dizziness · headache · myalgia · nausea · palpitation · paraesthesia · prolonged QT interval · pruritus · rash · sleep disturbances · vomiting
- ▶ **Uncommon** Ataxia · clonus · hypoaesthesia
- **PREGNANCY** Toxicity in *animal* studies with artemether. Manufacturer advises use only if potential benefit outweighs risk.
- **BREAST FEEDING** Manufacturer advises avoid breastfeeding for at least 1 week after last dose. Present in milk in *animal* studies.
- **HEPATIC IMPAIRMENT** Manufacturer advises caution in severe impairment.
- **RENAL IMPAIRMENT** Manufacturer advises caution in severe impairment. In severe renal impairment monitor ECG and plasma potassium concentration.
- **MONITORING REQUIREMENTS** Monitor patients unable to take food (greater risk of recrudescence).
- **DIRECTIONS FOR ADMINISTRATION** Tablets may be crushed just before administration.
- **PATIENT AND CARER ADVICE**
  Driving and skilled tasks
  Dizziness may affect performance of skilled tasks (e.g. driving).

- **MEDICINAL FORMS**
  There can be variation in the licensing of different medicines containing the same drug.
  Tablet
  CAUTIONARY AND ADVISORY LABELS 21
  ▶ Riamet (Novartis Pharmaceuticals UK Ltd)
    Artemether 20 mg, Lumefantrine 120 mg Riamet tablets |
    24 tablet PoM £22.50

Artenimol with piperaquine phosphate

(Piperaquine tetraphosphate with dihydroartemisinin)

- **INDICATIONS AND DOSE**
  Treatment of uncomplicated falciparum malaria
  ▶ BY MOUTH
  ▶ Child 6 months-17 years (body-weight 7-12 kg): 0.5 tablet once daily for 3 days, max. 2 courses in 12 months; second course given at least 2 months after first course
  ▶ Child 6 months-17 years (body-weight 13-23 kg): 1 tablet once daily for 3 days, max. 2 courses in 12 months; second course given at least 2 months after first course
  ▶ Child 6 months-17 years (body-weight 24-35 kg): 2 tablets once daily for 3 days, max. 2 courses in 12 months; second course given at least 2 months after first course
  ▶ Child 6 months-17 years (body-weight 36-74 kg): 3 tablets once daily for 3 days, max. 2 courses in 12 months; second course given at least 2 months after first course
  ▶ Child 6 months-17 years (body-weight 75-99 kg): 4 tablets once daily for 3 days, max. 2 courses in 12 months; second course given at least 2 months after first course

- **CONTRA-INDICATIONS** Acute myocardial infarction · bradycardia · congenital long QT syndrome · electrolyte disturbances · family history of sudden death · heart failure with reduced left ventricular ejection fraction · history of symptomatic arrhythmias · left ventricular hypertrophy · risk factors for QT interval prolongation · severe hypertension
- **INTERACTIONS** → Appendix 1 (artenimol with piperaquine).

Piperaquine has a long half-life; there is a potential for drug interactions to occur for up to 3 months after treatment has been stopped.
Concomitant use with other drugs known to prolong the QT interval contra-indicated.

- **SIDE-EFFECTS**
- ▶ **Common or very common** Abdominal pain · anaemia · blood disorders · conjunctivitis · cough · diarrhoea · irregular heart rate · leucopenia · malaise · QT interval prolonged · rash · thrombocytopenia · vomiting
- ▶ **Uncommon** Acanthosis · arrhythmias · arthralgia · convulsions · headache · heart murmur · hepatitis · hepatomegaly · influenza-like symptoms · jaundice · nausea · stomatitis
- **PREGNANCY** Teratogenic in *animal* studies—manufacturer advises use only if other antimalarials cannot be used.
- **BREAST FEEDING** Manufacturer advises avoid—present in milk in *animal* studies.
- **HEPATIC IMPAIRMENT** No information available in moderate to severe impairment. Manufacturer advises monitor ECG and plasma-potassium concentration in moderate to severe hepatic impairment.
- **RENAL IMPAIRMENT** No information available in moderate to severe impairment. Manufacturer advises monitor ECG and plasma-potassium concentration in moderate to severe renal impairment.
- **MONITORING REQUIREMENTS**
  ▶ Consider obtaining ECG in all patients before third dose and 4–6 hours after third dose. If QT_C interval more than 500 milliseconds, discontinue treatment and monitor ECG for a further 24–48 hours.
  ▶ Obtain ECG as soon as possible after starting treatment then continue monitoring in those taking medicines that increase plasma-piperaquine concentration, in children who are vomiting or in females.
- **DIRECTIONS FOR ADMINISTRATION** Tablets to be taken at least 3 hours before and at least 3 hours after food. Tablets may be crushed and mixed with water immediately before administration.
- **PATIENT AND CARER ADVICE** Patients or carers should be given advice on how to administer tablets containing piperaquine phosphate with artenimol.

- **MEDICINAL FORMS**
  There can be variation in the licensing of different medicines containing the same drug.
  Tablet
  ▶ Eurartesim (Sigma-Tau Pharma Ltd) ▼
    Artenimol 40 mg, Piperaquine phosphate 320 mg Eurartesim
    320mg/40mg tablets | 12 tablet PoM £40.00

Atovaquone with proguanil hydrochloride

- **INDICATIONS AND DOSE**
  MALARONE®
  Prophylaxis of falciparum malaria, particularly where resistance to other antimalarial drugs suspected
  ▶ BY MOUTH
  ▶ Child (body-weight 41 kg and above): 1 tablet daily, to be started 1–2 days before entering endemic area and continued for 1 week after leaving
  **Treatment of acute uncomplicated falciparum malaria |
  Treatment of non-falciparum malaria**
  ▶ BY MOUTH
  ▶ Child (body-weight 11-20 kg): 1 tablet once daily for 3 days
  ▶ Child (body-weight 21-30 kg): 2 tablets once daily for 3 days
  continued →

5

Infection

- Child (body-weight 31–40 kg): 3 tablets once daily for 3 days
- Child (body-weight 41 kg and above): 4 tablets once daily for 3 days

MALARONE® PAEDIATRIC

Prophylaxis of falciparum malaria, particularly where resistance to other antimalarial drugs suspected

▸ BY MOUTH
- Child (body-weight 5–8 kg): 0.5 tablet once daily, to be started 1–2 days before entering endemic area and continued for 1 week after leaving
- Child (body-weight 9–10 kg): 0.75 tablet once daily, to be started 1–2 days before entering endemic area and continued for 1 week after leaving
- Child (body-weight 11–20 kg): 1 tablet once daily, to be started 1–2 days before entering endemic area and continued for 1 week after leaving
- Child (body-weight 21–30 kg): 2 tablets once daily, to be started 1–2 days before entering endemic area and continued for 1 week after leaving
- Child (body-weight 31–40 kg): 3 tablets once daily, to be started 1–2 days before entering endemic area and continued for 1 week after leaving
- Child (body-weight 41 kg and above): Use *Malarone*® (standard) tablets.

Treatment of acute uncomplicated falciparum malaria | Treatment of non-falciparum malaria

▸ BY MOUTH
- Child (body-weight 5–8 kg): 2 tablets once daily for 3 days
- Child (body-weight 9–10 kg): 3 tablets once daily for 3 days
- Child (body-weight 11 kg and above): Use *Malarone*® (standard) tablets.

- UNLICENSED USE Not licensed for treatment of non-falciparum malaria. Not licensed for prophylaxis of malaria in children under 11 kg.

- CAUTIONS Diarrhoea or vomiting (reduced absorption of atovaquone) · efficacy not evaluated in cerebral or complicated malaria (including hyperparasitaemia, pulmonary oedema or renal failure)

- INTERACTIONS → Appendix 1 (proguanil, atovaquone).

- SIDE-EFFECTS
▸ **Common or very common** Abdominal pain · abnormal dreams · anorexia · cough · depression · diarrhoea · dizziness · fever · headache · insomnia · nausea · pruritus · rash · vomiting
▸ **Uncommon** Anxiety · blood disorders · hair loss · hyponatraemia · palpitation · stomatitis
▸ **Frequency not known** Cholestasis · hallucinations · hepatitis · mouth ulcers · photosensitivity · seizures · Stevens-Johnson syndrome · tachycardia · vasculitis

- PREGNANCY Manufacturer advises avoid unless essential.

- BREAST FEEDING Use only if no suitable alternative available.

- RENAL IMPAIRMENT Avoid for malaria prophylaxis and, if possible, for treatment if estimated glomerular filtration rate less than 30 mL/minute/1.73 m².

- DIRECTIONS FOR ADMINISTRATION
MALARONE® PAEDIATRIC ▸ With oral use Tablets may be crushed and mixed with food or milky drink just before administration.

- PATIENT AND CARER ADVICE
Medicines for Children leaflet: Malarone for prevention of malaria www.medicinesforchildren.org.uk/malarone-for-prevention-of-malaria
Warn travellers about **importance** of avoiding mosquito bites, **importance** of taking prophylaxis regularly, and **importance** of immediate visit to doctor if ill within 1 year and **especially** within 3 months of return.

- NATIONAL FUNDING/ACCESS DECISIONS
NHS restrictions Drugs for malaria prophylaxis not prescribable on the NHS; health authorities may investigate circumstances under which antimalarials prescribed

- MEDICINAL FORMS
There can be variation in the licensing of different medicines containing the same drug.
Tablet
CAUTIONARY AND ADVISORY LABELS 21
▸ Malarone (GlaxoSmithKline UK Ltd)
Proguanil hydrochloride 25 mg, Atovaquone 62.5 mg Malarone Paediatric tablets | 12 tablet [PoM] £6.26
Proguanil hydrochloride 100 mg, Atovaquone 250 mg Malarone tablets | 12 tablet [PoM] £25.21 DT price = £25.21

| Chloroquine

- INDICATIONS AND DOSE

Prophylaxis of malaria

▸ INITIALLY BY MOUTH USING SYRUP
- Child up to 6 weeks (body-weight up to 4.5 kg): 25 mg once weekly, started 1 week before entering endemic area and continued for 4 weeks after leaving
- Child 6 weeks–5 months (body-weight 4.5–7 kg): 50 mg once weekly, started 1 week before entering endemic area and continued for 4 weeks after leaving
- Child 6–11 months (body-weight 8–10 kg): 75 mg once weekly, started 1 week before entering endemic area and continued for 4 weeks after leaving
- Child 1–2 years (body-weight 11–14 kg): 100 mg once weekly, started 1 week before entering endemic area and continued for 4 weeks after leaving
- Child 3–4 years (body-weight 15–16.4 kg): 125 mg once weekly, started 1 week before entering endemic area and continued for 4 weeks after leaving
- Child 4–7 years (body-weight 16.5–24 kg): 150 mg once weekly, alternatively (by mouth using tablets) 155 mg once weekly, started 1 week before entering endemic area and continued for 4 weeks after leaving
- Child 8–13 years (body-weight 25–44 kg): 225 mg once weekly, alternatively (by mouth using tablets) 232.5 mg once weekly, started 1 week before entering endemic area and continued for 4 weeks after leaving
▸ INITIALLY BY MOUTH USING TABLETS
- Child 14–17 years (body-weight 45 kg and above): 310 mg once weekly, alternatively (by mouth using syrup) 300 mg once weekly, started 1 week before entering endemic area and continued for 4 weeks after leaving

Treatment of non-falciparum malaria
▸ BY MOUTH
- Child: Initially 10 mg/kg (max. per dose 620 mg), then 5 mg/kg after 6–8 hours (max. per dose 310 mg), then 5 mg/kg daily (max. per dose 310 mg) for 2 days

***P. vivax* or *P. ovale* infection during pregnancy while radical cure is postponed**
▸ BY MOUTH
- Child: 10 mg/kg once weekly (max. per dose 310 mg)

DOSE EQUIVALENCE AND CONVERSION
Doses expressed as chloroquine base. Chloroquine base 150 mg = chloroquine sulfate 200 mg = chloroquine phosphate 250 mg (approx.)

- UNLICENSED USE Chloroquine doses for the treatment and prophylaxis of malaria in BNF publications may differ from those in product literature.

- CAUTIONS Acute porphyrias p. 562 · G6PD deficiency · long-term therapy (regular ophthalmic examination recommended by manufacturers) · may aggravate myasthenia gravis · may exacerbate psoriasis · neurological disorders, especially epilepsy (avoid for prophylaxis of malaria if history of epilepsy) · severe gastro-intestinal disorders

● **INTERACTIONS** → Appendix 1 (chloroquine).
Avoid concurrent therapy with hepatotoxic drugs.

● **SIDE-EFFECTS**
▸ **Common or very common** Gastro-intestinal disturbances · headache · pruritus · rashes · skin reactions
▸ **Uncommon** Convulsions · discoloration of mucous membranes · discoloration of nails · discoloration of skin · ECG changes · hair depigmentation · hair loss · keratopathy · ototoxicity · retinal damage · visual changes
▸ **Rare** Acute generalised exanthematous pustulosis · agranulocytosis · angioedema · aplastic anaemia · blood disorders · bone marrow suppression · cardiomyopathy · emotional disturbances · exfoliative dermatitis · hepatic damage · hypersensitivity reactions · mental changes · myopathy · neuromyopathy · photosensitivity · psychosis · Stevens-Johnson syndrome · thrombocytopenia · urticaria
▸ **Frequency not known** Bronchospasm · diffuse parenchymal lung disease · drug rash with eosinophilia and systemic symptoms · extrapyramidal symptoms (associated with use in malaria) · hypotension · visual disturbances

SIDE-EFFECTS, FURTHER INFORMATION
▸ Malaria prophylaxis and treatment Serious skin reactions, ECG changes, visual effects, ototoxicity, blood disorders, mental changes, myopathies and hepatic damage are not usually associated with malaria prophylaxis or treatment.

Overdose
Chloroquine is very toxic in overdosage; overdosage is extremely hazardous and difficult to treat. Urgent advice from the National Poisons Information Service is essential. Life-threatening features include arrhythmias (which can have a very rapid onset) and convulsions (which can be intractable).

● **PREGNANCY** Benefit of use in prophylaxis and treatment in malaria outweighs risk. For rheumatoid disease, it is not necessary to withdraw an antimalarial drug during pregnancy if the disease is well controlled.

● **BREAST FEEDING** Present in breast milk and breast-feeding should be avoided when used to treat rheumatic disease. Amount in milk probably too small to be harmful when used for malaria.

● **HEPATIC IMPAIRMENT** Use with caution in moderate to severe impairment.

● **RENAL IMPAIRMENT** Only partially excreted by the kidneys and reduction of the dose is not required for prophylaxis of malaria except in severe impairment. For rheumatoid arthritis and lupus erythematosus, reduce dose. Manufacturers advise caution.

● **MONITORING REQUIREMENTS** Ophthalmic examination with long-term therapy.

● **PATIENT AND CARER ADVICE** Warn travellers going to malarious areas about **importance** of avoiding mosquito bites, **importance** of taking prophylaxis regularly, and **importance** of immediate visit to doctor if ill within 1 year and **especially** within 3 months of return.

● **NATIONAL FUNDING/ACCESS DECISIONS**
NHS restrictions Drugs for malaria prophylaxis not prescribable on the NHS; health authorities may investigate circumstances under which antimalarials prescribed

● **EXCEPTIONS TO LEGAL CATEGORY** Can be sold to the public provided it is licensed and labelled for the prophylaxis of malaria.

● **MEDICINAL FORMS**
There can be variation in the licensing of different medicines containing the same drug. Forms available from special-order manufacturers include: oral solution

Tablet
CAUTIONARY AND ADVISORY LABELS 5
▸ **Avloclor** (Alliance Pharmaceuticals Ltd)
Chloroquine phosphate 250 mg Avloclor 250mg tablets | 20 tablet [PoM] £7.95 DT price = £7.95

Oral solution
CAUTIONARY AND ADVISORY LABELS 5
▸ **Malarivon** (Wallace Manufacturing Chemists Ltd)
Chloroquine phosphate 16 mg per 1 ml Malarivon 80mg/5ml syrup | 75 ml [PoM] £30.00

Chloroquine with proguanil

The properties listed below are those particular to the combination only. For the properties of the components please consider, chloroquine p. 372, proguanil hydrochloride p. 375.

● **INDICATIONS AND DOSE**
Prophylaxis of malaria
▸ BY MOUTH
▸ Child: (consult product literature)

● **EXCEPTIONS TO LEGAL CATEGORY** Can be sold to the public provided it is licensed and labelled for the prophylaxis of malaria.

● **MEDICINAL FORMS**
There can be variation in the licensing of different medicines containing the same drug.

Tablet
▸ **Paludrine/Avloclor** (Alliance Pharmaceuticals Ltd)
Paludrine/Avloclor tablets anti-malarial travel pack | 112 tablet [P] £13.50

Mefloquine

● **INDICATIONS AND DOSE**
Treatment of malaria
▸ BY MOUTH
▸ Child: (consult product literature)
Prophylaxis of malaria
▸ BY MOUTH
▸ Child (body-weight 5-15 kg): 62.5 mg once weekly, dose to be started 2–3 weeks before entering endemic area and continued for 4 weeks after leaving
▸ Child (body-weight 16-24 kg): 125 mg once weekly, dose to be started 2–3 weeks before entering endemic area and continued for 4 weeks after leaving
▸ Child (body-weight 25-44 kg): 187.5 mg once weekly, dose to be started 2–3 weeks before entering endemic area and continued for 4 weeks after leaving
▸ Child (body-weight 45 kg and above): 250 mg once weekly, dose to be started 2–3 weeks before entering endemic area and continued for 4 weeks after leaving

● **UNLICENSED USE** Mefloquine doses in BNF Publications may differ from those in product literature. Not licensed for use in children under 5 kg body-weight and under 3 months.

● **CONTRA-INDICATIONS** Avoid for prophylaxis if history of psychiatric disorders (including depression) or convulsions · avoid for standby treatment if history of convulsions · history of blackwater fever

● **CAUTIONS** Cardiac conduction disorders · epilepsy (avoid for prophylaxis) · not recommended in infants under 3 months (5 kg) · traumatic brain injury

5

Infection

CAUTIONS, FURTHER INFORMATION

▶ **Neuropsychiatric reactions** Mefloquine is associated with potentially serious neuropsychiatric reactions. Abnormal dreams, insomnia, anxiety, and depression occur commonly. Psychosis, suicidal ideation, and suicide have also been reported. Psychiatric symptoms such as nightmares, acute anxiety, depression, restlessness, or confusion should be regarded as potentially prodromal for a more serious event. If neuropsychiatric symptoms occur, patients should be advised to discontinue mefloquine and to seek immediate medical attention so that mefloquine can be replaced with an alternative antimalarial. Adverse reactions may occur and persist up to several months after discontinuation because mefloquine has a long half-life. Mefloquine is contra-indicated for malaria prophylaxis in those with a history of psychiatric disorders or convulsions.

● INTERACTIONS → Appendix 1 (mefloquine).

● SIDE-EFFECTS

▶ **Common or very common** Abdominal pain · diarrhoea · dizziness · headache · nausea · neuropsychiatric reactions · pruritus · visual disturbances · vomiting

▶ **Very rare** Optic neuropathy

▶ **Frequency not known** Alopecia · amnesia · anorexia · arrhythmias · arthralgia · ataxia · blood disorders · bradycardia · cataract · chest pain · confusion · drowsiness · dyspepsia · dyspnoea · encephalopathy · fever · flushing · hepatic failure · hyperhidrosis · hypertension · hypotension · leucocytosis · leucopenia · malaise · motor neuropathies · muscle weakness · myalgia · oedema · palpitation · panic attacks · pneumonitis · rash · seizures · sensory neuropathies · speech disturbances · Stevens-Johnson syndrome · syncope · tachycardia · thrombocytopenia · tremor · vestibular disorders

● ALLERGY AND CROSS-SENSITIVITY Contra-indicated in patients with hypersensitivity to quinine.

● CONCEPTION AND CONTRACEPTION Manufacturer advises adequate contraception during prophylaxis and for 3 months after stopping (teratogenicity in *animal* studies).

● PREGNANCY Manufacturer advises avoid (particularly in the first trimester) unless the potential benefit outweighs the risk; however, studies of mefloquine in pregnancy (including use in the first trimester) indicate that it can be considered for travel to chloroquine-resistant areas.

● BREAST FEEDING Present in milk but risk to infant minimal.

● HEPATIC IMPAIRMENT Elimination may be prolonged; avoid in severe impairment.

● RENAL IMPAIRMENT Manufacturer advises caution.

● DIRECTIONS FOR ADMINISTRATION Tablet may be crushed and mixed with food such as jam or honey just before administration.

● PATIENT AND CARER ADVICE
Inform travellers about adverse reactions of mefloquine and, if they occur, to seek medical advice on alternative antimalarials before the next dose is due. Also warn travellers about **importance** of avoiding mosquito bites, **importance** of taking prophylaxis regularly, and **importance** of immediate visit to doctor if ill within 1 year and especially within 3 months of return.

Driving and skilled tasks
Dizziness or a disturbed sense of balance may affect performance of skilled tasks (e.g. driving); effects may occur and persist up to several months after stopping mefloquine.

● NATIONAL FUNDING/ACCESS DECISIONS
NHS restrictions Drugs for malaria prophylaxis not prescribable on the NHS; health authorities may investigate circumstances under which antimalarials prescribed

● MEDICINAL FORMS
There can be variation in the licensing of different medicines containing the same drug.
Tablet
CAUTIONARY AND ADVISORY LABELS 21, 27
▶ Lariam (Roche Products Ltd)
Mefloquine (as Mefloquine hydrochloride) 250 mg Lariam 250mg tablets | 8 tablet [PoM] £14.53

❙ Primaquine

● INDICATIONS AND DOSE

Adjunct in the treatment of non-falciparum malaria caused by *P.vivax* infection
▶ BY MOUTH
▸ Child 6 months–17 years: 500 micrograms/kg daily (max. per dose 30 mg) for 14 days

Adjunct in the treatment of non-falciparum malaria caused by *P.ovale* infection
▶ BY MOUTH
▸ Child 6 months–17 years: 250 micrograms/kg daily (max. per dose 15 mg) for 14 days

Adjunct in the treatment of non-falciparum malaria caused by *P.vivax* infection in patients with mild G6PD deficiency (administered on expert advice) | Adjunct in the treatment of non-falciparum malaria caused by *P.ovale* infection in patients with mild G6PD deficiency (administered on expert advice)
▶ BY MOUTH
▸ Child: 750 micrograms/kg once weekly for 8 weeks; maximum 45 mg per week

Treatment of mild to moderate pneumocystis infection (in combination with clindamycin)
▶ BY MOUTH
▸ Child: This combination is associated with considerable toxicity (consult product literature)

● UNLICENSED USE Not licensed.

● CAUTIONS G6PD deficiency · systemic diseases associated with granulocytopenia (e.g. juvenile idiopathic arthritis, rheumatoid arthritis, lupus erythematosus)

● INTERACTIONS → Appendix 1 (primaquine).

● SIDE-EFFECTS
▶ **Common or very common** Abdominal pain · anorexia · nausea · vomiting
▶ **Uncommon** Haemolytic anaemia especially in G6PD deficiency · leucopenia · methaemoglobinaemia

● PREGNANCY Risk of neonatal haemolysis and methaemoglobinaemia in third trimester.

● BREAST FEEDING No information available; theoretical risk of haemolysis in G6PD-deficient infants.

● PRE-TREATMENT SCREENING Before starting primaquine, blood should be tested for glucose-6-phosphate dehydrogenase (G6PD) activity since the drug can cause haemolysis in G6PD-deficient patients. Specialist advice should be obtained in G6PD deficiency.

● MEDICINAL FORMS
There can be variation in the licensing of different medicines containing the same drug. Forms available from special-order manufacturers include: oral suspension
Tablet
▶ Primaquine (Non-proprietary)
Primaquine (as Primaquine phosphate) 15 mg Primaquine 15mg tablets | 100 tablet [PoM] no price available

Proguanil hydrochloride

● **INDICATIONS AND DOSE**

Prophylaxis of malaria

▶ BY MOUTH

▸ Child 4–11 weeks (body-weight up to 6 kg): 25 mg once daily, dose to be started 1 week before entering endemic area and continued for 4 weeks after leaving

▸ Child 3–11 months (body-weight 6–9 kg): 50 mg once daily, dose to be started 1 week before entering endemic area and continued for 4 weeks after leaving

▸ Child 1–3 years (body-weight 10–15 kg): 75 mg once daily, dose to be started 1 week before entering endemic area and continued for 4 weeks after leaving

▸ Child 4–7 years (body-weight 16–24 kg): 100 mg once daily, dose to be started 1 week before entering endemic area and continued for 4 weeks after leaving

▸ Child 8–12 years (body-weight 25–44 kg): 150 mg once daily, dose to be started 1 week before entering endemic area and continued for 4 weeks after leaving

▸ Child 13–17 years (body-weight 45 kg and above): 200 mg once daily, dose to be started 1 week before entering endemic area and continued for 4 weeks after leaving

● **UNLICENSED USE** Proguanil doses in BNF Publications may differ from those in product literature.

● **INTERACTIONS** → Appendix 1 (proguanil).

● **SIDE-EFFECTS**

▶ **Common or very common** Constipation · diarrhoea · mild gastric intolerance

▶ **Very rare** Cholestasis · hair loss · skin reactions · vasculitis

▶ **Frequency not known** Mouth ulcers · stomatitis

● **PREGNANCY** Benefit of prophylaxis in malaria outweighs risk. Adequate folate supplements should be given to mother.

● **BREAST FEEDING** Amount in milk probably too small to be harmful when used for malaria prophylaxis.

● **RENAL IMPAIRMENT** Use half normal dose if estimated glomerular filtration rate 20–60 mL/minute/1.73m^2. Use one-quarter normal dose on alternate days if estimated glomerular filtration rate 10–20 mL/minute/1.73m^2. Use one-quarter normal dose once weekly if estimated glomerular filtration rate less than 10 mL/minute/1.73m^2; increased risk of haematological toxicity in severe impairment.

● **DIRECTIONS FOR ADMINISTRATION** Tablet may be crushed and mixed with food such as milk, jam, or honey just before administration.

● **PATIENT AND CARER ADVICE** Warn travellers about **importance** of avoiding mosquito bites, **importance** of taking prophylaxis regularly, and **importance** of immediate visit to doctor if ill within 1 year and **especially** within 3 months of return.

● **NATIONAL FUNDING/ACCESS DECISIONS**

NHS restrictions Drugs for malaria prophylaxis not prescribable on the NHS; health authorities may investigate circumstances under which antimalarials prescribed

● **EXCEPTIONS TO LEGAL CATEGORY** Can be sold to the public provided it is licensed and labelled for the prophylaxis of malaria.

● **MEDICINAL FORMS**

There can be variation in the licensing of different medicines containing the same drug. Forms available from special-order manufacturers include: oral suspension, oral solution

Tablet

CAUTIONARY AND ADVISORY LABELS 21

▸ Paludrine (Alliance Pharmaceuticals Ltd)
Proguanil hydrochloride 100 mg Paludrine 100mg tablets | 98 tablet P £11.95 DT price = £11.95

Pyrimethamine

● **INDICATIONS AND DOSE**

Toxoplasmosis in pregnancy (in combination with sulfadiazine and folinic acid)

▶ BY MOUTH

▸ Child 12–17 years: 50 mg once daily until delivery

Congenital toxoplasmosis (in combination with sulfadiazine and folinic acid)

▶ BY MOUTH

▸ Neonate: 1 mg/kg twice daily for 2 days, then 1 mg/kg once daily for 6 months, then 1 mg/kg 3 times a week for 6 months.

Malaria

▶ BY MOUTH

▸ Child: No dose stated because not recommended alone

● **UNLICENSED USE** Not licensed for use in children under 5 years.

● **CAUTIONS** History of seizures—avoid large loading doses · predisposition to folate deficiency

● **INTERACTIONS** → Appendix 1 (pyrimethamine).

● **SIDE-EFFECTS**

▶ **Common or very common** Anaemia (with high doses) · blood disorders (with high doses) · diarrhoea · dizziness · headache · leucopenia (with high doses) · nausea · rash · thrombocytopenia (with high doses) · vomiting

▶ **Uncommon** Abnormal skin pigmentation · fever

▶ **Very rare** Buccal ulceration · colic · convulsions

● **PREGNANCY** Theoretical teratogenic risk in *first trimester* (folate antagonist). Adequate folate supplements should be given to the mother.

● **BREAST FEEDING** Significant amount in milk—avoid administration of other folate antagonists to infant. Avoid breast-feeding during toxoplasmosis treatment.

● **HEPATIC IMPAIRMENT** Manufacturer advises caution.

● **RENAL IMPAIRMENT** Manufacturer advises caution.

● **MONITORING REQUIREMENTS** Blood counts required with prolonged treatment.

● **LESS SUITABLE FOR PRESCRIBING** Pyrimethamine should not be used alone for malaria, but is used with sulfadoxine.

● **MEDICINAL FORMS**

There can be variation in the licensing of different medicines containing the same drug. Forms available from special-order manufacturers include: oral suspension

Tablet

▸ Daraprim (GlaxoSmithKline UK Ltd)
Pyrimethamine 25 mg Daraprim 25mg tablets | 30 tablet PoM £13.00

Pyrimethamine with sulfadoxine

● **INDICATIONS AND DOSE**

Adjunct to quinine in treatment of Plasmodium falciparum malaria

▶ BY MOUTH

▸ Child 1 month–4 years (body-weight 5 kg and above): 12.5/250 mg for 1 dose

▸ Child 5–6 years: 25/500 mg for 1 dose

▸ Child 7–9 years: 37.5/750 mg for 1 dose

▸ Child 10–13 years: 50/1000 mg for 1 dose

▸ Child 14–17 years: 75/1500 mg for 1 dose

Malaria prophylaxis

▶ BY MOUTH

▸ Child: Not recommended by UK malaria experts

continued →

5

Infection

Infection

5

DOSE EQUIVALENCE AND CONVERSION Dose quantities are expressed in the form x/y where x and y are the strengths in milligrams of pyrimethamine and sulfadoxine respectively.

- **UNLICENSED USE** Not licensed for use in children of body-weight under 5 kg.
- **CONTRA-INDICATIONS** Acute porphyrias p. 562
- **CAUTIONS** Asthma · avoid in blood disorders (unless under specialist supervision) · avoid in infants under 6 weeks · G6PD deficiency · history of seizures—avoid large loading doses · not recommended for prophylaxis (severe side-effects on long-term use) · predisposition to folate deficiency
- **INTERACTIONS** → Appendix 1 (pyrimethamine, sulfonamides).
- **SIDE-EFFECTS**
  ‣ **Common or very common** Diarrhoea · headache · hyperkalaemia · nausea · rash
  ‣ **Uncommon** Vomiting
  ‣ **Very rare** Anorexia · antibiotic-associated colitis · arthralgia · aseptic meningitis · ataxia · blood disorders · convulsions · cough · depression · eosinophilia · glossitis · hallucinations · hepatic necrosis · hypoglycaemia · hyponatraemia · interstitial nephritis · jaundice · leucopenia · liver damage · megaloblastic anaemia · myalgia · myocarditis · pancreatitis · peripheral neuropathy · photosensitivity · renal disorders · rhabdomyolysis reported in HIV-infected patients · shortness of breath · Stevens-Johnson syndrome · stomatitis · systemic lupus erythematosus · thrombocytopenia · tinnitus · toxic epidermal necrolysis · uveitis · vasculitis · vertigo
  ‣ **Frequency not known** Allergic alveolitis · eosinophilic alveolitis · pulmonary infiltrates

  SIDE-EFFECTS, FURTHER INFORMATION
  Discontinue immediately if blood disorders or rash occur. Discontinue if cough or shortness of breath occur.

- **ALLERGY AND CROSS-SENSITIVITY** Contra-indicated in patients with sulfonamide allergy.
- **PREGNANCY** Possible teratogenic risk in *first trimester* (pyrimethamine a folate antagonist); in *third trimester*— risk of neonatal haemolysis and methaemoglobinaemia. Fear of increased risk of kernicterus in neonates appears to be unfounded.
- **BREAST FEEDING** Small risk of kernicterus in jaundiced infants; risk of haemolysis in G6PD-deficient infants (due to sulfadoxine).
- **MONITORING REQUIREMENTS** Monitor blood counts on prolonged treatment.
- **PRESCRIBING AND DISPENSING INFORMATION** Also known as *Fansidar*®.
- **PATIENT AND CARER ADVICE** Patients should be advised to maintain adequate fluid intake.

- **MEDICINAL FORMS**
  There can be variation in the licensing of different medicines containing the same drug.
  No licensed medicines listed.

▌Quinine

- **INDICATIONS AND DOSE**
Non-falciparum malaria
  ‣ BY INTRAVENOUS INFUSION
  ‣ **Child:** 10 mg/kg every 8 hours (max. per dose 700 mg), infused over 4 hours, given if patient is unable to take oral therapy. Changed to oral chloroquine as soon as the patient's condition permits

Falciparum malaria
‣ BY MOUTH
‣ **Child:** 10 mg/kg every 8 hours (max. per dose 600 mg) for 7 days, together with or followed by either doxycycline (in children over 12 years), or clindamycin
‣ BY INTRAVENOUS INFUSION
‣ **Neonate:** Loading dose 20 mg/kg (max. per dose 1.4 g), infused over 4 hours, the loading dose of 20 mg/kg should **not** be used if the patient has received quinine or mefloquine during the previous 12 hours, then maintenance 10 mg/kg every 8 hours (max. per dose 700 mg) until patient can tolerate oral medication to complete the 7-day course, maintenance dose to be given 8 hours after the start of the loading dose and infused over 4 hours, the quinine should be given together with or followed by clindamycin.

‣ **Child:** Loading dose 20 mg/kg (max. per dose 1.4 g), infused over 4 hours, the loading dose of 20 mg/kg should **not** be used if the patient has received quinine or mefloquine during the previous 12 hours, then maintenance 10 mg/kg every 8 hours (max. per dose 700 mg) until patient can swallow tablets to complete the 7-day course, maintenance dose to be given 8 hours after the start of the loading dose and infused over 4 hours, the quinine should be given together with or followed by either doxycycline (in children over 12 years), or clindamycin

Falciparum malaria (in intensive care unit)
‣ BY INTRAVENOUS INFUSION
‣ **Neonate:** Loading dose 7 mg/kg, infused over 30 minutes, followed immediately by 10 mg/kg, infused over 4 hours, then maintenance 10 mg/kg every 8 hours (max. per dose 700 mg) until patient can swallow tablets to complete the 7-day course, maintenance dose to be given 8 hours after the start of the loading dose and infused over 4 hours, the quinine should be given together with or followed by clindamycin.

‣ **Child:** Loading dose 7 mg/kg, infused over 30 minutes, followed immediately by 10 mg/kg, infused over 4 hours, then maintenance 10 mg/kg every 8 hours (max. per dose 700 mg) until patient can swallow tablets to complete the 7-day course, maintenance dose to be given 8 hours after the start of the loading dose and infused over 4 hours, the quinine should be given together with or followed by either doxycycline (in children over 12 years), or clindamycin

DOSE EQUIVALENCE AND CONVERSION
When using quinine for malaria, doses are valid for quinine hydrochloride, dihydrochloride, and sulfate; they are **not valid** for quinine bisulfate which contains a correspondingly smaller amount of quinine. Quinine (anhydrous base) 100 mg = quinine bisulfate 169 mg; quinine dihydrochloride 122 mg; quinine hydrochloride 122 mg; and quinine sulfate 121 mg. Quinine bisulfate 300 mg tablets are available but provide less quinine than 300 mg of the dihydrochloride, hydrochloride, or sulfate.

- **UNLICENSED USE** Injection not licensed.
- **CONTRA-INDICATIONS** Haemoglobinuria · myasthenia gravis · optic neuritis · tinnitus
- **CAUTIONS** Atrial fibrillation (monitor ECG during parenteral treatment) · cardiac disease (monitor ECG during parenteral treatment) · conduction defects (monitor ECG during parenteral treatment) · G6PD deficiency · heart block (monitor ECG during parenteral treatment)
- **INTERACTIONS** → Appendix 1 (quinine).
- **SIDE-EFFECTS** Agitation · tinnitus · abdominal pain · acute renal failure · angioedema · blood disorders · cardiovascular effects · cinchonism · confusion · diarrhoea · dyspnoea ·

flushed skin · headache · hearing impairment · hot skin · hypersensitivity reactions · hypoglycaemia (especially after parenteral administration) · intravascular coagulation · muscle weakness · nausea · photosensitivity · rashes · temporary blindness · thrombocytopenia · vertigo · visual disturbances · vomiting

Overdose
Quinine is very toxic in overdosage; life-threatening features include arrhythmias (which can have a very rapid onset) and convulsions (which can be intractable).

For details on the management of poisoning, see Emergency treatment of poisoning p. 786.

● **PREGNANCY** High doses are teratogenic in *first trimester*, but in malaria benefit of treatment outweighs risk.

● **BREAST FEEDING** Present in milk but not known to be harmful.

● **HEPATIC IMPAIRMENT**
▶ With intravenous use For treatment of malaria in severe impairment, reduce parenteral maintenance dose to 5–7 mg/kg of quinine salt.

● **RENAL IMPAIRMENT**
▶ With intravenous use For treatment of malaria in severe impairment, reduce parenteral maintenance dose to 5–7 mg/kg of quinine salt.

● **MONITORING REQUIREMENTS**
▶ With intravenous use Monitor blood glucose and electrolyte concentration during parenteral treatment.

● **DIRECTIONS FOR ADMINISTRATION**
▶ With intravenous use For *intravenous infusion*, dilute to a concentration of 2 mg/mL (max. 30 mg/mL in fluid restriction) with Glucose 5% *or* Sodium Chloride 0.9% and give over 4 hours.

● **PRESCRIBING AND DISPENSING INFORMATION**
▶ With intravenous use Intravenous injection of quinine is so hazardous that it has been superseded by infusion.

● **MEDICINAL FORMS**
There can be variation in the licensing of different medicines containing the same drug. Forms available from special-order manufacturers include: capsule, oral suspension, oral solution, solution for infusion

Tablet
▶ Quinine (Non-proprietary)
Quinine sulfate 200 mg Quinine sulfate 200mg tablets | 28 tablet [PoM] £6.05 DT price = £1.67
Quinine bisulfate 300 mg Quinine bisulfate 300mg tablets | 28 tablet [PoM] £4.80 DT price = £1.91
Quinine sulfate 300 mg Quinine sulfate 300mg tablets | 28 tablet [PoM] £5.05 DT price = £1.97 | 500 tablet [PoM] no price available

5.3 Toxoplasmosis

Drugs used for Toxoplasmosis not listed below
Pyrimethamine p. 375

ANTIBACTERIALS > MACROLIDES

Spiramycin

● **INDICATIONS AND DOSE**
Toxoplasmosis in pregnancy
▶ BY MOUTH
▶ Child 12–17 years: 1.5 g twice daily until delivery
Chemoprophylaxis of congenital toxoplasmosis
▶ BY MOUTH
▶ Neonate: 50 mg/kg twice daily.

DOSE EQUIVALENCE AND CONVERSION
3000 units ≡ 1 mg spiramycin.

● **UNLICENSED USE** Not licensed.

● **CAUTIONS** Arrhythmias · cardiac disease · predisposition to QT interval prolongation

● **SIDE-EFFECTS**
▶ **Rare** Prolongation of QT interval · thrombocytopenia · vasculitis
▶ **Frequency not known** Diarrhoea · dizziness · gastro-intestinal disturbances · headache · hepatotoxicity · nausea · rash · vomiting

● **ALLERGY AND CROSS-SENSITIVITY** Sensitivity to other macrolides.

● **BREAST FEEDING** Present in breast milk.

● **HEPATIC IMPAIRMENT** Use with caution.

● **MEDICINAL FORMS**
There can be variation in the licensing of different medicines containing the same drug.
Tablet
▶ Spiramycin (Non-proprietary)
Spiramycin 1500000 unit Rovamycine 1.5million unit tablets | 16 tablet [PoM] no price available
Spiramycin 3000000 unit Rovamycine 3million unit tablets | 10 tablet [PoM] no price available | 16 tablet [PoM] no price available
Oral solution
▶ Spiramycin (Non-proprietary)
Spiramycin 75000 unit per 1 ml Rovamycine 375,000units/5ml syrup | 150 ml [PoM] no price available

6 Viral infection
6.1 Hepatitis

Hepatitis

Overview

Treatment for viral hepatitis should be initiated by a specialist in hepatology or infectious diseases. The management of uncomplicated acute viral hepatitis is largely symptomatic. Hepatitis B and hepatitis C viruses are major causes of chronic hepatitis. Active or passive immunisation against hepatitis A and B infections can be given.

Chronic hepatitis B

Interferon alfa p. 517, **peginterferon alfa-2a**, lamivudine p. 393, adefovir dipivoxil, entecavir, and tenofovir disoproxil p. 394 have a role in the treatment of chronic hepatitis B in adults, but their role in children has not been well established. Specialist supervision is required for the management of chronic hepatitis B.

Tenofovir disoproxil, or a combination of tenofovir disoproxil with either emtricitabine p. 392 or lamivudine, may be used with other antiretrovirals, as part of 'highly active antiretroviral therapy' in children who require treatment for both HIV and chronic hepatitis B. If children infected with both HIV and chronic hepatitis B only require treatment for chronic hepatitis B, they should receive antivirals that are not active against HIV. Management of these children should be co-ordinated between HIV and hepatology specialists.

Chronic hepatitis C

Treatment should be considered for children with moderate or severe liver disease. Specialist supervision is required and the regimen is chosen according to the genotype of the infecting virus and the viral load. A combination of ribavirin p. 378 with either interferon alfa or **peginterferon alfa-2b** is licensed for use in children over 3 years with chronic hepatitis C. A combination of peginterferon alfa p. 379 and ribavirin is preferred.

5

Infection

6.2 Hepatitis infections
6.2a Chronic hepatitis C

> **Drugs used for Chronic hepatitis C not listed below**
> Interferon alfa, p. 517 · Peginterferon alfa, p. 379

ANTIVIRALS > NUCLEOSIDE ANALOGUES

Ribavirin
(Tribavirin)

● **INDICATIONS AND DOSE**

Bronchiolitis

▶ BY INHALATION OF AEROSOL, OR BY INHALATION OF NEBULISED SOLUTION

▸ **Child 1-23 months:** Inhale a solution containing 20 mg/mL for 12–18 hours for at least 3 days, maximum of 7 days, to be administered via small particle aerosol generator

Life-threatening RSV, parainfluenza virus, and adenovirus infection in immunocompromised children (administered on expert advice)

▶ BY INTRAVENOUS INFUSION

▸ **Child:** 33 mg/kg for 1 dose, to be administered over 15 minutes, then 16 mg/kg every 6 hours for 4 days, then 8 mg/kg every 8 hours for 3 days

REBETOL® CAPSULES

Chronic hepatitis C (in combination with interferon alfa or peginterferon alfa) in previously untreated children without liver decompensation

▶ BY MOUTH

▸ **Child 3-17 years (body-weight up to 47 kg):** 15 mg/kg daily in 2 divided doses

▸ **Child 3-17 years (body-weight 47-49 kg):** 200 mg, dose to be given in the morning and 400 mg, dose to be given in the evening

▸ **Child 3-17 years (body-weight 50-64 kg):** 400 mg twice daily

▸ **Child 3-17 years (body-weight 65-80 kg):** 400 mg, dose to be given in the morning and 600 mg, dose to be given in the evening

▸ **Child 3-17 years (body-weight 81-104 kg):** 600 mg twice daily

▸ **Child 3-17 years (body-weight 105 kg and above):** 600 mg, dose to be given in the morning and 800 mg, dose to be given in the evening

REBETOL® ORAL SOLUTION

Chronic hepatitis C (in combination with interferon alfa or peginterferon alfa) in previously untreated children without liver decompensation

▶ BY MOUTH

▸ **Child 3-17 years (body-weight up to 47 kg):** 15 mg/kg daily in 2 divided doses

▸ **Child 3-17 years (body-weight 47-49 kg):** 200 mg daily, dose to be given in the morning and 400 mg daily, dose to be given in the evening

▸ **Child 3-17 years (body-weight 50-64 kg):** 400 mg twice daily

▸ **Child 3-17 years (body-weight 65-80 kg):** 400 mg daily, dose to be given in the morning and 600 mg daily, dose to be given in the evening

▸ **Child 3-17 years (body-weight 81-104 kg):** 600 mg twice daily

▸ **Child 3-17 years (body-weight 105 kg and above):** 600 mg daily, dose to be given in the morning and 800 mg daily, dose to be given in the evening

● **UNLICENSED USE**

▸ When used by inhalation Inhalation licensed for use in children (age range not specified by manufacturer).

▸ With intravenous use Intravenous preparation not licensed.

● **CONTRA-INDICATIONS**

▸ With systemic use Active severe psychiatric condition · autoimmune disease · autoimmune hepatitis · consult product literature for specific contra-indications when ribavirin above used in combination with other medicinal products · haemoglobinopathies · history of severe psychiatric condition · severe debilitating medical conditions · severe, uncontrolled cardiac disease in children with chronic hepatitis C

● **CAUTIONS**

▸ When used by inhalation Maintain standard supportive respiratory and fluid management therapy

▸ With systemic use Cardiac disease (assessment including ECG recommended before and during treatment—discontinue if deterioration) · consult product literature for specific cautions when ribavirin above used in combination with other medicinal products · patients with a transplant—risk of rejection · risk of growth retardation the reversibility of which is uncertain—if possible, consider starting treatment after pubertal growth spurt

● **INTERACTIONS** → Appendix 1 (ribavirin).

● **SIDE-EFFECTS**

▸ When used by inhalation Bacterial pneumonia · haemolysis · non-specific anaemia · pneumothorax · worsening respiration

▸ With oral use Abdominal pain · abnormal dreams · acne · alopecia · anxiety · aplastic anaemia · arrhythmias · arthralgia · asthenia · asthenia · ataxia · breast pain · cardiomyopathy · changes in blood pressure · cheilitis · chest pain · colitis · constipation · cough · dehydration · depression · diarrhoea · dizziness · dry eyes · dry mouth · dry skin · dyspepsia · dysphagia · dysphonia · dyspnoea · earache · epistaxis · eye pain · flatulence · flushing · gastrointestinal bleeding · gastroesophageal reflux · gingivitis · glossitis · growth retardation (including decrease in height and weight) · haemolytic anaemia (anaemia may be improved by epoetin) · hallucination · headache · hearing impairment · hyperaesthesia · hyperglycaemia · hyperkinesia · hypertonia · hypertriglyceridaemia · hyperuricaemia · hypoaesthesia · hypocalcaemia · impaired concentration and memory · increased sweating · influenza-like symptoms · interstitial pneumonitis · leucopenia · loose stools · lymphadenopathy · menstrual disturbance · micturition disorders · mood disorders · mouth ulcers · musculoskeletal pain · myalgia · myocardial infarction · nasal congestion · nausea · neutropenia · optic neuropathy · oral candidiasis · pallor · palpitation · pancreatitis · panic attack · paraesthesia · peptic ulcer · pericarditis · peripheral ischaemia · peripheral neuropathy · peripheral oedema · photosensitivity · pruritus · psoriasis · psychotic disorders · pulmonary embolism · rash · renal failure · respiratory infections · retinal haemorrhage · rheumatoid arthritis · sarcoidosis · seizures · sexual dysfunction · sinus congestion · skin discolouration · sleep disturbances · sore throat · Stevens-Johnson syndrome · stomatitis · stroke · suicidal ideation · syncope · systemic lupus erythematosus · tachycardia · tachypnoea · taste disturbance · testicular pain · thrombocytopenia · thyroid disorders · tinnitus · tooth disorder · toxic epidermal necrolysis · urinary tract infections · vertigo · virilism · visual disturbances · vomiting · weight loss · wheezing

SIDE-EFFECTS, FURTHER INFORMATION

▸ With oral use Side effects listed are reported when oral ribavirin is used in combination with peginterferon alfa or interferon alfa, consult product literature for details.

- **CONCEPTION AND CONTRACEPTION**
- ▸ With systemic use Exclude pregnancy before treatment in females of childbearing age. Effective contraception essential during treatment and for 4 months after treatment in females and for 7 months after treatment in males of childbearing age. Routine monthly pregnancy tests recommended. Condoms must be used if partner of male patient is pregnant (ribavirin excreted in semen).
- ▸ When used by inhalation Women planning pregnancy should avoid exposure to aerosol.
- **PREGNANCY** Avoid; teratogenicity in *animal* studies.
- ▸ When used by inhalation Pregnant women should avoid exposure to aerosol.
- **BREAST FEEDING** Avoid—no information available.
- **HEPATIC IMPAIRMENT** No dosage adjustment required. Avoid oral ribavirin in severe hepatic dysfunction or decompensated cirrhosis.
- **RENAL IMPAIRMENT** Plasma-ribavirin concentration increased. Manufacturer advises avoid oral ribavirin if estimated glomerular filtration rate less than 50 mL/minute/1.73 m^2—monitor haemoglobin concentration closely.

  Manufacturer advises use intravenous preparation with caution if estimated glomerular filtration rate less than 30 mL/minute/1.73 m^2.
- **MONITORING REQUIREMENTS**
- ▸ When used by inhalation Monitor electrolytes closely. Monitor equipment for precipitation.
- ▸ With systemic use Determine full blood count, platelets, electrolytes, serum creatinine, liver function tests and uric acid before starting treatment and then on weeks 2 and 4 of treatment, then as indicated clinically—adjust dose if adverse reactions or laboratory abnormalities develop (consult product literature). Test thyroid function before treatment and then every 3 months.
- ▸ With oral use Eye examination recommended before treatment. Eye examination also recommended during treatment if pre-existing ophthalmological disorder or if decrease in vision reported—discontinue treatment if ophthalmological disorder deteriorates or if new ophthalmological disorder develops.
- **PRESCRIBING AND DISPENSING INFORMATION** Flavours of oral liquid formulations may include bubble-gum.
- **NATIONAL FUNDING/ACCESS DECISIONS**

  NICE technology appraisals (TAs)
- ▸ **Peginterferon alfa and ribavirin for chronic hepatitis C (November 2013)** NICE TA300 Peginterferon alfa in combination with ribavirin is recommended (within the marketing authorisation) as an option for treating chronic hepatitis C in children. www.nice.org.uk/TA300
- **LESS SUITABLE FOR PRESCRIBING** Ribavirin inhalation is less suitable for prescribing.

- **MEDICINAL FORMS**
  There can be variation in the licensing of different medicines containing the same drug. No licensed solution for injection listed.

  Capsule
  CAUTIONARY AND ADVISORY LABELS 21
- ▸ **Rebetol** (Merck Sharp & Dohme Ltd)
  Ribavirin 200 mg Rebetol 200mg capsules | 84 capsule PoM £160.69 | 140 capsule PoM £267.81 | 168 capsule PoM £321.38

  Oral solution
  CAUTIONARY AND ADVISORY LABELS 21
- ▸ **Rebetol** (Merck Sharp & Dohme Ltd)
  Ribavirin 40 mg per 1 ml Rebetol 40mg/ml oral solution | 100 ml PoM £67.08

IMMUNOSTIMULANTS ❯ INTERFERONS

Peginterferon alfa

- **DRUG ACTION** Polyethylene glycol-conjugated ('pegylated') derivatives of interferon alfa (**peginterferon alfa-2a** and **peginterferon alfa-2b**) are available; pegylation increases the persistence of the interferon in the blood.

- ● **INDICATIONS AND DOSE**

  PEGASYS®

  Chronic hepatitis C (in combination with ribavirin) in previously untreated children without liver decompensation
  - ▸ BY SUBCUTANEOUS INJECTION
  - ▸ Child 5-17 years: (consult product literature)

  VIRAFERONPEG®

  Chronic hepatitis C (in combination with ribavirin) in previously untreated children without liver decompensation
  - ▸ BY SUBCUTANEOUS INJECTION
  - ▸ Child 3-17 years: (consult product literature)

- **CONTRA-INDICATIONS** Severe psychiatric illness
  CONTRA-INDICATIONS, FURTHER INFORMATION
  For contra-indications consult product literature.
- **CAUTIONS**
  CAUTIONS, FURTHER INFORMATION
  For cautions consult product literature.
- **INTERACTIONS** → Appendix 1 (interferons).
- **SIDE-EFFECTS**
- ▸ **Common or very common** Anorexia · influenza-like symptoms · lethargy · nausea
- ▸ **Frequency not known** Alopecia · arrhythmias · cardiovascular problems · coma · confusion · depression · hepatotoxicity · hyperglycaemia · hypersensitivity reactions · hypertension · hypertriglyceridaemia (sometimes severe) · hypotension · myelosuppression (particularly affecting granulocyte counts) · nephrotoxicity · ocular side-effects · pneumonia · pneumonitis · psoriasiform rash · pulmonary infiltrates · reversible motor problems in young children · seizures · suicidal behaviour · thyroid abnormalities
  SIDE-EFFECTS, FURTHER INFORMATION
  For information on side effects consult product literature.
- ▸ Respiratory symptoms Respiratory symptoms should be investigated and if pulmonary infiltrates are suspected or lung function is impaired the discontinuation of peginterferon alfa should be considered.
- **CONCEPTION AND CONTRACEPTION** Effective contraception required during treatment—consult product literature.
- **PREGNANCY** Manufacturers recommend avoid unless potential benefit outweighs risk (toxicity in *animal* studies).
- **BREAST FEEDING** Manufacturers advise avoid—no information available.
- **HEPATIC IMPAIRMENT** Avoid in severe impairment.
- **RENAL IMPAIRMENT** Reduce dose in moderate to severe impairment. For information on peginterferon alfa use in renal impairment consult product literature. Close monitoring required in renal impairment.
- **MONITORING REQUIREMENTS**
- ▸ Monitoring of lipid concentration is recommended.
- ▸ Monitoring of hepatic function is recommended.

5

Infection

Infection

5

● NATIONAL FUNDING/ACCESS DECISIONS

NICE technology appraisals (TAs)

▶ **Peginterferon alfa and ribavirin for chronic hepatitis C (November 2013)** NICE TA300

Peginterferon alfa in combination with ribavirin is recommended (within the marketing authorisation) as an option for treating chronic hepatitis C in children. www.nice.org.uk/TA300

● MEDICINAL FORMS
There can be variation in the licensing of different medicines containing the same drug.

Solution for injection
EXCIPIENTS: May contain Benzyl alcohol

▶ Pegasys (Roche Products Ltd)
Peginterferon alfa-2a 180 microgram per 1 ml Pegasys 90micrograms/0.5ml solution for injection pre-filled syringes | 1 pre-filled disposable injection [PoM] £76.51
Peginterferon alfa-2a 270 microgram per 1 ml Pegasys 135micrograms/0.5ml solution for injection pre-filled syringes | 1 pre-filled disposable injection [PoM] £107.76
Pegasys 135micrograms/0.5ml solution for injection pre-filled pen | 1 pre-filled disposable injection [PoM] £107.76
Peginterferon alfa-2a 360 microgram per 1 ml Pegasys 180micrograms/0.5ml solution for injection pre-filled syringes | 4 pre-filled disposable injection [PoM] £497.60
Pegasys 180micrograms/0.5ml solution for injection pre-filled pen | 4 pre-filled disposable injection [PoM] £497.60

Powder and solvent for solution for injection

▶ ViraferonPeg (Merck Sharp & Dohme Ltd)
Peginterferon alfa-2b 50 microgram ViraferonPeg 50microgram powder and solvent for solution for injection pre-filled disposable devices | 1 pre-filled disposable injection [PoM] £66.46
Peginterferon alfa-2b 80 microgram ViraferonPeg 80microgram powder and solvent for solution for injection pre-filled disposable devices | 1 pre-filled disposable injection [PoM] £106.34
Peginterferon alfa-2b 100 microgram ViraferonPeg 100microgram powder and solvent for solution for injection pre-filled disposable devices | 1 pre-filled disposable injection [PoM] £132.92
Peginterferon alfa-2b 120 microgram ViraferonPeg 120microgram powder and solvent for solution for injection pre-filled disposable devices | 1 pre-filled disposable injection [PoM] £159.51
Peginterferon alfa-2b 150 microgram ViraferonPeg 150microgram powder and solvent for solution for injection pre-filled disposable devices | 1 pre-filled disposable injection [PoM] £199.38

▶ ViraferonPeg CLEARCLICK (Merck Sharp & Dohme Ltd)
Peginterferon alfa-2b 50 microgram ViraferonPeg 50microgram powder and solvent for solution for injection pre-filled disposable devices CLEARCLICK | 1 pre-filled disposable injection [PoM] £66.46
Peginterferon alfa-2b 80 microgram ViraferonPeg 80microgram powder and solvent for solution for injection pre-filled disposable devices CLEARCLICK | 1 pre-filled disposable injection [PoM] £106.34
Peginterferon alfa-2b 100 microgram ViraferonPeg 100microgram powder and solvent for solution for injection pre-filled disposable devices CLEARCLICK | 1 pre-filled disposable injection [PoM] £132.92
Peginterferon alfa-2b 120 microgram ViraferonPeg 120microgram powder and solvent for solution for injection pre-filled disposable devices CLEARCLICK | 1 pre-filled disposable injection [PoM] £159.51
Peginterferon alfa-2b 150 microgram ViraferonPeg 150microgram powder and solvent for solution for injection pre-filled disposable devices CLEARCLICK | 1 pre-filled disposable injection [PoM] £199.38

6.3 Herpesvirus infections

Herpesvirus infections

Herpes simplex and varicella–zoster infection

The two most important herpesvirus pathogens are herpes simplex virus (herpesvirus hominis) and varicella–zoster virus.

Herpes simplex infections

Herpes infection of the mouth and lips and in the eye is generally associated with herpes simplex virus serotype 1 (HSV-1); other areas of the skin may also be infected, especially in immunodeficiency. Genital infection is most

often associated with HSV-2 and also HSV-1. Treatment of herpes simplex infection should start as early as possible and usually within 5 days of the appearance of the infection.

In individuals with good immune function, mild infection of the eye (ocular herpes) and of the lips (herpes labialis or cold sores) is treated with a topical antiviral drug. Primary herpetic gingivostomatitis is managed by changes to diet and with analgesics. Severe infection, neonatal herpes infection or infection in immunocompromised individuals requires treatment with a systemic antiviral drug. After completing parenteral treatment of neonatal herpes simplex encephalitis, oral suppression therapy with aciclovir p. 381 for 6 months can be considered on specialist advice. Primary or recurrent genital herpes simplex infection is treated with an antiviral drug given by mouth. Persistence of a lesion or recurrence in an immunocompromised patient may signal the development of resistance.

Specialist advice should be sought for systemic treatment of herpes simplex infection in pregnancy.

Varicella-zoster infections
Regardless of immune function and the use of any immunoglobulins, neonates with *chickenpox* should be treated with a parenteral antiviral to reduce the risk of severe disease. Oral therapy in children is not recommended as absorption is variable. Chickenpox in otherwise healthy children between 1 month and 12 years is usually mild and antiviral treatment is not usually required.

Chickenpox is more severe in adolescents than in children; antiviral treatment started within 24 hours of the onset of rash may reduce the duration and severity of symptoms in otherwise healthy adolescents. Antiviral treatment is generally recommended in immunocompromised patients and those at special risk (e.g. because of severe cardiovascular or respiratory disease or chronic skin disorder); in such cases, an antiviral is given for 10 days with at least 7 days of parenteral treatment.

In pregnancy severe chickenpox may cause complications, especially varicella pneumonia. Specialist advice should be sought for the treatment of chickenpox during pregnancy.

Neonates and children who have been exposed to chickenpox and are at special risk of complications may require prophylaxis with varicella-zoster immunoglobulin (see under Disease-specific Immunoglobulins). Prophylactic intravenous aciclovir should be considered for neonates whose mothers develop chickenpox 4 days before to 2 days after delivery.

In *herpes zoster* (shingles) systemic antiviral treatment can reduce the severity and duration of pain, reduce complications, and reduce viral shedding. Treatment with the antiviral should be started within 72 hours of the onset of rash and is usually continued for 7–10 days. Immunocompromised patients at high risk of disseminated or severe infection should be treated with a parenteral antiviral drug.

Chronic pain which persists after the rash has healed (postherpetic neuralgia) requires specific management.

Choice
Aciclovir is active against herpesviruses but does not eradicate them. Uses of aciclovir include systemic treatment of varicella–zoster and the systemic and topical treatment of herpes simplex infections of the skin and mucous membranes. It is used by mouth for severe herpetic stomatitis. Aciclovir eye ointment is used for herpes simplex infections of the eye; it is combined with systemic treatment for ophthalmic zoster.

Famciclovir, a prodrug of penciclovir, is similar to aciclovir and is licensed in adults for use in herpes zoster and genital herpes; there is limited information available on use in children.

Valaciclovir p. 383 is an ester of aciclovir, licensed in adults for herpes zoster and herpes simplex infections of the skin and mucous membranes (including genital herpes); it is also licensed in children over 12 years for preventing cytomegalovirus disease following solid organ transplantation. Valaciclovir may be used for the treatment of mild herpes zoster in immunocompromised children over 12 years; treatment should be initiated under specialist supervision.

Cytomegalovirus infection

Ganciclovir p. 383 is related to aciclovir but it is more active against cytomegalovirus (CMV); it is also much more toxic than aciclovir and should therefore be prescribed under specialist supervision and only when the potential benefit outweighs the risks. Ganciclovir is administered by intravenous infusion for the *initial treatment* of CMV infection. The use of ganciclovir may also be considered for symptomatic congenital CMV infection. Ganciclovir causes profound myelosuppression when given with zidovudine p. 394; the two should not normally be given together particularly during initial ganciclovir therapy. The likelihood of ganciclovir resistance increases in patients with a high viral load or in those who receive the drug over a long duration.

Valaciclovir is licensed for use in children over 12 years for prevention of cytomegalovirus disease following renal transplantation.

Foscarnet sodium p. 384 is also active against cytomegalovirus; it is toxic and can cause renal impairment. It is deposited in teeth, bone and cartilage, and *animal* studies have shown that deposition is greater in young animals. Its effect on skeletal development in children is not known. Foscarnet sodium should be prescribed under specialist supervision.

ANTIVIRALS > NUCLEOSIDE ANALOGUES

Aciclovir
(Acyclovir)

● **INDICATIONS AND DOSE**
Herpes simplex, suppression
▸ BY MOUTH
▸ Child 12-17 years: 400 mg twice daily, alternatively 200 mg 4 times a day; increased to 400 mg 3 times a day, dose may be increased if recurrences occur on standard suppressive therapy or for suppression of genital herpes during late pregnancy (from 36 weeks gestation), therapy interrupted every 6–12 months to reassess recurrence frequency—consider restarting after two or more recurrences

Herpes simplex, prophylaxis in the immunocompromised
▸ BY MOUTH
▸ Child 1-23 months: 100–200 mg 4 times a day
▸ Child 2-17 years: 200–400 mg 4 times a day

Herpes Simplex, treatment
▸ BY MOUTH
▸ Child 1-23 months: 100 mg 5 times a day usually for 5 days (longer if new lesions appear during treatment or if healing incomplete)
▸ Child 2-17 years: 200 mg 5 times a day usually for 5 days (longer if new lesions appear during treatment or if healing incomplete)
▸ BY INTRAVENOUS INFUSION
▸ Neonate: 20 mg/kg every 8 hours for 14 days (for at least 21 days if CNS involvement—confirm cerebrospinal fluid negative for herpes simplex virus before stopping treatment).
▸ Child 1-2 months: 20 mg/kg every 8 hours for 14 days (for at least 21 days if CNS involvement—confirm cerebrospinal fluid negative for herpes simplex virus before stopping treatment)

▸ Child 3 months-11 years: 250 mg/m^2 every 8 hours usually for 5 days
▸ Child 12-17 years: 5 mg/kg every 8 hours usually for 5 days

Herpes Simplex, treatment, in immunocompromised or if absorption impaired
▸ BY MOUTH
▸ Child 1-23 months: 200 mg 5 times a day usually for 5 days (longer if new lesions appear during treatment or if healing incomplete)
▸ Child 2-17 years: 400 mg 5 times a day usually for 5 days (longer if new lesions appear during treatment or if healing incomplete)

Herpes Simplex, treatment, in immunocompromised or in simplex encephalitis
▸ BY INTRAVENOUS INFUSION
▸ Child 3 months-11 years: 500 mg/m^2 every 8 hours usually for 5 days (given for at least 14 days in encephalitis—confirm cerebrospinal fluid negative for herpes simplex virus before stopping treatment)
▸ Child 12-17 years: 10 mg/kg every 8 hours usually for 5 days (given for at least 14 days in encephalitis and for at least 21 days if also immunocompromised—confirm cerebrospinal fluid negative for herpes simplex virus before stopping treatment)

Varicella zoster (chickenpox), treatment | Herpes zoster (shingles), treatment
▸ BY MOUTH
▸ Child 1-23 months: 200 mg 4 times a day for 5 days
▸ Child 2-5 years: 400 mg 4 times a day for 5 days
▸ Child 6-11 years: 800 mg 4 times a day for 5 days
▸ Child 12-17 years: 800 mg 5 times a day for 7 days
▸ BY INTRAVENOUS INFUSION
▸ Neonate: 10–20 mg/kg every 8 hours for at least 7 days.
▸ Child 1-2 months: 10–20 mg/kg every 8 hours for at least 7 days
▸ Child 3 months-11 years: 250 mg/m^2 every 8 hours usually for 5 days
▸ Child 12-17 years: 5 mg/kg every 8 hours usually for 5 days

Varicella zoster (chickenpox), treatment in immunocompromised | Herpes zoster (shingles), treatment in immunocompromised
▸ BY INTRAVENOUS INFUSION
▸ Child 3 months-11 years: 500 mg/m^2 every 8 hours usually for 5 days
▸ Child 12-17 years: 10 mg/kg every 8 hours usually for 5 days

Herpes zoster (shingles), treatment in immunocompromised
▸ BY MOUTH
▸ Child 1-23 months: 200 mg 4 times a day continued for 2 days after crusting of lesions
▸ Child 2-5 years: 400 mg 4 times a day continued for 2 days after crusting of lesions
▸ Child 6-11 years: 800 mg 4 times a day continued for 2 days after crusting of lesions
▸ Child 12-17 years: 800 mg 5 times a day continued for 2 days after crusting of lesions

Herpes zoster, treatment in encephalitis | Varicella zoster, treatment in encephalitis
▸ BY INTRAVENOUS INFUSION
▸ Neonate: 10–20 mg/kg every 8 hours given for 10–14 days in encephalitis, possibly longer if also immunocompromised.
▸ Child 1-2 months: 10–20 mg/kg every 8 hours given for 10–14 days in encephalitis, possibly longer if also immunocompromised

continued →

5

Infection

▸ Child 3 months–11 years: 500 mg/m^2 every 8 hours given for 10–14 days in encephalitis, possibly longer if also immunocompromised

▸ Child 12–17 years: 10 mg/kg every 8 hours given for 10–14 days in encephalitis, possibly longer if also immunocompromised

Varicella zoster (chickenpox), attenuation of infection if varicella–zoster immunoglobulin not indicated
▸ BY MOUTH
▸ Child: 10 mg/kg 4 times a day for 7 days, to be started 1 week after exposure

Varicella zoster (chickenpox), prophylaxis after delivery
▸ BY INTRAVENOUS INFUSION
▸ Neonate: 10 mg/kg every 8 hours continued until serological tests confirm absence of virus.

DOSES AT EXTREMES OF BODY-WEIGHT
▸ With intravenous use To avoid excessive dosage in obese patients parenteral dose should be calculated on the basis of ideal weight for height.

● **UNLICENSED USE**
▸ With oral use Tablets and suspension not licensed for suppression of herpes simplex or for treatment of herpes zoster in children (age range not specified by manufacturer). Aciclovir doses in BNF may differ from those in product literature. Attenuation of chickenpox is an unlicensed indication.
▸ With intravenous use Intravenous infusion not licensed for herpes zoster in children under 18 years.

● **CAUTIONS** Maintain adequate hydration (especially with infusion or high doses)

● **INTERACTIONS** → Appendix 1 (aciclovir).

● **SIDE-EFFECTS**
▸ Common or very common Abdominal pain · diarrhoea · fatigue · headache · nausea · photosensitivity · pruritus · rash · urticaria · vomiting
▸ Very rare
▸ With intravenous use Agitation · fever · psychosis · severe local inflammation (sometimes leading to ulceration) · tremors
▸ With systemic use Acute renal failure · anaemia · ataxia · confusion · convulsions · dizziness · drowsiness · dysarthria · dyspnoea · hallucinations · hepatitis · jaundice · leucopenia · neurological reactions · thrombocytopenia

● **PREGNANCY** Not known to be harmful—manufacturers advise use only when potential benefit outweighs risk.

● **BREAST FEEDING** Significant amount in milk after systemic administration—not known to be harmful but manufacturer advises caution.

● **RENAL IMPAIRMENT**
▸ With intravenous use Use *normal intravenous dose* every 12 hours if estimated glomerular filtration rate 25–50 mL/minute/1.73m^2 (every 24 hours if estimated glomerular filtration rate 10–25 mL/minute/1.73m^2. Consult product literature for intravenous dose if estimated glomerular filtration rate less than 10 mL/minute/1.73^2.
▸ With oral use For *herpes zoster*, use normal oral dose every 8 hours if estimated glomerular filtration rate 10–25 mL/minute/1.73m^2 (every 12 hours if estimated glomerular filtration rate less than 10 mL/minute/1.73m^2. For *herpes simplex*, use normal dose every 12 hours if estimated glomerular filtration rate less than 10 mL/minute/1.73^2.
▸ With systemic use Risk of neurological reactions increased. Maintain adequate hydration (especially during renal impairment).

● **DIRECTIONS FOR ADMINISTRATION** For *intravenous infusion*, reconstitute to 25 mg/mL with Water for Injections or Sodium Chloride 0.9% then dilute to

concentration of 5 mg/mL with Sodium Chloride 0.9% or Sodium Chloride and Glucose and give over 1 hour; alternatively, may be administered in a concentration of 25 mg/mL using a suitable infusion pump and central venous access and given over 1 hour.

● **PRESCRIBING AND DISPENSING INFORMATION** Flavours of oral liquid preparations may include banana, or orange.

● **PATIENT AND CARER ADVICE**
Medicines for Children leaflet: Aciclovir (oral) for viral infections
www.medicinesforchildren.org.uk/aciclovir-for-viral-infections

● **PROFESSION SPECIFIC INFORMATION**
Dental practitioners' formulary
▸ With oral use Aciclovir Tablets 200 mg or 800 mg may be prescribed. Aciclovir Oral Suspension 200 mg/5mL may be prescribed.

● **MEDICINAL FORMS**
There can be variation in the licensing of different medicines containing the same drug.
Tablet
CAUTIONARY AND ADVISORY LABELS 9
▸ Aciclovir (Non-proprietary)
Aciclovir 200 mg Aciclovir 200mg tablets | 25 tablet [PoM] £10.00 DT price = £1.44
Aciclovir 400 mg Aciclovir 400mg tablets | 56 tablet [PoM] £15.00 DT price = £3.20
Aciclovir 800 mg Aciclovir 800mg tablets | 35 tablet [PoM] £20.00 DT price = £3.48

Dispersible tablet
CAUTIONARY AND ADVISORY LABELS 9
▸ Aciclovir (Non-proprietary)
Aciclovir 200 mg Aciclovir 200mg dispersible tablets | 25 tablet [PoM] £17.50 DT price = £1.77
Aciclovir 400 mg Aciclovir 400mg dispersible tablets | 56 tablet [PoM] £20.00 DT price = £11.95
Aciclovir 800 mg Aciclovir 800mg dispersible tablets | 35 tablet [PoM] £65.00 DT price = £10.96
▸ Zovirax (GlaxoSmithKline UK Ltd)
Aciclovir 200 mg Zovirax 200mg dispersible tablets | 25 tablet [PoM] £2.85 DT price = £1.77
Aciclovir 800 mg Zovirax 800mg dispersible tablets | 35 tablet [PoM] £10.50 DT price = £10.96

Oral suspension
CAUTIONARY AND ADVISORY LABELS 9
▸ Aciclovir (Non-proprietary)
Aciclovir 40 mg per 1 ml Aciclovir 200mg/5ml oral suspension sugar free sugar-free | 125 ml [PoM] £35.76 DT price = £35.76
Aciclovir 80 mg per 1 ml Aciclovir 400mg/5ml oral suspension sugar free sugar-free | 100 ml [PoM] £39.47 DT price = £39.47
▸ Zovirax (GlaxoSmithKline UK Ltd)
Aciclovir 40 mg per 1 ml Zovirax 200mg/5ml oral suspension sugar-free | 125 ml [PoM] £29.56 DT price = £35.76
Aciclovir 80 mg per 1 ml Zovirax Double Strength 400mg/5ml oral suspension sugar-free | 100 ml [PoM] £33.02 DT price = £39.47

Solution for infusion
ELECTROLYTES: May contain Sodium
▸ Aciclovir (Non-proprietary)
Aciclovir (as Aciclovir sodium) 25 mg per 1 ml Aciclovir 1g/40ml solution for infusion vials | 1 vial [PoM] £40.00
Aciclovir 500mg/20ml solution for infusion vials | 5 vial [PoM] £100.00
Aciclovir 250mg/10ml solution for infusion vials | 5 vial [PoM] £50.00

Powder for solution for infusion
ELECTROLYTES: May contain Sodium
▸ Aciclovir (Non-proprietary)
Aciclovir (as Aciclovir sodium) 250 mg Aciclovir 250mg powder for solution for infusion vials | 5 vial [PoM] £45.66
▸ Zovirax (GlaxoSmithKline UK Ltd)
Aciclovir (as Aciclovir sodium) 250 mg Zovirax I.V. 250mg powder for solution for infusion vials | 5 vial [PoM] £16.70
Aciclovir (as Aciclovir sodium) 500 mg Zovirax I.V. 500mg powder for solution for infusion vials | 5 vial [PoM] £17.00

Valaciclovir

- **INDICATIONS AND DOSE**

Herpes zoster infection, treatment in immunocompromised patients
▸ BY MOUTH
▸ Child 12–17 years: 1 g 3 times a day for at least 7 days and continued for 2 days after crusting of lesions

Herpes simplex, treatment of first infective episode
▸ BY MOUTH
▸ Child 12–17 years: 500 mg twice daily for 5 days (longer if new lesions appear during treatment or healing is incomplete)

Herpes simplex infections treatment of first episode in immunocompromised or HIV-positive patients
▸ BY MOUTH
▸ Child 12–17 years: 1 g twice daily for 10 days

Herpes simplex, treatment of recurrent infections
▸ BY MOUTH
▸ Child 12–17 years: 500 mg twice daily for 3–5 days

Treatment of recurrent herpes simplex infections in immunocompromised or HIV-positive patients
▸ BY MOUTH
▸ Child 12–17 years: 1 g twice daily for 5–10 days

Herpes labialis treatment
▸ BY MOUTH
▸ Child 12–17 years: Initially 2 g, then 2 g after 12 hours

Herpes simplex, suppression of infections
▸ BY MOUTH
▸ Child 12–17 years: 500 mg daily in 1–2 divided doses, therapy to be interrupted every 6–12 months to reassess recurrence frequency—consider restarting after two or more recurrences

Herpes simplex, suppression of infections in immunocompromised or HIV-positive patients
▸ BY MOUTH
▸ Child 12–17 years: 500 mg twice daily, therapy to be interrupted every 6–12 months to reassess recurrence frequency—consider restarting after two or more recurrences

Prevention of cytomegalovirus disease following solid organ transplantation when valganciclovir or ganciclovir cannot be used
▸ BY MOUTH
▸ Child 12–17 years: 2 g 4 times a day usually for 90 days, preferably starting within 72 hours of transplantation

- **UNLICENSED USE** Not licensed for treatment of herpes zoster in children. Not licensed for treatment or suppression of herpes simplex infection in immunocompromised or HIV-positive children.
- **CAUTIONS** Maintain adequate hydration (especially with high doses)
- **INTERACTIONS** → Appendix 1 (valaciclovir).
- **SIDE-EFFECTS**
▸ **Very rare** Acute renal failure · anaemia · ataxia · confusion · convulsions · dizziness · drowsiness · dysarthria · dyspnoea · hallucinations · hepatitis · jaundice · leucopenia · neurological reactions · thrombocytopenia
▸ **Frequency not known** Abdominal pain · diarrhoea · fatigue · headache · nausea · photosensitivity · pruritus · rash · urticaria · vomiting
  SIDE-EFFECTS, FURTHER INFORMATION
▸ Neurological reactions Neurological reactions (including dizziness, confusion, hallucinations, convulsions, ataxia, dysarthria, and drowsiness) more frequent with higher doses.
- **PREGNANCY** Not known to be harmful—manufacturers advise use only when potential benefit outweighs risk.

- **BREAST FEEDING** Significant amount in milk after systemic administration—not known to be harmful but manufacturer advises caution.
- **HEPATIC IMPAIRMENT** Manufacturer advises caution with high doses used for preventing cytomegalovirus disease—no information available in children.
- **RENAL IMPAIRMENT** For *herpes zoster*, 1 g every 12 hours if estimated glomerular filtration rate 30–50 mL/minute/1.73 m^2 (1 g every 24 hours if estimated glomerular filtration rate 10–30 mL/minute/1.73 m^2; 500 mg every 24 hours if estimated glomerular filtration rate less than 10 mL/minute/1.73 m^2). For *treatment of herpes simplex*, 500 mg (1 g in immunocompromised or HIV-positive children) every 24 hours if estimated glomerular filtration rate less than 30 mL/minute/1.73 m^2. For *treatment of herpes labialis*, if estimated glomerular filtration rate 30–50 mL/minute/1.73 m^2, initially 1 g, then 1 g 12 hours after initial dose (if estimated glomerular filtration rate 10–30 mL/minute/1.73 m^2, initially 500 mg, then 500 mg 12 hours after initial dose; if estimated glomerular filtration rate less than 10 mL/minute/1.73 m^2, 500 mg as a single dose). For *suppression of herpes simplex*, 250 mg (500 mg in immunocompromised or HIV-positive children) every 24 hours if estimated glomerular filtration rate less than 30 mL/minute/1.73 m^2. Reduce dose according to estimated glomerular filtration rate for *cytomegalovirus prophylaxis* following solid organ transplantation (consult product literature). Maintain adequate hydration.
- **PRESCRIBING AND DISPENSING INFORMATION** Valaciclovir is a pro-drug of aciclovir.

- **MEDICINAL FORMS**
There can be variation in the licensing of different medicines containing the same drug. Forms available from special-order manufacturers include: oral suspension
Tablet
CAUTIONARY AND ADVISORY LABELS 9
▸ Valaciclovir (Non-proprietary)
  Valaciclovir (as Valaciclovir hydrochloride) 500 mg Valaciclovir 500mg tablets | 10 tablet [PoM] £20.59 DT price = £3.04 | 42 tablet [PoM] £86.30
▸ Valtrex (GlaxoSmithKline UK Ltd)
  Valaciclovir (as Valaciclovir hydrochloride) 250 mg Valtrex 250mg tablets | 60 tablet [PoM] £123.28 DT price = £123.28
  Valaciclovir (as Valaciclovir hydrochloride) 500 mg Valtrex 500mg tablets | 10 tablet [PoM] £20.59 DT price = £3.04 | 42 tablet [PoM] £86.30

6.3a Cytomegalovirus infections

ANTIVIRALS › NUCLEOSIDE ANALOGUES

Ganciclovir

- **INDICATIONS AND DOSE**

Prevention of cytomegalovirus disease during immunosuppressive therapy following organ transplantation
▸ BY INTRAVENOUS INFUSION
▸ Child: 5 mg/kg every 12 hours for 7–14 days

Treatment of life-threatening or sight-threatening cytomegalovirus infections in immunocompromised patients only
▸ BY INTRAVENOUS INFUSION
▸ Child: Initially 5 mg/kg every 12 hours for 14–21 days, followed by maintenance 6 mg/kg daily on 5 days of the week, alternatively 5 mg/kg daily until adequate recovery of immunity, maintenance only for patients at risk of relapse of retinitis, if retinitis progresses initial induction treatment may be repeated continued →

5

Infection

5

Infection

Congenital cytomegalovirus infection of the CNS
▶ BY INTRAVENOUS INFUSION
▷ Neonate: 6 mg/kg every 12 hours for 6 weeks.

- **UNLICENSED USE** Not licensed for use in children.
- **CONTRA-INDICATIONS** Abnormally low haemoglobin count (consult product literature) · abnormally low neutrophil count (consult product literature) · abnormally low platelet count (consult product literature)
- **CAUTIONS** Children (possible risk of long-term carcinogenic or reproductive toxicity) · ensure adequate hydration · history of cytopenia · potential carcinogen · potential teratogen · radiotherapy · vesicant
- **INTERACTIONS** → Appendix 1 (ganciclovir). Increased risk of myelosuppression with other myelosuppressive drugs—consult product literature.
- **SIDE-EFFECTS**
▶ **Common or very common** Abdominal pain · abnormal thinking · anaemia · anorexia · anxiety · arthralgia · chest pain · confusion · constipation · convulsions · cough · depression · dermatitis · diarrhoea · dizziness · dyspepsia · dysphagia · dyspnoea · ear pain · eye pain · fatigue · flatulence · headache · hepatic dysfunction · infection · injection-site reactions · insomnia · leucopenia · macular oedema · myalgia · nausea · night sweats · pancytopenia · peripheral neuropathy · pruritus · pyrexia · renal impairment · retinal detachment · taste disturbance · thrombocytopenia · vitreous floaters · vomiting · weight loss
▶ **Uncommon** Alopecia · anaphylactic reactions · arrhythmias · disturbances in hearing and vision · haematuria · hypotension · male infertility · mouth ulcers · pancreatitis · psychosis · tremor
- **ALLERGY AND CROSS-SENSITIVITY** Contra-indicated in patients hypersensitive to valganciclovir, aciclovir, or valaciclovir.
- **CONCEPTION AND CONTRACEPTION** Ensure effective contraception during treatment and barrier contraception for men during and for at least 90 days after treatment.
- **PREGNANCY** Avoid—teratogenic risk.
- **BREAST FEEDING** Avoid—no information available.
- **RENAL IMPAIRMENT** Reduce dose if estimated glomerular filtration rate less than 70 mL/minute/1.73 m^2; consult product literature.
- **MONITORING REQUIREMENTS** Monitor full blood count closely (severe deterioration may require correction and possibly treatment interruption).
- **DIRECTIONS FOR ADMINISTRATION** Infuse into vein with adequate flow preferably using plastic cannula. For *intravenous infusion*, reconstitute with Water for Injections (500 mg/10 mL) then dilute to a concentration of not more than 10 mg/mL with Glucose 5% *or* Sodium Chloride 0.9% and give over 1 hour.
- **HANDLING AND STORAGE**
Caution in handling
Ganciclovir is toxic and personnel should be adequately protected during handling and administration; if solution comes into contact with skin or mucosa, wash off immediately with soap and water.

- **MEDICINAL FORMS**
There can be variation in the licensing of different medicines containing the same drug.
Powder for solution for infusion
ELECTROLYTES: May contain Sodium
▶ Cymevene (Roche Products Ltd)
Ganciclovir (as Ganciclovir sodium) 500 mg Cymevene 500mg powder for solution for infusion vials | 5 vial [PoM] £148.83

ANTIVIRALS 〉 OTHER

Foscarnet sodium

- **INDICATIONS AND DOSE**
Cytomegalovirus disease
▶ BY INTRAVENOUS INFUSION
▷ Child (under expert supervision): Initially 60 mg/kg every 8 hours 2–3 weeks, then maintenance 60 mg/kg daily, increased if tolerated to 90–120 mg/kg daily, if disease progresses on maintenance dose, repeat induction regimen

Mucocutaneous herpes simplex virus infections unresponsive to aciclovir in immunocompromised patients
▶ BY INTRAVENOUS INFUSION
▷ Child (under expert supervision): 40 mg/kg every 8 hours for 2–3 weeks or until lesions heal

- **UNLICENSED USE** Not licensed for use in children.
- **CAUTIONS** Ensure adequate hydration
- **INTERACTIONS** → Appendix 1 (foscarnet).
- **SIDE-EFFECTS**
▶ **Common or very common** Abdominal pain · acute renal failure · aggression · agitation · anaemia · anorexia · anxiety · changes in blood pressure · changes in ECG · confusion · constipation · convulsions · depression · diarrhoea · dizziness · dyspepsia · dysuria · electrolyte disturbances · genital irritation and ulceration (due to high concentrations excreted in urine) · granulocytopenia · headache · hepatic dysfunction · hypocalcaemia · hypokalaemia · hypomagnesaemia · leucopenia · malaise · myalgia · nausea (reduce infusion rate) · neurological disorders · oedema · palpitation · pancreatitis · paraesthesia (reduce infusion rate) · polyuria · pruritus · rash · renal impairment · thrombocytopenia · thrombophlebitis if given undiluted by peripheral vein · tremor · vomiting
▶ **Uncommon** Acidosis
▶ **Frequency not known** Diabetes insipidus · myasthenia · myositis · oesophageal ulceration · rhabdomyolysis · ventricular arrhythmias
- **CONCEPTION AND CONTRACEPTION** Men should avoid fathering a child during and for 6 months after treatment.
- **PREGNANCY** Manufacturer advises avoid.
- **BREAST FEEDING** Avoid—present in milk in *animal* studies.
- **RENAL IMPAIRMENT** Reduce dose; consult product literature.
- **MONITORING REQUIREMENTS**
▶ Monitor electrolytes, particularly calcium and magnesium.
▶ Monitor serum creatinine every second day during induction and every week during maintenance.
- **DIRECTIONS FOR ADMINISTRATION** Avoid rapid infusion. For *intravenous infusion*, give undiluted solution via a central venous catheter; alternatively dilute to a concentration of 12 mg/mL with Glucose 5% *or* Sodium Chloride 0.9% for administration via a peripheral vein; give over at least 1 hour (give doses greater than 60 mg/kg over 2 hours).

- **MEDICINAL FORMS**
There can be variation in the licensing of different medicines containing the same drug.
Solution for infusion
ELECTROLYTES: May contain Sodium
▶ Foscavir (Clinigen Healthcare Ltd)
Foscarnet sodium 24 mg per 1 ml Foscavir 6g/250ml solution for infusion bottles | 1 bottle [PoM] £119.85 (Hospital only)

6.4 HIV infection

HIV infection

Overview

There is no cure for infection caused by the human immunodeficiency virus (HIV) but a number of drugs slow or halt disease progression. Drugs for HIV infection (antiretrovirals) may be associated with serious side-effects. Although antiretrovirals increase life expectancy considerably and decrease the risk of complications associated with premature ageing, mortality and morbidity remain slightly higher than in uninfected individuals.

The natural progression of HIV disease is different in children compared to adults; drug treatment should only be undertaken by specialists within a formal paediatric HIV clinical network. Guidelines and dose regimens are under constant review and for this reason some dose recommendations have not been included in *BNF for Children*.

Further information on the management of children with HIV can be obtained from the Children's HIV Association (CHIVA) www.chiva.org.uk; and further information on antiretroviral use and toxicity can be obtained from the Paediatric European Network for Treatment of AIDS (PENTA) website www.pentatrials.org.

Principles of treatment

Treatment is aimed at suppressing viral replication for as long as possible; it should be started before the immune system is irreversibly damaged. The need for early drug treatment should, however, be balanced against the risk of toxicity. Commitment to treatment and strict adherence over many years are required; the regimen chosen should take into account convenience and the child's tolerance of treatment. The development of drug resistance is reduced by using a combination of drugs; such combinations should have synergistic or additive activity while ensuring that their toxicity is not additive. It is recommended that viral sensitivity to antiretroviral drugs is established before starting treatment or before switching drugs if the infection is not responding.

Initiation of treatment

Treatment is started in all HIV infected children under 1 year of age regardless of clinical and immunological parameters. In children over 1 year of age, treatment is based on the child's age, CD4 cell count, viral load, and symptoms. The choice of antiviral treatment for children should take into account the method and frequency of administration, risk of side-effects, compatibility of drugs with food, palatability, and the appropriateness of the formulation. Initiating treatment with a combination of drugs ('highly active antiretroviral therapy' which includes 2 nucleoside reverse transcriptase inhibitors with *either* a non-nucleoside reverse transcriptase inhibitor *or* a boosted protease inhibitor) is recommended. Abacavir p. 390 and lamivudine p. 393 are the nucleoside reverse transcriptase inhibitors of choice for initial therapy; however, zidovudine p. 394 and lamivudine are used in children who are positive for the HLA-B*5701 allele. Nevirapine p. 389 is the preferred non-nucleoside reverse transcriptase inhibitor in children under 3 years of age, but efavirenz p. 388 is preferred in older children. Lopinavir with ritonavir p. 397 is the preferred boosted protease inhibitor for initial therapy. The metabolism of many antiretrovirals varies in young children; it may therefore be necessary to adjust the dose according to the plasma-drug concentration. Children who require treatment for both HIV and chronic hepatitis B should receive antivirals that are active against both diseases.

Switching therapy

Deterioration of the condition (including clinical, virological changes, and CD4 cell changes) may require a complete change of therapy. The choice of an alternative regimen depends on factors such as the response to previous treatment, tolerance, and the possibility of cross-resistance.

Pregnancy

Treatment of HIV infection in pregnancy aims to reduce the risk of toxicity to the fetus (although information on the teratogenic potential of most antiretroviral drugs is limited), to minimise the viral load and disease progression in the mother, and to prevent transmission of infection to the neonate. **All treatment options require careful assessment by a specialist.** Combination antiretroviral therapy maximises the chance of preventing transmission and represents optimal therapy for the mother. However, it may be associated with a greater risk of preterm delivery. Local protocols and national guidelines (www.bhiva.org) should be consulted for recommendations on treatment during pregnancy and the perinatal period. Pregnancies in HIV-positive women and babies born to them should be reported prospectively to the National Study of HIV in Pregnancy and Childhood at www.ucl.ac.uk/nshpc/ and to the Antiretroviral Pregnancy Registry at www.apregistry.com.

Breast-feeding

Breast-feeding by HIV-positive mothers may cause HIV infection in the infant and should be avoided.

Post-exposure prophylaxis

Children exposed to HIV infection through needlestick injury or by another route should be sent immediately to an accident and emergency department for post-exposure prophylaxis [unlicensed indication]. Antiretrovirals for prophylaxis are chosen on the basis of efficacy and potential for toxicity. Recommendations have been developed by the Children's HIV Association, www.chiva.org.uk.

Drugs used for HIV infection

Zidovudine, a nucleoside reverse transcriptase inhibitor (or 'nucleoside analogue'), was the first anti-HIV drug to be introduced. Other nucleoside reverse transcriptase inhibitors include abacavir, didanosine p. 392, emtricitabine p. 392, lamivudine, stavudine p. 393, and tenofovir disoproxil p. 394. There are concerns about renal toxicity and effects on bone mineralisation when tenofovir disoproxil is used in prepubertal children.

The protease inhibitors include atazanavir p. 396, darunavir p. 396, fosamprenavir p. 397 (a pro-drug of amprenavir), indinavir, lopinavir (available as lopinavir with ritonavir), ritonavir p. 397, and tipranavir p. 398. Indinavir is no longer recommended because it is associated with nephrolithiasis. Ritonavir in low doses boosts the activity of atazanavir, darunavir, fosamprenavir, lopinavir (available as lopinavir with ritonavir), and tipranavir increasing the persistence of plasma concentrations of these drugs; at such a low dose, ritonavir has no intrinsic antiviral activity. The protease inhibitors are metabolised by cytochrome P450 enzyme systems and therefore have a significant potential for drug interactions. Protease inhibitors are associated with lipodystrophy and metabolic effects.

The non-nucleoside reverse transcriptase inhibitors efavirenz, etravirine p. 389, and nevirapine are active against the subtype HIV-1 but not HIV-2, a subtype that is rare in the UK. These drugs may interact with a number of drugs metabolised in the liver. Nevirapine is associated with a high incidence of rash (including Stevens-Johnson syndrome) and rarely fatal hepatitis. Rash is also associated with efavirenz and etravirine but it is usually milder. Psychiatric or CNS disturbances are common with efavirenz. CNS disturbances are often self-limiting and can be reduced by taking the dose at bedtime (especially in the first 2–4 weeks of treatment). Efavirenz has also been associated with an increased plasma cholesterol concentration. Etravirine is used in regimens containing a boosted protease inhibitor for HIV infection resistant to other non-nucleoside reverse transcriptase inhibitors and protease inhibitors.

Enfuvirtide below, which inhibits the fusion of HIV to the host cell, is licensed for managing infection that has failed to respond to a regimen of other antiretroviral drugs. Enfuvirtide should be combined with other potentially active antiretroviral drugs; it is given by subcutaneous injection.

Maraviroc p. 399 is an antagonist of the CCR5 chemokine receptor. It is used in patients exclusively infected with CCR5–tropic HIV.

Dolutegravir p. 387 and raltegravir p. 387 are inhibitors of HIV integrase. They are used for the treatment of HIV infection when non-nucleoside reverse transcriptase inhibitors or protease inhibitors cannot be used because of intolerance, drug interactions, or resistance.

Immune reconstitution syndrome

Improvement in immune function as a result of antiretroviral treatment may provoke a marked inflammatory reaction against residual opportunistic organisms; these reactions may occur within the first few weeks or months of initiating treatment. Autoimmune disorders (such as Graves' disease) have also been reported many months after initiation of treatment.

Lipodystrophy syndrome

Metabolic effects associated with antiretroviral treatment include *fat redistribution*, *insulin resistance*, and *dyslipidaemia*; collectively these have been termed *lipodystrophy syndrome*. Children should be encouraged to lead a healthy lifestyle that reduces their long-term cardiovascular risk. Plasma lipids and blood glucose should be measured before starting antiretroviral therapy, after 3–6 months of treatment, and then at least annually. Insulin resistance and hyperglycaemia occur only rarely in children.

Fat redistribution (with loss of subcutaneous fat, increased abdominal fat, 'buffalo hump' and breast enlargement) is associated with regimens containing protease inhibitors and nucleoside reverse transcriptase inhibitors. Stavudine, and to a lesser extent zidovudine, are associated with a higher risk of lipoatrophy and should be used only if alternative regimens are not suitable.

Dyslipidaemia is associated with antiretroviral treatment, particularly with protease inhibitors; in children, hypercholesterolaemia appears to be more common than hypertriglyceridaemia. Protease inhibitors and some nucleoside reverse transcriptase inhibitors are associated with insulin resistance and hyperglycaemia, but they occur rarely in children. Of the protease inhibitors, atazanavir and darunavir are less likely to cause dyslipidaemia, while atazanavir is less likely to impair glucose tolerance.

Osteonecrosis

Osteonecrosis has been reported in children with advanced HIV disease or following long-term exposure to combination antiretroviral therapy.

Neonates

In order to prevent transmission of infection, neonates born to HIV-positive mothers should be given post-exposure prophylaxis as soon as possible after birth, but starting no later than 72 hours after birth. Zidovudine p. 394 alone should be given to neonates whose mothers had a viral load less than 50 HIV RNA copies/mL between 36 weeks' gestation and delivery, or whose mothers underwent caesarean section while taking zidovudine monotherapy. Combination antiretroviral therapy should be given to neonates whose mothers had a viral load over 50 HIV RNA copies/mL at delivery or whose mothers are found to be HIV positive after delivery. Prophylaxis is continued for 4 weeks.

ANTIVIRALS ⟩ HIV-FUSION INHIBITORS

▌Enfuvirtide

- **DRUG ACTION** Enfuvirtide inhibits the fusion of HIV to the host cell.

- **INDICATIONS AND DOSE**

  HIV infection in combination with other antiretroviral drugs for resistant infection or for patients intolerant to other antiretroviral regimens
  - ▸ BY SUBCUTANEOUS INJECTION
  - ▸ Child 6–15 years: 2 mg/kg twice daily (max. per dose 90 mg)
  - ▸ Child 16–17 years: 90 mg twice daily

- **INTERACTIONS** → Appendix 1 (enfuvirtide).
- **SIDE-EFFECTS**
  - ▸ **Common or very common** Acne · anorexia · anxiety · asthenia · conjunctivitis · diabetes mellitus · dry skin · erythema · gastro-oesophageal reflux disease · haematuria · hypertriglyceridaemia · impaired concentration · influenza-like illness · injection-site reactions · irritability · lymphadenopathy · myalgia · nightmares · pancreatitis · peripheral neuropathy · pneumonia · renal calculi · sinusitis · skin papilloma · tremor · vertigo · weight loss
  - ▸ **Uncommon** Hypersensitivity reactions
  - ▸ **Frequency not known** Osteonecrosis

  SIDE-EFFECTS, FURTHER INFORMATION
  - ▸ **Hypersensitivity reactions** Hypersensitivity reactions including rash, fever, nausea, vomiting, chills, rigors, low blood pressure, respiratory distress, glomerulonephritis, and raised liver enzymes reported; discontinue immediately if any signs or symptoms of systemic hypersensitivity develop and do not rechallenge.
  - ▸ **Osteonecrosis** For further information see HIV infection p. 385.

- **PREGNANCY** Manufacturer advises use only if potential benefit outweighs risk.

- **HEPATIC IMPAIRMENT** Manufacturer advises caution— no information available; chronic hepatitis B or C (possibly greater risk of hepatic side-effects).

- **DIRECTIONS FOR ADMINISTRATION** For *subcutaneous injection*, reconstitute with 1.1 mL Water for Injections and allow to stand (for up to 45 minutes) to dissolve; do **not** shake or invert vial.

- **PATIENT AND CARER ADVICE**
  Hypersensitivity reactions Patients or carers should be told how to recognise signs of hypersensitivity, and advised to discontinue treatment and seek immediate medical attention if symptoms develop.

- **MEDICINAL FORMS**
  There can be variation in the licensing of different medicines containing the same drug.
  Powder and solvent for solution for injection
  ELECTROLYTES: May contain Sodium
  - ▸ **Fuzeon** (Roche Products Ltd)
    Enfuvirtide 108 mg Fuzeon 108mg powder and solvent for solution for injection vials | 60 vial [PoM] £1,081.57

ANTIVIRALS > HIV-INTEGRASE INHIBITORS

Dolutegravir

- **DRUG ACTION** Dolutegravir is an inhibitor of HIV integrase.

- **INDICATIONS AND DOSE**

HIV infection without resistance to other inhibitors of HIV integrase, in combination with other antiretroviral drugs
▸ BY MOUTH
  ▸ Child 12–17 years (body-weight 40 kg and above): 50 mg once daily

HIV infection in combination with other antiretroviral drugs (with concomitant carbamazepine, efavirenz, etravirine (without boosted protease inhibitors, but see also Interactions), fosphenytoin, phenobarbital, phenytoin, primidone, nevirapine, oxcarbazepine, St John's wort, rifampicin, or tipranavir)
▸ BY MOUTH
  ▸ Child 12–17 years (body-weight 40 kg and above): 50 mg twice daily, avoid concomitant use with these drugs if resistance to other inhibitors of HIV integrase suspected

- **INTERACTIONS** → Appendix 1 (dolutegravir). Caution—avoid concomitant use with etravirine, unless used in combination with atazanavir, darunavir, or lopinavir.

- **SIDE-EFFECTS**
▸ **Common or very common** Abdominal pain · abnormal dreams · diarrhoea · dizziness · fatigue · flatulence · headache · insomnia · nausea · pruritus · raised creatine kinase · rash · vomiting
▸ **Uncommon** Hepatitis · hypersensitivity reactions
▸ **Frequency not known** Osteonecrosis

  SIDE-EFFECTS, FURTHER INFORMATION
▸ Hypersensitivity reactions Hypersensitivity reactions (including severe rash, or rash accompanied by fever, malaise, arthralgia, myalgia, blistering, oral lesions, conjunctivitis, angioedema, eosinophilia, or raised liver enzymes) reported uncommonly. Discontinue immediately if any sign or symptoms of hypersensitivity reactions develop.
▸ Osteonecrosis For further information see HIV infection p. 385.

- **PREGNANCY** Manufacturer advises use only if potential benefit outweighs risk.

- **HEPATIC IMPAIRMENT** Manufacturer advises caution in severe impairment—no information available.

- **DIRECTIONS FOR ADMINISTRATION** Avoid antacids 6 hours before or 2 hours after taking dolutegravir.

- **PATIENT AND CARER ADVICE**
Patients or carers should be given advice on how to administer dolutegravir tablets.

  Missed doses
  If a dose is more than 20 hours late on the once daily regimen (or more than 8 hours late on the twice daily regimen), the missed dose should not be taken and the next dose should be taken at the normal time.

- **MEDICINAL FORMS**
There can be variation in the licensing of different medicines containing the same drug.
  Tablet
  ▸ Tivicay (ViiV Healthcare UK Ltd) ▼
    Dolutegravir (as Dolutegravir sodium) 50 mg Tivicay 50mg tablets | 30 tablet PoM £498.75

  Combinations available: *Abacavir with dolutegravir and lamivudine*, p. 391

Raltegravir

- **DRUG ACTION** Raltegravir is an inhibitor of HIV integrase.

- **INDICATIONS AND DOSE**

HIV infection resistant to multiple antiretrovirals, in combination with other antiretroviral drugs
▸ BY MOUTH USING TABLETS
  ▸ Child 6–17 years (body-weight 25 kg and above): 400 mg twice daily
▸ BY MOUTH USING CHEWABLE TABLETS
  ▸ Child 2–11 years (body-weight 12–13 kg): 75 mg twice daily
  ▸ Child 2–11 years (body-weight 14–19 kg): 100 mg twice daily
  ▸ Child 2–11 years (body-weight 20–27 kg): 150 mg twice daily
  ▸ Child 2–11 years (body-weight 28–39 kg): 200 mg twice daily
  ▸ Child 2–11 years (body-weight 40 kg and above): 300 mg twice daily

DOSE EQUIVALENCE AND CONVERSION
The bioavailability of *Isentress*® chewable tablets is higher than that of the 'standard' 400 mg tablets; the chewable tablets are **not** interchangeable with the 'standard' tablets on a milligram-for-milligram basis.

- **CAUTIONS** Psychiatric illness (may exacerbate underlying illness including depression) · risk factors for myopathy · risk factors for rhabdomyolysis

- **INTERACTIONS** → Appendix 1 (raltegravir).

- **SIDE-EFFECTS**
▸ **Common or very common** Abdominal pain · abnormal dreams · asthenia · depression · diarrhoea · dizziness · dyspepsia · flatulence · headache · hyperactivity · hypertriglyceridaemia · insomnia · nausea · rash · vomiting
▸ **Uncommon** Acne · alopecia · anaemia · anxiety · appetite changes · arthralgia · bradycardia · carpal tunnel syndrome · chest pain · chills · confusion · constipation · drowsiness · dry mouth · dry skin · dysphonia · epistaxis · erectile dysfunction · flushing · gastritis · glossitis · gynaecomastia · hepatitis · hyperhidrosis · hypertension · impaired memory and attention · lipodystrophy · Lipodystrophy Syndrome · menopausal symptoms · myalgia · nasal congestion · neutropenia · nocturia · oedema · osteopenia · pain on swallowing · palpitation · pancreatitis · peptic ulcer · peripheral neuropathy · polydipsia · pruritus · pyrexia · rash with eosinophilia and systemic symptoms · rectal bleeding · renal failure · rhabdomyolysis · skin papilloma · Stevens-Johnson syndrome · suicidal ideation · taste disturbances · thrombocytopenia · tinnitus · tremor · ventricular extrasystoles · visual disturbances
▸ **Frequency not known** Osteonecrosis

  SIDE-EFFECTS, FURTHER INFORMATION
▸ Rash Rash occurs commonly. Discontinue if severe rash or rash accompanied by fever, malaise, arthralgia, myalgia, blistering, mouth ulceration, conjunctivitis, angioedema, hepatitis, or eosinophilia.
▸ Lipodystrophy syndrome For further information see HIV infection p. 385.
▸ Osteonecrosis For further information see HIV infection p. 385.

- **PREGNANCY** Manufacturer advises avoid—toxicity in *animal* studies.

- **HEPATIC IMPAIRMENT** Manufacturer advises caution in severe impairment—no information available. Use with caution in patients with chronic hepatitis B or C (at greater risk of hepatic side-effects).

- **PRESCRIBING AND DISPENSING INFORMATION** Dispense raltegravir chewable tablets in original container (contains desiccant).

Infection

5

● **MEDICINAL FORMS**
There can be variation in the licensing of different medicines containing the same drug.

Tablet

CAUTIONARY AND ADVISORY LABELS 25
▸ Isentress (Merck Sharp & Dohme Ltd)
Raltegravir 400 mg Isentress 400mg tablets | 60 tablet [PoM] £471.41

Chewable tablet

CAUTIONARY AND ADVISORY LABELS 24
EXCIPIENTS: May contain Aspartame
▸ Isentress (Merck Sharp & Dohme Ltd)
Raltegravir 25 mg Isentress 25mg chewable tablets | 60 tablet [PoM] £29.46 DT price = £29.46
Raltegravir 100 mg Isentress 100mg chewable tablets | 60 tablet [PoM] £117.85 DT price = £117.85

ANTIVIRALS > NON-NUCLEOSIDE REVERSE TRANSCRIPTASE INHIBITORS

Efavirenz

● **INDICATIONS AND DOSE**

HIV infection in combination with other antiretroviral drugs

▸ BY MOUTH USING CAPSULES
▸ Child 3 months–17 years (body-weight 3.5–4 kg): 100 mg once daily
▸ Child 3 months–17 years (body-weight 5–7.4 kg): 150 mg once daily
▸ Child 3 months–17 years (body-weight 7.5–14 kg): 200 mg once daily
▸ Child 3 months–17 years (body-weight 15–19 kg): 250 mg once daily
▸ Child 3 months–17 years (body-weight 20–24 kg): 300 mg once daily
▸ Child 3 months–17 years (body-weight 25–32.4 kg): 350 mg once daily
▸ Child 3 months–17 years (body-weight 32.5–39 kg): 400 mg once daily
▸ Child 3 months–17 years (body-weight 40 kg and above): 600 mg once daily
▸ BY MOUTH USING TABLETS
▸ Child (body-weight 40 kg and above): 600 mg once daily
▸ BY MOUTH USING ORAL SOLUTION
▸ Child 3–4 years (body-weight 13–14 kg): 360 mg once daily
▸ Child 3–4 years (body-weight 15–19 kg): 390 mg once daily
▸ Child 3–4 years (body-weight 20–24 kg): 450 mg once daily
▸ Child 3–4 years (body-weight 25–32.5 kg): 510 mg once daily
▸ Child 5–17 years (body-weight 13–14 kg): 270 mg once daily
▸ Child 5–17 years (body-weight 15–19 kg): 300 mg once daily
▸ Child 5–17 years (body-weight 20–24 kg): 360 mg once daily
▸ Child 5–17 years (body-weight 25–32.4 kg): 450 mg once daily
▸ Child 5–17 years (body-weight 32.5–39 kg): 510 mg once daily
▸ Child 5–17 years (body-weight 40 kg and above): 720 mg once daily

DOSE EQUIVALENCE AND CONVERSION

The bioavailability of *Sustiva*® oral solution is lower than that of the capsules and tablets; the oral solution is **not** interchangeable with either capsules or tablets on a milligram-for-milligram basis.

● **UNLICENSED USE** Opening capsules and adding contents to food is an unlicensed method of administration.

● CAUTIONS Acute porphyrias p. 562 · history of psychiatric disorders · history of seizures

● INTERACTIONS → Appendix 1 (efavirenz).

● SIDE-EFFECTS
▸ **Common or very common** Abdominal pain · abnormal dreams · anxiety · depression · diarrhoea · dizziness · fatigue · headache · impaired concentration · nausea · pruritus · rash · sleep disturbances · Stevens-Johnson syndrome · vomiting
▸ **Uncommon** Amnesia · ataxia · blurred vision · convulsions · flushing · gynaecomastia · hepatitis · hypersensitivity · mania · pancreatitis · psychosis · suicidal ideation · tinnitus · tremor · vertigo
▸ **Rare** Hepatic failure · photosensitivity · suicide
▸ **Frequency not known** Lipodystrophy syndrome · osteonecrosis · raised serum cholesterol

SIDE-EFFECTS, FURTHER INFORMATION
▸ Rash Rash, usually in the first 2 weeks, is the most common side-effect; discontinue if severe rash with blistering, desquamation, mucosal involvement or fever; if rash mild or moderate, may continue without interruption—usually resolves within 1 month.
▸ CNS effects Administration at bedtime especially in first 2–4 weeks reduces CNS effects.
▸ Lipodystrophy syndrome For further information see HIV infection p. 385.
▸ Osteonecrosis For further information see HIV infection p. 385.
▸ Immune Reconstitution Syndrome For further information see HIV infection p. 385.

● PREGNANCY Reports of neural tube defects when used in first trimester.

● HEPATIC IMPAIRMENT Greater risk of hepatic side-effects in chronic hepatitis B or C. Avoid in severe impairment. In mild to moderate liver disease, monitor for dose-related side-effects (e.g. CNS effects) and liver function.

● RENAL IMPAIRMENT Manufacturer advises caution in severe renal failure—no information available.

● MONITORING REQUIREMENTS Monitor liver function if receiving other hepatotoxic drugs.

● DIRECTIONS FOR ADMINISTRATION Capsules may be opened and contents added to food (contents have a peppery taste).

● PRESCRIBING AND DISPENSING INFORMATION Flavours of oral liquid formulations may include strawberry and mint.

● PATIENT AND CARER ADVICE
Psychiatric disorders Patients or their carers should be advised to seek immediate medical attention if symptoms such as severe depression, psychosis or suicidal ideation occur.

● MEDICINAL FORMS
There can be variation in the licensing of different medicines containing the same drug.

Tablet

CAUTIONARY AND ADVISORY LABELS 23
▸ Efavirenz (Non-proprietary)
Efavirenz 600 mg Efavirenz 600mg tablets | 30 tablet [PoM] £190.26–£200.27 | 30 tablet [PoM] £90.43 (Hospital only)
▸ Sustiva (Bristol-Myers Squibb Pharmaceuticals Ltd)
Efavirenz 600 mg Sustiva 600mg tablets | 30 tablet [PoM] £200.27 (Hospital only)

Capsule

CAUTIONARY AND ADVISORY LABELS 23
▸ Sustiva (Bristol-Myers Squibb Pharmaceuticals Ltd)
Efavirenz 50 mg Sustiva 50mg capsules | 30 capsule [PoM] £16.73 (Hospital only)
Efavirenz 100 mg Sustiva 100mg capsules | 30 capsule [PoM] £33.41 (Hospital only)
Efavirenz 200 mg Sustiva 200mg capsules | 90 capsule [PoM] £200.27 (Hospital only)

Etravirine

● **INDICATIONS AND DOSE**

HIV infection resistant to other non-nucleoside reverse transcriptase inhibitor and protease inhibitors in combination with other antiretroviral drugs (including a boosted protease inhibitor)
▸ BY MOUTH
▸ Child 6–17 years (body-weight 16–19 kg): 100 mg twice daily
▸ Child 6–17 years (body-weight 20–24 kg): 125 mg twice daily
▸ Child 6–17 years (body-weight 25–29 kg): 150 mg twice daily
▸ Child 6–17 years (body-weight 30 kg and above): 200 mg twice daily

● **CONTRA-INDICATIONS** Acute porphyrias p. 562

● **INTERACTIONS** → Appendix 1 (etravirine).

● **SIDE-EFFECTS**
▸ **Common or very common** Abdominal pain · anaemia · diabetes · flatulence · gastritis · gastro-oesophageal reflux · hyperlipidaemia · hypertension · Lipodystrophy Syndrome · nausea · peripheral neuropathy · rash · renal failure
▸ **Uncommon** Blurred vision · bronchospasm · chest pain · drowsiness · dry mouth · gynaecomastia · haematemesis · hepatitis · malaise · pancreatitis · sweating
▸ **Rare** Stevens-Johnson syndrome
▸ **Very rare** Toxic epidermal necrolysis
▸ **Frequency not known** Haemorrhagic stroke · hypersensitivity reactions · osteonecrosis

SIDE-EFFECTS, FURTHER INFORMATION
▸ Hypersensitivity reactions Rash, usually in the second week, is the most common side-effect and appears more frequently in females. Life-threatening hypersensitivity reactions reported usually during week 3–6 of treatment and characterised by rash, eosinophilia, and systemic symptoms (including fever, general malaise, myalgia, arthralgia, blistering, oral lesions, conjunctivitis, and hepatitis). Discontinue permanently if hypersensitivity reaction or severe rash develop. If rash mild or moderate (without signs of hypersensitivity reaction), may continue without interruption—usually resolves within 2 weeks.
▸ Lipodystrophy For further information see HIV infection p. 385.
▸ Osteonecrosis For further information see HIV infection p. 385.

● **HEPATIC IMPAIRMENT** Manufacturer advises caution in moderate impairment; avoid in severe impairment— no information available; greater risk of hepatic side-effects in chronic hepatitis B or C.

● **DIRECTIONS FOR ADMINISTRATION** Patients with swallowing difficulties may disperse tablets in a glass of water just before administration.

● **PRESCRIBING AND DISPENSING INFORMATION** Dispense in original container (contains desiccant).

● **PATIENT AND CARER ADVICE**
Hypersensitivity reactions Patients or carers should be told how to recognise hypersensitivity reactions and advised to seek immediate medical attention if hypersensitivity reaction or severe rash develop.
Missed doses
If a dose is more than 6 hours late, the missed dose should not be taken and the next dose should be taken at the normal time.

● **MEDICINAL FORMS**
There can be variation in the licensing of different medicines containing the same drug.
Tablet
CAUTIONARY AND ADVISORY LABELS 21
▸ **Intelence** (Janssen-Cilag Ltd)
Etravirine 25 mg Intelence 25mg tablets | 120 tablet [PoM] £75.32
Etravirine 100 mg Intelence 100mg tablets | 120 tablet [PoM] £301.27
Etravirine 200 mg Intelence 200mg tablets | 60 tablet [PoM] £301.27

Nevirapine

● **INDICATIONS AND DOSE**

HIV infection in combination with other antiretroviral drugs (initial dose)
▸ BY MOUTH USING IMMEDIATE-RELEASE MEDICINES
▸ Child: Initially 150–200 mg/m^2 once daily (max. per dose 200 mg) for first 14 days, initial dose titration using 'immediate-release' preparation should not exceed 28 days; if rash occurs and is not resolved within 28 days, alternative treatment should be sought. If treatment interrupted for more than 7 days, restart using the lower dose of the 'immediate-release' preparation for the first 14 days as for new treatment

HIV infection in combination with other antiretroviral drugs (maintenance dose following initial dose titration if no rash present)
▸ BY MOUTH USING IMMEDIATE-RELEASE MEDICINES
▸ Child 1 month–2 years: 150–200 mg/m^2 twice daily (max. per dose 200 mg), alternatively 300–400 mg/m^2 once daily (max. per dose 400 mg)
▸ Child 3–17 years: 150–200 mg/m^2 twice daily (max. per dose 200 mg)

HIV infection in combination with other antiretroviral drugs (maintenance dose following initial dose titration if no rash present)
▸ BY MOUTH USING IMMEDIATE-RELEASE MEDICINES
▸ Child 3–17 years (body surface area 0.58–0.83 m^2): 200 mg once daily
▸ Child 3–17 years (body surface area 0.84–1.17 m^2): 300 mg once daily
▸ Child 3–17 years (body surface area 1.18 m^2 and above): 400 mg once daily
▸ BY MOUTH USING MODIFIED-RELEASE MEDICINES
▸ Child 3–17 years (body surface area 0.58–0.83 m^2): 200 mg once daily
▸ Child 3–17 years (body surface area 0.84–1.17 m^2): 300 mg once daily
▸ Child 3–17 years (body surface area 1.18 m^2 and above): 400 mg once daily

● **UNLICENSED USE** 'Immediate-release' tablets not licensed for use in children weighing less than 50 kg or with body surface area less than 1.25 m^2; 'immediate-release' tablets and suspension not licensed for once daily dose after the initial dose titration.

● **CONTRA-INDICATIONS** Acute porphyrias p. 562 · post-exposure prophylaxis

● **CAUTIONS** Females (at greater risk of hepatic side effects) · high CD4 cell count (at greater risk of hepatic side effects)

● **INTERACTIONS** → Appendix 1 (nevirapine).

● **SIDE-EFFECTS**
▸ **Common or very common** Abdominal pain · diarrhoea · fatigue · fever · granulocytopenia · headache · hepatitis · hypersensitivity reactions (may involve hepatic reactions and rash) · nausea · rash · Stevens-Johnson syndrome · toxic epidermal necrolysis · vomiting
▸ **Uncommon** Anaemia · arthralgia · myalgia
▸ **Frequency not known** Osteonecrosis

SIDE-EFFECTS, FURTHER INFORMATION

▸ Hepatic effects Potentially life-threatening hepatotoxicity including fatal fulminant hepatitis reported usually in first 6 weeks; discontinue permanently if abnormalities in liver function tests accompanied by hypersensitivity reaction (rash, fever, arthralgia, myalgia, lymphadenopathy, hepatitis, renal impairment, eosinophilia, granulocytopenia); suspend if severe abnormalities in liver function tests but no hypersensitivity reaction—discontinue permanently if significant liver function abnormalities recur; monitor patient closely if mild to moderate abnormalities in liver function tests with no hypersensitivity reaction.

▸ Rash Rash, usually in first 6 weeks, is most common side-effect; incidence reduced if introduced at low dose and dose increased gradually (after 14 days); Discontinue permanently if severe rash or if rash accompanied by blistering, oral lesions, conjunctivitis, facial oedema, general malaise or hypersensitivity reactions; if rash mild or moderate may continue without interruption but dose should not be increased until rash resolves.

▸ Osteonecrosis For more information see HIV infection p. 385.

● HEPATIC IMPAIRMENT Manufacturer advises avoid modified-release preparation—no information available; use 'immediate-release' preparation with caution in moderate impairment and avoid in severe impairment. Use with caution in patients with chronic hepatitis B or C (at greater risk of hepatic side effects).

● RENAL IMPAIRMENT Manufacturer advises avoid modified-release preparation—no information available.

● MONITORING REQUIREMENTS

▸ Hepatic disease Close monitoring of liver function required during first 18 weeks; monitor liver function before treatment then every 2 weeks for 2 months then after 1 month and then regularly.

▸ Rash Monitor closely for skin reactions during first 18 weeks.

● PATIENT AND CARER ADVICE
Hypersensitivity reactions Patients or carers should be told how to recognise hypersensitivity reactions and advised to discontinue treatment and seek immediate medical attention if severe skin reaction, hypersensitivity reactions, or symptoms of hepatitis develop.

● MEDICINAL FORMS
There can be variation in the licensing of different medicines containing the same drug.

Tablet

▸ Nevirapine (Non-proprietary)
Nevirapine 200 mg Nevirapine 200mg tablets | 60 tablet PoM
£28.60–£170.00

▸ Viramune (Boehringer Ingelheim Ltd)
Nevirapine 200 mg Viramune 200mg tablets | 14 tablet PoM
£39.67 | 60 tablet PoM £170.00

Oral suspension

▸ Viramune (Boehringer Ingelheim Ltd)
Nevirapine (as Nevirapine hemihydrate) 10 mg per 1 ml Viramune 50mg/5ml oral suspension | 240 ml PoM £50.40

ANTIVIRALS ⟩ NUCLEOSIDE REVERSE TRANSCRIPTASE INHIBITORS

Nucleoside reverse transcriptase inhibitors

● CAUTIONS Patients at risk of lactic acidosis

CAUTIONS, FURTHER INFORMATION

▸ Lactic acidosis Life-threatening lactic acidosis associated with hepatomegaly and hepatic steatosis has been reported with nucleoside reverse transcriptase inhibitors.

They should be used with caution in patients with hepatomegaly, hepatitis (especially hepatitis C treated with interferon alfa and ribavirin), liver-enzyme abnormalities and with other risk factors for liver disease and hepatic steatosis. Treatment with the nucleoside reverse transcriptase inhibitor should be **discontinued** in case of symptomatic hyperlactataemia, lactic acidosis, progressive hepatomegaly or rapid deterioration of liver function.

● SIDE-EFFECTS Abdominal pain · anaemia · anorexia · arthralgia · blood disorders · cough · diarrhoea · dizziness · dyspnoea · fatigue · fever · flatulence · gastro-intestinal disturbances · headache · insomnia · lactic acidosis · lipodystrophy (Lipodystrophy Syndrome) · liver damage · metabolic effects · myalgia · nausea · neutropenia · osteonecrosis · pancreatitis · rash · thrombocytopenia · urticaria · vomiting

SIDE-EFFECTS, FURTHER INFORMATION

▸ Lipodystrophy syndrome For further information see HIV infection p. 385.

▸ Osteonecrosis For further information see HIV infection p. 385.

● PREGNANCY Mitochondrial dysfunction has been reported in infants exposed to nucleoside reverse transcriptase inhibitors in utero; the main effects include haematological, metabolic, and neurological disorders; all infants whose mothers received nucleoside reverse transcriptase inhibitors during pregnancy should be monitored for relevant signs or symptoms.

● HEPATIC IMPAIRMENT Use with caution in children with hepatic impairment (greater risk of hepatic side effects). However, some nucleoside reverse transcriptase inhibitors are used in children who also have chronic hepatitis B.

🖝 above

Abacavir

● INDICATIONS AND DOSE

HIV infection in combination with other antiretroviral drugs

▸ BY MOUTH

▸ Child 3 months-11 years: 8 mg/kg twice daily (max. per dose 300 mg), alternatively 16 mg/kg once daily (max. per dose 600 mg)

▸ Child 3 months-11 years (body-weight 14-20 kg): 150 mg twice daily, alternatively 300 mg once daily

▸ Child 3 months-11 years (body-weight 21-29 kg): 150 mg, taken in the morning and 300 mg, taken in the evening, alternatively 450 mg once daily

▸ Child 3 months-11 years (body-weight 30 kg and above): 300 mg twice daily, alternatively 600 mg once daily

▸ Child 12-17 years: 300 mg twice daily, alternatively 600 mg once daily

● INTERACTIONS → Appendix 1 (abacavir).

● SIDE-EFFECTS

▸ Very rare Stevens-Johnson syndrome · toxic epidermal necrolysis

▸ Frequency not known Hypersensitivity reactions

SIDE-EFFECTS, FURTHER INFORMATION

▸ Hypersensitivity reactions Life-threatening hypersensitivity reactions reported—characterised by fever or rash and possibly nausea, vomiting, diarrhoea, abdominal pain, dyspnoea, cough, lethargy, malaise, headache, and myalgia; less frequently mouth ulceration, oedema, hypotension, sore throat, acute respiratory distress syndrome, anaphylaxis, paraesthesia, arthralgia, conjunctivitis, lymphadenopathy, lymphocytopenia and renal failure; rarely myolysis; laboratory abnormalities may include raised liver function tests and creatine kinase;

symptoms usually appear in the first 6 weeks, but may occur at any time.

Discontinue immediately if any symptom of hypersensitivity develops and do not rechallenge (risk of more severe hypersensitivity reaction); discontinue if hypersensitivity cannot be ruled out, even when other diagnoses possible—if rechallenge necessary it must be carried out in hospital setting; if abacavir is stopped for any reason other than hypersensitivity, exclude hypersensitivity reaction as the cause and rechallenge only if medical assistance is readily available; care needed with concomitant use of drugs which cause skin toxicity.

‣ Gastro-intestinal disturbances More common in children.

‣ Rash More common in children.

● **ALLERGY AND CROSS-SENSITIVITY** Caution—increased risk of hypersensitivity reaction in presence of HLA-B*5701 allele.

● **HEPATIC IMPAIRMENT** Monitor closely in mild impairment (combination preparations not recommended as reduced abacavir dose may be required). Avoid in moderate impairment unless essential—close monitoring recommended. Avoid in severe impairment.

● **RENAL IMPAIRMENT** Manufacturer advises avoid in end-stage renal disease.

● **PRE-TREATMENT SCREENING** Test for HLA-B*5701 allele before treatment or if restarting treatment and HLA-B*5701 status not known.

● **MONITORING REQUIREMENTS** Monitor for symptoms of hypersensitivity reaction every 2 weeks for 2 months.

● **PRESCRIBING AND DISPENSING INFORMATION** Flavours of oral liquid formulations may include banana, or strawberry.

● **PATIENT AND CARER ADVICE** Patients should be provided with an alert card and advised to keep it with them at all times.

Patients and their carers should be told the importance of regular dosing (intermittent therapy may increase the risk of sensitisation), how to recognise signs of hypersensitivity, and advised to seek immediate medical attention if symptoms develop or before re-starting treatment.

● **MEDICINAL FORMS** There can be variation in the licensing of different medicines containing the same drug.

Tablet
‣ Ziagen (ViiV Healthcare UK Ltd)
  Abacavir (as Abacavir sulfate) 300 mg Ziagen 300mg tablets | 60 tablet PoM £177.60

Oral solution
EXCIPIENTS: May contain Propylene glycol
‣ Ziagen (ViiV Healthcare UK Ltd)
  Abacavir (as Abacavir sulfate) 20 mg per 1 ml Ziagen 20mg/ml oral solution sugar-free | 240 ml PoM £47.36

Abacavir with dolutegravir and lamivudine

The properties listed below are those particular to the combination only. For the properties of the components please consider, abacavir p. 390, lamivudine p. 393, dolutegravir p. 387.

● **INDICATIONS AND DOSE**
HIV infection
▸ BY MOUTH
▸ Child 12-17 years (body-weight 40 kg and above): 1 tablet once daily

● **RENAL IMPAIRMENT** Avoid *Triumeq*® if estimated glomerular filtration rate less than 50 mL/minute/1.73 m².

● **PATIENT AND CARER ADVICE**
Missed doses
If a dose is more than 20 hours late, the missed dose should not be taken and the next dose should be taken at the normal time.

● **MEDICINAL FORMS** There can be variation in the licensing of different medicines containing the same drug.

Tablet
▸ Triumeq (ViiV Healthcare UK Ltd) ▼
  Dolutegravir (as Dolutegravir sodium) 50 mg, Lamivudine 300 mg, Abacavir (as Abacavir sulfate) 600 mg Triumeq 50mg/600mg/300mg tablets | 30 tablet PoM £798.16

Abacavir with lamivudine

The properties listed below are those particular to the combination only. For the properties of the components please consider, abacavir p. 390, lamivudine p. 393.

● **INDICATIONS AND DOSE**
HIV infection in combination with other antiretrovirals
▸ BY MOUTH
▸ Child 12-17 years (body-weight 40 kg and above): 1 tablet once daily

● **RENAL IMPAIRMENT** Avoid *Kivexa*® if estimated glomerular filtration rate less than 50 mL/minute/1.73 m².

● **MEDICINAL FORMS** There can be variation in the licensing of different medicines containing the same drug.

Tablet
▸ Abacavir with lamivudine (Non-proprietary)
  Lamivudine 300 mg, Abacavir (as Abacavir sulfate) 600 mg Abacavir 600mg / Lamivudine 300mg tablets | 30 tablet PoM £194.62
▸ Kivexa (ViiV Healthcare UK Ltd)
  Lamivudine 300 mg, Abacavir (as Abacavir sulfate) 600 mg Kivexa 600mg/300mg tablets | 30 tablet PoM £299.41

Abacavir with lamivudine and zidovudine

The properties listed below are those particular to the combination only. For the properties of the components please consider, abacavir p. 390, lamivudine p. 393, zidovudine p. 394.

● **INDICATIONS AND DOSE**
HIV infection (use only if patient is stabilised for 6–8 weeks on the individual components in the same proportions)
▸ BY MOUTH
▸ Child (body-weight 30 kg and above): 1 tablet twice daily

● **UNLICENSED USE** *Trizivir*® not licensed for use in children.

● **RENAL IMPAIRMENT** Avoid *Trizivir*® if estimated glomerular filtration rate less than 50 mL/minute/1.73 m².

● **MEDICINAL FORMS** There can be variation in the licensing of different medicines containing the same drug.

Tablet
▸ Trizivir (ViiV Healthcare UK Ltd)
  Lamivudine 150 mg, Abacavir (as Abacavir sulfate) 300 mg, Zidovudine 300 mg Trizivir tablets | 60 tablet PoM £432.70

↞ 390

Didanosine

(ddI; DDI)

- **INDICATIONS AND DOSE**

HIV infection in combination with other antiretroviral drugs
  - ▸ BY MOUTH
  - ▸ Child 1-7 months: 50–100 mg/m^2 twice daily
  - ▸ Child 8 months-17 years: 180–240 mg/m^2 once daily; usual dose 200 mg/m^2 once daily; maximum 400 mg per day

- **UNLICENSED USE** Tablets not licensed for use in children under 3 months. EC capsules not licensed for use in children under 6 years.
- **CAUTIONS** History of pancreatitis (preferably avoid, otherwise extreme caution) · hyperuricaemia · peripheral neuropathy
- **INTERACTIONS** → Appendix 1 (didanosine). Antacids in tablet formulation might affect absorption of other drugs—give at least 2 hours apart.
- **SIDE-EFFECTS** Acute renal failure · alopecia · anaphylactic reactions · diabetes mellitus · dry eyes · dry mouth · hyperuricaemia (suspend if raised significantly) · hypoglycaemia · liver failure · non-cirrhotic portal hypertension · optic nerve changes · pancreatitis (less common in children) · parotid gland enlargement · peripheral neuropathy (switch to another antiretroviral if peripheral neuropathy develops) · retinal changes · rhabdomyolysis · sialadenitis

  SIDE-EFFECTS, FURTHER INFORMATION
  - ▸ Pancreatitis Suspend treatment if serum lipase raised (even if asymptomatic) or if symptoms of pancreatitis develop; discontinue if pancreatitis confirmed. Whenever possible avoid concomitant treatment with other drugs known to cause pancreatic toxicity (e.g. intravenous pentamidine isetionate); monitor closely if concomitant therapy unavoidable. Since significant elevations of triglycerides cause pancreatitis monitor closely if elevated.

- **PREGNANCY** Manufacturer advises use only if potential benefit outweighs risk.
- **HEPATIC IMPAIRMENT** In hepatic impairment, monitor for toxicity.
- **RENAL IMPAIRMENT** Reduce dose if estimated glomerular filtration rate less than 60 mL/minute/1.73 m^2; consult product literature.
- **MONITORING REQUIREMENTS** Ophthalmological examination (including visual acuity, colour vision, and dilated fundus examination) recommended annually or if visual changes occur.
- **DIRECTIONS FOR ADMINISTRATION** Capsules should be swallowed whole and taken at least 2 hours before or 2 hours after food.

  With chewable tablets, to ensure sufficient antacid, each dose to be taken as at least 2 tablets (child under 1 year 1 tablet) chewed thoroughly, crushed or dispersed in water; clear apple juice may be added for flavouring; tablets to be taken 2 hours after lopinavir with ritonavir capsules and oral solution or atazanavir with ritonavir.

- **PATIENT AND CARER ADVICE** Patients or carers should be given advice on how to administer didanosine capsules and chewable tablets.

- **MEDICINAL FORMS**
  There can be variation in the licensing of different medicines containing the same drug.

  Chewable tablet
  CAUTIONARY AND ADVISORY LABELS 23
  EXCIPIENTS: May contain Aspartame
  - ▸ Videx (Bristol-Myers Squibb Pharmaceuticals Ltd)
    Didanosine 25 mg Videx 25mg chewable dispersible tablets sugar-free | 60 tablet [PoM] £25.06 (Hospital only)

  Gastro-resistant capsule
  CAUTIONARY AND ADVISORY LABELS 25
  - ▸ Videx EC (Bristol-Myers Squibb Pharmaceuticals Ltd)
    Didanosine 125 mg Videx EC 125mg capsules | 30 capsule [PoM] £48.18 (Hospital only)
    Didanosine 200 mg Videx EC 200mg capsules | 30 capsule [PoM] £77.09 (Hospital only)
    Didanosine 250 mg Videx EC 250mg capsules | 30 capsule [PoM] £96.37 (Hospital only)
    Didanosine 400 mg Videx EC 400mg capsules | 30 capsule [PoM] £154.19 (Hospital only)

↞ 390

Emtricitabine

(FTC)

- **INDICATIONS AND DOSE**

HIV infection in combination with other antiretroviral drugs
  - ▸ BY MOUTH USING CAPSULES
  - ▸ Child (body-weight 33 kg and above): 200 mg once daily
  - ▸ BY MOUTH USING ORAL SOLUTION
  - ▸ Child 4 months-17 years (body-weight up to 33 kg): 6 mg/kg once daily
  - ▸ Child 4 months-17 years (body-weight 33 kg and above): 240 mg once daily

DOSE EQUIVALENCE AND CONVERSION
240 mg oral solution ≡ 200 mg capsule; where appropriate the capsule may be used instead of the oral solution.

- **INTERACTIONS** → Appendix 1 (emtricitabine).
- **SIDE-EFFECTS** Abnormal dreams · hyperpigmentation · pruritus
- **HEPATIC IMPAIRMENT** On discontinuation, monitor patients with hepatitis B (risk of exacerbation of hepatitis).
- **RENAL IMPAIRMENT** Reduce dose or increase dosage interval if estimated glomerular filtration rate less than 50 mL/minute/1.73 m^2; consult product literature.
- **PRESCRIBING AND DISPENSING INFORMATION** Flavours of oral liquid formulations may include candy.
- **PATIENT AND CARER ADVICE**

  Missed doses
  If a dose is more than 12 hours late, the missed dose should not be taken and the next dose should be taken at the normal time.

- **MEDICINAL FORMS**
  There can be variation in the licensing of different medicines containing the same drug.

  Capsule
  - ▸ Emtriva (Gilead Sciences International Ltd)
    Emtricitabine 200 mg Emtriva 200mg capsules | 30 capsule [PoM] £138.98

  Oral solution
  ELECTROLYTES: May contain Sodium
  - ▸ Emtriva (Gilead Sciences International Ltd)
    Emtricitabine 10 mg per 1 ml Emtriva 10mg/ml oral solution sugar-free | 170 ml [PoM] £39.53

Lamivudine

(3TC)

⚑ 390

● INDICATIONS AND DOSE

EPIVIR® ORAL SOLUTION

HIV infection in combination with other antiretroviral drugs

▸ BY MOUTH

- Child 1–2 months: 4 mg/kg twice daily
- Child 3 months–11 years (body-weight up to 14 kg): 4 mg/kg twice daily (max. per dose 150 mg), alternatively 8 mg/kg once daily (max. per dose 300 mg)
- Child 3 months–11 years (body-weight 14–20 kg): 4 mg/kg twice daily (max. per dose 150 mg), alternatively 8 mg/kg once daily (max. per dose 300 mg), alternatively 75 mg twice daily, alternatively 150 mg once daily
- Child 3 months–11 years (body-weight 21–29 kg): 4 mg/kg twice daily (max. per dose 150 mg), alternatively 8 mg/kg once daily (max. per dose 300 mg), alternatively 75 mg daily, dose to be taken in the morning and 150 mg daily, dose to be taken in the evening, alternatively 225 mg once daily
- Child 3 months–11 years (body-weight 30 kg and above): 4 mg/kg twice daily (max. per dose 150 mg), alternatively 8 mg/kg once daily (max. per dose 300 mg), alternatively 150 mg twice daily, alternatively 300 mg once daily
- Child 12–17 years: 150 mg twice daily, alternatively 300 mg once daily

EPIVIR® TABLETS

HIV infection in combination with other antiretroviral drugs

▸ BY MOUTH

- Child 1–2 months: 4 mg/kg twice daily
- Child 3 months–11 years (body-weight up to 14 kg): 4 mg/kg twice daily, alternatively 8 mg/kg once daily
- Child 3 months–11 years (body-weight 14–20 kg): 4 mg/kg twice daily (max. per dose 150 mg), alternatively 8 mg/kg once daily (max. per dose 300 mg), alternatively 75 mg twice daily, alternatively 150 mg once daily
- Child 3 months–11 years (body-weight 21–29 kg): 4 mg/kg twice daily (max. per dose 150 mg), alternatively 8 mg/kg once daily (max. per dose 300 mg), alternatively 75 mg daily, dose to be taken in the morning and 150 mg daily, dose to be taken in the evening, alternatively 225 mg once daily
- Child 3 months–11 years (body-weight 30 kg and above): 4 mg/kg twice daily (max. per dose 150 mg), alternatively 8 mg/kg once daily (max. per dose 300 mg), alternatively 150 mg twice daily, alternatively 300 mg once daily
- Child 12–17 years: 150 mg twice daily, alternatively 300 mg once daily

ZEFFIX®

Chronic hepatitis B infection either with compensated liver disease (with evidence of viral replication and histology of active liver inflammation or fibrosis) when first-line treatments cannot be used, or (in combination with another antiviral drug without cross-resistance to lamivudine) with decompensated liver disease

▸ BY MOUTH

- Child 2–11 years: 3 mg/kg once daily (max. per dose 100 mg), children receiving lamivudine for concomitant HIV infection should continue to receive lamivudine in a dose appropriate for HIV infection

- Child 12–17 years: 100 mg once daily, patients receiving lamivudine for concomitant HIV infection should continue to receive lamivudine in a dose appropriate for HIV infection

● UNLICENSED USE

EPIVIR® ORAL SOLUTION Not licensed for use in children under 3 months.

ZEFFIX® Not licensed for use in children.

EPIVIR® TABLETS Not licensed for use in children under 3 months.

● CAUTIONS Recurrent hepatitis in patients with chronic hepatitis B may occur on discontinuation of lamivudine

● INTERACTIONS → Appendix 1 (lamivudine).

● SIDE-EFFECTS Alopecia · muscle disorders · nasal symptoms · peripheral neuropathy · rhabdomyolysis

● BREAST FEEDING Can be used with caution in women infected with chronic hepatitis B alone, providing that adequate measures are taken to prevent hepatitis B infection in infants.

● RENAL IMPAIRMENT Reduce dose if estimated glomerular filtration rate less than 50 mL/minute/1.73 m^2; consult product literature.

● MONITORING REQUIREMENTS When treating chronic hepatitis B with lamivudine, monitor liver function tests every 3 months, and viral markers of hepatitis B every 3–6 months, more frequently in patients with advanced liver disease or following transplantation (monitoring to continue for at least 1 year after discontinuation—recurrent hepatitis may occur on discontinuation).

● PRESCRIBING AND DISPENSING INFORMATION Flavours of oral liquid formulations may include banana and strawberry.

● MEDICINAL FORMS
There can be variation in the licensing of different medicines containing the same drug.

Tablet
▸ Epivir (ViiV Healthcare UK Ltd)
  Lamivudine 150 mg Epivir 150mg tablets | 60 tablet PoM £121.82
  Lamivudine 300 mg Epivir 300mg tablets | 30 tablet PoM £133.89
▸ Zeffix (GlaxoSmithKline UK Ltd)
  Lamivudine 100 mg Zeffix 100mg tablets | 28 tablet PoM £78.09
  DT price = £67.75

Oral solution
EXCIPIENTS: May contain Sucrose
▸ Epivir (ViiV Healthcare UK Ltd)
  Lamivudine 10 mg per 1 ml Epivir 50mg/5ml oral solution | 240 ml PoM £33.16

⚑ 390

Stavudine

(d4T)

● INDICATIONS AND DOSE

HIV infection in combination with other antiretroviral drugs when no suitable alternative available and when prescribed for shortest period possible

▸ BY MOUTH

- Child (body-weight up to 30 kg): 1 mg/kg twice daily, to be taken preferably at least 1 hour before food
- Child (body-weight 30–59 kg): 30 mg twice daily, to be taken preferably at least 1 hour before food
- Child (body-weight 60 kg and above): 40 mg twice daily, to be taken preferably at least 1 hour before food

● UNLICENSED USE Capsules not licensed for use in children under 3 months.

● CAUTIONS Excessive alcohol intake · higher risk of lactic acidosis than other nucleoside reverse transcriptase inhibitors (especially when used in combination with

Infection
5

didanosine)—use only if alternative regimens are not suitable · history of pancreatitis · history of peripheral neuropathy

- **INTERACTIONS** → Appendix 1 (stavudine).
Caution with concomitant use of isoniazid—risk of peripheral neuropathy.
Caution with concomitant use with other drugs associated with pancreatitis.
- **SIDE-EFFECTS**
- ▶ **Common or very common** Abnormal dreams · cognitive dysfunction · depression · drowsiness · peripheral neuropathy (switch to another antiretroviral if peripheral neuropathy develops) · pruritus
- ▶ **Uncommon** Anxiety · gynaecomastia
- **PREGNANCY** Manufacturer advises use only if potential benefit outweighs risk.
- **RENAL IMPAIRMENT** Reduce dose to 50% if estimated glomerular filtration rate 25–50 mL/minute/1.73 m²; reduce dose to 25% if estimated glomerular filtration rate less than 25 mL/minute/1.73 m². Risk of peripheral neuropathy.
- **PRESCRIBING AND DISPENSING INFORMATION** Flavours of oral liquid formulations may include cherry.
- **LESS SUITABLE FOR PRESCRIBING** Stavudine (especially in combination with didanosine) is associated with a higher risk of lipoatrophy and should be used only if alternative regimens are not suitable; it is considered to be less suitable for prescribing.

- **MEDICINAL FORMS**
There can be variation in the licensing of different medicines containing the same drug.

Capsule
- ▶ Zerit (Bristol-Myers Squibb Pharmaceuticals Ltd)
Stavudine 20 mg Zerit 20mg capsules | 56 capsule [PoM] £139.46 (Hospital only)
Stavudine 30 mg Zerit 30mg capsules | 56 capsule [PoM] £146.25 (Hospital only)
Stavudine 40 mg Zerit 40mg capsules | 56 capsule [PoM] £150.66 (Hospital only)

Oral solution
- ▶ Zerit (Bristol-Myers Squibb Pharmaceuticals Ltd)
Stavudine 1 mg per 1 ml Zerit 1mg/ml oral solution | 200 ml [PoM] £22.94 (Hospital only)

F 390

Tenofovir disoproxil

- **INDICATIONS AND DOSE**

HIV infection in combination with other antiretroviral drugs when first-line nucleoside reverse transcriptase inhibitors cannot be used because of resistance or contra-indications
- ▶ BY MOUTH
- ▶ Child 2–17 years: 6.5 mg/kg once daily (max. per dose 245 mg)
- ▶ Child 6–17 years (body-weight 17–21 kg): 123 mg once daily
- ▶ Child 6–17 years (body-weight 22–27 kg): 163 mg once daily
- ▶ Child 6–17 years (body-weight 28–34 kg): 204 mg once daily
- ▶ Child 6–17 years (body-weight 35 kg and above): 245 mg once daily

Chronic hepatitis B infection with compensated liver disease (with evidence of viral replication, and histology of active liver inflammation or fibrosis)
- ▶ BY MOUTH
- ▶ Child 12–17 years (body-weight 35 kg and above): 245 mg once daily

DOSE EQUIVALENCE AND CONVERSION
7.5 scoops of granules contains approx. 245 mg tenofovir disoproxil (as fumarate).

- **INTERACTIONS** → Appendix 1 (tenofovir).
Use with caution if concomitant or recent use of nephrotoxic drugs.
- **SIDE-EFFECTS**
- ▶ **Rare** Nephrogenic diabetes insipidus · proximal renal tubulopathy · renal failure
- ▶ **Frequency not known** Hypophosphataemia · reduced bone density
- **RENAL IMPAIRMENT** Manufacturer advises avoid—no information available.
- **MONITORING REQUIREMENTS**
- ▶ Test renal function and serum phosphate before treatment, then every 4 weeks (more frequently if at increased risk of renal impairment) for 1 year and then every 3 months, interrupt treatment if renal function deteriorates or serum phosphate decreases.
- ▶ When treating chronic hepatitis B with tenofovir, monitor liver function tests every 3 months and viral markers for hepatitis B every 3–6 months during treatment (continue monitoring for at least 1 year after discontinuation—recurrent hepatitis may occur on discontinuation).
- **DIRECTIONS FOR ADMINISTRATION** *Granules*: mix 1 scoop of granules with 1 tablespoon of soft food (e.g. yoghurt, apple sauce) and take immediately without chewing. Do **not** mix granules with liquids.
- **PATIENT AND CARER ADVICE**
Patients or carers should be given advice on how to administer tenofovir granules.

Missed doses
If a dose is more than 12 hours late, the missed dose should not be taken and the next dose should be taken at the normal time.

- **MEDICINAL FORMS**
There can be variation in the licensing of different medicines containing the same drug.

Tablet
CAUTIONARY AND ADVISORY LABELS 21
- ▶ Viread (Gilead Sciences International Ltd)
Tenofovir disoproxil (as Tenofovir disoproxil fumarate) 123 mg Viread 123mg tablets | 30 tablet [PoM] £102.60
Tenofovir disoproxil (as Tenofovir disoproxil fumarate) 163 mg Viread 163mg tablets | 30 tablet [PoM] £135.98
Tenofovir disoproxil (as Tenofovir disoproxil fumarate) 204 mg Viread 204mg tablets | 30 tablet [PoM] £170.19
Tenofovir disoproxil (as Tenofovir disoproxil fumarate) 245 mg Viread 245mg tablets | 30 tablet [PoM] £204.39

Granules
CAUTIONARY AND ADVISORY LABELS 21
- ▶ Viread (Gilead Sciences International Ltd)
Tenofovir disoproxil (as Tenofovir disoproxil fumarate) 33 mg per 1 gram Viread 33mg/g granules | 60 gram [PoM] £54.50

F 390

Zidovudine

(Azidothymidine; AZT)

- **INDICATIONS AND DOSE**

HIV infection in combination with other antiretroviral drugs
- ▶ BY MOUTH
- ▶ Child: 180 mg/m² twice daily (max. per dose 300 mg)
- ▶ Child (body-weight 8–13 kg): 100 mg twice daily
- ▶ Child (body-weight 14–20 kg): 100 mg, to be taken in the morning and 200 mg, to be taken in the evening
- ▶ Child (body-weight 21–27 kg): 200 mg twice daily
- ▶ Child (body-weight 28–29 kg): 200–250 mg twice daily

▸ Child (body-weight 30 kg and above): 250–300 mg twice daily

HIV infection in combination with other antiretroviral drugs (dose expressed in mg/kg)
▸ BY MOUTH
▸ Child (body-weight 4–8 kg): 12 mg/kg twice daily
▸ Child (body-weight 9–29 kg): 9 mg/kg twice daily

Prevention of maternal-fetal HIV transmission
▸ BY MOUTH, OR BY INTRAVENOUS INFUSION
▸ Child: Seek specialist advice (combination therapy preferred) (consult local protocol)

HIV infection in combination with other antiretroviral drugs in patients temporarily unable to take zidovudine by mouth
▸ BY INTRAVENOUS INFUSION
▸ Child 3 months–11 years: 60–80 mg/m^2 every 6 hours usually for not more than 2 weeks, dose approximating to 9–12 mg/kg twice daily by mouth
▸ Child 12–17 years: 0.8–1 mg/kg every 4 hours usually for not more than 2 weeks, dose approximating to 1.2–1.5 mg/kg every 4 hours by mouth

● **CONTRA-INDICATIONS** Abnormally low haemoglobin concentration (consult product literature) · abnormally low neutrophil counts (consult product literature) · Acute porphyrias p. 562 · neonates with hyperbilirubinaemia requiring treatment other than phototherapy, or with raised transaminase (consult product literature)

● **CAUTIONS** Risk of haematological toxicity particularly with high dose and advanced disease · vitamin B$_{12}$ deficiency (increased risk of neutropenia)

● **INTERACTIONS** → Appendix 1 (zidovudine). Increased risk of toxicity with nephrotoxic and myelosuppressive drugs—for further details consult product literature.

● **SIDE-EFFECTS** Anaemia (may require transfusion) · anxiety · chest pain · convulsions · depression · dizziness · drowsiness · gynaecomastia · influenza-like symptoms · loss of mental acuity · myopathy · neuropathy · paraesthesia · pigmentation of nails · pigmentation of oral mucosa · pigmentation of skin · pruritus · sweating · taste disturbance · urinary frequency

SIDE-EFFECTS, FURTHER INFORMATION
▸ Anaemia and myelosuppression If anaemia or myelosuppression occur, reduce dose or interrupt treatment according to product literature, or consider other treatment
▸ Lipoatrophy Zidovudine is associated with a higher risk of lipoatrophy than other antiretrovirals and should be used only if alternative regimens are not suitable.

● **HEPATIC IMPAIRMENT** Accumulation may occur.

● **RENAL IMPAIRMENT** Reduce dose if estimated glomerular filtration rate less than 10 mL/minute/1.73 m^2—consult product literature.

● **MONITORING REQUIREMENTS** Monitor full blood count after 4 weeks of treatment, then every 3 months.

● **DIRECTIONS FOR ADMINISTRATION**
▸ With intravenous use For *intermittent intravenous infusion*, dilute to a concentration of 2 mg/mL or 4 mg/mL with Glucose 5% and give over 1 hour.

● **PRESCRIBING AND DISPENSING INFORMATION** The abbreviation AZT which is sometimes used for zidovudine has also been used for another drug.

● **MEDICINAL FORMS**
There can be variation in the licensing of different medicines containing the same drug.
Capsule
▸ Zidovudine (Non-proprietary)
Zidovudine 100 mg Zidovudine 100mg capsules | 60 capsule PoM
£40.41

Zidovudine 250 mg Zidovudine 250mg capsules | 60 capsule PoM
£96.36
▸ Retrovir (ViiV Healthcare UK Ltd)
Zidovudine 100 mg Retrovir 100mg capsules | 100 capsule PoM
£88.86
Zidovudine 250 mg Retrovir 250mg capsules | 40 capsule PoM
£88.86

Oral solution
▸ Retrovir (ViiV Healthcare UK Ltd)
Zidovudine 10 mg per 1 ml Retrovir 50mg/5ml oral solution sugar-free | 200 ml PoM £17.78

Solution for infusion
▸ Retrovir (ViiV Healthcare UK Ltd)
Zidovudine 10 mg per 1 ml Retrovir IV 200mg/20ml concentrate for solution for infusion vials | 5 vial PoM £44.61

Zidovudine with lamivudine

The properties listed below are those particular to the combination only. For the properties of the components please consider, zidovudine p. 394, lamivudine p. 393.

● **INDICATIONS AND DOSE**

HIV infection in combination with other antiretroviral drugs
▸ BY MOUTH
▸ Child (body-weight 14–20 kg): 0.5 tablet twice daily
▸ Child (body-weight 21–29 kg): 0.5 tablet daily, to be given in the morning and 1 tablet daily, to be given in the evening
▸ Child (body-weight 30 kg and above): 1 tablet twice daily

● **RENAL IMPAIRMENT** Avoid if estimated glomerular filtration rate less than 50 mL/minute/1.73 m^2.

● **DIRECTIONS FOR ADMINISTRATION**
COMBIVIR® TABLETS Tablets may be crushed and mixed with semi-solid food or liquid just before administration.

● **MEDICINAL FORMS**
There can be variation in the licensing of different medicines containing the same drug.
Tablet
▸ Zidovudine with lamivudine (Non-proprietary)
Lamivudine 150 mg, Zidovudine 300 mg Zidovudine 300mg / Lamivudine 150mg tablets | 60 tablet PoM £70.61–£285.11
▸ Combivir (ViiV Healthcare UK Ltd)
Lamivudine 150 mg, Zidovudine 300 mg Combivir 150mg/300mg tablets | 60 tablet PoM £255.10

ANTIVIRALS 〉 PROTEASE INHIBITORS, HIV

Protease inhibitors

● **CONTRA-INDICATIONS** Acute porphyrias p. 562

● **CAUTIONS** Diabetes · haemophilia (increased risk of bleeding)

● **SIDE-EFFECTS** Abdominal pain · anaemia · anaphylaxis · anorexia · blood disorders · diarrhoea · dizziness · fatigue · flatulence · gastro-intestinal disturbances · headache · hepatic dysfunction · hypersensitivity reactions · lipodystrophy · Lipodystrophy Syndrome · myalgia · myositis · nausea · neutropenia · osteonecrosis · pancreatitis · paraesthesia · pruritus · rash · rhabdomyolysis · sleep disturbances · Stevens-Johnson syndrome · taste disturbances · thrombocytopenia · vomiting

SIDE-EFFECTS, FURTHER INFORMATION
▸ Lipodystrophy Syndrome For further information see HIV infection p. 385.
▸ Osteonecrosis For further information see HIV infection p. 385.

● **HEPATIC IMPAIRMENT** Use with caution in patients with chronic hepatitis B or C (increased risk of hepatic side-effects).

Infection

5

☞ 395

Atazanavir

- **INDICATIONS AND DOSE**

HIV infection in combination with other antiretroviral drugs—with low-dose ritonavir
- ▸ BY MOUTH
- ▸ Child 6-17 years (body-weight 15-19 kg): 150 mg once daily
- ▸ Child 6-17 years (body-weight 20-39 kg): 200 mg once daily
- ▸ Child 6-17 years (body-weight 40 kg and above): 300 mg once daily

- **CAUTIONS** Cardiac conduction disorders · electrolyte disturbances · predisposition to QT interval prolongation
- **INTERACTIONS** → Appendix 1 (atazanavir).
  Caution if concomitant use with drugs that prolong PR interval.
  Caution with concomitant use of drugs that prolong QT interval.
- **SIDE-EFFECTS**
- ▸ **Common or very common** AV block
- ▸ **Uncommon** Abnormal dreams · alopecia · amnesia · anxiety · arthralgia · chest pain · cholelithiasis · depression · disorientation · dry mouth · dyspnoea · gynaecomastia · haematuria · hypertension · increased appetite · mouth ulcers · nephrolithiasis · peripheral neuropathy · proteinuria · syncope · torsade de pointes · urinary frequency · weight changes
- ▸ **Rare** Abnormal gait · cholecystitis · hepatosplenomegaly · oedema · palpitation
  SIDE-EFFECTS, FURTHER INFORMATION
- ▸ **Rash** Mild to moderate rash occurs commonly, usually within the first 3 weeks of therapy. Severe rash occurs less frequently and may be accompanied by systemic symptoms. Discontinue if severe rash develops.
- **PREGNANCY** Theoretical risk of hyperbilirubinaemia in neonate if used at term.
  In pregnancy, monitor viral load and plasma-atazanavir concentration during third trimester.
- **HEPATIC IMPAIRMENT** Manufacturer advises caution in mild impairment; avoid in moderate to severe impairment.

- **MEDICINAL FORMS**
  There can be variation in the licensing of different medicines containing the same drug.
  Capsule
  CAUTIONARY AND ADVISORY LABELS 5, 21
  - ▸ Reyataz (Bristol-Myers Squibb Pharmaceuticals Ltd)
    Atazanavir (as Atazanavir sulfate) 150 mg Reyataz 150mg capsules | 60 capsule PoM £303.38 (Hospital only)
    Atazanavir (as Atazanavir sulfate) 200 mg Reyataz 200mg capsules | 60 capsule PoM £303.38 (Hospital only)
    Atazanavir (as Atazanavir sulfate) 300 mg Reyataz 300mg capsules | 30 capsule PoM £303.38 (Hospital only)

☞ 395

Darunavir

- **INDICATIONS AND DOSE**

HIV infection in combination with other antiretroviral drugs in patients previously treated with antiretroviral therapy—with low-dose ritonavir
- ▸ BY MOUTH
- ▸ Child 3-17 years (body-weight 15-29 kg): 375 mg twice daily
- ▸ Child 3-17 years (body-weight 30-39 kg): 450 mg twice daily
- ▸ Child 3-17 years (body-weight 40 kg and above): 600 mg twice daily

- ▸ Child 12-17 years: 800 mg once daily, once daily dose only to be used if no resistance to darunavir, if plasma HIV-RNA concentration less than 100 000 copies/mL, and if CD4 cell count greater than 100 cells × 10^6/litre

HIV infection in combination with other antiretroviral drugs in patients not previously treated with antiretroviral therapy—with low-dose ritonavir
- ▸ BY MOUTH
- ▸ Child 12-17 years (body-weight 40 kg and above): 800 mg once daily

- **INTERACTIONS** → Appendix 1 (darunavir).
- **SIDE-EFFECTS**
- ▸ **Common or very common** Peripheral neuropathy · rash
- ▸ **Uncommon** Abnormal dreams · acne · alopecia · anxiety · arthralgia · chest pain · conjunctival hyperaemia · cough · depression · dry eyes · dry mouth · dyspnoea · dysuria · eczema · erectile dysfunction · flushing · gynaecomastia · hypertension · hypothyroidism · increased appetite · increased sweating · memory impairment · myocardial infarction · nail discoloration · nephrolithiasis · osteoporosis · peripheral oedema · polyuria · pyrexia · QT interval prolongation · reduced libido · renal failure · severe skin rash · Stevens-Johnson syndrome · stomatitis · tachycardia · throat irritation · toxic epidermal necrolysis · weight changes
- ▸ **Rare** Bradycardia · confusion · convulsions · haematemesis · palpitation · rhinorrhoea · seborrhoeic dermatitis · syncope · visual disturbances
  SIDE-EFFECTS, FURTHER INFORMATION
- ▸ **Rash** Mild to moderate rash occurs commonly, usually within the first 4 weeks of therapy and resolves without stopping treatment. Severe skin rash (including Stevens-Johnson syndrome and toxic epidermal necrolysis) occurs less frequently and may be accompanied by fever, malaise, arthralgia, myalgia, oral lesions, conjunctivitis, hepatitis, or eosinophilia; treatment should be stopped if severe rash develops.
- **ALLERGY AND CROSS-SENSITIVITY** Use with caution in patients with sulfonamide sensitivity.
- **PREGNANCY** Manufacturer advises use only if potential benefit outweighs risk; if required, use the twice daily dose regimen.
- **HEPATIC IMPAIRMENT** Manufacturer advises caution in mild to moderate impairment; avoid in severe impairment—no information available.
- **MONITORING REQUIREMENTS** Monitor liver function before and during treatment.
- **PRESCRIBING AND DISPENSING INFORMATION** Flavours of oral liquid formulations may include strawberry.
- **PATIENT AND CARER ADVICE**
  Missed doses
  If a dose is more than 6 hours late on the twice daily regimen (or more than 12 hours late on the once daily regimen), the missed dose should not be taken and the next dose should be taken at the normal time.

- **MEDICINAL FORMS**
  There can be variation in the licensing of different medicines containing the same drug.
  Tablet
  CAUTIONARY AND ADVISORY LABELS 21
  - ▸ Prezista (Janssen-Cilag Ltd)
    Darunavir (as Darunavir ethanolate) 75 mg Prezista 75mg tablets | 480 tablet PoM £446.70
    Darunavir (as Darunavir ethanolate) 150 mg Prezista 150mg tablets | 240 tablet PoM £446.70
    Darunavir (as Darunavir ethanolate) 400 mg Prezista 400mg tablets | 60 tablet PoM £297.80
    Darunavir (as Darunavir ethanolate) 600 mg Prezista 600mg tablets | 60 tablet PoM £446.70

Darunavir (as Darunavir ethanolate) 800 mg Prezista 800mg
tablets | 30 tablet PoM £297.80
Oral suspension
CAUTIONARY AND ADVISORY LABELS 21
▸ Prezista (Janssen-Cilag Ltd)
Darunavir (as Darunavir ethanolate) 100 mg per 1 ml Prezista
100mg/ml oral suspension sugar-free | 200 ml PoM £248.17

⚑ 395

Fosamprenavir

● DRUG ACTION Fosamprenavir is a pro-drug of amprenavir.

● **INDICATIONS AND DOSE**

**HIV infection in combination with other antiretroviral
drugs—with low-dose ritonavir**
▸ BY MOUTH
▸ Child 6–17 years (body-weight 25–39 kg): 18 mg/kg twice
daily (max. per dose 700 mg)
▸ Child 6–17 years (body-weight 40 kg and above): 700 mg
twice daily

DOSE EQUIVALENCE AND CONVERSION
700 mg fosamprenavir is equivalent to approximately
600 mg amprenavir.

● INTERACTIONS → Appendix 1 (fosamprenavir).

● SIDE-EFFECTS
▸ **Rare** Stevens-Johnson syndrome
▸ **Frequency not known** Rash

SIDE-EFFECTS, FURTHER INFORMATION
▸ Rash Rash may occur, usually in the second week of
therapy; discontinue permanently if severe rash with
systemic or allergic symptoms or, mucosal involvement; if
rash mild or moderate, may continue without
interruption—usually resolves within 2 weeks and may
respond to antihistamines.

● PREGNANCY Toxicity in *animal* studies; manufacturer
advises use only if potential benefit outweighs risk.

● HEPATIC IMPAIRMENT Reduce dose in moderate to severe
impairment. Manufacturer advises caution in mild
impairment.

● DIRECTIONS FOR ADMINISTRATION In children, oral
suspension should be taken with food.

● PRESCRIBING AND DISPENSING INFORMATION Flavours of
oral liquid formulations may include grape, bubblegum, or
peppermint.

● PATIENT AND CARER ADVICE Patients or carers should be
given advice on how to administer fosamprenavir oral
suspension.

● MEDICINAL FORMS
There can be variation in the licensing of different medicines
containing the same drug.
Tablet
▸ Telzir (ViiV Healthcare UK Ltd)
Fosamprenavir (as Fosamprenavir calcium) 700 mg Telzir 700mg
tablets | 60 tablet PoM £220.13
Oral suspension
EXCIPIENTS: May contain Propylene glycol
▸ Telzir (ViiV Healthcare UK Ltd)
Fosamprenavir (as Fosamprenavir calcium) 50 mg per 1 ml Telzir
50mg/ml oral suspension | 225 ml PoM £58.70

⚑ 395

Lopinavir with ritonavir

● **INDICATIONS AND DOSE**

**HIV infection in combination with other antiretroviral
drugs**
▸ BY MOUTH USING TABLETS
▸ Child 2–17 years (body-weight up to 40 kg and body surface
area 0.5–0.7 m²): 200/50 mg twice daily

▸ Child 2–17 years (body-weight up to 40 kg and body surface
area 0.8–1.1 m²): 300/75 mg twice daily
▸ Child 2–17 years (body-weight 40 kg and above and body
surface area 1.2 m² and above): 400/100 mg twice daily
▸ BY MOUTH USING ORAL SOLUTION
▸ Child 2–17 years: 2.9 mL/m² twice daily (max. per dose
5 mL), to be taken with food, oral solution contains
400 mg lopinavir, 100 mg ritonavir/5 mL

● CAUTIONS Cardiac conduction disorders · pancreatitis ·
structural heart disease

● INTERACTIONS → Appendix 1 (lopinavir, ritonavir).
Caution if concomitant use with drugs that prolong QT or
PR interval.

● SIDE-EFFECTS
▸ **Common or very common** Amenorrhoea · anxiety ·
arthralgia · colitis · hypertension · menorrhagia ·
neuropathy · night sweats · sexual dysfunction · weight
changes
▸ **Uncommon** Abnormal dreams · alopecia · artherosclerosis ·
AV block · cerebrovascular accident · convulsions · deep
vein thrombosis · dry mouth · gastro-intestinal ulcer ·
haematuria · nephritis · rectal bleeding · stomatitis ·
tinnitus · tremor · visual disturbances

SIDE-EFFECTS, FURTHER INFORMATION
▸ Pancreatitis Signs and symptoms suggestive of pancreatitis
(including raised serum lipase) should be evaluated—
discontinue if pancreatitis diagnosed

● PREGNANCY Avoid oral solution due to high propylene
glycol content; use tablets only if potential benefit
outweighs risk (toxicity in *animal* studies).

● HEPATIC IMPAIRMENT Avoid oral solution due to
propylene glycol content; manufacturer advises avoid
tablets in severe impairment.

● RENAL IMPAIRMENT Avoid oral solution due to high
propylene glycol content.

● MONITORING REQUIREMENTS Monitor liver function
before and during treatment.

● PATIENT AND CARER ADVICE Oral solution tastes bitter.

● MEDICINAL FORMS
There can be variation in the licensing of different medicines
containing the same drug.
Tablet
CAUTIONARY AND ADVISORY LABELS 25
▸ Kaletra (AbbVie Ltd)
Ritonavir 25 mg, Lopinavir 100 mg Kaletra 100mg/25mg tablets |
60 tablet PoM £76.85
Ritonavir 50 mg, Lopinavir 200 mg Kaletra 200mg/50mg tablets |
120 tablet PoM £285.41
Oral solution
CAUTIONARY AND ADVISORY LABELS 21
EXCIPIENTS: May contain Alcohol, propylene glycol
▸ Kaletra (AbbVie Ltd)
Ritonavir 20 mg per 1 ml, Lopinavir 80 mg per 1 ml Kaletra
80mg/20mg/1ml oral solution | 300 ml PoM £307.39

⚑ 395

Ritonavir

● **INDICATIONS AND DOSE**

**HIV infection in combination with other antiretroviral
drugs (high-dose ritonavir)**
▸ BY MOUTH
▸ Child 2–17 years: Initially 250 mg/m² twice daily,
increased in steps of 50 mg/m² every 2–3 days;
increased to 350 mg/m² twice daily (max. per dose
600 mg twice daily), tolerability of this
regimen is poor continued →

5

Infection

395

Low-dose ritonavir to increase the effect of atazanavir
▸ BY MOUTH
▸ Child 6-17 years (body-weight 15-19 kg): 80—100 mg once daily
▸ Child 6-17 years (body-weight 20 kg and above): 100 mg once daily

Low-dose ritonavir to increase the effect of darunavir
▸ BY MOUTH
▸ Child 3-17 years (body-weight 15-29 kg): 50 mg twice daily
▸ Child 3-17 years (body-weight 30-39 kg): 60 mg twice daily
▸ Child 3-17 years (body-weight 40 kg and above): 100 mg twice daily
▸ Child 12-17 years (body-weight 40 kg and above): 100 mg once daily for use in patients taking darunavir once daily

Low-dose ritonavir to increase the effect of fosamprenavir
▸ BY MOUTH
▸ Child 6-17 years (body-weight 25-32 kg): 3 mg/kg twice daily
▸ Child 6-17 years (body-weight 33 kg and above): 100 mg twice daily

Low-dose ritonavir to increase the effect of tipranavir
▸ BY MOUTH
▸ Child 2-11 years: 150 mg/m^2 twice daily (max. per dose 200 mg)
▸ Child 12-17 years: 200 mg twice daily

● **CAUTIONS** Cardiac conduction disorders · pancreatitis · structural heart disease
● **INTERACTIONS** → Appendix 1 (ritonavir). Caution if concomitant use with drugs that prolong PR interval.
● **SIDE-EFFECTS**
▸ **Common or very common** Acne · anxiety · arthralgia · blood pressure changes · blurred vision · confusion · cough · decreased blood thyroxine concentration · fever · flushing · gastro-intestinal haemorrhage · menorrhagia · mouth ulcers · oedema · peripheral neuropathy · pharyngitis · renal impairment · seizures · syncope
▸ **Uncommon** Electrolyte disturbances · myocardial infarction
▸ **Rare** Toxic epidermal necrolysis
  SIDE-EFFECTS, FURTHER INFORMATION
▸ Pancreatitis Signs and symptoms suggestive of pancreatitis (including raised serum lipase) should be evaluated—discontinue if pancreatitis diagnosed.
● **PREGNANCY** Only use low-dose booster to increase the effect of other protease inhibitors.
● **HEPATIC IMPAIRMENT** Avoid in decompensated liver disease; in severe impairment without decompensation, use 'booster' doses with caution (avoid treatment doses).
● **DIRECTIONS FOR ADMINISTRATION** Bitter taste of oral solution can be masked by mixing with chocolate milk; do not mix with water, measuring cup must be dry.
● **PATIENT AND CARER ADVICE** Patients or carers should be given advice on how to administer ritonavir oral solution.

● **MEDICINAL FORMS**
There can be variation in the licensing of different medicines containing the same drug.
Tablet
CAUTIONARY AND ADVISORY LABELS 21, 25
▸ Norvir (AbbVie Ltd)
  Ritonavir 100 mg Norvir 100mg tablets | 30 tablet PoM £19.44
Oral solution
CAUTIONARY AND ADVISORY LABELS 21
EXCIPIENTS: May contain Alcohol, propylene glycol
▸ Norvir (AbbVie Ltd)
  Ritonavir 80 mg per 1 ml Norvir 80mg/ml oral solution sugar-free | 450 ml PoM £403.20

Tipranavir

● **INDICATIONS AND DOSE**
HIV infection resistant to other protease inhibitors, in combination with other antiretroviral drugs in patients previously treated with antiretrovirals–with low-dose ritonavir
▸ BY MOUTH USING CAPSULES
▸ Child 12-17 years: 500 mg twice daily
▸ BY MOUTH USING ORAL SOLUTION
▸ Child 2-11 years: 375 mg/m^2 twice daily (max. per dose 500 mg)

DOSE EQUIVALENCE AND CONVERSION
The bioavailability of tipranavir oral solution is higher than that of the capsules; the oral solution is not interchangeable with the capsules on a milligram-for-milligram basis.

● **CAUTIONS** Patients at risk of increased bleeding from trauma, surgery or other pathological conditions
● **INTERACTIONS** → Appendix 1 (tipranavir). Caution with concomitant use of drugs that increase risk of bleeding.
● **SIDE-EFFECTS**
▸ **Rare** Dehydration
▸ **Frequency not known** Anorexia · dyspnoea · influenza-like symptoms · peripheral neuropathy · photosensitivity · renal impairment
  SIDE-EFFECTS, FURTHER INFORMATION
▸ Hepatotoxicity Potentially life-threatening hepatotoxicity reported. Discontinue if signs or symptoms of hepatitis develop or if liver-function abnormality develops (consult product literature).
● **PREGNANCY** Manufacturer advises use only if potential benefit outweighs risk—toxicity in *animal* studies.
● **HEPATIC IMPAIRMENT** Manufacturer advises caution in mild impairment; avoid in moderate or severe impairment—no information available.
● **MONITORING REQUIREMENTS** Monitor liver function before treatment then every 2 weeks for 1 month, then every 3 months.
● **PRESCRIBING AND DISPENSING INFORMATION** Flavours of oral liquid formulations may include toffee and mint.
● **PATIENT AND CARER ADVICE** Patients or carers should be told to observe the oral solution for crystallisation; the bottle should be replaced if more than a thin layer of crystals form (doses should continue to be taken at the normal time until the bottle is replaced).

● **MEDICINAL FORMS**
There can be variation in the licensing of different medicines containing the same drug.
Capsule
CAUTIONARY AND ADVISORY LABELS 5, 21
EXCIPIENTS: May contain Ethanol
▸ Aptivus (Boehringer Ingelheim Ltd)
  Tipranavir 250 mg Aptivus 250mg capsules | 120 capsule PoM £441.00
Oral solution
CAUTIONARY AND ADVISORY LABELS 5, 21
EXCIPIENTS: May contain Vitamin e
▸ Aptivus (Boehringer Ingelheim Ltd)
  Tipranavir 100 mg per 1 ml Aptivus 100mg/ml oral solution sugar-free | 95 ml PoM £129.65

ANTIVIRALS > OTHER

Maraviroc

- **DRUG ACTION** Maraviroc is an antagonist of the CCR5 chemokine receptor.

- **INDICATIONS AND DOSE**
  CCR5-tropic HIV infection in combination with other antiretroviral drugs in patients previously treated with antiretrovirals
  ‣ BY MOUTH
  ‣ Child: (consult local protocol)

- **UNLICENSED USE** Not licensed for use in children.
- **CAUTIONS** Cardiovascular disease
- **INTERACTIONS** → Appendix 1 (maraviroc).
- **SIDE-EFFECTS**
  ‣ **Common or very common** Abdominal pain · anaemia · anorexia · depression · diarrhoea · flatulence · headache · insomnia · malaise · nausea · rash
  ‣ **Uncommon** Myositis · proteinuria · renal failure · seizures
  ‣ **Rare** Angina · granulocytopenia · hepatitis · pancytopenia · Stevens-Johnson syndrome · toxic epidermal necrolysis
  ‣ **Frequency not known** Eosinophilia · fever · hepatic reactions · hypersensitivity reactions · osteonecrosis · rash
  SIDE-EFFECTS, FURTHER INFORMATION
- Osteonecrosis For further information see HIV infection p. 385.
- **PREGNANCY** Manufacturer advises use only if potential benefit outweighs risk—toxicity in *animal* studies.
- **HEPATIC IMPAIRMENT** Manufacturer advises caution in hepatic impairment, including patients with chronic hepatitis B or C.
- **RENAL IMPAIRMENT** If estimated glomerular filtration rate less than 80 mL/minute/1.73 m^2, consult product literature.

- **MEDICINAL FORMS**
  There can be variation in the licensing of different medicines containing the same drug.
  Tablet
  ‣ Celsentri (ViiV Healthcare UK Ltd)
  Maraviroc 150 mg Celsentri 150mg tablets | 60 tablet PoM £441.27
  Maraviroc 300 mg Celsentri 300mg tablets | 60 tablet PoM £441.27

6.5 Influenza

Influenza

Management

Oseltamivir below and zanamivir p. 401 are most effective for the treatment of influenza if started within a few hours of the onset of symptoms; oseltamivir is licensed for use within 48 hours of the first symptoms while zanamivir is licensed for use within 36 hours of the first symptoms. In otherwise healthy individuals they reduce the duration of symptoms by about 1–1.5 days.

Oseltamivir and zanamivir are licensed for post-exposure prophylaxis of influenza when influenza is circulating in the community. Oseltamivir should be given within 48 hours of exposure to influenza while zanamivir should be given within 36 hours of exposure to influenza. However, in children with severe influenza or in those who are immunocompromised, antivirals may still be effective after this time if viral shedding continues [unlicensed use]. Oseltamivir and zanamivir are also licensed for use in exceptional circumstances (e.g. when vaccination does not

cover the infecting strain) to prevent influenza in an epidemic.

There is evidence that some strains of influenza A virus have reduced susceptibility to oseltamivir, but may retain susceptibility to zanamivir. Resistance to oseltamivir may be greater in severely immunocompromised children.

Zanamivir should be reserved for patients who are severely immunocompromised, or when oseltamivir cannot be used, or when resistance to oseltamivir is suspected. For those unable to use the dry powder for inhalation, zanamivir is available as a solution that can be administered by nebuliser or intravenously [unlicensed].

Information on pandemic influenza, avian influenza, and swine influenza may be found at www.gov.uk/phe.

Immunisation against influenza is recommended for persons at high risk, and to reduce transmission of infection.

Oseltamivir in children under 1 year of age

Data on the use of oseltamivir in children under 1 year of age is limited. Furthermore, oseltamivir may be ineffective in neonates because they may not be able to metabolise oseltamivir to its active form. However, oseltamivir can be used (under specialist supervision) for the treatment and post-exposure prophylaxis of influenza in children under 1 year of age. The Department of Health has advised (May 2009) that during a pandemic, treatment with oseltamivir can be overseen by healthcare professionals experienced in assessing children.

Amantadine hydrochloride is licensed for prophylaxis and treatment of influenza A in children over 10 years of age, but it is no longer recommended.

ANTIVIRALS > NEURAMINIDASE INHIBITORS

Oseltamivir

- **DRUG ACTION** Reduces replication of influenza A and B viruses by inhibiting viral neuraminidase.

- **INDICATIONS AND DOSE**
  Prevention of influenza
  ‣ BY MOUTH
  ‣ Neonate: 3 mg/kg once daily for 10 days for post-exposure prophylaxis.
  ‣ Child 1–11 months: 3 mg/kg once daily for 10 days for post-exposure prophylaxis
  ‣ Child 1–12 years (body-weight 10–15 kg): 30 mg once daily for 10 days for post-exposure prophylaxis; for up to 6 weeks during an epidemic
  ‣ Child 1–12 years (body-weight 15–23 kg): 45 mg once daily for 10 days for post-exposure prophylaxis; for up to 6 weeks during an epidemic
  ‣ Child 1–12 years (body-weight 23–40 kg): 60 mg once daily for 10 days for post-exposure prophylaxis; for up to 6 weeks during an epidemic
  ‣ Child 1–12 years (body-weight 40 kg and above): 75 mg once daily for 10 days for post-exposure prophylaxis; for up to 6 weeks during an epidemic
  ‣ Child 13–17 years: 75 mg once daily for 10 days for post-exposure prophylaxis; for up to 6 weeks during an epidemic

  Treatment of influenza
  ‣ BY MOUTH
  ‣ Neonate: 3 mg/kg twice daily for 5 days.
  ‣ Child 1–11 months: 3 mg/kg twice daily for 5 days
  ‣ Child 1–12 years (body-weight 10–15 kg): 30 mg twice daily for 5 days
  ‣ Child 1–12 years (body-weight 15–23 kg): 45 mg twice daily for 5 days
  ‣ Child 1–12 years (body-weight 23–40 kg): 60 mg twice daily for 5 days

continued →

Infection
5

▸ Child 1-12 years (body-weight 40 kg and above): 75 mg twice daily for 5 days
▸ Child 13-17 years: 75 mg twice daily for 5 days

● **UNLICENSED USE** Not licensed for use in premature infants.

● **SIDE-EFFECTS**
▸ **Common or very common** Abdominal pain · dyspepsia · headache · nausea · vomiting
▸ **Uncommon** Altered consciousness · arrhythmias · convulsions · eczema · rash
▸ **Rare** Gastro-intestinal bleeding · hepatitis · neuropsychiatric disorders · Stevens-Johnson syndrome · thrombocytopenia · toxic epidermal necrolysis · visual disturbances

● **PREGNANCY** Although safety data are limited, oseltamivir can be used in women who are pregnant when the potential benefit outweighs the risk (e.g. during a pandemic). Use only if potential benefit outweighs risk (e.g. during a pandemic).

● **BREAST FEEDING** Although safety data are limited, oseltamivir can be used in women who are breast-feeding when the potential benefit outweighs the risk (e.g. during a pandemic). Oseltamivir is the preferred drug in women who are breast-feeding. Amount probably too small to be harmful; use only if potential benefit outweighs risk (e.g. during a pandemic).

● **RENAL IMPAIRMENT** For *treatment*, use 40% of normal dose twice daily if estimated glomerular filtration rate 30–60 mL/minute/1.73 m² (40% of normal dose once daily if estimated glomerular filtration rate 10–30 mL/minute/1.73 m²). For *prevention*, use 40% of normal dose once daily if estimated glomerular filtration rate 30–60 mL/minute/1.73 m² (40% of normal dose every 48 hours if estimated glomerular filtration rate 10–30 mL/minute/1.73 m²). Avoid for *treatment* and *prevention* if estimated glomerular filtration rate less than 10 mL/minute/1.73 m².

● **DIRECTIONS FOR ADMINISTRATION** If suspension not available, capsules can be opened and the contents mixed with a small amount of sweetened food, such as sugar water or chocolate syrup, just before administration.

● **PRESCRIBING AND DISPENSING INFORMATION** Flavours of oral liquid formulations may include tutti-frutti.

● **PATIENT AND CARER ADVICE**
Medicines for Children leaflet: Oseltamivir for influenza (flu)
www.medicinesforchildren.org.uk/oseltamivir-for-influenza

● **NATIONAL FUNDING/ACCESS DECISIONS**
NICE technology appraisals (TAs)
▸ **Oseltamivir, zanamivir, and amantadine for prophylaxis of influenza (September 2008)** NICE TA158
Oseltamivir is **not** a substitute for vaccination, which remains the most effective way of preventing illness from influenza.
● Oseltamivir is **not** recommended for seasonal prophylaxis against influenza.
● When influenza is circulating in the community, oseltamivir is a treatment option recommended (in accordance with UK licensing) for post-exposure prophylaxis in at-risk patients who are not effectively protected by influenza vaccine, and who have been in close contact with someone suffering from influenza-like illness in the same household or residential setting. Oseltamivir should be given within 48 hours of exposure to influenza. (National surveillance schemes, including those run by Public Health England, should be used to indicate when influenza is circulating in the community.)
● During local outbreaks of influenza-like illness, when there is a high level of certainty that influenza is present, oseltamivir may be used for post-exposure

prophylaxis in at-risk patients (regardless of influenza vaccination) living in long-term residential or nursing homes.
At risk patients are those who have one or more of the following conditions:
● chronic respiratory disease (including asthma);
● chronic heart disease;
● chronic renal disease;
● chronic liver disease;
● chronic neurological disease;
● immunosuppression;
● diabetes mellitus.
The Department of Health in England has advised (November 2010 and April 2011) that 'at risk patients' also includes children who are at risk of developing medical complications from influenza (treatment only) or females who are pregnant.
   This guidance does not cover the circumstances of a pandemic, an impending pandemic, or a widespread epidemic of a new strain of influenza to which there is little or no immunity in the community.
www.nice.org.uk/TA158

▸ **Oseltamivir, zanamivir, and amantadine for treatment of influenza (February 2009)** NICE TA168
Oseltamivir is **not** a substitute for vaccination, which remains the most effective way of preventing illness from influenza.
● When influenza is circulating in the community, oseltamivir is an option recommended (in accordance with UK licensing) for the treatment of influenza in at-risk patients who can start treatment within 48 hours of the onset of symptoms. (National surveillance schemes, including those run by Public Health England, should be used to indicate when influenza is circulating in the community.)
● During local outbreaks of influenza-like illness, when there is a high level of certainty that influenza is present, oseltamivir may be used for treatment in at-risk patients living in long-term residential or nursing homes.
At risk patients are those who have one or more of the following conditions:
● chronic respiratory disease (including asthma and chronic obstructive pulmonary disease);
● chronic heart disease;
● chronic renal disease;
● chronic liver disease;
● chronic neurological disease;
● immunosuppression;
● diabetes mellitus.
The Department of Health in England has advised (November 2010 and April 2011) that 'at risk patients' also includes children who are at risk of developing medical complications from influenza (treatment only) or females who are pregnant.
   This guidance does not cover the circumstances of a pandemic, an impending pandemic, or a widespread epidemic of a new strain of influenza to which there is little or no immunity in the community.
www.nice.org.uk/TA168

NHS restrictions Except for the treatment and prophylaxis of influenza as indicated in the NICE guidance; endorse prescription 'SLS'.

● **MEDICINAL FORMS**
There can be variation in the licensing of different medicines containing the same drug. Forms available from special-order manufacturers include: oral suspension, oral solution
Capsule
CAUTIONARY AND ADVISORY LABELS 9
▸ **Tamiflu** (Roche Products Ltd)
Oseltamivir (as Oseltamivir phosphate) 30 mg Tamiflu 30mg capsules | 10 capsule PoM £7.71

Oseltamivir (as Oseltamivir phosphate) 45 mg Tamiflu 45mg capsules | 10 capsule PoM £15.41

Oseltamivir (as Oseltamivir phosphate) 75 mg Tamiflu 75mg capsules | 10 capsule PoM £15.41

Oral suspension

CAUTIONARY AND ADVISORY LABELS 9

EXCIPIENTS: May contain Sorbitol

▸ **Tamiflu** (Roche Products Ltd)

Oseltamivir (as Oseltamivir phosphate) 6 mg per 1 ml Tamiflu 6mg/ml oral suspension sugar-free | 65 ml PoM £10.27

Oral solution

CAUTIONARY AND ADVISORY LABELS 9

▸ **Oseltamivir** (Non-proprietary)

Oseltamivir (as Oseltamivir phosphate) 15 mg per 1 ml Oseltamivir 15mg/ml oral solution sugar free sugar-free | 20 ml PoM £10.00

Zanamivir

- **DRUG ACTION** Reduces replication of influenza A and B viruses by inhibiting viral neuraminidase.

- **INDICATIONS AND DOSE**

Post-exposure prophylaxis of influenza

▸ BY INHALATION OF POWDER

▸ Child 5-17 years: 10 mg once daily for 10 days

Prevention of influenza during an epidemic

▸ BY INHALATION OF POWDER

▸ Child 5-17 years: 10 mg once daily for up to 28 days

Treatment of influenza

▸ BY INHALATION OF POWDER

▸ Child 5-17 years: 10 mg twice daily for 5 days (for up to 10 days if resistance to oseltamivir suspected)

- **UNLICENSED USE** Use of zanamivir for up to 10 days if resistance to oseltamivir suspected is an unlicensed duration.

- **CAUTIONS** Asthma · chronic pulmonary disease · uncontrolled chronic illness

CAUTIONS, FURTHER INFORMATION

▸ Asthma and chronic pulmonary disease Risk of bronchospasm—short-acting bronchodilator should be available.

Avoid in severe asthma unless close monitoring possible and appropriate facilities available to treat bronchospasm.

- **SIDE-EFFECTS**

- **Common or very common** Rash

▸ **Uncommon** Angioedema · bronchospasm · dyspnoea · urticaria

▸ **Rare** Neuropsychiatric disorders · Stevens-Johnson syndrome · toxic epidermal necrolysis

- **PREGNANCY** Although safety data are limited, zanamivir can be used in women who are pregnant when the potential benefit outweighs the risk (e.g. during a pandemic). Use only if potential benefit outweighs risk (e.g. during a pandemic).

- **BREAST FEEDING** Although safety data are limited, zanamivir can be used in women who are breast-feeding when the potential benefit outweighs the risk (e.g. during a pandemic). Amount probably too small to be harmful; use only if potential benefit outweighs risk (e.g. during a pandemic).

- **DIRECTIONS FOR ADMINISTRATION** Other inhaled drugs should be administered before zanamivir.

- **PRESCRIBING AND DISPENSING INFORMATION** Except for the treatment and prophylaxis of influenza as indicated in the NICE guidance; endorse prescription 'SLS'.

- **NATIONAL FUNDING/ACCESS DECISIONS**

NICE technology appraisals (TAs)

▸ Oseltamivir, zanamivir, and amantadine for prophylaxis of influenza (September 2008) NICE TA158

Zanamivir is not a substitute for vaccination, which remains the most effective way of preventing illness from influenza.

- Zanamivir is not recommended for seasonal prophylaxis against influenza.

- When influenza is circulating in the community, zanamivir is an option recommended (in accordance with UK licensing) for post-exposure prophylaxis in at-risk patients who are not effectively protected by influenza vaccine, and who have been in close contact with someone suffering from influenza-like illness in the same household or residential setting. Zanamivir should be given within 36 hours of exposure to influenza. (National surveillance schemes, including those run by Public Health England, should be used to indicate when influenza is circulating in the community.)

- During local outbreaks of influenza-like illness, when there is a high level of certainty that influenza is present, zanamivir may be used for post-exposure prophylaxis in at-risk patients (regardless of influenza vaccination) living in long-term residential or nursing homes.

At risk patients are those who have one or more of the following conditions:

- chronic respiratory disease (including asthma and chronic obstructive pulmonary disease);
- chronic heart disease;
- chronic renal disease;
- chronic liver disease;
- chronic neurological disease;
- immunosuppression;
- diabetes mellitus.

The Department of Health in England has advised (November 2010 and April 2011) that 'at risk patients' also includes children who are at risk of developing medical complications from influenza (treatment only) or females who are pregnant.

This guidance does not cover the circumstances of a pandemic, an impending pandemic, or a widespread epidemic of a new strain of influenza to which there is little or no immunity in the community.

www.nice.org.uk/TA158

▸ Oseltamivir, zanamivir, and amantadine for treatment of influenza (February 2009) NICE TA168

Zanamivir is not a substitute for vaccination, which remains the most effective way of preventing illness from influenza.

- When influenza is circulating in the community, zanamivir is an option recommended (in accordance with UK licensing) for the treatment of influenza in at-risk patients who can start treatment within 36 hours of the onset of symptoms. (National surveillance schemes, including those run by Public Health England, should be used to indicate when influenza is circulating in the community.)

- During local outbreaks of influenza-like illness, when there is a high level of certainty that influenza is present, zanamivir may be used for treatment in at-risk patients living in long-term residential or nursing homes.

At risk patients are those who have one or more of the following conditions:

- chronic respiratory disease (including asthma and chronic obstructive pulmonary disease);
- chronic heart disease;
- chronic renal disease;
- chronic liver disease;
- chronic neurological disease;
- immunosuppression;
- diabetes mellitus.

The Department of Health in England has advised (November 2010 and April 2011) that 'at risk patients' also includes children who are at risk of developing medical complications from influenza (treatment only) or females who are pregnant.

This guidance does not cover the circumstances of a pandemic, an impending pandemic, or a widespread epidemic of a new strain of influenza to which there is little or no immunity in the community. www.nice.org.uk/TA168

- **MEDICINAL FORMS**
There can be variation in the licensing of different medicines containing the same drug.
Inhalation powder
  ▸ **Relenza** (GlaxoSmithKline UK Ltd)
    Zanamivir 5 mg Relenza 5mg inhalation powder blisters with Diskhaler | 20 blister [PoM] £16.36

6.6 Respiratory syncytial virus

Respiratory syncytial virus

Management
Ribavirin p. 378 inhibits a wide range of DNA and RNA viruses. It is licensed for administration by inhalation for the treatment of severe bronchiolitis caused by the respiratory syncytial virus (RSV) in infants, especially when they have other serious diseases. However, there is no evidence that ribavirin produces clinically relevant benefit in RSV bronchiolitis. Ribavirin is given by mouth with peginterferon alfa p. 379 or interferon alfa p. 517 for the treatment of chronic hepatitis C infection. Ribavirin is also effective in Lassa fever and has also been used parenterally in the treatment of life-threatening RSV, parainfluenza virus, and adenovirus infections in immunocompromised children [unlicensed indications].

Palivizumab below is a monoclonal antibody licensed for preventing serious lower respiratory-tract disease caused by respiratory syncytial virus in children at high risk of the disease; it should be prescribed under specialist supervision and on the basis of the likelihood of hospitalisation. Palivizumab is recommended for:

- children under 9 months of age with chronic lung disease (defined as requiring oxygen for at least 28 days from birth) and who were born preterm;
- children under 6 months of age with haemodynamically significant, acyanotic congenital heart disease who were born preterm.

Palivizumab should be considered for:

- children under 2 years of age with severe combined immunodeficiency syndrome;
- children under 1 year of age who require long-term ventilation;
- children 1–2 years of age who require long-term ventilation and have an additional co-morbidity (including cardiac disease or pulmonary hypertension).

For details of the preterm age groups included in the recommendations, see *Immunisation against Infectious Disease* (2006), available at www.gov.uk/dh.

DRUGS FOR RESPIRATORY DISEASES ›
MONOCLONAL ANTIBODIES

▌ Palivizumab

- **INDICATIONS AND DOSE**
Prevention of serious lower respiratory-tract disease caused by respiratory syncytial virus in children at high risk of the disease (under expert supervision)
  ▸ BY INTRAMUSCULAR INJECTION

  ▸ Neonate: 15 mg/kg once a month, preferably injected in the anterolateral thigh, to be administered during season of RSV risk.

  ▸ Child 1–23 months: 15 mg/kg once a month, preferably injected in the anterolateral thigh, to be administered during season of RSV risk, injection volume over 1 mL should be divided between 2 or more sites

Prevention of serious lower respiratory-tract disease caused by respiratory syncytial virus in children at high risk of the disease and undergoing cardiac bypass surgery (under expert supervision)
  ▸ BY INTRAMUSCULAR INJECTION
  ▸ Child 1–23 months: Initially 15 mg/kg, to be administered as soon as stable after surgery, preferably in the anterolateral thigh, then 15 mg/kg once a month, preferably injected in the anterolateral thigh, to be administered during season of RSV risk, injection volume over 1 mL should be divided between 2 or more sites

- **UNLICENSED USE** Licensed for the prevention of serious lower respiratory-tract disease caused by respiratory syncytial virus (RSV) in children under 6 months of age (at the start of the RSV season) and born at less than 35 weeks corrected gestational age, or in children under 2 years of age who have received treatment for bronchopulmonary dysplasia in the last 6 months, or in children under 2 years of age with haemodynamically significant congenital heart disease.

- **CAUTIONS** Moderate to severe acute infection · moderate to severe febrile illness · serum-palivizumab concentration may be reduced after cardiac surgery · thrombocytopenia

- **SIDE-EFFECTS**
  ▸ **Common or very common** Fever · injection-site reactions · nervousness
  ▸ **Uncommon** Asthenia · constipation · cough · diarrhoea · drowsiness · haemorrhage · hyperkinesia · leucopenia · pain · rash · rhinitis · vomiting · wheeze
  ▸ **Frequency not known** Anaphylaxis · apnoea · convulsions · hypersensitivity reactions · thrombocytopenia

- **ALLERGY AND CROSS-SENSITIVITY** Hypersensitivity to humanised monoclonal antibodies.

- **MEDICINAL FORMS**
There can be variation in the licensing of different medicines containing the same drug.
Solution for injection
  ▸ **Synagis** (AbbVie Ltd)
    Palivizumab 100 mg per 1 ml Synagis 100mg/1ml solution for injection vials | 1 vial [PoM] £563.64
    Synagis 50mg/0.5ml solution for injection vials | 1 vial [PoM] £306.34
Powder and solvent for solution for injection
  ▸ **Synagis** (AbbVie Ltd)
    Palivizumab 50 mg Synagis 50mg powder and solvent for solution for injection vials | 1 vial [PoM] £306.34
    Palivizumab 100 mg Synagis 100mg powder and solvent for solution for injection vials | 1 vial [PoM] £563.64

Chapter 6
Endocrine system

CONTENTS

1	**Antidiuretic hormone disorders**	page 403
1.1	Diabetes insipidus	403
2	**Corticosteroid responsive conditions**	405
2.1	Cushing's syndrome and disease	414
3	**Diabetes mellitus and hypoglycaemia**	415
3.1	Diabetes mellitus	415
	3.1a　Diabetes, diagnosis and monitoring	428
3.2	Hypoglycaemia	433
	3.2a　Chronic hypoglycaemia	434
4	**Disorders of bone metabolism**	435
5	**Gonadotrophin responsive conditions**	439
6	**Hypothalamic and anterior pituitary hormone related disorders**	441
6.1	Adrenocortical function testing	441

6.2	Assessment of pituitary function	page 442
6.3	Gonadotrophin replacement therapy	443
6.4	Growth hormone disorders	443
	6.4a　Insulin-like growth factor-I Deficiency	445
7	**Sex hormone responsive conditions**	445
7.1	Female sex hormone responsive conditions	446
7.2	Male sex hormone responsive conditions	449
	7.2a　Male sex hormone antagonism	450
	7.2b　Precocious puberty	451
8	**Thyroid disorders**	451
8.1	Hyperthyroidism	451
8.2	Hypothyroidism	453

1 Antidiuretic hormone disorders

Posterior pituitary hormones and antagonists

Posterior pituitary hormones

Diabetes insipidus

Diabetes insipidus is caused by either a deficiency of anti-diuretic hormone (ADH, vasopressin p. 62) secretion (cranial, neurogenic, or pituitary diabetes insipidus) or by failure of the renal tubules to react to secreted antidiuretic hormone (nephrogenic diabetes insipidus).

Vasopressin (antidiuretic hormone, ADH) is used in the treatment of *pituitary diabetes insipidus* as is its analogue desmopressin below. Dosage is tailored to produce a regular diuresis every 24 hours to avoid water intoxication. Treatment may be required permanently or for a limited period only in diabetes insipidus following trauma or pituitary surgery.

Desmopressin is more potent and has a longer duration of action than vasopressin; unlike vasopressin it has no vasoconstrictor effect. It is given by mouth or intranasally for maintenance therapy, and by injection in the postoperative period or in unconscious patients. Desmopressin is also used in the differential diagnosis of diabetes insipidus; following an intramuscular or intranasal dose, restoration of the ability to concentrate urine after water deprivation confirms a diagnosis of pituitary diabetes insipidus. Failure to respond suggests nephrogenic diabetes insipidus. Fluid input must be managed carefully to avoid hyponatraemia; this test is not usually recommended in young children.

In *nephrogenic* and *partial pituitary diabetes insipidus* benefit may be gained from the paradoxical antidiuretic effect of thiazides.

Other uses

Desmopressin is also used to boost factor VIII concentration in mild to moderate haemophilia and in von Willebrand's disease; it is also used to test fibrinolytic response. Desmopressin also has a role in nocturnal enuresis.

Vasopressin infusion is used to control variceal bleeding in portal hypertension, before introducing more definitive treatment. Terlipressin acetate, a derivative of vasopressin with reportedly less pressor and antidiuretic activity, and octreotide are used similarly but experience in children is limited.

1.1 Diabetes insipidus

> **Drugs used for Diabetes insipidus not listed below**
> Chlorothiazide, p. 103

PITUITARY AND HYPOTHALAMIC HORMONES AND ANALOGUES › VASOPRESSIN AND ANALOGUES

Desmopressin

- **DRUG ACTION** Desmopressin is an analogue of vasopressin.

- **INDICATIONS AND DOSE**

Diabetes insipidus, treatment
▸ BY MOUTH

▸ Neonate: Initially 1–4 micrograms 2–3 times a day, adjusted according to response.

▸ Child 1–23 months: Initially 10 micrograms 2–3 times a day, adjusted according to response; usual dose 30–150 micrograms daily

▸ Child 2–11 years: Initially 50 micrograms 2–3 times a day, adjusted according to response; usual dose 100–800 micrograms daily

▸ Child 12–17 years: Initially 100 micrograms 2–3 times a day, adjusted according to response; usual dose 0.2–1.2 mg daily

continued →

▸ BY SUBLINGUAL ADMINISTRATION
▹ Child 2–17 years: Initially 60 micrograms 3 times a day, adjusted according to response; usual dose 40–240 micrograms 3 times a day
▸ BY INTRANASAL ADMINISTRATION
▹ Neonate: Initially 100–500 nanograms, adjusted according to response; usual dose 1.25–10 micrograms daily in 1–2 divided doses.
▹ Child 1–23 months: Initially 2.5–5 micrograms 1–2 times a day, adjusted according to response
▹ Child 2–11 years: Initially 5–20 micrograms 1–2 times a day, adjusted according to response
▹ Child 12–17 years: Initially 10–20 micrograms 1–2 times a day, adjusted according to response
▸ BY INTRAMUSCULAR INJECTION
▹ Neonate: Initially 100 nanograms once daily, adjusted according to response.
▸ BY SUBCUTANEOUS INJECTION, OR BY INTRAMUSCULAR INJECTION
▹ Child 1 month–11 years: Initially 400 nanograms once daily, adjusted according to response
▹ Child 12–17 years: Initially 1–4 micrograms once daily, adjusted according to response

Primary nocturnal enuresis
▸ BY MOUTH
▹ Child 5–17 years: 200 micrograms once daily, only increased to 400 micrograms if lower dose not effective; withdraw for at least 1 week for reassessment after 3 months, dose to be taken at bedtime, limit fluid intake from 1 hour before to 8 hours after administration
▸ BY SUBLINGUAL ADMINISTRATION
▹ Child 5–17 years: 120 micrograms once daily, increased if necessary to 240 micrograms once daily, dose to be taken at bedtime, limit fluid intake from 1 hour before to 8 hours after administration, dose to be increased only if lower dose not effective, reassess after 3 months by withdrawing treatment for at least 1 week

Diabetes insipidus, diagnosis (water deprivation test)
▸ BY INTRANASAL ADMINISTRATION
▹ Neonate: Not recommended, use trial of treatment.
▹ Child 1–23 months: 5–10 micrograms for 1 dose, manage fluid input carefully to avoid hyponatraemia, not usually recommended
▹ Child 2–11 years: 10–20 micrograms for 1 dose, manage fluid input carefully to avoid hyponatraemia
▹ Child 12–17 years: 20 micrograms for 1 dose, manage fluid input carefully to avoid hyponatraemia
▸ BY INTRAMUSCULAR INJECTION, OR BY SUBCUTANEOUS INJECTION
▹ Neonate: Not recommended, use trial of treatment.
▹ Child 1–23 months: 400 nanograms for 1 dose, manage fluid input carefully to avoid hyponatraemia, not usually recommended
▹ Child 2–11 years: 0.5–1 microgram for 1 dose, manage fluid input carefully to avoid hyponatraemia
▹ Child 12–17 years: 1–2 micrograms for 1 dose, manage fluid input carefully to avoid hyponatraemia

Renal function testing
▸ BY INTRANASAL ADMINISTRATION
▹ Child 1–11 months: 10 micrograms, empty bladder at time of administration and restrict fluid intake to 50% at next 2 feeds to avoid fluid overload
▹ Child 1–14 years: 20 micrograms, empty bladder at time of administration and restrict fluid intake to 500 mL from 1 hour before until 8 hours after administration to avoid fluid overload

▹ Child 15–17 years: 40 micrograms, empty bladder at time of administration and limit fluid intake to 500 mL from 1 hour before until 8 hours after administration to avoid fluid overload
▸ BY SUBCUTANEOUS INJECTION, OR BY INTRAMUSCULAR INJECTION
▹ Child 1–11 months: 400 nanograms, empty bladder at time of administration and restrict fluid intake to 50% at next 2 feeds to avoid fluid overload
▹ Child 1–17 years: 2 micrograms, empty bladder at time of administration and restrict fluid intake to 500 mL from 1 hour before until 8 hours after administration to avoid fluid overload

Mild to moderate haemophilia and von Willebrand's disease
▸ BY INTRANASAL ADMINISTRATION
▹ Child 1–17 years: 4 micrograms/kg for 1 dose, for pre-operative use give 2 hours before procedure
▸ BY INTRAVENOUS INFUSION, OR BY SUBCUTANEOUS INJECTION
▹ Child: 300 nanograms/kg for 1 dose, to be administered immediately before surgery or after trauma; may be repeated at intervals of 12 hours if no tachycardia

Fibrinolytic response testing
▸ BY SUBCUTANEOUS INJECTION, OR BY INTRAVENOUS INJECTION
▹ Child 2–17 years: 300 nanograms/kg for 1 dose, blood to be sampled after 20 minutes for fibrinolytic activity

Assessment of antidiuretic hormone secretion (congenital deficiency suspected) (specialist use only)
▸ BY INTRANASAL ADMINISTRATION
▹ Child 1–23 months: Initially 100–500 nanograms for 1 dose

Assessment of antidiuretic hormone secretion (congenital deficiency not suspected) (specialist use only)
▸ BY INTRANASAL ADMINISTRATION
▹ Child 1–23 months: 1–5 micrograms for 1 dose

● **UNLICENSED USE** Consult product literature for individual preparations. Not licensed for assessment of antidiuretic hormone secretion. Oral use of *DDAVP* intravenous injection is not licensed.
● **CONTRA-INDICATIONS** Cardiac insufficiency · conditions treated with diuretics · polydipsia in alcohol dependence · psychogenic polydipsia
● **CAUTIONS**
GENERAL CAUTIONS
Asthma · avoid fluid overload · cardiovascular disease (not indicated for nocturnal enuresis or nocturia) · conditions which might be aggravated by water retention · cystic fibrosis · epilepsy · heart failure · hypertension (not indicated for nocturnal enuresis or nocturia) · migraine · nocturia—limit fluid intake to minimum from 1 hour before dose until 8 hours afterwards · nocturnal enuresis—limit fluid intake to minimum from 1 hour before dose until 8 hours afterwards
SPECIFIC CAUTIONS
▸ With intranasal use Should not be given intranasally for nocturnal enuresis due to an increased incidence of side-effects
● **INTERACTIONS** → Appendix 1 (desmopressin).
● **SIDE-EFFECTS**
GENERAL SIDE-EFFECTS
Allergic reactions · emotional disturbance in children · epistaxis · fluid retention · headache · hyponatraemia (in more serious cases with convulsions) on administration without restricting fluid intake · nasal congestion · nausea · stomach pain · vomiting
SPECIFIC SIDE-EFFECTS
▸ With intranasal use Rhinitis

SIDE-EFFECTS, FURTHER INFORMATION

▶ Hyponatraemic convulsions The risk of hyponatraemic convulsions can be minimised by keeping to the recommended starting doses and by avoiding concomitant use of drugs which increase secretion of vasopressin (e.g. tricyclic antidepressants).

● PREGNANCY Small oxytocic effect in third trimester; increased risk of pre-eclampsia.

● BREAST FEEDING Amount too small to be harmful.

● RENAL IMPAIRMENT Use with caution; antidiuretic effect may be reduced.

● MONITORING REQUIREMENTS In *nocturia*, periodic blood pressure and weight checks are needed to monitor for fluid overload.

● DIRECTIONS FOR ADMINISTRATION *DDVAP*® and *Desmotabs*® tablets may be crushed.

    DDAVP® intranasal solution may be diluted with Sodium Chloride 0.9% to a concentration of 10 micrograms/mL.

    DDAVP® injection may be administered orally.

    Desmopressin oral lyophilisates are for sublingual administration.

▶ With intravenous use Higher doses of *DDAVP*® by *intravenous infusion*, used in mild to moderate haemophilia and von Willebrand's disease, may be diluted with 30–50 mL Sodium Chloride 0.9% intravenous infusion.

    For *intravenous infusion* (*Octim*®), dilute with 50 mL of Sodium Chloride 0.9% and give over 20 minutes.

● PRESCRIBING AND DISPENSING INFORMATION Oral, intranasal, intravenous, subcutaneous and intramuscular doses are expressed as desmopressin acetate; sublingual doses are expressed as desmopressin base.

    Children requiring an intranasal dose of less than 10 micrograms should be given *DDAVP*® intranasal solution.

● PATIENT AND CARER ADVICE

Hyponatraemic convulsions Patients being treated for primary nocturnal enuresis should be warned to avoid fluid overload (including during swimming) and to stop taking desmopressin during an episode of vomiting or diarrhoea (until fluid balance normal).

Medicines for Children leaflet: Desmopressin for bedwetting www.medicinesforchildren.org.uk/desmopressin-bedwetting-0

● MEDICINAL FORMS

There can be variation in the licensing of different medicines containing the same drug. Forms available from special-order manufacturers include: capsule, oral suspension, oral solution, spray, nasal drops

Tablet

▶ Desmopressin (Non-proprietary)

Desmopressin acetate 100 microgram Desmopressin 100microgram tablets | 90 tablet PoM £76.62 DT price = £62.88

Desmopressin acetate 200 microgram Desmopressin 200microgram tablets | 30 tablet PoM £35.23 DT price = £7.58 | 90 tablet PoM £87.50

▶ DDAVP (Ferring Pharmaceuticals Ltd)

Desmopressin acetate 100 microgram DDAVP 0.1mg tablets | 90 tablet PoM £44.12 DT price = £62.88

Desmopressin acetate 200 microgram DDAVP 0.2mg tablets | 90 tablet PoM £88.23

▶ Desmotabs (Ferring Pharmaceuticals Ltd)

Desmopressin acetate 200 microgram Desmotabs 0.2mg tablets | 30 tablet PoM £29.43 DT price = £7.58

Oral solution

▶ Desmopressin (Non-proprietary)

Desmopressin (as Desmopressin acetate) 360 microgram per 1 ml Desmopressin 360micrograms/ml oral solution | 15 ml PoM £30.00

Oral lyophilisate

CAUTIONARY AND ADVISORY LABELS 26

▶ Desmopressin (Non-proprietary)

Desmopressin (as Desmopressin acetate)

120 microgram Desmopressin 120microgram oral lyophilisates sugar free sugar-free | 30 tablet PoM no price available DT price = £30.34

Desmopressin (as Desmopressin acetate)

240 microgram Desmopressin 240microgram oral lyophilisates sugar free sugar-free | 30 tablet PoM no price available DT price = £60.68

▶ DDAVP (Ferring Pharmaceuticals Ltd)

Desmopressin (as Desmopressin acetate) 60 microgram DDAVP Melt 60microgram oral lyophilisates sugar-free | 100 tablet PoM £50.53 DT price = £50.53

Desmopressin (as Desmopressin acetate) 120 microgram DDAVP Melt 120microgram oral lyophilisates sugar-free | 100 tablet PoM £101.07 DT price = £101.07

Desmopressin (as Desmopressin acetate) 240 microgram DDAVP Melt 240microgram oral lyophilisates sugar-free | 100 tablet PoM £202.14

▶ DesmoMelt (Ferring Pharmaceuticals Ltd)

Desmopressin (as Desmopressin acetate)

120 microgram DesmoMelt 120microgram oral lyophilisates sugar-free | 30 tablet PoM £30.34 DT price = £30.34

Desmopressin (as Desmopressin acetate)

240 microgram DesmoMelt 240microgram oral lyophilisates sugar-free | 30 tablet PoM £60.68 DT price = £60.68

Solution for injection

▶ DDAVP (Ferring Pharmaceuticals Ltd)

Desmopressin acetate 4 microgram per 1 ml DDAVP 4micrograms/1ml solution for injection ampoules | 10 ampoule PoM £13.16

▶ Octim (Ferring Pharmaceuticals Ltd)

Desmopressin acetate 15 microgram per 1 ml Octim 15micrograms/1ml solution for injection ampoules | 10 ampoule PoM £192.20

Spray

▶ Desmopressin (Non-proprietary)

Desmopressin acetate 2.5 microgram per 1 dose Minirin 2.5micrograms/dose nasal spray | 50 dose PoM no price available

Desmopressin acetate 10 microgram per 1 dose Desmopressin 10micrograms/dose nasal spray | 60 dose PoM £30.00 DT price = £12.41

▶ Desmospray (Ferring Pharmaceuticals Ltd)

Desmopressin acetate 2.5 microgram per 1 dose Desmospray 2.5micrograms/dose nasal spray | 50 dose no price available

Desmopressin acetate 10 microgram per 1 dose Desmospray 10micrograms/dose nasal spray | 60 dose PoM £25.02 DT price = £12.41

▶ Octim (Ferring Pharmaceuticals Ltd)

Desmopressin acetate 150 microgram per 1 dose Octim 150micrograms/dose nasal spray | 25 dose PoM £576.60

Nasal drops

▶ DDAVP (Ferring Pharmaceuticals Ltd)

Desmopressin acetate 100 microgram per 1 ml DDAVP 100micrograms/ml intranasal solution | 2.5 ml PoM £9.72 DT price = £9.72

2   Corticosteroid responsive conditions

CORTICOSTEROIDS

Corticosteroids, general use

Overview

Dosages of corticosteroids vary widely in different diseases and in different patients. If the use of a corticosteroid can save or prolong life, as in exfoliative dermatitis, pemphigus, acute leukaemia or acute transplant rejection, high doses may need to be given, because the complications of therapy are likely to be less serious than the effects of the disease itself.

When long-term corticosteroid therapy is used in some chronic diseases, the adverse effects of treatment may become greater than the disabilities caused by the disease. To minimise side-effects the maintenance dose should be kept as low as possible.

When potentially less harmful measures are ineffective corticosteroids are used topically for the treatment of inflammatory conditions of the skin. Corticosteroids should be avoided or used only under specialist supervision in psoriasis.

Corticosteroids are used both topically (by rectum) and systemically (by mouth or intravenously) in the management of ulcerative colitis and Crohn's disease.

Use can be made of the mineralocorticoid activity of fludrocortisone acetate p. 411 to treat postural hypotension in autonomic neuropathy.

High-dose corticosteroids should be avoided for the management of septic shock. However, low-dose hydrocortisone p. 411 can be used in septic shock that is resistant to volume expansion and catecholamines, and is accompanied by suspected or proven adrenal insufficiency.

The suppressive action of glucocorticoids on the hypothalamic-pituitary-adrenal axis is greatest and most prolonged when they are given at night. In most adults a single dose of dexamethasone at night is sufficient to inhibit corticotropin secretion for 24 hours. This is the basis of the 'overnight dexamethasone suppression test' for diagnosing Cushing's syndrome.

Betamethasone p. 409 and dexamethasone are also appropriate for conditions where water retention would be a disadvantage.

A corticosteroid may be used in the management of raised intracranial pressure or cerebral oedema that occurs as a result of malignancy (see Prescribing in palliative care p. 18); high doses of betamethasone or dexamethasone are generally used. However, a corticosteroid should **not** be used for the management of head injury or stroke because it is unlikely to be of benefit and may even be harmful.

In acute hypersensitivity reactions, such as angioedema of the upper respiratory tract and anaphylaxis, corticosteroids are indicated as an adjunct to emergency treatment with adrenaline/epinephrine p. 128. In such cases hydrocortisone (as sodium succinate) by intravenous injection may be required.

In the management of asthma, corticosteroids are preferably used by inhalation but systemic therapy along with bronchodilators is required for the emergency treatment of severe acute asthma.

Betamethasone is used in women at risk of preterm delivery to reduce the incidence of neonatal respiratory distress syndrome [unlicensed use].

Dexamethasone should not be used routinely for the prophylaxis and treatment of chronic lung disease in neonates because of an association with adverse neurological effects.

Corticosteroids may be useful in conditions such as auto-immune hepatitis, rheumatoid arthritis, and sarcoidosis; they may also lead to remissions of acquired haemolytic anaemia and thrombocytopenic purpura.

High doses of a corticosteroid (usually prednisolone p. 413) are used in the treatment of *glomerular kidney disease*, including *nephrotic syndrome*. The condition frequently recurs; a corticosteroid given in high doses and for prolonged periods may delay relapse but the higher incidence of adverse effects limits the overall benefit. Those who suffer frequent relapses may be treated with prednisolone given in a low dose (daily or on alternate days) for 3–6 months; the dose should be adjusted to minimise effects on growth and development. Other drugs used in the treatment of glomerular kidney disease include levamisole p. 361, cyclophosphamide p. 498, chlorambucil p. 498, and ciclosporin p. 486. *Congenital nephrotic syndrome* may be resistant to corticosteroids and immunosuppressants; indometacin p. 611 and an ACE inhibitor such as captopril p. 103 have been used.

Corticosteroids can improve the prognosis of serious conditions such as systemic lupus erythematosus and polyarteritis nodosa; the effects of the disease process may be suppressed and symptoms relieved, but the underlying condition is not cured, although it may ultimately remit. It is usual to begin therapy in these conditions at fairly high dose and then to reduce the dose to the lowest commensurate with disease control.

For other references to the use of corticosteroids see: Prescribing in Palliative Care, immunosuppression, rheumatic diseases, eye, otitis externa, allergic rhinitis, and aphthous ulcers.

Side-effects

Overdosage or prolonged use can exaggerate some of the normal physiological actions of corticosteroids leading to mineralocorticoid and glucocorticoid side-effects.

Mineralocorticoid side effects

- hypertension
- sodium retention
- water retention
- potassium loss
- calcium loss

Mineralocorticoid side effects are most marked with fludrocortisone acetate, but are significant with hydrocortisone, corticotropin, and tetracosactide p. 441. Mineralocorticoid actions are negligible with the high potency glucocorticoids, betamethasone and dexamethasone, and occur only slightly with methylprednisolone p. 412, prednisolone, and triamcinolone.

Glucocorticoid side effects

- diabetes
- osteoporosis
- in addition high doses are associated with avascular necrosis of the femoral head.
- Muscle wasting (proximal myopathy) can also occur.
- Corticosteroid therapy is also weakly linked with peptic ulceration and perforation.
- Psychiatric reactions may also occur.

Managing side-effects

Side-effects can be minimised by using lowest effective dose for minimum period possible. The suppressive action of a corticosteroid on cortisol secretion is least when it is given as a single dose in the morning. In an attempt to reduce pituitary-adrenal suppression further, the total dose for two days can sometimes be taken as a single dose on alternate days; alternate-day administration has not been very successful in the management of asthma. Pituitary-adrenal suppression can also be reduced by means of intermittent therapy with short courses. In some conditions it may be possible to reduce the dose of corticosteroid by adding a small dose of an immunosuppressive drug.

Whenever possible *local treatment* with creams, intra-articular injections, inhalations, eye-drops, or enemas should be used in preference to *systemic treatment*.

Inhaled corticosteroids have considerably fewer systemic effects than oral corticosteroids, but adverse effects including adrenal suppression have been reported. Use of other corticosteroid therapy (including topical) or concurrent use of drugs which inhibit corticosteroid metabolism should be taken into account when assessing systemic risk. In children, growth restriction associated with systemic corticosteroid therapy does not seem to occur with recommended doses of inhaled therapy; although initial growth velocity may be reduced, there appears to be no effect on achieving normal adult height. Large-volume spacer devices should be used for administering inhaled corticosteroids in children under 15 years; they are also useful in older children and adults, particularly if high doses are required. Spacer devices increase airway deposition and reduce oropharyngeal deposition.

Corticosteroids, replacement therapy

Overview

The adrenal cortex normally secretes hydrocortisone p. 411 (cortisol) which has glucocorticoid activity and weak mineralocorticoid activity. It also secretes the mineralocorticoid aldosterone.

In deficiency states, physiological replacement is best achieved with a combination of hydrocortisone and the mineralocorticoid fludrocortisone acetate p. 411; hydrocortisone alone does not usually provide sufficient mineralocorticoid activity for complete replacement.

In *Addison's disease* or following adrenalectomy, hydrocortisone by mouth is usually required. This is given in 2–3 divided doses, the larger in the morning and the smaller in the evening, mimicking the normal diurnal rhythm of cortisol secretion. The optimum daily dose is determined on the basis of clinical response. Glucocorticoid therapy is supplemented by fludrocortisone acetate.

In *acute adrenocortical insufficiency*, hydrocortisone is given intravenously (preferably as sodium succinate) every 6 to 8 hours in sodium chloride intravenous infusion 0.9%.

In *hypopituitarism*, glucocorticoids should be given as in adrenocortical insufficiency, but since production of aldosterone is also regulated by the renin-angiotensin system a mineralocorticoid is not usually required. Additional replacement therapy with levothyroxine sodium p. 454 and sex hormones should be given as indicated by the pattern of hormone deficiency.

In *congenital adrenal hyperplasia*, the pituitary gland increases production of corticotropin to compensate for reduced formation of cortisol; this results in excessive adrenal androgen production. Treatment is aimed at suppressing corticotropin using hydrocortisone. Careful and continual dose titration is required to avoid growth retardation and toxicity; for this reason potent, synthetic glucocorticoids such as dexamethasone are usually reserved for use in adolescents. The dose is adjusted according to clinical response and measurement of adrenal androgens and 17-hydroxyprogesterone. Salt-losing forms of congenital adrenal hyperplasia (where there is a lack of aldosterone production) also require mineralocorticoid replacement and salt supplementation (particularly in early life). The dose of mineralocorticoid is adjusted according to electrolyte concentration and plasma-renin activity.

Glucocorticoid therapy

Glucocorticoid and mineralocorticoid activity

In comparing the relative potencies of corticosteroids in terms of their anti-inflammatory (glucocorticoid) effects it should be borne in mind that high glucocorticoid activity in itself is of no advantage unless it is accompanied by relatively low mineralocorticoid activity (see Disadvantages of Corticosteroids). The mineralocorticoid activity of fludrocortisone acetate p. 411 is so high that its anti-inflammatory activity is of no clinical relevance.

Equivalent anti-inflammatory doses of corticosteroids

This table takes no account of mineralocorticoid effects, nor does it take account of variations in duration of action		
Prednisolone 1 mg	≡	Betamethasone 150 micrograms
	≡	Deflazacort 1.2 mg
	≡	Dexamethasone 150 micrograms
	≡	Hydrocortisone 4 mg
	≡	Methylprednisolone 800 micrograms
	≡	Triamcinolone 800 micrograms

The relatively high mineralocorticoid activity of hydrocortisone p. 411, and the resulting fluid retention, makes it unsuitable for disease suppression on a long-term basis. However, hydrocortisone can be used for adrenal replacement therapy. Hydrocortisone is used on a short-term basis by intravenous injection for the emergency management of some conditions. The relatively moderate anti-inflammatory potency of hydrocortisone also makes it a useful topical corticosteroid for the management of inflammatory skin conditions because side-effects (both topical and systemic) are less marked.

Prednisolone p. 413 has predominantly glucocorticoid activity and is the corticosteroid most commonly used by mouth for long-term disease suppression.

Betamethasone p. 409 and dexamethasone p. 410 have very high glucocorticoid activity in conjunction with insignificant mineralocorticoid activity. This makes them particularly suitable for high-dose therapy in conditions where fluid retention would be a disadvantage.

Betamethasone and dexamethasone also have a long duration of action and this, coupled with their lack of mineralocorticoid action makes them particularly suitable for conditions which require suppression of corticotropin (corticotrophin) secretion.

Some esters of betamethasone and of beclometasone dipropionate (beclomethasone) p. 652 exert a considerably more marked topical effect (e.g. on the skin or the lungs) than when given by mouth; use is made of this to obtain topical effects whilst minimising systemic side-effects (e.g. for skin applications and asthma inhalations).

Deflazacort p. 409 has a high glucocorticoid activity; it is derived from prednisolone.

Corticosteroids (systemic)

- **CONTRA-INDICATIONS** Avoid injections containing benzyl alcohol in neonates (in neonates) · avoid live virus vaccines in those receiving immunosuppressive doses (serum antibody response diminished) · systemic infection (unless specific therapy given)

  CONTRA-INDICATIONS, FURTHER INFORMATION
  ▸ With intra-articular use or intradermal use or intralesional use For further information on contra-indications associated with intra-articular, intradermal and intralesional preparations, consult product literature.

- **CAUTIONS** Congestive heart failure · diabetes mellitus (including a family history of) · diverticulitis · epilepsy · glaucoma (including a family history of or susceptibility to) · history of steroid myopathy · history of tuberculosis or X-ray changes (frequent monitoring required) · hypertension · hypothyroidism · infection (particularly untreated) · myasthenia gravis · ocular herpes simplex (risk of corneal perforation) · osteoporosis · peptic ulcer · psychiatric reactions · recent intestinal anastomoses · recent myocardial infarction (rupture reported) · severe affective disorders (particularly if history of steroid-induced psychosis) · should not be used long-term · thromboembolic disorders · ulcerative colitis

CAUTIONS, FURTHER INFORMATION

▸ With intra-articular use or intradermal use or intralesional use For further information on cautions associated with intra-articular, intradermal and intralesional preparations, consult product literature.

● INTERACTIONS → Appendix 1 (corticosteroids).

● SIDE-EFFECTS

GENERAL SIDE-EFFECTS
Abdominal distension · acute pancreatitis · aggravation of epilepsy · aggravation of schizophrenia · amenorrhoea · anaphylaxis · bruising · candidiasis · congestive heart failure · corneal thinning · Cushing's syndrome (with moon face, striae and acne) · dyspepsia · ecchymoses · exacerbation of ophthalmic fungal disease · exacerbation of ophthalmic viral disease · exophthalmos · facial erythema · glaucoma · headache · hiccups · hirsutism · hypercholesterolaemia · hyperglycaemia · hyperhidrosis · hyperlipidaemia · hypersensitivity reactions · impaired healing · increased appetite · increased intra-ocular pressure · increased intracranial pressure with papilloedema (usually after withdrawal) · increased susceptibility to and severity of infection · insomnia · leucocytosis · long bone fractures · malaise · menstrual irregularities · muscle weakness · myocardial rupture following recent myocardial infarction · nausea · negative calcium balance · negative nitrogen balance · oesophageal ulceration · petechiae · posterior subcapsular cataracts · potassium loss · psychological dependence · reactivation of dormant tuberculosis · scleral thinning · skin atrophy · sodium retention · suppression of growth · telangiectasia · tendon rupture · thromboembolism · urticaria · vertebral fractures · vertigo · water retention · weight gain

SPECIFIC SIDE-EFFECTS

▸ With intra-articular use Flushing · may affect the hyaline cartilage

SIDE-EFFECTS, FURTHER INFORMATION
Side effects can be managed by choice of route and duration of course. For further detail see Corticosteroids, general use p. 405

▸ Adrenal suppression During prolonged therapy with corticosteroids, particularly with systemic use, adrenal atrophy develops and can persist for years after stopping. Abrupt withdrawal after a prolonged period can lead to acute adrenal insufficiency, hypotension, or death.

To compensate for a diminished adrenocortical response caused by prolonged corticosteroid treatment, any significant intercurrent illness, trauma, or surgical procedure requires a temporary increase in corticosteroid dose, or if already stopped, a temporary reintroduction of corticosteroid treatment. To avoid a precipitous fall in blood pressure during anaesthesia or in the immediate postoperative period, anaesthetists **must** know whether a patient is taking or has been taking a corticosteroid. A suitable regimen for corticosteroid replacement, in patients who have taken more than 10 mg prednisolone daily (or equivalent) within 3 months of surgery, is:

● Minor surgery under general anaesthesia—usual oral corticosteroid dose on the morning of surgery or hydrocortisone (usually the sodium succinate) intravenously at induction; the usual oral corticosteroid dose is recommenced after surgery.

● Moderate or major surgery—usual oral corticosteroid dose on the morning of surgery and hydrocortisone intravenously at induction, followed by hydrocortisone 3 times a day by intravenous injection for 24 hours after moderate surgery or for 48–72 hours after major surgery; the usual pre-operative oral corticosteroid dose is recommenced on stopping hydrocortisone injections.

Patients on long-term corticosteroid treatment should carry a steroid treatment card which gives guidance on minimising risk and provides details of prescriber, drug, dosage and duration of treatment.

▸ Infections Prolonged courses of corticosteroids increase susceptibility to infections and severity of infections; clinical presentation of infections may also be atypical. Serious infections e.g. *septicaemia* and *tuberculosis* may reach an advanced stage before being recognised, and *amoebiasis* or *strongyloidiasis* may be activated or exacerbated (exclude before initiating a corticosteroid in those at risk or with suggestive symptoms). Fungal or viral *ocular infections* may also be exacerbated.

▸ Chickenpox Unless they have had chickenpox, patients receiving oral or parenteral corticosteroids for purposes other than replacement should be regarded as being *at risk of severe chickenpox* (see Steroid Treatment Card). Manifestations of fulminant illness include pneumonia, hepatitis and disseminated intravascular coagulation; rash is not necessarily a prominent feature.

Passive immunisation with varicella–zoster immunoglobulin is needed for exposed non–immune patients receiving systemic corticosteroids or for those who have used them within the previous 3 months. Confirmed chickenpox warrants specialist care and urgent treatment. Corticosteroids should not be stopped and dosage may need to be increased.

Topical, inhaled or rectal corticosteroids are less likely to be associated with an increased risk of severe chickenpox.

▸ Measles Patients taking corticosteroids should be advised to take particular care to avoid exposure to measles and to seek immediate medical advice if exposure occurs. Prophylaxis with intramuscular normal immunoglobulin may be needed.

▸ Psychiatric reactions Systemic corticosteroids, particularly in high doses, are linked to psychiatric reactions including euphoria, nightmares, insomnia, irritability, mood lability, suicidal thoughts, psychotic reactions, and behavioural disturbances. A serious paranoid state or depression with risk of suicide can be induced, particularly in patients with a history of mental disorder. These reactions frequently subside on reducing the dose or discontinuing the corticosteroid but they may also require specific management. Patients should be advised to seek medical advice if psychiatric symptoms (especially depression and suicidal thoughts) occur and they should also be alert to the rare possibility of such reactions during withdrawal of corticosteroid treatment.

Systemic corticosteroids should be prescribed with care in those predisposed to psychiatric reactions, including those who have previously suffered corticosteroid–induced psychosis, or who have a personal or family history of psychiatric disorders.

● PREGNANCY The benefit of treatment with corticosteroids during pregnancy outweighs the risk. Corticosteroid cover is required during labour. Following a review of the data on the safety of systemic corticosteroids used in pregnancy and breast-feeding the CSM (May 1998) concluded that corticosteroids vary in their ability to cross the placenta but there is no convincing evidence that systemic corticosteroids increase the incidence of congenital abnormalities such as cleft palate or lip. When administration is prolonged or repeated during pregnancy, systemic corticosteroids increase the risk of intra-uterine growth restriction; there is no evidence of intra-uterine growth restriction following short-term treatment (e.g. prophylactic treatment for neonatal respiratory distress syndrome). Any adrenal suppression in the neonate following prenatal exposure usually resolves spontaneously after birth and is rarely clinically important.

Pregnant women with fluid retention should be monitored closely when given systemic corticosteroids.

- **BREAST FEEDING** The benefit of treatment with corticosteroids during breast-feeding outweighs the risk.
- **HEPATIC IMPAIRMENT** The plasma-drug concentration may be increased (particularly on systemic use). Oral and parenteral use should be undertaken with caution.
- **RENAL IMPAIRMENT** Use by oral and injectable routes should be undertaken with caution.
- **MONITORING REQUIREMENTS** The height and weight of children receiving prolonged treatment with corticosteroids should be monitored annually; if growth is slowed, referral to a paediatrician should be considered.
- **EFFECT ON LABORATORY TESTS** Suppression of skin test reactions.
- **TREATMENT CESSATION** The magnitude and speed of dose reduction in corticosteroid withdrawal should be determined on a case-by-case basis, taking into consideration the underlying condition that is being treated, and individual patient factors such as the likelihood of relapse and the duration of corticosteroid treatment. *Gradual* withdrawal of systemic corticosteroids should be considered in those whose disease is unlikely to relapse and have:
  - received more than 40 mg prednisolone (or equivalent) daily for more than 1 week *or* 2 mg/kg daily for 1 week *or* 1 mg/kg daily for 1 month;
  - been given repeat doses in the evening;
  - received more than 3 weeks' treatment;
  - recently received repeated courses (particularly if taken for longer than 3 weeks);
  - taken a short course within 1 year of stopping long-term therapy;
  - other possible causes of adrenal suppression.

Systemic corticosteroids may be stopped abruptly in those whose disease is unlikely to relapse *and* who have received treatment for 3 weeks or less *and* who are not included in the patient groups described above.

During corticosteroid withdrawal the dose may be reduced rapidly down to physiological doses (equivalent to prednisolone 2–2.5 mg/m² daily) and then reduced more slowly. Assessment of the disease may be needed during withdrawal to ensure that relapse does not occur.

- **PATIENT AND CARER ADVICE**

Advice for patients Patients on long-term corticosteroid treatment should carry a Steroid Treatment Card which gives guidance on minimising risk and provides details of prescriber, drug, dosage and duration of treatment.

A patient information leaflet should be supplied to every patient when a systemic corticosteroid is prescribed. Patients should especially be advised of the following:

- **Immunosuppression** Prolonged courses of corticosteroids can increase susceptibility to infection and serious infections can go unrecognised. Unless already immune, patients are at risk of severe **chickenpox** and should avoid close contact with people who have chickenpox or shingles. Similarly, precautions should also be taken against contracting **measles**;
- **Adrenal suppression** If the corticosteroid is given for longer than 3 weeks, treatment must not be stopped abruptly. Adrenal suppression can last for a year or more after stopping treatment and the patient must mention the course of corticosteroid when receiving treatment for any illness or injury;
- **Mood and behaviour changes** Corticosteroid treatment, especially with high doses, can alter mood and behaviour early in treatment—the patient can become confused, irritable and suffer from delusion and suicidal thoughts. These effects can also occur when corticosteroid treatment is being withdrawn. Medical advice should be sought if worrying psychological changes occur;

- **Other serious effects** Serious gastro-intestinal, musculoskeletal, and ophthalmic effects which require medical help can also occur.

Steroid treatment cards Steroid treatment cards should be issued where appropriate. Consider giving a 'steroid card' to support communication of the risks associated with treatment, and specific written advice to consider corticosteroid replacement during an episode of stress, such as severe intercurrent illness or an operation, to patients using greater than maximum licensed doses of inhaled corticosteroids. Steroid treatment cards are available for purchase from:

Gorse Street, Chadderton, Oldham, OL9 9QH
Tel: 0845 610 1112

GP practices can obtain supplies through their Local Area Team Stores. NHS Trusts can order supplies from www.nhsforms.co.uk or by emailing nhsforms@mmm.com.

In **Scotland**, steroid treatment cards can be obtained from APS Group Scotland by emailing stockorders.dppas@theapsgroup.com or by fax on 0131 629 9967.

F 407

Betamethasone

- **INDICATIONS AND DOSE**

Suppression of inflammatory and allergic disorders | Congenital adrenal hyperplasia
- ▶ BY SLOW INTRAVENOUS INJECTION, OR BY INTRAVENOUS INFUSION
- ▶ Child 1–11 months: Initially 1 mg, repeated up to 4 times in 24 hours according to response
- ▶ Child 1–5 years: Initially 2 mg, repeated up to 4 times in 24 hours according to response
- ▶ Child 6–11 years: Initially 4 mg, repeated up to 4 times in 24 hours according to response
- ▶ Child 12–17 years: 4–20 mg, repeated up to 4 times in 24 hours according to response

- **PREGNANCY** Readily crosses the placenta. Transient effect on fetal movements and heart rate.

- **DIRECTIONS FOR ADMINISTRATION** For *intravenous infusion*, dilute with Glucose 5% or Sodium Chloride 0.9%.

- **MEDICINAL FORMS**
There can be variation in the licensing of different medicines containing the same drug.
Solution for injection
CAUTIONARY AND ADVISORY LABELS 10
- ▶ Betamethasone (Non-proprietary)
  Betamethasone (as Betamethasone sodium phosphate) 4 mg per 1 ml Betamethasone 4mg/1ml solution for injection ampoules | 5 ampoule [PoM] £13.06

F 407

Deflazacort

- **INDICATIONS AND DOSE**

Inflammatory and allergic disorders
- ▶ BY MOUTH
- ▶ Child 1 month–11 years: 0.25–1.5 mg/kg once daily or on alternate days; increased if necessary up to 2.4 mg/kg daily (max. per dose 120 mg), in emergency situations
- ▶ Child 12–17 years: 3–18 mg once daily or on alternate days; increased if necessary up to 2.4 mg/kg daily (max. per dose 120 mg), in emergency situations　continued →

Nephrotic syndrome

▸ BY MOUTH

▸ Child: Initially 1.5 mg/kg once daily (max. per dose 120 mg), reduced to the lowest effective dose for maintenance

● **RENAL IMPAIRMENT** Use with caution.

● **PATIENT AND CARER ADVICE** Patient counselling is advised for deflazacort tablets (steroid card).

● **MEDICINAL FORMS**
There can be variation in the licensing of different medicines containing the same drug. Forms available from special-order manufacturers include: tablet

Tablet
CAUTIONARY AND ADVISORY LABELS 5, 10

▸ Calcort (Sanofi)
  Deflazacort 6 mg Calcort 6mg tablets | 60 tablet PoM £15.82

⌐ 407

Dexamethasone
6.6.2016

● **INDICATIONS AND DOSE**

Physiological replacement

▸ BY MOUTH, OR BY SLOW INTRAVENOUS INJECTION

▸ Child: 250–500 micrograms/m^2 every 12 hours, adjusted according to response

Suppression of inflammatory and allergic disorders

▸ BY MOUTH

▸ Child: 10–100 micrograms/kg daily in 1–2 divided doses, adjusted according to response; up to 300 micrograms/kg daily may be required in emergency situations

▸ BY INTRAMUSCULAR INJECTION, OR BY SLOW INTRAVENOUS INJECTION, OR BY INTRAVENOUS INFUSION

▸ Child 1 month–11 years: 83–333 micrograms/kg daily in 1–2 divided doses; maximum 20 mg per day

▸ Child 12–17 years: Initially 0.4–20 mg daily

Mild croup

▸ BY MOUTH

▸ Child: 150 micrograms/kg for 1 dose

Severe croup (or mild croup that might cause complications)

▸ INITIALLY BY MOUTH

▸ Child: Initially 150 micrograms/kg for 1 dose, to be given before transfer to hospital, then (by mouth or by intravenous injection) 150 micrograms/kg, then (by mouth or by intravenous injection) 150 micrograms/kg after 12 hours if required

Adjunctive treatment of bacterial meningitis (starting before or with first dose of antibacterial)

▸ BY SLOW INTRAVENOUS INJECTION

▸ Child 3 months–17 years: 150 micrograms/kg every 6 hours (max. per dose 10 mg) for 4 days

Life-threatening cerebral oedema

▸ BY INTRAVENOUS INJECTION

▸ Child (body-weight up to 35 kg): Initially 16.7 mg, then 3.3 mg every 3 hours for 3 days, then 3.3 mg every 6 hours for 1 day, then 1.7 mg every 6 hours for 4 days, then reduced in steps of 0.8 mg daily

▸ Child (body-weight 35 kg and above): Initially 20.8 mg, then 3.3 mg every 2 hours for 3 days, then 3.3 mg every 4 hours for 1 day, then 3.3 mg every 6 hours for 4 days, then reduced in steps of 1.7 mg daily

● **UNLICENSED USE**

▸ With intravenous use Consult product literature; not licensed for use in bacterial meningitis.

● **SIDE-EFFECTS**

▸ With intravenous use Perineal irritation may follow intravenous administration of the phosphate ester

● **PREGNANCY** Dexamethasone readily crosses the placenta.

● **DIRECTIONS FOR ADMINISTRATION**

▸ With oral use For administration *by mouth* tablets may be dispersed in water or injection solution given by mouth.

▸ With intravenous use For *intravenous infusion* dilute with Glucose 5% or Sodium Chloride 0.9%; give over 15–20 minutes.

● **PRESCRIBING AND DISPENSING INFORMATION**
Dexamethasone 3.8 mg/mL Injection has replaced Dexamethasone 4 mg/mL Injection. All dosage recommendations for intravenous, intramuscular, intrarticular use or local infiltration; are given in units of dexamethasone base.

● **PATIENT AND CARER ADVICE**
Medicines for Children leaflet: Dexamethasone for croup www.medicinesforchildren.org.uk/dexamethasone-croup-0

▸ With systemic use Patient counselling is advised for dexamethasone tablet, oral solution and injection (steroid card).

● **MEDICINAL FORMS**
There can be variation in the licensing of different medicines containing the same drug. Forms available from special-order manufacturers include: capsule, oral suspension, oral solution

Tablet
CAUTIONARY AND ADVISORY LABELS 10, 21

▸ Dexamethasone (Non-proprietary)
  Dexamethasone 500 microgram Dexamethasone 500microgram tablets | 28 tablet PoM £54.48 DT price = £54.09 | 30 tablet PoM £64.82

  Dexamethasone 2 mg Dexamethasone 2mg tablets | 50 tablet PoM £49.04 DT price = £49.00 | 100 tablet PoM £98.08 | 500 tablet PoM £490.00

Soluble tablet

▸ Dexamethasone (Non-proprietary)
  Dexamethasone (as Dexamethasone sodium phosphate)
  2 mg Dexamethasone 2mg soluble tablets sugar free sugar-free | 50 tablet PoM £30.00

  Dexamethasone (as Dexamethasone sodium phosphate)
  4 mg Dexamethasone 4mg soluble tablets sugar free sugar-free | 50 tablet PoM £60.00

  Dexamethasone (as Dexamethasone sodium phosphate)
  8 mg Dexamethasone 8mg soluble tablets sugar free sugar-free | 50 tablet PoM £120.00

Oral solution
CAUTIONARY AND ADVISORY LABELS 10, 21

▸ Dexamethasone (Non-proprietary)
  Dexamethasone (as Dexamethasone sodium phosphate)
  400 microgram per 1 ml Dexamethasone 2mg/5ml oral solution sugar free sugar-free | 75 ml PoM no price available sugar-free | 150 ml PoM £42.30 DT price = £42.30

  Dexamethasone (as Dexamethasone sodium phosphate) 2 mg per 1 ml Dexamethasone 10mg/5ml oral solution sugar free sugar-free | 50 ml PoM £24.50–£24.95 sugar-free | 150 ml PoM £101.40 DT price = £94.44

  Dexamethasone (as Dexamethasone sodium phosphate) 4 mg per 1 ml Dexamethasone 20mg/5ml oral solution sugar free sugar-free | 50 ml PoM £49.50

▸ Dexsol (Rosemont Pharmaceuticals Ltd)
  Dexamethasone (as Dexamethasone sodium phosphate)
  400 microgram per 1 ml Dexsol 2mg/5ml oral solution sugar-free | 75 ml PoM £21.15 sugar-free | 150 ml PoM £42.30 DT price = £42.30

▸ Martapan (Martindale Pharmaceuticals Ltd)
  Dexamethasone (as Dexamethasone sodium phosphate)
  400 microgram per 1 ml Martapan 2mg/5ml oral solution sugar-free | 150 ml PoM £42.30 DT price = £42.30

Solution for injection
CAUTIONARY AND ADVISORY LABELS 10

▸ Dexamethasone (Non-proprietary)
  Dexamethasone (as Dexamethasone sodium phosphate) 3.3 mg per 1 ml Dexamethasone 6.6mg/2ml solution for injection vials | 5 vial PoM £24.00
  Dexamethasone 6.6mg/2ml solution for injection ampoules | 5 ampoule PoM £11.00
  Dexamethasone 3.3mg/1ml solution for injection ampoules | 5 ampoule PoM £12.00 | 10 ampoule PoM £12.00

Dexamethasone (as Dexamethasone sodium phosphate) 3.8 mg
per 1 ml Dexamethasone 3.8mg/1ml solution for injection vials |
10 vial [PoM] £19.99 DT price = £19.99

▶ 407

Fludrocortisone acetate

● INDICATIONS AND DOSE

Mineralocorticoid replacement in adrenocortical insufficiency
▶ BY MOUTH

▸ Neonate: Initially 50 micrograms once daily, adjusted
according to response; usual dose 50–200 micrograms
once daily, higher doses may be required, dose
adjustment may be required if salt supplements are
administered.

▸ Child: Initially 50–100 micrograms once daily;
maintenance 50–300 micrograms once daily, adjusted
according to response, dose adjustment may be
required if salt supplements are administered

● HEPATIC IMPAIRMENT Monitor patient closely in hepatic
impairment.

● PATIENT AND CARER ADVICE
Medicines for Children leaflet: Fludrocortisone for hormone
replacement www.medicinesforchildren.org.uk/
fludrocortisone-for-hormone-replacement

● MEDICINAL FORMS
There can be variation in the licensing of different medicines
containing the same drug. Forms available from special-order
manufacturers include: capsule, oral suspension

Tablet
CAUTIONARY AND ADVISORY LABELS 10
▸ Fludrocortisone acetate (Non-proprietary)
Fludrocortisone acetate 100 microgram Fludrocortisone
100microgram tablets | 30 tablet [PoM] £30.00 DT price = £30.00

▶ 407

Hydrocortisone

● INDICATIONS AND DOSE

Acute adrenocortical insufficiency (Addisonian crisis)
▶ INITIALLY BY SLOW INTRAVENOUS INJECTION

▸ Neonate: Initially 10 mg, then (by continuous
intravenous infusion) 100 mg/m^2 daily, alternatively (by
intravenous infusion) 100 mg/m^2 daily in divided doses,
to be given every 6–8 hours; adjusted according to
response, when stable reduce over 4–5 days to oral
maintenance dose.

▶ BY SLOW INTRAVENOUS INJECTION, OR BY INTRAVENOUS
INFUSION
▸ Child 1 month–11 years: Initially 2–4 mg/kg, then
2–4 mg/kg every 6 hours, adjusted according to
response, when stable reduce over 4–5 days to oral
maintenance dose
▸ Child 12–17 years: 100 mg every 6–8 hours

Congenital adrenal hyperplasia
▶ BY MOUTH USING IMMEDIATE-RELEASE MEDICINES
▸ Neonate: 9–15 mg/m^2 in 3 divided doses, adjusted
according to response.
▸ Child: 9–15 mg/m^2 in 3 divided doses, adjusted
according to response

**Adrenal hypoplasia | Addison's disease, chronic
maintenance or replacement therapy**
▶ BY MOUTH USING IMMEDIATE-RELEASE MEDICINES
▸ Neonate: 8–10 mg/m^2 daily in 3 divided doses, the larger
dose to be given in the morning and the smaller in the
evening, higher doses may be needed.

▸ Child: 8–10 mg/m^2 daily in 3 divided doses, the larger
dose to be given in the morning and the smaller in the
evening, higher doses may be needed

Inflammatory bowel disease—induction of remission
▶ BY INTRAVENOUS INJECTION
▸ Child 2–17 years: 2.5 mg/kg every 6 hours (max. per dose
100 mg)
▶ BY CONTINUOUS INTRAVENOUS INFUSION
▸ Child 2–17 years: 10 mg/kg daily; maximum 400 mg per
day

Ulcerative colitis | Proctitis | Proctosigmoiditis
▶ BY RECTUM USING RECTAL FOAM
▸ Child 2–17 years: Initially 1 metered application
1–2 times a day for 2–3 weeks, then reduced to
1 metered application once daily on alternate days, to
be inserted into the rectum

Acute hypersensitivity reactions | Angioedema
▶ BY INTRAMUSCULAR INJECTION, OR BY INTRAVENOUS
INJECTION
▸ Child 1–5 months: Initially 25 mg 3 times a day, adjusted
according to response
▸ Child 6 months–5 years: Initially 50 mg 3 times a day,
adjusted according to response
▸ Child 6–11 years: Initially 100 mg 3 times a day, adjusted
according to response
▸ Child 12–17 years: Initially 200 mg 3 times a day,
adjusted according to response

**Hypotension resistant to inotropic treatment and volume
replacement (limited evidence)**
▶ BY INTRAVENOUS INJECTION

▸ Neonate: Initially 2.5 mg/kg, then 2.5 mg/kg after
4 hours if required, followed by 2.5 mg/kg every 6 hours
for 48 hours or until blood pressure recovers, dose to
then be reduced gradually over at least 48 hours.

▸ Child: 1 mg/kg every 6 hours (max. per dose 100 mg)

Severe acute asthma | Life-threatening acute asthma
▶ BY INTRAVENOUS INJECTION
▸ Child 1 month–1 year: 4 mg/kg every 6 hours (max. per
dose 100 mg), alternatively 25 mg every 6 hours until
conversion to oral prednisolone is possible, dose given,
preferably, as sodium succinate
▸ Child 2–4 years: 4 mg/kg every 6 hours (max. per dose
100 mg), alternatively 50 mg every 6 hours until
conversion to oral prednisolone is possible, dose given,
preferably, as sodium succinate
▸ Child 5–11 years: 4 mg/kg every 6 hours (max. per dose
100 mg), alternatively 100 mg every 6 hours until
conversion to oral prednisolone is possible, dose given,
preferably, as sodium succinate
▸ Child 12–17 years: 4 mg/kg every 6 hours (max. per dose
100 mg), alternatively 100 mg every 6 hours until
conversion to oral prednisolone is possible, dose given,
preferably, as sodium succinate

● UNLICENSED USE Use of injection by mouth is unlicensed.

● CONTRA-INDICATIONS
▸ When used by ear Avoid alone in the presence of untreated
infection (combine with suitable anti-infective)
▸ With rectal use Bowel perforation · extensive fistulas ·
intestinal obstruction · recent intestinal anastomoses

● CAUTIONS
▸ With rectal use Systemic absorption may occur

● SIDE-EFFECTS
▸ With intravenous use Phosphate ester associated with pain
and paraesthesia (particularly in the perineal region)
▸ With rectal use Local irritation

6

Endocrine system

- **DIRECTIONS FOR ADMINISTRATION**
- With intravenous use For *intravenous administration*, dilute with Glucose 5% or Sodium Chloride 0.9%. For *intermittent infusion* give over 20–30 minutes.
- With oral use For administration *by mouth*, injection solution may be swallowed [unlicensed use] but consider phosphate content.

- **PATIENT AND CARER ADVICE**
- With systemic use Patient counselling is advised for hydrocortisone tablets and injections (steroid card).

- **LESS SUITABLE FOR PRESCRIBING**
- With intravenous use Hydrocortisone as the sodium phosphate is less suitable for prescribing as paraesthesia and pain (particularly in the perineal region) may follow intravenous injection.

- **EXCEPTIONS TO LEGAL CATEGORY**
- With intramuscular use or intravenous use Prescription only medicine restriction does not apply where administration is for saving life in emergency.

- **MEDICINAL FORMS**
There can be variation in the licensing of different medicines containing the same drug. Forms available from special-order manufacturers include: capsule, oral suspension, oral solution

Tablet
CAUTIONARY AND ADVISORY LABELS 10, 21
- Hydrocortisone (Non-proprietary)
  Hydrocortisone 10 mg Hydrocortisone 10mg tablets | 30 tablet PoM £113.00 DT price = £76.07
  Hydrocortisone 20 mg Hydrocortisone 20mg tablets | 30 tablet PoM £100.86 DT price = £101.40

Solution for injection
CAUTIONARY AND ADVISORY LABELS 10
- Hydrocortisone (Non-proprietary)
  Hydrocortisone (as Hydrocortisone sodium phosphate) 100 mg per 1 ml Hydrocortisone sodium phosphate 100mg/1ml solution for injection ampoules | 5 ampoule PoM £8.33
  Hydrocortisone sodium phosphate 500mg/5ml solution for injection ampoules | 5 ampoule PoM £36.45

Powder for solution for injection
- Solu-Cortef (Pfizer Ltd)
  Hydrocortisone (as Hydrocortisone sodium succinate) 100 mg Solu-Cortef 100mg powder for solution for injection vials | 10 vial PoM £9.17

Powder and solvent for solution for injection
CAUTIONARY AND ADVISORY LABELS 10
- Solu-Cortef (Pfizer Ltd)
  Hydrocortisone (as Hydrocortisone sodium succinate) 100 mg Solu-Cortef 100mg powder and solvent for solution for injection vials | 1 vial PoM £1.16 DT price = £1.16

Foam
EXCIPIENTS: May contain Cetostearyl alcohol (including cetyl and stearyl alcohol), hydroxybenzoates (parabens), propylene glycol
- Colifoam (Meda Pharmaceuticals Ltd)
  Hydrocortisone acetate 100 mg per 1 gram Colifoam 10% aerosol | 14 dose PoM £9.33 DT price = £9.33

F 407

Methylprednisolone

- **INDICATIONS AND DOSE**
Inflammatory and allergic disorders
- BY MOUTH, OR BY SLOW INTRAVENOUS INJECTION, OR BY INTRAVENOUS INFUSION
- Child: 0.5–1.7 mg/kg daily in 2–4 divided doses, divide doses depending on condition and response

Treatment of graft rejection reactions
- BY INTRAVENOUS INJECTION
- Child: 10–20 mg/kg once daily for 3 days, alternatively 400–600 mg/m^2 once daily (max. per dose 1 g) for 3 days

Severe erythema multiforme | Lupus nephritis | Systemic onset juvenile idiopathic arthritis
- BY INTRAVENOUS INJECTION
- Child: 10–30 mg/kg once daily or on alternate days (max. per dose 1 g) for up to 3 doses

DEPO-MEDRONE®
Suppression of inflammatory and allergic disorders
- BY DEEP INTRAMUSCULAR INJECTION
- Child: Seek specialist advice, to be injected into the gluteal muscle

- **CAUTIONS**
- With intravenous use Rapid intravenous administration of large doses associated with cardiovascular collapse

- **DIRECTIONS FOR ADMINISTRATION**
- With intravenous use Intravenous injection given over 30 minutes. For intravenous infusion, may be diluted with sodium chloride intravenous infusion 0.9% or 0.45%, or glucose intravenous infusion 5% or 10%.

- **PATIENT AND CARER ADVICE** Patient counselling is advised for methylprednisolone tablets and injections (steroid card).

- **MEDICINAL FORMS**
There can be variation in the licensing of different medicines containing the same drug. Forms available from special-order manufacturers include: oral suspension

Tablet
CAUTIONARY AND ADVISORY LABELS 10, 21
- Medrone (Pfizer Ltd)
  Methylprednisolone 2 mg Medrone 2mg tablets | 30 tablet PoM £3.88
  Methylprednisolone 4 mg Medrone 4mg tablets | 30 tablet PoM £6.19
  Methylprednisolone 16 mg Medrone 16mg tablets | 30 tablet PoM £17.17
  Methylprednisolone 100 mg Medrone 100mg tablets | 20 tablet PoM £48.32

Powder and solvent for solution for injection
CAUTIONARY AND ADVISORY LABELS 10
- Methylprednisolone (Non-proprietary)
  Methylprednisolone (as Methylprednisolone sodium succinate) 500 mg Methylprednisolone sodium succinate 500mg powder and solvent for solution for injection vials | 1 vial PoM £9.60
  Methylprednisolone (as Methylprednisolone sodium succinate) 1 gram Methylprednisolone sodium succinate 1g powder and solvent for solution for injection vials | 1 vial PoM £17.30
- Solu-Medrone (Pfizer Ltd)
  Methylprednisolone (as Methylprednisolone sodium succinate) 40 mg Solu-Medrone 40mg powder and solvent for solution for injection vials | 1 vial PoM £1.58
  Methylprednisolone (as Methylprednisolone sodium succinate) 125 mg Solu-Medrone 125mg powder and solvent for solution for injection vials | 1 vial PoM £4.75
  Methylprednisolone (as Methylprednisolone sodium succinate) 500 mg Solu-Medrone 500mg powder and solvent for solution for injection vials | 1 vial PoM £9.60
  Methylprednisolone (as Methylprednisolone sodium succinate) 1 gram Solu-Medrone 1g powder and solvent for solution for injection vials | 1 vial PoM £17.30
  Methylprednisolone (as Methylprednisolone sodium succinate) 2 gram Solu-Medrone 2g powder and solvent for solution for injection vials | 1 vial PoM £32.86

Suspension for injection
CAUTIONARY AND ADVISORY LABELS 10
- Depo-Medrone (Pfizer Ltd)
  Methylprednisolone acetate 40 mg per 1 ml Depo-Medrone 40mg/1ml suspension for injection vials | 1 vial PoM £3.44 DT price = £3.44 | 10 vial PoM £34.04
  Depo-Medrone 80mg/2ml suspension for injection vials | 1 vial PoM £6.18 DT price = £6.18 | 10 vial PoM £61.39
  Depo-Medrone 120mg/3ml suspension for injection vials | 1 vial PoM £8.96 DT price = £8.96 | 10 vial PoM £88.81

Prednisolone

📖 407

- ● **INDICATIONS AND DOSE**

Severe croup (before transfer to hospital) | Mild croup that might cause complications (before transfer to hospital)
- ▶ BY MOUTH
- ▸ Child: 1–2 mg/kg

Mild to moderate acute asthma (when oral corticosteroid taken for more than a few days) | Severe or life-threatening acute asthma (when oral corticosteroid taken for more than a few days)
- ▶ BY MOUTH
- ▸ Child 1 month–11 years: 2 mg/kg once daily (max. per dose 60 mg) for up to 3 days, longer if necessary

Mild to moderate acute asthma | Severe or life-threatening acute asthma
- ▶ BY MOUTH
- ▸ Child 1 month–11 years: 1–2 mg/kg once daily (max. per dose 40 mg) for up to 3 days, longer if necessary
- ▸ Child 12–17 years: 40–50 mg daily for at least 5 days

Autoimmune inflammatory disorders (including juvenile idiopathic arthritis, connective tissue disorders and systemic lupus erythematosus)
- ▶ BY MOUTH
- ▸ Child: Initially 1–2 mg/kg once daily, to be reduced after a few days if appropriate; maximum 60 mg per day

Autoimmune hepatitis
- ▶ BY MOUTH
- ▸ Child: Initially 2 mg/kg once daily, to then be reduced to minimum effective dose; maximum 40 mg per day

Corticosteroid replacement therapy
- ▶ BY MOUTH
- ▸ Child 12–17 years: 2–2.5 mg/m^2 daily in 1–2 divided doses, adjusted according to response

Infantile spasms
- ▶ BY MOUTH
- ▸ Child 1 month–1 year: Initially 10 mg 4 times a day for 14 days; increased to 20 mg 3 times a day for 7 days if seizures not controlled after initial 7 days, reduce dose gradually over 15 days until stopped

Infantile spasms (dose reduction in patient taking 40 mg daily)
- ▶ BY MOUTH
- ▸ Child 1 month–1 year: Reduced in steps of 10 mg every 5 days, reduce gradually over 20 days until stopped

Infantile spasms (dose reduction in patient taking 60 mg daily)
- ▶ BY MOUTH
- ▸ Child 1 month–1 year: Reduced to 40 mg daily for 5 days, then reduced to 20 mg daily for 5 days, then reduced to 10 mg daily for 5 days and then stop

Idiopathic thrombocytopenic purpura
- ▶ BY MOUTH
- ▸ Child 1–9 years: 1–2 mg/kg daily for maximum of 14 days, alternatively 4 mg/kg daily for a maximum of 4 days

Nephrotic syndrome
- ▶ BY MOUTH
- ▸ Child: Initially 60 mg/m^2 once daily for 4–6 weeks until proteinuria ceases, then reduced to 40 mg/m^2 once daily on alternate days for 4–6 weeks, then withdraw by reducing dose gradually; maximum 80 mg per day

Nephrotic syndrome (prevention of relapse)
- ▶ BY MOUTH
- ▸ Child: 0.5–1 mg/kg once daily or on alternate days for 3–6 months

Ulcerative colitis | Crohn's disease
- ▶ BY MOUTH
- ▸ Child 2–17 years: 2 mg/kg once daily (max. per dose 60 mg) until remission occurs, followed by reducing doses

Pneumocystis pneumonia in moderate to severe infections associated with HIV infection
- ▶ BY MOUTH
- ▸ Child: 2 mg/kg daily for 5 days, the dose is then reduced over the next 16 days and then stopped, corticosteroid treatment should ideally be started at the same time as the anti-pneumocystis therapy and certainly no later than 24–72 hours afterwards, the corticosteroid should be withdrawn before anti-pneumocystis treatment is complete; maximum 80 mg per day

Proctitis
- ▶ BY RECTUM USING RECTAL FOAM
- ▸ Child 12–17 years: 1 metered application 1–2 times a day for 2 weeks, continued for further 2 weeks if good response, to be inserted into the rectum, 1 metered application contains 20 mg prednisolone
- ▶ BY RECTUM USING SUPPOSITORIES
- ▸ Child 2–17 years: 5 mg twice daily, to be inserted in to the rectum morning and night, after a bowel movement

Distal ulcerative colitis
- ▶ BY RECTUM USING RECTAL FOAM
- ▸ Child 12–17 years: 1 metered application 1–2 times a day for 2 weeks, continued for further 2 weeks if good response, to be inserted into the rectum, 1 metered application contains 20 mg prednisolone

Rectal complications of Crohn's disease
- ▶ BY RECTUM USING SUPPOSITORIES
- ▸ Child 2–17 years: 5 mg twice daily, to be inserted in to the rectum morning and night, after a bowel movement

- ● **UNLICENSED USE**
- ▶ With rectal use Prednisolone rectal foam not licensed for use in children (age range not specified by manufacturer).

- ● **CONTRA-INDICATIONS**
- ▶ With rectal use Bowel perforation · extensive fistulas · intestinal obstruction · recent intestinal anastomoses

- ● **CAUTIONS**
- ▶ With rectal use Systemic absorption may occur with rectal preparations
- ▶ With systemic use Duchenne's muscular dystrophy (possible transient rhabdomyolysis and myoglobinuria following strenuous physical activity)

- ● **PREGNANCY** As it crosses the placenta 88% of prednisolone is inactivated.
- ▶ With systemic use Pregnant women with fluid retention should be monitored closely.

- ● **BREAST FEEDING** Prednisolone appears in small amounts in breast milk but maternal doses of up to 40 mg daily are unlikely to cause systemic effects in the infant.
- ▶ With systemic use Infant should be monitored for adrenal suppression if mother is taking a dose higher than 40 mg.

- ● **PATIENT AND CARER ADVICE**
Prednisolone (oral) for nephrotic syndrome
- ▶ With oral use www.medicinesforchildren.org.uk/prednisolone-oral-for-nephrotic-syndrome
Medicines for Children leaflet: Prednisolone for asthma
- ▶ With oral use www.medicinesforchildren.org.uk/prednisolone-for-asthma
- ▶ With oral use Patient counselling is advised for prednisolone tablets (steroid card).

6

Endocrine system

● MEDICINAL FORMS

There can be variation in the licensing of different medicines containing the same drug. Forms available from special-order manufacturers include: oral suspension, oral solution, enema

Tablet

CAUTIONARY AND ADVISORY LABELS 10, 21

▶ Prednisolone (Non-proprietary)

Prednisolone 1 mg Prednisolone 1mg tablets | 28 tablet PoM £4.00 DT price = £0.78 | 100 tablet PoM no price available

Prednisolone 2.5 mg Prednisolone 2.5mg tablets | 28 tablet PoM £0.68

Prednisolone 5 mg Prednisolone 5mg tablets | 28 tablet PoM £11.00 DT price = £0.88 | 100 tablet PoM no price available

Prednisolone 10 mg Prednisolone 10mg tablets | 28 tablet PoM £2.72

Prednisolone 20 mg Prednisolone 20mg tablets | 28 tablet PoM £5.43

Prednisolone 25 mg Prednisolone 25mg tablets | 56 tablet PoM £75.00 DT price = £75.00

Prednisolone 30 mg Prednisolone 30mg tablets | 28 tablet PoM £8.15

▶ Pevanti (AMCo)

Prednisolone 2.5 mg Pevanti 2.5mg tablets | 30 tablet PoM £1.42 DT price = £1.42

Prednisolone 5 mg Pevanti 5mg tablets | 30 tablet PoM £0.95

Prednisolone 10 mg Pevanti 10mg tablets | 30 tablet PoM £1.90 DT price = £1.90

Prednisolone 20 mg Pevanti 20mg tablets | 30 tablet PoM £3.80 DT price = £3.80

Prednisolone 25 mg Pevanti 25mg tablets | 56 tablet PoM £40.00 DT price = £75.00

Soluble tablet

CAUTIONARY AND ADVISORY LABELS 10, 13, 21

▶ Prednisolone (Non-proprietary)

Prednisolone (as Prednisolone sodium phosphate)

5 mg Prednisolone 5mg soluble tablets | 30 tablet PoM £75.00 DT price = £53.48

Gastro-resistant tablet

CAUTIONARY AND ADVISORY LABELS 5, 10, 25

▶ Prednisolone (Non-proprietary)

Prednisolone 1 mg Prednisolone 1mg gastro-resistant tablets | 30 tablet PoM £1.60

Prednisolone 2.5 mg Prednisolone 2.5mg gastro-resistant tablets | 28 tablet PoM £15.45 DT price = £1.26 | 30 tablet PoM £6.15 | 100 tablet PoM £4.96

Prednisolone 5 mg Prednisolone 5mg gastro-resistant tablets | 28 tablet PoM £13.50 DT price = £1.31 | 30 tablet PoM £6.29 | 100 tablet PoM £5.18

▶ Deltacortril Enteric (Alliance Pharmaceuticals Ltd)

Prednisolone 2.5 mg Deltacortril 2.5mg gastro-resistant tablets | 30 tablet PoM £1.16

Prednisolone 5 mg Deltacortril 5mg gastro-resistant tablets | 30 tablet PoM £1.19

▶ Dilacort (Crescent Pharma Ltd)

Prednisolone 2.5 mg Dilacort 2.5mg gastro-resistant tablets | 28 tablet PoM £1.39 DT price = £1.26

Prednisolone 5 mg Dilacort 5mg gastro-resistant tablets | 28 tablet PoM £1.45 DT price = £1.31

Oral solution

▶ Prednisolone (Non-proprietary)

Prednisolone 1 mg per 1 ml Prednisolone 5mg/5ml oral solution unit dose | 10 unit dose PoM £11.41 DT price = £11.41

Prednisolone 10 mg per 1 ml Prednisolone 10mg/ml oral solution sugar free sugar-free | 30 ml PoM £55.00–£55.50

Foam

▶ Prednisolone (Non-proprietary)

Prednisolone (as Prednisolone sodium metasulfobenzoate)

20 mg per 1 application Prednisolone 20mg/application foam enema | 14 dose PoM £78.00 DT price = £78.00

Suppository

▶ Prednisolone (Non-proprietary)

Prednisolone (as Prednisolone sodium phosphate)

5 mg Prednisolone sodium phosphate 5mg suppositories | 10 suppository PoM £38.63 DT price = £37.89

2.1 Cushing's syndrome and disease

Cushing's Syndrome

Management

Most types of *Cushing's syndrome* are treated surgically. Metyrapone p. 415 may be useful to control the symptoms of the disease or to prepare the child for surgery. The dosages of metyrapone used are either low, and tailored to cortisol production, or high, in which case corticosteroid replacement therapy is also needed.

Ketoconazole below may have a direct effect on corticotropic tumour cells in patients with Cushing's disease. It is used under specialist supervision in children over 12 years for treatment of endogenous Cushing's syndrome.

ENZYME INHIBITORS

Ketoconazole

● DRUG ACTION

▶ With oral use An imidazole derivative which acts as a potent inhibitor of cortisol and aldosterone synthesis by inhibiting the activity of 17α-hydroxylase, 11-hydroxylation steps and at higher doses the cholesterol side-chain cleavage enzyme. It also inhibits the activity of adrenal C17-20 lyase enzymes resulting in androgen synthesis inhibition, and may have a direct effect on corticotropic tumour cells in patients with Cushing's disease.

● INDICATIONS AND DOSE

Endogenous Cushing's syndrome (specialist use only)

▶ BY MOUTH

▶ Child 12–17 years: Initially 400–600 mg daily in 2–3 divided doses, increased to 800–1200 mg daily; maintenance 400–800 mg daily in 2–3 divided doses, for dose titrations in patients with established dose, adjustments in adrenal insufficiency, or concomitant corticosteroid replacement therapy, consult product literature; maximum 1200 mg per day

IMPORTANT SAFETY INFORMATION

CHMP ADVICE: KETOCONAZOLE (JULY 2013)

The CHMP has recommended that the marketing authorisation for oral ketoconazole to treat fungal infections should be suspended. The CHMP concluded that the risk of hepatotoxicity associated with oral ketoconazole is greater than the benefit in treating fungal infections. Doctors should review patients who are being treated with oral ketoconazole for fungal infections, with a view to stopping treatment or choosing an alternative treatment. Patients with a prescription of oral ketoconazole for fungal infections should be referred back to their doctors.

Oral ketoconazole for Cushing's syndrome and topical products containing ketoconazole are not affected by this advice.

● CONTRA-INDICATIONS Acquired QTc prolongation · avoid concomitant use of hepatotoxic drugs · congenital QTc prolongation

● CAUTIONS Risk of adrenal insufficiency

● INTERACTIONS → Appendix 1 (antifungals, imidazole).

- **SIDE-EFFECTS**
- ▶ **Common or very common** Abdominal pain · adrenal insufficiency · diarrhoea · hepatic enzymes increased · nausea · pruritus · rash · vomiting
- ▶ **Uncommon** Alopecia · dizziness · headache · malaise · somnolence · thrombocytopenia · urticaria
- ▶ **Rare** Hepatic failure · hepatitis · jaundice · liver damage
- ▶ **Very rare** Pyrexia
- ▶ **Frequency not known** Alcohol intolerance · anorexia · arthralgia · azoospermia · dermatitis · dry mouth · dysgeusia · dyspepsia · epistaxis · erectile dysfunction · erythema · flatulence · gynaecomastia · hot flush · increased appetite · insomnia · menstrual disorder · myalgia · nervousness · paraesthesia · peripheral oedema · photophobia · photosensitivity · raised intracranial pressure · reduced testosterone concentrations · tongue discoloration · xeroderma

SIDE-EFFECTS, FURTHER INFORMATION
- ▶ Hepatotoxicity Potentially life-threatening hepatotoxicity reported rarely.
- **CONCEPTION AND CONTRACEPTION** Effective contraception must be used in women of child-bearing potential.
- **PREGNANCY** Manufacturer advises avoid—teratogenic in *animal* studies.
- **BREAST FEEDING** Manufacturer advises avoid—present in breast milk.
- **HEPATIC IMPAIRMENT** Avoid in acute or chronic impairment. Do not initiate treatment if liver enzymes greater than 2 times the normal upper limit.
- **MONITORING REQUIREMENTS**
- ▶ Monitor ECG before and one week after initiation, and then as clinically indicated thereafter.
- ▶ Adrenal insufficiency Monitor adrenal function within one week of initiation, then regularly thereafter. When cortisol levels are normalised or close to target and effective dose established, monitor every 3–6 months as there is a risk of autoimmune disease development or exacerbation after normalisation of cortisol levels. If symptoms suggestive of adrenal insufficiency such as fatigue, anorexia, nausea, vomiting, hypotension, hyponatraemia, hyperkalaemia, and/or hypoglycaemia occur, measure cortisol levels and discontinue treatment temporarily (can be resumed thereafter at lower dose) or reduce dose and if necessary, initiate corticosteroid substitution.
- ▶ Hepatotoxicity Monitor liver function before initiation of treatment, then weekly for 1 month after initiation, then monthly for 6 months—more frequently if dose adjusted or abnormal liver function detected. Reduce dose if liver enzymes increase less than 3 times the normal upper limit—consult product literature; if liver enzymes are raised to 3 times or greater the normal upper limit, discontinue treatment permanently.
- **PATIENT AND CARER ADVICE** Dizziness and somnolence may affect the performance of skilled tasks (e.g. driving). Patients or their carers should be told how to recognise signs of liver disorder, and advised to discontinue treatment and seek prompt medical attention if symptoms such as anorexia, nausea, vomiting, fatigue, jaundice, abdominal pain, or dark urine develop. Patients or their carers should also be told how to recognise signs of adrenal insufficiency.

- **MEDICINAL FORMS**
There can be variation in the licensing of different medicines containing the same drug. Forms available from special-order manufacturers include: oral suspension
Tablet
CAUTIONARY AND ADVISORY LABELS 2, 5, 21
- ▶ Ketoconazole (Non-proprietary) ▼
Ketoconazole 200 mg Ketoconazole 200mg tablets |
60 tablet [PoM] £480.00

Metyrapone

- **DRUG ACTION** Metyrapone is a competitive inhibitor of 11β-hydroxylation in the adrenal cortex; the resulting inhibition of cortisol (and to a lesser extent aldosterone) production leads to an increase in ACTH production which, in turn, leads to increased synthesis and release of cortisol precursors. Metyrapone may be used as a test of anterior pituitary function.

- **INDICATIONS AND DOSE**
Differential diagnosis of ACTH-dependent Cushing's syndrome (specialist supervision in hospital)
- ▶ BY MOUTH
- ▶ Child: 15 mg/kg every 4 hours for 6 doses, alternatively 300 mg/m^2 every 4 hours for 6 doses; usual dose 250–750 mg every 4 hours
Management of Cushing's syndrome (specialist supervision in hospital)
- ▶ BY MOUTH
- ▶ Child: Usual dose 0.25–6 g daily, dose to be tailored to cortisol production, dose is either low, and tailored to cortisol production, or high, in which case corticosteroid replacement therapy is also needed

- **CONTRA-INDICATIONS** Adrenocortical insufficiency
- **CAUTIONS** Avoid in Acute porphyrias p. 562 · gross hypopituitarism (risk of precipitating acute adrenal failure) · hypertension on long-term administration · hypothyroidism (delayed response)
- **INTERACTIONS** Many drugs interfere with diagnostic estimation of steroids.
- **SIDE-EFFECTS**
- ▶ **Rare** Abdominal pain · allergic skin reactions · hirsutism · hypoadrenalism
- ▶ **Frequency not known** Dizziness · headache · hypotension · nausea · sedation · vomiting
- **PREGNANCY** Avoid (may impair biosynthesis of fetal-placental steroids).
- **BREAST FEEDING** Avoid—no information available.
- **HEPATIC IMPAIRMENT** Use with caution in hepatic impairment (delayed response).
- **PATIENT AND CARER ADVICE**
Driving and skilled tasks
Drowsiness may affect the performance of skilled tasks (e.g. driving).

- **MEDICINAL FORMS**
There can be variation in the licensing of different medicines containing the same drug.
Capsule
CAUTIONARY AND ADVISORY LABELS 21
- ▶ Metopirone (HRA Pharma UK Ltd)
Metyrapone 250 mg Metopirone 250mg capsules |
100 capsule [PoM] £363.66

3 Diabetes mellitus and hypoglycaemia
3.1 Diabetes mellitus

Diabetes

Overview

Diabetes mellitus occurs because of a lack of insulin or resistance to its action. It is diagnosed by measuring fasting or random blood-glucose concentration (and occasionally by oral glucose tolerance test). Although there are many subtypes, the two principle classes of diabetes are type 1 diabetes and type 2 diabetes.

Type 1 diabetes, (formerly referred to as insulin-dependent diabetes mellitus (IDDM)), is due to a deficiency of insulin following autoimmune destruction of pancreatic beta cells and is the most common form of diabetes in children. Children with type 1 diabetes require administration of insulin.

Type 2 diabetes, (formerly referred to as non-insulin dependent diabetes mellitus (NIDDM)), is rare in children but the incidence is increasing, particularly in adolescents, as obesity increases. It results from reduced secretion of insulin or from peripheral resistance to the action of insulin, or from a combination of both. Although children may be controlled on diet alone, many require oral antidiabetic drugs or insulin to maintain satisfactory control. There is limited information available on the use of oral antidiabetic drugs in children. In overweight individuals, type 2 diabetes may be prevented by losing weight and increasing physical activity.

Genetic defects of beta-cell function (formerly referred to as maturity-onset diabetes of the young (MODY)), describes a number of rare disease states, characterised by onset of mild hyperglycaemia, generally before 25 years of age. A sulfonylurea, such as gliclazide p. 421, may be effective in these patients.

Treatment of diabetes

Treatment should be aimed at alleviating symptoms and minimising the risk of long-term complications.

Diabetes is a strong risk factor for cardiovascular disease later in life. Other risk factors for cardiovascular disease (smoking, hypertension, obesity and hyperlipidaemia) should be addressed. The use of an ACE inhibitor and of a lipid-regulating drug can be beneficial in children with diabetes and a high cardiovascular disease risk. (ACE inhibitors may also have a role in the management of diabetic nephropathy).

Prevention of diabetic complications

Although rare, retinopathy, neuropathy and nephropathy can occur in children with diabetes. Screening for complications should begin 5 years after diagnosis of diabetes or from 12 years of age. Optimal glycaemic control in both type 1 diabetes and type 2 diabetes reduces, in the long term, the risk of microvascular complications including retinopathy, development of proteinuria and to some extent neuropathy.

A measure of the total glycosylated (or glycated) haemoglobin (HbA_1) or a specific fraction (HbA_{1c}) provides a good indication of long-term glycaemic control. Overall it is ideal to aim for an HbA_{1c} concentration of 48–59 mmol/mol or less (reference range 20–42 mmol/mol), but this cannot always be achieved and for those using insulin there is a significantly increased risk of disabling hypoglycaemia.

Measurement of HbA_{1c}

HbA_{1c} values are expressed in *mmol of glycosylated haemoglobin per mol of haemoglobin (mmol/mol)*, a standardised unit specific for HbA_{1c} created by the International Federation of Clinical Chemistry and Laboratory Medicine (IFCC). HbA_{1c} values were previously aligned to the assay used in the Diabetes Control and Complications Trial (DCCT) and expressed as a percentage.

Equivalent values	
IFCC-HbA_{1c} (mmol/mol)	DCCT-HbA_{1c} (%)
42	6.0
48	6.5
53	7.0
59	7.5
64	8.0
75	9.0

Laboratory measurement of serum-fructosamine concentration is technically simpler and cheaper than the measurement of HbA_{1c} and can be used to assess control over short periods of time, particularly when HbA_{1c} monitoring is invalid (e.g. disturbed erythrocyte turnover or abnormal haemoglobin type).

Tight control of blood pressure in hypertensive children with type 2 diabetes may reduce mortality significantly and protects visual acuity (by reducing considerably the risks of maculopathy and retinal photocoagulation).

Driving

Information on the requirements for driving vehicles by individuals receiving treatment for diabetes is available in the BNF or from the DVLA at www.gov.uk/government/publications/at-a-glance.

Diabetic nephropathy

Regular review of diabetic children over 12 years of age should include an annual test for microalbuminuria (the earliest sign of nephropathy). If reagent strip tests (*Micral-Test II*® or *Microbumintest*®) are used and prove positive, the result should be confirmed by laboratory analysis of a urine sample. Microalbuminuria can occur transiently during puberty; if it persists (at least 3 positive tests) treatment with an ACE inhibitor or an angiotensin-II receptor antagonist under specialist guidance should be considered; to minimise the risk of renal deterioration, blood pressure should be carefully controlled.

ACE inhibitors can potentiate the hypoglycaemic effect of insulin and oral antidiabetic drugs; this effect is more likely during the first weeks of combined treatment and in children with renal impairment.

See also treatment of hypertension in diabetes.

Neuropathy

Clinical neuropathy is rare in children whose diabetes is well controlled.

Diabetic ketoacidosis

Management

The management of diabetic ketoacidosis involves the replacement of fluid and electrolytes and the administration of insulin. Guidelines for the Management of Diabetic Ketoacidosis, published by the British Society of Paediatric Endocrinology and Diabetes, (available at www.bsped.org.uk) should be followed. Clinically well children with mild ketoacidosis who are dehydrated up to 5% usually respond to oral rehydration and subcutaneous insulin. For those who do not respond, or are clinically unwell, or are dehydrated by more than 5%, insulin and replacement fluids are best given by intravenous infusion.

- To restore circulating volume for children in *shock*, give 10 mL/kg **sodium chloride 0.9%** as a rapid infusion, repeat as necessary up to a maximum of 30 mL/kg.
- Further fluid should be given by intravenous infusion at a rate that replaces deficit and provides maintenance over

48 hours; initially use **sodium chloride 0.9%**, changing to **sodium chloride 0.45%** and **glucose 5%** after 12 hours if response is adequate and plasma-sodium concentration is stable.

- Include **potassium chloride** in the fluids unless anuria is suspected, adjust according to plasma-potassium concentration.
- Insulin infusion is necessary to switch off ketogenesis and reverse acidosis; it should not be started until at least 1 hour after the start of intravenous rehydration fluids.
- **Soluble insulin** should be diluted (and **mixed thoroughly**) with **sodium chloride 0.9%** intravenous infusion to a concentration of 1 unit/mL and infused at a rate of 0.1 units/kg/hour.
- **Sodium bicarbonate** infusion (1.26% or 2.74%) is rarely necessary and is used only in cases of extreme acidosis (blood pH less than 6.9) and shock, since the acid-base disturbance is normally corrected by treatment with insulin.
- Once blood glucose falls to 14 mmol/litre, **glucose intravenous infusion 5%** *or* **10%** should be added to the fluids.
- The insulin infusion rate can be reduced to no less than 0.05 units/kg/hour when blood-glucose concentration has fallen to 14 mmol/litre *and* blood pH is greater than 7.3 *and* a glucose infusion has been started; it is continued until the child is ready to take food by mouth. Subcutaneous insulin can then be started.
- The insulin infusion should not be stopped until 1 hour after starting subcutaneous soluble or long acting insulin, or 10 minutes after starting subcutaneous insulin aspart p. 426, or insulin glulisine p. 427, or insulin lispro p. 427.

Hyperosmolar hyperglycaemic state or hyperosmolar hyperglycaemic nonketotic coma occurs rarely in children. Treatment is similar to that of diabetic ketoacidosis, although lower rates of insulin infusion and slower rehydration may be required.

Insulins and anti-diabetic drugs

Insulin

Insulin is a polypeptide hormone that plays a key role in the regulation of carbohydrate, fat, and protein metabolism. There are differences in the amino-acid sequence of animal insulins, human insulins, and the human insulin analogues. Human sequence insulin may be produced semisynthetically by enzymatic modification of porcine insulin (emp) or biosynthetically by recombinant DNA technology using bacteria (crb, prb) or yeast (pyr).

Immunological resistance to insulin action is uncommon. Preparations of human sequence insulin should theoretically be less immunogenic than other insulin preparations, but no real advantage has been shown in trials.

Insulin is inactivated by gastro-intestinal enzymes, and must therefore be given by injection; the subcutaneous route is ideal in most circumstances. Insulin is usually injected into the thighs, buttocks, or abdomen; absorption from a limb site can be increased if the limb is used in strenuous exercise after the injection. Generally, subcutaneous insulin injections cause few problems; lipodystrophy may occur and is a factor in poor glycaemic control. Lipodystrophy can be minimised by using different injection sites in rotation. Local allergic reactions are rare.

Insulin should be given to all children with type 1 diabetes; it may also be needed to treat type 2 diabetes either when other methods cannot control the condition or during periods of acute illness or peri-operatively. Insulin is required in all instances of ketoacidosis (see Diabetic ketoacidosis p. 416), which can develop rapidly in children.

Safe and Effective Use of Insulin in Hospitalised Patients (March 2010)
NHS diabetes guidance available at www.diabetes.nhs.uk.

Management of diabetes with insulin
The aim of treatment is to achieve the best possible control of blood-glucose concentration without making the child or carer obsessional and to avoid disabling hypoglycaemia; close co-operation is needed between the child or carer and the medical team to achieve good control and thereby reduce the risk of complications.

Insulin preparations can be divided into 3 types:

- those of **short** duration which have a relatively rapid onset of action, namely soluble insulin and the rapid-acting insulin analogues, insulin aspart p. 426, insulin glulisine p. 427, and insulin lispro p. 427;
- those with an **intermediate** action, e.g. isophane insulin p. 423; and
- those whose action is slower in onset and lasts for **long** periods, e.g. protamine zinc insulin p. 425, insulin detemir p. 424, and insulin glargine p. 424.

The duration of action of a particular type of insulin can vary from one child to another, and needs to be assessed individually.

Mixtures of insulin preparations may be required and appropriate combinations have to be determined for the individual child. Treatment should be started with several doses of short-acting insulin (soluble insulin or a rapid-acting insulin analogue) given throughout the day with a longer-acting insulin given once or twice daily. Alternatively, for those who have difficulty with, or prefer not to use, multiple daily injection regimens or in whom such regimens fail to achieve adequate glycaemic control, a mixture of premixed short- and intermediate- acting insulins (most commonly in a proportion of 30% soluble insulin and 70% isophane insulin) can be given twice daily. The dose of short-acting or rapid-acting insulin (or the proportion of the short-acting soluble insulin component in premixed insulin) can be increased in those with excessive postprandial hyperglycaemia. The dose of insulin is increased gradually according to the child's individual requirements, taking care to avoid troublesome hypoglycaemia. Initiation of insulin may be followed by a partial remission phase or 'honeymoon period' when lower doses of insulin are required than are subsequently necessary to maintain glycaemic control.

Examples of insulin regimens

- Multiple injection regimen: short-acting insulin or rapid-acting insulin analogue, before meals. With intermediate-acting or long-acting insulin, once or twice daily;
- Short-acting insulin or rapid-acting insulin analogue mixed with intermediate-acting insulin, twice daily (before breakfast and the main evening meal);
- Short-acting insulin or rapid-acting insulin analogue mixed with intermediate-acting insulin, before breakfast. With short-acting or rapid-acting insulin analogue alone, before afternoon snack or the main evening meal, and intermediate-acting insulin or long-acting insulin, at bedtime;
- Continuous subcutaneous insulin infusion.

Insulin requirements
Most prepubertal children require around 0.6–0.8 units/kg/day of insulin after the initial temporary remission phase. Unless the child has a very sedentary life-style, a requirement for higher doses may indicate poor compliance, poor absorption of insulin from the injection site (e.g. because of lipohypertrophic sites), or the beginning of puberty. During puberty up to 1.5–2 units/kg/day of insulin may be required, especially during growth spurts. Around 1 year after menarche or after the growth spurt in boys, the dose may need to be adjusted to avoid excessive weight gain. Insulin requirements can be *increased* by

infection, stress, and accidental or surgical trauma. Insulin requirements can be *reduced* in very active individuals, in those with certain endocrine disorders (e.g. Addison's disease, hypopituitarism), or in coeliac disease. Insulin requirements should be assessed frequently in all these circumstances.

Hypoglycaemia

Very tight control of diabetes lowers the blood-glucose concentration needed to trigger hypoglycaemic symptoms; an increase in the frequency of hypoglycaemic episodes may reduce the warning symptoms experienced by the child. Loss of warning of hypoglycaemia among insulin-treated children can be a serious hazard, especially for cyclists and drivers.

To restore the warning signs, episodes of hypoglycaemia must be minimised; this involves appropriate adjustment of insulin type, dose, and frequency, together with suitable timing and quantity of meals and snacks.

Diabetes and surgery

Children with type 1 diabetes should undergo surgery in centres with facilities for, and expertise in, the care of children with diabetes. Detailed local protocols should be available to all healthcare professionals involved in the treatment of these children.

Children with type 1 diabetes who require surgery:

- should be admitted to hospital for general anaesthesia;
- should receive insulin, even if they are fasting, to avoid ketoacidosis;
- should receive glucose infusion when fasting before an anaesthetic to prevent hypoglycaemia;
- should have careful monitoring of blood-glucose concentration because surgery may cause hyperglycaemia.

Elective surgery

Surgery in children with diabetes is best scheduled early on the list, preferably in the morning. If glycaemic control is poor it is advisable to admit the child well in advance of surgery. On the *evening before surgery*, blood-glucose should be measured frequently, especially before meals and snacks and at bedtime; urine should be tested for ketones. The usual evening or bedtime insulin and bedtime snack should be given. Ketosis or severe hypoglycaemia require correction, preferably by overnight intravenous infusion, and the surgery may need to be postponed.

For *minor procedures that require fasting*, a slight modification of the usual regimen may be all that is necessary e.g. for early morning procedures delay insulin and food until immediately after the procedure.

For *other types of elective surgery*, consult local treatment protocols.

Emergency surgery

Intravenous fluids and an insulin infusion should be started immediately. If ketoacidosis is present the recommendations for diabetic ketoacidosis should be followed.

Intravenous fluids and continuous insulin infusion

Blood-glucose and plasma-electrolyte concentrations must be measured frequently in a child receiving intravenous support. Intravenous infusion should be continued until after the child starts to eat and drink. The following infusions should be used and adjusted according to the child's fluid and electrolyte requirements:

- Constant infusion of sodium chloride 0.45% and glucose 5% intravenous infusion together with potassium chloride 20 mmol/litre (provided that plasma-potassium concentration is not raised) at a rate determined by factors such as volume depletion and age; the amount of potassium chloride infused is adjusted according to plasma electrolyte measurements;
- Constant infusion of soluble insulin 1 unit/mL in sodium chloride 0.9% intravenous initially at a rate of 0.025 units/kg/hour (up to 0.05 units/kg/hour if the child is unwell), then adjusted according to blood-glucose

concentration (frequent monitoring necessary) in line with locally agreed protocols and the child's volume depletion and age;

- Blood-glucose concentration should be maintained between 5 and 10 mmol/litre. If the glucose concentration falls below 5 mmol/litre, glucose 10% intravenous infusion may be required; conversely, if the glucose concentration persistently exceeds 14 mmol/litre, sodium chloride 0.9% intravenous infusion should be substituted;
- The insulin infusion may be stopped temporarily for 10–15 minutes if blood-glucose concentration falls below 4 mmol/litre.

The usual subcutaneous insulin regimen should be started before the first meal (but the dose may need to be 10–20% higher than usual if the child is still bed bound or unwell) and the intravenous insulin infusion stopped 1 hour later. If glycaemic control is not adequately achieved, additional insulin can be given in the following ways:

- additional doses of soluble insulin at any of the 4 injection times (before meals or bedtime) *or*
- temporary addition of intravenous insulin infusion to subcutaneous regimen *or*
- complete reversion to intravenous insulin infusion (particularly if the child is unwell).

Short-acting insulins

Soluble insulin is a short-acting form of insulin. For maintenance regimens it is usual to inject it 15 to 30 minutes before meals.

Soluble insulin is the most appropriate form of insulin for use in diabetic emergencies and at the time of surgery. It can be given intravenously and intramuscularly, as well as subcutaneously.

When injected subcutaneously, soluble insulin has a rapid onset of action (30 to 60 minutes), a peak action between 2 and 4 hours, and a duration of action of up to 8 hours.

When injected intravenously, soluble insulin has a very short half-life of only about 5 minutes and its effect disappears within 30 minutes.

The rapid-acting human insulin analogues, insulin aspart p. 426, insulin glulisine p. 427, and insulin lispro p. 427, have a faster onset (10–20 minutes) and shorter duration of action (2–5 hours) than soluble insulin; as a result, fasting and preprandial blood-glucose concentrations are a little higher, postprandial blood-glucose concentration is a little lower, and hypoglycaemia occurs slightly less frequently. These rapid-acting insulins are ideal for prandial dosing in a multiple injection regimen in combination with a long-acting insulin once or twice daily. Insulin aspart, insulin glulisine, and insulin lispro can be administered by subcutaneous infusion. Insulin aspart and insulin lispro can also be administered intravenously and can be used as alternatives to soluble insulin for diabetic emergencies and at the time of surgery.

Intermediate- and long-acting insulins

When given by subcutaneous injection, intermediate- and long-acting insulins have an onset of action of approximately 1–2 hours, a maximal effect at 4–12 hours, and a duration of 16–35 hours. Some are given twice daily in conjunction with short-acting (soluble) insulin, and others are given once daily. Soluble insulin can be mixed with intermediate and long-acting insulins (except insulin detemir p. 424, insulin glargine p. 424, and insulin degludec p. 424) in the syringe, essentially retaining the properties of the two components, although there may be some blunting of the initial effect of the soluble insulin component (especially on mixing with protamine zinc insulin p. 425).

Close monitoring of blood glucose is essential when introducing a change to the insulin regimen; the total daily dose as well as any concomitant treatment may need to be adjusted.

Isophane insulin p. 423 is a suspension of insulin with protamine; it is of particular value for initiation of twice-daily insulin regimens. Isophane can be mixed with soluble insulin before injection but ready-mixed preparations may be appropriate (biphasic isophane insulin p. 422, biphasic insulin aspart p. 423, or biphasic insulin lispro p. 423).

Insulin zinc suspension p. 425 (30% amorphous, 70% crystalline) has a more prolonged duration of action.

Protamine zinc insulin is usually given once daily with short-acting (soluble) insulin. It has the drawback of binding with the soluble insulin when mixed in the same syringe and is now rarely used.

Insulin detemir and insulin glargine are long-acting human insulin analogues with a prolonged duration of action; insulin detemir is given once or twice daily and insulin glargine is given once daily. These long-acting insulins are ideal for once or twice daily dosing in a multiple injection regimen in combination with a short-acting insulin before meals. NICE (December 2002) has recommended that insulin glargine should be available as an option for patients with type 1 diabetes.

NICE (May 2009) has recommended that, if insulin is required in patients with type 2 diabetes, insulin detemir or insulin glargine may be considered for those:

- who require assistance with injecting insulin *or*
- whose lifestyle is significantly restricted by recurrent symptomatic hypoglycaemia *or*
- who would otherwise need twice-daily basal insulin injections in combination with oral antidiabetic drugs *or*
- who cannot use the device needed to inject isophane insulin.

Insulin degludec is a long-acting human insulin analogue for once daily subcutaneous administration.

Biphasic insulins
Biphasic insulins are pre-mixed insulin preparations containing various combinations of short-acting (soluble) or rapid-acting (analogue) insulin and an intermediate-acting insulin.

The percentage of short-acting insulin varies from 10% to 50%. These preparations should be administered by subcutaneous injection up to 15 minutes before or soon after a meal.

Hypodermic equipment
Carers and children should be advised on the safe disposal of lancets, single-use syringes, and needles. Suitable arrangements for the safe disposal of contaminated waste must be made before these products are prescribed for patients who are carriers of infectious diseases.

Antidiabetic drugs

Oral antidiabetic drugs are used for the treatment of type 2 diabetes mellitus. They should be prescribed only if the child fails to respond adequately to restriction of energy and carbohydrate intake and an increase in physical activity. They should be used to augment the effect of diet and exercise, and not to replace them.

In children, type 2 diabetes does not usually occur until adolescence and information on the use of oral antidiabetic drugs in children is limited. Treatment with oral antidiabetic drugs should be initiated under specialist supervision **only**; the initial dose should be at the lower end of the adult dose range and then adjusted according to response.

Metformin hydrochloride p. 420 is the oral antidiabetic drug of choice because there is most experience with this drug in children. If dietary changes and metformin hydrochloride do not control the diabetes adequately, either a sulfonylurea or insulin can be added.

Alternatively, oral therapy may be substituted with insulin.

When insulin is added to oral therapy, it is generally given at bedtime as isophane or long-acting insulin, and when insulin replaces an oral regimen it may be given as twice-daily injections of a biphasic insulin (or isophane insulin p. 423 mixed with soluble insulin), or a multiple injection regimen. Weight gain and hypoglycaemia may be complications of insulin therapy but weight gain can be reduced if the insulin is given in combination with metformin hydrochloride.

Pregnancy and breast-feeding
During pregnancy, women with *pre-existing diabetes* can be treated with metformin hydrochloride [unlicensed use], either alone or in combination with insulin p. 425. Metformin hydrochloride can be continued, or glibenclamide p. 421 resumed, during breast-feeding for those with pre-existing diabetes. Women with *gestational diabetes* may be treated, with or without concomitant insulin, with glibenclamide from 11 weeks gestation (after organogenesis) [unlicensed use] or with metformin hydrochloride [unlicensed use]. Women with gestational diabetes should discontinue hypoglycaemic treatment after giving birth.

Sulfonylureas
The sulfonylureas are not the first choice oral antidiabetics in children.

Sulfonylureas are considered for children in whom metformin hydrochloride is contra-indicated or not tolerated. Several sulfonylureas are available but experience in children is limited; choice is determined by side-effects and the duration of action as well as the child's age and renal function. Glibenclamide, a long-acting sulfonylurea, is associated with a greater risk of hypoglycaemia and for this reason is generally avoided in children. Shorter-acting alternatives, such as tolbutamide p. 421, may be preferred.

Insulin therapy should be instituted temporarily during intercurrent illness (such as coma, infection, and trauma). Sulfonylureas should be omitted on the morning of surgery; insulin is often required because of the ensuing hyperglycaemia in these circumstances.

Sulfonylureas can be useful in the management of certain forms of diabetes that result from genetic defects of beta-cell function; there is most experience with gliclazide p. 421.

Biguanides
Metformin hydrochloride, the only available biguanide, has a different mode of action from the sulfonylureas, and is not interchangeable with them.

Metformin hydrochloride is the drug of first choice in children with type 2 diabetes, in whom strict dieting has failed to control diabetes. When the combination of strict diet and metformin hydrochloride treatment fails, other options to be considered under specialist management only, include:

- combining with insulin but weight gain and hypoglycaemia can be problems (weight gain minimised if insulin given at night);
- combining with a sulfonylurea (reports of increased hazard with this combination remain unconfirmed).

Insulin treatment is almost always required in medical and surgical emergencies; insulin should also be substituted before elective surgery (omit metformin hydrochloride on the morning of surgery and give insulin if required).

Hypoglycaemia does not usually occur with metformin hydrochloride; other advantages are the lower incidence of weight gain and lower plasma-insulin concentration. It does not exert a hypoglycaemic action in non-diabetic subjects unless given in overdose.

Other antidiabetic drugs
There is little experience of the use of acarbose in children. It has been used in older children; therapy should be initiated by an appropriate expert.

The use of nateglinide in combination with a sulfonylurea is generally reserved for the management of some subtypes of diabetes resulting from genetic defects of beta-cell function or other syndromes of diabetes and requires specialist management.

Insulin and glucose

Neonatal hyperglycaemia
Newborn babies are relatively intolerant of glucose, especially in the first week of life and if premature. If intravenous glucose is necessary e.g. for total parenteral nutrition, infuse at a lower rate for 6–12 hours and the glucose intolerance should resolve. Insulin is not needed for such transient glucose intolerance, but may be needed if blood-glucose concentration is persistently high.

Neonatal diabetes
Neonatal diabetes is a rare condition that presents with acidosis, dehydration, hyperglycaemia, and rarely ketosis; it responds to continuous insulin infusion. When the neonate is stable, treatment can be switched to subcutaneous insulin given once or twice a day. Treatment is normally required for 4–6 weeks in transient forms, but may be required permanently in some cases.

BLOOD GLUCOSE LOWERING DRUGS ›
BIGUANIDES

| Metformin hydrochloride

- **DRUG ACTION** Metformin exerts its effect mainly by decreasing gluconeogenesis and by increasing peripheral utilisation of glucose; since it acts only in the presence of endogenous insulin it is effective only if there are some residual functioning pancreatic islet cells.

- ● **INDICATIONS AND DOSE**

  Diabetes mellitus
  ▸ BY MOUTH USING IMMEDIATE-RELEASE MEDICINES
  ▸ Child 8-9 years (specialist use only): Initially 200 mg once daily, dose to be adjusted according to response at intervals of at least 1 week, maximum daily dose to be given in 2–3 divided doses; maximum 2 g per day
  ▸ Child 10-17 years (specialist use only): Initially 500 mg once daily, dose to be adjusted according to response at intervals of at least 1 week, maximum daily dose to be given in 2–3 divided doses; maximum 2 g per day

- **UNLICENSED USE** Not licensed for use in children under 10 years.

- **CONTRA-INDICATIONS** Ketoacidosis · use of general anaesthesia (suspend metformin on the morning of surgery and restart when renal function returns to baseline)

  CONTRA-INDICATIONS, FURTHER INFORMATION
  ▸ Iodine-containing X-ray contrast media Intravascular administration of iodinated contrast agents can cause renal failure, which can increase the risk of lactic acidosis with metformin. Suspend metformin prior to the test; restart no earlier than 48 hours after the test if renal function has returned to baseline.

- **CAUTIONS** Can provoke lactic acidosis

- **INTERACTIONS** → Appendix 1 (antidiabetics).

- **SIDE-EFFECTS**
  ▸ Common or very common Abdominal pain · anorexia · diarrhoea (usually transient) · nausea · taste disturbance · vomiting
  ▸ Rare Decreased vitamin-B_{12} absorption · erythema · lactic acidosis (withdraw treatment) · pruritus · urticaria
  ▸ Frequency not known Hepatitis
  SIDE-EFFECTS, FURTHER INFORMATION
  ▸ Gastro-intestinal effects Gastro-intestinal side-effects are initially common with metformin, and may persist in some patients, particularly when very high doses are given. A slow increase in dose may improve tolerability.

- **PREGNANCY** Can be used in pregnancy for both preexisting and gestational diabetes. Women with gestational diabetes should discontinue treatment after giving birth.

- **BREAST FEEDING** May be used during breast-feeding in women with pre-existing diabetes.

- **HEPATIC IMPAIRMENT** Withdraw if tissue hypoxia likely.

- **RENAL IMPAIRMENT** Use with caution in renal impairment— increased risk of lactic acidosis.
  Lactic acidosis Withdraw or interrupt treatment in those at risk of tissue hypoxia or sudden deterioration in renal function, such as those with dehydration, severe infection, shock, sepsis, acute heart failure, respiratory failure or hepatic impairment, or those who have recently had a myocardial infarction.
  Avoid in significant renal impairment.

- **MONITORING REQUIREMENTS** Determine renal function before treatment and at least annually (at least twice a year in patients with additional risk factors for renal impairment, or if deterioration suspected).

- **PATIENT AND CARER ADVICE**
  Medicines for Children leaflet: Metformin for diabetes
  www.medicinesforchildren.org.uk/metformin-diabetes

- **MEDICINAL FORMS**
  There can be variation in the licensing of different medicines containing the same drug. Forms available from special-order manufacturers include: capsule, oral suspension, oral solution

  Tablet
  CAUTIONARY AND ADVISORY LABELS 21
  ▸ Metformin hydrochloride (Non-proprietary)
  Metformin hydrochloride 500 mg Metformin 500mg tablets | 28 tablet PoM £1.55 DT price = £0.86 | 84 tablet PoM £3.81 | 500 tablet PoM £16.96
  Metformin hydrochloride 850 mg Metformin 850mg tablets | 56 tablet PoM £2.48 DT price = £1.30 | 60 tablet PoM no price available | 300 tablet PoM £10.00
  ▸ Glucophage (Merck Serono Ltd)
  Metformin hydrochloride 500 mg Glucophage 500mg tablets | 84 tablet PoM £2.88
  Metformin hydrochloride 850 mg Glucophage 850mg tablets | 56 tablet PoM £3.20 DT price = £1.30

  Oral solution
  CAUTIONARY AND ADVISORY LABELS 21
  ▸ Metformin hydrochloride (Non-proprietary)
  Metformin hydrochloride 100 mg per 1 ml Metformin 500mg/5ml oral solution sugar free sugar-free | 100 ml PoM £15.00 sugar-free | 150 ml PoM £60.00 DT price = £17.24

  Powder
  ▸ Metformin hydrochloride (Non-proprietary)
  Metformin hydrochloride 1 gram Metformin 1g oral powder sachets sugar free sugar-free | 30 sachet PoM no price available

BLOOD GLUCOSE LOWERING DRUGS ›
SULFONYLUREAS

Sulfonylureas

- **DRUG ACTION** The sulfonylureas act mainly by augmenting insulin secretion and consequently are effective only when some residual pancreatic beta-cell activity is present; during long-term administration they also have an extrapancreatic action.

- **CONTRA-INDICATIONS** Presence of ketoacidosis

- **CAUTIONS** Can encourage weight gain (should be prescribed only if poor control and symptoms persist despite adequate attempts at dieting) · G6PD deficiency

- **SIDE-EFFECTS**
  ▸ Uncommon Hypoglycaemia
  ▸ Rare Agranulocytosis · aplastic anaemia · blood disorders · cholestatic jaundice · haemolytic anaemia · hepatic failure · hepatitis · leucopenia · pancytopenia · thrombocytopenia
  ▸ Frequency not known Allergic skin reactions (usually in the first 6–8 weeks of therapy) · constipation · diarrhoea ·

disturbance in liver function · erythema multiforme (usually in the first 6–8 weeks of therapy) · exfoliative dermatitis (usually in the first 6–8 weeks of therapy) · fever (usually in the first 6–8 weeks of therapy) · gastro-intestinal disturbances · hypersensitivity reactions (usually in the first 6–8 weeks of therapy) · jaundice (usually in the first 6–8 weeks of therapy) · nausea · vomiting

SIDE-EFFECTS, FURTHER INFORMATION

▸ Hypoglycaemia This is uncommon and usually indicates excessive dosage. Sulfonylurea-induced hypoglycaemia may persist for many hours and must always be treated in hospital.

● HEPATIC IMPAIRMENT Sulfonylureas should be avoided or a reduced dose should be used in severe hepatic impairment, because there is an increased risk of hypoglycaemia. Jaundice may occur.

● RENAL IMPAIRMENT Sulfonylureas should be used with care in those with mild to moderate renal impairment, because of the hazard of hypoglycaemia. Care is required to use the lowest dose that adequately controls blood glucose. Avoid where possible in severe renal impairment.

● PATIENT AND CARER ADVICE

Driving and skilled tasks

Driving Drivers need to be particularly careful to avoid hypoglycaemia and should be warned of the problems.

Glibenclamide ▸ 420

● **INDICATIONS AND DOSE**

Type 2 diabetes mellitus

▸ BY MOUTH
  ▸ Child 12–17 years: Initially 2.5 mg daily, adjusted according to response, dose to be taken with or immediately after breakfast; maximum 15 mg per day

Maturity-onset diabetes of the young (specialist use only)

▸ BY MOUTH
  ▸ Child 12–17 years: Initially 2.5 mg daily, adjusted according to response, dose to be taken with or immediately after breakfast; maximum 15 mg per day

● UNLICENSED USE Not licensed for use in breast feeding women with pre-existing diabetes. Not licensed for use in gestational diabetes.
  Not licensed for use in children.

● CONTRA-INDICATIONS Avoid where possible in Acute porphyrias p. 562

● INTERACTIONS → Appendix 1 (antidiabetics).

● PREGNANCY The use of sulfonylureas in pregnancy should generally be avoided because of the risk of neonatal hypoglycaemia; however, glibenclamide can be used during the second and third trimesters of pregnancy in women with gestational diabetes.

● BREAST FEEDING Glibenclamide can be used during breast-feeding in women with pre-existing diabetes.

● MEDICINAL FORMS
There can be variation in the licensing of different medicines containing the same drug. Forms available from special-order manufacturers include: oral suspension, oral solution

Tablet

▸ Glibenclamide (Non-proprietary)
  Glibenclamide 2.5 mg Glibenclamide 2.5mg tablets | 28 tablet [PoM] £7.21 DT price = £6.95
  Glibenclamide 5 mg Glibenclamide 5mg tablets | 28 tablet £19.99 DT price = £0.85

Gliclazide ▸ 420

● **INDICATIONS AND DOSE**

Type 2 diabetes mellitus

▸ BY MOUTH USING IMMEDIATE-RELEASE MEDICINES
  ▸ Child 12–17 years: Initially 20 mg once daily, adjusted according to response, increased if necessary up to 160 mg once daily (max. per dose 160 mg twice daily), dose to be taken with breakfast

Maturity-onset diabetes of the young (specialist use only)

▸ BY MOUTH USING IMMEDIATE-RELEASE MEDICINES
  ▸ Child 12–17 years: Initially 20 mg once daily, adjusted according to response, increased if necessary up to 160 mg once daily (max. per dose 160 mg twice daily), dose to be taken with breakfast

● UNLICENSED USE Not licensed for use in children.

● CONTRA-INDICATIONS Avoid where possible in Acute porphyrias p. 562

● INTERACTIONS → Appendix 1 (antidiabetics).

● PREGNANCY The use of sulfonylureas in pregnancy should generally be avoided because of the risk of neonatal hypoglycaemia.

● BREAST FEEDING Avoid—theoretical possibility of hypoglycaemia in the infant.

● RENAL IMPAIRMENT If necessary, gliclazide which is principally metabolised in the liver, can be used in renal impairment but careful monitoring of blood-glucose concentration is essential.

● MEDICINAL FORMS
There can be variation in the licensing of different medicines containing the same drug. Forms available from special-order manufacturers include: oral suspension

Tablet

▸ Gliclazide (Non-proprietary)
  Gliclazide 40 mg Gliclazide 40mg tablets | 28 tablet [PoM] £3.66 DT price = £3.36
  Gliclazide 80 mg Gliclazide 80mg tablets | 28 tablet [PoM] £12.74 DT price = £0.85 | 60 tablet [PoM] £19.85
▸ Diamicron (Servier Laboratories Ltd)
  Gliclazide 80 mg Diamicron 80mg tablets | 60 tablet [PoM] £4.38
▸ Zicron (Bristol Laboratories Ltd)
  Gliclazide 40 mg Zicron 40mg tablets | 28 tablet [PoM] £3.36 DT price = £3.36

Tolbutamide ▸ 420

● **INDICATIONS AND DOSE**

Type 2 diabetes mellitus

▸ BY MOUTH
  ▸ Child 12–17 years (specialist use only): 0.5–1.5 g daily in divided doses, dose to be taken with or immediately after meals, alternatively 0.5–1.5 g once daily, dose to be taken with or immediately after breakfast; maximum 2 g per day

● UNLICENSED USE Not licensed for use in children.

● CONTRA-INDICATIONS Avoid where possible in Acute porphyrias p. 562

● INTERACTIONS → Appendix 1 (antidiabetics).

● SIDE-EFFECTS Headache · tinnitus

● PREGNANCY The use of sulfonylureas in pregnancy should generally be avoided because of the risk of neonatal hypoglycaemia.

● BREAST FEEDING The use of sulfonylureas in breast-feeding should be avoided because there is a theoretical possibility of hypoglycaemia in the infant.

- **RENAL IMPAIRMENT** If necessary, the short-acting drug tolbutamide can be used in renal impairment but careful monitoring of blood-glucose concentration is essential.

- **MEDICINAL FORMS**
There can be variation in the licensing of different medicines containing the same drug. Forms available from special-order manufacturers include: oral suspension

Tablet
▸ **Tolbutamide (Non-proprietary)**
Tolbutamide 500 mg Tolbutamide 500mg tablets | 28 tablet PoM £42.50 DT price = £11.12 | 112 tablet PoM £57.28

INSULINS

Insulins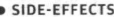

- **SIDE-EFFECTS**
▸ **Common or very common** Fat hypertrophy at injection site · local reactions at injection site · transient oedema
▸ **Rare** Hypersensitivity reactions · rash · urticaria
Overdose
Overdose causes hypoglycaemia.

- **PREGNANCY** During pregnancy, insulin requirements may alter and doses should be assessed frequently by an experienced diabetes physician. The dose of insulin generally needs to be increased in the second and third trimesters of pregnancy.

- **BREAST FEEDING**
During breast-feeding, insulin requirements may alter and doses should be assessed frequently by an experienced diabetes physician.

- **HEPATIC IMPAIRMENT** Insulin requirements may be decreased in patients with hepatic impairment.

- **RENAL IMPAIRMENT** Insulin requirements may decrease in patients with renal impairment and therefore dose reduction may be necessary. The compensatory response to hypoglycaemia is impaired in renal impairment.

- **MONITORING REQUIREMENTS**
▸ Many patients now monitor their own blood-glucose concentrations; all carers and children need to be trained to do this.
▸ Since blood-glucose concentration varies substantially throughout the day, 'normoglycaemia' cannot always be achieved throughout a 24-hour period without causing damaging hypoglycaemia.
▸ It is therefore best to recommend that children should maintain a blood-glucose concentration of between 4 and 10 mmol/litre for most of the time (4–8 mmol/litre before meals and less than 10 mmol/litre after meals).
▸ While accepting that on occasions, for brief periods, the blood-glucose concentration will be above these values; strenuous efforts should be made to prevent it from falling below 4 mmol/litre. Patients using multiple injection regimens should understand how to adjust their insulin dose according to their carbohydrate intake. With fixed-dose insulin regimens, the carbohydrate intake needs to be regulated, and should be distributed throughout the day to match the insulin regimen. The intake of energy and of simple and complex carbohydrates should be adequate to allow normal growth and development but obesity must be avoided.

- **DIRECTIONS FOR ADMINISTRATION** Insulin is generally given by *subcutaneous injection*; the injection site should be rotated to prevent lipodystrophy. Injection devices ('pens'), which hold the insulin in a cartridge and meter the required dose, are convenient to use. Insulin syringes (for use with needles) are required for insulins not available in cartridge form, but are less popular with children and carers. For intensive insulin regimens multiple subcutaneous injections (3 or more times daily) are usually recommended.

- **PRESCRIBING AND DISPENSING INFORMATION**
Units The word 'unit' should **not** be abbreviated.
Show container to patient or carer and confirm the expected version is dispensed.

- **PATIENT AND CARER ADVICE** Drivers need to be particularly careful to avoid hypoglycaemia and should be warned of the problems.
Insulin Passport Insulin Passports and patient information booklets should be offered to patients receiving insulin. The Insulin Passport provides a record of the patient's current insulin preparations and contains a section for emergency information. The patient information booklet provides advice on the safe use of insulin. They are available for purchase from:
3M Security Print and Systems Limited
Gorse Street, Chadderton
Oldham
OL9 9QH
Tel: 0845 610 1112
GP practices can obtain supplies through their Local Area Team stores.
NHS Trusts can order supplies from www.nhsforms.co.uk or by emailing nhsforms@mmm.com. Further information is available at www.npsa.nhs.uk.
Hypoglycaemia Hypoglycaemia is a potential problem with insulin therapy. All patients must be carefully instructed on how to avoid it; this involves appropriate adjustment of insulin type, dose and frequency together with suitable timing and quantity of meals and snacks.

INSULINS > INTERMEDIATE-ACTING

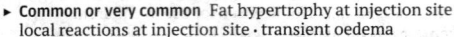 ☞ above

Biphasic isophane insulin

(Biphasic Isophane Insulin Injection— intermediate acting)

- **INDICATIONS AND DOSE**
Diabetes mellitus
▸ BY SUBCUTANEOUS INJECTION
▹ **Child:** According to requirements

- **INTERACTIONS** → Appendix 1 (antidiabetics).

- **SIDE-EFFECTS** Protamine may cause allergic reactions

- **PRESCRIBING AND DISPENSING INFORMATION** A sterile buffered suspension of either porcine or human insulin complexed with protamine sulfate (or another suitable protamine) in a solution of insulin of the same species.
Check product container—the proportions of the two components should be checked carefully (the order in which the proportions are stated may not be the same in other countries).

- **MEDICINAL FORMS**
There can be variation in the licensing of different medicines containing the same drug.
Suspension for injection
▸ **Humulin M3** (Eli Lilly and Company Ltd)
Insulin human (as Insulin soluble human) 30 unit per 1 ml, Insulin human (as Insulin isophane human) 70 unit per 1 ml Humulin M3 100units/ml suspension for injection 3ml cartridges | 5 cartridge PoM £19.08
Humulin M3 100units/ml suspension for injection 10ml vials | 1 vial PoM £15.68
▸ **Humulin M3 KwikPen** (Eli Lilly and Company Ltd)
Insulin human (as Insulin soluble human) 30 unit per 1 ml, Insulin human (as Insulin isophane human) 70 unit per 1 ml Humulin M3 KwikPen 100units/ml suspension for injection 3ml pre-filled pen | 5 pre-filled disposable injection PoM £21.70

▸ **Hypurin Porcine 30/70 Mix** (Wockhardt UK Ltd)
Insulin porcine (as Insulin soluble porcine) 30 unit per 1 ml, Insulin porcine (as Insulin isophane porcine) 70 unit per 1 ml Hypurin Porcine 30/70 Mix 100units/ml suspension for injection 3ml cartridges | 5 cartridge PoM £37.80
Hypurin Porcine 30/70 Mix 100units/ml suspension for injection 10ml vials | 1 vial PoM £25.20

▸ **Insuman Comb 15** (Sanofi)
Insulin human (as Insulin soluble human) 15 unit per 1 ml, Insulin human (as Insulin isophane human) 85 unit per 1 ml Insuman Comb 15 100units/ml suspension for injection 3ml cartridges | 5 cartridge PoM £17.50

▸ **Insuman Comb 25** (Sanofi)
Insulin human (as Insulin soluble human) 25 unit per 1 ml, Insulin human (as Insulin isophane human) 75 unit per 1 ml Insuman Comb 25 100units/ml suspension for injection 5ml vials | 1 vial PoM £5.61
Insuman Comb 25 100units/ml suspension for injection 3ml cartridges | 5 cartridge PoM £17.50

▸ **Insuman Comb 25 SoloStar** (Sanofi)
Insulin human (as Insulin soluble human) 25 unit per 1 ml, Insulin human (as Insulin isophane human) 75 unit per 1 ml Insuman Comb 25 100units/ml suspension for injection 3ml pre-filled SoloStar pen | 5 pre-filled disposable injection PoM £19.80

▸ **Insuman Comb 50** (Sanofi)
Insulin human (as Insulin isophane human) 50 unit per 1 ml, Insulin human (as Insulin soluble human) 50 unit per 1 ml Insuman Comb 50 100units/ml suspension for injection 3ml cartridges | 5 cartridge PoM £17.50

F 422

Isophane insulin

(Isophane Insulin Injection; Isophane Protamine Insulin Injection; Isophane Insulin (NPH)— intermediate acting)

● **INDICATIONS AND DOSE**
Diabetes mellitus
▸ BY SUBCUTANEOUS INJECTION
▸ Child: According to requirements

● **INTERACTIONS** → Appendix 1 (antidiabetics).
● **SIDE-EFFECTS** Protamine may cause allergic reactions
● **PREGNANCY** Recommended where longer-acting insulins are needed.
● **PRESCRIBING AND DISPENSING INFORMATION** A sterile suspension of bovine or porcine insulin or of human insulin in the form of a complex obtained by the addition of protamine sulfate or another suitable protamine.

● **MEDICINAL FORMS**
There can be variation in the licensing of different medicines containing the same drug.
Suspension for injection
▸ **Humulin I** (Eli Lilly and Company Ltd)
Insulin human (as Insulin isophane human) 100 unit per 1 ml Humulin I 100units/ml suspension for injection 10ml vials | 1 vial PoM £15.68
Humulin I 100units/ml suspension for injection 3ml cartridges | 5 cartridge PoM £19.08

▸ **Humulin I KwikPen** (Eli Lilly and Company Ltd)
Insulin human (as Insulin isophane human) 100 unit per 1 ml Humulin I KwikPen 100units/ml suspension for injection 3ml pre-filled pen | 5 pre-filled disposable injection PoM £21.70

▸ **Hypurin Bovine Isophane** (Wockhardt UK Ltd)
Insulin bovine (as Insulin isophane bovine) 100 unit per 1 ml Hypurin Bovine Isophane 100units/ml suspension for injection 10ml vials | 1 vial PoM £27.72
Hypurin Bovine Isophane 100units/ml suspension for injection 3ml cartridges | 5 cartridge PoM £41.58

▸ **Hypurin Porcine Isophane** (Wockhardt UK Ltd)
Insulin porcine (as Insulin isophane porcine) 100 unit per 1 ml Hypurin Porcine Isophane 100units/ml suspension for injection 10ml vials | 1 vial PoM £25.20
Hypurin Porcine Isophane 100units/ml suspension for injection 3ml cartridges | 5 cartridge PoM £37.80

▸ **Insulatard** (Novo Nordisk Ltd)
Insulin human (as Insulin isophane human) 100 unit per 1 ml Insulatard 100units/ml suspension for injection 10ml vials | 1 vial PoM £7.48

▸ **Insulatard InnoLet** (Novo Nordisk Ltd)
Insulin human (as Insulin isophane human) 100 unit per 1 ml Insulatard InnoLet 100units/ml suspension for injection 3ml pre-filled pen | 5 pre-filled disposable injection PoM £20.40

▸ **Insulatard Penfill** (Novo Nordisk Ltd)
Insulin human (as Insulin isophane human) 100 unit per 1 ml Insulatard Penfill 100units/ml suspension for injection 3ml cartridges | 5 cartridge PoM £22.90

▸ **Insuman Basal** (Sanofi)
Insulin human (as Insulin isophane human) 100 unit per 1 ml Insuman Basal 100units/ml suspension for injection 5ml vials | 1 vial PoM £5.61
Insuman Basal 100units/ml suspension for injection 3ml cartridges | 5 cartridge PoM £17.50

▸ **Insuman Basal SoloStar** (Sanofi)
Insulin human (as Insulin isophane human) 100 unit per 1 ml Insuman Basal 100units/ml suspension for injection 3ml pre-filled SoloStar pen | 5 pre-filled disposable injection PoM £19.80

INSULINS > INTERMEDIATE-ACTING COMBINED WITH RAPID-ACTING

F 422

Biphasic insulin aspart

(Intermediate-acting insulin)

● **INDICATIONS AND DOSE**
Diabetes mellitus
▸ BY SUBCUTANEOUS INJECTION
▸ Child: Administer up to 10 minutes before or soon after a meal, according to requirements

● **INTERACTIONS** → Appendix 1 (antidiabetics).
● **SIDE-EFFECTS** Protamine may cause allergic reactions
● **PRESCRIBING AND DISPENSING INFORMATION** Check product container—the proportions of the two components should be checked carefully (the order in which the proportions are stated may not be the same in other countries).

● **MEDICINAL FORMS**
There can be variation in the licensing of different medicines containing the same drug.
Suspension for injection
▸ **NovoMix 30 FlexPen** (Novo Nordisk Ltd)
Insulin aspart 30 unit per 1 ml, Insulin aspart (as Insulin aspart protamine) 70 unit per 1 ml NovoMix 30 FlexPen 100units/ml suspension for injection 3ml pre-filled pen | 5 pre-filled disposable injection PoM £29.89

▸ **NovoMix 30 Penfill** (Novo Nordisk Ltd)
Insulin aspart 30 unit per 1 ml, Insulin aspart (as Insulin aspart protamine) 70 unit per 1 ml NovoMix 30 Penfill 100units/ml suspension for injection 3ml cartridges | 5 cartridge PoM £28.79

F 422

Biphasic insulin lispro

(Intermediate-acting insulin)

● **INDICATIONS AND DOSE**
Diabetes mellitus
▸ BY SUBCUTANEOUS INJECTION
▸ Child: Administer up to 15 minutes before or soon after a meal, according to requirements

● **CAUTIONS** Children under 12 years (use only if benefit likely compared to soluble insulin)
● **INTERACTIONS** → Appendix 1 (antidiabetics).
● **SIDE-EFFECTS** Protamine may cause allergic reactions
● **PRESCRIBING AND DISPENSING INFORMATION** Check product container—the proportions of the two

components should be checked carefully (the order in which the proportions are stated may not be the same in other countries).

● MEDICINAL FORMS
There can be variation in the licensing of different medicines containing the same drug.
Suspension for injection
▸ Humalog Mix25 (Eli Lilly and Company Ltd)
  Insulin lispro 25 unit per 1 ml, Insulin lispro protamine) 75 unit per 1 ml Humalog Mix25 100units/ml suspension for injection 10ml vials | 1 vial PoM £16.61
  Humalog Mix25 100units/ml suspension for injection 3ml cartridges | 5 cartridge PoM £29.46
▸ Humalog Mix25 KwikPen (Eli Lilly and Company Ltd)
  Insulin lispro 25 unit per 1 ml, Insulin lispro (as Insulin lispro protamine) 75 unit per 1 ml Humalog Mix25 KwikPen 100units/ml suspension for injection 3ml pre-filled pen | 5 pre-filled disposable injection PoM £30.98
▸ Humalog Mix50 (Eli Lilly and Company Ltd)
  Insulin lispro 50 unit per 1 ml, Insulin lispro (as Insulin lispro protamine) 50 unit per 1 ml Humalog Mix50 100units/ml suspension for injection 3ml cartridges | 5 cartridge PoM £29.46
▸ Humalog Mix50 KwikPen (Eli Lilly and Company Ltd)
  Insulin lispro 50 unit per 1 ml, Insulin lispro (as Insulin lispro protamine) 50 unit per 1 ml Humalog Mix50 KwikPen 100units/ml suspension for injection 3ml pre-filled pen | 5 pre-filled disposable injection PoM £30.98

INSULINS > LONG-ACTING

F 422

Insulin degludec

(Recombinant human insulin analogue—long acting)

● INDICATIONS AND DOSE
Diabetes mellitus
▸ BY SUBCUTANEOUS INJECTION
▸ Child 1-17 years: Dose to be given according to requirements

● INTERACTIONS → Appendix 1 (antidiabetics).

● PREGNANCY Evidence of the safety of long-acting insulin analogues in pregnancy is limited, therefore isophane insulin is recommended where longer-acting insulins are needed; insulin detemir may also be considered.

● PRESCRIBING AND DISPENSING INFORMATION Insulin degludec (*Tresiba*®) is available in strengths of 100 units/mL (allows 1-unit dose adjustment) and 200 units/mL (allows 2-unit dose adjustment)—ensure correct strength prescribed.

● MEDICINAL FORMS
There can be variation in the licensing of different medicines containing the same drug.
Solution for injection
▸ Tresiba FlexTouch (Novo Nordisk Ltd) ▼
  Insulin human (as Insulin degludec) 100 unit per 1 ml Tresiba FlexTouch 100units/ml solution for injection 3ml pre-filled pen | 5 pre-filled disposable injection PoM £72.00
  Insulin human (as Insulin degludec) 200 unit per 1 ml Tresiba FlexTouch 200units/ml solution for injection 3ml pre-filled pen | 3 pre-filled disposable injection PoM £86.40
▸ Tresiba Penfill (Novo Nordisk Ltd) ▼
  Insulin human (as Insulin degludec) 100 unit per 1 ml Tresiba Penfill 100units/ml solution for injection 3ml cartridges | 5 cartridge PoM £72.00

F 422

Insulin detemir

(Recombinant human insulin analogue—long acting)

● INDICATIONS AND DOSE
Diabetes mellitus
▸ BY SUBCUTANEOUS INJECTION
▸ Child 2-17 years: According to requirements

● INTERACTIONS → Appendix 1 (antidiabetics).

● PREGNANCY Evidence of the safety of long-acting insulin analogues in pregnancy is limited, therefore isophane insulin p. 423 is recommended where longer-acting insulins are needed; insulin detemir may also be considered where longer-acting insulins are needed.

● MEDICINAL FORMS
There can be variation in the licensing of different medicines containing the same drug.
Solution for injection
▸ Levemir FlexPen (Novo Nordisk Ltd)
  Insulin human (as Insulin detemir) 100 unit per 1 ml Levemir FlexPen 100units/ml solution for injection 3ml pre-filled pen | 5 pre-filled disposable injection PoM £42.00
▸ Levemir InnoLet (Novo Nordisk Ltd)
  Insulin human (as Insulin detemir) 100 unit per 1 ml Levemir InnoLet 100units/ml solution for injection 3ml pre-filled pen | 5 pre-filled disposable injection PoM £44.85
▸ Levemir Penfill (Novo Nordisk Ltd)
  Insulin human (as Insulin detemir) 100 unit per 1 ml Levemir Penfill 100units/ml solution for injection 3ml cartridges | 5 cartridge PoM £42.00

F 422

Insulin glargine

(Recombinant human insulin analogue—long acting)

● INDICATIONS AND DOSE
Diabetes mellitus
▸ BY SUBCUTANEOUS INJECTION
▸ Child 2-17 years: According to requirements

● INTERACTIONS → Appendix 1 (antidiabetics).

● PREGNANCY Evidence of the safety of long-acting insulin analogues in pregnancy is limited, therefore isophane insulin is recommended where longer-acting insulins are needed; insulin detemir may also be considered.

● PRESCRIBING AND DISPENSING INFORMATION Products containing insulin glargine are not identical and although there should be no important differences in terms of safety and efficacy, when prescribing biological products it is good practice to use the brand name see *Biosimilar medicines*, under Guidance on prescribing p. 1. Dose adjustments and close metabolic monitoring is recommended if switching between insulin glargine preparations.

● NATIONAL FUNDING/ACCESS DECISIONS
Scottish Medicines Consortium (SMC) Decisions
The *Scottish Medicines Consortium* has advised that *Lantus*® preparations (April 2013) and *Toujeo*® (August 2015) are accepted for restricted use within NHS Scotland for the treatment of type 1 diabetes:
● in those who are at risk of or experience unacceptable frequency or severity of nocturnal hypoglycaemia on attempting to achieve better hypoglycaemic control during treatment with other insulins
● as a once daily insulin therapy for patients who require a carer to administer their insulin
  It is **not** recommended for routine use in patients with type 2 diabetes unless they suffer from recurrent

episodes of hypoglycaemia or require assistance with their insulin injections.

● **MEDICINAL FORMS**
There can be variation in the licensing of different medicines containing the same drug.

Solution for injection

▶ **Abasaglar** (Eli Lilly and Company Ltd) ▼
  Insulin human (as Insulin glargine) 100 unit per 1 ml Abasaglar 100units/ml solution for injection 3ml cartridges | 5 cartridge PoM £35.28

▶ **Abasaglar KwikPen** (Eli Lilly and Company Ltd) ▼
  Insulin human (as Insulin glargine) 100 unit per 1 ml Abasaglar KwikPen 100units/ml solution for injection 3ml pre-filled pen | 5 pre-filled disposable injection PoM £35.28

▶ **Lantus** (Sanofi)
  Insulin human (as Insulin glargine) 100 unit per 1 ml Lantus 100units/ml solution for injection 3ml cartridges | 5 cartridge PoM £41.50
  Lantus 100units/ml solution for injection 10ml vials | 1 vial PoM £30.68

▶ **Lantus SoloStar** (Sanofi)
  Insulin human (as Insulin glargine) 100 unit per 1 ml Lantus 100units/ml solution for injection 3ml pre-filled SoloStar pen | 5 pre-filled disposable injection PoM £41.50

▶ **Toujeo** (Sanofi)
  Insulin human (as Insulin glargine) 300 unit per 1 ml Toujeo 300units/ml solution for injection 1.5ml pre-filled SoloStar pen | 3 pre-filled disposable injection PoM £33.13

⌲ 422

Insulin zinc suspension

(Insulin zinc suspension (mixed)—long acting)

● **INDICATIONS AND DOSE**

Diabetes mellitus
▶ BY SUBCUTANEOUS INJECTION
▷ Child: According to requirements

● **INTERACTIONS** → Appendix 1 (antidiabetics).

● **PREGNANCY** Evidence of the safety of long-acting insulin analogues in pregnancy is limited, therefore isophane insulin p. 423 is recommended where longer-acting insulins are needed; insulin detemir p. 424 may also be considered.

● **PRESCRIBING AND DISPENSING INFORMATION** A sterile neutral suspension of bovine and/or porcine insulin or of human insulin in the form of a complex obtained by the addition of a suitable zinc salt; consists of rhombohedral crystals (10–40 microns) and of particles of no uniform shape (not exceeding 2 microns).

● **MEDICINAL FORMS**
There can be variation in the licensing of different medicines containing the same drug.

Suspension for injection

▶ **Hypurin Bovine Lente** (Wockhardt UK Ltd)
  Insulin bovine (as Insulin zinc suspension mixed bovine) 100 unit per 1 ml Hypurin Bovine Lente 100units/ml suspension for injection 10ml vials | 1 vial PoM £27.72

⌲ 422

Protamine zinc insulin

(Protamine zinc insulin injection—long acting)

● **INDICATIONS AND DOSE**

Diabetes mellitus
▶ BY SUBCUTANEOUS INJECTION
▷ Child: According to requirements

● **INTERACTIONS** → Appendix 1 (antidiabetics).

● **SIDE-EFFECTS** Protamine may cause allergic reactions

● **PREGNANCY** Evidence of the safety of long-acting insulin analogues in pregnancy is limited, therefore isophane

insulin p. 423 is recommended where longer-acting insulins are needed; insulin detemir p. 424 may also be considered.

● **PRESCRIBING AND DISPENSING INFORMATION** A sterile suspension of insulin in the form of a complex obtained by the addition of a suitable protamine and zinc chloride; this preparation was included in BP 1980 but is not included in BP 1988.

● **MEDICINAL FORMS**
There can be variation in the licensing of different medicines containing the same drug.

Suspension for injection

▶ **Hypurin Bovine Protamine Zinc** (Wockhardt UK Ltd)
  Insulin bovine (as Insulin protamine zinc bovine) 100 unit per 1 ml Hypurin Bovine Protamine Zinc 100units/ml suspension for injection 10ml vials | 1 vial PoM £27.72

INSULINS 〉 RAPID-ACTING

⌲ 422

Insulin

(Insulin Injection; Neutral Insulin; Soluble Insulin—short acting)

● **INDICATIONS AND DOSE**

Diabetes mellitus
▶ BY SUBCUTANEOUS INJECTION
▷ Child: According to requirements

Hyperglycaemia during illness
▶ BY INTRAVENOUS INFUSION
▷ Neonate: 0.02–0.125 unit/kg/hour, dose to be adjusted according to blood-glucose concentration.

▷ Child: 0.025–0.1 unit/kg/hour, dose to be adjusted according to blood-glucose concentration.

Neonatal hyperglycaemia | Neonatal diabetes
▶ BY INTRAVENOUS INFUSION
▷ Neonate: 0.02–0.125 unit/kg/hour, dose to be adjusted according to blood-glucose concentration.

Diabetic ketoacidosis | Diabetes during surgery
▶ BY INTRAVENOUS INFUSION
▷ Child: (consult local protocol)

● **INTERACTIONS** → Appendix 1 (antidiabetics).

● **DIRECTIONS FOR ADMINISTRATION** Short-acting injectable insulins can be given by continuous subcutaneous infusion using a portable infusion pump. This device delivers a continuous basal insulin infusion and patient-activated bolus doses at meal times. This technique can be useful for patients who suffer recurrent hypoglycaemia or marked morning rise in blood-glucose concentration despite optimised multiple-injection regimens. Patients on subcutaneous insulin infusion must be highly motivated, able to monitor their blood-glucose concentration, and have expert training, advice and supervision from an experienced healthcare team. Some insulin preparations are not recommended for use in subcutaneous insulin infusion pumps—may precipitate in catheter or needle—consult product literature.

▷ With intravenous use For *intravenous infusion*, dilute to a concentration of 1 unit/mL with Sodium Chloride 0.9% and mix thoroughly; insulin may be adsorbed by plastics, flush giving set with 5 mL of infusion fluid containing insulin. *For intravenous infusion in neonatal intensive care*, dilute 5 units to a final volume of 50 mL with Sodium Chloride 0.9% and mix thoroughly; an intravenous infusion rate of 0.1 mL/kg/hour provides a dose of 0.01 units/kg/hour.

● **PRESCRIBING AND DISPENSING INFORMATION** A sterile solution of insulin (i.e. bovine or porcine) or of human insulin; pH 6.6–8.0.

- **NATIONAL FUNDING/ACCESS DECISIONS**

NICE technology appraisals (TAs)

▸ Continuous subcutaneous insulin infusion for the treatment of diabetes mellitus (type 1) (July 2008) NICE TA151

Continuous subcutaneous insulin infusion is recommended as an option in children over 12 years with type 1 diabetes:

- who suffer repeated or unpredictable hypoglycaemia, whilst attempting to achieve optimal glycaemic control with multiple-injection regimens, **or**
- whose glycaemic control remains inadequate (HbA$_{1c}$ over 8.5% [69 mmol/mol]) despite optimised multiple-injection regimens (including the use of long-acting insulin analogues where appropriate).

Continuous subcutaneous insulin infusion is also recommended as an option for children under 12 years with type 1 diabetes for whom multiple-injection regimens are considered impractical or inappropriate. Children on insulin pumps should undergo a trial of multiple-injection therapy between the ages of 12 and 18 years.
www.nice.org.uk/TA151

- **MEDICINAL FORMS**
There can be variation in the licensing of different medicines containing the same drug. Forms available from special-order manufacturers include: solution for injection, solution for infusion

Solution for injection

▸ Insulin (Non-proprietary)

Insulin human 100 unit per 1 ml Humulin R 100units/ml solution for injection 10ml vials | 1 vial PoM no price available

Insulin human 500 unit per 1 ml Humulin R 500units/ml solution for injection 20ml vials | 1 vial PoM no price available

▸ Actrapid (Novo Nordisk Ltd)

Insulin human (as Insulin soluble human) 100 unit per 1 ml Actrapid 100units/ml solution for injection 10ml vials | 1 vial PoM £7.48

▸ Humulin S (Eli Lilly and Company Ltd)

Insulin human (as Insulin soluble human) 100 unit per 1 ml Humulin S 100units/ml solution for injection 10ml vials | 1 vial PoM £15.68

Humulin S 100units/ml solution for injection 3ml cartridges | 5 cartridge PoM £19.08

▸ Hypurin Bovine Neutral (Wockhardt UK Ltd)

Insulin bovine (as Insulin soluble bovine) 100 unit per 1 ml Hypurin Bovine Neutral 100units/ml solution for injection 10ml vials | 1 vial PoM £27.72

Hypurin Bovine Neutral 100units/ml solution for injection 3ml cartridges | 5 cartridge PoM £41.58

▸ Hypurin Porcine Neutral (Wockhardt UK Ltd)

Insulin porcine (as Insulin soluble porcine) 100 unit per 1 ml Hypurin Porcine Neutral 100units/ml solution for injection 10ml vials | 1 vial PoM £25.20

Hypurin Porcine Neutral 100units/ml solution for injection 3ml cartridges | 5 cartridge PoM £37.80

▸ Insuman Infusat (Sanofi)

Insulin human 100 unit per 1 ml Insuman Infusat 100units/ml solution for injection 3.15ml cartridges | 5 cartridge PoM £250.00

Insuman Infusat 100units/ml solution for injection 10ml vials | 3 vial PoM £250.00

▸ Insuman Rapid (Sanofi)

Insulin human (as Insulin soluble human) 100 unit per 1 ml Insuman Rapid 100units/ml solution for injection 3ml cartridges | 5 cartridge PoM £17.50

▸ 422

Insulin aspart

(Recombinant human insulin analogue—short acting)

- **INDICATIONS AND DOSE**

Diabetes mellitus

▸ BY SUBCUTANEOUS INJECTION

▸ Child 1 month–1 year: Administer immediately before meals or when necessary shortly after meals, according to requirements

▸ Child 2–17 years: Administer immediately before meals or when necessary shortly after meals, according to requirements

▸ BY SUBCUTANEOUS INFUSION, OR BY INTRAVENOUS INFUSION, OR BY INTRAVENOUS INJECTION

▸ Child 1 month–1 year: According to requirements

▸ Child 2–17 years: According to requirements

- **UNLICENSED USE** Not licensed for use in children under 2 years.

- **INTERACTIONS** → Appendix 1 (antidiabetics).

- **PREGNANCY** Not known to be harmful—may be used during pregnancy.

- **BREAST FEEDING** Not known to be harmful—may be used during lactation.

- **DIRECTIONS FOR ADMINISTRATION** Short-acting injectable insulins can be given by continuous subcutaneous infusion using a portable infusion pump. This device delivers a continuous basal insulin infusion and patient-activated bolus doses at meal times. This technique can be useful for patients who suffer recurrent hypoglycaemia or marked morning rise in blood-glucose concentration despite optimised multiple-injection regimens. Patients on subcutaneous insulin infusion must be highly motivated, able to monitor their blood-glucose concentration, and have expert training, advice and supervision from an experienced healthcare team.

▸ With intravenous use For *intravenous infusion*, dilute to a concentration of 0.05–1 unit/mL with Glucose 5% or Sodium Chloride 0.9% and mix thoroughly; insulin may be adsorbed by plastics, flush giving set with 5 mL of infusion fluid containing insulin.

- **NATIONAL FUNDING/ACCESS DECISIONS**

NICE technology appraisals (TAs)

▸ Continuous subcutaneous insulin infusion for the treatment of diabetes mellitus (type 1) (July 2008) NICE TA151

Continuous subcutaneous insulin infusion is recommended as an option in children over 12 years with type 1 diabetes:

- who suffer repeated or unpredictable hypoglycaemia, whilst attempting to achieve optimal glycaemic control with multiple-injection regimens, **or**
- whose glycaemic control remains inadequate (HbA$_{1c}$ over 8.5% [69 mmol/mol]) despite optimised multiple-injection regimens (including the use of long-acting insulin analogues where appropriate).

Continuous subcutaneous insulin infusion is also recommended as an option for children under 12 years with type 1 diabetes for whom multiple-injection regimens are considered impractical or inappropriate. Children on insulin pumps should undergo a trial of multiple-injection therapy between the ages of 12 and 18 years.
www.nice.org.uk/TA151

● **MEDICINAL FORMS**
There can be variation in the licensing of different medicines containing the same drug.

Solution for injection

▸ **NovoRapid** (Novo Nordisk Ltd)
Insulin aspart 100 unit per 1 ml NovoRapid 100units/ml solution for injection 10ml vials | 1 vial PoM £14.08

▸ **NovoRapid FlexPen** (Novo Nordisk Ltd)
Insulin aspart 100 unit per 1 ml NovoRapid FlexPen 100units/ml solution for injection 3ml pre-filled pen | 5 pre-filled disposable injection PoM £30.60

▸ **NovoRapid FlexTouch** (Novo Nordisk Ltd)
Insulin aspart 100 unit per 1 ml NovoRapid FlexTouch 100units/ml solution for injection 3ml pre-filled pen | 5 pre-filled disposable injection PoM £32.13

▸ **NovoRapid Penfill** (Novo Nordisk Ltd)
Insulin aspart 100 unit per 1 ml NovoRapid Penfill 100units/ml solution for injection 3ml cartridges | 5 cartridge PoM £28.31

▸ **NovoRapid PumpCart** (Novo Nordisk Ltd)
Insulin aspart 100 unit per 1 ml NovoRapid PumpCart 100units/ml solution for injection 1.6ml cartridges | 5 cartridge PoM £15.10

⬥ 422

Insulin glulisine

(Recombinant human insulin analogue–short acting)

● **INDICATIONS AND DOSE**

Diabetes mellitus

▸ BY SUBCUTANEOUS INJECTION

▸ Child: Administer immediately before meals or when necessary shortly after meals, according to requirements

▸ BY SUBCUTANEOUS INFUSION, OR BY INTRAVENOUS INFUSION

▸ Child: According to requirements

● **UNLICENSED USE** Not licensed for children under 6 years.

● **INTERACTIONS** → Appendix 1 (antidiabetics).

● **DIRECTIONS FOR ADMINISTRATION** Short-acting injectable insulins can be given by continuous subcutaneous infusion using a portable infusion pump. This device delivers a continuous basal insulin infusion and patient-activated bolus doses at meal times. This technique can be useful for patients who suffer recurrent hypoglycaemia or marked morning rise in blood-glucose concentration despite optimised multiple-injection regimens. Patients on subcutaneous insulin infusion must be highly motivated, able to monitor their blood-glucose concentration, and have expert training, advice and supervision from an experienced healthcare team.

● **NATIONAL FUNDING/ACCESS DECISIONS**

NICE technology appraisals (TAs)

▸ Continuous subcutaneous insulin infusion for the treatment of diabetes mellitus (type 1) (July 2008) NICE TA151
Continuous subcutaneous insulin infusion is recommended as an option in children over 12 years with type 1 diabetes:

● who suffer repeated or unpredictable hypoglycaemia, whilst attempting to achieve optimal glycaemic control with multiple-injection regimens, **or**

● whose glycaemic control remains inadequate (HbA$_{1c}$ over 8.5% [69 mmol/mol]) despite optimised multiple-injection regimens (including the use of long-acting insulin analogues where appropriate).

Continuous subcutaneous insulin infusion is also recommended as an option for children under 12 years with type 1 diabetes for whom multiple-injection regimens are considered impractical or inappropriate. Children on insulin pumps should undergo a trial of multiple-injection therapy between the ages of 12 and 18 years.
www.nice.org.uk/TA151

Scottish Medicines Consortium (SMC) Decisions
The *Scottish Medicines Consortium* has advised (October 2008) that *Apidra*® is accepted for restricted use within NHS Scotland for the treatment of adults and children over 6 years with diabetes mellitus in whom the use of a short-acting insulin analogue is appropriate.

● **MEDICINAL FORMS**
There can be variation in the licensing of different medicines containing the same drug.

Solution for injection

▸ **Apidra** (Sanofi)
Insulin glulisine 100 unit per 1 ml Apidra 100units/ml solution for injection 10ml vials | 1 vial PoM £16.00
Apidra 100units/ml solution for injection 3ml cartridges | 5 cartridge PoM £28.30

▸ **Apidra SoloStar** (Sanofi)
Insulin glulisine 100 unit per 1 ml Apidra 100units/ml solution for injection 3ml pre-filled SoloStar pen | 5 pre-filled disposable injection PoM £28.30

⬥ 422

Insulin lispro

(Recombinant human insulin analogue–short acting)

● **INDICATIONS AND DOSE**

Diabetes mellitus

▸ BY SUBCUTANEOUS INJECTION

▸ Child 1 month–1 year: Administer shortly before meals or when necessary shortly after meals, according to requirements

▸ Child 2–17 years: Administer shortly before meals or when necessary shortly after meals, according to requirements

▸ BY SUBCUTANEOUS INFUSION, OR BY INTRAVENOUS INFUSION, OR BY INTRAVENOUS INJECTION

▸ Child 1 month–1 year: According to requirements

▸ Child 2–17 years: According to requirements

● **UNLICENSED USE** Not licensed for use in children under 2 years.

● **CAUTIONS** Children under 12 years (use only if benefit likely compared to soluble insulin)

● **INTERACTIONS** → Appendix 1 (antidiabetics).

● **PREGNANCY** Not known to be harmful—may be used during pregnancy.

● **BREAST FEEDING** Not known to be harmful—may be used during lactation.

● **DIRECTIONS FOR ADMINISTRATION** Short-acting injectable insulins can be given by continuous subcutaneous infusion using a portable infusion pump. This device delivers a continuous basal insulin infusion and patient-activated bolus doses at meal times. This technique can be useful for patients who suffer recurrent hypoglycaemia or marked morning rise in blood-glucose concentration despite optimised multiple-injection regimens (see also NICE guidance, below). Patients on subcutaneous insulin infusion must be highly motivated, able to monitor their blood-glucose concentration, and have expert training, advice and supervision from an experienced healthcare team.

▸ With intravenous use For *intravenous infusion*, dilute to a concentration of 0.1–1 unit/mL with Glucose 5% or Sodium Chloride 0.9% and mix thoroughly; insulin may be adsorbed by plastics, flush giving set with 5 mL of infusion fluid containing insulin.

● NATIONAL FUNDING/ACCESS DECISIONS
NICE technology appraisals (TAs)
▶ **Continuous subcutaneous insulin infusion for the treatment of diabetes mellitus (type 1) (July 2008)** NICE TA151

Continuous subcutaneous insulin infusion is recommended as an option in children over 12 years with type 1 diabetes:

- who suffer repeated or unpredictable hypoglycaemia, whilst attempting to achieve optimal glycaemic control with multiple-injection regimens, **or**
- whose glycaemic control remains inadequate (HbA$_{1c}$ over 8.5% [69 mmol/mol]) despite optimised multiple-injection regimens (including the use of long-acting insulin analogues where appropriate).

Continuous subcutaneous insulin infusion is also recommended as an option for children under 12 years with type 1 diabetes for whom multiple-injection regimens are considered impractical or inappropriate. Children on insulin pumps should undergo a trial of multiple-injection therapy between the ages of 12 and 18 years.
www.nice.org.uk/TA151

● MEDICINAL FORMS
There can be variation in the licensing of different medicines containing the same drug.

Solution for injection
▶ Humalog (Eli Lilly and Company Ltd)
Insulin lispro 100 unit per 1 ml Humalog 100units/ml solution for injection 10ml vials | 1 vial PoM £16.61
Humalog 100units/ml solution for injection 3ml cartridges | 5 cartridge PoM £28.31
▶ Humalog KwikPen (Eli Lilly and Company Ltd)
Insulin lispro 100 unit per 1 ml Humalog KwikPen 100units/ml solution for injection 3ml pre-filled pen | 5 pre-filled disposable injection PoM £29.46
Insulin lispro 200 unit per 1 ml Humalog KwikPen 200units/ml solution for injection 3ml pre-filled pen | 5 pre-filled disposable injection PoM £58.92

3.1a Diabetes, diagnosis and monitoring

Diabetes mellitus, diagnostic and monitoring devices

Urinalysis

Reagent strips are available for measuring for glucose in the urine. Tests for ketones by patients are rarely required unless they become unwell—see Blood Monitoring.

Microalbuminuria can be detected with *Micral-Test II* ® but this should be followed by confirmation in the laboratory, since false positive results are common.

Blood monitoring

Blood glucose monitoring using a meter gives a direct measure of the glucose concentration at the time of the test and can detect hypoglycaemia as well as hyperglycaemia. Carers and children should be properly trained in the use of blood glucose monitoring systems and the appropriate action to take on the results obtained. Inadequate understanding of the normal fluctuations in blood glucose can lead to confusion and inappropriate action.

Children using multiple injection regimens should understand how to adjust their insulin dose according to their carbohydrate intake. With fixed-dose insulin regimens, the carbohydrate intake needs to be regulated, and should be distributed throughout the day to match the insulin regimen.

In the UK blood-glucose concentration is expressed in mmol/litre and Diabetes UK advises that these units should be used for self-monitoring of blood glucose. In other European countries units of mg/100 mL (or mg/dL) are commonly used.

It is advisable to check that the meter is pre-set in the correct units.

If the blood glucose level is high or if the child is unwell, blood **ketones** should be measured according to local guidelines in order to detect diabetic ketoacidosis. Children and their carers should be trained in the use of blood ketone monitoring systems and to take appropriate action on the results obtained, including when to seek medical attention.

Oral glucose tolerance test

The oral glucose tolerance test is used mainly for diagnosis of impaired glucose tolerance; it is not recommended or necessary for routine diagnostic use when severe symptoms of hyperglycaemia are present. However, it is used for the investigation of insulin resistance, glycogen storage disease, and excessive growth hormone secretion. In children who have less severe symptoms and blood-glucose concentrations that do not establish or exclude diabetes (e.g. impaired fasting glycaemia), an oral glucose tolerance test may be required.Glucose is used to establish the presence of gestational diabetes; this generally involves giving anhydrous glucose by mouth to the fasting patient, and measuring blood-glucose concentration at intervals. The appropriate amount of glucose should be given with 200–300 mL fluid. Alternatively anhydrous glucose can be given as 113 mL *Polycal* ® with extra fluid to administer a total volume of 200–300 mL, or as *Rapilose* ® *OGTT* oral solution.

▌ Blood monitoring test strips

● BLOOD GLUCOSE TESTING STRIPS

Active testing strips (Roche Diabetes Care Ltd)
50 strip · NHS indicative price = £9.95 · Drug Tariff (Part IXr)

Advocate Redi-Code+ testing strips (Diabetes Care Technology Ltd)
50 strip · NHS indicative price = £9.95 · Drug Tariff (Part IXr)

AutoSense testing strips (Advance Diagnostic Products (NI) Ltd)
25 strip · NHS indicative price = £4.50 · Drug Tariff (Part IXr)

Aviva testing strips (Roche Diabetes Care Ltd)
50 strip · NHS indicative price = £15.79 · Drug Tariff (Part IXr)

BGStar testing strips (Sanofi)
50 strip · NHS indicative price = £14.73 · Drug Tariff (Part IXr)

Betachek C50 cassette (National Diagnostic Products)
100 device · NHS indicative price = £29.98 · Drug Tariff (Part IXr)

Betachek G5 testing strips (National Diagnostic Products)
50 strip · NHS indicative price = £14.19 · Drug Tariff (Part IXr)

Betachek Visual testing strips (National Diagnostic Products)
50 strip · NHS indicative price = £6.80 · Drug Tariff (Part IXr)

Breeze 2 testing discs (Bayer Plc)
50 strip · NHS indicative price = £15.00 · Drug Tariff (Part IXr)

CareSens N testing strips (Spirit Healthcare Ltd)
50 strip · NHS indicative price = £12.75 · Drug Tariff (Part IXr)

Compact testing strips (Roche Diabetes Care Ltd)
51 strip · NHS indicative price = £16.22 · Drug Tariff (Part IXr)

Contour Next testing strips (Bayer Diagnostics Manufacturing Ltd)
50 strip · NHS indicative price = £15.04 · Drug Tariff (Part IXr)

Contour TS testing strips (Bayer Diagnostics Manufacturing Ltd)
50 strip · NHS indicative price = £9.50 · Drug Tariff (Part IXr)

Contour testing strips (Bayer Diagnostics Manufacturing Ltd)
50 strip · NHS indicative price = £9.95 · Drug Tariff (Part IXr)

Dario Lite testing strips (LabStyle Innovations Ltd)
50 strip · NHS indicative price = £9.95 · Drug Tariff (Part IXr)

Dario testing strips (LabStyle Innovations Ltd)
50 strip · NHS indicative price = £14.95 · Drug Tariff (Part IXr)

Diastix testing strips (Bayer Diagnostics Manufacturing Ltd)
50 strip · NHS indicative price = £2.89 · Drug Tariff (Part IXr)

Element testing strips (Neon Diagnostics Ltd)
50 strip · NHS indicative price = £9.89 · Drug Tariff (Part IXr)

Meters and test strips

Meter (all [NHS])	Type of monitoring	Compatible test strips	Test strip net price	Sensitivity range (mmol/litre)	Manufacturer
Accu-Chek® Active	Blood glucose	Active®	50 strip = £9.95	0.6-33.3 mmol/litre	Roche Diabetes Care Ltd
Accu-Chek® Advantage Meter no longer available	Blood glucose	Advantage Plus®	50 strip = £0.00	0.6-33.3 mmol/litre	Roche Diabetes Care Ltd
Accu-Chek® Aviva	Blood glucose	Aviva®	50 strip = £15.79	0.6-33.3 mmol/litre	Roche Diabetes Care Ltd
Accu-Chek® Aviva Expert	Blood glucose	Aviva®	50 strip = £15.79	0.6-33.3 mmol/litre	Roche Diabetes Care Ltd
Accu-Chek® Compact Plus Meter no longer available	Blood glucose	Compact®	3 × 17 strips = £16.22	0.6-33.3 mmol/litre	Roche Diabetes Care Ltd
Accu-Chek® Mobile	Blood glucose	Mobile®	100 device = £32.48	0.3-33.3 mmol/litre	Roche Diabetes Care Ltd
Accu-Chek® Aviva Nano	Blood glucose	Aviva®	50 strip = £15.79	0.6-33.3 mmol/litre	Roche Diabetes Care Ltd
BGStar® Free of charge from diabetes healthcare professionals	Blood glucose	BGStar®	50 strip = £14.73	1.1-33.3 mmol/litre	Sanofi
Breeze 2®	Blood glucose	Breeze 2®	50 strip = £15.00	0.6-33.3 mmol/litre	Bayer Plc
CareSens N® Free of charge from diabetes healthcare professionals	Blood glucose	CareSens N®	50 strip = £12.75	1.1-33.3 mmol/litre	Spirit Healthcare Ltd
Contour®	Blood glucose	Contour®	50 strip = £9.95	0.6-33.3 mmol/litre	Bayer Diagnostics Manufacturing Ltd
Contour® XT	Blood glucose	Contour® Next	50 strip = £15.04	0.6-33.3 mmol/litre	Bayer Diagnostics Manufacturing Ltd
Element®	Blood glucose	Element®	50 strip = £9.89	0.55-33.3 mmol/litre	Neon Diagnostics Ltd
FreeStyle® Meter no longer available	Blood glucose	FreeStyle®	50 strip = £15.81	1.1-27.8 mmol/litre	Abbott Laboratories Ltd
FreeStyle Freedom® Meter no longer available	Blood glucose	FreeStyle®	50 strip = £15.81	1.1-27.8 mmol/litre	Abbott Laboratories Ltd
FreeStyle Freedom Lite®	Blood glucose	FreeStyle Lite®	50 strip = £15.80	1.1-27.8 mmol/litre	Abbott Laboratories Ltd
FreeStyle InsuLinx®	Blood glucose	FreeStyle Lite®	50 strip = £15.80	1.1-27.8 mmol/litre	Abbott Laboratories Ltd
FreeStyle Lite®	Blood glucose	FreeStyle Lite®	50 strip = £15.80	1.1-27.8 mmol/litre	Abbott Laboratories Ltd
FreeStyle Mini® Meter no longer available	Blood glucose	FreeStyle®	50 strip = £15.81	1.1-27.8 mmol/litre	Abbott Laboratories Ltd
FreeStyle Optium®	Blood glucose	FreeStyle Optium®	50 strip = £15.71	1.1-27.8 mmol/litre	Abbott Laboratories Ltd
FreeStyle Optium®	Blood ketones	FreeStyle Optium® β-ketone	10 strip = £21.14	0-8.0 mmol/litre	Abbott Laboratories Ltd
FreeStyle Optium Neo®	Blood glucose	FreeStyle Optium®	50 strip = £15.71	1.1-27.8 mmol/litre	Abbott Laboratories Ltd
FreeStyle Optium Neo®	Blood ketones	FreeStyle Optium® β-ketone	10 strip = £21.14	0-8.0 mmol/litre	Abbott Laboratories Ltd
GlucoDock® module For use with iPhone®, iPod touch®, and iPad®	Blood glucose	GlucoDock®	50 strip = £14.90	1.1-33.3 mmol/litre	Medisana Healthcare (UK) Ltd

6

Endocrine system

Endocrine system

6

Meter (all [NHS])	Type of monitoring	Compatible test strips	Test strip net price	Sensitivity range (mmol/litre)	Manufacturer
GlucoLab®	Blood glucose	GlucoLab®	50 strip = £9.89	0.55–33.3 mmol/litre	Neon Diagnostics Ltd
GlucoMen® GM	Blood glucose	GlucoMen® GM	50 strip = £9.95	0.6–33.3 mmol/litre	A Menarini Diagnostics Ltd
GlucoMen® LX	Blood glucose	GlucoMen® LX Sensor	50 strip = £15.59	1.1–33.3 mmol/litre	A Menarini Diagnostics Ltd
GlucoMen® LX Plus	Blood glucose	GlucoMen® LX Sensor	50 strip = £15.59	1.1–33.3 mmol/litre	A Menarini Diagnostics Ltd
GlucoMen® LX Plus	Blood ketones	GlucoMen® LX Ketone	10 strip = £20.84	0–0.8 mmol/litre	A Menarini Diagnostics Ltd
GlucoMen® Visio	Blood glucose	GlucoMen® Visio Sensor	50 strip = £15.75	1.1–33.3 mmol/litre	A Menarini Diagnostics Ltd
GlucoRx® Free of charge from diabetes healthcare professionals	Blood glucose	GlucoRx®	50 strip = £9.45	1.1–33.3 mmol/litre	GlucoRx Ltd
GlucoRx Nexus® Free of charge from diabetes healthcare professionals	Blood glucose	GlucoRx Nexus®	50 strip = £9.95	1.1–33.3 mmol/litre	GlucoRx Ltd
Glucotrend® Meter no longer available	Blood glucose	Active®	50 strip = £9.95	0.6–33.3 mmol/litre	Roche Diabetes Care Ltd
iBGStar®	Blood glucose	BGStar®	50 strip = £14.73	1.1–33.3 mmol/litre	Sanofi
IME-DC®	Blood glucose	IME-DC®	50 strip = £14.10	1.1–33.3 mmol/litre	Arctic Medical Ltd
Mendor Discreet®	Blood glucose	Mendor Discreet®	50 strip = £14.75	1.1–33.3 mmol/litre	SpringMed Solutions Ltd
Microdot®+ Free of charge from diabetes healthcare professionals	Blood glucose	Microdot®+	50 strip = £9.49	1.1–29.2 mmol/litre	Cambridge Sensors Ltd
MyGlucoHealth®	Blood glucose	MyGlucoHealth®	50 strip = £15.50	0.6–33.3 mmol/litre	Entra Health Systems Ltd
Omnitest® 3	Blood glucose	Omnitest® 3	50 strip = £9.89	0.6–33.3 mmol/litre	B.Braun Medical Ltd
One Touch Ultra® Meter no longer available	Blood glucose	One Touch Ultra®	50 strip = £9.99	1.1–33.3 mmol/litre	LifeScan
One Touch Ultra 2® Free of charge from diabetes healthcare professionals	Blood glucose	One Touch Ultra®	50 strip = £9.99	1.1–33.3 mmol/litre	LifeScan
One Touch UltraEasy® Free of charge from diabetes healthcare professionals	Blood glucose	One Touch Ultra®	50 strip = £9.99	1.1–33.3 mmol/litre	LifeScan
One Touch UltraSmart® Free of charge from diabetes healthcare professionals	Blood glucose	One Touch Ultra®	50 strip = £9.99	1.1–33.3 mmol/litre	LifeScan
One Touch® VerioPro Free of charge from diabetes healthcare professionals	Blood glucose	One Touch® Verio	50 strip = £15.12	1.1–33.3 mmol/litre	LifeScan
One Touch® Vita Free of charge from diabetes healthcare professionals	Blood glucose	One Touch® Vita	50 strip = £15.07	1.1–33.3 mmol/litre	LifeScan
SD CodeFree®	Blood glucose	SD CodeFree®	50 strip = £6.99	0.6–33.3 mmol/litre	SD Biosensor Inc
Sensocard Plus® Meter no longer available	Blood glucose	Sensocard®	50 strip = £16.30	1.1–33.3 mmol/litre	BBI Healthcare Ltd

Meter (all NHS)	Type of monitoring	Compatible test strips	Test strip net price	Sensitivity range (mmol/litre)	Manufacturer
SuperCheck2® Free of charge from diabetes healthcare professionals	Blood glucose	SuperCheck2®	50 strip = £8.49	1.1–33.3 mmol/litre	Apollo Medical Technologies Ltd
TRUEone® All-in-one test strips and meter	Blood glucose	TRUEone®	50 strip = £14.99	1.1–33.3 mmol/litre	Nipro Diagnostics (UK) Ltd
TRUEresult® Free of charge from diabetes healthcare professionals	Blood glucose	TRUEresult®	50 strip = £14.99	1.1–33.3 mmol/litre	Nipro Diagnostics (UK) Ltd
TRUEresult twist® Free of charge from diabetes healthcare professionals	Blood glucose	TRUEresult®	50 strip = £14.99	1.1–33.3 mmol/litre	Nipro Diagnostics (UK) Ltd
TRUEtrack® Free of charge from diabetes healthcare professionals	Blood glucose	TRUEtrack®	50 strip = £14.99	1.1–33.3 mmol/litre	Nipro Diagnostics (UK) Ltd
TRUEyou mini®	Blood glucose	TRUEyou®	50 strip = £9.92	1.1–33.3 mmol/litre	Nipro Diagnostics (UK) Ltd
WaveSense JAZZ® Free of charge from diabetes healthcare professionals	Blood glucose	WaveSense JAZZ®	50 strip = £9.87	1.1–33.3 mmol/litre	AgaMatrix Europe Ltd

6

Endocrine system

Finetest Lite testing strips (Neon Diagnostics Ltd)
50 strip · NHS indicative price = £7.86 · Drug Tariff (Part IXr)

FreeStyle Lite testing strips (Abbott Laboratories Ltd)
50 strip · NHS indicative price = £15.80 · Drug Tariff (Part IXr)

FreeStyle Optium testing strips (Abbott Laboratories Ltd)
50 strip · NHS indicative price = £15.71 · Drug Tariff (Part IXr)

FreeStyle testing strips (Abbott Laboratories Ltd)
50 strip · NHS indicative price = £15.81 · Drug Tariff (Part IXr)

GluNEO testing strips (Neon Diagnostics Ltd)
50 strip · NHS indicative price = £9.89 · Drug Tariff (Part IXr)

GlucoDock testing strips (Medisana Healthcare (UK) Ltd)
50 strip · NHS indicative price = £14.90 · Drug Tariff (Part IXr)

GlucoLab testing strips (Neon Diagnostics Ltd)
50 strip · NHS indicative price = £9.89 · Drug Tariff (Part IXr)

GlucoMen GM testing strips (A Menarini Diagnostics Ltd)
50 strip · NHS indicative price = £9.95 · Drug Tariff (Part IXr)

GlucoMen LX Sensor testing strips (A Menarini Diagnostics Ltd)
50 strip · NHS indicative price = £15.59 · Drug Tariff (Part IXr)

GlucoMen Sensor testing strips (A Menarini Diagnostics Ltd)
50 strip · NHS indicative price = £14.83 · Drug Tariff (Part IXr)

GlucoMen Visio testing strips (A Menarini Diagnostics Ltd)
50 strip · NHS indicative price = £15.75 · Drug Tariff (Part IXr)

GlucoMen areo Sensor testing strips (A Menarini Diagnostics Ltd)
50 strip · NHS indicative price = £9.95 · Drug Tariff (Part IXr)

GlucoNavii testing strips (Neon Diagnostics Ltd)
50 strip · NHS indicative price = £8.95 · Drug Tariff (Part IXr)

GlucoRx GO testing strips (GlucoRx Ltd)
50 strip · NHS indicative price = £9.95 · Drug Tariff (Part IXr)

GlucoRx HCT Glucose testing strips (GlucoRx Ltd)
50 strip · NHS indicative price = £13.95 · Drug Tariff (Part IXr)

GlucoRx Nexus testing strips (GlucoRx Ltd)
50 strip · NHS indicative price = £9.95 · Drug Tariff (Part IXr)

GlucoRx Original testing strips (GlucoRx Ltd)
50 strip · NHS indicative price = £9.45 · Drug Tariff (Part IXr)

GlucoZen.auto testing strips (GlucoZen Ltd)
50 strip · NHS indicative price = £7.64 · Drug Tariff (Part IXr)

Glucoflex-R testing strips (Bio-Diagnostics Ltd)
50 strip · NHS indicative price = £6.75 · Drug Tariff (Part IXr)

IME-DC testing strips (Arctic Medical Ltd)
50 strip · NHS indicative price = £14.10 · Drug Tariff (Part IXr)

MODZ testing strips (Modz Oy)
50 strip · NHS indicative price = £14.00 · Drug Tariff (Part IXr)

Medi-Test Glucose testing strips (BHR Pharmaceuticals Ltd)
50 strip · NHS indicative price = £2.33 · Drug Tariff (Part IXr)

MediSense SoftSense testing strips (Abbott Laboratories Ltd)
50 strip · NHS indicative price = £15.05 · Drug Tariff (Part IXr)

MediTouch 2 testing strips (Medisana Healthcare (UK) Ltd)
50 strip · NHS indicative price = £12.49 · Drug Tariff (Part IXr)

MediTouch testing strips (Medisana Healthcare (UK) Ltd)
50 strip · NHS indicative price = £14.90 · Drug Tariff (Part IXr)

Mendor Discreet testing strips (SpringMed Solutions Ltd)
50 strip · NHS indicative price = £14.75 · Drug Tariff (Part IXr)

Microdot+ testing strips (Cambridge Sensors Ltd)
50 strip · NHS indicative price = £9.49 · Drug Tariff (Part IXr)

Mission Glucose testing strips (Spirit Healthcare Ltd)
50 strip · NHS indicative price = £2.29 · Drug Tariff (Part IXr)

Mobile cassette (Roche Diabetes Care Ltd)
100 device · NHS indicative price = £32.48 · Drug Tariff (Part IXr)

Myglucohealth testing strips (Entra Health Systems Ltd)
50 strip · NHS indicative price = £15.50 · Drug Tariff (Part IXr)

Mylife Pura testing strips (Ypsomed Ltd)
50 strip · NHS indicative price = £9.50 · Drug Tariff (Part IXr)

Mylife Unio testing strips (Ypsomed Ltd)
50 strip · NHS indicative price = £9.50 · Drug Tariff (Part IXr)

Omnitest 3 testing strips (B.Braun Medical Ltd)
50 strip · NHS indicative price = £9.89 · Drug Tariff (Part IXr)

On-Call Advanced testing strips (Point Of Care Testing Ltd)
50 strip · NHS indicative price = £13.65 · Drug Tariff (Part IXr)

OneTouch Select Plus testing strips (LifeScan)
50 strip · NHS indicative price = £9.99 · Drug Tariff (Part IXr)

OneTouch Ultra testing strips (LifeScan)
50 strip · NHS indicative price = £9.99 · Drug Tariff (Part IXr)

OneTouch Verio testing strips (LifeScan)
50 strip · NHS indicative price = £15.12 · Drug Tariff (Part IXr)

OneTouch Vita testing strips (LifeScan)
50 strip · NHS indicative price = £15.07 · Drug Tariff (Part IXr)

Performa testing strips (Roche Diabetes Care Ltd)
50 strip · NHS indicative price = £9.95 · Drug Tariff (Part IXr)

SD CodeFree testing strips (SD Biosensor Inc)
50 strip · NHS indicative price = £6.99 · Drug Tariff (Part IXr)

SURESIGN Resure testing strips (Ciga Healthcare Ltd)
50 strip · NHS indicative price = £9.99 · Drug Tariff (Part IXr)

Sensocard testing strips (BBI Healthcare Ltd)
50 strip · NHS indicative price = £16.30 · Drug Tariff (Part IXr)

SuperCheck 2 testing strips (Apollo Medical Technologies Ltd)
50 strip · NHS indicative price = £8.49 · Drug Tariff (Part IXr)

SuperCheck Plus testing strips (Apollo Medical Technologies Ltd)
50 strip · NHS indicative price = £9.45 · Drug Tariff (Part IXr)

TEE2 testing strips (Spirit Healthcare Ltd)
50 strip · NHS indicative price = £7.75 · Drug Tariff (Part IXr)

TRUEone testing strips (Nipro Diagnostics (UK) Ltd)
50 strip · NHS indicative price = £14.99 · Drug Tariff (Part IXr)

TRUEresult testing strips (Nipro Diagnostics (UK) Ltd)
50 strip · NHS indicative price = £14.99 · Drug Tariff (Part IXr)

TRUEyou testing strips (Nipro Diagnostics (UK) Ltd)
50 strip · NHS indicative price = £9.92 · Drug Tariff (Part IXr)

TrueTrack System testing strips (Nipro Diagnostics (UK) Ltd)
50 strip · NHS indicative price = £14.99 · Drug Tariff (Part IXr)

WaveSense JAZZ Duo testing strips (AgaMatrix Europe Ltd)
50 strip · NHS indicative price = £9.95 · Drug Tariff (Part IXr)

WaveSense JAZZ testing strips (AgaMatrix Europe Ltd)
50 strip · NHS indicative price = £9.87 · Drug Tariff (Part IXr)

eBchek testing strips (IRASCO Ltd)
50 strip · NHS indicative price = £15.89 · Drug Tariff (Part IXr)

iHealth testing strips (Technomed Ltd)
50 strip · NHS indicative price = £9.49 · Drug Tariff (Part IXr)

palmdoc iCare Advanced Solo testing strips (Palmdoc Ltd)
50 strip · NHS indicative price = £13.50 · Drug Tariff (Part IXr)

palmdoc iCare Advanced testing strips (Palmdoc Ltd)
50 strip · NHS indicative price = £9.70 · Drug Tariff (Part IXr)

palmdoc testing strips (Palmdoc Ltd)
50 strip · NHS indicative price = £9.40 · Drug Tariff (Part IXr)

● BLOOD KETONES TESTING STRIPS

FreeStyle Optium beta-ketone testing strips (Abbott Laboratories Ltd) | 10 strip · NHS indicative price = £21.14 · Drug Tariff (Part IXr)

GlucoMen LX beta-ketone testing strips (A Menarini Diagnostics Ltd) | 10 strip · NHS indicative price = £20.84 · Drug Tariff (Part IXr)

GlucoRx HCT Ketone testing strips (GlucoRx Ltd) | 10 strip · NHS indicative price = £14.95 · Drug Tariff (Part IXr)

Hypodermic insulin injection pens

● HYPODERMIC INSULIN INJECTION PENS
AUTOPEN® 24
Autopen®24 (for use with Sanofi- Aventis 3-mL insulin cartridges), allowing 1-unit dosage adjustment, max. 21 units (single-unit version) or 2-unit dosage adjustment, max. 42 units (2- unit version).

Autopen 24 hypodermic insulin injection pen reusable for 3ml cartridge 1 unit dial up / range 1-21 units (Owen Mumford Ltd)
1 device · NHS indicative price = £16.47 · Drug Tariff (Part IXa)

Autopen 24 hypodermic insulin injection pen reusable for 3ml cartridge 2 unit dial up / range 2-42 units (Owen Mumford Ltd)
1 device · NHS indicative price = £16.47 · Drug Tariff (Part IXa)

AUTOPEN® CLASSIC
Autopen® Classic (for use with Lilly and Wockhardt 3-mL insulin cartridges), allowing 1-unit dosage adjustment, max. 21 units (single-unit version) or 2-unit dosage adjustment, max. 42 units (2-unit version).

Autopen Classic hypodermic insulin injection pen reusable for 3ml cartridge 1 unit dial up / range 1-21 units (Owen Mumford Ltd)
1 device · NHS indicative price = £16.72 · Drug Tariff (Part IXa)

Autopen Classic hypodermic insulin injection pen reusable for 3ml cartridge 2 unit dial up / range 2-42 units (Owen Mumford Ltd)
1 device · NHS indicative price = £16.72 · Drug Tariff (Part IXa)

CLIKSTAR®
For use with *Lantus*®, *Apidra*®, and *Insuman*® 3-mL insulin cartridges; allowing 1-unit dose adjustment, max. 80 units.

ClikSTAR hypodermic insulin injection pen reusable for 3ml cartridge 1 unit dial up / range 1-80 units (Sanofi)
1 device · NHS indicative price = £25.00 · Drug Tariff (Part IXa)

ClikSTAR hypodermic insulin injection pen reusable for 3ml cartridge 1 unit dial up / range 1-80 units (Sanofi)
1 device · NHS indicative price = £25.00 · Drug Tariff (Part IXa)

HUMAPEN® LUXURA HD
For use with *Humulin*® and *Humalog*® 3-mL cartridges; allowing 0.5-unit dosage adjustment, max. 30 units.

HumaPen Luxura HD hypodermic insulin injection pen reusable for 3ml cartridge 0.5 unit dial up / range 1-30 units (Eli Lilly and Company Ltd)
1 device · NHS indicative price = £26.82 · Drug Tariff (Part IXa)

NOVOPEN® 4
For use with *Penfill*® 3-mL insulin cartridges; allowing 1-unit dosage adjustment, max. 60 units.

NovoPen 4 hypodermic insulin injection pen reusable for 3ml cartridge 1 unit dial up / range 1-60 units (Novo Nordisk Ltd)
1 device · NHS indicative price = £26.86 · Drug Tariff (Part IXa)

NovoPen 4 hypodermic insulin injection pen reusable for 3ml cartridge 1 unit dial up / range 1-60 units (Novo Nordisk Ltd)
1 device · NHS indicative price = £26.86 · Drug Tariff (Part IXa)

Needle free Insulin delivery systems

● NEEDLE FREE INSULIN DELIVERY SYSTEMS
INSUJET®
For use with any 10-mL vial or 3-mL cartridge of insulin, allowing 1-unit dosage adjustment, max 40 units. Available as *starter set* (*InsuJet*® device, nozzle cap, nozzle and piston, 1 × 10-mL adaptor, 1 × 3-mL adaptor, 1 cartridge cap removal key), *nozzle pack* (15 nozzles), *cartridge adaptor pack* (15 adaptors), or *vial adaptor pack* (15 adaptors).

InsuJet starter set (Spirit Healthcare Ltd)
1 pack · NHS indicative price = £90.00 · Drug Tariff (Part IXa)

Urinanalysis reagent strips

● PRESCRIBING AND DISPENSING INFORMATION
Other reagent strips available for urinalysis
Include: *Combur-3 Test*® (glucose and protein—Roche Diagnostics); *Clinitek Microalbumin*® (albumin and creatinine—Siemens); *Ketodiastix*® (glucose and ketones—Bayer Diagnostics); *Medi-Test Combi 2*® (glucose and protein—BHR); *Micral-Test II*®, used to detect microalbuminuria but this should be followed by confirmation in the laboratory—false positive results are common (albumin—Roche Diagnostics); *Microalbustix*® (albumin and creatinine—Siemens); *Uristix*® (glucose and protein—Siemens).
These reagent strips are not prescribable under National Health Service (NHS).

● URINE GLUCOSE TESTING STRIPS

Diastix testing strips (Bayer Diagnostics Manufacturing Ltd)
50 strip · NHS indicative price = £2.89 · Drug Tariff (Part IXr)

Medi-Test Glucose testing strips (BHR Pharmaceuticals Ltd)
50 strip · NHS indicative price = £2.33 · Drug Tariff (Part IXr)

Mission Glucose testing strips (Spirit Healthcare Ltd)
50 strip · NHS indicative price = £2.29 · Drug Tariff (Part IXr)

● URINE PROTEIN TESTING STRIPS

Albustix testing strips (Siemens Medical Solutions Diagnostics Ltd)
50 strip · NHS indicative price = £4.10 · Drug Tariff (Part IXr)

Medi-Test Protein 2 testing strips (BHR Pharmaceuticals Ltd)
50 strip · NHS indicative price = £3.27 · Drug Tariff (Part IXr)

- **URINE KETONES TESTING STRIPS**

  GlucoRx KetoRx Sticks 2GK testing strips (GlucoRx Ltd)
  50 strip · NHS indicative price = £2.25 · Drug Tariff (Part IXr)

  Ketostix testing strips (Bayer Diagnostics Manufacturing Ltd)
  50 strip · NHS indicative price = £3.06 · Drug Tariff (Part IXr)

  Mission Ketone testing strips (Spirit Healthcare Ltd)
  50 strip · NHS indicative price = £2.50 · Drug Tariff (Part IXr)

3.2 Hypoglycaemia

Hypoglycaemia

Treatment of hypoglycaemia

Prompt treatment of hypoglycaemia in children from any cause is essential as severe hypoglycaemia may cause subsequent neurological damage. Hyperinsulinism, fatty acid oxidation disorders and glycogen storage disease are less common causes of acute hypoglycaemia in children.

Initially glucose 10–20 g is given by mouth either in liquid form or as granulated sugar or sugar lumps. Approximately 10 g of glucose is available from non-diet versions of *Lucozade® Energy Original* 55 mL, *Coca-Cola®* 100 mL, and *Ribena Blackcurrant* 19 mL (to be diluted), 2 teaspoons of sugar, and also from 3 sugar lumps. Proprietary products of quick-acting carbohydrate (e.g. *GlucoGel®*, *Dextrogel®*, *GSF-Syrup®*, *Rapilose®* gel) are available on prescription for the patient to keep to hand in case of hypoglycaemia. If necessary this can be repeated in 10–15 minutes. After initial treatment, a snack providing sustained availability of carbohydrate (e.g. a sandwich, fruit, milk, or biscuits) or the next meal, if it is due, can prevent blood-glucose concentration from falling again.

Hypoglycaemia which causes unconsciousness or seizures is an emergency. Glucagon below, a polypeptide hormone produced by the alpha cells of the islets of Langerhans, increases blood-glucose concentration by mobilising glycogen stored in the liver. In hypoglycaemia, if sugar cannot be given by mouth, glucagon can be given by injection. Carbohydrates should be given as soon as possible to restore liver glycogen; glucagon is not appropriate for chronic hypoglycaemia. Glucagon can be issued to parents or carers of insulin-treated children for emergency use in hypoglycaemic attacks. It is often advisable to prescribe it on an 'if necessary' basis for hospitalised insulin-treated children, so that it can be given rapidly by the nurses during a hypoglycaemic emergency. If not effective in 10 minutes intravenous glucose should be given.

Alternatively, glucose intravenous infusion 10% can be given intravenously into a large vein through a large-gauge needle; care is required since this concentration is irritant especially if extravasation occurs. Glucose intravenous infusion 50% is **not** recommended, as it is very viscous and hypertonic. Close monitoring is necessary, particularly in the case of an overdose with a long-acting insulin because further administration of glucose may be required. Children whose hypoglycaemia is caused by an oral antidiabetic drug should be transferred to hospital because the hypoglycaemic effects of these drugs can persist for many hours.

Glucagon is not effective in the treatment of hypoglycaemia due to fatty acid oxidation or glycogen storage disorders.

Chronic hypoglycaemia

Diazoxide p. 434 is useful in the management of chronic hypoglycaemia due to excessive insulin secretion, either from a tumour involving the islets of Langerhans or from persisting hyperinsulinaemic hypoglycaemia of infancy (nesidioblastosis). Diazoxide has no place in the management of acute hypoglycaemia. Chlorothiazide p. 103 reduces diazoxide-induced sodium and water retention and

has the added benefit of potentiating the glycaemic effect of diazoxide.

If diazoxide and chlorothiazide fail to suppress excessive glucose requirements in chronic hypoglycaemia then octreotide p. 434 or nifedipine p. 100 can be added. Octreotide suppresses secretion of growth hormone, but growth is unlikely to be affected in the long term.

Neonatal hypoglycaemia

Neonatal hypoglycaemia at birth is treated with glucose **intravenous infusion 10%**. Mild asymptomatic persistent hypoglycaemia may respond to a single dose of glucagon. Glucagon has also been used in the short-term management of endogenous hyperinsulinism.

GLYCOGENOLYTIC HORMONES

▍ Glucagon

- **● INDICATIONS AND DOSE**

  Insulin-induced hypoglycaemia

  ▸ BY SUBCUTANEOUS INJECTION, OR BY INTRAMUSCULAR INJECTION

  ▸ Neonate: 20 micrograms/kg.

  ▸ Child 1 month–1 year: 500 micrograms

  ▸ Child 2–17 years (body-weight up to 25 kg): 500 micrograms, if no response within 10 minutes intravenous glucose must be given

  ▸ Child 2–17 years (body-weight 25 kg and above): 1 mg, if no response within 10 minutes intravenous glucose must be given

  Endogenous hyperinsulinism

  ▸ BY INTRAMUSCULAR INJECTION, OR BY INTRAVENOUS INJECTION

  ▸ Neonate: 200 micrograms/kg (max. per dose 1 mg) for 1 dose.

  ▸ Child 1 month–1 year: 1 mg for 1 dose

  ▸ BY CONTINUOUS INTRAVENOUS INFUSION

  ▸ Neonate: 1–18 micrograms/kg/hour (max. per dose 50 micrograms/kg/hour), adjusted according to response.

  ▸ Child 1 month–1 year: 1–10 micrograms/kg/hour, dose to be adjusted as necessary

  Diagnosis of growth hormone secretion (specialist use only)

  ▸ BY INTRAMUSCULAR INJECTION

  ▸ Child: 100 micrograms/kg (max. per dose 1 mg) for 1 dose, dose may vary, consult local guidelines

  Beta-blocker poisoning (cardiogenic shock unresponsive to atropine)

  ▸ INITIALLY BY INTRAVENOUS INJECTION

  ▸ Child: 50–150 micrograms/kg (max. per dose 10 mg), to be administered in glucose 5% (with precautions to protect the airway in case of vomiting), followed by (by intravenous infusion) 50 micrograms/kg/hour

  DOSE EQUIVALENCE AND CONVERSION
  1 unit of glucagon = 1 mg of glucagon.

- **● UNLICENSED USE** Dose and indication for cardiogenic shock unresponsive to atropine in beta-blocker overdose not licensed. Unlicensed for growth hormone test and hyperinsulinism.

- **● CONTRA-INDICATIONS** Phaeochromocytoma

- **● CAUTIONS** Glucagonoma · ineffective in chronic hypoglycaemia, starvation, and adrenal insufficiency · insulinoma · when used in the diagnosis of growth hormone secretion, delayed hypoglycaemia may result—deaths reported (ensure a meal is eaten before discharge)

6

Endocrine system

- **SIDE-EFFECTS**
- ▶ **Rare** Hypersensitivity reactions
- ▶ **Frequency not known** Diarrhoea · hypokalaemia · nausea · vomiting
- **DIRECTIONS FOR ADMINISTRATION**
- ▶ With intravenous use When administered by *continuous intravenous infusion*, do not add to infusion fluids containing calcium—precipitation may occur.
- **PATIENT AND CARER ADVICE** Medicines for Children leaflet: Glucagon for hypoglycaemia www.medicinesforchildren.org.uk/glucagon-for-hypoglycaemia
- **EXCEPTIONS TO LEGAL CATEGORY** Prescription-only medicine restriction does not apply where administration is for saving life in emergency.

- **MEDICINAL FORMS** There can be variation in the licensing of different medicines containing the same drug.
  Powder and solvent for solution for injection
  - ▶ GlucaGen Hypokit (Novo Nordisk Ltd)
    Glucagon hydrochloride 1 mg GlucaGen Hypokit 1mg powder and solvent for solution for injection | 1 vial PoM £11.52 DT price = £11.52

3.2a Chronic hypoglycaemia

GLYCOGENOLYTIC HORMONES

Diazoxide

- **INDICATIONS AND DOSE**
  Resistant hypertension
  - ▶ BY MOUTH
  - ▶ Neonate: Initially 1.7 mg/kg 3 times a day, adjusted according to response; maximum 15 mg/kg per day.
  - ▶ Child: Initially 1.7 mg/kg 3 times a day, adjusted according to response; maximum 15 mg/kg per day

  Chronic intractable hypoglycaemia
  - ▶ BY MOUTH
  - ▶ Neonate: Initially 5 mg/kg twice daily, adjusted according to response, initial dose used to establish response; maintenance 1.5–3 mg/kg 2–3 times a day; increased if necessary up to 7 mg/kg 3 times a day, higher doses are unlikely to be beneficial, but may be required in some cases.
  - ▶ Child: Initially 1.7 mg/kg 3 times a day, adjusted according to response; maintenance 1.5–3 mg/kg 2–3 times a day, increased if necessary up to 5 mg/kg 3 times a day, doses up to 5 mg/kg may be required in some cases, but higher doses are unlikely to be beneficial

- **UNLICENSED USE** Not licensed for resistant hypertension.
- **CAUTIONS** Aortic coarctation · aortic stenosis · arteriovenous shunt · heart failure · hyperuricaemia · impaired cardiac circulation · impaired cerebral circulation
- **INTERACTIONS** → Appendix 1 (diazoxide).
- **SIDE-EFFECTS** Taste disturbance · abdominal pain · anaemia · anorexia (prolonged use) · bleeding · constipation · decreased libido · dermatitis · diarrhoea · dizziness · dyspnoea · eosinophilia · extrapyramidal effects · galactorrhoea · headache · heart failure · hyperglycaemia · hyperosmolar non-ketotic coma · hypertrichosis · hyperuricaemia (prolonged use) · hypotension · ileus · lacrimation · leucopenia · lichenoid eruption · musculoskeletal pain · nausea · pancreatitis · pruritus · pulmonary hypertension · raised serum creatinine · raised serum urea · reversible nephritic syndrome · sodium and fluid retention · thrombocytopenia · tinnitus · transient

cataracts · visual disturbances · voice changes (prolonged use) · vomiting
- **PREGNANCY** Use only if essential; alopecia and hypertrichosis reported in neonates with prolonged use; may inhibit uterine activity during labour.
- **BREAST FEEDING** Manufacturer advises avoid—no information available.
- **RENAL IMPAIRMENT** Dose reduction may be required.
- **MONITORING REQUIREMENTS**
  - ▶ Monitor blood pressure.
  - ▶ Monitor white cell and platelet count during prolonged use.
  - ▶ Regularly assess growth, bone, and psychological development during prolonged use.

- **MEDICINAL FORMS** There can be variation in the licensing of different medicines containing the same drug. Forms available from special-order manufacturers include: capsule, oral suspension, oral solution
  Tablet
  - ▶ Eudemine (Focus Pharmaceuticals Ltd)
    Diazoxide 50 mg Eudemine 50mg tablets | 100 tablet PoM £46.45
  Capsule
  - ▶ Diazoxide (Non-proprietary)
    Diazoxide 25 mg Proglycem 25 capsules | 100 capsule PoM no price available
  Oral suspension
  - ▶ Diazoxide (Non-proprietary)
    Diazoxide 50 mg per 1 ml Proglycem 250mg/5ml oral suspension | 30 ml PoM no price available DT price = £126.47

PITUITARY AND HYPOTHALAMIC HORMONES AND ANALOGUES 〉 SOMATOSTATIN ANALOGUES

Somatostatin analogues ⬛

- **CAUTIONS** Diabetes mellitus (antidiabetic requirements may be reduced) · insulinoma (increased depth and duration of hypoglycaemia may occur—observe patients and monitor blood glucose levels when initiating treatment and changing doses)
- **SIDE-EFFECTS**
  - ▶ **Rare** Pancreatitis (shortly after administration)
  - ▶ **Frequency not known** Abdominal pain · anorexia · bloating · diarrhoea · flatulence · gallstones (after long-term treatment) · gastro-intestinal disturbances · hyperglycaemia (with chronic administration) · hypoglycaemia · impaired postprandial glucose tolerance (with chronic administration) · irritation at the injection site · nausea · pain at the injection site · steatorrhoea · vomiting
- **DIRECTIONS FOR ADMINISTRATION** Injection sites should be rotated.

⬛ above

Octreotide

- **INDICATIONS AND DOSE**
  Persistent hyperinsulinaemic hypoglycaemia unresponsive to diazoxide and glucose
  - ▶ BY SUBCUTANEOUS INJECTION
  - ▶ Neonate: Initially 2–5 micrograms/kg every 6–8 hours, adjusted according to response; increased if necessary up to 7 micrograms/kg every 4 hours, dosing up to 7 micrograms/kg may rarely be required.
  - ▶ Child: Initially 1–2 micrograms/kg every 4–6 hours, adjusted according to response; increased if necessary up to 7 micrograms/kg every 4 hours, dosing up to 7 micrograms/kg may rarely be required

Bleeding from oesophageal or gastric varices
▶ BY CONTINUOUS INTRAVENOUS INFUSION
▶ Child: 1 microgram/kg/hour, higher doses may be required initially, when no active bleeding reduce dose over 24 hours; Usual maximum 50 micrograms/hour

- **UNLICENSED USE** Not licensed in children.
- **INTERACTIONS** → Appendix 1 (octreotide).
- **SIDE-EFFECTS** Alopecia · arrhythmias · biliary colic (associated with abrupt withdrawal of subcutaneous octreotide) · bradycardia · constipation · dizziness · dyspnoea · headache · hepatitis · pancreatitis (associated with abrupt withdrawal of subcutaneous octreotide) · rash · reduced bile flow · reduced gall bladder motility
  SIDE-EFFECTS, FURTHER INFORMATION
  ▶ Gastro-intestinal side-effects Administering non-depot injections of octreotide between meals and at bedtime may reduce gastro-intestinal side-effects.
- **CONCEPTION AND CONTRACEPTION** Effective contraception required during treatment.
- **PREGNANCY** Possible effect on fetal growth; manufacturer advises use only if potential benefit outweighs risk.
- **BREAST FEEDING** Manufacturer advises avoid—present in milk in *animal* studies.
- **MONITORING REQUIREMENTS**
  ▶ Monitor thyroid function on long-term therapy.
  ▶ Monitor liver function.
- **TREATMENT CESSATION** Avoid abrupt withdrawal of short-acting subcutaneous octreotide (associated with biliary colic and pancreatitis).
- **DIRECTIONS FOR ADMINISTRATION** For *intravenous injection* or *intravenous infusion*, dilute with Sodium Chloride 0.9% to a concentration of 10–50%.

- **MEDICINAL FORMS**
  There can be variation in the licensing of different medicines containing the same drug.
  Solution for injection
  ▶ Octreotide (Non-proprietary)
  Octreotide (as Octreotide acetate) 50 microgram per 1 ml Octreotide 50micrograms/1ml solution for injection pre-filled syringes | 5 pre-filled disposable injection [PoM] £15.85
  Octreotide 50micrograms/1ml solution for injection vials | 5 vial [PoM] £14.87–£22.00
  Octreotide 50micrograms/1ml solution for injection ampoules | 5 ampoule [PoM] £4.60–£18.60
  Octreotide (as Octreotide acetate) 100 microgram per 1 ml Octreotide 100micrograms/1ml solution for injection ampoules | 5 ampoule [PoM] £7.24–£32.65
  Octreotide 100micrograms/1ml solution for injection pre-filled syringes | 5 pre-filled disposable injection [PoM] £28.90
  Octreotide 100micrograms/1ml solution for injection vials | 5 vial [PoM] £27.97–£32.65
  Octreotide (as Octreotide acetate) 200 microgram per 1 ml Octreotide 1mg/5ml solution for injection vials | 1 vial [PoM] £65.00–£69.66
  Octreotide (as Octreotide acetate) 500 microgram per 1 ml Octreotide 500micrograms/1ml solution for injection vials | 5 vial [PoM] £135.47–£158.25
  Octreotide 500micrograms/1ml solution for injection pre-filled syringes | 5 pre-filled disposable injection [PoM] £135.47–£149.00
  Octreotide 500micrograms/1ml solution for injection ampoules | 5 ampoule [PoM] £14.12–£169.35 DT price = £135.47
  ▶ Sandostatin (Novartis Pharmaceuticals UK Ltd)
  Octreotide (as Octreotide acetate) 50 microgram per 1 ml Sandostatin 50micrograms/1ml solution for injection ampoules | 5 ampoule [PoM] £14.87
  Octreotide (as Octreotide acetate) 100 microgram per 1 ml Sandostatin 100micrograms/1ml solution for injection ampoules | 5 ampoule [PoM] £27.97
  Octreotide (as Octreotide acetate) 200 microgram per 1 ml Sandostatin 1mg/5ml solution for injection vials | 1 vial [PoM] £55.73

Octreotide (as Octreotide acetate) 500 microgram per 1 ml Sandostatin 500micrograms/1ml solution for injection ampoules | 5 ampoule [PoM] £135.47 DT price = £135.47

Powder and solvent for suspension for injection
▶ Sandostatin LAR (Novartis Pharmaceuticals UK Ltd)
Octreotide (as Octreotide acetate) 10 mg Sandostatin LAR 10mg powder and solvent for suspension for injection vials | 1 vial [PoM] £549.71
Octreotide (as Octreotide acetate) 20 mg Sandostatin LAR 20mg powder and solvent for suspension for injection vials | 1 vial [PoM] £799.33
Octreotide (as Octreotide acetate) 30 mg Sandostatin LAR 30mg powder and solvent for suspension for injection vials | 1 vial [PoM] £998.41

4 Disorders of bone metabolism

Bone metabolism

Disorders of bone metabolism

The two main disorders of bone metabolism that occur in children are rickets and osteoporosis. The two most common forms of rickets are Vitamin D deficiency rickets and hypophosphataemic rickets. See also calcium.

Osteoporosis

Osteoporosis in children may be primary (e.g. *osteogenesis imperfecta* and *idiopathic juvenile osteoporosis*), or secondary (e.g. due to inflammatory disorders, immobilisation, or corticosteroids); specialist management is required.

Corticosteroid-induced osteoporosis
To reduce the risk of osteoporosis doses of oral corticosteroids should be as low as possible and courses of treatment as short as possible.

Calcitonin

Calcitonin is involved with parathyroid hormone in the regulation of bone turnover and hence in the maintenance of calcium balance and homoeostasis. Calcitonin (salmon) p. 439 (synthetic or recombinant salmon calcitonin) is used by specialists to lower the plasma-calcium concentration in children with hypercalcaemia associated with malignancy.

Bisphosphonates

A bisphosphonate such as pamidronate disodium p. 437 is used in the management of severe forms of *osteogenesis imperfecta* and other causes of osteoporosis in children to reduce the number of fractures; the long-term effects of bisphosphonates in children have not been established. Single doses of biphosphonates are also used to manage hypercalaemia. Treatment should be initiated under specialist advice **only**.

BISPHOSPHONATES

Bisphosphonates

- **DRUG ACTION** Bisphosphonates are adsorbed onto hydroxyapatite crystals in bone, slowing both their rate of growth and dissolution, and therefore reducing the rate of bone turnover.

IMPORTANT SAFETY INFORMATION
MHRA/CHM ADVICE: BISPHOSPHONATES: ATYPICAL FEMORAL FRACTURES (JUNE 2011)
Atypical femoral fractures have been reported rarely with bisphosphonate treatment, mainly in patients receiving long-term treatment for osteoporosis.

6

Endocrine system

The need to continue bisphosphonate treatment for osteoporosis should be re-evaluated periodically based on an assessment of the benefits and risks of treatment for individual patients, particularly after 5 or more years of use.

Patients should be advised to report any thigh, hip, or groin pain during treatment with a bisphosphonate.

Discontinuation of bisphosphonate treatment in patients suspected to have an atypical femoral fracture should be considered after an assessment of the benefits and risks of continued treatment.

MHRA/CHM ADVICE: BISPHOSPHONATES: OSTEONECROSIS OF THE JAW (NOVEMBER 2009) AND INTRAVENOUS BISPHOSPHONATES: OSTEONECROSIS OF THE JAW—FURTHER MEASURES TO MINIMISE RISK (JULY 2015)

The risk of osteonecrosis of the jaw is substantially greater for patients receiving intravenous bisphosphonates in the treatment of cancer than for patients receiving oral bisphosphonates for osteoporosis or Paget's disease.

Risk factors for developing osteonecrosis of the jaw that should be considered are: potency of bisphosphonate (highest for zoledronate), route of administration, cumulative dose, duration and type of malignant disease, concomitant treatment, smoking, comorbid conditions, and history of dental disease.

All patients should have a dental check-up (and any necessary remedial work should be performed) before bisphosphonate treatment, or as soon as possible after starting treatment. Patients should also maintain good oral hygiene, receive routine dental check-ups, and report any oral symptoms such as dental mobility, pain, or swelling, non-healing sores or discharge to a doctor and dentist during treatment.

Before prescribing an intravenous bisphosphonate, patients should be given a patient reminder card and informed of the risk of osteonecrosis of the jaw. Advise patients to tell their doctor if they have any problems with their mouth or teeth before starting treatment, and if the patient wears dentures, they should make sure their dentures fit properly. Patients should tell their doctor and dentist that they are receiving an intravenous bisphosphonate if they need dental treatment or dental surgery.

Guidance for dentists in primary care is included in *Oral Health Management of Patients Prescribed Bisphosphonates: Dental Clinical Guidance*, Scottish Dental Clinical Effectiveness Programme, April 2011 (available at www.sdcep.org.uk).

MHRA/CHM ADVICE: BISPHOSPHONATES: OSTEONECROSIS OF THE EXTERNAL AUDITORY CANAL (DECEMBER 2015)

Benign idiopathic osteonecrosis of the external auditory canal has been reported very rarely with bisphosphonate treatment, mainly in patients receiving long-term therapy (2 years or longer).

The possibility of osteonecrosis of the external auditory canal should be considered in patients receiving bisphosphonates who present with ear symptoms, including chronic ear infections, or suspected cholesteatoma.

Risk factors for developing osteonecrosis of the external auditory canal include: steroid use, chemotherapy, infection, an ear operation, or cotton-bud use.

Patients should be advised to report any ear pain, discharge from the ear, or an ear infection during treatment with a bisphosphonate.

● PATIENT AND CARER ADVICE

Atypical femoral fractures Patients should be advised to report any thigh, hip, or groin pain during treatment with a bisphosphonate.

Osteonecrosis of the jaw During bisphosphonate treatment patients should maintain good oral hygiene, receive routine dental check-ups, and report any oral symptoms. Osteonecrosis of the external auditory canal Patients should be advised to report any ear pain, discharge from ear or an ear infection during treatment with a bisphosphonate.

F 435

Alendronic acid

10.6.2016

(Alendronate)

● INDICATIONS AND DOSE

Osteoporosis (due to osteogenesis imperfecta and other causes) (initiated under specialist supervision) | Hypercalcaemia (initiated under specialist supervision)
▸ BY MOUTH
  ▸ Child: (consult local protocol)

● UNLICENSED USE Not licensed for use in children.

● CONTRA-INDICATIONS Abnormalities of oesophagus · hypocalcaemia · other factors which delay emptying (e.g. stricture or achalasia)

● CAUTIONS Active gastro-intestinal bleeding · atypical femoral fractures · duodenitis · dysphagia · exclude other causes of osteoporosis · gastritis · history (within 1 year) of ulcers · surgery of the upper gastro-intestinal tract · symptomatic oesophageal disease · ulcers · upper gastro-intestinal disorders

● INTERACTIONS → Appendix 1 (bisphosphonates).

● SIDE-EFFECTS

▸ **Common or very common** Abdominal distension · abdominal pain · alopecia · asthenia · constipation · diarrhoea · dizziness · dyspepsia · flatulence · headache · joint swelling · musculoskeletal pain · oesophageal reactions · peripheral oedema · pruritus · regurgitation · vertigo

▸ **Uncommon** Dysgeusia · episcleritis · erythema · gastritis · malaise (on initiation) · melena · myalgia (on initiation) · nausea · rash · scleritis · uveitis · vomiting

▸ **Rare** Atypical femoral fractures with long-term use · fever (on initiation) · hypocalcaemia · osteonecrosis of the jaw · photosensitivity · severe skin reactions · Stevens-Johnson syndrome · toxic epidermal necrolysis

▸ **Very rare** Osteonecrosis of the external auditory canal

SIDE-EFFECTS, FURTHER INFORMATION

▸ Oesophageal reactions Severe oesophageal reactions (oesophagitis, oesophageal ulcers, oesophageal stricture and oesophageal erosions) have been reported; patients should be advised to stop taking the tablets and to seek medical attention if they develop symptoms of oesophageal irritation such as dysphagia, new or worsening heartburn, pain on swallowing or retrosternal pain.

● PREGNANCY Avoid.

● BREAST FEEDING Manufacturer advises avoid—no information available.

● RENAL IMPAIRMENT Avoid if estimated glomerular filtration rate is less than 35 mL/minute/1.73 m^2.

● MONITORING REQUIREMENTS Correct disturbances of calcium and mineral metabolism (e.g. vitamin-D deficiency, hypocalcaemia) before starting treatment. Monitor serum-calcium concentration during treatment.

● DIRECTIONS FOR ADMINISTRATION Tablets should be swallowed whole and oral solution should be swallowed as a single 100 mL dose. Doses should be taken with plenty of water while sitting or standing, on an empty stomach at least 30 minutes before breakfast (or another oral medicine); patient should stand or sit upright for at least 30 minutes after administration.

- **PATIENT AND CARER ADVICE** Patients or their carers should be given advice on how to administer alendronic acid tablets and oral solution.
  Oesophageal reactions Patients (or their carers) should be advised to stop taking alendronic acid and to seek medical attention if they develop symptoms of oesophageal irritation such as dysphagia, new or worsening heartburn, pain on swallowing or retrosternal pain.
- **NATIONAL FUNDING/ACCESS DECISIONS**
  Scottish Medicines Consortium (SMC) Decisions
  The *Scottish Medicines Consortium* has advised (April 2016) that alendronic acid (*Binosto®*) is accepted for restricted use within NHS Scotland for the treatment of postmenopausal osteoporosis where alendronic acid is the appropriate treatment choice, but the patient is unable to swallow tablets.

- **MEDICINAL FORMS**
  There can be variation in the licensing of different medicines containing the same drug. Forms available from special-order manufacturers include: oral solution
  Tablet
  ▸ Alendronic acid (Non-proprietary)
  Alendronic acid (as Alendronate sodium) 10 mg Alendronic acid 10mg tablets | 28 tablet [PoM] £3.25 DT price = £1.78
  Alendronic acid (as Alendronate sodium) 70 mg Alendronic acid 70mg tablets | 4 tablet [PoM] £22.80 DT price = £0.79
  ▸ Fosamax (Merck Sharp & Dohme Ltd)
  Alendronic acid (as Alendronate sodium) 10 mg Fosamax 10mg tablets | 28 tablet [PoM] £23.12 DT price = £1.78
  Alendronic acid (as Alendronate sodium) 70 mg Fosamax Once Weekly 70mg tablets | 4 tablet [PoM] £22.80 DT price = £0.79
  Effervescent tablet
  ▸ Binosto (Internis Pharmaceuticals Ltd)
  Alendronic acid (as Alendronate sodium) 70 mg Binosto 70mg effervescent tablets sugar-free | 4 tablet [PoM] £22.80 DT price = £22.80
  Oral solution
  ▸ Alendronic acid (Non-proprietary)
  Alendronic acid 700 microgram per 1 ml Alendronic acid 70mg/100ml oral solution unit dose sugar free sugar-free | 4 unit dose [PoM] £27.36 DT price = £27.36

▸ 435

Pamidronate disodium

(Formerly called aminohydroxypropylidenediphosphonate disodium (APD))

- **INDICATIONS AND DOSE**
  Osteoporosis (due to osteogenesis imperfecta and other causes) (specialist use only) | Hypercalcaemia (specialist use only)
  ▸ BY INTRAVENOUS INFUSION
  ▸ Child: (consult product literature)

- **UNLICENSED USE** Not licensed for use in children.
- **CAUTIONS** Atypical femoral fractures · cardiac disease · ensure adequate hydration · previous thyroid surgery (risk of hypocalcaemia)
- **INTERACTIONS** → Appendix 1 (bisphosphonates). Avoid concurrent use with other bisphosphonates.
- **SIDE-EFFECTS**
▸ **Common or very common** Arthralgia · bone pain · fever · headache · hypomagnesaemia · hypophosphataemia · influenza- like symptoms (sometimes accompanied by malaise, rigors, fatigue and flushes) · lymphocytopenia · myalgia · nausea · transient rise in body temperature · vomiting
▸ **Rare** Abdominal pain · acute renal failure · agitation · anaemia · anorexia · atypical femoral fractures · confusion · conjunctivitis · constipation · deterioration of renal disease · diarrhoea · dizziness · dyspepsia · haematuria ·

hallucinations · hyperkalaemia · hypernatraemia · hypertension · hypokalaemia · hypotension · insomnia · isolated cases of seizures · lethargy · leucopenia · muscle cramps · osteonecrosis of the jaw · other ocular symptoms · paraesthesia · pruritus · rash · somnolence · symptomatic hypocalcaemia · tetany · thrombocytopenia
▸ **Very rare** Osteonecrosis of the external auditory canal
▸ **Frequency not known** Atrial fibrillation · injection-site reactions · reactivation of herpes simplex · reactivation of herpes zoster

- **PREGNANCY** Avoid—toxicity in *animal* studies.
- **BREAST FEEDING** Avoid.
- **HEPATIC IMPAIRMENT** Caution in severe hepatic impairment—no information available.
- **RENAL IMPAIRMENT** Monitor renal function in renal disease or predisposition to renal impairment (e.g. in tumour-induced hypercalcaemia).
- **DIRECTIONS FOR ADMINISTRATION** For *slow intravenous infusion* (*Aredia®*; *Pamidronate disodium*, Hospira, Medac, Wockhardt), give intermittently in Glucose 5% or Sodium chloride 0.9%; give at a rate not exceeding 1 mg/minute; not to be given with infusion fluids containing calcium. For *Aredia®*, reconstitute initially with water for injections (15 mg in 5 mL, 30 mg or 90 mg in 10 mL), then dilute with infusion fluid to a concentration of not more than 90 mg in 250 mL. For *Pamidronate disodium* (Medac, Hospira, Wockhardt) dilute with infusion fluid to a concentration of not more than 90 mg in 250 mL
- **PATIENT AND CARER ADVICE**
  Driving and skilled tasks
  Patients should be warned against performing skilled tasks (e.g. cycling, driving or operating machinery) immediately after treatment (somnolence or dizziness can occur).
  A patient reminder card should be provided (risk of osteonecrosis of the jaw).

- **MEDICINAL FORMS**
  There can be variation in the licensing of different medicines containing the same drug.
  Solution for infusion
  ▸ Pamidronate disodium (Non-proprietary)
  Pamidronate disodium 3 mg per 1 ml Pamidronate disodium 15mg/5ml solution for infusion vials | 1 vial [PoM] £27.50 (Hospital only) | 5 vial [PoM] £149.15
  Pamidronate disodium 30mg/10ml solution for infusion vials | 1 vial [PoM] £55.00 (Hospital only) | 1 vial [PoM] £59.66
  Pamidronate disodium 60mg/20ml solution for infusion vials | 1 vial [PoM] £110.00 (Hospital only)
  Pamidronate disodium 90mg/30ml solution for infusion vials | 1 vial [PoM] £165.00 (Hospital only)
  Pamidronate disodium 6 mg per 1 ml Pamidronate disodium 60mg/10ml solution for infusion vials | 1 vial [PoM] £115.25
  Pamidronate disodium 9 mg per 1 ml Pamidronate disodium 90mg/10ml solution for infusion vials | 1 vial [PoM] £170.45
  Pamidronate disodium 15 mg per 1 ml Pamidronate disodium 60mg/4ml solution for infusion ampoules | 1 ampoule [PoM] £119.32
  Pamidronate disodium 15mg/1ml solution for infusion ampoules | 4 ampoule [PoM] £119.32
  Pamidronate disodium 90mg/6ml solution for infusion ampoules | 1 ampoule [PoM] £170.46
  Pamidronate disodium 30mg/2ml solution for infusion ampoules | 2 ampoule [PoM] £119.32

▸ 435

Risedronate sodium

- **INDICATIONS AND DOSE**
  Osteoporosis (due to osteogenesis imperfecta and other causes) (specialist use only) | Hypercalcaemia (specialist use only)
  ▸ BY MOUTH
  ▸ Child: (consult local protocol)

- **UNLICENSED USE** Not licensed for use in children.

- **CONTRA-INDICATIONS** Hypocalcaemia
- **CAUTIONS** Atypical femoral fractures · oesophageal abnormalities · other factors which delay transit or emptying (e.g. stricture or achalasia
- **INTERACTIONS** → Appendix 1 (bisphosphonates).
- **SIDE-EFFECTS**
  ‣ **Common or very common** Abdominal pain · constipation · diarrhoea · dyspepsia · headache · musculoskeletal pain · nausea
  ‣ **Uncommon** Duodenitis · dysphagia · gastritis · oesophageal ulcer · oesophagitis · uveitis
  ‣ **Rare** Atypical femoral fractures · glossitis · oesophageal stricture
  ‣ **Very rare** Osteonecrosis of the external auditory canal
  ‣ **Frequency not known** Cutaneous vasculitis · gastroduodenal ulceration · hair loss · hepatic disorders · osteonecrosis of the jaw · Stevens-Johnson syndrome · toxic epidermal necrolysis
- **PREGNANCY** Avoid.
- **BREAST FEEDING** Avoid.
- **RENAL IMPAIRMENT** Avoid if estimated glomerular filtration rate is less than 30 mL/minute/1.73 m^2.
- **MONITORING REQUIREMENTS**
  ‣ Correct hypocalcaemia before starting.
  ‣ Correct other disturbances of bone and mineral metabolism (e.g. vitamin- D deficiency) at onset of treatment.
- **DIRECTIONS FOR ADMINISTRATION** Swallow tablets whole with full glass of water; on rising, take on an empty stomach at least 30 minutes before first food or drink of the day **or**, if taking at any other time of the day, avoid food and drink for at least 2 hours before or after risedronate (particularly avoid calcium-containing products e.g. milk; also avoid iron and mineral supplements and antacids); stand or sit upright for at least 30 minutes; do not take tablets at bedtime or before rising.
- **PATIENT AND CARER ADVICE**
  Patients or carers should be given advice on how to administer risedronate sodium tablets.
  Oesophageal reactions Patients should be advised to stop taking the tablets and seek medical attention if they develop symptoms of oesophageal irritation such as dysphagia, pain on swallowing, retrosternal pain, or heartburn.
  Medicines for Children leaflet: Risedronate for brittle bones www.medicinesforchildren.org.uk/risedronate-for-brittle-bones
- **MEDICINAL FORMS**
  There can be variation in the licensing of different medicines containing the same drug. Forms available from special-order manufacturers include: oral suspension, oral solution

Tablet
  ‣ Risedronate sodium (Non-proprietary)
  Risedronate sodium 5 mg Risedronate sodium 5mg tablets | 28 tablet PoM £24.78 DT price = £18.87
  Risedronate sodium 30 mg Risedronate sodium 30mg tablets | 28 tablet PoM £143.95 DT price = £143.89
  Risedronate sodium 35 mg Risedronate sodium 35mg tablets | 4 tablet PoM £19.12 DT price = £0.88
  ‣ Actonel (Warner Chilcott UK Ltd)
  Risedronate sodium 5 mg Actonel 5mg tablets | 28 tablet PoM £17.99 DT price = £18.87
  Risedronate sodium 30 mg Actonel 30mg tablets | 28 tablet PoM £143.95 DT price = £143.89
  Risedronate sodium 35 mg Actonel Once a Week 35mg tablets | 4 tablet PoM £19.12 DT price = £0.88
  Actonel 35mg tablets | 4 tablet PoM no price available DT price = £0.88

⌐ 435

Sodium clodronate

- **INDICATIONS AND DOSE**

Osteoporosis (due to osteogenesis imperfecta or other causes) (specialist use only) | Hypercalcaemia (specialist use only)
  ‣ BY MOUTH
  ‣ **Child:** (consult local protocol)

- **UNLICENSED USE** Not licensed for use in children.
- **CONTRA-INDICATIONS** Acute gastro-intestinal inflammatory conditions
- **CAUTIONS** Atypical femoral fractures · maintain adequate fluid intake during treatment
- **INTERACTIONS** → Appendix 1 (bisphosphonates). Renal dysfunction reported in patients receiving concomitant NSAIDs.
- **SIDE-EFFECTS**
  ‣ **Common or very common** Bronchospasm · diarrhoea · nausea · skin reactions · vomiting
  ‣ **Rare** Atypical femoral fractures
  ‣ **Very rare** Osteonecrosis of the external auditory canal · osteonecrosis of the jaw
  ‣ **Frequency not known** Renal impairment · uveitis
- **PREGNANCY** Avoid.
- **BREAST FEEDING** Manufacturer advises avoid—no information available.
- **RENAL IMPAIRMENT** Reduce dose if estimated glomerular filtration rate 30—50 mL/minute/1.73m^2. Use half normal dose if estimated glomerular filtration rate 10–30 mL/minute/1.73 m^2. Avoid if estimated filtration rate less than 10 mL/minute/1.73 m^2.
- **MONITORING REQUIREMENTS** Monitor renal function, serum calcium and serum phosphate before and during treatment.
- **DIRECTIONS FOR ADMINISTRATION** Avoid food for 2 hours before and 1 hour after treatment, particularly calcium-containing products e.g. milk; also avoid iron and mineral supplements and antacids; maintain adequate fluid intake.
- **PATIENT AND CARER ADVICE** Patients or carers should be given advice on how to administer sodium clodronate capsules and tablets.

- **MEDICINAL FORMS**
  There can be variation in the licensing of different medicines containing the same drug.

Tablet
  CAUTIONARY AND ADVISORY LABELS 10
  ‣ Sodium clodronate (Non-proprietary)
  Sodium clodronate 800 mg Sodium clodronate 800mg tablets | 60 tablet PoM £116.72 DT price = £146.43
  ‣ Bonefos (Bayer Plc)
  Sodium clodronate 800 mg Bonefos 800mg tablets | 60 tablet PoM £146.43 DT price = £146.43
  ‣ Clasteon (Beacon Pharmaceuticals Ltd)
  Sodium clodronate 800 mg Clasteon 800mg tablets | 60 tablet PoM £146.43 DT price = £146.43
  ‣ Loron (Intrapharm Laboratories Ltd)
  Sodium clodronate 520 mg Loron 520mg tablets | 60 tablet PoM £152.59 DT price = £152.59

Capsule
  ‣ Sodium clodronate (Non-proprietary)
  Sodium clodronate 400 mg Sodium clodronate 400mg capsules | 30 capsule PoM £40.49 | 120 capsule PoM £161.97 DT price = £139.83
  ‣ Bonefos (Bayer Plc)
  Sodium clodronate 400 mg Bonefos 400mg capsules | 120 capsule PoM £139.83 DT price = £139.83
  ‣ Clasteon (Beacon Pharmaceuticals Ltd)
  Sodium clodronate 400 mg Clasteon 400mg capsules | 30 capsule PoM £34.96 | 120 capsule PoM £139.83 DT price = £139.83

CALCIUM REGULATING DRUGS > BONE
RESORPTION INHIBITORS

Calcitonin (salmon)

(Salcatonin)

- **INDICATIONS AND DOSE**

Hypercalcaemia (limited experience in children) (specialist use only)
▸ BY SUBCUTANEOUS INJECTION, OR BY INTRAMUSCULAR INJECTION
  ▸ Child: 2.5–5 units/kg every 12 hours (max. per dose 400 units every 6–8 hours), adjusted according to response, no additional benefit with doses over 8 units/kg every 6 hours
▸ BY INTRAVENOUS INFUSION
  ▸ Child: 5–10 units/kg, to be administered by slow intravenous infusion over at least 6 hours

Osteoporosis (specialist use only)
▸ BY INTRAMUSCULAR INJECTION, OR BY SUBCUTANEOUS INJECTION
  ▸ Child: Refer for specialist advice, experience very limited

- **UNLICENSED USE** Not licensed in children.
- **CONTRA-INDICATIONS** Hypocalcaemia
- **CAUTIONS** Heart failure · history of allergy (skin test advised) · risk of malignancy—avoid prolonged use (use lowest effective dose for shortest possible time)
- **SIDE-EFFECTS**
  ▸ **Common or very common** Abdominal pain · diarrhoea · dizziness · fatigue · flushing · headache · malignancy (with long-term use) · musculoskeletal pain · nausea · taste disturbances · vomiting
  ▸ **Uncommon** Cough · hypersensitivity reactions · hypertension · injection-site reactions · oedema · polyuria · pruritus · rash · visual disturbances
  ▸ **Frequency not known** Tremor
- **PREGNANCY** Avoid unless potential benefit outweighs risk (toxicity in *animal* studies).
- **BREAST FEEDING** Avoid; inhibits lactation in *animals*.
- **RENAL IMPAIRMENT** Use with caution.
- **MONITORING REQUIREMENTS** Monitor bone growth.
- **DIRECTIONS FOR ADMINISTRATION** For *intravenous infusion*, dilute injection solution (e.g. 400 units in 500 mL) with Sodium Chloride 0.9% and give over at least 6 hours; glass or hard plastic containers should not be used; some loss of potency on dilution and administration—use diluted solution without delay.

- **MEDICINAL FORMS**
  There can be variation in the licensing of different medicines containing the same drug.
  Solution for injection
  ▸ Miacalcic (Novartis Pharmaceuticals UK Ltd)
    Calcitonin (salmon) 50 unit per 1 ml Miacalcic 50units/1ml solution for injection ampoules | 5 ampoule PoM £17.10
    Calcitonin (salmon) 100 unit per 1 ml Miacalcic 100units/1ml solution for injection ampoules | 5 ampoule PoM £34.21
    Calcitonin (salmon) 200 unit per 1 ml Miacalcic 400units/2ml multidose solution for injection vials | 1 vial PoM £24.60

5　Gonadotrophin responsive conditions

PITUITARY AND HYPOTHALAMIC HORMONES AND ANALOGUES > GONADOTROPIN-RELEASING HORMONES

Goserelin

- **DRUG ACTION** Administration of gonadorelin analogues produces an initial phase of stimulation; continued administration is followed by down-regulation of gonadotrophin-releasing hormone receptors, thereby reducing the release of gonadotrophins (follicle stimulating hormone and luteinising hormone) which in turn leads to inhibition of androgen and oestrogen production.

- **INDICATIONS AND DOSE**

ZOLADEX LA®

Gonadotrophin-dependent precocious puberty
▸ BY SUBCUTANEOUS INJECTION
  ▸ Child: 10.8 mg every 12 weeks, to be administered into the anterior abdominal wall, injections may be required more frequently in some cases

ZOLADEX®

Gonadotrophin-dependent precocious puberty
▸ BY SUBCUTANEOUS INJECTION
  ▸ Child: 3.6 mg every 28 days, to be administered into the anterior abdominal wall, injections may be required more frequently in some cases

- **UNLICENSED USE** Not licensed for use in children.
- **CONTRA-INDICATIONS** Undiagnosed vaginal bleeding
- **CAUTIONS** Depression · patients with metabolic bone disease (decrease in bone mineral density can occur)
- **SIDE-EFFECTS** Anaphylaxis · asthma · breast tenderness · changes in blood pressure · changes in breast size · changes in scalp and body hair · depression · headache · hypersensitivity reactions · local reactions at injection site · mood changes · ovarian cysts (may require withdrawal) · paraesthesia · pruritus · rash · urticaria · vaginal bleeding · visual disturbances · weight change · withdrawal bleeding
- **CONCEPTION AND CONTRACEPTION** Non-hormonal, barrier methods of contraception should be used during entire treatment period. Pregnancy should be excluded before treatment, the first injection should be given during menstruation or shortly afterwards or use barrier contraception for 1 month beforehand.
- **PREGNANCY** Avoid.
- **BREAST FEEDING** Avoid.
- **MONITORING REQUIREMENTS** Monitor bone mineral density.
- **DIRECTIONS FOR ADMINISTRATION** Rotate injection site to prevent atrophy and nodule formation.

- **MEDICINAL FORMS**
  There can be variation in the licensing of different medicines containing the same drug.
  Implant
  ▸ Zoladex (AstraZeneca UK Ltd)
    Goserelin (as Goserelin acetate) 3.6 mg Zoladex 3.6mg implant SafeSystem pre-filled syringes | 1 pre-filled disposable injection PoM £65.00 DT price = £65.00
  ▸ Zoladex LA (AstraZeneca UK Ltd)
    Goserelin (as Goserelin acetate) 10.8 mg Zoladex LA 10.8mg implant SafeSystem pre-filled syringes | 1 pre-filled disposable injection PoM £235.00 DT price = £235.00

6

Endocrine system

Leuprorelin acetate

- **DRUG ACTION** Administration of gonadorelin analogues produces an initial phase of stimulation; continued administration is followed by down-regulation of gonadotrophin-releasing hormone receptors, thereby reducing the release of gonadotrophins (follicle stimulating hormone and luteinising hormone) which in turn leads to inhibition of androgen and oestrogen production.

- **INDICATIONS AND DOSE**

PROSTAP 3 DCS®

Gonadotrophin-dependent precocious puberty

 ▸ BY SUBCUTANEOUS INJECTION, OR BY INTRAMUSCULAR INJECTION

 ▸ **Child:** 11.25 mg every 12 weeks, injections may be required more frequently in some cases

PROSTAP SR DCS®

Gonadotrophin-dependent precocious puberty

 ▸ BY SUBCUTANEOUS INJECTION, OR BY INTRAMUSCULAR INJECTION

 ▸ **Child:** 3.75 mg every 4 weeks, half this dose is sometimes used in children with body-weight under 20 kg, injections may be required more frequently in some cases

- **UNLICENSED USE** Not licensed for use in children.
- **CONTRA-INDICATIONS** Undiagnosed vaginal bleeding
- **CAUTIONS** Patients with metabolic bone disease (decrease in bone mineral density can occur)
- **SIDE-EFFECTS** Abdominal pain · acne · anaphylaxis · asthma · breast tenderness (males and females) · changes in blood pressure · changes in breast size · changes in scalp and body hair · depression · headache · hypersensitivity reactions · local reactions at injection site · mood changes · paraesthesia · pruritus · rash · urticaria · visual disturbances · weight changes · withdrawal bleeding
- **PREGNANCY** Avoid—teratogenic in *animal* studies.
- **BREAST FEEDING** Avoid.
- **MONITORING REQUIREMENTS** Monitor bone mineral density.
- **DIRECTIONS FOR ADMINISTRATION** Rotate injection site to prevent atrophy and nodule formation.

- **MEDICINAL FORMS**
  There can be variation in the licensing of different medicines containing the same drug.
  Powder and solvent for suspension for injection
   ▸ Prostap 3 DCS (Takeda UK Ltd)
   Leuprorelin acetate 11.25 mg Prostap 3 DCS 11.25mg powder and solvent for suspension for injection pre-filled syringes | 1 pre-filled disposable injection PoM £225.72 DT price = £225.72
   ▸ Prostap SR DCS (Takeda UK Ltd)
   Leuprorelin acetate 3.75 mg Prostap SR DCS 3.75mg powder and solvent for suspension for injection pre-filled syringes | 1 pre-filled disposable injection PoM £75.24 DT price = £75.24

Triptorelin

- **DRUG ACTION** Administration of gonadorelin analogues produces an initial phase of stimulation; continued administration is followed by down-regulation of gonadotrophin-releasing hormone receptors, thereby reducing the release of gonadotrophins (follicle stimulating hormone and luteinising hormone) which in turn leads to inhibition of androgen and oestrogen production.

- **INDICATIONS AND DOSE**

DECAPEPTYL® SR 11.25MG

Gonadotrophin-dependent precocious puberty

 ▸ BY INTRAMUSCULAR INJECTION

 ▸ **Child:** 11.25 mg every 3 months, discontinue when bone maturation consistent with age of 12 years in girls or 13–14 years in boys

GONAPEPTYL DEPOT®

Gonadotrophin-dependent precocious puberty

 ▸ BY SUBCUTANEOUS INJECTION, OR BY DEEP INTRAMUSCULAR INJECTION

 ▸ **Child (body-weight up to 20 kg):** Initially 1.875 mg every 2 weeks for 3 doses, to be administered on days 0, 14, and 28 of treatment, then 1.875 mg every 3–4 weeks, discontinue when bone maturation consistent with age over 12 years in girls and over 13 years in boys

 ▸ **Child (body-weight 20-30 kg):** Initially 2.5 mg every 2 weeks for 3 doses, to be administered on days 0, 14, and 28 of treatment, then 2.5 mg every 3–4 weeks, discontinue when bone maturation consistent with age over 12 years in girls and over 13 years in boys

 ▸ **Child (body-weight 31 kg and above):** Initially 3.75 mg every 2 weeks for 3 doses, to be administered on days 0, 14, and 28 of treatment, then 3.75 mg every 3–4 weeks, discontinue when bone maturation consistent with age over 12 years in girls and over 13 years in boys

- **CONTRA-INDICATIONS** Undiagnosed vaginal bleeding
- **SIDE-EFFECTS** Anaphylaxis · arthralgia · asthenia · asthma · breast tenderness (males and females) · changes in blood pressure · changes in breast size · changes in scalp and body hair · depression · gastro-intestinal disturbances · headache · hypersensitivity reactions · local reactions at injection site · mood changes · ovarian cysts (may require withdrawal) · paraesthesia · pruritus · rash · urticaria · visual disturbances · weight changes · withdrawal bleeding (may occur in the first month of treatment)
- **CONCEPTION AND CONTRACEPTION** Non-hormonal, barrier methods of contraception should be used during entire treatment period. Pregnancy should be excluded before treatment, the first injection should be given during menstruation or shortly afterwards or use barrier contraception for 1 month beforehand.
- **PREGNANCY** Avoid.
- **BREAST FEEDING** Avoid.
- **MONITORING REQUIREMENTS** Monitor bone mineral density.
- **DIRECTIONS FOR ADMINISTRATION** Rotate injection site to prevent atrophy and nodule formation.
- **PRESCRIBING AND DISPENSING INFORMATION**
  DECAPEPTYL® SR 11.25MG Each vial includes an overage to allow accurate administration of an 11.25 mg dose.

- **MEDICINAL FORMS**
There can be variation in the licensing of different medicines containing the same drug.

Powder and solvent for suspension for injection

▶ Decapeptyl SR (Ipsen Ltd)
Triptorelin (as Triptorelin acetate) **11.25 mg** Decapeptyl SR 11.25mg powder and solvent for suspension for injection vials | 1 vial PoM £207.00

▶ Gonapeptyl Depot (Ferring Pharmaceuticals Ltd)
Triptorelin (as Triptorelin acetate) **3.75 mg** Gonapeptyl Depot 3.75mg powder and solvent for suspension for injection pre-filled disposable devices | 1 pre-filled disposable injection PoM £81.69

6   Hypothalamic and anterior pituitary hormone related disorders

Hypothalamic and anterior pituitary hormones

Anterior pituitary hormones

Corticotrophins

Tetracosactide below(tetracosactrin), an analogue of corticotropin (adrenocorticotrophic hormone, ACTH), is used to test adrenocortical function; failure of plasma-cortisol concentration to rise after administration of tetracosactide indicates adrenocortical insufficiency. A low-dose test is considered by some clinicians to be more sensitive when used to confirm established, partial adrenal suppression.

Tetracosactide should be given only if no other ACTH preparations have been given previously. Tetracosactide depot injection (*Synacthen Depot*®) is also used in the treatment of infantile spasms but it is contra-indicated in neonates because of the presence of benzyl alcohol in the injection. Corticotropin-releasing factor, corticorelin p. 442, (also known as corticotropin-releasing hormone, CRH) is used to test anterior pituitary function and secretion of corticotropin.

Gonadotrophins

Gonadotrophins are occasionally used in the treatment of hypogonadotrophic hypogonadism and associated oligospermia. There is no justification for their use in primary gonadal failure.

Chorionic gonadotrophin p. 443 is used in the investigation of testicular function in suspected primary hypogonadism and incomplete masculinisation. It has also been used in delayed puberty in boys to stimulate endogenous testosterone production, but it has little advantage over testosterone.

Growth hormone

Growth hormone is used to treat proven deficiency of the hormone, Prader-Willi syndrome, Turner's syndrome, growth disturbance in children born small for corrected gestational age, chronic renal insufficiency, and short stature homeobox-containing gene (SHOX) deficiency. Growth hormone is also used in Noonan syndrome and idiopathic short stature [unlicensed indications] under specialist management. Treatment should be initiated and monitored by a paediatrician with expertise in managing growth-hormone disorders; treatment can be continued under a shared-care protocol by a general practitioner.

Growth hormone of human origin (HGH; somatotrophin) has been replaced by a growth hormone of human sequence, somatropin p. 443, produced using recombinant DNA technology.

Mecasermin p. 445, a human insulin-like growth factor-I (rhIGF-I), is licensed to treat growth failure in children with severe primary insulin-like growth factor-I deficiency.

Hypothalamic hormones

Gonadorelin p. 442 when injected intravenously in post-pubertal girls leads to a rapid rise in plasma concentrations of both luteinising hormone (LH) and follicle-stimulating hormone (FSH). It has not proved to be very helpful, however, in distinguishing hypothalamic from pituitary lesions. It is used in the assessment of delayed or precocious puberty.

Other growth hormone stimulation tests involve the use of insulin, glucagon p. 433, arginine p. 571, and clonidine hydrochloride p. 93 [all unlicensed uses]. The tests should be carried out in specialist centres.

6.1   Adrenocortical function testing

PITUITARY AND HYPOTHALAMIC HORMONES AND ANALOGUES > CORTICOTROPHINS

▌Tetracosactide

(Tetracosactrin)

- **INDICATIONS AND DOSE**

Diagnosis of adrenocortical insufficiency (diagnostic 30-minute test), standard-dose test

▶ BY INTRAMUSCULAR INJECTION, OR BY INTRAVENOUS INJECTION
▶ Child: 145 micrograms/m^2 (max. per dose 250 micrograms) for 1 dose

Diagnosis of adrenocortical insufficiency (diagnostic 30-minute test), low-dose test

▶ BY INTRAMUSCULAR INJECTION, OR BY INTRAVENOUS INJECTION
▶ Child: 0.3 microgram/m^2 for 1 dose

Infantile spasm

▶ BY INTRAMUSCULAR INJECTION USING DEPOT INJECTION
▶ Child 1–23 months: Initially 500 micrograms once daily on alternate days, adjusted according to response

- **UNLICENSED USE** Not licensed for low-dose test for adrenocortical insufficiency. Not licensed for treatment of infantile spasms.

- **CONTRA-INDICATIONS** Acute psychosis · adrenogenital syndrome · allergic disorders · asthma · avoid injections containing benzyl alcohol in neonates · Cushing's syndrome · infectious diseases · peptic ulcer · primary adrenocortical insufficiency · refractory heart failure

- **CAUTIONS** Active infectious diseases (should not be used unless adequate disease-specific therapy is being given) · active systemic diseases (should not be used unless adequate disease-specific therapy is being given) · diabetes mellitus · diverticulitis · history of asthma · history of atopic allergy · history of eczema · history of hayfever · history of hypersensitivity · hypertension · latent amoebiasis (may become activated) · latent tuberculosis (may become activated) · myasthenia gravis · ocular herpes simplex · osteoporosis · predisposition to thromboembolic · pscyhological disturbances may be triggered · recent intestinal anastomosis · reduced immune response (should not be used unless adequate disease-specific therapy is being given) · ulcerative colitis

CAUTIONS, FURTHER INFORMATION
▶ **Risk of anaphylaxis** Should only be administered under medical supervision. Consult product literature.

6

Endocrine system

▸ **Hypertension** Patients already receiving medication for moderate to severe hypertension must have their dosage adjusted if treatment started.

▸ **Diabetes mellitus** Patients already receiving medication for diabetes mellitus must have their dosage adjusted if treatment started.

● **INTERACTIONS** → Appendix 1 (corticosteroids).

● **SIDE-EFFECTS** Abdominal distention · abscess · acne · anaphylactic shock · anaphylactoid reactions in children aged under 3 years (benzyl alcohol-containing injections) · angioneurotic oedema · aseptic necrosis of femoral and humeral heads · benign intracranial pressure increased with papilloedema · calcium deficiency · cardiac disorders · convulsions · Cushing's syndrome · decreased carbohydrate tolerance · dizziness · dysponea · ecchymosis · erythema · euphoria · fluid retention · flushing · glaucoma · growth retardation · headache · hirsutism · hyperglycaemia · hyperhidrosis · hypersensitivity reactions (tend to be more severe in patients susceptible to allergies, especially asthma) · hypertension · hypokalaemia · hypokalaemic alkalosis · impaired healing · increased appetite · increased intraocular pressure · infection susceptibility increased · insomnia · irregular menstruation · leukocytosis · malaise · manifestations of latent diabetes mellitus · mood swings · muscle atrophy · muscular weakness · myopathy · nausea · necrotising vasculitis · negative nitrogen balance · osteoporosis · pancreatitis · pathological fracture of long bones · peptic ulcer · personality changes · petechiae · posterior subcapsular cataracts · pruritus · psychotic manifestations · Quincke's oedema · secondary adrenocortical unresponsiveness · secondary pituitary unresponsiveness · severe depression · skin atrophy · skin hyperpigmentation · skin reactions at injection site · sodium retention · spinal compression fractures · tendon rupture · thromboembolism · toxic reactions in children aged under 3 years (benzyl alcohol-containing injections) · ulcerative oesophagitis · urticaria · vertigo · vomiting · weight increase

● **ALLERGY AND CROSS-SENSITIVITY** Contra-indicated in patients with history of hypersensitivity to tetracosactide/corticotrophins or excipients.

● **PREGNANCY** Avoid (but may be used diagnostically if essential).

● **BREAST FEEDING** Avoid (but may be used diagnostically if essential).

● **HEPATIC IMPAIRMENT** An enhanced effect of tetracosactide therapy may occur in patients with cirrhosis of the liver. Use with caution in hepatic impairment. Monitor hepatic function closely during treatment.

● **RENAL IMPAIRMENT** Use with caution in patients with renal impairment.

● **EFFECT ON LABORATORY TESTS** May suppress skin test reactions.

Post administration total plasma cortisol levels during 30-minute test for diagnosis of adrenocotical insufficiency might be misleading due to altered cortisol binding globulin levels in some special clinical situations including, patients on oral contraceptives, post-operative patients, critical illness, severe liver disease and nephrotic syndrome.

● **DIRECTIONS FOR ADMINISTRATION** For *intramuscular* or *intravenous injection*, may be diluted in sodium chloride 0.9% to 250 nanograms/mL.

● **MEDICINAL FORMS**
There can be variation in the licensing of different medicines containing the same drug.

Solution for injection
▸ Synacthen (Mallinckrodt Specialty Pharmaceuticals Ireland Ltd)
Tetracosactide acetate 250 microgram per 1 ml Synacthen 250micrograms/1ml solution for injection ampoules | 1 ampoule PoM £38.00

Suspension for injection
EXCIPIENTS: May contain Benzyl alcohol
▸ Synacthen Depot (Mallinckrodt Specialty Pharmaceuticals Ireland Ltd)
Tetracosactide acetate 1 mg per 1 ml Synacthen Depot 1mg/1ml suspension for injection ampoules | 1 ampoule PoM £346.28

6.2 Assessment of pituitary function

DIAGNOSTIC AGENTS

Corticorelin

(Corticotrophin-releasing hormone; CRH)

● **INDICATIONS AND DOSE**
Test of anterior pituitary function
▸ BY INTRAVENOUS INJECTION
▸ Child: 1 microgram/kg (max. per dose 100 micrograms) for 1 dose, to be administered over 30 seconds

● **UNLICENSED USE** Not licensed.

● **SIDE-EFFECTS** Flushing of face · flushing of neck · flushing of upper body · hypotension · mild sensation of smell · mild sensation of taste

● **PREGNANCY** Avoid.

● **BREAST FEEDING** Avoid.

● **MEDICINAL FORMS**
There can be variation in the licensing of different medicines containing the same drug.
No licensed medicines listed.

Gonadorelin

(Gonadotrophin-releasing hormone; GnRH; LH–RH)

● **INDICATIONS AND DOSE**
Assessment of anterior pituitary function | Assessment of delayed puberty
▸ BY INTRAVENOUS INJECTION, OR BY SUBCUTANEOUS INJECTION
▸ Child 1–17 years: 2.5 micrograms/kg (max. per dose 100 micrograms) for 1 dose

● **UNLICENSED USE** Not licensed for use in children under 1 year.

● **CAUTIONS** Pituitary adenoma

● **SIDE-EFFECTS** Abdominal pain · headache · hypersensitivity reaction on repeated administration of large doses · increased menstrual bleeding · irritation at injection site · nausea

● **PREGNANCY** Avoid.

● **BREAST FEEDING** Avoid.

- **MEDICINAL FORMS**
  There can be variation in the licensing of different medicines containing the same drug.
  Powder and solvent for solution for injection
  EXCIPIENTS: May contain Benzyl alcohol
  ▸ Gonadorelin (Non-proprietary)
    Gonadorelin (as Gonadorelin hydrochloride)
    100 microgram Gonadorelin 100microgram powder and solvent for solution for injection vials | 1 vial [PoM] £75.00 (Hospital only)

6.3 Gonadotrophin replacement therapy

GONADOTROPHINS

▌Chorionic gonadotrophin

(Human chorionic gonadotrophin; HCG)

- **DRUG ACTION** A preparation of a glycoprotein fraction secreted by the placenta and obtained from the urine of pregnant women having the action of the pituitary luteinising hormone.

- **INDICATIONS AND DOSE**

  Delayed puberty in the male to stimulate endogenous testosterone production
  ▸ BY INTRAMUSCULAR INJECTION, OR BY SUBCUTANEOUS INJECTION
  ▸ Child: (consult product literature)

  Test of testicular function, short stimulation test
  ▸ BY INTRAMUSCULAR INJECTION
  ▸ Child: 1500–2000 units once daily for 3 days

  Test of testicular function, prolonged stimulation test
  ▸ BY INTRAMUSCULAR INJECTION
  ▸ Child: 1500–2000 units twice weekly for 3 weeks

  Hypogonadotrophic hypogonadism
  ▸ BY INTRAMUSCULAR INJECTION
  ▸ Child: 1000–2000 units twice weekly, adjusted according to response

  Undescended testes
  ▸ BY INTRAMUSCULAR INJECTION
  ▸ Child 7-16 years: Initially 500 units 3 times a week, adjusted according to response to up to 4000 units 3 times a week continue for 1–2 months after testicular descent
  ▸ Child 17 years: Initially 1000 units twice weekly, adjusted according to response to up to 4000 units 3 times a week continue for 1–2 months after testicular descent

- **UNLICENSED USE** Unlicensed in children for test of testicular function.
- **CONTRA-INDICATIONS** Androgen-dependent tumours
- **CAUTIONS** Asthma · cardiac impairment · epilepsy · migraine · prepubertal boys (risk of premature epiphyseal closure or precocious puberty)
- **SIDE-EFFECTS** Gynaecomastia · headache · local reactions · mood changes · oedema (particularly in males—reduce dose) · tiredness
- **RENAL IMPAIRMENT** Use with caution.

- **MEDICINAL FORMS**
  There can be variation in the licensing of different medicines containing the same drug.
  Powder and solvent for solution for injection
  ▸ Choragon (Ferring Pharmaceuticals Ltd)
    Chorionic gonadotrophin human 5000 unit Choragon 5,000unit powder and solvent for solution for injection ampoules | 3 ampoule [PoM] £9.77 [CD4-2]

▸ Pregnyl (Merck Sharp & Dohme Ltd)
  Chorionic gonadotrophin human 1500 unit Pregnyl 1,500unit powder and solvent for solution for injection ampoules | 1 ampoule [PoM] £2.12 [CD4-2]
  Chorionic gonadotrophin human 5000 unit Pregnyl 5,000unit powder and solvent for solution for injection ampoules | 1 ampoule [PoM] £3.15 [CD4-2]

6.4 Growth hormone disorders

PITUITARY AND HYPOTHALAMIC HORMONES AND ANALOGUES ⟩ HUMAN GROWTH HORMONES

▌Somatropin

(Recombinant Human Growth Hormone)

- **INDICATIONS AND DOSE**

  Gonadal dysgenesis (Turner syndrome)
  ▸ BY SUBCUTANEOUS INJECTION
  ▸ Child: 1.4 mg/m^2 daily, alternatively 45–50 micrograms/kg daily

  Deficiency of growth hormone
  ▸ BY SUBCUTANEOUS INJECTION, OR BY INTRAMUSCULAR INJECTION
  ▸ Child: 23–39 micrograms/kg daily, alternatively 0.7–1 mg/m^2 daily

  Growth disturbance in children born small for gestational age whose growth has not caught up by 4 years or later | Noonan syndrome
  ▸ BY SUBCUTANEOUS INJECTION
  ▸ Child 4-17 years: 35 micrograms/kg daily, alternatively 1 mg/m^2 daily

  Prader-Willi syndrome, in children with growth velocity greater than 1 cm/year, in combination with energy-restricted diet
  ▸ BY SUBCUTANEOUS INJECTION
  ▸ Child: 1 mg/m^2 daily, alternatively 35 micrograms/kg daily; maximum 2.7 mg per day

  Chronic renal insufficiency (renal function decreased to less than 50%)
  ▸ BY SUBCUTANEOUS INJECTION
  ▸ Child: 45–50 micrograms/kg daily, alternatively 1.4 mg/m^2 daily, higher doses may be needed, adjust if necessary after 6 months

  SHOX deficiency
  ▸ BY SUBCUTANEOUS INJECTION
  ▸ Child: 45–50 micrograms/kg daily

  DOSE EQUIVALENCE AND CONVERSION
  Dose formerly expressed in units; somatropin 1 mg ≡ 3 units.

- **UNLICENSED USE** Not licensed for use in Noonan syndrome.
- **CONTRA-INDICATIONS** Avoid injections containing benzyl alcohol in neonates · evidence of tumour activity (complete antitumour therapy and ensure intracranial lesions inactive before starting) · not to be used after renal transplantation · not to be used for growth promotion in children with closed epiphyses (or near closure in Prader-Willi syndrome) · severe obesity in Prader-Willi syndrome · severe respiratory impairment in Prader-Willi syndrome
- **CAUTIONS** Diabetes mellitus (adjustment of antidiabetic therapy may be necessary) · disorders of the epiphysis of the hip (monitor for limping) · history of malignant disease · hypothyroidism—manufacturers recommend periodic thyroid function tests but limited evidence of clinical value · initiation of treatment close to puberty not recommended in child born small for corrected gestational age · papilloedema · relative deficiencies of other pituitary

6

Endocrine system

hormones · resolved intracranial hypertension (monitor closely) · Silver-Russell syndrome

● INTERACTIONS → Appendix 1 (somatropin).

● SIDE-EFFECTS Antibody formation · arthralgia · benign intracranial hypertension · carpal tunnel syndrome · fluid retention (peripheral oedema) · headache · hyperglycaemia · hypoglycaemia · hypothyroidism · insulin resistance · leukaemia in children with growth hormone deficiency · myalgia · nausea · papilloedema · paraesthesia · reactions at injection site · visual problems · vomiting

SIDE-EFFECTS, FURTHER INFORMATION
▸ Papilloedema Funduscopy for papilloedema recommended if severe or recurrent headache, visual problems, nausea and vomiting occur—if papilloedema confirmed consider benign intracranial hypertension (rare cases reported).

● PREGNANCY Discontinue if pregnancy occurs—no information available.

● BREAST FEEDING No information available. Absorption from milk unlikely.

● DIRECTIONS FOR ADMINISTRATION Rotate subcutaneous injection sites to prevent lipoatrophy.
NUTROPINAQ®, GENOTROPIN®, NORDITROPIN®, OMNITROPE®, SAIZEN® and ZOMACTON® PREPARATIONS For use by subcutaneous injection.
HUMATROPE® Cartridges for use by subcutaneous injection. Powder for reconstitution for use by subcutaneous or intramuscular injection.

● PRESCRIBING AND DISPENSING INFORMATION Medicinal products containing somatropin are not identical and although there should be no important differences in terms of safety and efficacy, when prescribing biological products it is good practice to use the brand name, see *Biosimilar medicines*, under Guidance on prescribing p. 1.
SAIZEN® SOLUTION FOR INJECTION For use with *cool.click®* needle-free autoinjector device or *easypod®* autoinjector device (non-NHS but available free of charge from clinics).
NUTROPINAQ® For use with *NutropinAq®* Pen device (non-NHS but available free of charge from clinics).
OMNITROPE® For use with *Omnitrope Pen 5®* and *Omnitrope Pen 10®* devices (non-NHS but available free of charge from clinics).
NORDITROPIN® PREPARATIONS Cartridges for use with appropriate *NordiPen®* device (non-NHS but available free of charge from clinics).
  Multidose disposable prefilled pens for use with *NovoFine®* or *NovoTwist®* needles.
ZOMACTON® 4 mg vial for use with *ZomaJet 2® Vision* needle-free device (non-NHS but available free of charge from clinics) or with needles and syringes.
  10 mg vial for use with *ZomaJet Vision X®* needle-free device (non-NHS but available free of charge from clinics) or with needles and syringes.
GENOTROPIN® PREPARATIONS Cartridges are for use with *Genotropin®* Pen device (non-NHS but available free of charge from clinics).
SAIZEN® POWDER AND SOLVENT FOR SOLUTION FOR INJECTION For use with *one. click®* autoinjector device or *cool.click®* needle-free autoinjector device or *easypod®* autoinjector device (non-NHS but available free of charge from clinics).

● NATIONAL FUNDING/ACCESS DECISIONS
NICE technology appraisals (TAs)
▸ **Somatropin for the treatment of growth failure in children (May 2010)** NICE TA188
Somatropin is recommended for children with growth failure who:
  ● have growth-hormone deficiency
  ● have Turner syndrome
  ● have Prader-Willi syndrome

  ● have chronic renal insufficiency
  ● are born small for gestational age with subsequent growth failure at 4 years of age or later
  ● have short stature homeobox-containing gene (SHOX) deficiency.
Treatment should be discontinued if growth velocity increases by less than 50% from baseline in the first year of treatment.
www.nice.org.uk/TA188

● MEDICINAL FORMS
There can be variation in the licensing of different medicines containing the same drug.

Solution for injection
EXCIPIENTS: May contain Benzyl alcohol
▸ **Norditropin NordiFlex** (Novo Nordisk Ltd)
Somatropin (epr) 3.3 mg per 1 ml Norditropin NordiFlex 5mg/1.5ml solution for injection pre-filled pen | 1 pre-filled disposable injection PoM £115.90 CD4-2
Somatropin (epr) 6.7 mg per 1 ml Norditropin NordiFlex 10mg/1.5ml solution for injection pre-filled pen | 1 pre-filled disposable injection PoM £231.80 CD4-2
Somatropin (epr) 10 mg per 1 ml Norditropin NordiFlex 15mg/1.5ml solution for injection pre-filled pen | 1 pre-filled disposable injection PoM £347.70 CD4-2
▸ **Norditropin SimpleXx** (Novo Nordisk Ltd)
Somatropin (epr) 3.3 mg per 1 ml Norditropin SimpleXx 5mg/1.5ml solution for injection cartridges | 1 cartridge PoM £106.35 CD4-2
Somatropin (epr) 6.7 mg per 1 ml Norditropin SimpleXx 10mg/1.5ml solution for injection cartridges | 1 cartridge PoM £212.70 CD4-2
Somatropin (epr) 10 mg per 1 ml Norditropin SimpleXx 15mg/1.5ml solution for injection cartridges | 1 cartridge PoM £319.05 CD4-2
▸ **NutropinAq** (Ipsen Ltd)
Somatropin (rbe) 5 mg per 1 ml NutropinAq 10mg/2ml solution for injection cartridges | 1 cartridge PoM £203.00 CD4-2 | 3 cartridge PoM £609.00 CD4-2
▸ **Omnitrope Pen** (Sandoz Ltd)
Somatropin (rbe) 3.333 mg per 1 ml Omnitrope Pen 5 5mg/1.5ml solution for injection cartridges | 5 cartridge PoM £368.74 CD4-2
Somatropin (rbe) 6.667 mg per 1 ml Omnitrope Pen 10 10mg/1.5ml solution for injection cartridges | 5 cartridge PoM £737.49 CD4-2
▸ **Omnitrope SurePal** (Sandoz Ltd)
Somatropin (rbe) 3.333 mg per 1 ml Omnitrope SurePal 5 5mg/1.5ml solution for injection cartridges | 5 cartridge PoM £368.74 CD4-2
Somatropin (rbe) 6.667 mg per 1 ml Omnitrope SurePal 10 10mg/1.5ml solution for injection cartridges | 5 cartridge PoM £737.49 CD4-2
Somatropin (rbe) 10 mg per 1 ml Omnitrope SurePal 15 15mg/1.5ml solution for injection cartridges | 5 cartridge PoM £1,106.22 CD4-2
▸ **Saizen** (Merck Serono Ltd)
Somatropin (rmc) 5.825 mg per 1 ml Saizen 6mg/1.03ml solution for injection cartridges | 1 cartridge PoM £139.08 CD4-2
Somatropin (rmc) 8 mg per 1 ml Saizen 20mg/2.5ml solution for injection cartridges | 1 cartridge PoM £463.60 CD4-2
Saizen 12mg/1.5ml solution for injection cartridges | 1 cartridge PoM £278.16 CD4-2

Powder and solvent for solution for injection
EXCIPIENTS: May contain Benzyl alcohol
▸ **Genotropin** (Pfizer Ltd)
Somatropin (rbe) 5.3 mg Genotropin 5.3mg powder and solvent for solution for injection cartridges | 1 cartridge PoM £92.15 CD4-2
Somatropin (rbe) 12 mg Genotropin 12mg powder and solvent for solution for injection cartridges | 1 cartridge PoM £208.65 CD4-2
▸ **Genotropin GoQuick** (Pfizer Ltd)
Somatropin (rbe) 5.3 mg Genotropin GoQuick 5.3mg powder and solvent for solution for injection pre-filled disposable devices | 1 pre-filled disposable injection PoM £92.15 CD4-2
Somatropin (rbe) 12 mg Genotropin GoQuick 12mg powder and solvent for solution for injection pre-filled disposable devices | 1 pre-filled disposable injection PoM £208.65 CD4-2
▸ **Genotropin MiniQuick** (Pfizer Ltd)
Somatropin (rbe) 200 microgram Genotropin MiniQuick 200microgram powder and solvent for solution for injection pre-filled disposable devices | 7 pre-filled disposable injection PoM £24.35 CD4-2

Somatropin (rbe) 400 microgram Genotropin MiniQuick 400microgram powder and solvent for solution for injection pre-filled disposable devices | 7 pre-filled disposable injection PoM £48.68 CD4-2

Somatropin (rbe) 600 microgram Genotropin MiniQuick 600microgram powder and solvent for solution for injection pre-filled disposable devices | 7 pre-filled disposable injection PoM £73.03 CD4-2

Somatropin (rbe) 800 microgram Genotropin MiniQuick 800microgram powder and solvent for solution for injection pre-filled disposable devices | 7 pre-filled disposable injection PoM £97.37 CD4-2

Somatropin (rbe) 1 mg Genotropin MiniQuick 1mg powder and solvent for solution for injection pre-filled disposable devices | 7 pre-filled disposable injection PoM £121.71 CD4-2

Somatropin (rbe) 1.2 mg Genotropin MiniQuick 1.2mg powder and solvent for solution for injection pre-filled disposable devices | 7 pre-filled disposable injection PoM £146.06 CD4-2

Somatropin (rbe) 1.4 mg Genotropin MiniQuick 1.4mg powder and solvent for solution for injection pre-filled disposable devices | 7 pre-filled disposable injection PoM £170.39 CD4-2

Somatropin (rbe) 1.6 mg Genotropin MiniQuick 1.6mg powder and solvent for solution for injection pre-filled disposable devices | 7 pre-filled disposable injection PoM £194.74 CD4-2

Somatropin (rbe) 1.8 mg Genotropin MiniQuick 1.8mg powder and solvent for solution for injection pre-filled disposable devices | 7 pre-filled disposable injection PoM £219.08 CD4-2

Somatropin (rbe) 2 mg Genotropin MiniQuick 2mg powder and solvent for solution for injection pre-filled disposable devices | 7 pre-filled disposable injection PoM £243.42 CD4-2

▸ **Humatrope** (Eli Lilly and Company Ltd)

Somatropin (rbe) 6 mg Humatrope 6mg powder and solvent for solution for injection cartridges | 1 cartridge PoM £108.00 CD4-2

Somatropin (rbe) 12 mg Humatrope 12mg powder and solvent for solution for injection cartridges | 1 cartridge PoM £216.00 CD4-2

Somatropin (rbe) 24 mg Humatrope 24mg powder and solvent for solution for injection cartridges | 1 cartridge PoM £432.00 CD4-2

▸ **Saizen** (Merck Serono Ltd)

Somatropin (rmc) 8 mg Saizen 8mg click.easy powder and solvent for solution for injection vials | 1 vial PoM £185.44 CD4-2

▸ **Zomacton** (Ferring Pharmaceuticals Ltd)

Somatropin (rbe) 4 mg Zomacton 4mg powder and solvent for solution for injection vials | 1 vial PoM £79.69 CD4-2

Somatropin (rbe) 10 mg Zomacton 10mg powder and solvent for solution for injection vials | 1 vial PoM £199.23 CD4-2

6.4a Insulin-like growth factor-I deficiency

PITUITARY AND HYPOTHALAMIC HORMONES AND ANALOGUES > SOMATOMEDINS

Mecasermin

(Recombinant human factor-I; rhIGF-I)

● **DRUG ACTION** Somatomedins are a group of polypeptide hormones structurally related to insulin and commonly known as insulin-like growth factors (IGFs). Mecasermin, a human insulin-like growth factor-I (rhIGF-I), is the principal mediator of the somatotropic effects of human growth hormone.

● **INDICATIONS AND DOSE**

Treatment of growth failure in children with severe primary insulin-like growth factor-I deficiency

▸ BY SUBCUTANEOUS INJECTION

▸ Child 2–17 years: Initially 40 micrograms/kg twice daily for 1 week, increased, if tolerated, in steps of 40 micrograms/kg (max. per dose 120 micrograms/kg twice daily), discontinue if no response within 1 year, reduce dose if hypoglycaemia occurs despite adequate food intake; withhold injection if patient unable to eat

● **CONTRA-INDICATIONS** Evidence of tumour activity (discontinue treatment)

● **CAUTIONS** Correct hypothyroidism before initiating treatment · diabetes mellitus (adjustment of antidiabetic therapy may be necessary) · papilloedema

● **SIDE-EFFECTS** Antibody formation · arthralgia · cardiomegaly · convulsions · dizziness · gynaecomastia · headache · hyperglycaemia · hypoglycaemia (especially in first month, and in younger children) · impaired hearing · injection-site reactions (rotate site) · myalgia · nausea · nervousness · night terrors · severe or recurrent headache · sleep apnoea · tachycardia · tonsillar hypertrophy · ventricular hypertrophy · visual disturbance · visual problems · vomiting

SIDE-EFFECTS, FURTHER INFORMATION

▸ Papilloedema Funduscopy for papilloedema recommended if severe or recurrent headache, visual problems, nausea and vomiting occur—if papilloedema confirmed consider benign intracranial hypertension (rare cases reported).

● **CONCEPTION AND CONTRACEPTION** Contraception advised in women of child-bearing potential.

● **PREGNANCY** Avoid unless essential.

● **BREAST FEEDING** Avoid.

● **MONITORING REQUIREMENTS**

▸ Monitor ECG before and on termination of treatment (and during treatment if ECG abnormal).

▸ Monitor for disorders of the epiphysis of the hip (monitor for limping).

▸ Monitor for signs of tonsillar hypertrophy (snoring, sleep apnoea, and chronic middle ear effusions).

● **DIRECTIONS FOR ADMINISTRATION** Dose should be administered just before or after food.

● **PATIENT AND CARER ADVICE**

Patients or carers should be given advice on how to administer mecasermin injection.

Missed doses

Patients or carers should be advised not to increase dose if a dose is missed.

● **MEDICINAL FORMS**

There can be variation in the licensing of different medicines containing the same drug.

Solution for injection

EXCIPIENTS: May contain Benzyl alcohol

▸ Increlex (Ipsen Ltd) ▼

Mecasermin 10 mg per 1 ml Increlex 40mg/4ml solution for injection vials | 1 vial PoM £605.00

7 Sex hormone responsive conditions

Sex hormones

Hormone replacement therapy

Sex hormone replacement therapy is indicated in children for the treatment of gonadotrophin deficiency, gonadal disorders, or delayed puberty that interferes with quality of life. Indications include constitutional delay in puberty, congenital or acquired hypogonadotrophic hypogonadism, hypergonadotrophic hypogonadism (Turner's syndrome, Klinefelter's syndrome), endocrine disorders (Cushing's syndrome or hyperprolactinaemia), and chronic illnesses, such as cystic fibrosis or sickle-cell disease, that may affect the onset of puberty.

Replacement therapy is generally started at the appropriate age for the development of puberty and should be managed by a paediatric endocrinologist. Patients with constitutional delay, chronic illness, or eating disorders may need only small doses of hormone supplements for 4 to 6 months to induce puberty and endogenous sex hormone production, which is then sustained. Patients with organic causes of hormone deficiency will require life-long replacement, adjusted to allow normal development.

Inadequate treatment may lead to poor bone mineralisation, resulting in fractures and osteoporosis.

Female sex hormones

Oestrogens

Oestrogens are necessary for the development of female secondary sexual characteristics. If onset of puberty is delayed because of organic pathology, puberty can be induced with ethinylestradiol below in increasing doses, guided by breast staging and uterine scans. Cyclical progestogen replacement is added after 12–18 months of oestrogen treatment. Once the adult dosage of oestrogen has been reached, it may be more convenient to provide replacement either as a low-dose oestrogen containing oral contraceptive formulation [unlicensed indication] or as a combined oestrogen and progestogen hormone replacement therapy preparation [unlicensed indication]. There is limited experience in the use of transdermal patches or gels in children; compliance and skin irritation are sometimes a problem.

Ethinylestradiol is occasionally used, under **specialist supervision**, for the management of hereditary haemorrhagic telangiectasia (but evidence of benefit is limited), for the prevention of tall stature, and in tests of growth hormone secretion.

Topical oestrogen creams are used in the treatment of labial adhesions.

Progestogens

There are two main groups of progestogen, *progesterone and its analogues* (dydrogesterone and medroxyprogesterone acetate p. 478) and *testosterone analogues* (norethisterone p. 447 and norgestrel). The newer progestogens (desogestrel p. 474, norgestimate, and gestodene) are all derivatives of norgestrel; levonorgestrel p. 475 is the active isomer of norgestrel and has twice its potency. Progesterone and its analogues are less androgenic than the testosterone derivatives and neither progesterone nor dydrogesterone causes virilisation.

In delayed puberty cyclical progestogen is added after 12–18 months of oestrogen therapy to establish a menstrual cycle.

Norethisterone is also used to postpone menstruation during a cycle; treatment is started 3 days before the expected onset of menstruation.

7.1 Female sex hormone responsive conditions

OESTROGENS

Ethinylestradiol

(Ethinyloestradiol)

- ● **INDICATIONS AND DOSE**

Induction of sexual maturation in girls
- ▶ BY MOUTH
- ▶ Child (female): Initially 2 micrograms daily for 6 months, then increased to 5 micrograms daily for 6 months, then increased to 10 micrograms daily for 6 months, then increased to 20 micrograms daily, after 12–18 months of treatment give progestogen for 7 days of each 28-day cycle.

Maintenance of sexual maturation in girls
- ▶ BY MOUTH
- ▶ Child (female): 20 micrograms daily, to be given with cyclical progestogen for 7 days of each 28-day cycle.

Prevention of tall stature in girls
- ▶ BY MOUTH
- ▶ Child 2–11 years (female): 20–50 micrograms daily.

Pituitary priming before growth hormone secretion test in girls with bone age over 10 years
- ▶ BY MOUTH
- ▶ Child (female): 100 micrograms daily for 3 days before test.

- ● **UNLICENSED USE** Unlicensed for use in children.
- ● **CONTRA-INDICATIONS** Acute porphyrias p. 562 · cardiovascular disease (sodium retention with oedema) · family history of thromboembolism · gallstones · heart disease associated with pulmonary hypertension · heart disease associated with risk of embolus · history during pregnancy of cholestatic jaundice · history during pregnancy of chorea · history during pregnancy of pemphigoid gestationis · history during pregnancy of pruritus · history of breast cancer · history of haemolytic uraemic syndrome · migraine with aura · sclerosing treatment for varicose veins · severe or multiple risk factors for arterial disease · severe or multiple risk factors for venous thromboembolism · systemic lupus erythematosus · transient cerebral ischaemic attacks without headaches · undiagnosed vaginal bleeding · venous thromboembolism, or history of recurrent venous thromboembolism (unless already on anticoagulant treatment)
- ● **CAUTIONS** Active trophoblastic disease (until return to normal of urine- and plasma-gonadotrophin concentration)—seek specialist advice · Crohn's disease · gene mutations associated with breast cancer (e.g. BRCA 1) · history of severe depression (especially if induced by hormonal contraceptive) · hyperprolactinaemia (seek specialist advice) · inflammatory bowel disease · migraine (migraine-like headaches) · personal or family history of hypertriglyceridaemia (increased risk of pancreatitis) · risk factors for arterial disease · risk factors for migraine · risk factors for venous thromboembolism · sickle-cell disease · undiagnosed breast mass

CAUTIONS, FURTHER INFORMATION
- ▶ Other conditions The product literature advises caution in other conditions including hypertension, renal disease, asthma, epilepsy, sickle-cell disease, melanoma, otosclerosis, multiple sclerosis, and systemic lupus erythematosus (but care required if antiphospholipid antibodies present, see above). Evidence for caution in these conditions is unsatisfactory and many women with these conditions may stand to benefit from treatment.
- ▶ Risk of venous thromboembolism Use with **caution** if any of following factors present but **avoid** if two or more factors present:
  - *family history of venous thromboembolism* in first-degree relative aged under 45 years (avoid if known prothrombotic coagulation abnormality e.g. factor V Leiden or antiphospholipid antibodies (including lupus anticoagulant));
  - *obesity*—body mass index $\geq$30 kg/m^2 (avoid if body mass index $\geq$35 kg/m^2 unless no suitable alternative); (In adolescents, caution if obese according to BMI (adjusted for age and gender); in those who are markedly obese, avoid unless no suitable alternative);
  - *long-term immobilisation* e.g. in a wheelchair (avoid if confined to bed or leg in plaster cast);
  - *history of superficial thrombophlebitis;*
  - *age* over 35 years (avoid if over 50 years);
  - *smoking.*

▸ **Risk factors for arterial disease** Use with **caution** if any one of following factors present but **avoid** if two or more factors present:

- *family history of arterial disease* in first degree relative aged under 45 years (avoid if atherogenic lipid profile);
- *diabetes mellitus* (avoid if diabetes complications present);
- *hypertension*—blood pressure above *systolic* 140 *mmHg* or *diastolic* 90 *mmHg* (avoid if blood pressure above *systolic* 160 *mmHg* or *diastolic* 95 *mmHg*); (In adolescents, avoid if blood pressure very high);
- *smoking* (avoid if smoking 40 or more cigarettes daily);
- *age* over 35 years (avoid if over 50 years);
- *obesity* (avoid if body mass index $\geq$35 kg/m^2 unless no suitable alternative); (In adolescents, caution if obese according to BMI (adjusted for age and gender); in those who are markedly obese, avoid unless no suitable alternative);
- *migraine without aura* (avoid if *migraine with aura* (focal symptoms), *or* severe migraine frequently lasting over 72 hours despite treatment, *or* migraine treated with ergot derivatives).

▸ **Migraine** Women should report any increase in headache frequency or onset of focal symptoms (discontinue immediately and refer urgently to neurology expert if focal neurological symptoms not typical of aura persist for more than 1 hour).

● **INTERACTIONS** → Appendix 1 (oestrogens).

● **SIDE-EFFECTS**

▸ **Rare** Gallstones · systemic lupus erythematosus

▸ **Frequency not known** Abdominal cramps · absence of withdrawal bleeding · amenorrhoea after discontinuation · breast enlargement · breast secretion · breast tenderness · cervical erosion · changes in libido · changes in lipid metabolism · changes in vaginal discharge · chloasma · chorea · contact lenses may irritate · depression · fluid retention · headache · hepatic tumours · hypertension · irritability · leg cramps (rule out venous thrombosis) · liver impairment · nausea · nervousness · photosensitivity · reduced menstrual loss · skin reactions · symptoms of endometriosis may be exacerbated · thrombosis (more common when factor V Leiden present or in blood groups A, B, and AB) · uterine fibroids may increase in size · visual disturbances · vomiting · weight changes · 'spotting' in early cycles

SIDE-EFFECTS, FURTHER INFORMATION

● **PREGNANCY** Avoid.

● **BREAST FEEDING** Avoid.

● **HEPATIC IMPAIRMENT** Avoid in liver disease including disorders of hepatic excretion (e.g. Dubin-Johnson or Rotor syndromes), infective hepatitis (until liver function returns to normal), and jaundice.

● **MEDICINAL FORMS**
There can be variation in the licensing of different medicines containing the same drug. Forms available from special-order manufacturers include: tablet, capsule, oral suspension

Tablet
▸ Ethinylestradiol (Non-proprietary)
Ethinylestradiol 10 microgram Ethinylestradiol 10microgram tablets | 21 tablet [PoM] £200.00 DT price = £200.00
Ethinylestradiol 50 microgram Ethinylestradiol 50microgram tablets | 21 tablet [PoM] £200.00 DT price = £200.00
Ethinylestradiol 1 mg Ethinylestradiol 1mg tablets | 28 tablet [PoM] £200.00 DT price = £200.00

PROGESTOGENS

Norethisterone

● **INDICATIONS AND DOSE**

Postponement of menstruation
▸ BY MOUTH
▸ Females of childbearing potential: 5 mg 3 times a day, to be started 3 days before expected onset (menstruation occurs 2–3 days after stopping)

Induction and maintenance of sexual maturation in females (combined with an oestrogen after 12–18 months oestrogen therapy)
▸ BY MOUTH
▸ Child: 5 mg once daily for the last 7 days of 28-day cycle

Short-term contraception
▸ BY DEEP INTRAMUSCULAR INJECTION
▸ Females of childbearing potential: 200 mg, to be administered within first 5 days of cycle or immediately after parturition (duration 8 weeks). To be injected into the gluteal muscle, then 200 mg after 8 weeks if required

Contraception
▸ BY MOUTH
▸ Females of childbearing potential: 350 micrograms daily, dose to be taken at same time each day, starting on day 1 of cycle then continuously, if administration delayed for 3 hours or more it should be regarded as a 'missed pill'

● **UNLICENSED USE**
▸ When used for Induction and maintenance of sexual maturation in females or Postponement of menstruation Not licensed for use in children.
▸ When used for Contraception Consult product literature for the licensing status of individual preparations.

● **CONTRA-INDICATIONS**
GENERAL CONTRA-INDICATIONS
Avoid in patients with a history of liver tumours · breast cancer (unless progestogens are being used in the management of this condition) · genital cancer (unless progestogens are being used in the management of this condition) · history during pregnancy of idiopathic jaundice · history during pregnancy of pemphigoid gestationis (non-contraceptive indications) · history during pregnancy of severe pruritus (non-contraceptive indications) · when used as a contraceptive, history of breast cancer (can be used after 5 years if no evidence of disease and non-hormonal contraceptive methods unacceptable)

SPECIFIC CONTRA-INDICATIONS
▸ With oral use Acute porphyrias p. 562 · severe arterial disease · undiagnosed vaginal bleeding

● **CAUTIONS**
GENERAL CAUTIONS
Asthma · cardiac dysfunction · conditions that may worsen with fluid retention · diabetes (progestogens can decrease glucose tolerance—monitor patient closely) · epilepsy · history of depression · hypertension · migraine · susceptibility to thromboembolism (particular caution with high dose)

SPECIFIC CAUTIONS
▸ When used for contraception Active trophoblastic disease (until return to normal of urine- and plasma-gonadotrophin concentration)—seek specialist advice · arterial disease · functional ovarian cysts · history of jaundice in pregnancy · malabsorption syndromes · past ectopic pregnancy · sex-steroid dependent cancer · systemic lupus erythematosus with positive (or unknown) anti-phospholipid antibodies

6

Endocrine system

▸ With intramuscular use for contraception Disturbances of lipid metabolism · history during pregnancy of deterioration of otosclerosis · history during pregnancy of pruritus · possible risk of breast cancer

CAUTIONS, FURTHER INFORMATION

▸ Use as a contraceptive in co-morbidities The product literature advises caution in patients with history of thromboembolism, hypertension, diabetes mellitus and migraine; evidence for caution in these conditions is unsatisfactory.

▸ Breast cancer risk with contraceptive use There is a small increase in the risk of having breast cancer diagnosed in women using, or who have recently used, a progestogen-only contraceptive pill; this relative risk may be due to an earlier diagnosis. The most important risk factor appears to be the age at which the contraceptive is stopped rather than the duration of use; the risk disappears gradually during the 10 years after stopping and there is no excess risk by 10 years. A possible small increase in the risk of breast cancer should be weighed against the benefits.

● INTERACTIONS → Appendix 1 (progestogens).

▸ With intramuscular use Effectiveness of parenteral progestogen-only contraceptives is not affected by antibacterials that do not induce liver enzymes. The effectiveness of norethisterone intramuscular injection is not affected by enzyme-inducing drugs and may be continued as normal during courses of these drugs.

● SIDE-EFFECTS

GENERAL SIDE-EFFECTS

Acne · alopecia · anaphylactoid reactions · breast tenderness · change in libido · depression · disturbance of appetite · dizziness · fluid retention · headache · hirsutism · insomnia (non-contraceptive indications) · jaundice · menstrual disturbances · nausea · premenstrual-like syndrome · pruritus · rash · skin reactions · urticaria · vomiting · weight change

SPECIFIC SIDE-EFFECTS

▸ With intramuscular use Injection-site reactions

SIDE-EFFECTS, FURTHER INFORMATION

▸ Cervical cancer Use of injectable progestogen-only contraceptives may be associated with a small increased risk of cervical cancer, similar to that seen with combined oral contraceptives (use of combined oral contraceptives for 5 years or longer is associated with a small increased risk of cervical cancer; the risk diminishes after stopping and disappears by about 10 years). The risk of cervical cancer with other progestogen-only contraceptives is not yet known.

● PREGNANCY Not known to be harmful in contraceptive doses. Avoid in other indications.

● BREAST FEEDING Progestogen-only contraceptives do not affect lactation.

▸ With intramuscular use Withhold breast-feeding for neonates with severe or persistent jaundice requiring medical treatment.

● HEPATIC IMPAIRMENT When used as a contraceptive; caution in severe liver disease and recurrent cholestatic jaundice, avoid in liver tumour. Caution when used for sexual maturation and to postpone menstruation; avoid if severe.

● RENAL IMPAIRMENT Use with caution in non-contraceptive indications.

● PATIENT AND CARER ADVICE

Missed doses

Missed oral contraceptive pill The following advice is recommended: 'If you forget a pill, take it as soon as you remember and carry on with the next pill at the right time. If the pill was more than 3 hours overdue you are not protected. Continue normal pill-taking but you must also use another method, such as the condom, for the next 2 days.'

The Faculty of Sexual and Reproductive Healthcare recommends emergency contraception if one or more progestogen-only contraceptive tablets are missed or taken more than 3 hours late and unprotected intercourse has occurred before 2 further tablets have been correctly taken.

Diarrhoea and vomiting with oral contraceptives Vomiting and persistent, severe diarrhoea can interfere with the absorption of oral progestogen-only contraceptives. If vomiting occurs within 2 hours of taking an oral progestogen-only contraceptive, another pill should be taken as soon as possible. If a replacement pill is not taken within 3 hours of the normal time for taking the progestogen-only pill, or in cases of persistent vomiting or very severe diarrhoea, additional precautions should be used during illness and for 2 days after recovery.

Starting routine for oral contraceptives One tablet daily, on a continuous basis, starting on day 1 of cycle and taken at the same time each day (if delayed by longer than 3 hours contraceptive protection may be lost). Additional contraceptive precautions are not required if norethisterone is started up to and including day 5 of the menstrual cycle; if started after this time, additional contraceptive precautions are required for 2 days.

Changing from a combined oral contraceptive Start on the day following completion of the combined oral contraceptive course without a break (or in the case of ED tablets omitting the inactive ones).

After childbirth Oral progestogen-only contraceptives can be started up to and including day 21 postpartum without the need for additional contraceptive precautions. If started more than 21 days postpartum, additional contraceptive precautions are required for 2 days.

Contraceptives by injection Full counselling backed by *patient information leaflet* required before administration—likelihood of menstrual disturbance and the potential for a delay in return to full fertility. Delayed return of fertility and irregular cycles may occur after discontinuation of treatment but there is no evidence of permanent infertility.

● MEDICINAL FORMS

There can be variation in the licensing of different medicines containing the same drug. Forms available from special-order manufacturers include: oral suspension

Tablet

▸ Norethisterone (Non-proprietary)

Norethisterone 5 mg Norethisterone 5mg tablets | 30 tablet PoM £4.50 DT price = £2.18

▸ Micronor (Janssen-Cilag Ltd)

Norethisterone 350 microgram Micronor 350microgram tablets | 84 tablet PoM £1.80 DT price = £1.80

▸ Noriday (Pfizer Ltd)

Norethisterone 350 microgram Noriday 350microgram tablets | 84 tablet PoM £2.10 DT price = £1.80

▸ Primolut N (Bayer Plc)

Norethisterone 5 mg Primolut N 5mg tablets | 30 tablet PoM £2.26 DT price = £2.18

▸ Utovlan (Pfizer Ltd)

Norethisterone 5 mg Utovlan 5mg tablets | 30 tablet PoM £1.40 DT price = £2.18 | 90 tablet PoM £4.21

Solution for injection

▸ Noristerat (Bayer Plc)

Norethisterone enantate 200 mg per 1 ml Noristerat 200mg/1ml solution for injection ampoules | 1 ampoule PoM £4.05

7.2   Male sex hormone responsive conditions

Androgens, anti-androgens and anabolic steroids

Androgens

Androgens cause masculinisation; they are used as replacement therapy in androgen deficiency, in delayed puberty, and in those who are hypogonadal due to either pituitary or testicular disease.

When given to patients with hypopituitarism androgens can lead to normal sexual development and potency but not to fertility. If fertility is desired, the usual treatment is with gonadotrophins or pulsatile gonadotrophin-releasing hormone which stimulates spermatogenesis as well as androgen production.

Intramuscular depot preparations of **testosterone esters** are preferred for replacement therapy. Testosterone enantate or propionate or alternatively *Sustanon*®, which consists of a mixture of testosterone esters and has a longer duration of action, can be used. For induction of puberty, depot testosterone injections are given monthly and the doses increased every 6 to 12 months according to response. Single ester testosterone injections may need to be given more frequently.

Oral **testosterone undecanoate** is used for induction of puberty. An alternative approach that promotes growth rather than sexual maturation uses oral oxandrolone below.

Chorionic gonadotrophin has also been used in delayed puberty in the male to stimulate endogenous testosterone production, but has little advantage over testosterone.

Testosterone topical gel is also available but experience of use in children under 15 years is limited. Topical testosterone is applied to the penis in the treatment of microphallus; an extemporaneously prepared cream should be used because the alcohol in proprietary gel formulations causes irritation.

Anti-androgens and precocious puberty

The gonadorelin stimulation test is used to distinguish between *gonadotrophin-dependent (central) precocious puberty* and *gonadotrophin-independent precocious puberty.* Treatment requires specialist management.

Gonadorelin analogues, used in the management of gonadotrophin-dependent precocious puberty, delay development of secondary sexual characteristics and growth velocity.

Testolactone p. 451 and cyproterone acetate p. 450 are used in the management of gonadotrophin-independent precocious puberty, resulting from McCune-Albright syndrome, familial male precocious puberty (testotoxicosis), hormone-secreting tumours, and ovarian and testicular disorders. Testolactone inhibits the aromatisation of testosterone, the rate limiting step in oestrogen synthesis. Cyproterone acetate is a progestogen with anti-androgen properties.

Spironolactone is sometimes used in combination with testolactone because it has some androgen receptor blocking properties.

High blood concentration of sex hormones may activate release of gonadotrophin releasing hormone, leading to development of secondary, central gonadotrophin-dependent precocious puberty. This may require the addition of gonadorelin analogues to prevent progression of pubertal development and skeletal maturation.

Anabolic steroids have some androgenic activity but they cause less virilisation than androgens in girls. They are used in the treatment of some *aplastic anaemias.*

Oxandrolone is used to stimulate late pre-pubertal growth prior to induction of sexual maturation in boys with short stature and in girls with Turner's syndrome; specialist management is required.

ANABOLIC STEROIDS › ANDROSTAN DERIVATIVES

Oxandrolone

- **INDICATIONS AND DOSE**
  Stimulation of late pre-pubertal growth in boys (of appropriate age) with short stature
  ▸ BY MOUTH
  ▸ Child 10-17 years (male): 1.25–2.5 mg daily for 3–6 months.
  Stimulation of late pre-pubertal growth in girls with Turner's syndrome
  ▸ BY MOUTH
  ▸ Child (female): 0.625–2.5 mg daily, to be taken in combination with growth hormone.

- **CONTRA-INDICATIONS** History of primary liver tumours · hypercalcaemia · nephrosis

- **CAUTIONS** Cardiac impairment · diabetes mellitus · epilepsy · hypertension · migraine · skeletal metastases (risk of hypercalcaemia)

- **INTERACTIONS** → Appendix 1 (oxandrolone).

- **SIDE-EFFECTS**
  ▸ **Common or very common** Virilism in females · acne · androgenic effects · anxiety · asthenia · changes in libido · cholestatic jaundice · depression · electrolyte disturbances · excessive duration of penile erection · excessive frequency of penile erection · gastro-intestinal bleeding · gynaecomastia · headache · hirsutism · hypercalcaemia · hypertension · increased bone growth · male-pattern baldness · nausea · oedema · paraesthesia · polycythaemia · precocious sexual development in pre-pubertal males · premature closure of epiphyses in pre-pubertal males · pruritus · seborrhoea · sodium retention · suppression of spermatogenesis in males · weight gain
  ▸ **Rare** Liver tumours
  ▸ **Frequency not known** Sleep apnoea

- **PREGNANCY** Avoid—causes masculinisation of female fetus.

- **BREAST FEEDING** Avoid; may cause masculinisation in the female infant or precocious development in the male infant. High doses suppress lactation.

- **HEPATIC IMPAIRMENT** Avoid if possible—fluid retention and dose-related toxicity.

- **RENAL IMPAIRMENT** Use with caution—potential for fluid retention.

- **MEDICINAL FORMS**
  There can be variation in the licensing of different medicines containing the same drug. Forms available from special-order manufacturers include: tablet
  Tablet
  ▸ Oxandrolone (Non-proprietary)
    Oxandrolone 2.5 mg Oxandrin 2.5mg tablets | 100 tablet [PoM] no price available [CD4-2]

6

Endocrine system

ANDROGENS

Androgens ⊘

- **CONTRA-INDICATIONS** Breast cancer in males · history of liver tumours · hypercalcaemia · prostate cancer
- **CAUTIONS** Cardiac impairment · diabetes mellitus · epilepsy · hypertension · migraine · pre-pubertal boys (fusion of epiphyses is hastened and may result in short stature)—statural growth and sexual development should be monitored · skeletal metastases—risk of hypercalcaemia or hypercalciuria (if this occurs, treat appropriately and restart treatment once normal serum calcium concentration restored) · sleep apnoea · stop treatment or reduce dose if severe polycythaemia occurs · tumours—risk of hypercalcaemia or hypercalciuria (if this occurs, treat appropriately and restart treatment once normal serum calcium concentration restored)
- **INTERACTIONS** → Appendix 1 (testosterone).
- **SIDE-EFFECTS**
  - **Common or very common** Acne · androgenic effects (to be assessed regularly in women) · anxiety · asthenia · changes in libido · cholestatic jaundice · depression · electrolyte disturbances · excessive duration of penile erection · excessive frequency of penile erection · gastro-intestinal bleeding · gynaecomastia · headache · hirsutism · hypercalcaemia · hypertension · increased bone growth · male-pattern baldness · nausea · oedema · paraesthesia · polycythaemia · precocious sexual development in pre-pubertal males · premature closure of epiphyses in pre-pubertal males · pruritus · seborrhoea · sodium retention · suppression of virilism in women · weight gain
  - **Rare** Liver tumours
  - **Frequency not known** Sleep apnoea
    SIDE-EFFECTS, FURTHER INFORMATION
  - Polycythaemia Stop treatment or reduce dose if severe polycythaemia occurs.
- **PREGNANCY** Avoid—causes masculinisation of female fetus.
- **BREAST FEEDING** Avoid.
- **HEPATIC IMPAIRMENT** Avoid if possible—fluid retention and dose-related toxicity.
- **RENAL IMPAIRMENT** Caution—potential for fluid retention.
- **MONITORING REQUIREMENTS** Monitor haematocrit and haemoglobulin before treatment, every three months for the first year, and yearly thereafter.

⌐ above

Testosterone enantate

- **INDICATIONS AND DOSE**
  Induction and maintenance of sexual maturation in males (specialist use only)
  - ▸ BY DEEP INTRAMUSCULAR INJECTION
  - ▸ Child 12–17 years: 25–50 mg/m² every 1 month, increase dose every 6–12 months according to response
- **UNLICENSED USE** Not licensed for use in children.
- **SIDE-EFFECTS** Suppression of spermatogenesis
- **MEDICINAL FORMS**
  There can be variation in the licensing of different medicines containing the same drug.
  Solution for injection
  - ▸ Testosterone enantate (Non-proprietary)
    Testosterone enantate 250 mg per 1 ml Testosterone enantate 250mg/1ml solution for injection ampoules | 3 ampoule [PoM] £72.50 DT price = £72.50 [CD4-2]

⌐ above

Testosterone propionate

- **INDICATIONS AND DOSE**
  Delayed puberty in males
  - ▸ BY INTRAMUSCULAR INJECTION
  - ▸ Child: 50 mg once weekly
  Treatment of microphallus (specialist use only)
  - ▸ TO THE SKIN USING CREAM
  - ▸ Child: Apply 3 times a day for 3 weeks
- **SIDE-EFFECTS** Suppression of spermatogenesis
- **MEDICINAL FORMS**
  There can be variation in the licensing of different medicines containing the same drug. Forms available from special-order manufacturers include: solution for injection, cream

⌐ above

Testosterone undecanoate

- **INDICATIONS AND DOSE**
  Induction and maintenance of sexual maturation in males (specialist use only)
  - ▸ BY MOUTH
  - ▸ Child 12–17 years: 40 mg once daily on alternate days, adjusted according to response to 120 mg daily
- **SIDE-EFFECTS** Suppression of spermatogenesis
- **MEDICINAL FORMS**
  There can be variation in the licensing of different medicines containing the same drug.
  Capsule
  CAUTIONARY AND ADVISORY LABELS 21, 25
  - ▸ Restandol (Merck Sharp & Dohme Ltd)
    Testosterone undecanoate 40 mg Restandol 40mg Testocaps | 30 capsule [PoM] £8.55 [CD4-2] | 60 capsule [PoM] £17.10 DT price = £17.10 [CD4-2]

7.2a Male sex hormone antagonism

ANTI-ANDROGENS

Cyproterone acetate

- **INDICATIONS AND DOSE**
  Gonadotrophin-independent precocious puberty (specialist use only)
  - ▸ BY MOUTH
  - ▸ Child: Initially 25 mg twice daily, adjusted according to response
- **UNLICENSED USE** Unlicensed for use in children.
- **CONTRA-INDICATIONS** Dubin-Johnson syndrome · history of thromboembolic disorders · liver-disease · malignant diseases · meningioma or history of meningioma · previous or existing liver tumours · Rotor syndrome · severe depression · severe diabetes (with vascular changes) · sickle-cell anaemia · wasting diseases · youths under 18 years (may arrest bone maturation and testicular development)
- **CAUTIONS** Diabetes mellitus · in prostate cancer, severe depression · in prostate cancer, sickle-cell anaemia · ineffective for male hypersexuality in chronic alcoholism (relevance to prostate cancer not known)
- **SIDE-EFFECTS**
  - **Rare** Hypersensitivity reactions · osteoporosis · rash
  - **Frequency not known** Breathlessness · changes in hair pattern · fatigue · gynaecomastia (rarely leading to

galactorrhoea and benign breast nodules · hepatic failure · hepatitis · hepatotoxicity · inhibition of spermatogenesis · jaundice · lassitude · reduced sebum production (may clear acne) · risk of recurrence of thromboembolic disease · weight changes

SIDE-EFFECTS, FURTHER INFORMATION

▸ **Hepatotoxicity** Direct hepatic toxicity including jaundice, hepatitis and hepatic failure have been reported (fatalities reported, usually after several months, at dosages of 100 mg and above). If hepatotoxicity is confirmed, cyproterone should normally be withdrawn unless the hepatotoxicity can be explained by another cause such as metastatic disease (in which case cyproterone should be continued only if the perceived benefit exceeds the risk).

● **HEPATIC IMPAIRMENT** Avoid—dose-related toxicity.

● **MONITORING REQUIREMENTS**
▸ Monitor blood counts initially and throughout treatment.
▸ Monitor adrenocortical function regularly.
▸ Monitor hepatic function regularly—liver function tests should be performed before and regularly during treatment and whenever symptoms suggestive of hepatotoxicity occur.

● **PATIENT AND CARER ADVICE**
Driving and skilled tasks
Fatigue and lassitude may impair performance of skilled tasks (e.g. driving).

● **MEDICINAL FORMS**
There can be variation in the licensing of different medicines containing the same drug. Forms available from special-order manufacturers include: tablet, capsule, oral suspension, oral solution
Tablet
CAUTIONARY AND ADVISORY LABELS 21
▸ Cyproterone acetate (Non-proprietary)
Cyproterone acetate 50 mg Cyproterone 50mg tablets | 56 tablet [PoM] £48.95 | 168 tablet [PoM] £87.00 DT price = £87.00
Cyproterone acetate 100 mg Cyproterone 100mg tablets | 84 tablet [PoM] £132.57 DT price = £55.19
▸ Androcur (Bayer Plc)
Cyproterone acetate 50 mg Androcur 50mg tablets | 56 tablet [PoM] £29.25
▸ Cyprostat (Bayer Plc)
Cyproterone acetate 50 mg Cyprostat 50mg tablets | 168 tablet [PoM] £87.00 DT price = £87.00
Cyproterone acetate 100 mg Cyprostat 100mg tablets | 84 tablet [PoM] £87.00 DT price = £55.19

7.2b Precocious puberty

Drugs used for Precocious puberty not listed below
Goserelin p. 439 · Leuprorelin acetate p. 440 · Triptorelin p. 440

HORMONE ANTAGONISTS AND RELATED AGENTS ⟩ AROMATASE INHIBITORS

❙ Testolactone

● **INDICATIONS AND DOSE**
Gonadotrophin-independent precocious puberty (specialist use only)
▸ BY MOUTH
▸ Child: 5 mg/kg 3–4 times a day; increased if necessary up to 10 mg/kg 4 times a day

● **INTERACTIONS** → Appendix 1 (testolactone).

● **SIDE-EFFECTS**
● **Common or very common** Anorexia · changes in hair pattern · diarrhoea · hypertension · nausea · peripheral neuropathy · vomiting · weight changes

▸ **Rare** Hypersensitivity reactions · rash
● **PREGNANCY** Avoid.
● **BREAST FEEDING** No information available.

● **MEDICINAL FORMS**
There can be variation in the licensing of different medicines containing the same drug.
Tablet
▸ Testolactone (Non-proprietary)
Testolactone 50 mg Teslac 50mg tablets | 100 tablet [PoM] no price available

8   Thyroid disorders
8.1   Hyperthyroidism

Antithyroid drugs

Overview

Antithyroid drugs are used for hyperthyroidism either to prepare children for thyroidectomy or for long-term management. In the UK carbimazole p. 452 is the most commonly used drug. Propylthiouracil p. 452 should be reserved for children who are intolerant of, or for those who experience sensitivity reactions to carbimazole (sensitivity is not necessarily displayed to both drugs), and for whom other treatments are inappropriate. Both drugs act primarily by interfering with the synthesis of thyroid hormones.

Treatment in children should be undertaken by a specialist.

Carbimazole or propylthiouracil are initially given in large doses to block thyroid function. This dose is continued until the child becomes euthyroid, usually after 4 to 8 weeks, and is then gradually reduced to a maintenance dose of 30–60% of the initial dose. Alternatively high-dose treatment is continued in combination with levothyroxine sodium p. 454 replacement (*blocking-replacement regimen*); this is particularly useful when dose adjustment proves difficult. Treatment is usually continued for 12 to 24 months. The blocking-replacement regimen is **not** suitable during pregnancy. Hypothyroidism should be avoided particularly during pregnancy as it can cause fetal goitre.

Iodine has been used as an adjunct to antithyroid drugs for 10 to 14 days before partial thyroidectomy; however, there is little evidence of a beneficial effect. Iodine should not be used for long-term treatment because its antithyroid action tends to diminish.

Radioactive sodium iodide (^{131}I) solution is used increasingly for the treatment of thyrotoxicosis at all ages, particularly where medical therapy or compliance is a problem, in patients with cardiac disease, and in patients who relapse after thyroidectomy.

Propranolol hydrochloride p. 96 is useful for rapid relief of thyrotoxic symptoms and can be used in conjunction with antithyroid drugs or as an adjunct to radioactive iodine. Beta-blockers are also useful in neonatal thyrotoxicosis and in supraventricular arrhythmias due to hyperthyroidism. Propranolol hydrochloride has been used in conjunction with iodine to prepare mildly thyrotoxic patients for surgery but it is preferable to make the patient euthyroid with carbimazole. Laboratory tests of thyroid function are not altered by beta-blockers. Most experience in treating thyrotoxicosis has been gained with propranolol but atenolol is also used.

Thyrotoxic crisis ('thyroid storm') requires emergency treatment with intravenous administration of fluids, propranolol hydrochloride and hydrocortisone as sodium succinate, as well as oral iodine solution and carbimazole or propylthiouracil which may need to be administered by nasogastric tube.

Pregnancy

Radioactive iodine therapy is contra-indicated during pregnancy. Propylthiouracil and carbimazole can be given but the blocking-replacement regimen is **not** suitable. Rarely, carbimazole has been associated with congenital defects, including aplasia cutis of the neonate, therefore propylthiouracil remains the drug of choice during the first trimester of pregnancy. In the second trimester, consider switching to carbimazole because of the potential risk of hepatotoxicity with propylthiouracil. Both propylthiouracil and carbimazole cross the placenta and in high doses may cause fetal goitre and hypothyroidism—the lowest dose that will control the hyperthyroid state should be used (requirements in Graves' disease tend to fall during pregnancy).

Neonates

Neonatal hyperthyroidism is treated with carbimazole or propylthiouracil, usually for 8 to 12 weeks. In severe symptomatic disease iodine may be needed to block the thyroid and propranolol required to treat peripheral symptoms.

ANTITHYROID DRUGS > SULFUR-CONTAINING IMIDAZOLES

Carbimazole

● **INDICATIONS AND DOSE**

Hyperthyroidism (blocking-replacement regimen) in combination with levothyroxine
▸ BY MOUTH
▸ Child: Therapy usually given for 12 to 24 months (consult product literature or local protocols)

Hyperthyroidism (including Graves' disease)
▸ BY MOUTH

▸ Neonate: Initially 750 micrograms/kg daily until patient is euthyroid, usually after 8 to 12 weeks, then gradually reduce to a maintenance dose of 30–60% of the initial dose; higher initial doses (up to 1 mg/kg daily) are occasionally required, particularly in thyrotoxic crisis, dose may be given in single or divided doses.

▸ Child 1 month–11 years: Initially 750 micrograms/kg daily until patient is euthyroid, usually after 4–8 weeks, then gradually reduce to a maintenance dose of 30–60% of the initial dose; higher initial doses are occasionally required, particularly in thyrotoxic crisis, dose may be given in single or divided doses; maximum 30 mg per day

▸ Child 12–17 years: Initially 30 mg daily until euthyroid, usually after 4–8 weeks, then gradually reduce to a maintenance dose of 30–60% of the initial dose; higher initial doses are occasionally required, particularly in thyrotoxic crisis, dose may be given in single or divided doses

DOSE EQUIVALENCE AND CONVERSION
When substituting, carbimazole 1 mg is considered equivalent to propylthiouracil 10 mg but the dose may need adjusting according to response.

IMPORTANT SAFETY INFORMATION
NEUTROPENIA AND AGRANULOCYTOSIS
Doctors are reminded of the importance of recognising bone marrow suppression induced by carbimazole and the need to stop treatment promptly.
● Patient should be asked to report symptoms and signs suggestive of infection, especially sore throat.
● A white blood cell count should be performed if there is any clinical evidence of infection.

● Carbimazole should be stopped promptly if there is clinical or laboratory evidence of neutropenia.

● INTERACTIONS → Appendix 1 (carbimazole).

● SIDE-EFFECTS
▸ **Common or very common** Arthralgia · fever · headache · hepatic disorders · hepatitis · jaundice · malaise · mild gastro-intestinal disturbances · nausea · pruritus · rash · taste disturbance
▸ **Rare** Agranulocytosis · alopecia · bone marrow suppression · hypersensitivity reactions · jaundice · myopathy · pancytopenia

SIDE-EFFECTS, FURTHER INFORMATION
Rashes and pruritus are common with carbimazole but they can be treated with antihistamines without discontinuing therapy; alternatively propylthiouracil can be substituted.

● PREGNANCY Carbimazole can be given but the blocking-replacement regimen is **not** suitable. Rarely, carbimazole has been associated with congenital defects, including aplasia cutis of the neonate. Carbimazole cross the placenta and in high doses may cause fetal goitre and hypothyroidism—the lowest dose that will control the hyperthyroid state should be used (requirements in Graves' disease tend to fall during pregnancy).

● BREAST FEEDING Present in breast milk but this does not preclude breast-feeding as long as neonatal development is closely monitored and the lowest effective dose is used. Amount in milk may be sufficient to affect neonatal thyroid function therefore lowest effective dose should be used.

● HEPATIC IMPAIRMENT Use with caution in mild to moderate impairment. Avoid in severe impairment.

● PATIENT AND CARER ADVICE Warn patient or carers to tell doctor **immediately** if sore throat, mouth ulcers, bruising, fever, malaise, or non-specific illness develops.

● MEDICINAL FORMS
There can be variation in the licensing of different medicines containing the same drug. Forms available from special-order manufacturers include: capsule, oral suspension, oral solution
Tablet
▸ Carbimazole (Non-proprietary)
Carbimazole 5 mg Carbimazole 5mg tablets | 100 tablet PoM
£90.00 DT price = £78.83
Carbimazole 20 mg Carbimazole 20mg tablets | 100 tablet PoM
£240.00 DT price = £197.14

ANTITHYROID DRUGS > THIOURACILS

Propylthiouracil

● **INDICATIONS AND DOSE**

Hyperthyroidism (including Graves' disease)
▸ BY MOUTH

▸ Neonate: Initially 2.5–5 mg/kg twice daily until euthyroid, usually after 8 to 12 weeks, then gradually reduce to a maintenance dose of 30–60% of the initial dose; higher initial doses are occasionally required, particularly in thyrotoxic crisis.

▸ Child 1–11 months: Initially 2.5 mg/kg 3 times a day until euthyroid, usually after 4 to 8 weeks, then gradually reduce to a maintenance dose of 30–60% of the initial dose; higher initial doses are occasionally required, particularly in thyrotoxic crisis

▸ Child 1–4 years: Initially 25 mg 3 times a day until euthyroid, usually after 4 to 8 weeks, then gradually reduce to a maintenance dose of 30–60% of the initial dose; higher initial doses are occasionally required, particularly in thyrotoxic crisis

▸ **Child 5–11 years:** Initially 50 mg 3 times a day until euthyroid, usually after 4 to 8 weeks, then gradually reduce to a maintenance dose of 30–60% of the initial dose; higher initial doses are occasionally required, particularly in thyrotoxic crisis

▸ **Child 12–17 years:** Initially 100 mg 3 times a day until euthyroid, usually after 4 to 8 weeks, then gradually reduce to a maintenance dose of 30–60% of the initial dose; higher initial doses are occasionally required, particularly in thyrotoxic crisis

DOSE EQUIVALENCE AND CONVERSION
When substituting, carbimazole 1 mg is considered equivalent to propylthiouracil 10 mg but the dose may need adjusting according to response.

● **UNLICENSED USE** Not licensed for use in children under 6 years of age.

● **SIDE-EFFECTS**
▸ **Common or very common** Arthralgia · fever · headache · jaundice · leucopenia · malaise · mild gastro-intestinal disturbances · nausea · pruritus · rash · taste disturbance
▸ **Rare** Agranulocytosis · alopecia · aplastic anaemia · bone marrow suppression · cutaneous vasculitis · encephalopathy · hepatic disorders · hepatic failure · hepatic necrosis · hepatitis · hypersensitivity reactions · hypoprothrombinaemia · jaundice · lupus erythematous-like syndromes · myopathy · nephritis · pancytopenia · thrombocytopenia

SIDE-EFFECTS, FURTHER INFORMATION
▸ Hepatotoxicity Severe hepatic reactions have been reported, including fatal cases and cases requiring liver transplant—discontinue if significant liver-enzyme abnormalities develop.

● **PREGNANCY** Propylthiouracil can be given but the blocking-replacement regimen is **not** advisable. Propylthiouracil crosses the placenta and in high doses may cause fetal goitre and hypothyroidism—the lowest dose that will control the hyperthyroid state should be used (requirements in Graves' disease tend to fall during pregnancy).

● **BREAST FEEDING** Present in breast milk but this does not preclude breast-feeding as long as neonatal development is closely monitored and the lowest effective dose is used. Amount in milk probably too small to affect infant; high doses may affect neonatal thyroid function. Monitor infant's thyroid status.

● **HEPATIC IMPAIRMENT** Reduce dose.

● **RENAL IMPAIRMENT** Use 75% of normal dose if estimated glomerular filtration rate 10–50 mL/minute/1.73 m². Use 50% of normal dose if estimated glomerular filtration rate less than 10 mL/minute/1.73 m².

● **MONITORING REQUIREMENTS** Monitor for hepatotoxicity.

● **PATIENT AND CARER ADVICE** Patients should be told how to recognise signs of liver disorder and advised to seek prompt medical attention if symptoms such as anorexia, nausea, vomiting, fatigue, abdominal pain, jaundice, dark urine, or pruritus develop.

● **MEDICINAL FORMS**
There can be variation in the licensing of different medicines containing the same drug. Forms available from special-order manufacturers include: oral suspension, oral solution
Tablet
▸ Propylthiouracil (Non-proprietary)
　Propylthiouracil 50 mg Propylthiouracil 50mg tablets |
　56 tablet PoM £73.50 DT price = £57.72 | 100 tablet PoM £131.25

VITAMINS AND TRACE ELEMENTS

Iodide with iodine

● **INDICATIONS AND DOSE**
Thyrotoxicosis (pre-operative)
▸ BY MOUTH USING ORAL SOLUTION
▸ **Neonate:** 0.1–0.3 mL 3 times a day.
▸ **Child:** 0.1–0.3 mL 3 times a day
Neonatal thyrotoxicosis
▸ BY MOUTH USING ORAL SOLUTION
▸ **Neonate:** 0.05–0.1 mL 3 times a day.
Thyrotoxic crisis
▸ BY MOUTH USING ORAL SOLUTION
▸ **Child 1 month–1 year:** 0.2–0.3 mL 3 times a day

● **CAUTIONS** Children · not for long-term treatment
● **SIDE-EFFECTS** Bronchitis · conjunctivitis · coryza-like symptoms · depression (on prolonged treatment) · goitre in infants of mothers taking iodides · headache · hypersensitivity reactions · impotence (on prolonged treatment) · insomnia (on prolonged treatment) · lacrimation · laryngitis · pain in salivary glands · rashes
● **PREGNANCY** Neonatal goitre and hypothyroidism.
● **BREAST FEEDING** Stop breast-feeding. Danger of neonatal hypothyroidism or goitre. Appears to be concentrated in milk.
● **DIRECTIONS FOR ADMINISTRATION** For oral solution, dilute well with milk or water.

● **MEDICINAL FORMS**
There can be variation in the licensing of different medicines containing the same drug.
Oral solution
CAUTIONARY AND ADVISORY LABELS 27
▸ Iodide with iodine (Non-proprietary)
　Iodine 50 mg per 1 ml, Potassium iodide 100 mg per 1 ml Iodine aqueous oral solution | 500 ml P £9.58

8.2 Hypothyroidism

Thyroid hormones

Overview

Thyroid hormones are used in hypothyroidism (juvenile myxoedema), and also in diffuse non-toxic goitre, congenital or neonatal hypothyroidism, and Hashimoto's thyroiditis (lymphadenoid goitre). Neonatal hypothyroidism requires prompt treatment to facilitate normal development.

Levothyroxine sodium p. 454 (thyroxine sodium) is the treatment of choice for *maintenance* therapy.

Doses for congenital hypothyroidism and juvenile myxoedema should be titrated according to clinical response, growth assessment, and measurement of plasma thyroxine and thyroid-stimulating hormone concentrations. In congenital hypothyroidism higher initial doses may normalise metabolism more quickly, with associated beneficial effects on mental development.

Liothyronine sodium p. 455 has a similar action to levothyroxine sodium but is more rapidly metabolised and has a more rapid effect. Its effects develop after a few hours and disappear within 24 to 48 hours of discontinuing treatment. It may be used in *severe hypothyroid states* when a rapid response is desired.

Liothyronine sodium by intravenous injection is the treatment of choice in *hypothyroid coma*. Adjunctive therapy includes intravenous fluids, hydrocortisone, and treatment of infection; assisted ventilation is often required.

6

Endocrine system

THYROID HORMONES

▌Levothyroxine sodium

(Thyroxine sodium)

- **INDICATIONS AND DOSE**

Hypothyroidism
- ▸ BY MOUTH
- ▸ **Neonate:** Initially 10–15 micrograms/kg once daily (max. per dose 50 micrograms); adjusted in steps of 5 micrograms/kg every 2 weeks, alternatively adjusted in steps of 5 micrograms/kg as required; maintenance 20–50 micrograms daily, levothyroxine should be taken at the same time each day, preferably 30 minutes before meals, caffeine-containing drinks, or other medicines; this could be before breakfast or another more convenient time.
- ▸ **Child 1 month–1 year:** Initially 5 micrograms/kg once daily (max. per dose 50 micrograms); adjusted in steps of 10–25 micrograms every 2–4 weeks until metabolism normalised; maintenance 25–75 micrograms daily, levothyroxine should be taken at the same time each day, preferably 30 minutes before meals, caffeine-containing drinks, or other medicines; this could be before breakfast or another more convenient time
- ▸ **Child 2–11 years:** Initially 50 micrograms once daily; adjusted in steps of 25 micrograms every 2–4 weeks until metabolism normalised; maintenance 75–100 micrograms daily, levothyroxine should be taken at the same time each day, preferably 30 minutes before meals, caffeine-containing drinks, or other medicines; this could be before breakfast or another more convenient time
- ▸ **Child 12–17 years:** Initially 50 micrograms once daily; adjusted in steps of 25–50 micrograms every 3–4 weeks until metabolism normalised; maintenance 100–200 micrograms daily, levothyroxine should be taken at the same time each day, preferably 30 minutes before meals, caffeine-containing drinks, or other medicines; this could be before breakfast or another more convenient time

Hyperthyroidism (blocking-replacement regimen) in combination with carbimazole
- ▸ BY MOUTH
- ▸ **Child:** Therapy usually given for 12 to 24 months (consult product literature or local protocols)

- **CAUTIONS** Cardiac disorders (monitor ECG; start at low dose and carefully titrate) · diabetes insipidus · diabetes mellitus (dose of antidiabetic drugs including insulin may need to be increased) · long-standing hypothyroidism · panhypopituitarism (initiate corticosteroid therapy before starting levothyroxine) · predisposition to adrenal insufficiency (initiate corticosteroid therapy before starting levothyroxine)
- **INTERACTIONS** → Appendix 1 (thyroid hormones).
- **SIDE-EFFECTS** Anginal pain (usually at excessive dosage) · arrhythmias (usually at excessive dosage) · benign intracranial hypertension (usually at excessive dosage) · craniosynostosis · diarrhoea (usually at excessive dosage) · eosinophilia · excitability (usually at excessive dosage) · fever · flushing · headache · heat intolerance · hypersensitivity reactions · insomnia (usually at excessive dosage) · liver dysfunction · menstrual irregularities · muscle cramp · muscular weakness · nervousness · oedema · palpitation (usually at excessive dosage) · premature closure of epiphyses · pruritus · rash · restlessness (usually at excessive dosage) · sweating · tachycardia (usually at excessive dosage) · transient hair loss · tremor (usually at

excessive dosage) · vomiting (usually at excessive dosage) · weight-loss
- **PREGNANCY** Levothyroxine requirement may increase during pregnancy. Levothyroxine may cross the placenta. Excessive or insufficient maternal thyroid hormones can be detrimental to fetus.

  Assess maternal thyroid function before conception (if possible), at diagnosis of pregnancy, at antenatal booking, during both the second and third trimesters, and after delivery (more frequent monitoring required on initiation or adjustment of levothyroxine).
- **BREAST FEEDING** Amount too small to affect tests for neonatal hypothyroidism.
- **PRESCRIBING AND DISPENSING INFORMATION** Levothyroxine equivalent to 100 micrograms/m^2/day can be used as a guide to the requirements in children.
- **PATIENT AND CARER ADVICE** Medicines for Children leaflet: Levothyroxine for hypothyroidism www.medicinesforchildren.org.uk/levothyroxine-for-hypothyroidism

- **MEDICINAL FORMS** There can be variation in the licensing of different medicines containing the same drug. Forms available from special-order manufacturers include: capsule, oral suspension, oral solution

Tablet
- ▸ **Levothyroxine sodium** (Non-proprietary)
  Levothyroxine sodium anhydrous 25 microgram Levothyroxine sodium 25microgram tablets | 28 tablet [PoM] £4.00 DT price = £2.46 | 500 tablet [PoM] £56.25
  Levothyroxine sodium 25microgram tablets lactose free | 100 tablet [PoM] no price available
  Levothyroxine sodium anhydrous 50 microgram Levothyroxine sodium 50microgram tablets lactose free | 100 tablet [PoM] no price available
  Levothyroxine sodium 50microgram tablets | 28 tablet [PoM] £3.00 DT price = £1.73 | 1000 tablet [PoM] £68.21
  Levothyroxine sodium anhydrous 100 microgram Levothyroxine sodium 100microgram tablets lactose free | 100 tablet [PoM] no price available
  Levothyroxine sodium 100microgram tablets | 28 tablet [PoM] £3.00 DT price = £1.73 | 1000 tablet [PoM] £68.57
- ▸ **Eltroxin** (AMCo)
  Levothyroxine sodium anhydrous 25 microgram Eltroxin 25microgram tablets | 28 tablet [PoM] £2.54 DT price = £2.46
  Levothyroxine sodium anhydrous 50 microgram Eltroxin 50microgram tablets | 28 tablet [PoM] £1.77 DT price = £1.73
  Levothyroxine sodium anhydrous 100 microgram Eltroxin 100microgram tablets | 28 tablet [PoM] £1.78 DT price = £1.73

Capsule
- ▸ **Levothyroxine sodium** (Non-proprietary)
  Levothyroxine sodium anhydrous 25 microgram Tirosint 25microgram capsules | 28 capsule [PoM] no price available
  Levothyroxine sodium anhydrous 50 microgram Tirosint 50microgram capsules | 28 capsule [PoM] no price available
  Levothyroxine sodium anhydrous 100 microgram Tirosint 100microgram capsules | 28 capsule [PoM] no price available

Oral solution
- ▸ **Levothyroxine sodium** (Non-proprietary)
  Levothyroxine sodium anhydrous 5 microgram per 1 ml Levothyroxine sodium 25micrograms/5ml oral solution sugar free sugar-free | 100 ml [PoM] £95.00 DT price = £93.45
  Levothyroxine sodium anhydrous 10 microgram per 1 ml Levothyroxine sodium 50micrograms/5ml oral solution sugar free sugar-free | 100 ml [PoM] £101.79 DT price = £97.52
  Levothyroxine sodium anhydrous 20 microgram per 1 ml Levothyroxine sodium 100micrograms/5ml oral solution sugar free sugar-free | 100 ml [PoM] £165.00 DT price = £161.77

Liothyronine sodium

(L-Tri-iodothyronine sodium)

- **INDICATIONS AND DOSE**

Hypothyroidism

▸ BY MOUTH
▸ Child 12-17 years: Initially 10–20 micrograms daily; increased to 60 micrograms daily in 2–3 divided doses

Hypothyroid coma

▸ BY SLOW INTRAVENOUS INJECTION
▸ Child 12-17 years: 5–20 micrograms every 12 hours, increased to 5–20 micrograms every 4 hours if required, alternatively initially 50 micrograms for 1 dose, then 25 micrograms every 8 hours, reduced to 25 micrograms twice daily

Hypothyroidism (replacement for oral levothyroxine)

▸ BY SLOW INTRAVENOUS INJECTION
▸ Child: Convert daily levothyroxine dose to liothyronine and give in 2–3 divided doses, adjusted according to response

DOSE EQUIVALENCE AND CONVERSION
20–25 micrograms of liothyronine sodium is equivalent to approximately 100 micrograms of levothyroxine sodium.
Brands without a UK licence may not be bioequivalent and dose adjustment may be necessary.

- **CAUTIONS** Cardiac disorders (monitor ECG; start at low dose and carefully titrate) · diabetes insipidus · diabetes mellitus (dose of antidiabetic drugs including insulin may need to be increased) · prolonged hypothyroidism (initiate corticosteroid therapy in adrenal insufficiency) · severe hypothyroidism (initiate corticosteroid therapy in adrenal insufficiency)

- **INTERACTIONS** → Appendix 1 (thyroid hormones).

- **SIDE-EFFECTS** Anginal pain (usually at excessive dosage) · arrhythmias (usually at excessive dosage) · diarrhoea (usually at excessive dosage) · excitability (usually at excessive dosage) · flushing · headache · muscle cramp · muscular weakness · palpitation (usually at excessive dosage) · restlessness (usually at excessive dosage) · sweating · tachycardia (usually at excessive dosage) · weight-loss

- **PREGNANCY** Liothyronine requirement may increase during pregnancy. Does not cross the placenta in significant amounts. Excessive or insufficient maternal thyroid hormones can be detrimental to fetus.
  Assess maternal thyroid function before conception (if possible), at diagnosis of pregnancy, at antenatal booking, during both the second and third trimesters, and after delivery (more frequent monitoring required on initiation or adjustment of liothyronine).

- **BREAST FEEDING** Amount too small to affect tests for neonatal hypothyroidism.

- **PRESCRIBING AND DISPENSING INFORMATION**
  Switching to a different brand Patients switched to a different brand should be monitored (particularly if pregnant or if heart disease present) as brands without a UK licence may not be bioequivalent. Pregnant women or those with heart disease should undergo an early review of thyroid status, and other patients should have thyroid function assessed if experiencing a significant change in symptoms. If liothyronine is continued long-term, thyroid function tests should be repeated 1–2 months after any change in brand.

- **MEDICINAL FORMS**
  There can be variation in the licensing of different medicines containing the same drug. Forms available from special-order manufacturers include: tablet, capsule, oral suspension, oral solution, solution for injection

Tablet

▸ Liothyronine sodium (Non-proprietary)
  Liothyronine sodium 5 microgram Cytomel 5microgram tablets | 100 tablet [PoM] no price available
  Liothyronine sodium 20 microgram Liothyronine 20microgram tablets | 28 tablet [PoM] £258.20 DT price = £258.20
  Liothyronine sodium 25 microgram Cytomel 25microgram tablets | 100 tablet [PoM] no price available

Powder for solution for injection

▸ Liothyronine sodium (Non-proprietary)
  Liothyronine sodium 20 microgram Liothyronine 20microgram powder for solution for injection vials | 5 vial [PoM] £1,425.00

6

Endocrine system

Chapter 7
Genito-urinary system

CONTENTS

1	**Bladder and urinary disorders**	page 456
1.1	Urinary frequency, enuresis, and incontinence	456
1.2	Urinary retention	458
1.3	Urological pain	460
2	**Bladder instillations and urological surgery**	460
3	**Contraception**	461
3.1	Contraception, combined	465
3.2	Contraception, devices	471
3.3	Contraception, emergency	473

3.4	Contraception, oral progestogen-only	page 474
3.5	Contraception, parenteral progestogen-only	477
3.6	Contraception, spermicidal	479
4	**Erectile and ejaculatory conditions**	479
4.1	Erectile dysfunction	479
5	**Vaginal and vulval conditions**	479
5.1	Vaginal and vulval infections	480
5.1a	Vaginal and vulval bacterial infections	480
5.1b	Vaginal and vulval fungal infections	481

1   Bladder and urinary disorders

1.1   Urinary frequency, enuresis, and incontinence

Urinary frequency, enuresis and incontinence

Urinary incontinence

Antimuscarinic drugs reduce symptoms of urgency and urge incontinence and increase bladder capacity; oxybutynin hydrochloride p. 457 also has a direct relaxant effect on urinary smooth muscle. Oxybutynin hydrochloride can be considered first for children under 12 years. Side-effects limit the use of oxybutynin hydrochloride, but they may be reduced by starting at a lower dose and then slowly titrating upwards; alternatively oxybutynin hydrochloride can be given by intravesicular instillation. Tolterodine tartrate p. 458 is also effective for urinary incontinence; it can be considered for children over 12 years, or for younger children who have failed to respond to oxybutynin hydrochloride. Modified-release preparations of oxybutynin hydrochloride and tolterodine tartrate are available; they may have fewer side-effects. Antimuscarinic treatment should be reviewed soon after it is commenced, and then at regular intervals; a response generally occurs within 6 months but occasionally may take longer. Children with nocturnal enuresis may require specific additional measures if night-time symptoms also need to be controlled.

Nocturnal enuresis in children

Nocturnal enuresis is common in young children, but persists in a small proportion by 10 years of age. For children under 5 years, reassurance and advice on the management of nocturnal enuresis can be useful for some families. Treatment may be considered in children over 5 years depending on their maturity and motivation, the frequency of nocturnal enuresis, and the needs of the child and their family.

Initially, advice should be given on fluid intake, diet, toileting behaviour, and reward systems; for children who do not respond to this advice, further treatment may be necessary. An **enuresis alarm** should be first line treatment for motivated, well-supported children; alarms have a lower relapse rate than drug treatment when discontinued. Treatment should be reviewed after 4 weeks, and, if there are early signs of response, continued until a minimum of 2 weeks' uninterrupted dry nights have been achieved. If complete dryness is not achieved after 3 months, only continue if the condition is still improving and the child remains motivated to use the alarm. If initial alarm treatment is unsuccessful, consider combination treatment with **desmopressin p. 403**, or desmopressin alone if the alarm is no longer appropriate or desirable.

Desmopressin is given by oral or by sublingual administration. Desmopressin alone can be offered to children over 5 years of age if an alarm is inappropriate or undesirable, or when rapid or short-term results are the priority (for example to cover periods away from home); desmopressin alone can also be used if there has been a partial response to a combination of desmopressin and an alarm following initial treatment with an alarm. Treatment should be assessed after 4 weeks and continued for 3 months if there are signs of response. Desmopressin should be withdrawn at regular intervals (for 1 week every 3 months) for full reassessment. When stopping treatment with desmopressin, gradual withdrawal should be considered.

Nocturnal enuresis associated with daytime symptoms (overactive bladder) can be managed with antimuscarinic drugs in combination with desmopressin. Treatment should be prescribed only after specialist assessment and should be continued for 3 months; the course can be repeated if necessary.

The tricyclic antidepressant imipramine hydrochloride p. 226 may be considered for children who have not responded to all other treatments and have undergone specialist assessment, however, behavioural disturbances can occur and relapse is common after withdrawal. Treatment should not normally exceed 3 months unless a physical examination is made and the child is fully reassessed; toxicity following overdosage with tricyclics is of particular concern.

ANTIMUSCARINICS

Antimuscarinics (systemic)

- **CONTRA-INDICATIONS** Gastro-intestinal obstruction · intestinal atony · myasthenia gravis (but some antimuscarinics may be used to decrease muscarinic side-effects of anticholinesterases) · paralytic ileus · pyloric stenosis · severe ulcerative colitis · significant bladder outflow obstruction · toxic megacolon · urinary retention

- **CAUTIONS** Arrhythmias (may be worsened) · autonomic neuropathy · cardiac insufficiency (due to association with tachycardia) · cardiac surgery (due to association with tachycardia) · children (increased risk of side-effects) · conditions characterised by tachycardia · congestive heart failure (may be worsened) · coronary artery disease (may be worsened) · diarrhoea · gastro-oesophageal reflux disease · hiatus hernia with reflux oesophagitis · hypertension · hyperthyroidism (due to association with tachycardia) · individuals susceptible to angle-closure glaucoma · pyrexia · ulcerative colitis

- **INTERACTIONS** → Appendix 1 (antimuscarinics).
  Many drugs have antimuscarinic effects; concomitant use of two or more such drugs can increase side-effects such as dry mouth, urine retention, and constipation.

- **SIDE-EFFECTS**
  ▸ **Common or very common** Constipation · dilation of pupils with loss of accommodation · dry mouth · photophobia · reduced bronchial secretions · skin dryness · skin flushing · transient bradycardia (followed by tachycardia, palpitation and arrhythmias) · urinary retention · urinary urgency
  ▸ **Uncommon** Confusion · giddiness · nausea · vomiting
  ▸ **Very rare** Angle-closure glaucoma
  ▸ **Frequency not known** Angioedema · blurred vision · blurred vision · central nervous system stimulation · convulsion · diarrhoea · difficulty in micturition · disorientation · dizziness · drowsiness · dry eyes · euphoria · fatigue · flatulence · hallucinations · giddiness · headache · impaired memory · palpitation · photosensitivity · rash · reduced sweating (may lead to heat sensations and fainting in hot environments or patients with fever) · restlessness · taste disturbances

- **PATIENT AND CARER ADVICE**
  Driving and skilled tasks
  Antimuscarinics can affect the performance of skilled tasks (e.g. driving).

ANTIMUSCARINICS

☛ above

Oxybutynin hydrochloride

- **INDICATIONS AND DOSE**
  Urinary frequency | Urinary urgency | Urinary incontinence | Neurogenic bladder instability
  ▸ BY MOUTH USING IMMEDIATE-RELEASE MEDICINES
  ▸ **Child 2-4 years:** 1.25–2.5 mg 2–3 times a day
  ▸ **Child 5-11 years:** Initially 2.5–3 mg twice daily, increased to 5 mg 2–3 times a day
  ▸ **Child 12-17 years:** Initially 5 mg 2–3 times a day, increased if necessary up to 5 mg 4 times a day
  ▸ BY INTRAVESICAL INSTILLATION
  ▸ **Child 2-17 years:** 5 mg 2–3 times a day
  ▸ BY MOUTH USING MODIFIED-RELEASE TABLETS
  ▸ **Child 5-17 years:** Initially 5 mg once daily, adjusted in steps of 5 mg every 1 week, adjusted according to response; maximum 15 mg per day

Nocturnal enuresis associated with overactive bladder
  ▸ BY MOUTH USING IMMEDIATE-RELEASE MEDICINES
  ▸ **Child 5-17 years:** 2.5–3 mg twice daily, increased to 5 mg 2–3 times a day, last dose to be taken before bedtime
  ▸ BY MOUTH USING MODIFIED-RELEASE TABLETS
  ▸ **Child 5-17 years:** Initially 5 mg once daily, adjusted in steps of 5 mg every 1 week, adjusted according to response; maximum 15 mg per day

DOSE EQUIVALENCE AND CONVERSION
Patients taking immediate-release oxybutynin may be transferred to the nearest equivalent daily dose of *Lyrinel® XL*

- **UNLICENSED USE** Not licensed for use in children under 5 years. Intravesical instillation not licensed for use in children.

- **CAUTIONS** Acute porphyrias p. 562

- **SIDE-EFFECTS**
  ▸ **Uncommon** Anorexia · facial flushing
  ▸ **Rare** Night terrors

- **PREGNANCY** Manufacturers advise avoid unless essential—toxicity in *animal* studies.

- **BREAST FEEDING** Manufacturers advise avoid—present in milk in *animal* studies.

- **HEPATIC IMPAIRMENT** Manufacturer advises caution.

- **RENAL IMPAIRMENT** Manufacturer advises caution.

- **PRESCRIBING AND DISPENSING INFORMATION** The need for therapy for urinary indications should be reviewed soon after it has been commenced and then at regular intervals; a response usually occurs within 6 months but may take longer.

  Intravesical instillation may be available from 'special-order' manufacturers or specialist importing companies.

- **PATIENT AND CARER ADVICE**
  Medicines for Children leaflet: Oxybutynin for daytime urinary symptoms www.medicinesforchildren.org.uk/oxybutynin-for-daytime-urinary-symptoms

- **MEDICINAL FORMS**
  There can be variation in the licensing of different medicines containing the same drug. Forms available from special-order manufacturers include: oral suspension, oral solution, bladder irrigation

Tablet
CAUTIONARY AND ADVISORY LABELS 3
  ▸ **Oxybutynin hydrochloride (Non-proprietary)**
    Oxybutynin hydrochloride 2.5 mg Oxybutynin 2.5mg tablets | 56 tablet PoM £6.58 DT price = £1.44 | 84 tablet PoM £10.75
    Oxybutynin hydrochloride 3 mg Oxybutynin 3mg tablets | 56 tablet PoM £16.80 DT price = £16.80
    Oxybutynin hydrochloride 5 mg Oxybutynin 5mg tablets | 56 tablet PoM £14.00 DT price = £1.91 | 84 tablet PoM £20.77
  ▸ **Cystrin** (Zentiva)
    Oxybutynin hydrochloride 5 mg Cystrin 5mg tablets | 84 tablet PoM £21.99
  ▸ **Ditropan** (Sanofi)
    Oxybutynin hydrochloride 2.5 mg Ditropan 2.5mg tablets | 84 tablet PoM £1.60
    Oxybutynin hydrochloride 5 mg Ditropan 5mg tablets | 84 tablet PoM £2.90

Modified-release tablet
CAUTIONARY AND ADVISORY LABELS 3, 25
  ▸ **Lyrinel XL** (Janssen-Cilag Ltd)
    Oxybutynin hydrochloride 5 mg Lyrinel XL 5mg tablets | 30 tablet PoM £13.77 DT price = £13.77
    Oxybutynin hydrochloride 10 mg Lyrinel XL 10mg tablets | 30 tablet PoM £27.54 DT price = £27.54

Oral solution
CAUTIONARY AND ADVISORY LABELS 3
- ▶ Oxybutynin hydrochloride (Non-proprietary)
  Oxybutynin hydrochloride 500 microgram per 1 ml Oxybutynin 2.5mg/5ml oral solution sugar free sugar-free | 150 ml [PoM] £144.50–£167.40 DT price = £144.50
  Oxybutynin hydrochloride 1 mg per 1 ml Oxybutynin 5mg/5ml oral solution sugar free sugar-free | 150 ml [PoM] £199.20–£234.36 DT price = £199.20

F 457

Tolterodine tartrate

- ● **INDICATIONS AND DOSE**
  Urinary frequency | Urinary urgency | Urinary incontinence
  - ▶ BY MOUTH USING IMMEDIATE-RELEASE MEDICINES
  - ▶ **Child 2-17 years:** 1 mg once daily, then increased if necessary up to 2 mg twice daily, adjusted according to response
  - ▶ BY MOUTH USING MODIFIED-RELEASE CAPSULES
  - ▶ **Child 2-17 years:** 4 mg once daily

  Nocturnal enuresis associated with overactive bladder
  - ▶ BY MOUTH USING IMMEDIATE-RELEASE MEDICINES
  - ▶ **Child 5-17 years:** 1 mg once daily, dose to be taken at bedtime, then increased if necessary up to 2 mg twice daily, adjusted according to response

  DOSE EQUIVALENCE AND CONVERSION
  Children stabilised on immediate-release tolterodine tartrate 2 mg twice daily may be transferred to modified-release tolterodine tartrate 4 mg once daily.

- ● UNLICENSED USE Not licensed for use in children.
- ● CAUTIONS History of QT-interval prolongation
- ● INTERACTIONS Caution with concomitant use with other drugs known to prolong QT interval.
- ● SIDE-EFFECTS
  - ▶ **Common or very common** Bronchitis · chest pain · fatigue · paraesthesia · peripheral oedema · sinusitis · vertigo · weight gain
  - ▶ **Uncommon** Memory impairment
  - ▶ **Frequency not known** Flushing
- ● PREGNANCY Manufacturer advises avoid—toxicity in *animal* studies.
- ● BREAST FEEDING Manufacturer advises avoid—no information available.
- ● HEPATIC IMPAIRMENT Reduce dose. Avoid modified-release preparations.
- ● RENAL IMPAIRMENT Reduce dose if estimated glomerular filtration less than 30 mL/minute/1.73m^2. Avoid modified-release preparations if estimated glomerular filtration rate less than 30 mL/minute/1.73m^2.
- ● PRESCRIBING AND DISPENSING INFORMATION The need for therapy for urinary indications should be reviewed soon after it has been commenced and then at regular intervals; a response usually occurs within 6 months but may take longer.
- ● MEDICINAL FORMS
  There can be variation in the licensing of different medicines containing the same drug. Forms available from special-order manufacturers include: oral suspension, oral solution, powder

  ### Tablet
  CAUTIONARY AND ADVISORY LABELS 3
  - ▶ Tolterodine tartrate (Non-proprietary)
    Tolterodine tartrate 1 mg Tolterodine 1mg tablets | 56 tablet [PoM] £29.03 DT price = £1.95
    Tolterodine tartrate 2 mg Tolterodine 2mg tablets | 56 tablet [PoM] £30.56 DT price = £2.22
  - ▶ Detrusitol (Pfizer Ltd)
    Tolterodine tartrate 1 mg Detrusitol 1mg tablets | 56 tablet [PoM] £29.03 DT price = £1.95
    Tolterodine tartrate 2 mg Detrusitol 2mg tablets | 56 tablet [PoM] £30.56 DT price = £2.22

Modified-release capsule
CAUTIONARY AND ADVISORY LABELS 3, 25
- ▶ Tolterodine tartrate (Non-proprietary)
  Tolterodine tartrate 2 mg Tolterodine 2mg modified-release capsules | 28 capsule [PoM] no price available
- ▶ Blerone XL (Zentiva)
  Tolterodine tartrate 4 mg Blerone XL 4mg capsules | 28 capsule [PoM] £25.78 DT price = £25.78
- ▶ Detrusitol XL (Pfizer Ltd)
  Tolterodine tartrate 4 mg Detrusitol XL 4mg capsules | 28 capsule [PoM] £25.78 DT price = £25.78
- ▶ Efflosomyl XL (Mylan Ltd)
  Tolterodine tartrate 4 mg Efflosomyl XL 4mg capsules | 28 capsule [PoM] £20.62 DT price = £25.78
- ▶ Inconex XL (Sandoz Ltd)
  Tolterodine tartrate 4 mg Inconex XL 4mg capsules | 28 capsule [PoM] £21.91 DT price = £25.78
- ▶ Mariosea XL (Teva UK Ltd)
  Tolterodine tartrate 2 mg Mariosea XL 2mg capsules | 28 capsule [PoM] £11.59
  Tolterodine tartrate 4 mg Mariosea XL 4mg capsules | 28 capsule [PoM] £12.88 DT price = £25.78
- ▶ Neditol XL (Aspire Pharma Ltd)
  Tolterodine tartrate 2 mg Neditol XL 2mg capsules | 28 capsule [PoM] £11.60
  Tolterodine tartrate 4 mg Neditol XL 4mg capsules | 28 capsule [PoM] £12.89 DT price = £25.78
- ▶ Preblacon XL (Actavis UK Ltd)
  Tolterodine tartrate 4 mg Preblacon XL 4mg capsules | 28 capsule [PoM] £25.78 DT price = £25.78
- ▶ Santizor XL (Pfizer Ltd)
  Tolterodine tartrate 4 mg Santizor XL 4mg capsules | 28 capsule [PoM] £25.78 DT price = £25.78

1.2 Urinary retention

Drugs for urinary retention

Overview

Acute retention is painful and is treated by catheterisation.

Chronic retention is painless and often long-standing. Clean intermittent catheterisation may be considered. After the cause has been established and treated, drugs may be required to increase detrusor muscle tone.

Alpha-blockers such as doxazosin below and tamsulosin hydrochloride p. 459 can be used in some cases of dysfunctional voiding.

Alpha-blockers

The selective alpha-blockers doxazosin and tamsulosin hydrochloride can be used to improve bladder emptying in children with dysfunctional voiding where the post-void residual urine volume is significant; treatment should be under specialist advice only. Alpha-blockers can reduce blood pressure rapidly after the first dose and should be introduced with caution.

ALPHA-ADRENOCEPTOR BLOCKERS

Doxazosin

- ● **INDICATIONS AND DOSE**
  Hypertension
  - ▶ BY MOUTH USING IMMEDIATE-RELEASE MEDICINES
  - ▶ **Child 6-11 years:** Initially 500 micrograms once daily, then increased to 2–4 mg once daily, dose should be increased at intervals of 1 week
  - ▶ **Child 12-17 years:** Initially 1 mg once daily for 1–2 weeks, then increased to 2 mg once daily, then increased if necessary to 4 mg once daily, rarely doses of up to 16 mg daily may be required

Dysfunctional voiding (initiated under specialist supervision)

▶ BY MOUTH USING IMMEDIATE-RELEASE MEDICINES
▶ Child 4–11 years: Initially 0.5 mg daily, adjusted according to response, dose should be increased at monthly intervals; maximum 2 mg per day
▶ Child 12–17 years: Initially 1 mg daily, adjusted according to response, dose may be doubled at intervals of 1 month; usual maintenance 2–4 mg daily; maximum 8 mg per day

DOSE EQUIVALENCE AND CONVERSION
Patients stabilised on immediate-release doxazosin can be transferred to the equivalent dose of modified-release doxazosin.

● UNLICENSED USE Not licensed for use in children.
● CONTRA-INDICATIONS History of postural hypotension
● CAUTIONS Care with initial dose (postural hypotension) · cataract surgery (risk of intra-operative floppy iris syndrome) · heart failure · pulmonary oedema due to aortic or mitral stenosis
● INTERACTIONS → Appendix 1 (alpha-blockers).
● SIDE-EFFECTS
▶ **Common or very common** Anxiety · back pain · coughing · dyspnoea · fatigue · influenza-like symptoms · myalgia · paraesthesia · sleep disturbance · vertigo
▶ **Uncommon** Agitation · angina · arthralgia · epistaxis · gout · hypoaesthesia · impotence · micturition disturbance · myocardial infarction · purpura · tinnitus · tremor · weight changes
▶ **Very rare** Abnormal ejaculation · alopecia · arrhythmias · bradycardia · bronchospasm · cholestasis · gynaecomastia · hepatitis · hot flushes · jaundice · leucopenia · thrombocytopenia
▶ **Frequency not known** Asthenia · blurred vision · depression · dizziness · gastro-intestinal disturbances · headache · hypersensitivity · hypotension · oedema · palpitations · postural hypotension · priapism · pruritus · rash · rhinitis · syncope · tachycardia
● PREGNANCY No evidence of teratogenicity; manufacturers advise use only when potential benefit outweighs risk.
● BREAST FEEDING Accumulates in milk in *animal* studies—manufacturer advises avoid.
● HEPATIC IMPAIRMENT Use with caution. Manufacturer advises avoid in severe impairment—no information available.
● PATIENT AND CARER ADVICE
Patient counselling is advised for doxazosin tablets (initial dose).

Driving and skilled tasks
May affect performance of skilled tasks e.g. driving.

● MEDICINAL FORMS
There can be variation in the licensing of different medicines containing the same drug. Forms available from special-order manufacturers include: capsule, oral suspension, oral solution
Tablet
▶ Doxazosin (Non-proprietary)
Doxazosin (as Doxazosin mesilate) 1 mg Doxazosin 1mg tablets | 28 tablet [PoM] £10.56 DT price = £0.71
Doxazosin (as Doxazosin mesilate) 2 mg Doxazosin 2mg tablets | 28 tablet [PoM] £14.08 DT price = £0.73
Doxazosin (as Doxazosin mesilate) 4 mg Doxazosin 4mg tablets | 28 tablet [PoM] £14.08 DT price = £0.81
▶ Cardura (Pfizer Ltd)
Doxazosin (as Doxazosin mesilate) 1 mg Cardura 1mg tablets | 28 tablet [PoM] £10.56 DT price = £0.71
Doxazosin (as Doxazosin mesilate) 2 mg Cardura 2mg tablets | 28 tablet [PoM] £14.08 DT price = £0.73
▶ Doxadura (Discovery Pharmaceuticals)
Doxazosin (as Doxazosin mesilate) 1 mg Doxadura 1mg tablets | 28 tablet [PoM] £0.71 DT price = £0.71

Doxazosin (as Doxazosin mesilate) 2 mg Doxadura 2mg tablets | 28 tablet [PoM] £0.73 DT price = £0.73
Doxazosin (as Doxazosin mesilate) 4 mg Doxadura 4mg tablets | 28 tablet [PoM] £0.80 DT price = £0.81
Modified-release tablet
CAUTIONARY AND ADVISORY LABELS 25
▶ Cardozin XL (Almus Pharmaceuticals Ltd)
Doxazosin (as Doxazosin mesilate) 4 mg Cardozin XL 4mg tablets | 28 tablet [PoM] £6.33 DT price = £5.00
▶ Cardura XL (Pfizer Ltd)
Doxazosin (as Doxazosin mesilate) 4 mg Cardura XL 4mg tablets | 28 tablet [PoM] £5.00 DT price = £5.00
Doxazosin (as Doxazosin mesilate) 8 mg Cardura XL 8mg tablets | 28 tablet [PoM] £9.98 DT price = £9.98
▶ Doxadura XL (Discovery Pharmaceuticals)
Doxazosin (as Doxazosin mesilate) 4 mg Doxadura XL 4mg tablets | 28 tablet [PoM] £4.50 DT price = £5.00
▶ Doxzogen XL (Mylan Ltd)
Doxazosin (as Doxazosin mesilate) 4 mg Doxzogen XL 4mg tablets | 28 tablet [PoM] £5.70 DT price = £5.00
▶ Larbex XL (Teva UK Ltd)
Doxazosin (as Doxazosin mesilate) 4 mg Larbex XL 4mg tablets | 28 tablet [PoM] £6.08 DT price = £5.00
▶ Raporsin XL (Actavis UK Ltd)
Doxazosin (as Doxazosin mesilate) 4 mg Raporsin XL 4mg tablets | 28 tablet [PoM] £5.70 DT price = £5.00
▶ Slocinx XL (Zentiva)
Doxazosin (as Doxazosin mesilate) 4 mg Slocinx XL 4mg tablets | 28 tablet [PoM] £5.96 DT price = £5.00

Tamsulosin hydrochloride

● INDICATIONS AND DOSE
Dysfunctional voiding (administered on expert advice)
▶ BY MOUTH USING MODIFIED-RELEASE MEDICINES
▶ Child 12–17 years: 400 micrograms once daily

● UNLICENSED USE Not licensed for use in children.
● CONTRA-INDICATIONS History of postural hypotension
● CAUTIONS Care with initial dose (postural hypotension) · cataract surgery (risk of intra-operative floppy iris syndrome)
● INTERACTIONS → Appendix 1 (alpha-blockers).
● SIDE-EFFECTS Abnormal ejaculation · angioedema · asthenia · blurred vision · constipation · diarrhoea · dizziness · drowsiness · dry mouth · headache · hypersensitivity reactions · hypotension (notably postural hypotension) · intra-operative floppy iris syndrome · nausea · oedema · palpitations · priapism · pruritus · rash · rhinitis · syncope · urticaria · vomiting
● HEPATIC IMPAIRMENT Avoid in severe impairment.
● RENAL IMPAIRMENT Use with caution if estimated glomerular filtration rate less than 10 mL/minute/1.73 m^2.
● PATIENT AND CARER ADVICE
Driving and skilled tasks
May affect performance of skilled tasks e.g. driving.

● MEDICINAL FORMS
There can be variation in the licensing of different medicines containing the same drug. Forms available from special-order manufacturers include: oral suspension, oral solution, powder
Modified-release tablet
CAUTIONARY AND ADVISORY LABELS 25
▶ Tamsulosin hydrochloride (Non-proprietary)
Tamsulosin hydrochloride 400 microgram Tamsulosin 400microgram modified-release tablets | 30 tablet [PoM] £10.47 DT price = £10.47
▶ Cositam XL (Consilient Health Ltd)
Tamsulosin hydrochloride 400 microgram Cositam XL 400microgram tablets | 30 tablet [PoM] £8.89 DT price = £10.47
▶ Faramsil (Sandoz Ltd)
Tamsulosin hydrochloride 400 microgram Faramsil 400microgram modified-release tablets | 30 tablet [PoM] £8.89 DT price = £10.47

▸ Flectone XL (Teva UK Ltd)
Tamsulosin hydrochloride 400 microgram Flectone XL
400microgram tablets | 30 tablet [PoM] £9.95 DT price = £10.47
▸ Flomaxtra XL (Astellas Pharma Ltd)
Tamsulosin hydrochloride 400 microgram Flomaxtra XL
400microgram tablets | 30 tablet [PoM] £10.47 DT price = £10.47

Modified-release capsule
CAUTIONARY AND ADVISORY LABELS 25
▸ **Tamsulosin hydrochloride** (Non-proprietary)
Tamsulosin hydrochloride 400 microgram Tamsulosin
400microgram modified-release capsules | 30 capsule [PoM] £5.07 DT
price = £4.05
▸ Contiflo XL (Ranbaxy (UK) Ltd)
Tamsulosin hydrochloride 400 microgram Contiflo XL
400microgram capsules | 30 capsule [PoM] £7.44 DT price = £4.05
▸ Diffundox XL (Zentiva)
Tamsulosin hydrochloride 400 microgram Diffundox XL
400microgram capsules | 30 capsule [PoM] £9.55 DT price = £4.05
▸ Flomax MR (Boehringer Ingelheim Self-Medication Division)
Tamsulosin hydrochloride 400 microgram Flomax Relief MR
400microgram capsules | 14 capsule [P] £5.58 | 28 capsule [P]
£10.55
▸ Galebon (Consilient Health Ltd)
Tamsulosin hydrochloride 400 microgram Galebon 400microgram
modified-release capsules | 30 capsule [PoM] £3.78 DT price = £4.05
▸ Losinate MR (Aspire Pharma Ltd)
Tamsulosin hydrochloride 400 microgram Losinate MR
400microgram capsules | 30 capsule [PoM] £10.14 DT price = £4.05
▸ Pamsvax XL (Almus Pharmaceuticals Ltd, Actavis UK Ltd)
Tamsulosin hydrochloride 400 microgram Pamsvax XL
400microgram capsules | 30 capsule [PoM] £1.28–£4.42 DT price =
£4.05
▸ Petyme MR (Teva UK Ltd)
Tamsulosin hydrochloride 400 microgram Petyme 400microgram
MR capsules | 30 capsule [PoM] £4.06 DT price = £4.05
▸ Pinexel PR (Wockhardt UK Ltd)
Tamsulosin hydrochloride 400 microgram Pinexel PR
400microgram capsules | 30 capsule [PoM] £2.50 DT price = £4.05
▸ Prosurin XL (Mylan Ltd)
Tamsulosin hydrochloride 400 microgram Prosurin XL
400microgram capsules | 30 capsule [PoM] £4.28 DT price = £4.05
▸ Tabphyn MR (ProStrakan Ltd)
Tamsulosin hydrochloride 400 microgram Tabphyn MR
400microgram capsules | 30 capsule [PoM] £4.39 DT price = £4.05
▸ Tamfrex XL (Milpharm Ltd)
Tamsulosin hydrochloride 400 microgram Tamfrex XL
400microgram capsules | 30 capsule [PoM] no price available DT price
= £4.05
▸ Tamurex (Somex Pharma)
Tamsulosin hydrochloride 400 microgram Tamurex
400microgram modified-release capsules | 30 capsule [PoM] £3.50 DT
price = £4.05

1.3 Urological pain

Urological pain

Treatment

Lidocaine hydrochloride **gel** p. 780 is a useful topical
application in *urethral pain* or to relieve the discomfort of
catheterisation.

Alkalinisation of urine

Alkalinisation of urine can be undertaken with potassium
citrate. The alkalinising action may relieve the discomfort of
cystitis caused by lower urinary tract infections.

ALKALISING DRUGS 〉 ALKALISING DRUGS,
URINARY

Citric acid with potassium citrate

● **INDICATIONS AND DOSE**
Relief of discomfort in mild urinary-tract infections |
Alkalinisation of urine
▸ BY MOUTH USING ORAL SOLUTION
▸ **Child 1–5 years:** 5 mL 3 times a day, diluted well with
water
▸ **Child 6–17 years:** 10 mL 3 times a day, diluted well with
water

● **CAUTIONS** Cardiac disease

● **INTERACTIONS** → Appendix 1 (potassium salts).

● **SIDE-EFFECTS** Hyperkalaemia on prolonged high dosage ·
mild diuresis

● **RENAL IMPAIRMENT** Avoid in severe impairment. Close
monitoring required in renal impairment—high risk of
hyperkalaemia.

● **PRESCRIBING AND DISPENSING INFORMATION** When
prepared extemporaneously, the BP states Potassium
Citrate Mixture BP consists of potassium citrate 30%, citric
acid monohydrate 5% in a suitable vehicle with a lemon
flavour. Extemporaneous preparations should be recently
prepared according to the following formula: potassium
citrate 3 g, citric acid monohydrate 500 mg, syrup 2.5 mL,
quillaia tincture 0.1 mL, lemon spirit 0.05 mL, double-
strength chloroform water 3 mL, water to 10 mL. Contains
about 28 mmol K^+/10 mL.

● **EXCEPTIONS TO LEGAL CATEGORY** Proprietary brands of
potassium citrate are on sale to the public for the relief of
discomfort in mild urinary-tract infections.

● **MEDICINAL FORMS**
There can be variation in the licensing of different medicines
containing the same drug.
Oral solution
CAUTIONARY AND ADVISORY LABELS 27
▸ Citric acid with potassium citrate (Non-proprietary)
**Citric acid monohydrate 50 mg per 1 ml, Potassium citrate
300 mg per 1 ml** Potassium citrate mixture | 200 ml [GSL] £1.33 DT
price = £1.33 | 200 ml [P] £1.33 DT price = £1.33

2 Bladder instillations and urological surgery

Bladder instillations and urological surgery

Bladder infection

Various solutions are available as irrigations or washouts.
Aqueous chlorhexidine p. 656 can be used in the
management of common infections of the bladder but it is
ineffective against most *Pseudomonas spp.* Solutions
containing chlorhexidine 1 in 5000 (0.02%) are used but they
may irritate the mucosa and cause burning and haematuria
(in which case they should be discontinued); sterile sodium
chloride **solution 0.9%** p. 547 (physiological saline) is
usually adequate and is preferred as a mechanical irrigant.

Dissolution of blood clots

Clot retention is usually treated by irrigation with sterile
sodium chloride solution 0.9% but sterile sodium citrate
solution for bladder irrigation 3% may also be helpful.

Maintenance of indwelling urinary catheters

The deposition which occurs in catheterised patients is usually chiefly composed of phosphate and to minimise this the catheter (if latex) should be changed at least as often as every 6 weeks. If the catheter is to be left for longer periods a silicone catheter should be used together with the appropriate use of catheter maintenance solutions. Repeated blockage usually indicates that the catheter needs to be changed.

▌Catheter maintenance solutions

● CATHETER MAINTENANCE SOLUTIONS

OptiFlo R citric acid 6% catheter maintenance solution (Bard Ltd) 50 ml · NHS indicative price = £3.56 · Drug Tariff (Part IXa) 100 ml · NHS indicative price = £3.56 · Drug Tariff (Part IXa)

Uro-Tainer Twin Solutio R citric acid 6% catheter maintenance solution (B.Braun Medical Ltd) 60 ml · NHS indicative price = £4.81 · Drug Tariff (Part IXa)

OptiFlo S saline 0.9% catheter maintenance solution (Bard Ltd) Sodium chloride 9 mg per 1 ml 50 ml · NHS indicative price = £3.36 · Drug Tariff (Part IXa) 100 ml · NHS indicative price = £3.36 · Drug Tariff (Part IXa)

Uro-Tainer M sodium chloride 0.9% catheter maintenance solution (B.Braun Medical Ltd) Sodium chloride 9 mg per 1 ml 50 ml · No NHS indicative price available · Drug Tariff (Part IXa) 100 ml · No NHS indicative price available · Drug Tariff (Part IXa)

Uro-Tainer sodium chloride 0.9% catheter maintenance solution (B.Braun Medical Ltd) Sodium chloride 9 mg per 1 ml 50 ml · NHS indicative price = £3.51 · Drug Tariff (Part IXa) 100 ml · NHS indicative price = £3.51 · Drug Tariff (Part IXa)

3   Contraception

Contraceptives, hormonal

Overview

The Fraser Guidelines (Department of Health Guidance (July 2004): Best practice guidance for doctors and other health professionals on the provision of advice and treatment to young people under 16 on contraception, sexual and reproductive health, available at www.tinyurl.com/bpg16) should be followed when prescribing contraception for women under 16 years. The UK Medical Eligibility Criteria for Contraceptive Use (available at www.fsrh.org) is published by the Faculty of Sexual and Reproductive Healthcare; it categorises the risks of using contraceptive methods with pre-existing medical conditions.

Hormonal contraception is the most effective method of fertility control, but can have major and minor side-effects, especially for certain groups of women. Hormonal contraception should only be used by adolescents after menarche.

Intra-uterine devices are a highly effective method of contraception but may produce undesirable local side-effects. They may be used in women of all ages irrespective of parity, but are less appropriate for those with an increased risk of pelvic inflammatory disease.

Barrier methods alone (condoms, diaphragms, and caps) are less effective but can be reliable for well-motivated couples if used in conjunction with a **spermicide**. Occasionally sensitivity reactions occur. A female condom (*Femidom*®) is also available; it is pre-lubricated but does not contain a spermicide.

Combined hormonal contraceptives

Oral contraceptives containing an oestrogen and a progestogen ('combined oral contraceptives') are effective preparations for general use. Advantages of combined oral contraceptives include:

- reliable and reversible;
- reduced dysmenorrhoea and menorrhagia;
- reduced incidence of premenstrual tension;
- less symptomatic fibroids and functional ovarian cysts;
- less benign breast disease;
- reduced risk of ovarian and endometrial cancer;
- reduced risk of pelvic inflammatory disease.

Combined oral contraceptives containing a fixed amount of an oestrogen and a progestogen in each active tablet are termed 'monophasic'; those with varying amounts of the two hormones are termed 'phasic'. A transdermal patch and a vaginal ring, both containing an oestrogen with a progestogen, are also available.

Combined Oral Contraceptives Monophasic 21-day preparations		
Oestrogen content	**Progestogen content**	**Brand**
Ethinylestradiol 20 micrograms	Desogestrel 150 micrograms	Gedarel® 20/150
Ethinylestradiol 20 micrograms	Desogestrel 150 micrograms	Mercilon®
Ethinylestradiol 20 micrograms	Gestodene 75 micrograms	Femodette®
Ethinylestradiol 20 micrograms	Gestodene 75 micrograms	Millinette® 20/75
Ethinylestradiol 20 micrograms	Gestodene 75 micrograms	Sunya 20/75®
Ethinylestradiol 20 micrograms	Norethisterone acetate 1 mg	Loestrin 20®
Ethinylestradiol 30 micrograms	Desogestrel 150 micrograms	Gedarel® 30/150
Ethinylestradiol 30 micrograms	Desogestrel 150 micrograms	Marvelon®
Ethinylestradiol 30 micrograms	Drospirenone 3 mg	Yasmin®
Ethinylestradiol 30 micrograms	Gestodene 75 micrograms	Femodene®
Ethinylestradiol 30 micrograms	Gestodene 75 micrograms	Katya 30/75®
Ethinylestradiol 30 micrograms	Gestodene 75 micrograms	Millinette® 30/75
Ethinylestradiol 30 micrograms	Levonorgestrel 150 micrograms	Levest®
Ethinylestradiol 30 micrograms	Levonorgestrel 150 micrograms	Microgynon 30®
Ethinylestradiol 30 micrograms	Levonorgestrel 150 micrograms	Ovranette®
Ethinylestradiol 30 micrograms	Levonorgestrel 150 micrograms	Rigevidon®
Ethinylestradiol 30 micrograms	Norethisterone acetate 1.5 mg	Loestrin 30®
Ethinylestradiol 35 micrograms	Norgestimate 250 micrograms	Cilest®
Ethinylestradiol 35 micrograms	Norethisterone 500 micrograms	Brevinor®
Ethinylestradiol 35 micrograms	Norethisterone 500 micrograms	Ovysmen®
Ethinylestradiol 35 micrograms	Norethisterone 1 mg	Norimin®
Mestranol 50 micrograms	Norethisterone 1 mg	Norinyl-1®

7

Genito-urinary system

Combined Oral Contraceptives Monophasic 28-day preparations

Oestrogen content	Progestogen content	Brand
Ethinylestradiol 30 micrograms	Gestodene 75 micrograms	Femodene® ED
Ethinylestradiol 30 micrograms	Levonorgestrel 150 micrograms	Microgynon 30 ED®
Estradiol (as hemihydrate) 1.5 mg	Nomegestrol acetate 2.5 mg	Zoely®

Combined Oral Contraceptives Phasic 21-day preparations

Oestrogen content	Progestogen content	Brand
Ethinylestradiol 30 micrograms	Gestodene 50 micrograms	
Ethinylestradiol 40 micrograms	Gestodene 70 micrograms	Triadene®
Ethinylestradiol 30 micrograms	Gestodene 100 micrograms	
Ethinylestradiol 30 micrograms	Levonorgestrel 50 micrograms	
Ethinylestradiol 40 micrograms	Levonorgestrel 75 micrograms	Logynon®
Ethinylestradiol 30 micrograms	Levonorgestrel 125 micrograms	
Ethinylestradiol 30 micrograms	Levonorgestrel 50 micrograms	
Ethinylestradiol 40 micrograms	Levonorgestrel 75 micrograms	TriRegol®
Ethinylestradiol 30 micrograms	Levonorgestrel 125 micrograms	
Ethinylestradiol 35 micrograms	Norethisterone 500 micrograms	BiNovum®
Ethinylestradiol 35 micrograms	Norethisterone 1 mg	
Ethinylestradiol 35 micrograms	Norethisterone 500 micrograms	
Ethinylestradiol 35 micrograms	Norethisterone 1 mg	Synphase®
Ethinylestradiol 35 micrograms	Norethisterone 500 micrograms	

Combined Oral Contraceptives Phasic 28-day preparations

Oestrogen content	Progestogen content	Brand
Ethinylestradiol 30 micrograms	Levonorgestrel 50 micrograms	
Ethinylestradiol 40 micrograms	Levonorgestrel 75 micrograms	Logynon ED®
Ethinylestradiol 30 micrograms	Levonorgestrel 125 micrograms	
Estradiol valerate 3 mg		
Estradiol valerate 2 mg	Dienogest 2 mg	
Estradiol valerate 2 mg	Dienogest 3 mg	Qlaira®
Estradiol valerate 1 mg		

Choice

The majority of combined oral contraceptives contain ethinylestradiol p. 446 as the oestrogen component; mestranol and estradiol are also used. The ethinylestradiol content of combined oral contraceptives ranges from 20 to 40 micrograms. Generally a preparation with the lowest oestrogen and progestogen content which gives good cycle control and minimal side-effects in the individual woman is chosen. It is recommended that combined hormonal contraceptives are not continued beyond 50 years of age since more suitable alternatives exist.

- *Low strength preparations* (containing ethinylestradiol 20 micrograms) are particularly appropriate for women with risk factors for circulatory disease, provided a combined oral contraceptive is otherwise suitable.
- *Standard strength preparations* (containing ethinylestradiol 30 or 35 micrograms or in 30–40 microgram *phased* preparations) are appropriate for standard use. Phased preparations are generally reserved for women who *either* do not have withdrawal bleeding or who have breakthrough bleeding with monophasic products.

The progestogens ethinylestradiol with desogestrel p. 467, ethinylestradiol with drospirenone p. 468, and ethinylestradiol with gestodene p. 469 may be considered for women who have side-effects (such as acne, headache, depression, breast symptoms, and breakthrough bleeding) with other progestogens. Drospirenone, a derivative of spironolactone, has anti-androgenic and anti-mineralocorticoid activity; it should be used with care if an increased plasma-potassium concentration might be hazardous.

Dienogest with estradiol valerate p. 467 is in the combined oral contraceptive *Qlaira*®. Nomegestrol is the progestogen contained in the combined oral contraceptive *Zoely*®, in combination with estradiol.

The progestogen norelgestromin is combined with ethinylestradiol in a transdermal patch (*Evra*®). The vaginal contraceptive ring contains the progestogen etonogestrel combined with ethinylestradiol (*NuvaRing*®).

Surgery

Oestrogen-containing contraceptives should preferably be discontinued (and adequate alternative contraceptive arrangements made) 4 weeks before major elective surgery and all surgery to the legs or surgery which involves prolonged immobilisation of a lower limb; they should normally be recommenced at the first menses occurring at least 2 weeks after full mobilisation. A progestogen-only contraceptive may be offered as an alternative and the oestrogen-containing contraceptive restarted after mobilisation. When discontinuation of an oestrogen-containing contraceptive is not possible, e.g. after trauma or if a patient admitted for an elective procedure is still on an oestrogen- containing contraceptive, thromboprophylaxis (with unfractionated or low molecular weight heparin and graduated compression hosiery) is advised. These recommendations do not apply to minor surgery with short duration of anaesthesia, e.g. laparoscopic sterilisation or tooth extraction, or to women using oestrogen-free hormonal contraceptives.

Reason to stop immediately

Combined hormonal contraceptives or hormone replacement therapy (HRT) should be stopped (pending investigation and treatment), if any of the following occur:

- sudden severe chest pain (even if not radiating to left arm);
- sudden breathlessness (or cough with blood-stained sputum);
- unexplained swelling or severe pain in calf of one leg;
- severe stomach pain;
- serious neurological effects including unusual severe, prolonged headache especially if first time or getting

progressively worse *or* sudden partial *or* complete loss of vision *or* sudden disturbance of hearing or other perceptual disorders *or* dysphasia *or* bad fainting attack or collapse *or* first unexplained epileptic seizure *or* weakness, motor disturbances, very marked numbness suddenly affecting one side or one part of body;

- hepatitis, jaundice, liver enlargement;
- blood pressure above systolic 160 mmHg or diastolic 95 mmHg; (in adolescents stop if blood pressure very high);
- prolonged immobility after surgery or leg injury;
- detection of a risk factor which contra-indicates treatment.

Progestogen-only contraceptives

Oral progestogen-only contraceptives

Oral progestogen-only preparations alter cervical mucus to prevent sperm penetration and may inhibit ovulation in some women; oral desogestrel-only preparations consistently inhibit ovulation and this is their primary mechanism of action. There is insufficient clinical trial evidence to compare the efficacy of oral progestogen-only contraceptives with each other or with combined hormonal contraceptives. Progestogen-only contraceptives offer a suitable alternative to combined hormonal contraceptives when oestrogens are contra-indicated (including those with venous thrombosis or a past history or predisposition to venous thrombosis, heavy smokers, those with hypertension above systolic 160 mmHg or diastolic 95 mmHg, valvular heart disease, diabetes mellitus with complications, and migraine with aura).

Parenteral progestogen-only contraceptives

Medroxyprogesterone acetate (*Depo-Provera®, SAYANA PRESS®*) p. 478 is a long-acting progestogen given by injection; it is at least as effective as the combined oral preparations but because of its prolonged action it should never be given without *full counselling backed by the patient information leaflet*. It may be used as a short-term or long-term contraceptive for women who have been counselled about the likelihood of menstrual disturbance and the potential for a delay in return to full fertility. Delayed return of fertility and irregular cycles may occur after discontinuation of treatment but there is no evidence of permanent infertility. Troublesome bleeding has been reported in patients given medroxyprogesterone acetate in the immediate puerperium; delaying the first injection until 6 weeks after birth may minimise bleeding problems. If the woman is not breast-feeding, the first injection may be given within 5 days postpartum (she should be warned that the risk of troublesome bleeding may be increased).

- In adolescents, medroxyprogesterone acetate (*Depo-Provera®, SAYANA PRESS®*) should be used only when other methods of contraception are inappropriate;
- in all women, the benefits of using medroxyprogesterone acetate beyond 2 years should be evaluated against the risks;
- in women with risk factors for osteoporosis, a method of contraception other than medroxyprogesterone acetate should be considered.

Norethisterone enantate (*Noristerat®*) is a long-acting progestogen given as an oily injection which provides contraception for 8 weeks; it is used as short-term interim contraception e.g. before vasectomy becomes effective.

An **etonogestrel-releasing implant** (*Nexplanon®*) is also available. It is a highly effective long-acting contraceptive, consisting of a single flexible rod that is inserted subdermally into the lower surface of the upper arm and provides contraception for up to 3 years. The manufacturer advises that in heavier women, blood-etonogestrel concentrations are lower and therefore the implant may not provide effective contraception during the third year; they advise that earlier replacement may be considered in such

patients—however, evidence to support this recommendation is lacking. Local reactions such as bruising and itching can occur at the insertion site. The contraceptive effect of etonogestrel is rapidly reversed on removal of the implant.

Intra-uterine progestogen-only device

The progestogen-only intra-uterine systems *Mirena®, Jaydess®* and *Levosert®* release levonorgestrel p. 475 directly into the uterine cavity. *Mirena®* is licensed for use as a contraceptive, for the treatment of primary menorrhagia and for the prevention of endometrial hyperplasia during oestrogen replacement therapy. *Jaydess®* and *Levosert®* are licensed for contraception, and *Levosert®* is additionally licensed for the treatment of menorrhagia. These may therefore be a contraceptive method of choice for women who have excessively heavy menses.

The effects of the progestogen-only intra-uterine system are mainly local and hormonal including prevention of endometrial proliferation, thickening of cervical mucus, and suppression of ovulation in some women (in some cycles). In addition to the progestogenic activity, the intra-uterine system itself may contribute slightly to the contraceptive effect. Return of fertility after removal is rapid and appears to be complete.

Advantages of the progestogen-only intra-uterine system over copper intra-uterine devices are that there may be an improvement in any dysmenorrhoea and a reduction in blood loss; there is also evidence that the frequency of pelvic inflammatory disease may be reduced (particularly in the youngest age groups who are most at risk).

In primary menorrhagia, menstrual bleeding is reduced significantly within 3–6 months of inserting the progestogen-only intra-uterine system, probably because it prevents endometrial proliferation. Another treatment should be considered if menorrhagia does not improve within this time.

Surgery

All progestogen-only contraceptives (including those given by injection) are suitable for use as an alternative to combined hormonal contraceptives before major elective surgery, before all surgery to the legs, or before surgery which involves prolonged immobilisation of a lower limb.

Emergency contraception

Hormonal methods

Hormonal emergency contraceptives include levonorgestrel and ulipristal acetate p. 473; either drug should be taken as soon as possible after unprotected intercourse to increase efficacy.

Levonorgestrel is effective if taken within 72 hours (3 days) of unprotected intercourse and may also be used between 72 and 96 hours after unprotected intercourse [unlicensed use], but efficacy decreases with time. Ulipristal acetate, a progesterone receptor modulator, is effective if taken within 120 hours (5 days) of unprotected intercourse.

Levonorgestrel is less effective than insertion of an intra-uterine device. Ulipristal acetate is as effective as levonorgestrel, but its efficacy compared to an intra-uterine device is not yet known.

Intra-uterine device

Insertion of an intra-uterine device is more effective than oral levonorgestrel for emergency contraception. A copper intra-uterine contraceptive device can be inserted up to 120 hours (5 days) after unprotected intercourse; sexually transmitted infections should be tested for and insertion of the device should usually be covered by antibacterial prophylaxis (e.g. azithromycin p. 308). If intercourse has occurred more than 5 days previously, the device can still be inserted up to 5 days after the earliest likely calculated ovulation (i.e. within the minimum period before implantation), regardless of the number of episodes of unprotected intercourse earlier in the cycle.

Contraceptives, interactions

Combined hormonal contraceptives interactions

The effectiveness of *combined* oral contraceptives, *progestogen-only* oral contraceptives, contraceptive patches, and vaginal rings can be considerably reduced by interaction with drugs that induce hepatic enzyme activity (e.g. carbamazepine p. 184, nevirapine p. 389, oxcarbazepine p. 192, phenytoin p. 193, phenobarbital p. 203, primidone p. 204, ritonavir p. 397, **St John's Wort**, topiramate p. 199 and, above all, rifabutin p. 341 and rifampicin p. 342). A condom together with a long-acting method, such as an injectable contraceptive, may be more suitable for patients with HIV infection or at risk of HIV infection; advice on the possibility of interaction with antiretroviral drugs should be sought from HIV specialists.

Women taking combined hormonal contraceptives who require enzyme-inducing drugs should be advised to change to a contraceptive method that is unaffected by enzyme-inducers (e.g. some parenteral progestogen-only contraceptives, intra-uterine devices) for the duration of treatment and for 4 weeks after stopping. If a change in contraceptive method is undesirable or inappropriate the following options should be discussed:

- For a *short course (2 months or less) of an enzyme-inducing drug*, continue with a combined oral contraceptive providing ethinylestradiol 30 micrograms or more daily and use a 'tricycling' regimen (i.e. taking 3 packets of monophasic tablets without a break followed by a shortened tablet-free interval of 4 days [unlicensed use]). Additional contraceptive precautions should also be used whilst taking the enzyme-inducing drug and for 4 weeks after stopping. Another option (except for rifampicin or rifabutin) is to follow the advice for long-term courses, below.

For women using combined hormonal contraceptive patches or vaginal rings, additional contraceptive precautions are also required whilst taking the enzyme-inducing drug and for 4 weeks after stopping. If concomitant administration runs beyond the 3 weeks of patch or vaginal ring use, a new treatment cycle should be started immediately, without a patch-free or ring-free break.

- For a *long-term course (over 2 months) of an enzyme-inducing drug* (except rifampicin or rifabutin), adjust the dose of combined oral contraceptive to provide ethinylestradiol 50 micrograms or more daily [unlicensed use] and use a 'tricycling' regimen; continue for the duration of treatment with the enzyme-inducing drug and for 4 weeks after stopping.

If breakthrough bleeding occurs (and all other causes are ruled out) it is recommended that the dose of ethinylestradiol is increased by increments of 10 micrograms up to a maximum of 70 micrograms daily [unlicensed use], or to use additional precautions, or to change to a method unaffected by enzyme-inducing drugs.

Contraceptive patches and vaginal rings are not recommended for women taking enzyme-inducing drugs over a period.

- For a *long-term course (over 2 months) of rifampicin or rifabutin*, an alternative method of contraception (such as an IUD) is **always** recommended because they are such potent enzyme-inducing drugs; the alternative method of contraception should be continued for 4 weeks after stopping the enzyme-inducing drug.

Antibacterials that do not induce liver enzymes

Latest recommendations are that no additional contraceptive precautions are required when *combined* oral

contraceptives are used with antibacterials that do not induce liver enzymes (e.g. ampicillin p. 321, doxycycline p. 332), unless diarrhoea or vomiting occur. These recommendations should be discussed with the woman, who should also be advised that guidance in patient information leaflets may differ.

It is also currently recommended that no additional contraceptive precautions are required when contraceptive patches or vaginal rings are used with antibacterials that do not induce liver enzymes. There have been concerns that some antibacterials that do not induce liver enzymes reduce the efficacy of *combined* oral contraceptives by impairing the bacterial flora responsible for recycling ethinylestradiol from the large bowel; however, there is a lack of evidence to support this interaction.

Oral progestogen-only contraceptives interactions

Effectiveness of oral progestogen-only preparations is not affected by antibacterials that do not induce liver enzymes. The efficacy of oral progestogen-only preparations is, however, reduced by enzyme-inducing drugs and an alternative contraceptive method, unaffected by the interacting drug, is recommended during treatment with an enzyme-inducing drug and for at least 4 weeks afterwards. For a short course of an enzyme-inducing drug, if a change in contraceptive method is undesirable or inappropriate, the progestogen-only oral method may be continued in combination with additional contraceptive precautions (e.g. barrier methods) for the duration of treatment with the enzyme-inducing drug and for 4 weeks after stopping.

Parenteral progestogen-only contraceptives interactions

Effectiveness of parenteral progestogen-only contraceptives is not affected by antibacterials that do not induce liver enzymes. The effectiveness of norethisterone intramuscular injection p. 447 and medroxyprogesterone acetate intramuscular and subcutaneous injections p. 478 is not affected by enzyme-inducing drugs and they may be continued as normal during courses of these drugs. However, effectiveness of the etonogestrel-releasing implant p. 477 may be reduced by enzyme-inducing drugs and an alternative contraceptive method, unaffected by the interacting drug, is recommended during treatment with the enzyme-inducing drug and for at least 4 weeks after stopping. For a short course of an enzyme-inducing drug, if a change in contraceptive method is undesirable or inappropriate, the implant may be continued in combination with additional contraceptive precautions (e.g. condom) for the duration of treatment with the enzyme-inducing drug and for 4 weeks after stopping it.

Hormonal emergency contraception interactions

The effectiveness of levonorgestrel p. 475, and possibly ulipristal acetate p. 473, is reduced in women taking enzyme-inducing drugs (and possibly for 4 weeks after stopping); a copper intra-uterine device can be offered instead. If the copper intra-uterine device is undesirable or inappropriate, the dose of levonorgestrel should be increased to a total of 3 mg taken as a single dose [unlicensed dose—advise women accordingly]. There is no need to increase the dose for emergency contraception if the patient is taking antibacterials that are not enzyme inducers.

Contraceptives, non-hormonal

Spermicidal contraceptives

Spermicidal contraceptives are useful additional safeguards but do **not** give adequate protection if used alone unless fertility is already significantly diminished. They have two components: a spermicide and a vehicle which itself may have some inhibiting effect on sperm activity. They are suitable for use with barrier methods, such as diaphragms or caps; however, spermicidal contraceptives are not generally recommended for use with condoms, as there is no evidence of any additional protection compared with non-spermicidal lubricants.

Spermicidal contraceptives are not suitable for use in those with or at high risk of sexually transmitted infections (including HIV); high frequency use of the spermicide nonoxinol '9' p. 479 has been associated with genital lesions, which may increase the risk of acquiring these infections.

Products such as petroleum jelly (*Vaseline®*), baby oil and oil-based vaginal and rectal preparations are likely to damage condoms and contraceptive diaphragms made from latex rubber, and may render them less effective as a barrier method of contraception and as a protection from sexually transmitted infections (including HIV).

Contraceptive devices

Intra-uterine devices

The intra-uterine device (IUD) is a suitable contraceptive for women of all ages irrespective of parity; however, it is less appropriate for those with an increased risk of pelvic inflammatory disease e.g. women under 25 years.

The most effective intra-uterine devices have at least 380 mm^2 of copper and have banded copper on the arms. Smaller devices have been introduced to minimise side-effects; these consist of a plastic carrier wound with copper wire or fitted with copper bands; some also have a central core of silver to prevent fragmentation of the copper.

Fertility declines with age and therefore a copper intra-uterine device which is fitted in a woman over the age of 40, may remain in the uterus until menopause.

A frameless, copper-bearing intra-uterine device (*Gyne Fix®*) is also available. It consists of a knotted, polypropylene thread with 6 copper sleeves; the device is anchored in the uterus by inserting the knot into the uterine fundus.

3.1   Contraception, combined

OESTROGENS COMBINED WITH PROGESTOGENS

Combined hormonal contraceptives 🅟

- **CONTRA-INDICATIONS** Acute porphyrias p. 562 · gallstones · heart disease associated with pulmonary hypertension or risk of embolus · history during pregnancy of cholestatic jaundice · history during pregnancy of chorea · history during pregnancy of pemphigoid gestationis · history during pregnancy of pruritus · history of breast cancer (but can be used after 5 years if no evidence of disease and non-hormonal methods unacceptable) · history of haemolytic uraemic syndrome · migraine with aura · personal history of venous or arterial thrombosis · sclerosing treatment for varicose veins · severe or multiple risk factors for arterial disease · severe or multiple risk factors for venous thromboembolism · systemic lupus erythematosus · transient cerebral ischaemic attacks without headaches · undiagnosed vaginal bleeding
- **CAUTIONS** Active trophoblastic disease (until return to normal of urine- and plasma-gonadotrophin concentration)—seek specialist advice · Crohn's disease · gene mutations associated with breast cancer (e.g. BRCA 1) · history of severe depression especially if induced by hormonal contraceptive · hyperprolactinaemia (seek specialist advice) · inflammatory bowel disease · migraine · personal or family history of hypertriglyceridaemia

(increased risk of pancreatitis) · risk factors for arterial disease · risk factors for venous thromboembolism · sickle-cell disease · undiagnosed breast mass

CAUTIONS, FURTHER INFORMATION

▸ **Risk of venous thromboembolism** There is an increased risk of venous thromboembolic disease in users of combined hormonal contraceptives particularly during the first year and possibly after restarting combined hormonal contraceptives following a break of four weeks or more. This risk is considerably smaller than that associated with pregnancy (about 60 cases of venous thromboembolic disease per 100 000 pregnancies). In all cases the risk of venous thromboembolism increases with age and in the presence of other risk factors, such as obesity. The risk also varies depending on the type of progestogen.

Provided that women are informed of the relative risks of venous thromboembolism and accept them, the choice of oral contraceptive is for the woman together with the prescriber jointly to make in light of her individual medical history and any contra-indications.

Combined hormonal contraceptives also slightly increase the risk of *arterial* thromboembolism; however, there is no evidence to suggest that this risk varies between different preparations.

▸ **Risk factors for venous thromboembolism** Use with **caution** if any of following factors present but **avoid** if two or more factors present:

- *family history of venous thromboembolism* in first-degree relative aged under 45 years (avoid contraceptive containing desogestrel or gestodene, *or* avoid if known prothrombotic coagulation abnormality e.g. factor V Leiden or antiphospholipid antibodies (including lupus anticoagulant));
- *obesity*; body mass index ≥ 30 kg/m^2 (avoid if body mass index ≥ 35 kg/m^2 unless no suitable alternative); (in adolescents, caution if obese according to BMI (adjusted for age and gender); in those who are markedly obese, avoid unless no suitable alternative);
- *long-term immobilisation* e.g. in a wheelchair (avoid if confined to bed or leg in plaster cast);
- *history of superficial thrombophlebitis;*
- *age* over 35 years (avoid if over 50 years);
- *smoking.*

Combined Hormonal Contraception and Risk of Venous Thromboembolism

Progestogen in Combined Hormonal Contraceptive	Estimated incidence per 10 000 women per year of use
Non-pregnant, not using combined hormonal contraception	2
Levonorgesterol[1]	5–7
Norgestimate[1]	5–7
Norethisterone[1]	5–7
Etonogestrel[1]	6–12
Norelgestromin[1]	6–12
Gestodene[1]	9–12
Desogestrel[1]	9–12
Drospirenone[1]	9–12
Dienogest[2]	Not known–insufficient data
Nomegestrol[2]	Not known–insufficient data
[1]Combined with ethinylestradiol [2]Combined with estradiol	

▸ **Risk factors for arterial disease** Use with **caution** if any one of following factors present but **avoid** if two or more factors present:

Genito-urinary system

7

- *family history of arterial disease* in first degree relative aged under 45 years (avoid if atherogenic lipid profile);
- *diabetes mellitus* (avoid if diabetes complications present);
- *hypertension*; blood pressure above *systolic* 140 *mmHg* or *diastolic* 90 *mmHg* (avoid if blood pressure above *systolic* 160 *mmHg* or *diastolic* 95 *mmHg*); (in adolescents, avoid if blood pressure very high);
- *smoking* (avoid if smoking 40 or more cigarettes daily);
- *age* over 35 years (avoid if over 50 years);
- *obesity* (avoid if body mass index $\geq$ 35 kg/m^2 unless no suitable alternative); (in adolescents, caution if obese according to BMI (adjusted for age and gender); in those who are markedly obese, avoid unless no suitable alternative);
- *migraine without aura* (avoid if *migraine with aura* (focal symptoms), *or* severe migraine frequently lasting over 72 hours despite treatment, *or* migraine treated with ergot derivatives).

▸ Migraine Women should report any increase in headache frequency or onset of focal symptoms (discontinue immediately and refer urgently to neurology expert if focal neurological symptoms not typical of aura persist for more than 1 hour).

Combined hormonal contraceptives should be stopped (pending investigation and treatment), if serious neurological effects occur, including unusual severe, prolonged headache especially if first time or getting progressively worse *or* sudden partial or complete loss of vision *or* sudden disturbance of hearing or other perceptual disorders *or* dysphasia *or* bad fainting attack or collapse *or* first unexplained epileptic seizure *or* weakness, motor disturbances, very marked numbness suddenly affecting one side or one part of body.

● INTERACTIONS → Appendix 1 (oestrogens, progestogens).

● SIDE-EFFECTS

▸ **Rare** Gallstones · systemic lupus erythematosus
▸ **Frequency not known** Abdominal cramps · absence of withdrawal bleeding · amenorrhoea after discontinuation · breast enlargement · breast secretion · breast tenderness · cervical erosion · changes in libido · changes in lipid metabolism · changes in vaginal discharge · chloasma · chorea · contact lenses may irritate · depression · fluid retention · headache · hepatic tumours · hypertension · irritability · leg cramps · liver impairment · nausea · nervousness · photosensitivity · reduced menstrual loss · skin reactions · thrombosis (more common when factor V Leiden present or in blood groups A, B, and AB) · visual disturbances · vomiting · 'spotting' in early cycles

SIDE-EFFECTS, FURTHER INFORMATION

▸ Breast cancer There is a small increase in the risk of having breast cancer diagnosed in women taking the combined oral contraceptive pill; this relative risk may be due to an earlier diagnosis. In users of combined oral contraceptive pills the cancers are more likely to be localised to the breast. The most important factor for diagnosing breast cancer appears to be the age at which the contraceptive is stopped rather than the duration of use; any increase in the rate of diagnosis diminishes gradually during the 10 years after stopping and disappears by 10 years.

▸ Cervical cancer Use of combined oral contraceptives for 5 years or longer is associated with a small increased risk of cervical cancer; the risk diminishes after stopping and disappears by about 10 years.

The possible small increase in the risk of breast cancer and cervical cancer should be weighed against the protective effect against cancers of the ovary and endometrium.

● PREGNANCY Not known to be harmful.

● BREAST FEEDING Avoid until weaning or for 6 months after birth (adverse effects on lactation).

● HEPATIC IMPAIRMENT Avoid in active liver disease including disorders of hepatic excretion (e.g. Dubin-Johnson or Rotor syndromes), infective hepatitis (until liver function returns to normal), liver tumours.

● DIRECTIONS FOR ADMINISTRATION

▸ With oral use Each tablet should be taken at approximately same time each day; if delayed, contraceptive protection may be lost. 21-*day combined preparations*, 1 tablet daily for 21 days; subsequent courses repeated after a 7-day interval (during which withdrawal bleeding occurs); if reasonably certain woman is not pregnant, first course can be started on any day of cycle—if starting on day 6 of cycle or later, additional precautions (barrier methods) necessary during first 7 days. *Every day (ED) combined preparations*, 1 *active* tablet daily for 21 days, followed by 1 *inactive* tablet daily for 7 days; subsequent courses repeated without interval (withdrawal bleeding occurs when *inactive* tablets being taken); if reasonably certain woman is not pregnant, first course can be started on any day of cycle—if starting on day 6 of cycle or later, additional precautions (barrier methods) necessary during first 7 days.

Changing to combined preparation containing different progestogen If previous contraceptive used correctly, or pregnancy can reasonably be excluded, start the first active tablet of new brand immediately. See individual monographs for requirements of specific preparations.

Changing from progestogen-only tablet If previous contraceptive used correctly, or pregnancy can reasonably be excluded, start new brand immediately, additional precautions (barrier methods) necessary for first 7 days.

Secondary amenorrhoea (exclude pregnancy) Start any day, additional precautions (barrier methods) necessary during first 7 days (9 days for *Qlaira*®).

After childbirth (not breast-feeding) Start 3 weeks after birth (increased risk of thrombosis if started earlier); later than 3 weeks postpartum additional precautions (barrier methods) necessary for first 7 days (9 days for *Qlaira*®).

After abortion or miscarriage Start same day.

● PATIENT AND CARER ADVICE

Missed doses

Missed pill The critical time for loss of contraceptive protection is when a pill is omitted at the *beginning* or *end* of a cycle (which lengthens the pill-free interval).

If a woman forgets to take a pill, it should be taken as soon as she remembers, and the next one taken at the normal time (even if this means taking 2 pills together). A missed pill is one that is 24 or more hours late. If a woman misses only one pill, she should take an active pill as soon as she remembers and then resume normal pill-taking. No additional precautions are necessary.

If a woman misses 2 or more pills (especially from the first 7 in a packet), she may not be protected. She should take an active pill as soon as she remembers and then resume normal pill-taking. In addition, she must either abstain from sex or use an additional method of contraception such as a condom for the next 7 days. If these 7 days run beyond the end of the packet, the next packet should be started at once, omitting the pill-free interval (or, in the case of *everyday* (ED) pills, omitting the 7 inactive tablets).

Emergency contraception is recommended if 2 or more combined oral contraceptive tablets are missed from the first 7 tablets in a packet and unprotected intercourse has occurred since finishing the last packet.

Travel Women taking oral contraceptives are at an increased risk of deep vein thrombosis during travel involving long periods of immobility (over 3 hours). The risk may be reduced by appropriate exercise during the journey and possibly by wearing graduated compression hosiery.

Diarrhoea and vomiting Vomiting and persistent, severe diarrhoea can interfere with the absorption of combined oral contraceptives. If vomiting occurs within 2 hours of taking a combined oral contraceptive another pill should be taken as soon as possible. In cases of persistent vomiting or severe diarrhoea lasting more than 24 hours, additional precautions should be used during and for 7 days after recovery. If the vomiting and diarrhoea occurs during the last 7 tablets, the next pill-free interval should be omitted (in the case of ED tablets the inactive ones should be omitted).

▶ 465

Dienogest with estradiol valerate

● **INDICATIONS AND DOSE**

Contraception with 28-day combined preparations | Menstrual symptoms with 28-day combined preparations

▶ BY MOUTH

▶ Females of childbearing potential: 1 active tablet once daily for 26 days, followed by 1 inactive tablet daily for 2 days, withdrawal bleeding may occur during the 2-day interval of *inactive* tablets, tablets should be taken at approximately the same time each day

● **UNLICENSED USE** Consult product literature for the licensing status.

● **DIRECTIONS FOR ADMINISTRATION**
● Changing to *Qlaira®*: start the first active *Qlaira®* tablet on the day after taking the last active tablet of the previous brand

● **PATIENT AND CARER ADVICE**

Missed doses

A missed pill for a patient taking *Qlaira®* is one that is 12 hours or more late; for information on how to manage missed pills in women taking *Qlaira®*, refer to product literature.

Diarrhoea and vomiting In cases of persistent vomiting or severe diarrhoea lasting more than 12 hours in women taking *Qlaira®*, refer to product literature.

● **MEDICINAL FORMS**
There can be variation in the licensing of different medicines containing the same drug.

Tablet

▶ Dienogest with estradiol valerate (Non-proprietary)
Dienogest 2 mg, Estradiol valerate 2 mg Estradiol valerate 2mg / Dienogest 2mg tablets | 15 tablet [PoM] no price available
Estradiol valerate 2 mg, Dienogest 3 mg Estradiol valerate 2mg / Dienogest 3mg tablets | 51 tablet [PoM] no price available

▶ Qlaira (Bayer Plc)
Qlaira tablets | 84 tablet [PoM] £25.18

▶ 465

Estradiol with nomegestrol

● **INDICATIONS AND DOSE**

Contraception

▶ BY MOUTH

▶ Females of childbearing potential: 1 active tablet daily for 24 days, followed by 1 inactive tablet daily for 4 days, to be started on day 1 of cycle with first active tablet (withdrawal bleeding occurs when inactive tablets being taken); subsequent courses repeated without interval

● **PREGNANCY** Toxicity in *animal* studies.

● **DIRECTIONS FOR ADMINISTRATION**
● Changing to *Zoely®*: start the first active *Zoely®* tablet on the day after taking the last active tablet of the previous brand or, at the latest, the day after the tablet-free or inactive tablet interval of the previous brand

● **PATIENT AND CARER ADVICE**

Missed doses A missed pill for a patient taking *Zoely®* is one that is 12 hours or more late; for information on how to manage missed pills in women taking *Zoely®*, refer to product literature.

Diarrhoea and vomiting In cases of persistent vomiting or severe diarrhoea lasting more than 12 hours in women taking *Zoely®*, refer to product literature.

● **MEDICINAL FORMS**
There can be variation in the licensing of different medicines containing the same drug.

Tablet

▶ Zoely (Merck Sharp & Dohme Ltd) ▼
Estradiol (as Estradiol hemihydrate) 1.5 mg, Nomegestrol 2.5 mg Zoely 2.5mg/1.5mg tablets | 84 tablet [PoM] £19.80 DT price = £19.80

▶ 465

Ethinylestradiol with desogestrel

● **INDICATIONS AND DOSE**

Contraception with 21-day combined preparations | Menstrual symptoms with 21-day combined preparations

▶ BY MOUTH

▶ Females of childbearing potential: 1 tablet once daily for 21 days; subsequent courses repeated after 7-day interval, withdrawal bleeding occurs during the 7-day interval, if reasonably certain woman is not pregnant, first course can be started on any day of cycle—if starting on day 6 of cycle or later, additional precautions (barrier methods) necessary during first 7 days, tablets should be taken at approximately the same time each day

● **UNLICENSED USE** Consult product literature for the licensing status.

● **MEDICINAL FORMS**
There can be variation in the licensing of different medicines containing the same drug.

Tablet

▶ Ethinylestradiol with desogestrel (Non-proprietary)
Ethinylestradiol 20 microgram, Desogestrel 150 microgram Ethinylestradiol 20microgram / Desogestrel 150microgram tablets | 63 tablet [PoM] no price available
Ethinylestradiol 30 microgram, Desogestrel 150 microgram Ethinylestradiol 30microgram / Desogestrel 150microgram tablets | 63 tablet [PoM] no price available

▶ Alenini (Actavis UK Ltd)
Ethinylestradiol 20 microgram, Desogestrel 150 microgram Alenini 150microgram/20microgram tablets | 63 tablet [PoM] £8.44

▶ Alenvona (Actavis UK Ltd)
Ethinylestradiol 30 microgram, Desogestrel 150 microgram Alenvona 150microgram/30microgram tablets | 63 tablet [PoM] £6.45

▶ Bimizza (Morningside Healthcare Ltd)
Ethinylestradiol 20 microgram, Desogestrel 150 microgram Bimizza 150microgram/20microgram tablets | 63 tablet [PoM] £5.04

▶ Cimizt (Morningside Healthcare Ltd)
Ethinylestradiol 30 microgram, Desogestrel 150 microgram Cimizt 30microgram/150microgram tablets | 63 tablet [PoM] £3.80

▶ Gedarel (Consilient Health Ltd)
Ethinylestradiol 20 microgram, Desogestrel 150 microgram Gedarel 20microgram/150microgram tablets | 63 tablet [PoM] £5.08
Ethinylestradiol 30 microgram, Desogestrel 150 microgram Gedarel 30microgram/150microgram tablets | 63 tablet [PoM] £4.19

F 465

► Lestramyl (Mylan Ltd)
Ethinylestradiol 20 microgram, Desogestrel
150 microgram Lestramyl 20microgram/150microgram tablets |
63 tablet [PoM] £4.30
Ethinylestradiol 30 microgram, Desogestrel
150 microgram Lestramyl 30microgram/150microgram tablets |
63 tablet [PoM] £3.80
► Marvelon (Merck Sharp & Dohme Ltd)
Ethinylestradiol 30 microgram, Desogestrel
150 microgram Marvelon tablets | 63 tablet [PoM] £7.10
► Mercilon (Merck Sharp & Dohme Ltd)
Ethinylestradiol 20 microgram, Desogestrel
150 microgram Mercilon 150microgram/20microgram tablets |
63 tablet [PoM] £8.44
► Munalea (Lupin (Europe) Ltd)
Ethinylestradiol 20 microgram, Desogestrel
150 microgram Munalea 150microgram/20microgram tablets |
63 tablet [PoM] £6.45
Ethinylestradiol 30 microgram, Desogestrel
150 microgram Munalea 150microgram/30microgram tablets |
63 tablet [PoM] £7.67

F 465

Ethinylestradiol with drospirenone

● **INDICATIONS AND DOSE**

Contraception with 21-day combined preparations |
Menstrual symptoms with 21-day combined
preparations
► BY MOUTH
► Females of childbearing potential: 1 tablet once daily for
21 days; subsequent courses repeated after 7-day
interval, withdrawal bleeding occurs during the 7-day
interval

● **UNLICENSED USE** Consult product literature for the
licensing status.

● **MEDICINAL FORMS**
There can be variation in the licensing of different medicines
containing the same drug.

Tablet
► Ethinylestradiol with drospirenone (Non-proprietary)
Ethinylestradiol 20 microgram, Drospirenone 3 mg Yaz tablets |
84 tablet [PoM] no price available
Ethinylestradiol 30 microgram, Drospirenone
3 mg Ethinylestradiol 30microgram / Drospirenone 3mg tablets |
63 tablet [PoM] no price available
► Acondro (Mylan Ltd)
Ethinylestradiol 30 microgram, Drospirenone 3 mg Acondro
0.03mg/3mg tablets | 63 tablet [PoM] £8.35
► Cleosensa (Actavis UK Ltd)
Ethinylestradiol 30 microgram, Drospirenone 3 mg Cleosensa
0.03mg/3mg tablets | 63 tablet [PoM] £14.70
► Daylette (Consilient Health Ltd)
Ethinylestradiol 20 microgram, Drospirenone 3 mg Daylette
0.02mg/3mg tablets | 84 tablet [PoM] £10.50
► Dretine (Teva UK Ltd)
Ethinylestradiol 30 microgram, Drospirenone 3 mg Dretine
0.03mg/3mg tablets | 63 tablet [PoM] £8.30
► ELOINE (Bayer Plc)
Ethinylestradiol 20 microgram, Drospirenone 3 mg Eloine
0.02mg/3mg tablets | 84 tablet [PoM] £14.70
► Lucette (Consilient Health Ltd)
Ethinylestradiol 30 microgram, Drospirenone 3 mg Lucette
0.03mg/3mg tablets | 63 tablet [PoM] £9.35
► Yacella (Morningside Healthcare Ltd)
Ethinylestradiol 30 microgram, Drospirenone 3 mg Yacella
0.03mg/3mg tablets | 63 tablet [PoM] £8.30
► Yasmin (Bayer Plc)
Ethinylestradiol 30 microgram, Drospirenone 3 mg Yasmin
tablets | 63 tablet [PoM] £14.70

F 465

Ethinylestradiol with etonogestrel

● **INDICATIONS AND DOSE**

Contraception | **Menstrual symptoms**
► BY VAGINA
► Females of childbearing potential: 1 unit, insert the ring
into the vagina on day 1 of cycle and leave in for
3 weeks; remove ring on day 22; subsequent courses
repeated after 7-day ring free interval (during which
withdrawal bleeding occurs)

● **DIRECTIONS FOR ADMINISTRATION**
Changing method of contraception to vaginal ring
Changing from combined hormonal contraception Insert ring at
the latest on the day after the usual tablet-free, patch-free,
or inactive-tablet interval. If previous contraceptive used
correctly, or pregnancy can reasonably be excluded, can
switch to ring on any day of cycle.
Changing from progestogen-only method From an implant or
intra-uterine progestogen-only device, insert ring on the
day implant or intra-uterine progestogen-only device
removed; from an injection, insert ring when next
injection due; from oral preparation, first ring may be
inserted on any day after stopping pill. For all methods
additional precautions (barrier methods) should be used
concurrently for first 7 days.

● **PATIENT AND CARER ADVICE**
Patients or carers should be given advice on how to
administer vaginal ring.
Counselling The presence of the ring should be checked
regularly.

Missed doses
Expulsion, delayed insertion or removal, or broken vaginal
ring If the vaginal ring is expelled for *less than* 3 *hours*,
rinse the ring with cool water and reinsert immediately; no
additional contraception is needed.

If the ring remains outside the vagina for *more than*
3 *hours* or if the user does not know when the ring was
expelled, contraceptive protection may be reduced:
● If ring expelled during week 1 or 2 of cycle, rinse ring
with cool water and reinsert; use additional precautions
(barrier methods) for next 7 days;
● If ring expelled during week 3 of cycle, either insert a
new ring to start a new cycle *or* allow a withdrawal bleed
and insert a new ring no later than 7 days after ring was
expelled; latter option only available if ring was used
continuously for at least 7 days before expulsion.
If insertion of a new ring at the start of a new cycle is
delayed, contraceptive protection is lost. A new ring
should be inserted as soon as possible; additional
precautions (barrier methods) should be used for the first
7 days of the new cycle. If intercourse occurred during the
extended ring-free interval, pregnancy should be
considered.

No additional contraception is required if removal of the
ring is delayed by up to 1 week (4 weeks of continuous
use). The 7-day ring-free interval should be observed and
subsequently a new ring should be inserted. Contraceptive
protection may be reduced with continuous use of the ring
for more than 4 weeks—pregnancy should be ruled out
before inserting a new ring.

If the ring breaks during use, remove it and insert a new
ring immediately; additional precautions (barrier
methods) should be used for the first 7 days of the new
cycle.

● MEDICINAL FORMS
There can be variation in the licensing of different medicines containing the same drug.

Vaginal delivery system

▸ Ethinylestradiol with etonogestrel (Non-proprietary)
Ethinylestradiol 2.7 mg, Etonogestrel 11.7 mg Ethinylestradiol 2.7mg / Etonogestrel 11.7mg vaginal delivery system | 3 system [PoM] no price available

▸ NuvaRing (Merck Sharp & Dohme Ltd)
Ethinylestradiol 2.7 mg, Etonogestrel 11.7 mg NuvaRing 0.12mg/0.015mg per day vaginal delivery system | 3 system [PoM] £29.70

⚑ 465

Ethinylestradiol with gestodene

● **INDICATIONS AND DOSE**

Contraception with 21-day combined preparations | Menstrual symptoms with 21-day combined preparations

▸ BY MOUTH

▸ Females of childbearing potential: 1 tablet once daily for 21 days; subsequent courses repeated after 7-day interval, withdrawal bleeding occurs during the 7-day interval, if reasonably certain woman is not pregnant, first course can be started on any day of cycle—if starting on day 6 of cycle or later, additional precautions (barrier methods) necessary during first 7 days, tablets should be taken at approximately the same time each day

Contraception with 28-day combined preparations | Menstrual symptoms with 28-day combined preparations

▸ BY MOUTH

▸ Females of childbearing potential: 1 active tablet once daily for 21 days, followed by 1 inactive tablet daily for 7 days; subsequent courses repeated without interval, withdrawal bleeding occurs during the 7-day interval of *inactive* tablets being taken, if reasonably certain woman is not pregnant, first course can be started on any day of cycle—if starting on day 6 of cycle or later, additional precautions (barrier methods) necessary during first 7 days, tablets should be taken at approximately the same time each day

● UNLICENSED USE Consult product literature for the licensing status.

● MEDICINAL FORMS
There can be variation in the licensing of different medicines containing the same drug.

Tablet

▸ Ethinylestradiol with gestodene (Non-proprietary)
Ethinylestradiol 30 microgram, Gestodene 50 microgram Ethinylestradiol 30microgram / Gestodene 50microgram tablets | 18 tablet [PoM] no price available
Ethinylestradiol 40 microgram, Gestodene 70 microgram Ethinylestradiol 40microgram / Gestodene 70microgram tablets | 15 tablet [PoM] no price available
Ethinylestradiol 20 microgram, Gestodene 75 microgram Ethinylestradiol 20microgram / Gestodene 75microgram tablets | 63 tablet [PoM] no price available
Ethinylestradiol 30 microgram, Gestodene 75 microgram Ethinylestradiol 30microgram / Gestodene 75microgram tablets | 63 tablet [PoM] no price available
Ethinylestradiol 30 microgram, Gestodene 100 microgram Ethinylestradiol 30microgram / Gestodene 100microgram tablets | 30 tablet [PoM] no price available

▸ Aidulan (Lupin (Europe) Ltd)
Ethinylestradiol 30 microgram, Gestodene 75 microgram Aidulan 30microgram/75microgram tablets | 63 tablet [PoM] £6.04
Ethinylestradiol 20 microgram, Gestodene 75 microgram Aidulan 20microgram/75microgram tablets | 63 tablet [PoM] £5.41

▸ Femodene (Bayer Plc)
Ethinylestradiol 30 microgram, Gestodene 75 microgram Femodene tablets | 63 tablet [PoM] £6.73

▸ Femodette (Bayer Plc)
Ethinylestradiol 20 microgram, Gestodene 75 microgram Femodette tablets | 63 tablet [PoM] £8.85

▸ Juliperla (Actavis UK Ltd)
Ethinylestradiol 20 microgram, Gestodene 75 microgram Juliperla 75microgram/20microgram tablets | 63 tablet [PoM] £5.41

▸ Katya (Stragen UK Ltd)
Ethinylestradiol 30 microgram, Gestodene 75 microgram Katya 30/75 tablets | 63 tablet [PoM] £5.03

▸ Millinette (Consilient Health Ltd)
Ethinylestradiol 30 microgram, Gestodene 75 microgram Millinette 30microgram/75microgram tablets | 63 tablet [PoM] £4.12
Ethinylestradiol 20 microgram, Gestodene 75 microgram Millinette 20microgram/75microgram tablets | 63 tablet [PoM] £5.41

▸ Sofiperla (Actavis UK Ltd)
Ethinylestradiol 30 microgram, Gestodene 75 microgram Sofiperla 75microgram/30microgram tablets | 63 tablet [PoM] £4.12

▸ Sunya (Stragen UK Ltd)
Ethinylestradiol 20 microgram, Gestodene 75 microgram Sunya 20/75 tablets | 63 tablet [PoM] £6.62

⚑ 465

Ethinylestradiol with levonorgestrel

● **INDICATIONS AND DOSE**

Contraception with 21-day combined preparations | Menstrual symptoms with 21-day combined preparations

▸ BY MOUTH

▸ Females of childbearing potential: 1 tablet once daily for 21 days; subsequent courses repeated after 7-day interval, withdrawal bleeding occurs during the 7-day interval, if reasonably certain woman is not pregnant, first course can be started on any day of cycle—if starting on day 6 of cycle or later, additional precautions (barrier methods) necessary during first 7 days, tablets should be taken at approximately the same time each day

Contraception with 28-day combined preparations | Menstrual symptoms with 28-day combined preparations

▸ BY MOUTH

▸ Females of childbearing potential: 1 active tablet once daily for 21 days, followed by 1 inactive tablet once daily for 7 days, withdrawal bleeding occurs during the 7-day interval of *inactive* tablets being taken, if reasonably certain woman is not pregnant, first course can be started on any day of cycle—if starting on day 6 of cycle or later, additional precautions (barrier methods) necessary during first 7 days, tablets should be taken at approximately the same time each day. Subsequent courses repeated without interval

● UNLICENSED USE Consult product literature for the licensing status of individual preparations.

● MEDICINAL FORMS
There can be variation in the licensing of different medicines containing the same drug.

Tablet

▸ Ethinylestradiol with levonorgestrel (Non-proprietary)
Ethinylestradiol 30 microgram, Levonorgestrel 50 microgram Ethinylestradiol 30microgram / Levonorgestrel 50microgram tablets | 6 tablet [PoM] no price available | 18 tablet [PoM] no price available
Ethinylestradiol 40 microgram, Levonorgestrel 75 microgram Ethinylestradiol 40microgram / Levonorgestrel 75microgram tablets | 5 tablet [PoM] no price available | 15 tablet [PoM] no price available

Genito-urinary system

7

Ethinylestradiol 30 microgram, Levonorgestrel
125 microgram Ethinylestradiol 30microgram / Levonorgestrel
125microgram tablets | 10 tablet [PoM] no price available |
30 tablet [PoM] no price available
▸ Elevin (MedRx Healthcare LLP)
Ethinylestradiol 30 microgram, Levonorgestrel
150 microgram Elevin 150microgram/30microgram tablets |
63 tablet [PoM] £29.25 DT price = £2.82
▸ Erlibelle (Actavis UK Ltd)
Ethinylestradiol 30 microgram, Levonorgestrel
150 microgram Erlibelle 30microgram/150microgram tablets |
63 tablet [PoM] £2.82 DT price = £2.82
▸ Levest (Morningside Healthcare Ltd)
Ethinylestradiol 30 microgram, Levonorgestrel
150 microgram Levest 150/30 tablets | 21 tablet [PoM] £0.85
(Hospital only) | 63 tablet [PoM] £1.80 DT price = £2.82
▸ Maexeni (Lupin (Europe) Ltd)
Ethinylestradiol 30 microgram, Levonorgestrel
150 microgram Maexeni 150microgram/30microgram tablets |
63 tablet [PoM] £2.82 DT price = £2.82
▸ Microgynon 30 (Bayer Plc)
Ethinylestradiol 30 microgram, Levonorgestrel
150 microgram Microgynon 30 tablets | 63 tablet [PoM] £2.82 DT
price = £2.82
▸ Ovranette (Pfizer Ltd)
Ethinylestradiol 30 microgram, Levonorgestrel
150 microgram Ovranette 150microgram/30microgram tablets |
63 tablet [PoM] £2.20 DT price = £2.82
▸ Rigevidon (Consilient Health Ltd)
Ethinylestradiol 30 microgram, Levonorgestrel
150 microgram Rigevidon tablets | 63 tablet [PoM] £1.89 DT price =
£2.82

F 465

Ethinylestradiol with norelgestromin

● **INDICATIONS AND DOSE**
Contraception | Menstrual symptoms
▸ BY TRANSDERMAL APPLICATION
▸ Females of childbearing potential: Apply 1 patch once
weekly for 3 weeks, apply first patch on day 1 of cycle,
change patch on days 8 and 15; remove third patch on
day 22 and apply new patch after 7-day patch-free
interval to start subsequent contraceptive cycle,
subsequent courses repeated after a 7-day patch free
interval (during which withdrawal bleeding occurs)

● **UNLICENSED USE** Consult product literature for the
licensing status of individual preparations.

● **DIRECTIONS FOR ADMINISTRATION** Adhesives or bandages
should not be used to hold patch in place. If no longer
sticky do not reapply but use a new patch.
Changing to a transdermal combined hormonal contraceptive
Changing from combined oral contraception Apply
patch on the first day of withdrawal bleeding; if no
withdrawal bleeding within 5 days of taking last *active*
tablet, rule out pregnancy before applying first patch.
Unless patch is applied on first day of withdrawal bleeding,
additional precautions (barrier methods) should be used
concurrently for first 7 days.
Changing from progestogen-only method
● from an implant, apply first patch on the day implant
removed
● from an injection, apply first patch when next injection
due
● from oral progestogen, first patch may be applied on any
day after stopping pill
For all methods additional precautions (barrier methods)
should be used concurrently for first 7 days.
After childbirth (not breast-feeding) Start 4 weeks
after birth; if started later than 4 weeks after birth
additional precautions (barrier methods) should be used
for first 7 days.

After abortion or miscarriage Before 20 weeks'
gestation start immediately; no additional contraception
required if started immediately. After 20 weeks' gestation
start on day 21 after abortion or on the first day of first
spontaneous menstruation; additional precautions (barrier
methods) should be used for first 7 days after applying the
patch.

● **PATIENT AND CARER ADVICE**
Patients and carers should be given advice on how to
administer patches.

Missed doses
Delayed application or detached patch If a patch is partly
detached for less than 24 hours, reapply to the same site or
replace with a new patch immediately; no additional
contraception is needed and the next patch should be
applied on the usual 'change day'. If a patch remains
detached for more than 24 hours or if the user is not aware
when the patch became detached, then stop the current
contraceptive cycle and start a new cycle by applying a new
patch, giving a new 'Day 1'; an additional non-hormonal
contraceptive must be used concurrently for the first
7 days of the new cycle.
If application of a new patch at the start of a new cycle is
delayed, contraceptive protection is lost. A new patch
should be applied as soon as remembered giving a new
'Day 1'; additional non-hormonal methods of
contraception should be used for the first 7 days of the new
cycle. If application of a patch in the middle of the cycle is
delayed (i.e. the patch is not changed on day 8 or day 15):
● for up to 48 hours, apply a new patch immediately; next
patch 'change day' remains the same and no additional
contraception is required;
● for more than 48 hours, contraceptive protection may
have been lost. Stop the current cycle and start a new
4-week cycle immediately by applying a new patch
giving a new 'Day 1'; additional non-hormonal
contraception should be used for the first 7 days of the
new cycle.
If the patch is not removed at the end of the cycle (day 22),
remove it as soon as possible and start the next cycle on
the usual 'change day', the day after day 28; no additional
contraception is required.
Travel Women using patches are at an increased risk of
deep vein thrombosis during travel involving long periods
of immobility (over 3 hours). The risk may be reduced by
appropriate exercise during the journey and possibly by
wearing graduated compression hosiery.

● **NATIONAL FUNDING/ACCESS DECISIONS**
Scottish Medicines Consortium (SMC) Decisions
The *Scottish Medicines Consortium* has advised (September
2003) that *Evra®* patches should be restricted for use in
women who are likely to comply poorly with combined oral
contraceptives.

● **MEDICINAL FORMS**
There can be variation in the licensing of different medicines
containing the same drug.
Transdermal patch
▸ Evra (Janssen-Cilag Ltd)
**Ethinylestradiol 33.9 microgram per 24 hour, Norelgestromin
203 microgram per 24 hour** Evra transdermal patches |
9 patch [PoM] £19.51 DT price = £19.51

Ethinylestradiol with norethisterone

● **INDICATIONS AND DOSE**

Contraception with 21-day combined preparations | Menstrual symptoms with 21-day combined preparations
‣ BY MOUTH
‣ Females of childbearing potential: 1 tablet once daily for 21 days; subsequent courses repeated after 7-day interval, withdrawal bleeding occurs during the 7-day interval, if reasonably certain woman is not pregnant, first course can be started on any day of cycle—if starting on day 6 of cycle or later, additional precautions (barrier methods) necessary during first 7 days, tablets should be taken at approximately the same time each day

● **UNLICENSED USE** Consult product literature for the licensing status.

● **MEDICINAL FORMS**
There can be variation in the licensing of different medicines containing the same drug.
Tablet
‣ Ethinylestradiol with norethisterone (Non-proprietary)
Ethinylestradiol 35 microgram, Norethisterone
500 microgram Ethinylestradiol 35microgram / Norethisterone 500microgram tablets | 5 tablet [PoM] no price available | 7 tablet [PoM] no price available | 21 tablet [PoM] no price available
Ethinylestradiol 35 microgram, Norethisterone
750 microgram Ethinylestradiol 35microgram / Norethisterone 750microgram tablets | 21 tablet [PoM] no price available
Ethinylestradiol 35 microgram, Norethisterone
1 mg Ethinylestradiol 35microgram / Norethisterone 1mg tablets | 9 tablet [PoM] no price available | 21 tablet [PoM] no price available | 42 tablet [PoM] no price available
‣ Brevinor (Pfizer Ltd)
Ethinylestradiol 35 microgram, Norethisterone
500 microgram Brevinor 500microgram/35microgram tablets | 63 tablet [PoM] £1.99
‣ Loestrin 20 (Galen Ltd)
Ethinylestradiol 20 microgram, Norethisterone acetate
1 mg Loestrin 20 tablets | 63 tablet [PoM] £2.30
‣ Loestrin 30 (Galen Ltd)
Ethinylestradiol 30 microgram, Norethisterone acetate
1.5 mg Loestrin 30 tablets | 63 tablet [PoM] £3.32
‣ Norimin (Pfizer Ltd)
Ethinylestradiol 35 microgram, Norethisterone 1 mg Norimin 1mg/35microgram tablets | 63 tablet [PoM] £2.28 DT price = £2.28

Ethinylestradiol with norgestimate

● **INDICATIONS AND DOSE**

Contraception with 21-day combined preparations | Menstrual symptoms with 21-day combined preparations
‣ BY MOUTH
‣ Females of childbearing potential: 1 tablet once daily for 21 days; subsequent courses repeated after 7-day interval, withdrawal bleeding occurs during the 7-day interval, if reasonably certain woman is not pregnant, first course can be started on any day of cycle—if starting on day 6 of cycle or later, additional precautions (barrier methods) necessary during first 7 days, tablets should be taken at approximately the same time each day

● **UNLICENSED USE** Consult product literature for the licensing status.

● **MEDICINAL FORMS**
There can be variation in the licensing of different medicines containing the same drug.
Tablet
‣ Ethinylestradiol with norgestimate (Non-proprietary)
Ethinylestradiol 35 microgram, Norgestimate
250 microgram Ethinylestradiol 35microgram / Norgestimate 250microgram tablets | 63 tablet [PoM] no price available
‣ Cilest (Janssen-Cilag Ltd)
Ethinylestradiol 35 microgram, Norgestimate
250 microgram Cilest 35microgram/250microgram tablets | 63 tablet [PoM] £7.16 | 126 tablet [PoM] £14.32
‣ Cilique (Consilient Health Ltd)
Ethinylestradiol 35 microgram, Norgestimate
250 microgram Cilique 250microgram/35microgram tablets | 63 tablet [PoM] £4.65
‣ Lizinna (Morningside Healthcare Ltd)
Ethinylestradiol 35 microgram, Norgestimate
250 microgram Lizinna 250microgram/35microgram tablets | 63 tablet [PoM] £5.37

Norethisterone with mestranol

● **INDICATIONS AND DOSE**

Contraception | Menstrual symptoms
‣ BY MOUTH
‣ Females of childbearing potential: 1 tablet once daily for 21 days; subsequent courses repeated after 7-day interval, withdrawal bleeding can occur during the 7-day interval, if reasonably certain woman is not pregnant, first course can be started on any day of cycle—if starting on day 6 of cycle or later, additional precautions (barrier methods) necessary during first 7 days, tablets should be taken at the same time each day

● **UNLICENSED USE** Consult product literature for the licensing status of individual preparations.

● **MEDICINAL FORMS**
There can be variation in the licensing of different medicines containing the same drug.
Tablet
‣ Norinyl-1 (Pfizer Ltd)
Mestranol 50 microgram, Norethisterone 1 mg Norinyl-1 tablets | 63 tablet [PoM] £2.19 DT price = £2.19

3.2 Contraception, devices

Drugs used for contraception, devices not listed below
Levonorgestrel p. 475

CONTRACEPTIVE DEVICES

Intra-uterine contraceptive devices (copper)

● **INDICATIONS AND DOSE**

Contraception
‣ BY INTRA-UTERINE ADMINISTRATION
‣ Females of childbearing potential: (consult product literature)

IMPORTANT SAFETY INFORMATION
MHRA/CHM ADVICE (JUNE 2015) INTRA-UTERINE CONTRACEPTION: UTERINE PERFORATION—UPDATED INFORMATION ON RISK FACTORS
Uterine perforation most often occurs during insertion, but might not be detected until sometime later. The risk of uterine perforation is increased when the device is inserted up to 36 weeks postpartum or in patients who

7

Genito-urinary system

are breastfeeding. Before inserting an intra-uterine contraceptive device, inform patients that perforation occurs in approximately 1 in every 1000 insertions and signs and symptoms include:

- severe pelvic pain after insertion (worse than period cramps);
- pain or increased bleeding after insertion which continues for more than a few weeks;
- sudden changes in periods;
- pain during intercourse;
- unable to feel the threads.

Patients should be informed on how to check their threads and to arrange a check-up if threads cannot be felt, especially if they also have significant pain. Partial perforation may occur even if the threads can be seen; consider this if there is severe pain following insertion and perform an ultrasound.

- **CONTRA-INDICATIONS** Active trophoblastic disease (until return to normal of urine and plasma-gonadotrophin concentration) · distorted uterine cavity · established or marked immunosuppression · genital malignancy · medical diathermy · pelvic inflammatory disease · recent sexually transmitted infection (if not fully investigated and treated) · severe anaemia · small uterine cavity · unexplained uterine bleeding · Wilson's disease

- **CAUTIONS** Anaemia · anticoagulant therapy (avoid if possible) · diabetes · disease-induced immunosuppression (risk of infection—avoid if marked immunosuppression) · drug-induced immunosuppression (risk of infection—avoid if marked immunosuppression) · endometriosis · epilepsy (risk of seizure at time of insertion) · fertility problems · history of pelvic inflammatory disease · increased risk of expulsion if inserted before uterine involution · menorrhagia (progestogen intra-uterine system might be preferable) · nulliparity · severe cervical stenosis · severe primary dysmenorrhoea · severely scarred uterus (including after endometrial resection) · young age

CAUTIONS, FURTHER INFORMATION
An intra-uterine device should not be removed in mid-cycle unless an additional contraceptive was used for the previous 7 days. If removal is essential post-coital contraception should be considered.

▸ **Risk of infection** The main excess risk of infection occurs in the first 20 days after insertion and is believed to be related to existing carriage of a sexually transmitted infection. Women are considered to be at a higher risk of sexually transmitted infections if:

- they are under 25 years old *or*
- they are over 25 years old *and* ● have a new partner *or*
- have had more than one partner in the past year *or*
- their regular partner has other partners.

In these women, pre-insertion screening (for chlamydia and, depending on sexual history and local prevalence of disease, *Neisseria gonorrhoeae*) should be performed. If results are unavailable at the time of fitting an intra-uterine device for emergency contraception, appropriate prophylactic antibacterial cover should be given. The woman should be advised to attend *as an emergency* if she experiences sustained pain during the next 20 days.

- **SIDE-EFFECTS** Allergy · bleeding (on insertion) · cervical perforation · displacement · dysmenorrhoea · expulsion · menorrhagia · occasionally epileptic seizure (on insertion) · pain (on insertion, alleviated by NSAID such as ibuprofen 30 minutes before insertion) · pelvic infection may be exacerbated · uterine perforation · vasovagal attack (on insertion)

SIDE-EFFECTS, FURTHER INFORMATION
▸ Presence of significant symptoms (especially pain) Advise the patient to seek medical attention promptly in case of significant symptoms.

- **ALLERGY AND CROSS-SENSITIVITY** Contra-indicated if patient has a copper allergy.

- **PREGNANCY** If an intra-uterine device fails and the woman wishes to continue to full-term the device should be removed in the first trimester if possible. Remove device; if pregnancy occurs, increased likelihood that it may be ectopic.

- **BREAST FEEDING** Not known to be harmful.

- **MONITORING REQUIREMENTS** Gynaecological examination before insertion, 6–8 weeks after insertion, then annually.

- **DIRECTIONS FOR ADMINISTRATION** The timing and technique of fitting an intra-uterine device are critical for its subsequent performance. *The healthcare professional inserting (or removing) the device should be fully trained in the technique and should provide full counselling backed, where available, by the patient information leaflet.* Devices should not be fitted during the heavy days of the period; they are best fitted after the end of menstruation and before the calculated time of implantation.

- **PRESCRIBING AND DISPENSING INFORMATION**

UT380 STANDARD® For uterine length 6.5–9 cm; replacement every 5 years.

NOVAPLUS T 380® AG 'Mini' size for minimum uterine length 5 cm; 'Normal' size for uterine length 6.5–9 cm; replacement every 5 years.

GYNEFIX® Suitable for all uterine sizes; replacement every 5 years.

UT380 SHORT® For uterine length 5–7 cm; replacement every 5 years.

NOVA-T® 380 For uterine length 6.5–9 cm; replacement every 5 years.

FLEXI-T®+ 380 For uterine length over 6 cm; replacement every 5 years.

NOVAPLUS T 380® CU 'Mini' size for minimum uterine length 5 cm; 'Normal' size for uterine length 6.5–9 cm; replacement every 5 years.

LOAD® 375 For uterine length over 7 cm; replacement every 5 years.

ANCORA® 375 CU For uterine length over 6.5 cm; replacement every 5 years.

T-SAFE® 380A QL For uterine length 6.5–9 cm; replacement every 10 years.

MULTILOAD® CU375 For uterine length 6–9 cm; replacement every 5 years.

MINI TT380® SLIMLINE For minimum uterine length 5 cm; replacement every 5 years.

COPPER T380 A® For uterine length 6.5–9 cm; replacement every 10 years.

TT380® SLIMLINE For uterine length 6.5–9 cm; replacement every 10 years.

NEO-SAFE® T380 For uterine length 6.5–9 cm; replacement every 5 years.

MULTI-SAFE® 375 For uterine length 6–9 cm; replacement every 5 years.

FLEXI-T® 300 For uterine length over 5 cm; replacement every 5 years.

- **MEDICINAL FORMS**
There can be variation in the licensing of different medicines containing the same drug.

Intra-uterine devices

▸ **Intra-uterine contraceptive devices** (R.F. Medical Supplies Ltd, Farla Medical Ltd, Durbin Plc, Williams Medical Supplies Ltd, Bayer Plc, Organon Laboratories Ltd)
Copper T380 A intra-uterine contraceptive device | 1 device £8.95
Steriload intra-uterine contraceptive device | 1 device £9.65
Load 375 intra-uterine contraceptive device | 1 device £8.52
Novaplus T 380 Ag intra-uterine contraceptive device mini | 1 device £12.50

T-Safe 380A QL intra-uterine contraceptive device | 1 device £10.47
UT380 Standard intra-uterine contraceptive device | 1 device £11.22
Nova-T 380 intra-uterine contraceptive device | 1 device £15.20
Flexi-T+ 380 intra-uterine contraceptive device | 1 device £10.06
Mini TT380 Slimline intra-uterine contraceptive device | 1 device
£12.46
Flexi-T 300 intra-uterine contraceptive device | 1 device £9.47
Multi-Safe 375 intra-uterine contraceptive device | 1 device £8.96
Multiload Cu375 intra-uterine contraceptive device | 1 device £9.24
Optima TCu 380A intra-uterine contraceptive device | 1 device £9.65
Novaplus T 380 intra-uterine contraceptive device normal |
1 device £12.50
GyneFix intra-uterine contraceptive device | 1 device £27.11
Novaplus T 380 Cu intra-uterine contraceptive device mini | 1 device
£10.95
TT380 Slimline intra-uterine contraceptive device | 1 device £12.46
Ancora 375 Cu intra-uterine contraceptive device | 1 device £7.95
Novaplus T 380 Cu intra-uterine contraceptive device normal |
1 device £10.95
Neo-Safe T380 intra-uterine contraceptive device | 1 device £13.31
UT380 Short intra-uterine contraceptive device | 1 device £11.22

Vaginal contraceptives

● SILICONE CONTRACEPTIVE DIAPHRAGMS

Milex arcing spring silicone diaphragm 60mm (Durbin Plc)
1 device · NHS indicative price = £9.31 · Drug Tariff (Part IXa)
Milex arcing spring silicone diaphragm 65mm (Durbin Plc)
1 device · NHS indicative price = £9.31 · Drug Tariff (Part IXa)
Milex arcing spring silicone diaphragm 70mm (Durbin Plc)
1 device · NHS indicative price = £9.31 · Drug Tariff (Part IXa)
Milex arcing spring silicone diaphragm 75mm (Durbin Plc)
1 device · NHS indicative price = £9.31 · Drug Tariff (Part IXa)
Milex arcing spring silicone diaphragm 80mm (Durbin Plc)
1 device · NHS indicative price = £9.31 · Drug Tariff (Part IXa)
Milex arcing spring silicone diaphragm 85mm (Durbin Plc)
1 device · NHS indicative price = £9.31 · Drug Tariff (Part IXa)
Milex arcing spring silicone diaphragm 90mm (Durbin Plc)
1 device · NHS indicative price = £9.31 · Drug Tariff (Part IXa)
Milex omniflex coil spring silicone diaphragm 60mm (Durbin
Plc)
1 device · NHS indicative price = £9.31 · Drug Tariff (Part IXa)
Milex omniflex coil spring silicone diaphragm 65mm (Durbin Plc)
1 device · NHS indicative price = £9.31 · Drug Tariff (Part IXa)
Milex omniflex coil spring silicone diaphragm 70mm (Durbin
Plc)
1 device · NHS indicative price = £9.31 · Drug Tariff (Part IXa)
Milex omniflex coil spring silicone diaphragm 75mm (Durbin Plc)
1 device · NHS indicative price = £9.31 · Drug Tariff (Part IXa)
Milex omniflex coil spring silicone diaphragm 80mm (Durbin
Plc)
1 device · NHS indicative price = £9.31 · Drug Tariff (Part IXa)
Milex omniflex coil spring silicone diaphragm 85mm (Durbin Plc)
1 device · NHS indicative price = £9.31 · Drug Tariff (Part IXa)
Milex omniflex coil spring silicone diaphragm 90mm (Durbin
Plc)
1 device · NHS indicative price = £9.31 · Drug Tariff (Part IXa)
Ortho All-Flex arcing spring silicone diaphragm 65mm (Janssen-
Cilag Ltd)
1 device · NHS indicative price = £8.35 · Drug Tariff (Part IXa)
Ortho All-Flex arcing spring silicone diaphragm 70mm (Janssen-
Cilag Ltd)
1 device · NHS indicative price = £8.35 · Drug Tariff (Part IXa)
Ortho All-Flex arcing spring silicone diaphragm 75mm (Janssen-
Cilag Ltd)
1 device · NHS indicative price = £8.35 · Drug Tariff (Part IXa)
Ortho All-Flex arcing spring silicone diaphragm 80mm
(Janssen-Cilag Ltd)
1 device · NHS indicative price = £8.35 · Drug Tariff (Part IXa)

● SILICONE CONTRACEPTIVE PESSARIES

FemCap 22mm (Durbin Plc)
1 device · NHS indicative price = £15.29 · Drug Tariff (Part IXa)
FemCap 26mm (Durbin Plc)
1 device · NHS indicative price = £15.29 · Drug Tariff (Part IXa)
FemCap 30mm (Durbin Plc)
1 device · NHS indicative price = £15.29 · Drug Tariff (Part IXa)

3.3 Contraception, emergency

**Drugs used for Contraception, emergency not listed
below** Intra-uterine contraceptive devices (copper), p. 471 ·
Levonorgestrel p. 475

PROGESTERONE RECEPTOR MODULATORS

Ulipristal acetate

● **DRUG ACTION** Ulipristal acetate is a progesterone receptor
modulator with a partial progesterone antagonist effect.

● **INDICATIONS AND DOSE**
Emergency contraception
▸ BY MOUTH
  ▸ Females of childbearing potential: 30 mg for 1 dose, to be
    taken as soon as possible after coitus, but no later than
    after 120 hours

● **CONTRA-INDICATIONS** Repeated use as an emergency
contraceptive within a menstrual cycle

● **CAUTIONS** Uncontrolled severe asthma

● **INTERACTIONS** → Appendix 1 (ulipristal).
The effectiveness of ulipristal as an emergency
contraceptive is possibly reduced in women taking
enzyme-inducing drugs (and possibly for 4 weeks after
stopping); a copper intra-uterine device can be offered
instead. There is no need to increase the dose for
emergency contraception if the patient is taking
antibacterials that are not enzyme inducers.

● **SIDE-EFFECTS**
▸ **Common or very common** Abdominal pain · back pain ·
  diarrhoea · dizziness · fatigue · gastro-intestinal
  disturbances · headache · menstrual irregularities · muscle
  spasms · nausea · vomiting
▸ **Uncommon** Blurred vision · breast tenderness · dry mouth ·
  hot flushes · pruritus · rash · tremor · uterine spasm

● **CONCEPTION AND CONTRACEPTION** When ulipristal is
given as an emergency contraceptive the effectiveness of
combined hormonal and progestogen-only contraceptives
may be reduced—additional precautions (barrier methods)
required for 14 days for combined and parenteral
progestogen-only hormonal contraceptives (16 days for
Qlaira®) and 9 days for oral progestogen-only
contraceptives.

● **PREGNANCY** Limited information available when used as
an emergency contraceptive.

● **BREAST FEEDING** In emergency contraception
manufacturer advises avoid for 1 week after
administration—present in milk.

● **HEPATIC IMPAIRMENT** Manufacturer advises avoid in
severe impairment—no information available.

● **MEDICINAL FORMS**
There can be variation in the licensing of different medicines
containing the same drug.
Tablet
▸ Ellaone (HRA Pharma UK Ltd)
  Ulipristal acetate 30 mg EllaOne 30mg tablets | 1 tablet Ⓟ £14.05
▸ Esmya (Gedeon Richter (UK) Ltd)
  Ulipristal acetate 5 mg Esmya 5mg tablets | 28 tablet PoM
  £114.13

3.4 Contraception, oral progestogen-only

Drugs used for Contraception, oral progestogen-only not listed below Norethisterone p. 447

PROGESTOGENS

Desogestrel

- **INDICATIONS AND DOSE**

Contraception
▶ BY MOUTH
▸ Females of childbearing potential: 75 micrograms daily, dose to be taken at same time each day, starting on day 1 of cycle then continuously, if administration delayed for 12 hours or more it should be regarded as a 'missed pill'

- **UNLICENSED USE** Consult product literature for the licensing status of individual preparations.
- **CONTRA-INDICATIONS** Acute porphyrias p. 562 · history of breast cancer but can be used after 5 years if no evidence of disease and non-hormonal contraceptive methods unacceptable · severe arterial disease · undiagnosed vaginal bleeding
- **CAUTIONS** Active trophoblastic disease (until return to normal of urine- and plasma-gonadotrophin concentration)—seek specialist advice · arterial disease · functional ovarian cysts · history of jaundice in pregnancy · malabsorption syndromes · past ectopic pregnancy · sex-steroid dependent cancer · systemic lupus erythematosus with positive (or unknown) antiphospholipid antibodies
 CAUTIONS, FURTHER INFORMATION
▸ Other conditions The product literature advises caution in patients with history of thromboembolism, hypertension, diabetes mellitus and migraine; evidence for caution in these conditions is unsatisfactory.
- **INTERACTIONS** → Appendix 1 (progestogens).
- **SIDE-EFFECTS** Breast discomfort · changes in libido · depression · disturbance of appetite · dizziness · headache · menstrual irregularities · nausea · skin disorders · vomiting
 SIDE-EFFECTS, FURTHER INFORMATION
▸ Breast cancer There is a small increase in the risk of having breast cancer diagnosed in women using, or who have recently used, a progestogen-only contraceptive pill; this relative risk may be due to an earlier diagnosis. The most important risk factor appears to be the age at which the contraceptive is stopped rather than the duration of use; the risk disappears gradually during the 10 years after stopping and there is no excess risk by 10 years. A possible small increase in the risk of breast cancer should be weighed against the benefits.
- **PREGNANCY** Not known to be harmful.
- **BREAST FEEDING** Progestogen-only contraceptives do not affect lactation.
- **HEPATIC IMPAIRMENT** Caution in severe liver disease and recurrent cholestatic jaundice. Avoid in liver tumour.
- **PATIENT AND CARER ADVICE**
 Missed doses
 Missed pill The following advice is recommended: 'If you forget a pill, take it as soon as you remember and carry on with the next pill at the right time. If the pill was more than 12 hours overdue you are not protected. Continue normal pill-taking but you must also use another method, such as the condom, for the next 2 days'.
 The Faculty of Sexual and Reproductive Healthcare

recommends emergency contraception if one or more tablets are missed or taken more than 12 hours late and unprotected intercourse has occurred before 2 further tablets have been correctly taken.
Surgery All progestogen-only contraceptives are suitable for use as an alternative to combined hormonal contraceptives before major elective surgery, before all surgery to the legs, or before surgery which involves prolonged immobilisation of a lower limb.
Starting routine One tablet daily, on a continuous basis, starting on day 1 of cycle and taken at the same time each day (if delayed by longer than 12 hours contraceptive protection may be lost). Additional contraceptive precautions are not required if desogestrel is started up to and including day 5 of the menstrual cycle; if started after this time, additional contraceptive precautions are required for 2 days.
Changing from a combined oral contraceptive Start on the day following completion of the combined oral contraceptive course without a break (or in the case of ED tablets omitting the inactive ones).
After childbirth Oral progestogen-only contraceptives can be started up to and including day 21 postpartum without the need for additional contraceptive precautions. If started more than 21 days postpartum, additional contraceptive precautions are required for 2 days.
Diarrhoea and vomiting Vomiting and persistent, severe diarrhoea can interfere with the absorption of oral progestogen-only contraceptives. If vomiting occurs within 2 hours of taking desogestrel, another pill should be taken as soon as possible. If a replacement pill is not taken within 12 hours of the normal time for taking desogestrel, or in cases of persistent vomiting or very severe diarrhoea, additional precautions should be used during illness and for 2 days after recovery.

- **NATIONAL FUNDING/ACCESS DECISIONS**
 Scottish Medicines Consortium (SMC) Decisions
 The *Scottish Medicines Consortium* has advised (September 2003) that *Cerazette®* should be restricted for use in women who cannot tolerate oestrogen-containing contraceptives or in whom such preparations are contra-indicated.

- **MEDICINAL FORMS**
 There can be variation in the licensing of different medicines containing the same drug.
 Tablet
 ▸ Desogestrel (Non-proprietary)
  Desogestrel 75 microgram Desogestrel 75microgram tablets | 84 tablet PoM £9.55 DT price = £2.30
 ▸ Aizea (Besins Healthcare (UK) Ltd)
  Desogestrel 75 microgram Aizea 75microgram tablets | 84 tablet PoM £5.21 DT price = £2.30
 ▸ Cerazette (Merck Sharp & Dohme Ltd)
  Desogestrel 75 microgram Cerazette 75microgram tablets | 84 tablet PoM £9.55 DT price = £2.30
 ▸ Cerelle (Consilient Health Ltd)
  Desogestrel 75 microgram Cerelle 75microgram tablets | 84 tablet PoM £3.50 DT price = £2.30
 ▸ Desomono (MedRx Developments Ltd)
  Desogestrel 75 microgram Desomono 75microgram tablets | 84 tablet PoM £7.49 DT price = £2.30
 ▸ Desorex (Somex Pharma)
  Desogestrel 75 microgram Desorex 75microgram tablets | 84 tablet PoM £6.70 DT price = £2.30
 ▸ Feanolla (Lupin (Europe) Ltd)
  Desogestrel 75 microgram Feanolla 75microgram tablets | 84 tablet PoM £7.37 DT price = £2.30
 ▸ Nacrez (Teva UK Ltd)
  Desogestrel 75 microgram Nacrez 75microgram tablets | 84 tablet PoM £3.50 DT price = £2.30
 ▸ Zeleta (Morningside Healthcare Ltd)
  Desogestrel 75 microgram Zeleta 75microgram tablets | 84 tablet PoM £3.35 DT price = £2.30

Levonorgestrel

18.2.2016

● **INDICATIONS AND DOSE**

Emergency contraception
▶ BY MOUTH
▶ Females of childbearing potential: 1.5 mg for 1 dose, taken as soon as possible after coitus, preferably within 12 hours but no later than after 72 hours

Contraception
▶ BY MOUTH
▶ Females of childbearing potential: 1 tablet daily starting on day 1 of the cycle then continuously, dose is to be taken at the same time each day, if administration delayed for 3 hours or more it should be regarded as a "missed pill"

JAYDESS ® 13.5MG INTRA-UTERINE DEVICE

Contraception
▶ BY VAGINA
▶ Females of childbearing potential: Insert into uterine cavity within 7 days of onset of menstruation, or any time if replacement, or immediately after first-trimester termination; postpartum insertions should be delayed until at least 6 weeks after delivery (12 weeks if uterus involution is substantially delayed); effective for 3 years

LEVOSERT ® 20MICROGRAMS/24HOURS INTRA-UTERINE DEVICE

Contraception | Menorrhagia
▶ BY INTRA-UTERINE ADMINISTRATION
▶ Females of childbearing potential: Insert into uterine cavity within 7 days of onset of menstruation, or any time if replacement, or immediately after first-trimester abortion; postpartum insertions should be delayed until at least 6 weeks after delivery; effective for 3 years

MIRENA®20MICROGRAMS/24HOURS INTRA-UTERINE DEVICE

Contraception | Menorrhagia
▶ BY INTRA-UTERINE ADMINISTRATION
▶ Females of childbearing potential: Insert into uterine cavity within 7 days of onset of menstruation, or any time if replacement, or any time if reasonably certain woman is not pregnant and there is no risk of conception (additional precautions (e.g. barrier methods) necessary for next 7 days), or immediately after first-trimester termination by curettage; postpartum insertions should be delayed until at least 4 weeks after delivery; effective for 5 years

Prevention of endometrial hyperplasia during oestrogen replacement therapy
▶ BY INTRA-UTERINE ADMINISTRATION
▶ Females of childbearing potential: Insert during last days of menstruation or withdrawal bleeding or at any time if amenorrhoeic; effective for 4 years

● **UNLICENSED USE**
▶ With oral use Consult product literature for licensing status of individual preparations.
▶ With vaginal use Not licensed for use in women under 18 years.

IMPORTANT SAFETY INFORMATION

MHRA/CHM ADVICE (JUNE 2015) INTRA-UTERINE CONTRACEPTION: UTERINE PERFORATION–UPDATED INFORMATION ON RISK FACTORS
Uterine perforation most often occurs during insertion, but might not be detected until sometime later. The risk of uterine perforation is increased when the device is inserted up to 36 weeks postpartum or in patients who are breastfeeding. Before inserting an intra-uterine

contraceptive device, inform patients that perforation occurs in approximately 1 in every 1000 insertions and signs and symptoms include:
● severe pelvic pain after insertion (worse than period cramps);
● pain or increased bleeding after insertion which continues for more than a few weeks;
● sudden changes in periods;
● pain during intercourse;
● unable to feel the threads.
Patients should be informed on how to check their threads and to arrange a check-up if threads cannot be felt, especially if they also have significant pain. Partial perforation may occur even if the threads can be seen; consider this if there is severe pain following insertion and perform an ultrasound.

● **CONTRA-INDICATIONS**
▶ With intra-uterine use Active trophoblastic disease (until return to normal of urine- and plasma-gonadotrophin concentration · acute cervicitis · acute vaginitis · distorted uterine cavity · established immunosuppression · genital malignancy · history of breast cancer but can be considered for a woman in long-term remission who has menorrhagia and requires effective contraception · infected abortion during the previous three months · marked immunosuppression · not suitable for emergency contraception · pelvic inflammatory disease · postpartum endometritis · recent sexually transmitted infection (if not fully investigated and treated) · severe anaemia · small uterine cavity · unexplained uterine bleeding
▶ With oral use Acute porphyrias p. 562
▶ When used for contraception With oral use for contraception history of breast cancer but can be used after 5 years if no evidence of disease and non-hormonal contraceptive methods unacceptable · severe arterial disease · undiagnosed vaginal bleeding

● **CAUTIONS**
▶ With intra-uterine use Disease-induced immunosuppression (risk of infection—avoid if marked immunosuppression) · anaemia · anticoagulant therapy (avoid if possible) · diabetes · drug-induced immunosuppression (risk of infection—avoid if marked immunosuppression) · endometriosis · epilepsy (risk of seizure at time of insertion) · fertility problems · history of pelvic inflammatory disease · increased risk of expulsion if inserted before uterine involution · menorrhagia (progestogen intra-uterine system might be preferable) · nulliparity · severe cervical stenosis · severe primary dysmenorrhoea · severely scarred uterus (including after endometrial resection) · young age
▶ When used for contraception With oral use for contraception active trophoblastic disease (until return to normal of urine- and plasma-gonadotrophin concentration)—seek specialist advice · arterial disease · functional ovarian cysts · history of jaundice in pregnancy · malabsorption syndromes · past ectopic pregnancy · sex-steroid dependent cancer · systemic lupus erythematosus with positive (or unknown) antiphospholipid antibodies
▶ When used for emergency contraception With oral use for emergency contraception active trophoblastic disease (until return to normal of urine- and plasma-gonadotrophin concentration)—seek specialist advice · past ectopic pregnancy · severe malabsorption syndromes

CAUTIONS, FURTHER INFORMATION
An intra-uterine device should not be removed in mid-cycle unless an additional contraceptive was used for the previous 7 days. If removal is essential post-coital contraception should be considered.
▶ Risk of infection with intra-uterine devices The main excess risk of infection occurs in the first 20 days after insertion and is believed to be related to existing carriage of a sexually

7

Genito-urinary system

transmitted infection. Women are considered to be at a higher risk of sexually transmitted infections if:

- they are under 25 years old *or*
- they are over 25 years old *and*
- have a new partner *or*
- have had more than one partner in the past year *or*
- their regular partner has other partners.

In these women, pre-insertion screening (for chlamydia and, depending on sexual history and local prevalence of disease, *Neisseria gonorrhoeae*) should be performed. If results are unavailable at the time of fitting an intra-uterine device for emergency contraception, appropriate prophylactic antibacterial cover should be given. The woman should be advised to attend *as an emergency* if she experiences sustained pain during the next 20 days.

▸ Use as a contraceptive in co-morbidities

▸ With oral use The product literature advises caution in patients with history of thromboembolism, hypertension, diabetes mellitus and migraine; evidence for caution in these conditions is unsatisfactory.

MIRENA®20MICROGRAMS/24HOURS INTRA-UTERINE DEVICE Advanced uterine atrophy

- INTERACTIONS → Appendix 1 (progestogens). When used orally as an emergency contraceptive, the effectiveness of levonorgestrel is reduced in women taking enzyme-inducing drugs (and possibly for 4 weeks after stopping); a copper intra-uterine device can be offered instead. If the copper intra-uterine device is undesirable or inappropriate, the dose of levonorgestrel should be increased to a total of 3 mg taken as a single dose [unlicensed dose—advise women accordingly]. There is no need to increase the dose for emergency contraception if the patient is taking antibacterials that are not enzyme inducers.
With the progestogen-only intra-uterine device, levonorgestrel is released close to the site of the main contraceptive action (on cervical mucus and endometrium) and therefore progestogenic side-effects and interactions are less likely; in particular, enzyme-inducing drugs are unlikely to significantly reduce the contraceptive effect of the progestogen-only intra-uterine system and additional contraceptive precautions are not required.

- SIDE-EFFECTS
GENERAL SIDE-EFFECTS
▸ **Common or very common** Depression (sometimes severe) · headache · nausea
▸ **Frequency not known** Vomiting
SPECIFIC SIDE-EFFECTS
▸ **Common or very common**
▸ With intra-uterine use Changes in the pattern and duration of menstrual bleeding (spotting or prolonged bleeding) · abdominal pain · acne · alopecia · back pain · breast pain · expulsion · hirsutism · migraine · nervousness · pelvic pain · peripheral oedema · salpingitis
▸ **Uncommon**
▸ With intra-uterine use Abdominal distension · cervicitis · eczema · pelvic inflammatory disease · pruritus · skin hyperpigmentation
▸ **Rare**
▸ With intra-uterine use Rash · uterine perforation
▸ **Frequency not known**
▸ With intra-uterine use Functional ovarian cysts (usually asymptomatic and usually resolve spontaneously— ultrasound monitoring recommended) · allergy · bleeding (on insertion) · cervical perforation · displacement · dysmenorrhoea · epileptic seizures (on insertion) · menorrhagia · pain (on insertion, alleviated by NSAID such as ibuprofen 30 minutes before insertion) · pelvic infection may be exacerbated · vasovagal attack (on insertion)

▸ With oral use Breast discomfort · breast tenderness · changes in libido · disturbances of appetite · dizziness · fatigue · menstrual irregularities · skin disorders
SIDE-EFFECTS, FURTHER INFORMATION
▸ Breast cancer There is a small increase in the risk of having breast cancer diagnosed in women using, or who have recently used, a progestogen-only contraceptive pill; this relative risk may be due to an earlier diagnosis. The most important risk factor appears to be the age at which the contraceptive is stopped rather than the duration of use; the risk disappears gradually during the 10 years after stopping and there is no excess risk by 10 years. A possible small increase in the risk of breast cancer should be weighed against the benefits.

Although the progestogen-only intra-uterine system produces little systemic progestogenic activity, it is usually avoided for 5 years after any evidence of breast cancer. However, the system can be considered for a woman in long-term remission from breast cancer who has menorrhagia and requires effective contraception.

▸ With intra-uterine use Endometrial disorders should be ruled out before insertion and the patient should be fully counselled (and provided with a patient information leaflet). Improvement in progestogenic side-effects, such as mastalgia and in the bleeding pattern may often become very light or absent. Removal of the intra-uterine system should be considered if the patient experiences migraine or severe headache, jaundice, marked increase of blood pressure, or severe arterial disease.

- PREGNANCY
▸ With oral use Not known to be harmful.
▸ With vaginal use If an intra-uterine device fails and the woman wishes to continue to full-term the device should be removed in the first trimester if possible. Avoid; if pregnancy occurs remove intra-uterine system.

- BREAST FEEDING Progestogen-only contraceptives do not affect lactation.

- HEPATIC IMPAIRMENT Caution in severe liver disease and recurrent cholestatic jaundice. Avoid in liver tumour.

- MONITORING REQUIREMENTS
▸ With intra-uterine use Gynaecological examination before insertion, 4–6 weeks after insertion, then annually.

- DIRECTIONS FOR ADMINISTRATION
▸ With intra-uterine use *The doctor or nurse administering (or removing) the system should be fully trained in the technique and should provide full counselling reinforced by the patient information leaflet.*

- PRESCRIBING AND DISPENSING INFORMATION
▸ With intra-uterine use Levonorgestrel-releasing intra-uterine devices vary in licensed indication, duration of use and insertion technique—the MHRA recommends to prescribe and dispense by brand name to avoid inadvertent switching.

MIRENA®20MICROGRAMS/24HOURS INTRA-UTERINE DEVICE When system is removed (and not immediately replaced) and pregnancy is not desired, remove during the first few days of menstruation, otherwise additional precautions (e.g. barrier methods) should be used for at least 7 days before removal.

JAYDESS® 13.5MG INTRA-UTERINE DEVICE When system is removed (and not immediately replaced) and pregnancy is not desired, remove within 7 days of the onset of menstruation; additional precautions (e.g. barrier methods) should be used if the system is removed at some other time during the cycle and there is intercourse within 7 days.

LEVONELLE® ONE STEP Can be sold to women over 16 years; when supplying emergency contraception to the public, pharmacists should refer to guidance issued by the Royal Pharmaceutical Society.

- **PATIENT AND CARER ADVICE**
Missed doses
When used as an oral contraceptive, the following advice is recommended 'If you forget a pill, take it as soon as you remember and carry on with the next pill at the right time. If the pill was more than 3 hours overdue you are not protected. Continue normal pill-taking but you must also use another method, such as the condom, for the next 2 days'.

The Faculty of Sexual and Reproductive Healthcare recommends emergency contraception if one or more progestogen-only contraceptive tablets are missed or taken more than 3 hours late and unprotected intercourse has occurred before 2 further tablets have been correctly taken.

Diarrhoea and vomiting with use as an oral contraceptive Vomiting and persistent, severe diarrhoea can interfere with the absorption of oral progestogen-only contraceptives. If vomiting occurs within 2 hours of taking an oral progestogen-only contraceptive, another pill should be taken as soon as possible. If a replacement pill is not taken within 3 hours of the normal time for taking the progestogen-only pill, or in cases of persistent vomiting or very severe diarrhoea, additional precautions should be used during illness and for 2 days after recovery.

Starting routine

▸ With oral use for Contraception One tablet daily, on a continuous basis, starting on day 1 of cycle and taken at the same time each day (if delayed by longer than 3 hours contraceptive protection may be lost). Additional contraceptive precautions are not required if levonorgestrel is started up to and including day 5 of the menstrual cycle; if started after this time, additional contraceptive precautions are required for 2 days.
Changing from a combined oral contraceptive Start on the day following completion of the combined oral contraceptive course without a break (or in the case of ED tablets omitting the inactive ones).
After childbirth Oral progestogen-only contraceptives can be started up to and including day 21 postpartum without the need for additional contraceptive precautions. If started more than 21 days postpartum, additional contraceptive precautions are required for 2 days.

▸ With intra-uterine use Counsel women to seek medical attention promptly in case of significant symptoms, especially pain. Patient counselling advised. Patient information leaflet to be provided.

▸ With oral use for Emergency contraception If vomiting occurs within 2 hours of taking levonorgestrel, a replacement dose should be given.

▸ With oral use for Emergency contraception
  • When prescribing or supplying hormonal emergency contraception, women should be advised:
  • that their next period may be early or late;
  • that a barrier method of contraception needs to be used until the next period;
  • to seek medical attention promptly if any lower abdominal pain occurs because this could signify an ectopic pregnancy;
  • to return in 3 to 4 weeks if the subsequent menstrual bleed is abnormally light, heavy or brief, or is absent, or if she is otherwise concerned (if there is any doubt as to whether menstruation has occurred, a pregnancy test should be performed at least 3 weeks after unprotected intercourse).

- **EXCEPTIONS TO LEGAL CATEGORY** *Levonelle*® *One Step* can be sold to women over 16 years; when supplying emergency contraception to the public, pharmacists should refer to guidance issued by the Royal Pharmaceutical Society.

- **MEDICINAL FORMS**
There can be variation in the licensing of different medicines containing the same drug.

Tablet
▸ Levonorgestrel (Non-proprietary)
  Levonorgestrel 1.5 mg Levonorgestrel 1.5mg tablets | 1 tablet [P]
  £13.83 DT price = £5.20 | 1 tablet [PoM] £3.86–£5.20 DT price = £5.20
▸ Emerres (Morningside Healthcare Ltd)
  Levonorgestrel 1.5 mg Emerres Una 1.5mg tablets | 1 tablet [P]
  £13.83 DT price = £5.20
  Emerres 1.5mg tablets | 1 tablet [PoM] £3.65 DT price = £5.20
▸ Isteranda (Sandoz Ltd)
  Levonorgestrel 1.5 mg Isteranda 1.5mg tablets | 1 tablet [PoM]
  £5.20 DT price = £5.20
▸ Levonelle (Bayer Plc)
  Levonorgestrel 1.5 mg Levonelle 1500microgram tablets |
  1 tablet [PoM] £5.20 DT price = £5.20
  Levonelle One Step 1.5mg tablets | 1 tablet [P] £13.83 DT price = £5.20
▸ Norgeston (Bayer Plc)
  Levonorgestrel 30 microgram Norgeston 30microgram tablets |
  35 tablet [PoM] £0.92 DT price = £0.92
▸ Upostelle (Consilient Health Ltd)
  Levonorgestrel 1.5 mg Upostelle 1500microgram tablets |
  1 tablet [PoM] £3.75 DT price = £5.20

Intra-uterine device
▸ Jaydess (Bayer Plc) ▼
  Levonorgestrel 13.5 mg Jaydess 13.5mg intra-uterine device |
  1 device [PoM] £69.22
▸ Levosert (Allergan Ltd)
  Levonorgestrel 20 microgram per 24 hour Levosert
  20micrograms/24hours intra-uterine device | 1 device [PoM] £66.00
▸ Mirena (Bayer Plc)
  Levonorgestrel 20 microgram per 24 hour Mirena
  20micrograms/24hours intra-uterine device | 1 device [PoM] £88.00

3.5 Contraception, parenteral progestogen-only

> **Drugs used for Contraception, parenteral progestogen-only not listed below** Norethisterone p. 447

PROGESTOGENS

Etonogestrel

2.6.2016

- **INDICATIONS AND DOSE**

Contraception (no hormonal contraceptive use in previous month)
▸ BY SUBDERMAL IMPLANTATION
▸ Females of childbearing potential: 1 implant inserted during first 5 days of cycle, implant should be removed within 3 years of insertion

Contraception (postpartum)
▸ BY SUBDERMAL IMPLANTATION
▸ Females of childbearing potential: 1 implant to be inserted 21–28 days after delivery, 1 implant to be inserted after 28 days postpartum in breast-feeding mothers, implant should be removed within 3 years of insertion

Contraception following abortion or miscarriage in the second trimester
▸ BY SUBDERMAL IMPLANTATION
▸ Females of childbearing potential: 1 implant to be inserted 21–28 days after abortion or miscarriage, implant should be removed within 3 years of insertion

continued →

7

Genito-urinary system

Contraception following abortion or miscarriage in the first trimester
▶ BY SUBDERMAL IMPLANTATION
▸ Females of childbearing potential: 1 implant to be inserted within 5 days, implant should be removed within 3 years of insertion

Contraception (changing from other hormonal contraceptive)
▶ BY SUBDERMAL IMPLANTATION
▸ Females of childbearing potential: Implant should be removed within 3 years of insertion (consult product literature)

● CONTRA-INDICATIONS Acute porphyria · history of breast cancer but can be used after 5 years if no evidence of disease and non-hormonal contraceptive methods unacceptable · severe arterial disease · undiagnosed vaginal bleeding

● CAUTIONS Active trophoblastic disease (until return to normal of urine- and plasma-gonadotrophin concentration)—seek specialist advice · arterial disease · disturbances of lipid metabolism · history during pregnancy of deterioration of otosclerosis · history during pregnancy of pruritus · history of jaundice in pregnancy · malabsorption syndromes · possible risk of breast cancer · sex-steroid dependent cancer · systemic lupus erythematosus with positive (or unknown) antiphospholipid antibodies

● INTERACTIONS → Appendix 1 (progestogens). Effectiveness of parenteral progestogen-only contraceptives is not affected by antibacterials that do not induce liver enzymes. Effectiveness of the etonogestrel-releasing implant may be reduced by enzyme-inducing drugs and an alternative contraceptive method, unaffected by the interacting drug, is recommended during treatment with the enzyme-inducing drug and for at least 4 weeks after stopping. For a short course of an enzyme-inducing drug, if a change in contraceptive method is undesirable or inappropriate, the implant may be continued in combination with additional contraceptive precautions (e.g. condom) for the duration of treatment with the enzyme-inducing drug and for 4 weeks after stopping it.

● SIDE-EFFECTS Breast discomfort · changes in libido · depression · disturbance of appetite · dizziness · headache · injection-site reactions · menstrual irregularities · nausea · vomiting
SIDE-EFFECTS, FURTHER INFORMATION
▸ Cervical cancer Use of injectable progestogen-only contraceptives may be associated with a small increased risk of cervical cancer, similar to that seen with combined oral contraceptives. The risk of cervical cancer with other progestogen-only contraceptives is not yet known.
▸ Breast cancer There is a small increase in the risk of having breast cancer diagnosed in women using, or who have recently used, a progestogen-only contraceptive pill; this relative risk may be due to an earlier diagnosis. The most important risk factor appears to be the age at which the contraceptive is stopped rather than the duration of use; the risk disappears gradually during the 10 years after stopping and there is no excess risk by 10 years. A possible small increase in the risk of breast cancer should be weighed against the benefits.

● PREGNANCY Not known to be harmful, remove implant if pregnancy occurs.

● BREAST FEEDING Progestogen-only contraceptives do not affect lactation.

● DIRECTIONS FOR ADMINISTRATION The doctor or nurse administering (or removing) the system should be fully trained in the technique and should provide full counselling reinforced by the patient information leaflet.

● PATIENT AND CARER ADVICE Full counselling backed by patient information leaflet required before administration.

● MEDICINAL FORMS
There can be variation in the licensing of different medicines containing the same drug.
Implant
▸ Etonogestrel (Non-proprietary)
Etonogestrel 68 mg Etonogestrel 68mg implant | 1 device [PoM] no price available DT price = £83.43
▸ Nexplanon (Merck Sharp & Dohme Ltd)
Etonogestrel 68 mg Nexplanon 68mg implant | 1 device [PoM] £83.43 DT price = £83.43

❙ Medroxyprogesterone acetate

● INDICATIONS AND DOSE
Contraception
▶ BY DEEP INTRAMUSCULAR INJECTION
▸ Females of childbearing potential: 150 mg, to be administered within the first 5 days of cycle or within first 5 days after parturition (delay until 6 weeks after parturition if breast-feeding)
▶ BY SUBCUTANEOUS INJECTION
▸ Females of childbearing potential: 104 mg, to be administered within first 5 days of cycle or within 5 days postpartum (delay until 6 weeks postpartum if breast-feeding), injected into anterior thigh or abdomen, dose only suitable if no hormonal contraceptive use in previous month
Long-term contraception
▶ BY DEEP INTRAMUSCULAR INJECTION
▸ Females of childbearing potential: 150 mg every 12 weeks, to be administered within the first 5 days of cycle or within first 5 days after parturition (delay until 6 weeks after parturition if breast-feeding)
▶ BY SUBCUTANEOUS INJECTION
▸ Females of childbearing potential: 104 mg every 13 weeks, to be administered within first 5 days of cycle or within 5 days postpartum (delay until 6 weeks postpartum if breast-feeding), injected into anterior thigh or abdomen, dose only suitable if no hormonal contraceptive use in previous month
Contraception (when patient changing from other hormonal contraception)
▶ BY SUBCUTANEOUS INJECTION
▸ Females of childbearing potential: (consult product literature)

● CONTRA-INDICATIONS Acute porphyrias p. 562 · history of breast cancer but can be used after 5 years if no evidence of disease and non-hormonal contraceptive methods unacceptable · severe arterial disease · undiagnosed vaginal bleeding

● CAUTIONS History during pregnancy of disturbances in lipid metabolism · history during pregnancy of deterioration of otosclerosis · history during pregnancy of pruritus · possible risk of breast cancer

● INTERACTIONS → Appendix 1 (progestogens). Effectiveness of parenteral progestogen-only contraceptives is not affected by antibacterials that do not induce liver enzymes. The effectiveness of medroxyprogesterone acetate intramuscular and subcutaneous injections is not affected by enzyme-inducing drugs and they may be continued as normal during courses of these drugs.

● SIDE-EFFECTS
▸ Rare Osteoporosis · osteoporotic fractures
▸ **Frequency not known** Breast discomfort · changes in libido · depression · dizziness · disturbance of appetite · headache · indigestion · injection site reactions · loss of vision during

treatment (discontinue treatment if papilloedema or retinal vascular lesions) · menstrual irregularities · nausea · reduced bone mineral density · skin disorders · vomiting · weight gain

SIDE-EFFECTS, FURTHER INFORMATION
Use of injectable progestogen-only contraceptives may be associated with a small increased risk of cervical cancer, similar to that seen with combined oral contraceptives. The risk of cervical cancer with other progestogen-only contraceptives is not yet known.

Reduction in bone mineral density occurs in the first 2–3 years of use then stabilises.

- **CONCEPTION AND CONTRACEPTION**
  - With intramuscular use If interval between dose is greater than 12 weeks and 5 days (in long-term contraception), rule out pregnancy before next injection and advise patient to use additional contraceptive measures (e.g. barrier) for 14 days after the injection.
  - With subcutaneous use If interval between dose is greater than 13 weeks and 7 days (in long-term contraception), rule out pregnancy before next injection.
- **PREGNANCY** Not known to be harmful.
- **BREAST FEEDING** Present in milk—no adverse effects reported. Progestogen-only contraceptives do not affect lactation.

  The manufacturers advise that in women who are breast-feeding, the first dose should be delayed until 6 weeks after birth; however, evidence suggests no harmful effect to infant if given earlier. The benefits of using medroxyprogesterone acetate in breast-feeding women outweigh any risks.
- **HEPATIC IMPAIRMENT** Avoid in liver tumour. Caution in severe liver disease and recurrent cholestatic jaundice.
- **PATIENT AND CARER ADVICE**
  Full counselling backed by *patient information leaflet* required before administration—likelihood of menstrual disturbance and the potential for a delay in return to full fertility. Delayed return of fertility and irregular cycles may occur after discontinuation of treatment but there is no evidence of permanent infertility.

- **MEDICINAL FORMS**
  There can be variation in the licensing of different medicines containing the same drug.

  Suspension for injection
  - Depo-Provera (Pfizer Ltd)
    Medroxyprogesterone acetate 150 mg per 1 ml Depo-Provera 150mg/1ml suspension for injection pre-filled syringes | 1 pre-filled disposable injection PoM £6.01 DT price = £6.01
  - Sayana Press (Pfizer Ltd)
    Medroxyprogesterone acetate 160 mg per 1 ml Sayana Press 104mg/0.65 ml suspension for injection pre-filled disposable devices | 1 pre-filled disposable injection PoM £6.90

3.6 Contraception, spermicidal

SPERMICIDALS

Nonoxinol

- **INDICATIONS AND DOSE**
  Spermicidal contraceptive in conjunction with barrier methods of contraception such as diaphragms or caps
  - BY VAGINA
  - Females of childbearing potential: (consult product literature)

- **SIDE-EFFECTS** Genital lesions
  SIDE-EFFECTS, FURTHER INFORMATION
  High frequency use of the spermicide nonoxinol '9' has been associated with genital lesions, which may increase the risk of acquiring these infections.
- **CONCEPTION AND CONTRACEPTION** No evidence of harm to latex condoms and diaphragms.
- **PREGNANCY** Toxicity in *animal* studies.
- **BREAST FEEDING** Present in milk in *animal* studies.

- **MEDICINAL FORMS**
  There can be variation in the licensing of different medicines containing the same drug.
  Gel
  EXCIPIENTS: May contain Hydroxybenzoates (parabens), propylene glycol, sorbic acid
  - Gygel (Marlborough Pharmaceuticals Ltd)
    Nonoxinol-9 20 mg per 1 ml Gygel 2% contraceptive jelly | 30 gram GSL £4.25 | 81 gram GSL £11.00

4 Erectile and ejaculatory conditions
4.1 Erectile dysfunction

Erectile dysfunction

Adolescents presenting with erectile dysfunction should be referred to a specialist.

5 Vaginal and vulval conditions

Vaginal and vulval conditions

Management

Pre-pubertal girls may be particularly susceptible to vulvovaginitis. Barrier preparations applied after cleansing can be useful when the symptoms are due to non-specific irritation, but systemic drugs are required in the treatment of bacterial infection or threadworm infestation. Intravaginal preparations, particularly those that require the use of an applicator, are not generally suitable for young girls; topical preparations may be useful in some adolescent girls.

In older girls symptoms are often restricted to the vulva, but infections almost invariably involve the vagina, which should also be treated; treatment should be as for adults.

Preparations for vaginal and vulval changes

Topical oestrogen creams containing **estriol** 0.01% (*Gynest*®) are used in the treatment of labial adhesions;

treatment is usually restricted to symptomatic cases. Estriol cream should be applied to the adhesions once or twice daily for 2–6 weeks; adhesions may recur following treatment.

Vaginal and vulval infections

Effective specific treatments are available for the common vaginal infections.

Fungal infections

Vaginal fungal infections are not normally a problem in younger girls but can occur in adolescents. *Candidal vulvitis* can be treated locally with cream, but is almost invariably associated with vaginal infection which should also be treated. *Vaginal candidiasis*, rare in girls before puberty, can be treated with antifungal pessaries or cream inserted high into the vagina (including during menstruation), however, these are not recommended for pre-pubertal girls and treatment with an external cream may be more appropriate. Single-dose intravaginal preparations offer an advantage when compliance is a problem. Local irritation can occur on application of vaginal antifungal products.

Imidazole drugs (clotrimazole p. 481, econazole nitrate p. 481, fenticonazole nitrate p. 482, and miconazole p. 482) are effective against candida in short courses of 1 to 3 days according to the preparation used; treatment can be repeated if initial course fails to control symptoms or if symptoms recur. Vaginal applications may be supplemented with antifungal cream for vulvitis and to treat other superficial sites of infection.

Oral treatment of vaginal infection with fluconazole p. 352 may be considered for girls post-puberty.

Vulvovaginal candidiasis in pregnancy

Vulvovaginal candidiasis is common during pregnancy and can be treated with vaginal application of an imidazole (such as clotrimazole), and a topical imidazole cream for vulvitis. Pregnant women need a longer duration of treatment, usually about 7 days, to clear the infection. There is limited absorption of imidazoles from the skin and vagina. Oral antifungal treatment should be avoided during pregnancy.

Recurrent vulvovaginal candidiasis

Recurrent vulvovaginal candidiasis is very rare in children, but can occur if there are predisposing factors such as antibacterial therapy, pregnancy, diabetes mellitus, or possibly oral contraceptive use. Reservoirs of infection can also lead to recontamination and should be treated; these include other skin sites such as the digits, nail beds, and umbilicus, as well as the gastro-intestinal tract and the bladder. The sexual partner may also be the source of re-infection and, if symptomatic, should be treated with a topical imidazole cream at the same time.

Treatment against candida may need to be extended for 6 months in recurrent vulvovaginal candidiasis.

Other infections

Trichomonal infections commonly involve the lower urinary tract as well as the genital system and need systemic treatment with metronidazole p. 313 or tinidazole p. 315.

Bacterial infections with Gram-negative organisms are particularly common in association with gynaecological operations and trauma. Metronidazole is effective against certain Gram-negative organisms, especially *Bacteroides* spp. and can be used prophylactically in gynaecological surgery.

Clindamycin below cream and metronidazole gel are indicated for bacterial vaginosis.

The antiviral drugs aciclovir p. 381 and valaciclovir p. 383 can be used in the treatment of genital infection due to *herpes simplex virus*, the HSV type 2 being a major cause of genital ulceration. They have a beneficial effect on virus shedding and healing, generally giving relief from pain and other symptoms.

5.1 Vaginal and vulval infections

5.1a Vaginal and vulval bacterial infections

ANTIBACTERIALS > LINCOSAMIDES

Clindamycin

- **INDICATIONS AND DOSE**

  DALACIN® 2% CREAM

  Bacterial vaginosis
  - ▸ BY VAGINA
  - ▸ Child: 1 applicatorful daily for 3–7 nights, dose to be administered at night

  DOSE EQUIVALENCE AND CONVERSION
  1 applicatorful delivers a 5 g dose of clindamycin 2%.

- **UNLICENSED USE** Not licensed for use in children.

- **CAUTIONS** Avoid intravaginal preparations (particularly those that require the use of an applicator) in young girls who are not sexually active, unless there is no alternative

- **SIDE-EFFECTS** Cervicitis · irritation · vaginitis

  SIDE-EFFECTS, FURTHER INFORMATION
  Clindamycin 2% cream is poorly absorbed into the blood—low risk of systemic effects.

- **CONCEPTION AND CONTRACEPTION** Damages latex condoms and diaphragms.

- **MEDICINAL FORMS**
  There can be variation in the licensing of different medicines containing the same drug.

  Cream
  EXCIPIENTS: May contain Benzyl alcohol, cetostearyl alcohol (including cetyl and stearyl alcohol), polysorbates, propylene glycol
  - ▸ Dalacin (Pfizer Ltd)
    Clindamycin (as Clindamycin phosphate) 20 mg per
    1 gram Dalacin 2% cream | 40 gram [PoM] £10.86 DT price = £10.86

ANTIBACTERIALS > NITROIMIDAZOLE DERIVATIVES

Metronidazole

- **DRUG ACTION** Metronidazole is an antimicrobial drug with high activity against anaerobic bacteria and protozoa.

- **INDICATIONS AND DOSE**

  Bacterial vaginosis
  - ▸ BY VAGINA USING VAGINAL GEL
  - ▸ Child: 1 applicatorful daily for 5 days, dose to be administered at night

  DOSE EQUIVALENCE AND CONVERSION
  1 applicatorful delivers a 5 g dose of metronidazole 0.75%.

- **UNLICENSED USE** Metronidazole vaginal gel not licensed for use in children under 18 years.

- **CAUTIONS** Avoid intravaginal preparations (particularly those that require the use of an applicator) in young girls who are not sexually active, unless there is no alternative · not recommended during menstruation · some systemic absorption may occur with vaginal gel

- **SIDE-EFFECTS** Abnormal vaginal discharge · local irritation · pelvic discomfort · vaginal candidiasis

- **PATIENT AND CARER ADVICE**
  Medicines for Children leaflet: Metronidazole for bacterial infections www.medicinesforchildren.org.uk/metronidazole-for-bacterial-infections

- MEDICINAL FORMS
  There can be variation in the licensing of different medicines containing the same drug.
  Vaginal gel
  EXCIPIENTS: May contain Disodium edetate, hydroxybenzoates (parabens), propylene glycol
  ▸ Metronidazole (Non-proprietary)
    Metronidazole 7.5 mg per 1 gram Metronidazole 0.75% vaginal gel | 40 gram PoM no price available
  ▸ Zidoval (Meda Pharmaceuticals Ltd)
    Metronidazole 7.5 mg per 1 gram Zidoval 0.75% vaginal gel | 40 gram PoM £4.31

CARBOXYLIC ACIDS

Lactic acid

- INDICATIONS AND DOSE
  BALANCE ACTIV RX® GEL
  Prevention of bacterial vaginosis
  ▸ BY VAGINA
  ▸ Child: 5 mL 1–2 times a week, insert the content of 1 tube (5 mL)

- MEDICINAL FORMS
  There can be variation in the licensing of different medicines containing the same drug.
  Vaginal gel
  EXCIPIENTS: May contain Propylene glycol
  ▸ Balance Activ (BBI Healthcare Ltd)
    Balance Activ BV vaginal pH correction gel | 7 device £5.25
    Balance Activ pessaries | 7 pessary £5.25

5.1b Vaginal and vulval fungal infections

ANTIFUNGALS ⟩ IMIDAZOLE ANTIFUNGALS

Clotrimazole

- INDICATIONS AND DOSE
  Superficial sites of infection in vaginal and vulval candidiasis (dose for 1% or 2% cream)
  ▸ BY VAGINA USING CREAM
  ▸ Child: Apply 2–3 times a day, to be applied to anogenital area
  Vaginal candidiasis (dose for 10% intravaginal cream)
  ▸ BY VAGINA USING VAGINAL CREAM
  ▸ Child: 5 g for 1 dose, one applicatorful to be inserted into the vagina at night, dose can be repeated once if necessary
  Vaginal candidiasis
  ▸ BY VAGINA USING PESSARIES
  ▸ Child: 200 mg for 3 nights, course can be repeated once if necessary, alternatively 500 mg for 1 night, dose can be repeated once if necessary
  Recurrent vulvovaginal candidiasis
  ▸ BY VAGINA USING PESSARIES
  ▸ Child: 500 mg every 1 week for 6 months, dose to be administered following topical imidazole for 10–14 days

- UNLICENSED USE Consult product literature for individual preparations.
- CAUTIONS Avoid intravaginal preparations (particularly those that require use of an applicator) in young girls who are not sexually active, unless there is no alternative
- SIDE-EFFECTS Local irritation

- CONCEPTION AND CONTRACEPTION Cream and pessaries may damage latex condoms and diaphragms.
- PREGNANCY Pregnant women need a longer duration of treatment, usually about 7 days, to clear the infection. Oral antifungal treatment should be avoided during pregnancy.
- EXCEPTIONS TO LEGAL CATEGORY Brands for sale to the public include *Canesten*® Internal Cream.

- MEDICINAL FORMS
  There can be variation in the licensing of different medicines containing the same drug.
  Pessary
  EXCIPIENTS: May contain Benzyl alcohol, cetostearyl alcohol (including cetyl and stearyl alcohol), polysorbates
  ▸ Clotrimazole (Non-proprietary)
    Clotrimazole 500 mg Clotrimazole 500mg pessaries | 1 pessary P £6.60 DT price = £2.91
  ▸ Canesten (clotrimazole) (Bayer Plc)
    Clotrimazole 100 mg Canesten 100mg pessaries | 6 pessary P £3.50 DT price = £3.50
    Clotrimazole 200 mg Canesten 200mg pessaries | 3 pessary P £3.10 DT price = £3.10
    Clotrimazole 500 mg Canesten 500mg Soft Gel pessaries | 1 pessary P £6.41 DT price = £2.91
    Canesten 500mg pessaries | 1 pessary P no price available DT price = £2.91
    Canesten Vaginal 500mg pessaries | 1 pessary PoM £2.00 DT price = £2.91
  Cream
  EXCIPIENTS: May contain Benzyl alcohol, cetostearyl alcohol (including cetyl and stearyl alcohol), polysorbates
  ▸ Clotrimazole (Non-proprietary)
    Clotrimazole 10 mg per 1 gram Clotrimazole 1% cream | 20 gram P £2.79 DT price = £1.04 | 50 gram P £5.45 DT price = £2.60
  ▸ Canesten (clotrimazole) (Bayer Plc)
    Clotrimazole 10 mg per 1 gram Canesten 1% cream | 20 gram P £2.14 DT price = £1.04 | 50 gram P £3.50 DT price = £2.60
    Canesten Antifungal 1% cream | 20 gram P £1.85 DT price = £1.04
    Clotrimazole 20 mg per 1 gram Canesten 2% thrush cream | 10 gram P no price available | 20 gram P £4.46 DT price = £4.46
    Clotrimazole 100 mg per 1 gram Canesten Internal 10% cream | 5 gram P £6.23 DT price = £6.23
    Canesten 10% VC cream | 5 gram PoM £4.50 DT price = £6.23

Econazole nitrate

- INDICATIONS AND DOSE
  GYNO-PEVARYL® ONCE
  Vaginal and vulval candidiasis
  ▸ BY VAGINA
  ▸ Child: 1 pessary for 1 dose, pessary to be inserted at night, dose to be repeated once if necessary
  GYNO-PEVARYL® PESSARY
  Vaginal and vulval candidiasis
  ▸ BY VAGINA
  ▸ Child: 1 pessary daily for 3 days, pessary to be inserted at night, course can be repeated once if necessary

- CAUTIONS Avoid intravaginal preparations (particularly those that require use of an applicator) in young girls who are not sexually active, unless there is no alternative
- SIDE-EFFECTS Occasional local irritation
- CONCEPTION AND CONTRACEPTION Cream and pessaries damage latex condoms and diaphragms.
- PREGNANCY Pregnant women need a longer duration of treatment, usually about 7 days, to clear the infection.

● MEDICINAL FORMS
There can be variation in the licensing of different medicines containing the same drug.

Pessary
▸ Gyno-Pevaryl (Janssen-Cilag Ltd)
 Econazole nitrate 150 mg Gyno-Pevaryl Once 150mg vaginal pessary | 1 pessary PoM £3.69
 Gyno-Pevaryl 150mg vaginal pessaries | 3 pessary PoM £4.17

Fenticonazole nitrate

● **INDICATIONS AND DOSE**

Vaginal and vulva candidiasis
▸ BY VAGINA USING CAPSULES
▸ Child: 200 mg daily for 3 days, alternatively 600 mg daily for 1 dose, to be inserted at night
▸ BY VAGINA USING CREAM
▸ Child: 1 applicatorful twice daily for 3 days

DOSE EQUIVALENCE AND CONVERSION
▸ With topical use 1 applicatorful delivers a 5 g dose of fenticonazole 2 %.

● CAUTIONS Avoid intravaginal preparations (particularly those that require use of an applicator) in young girls who are not sexually active, unless there is no alternative

● SIDE-EFFECTS Local irritation

● CONCEPTION AND CONTRACEPTION Intravaginal cream and vaginal capsules damage latex condoms and diaphragms.

● MEDICINAL FORMS
There can be variation in the licensing of different medicines containing the same drug.

Capsule
EXCIPIENTS: May contain Hydroxybenzoates (parabens)
▸ Gynoxin (Recordati Pharmaceuticals Ltd)
 Fenticonazole nitrate 200 mg Gynoxin 200mg vaginal capsules | 3 capsule PoM £2.42
 Fenticonazole nitrate 600 mg Gynoxin 600mg vaginal capsules | 1 capsule PoM £2.62

Cream
EXCIPIENTS: May contain Cetostearyl alcohol (including cetyl and stearyl alcohol), propylene glycol, wool fat and related substances including lanolin
▸ Gynoxin (Recordati Pharmaceuticals Ltd)
 Fenticonazole nitrate 20 mg per 1 gram Gynoxin 2% vaginal cream | 30 gram PoM £3.74

Miconazole

● **INDICATIONS AND DOSE**

Vaginal and vulval candidiasis
▸ BY VAGINA USING CAPSULES
▸ Child: 1 capsule daily, ovule to be inserted at night as a single dose, dose can be repeated once if necessary

● CAUTIONS Avoid in Acute porphyrias p. 562 · avoid intravaginal preparations (particularly those that require use of an applicator) in young girls who are not sexually active, unless there is no alternative

● INTERACTIONS → Appendix 1 (antifungals, imidazole).

● SIDE-EFFECTS
▸ Common or very common Nausea · rash · vomiting
▸ Frequency not known Occasional local irritation

● CONCEPTION AND CONTRACEPTION *Gyno-Daktarin*® damages latex condoms and diaphragms.

● PREGNANCY Pregnant women need a longer duration of treatment, usually about 7 days, to clear the infection.

● BREAST FEEDING Manufacturer advises caution—no information available.

● MEDICINAL FORMS
There can be variation in the licensing of different medicines containing the same drug.

Capsule
EXCIPIENTS: May contain Hydroxybenzoates (parabens)
▸ Gyno-Daktarin (Janssen-Cilag Ltd)
 Miconazole nitrate 1.2 gram Gyno-Daktarin 1200mg vaginal capsules | 1 capsule PoM £2.94 DT price = £2.94

Chapter 8
Immune system and malignant disease

CONTENTS

Immune system		page 483
1	Immune system disorders and transplantation	483
Malignant disease		493
1	Antibody responsive malignancy	493
2	Cytotoxic responsive malignancy	494
2.1	Cytotoxic drug-induced side effects	515

2.1a	Hyperuricaemia associated with cytotoxic drugs	page 516
3	Immunotherapy responsive malignancy	517
4	Targeted therapy responsive malignancy	519

8

Immune system

1   Immune system disorders and transplantation

Immune response

Inflammatory bowel disease

Azathioprine p. 485, mercaptopurine p. 505, or once weekly methotrexate p. 506 are used to induce remission in unresponsive or chronically active Crohn's disease. Azathioprine or mercaptopurine may also be helpful for retaining remission in frequently relapsing inflammatory bowel disease; once weekly methotrexate is used in Crohn's disease when azathioprine or mercaptopurine are ineffective or not tolerated. Response to azathioprine or mercaptopurine may not become apparent for several months. Folic acid p. 533 should be given to reduce the possibility of methotrexate toxicity. Folic acid is usually given weekly on a different day to the methotrexate; alternative regimens may be used in some settings.

Ciclosporin (cyclosporin) p. 486 is a potent immunosuppressant and is markedly nephrotoxic. In children with severe ulcerative colitis unresponsive to other treatment, ciclosporin may reduce the need for urgent colorectal surgery.

Immunosuppressant therapy

Immunosuppressants are used to suppress rejection in organ transplant recipients and to treat a variety of chronic inflammatory and autoimmune diseases. Solid organ transplant patients are maintained on drug regimens, which may include antiproliferative drugs (azathioprine or mycophenolate mofetil p. 492), calcineurin inhibitors (ciclosporin or tacrolimus p. 488), corticosteroids, or sirolimus p. 487. Choice is dependent on the type of organ, time after transplant, and clinical condition of the patient. Specialist management is required and other immunomodulators may be used to initiate treatment or to treat rejection.

Impaired immune responsiveness

Infections in the immunocompromised child can be severe and show atypical features. Specific local protocols should be followed for the management of infection. Corticosteroids may suppress clinical signs of infection and allow diseases such as septicaemia or tuberculosis to reach an advanced stage before being recognised. Children should be up-to-date with their childhood vaccinations before initiation of immunosuppressant therapy (e.g. before transplantation); vaccination with varicella-zoster vaccine is also necessary during this period—**important**: normal immunoglobulin administration should be considered as soon as possible after measles exposure, and varicella–zoster immunoglobulin (VZIG) is recommended for individuals who have significant chickenpox (varicella) exposure. Specialist advice should be sought on the use of live vaccines for those being treated with immunosuppressive drugs.

Antiproliferative immunosuppressants

Azathioprine is widely used for transplant recipients and it is also used to treat a number of auto-immune conditions, usually when corticosteroid therapy alone provides inadequate control. It is metabolised to mercaptopurine, and doses should be reduced (to one quarter of the original dose in children) when allopurinol p. 516 is given concurrently.

Mycophenolate mofetil is metabolised to mycophenolic acid which has a more selective mode of action than azathioprine.

There is evidence that compared with similar regimens incorporating azathioprine, mycophenolate mofetil may reduce the risk of acute rejection episodes; the risk of opportunistic infections (particularly due to tissue-invasive cytomegalovirus) and the occurrence of blood disorders such as leucopenia may be higher. Children may suffer a high incidence of side-effects, particularly gastrointestinal effects, calling for temporary reduction in dose or interruption of treatment.

Cyclophosphamide p. 498 is less commonly prescribed as an immunosuppressant.

Corticosteroids and other immunosuppressants

The corticosteroids prednisolone p. 413 and dexamethasone p. 410 are widely used in paediatric oncology; they have a marked antitumour effect. Dexamethasone is preferred for acute lymphoblastic leukaemia whilst prednisolone may be used for Hodgkin's disease, non-Hodgkin's lymphoma, and B-cell lymphoma and leukaemia.

Dexamethasone is the corticosteroid of choice in paediatric supportive and palliative care. For children who are not receiving a corticosteroid as a component of their chemotherapy, dexamethasone may be used to reduce raised intracranial pressure, or to help control emesis when combined with an appropriate anti-emetic.

The corticosteroids are also powerful immunosuppressants. They are used to prevent organ transplant rejection, and in high dose to treat rejection episodes.

Ciclosporin (cyclosporin), a calcineurin inhibitor, is a potent immunosuppressant which is virtually nonmyelotoxic but markedly nephrotoxic. It may be used in organ and tissue transplantation, for prevention of graft rejection following bone marrow, kidney, liver, pancreas, heart, lung, and heart-lung transplantation, and for prophylaxis and treatment of graft-versus-host disease. Ciclosporin also has a role in steroid-sensitive and steroid-resistant nephrotic syndrome; in corticosteroid-sensitive nephrotic syndrome it may be given with prednisolone.

Tacrolimus is also a calcineurin inhibitor. Although not chemically related to ciclosporin it has a similar mode of action and side-effects.

NICE technology appraisals (TAs)
Immunosuppressive therapy for renal transplantation in adults (September 2004) Immunosuppressive therapy for renal transplantation in children and adolescents (April 2006) NICE TA85
For induction therapy in the prophylaxis of organ rejection, either basiliximab or daclizumab [discontinued] are options for combining with a calcineurin inhibitor. For each individual, ciclosporin or tacrolimus is chosen as the calcineurin inhibitor on the basis of side-effects.

Mycophenolate mofetil [mycophenolic acid also available but not licensed for use in children] is recommended as part of an immunosuppressive regimen only if:

- the calcineurin inhibitor is not tolerated, particularly if nephrotoxicity endangers the transplanted kidney; or
- there is very high risk of nephrotoxicity from the calcineurin inhibitor, requiring a reduction in the dose of the calcineurin inhibitor or its avoidance.

Sirolimus is recommended as a component of immunosuppressive regimen **only if** intolerance necessitates the withdrawal of a calcineurin inhibitor. These recommendations may not be consistent with the marketing authorisation of some of the products.
www.nice.org.uk/TA85

Immunosuppressive therapy for renal transplantation in children and adolescents (April 2006) NICE TA99
NICE has recommended that for induction therapy in the prophylaxis of organ rejection, either basiliximab or daclizumab [discontinued] are options for combining with a calcineurin inhibitor. For each individual, ciclosporin or tacrolimus is chosen as the calcineurin inhibitor on the basis of side-effects. Mycophenolate mofetil is recommended as part of an immunosuppressive regimen **only if**:

- the calcineurin inhibitor is not tolerated, particularly if nephrotoxicity endangers the transplanted kidney; or
- there is very high risk of nephrotoxicity from the calcineurin inhibitor, requiring a reduction in the dose of the calcineurin inhibitor or its avoidance.

Mycophenolic acid is not recommended as part of an immunosuppressive regimen for renal transplantation in children or adolescents.

Sirolimus [not licensed for use in children] is recommended as a component of immunosuppressive regimen **only if** intolerance necessitates the withdrawal of a calcineurin inhibitor.

These recommendations may not be consistent with the marketing authorisation of some of the products.
www.nice.org.uk/TA99

> **Drugs used for Immune system disorders and transplantation not listed below** Hydroxychloroquine sulfate, p. 596

IMMUNE SERA AND IMMUNOGLOBULINS 〉
IMMUNOGLOBULINS

Antithymocyte immunoglobulin (rabbit)

- **INDICATIONS AND DOSE**

Prophylaxis of organ rejection in heart allograft recipients
▸ BY INTRAVENOUS INFUSION
▸ Child: 1–2.5 mg/kg daily for 3–5 days, start treatment on day of transplantation, to be given over at least 6 hours

Prophylaxis of organ rejection in renal allograft recipients
▸ BY INTRAVENOUS INFUSION
▸ Child 1–17 years: 1–1.5 mg/kg daily for 3–9 days, start treatment on day of transplantation, to be given over at least 6 hours

Treatment of corticosteroid-resistant allograft rejection in renal transplantation
▸ BY INTRAVENOUS INFUSION
▸ Child 1-17 years: 1.5 mg/kg daily for 7–14 days, to be given over at least 6 hours

DOSES AT EXTREMES OF BODY-WEIGHT
To avoid excessive dosage in obese patients, calculate dose on the basis of ideal body weight.

- **CONTRA-INDICATIONS** Infection
- **SIDE-EFFECTS** Anaphylaxis · cytokine release syndrome · diarrhoea · dysphagia · fever · hypotension · increased susceptibility to infection · increased susceptibility to malignancy · infusion-related reactions · lymphopenia · myalgia · nausea · neutropenia · pruritus · rash · serum sickness · shivering · thrombocytopenia · vomiting

SIDE-EFFECTS, FURTHER INFORMATION
Tolerability is increased by pretreatment with an intravenous corticosteroid and antihistamine; an antipyretic drug such as paracetamol may also be beneficial.

- **PREGNANCY** Manufacturer advises use only if potential benefit outweighs risk—no information available.
- **BREAST FEEDING** Manufacturer advises avoid—no information available.
- **MONITORING REQUIREMENTS** Monitor blood count.
- **DIRECTIONS FOR ADMINISTRATION**
▸ With intravenous use For *continuous intravenous infusion* reconstitute each vial with 5 mL water for injections to produce a solution of 5 mg/mL; gently rotate to dissolve. Dilute requisite dose with Glucose 5% or Sodium Chloride 0.9% to an approx. concentration of 0.5 mg/mL; begin infusion immediately after dilution; give through an in-line filter (pore size 0.22 micron); incompatible with unfractionated heparin and hydrocortisone in glucose infusion—precipitation reported.

- **MEDICINAL FORMS**
There can be variation in the licensing of different medicines containing the same drug.
Solution for infusion
▸ Antithymocyte immunoglobulin (rabbit) (Non-proprietary)
Antithymocyte immunoglobulin (rabbit) 20 mg per 1 ml Grafalon 100mg/5ml concentrate for solution for infusion vials | 1 vial PoM no price available
Powder and solvent for solution for infusion
▸ Thymoglobulin (Sanofi)
Antithymocyte immunoglobulin (rabbit) 25 mg Thymoglobuline 25mg powder and solvent for solution for infusion vials | 1 vial PoM £158.77 (Hospital only)

IMMUNOSUPPRESSANTS > ANTIMETABOLITES

Azathioprine

- **DRUG ACTION** Azathioprine is metabolised to mercaptopurine.

- **INDICATIONS AND DOSE**

Severe ulcerative colitis | Severe Crohn's disease
- ▸ BY MOUTH
  - ▸ Child 2-17 years: Initially 2 mg/kg once daily, then increased if necessary up to 2.5 mg/kg once daily

Systemic lupus erythematosus | Vasculitis | Autoimmune conditions usually when corticosteroid therapy alone has proved inadequate
- ▸ BY MOUTH
  - ▸ Child: Initially 1 mg/kg daily, then adjusted according to response to 3 mg/kg daily, consider withdrawal if no improvement within 3 months; maximum 3 mg/kg per day

Suppression of transplant rejection
- ▸ BY MOUTH, OR BY INTRAVENOUS INFUSION
  - ▸ Child: Maintenance 1-3 mg/kg daily, adjusted according to response, consult local treatment protocol for details, oral route preferred, but if oral route is not possible then can be given by intravenous infusion, the total daily dose may alternatively be given in 2 divided doses

- **CAUTIONS** Reduced thiopurine methyltransferase activity

- **INTERACTIONS** → Appendix 1 (azathioprine).

- **SIDE-EFFECTS**
- ▸ **Rare** Hepatic veno-occlusive disease · lymphoma · pancreatitis · pneumonitis · red cell aplasia
- ▸ **Frequency not known** Arthralgia · cholestatic jaundice · colitis in patients also receiving corticosteroids · diarrhoea · dizziness · dose-related bone marrow suppression · fever · hair loss · herpes zoster infection · hypersensitivity reactions · hypotension · increased susceptibility to infections in patients also receiving corticosteroids · interstitial nephritis · liver impairment · malaise · myalgia · nausea · neutropenia · rash · rigors · thrombocytopenia · vomiting

SIDE-EFFECTS, FURTHER INFORMATION
- ▸ **Red cell aplasia** Cases of pure red cell aplasia have been reported with azathioprine; dose reduction or discontinuation should be considered under specialist supervision.
- ▸ **Neutropenia and thrombocytopenia** Usually resolved by reducing the dose.
- ▸ **Hypersensitivity reactions** Hypersensitivity reactions (including malaise, dizziness, vomiting, diarrhoea, fever, rigors, myalgia, arthralgia, rash, hypotension and interstitial nephritis) call for immediate withdrawal.

- **ALLERGY AND CROSS-SENSITIVITY** Contra-indicated in hypersensitivity to mercaptopurine.

- **PREGNANCY** Transplant patients immunosuppressed with azathioprine should not discontinue it on becoming pregnant. However, there have been reports of premature birth and low birth-weight following exposure to azathioprine, particularly in combination with corticosteroids. Spontaneous abortion has been reported following maternal or paternal exposure. Azathioprine is teratogenic in *animal* studies. The use of azathioprine during pregnancy needs to be supervised in specialist units. Treatment should not generally be initiated during pregnancy.

- **BREAST FEEDING** Present in milk in low concentration. No evidence of harm in small studies—use if potential benefit outweighs risk.

- **HEPATIC IMPAIRMENT** Reduce dose. Monitor liver function.

- **RENAL IMPAIRMENT** Reduce dose.

- **PRE-TREATMENT SCREENING**
Thiopurine methyltransferase The enzyme thiopurine methyltransferase (TPMT) metabolises thiopurine drugs (azathioprine, mercaptopurine, tioguanine); the risk of myelosuppression is increased in patients with reduced activity of the enzyme, particularly for the few individuals in whom TPMT activity is undetectable. Consider measuring TPMT activity before starting azathioprine, mercaptopurine, or tioguanine therapy. Patients with absent TPMT activity should not receive thiopurine drugs; those with reduced TPMT activity may be treated under specialist supervision.

- **MONITORING REQUIREMENTS**
- ▸ Monitor for toxicity throughout treatment.
- ▸ Monitor full blood count weekly (more frequently with higher doses or if severe hepatic or renal impairment) for first 4 weeks (manufacturer advises weekly monitoring for 8 weeks but evidence of practical value unsatisfactory), thereafter reduce frequency of monitoring to at least every 3 months.
- ▸ Blood tests and monitoring for signs of myelosuppression are essential in long-term treatment.

- **DIRECTIONS FOR ADMINISTRATION**
- ▸ With intravenous use Consult local treatment protocol for details. For *intravenous injection*, reconstitute 50 mg with 5–15 mL Water for Injections; give over at least 1 minute. For *intravenous infusion*, reconstitute 50 mg with 5–15 mL Water for Injections; dilute requisite dose to a concentration of 0.25–2.5 mg/mL in Glucose 5% *or* Sodium Chloride 0.9%. Intravenous injection is alkaline and very irritant. Intravenous route should therefore be used **only** if oral route not feasible and discontinued as soon as oral route can be tolerated. To reduce irritation flush line with infusion fluid.

- **PATIENT AND CARER ADVICE**
Medicines for Children leaflet: Azathioprine for inflammatory bowel disease www.medicinesforchildren.org.uk/azathioprine-inflammatory-bowel-disease-0
Medicines for Children leaflet: Azathioprine for renal (kidney) transplant www.medicinesforchildren.org.uk/azathioprine-renal-kidney-transplant-0
Bone marrow suppression Patients and their carers should be warned to report immediately any signs or symptoms of bone marrow suppression e.g. inexplicable bruising or bleeding, infection.

- **MEDICINAL FORMS**
There can be variation in the licensing of different medicines containing the same drug. Forms available from special-order manufacturers include: capsule, oral suspension, oral solution

Tablet
CAUTIONARY AND ADVISORY LABELS 21
- ▸ **Azathioprine (Non-proprietary)**
  Azathioprine 25 mg Azathioprine 25mg tablets | 28 tablet PoM £8.41 DT price = £2.24 | 100 tablet PoM £33.26
  Azathioprine 50 mg Azathioprine 50mg tablets | 56 tablet PoM £15.85 DT price = £2.43 | 100 tablet PoM £29.00
- ▸ **Azapress** (Ennogen Pharma Ltd)
  Azathioprine 50 mg Azapress 50mg tablets | 56 tablet PoM £2.83 DT price = £2.43
- ▸ **Imuran** (Aspen Pharma Trading Ltd)
  Azathioprine 25 mg Imuran 25mg tablets | 100 tablet PoM £10.99
  Azathioprine 50 mg Imuran 50mg tablets | 100 tablet PoM £7.99

Powder for solution for injection
- ▸ **Imuran** (Aspen Pharma Trading Ltd)
  Azathioprine 50 mg Imuran 50mg powder for solution for injection vials | 1 vial PoM £15.38

8

Immune system and malignant disease

IMMUNOSUPPRESSANTS ⟩ CALCINEURIN INHIBITORS AND RELATED DRUGS

| Ciclosporin

(Cyclosporin)

- **DRUG ACTION** Ciclosporin is a calcineurin inhibitor.

● **INDICATIONS AND DOSE**

Refractory ulcerative colitis
▸ BY MOUTH
- ▸ Child 2–17 years: Initially 2 mg/kg twice daily (max. per dose 5 mg/kg twice daily), dose adjusted according to blood-ciclosporin concentration and response
▸ BY INTRAVENOUS INFUSION
- ▸ Child 3–17 years: Initially 0.5–1 mg/kg twice daily, dose adjusted according to blood-ciclosporin concentration and response

Short-term treatment of severe atopic dermatitis where conventional therapy ineffective or inappropriate (administered on expert advice)
▸ BY MOUTH
- ▸ Child: Initially 1.25 mg/kg twice daily (max. per dose 2.5 mg/kg twice daily) usual maximum duration of 8 weeks but may be used for longer under specialist supervision, if good initial response not achieved within 2 weeks, increase dose rapidly up to maximum

Short-term treatment of very severe atopic dermatitis where conventional therapy ineffective or inappropriate (administered on expert advice)
▸ BY MOUTH
- ▸ Child: 2.5 mg/kg twice daily usual maximum duration of 8 weeks but may be used for longer under specialist supervision

Severe psoriasis where conventional therapy ineffective or inappropriate (administered on expert advice)
▸ BY MOUTH
- ▸ Child: Initially 1.25 mg/kg twice daily (max. per dose 2.5 mg/kg twice daily), increased gradually to maximum if no improvement within 1 month, initial dose of 2.5 mg/kg twice daily justified if condition requires rapid improvement; discontinue if inadequate response after 3 months at the optimum dose; max. duration of treatment usually 1 year unless other treatments cannot be used

Prevention of graft rejection following bone-marrow, kidney, liver, pancreas, heart, lung, and heart-lung transplantation | Prevention and treatment of graft-versus-host disease
▸ BY MOUTH, OR BY INTRAVENOUS INFUSION
- ▸ Child: (consult local protocol)

Nephrotic syndrome
▸ BY MOUTH
- ▸ Child: 3 mg/kg twice daily, dose can be increased if necessary in corticosteroid-resistant disease; for maintenance reduce to lowest effective dose according to whole blood-ciclosporin concentrations, proteinuria, and renal function

- **UNLICENSED USE** Not licensed for use in children under 3 months. Not licensed for use in children under 16 years for atopic eczema (dermatitis) or psoriasis. Not licensed for use in ulcerative colitis.

┌───┐
IMPORTANT SAFETY INFORMATION
Patients should be stabilised on a particular brand of oral ciclosporin because switching between formulations without close monitoring may lead to clinically important changes in blood-ciclosporin concentration.
└───┘

- **CONTRA-INDICATIONS** Abnormal renal function (in non-transplant indications) · malignancy (in non-transplant indications) · uncontrolled hypertension (in non-transplant indications) · uncontrolled infections (in non-transplant indications) · use with tacrolimus specifically contra-indicated

- **CAUTIONS** Hyperuricaemia · in atopic dermatitis allow herpes simplex infections to clear before starting (if they occur during treatment withdraw if severe) · in atopic dermatitis and psoriasis discontinue if lymphoproliferative disorder develops · in atopic dermatitis *Staphylococcus aureus* skin infections—not absolute contra-indication providing controlled (but avoid erythromycin unless no other alternative) · in psoriasis treat patients with malignant or pre-malignant conditions of skin only after appropriate treatment (and if no other option)

- **INTERACTIONS** → Appendix 1 (ciclosporin).
For patients other than transplant recipients, preferably avoid other immunosuppressants (increased risk of infection and malignancies, including lymphoma and skin cancer).

- **SIDE-EFFECTS**
GENERAL SIDE-EFFECTS
- ▸ **Common or very common** Abdominal pain · anorexia · diarrhoea · fatigue · gingival hyperplasia · headache · hepatic dysfunction · hypercholesterolaemia · hyperkalaemia · hyperlipidaemia · hypertension · hypertrichosis · hyperuricaemia · hypomagnesaemia · muscle cramps · myalgia · nausea · paraesthesia · renal dysfunction (renal structural changes on long-term administration) · tremor · vomiting
- ▸ **Uncommon** Anaemia · oedema · signs of encephalopathy · thrombocytopenia · weight gain
- ▸ **Rare** Gynaecomastia · haemolytic uraemic syndrome · hyperglycaemia · menstrual disturbances · micro-angiopathic haemolytic anaemia · motor polyneuropathy · muscle weakness · myopathy · pancreatitis · visual disturbances secondary to benign intracranial hypertension

SPECIFIC SIDE-EFFECTS
- ▸ With intravenous use Anaphylaxis
SIDE-EFFECTS, FURTHER INFORMATION
- ▸ Visual disturbances Discontinue if visual disturbances secondary to benign intracranial hypertension occur.

- **PREGNANCY** Crosses placenta. There is less experience of ciclosporin in pregnancy but it does not appear to be any more harmful than azathioprine. The use of ciclosporin during pregnancy needs to be supervised in specialist units.

- **BREAST FEEDING** Present in milk—manufacturer advises avoid.

- **HEPATIC IMPAIRMENT** Dosage adjustment based on bilirubin and liver enzymes may be needed.

- **RENAL IMPAIRMENT** In patients with nephrotic syndrome and renal impairment initially 2.5 mg/kg daily. Reduce dose by 25–50% if serum creatinine more than 30% above baseline on more than one measurement.
In psoriasis and atopic dermatitis, reduce dose by 25–50% if serum creatinine increases more than 30% above baseline (even if within normal range) and discontinue if reduction not successful within 1 month.

- **PRE-TREATMENT SCREENING** In psoriasis, exclude malignancies (including those of skin and cervix) before starting (biopsy any lesions not typical of psoriasis).

- **MONITORING REQUIREMENTS**
- ▸ Monitor whole blood ciclosporin concentration (trough level dependent on indication—consult local treatment protocol for details).
- ▸ Dermatological and physical examination, including blood pressure and renal function measurements required at

least twice before starting treatment for psoriasis or atopic dermatitis.

▸ Monitor liver function.

▸ Monitor serum potassium especially in renal dysfunction (risk of hyperkalaemia).

▸ Monitor serum magnesium.

▸ Measure blood lipids before treatment and after the first month of treatment.

▸ In psoriasis and atopic dermatitis monitor serum creatinine every 2 weeks for first 3 months then every month.

▸ Investigate lymphadenopathy that persists despite improvement in atopic dermatitis.

▸ Monitor kidney function—dose dependent increase in serum creatinine and urea during first few weeks may necessitate discontinuation (exclude rejection of kidney transplant).

▸ Monitor blood pressure—discontinue if hypertension develops that cannot be controlled by antihypertensives.

▸ In long-term management of nephrotic syndrome, perform renal biopsies every 1–2 years.

● DIRECTIONS FOR ADMINISTRATION

▸ With oral use Mix solution with orange juice (or squash) or apple juice (to improve taste) or with water immediately before taking (and rinse with more to ensure total dose). Do not mix with grapefruit juice. With capsules and oral solution, total daily dose should be taken in 2 divided doses.

▸ With intravenous use For intermittent *intravenous infusion*, dilute to a concentration of 0.5–2.5 mg/mL with Glucose 5% *or* Sodium Chloride 0.9%; give over 2–6 hours; not to be used with PVC equipment. Observe patient for signs of anaphylaxis for at least 30 minutes after starting infusion and at frequent intervals thereafter.

● PRESCRIBING AND DISPENSING INFORMATION
Brand name prescribing Prescribing and dispensing of ciclosporin should be by brand name to avoid inadvertent switching. If it is necessary to switch a patient to a different brand of ciclosporin, the patient should be monitored closely for changes in blood-ciclosporin concentration, serum creatinine, blood pressure, and transplant function.

▸ With oral use *Sandimmun*® capsules and oral solution are available direct from Novartis for patients who cannot be transferred to a different oral preparation.

● HANDLING AND STORAGE Keep medicine measure away from other liquids (including water).

● PATIENT AND CARER ADVICE
Avoid excessive exposure to UV light, including sunlight. In psoriasis and atopic dermatitis, avoid use of UVB or PUVA.

Medicines for Children leaflet: Ciclosporin for nephrotic syndrome www.medicinesforchildren.org.uk/ciclosporin-nephrotic-syndrome-0

▸ With oral use Patients and carers should be counselled on the administration of ciclosporin capsules and oral solution.

● MEDICINAL FORMS
There can be variation in the licensing of different medicines containing the same drug.

Capsule
EXCIPIENTS: May contain Ethanol, ethyl lactate, propylene glycol
▸ Ciclosporin (Non-proprietary)
Ciclosporin 25 mg Ciclosporin 25mg capsules | 30 capsule PoM no price available DT price = £18.37
Ciclosporin 50 mg Ciclosporin 50mg capsules | 30 capsule PoM no price available DT price = £35.97
Ciclosporin 100 mg Ciclosporin 100mg capsules | 30 capsule PoM no price available DT price = £68.28
▸ Capimune (Mylan Ltd)
Ciclosporin 25 mg Capimune 25mg capsules | 30 capsule PoM £13.05 DT price = £18.37

Ciclosporin 50 mg Capimune 50mg capsules | 30 capsule PoM £25.50 DT price = £35.97
Ciclosporin 100 mg Capimune 100mg capsules | 30 capsule PoM £48.50 DT price = £68.28
▸ Capsorin (Morningside Healthcare Ltd)
Ciclosporin 25 mg Capsorin 25mg capsules | 30 capsule PoM £13.05 DT price = £18.37
Ciclosporin 50 mg Capsorin 50mg capsules | 30 capsule PoM £25.59 DT price = £35.97
Ciclosporin 100 mg Capsorin 100mg capsules | 30 capsule PoM £48.89 DT price = £68.28
▸ Deximune (Dexcel-Pharma Ltd)
Ciclosporin 25 mg Deximune 25mg capsules | 30 capsule PoM £13.06 DT price = £18.37
Ciclosporin 50 mg Deximune 50mg capsules | 30 capsule PoM £25.60 DT price = £35.97
Ciclosporin 100 mg Deximune 100mg capsules | 30 capsule PoM £48.90 DT price = £68.28
▸ Neoral (Novartis Pharmaceuticals UK Ltd)
Ciclosporin 10 mg Neoral 10mg capsules | 60 capsule PoM £18.25 DT price = £18.25
Ciclosporin 25 mg Neoral 25mg capsules | 30 capsule PoM £18.37 DT price = £18.37
Ciclosporin 50 mg Neoral 50mg capsules | 30 capsule PoM £35.97 DT price = £35.97
Ciclosporin 100 mg Neoral 100mg capsules | 30 capsule PoM £68.28 DT price = £68.28
▸ Vanquoral (Teva UK Ltd)
Ciclosporin 10 mg Vanquoral 10mg capsules | 30 capsule PoM £12.75 | 60 capsule PoM £12.75 DT price = £18.25
Ciclosporin 25 mg Vanquoral 25mg capsules | 30 capsule PoM £13.05 DT price = £18.37
Ciclosporin 50 mg Vanquoral 50mg capsules | 30 capsule PoM £25.59 DT price = £35.97
Ciclosporin 100 mg Vanquoral 100mg capsules | 30 capsule PoM £48.89 DT price = £68.28

Oral solution
EXCIPIENTS: May contain Alcohol, propylene glycol
▸ Neoral (Novartis Pharmaceuticals UK Ltd)
Ciclosporin 100 mg per 1 ml Neoral 100mg/ml oral solution sugar-free | 50 ml PoM £102.30

Solution for infusion
EXCIPIENTS: May contain Alcohol, polyoxyl castor oils
▸ Sandimmun (Novartis Pharmaceuticals UK Ltd)
Ciclosporin 50 mg per 1 ml Sandimmun 250mg/5ml concentrate for solution for infusion ampoules | 10 ampoule PoM £110.05 Sandimmun 50mg/1ml concentrate for solution for infusion ampoules | 10 ampoule PoM £23.23

Sirolimus

● DRUG ACTION Sirolimus is a non-calcineurin inhibiting immunosuppressant.

● INDICATIONS AND DOSE

As a component of immunosuppressive therapy for renal transplantation in children and adolescents only if intolerance necessitates the withdrawal of a calcineurin inhibitor
▸ BY MOUTH
▸ Child: (consult local protocol)

DOSE EQUIVALENCE AND CONVERSION
The 500 microgram tablet is not bioequivalent to the 1 mg and 2 mg tablets. Multiples of 500 microgram tablets should **not** be used as a substitute for other tablet strengths.

● UNLICENSED USE Not licensed for use in children.

● CAUTIONS Hyperlipidaemia · increased susceptibility to infection (especially urinary-tract infection) · increased susceptibility to lymphoma and other malignancies, particularly of the skin (limit exposure to UV light)

● INTERACTIONS → Appendix 1 (sirolimus).

8

Immune system and malignant disease

- **SIDE-EFFECTS**
  - **Common or very common** Abdominal pain · acne · anaemia · arthralgia · ascites · constipation · diarrhoea · epistaxis · haemolytic uraemic syndrome · headache · hypercholesterolaemia · hyperglycaemia · hypertension · hypertriglyceridaemia · hypokalaemia · hypophosphataemia · impaired healing · leucopenia · lymphocele · nausea · neutropenia · oedema · osteonecrosis · pleural effusion · pneumonitis · proteinuria · pyrexia · rash · stomatitis · tachycardia · thrombocytopenia · thrombotic thrombocytopenic purpura · venous thromboembolism
  - **Uncommon** Nephrotic syndrome · pancreatitis · pancytopenia · pericardial effusion · pulmonary embolism · pulmonary haemorrhage
  - **Rare** Alveolar proteinosis · anaphylactic reactions · angioedema · exfoliative dermatitis · hepatic necrosis · hypersensitivity reactions · hypersensitivity vasculitis · interstitial lung disease · lymphoedema
  - **Frequency not known** Focal segmental glomerulosclerosis · reversible impairment of male fertility
- **CONCEPTION AND CONTRACEPTION** Effective contraception must be used during treatment and for 12 weeks after stopping.
- **PREGNANCY** Avoid unless essential—toxicity in *animal* studies.
- **BREAST FEEDING** Discontinue breast-feeding.
- **HEPATIC IMPAIRMENT** Dose reduction may be necessary, consult local treatment protocols for details. Monitor whole blood-sirolimus level closely and consult local treatment protocol in hepatic impairment.
- **MONITORING REQUIREMENTS**
  - Monitor whole blood-sirolimus trough concentration (Afro-Caribbean patients may require higher doses).
  - Monitor kidney function when given with ciclosporin; monitor lipids; monitor urine proteins.
- **DIRECTIONS FOR ADMINISTRATION** Food may affect absorption (take at the same time with respect to food). Sirolimus oral solution should be mixed with at least 60 mL water or orange juice in a glass or plastic container immediately before taking; refill container with at least 120 mL of water or orange juice and drink immediately (to ensure total dose). Do not mix with any other liquids.
- **PATIENT AND CARER ADVICE** Patient or carers should be given advice on how to administer sirolimus.
  Patients should be advised to avoid excessive exposure to UV light.

- **MEDICINAL FORMS**
  There can be variation in the licensing of different medicines containing the same drug.
  Tablet
  - Rapamune (Pfizer Ltd)
    Sirolimus 500 microgram Rapamune 0.5mg tablets | 30 tablet [PoM] £69.00 DT price = £69.00
    Sirolimus 1 mg Rapamune 1mg tablets | 30 tablet [PoM] £86.49 DT price = £86.49
    Sirolimus 2 mg Rapamune 2mg tablets | 30 tablet [PoM] £172.98 DT price = £172.98
  Oral solution
  EXCIPIENTS: May contain Ethanol
  - Rapamune (Pfizer Ltd)
    Sirolimus 1 mg per 1 ml Rapamune 1mg/ml oral solution sugar-free | 60 ml [PoM] £162.41

Tacrolimus

- **DRUG ACTION** Tacrolimus is a calcineurin inhibitor.

- **INDICATIONS AND DOSE**
  ADOPORT®
  Prophylaxis of graft rejection following liver transplantation, starting 12 hours after transplantation
  - BY MOUTH
  - Neonate: Initially 150 micrograms/kg twice daily.
  - Child: Initially 150 micrograms/kg twice daily
  Prophylaxis of graft rejection following kidney transplantation, starting within 24 hours of transplantation
  - BY MOUTH
  - Neonate: Initially 150 micrograms/kg twice daily.
  - Child: Initially 150 micrograms/kg twice daily, a lower initial dose of 100 micrograms/kg twice daily has been used in adolescents to prevent very high 'trough' concentrations
  Prophylaxis of graft rejection following heart transplantation following antibody induction, starting within 5 days of transplantation
  - BY MOUTH
  - Neonate: Initially 50–150 micrograms/kg twice daily.
  - Child: Initially 50–150 micrograms/kg twice daily
  Prophylaxis of graft rejection following heart transplantation without antibody induction, starting within 12 hours of transplantation
  - BY MOUTH
  - Neonate: Initially 150 micrograms/kg twice daily, dose to be given as soon as clinically possible (8–12 hours after discontinuation of intravenous infusion).
  - Child: Initially 150 micrograms/kg twice daily, dose to be given as soon as clinically possible (8–12 hours after discontinuation of intravenous infusion)
  Allograft rejection resistant to conventional immunosuppressive therapy
  - BY MOUTH
  - Child: Seek specialist advice
  CAPEXION®
  Prophylaxis of graft rejection following liver transplantation, starting 12 hours after transplantation
  - BY MOUTH
  - Neonate: Initially 150 micrograms/kg twice daily.
  - Child: Initially 150 micrograms/kg twice daily
  Prophylaxis of graft rejection following kidney transplantation, starting within 24 hours of transplantation
  - BY MOUTH
  - Neonate: Initially 150 micrograms/kg twice daily.
  - Child: Initially 150 micrograms/kg twice daily, a lower initial dose of 100 micrograms/kg twice daily has been used in adolescents to prevent very high 'trough' concentrations
  Prophylaxis of graft rejection following heart transplantation following antibody induction, starting within 5 days of transplantation
  - BY MOUTH
  - Neonate: Initially 50–150 micrograms/kg twice daily.
  - Child: Initially 50–150 micrograms/kg twice daily

Prophylaxis of graft rejection following heart transplantation without antibody induction, starting within 12 hours of transplantation
▸ BY MOUTH

▸ Neonate: Initially 150 micrograms/kg twice daily, dose to be given as soon as clinically possible (8–12 hours after discontinuation of intravenous infusion).

▸ Child: Initially 150 micrograms/kg twice daily, dose to be given as soon as clinically possible (8–12 hours after discontinuation of intravenous infusion)

Allograft rejection resistant to conventional immunosuppressive therapy
▸ BY MOUTH
▸ Child: Seek specialist advice

MODIGRAF®

Prophylaxis of graft rejection following liver transplantation, starting 12 hours after transplantation
▸ BY MOUTH

▸ Neonate: Initially 150 micrograms/kg twice daily.

▸ Child: Initially 150 micrograms/kg twice daily

Prophylaxis of graft rejection following kidney transplantation, starting within 24 hours of transplantation
▸ BY MOUTH

▸ Neonate: Initially 150 micrograms/kg twice daily.

▸ Child: Initially 150 micrograms/kg twice daily, a lower initial dose of 100 micrograms/kg twice daily has been used in adolescents to prevent very high 'trough' concentrations

Prophylaxis of graft rejection following heart transplantation following antibody induction, starting within 5 days of transplantation
▸ BY MOUTH

▸ Neonate: Initially 50–150 micrograms/kg twice daily.

▸ Child: Initially 50–150 micrograms/kg twice daily

Prophylaxis of graft rejection following heart transplantation without antibody induction, starting within 12 hours of transplantation
▸ BY MOUTH

▸ Neonate: Initially 150 micrograms/kg twice daily, dose to be given as soon as clinically possible (8–12 hours after discontinuation of intravenous infusion).

▸ Child: Initially 150 micrograms/kg twice daily, dose to be given as soon as clinically possible (8–12 hours after discontinuation of intravenous infusion)

Allograft rejection resistant to conventional immunosuppressive therapy
▸ BY MOUTH
▸ Child: Seek specialist advice

PROGRAF® CAPSULES

Prophylaxis of graft rejection following liver transplantation, starting 12 hours after transplantation
▸ BY MOUTH

▸ Neonate: Initially 150 micrograms/kg twice daily.

▸ Child: Initially 150 micrograms/kg twice daily

Prophylaxis of graft rejection following kidney transplantation, starting within 24 hours of transplantation
▸ BY MOUTH

▸ Neonate: Initially 150 micrograms/kg twice daily.

▸ Child: Initially 150 micrograms/kg twice daily, a lower initial dose of 100 micrograms/kg twice daily has been used in adolescents to prevent very high 'trough' concentrations

Prophylaxis of graft rejection following heart transplantation following antibody induction, starting within 5 days of transplantation
▸ BY MOUTH

▸ Neonate: Initially 50–150 micrograms/kg twice daily.

▸ Child: Initially 50–150 micrograms/kg twice daily

Prophylaxis of graft rejection following heart transplantation without antibody induction, starting within 12 hours of transplantation
▸ BY MOUTH

▸ Neonate: Initially 150 micrograms/kg twice daily, dose to be given as soon as clinically possible (8–12 hours after discontinuation of intravenous infusion).

▸ Child: Initially 150 micrograms/kg twice daily, dose to be given as soon as clinically possible (8–12 hours after discontinuation of intravenous infusion)

Allograft rejection resistant to conventional immunosuppressive therapy
▸ BY MOUTH
▸ Child: Seek specialist advice

PROGRAF® INFUSION

Prophylaxis of graft rejection following liver transplantation, starting 12 hours after transplantation when oral route not appropriate
▸ BY CONTINUOUS INTRAVENOUS INFUSION

▸ Neonate: Initially 50 micrograms/kg daily for up to 7 days (then transfer to oral therapy), dose to be administered over 24 hours.

▸ Child: Initially 50 micrograms/kg daily for up to 7 days (then transfer to oral therapy), dose to be administered over 24 hours

Prophylaxis of graft rejection following kidney transplantation, starting within 24 hours of transplantation when oral route not appropriate
▸ BY CONTINUOUS INTRAVENOUS INFUSION

▸ Neonate: Initially 75–100 micrograms/kg daily for up to 7 days (then transfer to oral therapy), dose to be administered over 24 hours.

▸ Child: Initially 75–100 micrograms/kg daily for up to 7 days (then transfer to oral therapy), dose to be administered over 24 hours

Prophylaxis of graft rejection following heart transplantation without antibody induction, starting within 12 hours of transplantation
▸ BY CONTINUOUS INTRAVENOUS INFUSION

▸ Neonate: Initially 30–50 micrograms/kg daily for up to 7 days (then transfer to oral therapy), dose to be administered over 24 hours.

▸ Child: Initially 30–50 micrograms/kg daily for up to 7 days (then transfer to oral therapy), dose to be administered over 24 hours

Allograft rejection resistant to conventional immunosuppressive therapy
▸ BY CONTINUOUS INTRAVENOUS INFUSION
▸ Child: Seek specialist advice (consult local protocol)

TACNI®

Prophylaxis of graft rejection following liver transplantation, starting 12 hours after transplantation
▸ BY MOUTH

▸ Neonate: Initially 150 micrograms/kg twice daily.

▸ Child: Initially 150 micrograms/kg twice daily

continued →

8

Immune system and malignant disease

Prophylaxis of graft rejection following kidney transplantation, starting within 24 hours of transplantation

▸ BY MOUTH

▸ Neonate: Initially 150 micrograms/kg twice daily.

▸ Child: Initially 150 micrograms/kg twice daily, a lower initial dose of 100 micrograms/kg twice daily has been used in adolescents to prevent very high 'trough' concentrations

Prophylaxis of graft rejection following heart transplantation following antibody induction, starting within 5 days of transplantation

▸ BY MOUTH

▸ Neonate: Initially 50–150 micrograms/kg twice daily.

▸ Child: Initially 50–150 micrograms/kg twice daily

Prophylaxis of graft rejection following heart transplantation without antibody induction, starting within 12 hours of transplantation

▸ BY MOUTH

▸ Neonate: Initially 150 micrograms/kg twice daily, dose to be given as soon as clinically possible (8–12 hours after discontinuation of intravenous infusion).

▸ Child: Initially 150 micrograms/kg twice daily, dose to be given as soon as clinically possible (8–12 hours after discontinuation of intravenous infusion)

Allograft rejection resistant to conventional immunosuppressive therapy

▸ BY MOUTH

▸ Child: Seek specialist advice

VIVADEX®

Prophylaxis of graft rejection following liver transplantation, starting 12 hours after transplantation

▸ BY MOUTH

▸ Neonate: Initially 150 micrograms/kg twice daily.

▸ Child: Initially 150 micrograms/kg twice daily

Prophylaxis of graft rejection following kidney transplantation, starting within 24 hours of transplantation

▸ BY MOUTH

▸ Neonate: Initially 150 micrograms/kg twice daily.

▸ Child: Initially 150 micrograms/kg twice daily, a lower initial dose of 100 micrograms/kg twice daily has been used in adolescents to prevent very high 'trough' concentrations

Prophylaxis of graft rejection following heart transplantation following antibody induction, starting within 5 days of transplantation

▸ BY MOUTH

▸ Neonate: Initially 50–150 micrograms/kg twice daily.

▸ Child: Initially 50–150 micrograms/kg twice daily

Prophylaxis of graft rejection following heart transplantation without antibody induction, starting within 12 hours of transplantation

▸ BY MOUTH

▸ Neonate: Initially 150 micrograms/kg twice daily, dose to be given as soon as clinically possible (8–12 hours after discontinuation of intravenous infusion).

▸ Child: Initially 150 micrograms/kg twice daily, dose to be given as soon as clinically possible (8–12 hours after discontinuation of intravenous infusion)

Allograft rejection resistant to conventional immunosuppressive therapy

▸ BY MOUTH

▸ Child: Seek specialist advice

> **IMPORTANT SAFETY INFORMATION**
>
> MHRA/CHM ADVICE: ORAL TACROLIMUS PRODUCTS: PRESCRIBE AND DISPENSE BY BRAND NAME ONLY, TO MINIMISE THE RISK OF INADVERTENT SWITCHING BETWEEN PRODUCTS, WHICH HAS BEEN ASSOCIATED WITH REPORTS OF TOXICITY AND GRAFT REJECTION (JUNE 2012)
>
> Inadvertent switching between oral tacrolimus products has been associated with reports of toxicity and graft rejection. To ensure maintenance of therapeutic response when a patient is stabilised on a particular brand, oral tacrolimus products should be prescribed and dispensed by brand name only.
>
> - *Adoport*®, *Prograf*®, *Capexion*®, *Tacni*®, and *Vivadex*® are immediate-release capsules that are taken twice daily, once in the morning and once in the evening;
> - *Modigraf*® granules are used to prepare an immediate-release oral suspension which is taken twice daily, once in the morning and once in the evening;
> - *Advagraf*® is a prolonged-release capsule that is taken once daily in the morning.
>
> Switching between tacrolimus brands requires careful supervision and therapeutic monitoring by an appropriate specialist.
>
> Important: *Envarsus*® is not interchangeable with other oral tacrolimus containing products; the MHRA has advised (June 2012) that oral tacrolimus products should be prescribed and dispensed by brand only.

● CAUTIONS Increased risk of infections · lymphoproliferative disorders · malignancies · neurotoxicity · QT-interval prolongation · UV light (avoid excessive exposure to sunlight and sunlamps)

● INTERACTIONS Appendix 1 (tacrolimus). Contra-indication—avoid concurrent administration with ciclosporin (care if patient has previously received ciclosporin).

● SIDE-EFFECTS

▸ **Common or very common** Acne · alopecia · anaemia · anorexia · anxiety · arthralgia · ascites · bile-duct abnormalities · bloating · blood disorders · cholestasis · confusion · constipation · depression · diarrhoea · dizziness · dyspepsia · dyspnoea · electrolyte disturbances · flatulence · gastro-intestinal inflammation · gastro-intestinal perforation · gastro-intestinal ulceration · haemorrhage · headache · hepatic dysfunction · hyperglycaemia · hyperkalaemia · hypertension · hyperuricaemia · hypokalaemia · impaired hearing · ischaemic events · jaundice · leucopenia · mood changes · muscle cramp · nausea · oedema · pancytopenia · paraesthesia · parenchymal lung disorders · peripheral neuropathy · photophobia · pleural effusion · psychosis · renal failure · renal impairment · renal tubular necrosis · seizures · sleep disturbances · sweating · tachycardia · thrombocytopenia · thromboembolic events · tinnitus · tremor · urinary abnormalities · visual disturbances · vomiting · weight changes

▸ **Uncommon** Amnesia · arrhythmia · cardiac arrest · cardiomyopathy · cataract · cerebrovascular accident · coagulation disorders · coma · dermatitis · dysmenorrhoea · encephalopathy · gastro-intestinal reflux disease · heart failure · hypertonia · hypoglycaemia · influenza-like symptoms · palpitation · pancreatitis · paralysis · paralytic ileus · peritonitis · photosensitivity · respiratory failure · speech disorder

▸ **Rare** Blindness · dehydration · hirsutism · pericardial effusion · posterior reversible encephalopathy syndrome respiratory distress syndrome · thrombotic thrombocytopenic purpura · toxic epidermal necrolysis

▸ **Very rare** Haemorrhagic cystitis · myasthenia · Stevens-Johnson syndrome

▸ **Frequency not known** Agranulocytosis · haemolytic anaemia · pure red cell aplasia

SIDE-EFFECTS, FURTHER INFORMATION

▸ Cardiomyopathy
Cardiomyopathy has been reported in children. Patients should be monitored by echocardiography for hypertrophic changes—consider dose reduction or discontinuation if these occur.

● **ALLERGY AND CROSS-SENSITIVITY** Contra-indicated if history of hypersensitivity to macrolides.

● **CONCEPTION AND CONTRACEPTION** Exclude pregnancy before treatment.

● **PREGNANCY** Avoid unless potential benefit outweighs risk—crosses the placenta and risk of premature delivery, intra-uterine growth restriction, and hyperkalaemia.

● **BREAST FEEDING** Avoid—present in breast milk (following systemic administration).

● **HEPATIC IMPAIRMENT** Dose reduction may be necessary in severe impairment.

● **MONITORING REQUIREMENTS**

▸ After initial dosing, and for maintenance treatment, tacrolimus doses should be adjusted according to whole-blood concentration. Monitor whole blood-tacrolimus trough concentration (especially during episodes of diarrhoea)—consult local treatment protocol for details.

▸ Monitor blood pressure, ECG (for hypertrophic changes—risk of cardiomyopathy), fasting blood-glucose concentration, haematological and neurological (including visual) and coagulation parameters, electrolytes, hepatic and renal function.

● **DIRECTIONS FOR ADMINISTRATION**

▸ With intravenous use For *continuous intravenous infusion* over 24 hours, dilute to a concentration of 4–100 micrograms/mL with Glucose 5% *or* Sodium Chloride 0.9%, to a total volume between 20–500mL. Tacrolimus is incompatible with PVC.

● **PRESCRIBING AND DISPENSING INFORMATION**
PROGRAF® INFUSION ▸ With intravenous use Intravenous route should only be used if oral route is inappropriate.

● **PATIENT AND CARER ADVICE**
Avoid excessive exposure to UV light including sunlight.

Driving and skilled tasks
May affect performance of skilled tasks (e.g. driving). Medicines for Children leaflet: Tacrolimus for prevention of transplant rejection www.medicinesforchildren.org.uk/tacrolimus-for-prevention-of-transplant-rejection

● **NATIONAL FUNDING/ACCESS DECISIONS**

Scottish Medicines Consortium (SMC) Decisions
The *Scottish Medicines Consortium* has advised (November 2010) that tacrolimus granules for oral suspension (*Modigraf®*) are accepted for restricted use within NHS Scotland in patients for whom tacrolimus is an appropriate choice of immunosuppressive therapy and where small changes (less than 500 micrograms) in dosing increments are required (such as, in paediatric patients) or in seriously ill patients who are unable to swallow tacrolimus capsules.

● **MEDICINAL FORMS**
There can be variation in the licensing of different medicines containing the same drug.

Capsule
CAUTIONARY AND ADVISORY LABELS 23

▸ **Adoport** (Sandoz Ltd)
Tacrolimus 500 microgram Adoport 0.5mg capsules | 50 capsule PoM £42.92 DT price = £61.88

Tacrolimus 750 microgram Adoport 0.75mg capsules | 50 capsule PoM £51.75
Tacrolimus 1 mg Adoport 1mg capsules | 50 capsule PoM £55.69 DT price = £80.28 | 100 capsule PoM £111.36
Tacrolimus 2 mg Adoport 2mg capsules | 50 capsule PoM £111.00
Tacrolimus 5 mg Adoport 5mg capsules | 50 capsule PoM £205.74 DT price = £296.58

▸ **Capexion** (Mylan Ltd)
Tacrolimus 500 microgram Capexion 0.5mg capsules | 50 capsule PoM £52.50 DT price = £61.88
Tacrolimus 1 mg Capexion 1mg capsules | 50 capsule PoM £68.20 DT price = £80.28 | 100 capsule PoM £136.20
Tacrolimus 5 mg Capexion 5mg capsules | 50 capsule PoM £252.00 DT price = £296.58

▸ **Prograf** (Astellas Pharma Ltd)
Tacrolimus 500 microgram Prograf 500microgram capsules | 50 capsule PoM £61.88 DT price = £61.88
Tacrolimus 1 mg Prograf 1mg capsules | 50 capsule PoM £80.28 DT price = £80.28 | 100 capsule PoM £160.54
Tacrolimus 5 mg Prograf 5mg capsules | 50 capsule PoM £296.58 DT price = £296.58

Granules
CAUTIONARY AND ADVISORY LABELS 13, 23

▸ **Modigraf** (Astellas Pharma Ltd)
Tacrolimus (as Tacrolimus monohydrate)
200 microgram Modigraf 0.2mg granules sachets sugar-free | 50 sachet PoM £71.30 DT price = £71.30
Tacrolimus (as Tacrolimus monohydrate) 1 mg Modigraf 1mg granules sachets sugar-free | 50 sachet PoM £356.65 DT price = £356.65

Solution for infusion
EXCIPIENTS: May contain Polyoxyl castor oils

▸ **Prograf** (Astellas Pharma Ltd)
Tacrolimus 5 mg per 1 ml Prograf 5mg/1ml solution for infusion ampoules | 10 ampoule PoM £584.51

IMMUNOSUPPRESSANTS ⟩ MONOCLONAL ANTIBODIES

Canakinumab

● **DRUG ACTION** Canakinumab is a recombinant human monoclonal antibody that selectively inhibits interleukin-1 beta receptor binding.

● **INDICATIONS AND DOSE**

Treatment of cryopyrin-associated periodic syndromes, including severe forms of familial cold auto-inflammatory syndrome (or familial cold urticaria), Muckle-Wells syndrome, and neonatal-onset multisystem inflammatory disease (also known as chronic infantile neurological cutaneous and articular syndrome)

▸ BY SUBCUTANEOUS INJECTION

▸ Child: (consult product literature)

Active systemic juvenile idiopathic arthritis (in combination with methotrexate or alone) in children who have had an inadequate response to NSAIDs and systemic corticosteroids

▸ BY SUBCUTANEOUS INJECTION

▸ Child 2–17 years (body-weight 7.5 kg and above): 4 mg/kg every 4 weeks (max. per dose 300 mg)

● **CONTRA-INDICATIONS** Active infection · leucopenia · neutropenia

● **CAUTIONS** History of recurrent infection · latent and active tuberculosis · predisposition to infection

CAUTIONS, FURTHER INFORMATION

▸ Vaccinations Patients should receive all recommended vaccinations (including pneumococcal and inactivated influenza vaccine) before starting treatment; avoid live vaccines unless potential benefit outweighs risk—consult product literature for further information.

8

Immune system and malignant disease

- **INTERACTIONS** → Appendix 1 (canakinumab). Contra-indicated with concomitant use with tumour necrosis factor inhibitors (possible increased risk of infections).
- **SIDE-EFFECTS**
  GENERAL SIDE-EFFECTS
  ▸ **Common or very common** Back pain · increased susceptibility to infection (including serious infection) · injection-site reactions · malaise · neutropenia · vertigo
  ▸ **Uncommon** Gastro-oesophageal reflux
  ▸ **Frequency not known** Malignancy · vomiting
  SPECIFIC SIDE-EFFECTS
  ▸ When used for active systemic juvenile idiopathic arthritis (in combination with methotrexate or alone) in children who have had an inadequate response to nsaids and systemic corticosteroids Abdominal pain · arthralgia · musculoskeletal pain · rhinitis
- **CONCEPTION AND CONTRACEPTION** Effective contraception required during treatment and for up to 3 months after last dose.
- **PREGNANCY** Manufacturer advises avoid unless potential benefit outweighs risk.
- **BREAST FEEDING** Consider if benefit outweighs risk—not known if present in human milk.
- **HEPATIC IMPAIRMENT** No information available.
- **RENAL IMPAIRMENT** Limited information available but manufacturer advises no dose adjustment required.
- **PRE-TREATMENT SCREENING** Patients should be evaluated for latent and active tuberculosis before starting treatment.
- **MONITORING REQUIREMENTS**
  ▸ Monitor full blood count including neutrophil count before starting treatment, 1–2 months after starting treatment, and periodically thereafter.
  ▸ Monitor for signs and symptoms of tuberculosis during and after treatment.
- **MEDICINAL FORMS**
  There can be variation in the licensing of different medicines containing the same drug.
  Powder for solution for injection
  ▸ Ilaris (Novartis Pharmaceuticals UK Ltd) ▼
  Canakinumab 150 mg Ilaris 150mg powder for solution for injection vials | 1 vial [PoM] £9,927.80

IMMUNOSUPPRESSANTS > MONOCLONAL ANTIBODIES > MONOCLONAL ANTIBODIES, ANTI-LYMPHOCYTE

Basiliximab

- **DRUG ACTION** Basiliximab is a monoclonal antibody that acts as an interleukin-2 receptor antagonist and prevents T-lymphocyte proliferation.

- **INDICATIONS AND DOSE**
  Prophylaxis of acute rejection in allogeneic renal transplantation used in combination with ciclosporin and corticosteroid-containing immunosuppression regimens (specialist use only)
  ▸ BY INTRAVENOUS INJECTION, OR BY INTRAVENOUS INFUSION
  ▸ Child 1-17 years (body-weight up to 35 kg): Initially 10 mg, dose to be administered within 2 hours before transplant surgery, followed by 10 mg after 4 days, dose administered after transplant surgery, withhold second dose if severe hypersensitivity or graft loss occurs
  ▸ Child 1-17 years (body-weight 35 kg and above): Initially 20 mg, administered within 2 hours before transplant surgery, followed by 20 mg after 4 days, dose to be administered after surgery, withhold second dose if severe hypersensitivity or graft loss occurs

- **CAUTIONS** Off-label use in cardiac transplantation—increased risk of serious cardiac side-effects
- **INTERACTIONS** → Appendix 1 (basiliximab).
- **SIDE-EFFECTS** Atrial flutter · cardiac arrest · cytokine release syndrome · palpitations · severe hypersensitivity reactions
- **CONCEPTION AND CONTRACEPTION** Adequate contraception must be used during treatment and for 16 weeks after last dose.
- **PREGNANCY** Manufacturer advises avoid—no information available.
- **BREAST FEEDING** Manufacturer advises avoid—no information available.
- **DIRECTIONS FOR ADMINISTRATION**
  ▸ With intravenous use For *intravenous infusion*, dilute reconstituted solution to a concentration not exceeding 400 micrograms/mL, with Glucose 5% or Sodium Chloride 0.9%; give over 20–30 minutes.

- **MEDICINAL FORMS**
  There can be variation in the licensing of different medicines containing the same drug.
  Powder and solvent for solution for injection
  ▸ Simulect (Novartis Pharmaceuticals UK Ltd)
  Basiliximab 10 mg Simulect 10mg powder and solvent for solution for injection vials | 1 vial [PoM] £758.69 (Hospital only)
  Basiliximab 20 mg Simulect 20mg powder and solvent for solution for injection vials | 1 vial [PoM] £842.38 (Hospital only)

IMMUNOSUPPRESSANTS > PURINE SYNTHESIS INHIBITORS

Mycophenolate mofetil

- **INDICATIONS AND DOSE**
  Prophylaxis of acute rejection in renal transplantation (in combination with a corticosteroid and ciclosporin) (under expert supervision)
  ▸ BY MOUTH
  ▸ Child: 600 mg/m^2 twice daily, consult local protocol for details; maximum 2 g per day
  Prophylaxis of acute rejection in renal transplantation (in combination with a corticosteroid and tacrolimus) (under expert supervision)
  ▸ BY MOUTH
  ▸ Child: 300 mg/m^2 twice daily, consult local protocol for details; maximum 2 g per day
  Prophylaxis of acute rejection in hepatic transplantation (in combination with a corticosteroid and ciclosporin or tacrolimus) (under expert supervision)
  ▸ BY MOUTH
  ▸ Child: 10 mg/kg twice daily, increased to 20 mg/kg twice daily, consult local protocol for details; maximum 2 g per day

  DOSE EQUIVALENCE AND CONVERSION
  MYFORTIC®
  Mycophenolic acid 720 mg is approximately equivalent to mycophenolate mofetil 1 g but avoid unnecessary switching because of pharmacokinetic differences.

- **UNLICENSED USE** Not licensed for use in children under 2 years for the prophylaxis of acute rejection in renal transplantation. Not licensed for use in children for the prophylaxis of acute rejection in hepatic transplantation.
- **CAUTIONS** Active serious gastro-intestinal disease (risk of haemorrhage, ulceration and perforation) · children (higher incidence of side-effects may call for temporary reduction of dose or interruption) · delayed graft function · increased susceptibility to skin cancer (avoid exposure to strong sunlight) · risk of hypogammaglobulinaemia or

bronchiectasis when used in combination with other immunosuppressants

CAUTIONS, FURTHER INFORMATION
▶ Hypogammaglobulinaemia or bronchiectasis Measure serum immunoglobulin levels if recurrent infections develop, and consider bronchiectasis or pulmonary fibrosis if persistent respiratory symptoms such as cough and dyspnoea develop.

● INTERACTIONS → Appendix 1 (mycophenolate). Possible decreased effectiveness of vaccination— avoid live vaccines.

● SIDE-EFFECTS
▶ Common or very common Abdominal pain · acne · agitation · alopecia · anaemia · anorexia · anxiety · arthralgia · blood disorders · confusion · constipation · convulsions · cough · depression · diarrhoea · disturbances of blood lipids · disturbances of electrolytes and blood lipids · dizziness · dyspnoea · flatulence · gastro-intestinal bleeding · gastro-intestinal inflammation · gastro-intestinal ulceration · gingival hyperplasia · headache · hepatitis · hyperglycaemia · hypertension · hypotension · ileus · infections · influenza-like syndrome · insomnia · jaundice · leucopenia · malignancy (particularly of the skin) · myasthenic syndrome · nausea · oedema · pancreatitis · pancytopenia · paraesthesia · pleural effusion · rash · red cell aplasia · renal impairment · skin hypertrophy · stomatitis · tachycardia · taste disturbance · thrombocytopenia · tremor · vasodilatation · vomiting · weight loss
▶ Frequency not known Interstitial lung disease · intestinal villous atrophy · progressive multifocal leucoencephalopathy · pulmonary fibrosis

SIDE-EFFECTS, FURTHER INFORMATION
▶ Cases of pure red cell aplasia have been reported with mycophenolate mofetil; dose reduction or discontinuation should be considered under specialist supervision.

● CONCEPTION AND CONTRACEPTION
Pregnancy prevention In females of child-bearing potential, exclude pregnancy immediately before and during treatment.
  Women should use 2 methods of effective contraception during treatment, and for 6 weeks after discontinuation. Men should use condoms during treatment and for at least 90 days after discontinuation of treatment; female partners of male patients should also use effective contraception during treatment and for 90 days after discontinuation.

● PREGNANCY Avoid unless no suitable alternative— congenital malformations and spontaneous abortions reported.

● BREAST FEEDING Manufacturer advises avoid—present in milk in *animal* studies.

● RENAL IMPAIRMENT Manufacturer advises consider dose reduction if estimated glomerular filtration rate less than 25 mL/minute/1.73 m².

● MONITORING REQUIREMENTS Monitor full blood count every week for 4 weeks then twice a month for 2 months then every month in the first year (consider interrupting treatment if neutropenia develops).

● PRESCRIBING AND DISPENSING INFORMATION Tablets and capsules not appropriate for dose titration in children with body surface are less than 1.25 m².

● PATIENT AND CARER ADVICE
Bone marrow suppression Patients should be warned to report immediately any signs or symptoms of bone marrow suppression e.g. infection or inexplicable bruising or bleeding.

● MEDICINAL FORMS
There can be variation in the licensing of different medicines containing the same drug. Forms available from special-order manufacturers include: oral suspension

Tablet
▶ Mycophenolate mofetil (Non-proprietary)
  Mycophenolate mofetil 500 mg Mycophenolate mofetil 500mg tablets | 50 tablet [PoM] £82.26 DT price = £8.05
▶ CellCept (Roche Products Ltd)
  Mycophenolate mofetil 500 mg CellCept 500mg tablets | 50 tablet [PoM] £82.26 DT price = £8.05
▶ Myfenax (Teva UK Ltd)
  Mycophenolate mofetil 500 mg Myfenax 500mg tablets | 50 tablet [PoM] £78.15 DT price = £8.05

Gastro-resistant tablet
CAUTIONARY AND ADVISORY LABELS 25
▶ Myfortic (Novartis Pharmaceuticals UK Ltd)
  Mycophenolic acid (as Mycophenolate sodium) 180 mg Myfortic 180mg gastro-resistant tablets | 120 tablet [PoM] £96.72
  Mycophenolic acid (as Mycophenolate sodium) 360 mg Myfortic 360mg gastro-resistant tablets | 120 tablet [PoM] £193.43

Capsule
▶ Mycophenolate mofetil (Non-proprietary)
  Mycophenolate mofetil 250 mg Mycophenolate mofetil 250mg capsules | 100 capsule [PoM] £82.26 DT price = £82.26
▶ CellCept (Roche Products Ltd)
  Mycophenolate mofetil 250 mg CellCept 250mg capsules | 100 capsule [PoM] £82.26 DT price = £82.26
▶ Myfenax (Teva UK Ltd)
  Mycophenolate mofetil 250 mg Myfenax 250mg capsules | 100 capsule [PoM] £78.15 DT price = £82.26

Oral suspension
EXCIPIENTS: May contain Aspartame
▶ CellCept (Roche Products Ltd)
  Mycophenolate mofetil 200 mg per 1 ml CellCept 1g/5ml oral suspension sugar-free | 175 ml [PoM] £115.16

Malignant disease

1 Antibody responsive malignancy

IMMUNOSUPPRESSANTS › MONOCLONAL ANTIBODIES › MONOCLONAL ANTIBODIES, ANTI-LYMPHOCYTE

Anti-lymphocyte monoclonal antibodies

● DRUG ACTION The anti-lymphocyte monoclonal antibodies cause lysis of B lymphocytes.

IMPORTANT SAFETY INFORMATION
All anti-lymphocyte monoclonal antibodies should be given under the supervision of an experienced specialist, in an environment where full resuscitation facilities are immediately available.

● SIDE-EFFECTS
▶ Common or very common Allergic reactions · angioedema · bronchospasm · chills · cytokine release syndrome · dyspnoea · fever · flushing · nausea · pruritus · rash · tumour pain · vomiting

SIDE-EFFECTS, FURTHER INFORMATION
▶ Infusion-related side-effects Infusion-related side-effects occur predominantly during the first infusion. Patients should be given paracetamol and an antihistamine before each dose of anti-lymphocyte monoclonal antibodies to reduce infusion-related side-effects. Premedication with a

corticosteroid should also be considered.

The infusion may have to be stopped temporarily and the infusion-related effects treated—consult product literature for appropriate management.

Evidence of pulmonary infiltration and features of tumour lysis syndrome should be sought if infusion-related effects occur.

‣ Cytokine release syndrome Fatalities following **severe** cytokine release syndrome (characterised by severe dyspnoea) and associated with features of tumour lysis syndrome have occurred after infusions of anti-lymphocyte monoclonal antibodies. Patients with a high tumour burden as well as those with pulmonary insufficiency or infiltration are at increased risk and should be monitored **very closely** (and a slower rate of infusion considered).

● PRE-TREATMENT SCREENING All patients should be screened for hepatitis B before treatment.

F 493

Rituximab

● **INDICATIONS AND DOSE**

Post-transplantation lymphoproliferative disease (under expert supervision) | Non-Hodgkin's lymphoma (under expert supervision) | Hodgkin's lymphoma (under expert supervision) | Severe cases of resistant immune modulated disease including idiopathic thrombocytopenia purpura, haemolytic anaemia, and systemic lupus erythematosus (under expert supervision)

 ‣ BY INTRAVENOUS INFUSION
 ‣ Child: Patients should receive premedication before each dose (consult product literature for details) (consult local protocol)

● UNLICENSED USE Not licensed for use in children.

● CAUTIONS History of cardiovascular disease; in adults exacerbation of angina, arrhythmia, and heart failure have been reported · transient hypotension occurs frequently during infusion (anti-hypertensives may need to be withheld for 12 hours before infusion)

CAUTIONS, FURTHER INFORMATION

 ‣ Hepatitis B infection and reactivation Hepatitis B infection and reactivation (including fatal cases) have been reported in patients taking **rituximab**. Patients with positive hepatitis B serology should be referred to a liver specialist for monitoring and initiation of antiviral therapy before treatment initiation; treatment should not be initiated in patients with evidence of current hepatitis B infection until the infection has been adequately treated. Patients should be closely monitored for clinical and laboratory signs of active hepatitis B infection during treatment and for up to a year following the last infusion (consult product literature).

For full details on cautions, consult product literature or local treatment protocol.

● INTERACTIONS → Appendix 1 (rituximab).

● SIDE-EFFECTS Abdominal pain · anaemia · antibody formation · aplastic anaemia · arthralgia · asthenia · blood disorders · depression · dyspepsia · headache · hypertension · hypotension · injection-site reactions · leucopenia · lupus erythematosus-like syndrome · migraine · muscle spasm · pancytopenia · paraesthesia · progressive multifocal leucoencephalopathy · pruritus · rhinitis · severe fatal skin reactions · severe skin reactions (permanently discontinue treatment if occurs) · sore throat · Stevens-Johnson syndrome (permanently discontinue treatment if occurs) · thrombocytopenia · toxic epidermal necrolysis (permanently discontinue treatment if occurs) · urticaria · worsening heart failure

SIDE-EFFECTS, FURTHER INFORMATION

Associated with infections, sometimes severe, including tuberculosis, septicaemia, and hepatitis B reactivation.

 ‣ Progressive multifocal leucoencephalopathy Progressive multifocal leucoencephalopathy (which is usually fatal or causes severe disability) has been reported in association with rituximab; patients should be monitored for cognitive, neurological, or psychiatric signs and symptoms. If progressive multifocal leucoencephalopathy is suspected, suspend treatment until it has been excluded.

For full details, including management of side-effects, consult product literature.

● CONCEPTION AND CONTRACEPTION Effective contraception (in both sexes) required during and for 12 months after treatment.

● PREGNANCY Avoid unless potential benefit to mother outweighs risk of B-lymphocyte depletion in fetus.

● BREAST FEEDING Avoid breast-feeding during and for 12 months after treatment.

● MONITORING REQUIREMENTS For full details on monitoring requirements consult product literature.

● MEDICINAL FORMS
There can be variation in the licensing of different medicines containing the same drug.
Solution for infusion
 ‣ MabThera (Roche Products Ltd)
 Rituximab 10 mg per 1 ml MabThera 100mg/10ml concentrate for solution for infusion vials | 2 vial [PoM] £349.25
 MabThera 500mg/50ml concentrate for solution for infusion vials | 1 vial [PoM] £873.15

2 Cytotoxic responsive malignancy

Cytotoxic drugs

Overview

The management of childhood cancer is complex and is generally confined to specialist regional centres and some associated shared-care units.

Cytotoxic drugs have both anti-cancer activity and the potential for damage to normal tissue. In children, chemotherapy is almost always started with curative intent, but may be continued as palliation if the disease is refractory.

Chemotherapy with a combination of two or more cytotoxic drugs aims to reduce the development of resistance and to improve cytotoxic effect. Treatment protocols generally incorporate a series of treatment courses at defined intervals with clear criteria for starting each course, such as adequate bone-marrow recovery and renal or cardiac function. The principal component of treatment for leukaemias in children is cytotoxic therapy, whereas solid tumours may be managed with surgery or radiotherapy in addition to chemotherapy.

Only medical or nursing staff who have received appropriate training should administer parenteral cytotoxics. In most instances central venous access will be required for the intravenous administration of cytotoxics to children; care is required to avoid the risk of extravasation (see Side-effects of Cytotoxic Drugs and their Management).

Guidelines for handling cytotoxic drugs

● Trained personnel should reconstitute cytotoxics
● Reconstitution should be carried out in designated pharmacy areas

- Protective clothing (including gloves, gowns, and masks) should be worn
- The eyes should be protected and means of first aid should be specified
- Pregnant staff should avoid exposure to cytotoxic drugs (all females of child-bearing age should be informed of the reproductive hazard)
- Use local procedures for dealing with spillages and safe disposal of waste material, including syringes, containers, and absorbent material
- Staff exposure to cytotoxic drugs should be monitored

Intrathecal chemotherapy

A Health Service Circular (HSC 2008/001) provides guidance on the introduction of safe practice in NHS Trusts where intrathecal chemotherapy is administered; written local guidance covering all aspects of national guidance should be available. Support for training programmes is also available.

Copies, and further information may be obtained from:
Department of Health
PO Box 777
London
SE1 6XH
Fax: 01623 724524

It is also available from the Department of Health website (www.dh.gov.uk).

Safe systems for cytotoxic medicines:

Safe system requirements for cytotoxic medicines:

- Cytotoxic drugs for the treatment of cancer should be given as part of a wider pathway of care that is co-ordinated by a multi-disciplinary team
- Cytotoxic drugs should be prescribed, dispensed and administered only in the context of a written protocol or treatment plan
- Injectable cytotoxic drugs should only be dispensed if they are prepared for administration
- Oral cytotoxic medicines should be dispensed with clear directions for use

---

IMPORTANT SAFETY INFORMATION

RISKS OF INCORRECT DOSING OF ORAL ANTI-CANCER MEDICINES
The National Patient Safety Agency has advised (January 2008) that the prescribing and use of oral cytotoxic medicines should be carried out to the same standard as parenteral cytotoxic therapy. Standards to be followed to achieve this include:

- non-specialists who prescribe or administer on-going oral cytotoxic medication should have access to written protocols and treatment plans, including guidance on the monitoring and treatment of toxicity;
- staff dispensing oral cytotoxic medicines should confirm that the prescribed dose is appropriate for the patient. Patients should have written information that includes details of the intended oral anti-cancer regimen, the treatment plan, and arrangements for monitoring, taken from the original protocol from the initiating hospital. Staff dispensing oral cytotoxic medicines should also have access to this information, and to advice from an experienced cancer pharmacist in the initiating hospital.

Doses

Doses of cytotoxic drugs are determined using a variety of different methods including age, body-surface area, or body-weight. Alternatively, doses may be fixed. Doses may be further adjusted following consideration of a patient's neutrophil count, renal and hepatic function, and history of previous adverse effects to the cytotoxic drug. Doses may also differ depending on whether a drug is used alone or in combination.

Because of the complexity of dosage regimens in the treatment of malignant disease, dose statements have been omitted from many of the drug entries in this chapter.

Pregnancy and reproductive function

Most cytotoxic drugs are teratogenic and should not be administered during pregnancy, especially during the first trimester. Exclude pregnancy before treatment with cytotoxic drugs. Considerable caution is necessary if a pregnant woman presents with cancer requiring chemotherapy, and specialist advice should always be sought.

Contraceptive advice should be given to men and women before cytotoxic therapy begins (and should cover the duration of contraception required after therapy has ended).

Alkylating drugs can have an adverse effect on gametogenesis, which may be reversible particularly in females. Regimens that do not contain an alkylating drug or procarbazine may have less effect on fertility, but those with an alkylating drug or procarbazine carry the risk of causing permanent male sterility (there is no effect on potency). Pretreatment counselling and consideration of sperm storage may be appropriate. Women are less severely affected, though the span of reproductive life may be shortened by the onset of a premature menopause. No increase in fetal abnormalities or abortion rate has been recorded in patients who remain fertile after cytotoxic chemotherapy. Amenorrhoea may occur, which may also be reversible.

Side-effects of cytotoxic drugs and their management

Gastro-intestinal effects

Management of gastrointestinal effects of cytotoxic drugs includes the use of antacids, H_2-receptor antagonists, and proton pump inhibitors to protect the gastric mucosa, laxatives to treat constipation, and enteral and parenteral nutritional support.

Oral mucositis

Good oral hygiene keeps the mouth clean and moist and helps to prevent mucositis; prevention is more effective than treatment of the complication. Good oral hygiene measures for children over 6 months include brushing teeth with a soft small brush with fluoride toothpaste 2–3 times daily, and rinsing the mouth frequently. Daily fluoride supplements can be used on the advice of the child's dental team. For children under 6 months or when it is not possible to brush teeth, carers should be instructed how to clean the mouth using an oral sponge moistened with water or with an antimicrobial solution such as diluted chlorhexidine. Mucositis related to chemotherapy can be extremely painful and may, in some circumstances, require opioid analgesia. Secondary infection with candida is frequent; treatment with a systemically absorbed antifungal, such as fluconazole p. 352, is effective.

Nausea and vomiting

Nausea and vomiting cause considerable distress to many children who receive chemotherapy, and to a lesser extent abdominal radiotherapy, and may lead to refusal of further treatment; prophylaxis of nausea and vomiting is therefore extremely important. Symptoms may be acute (occurring within 24 hours of treatment), delayed (first occurring more than 24 hours after treatment), or anticipatory (occurring prior to subsequent doses). Delayed and anticipatory symptoms are more difficult to control than acute symptoms and require different management.

Susceptibility to nausea and vomiting may increase with repeated exposure to the cytotoxic drug.

Drugs may be divided according to their emetogenic potential and some examples are given below, but the symptoms vary according to the dose, to other drugs administered, and to the individual's susceptibility to emetogenic stimuli.

Mildly emetogenic treatment— fluorouracil, etoposide p. 510, low doses of methotrexate p. 506, the vinca alkaloids, and abdominal radiotherapy.

Moderately emetogenic treatment—carboplatin p. 509, doxorubicin hydrochloride p. 502, intermediate and low doses of cyclophosphamide p. 498, mitoxantrone p. 503, and high doses of methotrexate.

Highly emetogenic treatment—cisplatin p. 510, dacarbazine p. 499, and high doses of alkylating drugs.

Anti-emetic drugs, when given regularly, help prevent or ameliorate emesis associated with chemotherapy in children.

Prevention of acute symptoms: For patients at low risk of emesis, pretreatment with a 5HT$_3$-receptor antagonist may be of benefit.

For patients at high risk of *emesis* or when other treatment is inadequate, a 5HT$_3$-receptor antagonist is often highly effective. The addition of dexamethasone p. 410 and other anti-emetics may also be required.

Prevention of delayed symptoms: dexamethasone, given by mouth, is the drug of choice for preventing delayed symptoms; it is used alone or with metoclopramide hydrochloride p. 246. Due to the risks of neurological side-effects, metoclopramide hydrochloride should only be used in children as a second-line option. The 5HT$_3$-receptor antagonists may have a role in preventing uncontrolled symptoms.

Prevention of anticipatory symptoms: Good symptom control is the best way to prevent anticipatory symptoms. Lorazepam p. 209 can be helpful for its amnesiac, sedative, and anxiolytic effects.

Bone-marrow suppression

All cytotoxic drugs except vincristine sulfate p. 511 and bleomycin p. 509 cause bone-marrow suppression. This commonly occurs 7 to 10 days after administration, but is delayed for certain drugs, such as melphalan p. 500. Peripheral blood counts must be checked before each treatment. The duration and severity of neutropenia can be reduced by the use of granulocyte-colony stimulating factors; their use should be reserved for children who have previously experienced severe neutropenia.

Cytotoxic drugs may be contra-indicated in children with acute infection; any infection should be treated before, or when starting, cytotoxic drugs.

Infection in a child with neutropenia requires immediate broad-spectrum antibacterial treatment that covers all likely pathogens. Appropriate bacteriological investigations should be conducted as soon as possible. Children taking cytotoxic drugs who have signs or symptoms of infection (or their carers) should be advised to seek prompt medical attention. All children should be investigated and treated under the supervision of an appropriate oncology or haematology specialist. Antifungal treatment may be required in a child with prolonged neutropenia or fever lasting longer than 4–5 days. Chickenpox and measles can be particularly hazardous in immunocompromised children. Varicella-zoster immunoglobulin p. 730 is indicated if the child does not have immunity against varicella and has had close contact with infectious chickenpox or herpes zoster. Antiviral prophylaxis can be considered in addition to varicella-zoster immunoglobulin or as an alternative if varicella–zoster immunoglobulin is inappropriate. If an immunocompromised child has come into close contact with an infectious individual with measles, normal immunoglobulin p. 727 should be given.

For advice on the use of live vaccines in individuals with impaired immune response, see Vaccines.

Alopecia

Reversible hair loss is a common complication, although it varies in degree between drugs and individual patients.

Long-term and delayed toxicity

Cytotoxic drugs may produce specific organ-related toxicity in children (e.g. cardiotoxicity with doxorubicin hydrochloride or nephrotoxicity with cisplatin and ifosfamide p. 499). Manifestations of such toxicity may not appear for several months or even years after cancer treatment. Careful follow-up of survivors of childhood cancer is therefore vital; national and local guidelines have been developed to facilitate this.

Thromboembolism

Venous thromboembolism can be a complication of cancer itself, but chemotherapy increases the risk.

Tumour lysis syndrome

Tumour lysis syndrome occurs secondary to spontaneous or treatment related rapid destruction of malignant cells. Patients at risk of tumour lysis syndrome include those with non- Hodgkin's lymphoma (especially if high grade and bulky disease), Burkitt's lymphoma, acute lymphoblastic leukaemia and acute myeloid leukaemia (particularly if high white blood cell counts or bulky disease), and occasionally those with solid tumours. Pre-existing hyperuricaemia, dehydration and renal impairment are also predisposing factors. Features, include hyperkalaemia, hyperuricaemia, and hyperphosphataemia with hypocalcaemia; renal damage and arrhythmias can follow. Early recognition of patients at risk, and initiation of prophylaxis or therapy for tumour lysis syndrome, is essential.

Treatment for cytotoxic-induced side effects

Hyperuricaemia

Hyperuricaemia, which may be present in high-grade lymphoma and leukaemia, can be markedly worsened by chemotherapy and is associated with acute renal failure.

Allopurinol p. 516 is used routinely in children at low to moderate risk of hyperuricaemia. It should be started 24 hours before treatment; patients should be adequately hydrated (consideration should be given to omitting phosphate and potassium from hydration fluids). The dose of mercaptopurine p. 505 or azathioprine p. 485 should be reduced if allopurinol is given concomitantly.

Rasburicase p. 516 is a recombinant urate oxidase used in children who are at high-risk of developing hyperuricaemia. It rapidly reduces plasma-uric acid concentration and may be of particular value in preventing complications following treatment of leukaemias or bulky lymphomas.

Methotrexate-induced mucositis and myelosuppression

Folinic acid p. 515 (given as calcium folinate) is used to counteract the folate-antagonist action of methotrexate and thus speed recovery from methotrexate-induced mucositis or myelosuppression ('folinic acid rescue').

The calcium salt of levofolinic acid p. 516, a single isomer of folinic acid, is also used following methotrexate administration. The dose of calcium levofolinate is generally half that of calcium folinate.

The disodium salts of folinic acid and levofolinic acid are also used for rescue therapy following methotrexate administration.

The efficacy of high dose methotrexate is enhanced by delaying initiation of folinic acid for at least 24 hours, local protocols define the correct time. Folinic acid is normally continued until the plasma-methotrexate concentration falls to 45–90 nanograms/mL (100–200 nanomol/litre).

In the treatment of methotrexate p. 506 overdose, folinate should be administered immediately; other measures to enhance the elimination of methotrexate are also necessary.

Urothelial toxicity

Haemorrhagic cystitis is a common manifestation of urothelial toxicity which occurs with the oxazaphosphorines, cyclophosphamide p. 498 and ifosfamide p. 499; it is caused by the metabolite acrolein. Adequate hydration is essential to reduce the risk of urothelial toxicity. Mesna p. 515 reacts specifically with acrolein in the urinary tract, preventing toxicity. Mesna is given for the same duration as cyclophosphamide or ifosfamide. It is generally given intravenously; the dose of mesna is equal to or greater than that of the oxazaphosphorine. See the role of nebulised mesna as a mucolytic in cystic fibrosis.

Cytotoxic antibiotics

Cytotoxic antibiotics are widely used. Many act as radiomimetics and simultaneous use of radiotherapy should be **avoided** because it may markedly increase toxicity.
Daunorubicin p. 501, doxorubicin hydrochloride p. 502, and epirubicin hydrochloride p. 502 are anthracycline antibiotics. Mitoxantrone p. 503 (mitozantrone) is an anthracycline derivative.
Epirubicin hydrochloride and mitoxantrone are considered less toxic than the other anthracycline antibiotics, and may be suitable for children who have received high cumulative doses of other anthracyclines.

Vinca alkaloids

The vinca alkaloids, vinblastine sulfate p. 511 and vincristine sulfate p. 511 are used to treat a variety of cancers including leukaemias, lymphomas, and some solid tumours.

Antimetabolites

Antimetabolites are incorporated into new nuclear material or they combine irreversibly with cellular enzymes and prevent normal cellular division. Cytarabine p. 504, fludarabine phosphate p. 505, mercaptopurine p. 505, methotrexate, and tioguanine p. 508 are commonly used in paediatric chemotherapy.

Other antineoplastic drugs

Asparaginase

Asparaginase is used almost exclusively in the treatment of acute lymphoblastic leukaemia. Hypersensitivity reactions may occur and facilities for the management of anaphylaxis should be available. A number of different preparations of asparaginase exist and only the product specified in the treatment protocol should be used.

ANTINEOPLASTIC DRUGS > ALKYLATING AGENTS

| Busulfan

(Busulphan)

● INDICATIONS AND DOSE

Conditioning treatment before haematopoietic progenitor cell transplantation
▸ BY MOUTH, OR BY INTRAVENOUS INFUSION
▸ **Child:** (consult local protocol)

DOSES AT EXTREMES OF BODY-WEIGHT
Dose may need to be calculated based on body surface area or adjusted ideal body weight in obese patients—consult product literature.

IMPORTANT SAFETY INFORMATION
RISKS OF INCORRECT DOSING OF ORAL ANTI-CANCER MEDICINES
See Cytotoxic drugs p. 494.

● **CAUTIONS** Avoid in Acute porphyrias p. 562 · high dose (antiepileptic prophylaxis required) · history of seizures (antiepileptic prophylaxis required) · ineffective once in blast crisis phase · previous progenitor cell transplant (increased risk of hepatic veno-occlusive disease) · previous radiation therapy (increased risk of hepatic veno-occlusive disease) · risk of second malignancy · three or more cycles of chemotherapy (increased risk of hepatic veno-occlusive disease)

● **INTERACTIONS** → Appendix 1 (busulfan).
● **SIDE-EFFECTS**
GENERAL SIDE-EFFECTS
▸ **Common or very common** Cardiac tamponade in thalassaemia · hepatic fibrosis · hepatic veno-occlusive disease · hepatotoxicity · hyperbilirubinaemia · jaundice · pneumonia · skin hyperpigmentation
▸ **Rare** Aplastic anaemia · erythema · hypersensitivity reactions · progressive pulmonary fibrosis · seizures · urticaria · visual disturbances
▸ **Very rare** Gynaecomastia · myasthenia gravis
▸ **Frequency not known** Alopecia · amenorrhoea (may be reversible) · bone-marrow suppression · dilutional hyponatraemia · fluid retention · gastro-intestinal effects · hyperuricaemia · irreversible bone-marrow aplasia · lung toxicity · male sterility · nausea · oedema · oral mucositis · organ-related toxicity (long-term and delayed) · premature menopause · secondary malignancy · thromboembolism · tumour lysis syndrome · vomiting
SPECIFIC SIDE-EFFECTS
▸ With intravenous use Extravasation
SIDE-EFFECTS, FURTHER INFORMATION
▸ Lung toxicity Discontinue if lung toxicity develops.
▸ Secondary malignancy Alkylating drugs are associated with a marked increase in the incidence of secondary tumours and leukaemia, particularly when they are combined with extensive irradiation.
▸ Fluid retention Alkylating drugs can cause fluid retention with oedema and dilutional hyponatraemia in younger children; the risk of this complication is higher in the first 2 days and also when given with concomitant vinca alkaloids.
● **CONCEPTION AND CONTRACEPTION** Manufacturers advise effective contraception during and for 6 months after treatment in men or women. See also *Pregnancy and reproductive function* in Cytotoxic drugs p. 494.
● **PREGNANCY** Avoid (teratogenic in *animals*). See also *Pregnancy and reproductive function* in Cytotoxic drugs p. 494.
● **BREAST FEEDING** Discontinue breast-feeding.
● **HEPATIC IMPAIRMENT** Manufacturer advises caution. In patients with hepatic impairment, manufacturer advises regular liver function tests—consult product literature.
● **MONITORING REQUIREMENTS**
▸ Monitor cardiac and liver function.
▸ Monitor full blood count regularly throughout treatment.

● **MEDICINAL FORMS**
There can be variation in the licensing of different medicines containing the same drug. Forms available from special-order manufacturers include: capsule, oral suspension, oral solution
Tablet
▸ Busulfan (Non-proprietary)
 Busulfan 2 mg Busulfan 2mg tablets | 25 tablet PoM £69.02
Solution for infusion
▸ Busilvex (Pierre Fabre Ltd)
 Busulfan 6 mg per 1 ml Busilvex 60mg/10ml concentrate for solution for infusion ampoules | 8 ampoule PoM £1,610.00 (Hospital only)

8

Immune system and malignant disease

Chlorambucil

- ● **INDICATIONS AND DOSE**

Hodgkin's disease | Non-Hodgkin's lymphoma
- ▶ BY MOUTH
- ▶ Child: (consult local protocol)

Relapsing steroid-sensitive nephrotic syndrome (initiated in specialist centres)
- ▶ BY MOUTH
- ▶ Child 3 months–17 years: 200 micrograms/kg daily for 8 weeks

- ● **UNLICENSED USE** Not licensed for use in nephrotic syndrome.

IMPORTANT SAFETY INFORMATION
RISKS OF INCORRECT DOSING OF ORAL ANTI-CANCER MEDICINES
See Cytotoxic drugs p. 494.

- ● **CAUTIONS** Avoid in Acute porphyrias p. 562 · children with nephrotic syndrome (increased seizure risk) · history of epilepsy (increased seizure risk)
- ● **SIDE-EFFECTS**
- ▶ **Uncommon** Skin rash
- ▶ **Rare** Hepatotoxicity · jaundice · seizures
- ▶ **Very rare** Irreversible bone-marrow suppression · male sterility (in prepubertal and pubertal males) · peripheral neuropathy · pulmonary fibrosis · sterile cystitis · tremor
- ▶ **Frequency not known** Alopecia · amenorrhoea · bone-marrow suppression · dilutional hyponatraemia · fluid retention · gastro-intestinal effects · hyperuricaemia · nausea · oedema · oral mucositis · organ-related toxicity (long-term and delayed) · premature menopause · secondary malignancy · Stevens-Johnson syndrome · thromboembolism · toxic epidermal necrolysis · tumour lysis syndrome · vomiting

SIDE-EFFECTS, FURTHER INFORMATION
- ▶ Secondary malignancy Alkylating drugs are associated with a marked increase in the incidence of secondary tumours and leukaemia, particularly when they are combined with extensive irradiation.
- ▶ Fluid retention Alkylating drugs can cause fluid retention with oedema and dilutional hyponatraemia in younger children; the risk of this complication is higher in the first 2 days and also when given with concomitant vinca alkaloids.

- ● **CONCEPTION AND CONTRACEPTION** Contraceptive advice required, see *Pregnancy and reproductive function* in Cytotoxic drugs p. 494.
- ● **PREGNANCY** Avoid. See also *Pregnancy and reproductive function* in Cytotoxic drugs p. 494.
- ● **BREAST FEEDING** Discontinue breast-feeding.
- ● **HEPATIC IMPAIRMENT** Manufacturer advises consider dose reduction in severe impairment—limited information available.
- ● **MONITORING REQUIREMENTS** Monitor full blood count regularly throughout treatment.
- ● **PATIENT AND CARER ADVICE**
Medicines for Children leaflet: Chlorambucil for nephrotic syndrome www.medicinesforchildren.org.uk/chlorambucil-nephrotic-syndrome-0

- ● **MEDICINAL FORMS**
There can be variation in the licensing of different medicines containing the same drug.

Tablet
- ▶ Chlorambucil (Non-proprietary)
  Chlorambucil 2 mg Chlorambucil 2mg tablets | 25 tablet PoM
  £42.87 DT price = £42.87

Cyclophosphamide

- ● **INDICATIONS AND DOSE**

Acute lymphoblastic leukaemia, non-Hodgkin's lymphoma, retinoblastoma, neuroblastoma, rhabdomyosarcoma, soft-tissue sarcomas, Ewing tumour, neuroectodermal tumours (including medulloblastoma), infant brain tumours, ependymona, high-dose conditioning for bone marrow transplantation, lupus nephritis
- ▶ BY MOUTH, OR BY INTRAVENOUS INFUSION
- ▶ Child: (consult local protocol)

Steroid-sensitive nephrotic syndrome
- ▶ BY MOUTH
- ▶ Child 3 months–17 years: 2–3 mg/kg daily for 8 weeks
- ▶ BY INTRAVENOUS INFUSION
- ▶ Child 3 months–17 years: 500 mg/m^2 once a month for 6 months

- ● **UNLICENSED USE** Not licensed for use in children.

IMPORTANT SAFETY INFORMATION
RISKS OF INCORRECT DOSING OF ORAL ANTI-CANCER MEDICINES
See Cytotoxic drugs p. 494.

- ● **CONTRA-INDICATIONS** Haemorrhagic cystitis
- ● **CAUTIONS** Avoid in Acute porphyrias p. 562 · diabetes mellitus · previous or concurrent mediastinal irradiation— risk of cardiotoxicity
- ● **INTERACTIONS** → Appendix 1 (cyclophosphamide).
- ● **SIDE-EFFECTS**
GENERAL SIDE-EFFECTS
- ▶ **Common or very common** Anorexia · cardiotoxicity at high doses · disturbances of carbohydrate metabolism · inappropriate secretion of anti-diuretic hormone · interstitial pulmonary fibrosis · pancreatitis · pigmentation of nails · pigmentation of palms · pigmentation of soles · urothelial toxicity
- ▶ **Rare** Hepatotoxicity · renal dysfunction
- ▶ **Frequency not known** Alopecia · amenorrhoea · bone-marrow suppression · dilutional hyponatraemia · fluid retention · gastro-intestinal effects · haemorrhagic cystitis · hyperuricaemia · male sterility · nausea · oedema · oral mucositis · organ-related toxicity (long-term and delayed) · premature menopause · secondary malignancy · thromboembolism · tumour lysis syndrome · vomiting
SPECIFIC SIDE-EFFECTS
- ▶ With intravenous use Extravasation
SIDE-EFFECTS, FURTHER INFORMATION
- ▶ Haemorrhagic cystitis and urothelial toxicity Haemorrhagic cystitis is a common manifestation of urothelial toxicity; adequate hydration is essential to reduce the risk of urothelial toxicity with intravenous use of cyclophosphamide; mesna provides further protection against urotoxic effects.
- ▶ Secondary malignancy Alkylating drugs are associated with a marked increase in the incidence of secondary tumours and leukaemia, particularly when they are combined with extensive irradiation.
- ▶ Fluid retention Alkylating drugs can cause fluid retention with oedema and dilutional hyponatraemia in younger children; the risk of this complication is higher in the first 2 days and also when given with concomitant vinca alkaloids.

- ● **CONCEPTION AND CONTRACEPTION** Manufacturer advises effective contraception during and for at least 3 months after treatment in men or women. See also *Pregnancy and reproductive function* in Cytotoxic drugs p. 494.
- ● **PREGNANCY** Avoid. See also *Pregnancy and reproductive function* in Cytotoxic drugs p. 494.

- **BREAST FEEDING** Discontinue breast-feeding during and for 36 hours after stopping treatment.
- **HEPATIC IMPAIRMENT** Reduce dose—consult local treatment protocol for details.
- **RENAL IMPAIRMENT** Reduce dose—consult local treatment protocol for details.
- **DIRECTIONS FOR ADMINISTRATION** Consult local treatment protocol for details.
- **PATIENT AND CARER ADVICE**
Medicines for Children leaflet: Cyclophosphamide for nephrotic syndrome www.medicinesforchildren.org.uk/cyclophosphamide-nephrotic-syndrome-0

- **MEDICINAL FORMS**
There can be variation in the licensing of different medicines containing the same drug. Forms available from special-order manufacturers include: tablet, oral suspension, oral solution, solution for injection, solution for infusion

Tablet
CAUTIONARY AND ADVISORY LABELS 25, 27
- Cyclophosphamide (Non-proprietary)
Cyclophosphamide (as Cyclophosphamide monohydrate)
50 mg Cyclophosphamide 50mg tablets | 100 tablet [PoM] £139.00
DT price = £139.00
- Cytoxan (Imported (United States))
Cyclophosphamide 25 mg Cytoxan 25mg tablets | 100 tablet [PoM] no price available

Powder for solution for injection
- Cyclophosphamide (Non-proprietary)
Cyclophosphamide (as Cyclophosphamide monohydrate)
500 mg Cyclophosphamide 500mg powder for solution for injection vials | 1 vial [PoM] £9.66-£9.95
Cyclophosphamide (as Cyclophosphamide monohydrate)
1 gram Cyclophosphamide 1g powder for solution for injection vials | 1 vial [PoM] £17.06-£18.47
Cyclophosphamide (as Cyclophosphamide monohydrate)
2 gram Cyclophosphamide 2g powder for solution for injection vials | 1 vial [PoM] £34.12

Dacarbazine

- **INDICATIONS AND DOSE**

Hodgkin's disease | Paediatric solid tumours
- BY INTRAVENOUS INJECTION, OR BY INTRAVENOUS INFUSION
- Child: (consult local protocol)

- **CAUTIONS** Caution in handling—irritant to tissues
- **INTERACTIONS** → Appendix 1 (dacarbazine).
- **SIDE-EFFECTS**
- **Common or very common** Anorexia
- **Uncommon** Blurred vision · confusion · facial flushing · facial paraesthesia · headache · influenza-like symptoms · rash · renal impairment · seizures
- **Rare** Diarrhoea · hepatic vein thrombosis · hepatotoxicity · injection-site reactions · irritant to skin · irritant to tissues · liver necrosis · photosensitivity
- **Frequency not known** Alopecia · bone-marrow suppression · extravasation · gastro-intestinal effects · hyperuricaemia · nausea · oral mucositis · organ-related toxicity (long-term and delayed) · thromboembolism · tumour lysis syndrome · vomiting
- **CONCEPTION AND CONTRACEPTION** Ensure effective contraception during and for at least 6 months after treatment in men or women. See also *Pregnancy and reproductive function* in Cytotoxic drugs p. 494.
- **PREGNANCY** Avoid (carcinogenic and teratogenic in *animal* studies). See also *Pregnancy and reproductive function* in Cytotoxic drugs p. 494.
- **BREAST FEEDING** Discontinue breast-feeding.
- **HEPATIC IMPAIRMENT** Dose reduction may be required in combined renal and hepatic impairment. Avoid in severe impairment.

- **RENAL IMPAIRMENT** Dose reduction may be required in combined renal and hepatic impairment. Avoid in severe impairment.
- **PRESCRIBING AND DISPENSING INFORMATION** Dacarbazine is a component of a commonly used combination for Hodgkin's disease (ABVD—doxorubicin [previously *Adriamycin ®*], bleomycin, vinblastine, and dacarbazine).

- **MEDICINAL FORMS**
There can be variation in the licensing of different medicines containing the same drug.
Powder for solution for injection
- Dacarbazine (Non-proprietary)
Dacarbazine (as Dacarbazine citrate) 100 mg Dacarbazine 100mg powder for solution for injection vials | 10 vial [PoM] £90.00
Dacarbazine (as Dacarbazine citrate) 200 mg Dacarbazine 200mg powder for solution for injection vials | 10 vial [PoM] £160.00
Powder for solution for infusion
- Dacarbazine (Non-proprietary)
Dacarbazine (as Dacarbazine citrate) 500 mg Dacarbazine 500mg powder for solution for infusion vials | 1 vial [PoM] £37.50
Dacarbazine (as Dacarbazine citrate) 1 gram Dacarbazine 1g powder for solution for infusion vials | 1 vial [PoM] £70.00

Ifosfamide

- **INDICATIONS AND DOSE**

Rhabdomyosarcoma | Soft-tissue sarcomas | Ewing tumour | Germ cell tumour | Osteogenic sarcoma
- BY INTRAVENOUS INFUSION
- Child: (consult local protocol)

- **CONTRA-INDICATIONS** Acute infection · urinary-tract infection · urinary-tract obstruction · urothelial damage
- **CAUTIONS** Avoid in Acute porphyrias p. 562
- **INTERACTIONS** → Appendix 1 (ifosfamide).
- **SIDE-EFFECTS**
- **Common or very common** Confusion · disorientation · drowsiness · psychosis · renal toxicity (may lead to tubular dysfunction, Fanconi's syndrome, or diabetes insipidus) · restlessness · urothelial toxicity causing haemorrhagic cystitis and dysuria
- **Uncommon** Severe encephalopathy
- **Rare** Anorexia · constipation · convulsions · diarrhoea
- **Very rare** Jaundice · syndrome of inappropriate antidiuretic hormone secretion · thrombophlebitis
- **Frequency not known** Alopecia · amenorrhoea · bone-marrow suppression · dilutional hyponatraemia · extravasation · fluid retention · gastro-intestinal effects · hyperuricaemia · male sterility · nausea · oedema · oral mucositis · organ-related toxicity (long-term and delayed) · premature menopause · secondary malignancy · thromboembolism · tumour lysis syndrome · vomiting
SIDE-EFFECTS, FURTHER INFORMATION
- Urothelial toxicity Adequate hydration may reduce the risk of urothelial toxicity with intravenous use of ifosfamide; mesna provides further protection against urotoxic effects.
- Secondary malignancy Alkylating drugs are associated with a marked increase in the incidence of secondary tumours and leukaemia, particularly when they are combined with extensive irradiation.
- Fluid retention Alkylating drugs can cause fluid retention with oedema and dilutional hyponatraemia in younger children; the risk of this complication is higher in the first 2 days and also when given with concomitant vinca alkaloids.
- **CONCEPTION AND CONTRACEPTION** Manufacturer advises adequate contraception during and for at least 6 months after treatment in men or women. See also *Pregnancy and reproductive function* in Cytotoxic drugs p. 494.

- **PREGNANCY** Avoid (teratogenic and carcinogenic in *animals*). See also *Pregnancy and reproductive function* in Cytotoxic drugs p. 494.
- **BREAST FEEDING** Discontinue breast-feeding.
- **HEPATIC IMPAIRMENT** Avoid.
- **RENAL IMPAIRMENT** Avoid.
- **MONITORING REQUIREMENTS** Ensure satisfactory electrolyte balance and renal function before each course (risk of tubular dysfunction, Fanconi's syndrome or diabetes insipidus if renal toxicity not treated promptly).

- **MEDICINAL FORMS**
  There can be variation in the licensing of different medicines containing the same drug.
  Powder for solution for injection
  ‣ Ifosfamide (Non-proprietary)
    Ifosfamide 1 gram Ifosfamide 1g powder for concentrate for solution for injection vials | 1 vial [PoM] £91.32
    Ifosfamide 2 gram Ifosfamide 2g powder for concentrate for solution for injection vials | 1 vial [PoM] £179.88

Melphalan

- **INDICATIONS AND DOSE**
  High intravenous dose with haematopoietic stem cell transplantation in the treatment of childhood neuroblastoma and some other advanced embryonal tumours
  ‣ BY INTRAVENOUS INFUSION
  ‣ Child: (consult local protocol)

- **UNLICENSED USE** Not licensed for use in embryonal tumours.
- **CAUTIONS** Avoid in Acute porphyrias p. 562 · consider use of prophylactic anti-infective agents · for high-dose intravenous administration establish adequate hydration · haematopoietic stem cell transplantation essential for high dose treatment (consult local treatment protocol for details)
- **INTERACTIONS** → Appendix 1 (melphalan).
- **SIDE-EFFECTS**
  ‣ **Rare** Interstitial pneumonitis · life threatening pulmonary fibrosis
  ‣ **Frequency not known** Alopecia · amenorrhoea · bone-marrow suppression (delayed) · dilutional hyponatraemia · extravasation · fluid retention · gastro-intestinal effects · hyperuricaemia · male sterility · nausea · oedema · oral mucositis · organ-related toxicity (long-term and delayed) · premature menopause · secondary malignancy · thromboembolism · tumour lysis syndrome · vomiting
  SIDE-EFFECTS, FURTHER INFORMATION
  ‣ Secondary malignancy Alkylating drugs are associated with a marked increase in the incidence of secondary tumours and leukaemia, particularly when they are combined with extensive irradiation.
  ‣ Fluid retention Alkylating drugs can cause fluid retention with oedema and dilutional hyponatraemia in younger children; the risk of this complication is higher in the first 2 days and also when given with concomitant vinca alkaloids.
- **CONCEPTION AND CONTRACEPTION** Manufacturer advises adequate contraception during treatment in men or women. See also *Pregnancy and reproductive function* in Cytotoxic drugs p. 494.
- **PREGNANCY** Avoid. See also *Pregnancy and reproductive function* in Cytotoxic drugs p. 494.
- **BREAST FEEDING** Discontinue breast-feeding.
- **RENAL IMPAIRMENT** Reduce dose initially (consult product literature).

- **MONITORING REQUIREMENTS** Monitor full blood count before and throughout treatment.

- **MEDICINAL FORMS**
  There can be variation in the licensing of different medicines containing the same drug.
  Powder and solvent for solution for injection
  ‣ Melphalan (Non-proprietary)
    Melphalan (as Melphalan hydrochloride) 50 mg Melphalan 50mg powder and solvent for solution for injection vials | 1 vial [PoM] £137.37

Temozolomide

- **DRUG ACTION** Temozolomide is structurally related to dacarbazine.

- **INDICATIONS AND DOSE**
  Treatment of recurrent or progressive malignant glioma
  ‣ BY MOUTH
  ‣ Child 3–17 years: (consult local protocol)

> IMPORTANT SAFETY INFORMATION
> RISKS OF INCORRECT DOSING OF ORAL ANTI-CANCER MEDICINES
> See Cytotoxic drugs p. 494.

- **CAUTIONS** *Pneumocystis jirovecii* pneumonia—consult product literature for monitoring and prophylaxis requirements
- **INTERACTIONS** → Appendix 1 (temozolomide).
- **SIDE-EFFECTS** Alopecia · bone-marrow suppression · gastro-intestinal effects · hyperuricaemia · nausea · oral mucositis · organ-related toxicity (long-term and delayed) · thromboembolism · tumour lysis syndrome · vomiting
  SIDE-EFFECTS, FURTHER INFORMATION
  For further information on side-effects consult product literature.
- **CONCEPTION AND CONTRACEPTION** Manufacturer advises adequate contraception during treatment. Men should avoid fathering a child during and for at least 6 months after treatment. See also *Pregnancy and reproductive function* in Cytotoxic drugs p. 494.
- **PREGNANCY** Avoid (teratogenic and embryotoxic in *animal* studies). See also *Pregnancy and reproductive function* in Cytotoxic drugs p. 494.
- **BREAST FEEDING** Discontinue breast-feeding.
- **HEPATIC IMPAIRMENT** Use with caution in severe impairment—no information available.
- **RENAL IMPAIRMENT** Manufacturer advises caution—no information available.
- **MONITORING REQUIREMENTS**
  ‣ Monitor liver function before treatment initiation, after each treatment cycle and midway through 42-day treatment cycles—consider the balance of benefits and risks of treatment if results are abnormal at any point (fatal liver injury reported).
  ‣ Monitor for myelodysplastic syndrome.
  ‣ Monitor for secondary malignancies.

- **MEDICINAL FORMS**
  There can be variation in the licensing of different medicines containing the same drug. Forms available from special-order manufacturers include: oral suspension
  Capsule
  CAUTIONARY AND ADVISORY LABELS 23, 25
  ‣ Temozolomide (Non-proprietary)
    Temozolomide 5 mg Temozolomide 5mg capsules | 5 capsule [PoM] £16.44 | 5 capsule [PoM] £17.30 (Hospital only)
    Temozolomide 20 mg Temozolomide 20mg capsules | 5 capsule [PoM] £67.88 | 5 capsule [PoM] £69.20 (Hospital only)
    Temozolomide 100 mg Temozolomide 100mg capsules | 5 capsule [PoM] £328.70 | 5 capsule [PoM] £346.00 (Hospital only)

Temozolomide 140 mg Temozolomide 140mg capsules |
5 capsule PoM £465.00 | 5 capsule PoM £484.49 (Hospital only)
Temozolomide 180 mg Temozolomide 180mg capsules |
5 capsule PoM £610.92 | 5 capsule PoM £622.80 (Hospital only)
Temozolomide 250 mg Temozolomide 250mg capsules |
5 capsule PoM £814.00 | 5 capsule PoM £865.00 (Hospital only)
▸ **Temodal** (Merck Sharp & Dohme Ltd)
Temozolomide 5 mg Temodal 5mg capsules | 5 capsule PoM
£10.59 (Hospital only)
Temozolomide 20 mg Temodal 20mg capsules | 5 capsule PoM
£42.35 (Hospital only)
Temozolomide 100 mg Temodal 100mg capsules | 5 capsule PoM
£211.77 (Hospital only)
Temozolomide 140 mg Temodal 140mg capsules | 5 capsule PoM
£296.48 (Hospital only)
Temozolomide 180 mg Temodal 180mg capsules | 5 capsule PoM
£381.19 (Hospital only)
Temozolomide 250 mg Temodal 250mg capsules | 5 capsule PoM
£529.43 (Hospital only)
▸ **Temomedac** (medac UK)
Temozolomide 5 mg Temomedac 5mg capsules | 5 capsule PoM
£16.12
Temozolomide 20 mg Temomedac 20mg capsules | 5 capsule PoM
£64.49
Temozolomide 100 mg Temomedac 100mg capsules |
5 capsule PoM £322.43
Temozolomide 140 mg Temomedac 140mg capsules |
5 capsule PoM £451.40
Temozolomide 180 mg Temomedac 180mg capsules |
5 capsule PoM £580.37
Temozolomide 250 mg Temomedac 250mg capsules |
5 capsule PoM £806.08

Thiotepa

- ● **INDICATIONS AND DOSE**
**Conditioning treatment before haematopoietic stem cell
transplantation in the treatment of haematological
disease or solid tumours, in combination with other
chemotherapy**
  ▸ BY INTRAVENOUS INFUSION
  ▸ **Child:** (consult local protocol)

- ● **CAUTIONS** Avoid in Acute porphyrias p. 562
- ● **INTERACTIONS** → Appendix 1 (thiotepa).
- ● **SIDE-EFFECTS** Alopecia · amenorrhoea · bone-marrow
suppression · dilutional hyponatraemia · extravasation ·
fluid retention · gastro-intestinal effects · hyperuricaemia ·
male sterility · nausea · oedema · oral mucositis · organ-
related toxicity (long-term and delayed) · premature
menopause · secondary malignancy · thromboembolism ·
tumour lysis syndrome · vomiting
  SIDE-EFFECTS, FURTHER INFORMATION
  ▸ Secondary malignancy Alkylating drugs are associated with a
marked increase in the incidence of secondary tumours
and leukaemia, particularly when they are combined with
extensive irradiation.
  ▸ Fluid retention Alkylating drugs can cause fluid retention
with oedema and dilutional hyponatraemia in younger
children; the risk of this complication is higher in the first
2 days and also when given with concomitant vinca
alkaloids.
- ● **CONCEPTION AND CONTRACEPTION** Contraceptive advice
required, see *Pregnancy and reproductive function* in
Cytotoxic drugs p. 494.
- ● **PREGNANCY** Avoid (teratogenic and embryotoxic in
animals). See also *Pregnancy and reproductive function* in
Cytotoxic drugs p. 494.
- ● **BREAST FEEDING** Discontinue breast-feeding.
- ● **NATIONAL FUNDING/ACCESS DECISIONS**
  Scottish Medicines Consortium (SMC) Decisions
  The *Scottish Medicines Consortium* has advised (June 2012)
that thiotepa (*Tepadina®*) is **not** recommended for use

within NHS Scotland in combination with other
chemotherapy as conditioning treatment in adults or
children with haematological diseases, or solid tumours
prior to haematopoietic stem cell transplantation.

- ● **MEDICINAL FORMS**
There can be variation in the licensing of different medicines
containing the same drug.
  Powder for solution for infusion
  ▸ **Tepadina** (Adienne Pharma & Biotech)
Thiotepa 15 mg Tepadina 15mg powder for concentrate for solution
for infusion vials | 1 vial PoM no price available
Thiotepa 100 mg Tepadina 100mg powder for concentrate for
solution for infusion vials | 1 vial PoM no price available

ANTINEOPLASTIC DRUGS › ANTHRACYCLINES AND RELATED DRUGS

Daunorubicin

- ● **INDICATIONS AND DOSE**
**Acute myelogenous leukaemia | Acute lymphocytic
leukaemia**
  ▸ BY INTRAVENOUS INFUSION
  ▸ **Child:** (consult local protocol)

- ● **UNLICENSED USE** *DaunoXome®* is not licensed for use in
children.
- ● **CONTRA-INDICATIONS** Myocardial insufficiency · previous
treatment with maximum cumulative doses of
daunorubicin or other anthracycline · recent myocardial
infarction · severe arrhythmia
  CONTRA-INDICATIONS, FURTHER INFORMATION
  Anthracycline antibiotics should not normally be used in
children with left ventricular dysfunction.
- ● **CAUTIONS** Caution in handling—irritant to tissues
- ● **INTERACTIONS** → Appendix 1 (daunorubicin).
Caution is necessary with concomitant use of cardiotoxic
drugs, or drugs that reduce cardiac contractility. Cardiac
function should be monitored closely on the concomitant
use of anthracyclines with trastuzumab.
- ● **SIDE-EFFECTS**
  ▸ **Common or very common** Leucopenia
  ▸ **Uncommon** Mucositis
  ▸ **Frequency not known** Alopecia · bone-marrow suppression
· cardiac toxicity (usually 1–6 months after initiation of
therapy) · extravasation · fever · gastro-intestinal effects ·
hyperuricaemia · nausea · oral mucositis · organ-related
toxicity (long-term and delayed) · red urine discolouration
· thromboembolism · tumour lysis syndrome · vomiting
  SIDE-EFFECTS, FURTHER INFORMATION
  ▸ Cardiotoxicity All anthracycline antibiotics have been
associated with varying degrees of cardiac toxicity—this
may be idiosyncratic and reversible, but is commonly
related to total cumulative dose and is irreversible
- ● **CONCEPTION AND CONTRACEPTION** Contraceptive advice
required, see *Pregnancy and reproductive function* in
Cytotoxic drugs p. 494.
- ● **PREGNANCY** Avoid (teratogenic and carcinogenic in
animal studies). See also *Pregnancy and reproductive
function* in Cytotoxic drugs p. 494.
- ● **BREAST FEEDING** Discontinue breast-feeding.
- ● **HEPATIC IMPAIRMENT** Reduce dose according to serum
bilirubin concentration—consult local protocol for details.
Avoid in severe impairment.
- ● **RENAL IMPAIRMENT** Reduce dose—consult local treatment
protocol for details. Avoid in severe impairment.

8

Immune system and malignant disease

- **MONITORING REQUIREMENTS**
- Cardiac monitoring essential.
- Cardiac function should be monitored before and at regular intervals throughout treatment and afterwards.

- **MEDICINAL FORMS**
There can be variation in the licensing of different medicines containing the same drug.
Powder for solution for infusion
- Daunorubicin (Non-proprietary)
  Daunorubicin (as Daunorubicin hydrochloride)
  20 mg Daunorubicin 20mg powder for solution for infusion vials | 10 vial [PoM] £650.00 (Hospital only)
Emulsion for infusion
- DaunoXome (Galen Ltd)
  Daunorubicin (as Daunorubicin hydrochloride citrate)
  50 mg DaunoXome 50mg emulsion for infusion vials | 1 vial [PoM] £250.00

Doxorubicin hydrochloride

10.6.2016

- **INDICATIONS AND DOSE**

Some paediatric malignancies | Ewing's sarcoma | Osteogenic sarcoma | Wilm's tumour | Neuroblastoma | Retinoblastoma | Some liver tumours | Acute lymphoblastic leukaemia | Hodgkin's lymphoma | Non-Hodgkin's lymphoma
  ▸ BY INTRAVENOUS INFUSION
- Child: (consult local protocol)

- **CONTRA-INDICATIONS** Acute inflammatory heart disease · consult product literature · increased haemorrhagic tendency · marked persisting myelosuppression induced by previous treatment · marked persisting stomatitis induced by previous treatment · previous myocardial infarction · previous treatment with maximum cumulative doses of doxorubicin · previous treatment with maximum cumulative doses of other anthracycline · severe arrhythmia · severe myocardial insufficiency
  CONTRA-INDICATIONS, FURTHER INFORMATION
  Anthracycline antibiotics should not normally be used in children with left ventricular dysfunction.

- **CAUTIONS** Caution in handling—irritant to tissues · consult product literature

- **INTERACTIONS** → Appendix 1 (doxorubicin). Caution is necessary with concomitant use of cardiotoxic drugs, or drugs that reduce cardiac contractility. Cardiac function should be monitored closely on the concomitant use of anthracyclines with trastuzumab.

- **SIDE-EFFECTS**
- **Common or very common** Red colouration of the urine
- **Frequency not known** Alopecia · bone-marrow suppression · consult product literature · extravasation · gastro-intestinal effects · hyperuricaemia · nausea · oral mucositis · organ-related toxicity (long-term and delayed) · thromboembolism · tumour lysis syndrome · vomiting
  SIDE-EFFECTS, FURTHER INFORMATION
- Extravasation Extravasation can cause severe tissue necrosis.
- Cardiotoxic All anthracycline antibiotics have been associated with varying degrees of cardiac toxicity—this may be idiosyncratic and reversible, but is commonly related to total cumulative dose and is irreversible.

- **CONCEPTION AND CONTRACEPTION** Manufacturer advises effective contraception during and for at least 6 months after treatment in men or women.

- **PREGNANCY** Avoid (teratogenic and toxic in *animal* studies). See also *Pregnancy and reproductive function* in Cytotoxic drugs p. 494.

- **BREAST FEEDING** Discontinue breast-feeding.

- **HEPATIC IMPAIRMENT** Reduce dose according to bilirubin concentration—consult product literature or local treatment protocol for details. Avoid in severe impairment.

- **RENAL IMPAIRMENT** Consult product literature in severe impairment.

- **MONITORING REQUIREMENTS** Cardiac function should be monitored before and at regular intervals throughout treatment and afterwards.

- **MEDICINAL FORMS**
There can be variation in the licensing of different medicines containing the same drug. Forms available from special-order manufacturers include: solution for infusion
Solution for injection
- Doxorubicin hydrochloride (Non-proprietary)
  Doxorubicin hydrochloride 2 mg per 1 ml Doxorubicin 10mg/5ml solution for injection vials | 1 vial [PoM] £18.54 (Hospital only)
  Doxorubicin 50mg/25ml solution for injection Cytosafe vials | 1 vial [PoM] £103.00
  Doxorubicin 50mg/25ml solution for infusion vials | 1 vial [PoM] £103.00 (Hospital only)
  Doxorubicin 10mg/5ml solution for injection Cytosafe vials | 1 vial [PoM] £20.60
  Doxorubicin 10mg/5ml concentrate for solution for infusion vials | 1 vial [PoM] no price available
  Doxorubicin 10mg/5ml solution for infusion vials | 1 vial [PoM] £20.60 (Hospital only)
  Doxorubicin 50mg/25ml solution for injection vials | 1 vial [PoM] £92.70 (Hospital only)
  Doxorubicin 50mg/25ml concentrate for solution for infusion vials | 1 vial [PoM] no price available
Powder for solution for injection
- Doxorubin (medac UK)
  Doxorubicin hydrochloride 10 mg Doxorubin 10mg powder for solution for injection vials | 10 vial [PoM] £182.80
  Doxorubicin hydrochloride 50 mg Doxorubin 50mg powder for solution for injection vials | 10 vial [PoM] £914.00
Solution for infusion
- Doxorubicin hydrochloride (Non-proprietary)
  Doxorubicin hydrochloride 2 mg per 1 ml Doxorubicin 200mg/100ml solution for injection Cytosafe vials | 1 vial [PoM] £412.00
  Doxorubicin 200mg/100ml solution for infusion vials | 1 vial [PoM] £370.80–£412.00 (Hospital only)
  Doxorubicin 200mg/100ml concentrate for solution for infusion vials | 1 vial [PoM] no price available
- Caelyx (Janssen-Cilag Ltd)
  Doxorubicin hydrochloride (as Doxorubicin hydrochloride liposomal pegylated) 2 mg per 1 ml Caelyx 50mg/25ml concentrate for solution for infusion vials | 1 vial [PoM] £712.49
  Caelyx 20mg/10ml concentrate for solution for infusion vials | 1 vial [PoM] £360.23
Powder and solvent for suspension for infusion
ELECTROLYTES: May contain Sodium
- Myocet (Teva UK Ltd)
  Doxorubicin hydrochloride 50 mg Myocet 50mg powder and solvent for suspension for infusion vials | 2 vial [PoM] £912.26 (Hospital only)

Epirubicin hydrochloride

- **INDICATIONS AND DOSE**

Recurrent acute lymphoblastic leukaemia | Rhabdomyosarcoma | Other soft-tissue tumours of childhood
  ▸ BY INTRAVENOUS INFUSION
- Child: (consult local protocol)

- **UNLICENSED USE** Not licensed for use in children.

- **CONTRA-INDICATIONS** Bladder inflammation or contraction (when used as a bladder instillation) · catheterisation difficulties (when used as a bladder instillation) · haematuria (when used as a bladder instillation) · invasive tumours penetrating the bladder (when used as a bladder instillation) · myocardiopathy ·

previous treatment with maximum cumulative doses of epirubicin or other anthracycline · recent myocardial infarction · severe arrhythmia · severe myocardial insufficiency · unstable angina · urinary tract infections (when used as a bladder instillation)

CONTRA-INDICATIONS, FURTHER INFORMATION
Anthracycline antibiotics should not normally be used in children with left ventricular dysfunction.

● CAUTIONS Caution in handling—irritant to tissues
● INTERACTIONS → Appendix 1 (epirubicin).
Caution is necessary with concomitant use of cardiotoxic drugs, or drugs that reduce cardiac contractility. Cardiac function should be monitored closely on the concomitant use of anthracyclines with trastuzumab.

● SIDE-EFFECTS Alopecia · anaphylaxis · bone-marrow suppression · cardiotoxicity · extravasation · gastro-intestinal effects · hyperuricaemia · nausea · oral mucositis · organ-related toxicity (long-term and delayed) · red colouration of the urine · thromboembolism · tumour lysis syndrome · vomiting

SIDE-EFFECTS, FURTHER INFORMATION
▸ Cardiotoxicity All anthracycline antibiotics have been associated with varying degrees of cardiac toxicity—this may be idiosyncratic and reversible, but is commonly related to total cumulative dose and is irreversible.
▸ Cumulative doses of other anthracycline Epirubicin is considered less toxic than other anthracyline antibiotics, and may be suitable for children who have received high cumulative doses of other anthracyclines.

● CONCEPTION AND CONTRACEPTION Contraceptive advice required, see *Pregnancy and reproductive function* in Cytotoxic drugs p. 494.
● PREGNANCY Avoid (carcinogenic in *animal* studies). See also *Pregnancy and reproductive function* in Cytotoxic drugs p. 494.
● BREAST FEEDING Discontinue breast-feeding.
● HEPATIC IMPAIRMENT Reduce dose according to bilirubin concentration—consult local treatment protocol for details. Avoid in severe impairment.
● RENAL IMPAIRMENT Dose reduction may be necessary in severe impairment.
● MONITORING REQUIREMENTS
▸ Cardiac toxicity Cardiac function should be monitored before and at regular intervals throughout treatment and afterwards.

● MEDICINAL FORMS
There can be variation in the licensing of different medicines containing the same drug. Forms available from special-order manufacturers include: solution for injection, solution for infusion

Solution for injection
▸ **Epirubicin hydrochloride** (Non-proprietary)
Epirubicin hydrochloride 2 mg per 1 ml Epirubicin 50mg/25ml solution for injection vials | 1 vial [PoM] £100.88
Epirubicin 10mg/5ml solution for injection vials | 1 vial [PoM] £21.24
▸ **Pharmorubicin** (Pfizer Ltd)
Epirubicin hydrochloride 2 mg per 1 ml Pharmorubicin 50mg/25ml solution for injection Cytosafe vials | 1 vial [PoM] £106.19
Pharmorubicin 10mg/5ml solution for injection Cytosafe vials | 1 vial [PoM] £21.24

Solution for infusion
▸ **Epirubicin hydrochloride** (Non-proprietary)
Epirubicin hydrochloride 2 mg per 1 ml Epirubicin 100mg/50ml solution for infusion vials | 1 vial [PoM] £169.92
Epirubicin 200mg/100ml solution for infusion vials | 1 vial [PoM] £386.16
▸ **Pharmorubicin** (Pfizer Ltd)
Epirubicin hydrochloride 2 mg per 1 ml Pharmorubicin 200mg/100ml solution for infusion Cytosafe vials | 1 vial [PoM] £386.16

Mitoxantrone
(Mitozantrone)

● **INDICATIONS AND DOSE**
Acute myeloid leukaemia | Recurrent acute lymphoblastic leukaemia
▸ BY INTRAVENOUS INFUSION
▸ Child: (consult local protocol)

● UNLICENSED USE Not licensed for use in children.
● CONTRA-INDICATIONS

CONTRA-INDICATIONS, FURTHER INFORMATION
Anthracycline antibiotics should not normally be used in children with left ventricular dysfunction.

● INTERACTIONS → Appendix 1 (mitoxantrone).
Caution is necessary with concomitant use of cardiotoxic drugs, or drugs that reduce cardiac contractility. Cardiac function should be monitored closely on the concomitant use of anthracyclines with trastuzumab.

● SIDE-EFFECTS
▸ **Common or very common** Transient blue-green discoloration of urine
▸ **Uncommon** Allergic reactions · amenorrhoea · anorexia · dyspnoea · fatigue · fever · gastro-intestinal bleeding · transient blue discoloration of nails · transient blue discoloration of skin
▸ **Frequency not known** Alopecia · bone-marrow suppression · dose-related cardiotoxicity · extravasation · gastro-intestinal effects · hyperuricaemia · myelosuppression · nausea · oral mucositis · organ-related toxicity (long-term and delayed) · thromboembolism · tumour lysis syndrome · vomiting

SIDE-EFFECTS, FURTHER INFORMATION
▸ Cardiotoxicity All anthracycline antibiotics have been associated with varying degrees of cardiac toxicity—this may be idiosyncratic and reversible, but is commonly related to total cumulative dose and is irreversible.

● CONCEPTION AND CONTRACEPTION Manufacturer advises effective contraception during and for at least 6 months after treatment in men or women.
● PREGNANCY Avoid. See also *Pregnancy and reproductive function* in Cytotoxic drugs p. 494.
● BREAST FEEDING Discontinue breast-feeding.
● HEPATIC IMPAIRMENT Use with caution—consult local treatment protocol.
● MONITORING REQUIREMENTS
▸ Cardiac toxicity Cardiac function should be monitored before and at regular intervals throughout treatment and afterwards.

● MEDICINAL FORMS
There can be variation in the licensing of different medicines containing the same drug.
Solution for infusion
▸ **Mitoxantrone** (Non-proprietary)
Mitoxantrone (as Mitoxantrone hydrochloride) 2 mg per 1 ml Mitoxantrone 20mg/10ml concentrate for solution for infusion vials | 1 vial [PoM] £121.85
▸ **Onkotrone** (Baxter Healthcare Ltd)
Mitoxantrone (as Mitoxantrone hydrochloride) 2 mg per 1 ml Onkotrone 20mg/10ml solution for infusion vials | 1 vial [PoM] no price available
Onkotrone 25mg/12.5ml solution for infusion vials | 1 vial [PoM] no price available

ANTINEOPLASTIC DRUGS › ANTIMETABOLITES

Clofarabine

- **INDICATIONS AND DOSE**
Relapsed or refractory acute lymphoblastic leukaemia in patients who have received at least two previous regimens
  - ▸ BY INTRAVENOUS INFUSION
  - ▸ Child 1-17 years: (consult local protocol)

- **UNLICENSED USE** Not licensed for use in children under 1 year.
- **CAUTIONS** Cardiac disease
- **SIDE-EFFECTS** Abdominal pain · agitation · alopecia · anxiety · arthralgia · bone-marrow suppression · cough · diarrhoea · dizziness · drowsiness · dyspnoea · extravasation · flushing · gastro-intestinal effects · haematoma · haematuria · hand-foot (desquamative) syndrome · headache · hyperuricaemia · hypotension · increased sweating · jaundice · myalgia · nausea · oedema · oral mucositis · organ-related toxicity (long-term and delayed) · pancreatitis · paraesthesia · pericardial effusion · peripheral neuropathy · pruritus · rash · restlessness · tachycardia · thromboembolism · tumour lysis syndrome · vomiting
- **CONCEPTION AND CONTRACEPTION** Contraceptive advice required, see *Pregnancy and reproductive function* in Cytotoxic drugs p. 494.
- **PREGNANCY** Manufacturer advises avoid (teratogenic in *animal* studies). See also *Pregnancy and reproductive function* in Cytotoxic drugs p. 494.
- **BREAST FEEDING** Discontinue breast-feeding.
- **HEPATIC IMPAIRMENT** Manufacturer advises caution in mild to moderate impairment. Avoid in severe impairment.
- **RENAL IMPAIRMENT** Manufacturer advises caution in mild to moderate impairment. Avoid in severe impairment.

- **MEDICINAL FORMS**
There can be variation in the licensing of different medicines containing the same drug.
Solution for infusion
ELECTROLYTES: May contain Sodium
  - ▸ Evoltra (Sanofi) ▼
  Clofarabine 1 mg per 1 ml Evoltra 20mg/20ml concentrate for solution for infusion vials | 4 vial PoM £5,304.72 (Hospital only)

Cytarabine

- **DRUG ACTION** Cytarabine acts by interfering with pyrimidine synthesis.

- **INDICATIONS AND DOSE**
Acute lymphoblastic leukaemia | Acute myeloid leukaemia | Non-Hodgkin's lymphoma
  - ▸ BY INTRAVENOUS INJECTION, OR BY INTRAVENOUS INFUSION, OR BY SUBCUTANEOUS INJECTION
  - ▸ Child: (consult local protocol)
Meningeal leukaemia | Meningeal neoplasms
  - ▸ BY INTRATHECAL INJECTION
  - ▸ Child: (consult local protocol)

- **UNLICENSED USE** *Depocyte* ® intrathecal injection not licensed for use in children.

IMPORTANT SAFETY INFORMATION
Not all cytarabine preparations can be given by intrathecal injection—consult product literature.

- **INTERACTIONS** → Appendix 1 (cytarabine).

- **SIDE-EFFECTS**
GENERAL SIDE-EFFECTS
- **Common or very common** Bone pain · maculopapular rash · myalgia
- **Uncommon** Conjunctivitis (consider prophylactic corticosteroid eye drops) · hepatic dysfunction · jaundice · neurotoxicity · renal dysfuncton
- **Frequency not known** Alopecia · bone-marrow suppression · chest pain · extravasation · gastro-intestinal effects · hyperuricaemia · nausea · oral mucositis · organ-related toxicity (long-term and delayed) · thromboembolism · tumour lysis syndrome · vomiting
SPECIFIC SIDE-EFFECTS
- **Common or very common**
  - ▸ With intravenous use 'cytarabine syndrome' (6–12 hours after intravenous administration—characterised by fever and malaise)
- **Rare**
  - ▸ With intrathecal use Severe spinal cord toxicity following intrathecal administration

- **CONCEPTION AND CONTRACEPTION** Contraceptive advice required, see *Pregnancy and reproductive function* in Cytotoxic drugs p. 494.
- **PREGNANCY** Avoid (teratogenic in *animal* studies). See also *Pregnancy and reproductive function* in Cytotoxic drugs p. 494.
- **BREAST FEEDING** Discontinue breast-feeding.
- **HEPATIC IMPAIRMENT** Reduce dose—consult product literature.
- **RENAL IMPAIRMENT** Consult local treatment protocols.
- **MONITORING REQUIREMENTS**
- Haematological monitoring Cytarabine is a potent myelosuppressant and requires careful haematological monitoring.
- **PRESCRIBING AND DISPENSING INFORMATION** Dose is based on weight or body-surface area, children may tolerate higher doses of cytarabine than adults.
- **NATIONAL FUNDING/ACCESS DECISIONS**
DEPOCYTE®
Scottish Medicines Consortium (SMC) Decisions
The *Scottish Medicines Consortium* has advised (July 2007) that liposomal cytarabine suspension (*DepoCyte* ®) is not recommended for use within NHS Scotland for the intrathecal treatment of lymphomatous meningitis.

- **MEDICINAL FORMS**
There can be variation in the licensing of different medicines containing the same drug. Forms available from special-order manufacturers include: solution for injection
Solution for injection
  - ▸ Cytarabine (Non-proprietary)
  Cytarabine 20 mg per 1 ml Cytarabine 500mg/25ml solution for injection vials | 1 vial PoM £19.50
  Cytarabine 100mg/5ml solution for injection vials | 5 vial PoM £20.98–£30.00
  Cytarabine 100 mg per 1 ml Cytarabine 500mg/5ml solution for injection vials | 5 vial PoM £100.00
  Cytarabine 100mg/1ml solution for injection vials | 5 vial PoM £30.00
  Cytarabine 2g/20ml solution for injection vials | 1 vial PoM £79.00
  Cytarabine 1g/10ml solution for injection vials | 1 vial PoM £40.00
Suspension for injection
  - ▸ DepoCyte (Napp Pharmaceuticals Ltd)
  Cytarabine 10 mg per 1 ml DepoCyte 50mg/5ml suspension for injection vials | 1 vial PoM £1,223.75 (Hospital only)

Fludarabine phosphate

● **INDICATIONS AND DOSE**

Poor prognosis or relapsed acute myeloid leukaemia | Relapsed acute lymphoblastic leukaemia | Conditioning before bone marrow transplantation

▸ BY MOUTH, OR BY INTRAVENOUS INJECTION, OR BY INTRAVENOUS INFUSION

▸ Child: (consult local protocol)

● **UNLICENSED USE** Not licensed for use in children.

> **IMPORTANT SAFETY INFORMATION**
> RISKS OF INCORRECT DOSING OF ORAL ANTI-CANCER MEDICINES
> See Cytotoxic drugs p. 494.

● **CONTRA-INDICATIONS** Haemolytic anaemia

● **CAUTIONS** Increased susceptibility to skin cancer · worsening of existing skin cancer

CAUTIONS, FURTHER INFORMATION

▸ Immunosuppression Fludarabine has a potent and prolonged immunosuppresive effect. Patients treated with fludarabine are more prone to serious bacterial, opportunistic fungal, and viral infections, and prophylactic therapy is recommended in those at risk. To prevent potentially fatal transfusion-related graft-versus-host reaction, only irradiated blood products should be administered. Prescribers should consult specialist literature when using highly immunosuppressive drugs.

● **INTERACTIONS** → Appendix 1 (fludarabine).

● **SIDE-EFFECTS**

▸ **Common or very common** Acute myeloid leukaemia · anorexia · chills · cough · diarrhoea · fever · immunosuppression · malaise · myelodysplastic syndrome · myelosupression (may be cumulative) · oedema · peripheral neuropathy · pneumonia · rash · visual disturbances · weakness

▸ **Uncommon** Autoimmune disorder · confusion · fibrosis · haemorrhage · pneumonitis · pulmonary toxicity

▸ **Rare** Agitation · arrhythmia · blindness · coma · heart failure · optic neuropathy · seizures · skin cancer · Stevens-Johnson syndrome · toxic epidermal necrolysis

▸ **Frequency not known** Alopecia · bone-marrow suppression · extravasation · gastro-intestinal effects · haemorrhagic cystitis · hyperuricaemia · nausea · oral mucositis · organ-related toxicity (long-term and delayed) · thromboembolism · tumour lysis syndrome · vomiting

● **CONCEPTION AND CONTRACEPTION** Manufacturer advises effective contraception during and for at least 6 months after treatment in men or women.

● **PREGNANCY** Avoid (embryotoxic and teratogenic in *animal* studies). See also *Pregnancy and reproductive function* in Cytotoxic drugs p. 494.

● **BREAST FEEDING** Discontinue breast-feeding.

● **RENAL IMPAIRMENT** Reduce dose by up to 50% if creatinine clearance 30–70 mL/minute/1.73 m^2. Avoid if creatinine clearance less than 30 mL/minute/1.73 m^2.

● **MONITORING REQUIREMENTS**

▸ Monitor for signs of haemolysis.

▸ Monitor for neurological toxicity.

● **DIRECTIONS FOR ADMINISTRATION** Concentrate for intravenous injection or infusion must be diluted before administration (consult product literature).

● **MEDICINAL FORMS**

There can be variation in the licensing of different medicines containing the same drug.

Tablet

▸ Fludara (Sanofi)

Fludarabine phosphate 10 mg Fludara 10mg tablets | 15 tablet [PoM] £302.48 (Hospital only) | 20 tablet [PoM] £403.31 (Hospital only)

Solution for injection

▸ Fludarabine phosphate (Non-proprietary)

Fludarabine phosphate 25 mg per 1 ml Fludarabine phosphate 50mg/2ml solution for injection vials | 1 vial [PoM] £117.75
Fludarabine phosphate 50mg/2ml concentrate for solution for injection vials | 1 vial [PoM] £156.00 (Hospital only) | 1 vial [PoM] £155.00

Powder for solution for injection

▸ Fludarabine phosphate (Non-proprietary)

Fludarabine phosphate 50 mg Fludarabine phosphate 50mg powder for solution for injection vials | 1 vial [PoM] £155.00 (Hospital only) | 1 vial [PoM] £155.00 | 5 vial [PoM] £735.35 (Hospital only)

▸ Fludara (Sanofi)

Fludarabine phosphate 50 mg Fludara 50mg powder for solution for injection vials | 5 vial [PoM] £735.34 (Hospital only)

Mercaptopurine

(6-Mercaptopurine)

● **INDICATIONS AND DOSE**

Severe ulcerative colitis | Severe Crohn's disease

▸ BY MOUTH

▸ Child 2–17 years: Initially 1–1.5 mg/kg once daily (max. per dose 50 mg), then increased if necessary up to 75 mg once daily

Acute lymphoblastic leukaemia | Lymphoblastic lymphomas

▸ BY MOUTH

▸ Child: (consult local protocol)

DOSE EQUIVALENCE AND CONVERSION

Mercaptopurine tablets and *Xaluprine*® oral suspension are **not** bioequivalent, haematological monitoring is advised when switching formulations.

● **UNLICENSED USE** Not licensed for use in severe ulcerative colitis and Crohn's disease.

Not licensed for use in children for acute lymphoblastic lymphoma or T-cell non-Hodgkins lymphoma.

> **IMPORTANT SAFETY INFORMATION**
> RISKS OF INCORRECT DOSING OF ORAL ANTI-CANCER MEDICINES
> See Cytotoxic drugs p. 494.

● **CONTRA-INDICATIONS** Absent thiopurine methyltransferase activity

● **CAUTIONS** Reduced thiopurine methyltransferase activity

CAUTIONS, FURTHER INFORMATION

▸ Thiopurine methyltransferase The enzyme thiopurine methyltransferase (TPMT) metabolises thiopurine drugs (azathioprine, mercaptopurine, tioguanine); the risk of myelosuppression is increased in patients with reduced activity of the enzyme, particularly for the few individuals in whom TPMT activity is undetectable. Patients with absent TPMT activity should not receive thiopurine drugs; those with reduced TPMT activity may be treated under specialist supervision.

● **INTERACTIONS** → Appendix 1 (mercaptopurine).

● **SIDE-EFFECTS**

▸ **Rare** Crystalluria with haematuria · fever · hyperpigmentation · intestinal ulceration · pancreatitis · rash

▸ **Very rare** Lymphoma

▸ **Frequency not known** Alopecia · bone-marrow suppression · gastro-intestinal effects · hepatotoxicity (more frequent at higher doses) · hyperuricaemia · nausea · oral mucositis · organ-related toxicity (long-term and delayed) · thromboembolism · tumour lysis syndrome · vomiting

SIDE-EFFECTS, FURTHER INFORMATION

▸ **Gastro-intestinal side-effects** Tioguanine has a lower incidence of gastrointestinal side-effects than mercaptopurine.

● **CONCEPTION AND CONTRACEPTION** Contraceptive advice required, see *Pregnancy and reproductive function* in Cytotoxic drugs p. 494.

● **PREGNANCY** Avoid (teratogenic). See also *Pregnancy and reproductive function* in Cytotoxic drugs p. 494.

● **BREAST FEEDING** Discontinue breast-feeding.

● **HEPATIC IMPAIRMENT** May need dose reduction.

● **RENAL IMPAIRMENT** Manufacturer advises consider reducing dose.

● **PRE-TREATMENT SCREENING** Consider measuring thiopurine methyltransferase (TPMT) activity before starting mercaptopurine therapy.

● **MONITORING REQUIREMENTS**

▸ Monitor liver function—discontinue if jaundice develops.

▸ When used for Severe ulcerative colitis or Severe Crohn's disease Monitor for toxicity throughout treatment. Monitor full blood count weekly (more frequently with higher doses or if severe hepatic or renal impairment) for first 4 weeks (manufacturer advises weekly monitoring for 8 weeks but evidence of practical value unsatisfactory), thereafter reduce frequency of monitoring to at least every 3 months.

● **PRESCRIBING AND DISPENSING INFORMATION** Flavours of oral liquid formulations may include raspberry.

● **MEDICINAL FORMS**
There can be variation in the licensing of different medicines containing the same drug. Forms available from special-order manufacturers include: tablet, capsule, oral suspension

Tablet

▸ Mercaptopurine (Non-proprietary)
Mercaptopurine 50 mg Mercaptopurine 50mg tablets | 25 tablet PoM £49.15 DT price = £49.15

Oral suspension
EXCIPIENTS: May contain Aspartame

▸ Xaluprine (Nova Laboratories Ltd)
Mercaptopurine 20 mg per 1 ml Xaluprine 20mg/ml oral suspension | 100 ml PoM £170.00

Methotrexate

● **DRUG ACTION** Methotrexate inhibits the enzyme dihydrofolate reductase, essential for the synthesis of purines and pyrimidines.

● **INDICATIONS AND DOSE**

Severe Crohn's disease

▸ BY SUBCUTANEOUS INJECTION, OR BY INTRAMUSCULAR INJECTION

▸ Child 7-17 years: 15 mg/m^2 once weekly (max. per dose 25 mg)

Maintenance of remission of severe Crohn's disease

▸ BY MOUTH, OR BY SUBCUTANEOUS INJECTION, OR BY INTRAMUSCULAR INJECTION

▸ Child 7-17 years: 15 mg/m^2 once weekly (max. per dose 25 mg), dose reduced according to response to lowest effective dose

Juvenile idiopathic arthritis | Juvenile dermatomyositis | Vasculitis | Uveitis | Systemic lupus erythematosus | Localised scleroderma | Sarcoidosis

▸ BY MOUTH, OR BY SUBCUTANEOUS INJECTION, OR BY INTRAMUSCULAR INJECTION

▸ Child: Initially 10–15 mg/m^2 once weekly, then increased if necessary up to 25 mg/m^2 once weekly

Maintenance and remission of acute lymphoblastic leukaemia, lymphoblastic lymphoma

▸ BY MOUTH

▸ Child: (consult local protocol)

Treatment of early stage Burkitt's lymphoma, non-Hodgkin's lymphoma, osteogenic sarcoma, some CNS tumours including infant brain tumours, acute lymphoblastic leukaemia

▸ BY INTRAVENOUS INJECTION, OR BY INTRAVENOUS INFUSION

▸ Child: (consult local protocol)

Meningeal leukaemia, treatment and prevention of CNS involvement of leukaemia

▸ BY INTRATHECAL INJECTION

▸ Child: (consult local protocol)

Severe psoriasis unresponsive to conventional therapy (specialist use only)

▸ BY MOUTH

▸ Child 2-17 years: Initially 200 micrograms/kg once weekly (max. per dose 10 mg), then increased if necessary to 400 micrograms/kg once weekly (max. per dose 25 mg), adjusted according to response, stop treatment if inadequate response after 3 months at the optimum dose

● **UNLICENSED USE** *Metoject*® is licensed for use in children over 3 years for polyarticular forms of juvenile idiopathic arthritis; other preparations not licensed for use in children for non-malignant conditions.

> **IMPORTANT SAFETY INFORMATION**
> Note that the dose is a **weekly** dose. To avoid error with low-dose methotrexate, it is recommended that:
> - the child or their carer is carefully advised of the **dose** and **frequency** and the reason for taking methotrexate and any other prescribed medication (e.g. folic acid);
> - only one strength of methotrexate tablet (usually 2.5 mg) is prescribed and dispensed;
> - the prescription and the dispensing label clearly show the dose and frequency of methotrexate administration;
> - the child or their carer is warned to report immediately the onset of any feature of blood disorders (e.g. sore throat, bruising, and mouth ulcers), liver toxicity (e.g. nausea, vomiting, abdominal discomfort, and dark urine), and respiratory effects (e.g. shortness of breath).

● **CONTRA-INDICATIONS** Active infection (in non-malignant conditions) · ascites · immunodeficiency syndromes (in non-malignant conditions) · significant pleural effusion

● **CAUTIONS** Acute porphyrias p. 562 · photosensitivity—psoriasis lesions aggravated by UV radiation (skin ulceration reported) · diarrhoea · extreme caution in blood disorders (avoid if severe) · peptic ulceration · risk of accumulation in pleural effusion or ascites—drain before treatment · ulcerative colitis · ulcerative stomatitis

CAUTIONS, FURTHER INFORMATION

▸ **Blood count** Bone marrow suppression can occur abruptly; factors likely to increase toxicity include advanced age, renal impairment, and concomitant use with another anti-folate drug (e.g. trimethoprim). A clinically significant drop in white cell count or platelet count calls for immediate withdrawal of methotrexate and introduction of supportive therapy.

- Gastro-intestinal toxicity Withdraw treatment if stomatitis develops—may be first sign of gastro-intestinal toxicity.
- Liver toxicity Persistent 2–fold rise in liver transaminases may necessitate dose reduction or rarely discontinuation; abrupt withdrawal should be avoided as this can lead to disease flare.
- Pulmonary toxicity Acute pulmonary toxicity is rare in children treated for juvenile idiopathic arthritis, but children and carers should seek medical attention if dyspnoea, cough or fever develops; discontinue if pneumonitis suspected.

● INTERACTIONS → Appendix 1 (methotrexate).
If aspirin or other NSAIDs are given concurrently the dose of methotrexate should be carefully monitored.

● SIDE-EFFECTS
▶ Rare Pneumonitis
▶ Frequency not known Abdominal discomfort · abnormal cranial sensations · acne · alopecia · anaphylactic reactions · anorexia · arthralgia · blepharitis · blood dyscrasias (including fatalities) · cerebral oedema · changes in nail pigmentation · changes in skin pigmentation · chills · chronic pulmonary fibrosis · confusion · conjunctivitis · cystitis · diarrhoea · dizziness · drowsiness · dyspepsia · dysuria · ecchymosis · fever · furunculosis · gastro-intestinal bleeding · gastro-intestinal ulceration · haematuria · headache · hepatotoxicity · hypotension · impotence · injection-site reactions · insomnia · interstitial pneumonitis · liver cirrhosis · malaise · menstrual disturbances · mood changes · mucositis · myalgia · myelosuppression · nausea · neurotoxicity · osteoporosis · paraesthesia · pericardial tamponade · pericarditis · photosensitivity · pleuritic pain · precipitation of diabetes · pruritus · psychosis · pulmonary fibrosis · pulmonary oedema · rash · reduced libido · renal failure · Stevens-Johnson syndrome · telangiectasia · thrombosis · toxic epidermal necrolysis · toxic megacolon · urticaria · vaginitis · vasculitis · visual disturbance · vomiting

SIDE-EFFECTS, FURTHER INFORMATION
In patients taking methotrexate for non-malignant conditions who experience side-effects, folic acid given on a different day from the methotrexate, may help to reduce the frequency of such side-effects.

Withdraw treatment if stomatitis develops—may be first sign of gastro-intestinal toxicity.

Treatment with folinic acid (as calcium folinate) may be required in acute toxicity.

● CONCEPTION AND CONTRACEPTION Effective contraception required during and for at least 3 months after treatment in men or women.

● PREGNANCY Avoid (teratogenic; fertility may be reduced during therapy but this may be reversible).

● BREAST FEEDING Discontinue breast-feeding—present in milk.

● HEPATIC IMPAIRMENT When used for malignancy, avoid in severe hepatic impairment—consult local treatment protocol for details. Avoid with hepatic impairment in non-malignant conditions—dose-related toxicity.

● RENAL IMPAIRMENT Reduce dose. Risk of nephrotoxicity at high doses. Avoid in severe impairment.

● PRE-TREATMENT SCREENING Exclude pregnancy before treatment.
Patients should have full blood count and renal and liver function tests before starting treatment.
Check immunity to varicella-zoster and consider vaccination before initiating therapy.

● MONITORING REQUIREMENTS Full blood count and liver function tests repeated fortnightly for at least the first 4 weeks of treatment and at this frequency after any change in dose until therapy stabilised, thereafter

monthly; renal function tests should be performed regularly during treatment.

● PRESCRIBING AND DISPENSING INFORMATION Folinic acid following methotrexate administration helps to prevent methotrexate-induced mucositis and myelosuppression.

● PATIENT AND CARER ADVICE
Patients and their carers should be warned to report immediately the onset of any feature of blood disorders (e.g. sore throat, bruising, and mouth ulcers), liver toxicity (e.g. nausea, vomiting, abdominal discomfort and dark urine), and respiratory effects (e.g. shortness of breath).
Children and carers should be advised to avoid self-medication with over-the-counter ibuprofen
Children and their carers should be counselled on the dose and use of NSAIDs.

Medicines for Children leaflet: Methotrexate for skin conditions www.medicinesforchildren.org.uk/methotrexate-for-skin-conditions

● MEDICINAL FORMS
There can be variation in the licensing of different medicines containing the same drug. Forms available from special-order manufacturers include: oral suspension, oral solution, solution for injection

Tablet
▶ **Methotrexate** (Non-proprietary)
Methotrexate 2.5 mg Methotrexate 2.5mg tablets | 24 tablet [PoM] £3.75 | 28 tablet [PoM] £3.82 DT price = £1.97 | 100 tablet [PoM] £14.19
Methotrexate 10 mg Methotrexate 10mg tablets | 100 tablet [PoM] £57.21 DT price = £37.75
▶ Maxtrex (Pfizer Ltd)
Methotrexate 2.5 mg Maxtrex 2.5mg tablets | 24 tablet [PoM] £2.39 | 100 tablet [PoM] £9.96
Methotrexate 10 mg Maxtrex 10mg tablets | 100 tablet [PoM] £45.16 DT price = £37.75

Oral solution
▶ **Methotrexate** (Non-proprietary)
Methotrexate (as Methotrexate sodium) 2 mg per
1 ml Methotrexate 2mg/ml oral solution sugar free sugar-free | 35 ml [PoM] £95.00-£114.00 DT price = £95.00 sugar-free | 65 ml [PoM] £125.00-£150.00 DT price = £125.00

Solution for injection
▶ **Methotrexate** (Non-proprietary)
Methotrexate (as Methotrexate sodium) 2.5 mg per
1 ml Methotrexate 5mg/2ml solution for injection vials | 5 vial [PoM] £30.00
Methotrexate (as Methotrexate sodium) 25 mg per
1 ml Methotrexate 1g/40ml solution for injection vials | 1 vial [PoM] £43.68 (Hospital only) | 1 vial [PoM] £44.57-£67.50
Methotrexate 500mg/20ml solution for injection vials | 1 vial [PoM] £38.30 (Hospital only) | 1 vial [PoM] £22.56-£48.00
Methotrexate 50mg/2ml solution for injection vials | 1 vial [PoM] £4.49 (Hospital only) | 1 vial [PoM] £3.00 | 5 vial [PoM] £35.00
Methotrexate 200mg/8ml solution for injection vials | 1 vial [PoM] £10.02
Methotrexate (as Methotrexate sodium) 100 mg per
1 ml Methotrexate 1g/10ml solution for injection vials | 1 vial [PoM] £85.00
▶ Metoject PEN (medac UK)
Methotrexate 50 mg per 1 ml Metoject PEN 30mg/0.6ml solution for injection pre-filled pen | 1 pre-filled disposable injection [PoM] £18.95
Metoject PEN 22.5mg/0.45ml solution for injection pre-filled pen | 1 pre-filled disposable injection [PoM] £18.45
Metoject PEN 12.5mg/0.25ml solution for injection pre-filled pen | 1 pre-filled disposable injection [PoM] £16.50
Metoject PEN 20mg/0.4ml solution for injection pre-filled pen | 1 pre-filled disposable injection [PoM] £17.84
Metoject PEN 17.5mg/0.35ml solution for injection pre-filled pen | 1 pre-filled disposable injection [PoM] £17.50
Metoject PEN 7.5mg/0.15ml solution for injection pre-filled pen | 1 pre-filled disposable injection [PoM] £14.85
Metoject PEN 10mg/0.2ml solution for injection pre-filled pen | 1 pre-filled disposable injection [PoM] £15.29
Metoject PEN 27.5mg/0.55ml solution for injection pre-filled pen | 1 pre-filled disposable injection [PoM] £18.89
Metoject PEN 25mg/0.5ml solution for injection pre-filled pen | 1 pre-filled disposable injection [PoM] £18.48

8

Immune system and malignant disease

Metoject PEN 15mg/0.3ml solution for injection pre-filled pen | 1 pre-filled disposable injection [PoM] £16.57

▸ **Zlatal** (Nordic Pharma Ltd)

Methotrexate (as Methotrexate sodium) 25 mg per 1 ml Zlatal 17.5mg/0.7ml solution for injection pre-filled syringes | 1 pre-filled disposable injection [PoM] £15.75

Zlatal 10mg/0.4ml solution for injection pre-filled syringes | 1 pre-filled disposable injection [PoM] £13.77

Zlatal 25mg/1ml solution for injection pre-filled syringes | 1 pre-filled disposable injection [PoM] £16.64

Zlatal 20mg/0.8ml solution for injection pre-filled syringes | 1 pre-filled disposable injection [PoM] £16.06

Zlatal 12.5mg/0.5ml solution for injection pre-filled syringes | 1 pre-filled disposable injection [PoM] £14.85

Zlatal 7.5mg/0.3ml solution for injection pre-filled syringes | 1 pre-filled disposable injection [PoM] £13.37

Zlatal 22.5mg/0.9ml solution for injection pre-filled syringes | 1 pre-filled disposable injection [PoM] £16.61

Zlatal 15mg/0.6ml solution for injection pre-filled syringes | 1 pre-filled disposable injection [PoM] £14.92

Solution for infusion

▸ **Methotrexate** (Non-proprietary)

Methotrexate (as Methotrexate sodium) 25 mg per 1 ml Methotrexate 5g/200ml solution for infusion vials | 1 vial [PoM] £200.57

Methotrexate (as Methotrexate sodium) 100 mg per 1 ml Methotrexate 5g/50ml solution for infusion vials | 1 vial [PoM] £400.00

Nelarabine

● **INDICATIONS AND DOSE**

T-cell acute lymphoblastic leukaemia and T-cell lymphoblastic lymphoma in children who have relapsed or who are refractory after receiving at least two previous regimens

▸ BY INTRAVENOUS INFUSION

▸ Child: (consult local protocol)

● **CAUTIONS** Previous or concurrent craniospinal irradiation (increased risk of neurotoxicity) · previous or concurrent intrathecal chemotherapy (increased risk of neurotoxicity)

● **SIDE-EFFECTS**

▸ **Common or very common** Neurotoxicity (discontinue)

▸ **Frequency not known** Alopecia · arthralgia · asthenia · ataxia · benign and malignant tumours · bone-marrow suppression · confusion · constipation · demyelination · diarrhoea · drowsiness · electrolyte disturbances · extravasation · fatigue · gastro-intestinal effects · headache · hyperuricaemia · hypoaesthesia · hypoglycaemia · nausea · oral mucositis · organ-related toxicity (long-term and delayed) · paraesthesia · peripheral neurological disorders · pyrexia · seizures · thromboembolism · tremor · tumour lysis syndrome · vomiting

● **CONCEPTION AND CONTRACEPTION** Manufacturer advises effective contraception during and for at least 3 months after treatment in men and women.

● **PREGNANCY** Avoid (toxicity in *animal* studies). See also *Pregnancy and reproductive function* in Cytotoxic drugs p. 494.

● **BREAST FEEDING** Discontinue breast-feeding.

● **MONITORING REQUIREMENTS**

▸ Neurotoxicity Close monitoring for neurological events is strongly recommended—discontinue if neurotoxicty occurs.

● **PATIENT AND CARER ADVICE**

Driving and skilled tasks

Drowsiness may affect performance of skilled tasks (e.g. cycling or driving).

● **MEDICINAL FORMS**

There can be variation in the licensing of different medicines containing the same drug.

Solution for infusion

ELECTROLYTES: May contain Sodium

▸ **Atriance** (Novartis Pharmaceuticals UK Ltd) ▼

Nelarabine 5 mg per 1 ml Atriance 250mg/50ml solution for infusion vials | 6 vial [PoM] £1,332.00

Tioguanine

(Thioguanine)

● **INDICATIONS AND DOSE**

Infant acute lymphoblastic leukaemia

▸ BY MOUTH

▸ Child: Can be given at various stages of treatment in short-term cycles (consult local protocol)

IMPORTANT SAFETY INFORMATION

RISKS OF INCORRECT DOSING OF ORAL ANTI-CANCER MEDICINES
See Cytotoxic drugs p. 494.

● **CONTRA-INDICATIONS** Absent thiopurine methyltransferase activity

● **CAUTIONS** Thiopurine methyltransferase status

CAUTIONS, FURTHER INFORMATION

▸ Thiopurine methyltransferase The enzyme thiopurine methyltransferase (TPMT) metabolises thiopurine drugs (azathioprine, mercaptopurine, tioguanine); the risk of myelosuppression is increased in patients with reduced activity of the enzyme, particularly for the few individuals in whom TPMT activity is undetectable. Patients with absent TPMT activity should not receive thiopurine drugs; those with reduced TPMT activity may be treated under specialist supervision.

▸ Long-term therapy Long-term therapy is no longer recommended because of the high risk of liver toxicity.

● **INTERACTIONS** → Appendix 1 (tioguanine).

● **SIDE-EFFECTS**

▸ **Rare** Intestinal necrosis · intestinal perforation

▸ **Frequency not known** Alopecia · bone-marrow suppression · gastro-intestinal effects · hepatotoxicity (discontinue) · hyperuricaemia · nausea · oral mucositis · organ-related toxicity (long-term and delayed) · stomatitis · thromboembolism · tumour lysis syndrome · vomiting · vomiting

SIDE-EFFECTS, FURTHER INFORMATION

▸ Gastro-intestinal side-effects Tioguanine has a lower incidence of gastrointestinal side-effects than mercaptopurine.

● **CONCEPTION AND CONTRACEPTION** Ensure effective contraception during treatment in men or women.

● **PREGNANCY** Avoid (teratogenicity reported when men receiving tioguanine have fathered children). See also *Pregnancy and reproductive function* in Cytotoxic drugs p. 494.

● **BREAST FEEDING** Discontinue breast-feeding.

● **HEPATIC IMPAIRMENT** Reduce dose.

● **RENAL IMPAIRMENT** Reduce dose.

● **PRE-TREATMENT SCREENING** Consider measuring thiopurine methyltransferase (TPMT) activity before starting tioguanine therapy.

● **MONITORING REQUIREMENTS** Monitor liver function weekly—discontinue if liver toxicity develops.

● **MEDICINAL FORMS**
There can be variation in the licensing of different medicines containing the same drug. Forms available from special-order manufacturers include: capsule

Tablet
▸ Tioguanine (Non-proprietary)
Tioguanine 40 mg Tioguanine 40mg tablets | 25 tablet PoM
£109.57

ANTINEOPLASTIC DRUGS > CYTOTOXIC ANTIBIOTICS AND RELATED SUBSTANCES

Bleomycin

● **INDICATIONS AND DOSE**
Some germ cell tumours | Hodgkin's lymphoma
▸ BY INTRAVENOUS INFUSION
▸ Child: (consult local protocol)

● **UNLICENSED USE** Not licensed for use in children.
● **CONTRA-INDICATIONS** Acute pulmonary infection · significantly reduced lung function
● **CAUTIONS** Caution in handling—irritant to tissues
● **INTERACTIONS** → Appendix 1 (bleomycin).
● **SIDE-EFFECTS**
▸ **Common or very common** Dermatological toxicity · mucositis
▸ **Rare** Cardiorespiratory collapse · hyperpyrexia
▸ **Frequency not known** Alopecia · anorexia · chills (after drug administration) · extravasation · fatigue · fever (after drug administration) · gastro-intestinal effects · hypersensitivity reactions · hyperuricaemia · increased pigmentation particularly affecting the flexures and subcutaneous sclerotic plaques · less bone marrow suppression · nausea · oral mucositis · organ-related toxicity (long-term and delayed) · progressive pulmonary fibrosis (dose-related) · pulmonary toxicity · thromboembolism · tumour lysis syndrome · vomiting
● **CONCEPTION AND CONTRACEPTION** Contraceptive advice required, see *Pregnancy and reproductive function* in Cytotoxic drugs p. 494.
● **PREGNANCY** Avoid (teratogenic and carcinogenic in *animal* studies). See also *Pregnancy and reproductive function* in Cytotoxic drugs p. 494
● **BREAST FEEDING** Discontinue breast feeding.
● **RENAL IMPAIRMENT** Reduce dose—consult local treatment protocol for details.
● **MONITORING REQUIREMENTS** Ensure monitoring of pulmonary function—investigate any shortness of breath before initiation.
● **PRESCRIBING AND DISPENSING INFORMATION** To conform to the European Pharmacopoeia vials previously labelled as containing '15 units' of bleomycin are now labelled as containing 15 000 units. The amount of bleomycin in the vial has not changed.

● **MEDICINAL FORMS**
There can be variation in the licensing of different medicines containing the same drug.
Powder for solution for injection
▸ Bleo-Kyowa (ProStrakan Ltd)
Bleomycin (as Bleomycin sulfate) 15000 unit Bleo-Kyowa 15,000unit powder for solution for injection vials | 10 vial PoM
£190.60

Dactinomycin
(Actinomycin D)

● **INDICATIONS AND DOSE**
Wilms' tumour | Childhood rhabdomyosarcoma and other soft-tissue sarcomas | Ewing's sarcoma
▸ BY INTRAVENOUS INJECTION
▸ Child: (consult local protocol)

● **UNLICENSED USE** Not licensed for use in children under 12 years.
● **CAUTIONS** Caution in handling—irritant to tissues
● **INTERACTIONS** → Appendix 1 (dactinomycin).
● **SIDE-EFFECTS**
▸ **Uncommon** Acne · anaemia · cheilitis · dysphagia · fever · hypoglycaemia · lethargy · malaise · myalgia
▸ **Rare** Hepatotoxicity (possibly dose-related)
▸ **Frequency not known** Alopecia · bone-marrow suppression · extravasation · gastro-intestinal effects · hyperuricaemia · nausea · oral mucositis · organ-related toxicity · thromboembolism · tumour lysis syndrome · vomiting
● **CONCEPTION AND CONTRACEPTION** Exclude pregnancy before treatment with cytotoxic drugs. Contraceptive advice should be given to men and women before cytotoxic therapy begins (and should cover the duration of contraception required after therapy has ended). Regimens that do not contain an alkylating drug or procarbazine may have less effect on fertility, but those with an alkylating drug or procarbazine carry the risk of causing permanent male sterility (there is no effect on potency). Pretreatment counselling and consideration of sperm storage may be appropriate. Women are less severely affected, though the span of reproductive life may be shortened by the onset of a premature menopause. No increase in fetal abnormalities or abortion rate has been recorded in patients who remain fertile after cytotoxic chemotherapy.
● **PREGNANCY** Avoid (teratogenic in *animal* studies). Most cytotoxic drugs are teratogenic and should not be administered during pregnancy, especially during the first trimester. Considerable caution is necessary if a pregnant woman presents with cancer requiring chemotherapy, and specialist advice should always be sought.
● **BREAST FEEDING** Discontinue breast-feeding.
● **HEPATIC IMPAIRMENT** Consider dose reduction if raised serum bilirubin or biliary obstruction; consult local treatment protocols.

● **MEDICINAL FORMS**
There can be variation in the licensing of different medicines containing the same drug.
Powder for solution for injection
▸ Cosmegen (Orphan Europe (UK) Ltd)
Dactinomycin 500 microgram Cosmegen Lyovac 500microgram powder for solution for injection vials | 1 vial PoM £52.58

ANTINEOPLASTIC DRUGS > PLATINUM COMPOUNDS

Carboplatin   10.6.2016

● **INDICATIONS AND DOSE**
Stage 4 neuroblastoma | Germ cell tumours | Low-grade gliomas (including astrocytomas) | Neuroectodermal tumours (including medulloblastoma) | Rhabdomyosarcoma (metastatic and non-metastatic disease) | Soft-tissue sarcomas | Retinoblastoma | High risk Wilms' tumour | Some liver tumours
▸ BY INTRAVENOUS INFUSION
▸ Child: (consult local protocol)

8

Immune system and malignant disease

- **UNLICENSED USE** Not licensed for use in children.
- **INTERACTIONS** → Appendix 1 (platinum compounds).
- **SIDE-EFFECTS** Alopecia · bone-marrow suppression · extravasation · gastro-intestinal effects · hyperuricaemia · myelosuppression · nausea · nausea · nephrotoxicity · neurotoxicity · oral mucositis · organ-related toxicity (long-term and delayed) · ototoxicity · thromboembolism · tumour lysis syndrome · vomiting · vomiting

  SIDE-EFFECTS, FURTHER INFORMATION
  Carboplatin is better tolerated than cisplatin; nausea and vomiting are reduced in severity and nephrotoxicity, neurotoxicity, and ototoxicity are much less of a problem than with cisplatin. It is, however, more myelosuppressive than cisplatin.

- **CONCEPTION AND CONTRACEPTION** Contraceptive advice required, see *Pregnancy and reproductive function* in Cytotoxic drugs p. 494.
- **PREGNANCY** Avoid (teratogenic and embryotoxic in *animal* studies). See also *Pregnancy and reproductive function* in Cytotoxic drugs p. 494.
- **BREAST FEEDING** Discontinue breast-feeding.
- **RENAL IMPAIRMENT** Reduce dose. Avoid if creatinine clearance less than 20 mL/minute/1.73 m^2. Monitor haematological parameters in renal impairment.
  Monitor renal function in renal impairment.
- **MONITORING REQUIREMENTS**
  ▸ Consider therapeutic drug monitoring.
- **PRESCRIBING AND DISPENSING INFORMATION** Carboplatin can be given in an outpatient setting.

- **MEDICINAL FORMS**
  There can be variation in the licensing of different medicines containing the same drug.
  Solution for infusion
  ▸ Carboplatin (Non-proprietary)
  Carboplatin 10 mg per 1 ml Carboplatin 50mg/5ml concentrate for solution for infusion vials | 1 vial [PoM] £22.04 (Hospital only) | 1 vial [PoM] £20.00
  Carboplatin 150mg/15ml concentrate for solution for infusion vials | 1 vial [PoM] £56.92 (Hospital only) | 1 vial [PoM] £50.00
  Carboplatin 600mg/60ml concentrate for solution for infusion vials | 1 vial [PoM] £260.00
  Carboplatin 600mg/60ml solution for infusion vials | 1 vial [PoM] £260.00
  Carboplatin 450mg/45ml concentrate for solution for infusion vials | 1 vial [PoM] £168.85 (Hospital only) | 1 vial [PoM] £160.00
  Carboplatin 450mg/45ml solution for infusion vials | 1 vial [PoM] £197.48
  Carboplatin 150mg/15ml solution for infusion vials | 1 vial [PoM] £65.83
  Carboplatin 50mg/5ml solution for infusion vials | 1 vial [PoM] £22.86

Cisplatin

- **INDICATIONS AND DOSE**
  Osteogenic sarcoma | Stage 4 neuroblastoma | Some liver tumours | Infant brain tumours | Intra-cranial germ-cell tumours
  ▸ BY INTRAVENOUS INFUSION
  ▸ Child: (consult local protocol)

- **UNLICENSED USE** Not licensed for use in children.
- **CAUTIONS**

  CAUTIONS, FURTHER INFORMATION
  ▸ Hydration Cisplatin requires intensive intravenous hydration; routine use of intravenous fluids containing potassium or magnesium may also be required to help control hypokalaemia and hypomagnesaemia. Treatment may be complicated by severe nausea and vomiting; delayed vomiting may occur and is difficult to control.

- **INTERACTIONS** → Appendix 1 (platinum compounds).

- **SIDE-EFFECTS** Alopecia · bone-marrow suppression · extravasation · gastro-intestinal effects · hyperuricaemia · hyperuricaemia · hypocalcaemia · hypokalaemia · hypomagnesaemia · hypophosphataemia · nephrotoxicity (dose-related and potentially cumulative) · neurotoxicity (dose-related and potentially cumulative) · oral mucositis · organ-related toxicity (long-term and delayed) · ototoxicity (dose-related and potentially cumulative) · peripheral neuropathy · severe nausea · severe vomiting (may be delayed and difficult to control) · thromboembolism · tumour lysis syndrome
- **CONCEPTION AND CONTRACEPTION** Manufacturer advises effective contraception during and for at least 6 months after treatment in men or women.
- **PREGNANCY** Avoid (teratogenic and toxic in *animal* studies. See also *Pregnancy and reproductive function* in Cytotoxic drugs p. 494.
- **BREAST FEEDING** Discontinue breast-feeding.
- **RENAL IMPAIRMENT** Avoid if possible—nephrotoxic. Baseline testing of renal function is required; for children with pre-existing renal impairment, consideration should be given to withholding treatment or using another drug.
- **MONITORING REQUIREMENTS**
  ▸ Monitor full blood count.
  ▸ Monitor audiology.
  ▸ Monitor plasma electrolytes.
  ▸ Baseline testing of hearing is required; for children with pre-existing hearing impairment, consideration should be given to withholding treatment or using another drug.
  ▸ For children with pre-existing marked bone-marrow suppression, consideration should be given to withholding treatment or using another drug.
  ▸ Monitor renal function.

- **MEDICINAL FORMS**
  There can be variation in the licensing of different medicines containing the same drug.
  Solution for infusion
  ▸ Cisplatin (Non-proprietary)
  Cisplatin 1 mg per 1 ml Cisplatin 50mg/50ml concentrate for solution for infusion vials | 1 vial [PoM] no price available
  Cisplatin 100mg/100ml solution for infusion vials | 1 vial [PoM] £50.22 (Hospital only) | 1 vial [PoM] £50.22–£55.64
  Cisplatin 10mg/10ml solution for infusion vials | 1 vial [PoM] £5.90 (Hospital only) | 1 vial [PoM] £5.90
  Cisplatin 50mg/50ml solution for infusion vials | 1 vial [PoM] £25.37 (Hospital only) | 1 vial [PoM] £25.37–£28.11
  Cisplatin 10mg/10ml concentrate for solution for infusion vials | 1 vial [PoM] no price available
  Cisplatin 100mg/100ml concentrate for solution for infusion vials | 1 vial [PoM] £50.22 (Hospital only) | 1 vial [PoM] no price available

ANTINEOPLASTIC DRUGS > PODOPHYLLOTIXIN DERIVATIVES

Etoposide

- **INDICATIONS AND DOSE**
  Stage 4 neuroblastoma | Germ-cell tumours | Intracranial germ-cell tumours | Rhabdomyosarcoma | Soft-tissue sarcomas | Neuroectodermal tumours (including medulloblastoma) | Relapsed Hodgkin's disease | Non-Hodgkin's lymphoma | Ewing tumour | Acute lymphoblastic leukaemia | Acute myeloid leukaemia
  ▸ BY MOUTH, OR BY INTRAVENOUS INFUSION
  ▸ Child: (consult local protocol)

- **UNLICENSED USE** Not licensed for use in children.

  IMPORTANT SAFETY INFORMATION
  RISKS OF INCORRECT DOSING OF ORAL ANTI-CANCER MEDICINES
  See Cytotoxic drugs p. 494.

- **INTERACTIONS** → Appendix 1 (etoposide).
- **SIDE-EFFECTS**
  GENERAL SIDE-EFFECTS
  Alopecia · bone-marrow suppression · dose limiting myelosuppression · gastro-intestinal effects · hyperuricaemia · irritant to tissues · nausea · oral mucositis (more common if given with doxorubicin) · organ-related toxicity (long-term and delayed) · thromboembolism · tumour lysis syndrome · vomiting
  SPECIFIC SIDE-EFFECTS
  - With intravenous use Anaphylaxis (associated with concentrated infusions) · hypotension associated with rapid infusion · irritant to tissues (if extravasated)
- **CONCEPTION AND CONTRACEPTION** Contraceptive advice required, see *Pregnancy and reproductive function* in Cytotoxic drugs p. 494.
- **PREGNANCY** Avoid (teratogenic in *animal* studies). See also *Pregnancy and reproductive function* in Cytotoxic drugs p. 494.
- **BREAST FEEDING** Discontinue breast-feeding.
- **HEPATIC IMPAIRMENT** Avoid in severe impairment.
- **RENAL IMPAIRMENT** Consider dose reduction—consult local treatment protocol for details.
- **DIRECTIONS FOR ADMINISTRATION** Etoposide is usually given by slow intravenous infusion. It may also be given by mouth, but it is unpredictably absorbed.

- **MEDICINAL FORMS**
  There can be variation in the licensing of different medicines containing the same drug.
  Capsule
  CAUTIONARY AND ADVISORY LABELS 23
  - Vepesid (Bristol-Myers Squibb Pharmaceuticals Ltd)
    Etoposide 50 mg Vepesid 50mg capsules | 20 capsule PoM £99.82 (Hospital only)
    Etoposide 100 mg Vepesid 100mg capsules | 10 capsule PoM £87.23 (Hospital only)
  Powder for solution for injection
  - Etopophos (Bristol-Myers Squibb Pharmaceuticals Ltd)
    Etoposide (as Etoposide phosphate) 100 mg Etopophos 100mg powder for solution for injection vials | 10 vial PoM £261.68 (Hospital only)
  Solution for infusion
  - Etoposide (Non-proprietary)
    Etoposide 20 mg per 1 ml Etoposide 100mg/5ml concentrate for solution for infusion vials | 1 vial PoM no price available (Hospital only) | 1 vial PoM £11.50 | 10 vial PoM £115.00
    Etoposide 500mg/25ml concentrate for solution for infusion vials | 1 vial PoM £60.75 (Hospital only)
  - Eposin (medac UK)
    Etoposide 20 mg per 1 ml Eposin 500mg/25ml concentrate for solution for infusion vials | 1 vial PoM £67.50 (Hospital only)
    Eposin 100mg/5ml concentrate for solution for infusion vials | 1 vial PoM £13.50 (Hospital only)

ANTINEOPLASTIC DRUGS > VINCA ALKALOIDS

Vinblastine sulfate

- **INDICATIONS AND DOSE**
  Hodgkin's disease and other lymphomas
  - BY INTRAVENOUS INJECTION
  - Child: (consult local protocol)

- **UNLICENSED USE** Licensed for use in children (age range not specified by manufacturer).

  IMPORTANT SAFETY INFORMATION
  Vinblastine is for **intravenous administration only**. Inadvertent intrathecal administration can cause severe neurotoxicity, which is usually fatal.
  The National Patient Safety Agency has advised (August 2008) that adult and teenage patients treated in

an adult or adolescent unit should receive their vinca alkaloid dose in a 50 mL minibag. Teenagers and children treated in a child unit may receive their vinca alkaloid dose in a syringe.

- **CONTRA-INDICATIONS** Intrathecal injection **contra-indicated**.
- **CAUTIONS** Caution in handling—irritant to tissues
- **INTERACTIONS** → Appendix 1 (vinblastine).
- **SIDE-EFFECTS**
  - **Common or very common** Abdominal pain · constipation · leucopenia · muscle pain
  - **Uncommon** Peripheral neuropathy
  - **Rare** Paralytic ileus
  - **Frequency not known** Alopecia (reversible) · autonomic neuropathy · gastro-intestinal effects · hyperuricaemia · loss of deep tendon reflexes · motor weakness · myelosuppression (dose-limiting) · nausea · neurotoxicity · oral mucositis · organ-related toxicity (long-term and delayed) · ototoxicity · peripheral neuropathy · peripheral paraesthesia · severe local irritation (care must be taken to avoid extravasation) · thromboembolism · tumour lysis syndrome · vomiting
  SIDE-EFFECTS, FURTHER INFORMATION
  - Neurotoxicity Neurotoxicity, usually as peripheral or autonomic neuropathy, occurs with all vinca alkaloids; it occurs less often with vinblastine than with vincristine. Patients with neurotoxicity commonly have peripheral paraesthesia, loss of deep tendon reflexes, abdominal pain, and constipation; ototoxicity has been reported. If symptoms of neurotoxicity are severe, doses should be reduced.
    Motor weakness can also occur and dose reduction or discontinuation of therapy may be appropriate if motor weakness increases. Recovery from neurotoxic effects is usually slow but complete.
  - Constipation Prophylactic use of laxatives may be considered.
- **CONCEPTION AND CONTRACEPTION** Contraceptive advice required, see *Pregnancy and reproductive function* in Cytotoxic drugs p. 494.
- **PREGNANCY** Avoid (limited experience suggests fetal harm; teratogenic in *animal* studies). See also *Pregnancy and reproductive function* in Cytotoxic drugs p. 494.
- **BREAST FEEDING** Discontinue breast-feeding.
- **HEPATIC IMPAIRMENT** Dose reduction may be necessary—consult local treatment protocol for details.

- **MEDICINAL FORMS**
  There can be variation in the licensing of different medicines containing the same drug.
  Solution for injection
  - Vinblastine sulfate (Non-proprietary)
    Vinblastine sulfate 1 mg per 1 ml Vinblastine 10mg/10ml solution for injection vials | 5 vial PoM £85.00

Vincristine sulfate

- **INDICATIONS AND DOSE**
  Acute leukaemias | Lymphomas | Paediatric solid tumours
  - BY INTRAVENOUS INJECTION
  - Child: (consult local protocol)

- **UNLICENSED USE** Licensed for use in children (age range not specified by manufacturer).

  IMPORTANT SAFETY INFORMATION
  Vincristine injections are for **intravenous administration only**. Inadvertent intrathecal administration can cause severe neurotoxicity, which is usually fatal.

The National Patient Safety Agency has advised (August 2008) that adult and teenage patients treated in an adult or adolescent unit should receive their vinca alkaloid dose in a 50 mL minibag. Teenagers and children treated in a child unit may receive their vinca alkaloid dose in a syringe.

- **CONTRA-INDICATIONS**
  CONTRA-INDICATIONS, FURTHER INFORMATION
  Intrathecal injection **contra-indicated**.
- **CAUTIONS** Caution in handling—irritant to tissues · ileus · neuromuscular disease
- **INTERACTIONS** → Appendix 1 (vincristine).
- **SIDE-EFFECTS**
  ‣ **Common or very common** Constipation
  ‣ **Rare** Convulsions followed by coma · inappropriate secretion of antidiuretic hormone
  ‣ **Frequency not known** Abdominal pain · alopecia (reversible) · autonomic neuropathy · diarrhoea · extravasation · gastro-intestinal effects · hyperuricaemia · intestinal necrosis · loss of deep tendon reflexes · motor weakness · myelosuppression (negligible) · nausea · neuromuscular effects (dose-limiting) · neurotoxicity · oral mucositis · organ-related toxicity (long-term and delayed) · ototoxicity · paralytic ileus (in young children) · peripheral neuropathy · peripheral paraesthesia · severe local irritation (care must be taken to avoid extravasation) · thromboembolism · tumour lysis syndrome · urinary retention · vomiting
  SIDE-EFFECTS, FURTHER INFORMATION
  ‣ Neurotoxicity Neurotoxicity, usually as peripheral or autonomic neuropathy, occurs with all vinca alkaloids and is a limiting side-effect of vincristine. Children with neurotoxicity commonly have peripheral paraesthesia, loss of deep tendon reflexes, abdominal pain, and constipation; ototoxicity has been reported. If symptoms of neurotoxicity are severe, doses should be reduced, but children generally tolerate vincristine better than adults.
    Motor weakness can also occur and dose reduction or discontinuation of therapy may be appropriate if motor weakness increases. Recovery from neurotoxic effects is usually slow but complete.
  ‣ Constipation Prophylactic use of laxatives may be considered.
- **CONCEPTION AND CONTRACEPTION** Contraceptive advice required, see *Pregnancy and reproductive function* in Cytotoxic drugs p. 494.
- **PREGNANCY** Avoid (teratogenicity and fetal loss in *animal* studies). See also *Pregnancy and reproductive function* in Cytotoxic drugs p. 494.
- **BREAST FEEDING** Discontinue breast-feeding.
- **HEPATIC IMPAIRMENT** Dose reduction may be necessary—consult local treatment protocol for details.

- **MEDICINAL FORMS**
  There can be variation in the licensing of different medicines containing the same drug.
  Solution for injection
  ‣ Vincristine sulfate (Non-proprietary)
    Vincristine sulfate 1 mg per 1 ml Vincristine 1mg/1ml solution for injection vials | 1 vial [PoM] £13.47 (Hospital only) | 5 vial [PoM] £67.35
    Vincristine 2mg/2ml solution for injection vials | 1 vial [PoM] £26.66 (Hospital only) | 5 vial [PoM] £133.30
    Vincristine 5mg/5ml solution for injection vials | 5 vial [PoM] £329.50

ANTINEOPLASTIC DRUGS 〉 OTHER

Crisantaspase

- **DRUG ACTION** Crisantaspase is the enzyme asparaginase produced by *Erwinia chrysanthemi*.

- **INDICATIONS AND DOSE**
  Acute lymphoblastic leukaemia | Acute myeloid leukaemia | Non-Hodgkin's lymphoma
  ‣ BY INTRAVENOUS INJECTION, OR BY INTRAMUSCULAR INJECTION, OR BY SUBCUTANEOUS INJECTION
  ‣ Child: (consult local protocol)

- **UNLICENSED USE** Preparations of asparaginase derived from *Escherichia coli* are available but they are not licensed, they include: *Medac*® asparaginase, *Elspar*® asparaginase, and *Oncaspar*® pegaspargase.
- **CONTRA-INDICATIONS** History of pancreatitis related to asparaginase therapy
- **SIDE-EFFECTS**
  ‣ **Common or very common** Coagulation disorders · confusion · convulsions · diarrhoea · dizziness · drowsiness · headache · lethargy · liver dysfunction · neurotoxicity · pancreatitis
  ‣ **Uncommon** Anaphylaxis · changes in blood lipids · hyperglycaemia
  ‣ **Rare** CNS depression
  ‣ **Very rare** Abdominal pain · hypertension · myalgia
  ‣ **Frequency not known** Alopecia · bone-marrow suppression · extravasation · gastro-intestinal effects · hyperuricaemia · nausea · oral mucositis · organ-related toxicity (long-term and delayed) · thromboembolism · tumour lysis syndrome · vomiting
- **ALLERGY AND CROSS-SENSITIVITY** Children who are hypersensitive to asparaginase derived from one organism may tolerate asparaginase derived from another organism but cross-sensitivity occurs in about 20–30% of individuals.
- **CONCEPTION AND CONTRACEPTION** Contraceptive advice required, see *Pregnancy and reproductive function* in Cytotoxic drugs p. 494.
- **PREGNANCY** Avoid. See also, *Pregnancy and reproductive function* in Cytotoxic drugs p. 494.
- **BREAST FEEDING** Discontinue breast-feeding.
- **DIRECTIONS FOR ADMINISTRATION** Facilities for the management of anaphylaxis should be available.

- **MEDICINAL FORMS**
  There can be variation in the licensing of different medicines containing the same drug.
  Powder for solution for injection
  ‣ Erwinase (EUSA Pharma Ltd)
    Crisantaspase 10000 unit Erwinase 10,000unit powder for solution for injection vials | 5 vial [PoM] £3,065.00

Hydroxycarbamide
(Hydroxyurea)

- **INDICATIONS AND DOSE**
  Sickle-cell disease in children who have recurrent episodes of acute pain (more than 3 admissions in the previous 12 months, or who are very symptomatic in the community) or who have had 2 or more episodes of acute sickle chest syndrome in the last 2 years (or 1 episode requiring ventilatory support)—consult with a specialist centre
  ‣ BY MOUTH
  ‣ Child 2–17 years: Initially 10–15 mg/kg once daily, increased in steps of 2.5–5 mg/kg daily, dose to be

increased every 12 weeks according to response; usual dose 15–30 mg/kg daily; maximum 35 mg/kg per day

> **IMPORTANT SAFETY INFORMATION**
> RISKS OF INCORRECT DOSING OF ORAL ANTI-CANCER MEDICINES
> See Cytotoxic drugs p. 494.

- **CAUTIONS** Leg ulcers (review treatment if cutaneous vasculitic ulcerations develop)
- **INTERACTIONS** → Appendix 1 (hydroxycarbamide).
- **SIDE-EFFECTS**
  - **Common or very common** Headache · myelosuppression · skin reactions
  - **Rare** Amenorrhoea (in sickle-cell disease) · fever (in sickle-cell disease)
  - **Frequency not known** Alopecia · bleeding (in sickle-cell disease) · bone-marrow suppression · dizziness · hyperuricaemia · hypomagnesaemia (in sickle-cell disease) · nausea · oral mucositis · rash · reduced sperm count and activity · thromboembolism · tumour lysis syndrome · vomiting
- **CONCEPTION AND CONTRACEPTION** Manufacturer advises effective contraception before and during treatment.
- **PREGNANCY** Avoid (teratogenic in *animal* studies). See also *Pregnancy and reproductive function* in Cytotoxic drugs p. 494.
- **BREAST FEEDING** Discontinue breast-feeding.
- **HEPATIC IMPAIRMENT** Manufacturer advises caution in mild to moderate impairment. Avoid in severe impairment, unless used for malignant conditions.
- **RENAL IMPAIRMENT** In sickle-cell disease, reduce initial dose by 50% if estimated glomerular filtration rate less than 60 mL/minute/1.73 m². In sickle-cell disease, avoid if estimated glomerular filtration rate less than 30 mL/minute/1.73 m².
- **MONITORING REQUIREMENTS**
  - Monitor renal and hepatic function before and during treatment.
  - Monitor full blood count before treatment, and repeatedly throughout use; in sickle-cell disease monitor every 2 weeks for the first 2 months and then every 2 months thereafter (or every 2 weeks if on maximum dose).
  - Patients receiving long-term therapy for malignant disease should be monitored for secondary malignancies.
- **PATIENT AND CARER ADVICE**
  Medicines for Children leaflet: Hydroxycarbamide for sickle cell disease www.medicinesforchildren.org.uk/hydroxycarbamide-for-sickle-cell-disease

  Patients receiving long-term therapy with hydroxycarbamide should be advised to protect skin from sun exposure.

- **MEDICINAL FORMS**
  There can be variation in the licensing of different medicines containing the same drug. Forms available from special-order manufacturers include: capsule, oral suspension, oral solution
  Tablet
  - Siklos (Nordic Pharma Ltd)
    Hydroxycarbamide 100 mg Siklos 100mg tablets | 60 tablet [PoM] £100.00 DT price = £100.00
    Hydroxycarbamide 1 gram Siklos 1000mg tablets | 30 tablet [PoM] £500.00
  Capsule
  - Hydroxycarbamide (Non-proprietary)
    Hydroxycarbamide 500 mg Hydroxycarbamide 500mg capsules | 100 capsule [PoM] £86.00 DT price = £11.70
  - Droxia (Imported (United States))
    Hydroxycarbamide 300 mg Droxia 300mg capsules | 60 capsule [PoM] no price available

- Hydrea (Bristol-Myers Squibb Pharmaceuticals Ltd)
  Hydroxycarbamide 500 mg Hydrea 500mg capsules | 100 capsule [PoM] £10.47 DT price = £11.70

Mitotane

- **DRUG ACTION** Mitotane selectively inhibits the activity of the adrenal cortex, necessitating corticosteroid replacement therapy.

- **INDICATIONS AND DOSE**
  Symptomatic treatment of advanced or inoperable adrenocortical carcinoma
  - BY MOUTH
  - Child: (consult local protocol)

- **UNLICENSED USE** Not licensed for use in children.

> **IMPORTANT SAFETY INFORMATION**
> RISKS OF INCORRECT DOSING OF ORAL ANTI-CANCER MEDICINES
> See Cytotoxic drugs p. 494.

- **CAUTIONS** Avoid in Acute porphyrias p. 562 · risk of accumulation in overweight patients
- **INTERACTIONS** → Appendix 1 (mitotane).
- **SIDE-EFFECTS**
  - **Common or very common** Anaemia · anorexia · asthenia · ataxia · cognitive impairment · confusion · diarrhoea · dizziness · drowsiness · epigastric discomfort · gastro-intestinal disturbances · gynaecomastia · headache · hypercholesterolaemia · hypertriglyceridaemia · leucopenia · liver disorders · movement disorder · myasthenia · nausea · neuropathy · paraesthesia · prolonged bleeding time · rash · thrombocytopenia · vomiting
  - **Rare** Flushing · haematuria · haemorrhagic cystitis · hypersalivation · hypertension · hypouricaemia · ocular disorders · postural hypotension · proteinuria · pyrexia · visual disturbances
  - **Frequency not known** Alopecia · bone-marrow suppression · gastro-intestinal effects · hyperuricaemia · nausea · neuropsychological impairment (possibly secondary to hypothyroidism, and growth retardation) · oral mucositis · organ-related toxicity (long-term and delayed) · thromboembolism · tumour lysis syndrome · vomiting
- **CONCEPTION AND CONTRACEPTION** Contraceptive advice required, see *Pregnancy and reproductive* function in Cytotoxic drugs p. 494.
- **PREGNANCY** Manufacturer advises avoid. See also *Pregnancy and reproductive function* in Cytotoxic drugs p. 494.
- **BREAST FEEDING** Discontinue breast-feeding.
- **HEPATIC IMPAIRMENT** Manufacturer advises caution in mild to moderate impairment. Avoid in severe impairment. In mild to moderate hepatic impairment, monitoring of plasma-mitotane concentration is recommended.
- **RENAL IMPAIRMENT** Manufacturer advises caution in mild to moderate impairment. Avoid in severe impairment. In mild to moderate renal impairment, monitoring of plasma-mitotane concentration is recommended.
- **MONITORING REQUIREMENTS**
  - Monitor plasma-mitotane concentration—consult product literature.
- **PRESCRIBING AND DISPENSING INFORMATION**
  Corticosteroid replacement therapy Corticosteroid replacement therapy is necessary with treatment with mitotane. The dose of glucocorticoid should be increased in case of shock, trauma, or infection.

- **PATIENT AND CARER ADVICE**
Patients should be warned to contact doctor immediately if injury, infection, or illness occurs (because of risk of acute adrenal insufficiency).

Driving and skilled tasks
Central nervous system toxicity may affect performance of skilled tasks (e.g. driving).

- **MEDICINAL FORMS**
There can be variation in the licensing of different medicines containing the same drug.

Tablet
CAUTIONARY AND ADVISORY LABELS 2, 10, 21
▸ Lysodren (HRA Pharma UK Ltd)
Mitotane 500 mg Lysodren 500mg tablets | 100 tablet PoM £590.97

Procarbazine

- **DRUG ACTION** Procarbazine is a mild monoamine-oxidase inhibitor.

- **INDICATIONS AND DOSE**
Hodgkin's lymphoma
▸ BY MOUTH
▸ Child: (consult local protocol)

IMPORTANT SAFETY INFORMATION
RISKS OF INCORRECT DOSING OF ORAL ANTI-CANCER MEDICINES
See Cytotoxic drugs p. 494.

- **CONTRA-INDICATIONS** Pre-existing severe leucopenia · pre-existing severe thrombocytopenia
- **CAUTIONS** Cardiovascular disease · cerebrovascular disease · epilepsy · phaeochromocytoma · procarbazine is a mild monoamineoxidase inhibitor (dietary restriction is rarely considered necessary)
- **INTERACTIONS** → Appendix 1 (procarbazine).
Alcohol ingestion may cause a disulfiram-like reaction.
- **SIDE-EFFECTS**
▸ **Common or very common** Loss of appetite
▸ **Frequency not known** Alopecia · bone-marrow suppression · gastro-intestinal effects · hypersensitivity rash (discontinue treatment) · hyperuricaemia · jaundice · nausea · oral mucositis · organ-related toxicity (long-term and delayed) · thromboembolism · tumour lysis syndrome · vomiting
- **CONCEPTION AND CONTRACEPTION** Contraceptive advice required, see *Pregnancy and reproductive function* in Cytotoxic drugs p. 494.
- **PREGNANCY** Avoid (teratogenic in *animal* studies and isolated reports in humans). See also *Pregnancy and reproductive function* in Cytotoxic drugs p. 494.
- **BREAST FEEDING** Discontinue breast-feeding.
- **HEPATIC IMPAIRMENT** Caution in mild to moderate impairment. Avoid in severe impairment.
- **RENAL IMPAIRMENT** Caution in mild to moderate impairment. Avoid in severe impairment.

- **MEDICINAL FORMS**
There can be variation in the licensing of different medicines containing the same drug.
Capsule
CAUTIONARY AND ADVISORY LABELS 4
▸ Procarbazine (Non-proprietary)
Procarbazine (as Procarbazine hydrochloride)
50 mg Procarbazine 50mg capsules | 50 capsule PoM £339.95

RETINOID AND RELATED DRUGS

Tretinoin

- **INDICATIONS AND DOSE**
Induction of remission in acute promyelocytic leukaemia (used in previously untreated patients as well as in those who have relapsed after standard chemotherapy or who are refractory to it)
▸ BY MOUTH
▸ Child: (consult local protocol)

- **CAUTIONS** Increased risk of thromboembolism during first month of treatment
- **INTERACTIONS** → Appendix 1 (retinoids).
- **SIDE-EFFECTS** Alopecia · anxiety · arrhythmias · benign intracranial hypertension (children particularly susceptible—consider dose reduction if intractable headache in children) · bone pain · cheilitis · chest pain · confusion · depression · dizziness · dry mucous membranes · dry skin · erythema · flushing · gastro-intestinal disturbances · genital ulceration · headache · hearing disturbances · hypercalcaemia · insomnia · oedema · pancreatitis · paraesthesia · pruritus · raised lipids · raised liver enzymes · raised serum creatinine · rash · retinoic acid syndrome · shivering · sweating · thromboembolism · visual disturbances

SIDE-EFFECTS, FURTHER INFORMATION
▸ Retinoic acid syndrome Fever, dyspnoea, acute respiratory distress, pulmonary infiltrates, pleural effusion, hyperleucocytosis, hypotension, oedema, weight gain, hepatic, renal and multi-organ failure requires immediate treatment—consult product literature.
▸ Nervous system effects Children particularly susceptible to nervous system effects.

- **CONCEPTION AND CONTRACEPTION** Effective contraception must be used for at least 1 month before oral treatment, during treatment and for at least 1 month after stopping (oral progestogen-only contraceptives not considered effective).
- **PREGNANCY** Teratogenic. See *Pregnancy and reproductive function* in Cytotoxic drugs p. 494.
- **BREAST FEEDING** Avoid (discontinue breast-feeding).
- **HEPATIC IMPAIRMENT** Reduce dose—consult local treatment protocol for details.
- **RENAL IMPAIRMENT** Reduce dose—consult local treatment protocol for details.
- **MONITORING REQUIREMENTS** Monitor haematological and coagulation profile, liver function, serum calcium and plasma lipids before and during treatment.
- **PRESCRIBING AND DISPENSING INFORMATION** Tretinoin is the acid form of vitamin A.

- **MEDICINAL FORMS**
There can be variation in the licensing of different medicines containing the same drug.
Capsule
CAUTIONARY AND ADVISORY LABELS 21, 25
▸ Tretinoin (Non-proprietary)
Tretinoin 10 mg Tretinoin 10mg capsules | 100 capsule PoM £240.00 DT price = £240.00

2.1 Cytotoxic drug-induced side effects

DETOXIFYING DRUGS › UROPROTECTIVE DRUGS

Mesna

- **INDICATIONS AND DOSE**

Urothelial toxicity following oxazaphosphorine therapy
▸ BY INTRAVENOUS INJECTION, OR BY CONTINUOUS INTRAVENOUS INFUSION
▸ Child: (consult local protocol)

Mucolytic in cystic fibrosis
▸ BY INHALATION OF NEBULISED SOLUTION
▸ Child: 3–6 mL twice daily, use a 20% solution

- **UNLICENSED USE** Not licensed for use in children.
- **SIDE-EFFECTS**
▸ **Common or very common** Colic · depression · diarrhoea · fatigue · headache · hypotension · irritability · joint pains · limb pains · nausea · rash · tachycardia · vomiting
▸ **Rare** Hypersensitivity reactions (more common in patients with auto-immune disorders)
- **ALLERGY AND CROSS-SENSITIVITY** Contra-indicated if history of hypersensitivity to thiol-containing compounds.
- **PREGNANCY** Not known to be harmful. See also *Pregnancy and reproductive function* in Cytotoxic drugs p. 494.
- **DIRECTIONS FOR ADMINISTRATION** For oral administration of the injection, contents of ampoule are taken in a flavoured drink such as orange juice or cola which may be stored in a refrigerator for up to 24 hours in a sealed container.

- **MEDICINAL FORMS**
There can be variation in the licensing of different medicines containing the same drug. Forms available from special-order manufacturers include: oral solution
Tablet
▸ Mesna (Non-proprietary)
Mesna 400 mg Mesna 400mg tablets | 10 tablet PoM £134.30–£134.40
Mesna 600 mg Mesna 600mg tablets | 10 tablet PoM £190.60
Solution for injection
▸ Mesna (Non-proprietary)
Mesna 100 mg per 1 ml Mesna 1g/10ml solution for injection ampoules | 15 ampoule PoM £441.15
Mesna 400mg/4ml solution for injection ampoules | 15 ampoule PoM £201.15

VITAMINS AND TRACE ELEMENTS › FOLATES

Folinic acid

- **INDICATIONS AND DOSE**

Reduction of methotrexate-induced toxicity
▸ BY MOUTH, OR BY INTRAVENOUS INFUSION, OR BY INTRAVENOUS INJECTION
▸ Child: (consult local protocol)

Methotrexate overdose
▸ BY INTRAVENOUS INFUSION, OR BY INTRAVENOUS INJECTION
▸ Child: (consult local protocol)

Megaloblastic anaemia due to folate deficiency
▸ BY MOUTH
▸ Child 1 month–11 years: 250 micrograms/kg once daily
▸ Child 12–17 years: 15 mg once daily

Metabolic disorders leading to folate deficiency
▸ BY MOUTH, OR BY INTRAVENOUS INFUSION
▸ Child: 15 mg once daily, larger doses may be required in older children

Prevention of megaloblastic anaemia associated with pyrimethamine and sulfadiazine treatment of congenital toxoplasmosis
▸ BY MOUTH
▸ Neonate: 5 mg 3 times a week; increased if necessary up to 20 mg 3 times a week, if the patient is neutropenic.
▸ Child 1–11 months: 10 mg 3 times a week

SODIOFOLIN®

As an antidote to methotrexate
▸ BY INTRAVENOUS INFUSION, OR BY INTRAVENOUS INJECTION
▸ Child: (consult product literature)

- **UNLICENSED USE** Consult product literature for licensing status of individual preparations.
- **CONTRA-INDICATIONS** Intrathecal injection
- **CAUTIONS** Avoid simultaneous administration of methotrexate · **not** indicated for pernicious anaemia or other megaloblastic anaemias caused by vitamin B_{12} deficiency
- **INTERACTIONS** → Appendix 1 (folates).
- **SIDE-EFFECTS**
▸ **Rare** Agitation (after high doses) · depression (after high doses) · gastro-intestinal disturbances (after high doses) · insomnia (after high doses) · pyrexia (after parenteral use)
- **PREGNANCY** Not known to be harmful; benefit outweighs risk.
- **BREAST FEEDING** Presence in milk unknown but benefit outweighs risk.

- **MEDICINAL FORMS**
There can be variation in the licensing of different medicines containing the same drug. Forms available from special-order manufacturers include: oral suspension, oral solution
Tablet
▸ Folinic acid (Non-proprietary)
Folinic acid (as Calcium folinate) 15 mg Calcium folinate 15mg tablets | 10 tablet PoM £49.10 DT price = £49.11
▸ Refolinon (Pfizer Ltd)
Folinic acid (as Calcium folinate) 15 mg Refolinon 15mg tablets | 30 tablet PoM £85.74
Solution for injection
▸ Folinic acid (Non-proprietary)
Folinic acid (as Calcium folinate) 3 mg per 1 ml Calcium folinate 3mg/1ml solution for injection ampoules | 5 ampoule PoM £30.00
Folinic acid (as Calcium folinate) 7.5 mg per 1 ml Calcium folinate 15mg/2ml solution for injection ampoules | 5 ampoule PoM £38.99–£39.00
Folinic acid (as Calcium folinate) 10 mg per 1 ml Calcium folinate 50mg/5ml solution for injection vials | 1 vial PoM £18.44 (Hospital only) | 1 vial PoM £20.00
Calcium folinate 300mg/30ml solution for injection vials | 1 vial PoM £89.95 (Hospital only) | 1 vial PoM £100.00
Calcium folinate 100mg/10ml solution for injection vials | 1 vial PoM £34.94 (Hospital only) | 1 vial PoM £37.50
Folinic acid (as Disodium folinate) 50 mg per 1 ml Disodium folinate 50mg/1ml solution for injection vials | 1 vial PoM £24.70
Disodium folinate 200mg/4ml solution for injection vials | 1 vial PoM £80.40
▸ Refolinon (Pfizer Ltd)
Folinic acid (as Calcium folinate) 3 mg per 1 ml Refolinon 30mg/10ml solution for injection ampoules | 5 ampoule PoM £23.12
▸ Sodiofolin (medac UK)
Folinic acid (as Disodium folinate) 50 mg per 1 ml Sodiofolin 400mg/8ml solution for injection vials | 1 vial PoM £126.25 (Hospital only)
Sodiofolin 100mg/2ml solution for injection vials | 1 vial PoM £35.09 (Hospital only)

Levofolinic acid

- **DRUG ACTION** Levofolinic acid is an isomer of folinic acid.

- **INDICATIONS AND DOSE**

Reduction of methotrexate-induced toxicity
- ▶ BY INTRAMUSCULAR INJECTION, OR BY INTRAVENOUS INJECTION, OR BY INTRAVENOUS INFUSION
- ▶ Child: (consult local protocol)

Methotrexate overdose
- ▶ BY INTRAMUSCULAR INJECTION, OR BY INTRAVENOUS INJECTION, OR BY INTRAVENOUS INFUSION
- ▶ Child: (consult local protocol)

- **CONTRA-INDICATIONS** Intrathecal injection
- **CAUTIONS** Avoid simultaneous administration of methotrexate · **not** indicated for pernicious anaemia or other megaloblastic anaemias caused by vitamin B_{12} deficiency
- **INTERACTIONS** → Appendix 1 (folates).
- **SIDE-EFFECTS**
- ▶ Rare Agitation (after high doses) · depression (after high doses) · gastro-intestinal disturbances (after high doses) · insomnia (after high doses) · pyrexia (after parenteral use)
- **PREGNANCY** Not known to be harmful; benefit outweighs risk.
- **BREAST FEEDING** Presence in milk unknown but benefit outweighs risk.

- **MEDICINAL FORMS**
There can be variation in the licensing of different medicines containing the same drug.
Solution for injection
- ▶ Isovorin (Pfizer Ltd)
Levofolinic acid (as Calcium levofolinate) 10 mg per 1 ml Isovorin 175mg/17.5ml solution for injection vials | 1 vial PoM £81.33 (Hospital only)
Isovorin 25mg/2.5ml solution for injection vials | 1 vial PoM £11.62 (Hospital only)

2.1a Hyperuricaemia associated with cytotoxic drugs

DETOXIFYING DRUGS › URATE OXIDASES

Rasburicase

- **INDICATIONS AND DOSE**
Prophylaxis and treatment of acute hyperuricaemia with initial chemotherapy for haematological malignancy
- ▶ BY INTRAVENOUS INFUSION
- ▶ Child: (consult local protocol)

- **UNLICENSED USE** Not licensed for use in children.
- **CONTRA-INDICATIONS** G6PD deficiency
- **CAUTIONS** Atopic allergies
- **SIDE-EFFECTS**
- ▶ **Common or very common** Fever · nausea · vomiting
- ▶ **Uncommon** Anaphylaxis · bronchospasm · diarrhoea · haemolytic anaemia · headache · hypersensitivity reactions · methaemoglobinaemia · rash
- **PREGNANCY** Manufacturer advises avoid—no information available.
- **BREAST FEEDING** Manufacturer advises avoid—no information available.
- **MONITORING REQUIREMENTS** Monitor closely for hypersensitivity.
- **EFFECT ON LABORATORY TESTS** May interfere with test for uric acid—consult product literature.

- **MEDICINAL FORMS**
There can be variation in the licensing of different medicines containing the same drug.
Powder and solvent for solution for infusion
- ▶ Fasturtec (Sanofi)
Rasburicase 1.5 mg Fasturtec 1.5mg powder and solvent for solution for infusion vials | 3 vial PoM £208.39 (Hospital only)
Rasburicase 7.5 mg Fasturtec 7.5mg powder and solvent for solution for infusion vials | 1 vial PoM £347.32 (Hospital only)

XANTHINE OXIDASE INHIBITORS

Allopurinol

- **INDICATIONS AND DOSE**
Prophylaxis of hyperuricaemia associated with cancer chemotherapy | Prophylaxis of hyperuricaemic nephropathy, enzyme disorders causing increased serum urate e.g Lesch-Nyhan syndrome
- ▶ BY MOUTH
- ▶ Child 1 month–14 years: 10–20 mg/kg daily, dose to be taken preferably after food; maximum 400 mg per day
- ▶ Child 15–17 years: Initially 100 mg daily, taken preferably after food; dose to be increased according to response, up to 900 mg daily in divided doses (max. per dose 300 mg)

- **CAUTIONS** Ensure adequate fluid intake · for hyperuricaemia associated with cancer therapy, allopurinol treatment should be started before cancer therapy
- **INTERACTIONS** → Appendix 1 (allopurinol).
- **SIDE-EFFECTS**
- ▶ **Common or very common** Gastro-intestinal disorders · rashes (**withdraw** therapy; if rash mild re-introduce cautiously but **discontinue** immediately if recurrence)
- ▶ **Rare** Alopecia · aplastic anaemia · arthralgia · blood disorders · drowsiness · eosinophilia resembling Stevens-Johnson syndrome · eosinophilia resembling toxic epidermal necrolysis · exfoliation · fever · haemolytic anaemia · headache · hepatitis · hepatotoxicity · hypersensitivity reactions · hypertension · leucopenia · lymphadenopathy · malaise · neuropathy · paraesthesia · renal impairment · taste disturbances · thrombocytopenia · vasculitis · vertigo · visual disturbances
- ▶ **Very rare** Seizures
- **PREGNANCY** Toxicity not reported. Manufacturer advises use only if no safer alternative and disease carries risk for mother or child.
- **BREAST FEEDING** Present in milk—not known to be harmful.
- **HEPATIC IMPAIRMENT** Reduce dose. Monitor hepatic function.
- **RENAL IMPAIRMENT** Manufacturer advises reduce dose or increase dose interval in severe impairment; adjust dose to maintain plasma-oxipurinol concentration below 100 micromol/litre.
- **PATIENT AND CARER ADVICE**
Medicines for Children leaflet: Allopurinol for hyperuricaemia www.medicinesforchildren.org.uk/allopurinol-for-hyperuricaemia

- **MEDICINAL FORMS**
There can be variation in the licensing of different medicines containing the same drug. Forms available from special-order manufacturers include: oral suspension, oral solution
Tablet
CAUTIONARY AND ADVISORY LABELS 8, 21, 27
- ▶ Allopurinol (Non-proprietary)
Allopurinol 100 mg Allopurinol 100mg tablets | 28 tablet PoM £1.64 DT price = £0.80

Allopurinol 300 mg Allopurinol 300mg tablets | 28 tablet [PoM] £1.72 DT price = £0.90

▸ **Urico** (Ennogen Pharma Ltd)
Allopurinol 100 mg Urico 100mg tablets | 28 tablet [PoM] £1.25 DT price = £0.80
Allopurinol 300 mg Urico 300mg tablets | 28 tablet [PoM] £0.94 DT price = £0.90

▸ **Zyloric** (Aspen Pharma Trading Ltd)
Allopurinol 100 mg Zyloric 100mg tablets | 100 tablet [PoM] £10.19
Allopurinol 300 mg Zyloric 300mg tablets | 28 tablet [PoM] £7.31 DT price = £0.90

3   Immunotherapy responsive malignancy

IMMUNOSTIMULANTS ⟩ INTERFERONS

Interferon alfa

● **DRUG ACTION** Interferon alfa has shown some antitumour effect in certain lymphomas and solid tumours.

● **INDICATIONS AND DOSE**

Induction of early regression of life-threatening corticosteroid resistant haemangiomata of infancy
▸ BY SUBCUTANEOUS INJECTION
▸ Child: (consult local protocol)

INTRONA® PEN

Chronic active hepatitis B
▸ BY SUBCUTANEOUS INJECTION
▸ Child 2-17 years: 5 000 000–10 000 000 units/m^2 3 times a week

Chronic active hepatitis C (in combination with oral ribavirin)
▸ BY SUBCUTANEOUS INJECTION
▸ Child 3-17 years: 3 000 000 units/m^2 3 times a week

INTRONA® VIALS

Chronic active hepatitis B
▸ BY SUBCUTANEOUS INJECTION
▸ Child 2-17 years: 5 000 000–10 000 000 units/m^2 3 times a week

Chronic active hepatitis C (in combination with ribavirin)
▸ BY SUBCUTANEOUS INJECTION
▸ Child 3-17 years: 3 000 000 units/m^2 3 times a week

ROFERON-A®

Chronic active hepatitis B
▸ BY SUBCUTANEOUS INJECTION
▸ Child 2-17 years: 2 500 000–5 000 000 units/m^2 3 times a week, up to 10 000 000 units/m^2 has been used 3 times a week

● **UNLICENSED USE** Not licensed for use in children for chronic active hepatitis B.
ROFERON-A® *Roferon-A®* not licensed for use in children.

● **CONTRA-INDICATIONS** Avoid injections containing benzyl alcohol in neonates · history of severe psychiatric illness
CONTRA-INDICATIONS, FURTHER INFORMATION
For contra-indications consult product literature and local treatment protocol.

● **CAUTIONS**
CAUTIONS, FURTHER INFORMATION
For cautions consult product literature and local treatment protocol.
    Interferon alfa should always be used under the close supervision of a specialist; the decision to treat should be made only after careful assessment of the expected benefits versus the potential risks, in particular the risk of growth inhibition caused by combination therapy.

● **INTERACTIONS** → Appendix 1 (interferons).

● **SIDE-EFFECTS**
▸ **Common or very common** Anorexia · influenza-like symptoms · lethargy · nausea
▸ **Rare** Pneumonia · pneumonitis · pulmonary infiltrates
▸ **Frequency not known** Alopecia · arrhythmias · cardiovascular problems · coma · confusion · depression · hepatotoxicity · hyperglycaemia · hypersensitivity reactions · hypertension · hypertriglyceridaemia (sometimes severe) · hypotension · myelosuppression (particularly affecting granulocyte counts) · nephrotoxicity · ocular side-effects · psoriasiform rash · reversible motor problems in young children · seizures · suicidal behaviour · thyroid abnormalities
SIDE-EFFECTS, FURTHER INFORMATION
Consult product literature and local treatment protocols for information on side-effects.
    Respiratory symptoms should be investigated and if pulmonary infiltrates are suspected or lung function is impaired the discontinuation of interferon alfa should be considered.

● **CONCEPTION AND CONTRACEPTION** Effective contraception required during treatment—consult product literature.

● **PREGNANCY** Avoid unless potential benefit outweighs risk (toxicity in *animal* studies).

● **BREAST FEEDING** Unlikely to be harmful.

● **HEPATIC IMPAIRMENT** Avoid in severe hepatic impairment. Close monitoring required in mild to moderate hepatic impairment.

● **RENAL IMPAIRMENT** Avoid in severe renal impairment. Close monitoring required in mild to moderate renal impairment.

● **MONITORING REQUIREMENTS**
▸ Monitoring of lipid concentration is recommended.
▸ Monitoring of hepatic function is recommended.

● **MEDICINAL FORMS**
There can be variation in the licensing of different medicines containing the same drug.
Solution for injection
EXCIPIENTS: May contain Benzyl alcohol
▸ **IntronA** (Merck Sharp & Dohme Ltd)
Interferon alfa-2b 10 mega u per 1 ml IntronA 10million units/1ml solution for injection vials | 1 vial [PoM] no price available
IntronA 25million units/2.5ml solution for injection multidose vials | 1 vial [PoM] £103.94
Interferon alfa-2b 15 mega u per 1 ml IntronA 18million units/1.2ml solution for injection multidose pens | 1 pre-filled disposable injection [PoM] £74.83
Interferon alfa-2b 25 mega u per 1 ml IntronA 30million units/1.2ml solution for injection multidose pens | 1 pre-filled disposable injection [PoM] £124.72
Interferon alfa-2b 50 mega u per 1 ml IntronA 60million units/1.2ml solution for injection multidose pens | 1 pre-filled disposable injection [PoM] £249.45
▸ **Roferon-A** (Roche Products Ltd)
Interferon alfa-2a 6 mega u per 1 ml Roferon-A 3million units/0.5ml solution for injection pre-filled syringes | 1 pre-filled disposable injection [PoM] £14.20
Interferon alfa-2a 9 mega u per 1 ml Roferon-A 4.5million units/0.5ml solution for injection pre-filled syringes | 1 pre-filled disposable injection [PoM] £21.29
Interferon alfa-2a 12 mega u per 1 ml Roferon-A 6million units/0.5ml solution for injection pre-filled syringes | 1 pre-filled disposable injection [PoM] £28.37
Interferon alfa-2a 18 mega u per 1 ml Roferon-A 9million units/0.5ml solution for injection pre-filled syringes | 1 pre-filled disposable injection [PoM] £42.57

8

Immune system and malignant disease

Interferon gamma-1b

(Immune interferon)

- **INDICATIONS AND DOSE**

To reduce the frequency of serious infection in chronic granulomatous disease
- ▶ BY SUBCUTANEOUS INJECTION
- ▶ Child 6 months–17 years (body surface area up to 0.6 m²): 1.5 micrograms/kg 3 times a week
- ▶ Child 6 months–17 years (body surface area 0.6 m² and above): 50 micrograms/m² 3 times a week

To reduce the frequency of serious infection in severe malignant osteoporosis
- ▶ BY SUBCUTANEOUS INJECTION
- ▶ Child (body surface area up to 0.6 m²): 1.5 micrograms/kg 3 times a week
- ▶ Child (body surface area 0.6 m² and above): 50 micrograms/m² 3 times a week

- **CAUTIONS** Arrhythmias · cardiac disease · congestive heart failure · ischaemia · seizure disorders (including seizures associated with fever)
- **INTERACTIONS** → Appendix 1 (interferons). Avoid simultaneous administration of foreign proteins including immunological products (risk of exaggerated immune response).
- **SIDE-EFFECTS**
  - ▶ **Common or very common** Abdominal pain · arthralgia · chills · depression · diarrhoea · fatigue · fever · headache · injection-site reactions · myalgia · nausea · rash · vomiting
  - ▶ **Rare** Confusion · systemic lupus erythematosus
  - ▶ **Frequency not known** Neutropenia · proteinuria · raised liver enzymes · thrombocytopenia
- **CONCEPTION AND CONTRACEPTION** Effective contraception required during treatment—consult product literature.
- **PREGNANCY** Manufacturers recommend avoid unless potential benefit outweighs risk (toxicity in *animal* studies).
- **BREAST FEEDING** Manufacturers advise avoid—no information available.
- **HEPATIC IMPAIRMENT** Manufacturer advises caution in severe impairment—risk of accumulation.
- **RENAL IMPAIRMENT** Manufacturer advises caution in severe impairment—risk of accumulation.
- **MONITORING REQUIREMENTS** Monitor before and during treatment: haematological tests (including full blood count, differential white cell count, and platelet count), blood chemistry tests (including renal and liver function tests) and urinalysis.

- **MEDICINAL FORMS**
  There can be variation in the licensing of different medicines containing the same drug.
  Solution for injection
  - ▶ Immukin (Boehringer Ingelheim Ltd)
    Interferon gamma-1b (recombinant human) 200 microgram per 1 ml Immukin 100micrograms/0.5ml solution for injection vials | 6 vial [PoM] £450.00

IMMUNOSTIMULANTS > IMMUNOSTIMULANTS, OTHER

Mifamurtide

- **INDICATIONS AND DOSE**

Treatment of high-grade, resectable, non-metastatic osteosarcoma after complete surgical resection (in combination with chemotherapy)
- ▶ BY INTRAVENOUS INFUSION
- ▶ Child 2–17 years: Infusion to be given over 1 hour (consult product literature or local protocols)

- **UNLICENSED USE** Not licensed for use in patients under 2 years of age at initial diagnosis.
- **CAUTIONS** Asthma—consider prophylactic bronchodilator therapy · chronic obstructive pulmonary disease—consider prophylactic bronchodilator therapy · history of autoimmune disease · history of collagen disease · history of inflammatory disease
- **INTERACTIONS** → Appendix 1 (mifamurtide).
- **SIDE-EFFECTS** Abdominal pain · alopecia · anaemia · anorexia · anxiety · blurred vision · confusion · constipation · cough · depression · diarrhoea · dizziness · drowsiness · dry skin · dyspepsia · dyspnoea · dysuria · epistaxis · flushing · gastro-intestinal disturbances · granulocytopenia · haematuria · haemoptysis · headache · hearing loss · hypertension · hypoaesthesia · hypokalaemia · hypotension · insomnia · leucopenia · musculoskeletal pain · nausea · oedema · palpitations · paraesthesia · phlebitis · pleural effusion · pollakiuria · rash · respiratory disorders · sweating · tachycardia · tachypnoea · thrombocytopenia · tinnitus · tremor · vertigo · vomiting
- **CONCEPTION AND CONTRACEPTION** Effective contraception required.
- **PREGNANCY** Avoid.
- **BREAST FEEDING** Avoid—no information available.
- **HEPATIC IMPAIRMENT** Use with caution—no information available.
- **RENAL IMPAIRMENT** Use with caution—no information available.
- **MONITORING REQUIREMENTS**
  - ▶ Monitor renal function, hepatic function and clotting parameters.
  - ▶ Monitor patients with history of venous thrombosis, vasculitis, or unstable cardiovascular disorders for persistent or worsening symptoms during administration—consult product literature.
- **NATIONAL FUNDING/ACCESS DECISIONS**
  NICE technology appraisals (TAs)
  - ▶ **Mifamurtide for the treatment of osteosarcoma (October 2011)** NICE TA235
    Mifamurtide in combination with postoperative multi-agent chemotherapy is recommended (within its licensed indication), as an option for the treatment of high-grade resectable non-metastatic osteosarcoma after macroscopically complete surgical resection in children, adolescents and young adults and when mifamurtide is made available at a reduced cost to the NHS under the patient access scheme.
    www.nice.org.uk/TA235

- **MEDICINAL FORMS**
  There can be variation in the licensing of different medicines containing the same drug.
  Powder for suspension for infusion
  - ▶ Mepact (Takeda UK Ltd)
    Mifamurtide 4 mg Mepact 4mg powder for suspension for infusion vials | 1 vial [PoM] no price available

4 Targeted therapy responsive malignancy

ANTINEOPLASTIC DRUGS > PROTEIN KINASE INHIBITORS

Everolimus

● **DRUG ACTION** Everolimus is a protein kinase inhibitor.

● INDICATIONS AND DOSE

VOTUBIA®

Subependymal giant cell astrocytoma associated with tuberous sclerosis complex
▸ BY MOUTH
▸ Child: (consult product literature)

IMPORTANT SAFETY INFORMATION
RISKS OF INCORRECT DOSING OF ORAL ANTI-CANCER MEDICINES
See Cytotoxic drugs p. 494.

● **CAUTIONS** History of bleeding disorders
● **INTERACTIONS** → Appendix 1 (everolimus).
Caution with concomitant use of drugs that increase risk of bleeding.
● **SIDE-EFFECTS**
▸ **Common or very common** Abdominal pain · anorexia · arthralgia · asthenia · chest pain · convulsions · dehydration · diarrhoea · dry mouth · dysphagia · electrolyte disturbance · epistaxis · eyelid oedema · fatigue · hand-foot syndrome · headache · hypercholesterolaemia · hyperglycaemia · hyperlipidaemia · hypertension · hypoglycaemia · increased susceptibility to aspergillosis · increased susceptibility to candidiasis · increased susceptibility to infections · increased susceptibility to pneumonia · insomnia · interstitial lung disease · irritability · nail disorders · peripheral oedema · pneumonitis · renal failure · skin disorders · taste disturbance
▸ **Uncommon** Aggression · agitation · congestive heart failure · flushing · impaired wound healing · rhabdomyolysis
▸ **Frequency not known** Alopecia · bone-marrow suppression · gastro-intestinal effects · haemorrhage · hepatitis B reactivation · hyperuricaemia · nausea · oral mucositis · organ-related toxicity (long-term and delayed) · thromboembolism · tumour lysis syndrome · vomiting
SIDE-EFFECTS, FURTHER INFORMATION
Reduce dose or discontinue if severe side-effects occur—consult product literature.
● **CONCEPTION AND CONTRACEPTION** Effective contraception must be used during and for up to 8 weeks after treatment.
● **PREGNANCY** Manufacturer advises avoid (toxicity in *animal* studies). See also *Pregnancy and reproductive function* in Cytotoxic drugs p. 494.
● **BREAST FEEDING** Manufacturer advises avoid.
● **HEPATIC IMPAIRMENT** Consult product literature.
● **MONITORING REQUIREMENTS**
▸ Monitor blood-glucose concentration, serum-triglycerides and serum-cholesterol before treatment and periodically thereafter.
▸ Monitor renal function before treatment and periodically thereafter.
● **DIRECTIONS FOR ADMINISTRATION**
VOTUBIA® Tablets may be dispersed in approximately 30 mL of water by gently stirring, immediately before drinking. After solution has been swallowed, any residue must be re-dispersed in the same volume of water and swallowed.
● **PATIENT AND CARER ADVICE**
Pneumonitis Non-infectious pneumonitis reported. Patients should be advised to seek urgent medical advice if new or worsening respiratory symptoms occur.
● **MEDICINAL FORMS**
There can be variation in the licensing of different medicines containing the same drug.
Tablet
CAUTIONARY AND ADVISORY LABELS 25
▸ Votubia (Novartis Pharmaceuticals UK Ltd)
 Everolimus **2.5 mg** Votubia 2.5mg tablets | 30 tablet PoM
 £1,200.00
 Everolimus **5 mg** Votubia 5mg tablets | 30 tablet PoM £2,250.00
 Everolimus **10 mg** Votubia 10mg tablets | 30 tablet PoM £2,970.00

Imatinib

● **DRUG ACTION** Imatinib is a tyrosine kinase inhibitor.

● INDICATIONS AND DOSE

Treatment of newly diagnosed Philadelphia-chromosome-positive chronic myeloid leukaemia when bone marrow transplantation is not considered first line treatment | Treatment of Philadelphia-chromosome-positive chronic myeloid leukaemia in chronic phase after failure of interferon alfa, or in accelerated phase, or in blast crisis | Treatment of newly diagnosed Philadelphia-chromosome-positive acute lymphoblastic leukaemia in combination with chemotherapy
▸ BY MOUTH
▸ Child: (consult local protocol)

IMPORTANT SAFETY INFORMATION
RISKS OF INCORRECT DOSING OF ORAL ANTI-CANCER MEDICINES
See Cytotoxic drugs p. 494.

● **CAUTIONS** Cardiac disease · history of renal failure · risk factors for heart failure
● **INTERACTIONS** → Appendix 1 (imatinib).
● **SIDE-EFFECTS**
▸ **Common or very common** Abdominal pain · appetite changes · arthralgia · ascites · conjunctivitis · constipation · cough · cramps · diarrhoea · dizziness · dry eyes · dry mouth · dry skin · dyspnoea · epistaxis · fatigue · flatulence · flushing · gastro-oesophageal reflux · haemorrhage · headache · hypoaesthesia · increased lacrimation · influenza-like symptoms · insomnia · oedema · paraesthesia · photosensitivity · pleural effusion · pruritus · pulmonary oedema · rash · sweating · taste disturbance · visual disturbances · weight changes
▸ **Uncommon** Acute respiratory failure · anxiety · cold extremities · cough · depression · drowsiness · dysphagia · electrolyte disturbances · gastric ulceration · gout · gynaecomastia · haematoma · hearing loss · heart failure · hepatic dysfunction · hypertension · hypotension · impaired memory · irregular menstruation · menorrhagia · migraine · palpitation · pancreatitis · peripheral neuropathy · renal failure · sexual dysfunction · skin hyperpigmentation · syncope · tachycardia · tinnitus · tremor · urinary frequency · vertigo
▸ **Rare** Angina · angioedema · arrhythmia · aseptic necrosis of bone · atrial fibrillation · cataract · convulsions · exfoliative dermatitis · gastro-intestinal perforation · glaucoma · haemolytic anaemia · hepatic failure · hepatic necrosis · increased intracranial pressure · inflammatory bowel disease · intestinal obstruction · myocardial infarction · myopathy · pulmonary fibrosis · pulmonary hypertension · rhabdomyolysis · Stevens-Johnson syndrome

Immune system and malignant disease

8

- ▸ **Frequency not known** Alopecia · bone-marrow suppression · drug rash with eosinophilia and systemic symptoms (DRESS) · gastro-intestinal effects · growth retardation in children · hyperuricaemia · nausea · oral mucositis · organ-related toxicity (long-term and delayed) · thromboembolism · tumour lysis syndrome · vomiting
- ● **CONCEPTION AND CONTRACEPTION** Effective contraception required during treatment.
- ● **PREGNANCY** Manufacturer advises avoid unless potential benefit outweighs risk. See also *Pregnancy and reproductive function* in Cytotoxic drugs p. 494.
- ● **BREAST FEEDING** Discontinue breast-feeding.
- ● **HEPATIC IMPAIRMENT** Start with minimum recommended dose; reduce dose further if not tolerated; consult local treatment protocol.
- ● **RENAL IMPAIRMENT** Start with minimum recommended dose; reduce dose further if not tolerated; consult local treatment protocol.
- ● **MONITORING REQUIREMENTS**
- ▸ Monitor for gastrointestinal haemorrhage.
- ▸ Monitor complete blood counts regularly.
- ▸ Monitor for fluid retention.
- ▸ Monitor liver function.
- ▸ Monitor growth in children (may cause growth retardation).
- ● **DIRECTIONS FOR ADMINISTRATION** Tablets may be dispersed in water or apple juice.
- ● **PATIENT AND CARER ADVICE** Patients or carers should be given advice on how to administer imatinib tablets.

- ● **MEDICINAL FORMS**
  There can be variation in the licensing of different medicines containing the same drug.

  Tablet
  CAUTIONARY AND ADVISORY LABELS 21, 27
  - ▸ Glivec (Novartis Pharmaceuticals UK Ltd) ▼
    Imatinib (as Imatinib mesilate) 100 mg Glivec 100mg tablets | 60 tablet PoM £973.32
    Imatinib (as Imatinib mesilate) 400 mg Glivec 400mg tablets | 30 tablet PoM £1,946.67

Chapter 9
Blood and nutrition

CONTENTS

Blood and blood-forming organs		page 521
1	**Anaemias**	521
1.1	Hypoplastic, haemolytic, and renal anaemias	522
	1.1a Atypical haemolytic uraemic syndrome and paroxysmal nocturnal haemoglobinuria	527
1.2	Iron deficiency anaemia	527
1.3	Megaloblastic anaemia	532
2	**Iron overload**	535
3	**Neutropenia and stem cell mobilisation**	537
3.1	Neutropenia	537
4	**Platelet disorders**	539
4.1	Essential thrombocythaemia	540
Nutrition and metabolic disorders		540
1	**Acid-base imbalance**	540
1.1	Metabolic acidosis	540
2	**Fluid and electrolyte imbalances**	541
2.1	Calcium imbalance	551
	2.1a Hypocalcaemia	552
2.2	Low blood volume	554
2.3	Magnesium imbalance	555
	2.3a Hypomagnesaemia	556
2.4	Phosphate imbalance	557
	2.4a Hyperphosphataemia	558
	2.4b Hypophosphataemia	559
2.5	Potassium imbalance	559

	2.5a Hyperkalaemia	page 559
	2.5b Hypokalaemia	561
3	**Metabolic disorders**	562
3.1	Acute porphyrias	562
3.2	Carnitine deficiency	564
3.3	Fabry's disease	565
3.4	Gaucher's disease	566
3.5	Homocystinuria	566
3.6	Mitochondrial disorders	567
3.7	Mucopolysaccharidosis	567
3.8	Nephropathic cystinosis	569
3.9	Niemann-pick type C disease	569
3.10	Pompe disease	570
3.11	Tyrosinaemia type I	570
3.12	Urea cycle disorders	571
3.13	Wilson's disease	573
4	**Mineral and trace elements deficiencies**	575
4.1	Zinc deficiency	575
5	**Nutrition (intravenous)**	575
6	**Nutrition (oral)**	578
6.1	Special diets	580
	6.1a Phenylketonuria	580
7	**Vitamin deficiency**	581
7.1	Neural tube defects (prevention in pregnancy)	594

9

Blood and nutrition

Blood and blood-forming organs

1 Anaemias

Anaemias

Initiation of treatment

Before initiating treatment for anaemia it is essential to determine which type is present. Iron salts may be harmful and result in iron overload if given alone to patients with anaemias other than those due to iron deficiency.

Sickle-cell anaemia

Sickle-cell disease is caused by a structural abnormality of haemoglobin resulting in deformed, less flexible red blood cells. Acute complications in the more severe forms include sickle-cell crisis, where infarction of the microvasculature and blood supply to organs results in severe pain. Sickle-cell crisis requires hospitalisation, intravenous fluids, analgesia and treatment of any concurrent infection. Chronic complications include skin ulceration, renal failure, and increased susceptibility to infection. Pneumococcal vaccine, haemophilus influenzae type b vaccine, an annual influenza vaccine and prophylactic penicillin reduce the risk of infection. Hepatitis B vaccine should be considered if the patient is not immune.

In most forms of sickle-cell disease, varying degrees of haemolytic anaemia are present accompanied by increased erythropoiesis; this may increase folate requirements and folate supplementation may be necessary.

Hydroxycarbamide p. 512 can reduce the frequency of crises and the need for blood transfusions in sickle-cell disease. The beneficial effects of hydroxycarbamide may not become evident for several months.

G6PD deficiency

Glucose 6-phosphate dehydrogenase (G6PD) deficiency is highly prevalent in individuals originating from most parts of Africa, from most parts of Asia, from Oceania, and from Southern Europe; it can also occur, rarely, in any other individuals. G6PD deficiency is more common in males than it is in females.

Individuals with G6PD deficiency are susceptible to developing acute haemolytic anaemia when they take a number of common drugs. They are also susceptible to developing acute haemolytic anaemia when they eat fava beans (broad beans, *Vicia faba*); this is termed *favism* and can be more severe in children or when the fresh fava beans are eaten raw.

When prescribing drugs for patients with G6PD deficiency, the following three points should be kept in mind:

- G6PD deficiency is genetically heterogeneous; susceptibility to the haemolytic risk from drugs varies;

thus, a drug found to be safe in some G6PD-deficient individuals may not be equally safe in others;

- manufacturers do not routinely test drugs for their effects in G6PD-deficient individuals;
- the risk and severity of haemolysis is almost always dose-related.

The lists below should be read with these points in mind. Ideally, information about G6PD deficiency should be available before prescribing a drug listed below. However, in the absence of this information, the possibility of haemolysis should be considered, especially if the patient belongs to a group in which G6PD deficiency is common.

A very few G6PD-deficient individuals with chronic non-spherocytic haemolytic anaemia have haemolysis even in the absence of an exogenous trigger. These patients must be regarded as being at high risk of severe exacerbation of haemolysis following administration of any of the drugs listed below.

Drugs with definite risk of haemolysis in most G6PD-deficient individuals

- Dapsone and other sulfones (higher doses for dermatitis herpetiformis more likely to cause problems)
- Methylthioninium chloride
- Niridazole [not on UK market]
- Nitrofurantoin
- Pamaquin [not on UK market]
- Primaquine (30 mg weekly for 8 weeks has been found to be without undue harmful effects in African and Asian people)
- Quinolones (including ciprofloxacin, moxifloxacin, nalidixic acid, norfloxacin, and ofloxacin)
- Rasburicase
- Sulfonamides (including co-trimoxazole; some sulfonamides, e.g. sulfadiazine, have been tested and found not to be haemolytic in many G6PD-deficient individuals)

Drugs with possible risk of haemolysis in some G6PD-deficient individuals

- Aspirin (acceptable up to a dose of at least 1 g daily in most G6PD-deficient individuals)
- Chloroquine (acceptable in acute malaria and malaria chemoprophylaxis)
- Menadione, water-soluble derivatives (e.g. menadiol sodium phosphate)
- Quinidine (acceptable in acute malaria) [not on UK market]
- Quinine (acceptable in acute malaria)
- Sulfonylureas

Naphthalene in mothballs also causes haemolysis in individuals with Gana6PD deficiency.

Drugs used in hypoplastic, haemolytic, and renal anaemias

Anabolic steroids, pyridoxine hydrochloride p. 585, antilymphocyte immunoglobulin, and corticosteroids are used in hypoplastic and haemolytic anaemias.

Antilymphocyte immunoglobulin given intravenously through a central line over 12–18 hours each day for 5 days produces a response in about 50% of cases of acquired *aplastic anaemia*; the response rate may be increased when ciclosporin p. 486 is given as well. Severe reactions are common in the first 2 days and profound immunosuppression can occur; antilymphocyte immunoglobulin should be given under specialist supervision with appropriate resuscitation facilities. Alternatively, oxymetholone tablets (available from 'special order' manufacturers or specialist importing companies) can be used in aplastic anaemia for 3 to 6 months.

It is unlikely that dietary deprivation of pyridoxine hydrochloride produces clinically relevant haematological effects. However, certain forms of *sideroblastic anaemia*

respond to pharmacological doses, possibly reflecting its role as a co-enzyme during haemoglobin synthesis. Pyridoxine hydrochloride is indicated in both *idiopathic acquired* and *hereditary sideroblastic anaemias*. Although complete cures have not been reported, some increase in haemoglobin can occur with high doses. *Reversible sideroblastic anaemias* respond to treatment of the underlying cause but pyridoxine hydrochloride is indicated in pregnancy, haemolytic anaemias, or during isoniazid p. 345 treatment.

Corticosteroids have an important place in the management of haematological disorders including *autoimmune haemolytic anaemia, idiopathic thrombocytopenias* and *neutropenias*, and *major transfusion reactions*. They are also used in chemotherapy schedules for many types of *lymphoma, lymphoid leukaemias*, and *paraproteinaemias*, including *multiple myeloma*.

Erythropoietins

Epoetins (recombinant human erythropoietins) are used to treat the anaemia associated with erythropoietin deficiency in chronic renal failure.

Epoetin beta p. 525 is also used for the prevention of anaemia in preterm neonates of low birth-weight; a therapeutic response may take several weeks.

There is insufficient information to support the use of erythropoietins in children with leukaemia or in those receiving cancer chemotherapy.

Darbepoetin is a glycosylated derivative of epoetin; it persists longer in the body and can be administered less frequently than epoetin.

1.1 Hypoplastic, haemolytic, and renal anaemias

ANABOLIC STEROIDS › ANDROSTAN DERIVATIVES

| Oxymetholone

- **INDICATIONS AND DOSE**

Aplastic anaemia

▸ BY MOUTH
▸ Child: 1–5 mg/kg daily for 3 to 6 months

- **MEDICINAL FORMS**
There can be variation in the licensing of different medicines containing the same drug. Forms available from special-order manufacturers include: oral suspension

Capsule

▸ Oxymetholone (Non-proprietary)
Oxymetholone 50 mg Oxymetholone 50mg capsules | 50 capsule PoM £475.00 CD4-2

EPOETINS

Epoetins

IMPORTANT SAFETY INFORMATION

ERYTHROPOIETINS–HAEMOGLOBIN CONCENTRATION

In chronic kidney disease, the use of erythropoietins can be considered in a child with anaemia. The aim of treatment is to relieve symptoms of anaemia and to avoid the need for blood transfusion. The optimum haemoglobin concentration is dependent on the child's age and factors such as comorbidities, and patient preferences. The haemoglobin concentration should not be increased beyond that which provides adequate control of symptoms of anaemia. In *adults*, overcorrection of haemoglobin concentration with erythropoietins in those with chronic kidney disease may increase the risk of serious cardiovascular events and death; haemoglobin concentrations higher than 12 g/100 mL should be avoided in children.

- **CONTRA-INDICATIONS** Avoid injections containing benzyl alcohol in neonates · pure red cell aplasia following erythropoietin therapy · uncontrolled hypertension

- **CAUTIONS** Aluminium toxicity (can impair the response to erythropoietin) · concurrent infection (can impair the response to erythropoietin) · correct factors that contribute to the anaemia of chronic renal failure, such as iron or folate deficiency, before treatment. · during dialysis (increase in unfractionated or low molecular weight heparin dose may be needed) · epilepsy · inadequately treated or poorly controlled blood pressure—interrupt treatment if blood pressure uncontrolled · ischaemic vascular disease · malignant disease · other inflammatory disease (can impair the response to erythropoietin) · sickle-cell disease (lower target haemoglobin concentration may be appropriate) · sudden stabbing migraine-like pain (warning of a hypertensive crisis) · thrombocytosis (monitor platelet count for first 8 weeks)

- **SIDE-EFFECTS**
- **Common or very common** Aggravation of hypertension (dose-dependent) · cardiovascular events · diarrhoea · dose-dependent increase in platelet count regressing during treatment (but thrombocytosis rare) · headache · hypertensive crisis (in isolated patients with normal or low blood pressure) · increase in blood pressure (dose-dependent) · influenza-like symptoms (may be reduced if intravenous injection given over 5 minutes) · nausea · shunt thrombosis especially if tendency to hypotension or arteriovenous shunt complications · vomiting
- **Very rare** Sudden loss of efficacy because of pure red cell aplasia, particularly following subcutaneous administration in patients with chronic renal failure
- **Frequency not known** Anaphylaxis · angioedema · hyperkalaemia · hypersensitivity reactions · injection-site reactions · peripheral oedema · skin reactions

SIDE-EFFECTS, FURTHER INFORMATION
Hypertensive crisis In isolated patients with normal or low blood pressure, hypertensive crisis with encephalopathy-like symptoms and generalised tonic-clonic seizures requiring immediate medical attention has occured with epoetin.
Pure red cell aplasia There have been very rare reports of pure red cell aplasia in patients treated with erythropoietins. In patients who develop a lack of efficacy with erythropoietin therapy and a diagnosis of pure red cell aplasia, treatment with erythropoietins must be discontinued and testing for erythropoietin antibodies considered. Patients who develop pure red cell aplasia should **not** be switched to another form of erythropoietin.

- **MONITORING REQUIREMENTS**
- Monitor closely blood pressure, reticulocyte counts, haemoglobin, and electrolytes—interrupt treatment if blood pressure uncontrolled.
Other factors, such as iron or folate deficiency, that contribute to the anaemia of chronic renal failure should be corrected before treatment and monitored during therapy. Supplemental iron may improve the response in resistant patients and in preterm neonates.

▸ 522

Darbepoetin alfa

- **INDICATIONS AND DOSE**

Symptomatic anaemia associated with chronic renal failure in patients on dialysis
- BY SUBCUTANEOUS INJECTION, OR BY INTRAVENOUS INJECTION
- Child 11–17 years: Initially 450 nanograms/kg once weekly, dose to be adjusted according to response by approximately 25% at intervals of at least 4 weeks, maintenance dose to be given once weekly or once every 2 weeks, reduce dose by approximately 25% if rise in haemoglobin concentration exceeds 2 g/100 mL over 4 weeks or if haemoglobin concentration exceeds 12 g/100 mL; if haemoglobin concentration continues to rise, despite dose reduction, suspend treatment until haemoglobin concentration decreases and then restart at a dose approximately 25% lower than the previous dose, when changing route give same dose then adjust according to weekly or fortnightly haemoglobin measurements, adjust doses not more frequently than every 2 weeks during maintenance treatment

Symptomatic anaemia associated with chronic renal failure in patients not on dialysis
- BY SUBCUTANEOUS INJECTION
- Child 11–17 years: Initially 450 nanograms/kg once weekly, alternatively initially 750 nanograms/kg every 2 weeks, dose to be adjusted according to response by approximately 25% at intervals of at least 4 weeks, maintenance dose can be given once weekly, every 2 weeks, or once a month, subcutaneous route preferred in patients not on haemodialysis, reduce dose by approximately 25% if rise in haemoglobin concentration exceeds 2 g/100 mL over 4 weeks or if haemoglobin concentration exceeds 12 g/100 mL; if haemoglobin concentration continues to rise, despite dose reduction, suspend treatment until haemoglobin concentration decreases and then restart at a dose approximately 25% lower than the previous dose, when changing route give same dose then adjust according to weekly or fortnightly haemoglobin measurements, adjust doses not more frequently than every 2 weeks during maintenance treatment

Symptomatic anaemia associated with chronic renal failure in patients not on dialysis
- BY INTRAVENOUS INJECTION
- Child 11–17 years: Initially 450 nanograms/kg once weekly, dose to be adjusted according to response by approximately 25% at intervals of at least 4 weeks, maintenance dose given once weekly, subcutaneous route preferred in patients not on haemodialysis, reduce dose by approximately 25% if rise in haemoglobin concentration exceeds 2 g/100 mL over 4 weeks or if haemoglobin concentration exceeds 12 g/100 mL; if haemoglobin concentration continues to rise, despite dose reduction, suspend treatment until haemoglobin concentration decreases and then restart at a dose approximately 25% lower than the previous dose, when changing route give same dose then adjust according to weekly or fortnightly haemoglobin measurements, adjust doses not more frequently than every 2 weeks during maintenance treatment

- **SIDE-EFFECTS** Injection-site pain · oedema
- **PREGNANCY** No evidence of harm in *animal* studies—manufacturer advises caution.
- **BREAST FEEDING** Manufacturer advises avoid—no information available.
- **HEPATIC IMPAIRMENT** Manufacturer advises caution.

9

Blood and nutrition

● MEDICINAL FORMS
There can be variation in the licensing of different medicines containing the same drug.

Solution for injection

▸ Aranesp (Amgen Ltd)

Darbepoetin alfa 25 microgram per 1 ml Aranesp 10micrograms/0.4ml solution for injection pre-filled syringes | 4 pre-filled disposable injection PoM £58.72

Darbepoetin alfa 40 microgram per 1 ml Aranesp 20micrograms/0.5ml solution for injection pre-filled syringes | 4 pre-filled disposable injection PoM £117.45

Darbepoetin alfa 100 microgram per 1 ml Aranesp 50micrograms/0.5ml solution for injection pre-filled syringes | 4 pre-filled disposable injection PoM £293.62
Aranesp 40micrograms/0.4ml solution for injection pre-filled syringes | 4 pre-filled disposable injection PoM £234.90
Aranesp 30micrograms/0.3ml solution for injection pre-filled syringes | 4 pre-filled disposable injection PoM £176.17

Darbepoetin alfa 200 microgram per 1 ml Aranesp 130micrograms/0.65ml solution for injection pre-filled syringes | 4 pre-filled disposable injection PoM £763.42
Aranesp 100micrograms/0.5ml solution for injection pre-filled syringes | 4 pre-filled disposable injection PoM £587.24
Aranesp 80micrograms/0.4ml solution for injection pre-filled syringes | 4 pre-filled disposable injection PoM £469.79
Aranesp 60micrograms/0.3ml solution for injection pre-filled syringes | 4 pre-filled disposable injection PoM £352.35

Darbepoetin alfa 500 microgram per 1 ml Aranesp 300micrograms/0.6ml solution for injection pre-filled syringes | 1 pre-filled disposable injection PoM £440.43
Aranesp 500micrograms/1ml solution for injection pre-filled syringes | 1 pre-filled disposable injection PoM £734.05
Aranesp 150micrograms/0.3ml solution for injection pre-filled syringes | 4 pre-filled disposable injection PoM £880.86

▸ Aranesp SureClick (Amgen Ltd)

Darbepoetin alfa 40 microgram per 1 ml Aranesp SureClick 20micrograms/0.5ml solution for injection pre-filled disposable devices | 1 pre-filled disposable injection PoM £29.36

Darbepoetin alfa 100 microgram per 1 ml Aranesp SureClick 40micrograms/0.4ml solution for injection pre-filled disposable devices | 1 pre-filled disposable injection PoM £58.72
Aranesp SureClick 80micrograms/0.4ml solution for injection pre-filled disposable devices | 1 pre-filled disposable injection PoM £117.45

Darbepoetin alfa 200 microgram per 1 ml Aranesp SureClick 60micrograms/0.3ml solution for injection pre-filled disposable devices | 1 pre-filled disposable injection PoM £88.09
Aranesp SureClick 100micrograms/0.5ml solution for injection pre-filled disposable devices | 1 pre-filled disposable injection PoM £146.81

Darbepoetin alfa 500 microgram per 1 ml Aranesp SureClick 150micrograms/0.3ml solution for injection pre-filled disposable devices | 1 pre-filled disposable injection PoM £220.22
Aranesp SureClick 300micrograms/0.6ml solution for injection pre-filled disposable devices | 1 pre-filled disposable injection PoM £440.43
Aranesp SureClick 500micrograms/1ml solution for injection pre-filled disposable devices | 1 pre-filled disposable injection PoM £734.05

◀ 522

▌Epoetin alfa

● INDICATIONS AND DOSE

BINOCRIT® PRE-FILLED SYRINGES

Symptomatic anaemia associated with chronic renal failure in patients on haemodialysis

▸ BY INTRAVENOUS INJECTION

▸ **Child (body-weight up to 10 kg):** Initially 50 units/kg 3 times a week, adjusted in steps of 25 units/kg 3 times a week, dose adjusted according to response at intervals of at least 4 weeks; maintenance 75–150 units/kg 3 times a week, intravenous injection to be given over 1–5 minutes, reduce dose by approximately 25% if rise in haemoglobin concentration exceeds 2 g/100 mL over 4 weeks or if haemoglobin concentration exceeds 12 g/100 mL; if haemoglobin concentration continues to rise, despite dose reduction, suspend treatment until haemoglobin

concentration decreases and then restart at a dose approximately 25% lower than the previous dose

▸ **Child (body-weight 10–30 kg):** Initially 50 units/kg 3 times a week, adjusted in steps of 25 units/kg 3 times a week, dose adjusted according to response at intervals of at least 4 weeks; maintenance 60–150 units/kg 3 times a week, intravenous injection to be given over 1–5 minutes, reduce dose by approximately 25% if rise in haemoglobin concentration exceeds 2 g/100 mL over 4 weeks or if haemoglobin concentration exceeds 12 g/100 mL; if haemoglobin concentration continues to rise, despite dose reduction, suspend treatment until haemoglobin concentration decreases and then restart at a dose approximately 25% lower than the previous dose

▸ **Child (body-weight 31 kg and above):** Initially 50 units/kg 3 times a week, adjusted in steps of 25 units/kg 3 times a week, dose adjusted according to response at intervals of at least 4 weeks; maintenance 30–100 units/kg 3 times a week, intravenous injection to be given over 1–5 minutes, reduce dose by approximately 25% if rise in haemoglobin concentration exceeds 2 g/100 mL over 4 weeks or if haemoglobin concentration exceeds 12 g/100 mL; if haemoglobin concentration continues to rise, despite dose reduction, suspend treatment until haemoglobin concentration decreases and then restart at a dose approximately 25% lower than the previous dose

EPREX® PRE-FILLED SYRINGES

Symptomatic anaemia associated with chronic renal failure in patients on haemodialysis

▸ BY INTRAVENOUS INJECTION

▸ **Child (body-weight up to 10 kg):** Initially 50 units/kg 3 times a week, adjusted in steps of 25 units/kg 3 times a week, dose adjusted according to response at intervals of at least 4 weeks; maintenance 75–150 units/kg 3 times a week, intravenous injection to be given over 1–5 minutes, reduce dose by approximately 25% if rise in haemoglobin concentration exceeds 2 g/100 mL over 4 weeks or if haemoglobin concentration exceeds 12 g/100 mL; if haemoglobin concentration continues to rise, despite dose reduction, suspend treatment until haemoglobin concentration decreases and then restart at a dose approximately 25% lower than the previous dose

▸ **Child (body-weight 10–30 kg):** Initially 50 units/kg 3 times a week, adjusted in steps of 25 units/kg 3 times a week, dose adjusted according to response at intervals of at least 4 weeks; maintenance 60–150 units/kg 3 times a week, intravenous injection to be given over 1–5 minutes, reduce dose by approximately 25% if rise in haemoglobin concentration exceeds 2 g/100 mL over 4 weeks or if haemoglobin concentration exceeds 12 g/100 mL; if haemoglobin concentration continues to rise, despite dose reduction, suspend treatment until haemoglobin concentration decreases and then restart at a dose approximately 25% lower than the previous dose

▸ **Child (body-weight 31–60 kg):** Initially 50 units/kg 3 times a week, adjusted in steps of 25 units/kg 3 times a week, dose adjusted according to response at intervals of at least 4 weeks; maintenance 30–100 units/kg 3 times a week, intravenous injection to be given over 1–5 minutes, reduce dose by approximately 25% if rise in haemoglobin concentration exceeds 2 g/100 mL over 4 weeks or if haemoglobin concentration exceeds 12 g/100 mL; if haemoglobin concentration continues to rise, despite dose reduction, suspend treatment until haemoglobin concentration decreases and then restart at a dose approximately 25% lower than the previous dose

▸ **Child (body-weight 61 kg and above):** Initially 50 units/kg 3 times a week, adjusted in steps of 25 units/kg 3 times a week, dose adjusted according to response at intervals of at least 4 weeks; maintenance 75–300 units/kg once weekly, maintenance dose can be given as a single dose or in divided doses, intravenous injection to be given over 1–5 minutes, reduce dose by approximately 25% if rise in haemoglobin concentration exceeds 2 g/100 mL over 4 weeks or if haemoglobin concentration exceeds 12 g/100 mL; if haemoglobin concentration continues to rise, despite dose reduction, suspend treatment until haemoglobin concentration decreases and then restart at a dose approximately 25% lower than the previous dose

● **PREGNANCY** No evidence of harm. Benefits probably outweigh risk of anaemia and of blood transfusion in pregnancy.

● **BREAST FEEDING** Unlikely to be present in milk. Minimal effect on infant.

● **HEPATIC IMPAIRMENT** Manufacturers advise caution in chronic hepatic failure.

● **PRESCRIBING AND DISPENSING INFORMATION** Products containing epoetin alfa are not identical and although there should be no important differences in terms of safety and efficacy, when prescribing biological products it is good practice to use the brand name, see *Biosimilar medicines*, under Guidance on prescribing p. 1.

● **MEDICINAL FORMS**
There can be variation in the licensing of different medicines containing the same drug.

Solution for injection

▸ Eprex (Janssen-Cilag Ltd)
Epoetin alfa 2000 unit per 1 ml Eprex 1,000units/0.5ml solution for injection pre-filled syringes | 6 pre-filled disposable injection PoM £33.18
Epoetin alfa 4000 unit per 1 ml Eprex 2,000units/0.5ml solution for injection pre-filled syringes | 6 pre-filled disposable injection PoM £66.37
Epoetin alfa 10000 unit per 1 ml Eprex 6,000units/0.6ml solution for injection pre-filled syringes | 6 pre-filled disposable injection PoM £199.11
Eprex 4,000units/0.4ml solution for injection pre-filled syringes | 6 pre-filled disposable injection PoM £132.74
Eprex 5,000units/0.5ml solution for injection pre-filled syringes | 6 pre-filled disposable injection PoM £165.92
Eprex 3,000units/0.3ml solution for injection pre-filled syringes | 6 pre-filled disposable injection PoM £99.55
Eprex 10,000units/1ml solution for injection pre-filled syringes | 6 pre-filled disposable injection PoM £331.85
Eprex 8,000units/0.8ml solution for injection pre-filled syringes | 6 pre-filled disposable injection PoM £265.48
Epoetin alfa 40000 unit per 1 ml Eprex 20,000units/0.5ml solution for injection pre-filled syringes | 1 pre-filled disposable injection PoM £110.62
Eprex 30,000units/0.75ml solution for injection pre-filled syringes | 1 pre-filled disposable injection PoM £199.11
Eprex 40,000units/1ml solution for injection pre-filled syringes | 1 pre-filled disposable injection PoM £265.48

Epoetin beta

F 522

● **INDICATIONS AND DOSE**

Symptomatic anaemia associated with chronic renal failure
▸ BY SUBCUTANEOUS INJECTION

▸ **Neonate:** Initially 20 units/kg 3 times a week for 4 weeks, increased in steps of 20 units/kg 3 times a week, according to response at intervals of 1–2 weeks, total weekly dose may be divided into daily doses; maintenance dose, initially reduce dose by half then adjust according to response at intervals of 1–2 weeks, total weekly maintenance dose may be given as a single dose or in 3 or 7 divided doses. Subcutaneous route preferred in patients not on haemodialysis. Reduce dose by approximately 25% if rise in haemoglobin concentration exceeds 2 g/100 mL over 4 weeks or if haemoglobin concentration approaches or exceeds 12 g/100 mL; if haemoglobin concentration continues to rise, despite dose reduction, suspend treatment until haemoglobin concentration decreases and then restart at a dose approximately 25% lower than the previous dose; maximum 720 units/kg per week.

▸ **Child:** Initially 20 units/kg 3 times a week for 4 weeks, increased in steps of 20 units/kg 3 times a week, according to response at intervals of 4 weeks, total weekly dose may be divided into daily doses; maintenance dose, initially reduce dose by half then adjust according to response at intervals of 1–2 weeks, total weekly maintenance dose may be given as a single dose or in 3 or 7 divided doses. Subcutaneous route preferred in patients not on haemodialysis. Reduce dose by approximately 25% if rise in haemoglobin concentration exceeds 2 g/100 mL over 4 weeks or if haemoglobin concentration approaches or exceeds 12 g/100 mL; if haemoglobin concentration continues to rise, despite dose reduction, suspend treatment until haemoglobin concentration decreases and then restart at a dose approximately 25% lower than the previous dose; maximum 720 units/kg per week
▸ BY INTRAVENOUS INJECTION

▸ **Neonate:** Initially 40 units/kg 3 times a week for 4 weeks, then increased to 80 units/kg 3 times a week, then increased in steps of 20 units/kg 3 times a week if required, at intervals of 4 weeks; maintenance dose, initially reduce dose by half then adjust according to response at intervals of 1–2 weeks. Intravenous injection to be administered over 2 minutes. Subcutaneous route preferred in patients not on haemodialysis. Reduce dose by approximately 25% if rise in haemoglobin concentration exceeds 2 g/100 mL over 4 weeks or if haemoglobin concentration approaches or exceeds 12 g/100 mL; if haemoglobin concentration continues to rise, despite dose reduction, suspend treatment until haemoglobin concentration decreases and then restart at a dose approximately 25% lower than the previous dose; maximum 720 units/kg per week.

▸ **Child:** Initially 40 units/kg 3 times a week for 4 weeks, then increased to 80 units/kg 3 times a week, then increased in steps of 20 units/kg 3 times a week if required, at intervals of 4 weeks; maintenance dose, initially reduce dose by half then adjust according to response at intervals of 1–2 weeks. Intravenous injection to be administered over 2 minutes. Subcutaneous route preferred in patients not on haemodialysis. Reduce dose by approximately 25% if rise in haemoglobin concentration exceeds 2 g/100 mL over 4 weeks or if haemoglobin continued →

9

Blood and nutrition

concentration approaches or exceeds 12 g/100 mL; if haemoglobin concentration continues to rise, despite dose reduction, suspend treatment until haemoglobin concentration decreases and then restart at a dose approximately 25% lower than the previous dose; maximum 720 units/kg per week

Prevention of anaemias of prematurity in neonates
▸ BY SUBCUTANEOUS INJECTION

▸ Neonate up to 33 weeks corrected gestational age (body-weight 0.75-1.5 kg): 250 units/kg 3 times a week preferably started within 3 days of birth and continued for 6 weeks, using single-dose unpreserved injection.

IMPORTANT SAFETY INFORMATION

MHRA/CHM ADVICE (MAY 2015) EPOETIN BETA (NEORECORMON): INCREASED RISK OF RETINOPATHY IN PRETERM INFANTS CANNOT BE EXCLUDED

There is a possible increased risk of retinopathy in premature infants, when epoetin beta is used for preventing anaemia of prematurity. When using epoetin beta in preterm infants:
- consider the benefits and risks of treatment, including the possible risk of retinopathy,
- monitor the infant for features of retinopathy, and
- advise parents or carers that their baby's eyes will be carefully monitored for any ill effects.

- **PREGNANCY** No evidence of harm. Benefits probably outweigh risk of anaemia and of blood transfusion in pregnancy.
- **BREAST FEEDING** Unlikely to be present in milk. Minimal effect on infant.
- **HEPATIC IMPAIRMENT** Manufacturers advise caution in chronic hepatic failure.

- **MEDICINAL FORMS**
There can be variation in the licensing of different medicines containing the same drug.
Solution for injection
EXCIPIENTS: May contain Phenylalanine
▸ **NeoRecormon** (Roche Products Ltd)
Epoetin beta 1667 unit per 1 ml NeoRecormon 500units/0.3ml solution for injection pre-filled syringes | 6 pre-filled disposable injection [PoM] £21.05
Epoetin beta 6667 unit per 1 ml NeoRecormon 2,000units/0.3ml solution for injection pre-filled syringes | 6 pre-filled disposable injection [PoM] £84.17
Epoetin beta 10000 unit per 1 ml NeoRecormon 3,000units/0.3ml solution for injection pre-filled syringes | 6 pre-filled disposable injection [PoM] £126.25
Epoetin beta 13333 unit per 1 ml NeoRecormon 4,000units/0.3ml solution for injection pre-filled syringes | 6 pre-filled disposable injection [PoM] £168.34
Epoetin beta 16667 unit per 1 ml NeoRecormon 10,000units/0.6ml solution for injection pre-filled syringes | 6 pre-filled disposable injection [PoM] £420.85
NeoRecormon 5,000units/0.3ml solution for injection pre-filled syringes | 6 pre-filled disposable injection [PoM] £210.42
Epoetin beta 20000 unit per 1 ml NeoRecormon 6,000units/0.3ml solution for injection pre-filled syringes | 6 pre-filled disposable injection [PoM] £252.50
Epoetin beta 33333 unit per 1 ml NeoRecormon 20,000units/0.6ml solution for injection pre-filled syringes | 6 pre-filled disposable injection [PoM] £841.71
Epoetin beta 50000 unit per 1 ml NeoRecormon 30,000units/0.6ml solution for injection pre-filled syringes | 4 pre-filled disposable injection [PoM] £841.71

F 522

Epoetin zeta

- **INDICATIONS AND DOSE**

Symptomatic anaemia associated with chronic renal failure in patients on haemodialysis
▸ BY INTRAVENOUS INJECTION
▸ Child (body-weight up to 10 kg): Initially 50 units/kg 3 times a week, adjusted according to response, adjusted in steps of 25 units/kg 3 times a week, dose to be adjusted at intervals of at least 4 weeks; maintenance 75–150 units/kg 3 times a week, to be administered over 1–5 minutes, avoid increasing haemoglobin concentration at a rate exceeding 2 g/100 mL over 4 weeks
▸ Child (body-weight 10-30 kg): Initially 50 units/kg 3 times a week, adjusted according to response, adjusted in steps of 25 units/kg 3 times a week, dose to be adjusted at intervals of at least 4 weeks; maintenance 60–150 units/kg 3 times a week, to be administered over 1–5 minutes, avoid increasing haemoglobin concentration at a rate exceeding 2 g/100 mL over 4 weeks
▸ Child (body-weight 31 kg and above): Initially 50 units/kg 3 times a week, adjusted according to response, adjusted in steps of 25 units/kg 3 times a week, dose to be adjusted at intervals of at least 4 weeks; maintenance 30–100 units/kg 3 times a week, to be administered over 1–5 minutes, avoid increasing haemoglobin concentration at a rate exceeding 2 g/100 mL over 4 weeks

- **PREGNANCY** No evidence of harm. Benefits probably outweigh risk of anaemia and of blood transfusion in pregnancy.
- **BREAST FEEDING** Unlikely to be present in milk. Minimal effect on infant.
- **HEPATIC IMPAIRMENT** Manufacturers advise caution in chronic hepatic failure.
- **PRESCRIBING AND DISPENSING INFORMATION** Products containing epoetin zeta are not identical and although there should be no important differences in terms of safety and efficacy, when prescribing biological products it is good practice to use the brand name, see *Biosimilar medicines*, under Guidance on prescribing p. 1.

- **MEDICINAL FORMS**
There can be variation in the licensing of different medicines containing the same drug.
Solution for injection
EXCIPIENTS: May contain Phenylalanine
▸ **Retacrit** (Hospira UK Ltd)
Epoetin zeta 3333 unit per 1 ml Retacrit 2,000units/0.6ml solution for injection pre-filled syringes | 6 pre-filled disposable injection [PoM] £67.88 (Hospital only)
Retacrit 3,000units/0.9ml solution for injection pre-filled syringes | 6 pre-filled disposable injection [PoM] £101.82 (Hospital only)
Retacrit 1,000units/0.3ml solution for injection pre-filled syringes | 6 pre-filled disposable injection [PoM] £33.94 (Hospital only)
Epoetin zeta 10000 unit per 1 ml Retacrit 6,000units/0.6ml solution for injection pre-filled syringes | 6 pre-filled disposable injection [PoM] £203.63 (Hospital only)
Retacrit 10,000units/1ml solution for injection pre-filled syringes | 6 pre-filled disposable injection [PoM] £339.39 (Hospital only)
Retacrit 8,000units/0.8ml solution for injection pre-filled syringes | 6 pre-filled disposable injection [PoM] £271.52 (Hospital only)
Retacrit 4,000units/0.4ml solution for injection pre-filled syringes | 6 pre-filled disposable injection [PoM] £135.76 (Hospital only)
Retacrit 5,000units/0.5ml solution for injection pre-filled syringes | 6 pre-filled disposable injection [PoM] £169.70 (Hospital only)
Epoetin zeta 40000 unit per 1 ml Retacrit 20,000units/0.5ml solution for injection pre-filled syringes | 1 pre-filled disposable injection [PoM] £96.16 (Hospital only)
Retacrit 40,000units/1ml solution for injection pre-filled syringes | 1 pre-filled disposable injection [PoM] £226.26 (Hospital only)
Retacrit 30,000units/0.75ml solution for injection pre-filled syringes | 1 pre-filled disposable injection [PoM] £169.70 (Hospital only)

1.1a Atypical haemolytic uraemic syndrome and paroxysmal nocturnal haemoglobinuria

IMMUNOSUPPRESSANTS > MONOCLONAL ANTIBODIES

Eculizumab

- **DRUG ACTION** Eculizumab, a recombinant monoclonal antibody, inhibits terminal complement activation at the C5 protein and thereby reduces haemolysis and thrombotic microangiopathy.

- **INDICATIONS AND DOSE**

  Reduce haemolysis in paroxysmal nocturnal haemoglobinuria (PNH), in those with a history of blood transfusions (under expert supervision)
  - ▸ BY INTRAVENOUS INFUSION
  - ▸ Child: Refer for specialist advice, experience very limited

  Reduce thrombotic microangiopathy in atypical haemolytic uraemic syndrome (aHUS) (specialist use only)
  - ▸ BY INTRAVENOUS INFUSION
  - ▸ Child 2 months–17 years (body-weight 5–9 kg): Initially 300 mg once weekly for 2 weeks, followed by 300 mg every 3 weeks
  - ▸ Child 2 months–17 years (body-weight 10–19 kg): Initially 600 mg once weekly for 1 week, then reduced to 300 mg once weekly for 1 week, followed by 300 mg every 2 weeks
  - ▸ Child 2 months–17 years (body-weight 20–29 kg): Initially 600 mg once weekly for 3 weeks, followed by 600 mg every 2 weeks
  - ▸ Child 2 months–17 years (body-weight 30–39 kg): Initially 600 mg once weekly for 2 weeks, then increased to 900 mg once weekly for 1 week, followed by 900 mg every 2 weeks
  - ▸ Child 2 months–17 years (body-weight 40 kg and above): Initially 900 mg once weekly for 4 weeks, then increased to 1.2 g once weekly for 1 week, followed by 1.2 g every 2 weeks

- **UNLICENSED USE** Not licensed for use in children for paroxysmal nocturnal haemoglobinuria.

- **CONTRA-INDICATIONS** Patients unvaccinated against *Neisseria meningitidis* · unresolved *Neisseria meningitidis* infection

- **CAUTIONS** Active systemic infection

  CAUTIONS, FURTHER INFORMATION
  - ▸ Meningococcal infection Vaccinate against *Neisseria meningitidis* at least 2 weeks before treatment (tetravalent vaccine against serotypes A, C, W135 and Y recommended); revaccinate according to current medical guidelines. Patients receiving eculizumab less than 2 weeks after receiving meningococcal vaccine must be given prophylactic antibiotics until 2 weeks after vaccination. Advise patient to report promptly any signs of meningococcal infection. Other immunisations should also be up to date.

- **SIDE-EFFECTS**
  - ▸ Common or very common Alopecia · arthralgia · blood disorders · cough · dizziness · dysgeusia · dysuria · fatigue · gastro-intestinal disturbances · headache · infection (including meningococcal infection) · influenza-like symptoms · infusion-related reactions · leucopenia · myalgia · nasopharyngitis · oedema · paraesthesia · pruritus · rash · spontaneous erection · thrombocytopenia · vertigo
  - ▸ Uncommon Anorexia · anxiety · chest pain · depression · epistaxis · gingival pain · Graves' disease · haematoma · hot flushing · hyperhidrosis · hypotension · jaundice · malignant melanoma · menstrual disorders · mood changes · muscle spasms · myelodysplastic syndrome · palpitation · petechiae · renal impairment · skin depigmentation · sleep disturbances · syncope · tinnitus · tremor · visual disturbances

- **CONCEPTION AND CONTRACEPTION** Manufacturer advises effective contraception during and for 5 months after treatment.

- **PREGNANCY** No information available—use only if potential benefit outweighs risk. Human IgG antibodies known to cross placenta.

- **BREAST FEEDING** No information available—manufacturer advises avoid breast-feeding during and for 5 months after treatment.

- **MONITORING REQUIREMENTS**
  - ▸ Monitor for 1 hour after infusion.
  - ▸ For *paroxysmal nocturnal haemoglobinuria*, monitor for intravascular haemolysis (including serum-lactate dehydrogenase concentration) during treatment and for at least 8 weeks after discontinuation.
  - ▸ For *atypical haemolytic uraemic syndrome*, monitor for thrombotic microangiopathy (measure platelet count, serum-lactate dehydrogenase concentration, and serum creatinine) during treatment and for at least 12 weeks after discontinuation.

- **DIRECTIONS FOR ADMINISTRATION**
  - ▸ With intravenous use Dilute requisite dose to a concentration of 5 mg/mL with Glucose 5% or Sodium Chloride 0.9% and mix gently; give over 25–45 minutes. If infusion-related reactions occur, infusion time may be increased to 4 hours in child under 12 years or 2 hours in child over 12 years.

- **PRESCRIBING AND DISPENSING INFORMATION** Consult product literature for details of supplemental doses with concomitant plasmapheresis, plasma exchange, or plasma infusion.

- **PATIENT AND CARER ADVICE** A patient information card should be provided.

  Patient or carers should be advised to report promptly any signs of meningococcal infection.

- **MEDICINAL FORMS**
  There can be variation in the licensing of different medicines containing the same drug.

  Solution for infusion
  ELECTROLYTES: May contain Sodium
  - ▸ Soliris (Alexion Pharma UK Ltd)
    Eculizumab 10 mg per 1 ml Soliris 300mg/30ml concentrate for solution for infusion vials | 1 vial [PoM] £3,150.00 (Hospital only)

1.2 Iron deficiency anaemia

Anaemia, iron deficiency

Treatment and prophylaxis

Treatment with an iron preparation is justified only in the presence of a demonstrable iron-deficiency state. Before starting treatment, it is important to exclude any serious underlying cause of the anaemia (e.g. gastro-intestinal bleeding). The possibility of thalassaemia should be considered in children of Mediterranean or Indian subcontinent descent.

Prophylaxis with an iron preparation may be appropriate in those with a poor diet, malabsorption, menorrhagia, pregnancy, in haemodialysis patients, and in the management of low birth-weight infants such as preterm neonates.

Oral iron
Iron salts should be given by mouth unless there are good reasons for using another route.

Ferrous salts show only marginal differences between one another in efficiency of absorption of iron. Haemoglobin regeneration rate is little affected by the type of salt used provided sufficient iron is given, and in most patients the speed of response is not critical. Choice of preparation is thus usually decided by formulation, palatability, incidence of side-effects, and cost.

Treatment of iron-deficiency anaemia
The oral dose of elemental iron to treat deficiency is 3–6 mg/kg (max. 200 mg) daily given in 2–3 divided doses. Iron supplementation may also be required to produce an optimum response to erythropoietins in iron-deficient children with chronic renal failure or in preterm neonates.

When prescribing, express the dose in terms of elemental iron and iron salt and select the most appropriate preparation; specify both the iron salt and formulation on the prescription. The iron content of artificial formula feeds should also be considered.

Iron content of different iron salts

Iron salt/amount	Content of ferrous iron
ferrous fumarate 200 mg	65 mg
ferrous gluconate 300 mg	35 mg
ferrous sulfate 300 mg	60 mg
ferrous sulfate dried 200 mg	65 mg
sodium feredetate 190 mg	27.5 mg

Prophylaxis of iron deficiency
In neonates, haemoglobin and haematocrit concentrations change rapidly. These changes are not due to iron deficiency and cannot be corrected by iron supplementation. Similarly, neonatal anaemia resulting from repeated blood sampling does not respond to iron therapy.

All babies, including preterm neonates, are born with substantial iron stores but these stores can become depleted unless dietary intake is adequate. All babies require an iron intake of 400–700 nanograms daily to maintain body stores. Iron in breast milk is well absorbed but that in artificial feeds or in cow's milk is less so. Most artificial formula feeds are sufficiently fortified with iron to prevent deficiency and their iron content should be taken into account when considering further iron supplementation.

Prophylactic iron supplementation may be required in babies of low birth-weight who are solely breast-fed; supplementation is started 4–6 weeks after birth and continued until mixed feeding is established.

Infants with a poor diet may become anaemic in the second year of life, particularly if cow's milk, rather than fortified formula feed, is a major part of the diet.

Compound preparations
Some oral preparations contain ascorbic acid p. 587 to aid absorption of the iron, but the therapeutic advantage of such preparations is minimal and cost may be increased.

There is no justification for the inclusion of other ingredients, such as the **B group of vitamins**, except folic acid for pregnant women.

Parenteral iron
Iron can be administered parenterally as iron dextran p. 529, iron sucrose p. 529 or ferric carboxymaltose p. 529. Parenteral iron is generally reserved for use when oral therapy is unsuccessful because the child cannot tolerate

oral iron, or does not take it reliably, or if there is continuing blood loss, or in malabsorption.

Many children with chronic renal failure who are receiving haemodialysis (and some who are receiving peritoneal dialysis) also require iron by the intravenous route on a regular basis.

With the exception of children with severe renal failure receiving haemodialysis, parenteral iron does not produce a faster haemoglobin response than oral iron provided that the oral iron preparation is taken reliably and is absorbed adequately. If parenteral iron is necessary, the dose should be calculated according to the child's body-weight and total iron deficit. Depending on the preparation used, parenteral iron is given as a total dose or in divided doses. Further treatment should be guided by monitoring haemoglobin and serum iron concentrations.

MINERALS AND TRACE ELEMENTS > IRON, INJECTABLE

Iron (injectable)

IMPORTANT SAFETY INFORMATION

MHRA/CHM ADVICE: SERIOUS HYPERSENSITIVITY REACTIONS WITH INTRAVENOUS IRON (AUGUST 2013)

Serious hypersensitivity reactions, including life-threatening and fatal anaphylactic reactions, have been reported in patients receiving intravenous iron. These reactions can occur even when a previous administration has been tolerated (including a negative test dose). Test doses are no longer recommended and caution is needed with every dose of intravenous iron.

Intravenous iron products should only be administered when appropriately trained staff and resuscitation facilities are immediately available; patients should be closely monitored for signs of hypersensitivity during and for at least 30 minutes after every administration. In the event of a hypersensitivity reaction, treatment should be stopped immediately and appropriate management initiated.

The risk of hypersensitivity is increased in patients with known allergies, immune or inflammatory conditions, or those with a history of severe asthma, eczema, or other atopic allergy; in these patients, intravenous iron should only be used if the benefits outweigh the risks.

Intravenous iron should be avoided in the first trimester of pregnancy and used in the second or third trimesters only if the benefit outweighs the potential risks for both mother and fetus.

● **SIDE-EFFECTS** Hypersensitivity reactions
SIDE-EFFECTS, FURTHER INFORMATION

▸ Anaphylactic reactions Anaphylactic reactions can occur with parenteral administration of iron complexes and facilities for cardiopulmonary resuscitation must be available. If children complain of acute symptoms particularly nausea, back pain, breathlessness, or develop hypotension, the infusion should be stopped.

Overdose
For details on the management of poisoning, see Iron salts, under Emergency treatment of poisoning p. 786.

Ferric carboxymaltose

🔖 528

- **INDICATIONS AND DOSE**

Iron-deficiency anaemia
- ▸ BY SLOW INTRAVENOUS INJECTION, OR BY INTRAVENOUS INFUSION
- ▸ Child: Dose calculated according to body-weight and iron deficit (consult product literature)

- **UNLICENSED USE** Not licensed for use in children under 14 years.
- **CAUTIONS** Allergic disorders · asthma · eczema · hypersensitivity can occur with parenteral iron and facilities for cardiopulmonary resuscitation must be available · infection (discontinue if ongoing bacteraemia) · oral iron should not be given until 5 days after last injection
- **SIDE-EFFECTS**
- ▸ **Common or very common** Dizziness · gastro-intestinal disturbances · headache · injection-site reactions · rash
- ▸ **Uncommon** Anaphylaxis · arthralgia · back pain · chest pain · fatigue · flushing · hypertension · hypotension · malaise · myalgia · paraesthesia · peripheral oedema · pruritus · pyrexia · rigors · urticaria
- ▸ **Rare** Dyspnoea
- **PREGNANCY** Avoid in first trimester; crosses the placenta in *animal* studies. May influence skeletal development.
- **HEPATIC IMPAIRMENT** Use with caution. Avoid in conditions where iron overload increases risk of impairment.
- **PRESCRIBING AND DISPENSING INFORMATION** A ferric carboxymaltose complex containing 5% (50 mg/mL) of iron.

- **MEDICINAL FORMS**
There can be variation in the licensing of different medicines containing the same drug.
Solution for injection
ELECTROLYTES: May contain Sodium
- ▸ Ferinject (Vifor Pharma UK Ltd) ▼
Iron (as Ferric carboxymaltose) 50 mg per 1 ml Ferinject 1000mg/20ml solution for injection vials | 1 vial [PoM] £154.23
Ferinject 100mg/2ml solution for injection vials | 5 vial [PoM] £81.18
Ferinject 500mg/10ml solution for injection vials | 5 vial [PoM] £405.88

Iron dextran

🔖 528

- **INDICATIONS AND DOSE**

Iron-deficiency anaemia
- ▸ BY DEEP INTRAMUSCULAR INJECTION
- ▸ Child 14–17 years: Intramuscular injection to be administered into the gluteal muscle, doses calculated according to body-weight and iron deficit (consult product literature)
- ▸ BY SLOW INTRAVENOUS INJECTION, OR BY INTRAVENOUS INFUSION
- ▸ Child: Doses calculated according to body-weight and iron deficit (consult product literature)

- **UNLICENSED USE** Not licensed for use in children under 14 years.
- **CONTRA-INDICATIONS** Active rheumatoid arthritis · asthma · eczema · history of allergic disorders · infection
- **CAUTIONS** Hypersensitivity can occur with parenteral iron and facilities for cardiopulmonary resuscitation must be available · oral iron should not be given until 5 days after last injection

- **SIDE-EFFECTS**
- ▸ **Uncommon** Abdominal pain · anaphylaxis · blurred vision · cramps · dyspnoea · flushing · nausea · numbness · pruritus · rash · vomiting
- ▸ **Rare** Angioedema · arrhythmias · arthralgia · chest pain · diarrhoea · dizziness · fatigue · hypotension · impaired consciousness · injection-site reactions · myalgia · restlessness · seizures · sweating · tachycardia · tremor
- ▸ **Very rare** Haemolysis · headache · hypertension · palpitation · paraesthesia · transient deafness
- **PREGNANCY** Avoid in first trimester.
- **HEPATIC IMPAIRMENT** Avoid in severe impairment.
- **RENAL IMPAIRMENT** Avoid in acute renal failure.
- **PRESCRIBING AND DISPENSING INFORMATION** A complex of ferric hydroxide with dextran containing 5% (50 mg/mL) of iron.

- **MEDICINAL FORMS**
There can be variation in the licensing of different medicines containing the same drug.
Solution for injection
- ▸ CosmoFer (Pharmacosmos UK Ltd) ▼
Iron (as Iron dextran) 50 mg per 1 ml CosmoFer 500mg/10ml solution for injection ampoules | 2 ampoule [PoM] £79.70
CosmoFer 100mg/2ml solution for injection ampoules | 5 ampoule [PoM] £39.85

Iron sucrose

🔖 528

- **INDICATIONS AND DOSE**

Iron-deficiency anaemia
- ▸ BY SLOW INTRAVENOUS INJECTION, OR BY INTRAVENOUS INFUSION
- ▸ Child (body-weight up to 67 kg): Dose calculated according to body-weight and iron deficit, each divided dose should not exceed 3 mg/kg/dose (consult product literature)
- ▸ Child (body-weight 67 kg and above): Dose calculated according to body-weight and iron deficit, each divided dose should not exceed max. 200 mg/dose (consult product literature)

- **UNLICENSED USE** Not licensed for use in children.
- **CONTRA-INDICATIONS** Anaphylaxis · asthma · eczema · history of allergic disorders
- **CAUTIONS** Hypersensitivity reactions can occur with parenteral iron and facilities for cardiopulmonary resuscitation must be available · infection (discontinue if ongoing bacteraemia · oral iron should not be given until 5 days after last injection

- **SIDE-EFFECTS**
- ▸ **Common or very common** Taste disturbances
- ▸ **Uncommon** Abdominal pain · bronchospasm · chest pain · diarrhoea · dizziness · dyspnoea · fever · flushing · headache · hypotension · injection-site reactions · myalgia · nausea · palpitation · pruritus · rash · tachycardia · vomiting
- ▸ **Rare** Anaphylaxis · asthenia · fatigue · hypertension · paraesthesia · peripheral oedema
- ▸ **Frequency not known** Arthralgia · bradycardia · confusion · increased sweating
- **PREGNANCY** Avoid in first trimester.
- **HEPATIC IMPAIRMENT** Use with caution. Avoid in conditions where iron overload increases risk of impairment.
- **PRESCRIBING AND DISPENSING INFORMATION** A complex of ferric hydroxide with sucrose containing 2% (20 mg/mL) of iron.

9

Blood and nutrition

- **MEDICINAL FORMS**
  There can be variation in the licensing of different medicines containing the same drug.
  Solution for injection
  - Venofer (Vifor Pharma UK Ltd, Imported (United States)) ▼
    Iron (as Iron sucrose) 20 mg per 1 ml Venofer 100mg/5ml solution for injection vials | 5 vial [PoM] £43.52
    Venofer 50mg/2.5ml solution for injection vials | 5 vial [PoM] no price available

MINERALS AND TRACE ELEMENTS > IRON, ORAL

Iron (oral)

- **SIDE-EFFECTS** Constipation · diarrhoea · epigastric pain (dose related) · faecal impaction · gastro-intestinal irritation · nausea (dose related)
  SIDE-EFFECTS, FURTHER INFORMATION
  - Managing side-effects If side-effects occur, the dose may be reduced; alternatively, another iron salt may be used, but an improvement in tolerance may simply be a result of a lower content of elemental iron. The incidence of side-effects due to ferrous sulfate is no greater than with other iron salts when compared on the basis of equivalent amounts of elemental iron.
  - Altered bowel habit Iron preparations taken orally can be constipating and occasionally lead to faecal impaction.
    Oral iron, particularly modified-release preparations, can exacerbate diarrhoea in patients with inflammatory bowel disease; care is also needed in patients with intestinal strictures and diverticular disease.
    The relationship between dose and altered bowel habit (constipation or diarrhoea) is less clear than for nausea and epigastric pain.
  Overdose
  For details on the management of poisoning, see Iron salts, under Emergency treatment of poisoning p. 786.
    Iron preparations are an important cause of accidental overdose in children and as little as 20 mg/kg of elemental iron can lead to symptoms of toxicity.
- **MONITORING REQUIREMENTS**
  - Therapeutic response The haemoglobin concentration should rise by about 100–200 mg/100 mL (1–2 g/litre) per day or 2 g/100 mL (20 g/litre) over 3–4 weeks. When the haemoglobin is in the normal range, treatment should be continued for a further 3 months to replenish the iron stores. Epithelial tissue changes such as atrophic glossitis and koilonychia are usually improved, but the response is often slow.
- **PRESCRIBING AND DISPENSING INFORMATION** Express the dose in terms of elemental iron and iron salt and select the most appropriate preparation; specify both the iron salt and formulation on the prescription.
    The iron content of artificial formula feeds should also be considered.
    The most common reason for lack of response in children is poor compliance; poor absorption is rare in children.
- **PATIENT AND CARER ADVICE** Although iron preparations are best absorbed on an empty stomach they can be taken after food to reduce gastro-intestinal side-effects. May discolour stools.

  ⬈ above

| Ferrous fumarate

- **INDICATIONS AND DOSE**
  Iron-deficiency anaemia (prophylactic)
  - BY MOUTH USING TABLETS
  - Child 12–17 years: 210 mg 1–2 times a day

- BY MOUTH USING SYRUP
  - Child 12–17 years: 140 mg twice daily
  Iron-deficiency anaemia (therapeutic)
  - BY MOUTH USING TABLETS
  - Child 12–17 years: 210 mg 2–3 times a day
  - BY MOUTH USING SYRUP
  - Child 12–17 years: 280 mg twice daily

FERSADAY®
Iron-deficiency anaemia (prophylactic)
- BY MOUTH
  - Child 12–17 years: 322 mg daily
Iron-deficiency anaemia (therapeutic)
- BY MOUTH
  - Child 12–17 years: 322 mg twice daily

GALFER® CAPSULES
Iron-deficiency anaemia (prophylactic)
- BY MOUTH
  - Child 12–17 years: 305 mg daily
Iron-deficiency anaemia (therapeutic)
- BY MOUTH
  - Child 12–17 years: 305 mg twice daily

GALFER® SYRUP
Iron-deficiency anaemia (prophylaxis)
- BY MOUTH
  - Neonate up to 36 weeks corrected gestational age (body-weight up to 3 kg): 0.5 mL daily, prophylactic iron supplementation may be required in babies of low birth-weight who are solely breast-fed; supplementation is started 4–6 weeks after birth and continued until mixed feeding is established.

  - Neonate: 0.25 mL/kilogram twice daily, the total daily dose may alternatively be given in 3 divided doses, prophylactic iron supplementation may be required in babies of low birth-weight who are solely breast-fed; supplementation is started 4–6 weeks after birth and continued until mixed feeding is established.

  - Child 1 month–11 years: 0.25 mL/kilogram twice daily, the total daily dose may alternatively be given in 3 divided doses, prophylactic iron supplementation may be required in babies of low birth-weight who are solely breast-fed; supplementation is started 4–6 weeks after birth and continued until mixed feeding is established; maximum 20 mL per day
  - Child 12–17 years: 10 mL once daily
  Iron-deficiency anaemia (therapeutic)
  - BY MOUTH
  - Neonate: 0.25 mL/kilogram twice daily, the total daily dose may alternatively be given in 3 divided doses.

  - Child 1 month–11 years: 0.25 mL/kilogram twice daily, the total daily dose may alternatively be given in 3 divided doses; maximum 20 mL per day
  - Child 12–17 years: 10 mL 1–2 times a day

- **INTERACTIONS** → Appendix 1 (iron salts).
- **PRESCRIBING AND DISPENSING INFORMATION** Non-proprietary ferrous fumarate tablets may contain 210 mg (68 mg iron), syrup may contain approx. 140 mg (45 mg iron)/5 mL; Galfer® capsules contain ferrous fumarate 305 mg (100 mg iron); Fersaday® tablets contain ferrous fumarate 322 mg (100 mg iron).
- **PATIENT AND CARER ADVICE**
  Medicines for Children leaflet: Ferrous fumarate for iron-deficiency anaemia www.medicinesforchildren.org.uk/ferrous-fumarate-for-iron-deficiency-anaemia

● **MEDICINAL FORMS**
There can be variation in the licensing of different medicines containing the same drug.

Tablet
▸ Ferrous fumarate (Non-proprietary)
Ferrous fumarate 210 mg Ferrous fumarate 210mg tablets | 84 tablet no price available DT price = £2.75 | 84 tablet P £2.75 DT price = £2.75
Ferrous fumarate 322 mg Ferrous fumarate 322mg tablets | 28 tablet no price available DT price = £0.95 | 28 tablet P £0.95–£1.00 DT price = £0.95
▸ Fersaday (AMCo)
Ferrous fumarate 322 mg Fersaday 322mg tablets | 28 tablet P £0.95 DT price = £0.95

Capsule
▸ Galfer (Thornton & Ross Ltd)
Ferrous fumarate 305 mg Galfer 305mg capsules | 100 capsule P £2.33 DT price = £2.33 | 250 capsule P £5.00

Oral solution
▸ Ferrous fumarate (Non-proprietary)
Ferrous fumarate 28 mg per 1 ml Ferrous fumarate 140mg/5ml oral solution | 200 ml P £3.73 DT price = £3.73
▸ Galfer (Thornton & Ross Ltd)
Ferrous fumarate 28 mg per 1 ml Galfer 140mg/5ml syrup sugar-free | 300 ml P £5.33 DT price = £5.33

F 530

Ferrous gluconate

● **INDICATIONS AND DOSE**

Prophylaxis of iron-deficiency anaemia
▸ BY MOUTH USING TABLETS
▸ Child 6–11 years: 300–900 mg daily
▸ Child 12–17 years: 600 mg daily

Treatment of iron-deficiency anaemia
▸ BY MOUTH USING TABLETS
▸ Child 6–11 years: 300–900 mg daily
▸ Child 12–17 years: 1.2–1.8 g daily in divided doses

● **INTERACTIONS** → Appendix 1 (iron salts).
● **PRESCRIBING AND DISPENSING INFORMATION** Ferrous gluconate 300 mg contains 35 mg iron.
● **PATIENT AND CARER ADVICE**
Medicines for Children leaflet: Ferrous gluconate for iron-deficiency anaemia www.medicinesforchildren.org.uk/ferrous-gluconate-for-iron-deficiency-anaemia

● **MEDICINAL FORMS**
There can be variation in the licensing of different medicines containing the same drug.

Tablet
▸ Ferrous gluconate (Non-proprietary)
Ferrous gluconate 300 mg Ferrous gluconate 300mg tablets | 28 tablet P £3.35 DT price = £1.95 | 1000 tablet P £119.64

F 530

Ferrous sulfate

● **INDICATIONS AND DOSE**

Iron-deficiency anaemia (prophylactic)
▸ BY MOUTH USING TABLETS
▸ Child 6–17 years: 200 mg daily

Iron-deficiency anaemia (therapeutic)
▸ BY MOUTH USING TABLETS
▸ Child 6–17 years: 200 mg 2–3 times a day

FEOSPAN®
Iron-deficiency anaemia
▸ BY MOUTH
▸ Child 1–17 years: 1 capsule daily, capsule can be opened and sprinkled on food

FERROGRAD®
Iron-deficiency anaemia (prophylactic and therapeutic)
▸ BY MOUTH
▸ Child 12–17 years: 1 tablet daily

IRONORM® DROPS
Iron-deficiency anaemia (prophylactic)
▸ BY MOUTH
▸ Child 1 month–5 years: 0.2 mL daily until mixed feeding established, higher doses up to max. 0.08 mL/kg daily may be needed, then 0.5–1.2 mL daily
▸ Child 6–11 years: 2.4 mL daily
▸ Child 12–17 years: 2.4–4.8 mL daily

Iron-deficiency anaemia (therapeutic)
▸ BY MOUTH
▸ Child 1 month–5 years: 0.12–0.24 mL/kilogram daily in 2–3 divided doses (max. per dose 8 mL)
▸ Child 6–11 years: 0.12–0.24 mL/kilogram daily in 2–3 divided doses (max. per dose 8 mL)
▸ Child 12–17 years: 4 mL 1–2 times a day

● **INTERACTIONS** → Appendix 1 (iron salts).
● **PRESCRIBING AND DISPENSING INFORMATION**
Iron content Ferrous sulfate 200 mg is equivalent to 65 mg iron; *Ironorm*® drops contain ferrous sulfate 125 mg (equivalent to 25 mg iron)/mL; *Feospan*® spansules contains ferrous sulfate 150 mg (47 mg iron) (spansule (= capsules m/r)); *Ferrograd*® tablets contain ferrous sulfate 325 mg (105 mg iron).
● **PATIENT AND CARER ADVICE**
Medicines for Children leaflet: Ferrous sulfate for iron-deficiency anaemia www.medicinesforchildren.org.uk/ferrous-sulfate-iron-deficiency-anaemia
● **NATIONAL FUNDING/ACCESS DECISIONS**
Feospan® is not prescribable under the National Health Service.
● **LESS SUITABLE FOR PRESCRIBING** *Feospan*® is less suitable for prescribing. *Ferrograd*® is less suitable for prescribing.
● **MEDICINAL FORMS**
There can be variation in the licensing of different medicines containing the same drug.

Tablet
▸ Ferrous sulfate (Non-proprietary)
Ferrous sulfate dried 200 mg Ferrous sulfate 200mg tablets | 28 tablet P £8.15 DT price = £2.75 | 60 tablet P £1.78 | 100 tablet P £14.96 | 1000 tablet P £108.93

Modified-release tablet
CAUTIONARY AND ADVISORY LABELS 25
▸ Ferrograd (Teofarma)
Ferrous sulfate dried 325 mg Ferrograd 325mg modified-release tablets | 30 tablet P £2.58 DT price = £2.58

Modified-release capsule
CAUTIONARY AND ADVISORY LABELS 25
▸ Feospan Spansules (Intrapharm Laboratories Ltd)
Ferrous sulfate dried 150 mg Feospan 150mg Spansules | 30 capsule P £3.95

Oral drops
▸ Ironorm (Wallace Manufacturing Chemists Ltd)
Ferrous sulfate 125 mg per 1 ml Ironorm 125mg/ml oral drops sugar-free | 15 ml P £30.00

Ferrous sulfate with folic acid

The properties listed below are those particular to the combination only. For the properties of the components please consider, ferrous sulfate above, folic acid p. 533.

● **INDICATIONS AND DOSE**

Iron-deficiency anaemia
▸ BY MOUTH USING MODIFIED-RELEASE TABLETS
▸ Child 12–17 years: 1 tablet daily, to be taken before food

9

Blood and nutrition

9

- LESS SUITABLE FOR PRESCRIBING *Ferrograd Folic*® is less suitable for prescribing.

- MEDICINAL FORMS
There can be variation in the licensing of different medicines containing the same drug.
Modified-release tablet
CAUTIONARY AND ADVISORY LABELS 25
▸ Ferrograd Folic (Teofarma)
Folic acid 350 microgram, Ferrous sulfate dried 325 mg Ferrograd Folic 325mg/350microgram modified-release tablets | 30 tablet P £2.64 DT price = £2.64

⟶ 530

Polysaccharide-iron complex

- INDICATIONS AND DOSE
Iron-deficiency anaemia (prophylactic)
▸ BY MOUTH

▸ Neonate: 1 drop (approximately 500 micrograms iron) per 450 g body-weight to be given 3 times a daily, dose to be administered from dropper bottle, prophylactic iron supplementation may be required in babies of low birth-weight who are solely breast-fed; supplementation is started 4–6 weeks after birth and continued until mixed feeding is established.

▸ Child 1 month–1 year: 1 drop (approximately 500 micrograms iron) per 450 g body-weight to be to be given 3 times a daily, dose to be administered from dropper bottle, prophylactic iron supplementation may be required in babies of low birth-weight who are solely breast-fed; supplementation is started 4–6 weeks after birth and continued until mixed feeding is established
▸ Child 12–17 years: 2.5 mL daily

Iron-deficiency anaemia (therapeutic)
▸ BY MOUTH
▸ Child 2–5 years: 2.5 mL daily
▸ Child 6–11 years: 5 mL daily
▸ Child 12–17 years: 5 mL 1–2 times a day

Iron-deficiency anaemia (therapeutic) if required during second and third trimester of pregnancy
▸ BY MOUTH
▸ Child 12–17 years: 5 mL once daily

- INTERACTIONS → Appendix 1 (iron salts).

- PATIENT AND CARER ADVICE Counselling on the use of the dropper advised.

- NATIONAL FUNDING/ACCESS DECISIONS
Niferex® is not available on prescription under NHS, except 30-mL paediatric dropper bottle for prophylaxis and treatment of iron deficiency in infants born prematurely; endorse prescription 'SLS'.

- MEDICINAL FORMS
There can be variation in the licensing of different medicines containing the same drug.
Oral solution
▸ Niferex (Tillomed Laboratories Ltd)
Iron (as Polysaccharide-iron complex) 100 mg Niferex 100mg/5ml elixir sugar-free | 30 ml P £2.16 sugar-free | 240 ml P £6.06

⟶ 530

Sodium feredetate

(Sodium ironedetate)

- INDICATIONS AND DOSE
Iron-deficiency anaemia (therapeutic)
▸ BY MOUTH USING ORAL SOLUTION
▸ Neonate: Up to 2.5 mL twice daily, smaller doses to be used initially.
▸ Child 1–11 months: Up to 2.5 mL twice daily, smaller doses to be used initially

▸ Child 1–4 years: 2.5 mL 3 times a day
▸ Child 5–11 years: 5 mL 3 times a day
▸ Child 12–17 years: 5 mL 3 times a day, increased to 10 mL 3 times a day, dose to be increased gradually

Iron-deficiency anaemia (prophylactic)
▸ BY MOUTH USING ORAL SOLUTION

▸ Neonate: 1 mL daily, prophylactic iron supplementation may be required in babies of low birth-weight who are solely breast-fed; supplementation is started 4–6 weeks after birth and continued until mixed feeding is established.

▸ Child 1–11 months: 1 mL daily, prophylactic iron supplementation may be required in babies of low birth-weight who are solely breast-fed; supplementation is started 4–6 weeks after birth and continued until mixed feeding is established

- UNLICENSED USE Not licensed for prophylaxis of iron deficiency.

- INTERACTIONS → Appendix 1 (iron salts).

- PRESCRIBING AND DISPENSING INFORMATION *Sytron*® contains 190 mg sodium feredetate, which is equivalent to 27.5 mg of iron/5 mL.

- PATIENT AND CARER ADVICE
Medicines for Children leaflet: Sytron (sodium feredetate) for the prevention of anaemia www.medicinesforchildren.org.uk/sytron-sodium-feredetate-for-prevention-of-anaemia
Medicines for Children leaflet: Sytron (sodium feredetate) for the treatment of anaemia www.medicinesforchildren.org.uk/sytron-sodium-feredetate-for-treatment-of-anaemia

- MEDICINAL FORMS
There can be variation in the licensing of different medicines containing the same drug.
Oral solution
▸ Sodium feredetate (Non-proprietary)
Sodium feredetate 38 mg per 1 ml Sodium feredetate 190mg/5ml oral solution sugar free sugar-free | 500 ml PoM £14.95–£17.94 DT price = £14.95
▸ Sytron (Forum Health Products Ltd)
Sodium feredetate 38 mg per 1 ml Sytron oral solution sugar-free | 500 ml P £14.95 DT price = £14.95

1.3 Megaloblastic anaemia

Anaemia, megaloblastic

Overview

Megaloblastic anaemias are rare in children; they may result from a lack of either vitamin B_{12} or folate and it is essential to establish in every case which deficiency is present and the underlying cause. In emergencies, when delay might be dangerous, it is sometimes necessary to administer both substances after the bone marrow test while plasma assay results are awaited. Normally, however, appropriate treatment should not be instituted until the results of tests are available.

Vitamin B_{12} is used in the treatment of megaloblastosis caused by *prolonged nitrous oxide anaesthesia*, which inactivates the vitamin, and in the rare disorders of *congenital transcobalamin II deficiency* and *homocystinuria*.

Vitamin B_{12} should be given prophylactically after *total ileal resection*.

Apart from dietary deficiency, all other causes of vitamin B_{12} deficiency are attributable to malabsorption. There is little place for the use of low-dose vitamin B_{12} orally and none for vitamin B_{12} intrinsic factor complexes given by mouth. Vitamin B_{12} in large oral doses [unlicensed] may be effective.

Hydroxocobalamin p. 534 has completely replaced cyanocobalamin p. 534 as the form of vitamin B_{12} of choice for therapy; it is retained in the body longer than cyanocobalamin and thus for maintenance therapy can be given at intervals of up to 3 months. Treatment is generally initiated with frequent administration of intramuscular injections to replenish the depleted body stores. Thereafter, maintenance treatment, which is usually for life, can be instituted. There is no evidence that doses larger than those recommended provide any additional benefit in vitamin B_{12} neuropathy.

Folic acid below has few indications for long-term therapy since most causes of folate deficiency are self-limiting or will yield to a short course of treatment. It should not be used in undiagnosed megaloblastic anaemia unless vitamin B_{12} is administered concurrently otherwise neuropathy may be precipitated.

In *folate-deficient megaloblastic anaemia* (e.g. because of poor nutrition, pregnancy, or antiepileptic drugs), daily folic acid supplementation for 4 months brings about haematological remission and replenishes body stores; higher doses may be necessary in malabsorption states. In pregnancy, folic acid daily is continued to term.

For prophylaxis in *chronic haemolytic states*, *malabsorption*, or *in renal dialysis*, folic acid is given daily or sometimes weekly, depending on the diet and the rate of haemolysis.

Folic acid is also used for the prevention of methotrexate-induced side-effects in juvenile idiopathic arthritis, severe Crohn's disease and severe psoriasis.

Folic acid is actively excreted in breast milk and is well absorbed by the infant. It is also present in cow's milk and artificial formula feeds but is heat labile. Serum and red cell folate concentrations fall after delivery and urinary losses are high, particularly in low birth-weight neonates. Although symptomatic deficiency is rare in the absence of malabsorption or prolonged diarrhoea, it is common for neonatal units to give supplements of folic acid to all preterm neonates from 2 weeks of age until full-term corrected age is reached, particularly if heated breast milk is used without an artificial formula fortifier.

Folinic acid p. 515 is also effective in the treatment of folate deficient megaloblastic anaemia but it is normally only used in association with cytotoxic drugs; it is given as calcium folinate.

There is **no** justification for prescribing multiple ingredient vitamin preparations containing vitamin B_{12} or folic acid.

For the use of folic acid before and during pregnancy, see Neural tube defects (prevention in pregnancy) p. 594.

VITAMINS AND TRACE ELEMENTS > FOLATES

Folic acid

9.6.2016

- **INDICATIONS AND DOSE**

Folate-deficient megaloblastic anaemia
▸ BY MOUTH

▸ Neonate: Initially 500 micrograms/kg once daily for up to 4 months.

▸ Child 1–11 months: Initially 500 micrograms/kg once daily (max. per dose 5 mg) for up to 4 months, doses up to 10 mg daily may be required in malabsorption states
▸ Child 1–17 years: 5 mg daily for 4 months (until term in pregnant women), doses up to 15 mg daily may be required in malabsorption states

Folate supplementation in neonates
▸ BY MOUTH

▸ Neonate: 50 micrograms once daily.

Prevention of neural tube defects (in those at a low risk of conceiving a child with a neural tube defect see p. 594)
▸ BY MOUTH

▸ Females of childbearing potential: 400 micrograms daily, to be taken before conception and until week 12 of pregnancy

Prevention of neural tube defects (in those in the high-risk group who wish to become pregnant or who are at risk of becoming pregnant see p. 594)
▸ BY MOUTH

▸ Females of childbearing potential: 5 mg daily, to be taken before conception and until week 12 of pregnancy

Prevention of neural tube defects (in those with sickle-cell disease)
▸ BY MOUTH

▸ Females of childbearing potential: 5 mg daily, patient should continue taking their normal dose of folic acid 5 mg daily (or increase the dose to 5 mg daily) before conception and continue this throughout pregnancy

Prevention of methotrexate side-effects in severe Crohn's disease | Prevention of methotrexate side-effects in severe psoriasis
▸ BY MOUTH

▸ Child: 5 mg once weekly, dose to be taken on a different day to methotrexate dose

Prophylaxis of folate deficiency in dialysis
▸ BY MOUTH

▸ Child 1 month–11 years: 250 micrograms/kg once daily (max. per dose 10 mg)
▸ Child 12–17 years: 5–10 mg once daily

Haemolytic anaemia | Metabolic disorders
▸ BY MOUTH

▸ Child 1 month–11 years: 2.5–5 mg once daily
▸ Child 12–17 years: 5–10 mg once daily

Prevention of methotrexate side-effects in juvenile idiopathic arthritis
▸ BY MOUTH

▸ Child: 1 mg daily, alternatively 5 mg once weekly, dose to be adjusted according to local guidelines, weekly dose to be taken on a different day to methotrexate dose

- **UNLICENSED USE** Unlicensed for limiting methotrexate toxicity.
- **CAUTIONS** Should never be given alone for pernicious anaemia (may precipitate subacute combined degeneration of the spinal cord)
- **INTERACTIONS** → Appendix 1 (folates).
- **SIDE-EFFECTS**
▸ **Rare** Gastro-intestinal disturbances
- **PATIENT AND CARER ADVICE**
Medicines for Children leaflet: Folic acid for megaloblastic anaemia caused by folate deficiency and haemolytic anaemia www.medicinesforchildren.org.uk/folic-acid-megaloblastic-anaemia-caused-folate-deficiency-and-haemolytic-anaemia

- **EXCEPTIONS TO LEGAL CATEGORY** Can be sold to the public provided daily doses do not exceed 500 micrograms.

- **MEDICINAL FORMS**
There can be variation in the licensing of different medicines containing the same drug. Forms available from special-order manufacturers include: capsule, oral suspension, oral solution

Tablet
▸ **Folic acid (Non-proprietary)**
Folic acid 400 microgram Folic acid 400microgram tablets | 90 tablet [PoM] no price available DT price = £2.71 | 90 tablet £2.71 DT price = £2.71
Folic acid 5 mg Folic acid 5mg tablets | 28 tablet [PoM] £2.00 DT price = £0.83 | 1000 tablet [PoM] £41.75

Oral solution

▸ Folic acid (Non-proprietary)
Folic acid 500 microgram per 1 ml Folic acid 2.5mg/5ml oral solution sugar free sugar-free | 150 ml [PoM] £9.16 DT price = £9.16 sugar-free | 150 ml [PoM] £9.16 DT price = £9.16

▸ Lexpec (Rosemont Pharmaceuticals Ltd)
Folic acid 500 microgram per 1 ml Lexpec Folic Acid 2.5mg/5ml oral solution sugar-free | 150 ml [PoM] £9.16 DT price = £9.16

VITAMINS AND TRACE ELEMENTS ❭ VITAMIN B GROUP

Cyanocobalamin

● **INDICATIONS AND DOSE**

Vitamin B$_{12}$ deficiency of dietary origin
▸ BY MOUTH
▸ Child: 50–105 micrograms daily in 1–3 divided doses

● **PRESCRIBING AND DISPENSING INFORMATION** The BP directs that when vitamin B$_{12}$ injection is prescribed or demanded hydroxocobalamin injection shall be dispensed or supplied.
 Currently available brands of the tablet may not be suitable for vegans.

● **NATIONAL FUNDING/ACCESS DECISIONS**
Cyanocobalamin liquid, *Cytacon*® tablets, and *Cytamen*® injection are not available on prescription under the NHS.

● **LESS SUITABLE FOR PRESCRIBING** Cyanocobalamin is less suitable for prescribing.

● **MEDICINAL FORMS**
There can be variation in the licensing of different medicines containing the same drug. Forms available from special-order manufacturers include: tablet

Tablet

▸ Cyanocobalamin (Non-proprietary)
Cyanocobalamin 50 microgram Cyanocobalamin 50microgram tablets | 50 tablet [P] £6.24 DT price = £8.99 | 50 tablet £8.99 DT price = £8.99 | 100 tablet no price available
Cyanocobalamin 1 mg Behepan 1mg tablets | 100 tablet [PoM] no price available

▸ Cytacon (AMCo)
Cyanocobalamin 50 microgram Cytacon 50microgram tablets | 50 tablet [P] £8.99 DT price = £8.99

Oral solution

▸ Cyanocobalamin (Non-proprietary)
Cyanocobalamin 7 microgram per 1 ml Cyanocobalamin 35micrograms/5ml oral solution | 200 ml [P] £8.75

Hydroxocobalamin

● **INDICATIONS AND DOSE**

Macrocytic anaemia without neurological involvement
▸ BY INTRAMUSCULAR INJECTION
▸ Child: Initially 0.25–1 mg 3 times a week for 2 weeks, then 0.25 mg once weekly until blood count normal, then 1 mg every 3 months

Macrocytic anaemia with neurological involvement
▸ BY INTRAMUSCULAR INJECTION
▸ Child: Initially 1 mg once daily on alternate days until no further improvement, then 1 mg every 2 months

Prophylaxis of macrocytic anaemias associated with vitamin B$_{12}$ deficiency
▸ BY INTRAMUSCULAR INJECTION
▸ Child: 1 mg every 2–3 months

Leber's optic atrophy
▸ BY INTRAMUSCULAR INJECTION
▸ Child: Initially 1 mg daily for 2 weeks, then 1 mg twice weekly until no further improvement, then 1 mg every 1–3 months

Congenital transcobalamin II deficiency
▸ BY INTRAMUSCULAR INJECTION
▸ Neonate: 1 mg 3 times a week for 1 year, then reduced to 1 mg once weekly, adjusted as appropriate.
▸ Child: 1 mg 3 times a week for 1 year, then reduced to 1 mg once weekly, adjusted as appropriate

Methylmalonic acidaemia and homocystinuria
▸ BY INTRAMUSCULAR INJECTION
▸ Child: Initially 1 mg daily for 5–7 days, then adjusted according to response to up to 1 mg 1–2 times a week, this is the maintenance dose

Methylmalonic acidaemia, maintenance once intramuscular response established
▸ BY MOUTH
▸ Child: 5–10 mg 1–2 times a week, some children do not respond to oral route

CYANOKIT®

Poisoning with cyanides
▸ BY INTRAVENOUS INFUSION
▸ Child (body-weight 5 kg and above): Initially 70 mg/kg (max. per dose 5 g), to be given over 15 minutes, then 70 mg/kg (max. per dose 5 g) if required, this second dose can be given over 15 minutes–2 hours depending on severity of poisoning and patient stability

● **UNLICENSED USE**
▸ With intramuscular use or oral use Licensed for use in children (age not specified by manufacturers). Not licensed for use in inborn errors of metabolism.

● **CAUTIONS**
▸ With intramuscular or oral use Should not be given before diagnosis fully established

● **INTERACTIONS** → Appendix 1 (hydroxocobalamin).

● **SIDE-EFFECTS**

GENERAL SIDE-EFFECTS
Dizziness · headache · pruritus

SPECIFIC SIDE-EFFECTS
▸ With intramuscular use Chromaturia · fever · hypersensitivity reactions · hypokalaemia (during initial treatment) · injection-site reactions · nausea · rash · thrombocytosis (during initial treatment)
▸ With intravenous use Dyspnoea · eye disorders · gastro-intestinal disturbances · hot flush · lymphocytopenia · memory impairment · peripheral oedema · pustular rashes · red coloration of urine · restlessness · reversible red coloration of skin and mucous membranes · throat disorders · transient hypertension
▸ With oral use Chromaturia · fever · hypersensitivity reactions · nausea

● **BREAST FEEDING** Present in milk but not known to be harmful.

● **EFFECT ON LABORATORY TESTS**
▸ With intravenous use Deep red colour of hydroxocobalamin may interfere with laboratory tests.

● **DIRECTIONS FOR ADMINISTRATION**
▸ With intravenous use For *intravenous infusion (Cyanokit)*®, given intermittently *in* Sodium chloride 0.9%, reconstitute 5 g vial with 200 mL Sodium Chloride 0.9%; gently invert vial for at least 1 minute to mix (do not shake).
▸ With oral use For administration by *mouth*, injection solution may be given orally; it will not have prolonged effect via this route.

● **PRESCRIBING AND DISPENSING INFORMATION**
▸ With intramuscular use The BP directs that when vitamin B$_{12}$ injection is prescribed or demanded, hydroxocobalamin injection shall be dispensed or supplied.
Poisoning by cyanides
▸ With intravenous use *Cyanokit*® is the only preparation of hydroxocobalamin that is suitable for use in victims of

smoke inhalation who show signs of significant cyanide poisoning.

- **NATIONAL FUNDING/ACCESS DECISIONS**
  Cobalin-H® is not prescribable under National Health Service (NHS). *Neo-Cytamen*® is not prescribable under National Health Service (NHS).

- **MEDICINAL FORMS**
  There can be variation in the licensing of different medicines containing the same drug. Forms available from special-order manufacturers include: oral suspension, oral solution

  Solution for injection
  ▸ Hydroxocobalamin (Non-proprietary)
    Hydroxocobalamin 1 mg per 1 ml Hydroxocobalamin 1mg/1ml solution for injection ampoules | 5 ampoule [PoM] £12.49 DT price = £7.18
    Hydroxocobalamin 2.5 mg per 1 ml Hepavit 5mg/2ml solution for injection ampoules | 2 ampoule [PoM] no price available
    Hydroxocobalamin 5 mg per 1 ml Megamilbedoce 10mg/2ml solution for injection ampoules | 10 ampoule [PoM] no price available
  ▸ Cobalin (AMCo)
    Hydroxocobalamin 1 mg per 1 ml Cobalin-H 1mg/1ml solution for injection ampoules | 5 ampoule [PoM] £9.50 DT price = £7.18
  ▸ Neo-Cytamen (Focus Pharmaceuticals Ltd)
    Hydroxocobalamin 1 mg per 1 ml Neo-Cytamen 1000micrograms/1ml solution for injection ampoules | 5 ampoule [PoM] £12.49 DT price = £7.18

  Powder for solution for infusion
  ▸ Cyanokit (Swedish Orphan Biovitrum Ltd)
    Hydroxocobalamin 5 gram Cyanokit 5g powder for solution for infusion vials | 1 vial [PoM] no price available

2 Iron overload

Iron overload

Overview

Severe tissue iron overload can occur in aplastic and other refractory anaemias, mainly as the result of repeated blood transfusions. It is a particular problem in refractory anaemias with hyperplastic bone marrow, especially *thalassaemia major*, where excessive iron absorption from the gut and inappropriate iron therapy can add to the tissue siderosis.

Iron overload associated with haemochromatosis can be treated with repeated venesection. Venesection may also be used for patients who have received multiple transfusions and whose bone marrow has recovered. Where venesection is contra-indicated, and in thalassaemia, the long-term administration of the iron chelating compound desferrioxamine mesilate p. 536 is useful. Desferrioxamine mesilate (up to 2 g per unit of blood) may also be given at the time of blood transfusion, provided that the desferrioxamine mesilate is **not** added to the blood and is **not** given through the same line as the blood (but the two may be given through the same cannula).

Iron excretion induced by desferrioxamine mesilate is enhanced by ascorbic acid p. 587 (vitamin C) daily by mouth; it should be given separately from food since it also enhances iron absorption. Ascorbic acid should not be given to children with cardiac dysfunction; in children with normal cardiac function ascorbic acid should be introduced 1 month after starting desferrioxamine mesilate.

Desferrioxamine mesilate infusion can be used to treat *aluminium overload* in dialysis patients; theoretically 100 mg of desferrioxamine binds with 4.1 mg of aluminium.

ANTIDOTES AND CHELATORS › IRON CHELATORS

Deferasirox

- **DRUG ACTION** Deferasirox is an oral iron chelator.

- **INDICATIONS AND DOSE**

  Transfusion-related chronic iron overload when desferrioxamine is contra-indicated or inadequate in children aged 2–5 years with thalassaemia major who receive frequent blood transfusions | Transfusion-related chronic iron overload when desferrioxamine is contra-indicated or inadequate in patients over 2 years with thalassaemia major who receive infrequent blood transfusions (less than 7 mL/kg/month of packed red blood cells) | Transfusion-related chronic iron overload when desferrioxamine is contra-indicated or inadequate in patients over 2 years with other anaemias | Treatment of chronic iron overload in patients over 6 years with thalassaemia major who receive frequent blood transfusions (more than 7 mL/kg/month of packed red blood cells)
  ▸ BY MOUTH
  ▸ Child 2–17 years: Initially 10–30 mg/kg once daily, dose adjusted according to serum-ferritin concentration and amount of transfused blood—consult product literature; adjusted in steps of 5–10 mg/kg every 3–6 months, maintenance dose adjusted according to serum-ferritin concentration; maximum 40 mg/kg per day; Usual maximum 30 micrograms/kg

  Treatment of chronic iron overload when desferrioxamine is contra-indicated or inadequate (with non-transfusion-dependent thalassaemia syndromes)
  ▸ BY MOUTH
  ▸ Child 10–17 years: Initially 10 mg/kg once daily, maintenance dose adjusted according to serum-ferritin concentration and liver-iron concentration (consult product literature); maximum 10 mg/kg per day

- **UNLICENSED USE** Not licensed for treatment of chronic iron overload in children under 6 years with thalassaemia major who receive frequent blood transfusions (more than 7 mL/kg/month of packed red blood cells).

- **CAUTIONS** History of liver cirrhosis · not recommended in conditions which may reduce life expectancy (e.g. high-risk myelodysplastic syndromes) · platelet count less than $50{\times}10^9$/litre · risk of gastro-intestinal ulceration and haemorrhage · unexplained cytopenia—consider treatment interruption

- **INTERACTIONS** → Appendix 1 (deferasirox).

- **SIDE-EFFECTS**
  ▸ **Common or very common** Fatal gastro-intestinal haemorrhage · gastro-intestinal disturbances · gastro-intestinal ulceration · headache · proteinuria · pruritus · rash
  ▸ **Uncommon** Anxiety · cholelithiasis · disturbances of hearing and vision · dizziness · fatigue · glucosuria · hepatitis · lens opacity · maculopathy · oedema · pharyngitis · pyrexia · renal tubulopathy · skin pigmentation · sleep disorder
  ▸ **Frequency not known** Acute renal failure · agranulocytosis · alopecia · anaemia · anaphylaxis · angioedema · blood disorders · hepatic failure · hypersensitivity reactions · neutropenia · pancytopenia · thrombocytopenia · tubulointerstitial nephritis

- **PREGNANCY** Manufacturer advises avoid unless essential— toxicity in *animal* studies.

- **BREAST FEEDING** Manufacturer advises avoid—present in milk in *animal* studies.

- **HEPATIC IMPAIRMENT** Use with caution in moderate impairment, reduce dose considerably then gradually

9

Blood and nutrition

increase to max. 50% of normal dose. Avoid in severe impairment.

- **RENAL IMPAIRMENT** Reduce dose by 10 mg/kg if serum-creatinine increased above age-appropriate limits or estimated glomerular filtration rate less than 90 mL/minute/1.73 m² on 2 consecutive occasions—interrupt treatment if deterioration in renal function persists after dose reduction. Avoid if estimated glomerular filtration rate less than 60 mL/minute/1.73 m².
- **MONITORING REQUIREMENTS**
  ‣ Eye and ear examinations required before treatment and annually during treatment.
  ‣ Monitor body-weight, height, and sexual development in children annually.
  ‣ Monitor serum-ferritin concentration monthly.
  ‣ Test liver function before treatment, then every 2 weeks during the first month, and then monthly.
  ‣ Measure baseline serum creatinine and monitor renal function weekly during the first month of treatment and monthly thereafter.
  ‣ Test for proteinuria monthly.
  ‣ Monitor liver-iron concentration every three months in children with non-transfusion-dependent thalassaemia syndromes when serum ferritin is ≤800 micrograms/litre.
- **DIRECTIONS FOR ADMINISTRATION** Tablets should be dispersed in water, orange juice, or apple juice; if necessary resuspend residue.
- **PATIENT AND CARER ADVICE**
  Medicines for Children leaflet: Deferasirox for removing excess iron www.medicinesforchildren.org.uk/deferasirox-for-removing-excess-iron

  Patient or carers should be given advice on how to administer deferasirox dispersible tablets.
- **MEDICINAL FORMS**
  There can be variation in the licensing of different medicines containing the same drug.
  Dispersible tablet
  CAUTIONARY AND ADVISORY LABELS 13, 22
  ‣ **Exjade** (Novartis Pharmaceuticals UK Ltd) ▼
    Deferasirox 125 mg Exjade 125mg dispersible tablets sugar-free | 28 tablet PoM £117.60
    Deferasirox 250 mg Exjade 250mg dispersible tablets sugar-free | 28 tablet PoM £235.20
    Deferasirox 500 mg Exjade 500mg dispersible tablets sugar-free | 28 tablet PoM £470.40

Deferiprone

- **DRUG ACTION** Deferiprone is an oral iron chelator.

- **INDICATIONS AND DOSE**
  Treatment of iron overload in patients with thalassaemia major in whom desferrioxamine is contra-indicated or is inadequate
  ‣ BY MOUTH
  ‣ Child 6–17 years: 25 mg/kg 3 times a day; maximum 100 mg/kg per day

- **UNLICENSED USE** Not licensed for use in children under 6 years.
- **CONTRA-INDICATIONS** History of agranulocytosis or recurrent neutropenia
- **INTERACTIONS** → Appendix 1 (deferiprone).
- **SIDE-EFFECTS** Agranulocytosis · arthropathy · blood dyscrasias · gastro-intestinal disturbances (reducing dose and increasing gradually may improve tolerance) · headache · increased appetite · neutropenia · red-brown urine discoloration · zinc deficiency
- **CONCEPTION AND CONTRACEPTION** Manufacturer advises avoid before intended conception—teratogenic and

embryotoxic in *animal* studies. Contraception advised in females of child-bearing potential.

- **PREGNANCY** Manufacturer advises avoid during pregnancy—teratogenic and embryotoxic in *animal* studies.
- **BREAST FEEDING** Manufacturer advises avoid—no information available.
- **HEPATIC IMPAIRMENT** Manufacturer advises monitor liver function—interrupt treatment if persistent elevation in serum alanine aminotransferase.
- **RENAL IMPAIRMENT** Manufacturer advises caution—no information available.
- **MONITORING REQUIREMENTS** Monitor neutrophil count weekly and discontinue treatment if neutropenia develops.
- **PATIENT AND CARER ADVICE**
  Blood disorders Patients or their carers should be told how to recognise signs of neutropenia and advised to seek immediate medical attention if symptoms such as fever or sore throat develop.

- **MEDICINAL FORMS**
  There can be variation in the licensing of different medicines containing the same drug. Forms available from special-order manufacturers include: capsule, oral suspension, oral solution
  Tablet
  CAUTIONARY AND ADVISORY LABELS 14
  ‣ **Ferriprox** (Swedish Orphan Biovitrum Ltd)
    Deferiprone 500 mg Ferriprox 500mg tablets | 100 tablet PoM £152.39
    Deferiprone 1 gram Ferriprox 1000mg tablets | 50 tablet PoM £175.25
  Oral solution
  CAUTIONARY AND ADVISORY LABELS 14
  ‣ **Ferriprox** (Swedish Orphan Biovitrum Ltd)
    Deferiprone 100 mg per 1 ml Ferriprox 100mg/ml oral solution sugar-free | 500 ml PoM £152.39

Desferrioxamine mesilate

(Deferoxamine Mesilate)

- **INDICATIONS AND DOSE**
  Iron poisoning
  ‣ BY CONTINUOUS INTRAVENOUS INFUSION
  ‣ Neonate: Initially up to 15 mg/kg/hour, max. 80 mg/kg in 24 hours, dose to be reduced after 4–6 hours, in severe cases, higher doses may be given on advice from the National Poisons Information Service.
  ‣ Child: Initially up to 15 mg/kg/hour, max. 80 mg/kg in 24 hours, dose to be reduced after 4–6 hours, in severe cases, higher doses may be given on advice from the National Poisons Information Service
  Aluminium overload in dialysis patients
  ‣ BY INTRAVENOUS INFUSION
  ‣ Child: 5 mg/kg once weekly
  Chronic iron overload (low iron overload)
  ‣ BY SUBCUTANEOUS INFUSION
  ‣ Child: Initially up to 30 mg/kg 3–7 times a week, to be given over 8–12 hours, the dose should reflect the degree of iron overload
  Chronic iron overload (established overload)
  ‣ BY SUBCUTANEOUS INFUSION
  ‣ Child: 20–50 mg/kg daily

- **UNLICENSED USE**
  ‣ When used for Iron poisoning Licensed for use in children (age range not specified by manufacturer).
- **CAUTIONS** Aluminium-related encephalopathy (may exacerbate neurological dysfunction)
- **INTERACTIONS** → Appendix 1 (desferrioxamine).

SIDE-EFFECTS

▶ **Common or very common** Abdominal pain · arthralgia · bone disorders · growth retardation · headache · hearing disturbances · injection-site reactions · myalgia · nausea · pyrexia · vomiting

▶ **Rare** Anaphylaxis · blood dyscrasias · bone pain · diarrhoea · hepatic impairment · hypotension (especially when given too rapidly by intravenous injection) · leg cramps · lens opacity · leucopenia · rash · retinopathy · thrombocytopenia · visual disturbances · Yersinia and mucormycosis infections

▶ **Very rare** Acute respiratory distress · convulsions · dizziness · neurological disturbances · neuropathy · paraesthesia · renal impairment

▶ **Frequency not known** Muscle spasms

● **PREGNANCY** Teratogenic in *animal* studies. Manufacturer advises use only if potential benefit outweighs risk.

● **BREAST FEEDING** Manufacturer advises use only if potential benefit outweighs risk—no information available.

● **RENAL IMPAIRMENT** Use with caution.

● **MONITORING REQUIREMENTS**

▶ Eye and ear examinations before treatment and at 3-month intervals during treatment.

▶ Monitor body-weight and height in children at 3-month intervals—risk of growth retardation with excessive doses.

● **DIRECTIONS FOR ADMINISTRATION** For full details and warnings relating to administration, consult product literature.

▶ When used for Chronic iron overload or Aluminium overload in dialysis patients For *intravenous* or *subcutaneous infusion*, reconstitute powder with Water for Injection to a concentration of 100 mg/mL; dilute with Glucose 5% or Sodium Chloride 0.9%. In *haemodialysis* or *haemo-filtration* administer over the last hour of dialysis (may be given via the dialysis fistula). *Intraperitoneal*: may be added to dialysis fluid. In CAPD give prior to the last exchange of the day.

● **PATIENT AND CARER ADVICE**
Medicines for Children leaflet: Deferasirox for removing excess iron www.medicinesforchildren.org.uk/deferasirox-removing-excess-iron-0

● **MEDICINAL FORMS**
There can be variation in the licensing of different medicines containing the same drug.

Powder for solution for injection

▶ Desferrioxamine mesilate (Non-proprietary)
Desferrioxamine mesilate 500 mg Desferrioxamine 500mg powder for solution for injection vials | 10 vial PoM £39.90–£50.00
Desferrioxamine mesilate 2 gram Desferrioxamine 2g powder for solution for injection vials | 1 vial PoM £17.95–£20.00

▶ Desferal (Novartis Pharmaceuticals UK Ltd)
Desferrioxamine mesilate 500 mg Desferal 500mg powder for solution for injection vials | 10 vial PoM £46.63
Desferrioxamine mesilate 2 gram Desferal 2g powder for solution for injection vials | 1 vial PoM £18.66

---

3 Neutropenia and stem cell mobilisation

3.1 Neutropenia

Neutropenia

Management

Recombinant human granulocyte-colony stimulating factor (rhG-CSF) stimulates the production of neutrophils and may reduce the duration of chemotherapy-induced neutropenia

and thereby reduce the incidence of associated sepsis; there is as yet no evidence that it improves overall survival. Filgrastim p. 538 (unglycosylated rhG-CSF) and lenograstim p. 539 (glycosylated rhG-CSF) have similar effects; both have been used in a variety of clinical settings, including cytotoxic-induced neutropenia, and neutropenia following bone marrow transplantation, but they do not have any clear-cut routine indications. In congenital neutropenia filgrastim usually increases the neutrophil count with an appropriate clinical response. Prolonged use may be associated with an increased risk of myeloid malignancy.

Treatment with granulocyte-colony stimulating factors should only be prescribed by those experienced in their use.

Neonatal neutropenia

Filgrastim has been used to treat sepsis-induced neutropenia in preterm neonates. There is no clear evidence that granulocyte–colony stimulating factors improve survival or long–term outcomes.

IMMUNOSTIMULANTS > GRANULOCYTE-COLONY STIMULATING FACTORS

Granulocyte-colony stimulating factors

● **DRUG ACTION** Recombinant human granulocyte-colony stimulating factor (rhG-CSF) stimulates the production of neutrophils.

● **CAUTIONS** Malignant myeloid conditions · pre-malignant myeloid conditions · risk of splenomegaly and rupture—spleen size should be monitored · sickle-cell disease

CAUTIONS, FURTHER INFORMATION

▶ Acute respiratory distress syndrome There have been reports of pulmonary infiltrates leading to acute respiratory distress syndrome—patients with a recent history of pulmonary infiltrates or pneumonia may be at higher risk.

● **SIDE-EFFECTS**

▶ **Common or very common** Alopecia · anorexia · asthenia · bone pain · chest pain · fever · gastro-intestinal disturbances · headache · injection-site reactions · leucocytosis · musculoskeletal pain · rash · thrombocytopenia

▶ **Rare** Acute febrile neutrophilic dermatosis · cutaneous vasculitis · pulmonary side-effects (particularly interstitial pneumonia)

SIDE-EFFECTS, FURTHER INFORMATION

▶ Pulmonary infiltration Treatment should be withdrawn in patients who develop signs of pulmonary infiltration.

● **PREGNANCY** There have been reports of toxicity in *animal* studies and manufacturers advise not to use granulocyte-colony stimulating factors during pregnancy unless the potential benefit outweighs the risk.

● **BREAST FEEDING** There is no evidence for the use of granulocyte-colony stimulating factors during breast-feeding and manufacturers advise avoiding their use.

● **MONITORING REQUIREMENTS**

▶ Full blood counts including differential white cell and platelet counts should be monitored.

▶ Spleen size should be monitored during treatment—risk of splenomegaly and rupture.

9

Blood and nutrition

Blood and nutrition

9

F 537

Filgrastim

(Recombinant human granulocyte-colony stimulating factor; G-CSF)

- **INDICATIONS AND DOSE**

Reduction in duration of neutropenia and incidence of febrile neutropenia in cytotoxic chemotherapy for malignancy (except chronic myeloid leukaemia and myelodysplastic syndromes) (specialist use only)
▶ BY SUBCUTANEOUS INJECTION, OR BY INTRAVENOUS INFUSION
▶ Child: 5 micrograms/kg daily until neutrophil count in normal range, usually for up to 14 days (up to 38 days in acute myeloid leukaemia), to be started at least 24 hours after cytotoxic chemotherapy. Preferably given by subcutaneous injection; if given by intravenous infusion, administer over 30 minutes

Reduction in duration of neutropenia (and associated sequelae) in myeloablative therapy followed by bone-marrow transplantation (specialist use only)
▶ BY SUBCUTANEOUS INFUSION, OR BY INTRAVENOUS INFUSION
▶ Child: 10 micrograms/kg daily, to be started at least 24 hours following cytotoxic chemotherapy and within 24 hours of bone-marrow infusion, then adjusted according to neutrophil count— consult product literature, doses administered over 30 minutes or 24 hours via intravenous route and over 24 hours via subcutaneous route

Mobilisation of peripheral blood progenitor cells for autologous infusion, used alone (specialist use only)
▶ BY SUBCUTANEOUS INFUSION, OR BY SUBCUTANEOUS INJECTION
▶ Child: 10 micrograms/kg daily for 5–7 days, to be administered over 24 hours if given by subcutaneous infusion

Mobilisation of peripheral blood progenitor cells for autologous infusion, used following adjunctive myelosuppressive chemotherapy—to improve yield (specialist use only)
▶ BY SUBCUTANEOUS INJECTION
▶ Child: 5 micrograms/kg daily until neutrophil count in normal range, to be started the day after completing chemotherapy, for timing of leucopheresis, consult product literature

Mobilisation of peripheral blood progenitor cells in normal donors for allogeneic infusion (specialist use only)
▶ BY SUBCUTANEOUS INJECTION
▶ Child 16–17 years: 10 micrograms/kg daily for 4–5 days, for timing of leucopheresis, consult product literature

Severe congenital neutropenia and history of severe or recurrent infections (distinguish carefully from other haematological disorders) (specialist use only)
▶ BY SUBCUTANEOUS INJECTION
▶ Child: Initially 12 micrograms/kg daily, adjusted according to response, can be given in single or divided doses, consult product literature and local protocol

Severe cyclic neutropenia, or idiopathic neutropenia and history of severe or recurrent infections (distinguish carefully from other haematological disorders) (specialist use only)
▶ BY SUBCUTANEOUS INJECTION
▶ Child: Initially 5 micrograms/kg daily, adjusted according to response, can be given in single or divided doses, consult product literature and local protocol

Persistent neutropenia in HIV infection (specialist use only)
▶ BY SUBCUTANEOUS INJECTION
▶ Child: Initially 1 microgram/kg daily, subsequent doses increased as necessary until neutrophil count in normal range, then adjusted to maintain neutrophil count in normal range—consult product literature; maximum 4 micrograms/kg per day

Neonatal neutropenia (specialist use only)
▶ BY SUBCUTANEOUS INJECTION
▶ Neonate: 10 micrograms/kg daily, to be discontinued if white cell count exceeds 50×10^9/litre.

Glycogen storage disease type 1b (specialist use only)
▶ BY SUBCUTANEOUS INJECTION
▶ Child: Initially 5 micrograms/kg daily, dose to be adjusted as necessary

- **UNLICENSED USE** Not licensed for treatment of glycogen storage disease or neonatal neutropenia.
- **CONTRA-INDICATIONS** Severe congenital neutropenia (Kostmann's syndrome) with abnormal cytogenetics
- **CAUTIONS** Osteoporotic bone disease (monitor bone density if given for more than 6 months) · secondary acute myeloid leukaemia
- **INTERACTIONS** → Appendix 1 (filgrastim).
- **SIDE-EFFECTS**
▶ **Common or very common** Anaemia · dysuria · epistaxis · exacerbation of rheumatoid arthritis · haematuria · hepatomegaly · mucositis · osteoporosis · proteinuria · pseudogout · raised uric acid · splenic enlargement · transient decrease in blood glucose · transient hypotension · urinary abnormalities
▶ **Uncommon** Capillary leak syndrome (including fatal cases)
▶ **Rare** Splenic rupture
- **MONITORING REQUIREMENTS** Regular morphological and cytogenetic bone-marrow examinations recommended in severe congenital neutropenia (possible risk of myelodysplastic syndromes or leukaemia).
- **DIRECTIONS FOR ADMINISTRATION**
▶ With intravenous use or subcutaneous use For *subcutaneous* or *intravenous infusion*, dilute with Glucose 5% to a concentration of not less than 15 micrograms/mL; to dilute to a concentration of 2–15 micrograms/mL, add albumin solution (human albumin solution) to produce a final albumin solution of 2 mg/mL; not compatible with Sodium Chloride solutions.
- **PRESCRIBING AND DISPENSING INFORMATION** Products containing filgrastim are not identical and although theoretically there should be no important differences in terms of safety and efficacy, when prescribing biological products it is good practice to use the brand name, see *Biosimilar medicines*, under Guidance on prescribing p. 1.
  1 million units of filgrastim solution for injection contains 10 micrograms filgrastim.

- **MEDICINAL FORMS**
There can be variation in the licensing of different medicines containing the same drug.
Solution for injection
▶ Accofil (Accord Healthcare Ltd) ▼
  Filgrastim 60 mega u per 1 ml Accofil 30million units/0.5ml solution for injection pre-filled syringes | 5 pre-filled disposable injection PoM £284.20
  Filgrastim 96 mega u per 1 ml Accofil 48million units/0.5ml solution for injection pre-filled syringes | 5 pre-filled disposable injection PoM £455.70
▶ Neupogen (Amgen Ltd)
  Filgrastim 30 mega u per 1 ml Neupogen 30million units/1ml solution for injection vials | 5 vial PoM £263.52

- **Neupogen Singleject** (Amgen Ltd)
  Filgrastim 60 mega u per 1 ml Neupogen Singleject 30million units/0.5ml solution for injection pre-filled syringes | 1 pre-filled disposable injection [PoM] £52.70 | 5 pre-filled disposable injection [PoM] £263.52
  Filgrastim 96 mega u per 1 ml Neupogen Singleject 48million units/0.5ml solution for injection pre-filled syringes | 1 pre-filled disposable injection [PoM] £84.06 | 5 pre-filled disposable injection [PoM] £420.29
- **Nivestim** (Hospira UK Ltd)
  Filgrastim 60 mega u per 1 ml Nivestim 30million units/0.5ml solution for injection pre-filled syringes | 5 pre-filled disposable injection [PoM] £290.00 (Hospital only)
  Nivestim 12million units/0.2ml solution for injection pre-filled syringes | 5 pre-filled disposable injection [PoM] £180.00 (Hospital only)
  Filgrastim 96 mega u per 1 ml Nivestim 48million units/0.5ml solution for injection pre-filled syringes | 5 pre-filled disposable injection [PoM] £465.00 (Hospital only)
- **Zarzio** (Sandoz Ltd)
  Filgrastim 60 mega u per 1 ml Zarzio 30million units/0.5ml solution for injection pre-filled syringes | 5 pre-filled disposable injection [PoM] £250.75
  Filgrastim 96 mega u per 1 ml Zarzio 48million units/0.5ml solution for injection pre-filled syringes | 5 pre-filled disposable injection [PoM] £399.50

F 537

Lenograstim

(Recombinant human granulocyte-colony stimulating factor; rHuG-CSF)

● **INDICATIONS AND DOSE**

Reduction in the duration of neutropenia and associated complications following bone-marrow transplantation for non-myeloid malignancy (specialist use only) | **Reduction in the duration of neutropenia and associated complications following peripheral stem cells transplantation for non-myeloid malignancy (specialist use only)**
▸ BY INTRAVENOUS INFUSION, OR BY SUBCUTANEOUS INJECTION
▸ **Child 2–17 years:** 150 micrograms/m^2 daily until neutrophil count stable in acceptable range (max. 28 days), to be started the day after transplantation. Intravenous infusion to be given over 30 minutes

Reduction in the duration of neutropenia and associated complications following treatment with cytotoxic chemotherapy associated with a significant incidence of febrile neutropenia (specialist use only)
▸ BY SUBCUTANEOUS INJECTION
▸ **Child 2–17 years:** 150 micrograms/m^2 daily until neutrophil count stable in acceptable range (max. 28 days), to be started on the day after completion of chemotherapy

Mobilisation of peripheral blood progenitor cells for harvesting and subsequent infusion, used alone (specialist use only)
▸ BY SUBCUTANEOUS INJECTION
▸ **Child 2–17 years:** 10 micrograms/kg daily for 4–6 days (5–6 days in healthy donors)

Mobilisation of peripheral blood progenitor cells, used following adjunctive myelosuppressive chemotherapy (to improve yield) (specialist use only)
▸ BY SUBCUTANEOUS INJECTION
▸ **Child 2–17 years:** 150 micrograms/m^2 daily until neutrophil count stable in acceptable range, to be started 1–5 days after completion of chemotherapy, for timing of leucopheresis, consult product literature

● **UNLICENSED USE** Not licensed for use in children for cytotoxic-induced neutropenia, mobilisation of peripheral blood progenitor cells (monotherapy or adjunctive therapy), or following peripheral stem cells transplantation.

● **SIDE-EFFECTS** Mucositis · splenic rupture · toxic epidermal necrolysis

● **DIRECTIONS FOR ADMINISTRATION** For *intravenous infusion*, dilute reconstituted solution to a concentration of not less than 2 micrograms/mL (*Granocyte*-13) or 2.5 micrograms/mL (*Granocyte*-34) with Sodium Chloride 0.9%.

● **PRESCRIBING AND DISPENSING INFORMATION** *Granocyte*® solution for injection contains 105 micrograms of lenograstim per 13.4 mega unit vial and 263 micrograms lenograstim per 33.6 mega unit vial.

● **MEDICINAL FORMS**
There can be variation in the licensing of different medicines containing the same drug.
Powder and solvent for solution for injection
EXCIPIENTS: May contain Phenylalanine
▸ **Granocyte** (Chugai Pharma UK Ltd)
  Lenograstim 13.4 mega u Granocyte-13 powder and solvent for solution for injection vials | 1 vial [PoM] £40.11 | 5 vial [PoM] £200.55
  Lenograstim 33.6 mega u Granocyte-34 powder and solvent for solution for injection vials | 1 vial [PoM] £62.54 | 5 vial [PoM] £312.69

4 Platelet disorders

Platelet disorders

Idiopathic thrombocytopenic purpura

Acute idiopathic thrombocytopenic purpura is usually self-limiting in children. A corticosteroid, such as prednisolone p. 413, is sometimes used if idiopathic thrombocytopenic purpura does not resolve spontaneously or if it is associated with severe cutaneous symptoms or mucous membrane bleeding; corticosteroid treatment should not be continued longer than 14 days regardless of the response.

Immunoglobulin preparations may be used in idiopathic thrombocytopenic purpura or where a temporary rapid rise in platelets is needed, as in pregnancy or pre-operatively; they are often used in preference to a corticosteroid. Anti-D (Rh$_0$) immunoglobulin p. 725 is licensed for the management of idiopathic thrombocytopenic purpura.

Other therapy that has been tried under specialist supervision in refractory idiopathic thrombocytopenic purpura includes azathioprine, cyclophosphamide, vincristine sulfate, and ciclosporin. Rituximab p. 494 is also used in specialist centres but experience of its use in children is limited. For patients with chronic severe thrombocytopenia refractory to other therapy, tranexamic acid p. 76 may be given to reduce the severity of haemorrhage.

Splenectomy is considered in chronic thrombocytopenic purpura if a satisfactory platelet count is not achieved with regular immunoglobulin infusions, if there is a relapse on withdrawing or reducing the dose of corticosteroid, and if other therapies are considered inappropriate.

Essential thrombocythaemia

Anagrelide p. 540 reduces platelets in essential thrombocythaemia in patients at risk of thrombo-haemorrhagic events who have not responded adequately to other drugs or who cannot tolerate other drugs.

9

Blood and nutrition

4.1 Essential thrombocythaemia

ANTITHROMBOTIC DRUGS > CYCLIC AMP PHOSPHODIESTERASE III INHIBITORS

Anagrelide

- **INDICATIONS AND DOSE**
  Essential thrombocythaemia in patients at risk of thrombo-haemorrhagic events who have not responded adequately to other drugs or who cannot tolerate other drugs (initiated under specialist supervision)
  ‣ BY MOUTH
  ‣ Child 7-17 years: Initially 500 micrograms daily, dose to be adjusted at weekly intervals according to response, increased in steps of 500 micrograms daily; usual dose 1–3 mg daily in divided doses (max. per dose 2.5 mg); maximum 10 mg per day

- **UNLICENSED USE** Not licensed for use in children.
- **CAUTIONS** Cardiovascular disease—assess cardiac function before and regularly during treatment · concomitant use of drugs that prolong QT-interval—assess cardiac function before and regularly during treatment · risk factors for QT-interval prolongation—assess cardiac function before and regularly during treatment
- **INTERACTIONS** → Appendix 1 (anagrelide). Caution with concomitant aspirin in patients at risk of haemorrhage.
- **SIDE-EFFECTS**
  ‣ **Common or very common** Anaemia · dizziness · fatigue · fluid retention · gastro-intestinal disturbances · headache · palpitation · rash · tachycardia
  ‣ **Uncommon** Alopecia · amnesia · anorexia · arrhythmias · arthralgia · back pain · blood disorders · chest pain · confusion · congestive heart failure · depression · dry mouth · dyspnoea · ecchymosis · epistaxis · fever · gastro-intestinal haemorrhage · haemorrhage · hypertension · hypoaesthesia · impotence · malaise · myalgia · nervousness · oedema · pancreatitis · paraesthesia · pneumonia pleural effusion · pruritus · skin discoloration · sleep disturbances · syncope · weight changes
  ‣ **Rare** Angina · asthenia · cardiomegaly · cardiomyopathy · colitis · dry skin · dysarthria · gastritis · gingival bleeding · impaired coordination · migraine · myocardial infarction · nocturia · pericardial effusion · postural hypotension · pulmonary hypertension · pulmonary infiltrates · renal failure · somnolence · tinnitus · vasodilatation · visual disturbances
  ‣ **Frequency not known** Hepatitis · interstitial lung disease · Torsade de pointes · tubulointerstitial nephritis
- **CONCEPTION AND CONTRACEPTION** Effective contraception required during treatment.
- **PREGNANCY** Manufacturer advises avoid (toxicity in *animal* studies).
- **BREAST FEEDING** Manufacturer advises avoid—present in milk in *animal* studies.
- **HEPATIC IMPAIRMENT** Manufacturer advises caution in mild impairment. Avoid in moderate to severe impairment.
- **RENAL IMPAIRMENT** Manufacturer advises avoid if estimated glomerular filtration rate less than 50 mL/minute/1.73 m^2
- **MONITORING REQUIREMENTS**
  ‣ Monitor full blood count (monitor platelet count every 2 days for 1 week, then weekly until maintenance dose established).
  ‣ Monitor liver function.
  ‣ Monitor serum creatinine.

‣ Monitor urea.
‣ Monitor electrolytes (including potassium, magnesium and calcium) before and during treatment.
‣ Monitor closely for further signs of disease progression such as malignant transformation.
- **PRESCRIBING AND DISPENSING INFORMATION** Initiate only when signs of disease progression or patient suffers from thrombosis. Consider stopping treatment after 3 months if inadequate response.
- **PATIENT AND CARER ADVICE**
  Driving and skilled tasks
  Dizziness may affect performance of skilled tasks (e.g. cycling, driving).
- **MEDICINAL FORMS**
  There can be variation in the licensing of different medicines containing the same drug.
  Capsule
  ‣ Xagrid (Shire Pharmaceuticals Ltd) ▼
  Anagrelide (as Anagrelide hydrochloride) 500 microgram Xagrid 500microgram capsules | 100 capsule PoM £404.57

Nutrition and metabolic disorders

1 Acid-base imbalance
1.1 Metabolic acidosis

ALKALISING DRUGS > OTHER

Trometamol

(Tris(hydroxymethyl)aminomethane, THAM)

- **INDICATIONS AND DOSE**
  Metabolic acidosis
  ‣ BY INTRAVENOUS INFUSION
  ‣ Child: To be administered at an amount appropriate to the body base deficit

- **UNLICENSED USE** Unlicensed preparation.
- **CONTRA-INDICATIONS** Anuria · chronic respiratory acidosis
- **CAUTIONS** Extravasation can cause severe tissue damage
- **SIDE-EFFECTS** Hyperkalaemia in renal impairment · hypoglycaemia · liver necrosis (following administration via umbilical vein) (in neonates) · respiratory depression

  SIDE-EFFECTS, FURTHER INFORMATION
  ‣ Respiratory depression Respiratory support may be required because trometamol induces respiratory depression.
- **PREGNANCY** Limited information available, hypoglycaemia may harm fetus.
- **BREAST FEEDING** No information available.
- **RENAL IMPAIRMENT** Use with caution, may cause hyperkalaemia.

- **MEDICINAL FORMS**
  There can be variation in the licensing of different medicines containing the same drug. Forms available from special-order manufacturers include: solution for infusion
  Solution for infusion
  ‣ Trometamol (Non-proprietary)
  Trometamol 363.4 mg per 1 ml Tris 36.34% solution for infusion 20ml ampoules | 10 ampoule PoM no price available

2 Fluid and electrolyte imbalances

Fluids and electrolytes

Electrolyte replacement therapy

The electrolyte concentrations (intravenous fluid) table and the electrolyte content (gastro-intestinal secretions) table may be helpful in planning replacement electrolyte therapy; faeces, vomit, or aspiration should be saved and analysed where possible if abnormal losses are suspected.

Oral preparations for fluid and electrolyte imbalance

Sodium and potassium salts, may be given by mouth to prevent deficiencies or to treat established deficiencies of mild or moderate degree.

Oral potassium

Compensation for potassium loss is especially necessary:
- in children in whom secondary hyperaldosteronism occurs, e.g. renal artery stenosis, renal tubule disorder, the nephrotic syndrome, and severe heart failure;
- in children with excessive losses of potassium in the faeces, e.g. chronic diarrhoea associated with intestinal malabsorption or laxative abuse;
- in those taking digoxin or anti-arrhythmic drugs, where potassium depletion may induce arrhythmias.

Measures to compensate for potassium loss may be required during long-term administration of drugs known to induce potassium loss (e.g. corticosteroids). Potassium supplements are **seldom required** with the small doses of diuretics given to treat hypertension; **potassium-sparing diuretics** (rather than potassium supplements) are recommended for prevention of hypokalaemia due to diuretics such as furosemide p. 132 or the thiazides when these are given to eliminate oedema.

If potassium salts are used for the *prevention of hypokalaemia*, then doses of potassium chloride p. 561 daily by mouth are suitable in patients taking a normal diet. Smaller doses must be used if there is renal insufficiency to reduce the risk of **hyperkalaemia**.

Potassium salts cause nausea and vomiting and poor compliance is a major limitation to their effectiveness (small divided doses may minimise gastric irritation); when appropriate, potassium-sparing diuretics are preferable. When there is *established potassium depletion* larger doses may be necessary, the quantity depending on the severity of any continuing potassium loss (monitoring of plasma-potassium concentration and specialist advice would be required). Potassium depletion is frequently associated with chloride depletion and with metabolic alkalosis, and these disorders require correction.

Management of hyperkalaemia

Acute severe hyperkalaemia calls for urgent treatment with intravenous infusion of **soluble insulin** 0.3–0.6 units/kg/hour in neonates and 0.05–0.2 units/kg/hour in children over 1 month) with glucose 0.5–1 g/kg/hour (5–10 mL/kg of glucose 10%; 2.5–5 mL/kg of glucose 20% via a central venous catheter may also be considered). If insulin cannot be used, albutamol p. 146 can be given by intravenous injection, but it has a slower onset of action and may be less effective for reducing plasma-potassium concentration.

Calcium gluconate p. 553 is given by slow intravenous injection to manage cardiac excitability caused by hyperkalaemia.

The correction of causal or compounding acidosis with sodium bicarbonate infusion p. 544 should be considered (**important**: preparations of sodium bicarbonate and calcium salts should not be administered in the same line—risk of precipitation). Intravenous furosemide can also be given but is less effective in children with renal impairment. Drugs exacerbating hyperkalaemia should be reviewed and stopped as appropriate; dialysis may occasionally be required.

Ion-exchange resins may be used to remove excess potassium in *mild hyperkalaemia* or in *moderate hyperkalaemia* when there are no ECG changes. Calcium polystyrene sulfonate is preferred unless plasma-calcium concentrations are high.

Oral sodium and water

Sodium chloride p. 547 is indicated in states of sodium depletion. In preterm neonates in the first few weeks of life and in chronic conditions associated with mild or moderate degrees of sodium depletion, e.g. in salt-losing bowel or renal disease, oral supplements of sodium chloride may be sufficient. Sodium chloride solutions suitable for use by mouth in neonates are available from 'special-order' manufacturers or specialist importing companies, they should be used with care because they are hypertonic. Supplementation with sodium chloride may be required to replace losses in children with cystic fibrosis particularly in warm weather.

Oral rehydration therapy (ORT)

Diarrhoea in children is usually self-limiting, however, in children under 6 months of age, and more particularly in those under 3 months, symptoms of dehydration may be less obvious and there is a risk of rapid and severe deterioration. Intestinal absorption of sodium and water is enhanced by glucose (and other carbohydrates). Replacement of fluid and electrolytes lost through diarrhoea can therefore be achieved by giving solutions containing sodium, potassium, and glucose or another carbohydrate such as rice starch.

Oral rehydration solutions should:
- enhance the absorption of water and electrolytes;
- replace the electrolyte deficit adequately and safely;
- contain an alkalinising agent to counter acidosis;
- be slightly hypo-osmolar (about 250 mmol/litre) to prevent the possible induction of osmotic diarrhoea;
- be simple to use in hospital and at home;
- be palatable and acceptable, especially to children;
- be readily available.

It is the policy of the World Health Organization (WHO) to promote a single oral rehydration solution but to use it flexibly (e.g. by giving extra water between drinks of oral rehydration solution to moderately dehydrated infants).

The WHO oral rehydration salts formulation contains sodium chloride 2.6 g, potassium chloride 1.5 g, sodium citrate 2.9 g, anhydrous glucose 13.5 g. It is dissolved in sufficient water to produce 1 litre (providing Na^+ 75 mmol, K^+ 20 mmol, Cl^- 65 mmol, citrate 10 mmol, glucose 75 mmol/litre). This formulation is recommended by the WHO and the United Nations Children's fund, but it is not commonly used in the UK.

Oral rehydration solutions used in the UK are lower in sodium (50–60 mmol/litre) than the WHO formulation since, in general, patients suffer less severe sodium loss.

Rehydration should be rapid over 3 to 4 hours (except in hypernatraemic dehydration in which case rehydration should occur more slowly over 12 hours). The patient should be reassessed after initial rehydration and if still dehydrated rapid fluid replacement should continue.

Once rehydration is complete further dehydration is prevented by encouraging the patient to drink normal volumes of an appropriate fluid and by replacing continuing losses with an oral rehydration solution; in infants, breast-feeding or formula feeds should be offered between oral rehydration drinks.

Oral bicarbonate

Sodium bicarbonate is given by mouth for *chronic acidotic states* such as uraemic acidosis or renal tubular acidosis. The dose for correction of metabolic acidosis is not predictable and the response must be assessed. For severe *metabolic acidosis*, sodium bicarbonate can be given intravenously.

Sodium supplements may increase blood pressure or cause fluid retention and pulmonary oedema in those at risk; hypokalaemia may be exacerbated.

Sodium bicarbonate may affect the stability or absorption of other drugs if administered at the same time. If possible, allow 1–2 hours before administering other drugs orally.

Where *hyperchloraemic acidosis* is associated with potassium deficiency, as in some renal tubular and gastrointestinal disorders it may be appropriate to give oral **potassium bicarbonate**, although acute or severe deficiency should be managed by intravenous therapy.

Parenteral preparations for fluid and electrolyte imbalance

Electrolytes and water

Solutions of electrolytes are given intravenously, to meet normal fluid and electrolyte requirements or to replenish substantial deficits or continuing losses when it is not possible or desirable to use the oral route. When intravenous administration is not possible, fluid (as sodium chloride 0.9% p. 547 or glucose 5% p. 549) can also be given subcutaneously by hypodermoclysis.

In an individual patient the nature and severity of the electrolyte imbalance must be assessed from the history and clinical and biochemical examination. Sodium, potassium, chloride, magnesium, phosphate, and water depletion can occur singly and in combination with or without disturbances of acid-base balance.

Isotonic solutions may be infused safely into a peripheral vein. Solutions more concentrated than plasma, for example 15% glucose, are best given through an indwelling catheter positioned in a large vein.

Maintenance fluid requirements in children are usually derived from the relationship that exists between body-weight and metabolic rate; the figures in the table below may be used as a guide outside the neonatal period. The glucose requirement is that needed to minimise gluconeogenesis from amino acids obtained as substrate from muscle breakdown. Maintenance fluids are intended only to provide hydration for a short period until enteral or parenteral nutrition can be established.

It is usual to meet these requirements by using a standard solution of sodium chloride with glucose. Solutions containing 20 mmol/litre of potassium chloride meet usual potassium requirements when given in the suggested volumes; adjustments may be needed if there is an inability to excrete fluids or electrolytes, excessive renal loss or continuing extra-renal losses. The exact requirements depend upon the nature of the clinical situation and types of losses incurred.

Fluid requirements for children over 1 month:	
Body-weight	**24-hour fluid requirement**
Under 10 kg	100 mL/kg
10–20 kg	100 mL/kg for the first 10 kg + 50 mL/kg for each 1 kg body-weight over 10 kg
Over 20 kg	100 mL/kg for the first 10 kg + 50 mL/kg for each 1 kg body-weight between 10–20 kg + 20 mL/kg for each 1 kg body-weight over 20 kg (max. 2 litres in females, 2.5 litres in males)

Important The baseline fluid requirements shown in the table should be adjusted to take account of factors that reduce water loss (e.g. increased antidiuretic hormone, renal failure, hypothermia, and high ambient humidity) or increase water loss (e.g. pyrexia or burns).

Replacement therapy: initial intravenous replacement fluid is generally required if the child is over 10% dehydrated, or if 5–10% dehydrated and oral or enteral rehydration is not tolerated or possible. Oral rehydration is adequate, if tolerated, in the majority of those less than 10% dehydrated. Subsequent fluid and electrolyte requirements are determined by clinical assessment of fluid balance.

Intravenous sodium

Intravenous sodium chloride in isotonic (0.9%) solution provides the most important extracellular ions in near physiological concentrations and is indicated in *sodium depletion*. It may be given for initial treatment of acute fluid loss and to replace ongoing gastro-intestinal losses from the upper gastro-intestinal tract. Intravenous sodium chloride is commonly given as a component of maintenance and replacement therapy, usually in combination with other electrolytes and glucose.

Chronic hyponatraemia should ideally be corrected by fluid restriction. However, if sodium chloride is required, the deficit should be corrected slowly to avoid the risk of osmotic demyelination syndrome; the rise in plasma sodium concentration should be no more than 10 mmol/litre in 24 hours.

Sodium chloride with glucose solutions are indicated when there is combined *water and sodium depletion*. A 1:1 mixture of isotonic sodium chloride and 5% glucose allows some of the water (free of sodium) to enter body cells which suffer most from dehydration while the sodium salt with a volume of water determined by the normal plasma Na$^+$ remains extracellular.

Combined sodium, potassium, chloride, and water depletion may occur, for example, with severe diarrhoea or persistent vomiting; replacement is carried out with sodium chloride intravenous infusion 0.9% and glucose intravenous infusion 5% with potassium as appropriate

Compound sodium lactate (Hartmann's solution) can be used instead of isotonic sodium chloride solution during or after surgery, or in the initial management of the injured or wounded.

Intravenous glucose

Glucose solutions are used mainly to replace water deficit. Water depletion (dehydration) tends to occur when losses are not matched by a comparable intake, as may occur in coma or dysphagia.

Water loss rarely exceeds electrolyte losses but this can occur in fevers, hyperthyroidism, and in uncommon water-losing renal states such as diabetes insipidus or hypercalcaemia. The volume of glucose solution needed to replace deficits varies with the severity of the disorder; the rate of infusion should be adjusted to return the plasma-sodium concentration to normal over 48 hours.

Glucose solutions are also used to correct and prevent hypoglycaemia and to provide a source of energy in those

Electrolyte concentrations—intravenous fluids

Intravenous infusion	Millimoles per litre				
	Na^+	K^+	HCO_3^-	Cl^-	Ca^{2+}
Normal plasma values	142	4.5	26	103	2.5
Sodium Chloride 0.9%	150	–	–	150	–
Compound Sodium Lactate (Hartmann's)	131	5	29	111	2
Sodium Chloride 0.18% and Glucose 4% (Adults only)	30	–	–	30	–
Sodium Chloride 0.45% and Glucose 5% (Children only)	75	–	–	75	–
Potassium Chloride 0.15% and Glucose 5% (Children only)	–	20	–	20	–
Potassium Chloride 0.15% and Sodium Chloride 0.9% (Children only)	150	20	–	170	–
Potassium Chloride 0.3% and Glucose 5%	–	40	–	40	–
Potassium Chloride 0.3% and Sodium Chloride 0.9%	150	40	–	190	–
To correct metabolic acidosis					
Sodium Bicarbonate 1.26%	150	–	150	–	–
Sodium Bicarbonate 8.4% for cardiac arrest	1000	–	1000	–	–
Sodium Lactate (m/6)	167	–	167	–	–

Electrolyte content—gastro-intestinal secretions

Type of fluid	Millimoles per litre				
	H^+	Na^+	K^+	HCO_3^-	Cl^-
Gastric	40–60	20–80	5–20	–	100–150
Biliary	–	120–140	5–15	30–50	80–120
Pancreatic	–	120–140	5–15	70–110	40–80
Small bowel	–	120–140	5–15	20–40	90–130

too ill to be fed adequately by mouth; glucose solutions are a key component of parenteral nutrition.

Glucose solutions are given with insulin for the emergency management of *hyperkalaemia*. They are also given, after correction of hyperglycaemia, during treatment of diabetic ketoacidosis, when they must be accompanied by continuous insulin infusion.

Intravenous potassium

Potassium chloride with sodium chloride intravenous infusion is the initial treatment for the correction of *severe hypokalaemia* and when sufficient potassium cannot be taken by mouth.

Repeated measurements of plasma-potassium concentration are necessary to determine whether further infusions are required and to avoid the development of hyperkalaemia, which is especially likely in renal impairment.

Initial potassium replacement therapy should **not** involve glucose infusions, because glucose may cause a further decrease in the plasma-potassium concentration.

Bicarbonate and trometamol

Sodium bicarbonate is used to control severe *metabolic acidosis* (pH < 7.1) particularly that caused by loss of bicarbonate (as in renal tubular acidosis or from excessive gastro-intestinal losses). Mild metabolic acidosis associated with volume depletion should first be managed by appropriate fluid replacement because acidosis usually resolves as tissue and renal perfusion are restored. In more severe metabolic acidosis or when the acidosis remains unresponsive to correction of anoxia or hypovolaemia, sodium bicarbonate (1.26%) p. 544 can be infused over 3–4 hours with plasma-pH and electrolyte monitoring. In

severe shock, for example in cardiac arrest, metabolic acidosis can develop without sodium depletion; in these circumstances sodium bicarbonate is best given intravenously as a small volume of hypertonic solution, such as 8.4%; plasma pH and electrolytes should be monitored. For *chronic acidotic states*, sodium bicarbonate can be given by mouth.

Trometamol (tris(hydroxymethyl)aminomethane, THAM) p. 540, an organic buffer, corrects metabolic acidosis by causing an increase in urinary pH and an osmotic diuresis. It is indicated when sodium bicarbonate is unsuitable as in carbon dioxide retention, hypernatraemia, or renal impairment. It is also used during cardiac bypass surgery and, very rarely, in cardiac arrest.

Plasma and plasma substitutes

Albumin solution p. 554, prepared from whole blood, contain soluble proteins and electrolytes but no clotting factors, blood group antibodies, or plasma cholinesterases; they may be given without regard to the recipient's blood group.

Albumin is usually used after the acute phase of illness to correct a plasma-volume deficit; hypoalbuminaemia itself is not an appropriate indication. The use of albumin solution in acute plasma or blood loss may be wasteful; plasma substitutes are more appropriate. Concentrated albumin solution may also be used to obtain a diuresis in hypoalbuminaemic patients (e.g. in nephrotic syndrome).

Recent evidence does not support the previous view that the use of albumin increases mortality.

Plasma substitutes

Gelatin p. 555 is a macromolecular substance that is metabolised slowly. Gelatin may be used at the outset to expand and maintain blood volume in shock arising from conditions such as burns or septicaemia; it may also be used as an immediate short-term measure to treat haemorrhage until blood is available. Gelatin is rarely needed when shock is due to sodium and water depletion because, in these circumstances, the shock responds to water and electrolyte repletion; see also the management of shock.

Plasma substitutes should **not** be used to maintain plasma volume in conditions such as burns or peritonitis where there is loss of plasma protein, water, and electrolytes over periods of several days or weeks. In these situations, plasma or plasma protein fractions containing large amounts of albumin should be given.

Large volumes of *some* plasma substitutes can increase the risk of bleeding through depletion of coagulation factors.

Parenteral preparations for fluid and electrolyte imbalance in neonates

Electrolytes and water

Neonates lose water through the skin and nose, particularly if preterm or if the skin is damaged. The basic fluid requirement for a term baby in average ambient humidity is 40–60 mL/kg/day. Preterm babies have very high transepidermal losses particularly in the first few days of life; they may need more fluid replacement than full term babies and up to 180 mL/kg/day may be required. Local guidelines for fluid management in the neonatal period should be consulted.

Intravenous sodium

The sodium requirement for most healthy neonates is 3 mmol/kg daily. Preterm neonates, particularly below 30 weeks gestation, may require up to 6 mmol/kg daily. *Hyponatraemia* may be caused by excessive renal loss of sodium; it may also be dilutional and restriction of fluid intake may be appropriate. Sodium supplementation is likely to be required if the serum sodium concentration is significantly reduced.

Hypernatraemia may also occur, most often due to dehydration (e.g. breast milk insufficiency). Severe hypernatraemia and hyponatraemia can cause fits and rarely brain damage. Sodium in drug preparations, delivered via continuous infusions, or in infusions to maintain the patency of intravascular or umbilical lines, can result in significant amounts of sodium being delivered, (e.g. 1 mL/hour of 0.9% sodium chloride infused over 24 hours is equivalent to 3.6 mmol/day of sodium).

BICARBONATE

Sodium bicarbonate

● **INDICATIONS AND DOSE**

Chronic acidotic states such as uraemic acidosis or renal tubular acidosis
▶ BY MOUTH
▶ Neonate: Initially 1–2 mmol/kg daily in divided doses, adjusted according to response.
▶ Child: Initially 1–2 mmol/kg daily in divided doses, adjusted according to response

Severe metabolic acidosis
▶ BY SLOW INTRAVENOUS INJECTION, OR BY INTRAVENOUS INFUSION
▶ Child: Administer an amount appropriate to the body base deficit, to be given by slow intravenous injection of a strong solution (up to 8.4%), or by continuous intravenous infusion of a weaker solution (usually 1.26%)

Renal hyperkalaemia
▶ BY SLOW INTRAVENOUS INJECTION
▶ Neonate: 1 mmol/kg daily.
▶ Child: 1 mmol/kg daily

Persistent cyanotic spell in a child with congenital heart disease despite optimal use of 100% oxygen and propranolol
▶ BY INTRAVENOUS INFUSION
▶ Child: 1 mmol/kg, dose given to correct acidosis (or dose calculated according to arterial blood gas results), sodium bicarbonate 4.2% intravenous infusion is appropriate for a child under 1 year and sodium bicarbonate 8.4% intravenous infusion in children over 1 year

● **CONTRA-INDICATIONS**
▶ With oral use Salt restricted diet
● **CAUTIONS**
▶ With systemic use Respiratory acidosis
● **INTERACTIONS** → Appendix 1 (antacids).
● **SIDE-EFFECTS**
▶ When used for chronic acidotic states such as uraemic acidosis or renal tubular acidosis With oral use for chronic acidotic states such as uraemic acidosis or renal tubular acidosis fluid retention (in those at risk) · hypokalaemia may be exacerbated · increase blood pressure · pulmonary oedema (in those at risk)

● **MONITORING REQUIREMENTS**
▶ With intravenous use Plasma-pH and electrolytes should be monitored.

● **DIRECTIONS FOR ADMINISTRATION**
▶ With intravenous use For *peripheral infusion* dilute 8.4% solution at least 1 in 10. For *central line infusion* dilute 1 in 5 with Glucose 5% or 10% *or* Sodium Chloride 0.9%. Extravasation can cause severe tissue damage.
▶ With oral use Sodium bicarbonate may affect the stability or absorption of other drugs if administered at the same time. If possible, allow 1–2 hours before administering other drugs orally.

● **PRESCRIBING AND DISPENSING INFORMATION**
▶ With oral use *Sodium bicarbonate* 500*mg* capsules contain approximately 6 mmol each of Na^+ and HCO_3^-; *Sodium bicarbonate* 600*mg* capsules contain approximately 7 mmol each of Na^+ and HCO_3^-. Oral solutions of sodium bicarbonate are required occasionally; these are available from 'special-order' manufacturers or specialist importing companies; the strength of sodium bicarbonate should be stated on the prescription.
▶ With intravenous use Usual strength Sodium bicarbonate 1.26% (12.6 g, 150 mmol each of Na^+ and HCO_3^-/litre), various other strengths available.

● **PATIENT AND CARER ADVICE**
Medicines for Children leaflet: Sodium bicarbonate for acidosis www.medicinesforchildren.org.uk/ sodium-bicarbonate-for-acidosis
▶ With oral use Patients or carers should be given advice on the administration of sodium bicarbonate oral medicines.

● **MEDICINAL FORMS**
There can be variation in the licensing of different medicines containing the same drug. Forms available from special-order manufacturers include: capsule, oral suspension, oral solution, solution for injection

Tablet
▶ Sodium bicarbonate (Non-proprietary)
Sodium bicarbonate **600 mg** Sodium bicarbonate 600mg tablets | 100 tablet £125.50 | 100 tablet GSL £29.75
S-Bicarb 600mg tablets | 100 tablet £125.50

Capsule
▶ Sodium bicarbonate (Non-proprietary)
Sodium bicarbonate **500 mg** Sodium bicarbonate 500mg capsules | 56 capsule P £17.56 DT price = £2.23 | 100 capsule PoM no price available

Oral solution
▶ Sodium bicarbonate (Non-proprietary)
Sodium bicarbonate **10 mg per 1 ml**

Sodium bicarbonate 84 mg per 1 ml S-Bicarb SF 420mg/5ml (1mmol/ml) oral solution sugar-free | 100 ml £26.25 DT price = £39.80

S-Bicarb 420mg/5ml (1mmol/ml) oral solution | 100 ml no price available

SodiBic 420mg/5ml (1mmol/ml) oral solution sugar-free | 100 ml £17.71 DT price = £39.80

▸ **Thamicarb** (Thame Laboratories Ltd)

Sodium bicarbonate 84 mg per 1 ml Thamicarb 84mg/1ml (1mmol/ml) oral solution sugar-free | 100 ml P £39.80 DT price = £39.80 sugar-free | 500 ml P £199.20 DT price = £199.20

Solution for injection

▸ **Sodium bicarbonate** (Non-proprietary)

Sodium bicarbonate 84 mg per 1 ml Sodium bicarbonate 8.4% (1mmol/ml) solution for injection 10ml ampoules | 10 ampoule PoM £77.40

Sodium bicarbonate 8.4% solution for injection 10ml Minijet pre-filled syringes | 1 pre-filled disposable injection PoM £9.71

Sodium bicarbonate 8.4% (1mmol/ml) solution for injection 250ml bottles | 10 bottle PoM £65.34

Sodium bicarbonate 8.4% (1mmol/ml) solution for injection 100ml bottles | 10 bottle PoM £62.04

Infusion

▸ **Sodium bicarbonate** (Non-proprietary)

Sodium bicarbonate 12.6 mg per 1 ml Polyfusor BC sodium bicarbonate 1.26% infusion 500ml bottles | 1 bottle PoM £9.86 | 12 bottle PoM no price available

Sodium bicarbonate 14 mg per 1 ml Polyfusor BD sodium bicarbonate 1.4% infusion 500ml bottles | 1 bottle PoM £9.86 | 12 bottle PoM no price available

Sodium bicarbonate 27.4 mg per 1 ml Polyfusor V sodium bicarbonate 2.74% infusion 500ml bottles | 1 bottle PoM £9.86 | 12 bottle PoM no price available

Sodium bicarbonate 42 mg per 1 ml Polyfusor BE sodium bicarbonate 4.2% infusion 500ml bottles | 1 bottle PoM £9.86 | 12 bottle PoM no price available

Sodium bicarbonate 84 mg per 1 ml Polyfusor B sodium bicarbonate 8.4% infusion 200ml bottles | 1 bottle PoM £9.86 | 12 bottle PoM no price available

ELECTROLYTES AND MINERALS > POTASSIUM

Potassium chloride with calcium chloride and sodium chloride and sodium lactate

(Sodium Lactate Intravenous Infusion, Compound; Compound, Hartmann's Solution for Injection; Ringer-Lactate Solution for Injection)

The properties listed below are those particular to the combination only. For the properties of the components please consider, potassium chloride p. 561, sodium chloride p. 547, calcium chloride p. 553.

● **INDICATIONS AND DOSE**

For prophylaxis, and replacement therapy, requiring the use of sodium chloride and lactate, with minimal amounts of calcium and potassium

▸ BY INTRAVENOUS INFUSION

▸ Child: (consult product literature)

● PRESCRIBING AND DISPENSING INFORMATION Compound sodium lactate intravenous infusion contains Na^+ 131 mmol, K^+ 5 mmol, Ca^{2+} 2 mmol, HCO_3^- (as lactate) 29 mmol, Cl^- 111 mmol/litre.

● MEDICINAL FORMS
There can be variation in the licensing of different medicines containing the same drug.

Infusion

▸ Potassium chloride with calcium chloride and sodium chloride and sodium lactate (Non-proprietary)

Calcium chloride 270 microgram per 1 ml, Potassium chloride 400 microgram per 1 ml, Sodium lactate 3.17 mg per 1 ml, Sodium chloride 6 mg per 1 ml Sodium lactate compound infusion

1litre Macoflex N bags | 1 bag PoM no price available | 10 bag PoM no price available

Sodium lactate compound infusion 1litre Viaflex bags | 1 bag PoM no price available | 10 bag PoM no price available

Sodium lactate compound infusion 1litre Macoflex bags | 1 bag PoM no price available | 12 bag PoM no price available

Sodium lactate compound infusion 1litre Viaflo bags | 1 bag PoM no price available | 10 bag PoM no price available

Ringer lactate infusion 1litre Viaflo bags | 1 bag PoM no price available | 10 bag PoM no price available

Potassium chloride with calcium chloride dihydrate and sodium chloride

(Ringer's solution)

The properties listed below are those particular to the combination only. For the properties of the components please consider, potassium chloride p. 561, sodium chloride p. 547.

● **INDICATIONS AND DOSE**

Electrolyte imbalance

▸ BY INTRAVENOUS INFUSION

▸ Child: Dosed according to the deficit or daily maintenance requirements (consult product literature)

● PRESCRIBING AND DISPENSING INFORMATION Ringer's solution for injection provides the following ions (in mmol/litre), Ca^{2+} 2.2, K^+ 4, Na^+ 147, Cl^- 156.

● MEDICINAL FORMS
There can be variation in the licensing of different medicines containing the same drug.

Infusion

▸ Potassium chloride with calcium chloride dihydrate and sodium chloride (Non-proprietary)

Potassium chloride 300 microgram per 1 ml, Calcium chloride 320 microgram per 1 ml, Sodium chloride 8.6 mg per 1 ml Polyfusor C ringers infusion 500ml bottles | 1 bottle PoM £2.95 | 12 bottle PoM no price available

Steriflex No.9 ringers infusion 1litre bags | 1 bag PoM £2.22 | 10 bag PoM no price available

Steriflex No.9 ringers infusion 500ml bags | 1 bag PoM £1.96 | 15 bag PoM no price available

Potassium chloride with glucose

The properties listed below are those particular to the combination only. For the properties of the components please consider, potassium chloride p. 561, glucose p. 549.

● **INDICATIONS AND DOSE**

Electrolyte imbalance

▸ BY INTRAVENOUS INFUSION

▸ Child: Dosed according to the deficit or daily maintenance requirements

● PRESCRIBING AND DISPENSING INFORMATION Potassium chloride 0.3% contains 40 mmol each of K^+ and Cl^-/litre or 0.15% contains 20 mmol each of K^+ and Cl^-/litre with 5% of anhydrous glucose.

● MEDICINAL FORMS
There can be variation in the licensing of different medicines containing the same drug. Forms available from special-order manufacturers include: infusion, solution for infusion

Infusion

▸ Potassium chloride with glucose (Non-proprietary)

Potassium chloride 3 mg per 1 ml, Glucose anhydrous 50 per 1 ml Potassium chloride 0.3% (potassium 40mmol/1litre) / Glucose 5% infusion 1litre Macoflex bags | 1 bag PoM no price available | 12 bag PoM no price available

Steriflex No.16 potassium chloride 0.3% (potassium 20mmol/500ml) / glucose 5% infusion 500ml bags | 1 bag [PoM] £1.67 | 15 bag [PoM] no price available

Potassium chloride 0.3% (potassium 20mmol/500ml) / Glucose 5% infusion 500ml Macoflex bags | 1 bag [PoM] no price available | 20 bag [PoM] no price available

Potassium chloride 0.3% (potassium 40mmol/1litre) / Glucose 5% infusion 1litre bags | 1 bag [PoM] £1.79

Steriflex No.16 potassium chloride 0.3% (potassium 40mmol/1litre) / glucose 5% infusion 1litre bags | 1 bag [PoM] £2.20 | 10 bag [PoM] no price available

Potassium chloride 0.3% (potassium 20mmol/500ml) / Glucose 5% infusion 500ml Viaflo bags | 1 bag [PoM] no price available | 20 bag [PoM] no price available

Potassium chloride 0.3% (potassium 40mmol/1litre) / Glucose 5% infusion 1litre Viaflo bags | 1 bag [PoM] no price available | 10 bag [PoM] no price available

Potassium chloride 2 mg per 1 ml, Glucose anhydrous 50 mg per 1 ml Steriflex No.29 potassium chloride 0.2% (potassium 27mmol/1litre) / glucose 5% infusion 1litre bags | 1 bag [PoM] £2.20 | 10 bag [PoM] no price available

Steriflex No.29 potassium chloride 0.2% (potassium 13.3mmol/500ml) / glucose 5% infusion 500ml bags | 1 bag [PoM] £1.67 | 15 bag [PoM] no price available

Potassium chloride 1.5 mg per 1 ml, Glucose anhydrous 50 mg per 1 ml Steriflex No.13 potassium chloride 0.15% (potassium 10mmol/500ml) / glucose 5% infusion 500ml bags | 1 bag [PoM] £1.67 | 15 bag [PoM] no price available

Steriflex No.13 potassium chloride 0.15% (potassium 20mmol/1litre) / glucose 5% infusion 1litre bags | 1 bag [PoM] £2.20 | 10 bag [PoM] no price available

Potassium chloride 0.15% (potassium 20mmol/1litre) / Glucose 5% infusion 1litre Macoflex bags | 1 bag [PoM] no price available | 12 bag [PoM] no price available

Potassium chloride 0.15% (potassium 10mmol/500ml) / Glucose 5% infusion 500ml Macoflex bags | 1 bag [PoM] no price available | 20 bag [PoM] no price available

Potassium chloride 0.15% (potassium 20mmol/1litre) / Glucose 5% infusion 1litre Viaflo bags | 1 bag [PoM] no price available

Potassium chloride 0.15% (potassium 20mmol/1litre) / Glucose 5% infusion 1litre Viaflex bags | 1 bag [PoM] no price available | 10 bag [PoM] no price available

Potassium chloride with glucose and sodium chloride

The properties listed below are those particular to the combination only. For the properties of the components please consider, potassium chloride p. 561, glucose p. 549, sodium chloride p. 547.

● **INDICATIONS AND DOSE**

Electrolyte imbalance

▸ BY INTRAVENOUS INFUSION

▸ Child: Dosed according to the deficit or daily maintenance requirements

● PRESCRIBING AND DISPENSING INFORMATION Concentration of potassium chloride to be specified by the prescriber (usually K^+ 10–40 mmol/litre).

● MEDICINAL FORMS
There can be variation in the licensing of different medicines containing the same drug. Forms available from special-order manufacturers include: infusion, solution for infusion
Infusion

▸ Potassium chloride with glucose and sodium chloride (Non-proprietary)
Sodium chloride 1.8 mg per 1 ml, Potassium chloride 3 mg per 1 ml, Glucose anhydrous 40 mg per 1 ml Steriflex No.17 potassium chloride 0.3% (potassium 40mmol/1litre) / glucose 4% / sodium chloride 0.18% infusion 1litre bags | 1 bag [PoM] £2.20 | 10 bag [PoM] no price available
Steriflex No.17 potassium chloride 0.3% (potassium 20mmol/500ml) / glucose 4% / sodium chloride 0.18% infusion 500ml bags | 1 bag [PoM] £1.67 | 15 bag [PoM] no price available
Potassium chloride 0.3% (potassium 20mmol/500ml) / Glucose 4% / Sodium chloride 0.18% infusion 500ml Macoflex bags | 1 bag [PoM] no price available | 20 bag [PoM] no price available

Potassium chloride 0.3% (potassium 40mmol/1litre) / Glucose 4% / Sodium chloride 0.18% infusion 1litre Macoflex bags | 1 bag [PoM] no price available | 12 bag [PoM] no price available

Potassium chloride 0.3% (potassium 40mmol/1litre) / Glucose 4% / Sodium chloride 0.18% infusion 1litre Viaflo bags | 1 bag [PoM] no price available | 10 bag [PoM] no price available

Potassium chloride 1.5 mg per 1 ml, Sodium chloride 1.8 mg per 1 ml, Glucose anhydrous 40 mg per 1 ml Potassium chloride 0.15% (potassium 20mmol/1litre) / Glucose 4% / Sodium chloride 0.18% infusion 1litre Viaflo bags | 1 bag [PoM] no price available | 10 bag [PoM] no price available

Steriflex No.14 potassium chloride 0.15% (potassium 20mmol/1litre) / glucose 4% / sodium chloride 0.18% infusion 1litre bags | 1 bag [PoM] £2.20 | 10 bag [PoM] no price available

Potassium chloride 0.15% (potassium 20mmol/1litre) / Glucose 4% / Sodium chloride 0.18% infusion 1litre Macoflex bags | 1 bag [PoM] no price available | 12 bag [PoM] no price available

Potassium chloride 0.15% (potassium 10mmol/500ml) / Glucose 4% / Sodium chloride 0.18% infusion 500ml Macoflex bags | 1 bag [PoM] no price available | 20 bag [PoM] no price available

Steriflex No.14 potassium chloride 0.15% (potassium 10mmol/500ml) / glucose 4% / sodium chloride 0.18% infusion 500ml bags | 1 bag [PoM] £1.67 | 15 bag [PoM] no price available

Sodium chloride 1.8 mg per 1 ml, Potassium chloride 2 mg per 1 ml, Glucose anhydrous 40 mg per 1 ml Steriflex No.30 potassium chloride 0.2% (potassium 13.3mmol/500ml) / glucose 4% / sodium chloride 0.18% infusion 500ml bags | 1 bag [PoM] £1.67 | 15 bag [PoM] no price available

Steriflex No.30 potassium chloride 0.2% (potassium 27mmol/1litre) / glucose 4% / sodium chloride 0.18% infusion 1litre bags | 1 bag [PoM] £2.20 | 10 bag [PoM] no price available

Potassium chloride 1.5 mg per 1 ml, Sodium chloride 4.5 per 1 ml, Glucose anhydrous 50 mg per 1 ml Intraven potassium chloride 0.15% (potassium 10mmol/500ml) / glucose 5% / sodium chloride 0.45% infusion 500ml bags | 1 bag [PoM] £3.12

Potassium chloride with potassium bicarbonate

The properties listed below are those particular to the combination only. For the properties of the components please consider, potassium chloride p. 561.

● **INDICATIONS AND DOSE**

Potassium depletion

▸ BY MOUTH

▸ Child: Dosed according to the deficit or daily maintenance requirements (consult product literature)

● PRESCRIBING AND DISPENSING INFORMATION Each *Sando-K®* tablet contains potassium 470 mg (12 mmol of K^+) and chloride 285mg (8 mmol of Cl^-).

● MEDICINAL FORMS
There can be variation in the licensing of different medicines containing the same drug.
Effervescent tablet
CAUTIONARY AND ADVISORY LABELS 13, 21

▸ Sando-K (HK Pharma Ltd)
Potassium bicarbonate 400 mg, Potassium chloride 600 mg Sando-K effervescent tablets | 100 tablet [P] £7.65 DT price = £7.65

Potassium chloride with sodium chloride

The properties listed below are those particular to the combination only. For the properties of the components please consider, potassium chloride p. 561, sodium chloride p. 547.

● **INDICATIONS AND DOSE**

Electrolyte imbalance

▸ BY INTRAVENOUS INFUSION

▸ Child: Depending on the deficit or the daily maintenance requirements (consult product literature)

- **PRESCRIBING AND DISPENSING INFORMATION** Potassium chloride 0.15% with sodium chloride 0.9% contains K^+ 20 mmol, Na^+ 150 mmol, and Cl^- 170 mmol/litre or potassium chloride 0.3% with sodium chloride 0.9% contains K^+ 40 mmol, Na^+ 150 mmol, and Cl^- 190 mmol/litre.

- **MEDICINAL FORMS**
There can be variation in the licensing of different medicines containing the same drug. Forms available from special-order manufacturers include: infusion, solution for infusion

Infusion

▶ **Potassium chloride with sodium chloride (Non-proprietary)**
Potassium chloride 3 mg per 1 ml, Sodium chloride 9 mg per 1 ml Steriflex No.15 potassium chloride 0.3% (potassium 20mmol/500ml) / sodium chloride 0.9% infusion 500ml bags | 1 bag [PoM] £1.67 | 15 bag [PoM] no price available
Potassium chloride 0.3% (potassium 20mmol/500ml) / Sodium chloride 0.9% infusion 500ml Macoflex bags | 1 bag [PoM] no price available | 20 bag [PoM] no price available
Potassium chloride 0.3% (potassium 20mmol/500ml) / Sodium chloride 0.9% infusion 500ml bags | 1 bag [PoM] £1.42
Potassium chloride 0.3% (potassium 20mmol/500ml) / Sodium chloride 0.9% infusion 500ml Viaflo bags | 1 bag [PoM] no price available | 20 bag [PoM] no price available
Potassium chloride 0.3% (potassium 40mmol/1litre) / Sodium chloride 0.9% infusion 1litre Macoflex bags | 1 bag [PoM] no price available | 12 bag [PoM] no price available
Potassium chloride 0.3% (potassium 40mmol/1litre) / Sodium chloride 0.9% infusion 1litre Viaflo bags | 1 bag [PoM] no price available | 10 bag [PoM] no price available
Steriflex No.15 potassium chloride 0.3% (potassium 40mmol/1litre) / sodium chloride 0.9% infusion 1litre bags | 1 bag [PoM] £2.20 | 10 bag [PoM] no price available
Potassium chloride 1.5 mg per 1 ml, Sodium chloride 9 mg per 1 ml Steriflex No.12 potassium chloride 0.15% (potassium 20mmol/1litre) / sodium chloride 0.9% infusion 1litre bags | 1 bag [PoM] £2.20 | 10 bag [PoM] no price available
Steriflex No.12 potassium chloride 0.15% (potassium 10mmol/500ml) / sodium chloride 0.9% infusion 500ml bags | 1 bag [PoM] £1.67 | 15 bag [PoM] no price available
Potassium chloride 0.15% (potassium 10mmol/500ml) / Sodium chloride 0.9% infusion 500ml Viaflo bags | 1 bag [PoM] no price available | 20 bag [PoM] no price available
Potassium chloride 0.15% (potassium 20mmol/1litre) / Sodium chloride 0.9% infusion 1litre Viaflo bags | 1 bag [PoM] no price available | 10 bag [PoM] no price available
Potassium chloride 0.15% (potassium 10mmol/500ml) / Sodium chloride 0.9% infusion 500ml Viaflex bags | 1 bag [PoM] no price available | 20 bag [PoM] no price available
Potassium chloride 0.15% (potassium 10mmol/500ml) / Sodium chloride 0.9% infusion 500ml Macoflex bags | 1 bag [PoM] no price available | 20 bag [PoM] no price available
Potassium chloride 0.15% (potassium 20mmol/1litre) / Sodium chloride 0.9% infusion 1litre Viaflo bags | 1 bag [PoM] no price available | 10 bag [PoM] no price available
Potassium chloride 0.15% (potassium 20mmol/1litre) / Sodium chloride 0.9% infusion 1litre Macoflex bags | 1 bag [PoM] no price available | 12 bag [PoM] no price available
Potassium chloride 2 mg per 1 ml, Sodium chloride 9 mg per 1 ml Steriflex No.28 potassium chloride 0.2% (potassium 13.3mmol/500ml) / sodium chloride 0.9% infusion 500ml bags | 1 bag [PoM] £1.67 | 15 bag [PoM] no price available
Steriflex No.28 potassium chloride 0.2% (potassium 27mmol/1litre) / sodium chloride 0.9% infusion 1litre bags | 1 bag [PoM] £2.20 | 10 bag [PoM] no price available

ELECTROLYTES AND MINERALS › SODIUM CHLORIDE

Sodium chloride

- **INDICATIONS AND DOSE**
Chronic renal salt wasting
▶ BY MOUTH
▶ Child: 1–2 mmol/kg daily in divided doses, adjusted according to requirements

Sodium supplementation in neonates
▶ INITIALLY BY MOUTH

▶ Neonate up to 36 weeks corrected gestational age: 2 mmol, dose to be administered in 100 ml of formula feed (consult dietician), alternatively (by mouth using modified-release tablets) 3–4 mmol, dose to be administered in 100 ml of breast milk (consult dietician).

Sodium replacement
▶ BY MOUTH USING MODIFIED-RELEASE TABLETS
▶ Child: 1–2 mmol/kg daily in divided doses, adjusted according to requirements, higher doses may be needed in severe depletion

Management of diabetic ketoacidosis (to restore circulating volume if systolic blood pressure is below 90 mmHg and adjusted for age, sex, and medication as appropriate)
▶ BY INTRAVENOUS INFUSION
▶ Child: (consult local protocol)

Diluent for instillation of drugs to the bladder
▶ BY INTRAVESICAL INSTILLATION
▶ Child: (consult product literature)

- **CAUTIONS**
▶ With intravenous use Avoid excessive administration · cardiac failure · cardio-respiratory diseases · children receiving glucocorticoids · dilutional hyponatraemia · hepatic cirrhosis · hypertension · peripheral oedema · pulmonary oedema · reduced fluid loss · renal insufficiency · restrict intake in impaired renal function · toxaemia of pregnancy

CAUTIONS, FURTHER INFORMATION
▶ Reduced fluid loss
▶ With intravenous use The volume of fluid infused should take into account the possibility of reduced fluid loss owing to increased antidiuretic hormone and factors such as renal failure, hypothermia, and high humidity.
▶ Dilutional hyponatraemia
▶ With intravenous use Dilutional hyponatraemia is a rare but potentially fatal risk of parenteral hydration. It may be caused by inappropriate use of hypotonic fluids such as sodium chloride 0.18% and glucose 4% intravenous infusion, especially in the postoperative period when antidiuretic hormone secretion is increased. Dilutional hyponatraemia is characterized by a rapid fall in plasma-sodium concentration leading to cerebral oedema and seizures; any child with severe hyponatraemia or rapidly changing plasma-sodium concentration should be referred urgently to a paediatric high dependency facility.

- **SIDE-EFFECTS**
▶ With intravenous use Administration of large doses may give rise to sodium accumulation · oedema

- **MONITORING REQUIREMENTS**
▶ With intravenous use During parenteral hydration, fluids and electrolytes should be monitored closely and any disturbance corrected by slow infusion of an appropriate solution.

- **PRESCRIBING AND DISPENSING INFORMATION**
▶ With intravenous use Sodium chloride 0.9% intravenous infusion contains Na^+ and Cl^- each 150 mmol/litre. The term 'normal saline' should not be used to describe sodium chloride intravenous infusion 0.9%; the term 'physiological saline' is acceptable but it is preferable to give the composition (i.e. sodium chloride intravenous infusion 0.9%).
▶ With oral use Each *Slow Sodium*® tablet contains approximately 10 mmol each of Na^+ and Cl^-; tablets can be crushed before administration.

9

Blood and nutrition

- **PATIENT AND CARER ADVICE**
  Medicines for Children leaflet: Sodium chloride for hyponatraemia
  www.medicinesforchildren.org.uk/
  sodium-chloride-for-hyponatraemia

- **MEDICINAL FORMS**
  There can be variation in the licensing of different medicines containing the same drug. Forms available from special-order manufacturers include: capsule, solution for injection, infusion, solution for infusion, irrigation

Modified-release tablet

CAUTIONARY AND ADVISORY LABELS 25

▸ Slow Sodium (HK Pharma Ltd)
  Sodium chloride 600 mg Slow Sodium 600mg tablets |
  100 tablet [GSL] £6.05 DT price = £6.05

Solution for injection

▸ Sodium chloride (Non-proprietary)
  Sodium chloride 9 mg per 1 ml Sodium chloride 0.9% solution for injection 5ml Sure-Amp ampoules | 20 ampoule [PoM] £7.15
  Sodium chloride 0.9% solution for injection 50ml vials | 1 vial [PoM] £3.41 DT price = £3.41 | 25 vial [PoM] £75.00–£85.00
  Sodium chloride 0.9% solution for injection 10ml ampoules | 10 ampoule [PoM] £2.30–£2.96 DT price = £2.96 | 50 ampoule [PoM] £14.75
  Sodium chloride 0.9% solution for injection 20ml Mini-Plasco ampoules | 20 ampoule [PoM] £18.93
  Sodium chloride 0.9% solution for injection 5ml Mini-Plasco ampoules | 20 ampoule [PoM] £8.96
  Sodium chloride 0.9% solution for injection 2ml Sure-Amp ampoules | 20 ampoule [PoM] £7.15
  Sodium chloride 0.9% solution for injection 20ml ampoules | 20 ampoule [PoM] £15.75
  Sodium chloride 0.9% solution for injection 2ml ampoules | 10 ampoule [PoM] £1.80–£2.57 DT price = £2.07
  Sodium chloride 0.9% solution for injection 5ml ampoules | 10 ampoule [PoM] £2.00–£2.11 DT price = £2.11 | 50 ampoule [PoM] £10.50
  Sodium chloride 0.9% solution for injection 10ml Sure-Amp ampoules | 20 ampoule [PoM] £8.15
  Sodium chloride 0.9% solution for injection 10ml Mini-Plasco ampoules | 20 ampoule [PoM] £10.21
  Sodium chloride 300 mg per 1 ml Sodium chloride 30% solution for injection 10ml ampoules | 10 ampoule [PoM] £67.46
  Sodium chloride 30% solution for injection 50ml vials | 1 vial [PoM] £12.09

▸ Drytec saline (GE Healthcare Biosciences)
  Sodium chloride 9 mg per 1 ml Drytec saline eluent 5ml vials | 20 vial [PoM] no price available (Hospital only) | 100 vial [PoM] no price available (Hospital only)
  Drytec saline eluent 10ml vials | 20 vial [PoM] no price available (Hospital only) | 100 vial [PoM] no price available (Hospital only)
  Drytec saline eluent 20ml vials | 20 vial [PoM] no price available (Hospital only) | 100 vial [PoM] no price available (Hospital only)

Infusion

▸ Sodium chloride (Non-proprietary)
  Sodium chloride 1.8 mg per 1 ml Polyfusor O sodium chloride 0.18% infusion 500ml bottles | 1 bottle [PoM] £3.44 | 12 bottle [PoM] no price available
  Sodium chloride 4.5 mg per 1 ml Sodium chloride 0.45% infusion 500ml Viaflo bags | 1 bag [PoM] no price available | 20 bag [PoM] no price available
  Polyfusor SB sodium chloride 0.45% infusion 500ml bottles | 1 bottle [PoM] £3.44 | 12 bottle [PoM] no price available
  Sodium chloride 0.45% infusion 500ml Viaflex bags | 1 bag [PoM] no price available | 20 bag [PoM] no price available
  Steriflex No.2 sodium chloride 0.45% infusion 500ml bags | 1 bag [PoM] £1.38 | 15 bag [PoM] no price available
  Sodium chloride 9 mg per 1 ml Sodium chloride 0.9% infusion 100ml bags | 1 bag [PoM] £1.27
  Sodium chloride 0.9% infusion 250ml Macoflex N bags | 1 bag [PoM] no price available | 30 bag [PoM] no price available
  Sodium chloride 0.9% infusion 1litre Macoflex N bags | 1 bag [PoM] no price available | 10 bag [PoM] no price available
  Sodium chloride 0.9% infusion 100ml Viaflo bags | 1 bag [PoM] no price available | 50 bag [PoM] no price available
  Sodium chloride 0.9% infusion 500ml Viaflo bags | 1 bag [PoM] no price available | 20 bag [PoM] no price available
  Sodium chloride 0.9% infusion 50ml Viaflex bags | 1 bag [PoM] no price available | 50 bag [PoM] no price available
  Intraven sodium chloride 0.9% infusion 2litre bags | 1 bag [PoM] £3.01

Sodium chloride 0.9% infusion 500ml Macoflex N bags | 1 bag [PoM] no price available | 18 bag [PoM] no price available
Sodium chloride 0.9% infusion 50ml Easyflex N bags | 1 bag [PoM] no price available | 70 bag [PoM] no price available
Sodium chloride 0.9% infusion 250ml Viaflo bags | 1 bag [PoM] no price available | 30 bag [PoM] no price available
Sodium chloride 0.9% infusion 1litre Easyflex N bags | 1 bag [PoM] no price available | 10 bag [PoM] no price available
Sodium chloride 0.9% infusion 100ml polyethylene bottles | 1 bottle [PoM] £0.55 | 20 bottle [PoM] £11.00
Sodium chloride 0.9% infusion 100ml Macoflex N bags | 1 bag [PoM] no price available | 60 bag [PoM] no price available
Sodium chloride 0.9% infusion 250ml bags | 1 bag [PoM] £1.33
Sodium chloride 0.9% infusion 250ml Viaflex bags | 1 bag [PoM] no price available | 30 bag [PoM] no price available
Intraven sodium chloride 0.9% infusion 500ml bags | 1 bag [PoM] £1.61
Sodium chloride 0.9% infusion 500ml Easyflex N bags | 1 bag [PoM] no price available | 18 bag [PoM] no price available
Sodium chloride 0.9% infusion 50ml Mini-Bag Plus Viaflex bags | 1 bag [PoM] no price available | 30 bag [PoM] no price available
Sodium chloride 0.9% infusion 250ml Macoflex bags | 1 bag [PoM] no price available | 30 bag [PoM] no price available
Sodium chloride 0.9% infusion 500ml Viaflex bags | 1 bag [PoM] no price available | 20 bag [PoM] no price available
Sodium chloride 0.9% infusion 100ml Mini-Bag Plus Viaflex bags | 1 bag [PoM] no price available | 30 bag [PoM] no price available
Sodium chloride 0.9% infusion 500ml Macoflex bags | 1 bag [PoM] no price available | 20 bag [PoM] no price available
Sodium chloride 0.9% infusion 50ml Macoflex N bags | 1 bag [PoM] no price available | 70 bag [PoM] no price available
Sodium chloride 0.9% infusion 1litre Macoflex bags | 1 bag [PoM] no price available | 12 bag [PoM] no price available
Sodium chloride 0.9% infusion 50ml Viaflo bags | 1 bag [PoM] no price available | 50 bag [PoM] no price available
Sodium chloride 0.9% infusion 1litre Viaflo bags | 1 bag [PoM] no price available | 10 bag [PoM] no price available
Intraven sodium chloride 0.9% infusion 50ml bags | 1 bag [PoM] £1.49
Sodium chloride 0.9% infusion 50ml Macoflex bags | 1 bag [PoM] no price available | 70 bag [PoM] no price available
Intraven sodium chloride 0.9% infusion 250ml bags | 1 bag [PoM] £1.61
Sodium chloride 0.9% infusion 1litre Viaflex bags | 1 bag [PoM] no price available | 10 bag [PoM] no price available
Intraven sodium chloride 0.9% infusion 100ml bags | 1 bag [PoM] £1.49
Polyfusor S sodium chloride 0.9% infusion 500ml bottles | 1 bottle [PoM] £2.33 | 12 bottle [PoM] no price available
Sodium chloride 0.9% infusion 100ml Easyflex N bags | 1 bag [PoM] no price available | 60 bag [PoM] no price available
Sodium chloride 0.9% infusion 250ml Easyflex N bags | 1 bag [PoM] no price available | 30 bag [PoM] no price available
Intraven sodium chloride 0.9% infusion 1litre bags | 1 bag [PoM] £2.33
Polyfusor S sodium chloride 0.9% infusion 1litre bottles | 1 bottle [PoM] £3.10 | 6 bottle [PoM] no price available
Sodium chloride 0.9% infusion 100ml Macoflex bags | 1 bag [PoM] no price available | 60 bag [PoM] no price available
Sodium chloride 18 mg per 1 ml Polyfusor SC sodium chloride 1.8% infusion 500ml bottles | 1 bottle [PoM] £3.44 | 12 bottle [PoM] no price available
Sodium chloride 27 mg per 1 ml Polyfusor SD sodium chloride 2.7% infusion 500ml bottles | 1 bottle [PoM] £3.44 | 12 bottle [PoM] no price available
Sodium chloride 50 mg per 1 ml Polyfusor SE sodium chloride 5% infusion 500ml bottles | 1 bottle [PoM] £3.44 | 12 bottle [PoM] no price available

Solution for infusion

▸ Sodium chloride (Non-proprietary)
  Sodium chloride 300 mg per 1 ml Sodium chloride 30% concentrat for solution for infusion 100ml vials | 10 vial [PoM] £44.20
  Sodium chloride 30% concentrate for solution for infusion 50ml vials | 10 vial [PoM] £27.70
  Sodium chloride 30% concentrate for solution for infusion 10ml ampoules | 10 ampoule [PoM] £16.40

Intravesical solution

▸ Sodium chloride (Non-proprietary)
  Sodium chloride 9 mg per 1 ml Sodium chloride 0.9% intravesical solution 50ml bags | 1 bag [P] £5.00

Combinations available: *Potassium chloride with calcium* *chloride and sodium chloride and sodium lactate*, p. 545 · *Potassium chloride with calcium chloride dihydrate and sodium chloride*, p. 545 · *Potassium chloride with glucose and sodium chloride*, p. 546 · *Potassium chloride with sodium chloride*, p. 546

Sodium chloride with glucose

The properties listed below are those particular to the combination only. For the properties of the components please consider, sodium chloride p. 547, glucose below.

● **INDICATIONS AND DOSE**

Combined water and sodium depletion
▶ BY INTRAVENOUS INFUSION
▶ Child: (consult product literature)

● **CAUTIONS**

CAUTIONS, FURTHER INFORMATION
Sodium chloride 0.18% and glucose 4% intravenous infusion fluid should not be used for fluid replacement in children aged 16 years or less because of the risk of hyponatraemia; availability of this infusion should be restricted to high dependency and intensive care units, and specialist wards, such as renal, liver, and cardiac units. Local guidelines on intravenous fluids should be consulted.

● **MONITORING REQUIREMENTS**
▶ Maintenance fluid should accurately reflect daily requirements and close monitoring is required to avoid fluid and electrolyte imbalance.
▶ During parenteral hydration, fluids and electrolytes should be monitored closely and any disturbance corrected by slow infusion of an appropriate solution.

● **MEDICINAL FORMS**
There can be variation in the licensing of different medicines containing the same drug. Forms available from special-order manufacturers include: solution for infusion
Infusion
▶ **Sodium chloride with glucose (Non-proprietary)**
Sodium chloride 4.5 mg per 1 ml, Glucose anhydrous 25 mg per 1 ml Sodium chloride 0.45% / Glucose 2.5% infusion 500ml Viaflex bags | 1 bag [PoM] no price available | 20 bag [PoM] no price available
Sodium chloride 0.45% / Glucose 2.5% infusion 500ml Viaflo bags | 1 bag [PoM] no price available | 20 bag [PoM] no price available
Sodium chloride 1.8 mg per 1 ml, Glucose anhydrous 40 mg per 1 ml Polyfusor T glucose 4% / sodium chloride 0.18% infusion 500ml bottles | 1 bottle [PoM] £2.40 | 12 bottle [PoM] no price available
Sodium chloride 0.18% / Glucose 4% infusion 500ml Macoflex bags | 1 bag [PoM] no price available | 20 bag [PoM] no price available
Sodium chloride 0.18% / Glucose 4% infusion 500ml Viaflo bags | 1 bag [PoM] no price available | 20 bag [PoM] no price available
Sodium chloride 0.18% / Glucose 4% infusion 1litre Macoflex bags | 1 bag [PoM] no price available | 12 bag [PoM] no price available
Sodium chloride 0.18% / Glucose 4% infusion 500ml Viaflex bags | 1 bag [PoM] no price available | 20 bag [PoM] no price available
Sodium chloride 0.18% / Glucose 4% infusion 1litre Viaflo bags | 1 bag [PoM] no price available | 10 bag [PoM] no price available
Sodium chloride 9 mg per 1 ml, Glucose 50 mg per 1 ml Steriflex No.3 glucose 5% / sodium chloride 0.9% infusion 500ml bags | 1 bag [PoM] £1.47 | 15 bag [PoM] no price available
Sodium chloride 0.9% / Glucose 5% infusion 500ml bags | 1 bag [PoM] £1.27
Sodium chloride 0.9% / Glucose 5% infusion 500ml Viaflex bags | 1 bag [PoM] no price available | 20 bag [PoM] no price available
Steriflex No.3 glucose 5% / sodium chloride 0.9% infusion 1litre bags | 1 bag [PoM] £2.10 | 10 bag [PoM] no price available
Sodium chloride 4.5 mg per 1 ml, Glucose anhydrous 50 mg per 1 ml Sodium chloride 0.45% / Glucose 5% infusion 500ml Viaflex bags | 1 bag [PoM] no price available | 20 bag [PoM] no price available
Steriflex No.45 Glucose 5% / sodium chloride 0.45% infusion 500ml bags | 1 bag [PoM] £2.02 | 15 bag [PoM] no price available
Sodium chloride 1.8 mg per 1 ml, Glucose anhydrous 100 mg per 1 ml Steriflex No.19 glucose 10% / sodium chloride 0.18% infusion 500ml bags | 1 bag [PoM] £2.02 | 15 bag [PoM] no price available

NUTRIENTS › SUGARS

Glucose

(Dextrose Monohydrate)

● **INDICATIONS AND DOSE**

Establish presence of gestational diabetes
▶ BY MOUTH
▶ Child: Test dose 75 g, anhydrous glucose to be given to the fasting patient and blood-glucose concentrations measured at intervals, to be given with 200–300 mL fluid

Oral glucose tolerance test
▶ BY MOUTH
▶ Child: Test dose 1.75 g/kg (max. per dose 75 g), anhydrous glucose to be given to the fasting patient and blood-glucose concentrations measured at intervals. To be given with 200–300 mL fluid

Neonatal hypoglycaemia
▶ BY INTRAVENOUS INFUSION
▶ Neonate: 500 mg/kg/hour, to be administered as Glucose 10% intravenous infusion, an initial dose of 250 mg/kg over 5 minutes may be required if hypoglycaemia is severe enough to cause loss of consciousness or seizures.

Hypoglycaemia
▶ BY INTRAVENOUS INFUSION
▶ Child: 500 mg/kg, to be administered as Glucose 10% intravenous infusion into a large vein through a large-gauge needle; care is required since this concentration is irritant especially if extravasation occurs

Energy source
▶ BY INTRAVENOUS INFUSION
▶ Child: (consult product literature)

Water replacement
▶ BY INTRAVENOUS INFUSION
▶ Child: The volume of glucose solution needed to replace deficits may vary (consult product literature)

Persistent cyanosis (in combination with propranolol) when blood glucose less than 3 mmol/litre (followed by morphine)
▶ BY INTRAVENOUS INFUSION
▶ Child: 200 mg/kg, to be administered as Glucose 10% intravenous infusion over 10 minutes

Management of diabetic ketoacidosis
▶ BY INTRAVENOUS INFUSION
▶ Child: Glucose 5% or 10% should be added to replacement fluid once blood-glucose concentration falls below 14 mmol/litre

DOSE EQUIVALENCE AND CONVERSION
75 g anhydrous glucose is equivalent to Glucose BP 82.5 g.

● **CAUTIONS** Do not give alone except when there is no significant loss of electrolytes · prolonged administration of glucose solutions without electrolytes can lead to hyponatreamia and other electrolyte disturbances

● **SIDE-EFFECTS** Glucose injections especially if hypertonic may have a low pH and may cause venous irritation and thrombophlebitis

● **DIRECTIONS FOR ADMINISTRATION**
▶ With intravenous use Injections containing more than 10% glucose can be irritant and should be given into a central venous line; however, solutions containing up to 12.5% can be administered for a short period into a peripheral line.

● **PRESCRIBING AND DISPENSING INFORMATION** Glucose BP is the monohydrate but Glucose Intravenous Infusion BP is a sterile solution of anhydrous glucose or glucose

9

Blood and nutrition

monohydrate, potency being expressed in terms of anhydrous glucose.

- **EXCEPTIONS TO LEGAL CATEGORY**
  ‣ With intravenous use Prescription only medicine restriction does not apply to 50% solution where administration is for saving life in emergency.

- **MEDICINAL FORMS**
  There can be variation in the licensing of different medicines containing the same drug. Forms available from special-order manufacturers include: solution for injection, solution for infusion

Oral solution
‣ **Rapilose OGTT** (Aspire Pharma Ltd)
  Glucose 250 mg per 1 ml Rapilose OGTT solution | 300 ml £3.48

Oral gel
‣ **Dextrogel** (Neoceuticals Ltd)
  Glucose 400 mg per 1 gram Dextrogel 40% gel | 75 gram £7.16 DT price = £7.16 | 80 gram £6.84
‣ **GlucoBoost** (Ennogen Healthcare Ltd)
  Glucose 400 mg per 1 gram GlucoBoost 40% gel | 75 gram £7.16 DT price = £7.16 | 80 gram £6.84
‣ **GlucoGel** (BBI Healthcare Ltd)
  Glucose 400 mg per 1 gram GlucoGel 40% gel original | 75 gram [GSL] £7.16 DT price = £7.16 | 80 gram [GSL] £6.84
‣ **Rapilose** (Galen Ltd)
  Glucose 400 mg per 1 gram Rapilose 40% gel | 75 gram £5.49 DT price = £7.16

Infusion
‣ **Glucose** (Non-proprietary)
  Glucose anhydrous 50 mg per 1 ml Glucose 5% infusion 1litre Macoflex bags | 1 bag [PoM] no price available | 12 bag [PoM] no price available
  Glucose 5% infusion 500ml bags | 1 bag [PoM] £1.27
  Glucose 5% infusion 500ml Macoflex N bags | 1 bag [PoM] no price available | 18 bag [PoM] no price available
  Glucose 5% infusion 100ml bags | 1 bag [PoM] £1.27
  Glucose 5% infusion 1litre Easyflex N bags | 1 bag [PoM] no price available | 10 bag [PoM] no price available
  Glucose 5% infusion 100ml Easyflex N bags | 1 bag [PoM] no price available | 60 bag [PoM] no price available
  Glucose 5% infusion 500ml Viaflo bags | 1 bag [PoM] no price available | 20 bag [PoM] no price available
  Glucose 5% infusion 100ml Macoflex N bags | 1 bag [PoM] no price available | 60 bag [PoM] no price available
  Glucose 5% infusion 500ml Viaflex bags | 1 bag [PoM] no price available | 20 bag [PoM] no price available
  Glucose 5% infusion 250ml Macoflex N bags | 1 bag [PoM] no price available | 30 bag [PoM] no price available
  Glucose 5% infusion 500ml Macoflex bags | 1 bag [PoM] no price available | 20 bag [PoM] no price available
  Polyfusor D glucose 5% infusion 1litre bottles | 1 bottle [PoM] £3.02 | 6 bottle [PoM] no price available
  Glucose 5% infusion 500ml Easyflex N bags | 1 bag [PoM] no price available | 18 bag [PoM] no price available
  Glucose 5% infusion 1litre Viaflo bags | 1 bag [PoM] no price available | 10 bag [PoM] no price available
  Glucose 5% infusion 50ml Viaflo bags | 1 bag [PoM] no price available | 50 bag [PoM] no price available
  Glucose 5% infusion 250ml Easyflex N bags | 1 bag [PoM] no price available | 30 bag [PoM] no price available
  Glucose 5% infusion 100ml Macoflex bags | 1 bag [PoM] no price available | 60 bag [PoM] no price available
  Glucose 5% infusion 50ml Easyflex N bags | 1 bag [PoM] no price available | 70 bag [PoM] no price available
  Glucose 5% infusion 50ml Macoflex N bags | 1 bag [PoM] no price available | 70 bag [PoM] no price available
  Glucose 5% infusion 250ml Viaflex bags | 1 bag [PoM] no price available | 30 bag [PoM] no price available
  Polyfusor D glucose 5% infusion 500ml bottles | 1 bottle [PoM] £2.25 | 12 bottle [PoM] no price available
  Glucose 5% infusion 50ml Viaflex bags | 1 bag [PoM] no price available | 50 bag [PoM] no price available
  Glucose 5% infusion 100ml Viaflex bags | 1 bag [PoM] no price available | 50 bag [PoM] no price available
  Glucose 5% infusion 100ml Viaflo bags | 1 bag [PoM] no price available | 50 bag [PoM] no price available
  Glucose 5% infusion 1litre Macoflex N bags | 1 bag [PoM] no price available | 10 bag [PoM] no price available
  Glucose 5% infusion 250ml Macoflex bags | 1 bag [PoM] no price available | 30 bag [PoM] no price available

Glucose 5% infusion 50ml Macoflex bags | 1 bag [PoM] no price available | 70 bag [PoM] no price available
Glucose 5% infusion 250ml Viaflo bags | 1 bag [PoM] no price available | 30 bag [PoM] no price available
Glucose anhydrous 100 mg per 1 ml Steriflex No.7 glucose 10% infusion 1litre bags | 1 bag [PoM] £2.54 | 10 bag [PoM] no price available
Glucose 10% infusion 1litre Viaflo bags | 1 bag [PoM] no price available | 10 bag [PoM] no price available
Glucose 10% infusion 500ml Macoflex bags | 1 bag [PoM] no price available | 20 bag [PoM] no price available
Glucose 10% infusion 500ml Viaflo bags | 1 bag [PoM] no price available | 20 bag [PoM] no price available
Glucose 10% infusion 1litre Macoflex bags | 1 bag [PoM] no price available | 12 bag [PoM] no price available
Steriflex No.7 glucose 10% infusion 500ml bags | 1 bag [PoM] £1.85 | 15 bag [PoM] no price available
Glucose anhydrous 200 mg per 1 ml Steriflex No.31 glucose 20% infusion 500ml bags | 1 bag [PoM] £2.64 | 15 bag [PoM] no price available
Glucose 20% infusion 500ml bags | 1 bag [PoM] £2.31
Glucose (as Glucose monohydrate) 300 mg per 1 ml Glucose 30% infusion 500ml polyethylene bottles | 10 bottle [PoM] no price available
Glucose anhydrous 400 mg per 1 ml Steriflex No.33 glucose 40% infusion 500ml bags | 1 bag [PoM] £2.81 | 15 bag [PoM] no price available
Glucose anhydrous 500 mg per 1 ml Steriflex No.34 glucose 50% infusion 500ml bags | 1 bag [PoM] £3.11 | 15 bag [PoM] no price available
Glucose 50% infusion 500ml polyethylene bottles | 1 bottle [PoM] £2.94
Glucose anhydrous 700 mg per 1 ml Glucose 70% concentrate for solution for infusion 500ml Viaflex bags | 1 bag [PoM] no price available

Solution for infusion
‣ **Glucose** (Non-proprietary)
  Glucose anhydrous 200 mg per 1 ml Glucose 20% solution for infusion 100ml vials | 1 vial [PoM] £3.50
  Glucose anhydrous 500 mg per 1 ml Glucose 50% solution for infusion 20ml ampoules | 10 ampoule [PoM] £10.00-£12.50
  Glucose 50% solution for infusion 500ml vials | 1 vial [PoM] £2.01 DT price = £2.01 | 25 vial [PoM] £45.00-£50.00

Combinations available: *Potassium chloride with glucose,* p. 545 · *Potassium chloride with glucose and sodium chloride,* p. 546 · *Sodium chloride with glucose,* p. 549

ORAL REHYDRATION SALTS

Disodium hydrogen citrate with glucose, potassium chloride and sodium chloride

(Formulated as oral rehydration salts)

- **INDICATIONS AND DOSE**
  Fluid and electrolyte loss in diarrhoea
  ‣ BY MOUTH
  ‣ Child 1-11 months: 1-1½ times usual feed volume to be given
  ‣ Child 1-11 years: 200 mL, to be given after every loose motion
  ‣ Child 12-17 years: 200-400 mL, to be given after every loose motion, dose according to fluid loss

- **DIRECTIONS FOR ADMINISTRATION** Reconstitute 1 sachet with 200mL of water (freshly boiled and cooled for infants); 5 sachets reconstituted with 1 litre of water provide Na^+ 60 mmol, K^+ 20 mmol, Cl^- 60 mmol, citrate 10 mmol, and glucose 90 mmol.

- **PRESCRIBING AND DISPENSING INFORMATION** Flavours of oral powder formulations may include black currant, citrus, or natural.

- **PATIENT AND CARER ADVICE**
  Medicines for Children leaflet: Oral rehydration salts
  www.medicinesforchildren.org.uk/oral-rehydration-salts

After reconstitution any unused solution should be discarded no later than 1 hour after preparation unless stored in a refrigerator when it may be kept for up to 24 hours.

- **MEDICINAL FORMS**
There can be variation in the licensing of different medicines containing the same drug.
  Powder
  ▸ Dioralyte (Sanofi)
  Potassium chloride 300 mg, Sodium chloride 470 mg, Disodium hydrogen citrate 530 mg, Glucose 3.56 gram Dioralyte oral powder sachets citrus | 20 sachet P £6.72
  Dioralyte oral powder sachets plain | 20 sachet P £6.72
  Dioralyte oral powder sachets blackcurrant | 20 sachet P £6.72

Glucose with potassium chloride, sodium bicarbonate and sodium chloride

(Formulated as oral rehydration salts)

- **INDICATIONS AND DOSE**
Fluid and electrolyte loss in diarrhoea
  ▸ BY MOUTH
  ▸ Child 1–11 months: 1–1½ times usual feed volume to be given
  ▸ Child 1–11 years: 200 mL, to be given after every loose motion
  ▸ Child 12–17 years: 200–400 mL, to be given after every loose motion, dose according to fluid loss

- **DIRECTIONS FOR ADMINISTRATION** Reconstitute 1 sachet with 200 mL of water (freshly boiled and cooled for infants); 5 sachets when reconstituted with 1 litre of water provide Na^+ 50 mmol, K^+ 20 mmol, Cl^- 40 mmol, HCO_3^- 30 mmol, and glucose 111 mmol.

- **PRESCRIBING AND DISPENSING INFORMATION** Flavours of oral powder formulations may include banana, orange, black current, lemon and lime, plain, or multiflavoured.

- **PATIENT AND CARER ADVICE** Patients and carers should be advised how to reconstitute *Electrolade*® oral powder. After reconstitution any unused solution should be discarded no later than 1 hour after preparation unless stored in a refrigerator when it may be kept for up to 24 hours.

- **MEDICINAL FORMS**
There can be variation in the licensing of different medicines containing the same drug.
No licensed medicines listed.

Potassium chloride with rice powder, sodium chloride and sodium citrate

(Formulated as oral rehydation salts)

- **INDICATIONS AND DOSE**
Fluid and electrolyte loss in diarrhoea
  ▸ BY MOUTH
  ▸ Child 1–11 months: 1–1½ times usual feed volume to be given
  ▸ Child 1–11 years: 200 mL, to be given after every loose motion
  ▸ Child 12–17 years: 200–400 mL, to be given after every loose motion, dose according to fluid loss

- **UNLICENSED USE** *Dioralyte Relief*® not licensed for use in children under 3 months.

- **DIRECTIONS FOR ADMINISTRATION** Reconstitute 1 sachet with 200 mL of water (freshly boiled and cooled for infants); 5 sachets when reconstituted with 1 litre of water provide Na^+ 60 mmol, K^+ 20 mmol, Cl^- 50 mmol and citrate 10 mmol.

- **PRESCRIBING AND DISPENSING INFORMATION** Flavours of oral powder formulations may include apricot, black currant, or raspberry.

- **PATIENT AND CARER ADVICE**
Patients and carers should be advised how to reconstitute *Dioralyte*® Relief oral powder.
After reconstitution any unused solution should be discarded no later than 1 hour after preparation unless stored in a refrigerator when it may be kept for up to 24 hours.

Medicines for Children leaflet: Oral rehydration salts
www.medicinesforchildren.org.uk/oral-rehydration-salts

- **MEDICINAL FORMS**
There can be variation in the licensing of different medicines containing the same drug.
  Powder
  EXCIPIENTS: May contain Aspartame
  ▸ Dioralyte Relief (Sanofi)
  Potassium chloride 300 mg, Sodium chloride 350 mg, Sodium citrate 580 mg, Rice powder pre-cooked 6 gram Dioralyte Relief oral powder sachets raspberry sugar-free | 6 sachet GSL £2.50
  Dioralyte Relief oral powder sachets blackcurrant sugar-free | 20 sachet P £7.13

2.1 Calcium imbalance

Calcium

Calcium supplements

Calcium supplements are usually only required where dietary calcium intake is deficient. This dietary requirement varies with age and is relatively greater in childhood, pregnancy, and lactation, due to an increased demand. Hypocalcaemia may be caused by vitamin D deficiency (see Vitamin D under Vitamins p. 581), impaired metabolism, a failure of secretion (hypoparathyroidism), or resistance to parathyroid hormone (pseudohypoparathyroidism).

Mild asymptomatic hypocalcaemia may be managed with oral calcium supplements. *Severe symptomatic hypocalcaemia* requires an intravenous infusion of calcium gluconate 10% p. 553 over 5 to 10 minutes, repeating the dose if symptoms persist; in exceptional cases it may be necessary to maintain a continuous calcium infusion over a day or more. Calcium chloride injection p. 553 is also available, but is more irritant; care should be taken to prevent extravasation.

See the role of calcium gluconate in temporarily reducing the toxic effects of *hyperkalaemia*.

Persistent hypocalcaemia requires oral calcium supplements and either a vitamin D analogue (alfacalcidol p. 588 or calcitriol p. 588) for hypoparathyroidism and pseudohypoparathyroidism or natural vitamin D (calciferol) if due to vitamin D deficiency. It is important to monitor plasma and urinary calcium during long-term maintenance therapy.

Severe hypercalcaemia

Severe hypercalcaemia calls for urgent treatment before detailed investigation of the cause. Dehydration should be corrected first with intravenous infusion of sodium chloride 0.9% p. 547. Drugs (such as thiazides and vitamin D compounds) which promote hypercalcaemia, should be discontinued and dietary calcium should be restricted.

If *severe hypercalcaemia persists* drugs which inhibit mobilisation of calcium from the skeleton may be required. The **bisphosphonates** are useful and pamidronate disodium p. 437 is probably the most effective.

9

Blood and nutrition

Corticosteroids are widely given, but may only be useful where hypercalcaemia is due to sarcoidosis or vitamin D intoxication; they often take several days to achieve the desired effect.

Calcitonin (salmon) p. 439 can be used by specialists for the treatment of hypercalcaemia associated with malignancy; it is rarely effective where bisphosphonates have failed to reduce serum calcium adequately.

After treatment of severe hypercalcaemia the underlying cause must be established. *Further treatment* is governed by the same principles as for initial therapy. Salt and water depletion and drugs promoting hypercalcaemia should be avoided; oral administration of a bisphosphonate may be useful. Parathyroidectomy may be indicated for hyperparathyroidism.

Hypercalciuria

Hypercalciuria should be investigated for an underlying cause, which should be treated. Reducing dietary calcium intake may be beneficial but severe restriction of calcium intake has not proved beneficial and may even be harmful.

Neonates

Calcium supplements

Hypocalcaemia is common in the first few days of life, particularly following birth asphyxia or respiratory distress. Late onset at 4–10 days after birth may be secondary to vitamin D deficiency, hypoparathyroidism or hypomagnesaemia and may be associated with seizures.

2.1a Hypocalcaemia

ELECTROLYTES AND MINERALS ⟩ CALCIUM

Calcium salts

- **CONTRA-INDICATIONS** Conditions associated with hypercalcaemia (e.g. some forms of malignant disease) · conditions associated with hypercalciuria (e.g. some forms of malignant disease)
- **CAUTIONS** History of nephrolithiasis · sarcoidosis
- **INTERACTIONS** → Appendix 1 (antacids, calcium salts).
- **SIDE-EFFECTS**
  GENERAL SIDE-EFFECTS
- Rare Gastro-intestinal disturbances
- **Frequency not known** Hypercalcaemia
  SPECIFIC SIDE-EFFECTS
- With intravenous use Arrhythmias · bradycardia · fall in blood pressure · injection-site reactions · peripheral vasodilatation · severe tissue damage with extravasation · sweating
- **RENAL IMPAIRMENT** Use with caution. Risk of hypercalcaemia and renal calculi.

↱ above

Calcium carbonate

- **INDICATIONS AND DOSE**

Phosphate binding in renal failure and hyper-phosphataemia
- BY MOUTH
- Child 1–11 months: 120 mg 3–4 times a day, dose to be adjusted as necessary, to be taken with feeds
- Child 1–5 years: 300 mg 3–4 times a day, dose to be adjusted as necessary, to be taken prior to or with meals
- Child 6–11 years: 600 mg 3–4 times a day, dose to be adjusted as necessary, to be taken prior to or with meals

- Child 12–17 years: 1.25 g 3–4 times a day, dose to be adjusted as necessary, to be taken prior to or with meals

Calcium deficiency
- BY MOUTH
- Neonate: 0.25 mmol/kg 4 times a day, adjusted according to response

- Child 1 month–4 years: 0.25 mmol/kg 4 times a day, adjusted according to response
- Child 5–11 years: 0.2 mmol/kg 4 times a day, adjusted according to response
- Child 12–17 years: 10 mmol 4 times a day, adjusted according to response

- **PRESCRIBING AND DISPENSING INFORMATION** *Adcal*® contains calcium carbonate 1.5 g (calcium 600 mg or Ca^{2+} 15 mmol); *Calcichew*® contains calcium carbonate 1.25 g (calcium 500 mg or Ca^{2+} 12.5 mmol);*Calcichew Forte*® contains calcium carbonate 2.5 g (calcium 1 g or Ca^{2+} 25 mmol);*Cacit*® contains calcium carbonate 1.25 g, providing calcium citrate when dispersed in water (calcium 500 mg or Ca^{2+} 12.5 mmol); consult product literature for details of other available products.

  Flavours of chewable tablet formulations may include orange or fruit flavour.

- **PATIENT AND CARER ADVICE**
  Medicines for Children leaflet: Calcium salts for kidney disease www.medicinesforchildren.org.uk/calcium-salts-kidney-disease-0

- **MEDICINAL FORMS**
  There can be variation in the licensing of different medicines containing the same drug. Forms available from special-order manufacturers include: tablet, capsule, oral suspension

Tablet
CAUTIONARY AND ADVISORY LABELS 25
- Calcium carbonate (Non-proprietary)
  Calcium carbonate 1.25 gram Calcium carbonate 1.25g tablets | 100 tablet no price available

Chewable tablet
CAUTIONARY AND ADVISORY LABELS 24
EXCIPIENTS: May contain Aspartame
- Calcium carbonate (Non-proprietary)
  Calcium carbonate 1.25 gram Calcium carbonate 1.25g chewable tablets sugar free sugar-free | 100 tablet £12.50 DT price = £9.33
- Adcal (ProStrakan Ltd)
  Calcium carbonate 1.5 gram Adcal 1500mg chewable tablets sugar-free | 100 tablet Ⓟ £8.70 DT price = £8.70
- Calcichew (Forum Health Products Ltd)
  Calcium carbonate 1.25 gram Calcichew 500mg chewable tablets sugar-free | 100 tablet Ⓟ £9.33 DT price = £9.33
  Calcium carbonate 2.5 gram Calcichew Forte chewable tablets sugar-free | 60 tablet Ⓟ £13.16 DT price = £13.16

Effervescent tablet
CAUTIONARY AND ADVISORY LABELS 13
- Cacit (Warner Chilcott UK Ltd)
  Calcium carbonate 1.25 gram Cacit 500mg effervescent tablets sugar-free | 76 tablet Ⓟ £11.81 DT price = £11.81

Calcium carbonate with calcium lactate gluconate

The properties listed below are those particular to the combination only. For the properties of the components please consider, calcium carbonate above.

- **INDICATIONS AND DOSE**

Calcium deficiency
- BY MOUTH
- Neonate: 0.25 mmol/kg 4 times a day, adjusted according to response.

- Child 1 month–4 years: 0.25 mmol/kg 4 times a day, adjusted according to response

‣ Child 5–11 years: 0.2 mmol/kg 4 times a day, adjusted according to response
‣ Child 12–17 years: 10 mmol 4 times a day, adjusted according to response

● PRESCRIBING AND DISPENSING INFORMATION Each *Sandocal®* tablet contains 1 g calcium (Ca²⁺ 25 mmol); flavours of soluble tablet formulations may include orange.

● MEDICINAL FORMS
There can be variation in the licensing of different medicines containing the same drug.
Effervescent tablet
CAUTIONARY AND ADVISORY LABELS 13
EXCIPIENTS: May contain Aspartame
‣ Sandocal (Novartis Consumer Health UK Ltd)
  Calcium carbonate 1.75 gram, Calcium lactate gluconate 2.263 gram Sandocal 1000 effervescent tablets sugar-free | 30 tablet P £7.95 DT price = £7.95

⯌ 552

Calcium chloride

● INDICATIONS AND DOSE
Acute hypocalcaemia
▶ BY INTRAVENOUS INJECTION
‣ Child: (consult product literature)

● CAUTIONS Avoid in respiratory acidosis · avoid in respiratory failure

● DIRECTIONS FOR ADMINISTRATION Care should be taken to avoid extravasation.

● PRESCRIBING AND DISPENSING INFORMATION Non-proprietary *Calcium chloride dihydrate 7.35%* (calcium 20 mg or Ca²⁺ 500 micromol/mL); *Calcium chloride dihydrate 10%* (calcium 27.3 mg or Ca²⁺ 680 micromol/mL); *Calcium chloride dihydrate 14.7%* (calcium 40.1 mg or Ca²⁺ 1000 micromol/mL).

● MEDICINAL FORMS
There can be variation in the licensing of different medicines containing the same drug. Forms available from special-order manufacturers include: solution for infusion
Solution for injection
▶ Calcium chloride (Non-proprietary)
  Calcium chloride dihydrate 73.5 mg per 1 ml Calcium chloride 7.35% solution for injection 10ml ampoules | 10 ampoule PoM £66.38
  Calcium chloride dihydrate 100 mg per 1 ml Calcium chloride 10% solution for injection 10ml pre-filled syringes | 1 pre-filled disposable injection PoM £9.42
  Calcium chloride dihydrate 147 mg per 1 ml Calcium chloride 14.7% solution for injection 5ml ampoules | 10 ampoule PoM £95.22
  Calcium chloride 14.7% solution for injection 10ml ampoules | 10 ampoule PoM £64.69-£66.38

⯌ 552

Calcium gluconate

● INDICATIONS AND DOSE
Calcium deficiency | Mild asymptomatic hypocalcaemia
▶ BY MOUTH
‣ Neonate: 0.25 mmol/kg 4 times a day, adjusted according to response.
‣ Child 1 month–4 years: 0.25 mmol/kg 4 times a day, adjusted according to response
‣ Child 5–11 years: 0.2 mmol/kg 4 times a day, adjusted according to response
‣ Child 12–17 years: 10 mmol 4 times a day, adjusted according to response

Acute hypocalcaemia, urgent correction | Hyperkalaemia (prevention of arrhythmias)
▶ BY SLOW INTRAVENOUS INJECTION
‣ Neonate: 0.11 mmol/kg for 1 dose, to be given over 5–10 minutes, some units use a dose of 0.46 mmol/kg (2 mL/kg calcium gluconate 10%) for hypocalcaemia in line with US practice.
‣ Child: 0.11 mmol/kg, to be given over 5–10 minutes, maximum 4.5 mmol (20 mL calcium gluconate 10%)

Acute hypocalcaemia, maintenance
▶ BY CONTINUOUS INTRAVENOUS INFUSION
‣ Neonate: 0.5 mmol/kg daily, adjusted according to response, dose to be given over 24 hours, use oral route as soon as possible due to risk of extravasation.
‣ Child 1 month–1 year: 1 mmol/kg daily, adjusted according to response, dose to be given over 24 hours, use oral route as soon as possible due to risk of extravasation; Usual maximum 8.8 mmol
‣ Child 2–17 years: 8.8 mmol daily, adjusted according to response, dose to be given over 24 hours, use oral route as soon as possible due to risk of extravasation

DOSE EQUIVALENCE AND CONVERSION
0.11 mmol/kg is equivalent to 0.5 mL/kg of calcium gluconate 10%.

┌───┐
IMPORTANT SAFETY INFORMATION
The MHRA has advised that repeated or prolonged administration of calcium gluconate injection packaged in 10 mL glass containers is contra-indicated in children under 18 years and in patients with renal impairment owing to the risk of aluminium accumulation; in these patients the use of calcium gluconate injection packaged in plastic containers is recommended.
└───┘

● MONITORING REQUIREMENTS
▶ With intravenous use Plasma-calcium and ECG monitoring required for administration by slow intravenous injection (risk of arrhythmias if given too rapidly).

● DIRECTIONS FOR ADMINISTRATION
▶ With intravenous use For intravenous infusion dilute to at least 45 micromol/mL with Glucose 5% *or* Sodium Chloride 0.9%. Maximum administration rate 45 micromol/kg/hour (or in neonates max. 22 micromol/kg/hour). May be given more concentrated via a central venous catheter. May be used undiluted (10% calcium gluconate) in emergencies. Avoid extravasation; should not be given by intramuscular injection. Incompatible with sodium bicarbonate and phosphate solutions.

● PRESCRIBING AND DISPENSING INFORMATION Calcium gluconate 1 g contains calcium 89 mg or Ca²⁺ 2.23 mmol.

● MEDICINAL FORMS
There can be variation in the licensing of different medicines containing the same drug. Forms available from special-order manufacturers include: tablet, capsule, oral suspension, oral solution, solution for infusion
Effervescent tablet
CAUTIONARY AND ADVISORY LABELS 13
ELECTROLYTES: May contain Sodium
▶ Calcium gluconate (Non-proprietary)
  Calcium gluconate 1 gram Calcium gluconate 1g effervescent tablets | 28 tablet GSL £15.68 DT price = £15.68
Solution for injection
▶ Calcium gluconate (Non-proprietary)
  Calcium gluconate 100 mg per 1 ml Calcium gluconate 10% solution for injection 10ml ampoules | 10 ampoule PoM £6.50-£7.50

Calcium lactate

F 552

- **INDICATIONS AND DOSE**

Calcium deficiency
  ▶ BY MOUTH
  ▶ Neonate: 0.25 mmol/kg 4 times a day, adjusted according to response.
  ▶ Child 1 month-4 years: 0.25 mmol/kg 4 times a day, adjusted according to response
  ▶ Child 5-11 years: 0.2 mmol/kg 4 times a day, adjusted according to response
  ▶ Child 12-17 years: 10 mmol 4 times a day, adjusted according to response

- **MEDICINAL FORMS**
There can be variation in the licensing of different medicines containing the same drug.
Tablet
  ▶ Calcium lactate (Non-proprietary)
    Calcium lactate 300 mg Calcium lactate 300mg tablets | 84 tablet no price available DT price = £4.57 | 84 tablet GSL £4.57 DT price = £4.57

Calcium phosphate

F 552

- **INDICATIONS AND DOSE**

Indications listed in combination monographs (available in the UK only in combination with other drugs)
  ▶ BY MOUTH
  ▶ Child: Doses listed in combination monographs

- **MEDICINAL FORMS**
There can be variation in the licensing of different medicines containing the same drug.
No licensed medicines listed.

2.2   Low blood volume

BLOOD AND RELATED PRODUCTS ⟩ PLASMA PRODUCTS

Albumin solution

(Human Albumin Solution)

- **INDICATIONS AND DOSE**

Acute or sub-acute loss of plasma volume e.g. in burns, pancreatitis, trauma, and complications of surgery (with isotonic solutions) | Plasma exchange (with isotonic solutions) | Severe hypoalbuminaemia associated with low plasma volume and generalised oedema where salt and water restriction with plasma volume expansion are required (with concentrated solutions 20%) | Paracentesis of large volume ascites associated with portal hypertension (with concentrated solutions 20%)
  ▶ BY INTRAVENOUS INFUSION
  ▶ Child: (consult product literature)

Adjunct in the treatment of hyperbilirubinaemia by exchange transfusion in the newborn (with concentrated solutions 20%)
  ▶ BY INTRAVENOUS INFUSION
  ▶ Child: (consult product literature)

- **CONTRA-INDICATIONS** Cardiac failure · severe anaemia
- **CAUTIONS** Correct dehydration when administering concentrated solution · history of cardiac disease (administer slowly to avoid rapid rise in blood pressure and cardiac failure, and monitor cardiovascular and respiratory function) · history of circulatory disease (administer slowly to avoid rapid rise in blood pressure and cardiac failure, and monitor cardiovascular and respiratory function) · increased capillary permeability

- **SIDE-EFFECTS** Anaphylaxis · chills · fever · hypersensitivity reactions · hypotension · increased salivation · nausea · tachycardia · vomiting

- **MONITORING REQUIREMENTS** Plasma and plasma substitutes are often used in very ill patients whose condition is unstable. Therefore, close monitoring is required and fluid and electrolyte therapy should be adjusted according to the patient's condition at all times.

- **PRESCRIBING AND DISPENSING INFORMATION** A solution containing protein derived from plasma, serum, or normal placentas; at least 95% of the protein is albumin. The solution may be isotonic (containing 3.5–5% protein) or concentrated (containing 15–25% protein).

- **MEDICINAL FORMS**
There can be variation in the licensing of different medicines containing the same drug.
Infusion
  ▶ Flexbumin (Baxalta UK Ltd)
    Albumin solution human 200 gram per 1 litre Flexbumin 20% infusion 100ml bags | 1 bag PoM no price available | 12 bag PoM no price available
    Flexbumin 20% infusion 50ml bags | 1 bag PoM no price available | 24 bag PoM no price available
Solution for infusion
  ▶ Albunorm (Octapharma Ltd)
    Albumin solution human 50 mg per 1 ml Albunorm 5% solution for infusion 250ml bottles | 1 bottle PoM £25.50
    Albunorm 5% solution for infusion 100ml bottles | 1 bottle PoM £10.20
    Albunorm 5% solution for infusion 500ml bottles | 1 bottle PoM £51.00
    Albumin solution human 200 mg per 1 ml Albunorm 20% solution for infusion 100ml bottles | 1 bottle PoM £40.80
  ▶ Alburex (CSL Behring UK Ltd)
    Albumin solution human 50 mg per 1 ml Alburex 5% solution for infusion 500ml vials | 1 vial PoM £42.50
    Albumin solution human 200 mg per 1 ml Alburex 20% solution for infusion 100ml vials | 1 vial PoM £34.00
  ▶ Albutein (Grifols UK Ltd)
    Albumin solution human 50 mg per 1 ml Albutein 5% solution for infusion 500ml vials | 1 vial PoM no price available
    Albutein 5% solution for infusion 250ml vials | 1 vial PoM no price available
    Albumin solution human 200 mg per 1 ml Albutein 20% solution for infusion 100ml vials | 1 vial PoM no price available
    Albutein 20% solution for infusion 50ml vials | 1 vial PoM no price available
    Albumin solution human 250 mg per 1 ml Albutein 25% solution for infusion 100ml vials | 1 vial PoM no price available
    Albutein 25% solution for infusion 20ml vials | 1 vial PoM no price available
    Albutein 25% solution for infusion 50ml vials | 1 vial PoM no price available
  ▶ Biotest (Biotest (UK) Ltd)
    Albumin solution human 50 mg per 1 ml Human Albumin Biotest 5% solution for infusion 250ml vials | 1 vial PoM £29.75
    Albumin solution human 200 mg per 1 ml Human Albumin Biotest 20% solution for infusion 50ml vials | 1 vial PoM £23.80
    Human Albumin Biotest 20% solution for infusion 100ml vials | 1 vial PoM £47.60
  ▶ Grifols (Grifols UK Ltd)
    Albumin solution human 50 mg per 1 ml Human albumin Grifols 5% solution for infusion 500ml bottles | 1 bottle PoM £49.50 | 6 bottle PoM no price available
    Human albumin Grifols 5% solution for infusion 250ml bottles | 1 bottle PoM £24.75 | 10 bottle PoM no price available
    Human albumin Grifols 5% solution for infusion 100ml bottles | 1 bottle PoM £9.90 | 10 bottle PoM no price available
  ▶ Zenalb (Bio Products Laboratory Ltd)
    Albumin solution human 45 mg per 1 ml Zenalb 4.5% solution for infusion 250ml bottles | 1 bottle PoM £26.31 | 10 bottle PoM no price available

Zenalb 4.5% solution for infusion 100ml bottles | 1 bottle PoM £11.15
Zenalb 4.5% solution for infusion 500ml bottles | 1 bottle PoM £52.61 | 20 bottle PoM no price available
Albumin solution human 200 mg per 1 ml Zenalb 20% solution for infusion 100ml bottles | 1 bottle PoM £50.07 | 20 bottle PoM no price available
Zenalb 20% solution for infusion 50ml bottles | 1 bottle PoM £24.72 | 20 bottle PoM no price available

PLASMA SUBSTITUTES

Gelatin

- ● **INDICATIONS AND DOSE**
  Low blood volume in hypovolaemic shock, burns and cardiopulmonary bypass
  - ▶ BY INTRAVENOUS INFUSION
  - ▶ **Child:** Initially 10–20 mL/kilogram, use 3.5–4% solution

- ● CAUTIONS Cardiac disease · severe liver disease
  CAUTIONS, FURTHER INFORMATION
  The use of plasma substitutes in children requires specialist supervision due to the risk of fluid overload; use is best restricted to an intensive care setting.
- ● **SIDE-EFFECTS**
  - ▶ **Rare** Severe anaphylactic reactions
  - ▶ **Frequency not known** Hypersensitivity reactions · transient increase in bleeding time
- ● PREGNANCY Manufacturer of *Geloplasma*® advises avoid at the end of pregnancy.
- ● HEPATIC IMPAIRMENT Use with caution in severe impairment.
- ● RENAL IMPAIRMENT Use with caution in renal impairment.
- ● MONITORING REQUIREMENTS
  - ▶ Urine output should be monitored. Care should be taken to avoid haematocrit concentration from falling below 25–30% and the patient should be monitored for hypersensitivity reactions.
  - ▶ Plasma and plasma substitutes are often used in very ill patients whose condition is unstable. Therefore, close monitoring is required and fluid and electrolyte therapy should be adjusted according to the patient's condition at all times.
- ● PRESCRIBING AND DISPENSING INFORMATION The gelatin is partially degraded.
  Gelaspan® contains succinylated gelatin (modified fluid gelatin, average molecular weight 26 500) 40 g, Na^+ 151 mmol, K^+ 4 mmol, Mg^{2+} 1 mmol, Cl^- 103 mmol, Ca^{2+} 1 mmol, acetate 24 mmol/litre; *Gelofusine*® contains succinylated gelatin (modified fluid gelatin, average molecular weight 30 000) 40 g (4%), Na^+ 154 mmol, Cl^- 124 mmol/litre; *Geloplasma*® contains partially hydrolysed and succinylated gelatin (modified liquid gelatin) (as anhydrous gelatin) 30 g (3%), Na^+ 150 mmol, K^+ 5 mmol, Mg^{2+} 1.5mmol, Cl^- 100 mmol, lactate 30 mmol/litre; *Isoplex*® contains succinylated gelatin (modified fluid gelatin, average molecular weight 30 000) 40g (4%), Na^+ 145 mmol, K^+ 4 mmol, Mg^{2+} 0.9 mmol, Cl^- 105 mmol, lactate 25mmol/litre; *Volplex*® contains succinylated gelatin (modified fluid gelatin, average molecular weight 30 000) 40 g (4%), Na^+ 154 mmol, Cl^- 125 mmol/litre.

- ● MEDICINAL FORMS
  There can be variation in the licensing of different medicines containing the same drug.
  Infusion
  - ▶ **Gelaspan** (B.Braun Medical Ltd)
    Gelatin 40 mg per 1 ml Gelaspan 4% infusion 500ml Ecobags | 1 bag PoM £5.78 (Hospital only) | 20 bag PoM no price available (Hospital only)

- ▶ **Gelofusine** (B.Braun Medical Ltd)
  Gelatin 40 mg per 1 ml Gelofusine 4% infusion 1litre Ecobags | 1 bag PoM £9.04 | 10 bag PoM no price available
  Gelofusine 4% infusion 500ml Ecobags | 1 bag PoM £4.83 | 20 bag PoM no price available
- ▶ **Geloplasma** (Fresenius Kabi Ltd)
  Gelatin 30 mg per 1 ml Geloplasma 3% infusion 500ml Freeflex bags | 15 bag PoM no price available (Hospital only)
- ▶ **Isoplex** (Beacon Pharmaceuticals Ltd)
  Gelatin 40 mg per 1 ml Isoplex 4% infusion 500ml bags | 10 bag PoM £75.30 (Hospital only)
- ▶ **Volplex** (Beacon Pharmaceuticals Ltd)
  Gelatin 40 mg per 1 ml Volplex 4% infusion 500ml bags | 10 bag PoM £47.00 (Hospital only)
  Volplex 4% infusion 1litre bags | 6 bag PoM £54.54 (Hospital only)

2.3 Magnesium imbalance

Magnesium

Magnesium is an essential constituent of many enzyme systems, particularly those involved in energy generation; the largest stores are in the skeleton.

Magnesium salts are not well absorbed from the gastrointestinal tract, which explains the use of magnesium sulfate as an osmotic laxative.

Magnesium is excreted mainly by the kidneys and is therefore retained in renal failure, but significant *hypermagnesaemia* (causing muscle weakness and arrhythmias) is rare.

Hypomagnesaemia

Since magnesium is secreted in large amounts in the gastro-intestinal fluid, excessive losses in diarrhoea, stoma or fistula are the most common causes of *hypomagnesaemia*; deficiency may also occur as a result of treatment with certain drugs. Hypomagnesaemia often causes secondary hypocalcaemia (with which it may be confused), particularly in neonates, and also hypokalaemia and hyponatraemia.

Symptomatic *hypomagnesaemia* is associated with a deficit of 0.5–1 mmol/kg. Magnesium is given initially by intravenous infusion or by intramuscular injection of magnesium sulfate; the intramuscular injection is painful. Plasma magnesium concentration should be measured to determine the rate and duration of infusion and the dose should be reduced in renal impairment. To prevent *recurrence of the deficit*, magnesium may be given by mouth in divided doses, but there is limited evidence of benefit. Magnesium aspartate powder for oral solution p. 556 is available as a licensed preparation.

Arrhythmias

Magnesium sulfate injection has also been recommended for the emergency treatment of *serious arrhythmias*, especially in the presence of hypokalaemia (when hypomagnesaemia may also be present) and when salvos of rapid ventricular tachycardia show the characteristic twisting wave front known as *torsade de pointes*.

9

Blood and nutrition

2.3a Hypomagnesaemia

ELECTROLYTES AND MINERALS > MAGNESIUM

Magnesium aspartate

● INDICATIONS AND DOSE
Treatment and prevention of magnesium deficiency
▸ BY MOUTH
▸ Child 2-3 years: 4.5 mmol daily, given as one level 5 mL spoonful of *Magnaspartate*® powder.
▸ Child 4-9 years: 4.5 mmol daily, given as a 5 mL level spoonful of *Magnaspartate*® powder, alternatively 10 mmol daily, given as 1 sachet of *Magnaspartate*® powder.
▸ Child 10-17 years: 10 mmol daily, given as 1 sachet of *Magnaspartate*® powder.

● CONTRA-INDICATIONS Disorders of cardiac conduction
● INTERACTIONS → Appendix 1 (magnesium salts, oral).
● SIDE-EFFECTS
▸ **Uncommon** Diarrhoea
▸ **Rare** Hypermagnesaemia
▸ **Frequency not known** Dental caries (on long term use) · gastrointestinal irritation

SIDE-EFFECTS, FURTHER INFORMATION
Side-effects generally occur at higher doses; if side-effects (such as diarrhoea) occur, consider interrupting treatment and restarting at a reduced dose.

Overdose
Symptoms of hypermagnesaemia may include nausea, vomiting, flushing of the skin, thirst, hypotension due to peripheral vasodilatation, drowsiness, confusion, loss of tendon reflexes and respiratory depression due to neuromuscular blockade, slurred speech, double vision, muscle weakness, bradycardia, cardiac arrhythmias, coma, and cardiac arrest.

● RENAL IMPAIRMENT Avoid in severe impairment (estimated glomerular filtration rate less than 30 mL/minute/1.73^2).

● DIRECTIONS FOR ADMINISTRATION Dissolve sachet contents in 50–200 mL water, tea or orange juice and take immediately.

● PRESCRIBING AND DISPENSING INFORMATION *Magnaspartate*® contains magnesium aspartate 6.5 g (10 mmol Mg^{2+})/sachet.

● PATIENT AND CARER ADVICE Patients and carers should be given advice on how to administer magnesium aspartate powder.

● MEDICINAL FORMS
There can be variation in the licensing of different medicines containing the same drug.
Powder
EXCIPIENTS: May contain Sucrose
▸ **Magnesium aspartate (Non-proprietary)**
Magnesium (as Magnesium aspartate) 243 mg Magnaspartate 243mg (magnesium 10mmol) oral powder sachets | 10 sachet [PoM] £8.95

Magnesium glycerophosphate

● INDICATIONS AND DOSE
Hypomagnesaemia
▸ BY MOUTH
▸ Child 1 month-11 years: Initially 50 mg/kg 3 times a day, dose to be adjusted as necessary
▸ Child 12-17 years: Initially 1–2 g 3 times a day, dose to be adjusted as necessary

DOSE EQUIVALENCE AND CONVERSION
Magnesium glycerophosphate 1 g is equivalent to approximately magnesium 97 mg or Mg^{2+} 4 mmol.

● UNLICENSED USE Not licensed.
● INTERACTIONS → Appendix 1 (magnesium salts, oral).
● SIDE-EFFECTS Arrhythmias · colic · coma · confusion · diarrhoea · drowsiness · flushing of skin · hypermagnesaemia associated side-effects · hypotension · loss of tendon reflexes · muscle weakness · nausea · respiratory depression · thirst · vomiting
● RENAL IMPAIRMENT Avoid or reduce dose. Increased risk of toxicity.
● MONITORING REQUIREMENTS Monitor blood pressure, respiratory rate, urinary output and for signs of overdosage (loss of patellar reflexes, weakness, nausea, sensation of warmth, flushing, drowsiness, double vision, and slurred speech).
● DIRECTIONS FOR ADMINISTRATION Tablets may be dispersed in water.

● MEDICINAL FORMS
There can be variation in the licensing of different medicines containing the same drug. Forms available from special-order manufacturers include: tablet, chewable tablet, capsule, oral suspension, oral solution, powder
Tablet
▸ **Magnesium glycerophosphate (Non-proprietary)**
Magnesium (as Magnesium glycerophosphate) 97.2 mg Mag-4 (magnesium 97.2mg (4mmol)) tablets | 30 tablet £84.50
Chewable tablet
▸ **Magnesium glycerophosphate (Non-proprietary)**
Magnesium (as Magnesium glycerophosphate) 97.2 mg YourMAG (magnesium 97.2mg (4mmol)) chewable tablets | 50 tablet £20.00
Mag-4 (magnesium 97.2mg (4mmol)) chewable tablets sugar-free | 30 tablet £84.50
Neomag (magnesium 97mg (4mmol)) chewable tablets sugar-free | 50 tablet £20.00
▸ **MagnaPhate** (Arjun Products Ltd)
Magnesium (as Magnesium glycerophosphate)
97.2 mg MagnaPhate (magnesium 97.2mg (4mmol)) chewable tablets sugar-free | 50 tablet £22.64
Capsule
▸ **Magnesium glycerophosphate (Non-proprietary)**
Magnesium (as Magnesium glycerophosphate) 48.6 mg Mag-4 (magnesium 48.6mg (2mmol)) capsules | 30 capsule £85.70
Magnesium (as Magnesium glycerophosphate) 97.2 mg Mag-4 (magnesium 97.2mg (4mmol)) capsules | 30 capsule £89.30
Oral solution
▸ **LiquaMag GP** (Fontus Health Ltd)
Magnesium (as Magnesium glycerophosphate) 24.25 mg per 1 ml LiquaMag GP (magnesium 121.25mg/5ml (5mmol/5ml)) oral solution sugar-free | 250 ml £55.00

Magnesium sulfate

● INDICATIONS AND DOSE
Severe acute asthma | Continuing respiratory deterioration in anaphylaxis
▸ BY INTRAVENOUS INFUSION
▸ Child 2-17 years: 40 mg/kg (max. per dose 2 g), to be given over 20 minutes

Persistent pulmonary hypertension of the newborn
▸ INITIALLY BY INTRAVENOUS INFUSION

▸ **Neonate:** Initially 200 mg/kg, to be given over 20–30 minutes, then (by continuous intravenous infusion) 20–75 mg/kg/hour for up to 5 days if response occurs after initial dose (to maintain plasma magnesium concentration between 3.5–5.5 mmol/litre).

Hypomagnesaemia
▸ BY INTRAVENOUS INJECTION

▸ **Neonate:** 100 mg/kg every 6–12 hours as required, to be given over at least 10 minutes.

▸ **Child 1 month–11 years:** 50 mg/kg every 12 hours as required, to be given over at least 10 minutes

▸ **Child 12–17 years:** 1 g every 12 hours as required, to be given over at least 10 minutes

Hypomagnesaemia maintenance (e.g. in intravenous nutrition)
▸ BY INTRAVENOUS INFUSION, OR BY INTRAMUSCULAR INJECTION

▸ **Child:** 50–100 mg/kg daily; maximum 5 g per day

Neonatal hypocalaemia
▸ BY DEEP INTRAMUSCULAR INJECTION, OR BY INTRAVENOUS INFUSION

▸ **Neonate:** 100 mg/kg every 12 hours for 2–3 doses.

Torsade de pointes
▸ BY INTRAVENOUS INJECTION

▸ **Child:** 25–50 mg/kg (max. per dose 2 g), to be given over 10–15 minutes, dose may be repeated once if necessary (consult local protocol)

DOSE EQUIVALENCE AND CONVERSION
Magnesium sulfate heptahydrate 1 g equivalent to Mg^{2+} approx. 4 mmol.

● **UNLICENSED USE** Unlicensed indication in severe acute asthma. Continuing respiratory deterioration in anaphylaxis.

● **INTERACTIONS** → Appendix 1 (magnesium, parenteral).

● **SIDE-EFFECTS** Arrhythmias · colic · coma · confusion · diarrhoea · drowsiness · flushing of skin · hypermagnesaemia associated side-effects · hypotension · loss of tendon reflexes · muscle weakness · nausea · respiratory depression · thirst · vomiting

● **PREGNANCY**
▸ When used for Neonatal hypocalcaemia or Hypomagnesaemia or Torsade de pointes or Severe acute asthma or Continuing respiratory deterioration in anaphylaxis Sufficient amount may cross the placenta in mothers treated with high doses causing hypotonia and respiratory depression in newborns.

● **HEPATIC IMPAIRMENT** Avoid in hepatic coma if risk of renal failure.

● **RENAL IMPAIRMENT** Avoid or reduce dose. Increased risk of toxicity.

● **MONITORING REQUIREMENTS** Monitor blood pressure, respiratory rate, urinary output and for signs of overdosage (loss of patellar reflexes, weakness, nausea, sensation of warmth, flushing, drowsiness, double vision, and slurred speech).

● **DIRECTIONS FOR ADMINISTRATION**
▸ With intravenous use In severe hypomagnesaemia administer initially via controlled infusion device (preferably syringe pump).
▸ With intravenous use For *intravenous infusion*, in persistent pulmonary hypertension of the newborn, dilute to a max. concentration of 100 mg/mL (10%) (0.4 mmol/mL Mg^{2+}) magnesium sulfate heptahydrate (200 mg/mL (0.8 mmol/mL Mg^{2+}) if fluid restricted) with Glucose 5% *or* Sodium Chloride 0.9%.

▸ With intravenous use For neonatal hypocalcaemia, hypomagnaesemia, and torsade de pointes, dilute to 10% (100 mg magnesium sulfate heptahydrate (0.4 mmol Mg^{2+}) in 1 mL) with Glucose 5% *or* 10%, Sodium Chloride 0.45% *or* 0.9% *or* Glucose and Sodium Chloride combinations. Up to 20% solution may be given in fluid restriction. Rate of administration should not exceed 10 mg/kg/minute (0.04 mmol/kg/minute Mg^{2+}) of magnesium sulfate heptahydrate.

● **PRESCRIBING AND DISPENSING INFORMATION**
▸ With intramuscular use or intravenous use The BP directs that the label states the strength as the % w/v of magnesium sulfate heptahydrate and as the approximate concentration of magnesium ions (Mg^{2+}) in mmol/mL. Magnesium Sulfate Injection BP is a sterile solution of Magnesium Sulfate Heptahydrate.

● **MEDICINAL FORMS**
There can be variation in the licensing of different medicines containing the same drug. Forms available from special-order manufacturers include: solution for injection, infusion, solution for infusion

Solution for injection
▸ **Magnesium sulfate** (Non-proprietary)
Magnesium sulfate heptahydrate 500 mg per 1 ml Magnesium sulfate 50% (magnesium 2mmol/ml) solution for injection 10ml ampoules | 10 ampoule [PoM] £11.85–£35.25
Magnesium sulfate 50% (magnesium 2mmol/ml) solution for injection 20ml vials | 10 vial [PoM] £46.40
Magnesium sulfate 50% (magnesium 2mmol/ml) solution for injection 5ml ampoules | 10 ampoule [PoM] £21.80–£58.34
Magnesium sulfate 50% (magnesium 2mmol/ml) solution for injection 2ml ampoules | 10 ampoule [PoM] £11.72–£17.90 DT price = £11.85

Solution for infusion
▸ **Magnesium sulfate** (Non-proprietary)
Magnesium sulfate heptahydrate 100 mg per 1 ml Magnesium sulfate 10% (magnesium 0.4mmol/ml) solution for injection 10ml ampoules | 10 ampoule [PoM] £57.12–£58.80
Magnesium sulfate heptahydrate 500 mg per 1 ml Magnesium sulfate 50% (magnesium 2mmol/ml) solution for infusion 50ml vials | 10 vial [PoM] £63.70

2.4 Phosphate imbalance

Phosphorus

Phosphate supplements

Oral phosphate supplements p. 559 may be required in addition to vitamin D in children with hypophosphataemic vitamin D-resistant rickets, see also Vitamin D, under Vitamins p. 581.

Phosphate infusion is occasionally needed in phosphate deficiency arising from use of parenteral nutrition deficient in phosphate supplements; phosphate depletion also occurs in severe diabetic ketoacidosis. It is difficult to provide detailed guidelines for the treatment of *severe hypophosphatemia* because the extent of total body deficits and response to therapy are difficult to predict. High doses of phosphate may result in a transient serum elevation followed by redistribution into intracellular compartments or bone tissue. It is recommended that severe hypophosphataemia be treated intravenously as large doses of oral phosphate may cause diarrhoea; intestinal absorption may be unreliable and dose adjustment may be necessary.

Phosphate is not the first choice for the treatment of hypercalcaemia because of the risk of precipitation of calcium phosphate in the kidney and other tissues. If used, the child should be well hydrated and electrolytes monitored.

Neonates

Phosphate deficiency may occur in very low-birthweight infants and may compromise bone growth if not corrected. Parenterally fed infants may be at risk of phosphate deficiency due to the limited solubility of phosphate. Some units routinely supplement expressed breast milk with phosphate, although the effect on the osmolality of the milk should be considered.

Phosphate-binding agents

Calcium-containing preparations are used as phosphate-binding agents in the management of hyperphosphataemia complicating renal failure. Aluminium- containing preparations are rarely used as phosphate- binding agents and can cause aluminium accumulation.

Sevelamer hydrochloride is licensed for the treatment of hyperphosphataemia in adults on haemodialysis or peritoneal dialysis. Although experience is limited in children sevelamer hydrochloride may be useful when hypercalcaemia prevents the use of calcium carbonate p. 552.

2.4a Hyperphosphataemia

ELECTROLYTES AND MINERALS > ALUMINIUM

Aluminium hydroxide

- **INDICATIONS AND DOSE**

Hyperphosphataemia in renal failure
▶ BY MOUTH USING CAPSULES
▸ Child 5–11 years: 1–2 capsules 3–4 times a day, dose adjusted as necessary
▸ Child 12–17 years: 1–5 capsules 3–4 times a day, dose adjusted as necessary

- **CONTRA-INDICATIONS** Hypophosphataemia · infants · neonates

CONTRA-INDICATIONS, FURTHER INFORMATION
▶ Neonates and infants Aluminium-containing antacids should not be used because accumulation may lead to increased plasma-aluminium concentrations.

- **INTERACTIONS** → Appendix 1 (antacids).
Antacids should preferably not be taken at the same time as other drugs since they may impair absorption. Antacids may damage enteric coatings designed to prevent dissolution in the stomach.

- **SIDE-EFFECTS** Constipation · hyperaluminaemia

- **HEPATIC IMPAIRMENT** Avoid; can cause constipation which can precipitate coma.

- **RENAL IMPAIRMENT** There is a risk of accumulation and aluminium toxicity with antacids containing aluminium salts. Absorption of aluminium from aluminium salts is increased by citrates, which are contained in many effervescent preparations (such as effervescent analgesics).

- **MEDICINAL FORMS**
There can be variation in the licensing of different medicines containing the same drug.
Capsule
▸ Alu-Cap (Meda Pharmaceuticals Ltd)
Aluminium hydroxide 475 mg Alu-Cap 475mg capsules | 120 capsule [P] £13.71 DT price = £13.71

ELECTROLYTES AND MINERALS >
CALCIUM

☞ 552

Calcium acetate

- **INDICATIONS AND DOSE**

PHOSEX® TABLETS
Phosphate binding in renal failure and hyperphosphataemia
▶ BY MOUTH
▸ Child: Dose to be adjusted according to requirements of patient, dose to be taken with meals (consult product literature)

- **DIRECTIONS FOR ADMINISTRATION**
Phosex® tablets are taken with meals.
Tablets can be broken to aid swallowing, but not chewed (bitter taste).

- **PRESCRIBING AND DISPENSING INFORMATION** *Phosex*® tablets contain calcium acetate 1 g (equivalent to calcium 250 mg or Ca^{2+} 6.2 mmol).

- **PATIENT AND CARER ADVICE**
Medicines for Children leaflet: Calcium salts for kidney disease www.medicinesforchildren.org.uk/calcium-salts-kidney-disease-0

PHOSEX® TABLETS Patients or carers should be given advice on how to administer *Phosex*® tablets.

- **MEDICINAL FORMS**
There can be variation in the licensing of different medicines containing the same drug.
Tablet
CAUTIONARY AND ADVISORY LABELS 25
▸ Phosex (Pharmacosmos UK Ltd)
Calcium acetate 1 gram Phosex 1g tablets | 180 tablet [PoM] £19.79
DT price = £19.79

PHOSPHATE BINDERS

Sevelamer

- **INDICATIONS AND DOSE**

RENAGEL®
Hyperphosphataemia in patients on haemodialysis or peritoneal dialysis
▶ BY MOUTH
▸ Child 12–17 years: Initially 0.8–1.6 g 3 times a day, dose to be given with meals and adjusted according to serum-phosphate concentration

- **UNLICENSED USE** Not licensed for use in children under 18 years.

- **CONTRA-INDICATIONS** Bowel obstruction

- **CAUTIONS** Gastro-intestinal disorders

- **INTERACTIONS** → Appendix 1 (sevelamer).

- **SIDE-EFFECTS**
▸ **Common or very common** Abdominal pain · constipation · diarrhoea · dyspepsia · flatulence · nausea · vomiting
▸ **Frequency not known** Diverticulitis · ileus · intestinal obstruction (higher incidence with sevelamer hydrochloride salt) · intestinal perforation · pruritus · rash

- **PREGNANCY** Manufacturer advises use only if potential benefit outweighs risk.

- **BREAST FEEDING** Manufacturer advises use only if potential benefit outweighs risk.

- **PATIENT AND CARER ADVICE**
Medicines for Children leaflet: Sevelamer in dialysis www.medicinesforchildren.org.uk/sevelamer-in-dialysis

● **MEDICINAL FORMS**
There can be variation in the licensing of different medicines containing the same drug.

Tablet

CAUTIONARY AND ADVISORY LABELS 25
EXCIPIENTS: May contain Propylene glycol
▸ **Renagel** (Sanofi)
Sevelamer 800 mg Renagel 800mg tablets | 180 tablet [PoM]
£167.04 DT price = £87.00

2.4b Hypophosphataemia

PHOSPHATES

Phosphate

● **INDICATIONS AND DOSE**

Hypophosphataemia | Hypophosphataemic rickets | Osteomalacia
▸ BY MOUTH USING EFFERVESCENT TABLETS

▸ Neonate: 1 mmol/kg daily in 1–2 divided doses, dose can be taken as a supplement in breast milk—caution advised as solubility in breast milk is limited to 1.2 mmol in 100 mL if calcium also added, contact pharmacy department for details.

▸ Child 1 month-4 years: 2–3 mmol/kg daily in 2–4 divided doses, dose to be adjusted as necessary, dose can be taken as a supplement in breast milk—caution advised as solubility in breast milk is limited to 1.2 mmol in 100 mL if calcium also added, contact pharmacy department for details; maximum 48 mmol per day

▸ Child 5-17 years: 2–3 mmol/kg daily in 2–4 divided doses, dose to be adjusted as necessary; maximum 97 mmol per day

▸ BY INTRAVENOUS INFUSION

▸ Neonate: 1 mmol/kg daily, dose to be adjusted as necessary.

▸ Child 1 month-1 year: 0.7 mmol/kg daily, to be adjusted as necessary

▸ Child 2-17 years: 0.4 mmol/kg daily, dose to be adjusted as necessary

IMPORTANT SAFETY INFORMATION
▸ With intravenous use
Some phosphate injection preparations also contain potassium. For peripheral intravenous administration the *concentration* of potassium should not usually exceed 40 mmol/litre. The infusion solution should be **thoroughly mixed.** Local policies on avoiding inadvertent use of potassium concentrate should be followed. The potassium content of some phosphate preparations may also limit the *rate* at which they may be administered.

● **CAUTIONS**

GENERAL CAUTIONS
Cardiac disease · dehydration · diabetes mellitus · sodium and potassium concentrations of preparations

SPECIFIC CAUTIONS
▸ With intravenous use Avoid extravasation · severe tissue necrosis

● **SIDE-EFFECTS**
▸ **Common or very common** Diarrhoea
▸ **Frequency not known** Acute renal failure · hypocalcaemia · hypotension · metastatic calcification · nausea · oedema · phlebitis · tissue necrosis on extravasation

SIDE-EFFECTS, FURTHER INFORMATION
Diarrhoea is a common side-effect and should prompt a reduction in dosage.

● **RENAL IMPAIRMENT** Reduce dose. Monitor closely in renal impairment.

● **MONITORING REQUIREMENTS** It is essential to monitor closely plasma concentrations of calcium, phosphate, potassium, and other electrolytes—excessive doses of phosphates may cause hypocalcaemia and metastatic calcification.

● **DIRECTIONS FOR ADMINISTRATION**
▸ With intravenous use Dilute injection with Sodium Chloride 0.9% or 0.45% or Glucose 5% or 10%. Administration rate of phosphate should not exceed 0.05 mmol/kg/hour. In emergencies in intensive care faster rates may be used—seek specialist advice.

● **PRESCRIBING AND DISPENSING INFORMATION** *Phosphate Sandoz*® contains sodium dihydrogen phosphate anhydrous (anhydrous sodium acid phosphate) 1.936 g, sodium bicarbonate 350 mg, potassium bicarbonate 315 mg, equivalent to phosphorus 500 mg (phosphate 16.1 mmol), sodium 468.8 mg (Na^+ 20.4 mmol), potassium 123 mg (K^+ 3.1 mmol); *Polyfusor NA*® contains Na^+ 162 mmol/litre, K^+ 19 mmol/litre, PO_4^{3-} 100 mmol/litre; non-proprietary *potassium dihydrogen phosphate injection* (potassium acid phosphate)13.6% may contain 1 mmol/mL phosphate, 1 mmol/mL potassium.

● **PATIENT AND CARER ADVICE**
Medicines for Children leaflet: Phosphate supplements for low phosphate levels www.medicinesforchildren.org.uk/phosphate-supplements-low-phosphate-levels

● **MEDICINAL FORMS**
There can be variation in the licensing of different medicines containing the same drug. Forms available from special-order manufacturers include: infusion, solution for infusion

Tablet

Effervescent tablet
CAUTIONARY AND ADVISORY LABELS 13
▸ **Phosphate Sandoz** (HK Pharma Ltd)
Sodium dihydrogen phosphate anhydrous 1.936 gram Phosphate Sandoz effervescent tablets | 100 tablet [P] £16.43

Infusion
▸ **Phosphate** (Non-proprietary)
Potassium dihydrogen phosphate 1.295 gram per 1 litre, Disodium hydrogen phosphate anhydrous 5.75 gram per 1 litre Polyfusor NA phosphates infusion 500ml bottles | 1 bottle [PoM] £5.15

Solution for infusion
▸ **Phosphate** (Non-proprietary)
Potassium dihydrogen phosphate 136 mg per 1 ml Potassium dihydrogen phosphate 13.6% (potassium 10mmol/10ml) solution for infusion 10ml ampoules | 10 ampoule [PoM] £72.95–£80.25

2.5 Potassium imbalance
2.5a Hyperkalaemia

Drugs used for Hyperkalaemia not listed below Calcium gluconate p. 553

ANTIDOTES AND CHELATORS ⟩ CATION EXCHANGE RESINS

Calcium polystyrene sulfonate

● **INDICATIONS AND DOSE**

Hyperkalaemia associated with anuria or severe oliguria, and in dialysis patients
▸ BY MOUTH

▸ Child: 0.5–1 g/kg daily in divided doses; maximum 60 g per day continued →

▸ BY RECTUM

▸ Neonate: 0.5–1 g/kg daily, irrigate colon to remove resin after 8–12 hours.

▸ Child: 0.5–1 g/kg daily, irrigate colon to remove resin after 8–12 hours; maximum 30 g per day

SORBISTERIT® POWDER

Hyperkalaemia associated with anuria or severe oliguria, and in dialysis patients

▸ BY MOUTH

▸ Child: 0.5–1 g/kg daily, to be given in at least 3 divided doses; maximum 60 g per day

▸ BY RECTUM

▸ Neonate: 0.5–1 g/kg daily, retained for 6 hours followed by irrigation to remove resin from colon.

▸ Child: 0.5–1 g/kg daily, retained for 6 hours followed by irrigation to remove resin from colon; maximum 40 g per day

● CONTRA-INDICATIONS Hyperparathyroidism · metastatic carcinoma · multiple myeloma · obstructive bowel disease · reduced gut motility (in neonates) · sarcoidosis

● CAUTIONS Impaction of resin with excessive dosage or inadequate dilution

● INTERACTIONS → Appendix 1 (polystyrene sulfonate resins).

● SIDE-EFFECTS

GENERAL SIDE-EFFECTS

Anorexia · constipation (discontinue treatment—avoid magnesium-containing laxatives) · diarrhoea · gastric irritation · gastro-intestinal obstruction · hypercalcaemia (including in dialysed patients and occasionally in those with renal impairment) · hypomagnesaemia · intestinal necrosis (reported with concomitant sorbitol) · ischaemic colitis · nausea · necrosis · ulceration · vomiting

SPECIFIC SIDE-EFFECTS

▸ With oral use Gastro-intestinal concretions

▸ With rectal use Faecal impaction

● PREGNANCY Manufacturers advise use only if potential benefit outweighs risk—no information available.

● BREAST FEEDING Manufacturers advise use only if potential benefit outweighs risk—no information available.

● MONITORING REQUIREMENTS Monitor for electrolyte disturbances (stop if plasma-potassium concentration below 5 mmol/litre).

● DIRECTIONS FOR ADMINISTRATION

▸ With rectal use Mix each 1 g of resin with 5 mL of water or 10% glucose.

SORBISTERIT® POWDER *By mouth*, administer in a small amount of water or soft drink—do not give with fruit juice or squash, which have a high potassium content.
By rectum, mix each 1 g of resin with 4 mL of 5% glucose.

● MEDICINAL FORMS

There can be variation in the licensing of different medicines containing the same drug. Forms available from special-order manufacturers include: enema

Powder

CAUTIONARY AND ADVISORY LABELS 13, 21 (Sorbisterit® powder only)

EXCIPIENTS: May contain Sucrose

▸ Calcium Resonium (Sanofi)

Calcium polystyrene sulfonate 999.34 mg per 1 gram Calcium Resonium powder sugar-free | 300 gram Ⓟ £82.16

Sodium polystyrene sulfonate

● INDICATIONS AND DOSE

Hyperkalaemia associated with anuria or severe oliguria, and in dialysis patients

▸ BY MOUTH

▸ Child: 0.5–1 g/kg daily in divided doses; maximum 60 g per day

▸ BY RECTUM

▸ Neonate: 0.5–1 g/kg daily, irrigate colon to remove resin after 8–12 hours.

▸ Child: 0.5–1 g/kg daily, irrigate colon to remove resin after 8–12 hours; maximum 30 g per day

● CONTRA-INDICATIONS Obstructive bowel disease · reduced gut motility (in neonates)

● CAUTIONS Congestive heart failure · hypertension · impaction of resin with excessive dosage or inadequate dilution · oedema

● INTERACTIONS → Appendix 1 (polystyrene sulfonate resins).

● SIDE-EFFECTS

GENERAL SIDE-EFFECTS

Anorexia · constipation (discontinue treatment—avoid magnesium-containing laxatives) · diarrhoea · gastric irritation · gastro-intestinal obstruction · hypocalcaemia · hypomagnesaemia · intestinal necrosis (reported with concomitant use of sorbitol) · ischaemic colitis · nausea · necrosis · sodium retention · ulceration · vomiting

SPECIFIC SIDE-EFFECTS

▸ With oral use Gastro-intestinal concretions

▸ With rectal use Faecal impaction

● PREGNANCY Manufacturers advise use only if potential benefit outweighs risk—no information available.

● BREAST FEEDING Manufacturers advise use only if potential benefit outweighs risk—no information available.

● RENAL IMPAIRMENT Use with caution.

● MONITORING REQUIREMENTS Monitor for electrolyte disturbances (stop if plasma-potassium concentration below 5 mmol/litre).

● DIRECTIONS FOR ADMINISTRATION

▸ With rectal use Mix each 1 g of resin with 5 mL of water or 10% glucose.

▸ With oral use Administer dose (powder) in a small amount of water or honey—do not give with fruit juice or squash, which have a high potassium content.

● MEDICINAL FORMS

There can be variation in the licensing of different medicines containing the same drug. Forms available from special-order manufacturers include: oral suspension

Powder

CAUTIONARY AND ADVISORY LABELS 13

▸ Resonium A (Sanofi)

Sodium polystyrene sulfonate 999.34 mg per 1 gram Resonium A powder sugar-free | 454 gram Ⓟ £81.11

2.5b Hypokalaemia

ELECTROLYTES AND MINERALS > POTASSIUM

Potassium bicarbonate with potassium acid tartrate

- **INDICATIONS AND DOSE**

Hyperchloraemic acidosis associated with potassium deficiency (as in some renal tubular and gastro-intestinal disorders)
▸ BY MOUTH
▸ Child: (consult product literature)

- **CONTRA-INDICATIONS** Hypochloraemia · plasma-potassium concentration above 5 mmol/litre
- **CAUTIONS** Cardiac disease
- **INTERACTIONS** → Appendix 1 (potassium salts).
- **SIDE-EFFECTS** Abdominal pain · diarrhoea · flatulence · nausea · vomiting
- **RENAL IMPAIRMENT** Avoid in severe impairment. Close monitoring required in renal impairment—high risk of hyperkalaemia.
- **DIRECTIONS FOR ADMINISTRATION** To be dissolved in water before administration.
- **PRESCRIBING AND DISPENSING INFORMATION** These tablets do not contain chloride.

- **MEDICINAL FORMS**
There can be variation in the licensing of different medicines containing the same drug.
Effervescent tablet
CAUTIONARY AND ADVISORY LABELS 13, 21
▸ Potassium bicarbonate with potassium acid tartrate (Non-proprietary)
　Potassium acid tartrate 300 mg, Potassium bicarbonate 500 mg Potassium (potassium 6.5mmol) effervescent tablets BPC 1968 | 56 tablet GSL £77.77–£99.15 DT price = £92.02

Potassium chloride

- **INDICATIONS AND DOSE**

Prevention of hypokalaemia (patients with normal diet)
▸ BY MOUTH
▸ Child: 1–2 mmol/kg daily; Usual maximum 50 mmol
Electrolyte imbalance
▸ BY INTRAVENOUS INFUSION
▸ Neonate: 1–2 mmol/kg daily, dose dependent on deficit or the daily maintenance requirements.
▸ Child: 1–2 mmol/kg daily, dose dependent on deficit or the daily maintenance requirements
Potassium depletion
▸ BY MOUTH
▸ Neonate: 0.5–1 mmol/kg twice daily, total daily dose may alternatively be given in 3 divided doses, dose to be adjusted according to plasma-potassium concentration.
▸ Child: 0.5–1 mmol/kg twice daily, total daily dose may alternatively be given in 3 divided doses, dose to be adjusted according to plasma-potassium concentration

IMPORTANT SAFETY INFORMATION
SAFE PRACTICE
Potassium overdose can be fatal. Ready-mixed infusion solutions containing potassium should be used. Exceptionally, if potassium chloride concentrate is used for preparing an infusion, the infusion solution should be **thoroughly mixed**. Local policies on avoiding inadvertent use of potassium chloride concentrate should be followed.

- **CONTRA-INDICATIONS** Plasma-potassium concentration above 5 mmol/litre
- **CAUTIONS**
▸ With intravenous use Seek specialist advice in very severe potassium depletion or difficult cases
▸ With oral use Cardiac disease · hiatus hernia (*with modified-release preparations*) · history of peptic ulcer (*with modified-release preparations*) · intestinal stricture (*with modified-release preparations*)
- **INTERACTIONS** → Appendix 1 (potassium salts).
- **SIDE-EFFECTS**
▸ Common or very common
▸ With oral use Abdominal pain · diarrhoea · flatulence · nausea · vomiting
▸ Frequency not known
▸ With intravenous use Heart toxicity (with rapid infusion)
▸ With oral use Bleeding (*with modified-release preparations*) · gastro-intestinal obstruction (*with modified-release preparations*) · ulceration (*with modified-release preparations*)
- **RENAL IMPAIRMENT** Smaller doses must be used in the prevention of hypokalaemia, to reduce the risk of hyperkalaemia. Avoid in severe impairment. Close monitoring required in renal impairment—high risk of hyperkalaemia.
- **MONITORING REQUIREMENTS**
▸ Regular monitoring of plasma-potassium concentration is essential in those taking potassium supplements.
▸ With intravenous use ECG monitoring should be performed in difficult cases.
- **DIRECTIONS FOR ADMINISTRATION**
▸ With oral use in neonates Potassium chloride solutions suitable for use by mouth in neonates are available from 'special order' manufacturers or specialist importing companies; they should be used with care because they are hypertonic and can damage the gastric mucosa.
▸ With oral use Potassium salts are preferably given as a liquid (or effervescent) preparation, rather than modified-release tablets; they should be given as the chloride (the use of effervescent potassium tablets BPC 1968 should be restricted to *hyperchloraemic* states).
▸ With intravenous use Potassium chloride concentrate must be diluted with **not less** than 50 times its volume of sodium chloride intravenous infusion 0.9% or other suitable diluent and **mixed well**.
▸ With intravenous use Ready-mixed infusion solutions should be used when possible. For *peripheral intravenous infusion*, the concentration of potassium should not usually exceed 40 mmol/L. Potassium infusions should be given slowly over at least 2–3 hours and at a rate not exceeding 0.2 mmol/kg/hour with specialist advice and ECG monitoring in difficult cases. Higher concentrations of potassium chloride or faster infusion rates may be given in very severe depletion, but require specialist advice.
- **PRESCRIBING AND DISPENSING INFORMATION** Kay-Cee-L® contains 1 mmol/mL each of K+ and Cl−.
Potassium Tablets
▸ With oral use Do not confuse Effervescent Potassium Tablets BPC 1968 with effervescent potassium chloride tablets. Effervescent Potassium Tablets BPC 1968 do not contain chloride ions and their use should be restricted to hyperchloraemic states.
- **PATIENT AND CARER ADVICE**
Patient or carers should be given advice on how to administer potassium chloride modified-release tablets.
Salt substitutes A number of salt substitutes which contain significant amounts of potassium chloride are readily available as health food products (e.g. *LoSalt*® and

9

Blood and nutrition

Ruthmol®). These should not be used by patients with renal failure as potassium intoxication may result.

- LESS SUITABLE FOR PRESCRIBING Modified-release tablets are less suitable for prescribing. Modified-release preparations should be avoided unless effervescent tablets or liquid preparations inappropriate.

- MEDICINAL FORMS
There can be variation in the licensing of different medicines containing the same drug. Forms available from special-order manufacturers include: modified-release tablet, modified-release capsule, oral solution, solution for injection, infusion, solution for infusion

Modified-release tablet
CAUTIONARY AND ADVISORY LABELS 25, 27
▸ **Potassium chloride (Non-proprietary)**
Potassium chloride 600 mg Kaleorid LP 600mg tablets |
30 tablet [PoM] no price available
Duro-K 600mg tablets | 100 tablet [PoM] no price available

Oral solution
CAUTIONARY AND ADVISORY LABELS 21
▸ **Kay-Cee-L** (Geistlich Sons Ltd)
Potassium chloride 75 mg per 1 ml Kay-Cee-L syrup sugar-free |
500 ml [P] £7.57

Solution for infusion
▸ **Potassium chloride (Non-proprietary)**
Potassium chloride 150 mg per 1 ml Potassium chloride 15%
(potassium 20mmol/10ml) solution for infusion 10ml ampoules |
10 ampoule [PoM] £6.50 | 20 ampoule [PoM] £6.50
Potassium chloride 15% (potassium 20mmol/10ml) solution for
infusion 10ml Mini-Plasco ampoules | 20 ampoule [PoM] £10.70
Potassium chloride 200 mg per 1 ml Potassium chloride 20%
(potassium 13.3mmol/5ml) solution for infusion 5ml ampoules |
10 ampoule [PoM] £3.84–£4.00
Potassium chloride 20% (potassium 27mmol/10ml) solution for
infusion 10ml ampoules | 10 ampoule [PoM] £115.48

3 Metabolic disorders

Metabolic disorders

Use of medicines in metabolic disorders

Metabolic disorders should be managed under the guidance of a specialist. As many preparations are unlicensed and may be difficult to obtain, arrangements for continued prescribing and supply should be made in primary care.

General advice on the use of medicines in metabolic disorders can be obtained from:
Alder Hey Children's Hospital, Medicines Information Centre
(0151) 252 5381
and
Great Ormond Street Hospital for Children, pharmacy
(020) 7405 9200

Urea cycle disorders

Sodium benzoate p. 572 and sodium phenylbutyrate p. 573 are used in the management of urea cycle disorders. Both, either singly or in combination, are indicated as adjunctive therapy in all patients with neonatal-onset disease and in those with late-onset disease who have a history of hyperammonaemic encephalopathy. Sodium benzoate is also used in non-ketotic hyperglycinaemia.

The long-term management of urea cycle disorders includes oral maintenance treatment with sodium benzoate and sodium phenylbutyrate combined with a low protein diet and other drugs such as arginine p. 571 or citrulline p. 572, depending on the specific disorder.

Emergency management

For further information on the emergency management of urea cycle disorders consult the British Inherited Metabolic Disease Group (BIMDG) website at: www.bimdg.org.uk.

3.1 Acute porphyrias

Acute porphyrias

Overview

The acute porphyrias (acute intermittent porphyria, variegate porphyria, hereditary coproporphyria, and 5-aminolaevulinic acid dehydratase deficiency porphyria) are hereditary disorders of haem biosynthesis; they have a prevalence of about 1 in 10 000 of the population.

Great care must be taken when prescribing for patients with acute porphyria, since certain drugs can induce acute porphyric crises. Since acute porphyrias are hereditary, relatives of affected individuals should be screened and advised about the potential danger of certain drugs. Acute attacks of porphyria are exceptionally rare before puberty. When acute porphyria is suspected in a child, support from an expert porphyria service should be sought.

Treatment of serious or life-threatening conditions should not be withheld from patients with acute porphyria. When there is no safe alternative, treatment should be started and urinary porphobilinogen excretion should be measured regularly; if it increases or symptoms occur, the drug can be withdrawn and the acute attack treated. If an acute attack of porphyria occurs during pregnancy, contact an expert porphyria service for further advice.

Haem arginate p. 564 is administered by short intravenous infusion as haem replacement in moderate, severe, or unremitting acute porphyria crises.

In the United Kingdom the National Acute Porphyria Service (NAPS) provides clinical support and treatment with haem arginate from three centres (University Hospital of Wales, Addenbrooke's Hospital, and King's College Hospital). To access the service telephone (029) 2074 7747 and ask for the Acute Porphyria Service.

Drugs unsafe for use in acute porphyrias

The following list contains drugs on the UK market that have been classified as 'unsafe' in porphyria because they have been shown to be porphyrinogenic in animals or in vitro, or have been associated with acute attacks in patients. Absence of a drug from the following lists does not necessarily imply that the drug is safe. For many drugs no information about porphyria is available.

An up-to-date list of drugs considered **safe** in acute porphyrias is available at www.wmic.wales.nhs.uk/porphyria_info.php.

Further information may be obtained from:
www.porphyria-europe.org and also from:

Welsh Medicines Information Centre
University Hospital of Wales
CF14 4XW
Cardiff
(029) 2074 2979/3877

Quite modest changes in chemical structure can lead to changes in porphyrinogenicity but where possible general statements have been made about groups of drugs; these should be checked first.

Unsafe Drug Groups (check first)

- Alkylating drugs (contact Welsh Medicines Information Centre for further advice)
- Anabolic steroids
- Antidepressants (includes tricyclic (and related) antidepressants and MAOIs; fluoxetine, duloxetine, venlafaxine, and trazodone thought to be safe)
- Antihistamines (alimemazine, chlorphenamine, desloratadine, fexofenadine, ketotifen, loratadine, and promethazine thought to be safe)

- Barbiturates (includes primidone and thiopental)
- Calcium channel blockers (amlodipine, felodipine, and nifedipine thought to be safe)
- Contraceptives, hormonal (progestogens are more porphyrinogenic than oestrogens; oestrogens may be safe at least in replacement doses. Progestogens should be avoided whenever possible by all women susceptible to acute porphyria; however, when non-hormonal contraception is inappropriate, progestogens may be used with extreme caution if the potential benefit outweighs risk. The risk of an acute attack is greatest in young women who have had a previous attack. Long-acting progestogen preparations should **never** be used in those at risk of acute porphyria.
- Ergot derivatives (includes ergometrine (oxytocin probably safe) and pergolide)
- Imidazole antifungals (applies to oral and intravenous use; topical antifungals are thought to be safe due to low systemic exposure)
- Non-nucleoside reverse transcriptase inhibitors (contact Welsh Medicines Information Centre for further advice)
- Progestogens (progestogens are more porphyrinogenic than oestrogens; oestrogens may be safe at least in replacement doses. Progestogens should be avoided whenever possible by all women susceptible to acute porphyria; however, when non-hormonal contraception is inappropriate, progestogens may be used with extreme caution if the potential benefit outweighs risk. The risk of an acute attack is greatest in young women who have had a previous attack. Long-acting progestogen preparations should **never** be used in those at risk of acute porphyria.)
- Protease inhibitors (contact Welsh Medicines Information Centre for further advice)
- Sulfonamides (includes co-trimoxazole and sulfasalazine)
- Sulfonylureas (glipizide is thought to be safe)
- Taxanes (contact Welsh Medicines Information Centre for further advice)
- Thiazolidinediones (contact Welsh Medicines Information Centre for further advice)
- Triazole antifungals (applies to oral and intravenous use; topical antifungals are thought to be safe due to low systemic exposure)

Unsafe drugs (check groups above first)

- Aceclofenac
- Alcohol
- Amiodarone
- Aprepitant (contact Welsh Medicines Information Centre for further advice)
- Artemether with lumefantrine
- Bexarotene
- Bosentan
- Bromocriptine
- Buspirone
- Cabergoline
- Carbamazepine
- Chloral hydrate (although evidence of hazard is uncertain, manufacturer advises avoid)
- Chloramphenicol
- Chloroform (small amounts in medicines probably safe)
- Clindamycin
- Cocaine
- Colistimethate sodium
- Danazol
- Dapsone
- Dexfenfluramine
- Disopyramide
- Disulfiram
- Erythromycin
- Etamsylate
- Ethosuximide
- Etomidate

- Fenfluramine
- Flupentixol
- Flutamide
- Fosaprepitant (contact Welsh Medicines Information Centre for further advice)
- Fosphenytoin
- Griseofulvin
- Hydralazine
- Indapamide
- Isometheptene mucate
- Isoniazid (safety uncertain, contact Welsh Medicines Information Centre for further advice)
- Ketamine
- Mefenamic acid (may be used with caution if safer alternative not available)
- Meprobamate
- Methyldopa
- Metolazone
- Metyrapone
- Mifepristone
- Minoxidil (may be used with caution if safer alternative not available)
- Mitotane
- Nalidixic acid
- Nitrazepam
- Nitrofurantoin
- Orphenadrine
- Oxcarbazepine
- Oxybutynin
- Pentazocine (buprenorphine, codeine, diamorphine, dihydrocodeine, fentanyl, methadone, morphine, oxycodone, pethidine, and tramadol are thought to be safe)
- Pentoxifylline
- Phenoxybenzamine
- Phenytoin
- Pivmecillinam
- Porfimer
- Potassium canrenoate (evidence of hazard uncertain—contact Welsh Medicines Information Centre for further advice)
- Raloxifene
- Rifabutin (safety uncertain, contact Welsh Medicines Information Centre for further advice)
- Rifampicin
- Riluzole
- Risperidone
- Selegiline
- Spironolactone
- Sulfinpyrazone
- Tamoxifen
- Telithromycin
- Temoporfin
- Tiagabine
- Tibolone
- Tinidazole
- Topiramate
- Toremifene
- Trimethoprim
- Valproate
- Xipamide
- Zidovudine (contact Welsh Medicines Information Centre for further advice)
- Zuclopenthixol

9

Blood and nutrition

BLOOD AND RELATED PRODUCTS ⟩ HAEM DERIVATIVES

Haem arginate

(Human hemin)

● **INDICATIONS AND DOSE**

Acute porphyrias | Acute intermittent porphyria | Porphyria variegata | Hereditary coproporphyria
▸ BY INTRAVENOUS INFUSION
▸ **Child:** Initially 3 mg/kg once daily for 4 days, if response inadequate, repeat 4-day course with close biochemical monitoring; maximum 250 mg per day

● **SIDE-EFFECTS**
▸ **Common or very common** Pain at injection site · thrombophlebitis at injection site
▸ **Rare** Fever · hypersensitivity reactions
▸ **Frequency not known** Headache
● **PREGNANCY** Manufacturer advises avoid unless essential.
● **BREAST FEEDING** Manufacturer advises avoid unless essential—no information available.
● **DIRECTIONS FOR ADMINISTRATION**
▸ With intravenous use Administer over at least 30 minutes through a filter via large antebrachial or central vein; dilute requisite dose in 100 mL Sodium Chloride 0.9% in glass bottle; administer within 1 hour after dilution; max. concentration 2.5 mg/mL.

● **MEDICINAL FORMS**
There can be variation in the licensing of different medicines containing the same drug.
Solution for infusion
▸ **Normosang** (Orphan Europe (UK) Ltd)
Haem arginate 25 mg per 1 ml Normosang 250mg/10ml solution for infusion ampoules | 4 ampoule PoM £1,737.00

3.2 Carnitine deficiency

AMINO ACIDS AND DERIVATIVES

Levocarnitine

(Carnitine)

● **INDICATIONS AND DOSE**

Primary carnitine deficiency due to inborn errors of metabolism
▸ BY MOUTH
▸ **Neonate:** Up to 200 mg/kg daily in 2–4 divided doses.
▸ **Child:** Up to 200 mg/kg daily in 2–4 divided doses; maximum 3 g per day
▸ INITIALLY BY INTRAVENOUS INFUSION
▸ **Neonate:** Initially 100 mg/kg, to be administered over 30 minutes, followed by (by continuous intravenous infusion) 4 mg/kg/hour.
▸ **Child:** Initially 100 mg/kg, to be administered over 30 minutes, followed by (by continuous intravenous infusion) 4 mg/kg/hour
▸ BY SLOW INTRAVENOUS INJECTION
▸ **Neonate:** Up to 100 mg/kg daily in 2–4 divided doses, to be administered over 2–3 minutes.
▸ **Child:** Up to 100 mg/kg daily in 2–4 divided doses, to be administered over 2–3 minutes

Secondary carnitine deficiency in haemodialysis patients
▸ INITIALLY BY SLOW INTRAVENOUS INJECTION
▸ **Child:** 20 mg/kg, to be administered over 2–3 minutes, after each dialysis session, dosage adjusted according to plasma-carnitine concentration, then (by mouth) maintenance 1 g daily, administered if benefit is gained from first intravenous course
Organic acidaemias
▸ BY MOUTH
▸ **Neonate:** Up to 200 mg/kg daily in 2–4 divided doses.
▸ **Child:** Up to 200 mg/kg daily in 2–4 divided doses; maximum 3 g per day
▸ INITIALLY BY INTRAVENOUS INFUSION
▸ **Neonate:** Initially 100 mg/kg, to be administered over 30 minutes, followed by (by continuous intravenous infusion) 4 mg/kg/hour.
▸ **Child:** Initially 100 mg/kg, to be administered over 30 minutes, followed by (by continuous intravenous infusion) 4 mg/kg/hour
▸ BY SLOW INTRAVENOUS INJECTION
▸ **Neonate:** Up to 100 mg/kg daily in 2–4 divided doses, to be administered over 2–3 minutes.
▸ **Child:** Up to 100 mg/kg daily in 2–4 divided doses, to be administered over 2–3 minutes

● **UNLICENSED USE**
Not licensed for use in organic acidaemias.
▸ With intravenous use Not licensed for use by intravenous infusion.
▸ With oral use Tablets, chewable tablets, and oral liquid (10%) not licensed in children under 12 years. Paediatric oral solution (30%) not licensed in children over 12 years.
● **CAUTIONS** Diabetes mellitus
● **SIDE-EFFECTS** Abdominal pain · body odour · diarrhoea · nausea · vomiting

SIDE-EFFECTS, FURTHER INFORMATION
Side-effects may be dose-related—monitor tolerance during first week and after any dose increase.

● **PREGNANCY** Appropriate to use; no evidence of teratogenicity in *animal* studies.
● **RENAL IMPAIRMENT** Accumulation of metabolites may occur with chronic oral administration in severe impairment.
● **MONITORING REQUIREMENTS**
▸ Monitoring of free and acyl carnitine in blood and urine recommended.
● **DIRECTIONS FOR ADMINISTRATION**
▸ With intravenous use For *intravenous infusion*, dilute injection with Sodium Chloride 0.9% or Glucose 5% or 10%.
● **PRESCRIBING AND DISPENSING INFORMATION**
▸ When used for Organic acidaemias Levocarnitine is used in the treatment of some organic acidaemias; however, use in fatty acid oxidation is controversial.
● **PATIENT AND CARER ADVICE**
Medicines for Children leaflet: Carnitine for metabolic disorders www.medicinesforchildren.org.uk/carnitine-metabolic-disorders-0

● **MEDICINAL FORMS**
There can be variation in the licensing of different medicines containing the same drug. Forms available from special-order manufacturers include: capsule
Tablet
▸ **Carnitor** (Sigma-Tau Pharma Ltd)
L-Carnitine 330 mg Carnitor 330mg tablets | 90 tablet PoM £103.95

Chewable tablet

▸ **Carnitor** (Sigma-Tau Pharma Ltd)
  L-Carnitine 1 gram Carnitor 1g chewable tablets | 10 tablet PoM
  £35.00

Capsule

▸ **Levocarnitine** (Non-proprietary)
  L-Carnitine 250 mg Bio-Carnitine 250mg capsules | 125 capsule
  £11.06
  L-Carnitine 500 mg Lamberts L-Carnitine 500mg capsules |
  60 capsule £11.67

Oral solution

▸ **Levocarnitine** (Non-proprietary)
  L-Carnitine 300 mg per 1 ml Levocarnitine 1.5g/5ml (30%) oral
  solution paediatric | 20 ml PoM £71.40 DT price = £71.40
▸ **Carnitor** (Sigma-Tau Pharma Ltd)
  L-Carnitine 100 mg per 1 ml Carnitor oral single dose 1g solution
  sugar-free | 10 unit dose PoM £35.00

Solution for injection

▸ **Carnitor** (Sigma-Tau Pharma Ltd)
  L-Carnitine 200 mg per 1 ml Carnitor 1g/5ml solution for injection
  ampoules | 5 ampoule PoM £59.50

3.3 Fabry's disease

ENZYMES

Agalsidase alfa

● **DRUG ACTION** Agalsidase alfa, an enzyme produced by
recombinant DNA technology are licensed for long-term
enzyme replacement therapy in Fabry's disease (a
lysosomal storage disorder caused by deficiency of alpha-
galactosidase A).

● **INDICATIONS AND DOSE**

Fabry's disease (specialist use only)

▸ BY INTRAVENOUS INFUSION
▸ Child 7–17 years: 200 micrograms/kg every 2 weeks

● **INTERACTIONS** → Appendix 1 (agalsidase alfa and beta).

● **SIDE-EFFECTS**

▸ **Common or very common** Acne · angioedema · arthralgia ·
asthenia · bradycardia · chest pain · cough · dizziness ·
dyspnoea · eye irritation · fatigue · flushing · gastro-
intestinal disturbances · headache · hypersensitivity
reactions · hypertension · hypotension · influenza- like
symptoms · muscle spasms · myalgia · nasopharyngitis ·
neuropathic pain · oedema · palpitation · paraesthesia ·
pruritus · rash · rhinorrhoea · sleep disturbances · syncope ·
tachycardia · taste disturbances · tinnitus · tremor ·
urticaria

▸ **Uncommon** Cold extremities · ear pain · ear swelling ·
injection-site reactions · parosmia · skin discoloration

SIDE-EFFECTS, FURTHER INFORMATION
Infusion-related reactions Infusion-related reactions very
common; manage by slowing the infusion rate or
interrupting the infusion, or minimise by pre-treatment
with an antihistamine, antipyretic, or corticosteroid—
consult product literature.

● **PREGNANCY** Use with caution.

● **BREAST FEEDING** Use with caution—no information
available.

● **DIRECTIONS FOR ADMINISTRATION**
With intravenous use Administration for *intravenous infusion*,
dilute requisite dose with 100 mL Sodium Chloride 0.9%
and give over 40 minutes using an in-line filter; use within
3 hours of dilution.

● **MEDICINAL FORMS**
There can be variation in the licensing of different medicines
containing the same drug.

Solution for infusion

▸ **Replagal** (Shire Pharmaceuticals Ltd)
  Agalsidase alfa 1 mg per 1 ml Replagal 3.5mg/3.5ml solution for
  infusion vials | 1 vial PoM £1,068.64

Agalsidase beta

● **DRUG ACTION** Agalsidase beta, an enzyme produced by
recombinant DNA technology are licensed for long-term
enzyme replacement therapy in Fabry's disease (a
lysosomal storage disorder caused by deficiency of alpha-
galactosidase A).

● **INDICATIONS AND DOSE**

Fabry's disease (specialist use only)

▸ BY INTRAVENOUS INFUSION
▸ Child 8–17 years: 1 mg/kg every 2 weeks

● **INTERACTIONS** → Appendix 1 (agalsidase alfa and beta).

● **SIDE-EFFECTS**

▸ **Common or very common** Acne · angioedema · arthralgia ·
asthenia · bradycardia · chest pain · cough · dizziness ·
dyspnoea · eye irritation · fatigue · flushing · gastro-
intestinal disturbances · headache · hypersensitivity
reactions · hypertension · hypotension · influenza- like
symptoms · muscle spasms · myalgia · nasopharyngitis ·
neuropathic pain · oedema · palpitation · paraesthesia ·
pruritus · rash · rhinorrhoea · sleep disturbances · syncope ·
tachycardia · taste disturbances · tinnitus · tremor ·
urticaria

▸ **Uncommon** Cold extremities · ear pain · ear swelling ·
injection-site reactions · parosmia · skin discoloration

SIDE-EFFECTS, FURTHER INFORMATION
▸ Infusion-related reactions Infusion-related reactions very
common; manage by slowing the infusion rate or
interrupting the infusion, or minimise by pre-treatment
with an antihistamine, antipyretic, or corticosteroid—
consult product literature.

● **PREGNANCY** Use with caution.

● **BREAST FEEDING** Use with caution—no information
available.

● **DIRECTIONS FOR ADMINISTRATION** For *intravenous
infusion*, given intermittently in Sodium chloride 0.9%,
reconstitute initially with Water for Injections (5 mg in
1.1 mL, 35 mg in 7.2 mL) to produce a solution containing
5 mg/mL. Dilute with Sodium Chloride 0.9% (for doses less
than 35 mg dilute with at least 50 mL; doses 35–70 mg
dilute with at least 100 mL; doses 70–100 mg dilute with at
least 250 mL; doses greater than 100 mg dilute with
500 mL) and give through an in-line low protein-binding
0.2 micron filter at an initial rate of no more than
15 mg/hour; for subsequent infusions, infusion rate may
be increased gradually once tolerance has been
established.

● **MEDICINAL FORMS**
There can be variation in the licensing of different medicines
containing the same drug.

Powder for solution for infusion

▸ **Fabrazyme** (Genzyme Therapeutics Ltd)
  Agalsidase beta 5 mg Fabrazyme 5mg powder for solution for
  infusion vials | 1 vial PoM £315.08
  Agalsidase beta 35 mg Fabrazyme 35mg powder for solution for
  infusion vials | 1 vial PoM £2,196.59

9

Blood and nutrition

3.4 Gaucher's disease

ENZYMES

Imiglucerase

- **DRUG ACTION** Imiglucerase is an enzyme produced by recombinant DNA technology that is administered as enzyme replacement therapy for non-neurological manifestations of type I or type III Gaucher's disease, a familial disorder affecting principally the liver, spleen, bone marrow, and lymph nodes.

- **INDICATIONS AND DOSE**

Gaucher's disease type I (specialist use only)
▸ BY INTRAVENOUS INFUSION

  ▸ Neonate: Initially 60 units/kg every 2 weeks, adjusted according to response, doses as low as 30 units/kg once every 2 weeks may be appropriate

  ▸ Child: Initially 60 units/kg every 2 weeks, adjusted according to response, doses as low as 30 units/kg once every 2 weeks may be appropriate

Gaucher's disease type III (specialist use only)
▸ BY INTRAVENOUS INFUSION

  ▸ Neonate: Initially 60–120 units/kg every 2 weeks, adjusted according to response.

  ▸ Child: Initially 60–120 units/kg every 2 weeks, adjusted according to response

- **SIDE-EFFECTS**
▸ **Common or very common** Angioedema · backache · cyanosis · flushing · hypersensitivity reactions · hypotension · paraesthesia · tachycardia · urticaria
▸ **Uncommon** Abdominal cramps · arthralgia · diarrhoea · dizziness · fatigue · fever · headache · injection-site reactions · nausea · vomiting

- **PREGNANCY** Manufacturer advises use with caution—limited information available.

- **BREAST FEEDING** No information available.

- **MONITORING REQUIREMENTS**
▸ Monitor for immunoglobulin G (IgG) antibodies to imiglucerase.
▸ When stabilised, monitor all parameters and response to treatment at intervals of 6–12 months.

- **DIRECTIONS FOR ADMINISTRATION**
▸ With intravenous use For *intravenous infusion (Cerezyme ®)*, give intermittently in Sodium chloride 0.9%; initially reconstitute with water for injections (200 units in 5.1 mL, 400 units in 10.2 mL) to give 40 units/mL solution; dilute requisite dose with infusion fluid to a final volume of 100–200 mL and give initial dose at a rate not exceeding 0.5 units/kg/minute, subsequent doses to be given at a rate not exceeding 1 unit/kg/minute; administer within 3 hours after reconstitution.

- **MEDICINAL FORMS**
There can be variation in the licensing of different medicines containing the same drug.
Powder for solution for infusion
ELECTROLYTES: May contain Sodium
▸ Cerezyme (Genzyme Therapeutics Ltd)
  Imiglucerase 400 unit Cerezyme 400unit powder for solution for infusion vials | 1 vial [PoM] £1,071.29

Velaglucerase alfa

- **DRUG ACTION** Velaglucerase alfa is an enzyme produced by recombinant DNA technology that is administered as enzyme replacement therapy for the treatment of type I Gaucher's disease.

- **INDICATIONS AND DOSE**

Type I Gaucher's disease (specialist use only)
▸ BY INTRAVENOUS INFUSION

  ▸ Child 4-17 years: Initially 60 units/kg every 2 weeks; adjusted according to response to 15–60 units/kg every 2 weeks

- **SIDE-EFFECTS** Abdominal pain · arthralgia · back pain · bone pain · dizziness · flushing · headache · hypersensitivity reactions · hypertension · hypotension · malaise · nausea · pyrexia · rash · tachycardia · urticaria
SIDE-EFFECTS, FURTHER INFORMATION
▸ Infusion-related reactions Infusion-related reactions very common; manage by slowing the infusion rate, or interrupting the infusion, or minimise by pre-treatment with an antihistamine, antipyretic, or corticosteroid—consult product literature.

- **PREGNANCY** Manufacturer advises use with caution—limited information available.

- **BREAST FEEDING** Manufacturer advises use with caution—no information available.

- **MONITORING REQUIREMENTS** Monitor immunoglobulin G (IgG) antibody concentration in severe infusion-related reactions or if there is a lack or loss of effect with velaglucerase alfa.

- **DIRECTIONS FOR ADMINISTRATION**
▸ With intravenous use For *intravenous infusion*, reconstitute each 400-unit vial with 4.3 mL water for injections; dilute requisite dose in 100 mL Sodium Chloride 0.9% and give over 60 minutes through a 0.22 micron filter; start infusion within 24 hours of reconstitution.

- **MEDICINAL FORMS**
There can be variation in the licensing of different medicines containing the same drug.
Powder for solution for infusion
ELECTROLYTES: May contain Sodium
▸ VPRIV (Shire Pharmaceuticals Ltd)
  Velaglucerase alfa 400 unit VPRIV 400units powder for solution for infusion vials | 1 vial [PoM] £1,410.20

3.5 Homocystinuria

METHYL DONORS

Betaine

- **INDICATIONS AND DOSE**

Adjunctive treatment of homocystinuria involving deficiencies or defects in cystathionine beta-synthase, 5,10-methylene-tetrahydrofolate reductase, or cobalamin cofactor metabolism (specialist use only)
▸ BY MOUTH

  ▸ Neonate: Initially 50 mg/kg twice daily (max. per dose 75 mg/kg), adjusted according to response; maximum 150 mg/kg per day.

  ▸ Child 1 month-9 years: Initially 50 mg/kg twice daily (max. per dose 75 mg/kg), adjusted according to response; maximum 150 mg/kg per day

  ▸ Child 10-17 years: 3 g twice daily (max. per dose 10 g), adjusted according to response; maximum 20 g per day

- **SIDE-EFFECTS**
- ▶ **Uncommon** Agitation · alopecia · anorexia · depression · gastro-intestinal disorders · personality disorder · reversible cerebral oedema · sleep disturbances · urinary incontinence · urticaria
- **PREGNANCY** Manufacturer advises avoid unless essential—limited information available.
- **BREAST FEEDING** Manufacturer advises caution—no information available.
- **MONITORING REQUIREMENTS** Monitor plasma-methionine concentration before and during treatment—interrupt treatment if symptoms of cerebral oedema occur.
- **DIRECTIONS FOR ADMINISTRATION** Powder should be mixed with water, juice, milk, formula, or food until completely dissolved and taken immediately; measuring spoons are provided to measure 1 g, 150 mg, and 100 mg of *Cystadane®* powder.
- **PRESCRIBING AND DISPENSING INFORMATION** Betaine should be used in conjunction with dietary restrictions and may be given with supplements of Vitamin B_{12}, pyridoxine, and folate under specialist advice.
- **NATIONAL FUNDING/ACCESS DECISIONS**
  Scottish Medicines Consortium (SMC) Decisions
  The *Scottish Medicines Consortium* has advised (July 2010) that betaine anhydrous (Cystadane®) is accepted for restricted use within NHS Scotland for the adjunctive treatment of homocystinuria involving deficiencies or defects in cystathionine beta-synthase, 5,10-methylene-tetrahydrofolate reductase, or cobalamin cofactor metabolism in patients who are not responsive to pyridoxine treatment.
- **MEDICINAL FORMS**
  There can be variation in the licensing of different medicines containing the same drug. Forms available from special-order manufacturers include: tablet, oral solution

Powder
- ▶ **Cystadane** (Orphan Europe (UK) Ltd)
  Betaine 1 gram per 1 gram Cystadane oral powder | 180 gram PoM £347.00

3.6 Mitochondrial disorders

CO-ENZYMES

Ubidecarenone

(Ubiquinone; Co-enzyme Q10)

- **INDICATIONS AND DOSE**
  Mitochondrial disorders
  ▶ BY MOUTH
  ▶ **Neonate:** Initially 5 mg 1–2 times a day, adjusted according to response, dose too be taken with food, increased if necessary up to 200 mg daily.
  ▶ **Child:** Initially 5 mg 1–2 times a day, adjusted according to response, dose to be taken with food, increased if necessary up to 300 mg daily

- **UNLICENSED USE** Not licensed.
- **CAUTIONS** May reduce insulin requirement in diabetes mellitus
- **INTERACTIONS** → Appendix 1 (ubidecarenone).
- **SIDE-EFFECTS**
  Common or very common Diarrhoea · heartburn · nausea
  Rare Agitation · dizziness · headache · irritability
- **HEPATIC IMPAIRMENT** Reduce dose in moderate and severe impairment.

- **PATIENT AND CARER ADVICE**
  Medicines for Children leaflet: Ubidecarenone for mitochondrial disease www.medicinesforchildren.org.uk/ubidecarenone-for-mitochondrial-disease

- **MEDICINAL FORMS**
  There can be variation in the licensing of different medicines containing the same drug. Forms available from special-order manufacturers include: oral suspension, oral solution, oral drops

Tablet
- ▶ **Ubidecarenone** (Non-proprietary)
  Ubidecarenone 30 mg Higher Nature Co-enzyme Q10 30mg tablets | 30 tablet £6.42 | 90 tablet £17.87

Chewable tablet
- ▶ **Ubidecarenone** (Non-proprietary)
  Ubidecarenone 25 mg Kirkman Coenzyme Q10 25mg chewable tablets sugar-free | 250 tablet PoM no price available

Capsule
- ▶ **Ubidecarenone** (Non-proprietary)
  Ubidecarenone 30 mg BioActive Q10 Uniquinol 30mg capsules | 60 capsule £11.06 | 150 capsule £22.11
  Hunza Health Co-enzyme Q10 30mg capsules | 30 capsule no price available
  FSC Co-Q-10 30mg capsules | 30 capsule £2.38 | 90 capsule £6.46
  Natures Aid Co-Q-10 30mg capsules | 30 capsule £4.72 | 90 capsule £11.64
  Boots Co-enzyme Q10 30mg capsules | 30 capsule no price available
  Lamberts Co-Enzyme Q10 30mg capsules | 60 capsule £8.51 | 180 capsule £17.64
  Solgar CoQ-10 30mg capsules | 30 capsule no price available
  Vega Co-Enzyme Q10 30mg capsules | 30 capsule £6.96 | 60 capsule £12.17 | 120 capsule £21.78
  Superdrug Co-Enzyme Q10 30mg capsules | 30 capsule no price available
  Ubidecarenone 60 mg Solgar CoQ-10 60mg capsules | 30 capsule no price available
  Ubidecarenone 100 mg BioActive Q10 Uniquinol 100mg capsules | 60 capsule £26.57 | 150 capsule £53.14
  Myoquinone 100mg capsules | 60 capsule no price available
  Natures Aid Co-Q-10 100mg capsules | 30 capsule £9.42 | 90 capsule £22.69
  Solgar CoQ-10 100mg capsules | 30 capsule no price available
  Lamberts Co-Enzyme Q10 100mg capsules | 60 capsule £16.50
  Bio-Quinone Q10 GOLD 100mg capsules | 20 capsule £8.12 | 60 capsule £21.03 | 150 capsule £42.09
  Ubidecarenone 120 mg HealthAid Mega CO-Q-10 120mg capsules | 30 capsule £15.07
  Ubidecarenone 200 mg Lamberts Co-Enzyme Q10 200mg capsules | 60 capsule £19.93
  Ubidecarenone 300 mg Natures Aid Co-Q-10 300mg capsules | 60 capsule £22.21
- ▶ **Super Bio-Quinone** (Pharma Nord (UK) Ltd)
  Ubidecarenone 30 mg Super Bio-Quinone Q10 30mg capsules | 30 capsule £4.96 | 60 capsule £8.84 | 150 capsule £15.77

Oral drops
- ▶ **Ubidecarenone** (Non-proprietary)
  Ubidecarenone 5 mg per 1 ml Ubicor 5mg/ml oral drops | 10 ml PoM no price available

3.7 Mucopolysaccharidosis

ENZYMES

Galsulfase

- **DRUG ACTION** Galsulfase is a recombinant form of human N-acetylgalactosamine-4-sulfatase.

- **INDICATIONS AND DOSE**
  Mucopolysaccharidosis VI (specialist use only)
  ▶ BY INTRAVENOUS INFUSION
  ▶ **Child 5–17 years:** 1 mg/kg once weekly

- **CAUTIONS** Acute febrile illness (consider delaying treatment) · acute respiratory illness (consider delaying treatment) · infusion-related reactions can occur · respiratory disease

9

Blood and nutrition

- SIDE-EFFECTS Abdominal pain · apnoea · areflexia · chest pain · conjunctivitis · corneal opacity · dyspnoea · ear pain · facial oedema · gastroenteritis · hypertension · infusion-related reactions · malaise · nasal congestion · pharyngitis · rigors · umbilical hernia

SIDE-EFFECTS, FURTHER INFORMATION
‣ Infusion-related reactions Infusion-related reactions often occur, they can be managed by slowing the infusion rate or interrupting the infusion, and can be minimised by pre-treatment with an antihistamine and an antipyretic. Recurrent infusion-related reactions may require pre-treatment with a corticosteroid—consult product literature for details.

- PREGNANCY Manufacturer advises avoid unless essential.

- BREAST FEEDING Manufacturer advises avoid—no information available.

- DIRECTIONS FOR ADMINISTRATION
‣ With intravenous use For *intravenous infusion*, dilute requisite dose with Sodium Chloride 0.9% to a final volume of 250 mL and mix gently; infuse through a 0.2 micron in-line filter; give approx. 2.5% of the total volume over 1 hour, then infuse remaining volume over next 3 hours; if body-weight under 20 kg and at risk of fluid overload, dilute requisite dose in 100 mL Sodium Chloride 0.9% and give over at least 4 hours.

- MEDICINAL FORMS
There can be variation in the licensing of different medicines containing the same drug.
Solution for infusion
‣ Naglazyme (BioMarin Europe Ltd) ▼
Galsulfase 1 mg per 1 ml Naglazyme 5mg/5ml solution for infusion vials | 1 vial PoM £982.00

Idursulfase

- DRUG ACTION Idursulfase is an enzyme produced by recombinant DNA technology licensed for long-term replacement therapy in mucopolysaccharidosis II (Hunter syndrome), a lysosomal storage disorder caused by deficiency of iduronate-2-sulfatase.

- INDICATIONS AND DOSE
Mucopolysaccharidosis II (specialist use only)
‣ BY INTRAVENOUS INFUSION
‣ Child 5–17 years: 500 micrograms/kg once weekly

- CAUTIONS Acute febrile respiratory illness (consider delaying treatment) · infusion-related reactions can occur · severe respiratory disease

- SIDE-EFFECTS
‣ Common or very common Arrhythmia · arthralgia · bronchospasm · chest pain · cough · cyanosis · dizziness · dyspnoea · erythema · facial oedema · flushing · gastro-intestinal disturbances · headache · hypertension · hypotension · hypoxia · infusion-site swelling · peripheral oedema · pruritus · pyrexia · rash · swollen tongue · tachycardia · tachypnoea · tremor · urticaria · wheezing
‣ Frequency not known Anaphylaxis · infusion-related reactions · pulmonary embolism

SIDE-EFFECTS, FURTHER INFORMATION
‣ Infusion-related reactions Infusion-related reactions often occur, they can be managed by slowing the infusion rate or interrupting the infusion, and can be minimised by pre-treatment with an antihistamine and an antipyretic. Recurrent infusion-related reactions may require pre-treatment with a corticosteroid—consult product literature for details.

- CONCEPTION AND CONTRACEPTION Contra-indicated in women of child-bearing potential.

- PREGNANCY Manufacturer advises avoid.

- BREAST FEEDING Manufacturer advises avoid—present in milk in *animal* studies.

- DIRECTIONS FOR ADMINISTRATION
‣ With intravenous use For *intravenous infusion*, dilute requisite dose in 100 mL Sodium Chloride 0.9% and mix gently (do not shake); give over 3 hours (gradually reduced to 1 hour if no infusion-related reactions).

- MEDICINAL FORMS
There can be variation in the licensing of different medicines containing the same drug.
Solution for infusion
‣ Elaprase (Shire Pharmaceuticals Ltd) ▼
Idursulfase 2 mg per 1 ml Elaprase 6mg/3ml concentrate for solution for infusion vials | 1 vial PoM £1,985.00

Laronidase

- DRUG ACTION Laronidase is an enzyme produced by recombinant DNA technology licensed for long-term replacement therapy in the treatment of non-neurological manifestations of mucopolysaccharidosis I, a lysosomal storage disorder caused by deficiency of alpha-L-iduronidase.

- INDICATIONS AND DOSE
Non-neurological manifestations of mucopolysaccharidosis I (specialist use only)
‣ BY INTRAVENOUS INFUSION
‣ Child: 100 units/kg once weekly

- CAUTIONS Infusion-related reactions can occur

- INTERACTIONS → Appendix 1 (laronidase).

- SIDE-EFFECTS
‣ Common or very common Abdominal pain · alopecia · anaphylaxis · angioedema · blood pressure changes · cold extremities · cough · diarrhoea · dizziness · dyspnoea · fatigue · flushing · headache · influenza-like symptoms · infusion-site reactions · musculoskeletal pain · nausea · pain in extremities · pallor · paraesthesia · pruritus · rash · restlessness · tachycardia · urticaria · vomiting
‣ Frequency not known Bronchospasm · infusion-related reactions · respiratory arrest

SIDE-EFFECTS, FURTHER INFORMATION
‣ Infusion-related reactions Infusion-related reactions often occur, they can be managed by slowing the infusion rate or interrupting the infusion, and can be minimised by pre-treatment with an antihistamine and an antipyretic. Recurrent infusion-related reactions may require pre-treatment with a corticosteroid—consult product literature for details.

- PREGNANCY Manufacturer advises avoid unless essential—no information available.

- BREAST FEEDING Manufacturer advises avoid—no information available.

- MONITORING REQUIREMENTS Monitor immunoglobulin G (IgG) antibody concentration.

- DIRECTIONS FOR ADMINISTRATION
‣ With intravenous use For *intravenous infusion*, dilute with Sodium Chloride 0.9%; body-weight under 20 kg, dilute to 100 mL, body-weight over 20 kg dilute to 250 mL; give through in-line filter (0.22 micron) initially at a rate of 2 units/kg/hour then increase gradually every 15 minutes to max. 43 units/kg/hour.

- MEDICINAL FORMS
There can be variation in the licensing of different medicines containing the same drug.
Solution for infusion
ELECTROLYTES: May contain Sodium
‣ Aldurazyme (Genzyme Therapeutics Ltd)
Laronidase 100 unit per 1 ml Aldurazyme 500units/5ml solution for infusion vials | 1 vial PoM £444.70

3.8 Nephropathic cystinosis

AMINO ACIDS AND DERIVATIVES

Mercaptamine

(Cysteamine)

● **INDICATIONS AND DOSE**

Nephropathic cystinosis (specialist use only)
▶ BY MOUTH

▶ Neonate: Initially one-sixth to one-quarter of the expected maintenance dose, increased gradually over 4–6 weeks to avoid intolerance, maintenance 1.3 g/m² daily in 4 divided doses.

▶ Child 1 month–11 years (body-weight up to 50 kg): Initially one-sixth to one-quarter of the expected maintenance dose, increased gradually over 4–6 weeks to avoid intolerance, maintenance 1.3 g/m² daily in 4 divided doses

▶ Child 12–17 years (body-weight up to 50 kg): Initially one-sixth to one-quarter of the expected maintenance dose, increased gradually over 4–6 weeks to avoid intolerance, maintenance 1.3 g/m² daily in 4 divided doses

▶ Child 12–17 years (body-weight 50 kg and above): Initially one-sixth to one-quarter of the expected maintenance dose, increased gradually over 4–6 weeks to avoid intolerance, maintenance 2 g daily in 4 divided doses

DOSE EQUIVALENCE AND CONVERSION
1.3 g/m² is approximately equivalent to 50 mg/kg.

● **UNLICENSED USE**
When used by eye Mercaptamine eye drops for the management of ocular symptoms arising from the deposition of cystine crystals in the eye are not licensed.

IMPORTANT SAFETY INFORMATION
SAFE PRACTICE
Mercaptamine has been confused with mercaptopurine; care must be taken to ensure the correct drug is prescribed and dispensed.

● **CAUTIONS** Dose of phosphate supplement may need to be adjusted if transferring from phosphocysteamine to mercaptamine

SIDE-EFFECTS
Common or very common Abdominal pain · anorexia · breath and body odour · diarrhoea · dyspepsia · encephalopathy · fever · gastroenteritis · headache · malaise · nausea · rash · vomiting
Uncommon Drowsiness · gastro-intestinal ulcer · hallucinations · leucopenia · nephrotic syndrome · nervousness · seizures

ALLERGY AND CROSS-SENSITIVITY Contra-indicated if history of hypersensitivity to penicillamine.

PREGNANCY Avoid—teratogenic and toxic in *animal* studies.

BREAST FEEDING Avoid.

MONITORING REQUIREMENTS Leucocyte-cystine concentration and haematological monitoring required—consult product literature.
All patients receiving mercaptamine should be registered (contact local specialist centre for details).

DIRECTIONS FOR ADMINISTRATION
With oral use For children under 6 years at risk of aspiration, capsules can be opened and contents sprinkled on food (at a temperature suitable for eating); avoid adding to acidic drinks (e.g. orange juice).

● **PRESCRIBING AND DISPENSING INFORMATION**
Mercaptamine has a very unpleasant taste and smell, which can affect compliance.

● **PATIENT AND CARER ADVICE**
Medicines for Children leaflet: Mercaptamine eye drops for ocular symptoms of cystinosis www.medicinesforchildren.org.uk/nercaptamine-eye-drops-for-cystinosis

● **MEDICINAL FORMS**
There can be variation in the licensing of different medicines containing the same drug. Forms available from special-order manufacturers include: eye drops
Capsule
CAUTIONARY AND ADVISORY LABELS 21
▶ Cystagon (Orphan Europe (UK) Ltd)
Mercaptamine (as Mercaptamine bitartrate) 50 mg Cystagon 50mg capsules | 100 capsule [PoM] £70.00
Mercaptamine (as Mercaptamine bitartrate) 150 mg Cystagon 150mg capsules | 100 capsule [PoM] £190.00
Gastro-resistant capsule
▶ Procysbi (Raptor Pharmaceuticals)
Mercaptamine (as Mercaptamine bitartrate) 25 mg Procysbi 25mg gastro-resistant capsules | 60 capsule [PoM] £335.97
Mercaptamine (as Mercaptamine bitartrate) 75 mg Procysbi 75mg gastro-resistant capsules | 250 capsule [PoM] £4,199.65
Eye drops
▶ Mercaptamine (Non-proprietary)
Mercaptamine (as Mercaptamine hydrochloride) 4.4 mg per 1 ml Cystaran 0.44% eye drops | 15 ml [PoM] no price available

3.9 Niemann-pick type C disease

ENZYME INHIBITORS › GLUCOSYLCERAMIDE SYNTHASE INHIBITORS

Miglustat

● **DRUG ACTION** Miglustat is an inhibitor of glucosylceramide synthase.

● **INDICATIONS AND DOSE**

Treatment of progressive neurological manifestations of Niemann-Pick type C disease (under expert supervision)
▶ BY MOUTH

▶ Child 4–11 years (body surface area up to 0.48 m²): 100 mg once daily

▶ Child 4–11 years (body surface area 0.48–0.73 m²): 100 mg twice daily

▶ Child 4–11 years (body surface area 0.74–0.88 m²): 100 mg 3 times a day

▶ Child 4–11 years (body surface area 0.89–1.25 m²): 200 mg twice daily

▶ Child 4–11 years (body surface area 1.26 m² and above): 200 mg 3 times a day

▶ Child 12–17 years: 200 mg 3 times a day

● **SIDE-EFFECTS** Abdominal pain · amnesia · anorexia · ataxia · chills · constipation · decreased libido · depression · diarrhoea · dizziness · dyspepsia · flatulence · headache · hypoaesthesia · insomnia · malaise · muscle spasm · muscle weakness · nausea · paraesthesia · peripheral neuropathy · thrombocytopenia · tremor · vomiting · weight changes

● **CONCEPTION AND CONTRACEPTION** Effective contraception must be used during treatment. Men should avoid fathering a child during and for 3 months after treatment.

● **PREGNANCY** Manufacturer advises avoid—toxicity in *animal* studies.

● **BREAST FEEDING** Manufacturer advises avoid—no information available.

● **HEPATIC IMPAIRMENT** No information available—manufacturer advises caution.

9

Blood and nutrition

- **RENAL IMPAIRMENT** Child 12–17 years, initially 200 mg twice daily if estimated glomerular filtration rate 50–70 mL/minute/1.73 m^2. Child 12–17 years, initially 100 mg twice daily if estimated glomerular filtration rate 30–50 mL/minute/1.73 m^2. Avoid if estimated glomerular filtration less than 30 mL/minute/1.73 m^2.
  Child under 12 years—consult product literature.

- **MONITORING REQUIREMENTS**
  - Monitor cognitive and neurological function.
  - Monitor growth and platelet count in Niemann-Pick type C disease.

- **MEDICINAL FORMS**
  There can be variation in the licensing of different medicines containing the same drug.
  Capsule
  - Zavesca (Actelion Pharmaceuticals UK Ltd)
    Miglustat 100 mg Zavesca 100mg capsules | 84 capsule [PoM] £3,934.17 (Hospital only)

3.10 Pompe disease

ENZYMES

Alglucosidase alfa

- **DRUG ACTION** Alglucosidase alfa is an enzyme produced by recombinant DNA technology licensed for long-term replacement therapy in Pompe disease, a lysosomal storage disorder caused by deficiency of acid alpha-glucosidase.

- **INDICATIONS AND DOSE**
  Pompe disease (specialist use only)
  - BY INTRAVENOUS INFUSION
    - Neonate: 20 mg/kg every 2 weeks.
    - Child: 20 mg/kg every 2 weeks

- **CAUTIONS** Cardiac dysfunction · infusion-related reactions—consult product literature · respiratory dysfunction

- **SIDE-EFFECTS**
  - **Common or very common** Agitation · anaphylaxis · antibody formation · blood pressure changes · bronchospasm · chest discomfort · cold extremities · cough · cyanosis · diarrhoea · dizziness · facial oedema · fatigue · flushing · headache · hypersensitivity reactions · injection-site reactions · irritability · muscle spasm · myalgia · nausea · paraesthesia · pruritus · pyrexia · rash · restlessness · sweating · tachycardia · tachypnoea · tremor · urticaria · vomiting
  - **Frequency not known** Infusion-related reactions · necrotising skin lesions · severe skin reactions · ulcerative skin lesions

  SIDE-EFFECTS, FURTHER INFORMATION
  - Infusion-related reactions Infusion-related reactions very common, calling for use of antihistamine, antipyretic, or corticosteroid; consult product literature for details.

- **PREGNANCY** Toxicity in *animal* studies, but treatment should not be withheld.

- **BREAST FEEDING** Manufacturer advises avoid—no information available.

- **MONITORING REQUIREMENTS**
  - Monitor closely if cardiac dysfunction.
  - Monitor closely if respiratory dysfunction.
  - Monitor immunoglobulin G (IgG) antibody concentration.

- **DIRECTIONS FOR ADMINISTRATION**
  - With intravenous use For *intravenous infusion*, reconstitute 50 mg with 10.3 mL water for injections to produce 5 mg/mL solution; gently rotate vial without shaking; dilute requisite dose with Sodium Chloride 0.9% to give a final concentration of 0.5–4 mg/mL; give through a low protein-binding in-line filter (0.2 micron) at an initial rate of 1 mg/kg/hour increased by 2 mg/kg/hour every 30 minutes to max. 7mg/kg/hour.

- **MEDICINAL FORMS**
  There can be variation in the licensing of different medicines containing the same drug.
  Powder for solution for infusion
  - Myozyme (Genzyme Therapeutics Ltd)
    Alglucosidase alfa 50 mg Myozyme 50mg powder for concentrate for solution for infusion vials | 1 vial [PoM] £356.06 (Hospital only)

3.11 Tyrosinaemia type I

ENZYME INHIBITORS › 4-HYDROXYPHENYLPYRUVATE DIOXYGENASE INHIBITORS

Nitisinone

(NTBC)

- **INDICATIONS AND DOSE**
  Hereditary tyrosinaemia type I (in combination with dietary restriction of tyrosine and phenylalanine) (specialist use only)
  - BY MOUTH
    - Neonate: Initially 500 micrograms/kg twice daily, adjusted according to response; maximum 2 mg/kg per day.
    - Child: Initially 500 micrograms/kg twice daily, adjusted according to response; maximum 2 mg/kg per day

- **SIDE-EFFECTS**
  - **Common or very common** Conjunctivitis · corneal opacity · eye pain · granulocytopenia · keratitis · leucopenia · photophobia · thrombocytopenia
  - **Uncommon** Blepharitis · erythematous rash · exfoliative dermatitis · leucocytosis · pruritus

- **PREGNANCY** Manufacturer advises avoid unless potential benefit outweighs risk—toxicity in *animal* studies.

- **BREAST FEEDING** Manufacturer advises avoid—adverse effects in *animal* studies.

- **PRE-TREATMENT SCREENING** Slit-lamp examination of eyes recommended before treatment.

- **MONITORING REQUIREMENTS**
  - Monitor liver function regularly.
  - Monitor platelet and white blood cell count every 6 months.

- **DIRECTIONS FOR ADMINISTRATION** Capsules can be opened and the contents suspended in a small amount of water or formula diet and taken immediately.

- **MEDICINAL FORMS**
  There can be variation in the licensing of different medicines containing the same drug.
  Capsule
  - Orfadin (Swedish Orphan Biovitrum Ltd)
    Nitisinone 2 mg Orfadin 2mg capsules | 60 capsule [PoM] £564.00
    Nitisinone 5 mg Orfadin 5mg capsules | 60 capsule [PoM] £1,127.00
    Nitisinone 10 mg Orfadin 10mg capsules | 60 capsule [PoM] £2,062.00
    Nitisinone 20 mg Orfadin 20mg capsules | 60 capsule [PoM] £4,512.00
  Oral suspension
  - Orfadin (Swedish Orphan Biovitrum Ltd)
    Nitisinone 4 mg per 1 ml Orfadin 4mg/1ml oral suspension sugar-free | 90 ml [PoM] £1,692.00

3.12 Urea cycle disorders

AMINO ACIDS AND DERIVATIVES

Arginine

- **INDICATIONS AND DOSE**

Acute hyperammonaemia in carbamylphosphate synthetase deficiency (specialist use only) | Acute hyperammonaemia in ornithine transcarbamylase deficiency (specialist use only)
- ▸ BY INTRAVENOUS INFUSION

- ▸ Neonate: 6 mg/kg/hour.

- ▸ Child (body-weight up to 40 kg): 6 mg/kg/hour
- ▸ Child (body-weight 40 kg and above): 4 mg/kg/hour

Maintenance treatment of hyperammonaemia in carbamylphosphate synthetase deficiency (specialist use only) | Maintenance treatment of hyperammonaemia in ornithine transcarbamylase deficiency (specialist use only)
- ▸ BY MOUTH

- ▸ Neonate: 100–200 mg/kg daily in 3–4 divided doses, dose to be taken with feeds.

- ▸ Child (body-weight up to 20 kg): 100–200 mg/kg daily in 3–4 divided doses, dose to be given with feeds or meals
- ▸ Child (body-weight 20 kg and above): 2.5–6 g/m^2 daily in 3–4 divided doses, dose to be taken with meals; maximum 6 g per day

Acute hyperammonaemia in citrullinaemia (specialist use only) | Acute hyperammonaemia in arginosuccinic aciduria (specialist use only)
- ▸ BY INTRAVENOUS INFUSION

- ▸ Neonate: Initially 300 mg/kg, to be administered over 90 minutes, followed by 12.5 mg/kg/hour, to be administered over 24 hours (maximum 25 mg/kg/hour thereafter).

- ▸ Child (body-weight up to 40 kg): Initially 300 mg/kg, to be administered over 90 minutes, followed by 12.5 mg/kg/hour, to be administered over 24 hours (maximum 25 mg/kg/hour thereafter)
- ▸ Child (body-weight 40 kg and above): 21 mg/kg/hour

Maintenance treatment of hyperammonaemia in citrullinaemia (specialist use only) | Maintenance treatment of hyperammonaemia in arginosuccinic aciduria (specialist use only)
- ▸ BY MOUTH

- ▸ Neonate: 100–300 mg/kg daily in 3–4 divided doses, dose to be taken with feeds.

- ▸ Child (body-weight up to 20 kg): 100–300 mg/kg daily in 3–4 divided doses, dose to be taken with feed or meals
- ▸ Child (body-weight 20 kg and above): 2.5–6 g/m^2 daily in 3–4 divided doses, doses to be taken with meals; maximum 6 g per day

- **UNLICENSED USE**
- ▸ With intravenous use Injection not licensed in children.
- ▸ With oral use Tablets not licensed in children. Powder licensed for urea cycle disorders in children.
- **CONTRA-INDICATIONS** Not to be used in the treatment of arginase deficiency
- **SIDE-EFFECTS**
- ▸ With intravenous use Flushing · headache · hyperchloraemic metabolic acidosis · hypotension · irritation at injection-site · nausea · numbness · vomiting
- **PREGNANCY** No information available.
- **BREAST FEEDING** No information available.

- **MONITORING REQUIREMENTS** Monitor plasma pH and chloride.
- **DIRECTIONS FOR ADMINISTRATION**
- ▸ With intravenous use For *intravenous infusion*, dilute to a max. concentration of 50 mg/mL with glucose 10%.
- **PRESCRIBING AND DISPENSING INFORMATION**
- ▸ With oral use Powder to be prescribed as a borderline substance (ACBS). For use as a supplement in urea cycle disorders other than arginase deficiency, such as hyperammonaemia types I and II, citrullinaemia, arginosuccinic aciduria, and deficiency of N-acetyl glutamate synthetase.
- **PATIENT AND CARER ADVICE**
Medicines for Children leaflet: Arginine for urea cycle disorders www.medicinesforchildren.org.uk/arginine-urea-cycle-disorders-0
- **MEDICINAL FORMS**
There can be variation in the licensing of different medicines containing the same drug. Forms available from special-order manufacturers include: tablet, capsule, oral solution, solution for infusion

Tablet
- ▸ Arginine (Non-proprietary)
  L-Arginine 500 mg HealthAid L-Arginine 500mg tablets | 60 tablet £5.30
  L-Arginine 1 gram Arginine 1g tablets | 90 tablet £10.58
Capsule
- ▸ Arginine (Non-proprietary)
  L-Arginine 500 mg Quest L-Arginine 500mg capsules | 30 capsule £3.06
  L-Arginine 500mg capsules | 100 capsule £13.21
Powder
- ▸ Arginine (Non-proprietary)
  L-Arginine 1 gram per 1 gram L-Arginine powder | 100 gram £41.89

Carglumic acid

- **INDICATIONS AND DOSE**

Hyperammonaemia due to N-acetylglutamate synthase deficiency (under expert supervision)
- ▸ BY MOUTH

- ▸ Neonate: Initially 50–125 mg/kg twice daily, to be taken immediately before feeds, dose adjusted according to plasma–ammonia concentration; maintenance 5–50 mg/kg twice daily, the total daily dose may alternatively be given in 3–4 divided doses.

- ▸ Child: Initially 50–125 mg/kg twice daily, to be taken immediately before food, dose adjusted according to plasma–ammonia concentration; maintenance 5–50 mg/kg twice daily, the total daily dose may alternatively be given in 3–4 divided doses

Hyperammonaemia due to organic acidaemia (under expert supervision)
- ▸ BY MOUTH

- ▸ Neonate: Initially 50–125 mg/kg twice daily, to be taken immediately before feeds, dose adjusted according to plasma-ammonia concentration, the total daily dose may alternatively be given in 3–4 divided doses.

- ▸ Child: Initially 50–125 mg/kg twice daily, to be taken immediately before food, dose adjusted according to plasma-ammonia concentration, the total daily dose may alternatively be given in 3–4 divided doses

---

IMPORTANT SAFETY INFORMATION
EMERGENCY MANAGEMENT OF UREA CYCLE DISORDERS
For further information on the emergency management of urea cycle disorders consult the British Inherited Metabolic Disease Group (BIMDG) website at www.bimdg.org.uk.

9

Blood and nutrition

- **SIDE-EFFECTS**
- ► **Common or very common** Sweating
- ► **Uncommon** Bradycardia · diarrhoea · pyrexia · vomiting
- **PREGNANCY** Manufacturer advises avoid unless essential—no information available.
- **BREAST FEEDING** Manufacturer advises avoid—present in milk in *animal* studies.
- **DIRECTIONS FOR ADMINISTRATION** Dispersible tablets must be dispersed in at least 5–10 mL of water and taken orally immediately, or administered via a nasogastric tube.
- **MEDICINAL FORMS**
  There can be variation in the licensing of different medicines containing the same drug.
  Dispersible tablet
  CAUTIONARY AND ADVISORY LABELS 13
  ► Carbaglu (Orphan Europe (UK) Ltd)
  Carglumic acid 200 mg Carbaglu 200mg dispersible tablets sugar-free | 5 tablet [PoM] £299.00 sugar-free | 60 tablet [PoM] £3,499.00

Citrulline

- **INDICATIONS AND DOSE**
  Carbamyl phosphate synthase deficiency | Ornithine carbamyl transferase deficiency
  ► BY MOUTH
  ► Neonate: 150 mg/kg daily in 3–4 divided doses, adjusted according to response.
  ► Child: 150 mg/kg daily in 3–4 divided doses, adjusted according to response

- **PREGNANCY** No information available.
- **BREAST FEEDING** No information available.
- **DIRECTIONS FOR ADMINISTRATION**
  ► With oral use Powder may be mixed with drinks or taken as a paste.

- **MEDICINAL FORMS**
  There can be variation in the licensing of different medicines containing the same drug. Forms available from special-order manufacturers include: tablet, oral solution, powder
  Powder
  ► Citrulline (Non-proprietary)
  L-citrulline 1 mg per 1 mg L-Citrulline powder | 100 gram £221.49

BENZOATES

Sodium benzoate

- **INDICATIONS AND DOSE**
  Acute hyperammonaemia due to urea cycle disorder (specialist use only)
  ► BY INTRAVENOUS INFUSION
  ► Neonate: Initially 250 mg/kg, to be administered over 90 minutes, followed by 10 mg/kg/hour, adjusted according to response.
  ► Child: Initially 250 mg/kg, to be administered over 90 minutes, followed by 10 mg/kg/hour, adjusted according to response
  Maintenance treatment of hyperammonaemia due to urea cycle disorders (specialist use only) | Non-ketotic hyperglycinaemia (specialist use only)
  ► BY MOUTH
  ► Neonate: Up to 250 mg/kg daily in 3–4 divided doses, dose to be taken with feeds.
  ► Child: Up to 250 mg/kg daily in 3–4 divided doses, dose to be taken with feeds or meals; maximum 12 g per day

- **UNLICENSED USE** Not licensed for use in children.

- **CAUTIONS** Conditions involving sodium retention with oedema (preparations contain significant amounts of sodium) · congestive heart failure (preparations contain significant amounts of sodium) · neonates (risk of kernicterus and increased side-effects)
- **INTERACTIONS** → Appendix 1 (sodium benzoate).
- **SIDE-EFFECTS** Anorexia · coma · irritability · lethargy · nausea · vomiting
  SIDE-EFFECTS, FURTHER INFORMATION
  Gastro-intestinal side-effects may be reduced by giving smaller doses more frequently.
- **PREGNANCY** No information available.
- **BREAST FEEDING** No information available.
- **RENAL IMPAIRMENT** Caution in renal insufficiency—preparations contain significant amounts of sodium.
- **DIRECTIONS FOR ADMINISTRATION**
  ► With oral use For administration *by mouth*, oral solution or powder may be administered in fruit drinks; less soluble in acidic drinks.
  ► With intravenous use For *intravenous infusion*, dilute to a max. concentration of 50 mg/mL with Glucose 10%.
- **PATIENT AND CARER ADVICE**
  Medicines for Children leaflet: Sodium benzoate for urea cycle disorders www.medicinesforchildren.org.uk/sodium-benzoate-for-urea-cycle-disorders
- **MEDICINAL FORMS**
  There can be variation in the licensing of different medicines containing the same drug. Forms available from special-order manufacturers include: tablet, capsule, oral solution, solution for infusion, powder

DRUGS FOR METABOLIC DISORDERS > ACETIC ACIDS

Sodium dichloroacetate

- **INDICATIONS AND DOSE**
  Pyruvate dehydrogenase defects
  ► BY MOUTH
  ► Neonate: Initially 12.5 mg/kg 4 times a day, adjusted according to response, increased if necessary up to 200 mg/kg daily.
  ► Child: Initially 12.5 mg/kg 4 times a day, adjusted according to response, increased if necessary up to 200 mg/kg daily

- **SIDE-EFFECTS** Abnormal oxalate metabolism · metabolic acidosis · polyneuropathy on prolonged use
- **PREGNANCY** No information available.
- **BREAST FEEDING** No information available.

- **MEDICINAL FORMS**
  There can be variation in the licensing of different medicines containing the same drug.
  No licensed medicines listed.

DRUGS FOR METABOLIC DISORDERS ⟩
AMMONIA LOWERING DRUGS

Sodium phenylbutyrate

● **INDICATIONS AND DOSE**
Acute hyperammonaemia due to urea cycle disorders (specialist use only)
▶ BY INTRAVENOUS INFUSION
▸ Neonate: Initially 250 mg/kg, to be administered over 90 minutes, followed by 10 mg/kg/hour, adjusted according to response.
▸ Child: Initially 250 mg/kg, to be administered over 90 minutes, followed by 10 mg/kg/hour, adjusted according to response
Maintenance treatment of hyperammonaemia due to urea cycle disorders (specialist use only)
▶ BY MOUTH
▸ Neonate: Up to 250 mg/kg daily in 3–4 divided doses, with feeds.
▸ Child (body-weight up to 20 kg): Up to 250 mg/kg daily in 3–4 divided doses, with feeds or meals
▸ Child (body-weight 20 kg and above): 5 g/m^2 daily in 3–4 divided doses, with meals; maximum 12 g per day

● UNLICENSED USE
▶ With intravenous use Injection not licensed for use in children.

> **IMPORTANT SAFETY INFORMATION**
> EMERGENCY MANAGEMENT OF UREA CYCLE DISORDERS
> For further information on the emergency management of urea cycle disorders consult the British Inherited Metabolic Disease Group (BIMDG) website at www.bimdg.org.uk.

● CAUTIONS Conditions involving sodium retention with oedema (preparations contain significant amounts of sodium) · congestive heart failure (preparations contain significant amounts of sodium)
● INTERACTIONS → Appendix 1 (sodium phenylbutyrate).
● SIDE-EFFECTS
▶ **Common or very common** Amenorrhoea · body odour · decreased appetite · depression · gastro-intestinal disturbances · headache · irregular menstrual cycles · oedema · rash · renal tubular acidosis · syncope · taste disturbance · weight gain
▶ **Uncommon** Abdominal pain · aplastic anaemia · arrhythmias · ecchymoses · nausea · oedema · pancreatitis · peptic ulcer · rectal bleeding · vomiting
SIDE-EFFECTS, FURTHER INFORMATION
Gastro-intestinal side-effects may be reduced by giving smaller doses more frequently.
● CONCEPTION AND CONTRACEPTION Manufacturer advises adequate contraception during administration in women of child-bearing potential.
● PREGNANCY Avoid—toxicity in *animal* studies.
● BREAST FEEDING Manufacturer advises avoid—no information available.
● HEPATIC IMPAIRMENT Manufacturer advises use with caution.
● RENAL IMPAIRMENT Manufacturer advises use with caution (preparations contain significant amounts of sodium).
● DIRECTIONS FOR ADMINISTRATION
▶ With oral use Oral dose may be mixed with fruit drinks, milk, or feeds.
▶ With oral use Granules should be mixed with food before taking. *Pheburane*® granules must not be administered by nasogastric or gastrostromy tubes.
▶ With intravenous use For *intravenous infusion*, dilute to a maximum concentration of 50 mg/mL with Glucose 10%.
● PATIENT AND CARER ADVICE
Medicines for Children leaflet: Sodium phenylbutyrate for urea cycle disorders www.medicinesforchildren.org.uk/sodium-phenylbutyrate-for-urea-cycle-disorders
● MEDICINAL FORMS
There can be variation in the licensing of different medicines containing the same drug. Forms available from special-order manufacturers include: capsule, oral suspension, oral solution, solution for infusion
Tablet
▸ Ammonaps (Swedish Orphan Biovitrum Ltd)
Sodium phenylbutyrate 500 mg Ammonaps 500mg tablets | 250 tablet PoM £493.00
Granules
▸ Ammonaps (Swedish Orphan Biovitrum Ltd)
Sodium phenylbutyrate 940 mg per 1 gram Ammonaps 940mg/g granules sugar-free | 266 gram PoM £860.00
▸ Pheburane (Lucane Pharma Ltd)
Sodium phenylbutyrate 483 mg per 1 gram Pheburane 483mg/g granules | 174 gram PoM £331.00

3.13 Wilson's disease

ANTIDOTES AND CHELATORS ⟩ COPPER ABSORPTION INHIBITORS

Zinc acetate

● **DRUG ACTION** Zinc prevents the absorption of copper in Wilson's disease.

● **INDICATIONS AND DOSE**
Wilson's disease (initiated under specialist supervision)
▶ BY MOUTH
▸ Child 1–5 years: 25 mg twice daily
▸ Child 6–15 years (body-weight up to 57 kg): 25 mg 3 times a day
▸ Child 6–15 years (body-weight 57 kg and above): 50 mg 3 times a day
▸ Child 16–17 years: 50 mg 3 times a day
DOSE EQUIVALENCE AND CONVERSION
Doses expressed as elemental zinc.
PHARMACOKINETICS
Symptomatic Wilson's disease patients should be treated initially with a chelating agent because zinc has a slow onset of action. When transferring from chelating treatment to zinc maintenance therapy, chelating treatment should be co-administered for 2–3 weeks until zinc produces its maximal effect.

● CAUTIONS Portal hypertension (risk of hepatic decompensation when switching from chelating agent)
● INTERACTIONS → Appendix 1 (zinc).
● SIDE-EFFECTS
▶ **Common or very common** Gastric irritation (usually transient)
▶ **Uncommon** Leucopenia · sideroblastic anaemia
SIDE-EFFECTS, FURTHER INFORMATION
Transient gastric irritation may be reduced if first dose is taken mid-morning or with a little protein.
● PREGNANCY Usual dose 25 mg 3 times daily adjusted according to plasma-copper concentration and urinary copper excretion.
● BREAST FEEDING Manufacturer advises avoid; present in milk—may cause zinc-induced copper deficiency in infant.

9

Blood and nutrition

9

Blood and nutrition

- **MONITORING REQUIREMENTS** Monitor full blood count and serum cholesterol.
- **DIRECTIONS FOR ADMINISTRATION** Capsules may be opened and the contents mixed with water.
- **MEDICINAL FORMS**
There can be variation in the licensing of different medicines containing the same drug.
Capsule
CAUTIONARY AND ADVISORY LABELS 23
▸ Wilzin (Orphan Europe (UK) Ltd)
Zinc (as Zinc acetate) 25 mg Wilzin 25mg capsules |
250 capsule PoM £132.00
Zinc (as Zinc acetate) 50 mg Wilzin 50mg capsules |
250 capsule PoM £242.00

ANTIDOTES AND CHELATORS ❭ COPPER CHELATORS

Penicillamine

- **DRUG ACTION** Penicillamine aids the elimination of copper ions in Wilson's disease (hepatolenticular degeneration).

- **INDICATIONS AND DOSE**
Wilson's disease
▸ BY MOUTH
▸ Child 1 month–11 years: 20 mg/kg daily in 2–3 divided doses, to be taken 1 hour before food; maximum 2 g per day
▸ Child 12–17 years: Initially 20 mg/kg daily in 2–3 divided doses. maintenance 0.75–1 g daily, to be taken 1 hour before food; maximum 2 g per day

Cystinuria
▸ BY MOUTH
▸ Child: 20–30 mg/kg daily in 2–3 divided doses, lower doses may be used initially and increased gradually, doses to be adjusted to maintain 24-hour urinary cystine below 1 mmol/litre, maintain adequate fluid intake, to be taken 1 hour before food; maximum 3 g per day

- **CONTRA-INDICATIONS** Lupus erythematosus
- **CAUTIONS** Neurological involvement in Wilson's disease
- **INTERACTIONS** → Appendix 1 (penicillamine). Caution with concomitant nephrotoxic drugs (increased risk of toxicity).
- **SIDE-EFFECTS**
▸ **Common or very common** Anorexia · fever · nausea · proteinuria · rash · thrombocytopenia
▸ **Rare** Alopecia · breast enlargement (male and female) · elastosis perforans · haematuria (withdraw immediately if cause unknown) · mouth ulceration · pseudoxanthoma elasticum · skin laxity · stomatitis
▸ **Frequency not known** Agranulocytosis · aplastic anaemia · blood disorders · bronchiolitis · cholestatic jaundice · dermatomyositis · glomerulonephritis · Goodpasture's syndrome · haemolytic anaemia · haemolytic leucopenia · late rashes (consider dose reduction) · lupus erythematosus · myasthenia gravis · nephrotic syndrome · neuropathy (especially if neurological involvement in Wilson's disease—prophylactic pyridoxine recommended) · neutropenia · pancreatitis · pemphigus · pneumonitis · polymyositis · pulmonary haemorrhage · rheumatoid arthritis · Stevens-Johnson syndrome · taste loss (mineral supplements not recommended) · urticaria · vomiting
- **ALLERGY AND CROSS-SENSITIVITY** Patients who are hypersensitive to penicillin may react rarely to penicillamine.
- **PREGNANCY** Fetal abnormalities reported rarely; avoid if possible.

- **BREAST FEEDING** Manufacturer advises avoid unless potential benefit outweighs risk—no information available.
- **RENAL IMPAIRMENT** Reduce dose and monitor renal function or avoid (consult product literature).
- **MONITORING REQUIREMENTS**
▸ Consider withdrawal if platelet count falls below 120 000/mm^3 or white blood cells below 2500/mm^3 or if 3 successive falls within reference range (can restart at reduced dose when counts return to within reference range but permanent withdrawal necessary if recurrence of leucopenia or thrombocytopenia).
▸ Monitor urine for proteinuria.
▸ Monitor blood and platelet count regularly.
- **PATIENT AND CARER ADVICE** Counselling on the symptoms of blood disorders is advised. Warn patient and carers to tell doctor immediately if sore throat, fever, infection, non-specific illness, unexplained bleeding and bruising, purpura, mouth ulcers, or rashes develop.

- **MEDICINAL FORMS**
There can be variation in the licensing of different medicines containing the same drug. Forms available from special-order manufacturers include: oral solution
Tablet
CAUTIONARY AND ADVISORY LABELS 6, 22
▸ Penicillamine (Non-proprietary)
Penicillamine 125 mg Penicillamine 125mg tablets | 56 tablet PoM £45.00 DT price = £44.03
Penicillamine 250 mg Penicillamine 250mg tablets | 56 tablet PoM £90.00 DT price = £86.25
▸ Distamine (Alliance Pharmaceuticals Ltd)
Penicillamine 125 mg Distamine 125mg tablets | 100 tablet PoM £10.34
Penicillamine 250 mg Distamine 250mg tablets | 100 tablet PoM £17.78

Trientine dihydrochloride

- **INDICATIONS AND DOSE**
Wilson's disease in patients intolerant of penicillamine
▸ BY MOUTH
▸ Child 2–11 years: Initially 0.6–1.5 g daily in 2–4 divided doses, adjusted according to response, to be taken before food
▸ Child 12–17 years: 1.2–2.4 g daily in 2–4 divided doses, adjusted according to response, to be taken before food

- **INTERACTIONS** → Appendix 1 (trientine).
- **SIDE-EFFECTS**
▸ **Common or very common** Nausea · rash
▸ **Very rare** Anaemia
▸ **Frequency not known** Colitis · duodenitis
- **PREGNANCY** Teratogenic in *animal* studies—use only if benefit outweighs risk. Monitor maternal and neonatal serum-copper concentrations.
- **PRESCRIBING AND DISPENSING INFORMATION** Trientine is **not** an alternative to penicillamine for rheumatoid arthritis or cystinuria. Penicillamine-induced systemic lupus erythematosus may not resolve on transfer to trientine.

- **MEDICINAL FORMS**
There can be variation in the licensing of different medicines containing the same drug.
Capsule
CAUTIONARY AND ADVISORY LABELS 6, 22
▸ Trientine dihydrochloride (Non-proprietary)
Trientine dihydrochloride 300 mg Trientine dihydrochloride 300mg capsules | 100 capsule PoM no price available

4 Mineral and trace elements deficiencies

4.1 Zinc deficiency

Zinc deficiency

Zinc supplements should not be given unless there is good evidence of deficiency (hypoproteinaemia spuriously lowers plasma-zinc concentration) or in zinc-losing conditions. Zinc deficiency can occur as a result of inadequate diet or malabsorption; excessive loss of zinc can occur in trauma, burns, and protein-losing conditions. A zinc supplement is given until clinical improvement occurs, but it may need to be continued in severe malabsorption, metabolic disease, or in zinc-losing states.

Zinc is used in the treatment of Wilson's disease and acrodermatitis enteropathica, a rare inherited abnormality of zinc absorption.

Parenteral nutrition regimens usually include trace amounts of zinc, see also Intravenous nutrition below. If necessary, further zinc can be added to intravenous feeding regimens.

ELECTROLYTES AND MINERALS > ZINC

Zinc sulfate

● **INDICATIONS AND DOSE**

Zinc deficiency or supplementation in zinc-losing conditions

▶ BY MOUTH USING EFFERVESCENT TABLETS

▶ **Neonate:** 1 mg/kg daily, dose expressed as elemental zinc, to be dissolved in water and taken after food.

▶ **Child (body-weight up to 10 kg):** 22.5 mg daily, dose to be adjusted as necessary, to be dissolved in water and taken after food, dose expressed as elemental zinc

▶ **Child (body-weight 10–30 kg):** 22.5 mg 1–3 times a day, dose to be adjusted as necessary, to be dissolved in water and taken after food, dose expressed as elemental zinc

▶ **Child (body-weight 30 kg and above):** 45 mg 1–3 times a day, dose to be adjusted as necessary, to be dissolved in water and taken after food, dose expressed as elemental zinc

Acrodermatitis enteropathica

▶ BY MOUTH USING EFFERVESCENT TABLETS

▶ **Neonate:** 0.5–1 mg/kg twice daily, dose to be adjusted as necessary, total daily dose may alternatively be given in 3 divided doses, dose expressed as elemental zinc.

▶ **Child:** 0.5–1 mg/kg twice daily, dose to be adjusted as necessary, total daily dose may alternatively be given in 3 divided doses, dose expressed as elemental zinc

● **UNLICENSED USE** Solvazinc® is not licensed for use in acrodermatitis enteropathica.

● **INTERACTIONS** → Appendix 1 (zinc).

● **SIDE-EFFECTS** Abdominal pain · diarrhoea · dyspepsia · gastric irritation · gastritis · headache · irritability · lethargy · nausea · vomiting

● **PREGNANCY** Crosses placenta; risk theoretically minimal, but no information available.

● **BREAST FEEDING** Present in milk; risk theoretically minimal, but no information available.

● **RENAL IMPAIRMENT** Accumulation may occur in acute renal failure.

● **PRESCRIBING AND DISPENSING INFORMATION** Each Solvazinc® tablet contains zinc sulfate monohydrate 125 mg (45 mg zinc).

● **MEDICINAL FORMS** There can be variation in the licensing of different medicines containing the same drug. Forms available from special-order manufacturers include: oral solution, solution for injection, liquid

Effervescent tablet

CAUTIONARY AND ADVISORY LABELS 13, 21

▶ Solvazinc (Galen Ltd)
Zinc sulfate monohydrate 125 mg   Solvazinc 125mg effervescent tablets sugar-free | 90 tablet P £14.95 DT price = £14.95

5 Nutrition (intravenous)

Intravenous nutrition

Overview

When adequate feeding through the alimentary tract is not possible, nutrients may be given by intravenous infusion. This may be in addition to oral or enteral tube feeding— **supplemental parenteral nutrition**, or may be the sole source of nutrition—**total parenteral nutrition** (TPN). Complete enteral starvation is undesirable and total parenteral nutrition is a last resort.

Indications for parenteral nutrition include prematurity; severe or prolonged disorders of the gastro-intestinal tract; preparation of undernourished patients for surgery, chemotherapy, or radiation therapy; major surgery, trauma, or burns; prolonged coma or inability to eat; and some patients with renal or hepatic failure. The composition of proprietary preparations used in children is given under Proprietary Infusion Fluids for Parenteral Feeding p. 576.

Parenteral nutrition requires the use of a solution containing amino acids, glucose, lipids, electrolytes, trace elements, and vitamins. This is now commonly provided by the pharmacy in the form of an amino-acid, glucose, electrolyte bag, and a separate lipid infusion or, in older children a single 'all-in-one' bag. If the patient is able to take small amounts by mouth, vitamins may be given orally.

The nutrition solution is infused through a central venous catheter inserted under full surgical precautions. Alternatively, infusion through a peripheral vein may be used for supplementary as well as total parenteral nutrition, depending on the availability of peripheral veins; factors prolonging cannula life and preventing thrombophlebitis include the use of soft polyurethane paediatric cannulas and use of nutritional solutions of low osmolality and neutral pH. Nutritional fluids should be given by a dedicated intravenous line; if not possible, compatibility with any drugs or fluids should be checked as precipitation of components may occur. Extravasation of parenteral nutrition solution can cause severe tissue damage and injury; the infusion site should be regularly monitored.

Before starting intravenous nutrition the patient should be clinically stable and renal function and acid-base status should be assessed. Appropriate biochemical tests should have been carried out beforehand and serious deficits corrected. Nutritional and electrolyte status must be monitored throughout treatment. The nutritional components of parenteral nutrition regimens are usually increased gradually over a number of days to prevent metabolic complications and to allow metabolic adaptation to the infused nutrients. The solutions are usually infused over 24 hours but this may be gradually reduced if long-term nutrition is required. Home parenteral nutrition is usually infused over 12 hours overnight.

9

Blood and nutrition

Proprietary Infusion Fluids for Parenteral Feeding

Preparation	Nitrogen g/litre	[1,2]Energy kJ/litre	Electrolytes					Other components/litre
			K⁺	Mg²⁺	Na⁺	Acet⁻	Cl⁻	
ClinOleic 20% (Baxter Healthcare Ltd) Net price 100 ml: no price available; Net price 250 ml: no price available; Net price 500 ml: no price available	–	8360	–	–	–	–	–	purified olive and soya oil 200 g, glycerol 22.5 g, egg phosphatides 12 g
Intralipid 10% (Fresenius Kabi Ltd) Net price 100 ml = £4.12; Net price 500 ml = £9.01	–	4600	–	–	–	–	–	soya oil 100 g, glycerol 22 g, purified egg phospholipids 12 g, phosphate 15 mmol
Intralipid 20% (Fresenius Kabi Ltd) Net price 100 ml = £6.21; Net price 250 ml = £10.16; Net price 500 ml = £13.52	–	8400	–	–	–	–	–	soya oil 200 g, glycerol 22 g, purified egg phospholipids 12 g, phosphate 15 mmol
Intralipid 30% (Fresenius Kabi Ltd) Net price 333 ml = £17.80	–	12600	–	–	–	–	–	soya oil 300 g, glycerol 16.7 g, purified egg phospholipids 12 g, phosphate 15 mmol
Lipofundin MCT/LCT 10% (B.Braun Medical Ltd) Net price 100 ml: no price available; Net price 500 ml = £13.70	–	4430	–	–	–	–	–	soya oil 50 g, medium-chain triglycerides 50 g
Lipofundin MCT/LCT 20% (B.Braun Medical Ltd) Net price 100 ml = £13.28; Net price 250 ml: no price available; Net price 500 ml = £20.36	–	8000	–	–	–	–	–	soya oil 100 g, medium-chain triglycerides 100 g
Primene 10% (Baxter Healthcare Ltd) Net price 100 ml: no price available; Net price 250 ml: no price available	15.0	–	–	–	–	–	19.0	
Synthamin 9 (Baxter Healthcare Ltd) Net price 500 ml: no price available; Net price 1 litre: no price available	9.1	–	60.0	5.0	70.0	100.0	70.0	acid phosphate 30 mmol
Synthamin 9 EF (electrolyte-free) (Baxter Healthcare Ltd) Net price 500 ml: no price available; Net price 1 litre: no price available	9.1	–	–	–	–	44.0	22.0	
Vamin 9 Glucose (Fresenius Kabi Ltd) Net price 100 ml = £3.90; Net price 500 ml = £7.95; Net price 1 litre = £13.80	9.4	1700	20.0	1.5	50.0	–	50.0	CA²⁺ 2.5 mmol, anhydrous glucose 100 g
Vaminolact (Fresenius Kabi Ltd) Net price 100 ml = £3.70; Net price 500 ml = £8.50	9.3	–	–	–	–	–	–	

1 1000 kcal = 4200kJ; 1000 kJ = 238.8 kcal. All entries are Prescription-only medicines.

2 Excludes protein- or amino acid-derived energy

Complications of long-term parenteral nutrition include gall bladder sludging, gall stones, cholestasis and abnormal liver function tests. For details of the prevention and management of parenteral nutrition complications, specialist literature should be consulted.

Protein (nitrogen) is given as mixtures of essential and non-essential synthetic L-amino acids. Ideally, all essential amino acids should be included with a wide variety of non-essential ones to provide sufficient nitrogen together with electrolytes. Solutions vary in their composition of amino acids; they often contain an energy source (usually glucose) and electrolytes. Solutions for use in neonates and children under 1 year of age are based on the amino acid profile of umbilical cord blood (*Primene®*) or breast milk (*Vaminolact®*) and contain amino acids that are essential in this age group; these amino acids may not be present in sufficient quantities in preparations designed for older children and adults.

Energy requirements must be met if amino acids are to be utilised for tissue maintenance. An appropriate energy to protein ratio is essential and requirements will vary depending on the child's age and condition. A mixture of carbohydrate and fat energy sources (usually 30–50% as fat) gives better utilisation of amino acids than glucose alone.

Glucose p. 549 is the preferred source of carbohydrate, but frequent monitoring of blood glucose is required particularly during initiation and build-up of the regimen; insulin may be necessary. Glucose above a concentration of 12.5% must be infused through a central venous catheter to avoid thrombosis; the maximum concentration of glucose that should normally be infused in fluid restricted children is 20–25%.

In parenteral nutrition regimens, it is necessary to provide adequate **phosphate** in order to allow phosphorylation of glucose and to prevent hypophosphataemia. Neonates, particularly preterm neonates, and young children also require phosphorus and calcium to ensure adequate bone mineralisation. The compatibility and solubility of calcium and phosphorus salts is complex and unpredictable; precipitation is a risk and specialist pharmacy advice should be sought.

Fat (lipid) emulsions have the advantages of a high energy to fluid volume ratio, neutral pH, and iso-osmolarity with plasma, and provide essential fatty acids. Several days of adaptation may be required to attain maximal utilisation. Reactions include occasional febrile episodes (usually only with 20% emulsions) and rare anaphylactic responses. Interference with biochemical measurements such as those for blood gases and calcium may occur if samples are taken before fat has been cleared. Regular monitoring of plasma cholesterol and triglyceride is necessary to ensure clearance from the plasma, particularly in conditions where fat metabolism may be disturbed e.g. infection. Emulsions containing 20% or 30% fat should be used in neonates as they are cleared more efficiently. **Additives should not be mixed with fat emulsions unless compatibility is known.**

Electrolytes are usually provided as the chloride salts of potassium and sodium. Acetate salts can be used to reduce the amount of chloride infused; hyperchloraemic acidosis or hypochloraemic alkalosis can occur in preterm neonates or children with renal impairment.

Adminstration
Because of the complex requirements relating to parenteral nutrition full details relating to administration have been omitted. In all cases *specialist pharmacy advice, product literature and other specialist literature should be consulted.*

NUTRIENTS ⟩ PARENTERAL NUTRITION

Parenteral nutrition supplements

- ● **INDICATIONS AND DOSE**
  DIPEPTIVEN 20G/100ML CONCENTRATE FOR SOLUTION FOR INFUSION BOTTLES

  Amino acid supplement for hypercatabolic or hypermetabolic states
  ▶ BY INTRAVENOUS INFUSION
  ▶ Child: 300–400 mg/kg daily, dose not to exceed 20% of total amino acid intake

- ● **CAUTIONS**
  PEDITRACE SOLUTION FOR INFUSION 10ML VIALS Reduced biliary excretion · reduced biliary excretion in cholestatic liver disease · reduced biliary excretion in markedly reduced urinary excretion (careful biochemical monitoring required) · total parenteral nutrition exceeding one month
  CAUTIONS, FURTHER INFORMATION
  ▶ Total parenteral nutrition exceeding one month Measure serum manganese concentration and check liver function before commencing treatment and regularly during treatment— discontinue if manganese concentration raised or if cholestasis develops.

- ● **DIRECTIONS FOR ADMINISTRATION** Because of the complex requirements relating to parenteral nutrition, full details relating to administration have been omitted. In all cases *specialist pharmacy advice, product literature, and other specialist literature should be consulted.* Compatibility with the infusion solution must be ascertained before adding supplementary preparations. **Additives should not be mixed with fat emulsions unless compatibility is known.**
  CERNEVIT SOLUTION FOR INJECTION VIALS AND DILUENT Dissolve in 5 mL water for injections.
  PEDITRACE SOLUTION FOR INFUSION 10ML VIALS For addition to *Vaminolact®*, *Vamin® 14 Electrolyte-Free* solutions, and glucose intravenous infusions.
  DECAN CONCENTRATE FOR SOLUTION FOR INFUSION 40ML BOTTLES For addition to infusion solutions.
  ADDIPHOS® VIALS For addition to *Vamin®* solutions and glucose intravenous infusions.
  DIPEPTIVEN 20G/100ML CONCENTRATE FOR SOLUTION FOR INFUSION BOTTLES For addition to infusion solutions containing amino acids.

ADDITRACE SOLUTION FOR INFUSION 10ML AMPOULES For addition to *Vamin®* solutions and glucose intravenous infusions.

GLYCOPHOS® VIALS For addition to *Vamin®* and *Vaminolact®* solutions, and glucose intravenous infusions.

SOLIVITO N POWDER FOR SOLUTION FOR INFUSION VIALS Dissolve in water for injections or glucose intravenous infusion for adding to glucose intravenous infusion or *Intralipid®*; dissolve in *Vitlipid N®* or *Intralipid®* for adding to *Intralipid®* only.

VITLIPID N INFANT EMULSION FOR INJECTION 10ML AMPOULES For addition to *Intralipid®*.

VITLIPID N ADULT EMULSION FOR INJECTION 10ML AMPOULES For addition to *Intralipid®*.

- ● **PRESCRIBING AND DISPENSING INFORMATION**
  CERNEVIT SOLUTION FOR INJECTION VIALS AND DILUENT *Cernevit®* solution contains *dl*-alpha tocopherol 11.2 units, ascorbic acid 125 mg, biotin 69 micrograms, colecalciferol 220 units, cyanocobalamin 6 micrograms, folic acid 414 micrograms, glycine 250 mg, nicotinamide 46 mg, pantothenic acid (as dexpanthenol) 17.25 mg, pyridoxine hydrochloride 5.5 mg, retinol (as palmitate) 3500 units, riboflavin (as dihydrated sodium phosphate) 4.14 mg, thiamine (as cocarboxylase tetrahydrate) 3.51 mg.

  PEDITRACE SOLUTION FOR INFUSION 10ML VIALS For use in neonates (when kidney function established, usually second day of life), infants, and children.
  Peditrace® solution contains traces of Zn^{2+}, Cu^{2+}, Mn^{2+}, Se^{4+}, F^-, I^-.

  DECAN CONCENTRATE FOR SOLUTION FOR INFUSION 40ML BOTTLES For patients over 40 kg.
  Decan® solution contains trace elements Fe^{2+}, Zn^{2+}, Cu^{2+}, Mn^{2+}, F^-, Co^{2+}, I^-, Se^{4+}, Mo^{6+}, Cr^{3+}.

  ADDIPHOS® VIALS *Addiphos®* sterile solution contains phosphate 40 mmol, K^+ 30 mmol, Na^+ 30 mmol/20 mL.

  DIPEPTIVEN 20G/100ML CONCENTRATE FOR SOLUTION FOR INFUSION BOTTLES *Dipeptiven®* solution contains N(2)-L-alanyl-L-glutamine 200 mg/mL (providing L-alanine 82 mg, L-glutamine 134.6 mg).

  ADDITRACE SOLUTION FOR INFUSION 10ML AMPOULES For patients over 40 kg. *Additrace®* solution contains traces of Fe^{3+}, Zn^{2+}, Mn^{2+}, Cu^{2+}, Cr^{3+}, Se^{4+}, Mo^{6+}, F^-, I^-.

  GLYCOPHOS® VIALS *Glycophos®* Sterile Concentrate solution contains phosphate 20 mmol, Na^+ 40 mmol/20 mL.

  SOLIVITO N POWDER FOR SOLUTION FOR INFUSION VIALS *Solivito N®* powder for reconstitution contains biotin 60 micrograms, cyanocobalamin 5 micrograms, folic acid 400 micrograms, glycine 300 mg, nicotinamide 40 mg, pyridoxine hydrochloride 4.9 mg, riboflavin sodium phosphate 4.9 mg, sodium ascorbate 113 mg, sodium pantothenate 16.5 mg, thiamine mononitrate 3.1 mg.

  VITLIPID N INFANT EMULSION FOR INJECTION 10ML AMPOULES *Vitlipid N®* infant emulsion contains vitamin A 230 units, ergocalciferol 40 units, *dl*-alpha tocopherol 0.7 unit, phytomenadione 20 micrograms/mL.

  VITLIPID N ADULT EMULSION FOR INJECTION 10ML AMPOULES *Vitlipid N®* adult emulsion contains vitamin A 330 units, ergocalciferol 20 units, *dl*-alpha tocopherol 1 unit, phytomenadione 15 micrograms/mL. For children over 11 years.

9

Blood and nutrition

● MEDICINAL FORMS
There can be variation in the licensing of different medicines containing the same drug. Forms available from special-order manufacturers include: solution for infusion

Solution for injection

▸ Cernevit (Baxter Healthcare Ltd)
Alpha tocopherol 11.2 unit, Cyanocobalamin 6 microgram, Biotin 69 microgram, Folic acid 414 microgram, Thiamine 3.51 mg, Riboflavin (as Riboflavin sodium phosphate) 4.14 mg, Pyridoxine (as Pyridoxine hydrochloride) 4.53 mg, Ascorbic acid 125 mg, Colecalciferol 220 unit, Pantothenic acid (as Dexpanthenol) 17.25 mg, Nicotinamide 46 mg, Retinol 3500 unit Cernevit solution for injection vials and diluent | 10 vial [PoM] no price available

Emulsion for injection

▸ Vitlipid N Adult (Fresenius Kabi Ltd)
Alpha tocopherol 910 microgram per 1 ml, Ergocalciferol 500 nanogram per 1 ml, Phytomenadione 15 microgram per 1 ml, Retinol palmitate 99 microgram per 1 ml Vitlipid N Adult emulsion for injection 10ml ampoules | 1 ampoule [PoM] £1.97 | 10 ampoule [PoM] no price available

▸ Vitlipid N Infant (Fresenius Kabi Ltd)
Ergocalciferol 1 microgram per 1 ml, Phytomenadione 20 microgram per 1 ml, Retinol palmitate 69 microgram per 1 ml, Alpha tocopherol 640 microgram per 1 ml Vitlipid N Infant emulsion for injection 10ml ampoules | 1 ampoule [PoM] £1.97 | 10 ampoule [PoM] no price available

Solution for infusion

▸ Parenteral nutrition supplements (Non-proprietary)
Sodium glycerophosphate 216 mg per 1 ml Sodium glycerophosphate 4.32g/20ml concentrate for solution for infusion vials | 1 vial [PoM] £4.83 | 10 vial [PoM] no price available

▸ Additrace (Fresenius Kabi Ltd)
Sodium molybdate 4.85 microgram per 1 ml, Chromic chloride 5.33 microgram per 1 ml, Sodium selenite 10.5 microgram per 1 ml, Potassium iodide 16.6 microgram per 1 ml, Manganese chloride 99 microgram per 1 ml, Sodium fluoride 210 microgram per 1 ml, Copper chloride 340 microgram per 1 ml, Ferric chloride 544 microgram per 1 ml, Zinc chloride 1.36 mg per 1 ml Additrace solution for infusion 10ml ampoules | 1 ampoule [PoM] £1.96 | 20 ampoule [PoM] no price available

▸ Dipeptiven (Fresenius Kabi Ltd)
N(2)-L-alanyl-L-glutamine 200 mg per 1 ml Dipeptiven 20g/100ml concentrate for solution for infusion bottles | 1 bottle [PoM] £25.93 | 10 bottle [PoM] no price available
Dipeptiven 10g/50ml concentrate for solution for infusion bottles | 1 bottle [PoM] £13.94 | 10 bottle [PoM] no price available

▸ Peditrace (Fresenius Kabi Ltd)
Manganese (as Manganese chloride) 1 microgram per 1 ml, Iodine (as Potassium iodide) 1 microgram per 1 ml, Selenium (as Sodium selenite) 2 microgram per 1 ml, Copper (as Copper chloride) 20 microgram per 1 ml, Fluoride (as Sodium fluoride) 57 microgram per 1 ml, Zinc (as Zinc chloride) 250 microgram per 1 ml Peditrace solution for infusion 10ml vials | 1 vial [PoM] £3.55 | 10 vial [PoM] no price available

▸ Tracutil (B.Braun Medical Ltd)
Sodium molybdate dihydrate 2.42 microgram per 1 ml, Chromic chloride 5.3 microgram per 1 ml, Sodium selenite pentahydrate 7.89 microgram per 1 ml, Potassium iodide 16.6 microgram per 1 ml, Sodium fluoride 126 microgram per 1 ml, Manganese chloride 197.9 microgram per 1 ml, Copper chloride 204.6 microgram per 1 ml, Zinc chloride 681.5 microgram per 1 ml, Ferrous chloride 695.8 microgram per 1 ml Tracutil concentrate for solution for infusion 10ml ampoules | 5 ampoule [PoM] £7.96

Powder for solution for infusion

▸ Solivito N (Fresenius Kabi Ltd)
Cyanocobalamin 5 microgram, Biotin 60 microgram, Folic acid 400 microgram, Thiamine nitrate 3.1 mg, Pyridoxine hydrochloride 4.9 mg, Riboflavin sodium phosphate 4.9 mg, Sodium pantothenate 16.5 mg, Nicotinamide 40 mg, Sodium ascorbate 113 mg Solivito N powder for solution for infusion vials | 1 vial [PoM] £1.97 | 10 vial [PoM] no price available

6   Nutrition (oral)

Enteral nutrition

Overview

Children have higher nutrient requirements per kg bodyweight, different metabolic rates, and physiological responses compared to adults. They have low nutritional stores and are particularly vulnerable to growth and nutritional problems during critical periods of development. Major illness, operations, or trauma impose increased metabolic demands and can rapidly exhaust nutritional reserves.

Every effort should be made to optimise oral food intake before beginning enteral tube feeding; this may include change of posture, special seating, feeding equipment, oral desensitisation, food texture changes, thickening of liquids, increasing energy density of food, treatment of reflux or oesophagitis, as well as using age-specific nutritional supplements.

Enteral tube feeding has a role in both short-term rehabilitation and long-term nutritional management in paediatrics. It can be used as supportive therapy, in which the enteral feed supplies a proportion of the required nutrients, or as primary therapy, in which the enteral feed delivers all the necessary nutrients. Most children receiving tube feeds should also be encouraged to take oral food and drink. Tube feeding should be considered in the following situations:

● unsafe swallowing and risk of aspiration
● inability to consume at least 60% of energy needs by mouth
● total feeding time of more than 4 hours per day
● weight loss or no weight gain for a period of 3 months (less for younger children and infants)
● weight for height (or length) less than 2nd percentile for age and sex

Most feeds for enteral use contain protein derived from cows' milk or soya. Elemental feeds containing protein hydrolysates or free amino acids can be used for children who have diminished ability to break down protein, for example in inflammatory bowel disease or pancreatic insufficiency.

Even when nutritionally complete feeds are given, water and electrolyte balance should be monitored. Haematological and biochemical parameters should also be monitored, particularly in the clinically unstable child. Extra minerals (e.g. magnesium and zinc) may be needed in patients where gastro-intestinal secretions are being lost. Additional vitamins may also be needed..

Choosing the best formula for children depends on several factors including: nutritional requirements, gastro-intestinal function, underlying disease, nutrient restrictions, age, and feed characteristics (nutritional composition, viscosity, osmolality, availability and cost). Children have specific dietary requirements and in many situations liquid feeds prepared for adults are totally unsuitable and should not be given. Expert advice from a dietician should be sought before prescribing enteral feeds for a child.

Infant formula feeds

Child 0–12 months. Term infants with normal gastro-intestinal function are given either breast milk or normal infant formula during the first year of life. The average intake is between 150 mL and 200 mL/kg/day. Infant milk formulas are based on whey- or casein-dominant protein, lactose with or without maltodextrin, amylose, vegetable oil and milk fat. The composition of all normal and soya infant formulas have to meet The Infant Formula and Follow-on Formula Regulations (England and Wales) 2007, which enact the European Community Regulations 2006/141/EC; the composition of other enteral and specialist feeds has to meet the Commission Directive (1999/21/EC) on Dietary Foods for Special Medical Purposes.

A high-energy feed, which contains 9–11% of energy derived from protein can be used for infants who fail to grow adequately. Alternatively, energy supplements may be added to normal infant formula to achieve a higher energy content (but this will reduce the protein to energy ratio) or the normal infant formula concentration may be increased slightly. Care should be taken not to present an osmotic load of more than 500 milliosmols/kg water to the normal functioning gut, otherwise osmotic diarrhoea will result. Concentrating or supplementing feeds should not be attempted without the advice of a paediatric dietician.

Enteral feeds
Child 1–6 years (body–weight 8–20 kg). Ready-to-use feeds based on caseinates, maltodextrin and vegetable oils (with or without added medium chain triglyceride (MCT) oil or fibre) are well tolerated and effective in improving nutritional status in this age group. Although originally designed for children 1–6 years (body–weight 8–20 kg), some products have ACBS approval for use in children weighing up to 30 kg (approx. 10 years of age). Enteral feeds formulated for children 1–6 years are low in sodium and potassium; electrolyte intake and biochemical status should be monitored. Older children in this age range taking small feed volumes may need to be given additional micronutrients. Fibre-enriched feeds may be helpful for children with chronic constipation or diarrhoea.

Child 7–12 years (body-weight 21–45 kg). Depending on age, weight, clinical condition and nutritional requirements, ready-to-use feeds formulated for 7–12 year olds may be given at appropriate rates.

Child over 12 years (body-weight over 45 kg). As there are no standard enteral feeds formulated for this age group, adult formulations are used. The intake of protein, electrolytes, vitamins, and trace minerals should be carefully assessed and monitored. Note: Adult feeds containing more than 6 g/100 mL protein or 2 g/100 mL fibre should be used with caution and expert advice.

Specialised formula
It is essential that any infant who is intolerant of breast milk or normal infant formula, or whose condition requires nutrient-specific adaptation, is prescribed an adequate volume of a nutritionally complete replacement formula. In the first 4 months of life, a volume of 150–200 mL/kg/day is recommended. After 6 months, should the formula still be required, a volume of 600 mL/day should be maintained, in addition to solid food.

Products for cow's milk protein intolerance or lactose intolerance. There are a number of infant formulas formulated for cow's milk protein intolerance or lactose intolerance; these feeds may contain a residual amount of lactose (less than 1 g/100 mL formula)—sometimes described as clinically lactose-free or 'lactose-free' by manufacturers. If the total daily intake of these formulas is low, it may be necessary to supplement with calcium, and a vitamin and mineral supplement.

Soya-based infant formulas have a high phytoestrogen content and this may be a long-term reproductive health risk. The Chief Medical Officer has advised that soya-based infant formulas should not be used as the first choice for the management of infants with proven cow's milk sensitivity, lactose intolerance, galactokinase deficiency and galactosaemia. Most UK paediatricians with expertise in inherited metabolic disease still advocate soya-based formulations for infants with galactosaemia as there are concerns about the residual lactose content of low lactose formulas and protein hydrolysates based on cow's milk protein.

Low lactose infant formulations, based on whole cow's milk protein, are unsuitable for children with cow's milk protein intolerance. Liquid soya milks purchased from supermarkets and health food stores are not nutritionally complete and should never be used for infants under 1 year of age.

Protein hydrolysate formulas. Non-milk, peptide-based feeds containing hydrolysates of casein, whey, meat and soya protein, are suitable for infants with disaccharide or whole protein intolerance. The total daily intake of electrolytes, vitamins and minerals should be carefully assessed and modified to meet the child's nutritional requirements; these feeds have a high osmolality when given at recommended dilution and need gradual and careful introduction.

Elemental (amino acid based formula). Specially formulated elemental feeds containing essential and nonessential amino acids are available for use in infants and children under 6 years with proven whole protein intolerance. Adult elemental formula may be used for children over 6 years; the intake of electrolytes, vitamins and minerals should be carefully assessed and modified to meet nutritional requirements. These feeds have a high osmolality when given at the recommended concentration and therefore need gradual and careful introduction.

Modular feeds. Modular feeds (see Specialised Formulas for Specific Clinical Conditions) are based on individual protein, fat, carbohydrate, vitamin and mineral components or modules which can be combined to meet the specific needs of a child. Modular feeds are used when nutritionally complete specialised formula are not tolerated, or if the fluid and nutrient requirements change e.g. in gastro-intestinal, renal or liver disease. The main advantage of modular feeds is their flexibility; disadvantages include their complexity and preparation difficulties. Modular feeds should not be used without the supervision of a paediatric dietician.

Specialised formula. Highly specialised formulas are designed to meet the specific requirements in various clinical conditions such as renal and liver diseases. When using these formulas, both the biochemical status of the child and their growth parameters need to be monitored.

Feed thickeners
Carob based thickeners may be used to thicken feeds for infants under 1 year with significant gastro-oesophageal reflux. Breast-fed infants can be given the thickener mixed to a paste with water or breast-milk prior to feeds.

Pre-thickened formula Milk-protein- or casein-dominant infant formula, which contains small quantities of pre-gelatinized starch, is recommended primarily for infants with mild gastro-oesophageal reflux. Pre-thickened formula is prepared in the same way as normal infant formula and flows through a standard teat. The feeds do not thicken on standing but thicken in the stomach when exposed to acid pH.

Starched based thickeners can be used to thicken liquids and feeds for children over 1 year of age with dysphagia.

Dietary supplements for oral use
Three types of prescribable fortified dietary supplements are available: fortified milk and non-milk tasting (juice-style) drinks, and fortified milk-based semi-solid preparations. The recommended daily quantity is age-dependent. The following is a useful guide: 1–2 years, 200 kcal (840 kJ); 3–5 years, 400 kcal (1680 kJ); 6–11 years, 600 kcal (2520 kJ); and over 12 years, 800 kcal (3360 kJ). Supplements containing 1.5 kcal/mL are high in protein and should not be used for children under 3 years of age. Many supplements are high in sugar or maltodextrin; care should be taken to prevent prolonged contact with teeth. Ideally supplements should be administered after meals or at bedtime so as not to affect appetite.

Products for metabolic diseases

There is a large range of disease-specific infant formulas and amino acid-based supplements available for use in children with metabolic diseases (see under specific metabolic diseases). Some of these formulas are nutritionally incomplete and supplementation with vitamins and other nutrients may be necessary. Many of the product names are similar; to prevent metabolic complications in children who cannot tolerate specific amino acids it is important to ensure the correct supplement is supplied.

Enteral feeding tubes

Care is required in choosing an appropriate formulation of a drug for administration through a nasogastric narrow-bore feeding tube or through a percutaneous endoscopic gastrostomy (PEG) or jejunostomy tube. Liquid preparations (or soluble tablets) are preferred; injection solutions may also be suitable for administration through an enteral tube.

If a solid formulation of a medicine needs to be given, it should be given as a suspension of particles fine enough to pass through the tube. It is possible to crush many immediate-release tablets but enteric-coated or modified-release preparations should **not** be crushed.

Enteral feeds may affect the absorption of drugs and it is therefore important to consider the timing of drug administration in relation to feeds. If more than one drug needs to be given, they should be given separately and the tube should be flushed with water after each drug has been given.

Clearing blockages

Carbonated (sugar-free) drinks may be marginally more effective than water in unblocking feeding tubes, but mildly acidic liquids (such as pineapple juice or cola-based drinks) can coagulate protein in feeds, causing further blockage. If these measures fail to clear the enteral feeding tube, an alkaline solution containing pancreatic enzymes may be introduced into the tube (followed after at least 5 minutes by water). Specific products designed to break up blockages caused by formula feeds are also available.

6.1 Special diets

Nutrition in special diets

Overview

These are preparations that have been modified to eliminate a particular constituent from a food or that are nutrient mixtures formulated as food substitutes for children who either cannot tolerate or cannot metabolise certain common constituents of food.

Coeliac disease

Intolerance to **gluten** in *coeliac disease* is managed by completely eliminating **gluten** from the diet. A range of gluten-free products is available for prescription.

Phenylketonuria

Phenylketonuria (hyperphenylalaninaemia, PKU), which results from the inability to metabolise **phenylalanine**, is managed by restricting dietary intake of **phenylalanine** to a small amount sufficient for tissue building and repair.

Aspartame (used as a sweetener in some foods and medicines) contributes to the **phenylalanine** intake and may affect control of *phenylketonuria*. If alternatives are unavailable, children with phenylketonuria should not be denied access to appropriate medication; the amount of **aspartame** consumed can be taken in to account in the management of the condition. Where the presence of **aspartame** in a preparation is specified in the product literature, **aspartame** is listed as an excipient in the relevant

product entry in *BNF for Children*; the child or carer should be informed of this.

Some rare forms *of phenylketonuria* are caused by a deficiency of **tetrahydrobiopterin**. Treatment involves oral supplementation of tetrahydrobiopterin p. 581; in some severe cases, the addition of the neurotransmitter precursors, levodopa and 5-hydroxytryptophan, is also necessary.

Sapropterin dihydrochloride below, a synthetic form of tetrahydrobiopterin p. 581, is licensed as an adjunct to dietary restriction of **phenylalanine** in the management of patients with *phenylketonuria* and *tetrahydrobiopterin deficiency*.

Products for metabolic diseases

There is a large range of disease-specific infant formulas and amino acid-based supplements available for use in children with metabolic diseases (see under specific metabolic diseases). Some of these formulas are nutritionally incomplete and supplementation with vitamins and other nutrients may be necessary. Many of the product names are similar; to prevent metabolic complications in children who cannot tolerate specific amino acids it is important to ensure the correct supplement is supplied.

6.1a Phenylketonuria

DRUGS FOR METABOLIC DISORDERS ›
TETRAHYDROBIOPTERIN AND DERIVATIVES

Sapropterin dihydrochloride

● **INDICATIONS AND DOSE**

Phenylketonuria (adjunct to dietary restriction of phenylalanine) (specialist use only)
▶ BY MOUTH
▸ Child 4-17 years: Initially 10 mg/kg once daily, adjusted according to response; usual dose 5–20 mg/kg once daily, dose to be taken preferably in the morning

Tetrahydrobiopterin deficiency (adjunct to dietary restriction of phenylalanine) (specialist use only)
▶ BY MOUTH
▸ Neonate: Initially 2–5 mg/kg once daily, adjusted according to response, dose to be taken preferably in the morning, the total daily dose may alternatively be given in 2–3 divided doses; maximum 20 mg/kg per day.

▸ Child: Initially 2–5 mg/kg once daily, adjusted according to response, dose to be taken preferably in the morning, the total daily dose may alternatively be given in 2–3 divided doses; maximum 20 mg/kg per day

● **CAUTIONS** History of convulsions

● **SIDE-EFFECTS**
▶ Common or very common Abdominal pain · cough · diarrhoea · headache · nasal congestion · pharyngolaryngeal pain · vomiting
▶ Frequency not known Hypersensitivity reactions

● **PREGNANCY** Manufacturer advises caution—consider only if strict dietary management inadequate.

● **BREAST FEEDING** Manufacturer advises avoid—no information available.

● **HEPATIC IMPAIRMENT** Manufacturer advises caution—no information available.

● **RENAL IMPAIRMENT** Manufacturer advises caution—no information available.

● **MONITORING REQUIREMENTS**
▶ Monitor blood-phenylalanine concentration before and after first week of treatment—if unsatisfactory response

increase dose at weekly intervals to max. dose and monitor blood-phenylalanine concentration weekly; discontinue treatment if unsatisfactory response after 1 month.
▸ Monitor blood-phenylalanine and tyrosine concentrations 1–2 weeks after dose adjustment and during treatment.

● **DIRECTIONS FOR ADMINISTRATION** Tablets should be dissolved in water and taken within 20 minutes.

● **PRESCRIBING AND DISPENSING INFORMATION** Sapropterin is a synthetic form of tetrahydrobiopterin.

● **PATIENT AND CARER ADVICE** Patient or carers should be given advice on how to administer sapropterin dihydrochloride dispersible tablets.

● **MEDICINAL FORMS**
There can be variation in the licensing of different medicines containing the same drug.

Tablet
▸ Sapropterin dihydrochloride (Non-proprietary)
  Sapropterin dihydrochloride 10 mg Tetrahydrobiopterin 10mg tablets | 100 tablet PoM no price available

Soluble tablet
CAUTIONARY AND ADVISORY LABELS 13, 21
▸ Kuvan (BioMarin Europe Ltd)
  Sapropterin dihydrochloride 100 mg Kuvan 100mg soluble tablets sugar-free | 30 tablet PoM £597.22

Tetrahydrobiopterin

● **INDICATIONS AND DOSE**

Monotherapy in tetrahydrobiopterin-sensitive phenylketonuria (specialist use only)
▸ BY MOUTH
▸ Child: 10 mg/kg twice daily, adjusted according to response, total daily dose may alternatively be given in 3 divided doses

In combination with neurotransmitter precursors for tetrahydrobiopterin-sensitive phenylketonuria (specialist use only)
▸ BY MOUTH
▸ Child 1 month-1 year: Initially 250–750 micrograms/kg 4 times a day, adjusted according to response, total daily dose may alternatively be given in 3 divided doses; maximum 7 mg/kg per day
▸ Child 2-17 years: Initially 250–750 micrograms/kg 4 times a day, adjusted according to response, total daily dose may alternatively be given in 3 divided doses; maximum 10 mg/kg per day

UNLICENSED USE Not licensed.

SIDE-EFFECTS Diarrhoea · disturbed sleep · urinary frequency

PREGNANCY Crosses the placenta; use only if benefit outweighs risk.

BREAST FEEDING Present in milk, effects unknown.

RENAL IMPAIRMENT Use with caution—accumulation of metabolites.

MEDICINAL FORMS
There can be variation in the licensing of different medicines containing the same drug.
No licensed medicines listed.

7 Vitamin deficiency

Vitamins

Overview

Vitamins are used for the prevention and treatment of specific deficiency states or where the diet is known to be inadequate; they may be prescribed in the NHS to prevent or treat deficiency but not as dietary supplements. Except for iron-deficiency anaemia, a primary vitamin or mineral deficiency due to simple dietary inadequacy is rare in the developed world. Some children may be at risk of developing deficiencies because of an inadequate intake, impaired vitamin synthesis or malabsorption in disease states such as cystic fibrosis and Crohn's disease.

The use of vitamins as general 'pick-me-ups' is of unproven value and, the 'fad' for mega-vitamin therapy with water-soluble vitamins, such as ascorbic acid and pyridoxine hydrochloride, is unscientific and can be harmful. Many vitamin supplements are described as 'multivitamin' but few contain the whole range of essential vitamins and many contain relatively high amounts of vitamins A and D. Care should be taken to ensure the correct dose is not exceeded.

Dietary reference values for vitamins are available in the Department of Health publication:

Dietary Reference Values for Food Energy and Nutrients for the United Kingdom: Report of the Panel on Dietary Reference Values of the Committee on Medical Aspects of Food Policy. *Report on Health and Social Subjects* 41. London: HMSO, 1991.

Dental patients

It is unjustifiable to treat stomatitis or glossitis with mixtures of vitamin preparations; this delays diagnosis and correct treatment.

Most patients who develop a nutritional deficiency despite an adequate intake of vitamins have malabsorption and if this is suspected the patient should be referred to a medical practitioner.

Vitamin A

Deficiency of vitamin A (retinol) p. 584 is associated with ocular defects (particularly xerophthalmia) and an increased susceptibility to infections, but deficiency is rare in the UK (even in disorders of fat absorption).

Vitamin A supplementation may be required in children with liver disease, particularly cholestatic liver disease, due to the malabsorption of fat soluble vitamins. In those with complete biliary obstruction an intramuscular dose once a month may be appropriate.

Preterm neonates have low plasma concentrations of vitamin A and are usually given vitamin A supplements, often as part of an oral multivitamin preparation once enteral feeding has been established.

Vitamin B group

Deficiency of the B vitamins, other than vitamin B_{12}, is rare in the UK and is usually treated by preparations containing thiamine (B_1) p. 586, and riboflavin (B_2). Other members (or substances traditionally classified as members) of the vitamin B complex such as aminobenzoic acid, biotin, choline, inositol nicotinate, and pantothenic acid or panthenol may be included in vitamin B preparations, but there is no evidence of their value as supplements; however, they can be used in the management of certain metabolic disorders. Anaphylaxis has been reported with parenteral B vitamins.

As with other vitamins of the B group, pyridoxine hydrochloride (B_6) deficiency is rare, but it may occur during isoniazid p. 345 therapy or penicillamine p. 574 treatment in

Wilson's disease and is characterised by peripheral neuritis. High doses of pyridoxine hydrochloride are given in some metabolic disorders, such as hyperoxaluria, cystathioninuria and homocystinuria; folic acid p. 533 supplementation may also be beneficial in these disorders. Pyridoxine hydrochloride is also used in sideroblastic anaemia. Rarely, seizures in the neonatal period or during infancy respond to pyridoxine hydrochloride treatment; pyridoxine hydrochloride should be tried in all cases of early-onset intractable seizures and status epilepticus. Pyridoxine hydrochloride has been tried for a wide variety of other disorders, but there is little sound evidence to support the claims of efficacy.

A number of mitochondrial disorders may respond to treatment with certain B vitamins but these disorders require specialist management. Thiamine is used in the treatment of maple syrup urine disease, mitochondrial respiratory chain defects and, together with riboflavin, in the treatment of congenital lactic acidosis; riboflavin is also used in glutaric acidaemias and cytochrome oxidase deficiencies; biotin is used in carboxylase defects.

Folic acid and vitamin B_{12} are used in the treatment of megaloblastic anaemia. Folinic acid p. 515 (available as calcium folinate) is used in association with cytotoxic therapy.

Vitamin C

Vitamin C (ascorbic acid) therapy is essential in scurvy, but less florid manifestations of vitamin C deficiency have been reported. Vitamin C is used to enhance the excretion of iron one month after starting desferrioxamine mesilate p. 536 therapy; it is given separately from food as it also enhances iron absorption. Vitamin C is also used in the treatment of some inherited metabolic disorders, particularly mitochondrial disorders; specialist management of these conditions is required.

Severe scurvy causes gingival swelling and bleeding margins as well as petechiae on the skin. This is, however, exceedingly rare and a child with these signs is more likely to have leukaemia. Investigation should not be delayed by a trial period of vitamin treatment.

Claims that vitamin C ameliorates colds or promotes wound healing have not been proved.

Vitamin D

The term Vitamin D is used for a range of compounds including ergocalciferol (calciferol, vitamin D_2) p. 591, colecalciferol (vitamin D_3) p. 589, dihydrotachysterol, alfacalcidol (1α-hydroxycholecalciferol) p. 588, and calcitriol (1,25- dihydroxycholecalciferol) p. 588.

Asymptomatic vitamin D deficiency is common in the United Kingdom; symptomatic deficiency may occur in certain ethnic groups, particularly as rickets or hypocalcaemia, and rarely in association with malabsorption. The amount of vitamin D required in infancy is related to the stores built up *in-utero* and subsequent exposure to sunlight. The amount of vitamin D in breast milk varies and some breast-fed babies, particularly if preterm or born to vitamin D deficient mothers, may become deficient. Most formula milk and supplement feeds contain adequate vitamin D to prevent deficiency.

Simple, nutritional vitamin D deficiency can be prevented by oral supplementation of ergocalciferol (calciferol, vitamin D_2) or colecalciferol (vitamin D_3) daily, using multi-vitamin drops, preparations of vitamins A and D, manufactured 'special' solutions, or as calcium and ergocalciferol tablets (although the calcium and other vitamins in supplements are unnecessary); excessive supplementation may cause hypercalcaemia.

Inadequate bone mineralisation can be caused by a deficiency, or a lack of action of vitamin D or its active metabolite. In childhood this causes bowing and distortion of bones (rickets). In nutritional vitamin D deficiency rickets, initial high doses of ergocalciferol or colecalciferol should be reduced to supplemental doses after 8–12 weeks, as there is a significant risk of hypercalcaemia. However, calcium supplements are recommended if there is hypocalcaemia or evidence of a poor dietary calcium intake. A single large dose of ergocalciferol p. 591 or colecalciferol p. 589 can also be effective for the treatment of nutritional vitamin D deficiency rickets.

Poor bone mineralisation in neonates and young children may also be due to inadequate intake of phosphate or calcium particularly during long-term parenteral nutrition— supplementation with phosphate or calcium may be required.

Hypophosphataemic rickets occurs due to abnormal phosphate excretion; treatment with high doses of oral phosphate, and hydroxylated (activated) forms of vitamin D allow bone mineralisation and optimise growth.

Nutritional deficiency of vitamin D is best treated with colecalciferol or ergocalciferol. Preparations containing calcium and colecalciferol are also occasionally used in children where there is evidence of combined calcium and vitamin D deficiency. Vitamin D deficiency caused by *intestinal malabsorption* or *chronic liver disease* usually requires vitamin D in pharmacological doses; the hypocalcaemia of *hypoparathyroidism* often requires higher doses in order to achieve normocalcaemia and alfacalcidol p. 588 is generally preferred.

Vitamin D supplementation is often given in combination with calcium supplements for persistent hypocalcaemia in neonates, and in chronic renal disease

Vitamin D requires hydroxylation, by the kidney and liver, to its active form therefore the hydroxylated derivatives alfacalcidol or calcitriol p. 588 should be prescribed if patients with *severe liver or renal impairment* require vitamin D therapy. Alfacalcidol is generally preferred in children as there is more experience of its use and appropriate formulations are available. Calcitriol is unlicensed for use in children and is generally reserved for those with severe liver disease.

Vitamin E

The daily requirement of vitamin E (tocopherol) has not been well defined. Vitamin E supplements are given to children with fat malabsorption such as in cystic fibrosis and cholestatic liver disease. In children with abetalipoproteinaemia abnormally low vitamin E concentrations may occur in association with neuromuscular problems; this usually responds to high doses of vitamin E. Some neonatal units still administer a single intramuscular dose of vitamin E at birth to preterm neonates to reduce the risk of complications; no trials of long-term outcome have been carried out. The intramuscular route should also be considered in children with severe liver disease when response to oral therapy is inadequate.

Vitamin E has been tried for various other conditions but there is little scientific evidence of its value.

Vitamin K

Vitamin K is necessary for the production of blood clotting factors and proteins necessary for the normal calcification of bone.

Because vitamin K is fat soluble, children with fat malabsorption, especially in biliary obstruction or hepatic disease, may become deficient. For oral administration to prevent vitamin K deficiency in malabsorption syndromes, a water-soluble synthetic vitamin K derivative, menadiol sodium phosphate p. 593 can be used if supplementation with phytomenadione p. 593 by mouth has been insufficient

Oral coumarin anticoagulants act by interfering with vitamin K metabolism in the hepatic cells and their effects can be antagonised by giving vitamin K; see advice on the use of vitamin K in haemorrhage.

Multivitamins

Multivitamin supplements are used in children with vitamin deficiencies and also in malabsorption conditions such as cystic fibrosis or liver disease. Supplementation is not required if nutrient enriched feeds are used; consult a dietician for further advice.

Vitamin K

▸ In neonates **Vitamin K deficiency bleeding**
Neonates are relatively deficient in vitamin K and those who do not receive supplements of vitamin K are at risk of serious bleeding including intracranial bleeding. The Chief Medical Officer and the Chief Nursing Officer have recommended that all newborn babies should receive vitamin K to prevent vitamin K deficiency bleeding (previously termed haemorrhagic disease of the newborn). An appropriate regimen should be selected after discussion with parents in the antenatal period.

Vitamin K (as phytomenadione) may be given by a single intramuscular injection at birth; this prevents vitamin K deficiency bleeding in virtually all babies.

Alternatively, in healthy babies who are not at particular risk of bleeding disorders, vitamin K may be given by mouth, and arrangements must be in place to ensure the appropriate regimen is followed. Two doses of a colloidal (mixed micelle) preparation of phytomenadione should be given by mouth in the first week, the first dose being given at birth and the second dose at 4–7 days. For exclusively breast-fed babies, a third dose of colloidal phytomenadione is given by mouth at 1 month of age; the third dose is omitted in formula-fed babies because formula feeds contain adequate vitamin K. An alternative regimen is to give one dose of phytomenadione by mouth at birth (using the contents of a phytomenadione capsule) to protect from the risk of vitamin K deficiency bleeding in the first week; for exclusively breast-fed babies, further doses of phytomenadione are given by mouth (using the contents of a phytomenadione capsule) at weekly intervals for 12 weeks.

VITAMINS AND TRACE ELEMENTS ›
MULTIVITAMINS

Vitamins A and D

- ● **INDICATIONS AND DOSE**
Prevention of vitamin A and D deficiency
▸ BY MOUTH
  ▸ Child: 1 capsule daily, 1 capsule contains 4000 units vitamin A and 400 units (10 micrograms) vitamin D

- ● **UNLICENSED USE** Not licensed in children under 6 months of age.
- ● **INTERACTIONS** → Appendix 1 (vitamins).
- ● **SIDE-EFFECTS**
Overdose
Excessive ingestion Prolonged excessive ingestion of vitamins A and D can lead to hypervitaminosis.
- ● **PRESCRIBING AND DISPENSING INFORMATION** This drug contains vitamin D; consult individual vitamin D monographs.
- ● **MEDICINAL FORMS**
There can be variation in the licensing of different medicines containing the same drug.
Capsule
▸ Vitamins A and D (Non-proprietary)
  Vitamin D 400 unit, Vitamin A 4000 unit Vitamins A and D capsules BPC 1973 | 28 capsule £2.81 | 28 capsule GSL £2.81 | 84 capsule £8.42 DT price = £8.42

Vitamins A, B group, C and D

- ● **INDICATIONS AND DOSE**
Prevention of deficiency
▸ BY MOUTH USING CAPSULES
  ▸ Child 1–11 years: 1 capsule daily
  ▸ Child 12–17 years: 2 capsules daily

Cystic Fibrosis: prevention of deficiency
▸ BY MOUTH USING CAPSULES
  ▸ Child 1–17 years: 2–3 capsules daily

ABIDEC MULTIVITAMIN DROPS®
Prevention of deficiency
▸ BY MOUTH USING ORAL DROPS

  ▸ Preterm neonate: 0.6 mL daily.

  ▸ Neonate: 0.3 mL daily.

  ▸ Child 1–11 months: 0.3 mL daily
  ▸ Child 1–17 years: 0.6 mL daily

Cystic Fibrosis: prevention of deficiency
▸ BY MOUTH USING ORAL DROPS
  ▸ Child 1–11 months: 0.6 mL daily
  ▸ Child 1–17 years: 1.2 mL daily

DALIVIT ORAL DROPS®
Prevention of deficiency
▸ BY MOUTH USING ORAL DROPS

  ▸ Preterm neonate: 0.3 mL daily.

  ▸ Neonate: 0.3 mL daily.

  ▸ Child 1–11 months: 0.3 mL daily
  ▸ Child 1–17 years: 0.6 mL daily

Cystic Fibrosis: prevention of deficiency
▸ BY MOUTH USING ORAL DROPS
  ▸ Child 1–11 months: 0.6 mL daily
  ▸ Child 1–17 years: 1 mL daily

- ● **UNLICENSED USE** *Dalivit* ® not licensed for use in children under 6 weeks.
- ● **PRESCRIBING AND DISPENSING INFORMATION** This drug contains vitamin D; consult individual vitamin D monographs.
  To avoid potential toxicity, the content of all vitamin preparations, particularly vitamin A, should be considered when used together with other supplements.
  Vitamin A concentration of preparations varies.
  ABIDEC MULTIVITAMIN DROPS® *Abidec* ® contains 1333 units of vitamin A (as palmitate) per 0.6 mL dose.
  DALIVIT ORAL DROPS® *Dalivit* ® contains 5000 units of vitamin A (as palmitate) per 0.6 mL dose.

- ● **MEDICINAL FORMS**
There can be variation in the licensing of different medicines containing the same drug.
Capsule
▸ Vitamins A, B group, C and D (Non-proprietary)
  Riboflavin 500 microgram, Thiamine hydrochloride 1 mg, Nicotinamide 7.5 mg, Ascorbic acid 15 mg, Vitamin D 300 unit, Vitamin A 2500 unit Vitamins capsules | 84 capsule no price available | 1000 capsule £48.20 DT price = £15.48
Oral drops
EXCIPIENTS: May contain Arachis (peanut) oil, sucrose
▸ Abidec Multivitamin (Omega Pharma Ltd)
  Ascorbic acid 66.7 mg per 1 ml, Ergocalciferol 667 iu per 1 ml, Nicotinamide 1333 microgram per 1 ml, Pyridoxine hydrochloride 1333 microgram per 1 ml, Riboflavin 1333 microgram per 1 ml, Thiamine hydrochloride 1.67 mg per 1 ml, Retinol (as Vitamin A palmitate) 2222 iu per 1 ml Abidec Multivitamin drops | 25 ml GSL £3.33

▸ Dalivit (Boston Healthcare Ltd)
Ascorbic acid 83 mg per 1 ml, Ergocalciferol 667 iu per 1 ml,
Riboflavin 667 microgram per 1 ml, Pyridoxine 833 microgram
per 1 ml, Thiamine 1667 microgram per 1 ml, Nicotinamide 8.3 mg
per 1 ml, Vitamin A 8333 iu per 1 ml Dalivit oral drops |
25 ml [GSL] £3.32 | 50 ml [GSL] £6.33

Vitamins A, C and D

The properties listed below are those particular to the
combination only. For the properties of the components
please consider, vitamin A below, ascorbic acid p. 587.

● **INDICATIONS AND DOSE**
Prevention of vitamin deficiency
▸ BY MOUTH
▸ Child 1 month–4 years: 5 drops daily, 5 drops contain
vitamin A approx. 700 units, vitamin D approx.
300 units (7.5 micrograms), ascorbic acid approx. 20 mg

● **PRESCRIBING AND DISPENSING INFORMATION** This drug
contains vitamin D; consult individual vitamin D
monographs.
    Available free of charge to children under 4 years in
families on the Healthy Start Scheme, or alternatively may
be available direct to the public—further information for
healthcare professionals can be accessed at
www.healthystart.nhs.uk. Beneficiaries can contact their
midwife or health visitor for further information on where
to obtain supplies.
    Healthy Start Vitamins for women (containing ascorbic
acid, vitamin D, and folic acid) are also available free of
charge to women on the Healthy Start Scheme during
pregnancy and until their baby is one year old, or
alternatively may be available direct to the public—further
information for healthcare professionals can be accessed
at www.healthystart.nhs.uk. Beneficiaries can contact their
midwife or health visitor for further information on where
to obtain supplies.

● **MEDICINAL FORMS**
There can be variation in the licensing of different medicines
containing the same drug.
Oral drops
▸ Healthy Start Children's Vitamin (Secretary of State for Health)
Vitamin A and D3 concentrate.55 mg per 1 ml, Sodium ascorbate
18.58 mg per 1 ml, Ascorbic acid 150 mg per 1 ml, Vitamin D
2000 iu per 1 ml, Vitamin A 5000 iu per 1 ml Healthy Start
Children's Vitamin drops | 10 ml no price available

VITAMINS AND TRACE ELEMENTS ❭ VITAMIN A

Vitamin A

(Retinol)

● **INDICATIONS AND DOSE**
Vitamin A deficiency
▸ BY MOUTH
▸ Neonate: 5000 units daily, higher doses may be used
initially for treatment of severe deficiency.
▸ Child 1–11 months: 5000 units daily, to be taken with or
after food, higher doses may be used initially for
treatment of severe deficiency
▸ Child 1–17 years: 10 000 units daily, to be taken with or
after food, higher doses may be used initially for
treatment of severe deficiency
Prevention of deficiency in complete biliary obstruction
▸ BY INTRAMUSCULAR INJECTION
▸ Neonate: 50 000 units once a month.
▸ Child 1–11 months: 50 000 units once a month

● **UNLICENSED USE** Preparations containing only vitamin A
are not licensed.

● **INTERACTIONS** → Appendix 1 (vitamins).

● **SIDE-EFFECTS**
Overdose
Massive overdose can cause rough skin, dry hair, an
enlarged liver, and a raised erythrocyte sedimentation rate
and raised serum calcium and serum alkaline phosphatase
concentrations.

● **PREGNANCY** Excessive doses may be teratogenic. In view
of evidence suggesting that high levels of vitamin A may
cause birth defects, women who are (or may become)
pregnant are advised not to take vitamin A supplements
(including tablets and fish liver oil drops), except on the
advice of a doctor or an antenatal clinic; nor should they
eat liver or products such as liver paté or liver sausage.

● **BREAST FEEDING** Theoretical risk of toxicity in infants of
mothers taking large doses.

● **MONITORING REQUIREMENTS** Treatment is sometimes
initiated with very high doses of vitamin A and the child
should be monitored closely; very high doses are
associated with acute toxicity.

● **MEDICINAL FORMS**
There can be variation in the licensing of different medicines
containing the same drug. Forms available from special-order
manufacturers include: drops, solution for injection
Drops
▸ Vitamin A (Non-proprietary)
Vitamin A 150000 unit per 1 ml Arovit 150,000units/ml drops |
7.5 ml [PoM] no price available
Solution for injection
▸ Vitamin A (Non-proprietary)
Retinol (as Vitamin A palmitate) 50000 unit per 1 ml Aquasol A
Parenteral 100,000units/2ml solution for injection vials | 1 vial [PoM]
no price available | 10 vial [PoM] no price available

Combinations available: *Vitamins A, C and D,* above

VITAMINS AND TRACE ELEMENTS ❭ VITAMIN B
GROUP

Biotin

(Vitamin H)

● **INDICATIONS AND DOSE**
Isolated carboxylase defects
▸ BY MOUTH, OR BY SLOW INTRAVENOUS INJECTION
▸ Neonate: 5 mg once daily, adjusted according to
response, maintenance 10–50 mg daily, higher doses
may be required.
▸ Child: 10 mg once daily, adjusted according to
response; maintenance 10–50 mg daily, increased if
necessary up to 100 mg daily
Defects of biotin metabolism
▸ BY MOUTH, OR BY SLOW INTRAVENOUS INJECTION
▸ Neonate: Initially 10 mg once daily, adjusted according
to response; maintenance 5–20 mg daily, higher doses
may be required.
▸ Child: Initially 10 mg once daily, adjusted according to
response; maintenance 5–20 mg daily, higher doses
may be required

● **PREGNANCY** No information available.

● **BREAST FEEDING** No information available.

● **DIRECTIONS FOR ADMINISTRATION**
▸ With oral use For administration *by mouth,* tablets may be
crushed and mixed with food or drink.

● PATIENT AND CARER ADVICE
Medicines for Children leaflet: Biotin for metabolic disorders www.medicinesforchildren.org.uk/biotin-metabolic-disorders-0

● MEDICINAL FORMS
There can be variation in the licensing of different medicines containing the same drug. Forms available from special-order manufacturers include: tablet, oral suspension, oral solution

Tablet
▸ Biotin (Non-proprietary)
   Biotin 5 mg tablets | 30 tablet PoM no price available
   Biotin 10 mg FORTE tablets | 30 tablet no price available

Solution for injection
▸ Biotin (Non-proprietary)
   Biotin 5 mg per 1 ml Biodermatin 5mg/1ml solution for injection vials | 10 vial PoM no price available

Pyridoxine hydrochloride

(Vitamin B₆)

● INDICATIONS AND DOSE
Isoniazid-induced neuropathy (prophylaxis)
▸ BY MOUTH

▸ Neonate: 5 mg daily.

▸ Child 1 month–11 years: 5–10 mg daily
▸ Child 12–17 years: 10 mg daily

Isoniazid-induced neuropathy (treatment)
▸ BY MOUTH

▸ Neonate: 5–10 mg daily.

▸ Child 1 month–11 years: 10–20 mg 2–3 times a day
▸ Child 12–17 years: 30–50 mg 2–3 times a day

Prevention of penicillamine-induced neuropathy in Wilson's disease
▸ BY MOUTH

▸ Child 1–11 years: 5–10 mg daily
▸ Child 12–17 years: 10 mg daily

Metabolic diseases | Cystathioninuria | Homocystinuria
▸ BY MOUTH

▸ Neonate: 50–100 mg 1–2 times a day.

▸ Child: 50–250 mg 1–2 times a day

Pyridoxine-dependent seizures
▸ INITIALLY BY INTRAVENOUS INJECTION

▸ Neonate: Test dose 50–100 mg, repeated if necessary, if responsive, followed by an oral maintenance dose; (by mouth) maintenance 50–100 mg once daily, dose to be adjusted as necessary.

▸ Child 1 month–11 years: Test dose 50–100 mg daily, if responsive, followed by an oral maintenance dose, (by mouth) maintenance 20–50 mg 1–2 times a day, dose to be adjusted as necessary, (by mouth) increased if necessary up to 30 mg/kg daily, alternatively (by mouth) increased if necessary up to 1 g daily

UNLICENSED USE Not licensed for prophylaxis of penicillamine-induced neuropathy in Wilson's disease. Not licensed for use in children.

CAUTIONS
With intravenous use Risk of cardiovascular collapse (with intravenous injection—resuscitation facilities must be available and monitor closely)

INTERACTIONS → Appendix 1 (vitamins).

SIDE-EFFECTS Sensory neuropathy (with high doses when given for extended periods)

Overdose
Overdosage induces toxic effects.

● MEDICINAL FORMS
There can be variation in the licensing of different medicines containing the same drug. Forms available from special-order manufacturers include: capsule, oral suspension, oral solution, solution for injection

Tablet
▸ Pyridoxine hydrochloride (Non-proprietary)
   Pyridoxine hydrochloride 10 mg Pyridoxine 10mg tablets | 28 tablet £12.95–£14.50 | 28 tablet GSL no price available | 30 tablet GSL no price available | 60 tablet GSL no price available | 60 tablet no price available | 500 tablet £8.48 | 500 tablet GSL no price available
   Pyridoxine (as Pyridoxine hydrochloride) 20 mg Pyridoxine 20mg tablets | 500 tablet GSL no price available | 500 tablet no price available
   Pyridoxine hydrochloride 50 mg Pyridoxine 50mg tablets | 28 tablet P no price available DT price = £5.95 | 28 tablet GSL £6.62 DT price = £5.95 | 500 tablet P no price available

Capsule
▸ Pyridoxine hydrochloride (Non-proprietary)
   Pyridoxine (as Pyridoxine hydrochloride) 100 mg capsules | 100 capsule no price available

Solution for injection
▸ Pyridoxine hydrochloride (Non-proprietary)
   Pyridoxine hydrochloride 50 mg per 1 ml Vitamin B6 Streuli 100mg/2ml solution for injection ampoules | 10 ampoule PoM no price available

Riboflavin

(Riboflavine; Vitamin B₂)

● INDICATIONS AND DOSE
Metabolic diseases
▸ BY MOUTH

▸ Neonate: 50 mg 1–2 times a day, adjusted according to response.

▸ Child: 50–100 mg 1–2 times a day, adjusted according to response to up to 400 mg daily

● UNLICENSED USE Not licensed in children.

● SIDE-EFFECTS Bright yellow urine

● PREGNANCY Crosses the placenta but no adverse effects reported, information at high doses limited.

● BREAST FEEDING Present in breast milk but no adverse effects reported, information at high doses limited.

● MEDICINAL FORMS
There can be variation in the licensing of different medicines containing the same drug. Forms available from special-order manufacturers include: tablet, modified-release tablet, capsule, oral suspension, oral solution

Tablet
▸ Riboflavin (Non-proprietary)
   Riboflavin 10 mg tablets | 20 tablet no price available
   Riboflavin 100 mg tablets | 100 tablet no price available

Modified-release tablet
▸ Riboflavin (Non-proprietary)
   Riboflavin 100 mg modified-release tablets | 60 tablet £4.18

Capsule
▸ Riboflavin (Non-proprietary)
   Riboflavin 50 mg Riboflavin 50mg capsules | 30 capsule £2.90 | 100 capsule £4.44
   Riboflavin 100 mg capsules | 100 capsule no price available

9

Blood and nutrition

Thiamine

(Vitamin B$_1$)

● **INDICATIONS AND DOSE**

Maple syrup urine disease

▸ BY MOUTH

▸ Neonate: 5 mg/kg daily, dose to be adjusted as necessary.

▸ Child: 5 mg/kg daily, dose to be adjusted as necessary

Metabolic disorders | Congenital lactic acidosis

▸ BY MOUTH, OR BY INTRAVENOUS INFUSION

▸ Neonate: 50–200 mg once daily, dose to be adjusted as necessary, the total dose may alternatively be given in 2–3 divided doses, administer intravenous infusion over 30 minutes.

▸ Child: 100–300 mg once daily, dose to be adjusted as necessary, the total dose may alternatively be given in 2–3 divided doses, administer intravenous infusion over 30 minutes, increased if necessary up to 2 g daily

● **UNLICENSED USE** Not licensed in children.

> **IMPORTANT SAFETY INFORMATION**
> MHRA/CHM ADVICE (SEPTEMBER 2007)
> Although potentially serious allergic adverse reactions may rarely occur during, or shortly after, parenteral administration, the CHM has recommended that:
> - This should not preclude the use of parenteral thiamine in patients where this route of administration is required, particularly in patients at risk of Wernicke-Korsakoff syndrome where treatment with thiamine is essential;
> - Intravenous administration should be by infusion over 30 minutes;
> - Facilities for treating anaphylaxis (including resuscitation facilities) should be available when parenteral thiamine is administered.

● **CAUTIONS** Anaphylaxis may occasionally follow injection

● **SIDE-EFFECTS**

▸ With intravenous use Hypersensitivity reactions

● **BREAST FEEDING** Severely thiamine-deficient mothers should avoid breast-feeding as toxic methyl-glyoxal present in milk.

● **PRESCRIBING AND DISPENSING INFORMATION**

▸ With intramuscular use or intravenous use Some preparations may contain phenol as a preservative.

● **MEDICINAL FORMS**
There can be variation in the licensing of different medicines containing the same drug. Forms available from special-order manufacturers include: oral suspension, oral solution

Tablet

▸ Thiamine (Non-proprietary)
Thiamine hydrochloride 50 mg Thiamine 50mg tablets | 28 tablet ⓟ £1.80–£2.00 | 100 tablet ⓟ £7.13 DT price = £7.13 | 100 tablet no price available DT price = £7.13
Thiamine hydrochloride 100 mg Thiamine 100mg tablets | 28 tablet ⓟ £2.50–£2.82 | 100 tablet no price available DT price = £9.99 | 100 tablet ⓟ £10.08 DT price = £9.99

▸ Tyvera (Auden McKenzie (Pharma Division) Ltd, Almus Pharmaceuticals Ltd, Teva UK Ltd)
Thiamine hydrochloride 50 mg Tyvera 50mg tablets | 100 tablet ⓟ £4.99–£7.13 DT price = £7.13
Thiamine hydrochloride 100 mg Tyvera 100mg tablets | 100 tablet ⓟ £6.99–£10.13 DT price = £9.99

Modified-release tablet

▸ Thiamine (Non-proprietary)
Thiamine hydrochloride 100 mg modified-release tablets | 90 tablet £4.18

Solution for injection

▸ Thiamine (Non-proprietary)
Thiamine hydrochloride 50 mg per 1 ml Betabion 100mg/2ml solution for injection ampoules | 5 ampoule [PoM] no price available Bevitine 100mg/2ml solution for injection ampoules | 5 ampoule [PoM] no price available
Thiamine hydrochloride 100 mg per 1 ml Vitamin B1 Streuli 100mg/1ml solution for injection ampoules | 10 ampoule [PoM] no price available

Vitamin B complex

● **INDICATIONS AND DOSE**

Treatment of deficiency

▸ BY MOUTH USING SYRUP

▸ Child 1–11 months: 5 mL 3 times a day, this dose is for *Vigranon B*® syrup.

▸ Child 1–11 years: 10 mL 3 times a day, this dose is for *Vigranon B*® syrup.

▸ Child 12–17 years: 10–15 mL 3 times a day, this dose is for *Vigranon B*® syrup.

Prophylaxis of deficiency

▸ BY MOUTH USING SYRUP

▸ Child 1–11 months: 5 mL once daily, this dose is for *Vigranon B*® syrup.

▸ Child 1–11 years: 5 mL twice daily, this dose is for *Vigranon B*® syrup.

▸ Child 12–17 years: 5 mL 3 times a day, this dose is for *Vigranon B*® syrup.

● **NATIONAL FUNDING/ACCESS DECISIONS**
Vigranon® syrup is not prescribable under the National Health Service (NHS).

● **LESS SUITABLE FOR PRESCRIBING** *Vigranon B*® syrup are less suitable for prescribing.

● **MEDICINAL FORMS**
There can be variation in the licensing of different medicines containing the same drug.

Oral solution

▸ Vigranon-B (Wallace Manufacturing Chemists Ltd)
Pyridoxine hydrochloride 400 microgram per 1 ml, Riboflavin sodium phosphate 548 microgram per 1 ml, Dexpanthenol 600 microgram per 1 ml, Thiamine hydrochloride 1 mg per 1 ml, Nicotinamide 4 mg per 1 ml Vigranon-B syrup sugar-free | 150 ml ⓟ £26.00

Vitamins with minerals and trace elements

● **INDICATIONS AND DOSE**

FORCEVAL® CAPSULES

Vitamin and mineral deficiency and as adjunct in synthetic diets

▸ BY MOUTH

▸ Child 12–17 years: 1 capsule daily, one hour after a meal

KETOVITE® LIQUID

Prevention of vitamin deficiency in disorders of carbohydrate or amino-acid metabolism | Adjunct in restricted, specialised, or synthetic diets

▸ BY MOUTH

▸ Child: 5 mL daily, dose adjusted according to condition, diet, or age, use with *Ketovite*® *Tablets* for complete vitamin supplementation.

KETOVITE® TABLETS

Prevention of vitamin deficiency in disorders of carbohydrate or amino-acid metabolism | Adjunct in restricted, specialised, or synthetic diets

▸ BY MOUTH

▸ Child: 1 tablet 3 times a day, dose adjusted according to condition, diet, or age, use with *Ketovite® Liquid* for complete vitamin supplementation.

● **PRESCRIBING AND DISPENSING INFORMATION** To avoid potential toxicity, the content of all vitamin preparations, particularly vitamin A, should be considered when used together with other supplements.

● **PATIENT AND CARER ADVICE**
Medicines for Children leaflet: Multivitamin preparations for vitamin deficiency www.medicinesforchildren.org.uk/multivitamin-preparations-vitamin-deficiency

KETOVITE® LIQUID *Ketovite®* liquid may be mixed with milk, cereal, or fruit juice.

KETOVITE® TABLETS Tablets may be crushed immediately before use.

● **MEDICINAL FORMS**
There can be variation in the licensing of different medicines containing the same drug.

Tablet

▸ Ketovite (Essential Pharmaceuticals Ltd)
Biotin 170 microgram, Folic acid 250 microgram, Pyridoxine hydrochloride 330 microgram, Acetomenaphthone 500 microgram, Riboflavin 1 mg, Thiamine hydrochloride 1 mg, Calcium pantothenate 1.16 mg, Nicotinamide 3.3 mg, Alpha tocopheryl acetate 5 mg, Ascorbic acid 16.6 mg, Inositol 50 mg Ketovite tablets | 100 tablet [PoM] £9.21

Capsule

▸ Forceval (Alliance Pharmaceuticals Ltd)
Cyanocobalamin 3 microgram, Selenium 50 microgram, Biotin 100 microgram, Iodine 140 microgram, Chromium 200 microgram, Molybdenum 250 microgram, Folic acid 400 microgram, Riboflavin 1.2 mg, Riboflavin 1.6 mg, Copper 2 mg, Pyridoxine 2 mg, Manganese 3 mg, Pantothenic acid 4 mg, Potassium 4 mg, Tocopheryl acetate 10 mg, Iron 12 mg, Zinc 15 mg, Nicotinamide 18 mg, Magnesium 30 mg, Ascorbic acid 60 mg, Phosphorus 77 mg, Calcium 100 mg, Ergocalciferol 400 unit, Vitamin A 2500 unit Forceval capsules | 15 capsule [P] £4.42 | 30 capsule [P] £7.71 | 90 capsule [P] £18.62

Oral emulsion

▸ Ketovite (Essential Pharmaceuticals Ltd)
Cyanocobalamin 2.5 microgram per 1 ml, Choline chloride 30 mg per 1 ml, Ergocalciferol 80 unit per 1 ml, Vitamin A 500 unit per 1 ml Ketovite liquid sugar-free | 150 ml [P] £19.10

VITAMINS AND TRACE ELEMENTS > VITAMIN C

Ascorbic acid
(Vitamin C)

● **INDICATIONS AND DOSE**
Treatment of scurvy

▸ BY MOUTH

▸ Child 1 month–3 years: 125–250 mg daily in 1–2 divided doses

▸ Child 4–11 years: 250–500 mg daily in 1–2 divided doses

▸ Child 12–17 years: 0.5–1 g daily in 1–2 divided doses

Adjunct to desferrioxamine (to enhance the excretion of iron 1 month after treatment)

▸ BY MOUTH

▸ Child: 100–200 mg daily, to be taken 1 hour before food

Metabolic disorders | Tyrosinaemia type III | Transient tyrosinaemia of the newborn | Glutathione synthase deficiency | Hawkinsinuria

▸ BY MOUTH

▸ Neonate: 50–200 mg daily, dose to be adjusted as necessary.

▸ Child: 200–400 mg daily in 1–2 divided doses, dose to be adjusted as necessary, increased if necessary up to 1 g daily

● **UNLICENSED USE** Not licensed for metabolic disorders.

● **CONTRA-INDICATIONS** Hyperoxaluria

● **CAUTIONS**

CAUTIONS, FURTHER INFORMATION

▸ Iron overload Ascorbic acid should not be given to patients with cardiac dysfunction.
In patients with normal cardiac function ascorbic acid should be introduced 1 month after starting desferrioxamine.

● **INTERACTIONS** → Appendix 1 (vitamins).

● **SIDE-EFFECTS** Diarrhoea · fatigue · headache · hyperoxaluria · nausea

● **PRESCRIBING AND DISPENSING INFORMATION** It is rarely necessary to prescribe more than 100 mg daily except early in the treatment of scurvy.

● **MEDICINAL FORMS**
There can be variation in the licensing of different medicines containing the same drug. Forms available from special-order manufacturers include: oral suspension, oral solution

Tablet

EXCIPIENTS: May contain Aspartame

▸ Ascorbic acid (Non-proprietary)
Ascorbic acid 50 mg Ascorbic acid 50mg tablets | 28 tablet [GSL] £15.10 DT price = £15.01 | 28 tablet no price available DT price = £15.01 | 500 tablet [GSL] no price available
Ascorbic acid 100 mg Ascorbic acid 100mg tablets | 28 tablet no price available DT price = £14.30 | 28 tablet [GSL] £14.30 DT price = £14.30
Ascorbic acid 200 mg Ascorbic acid 200mg tablets | 28 tablet no price available DT price = £19.89 | 28 tablet [GSL] £19.77 DT price = £19.89 | 100 tablet [GSL] no price available
Ascorbic acid 250 mg Ascorbic acid 250mg tablets | 1000 tablet [PoM] no price available
Ascorbic acid 500 mg Ascorbic acid 500mg tablets | 28 tablet [GSL] £26.87 DT price = £26.87 | 28 tablet no price available DT price = £26.87 | 100 tablet [GSL] no price available

Chewable tablet

CAUTIONARY AND ADVISORY LABELS 24
EXCIPIENTS: May contain Aspartame

▸ Ascorbic acid (Non-proprietary)
Ascorbic acid 60 mg chewable tablets | 60 tablet no price available | 180 tablet no price available
Ascorbic acid 500 mg chewable tablets | 60 tablet £3.90 | 100 tablet £5.58
Ascorbic acid 1 gram chewable tablets | 30 tablet £2.30 | 60 tablet £4.20

▸ Ascur (Ennogen Healthcare Ltd)
Ascorbic acid 100 mg Ascur 100mg chewable tablets | 30 tablet £3.95
Ascorbic acid (as Sodium ascorbate) 500 mg Ascur 500mg chewable tablets sugar-free | 30 tablet £2.99

Capsule

▸ Ascorbic acid (Non-proprietary)
Ascorbic acid 500 mg capsules | 100 capsule no price available
Ascorbic acid 1 gram capsules | 100 capsule no price available | 250 capsule no price available

Combinations available: *Vitamins A, C and D,* p. 584

9

Blood and nutrition

9

Blood and nutrition

Vitamin D and analogues (systemic)

- **CONTRA-INDICATIONS** Hypercalcaemia · metastatic calcification
- **INTERACTIONS** → Appendix 1 (vitamins).
- **SIDE-EFFECTS**

Overdose
Symptoms of overdosage include anorexia, lassitude, nausea and vomiting, diarrhoea, constipation, weight loss, polyuria, sweating, headache, thirst, vertigo, and raised concentrations of calcium and phosphate in plasma and urine.

- **PREGNANCY** High doses teratogenic in *animals* but therapeutic doses unlikely to be harmful.
- **BREAST FEEDING** Caution with high doses; may cause hypercalcaemia in infant—monitor serum-calcium concentration.
- **MONITORING REQUIREMENTS** **Important**: All patients receiving pharmacological doses of vitamin D should have their plasma-calcium concentration checked at intervals (initially once or twice weekly) and whenever nausea or vomiting occur.

▶ above

Alfacalcidol

(1α-Hydroxycholecalciferol)

- **INDICATIONS AND DOSE**

Hypophosphataemic rickets | Persistent hypocalcaemia due to hypoparathyroidism or pseudohypoparathyroidism
▶ BY MOUTH, OR BY INTRAVENOUS INJECTION
▶ Child 1 month–11 years: 25–50 nanograms/kg once daily, dose to be adjusted as necessary; maximum 1 microgram per day
▶ Child 12–17 years: 1 microgram once daily, dose to be adjusted as necessary

Persistent neonatal hypocalcaemia
▶ BY MOUTH, OR BY INTRAVENOUS INJECTION
▶ Neonate: 50–100 nanograms/kg once daily, dose to be adjusted as necessary, in resistant cases higher doses may be needed; increased if necessary up to 2 micrograms/kg daily.

Prevention of vitamin D deficiency in renal or cholestatic liver disease
▶ BY MOUTH, OR BY INTRAVENOUS INJECTION
▶ Neonate: 20 nanograms/kg once daily, dose to be adjusted as necessary.
▶ Child 1 month–11 years (body-weight up to 20 kg): 15–30 nanograms/kg once daily (max. per dose 500 nanograms)
▶ Child 1 month–11 years (body-weight 20 kg and above): 250–500 nanograms once daily, dose to be adjusted as necessary
▶ Child 12–17 years: 250–500 nanograms once daily, dose to be adjusted as necessary

DOSE EQUIVALENCE AND CONVERSION
One drop of alfacalcidol 2 microgram/mL oral drops contains approximately 100 nanograms alfacalcidol.

- **CAUTIONS** Nephrolithiasis · take care to ensure correct dose in infants

- **SIDE-EFFECTS**
- ▶ **Rare** Nephrocalcinosis · pruritus · rash · urticaria
- **RENAL IMPAIRMENT**

Monitoring
Monitor plasma-calcium concentration in renal impairment.

- **MONITORING REQUIREMENTS** Monitor plasma-calcium concentration in patients receiving high doses.
- **DIRECTIONS FOR ADMINISTRATION**
- ▶ With intravenous use For injection, shake ampoule for at least 5 seconds before use, and give over 30 seconds.

- **MEDICINAL FORMS**
There can be variation in the licensing of different medicines containing the same drug. Forms available from special-order manufacturers include: oral suspension, oral solution

Capsule
EXCIPIENTS: May contain Sesame oil
▶ **Alfacalcidol (Non-proprietary)**
Alfacalcidol 250 nanogram Alfacalcidol 250nanogram capsules | 30 capsule [PoM] £6.33 DT price = £1.82
Alfacalcidol 500 nanogram Alfacalcidol 500nanogram capsules | 30 capsule [PoM] £10.00 DT price = £3.96
Alfacalcidol 1 microgram Alfacalcidol 1microgram capsules | 30 capsule no price available DT price = £4.19 | 30 capsule [PoM] £14.03 DT price = £4.19
▶ **One-Alpha** (LEO Pharma)
Alfacalcidol 250 nanogram One-Alpha 250nanogram capsules | 30 capsule [PoM] £3.37 DT price = £1.82
Alfacalcidol 500 nanogram One-Alpha 0.5microgram capsules | 30 capsule [PoM] £6.27 DT price = £3.96
Alfacalcidol 1 microgram One-Alpha 1microgram capsules | 30 capsule [PoM] £8.75 DT price = £4.19

Oral drops
EXCIPIENTS: May contain Alcohol
▶ **One-Alpha** (LEO Pharma)
Alfacalcidol 2 microgram per 1 ml One-Alpha 2micrograms/ml oral drops sugar-free | 10 ml [PoM] £21.30 DT price = £21.30

Solution for injection
EXCIPIENTS: May contain Alcohol, propylene glycol
▶ **One-Alpha** (LEO Pharma)
Alfacalcidol 2 microgram per 1 ml One-Alpha 2micrograms/1ml solution for injection ampoules | 10 ampoule [PoM] £41.13
One-Alpha 1micrograms/0.5ml solution for injection ampoules | 10 ampoule [PoM] £21.57

▶ above

Calcitriol

(1,25-Dihydroxycholecalciferol)

- **INDICATIONS AND DOSE**

Vitamin D dependent rickets | Hypophosphataemic rickets | Persistent hypocalcaemia due to hypoparathyroidism | Pseudo-hypoparathyroidism (limited experience)
▶ BY MOUTH
▶ Child 1 month–11 years: Initially 15 nanograms/kg once daily (max. per dose 250 nanograms), increased in steps of 5 nanograms/kg daily (max. per dose 250 nanograms) if required, dose to be increased every 2–4 weeks
▶ Child 12–17 years: Initially 250 nanograms once daily, increased in steps of 5 nanograms/kg daily (max. per dose 250 nanograms) if required, dose to be increased every 2–4 weeks; usual dose 0.5–1 microgram daily

- **UNLICENSED USE** Not licensed for use in children.
- **CAUTIONS** Take care to ensure correct dose in infants
- **HEPATIC IMPAIRMENT** Manufacturer advises avoid—no information available.
- **RENAL IMPAIRMENT** Manufacturer advises avoid—no information available. Monitor plasma-calcium concentration in renal impairment.

- **MONITORING REQUIREMENTS** Monitor plasma calcium, phosphate, and creatinine during dosage titration. Monitor plasma-calcium concentration in patients receiving high doses.

- **DIRECTIONS FOR ADMINISTRATION** Contents of capsule may be administered by oral syringe.

- **MEDICINAL FORMS**
There can be variation in the licensing of different medicines containing the same drug. Forms available from special-order manufacturers include: oral suspension, oral solution

Capsule
- ▸ **Calcitriol (Non-proprietary)**
  Calcitriol 250 nanogram Calcitriol 250nanogram capsules | 30 capsule [PoM] £18.04 | 100 capsule [PoM] no price available DT price = £18.04
  Calcitriol 500 nanogram Calcitriol 500nanogram capsules | 30 capsule [PoM] £32.25 | 100 capsule [PoM] no price available DT price = £32.25
- ▸ **Rocaltrol (Roche Products Ltd)**
  Calcitriol 250 nanogram Rocaltrol 250nanogram capsules | 100 capsule [PoM] £18.04 DT price = £18.04
  Calcitriol 500 nanogram Rocaltrol 500nanogram capsules | 100 capsule [PoM] £32.25 DT price = £32.25

Oral solution
- ▸ **Calcitriol (Non-proprietary)**
  Calcitriol 1 microgram per 1 ml Rocaltrol 1micrograms/ml oral solution sugar-free | 10 ml [PoM] no price available

F 588

Colecalciferol

(Cholecalciferol; Vitamin D₃)

- **INDICATIONS AND DOSE**
Prevention of vitamin D deficiency
- ▸ BY MOUTH
- ▸ Child: 400 units daily

- **UNLICENSED USE** *Adcal-D3*®, *Calceos*®, and *Fultium-D₃*® 800 units and *Fultium-D₃*® 20000 units are not licensed for use in children under 12 years. *Cacit*®*D3*, *Calcichew-D₃*® *Forte, Calcichew-D₃*® 500 mg/400 unit, and *Kalcipos-D*® not licensed for use in children (age range not specified by manufacturers). *Accrete D3*®, *Calfovit D3*®, and *Natecal D3*® not licensed for use in children under 18 years.

- **CAUTIONS** Take care to ensure correct dose in infants

- **RENAL IMPAIRMENT**
Monitoring
Monitor plasma-calcium concentration in renal impairment.

- **MONITORING REQUIREMENTS** Monitor plasma-calcium concentration in patients receiving high doses.

- **DIRECTIONS FOR ADMINISTRATION**
INVITA D3® **25,000UNITS/1ML ORAL SOLUTION (CONSILIENT HEALTH LTD)** May be mixed with a small amount of milk or cold or lukewarm food immediately before administration.

- **MEDICINAL FORMS**
There can be variation in the licensing of different medicines containing the same drug. Forms available from special-order manufacturers include: tablet, capsule, oral suspension, oral solution, oral drops

Tablet
- ▸ **Colecalciferol (Non-proprietary)**
  Colecalciferol 400 unit Colecalciferol 400unit tablets | 30 tablet no price available | 60 tablet £15.50
  Colecalciferol 1000 unit Colecalciferol 1,000unit tablets | 28 tablet £20.95-£22.95 | 30 tablet no price available | 90 tablet £34.50 | 180 tablet no price available
  Colecalciferol 5000 unit tablets | 100 tablet £3.50
  Colecalciferol 10000 unit Colecalciferol 10,000unit tablets | 30 tablet £36.00
  Colecalciferol 20000 unit Colecalciferol 20,000unit tablets | 20 tablet £36.00 | 30 tablet no price available

- ▸ **Desunin (Meda Pharmaceuticals Ltd)**
  Colecalciferol 800 unit Desunin 800unit tablets | 30 tablet [PoM] £3.60 DT price = £3.60 | 90 tablet [PoM] £10.17
  Colecalciferol 4000 unit Desunin 4,000unit tablets | 70 tablet [PoM] £15.90
- ▸ **Stexerol-D3 (ProStrakan Ltd)**
  Colecalciferol 1000 unit Stexerol-D3 1,000unit tablets | 28 tablet [PoM] £2.95
  Colecalciferol 25000 unit Stexerol-D3 25,000unit tablets | 12 tablet [PoM] £17.00

Chewable tablet
- ▸ **Colecalciferol (Non-proprietary)**
  Colecalciferol 280 unit chewable tablets | 180 tablet £5.00
  Colecalciferol 1000 unit chewable tablets | 100 tablet no price available

Orodispersible tablet
- ▸ **Colecalciferol (Non-proprietary)**
  Colecalciferol 2000 unit tablets sugar-free | 120 tablet £4.88

Capsule
CAUTIONARY AND ADVISORY LABELS 25
- ▸ **Colecalciferol (Non-proprietary)**
  Colecalciferol 400 unit Colecalciferol 400unit capsules | 30 capsule no price available
  Colecalciferol 500 unit Vitamin D3 500IU capsules | 90 capsule [GSL] no price available
  Colecalciferol 600 unit Colecalciferol 600unit capsules | 30 capsule no price available
  Colecalciferol 800 unit Colecalciferol 800unit capsules | 30 capsule £3.60 DT price = £3.60
  Colecalciferol 1000 unit Colecalciferol 1,000unit capsules | 28 capsule £36.50 | 30 capsule £29.50
  Colecalciferol 2200 unit Colecalciferol 2,200unit capsules | 30 capsule no price available
  Colecalciferol 2500 unit Colecalciferol 2,500unit capsules | 30 capsule no price available
  Colecalciferol 3000 unit Colecalciferol 3,000unit capsules | 30 capsule no price available
  Colecalciferol 4000 unit capsules | 60 capsule no price available | 120 capsule no price available
  Colecalciferol 5000 unit Colecalciferol 5,000unit capsules | 30 capsule no price available | 40 capsule no price available | 100 capsule [PoM] no price available
  Colecalciferol 10000 unit Colecalciferol 10,000unit capsules | 30 capsule no price available
  Colecalciferol 20000 unit Colecalciferol 20,000unit capsules | 20 capsule £37.99 | 30 capsule £35.99 DT price = £29.00 | 30 capsule [PoM] £29.00 DT price = £29.00
  Colecalciferol 30000 unit Colecalciferol 30,000unit capsules | 10 capsule no price available
  Colecalciferol 50000 unit Colecalciferol 50,000unit capsules | 10 capsule £36.00 | 100 capsule [PoM] no price available
- ▸ **Aviticol (Colonis Pharma Ltd)**
  Colecalciferol 800 unit Aviticol 800unit capsules | 30 capsule [PoM] £3.60 DT price = £3.60
  Colecalciferol 1000 unit Aviticol 1,000unit capsules | 30 capsule [PoM] £3.16
  Colecalciferol 20000 unit Aviticol 20,000unit capsules | 30 capsule [PoM] £29.00 DT price = £29.00
- ▸ **Fultium-D3 (Internis Pharmaceuticals Ltd)**
  Colecalciferol 800 unit Fultium-D3 800unit capsules | 30 capsule [PoM] £3.60 DT price = £3.60 | 90 capsule [PoM] £8.85
  Colecalciferol 3200 unit Fultium-D3 3,200unit capsules | 30 capsule [PoM] £13.32 DT price = £13.32 | 90 capsule [PoM] £39.96
  Colecalciferol 20000 unit Fultium-D3 20,000unit capsules | 15 capsule [PoM] £17.04 DT price = £17.04 | 30 capsule [PoM] £29.00 DT price = £29.00
- ▸ **Plenachol (Auden McKenzie (Pharma Division) Ltd)**
  Colecalciferol 20000 unit Plenachol 20,000unit capsules | 10 capsule [PoM] £9.00
  Colecalciferol 40000 unit Plenachol 40,000unit capsules | 10 capsule [PoM] £15.00 DT price = £15.00
- ▸ **Strivit-D3 (Strides Arcolab International Ltd)**
  Colecalciferol 800 unit Strivit-D3 800unit capsules | 30 capsule [PoM] £2.34 DT price = £3.60

9

Blood and nutrition

Blood and nutrition

9

Oral solution
CAUTIONARY AND ADVISORY LABELS 21
▸ Colecalciferol (Non-proprietary)
Colecalciferol 3000 unit per 1 ml Colecalciferol 3,000units/ml oral solution | 100 ml PoM £119.70–£144.00 DT price = £144.00
Colecalciferol 10000 unit per 1 ml Colecalciferol 10,000units/ml oral solution | 10 ml no price available
▸ InVita D3 (Consilient Health Ltd)
Colecalciferol 25000 unit per 1 ml InVita D3 25,000units/1ml oral solution sugar-free | 3 ampoule PoM £4.45 DT price = £4.45
Colecalciferol 50000 unit per 1 ml InVita D3 50,000units/1ml oral solution sugar-free | 3 ampoule PoM £6.25 DT price = £6.25
▸ Thorens (Galen Ltd)
Colecalciferol 10000 unit per 1 ml Thorens 25,000units/2.5ml oral solution sugar-free | 2.5 ml PoM £1.55 DT price = £1.55 sugar-free | 10 ml PoM £5.85 DT price = £5.85

Oral drops
▸ Colecalciferol (Non-proprietary)
Colecalciferol 20000 unit per 1 ml Vigantol 20,000units/ml oral drops | 10 ml no price available
Colecalciferol 200 unit per 1 drop Natures Aid Vitamin D3 200units/drop for infants and children oral drops sugar-free | 50 ml £3.86
Healthaid Vitamin D3 200units/drop oral drops sugar-free | 15 ml £4.46
▸ Fultium-D3 (Internis Pharmaceuticals Ltd)
Colecalciferol 2740 unit per 1 ml Fultium-D3 2,740units/ml oral drops sugar-free | 25 ml PoM £10.70
▸ InVita D3 (Consilient Health Ltd)
Colecalciferol 2400 unit per 1 ml InVita D3 2,400units/ml oral drops sugar-free | 10 ml PoM £3.60
▸ Thorens (Galen Ltd)
Colecalciferol 10000 unit per 1 ml Thorens 10,000units/ml oral drops sugar-free | 10 ml PoM £5.85 DT price = £5.85

Colecalciferol with calcium carbonate

The properties listed below are those particular to the combination only. For the properties of the components please consider, colecalciferol p. 589, calcium carbonate p. 552.

● **INDICATIONS AND DOSE**

Prevention and treatment of vitamin D and calcium deficiency
▸ BY MOUTH
▸ Child: Dosed according to the deficit or daily maintenance requirements (consult product literature)

● UNLICENSED USE Adcal-D3 ® and Calceos ® are not licensed for use in children under 12 years. Cacit ®D3, Calcichew-D₃ ® Forte, Calcichew-D₃ ® and Kalcipos-D ® not licensed for use in children (age range not specified by manufacturers). Accrete D3 ® and Natecal D3 ® not licensed for use in children under 18 years.

● PRESCRIBING AND DISPENSING INFORMATION Accrete D3 ® contains calcium carbonate 1.5 g (calcium 600 mg or Ca^{2+} 15 mmol), colecalciferol 10 micrograms (400 units); Adcal-D3® tablets contain calcium carbonate 1.5 g (calcium 600 mg or Ca^{2+} 15 mmol), colecalciferol 10 micrograms (400 units); Cacit® D3 contains calcium carbonate 1.25 g (calcium 500 mg or Ca^{2+} 12.5 mmol), colecalciferol 11 micrograms (440 units)/sachet; Calceos ® contains calcium carbonate 1.25 g (calcium 500 mg or Ca^{2+} 12.5 mmol), colecalciferol 10 micrograms (400 units); Calcichew-D3 ® tablets contain calcium carbonate 1.25 g (calcium 500 mg or Ca^{2+} 12.5 mmol), colecalciferol 5 micrograms (200 units); Calcichew-D3® Forte tablets contain calcium carbonate 1.25 g (calcium 500 mg or Ca^{2+} 12.5 mmol), colecalciferol 10 micrograms (400 units); Calcichew-D3 ® 500 mg/400 unit caplets contain calcium carbonate (calcium 500 mg or Ca^{2+} 12.5 mmol), colecalciferol 10 micrograms (400 units); Kalcipos-D ® contains calcium carbonate (calcium 500 mg or Ca^{2+} 12.5 mmol), colecalciferol 20 micrograms (800 units);

Natecal D3 ® contains calcium carbonate 1.5 g (calcium 600 mg or Ca^{2+} 15 mmol), colecalciferol 10 micrograms (400 units); consult product literature for details of other available products.

Flavours of chewable and soluble forms may include orange, lemon, aniseed, peppermint, molasses, or tutti-frutti.

● **MEDICINAL FORMS**
There can be variation in the licensing of different medicines containing the same drug.

Tablet
EXCIPIENTS: May contain Propylene glycol
▸ Colecalciferol with calcium carbonate (Non-proprietary)
Calcium carbonate 400 mg, Colecalciferol 100 unit tablets | 30 tablet no price available | no price available
▸ Accrete D3 (Internis Pharmaceuticals Ltd)
Calcium carbonate 1.5 gram, Colecalciferol 400 unit Accrete D3 tablets | 60 tablet P £2.95 DT price = £2.95
▸ Adcal-D3 (ProStrakan Ltd)
Calcium carbonate 750 mg, Colecalciferol 200 unit Adcal-D3 750mg/200unit caplets | 112 tablet P £2.95 DT price = £2.95
▸ Calcichew D3 (Forum Health Products Ltd)
Calcium carbonate 1.25 gram, Colecalciferol 400 unit Calcichew D3 500mg/400unit caplets | 100 tablet P £7.43 DT price = £7.43
▸ Kalcipos-D (Meda Pharmaceuticals Ltd)
Calcium carbonate 1.25 gram, Colecalciferol 800 unit Kalcipos-D 500mg/800unit tablets | 30 tablet PoM £4.21 DT price = £4.21

Chewable tablet
CAUTIONARY AND ADVISORY LABELS 24
EXCIPIENTS: May contain Aspartame
▸ Colecalciferol with calcium carbonate (Non-proprietary)
Calcium carbonate 1.25 gram, Colecalciferol 400 unit Colecalciferol 400unit / Calcium carbonate 1.25g chewable tablets | 100 tablet £14.75
Calcium carbonate 1.5 gram, Colecalciferol 400 unit Colecalciferol 400unit / Calcium carbonate 1.5g chewable tablets | 60 tablet P £4.38
▸ Adcal-D3 (ProStrakan Ltd)
Calcium carbonate 1.5 gram, Colecalciferol 400 unit Adcal-D3 Lemon chewable tablets | 56 tablet P £3.65 DT price = £3.65 | 112 tablet P £7.49
Adcal-D3 chewable tablets tutti frutti | 56 tablet P £3.65 DT price = £3.65 | 112 tablet P £7.49
▸ Calceos (Galen Ltd)
Calcium carbonate 1.25 gram, Colecalciferol 400 unit Calceos 500mg/400unit chewable tablets | 60 tablet P £3.58 DT price = £4.24
▸ Calci-D (Consilient Health Ltd)
Calcium carbonate 2.5 gram, Colecalciferol 1000 iu Calci-D 1000mg/1,000unit chewable tablets | 28 tablet PoM £2.25
▸ Calcichew D3 (Forum Health Products Ltd)
Calcium carbonate 2.5 gram, Colecalciferol 800 iu Calcichew D3 1000mg/800unit Once Daily chewable tablets | 30 tablet P £6.75 DT price = £6.75
Calcium carbonate 1.25 gram, Colecalciferol 200 unit Calcichew D3 chewable tablets | 100 tablet P £7.68 DT price = £7.68
▸ Calcichew D3 Forte (Forum Health Products Ltd)
Calcium carbonate 1.25 gram, Colecalciferol 400 unit Calcichew D3 Forte chewable tablets | 60 tablet P £4.24 DT price = £4.24 | 100 tablet P £7.08
▸ Evacal D3 (Teva UK Ltd)
Calcium carbonate 1.5 gram, Colecalciferol 400 unit Evacal D3 1500mg/400unit chewable tablets | 56 tablet P £2.75 DT price = £3.65 | 112 tablet P £5.50
▸ Kalcipos-D (Meda Pharmaceuticals Ltd)
Calcium carbonate 1.25 gram, Colecalciferol 800 unit Kalcipos-D 500mg/800unit chewable tablets | 30 tablet PoM £4.21 DT price = £4.21
▸ Natecal (Chiesi Ltd)
Calcium carbonate 1.5 gram, Colecalciferol 400 unit Natecal D3 600mg/400unit chewable tablets | 60 tablet P £3.63
▸ TheiCal-D3 (Stirling Anglian Pharmaceuticals Ltd)
Calcium carbonate 2.5 gram, Colecalciferol 880 unit TheiCal-D3 1000mg/880unit chewable tablets | 30 tablet P £2.95 DT price = £2.95

Effervescent tablet

CAUTIONARY AND ADVISORY LABELS 13
- Adcal-D3 (ProStrakan Ltd)

  Calcium carbonate 1.5 gram, Colecalciferol 400 unit Adcal-D3 Dissolve 1500mg/400unit effervescent tablets | 56 tablet [P] £5.99 DT price = £5.99

Effervescent granules

CAUTIONARY AND ADVISORY LABELS 13
- Colecalciferol with calcium carbonate (Non-proprietary)

  Calcium carbonate 2.5 gram, Colecalciferol 880 unit Colecalciferol 880unit / Calcium carbonate 2.5g effervescent granules sachets | 24 sachet [PoM] no price available
- Cacit D3 (Warner Chilcott UK Ltd)

  Calcium carbonate 1.25 gram, Colecalciferol 440 unit Cacit D3 effervescent granules sachets | 30 sachet [P] £4.06 DT price = £4.06

Colecalciferol with calcium phosphate

The properties listed below are those particular to the combination only. For the properties of the components please consider, colecalciferol p. 589, calcium phosphate p. 554.

- **INDICATIONS AND DOSE**

Calcium and vitamin D deficiency
- BY MOUTH
- Child: (consult product literature)

- **MEDICINAL FORMS**
  There can be variation in the licensing of different medicines containing the same drug.

Powder

CAUTIONARY AND ADVISORY LABELS 13, 21
- Calfovit D3 (A. Menarini Farmaceutica Internazionale SRL)

  Calcium phosphate 3.1 gram, Colecalciferol 800 unit Calfovit D3 oral powder sachets | 30 sachet [P] £4.32 DT price = £4.32

F 588

Ergocalciferol

(Calciferol; Vitamin D₂)

- **INDICATIONS AND DOSE**

Nutritional vitamin-D deficiency rickets
- BY MOUTH
- Child 1–5 months: 3000 units daily, dose to be adjusted as necessary
- Child 6 months–11 years: 6000 units daily, dose to be adjusted as necessary
- Child 12–17 years: 10 000 units daily, dose to be adjusted as necessary

Nutritional or physiological supplement | Prevention of rickets
- BY MOUTH
- Neonate: 400 units daily.
- Child: 400–600 units daily

Vitamin D deficiency in intestinal malabsorption or in chronic liver disease
- BY MOUTH, OR BY INTRAMUSCULAR INJECTION
- Child 1–11 years: 10 000–25 000 units daily, dose to be adjusted as necessary
- Child 12–17 years: 10 000–40 000 units daily, dose to be adjusted as necessary

- CAUTIONS Take care to ensure correct dose in infants
- RENAL IMPAIRMENT

Monitoring
Monitor plasma-calcium concentration in renal impairment.

- MONITORING REQUIREMENTS Monitor plasma-calcium concentration in patients receiving high doses.

- PRESCRIBING AND DISPENSING INFORMATION The BP directs that when calciferol is prescribed or demanded, colecalciferol or ergocalciferol should be dispensed or supplied.

  When the strength of the tablets ordered or prescribed is not clear, the intention of the prescriber with respect to the strength (expressed in micrograms or milligrams per tablet) should be ascertained.

- MEDICINAL FORMS
  There can be variation in the licensing of different medicines containing the same drug. Forms available from special-order manufacturers include: tablet, oral suspension, oral solution, solution for injection

Tablet
- Ergocalciferol (Non-proprietary)

  Ergocalciferol 12.5 microgram Ergocalciferol 12.5microgram tablets | 30 tablet no price available
- Ergoral (Cubic Pharmaceuticals Ltd)

  Ergocalciferol 125 microgram Ergoral D2 5,000unit tablets | 30 tablet £19.95

  Ergocalciferol 250 microgram Ergoral D2 10,000unit tablets | 30 tablet £23.95

Capsule
- Ergocalciferol (Non-proprietary)

  Ergocalciferol 1.25 mg Ergocalciferol 1.25mg capsules | 30 capsule no price available | 50 capsule [PoM] £230.00
- Eciferol (Rhodes Pharma Ltd)

  Ergocalciferol 1.25 mg Eciferol D2 50,000unit capsules | 10 capsule £29.99
- Ergoral (Cubic Pharmaceuticals Ltd)

  Ergocalciferol 1.25 mg Ergoral D2 50,000unit capsules | 10 capsule £19.95

Oral solution
- Ergocalciferol (Non-proprietary)

  Ergocalciferol 1500 unit per 1 ml Uvesterol D 1,500units/ml oral solution sugar-free | 20 ml [PoM] no price available

  Ergocalciferol 20000 unit per 1 ml Sterogyl 100,000units/5ml oral solution | 20 ml [PoM] no price available DT price = £181.96
- Eciferol (Rhodes Pharma Ltd)

  Ergocalciferol 3000 unit per 1 ml Eciferol D2 3,000units/ml liquid | 60 ml £55.00 DT price = £111.25

Solution for injection
- Ergocalciferol (Non-proprietary)

  Ergocalciferol 300000 unit per 1 ml Ergocalciferol 300,000units/1ml solution for injection ampoules | 10 ampoule [PoM] £93.50

  Ergocalciferol 400000 unit per 1 ml Sterogyl 15H 600,000units/1.5ml solution for injection ampoules | 1 ampoule [PoM] no price available

Ergocalciferol with calcium lactate and calcium phosphate

(Calcium and vitamin D)

The properties listed below are those particular to the combination only. For the properties of the components please consider, ergocalciferol above, calcium lactate p. 554.

- **INDICATIONS AND DOSE**

Prevention of calcium and vitamin D deficiency | Treatment of calcium and vitamin D deficiency
- BY MOUTH
- Child: (consult product literature)

- UNLICENSED USE Calcium and Ergocalciferol tablets not licensed for use in children under 6 years.

- DIRECTIONS FOR ADMINISTRATION Tablets may be crushed before administration, or may be chewed.

- PRESCRIBING AND DISPENSING INFORMATION Each tablet contains calcium lactate 300 mg, calcium phosphate 150 mg (calcium 97 mg or Ca^{2+}2.4 mmol), ergocalciferol 10 micrograms (400 units).

9

- PATIENT AND CARER ADVICE Patient or carers should be given advice on how to administer calcium and ergocalciferol tablets.

- MEDICINAL FORMS
There can be variation in the licensing of different medicines containing the same drug.
Tablet
  ▸ Ergocalciferol with calcium lactate and calcium phosphate (Non-proprietary)
  Ergocalciferol 10 microgram, Calcium phosphate 150 mg, Calcium lactate 300 mg Calcium and Ergocalciferol tablets | 28 tablet no price available DT price = £15.43 | 28 tablet P £15.39 DT price = £15.43 | 500 tablet P no price available

VITAMINS AND TRACE ELEMENTS 〉 VITAMIN E

▌Alpha tocopherol

(Tocopherol)

- ● INDICATIONS AND DOSE
Vitamin E deficiency because of malabsorption in congenital or hereditary chronic cholestasis
  ▸ BY MOUTH USING ORAL SOLUTION
  ▸ Neonate: 17 mg/kg daily, dose to be adjusted as necessary.
  ▸ Child: 17 mg/kg daily, dose to be adjusted as necessary

- CONTRA-INDICATIONS Preterm neonates
- CAUTIONS Predisposition to thrombosis
- INTERACTIONS → Appendix 1 (Vitamin E).
- SIDE-EFFECTS
  ▸ Common or very common Diarrhoea
  ▸ Uncommon Alopecia · asthenia · disturbances in serum-potassium concentration · disturbances in serum-sodium concentration · headache · pruritus · rash
- PREGNANCY Manufacturer advises caution, no evidence of harm in *animal* studies.
- BREAST FEEDING Manufacturer advises use only if potential benefit outweighs risk—no information available.
- HEPATIC IMPAIRMENT Manufacturer advises caution—no information available. Manufacturer advises monitor closely in hepatic impairment.
- RENAL IMPAIRMENT Manufacturer advises caution. Risk of renal toxicity due to polyethylene glycol content. Manufacturer advises monitor closely in renal impairment.
- PRESCRIBING AND DISPENSING INFORMATION
Tocofersolan is a water-soluble form of D-alpha tocopherol.

- MEDICINAL FORMS
There can be variation in the licensing of different medicines containing the same drug.
Oral solution
  ▸ Vedrop (Orphan Europe (UK) Ltd) ▼
  D-alpha tocopherol (as Tocofersolan) 50 mg per 1 ml Vedrop 50mg/ml oral solution sugar-free | 20 ml PoM £54.55 sugar-free | 60 ml PoM £163.65

▌Alpha tocopheryl acetate

(Tocopherol)

- ● INDICATIONS AND DOSE
Vitamin E deficiency
  ▸ BY MOUTH
  ▸ Neonate: 10 mg/kg once daily.
  ▸ Child: 2–10 mg/kg daily, increased if necessary up to 20 mg/kg daily
Malabsorption in cystic fibrosis
  ▸ BY MOUTH
  ▸ Child 1–11 months: 50 mg once daily, dose to be adjusted as necessary, to be taken with food and pancreatic enzymes
  ▸ Child 1–11 years: 100 mg once daily, dose to be adjusted as necessary, to be taken with food and pancreatic enzymes
  ▸ Child 12–17 years: 100–200 mg once daily, dose to be adjusted as necessary, to be taken with food and pancreatic enzymes
Vitamin E deficiency in cholestasis and severe liver disease
  ▸ BY MOUTH
  ▸ Neonate: 10 mg/kg daily.
  ▸ Child 1 month–11 years: Initially 100 mg daily, adjusted according to response, increased if necessary up to 200 mg/kg daily
  ▸ Child 12–17 years: Initially 200 mg daily, adjusted according to response, increased if necessary up to 200 mg/kg daily
  ▸ BY INTRAMUSCULAR INJECTION
  ▸ Neonate: 10 mg/kg once a month.
  ▸ Child: 10 mg/kg once a month (max. per dose 100 mg)
Malabsorption in abetalipoproteinaemia
  ▸ BY MOUTH
  ▸ Neonate: 100 mg/kg once daily.
  ▸ Child: 50–100 mg/kg once daily

- CAUTIONS Increased risk of necrotising enterocolitis in neonate weighing less than 1.5 kg or in a preterm neonate · predisposition to thrombosis
- INTERACTIONS → Appendix 1 (Vitamins).
- SIDE-EFFECTS Abdominal pain (particularly with high doses) · diarrhoea (particularly with high doses)
- PREGNANCY No evidence of safety of high doses.
- BREAST FEEDING Excreted in milk; minimal risk, although caution with large doses.
- MONITORING REQUIREMENTS Increased bleeding tendency in vitamin-K deficient patients or those taking anticoagulants (prothrombin time and INR should be monitored).
- DIRECTIONS FOR ADMINISTRATION
  ▸ In neonates Consider dilution of oral suspension for use in neonates due to high osmolality.

- MEDICINAL FORMS
There can be variation in the licensing of different medicines containing the same drug. Forms available from special-order manufacturers include: chewable tablet
Chewable tablet
  ▸ Alpha tocopheryl acetate (Non-proprietary)
  Alpha tocopheryl acetate 100 mg Alpha tocopheryl acetate 100mg chewable tablets | 30 tablet no price available
  ▸ E-Tabs (Ennogen Healthcare Ltd)
  Alpha tocopheryl acetate 100 mg E-Tabs 100mg chewable tablets | 30 tablet £87.30

Capsule

▸ Alpha tocopheryl acetate (Non-proprietary)
   Alpha tocopherol 100 unit capsules | 30 capsule £0.59
   Alpha tocopherol 200 unit capsules | 100 capsule £6.60
   Alpha tocopherol 250 unit capsules | 100 capsule £6.11
   Alpha tocopherol 400 unit capsules | 30 capsule £6.69 |
   60 capsule £11.72
   Alpha tocopherol 500 unit capsules | 60 capsule £7.75
   Alpha tocopherol 600 unit capsules | 30 capsule no price
   available
   Alpha tocopherol 1000 unit Ncapsules | 30 capsule £6.64
▸ E-Caps (Ennogen Healthcare Ltd)
   Alpha tocopherol 75 unit E-Caps 75unit capsules | 100 capsule
   £109.50
   Alpha tocopherol 100 unit E-Caps 100unit capsules | 30 capsule
   £84.40
   Alpha tocopherol 200 unit E-Caps 200unit capsules | 30 capsule
   £89.50
   Alpha tocopherol 400 unit E-Caps 400unit capsules | 30 capsule
   £128.50
   Alpha tocopherol 1000 unit E-Caps 1,000unit capsules |
   30 capsule £130.20
▸ Vita-E (Typharm Ltd)
   Alpha tocopherol 75 unit Vita-E 75unit capsules | 100 capsule
   £3.69
   Alpha tocopherol 200 unit Vita-E 200unit capsules | 30 capsule
   £2.84 | 100 capsule £8.76
   Alpha tocopherol 400 unit Vita-E 400unit capsules | 30 capsule
   £4.27 | 100 capsule £13.93

Oral suspension
EXCIPIENTS: May contain Sucrose
▸ Alpha tocopheryl acetate (Non-proprietary)
   Alpha tocopheryl acetate 100 mg per 1 ml Alpha tocopheryl
   acetate 500mg/5ml oral suspension | 100 ml [GSL] £53.50 DT price =
   £53.50

Solution for injection
▸ Alpha tocopheryl acetate (Non-proprietary)
   Alpha tocopheryl acetate 50 mg per 1 ml E-Vicotrat 100mg/2ml
   solution for injection ampoules | 10 ampoule [PoM] no price available

VITAMINS AND TRACE ELEMENTS ⟩ VITAMIN K

Menadiol sodium phosphate

● **INDICATIONS AND DOSE**

Supplementation in vitamin K malabsorption
▸ BY MOUTH
▸ **Child 1-11 years:** 5–10 mg daily, dose to be adjusted as
   necessary
▸ **Child 12-17 years:** 10–20 mg daily, dose to be adjusted as
   necessary

● **CONTRA-INDICATIONS** Infants · neonates

● **CAUTIONS** G6PD deficiency (risk of haemolysis) · vitamin E
deficiency (risk of haemolysis)

● **INTERACTIONS** → Appendix 1 (Vitamins).

● **PREGNANCY** Avoid in late pregnancy and labour unless
benefit outweighs risk of neonatal haemolytic anaemia,
hyperbilirubinaemia, and kernicterus in neonate.

● **MEDICINAL FORMS**
There can be variation in the licensing of different medicines
containing the same drug. Forms available from special-order
manufacturers include: oral suspension, oral solution

Tablet
▸ Menadiol sodium phosphate (Non-proprietary)
   Menadiol phosphate (as Menadiol sodium phosphate)
   10 mg Menadiol 10mg tablets | 100 tablet [P] £169.00 DT price =
   £169.00

Phytomenadione

(Vitamin K₁)

● **INDICATIONS AND DOSE**

Neonatal prophylaxis of vitamin-K deficiency bleeding
▸ BY INTRAMUSCULAR INJECTION
▸ **Preterm neonate:** 400 micrograms/kg (max. per dose
   1 mg) for 1 dose, to be given at birth, the intravenous
   route may be used in preterm neonates with very low
   birth-weight if intramuscular injection is not possible,
   however, it may not provide the prolonged protection of
   the intramuscular injection, any neonate receiving
   intravenous vitamin K should be given subsequent oral
   doses.

▸ **Neonate:** 1 mg for 1 dose, to be given at birth.

**Neonatal prophylaxis of vitamin-K deficiency bleeding in
healthy babies who are not at particular risk of bleeding
disorders**
▸ BY MOUTH USING CAPSULES
▸ **Neonate:** 1 mg for 1 dose at birth (to protect from the risk
   of vitamin K deficiency bleeding in the first week).

**Neonatal prophylaxis of vitamin-K deficiency bleeding in
healthy babies who are not at particular risk of bleeding
disorders (exclusively breast-fed babies)**
▸ BY MOUTH USING CAPSULES
▸ **Neonate:** Initially 1 mg for 1 dose at birth, then 1 mg
   every 1 week for 12 weeks.

**Neonatal hypoprothrombinaemia | Vitamin-K deficiency
bleeding**
▸ BY INTRAVENOUS INJECTION
▸ **Neonate:** 1 mg every 8 hours if required.

Neonatal biliary atresia and liver disease
▸ BY MOUTH
▸ **Neonate:** 1 mg daily.

**Reversal of coumarin anticoagulation when continued
anticoagulation required or if no significant bleeding—
seek specialist advice**
▸ BY INTRAVENOUS INJECTION
▸ **Child:** 15–30 micrograms/kg (max. per dose 1 mg) for
   1 dose, dose may be repeated as necessary

**Reversal of coumarin anticoagulation when
anticoagulation not required or if significant bleeding—
seek specialist advice | Treatment of haemorrhage
associated with vitamin-K deficiency—seek specialist
advice**
▸ BY INTRAVENOUS INJECTION
▸ **Child:** 250–300 micrograms/kg (max. per dose 10 mg)
   for 1 dose

KONAKION® MM PAEDIATRIC
**Neonatal prophylaxis of vitamin-K deficiency bleeding in
healthy babies who are not at risk of bleeding disorders**
▸ BY MOUTH
▸ **Neonate:** Initially 2 mg for 1 dose at birth, then 2 mg
   after 4–7 days.

**Neonatal prophylaxis of vitamin-K deficiency bleeding in
healthy babies who are not at risk of bleeding disorders
(exclusively breast fed babies)**
▸ BY MOUTH
▸ **Neonate:** Initially 2 mg for 1 dose at birth, then 2 mg
   after 4–7 days for a further 1 dose, then 2 mg for a
   further 1 dose 1 month after birth.

9

Blood and nutrition

- CAUTIONS Intravenous injections should be given very slowly—risk of vascular collapse

KONAKION® MM PAEDIATRIC
▸ With intravenous use Parenteral administration in premature infant or neonate of less than 2.5 kg (increased risk of kernicterus)

- INTERACTIONS → Appendix 1 (Vitamins).

- SIDE-EFFECTS

KONAKION® MM Anaphylactoid reactions

- PREGNANCY Use if potential benefit outweighs risk.

- BREAST FEEDING Present in milk.

- HEPATIC IMPAIRMENT

KONAKION® MM Caution—glycocholic acid may displace bilirubin.

- DIRECTIONS FOR ADMINISTRATION
▸ With oral use in neonates The contents of one capsule should be administered by cutting the narrow tubular tip off and squeezing the liquid contents into the mouth; if the baby spits out the dose or is sick within three hours of administration a replacement dose should be given.

KONAKION® MM PAEDIATRIC *Konakion® MM Paediatric* may be administered *by mouth* or *by intramuscular injection* or *by intravenous injection.*
     For *intravenous injection*, may be diluted with Glucose 5% if necessary.

KONAKION® MM *Konakion® MM* may be administered by slow intravenous injection or by intravenous infusion in glucose 5%; **not** for intramuscular injection.

- MEDICINAL FORMS
There can be variation in the licensing of different medicines containing the same drug. Forms available from special-order manufacturers include: tablet, oral suspension, oral solution, drops

Capsule
▸ Neokay (Neoceuticals Ltd)
   Phytomenadione 1 mg NeoKay 1mg capsules | 12 capsule PoM
   £3.95 DT price = £3.95 | 100 capsule PoM £34.00

Drops
▸ Neokay (Neoceuticals Ltd)
   Phytomenadione 200 microgram per 1 ml NeoKay
   200micrograms/ml oral drops sugar-free | 25 ml £3.95

Solution for injection
EXCIPIENTS: May contain Glycocholic acid, lecithin
▸ Konakion MM (Roche Products Ltd)
   Phytomenadione 10 mg per 1 ml Konakion MM Paediatric
   2mg/0.2ml solution for injection ampoules | 5 ampoule PoM £4.71
   Konakion MM 10mg/1ml solution for injection ampoules |
   10 ampoule PoM £3.78 DT price = £3.78

7.1 Neural tube defects (prevention in pregnancy)

Neural tube defects (prevention in pregnancy)

Prevention in pregnancy

Folic acid supplements p. 533 taken before and during pregnancy can reduce the occurrence of neural tube defects. The risk of a neural tube defect occurring in a child should be assessed and folic acid given as follows:

- Women at a low risk of conceiving a child with a neural tube defect should be advised to take folic acid as a medicinal or food supplement daily (at low-risk group dose) before conception and until week 12 of pregnancy. Women who have not been taking folic acid and who suspect they are pregnant should start at once and continue until week 12 of pregnancy.

- Couples are at a high risk of conceiving a child with a neural tube defect if either partner has a neural tube defect (or either partner has a family history of neural tube defects), if they have had a previous pregnancy affected by a neural tube defect, or if the woman has *coeliac disease* (or other malabsorption state), diabetes mellitus, sickle-cell anaemia, or is taking **antiepileptic medicines**.

- Women in the high-risk group who wish to become pregnant (or who are at risk of becoming pregnant) should be advised to take folic acid daily (at high-risk group dose) and continue until week 12 of pregnancy (women with sickle-cell disease should continue taking their normal dose of folic acid (or to increase the dose to high-risk group daily dose) and continue this throughout pregnancy).

There is no justification for prescribing multiple-ingredient vitamin preparations containing vitamin B_{12} or folic acid.

Chapter 10
Musculoskeletal system

CONTENTS

1	**Arthritis**	page 595
2	**Neuromuscular disorders**	601
2.1	Myasthenia gravis	601
2.2	Spasticity	603

3	**Pain and inflammation in musculoskeletal disorders**	page 604
4	**Soft tissue and joint disorders**	616
4.1	Local inflammation of joints and soft tissue	616
4.2	Soft tissue disorders	617

1 Arthritis

Juvenile idiopathic arthritis

Management

Rheumatic diseases require symptomatic treatment to relieve pain, swelling, and stiffness, together with treatment to control and suppress disease activity. Treatment of juvenile idiopathic arthritis may involve Non-steroidal anti-inflammatory drugs (NSAIDs) p. 604, a disease modifying anti-rheumatic drug (DMARD) such as methotrexate p. 506 or a cytokine modulator, and intra-articular, intravenous, or oral corticosteroids.

Rheumatic disease, suppressing drugs

Overview

Certain drugs, such as methotrexate p. 506, cytokine modulators, and sulfasalazine p. 29, are used to suppress the disease process in *juvenile idiopathic arthritis* (juvenile chronic arthritis); these drugs are known as disease-modifying antirheumatic drugs (DMARDs). In children, disease modifying antirheumatic drugs should be used under specialist supervision.

Some children with juvenile idiopathic arthritis do not require disease-modifying antirheumatic drugs. Methotrexate is effective in juvenile idiopathic arthritis; sulfasalazine is an alternative but should be avoided in *systemic-onset juvenile idiopathic arthritis*. Gold and penicillamine p. 574 are no longer used. Cytokine modulators have a role in *polyarticular juvenile idiopathic arthritis*.

Unlike NSAIDs, disease-modifying antirheumatic drugs can affect the progression of disease but they may require 4–6 months of treatment for a full therapeutic response. Response to a disease-modifying antirheumatic drug may allow the dose of the NSAID to be reduced.

Disease-modifying antirheumatic drugs can improve not only the symptoms of inflammatory joint disease but also extra-articular manifestations. They reduce the erythrocyte sedimentation rate and C-reactive protein.

Antimalarials

The antimalarial hydroxychloroquine sulfate p. 596 is rarely used to treat juvenile idiopathic arthritis.

Hydroxychloroquine sulfate can also be useful for systemic or discoid lupus erythematosus, particularly involving the skin and joints, and in sarcoidosis.

Retinopathy rarely occurs provided that the recommended doses are not exceeded.

Mepacrine hydrochloride is used on rare occasions to treat discoid lupus erythematosus [unlicensed].

Drugs affecting the immune response

Methotrexate, given as a once weekly dose, is the disease-modifying antirheumatic drug of choice in the treatment of juvenile idiopathic arthritis and also has a role in juvenile dermatomyositis, vasculitis, uveitis, systemic lupus erythematosus, localised scleroderma, and sarcoidosis; for these indications it is given by the subcutaneous, oral, or rarely, the intramuscular route. Absorption from intramuscular or subcutaneous routes may be more predictable than from the oral route; if the oral route is ineffective subcutaneous administration is generally preferred. Folic acid may reduce mucosal or gastro-intestinal side-effects of methotrexate. The dosage regimen for folic acid p. 533 has not been established—in children over 2 years a weekly dose [unlicensed indication], may be given on a different day from the methotrexate.

Azathioprine p. 485 may be used in children for vasculitis which has failed to respond to other treatments, for the management of severe cases of *systemic lupus erythematosus* and other connective tissue disorders, in conjunction with corticosteroids for patients with severe or progressive renal disease, and in cases of *polymyositis* which are resistant to corticosteroids. Azathioprine has a corticosteroid-sparing effect in patients whose corticosteroid requirements are excessive.

Ciclosporin p. 486 is rarely used in juvenile idiopathic arthritis, connective tissue diseases, vasculitis, and uveitis; it may be considered if the condition has failed to respond to other treatments.

Cytokine modulators

Cytokine modulators should be used under specialist supervision.

Adalimumab p. 598, etanercept p. 600, and infliximab p. 30 inhibit the activity of tumour necrosis factor alpha (TNF-α). Adalimumab can be used for the management of active polyarticular juvenile idiopathic arthritis and enthesitis-related arthritis. Etanercept is licensed for the treatment of the following subtypes of juvenile idiopathic arthritis: polyarticular juvenile idiopathic arthritis in children who have had an inadequate response to methotrexate or who cannot tolerate it, oligoarthritis in children who have had an inadequate response to methotrexate or who cannot tolerate it, psoriatic arthritis in children over 12 years who have had an inadequate response to methotrexate or cannot tolerate it, and enthesitis-related arthritis in children over 12 years who have had an inadequate response to conventional therapy or cannot tolerate it. Infliximab has been used in refractory polyarticular juvenile idiopathic arthritis [unlicensed indication] when other treatments, such as etanercept, have failed.

Abatacept p. 598 prevents the full activation of T-lymphocytes; it can be used for the management of active polyarticular juvenile idiopathic arthritis. Abatacept is not recommended for use in combination with TNF inhibitors.

Canakinumab p. 491 inhibits the activity of interleukin-1 beta (IL-1β) and is licensed for the treatment of active systemic juvenile idiopathic arthritis in children over 2 years, when there has been an inadequate response to NSAIDs and systemic corticosteroids.

Tocilizumab p. 597 antagonises the actions of interleukin-6; it can be used for the management of active systemic juvenile idiopathic arthritis when there has been an inadequate response to NSAIDs and systemic corticosteroids and polyarticular juvenile idiopathic arthritis when there has been an inadequate response to methotrexate. Tocilizumab can be used in combination with methotrexate, or as monotherapy if methotrexate is not tolerated or is contra-indicated. Tocilizumab is not recommended for use with other cytokine modulators.

Sulfasalazine

Sulfasalazine has a beneficial effect in suppressing the inflammatory activity associated with some forms of juvenile idiopathic arthritis; it is generally not used in systemic-onset disease.

> **Drugs used for Arthritis not listed below** Diclofenac potassium, p. 605 · Diclofenac sodium, p. 605 · Etoricoxib, p. 607 · Flurbiprofen, p. 608 · Ibuprofen, p. 608 · Indometacin, p. 611 · Ketoprofen, p. 612 · Meloxicam, p. 613 · Naproxen, p. 614 · Piroxicam, p. 615

DISEASE-MODIFYING ANTI-RHEUMATIC DRUGS

▌ Hydroxychloroquine sulfate

● **INDICATIONS AND DOSE**

Active rheumatoid arthritis (including juvenile idiopathic arthritis) (administered on expert advice) | Systemic and discoid lupus erythematosus (administered on expert advice) | Dermatological conditions caused or aggravated by sunlight (administered on expert advice)
> ▸ BY MOUTH
> ▸ Child: 5–6.5 mg/kg once daily (max. per dose 400 mg), dose given based on ideal body-weight

● **UNLICENSED USE** *Plaquenil*® not licensed for use in children for dermatological conditions caused or aggravated by sunlight.

● **CAUTIONS** Acute porphyrias p. 562 · G6PD deficiency · may aggravate myasthenia gravis · may exacerbate psoriasis · neurological disorders (especially in those with a history of epilepsy) · severe gastro-intestinal disorders
CAUTIONS, FURTHER INFORMATION
> ▸ Screening for ocular toxicity Hydroxychloroquine is rarely associated with ocular toxicity. The British Society for Paediatric and Adolescent Rheumatology recommends that children should have their vision tested before long-term treatment with hydroxychloroquine and have an annual review of visual acuity. Children should be referred to an ophthalmologist if there is visual impairment, changes in visual acuity, or blurred vision. The Royal College of Ophthalmologists has recommended that a locally agreed protocol between the prescribing doctor and ophthalmologist be established to monitor the vision of these children. A review group convened by the Royal College of Ophthalmologists has updated guidelines for screening to prevent ocular toxicity on long-term

treatment with hydroxychloroquine (*Hydroxychloroquine and Ocular Toxicity: Recommendations on Screening* 2009); this includes the recommendation that a child treated for juvenile idiopathic arthritis should receive slit-lamp examination routinely to check for uveitis.

● **INTERACTIONS** → Appendix 1 (hydroxychloroquine). Concurrent use of hepatotoxic drugs should be avoided.

● **SIDE-EFFECTS**
> ▸ **Common or very common** Gastro-intestinal disturbances · headache · pruritus · rashes · skin reactions
> ▸ **Uncommon** Convulsions · discoloration of skin, nails, and mucous membranes · ECG changes · hair depigmentation · hair loss · keratopathy · ototoxicity · retinal damage · visual changes
> ▸ **Rare** Acute generalised exanthematous pustulosis · agranulocytosis · aplastic anaemia · blood disorders · cardiomyopathy · emotional disturbances · exfoliative dermatitis · hepatic damage · mental changes · myopathy · neuromyopathy · photosensitivity · psychosis · Stevens-Johnson syndrome · thrombocytopenia
> ▸ **Frequency not known** Angioedema · bronchospasm

Overdose
Hydroxychloroquine is very toxic in overdosage; overdosage is extremely hazardous and difficult to treat. Urgent advice from the National Poisons Information Service is essential. Life-threatening features include arrhythmias (which can have a very rapid onset) and convulsions (which can be intractable).

● **PREGNANCY** It is not necessary to withdraw an antimalarial drug during pregnancy if the rheumatic disease is well controlled; however, the manufacturer of hydroxychloroquine advises avoiding use.

● **BREAST FEEDING** Avoid—risk of toxicity in infant.

● **HEPATIC IMPAIRMENT** Caution in moderate to severe hepatic impairment.

● **RENAL IMPAIRMENT** Manufacturer advises caution. Monitor plasma-hydroxychloroquine concentration in severe renal impairment.

● **PRESCRIBING AND DISPENSING INFORMATION** To avoid excessive dosage in obese patients, the dose of hydroxychloroquine should be calculated on the basis of ideal body-weight.

● **PATIENT AND CARER ADVICE** Do not take antacids for at least 4 hours before or after hydroxychloroquine to reduce possible interference with hydroxychloroquine absorption

● **MEDICINAL FORMS**
There can be variation in the licensing of different medicines containing the same drug. Forms available from special-order manufacturers include: oral suspension, oral solution
Tablet
CAUTIONARY AND ADVISORY LABELS 21
> ▸ Hydroxychloroquine sulfate (Non-proprietary)
> Hydroxychloroquine sulfate 200 mg Hydroxychloroquine 200mg tablets | 60 tablet [PoM] £5.15 DT price = £3.83
> ▸ Plaquenil (Sanofi)
> Hydroxychloroquine sulfate 200 mg Plaquenil 200mg tablets | 60 tablet [PoM] £5.15 DT price = £3.83
> ▸ Quinoric (Bristol Laboratories Ltd)
> Hydroxychloroquine sulfate 200 mg Quinoric 200mg tablets | 60 tablet [PoM] £5.10 DT price = £3.83

IMMUNOSUPPRESSANTS > INTERLEUKIN INHIBITORS

Tocilizumab

31.5.2016

- **INDICATIONS AND DOSE**

Active systemic juvenile idiopathic arthritis (in combination with methotrexate or alone if methotrexate inappropriate) in children who have had an inadequate response to NSAIDs and systemic corticosteroids
- ▶ BY INTRAVENOUS INFUSION
- ▶ Child 2-17 years (body-weight up to 30 kg): 12 mg/kg every 2 weeks, review treatment if no improvement within 6 weeks
- ▶ Child 2-17 years (body-weight 30 kg and above): 8 mg/kg every 2 weeks, review treatment if no improvement within 6 weeks

Polyarticular juvenile idiopathic arthritis (in combination with methotrexate or alone if methotrexate inappropriate) in children who have had an inadequate response to methotrexate
- ▶ BY INTRAVENOUS INFUSION
- ▶ Child 2-17 years (body-weight up to 30 kg): 10 mg/kg every 4 weeks, review treatment if no improvement within 12 weeks
- ▶ Child 2-17 years (body-weight 30 kg and above): 8 mg/kg every 4 weeks, review treatment if no improvement within 12 weeks

- **CONTRA-INDICATIONS** Do not initiate if absolute neutrophil count less than 2×10^9/litre · severe active infection
- **CAUTIONS** History of diverticulitis · history of intestinal ulceration · history of recurrent or chronic infection (interrupt treatment if serious infection occurs) · low absolute neutrophil count · low platelet count · predisposition to infection (interrupt treatment if serious infection occurs)

CAUTIONS, FURTHER INFORMATION
- ▶ Tuberculosis Patients with latent tuberculosis should be treated with standard therapy before starting tocilizumab.
- **INTERACTIONS** → Appendix 1 (tocilizumab).
- **SIDE-EFFECTS**
- **Common or very common** Headache · hypercholesterolaemia · infection · neutropenia · raised hepatic transaminases · upper respiratory-tract infection
- **Frequency not known** Antibody formation · diarrhoea · infusion related reactions · nausea · thrombocytopenia

SIDE-EFFECTS, FURTHER INFORMATION
- ▶ Neutrophil and platelet counts Discontinue if absolute neutrophil count less than 0.5×10^9/litre or platelet count less than 50×10^3/microlitre).

- **CONCEPTION AND CONTRACEPTION** Effective contraception required during and for 3 months after treatment.
- **PREGNANCY** Manufacturer advises avoid unless essential—toxicity in *animal* studies.
- **BREAST FEEDING** Manufacturer advises use only if potential benefit outweighs risk—no information available.
- **HEPATIC IMPAIRMENT** Manufacturer advises caution—consult product literature.
- **RENAL IMPAIRMENT** Manufacturer advises monitor renal function closely in moderate or severe impairment.
- **PRE-TREATMENT SCREENING**
Tuberculosis Patients should be evaluated for tuberculosis before treatment.

- **MONITORING REQUIREMENTS**
- ▶ Monitor lipid profile 4–8 weeks after starting treatment and then as indicated.
- ▶ Monitor for demyelinating disorders.
- ▶ Monitor hepatic transaminases.
- ▶ Monitor neutrophil and platelet counts.
- **DIRECTIONS FOR ADMINISTRATION** For *intravenous infusion*; body-weight less than 30 kg, dilute requisite dose to a volume of 50 mL with Sodium chloride 0.9% and give over 1 hour; body-weight over 30 kg, dilute requisite dose to a volume of 100 mL with Sodium chloride 0.9% and give over 1 hour.
- **PATIENT AND CARER ADVICE** An alert card should be provided.

  Patients and their carers should be advised to seek immediate medical attention if symptoms of infection occur, or if symptoms of diverticular perforation such as abdominal pain, haemorrhage, or fever accompanying change in bowel habits occur.
- **NATIONAL FUNDING/ACCESS DECISIONS**

NICE technology appraisals (TAs)
- ▶ Tocilizumab for the treatment of systemic juvenile idiopathic arthritis (December 2011) NICE TA238
Tocilizumab is recommended for the treatment of systemic juvenile idiopathic arthritis in children aged over 2 years who have not responded adequately to NSAIDs, systemic corticosteroids and methotrexate, if the manufacturer makes tocilizumab available with the discount agreed as part of the patient access scheme.

  Tocilizumab is not recommended for the treatment of systemic juvenile idiopathic arthritis in children whose disease continues to respond to methotrexate or who have not been treated with methotrexate.

  Children currently receiving tocilizumab for systemic juvenile idiopathic arthritis who do not meet these criteria should have the option to continue treatment until it is considered appropriate to stop.
www.nice.org.uk/TA238
- ▶ **Abatacept, adalimumab, etanercept and tocilizumab for treating juvenile idiopathic arthritis (December 2015)** NICE TA373
Tocilizumab is recommended as an option for treatment of polyarticular juvenile idiopathic arthritis (JIA), including polyarticular-onset, polyarticular-course and extended oligoarticular JIA in children 2 years and older whose disease has responded inadequately to previous therapy with methotrexate and if the manufacturer provides tocilizumab with the discounts agreed in the patient access schemes.
www.nice.org.uk/TA373

- **MEDICINAL FORMS**
There can be variation in the licensing of different medicines containing the same drug.

Solution for infusion
- ▶ RoActemra (Roche Products Ltd)
Tocilizumab 20 mg per 1 ml RoActemra 400mg/20ml concentrate for solution for infusion vials | 1 vial POM £512.00 (Hospital only)
RoActemra 200mg/10ml concentrate for solution for infusion vials | 1 vial POM £256.00 (Hospital only)
RoActemra 80mg/4ml concentrate for solution for infusion vials | 1 vial POM £102.40 (Hospital only)

10

Musculoskeletal system

IMMUNOSUPPRESSANTS 〉 T-CELL ACTIVATION INHIBITORS

Abatacept
31.5.2016

- **INDICATIONS AND DOSE**

Moderate to severe active polyarticular juvenile idiopathic arthritis (in combination with methotrexate) in children who have not responded adequately to other disease-modifying antirheumatic drugs (including at least one tumour necrosis factor (TNF) inhibitor)
▸ BY INTRAVENOUS INFUSION
▸ Child 6–17 years (body-weight up to 75 kg): 10 mg/kg every 2 weeks for 3 doses, then 10 mg/kg every 4 weeks, review treatment if no response within 6 months
▸ Child 6–17 years (body-weight 75–100 kg): 750 mg every 2 weeks for 3 doses, then 750 mg every 4 weeks, review treatment if no response within 6 months
▸ Child 6–17 years (body-weight 101 kg and above): 1 g every 2 weeks for 3 doses, then 1 g every 4 weeks, review treatment if no response within 6 months

- **CONTRA-INDICATIONS** Severe infection
- **CAUTIONS** Children should be brought up to date with current immunisation schedule before initiating therapy · do not initiate until active infections are controlled · predisposition to infection (screen for latent tuberculosis and viral hepatitis) · progressive multifocal leucoencephalopathy (discontinue treatment if neurological symptoms present)
- **INTERACTIONS** → Appendix 1 (abatacept).
- **SIDE-EFFECTS**
- **Common or very common** Abdominal pain · conjunctivitis · cough · diarrhoea · dizziness · dyspepsia · fatigue · flushing · headache · hypertension · infection · leucopenia · nausea · pain in extremities · paraesthesia · stomatitis · vomiting
- **Uncommon** Psoriasis · alopecia · anxiety · arthralgia · basal and squamous cell carcinoma · bradycardia · bronchospasm · bruising · depression · dry eye · dry skin · dyspnoea · gastritis · hyperhidrosis · hypotension · menstrual disturbances · palpitation · skin papilloma · sleep disorder · tachycardia · thrombocytopenia · visual disturbance · weight gain
- **Frequency not known** Lung cancer · lymphoma
- **CONCEPTION AND CONTRACEPTION** Effective contraception required during treatment and for 14 weeks after last dose.
- **PREGNANCY** Manufacturer advises avoid unless essential.
- **BREAST FEEDING** Present in milk in *animal* studies—manufacturer advises avoid breast-feeding during treatment and for 14 weeks after last dose.
- **DIRECTIONS FOR ADMINISTRATION** For *intravenous infusion*, given intermittently *in* Sodium chloride 0.9%; reconstitute each vial with 10 mL water for injections using the silicone-free syringe provided; dilute requisite dose in Sodium Chloride 0.9% to 100 mL (using the same silicone-free syringe); give over 30 minutes through a low protein-binding filter (pore size 0.2–1.2 micron).
- **NATIONAL FUNDING/ACCESS DECISIONS**
  NICE technology appraisals (TAs)
  ▸ Abatacept, adalimumab, etanercept and tocilizumab for treating juvenile idiopathic arthritis (December 2015)
  NICE TA373
  Abatacept is recommended as options for treating polyarticular juvenile idiopathic arthritis (JIA), including polyarticular-onset, polyarticular-course and extended oligoarticular JIA in patients 6 years and older whose disease has responded inadequately to other disease-modifying anti-rheumatic drugs (DMARDs) including at least 1 tumour necrosis factor (TNF) inhibitor,

only if the manufacturer provides abatacept with the discounts agreed in the patient access schemes. www.nice.org.uk/TA373

- **MEDICINAL FORMS**
  There can be variation in the licensing of different medicines containing the same drug.
  Powder for solution for infusion
  ELECTROLYTES: May contain Sodium
  ▸ Orencia (Bristol-Myers Squibb Pharmaceuticals Ltd)
    Abatacept 250 mg Orencia 250mg powder for concentrate for solution for infusion vials | 1 vial [PoM] £302.40 (Hospital only)

IMMUNOSUPPRESSANTS 〉 TUMOR NECROSIS FACTOR ALPHA (TNF-α) INHIBITORS

Adalimumab
31.5.2016

- **INDICATIONS AND DOSE**

Severe chronic plaque psoriasis in children who have had an inadequate response to, or are inappropriate for topical therapy and phototherapies
▸ BY SUBCUTANEOUS INJECTION
▸ Child 4–17 years: Initially 0.8 mg/kg every 1 week (max. per dose 40 mg) for 2 doses, then 0.8 mg/kg every 2 weeks (max. per dose 40 mg), review treatment if no response within 16 weeks; for further information on dose banding, consult product literature

Active polyarticular juvenile idiopathic arthritis (in combination with methotrexate or alone if methotrexate inappropriate) in children who have not responded adequately to one or more disease-modifying antirheumatic drug
▸ BY SUBCUTANEOUS INJECTION
▸ Child 2–3 years: 24 mg/m² every 2 weeks (max. per dose 20 mg), review treatment if no response within 12 weeks; for further information on dose banding, consult product literature
▸ Child 4–12 years: 24 mg/m² every 2 weeks (max. per dose 40 mg), review treatment if no response within 12 weeks; for further information on dose banding, consult product literature
▸ Child 13–17 years: 40 mg every 2 weeks, review treatment if no response within 12 weeks; for further information on dose banding, consult product literature

Active enthesitis-related arthritis in children who have had an inadequate response to, or who are intolerant of, conventional therapy
▸ BY SUBCUTANEOUS INJECTION
▸ Child 6–17 years: 24 mg/m² every 2 weeks (max. per dose 40 mg), for further information on dose banding, consult product literature

Severe active Crohn's disease
▸ BY SUBCUTANEOUS INJECTION
▸ Child 6–17 years (body-weight up to 40 kg): Initially 40 mg, then 20 mg after 2 weeks; maintenance 20 mg every 2 weeks, increased if necessary to 20 mg once weekly, review treatment if no response within 12 weeks of initial dose
▸ Child 6–17 years (body-weight 40 kg and above): Initially 80 mg, then 40 mg after 2 weeks; maintenance 40 mg every 2 weeks, increased if necessary to 40 mg once weekly, maximum 40 mg administered at a single site, review treatment if no response within 12 weeks of initial dose

Severe active Crohn's disease (accelerated regimen)
▸ BY SUBCUTANEOUS INJECTION
▸ Child 6–17 years (body-weight up to 40 kg): Initially 80 mg, then 40 mg after 2 weeks; maintenance 20 mg every 2 weeks, increased if necessary to 20 mg once

weekly, maximum 40 mg administered at a single site, review treatment if no response within 12 weeks of initial dose

▶ Child 6–17 years (body-weight 40 kg and above): Initially 160 mg, dose can alternatively be given as divided injections over 2 days, then 80 mg after 2 weeks; maintenance 40 mg every 2 weeks, then increased if necessary to 40 mg once weekly, maximum 40 mg administered at a single site, review treatment if no response within 12 weeks of initial dose

- **CONTRA-INDICATIONS** Moderate or severe heart failure · severe infection

- **CAUTIONS** Children should be brought up to date with current immunisation schedule before initiating therapy · demyelinating disorders (risk of exacerbation) · development of malignancy · do not initiate until active infections are controlled (discontinue if new serious infection develops) · hepatitis B virus—monitor for active infection · history of malignancy · mild heart failure (discontinue if symptoms develop or worsen) · predisposition to infection

CAUTIONS, FURTHER INFORMATION

▶ Tuberculosis Active tuberculosis should be treated with standard treatment for at least 2 months before starting adalimumab. Patients who have previously received adequate treatment for tuberculosis can start adalimumab but should be monitored every 3 months for possible recurrence. In patients without active tuberculosis but who were previously not treated adequately, chemoprophylaxis should be completed before starting adalimumab. In patients at high risk of tuberculosis who cannot be assessed by tuberculin skin test, chemoprophylaxis can be given concurrently with adalimumab.

- **INTERACTIONS** → Appendix 1 (adalimumab).

- **SIDE-EFFECTS**

▶ **Common or very common** Anxiety · benign tumours · chest pain · cough · dehydration · dermatitis · dizziness · dyspepsia · dyspnoea · electrolyte disturbances · eye disorders · flushing · gastrointestinal haemorrhage · haematuria · hyperlipidaemia · hypertension · hyperuricaemia · impaired healing · mood changes · musculoskeletal pain · oedema · onycholysis · paraesthesia · rash · renal impairment · skin cancer · sleep disturbances · tachycardia · vomiting

▶ **Uncommon** Aortic aneurysm · arrhythmias · cholecystitis · cholelithiasis · dysphagia · erectile dysfunction · hearing loss · hepatic steatosis · interstitial lung disease · leukaemia · lymphoma · malignancy · neuropathy · nocturia · pancreatitis · pneumonitis · rhabdomyolysis · solid tumours · tinnitus · tremor · vascular occlusion

▶ **Rare** Autoimmune hepatitis · demyelinating disorders · myocardial infarction

▶ **Frequency not known** Abdominal pain · anaemia · antibody formation · aplastic anaemia · blood disorders · cutaneous vasculitis · depression · fever · headache · hypersensitivity reactions · injection-site reactions · leucopenia · lupus erythematosus-like syndrome · nausea · new onset psoriasis · pancytopenia · pleural effusion · pruritus · pulmonary embolism · sarcoidosis · Stevens-Johnson syndrome · thrombocytopenia · worsening heart failure · worsening of symptoms of dermatomyositis · worsening psoriasis

SIDE-EFFECTS, FURTHER INFORMATION
Associated with infections, sometimes severe, including tuberculosis, septicaemia, and hepatitis B reactivation.

- **CONCEPTION AND CONTRACEPTION** Manufacturer advises effective contraception required during treatment and for at least 5 months after last dose.

- **PREGNANCY** Avoid.

- **BREAST FEEDING** Avoid; manufacturer advises avoid for at least 5 months after last dose.

- **PRE-TREATMENT SCREENING**
Tuberculosis Patients should be evaluated for tuberculosis before treatment.

- **MONITORING REQUIREMENTS**
▶ Monitor for infection before, during, and for 4 months after treatment.
▶ Monitor for non-melanoma skin cancer before and during treatment, especially in patients with a history of PUVA treatment for psoriasis or extensive immunosuppressant therapy.

- **PATIENT AND CARER ADVICE** An alert card should be provided.
Tuberculosis Patients and their carers should be advised to seek medical attention if symptoms suggestive of tuberculosis (e.g. persistent cough, weight loss, and fever) develop.
Blood disorders Patients and their carers should be advised to seek medical attention if symptoms suggestive of blood disorders (such as fever, sore throat, bruising, or bleeding) develop.

- **NATIONAL FUNDING/ACCESS DECISIONS**
NICE technology appraisals (TAs)
▶ **Abatacept, adalimumab, etanercept and tocilizumab for treating juvenile idiopathic arthritis (December 2015)**
NICE TA373
Adalimumab is recommended as an option for treating polyarticular juvenile idiopathic arthritis (JIA), including polyarticular-onset, polyarticular-course and extended oligoarticular JIA in patients 2 years and older whose disease has responded inadequately to 1 or more disease-modifying antirheumatic drugs (DMARDs) and for treating enthesitis-related JIA in patients 6 years and older whose disease has responded inadequately to, or who are intolerant of, conventional therapy.
www.nice.org.uk/TA373

Scottish Medicines Consortium (SMC) Decisions
The *Scottish Medicines Consortium* has advised (April 2015) that adalimumab (*Humira*®) is accepted for restricted use within NHS Scotland for the treatment of active enthesitis-related arthritis in children over 6 years of age who have had an inadequate response to, or who are intolerant of, conventional therapy, and is used within specialist rheumatology services (including those working within the network for paediatric rheumatology).

The *Scottish Medicines Consortium* has advised (June 2015) that adalimumab (*Humira*®) is accepted for restricted use within NHS Scotland for the treatment of severe chronic plaque psoriasis in children over 4 years who have had an inadequate response to, or are inappropriate for, topical therapy and phototherapies, and have severe disease as defined by a total Psoriasis Area Severity Index (PASI) score of ≥10 and a Dermatology Life Quality Index (DLQI) of >10.

- **MEDICINAL FORMS**
There can be variation in the licensing of different medicines containing the same drug.
Solution for injection
CAUTIONARY AND ADVISORY LABELS 10
▶ Humira (AbbVie Ltd)
Adalimumab 50 mg per 1 ml Humira 40mg/0.8ml solution for injection pre-filled syringes | 2 pre-filled disposable injection [PoM] £704.28
Humira 40mg/0.8ml solution for injection vials | 2 vial [PoM] £704.28
Humira 40mg/0.8ml solution for injection pre-filled pen | 2 pre-filled disposable injection [PoM] £704.28

Etanercept

4.5.2016

- **INDICATIONS AND DOSE**

Polyarticular juvenile idiopathic arthritis in children who have had an inadequate response to methotrexate or who cannot tolerate it | Oligoarthritis in children who have had an inadequate response to methotrexate or who cannot tolerate it | Psoriatic arthritis in children who have had an inadequate response to methotrexate or cannot tolerate it | Enthesitis-related arthritis in children who have had an inadequate response to conventional therapy or cannot tolerate it

▶ BY SUBCUTANEOUS INJECTION

▶ Child 2-16 years: 400 micrograms/kg twice weekly (max. per dose 25 mg), to be given at an interval of 3–4 days between doses, alternatively 800 micrograms/kg once weekly (max. per dose 50 mg), consider discontinuation if no response after 4 months

Severe plaque psoriasis either refractory to at least 2 standard systemic treatments and photochemotherapy, or when standard treatments cannot be used because of intolerance or contra-indications

▶ BY SUBCUTANEOUS INJECTION

▶ Child 6-17 years: 800 micrograms/kg once weekly (max. per dose 50 mg) for up to 24 weeks, discontinue if no response after 12 weeks

- **CONTRA-INDICATIONS** Active infection
- **CAUTIONS** Children should be brought up to date with current immunisation schedule before initiating therapy · development of malignancy · diabetes mellitus · heart failure (risk of exacerbation) · hepatitis B virus—monitor for active infection · hepatitis C infection (monitor for worsening infection) · history of blood disorders · history of malignancy · history or increased risk of demyelinating disorders · predisposition to infection (avoid if predisposition to septicaemia) · significant exposure to herpes zoster virus—interrupt treatment and consider varicella–zoster immunoglobulin

CAUTIONS, FURTHER INFORMATION

▶ Tuberculosis Active tuberculosis should be treated with standard treatment for at least 2 months before starting etanercept. Patients who have previously received adequate treatment for tuberculosis can start etanercept but should be monitored every 3 months for possible recurrence. In patients without active tuberculosis but who were previously not treated adequately, chemoprophylaxis should ideally be completed before starting etanercept. In patients at high risk of tuberculosis who cannot be assessed by tuberculin skin test, chemoprophylaxis can be given concurrently with etanercept.

- **INTERACTIONS** → Appendix 1 (etanercept).

- **SIDE-EFFECTS**

▶ **Uncommon** Interstitial lung disease · new onset or worsening psoriasis · rash · skin cancer · uveitis

▶ **Rare** Demyelinating disorders · lymphoma · seizures · Stevens-Johnson syndrome · vasculitis

▶ **Very rare** Toxic epidermal necrolysis

▶ **Frequency not known** Abdominal pain · anaemia · antibody formation · aplastic anaemia · appendicitis · blood disorders · cutaneous ulcer · depression · diabetes mellitus · fever · gastritis · headache · hypersensitivity reactions · inflammatory bowel disease · injection-site reactions · leucopenia · leukaemia · lupus erythematosus-like syndrome · macrophage activation syndrome · malignancy · nausea · oesophagitis · pancytopenia · pruritus · solid tumours · thrombocytopenia · vomiting · worsening heart failure

SIDE-EFFECTS, FURTHER INFORMATION
Associated with infections, sometimes severe, including tuberculosis, septicaemia, and hepatitis B reactivation.

- **CONCEPTION AND CONTRACEPTION** Manufacturer advises effective contraception required during treatment and for 3 weeks after last dose.

- **PREGNANCY** Avoid—limited information available.

- **BREAST FEEDING** Manufacturer advises avoid—present in milk in *animal* studies.

- **HEPATIC IMPAIRMENT** Use with caution in moderate to severe alcoholic hepatitis.

- **PRE-TREATMENT SCREENING**
Tuberculosis Patients should be evaluated for tuberculosis before treatment.

- **MONITORING REQUIREMENTS** Monitor for skin cancer before and during treatment, particularly in those at risk (including patients with psoriasis or a history of PUVA treatment).

- **PRESCRIBING AND DISPENSING INFORMATION** Products containing etanercept are not identical and although there should be no important differences in terms of safety and efficacy, when prescribing biological products it is good practice to use the brand name, see *Biosimilar medicines*, under Guidance on prescribing p. 1.

- **PATIENT AND CARER ADVICE** An alert card should be provided.
Blood disorders Patients and their carers should be advised to seek medical attention if symptoms suggestive of blood disorders (such as fever, sore throat, bruising, or bleeding) develop.
Tuberculosis Patients and their carers should be advised to seek medical attention if symptoms suggestive of tuberculosis (e.g. persistent cough, weight loss, and fever) develop.

- **NATIONAL FUNDING/ACCESS DECISIONS**

NICE technology appraisals (TAs)
▶ Abatacept, adalimumab, etanercept and tocilizumab for treating juvenile idiopathic arthritis (December 2015)
NICE TA373
Etanercept is recommended as an option for treating:
- polyarticular juvenile idiopathic arthritis (JIA), including polyarticular-onset, polyarticular-course and extended oligoarticular JIA, in patients 2 years and over whose disease has responded inadequately to, or who are intolerant of, methotrexate;
- enthesitis-related JIA in patients 12 years and over whose disease has responded inadequately to, or who are intolerant of, conventional therapy;
- psoriatic JIA in patients 12 years and over whose disease has responded inadequately to, or who are intolerant of, methotrexate.
www.nice.org.uk/TA373

Scottish Medicines Consortium (SMC) Decisions
The *Scottish Medicines Consortium* issued similar advice to NICE TA103 on the use of etanercept for severe plaque psoriasis in adults (August 2009) and children over 6 years old (April 2012).

The *Scottish Medicines Consortium* has advised (January 2013) that etanercept (*Enbrel* ®) is accepted for restricted use within NHS Scotland for the treatment of polyarthritis (rheumatoid factor positive or negative) and extended oligoarthritis in children and adolescents from the age of 2 years who have had an inadequate response to or are intolerant of methotrexate, psoriatic arthritis in adolescents from the age of 12 years who have had an inadequate response to or are intolerant of methotrexate, and enthesitis-related arthritis in adolescents from the age of 12 years who have had an inadequate response to or intolerant of conventional therapy. It is further restricted to use within specialist rheumatology services (including those working within the network for paediatric rheumatology).

● **MEDICINAL FORMS**
There can be variation in the licensing of different medicines containing the same drug.

Solution for injection
CAUTIONARY AND ADVISORY LABELS 10
▸ **Benepali** (Biogen Idec Ltd) ▼
Etanercept 50 mg per 1 ml Benepali 50mg/1ml solution for injection pre-filled syringes | 4 pre-filled disposable injection PoM £656.00
Benepali 50mg/1ml solution for injection pre-filled pen | 4 pre-filled disposable injection PoM £656.00
▸ **Enbrel** (Pfizer Ltd)
Etanercept 50 mg per 1 ml Enbrel 50mg/1ml solution for injection pre-filled syringes | 4 pre-filled disposable injection PoM £715.00
Enbrel 25mg/0.5ml solution for injection pre-filled syringes | 4 pre-filled disposable injection PoM £357.50
▸ **Enbrel MyClic** (Pfizer Ltd)
Etanercept 50 mg per 1 ml Enbrel 50mg/1ml solution for injection pre-filled MyClic pen | 4 pre-filled disposable injection PoM £715.00

Powder and solvent for solution for injection
CAUTIONARY AND ADVISORY LABELS 10
EXCIPIENTS: May contain Benzyl alcohol
▸ **Enbrel** (Pfizer Ltd)
Etanercept 10 mg Enbrel Paediatric 10mg powder and solvent for solution for injection vials | 4 vial PoM £143.00
Etanercept 25 mg Enbrel 25mg powder and solvent for solution for injection vials | 4 vial PoM £357.50

---

2 Neuromuscular disorders

Neuromuscular disorders

Drugs that enhance neuromuscular transmission

Anticholinesterases are used as first-line treatment in *ocular myasthenia gravis* and as an adjunct to immunosuppressant therapy for *generalised myasthenia gravis*.

Corticosteroids are used when anticholinesterases do not control symptoms completely. A second-line immunosuppressant such as azathioprine p. 485 is frequently used to reduce the dose of corticosteroid.

Plasmapheresis or infusion of intravenous immunoglobulin [unlicensed indication] may induce temporary remission in severe relapses, particularly where bulbar or respiratory function is compromised or before thymectomy.

Anticholinesterases

Anticholinesterase drugs enhance neuromuscular transmission in voluntary and involuntary muscle in myasthenia gravis. Excessive dosage of these drugs can impair neuromuscular transmission and precipitate cholinergic crises by causing a depolarising block. This may be difficult to distinguish from a worsening myasthenic state.

Muscarinic side-effects of anticholinesterases include increased sweating, increased salivary and gastric secretions, increased gastro-intestinal and uterine motility, and bradycardia. These parasympathomimetic effects are antagonised by atropine sulfate p. 624.

Neostigmine p. 602 produces a therapeutic effect for up to 4 hours. Its pronounced muscarinic action is a disadvantage, and simultaneous administration of an antimuscarinic drug such as atropine sulfate or propantheline bromide p. 58 may be required to prevent colic, excessive salivation, or diarrhoea. In severe disease neostigmine can be given every 2 hours. In infants, neostigmine by either subcutaneous or intramuscular injection is preferred for the short-term management of myasthenia.

Pyridostigmine bromide p. 602 is less powerful and slower in action than neostigmine but it has a longer duration of action. It is preferable to neostigmine because of its smoother action and the need for less frequent dosage. It is particularly preferred in patients whose muscles are weak on waking. It has a comparatively mild gastrointestinal effect but an antimuscarinic drug may still be required. It is inadvisable to use excessive doses because acetylcholine receptor down regulation may occur. Immunosuppressant therapy may be considered if high doses of pyridostigmine bromide are needed.

Neostigmine and pyridostigmine bromide should be given to neonates 30 minutes before feeds to improve suckling.

Neostigmine is also used to reverse the actions of the non-depolarising neuromuscular blocking drugs.

Immunosuppressant therapy

A course of **corticosteroids** is an established treatment in severe cases of myasthenia gravis and may be particularly useful when antibodies to the acetylcholine receptor are present in high titre. Short courses of high-dose ('pulsed') methylprednisolone p. 412 followed by maintenance therapy with oral corticosteroids may also be useful.

Corticosteroid treatment is usually initiated under specialist supervision. Transient but very serious worsening of symptoms can occur in the first 2–3 weeks, especially if the corticosteroid is started at a high dose. Once remission has occurred (usually after 2– 6 months), the dose of prednisolone p. 413 should be reduced slowly to the minimum effective dose.

Skeletal muscle relaxants

The drugs described are used for the relief of chronic muscle spasm or spasticity associated with neurological damage; they are not indicated for spasm associated with minor injuries. They act principally on the central nervous system with the exception of dantrolene, which has a peripheral site of action. They differ in action from the muscle relaxants used in anaesthesia, which block transmission at the neuromuscular junction.

The underlying cause of spasticity should be treated and any aggravating factors (e.g. pressure sores, infection) remedied. Skeletal muscle relaxants are effective in most forms of spasticity except the rare alpha variety. The major disadvantage of treatment with these drugs is that reduction in muscle tone can cause a loss of splinting action of the spastic leg and trunk muscles and sometimes lead to an increase in disability.

Dantrolene sodium p. 775 acts directly on skeletal muscle and produces fewer central adverse effects. It is generally used in resistant cases. The dose should be increased slowly.

Baclofen p. 603 inhibits transmission at spinal level and also depresses the central nervous system. The dose should be increased slowly to avoid the major side-effects of sedation and muscular hypotonia (other adverse events are uncommon).

Diazepam p. 207 has undoubted efficacy in some children. Sedation and occasionally extensor hypotonus are disadvantages. Other benzodiazepines also have muscle-relaxant properties.

2.1 Myasthenia gravis

ANTICHOLINESTERASES ❭ OTHER

Anticholinesterases

● **DRUG ACTION** They prolong the action of acetylcholine by inhibiting the action of the enzyme acetylcholinesterase.

● **CONTRA-INDICATIONS** Intestinal obstruction · urinary obstruction

- **CAUTIONS** Arrhythmias · asthma (extreme caution) · atropine or other antidote to muscarinic effects may be necessary (particularly when neostigmine is given by injection) but not given routinely because it may mask signs of overdosage · bradycardia · epilepsy · hyperthyroidism · hypotension · parkinsonism · peptic ulceration · recent myocardial infarction · vagotonia
- **INTERACTIONS** → Appendix 1 (parasympathomimetics).
- **SIDE-EFFECTS** Abdominal cramps (more marked with higher doses) · diarrhoea · increased salivation · nausea · vomiting

  Overdose
  Signs of overdosage include bronchoconstriction, increased bronchial secretions, lacrimation, excessive sweating, involuntary defaecation, involuntary micturition, miosis, nystagmus, bradycardia, heart block, arrhythmias, hypotension, agitation, excessive dreaming, and weakness eventually leading to fasciculation and paralysis.
- **PREGNANCY** Manufacturer advises use only if potential benefit outweighs risk.
- **BREAST FEEDING** Amount probably too small to be harmful.

▶ 601

Neostigmine

(Neostigmine methylsulfate)

- **INDICATIONS AND DOSE**

  Treatment of myasthenia gravis
  ▶ BY MOUTH

  ▶ Neonate: Initially 1-2 mg, then 1-5 mg every 4 hours, given 30 minutes before feeds.

  ▶ Child 1 month-5 years: Initially 7.5 mg, dose repeated at suitable intervals throughout the day, total daily dose 15-90 mg

  ▶ Child 6-11 years: Initially 15 mg, dose repeated at suitable intervals throughout the day, total daily dose 15-90 mg

  ▶ Child 12-17 years: Initially 15-30 mg, dose repeated at suitable intervals throughout the day, total daily dose 75-300 mg, the maximum that most patients can tolerate is 180 mg daily

  ▶ BY SUBCUTANEOUS INJECTION, OR BY INTRAMUSCULAR INJECTION

  ▶ Neonate: 150 micrograms/kg every 6-8 hours, to be given 30 minutes before feeds, then increased if necessary up to 300 micrograms/kg every 4 hours.

  ▶ Child 1 month-11 years: 200-500 micrograms, dose repeated at suitable intervals throughout the day

  ▶ Child 12-17 years: 1-2.5 mg, dose repeated at suitable intervals throughout the day

  Reversal of non-depolarising (competitive) neuromuscular blockade
  ▶ BY INTRAVENOUS INJECTION

  ▶ Neonate: 50 micrograms/kg, to be given over 1 minute after or with glycopyrronium or atropine, followed by 25 micrograms/kg if required.

  ▶ Child 1 month-11 years: 50 micrograms/kg (max. per dose 2.5 mg), to be given over 1 minute after or with glycopyrronium or atropine, then 25 micrograms/kg if required

  ▶ Child 12-17 years: 50 micrograms/kg (max. per dose 2.5 mg), to be given over 1 minute after or with glycopyrronium or atropine, then 25 micrograms/kg (max. per dose 2.5 mg) if required

- **UNLICENSED USE**
  ▶ In neonates Dose for treatment of myasthenia gravis by subcutaneous or intramuscular injection is unlicensed.

- **CAUTIONS**
  ▶ With intravenous use Glycopyrronium or atropine should also be given when reversing neuromuscular blockade

- **INTERACTIONS** → Appendix 1 (parasympathomimetics).

- **RENAL IMPAIRMENT** May need dose reduction.

- **DIRECTIONS FOR ADMINISTRATION** For *intravenous injection*, give undiluted *or* dilute with Glucose 5% *or* Sodium Chloride 0.9%.

- **MEDICINAL FORMS**
  There can be variation in the licensing of different medicines containing the same drug. Forms available from special-order manufacturers include: oral solution

  Tablet
  ▶ Neostigmine (Non-proprietary)
    Neostigmine bromide 15 mg Prostigmin 15mg tablets | 100 tablet [PoM] no price available
    Neostigmine 15mg tablets | 140 tablet [PoM] £99.60

  Solution for injection
  ▶ Neostigmine (Non-proprietary)
    Neostigmine metilsulfate 2.5 mg per 1 ml Neostigmine 2.5mg/1ml solution for injection ampoules | 10 ampoule [PoM] £4.95-£5.06

▶ 601

Pyridostigmine bromide

- **DRUG ACTION** Pyridostigmine bromide has weaker muscarinic action than neostigmine.

- **INDICATIONS AND DOSE**

  Myasthenia gravis
  ▶ INITIALLY BY MOUTH

  ▶ Neonate: Initially 1-1.5 mg/kg, dose repeated throughout the day, then (by mouth using immediate-release medicines) increased if necessary up to 10 mg, to be increased gradually and given 30-60 minutes before feeds.

  ▶ Child 1 month-11 years: Initially 1-1.5 mg/kg daily, then (by mouth using immediate-release medicines) increased to 7 mg/kg daily in 6 divided doses, to be increased gradually; (by mouth using immediate-release medicines) usual dose 30-360 mg daily in divided doses

  ▶ Child 12-17 years: 30-120 mg, dose repeated throughout the day; (by mouth using immediate-release medicines) usual dose 300-600 mg daily in divided doses, consider immunosuppressant therapy if total daily dose exceeds 360 mg, down-regulation of acetylcholine receptors possible if total daily dose exceeds 450 mg

- **RENAL IMPAIRMENT** Reduce dose; excreted by kidney.

- **MEDICINAL FORMS**
  There can be variation in the licensing of different medicines containing the same drug. Forms available from special-order manufacturers include: oral suspension, oral solution

  Tablet
  ▶ Pyridostigmine bromide (Non-proprietary)
    Pyridostigmine bromide 60 mg Pyridostigmine bromide 60mg tablets | 200 tablet [PoM] £45.58 DT price = £45.58
  ▶ Mestinon (Meda Pharmaceuticals Ltd)
    Pyridostigmine bromide 60 mg Mestinon 60mg tablets | 200 tablet [PoM] £45.57 DT price = £45.58

2.2 Spasticity

MUSCLE RELAXANTS > CENTRALLY ACTING

Baclofen

- **INDICATIONS AND DOSE**

Chronic severe spasticity of voluntary muscle

▸ BY MOUTH

▸ Child 1 month-7 years: Initially 300 micrograms/kg daily in 4 divided doses, increased gradually at weekly intervals until satisfactory response; maintenance 0.75–2 mg/kg daily in divided doses, review treatment if no benefit within 6 weeks of achieving maximum dose; maximum 40 mg per day

▸ Child 8-17 years: Initially 300 micrograms/kg daily in 4 divided doses, increased gradually at weekly intervals until satisfactory response; maintenance 0.75–2 mg/kg daily in divided doses, review treatment if no benefit within 6 weeks of achieving maximum dose; maximum 60 mg per day

Severe chronic spasticity of cerebral or spinal origin unresponsive to oral antispastic drugs (or oral therapy not tolerated) (specialist use only)

▸ BY INTRATHECAL INJECTION

▸ Child 4-17 years: Test dose 25–50 micrograms, to be given over at least 1 minute via catheter or lumbar puncture, then increased in steps of 25 micrograms (max. per dose 100 micrograms), not more often than every 24 hours to determine initial maintenance dose; maintenance 25–200 micrograms daily, adjusted according to response, dose-titration phase, most often using infusion pump (implanted into chest wall or abdominal wall tissues) to establish maintenance dose retaining some spasticity to avoid sensation of paralysis

---

IMPORTANT SAFETY INFORMATION
Consult product literature for details on test dose and titration—important to monitor patients closely in appropriately equipped and staffed environment during screening and immediately after pump implantation. Resuscitation equipment must be available for immediate use. Treatment with continuous pump-administered intrathecal baclofen should be initiated within 3 months of a satisfactory response to intrathecal baclofen testing.

- **CONTRA-INDICATIONS**
▸ With intrathecal use Local infection · systemic infection
▸ With oral use Avoid oral route in active peptic ulceration

- **CAUTIONS**

GENERAL CAUTIONS

Diabetes · epilepsy · history of peptic ulcer · hypertonic bladder sphincter · psychiatric illness · respiratory impairment

SPECIFIC CAUTIONS

▸ With intrathecal use Coagulation disorders · malnutrition (increased risk of post-surgical complications) · previous spinal fusion procedure

- **INTERACTIONS** → Appendix 1 (muscle relaxants).

- **SIDE-EFFECTS**
▸ **Common or very common** Agitation · anxiety · ataxia · cardiovascular depression · confusion · depression · dizziness · drowsiness · dry mouth · euphoria · gastro-intestinal disturbances · hallucinations · headache · hyperhidrosis · hypotension · insomnia · myalgia · nightmares · rash · respiratory depression · sedation · seizure · tremor · urinary disturbances · visual disorders

▸ **Rare** Abdominal pain · changes in hepatic function · dysarthria · erectile dysfunction · paraesthesia · taste disturbances
▸ **Very rare** Hypothermia

- **PREGNANCY** Manufacturer advises use only if potential benefit outweighs risk (toxicity in *animal* studies).

- **BREAST FEEDING** Present in milk—amount probably too small to be harmful.

- **HEPATIC IMPAIRMENT**
▸ With oral use Manufacturer advises use with caution.

- **RENAL IMPAIRMENT**
▸ With oral use Risk of toxicity—use smaller oral doses and if necessary increase dosage interval; if estimated glomerular filtration rate less than 15 mL/minute/1.73 m^2 use by mouth only if potential benefit outweighs risk. Excreted by the kidney.

- **TREATMENT CESSATION** Avoid abrupt withdrawal (risk of hyperactive state, may exacerbate spasticity, and precipitate autonomic dysfunction including hyperthermia, psychiatric reactions and convulsions; to minimise risk, discontinue by gradual dose reduction over at least 1–2 weeks (longer if symptoms occur)).

- **PRESCRIBING AND DISPENSING INFORMATION** Flavours of oral liquid formulations may include raspberry.

- **PATIENT AND CARER ADVICE**

Driving and skilled tasks
Drowsiness may affect performance of skilled tasks (e.g. driving); effects of alcohol enhanced.

Medicines for Children leaflet: Baclofen for muscle spasm
www.medicinesforchildren.org.uk/baclofen-muscle-spasm

- **MEDICINAL FORMS**
There can be variation in the licensing of different medicines containing the same drug. Forms available from special-order manufacturers include: oral suspension, oral solution

Tablet
CAUTIONARY AND ADVISORY LABELS 2, 8, 21
EXCIPIENTS: May contain Gluten
▸ **Baclofen (Non-proprietary)**
Baclofen 10 mg Baclofen 10mg tablets | 84 tablet PoM £9.99 DT price = £2.69
▸ **Lioresal (Novartis Pharmaceuticals UK Ltd)**
Baclofen 10 mg Lioresal 10mg tablets | 100 tablet PoM £14.86

Oral solution
CAUTIONARY AND ADVISORY LABELS 2, 8, 21
▸ **Baclofen (Non-proprietary)**
Baclofen 1 mg per 1 ml Baclofen 5mg/5ml oral solution sugar free sugar-free | 300 ml PoM £22.45 DT price = £3.43
▸ **Lioresal (Novartis Pharmaceuticals UK Ltd)**
Baclofen 1 mg per 1 ml Lioresal 5mg/5ml liquid sugar-free | 300 ml PoM £10.31 DT price = £3.43
▸ **Lyflex (Chemidex Pharma Ltd)**
Baclofen 1 mg per 1 ml Lyflex 5mg/5ml oral solution sugar-free | 300 ml PoM £7.95 DT price = £3.43

Solution for injection
▸ **Baclofen (Non-proprietary)**
Baclofen 50 microgram per 1 ml Baclofen 50micrograms/1ml solution for injection ampoules | 5 ampoule PoM £10.95 | 10 ampoule PoM £25.00-£27.60
▸ **Lioresal (Novartis Pharmaceuticals UK Ltd)**
Baclofen 50 microgram per 1 ml Lioresal Intrathecal 50micrograms/1ml solution for injection ampoules | 1 ampoule PoM £3.16

Solution for infusion
▸ **Baclofen (Non-proprietary)**
Baclofen 500 microgram per 1 ml Baclofen 10mg/20ml solution for infusion ampoules | 1 ampoule PoM £48.62-£57.00
Baclofen 2 mg per 1 ml Baclofen 40mg/20ml solution for infusion ampoules | 1 ampoule PoM £228.00-£250.00
Baclofen 5mg/5ml solution for infusion ampoules | 5 ampoule PoM £243.10 | 10 ampoule PoM £500.00-£570.00

▶ Lioresal (Novartis Pharmaceuticals UK Ltd)
Baclofen 500 microgram per 1 ml Lioresal Intrathecal 10mg/20ml
solution for infusion ampoules | 1 ampoule [PoM] £70.01
Baclofen 2 mg per 1 ml Lioresal Intrathecal 10mg/5ml solution for
infusion ampoules | 1 ampoule [PoM] £70.01

3 Pain and inflammation in musculoskeletal disorders

Non-steroidal anti-inflammatory drugs

Therapeutic effects

In *single doses* non-steroidal anti-inflammatory drugs
(NSAIDs) have analgesic activity comparable to that of
paracetamol p. 254 but paracetamol is preferred.

In regular *full dosage* NSAIDs have both a lasting analgesic
and an anti-inflammatory effect which makes them
particularly useful for the treatment of continuous or regular
pain associated with inflammation.

Choice

Differences in anti-inflammatory activity between NSAIDs
are small, but there is considerable variation in individual
response and tolerance of these drugs. A large proportion of
children will respond to any NSAID; of the others, those who
do not respond to one may well respond to another. Pain
relief starts soon after taking the first dose and a full
analgesic effect should normally be obtained within a week,
whereas an anti-inflammatory effect may not be achieved (or
may not be clinically assessable) for up to 3 weeks. However,
in juvenile idiopathic arthritis NSAIDs may take 4–12 weeks
to be effective. If appropriate responses are not obtained
within these times, another NSAID should be tried. The
availability of appropriate formulations needs to be
considered when prescribing NSAIDs for children.

NSAIDs reduce the production of prostaglandins by
inhibiting the enzyme cyclo-oxygenase. They vary in their
selectivity for inhibiting different types of cyclo-oxygenase;
selective inhibition of cyclo-oxygenase-2 is associated with
less gastro-intestinal intolerance. However, in children
gastro-intestinal symptoms are rare in those taking NSAIDs
for short periods. The role of selective inhibitors of cyclo-
oxygenase-2 is undetermined in children.

Ibuprofen p. 608 and naproxen p. 614 are propionic acid
derivatives used in children.

Ibuprofen combines anti-inflammatory, analgesic, and
antipyretic properties. It has fewer side-effects than other
NSAIDs but its anti-inflammatory properties are weaker.

Naproxen combines good efficacy with a low incidence of
side-effects.

Diclofenac sodium p. 605, diclofenac potassium p. 605,
indometacin p. 611, mefenamic acid p. 612, and piroxicam
p. 615 have properties similar to those of propionic acid
derivatives:

Diclofenac sodium and diclofenac potassium are similar in
efficacy to naproxen.

Indometacin has an action equal to or superior to that of
naproxen, but with a high incidence of side-effects including
headache, dizziness, and gastro-intestinal disturbances. It is
rarely used in children and should be reserved for when
other NSAIDs have been unsuccessful.

Mefenamic acid has minor anti-inflammatory properties.
It has occasionally been associated with diarrhoea and
haemolytic anaemia which require discontinuation of
treatment.

Piroxicam is as effective as naproxen and has a long
duration of action which permits once-daily administration.
However, it has more gastro-intestinal side-effects than

most other NSAIDs, and is associated with more frequent
serious skin reactions.

Meloxicam p. 613 is a selective inhibitor of cyclo-
oxygenase-2. Its use may be considered in adolescents
intolerant to other NSAIDs.

Ketorolac trometamol p. 636 can be used for the short-
term management of postoperative pain.

Etoricoxib p. 607, a selective inhibitor of cyclo-oxygenase-
2, is licensed for the relief of pain in osteoarthritis,
rheumatoid arthritis, ankylosing spondylitis, and acute gout
in children aged 16 years and over.

Dental and orofacial pain

Most mild to moderate dental pain and inflammation is
effectively relieved by ibuprofen, diclofenac potassium or
diclofenac sodium.

NSAIDs and cardiovascular events

The risk of cardiovascular events secondary to NSAID use is
undetermined in children. In adults, all NSAID use
(including cyclo-oxygenase-2 selective inhibitors) can, to
varying degrees, be associated with a small increased risk of
thrombotic events (e.g. myocardial infarction and stroke)
independent of baseline cardiovascular risk factors or
duration of NSAID use; however, the greatest risk may be in
those patients receiving high doses long term. A small
increased thrombotic risk cannot be excluded in children.

In adults, cyclo-oxygenase-2 selective inhibitors,
diclofenac (150 mg daily) and ibuprofen (2.4 g daily) are
associated with an increased risk of thrombotic events. The
increased risk for diclofenac is similar to that of etoricoxib.
Naproxen (in adults, 1 g daily) is associated with a lower
thrombotic risk, and lower doses of ibuprofen (in adults,
1.2 g daily or less) have not been associated with an
increased risk of myocardial infarction.

The lowest effective dose of NSAID should be prescribed
for the shortest period of time to control symptoms, and the
need for long-term treatment should be reviewed
periodically.

NSAIDs and gastro-intestinal events

All NSAIDs are associated with gastro-intestinal toxicity. In
adults, evidence on the relative safety of NSAIDs indicates
differences in the risks of serious upper gastro-intestinal
side-effects—piroxicam and ketorolac trometamol are
associated with the highest risk; indometacin, diclofenac,
and naproxen are associated with intermediate risk, and
ibuprofen with the lowest risk (although high doses of
ibuprofen have been associated with intermediate risk).
Selective inhibitors of cyclo-oxygenase-2 are associated with
a *lower risk* of serious upper gastro-intestinal side-effects
than non-selective NSAIDs.

Children appear to tolerate NSAIDs better than adults and
gastro-intestinal side-effects are less common although they
do still occur and can be significant; use of gastro-protective
drugs may be necessary.

Asthma

All NSAIDs have the potential to worsen asthma, either
acutely or as a gradual worsening of symptoms; consider
both prescribed NSAIDs and those that are purchased over
the counter.

ANALGESICS > NON-STEROIDAL ANTI-INFLAMMATORY DRUGS

Diclofenac potassium

- **INDICATIONS AND DOSE**

Pain and inflammation in rheumatic disease and other musculoskeletal disorders
- ▸ BY MOUTH
- ▸ Child 14–17 years: 75–100 mg daily in 2–3 divided doses

Postoperative pain
- ▸ BY MOUTH
- ▸ Child 9–13 years (body-weight 35 kg and above): Up to 2 mg/kg daily in 3 divided doses; maximum 100 mg per day
- ▸ Child 14–17 years: 75–100 mg daily in 2–3 divided doses

Fever in ear, nose, or throat infection
- ▸ BY MOUTH
- ▸ Child 9–17 years (body-weight 35 kg and above): Up to 2 mg/kg daily in 3 divided doses; maximum 100 mg per day

- **UNLICENSED USE** *Voltarol® Rapid* not licensed for use in children under 14 years or in fever.

- **CONTRA-INDICATIONS** Active gastro-intestinal bleeding · active gastro-intestinal ulceration · cerebrovascular disease · history of gastro-intestinal bleeding related to previous NSAID therapy · history of gastro-intestinal perforation related to previous NSAID therapy · history of recurrent gastro-intestinal haemorrhage (two or more distinct episodes) · history of recurrent gastro-intestinal ulceration (two or more distinct episodes) · ischaemic heart disease · mild to severe heart failure · peripheral arterial disease

- **CAUTIONS** Allergic disorders · cardiac impairment (NSAIDs may impair renal function) · coagulation defects · connective-tissue disorders · Crohn's disease (may be exacerbated) · history of cardiac failure · hypertension · left ventricular dysfunction · oedema · risk factors for cardiovascular events · ulcerative colitis (may be exacerbated)

- **INTERACTIONS** → Appendix 1 (NSAIDs).

- **SIDE-EFFECTS**
- ▸ **Rare** Alveolitis · aseptic meningitis (patients with connective-tissue disorders such as systemic lupus erythematosus may be especially susceptible) · hepatic damage · interstitial fibrosis associated with NSAIDs can lead to renal failure · pancreatitis · papillary necrosis associated with NSAIDs can lead to renal failure · pulmonary eosinophilia · Stevens-Johnson syndrome · toxic epidermal necrolysis · visual disturbances
- ▸ **Frequency not known** Angioedema · blood disorders · bronchospasm · colitis (induction of or exacerbation of) · Crohn's disease (induction of or exacerbation of) · depression · diarrhoea · dizziness · drowsiness · fluid retention (rarely precipitating congestive heart failure) · gastro-intestinal bleeding · gastro-intestinal discomfort · gastro-intestinal disturbances · gastro-intestinal ulceration · haematuria · headache · hearing disturbances · hypersensitivity reactions · insomnia · nausea · nervousness · photosensitivity · raised blood pressure · rashes · renal failure (especially in patients with pre-existing renal impairment) · tinnitus · vertigo

- **ALLERGY AND CROSS-SENSITIVITY** Contra-indicated in patients with a history of hypersensitivity to aspirin or any other NSAID—which includes those in whom attacks of asthma, angioedema, urticaria or rhinitis have been precipitated by aspirin or any other NSAID.

- **PREGNANCY** Avoid unless the potential benefit outweighs the risk. Avoid during the third trimester (risk of closure of fetal ductus arteriosus *in utero* and possibly persistent pulmonary hypertension of the newborn); onset of labour may be delayed and duration may be increased.

- **BREAST FEEDING** Use with caution during breast-feeding. Amount in milk too small to be harmful.

- **HEPATIC IMPAIRMENT** Use with caution; there is an increased risk of gastro-intestinal bleeding and fluid retention. Avoid in severe liver disease.

- **RENAL IMPAIRMENT** The lowest effective dose should be used for the shortest possible duration. Avoid if possible or use with caution. Avoid in severe impairment. In renal impairment monitor renal function; sodium and water retention may occur and renal function may deteriorate, possibly leading to renal failure.

- **PATIENT AND CARER ADVICE**
Medicines for Children leaflet: Diclofenac for pain and inflammation www.medicinesforchildren.org.uk/diclofenac-for-pain-and-inflammation

- **MEDICINAL FORMS**
There can be variation in the licensing of different medicines containing the same drug.

Tablet
CAUTIONARY AND ADVISORY LABELS 21
- ▸ Diclofenac potassium (Non-proprietary)
  Diclofenac potassium 25 mg Diclofenac potassium 25mg tablets | 28 tablet PoM £3.87
  Diclofenac potassium 50 mg Diclofenac potassium 50mg tablets | 28 tablet PoM £7.41
- ▸ Voltarol Rapid (Novartis Pharmaceuticals UK Ltd)
  Diclofenac potassium 25 mg Voltarol Rapid 25mg tablets | 30 tablet PoM £4.15 DT price = £4.15
  Diclofenac potassium 50 mg Voltarol Rapid 50mg tablets | 30 tablet PoM £7.94 DT price = £7.94

Diclofenac sodium

- **INDICATIONS AND DOSE**

Pain and inflammation in rheumatic disease including juvenile idiopathic arthritis
- ▸ BY MOUTH USING IMMEDIATE-RELEASE MEDICINES
- ▸ Child 6 months–17 years: 1.5–2.5 mg/kg twice daily, total daily dose may alternatively be given in 3 divided doses; maximum 150 mg per day

Postoperative pain
- ▸ BY RECTUM
- ▸ Child 6 months–17 years (body-weight 8–11 kg): 12.5 mg twice daily for maximum 4 days
- ▸ Child 6 months–17 years (body-weight 12 kg and above): 1 mg/kg 3 times a day (max. per dose 50 mg) for maximum 4 days

Inflammation | Mild to moderate pain
- ▸ BY MOUTH USING IMMEDIATE-RELEASE MEDICINES, OR BY RECTUM
- ▸ Child 6 months–17 years: 0.3–1 mg/kg 3 times a day (max. per dose 50 mg)

DICLOMAX RETARD®
Pain and inflammation
- ▸ BY MOUTH
- ▸ Child 12–17 years: 1 capsule once daily

DICLOMAX SR®
Pain and inflammation
- ▸ BY MOUTH
- ▸ Child 12–17 years: 1 capsule 1–2 times a day

MOTIFENE®
Pain and inflammation
- ▸ BY MOUTH
- ▸ Child 12–17 years: 1 capsule 1–2 times a day continued →

10

Musculoskeletal system

VOLTAROL® 75MG SR TABLETS

Pain and inflammation
▶ BY MOUTH
▶ Child 12–17 years: 1 tablet 1–2 times a day

VOLTAROL® RETARD

Pain and inflammation
▶ BY MOUTH
▶ Child 12–17 years: 1 tablet once daily

VOLTAROL® SOLUTION FOR INJECTION

Postoperative pain
▶ BY INTRAVENOUS INFUSION, OR BY DEEP INTRAMUSCULAR INJECTION
▶ Child 2–17 years: 0.3–1 mg/kg 1–2 times a day for maximum 2 days, for intramuscular injection, to be injected into the gluteal muscle; maximum 150 mg per day

● UNLICENSED USE Not licensed for use in children under 1 year. *Suppositories* not licensed for use in children under 6 years except for use in children over 1 year for juvenile idiopathic arthritis. Solid dose forms containing more than 25 mg not licensed for use in children. *Injection* not licensed for use in children.

● CONTRA-INDICATIONS
GENERAL CONTRA-INDICATIONS
Active gastro-intestinal bleeding · active gastro-intestinal ulceration · avoid injections containing benzyl alcohol in neonates; avoid suppositories in proctitis · cerebrovascular disease · history of gastro-intestinal bleeding related to previous NSAID therapy · history of gastro-intestinal perforation related to previous NSAID therapy · history of recurrent gastro-intestinal haemorrhage (two or more distinct episodes) · history of recurrent gastro-intestinal ulceration (two or more distinct episodes) · ischaemic heart disease · mild to severe heart failure · peripheral arterial disease
SPECIFIC CONTRA-INDICATIONS
▶ With intravenous use Dehydration · history of asthma · history of confirmed or suspected cerebrovascular bleeding · history of haemorrhagic diathesis · hypovolaemia · operations with high risk of haemorrhage

● CAUTIONS
▶ With systemic use Allergic disorders · cardiac impairment (NSAIDs may impair renal function) · coagulation defects · connective-tissue disorders · Crohn's disease (may be exacerbated) · history of cardiac failure · hypertension · left ventricular dysfunction · oedema · risk factors for cardiovascular events · ulcerative colitis (may be exacerbated)

● INTERACTIONS → Appendix 1 (NSAIDs).
▶ With intravenous use Contra-indicated in concomitant NSAID use. Contra-indicated in concomitant anticoagulant use (including low-dose heparins).

● SIDE-EFFECTS
GENERAL SIDE-EFFECTS
▶ Rare Alveolitis · aseptic meningitis (patients with connective-tissue disorders such as systemic lupus erythematosus may be especially susceptible) · hepatic damage · interstitial fibrosis associated with NSAIDs can lead to renal failure · pancreatitis · papillary necrosis associated with NSAIDs can lead to renal failure · pulmonary eosinophilia · Stevens-Johnson syndrome · toxic epidermal necrolysis · visual disturbances
▶ Frequency not known Angioedema · blood disorders · bronchospasm · colitis (induction of or exacerbation of) · Crohn's disease (induction of or exacerbation of) · depression · diarrhoea · dizziness · drowsiness · fluid retention (rarely precipitating congestive heart failure) · gastro-intestinal bleeding · gastro-intestinal discomfort · gastro-intestinal disturbances · gastro-intestinal

ulceration · haematuria · headache · hearing disturbances · hypersensitivity reactions · insomnia · nausea · nervousness · photosensitivity · raised blood pressure · rashes · renal failure (especially in patients with pre-existing renal impairment) · tinnitus · vertigo
SPECIFIC SIDE-EFFECTS
▶ Frequency not known
▶ With intramuscular use or intravenous use Injection site reactions
▶ With rectal use Suppositories may cause rectal irritation
SIDE-EFFECTS, FURTHER INFORMATION
▶ Serious side-effects For information about cardiovascular and gastro-intestinal side-effects, and a possible exacerbation of symptoms in asthma, see Non-steroidal anti-inflammatory drugs p. 604.

● ALLERGY AND CROSS-SENSITIVITY Contra-indicated in patients with a history of hypersensitivity to aspirin or any other NSAID—which includes those in whom attacks of asthma, angioedema, urticaria or rhinitis have been precipitated by aspirin or any other NSAID.

● PREGNANCY Avoid unless the potential benefit outweighs the risk. Avoid during the third trimester (risk of closure of fetal ductus arteriosus *in utero* and possibly persistent pulmonary hypertension of the newborn); onset of labour may be delayed and duration may be increased.

● BREAST FEEDING Use with caution during breast-feeding. Amount in milk too small to be harmful.

● HEPATIC IMPAIRMENT Use with caution; there is an increased risk of gastro-intestinal bleeding and fluid retention. Avoid in severe liver disease.

● RENAL IMPAIRMENT Avoid if possible or use with caution. Avoid in severe impairment.If used, the lowest effective dose should be given for the shortest possible duration. Monitor renal function; sodium and water retention may occur and renal function may deteriorate, possibly leading to renal failure.
▶ With intravenous use Contra-indicated in moderate or severe renal impairment.

● DIRECTIONS FOR ADMINISTRATION
▶ With intravenous use For *intravenous infusion*, dilute 75 mg with 100–500 mL Glucose 5% *or* Sodium Chloride 0.9% (previously buffered with 0.5 mL Sodium Bicarbonate 8.4% solution *or* with 1 mL Sodium Bicarbonate 4.2% solution); give over 30–120 minutes.

● PATIENT AND CARER ADVICE
Medicines for Children leaflet: Diclofenac for pain and inflammation www.medicinesforchildren.org.uk/diclofenac-for-pain-and-inflammation

● MEDICINAL FORMS
There can be variation in the licensing of different medicines containing the same drug. Forms available from special-order manufacturers include: dispersible tablet, oral suspension, oral solution

Dispersible tablet
CAUTIONARY AND ADVISORY LABELS 13, 21
▶ Voltarol (Novartis Pharmaceuticals UK Ltd)
Diclofenac sodium 50 mg Voltarol 50mg dispersible tablets sugar-free | 21 tablet PoM £7.43 DT price = £7.43

Modified-release tablet
CAUTIONARY AND ADVISORY LABELS 21, 25
▶ Voltarol Retard (Novartis Pharmaceuticals UK Ltd)
Diclofenac sodium 100 mg Voltarol Retard 100mg tablets | 28 tablet PoM £11.36 DT price = £11.36
▶ Voltarol SR (Novartis Pharmaceuticals UK Ltd)
Diclofenac sodium 75 mg Voltarol 75mg SR tablets | 28 tablet PoM £7.75 | 56 tablet PoM £15.50 DT price = £15.50

Gastro-resistant tablet

CAUTIONARY AND ADVISORY LABELS 5, 25

▸ **Diclofenac sodium** (Non-proprietary)
Diclofenac sodium 25 mg Diclofenac sodium 25mg gastro-resistant tablets | 28 tablet [PoM] £2.25–£8.99 DT price = £2.45 | 84 tablet [PoM] £8.16
Diclofenac sodium 50 mg Diclofenac sodium 50mg gastro-resistant tablets | 28 tablet [PoM] £4.97 DT price = £3.29 | 84 tablet [PoM] £15.00 | 100 tablet [PoM] no price available

▸ **Dicloflex** (Dexcel-Pharma Ltd, Almus Pharmaceuticals Ltd)
Diclofenac sodium 25 mg Dicloflex 25mg gastro-resistant tablets | 84 tablet [PoM] £4.42
Diclofenac sodium 50 mg Dicloflex 50mg gastro-resistant tablets | 28 tablet [PoM] £2.75 DT price = £3.29 (Hospital only) | 84 tablet [PoM] £8.05–£8.85

▸ **Fenactol** (Discovery Pharmaceuticals)
Diclofenac sodium 50 mg Fenactol 50mg gastro-resistant tablets | 100 tablet [PoM] £3.70

▸ **Voltarol** (Novartis Pharmaceuticals UK Ltd)
Diclofenac sodium 25 mg Voltarol 25mg gastro-resistant tablets | 84 tablet [PoM] £2.94
Diclofenac sodium 50 mg Voltarol 50mg gastro-resistant tablets | 10 tablet [PoM] £0.91 (Hospital only) | 14 tablet [PoM] no price available (Hospital only) | 84 tablet [PoM] £4.57 | 90 tablet [PoM] £5.88

Modified-release capsule

CAUTIONARY AND ADVISORY LABELS 21 (does not apply to Motifene® 75 mg), 25
EXCIPIENTS: May contain Propylene glycol

▸ **Diclomax Retard** (Galen Ltd)
Diclofenac sodium 100 mg Diclomax Retard 100mg capsules | 28 capsule [PoM] £6.97 DT price = £6.97

▸ **Diclomax SR** (Galen Ltd)
Diclofenac sodium 75 mg Diclomax SR 75mg capsules | 56 capsule [PoM] £9.69 DT price = £9.69

▸ **Motifene** (Daiichi Sankyo UK Ltd)
Diclofenac sodium 75 mg Motifene 75mg modified-release capsules | 56 capsule [PoM] £8.00 DT price = £8.00

Solution for injection

EXCIPIENTS: May contain Benzyl alcohol, propylene glycol

▸ **Voltarol** (Novartis Pharmaceuticals UK Ltd)
Diclofenac sodium 25 mg per 1 ml Voltarol 75mg/3ml solution for injection ampoules | 10 ampoule [PoM] £9.91 DT price = £9.91

Suppository

▸ **Diclofenac sodium** (Non-proprietary)
Diclofenac sodium 100 mg Diclofenac 100mg suppositories | 10 suppository [PoM] £7.75 DT price = £3.64

▸ **Econac** (AMCo)
Diclofenac sodium 100 mg Econac 100mg suppositories | 10 suppository [PoM] £3.04 DT price = £3.64

▸ **Voltarol** (Novartis Pharmaceuticals UK Ltd)
Diclofenac sodium 12.5 mg Voltarol 12.5mg suppositories | 10 suppository [PoM] £0.70 DT price = £0.70
Diclofenac sodium 25 mg Voltarol 25mg suppositories | 10 suppository [PoM] £1.24 DT price = £1.24
Diclofenac sodium 50 mg Voltarol 50mg suppositories | 10 suppository [PoM] £2.04 DT price = £2.04
Diclofenac sodium 100 mg Voltarol 100mg suppositories | 10 suppository [PoM] £3.64 DT price = £3.64

Etoricoxib

● **INDICATIONS AND DOSE**

Pain and inflammation in osteoarthritis

▸ BY MOUTH
▸ Child 16–17 years: 30 mg once daily, then increased if necessary to 60 mg once daily

Pain and inflammation in rheumatoid arthritis | Ankylosing spondylitis

▸ BY MOUTH
▸ Child 16–17 years: 90 mg once daily

Acute gout

▸ BY MOUTH
▸ Child 16–17 years: 120 mg once daily for maximum 8 days

● **CONTRA-INDICATIONS** Active gastro-intestinal bleeding · active gastro-intestinal ulceration · cerebrovascular disease · inflammatory bowel disease · ischaemic heart disease · mild to severe heart failure · peripheral arterial disease · uncontrolled hypertension (persistently above 140/90 mmHg)

● **CAUTIONS** Allergic disorders · cardiac impairment (NSAIDs may impair renal function) · coagulation defects · connective-tissue disorders · Crohn's disease (may be exacerbated) · dehydration · history of cardiac failure · hypertension · left ventricular dysfunction · oedema · risk factors for cardiovascular events · ulcerative colitis (may be exacerbated)

● **INTERACTIONS** → Appendix 1 (NSAIDs).

● **SIDE-EFFECTS**

▸ **Common or very common** Ecchymosis · fatigue · influenza-like symptoms · palpitation

▸ **Uncommon** Anxiety · appetite change · arthralgia · atrial fibrillation · chest pain · cough · dry mouth · dyspnoea · electrolyte disturbance · epistaxis · flushing · mental acuity impaired · mouth ulcer · myalgia · paraesthesia · taste disturbance · transient ischaemic attack · weight change

▸ **Rare** Alveolitis · aseptic meningitis (patients with connective-tissue disorders such as systemic lupus erythematosus may be especially susceptible) · hepatic damage · interstitial fibrosis associated with NSAIDs can lead to renal failure · pancreatitis · papillary necrosis associated with NSAIDs can lead to renal failure · pulmonary eosinophilia · Stevens-Johnson syndrome · toxic epidermal necrolysis · visual disturbances

▸ **Very rare** Confusion · hallucinations

▸ **Frequency not known** Angioedema · blood disorders · bronchospasm · colitis (induction of or exacerbation of) · Crohn's disease (induction of or exacerbation of) · depression · diarrhoea · dizziness · drowsiness · fluid retention (rarely precipitating congestive heart failure) · gastro-intestinal bleeding · gastro-intestinal discomfort · gastro-intestinal disturbances · gastro-intestinal ulceration · haematuria · headache · hearing disturbances · hypersensitivity reactions · insomnia · nausea · nervousness · photosensitivity · raised blood pressure · rashes · renal failure (especially in patients with pre-existing renal impairment) · tinnitus · vertigo

SIDE-EFFECTS, FURTHER INFORMATION

▸ **Serious side-effects** For information about cardiovascular and gastro-intestinal side-effects, and a possible exacerbation of symptoms in asthma, see Non-steroidal anti-inflammatory drugs p. 604.

● **ALLERGY AND CROSS-SENSITIVITY** Contra-indicated in patients with a history of hypersensitivity to aspirin or any other NSAID—which includes those in whom attacks of asthma, angioedema, urticaria or rhinitis have been precipitated by aspirin or any other NSAID.

● **CONCEPTION AND CONTRACEPTION** Caution—long-term use of some NSAIDs is associated with reduced female fertility, which is reversible on stopping treatment.

● **PREGNANCY** Manufacturer advises avoid (teratogenic in *animal* studies). Avoid during the third trimester (risk of closure of fetal ductus arteriosus *in utero* and possibly persistent pulmonary hypertension of the newborn); onset of labour may be delayed and duration may be increased.

● **BREAST FEEDING** Use with caution during breast-feeding. Manufacturer advises avoid—present in milk in *animal* studies.

● **HEPATIC IMPAIRMENT** Max. 60 mg daily in mild impairment. Max. 60 mg on alternate days or 30 mg once daily in moderate impairment. Use with caution; there is an increased risk of gastro-intestinal bleeding and fluid retention. Avoid in severe liver disease.

10

Musculoskeletal system

10

Musculoskeletal system

- **RENAL IMPAIRMENT** Avoid if possible or use with caution. Avoid if estimated glomerular filtration rate less than 30 mL/minute/1.73 m². If used, the lowest effective dose should be given for the shortest possible duration. Monitor renal function; sodium and water retention may occur and renal function may deteriorate, possibly leading to renal failure.
- **MONITORING REQUIREMENTS** Monitor blood pressure before treatment, 2 weeks after initiation and periodically during treatment.

- **MEDICINAL FORMS**
There can be variation in the licensing of different medicines containing the same drug.

Tablet
- Arcoxia (Grunenthal Ltd)
  Etoricoxib 30 mg Arcoxia 30mg tablets | 28 tablet [PoM] £13.99 DT price = £13.99
  Etoricoxib 60 mg Arcoxia 60mg tablets | 28 tablet [PoM] £20.11 DT price = £20.11
  Etoricoxib 90 mg Arcoxia 90mg tablets | 5 tablet [PoM] £4.10 | 28 tablet [PoM] £22.96 DT price = £22.96
  Etoricoxib 120 mg Arcoxia 120mg tablets | 7 tablet [PoM] £6.03 | 28 tablet [PoM] £24.11 DT price = £24.11

Flurbiprofen

- **INDICATIONS AND DOSE**

Pain and inflammation in rheumatic disease and other musculoskeletal disorders | Migraine | Postoperative analgesia | Mild to moderate pain
▸ BY MOUTH
▸ Child 12–17 years: 150–200 mg daily in 2–4 divided doses, then increased to 300 mg daily, dose to be increased only in acute conditions

Dysmenorrhoea
▸ BY MOUTH
▸ Child 12–17 years: Initially 100 mg, then 50–100 mg every 4–6 hours; maximum 300 mg per day

- **CONTRA-INDICATIONS** Active gastro-intestinal bleeding · active gastro-intestinal ulceration · history of gastro-intestinal bleeding related to previous NSAID therapy · history of gastro-intestinal perforation related to previous NSAID therapy · history of recurrent gastro-intestinal haemorrhage (two or more distinct episodes) · history of recurrent gastro-intestinal ulceration (two or more distinct episodes) · severe heart failure
- **CAUTIONS** Allergic disorders · cardiac impairment (NSAIDs may impair renal function) · cerebrovascular disease · coagulation defects · connective-tissue disorders · Crohn's disease (may be exacerbated) · heart failure · ischaemic heart disease · peripheral arterial disease · risk factors for cardiovascular events · ulcerative colitis (may be exacerbated) · uncontrolled hypertension
- **INTERACTIONS** → Appendix 1 (NSAIDs).
- **SIDE-EFFECTS**
- **Common or very common** Stomatitis
- **Uncommon** Confusion · fatigue · hallucinations · paraesthesia
- **Rare** Alveolitis · aseptic meningitis (patients with connective-tissue disorders such as systemic lupus erythematosus may be especially susceptible) · hepatic damage · interstitial fibrosis associated with NSAIDs can lead to renal failure · pancreatitis · papillary necrosis associated with NSAIDs can lead to renal failure · pulmonary eosinophilia · Stevens-Johnson syndrome · toxic epidermal necrolysis · visual disturbances
- **Frequency not known** Angioedema · blood disorders · bronchospasm · colitis (induction of or exacerbation of) · Crohn's disease (induction of or exacerbation of) · depression · diarrhoea · dizziness · drowsiness · fluid

retention (rarely precipitating congestive heart failure) · gastro-intestinal bleeding · gastro-intestinal discomfort · gastro-intestinal disturbances · gastro-intestinal ulceration · haematuria · headache · hearing disturbances · hypersensitivity reactions · insomnia · nausea · nervousness · photosensitivity · raised blood pressure · rashes · renal failure (especially in patients with pre-existing renal impairment) · tinnitus · vertigo

SIDE-EFFECTS, FURTHER INFORMATION
▸ **Serious side-effects** For information about cardiovascular and gastro-intestinal side-effects, and a possible exacerbation of symptoms in asthma, see Non-steroidal anti-inflammatory drugs p. 604.

- **ALLERGY AND CROSS-SENSITIVITY** Contra-indicated in patients with a history of hypersensitivity to aspirin or any other NSAID—which includes those in whom attacks of asthma, angioedema, urticaria or rhinitis have been precipitated by aspirin or any other NSAID.
- **PREGNANCY** Avoid unless the potential benefit outweighs the risk. Avoid during the third trimester (risk of closure of fetal ductus arteriosus *in utero* and possibly persistent pulmonary hypertension of the newborn); onset of labour may be delayed and duration may be increased.
- **BREAST FEEDING** Use with caution during breast-feeding. Small amount present in milk—manufacturer advises avoid.
- **HEPATIC IMPAIRMENT** Use with caution; there is an increased risk of gastro-intestinal bleeding and fluid retention. Avoid in severe liver disease.
- **RENAL IMPAIRMENT** Avoid if possible or use with caution. Avoid in severe impairment. If used, the lowest effective dose should be given for the shortest possible duration. Monitor renal function; sodium and water retention may occur and renal function may deteriorate, possibly leading to renal failure.

- **MEDICINAL FORMS**
There can be variation in the licensing of different medicines containing the same drug.

Tablet
CAUTIONARY AND ADVISORY LABELS 21
▸ Flurbiprofen (Non-proprietary)
  Flurbiprofen 50 mg Flurbiprofen 50mg tablets | 100 tablet [PoM] £21.30–£35.97 DT price = £30.29
  Flurbiprofen 100 mg Flurbiprofen 100mg tablets | 100 tablet [PoM] £64.34 DT price = £54.18

Ibuprofen

- **INDICATIONS AND DOSE**

Closure of ductus arteriosus
▸ BY SLOW INTRAVENOUS INJECTION
▸ Neonate: Initially 10 mg/kg for 1 dose, followed by 5 mg/kg every 24 hours for 2 doses, the course may be repeated after 48 hours if necessary.

Mild to moderate pain | Pain and inflammation of soft-tissue injuries | Pyrexia with discomfort
▸ BY MOUTH USING IMMEDIATE-RELEASE MEDICINES
▸ Child 1–2 months: 5 mg/kg 3–4 times a day
▸ Child 3–5 months: 50 mg 3 times a day, maximum daily dose to be given in 3–4 divided doses; maximum 30 mg/kg per day
▸ Child 6–11 months: 50 mg 3–4 times a day, maximum daily dose to be given in 3–4 divided doses; maximum 30 mg/kg per day
▸ Child 1–3 years: 100 mg 3 times a day, maximum daily dose to be given in 3–4 divided doses; maximum 30 mg/kg per day

- Child 4–6 years: 150 mg 3 times a day, maximum daily dose to be given in 3–4 divided doses; maximum 30 mg/kg per day
- Child 7–9 years: 200 mg 3 times a day, maximum daily dose to be given in 3–4 divided doses; maximum 30 mg/kg per day; maximum 2.4 g per day
- Child 10–11 years: 300 mg 3 times a day, maximum daily dose to be given in 3–4 divided doses; maximum 30 mg/kg per day; maximum 2.4 g per day
- Child 12–17 years: Initially 300–400 mg 3–4 times a day; increased if necessary up to 600 mg 4 times a day; maintenance 200–400 mg 3 times a day, may be adequate

Pain and inflammation

- ▶ BY MOUTH USING MODIFIED-RELEASE MEDICINES
- Child 12–17 years: 1.6 g once daily, dose preferably taken in the early evening, increased to 2.4 g daily in 2 divided doses, dose to be increased only in severe cases

Pain and inflammation in rheumatic disease including juvenile idiopathic arthritis

- ▶ BY MOUTH USING IMMEDIATE-RELEASE MEDICINES
- Child 3 months–17 years: 30–40 mg/kg daily in 3–4 divided doses; maximum 2.4 g per day

Pain and inflammation in systemic juvenile idiopathic arthritis

- ▶ BY MOUTH USING IMMEDIATE-RELEASE MEDICINES
- Child 3 months–17 years: Up to 60 mg/kg daily in 4–6 divided doses; maximum 2.4 g per day

Post-immunisation pyrexia in infants (on doctor's advice only)

- ▶ BY MOUTH USING IMMEDIATE-RELEASE MEDICINES
- Child 2–3 months: 50 mg for 1 dose, followed by 50 mg after 6 hours if required

● UNLICENSED USE
With intravenous use in neonates Orphan licence for the injection for closure of ductus arteriosus in premature neonates less than 34 weeks corrected gestational age. With oral use Not licensed for use in children under 3 months or body-weight under 5 kg. Maximum dose for systemic juvenile idiopathic arthritis is unlicensed.

● CONTRA-INDICATIONS
With intravenous use in neonates Active bleeding (especially intracranial or gastro-intestinal) · coagulation defects · known or suspected necrotising enterocolitis · life-threatening infection · marked unconjugated hyperbilirubinaemia · pulmonary hypertension · thrombocytopenia
With oral use Active gastro-intestinal bleeding · active gastro-intestinal ulceration · history of gastro-intestinal bleeding related to previous NSAID therapy · history of gastro-intestinal perforation related to previous NSAID therapy · history of recurrent gastro-intestinal haemorrhage (two or more distinct episodes) · history of recurrent gastro-intestinal ulceration (two or more distinct episodes) · severe heart failure

● CAUTIONS
With intravenous use in neonates May mask symptoms of infection
With oral use Cardiac impairment (NSAIDs may impair renal function) · cerebrovascular disease · coagulation defects · connective-tissue disorders · Crohn's disease (may be exacerbated) · heart failure · ischaemic heart disease · peripheral arterial disease · risk factors for cardiovascular events · risk factors for cardiovascular events · ulcerative colitis (may be exacerbated) · uncontrolled hypertension

CAUTIONS, FURTHER INFORMATION
High-dose ibuprofen A small increase in cardiovascular risk, similar to the risk associated with cyclo-oxygenase-2

inhibitors and diclofenac, has been reported with high-dose ibuprofen (≥ 2.4 g daily); use should be avoided in patients with established ischaemic heart disease, peripheral arterial disease, cerebrovascular disease, congestive heart failure (New York Heart Association classification II-III), and uncontrolled hypertension.

● INTERACTIONS → Appendix 1 (NSAIDs).

● SIDE-EFFECTS
▶ **Common or very common**
▶ With intravenous use in neonates Bronchopulmonary dysplasia · fluid retention · haematuria · hyponatraemia · intestinal perforation · intraventricular haemorrhage · ischaemic brain injury · neutropenia · oliguria · pulmonary haemorrhage · thrombocytopenia
▶ **Uncommon**
▶ With intravenous use in neonates Gastrointestinal haemorrhage
▶ **Rare**
▶ With oral use Alveolitis · aseptic meningitis (patients with connective-tissue disorders such as systemic lupus erythematosus may be especially susceptible) · hepatic damage · interstitial fibrosis associated with NSAIDs can lead to renal failure · pancreatitis · papillary necrosis associated with NSAIDs can lead to renal failure · pulmonary eosinophilia · Stevens-Johnson syndrome · toxic epidermal necrolysis · visual disturbances
▶ **Frequency not known**
▶ With intravenous use in neonates Hypoxaemia
▶ With oral use Angioedema · blood disorders · bronchospasm · colitis (induction of or exacerbation of) · Crohn's disease (induction of or exacerbation of) · depression · diarrhoea · dizziness · drowsiness · fluid retention (rarely precipitating congestive heart failure) · gastro-intestinal bleeding · gastro-intestinal discomfort · gastro-intestinal disturbances · gastro-intestinal ulceration · haematuria · headache · hearing disturbances · hypersensitivity reactions · insomnia · nausea · nervousness · photosensitivity · raised blood pressure · rashes · renal failure (especially in patients with pre-existing renal impairment) · tinnitus · vertigo

SIDE-EFFECTS, FURTHER INFORMATION
▶ Serious side-effects For information about cardiovascular and gastro-intestinal side-effects, and a possible exacerbation of symptoms in asthma, see Non-steroidal anti-inflammatory drugs p. 604.

Overdose
Overdosage with ibuprofen may cause nausea, vomiting, epigastric pain, and tinnitus, but more serious toxicity is very uncommon. Charcoal, activated p. 793 followed by symptomatic measures are indicated if more than 100 mg/kg has been ingested within the preceding hour.
For details on the management of poisoning, see Emergency treatment of poisoning p. 786.

● ALLERGY AND CROSS-SENSITIVITY Contra-indicated in patients with a history of hypersensitivity to aspirin or any other NSAID—which includes those in whom attacks of asthma, angioedema, urticaria or rhinitis have been precipitated by aspirin or any other NSAID.

● PREGNANCY Avoid unless the potential benefit outweighs the risk. Avoid during the third trimester (risk of closure of fetal ductus arteriosus in utero and possibly persistent pulmonary hypertension of the newborn); onset of labour may be delayed and duration may be increased.

● BREAST FEEDING Use with caution during breast-feeding. Amount too small to be harmful but some manufacturers advise avoid.

● HEPATIC IMPAIRMENT
▶ With intravenous use in neonates Increased risk of gastro-

10

Musculoskeletal system

intestinal bleeding and fluid retention. Avoid in severe liver disease.

▸ With oral use Use with caution; there is an increased risk of gastro-intestinal bleeding and fluid retention. Avoid in severe liver disease.

● **RENAL IMPAIRMENT**
▸ With intravenous use in neonates Use lowest effective dose and monitor renal function; sodium and water retention may occur and renal function may deteriorate, possibly leading to renal failure. Avoid if possible in severe impairment.

▸ With oral use Avoid if possible or use with caution. Avoid in severe impairment. If used, the lowest effective dose should be given for the shortest possible duration. Monitor renal function; sodium and water retention may occur and renal function may deteriorate, possibly leading to renal failure.

● **MONITORING REQUIREMENTS**
▸ With intravenous use in neonates Monitor for bleeding. Monitor gastro-intestinal function.

● **DIRECTIONS FOR ADMINISTRATION**
▸ With intravenous use in neonates For *slow intravenous injection*, give over 15 minutes, preferably undiluted. May be diluted with Glucose 5% or Sodium Chloride 0.9%.

● **PRESCRIBING AND DISPENSING INFORMATION** Flavours of syrup may include orange.

● **PATIENT AND CARER ADVICE**
Medicines for Children leaflet: Ibuprofen for pain and inflammation www.medicinesforchildren.org.uk/ibuprofen-for-pain-and-inflammation

● **PROFESSION SPECIFIC INFORMATION**

Dental practitioners' formulary
Ibuprofen Oral Suspension Sugar-free may be prescribed. Ibuprofen Tablets may be prescribed.

● **EXCEPTIONS TO LEGAL CATEGORY** Oral preparations can be sold to the public in certain circumstances.

● **MEDICINAL FORMS**
There can be variation in the licensing of different medicines containing the same drug. Forms available from special-order manufacturers include: oral suspension

Tablet
CAUTIONARY AND ADVISORY LABELS 21
▸ **Ibuprofen (Non-proprietary)**
Ibuprofen 200 mg Ibuprofen 200mg tablets | 16 tablet Ⓟ £0.20 | 24 tablet Ⓟ £1.13 DT price = £0.82 | 48 tablet Ⓟ £1.93 | 84 tablet Ⓟ £3.57 DT price = £2.87 | 96 tablet Ⓟ £1.69
Ibuprofen 200mg tablets sugar coated | 84 tablet Ⓟ £3.92 DT price = £2.87
Ibuprofen 200mg tablets film coated | 84 tablet Ⓟ £1.38 DT price = £2.87
Ibuprofen 200mg caplets | 16 tablet Ⓟ £0.20 | 24 tablet Ⓟ no price available DT price = £0.82 | 48 tablet Ⓟ no price available | 96 tablet Ⓟ no price available | 100 tablet Ⓟ no price available
Ibuprofen 400 mg Ibuprofen 400mg tablets film coated | 24 tablet Ⓟ £1.02 DT price = £0.93 | 84 tablet Ⓟ £1.52 DT price = £3.26
Ibuprofen 400mg tablets | 24 tablet Ⓟ £1.39 DT price = £0.93 | 48 tablet Ⓟ £2.56 | 84 tablet Ⓟ £6.84 DT price = £3.26 | 96 tablet Ⓟ £2.46 | 250 tablet PoM £10.74
Ibuprofen 400mg caplets | 12 tablet Ⓟ no price available | 24 tablet Ⓟ no price available DT price = £0.93 | 48 tablet Ⓟ no price available | 96 tablet Ⓟ no price available
Ibuprofen 400mg tablets sugar coated | 24 tablet Ⓟ £1.50 DT price = £0.93 | 48 tablet Ⓟ £2.40
Ibuprofen 600 mg Ibuprofen 600mg tablets | 84 tablet PoM £6.95 DT price = £4.32
Ibuprofen 600mg tablets film coated | 84 tablet PoM £4.79 DT price = £4.32
▸ **Brufen** (BGP Products Ltd)
Ibuprofen 400 mg Brufen 400mg tablets | 60 tablet PoM £4.90
Ibuprofen 600 mg Brufen 600mg tablets | 60 tablet PoM £7.34

▸ **Cuprofen** (SSL International Plc)
Ibuprofen 400 mg Cuprofen Maximum Strength 400mg tablets | 12 tablet Ⓟ £1.03 | 24 tablet Ⓟ £1.61 DT price = £0.93 | 48 tablet Ⓟ £2.91 | 96 tablet Ⓟ £5.04
▸ **Ibucalm** (Aspar Pharmaceuticals Ltd)
Ibuprofen 200 mg Ibucalm 200mg tablets | 24 tablet Ⓟ £0.77 DT price = £0.82 | 48 tablet Ⓟ £1.43 | 96 tablet Ⓟ £2.43
Ibuprofen 400 mg Ibucalm 400mg tablets | 16 tablet Ⓟ £0.88 | 24 tablet Ⓟ £1.36 DT price = £0.93 | 48 tablet Ⓟ £2.44 | 96 tablet Ⓟ £4.19
▸ **Nurofen** (Reckitt Benckiser Healthcare (UK) Ltd)
Ibuprofen 200 mg Nurofen 200mg caplets | 24 tablet Ⓟ £2.48 DT price = £0.82
Nurofen 200mg tablets | 24 tablet Ⓟ £2.37 DT price = £0.82 | 48 tablet Ⓟ £4.36 | 96 tablet Ⓟ £7.20
Ibuprofen (as Ibuprofen lysine) 400 mg Nurofen Maximum Strength Migraine Pain 684mg caplets | 12 tablet Ⓟ £3.49

Modified-release tablet
CAUTIONARY AND ADVISORY LABELS 25, 27
▸ **Brufen Retard** (BGP Products Ltd)
Ibuprofen 800 mg Brufen Retard 800mg tablets | 56 tablet PoM £7.74 DT price = £7.74

Capsule
▸ **Ibuprofen (Non-proprietary)**
Ibuprofen 200 mg Ibuprofen 200mg capsules | 24 capsule Ⓟ £4.0 | 30 capsule Ⓟ no price available DT price = £4.40 | 32 capsule Ⓟ £0.79
Ibuprofen 400 mg Ibuprofen 400mg capsules | 10 capsule Ⓟ no price available | 20 capsule Ⓟ no price available

Chewable capsule
▸ **Nurofen** (Reckitt Benckiser Healthcare (UK) Ltd)
Ibuprofen 100 mg Nurofen for Children 100mg chewable capsules | 12 capsule Ⓟ £3.23

Effervescent granules
CAUTIONARY AND ADVISORY LABELS 13, 21
ELECTROLYTES: May contain Sodium
▸ **Brufen** (BGP Products Ltd)
Ibuprofen 600 mg Brufen 600mg effervescent granules sachets | 20 sachet PoM £6.80 DT price = £6.80

Oral suspension
CAUTIONARY AND ADVISORY LABELS 21
▸ **Ibuprofen (Non-proprietary)**
Ibuprofen 20 mg per 1 ml Ibuprofen 100mg/5ml oral suspension sugar free sugar-free | 100 ml Ⓟ £1.38 DT price = £1.25 sugar-free 150 ml Ⓟ no price available sugar-free | 500 ml PoM £7.55 sugar-free | 500 ml Ⓟ no price available
▸ **Brufen** (BGP Products Ltd)
Ibuprofen 20 mg per 1 ml Brufen 100mg/5ml syrup | 500 ml PoM £8.88 DT price = £8.88
▸ **Calprofen** (McNeil Products Ltd)
Ibuprofen 20 mg per 1 ml Calprofen 100mg/5ml oral suspension sugar-free | 200 ml Ⓟ £3.42
▸ **Mandafen** (M & A Pharmachem Ltd)
Ibuprofen 20 mg per 1 ml Mandafen for Children 100mg/5ml oral suspension sugar free sugar-free | 100 ml Ⓟ £0.69 DT price = £1.25
▸ **Nurofen** (Reckitt Benckiser Healthcare (UK) Ltd)
Ibuprofen 20 mg per 1 ml Nurofen for Children 100mg/5ml oral suspension orange sugar-free | 200 ml Ⓟ £4.20
Nurofen for Children 100mg/5ml oral suspension strawberry sugar-free | 200 ml Ⓟ £4.20
▸ **Orbifen** (Orbis Consumer Products Ltd)
Ibuprofen 20 mg per 1 ml Orbifen For Children 100mg/5ml oral suspension sugar-free | 100 ml Ⓟ £1.67 DT price = £1.25 sugar-free | 150 ml Ⓟ £2.71

Solution for infusion
▸ **Pedea** (Orphan Europe (UK) Ltd)
Ibuprofen 5 mg per 1 ml Pedea 10mg/2ml solution for infusion ampoules | 4 ampoule PoM £288.00 (Hospital only)

Indometacin

(Indomethacin)

● **INDICATIONS AND DOSE**

Symptomatic ductus arteriosus

▸ BY INTRAVENOUS INFUSION

▸ **Neonate:** Initially 100–200 micrograms/kg for 1 dose, followed by 100 micrograms/kg after 24 hours for 2 doses, at 24-hour intervals, doses to be given over 20–30 minutes, if residual patency present, 100 micrograms/kg to be given for a further 3 doses at 24-hour intervals.

Relief of pain and inflammation in rheumatic diseases including juvenile idiopathic arthritis

▸ BY MOUTH USING IMMEDIATE-RELEASE MEDICINES

▸ **Child:** 0.5–1 mg/kg twice daily, higher doses may be used under specialist supervision

● **UNLICENSED USE**
▸ With oral use Not licensed for use in children.

● **CONTRA-INDICATIONS**
▸ With intravenous use in neonates Bleeding (especially with active intracranial haemorrhage or gastro-intestinal bleeding) · coagulation defects · necrotising enterocolitis · thrombocytopenia · untreated infection
▸ With oral use Active gastro-intestinal bleeding · active gastro-intestinal ulceration · history of gastro-intestinal bleeding related to previous NSAID therapy · history of gastro-intestinal perforation related to previous NSAID therapy · history of recurrent gastro-intestinal haemorrhage (two or more distinct episodes) · history of recurrent gastro-intestinal ulceration (two or more distinct episodes) · severe heart failure

● **CAUTIONS**
GENERAL CAUTIONS
Heart failure
SPECIFIC CAUTIONS
▸ With intravenous use in neonates Inhibition of platelet aggregation (monitor for bleeding) · may induce hyponatraemia · may mask symptoms of infection · may reduce urine output by 50% or more and precipitate renal impairment especially if extracellular volume depleted · sepsis
With oral use Allergic disorders · cardiac impairment (NSAIDs may impair renal function) · cerebrovascular disease · coagulation defects · connective-tissue disorders · Crohn's disease (may be exacerbated) · epilepsy · ischaemic heart disease · peripheral arterial disease · psychiatric disturbances · risk factors for cardiovascular events · ulcerative colitis (may be exacerbated) · uncontrolled hypertension
▸ INTERACTIONS → Appendix 1 (NSAIDs).
With intravenous use in neonates Caution with concomitant use of nephrotoxic drugs.

● **SIDE-EFFECTS**
Rare
With oral use Alveolitis · aseptic meningitis (patients with connective-tissue disorders such as systemic lupus erythematosus may be especially susceptible) · blood disorders · confusion · convulsions · hepatic damage · hyperglycaemia · interstitial fibrosis associated with NSAIDs can lead to renal failure · intestinal strictures · pancreatitis · papillary necrosis associated with NSAIDs can lead to renal failure · peripheral neuropathy · psychiatric disturbances · pulmonary eosinophilia · Stevens-Johnson syndrome · syncope · thrombocytopenia · toxic epidermal necrolysis · visual disturbances

▸ Frequency not known
▸ With intravenous use in neonates Coagulation disorders · exacerbation of infection · fluid retention · gastro-intestinal disorders · haemorrhagic disorders · intracranial bleeding · metabolic disorders · pulmonary hypertension · renal disorders
▸ With oral use Angioedema · blood disorders · bronchospasm · colitis (induction of or exacerbation of) · Crohn's disease (induction of or exacerbation of) · depression · diarrhoea · dizziness · drowsiness · fluid retention (rarely precipitating congestive heart failure) · gastro-intestinal bleeding · gastro-intestinal discomfort · gastro-intestinal disturbances · gastro-intestinal ulceration · haematuria · headache · hearing disturbances · hyperkalaemia · hypersensitivity reactions · insomnia · nausea · nervousness · photosensitivity · raised blood pressure · rashes · renal failure (especially in patients with pre-existing renal impairment) · tinnitus · vertigo

SIDE-EFFECTS, FURTHER INFORMATION
▸ Serious side-effects For information about cardiovascular and gastro-intestinal side-effects, and a possible exacerbation of symptoms in asthma, see Non-steroidal anti-inflammatory drugs p. 604.

● **ALLERGY AND CROSS-SENSITIVITY** Contra-indicated in patients with a history of hypersensitivity to aspirin or any other NSAID—which includes those in whom attacks of asthma, angioedema, urticaria or rhinitis have been precipitated by aspirin or any other NSAID.

● **PREGNANCY** Avoid unless the potential benefit outweighs the risk. Avoid during the third trimester (risk of closure of fetal ductus arteriosus *in utero* and possibly persistent pulmonary hypertension of the newborn); onset of labour may be delayed and duration may be increased.

● **BREAST FEEDING** Amount probably too small to be harmful—manufacturers advise avoid. Use with caution during breast-feeding.

● **HEPATIC IMPAIRMENT**
▸ With intravenous use in neonates Increased risk of gastro-intestinal bleeding and fluid retention. Avoid in severe impairment.
▸ With oral use Use with caution; there is an increased risk of gastro-intestinal bleeding and fluid retention. Avoid in severe liver disease.

● **RENAL IMPAIRMENT**
▸ With intravenous use in neonates Use lowest effective dose. Avoid if possible in severe impairment.
▸ With oral use The lowest effective dose should be used for the shortest possible duration.
Anuria or oliguria
▸ With intravenous use in neonates If anuria or marked oliguria (urinary output less than 0.6 mL/kg/hour), delay further doses until renal function returns to normal.
▸ With oral use Avoid if possible or use with caution. Avoid in severe impairment. In renal impairment monitor renal function; sodium and water retention may occur and renal function may deteriorate, possibly leading to renal failure.

● **MONITORING REQUIREMENTS**
▸ With oral use During prolonged therapy ophthalmic and blood examinations particularly advisable.

● **DIRECTIONS FOR ADMINISTRATION**
▸ With intravenous use in neonates For *intravenous infusion*, dilute each vial with 1–2 mL Sodium Chloride 0.9% *or* Water for Injections.

● **PATIENT AND CARER ADVICE**
Driving and skilled tasks Dizziness may affect performance of skilled tasks (e.g. driving).

10

Musculoskeletal system

- **MEDICINAL FORMS**
There can be variation in the licensing of different medicines containing the same drug. Forms available from special-order manufacturers include: oral suspension, oral solution

Capsule
CAUTIONARY AND ADVISORY LABELS 21
▸ Indometacin (Non-proprietary)
Indometacin 25 mg Indometacin 25mg capsules | 28 capsule [PoM]
£5.00 DT price = £0.98
Indometacin 50 mg Indometacin 50mg capsules | 28 capsule [PoM]
£7.50 DT price = £1.39

Ketoprofen

- **INDICATIONS AND DOSE**
For use as a component of below
▸ BY MOUTH
▸ Child 15–17 years: (consult product literature)

- **CONTRA-INDICATIONS** Active gastro-intestinal bleeding · active gastro-intestinal ulceration · history of gastro-intestinal bleeding · history of gastro-intestinal perforation · history of gastro-intestinal ulceration · severe heart failure
- **CAUTIONS** Allergic disorders · cardiac impairment (NSAIDs may impair renal function) · cerebrovascular disease · coagulation defects · connective-tissue disorders · Crohn's disease (may be exacerbated) · heart failure · ischaemic heart disease · peripheral arterial disease · risk factors for cardiovascular events · ulcerative colitis (may be exacerbated) · uncontrolled hypertension
- **INTERACTIONS** → Appendix 1 (NSAIDs).
- **SIDE-EFFECTS**
▸ **Rare** Alveolitis · aseptic meningitis (patients with connective-tissue disorders such as systemic lupus erythematosus may be especially susceptible) · hepatic damage · interstitial fibrosis associated with NSAIDs can lead to renal failure · pancreatitis · papillary necrosis associated with NSAIDs can lead to renal failure · pulmonary eosinophilia · Stevens-Johnson syndrome · toxic epidermal necrolysis · visual disturbances
▸ **Frequency not known** Angioedema · blood disorders · bronchospasm · colitis (induction of or exacerbation of) · Crohn's disease (induction of or exacerbation of) · depression · diarrhoea · dizziness · drowsiness · fluid retention (rarely precipitating congestive heart failure) · gastro-intestinal bleeding · gastro-intestinal discomfort · gastro-intestinal disturbances · gastro-intestinal ulceration · haematuria · headache · hearing disturbances · hypersensitivity reactions · insomnia · nausea · nervousness · photosensitivity · raised blood pressure · rashes · renal failure (especially in patients with pre-existing renal impairment) · tinnitus · vertigo

SIDE-EFFECTS, FURTHER INFORMATION
▸ **Serious side-effects** For information about cardiovascular and gastro-intestinal side-effects, and a possible exacerbation of symptoms in asthma, see Non-steroidal anti-inflammatory drugs p. 604.

- **ALLERGY AND CROSS-SENSITIVITY** Contra-indicated in patients with a history of hypersensitivity to aspirin or any other NSAID—which includes those in whom attacks of asthma, angioedema, urticaria or rhinitis have been precipitated by aspirin or any other NSAID.
- **CONCEPTION AND CONTRACEPTION** Caution—long-term use of some NSAIDs is associated with reduced female fertility, which is reversible on stopping treatment.
- **PREGNANCY** Avoid unless the potential benefit outweighs the risk. Avoid during the third trimester (risk of closure of fetal ductus arteriosus *in utero* and possibly persistent pulmonary hypertension of the newborn); onset of labour may be delayed and duration may be increased.

- **BREAST FEEDING** Use with caution during breast-feeding. Amount probably too small to be harmful but manufacturers advise avoid.
- **HEPATIC IMPAIRMENT** Use with caution; there is an increased risk of gastro-intestinal bleeding and fluid retention. Should be avoided in severe liver disease.
- **RENAL IMPAIRMENT** Avoid if possible or use with caution. Avoid in severe impairment. If used, the lowest effective dose should be given for the shortest possible duration. Monitor renal function; sodium and water retention may occur and renal function may deteriorate, possibly leading to renal failure.
- **PRESCRIBING AND DISPENSING INFORMATION** Flavours of oral liquid formulations may include strawberry.
- **MEDICINAL FORMS**
There can be variation in the licensing of different medicines containing the same drug.

Ketoprofen with omeprazole

The properties listed below are those particular to the combination only. For the properties of the components please consider, ketoprofen above, omeprazole p. 54.

- **INDICATIONS AND DOSE**
Patients requiring ketoprofen for osteoarthritis, rheumatoid arthritis, and ankylosing spondylitis, who are at risk of NSAID associated duodenal or gastric ulcer or gastroduodenal erosions
▸ BY MOUTH USING MODIFIED-RELEASE MEDICINES
▸ Child 15–17 years: Initially 100/20 mg daily, increased if necessary to 200/20 mg daily, depending on severity of symptoms, dose expressed as x/y mg ketoprofen/omeprazole

- **PRESCRIBING AND DISPENSING INFORMATION** Capsules enclose microgranules containing modified-release ketoprofen and gastro-resistant omperazole.

- **MEDICINAL FORMS**
There can be variation in the licensing of different medicines containing the same drug.
Modified-release capsule
CAUTIONARY AND ADVISORY LABELS 21, 25
EXCIPIENTS: May contain Propylene glycol
▸ Axorid (Meda Pharmaceuticals Ltd)
Omeprazole 20 mg, Ketoprofen 100 mg Axorid 100mg/20mg modified-release capsules | 30 capsule [PoM] £13.80
Omeprazole 20 mg, Ketoprofen 200 mg Axorid 200mg/20mg modified-release capsules | 30 capsule [PoM] £13.80

Mefenamic acid

- **INDICATIONS AND DOSE**
Acute pain including dysmenorrhoea | Menorrhagia
▸ BY MOUTH
▸ Child 12–17 years: 500 mg 3 times a day

- **CONTRA-INDICATIONS** Active gastro-intestinal bleeding · active gastro-intestinal ulceration · history of gastro-intestinal bleeding related to previous NSAID therapy · history of gastro-intestinal perforation related to previous NSAID therapy · history of recurrent gastro-intestinal haemorrhage (two or more distinct episodes) · history of recurrent gastro-intestinal ulceration (two or more distinct episodes) · inflammatory bowel disease · severe heart failure
- **CAUTIONS** Acute porphyrias p. 562 · allergic disorders · cardiac impairment (NSAIDs may impair renal function) · cerebrovascular disease · coagulation defects · connective tissue disorders · Crohn's disease (may be exacerbated) ·

epilepsy · heart failure · ischaemic heart disease ·
peripheral arterial disease · risk factors for cardiovascular
events · ulcerative colitis (may be exacerbated) ·
uncontrolled hypertension
● **INTERACTIONS** → Appendix 1 (NSAIDs).
● **SIDE-EFFECTS**
▶ **Common or very common** Diarrhoea (withdraw treatment) ·
rashes (withdraw treatment) · stomatitis
▶ **Uncommon** Fatigue · paraesthesia
▶ **Rare** Alveolitis · aplastic anaemia · aseptic meningitis
(patients with connective-tissue disorders such as
systemic lupus erythematosus may be especially
susceptible) · glucose intolerance · haemolytic anaemia
(positive Coombs' test) · hepatic damage · hypotension ·
interstitial fibrosis associated with NSAIDs can lead to
renal failure · palpitation · pancreatitis · papillary necrosis
associated with NSAIDs can lead to renal failure ·
pulmonary eosinophilia · Stevens-Johnson syndrome ·
thrombocytopenia · toxic epidermal necrolysis · visual
disturbances
▶ **Frequency not known** Angioedema · blood disorders ·
bronchospasm · colitis (induction of or exacerbation of) ·
Crohn's disease (induction of or exacerbation of) ·
depression · dizziness · drowsiness · fluid retention (rarely
precipitating congestive heart failure) · gastro-intestinal
bleeding · gastro-intestinal discomfort · gastro-intestinal
disturbances · gastro-intestinal ulceration · haematuria ·
headache · hearing disturbances · hypersensitivity
reactions · insomnia · nausea · nervousness ·
photosensitivity · raised blood pressure · renal failure
(especially in patients with pre-existing renal impairment) ·
tinnitus · vertigo

SIDE-EFFECTS, FURTHER INFORMATION
▶ Serious side-effects For information about cardiovascular
and gastro-intestinal side-effects, and a possible
exacerbation of symptoms in asthma, see Non-steroidal
anti-inflammatory drugs p. 604.

Overdose
Mefenamic acid has important consequences in
overdosage because it can cause convulsions, which if
prolonged or recurrent, require treatment.
    For details on the management of poisoning, see
Emergency treatment of poisoning p. 786, in particular,
Convulsions.

● **ALLERGY AND CROSS-SENSITIVITY** Contra-indicated in
patients with a history of hypersensitivity to aspirin or any
other NSAID—which includes those in whom attacks of
asthma, angioedema, urticaria or rhinitis have been
precipitated by aspirin or any other NSAID.
● **PREGNANCY** Avoid unless the potential benefit outweighs
the risk. Avoid during the third trimester (risk of closure of
fetal ductus arteriosus *in utero* and possibly persistent
pulmonary hypertension of the newborn); onset of labour
may be delayed and duration may be increased.
● **BREAST FEEDING** Use with caution during breast-feeding.
Amount too small to be harmful but manufacturer advises
avoid.
● **HEPATIC IMPAIRMENT** Use with caution; there is an
increased risk of gastro-intestinal bleeding and fluid
retention. Avoid in severe liver disease.
● **RENAL IMPAIRMENT** Avoid if possible or use with caution.
Avoid in severe impairment. If used, the lowest effective
dose should be given for the shortest possible duration.
Monitor renal function; sodium and water retention may
occur and renal function may deteriorate, possibly leading
to renal failure.

● **MEDICINAL FORMS**
There can be variation in the licensing of different medicines
containing the same drug. Forms available from special-order
manufacturers include: oral suspension
Tablet
CAUTIONARY AND ADVISORY LABELS 21
▶ Mefenamic acid (Non-proprietary)
    Mefenamic acid 500 mg Mefenamic acid 500mg tablets |
    28 tablet [PoM] £18.00 DT price = £7.43 | 84 tablet [PoM] £44.99
▶ Ponstan (Chemidex Pharma Ltd)
    Mefenamic acid 500 mg Ponstan Forte 500mg tablets |
    100 tablet [PoM] £15.72
Capsule
CAUTIONARY AND ADVISORY LABELS 21
▶ Mefenamic acid (Non-proprietary)
    Mefenamic acid 250 mg Mefenamic acid 250mg capsules |
    100 capsule [PoM] £15.00 DT price = £12.04
▶ Ponstan (Chemidex Pharma Ltd)
    Mefenamic acid 250 mg Ponstan 250mg capsules |
    100 capsule [PoM] £8.17 DT price = £12.04
Oral suspension
CAUTIONARY AND ADVISORY LABELS 21
EXCIPIENTS: May contain Ethanol
▶ Mefenamic acid (Non-proprietary)
    Mefenamic acid 10 mg per 1 ml Mefenamic acid 50mg/5ml oral
    suspension | 125 ml [PoM] £79.98 DT price = £79.98

Meloxicam

● **INDICATIONS AND DOSE**
Exacerbation of osteoarthritis (short-term)
▶ BY MOUTH
▶ Child 16–17 years: 7.5 mg once daily, then increased if
  necessary up to 15 mg once daily
**Pain and inflammation in rheumatic disease | Ankylosing
spondylitis**
▶ BY MOUTH
▶ Child 16–17 years: 15 mg once daily, then reduced to
  7.5 mg once daily if required
**Relief of pain and inflammation in juvenile idiopathic
arthritis and other musculoskeletal disorders in children
intolerant to other NSAIDs**
▶ BY MOUTH
▶ Child 12–17 years (body-weight up to 50 kg): 7.5 mg once
  daily
▶ Child 12–17 years (body-weight 50 kg and above): 15 mg
  once daily

● **UNLICENSED USE** Not licensed for use in children under
16 years.
● **CONTRA-INDICATIONS** Active gastro-intestinal bleeding ·
active gastro-intestinal ulceration · history of gastro-
intestinal bleeding related to previous NSAID therapy ·
history of gastro-intestinal perforation related to previous
NSAID therapy · history of recurrent gastro-intestinal
haemorrhage (two or more distinct episodes) · history of
recurrent gastro-intestinal ulceration (two or more
distinct episodes) · severe heart failure
● **CAUTIONS** Allergic disorders · cardiac impairment (NSAIDs
may impair renal function) · cerebrovascular disease ·
coagulation defects · connective-tissue disorders · Crohn's
disease (may be exacerbated) · heart failure · ischaemic
heart disease · peripheral arterial disease · risk factors for
cardiovascular events · ulcerative colitis (may be
exacerbated) · uncontrolled hypertension
● **INTERACTIONS** → Appendix 1 (NSAIDs).
● **SIDE-EFFECTS**
▶ **Rare** Alveolitis · aseptic meningitis (patients with
connective-tissue disorders such as systemic lupus
erythematosus may be especially susceptible) · hepatic
damage · interstitial fibrosis associated with NSAIDs can
lead to renal failure · pancreatitis · papillary necrosis

10

Musculoskeletal system

associated with NSAIDs can lead to renal failure · pulmonary eosinophilia · Stevens-Johnson syndrome · toxic epidermal necrolysis · visual disturbances
▶ **Frequency not known** Angioedema · blood disorders · bronchospasm · colitis (induction of or exacerbation of) · Crohn's disease (induction of or exacerbation of) · depression · diarrhoea · dizziness · drowsiness · fluid retention (rarely precipitating congestive heart failure) · gastro-intestinal bleeding · gastro-intestinal discomfort · gastro-intestinal disturbances · gastro-intestinal ulceration · haematuria · headache · hearing disturbances · hypersensitivity reactions · insomnia · nausea · nervousness · photosensitivity · raised blood pressure · rashes · renal failure (especially in patients with pre-existing renal impairment) · tinnitus · vertigo

SIDE-EFFECTS, FURTHER INFORMATION
▶ **Serious side-effects** For information about cardiovascular and gastro-intestinal side-effects, and a possible exacerbation of symptoms in asthma, see Non-steroidal anti-inflammatory drugs p. 604.

● **ALLERGY AND CROSS-SENSITIVITY** Contra-indicated in patients with a history of hypersensitivity to aspirin or any other NSAID—which includes those in whom attacks of asthma, angioedema, urticaria or rhinitis have been precipitated by aspirin or any other NSAID.

● **PREGNANCY** Avoid unless the potential benefit outweighs the risk. Avoid during the third trimester (risk of closure of fetal ductus arteriosus *in utero* and possibly persistent pulmonary hypertension of the newborn); onset of labour may be delayed and duration may be increased.

● **BREAST FEEDING** Use with caution during breast-feeding. Present in milk in *animal* studies—manufacturer advises avoid.

● **HEPATIC IMPAIRMENT** Use with caution; there is an increased risk of gastro-intestinal bleeding and fluid retention. Avoid in severe liver disease.

● **RENAL IMPAIRMENT** Avoid if possible or use with caution. Avoid if estimated glomerular filtration rate less than 25 mL/minute/1.73 m^2. If used, the lowest effective dose should be given for the shortest possible duration. Monitor renal function; sodium and water retention may occur and renal function may deteriorate, possibly leading to renal failure.

● **MEDICINAL FORMS**
There can be variation in the licensing of different medicines containing the same drug. Forms available from special-order manufacturers include: oral suspension

Tablet
CAUTIONARY AND ADVISORY LABELS 21
▶ **Meloxicam (Non-proprietary)**
Meloxicam 7.5 mg Meloxicam 7.5mg tablets | 30 tablet [PoM] £8.20
DT price = £0.92
Meloxicam 15 mg Meloxicam 15mg tablets | 30 tablet [PoM] £4.00
DT price = £0.99

Orodispersible tablet
▶ **Meloxicam (Non-proprietary)**
Meloxicam 7.5 mg Meloxicam 7.5mg orodispersible tablets sugar free sugar-free | 30 tablet [PoM] £15.50
Meloxicam 15 mg Meloxicam 15mg orodispersible tablets sugar free sugar-free | 30 tablet [PoM] £15.50

Naproxen

● **INDICATIONS AND DOSE**
Pain and inflammation in musculoskeletal disorders | Dysmenorrhoea
▶ BY MOUTH
▶ Child: 5 mg/kg twice daily; maximum 1 g per day

Pain and inflammation in juvenile idiopathic arthritis
▶ BY MOUTH
▶ Child 2–17 years: 5–7.5 mg/kg twice daily; maximum 1 g per day

● **UNLICENSED USE** Not licensed for use in children under 5 years for juvenile idiopathic arthritis. Not licensed for use in children under 16 years for musculoskeletal disorders or dysmenorrhoea.

● **CONTRA-INDICATIONS** Active gastro-intestinal bleeding · active gastro-intestinal ulceration · history of gastro-intestinal bleeding related to previous NSAID therapy · history of gastro-intestinal perforation related to previous NSAID therapy · history of recurrent gastro-intestinal haemorrhage (two or more distinct episodes) · history of recurrent gastro-intestinal ulceration (two or more distinct episodes) · severe heart failure

● **CAUTIONS** Allergic disorders · cardiac impairment (NSAIDs may impair renal function) · cerebrovascular disease · coagulation defects · connective-tissue disorders · Crohn's disease (may be exacerbated) · heart failure · ischaemic heart disease · peripheral arterial disease · risk factors for cardiovascular events · ulcerative colitis (may be exacerbated) · uncontrolled hypertension

● **INTERACTIONS** → Appendix 1 (NSAIDs).

● **SIDE-EFFECTS**
▶ **Rare** Alveolitis · aseptic meningitis (patients with connective-tissue disorders such as systemic lupus erythematosus may be especially susceptible) · hepatic damage · interstitial fibrosis associated with NSAIDs can lead to renal failure · pancreatitis · papillary necrosis associated with NSAIDs can lead to renal failure · pulmonary eosinophilia · Stevens-Johnson syndrome · toxic epidermal necrolysis · visual disturbances
▶ **Frequency not known** Angioedema · blood disorders · bronchospasm · colitis (induction of or exacerbation of) · Crohn's disease (induction of or exacerbation of) · depression · diarrhoea · dizziness · drowsiness · fluid retention (rarely precipitating congestive heart failure) · gastro-intestinal bleeding · gastro-intestinal discomfort · gastro-intestinal disturbances · gastro-intestinal ulceration · haematuria · headache · hearing disturbances · hypersensitivity reactions · insomnia · nausea · nervousness · photosensitivity · raised blood pressure · rashes · renal failure (especially in patients with pre-existing renal impairment) · tinnitus · vertigo

SIDE-EFFECTS, FURTHER INFORMATION
▶ **Serious side-effects** For information about cardiovascular and gastro-intestinal side-effects, and a possible exacerbation of symptoms in asthma, see Non-steroidal anti-inflammatory drugs p. 604.

● **ALLERGY AND CROSS-SENSITIVITY** Contra-indicated in patients with a history of hypersensitivity to aspirin or any other NSAID—which includes those in whom attacks of asthma, angioedema, urticaria or rhinitis have been precipitated by aspirin or any other NSAID.

● **PREGNANCY** Avoid unless the potential benefit outweighs the risk. Avoid during the third trimester (risk of closure of fetal ductus arteriosus *in utero* and possibly persistent pulmonary hypertension of the newborn); onset of labour may be delayed and duration may be increased.

● **BREAST FEEDING** Use with caution during breast-feeding. Amount too small to be harmful but manufacturer advises avoid.

● **HEPATIC IMPAIRMENT** Use with caution; there is an increased risk of gastro-intestinal bleeding and fluid retention. Avoid in severe liver disease.

● **RENAL IMPAIRMENT** Avoid if possible or use with caution. Avoid if estimated glomerular filtration rate less than 30 mL/minute/1.73 m^2. If used, the lowest effective dose should be given for the shortest possible duration. Monitor renal function; sodium and water retention may occur and renal function may deteriorate, possibly leading to renal failure.

- **EXCEPTIONS TO LEGAL CATEGORY** Can be sold to the public for the treatment of primary dysmenorrhoea in women aged 15–50 years subject to max. single dose of 500 mg, max. daily dose of 750 mg for max. 3 days, and a max. pack size of 9 × 250 mg tablets.

- **MEDICINAL FORMS**
There can be variation in the licensing of different medicines containing the same drug. Forms available from special-order manufacturers include: oral suspension

Tablet
CAUTIONARY AND ADVISORY LABELS 21
▸ Naproxen (Non-proprietary)
Naproxen 250 mg Naproxen 250mg tablets | 28 tablet [PoM] £6.98 DT price = £0.91 | 56 tablet [PoM] £2.33
Naproxen 500 mg Naproxen 500mg tablets | 28 tablet [PoM] £8.76 DT price = £1.22 | 56 tablet [PoM] £3.99

Effervescent tablet
▸ Stirlescent (Stirling Anglian Pharmaceuticals Ltd)
Naproxen 250 mg Stirlescent 250mg effervescent tablets sugar-free | 20 tablet [PoM] £7.90

Gastro-resistant tablet
CAUTIONARY AND ADVISORY LABELS 5, 25
▸ Naproxen (Non-proprietary)
Naproxen 250 mg Naproxen 250mg gastro-resistant tablets | 56 tablet [PoM] £12.90 DT price = £3.27
Naproxen 375 mg Naproxen 375mg gastro-resistant tablets | 56 tablet [PoM] £26.82 DT price = £26.82
Naproxen 500 mg Naproxen 500mg gastro-resistant tablets | 56 tablet [PoM] £16.90 DT price = £7.91

Oral suspension
▸ Naproxen (Non-proprietary)
Naproxen 25 mg per 1 ml Naproxen 25mg/ml oral suspension sugar free sugar-free | 100 ml [PoM] £110.00
Naproxen 125mg/5ml oral suspension sugar free sugar-free | 100 ml [PoM] £110.00

Piroxicam

- **INDICATIONS AND DOSE**
Relief of pain and inflammation in juvenile idiopathic arthritis
▸ BY MOUTH
▸ Child 6–17 years (body-weight up to 15 kg): 5 mg daily
▸ Child 6–17 years (body-weight 15-25 kg): 10 mg daily
▸ Child 6–17 years (body-weight 26-45 kg): 15 mg daily
▸ Child 6–17 years (body-weight 46 kg and above): 20 mg daily

- **UNLICENSED USE** Not licensed for use in children.

IMPORTANT SAFETY INFORMATION
CHMP ADVICE–PIROXICAM (JUNE 2007)
The CHMP has recommended restrictions on the use of piroxicam because of the increased risk of gastro-intestinal side effects and serious skin reactions. The CHMP has advised that:
- piroxicam should be initiated only by physicians experienced in treating inflammatory or degenerative rheumatic diseases
- piroxicam should not be used as first-line treatment
- in adults, use of piroxicam should be limited to the symptomatic relief of osteoarthritis, rheumatoid arthritis, and ankylosing spondylitis
- piroxicam dose should not exceed 20 mg daily
- piroxicam should no longer be used for the treatment of acute painful and inflammatory conditions
- treatment should be reviewed 2 weeks after initiating piroxicam, and periodically thereafter

- concomitant administration of a gastro-protective agent should be considered.
Topical preparations containing piroxicam are not affected by these restrictions.

- **CONTRA-INDICATIONS** Active gastro-intestinal bleeding · active gastro-intestinal ulceration · history of gastro-intestinal bleeding · history of gastro-intestinal perforation · history of gastro-intestinal ulceration · inflammatory bowel disease · severe heart failure

- **CAUTIONS** Allergic disorders · cardiac impairment (NSAIDs may impair renal function) · cerebrovascular disease · coagulation defects · connective-tissue disorders · Crohn's disease (may be exacerbated) · heart failure · ischaemic heart disease · peripheral arterial disease · risk factors for cardiovascular events · ulcerative colitis (may be exacerbated) · uncontrolled hypertension

- **INTERACTIONS** → Appendix 1 (NSAIDs).

- **SIDE-EFFECTS**
▸ **Rare** Alveolitis · aseptic meningitis (patients with connective-tissue disorders such as systemic lupus erythematosus may be especially susceptible) · hepatic damage · interstitial fibrosis associated with NSAIDs can lead to renal failure · pancreatitis · papillary necrosis associated with NSAIDs can lead to renal failure · pulmonary eosinophilia · Stevens-Johnson syndrome · toxic epidermal necrolysis · visual disturbances
▸ **Frequency not known** Angioedema · blood disorders · bronchospasm · colitis (induction of or exacerbation of) · Crohn's disease (induction of or exacerbation of) · depression · diarrhoea · dizziness · drowsiness · fluid retention (rarely precipitating congestive heart failure) · gastro-intestinal bleeding · gastro-intestinal discomfort · gastro-intestinal disturbances · gastro-intestinal ulceration · haematuria · headache · hearing disturbances · hypersensitivity reactions · insomnia · nausea · nervousness · photosensitivity · raised blood pressure · rashes · renal failure (especially in patients with pre-existing renal impairment) · tinnitus · vertigo
SIDE-EFFECTS, FURTHER INFORMATION
▸ Serious side-effects For information about cardiovascular and gastro-intestinal side-effects, and a possible exacerbation of symptoms in asthma, see Non-steroidal anti-inflammatory drugs p. 604.

- **ALLERGY AND CROSS-SENSITIVITY** Contra-indicated in patients with a history of hypersensitivity to aspirin or any other NSAID—which includes those in whom attacks of asthma, angioedema, urticaria or rhinitis have been precipitated by aspirin or any other NSAID.

- **PREGNANCY** Avoid unless the potential benefit outweighs the risk. Avoid during the third trimester (risk of closure of fetal ductus arteriosus in utero and possibly persistent pulmonary hypertension of the newborn); onset of labour may be delayed and duration may be increased.

- **BREAST FEEDING** Use with caution during breast-feeding. Amount too small to be harmful.

- **HEPATIC IMPAIRMENT** Use with caution; there is an increased risk of gastro-intestinal bleeding and fluid retention. Avoid in severe liver disease.

- **RENAL IMPAIRMENT** Avoid if possible or use with caution. Avoid in severe impairment. If used, the lowest effective dose should be given for the shortest possible duration. Monitor renal function; sodium and water retention may occur and renal function may deteriorate, possibly leading to renal failure.

- **DIRECTIONS FOR ADMINISTRATION** Piroxicam orodispersible tablets can be taken by placing on the tongue and allowing to dissolve or by swallowing. Piroxicam orodispersible tablets may be halved to give 10 mg dose.

- **LESS SUITABLE FOR PRESCRIBING** Piroxicam is less suitable for prescribing.

- **MEDICINAL FORMS**
  There can be variation in the licensing of different medicines containing the same drug.
  Orodispersible tablet
  CAUTIONARY AND ADVISORY LABELS 10, 21
  EXCIPIENTS: May contain Aspartame
  ▶ **Feldene Melt** (Pfizer Ltd)
  Piroxicam 20 mg Feldene Melt 20mg tablets sugar-free |
  30 tablet PoM £10.53 DT price = £10.53
  Capsule
  CAUTIONARY AND ADVISORY LABELS 21
  ▶ **Piroxicam (Non-proprietary)**
  Piroxicam 10 mg Piroxicam 10mg capsules | 56 capsule PoM
  £16.82 DT price = £3.73
  Piroxicam 20 mg Piroxicam 20mg capsules | 28 capsule PoM
  £17.60 DT price = £3.13
  ▶ **Feldene** (Pfizer Ltd)
  Piroxicam 10 mg Feldene 10mg capsules | 30 capsule PoM £3.86
  Piroxicam 20 mg Feldene 20 capsules | 30 capsule PoM £7.71

4 Soft tissue and joint disorders

4.1 Local inflammation of joints and soft tissue

CORTICOSTEROIDS

Corticosteroids, inflammatory disorders

Systemic corticosteroids

In children with rheumatic diseases corticosteroids should be reserved for specific indications (e.g. when other therapies are unsuccessful or while waiting for DMARDs to take effect) and should be used only under the supervision of a specialist.

Systemic corticosteroids may be considered for the management of juvenile idiopathic arthritis in systemic disease or when several joints are affected. Systemic corticosteroids may also be considered in severe, possibly life-threatening conditions such as systemic lupus erythematosus, systemic vasculitis, juvenile dermatomyositis, Behçet's disease, and polyarticular joint disease.

In severe conditions, short courses ('pulses') of high dose intravenous methylprednisolone p. 617 or a pulsed oral corticosteroid may be particularly effective for providing rapid relief, and has fewer long-term adverse effects than continuous treatment.

Corticosteroid doses should be reduced with care because of the possibility of relapse if the reduction is too rapid. If complete discontinuation of corticosteroids is not possible, consideration should be given to alternate-day (or alternate high-dose, low-dose) administration; on days when no corticosteroid is given, or a lower dose is given, an additional dose of a NSAID may be helpful. In some conditions, alternative treatment using an antimalarial or concomitant use of an immunosuppressant drug, such as azathioprine p. 485, methotrexate p. 506 or cyclophosphamide p. 498 may prove useful; in less severe conditions treatment with a NSAID alone may be adequate.

Administration of corticosteroids may result in suppression of growth and may affect the development of puberty. The risk of corticosteroid-induced osteoporosis should be considered for those on long-term corticosteroid treatment; corticosteroids may also increase the risk of osteopenia in those unable to exercise. See the disadvantages of corticosteroid treatment.

Local corticosteroid injections

Corticosteroids are injected locally for an anti-inflammatory effect. In inflammatory conditions of the joints, including juvenile idiopathic arthritis, they are given by *intra-articular injection* as monotherapy, or as an adjunct to long-term therapy to reduce swelling and deformity in one or a few joints. Aseptic precautions (e.g. a no-touch technique) are essential, as is a clinician skilled in the technique; infected areas should be avoided and general anaesthesia, or local anaesthesia, or conscious sedation should be used. Occasionally an acute inflammatory reaction develops after an intra-articular or soft-tissue injection of a corticosteroid. This may be a reaction to the microcrystalline suspension of the corticosteroid used, but must be distinguished from sepsis introduced into the injection site.

Triamcinolone hexacetonide p. 617 [unlicensed] is preferred for intra-articular injection because it is almost insoluble and has a long-acting (depot) effect. Triamcinolone acetonide p. 617 and methylprednisolone may also be considered for intra-articular injection into larger joints, whilst hydrocortisone below acetate should be reserved for smaller joints or for soft-tissue injections. Intra-articular corticosteroid injections can cause flushing and, in adults, may affect the hyaline cartilage. Each joint should usually be treated no more than 3–4 times in one year.

A smaller amount of corticosteroid may also be injected directly into soft tissues for the relief of inflammation in conditions such as *tennis* or *golfer's elbow* or *compression neuropathies*, which occur rarely in children. In *tendinitis*, injections should be made into the tendon sheath and not directly into the tendon (due to the absence of a true tendon sheath and a high risk of rupture, the Achilles tendon should not be injected).

Corticosteroid injections are also injected into soft tissues for the treatment of skin lesions.

F 407

Hydrocortisone

- **INDICATIONS AND DOSE**
  HYDROCORTISTAB®
  Local inflammation of joints and soft-tissues
  ▶ BY INTRA-ARTICULAR INJECTION
  ▶ Child 1 month-11 years: 5–30 mg, select dose according to size of child and joint; where appropriate dose may be repeated at intervals of 21 days. Not more than 3 joints should be treated on any one day, for details consult product literature
  ▶ Child 12-17 years: 5–50 mg, select dose according to size of patient and joint; where appropriate dose may be repeated at intervals of 21 days. Not more than 3 joints should be treated on any one day, for details consult product literature

- **MEDICINAL FORMS**
  There can be variation in the licensing of different medicines containing the same drug.
  Suspension for injection
  ▶ Hydrocortistab (AMCo)
  Hydrocortisone acetate 25 mg per 1 ml Hydrocortistab 25mg/1ml suspension for injection ampoules | 10 ampoule PoM £68.72 DT price = £68.72

Methylprednisolone

F 407

● **INDICATIONS AND DOSE**

DEPO-MEDRONE®

Local inflammation of joints and soft tissues

▶ BY INTRA-ARTICULAR INJECTION

▸ Child: (consult product literature)

● **PATIENT AND CARER ADVICE** Patient counselling is advised for methylprednisolone tablets and injections (steroid card).

● **MEDICINAL FORMS**
There can be variation in the licensing of different medicines containing the same drug. Forms available from special-order manufacturers include: oral suspension

Suspension for injection

CAUTIONARY AND ADVISORY LABELS 10

▸ **Depo-Medrone** (Pfizer Ltd)
Methylprednisolone acetate 40 mg per 1 ml Depo-Medrone 40mg/1ml suspension for injection vials | 1 vial PoM £3.44 DT price = £3.44 | 10 vial PoM £34.04
Depo-Medrone 80mg/2ml suspension for injection vials | 1 vial PoM £6.18 DT price = £6.18 | 10 vial PoM £61.39
Depo-Medrone 120mg/3ml suspension for injection vials | 1 vial PoM £8.96 DT price = £8.96 | 10 vial PoM £88.81

Triamcinolone acetonide

F 407

● **INDICATIONS AND DOSE**

ADCORTYL® INTRA-ARTICULAR/INTRADERMAL

Local inflammation of joints and soft tissues

▶ BY INTRA-ARTICULAR INJECTION

▸ Child 1–17 years: 2 mg/kg (max. per dose 15 mg), for details consult product literature, dose applies for larger joints. For doses above 15 mg use *Kenalog® Intra-articular/Intramuscular*. If appropriate repeat treatment for relapse.

KENALOG® VIALS

Local inflammation of joints and soft tissues

▶ BY INTRA-ARTICULAR INJECTION

▸ Child 1–17 years: 2 mg/kg, for details consult product literature, if appropriate repeat treatment for relapse, higher doses than usual maximum have been used; Usual maximum 40 mg

● **UNLICENSED USE** Not licensed for use in children under 6 years.

● **MEDICINAL FORMS**
There can be variation in the licensing of different medicines containing the same drug.

Suspension for injection

CAUTIONARY AND ADVISORY LABELS 10

EXCIPIENTS: May contain Benzyl alcohol

▸ **Adcortyl Intra-articular / Intradermal** (Bristol-Myers Squibb Pharmaceuticals Ltd)
Triamcinolone acetonide 10 mg per 1 ml Adcortyl Intra-articular / Intradermal 50mg/5ml suspension for injection vials | 1 vial PoM £3.63
Adcortyl Intra-articular / Intradermal 10mg/1ml suspension for injection ampoules | 5 ampoule PoM £4.47 DT price = £4.47

▸ **Kenalog** (Bristol-Myers Squibb Pharmaceuticals Ltd)
Triamcinolone acetonide 40 mg per 1 ml Kenalog Intra-articular / Intramuscular 40mg/1ml suspension for injection vials | 5 vial PoM £7.45 DT price = £7.45

Triamcinolone hexacetonide

F 407

● **INDICATIONS AND DOSE**

Symptomatic treatment of subacute and chronic inflammatory joint diseases (for details, consult product literature)

▶ BY INTRA-ARTICULAR INJECTION

▸ Child 12–17 years: 2–20 mg, according to size of the joint; if appropriate repeat treatment at intervals of 3–4 weeks, no more than 2 joints should be treated on any one day

▶ BY PERI-ARTICULAR INJECTION

▸ Child 12–17 years: 10–20 mg, according to size of the joint, no more than 2 joints should be treated on any one day

Juvenile idiopathic arthritis

▶ BY INTRA-ARTICULAR INJECTION

▸ Child 3–11 years: (consult product literature)

● **CONTRA-INDICATIONS** Avoid injections containing benzyl alcohol in neonates · consult product literature

● **CAUTIONS** Consult product literature

● **SIDE-EFFECTS** Consult product literature

● **PRESCRIBING AND DISPENSING INFORMATION** Various strengths available from 'special order' manufacturers or specialist importing companies.

● **MEDICINAL FORMS**
There can be variation in the licensing of different medicines containing the same drug.

Suspension for injection

EXCIPIENTS: May contain Benzyl alcohol

▸ **Triamcinolone hexacetonide** (Non-proprietary)
Triamcinolone hexacetonide 20 mg per 1 ml Triamcinolone hexacetonide 20mg/1ml suspension for injection ampoules | 10 ampoule PoM £120.00

4.2 Soft tissue disorders

Soft-tissue disorders

Soft-tissue and musculoskeletal disorders

The management of children with soft-tissue injuries and strains, and musculoskeletal disorders, may include temporary rest together with the local application of heat or cold, local massage and physiotherapy. For pain relief, paracetamol p. 254 is often adequate and should be used first. Alternatively, the lowest effective dose of a **NSAID** (e.g. ibuprofen p. 608) can be used. If pain relief with either drug is inadequate, both paracetamol (in a full dose appropriate for the child) and a low dose of a NSAID may be required.

Extravasation

Local guidelines for the management of extravasation should be followed where they exist or specialist advice sought.

Extravasation injury follows leakage of drugs or intravenous fluids from the veins or inadvertent administration into the subcutaneous or subdermal tissue. It must be dealt with **promptly** to prevent tissue necrosis.

Acidic or alkaline preparations and those with an osmolarity greater than that of plasma can cause extravasation injury; excipients including alcohol and polyethylene glycol have also been implicated. Cytotoxic drugs commonly cause extravasation injury. Very young children are at increased risk. Those receiving anticoagulants are more likely to lose blood into surrounding tissues if extravasation occurs, while those receiving sedatives or

10

Musculoskeletal system

analgesics may not notice the early signs or symptoms of extravasation.

Prevention of extravasation

Precautions should be taken to avoid extravasation; ideally, drugs likely to cause extravasation injury should be given through a central line and children receiving repeated doses of hazardous drugs peripherally should have the cannula resited at regular intervals. Attention should be paid to the manufacturers' recommendations for administration. Placing a glyceryl trinitrate patch p. 127 or using glyceryl trinitrate ointment distal to the cannula may improve the patency of the vessel in children with small veins or in those whose veins are prone to collapse. Children or their carers should be asked to report any pain or burning at the site of injection immediately.

Management of extravasation

If extravasation is suspected the infusion should be stopped immediately but the cannula should not be removed until after an attempt has been made to aspirate the area (through the cannula) in order to remove as much of the drug as possible. Aspiration is sometimes possible if the extravasation presents with a raised bleb or blister at the injection site and is surrounded by hardened tissue, but it is often unsuccessful if the tissue is soft or soggy. **Corticosteroids** are usually given to treat inflammation, although there is little evidence to support their use in extravasation. Hydrocortisone p. 616 or dexamethasone p. 410 can be given either locally by subcutaneous injection or intravenously at a site distant from the injury. Antihistamines and analgesics may be required for symptom relief.

The management of extravasation beyond these measures is not well standardised and calls for specialist advice. Treatment depends on the nature of the offending substance; one approach is to localise and neutralise the substance whereas another is to spread and dilute it. The first method may be appropriate following extravasation of vesicant drugs and involves administration of an antidote (if available) and the application of cold compresses 3–4 times a day (consult specialist literature for details of specific antidotes). Spreading and diluting the offending substance involves infiltrating the area with physiological saline, applying warm compresses, elevating the affected limb, and administering hyaluronidase below. A saline flush-out technique (involving flushing the subcutaneous tissue with physiological saline) may be effective but requires specialist advice. Hyaluronidase should **not** be administered following extravasation of vesicant drugs (unless it is either specifically indicated or used in the saline flush-out technique).

Enzymes

Hyaluronidase is used for the management of extravasation.

ENZYMES

Hyaluronidase

● **INDICATIONS AND DOSE**

Extravasation

▶ BY LOCAL INFILTRATION

▶ Child: (consult product literature)

● **UNLICENSED USE** Licensed for use in children, but age range not specified by the manufacturer.

● **CONTRA-INDICATIONS** Avoid sites where infection is present · avoid sites where malignancy is present · do not apply direct to cornea · not for anaesthesia in unexplained premature labour · not for intravenous administration · not to be used to enhance the absorption and dispersion of dopamine and/or alpha-adrenoceptor agonists · not to be

used to reduce swelling of bites · not to be used to reduce swelling of stings

● **CAUTIONS** Infants (control speed and total volume and avoid overhydration especially in renal impairment)

● **SIDE-EFFECTS**

▶ **Common or very common** Oedema

▶ **Rare** Bleeding · bruising · infection · local irritation

▶ **Frequency not known** Anaphylaxis · severe allergy

● **MEDICINAL FORMS**
There can be variation in the licensing of different medicines containing the same drug.

Powder for solution for injection

▶ Hyaluronidase (Non-proprietary)
Hyaluronidase 1500 unit Hyaluronidase 1,500unit powder for solution for injection ampoules | 10 ampoule PoM £104.24

Chapter 11
Eye

CONTENTS

1 Allergic and inflammatory eye conditions	page 620
1.1 Allergic conjunctivitis	620
1.2 Inflammatory eye conditions	622
1.2a Anterior uveitis	624
2 Dry eye conditions	625
3 Eye infections	629
3.1 Bacterial eye infection	630

3.2 Viral eye infection	page 632
3.2a Ophthalmic herpes simplex	632
4 Eye procedures	633
4.1 Post-operative pain and inflammation	634
5 Glaucoma and ocular hypertension	636

Eye

Administration of drugs to the eye

Drugs are most commonly administered to the eye by topical application as eye drops or eye ointments. When a higher drug concentration is required within the eye, a local injection may be necessary.

Eye-drop dispenser devices are available to aid the instillation of eye drops from plastic bottles and some are prescribable on the NHS (consult Drug Tariff—see Appliances and Reagents). Product-specific devices may be supplied by manufacturers—contact individual manufacturers for further information. They are particularly useful for children in whom normal application is difficult, for the visually impaired, or otherwise physically limited patients.

Eye drops and eye ointments

Eye drops are generally instilled into the pocket formed by gently pulling down the lower eyelid and keeping the eye closed for as long as possible after application; in neonates and infants it may be more appropriate to administer the drop in the inner angle of the open eye. One drop is all that is needed; instillation of more than one drop at a time should be discouraged because it may increase systemic side-effects. A small amount of eye ointment is applied similarly; the ointment melts rapidly and blinking helps to spread it.

When two different eye-drop preparations are used at the same time of day, dilution and overflow can occur when one immediately follows the other. The carer or child should therefore leave an interval of at least 5 minutes between the two; the interval should be extended when eye drops with a prolonged contact time, such as gels and suspensions, are used. Eye ointment should be applied after drops. Both drops and ointment can cause transient blurred vision; children should be warned, where appropriate, not to perform skilled tasks (e.g. cycling or driving) until vision is clear.

Systemic effects may arise from absorption of drugs into the general circulation from conjunctival vessels or from the nasal mucosa after the excess preparation has drained down through the tear ducts. The extent of systemic absorption following ocular administration is highly variable; nasal drainage of drugs is associated with eye drops much more often than with eye ointments. Pressure on the lacrimal punctum for at least a minute after applying eye drops reduces nasolacrimal drainage and therefore decreases systemic absorption from the nasal mucosa.

Also see warnings relating to eye drops and contact lenses.

Eye lotions

These are solutions for the irrigation of the conjunctival sac. They act mechanically to flush out irritants or foreign bodies as a first-aid treatment. Sterile sodium chloride 0.9% p. 628 solution is usually used. Clean water will suffice in an emergency.

Other preparations administered to the eye

Subconjunctival injection may be used to administer anti-infective drugs, mydriatics, or corticosteroids for conditions not responding to topical therapy; intracameral and intravitreal routes can also be used to administer certain drugs, for example antibacterials. These injections should only be used under specialist supervision.

Drugs such as antimicrobials and corticosteroids may be administered systemically to treat susceptible eye conditions.

Ophthalmic Specials

The Royal College of Ophthalmologists and the UK Ophthalmic Pharmacy Group have produced the Ophthalmic Specials Guidance to help prescribers and pharmacists manage and restrict the use of unlicensed eye preparations. 'Specials' should only be prescribed in situations where a licensed product will not be suitable for a child's needs. The Ophthalmic Specials Guidance can be accessed on the Royal College of Ophthalmologists website (www.rcophth.ac.uk). The guidance will be reviewed every six months to ensure the most accurate and up-to-date information is available.

Preservatives and sensitisers

Information on preservatives and substances identified as skin sensitisers is provided under Excipients statements in preparation entries. Very rarely, cases of corneal calcification have been reported with the use of phosphate-containing eye drops in patients with significantly damaged corneas—consult product literature for further information.

Control of microbial contamination

Preparations for the eye should be sterile when issued. Care should be taken to avoid contamination of the contents during use.

Eye drops in multiple-application containers for *domiciliary use* should not be used for more than 4 weeks after first opening (unless otherwise stated by the manufacturer).

Multiple application eye drops for use in *hospital wards* are normally discarded 1 week after first opening—local practice may vary. Individual containers should be provided for each patient. A separate container should be supplied for each eye only if there are special concerns about contamination. Containers used before an eye operation should be discarded at the time of the operation and fresh containers supplied postoperatively. A fresh supply should also be provided upon discharge from hospital; in specialist ophthalmology units, it may be acceptable to issue containers that have been dispensed to the patient on the day of discharge.

In *out-patient departments* single-application containers should be used; if multiple-application containers are used, they should be discarded after single patient use within one clinical session.

In *eye surgery* single-application containers should be used if possible; if a multiple-application container is used, it should be discarded after single use. Preparations used during intra-ocular procedures and others that may penetrate into the anterior chamber must be isotonic and without preservatives and buffered if necessary to a neutral pH. Specially formulated fluids should be used for intra-ocular surgery; intravenous infusion preparations are not usually suitable for this purpose (Hartmann's solution may be used in some ocular surgery). For all surgical procedures, a previously unopened container is used for each patient.

Contact lenses

For cosmetic reasons many people prefer to wear contact lenses rather than spectacles; contact lenses are also sometimes required for medical indications. Visual defects are corrected by either rigid ('hard' or gas permeable) lenses or soft (hydrogel or silicone hydrogel—in adults only) lenses; soft lenses are the most popular type, because they are initially the most comfortable, but they may not give the best vision. Lenses should usually be worn for a specified number of hours each day and removed for sleeping. The risk of infectious and non-infectious keratitis is increased by extended continuous contact lens wear, which is not recommended, except when medically indicated.

Contact lenses require meticulous care. Poor compliance with directions for use, and with daily cleaning and disinfection, can result in complications including ulcerative keratitis or conjunctivitis. One-day disposable lenses, which are worn only once and therefore require no disinfection or cleaning, are becoming increasingly popular.

Acanthamoeba keratitis, a painful and sight-threatening condition, is associated with ineffective lens cleaning and disinfection, the use of contaminated lens cases, or tap water coming into contact with the lenses. The condition is especially associated with the use of soft lenses (including frequently replaced lenses) and should be treated by specialists.

Contact lenses and drug treatment

Special care is required in prescribing eye preparations for contact lens users. Some drugs and preservatives in eye preparations can accumulate in hydrogel lenses and may induce toxic and adverse reactions. Therefore, unless medically indicated, the lenses should be removed before instillation of the eye preparation and not worn during the period of treatment. Alternatively, unpreserved drops can be used. Eye drops may, however, be instilled while patients are wearing rigid corneal contact lenses. Ointment preparations should never be used in conjunction with contact lens wear; oily eye drops should also be avoided.

Many drugs given systemically can also have adverse effects on contact lens wear. These include oral contraceptives (particularly those with a higher oestrogen content), drugs which reduce blink rate (e.g. anxiolytics, hypnotics, antihistamines, and muscle relaxants), drugs which reduce lacrimation (e.g. antihistamines, antimuscarinics, phenothiazines and related drugs, some beta-blockers, diuretics, and tricyclic antidepressants), and drugs which increase lacrimation (including ephedrine hydrochloride p. 114 and hydralazine hydrochloride p. 108). Other drugs that may affect contact lens wear are isotretinoin p. 712 (can cause conjunctival inflammation), aspirin p. 83 (salicylic acid appears in tears and can be absorbed by contact lenses—leading to irritation), and rifampicin p. 342 and sulfasalazine p. 29 (can discolour lenses).

1 Allergic and inflammatory eye conditions

Eye, allergy and inflammation

Corticosteroids

Corticosteroids administered locally to the eye or given by mouth are effective for treating anterior segment inflammation, including that which results from surgery.

Topical corticosteroids should normally only be used under expert supervision; three main dangers are associated with their use:

- a 'red eye', when the diagnosis is unconfirmed, may be due to herpes simplex virus, and a corticosteroid may aggravate the condition, leading to corneal ulceration, with possible damage to vision and even loss of the eye. Bacterial, fungal, and amoebic infections pose a similar hazard;
- 'steroid glaucoma' can follow the use of corticosteroid eye preparations in susceptible individuals;
- a 'steroid cataract' can follow prolonged use.

Products combining a corticosteroid with an antimicrobial are used after ocular surgery to reduce inflammation and prevent infection: use of combination products is otherwise rarely justified.

Systemic corticosteroids may be useful for ocular conditions. The risk of producing a 'steroid cataract' increases with the dose and duration of corticosteroid use.

Other anti-inflammatory preparations

Eye drops containing **antihistamines**, such as **antazoline** (with xylometazoline hydrochloride p. 650 as *Otrivine-Antistin*®), azelastine hydrochloride p. 621, epinastine hydrochloride p. 621, ketotifen p. 621, and olopatadine p. 621, can be used for allergic conjunctivitis.

Sodium cromoglicate p. 622 and nedocromil sodium p. 622 eye drops may be useful for vernal keratoconjunctivitis and other allergic forms of conjunctivitis.

Lodoxamide eye drops p. 622 are used for allergic conjunctival conditions including seasonal allergic conjunctivitis.

Emedastine eye drops p. 621 are licensed for seasonal allergic conjunctivitis.

1.1 Allergic conjunctivitis

ANTIHISTAMINES

▌ Antazoline with xylometazoline

- **INDICATIONS AND DOSE**

  Allergic conjunctivitis
  ▸ TO THE EYE
  ▸ Child 12–17 years: Apply 2–3 times a day for maximum 7 days

- **CAUTIONS** Angle-closure glaucoma · cardiovascular disease · diabetes mellitus · hypertension · hyperthyroidism · phaeochromocytoma · urinary retention
- **INTERACTIONS** → Appendix 1 (antihistamines and sympathomimetics).

Absorption of antazoline and xylometazoline may result in the possibility of interaction with other drugs.

- SIDE-EFFECTS
- ▶ **Common or very common** Transient stinging
- ▶ **Frequency not known** Blurred vision · eye irritation · mydriasis

SIDE-EFFECTS, FURTHER INFORMATION
Absorption of antazoline and xylometazoline may result in systemic side-effects.

- MEDICINAL FORMS
There can be variation in the licensing of different medicines containing the same drug.

Eye drops
EXCIPIENTS: May contain Benzalkonium chloride, disodium edetate
- ▶ Otrivine Antistin (Thea Pharmaceuticals Ltd)
Xylometazoline hydrochloride 500 microgram per 1 ml, Antazoline sulfate 5 mg per 1 ml Otrivine Antistin 0.5%/0.05% eye drops | 10 ml P £2.35 DT price = £2.35

Azelastine hydrochloride

- INDICATIONS AND DOSE

Seasonal allergic conjunctivitis
- ▶ TO THE EYE
- ▶ Child 4–17 years: Apply twice daily, increased if necessary to 4 times a day

Perennial conjunctivitis
- ▶ TO THE EYE
- ▶ Child 12–17 years: Apply twice daily; increased if necessary to 4 times a day, maximum duration of treatment 6 weeks

- SIDE-EFFECTS
- ▶ **Frequency not known** Bitter taste · mild transient irritation

- MEDICINAL FORMS
There can be variation in the licensing of different medicines containing the same drug.

Eye drops
EXCIPIENTS: May contain Benzalkonium chloride, disodium edetate
- ▶ Optilast (Meda Pharmaceuticals Ltd)
Azelastine hydrochloride 500 microgram per 1 ml Optilast 0.05% eye drops | 8 ml PoM £6.40 DT price = £6.40

Emedastine

- INDICATIONS AND DOSE

Seasonal allergic conjunctivitis
- ▶ TO THE EYE
- ▶ Child 3–17 years: Apply twice daily

- SIDE-EFFECTS Blurred vision · corneal infiltrates (discontinue) · corneal staining · dry eye · headache · irritation · keratitis · lacrimation · local oedema · photophobia · rhinitis · transient burning · transient stinging

- MEDICINAL FORMS
There can be variation in the licensing of different medicines containing the same drug.

Eye drops
EXCIPIENTS: May contain Benzalkonium chloride
- ▶ Emadine (Alcon Laboratories (UK) Ltd)
Emedastine (as Emedastine difumarate) 500 microgram per 1 ml Emadine 0.5mg/ml eye drops | 5 ml PoM £7.31 DT price = £7.31

Epinastine hydrochloride

- INDICATIONS AND DOSE

Seasonal allergic conjunctivitis
- ▶ TO THE EYE
- ▶ Child 12–17 years: Apply twice daily for maximum 8 weeks

- SIDE-EFFECTS
- ▶ **Common or very common** Burning
- ▶ **Uncommon** Conjunctival hyperaemia · dry eye · eye pain · eye pruritus · headache · increased lacrimation · nasal irritation · rhinitis · taste disturbance · visual disturbance

- MEDICINAL FORMS
There can be variation in the licensing of different medicines containing the same drug.

Eye drops
EXCIPIENTS: May contain Benzalkonium chloride, disodium edetate
- ▶ Relestat (Allergan Ltd)
Epinastine hydrochloride 500 microgram per 1 ml Relestat 500micrograms/ml eye drops | 5 ml PoM £9.90 DT price = £9.90

Ketotifen

- INDICATIONS AND DOSE

Seasonal allergic conjunctivitis
- ▶ TO THE EYE
- ▶ Child 3–17 years: Apply twice daily

- INTERACTIONS Interactions do not generally apply to antihistamines used for topical action.

- SIDE-EFFECTS
- ▶ **Common or very common** Punctate corneal epithelial erosion · transient burning · transient stinging
- ▶ **Uncommon** Dry eye · photophobia · subconjunctival haemorrhage
- ▶ **Frequency not known** Drowsiness · dry mouth · headache · skin reactions

- MEDICINAL FORMS
There can be variation in the licensing of different medicines containing the same drug.

Eye drops
EXCIPIENTS: May contain Benzalkonium chloride
- ▶ Zaditen (Thea Pharmaceuticals Ltd)
Ketotifen (as Ketotifen fumarate) 250 microgram per 1 ml Zaditen 250micrograms/ml eye drops | 5 ml PoM £7.80 DT price = £7.80

Olopatadine

- INDICATIONS AND DOSE

Seasonal allergic conjunctivitis
- ▶ TO THE EYE
- ▶ Child 3–17 years: Apply twice daily for maximum 4 months

- SIDE-EFFECTS
- ▶ **Common or very common** Local irritation
- ▶ **Uncommon** Asthenia · dizziness · dry eye · headache · keratitis · local oedema · photophobia
- ▶ **Frequency not known** Dry nose

- MEDICINAL FORMS
There can be variation in the licensing of different medicines containing the same drug.

Eye drops
EXCIPIENTS: May contain Benzalkonium chloride
- ▶ Opatanol (Alcon Laboratories (UK) Ltd)
Olopatadine (as Olopatadine hydrochloride) 1 mg per 1 ml Opatanol 1mg/ml eye drops | 5 ml PoM £4.68 DT price = £4.68

11

Eye

MAST-CELL STABILISERS

Lodoxamide

- **INDICATIONS AND DOSE**

Allergic conjunctivitis

▸ TO THE EYE

▸ **Child 4-17 years:** Apply 4 times a day, improvement of symptoms may sometimes require treatment for up to 4 weeks

- **SIDE-EFFECTS**

▸ **Common or very common** Blurred vision · burning · itching · ocular discomfort · stinging · tear production disturbance

▸ **Uncommon** Blepharitis · dizziness · drowsiness · flushing · headache · keratitis · nasal dryness

- **EXCEPTIONS TO LEGAL CATEGORY** Lodoxamide 0.1% eye drops can be sold to the public for treatment of allergic conjunctivitis in adults and children over 4 years.

- **MEDICINAL FORMS**
There can be variation in the licensing of different medicines containing the same drug.

Eye drops

EXCIPIENTS: May contain Benzalkonium chloride, disodium edetate

▸ Alomide (Alcon Laboratories (UK) Ltd)
Lodoxamide (as Lodoxamide trometamol) 1 mg per 1 ml Alomide 0.1% eye drops | 10 ml [PoM] £5.21 DT price = £5.21
Alomide Allergy 0.1% eye drops | 5 ml [P] £3.12

Nedocromil sodium

- **INDICATIONS AND DOSE**

Seasonal and perennial conjunctivitis

▸ TO THE EYE

▸ **Child 6-17 years:** Apply twice daily, increased if necessary to 4 times a day, max.12 weeks duration of treatment for seasonal allergic conjunctivitis

Seasonal keratoconjunctivitis

▸ TO THE EYE

▸ **Child 6-17 years:** Apply 4 times a day

- **SIDE-EFFECTS** Distinctive taste · transient burning · transient stinging

- **MEDICINAL FORMS**
There can be variation in the licensing of different medicines containing the same drug.

Eye drops

EXCIPIENTS: May contain Benzalkonium chloride, disodium edetate

▸ Rapitil (Sanofi)
Nedocromil sodium 20 mg per 1 ml Rapitil 2% eye drops | 5 ml [PoM] £2.86 DT price = £2.86

Sodium cromoglicate

(Sodium cromoglycate)

- **INDICATIONS AND DOSE**

Allergic conjunctivitis | Seasonal keratoconjunctivitis

▸ TO THE EYE

▸ **Child:** Apply 4 times a day

- **SIDE-EFFECTS** Transient burning · transient stinging

- **EXCEPTIONS TO LEGAL CATEGORY** Sodium cromoglicate 2% eye drops can be sold to the public (in max. pack size of 10 mL) for treatment of acute seasonal and perennial allergic conjunctivitis.

- **MEDICINAL FORMS**
There can be variation in the licensing of different medicines containing the same drug. Forms available from special-order manufacturers include: eye drops

Eye drops

▸ Sodium cromoglicate (Non-proprietary)
Sodium cromoglicate 20 mg per 1 ml Sodium cromoglicate 2% eye drops | 13.5 ml [PoM] £3.85 DT price = £2.06

▸ Catacrom (Moorfields Pharmaceuticals)
Sodium cromoglicate 20 mg per 1 ml Catacrom 2% eye drops 0.3ml unit dose | 30 unit dose [P] £8.99 DT price = £8.99

▸ Cromolux (Tubilux Pharma Ltd)
Sodium cromoglicate 20 mg per 1 ml Cromolux 2% eye drops | 13.5 ml [PoM] £3.20 DT price = £2.06

▸ Opticrom (Sanofi)
Sodium cromoglicate 20 mg per 1 ml Opticrom Allergy 2% eye drops | 5 ml [P] £2.74 | 10 ml [P] £3.35
Opticrom Aqueous 2% eye drops | 13.5 ml [PoM] £8.03 DT price = £2.06

▸ Optrex Allergy (Reckitt Benckiser Healthcare (UK) Ltd)
Sodium cromoglicate 20 mg per 1 ml Optrex Allergy 2% eye drops | 10 ml [P] £3.88

▸ Pollenase (sodium cromoglicate) (E M Pharma)
Sodium cromoglicate 20 mg per 1 ml Pollenase Allergy 2% eye drops | 10 ml [P] £2.08

▸ Vividrin (Bausch & Lomb UK Ltd)
Sodium cromoglicate 20 mg per 1 ml Vividrin 2% eye drops | 13.5 ml [PoM] £10.95 DT price = £2.06

1.2 Inflammatory eye conditions

CORTICOSTEROIDS

Betamethasone

- **INDICATIONS AND DOSE**

Local treatment of inflammation (short term)

▸ TO THE EYE USING EYE DROP

▸ **Child:** Apply every 1–2 hours until controlled then reduce frequency

▸ TO THE EYE USING EYE OINTMENT

▸ **Child:** Apply 2–4 times a day, alternatively apply at night when used in combination with eye drops

- **SIDE-EFFECTS** Adrenal suppression following prolonged use in neonates · corneal thinning · scleral thinning

- **MEDICINAL FORMS**
There can be variation in the licensing of different medicines containing the same drug.

Ear/eye/nose drops solution

EXCIPIENTS: May contain Benzalkonium chloride, disodium edetate

▸ Betamethasone (Non-proprietary)
Betamethasone sodium phosphate 1 mg per 1 ml Betamethasone 0.1% ear/eye/nose drops | 5 ml [PoM] no price available

▸ Betnesol (Focus Pharmaceuticals Ltd)
Betamethasone sodium phosphate 1 mg per 1 ml Betnesol 0.1% eye/ear/nose drops | 10 ml [PoM] £2.32 DT price = £2.32

▸ Vistamethasone (Martindale Pharmaceuticals Ltd)
Betamethasone sodium phosphate 1 mg per 1 ml Vistamethasone 0.1% eye/ear/nose drops | 5 ml [PoM] £0.87 | 10 ml [PoM] £0.99 DT price = £2.32

Eye ointment

▸ Betnesol (Focus Pharmaceuticals Ltd)
Betamethasone sodium phosphate 1 mg per 1 gram Betnesol 0.1% eye ointment | 3 gram [PoM] £1.41 DT price = £1.41

Combinations available: *Betamethasone with neomycin*, p. 623

Dexamethasone

- **INDICATIONS AND DOSE**

Local treatment of inflammation (short-term)
▶ TO THE EYE USING EYE DROP
▶ Child: Apply 4–6 times a day

Short term local treatment of inflammation (severe conditions)
▶ TO THE EYE USING EYE DROP
▶ Child: Apply every 30–60 minutes until controlled, reduce frequency when control achieved

- **UNLICENSED USE** *Maxidex*® not licensed for use in children under 2 years. *Dropodex*® not licensed for use in children.
- **SIDE-EFFECTS** Adrenal suppression following prolonged use in neonates · corneal thinning · scleral thinning
- **PREGNANCY** Dexamethasone readily crosses the placenta.
- **PRESCRIBING AND DISPENSING INFORMATION** Although multi-dose Dexamethasone eye drops commonly contain preservatives, preservative-free unit dose vials may be available.
- **MEDICINAL FORMS**
There can be variation in the licensing of different medicines containing the same drug. Forms available from special-order manufacturers include:eye drops

Eye drops
EXCIPIENTS: May contain Benzalkonium chloride, disodium edetate, polysorbates
▶ **Dexamethasone (Non-proprietary)**
Dexamethasone sodium phosphate 1 mg per 1 ml Dexamethasone 0.1% eye drops 0.4ml unit dose preservative free | 20 unit dose [PoM] £9.75 DT price = £9.75
Minims dexamethasone 0.1% eye drops 0.5ml unit dose | 20 unit dose [PoM] £11.46 DT price = £11.46
▶ **Dexafree (Thea Pharmaceuticals Ltd)**
Dexamethasone sodium phosphate 1 mg per 1 ml Dexafree 1mg/1ml eye drops 0.4ml unit dose | 30 unit dose [PoM] £9.70
▶ **Dropodex (Moorfields Pharmaceuticals)**
Dexamethasone sodium phosphate 1 mg per 1 ml Dropodex 0.1% eye drops 0.4ml unit dose | 20 unit dose [PoM] £9.75 DT price = £9.75
▶ **Maxidex (Alcon Laboratories (UK) Ltd)**
Dexamethasone 1 mg per 1 ml Maxidex 0.1% eye drops | 5 ml [PoM] £1.42 DT price = £1.42 | 10 ml [PoM] £2.80 DT price = £2.80

Combinations available: *Dexamethasone with framycetin sulfate and gramicidin*, p. 624 · *Dexamethasone with hypromellose, neomycin and polymyxin B sulfate*, p. 624

Fluorometholone

- **INDICATIONS AND DOSE**

Local treatment of inflammation (short term)
▶ TO THE EYE
▶ Child 2-17 years: Apply every 1 hour for 24–48 hours, then reduced to 2–4 times a day

- **UNLICENSED USE** Not licensed for use in children under 2 years.
- **SIDE-EFFECTS** Adrenal suppression following prolonged use in neonates · corneal thinning · scleral thinning
- **MEDICINAL FORMS**
There can be variation in the licensing of different medicines containing the same drug.

Eye drops
EXCIPIENTS: May contain Benzalkonium chloride, disodium edetate, polysorbates
▶ **FML Liquifilm (Allergan Ltd)**
Fluorometholone 1 mg per 1 ml FML Liquifilm 0.1% ophthalmic suspension | 5 ml [PoM] £1.71 DT price = £1.71 | 10 ml [PoM] £2.95 DT price = £2.95

Prednisolone

- **INDICATIONS AND DOSE**

Local treatment of inflammation (short-term)
▶ TO THE EYE
▶ Child: Apply every 1–2 hours until controlled then reduce frequency

- **UNLICENSED USE** *Pred Forte*® not licensed for use in children (age range not specified by manufacturer).
- **SIDE-EFFECTS** Adrenal suppression following prolonged use in neonates · corneal thinning · scleral thinning
- **PRESCRIBING AND DISPENSING INFORMATION** Although multi-dose prednisolone eye drops commonly contain preservatives, preservative-free unit dose vials may be available.
- **MEDICINAL FORMS**
There can be variation in the licensing of different medicines containing the same drug. Forms available from special-order manufacturers include: eye drops

Ear/eye drops solution
EXCIPIENTS: May contain Benzalkonium chloride, disodium edetate
▶ **Predsol (Focus Pharmaceuticals Ltd)**
Prednisolone sodium phosphate 5 mg per 1 ml Predsol 0.5% ear/eye drops | 10 ml [PoM] £2.00 DT price = £2.00

Eye drops
EXCIPIENTS: May contain Benzalkonium chloride, disodium edetate, polysorbates
▶ **Prednisolone (Non-proprietary)**
Prednisolone sodium phosphate 300 microgram per 1 ml Prednisolone sodium phosphate 0.03% eye drops preservative free | 10 ml [PoM] £34.24 DT price = £34.24
Prednisolone sodium phosphate 1 mg per 1 ml Prednisolone sodium phosphate 0.1% eye drops preservative free | 10 ml [PoM] £27.10 DT price = £27.10
Prednisolone sodium phosphate 3 mg per 1 ml Prednisolone sodium phosphate 0.3% eye drops preservative free | 10 ml [PoM] £22.53 DT price = £22.53
Prednisolone sodium phosphate 5 mg per 1 ml Minims prednisolone sodium phosphate 0.5% eye drops 0.5ml unit dose | 20 unit dose [PoM] £11.78 DT price = £11.78
▶ **Pred Forte (Allergan Ltd)**
Prednisolone acetate 10 mg per 1 ml Pred Forte 1% eye drops | 5 ml [PoM] £1.82 DT price = £1.82 | 10 ml [PoM] £3.66 DT price = £3.66

CORTICOSTEROIDS > WITH ANTI-INFECTIVES

Betamethasone with neomycin

The properties listed below are those particular to the combination only. For the properties of the components please consider, betamethasone p. 622.

- **INDICATIONS AND DOSE**

Local treatment of eye inflammation and bacterial infection (short-term)
▶ TO THE EYE USING EYE DROP
▶ Child: (consult product literature)

- **LESS SUITABLE FOR PRESCRIBING** Betamethasone with neomycin eye-drops are less suitable for prescribing.
- **MEDICINAL FORMS**
There can be variation in the licensing of different medicines containing the same drug.

Ear/eye/nose drops solution
EXCIPIENTS: May contain Benzalkonium chloride, disodium edetate
▶ **Betnesol-N (Focus Pharmaceuticals Ltd)**
Betamethasone (as Betamethasone sodium phosphate) 1 mg per 1 ml, Neomycin sulfate 5 mg per 1 ml Betnesol-N ear/eye/nose drops | 10 ml [PoM] £2.39 DT price = £2.39

11

Eye

Dexamethasone with framycetin sulfate and gramicidin

The properties listed below are those particular to the combination only. For the properties of the components please consider, dexamethasone p. 623.

- **INDICATIONS AND DOSE**
  Local treatment of inflammation (short-term)
  ▸ TO THE EYE
  ▸ Child: Apply 4–6 times a day, may be administered every 30–60 minutes in severe conditions until controlled, then reduce frequency

- **LESS SUITABLE FOR PRESCRIBING** *Sofradex*® is less suitable for prescribing.

- **MEDICINAL FORMS**
  There can be variation in the licensing of different medicines containing the same drug.
  Ear/eye drops solution
  EXCIPIENTS: May contain Polysorbates
  ▸ Sofradex (Sanofi)
  Gramicidin 50 microgram per 1 ml, Dexamethasone (as Dexamethasone sodium metasulfobenzoate) 500 microgram per 1 ml, Framycetin sulfate 5 mg per 1 ml Sofradex ear/eye drops | 10 ml [PoM] £7.50

Dexamethasone with hypromellose, neomycin and polymyxin B sulfate

The properties listed below are those particular to the combination only. For the properties of the components please consider, dexamethasone p. 623.

- **INDICATIONS AND DOSE**
  Local treatment of inflammation (short-term)
  ▸ TO THE EYE USING EYE DROP
  ▸ Child: Apply every 30–60 minutes until controlled, then reduced to 4–6 times a day
  Local treatment of inflammation (short-term)
  ▸ TO THE EYE USING EYE OINTMENT
  ▸ Child: Apply 3–4 times a day, alternatively, apply at night when used with eye drops

- **LESS SUITABLE FOR PRESCRIBING** Dexamethasone with neomycin and polymixin B sulfate is less suitable for prescribing.

- **MEDICINAL FORMS**
  There can be variation in the licensing of different medicines containing the same drug.
  Eye drops
  EXCIPIENTS: May contain Benzalkonium chloride, polysorbates
  ▸ Maxitrol (Alcon Laboratories (UK) Ltd)
  Dexamethasone 1 mg per 1 ml, Neomycin (as Neomycin sulfate) 3.5 mg per 1 ml, Hypromellose 5 mg per 1 ml, Polymyxin B sulfate 6000 unit per 1 ml Maxitrol eye drops | 5 ml [PoM] £1.68
  Eye ointment
  EXCIPIENTS: May contain Hydroxybenzoates (parabens), wool fat and related substances including lanolin
  ▸ Maxitrol (Alcon Laboratories (UK) Ltd)
  Dexamethasone 1 mg per 1 gram, Neomycin (as Neomycin sulfate) 3500 unit per 1 gram, Polymyxin B sulfate 6000 unit per 1 gram Maxitrol eye ointment | 3.5 gram [PoM] £1.44

1.2a Anterior uveitis

ANTIMUSCARINICS

Antimuscarinics (eye)

- **CAUTIONS** Children under 3 months owing to the possible association between cycloplegia and the development of amblyopia · darkly pigmented iris is more resistant to pupillary dilatation and caution should be exercised to avoid overdosage · mydriasis can precipitate acute angle-closure glaucoma (usually in those who are predisposed to the condition because of a shallow anterior chamber) · neonates at increased risk of systemic toxicity

- **SIDE-EFFECTS** Conjunctivitis (on prolonged administration) · contact dermatitis · eye oedema (on prolonged administration) · hyperaemia (on prolonged administration) · local irritation (on prolonged administration) · raised intraocular pressure · transient stinging

- **PATIENT AND CARER ADVICE** Patients may not be able to undertake skilled tasks until vision clears after mydriasis.

◤ above

Atropine sulfate

- **INDICATIONS AND DOSE**
  Cycloplegia
  ▸ TO THE EYE USING EYE DROP
  ▸ Child 3 months-17 years: Apply twice daily for 3 days, before procedure
  Anterior uveitis
  ▸ TO THE EYE USING EYE DROP
  ▸ Child 2-17 years: Apply 1 drop up to 4 times a day

- **UNLICENSED USE** Not licensed for use in children for uveitis.

- **SIDE-EFFECTS**
  SIDE-EFFECTS, FURTHER INFORMATION
  Toxic systemic reactions can occur. Systemic side-effects can occur.

- **PRESCRIBING AND DISPENSING INFORMATION** Although multi-dose atropine sulfate eye drops commonly contain preservatives, preservative-free unit dose vials may be available.

- **MEDICINAL FORMS**
  There can be variation in the licensing of different medicines containing the same drug. Forms available from special-order manufacturers include: eye drops
  Eye drops
  ▸ Atropine sulfate (Non-proprietary)
  Atropine sulfate 10 mg per 1 ml Atropine 1% eye drops | 10 ml [PoM] £41.99 DT price = £35.15
  ▸ Atropine sulfate (Bausch & Lomb UK Ltd)
  Atropine sulfate 10 mg per 1 ml Minims atropine sulfate 1% eye drops 0.5ml unit dose | 20 unit dose [PoM] £15.10 DT price = £15.10

F 624

Cyclopentolate hydrochloride

● **INDICATIONS AND DOSE**

Cycloplegia

▶ TO THE EYE
▶ **Child 3 months–11 years:** Apply 1 drop, 30–60 minutes before examination, using 1% eye drops
▶ **Child 12–17 years:** Apply 1 drop, 30–60 minutes before examination, using 0.5% eye drops

Uveitis

▶ TO THE EYE
▶ **Child 3 months–17 years:** Apply 1 drop 2–4 times a day, using 0.5% eye drops (1% for deeply pigmented eyes)

● **SIDE-EFFECTS**

SIDE-EFFECTS, FURTHER INFORMATION
Toxic systemic reactions can occur . Systemic side-effects can occur.

● **PRESCRIBING AND DISPENSING INFORMATION** Although multi-dose cyclopentolate eye drops commonly contain preservatives, preservative-free unit dose vials may be available.

● **MEDICINAL FORMS**
There can be variation in the licensing of different medicines containing the same drug.

Eye drops
EXCIPIENTS: May contain Benzalkonium chloride
▶ **Cyclopentolate hydrochloride** (Bausch & Lomb UK Ltd)
Cyclopentolate hydrochloride 5 mg per 1 ml Minims cyclopentolate hydrochloride 0.5% eye drops 0.5ml unit dose | 20 unit dose PoM £10.97 DT price = £10.97
Cyclopentolate hydrochloride 10 mg per 1 ml Minims cyclopentolate hydrochloride 1% eye drops 0.5ml unit dose | 20 unit dose PoM £11.23 DT price = £11.23
▶ **Mydrilate** (Intrapharm Laboratories Ltd)
Cyclopentolate hydrochloride 5 mg per 1 ml Mydrilate 0.5% solution | 5 ml PoM £6.73 DT price = £6.73
Cyclopentolate hydrochloride 10 mg per 1 ml Mydrilate 1% solution | 5 ml PoM £6.73 DT price = £6.73

F 624

Homatropine hydrobromide

● **INDICATIONS AND DOSE**

Anterior uveitis

▶ TO THE EYE
▶ **Child 3 months–1 year:** Apply 1 drop daily, alternatively apply 1 drop once daily on alternate days, adjusted according to response, only 0.5% eye drops to be used
▶ **Child 2–17 years:** Apply 1 drop twice daily, adjusted according to response

● **UNLICENSED USE** Not licensed for use in children under 3 months.

● **MEDICINAL FORMS**
There can be variation in the licensing of different medicines containing the same drug. Forms available from special-order manufacturers include: eye drops

2   Dry eye conditions

Dry eye

Tear deficiency, ocular lubricants, and astringents

Chronic soreness of the eyes associated with reduced or abnormal tear secretion often responds to tear replacement therapy. The severity of the condition and child's preference will often guide the choice of preparation.

Hypromellose p. 626 is the traditional choice of treatment for tear deficiency. It may need to be instilled frequently (e.g. hourly) for adequate relief. Ocular surface mucin is often abnormal in tear deficiency and the combination of hypromellose with a mucolytic such as acetylcysteine below can be helpful.

The ability of **carbomers** to cling to the eye surface may help reduce frequency of application to 4 times daily.

Polyvinyl alcohol p. 627 increases the persistence of the tear film and is useful when the ocular surface mucin is reduced.

Sodium hyaluronate eye drops p. 628 are also used in the management of tear deficiency.

Sodium chloride 0.9% drops p. 628 are sometimes useful in tear deficiency, and can be used as 'comfort drops' by contact lens wearers, and to facilitate lens removal. Special presentations of sodium chloride 0.9% and other irrigation solutions are used routinely for intra-ocular surgery and in first aid for removal of harmful substances.

Eye ointments containing a paraffin can be used to lubricate the eye surface, especially in cases of recurrent corneal epithelial erosion. They may cause temporary visual disturbance and are best suited for application before sleep. Ointments should not be used during contact lens wear.

OCULAR LUBRICANTS

Acetylcysteine

● **INDICATIONS AND DOSE**

Tear deficiency | Impaired or abnormal mucus production

▶ TO THE EYE
▶ **Child:** Apply 3–4 times a day

● **MEDICINAL FORMS**
There can be variation in the licensing of different medicines containing the same drug. Forms available from special-order manufacturers include: eye drops

Eye drops
EXCIPIENTS: May contain Benzalkonium chloride, disodium edetate
▶ **Ilube** (Moorfields Pharmaceuticals)
Acetylcysteine 50 mg per 1 ml Ilube 5% eye drops | 10 ml PoM £14.93 DT price = £14.93

Carbomers

(Polyacrylic acid)

● **INDICATIONS AND DOSE**

Dry eyes including keratoconjunctivitis sicca, unstable tear film

▶ TO THE EYE
▶ **Child:** Apply 3–4 times a day or when required

● **UNLICENSED USE** Some preparations not licensed for use in children.

● **PRESCRIBING AND DISPENSING INFORMATION** Synthetic high molecular weight polymers of acrylic acid cross-linked with either allyl ethers of sucrose or allyl ethers of pentaerithrityl.

● **MEDICINAL FORMS**
There can be variation in the licensing of different medicines containing the same drug.
Eye drops
▶ **Carbomers** (Non-proprietary)
Carbomer 980 2 mg per 1 gram Carbomer '980' 0.2% eye drops | 10 gram P £2.80 DT price = £2.80
Carbomer 0.2% eye gel | 10 gram £2.80 DT price = £2.80
▶ **Artelac Nighttime** (Bausch & Lomb UK Ltd)
Carbomer 980 2 mg per 1 gram Artelac Nighttime 0.2% eye gel | 10 gram £2.96 DT price = £2.80

11

Eye

▸ **Clinitas Carbomer** (Altacor Ltd)
Carbomer 980 2 mg per 1 gram Clinitas Carbomer 0.2% eye gel | 10 gram £1.49 DT price = £2.80

▸ **GelTears** (Bausch & Lomb UK Ltd)
Carbomer 980 2 mg per 1 gram GelTears 0.2% gel | 10 gram P £2.80 DT price = £2.80

▸ **Lumecare Long Lasting** (Medicom Healthcare Ltd)
Carbomer 980 2 mg per 1 gram Lumecare Carbomer 0.2% eye gel | 10 gram £1.51 DT price = £2.80

▸ **Viscotears** (Alcon Laboratories (UK) Ltd)
Carbomer 980 2 mg per 1 gram Viscotears 2mg/g liquid gel | 10 gram P £1.59 DT price = £2.80
Viscotears 2mg/g eye gel 0.6ml unit dose | 30 unit dose P £5.42

▸ **Xailin** (Nicox Pharma)
Carbomer 980 2 mg per 1 gram Xailin 0.2% eye gel | 10 gram £3.25 DT price = £2.80

Eye gel

EXCIPIENTS: May contain Benzalkonium chloride, cetrimide, disodium edetate

▸ **Blephagel** (Thea Pharmaceuticals Ltd)
Carbomer 3.5 mg per 1 gram Blephagel 0.35% eye gel | 40 gram £6.66
Carbomer 3.6 mg per 1 gram Blephagel 0.36% eye gel preservative free | 30 gram £7.53

▸ **Liquivisc** (Thea Pharmaceuticals Ltd)
Carbomer 974P 2.5 mg per 1 gram Liquivisc 0.25% eye gel | 10 gram P £4.50 DT price = £4.50

Carmellose sodium

● **INDICATIONS AND DOSE**
Dry eye conditions
▸ TO THE EYE
▸ **Child:** Apply as required

● **PRESCRIBING AND DISPENSING INFORMATION** Some preparations are contained units which are resealable and may be used for up to 12 hours.

● **MEDICINAL FORMS**
There can be variation in the licensing of different medicines containing the same drug.
Eye drops
▸ **Carmellose sodium** (Non-proprietary)
Carmellose sodium 5 mg per 1 ml Carmellose 0.5% eye drops 0.4ml unit dose preservative free | 30 unit dose P no price available DT price = £4.80 | 30 unit dose £5.75 DT price = £4.80 | 90 unit dose P no price available
Carmellose 0.5% eye drops | 10 ml £7.49
Carmellose 1% eye drops 0.4ml unit dose preservative free | 30 unit dose PoM no price available DT price = £3.00 | 30 unit dose £3.00 DT price = £3.00 | 30 unit dose P no price available DT price = £3.00 | 60 unit dose P no price available

▸ **Carmeleze** (Martindale Pharmaceuticals Ltd)
Carmellose sodium 5 mg per 1 ml Melophthal 0.5% eye drops 0.4ml unit dose | 30 unit dose £5.75 DT price = £4.80
Melophthal 1% eye drops 0.4ml unit dose | 30 unit dose £3.00 DT price = £3.00

▸ **Carmize** (Aspire Pharma Ltd)
Carmellose sodium 5 mg per 1 ml Carmize 0.5% eye drops 0.4ml unit dose preservative free | 30 unit dose £5.75 DT price = £4.80 | 90 unit dose £15.53
Carmize 1% eye drops | 10 ml £8.49
Carmize 1% eye drops 0.4ml unit dose preservative free | 30 unit dose £3.00 DT price = £3.00 | 60 unit dose £6.00
Carmize 0.5% eye drops | 10 ml £7.49

▸ **Cellusan** (Farmigea S.p.A.)
Carmellose sodium 5 mg per 1 ml Cellusan Light 0.5% eye drops 0.4ml unit dose preservative free | 30 unit dose £5.75 DT price = £4.80
Cellusan 1% eye drops preservative free | 10 ml £4.80
Cellusan Light 0.5% eye drops preservative free | 10 ml £4.80
Cellusan 1% eye drops 0.4ml unit dose preservative free | 30 unit dose £3.00 DT price = £3.00

▸ **Celluvisc** (Allergan Ltd)
Carmellose sodium 5 mg per 1 ml Celluvisc 0.5% eye drops 0.4ml unit dose | 30 unit dose P £4.80 DT price = £4.80 | 90 unit dose P £15.53
Celluvisc 1% eye drops 0.4ml unit dose | 30 unit dose P £3.00 DT price = £3.00 | 60 unit dose P £10.99

▸ **Lumecare (Carmellose)** (Medicom Healthcare Ltd)
Carmellose sodium 5 mg per 1 ml Lumecare Singles Carmellose 0.5% eye drops 0.4ml unit dose | 30 unit dose £4.60 DT price = £4.80
Lumecare Advance Carmellose 0.5% eye drops | 10 ml £5.99

▸ **Optive** (Allergan Ltd)
Optive 0.5% eye drops | 10 ml £7.49

▸ **Optive Plus** (Allergan Ltd)
Optive Plus 0.5% eye drops | 10 ml £7.49

▸ **Xailin Fresh** (Nicox Pharma)
Carmellose sodium 5 mg per 1 ml Xailin Fresh 0.5% eye drops 0.4ml unit dose | 30 unit dose £3.84 DT price = £4.80

Hydroxyethylcellulose

● **INDICATIONS AND DOSE**
Tear deficiency
▸ TO THE EYE
▸ **Child:** Apply as required

● **PRESCRIBING AND DISPENSING INFORMATION** Although multi-dose hydroxyethylcellulose eye drops commonly contain preservatives, preservative-free unit dose vials may be available.

● **MEDICINAL FORMS**
There can be variation in the licensing of different medicines containing the same drug.
Eye drops
▸ **Artificial tears** (Bausch & Lomb UK Ltd)
Hydroxyethylcellulose 4.4 mg per 1 ml Minims artificial tears 0.44% eye drops 0.5ml unit dose | 20 unit dose P £8.97

Hydroxypropyl guar with polyethylene glycol and propylene glycol

(Formulated as an ocular lubricant)

● **INDICATIONS AND DOSE**
Dry eye conditions
▸ TO THE EYE
▸ **Child:** Apply as required

● **MEDICINAL FORMS**
There can be variation in the licensing of different medicines containing the same drug.
Eye drops
▸ **Systane** (Alcon Laboratories (UK) Ltd)
Systane Gel eye drops | 10 ml £7.49

Hypromellose

● **INDICATIONS AND DOSE**
Tear deficiency
▸ TO THE EYE
▸ **Child:** Apply as required

● **PRESCRIBING AND DISPENSING INFORMATION** The Royal Pharmaceutical Society has stated that where it is not possible to ascertain the strength of hypromellose prescribed, the prescriber should be contacted to clarify the strength intended.
Although multi-dose hypromellose eye drops commonly contain preservatives, preservative-free unit dose vials may be available.

- **MEDICINAL FORMS**
There can be variation in the licensing of different medicines containing the same drug. Forms available from special-order manufacturers include: eye drops
Eye drops
EXCIPIENTS: May contain Benzalkonium chloride, cetrimide, disodium edetate
▸ **Hypromellose (Non-proprietary)**
Hypromellose 2.5 mg per 1 ml Hypromellose 0.25% eye drops preservative free | 10 ml PoM £14.24 DT price = £14.24
Hypromellose 3 mg per 1 ml Hypromellose 0.3% eye drops preservative free | 10 ml £5.75
▸ **Artelac** (Bausch & Lomb UK Ltd)
Hypromellose 3.2 mg per 1 ml Artelac Single Dose Unit 0.32% eye drops 0.5ml unit dose | 30 unit dose P £16.95 | 60 unit dose P £32.85
Artelac 0.32% eye drops | 10 ml P £4.99
▸ **Brolene Cool** (Sanofi)
Hypromellose 3 mg per 1 ml Brolene Cool Eyes 0.3% eye drops | 10 ml GSL £2.38 DT price = £0.99
▸ **Hydromoor** (Moorfields Pharmaceuticals)
Hydromoor 0.3% eye drops 0.4ml unit dose preservative free | 30 unit dose £5.75
▸ **Hypromellose** (Moorfields Pharmaceuticals)
Hypromellose 3 mg per 1 ml PF Drops Hypromellose 0.3% eye drops preservative free | 10 ml £5.75
▸ **Hypromol** (Ennogen Healthcare Ltd)
Hypromellose 3 mg per 1 ml Hypromol 0.3% eye drops preservative free | 10 ml £4.55
▸ **Isopto Alkaline** (Alcon Laboratories (UK) Ltd)
Hypromellose 10 mg per 1 ml Isopto Alkaline 1% eye drops | 10 ml P £0.94 DT price = £0.94
▸ **Isopto Plain** (Alcon Laboratories (UK) Ltd)
Hypromellose 5 mg per 1 ml Isopto Plain 0.5% eye drops | 10 ml P £0.81 DT price = £0.81
▸ **Lumecare (Hypromellose)** (Medicom Healthcare Ltd)
Hypromellose 3 mg per 1 ml Lumecare Hypromellose 0.3% eye drops | 10 ml £1.67 DT price = £0.99
▸ **Lumecare Tear Drops** (Medicom Healthcare Ltd)
Hypromellose 3 mg per 1 ml Lumecare Tear Drops 0.3% eye drops | 10 ml £0.95 DT price = £0.99
▸ **Mandanol (Hydroxypropyl methylcellulose)** (M & A Pharmachem Ltd)
Hypromellose 3 mg per 1 ml Mandanol eye drops | 10 ml £1.33 DT price = £0.99
▸ **Ocu-Lube** (Sai-Meds Ltd)
Hypromellose 3 mg per 1 ml Ocu-Lube 0.3% eye drops preservative free | 10 ml £5.75
▸ **SoftDrops** (Farmigea S.p.A.)
Hypromellose 3 mg per 1 ml SoftDrops 0.3% eye drops | 10 ml £1.67 DT price = £0.99
▸ **Tear-Lac** (Scope Ophthalmics Ltd)
Hypromellose 3 mg per 1 ml Tear-Lac Hypromellose 0.3% eye drops preservative free | 10 ml £5.75
▸ **Xailin Hydrate** (Nicox Pharma)
Hypromellose 3 mg per 1 ml Xailin Hydrate 0.3% eye drops preservative free | 10 ml £4.60

Hypromellose with dextran 70

The properties listed below are those particular to the combination only. For the properties of the components please consider, hypromellose p. 626.

- **INDICATIONS AND DOSE**
Tear deficiency
▸ TO THE EYE
▸ Child: Apply as required

- **MEDICINAL FORMS**
There can be variation in the licensing of different medicines containing the same drug.
Eye drops
EXCIPIENTS: May contain Benzalkonium chloride, disodium edetate
▸ **Tears Naturale** (Alcon Laboratories (UK) Ltd)
Dextran 70 1 mg per 1 ml, Hypromellose 3 mg per 1 ml Tears Naturale eye drops | 15 ml P £1.89
Tears Naturale eye drops 0.4ml unit dose | 28 unit dose P £13.26

Liquid paraffin with white soft paraffin and wool alcohols

- **INDICATIONS AND DOSE**
Dry eye conditions
▸ TO THE EYE
▸ Child: Apply as required, best suited for application before sleep

- **PATIENT AND CARER ADVICE** May cause temporary visual disturbance. Should not be used during contact lens wear.

- **MEDICINAL FORMS**
There can be variation in the licensing of different medicines containing the same drug.
Eye ointment
▸ **Lacri-Lube** (Allergan Ltd)
Wool alcohols 2 mg per 1 gram, Liquid paraffin 425 mg per 1 gram, White soft paraffin 573 mg per 1 gram Lacri-lube eye ointment | 3.5 gram P £2.94 | 5 gram P £3.88

Paraffin, yellow, soft

- **INDICATIONS AND DOSE**
Eye surface lubrication
▸ TO THE EYE
▸ Child: Apply every 2 hours as required

- **PATIENT AND CARER ADVICE** Ophthalmic preparations may cause temporary visual disturbance. Should not be used during contact lens wear.

- **MEDICINAL FORMS**
There can be variation in the licensing of different medicines containing the same drug.
Eye ointment
▸ **Paraffin, yellow, soft (Non-proprietary)**
Liquid paraffin 100 mg per 1 gram, Wool fat 100 mg per 1 gram, Yellow soft paraffin 800 mg per 1 gram Simple eye ointment | 4 gram P £6.98 DT price = £5.82

Polyvinyl alcohol

- **INDICATIONS AND DOSE**
Tear deficiency
▸ TO THE EYE
▸ Child: Apply as required

- **PRESCRIBING AND DISPENSING INFORMATION** Although multi-dose polyvinyl alcohol eye drops commonly contain preservatives, preservative-free unit dose vials may be available.

- **MEDICINAL FORMS**
There can be variation in the licensing of different medicines containing the same drug. Forms available from special-order manufacturers include: eye drops
Eye drops
EXCIPIENTS: May contain Benzalkonium chloride, disodium edetate
▸ **Polyvinyl alcohol (Non-proprietary)**
Polyvinyl alcohol 14 mg per 1 ml Polyvinyl alcohol 1.4% eye drops 0.4ml unit dose preservative free | 30 unit dose P no price available
Polyvinyl alcohol 1.4% eye drops | 10 ml P no price available | 15 ml P no price available
▸ **Liquifilm Tears** (Allergan Ltd)
Polyvinyl alcohol 14 mg per 1 ml Liquifilm Tears 1.4% eye drops | 15 ml P £1.93
Liquifilm Tears 1.4% eye drops 0.4ml unit dose preservative free | 30 unit dose P £5.35
▸ **PVA** (Tubilux Pharma Ltd)
Polyvinyl alcohol 14 mg per 1 ml PVA 1.4% eye drops | 15 ml £1.63

11

Eye

▸ **Refresh Ophthalmic** (Allergan Ltd)
Polyvinyl alcohol 14 mg per 1 ml Refresh Ophthalmic 1.4% eye drops 0.4ml unit dose | 30 unit dose Ⓟ £2.25

▸ **Sno Tears** (Bausch & Lomb UK Ltd)
Polyvinyl alcohol 14 mg per 1 ml Sno Tears 1.4% eye drops | 10 ml Ⓟ £1.06

Retinol palmitate with white soft paraffin and light liquid paraffin and liquid paraffin and wool fat

(Formulated as an ocular lubricant)

● **INDICATIONS AND DOSE**
Dry eye conditions
▸ TO THE EYE
▸ Child: Apply as required

● **MEDICINAL FORMS**
There can be variation in the licensing of different medicines containing the same drug.
Eye ointment
▸ **VitA-POS** (Scope Ophthalmics Ltd)
VitA-POS eye ointment preservative free | 5 gram £2.75

Sodium chloride

● **INDICATIONS AND DOSE**
Tear deficiency | Ocular lubricants and astringents | Irrigation, including first-aid removal of harmful substances | Intra-ocular or topical irrigation during surgical procedures
▸ TO THE EYE USING 0.9% SOLUTION
▸ Child: Apply as required

Corneal oedema
▸ TO THE EYE USING 5% EYE DROPS OR EYE OINTMENT
▸ Child: Consult product literature

● **PRESCRIBING AND DISPENSING INFORMATION**
Although multi-dose sodium chloride eye drops commonly contain preservatives, preservative-free unit dose vials may be available.

● **MEDICINAL FORMS**
There can be variation in the licensing of different medicines containing the same drug. Forms available from special-order manufacturers include: eye drops, eye ointment
Eye drops
▸ **Sodium chloride** (Non-proprietary)
Sodium chloride 50 mg per 1 ml Sodium chloride 5% eye drops | 10 ml £25.25
▸ **Hypersal** (Ennogen Healthcare Ltd)
Sodium chloride 50 mg per 1 ml Hypersal 5% eye drops | 10 ml £25.25
▸ **ODM5** (Kestrel Ophthalmics Ltd)
Sodium chloride 50 mg per 1 ml ODM5 5% eye drops preservative free | 10 ml £24.00 DT price = £0.00
▸ **Saline** (Bausch & Lomb UK Ltd)
Sodium chloride 9 mg per 1 ml Minims saline 0.9% eye drops 0.5ml unit dose | 20 unit dose Ⓟ £7.14 DT price = £7.14
▸ **Sodium chloride** (Essential Pharmaceuticals Ltd, Moorfields Pharmaceuticals)
Sodium chloride 50 mg per 1 ml NaCl 5% eye drops 0.45ml unit dose preservative free | 20 unit dose £19.70
PF Drops Sodium Chloride 5% eye drops preservative free | 10 ml £25.20 DT price = £0.00
Eye ointment
▸ **Sodium chloride** (Non-proprietary)
Sodium chloride 50 mg per 1 ml Sodium chloride 5% eye ointment preservative free | 5 gram £22.50
Sodium chloride 50 mg per 1 gram Muro 128 5% eye ointment | 3.5 gram PoM no price available

Sodium hyaluronate

● **INDICATIONS AND DOSE**
Dry eye conditions
▸ TO THE EYE
▸ Child: Apply as required

● **PRESCRIBING AND DISPENSING INFORMATION** Some preparations are contained in units which are resealable and may be used for up to 12 hours.
Although multi-dose sodium hyaluronate eye drops commonly contain preservatives, preservative-free unit dose vials may be available.

● **MEDICINAL FORMS**
There can be variation in the licensing of different medicines containing the same drug.
Eye drops
▸ **Sodium hyaluronate** (Non-proprietary)
Vislube 0.18% eye drops 0.3ml unit dose preservative free | 20 unit dose no price available
▸ **Artelac Rebalance** (Bausch & Lomb UK Ltd)
Artelac Rebalance 0.15% eye drops | 10 ml £4.00
▸ **Artelac Splash** (Bausch & Lomb UK Ltd)
Artelac Splash 0.2% eye drops 0.5ml unit dose | 30 unit dose £7.00 | 60 unit dose £11.20
▸ **Blink Intensive** (AMO UK Ltd)
Blink Intensive Tears 0.2% eye drops 0.4ml unit dose | 20 unit dose £2.97
Blink Intensive Tears 0.2% eye drops | 10 ml £2.97
▸ **Clinitas** (Altacor Ltd)
Clinitas Multi 0.4% eye drops preservative free | 10 ml £6.99
Clinitas 0.4% eye drops 0.5ml unit dose | 30 unit dose £5.70
▸ **Evolve HA** (Medicom Healthcare Ltd)
Evolve HA 0.2% eye drops preservative free | 10 ml £5.99
▸ **Hy-Opti** (Alissa Healthcare Research Ltd)
Hy-Opti 0.1% eye drops preservative free | 10 ml £8.50
Hy-Opti 0.2% eye drops preservative free | 10 ml £9.50
▸ **Hyabak** (Thea Pharmaceuticals Ltd)
Hyabak UD 0.15% eye drops 0.4ml unit dose preservative free | 30 unit dose £4.99
Hyabak 0.15% eye drops | 10 ml £7.99
▸ **Hycosan** (Scope Ophthalmics Ltd)
Hycosan Extra 0.2% eye drops | 7.5 ml no price available
Hycosan 0.1% eye drops | 7.5 ml no price available
▸ **HydraMed** (Farmigea S.p.A.)
HydraMed 0.2% eye drops preservative free | 10 ml £5.60
HydraMed 0.2% eye drops 0.5ml unit dose preservative free | 30 unit dose £5.60
▸ **Hylo-Comod** (Scope Ophthalmics Ltd)
Hylo-Tear 0.1% eye drops preservative free | 10 ml £8.50
Hylo-Forte 0.2% eye drops preservative free | 10 ml £9.50
▸ **Hylo-fresh** (Scope Ophthalmics Ltd)
Hylo-Fresh 0.03% eye drops preservative free | 10 ml £4.95
▸ **Lubristil** (Moorfields Pharmaceuticals)
Lubristil 0.15% eye drops 0.3ml unit dose preservative free | 20 unit dose £4.99
▸ **Ocusan** (Agepha Pharma s.r.o.)
Ocusan 0.2% eye drops 0.5ml unit dose | 20 unit dose £5.31
▸ **Optive Fusion** (Allergan Ltd)
Optive Fusion 0.1% eye drops | 10 ml £7.49
▸ **Oxyal** (Bausch & Lomb UK Ltd)
Oxyal 0.15% eye drops | 10 ml £4.15
▸ **Vismed** (TRB Chemidica (UK) Ltd)
Vismed Gel Multi 0.3% eye drops preservative free | 10 ml £7.95
Vismed Multi 0.18% eye drops preservative free | 10 ml £6.81
Vismed 0.18% eye drops 0.3ml unit dose preservative free | 20 unit dose £5.10
▸ **Xailin HA** (Nicox Pharma)
Xailin HA 0.2% eye drops preservative free | 10 ml £7.13
Eye gel
▸ **Lubristil** (Moorfields Pharmaceuticals)
Lubristil 0.15% eye gel 0.4ml unit dose preservative free | 20 unit dose £6.49
▸ **Vismed** (TRB Chemidica (UK) Ltd)
Vismed 0.3% eye gel 0.45ml unit dose preservative free | 20 unit dose £5.98

Soybean oil

● **INDICATIONS AND DOSE**

Dry eye conditions

▶ TO THE EYE

▶ Child: Apply up to 4 times a day

● **MEDICINAL FORMS**
There can be variation in the licensing of different medicines containing the same drug.

Eye drops

▶ Emustil (Moorfields Pharmaceuticals)
Emustil eye drops 0.3ml unit dose preservative free | 20 unit dose
£6.22

3 Eye infections

Eye infections

Most acute superficial eye infections can be treated topically. Blepharitis and conjunctivitis are often caused by staphylococci; keratitis and endophthalmitis may be bacterial, viral, or fungal.

Bacterial *blepharitis* is treated by lid hygiene and application of antibacterial eye drops to the conjunctival sac or to the lid margins. Systemic treatment may be required and may be necessary for 3 months or longer.

Most cases of acute bacterial conjunctivitis are self-limiting; where treatment is appropriate, antibacterial eye drops or an eye ointment are used. A poor response might indicate viral or allergic conjunctivitis or antibiotic resistance.

Corneal *ulcer* and *keratitis* require specialist treatment, usually under inpatient care, and may call for intensive topical, subconjunctival, or systemic administration of antimicrobials.

Endophthalmitis is a medical emergency which also calls for specialist management and requires intravitreal administration of antimicrobials; concomitant systemic treatment is required in some cases. Surgical intervention, such as vitrectomy, is sometimes indicated.

See reference to the treatment of *crab lice of the eyelashes*.

Antibacterials

Bacterial eye infections are generally treated topically with eye drops and eye ointments. Systemic administration is sometimes appropriate in blepharitis.

Chloramphenicol p. 631 has a broad spectrum of activity and is the drug of choice for *superficial eye infections*. Chloramphenicol eye drops are well tolerated and the recommendation that chloramphenicol eye drops should be avoided because of an increased risk of aplastic anaemia is not well founded.

Other antibacterials with a broad spectrum of activity include the quinolones, ciprofloxacin p. 630, levofloxacin p. 631, moxifloxacin p. 631, and ofloxacin p. 631; the aminoglycosides, gentamicin p. 630 and tobramycin p. 630 are also active against a wide variety of bacteria. Gentamicin, tobramycin, quinolones (except moxifloxacin), and **polymyxin B** are effective for infections caused by *Pseudomonas aeruginosa*.

Ciprofloxacin eye drops are licensed for corneal ulcers; intensive application (especially in the first 2 days) is required throughout the day and night.

Azithromycin eye drops p. 630 are licensed for trachomatous conjunctivitis caused by *Chlamydia trachomatis* and for purulent bacterial conjunctivitis. *Trachoma* which results from chronic infection with *Chlamydia trachomatis* can be treated with azithromycin by mouth [unlicensed indication].

Fusidic acid is useful for staphylococcal infections.

Propamidine isetionate p. 632 is of little value in bacterial infections but is used by specialists to treat the rare, but potentially sight-threatening, condition of *acanthamoeba keratitis* [unlicensed indication].

Other antibacterial eye drops may be prepared aseptically in a specialist manufacturing unit from material supplied for injection.

With corticosteroids

Many antibacterial preparations also incorporate a corticosteroid but such mixtures should **not** be used unless a patient is under close specialist supervision. In particular they should not be prescribed for undiagnosed 'red eye' which is sometimes caused by the herpes simplex virus and may be difficult to diagnose.

Administration

Frequency of application depends on the severity of the infection and the potential for irreversible ocular damage; antibacterial eye preparations are usually administered as follows:

● *Eye drops*, apply 1 drop at least every 2 hours in severe infection then reduce frequency as infection is controlled and continue for 48 hours after healing. For less severe infection 3–4 times daily is generally sufficient.

● *Eye ointment*, apply *either* at night (if eye drops used during the day) *or* 3–4 times daily (if eye ointment used alone).

Antifungals

Fungal infections of the cornea are rare. Orbital mycosis is rarer, and when it occurs it is usually because of direct spread of infection from the paranasal sinuses. Debility or immunosuppression can encourage fungal proliferation. The spread of infection through blood occasionally produces metastatic endophthalmitis.

Many different fungi are capable of producing ocular infection; they can be identified by appropriate laboratory procedures.

Antifungal preparations for the eye are not generally available. Treatment will normally be carried out at specialist centres, but requests for information about supplies of preparations not available commercially should be addressed to the Strategic Health Authority (or equivalent in Scotland or Northern Ireland), or to the nearest hospital ophthalmology unit, or to Moorfields Eye Hospital, 162 City Road, London EC1V 2PD (Tel. (020) 7253 3411) or www.moorfields.nhs.uk.

Antivirals

Herpes simplex infections producing, for example, dendritic corneal ulcers can be treated with aciclovir p. 632. Aciclovir eye ointment is used in combination with systemic treatment for ophthalmic zoster.

Also see systemic treatment of CMV retinitis.

Antibacterials in neonates

Antibacterial eye drops are used to treat acute bacterial conjunctivitis in neonates (ophthalmia neonatorum); where possible the causative microorganism should be identified. Chloramphenicol eye drops are used to treat mild conjunctivitis; more serious infections also require a systemic antibacterial. Failure to respond to initial treatment requires further investigation; chlamydial infection is one of the most frequent causes of neonatal conjunctivitis and should be considered. Azithromycin eye drops are licensed to treat trachomatous conjunctivitis caused by *Chlamydia trachomatis* and purulent bacterial conjunctivitis in neonates. However, as there is a risk of simultaneous infection at other sites in neonates and children under 3 months presenting with conjunctivitis caused by *Chlamydia trachomatis*, systemic treatment with oral erythromycin p. 310 is required. *Gonococcal eye infections* are treated with a single-dose of parenteral cefotaxime p. 301 or

11

Eye

ceftriaxone p. 302. Gentamicin eye drops together with appropriate systemic antibacterials are used in the treatment of *pseudomonal eye infections*; high-strength gentamicin eye drops (1.5%) [unlicensed] are available for severe infections.

3.1 Bacterial eye infection

ANTIBACTERIALS › AMINOGLYCOSIDES

Gentamicin

● INDICATIONS AND DOSE

Bacterial eye infections
▸ TO THE EYE
▸ Child: Apply 1 drop at least every 2 hours in severe infection, reduce frequency as infection is controlled and continue for 48 hours after healing, frequency of eye drops depends on the severity of the infection and the potential for irreversible ocular damage; for less severe infection 3–4 times daily is generally sufficient

● PRESCRIBING AND DISPENSING INFORMATION Eye drops may be sourced as a manufactured special or from specialist importing companies.

● MEDICINAL FORMS
There can be variation in the licensing of different medicines containing the same drug. Forms available from special-order manufacturers include: eye drops
Ear/eye drops solution
EXCIPIENTS: May contain Benzalkonium chloride
▸ Gentamicin (Non-proprietary)
Gentamicin (as Gentamicin sulfate) 3 mg per 1 ml Gentamicin 0.3% ear/eye drops | 10 ml [PoM] £2.55 DT price = £2.13
Gentamicin 0.3% eye/ear drops | 10 ml [PoM] £2.13 DT price = £2.13

Tobramycin

● INDICATIONS AND DOSE

Local treatment of infections
▸ TO THE EYE
▸ Child 1-17 years: Apply twice daily for 6–8 days
Local treatment of infections (severe infection)
▸ TO THE EYE
▸ Child 1-17 years: Apply 4 times a day for first day, then apply twice daily for 5–7 days

● MEDICINAL FORMS
There can be variation in the licensing of different medicines containing the same drug.
Eye drops
EXCIPIENTS: May contain Benzododecinium bromide
▸ Tobravisc (Alcon Laboratories (UK) Ltd)
Tobramycin 3 mg per 1 ml Tobravisc 3mg/ml eye drops | 5 ml [PoM] £4.74

ANTIBACTERIALS › MACROLIDES

Azithromycin

● INDICATIONS AND DOSE

Trachomatous conjunctivitis caused by *Chlamydia trachomatis* | Purulent bacterial conjunctivitis
▸ TO THE EYE
▸ Child: Apply twice daily for 3 days, review if no improvement after 3 days of treatment

● INTERACTIONS → Appendix 1 (macrolides).
Caution with concomitant use of drugs that prolong the QT interval.

● SIDE-EFFECTS
▸ **Common or very common** Blurred vision · ocular burning · ocular discomfort · ocular pruritus
▸ **Uncommon** Conjunctival hyperaemia · eyelid eczema · eyelid erythema · eyelid oedema · keratitis

● MEDICINAL FORMS
There can be variation in the licensing of different medicines containing the same drug.
Eye drops
▸ Azyter (Thea Pharmaceuticals Ltd)
Azithromycin dihydrate 15 mg per 1 gram Azyter 15mg/g eye drops 0.25g unit dose | 6 unit dose [PoM] £6.99 DT price = £6.99

ANTIBACTERIALS › QUINOLONES

Ciprofloxacin

● INDICATIONS AND DOSE

Superficial bacterial eye infection
▸ TO THE EYE USING EYE DROP
▸ Child: Apply 4 times a day for maximum duration of treatment 21 days
▸ TO THE EYE USING EYE OINTMENT
▸ Child 1-17 years: Apply 1.25 centimetres 3 times a day for 2 days, then apply 1.25 centimetres twice daily for 5 days
Superficial bacterial eye infection (severe infection)
▸ TO THE EYE USING EYE DROP
▸ Child: Apply every 2 hours during waking hours for 2 days, then apply 4 times a day for maximum duration of treatment 21 days
Corneal ulcer
▸ TO THE EYE USING EYE DROP
▸ Child: Apply every 15 minutes for 6 hours, then apply every 30 minutes for the remainder of day 1, then apply every 1 hour on day 2, then apply every 4 hours on days 3–14, maximum duration of treatment 21 days, to be administered throughout the day and night
▸ TO THE EYE USING EYE OINTMENT
▸ Child 1-17 years: Apply 1.25 centimetres every 1–2 hours for 2 days, then apply 1.25 centimetres every 4 hours for the next 12 days, to be administered throughout the day and night

● UNLICENSED USE Eye ointment not licensed for use in children under 1 year.

● SIDE-EFFECTS
▸ **Common or very common** Corneal deposits (reversible after completion of treatment) · ocular discomfort · ocular hyperaemia · taste disturbance
▸ **Uncommon** Increased lacrimation · blurred vision · conjunctival hyperaemia · corneal infiltrates · corneal staining · eye dryness · eye irritation · eye pain · eye pruritus · eye swelling · eyelid disorders · eyelid erythema · eyelid exfoliation · eyelid oedema · headache · keratopathy · nausea · photophobia
▸ **Rare** Abdominal pain · asthenopia · corneal disorders · corneal epithelium defect · dermatitis · diarrhoea · diplopia · dizziness · ear pain · eye hypoaesthesia · keratitis · paranasal sinus hypersecretion · rhinitis

● PREGNANCY Manufacturer advises use only if potential benefit outweighs risk.

● BREAST FEEDING Manufacturer advises caution.

● **MEDICINAL FORMS**
There can be variation in the licensing of different medicines
containing the same drug. Forms available from special-order
manufacturers include: eye drops

Eye drops
EXCIPIENTS: May contain Benzalkonium chloride
▸ Ciloxan (Alcon Laboratories (UK) Ltd)
  **Ciprofloxacin (as Ciprofloxacin hydrochloride) 3 mg per
  1 ml** Ciloxan 0.3% eye drops | 5 ml PoM £4.70 DT price = £4.70

Eye ointment
▸ Ciloxan (Alcon Laboratories (UK) Ltd)
  **Ciprofloxacin (as Ciprofloxacin hydrochloride) 3 mg per
  1 gram** Ciloxan 3mg/g eye ointment | 3.5 gram PoM £5.22

Levofloxacin

● **INDICATIONS AND DOSE**

Local treatment of eye infections
▸ TO THE EYE
▸ **Child 1–17 years:** Apply every 2 hours for first 2 days, to
  be applied maximum 8 times a day, then apply 4 times
  a day for 3 days

● **SIDE-EFFECTS**
▸ **Common or very common** Ocular burning · visual
  disturbances
▸ **Uncommon** Conjunctival follicles · headache · lid erythema
  · lid oedema · ocular discomfort · ocular dryness · ocular
  itching · ocular pain · photophobia · rhinitis
● **PREGNANCY** Manufacturer advises use only if potential
  benefit outweighs risk.
● **BREAST FEEDING** Manufacturer advises use only if
  potential benefit outweighs risk.
● **PRESCRIBING AND DISPENSING INFORMATION** Although
  multi-dose levofloxacin eye drops commonly contain
  preservatives, preservative-free unit dose vials may be
  available.

● **MEDICINAL FORMS**
There can be variation in the licensing of different medicines
containing the same drug.

Eye drops
EXCIPIENTS: May contain Benzalkonium chloride
▸ Oftaquix (Santen UK Ltd)
  **Levofloxacin (as Levofloxacin hemihydrate) 5 mg per
  1 ml** Oftaquix 5mg/ml eye drops 0.5ml unit dose | 30 unit dose PoM
  £17.95
  Oftaquix 5mg/ml eye drops | 5 ml PoM £6.95

Moxifloxacin

● **INDICATIONS AND DOSE**

Local treatment of infections
▸ TO THE EYE
▸ **Child:** Apply 3 times a day continue treatment for
  2–3 days after infection improves; review if no
  improvement within 5 days

● **CAUTIONS** Not recommended for neonates
● **SIDE-EFFECTS**
Common or very common Hyperaemia · ocular discomfort ·
ocular dryness · ocular irritation · ocular pain · taste
disturbances
Uncommon Conjunctival haemorrhage · corneal disorders ·
corneal erosion · corneal keratitis · corneal staining · eyelid
erythema · headache · nasal discomfort · paraesthesia ·
pharyngolaryngeal pain · visual disturbances · vomiting
Frequency not known Dizziness · dyspnoea · nausea ·
palpitation · photophobia · pruritus · raised intra-ocular
pressure · rash

● **MEDICINAL FORMS**
There can be variation in the licensing of different medicines
containing the same drug.

Eye drops
▸ Moxivig (Alcon Laboratories (UK) Ltd)
  **Moxifloxacin (as Moxifloxacin hydrochloride) 5 mg per
  1 ml** Moxivig 0.5% eye drops | 5 ml PoM £9.80

Ofloxacin

● **INDICATIONS AND DOSE**

Local treatment of infections
▸ TO THE EYE
▸ **Child 1–17 years:** Apply every 2–4 hours for the first
  2 days, then reduced to 4 times a day for maximum
  10 days treatment

● **CAUTIONS** Corneal ulcer (risk of corneal perforation) ·
epithelial defect (risk of corneal perforation)
● **SIDE-EFFECTS**
▸ **Common or very common** Ocular discomfort
▸ **Frequency not known** Dry eyes · facial oedema · increased
  lacrimation · keratitis · ocular hyperaemia · ocular oedema ·
  photophobia · visual disturbances
● **PREGNANCY** Manufacturer advises use only if benefit
  outweighs risk (systemic quinolones have caused
  arthropathy in *animal* studies).
● **BREAST FEEDING** Manufacturer advises avoid.

● **MEDICINAL FORMS**
There can be variation in the licensing of different medicines
containing the same drug.

Eye drops
EXCIPIENTS: May contain Benzalkonium chloride
▸ Exocin (Allergan Ltd)
  Ofloxacin 3 mg per 1 ml Exocin 0.3% eye drops | 5 ml PoM £2.17
  DT price = £2.17

ANTIBACTERIALS > OTHER

Chloramphenicol

● **DRUG ACTION** Chloramphenicol is a potent broad-
spectrum antibiotic.

● **INDICATIONS AND DOSE**

Superficial eye infections
▸ TO THE EYE USING EYE DROP
▸ **Child:** Apply 1 drop every 2 hours then reduce
  frequency as infection is controlled and continue for
  48 hours after healing, frequency dependent on the
  severity of the infection. For less severe infection
  3–4 times daily is generally sufficient
▸ TO THE EYE USING EYE OINTMENT
▸ **Child:** Apply daily, to be applied at night (if eye drops
  used during the day), alternatively apply 3–4 times a
  day, if ointment used alone

● **SIDE-EFFECTS** Transient stinging
● **PREGNANCY** Avoid unless essential—no information on
  topical use but risk of 'neonatal grey-baby syndrome' with
  oral use in third trimester.
● **BREAST FEEDING** Avoid unless essential—*theoretical* risk
  of bone-marrow toxicity.
● **PRESCRIBING AND DISPENSING INFORMATION** Although
  multi-dose chloramphenicol eye drops commonly contain
  preservatives, preservative-free unit dose vials may be
  available.

11

Eye

- **PATIENT AND CARER ADVICE**
Medicines for Children leaflet: Chloramphenicol for eye infections www.medicinesforchildren.org.uk/
chloramphenicol-eye-infections-0
- **EXCEPTIONS TO LEGAL CATEGORY** Chloramphenicol 0.5% eye drops (in max. pack size 10 mL) and 1% eye ointment (in max. pack size 4 g) can be sold to the public for treatment of acute bacterial conjunctivitis in adults and children over 2 years; max. duration of treatment 5 days.

- **MEDICINAL FORMS**
There can be variation in the licensing of different medicines containing the same drug. Forms available from special-order manufacturers include: eye drops

Eye drops
EXCIPIENTS: May contain Phenylmercuric acetate
- **Chloramphenicol** (Non-proprietary)
Chloramphenicol 5 mg per 1 ml Minims chloramphenicol 0.5% eye drops 0.5ml unit dose | 20 unit dose PoM £10.99 DT price = £10.99
Chloramphenicol 0.5% eye drops | 10 ml PoM £2.20 DT price = £1.12
- **Brochlor** (Sanofi)
Chloramphenicol 5 mg per 1 ml Brochlor 0.5% eye drops | 10 ml P £2.83 DT price = £1.12
- **Brolene Antibiotic** (Sanofi)
Chloramphenicol 5 mg per 1 ml Brolene Antibiotic 0.5% eye drops | 10 ml P £3.00 DT price = £1.12
- **Chloromycetin** (AMCo)
Chloramphenicol 5 mg per 1 ml Chloromycetin Redidrops 0.5% | 10 ml PoM £0.90 DT price = £1.12
- **Optrex Infected Eyes** (Reckitt Benckiser Healthcare (UK) Ltd)
Chloramphenicol 5 mg per 1 ml Optrex Infected Eyes 0.5% eye drops | 10 ml P £3.88 DT price = £1.12

Eye ointment
- **Chloramphenicol** (Non-proprietary)
Chloramphenicol 10 mg per 1 gram Chloramphenicol 1% eye ointment | 4 gram PoM £4.25 DT price = £1.63
- **Brochlor** (Sanofi)
Chloramphenicol 10 mg per 1 gram Brochlor 1% eye ointment | 4 gram P £2.95 DT price = £1.63
- **Chloromycetin** (AMCo)
Chloramphenicol 10 mg per 1 gram Chloromycetin 1% eye ointment | 4 gram P £1.08 DT price = £1.63
- **Klorafect** (Blumont Pharma Ltd)
Chloramphenicol 10 mg per 1 gram Klorafect 1% eye ointment | 4 gram PoM £1.81 DT price = £1.63
- **Optrex Infected Eyes** (Reckitt Benckiser Healthcare (UK) Ltd)
Chloramphenicol 10 mg per 1 gram Optrex Infected Eyes 1% eye ointment | 4 gram P £3.88 DT price = £1.63

Fusidic acid

- **DRUG ACTION** Fusidic acid and its salts are narrow-spectrum antibiotics used for staphylococcal infections.

- **INDICATIONS AND DOSE**
Staphylococcal eye infections
- TO THE EYE
- Child: Apply twice daily

- **MEDICINAL FORMS**
There can be variation in the licensing of different medicines containing the same drug.
Modified-release drops
EXCIPIENTS: May contain Benzalkonium chloride, disodium edetate
- **Fusidic acid** (Non-proprietary)
Fusidic acid 10 mg per 1 gram Fusidic acid 1% modified-release eye drops | 5 gram PoM £29.06 DT price = £29.06

ANTIPROTOZOALS

Propamidine isetionate

- **INDICATIONS AND DOSE**
Acanthamoeba keratitis infections (specialist use only) |
Local treatment of eye infections
- TO THE EYE USING EYE OINTMENT
- Child: Apply 1–2 times a day
- TO THE EYE USING EYE DROP
- Child: Apply up to 4 times a day

- **UNLICENSED USE** Not licensed for *acanthamoeba keratitis* infections.
- **SIDE-EFFECTS** Eye irritation · eye pain
- **PREGNANCY** Manufacturer advises avoid unless essential—no information available.
- **BREAST FEEDING** Manufacturer advises avoid unless essential—no information available.

- **MEDICINAL FORMS**
There can be variation in the licensing of different medicines containing the same drug.
Eye drops
EXCIPIENTS: May contain Benzalkonium chloride
- **Brolene (Propamidine)** (Sanofi)
Propamidine isetionate 1 mg per 1 ml Brolene 0.1% eye drops | 10 ml P £2.80
- **Golden eye** (Cambridge Healthcare Supplies Ltd)
Propamidine isetionate 1 mg per 1 ml Golden Eye 0.1% drops | 10 ml P £3.26
Eye ointment
- **Brolene (Dibrompropamidine)** (Sanofi)
Dibrompropamidine isetionate 1.5 mg per 1 gram Brolene 0.15% eye ointment | 5 gram P £2.92 DT price = £3.49
- **Golden eye** (Cambridge Healthcare Supplies Ltd)
Dibrompropamidine isetionate 1.5 mg per 1 gram Golden Eye 0.15% ointment | 5 gram P £3.49 DT price = £3.49

3.2 Viral eye infection
3.2a Ophthalmic herpes simplex

ANTIVIRALS > NUCLEOSIDE ANALOGUES

Aciclovir
(Acyclovir)

- **INDICATIONS AND DOSE**
Herpes simplex infection (local treatment)
- TO THE EYE USING EYE OINTMENT
- Child: Apply 1 centimetre 5 times a day continue for at least 3 days after complete healing

- **SIDE-EFFECTS**
- **Common or very common** Local inflammation · local irritation · superficial punctate keratopathy
- **Rare** Blepharitis
- **Very rare** Angioedema · hypersensitivity reactions
- **PATIENT AND CARER ADVICE**
Medicines for Children leaflet: Aciclovir eye ointment for herpes simplex infections www.medicinesforchildren.org.uk/
aciclovir-eye-ointment-for-herpes-simplex-infection

- **MEDICINAL FORMS**
There can be variation in the licensing of different medicines containing the same drug.
Eye ointment
- **Zovirax** (GlaxoSmithKline UK Ltd)
Aciclovir 30 mg per 1 gram Zovirax 3% ophthalmic ointment | 4.5 gram PoM £9.34 DT price = £9.34

4 Eye procedures

Mydriatics and cycloplegics

Overview

Antimuscarinics dilate the pupil and paralyse the ciliary muscle; they vary in potency and duration of action.

Short-acting, relatively weak mydriatics, such as tropicamide 0.5% below (action lasts for 4–6 hours), facilitate the examination of the fundus of the eye. Cyclopentolate hydrochloride 1% p. 625 (action up to 24 hours) or atropine sulfate p. 624 (action up to 7 days) are preferable for producing cycloplegia for refraction in young children; tropicamide may be preferred in neonates.

Phenylephrine hydrochloride p. 634 is used for mydriasis in diagnostic or therapeutic procedures; mydriasis occurs within 60–90 minutes and lasts up to 5–7 hours.

Mydriatics and cycloplegics are used in the treatment of anterior uveitis, usually as an adjunct to corticosteroids. Atropine sulfate is used in anterior uveitis mainly to prevent posterior synechiae and to relieve ciliary spasm; cyclopentolate hydrochloride or homatropine hydrobromide p. 625 (action up to 3 days) can also be used and may be preferred because they have a shorter duration of action.

ANTIMUSCARINICS

F 624

Tropicamide

- **INDICATIONS AND DOSE**

Funduscopy
▶ TO THE EYE

- ▶ Neonate: 0.5% eye drops to be applied 20 minutes before examination.
- ▶ Child: 0.5% eye drops to be applied 20 minutes before examination

● **PRESCRIBING AND DISPENSING INFORMATION** Although multi-dose tropicamide eye drops commonly contain preservatives, preservative-free unit dose vials may be available.

● **MEDICINAL FORMS**
There can be variation in the licensing of different medicines containing the same drug.

Eye drops
EXCIPIENTS: May contain Benzalkonium chloride, edetic acid (edta)
▶ **Mydriacyl** (Alcon Laboratories (UK) Ltd)
   Tropicamide 5 mg per 1 ml Mydriacyl 0.5% eye drops | 5 ml PoM £1.29
   Tropicamide 10 mg per 1 ml Mydriacyl 1% eye drops | 5 ml PoM £1.60
▶ **Tropicamide** (Bausch & Lomb UK Ltd)
   Tropicamide 5 mg per 1 ml Minims tropicamide 0.5% eye drops 0.5ml unit dose | 20 unit dose PoM £10.75
   Tropicamide 10 mg per 1 ml Minims tropicamide 1% eye drops 0.5ml unit dose | 20 unit dose PoM £10.77

ANTISEPTICS AND DISINFECTANTS › IODINE PRODUCTS

Povidone-iodine

- **INDICATIONS AND DOSE**

Cutaneous peri-ocular and conjunctival antisepsis before ocular surgery
▶ TO THE EYE

- ▶ Neonate: Apply, leave for 2 minutes, then irrigate thoroughly with sodium chloride 0.9%.
- ▶ Child: Apply, leave for 2 minutes, then irrigate thoroughly with sodium chloride 0.9%

● **CONTRA-INDICATIONS** Concomitant use of ocular antimicrobial drugs · concomitant use of ocular formulations containing mercury-based preservatives · preterm neonates
● **SIDE-EFFECTS**
▶ **Rare** Conjunctival hyperaemia · superficial punctuate keratitis
▶ **Frequency not known** Cytotoxicity on deep tissue · cytotoxicity on mucous membranes · hypothyroidism in neonates · residual yellow coloration of the conjunctiva
● **PRESCRIBING AND DISPENSING INFORMATION** Although multi-dose povidone iodine eye drops commonly contain preservatives, preservative-free unit dose vials may be available.

● **MEDICINAL FORMS**
There can be variation in the licensing of different medicines containing the same drug. Forms available from special-order manufacturers include: eye drop
Eye drops
▶ **Povidone iodine** (Bausch & Lomb UK Ltd)
   Povidone iodine 50 mg per 1 ml Minims povidone iodine 5% eye drops 0.4ml unit dose | 20 unit dose PoM £16.00

DIAGNOSTIC AGENTS › DYES

Fluorescein sodium

- **INDICATIONS AND DOSE**

Detection of lesions and foreign bodies
▶ TO THE EYE USING EYE DROP
- ▶ Child: Use sufficient amount to stain damaged areas

● **PRESCRIBING AND DISPENSING INFORMATION** Although multi-dose fluorescein eye drops commonly contain preservatives, preservative-free unit dose vials may be available.

● **MEDICINAL FORMS**
There can be variation in the licensing of different medicines containing the same drug.
Eye drops
▶ **Fluorescein sodium** (Bausch & Lomb UK Ltd)
   Fluorescein sodium 10 mg per 1 ml Minims fluorescein sodium 1% eye drops 0.5ml unit dose | 20 unit dose P £8.89
   Fluorescein sodium 20 mg per 1 ml Minims fluorescein sodium 2% eye drops 0.5ml unit dose | 20 unit dose P £8.89

11

Eye

MIOTICS > PARASYMPATHOMIMETICS

Acetylcholine chloride

- **INDICATIONS AND DOSE**
Cataract surgery | Penetrating keratoplasty | Iridectomy | Anterior segment surgery requiring rapid complete miosis
  ▶ TO THE EYE
  ▶ Child: (consult product literature)

- **UNLICENSED USE** Not licensed for use in children.
- **CAUTIONS** Asthma · gastro-intestinal spasm · heart failure · hyperthyroidism · peptic ulcer · urinary-tract obstruction
- **PREGNANCY** Avoid unless potential benefit outweighs risk—no information available.
- **BREAST FEEDING** Avoid unless potential benefit outweighs risk—no information available.

- **MEDICINAL FORMS**
There can be variation in the licensing of different medicines containing the same drug.
Irrigation
  ▶ **Miochol-E** (Bausch & Lomb UK Ltd)
  Acetylcholine chloride 20 mg Miochol-E 20mg powder and solvent for solution for intraocular irrigation vials | 1 vial [PoM] £7.28
  ▶ **Miphtel** (Alan Pharmaceuticals)
  Acetylcholine chloride 20 mg Miphtel 20mg powder and solvent for solution for intraocular irrigation ampoules | 6 ampoule [PoM] £43.68 (Hospital only)

SYMPATHOMIMETICS > VASOCONSTRICTOR

Phenylephrine hydrochloride

- **INDICATIONS AND DOSE**
Mydriasis
  ▶ TO THE EYE
  ▶ Child: Apply 1 drop, to be administered before procedure, a drop of proxymetacaine topical anaesthetic may be applied to the eye a few minutes before using phenylephrine to prevent stinging

- **CONTRA-INDICATIONS** 10% strength eye drops · aneurysms · cardiovascular disease · hypertension · thyrotoxicosis
- **CAUTIONS** Asthma · corneal epithelial damage · darkly pigmented iris is more resistant to pupillary dilatation and caution should be exercised to avoid overdosage. · diabetes (avoid eye drops in long standing diabetes) · mydriasis can precipitate acute angle-closure glaucoma in the very few children who are predisposed to the condition because of a shallow anterior chamber · neonates are at an increased risk of systemic toxicity · ocular hyperaemia · susceptibility to angle-closure glaucoma
- **INTERACTIONS** → Appendix 1 (sympathomimetics). Phenylephrine may interact with systemically administered monoamine-oxidase inhibitors.
- **SIDE-EFFECTS** Arrhythmias · blurred vision · conjunctivitis on prolonged administration · coronary artery spasm · extrasystoles · hyperaemia on prolonged administration · local irritation on prolonged administration · hypertension · myocardial infarction (usually after use of 10% strength in patients with pre-existing cardiovascular disease) · oedema on prolonged administration · palpitation · photophobia · raised intraocular pressure · tachycardia · transient stinging
- **PREGNANCY** Use only if potential benefit outweighs risk.
- **BREAST FEEDING** Use only if potential benefit outweighs risk—no information available.
- **PRESCRIBING AND DISPENSING INFORMATION** Although multi-dose phenylephrine eye drops commonly contain

preservatives, preservative-free unit dose vials may be available.

- **PATIENT AND CARER ADVICE**
Driving and skilled tasks
Patients should be warned not to undertake skilled tasks (e.g. driving) until vision clears after mydriasis.

- **MEDICINAL FORMS**
There can be variation in the licensing of different medicines containing the same drug. Forms available from special-order manufacturers include: eye drops
Eye drops
EXCIPIENTS: May contain Disodium edetate, sodium metabisulfite
  ▶ **Phenylephrine hydrochloride** (Bausch & Lomb UK Ltd)
  Phenylephrine hydrochloride 25 mg per 1 ml Minims phenylephrine hydrochloride 2.5% eye drops 0.5ml unit dose | 20 unit dose [P] £11.41

4.1 Post-operative pain and inflammation

Eye, surgical and peri-operative drug use

Ocular peri-operative drugs

Drugs used to prepare the eye for surgery and drugs that are injected into the anterior chamber at the time of surgery are included here.

Sodium hyaluronate p. 628 is used during surgical procedures on the eye.

Apraclonidine p. 641, an alpha$_2$-adrenoceptor agonist, reduces intra-ocular pressure possibly by reducing the production of aqueous humour. It is used for short-term treatment only.

Balanced Salt Solution is used routinely in intra-ocular surgery.

Povidone-iodine p. 633 is used for peri-ocular and conjunctival antisepsis before ocular surgery to support postoperative infection control.

Local anaesthetics

Oxybuprocaine hydrochloride p. 635 and tetracaine p. 635 are widely used topical local anaesthetics. Proxymetacaine hydrochloride p. 635 causes less initial stinging and is useful for children. Oxybuprocaine hydrochloride or a combined preparation of lidocaine hydrochloride p. 780 and fluorescein sodium p. 633 is used for tonometry. Tetracaine produces a more profound anaesthesia and is suitable for use before minor surgical procedures, such as the removal of corneal sutures. It has a temporary disruptive effect on the corneal epithelium. Lidocaine hydrochloride, with or without adrenaline/epinephrine p. 128, is injected into the eyelids for minor surgery. Local anaesthetics should never be used for the management of ocular symptoms.

Local anaesthetic eye drops should be avoided in preterm neonates because of the immaturity of the metabolising enzyme system.

ANAESTHETICS, LOCAL

Fluorescein with lidocaine

- **INDICATIONS AND DOSE**
Local anaesthesia
  ▶ TO THE EYE
  ▶ Child: Apply as required

- **CONTRA-INDICATIONS** Avoid in pre-term neonate (immature metabolising enzyme system)

- **PRESCRIBING AND DISPENSING INFORMATION** Although multi-dose lidocaine and fluorescein eye drops commonly contain preservatives, preservative-free unit dose vials may be available.

- **MEDICINAL FORMS**
There can be variation in the licensing of different medicines containing the same drug.
Eye drops
  - Lidocaine and Fluorescein (Bausch & Lomb UK Ltd)
  Fluorescein sodium 2.5 mg per 1 ml, Lidocaine hydrochloride 40 mg per 1 ml Minims lidocaine and fluorescein eye drops 0.5ml unit dose | 20 unit dose PoM £11.24

Oxybuprocaine hydrochloride

(Benoxinate hydrochloride)

- **INDICATIONS AND DOSE**
Local anaesthetic
  - TO THE EYE
  - Child: Apply as required

- **CONTRA-INDICATIONS** Avoid in preterm neonates
- **PRESCRIBING AND DISPENSING INFORMATION** Although multi-dose oxybuprocaine eye drops commonly contain preservatives, preservative-free unit dose vials may be available.

- **MEDICINAL FORMS**
There can be variation in the licensing of different medicines containing the same drug.
Eye drops
  - Oxybuprocaine hydrochloride (Bausch & Lomb UK Ltd)
  Oxybuprocaine hydrochloride 4 mg per 1 ml Minims oxybuprocaine hydrochloride 0.4% eye drops 0.5ml unit dose | 20 unit dose PoM £10.15

Proxymetacaine hydrochloride

- **INDICATIONS AND DOSE**
Local anaesthetic
  - TO THE EYE
  - Child: Apply as required

- **CONTRA-INDICATIONS** Avoid in preterm neonates
- **PRESCRIBING AND DISPENSING INFORMATION** Although multi-dose proxymetacaine eye drops commonly contain preservatives, preservative-free unit dose vials may be available.

- **MEDICINAL FORMS**
There can be variation in the licensing of different medicines containing the same drug.
Eye drops
  - Proxymetacaine (Bausch & Lomb UK Ltd)
  Proxymetacaine hydrochloride 5 mg per 1 ml Minims proxymetacaine 0.5% eye drops 0.5ml unit dose | 20 unit dose PoM £11.54

Tetracaine

(Amethocaine)

- **INDICATIONS AND DOSE**
Local anaesthetic
  - TO THE EYE
  - Child: Apply as required

- **UNLICENSED USE** Not licensed for use in neonates.
- **CONTRA-INDICATIONS** Avoid in preterm neonates
- **SIDE-EFFECTS** Local skin reactions

SIDE-EFFECTS, FURTHER INFORMATION
The systemic toxicity of local anaesthetics mainly involves the central nervous and cardiovascular systems; systemic side effects unlikely as minimal absorption following topical application.

- **ALLERGY AND CROSS-SENSITIVITY**
  - Hypersensitivity and cross-sensitivity Hypersensitivity reactions occur mainly with the ester-type local anaesthetics, such as tetracaine and chloroprocaine; reactions are less frequent with the amide types, such as articaine, bupivacaine, levobupivacaine, lidocaine, mepivacaine, prilocaine, and ropivacaine. Cross-sensitivity reactions may be avoided by using the alternative chemical type.

- **PRESCRIBING AND DISPENSING INFORMATION** Although multi-dose tetracaine eye drops commonly contain preservatives, preservative-free unit dose vials may be available.

- **MEDICINAL FORMS**
There can be variation in the licensing of different medicines containing the same drug.
Eye drops
  - Tetracaine (Non-proprietary)
  Tetracaine hydrochloride 5 mg per 1 ml Minims tetracaine hydrochloride 0.5% eye drops 0.5ml unit dose | 20 unit dose PoM £10.16
  Tetracaine hydrochloride 10 mg per 1 ml Minims tetracaine hydrochloride 1% eye drops 0.5ml unit dose | 20 unit dose PoM £10.16

ANALGESICS > NON-STEROIDAL ANTI-INFLAMMATORY DRUGS

Diclofenac sodium

- **INDICATIONS AND DOSE**
Inhibition of intra-operative miosis during cataract surgery (but does not possess intrinsic mydriatic properties) | Postoperative inflammation in cataract surgery, strabismus surgery, argon laser trabeculoplasty
  - TO THE EYE
  - Child: (consult product literature)

- **UNLICENSED USE** Not licensed for use in children.
- **ALLERGY AND CROSS-SENSITIVITY** Contra-indicated in patients with a history of hypersensitivity to aspirin or any other NSAID—which includes those in whom attacks of asthma, angioedema, urticaria or rhinitis have been precipitated by aspirin or any other NSAID.

- **PRESCRIBING AND DISPENSING INFORMATION** Although multi-dose diclofenac sodium eye drops commonly contain preservatives, preservative-free unit dose vials may be available.

- **MEDICINAL FORMS**
There can be variation in the licensing of different medicines containing the same drug.
Eye drops
EXCIPIENTS: May contain Benzalkonium chloride, disodium edetate, propylene glycol
  - Voltarol Ophtha (Thea Pharmaceuticals Ltd)
  Diclofenac sodium 1 mg per 1 ml Voltarol Ophtha 0.1% eye drops 0.3ml unit dose | 5 unit dose PoM £4.00 | 40 unit dose PoM £32.00
  - Voltarol Ophtha Multidose (Thea Pharmaceuticals Ltd)
  Diclofenac sodium 1 mg per 1 ml Voltarol Ophtha Multidose 0.1% eye drops | 5 ml PoM £6.68

11

Eye

Flurbiprofen

- **INDICATIONS AND DOSE**

Inhibition of intra-operative miosis (but does not possess intrinsic mydriatic properties) | Control of anterior segment inflammation following postoperative and post-laser trabeculoplasty when corticosteroids contra-indicated
  - ▶ TO THE EYE
  - ▶ Child: (consult product literature)

- **UNLICENSED USE** Not licensed for use in children.

- **ALLERGY AND CROSS-SENSITIVITY** Contra-indicated in patients with a history of hypersensitivity to aspirin or any other NSAID—which includes those in whom attacks of asthma, angioedema, urticaria or rhinitis have been precipitated by aspirin or any other NSAID.

- **MEDICINAL FORMS**
There can be variation in the licensing of different medicines containing the same drug.
Eye drops
  - ▶ Ocufen (Allergan Ltd)
    Flurbiprofen sodium 300 microgram per 1 ml Ocufen 0.03% eye drops 0.4ml unit dose | 40 unit dose [PoM] £37.15

Ketorolac trometamol

- **INDICATIONS AND DOSE**

Prophylaxis and reduction of inflammation and associated symptoms following ocular surgery
  - ▶ TO THE EYE
  - ▶ Child: (consult product literature)

- **UNLICENSED USE** Not licensed for use in children.

- **ALLERGY AND CROSS-SENSITIVITY** Contra-indicated in patients with a history of hypersensitivity to aspirin or any other NSAID—which includes those in whom attacks of asthma, angioedema, urticaria or rhinitis have been precipitated by aspirin or any other NSAID.

- **MEDICINAL FORMS**
There can be variation in the licensing of different medicines containing the same drug.
Eye drops
EXCIPIENTS: May contain Benzalkonium chloride, disodium edetate
  - ▶ Acular (Allergan Ltd)
    Ketorolac trometamol 5 mg per 1 ml Acular 0.5% eye drops | 5 ml [PoM] £3.00 DT price = £3.00

5 Glaucoma and ocular hypertension

Glaucoma

Overview

Glaucoma describes a group of disorders characterised by a loss of visual field associated with cupping of the optic disc and optic nerve damage and is generally associated with raised intra-ocular pressure.

Glaucoma is rare in children and should always be managed by a specialist. *Primary congenital glaucoma* is the most common form of glaucoma in children, followed by *secondary glaucomas*, such as following hereditary anterior segment malformations; *juvenile open-angle glaucoma* is less common and usually occurs in older children.

Treatment of glaucoma is determined by the pathophysiology and usually involves controlling raised intra-ocular pressure with surgery. Drug therapy is generally supportive, and can be used temporarily, pre- or post-operatively, or both, to reduce intra-ocular pressure. In secondary glaucomas, drug therapy is often used first-line, and long-term treatment may be required. Drugs that reduce intra-ocular pressure by different mechanisms are available for managing glaucoma. A topical beta-blocker or a prostaglandin analogue can be used. It may be necessary to combine these drugs or add others, such as carbonic anhydrase inhibitors, or miotics to control intra-ocular pressure.

Children with an acute form of glaucoma (usually presenting with pain in older children, a cloudy cornea, and may be associated with a previous history of controlled glaucoma or recent intra-ocular surgery) need immediate referral for specialist ophthalmology assessment and treatment.

Beta-blockers

Topical application of a beta-blocker to the eye reduces intra-ocular pressure effectively in primary and secondary glaucomas, probably by reducing the rate of production of aqueous humour.

Prostaglandin analogues

The prostaglandin analogues latanoprost p. 641, and travoprost, and the synthetic prostamide, bimatoprost, increase uveoscleral outflow and subsequently reduce intra-ocular pressure. They are used to reduce intra-ocular pressure. Only latanoprost (*Xalatan*® and certain non-proprietary preparations of latanoprost) is licensed for use in children. Children receiving prostaglandin analogues should be managed by a specialist.

Sympathomimetics

Apraclonidine p. 641 is an alpha$_2$-adrenoceptor agonist that lowers intra-ocular pressure by reducing aqueous humour formation. Eye drops containing apraclonidine 0.5% are used for a short period to delay laser treatment or surgery for glaucoma in patients not adequately controlled by another drug; eye drops containing 1% are used for control of intra-ocular pressure after anterior segment laser surgery.

Brimonidine tartrate, an alpha$_2$-adrenoceptor agonist, is thought to lower intra-ocular pressure by reducing aqueous humour formation and increasing uveoscleral outflow.

Carbonic anhydrase inhibitors and systemic drugs

The **carbonic anhydrase inhibitors**, acetazolamide p. 638, brinzolamide p. 639, and dorzolamide p. 639, reduce intra-ocular pressure by reducing aqueous humour production. Systemic use of acetazolamide also produces weak diuresis.

Acetazolamide is given by mouth or, rarely in children, by intravenous injection (intramuscular injections are painful because of the alkaline pH of the solution). It is used as an adjunct to other treatment for reducing intra-ocular pressure. Acetazolamide is not generally recommended for long-term use.

Dorzolamide and brinzolamide are topical carbonic anhydrase inhibitors. They are unlicensed in children but are used in those resistant to beta-blockers or those in whom beta-blockers are contra-indicated. They are used alone or as an adjunct to a topical beta-blocker. Brinzolamide can also be used as an adjunct to a prostaglandin analogue. Systemic absorption can rarely cause sulfonamide-like side-effects and may require discontinuation if severe.

Metabolic acidosis can occur in children using topical carbonic anhydrase inhibitors; symptoms may include poor feeding and lack of weight gain.

Miotics

Miotics act by opening up the inefficient drainage channels in the trabecular meshwork. Pilocarpine p. 640 is a miotic used pre- and post-operatively in goniotomy and trabeculotomy; it is used occasionally for aphakic glaucoma.

BETA-ADRENOCEPTOR BLOCKERS

Betaxolol

- **INDICATIONS AND DOSE**
Primary and secondary glaucomas
  - ▸ TO THE EYE
  - ▸ Child: Apply twice daily

- **UNLICENSED USE** Not licensed for use in children.
- **CONTRA-INDICATIONS** Also consider contra-indications listed for systemically administered beta blockers · bradycardia · heart block
- **CAUTIONS** Patients with corneal disease
  CAUTIONS, FURTHER INFORMATION
  Systemic absorption can follow topical application to the eyes; consider cautions listed for systemically administered beta blockers.
- **INTERACTIONS** → Appendix 1 (beta-blockers).
  Since systemic absorption may follow topical application the possibility of interactions, in particular, with drugs such as verapamil should be borne in mind.
- **SIDE-EFFECTS** Anaphylaxis · blepharoconjunctivitis · burning · corneal disorders · cough, rather than wheeze, may occur · dry eyes · erythema · itching · ocular stinging · pain
  SIDE-EFFECTS, FURTHER INFORMATION
  Systemic absorption can follow topical application to the eyes; consider side effects listed for systemically administered beta blockers.
- **PRESCRIBING AND DISPENSING INFORMATION** Although multi-dose bextaxolol eye drops commonly contain preservatives, preservative-free unit dose vials may be available.

- **MEDICINAL FORMS**
  There can be variation in the licensing of different medicines containing the same drug.
  Eye drops
  EXCIPIENTS: May contain Benzalkonium chloride, disodium edetate
  - ▸ Betaxolol (Non-proprietary)
    Betaxolol (as Betaxolol hydrochloride) 2.5 mg per 1 ml Betaxolol 0.25% eye drops 0.25ml unit dose preservative free | 50 unit dose [PoM] no price available
    Betaxolol (as Betaxolol hydrochloride) 5 mg per 1 ml Betaxolol 0.5% eye drops | 5 ml [PoM] £1.90 DT price = £1.90
  - ▸ Betoptic (Alcon Laboratories (UK) Ltd)
    Betaxolol (as Betaxolol hydrochloride) 2.5 mg per 1 ml Betoptic 0.25% suspension eye drops | 5 ml [PoM] £2.66 DT price = £2.66
    Betoptic 0.25% eye drops suspension 0.25ml unit dose | 50 unit dose [PoM] £13.77
    Betaxolol (as Betaxolol hydrochloride) 5 mg per 1 ml Betoptic 0.5% eye drops | 5 ml [PoM] £1.90 DT price = £1.90

Carteolol hydrochloride

- **INDICATIONS AND DOSE**
Primary and secondary glaucomas
  - ▸ TO THE EYE
  - ▸ Child: Apply twice daily

- **UNLICENSED USE** Not licensed for use in children.
- **CONTRA-INDICATIONS** Also consider contra-indications listed for systemically administered beta blockers · bradycardia · heart block
- **CAUTIONS** Patients with corneal disease
  CAUTIONS, FURTHER INFORMATION
  Systemic absorption can follow topical application to the eyes; consider cautions listed for systemically administered beta blockers.

- **INTERACTIONS** → Appendix 1 (beta-blockers).
  Since systemic absorption may follow topical application the possibility of interactions, in particular, with drugs such as verapamil should be borne in mind.
- **SIDE-EFFECTS** Anaphylaxis · blepharoconjunctivitis · burning · corneal disorders · cough, rather than wheeze, may occur · dry eyes · erythema · itching · ocular stinging · pain
  SIDE-EFFECTS, FURTHER INFORMATION
  Systemic absorption can follow topical application to the eyes; consider side effects listed for systemically administered beta blockers.

- **MEDICINAL FORMS**
  There can be variation in the licensing of different medicines containing the same drug.
  Eye drops
  EXCIPIENTS: May contain Benzalkonium chloride
  - ▸ Teoptic (Thea Pharmaceuticals Ltd)
    Carteolol hydrochloride 10 mg per 1 ml Teoptic 1% eye drops | 5 ml [PoM] £7.60 DT price = £7.60
    Carteolol hydrochloride 20 mg per 1 ml Teoptic 2% eye drops | 5 ml [PoM] £8.40 DT price = £8.40

Levobunolol hydrochloride

- **INDICATIONS AND DOSE**
Primary and secondary glaucomas
  - ▸ TO THE EYE
  - ▸ Child: Apply 1–2 times a day

- **UNLICENSED USE** Not licensed for use in children.
- **CONTRA-INDICATIONS** Also consider contra-indications listed for systemically administered beta blockers · bradycardia · heart block
- **CAUTIONS** Patients with corneal disease
  CAUTIONS, FURTHER INFORMATION
  Systemic absorption can follow topical application to the eyes; consider cautions listed for systemically administered beta blockers.
- **INTERACTIONS** → Appendix 1 (beta-blockers).
  Since systemic absorption may follow topical application the possibility of interactions, in particular, with drugs such as verapamil should be borne in mind.
- **SIDE-EFFECTS** Anaphylaxis · anterior uveitis · blepharoconjunctivitis · burning · corneal disorders · cough, rather than wheeze, may occur · dry eyes · erythema · itching · ocular stinging · pain
  SIDE-EFFECTS, FURTHER INFORMATION
  Systemic absorption can follow topical application to the eyes; consider side effects listed for systemically administered beta blockers.
- **PRESCRIBING AND DISPENSING INFORMATION** Although multi-dose (Levobunolol) eye drops commonly contain preservatives, preservative-free unit dose vials may be available.

- **MEDICINAL FORMS**
  There can be variation in the licensing of different medicines containing the same drug.
  Eye drops
  EXCIPIENTS: May contain Benzalkonium chloride, disodium edetate, sodium metabisulfite
  - ▸ Betagan (Allergan Ltd)
    Levobunolol hydrochloride 5 mg per 1 ml Betagan 0.5% eye drops | 5 ml [PoM] £1.85 DT price = £1.85
    Betagan Unit Dose 0.5% eye drops 0.4ml unit dose | 30 unit dose [PoM] £9.98

11

Eye

Timolol maleate

- **INDICATIONS AND DOSE**

Primary congenital and primary juvenile glaucoma, for a transitional period, before surgery or following failed surgery
- ▸ TO THE EYE
- ▸ Child: (consult product literature)

TIMOPTOL-LA®

Reduction of intra-ocular pressure in primary and secondary glaucoma
- ▸ TO THE EYE
- ▸ Child: Apply once daily

TIOPEX®

Reduction of intra-ocular pressure primary and secondary glaucomas
- ▸ TO THE EYE
- ▸ Child: Apply once daily, to be applied in the morning

- **UNLICENSED USE** Not licensed for use in children.
- **CONTRA-INDICATIONS** Also consider contra-indications listed for systemically administered beta blockers · bradycardia · heart block
- **CAUTIONS** Consider also cautions listed for systemically administered beta blockers · patients with corneal disease
- **INTERACTIONS** Since systemic absorption may follow topical application the possibility of interactions, in particular, with drugs such as verapamil should be borne in mind.
- **SIDE-EFFECTS** Anaphylaxis · blepharoconjunctivitis · burning · corneal disorders · cough, rather than wheeze, may occur · dry eyes · erythema · itching · ocular stinging · pain

  SIDE-EFFECTS, FURTHER INFORMATION
  Systemic absorption can follow topical application to the eyes; consider side effects listed for systemically administered beta blockers.

- **NATIONAL FUNDING/ACCESS DECISIONS**

  TIOPEX®

  Scottish Medicines Consortium (SMC) Decisions
  The *Scottish Medicines Consortium* has advised (February 2014) that timolol gel eye drops (*Tiopex*®) are accepted for restricted use within NHS Scotland for the reduction of elevated intraocular pressure in patients with ocular hypertension or chronic open angle glaucoma who have proven sensitivity to preservatives.

- **MEDICINAL FORMS**
  There can be variation in the licensing of different medicines containing the same drug. Forms available from special-order manufacturers include: eye drops

  Eye drops
  EXCIPIENTS: May contain Benzalkonium chloride
  - ▸ Timolol maleate (Non-proprietary)
    Timolol (as Timolol maleate) 2.5 mg per 1 ml Timolol 0.25% eye drops | 5 ml [PoM] £1.80 DT price = £1.02
    Timolol (as Timolol maleate) 5 mg per 1 ml Timolol 0.5% eye drops | 5 ml [PoM] £1.95 DT price = £1.04
  - ▸ Timoptol (Santen UK Ltd)
    Timolol (as Timolol maleate) 2.5 mg per 1 ml Timoptol 0.25% eye drops | 5 ml [PoM] £3.12 DT price = £1.02
    Timoptol Unit Dose 0.25% ophthalmic solution 0.2ml unit dose | 30 unit dose [PoM] £8.45
    Timolol (as Timolol maleate) 5 mg per 1 ml Timoptol 0.5% eye drops | 5 ml [PoM] £3.12 DT price = £1.04
    Timoptol Unit Dose 0.5% ophthalmic solution 0.2ml unit dose | 30 unit dose [PoM] £9.65 DT price = £9.65
  - ▸ Tiopex (Thea Pharmaceuticals Ltd)
    Timolol (as Timolol maleate) 1 mg per 1 gram Tiopex 1mg/g eye gel 0.4g unit dose | 30 unit dose [PoM] £7.49 DT price = £7.49

Eye gel
EXCIPIENTS: May contain Benzododecinium bromide
- ▸ Timoptol-LA (Santen UK Ltd)
  Timolol (as Timolol maleate) 2.5 mg per 1 ml Timoptol-LA 0.25% ophthalmic gel-forming solution | 2.5 ml [PoM] £3.12 DT price = £3.12
  Timolol (as Timolol maleate) 5 mg per 1 ml Timoptol-LA 0.5% ophthalmic gel-forming solution | 2.5 ml [PoM] £3.12 DT price = £3.12

Combinations available: *Dorzolamide with timolol,* p. 640

CARBONIC ANHYDRASE INHIBITORS

Acetazolamide

- **INDICATIONS AND DOSE**

Glaucoma
- ▸ BY MOUTH USING MODIFIED-RELEASE MEDICINES
- ▸ Child 12–17 years: 250–500 mg daily

Epilepsy
- ▸ BY MOUTH USING IMMEDIATE-RELEASE MEDICINES, OR BY SLOW INTRAVENOUS INJECTION
- ▸ Neonate: Initially 2.5 mg/kg 2–3 times a day, followed by maintenance 5–7 mg/kg 2–3 times a day.
- ▸ Child 1 month–11 years: Initially 2.5 mg/kg 2–3 times a day, followed by maintenance 5–7 mg/kg 2–3 times a day; maximum 750 mg per day
- ▸ Child 12–17 years: 250 mg 2–3 times a day

Reduction of intra-ocular pressure in primary and secondary glaucoma (specialist use only)
- ▸ BY MOUTH USING IMMEDIATE-RELEASE MEDICINES, OR BY INTRAVENOUS INJECTION
- ▸ Child 1 month–11 years: 5 mg/kg 2–4 times a day, adjusted according to response; maximum 750 mg per day
- ▸ Child 12–17 years: 250 mg 2–4 times a day

Raised intracranial pressure
- ▸ BY MOUTH USING IMMEDIATE-RELEASE MEDICINES, OR BY SLOW INTRAVENOUS INJECTION
- ▸ Child 1 month–11 years: Initially 8 mg/kg 3 times a day, then increased if necessary up to 100 mg/kg daily

- **UNLICENSED USE** Not licensed for the treatment of glaucoma.
- **CONTRA-INDICATIONS** Adrenocortical insufficiency · hyperchloraemic acidosis · hypokalaemia · hyponatraemia · long-term administration in chronic angle-closure glaucoma
- **CAUTIONS** Avoid extravasation at injection site (risk of necrosis) · diabetes mellitus · impaired alveolar ventilation (risk of acidosis) · not generally recommended for long-term use · pulmonary obstruction (risk of acidosis) · renal calculi
- **INTERACTIONS** → Appendix 1 (diuretics).
- **SIDE-EFFECTS**
  - ▸ **Common or very common** Ataxia · depression · diarrhoea · dizziness · excitement · fatigue · flushing · headache · irritability · loss of appetite · nausea · paraesthesia · polyuria · taste disturbance · thirst · vomiting
  - ▸ **Uncommon** Blood disorders · bone marrow suppression · confusion · crystalluria · drowsiness · electrolyte disturbances on long-term therapy · fever · glycosuria · haematuria · hearing disturbances · melaena · metabolic acidosis · rash · renal calculi · renal colic · renal failure · renal lesions · Stevens-Johnson syndrome · toxic epidermal necrosis · ureteric colic
  - ▸ **Rare** Cholestatic jaundice · convulsions · flaccid paralysis · fulminant hepatic necrosis · hepatitis · photosensitivity
  - ▸ **Frequency not known** Transient myopia

  SIDE-EFFECTS, FURTHER INFORMATION
  Acetazolamide is a sulfonamide derivative; blood disorders, rashes, and other sulfonamide-related side-

effects occur occasionally—patients should be told to report any unusual skin rash.

If electrolyte disturbances and metabolic acidosis occur, these can be corrected by administering potassium bicarbonate (as effervescent potassium tablets).

- **ALLERGY AND CROSS-SENSITIVITY** Contra-indicated if history of sulfonamide hypersensitivity.
- **PREGNANCY** Manufacturer advises avoid, especially in first trimester (toxicity in *animal* studies).
- **BREAST FEEDING** Amount too small to be harmful.
- **HEPATIC IMPAIRMENT** Manufacturer advises avoid.
- **RENAL IMPAIRMENT** Avoid—risk of metabolic acidosis.
- **MONITORING REQUIREMENTS** Monitor blood count and plasma electrolyte concentrations with prolonged use.

- **MEDICINAL FORMS**
There can be variation in the licensing of different medicines containing the same drug. Forms available from special-order manufacturers include: oral suspension, oral solution

Tablet
CAUTIONARY AND ADVISORY LABELS 3
▸ Acetazolamide (Non-proprietary)
  Acetazolamide 250 mg Acetazolamide 250mg tablets |
  100 tablet [PoM] no price available | 112 tablet [PoM] £75.36 DT price = £64.00

Modified-release capsule
CAUTIONARY AND ADVISORY LABELS 3, 25
▸ Diamox SR (AMCo)
  Acetazolamide 250 mg Diamox SR 250mg capsules |
  30 capsule [PoM] £16.66 DT price = £16.66
▸ Eytazox (Auden McKenzie (Pharma Division) Ltd)
  Acetazolamide 250 mg Eytazox 250mg modified-release capsules |
  30 capsule [PoM] £16.60 DT price = £16.66

Powder for solution for injection
▸ Diamox (AMCo)
  Acetazolamide 500 mg Diamox Sodium Parenteral 500mg powder for solution for injection vials | 1 vial [PoM] £14.76

Brinzolamide

- **INDICATIONS AND DOSE**

Reduction of intra-ocular pressure in primary and secondary glaucoma either as adjunct to beta-blockers or prostaglandin analogues or used alone if unresponsive to beta-blockers or if beta-blockers contra-indicated
▸ TO THE EYE
▹ Child: Apply twice daily, then increased if necessary up to 3 times a day

- **UNLICENSED USE** Not licensed for use in children.
- **CONTRA-INDICATIONS** Hyperchloraemic acidosis
- **CAUTIONS** Renal tubular immaturity or abnormality—risk of metabolic acidosis · systemic absorption follows topical application
- **INTERACTIONS** → Appendix 1 (brinzolamide).
  When used by eye Since systemic absorption may follow topical application of brinzolamide to the eye, the possibility of interactions should be borne in mind.
- **SIDE-EFFECTS**
▸ **Common or very common** Corneal erosion · corneal oedema · dry mouth · headache · ocular disturbances · photophobia · reduced visual acuity · taste disturbances
▸ **Uncommon** Alopecia · amnesia · bradycardia · chest pain · cough · decreased libido · depression · diarrhoea · dizziness · drowsiness · dyspepsia · dyspnoea · epistaxis · erectile dysfunction · flatulence · malaise · nasal dryness · nausea · nervousness · oesophagitis · oral hypoaesthesia and paraesthesia · palpitation · paraesthesia · pharyngitis · renal pain · sinusitis · sleep disturbances · throat irritation · tinnitus · upper respiratory tract congestion · vomiting

▸ **Frequency not known** Arrhythmia · asthma · dermatitis · erythema · hypertension · peripheral oedema · pollakiuria · rhinitis · tachycardia · tremor · vertigo
  SIDE-EFFECTS, FURTHER INFORMATION
  Systemic absorption can rarely cause sulfonamide-like side-effects and may require discontinuation if severe.
- **ALLERGY AND CROSS-SENSITIVITY** Contra-indicated if history of sulfonamide hypersensitivity.
- **PREGNANCY** Avoid—toxicity in *animal* studies.
- **BREAST FEEDING** Use only if benefit outweighs risk.
- **HEPATIC IMPAIRMENT** Manufacturer advises avoid.
- **RENAL IMPAIRMENT** Avoid if estimated glomerular filtration rate less than 30 mL/minute/1.73 m^2.

- **MEDICINAL FORMS**
There can be variation in the licensing of different medicines containing the same drug.
Eye drops
EXCIPIENTS: May contain Benzalkonium chloride, disodium edetate
▸ Brinzolamide (Non-proprietary)
  Brinzolamide 10 mg per 1 ml Brinzolamide 10mg/ml eye drops |
  5 ml [PoM] £6.92 DT price = £3.36
▸ Azopt (Alcon Laboratories (UK) Ltd)
  Brinzolamide 10 mg per 1 ml Azopt 10mg/ml eye drops |
  5 ml [PoM] £6.92 DT price = £3.36

Dorzolamide

- **INDICATIONS AND DOSE**

Raised intra-ocular pressure in primary and secondary glaucoma used alone in patients unresponsive to beta-blockers or if beta-blockers contra-indicated
▸ TO THE EYE
▹ Child: Apply 3 times a day

Raised intra-ocular pressure in primary and secondary glaucoma as adjunct to a beta-blocker
▸ TO THE EYE
▹ Child: Apply twice daily

- **UNLICENSED USE** Not licensed for use in children.
- **CONTRA-INDICATIONS** Hyperchloraemic acidosis
- **CAUTIONS** Chronic corneal defects · history of intra-ocular surgery · history of renal calculi · immature renal tubules (neonates and infants)—risk of metabolic acidosis · low endothelial cell count · systemic absorption follows topical application
- **INTERACTIONS** → Appendix 1 (dorzolamide).
▸ When used by eye Since systemic absorption may follow topical application of dorzolamide to the eye, the possibility of interactions should be borne in mind.
- **SIDE-EFFECTS**
▸ **Common or very common** Asthenia · bitter taste · blurred vision · conjunctivitis · eyelid inflammation · headache · lacrimation · nausea · ocular irritation · superficial punctate keratitis
▸ **Uncommon** Iridocyclitis
▸ **Rare** Contact dermatitis · corneal oedema · dizziness · dry mouth · epistaxis · eyelid crusting · paraesthesia · Stevens-Johnson syndrome · throat irritation · toxic epidermal necrolysis · transient myopia · urolithiasis
▸ **Frequency not known** Metabolic acidosis
  SIDE-EFFECTS, FURTHER INFORMATION
  Systemic absorption can rarely cause sulfonamide-like side-effects and may require discontinuation if severe.
- **ALLERGY AND CROSS-SENSITIVITY** Contra-indicated if history of sulfonamide hypersensitivity.
- **PREGNANCY** Manufacturer advises avoid—toxicity in *animal* studies.
- **BREAST FEEDING** Manufacturer advises avoid—no information available.

11

Eye

- **HEPATIC IMPAIRMENT** Manufacturer advises caution— no information available.
- **RENAL IMPAIRMENT** Avoid if estimated glomerular filtration rate less than 30 mL/minute/1.73 m^2.
- **PRESCRIBING AND DISPENSING INFORMATION** Although multi-dose dorzolamide eye drops commonly contain preservatives, preservative-free unit dose vials may be available.

- **MEDICINAL FORMS**
  There can be variation in the licensing of different medicines containing the same drug.
  Eye drops
  EXCIPIENTS: May contain Benzalkonium chloride
  ▸ Dorzolamide (Non-proprietary)
    Dorzolamide (as Dorzolamide hydrochloride) 20 mg per 1 ml Dorzolamide 2% eye drops | 5 ml PoM £6.33 DT price = £1.92
  ▸ Trusopt (Santen UK Ltd)
    Dorzolamide (as Dorzolamide hydrochloride) 20 mg per 1 ml Trusopt 2% eye drops | 5 ml PoM £6.33 DT price = £1.92
    Trusopt 2% eye drops 0.2ml unit dose preservative free | 60 unit dose PoM £24.18 DT price = £24.18

Dorzolamide with timolol

The properties listed below are those particular to the combination only. For the properties of the components please consider, dorzolamide p. 639, timolol maleate p. 638.

- **INDICATIONS AND DOSE**
  Raised intra-ocular pressure in open-angle glaucoma when beta-blockers alone not adequate | Raised intra-ocular pressure in pseudo-exfoliative glaucoma when beta-blockers alone not adequate
  ▸ TO THE EYE
  ▸ Child: Apply twice daily

- **PRESCRIBING AND DISPENSING INFORMATION** Although multi-dose dorzolamide with timolol eye drops commonly contain preservatives, preservative-free unit dose vials may be available.

- **MEDICINAL FORMS**
  There can be variation in the licensing of different medicines containing the same drug.
  Eye drops
  EXCIPIENTS: May contain Benzalkonium chloride
  ▸ Dorzolamide with timolol (Non-proprietary)
    Timolol (as Timolol maleate) 5 mg per 1 ml, Dorzolamide (as Dorzolamide hydrochloride) 20 mg per 1 ml Dorzolamide 2% / Timolol 0.5% eye drops | 5 ml PoM £27.16 DT price = £2.20
    Dorzolamide 2% / Timolol 0.5% eye drops 0.2ml unit dose preservative free | 60 unit dose PoM £27.16 DT price = £28.59
  ▸ Cosopt (Santen UK Ltd)
    Timolol (as Timolol maleate) 5 mg per 1 ml, Dorzolamide (as Dorzolamide hydrochloride) 20 mg per 1 ml Cosopt eye drops 0.2ml unit dose preservative free | 60 unit dose PoM £28.59 DT price = £28.59
    Cosopt eye drops | 5 ml PoM £10.05 DT price = £2.20

MIOTICS › PARASYMPATHOMIMETICS

Pilocarpine

- **DRUG ACTION** Pilocarpine acts by opening the inefficient drainage channels in the trabecular meshwork.

- **INDICATIONS AND DOSE**
  Raised intra-ocular pressure
  ▸ TO THE EYE
  ▸ Child 1 month-1 year: Apply 1 drop 3 times a day, doses are for 0.5% or 1% solution
  ▸ Child 2-17 years: Apply 1 drop 4 times a day

Pre- and postoperatively in goniotomy and trabeculotomy
  ▸ TO THE EYE
  ▸ Child: Apply once daily, 1% or 2% solution to be applied

- **UNLICENSED USE** Not licensed for use in children.
- **CONTRA-INDICATIONS** Acute inflammatory disease of the anterior segment · acute iritis · anterior uveitis · conditions where pupillary constriction is undesirable · some forms of secondary glaucoma (where pupillary constriction is undesirable)
- **CAUTIONS** A darkly pigmented iris may require a higher concentration of the miotic or more frequent administration and care should be taken to avoid overdosage · asthma · cardiac disease · care in conjunctival damage · care in corneal damage · epilepsy · gastro-intestinal spasm · hypertension · hyperthyroidism · hypotension · peptic ulceration · retinal detachment has occurred in susceptible individuals and those with retinal disease · urinary-tract obstruction
- **INTERACTIONS →** Appendix 1 (parasympathomimetics). Systemic effects rare following application to the eye.
- **SIDE-EFFECTS**
  ▸ **Rare** Parasympathomimetics systemic side effects
  ▸ **Frequency not known** Blurred vision · ciliary spasm (leads to headache and browache which may be more severe in the initial 2–4 weeks of treatment—a particular disadvantage in patients under 40 years of age) · conjunctival vascular congestion · lens changes (with chronic use) · myopia · ocular burning · ocular itching · pupillary block · smarting · vitreous haemorrhage
- **PREGNANCY** Avoid unless the potential benefit outweighs risk—limited information available.
- **BREAST FEEDING** Avoid unless the potential benefit outweighs risk—no information available.
- **PRE-TREATMENT SCREENING** Fundus examination is advised before starting treatment with a miotic (retinal detachment has occurred).
- **MONITORING REQUIREMENTS** Intra-ocular pressure and visual fields should be monitored in those with chronic simple glaucoma and those receiving long-term treatment with a miotic.
- **PRESCRIBING AND DISPENSING INFORMATION** Although multi-dose pilocarpine eye drops commonly contain preservatives, preservative-free unit dose vials may be available.
- **PATIENT AND CARER ADVICE**
  Driving and skilled tasks
  Blurred vision may affect performance of skilled tasks (e.g. driving) particularly at night or in reduced lighting.

- **MEDICINAL FORMS**
  There can be variation in the licensing of different medicines containing the same drug. Forms available from special-order manufacturers include: eye drops
  Eye drops
  EXCIPIENTS: May contain Benzalkonium chloride
  ▸ Pilocarpine (Non-proprietary)
    Pilocarpine hydrochloride 10 mg per 1 ml Pilocarpine hydrochloride 1% eye drops | 10 ml PoM £6.30 DT price = £5.33
    Pilocarpine hydrochloride 20 mg per 1 ml Pilocarpine hydrochloride 2% eye drops | 10 ml PoM £7.74 DT price = £6.51
    Pilocarpine hydrochloride 40 mg per 1 ml Pilocarpine hydrochloride 4% eye drops | 10 ml PoM £8.70 DT price = £7.32
  ▸ Pilocarpine nitrate (Bausch & Lomb UK Ltd)
    Pilocarpine nitrate 20 mg per 1 ml Minims pilocarpine nitrate 2% eye drops 0.5ml unit dose | 20 unit dose PoM £11.99

PROSTAGLANDIN ANALOGUES AND PROSTAMIDES

Latanoprost

- **INDICATIONS AND DOSE**

Reduction of intra-ocular pressure in raised intra-ocular pressure and glaucoma

▶ TO THE EYE
- Child: Apply once daily, to be administered preferably in the evening

---

IMPORTANT SAFETY INFORMATION

MHRA/CHM ADVICE: LATANOPROST (*XALATAN* ®): INCREASED REPORTING OF EYE IRRITATION SINCE REFORMULATION (JULY 2015)

Following reformulation of *Xalatan* ®, to allow for long-term storage at room temperature, there has been an increase in the number of reports of eye irritation from across the EU. Patients should be advised to tell their health professional promptly (within a week) if they experience eye irritation (e.g. excessive watering) severe enough to make them consider stopping treatment. Review treatment and prescribe a different formulation if necessary.

- **CONTRA-INDICATIONS** Active herpes simplex keratitis · history of recurrent herpetic keratitis associated with prostaglandin analogues
- **CAUTIONS** Aphakia · asthma · children less than 1 year— limited information available · history of herpetic keratitis · history of significant ocular viral infections · peri-operative period of cataract surgery · preterm neonates less than 36 weeks gestational age—no information available · pseudophakia with torn posterior lens capsule or anterior chamber lenses · risk factors for cystoid macular oedema · risk factors for iritis · risk factors for uveitis
- **SIDE-EFFECTS**
▶ **Common or very common** Blepharitis · conjunctival hyperaemia · eye irritation · eye pain · eyelash and vellus hair changes · increased iris pigmentation · transient punctate epithelial erosion
▶ **Uncommon** Blurred vision · conjunctivitis · dry eye · eyelid oedema · keratitis · skin rash
▶ **Rare** Corneal erosion · corneal oedema · distichiasis · iritis · macular oedema · misdirected eyelashes · periorbital oedema · photophobia · uveitis
▶ **Very rare** Chest pain · darkening of palpebral skin of the eyelids · localised skin reaction on the eyelids · periorbital changes resulting in deepening of the eyelid sulcus
▶ **Frequency not known** Arthralgia · asthma · dizziness · dyspnoea · exacerbation of asthma · headache · herpetic keratitis · iris cyst · myalgia · nasopharyngitis · palpitation · pyrexia
- **PREGNANCY** Manufacturer advises avoid.
- **BREAST FEEDING** May be present in milk—manufacturer advises avoid.
- **MONITORING REQUIREMENTS** Monitor for changes to eye coloration.
- **PRESCRIBING AND DISPENSING INFORMATION** Although multi-dose latanoprost eye drops commonly contain preservatives, preservative-free unit dose vials may be available.
- **PATIENT AND CARER ADVICE**
Changes in eye colour Before initiating treatment, patients should be warned of a possible change in eye colour as an increase in the brown pigment in the iris can occur, which may be permanent; particular care is required in those with mixed coloured irides and those receiving treatment to one eye only. Changes in eyelashes and vellus hair can also occur, and patients should also be advised to avoid repeated contact of the eye drop solution with skin as this can lead to hair growth or skin pigmentation.

- **MEDICINAL FORMS**
There can be variation in the licensing of different medicines containing the same drug.
Eye drops
EXCIPIENTS: May contain Benzalkonium chloride
▶ Latanoprost (Non-proprietary)
Latanoprost 50 microgram per 1 ml Latanoprost 50micrograms/ml eye drops | 2.5 ml PoM £12.48 DT price = £1.56
▶ Monopost (Thea Pharmaceuticals Ltd)
Latanoprost 50 microgram per 1 ml Monopost 50micrograms/ml eye drops 0.2ml unit dose | 30 unit dose PoM £8.49 DT price = £8.49 | 90 unit dose PoM £25.47 DT price = £25.47
▶ Xalatan (Pfizer Ltd)
Latanoprost 50 microgram per 1 ml Xalatan 50micrograms/ml eye drops | 2.5 ml PoM £12.48 DT price = £1.56

SYMPATHOMIMETICS › ALPHA$_2$-ADRENOCEPTOR AGONISTS

Apraclonidine

- **DRUG ACTION** Apraclonidine is an alpha$_2$-adrenoceptor agonist that lowers intra-ocular pressure by reducing aqueous humour formation. It is a derivative of clonidine.

- **INDICATIONS AND DOSE**

Control or prevention of postoperative elevation of intra-ocular pressure after anterior segment laser surgery

▶ TO THE EYE
▶ Child: Apply 1 drop, 1 hour before laser procedure, then 1 drop, immediately after completion of procedure, 1% eye drops to be administered

Short-term adjunctive treatment of chronic glaucoma in patients not adequately controlled by another drug

▶ TO THE EYE
▶ Child 12–17 years: Apply 1 drop 3 times a day usually for maximum 1 month, 0.5% eye drops to be administered, may not provide additional benefit if patient already using two drugs that suppress the production of aqueous humour

- **UNLICENSED USE** 0.5% drops are not licensed for use in children under 12 years. 1% drops are not licensed for use in children.
- **CONTRA-INDICATIONS** History of severe or unstable and uncontrolled cardiovascular disease
- **CAUTIONS** Cerebrovascular disease · depression · heart failure · history of angina · hypertension · loss of effect may occur over time · Raynaud's syndrome · recent myocardial infarction · reduction in vision in end-stage glaucoma (suspend treatment) · severe coronary insufficiency · thromboangiitis obliterans · vasovagal attack
- **INTERACTIONS** → Appendix 1 (apraclonidine).
- **SIDE-EFFECTS**
▶ **Common or very common** Conjunctivitis · dry eye · ocular intolerance · rhinitis · taste disturbance
▶ **Uncommon** Asthma · blepharitis · blepharospasm · chest pain · conjunctival vascular disorders · corneal erosion and infiltrates · dyspnoea · eyelid ptosis or retraction · impaired co-ordination · irritability · keratitis · keratopathy · myalgia · mydriasis · nervousness · parosmia · photophobia · rhinorrhoea · throat irritation · visual impairment

SIDE-EFFECTS, FURTHER INFORMATION
▶ Ocular intolerance Withdraw if eye pruritus, ocular hyperaemia, increased lacrimation, or oedema of the eyelids and conjunctiva occur.
▶ Systemic effects Since absorption may follow topical application, see clonidine hydrochloride p. 93.
- **PREGNANCY** Manufacturer advises avoid—no information available.

● **BREAST FEEDING** Manufacturer advises avoid—no information available.

● **HEPATIC IMPAIRMENT** Manufacturer advises caution.

● **RENAL IMPAIRMENT** Use with caution in chronic renal failure.

● **MONITORING REQUIREMENTS**
▸ Monitor intra-ocular pressure and visual fields.
▸ Monitor for excessive reduction in intra-ocular pressure following peri-operative use.

● **PATIENT AND CARER ADVICE**

Driving and skilled tasks
Drowsiness may affect performance of skilled tasks (e.g. driving).

● **MEDICINAL FORMS**
There can be variation in the licensing of different medicines containing the same drug.

Eye drops
EXCIPIENTS: May contain Benzalkonium chloride
▸ **Iopidine** (Alcon Laboratories (UK) Ltd)
Apraclonidine (as Apraclonidine hydrochloride) 5 mg per 1 ml Iopidine 5mg/ml eye drops | 5 ml [PoM] £10.88 DT price = £10.88
Apraclonidine (as Apraclonidine hydrochloride) 10 mg per 1 ml Iopidine 1% eye drops 0.25ml unit dose | 24 unit dose [PoM] £77.85 DT price = £77.85

Chapter 12
Ear, nose and oropharynx

CONTENTS

Ear   page 643
  1 **Otitis externa**   644
  2 **Removal of earwax**   647
Nose   648
  1 **Nasal congestion**   649
  2 **Nasal infection**   650
  3 **Nasal inflammation, nasal polyps and rhinitis**   651
Oropharynx   654
  1 **Dry mouth**   654

  2 **Oral hygiene**   page 655
2.1 Dental caries   657
  3 **Oral ulceration and inflammation**   659
  4 **Oropharyngeal bacterial infections**   661
  5 **Oropharyngeal fungal infections**   662
  6 **Oropharyngeal viral infections**   663

12

Ear, nose and oropharynx

Ear

Ear

Otitis externa

Otitis externa is an inflammatory reaction of the lining of the ear canal usually associated with an underlying seborrhoeic dermatitis or eczema; it is important to exclude an underlying chronic otitis media before treatment is commenced. Many cases recover after thorough cleansing of the external ear canal by suction or dry mopping.

A frequent problem in resistant cases is the difficulty in applying lotions and ointments satisfactorily to the relatively inaccessible affected skin. The most effective method is to introduce a ribbon gauze dressing or sponge wick soaked with **corticosteroid** ear drops or with an astringent such as aluminium acetate solution p. 647. When this is not practical, the ear should be gently cleansed with a probe covered in cotton wool and the patient encouraged to lie with the affected ear uppermost for ten minutes after the canal has been filled with a liberal quantity of the appropriate solution.

Secondary infection in otitis externa may be of bacterial, fungal, or viral origin. If infection is present, a topical anti-infective which is not used systemically (such as neomycin sulfate p. 645 or **clioquinol**) may be used, but for only about a week because excessive use may result in fungal infections that are difficult to treat. Sensitivity to the anti-infective or solvent may occur and resistance to antibacterials is a possibility with prolonged use. Aluminium acetate ear drops are also effective against bacterial infection and inflammation of the ear. Chloramphenicol p. 645 may be used, but the ear drops contain propylene glycol and cause hypersensitivity reactions in about 10% of patients. Solutions containing an anti-infective and a corticosteroid are used for treating children when infection is present with inflammation and eczema. Clotrimazole 1% solution p. 645 is used topically to treat fungal infection in otitis externa.

In view of reports of ototoxicity, manufacturers contra-indicate treatment with topical **aminoglycosides** or **polymyxins** in children with a perforated tympanic membrane (eardrum) or patent grommet. However, some specialists do use these drops cautiously in the presence of a perforation or patent grommet in children with chronic suppurative otitis media and when other measures have failed for otitis externa; treatment should be considered only **by specialists** in the following circumstances:

- drops should only be used in the presence of obvious infection;
- treatment should be for no longer than 2 weeks;
- the carer and child should be counselled on the risk of ototoxicity and given justification for the use of these topical antibiotics;
- baseline audiometry should be performed, if possible, before treatment is commenced.

Clinical expertise and judgement should be used to assess the risk of treatment versus the benefit to the patient in such circumstances.

A solution of **acetic acid** 2% acts as an antifungal and antibacterial in the external ear canal. It may be used to treat mild otitis externa but in severe cases an anti-inflammatory preparation with or without an anti-infective drug is required. A proprietary preparation containing acetic acid 2% (*EarCalm*®️ spray) is on sale to the public for children over 12 years.

For severe pain associated with otitis externa, a simple analgesic, such as paracetamol p. 254 or ibuprofen p. 608, can be used. A systemic antibacterial can be used if there is spreading cellulitis or if the patient is systemically unwell. When a resistant staphylococcal infection (a boil) is present in the external auditory meatus, flucloxacillin p. 325 is the drug of choice; oral ciprofloxacin p. 328 or a systemic aminoglycoside may be needed for pseudomonal infections, particularly in children with diabetes or compromised immunity.

The skin of the pinna adjacent to the ear canal is often affected by eczema. Topical corticosteroid creams and ointments are then required, but prolonged use should be avoided.

Otitis media

Acute otitis media

Acute otitis media is the commonest cause of severe aural pain in young children and may occur with even minor upper respiratory tract infections. Children diagnosed with acute otitis media should not be prescribed antibacterials routinely as many infections, especially those accompanying coryza, are caused by viruses. Most uncomplicated cases resolve without antibacterial treatment and a **simple analgesic**, such as paracetamol, may be sufficient. In children without systemic features, a **systemic antibacterial** may be started after 72 hours if there is no improvement, or earlier if there is deterioration, if the child is systemically unwell, if the child is at high risk of serious complications (e.g. in immunosuppression, cystic fibrosis), if mastoiditis is present, or in children under 2 years of age with bilateral otitis media. Perforation of the tympanic membrane in children with *acute otitis media* usually heals spontaneously without treatment; if there is no improvement, e.g. pain or discharge persists, a systemic antibacterial can be given. Topical antibacterial treatment of acute otitis media is ineffective and there is no place for ear drops containing a local anaesthetic.

Otitis media with effusion
Otitis media with effusion (glue ear) occurs in about 10% of children and in 90% of children with cleft palates. Antimicrobials, corticosteroids, decongestants, and antihistamines have little place in the routine management of otitis media with effusion. If glue ear persists for more than a month or two, the child should be referred for assessment and follow up because of the risk of long-term hearing impairment which can delay language development. Untreated or resistant glue ear may be responsible for some types of *chronic otitis media.*

Chronic otitis media
Opportunistic organisms are often present in the debris, keratin, and necrotic bone of the middle ear and mastoid in children with chronic otitis media. The mainstay of treatment is thorough cleansing with aural microsuction, which may completely resolve long-standing infection. Cleansing may be followed by topical treatment as for otitis externa; this is particularly beneficial for discharging ears or infections of the mastoid cavity. Acute exacerbations of chronic infection may require treatment with an oral antibacterial; a swab should be taken to identify infecting organisms and antibacterial sensitivity.

In view of reports of ototoxicity, manufacturers contraindicate topical treatment with ototoxic antibacterials in the presence of a tympanic perforation or patent grommet. Ciprofloxacin or ofloxacin eye drops used in the ear [unlicensed use] or ear drops [both unlicensed; available from 'special-order' manufacturers or specialist importing companies] are an effective alternative to such ototoxic ear drops for chronic otitis media in patients with perforation of the tympanic membrane.

However, some specialists do use ear drops containing **aminoglycosides** or **polymyxins** [unlicensed indications] cautiously in children with chronic suppurative otitis media and perforation of the tympanic membrane, if the otitis media has failed to settle with systemic antibacterials; treatment should be considered only **by specialists** in the following circumstances:

- drops should only be used in the presence of obvious infection;
- treatment should be for no longer than 2 weeks;
- the carer and child should be counselled on the risk of ototoxicity and given justification for the use of these topical antibiotics;
- baseline audiometry should be performed, if possible, before treatment is commenced.

Clinical expertise and judgement should be used to assess the risk of treatment versus the benefit to the patient in such circumstances. It is considered that the pus in the middle ear associated with otitis media also carries a risk of ototoxicity.

Removal of ear wax
Ear wax (cerumen) is a normal bodily secretion which provides a protective film on the meatal skin and need only be removed if it causes hearing loss or interferes with a proper view of the ear drum.

Ear wax causing discomfort or impaired hearing may be softened using simple remedies such as **olive oil** ear drops or **almond oil** ear drops; sodium bicarbonate ear drops p. 647 are also effective, but may cause dryness of the ear canal. If the wax is hard and impacted, the drops can be used twice daily for several days and this may reduce the need for mechanical removal of the wax. The child should lie with the affected ear uppermost for 5 to 10 minutes after a generous amount of the softening remedy has been introduced into the ear. Proprietary preparations containing organic solvents can irritate the meatal skin, and in most cases the simple remedies indicated above are just as effective and less likely to cause irritation. Docusate sodium p. 647 or urea hydrogen peroxide p. 648 are ingredients in a number of proprietary preparations for softening ear wax.

If necessary, wax may be removed by irrigation with water (warmed to body temperature). Ear irrigation is generally best avoided in young children, in children unable to co-operate with the procedure, in children who have had otitis media in the last six weeks, in otitis externa, in children with cleft palate, a history of ear drum perforation, or previous ear surgery. A child who has hearing in one ear only should not have that ear irrigated because even a very slight risk of damage is unacceptable in this situation.

Administration
To administer ear drops, lay the child down with the head turned to one side; for an infant pull the earlobe back and down, for an older child pull the earlobe back and up.

1 Otitis externa

ANTIBACTERIALS › AMINOGLYCOSIDES

Framycetin sulfate

- **INDICATIONS AND DOSE**
Bacterial infection in otitis externa
  ▸ TO THE EAR
  ▸ Child: (consult product literature)

- **CONTRA-INDICATIONS** Perforated tympanic membrane

- **CAUTIONS** Avoid prolonged use

- **SIDE-EFFECTS** Local sensitivity

- **MEDICINAL FORMS**
  There can be variation in the licensing of different medicines containing the same drug.
  No licensed medicines listed.

  Combinations available: *Dexamethasone with framycetin sulfate and gramicidin,* p. 646

Gentamicin

- **INDICATIONS AND DOSE**
Bacterial infection in otitis externa
  ▸ TO THE EAR
  ▸ Child: Apply 2–3 drops 4–5 times a day, (including a dose at bedtime)

- **CONTRA-INDICATIONS** Patent grommet (although may be used by specialists (see Ear p. 643) · perforated tympanic membrane (although may be used by specialists (see Ear p. 643)

- **CAUTIONS** Avoid prolonged use

- **SIDE-EFFECTS** Local sensitivity

- **MEDICINAL FORMS**
There can be variation in the licensing of different medicines containing the same drug.
Ear/eye drops solution
EXCIPIENTS: May contain Benzalkonium chloride
 ▸ Gentamicin (Non-proprietary)
   Gentamicin (as Gentamicin sulfate) 3 mg per 1 ml Gentamicin 0.3% ear/eye drops | 10 ml PoM £2.55 DT price = £2.13
   Gentamicin 0.3% eye/ear drops | 10 ml PoM £2.13 DT price = £2.13

Gentamicin with hydrocortisone

- **INDICATIONS AND DOSE**

Eczematous inflammation in otitis externa
 ▸ TO THE EAR
 ▸ Child: Apply 2–4 drops 4–5 times a day, (including a dose at bedtime)

- **CONTRA-INDICATIONS** Patent grommet (although may be used by specialists, see Ear p. 643) · perforated tympanic membrane (although may be used by specialists, see Ear p. 643)
- **CAUTIONS** Avoid prolonged use
- **SIDE-EFFECTS** Local sensitivity reactions
- **PATIENT AND CARER ADVICE**
Medicines for Children leaflet: Gentamicin and hydrocortisone ear drops for inflammatory ear infections www.medicinesforchildren.org.uk/gentamicin-and-hydrocortisone-ear-drops-inflammatory-ear-infections

- **MEDICINAL FORMS**
There can be variation in the licensing of different medicines containing the same drug.
Ear drops
EXCIPIENTS: May contain Benzalkonium chloride, disodium edetate
 ▸ Gentamicin with hydrocortisone (Non-proprietary)
   Gentamicin (as Gentamicin sulfate) 3 mg per 1 ml, Hydrocortisone acetate 10 mg per 1 ml Gentamicin 0.3% / Hydrocortisone acetate 1% ear drops | 10 ml PoM £23.92 DT price = £23.92

Neomycin sulfate

- **INDICATIONS AND DOSE**

Bacterial infection in otitis externa
 ▸ TO THE EAR
 ▸ Child: (consult product literature)

- **CONTRA-INDICATIONS** Patent grommet (although may be used by specialists, see Ear p. 643) · perforated tympanic membrane (although may be used by specialists, see Ear p. 643)
- **SIDE-EFFECTS** Local sensitivity
- **MEDICINAL FORMS**
There can be variation in the licensing of different medicines containing the same drug. No licensed medicines listed.

   Combinations available: *Betamethasone with neomycin*, p. 646 · *Dexamethasone with glacial acetic acid and neomycin sulfate*, p. 646

ANTIBACTERIALS 〉 OTHER

Chloramphenicol

- **DRUG ACTION** Chloramphenicol is a potent broad-spectrum antibiotic.

- **INDICATIONS AND DOSE**

Bacterial infection in otitis externa
 ▸ TO THE EAR
 ▸ Child: Apply 2–3 drops 2–3 times a day

- **CAUTIONS** Avoid prolonged use
- **SIDE-EFFECTS**
 ▸ Common or very common High incidence of sensitivity reactions to vehicle
- **PATIENT AND CARER ADVICE**
Medicines for Children leaflet: Chloramphenicol ear drops for ear infections (otitis externa) www.medicinesforchildren.org.uk/chloramphenicol-ear-drops-ear-infections-otitis-externa-0
- **LESS SUITABLE FOR PRESCRIBING**
Chloramphenicol ear drops are less suitable for prescribing.

- **MEDICINAL FORMS**
There can be variation in the licensing of different medicines containing the same drug.
Ear drops
EXCIPIENTS: May contain Propylene glycol
 ▸ Chloramphenicol (Non-proprietary)
   Chloramphenicol 50 mg per 1 ml Chloramphenicol 5% ear drops | 10 ml PoM £75.99 DT price = £57.90
   Chloramphenicol 100 mg per 1 ml Chloramphenicol 10% ear drops | 10 ml PoM £42.18

ANTIFUNGALS 〉 IMIDAZOLE ANTIFUNGALS

Clotrimazole

- **INDICATIONS AND DOSE**

Fungal infection in otitis externa
 ▸ TO THE EAR
 ▸ Child: Apply 2–3 times a day continue for at least 14 days after disappearance of infection

- **SIDE-EFFECTS** Local irritation · local sensitivity
- **MEDICINAL FORMS**
There can be variation in the licensing of different medicines containing the same drug.
Liquid
 ▸ Canesten (clotrimazole) (Bayer Plc)
   Clotrimazole 10 mg per 1 ml Canesten 1% solution | 20 ml P £2.30 DT price = £2.30

CORTICOSTEROIDS

Betamethasone

- **INDICATIONS AND DOSE**
BETNESOL®

Eczematous inflammation in otitis externa
 ▸ TO THE EAR
 ▸ Child: Apply 2–3 drops every 2–3 hours, reduce frequency when relief obtained

VISTAMETHASONE®

Eczematous inflammation in otitis externa
 ▸ TO THE EAR
 ▸ Child: Apply 2–3 drops every 3–4 hours, reduce frequency when relief obtained

- **CONTRA-INDICATIONS** Avoid alone in the presence of untreated infection (combine with suitable anti-infective)
- **CAUTIONS** Avoid prolonged use
- **SIDE-EFFECTS** Local sensitivity reactions

- **MEDICINAL FORMS**
There can be variation in the licensing of different medicines containing the same drug.
Ear/eye/nose drops solution
EXCIPIENTS: May contain Benzalkonium chloride, disodium edetate
 ▸ Betnesol (Focus Pharmaceuticals Ltd)
   Betamethasone sodium phosphate 1 mg per 1 ml Betnesol 0.1% eye/ear/nose drops | 10 ml PoM £2.32 DT price = £2.32

12

Ear, nose and oropharynx

▶ Vistamethasone (Martindale Pharmaceuticals Ltd)
Betamethasone sodium phosphate 1 mg per 1 ml Vistamethasone
0.1% ear/eye/nose drops | 5 ml [PoM] £0.87 | 10 ml [PoM] £0.99 DT
price = £2.32

Combinations available: *Betamethasone with neomycin*, below

Clioquinol with flumetasone pivalate

● **INDICATIONS AND DOSE**

**Eczematous inflammation in otitis externa | Mild bacterial
or fungal infections in otitis externa**

▶ TO THE EAR
▶ Child 2-17 years: 2–3 drops twice daily for 7–10 days, to
be instilled into the ear

● **CONTRA-INDICATIONS** Iodine sensitivity
● **CAUTIONS** Avoid prolonged use · manufacturer advises
avoid in perforated tympanic membrane (but used by
specialists for short periods)
● **SIDE-EFFECTS** Local sensitivity
● **PATIENT AND CARER ADVICE** Clioquinol stains skin and
clothing

● **MEDICINAL FORMS**
There can be variation in the licensing of different medicines
containing the same drug.
Ear drops
▶ Clioquinol with flumetasone pivalate (Non-proprietary)
Flumetasone pivalate 200 microgram per 1 ml, Clioquinol 10 mg
per 1 ml Flumetasone 0.02% / Clioquinol 1% ear drops |
7.5 ml [PoM] £10.37 DT price = £10.37 | 10 ml [PoM] £13.82 DT price =
£13.82

Prednisolone

● **INDICATIONS AND DOSE**

Eczematous inflammation in otitis externa

▶ TO THE EAR
▶ Child: Apply 2–3 drops every 2–3 hours, frequency to
be reduced when relief obtained

● **CONTRA-INDICATIONS** Avoid alone in the presence of
untreated infection (combine with suitable anti-infective)
● **CAUTIONS** Avoid prolonged use
● **SIDE-EFFECTS** Local sensitivity reactions

● **MEDICINAL FORMS**
There can be variation in the licensing of different medicines
containing the same drug. Forms available from special-order
manufacturers include: ear drops
Ear/eye drops solution
EXCIPIENTS: May contain Benzalkonium chloride, disodium edetate
▶ Predsol (Focus Pharmaceuticals Ltd)
Prednisolone sodium phosphate 5 mg per 1 ml Predsol 0.5%
ear/eye drops | 10 ml [PoM] £2.00 DT price = £2.00

CORTICOSTEROIDS > CORTICOSTEROID
COMBINATIONS WITH ANTI-INFECTIVES

Betamethasone with neomycin

The properties listed below are those particular to the
combination only. For the properties of the components
please consider, betamethasone p. 645, neomycin sulfate
p. 645.

● **INDICATIONS AND DOSE**

Eczematous inflammation in otitis externa

▶ TO THE EAR USING EAR DROPS
▶ Child: Apply 2–3 drops 3–4 times a day

● **CONTRA-INDICATIONS** Patent grommet (although may be
used by specialists, see Ear p. 643) · perforated tympanic
membrane (although may be used by specialists, see Ear
p. 643)
● **CAUTIONS**
▶ When used by ear Avoid prolonged use
● **SIDE-EFFECTS**
▶ When used by ear Local sensitivity

● **MEDICINAL FORMS**
There can be variation in the licensing of different medicines
containing the same drug.
Ear/eye/nose drops solution
EXCIPIENTS: May contain Benzalkonium chloride, disodium edetate
▶ Betnesol-N (Focus Pharmaceuticals Ltd)
Betamethasone (as Betamethasone sodium phosphate) 1 mg per
1 ml, Neomycin sulfate 5 mg per 1 ml Betnesol-N ear/eye/nose
drops | 10 ml [PoM] £2.39 DT price = £2.39

Dexamethasone with framycetin sulfate and gramicidin

The properties listed below are those particular to the
combination only. For the properties of the components
please consider, framycetin sulfate p. 644.

● **INDICATIONS AND DOSE**

Eczematous inflammation in otitis externa

▶ TO THE EAR
▶ Child: 2–3 drops 3–4 times a day

● **LESS SUITABLE FOR PRESCRIBING** *Sofradex*® is less
suitable for prescribing.

● **MEDICINAL FORMS**
There can be variation in the licensing of different medicines
containing the same drug.
Ear/eye drops solution
EXCIPIENTS: May contain Polysorbates
▶ Sofradex (Sanofi)
Gramicidin 50 microgram per 1 ml, Dexamethasone (as
Dexamethasone sodium metasulfobenzoate) 500 microgram per
1 ml, Framycetin sulfate 5 mg per 1 ml Sofradex ear/eye drops |
10 ml [PoM] £7.50

Dexamethasone with glacial acetic acid and neomycin sulfate

● **INDICATIONS AND DOSE**

Eczematous inflammation in otitis externa

▶ TO THE EAR
▶ Child 2-17 years: Apply 1 spray 3 times a day

● **CONTRA-INDICATIONS** Patent grommet (although may be
used by specialists, see Ear p. 643) · perforated tympanic
membrane (although may be used by specialists, see Ear
p. 643)
● **CAUTIONS** Avoid prolonged use
● **SIDE-EFFECTS** Local sensitivity

● **MEDICINAL FORMS**
There can be variation in the licensing of different medicines
containing the same drug.
Spray
EXCIPIENTS: May contain Hydroxybenzoates (parabens)
▶ Otomize (Forest Laboratories UK Ltd)
Dexamethasone 1 mg per 1 gram, Neomycin sulfate 5 mg per
1 gram, Acetic acid glacial 20 mg per 1 gram Otomize ear spray |
5 ml [PoM] £3.27

DERMATOLOGICAL DRUGS > ASTRINGENTS

Aluminium acetate

- **INDICATIONS AND DOSE**

Inflammation in otitis externa
▶ TO THE EAR
▶ Child: To be inserted into meatus or apply on a ribbon gauze dressing or sponge wick which should be kept saturated with the ear drops

- **UNLICENSED USE** Not licensed for use in children.

- **DIRECTIONS FOR ADMINISTRATION** For ear drops 8%— dilute 8 parts aluminium acetate ear drops (13%) with 5 parts purified water. Must be freshly prepared.

- **MEDICINAL FORMS**
There can be variation in the licensing of different medicines containing the same drug. Forms available from special-order manufacturers include: ear drops

2   Removal of earwax

BICARBONATE

Sodium bicarbonate

- **INDICATIONS AND DOSE**

Removal of earwax (with 5% ear drop solution)
▶ TO THE EAR
▶ Child: (consult product literature)

- **SIDE-EFFECTS** Dryness of the ear canal

- **MEDICINAL FORMS**
There can be variation in the licensing of different medicines containing the same drug.
Ear drops
▶ Sodium bicarbonate (Non-proprietary)
Sodium bicarbonate 50 mg per 1 ml   Sodium bicarbonate 5% ear drops | 10 ml £1.23–£1.25

SOFTENING DRUGS

Almond oil

- **INDICATIONS AND DOSE**

Removal of earwax
▶ TO THE EAR
▶ Child: Allow drops to warm to room temperature before use (consult product literature)

- **DIRECTIONS FOR ADMINISTRATION** The patient should lie with the affected ear uppermost for 5 to 10 minutes after a generous amount of the softening remedy has been introduced into the ear.

- **MEDICINAL FORMS**
There can be variation in the licensing of different medicines containing the same drug.
Liquid
▶ Almond oil (Non-proprietary)
Almond oil 1 ml per 1 ml   Almond oil liquid | 50 ml £0.85 DT price = £0.85 | 70 ml £0.73 | 200 ml £2.01–£2.37 | 500 ml £11.67

Arachis oil with chlorobutanol

- **INDICATIONS AND DOSE**

Removal of earwax
▶ TO THE EAR
▶ Child 1–17 years: (consult product literature)

- **LESS SUITABLE FOR PRESCRIBING** Arachis (peanut) oil with chlorobutanol ear drops are less suitable for prescribing.

- **MEDICINAL FORMS**
There can be variation in the licensing of different medicines containing the same drug.
Ear drops
▶ Cerumol (Thornton & Ross Ltd)
Chlorobutanol 50 mg per 1 ml, Arachis oil 573 mg per 1 ml   Cerumol ear drops | 11 ml P £2.05

Docusate sodium

(Dioctyl sodium sulphosuccinate)

- **INDICATIONS AND DOSE**

Removal of ear wax
▶ TO THE EAR
▶ Child 1–17 years: (consult product literature)

- **LESS SUITABLE FOR PRESCRIBING** Ear drops less suitable for prescribing.

- **MEDICINAL FORMS**
There can be variation in the licensing of different medicines containing the same drug.
Ear drops
EXCIPIENTS: May contain Propylene glycol
▶ Molcer (Wallace Manufacturing Chemists Ltd)
Docusate sodium 50 mg per 1 ml   Molcer ear drops | 15 ml P £8.08
▶ Waxsol (Meda Pharmaceuticals Ltd)
Docusate sodium 5 mg per 1 ml   Waxsol ear drops | 10 ml P £1.95 DT price = £1.95

Olive oil

- **INDICATIONS AND DOSE**

Removal of earwax
▶ TO THE EAR
▶ Child: Apply twice daily for several days (if wax is hard and impacted)

- **DIRECTIONS FOR ADMINISTRATION** The patient should lie with the affected ear uppermost for 5 to 10 minutes after a generous amount of the softening remedy has been introduced into the ear. Allow ear drops to warm to room temperature before use.

- **MEDICINAL FORMS**
There can be variation in the licensing of different medicines containing the same drug.
Ear drops
▶ Olive oil (Non-proprietary)
Olive oil ear drops | 10 ml £1.42 | 20 ml £2.70
▶ Arjun (Arjun Products Ltd)
Arjun ear drops | 10 ml £1.25
▶ Cerumol (olive oil) (Thornton & Ross Ltd)
Cerumol olive oil ear drops | 10 ml no price available
▶ Oleax (JR Biomedical Ltd)
Oleax ear drops | 15 ml £1.40
▶ Olive oil (Thornton & Ross Ltd)
Care olive oil ear drops | 10 ml £1.42
Spray
▶ Earol (HL Healthcare Ltd)
Earol olive oil ear spray | 10 ml no price available

12

Ear, nose and oropharynx

Ear, nose and oropharynx 12

Urea hydrogen peroxide

● **INDICATIONS AND DOSE**

Softening and removal of earwax
▶ TO THE EAR
▶ Child: (consult product literature)

● **PATIENT AND CARER ADVICE** The patient should lie with the affected ear uppermost for 5 to 10 minutes after a generous amount of the softening remedy has been introduced into the ear.

● **LESS SUITABLE FOR PRESCRIBING** Urea-hydrogen peroxide ear drops are less suitable for prescribing.

● **MEDICINAL FORMS**
There can be variation in the licensing of different medicines containing the same drug.

Ear drops
▶ Exterol (Dermal Laboratories Ltd)
  Urea hydrogen peroxide 50 mg per 1 gram Exterol 5% ear drops | 8 ml ℗ £1.75 DT price = £2.89
▶ Otex (Dendron Ltd)
  Urea hydrogen peroxide 50 mg per 1 gram Otex 5% ear drops | 8 ml ℗ £2.89 DT price = £2.89

Nose

Nose

Rhinitis and bacterial sinusitis

Rhinitis is often self-limiting but bacterial sinusitis may require treatment with antibacterials. Many nasal preparations contain sympathomimetic drugs which can give rise to rebound congestion (*rhinitis medicamentosa*) and may damage the nasal cilia. Sodium chloride 0.9% solution p. 547 may be used as a douche or 'sniff' following endonasal surgery.

Administration
To administer nasal drops, lay the child face-upward with the neck extended, instil the drops, then sit the child up and tilt the head forward.

Drugs used in nasal allergy

Mild allergic rhinitis is controlled by **antihistamines** (see under Antihistamines, allergen immunotherapy and allergic emergencies p. 162) or topical **nasal corticosteroids**; systemic nasal decongestants are not recommended for use in children. Topical nasal decongestants can be used for a short period to relieve congestion and allow penetration of a topical nasal corticosteroid.

More persistent symptoms can be relieved by topical nasal **corticosteroids**; sodium cromoglicate p. 654 is an alternative, but may be less effective. The topical antihistamine, azelastine hydrochloride, is useful for controlling breakthrough symptoms in allergic rhinitis. Azelastine hydrochloride is less effective than nasal corticosteroids, but probably more effective than sodium cromoglicate. In seasonal allergic rhinitis (e.g. hay fever), treatment should begin 2 to 3 weeks before the season commences and may have to be continued for several months; continuous long-term treatment may be required in perennial rhinitis.

Montelukast p. 155 is less effective than topical nasal corticosteroids; it can be used in children with seasonal allergic rhinitis (unresponsive to other treatments) and concomitant asthma.

Children with disabling symptoms of seasonal rhinitis (e.g. students taking important examinations), may be treated with oral **corticosteroids** for short periods. Oral corticosteroids may also be used at the beginning of a course of treatment with a corticosteroid spray to relieve severe mucosal oedema and allow the spray to penetrate the nasal mucosa.

Sometimes allergic rhinitis is accompanied by vasomotor rhinitis. In this situation, the addition of topical nasal ipratropium bromide p. 651 can reduce watery rhinorrhoea.

Corticosteroids
Corticosteroid nasal preparations should be avoided in the presence of untreated nasal infections, after nasal surgery (until healing has occurred), and in pulmonary tuberculosis. Systemic absorption may follow nasal administration particularly if high doses are used or if treatment is prolonged; for cautions and side-effects of systemic corticosteroids. The risk of systemic effects may be greater with nasal drops than with nasal sprays; drops are administered incorrectly more often than sprays. The height of children receiving prolonged treatment with nasal corticosteroids should be monitored; if growth is slowed, referral to a paediatrician should be considered.

Nasal polyps
Short-term use of corticosteroid nasal drops helps to shrink nasal polyps; to be effective, the drops must be administered with the child in the 'head down' position. A short course of a systemic corticosteroid may be required initially to shrink large polyps. A corticosteroid nasal spray can be used to maintain the reduction in swelling and also for the initial treatment of small polyps.

Pregnancy
If a pregnant woman cannot tolerate the symptoms of allergic rhinitis, treatment with nasal beclometasone dipropionate p. 652, budesonide p. 652, fluticasone p. 652, or sodium cromoglicate may be considered.

Topical nasal decongestants

Sodium chloride 0.9% given as nasal drops or spray may relieve nasal congestion by helping to liquefy mucous secretions in children with rhinitis. In infants, 1–2 drops of sodium chloride 0.9% solution in each nostril before feeds will help relieve congestion and allow more effective suckling.

Inhalation of **warm moist air** is useful in the treatment of symptoms of acute nasal congestion in infants and children, but the use of boiling water for steam inhalation is dangerous for children and should **not** be recommended. Volatile substances such as menthol and eucalyptus may encourage inhalation of warm moist air (see also Aromatic inhalations, cough preparations and systemic nasal decongestants p. 176).

Topical nasal decongestants containing sympathomimetics can cause rebound congestion (*rhinitis medicamentosa*) following prolonged use (more than 7 days), and are therefore of limited value in the treatment of nasal congestion.

Ephedrine hydrochloride nasal drops p. 649 is the least likely of the sympathomimetic nasal decongestants to cause rebound congestion and can provide relief for several hours. The more potent sympathomimetic drugs **oxymetazoline** and xylometazoline hydrochloride p. 650 are more likely to cause a rebound effect.

Non-allergic watery rhinorrhoea often responds well to treatment with the antimuscarinic ipratropium bromide.

Recurrent, persistent bleeding may respond to the use of a sympathomimetic nasal spray; if infection is present, chlorhexidine and neomycin (*Naseptin*®) cream may be effective.

Sinusitis and oral pain

Sinusitis affecting the maxillary antrum can cause pain in the upper jaw. Where this is associated with blockage of the opening from the sinus into the nasal cavity, it may be helpful to relieve the congestion with inhalation of warm moist air or with ephedrine hydrochloride nasal drops.

Systemic antibacterials may sometimes be required for sinusitis (see under Nose infections, bacterial p. 289).

Nasal preparations for infection

There is **no** evidence that topical anti-infective nasal preparations have any therapeutic value in rhinitis or sinusitis; see elimination of nasal staphylococci. In children, acute complications such as periorbital cellulitis require hospital treatment.

Nasal staphylococci

Elimination of organisms such as staphylococci from the nasal vestibule can be achieved by the use of a cream containing **chlorhexidine** and **neomycin** (*Naseptin*®), but re-colonisation frequently occurs. Coagulase-positive staphylococci are present in the noses of 40% of the population.

A nasal ointment containing mupirocin p. 650 is also available; it should probably be held in reserve for resistant infections. In hospitals or in care establishments, mupirocin nasal ointment should be reserved for the eradication (in both patients and staff) of nasal carriage of meticillin-resistant *Staphylococcus aureus* (MRSA). A sample should be taken 2 days after treatment to confirm eradication. The course may be repeated if the sample is positive (and the throat is not colonised). To avoid the development of resistance, the treatment course should not exceed 7 days and the course should not be repeated on more than one occasion. If the MRSA strain is mupirocin-resistant or does not respond after 2 courses, consider alternative products such as chlorhexidine and neomycin cream.

For eradication of MRSA also consult local infection control policy. See also MRSA p. 339.

Nasal congestion

SYMPATHOMIMETICS > VASOCONSTRICTOR

Ephedrine hydrochloride

● **INDICATIONS AND DOSE**

Nasal congestion | Sinusitis affecting the maxillary antrum
▶ BY INTRANASAL ADMINISTRATION
▶ Child 12-17 years: Apply 1–2 drops up to 4 times a day as required for a maximum of 7 days, to be instilled into each nostril, administer ephedrine 0.5% nasal drops

---

IMPORTANT SAFETY INFORMATION

CHM/MHRA ADVICE
The CHM/MHRA has stated that non-prescription cough and cold medicines containing ephedrine can be considered for up to 5 days' treatment in children aged 6–12 years after basic principles of best care have been tried; these medicines should not be used in children under 6 years of age.

CAUTIONS Avoid excessive or prolonged use · cardiovascular disease · diabetes mellitus · hypertension · hyperthyroidism

INTERACTIONS → Appendix 1 (sympathomimetics).

SIDE-EFFECTS
Common or very common Headache · nausea
Frequency not known After excessive use tolerance with diminished effect · cardiovascular effect · local irritation · rebound congestion

PREGNANCY Manufacturer advises avoid.

BREAST FEEDING Present in milk; manufacturer advises avoid—irritability and disturbed sleep reported.

● **PRESCRIBING AND DISPENSING INFORMATION**
For nasal drops, the BP directs that if no strength is specified 0.5% drops should be supplied.

● **PROFESSION SPECIFIC INFORMATION**
Dental practitioners' formulary
Ephedrine nasal drops may be prescribed.

● **EXCEPTIONS TO LEGAL CATEGORY** Ephedrine nasal drops can be sold to the public provided no more than 180 mg of ephedrine base (or salts) are supplied at one time, and pseudoephedrine salts are not supplied at the same time; for conditions that apply to supplies made at the request of a patient, see *Medicines, Ethics and Practice*, London, Pharmaceutical Press (always consult latest edition).

● **MEDICINAL FORMS**
There can be variation in the licensing of different medicines containing the same drug. Forms available from special-order manufacturers include: nasal drops
Nasal drops
▶ Ephedrine hydrochloride (Non-proprietary)
  Ephedrine hydrochloride 5 mg per 1 ml Ephedrine 0.5% nasal drops | 10 ml Ⓟ £1.73–£1.75 DT price = £1.74
  Ephedrine hydrochloride 10 mg per 1 ml Ephedrine 1% nasal drops | 10 ml Ⓟ £1.79–£1.81 DT price = £1.80

Pseudoephedrine hydrochloride

● **INDICATIONS AND DOSE**

Congestion of mucous membranes of upper respiratory tract
▶ BY MOUTH
▶ Child 6-11 years: 30 mg 3–4 times a day
▶ Child 12-17 years: 60 mg 3–4 times a day

IMPORTANT SAFETY INFORMATION

MHRA/CHM ADVICE (MARCH 2008 AND FEBRUARY 2009): OVER-THE-COUNTER COUGH AND COLD MEDICINES FOR CHILDREN
Children under 6 years should not be given over-the-counter cough and cold medicines containing pseudoephedrine.

● **CAUTIONS** Diabetes · heart disease · hypertension · hyperthyroidism · raised intra-ocular pressure

● **INTERACTIONS** → Appendix 1 (sympathomimetics). Contra-indicated in patients taking monoamine oxidase inhibitors within the previous 2 weeks.

● **SIDE-EFFECTS**
▶ **Common or very common** Anxiety · headache · hypertension · insomnia · nausea · restlessness · tachycardia · vomiting
▶ **Rare** Hallucinations · rash
▶ **Very rare** Angle-closure glaucoma
▶ **Frequency not known** Urinary retention

● **PREGNANCY** Defective closure of the abdominal wall (gastroschisis) reported very rarely in newborns after first trimester exposure.

● **BREAST FEEDING** May suppress lactation; avoid if lactation not well established or if milk production insufficient.

● **HEPATIC IMPAIRMENT** Manufacturer advises use with caution in severe impairment.

● **RENAL IMPAIRMENT** Use with caution in mild to moderate renal impairment. Manufacturer advises avoid in severe renal impairment.

● **LESS SUITABLE FOR PRESCRIBING** Pseudoephedrine hydrochloride is less suitable for prescribing.

● **EXCEPTIONS TO LEGAL CATEGORY** *Galpseud*® and *Sudafed*® can be sold to the public provided no more than 720 mg of pseudoephedrine salts are supplied, and ephedrine base (or salts) are not supplied at the same time; for details see

12

Ear, nose and oropharynx

Medicines, Ethics and Practice, London, Pharmaceutical Press (always consult latest edition).

- **MEDICINAL FORMS**
  There can be variation in the licensing of different medicines containing the same drug.

  Tablet
  - ▸ Pseudoephedrine hydrochloride (Non-proprietary)
    Pseudoephedrine hydrochloride 60 mg tablets | 12 tablet P no price available
  - ▸ Galpseud (Thornton & Ross Ltd)
    Pseudoephedrine hydrochloride 60 mg Galpseud 60mg tablets | 24 tablet PoM £2.25 | 100 tablet PoM £5.42 DT price = £5.42
  - ▸ Sudafed Non-Drowsy Decongestant (pseudoephedrine) (McNeil Products Ltd)
    Pseudoephedrine hydrochloride 60 mg Sudafed Decongestant 60mg tablets | 12 tablet P £2.04

  Oral solution
  EXCIPIENTS: May contain Alcohol
  - ▸ Pseudoephedrine hydrochloride (Non-proprietary)
    Pseudoephedrine hydrochloride 6 mg per 1 ml Decongestant 30mg/5ml oral liquid sugar-free | 100 ml P £1.57 DT price = £1.57
  - ▸ Galpseud (Thornton & Ross Ltd)
    Pseudoephedrine hydrochloride 6 mg per 1 ml Galpseud 30mg/5ml linctus sugar-free | 2000 ml PoM £14.00
  - ▸ Sudafed Non-Drowsy Decongestant (pseudoephedrine) (McNeil Products Ltd)
    Pseudoephedrine hydrochloride 6 mg per 1 ml Sudafed Decongestant 30mg/5ml liquid | 100 ml P £1.92

Xylometazoline hydrochloride

- **DRUG ACTION** Xylometazoline is a sympathomimetic.

- **INDICATIONS AND DOSE**
  Nasal congestion
  - ▸ BY INTRANASAL ADMINISTRATION USING NASAL DROPS
  - ▸ Child 6–11 years: 1–2 drops 1–2 times a day as required for maximum duration of 5 days, 0.05% solution to be administered into each nostril
  - ▸ Child 12–17 years: 2–3 drops 2–3 times a day as required for maximum duration of 7 days, 0.1% solution to be administered into each nostril
  - ▸ BY INTRANASAL ADMINISTRATION USING NASAL SPRAY
  - ▸ Child 12–17 years: 1 spray 1–3 times a day as required for maximum duration of 7 days, to be administered into each nostril

  IMPORTANT SAFETY INFORMATION
  The CHM/MHRA has stated that non-prescription cough and cold medicines containing oxymetazoline or xylometazoline can be considered for up to 5 days' treatment in children aged 6–12 years after basic principles of best care have been tried; these medicines should not be used in children under 6 years of age.

- **CAUTIONS** Angle-closure glaucoma · avoid excessive or prolonged use · cardiovascular disease · diabetes mellitus · hypertension · hyperthyroidism · rebound congestion
  CAUTIONS, FURTHER INFORMATION
  - ▸ Rebound congestion Sympathomimetic drugs are of limited value in the treatment of nasal congestion because they can, following prolonged use (more than 7 days), give rise to a rebound congestion (rhinitis medicamentosa) on withdrawal, due to a secondary vasodilatation with a subsequent temporary increase in nasal congestion. This in turn tempts the further use of the decongestant, leading to a vicious cycle of events.

- **SIDE-EFFECTS** Cardiovascular effects · hallucinations in small children · headache · local irritation · nausea · rebound congestion · restlessness in small children · sleep disturbances in small children · tolerance with diminished effect (after excessive use) · transient visual disturbances

SIDE-EFFECTS, FURTHER INFORMATION
- ▸ Hallucinations (in small children) Discontinue treatment if the hallucinations occur.

- **PREGNANCY** Manufacturer advises avoid.
- **BREAST FEEDING** Manufacturer advises caution—no information available.

- **MEDICINAL FORMS**
  There can be variation in the licensing of different medicines containing the same drug.

  Spray
  - ▸ Otrivine (Novartis Consumer Health UK Ltd)
    Xylometazoline hydrochloride 1 mg per 1 ml Otrivine Congestion Relief 0.1% nasal spray | 10 ml GSL £3.05 DT price = £2.18
    Otrivine Allergy Relief 0.1% nasal spray | 10 ml GSL £2.62 DT price = £2.18
  - ▸ Sudafed Congestion Relief (McNeil Products Ltd)
    Xylometazoline hydrochloride 1 mg per 1 ml Sudafed Congestion Relief 0.1% nasal spray | 10 ml GSL £3.25 DT price = £2.18
  - ▸ Sudafed Mucus Relief (McNeil Products Ltd)
    Xylometazoline hydrochloride 1 mg per 1 ml Sudafed Mucus Relief 0.1% nasal spray | 15 ml GSL £2.37
  - ▸ Sudafed Non-Drowsy Decongestant (xylometazoline) (McNeil Products Ltd)
    Xylometazoline hydrochloride 1 mg per 1 ml Sudafed Blocked Nose 0.1% spray | 15 ml GSL £2.38

  Nasal drops
  - ▸ Otrivine (Novartis Consumer Health UK Ltd)
    Xylometazoline hydrochloride 500 microgram per 1 ml Otrivine Child nasal drops | 10 ml P £1.91 DT price = £1.91
    Xylometazoline hydrochloride 1 mg per 1 ml Otrivine Adult 0.1% nasal drops | 10 ml GSL £2.18 DT price = £2.18

2   Nasal infection

ANTIBACTERIALS ❭ AMINOGLYCOSIDES

Chlorhexidine with neomycin

- **INDICATIONS AND DOSE**
  Eradication of nasal carriage of staphylococci
  - ▸ BY INTRANASAL ADMINISTRATION
  - ▸ Child: Apply 4 times a day for 10 days

  Preventing nasal carriage of staphylococci
  - ▸ BY INTRANASAL ADMINISTRATION
  - ▸ Child: Apply twice daily

- **MEDICINAL FORMS**
  There can be variation in the licensing of different medicines containing the same drug.

  Cream
  EXCIPIENTS: May contain Arachis (peanut) oil, cetostearyl alcohol (including cetyl and stearyl alcohol)
  - ▸ Naseptin (Alliance Pharmaceuticals Ltd)
    Chlorhexidine hydrochloride 1 mg per 1 gram, Neomycin sulfate 5 mg per 1 gram Naseptin nasal cream | 15 gram PoM £2.24 DT price = £2.24

ANTIBACTERIALS ❭ OTHER

Mupirocin

- **INDICATIONS AND DOSE**
  BACTROBAN NASAL®
  For eradication of nasal carriage of staphylococci, including meticillin-resistant *Staphylococcus aureus* (MRSA)
  - ▸ BY INTRANASAL ADMINISTRATION
  - ▸ Child: Apply 2–3 times a day for 5 days; a sample should be taken 2 days after treatment to confirm eradication. Course may be repeated once if sample

positive (and throat not colonised), dose to be applied to the inner surface of each nostril

- **PREGNANCY** Manufacturer advises avoid unless potential benefit outweighs risk—no information available.
- **BREAST FEEDING** No information available.

- **MEDICINAL FORMS**
There can be variation in the licensing of different medicines containing the same drug.
Nasal ointment
  - Bactroban (GlaxoSmithKline UK Ltd)
  Mupirocin (as Mupirocin calcium) 20 mg per 1 gram Bactroban 2% nasal ointment | 3 gram [PoM] £3.89 DT price = £3.89

CORTICOSTEROIDS > CORTICOSTEROID COMBINATIONS WITH ANTI-INFECTIVES

Betamethasone with neomycin

The properties listed below are those particular to the combination only. For the properties of the components please consider, betamethasone p. 645, neomycin sulfate p. 645.

- **INDICATIONS AND DOSE**
Nasal infection
  - BY INTRANASAL ADMINISTRATION USING NASAL DROPS
  - Child: Apply 2–3 drops 2–3 times a day, to be applied into each nostril

- **LESS SUITABLE FOR PRESCRIBING** Betamethasone with neomycin nasal-drops are less suitable for prescribing; there is no evidence that topical anti-infective nasal preparations have any therapeutic value in rhinitis or sinusitis.

- **MEDICINAL FORMS**
There can be variation in the licensing of different medicines containing the same drug.
Ear/eye/nose drops solution
EXCIPIENTS: May contain Benzalkonium chloride, disodium edetate
  - Betnesol-N (Focus Pharmaceuticals Ltd)
  Betamethasone (as Betamethasone sodium phosphate) 1 mg per 1 ml, Neomycin sulfate 5 mg per 1 ml Betnesol-N ear/eye/nose drops | 10 ml [PoM] £2.39 DT price = £2.39

3   Nasal inflammation, nasal polyps and rhinitis

Drugs used for Nasal inflammation, nasal polyps and rhinitis not listed below Desloratadine, p. 165 · Fexofenadine hydrochloride, p. 165 · Ketotifen, p. 170

ANTIMUSCARINICS > OTHER

Ipratropium bromide   24.2.2016

- **INDICATIONS AND DOSE**
Rhinorrhoea associated with allergic and non-allergic rhinitis
  - BY INTRANASAL ADMINISTRATION
  - Child 12–17 years: 2 sprays 2–3 times a day, dose to be sprayed into each nostril

DOSE EQUIVALENCE AND CONVERSION
1 metered spray of nasal spray = 21 micrograms.

- **CAUTIONS** Avoid spraying near eyes · bladder outflow obstruction · cystic fibrosis · susceptibility to angle-closure glaucoma

- **SIDE-EFFECTS**
  - **Common or very common** Epistaxis · nasal dryness · nasal irritation
  - **Uncommon** Headache · nausea
  - **Very rare** Gastro-intestinal motility disturbances · palpitations · urinary retention

- **PREGNANCY** Manufacturer advises only use if potential benefit outweighs the risk.

- **BREAST FEEDING** No information available—manufacturer advises only use if potential benefit outweighs risk.

- **MEDICINAL FORMS**
There can be variation in the licensing of different medicines containing the same drug.
Spray
EXCIPIENTS: May contain Benzalkonium chloride, disodium edetate
  - Rinatec (Boehringer Ingelheim Ltd)
  Ipratropium bromide 21 microgram per 1 dose Rinatec 21micrograms/dose nasal spray | 180 dose [PoM] £6.54 DT price = £6.54

CORTICOSTEROIDS

Corticosteroids (intranasal) 🔄

- **CAUTIONS** Avoid after nasal surgery (until healing has occurred) · avoid in pulmonary tuberculosis · avoid in the presence of untreated nasal infections · patients transferred from systemic corticosteroids may experience exacerbation of some symptoms

  CAUTIONS, FURTHER INFORMATION
  - Systemic absorption Systemic absorption may follow nasal administration particularly if high doses are used or if treatment is prolonged; therefore also consider the cautions and side-effects of systemic corticosteroids. The risk of systemic effects may be greater with nasal drops than with nasal sprays; drops are administered incorrectly more often than sprays.

- **SIDE-EFFECTS**
  - **Rare** Glaucoma · raised intra-ocular pressure
  - **Very rare** Nasal septal perforation (usually following nasal surgery)
  - **Frequency not known** Aggression (particularly in children) · anxiety (particularly in children) · bronchospasm · depression (particularly in children) · dryness · epistaxis · headache · hyperactivity (particularly in children) · hypersensitivity reactions · nasal irritation · nasal ulceration · sleep disturbances (particularly in children) · smell disturbances · taste disturbances · throat irritation

  SIDE-EFFECTS, FURTHER INFORMATION
  - Systemic absorption Systemic absorption may follow nasal administration particularly if high doses are used or if treatment is prolonged. Therefore also consider the side-effects of systemic corticosteroids. The risk of systemic effects may be greater with nasal drops than with nasal sprays; drops are administered incorrectly more often than sprays.

- **MONITORING REQUIREMENTS** The height of children receiving prolonged treatment with nasal corticosteroids should be monitored; if growth is slowed, referral to a paediatrician should be considered.

F 651

Beclometasone dipropionate

(Beclomethasone dipropionate)

- **INDICATIONS AND DOSE**

Prophylaxis and treatment of allergic and vasomotor rhinitis
- ▸ BY INTRANASAL ADMINISTRATION
- ▸ Child 6–17 years: 100 micrograms twice daily, dose to be administered into each nostril, reduced to 50 micrograms twice daily, dose to be administered into each nostril, dose to be reduced when symptoms controlled; maximum 400 micrograms per day

- **MEDICINAL FORMS**
There can be variation in the licensing of different medicines containing the same drug.
Spray
EXCIPIENTS: May contain Benzalkonium chloride, polysorbates
- ▸ Beclometasone dipropionate (Non-proprietary)
Beclometasone dipropionate 50 microgram per 1 dose Beclometasone 50micrograms/dose nasal spray | 200 dose [PoM] no price available DT price = £2.02 | 200 dose [P] £5.70 DT price = £2.02
- ▸ Beconase (GlaxoSmithKline UK Ltd, Omega Pharma Ltd)
Beclometasone dipropionate 50 microgram per 1 dose Beconase Aqueous 50micrograms/dose nasal spray | 200 dose [PoM] £2.19 DT price = £2.02
Beconase Hayfever 50micrograms/dose nasal spray | 180 dose [P] £6.46
- ▸ Nasobec (Teva UK Ltd)
Beclometasone dipropionate 50 microgram per 1 dose Nasobec Aqueous 50micrograms/dose nasal spray | 200 dose [PoM] £3.06 DT price = £2.02
Nasobec Hayfever 50micrograms/dose nasal spray | 180 dose [P] £5.78
- ▸ Pollenase (beclometasone) (E M Pharma)
Beclometasone dipropionate 50 microgram per 1 dose Pollenase Hayfever 50micrograms/dose nasal spray | 200 dose [P] £3.36 DT price = £2.02

F 651

Betamethasone

- **INDICATIONS AND DOSE**

BETNESOL®
Non-infected inflammatory conditions of nose
- ▸ BY INTRANASAL ADMINISTRATION
- ▸ Child: Apply 2–3 drops 2–3 times a day, dose to be applied into each nostril

VISTAMETHASONE®
Non-infected inflammatory conditions of nose
- ▸ BY INTRANASAL ADMINISTRATION
- ▸ Child: Apply 2–3 drops twice daily, dose to be applied into each nostril

- **MEDICINAL FORMS**
There can be variation in the licensing of different medicines containing the same drug.
Ear/eye/nose drops solution
EXCIPIENTS: May contain Benzalkonium chloride, disodium edetate
- ▸ Betnesol (Focus Pharmaceuticals Ltd)
Betamethasone sodium phosphate 1 mg per 1 ml Betnesol 0.1% eye/ear/nose drops | 10 ml [PoM] £2.32 DT price = £2.32
- ▸ Vistamethasone (Martindale Pharmaceuticals Ltd)
Betamethasone sodium phosphate 1 mg per 1 ml Vistamethasone 0.1% ear/eye/nose drops | 5 ml [PoM] £0.87 | 10 ml [PoM] £0.99 DT price = £2.32

F 651

Budesonide

- **INDICATIONS AND DOSE**

Prophylaxis and treatment of allergic and vasomotor rhinitis
- ▸ BY INTRANASAL ADMINISTRATION
- ▸ Child 12–17 years: Initially 200 micrograms once daily, dose to be administered into each nostril in the morning, alternatively initially 100 micrograms twice daily, dose to be administered to each nostril; reduced to 100 micrograms once daily, dose to be administered into each nostril, dose can be reduced when control achieved

Nasal polyps
- ▸ BY INTRANASAL ADMINISTRATION
- ▸ Child 12–17 years: 100 micrograms twice daily for up to 3 months, dose to be administered into each nostril

RHINOCORT AQUA®
Rhinitis
- ▸ BY INTRANASAL ADMINISTRATION
- ▸ Child 12–17 years: 128 micrograms once daily, dose to be administered into each nostril in the morning, alternatively 64 micrograms twice daily, dose to be administered into each nostril; reduced to 64 micrograms once daily when control achieved. Use for maximum 3 months, doses to be administered into each nostril

Nasal polyps
- ▸ BY INTRANASAL ADMINISTRATION
- ▸ Child 12–17 years: 64 micrograms twice daily for up to 3 months, dose to be administered into each nostril

- **MEDICINAL FORMS**
There can be variation in the licensing of different medicines containing the same drug.
Spray
EXCIPIENTS: May contain Disodium edetate, polysorbates, potassium sorbate
- ▸ Budesonide (Non-proprietary)
Budesonide 100 microgram per 1 dose Budeflam Aquanase 100micrograms/dose nasal spray | 150 dose [PoM] no price available Aircort 100micrograms/dose nasal spray | 200 dose [PoM] no price available
- ▸ Rhinocort (AstraZeneca UK Ltd)
Budesonide 64 microgram per 1 dose Rhinocort Aqua 64 nasal spray | 120 dose [PoM] £3.49 DT price = £4.77

F 651

Fluticasone

4.1.2016

- **INDICATIONS AND DOSE**

Prophylaxis and treatment of allergic rhinitis and perennial rhinitis
- ▸ BY INTRANASAL ADMINISTRATION USING NASAL SPRAY
- ▸ Child 4–11 years: 50 micrograms once daily, to be administered into each nostril preferably in the morning, increased if necessary to 50 micrograms twice daily
- ▸ Child 12–17 years: 100 micrograms once daily, to be administered into each nostril preferably in the morning, increased if necessary to 100 micrograms twice daily; reduced to 50 micrograms once daily, dose to be administered into each nostril, dose to be reduced when control achieved

Nasal polyps
- ▸ BY INTRANASAL ADMINISTRATION USING NASAL DROPS
- ▸ Child 16–17 years: 200 micrograms 1–2 times a day, to be administered into each nostril, alternative

treatment should be considered if no improvement after 4–6 weeks, (200 micrograms is equivalent to approximately 6 drops)

AVAMYS® SPRAY

Prophylaxis and treatment of allergic rhinitis
- BY INTRANASAL ADMINISTRATION
- Child 6–11 years: 27.5 micrograms once daily, dose to be sprayed into each nostril, increased if necessary to 55 micrograms once daily if required, reduced to 27.5 micrograms once daily, dose to be reduced once control achieved; use minimum effective dose
- Child 12–17 years: 55 micrograms once daily, dose to be sprayed into each nostril, reduced to 27.5 micrograms once daily, to be sprayed into each nostril, dose to be reduced once control achieved; use minimum effective dose

DOSE EQUIVALENCE AND CONVERSION
For *Avamys*® spray: 1 spray equivalent to 27.5 micrograms.

- **SIDE-EFFECTS**
SIDE-EFFECTS, FURTHER INFORMATION
Nasal ulceration occurs commonly with nasal preparations containing fluticasone furoate.

- **MEDICINAL FORMS**
There can be variation in the licensing of different medicines containing the same drug.
Spray
EXCIPIENTS: May contain Benzalkonium chloride, disodium edetate, polysorbates
- ▸ **Fluticasone (Non-proprietary)**
  Fluticasone propionate 50 microgram per 1 dose Fluticasone propionate 50micrograms/dose nasal spray | 60 dose [PoM] no price available | 150 dose [PoM] £29.50 DT price = £11.01
- ▸ **Avamys** (GlaxoSmithKline UK Ltd)
  Fluticasone furoate 27.5 microgram per 1 dose Avamys 27.5micrograms/dose nasal spray | 120 dose [PoM] £6.44 DT price = £6.44
- ▸ **Flixonase** (GlaxoSmithKline UK Ltd)
  Fluticasone propionate 50 microgram per 1 dose Flixonase 50micrograms/dose aqueous nasal spray | 150 dose [PoM] £11.01 DT price = £11.01
- ▸ **Nasofan** (Teva UK Ltd)
  Fluticasone propionate 50 microgram per 1 dose Nasofan Allergy 50micrograms/dose nasal spray | 60 dose [P] £4.68 Nasofan 50micrograms/dose aqueous nasal spray | 150 dose [PoM] £8.04 DT price = £11.01
- ▸ **Pirinase Hayfever** (GlaxoSmithKline Consumer Healthcare)
  Fluticasone propionate 50 microgram per 1 dose Pirinase Hayfever 0.05% nasal spray | 60 dose [P] £4.59
Nasal drops
EXCIPIENTS: May contain Polysorbates
- ▸ **Flixonase** (GlaxoSmithKline UK Ltd)
  Fluticasone propionate 400 microgram Flixonase Nasule 400microgram/unit dose nasal drops | 28 unit dose [PoM] £12.99 DT price = £12.99

Fluticasone with azelastine

The properties listed below are those particular to the combination only. For the properties of the components please consider, fluticasone p. 652.

- **INDICATIONS AND DOSE**

Moderate to severe seasonal and perennial allergic rhinitis, if monotherapy with antihistamine or corticosteroid is inadequate
- BY INTRANASAL ADMINISTRATION
- Child 12–17 years: 1 spray twice daily, dose to be administered into each nostril

- **MEDICINAL FORMS**
There can be variation in the licensing of different medicines containing the same drug.
Spray
EXCIPIENTS: May contain Benzalkonium chloride, polysorbates
- ▸ **Fluticasone with azelastine (Non-proprietary)**
  Fluticasone propionate 50 microgram per 1 actuation, Azelastine hydrochloride 137 microgram per 1 actuation Fluticasone propionate 50micrograms/dose / Azelastine 137micrograms/dose nasal spray | 120 dose [PoM] no price available
- ▸ **Dymista** (Meda Pharmaceuticals Ltd)
  Fluticasone propionate 50 microgram per 1 actuation, Azelastine hydrochloride 137 microgram per 1 actuation Dymista 137micrograms/dose / 50micrograms/dose nasal spray | 120 dose [PoM] £14.80

F 651

Mometasone furoate

- **INDICATIONS AND DOSE**

Prophylaxis and treatment of allergic rhinitis
- BY INTRANASAL ADMINISTRATION
- Child 6–11 years: 50 micrograms daily, dose to be sprayed into each nostril
- Child 12–17 years: 100 micrograms daily, increased if necessary up to 200 micrograms daily, dose to be sprayed into each nostril; reduced to 50 micrograms daily, dose to be reduced when control achieved, dose to be sprayed into each nostril

- **SIDE-EFFECTS**
SIDE-EFFECTS, FURTHER INFORMATION
Nasal ulceration occurs commonly with preparations containing mometasone furoate.

- **MEDICINAL FORMS**
There can be variation in the licensing of different medicines containing the same drug.
Spray
EXCIPIENTS: May contain Benzalkonium chloride, polysorbates
- ▸ **Mometasone furoate (Non-proprietary)**
  Mometasone furoate 50 microgram per 1 dose Mometasone 50micrograms/dose nasal spray | 140 dose [PoM] £7.30 DT price = £2.01
- ▸ **Nasonex** (Merck Sharp & Dohme Ltd)
  Mometasone furoate 50 microgram per 1 dose Nasonex 50micrograms/dose nasal spray | 140 dose [PoM] £7.68 DT price = £2.01

F 651

Triamcinolone acetonide

- **INDICATIONS AND DOSE**

Prophylaxis and treatment of allergic rhinitis
- BY INTRANASAL ADMINISTRATION
- Child 2–5 years: 55 micrograms once daily for maximum 3 months, dose to be sprayed into each nostril
- Child 6–11 years: 55 micrograms once daily, dose to be sprayed into each nostril, increased if necessary to 110 micrograms once daily, dose to be sprayed into each nostril; reduced to 55 micrograms once daily, dose to be sprayed into each nostril, reduce dose when control achieved; maximum duration of treatment 3 months
- Child 12–17 years: 110 micrograms once daily, dose to be sprayed into each nostril, reduced to 55 micrograms once daily, dose to be sprayed into each nostril, reduce dose when control achieved

- **UNLICENSED USE** Not licensed for use in children under 6 years.

12

Ear, nose and oropharynx

- **MEDICINAL FORMS**
There can be variation in the licensing of different medicines containing the same drug.

Spray
EXCIPIENTS: May contain Benzalkonium chloride, disodium edetate, polysorbates
  - ▸ Nasacort (Sanofi)
    Triamcinolone acetonide 55 microgram per 1 dose Nasacort Allergy 55micrograms/dose nasal spray | 30 dose P £3.01
    Nasacort 55micrograms/dose nasal spray | 120 dose PoM £7.39 DT price = £7.39

MAST-CELL STABILISERS

Sodium cromoglicate

(Sodium cromoglycate)

- **INDICATIONS AND DOSE**
Prophylaxis of allergic rhinitis
  - ▸ BY INTRANASAL ADMINISTRATION
  - ▸ Child: 1 spray 2–4 times a day, to be administered into each nostril

- **UNLICENSED USE** Licensed for use in children (age range not specified by manufacturers).
- **SIDE-EFFECTS**
- ▸ **Rare** Transient bronchospasm
- ▸ **Frequency not known** Local irritation

- **MEDICINAL FORMS**
There can be variation in the licensing of different medicines containing the same drug.
No licensed medicines listed.

Oropharynx

1   Dry mouth

Treatment of dry mouth

Overview

Dry mouth (xerostomia) may be caused by drugs with antimuscarinic (anticholinergic) side-effects (e.g. antispasmodics and sedating antihistamines), by irradiation of the head and neck region or by damage to or disease of the salivary glands. Children with a persistently dry mouth may develop a burning or scalded sensation and have poor oral hygiene; they may develop dental caries, periodontal disease, and oral infections (particularly candidiasis). Dry mouth may be relieved in many patients by simple measures such as frequent sips of cool drinks or sucking pieces of ice or sugar-free fruit pastilles. Sugar-free chewing gum stimulates salivation in patients with residual salivary function.

Artificial saliva can provide useful relief of dry mouth. A properly balanced artificial saliva should be of a neutral pH and contain electrolytes (including fluoride) to correspond approximately to the composition of saliva. The acidic pH of some artificial saliva products may be inappropriate.

Artificial saliva products

- **ARTIFICIAL SALIVA PRODUCTS**
AS SALIVA ORTHANA® LOZENGES
Mucin 65 mg, xylitol 59 mg, in a sorbitol basis, pH neutral

- **INDICATIONS AND DOSE**
Dry mouth as a result of having (or having undergone) radiotherapy | Sicca syndrome
  - ▸ BY MOUTH
  - ▸ Child: 1 lozenge as required, allow to dissolve slowly in the mouth

- **PRESCRIBING AND DISPENSING INFORMATION** AS Saliva Orthana ® lozenges do not contain fluoride.
  - ▸ AS Saliva Orthana lozenges (A S Pharma Ltd)
    30 lozenge(ACBS) • NHS indicative price = £3.50

AS SALIVA ORTHANA® SPRAY
Gastric mucin (porcine) 3.5%, xylitol 2%, sodium fluoride 4.2 mg/litre, with preservatives and flavouring agents, pH neutral.

- **INDICATIONS AND DOSE**
Symptomatic treatment of dry mouth
  - ▸ BY MOUTH
  - ▸ Child: Apply 2–3 sprays as required, spray onto oral and pharyngeal mucosa

- **PROFESSION SPECIFIC INFORMATION**
Dental practitioners' formulary
AS Saliva Orthana ® Oral Spray may be prescribed.

BIOXTRA® GEL
Lactoperoxidase, lactoferrin, lysozyme, whey colostrum, xylitol and other ingredients.

- **INDICATIONS AND DOSE**
Dry mouth as a result of having (or having undergone) radiotherapy (ACBS) | Dry mouth as a result of sicca syndrome (ACBS)
  - ▸ BY MOUTH
  - ▸ Child: Apply as required, apply to oral mucosa

- **PROFESSION SPECIFIC INFORMATION**
Dental practitioners' formulary
BioXtra ® Gel may be prescribed.
  - ▸ BioXtra moisturising gel for dry mouths (R.I.S. Products Ltd)
    40 ml • NHS indicative price = £3.94

BIOTENE ORALBALANCE®
Lactoperoxidase, lactoferrin, lysozyme, glucose oxidase, xylitol in a gel basis

- **INDICATIONS AND DOSE**
Symptomatic treatment of dry mouth
  - ▸ BY MOUTH
  - ▸ Child: Apply as required, apply to gums and tongue

- **PATIENT AND CARER ADVICE** Avoid use with toothpastes containing detergents (including foaming agents).
- **PROFESSION SPECIFIC INFORMATION**
Dental practitioners' formulary
Biotene Oralbalance ® Saliva Replacement Gel may be prescribed as Artificial Saliva Gel.
  - ▸ Biotene Oralbalance dry mouth saliva replacement gel (GlaxoSmithKline Consumer Healthcare)
    Glucose oxidase 12000 unit, Lactoferrin 12 mg, Lactoperoxidase 12000 unit, Muramidase 12 mg 50 gram • NHS indicative price = £4.46 • Drug Tariff (Part IXa)

GLANDOSANE®

Carmellose sodium 500 mg, sorbitol 1.5 g, potassium chloride 60 mg, sodium chloride 42.2 mg, magnesium chloride 2.6 mg, calcium chloride 7.3 mg, and dipotassium hydrogen phosphate 17.1 mg/50 g, pH 5.75.

● **INDICATIONS AND DOSE**

Dry mouth as a result of having (or having undergone) radiotherapy (ACBS) | Dry mouth as a result of sicca syndrome (ACBS)
▸ BY MOUTH
▸ Child: Apply as required, spray onto oral and pharyngeal mucosa

● **PROFESSION SPECIFIC INFORMATION**

Dental practitioners' formulary
Glandosane® Aerosol Spray may be prescribed.
▸ **Glandosane synthetic saliva spray lemon** (Fresenius Kabi Ltd)
  50 ml(ACBS) · NHS indicative price = £5.58
▸ **Glandosane synthetic saliva spray natural** (Fresenius Kabi Ltd)
  50 ml(ACBS) · NHS indicative price = £5.58
▸ **Glandosane synthetic saliva spray peppermint** (Fresenius Kabi Ltd)
  50 ml(ACBS) · NHS indicative price = £5.58

ORALIEVE GEL

● **INDICATIONS AND DOSE**

Symptomatic treatment of dry mouth
▸ BY MOUTH
▸ Child: Apply as required, particularly at night, to oral mucosa

● **PRESCRIBING AND DISPENSING INFORMATION** Contains traces of milk protein and egg white protein.

SST®

Sugar-free, citric acid, malic acid and other ingredients in a sorbitol base.

● **INDICATIONS AND DOSE**

Symptomatic treatment of dry mouth in patients with impaired salivary gland function and patent salivary ducts
▸ BY MOUTH
▸ Child: 1 tablet as required, allow tablet to dissolve slowly in the mouth

● **PROFESSION SPECIFIC INFORMATION**

Dental practitioners' formulary
May be prescribed as Saliva Stimulating Tablets.
▸ **SST saliva stimulating tablets** (Sinclair IS Pharma Plc)
  100 tablet · NHS indicative price = £4.86 · Drug Tariff (Part IXa)

SALIVEZE®

Carmellose sodium (sodium carboxymethylcellulose), calcium chloride, magnesium chloride, potassium chloride, sodium chloride, and dibasic sodium phosphate, pH neutral

● **INDICATIONS AND DOSE**

Dry mouth as a result of having (or having undergone) radiotherapy (ACBS) | Dry mouth as a result of sicca syndrome (ACBS)
▸ BY MOUTH
▸ Child: Apply 1 spray as required, spray onto oral mucosa

● **PROFESSION SPECIFIC INFORMATION**

Dental practitioners' formulary
Saliveze® Oral Spray may be prescribed.
▸ **Saliveze mouth spray** (Wyvern Medical Ltd)
  50 ml(ACBS) · NHS indicative price = £3.50

SALIVIX®

Sugar-free, reddish-amber, acacia, malic acid and other ingredients.

● **INDICATIONS AND DOSE**

Symptomatic treatment of dry mouth
▸ BY MOUTH USING PASTILLES
▸ Child: 1 unit as required, suck pastille

● **PROFESSION SPECIFIC INFORMATION**

Dental practitioners' formulary
Salivix® Pastilles may be prescribed as Artificial Saliva Pastilles.
▸ **Salivix pastilles** (Galen Ltd)
  50 pastille · NHS indicative price = £3.55 · Drug Tariff (Part IXa)

XEROTIN®

Sugar-free, water, sorbitol, carmellose (carboxymethylcellulose), potassium chloride, sodium chloride, potassium phosphate, magnesium chloride, calcium chloride and other ingredients, pH neutral.

● **INDICATIONS AND DOSE**

Symptomatic treatment of dry mouth
▸ BY MOUTH
▸ Child: 1 spray as required

● **PROFESSION SPECIFIC INFORMATION**

Dental practitioners' formulary
Xerotin® Oral Spray may be prescribed as Artificial Saliva Oral Spray.
▸ **Xerotin spray** (SpePharm UK Ltd)
  100 ml · NHS indicative price = £6.86 · Drug Tariff (Part IXa)

2 Oral hygiene

Mouthwashes and other preparations for oropharyngeal use

Lozenges and sprays

There is no convincing evidence that antiseptic lozenges and sprays have a beneficial action and they sometimes irritate and cause sore tongue and sore lips. Some of these preparations also contain local anaesthetics which relieve pain but may cause sensitisation.

Mouthwashes and gargles

Superficial infections of the mouth are often helped by warm mouthwashes which have a mechanical cleansing effect and cause some local hyperaemia. However, to be effective, they must be used frequently and vigorously. Mouthwashes may not be suitable for children under 7 years (risk of the solution being swallowed); the mouthwash or dental gel may be applied using a cotton bud.

A warm saline mouthwash is ideal and can be prepared either by dissolving half a teaspoonful of salt in a glassful of warm water or by diluting compound sodium chloride mouthwash p. 657 with an equal volume of warm water.

Mouthwashes containing an oxidising agent, such as hydrogen peroxide p. 657, may be useful in the treatment of acute ulcerative gingivitis (Vincent's infection) since the organisms involved are anaerobes. It also has a mechanical cleansing effect arising from frothing when in contact with oral debris. Concentrations greater than 1.5% in children may cause ulceration and tissue damage.

Chlorhexidine p. 656 is an effective antiseptic which has the advantage of inhibiting plaque formation on the teeth. It does not, however, completely control plaque deposition and is not a substitute for effective toothbrushing. Moreover,

12

Ear, nose and oropharynx

chlorhexidine preparations do not penetrate significantly into stagnation areas and are therefore of little value in the control of dental caries or of periodontal disease once pocketing has developed. Chlorhexidine preparations are of little value in the control of acute necrotising ulcerative gingivitis. With prolonged use, chlorhexidine causes reversible brown staining of teeth and tongue. Chlorhexidine may be incompatible with some ingredients in toothpaste, causing an unpleasant taste in the mouth; rinse the mouth thoroughly with water between using toothpaste and chlorhexidine-containing products.

Chlorhexidine can be used as a mouthwash, spray or gel for secondary infection in mucosal ulceration and for controlling gingivitis, as an adjunct to other oral hygiene measures. These preparations may also be used instead of toothbrushing where there is a painful periodontal condition (e.g. primary herpetic stomatitis) or if the patient has a haemorrhagic disorder, or is disabled. Chlorhexidine mouthwash is used in the prevention of oral candidiasis in immunocompromised patients. Chlorhexidine mouthwash reduces the incidence of alveolar osteitis following tooth extraction. Chlorhexidine mouthwash should not be used for the prevention of endocarditis in children undergoing dental procedures.

ANTISEPTICS AND DISINFECTANTS > OTHER

Chlorhexidine

- **INDICATIONS AND DOSE**
  Oral hygiene and plaque inhibition | Oral candidiasis | Gingivitis | Management of aphthous ulcers
  ▸ BY MOUTH USING MOUTHWASH
  ▸ Child: Rinse or gargle 10 mL twice daily (rinse or gargle for about 1 minute)
  Oral hygiene and plaque inhibition and gingivitis
  ▸ BY MOUTH USING DENTAL GEL
  ▸ Child: Apply 1–2 times a day, to be brushed on the teeth
  Oral candidiasis | Management of aphthous ulcers
  ▸ BY MOUTH USING DENTAL GEL
  ▸ Child: Apply 1–2 times a day, to affected areas
  Oral hygiene and plaque inhibition | Oral candidiasis | Gingivitis | Management of aphthous ulcers
  ▸ BY MOUTH USING OROMUCOSAL SPRAY
  ▸ Child: Apply up to 12 sprays twice daily as required, to be applied tooth, gingival, or ulcer surfaces
  Bladder irrigation and catheter patency solutions
  ▸ BY INTRAVESICAL INSTILLATION
  ▸ Child: (consult product literature)

- **UNLICENSED USE** *Corsodyl*® not licensed for use in children under 12 years (unless on the advice of a healthcare professional).

- **SIDE-EFFECTS** Anaphylaxis · hypersensitivity · mucosal irritation · parotid gland swelling · reversible brown staining of composite restorations · reversible brown staining of silicate compositions · reversible brown staining of teeth · taste disturbance · tongue discolouration
  SIDE-EFFECTS, FURTHER INFORMATION
  If desquamation occurs with mucosal irritation, discontinue treatment or dilute mouthwash with an equal volume of water.

- **PATIENT AND CARER ADVICE** Chlorhexidine gluconate may be incompatible with some ingredients in toothpaste; rinse the mouth thoroughly with water between using toothpaste and chlorhexidine-containing product.

- **PROFESSION SPECIFIC INFORMATION**
  Dental practitioners' formulary
  Corsodyl® dental gel may be prescribed as Chlorhexidine Gluconate Gel; *Corsodyl*® mouthwash may be prescribed as Chlorhexidine Mouthwash; *Corsodyl*® oral spray may be prescribed as Chlorhexidine Oral Spray.

- **MEDICINAL FORMS**
  There can be variation in the licensing of different medicines containing the same drug.
  Dental gel
  ▸ Corsodyl (GlaxoSmithKline Consumer Healthcare)
  Chlorhexidine gluconate 10 mg per 1 gram Corsodyl 1% dental gel sugar-free | 50 gram Ⓟ £1.26 DT price = £1.26
  Mouthwash
  ▸ Chlorhexidine (Non-proprietary)
  Chlorhexidine gluconate 2 mg per 1 ml Chlorhexidine gluconate 0.2% mouthwash natural | 300 ml GSL £3.65 DT price = £3.48
  Chlorhexidine gluconate 0.2% mouthwash | 300 ml GSL £1.99–£2.09 DT price = £3.48
  Chlorhexidine gluconate 0.2% mouthwash plain | 300 ml GSL £3.48 DT price = £3.48
  Chlorhexidine gluconate 0.2% mouthwash peppermint | 300 ml GSL £3.65 DT price = £3.48
  Chlorhexidine gluconate 0.2% mouthwash original | 300 ml GSL £3.65 DT price = £3.48
  Chlorhexidine gluconate 0.2% mouthwash alcohol free | 300 ml GSL no price available DT price = £3.48 | 500 ml GSL no price available
  ▸ Corsodyl (GlaxoSmithKline Consumer Healthcare)
  Chlorhexidine gluconate 2 mg per 1 ml Corsodyl 0.2% mouthwash aniseed | 300 ml GSL £2.44 DT price = £3.48
  Corsodyl Mint 0.2% mouthwash | 300 ml GSL £2.44 DT price = £3.48 | 600 ml GSL £4.76
  Corsodyl 0.2% mouthwash alcohol free | 300 ml GSL £3.06 DT price = £3.48
  ▸ Curasept (Curaprox (UK) Ltd)
  Chlorhexidine gluconate 2 mg per 1 ml Curasept 0.2% oral rinse | 200 ml no price available
  Irrigation
  ▸ Chlorhexidine (Non-proprietary)
  Chlorhexidine acetate 200 microgram per 1 ml Chlorhexidine acetate 0.02% catheter maintenance solution | 100 ml Ⓟ no price available
  ▸ Uro-Tainer (chlorhexidine) (B.Braun Medical Ltd)
  Chlorhexidine acetate 200 microgram per 1 ml Uro-Tainer chlorhexidine 1:5000 catheter maintenance solution | 100 ml Ⓟ £2.70

Chlorhexidine with chlorobutanol

The properties listed below are those particular to the combination only. For the properties of the components please consider, chlorhexidine above.

- **INDICATIONS AND DOSE**
  Oral hygiene and plaque inhibition
  ▸ BY MOUTH USING MOUTHWASH
  ▸ Child 6–17 years: Rinse or gargle 10–15 mL 2–3 times a day, to be diluted with lukewarm water in measuring cup provided

- **PRESCRIBING AND DISPENSING INFORMATION** Flavours of mouthwash may include mint.

- **MEDICINAL FORMS**
  There can be variation in the licensing of different medicines containing the same drug.
  No licensed medicines listed.

Hexetidine

- **INDICATIONS AND DOSE**

Oral hygiene
- ▶ BY MOUTH USING MOUTHWASH
- ▸ **Child 6–17 years:** Rinse or gargle 15 mL 2–3 times a day, to be used undiluted

- **SIDE-EFFECTS**
- ▸ **Very rare** Taste disturbance · transient anaesthesia
- ▸ **Frequency not known** Local irritation

- **MEDICINAL FORMS**
There can be variation in the licensing of different medicines containing the same drug.
Mouthwash
- ▸ Oraldene (McNeil Products Ltd)
Hexetidine 1 mg per 1 ml Oraldene Icemint 0.1% mouthwash sugar-free | 200 ml [GSL] £2.21 DT price = £2.21
Oraldene 0.1% mouthwash peppermint sugar-free | 100 ml [GSL] £1.43 sugar-free | 200 ml [GSL] £2.21 DT price = £2.21

Hydrogen peroxide

- **DRUG ACTION** Hydrogen peroxide is an oxidising agent.

- **INDICATIONS AND DOSE**

Oral hygiene (with hydrogen peroxide 6%)
- ▶ BY MOUTH USING MOUTHWASH
- ▸ **Child:** Rinse or gargle 15 mL 2–3 times a day for 2–3 minutes, to be diluted in half a tumblerful of warm water

PEROXYL®

Oral hygiene
- ▶ BY MOUTH USING MOUTHWASH
- ▸ **Child 6–17 years:** Rinse or gargle 10 mL 3 times a day for about 1 minute, for maximum 7 days, to be used after meals and at bedtime

- **SIDE-EFFECTS** Hypertrophy of papillae of tongue on prolonged used

- **PRESCRIBING AND DISPENSING INFORMATION** When prepared extemporaneously, the BP states Hydrogen Peroxide Mouthwash, BP consists of hydrogen peroxide 6% solution (= approx. 20 volume) BP.

- **HANDLING AND STORAGE** Hydrogen peroxide bleaches fabric.

- **PROFESSION SPECIFIC INFORMATION**

Dental practitioners' formulary
Hydrogen Peroxide Mouthwash may be prescribed.

- **MEDICINAL FORMS**
There can be variation in the licensing of different medicines containing the same drug.
Mouthwash
- ▸ Peroxyl (Colgate-Palmolive (UK) Ltd)
Hydrogen peroxide 15 mg per 1 ml Peroxyl 1.5% mouthwash sugar-free | 300 ml [GSL] £2.94

Sodium bicarbonate with sodium chloride

- **INDICATIONS AND DOSE**

Oral hygiene
- ▶ BY MOUTH USING MOUTHWASH
- ▸ **Child:** (consult product literature)

- **DIRECTIONS FOR ADMINISTRATION** For mouthwash, extemporaneous preparations should be prepared according to the following formula: sodium chloride 1.5 g, sodium bicarbonate 1 g, concentrated peppermint

emulsion 2.5 mL, double-strength chloroform water 50 mL, water to 100 mL. To be diluted with an equal volume of warm water prior to administration.

- **PRESCRIBING AND DISPENSING INFORMATION** Flavours of mouthwash may include peppermint.

- **PROFESSION SPECIFIC INFORMATION**

Dental practitioners' formulary
Compound sodium chloride mouthwash may be prescribed.

- **MEDICINAL FORMS**
There can be variation in the licensing of different medicines containing the same drug. Forms available from special-order manufacturers include: mouthwash

Sodium chloride

- **INDICATIONS AND DOSE**

Oral hygiene
- ▶ BY MOUTH USING MOUTHWASH
- ▸ **Child:** Rinse or gargle as required

- **DIRECTIONS FOR ADMINISTRATION** Extemporaneous mouthwash preparations should be prepared according to the following formula: sodium chloride 1.5 g, sodium bicarbonate 1 g, concentrated peppermint emulsion 2.5 mL, double-strength chloroform water 50 mL, water to 100 mL. To be diluted with an equal volume of warm water.

- **PRESCRIBING AND DISPENSING INFORMATION** No mouthwash preparations available—when prepared extemporaneously, the BP states Sodium Chloride Mouthwash, Compound, BP consists of sodium bicarbonate 1%, sodium chloride 1.5% in a suitable vehicle with peppermint flavour.

- **PROFESSION SPECIFIC INFORMATION**

Dental practitioners' formulary
Compound Sodium Chloride Mouthwash may be prescribed.

- **MEDICINAL FORMS**
There can be variation in the licensing of different medicines containing the same drug. No licensed preparations listed.

2.1 Dental caries

Fluoride

Availability of adequate fluoride confers significant resistance to dental caries. It is now considered that the topical action of fluoride on enamel and plaque is more important than the systemic effect.

When the fluoride content of drinking water is less than 700 micrograms per litre (0.7 parts per million), daily administration of fluoride tablets or drops provides suitable supplementation. Systemic fluoride supplements should not be prescribed without reference to the fluoride content of the local water supply. Infants need not receive fluoride supplements until the age of 6 months.

Dentifrices which incorporate sodium fluoride or monofluorophosphate are also a convenient source of fluoride.

Individuals who are either particularly caries prone or medically compromised may be given additional protection by use of fluoride rinses or by application of fluoride gels. Rinses may be used daily or weekly; daily use of a less concentrated rinse is more effective than weekly use of a more concentrated one. High-strength gels must be applied regularly under professional supervision; extreme caution is necessary to prevent children from swallowing any excess.

12

Ear, nose and oropharynx

Less concentrated gels are available for home use. Varnishes are also available and are particularly valuable for young or disabled children since they adhere to the teeth and set in the presence of moisture.

VITAMINS AND TRACE ELEMENTS

Sodium fluoride

- **INDICATIONS AND DOSE**

Prophylaxis of dental caries for water content less than 300micrograms/litre (0.3 parts per million) of fluoride ion

▸ BY MOUTH USING TABLETS

▸ Child 6 months–2 years: 250 micrograms daily, doses expressed as fluoride ion (F⁻)
▸ Child 3–5 years: 500 micrograms daily, doses expressed as fluoride ion (F⁻)
▸ Child 6–17 years: 1 mg daily, doses expressed as fluoride ion (F⁻)

Prophylaxis of dental caries for water content between 300 and 700micrograms/litre (0.3–0.7 parts per million) of fluoride ion

▸ BY MOUTH USING TABLETS

▸ Child 3–5 years: 250 micrograms daily, doses expressed as fluoride ion (F⁻)
▸ Child 6–17 years: 500 micrograms daily, doses expressed as fluoride ion (F⁻)

Prophylaxis of dental caries for water content above 700micrograms/litre (0.7 parts per million) of fluoride ion

▸ Child 6 months–17 years: Supplements not advised

Prophylaxis of dental caries for individuals who are caries prone or medically compromised

▸ BY MOUTH USING MOUTHWASH

▸ Child 6–17 years: Rinse or gargle 10 mL daily

COLGATE DURAPHAT® 2800PPM FLUORIDE TOOTHPASTE

Prophylaxis of dental caries

▸ BY MOUTH USING PASTE

▸ Child 10–17 years: Apply 1 centimetre twice daily, to be applied using a toothbrush

COLGATE DURAPHAT® 5000PPM FLUORIDE TOOTHPASTE

Prophylaxis of dental caries

▸ BY MOUTH USING PASTE

▸ Child 16–17 years: Apply 2 centimetres 3 times a day, to be applied after meals using a toothbrush

EN-DE-KAY® FLUORINSE

Prophylaxis of dental carries for individuals who are caries prone or medically compromised

▸ BY MOUTH USING MOUTHWASH

▸ Child 8–17 years: 5 drops daily, dilute 5 drops to 10 mL of water, alternatively 20 drops once weekly, dilute 20 drops to 10 mL

DOSE EQUIVALENCE AND CONVERSION
Sodium fluoride 2.2 mg provides approx. 1 mg fluoride ion.
These doses reflect the recommendations of the British Dental Association, the British Society of Paediatric Dentistry and the British Association for the Study of Community Dentistry (*Br Dent J* 1997; **182**: 6–7).

- **CONTRA-INDICATIONS** Not for areas where drinking water is fluoridated
- **SIDE-EFFECTS**
▸ **Uncommon** Occasional white flecks on teeth with recommended doses
▸ **Rare** Yellowish-brown discoloration if recommended doses are exceeded

- **DIRECTIONS FOR ADMINISTRATION** Tablets should be sucked or dissolved in the mouth and taken preferably in the evening. For mouthwash, rinse mouth for 1 minute and then spit out.

COLGATE DURAPHAT® 2800PPM FLUORIDE TOOTHPASTE Brush teeth for 1 minute before spitting out.

COLGATE DURAPHAT® 5000PPM FLUORIDE TOOTHPASTE Brush teeth for 3 minutes before spitting out.

- **PRESCRIBING AND DISPENSING INFORMATION** Flavours of oral tablet formulations may include orange.
- **PATIENT AND CARER ADVICE**
Mouthwash Avoid eating, drinking, or rinsing mouth for 15 minutes after use.

COLGATE DURAPHAT® 2800PPM FLUORIDE TOOTHPASTE Patients or carers should be given advice on how to administer sodium fluoride toothpaste. Avoid drinking or rinsing mouth for 30 minutes after use.

COLGATE DURAPHAT® 5000PPM FLUORIDE TOOTHPASTE Patients or carers should be given advice on how to administer Sodium fluoride toothpaste.

- **PROFESSION SPECIFIC INFORMATION**
Dental practitioners' formulary
Tablets may be prescribed as Sodium Fluoride Tablets. Oral drops may be prescribed as Sodium Fluoride Oral Drops.
Mouthwashes may be prescribed as Sodium Fluoride Mouthwash 0.05% or Sodium Fluoride Mouthwash 2%.

COLGATE DURAPHAT® 2800PPM FLUORIDE TOOTHPASTE May be prescribed as Sodium Fluoride Toothpaste 0.619%.

COLGATE DURAPHAT® 5000PPM FLUORIDE TOOTHPASTE May be prescribed as Sodium Fluoride Toothpaste 1.1%.

Dental information
Fluoride mouthwash, oral drops, tablets and toothpaste are prescribable on form FP10D (GP14 in Scotland, WP10D in Wales.

There are also arrangements for health authorities to supply fluoride tablets in the course of pre-school dental schemes, and they may also be supplied in school dental schemes.

Fluoride gels are not prescribable on form FP10D (GP14 in Scotland, WP10D in Wales).

- **MEDICINAL FORMS**
There can be variation in the licensing of different medicines containing the same drug.

Tablet
▸ **Endekay** (Manx Healthcare Ltd)
Sodium fluoride 1.1 mg Endekay Fluotabs 3-6 Years 1.1mg tablets | 200 tablet P £2.38 DT price = £2.38
Sodium fluoride 2.2 mg Endekay Fluotabs 6+ Years 2.2mg tablets | 200 tablet P £2.38 DT price = £2.38

Chewable tablet
▸ **Fluor-a-day** (Dental Health Products Ltd)
Sodium fluoride 1.1 mg Fluor-a-day 1.1mg chewable tablets sugar-free | 200 tablet P £2.79 DT price = £2.79
Sodium fluoride 2.2 mg Fluor-a-day 2.2mg chewable tablets sugar-free | 200 tablet P £2.79 DT price = £2.79

Oral drops
▸ **Endekay** (Manx Healthcare Ltd)
Sodium fluoride 3.7 mg per 1 ml Endekay Fluodrops 0.37% drops paediatric sugar-free | 60 ml P £2.38 DT price = £2.38

Paste
▸ **Colgate Duraphat** (Colgate-Palmolive (UK) Ltd)
Fluoride (as Sodium fluoride) 2.8 mg per 1 gram Colgate Durapha 2800ppm fluoride toothpaste sugar-free | 75 ml PoM £3.26 DT price = £3.26
Fluoride (as Sodium fluoride) 5 mg per 1 gram Colgate Duraphat 5000ppm fluoride toothpaste sugar-free | 51 gram PoM £6.50 DT price = £6.50

Mouthwash

- **Sodium fluoride** (Non-proprietary)
  Sodium fluoride 500 microgram per 1 ml Sodium fluoride 0.05% mouthwash sugar free sugar-free | 250 ml [GSL] no price available sugar-free | 400 ml [GSL] no price available sugar-free | 500 ml [GSL] no price available
- **Colgate FluoriGard** (Colgate-Palmolive (UK) Ltd)
  Sodium fluoride 500 microgram per 1 ml Colgate FluoriGard 0.05% daily dental rinse alcohol free sugar-free | 400 ml £2.99
  Colgate FluoriGard 0.05% daily dental rinse sugar-free | 400 ml [GSL] £2.99
- **Endekay** (Manx Healthcare Ltd)
  Sodium fluoride 500 microgram per 1 ml Endekay 0.05% daily fluoride mouthrinse sugar-free | 250 ml [GSL] £1.50 sugar-free | 500 ml [GSL] £2.43
  Sodium fluoride 20 mg per 1 ml Endekay Fluorinse 2% mouthwash sugar-free | 100 ml [PoM] £4.97

3   Oral ulceration and inflammation

Oral ulceration and inflammation

Ulceration and inflammation

Ulceration of the oral mucosa may be caused by trauma (physical or chemical), recurrent aphthae, infections, carcinoma, dermatological disorders, nutritional deficiencies, gastro-intestinal disease, haematopoietic disorders, and drug therapy. It is important to establish the diagnosis in each case as the majority of these lesions require specific management in addition to local treatment. Local treatment aims to protect the ulcerated area, to relieve pain, to reduce inflammation, or to control secondary infection. Children with an unexplained mouth ulcer of more than 3 weeks' duration require urgent referral to hospital to exclude oral cancer in adults or secondary causes such as leukaemia.

Simple mouthwashes

A **saline** mouthwash may relieve the pain of traumatic ulceration. The mouthwash is made up with warm water and used at frequent intervals until the discomfort and swelling subsides.

Antiseptic mouthwashes

Secondary bacterial infection may be a feature of any mucosal ulceration; it can increase discomfort and delay healing. Use of chlorhexidine mouthwash p. 656 is often beneficial and may accelerate healing of recurrent aphthae.

Corticosteroids

Topical corticosteroid therapy may be used for some forms of oral ulceration. In the case of aphthous ulcers it is most effective if applied in the 'prodromal' phase. Thrush or other types of candidiasis are recognised complications of corticosteroid treatment.

Hydrocortisone **oromucosal tablets** p. 661 are allowed to dissolve next to an ulcer and are useful in recurrent aphthae and erosive lichenoid lesions.

Beclometasone dipropionate inhaler p. 150 sprayed on the oral mucosa is used to manage oral ulceration [unlicensed indication]. Alternatively, betamethasone soluble tablets p. 660 dissolved in water can be used as a mouthwash to treat oral ulceration [unlicensed indication].

Systemic corticosteroid therapy (see under Corticosteroids, inflammatory disorders p. 616) is reserved for severe conditions such as pemphigus vulgaris.

Local analgesics

Local analgesics have a limited role in the management of oral ulceration. When applied topically their action is of a relatively short duration so that analgesia cannot be maintained continuously throughout the day. When local anaesthetics are used in the mouth, care must be taken not to produce anaesthesia of the pharynx before meals as this might lead to choking.

Benzydamine hydrochloride p. 660 and flurbiprofen p. 660 are non-steroidal anti-inflammatory drugs (NSAIDs). Benzydamine hydrochloride mouthwash or spray may be useful in reducing the discomfort associated with a variety of ulcerative conditions. It has also been found to be effective in reducing the discomfort of tonsillectomy and post-irradiation mucositis. Some patients find the full-strength mouthwash causes some stinging and, for them, it should be diluted with an equal volume of water. Flurbiprofen lozenges are licensed for the relief of sore throat in adolescents.

Choline salicylate p. 661 is a derivative of salicylic acid and has some analgesic action. The dental gel may provide relief for recurrent aphthae, but excessive application or confinement under a denture irritates the mucosa and can itself cause ulceration in adults and children over 16 years of age.

Other preparations

Doxycycline p. 662 rinsed in the mouth may be of value for recurrent aphthous ulceration.

Periodontitis

Low-dose doxycycline (*Periostat*®) is licensed as an adjunct to scaling and root planing for the treatment of periodontitis; a low dose of doxycycline reduces collagenase activity without inhibiting bacteria associated with periodontitis.

For anti-infectives used in the treatment of destructive (refractory) forms of periodontal disease, see under Oropharyngeal bacterial infections p. 661. See also Mouthwashes and other preparations for oropharyngeal use p. 655 for mouthwashes used for oral hygiene and plaque inhibition.

ANAESTHETICS, LOCAL

Lidocaine hydrochloride

(Lignocaine hydrochloride)

- **INDICATIONS AND DOSE**

Dental practice
- ▸ BY BUCCAL ADMINISTRATION USING OINTMENT
- ▸ Child: Rub gently into dry gum

LARYNGOJET®

Anaesthesia of mucous membranes of oropharynx, trachea, or respiratory tract
- ▸ TO MUCOUS MEMBRANES
- ▸ Child: Up to 3 mg/kg (max. per dose 200 mg), to be given as a single dose sprayed, instilled (if a cavity) or applied with a swab; reduce dose according to size, age, and condition of child

XYLOCAINE®

Bronchoscopy | Laryngoscopy | Oesophagoscopy | Endotracheal intubation
- ▸ TO MUCOUS MEMBRANES
- ▸ Child: Up to 3 mg/kg

- **CAUTIONS** Can damage plastic cuffs of endotracheal tubes
- **INTERACTIONS** → Appendix 1 (lidocaine). Interactions less likely when lidocaine used topically.
- **SIDE-EFFECTS**

  SIDE-EFFECTS, FURTHER INFORMATION
  A single application of a topical lidocaine preparation does not generally cause systemic side-effects.
- **ALLERGY AND CROSS-SENSITIVITY**
- ▸ Hypersensitivity and cross-sensitivity Hypersensitivity reactions occur mainly with the ester-type local anaesthetics, such as tetracaine and chloroprocaine;

reactions are less frequent with the amide types, such as articaine, bupivacaine, levobupivacaine, lidocaine, mepivacaine, prilocaine, and ropivacaine. Cross-sensitivity reactions may be avoided by using the alternative chemical type.

● **PREGNANCY** Crosses the placenta but not known to be harmful in *animal* studies—use if benefit outweighs risk. When used as a local anaesthetic, large doses can cause fetal bradycardia; if given during delivery can also cause neonatal respiratory depression, hypotonia, or bradycardia after paracervical or epidural block.

● **BREAST FEEDING** Present in milk but amount too small to be harmful.

● **HEPATIC IMPAIRMENT** Caution—increased risk of side-effects.

● **RENAL IMPAIRMENT** Possible accumulation of lidocaine and active metabolite; caution in severe impairment.

● **PROFESSION SPECIFIC INFORMATION**
Dental practitioners' formulary
Lidocaine ointment 5% may be prescribed. Spray may be prescribed as Lidocaine Spray 10%
XYLOCAINE®
May be prescribed as lidocaine spray 10%.

● **MEDICINAL FORMS**
There can be variation in the licensing of different medicines containing the same drug.
Ointment
▸ Lidocaine hydrochloride (Non-proprietary)
Lidocaine hydrochloride 50 mg per 1 gram Lidocaine 5% ointment | 15 gram Ⓟ £6.50 DT price = £6.18
Spray
▸ Xylocaine (AstraZeneca UK Ltd)
Lidocaine 10 mg per 1 actuation Xylocaine 10mg/dose spray sugar-free | 50 ml Ⓟ £6.29
Liquid
▸ Laryngojet (UCB Pharma Ltd)
Lidocaine hydrochloride 40 mg per 1 mL Lidocaine 4% oromucosal solution | 1 pre-filled disposable injection PoM £5.10

ANALGESICS ❯ NON-STEROIDAL ANTI-INFLAMMATORY DRUGS

Benzydamine hydrochloride

● **INDICATIONS AND DOSE**
Painful inflammatory conditions of oropharynx
▸ **TO THE LESION USING MOUTHWASH**
▸ Child 13–17 years: Rinse or gargle 15 mL every 1.5–3 hours as required usually for not more than 7 days, dilute with an equal volume of water if stinging occurs
▸ **TO THE LESION USING OROMUCOSAL SPRAY**
▸ Child 1 month–5 years (body-weight 4–7 kg): 1 spray every 1.5–3 hours, to be administered onto the affected area
▸ Child 1 month–5 years (body-weight 8–11 kg): 2 sprays every 1.5–3 hours, to be administered onto the affected area
▸ Child 1 month–5 years (body-weight 12–15 kg): 3 sprays every 1.5–3 hours, to be administered onto the affected area
▸ Child 1 month–5 years (body-weight 16 kg and above): 4 sprays every 1.5–3 hours, to be administered onto the affected area
▸ Child 6–11 years: 4 sprays every 1.5–3 hours, to be administered onto affected area
▸ Child 12–17 years: 4–8 sprays every 1.5–3 hours, to be administered onto affected area

● **SIDE-EFFECTS**
▸ **Rare** Hypersensitivity reactions
▸ **Frequency not known** Occasional numbness or stinging

● **PROFESSION SPECIFIC INFORMATION**
Dental practitioners' formulary
Benzydamine Oromucosal Spray 0.15% may be prescribed. Benzydamine mouthwash may be prescribed as Benzydamine Mouthwash 0.15%.

● **MEDICINAL FORMS**
There can be variation in the licensing of different medicines containing the same drug.
Spray
▸ Benzydamine hydrochloride (Non-proprietary)
Benzydamine hydrochloride 1.5 mg per 1 ml Benzydamine 0.15% oromucosal spray sugar free sugar-free | 30 ml Ⓟ £4.64 DT price = £4.49
▸ Difflam (Meda Pharmaceuticals Ltd)
Benzydamine hydrochloride 1.5 mg per 1 ml Difflam 0.15% spray sugar-free | 30 ml Ⓟ £4.24 DT price = £4.49
Mouthwash
▸ Benzydamine hydrochloride (Non-proprietary)
Benzydamine hydrochloride 1.5 mg per 1 ml Benzydamine 0.15% mouthwash sugar free sugar-free | 300 ml Ⓟ £7.14 DT price = £6.01
▸ Difflam (Meda Pharmaceuticals Ltd)
Benzydamine hydrochloride 1.5 mg per 1 ml Difflam Oral Rinse 0.15% solution sugar-free | 300 ml Ⓟ £6.50 DT price = £6.01
Difflam 0.15% Sore Throat Rinse sugar-free | 200 ml Ⓟ £4.64

Flurbiprofen

● **INDICATIONS AND DOSE**
Relief of sore throat
▸ **BY MOUTH USING LOZENGES**
▸ Child 12–17 years: 1 lozenge every 3–6 hours for maximum 3 days, allow lozenge to dissolve slowly in the mouth; maximum 5 lozenges per day

● **INTERACTIONS** → Appendix 1 (NSAIDs).

● **SIDE-EFFECTS** Mouth ulcers (move lozenge around mouth) · taste disturbance

● **ALLERGY AND CROSS-SENSITIVITY** Contra-indicated in patients with a history of hypersensitivity to aspirin or any other NSAID—which includes those in whom attacks of asthma, angioedema, urticaria or rhinitis have been precipitated by aspirin or any other NSAID.

● **MEDICINAL FORMS**
There can be variation in the licensing of different medicines containing the same drug.
Lozenge
▸ Strefen (Reckitt Benckiser Healthcare (UK) Ltd)
Flurbiprofen 8.75 mg Strefen 8.75mg lozenges | 16 lozenge Ⓟ £2.58 DT price = £2.58

CORTICOSTEROIDS

Betamethasone

● **INDICATIONS AND DOSE**
Oral ulceration
▸ **BY MOUTH USING SOLUBLE TABLETS**
▸ Child 12–17 years: 500 micrograms 4 times a day, to be dissolved in 20 mL water and rinsed around the mouth; not to be swallowed

● **UNLICENSED USE** Betamethasone soluble tablets not licensed for use as mouthwash or in oral ulceration.

● **CONTRA-INDICATIONS** Untreated local infection

● **SIDE-EFFECTS** Candidal infection · exacerbation of local infection

● **PATIENT AND CARER ADVICE** Patient counselling is advised for betamethasone soluble tablets (administration).

● PROFESSION SPECIFIC INFORMATION

Dental practitioners' formulary
Betamethasone Soluble Tablets 500 micrograms may be prescribed for oral ulceration.

● MEDICINAL FORMS
There can be variation in the licensing of different medicines containing the same drug.
Soluble tablet
CAUTIONARY AND ADVISORY LABELS 10, 13, 21 (not for use as mouthwash for oral ulceration)
▸ Betamethasone (Non-proprietary)
  Betamethasone (as Betamethasone sodium phosphate)
  500 microgram Betamethasone 500microgram soluble tablets sugar free sugar-free | 100 tablet [PoM] £42.60 DT price = £42.04

Hydrocortisone

● INDICATIONS AND DOSE
Oral and perioral lesions
▸ TO THE LESION USING BUCCAL TABLET
▸ Child 1 month–11 years: Only on medical advice
▸ Child 12–17 years: 1 lozenge 4 times a day, allowed to dissolve slowly in the mouth in contact with the ulcer

● UNLICENSED USE *Hydrocortisone mucoadhesive buccal tablets* licensed for use in children (under 12 years—on medical advice only).
● CONTRA-INDICATIONS Untreated local infection
● SIDE-EFFECTS Candidal infection · exacerbation of local infection
● PROFESSION SPECIFIC INFORMATION

Dental practitioners' formulary
Mucoadhesive buccal tablets may be prescribed as Hydrocortisone Oromucosal Tablets.

● MEDICINAL FORMS
There can be variation in the licensing of different medicines containing the same drug.
Muco-adhesive buccal tablet
▸ Hydrocortisone (Non-proprietary)
  Hydrocortisone (as Hydrocortisone sodium succinate)
  2.5 mg Hydrocortisone 2.5mg muco-adhesive buccal tablets sugar free sugar-free | 20 tablet [P] £5.81 DT price = £5.05

SALICYLIC ACID AND DERIVATIVES

Choline salicylate

● INDICATIONS AND DOSE
Mild oral and perioral lesions
▸ TO THE LESION
▸ Child 16–17 years: Apply 0.5 inch, apply with gentle massage, not more often than every 3 hours

● CONTRA-INDICATIONS Children under 16 years
CONTRA-INDICATIONS, FURTHER INFORMATION
▸ Reye's syndrome The CHM has advised that topical oral pain relief products containing salicylate salts should not be used in children under 16 years, as a cautionary measure due to the theoretical risk of Reye's syndrome.
● CAUTIONS Frequent application, especially in children, may give rise to salicylate poisoning
● SIDE-EFFECTS Transient local burning sensation
● PRESCRIBING AND DISPENSING INFORMATION When prepared extemporaneously, the BP states Choline Salicylate Dental Gel, BP consists of choline salicylate 8.7% in a flavoured gel basis.
● PROFESSION SPECIFIC INFORMATION

Dental practitioners' formulary
Choline Salicylate Dental Gel may be prescribed.

● MEDICINAL FORMS
There can be variation in the licensing of different medicines containing the same drug.
Oromucosal gel
▸ Bonjela (Reckitt Benckiser Healthcare (UK) Ltd)
  Choline salicylate 87 mg per 1 gram Bonjela Cool Mint gel sugar-free | 15 gram [GSL] £3.07 DT price = £2.58
  Bonjela Original gel sugar-free | 15 gram [GSL] £2.58 DT price = £2.58

Salicylic acid with rhubarb extract

● INDICATIONS AND DOSE
Mild oral and perioral lesions
▸ TO THE LESION
▸ Child 16–17 years: Apply 3–4 times a day maximum duration 7 days

● CONTRA-INDICATIONS Children under 16 years
CONTRA-INDICATIONS, FURTHER INFORMATION
▸ Reye's syndrome The CHM has advised that topical oral pain relief products containing salicylate salts should not be used in children under 16 years, as a cautionary measure due to the theoretical risk of Reye's syndrome.
● CAUTIONS Frequent application, especially in children, may give rise to salicylate poisoning
● SIDE-EFFECTS Temporary discolouration of oral mucosa · temporary discolouration of teeth · transient local burning sensation
● PATIENT AND CARER ADVICE May cause temporary discolouration of teeth and oral mucosa.

● MEDICINAL FORMS
There can be variation in the licensing of different medicines containing the same drug.
Paint
EXCIPIENTS: May contain Ethanol
▸ Pyralvex (Meda Pharmaceuticals Ltd)
  Salicylic acid 10 mg per 1 ml, Rhubarb extract 50 mg per 1 ml Pyralvex solution | 10 ml [P] £3.25

4 Oropharyngeal bacterial infections

Oropharyngeal bacterial infections

Antibacterial therapy for pericoronitis

Antibacterial required only in presence of systemic features of infection, or of trismus, or persistent swelling despite local treatment.

● Metronidazole p. 313, or *alternatively*, amoxicillin p. 320
▸ *Suggested duration of treatment* 3 days or until symptoms resolve.

Antibacterial therapy for gingivitis: acute necrotising ulcerative

Antibacterial required only if systemic features of infection.

● Metronidazole, or *alternatively*, amoxicillin
▸ *Suggested duration of treatment* 3 days or until symptoms resolve.

Antibacterial therapy for periapical or periodontal abscess

Antibacterial required only in severe disease with cellulitis or if systemic features of infection.

● Amoxicillin, or *alternatively*, metronidazole
▸ *Suggested duration of treatment* 5 days.

Antibacterial therapy for periodontitis

Antibacterial used as an adjunct to debridement in severe disease or disease unresponsive to local treatment alone.

- Metronidazole, or *alternatively in children over 12 years*, doxycycline below

Antibacterial therapy for throat infections

Most throat infections are caused by viruses and many do not require antibacterial therapy. Consider antibacterial, if history of valvular heart disease, if marked systemic upset, if peritonsillar cellulitis or abscess, or if at increased risk from acute infection (e.g. in immunosuppression, cystic fibrosis); prescribe antibacterial for beta-haemolytic streptococcal pharyngitis.

- Phenoxymethylpenicillin p. 319
- ▸ In severe infection, initial parenteral therapy with benzylpenicillin sodium p. 318, then oral therapy with phenoxymethylpenicillin *or* amoxicillin (*or* ampicillin p. 321). **Avoid** amoxicillin if possibility of glandular fever.
- ▸ *Suggested duration of treatment* 10 days.
- *If penicillin-allergic*, clarithromycin p. 309 (*or* azithromycin p. 308 *or* erythromycin p. 310)
- ▸ *Suggested duration of treatment* 10 days

ANTIBACTERIALS ⟩ TETRACYCLINES AND RELATED DRUGS

▌ Doxycycline

- ● **INDICATIONS AND DOSE**
  Treatment of recurrent aphthous ulceration
  - ▸ BY MOUTH USING SOLUBLE TABLETS
  - ▸ Child 12–17 years: 100 mg 4 times a day usually for 3 days, dispersible tablet can be stirred into a small amount of water then rinsed around the mouth for 2–3 minutes, it should preferably not be swallowed

- ● **UNLICENSED USE** Not licensed for use in children under 12 years. Not licensed for severe aphthous ulceration.

- ● **CAUTIONS** Alcohol dependence

- ● **INTERACTIONS** The metabolism of doxycycline may be influenced by antiepileptics.

- ● **SIDE-EFFECTS** Anorexia · anxiety · dry mouth · flushing · tinnitus

- ● **RENAL IMPAIRMENT** Use with caution (avoid excessive doses).

- ● **PATIENT AND CARER ADVICE** Counselling on administration advised.
  Photosensitivity Patients should be advised to avoid exposure to sunlight or sun lamps.

- ● **PROFESSION SPECIFIC INFORMATION**
  Dental practitioners' formulary
  Dispersible tablets may be prescribed as Dispersible Doxycycline Tablets.

- ● **MEDICINAL FORMS**
  There can be variation in the licensing of different medicines containing the same drug.
  Dispersible tablet
  CAUTIONARY AND ADVISORY LABELS 6, 9, 11, 13
  - ▸ Vibramycin-D (Pfizer Ltd)
    Doxycycline (as Doxycycline monohydrate) 100 mg Vibramycin-D 100mg dispersible tablets sugar-free | 8 tablet [PoM] £4.91 DT price = £4.91

5 Oropharyngeal fungal infections

Oropharyngeal fungal infections

Overview

Fungal infections of the mouth are usually caused by *Candida* spp. (candidiasis or candidosis). Different types of oropharyngeal candidiasis are managed as follows:

Thrush

Acute pseudomembranous candidiasis (thrush), is usually an acute infection but it may persist for months in patients receiving inhaled corticosteroids, cytotoxics, or broad-spectrum antibacterials. Thrush also occurs in patients with serious systemic disease associated with reduced immunity such as leukaemia, other malignancies, and HIV infection. Any predisposing condition should be managed appropriately. When thrush is associated with corticosteroid inhalers, rinsing the mouth with water (or cleaning a child's teeth) immediately after using the inhaler may avoid the problem. Treatment with nystatin p. 663 or miconazole p. 663 may be needed. Fluconazole p. 352 is effective for unresponsive infections or if a topical antifungal drug cannot be used. Topical therapy may not be adequate in immunocompromised children and an oral triazole antifungal is preferred.

Acute erythematous candidiasis

Acute erythematous (atrophic) candidiasis is a relatively uncommon condition associated with corticosteroid and broad-spectrum antibacterial use and with HIV disease. It is usually treated with fluconazole.

Angular cheilitis

Angular cheilitis (angular stomatitis) is characterised by soreness, erythema and fissuring at the angles of the mouth. It may represent a nutritional deficiency or it may be related to orofacial granulomatosis or HIV infection. Both yeasts (*Candida* spp.) and bacteria (*Staphylococcus aureus* and beta-haemolytic streptococci) are commonly involved as interacting, infective factors. While the underlying cause is being identified and treated, it is often helpful to apply miconazole cream or fusidic acid ointment p. 336; if the angular cheilitis is unresponsive to treatment, hydrocortisone with miconazole cream or ointment p. 698 can be used.

Immunocompromised patients

See advice on prevention of fungal infections under *Immunocompromised children* in Antifungals, systemic use p. 349.

Antiseptic mouthwashes can have a role in the prevention of oral candidiasis in immunocompromised children.

Drugs used in oropharyngeal candidiasis

Nystatin is not absorbed from the gastro-intestinal tract and is applied locally (as a suspension) to the mouth for treating local fungal infections. Miconazole is used by local application (as an oral gel) in the mouth but it is also absorbed to the extent that potential interactions need to be considered. Miconazole also has some activity against Gram-positive bacteria including streptococci and staphylococci. In neonates, nystatin oral suspension or miconazole oral gel is used for the treatment of oropharyngeal candidiasis; to prevent re-infection it is important to ensure that the mother's breast nipples and the teats of feeding bottles are cleaned adequately.

Fluconazole given by mouth is reliably absorbed; it is used for infections that do not respond to topical therapy or when topical therapy cannot be used. Itraconazole p. 353 can be used for fluconazole-resistant infections.

If candidal infection fails to respond after 1 to 2 weeks of treatment with antifungal drugs the child should be sent for investigation to eliminate the possibility of underlying disease. Persistent infection may also be caused by re-infection from the genito-urinary or gastro-intestinal tract.

ANTIFUNGALS > IMIDAZOLE ANTIFUNGALS

Miconazole

- **INDICATIONS AND DOSE**

Prevention and treatment of oral candidiasis
▸ BY MOUTH USING ORAL GEL

▸ Neonate: 1 mL 2–4 times a day treatment should be continued for at least 7 days after lesions have healed or symptoms have cleared, to be smeared around the inside of the mouth after feeds.

▸ Child 1 month–1 year: 1.25 mL 4 times a day treatment should be continued for at least 7 days after lesions have healed or symptoms have cleared, to be smeared around the inside of the mouth after feeds

▸ Child 2–17 years: 2.5 mL 4 times a day treatment should be continued for at least 7 days after lesions have healed or symptoms have cleared, to be administered after meals, retain near oral lesions before swallowing (dental prostheses and orthodontic appliances should be removed at night and brushed with gel)

Prevention and treatment of intestinal candidiasis
▸ BY MOUTH USING ORAL GEL

▸ Child 4 months–17 years: 5 mg/kg 4 times a day (max. per dose 250 mg 4 times a day) treatment should be continued for at least 7 days after lesions have healed or symptoms have cleared

- **UNLICENSED USE** Not licensed for use in children under 4 months of age or during first 5–6 months of life of an infant born pre-term.

- **CONTRA-INDICATIONS** Infants with impaired swallowing reflex

- **CAUTIONS** Avoid in Acute porphyrias p. 562

- **INTERACTIONS** → Appendix 1 (antifungals, imidazole).

- **SIDE-EFFECTS**
- **Common or very common** Nausea · rash · vomiting
- **Very rare** Diarrhoea (usually on long term treatment) · hepatitis · rash · Stevens-Johnson syndrome · toxic epidermal necrolysis

- **PREGNANCY** Manufacturer advises avoid if possible—toxicity at high doses in *animal* studies.

- **BREAST FEEDING** Manufacturer advises caution—no information available.

- **HEPATIC IMPAIRMENT** Avoid.

- **DIRECTIONS FOR ADMINISTRATION** Oral gel should be held in mouth, after food.

- **PRESCRIBING AND DISPENSING INFORMATION** Flavours of oral gel may include orange.

- **PATIENT AND CARER ADVICE** Patients or carers should be given advice on how to administer miconazole oromucosal gel.

- **PROFESSION SPECIFIC INFORMATION**
Dental practitioners' formulary
Miconazole Oromucosal Gel may be prescribed.

- **EXCEPTIONS TO LEGAL CATEGORY** 15-g tube of oral gel can be sold to the public.

- **MEDICINAL FORMS**
There can be variation in the licensing of different medicines containing the same drug.
Oromucosal gel
CAUTIONARY AND ADVISORY LABELS 9
▸ Daktarin (McNeil Products Ltd, Janssen-Cilag Ltd)
Miconazole 20 mg per 1 gram Daktarin 20mg/g oromucosal gel sugar-free | 15 gram Ⓟ £3.23 DT price = £3.23 sugar-free | 80 gram PoM £4.38 DT price = £4.38

ANTIFUNGALS > POLYENE ANTIFUNGALS

Nystatin

6.6.2016

- **INDICATIONS AND DOSE**

Oral and perioral fungal infections
▸ BY MOUTH

▸ Neonate: 100 000 units 4 times a day usually for 7 days, and continued for 48 hours after lesions have resolved.

▸ Child 1 month–1 year: 200 000 units 4 times a day usually for 7 days, and continued for 48 hours after lesions have resolved, divide administration of the dose between both sides of the mouth

▸ Child 2–17 years: 400 000–600 000 units 4 times a day usually for 7 days, and continued for 48 hours after lesions have resolved, divide administration of the dose between both sides of the mouth

- **SIDE-EFFECTS** Nausea · local irritation · local sensitisation

- **PATIENT AND CARER ADVICE**
Medicines for Children leaflet: Nystatin for Candida infection www.medicinesforchildren.org.uk/nystatin-for-candida-infection

Counselling advised with oral suspension (use of pipette, hold in mouth, after food).

- **PROFESSION SPECIFIC INFORMATION**
Dental practitioners' formulary
Nystatin Oral Suspension may be prescribed.

- **MEDICINAL FORMS**
There can be variation in the licensing of different medicines containing the same drug. Forms available from special-order manufacturers include: oral suspension
Oral suspension
CAUTIONARY AND ADVISORY LABELS 9
EXCIPIENTS: May contain Ethanol
▸ Nystatin (Non-proprietary)
Nystatin 100000 unit per 1 ml Nystatin 100,000units/ml oral suspension | 30 ml PoM £22.44 DT price = £2.73
▸ Nystan (Bristol-Myers Squibb Pharmaceuticals Ltd)
Nystatin 100000 unit per 1 ml Nystan 100,000units/ml oral suspension (ready mixed) | 30 ml PoM £1.80 DT price = £2.73

6   Oropharyngeal viral infections

Oropharyngeal viral infections

Management

Viral infections are the most common cause of a sore throat. It is usually a self-limiting condition which does not benefit from anti-infective treatment. Adequate analgesia may be all that is required.

Children with varicella–zoster infection often develop painful lesions in the mouth and throat. Benzydamine hydrochloride p. 660 may be used to provide local analgesia. Chlorhexidine mouthwash or gel p. 656 will control plaque accumulation if toothbrushing is painful and will also help to control secondary infection in general.

12

Ear, nose and oropharynx

In severe herpetic stomatitis systemic aciclovir p. 381 or valaciclovir p. 383 may be used for oral lesions associated with herpes zoster. Aciclovir and valaciclovir are also used to prevent frequently recurring herpes simplex lesions of the mouth particularly when associated with the initiation of erythema multiforme. See the treatment of labial herpes simplex infections.

Chapter 13
Skin

CONTENTS

1	**Dry and scaling skin disorders**	page 666
2	**Infections of the skin**	673
2.1	Bacterial skin infections	675
2.2	Fungal skin infections	678
2.3	Parasitic skin infections	682
2.4	Viral skin infections	683
3	**Inflammatory skin conditions**	683
3.1	Eczema and psoriasis	683
4	**Perspiration**	705
4.1	Hyperhidrosis	705
5	**Photodamage**	706

6	**Pruritus**	page 707
7	**Rosacea and acne**	708
7.1	Acne	709
8	**Scalp and hair conditions**	714
9	**Skin cleansers, antiseptics and desloughing agents**	715
9.1	Minor cuts and abrasions	719
10	**Skin disfigurement**	719
11	**Superficial soft-tissue injuries and superficial thrombophlebitis**	720
12	**Warts and calluses**	720

13

Skin

Skin conditions, management

Topical preparations

When prescribing topical preparations for the treatment of skin conditions in children, the site of application, the condition being treated, and the child's (and carer's) preference for a particular vehicle all need to be taken into consideration.

Vehicles

The British Association of Dermatologists list of preferred unlicensed dermatological preparations (specials) is available at www.bad.org.uk.

The vehicle in topical preparations for the skin affects the degree of hydration, has a mild anti-inflammatory effect, and aids the penetration of the active drug. Therefore, the vehicle, as well as the active drug, should be chosen on the basis of their suitability for the child's skin condition.

Applications are usually viscous solutions, emulsions, or suspensions for application to the skin (including the scalp) or nails.

Collodions are painted on the skin and allowed to dry to leave a flexible film over the site of application.

Creams are emulsions of oil and water and are generally well absorbed into the skin. They may contain an antimicrobial preservative unless the active ingredient or basis is intrinsically bactericidal and fungicidal. Generally, creams are cosmetically more acceptable than ointments because they are less greasy and easier to apply.

Gels consist of active ingredients in suitable hydrophilic or hydrophobic bases; they generally have a high water content. Gels are particularly suitable for application to the face and scalp.

Lotions have a cooling effect and may be preferred to ointments or creams for application over a hairy area. Lotions in alcoholic basis can sting if used on broken skin. *Shake lotions* (such as calamine lotion) contain insoluble powders which leave a deposit on the skin surface.

Ointments are greasy preparations which are normally anhydrous and insoluble in water, and are more occlusive than creams. They are particularly suitable for chronic, dry lesions. The most commonly used ointment bases consist of soft paraffin or a combination of soft, liquid, and hard paraffin. Some ointment bases have both *hydrophilic and lipophilic* properties; they may have occlusive properties on the skin surface, encourage hydration, and also be miscible with water;

they often have a mild anti-inflammatory effect. *Water-soluble ointments* contain macrogols which are freely soluble in water and are therefore readily washed off; they have a limited but useful role where ready removal is desirable.

Pastes are stiff preparations containing a high proportion of finely powdered solids such as zinc oxide and starch suspended in an ointment. They are used for circumscribed lesions such as those which occur in lichen simplex, chronic eczema, or psoriasis. They are less occlusive than ointments and can be used to protect inflamed, lichenified, or excoriated skin.

Dusting powders are used only rarely. They reduce friction between opposing skin surfaces. Dusting powders should not be applied to moist areas because they can cake and abrade the skin. Talc is a lubricant but it does not absorb moisture; it can cause respiratory irritation. Starch is less lubricant but absorbs water.

Dilution

The BP directs that creams and ointments should **not** normally be diluted but that should dilution be necessary care should be taken, in particular, to prevent microbial contamination. The appropriate diluent should be used and heating should be avoided during mixing; excessive dilution may affect the stability of some creams. Diluted creams should normally be used within 2 weeks of preparation.

Suitable quantities for prescribing

Suitable quantities of dermatological preparations to be prescribed for specific areas of the body		
Area of body	Creams and Ointments	Lotions
Face	15–30 g	100 ml
Both hands	25–50 g	200 ml
Scalp	50–100 g	200 ml
Both arms or both legs	100–200 g	200 ml
Trunk	400 g	500 ml
Groins and genitalia	15–25 g	100 ml
These amounts are usually suitable for children 12-17 years for twice daily application for 1 week; smaller quantities will be required for children under 12 years. These recommendations **do not apply to corticosteroid preparations**.		

Excipients and sensitisation

Excipients in topical products rarely cause problems. If a patch test indicates allergy to an excipient, products containing the substance should be avoided (see also Anaphylaxis). The following excipients in topical preparations are associated, rarely, with sensitisation; the presence of these excipients is indicated in the entries for topical products. See also Excipients, under General Guidance.

- Beeswax
- Benzyl alcohol
- Butylated hydroxyanisole
- Butylated hydroxytoluene
- Cetostearyl alcohol (including cetyl and stearyl alcohol)
- Chlorocresol
- Edetic acid (EDTA)
- Ethylenediamine
- Fragrances
- Hydroxybenzoates (parabens)
- Imidurea
- Isopropyl palmitate
- N-(3-Chloroallyl)hexaminium chloride (quaternium 15)
- Polysorbates
- Propylene glycol
- Sodium metabisulfite
- Sorbic acid
- Wool fat and related substances including lanolin (purified versions of wool fat have reduced the problem)

Neonates

Caution is required when prescribing topical preparations for neonates—their large body surface area in relation to body mass increases susceptibility to toxicity from systemic absorption of substances applied to the skin. Topical preparations containing potentially sensitising substances such as corticosteroids, aminoglycosides, iodine, and parasiticidal drugs should be avoided. Preparations containing alcohol should be avoided because they can dehydrate the skin, cause pain if applied to raw areas, and the alcohol can cause necrosis. In *preterm neonates*, the skin is more fragile and offers a poor barrier, especially in the first fortnight after birth. Preterm infants, especially if below 32 weeks corrected gestational age, may also require special measures to maintain skin hydration.

1 Dry and scaling skin disorders

Emollient and barrier preparations

Borderline substances

The preparations marked 'ACBS' are regarded as drugs when prescribed in accordance with the advice of the Advisory Committee on Borderline Substances for the clinical conditions listed. Prescriptions issued in accordance with this advice and endorsed 'ACBS' will normally not be investigated.

Emollients

Emollients hydrate the skin, soften the skin, act as barrier to water and external irritants, and are indicated for all dry or scaling disorders. Their effects are short-lived and they should be applied frequently even after improvement occurs. They are useful in dry and eczematous disorders, and to a lesser extent in psoriasis; they should be applied immediately after washing or bathing to maximise the effect of skin hydration. The choice of an appropriate emollient will depend on the severity of the condition, the child's (or

carer's) preference, and the site of application. Ointments may exacerbate acne and folliculitis. Some ingredients rarely cause sensitisation and this should be suspected if an eczematous reaction occurs. The use of aqueous cream as a leave-on emollient may increase the risk of skin reactions, particularly in eczema.

Preparations such as **aqueous cream** and **emulsifying ointment** can be used as soap substitutes for handwashing and in the bath; the preparation is rubbed on the skin before rinsing off completely. The addition of a bath oil may also be helpful.

Urea is occasionally used with other topical agents such as corticosteroids to enhance penetration of the skin.

Emollient bath and shower preparations

In dry skin conditions soap should be avoided.

The quantities of bath additives recommended for older children are suitable for an adult-size bath. Proportionately less should be used for a child-size bath or a washbasin; recommended bath additive quantities for younger children reflect this.

Barrier preparations

Barrier preparations often contain water-repellent substances such as dimeticone p. 682, natural oils, and paraffins, to help protect the skin from abrasion and irritation; they are used to protect intact skin around stomas and pressure sores, and as a barrier against nappy rash. In neonates, barrier preparations which do not contain potentially sensitising excipients are preferred. Where the skin has broken down, barrier preparations have a limited role in protecting adjacent skin. Barrier preparations with zinc oxide or titanium salts are used to aid healing of uninfected, excoriated skin.

Nappy rash (Dermatitis)

The first line of treatment is to ensure that nappies are changed frequently and that tightly fitting water-proof pants are avoided. The rash may clear when left exposed to the air and a barrier preparation, applied with each nappy change, can be helpful. A mild corticosteroid such as hydrocortisone 0.5% or 1% p. 692 can be used if inflammation is causing discomfort, but it should be avoided in neonates. The barrier preparation should be applied after the corticosteroid preparation to prevent further damage. Preparations containing hydrocortisone should be applied for no more than a week; the hydrocortisone should be discontinued as soon as the inflammation subsides. The occlusive effect of nappies and waterproof pants may increase absorption of corticosteroids (see cautions). If the rash is associated with candidal infection, a topical antifungal such as clotrimazole cream p. 678 can be used. Topical antibacterial preparations can be used if bacterial infection is present; treatment with an oral antibacterial may occasionally be required in severe or recurrent infection. Hydrocortisone may be used in combination with antimicrobial preparations if there is considerable inflammation, erosion, and infection.

Emollients

In the *neonate*, a preservative-free paraffin-based emollient hydrates the skin without affecting the normal skin flora; substances such as olive oil are also used. The development of blisters (epidermolysis bullosa) or ichthyosis may be alleviated by applying liquid and white soft paraffin ointment while awaiting dermatological investigation.

DERMATOLOGICAL DRUGS > BARRIER PREPARATIONS

Barrier creams and ointments

- **INDICATIONS AND DOSE**

For use as a barrier preparation
- ▸ TO THE SKIN
- ▸ Child: (consult product literature)

- **MEDICINAL FORMS**
There can be variation in the licensing of different medicines containing the same drug.

Cream
EXCIPIENTS: May contain Beeswax, butylated hydroxyanisole, butylated hydroxytoluene, cetostearyl alcohol (including cetyl and stearyl alcohol), chlorocresol, fragrances, hydroxybenzoates (parabens), propylene glycol, wool fat and related substances including lanolin
- ▸ Conotrane (Astellas Pharma Ltd)
  Benzalkonium chloride 1 mg per 1 gram, Dimeticone 220 mg per 1 gram Conotrane cream | 100 gram GSL £0.88 DT price = £0.88 | 500 gram GSL £3.51
- ▸ Drapolene (Omega Pharma Ltd)
  Benzalkonium chloride 100 microgram per 1 gram, Cetrimide 2 mg per 1 gram Drapolene cream | 100 gram GSL £1.76 | 200 gram GSL £2.86 | 350 gram GSL £4.28
- ▸ Siopel (Derma UK Ltd)
  Cetrimide 3 mg per 1 gram, Dimeticone 1000 100 mg per 1 gram Siopel cream | 50 gram GSL £2.15
- ▸ Sudocrem (Forest Laboratories UK Ltd)
  Benzyl cinnamate 1.5 mg per 1 gram, Benzyl alcohol 3.9 mg per 1 gram, Benzyl benzoate 10.1 mg per 1 gram, Wool fat hydrous 40 mg per 1 gram, Zinc oxide 152.5 mg per 1 gram Sudocrem antiseptic healing cream | 60 gram GSL £1.45 | 125 gram GSL £2.15 | 250 gram GSL £3.67 | 400 gram GSL £5.25

Ointment
EXCIPIENTS: May contain Wool fat and related substances including lanolin
- ▸ Barrier creams and ointments (Non-proprietary)
  Cetostearyl alcohol 20 mg per 1 gram, Zinc oxide 75 mg per 1 gram, Beeswax white 100 mg per 1 gram, Arachis oil 305 mg per 1 gram, Castor oil 500 mg per 1 gram Zinc and Castor oil ointment | 15 gram GSL £1.08 | 50 gram GSL £2.01 | 100 gram GSL £1.41 | 500 gram GSL £4.99–£5.34 DT price = £5.34 Zinc and Castor oil cream | 100 gram GSL £1.41
- ▸ Brands may include Metanium

Spray
CAUTIONARY AND ADVISORY LABELS 15
EXCIPIENTS: May contain Cetostearyl alcohol (including cetyl and stearyl alcohol), hydroxybenzoates (parabens), wool fat and related substances including lanolin
- ▸ Sprilon (J M Loveridge Ltd)
  Dimeticone 10.4 mg per 1 gram, Zinc oxide 125 mg per 1 gram Sprilon aerosol spray | 115 gram GSL £8.90 DT price = £8.90

DERMATOLOGICAL DRUGS > EMOLLIENTS

Emollient bath and shower products, antimicrobial-containing

- **INDICATIONS AND DOSE**

DERMOL® 200 SHOWER EMOLLIENT
Dry and pruritic skin conditions including eczema and dermatitis
- ▸ TO THE SKIN
- ▸ Child: To be applied to the skin or used as a soap substitute

DERMOL® 600® BATH EMOLLIENT
Dry and pruritic skin conditions including eczema and dermatitis
- ▸ TO THE SKIN
- ▸ Child 1–23 months: 5–15 mL/bath, not to be used undiluted
- ▸ Child 2–17 years: 15–30 mL/bath, not to be used undiluted

DERMOL® WASH EMULSION
Dry and pruritic skin conditions including eczema and dermatitis
- ▸ TO THE SKIN
- ▸ Child: To be applied to the skin or used as a soap substitute

EMULSIDERM®
Dry skin conditions including eczema and ichthyosis
- ▸ TO THE SKIN
- ▸ Child 1–23 months: 5–10 mL/bath, alternatively, to be rubbed into dry skin until absorbed
- ▸ Child 2–17 years: 7–30 mL/bath, alternatively, to be rubbed into dry skin until absorbed

OILATUM® PLUS
Topical treatment of eczema, including eczema at risk from infection
- ▸ TO THE SKIN
- ▸ Child 6–11 months: 1 mL/bath, not to be used undiluted
- ▸ Child 1–17 years: 1–2 capfuls/bath, not to be used undiluted

---

IMPORTANT SAFETY INFORMATION

FIRE HAZARD WITH PARAFFIN-BASED EMOLLIENTS
Emulsifying ointment or 50% Liquid Paraffin and 50% White Soft Paraffin Ointment in contact with dressings and clothing is easily ignited by a naked flame. The risk is greater when these preparations are applied to large areas of the body, and clothing or dressings become soaked with the ointment. Patients should be told to keep away from fire or flames, and not to smoke when using these preparations. The risk of fire should be considered when using large quantities of any paraffin-based emollient.

These preparations make skin and surfaces slippery—particular care is needed when bathing.

- **DIRECTIONS FOR ADMINISTRATION** Emollient bath additives should be added to bath water; hydration can be improved by soaking in the bath for 10–20 minutes. Some bath emollients can be applied to wet skin undiluted and rinsed off. Emollient preparations contained in tubs should be removed with a clean spoon or spatula to reduce bacterial contamination of the emollient. Emollients should be applied in the direction of hair growth to reduce the risk of folliculitis.

- **PRESCRIBING AND DISPENSING INFORMATION** Preparations containing an antibacterial should be avoided unless infection is present or is a frequent complication.

- **MEDICINAL FORMS**
There can be variation in the licensing of different medicines containing the same drug.
Liquid
EXCIPIENTS: May contain Cetostearyl alcohol (including cetyl and stearyl alcohol)
- ▸ Dermol 200 (Dermal Laboratories Ltd)
  Benzalkonium chloride 1 mg per 1 gram, Chlorhexidine hydrochloride 1 mg per 1 gram, Isopropyl myristate 25 mg per 1 gram, Liquid paraffin 25 mg per 1 gram Dermol 200 shower emollient | 200 ml P £3.55

13

Skin

▸ Dermol Wash (Dermal Laboratories Ltd)
Benzalkonium chloride 1 mg per 1 gram, Chlorhexidine hydrochloride 1 mg per 1 gram, Isopropyl myristate 25 mg per 1 gram, Liquid paraffin 25 mg per 1 gram Dermol Wash cutaneous emulsion | 200 ml P £3.55
Bath additive
EXCIPIENTS: May contain Acetylated lanolin alcohols, isopropyl palmitate, polysorbates

▸ Dermol 600 (Dermal Laboratories Ltd)
Benzalkonium chloride 5 mg per 1 gram, Isopropyl myristate 250 mg per 1 gram, Liquid paraffin 250 mg per 1 gram Dermol 600 bath emollient | 600 ml P £7.55

▸ Emulsiderm (Dermal Laboratories Ltd)
Benzalkonium chloride 5 mg per 1 gram, Isopropyl myristate 250 mg per 1 gram, Liquid paraffin 250 mg per 1 gram Emulsiderm emollient | 300 ml P £3.85 | 1000 ml P £12.00

▸ Oilatum Plus (GlaxoSmithKline Consumer Healthcare)
Triclosan 20 mg per 1 gram, Benzalkonium chloride 60 mg per 1 gram, Liquid paraffin light 525 mg per 1 gram Oilatum Plus bath additive | 500 ml GSL £6.98

Emollient bath and shower products, colloidal oatmeal-containing

● **INDICATIONS AND DOSE**

Endogenous and exogenous eczema | Xeroderma | Ichthyosis
▸ TO THE SKIN
  ▸ Child 2-17 years: 20–30 mL/bath, alternatively apply to wet skin and rinse

---

IMPORTANT SAFETY INFORMATION
These preparations make skin and surfaces slippery—particular care is needed when bathing.

● **DIRECTIONS FOR ADMINISTRATION** Emollient bath additives should be added to bath water; hydration can be improved by soaking in the bath for 10–20 minutes. Some bath emollients can be applied to wet skin undiluted and rinsed off. Emollient preparations contained in tubs should be removed with a clean spoon or spatula to reduce bacterial contamination of the emollient. Emollients should be applied in the direction of hair growth to reduce the risk of folliculitis.

● **MEDICINAL FORMS**
There can be variation in the licensing of different medicines containing the same drug.
Bath additive
EXCIPIENTS: May contain Beeswax, fragrances
▸ Aveeno (Johnson & Johnson Ltd)
  Aveeno bath oil | 250 ml (ACBS) £4.49

Emollient bath and shower products, paraffin-containing

● **INDICATIONS AND DOSE**

AQUAMAX® WASH
Dry skin conditions
▸ TO THE SKIN
  ▸ Child: To be applied to wet or dry skin and rinse

CETRABEN® BATH
Dry skin conditions, including eczema
▸ TO THE SKIN
  ▸ Neonate: 0.5 capful/bath, alternatively, to be applied to wet skin and rinse.
  ▸ Child 1 month-11 years: 0.5–1 capful/bath, alternatively, to be applied to wet skin and rinse
  ▸ Child 12-17 years: 1–2 capfuls/bath, alternatively, to be applied to wet skin and rinse

DERMALO®
Dermatitis | Dry skin conditions, including ichthyosis
▸ TO THE SKIN
  ▸ Neonate: 5 mL/bath, alternatively, to be applied to wet skin and rinse.
  ▸ Child 1 month-11 years: 5–10 mL/bath, alternatively, to be applied to wet skin and rinse
  ▸ Child 12-17 years: 15–20 mL/bath, alternatively, to be applied to wet skin and rinse

DOUBLEBASE® EMOLLIENT BATH ADDITIVE
Dry skin conditions including dermatitis and ichthyosis
▸ TO THE SKIN
  ▸ Neonate: 5–10 mL/bath.
  ▸ Child 1 month-11 years: 5–10 mL/bath
  ▸ Child 12-17 years: 15–20 mL/bath

DOUBLEBASE® EMOLLIENT SHOWER GEL
Dry, chapped, or itchy skin conditions
▸ TO THE SKIN
  ▸ Child: To be applied to wet or dry skin and rinse, or apply to dry skin after showering

E45® BATH OIL
Endogenous and exogenous eczema, xeroderma, and ichthyosis
▸ TO THE SKIN
  ▸ Neonate: 5 mL/bath, alternatively, to be applied to wet skin and rinse.
  ▸ Child 1 month-11 years: 5–10 mL/bath, alternatively, to be applied to wet skin and rinse
  ▸ Child 12-17 years: 15 mL/bath, alternatively, to be applied to wet skin and rinse

E45® WASH CREAM
Endogenous and exogenous eczema, xeroderma, and ichthyosis
▸ TO THE SKIN
  ▸ Child: To be used as a soap substitute

HYDROMOL® BATH AND SHOWER EMOLLIENT
Dry skin conditions | Eczema | Ichthyosis
▸ TO THE SKIN
  ▸ Neonate: 0.5 capful/bath, alternatively apply to wet skin and rinse.
  ▸ Child 1 month-11 years: 0.5–2 capfuls/bath, alternatively apply to wet skin and rinse
  ▸ Child 12-17 years: 1–3 capfuls/bath, alternatively apply to wet skin and rinse

LPL 63.4®
Dry skin conditions
▸ TO THE SKIN
  ▸ Neonate: 0.5 capful/bath, alternatively, to be applied to wet skin and rinse.
  ▸ Child 1 month-11 years: 0.5–2 capfuls/bath, alternatively, to be applied to wet skin and rinse
  ▸ Child 12-17 years: 1–3 capfuls/bath, alternatively, to be applied to wet skin and rinse

OILATUM® EMOLLIENT BATH ADDITIVE
Dry skin conditions including dermatitis and ichthyosis
▸ TO THE SKIN
  ▸ Neonate: 0.5 capful/bath, alternatively, to be applied to wet skin and rinse.
  ▸ Child 1 month-11 years: Apply 0.5–2 capfuls/bath, alternatively, to be applied to wet skin and rinse
  ▸ Child 12-17 years: 1–3 capfuls/bath, alternatively, to be applied to wet skin and rinse

OILATUM® JUNIOR BATH ADDITIVE

Dry skin conditions including dermatitis and ichthyosis

▸ TO THE SKIN

▸ Neonate: 0.5 capful/bath, alternatively, apply to wet skin and rinse.

▸ Child 1 month–11 years: 0.5–2 capfuls/bath, alternatively, apply to wet skin and rinse

▸ Child 12–17 years: 1–3 capfuls/bath, alternatively, apply to wet skin and rinse

QV® BATH OIL

Dry skin conditions including eczema, psoriasis, ichthyosis, and pruritus

▸ TO THE SKIN

▸ Neonate: 5 mL/bath, alternatively, to be applied to wet skin and rinse.

▸ Child 1–11 months: 5 mL/bath, alternatively, to be applied to wet skin and rinse

▸ Child 1–17 years: 10 mL/bath, alternatively, to be applied to wet skin and rinse

QV® GENTLE WASH

Dry skin conditions including eczema, psoriasis, ichthyosis, and pruritus

▸ TO THE SKIN

▸ Child: To be used as a soap substitute

ZEROLATUM®

Dry skin conditions | Dermatitis | Ichthyosis

▸ TO THE SKIN

▸ Child 1 month–11 years: 5–10 mL/bath

▸ Child 12–17 years: 15–20 mL/bath

IMPORTANT SAFETY INFORMATION

FIRE HAZARD WITH PARAFFIN-BASED EMOLLIENTS

Emulsifying ointment or 50% Liquid Paraffin and 50% White Soft Paraffin Ointment in contact with dressings and clothing is easily ignited by a naked flame. The risk is greater when these preparations are applied to large areas of the body, and clothing or dressings become soaked with the ointment. Patients should be told to keep away from fire or flames, and not to smoke when using these preparations. The risk of fire should be considered when using large quantities of any paraffin-based emollient.

These preparations make the skin and surfaces slippery—particular care is needed when bathing.

● DIRECTIONS FOR ADMINISTRATION Emollient bath additives should be added to bath water; hydration can be improved by soaking in the bath for 10–20 minutes. Some bath emollients can be applied to wet skin undiluted and rinsed off. Emollient preparations contained in tubs should be removed with a clean spoon or spatula to reduce bacterial contamination of the emollient. Emollients should be applied in the direction of hair growth to reduce the risk of folliculitis.

● MEDICINAL FORMS
There can be variation in the licensing of different medicines containing the same drug.

Cream

EXCIPIENTS: May contain Cetostearyl alcohol (including cetyl and stearyl alcohol)

▸ **Emollient bath and shower products, paraffin-containing (Non-proprietary)**
Phenoxyethanol 10 mg per 1 gram, Liquid paraffin 60 mg per 1 gram, Emulsifying wax 90 mg per 1 gram, White soft paraffin 150 mg per 1 gram, Purified water 690 mg per 1 gram Aqueous cream | 30 gram GSL £1.35 | 100 gram GSL £2.15 DT price = £0.86 | 500 gram GSL £6.35 DT price = £4.30

Gel

EXCIPIENTS: May contain Cetostearyl alcohol (including cetyl and stearyl alcohol)

▸ **Doublebase** (Dermal Laboratories Ltd)
Isopropyl myristate 150 mg per 1 gram, Liquid paraffin 150 mg per 1 gram Doublebase Dayleve gel | 100 gram P £2.65 DT price = £2.65 | 500 gram P £6.29 DT price = £5.83
Doublebase gel | 100 gram P £2.65 DT price = £2.65 | 500 gram P £5.83 DT price = £5.83
Doublebase emollient wash gel | 200 gram P £5.21
Doublebase emollient shower gel | 200 gram P £5.21

Bath additive

EXCIPIENTS: May contain Acetylated lanolin alcohols, cetostearyl alcohol (including cetyl and stearyl alcohol), fragrances, isopropyl palmitate

▸ **Emollient bath and shower products, paraffin-containing (Non-proprietary)**
Liquid paraffin light 634 mg per 1 ml Liquid paraffin light 63.4% bath additive | 150 ml GSL no price available DT price = £2.84 | 250 ml GSL no price available DT price = £2.75 | 300 ml GSL no price available DT price = £4.88 | 500 ml GSL no price available DT price = £4.57

▸ **Cetraben** (Genus Pharmaceuticals Ltd)
Liquid paraffin light 828 mg per 1 gram Cetraben emollient 82.8% bath additive | 500 ml GSL £5.75

▸ **Dermalo** (Dermal Laboratories Ltd)
Acetylated wool alcohols 50 mg per 1 gram, Liquid paraffin 650 mg per 1 gram Dermalo bath emollient | 500 ml GSL £3.44

▸ **Doublebase emollient bath** (Dermal Laboratories Ltd)
Liquid paraffin 650 mg per 1 gram Doublebase emollient bath additive | 500 ml GSL £5.45

▸ **E45 emollient bath** (Forum Health Products Ltd)
E45 emollient bath oil | 250 ml (ACBS) £3.43 | 500 ml (ACBS) £5.32

▸ **Hydromol** (Alliance Pharmaceuticals Ltd)
Isopropyl myristate 130 mg per 1 ml, Liquid paraffin light 378 mg per 1 ml Hydromol Bath & Shower emollient | 350 ml GSL £3.88 | 500 ml GSL £4.42 | 1000 ml GSL £8.80

▸ **LPL** (Huxley Europe Ltd)
Liquid paraffin light 634 mg per 1 ml LPL 63.4 bath additive and emollient | 500 ml £3.10 DT price = £4.57

▸ **Oilatum** (GlaxoSmithKline Consumer Healthcare)
Liquid paraffin light 634 mg per 1 ml Oilatum Bath Formula | 150 ml GSL £2.84 DT price = £2.84 | 300 ml GSL £4.88 DT price = £4.88
Oilatum Emollient | 250 ml GSL £2.75 DT price = £2.75 | 500 ml GSL £4.57 DT price = £4.57

▸ **Oilatum junior** (GlaxoSmithKline Consumer Healthcare)
Liquid paraffin light 634 mg per 1 ml Oilatum Junior bath additive | 150 ml GSL £2.84 DT price = £2.84 | 250 ml GSL £4.05 DT price = £2.75 | 300 ml GSL £4.88 DT price = £4.88 | 600 ml GSL £5.89 DT price = £5.89

▸ **QV** (Crawford Healthcare Ltd)
Liquid paraffin light 850.9 mg per 1 gram QV 85.09% bath oil | 250 ml £2.91 | 500 ml £4.76

▸ **Zerolatum** (Thornton & Ross Ltd)
Acetylated wool alcohols 50 mg per 1 gram, Liquid paraffin 650 mg per 1 gram Zerolatum Emollient bath additive | 500 ml £4.79

Wash

EXCIPIENTS: May contain Cetostearyl alcohol (including cetyl and stearyl alcohol), polysorbates

▸ **Aquamax** (Intrapharm Laboratories Ltd)
Aquamax wash | 250 gram £2.99

▸ **E45 emollient wash** (Forum Health Products Ltd)
E45 emollient wash cream | 250 ml (ACBS) £3.43
EXCIPIENTS: May contain Hydroxybenzoates (parabens)

▸ **QV Gentle** (Crawford Healthcare Ltd)
QV Gentle wash | 250 ml £3.17 | 500 ml £5.29

13

Skin

Emollient bath and shower products, soya-bean oil-containing

● **INDICATIONS AND DOSE**

BALNEUM® BATH OIL

Dry skin conditions including those associated with dermatitis and eczema

▸ TO THE SKIN

▸ Neonate: 5–15 mL/bath, not to be used undiluted.

▸ Child 1-23 months: 5–15 mL/bath, not to be used undiluted

▸ Child 2-17 years: 20–60 mL/bath, not to be used undiluted

BALNEUM® PLUS BATH OIL

Dry skin conditions including those associated with dermatitis and eczema where pruritus also experienced

▸ TO THE SKIN

▸ Neonate: 5 mL/bath, alternatively, to be applied to wet skin and rinse.

▸ Child 1-23 months: 5 mL/bath, alternatively, to be applied to wet skin and rinse

▸ Child 2-17 years: 10–20 mL/bath, alternatively, to be applied to wet skin and rinse

ZERONEUM®

Dry skin conditions including eczema

▸ TO THE SKIN

▸ Child 1 month–11 years: 5 mL/bath

▸ Child 12-17 years: 20 mL/bath

● **IMPORTANT SAFETY INFORMATION**
These preparations make skin and surfaces slippery—particular care is needed when bathing.

● **DIRECTIONS FOR ADMINISTRATION** Emollient bath additives should be added to bath water; hydration can be improved by soaking in the bath for 10–20 minutes. Some bath emollients can be applied to wet skin undiluted and rinsed off. Emollient preparations contained in tubs should be removed with a clean spoon or spatula to reduce bacterial contamination of the emollient. Emollients should be applied in the direction of hair growth to reduce the risk of folliculitis.

● **MEDICINAL FORMS**
There can be variation in the licensing of different medicines containing the same drug.

Bath additive

EXCIPIENTS: May contain Butylated hydroxytoluene, fragrances, propylene glycol

▸ **Emollient bath and shower products, soya-bean oil-containing (Non-proprietary)**
Lauromacrogols 150 mg per 1 gram, Soya oil 829.5 mg per 1 gram Soya oil 82.95% / Lauromacrogols 15% bath oil | 500 ml GSL no price available
Soya oil 847.5 mg per 1 gram Soya oil 84.75% bath oil | 500 ml GSL no price available

▸ **Balneum** (Almirall Ltd)
Lauromacrogols 150 mg per 1 gram, Soya oil 829.5 mg per 1 gram Balneum Plus bath oil | 500 ml GSL £6.66
Soya oil 847.5 mg per 1 gram Balneum 84.75% bath oil | 200 ml GSL £2.48 | 500 ml GSL £5.38 | 1000 ml GSL £10.39

▸ **Zeroneum** (Thornton & Ross Ltd)
Soya oil 833.5 mg per 1 gram Zeroneum 83.35% bath additive | 500 ml £4.48

Emollient bath and shower products, tar-containing

● **INDICATIONS AND DOSE**

POLYTAR EMOLLIENT®

Psoriasis, eczema, atopic and pruritic dermatoses

▸ TO THE SKIN

▸ Child: 2–4 capfuls/bath, add 15–30 mL to an adult-size bath and proportionally less for a child's bath; soak for 20 minutes

PSORIDERM® EMULSION

Psoriasis

▸ TO THE SKIN

▸ Child: Up to 30 mL/bath, use 30mL in adult-size bath, and proportionately less for a child's bath, soak for 5 minutes

● **IMPORTANT SAFETY INFORMATION**

FIRE HAZARD WITH PARAFFIN-BASED EMOLLIENTS
Emulsifying ointment *or* 50% Liquid Paraffin and 50% White Soft Paraffin Ointment in contact with dressings and clothing is easily ignited by a naked flame. The risk is greater when these preparations are applied to large areas of the body, and clothing or dressings become soaked with the ointment. Patients should be told to keep away from fire or flames, and not to smoke when using these preparations. The risk of fire should be considered when using large quantities of any paraffin-based emollient.
These preparations make skin and surfaces slippery—particular care is needed when bathing.

● **DIRECTIONS FOR ADMINISTRATION** Emollient bath additives should be added to bath water; hydration can be improved by soaking in the bath for 10–20 minutes. Some bath emollients can be applied to wet skin undiluted and rinsed off. Emollient preparations contained in tubs should be removed with a clean spoon or spatula to reduce bacterial contamination of the emollient. Emollients should be applied in the direction of hair growth to reduce the risk of folliculitis.

● **MEDICINAL FORMS**
There can be variation in the licensing of different medicines containing the same drug.

Bath additive

EXCIPIENTS: May contain Isopropyl palmitate, polysorbates

▸ **Psoriderm** (Dermal Laboratories Ltd)
Coal tar distilled 400 mg per 1 ml Psoriderm Emulsion 40% bath additive | 200 ml P £2.74

Emollient creams and ointments, antimicrobial-containing

● **INDICATIONS AND DOSE**

Dry and pruritic skin conditions including eczema and dermatitis

▸ TO THE SKIN

▸ Child: To be applied to the skin or used as a soap substitute

● **IMPORTANT SAFETY INFORMATION**

FIRE HAZARD WITH PARAFFIN-BASED EMOLLIENTS
Emulsifying ointment *or* 50% Liquid Paraffin and 50% White Soft Paraffin Ointment in contact with dressings and clothing is easily ignited by a naked flame. The risk is greater when these preparations are applied to large areas of the body, and clothing or dressings become soaked with the ointment. Patients should be told to

keep away from fire or flames, and not to smoke when using these preparations. The risk of fire should be considered when using large quantities of any paraffin-based emollient.

These preparations make skin and surfaces slippery—particular care is needed when bathing.

- **DIRECTIONS FOR ADMINISTRATION** Emollients should be applied immediately after washing or bathing to maximise the effect of skin hydration. Emollient preparations contained in tubs should be removed with a clean spoon or spatula to reduce bacterial contamination of the emollient. Emollients should be applied in the direction of hair growth to reduce the risk of folliculitis.
- **PRESCRIBING AND DISPENSING INFORMATION** Preparations containing an antibacterial should be avoided unless infection is present or is a frequent complication.
- **MEDICINAL FORMS** There can be variation in the licensing of different medicines containing the same drug.

Liquid
EXCIPIENTS: May contain Cetostearyl alcohol (including cetyl and stearyl alcohol)
▶ Dermol 500 (Dermal Laboratories Ltd)
Benzalkonium chloride 1 mg per 1 gram, Chlorhexidine hydrochloride 1 mg per 1 gram, Isopropyl myristate 25 mg per 1 gram, Liquid paraffin 25 mg per 1 gram Dermol 500 lotion | 500 ml Ⓟ £6.04

Cream
EXCIPIENTS: May contain Cetostearyl alcohol (including cetyl and stearyl alcohol)
▶ Dermol (Dermal Laboratories Ltd)
Benzalkonium chloride 1 mg per 1 gram, Chlorhexidine hydrochloride 1 mg per 1 gram, Isopropyl myristate 100 mg per 1 gram, Liquid paraffin 100 mg per 1 gram Dermol cream | 100 gram Ⓟ £2.86 | 500 gram Ⓟ £6.63
▶ Eczmol (Genus Pharmaceuticals Ltd)
Chlorhexidine gluconate 10 mg per 1 gram Eczmol 1% cream | 250 ml GSL £3.70

Emollient creams and ointments, colloidal oatmeal-containing

- **INDICATIONS AND DOSE**
Endogenous and exogenous eczema | Xeroderma | Ichthyosis
▶ TO THE SKIN
▶ Child: (consult product literature)

- **DIRECTIONS FOR ADMINISTRATION** Emollients should be applied immediately after washing or bathing to maximise the effect of skin hydration. Emollient preparations contained in tubs should be removed with a clean spoon or spatula to reduce bacterial contamination of the emollient. Emollients should be applied in the direction of hair growth to reduce the risk of folliculitis.

- **MEDICINAL FORMS** There can be variation in the licensing of different medicines containing the same drug.
Cream and lotion
EXCIPIENTS: May contain Benzyl alcohol, cetostearyl alcohol (including cetyl and stearyl alcohol), isopropyl palmitate
▶ Aveeno (Johnson & Johnson Ltd)
Aveeno lotion | 500 ml (ACBS) £6.66
Aveeno cream | 100 ml (ACBS) £3.97 | 300 ml (ACBS) £6.80 | 500 ml (ACBS) £7.19

Emollient creams and ointments, paraffin-containing

- **INDICATIONS AND DOSE**
Dry skin conditions | Eczema | Psoriasis | Ichthyosis | Pruritus
▶ TO THE SKIN
▶ Child: (consult product literature)

IMPORTANT SAFETY INFORMATION
FIRE HAZARD WITH PARAFFIN-BASED EMOLLIENTS
Emulsifying ointment *or* 50% Liquid Paraffin and 50% White Soft Paraffin Ointment in contact with dressings and clothing is easily ignited by a naked flame. The risk is greater when these preparations are applied to large areas of the body, and clothing or dressings become soaked with the ointment. Patients should be told to keep away from fire or flames, and not to smoke when using these preparations. The risk of fire should be considered when using large quantities of any paraffin-based emollient.

- **DIRECTIONS FOR ADMINISTRATION** Emollients should be applied immediately after washing or bathing to maximise the effect of skin hydration. Emollient preparations contained in tubs should be removed with a clean spoon or spatula to reduce bacterial contamination of the emollient. Emollients should be applied in the direction of hair growth to reduce the risk of folliculitis.

- **MEDICINAL FORMS** There can be variation in the licensing of different medicines containing the same drug.
Liquid
EXCIPIENTS: May contain Benzyl alcohol, cetostearyl alcohol (including cetyl and stearyl alcohol), hydroxybenzoates (parabens), isopropyl palmitate
▶ Cetraben (Thornton & Ross Ltd)
Cetraben lotion | 200 ml £4.00 | 500 ml £5.64
▶ E45 (Forum Health Products Ltd)
E45 lotion | 200 ml £2.40 | 500 ml £4.50
▶ QV (Crawford Healthcare Ltd)
White soft paraffin 50 mg per 1 gram QV 5% skin lotion | 250 ml £3.17 | 500 ml £5.29

Cream
EXCIPIENTS: May contain Benzyl alcohol, cetostearyl alcohol (including cetyl and stearyl alcohol), chlorocresol, disodium edetate, fragrances, hydroxybenzoates (parabens), polysorbates, propylene glycol, sorbic acid, lanolin
▶ Emollient creams and ointments, paraffin-containing (Non-proprietary)
Liquid paraffin light 60 mg per 1 gram, White soft paraffin 150 mg per 1 gram White soft paraffin 15% / Liquid paraffin light 6% cream | 150 gram GSL no price available DT price = £3.06 | 500 ml GSL no price available DT price = £5.28 | 1050 ml GSL no price available DT price = £9.98
▶ Aquamax (Intrapharm Laboratories Ltd)
Aquamax cream | 100 gram £1.89 | 500 gram £3.99
▶ Aquamol (Thornton & Ross Ltd)
Aquamol cream | 50 gram £1.22 | 500 gram £6.40
▶ Cetraben (Thornton & Ross Ltd)
Liquid paraffin light 105 mg per 1 gram, White soft paraffin 132 mg per 1 gram Cetraben cream | 50 gram £1.40 | 150 gram £3.98 | 500 gram £5.99 | 1050 gram £11.62
▶ Diprobase (Bayer Plc)
Diprobase cream | 50 gram GSL £1.28 | 500 gram GSL £6.32
▶ E45 (Forum Health Products Ltd)
Wool fat 10 mg per 1 gram, Liquid paraffin light 126 mg per 1 gram, White soft paraffin 145 mg per 1 gram E45 cream | 50 gram GSL £1.61 | 125 gram GSL £2.90 | 350 gram GSL £5.17 | 500 gram GSL £5.62
▶ Enopen (Ennogen Healthcare Ltd)
Liquid paraffin light 105 mg per 1 gram, White soft paraffin 132 mg per 1 gram Enopen cream | 500 gram £5.99
▶ Epaderm (Molnlycke Health Care Ltd)
Epaderm cream | 50 gram £1.70 | 500 gram £6.95

13

Skin

▸ **Hydromol** (Alliance Pharmaceuticals Ltd)
Sodium lactate 10 mg per 1 gram, Sodium pidolate 25 mg per 1 gram, Isopropyl myristate 50 mg per 1 gram, Liquid paraffin 100 mg per 1 gram Hydromol 2.5% cream | 50 gram GSL £2.19 | 100 gram GSL £4.09 | 500 gram GSL £11.92

▸ **Lipobase** (Astellas Pharma Ltd)
Lipobase cream | 50 gram P £1.46

▸ **Oilatum** (GlaxoSmithKline Consumer Healthcare)
Liquid paraffin light 60 mg per 1 gram, White soft paraffin 150 mg per 1 gram Oilatum cream | 50 gram GSL £1.67 DT price = £1.67 | 150 gram GSL £3.06 DT price = £3.06 | 500 ml GSL £5.28 DT price = £5.28 | 1050 ml GSL £9.98 DT price = £9.98

▸ **Oilatum junior** (GlaxoSmithKline Consumer Healthcare)
Liquid paraffin light 60 mg per 1 gram, White soft paraffin 150 mg per 1 gram Oilatum Junior cream | 150 gram GSL £3.06 DT price = £3.06 | 350 ml GSL £4.65 DT price = £4.65 | 500 ml GSL £5.28 DT price = £5.28 | 1050 ml GSL £9.98 DT price = £9.98

▸ **QV** (Crawford Healthcare Ltd)
White soft paraffin 50 mg per 1 gram, Glycerol 100 mg per 1 gram, Liquid paraffin light 100 mg per 1 gram QV cream | 100 gram £2.06 | 500 gram £5.92 | 1050 gram £12.05

▸ **Soffen** (Vitame Ltd)
Liquid paraffin light 105 mg per 1 gram, White soft paraffin 132 mg per 1 gram Soffen cream | 500 gram £4.79

▸ **Unguentum M** (Almirall Ltd)
Unguentum M cream | 50 gram GSL £1.41 | 60 gram GSL no price available | 100 gram GSL £2.78 | 200 ml GSL £5.50 | 500 gram GSL £8.48

▸ **ZeroAQS** (Thornton & Ross Ltd)
ZeroAQS emollient cream | 500 gram £3.29

▸ **Zerobase** (Thornton & Ross Ltd)
Liquid paraffin 110 mg per 1 gram Zerobase 11% cream | 50 gram £1.04 | 500 gram £5.26

▸ **Zerocream** (Thornton & Ross Ltd)
Liquid paraffin 126 mg per 1 gram, White soft paraffin 145 mg per 1 gram Zerocream | 50 gram £1.17 | 500 gram £4.08

▸ **Zeroguent** (Thornton & Ross Ltd)
White soft paraffin 40 mg per 1 gram, Soya oil 50 mg per 1 gram, Liquid paraffin light 80 mg per 1 gram Zeroguent cream | 100 gram £2.33 | 500 gram £6.99

Ointment

EXCIPIENTS: May contain Cetostearyl alcohol (including cetyl and stearyl alcohol), polysorbates

▸ **Emollient creams and ointments, paraffin-containing (Non-proprietary)**
Cetraben ointment | 125 gram £3.49 | 450 gram £5.39

Liquid paraffin 200 mg per 1 gram, Emulsifying wax 300 mg per 1 gram, White soft paraffin 500 mg per 1 gram Emulsifying ointment | 100 gram GSL £2.82 | 500 gram GSL £3.26 DT price = £1.84 | 500 gram PoM no price available DT price = £1.84

White soft paraffin 1 mg per 1 mg White soft paraffin solid | 500 gram GSL £4.18 DT price = £3.23 | 4500 gram GSL £18.62–£29.07

Liquid paraffin 500 mg per 1 gram, White soft paraffin 500 mg per 1 gram Pure Health Liquid Paraffin 50% in White Soft Paraffin ointment | 500 gram £3.66 DT price = £4.57

Bell's Emollient 50 ointment | 250 gram £1.99 | 500 gram £3.17 DT price = £4.57

The 50:50 Ointment | 500 gram P £4.57 DT price = £4.57

White soft paraffin 50% / Liquid paraffin 50% ointment | 250 gram £1.87 | 500 gram £6.80 DT price = £4.57 | 500 gram P £4.57 DT price = £4.57

Magnesium sulfate dried 5 mg per 1 gram, Phenoxyethanol 10 mg per 1 gram, Wool alcohols ointment 500 mg per 1 gram Hydrous ointment | 500 gram GSL £4.89 DT price = £4.89

Yellow soft paraffin 1 mg per 1 mg Yellow soft paraffin solid | 15 gram GSL £1.16 | 500 gram GSL £13.02 DT price = £13.27 | 4500 gram GSL £18.29

▸ **Diprobase** (Bayer Plc)
Liquid paraffin 50 mg per 1 gram, White soft paraffin 950 mg per 1 gram Diprobase ointment | 50 gram GSL £1.28 DT price = £1.28 | 500 gram GSL £5.99 DT price = £5.99

▸ **Emelpin** (Vitame Ltd)
Emulsifying wax 300 mg per 1 gram, Yellow soft paraffin 300 mg per 1 gram Emelpin ointment | 125 gram £3.08 | 500 gram £5.22

▸ **Epaderm** (Molnlycke Health Care Ltd)
Emulsifying wax 300 mg per 1 gram, Yellow soft paraffin 300 mg per 1 gram Epaderm ointment | 125 gram £3.85 | 500 gram £6.53 | 1000 gram £12.02

▸ **Fifty:50** (Ennogen Healthcare Ltd)
Liquid paraffin 500 mg per 1 gram, White soft paraffin 500 mg per 1 gram Fifty:50 ointment | 250 gram £1.83 | 500 gram £3.66 DT price = £4.57

▸ **Hydromol** (Alliance Pharmaceuticals Ltd)
Emulsifying wax 300 mg per 1 gram, Yellow soft paraffin 300 mg per 1 gram Hydromol ointment | 125 gram £2.88 | 500 gram £4.89 | 1000 gram £9.09

▸ **QV intensive** (Crawford Healthcare Ltd)
QV Intensive ointment | 450 gram £5.71

▸ **Thirty:30** (Ennogen Healthcare Ltd)
Emulsifying wax 300 mg per 1 gram, Yellow soft paraffin 300 mg per 1 gram Thirty:30 ointment | 125 gram £3.81 | 250 gram £4.29 | 500 gram £6.47

▸ **Vaseline** (Unilever UK Home & Personal Care)
White soft paraffin 1 mg per 1 mg Vaseline Pure Petroleum jelly | 50 ml GSL no price available | 100 ml GSL no price available | 250 ml GSL no price available

Spray

CAUTIONARY AND ADVISORY LABELS 15

▸ **Dermamist** (Alliance Pharmaceuticals Ltd)
White soft paraffin 100 mg per 1 gram Dermamist 10% spray | 250 ml P £5.97

▸ **Emollin** (C D Medical Ltd)
Emollin aerosol spray | 150 ml £4.00 | 240 ml £6.39

Emollients, urea-containing

● **DRUG ACTION** Urea is a keratin softener and hydrating agent used in the treatment of dry, scaling conditions (including ichthyosis).

● **INDICATIONS AND DOSE**

AQUADRATE®

Dry, scaling, and itching skin
▸ TO THE SKIN
▸ Child: Apply twice daily, to be applied thinly

BALNEUM® CREAM

Dry skin conditions
▸ TO THE SKIN
▸ Child: Apply twice daily

BALNEUM® PLUS CREAM

Dry, scaling, and itching skin
▸ TO THE SKIN
▸ Child: Apply twice daily

CALMURID®

Dry, scaling, and itching skin
▸ TO THE SKIN
▸ Child: Apply twice daily, apply a thick layer for 3–5 minutes, massage into area, and remove excess. Can be diluted with aqueous cream (life of diluted cream is 14 days). Half-strength cream can be used for 1 week if stinging occurs

DERMATONICS ONCE HEEL BALM®

Dry skin on soles of feet
▸ TO THE SKIN
▸ Child 12–17 years: Apply once daily

E45® ITCH RELIEF CREAM

Dry, scaling, and itching skin
▸ TO THE SKIN
▸ Child: Apply twice daily

EUCERIN® INTENSIVE CREAM

Dry skin conditions including eczema, ichthyosis, xeroderma, and hyperkeratosis
▸ TO THE SKIN
▸ Child: Apply twice daily, to be applied thinly and rubbed into area

EUCERIN® INTENSIVE LOTION

Dry skin conditions including eczema, ichthyosis, xeroderma, and hyperkeratosis

▸ TO THE SKIN

▸ Child: Apply twice daily, to be applied sparingly and rubbed into area

FLEXITOL®

Dry skin on soles of feet and heels

▸ TO THE SKIN

▸ Child 12–17 years: Apply 1–2 times a day

HYDROMOL® INTENSIVE

Dry, scaling, and itching skin

▸ TO THE SKIN

▸ Child: Apply twice daily, to be applied thinly

IMUDERM® EMOLLIENT

Dry skin conditions including eczema, psoriasis or dermatitis

▸ TO THE SKIN

▸ Child: Apply to skin or use as a soap substitute

NUTRAPLUS®

Dry, scaling, and itching skin

▸ TO THE SKIN

▸ Child: Apply 2–3 times a day

● **DIRECTIONS FOR ADMINISTRATION** Emollients should be applied immediately after washing or bathing to maximise the effect of skin hydration. Emollient preparations contained in tubs should be removed with a clean spoon or spatula to reduce bacterial contamination of the emollient. Emollients should be applied in the direction of hair growth to reduce the risk of folliculitis.

● **MEDICINAL FORMS**
There can be variation in the licensing of different medicines containing the same drug.

Liquid
EXCIPIENTS: May contain Benzyl alcohol, isopropyl palmitate
▸ Eucerin (Beiersdorf Ltd)
Urea 100 mg per 1 gram Eucerin Intensive 10% lotion | 250 ml [GSL] £7.93

Cream
EXCIPIENTS: May contain Benzyl alcohol, cetostearyl alcohol (including cetyl and stearyl alcohol), hydroxybenzoates (parabens), isopropyl palmitate, polysorbates, propylene glycol, wool fat and isopropyl substances including lanolin
▸ Emollients, urea-containing (Non-proprietary)
Lauromacrogols 30 mg per 1 gram, Urea 50 mg per 1 gram Urea 5% / Lauromacrogols 3% cream | 500 gram no price available
Urea 100 mg per 1 gram Urea 10% cream | 100 gram [P] no price available
▸ Aquadrate (Alliance Pharmaceuticals Ltd)
Urea 100 mg per 1 gram Aquadrate 10% cream | 100 gram [P] £4.37
▸ Balneum (Almirall Ltd)
Balneum cream | 50 gram £2.85 | 500 gram £9.97
▸ Balneum Plus (Almirall Ltd)
Lauromacrogols 30 mg per 1 gram, Urea 50 mg per 1 gram Balneum Plus cream | 100 gram [GSL] £3.29 | 500 gram [GSL] £14.99
▸ Calmurid (Galderma (UK) Ltd)
Lactic acid 50 mg per 1 gram, Urea 100 mg per 1 gram Calmurid cream | 100 gram [P] £5.75 DT price = £5.75 | 500 gram [P] £33.40 DT price = £33.40
▸ E45 Itch Relief (Forum Health Products Ltd)
Lauromacrogols 30 mg per 1 gram, Urea 50 mg per 1 gram E45 Itch Relief cream | 50 gram [GSL] £2.81 | 100 gram [GSL] £3.74 | 500 gram [GSL] £14.99
▸ Eucerin (Beiersdorf UK Ltd)
Urea 100 mg per 1 gram Eucerin Intensive 10% cream | 100 ml [P] £7.59
▸ Hydromol Intensive (Alliance Pharmaceuticals Ltd)
Urea 100 mg per 1 gram Hydromol Intensive 10% cream | 30 gram [P] £1.64 | 100 gram [P] £4.37

▸ imuDERM emollient (CliniSupplies Ltd) 500 gram £6.50
▸ Nutraplus (Galderma (UK) Ltd)
Urea 100 mg per 1 gram Nutraplus 10% cream | 100 gram [P] £4.37

Balms
EXCIPIENTS: May contain Beeswax, benzyl alcohol, cetostearyl alcohol (including cetyl and stearyl alcohol), fragrances, lanolin
▸ Emollients, urea-containing (Non-proprietary)
imuDERM emollient | 500 gram £6.50
▸ Dermatonics once (Dermatonics Ltd)
Dermatonics Once Heel Balm | 75 ml £3.60 | 200 ml £8.50
▸ Flexitol (Thornton & Ross Ltd)
Flexitol Heel Balm | 40 gram £2.75 | 56 gram no price available | 75 gram £3.80 | 112 gram no price available | 200 gram £9.40 | 500 gram £14.75

2 Infections of the skin

Skin infections

Antibacterial preparations

Topical antibacterial preparations are used to treat localised bacterial skin infections caused by Gram-positive organisms (particularly by staphylococci or streptococci). Systemic antibacterial treatment is more appropriate for deep-seated skin infections.

Problems associated with the use of topical antibacterials include bacterial resistance, contact sensitisation, and superinfection. In order to minimise the development of resistance, antibacterials used systemically (e.g. fusidic acid p. 336) should not generally be chosen for topical use. *Resistant organisms* are more common in hospitals, and whenever possible swabs should be taken for bacteriological examination before beginning treatment.

Neomycin sulfate p. 675 applied topically may cause sensitisation and cross-sensitivity with other aminoglycoside antibacterials such as gentamicin p. 293 may occur. Topical antibacterials applied over large areas can cause systemic toxicity; ototoxicity with neomycin sulfate and with polymyxins p. 676 is a particular risk for neonates and children with renal impairment.

Superficial bacterial infection of the skin may be treated with a topical antiseptic such as povidone-iodine p. 633 which also softens crusts, or hydrogen peroxide p. 657 1% cream.

Bacterial infections such as *impetigo* and *folliculitis* can be treated with a short course of topical fusidic acid; mupirocin p. 677 should be used only to treat meticillin-resistant *Staphylococcus aureus*.

For extensive or long-standing impetigo, an oral antibacterial such as flucloxacillin p. 325 (or clarithromycin p. 309 in children with penicillin-allergy), should be used. A mild antiseptic may help to soften crusts. Mild antiseptics may be useful in reducing the spread of infection, but there is little evidence to support the use of topical antiseptics alone in the treatment of impetigo.

Cellulitis, a rapidly spreading deeply seated inflammation of the skin and subcutaneous tissue, requires systemic antibacterial treatment. Lower leg infections or infections spreading around wounds are almost always cellulitis. *Erysipelas*, a superficial infection with clearly defined edges (and often affecting the face), is also treated with a systemic antibacterial.

Staphylococcal scalded-skin syndrome requires urgent treatment with a systemic antibacterial, such as flucloxacillin.

Mupirocin is not related to any other antibacterial in use; it is effective for skin infections, particularly those due to Gram-positive organisms but it is not indicated for pseudomonal infection. Although *Staphylococcus aureus* strains with low-level resistance to mupirocin are emerging,

13

Skin

it is generally useful in infections resistant to other antibacterials. To avoid the development of resistance, mupirocin or fusidic acid should not be used for longer than 10 days and local microbiology advice should be sought before using it in hospital. In the presence of mupirocin-resistant MRSA infection, a topical antiseptic, such as povidone-iodine, chlorhexidine p. 656, or alcohol, can be used; their use should be discussed with the local microbiologist.

Mupirocin ointment contains macrogols; extensive absorption of macrogols through the mucous membranes or through application to thin or damaged skin may result in renal toxicity, especially in neonates. Mupirocin nasal ointment is formulated in a paraffin base and may be more suitable for the treatment of MRSA-infected open wound in neonates.

Metronidazole p. 676 gel is used topically in children to reduce the odour associated with anaerobic infections and for the treatment of periorificial rosacea; oral metronidazole is used to treat wounds infected with anaerobic bacteria.

Retapamulin p. 678 can be used for impetigo and other superficial bacterial skin infections caused by *Staphylococcus aureus* and *Streptococcus pyogenes* that are resistant to first-line topical antibacterials. However, it is not effective against MRSA.

Silver sulfadiazine p. 677 is licensed for the prevention and treatment of infection in burns but the use of appropriate dressings may be more effective. Systemic effects may occur following extensive application of silver sulfadiazine; its use is not recommended in neonates.

Antibacterial preparations also used systemically

Fusidic acid is a narrow-spectrum antibacterial used for staphylococcal infections. Fusidic acid has a role in the treatment of impetigo.

An ointment containing fusidic acid is used in the fissures of angular cheilitis when associated with staphylococcal infection. See Oropharyngeal fungal infections p. 662 for further information on angular cheilitis.

Metronidazole is used topically to treat rosacea and to reduce the odour associated with anaerobic infections; oral metronidazole is used to treat wounds infected with anaerobic bacteria.

Antifungal preparations

Most localised fungal infections are treated with topical preparations. To prevent relapse, local antifungal treatment should be continued for 1–2 weeks after the disappearance of all signs of infection. Systemic therapy is necessary for scalp infection or if the skin infection is widespread, disseminated or intractable; although topical therapy may be used to treat some nail infections, systemic therapy is more effective. Specimens of scale, nail or hair should be sent for mycological examination before starting treatment, unless the diagnosis is certain.

Dermatophytoses

Ringworm infection can affect the scalp (tinea capitis), body (tinea corporis), groin (tinea cruris), hand (tinea manuum), foot (tinea pedis, athlete's foot), or nail (tinea unguium, onychomycosis). Tinea capitis is a common childhood infection that requires systemic treatment with an oral antifungal; additional application of a topical antifungal, during the early stages of treatment, may reduce the risk of transmission. A topical antifungal can also be used to treat asymptomatic carriers of scalp ringworm.

Tinea corporis and tinea pedis infections in children respond to treatment with a topical **imidazole** (clotrimazole p. 678, econazole nitrate p. 678, or miconazole p. 679) or terbinafine cream p. 680. Nystatin p. 663 is less effective against tinea.

Compound benzoic acid ointment (Whitfield's ointment) has been used for ringworm infections but it is cosmetically less acceptable than proprietary preparations.

Antifungal dusting powders are of little therapeutic value in the treatment of fungal skin infections and may cause skin irritation; they may have some role in preventing re-infection.

Antifungal treatment may not be necessary in asymptomatic children with tinea infection of the nails. If treatment is necessary, a systemic antifungal is more effective than topical therapy. However, topical application of tioconazole p. 679 may be useful for treating early onychomycosis when involvement is limited to mild distal disease, or for superficial white onychomycosis, or where there are contra-indications to systemic therapy. Chronic paronychia on the fingers (usually due to a candidal infection) should be treated with topical clotrimazole or nystatin, but these preparations should be used with caution in children who suck their fingers. Chronic paronychia of the toes (usually due to dermatophyte infection) can be treated with topical terbinafine.

Pityriasis versicolor

Pityriasis (tinea) versicolor can be treated with ketoconazole shampoo p. 678 or **selenium sulfide** shampoo. Topical imidazole antifungals such as clotrimazole, econazole nitrateand miconazole or topical terbinafine are alternatives, but large quantities may be required.

If topical therapy fails, or if the infection is widespread, pityriasis versicolor is treated systemically with an azole antifungal. Relapse is common, especially in the immunocompromised.

Candidiasis

Candidal skin infections can be treated with topical imidazole antifungals clotrimazole p. 678, econazole nitrate p. 678, or miconazole p. 679; topical terbinafine p. 680 is an alternative. Topical application of nystatin p. 663 is also effective for candidiasis but it is ineffective against dermatophytosis. Refractory candidiasis requires systemic treatment generally with a triazole such as fluconazole p. 352; systemic treatment with griseofulvin p. 357 or terbinafine is **not appropriate** for refractory candidiasis. See the treatment of oral candiasis and for the management of nappy rash.

Angular cheilitis

Miconazole cream is used in the fissures of angular cheilitis when associated with *Candida*.

Compound topical preparations

Combination of an imidazole and a mild corticosteroid (such as hydrocortisone 1% p. 411) may be of value in the treatment of eczematous intertrigo and, in the first few days only, of a severely inflamed patch of ringworm. Combination of a mild corticosteroid with either an imidazole or nystatin may be of use in the treatment of *intertriginous eczema* associated with candida.

Antiviral preparations

Aciclovir p. 683 cream is used for the treatment of initial and recurrent labial, cutaneous, and genital *herpes simplex infections* in children; treatment should begin as early as possible. Systemic treatment is necessary for buccal or vaginal infections or if cold sores recur frequently.

Herpes labialis

Aciclovir cream can be used for the treatment of initial and recurrent labial herpes simplex infections (cold sores). It is best applied at the earliest possible stage, usually when prodromal changes of sensation are felt in the lip and before vesicles appear.

Penciclovir cream is also licensed for the treatment of herpes labialis; it needs to be applied more frequently than aciclovir cream.

Parasiticidal preparations

Suitable quantities of parasiticidal preparations

Area of body	Skin creams	Lotions	Cream rinses
Scalp (head lice)		50-100 mL	50-100 mL
Body (scabies)	30-60 g	100 mL	
Body (crab lice)	30-60 g	100 mL	

These amounts are usually suitable for a child 12-17 years for single application.

Scabies

Permethrin p. 683 is used for the treatment of *scabies* (*Sarcoptes scabiei*); malathion p. 682 can be used if permethrin is inappropriate.

Benzyl benzoate is an irritant and should be avoided in children; it is less effective than malathion and permethrin.

Ivermectin p. 361 (available from 'special-order' manufacturers or specialist importing companies) by mouth has been used, in combination with topical drugs, for the treatment of hyperkeratotic (crusted or 'Norwegian') scabies that does not respond to topical treatment alone.

Application

Although acaricides have traditionally been applied after a hot bath, this is **not** necessary and there is even evidence that a hot bath may increase absorption into the blood, removing them from their site of action on the skin.

All members of the affected household should be treated simultaneously. Treatment should be applied to the whole body including the scalp, neck, face, and ears. Particular attention should be paid to the webs of the fingers and toes and lotion brushed under the ends of nails. It is now recommended that malathion and permethrin should be applied twice, one week apart; in the case of benzyl benzoate in adults, up to 3 applications on consecutive days may be needed. It is important to warn users to reapply treatment to the hands if they are washed. Patients with hyperkeratotic scabies may require 2 or 3 applications of acaricide on consecutive days to ensure that enough penetrates the skin crusts to kill all the mites.

Itching

The *itch* and *eczema* of scabies persists for some weeks after the infestation has been eliminated and treatment for pruritus and eczema may be required. Application of crotamiton p. 707 can be used to control itching after treatment with more effective acaricides. A topical corticosteroid may help to reduce itch and inflammation after scabies has been treated successfully; however, persistent symptoms suggest that scabies eradication was not successful. Oral administration of a **sedating antihistamine** at night may also be useful.

Head lice

Dimeticone p. 682 is effective against head lice (*Pediculus humanus capitis*) and acts on the surface of the organism. Malathion, an organophosphorus insecticide, is an alternative, but resistance has been reported. Benzyl benzoate is licensed for the treatment of head lice but it is not recommended for use in children.

Head lice infestation (pediculosis) should be treated using lotion or liquid formulations only if live lice are present. A shampoos are diluted too much in use to be effective. A contact time of 8-12 hours or overnight treatment is recommended for lotions and liquids; a 2-hour treatment is not sufficient to kill eggs.

In general, a course of treatment for head lice should be 2 applications of product 7 days apart to kill lice emerging from any eggs that survive the first application. All affected household members should be treated at the same time.

Wet combing methods

Head lice can be mechanically removed by combing wet hair meticulously with a plastic detection comb (probably for at least 30 minutes each time) over the whole scalp at 4-day intervals for a minimum of 2 weeks, and continued until no lice are found on 3 consecutive sessions; hair conditioner or vegetable oil can be used to facilitate the process.

Several devices for the removal of head lice such as combs and topical solutions, are available and some are prescribable on the NHS.

The Drug Tariffs can be accessed online at:

- National Health Service Drug Tariff for England and Wales: www.ppa.org.uk/ppa/edt_intro.htm
- Health and Personal Social Services for Northern Ireland Drug Tariff: www.dhsspsni.gov.uk/pas-tariff
- Scottish Drug Tariff: www.isdscotland.org/Health-topics/Prescribing-and-Medicines/Scottish-Drug-Tariff/

Crab lice

Permethrin and malathion are used to eliminate *crab lice* (*Pthirus pubis*); permethrin is not licensed for treatment of crab lice in children under 18 years. An aqueous preparation should be applied, allowed to dry naturally and washed off after 12 hours; a second treatment is needed after 7 days to kill lice emerging from surviving eggs. All surfaces of the body should be treated, including the scalp, neck, and face (paying particular attention to the eyebrows and other facial hair). A different insecticide should be used if a course of treatment fails.

Parasiticidal preparations

Dimeticone coats head lice and interferes with water balance in lice by preventing the excretion of water; it is less active against eggs and treatment should be repeated after 7 days.

Malathion is recommended for *scabies*, *head lice* and *crab lice*. The risk of systemic effects associated with 1-2 applications of malathion p. 682 is considered to be very low; however, except in the treatment of hyperkeratotic scabies in children, applications of malathion liquid repeated at intervals of less than 1 week or application for more than 3 consecutive weeks should be **avoided** since the likelihood of eradication of lice is not increased.

Permethrin p. 683 is effective for *scabies*. It is also active against *head lice* but the formulation and licensed methods of application of the current products make them unsuitable for the treatment of head lice. Permethrin is also effective against *crab lice* but it is not licensed for this purpose in children under 18 years.

2.1 Bacterial skin infections

ANTIBACTERIALS > AMINOGLYCOSIDES

Neomycin sulfate

- **INDICATIONS AND DOSE**

Bacterial skin infections
- TO THE SKIN
  - Child: Apply up to 3 times a day, for short-term use only

- **UNLICENSED USE** *Neomycin Cream BPC*—no information available.
- **CONTRA-INDICATIONS** Neonates
- **CAUTIONS** If large areas of skin are being treated ototoxicity may be a hazard in children, particularly in those with renal impairment.
- **INTERACTIONS** → Appendix 1 (aminoglycosides).
- **SIDE-EFFECTS** Sensitisation (cross sensitivity with other aminoglycosides may occur)

- **RENAL IMPAIRMENT** Ototoxicity may be a hazard if large areas of skin are treated.
- **LESS SUITABLE FOR PRESCRIBING** Neomycin sulfate cream is less suitable for prescribing.

- **MEDICINAL FORMS**
  There can be variation in the licensing of different medicines containing the same drug. Forms available from special-order manufacturers include: cream

ANTIBACTERIALS > NITROIMIDAZOLE DERIVATIVES

Metronidazole

- **DRUG ACTION** Metronidazole is an antimicrobial drug with high activity against anaerobic bacteria and protozoa.

- **INDICATIONS AND DOSE**

ACEA®

Acute inflammatory exacerbation of rosacea
▸ TO THE SKIN
▸ Child 1–17 years: Apply twice daily, to be applied thinly

ANABACT®

Malodorous fungating tumours and malodorous gravitational and decubitus ulcers
▸ TO THE SKIN
▸ Child: Apply 1–2 times a day, to be applied to clean wound and covered with non-adherent dressing

METROGEL®

Acute inflammatory exacerbation of rosacea
▸ TO THE SKIN
▸ Child 1–17 years: Apply twice daily, to be applied thinly

Malodorous fungating tumours
▸ TO THE SKIN
▸ Child: Apply 1–2 times a day, to be applied to clean wound and covered with non-adherent dressing

METROSA®

Acute exacerbation of rosacea
▸ TO THE SKIN
▸ Child 1–17 years: Apply twice daily, to be applied thinly

ROSICED®

Inflammatory papules and pustules of rosacea
▸ TO THE SKIN
▸ Child 1–17 years: Apply twice daily for 6 weeks (longer if necessary)

ROZEX® CREAM

Inflammatory papules, pustules and erythema of rosacea
▸ TO THE SKIN
▸ Child 1–17 years: Apply twice daily

ROZEX® GEL

Inflammatory papules, pustules and erythema of rosacea
▸ TO THE SKIN
▸ Child 1–17 years: Apply twice daily

ZYOMET®

Acute inflammatory exacerbation of rosacea
▸ TO THE SKIN
▸ Child 1–17 years: Apply twice daily, to be applied thinly

- **UNLICENSED USE**
  METROSA® Not licensed for use in children.
  ANABACT® Not licensed for use in children under 12 years.
  ROZEX® GEL Not licensed for use in children.
  METROGEL® Not licensed for use in children.
  ZYOMET® Not licensed for use in children.
  ACEA® Not licensed for use in children under 12 years.

ROZEX® CREAM Not licensed for use in children.
ROSICED® Not licensed for use in children.

- **CAUTIONS** Avoid exposure to strong sunlight or UV light
- **SIDE-EFFECTS** Skin irritation
- **PATIENT AND CARER ADVICE**
  Medicines for Children leaflet: Metronidazole for bacterial infections www.medicinesforchildren.org.uk/metronidazole-for-bacterial-infections

- **MEDICINAL FORMS**
  There can be variation in the licensing of different medicines containing the same drug. Forms available from special-order manufacturers include: cream, gel

Cream
EXCIPIENTS: May contain Benzyl alcohol, isopropyl palmitate, propylene glycol
▸ **Rosiced** (Pierre Fabre Dermo-Cosmetique)
  Metronidazole 7.5 mg per 1 gram Rosiced 0.75% cream | 30 gram [PoM] £7.50 DT price = £6.60
▸ **Rozex** (Galderma (UK) Ltd)
  Metronidazole 7.5 mg per 1 gram Rozex 0.75% cream | 30 gram [PoM] £6.60 DT price = £6.60 | 40 gram [PoM] £9.88 DT price = £9.88

Gel
EXCIPIENTS: May contain Benzyl alcohol, disodium edetate, hydroxybenzoates (parabens), propylene glycol
▸ **Acea** (Ferndale Pharmaceuticals Ltd)
  Metronidazole 7.5 mg per 1 gram Acea 0.75% gel | 40 gram [PoM] £9.95
▸ **Anabact** (Cambridge Healthcare Supplies Ltd)
  Metronidazole 7.5 mg per 1 gram Anabact 0.75% gel | 15 gram [PoM] £4.47 | 30 gram [PoM] £7.89
▸ **Metrogel** (Galderma (UK) Ltd)
  Metronidazole 7.5 mg per 1 gram Metrogel 0.75% gel | 40 gram [PoM] £22.63
▸ **Metrosa** (M & A Pharmachem Ltd)
  Metronidazole 7.5 mg per 1 gram Metrosa 0.75% gel | 30 gram [PoM] £12.00 | 40 gram [PoM] £19.90
▸ **Rozex** (Galderma (UK) Ltd)
  Metronidazole 7.5 mg per 1 gram Rozex 0.75% gel | 30 gram [PoM] £6.60 | 40 gram [PoM] £9.88
▸ **Zyomet** (AMCo)
  Metronidazole 7.5 mg per 1 gram Zyomet 0.75% gel | 30 gram [PoM] £12.00

ANTIBACTERIALS > POLYMYXINS

Polymyxins

- **INDICATIONS AND DOSE**
Bacterial skin infections
▸ TO THE SKIN
▸ Child: Apply twice daily, may be applied more frequently if required

- **UNLICENSED USE** Licensed for use in children (age range not specified by manufacturer).
- **CAUTIONS**
  CAUTIONS, FURTHER INFORMATION
  ▸ Large areas If large areas of skin are being treated nephrotoxicity and neurotoxicity may be a hazard, particularly in children with renal impairment.
- **SIDE-EFFECTS** Sensitisation

- **MEDICINAL FORMS**
  There can be variation in the licensing of different medicines containing the same drug.
  No licensed medicines listed.

13

Skin

ANTIBACTERIALS > SULFONAMIDES

Silver sulfadiazine

- ● **INDICATIONS AND DOSE**

Prophylaxis and treatment of infection in burn wounds
- ▶ TO THE SKIN
- ▶ Child: Apply daily, may be applied more frequently if very exudative

For conservative management of finger-tip injuries
- ▶ TO THE SKIN
- ▶ Child: Apply every 2–3 days, consult product literature for details

Adjunct to prophylaxis of infection in skin graft donor sites and extensive abrasions
- ▶ TO THE SKIN
- ▶ Child: (consult product literature)

Adjunct to short-term treatment of infection in pressure sores
- ▶ TO THE SKIN
- ▶ Child: (consult product literature)

- ● **UNLICENSED USE** No age range specified by manufacturer.
- ● **CONTRA-INDICATIONS** Not recommended for neonates
- ● **CAUTIONS** G6PD deficiency

CAUTIONS, FURTHER INFORMATION
- ▶ Large areas Plasma-sulfadiazine concentrations may approach therapeutic levels with *side-effects* and *interactions* as for sulfonamides if large areas of skin are treated.

- ● **INTERACTIONS** → Appendix 1 (sulfonamides)—if large amounts given.

May inactivate enzymatic debriding agents—concomitant use may be inappropriate.

- ● **SIDE-EFFECTS** Allergic reactions · argyria (following treatment of large areas of skin or prolonged use) · burning · itching · leucopenia · rashes

SIDE-EFFECTS, FURTHER INFORMATION
- ▶ Severe blood and skin disorders Owing to the association of sulfonamides with severe blood and skin disorders, treatment should be stopped immediately if blood disorders or rashes develop.

Leucopenia developing 2–3 days after starting treatment of burns patients is reported usually to be self-limiting and silver sulfadiazine need not usually be discontinued provided blood counts are monitored carefully to ensure return to normality within a few days.

- ● **ALLERGY AND CROSS-SENSITIVITY** Contra-indicated in patients with sensitivity to sulfonamides.
- ● **PREGNANCY** Risk of neonatal haemolysis and methaemoglobinaemia in third trimester.
- ● **BREAST FEEDING** Small risk of kernicterus in jaundiced infants and of haemolysis in G6PD-deficient infants.
- ● **HEPATIC IMPAIRMENT** Manufacturer advises caution if significant impairment.
- ● **RENAL IMPAIRMENT** Manufacturer advises caution if significant impairment.
- ● **MONITORING REQUIREMENTS** Monitor for leucopenia.
- ● **DIRECTIONS FOR ADMINISTRATION** Apply with sterile applicator.

- ● **MEDICINAL FORMS**
There can be variation in the licensing of different medicines containing the same drug.

Cream
EXCIPIENTS: May contain Cetostearyl alcohol (including cetyl and stearyl alcohol), polysorbates, propylene glycol
- ▶ Flamazine (Smith & Nephew Healthcare Ltd)
Sulfadiazine silver 10 mg per 1 gram Flamazine 1% cream | 20 gram PoM £2.91 | 50 gram PoM £3.85 DT price = £3.85 | 250 gram PoM £10.32 DT price = £10.32 | 500 gram PoM £18.27 DT price = £18.27

ANTIBACTERIALS > OTHER

Bacitracin with polymyxin B

- ● **INDICATIONS AND DOSE**

Bacterial skin infections
- ▶ TO THE SKIN
- ▶ Child: Apply twice daily, can be applied more frequently if required

- ● **UNLICENSED USE** Licensed for use in children (age range not specified by manufacturer).
- ● **CAUTIONS** Nephrotoxicity · neurotoxicity

CAUTIONS, FURTHER INFORMATION
If large areas of skin are being treated nephrotoxicity and neurotoxicity may be a hazard, particularly in children with renal impairment.

- ● **SIDE-EFFECTS** Contact sensitisation
- ● **RENAL IMPAIRMENT** Renal impairment increases the risk of nephrotoxicity and neurotoxicity.

- ● **MEDICINAL FORMS**
There can be variation in the licensing of different medicines containing the same drug.

Ointment
- ▶ Polyfax (Teva UK Ltd)
Bacitracin zinc 500 unit per 1 gram, Polymyxin B sulfate 10000 unit per 1 gram Polyfax ointment | 4 gram PoM £3.26 | 20 gram PoM £4.62 DT price = £4.62

Mupirocin

- ● **INDICATIONS AND DOSE**

Bacterial skin infections, particularly those caused by Gram-positive organisms (except pseudomonal infection)
- ▶ TO THE SKIN
- ▶ Child: Apply up to 3 times a day for up to 10 days

- ● **UNLICENSED USE** Mupirocin ointment is licensed for use in children (age range not specified by manufacturer). *Bactroban* ® cream not recommended for use in children under 1 year.
- ● **SIDE-EFFECTS** Burning sensation · local reactions · pruritus · rash · urticaria
- ● **PREGNANCY** Manufacturer advises avoid unless potential benefit outweighs risk—no information available.
- ● **BREAST FEEDING** No information available.
- ● **RENAL IMPAIRMENT** Manufacturer advises caution when mupirocin ointment used in moderate or severe impairment because it contains macrogols (polyethylene glycol).

13

Skin

Skin

13

● **MEDICINAL FORMS**
There can be variation in the licensing of different medicines containing the same drug.

Cream
EXCIPIENTS: May contain Benzyl alcohol, cetostearyl alcohol (including cetyl and stearyl alcohol)
▸ Bactroban (GlaxoSmithKline UK Ltd)
Mupirocin (as Mupirocin calcium) 20 mg per 1 gram Bactroban 2% cream | 15 gram [PoM] £5.26 DT price = £5.26

Ointment
▸ Mupirocin (Non-proprietary)
Mupirocin 20 mg per 1 gram Mupirocin 2% ointment | 15 gram [PoM] £9.50 DT price = £4.38
▸ Bactroban (GlaxoSmithKline UK Ltd)
Mupirocin 20 mg per 1 gram Bactroban 2% ointment | 15 gram [PoM] £4.38 DT price = £4.38

Retapamulin

● **INDICATIONS AND DOSE**
Superficial bacterial skin infection caused by *Staphylococcus aureus* and *Streptococcus pyogenes* (if resistant to first line topical antibacterials)
▸ TO THE SKIN
▸ Child 9 months-17 years: Apply twice daily for 5 days, to be applied thinly, maximum area of skin treated 2% of body surface area, review treatment if no response within 2–3 days

● **CONTRA-INDICATIONS** Contact with eyes · contact with mucous membranes

● **SIDE-EFFECTS** Contact dermatitis · localised erythema · localised irritation · localised pain · pruritus

● **NATIONAL FUNDING/ACCESS DECISIONS**
Scottish Medicines Consortium (SMC) Decisions
The *Scottish Medicines Consortium* has advised (March 2008) that retapamulin (*Altargo®*) is **not** recommended for use within NHS Scotland for the treatment of superficial skin infections.

● **MEDICINAL FORMS**
There can be variation in the licensing of different medicines containing the same drug.
Ointment
CAUTIONARY AND ADVISORY LABELS 28
EXCIPIENTS: May contain Butylated hydroxytoluene
▸ Altargo (GlaxoSmithKline UK Ltd)
Retapamulin 10 mg per 1 gram Altargo 10mg/g ointment | 5 gram [PoM] £7.89

2.2 Fungal skin infections

ANTIFUNGALS > IMIDAZOLE ANTIFUNGALS

Clotrimazole

● **INDICATIONS AND DOSE**
Fungal skin infections
▸ TO THE SKIN
▸ Child: Apply 2–3 times a day

● **CAUTIONS** Contact with eyes and mucous membranes should be avoided

● **SIDE-EFFECTS** Local irritation · erythema · hypersensitivity reactions · itching · mild burning sensation
SIDE-EFFECTS, FURTHER INFORMATION
Treatment should be discontinued if side-effects are severe.

● **PREGNANCY** Minimal absorption from skin; not known to be harmful.

● **PRESCRIBING AND DISPENSING INFORMATION** Spray may be useful for application of clotrimazole to large or hairy areas of the skin.

● **MEDICINAL FORMS**
There can be variation in the licensing of different medicines containing the same drug. Forms available from special-order manufacturers include: powder

Liquid
▸ Canesten (clotrimazole) (Bayer Plc)
Clotrimazole 10 mg per 1 ml Canesten 1% solution | 20 ml [P] £2.30 DT price = £2.30

Cream
EXCIPIENTS: May contain Benzyl alcohol, cetostearyl alcohol (including cetyl and stearyl alcohol), polysorbates
▸ Clotrimazole (Non-proprietary)
Clotrimazole 10 mg per 1 gram Clotrimazole 1% cream | 20 gram [P] £2.79 DT price = £1.04 | 50 gram [P] £5.45 DT price = £2.60
▸ Canesten (clotrimazole) (Bayer Plc)
Clotrimazole 10 mg per 1 gram Canesten 1% cream | 20 gram [P] £2.14 DT price = £1.04 | 50 gram [P] £3.50 DT price = £2.60
Canesten Antifungal 1% cream | 20 gram [P] £1.85 DT price = £1.04

Combinations available: *Hydrocortisone with clotrimazole,* p. 697

Econazole nitrate

● **INDICATIONS AND DOSE**
Fungal skin infections
▸ TO THE SKIN
▸ Child: Apply twice daily
Fungal nail infections
▸ BY TRANSUNGUAL APPLICATION
▸ Child: Apply once daily, applied under occlusive dressing

● **CAUTIONS** Avoid contact with eyes and mucous membranes

● **SIDE-EFFECTS**
Burning sensation · erythema · hypersensitivity reactions · itching · occasional local irritation
SIDE-EFFECTS, FURTHER INFORMATION
Treatment should be discontinued if side-effects are severe.

● **PREGNANCY** Minimal absorption from skin; not known to be harmful.

● **MEDICINAL FORMS**
There can be variation in the licensing of different medicines containing the same drug.
Cream
EXCIPIENTS: May contain Butylated hydroxyanisole, fragrances
▸ Pevaryl (Janssen-Cilag Ltd)
Econazole nitrate 10 mg per 1 gram Pevaryl 1% cream | 30 gram [P] £3.71

Ketoconazole

● **INDICATIONS AND DOSE**
Treatment of seborrhoeic dermatitis and dandruff
▸ TO THE SKIN USING SHAMPOO
▸ Child 12-17 years: Apply twice weekly for 2–4 weeks, leave preparation on for 3–5 minutes before rinsing
Prophylaxis of seborrhoeic dermatitis and dandruff
▸ TO THE SKIN USING SHAMPOO
▸ Child 12-17 years: Apply every 1–2 weeks, leave preparation on for 3–5 minutes before rinsing

Treatment of pityriasis versicolor

▶ TO THE SKIN USING SHAMPOO

▸ Child 12–17 years: Apply once daily for maximum 5 days, leave preparation on for 3–5 minutes before rinsing

Prophylaxis of pityriasis versicolor

▶ TO THE SKIN USING SHAMPOO

▸ Child 12–17 years: Apply once daily for up to 3 days before sun exposure, leave preparation on for 3–5 minutes before rinsing

● CAUTIONS Avoid contact with eyes · avoid contact with mucous membranes

● INTERACTIONS → Appendix 1 (antifungals, imidazole).

● SIDE-EFFECTS Erythema · hypersensitivity reactions · itching · mild burning sensation · occasional local irritation

SIDE-EFFECTS, FURTHER INFORMATION

Treatment should be discontinued if side-effects are severe.

● NATIONAL FUNDING/ACCESS DECISIONS

NHS restrictions Ketoconazole cream is not prescribable on the NHS except for seborrhoeic dermatitis and pityriasis versicolor and endorsed 'SLS'

● EXCEPTIONS TO LEGAL CATEGORY Can be sold to the public for the prevention and treatment of dandruff and seborrhoeic dermatitis of the scalp as a shampoo formulation containing ketoconazole maximum 2%, in a pack containing maximum 120 mL and labelled to show a maximum frequency of application of once every 3 days.

● MEDICINAL FORMS

There can be variation in the licensing of different medicines containing the same drug.

Shampoo

EXCIPIENTS: May contain Imidurea

▸ Ketoconazole (Non-proprietary)

Ketoconazole 20 mg per 1 gram Ketoconazole 2% shampoo | 120 ml [PoM] £3.00 DT price = £2.71

▸ Dandrazol (Transdermal Ltd)

Ketoconazole 20 mg per 1 gram Dandrazol Anti-dandruff 2% shampoo | 60 ml [GSL] £3.42 | 100 ml [GSL] £5.28 Dandrazol 2% shampoo | 120 ml [PoM] £5.20 DT price = £2.71

▸ Nizoral (Janssen-Cilag Ltd, McNeil Products Ltd)

Ketoconazole 20 mg per 1 gram Nizoral 2% shampoo | 120 ml [PoM] £3.59 DT price = £2.71 Nizoral anti-dandruff 2% shampoo | 60 ml [GSL] £3.78 Nizoral Dandruff 2% shampoo | 100 ml [P] £5.68

Miconazole

● INDICATIONS AND DOSE

Fungal skin infections

▶ TO THE SKIN

▸ Neonate: Apply twice daily continuing for 10 days after lesions have healed.

▸ Child: Apply twice daily continuing for 10 days after lesions have healed

Fungal nail infections

▶ TO THE SKIN

▸ Child: Apply 1–2 times a day

● UNLICENSED USE Licensed for use in children (age range not specified by manufacturer).

● CAUTIONS Avoid in Acute porphyrias p. 562 · contact with eyes and mucous membranes should be avoided

● INTERACTIONS → Appendix 1 (antifungals, imidazole).

● SIDE-EFFECTS

SPECIFIC SIDE-EFFECTS

Burning sensation · erythema · hypersensitivity reactions · itching · occasional local irritation · rash

SIDE-EFFECTS, FURTHER INFORMATION

Treatment should be discontinued if side effects are severe.

● PREGNANCY Absorbed from the skin in small amounts; manufacturer advises caution.

● BREAST FEEDING Manufacturer advises caution—no information available.

● PROFESSION SPECIFIC INFORMATION

Dental practitioners' formulary

Miconazole cream may be prescribed.

● MEDICINAL FORMS

There can be variation in the licensing of different medicines containing the same drug.

Capsule

EXCIPIENTS: May contain Hydroxybenzoates (parabens)

▸ Gyno-Daktarin (Janssen-Cilag Ltd)

Miconazole nitrate 1.2 gram Gyno-Daktarin 1200mg vaginal capsules | 1 capsule [PoM] £2.94 DT price = £2.94

Cream

EXCIPIENTS: May contain Butylated hydroxyanisole

▸ Daktarin (McNeil Products Ltd, Janssen-Cilag Ltd)

Miconazole nitrate 20 mg per 1 gram Daktarin 2% cream | 15 gram [P] £2.14 | 30 gram [P] £1.82 DT price = £1.82 Daktarin Aktiv 2% cream | 15 gram [GSL] £2.16 | 30 gram [GSL] £3.22 DT price = £1.82

Powder

▸ Daktarin (McNeil Products Ltd)

Miconazole nitrate 20 mg per 1 gram Daktarin 2% powder | 20 gram [P] £2.58 DT price = £2.58

Tioconazole

● INDICATIONS AND DOSE

Fungal nail infection

▶ BY TRANSUNGUAL APPLICATION

▸ Child: Apply twice daily usually for up to 6 months (may be extended to 12 months), apply to nails and surrounding skin

● UNLICENSED USE Licensed for use in children (age range not specified by manufacturer).

● CAUTIONS

GENERAL CAUTIONS

Contact with eyes and mucous membranes should be avoided

SPECIFIC CAUTIONS

Use with caution if child likely to suck affected digits

● SIDE-EFFECTS Burning sensation · dry skin · erythema · exfoliation · hypersensitivity reactions · itching · local oedema · nail discoloration · nail pain · occasional local irritation · periungual inflammation · rash

SIDE-EFFECTS, FURTHER INFORMATION

Treatment should be discontinued if side-effects are severe.

● PREGNANCY Manufacturer advises avoid.

● MEDICINAL FORMS

There can be variation in the licensing of different medicines containing the same drug.

Paint

▸ Tioconazole (Non-proprietary)

Tioconazole 283 mg per 1 ml Tioconazole 283mg/ml medicated nail lacquer | 12 ml [PoM] £27.38–£28.74 DT price = £28.06

▸ Trosyl (Pfizer Ltd)

Tioconazole 283 mg per 1 ml Trosyl 283mg/ml nail solution | 12 ml [PoM] £27.38 DT price = £28.06

13

Skin

ANTIFUNGALS 〉 OTHER

Amorolfine

- **INDICATIONS AND DOSE**

Fungal nail infections
▶ BY TRANSUNGUAL APPLICATION
▶ Child 1 month-11 years: Apply 1-2 times a week for 6 months to treat finger nails and for toe nails 9-12 months (review at intervals of 3 months), apply to infected nails after filing and cleansing, allow to dry for approximately 3 minutes
▶ Child 12-17 years: Apply 1-2 times a week for 6 months to treat finger nails and for toe nails 9-12 months (review at intervals of 3 months), apply to infected nails after filing and cleansing, allow to dry for approximately 3 minutes

- **UNLICENSED USE** Not licensed for use in children under 12 years.
- **CAUTIONS** Avoid contact with ears · avoid contact with eyes and mucous membranes · use with caution in child likely to suck affected digits
- **SIDE-EFFECTS** Burning sensation · erythema · hypersensitivity reactions · itching · occasional local irritation
  SIDE-EFFECTS, FURTHER INFORMATION
  Treatment should be discontinued if side-effects are severe.
- **PATIENT AND CARER ADVICE** Avoid nail varnish or artificial nails during treatment.

- **MEDICINAL FORMS**
  There can be variation in the licensing of different medicines containing the same drug.
  Medicated nail lacquer
  CAUTIONARY AND ADVISORY LABELS 10
  ▶ Amorolfine (Non-proprietary)
  Amorolfine (as Amorolfine hydrochloride) 50 mg per 1 ml Amorolfine 5% medicated nail lacquer | 3 ml PoM no price available | 5 ml PoM £16.21 DT price = £7.45
  Boots Once Weekly Fungal Nail Treatment 5% medicated nail lacquer | 3 ml P no price available
  ▶ Loceryl (Galderma (UK) Ltd)
  Amorolfine (as Amorolfine hydrochloride) 50 mg per 1 ml Loceryl Curanail 5% medicated nail lacquer | 3 ml P £12.31
  Loceryl 5% medicated nail lacquer | 2.5 ml PoM £7.26 | 5 ml PoM £9.08 DT price = £7.45
  ▶ Omicur (Morningside Healthcare Ltd)
  Amorolfine (as Amorolfine hydrochloride) 50 mg per 1 ml Omicur 5% medicated nail lacquer | 2.5 ml PoM £9.09 | 5 ml PoM £9.09 DT price = £7.45

Terbinafine

- **INDICATIONS AND DOSE**

Tinea pedis
▶ TO THE SKIN USING CREAM
▶ Child: Apply 1-2 times a day for up to 1 week, to be applied thinly
▶ BY MOUTH USING TABLETS
▶ Child 1-17 years (body-weight 10-19 kg): 62.5 mg once daily for 2-6 weeks
▶ Child 1-17 years (body-weight 20-39 kg): 125 mg once daily for 2-6 weeks
▶ Child 1-17 years (body-weight 40 kg and above): 250 mg once daily for 2-6 weeks

Tinea corporis
▶ TO THE SKIN USING CREAM
▶ Child: Apply 1-2 times a day for up to 1-2 weeks, to be applied thinly, review treatment after 2 weeks

▶ BY MOUTH USING TABLETS
▶ Child 1-17 years (body-weight 10-19 kg): 62.5 mg once daily for 4 weeks
▶ Child 1-17 years (body-weight 20-39 kg): 125 mg once daily for 4 weeks
▶ Child 1-17 years (body-weight 40 kg and above): 250 mg once daily for 4 weeks

Tinea cruris
▶ TO THE SKIN USING CREAM
▶ Child: Apply 1-2 times a day for up to 1-2 weeks, to be applied thinly, review treatment after 2 weeks
▶ BY MOUTH USING TABLETS
▶ Child 1-17 years (body-weight 10-19 kg): 62.5 mg once daily for 2-4 weeks
▶ Child 1-17 years (body-weight 20-39 kg): 125 mg once daily for 2-4 weeks
▶ Child 1-17 years (body-weight 40 kg and above): 250 mg once daily for 2-4 weeks

Tinea capitis
▶ BY MOUTH USING TABLETS
▶ Child 1-17 years (body-weight 10-19 kg): 62.5 mg once daily for 4 weeks
▶ Child 1-17 years (body-weight 20-39 kg): 125 mg once daily for 4 weeks
▶ Child 1-17 years (body-weight 40 kg and above): 250 mg once daily for 4 weeks

Dermatophyte infections of the nails
▶ BY MOUTH USING TABLETS
▶ Child 1-17 years (body-weight 10-19 kg): 62.5 mg once daily for 6 weeks-3 months (occasionally longer in toenail infections)
▶ Child 1-17 years (body-weight 20-39 kg): 125 mg once daily for 6 weeks-3 months (occasionally longer in toenail infections)
▶ Child 1-17 years (body-weight 40 kg and above): 250 mg once daily for 6 weeks-3 months (occasionally longer in toenail infections)

Cutaneous candidiasis | Pityriasis versicolor
▶ TO THE SKIN USING CREAM
▶ Child: Apply 1-2 times a day for 2 weeks, to be applied thinly, review treatment after 2 weeks

- **UNLICENSED USE** Not licensed for use in children.
- **CAUTIONS**
  ▶ With oral use Autoimmune disease (risk of lupus-erythematosus-like effect) · psoriasis (risk of exacerbation)
  ▶ With topical use Contact with eyes and mucous membranes should be avoided
- **INTERACTIONS**
  ▶ With oral use Appendix 1 (terbinafine).
- **SIDE-EFFECTS**
  ▶ Common or very common
  ▶ With oral use Abdominal discomfort · anorexia · arthralgia · diarrhoea · dyspepsia · headache · myalgia · nausea · rash · urticaria
  ▶ Uncommon
  ▶ With oral use Taste disturbance
  ▶ Rare
  ▶ With oral use Cholestasis · dizziness · hepatitis · hypoaesthesia · jaundice · liver toxicity · malaise · paraesthesia
  ▶ Very rare
  ▶ With oral use Alopecia · blood disorders · lupus erythematosus-like effect · neutropenia · photosensitivity · serious skin reactions · Stevens-Johnson syndrome · thrombocytopenia · toxic epidermal necrolysis
  ▶ Frequency not known
  ▶ With oral use Disturbances in smell · exacerbation of psoriasis · hearing disturbances · influenza-like symptoms · pancreatitis · rhabdomyolysis · vasculitis

▶ With topical use Erythema · hypersensitivity reactions · itching · mild burning sensation · occasional local irritation
SIDE-EFFECTS, FURTHER INFORMATION
▶ Liver toxicity
▶ With oral use Discontinue treatment if liver toxicity develops (including jaundice, cholestasis and hepatitis).
▶ Serious skin reactions
▶ With oral use Discontinue treatment in progressive skin rash (including Stevens-Johnson syndrome and toxic epidermal necrolysis).
▶ Topical application
▶ With topical use Treatment should be discontinued if side effects are severe.
● PREGNANCY
▶ With topical use Manufacturer advises use only if potential benefit outweighs risk—*animal* studies suggest no adverse effects.
▶ With oral use Manufacturer advises use only if potential benefit outweighs risk—no information available.
● BREAST FEEDING
▶ With topical use Manufacturer advises avoid—present in milk. Less than 5% of the dose is absorbed after topical application of terbinafine; avoid application to mother's chest.
▶ With oral use Avoid—present in milk.
● HEPATIC IMPAIRMENT
▶ With oral use Manufacturer advises avoid—elimination reduced.
● RENAL IMPAIRMENT
▶ With oral use Use half normal dose if estimated glomerular filtration rate less than 50 mL/minute/1.73 m^2 and no suitable alternative available.
● MONITORING REQUIREMENTS
▶ With oral use Monitor hepatic function before treatment and then every 4–6 weeks during treatment—discontinue if abnormalities in liver function tests.
● EXCEPTIONS TO LEGAL CATEGORY
▶ With topical use Preparations of terbinafine hydrochloride (maximum 1%) can be sold to the public for use in those over 16 years for external use for the treatment of tinea pedis as a cream in a pack containing maximum 15 g, or for the treatment of tinea pedis and cruris as a cream in a pack containing maximum 15 g, or for the treatment of tinea pedis, cruris, and corporis as a spray in a pack containing maximum 30 mL spray or as a gel in a pack containing maximum 30 g gel.

● MEDICINAL FORMS
There can be variation in the licensing of different medicines containing the same drug.

Tablet
CAUTIONARY AND ADVISORY LABELS 9
▶ Terbinafine (Non-proprietary)
Terbinafine (as Terbinafine hydrochloride) 250 mg Terbinafine 250mg tablets | 14 tablet [PoM] £18.11 DT price = £1.22 | 28 tablet [PoM] £34.93
▶ Lamisil (Novartis Pharmaceuticals UK Ltd)
Terbinafine (as Terbinafine hydrochloride) 250 mg Lamisil 250mg tablets | 14 tablet [PoM] £21.30 DT price = £1.22 | 28 tablet [PoM] £41.09

Cream
EXCIPIENTS: May contain Benzyl alcohol, cetostearyl alcohol (including cetyl and stearyl alcohol), polysorbates
▶ Terbinafine (Non-proprietary)
Terbinafine hydrochloride 10 mg per 1 gram Terbinafine 1% cream | 7.5 gram [GSL] £5.50 | 7.5 gram [PoM] £1.06 | 15 gram [GSL] £4.59 DT price = £1.31 | 15 gram [PoM] £4.86 DT price = £1.31 | 30 gram [PoM] £8.76 DT price = £2.62
▶ Lamisil (Novartis Consumer Health UK Ltd)
Terbinafine hydrochloride 10 mg per 1 gram Lamisil 1% cream | 30 gram [PoM] £7.45 DT price = £2.62
Lamisil AT 1% cream | 7.5 gram [GSL] £2.39 | 15 gram [GSL] £3.60 DT price = £1.31

ANTISEPTICS AND DISINFECTANTS ›
UNDECENOATES

Undecenoic acid with zinc undecenoate

● INDICATIONS AND DOSE
Treatment of athletes foot
▶ TO THE SKIN
▶ Child: Apply twice daily, continue use for 7 days after lesions have healed
Prevention of athletes foot
▶ TO THE SKIN
▶ Child: Apply once daily

● UNLICENSED USE *Mycota*® licensed for use in children (age range not specified by manufacturer).
● CAUTIONS Avoid broken skin · contact with eyes should be avoided · contact with mucous membranes should be avoided
● SIDE-EFFECTS Erythema · hypersensitivity reactions · itching · local irritation · mild burning sensation
SIDE-EFFECTS, FURTHER INFORMATION
Treatment should be discontinued if side effects are severe.

● MEDICINAL FORMS
There can be variation in the licensing of different medicines containing the same drug.
Cream
EXCIPIENTS: May contain Cetostearyl alcohol (including cetyl and stearyl alcohol), fragrances
▶ Undecenoic acid with zinc undecenoate (Non-proprietary)
Undecenoic acid 50 mg per 1 gram, Zinc undecenoate 200 mg per 1 gram Mycota cream | 25 gram [GSL] £2.01
Powder
EXCIPIENTS: May contain Fragrances
▶ Undecenoic acid with zinc undecenoate (Non-proprietary)
Undecenoic acid 20 mg per 1 gram, Zinc undecenoate 200 mg per 1 gram Mycota powder | 70 gram [GSL] £2.71

ANTISEPTICS AND DISINFECTANTS › OTHER

Chlorhexidine with nystatin

● INDICATIONS AND DOSE
Skin infections due to Candida spp.
▶ TO THE SKIN
▶ Child: Apply 2–3 times a day, continuing for 7 days after lesions have healed

● UNLICENSED USE Licensed for use in children (age range not specified by manufacturer).
● CAUTIONS Avoid contact with eyes and mucous membranes
● SIDE-EFFECTS Burning sensation · erythema · hypersensitivity reactions · itching · occasional local irritation

SIDE-EFFECTS, FURTHER INFORMATION
Treatment should be discontinued if side-effects are severe.

● MEDICINAL FORMS
There can be variation in the licensing of different medicines containing the same drug.
Cream
EXCIPIENTS: May contain Benzyl alcohol, cetostearyl alcohol (including cetyl and stearyl alcohol), polysorbates
▶ Nystaform (Typharm Ltd)
Chlorhexidine hydrochloride 10 mg per 1 gram, Nystatin 100000 unit per 1 gram Nystaform cream | 30 gram [PoM] £2.62 DT price = £2.62

13

Skin

BENZOATES

Benzoic acid with salicylic acid

- **INDICATIONS AND DOSE**
Ringworm (tinea)
  - ▸ TO THE SKIN
  - ▸ Child: Apply twice daily

- **UNLICENSED USE** Licensed for use in children (age range not specified by manufacturer).
- **CAUTIONS** Avoid broken or inflamed skin · avoid contact with eyes · avoid contact with mucous membranes
  CAUTIONS, FURTHER INFORMATION
  - ▸ Salicylate toxicity Salicylate toxicity may occur particularly if applied on large areas of skin.
- **SIDE-EFFECTS** Erythema · hypersensitivity reactions · itching · mild burning sensation · occasional local irritation
  SIDE-EFFECTS, FURTHER INFORMATION
  Treatment should be discontinued if side effects are severe.
- **PRESCRIBING AND DISPENSING INFORMATION** Benzoic Acid Ointment, Compound, BP has also been referred to as Whitfield's ointment.

- **MEDICINAL FORMS**
  There can be variation in the licensing of different medicines containing the same drug. Forms available from special-order manufacturers include: cream, ointment

SALICYLIC ACID AND DERIVATIVES

Boric acid with salicylic acid and tannic acid

- **INDICATIONS AND DOSE**
Fungal nail infection, particularly tinea
  - ▸ BY TRANSUNGUAL APPLICATION
  - ▸ Child 5–17 years: Apply twice daily, and after washing

- **CAUTIONS** Avoid broken or inflamed skin · contact with eyes and mucous membranes should be avoided · use with caution in children likely to suck affected digits
  CAUTIONS, FURTHER INFORMATION
  - ▸ Salicylate toxicity Salicylate toxicity can occur particularly if applied on large areas of skin.
- **SIDE-EFFECTS** Burning sensation · erythema · hypersensitivity reactions · itching · occasional local irritation
  SIDE-EFFECTS, FURTHER INFORMATION
  Treatment should be discontinued if side-effects are severe.
- **PREGNANCY** Avoid.
- **LESS SUITABLE FOR PRESCRIBING** *Phytex* ® is less suitable for prescribing.

- **MEDICINAL FORMS**
  There can be variation in the licensing of different medicines containing the same drug.
  No licensed medicines listed.

2.3 Parasitic skin infections

PARASITICIDES

Dimeticone

- **INDICATIONS AND DOSE**
Head lice
  - ▸ TO THE SKIN
  - ▸ Child: Apply once weekly for 2 doses, rub into dry hair and scalp, allow to dry naturally, shampoo after minimum 8 hours (or overnight)

- **UNLICENSED USE** Not licensed for use in children under 6 months except under medical supervision.
- **CAUTIONS** Avoid contact with eyes · children under 6 months, medical supervision required
- **SIDE-EFFECTS** Skin irritation
- **PATIENT AND CARER ADVICE** Patients should be told to keep hair away from fire and flames during treatment.

- **MEDICINAL FORMS**
  There can be variation in the licensing of different medicines containing the same drug.
  Liquid
  - ▸ Hedrin (Thornton & Ross Ltd)
    Dimeticone 40 mg per 1 gram Hedrin 4% lotion | 50 ml Ⓟ £2.98
    DT price = £2.98 | 150 ml Ⓟ £6.92 DT price = £6.92
  Cutaneous spray solution
  - ▸ Hedrin (Thornton & Ross Ltd)
    Dimeticone 40 mg per 1 gram Hedrin 4% spray | 120 ml GSL £7.13
  Gel
  - ▸ Hedrin Once (Thornton & Ross Ltd)
    Hedrin Once spray gel | 60 ml £4.16 | 100 ml £6.83
    Hedrin Once liquid gel | 100 ml £5.95 | 250 ml £10.40

Malathion

- **INDICATIONS AND DOSE**
Head lice
  - ▸ TO THE SKIN
  - ▸ Child: Apply once weekly for 2 doses, rub preparation into dry hair and scalp, allow to dry naturally, remove by washing after 12 hours

Crab lice
  - ▸ TO THE SKIN
  - ▸ Child: Apply once weekly for 2 doses, apply preparation over whole body, allow to dry naturally, wash off after 12 hours or overnight

Scabies
  - ▸ TO THE SKIN
  - ▸ Child: Apply once weekly for 2 doses, apply preparation over whole body, and wash off after 24 hours, if hands are washed with soap within 24 hours, they should be retreated

- **UNLICENSED USE** Not licensed for use in children under 6 months except under medical supervision.
- **CAUTIONS** Alcoholic lotions **not** recommended for head lice in children with severe eczema or asthma, or for scabies or crab lice · avoid contact with eyes · children under 6 months, medical supervision required · do not use lotion more than once a week for 3 consecutive weeks · do not use on broken or secondarily infected skin
- **SIDE-EFFECTS** Chemical burns · hypersensitivity reactions · skin irritation
- **PRESCRIBING AND DISPENSING INFORMATION** For scabies, manufacturer recommends application to the body but no

necessarily to the head and neck. However, application should be extended to the scalp, neck, face, and ears.

● MEDICINAL FORMS
There can be variation in the licensing of different medicines containing the same drug.

Liquid
EXCIPIENTS: May contain Cetostearyl alcohol (including cetyl and stearyl alcohol), fragrances, hydroxybenzoates (parabens)
▸ Derbac-M (G.R. Lane Health Products Ltd)
Malathion 5 mg per 1 gram Derbac-M 0.5% liquid | 50 ml P £3.57 DT price = £3.57 | 200 ml P £8.44 DT price = £8.44

Permethrin

● INDICATIONS AND DOSE
Scabies
▸ TO THE SKIN
▸ Child: Apply once weekly for 2 doses, apply 5% preparation over whole body including face, neck, scalp and ears then wash off after 8–12 hours. If hands are washed with soap within 8 hours of application, they should be treated again with cream

● UNLICENSED USE *Dermal Cream* (scabies), not licensed for use in children under 2 months; not licensed for treatment of crab lice in children under 18 years. *Creme Rinse* (head lice) not licensed for use in children under 6 months except under medical supervision.

● CAUTIONS Avoid contact with eyes · children aged 2 months–2 years, medical supervision required for dermal cream (scabies) · children under 6 months, medical supervision required for cream rinse (head lice) · do not use on broken or secondarily infected skin

● SIDE-EFFECTS
▸ Rare Oedema · rashes
▸ Frequency not known Erythema · pruritus · stinging

● PRESCRIBING AND DISPENSING INFORMATION
Manufacturer recommends application to the body but to exclude head and neck. However, application should be extended to the scalp, neck, face, and ears.
    Larger patients may require up to two 30-g packs for adequate treatment.

● LESS SUITABLE FOR PRESCRIBING Lyclear® Creme Rinse is less suitable for prescribing.

● MEDICINAL FORMS
There can be variation in the licensing of different medicines containing the same drug.

Liquid
EXCIPIENTS: May contain Cetostearyl alcohol (including cetyl and stearyl alcohol)
▸ Lyclear (Omega Pharma Ltd)
Permethrin 10 mg per 1 gram Lyclear 1% creme rinse | 59 ml P £3.55 DT price = £3.55 | 118 ml P £6.46 DT price = £6.46

Cream
CAUTIONARY AND ADVISORY LABELS 10 (Dermal cream only)
EXCIPIENTS: May contain Butylated hydroxytoluene, wool fat and related substances including lanolin
▸ Permethrin (Non-proprietary)
Permethrin 50 mg per 1 gram Permethrin 5% cream | 30 gram P £7.46 DT price = £7.46
▸ Lyclear (Omega Pharma Ltd)
Permethrin 50 mg per 1 gram Lyclear 5% dermal cream | 30 gram P £5.71 DT price = £7.46

2.4 Viral skin infections

ANTIVIRALS 〉 NUCLEOSIDE ANALOGUES

Aciclovir

(Acyclovir)

● INDICATIONS AND DOSE
Herpes simplex infection (local treatment)
▸ TO THE SKIN
▸ Child: Apply 5 times a day for 5–10 days, to be applied to lesions approximately every 4 hours, starting at first sign of attack

● UNLICENSED USE Cream licensed for use in children (age range not specified by manufacturer).

● CAUTIONS Avoid cream coming in to contact with eyes and mucous membranes

● SIDE-EFFECTS Drying of the skin · erythema · itching of the skin · transient burning · transient stinging

● PREGNANCY Limited absorption from topical aciclovir preparations.

● PATIENT AND CARER ADVICE
Medicines for Children leaflet: Aciclovir cream for herpes www.medicinesforchildren.org.uk/aciclovir-cream-for-herpes

● PROFESSION SPECIFIC INFORMATION
Dental practitioners' formulary
Aciclovir Cream may be prescribed.

● EXCEPTIONS TO LEGAL CATEGORY A 2-g tube and a pump pack are on sale to the public for the treatment of cold sores.

● MEDICINAL FORMS
There can be variation in the licensing of different medicines containing the same drug.

Cream
EXCIPIENTS: May contain Cetostearyl alcohol (including cetyl and stearyl alcohol), propylene glycol
▸ Aciclovir (Non-proprietary)
Aciclovir 50 mg per 1 gram Aciclovir 5% cream | 2 gram GSL £0.83 DT price = £1.05 | 2 gram PoM £4.17 DT price = £1.05 | 10 gram PoM £12.56 DT price = £5.25
▸ Zovirax (GlaxoSmithKline Consumer Healthcare, GlaxoSmithKline UK Ltd)
Aciclovir 50 mg per 1 gram Zovirax Cold Sore 5% cream | 2 gram GSL £3.96–£4.28 DT price = £1.05
Zovirax 5% cream | 2 gram PoM £4.63 DT price = £1.05 | 10 gram PoM £13.96 DT price = £5.25

3 Inflammatory skin conditions

3.1 Eczema and psoriasis

Eczema

Types and management
The main types of eczema (dermatitis) in children are atopic, irritant and allergic contact; different types may co-exist. *Atopic eczema* is the most common type and it usually involves dry skin as well as infection and lichenification caused by scratching and rubbing. *Seborrhoeic dermatitis* is also common in infants.
    Management of eczema involves the removal or treatment of contributory factors; known or suspected irritants and contact allergens should be avoided. Rarely, ingredients in topical medicinal products may sensitise the skin; *BNF for*

Children lists active ingredients together with excipients that have been associated with skin sensitisation.

Skin dryness and the consequent irritant eczema requires **emollients** applied regularly (at least twice daily) and liberally to the affected area; this can be supplemented with bath or shower emollients. The use of emollients should continue even if the eczema improves or if other treatment is being used.

Topical corticosteroids are also required in the management of eczema; the potency of the corticosteroid should be appropriate to the severity and site of the condition, and the age of the child. Mild corticosteroids are generally used on the face and on flexures; the more potent corticosteroids are generally required for use on lichenified areas of eczema or for severe eczema on the scalp, limbs, and trunk. Treatment should be reviewed regularly, especially if a potent corticosteroid is required. In children with frequent flares (2–3 per month), a topical corticosteroid can be applied on 2 consecutive days each week to prevent further flares.

Bandages (including those containing ichthammol with zinc oxide p. 699) are sometimes applied over topical corticosteroids or emollients to treat eczema of the limbs. Dry-wrap dressings can be used to provide a physical barrier to help prevent scratching and improve retention of emollients. Wet elasticated viscose stockinette is used for 'wet-wrap' bandaging over topical corticosteroids or emollients to cool the skin and relieve itching, but there is an increased risk of infection and excessive absorption of the corticosteroid; 'wet-wrap' bandaging should be used under specialist supervision.

See *Wound management products and elasticated garments* for details of elasticated viscose stockinette tubular bandages and garments, and silk clothing.

See Eczema and psoriasis, drugs affecting the immune response below for the role of topical pimecrolimus p. 701 and tacrolimus p. 702 in atopic eczema.

Infection
Bacterial infection (commonly with *Staphylococcus aureus* and occasionally with *Streptococcus pyogenes*) can exacerbate eczema. A topical antibacterial may be used for small areas of mild infection; treatment should be limited to a short course (typically 1 week) to reduce the risk of drug resistance or skin sensitisation. Associated eczema is treated simultaneously with a topical corticosteroid which can be combined with a topical antimicrobial.

Eczema involving moderate to severe, widespread, or recurrent infection requires the use of a systemic antibacterial that is active against the infecting organism. Preparations that combine an antiseptic with an emollient application and with a bath emollient can also be used; antiseptic shampoos can be used on the scalp.

Intertriginous eczema commonly involves candida and bacteria; it is best treated with a mild or moderately potent topical corticosteroid combined with a suitable antimicrobial drug.

Widespread *herpes simplex infection* may complicate atopic eczema (eczema herpeticum) and treatment under specialist supervision with a systemic antiviral drug is indicated. Secondary bacterial infection often exacerbates eczema herpeticum.

Management of other features of eczema
Lichenification, which results from repeated scratching, is treated initially with a potent corticosteroid. Bandages containing ichthammol p. 699 (to reduce pruritus) and other substances such as **zinc oxide** can be applied over the corticosteroid or emollient. **Coal tar** and ichthammol can be useful in some cases of *chronic eczema*. *Discoid eczema*, with thickened plaques in chronic atopic eczema, is usually treated with a topical antiseptic preparation, a potent topical corticosteroid, and paste bandages containing ichthammol with zinc oxide.

A *non-sedating* antihistamine may be of some value in relieving severe itching or urticaria associated with eczema. A *sedating* antihistamine can be used at night if itching causes sleep disturbance, but a large dose may be needed and drowsiness may persist on the following day.

Exudative ('weeping') eczema requires a potent corticosteroid initially; infection may also be present and require specific treatment. Potassium permanganate solution (1 in 10,000) p. 716 can be used as a soak in exudating eczema for its antiseptic and astringent effects; treatment should be stopped when exudation stops.

Severe refractory eczema is best managed under specialist supervision; it may require phototherapy or drugs that act on the immune system.

Seborrhoeic dermatitis
Seborrhoeic dermatitis (seborrhoeic eczema) is associated with species of the yeast *Malassezia*. *Infantile seborrhoeic dermatitis* affects particularly the body folds, nappy area and scalp; it is treated with emollients and mild topical corticosteroids with suitable antimicrobials. Infantile seborrhoeic dermatitis affecting the scalp (*cradle cap*) is treated by hydrating the scalp using natural oils and the use of mild shampoo.

In older children, seborrhoeic dermatitis affects the scalp, paranasal areas, and eyebrows. Shampoos active against the yeast (including those containing ketoconazole p. 678 and coal tar) and combinations of mild topical corticosteroids with suitable antimicrobials are used to treat older children.

Medicated bandages
Zinc paste bandages (see *Wound management products and elasticated garments*) are used with **coal tar** or ichthammol in chronic lichenified skin conditions such as chronic eczema (ichthammol often being preferred since its action is considered to be milder). They are also used with calamine in milder eczematous skin conditions.

Eczema and psoriasis, drugs affecting the immune response

Overview

Drugs affecting the immune response are used for eczema or psoriasis. Pimecrolimus p. 701 by topical application is licensed for *mild to moderate atopic eczema*. Tacrolimus p. 702 is licensed for topical use in *moderate to severe atopic eczema*. Both are drugs whose long-term safety is still being evaluated and they should not usually be considered first-line treatment unless there is a specific reason to avoid or reduce the use of topical corticosteroids. Treatment with topical pimecrolimus or topical tacrolimus should be initiated only by prescribers experienced in treating atopic eczema.

Topical corticosteroids have a role in eczema and a limited role in psoriasis. A systemic corticosteroid such as prednisolone p. 413 may be used in severe refractory eczema.

Systemic drugs acting on the immune system are generally used by **specialists** in a hospital setting.

Ciclosporin p. 486 by mouth can be used for *severe psoriasis* and for *severe eczema*. Azathioprine p. 485 or mycophenolate mofetil p. 492 are also used for severe refractory eczema in children.

Methotrexate p. 506 can be used for *severe resistant* psoriasis; the dose is given **once weekly** and adjusted according to severity of the condition and haematological and biochemical measurements. Folic acid p. 533 should be given to reduce the possibility of methotrexate toxicity [unlicensed indication]. Folic acid can be given once weekly on a different day to the methotrexate; alternative regimens may be used in some settings.

Etanercept p. 600 (a cytokine modulator) is licensed in children over 6 years of age for the treatment of *severe plaque psoriasis* that is inadequately controlled by other systemic treatments and photochemotherapy, or when these other treatments cannot be used because of intolerance or contra-indications.

Adalimumab p. 598 (a cytokine modulator) is licensed in children over 4 years for the treatment of *severe chronic plaque psoriasis* that is inadequately controlled by other topical treatments and phototherapies, or when these treatments are inappropriate.

Psoriasis

Management

Psoriasis is characterised by epidermal thickening and scaling. It commonly affects extensor surfaces and the scalp. For mild psoriasis, reassurance and treatment with an emollient may be all that is necessary. *Guttate psoriasis* is a distinctive form of psoriasis that characteristically occurs in children and young adults, often following a streptococcal throat infection or tonsillitis.

Occasionally psoriasis is provoked or exacerbated by drugs such as lithium, chloroquine and hydroxychloroquine, beta-blockers, non-steroidal anti-inflammatory drugs, and ACE inhibitors. Psoriasis may not occur until the drug has been taken for weeks or months.

Emollients, in addition to their effects on dryness, scaling and cracking, may have an antiproliferative effect in psoriasis. They are particularly useful in *inflammatory psoriasis* and in *chronic stable plaque psoriasis*.

For *chronic stable plaque psoriasis* on extensor surfaces of trunk and limbs preparations containing **coal tar** are moderately effective, but the smell is unacceptable to some children. **Vitamin D** and its analogues are effective and cosmetically acceptable alternatives to preparations containing coal tar or dithranol p. 699. Dithranol is an effective topical antipsoriatic agent but it irritates and stains the skin and it should be used only under specialist supervision. Adverse effects of dithranol are minimised by using a 'short-contact technique' and by starting with low concentration preparations. Tazarotene, a topical retinoid for the treatment of mild to moderate plaque psoriasis, is not recommended for use in children under 18 years. These medications can irritate the skin particularly in the flexures and they are not suitable for the more inflammatory forms of psoriasis; their use should be suspended during an inflammatory phase of psoriasis. The efficacy and the irritancy of each substance varies between patients. If a substance irritates significantly, it should be stopped or the concentration reduced; if it is tolerated, its effects should be assessed after 4 to 6 weeks and treatment continued if it is effective.

Widespread *unstable psoriasis* of erythrodermic or generalised pustular type requires urgent specialist assessment. Initial topical treatment should be limited to using emollients frequently and generously. More localised acute or subacute *inflammatory psoriasis* with hot, spreading or itchy lesions, should be treated topically with emollients or with a corticosteroid of moderate potency.

Scalp psoriasis is usually scaly, and the scale may be thick and adherent. This requires softening with an emollient ointment, cream, or oil and usually combined with salicylic acid as a keratolytic.

Some preparations for psoriasis affecting the scalp combine salicylic acid with coal tar or **sulfur**. The preparation should be applied generously and left on for at least an hour, often more conveniently overnight, before washing it off. If a corticosteroid lotion or gel is required (e.g. for itch), it can be used in the morning.

Flexural psoriasis can be managed with short-term use of a mild potency topical corticosteroid. Calcitriol p. 704 or tacalcitol p. 705 can be used in the longer term; calcipotriol p. 704 is more likely to cause irritation in flexures and should be avoided. Low-strength tar preparations can also be used.

Facial psoriasis can be treated with short-term use of a mild topical corticosteroid; if this is ineffective, calcitriol, tacalcitol, or a low-strength tar preparation can be used.

Calcipotriol and tacalcitol are analogues of vitamin D that affect cell division and differentiation. Calcitriol is an active form of vitamin D. Vitamin D and its analogues are used as first-line treatment for plaque psoriasis; they do not smell or stain and they may be more acceptable than tar or dithranol products. Of the vitamin D analogues, tacalcitol and calcitriol are less likely to irritate.

Coal tar p. 700 has anti-inflammatory properties that are useful in chronic plaque psoriasis; it also has antiscaling properties. Contact of coal tar products with normal skin is not normally harmful and preparations containing coal tar can be used for widespread small lesions; however, irritation, contact allergy, and sterile folliculitis can occur. Leave-on preparations that remain in contact with the skin, such as creams or ointments, containing up to 6% coal tar may be used on children 1 month to 2 years; leave-on preparations containing coal tar 10% may be used on children over 2 years with more severe psoriasis. Tar baths and tar shampoos may also be helpful.

Dithranol is effective for chronic plaque psoriasis. Its major disadvantages are irritation (for which individual susceptibility varies) and staining of skin and of clothing. Dithranol is not generally suitable for widespread small lesions nor should it be used in the flexures or on the face. Proprietary preparations are more suitable for home use; they are usually washed off after 20–30 minutes ('short contact' technique). Specialist nurses may apply intensive treatment with dithranol paste which is covered by stockinette dressings and usually retained overnight. Dithranol should be discontinued if even a low concentration causes acute inflammation; continued use can result in the psoriasis becoming unstable.

A topical **corticosteroid** is not generally suitable for long-term use or as the sole treatment of extensive chronic plaque psoriasis; any early improvement is not usually maintained and there is a risk of the condition deteriorating or of precipitating an unstable form of psoriasis e.g. erythrodermic psoriasis or generalised pustular psoriasis on withdrawal. Topical use of potent corticosteroids on widespread psoriasis can also lead to systemic as well as local side-effects. However, topical corticosteroids used short-term may be appropriate to treat psoriasis in specific sites such as the face or flexures with a mild corticosteroid, and psoriasis of the scalp, palms, and soles with a potent corticosteroid. Very potent topical corticosteroids should only be used under specialist supervision.

Combining the use of a corticosteroid with another specific topical treatment may be beneficial in chronic plaque psoriasis; the drugs may be used separately at different times of the day or used together in a single formulation. *Eczema* co-existing with psoriasis may be treated with a corticosteroid, or coal tar, or both.

Phototherapy

Phototherapy is available in specialist centres under the supervision of a dermatologist. Narrow band ultraviolet B (UVB) radiation is usually effective for *chronic stable psoriasis* and for *guttate psoriasis*. It can be considered for children with moderately severe psoriasis in whom topical treatment has failed, but it may irritate inflammatory psoriasis. The use of phototherapy and photochemotherapy in children is limited by concerns over carcinogenicity and premature ageing.

13

Skin

Photochemotherapy combining long-wave ultraviolet A radiation with a psoralen (PUVA) is available in specialist centres under the supervision of a dermatologist. The psoralen, which enhances the effect of irradiation, is administered either by mouth or topically. PUVA is effective in most forms of psoriasis, including the *localised palmoplantar pustular psoriasis*. Early adverse effects include phototoxicity and pruritus. Higher cumulative doses exaggerate skin ageing, increase the risk of dysplastic and neoplastic skin lesions especially squamous cancer, and pose a theoretical risk of cataracts.

Phototherapy combined with coal tar, dithranol, topical vitamin D or vitamin D analogues, or oral acitretin, allows reduction of the cumulative dose of phototherapy required to treat psoriasis.

Systemic treatment

Systemic treatment is required for severe, resistant, unstable or complicated forms of psoriasis, and it should be initiated only under specialist supervision. Systemic drugs for psoriasis include acitretin and drugs that affect the immune response (see Eczema and psoriasis, drugs affecting the immune response p. 684).

Acitretin p. 703, a metabolite of etretinate, is a retinoid (vitamin A derivative); it is prescribed by specialists. The main indication of acitretin is severe psoriasis resistant to other forms of therapy. It is also used in disorders of keratinisation such as severe *Darier's disease* (keratosis follicularis), and some forms of *ichthyosis*. Although a minority of cases of psoriasis respond well to acitretin alone, it is only moderately effective in many cases; adverse effects are a limiting factor. A therapeutic effect occurs after 2 to 4 weeks and the maximum benefit after 4 months. Consideration should be given to stopping acitretin if the response is inadequate after 4 months at the optimum dose. Continuous treatment for longer than 6 months is not usually necessary in psoriasis. However, some patients, particularly those with severe ichthyosis, may benefit from longer treatment, provided that the lowest effective dose is used, patients are monitored carefully for adverse effects, and the need for treatment is reviewed regularly. Topical preparations containing keratolytics should normally be stopped before administration of acitretin. Liberal use of emollients should be encouraged and topical corticosteroids can be continued if necessary.

Acitretin is teratogenic; in females of child-bearing age, the possibility of pregnancy must be excluded before treatment and effective contraception must be used during treatment and for at least 3 years afterwards (oral progestogen-only contraceptives not considered effective).

Topical treatment

The vitamin D and analogues, calcipotriol p. 704, calcitriol p. 704, and tacalcitol p. 705 are used for the management of plaque psoriasis. They should be avoided by those with calcium metabolism disorders, and used with caution in generalised pustular or erythrodermic exfoliative psoriasis (enhanced risk of hypercalcaemia).

CORTICOSTEROIDS

Topical corticosteroids

Overview

Topical corticosteroids are used for the treatment of inflammatory conditions of the skin (other than those arising from an infection), particularly eczema, contact dermatitis, insect stings, and eczema of scabies. Corticosteroids suppress the inflammatory reaction during use; they are not curative and on discontinuation a rebound exacerbation of the condition may occur. They are generally used to relieve symptoms and suppress signs of the disorder when other measures such as emollients are ineffective.

Children, especially infants, are particularly susceptible to side-effects. However, concern about the safety of topical corticosteroids in children should not result in the child being undertreated. The aim is to control the condition as well as possible; inadequate treatment will perpetuate the condition. Carers of young children should be advised that treatment should **not** necessarily be reserved to 'treat only the worst areas' and they may need to be advised that patient information leaflets may contain inappropriate advice for the child's condition.

In an acute flare-up of atopic eczema, it may be appropriate to use more potent formulations of topical corticosteroids for a short period to regain control of the condition.

Topical corticosteroids are not recommended in the routine treatment of urticaria; treatment should only be initiated and supervised by a specialist. Topical corticosteroids may worsen ulcerated or secondarily infected lesions. They should not be used indiscriminately in pruritus (where they will only benefit if inflammation is causing the itch) and are **not** recommended for acne vulgaris.

Systemic or very potent topical corticosteroids should be avoided or given only under specialist supervision in psoriasis because, although they may suppress the psoriasis in the short term, relapse or vigorous rebound occurs on withdrawal (sometimes precipitating severe pustular psoriasis). Topical use of potent corticosteroids on widespread psoriasis can lead to systemic as well as to local side-effects. It is reasonable, however, to prescribe a mild topical corticosteroid for a short period (2–4 weeks) for *flexural* and *facial psoriasis*, and to use a more potent corticosteroid such as betamethasone p. 688 or fluocinonide p. 692 for *psoriasis* of the *scalp, palms,* or *soles*.

In general, the most potent topical corticosteroids should be reserved for recalcitrant dermatoses such as *chronic discoid lupus erythematosus, lichen simplex chronicus, hypertrophic lichen planus,* and *palmoplantar pustulosis*. Potent corticosteroids should generally be avoided on the face and skin flexures, but specialists occasionally prescribe them for use on these areas in certain circumstances.

When topical treatment has failed, intralesional corticosteroid injections may be used. These are more effective than the very potent topical corticosteroid preparations and should be reserved for severe cases where there are localised lesions such as *keloid scars, hypertrophic lichen planus,* or *localised alopecia areata*.

Perioral lesions

Hydrocortisone cream 1% p. 692 can be used for up to 7 days to treat uninfected inflammatory lesions on the lips. Hydrocortisone with miconazole cream or ointment p. 698 is useful where infection by susceptible organisms and inflammation co-exist, particularly for initial treatment (up to 7 days) e.g. in angular cheilitis. Organisms susceptible to miconazole include *Candida* spp. and many Gram-positive bacteria including streptococci and staphylococci.

Choice

Water-miscible corticosteroid creams are suitable for moist or weeping lesions whereas ointments are generally chosen for dry, lichenified or scaly lesions or where a more occlusive effect is required. Lotions may be useful when minimal application to a large or hair-bearing area is required or for the treatment of exudative lesions. *Occlusive polythene* or *hydrocolloid dressings* increase absorption, but also increase the risk of side-effects; they are therefore used only under supervision on a short-term basis for areas of very thick skin (such as the palms and soles). Disposable nappies and tight fitting pants also increase the risk of side-effects by increasing absorption of the corticosteroid. The inclusion of urea or salicylic acid also increases the penetration of the corticosteroid.

In the *BNF for Children*, topical corticosteroids for the skin are categorised as 'mild', 'moderately potent', 'potent' or 'very potent'; the least potent preparation which is effective should be chosen but dilution should be avoided whenever possible.

Topical hydrocortisone is usually used in children under 1 year of age. Moderately potent and potent topical corticosteroids should be used with great care in children and for short periods (1–2 weeks) only. A very potent corticosteroid should be initiated under the supervision of a specialist.

Appropriate topical corticosteroids for specific conditions are:

- *insect bites and stings*—mild corticosteroid such as hydrocortisone 1% cream;
- *inflamed nappy rash causing discomfort* in infant over 1 month—mild corticosteroid such as hydrocortisone 0.5% or 1% for up to 7 days (combined with antimicrobial if infected);
- *mild to moderate eczema, flexural and facial eczema or psoriasis*—mild corticosteroid such as hydrocortisone 1%;
- *severe eczema of the face and neck*—moderately potent corticosteroid for 3–5 days only, if not controlled by a mild corticosteroid;
- *severe eczema on the trunk and limbs*—moderately potent or potent corticosteroid for 1–2 weeks only, switching to a less potent preparation as the condition improves;
- *eczema affecting area with thickened skin (e.g. soles of feet)*— potent topical corticosteroid in combination with urea or salicylic acid (to increase penetration of corticosteroid).

Absorption through the skin

Mild and *moderately potent* topical corticosteroids are associated with few side-effects but particular care is required when treating neonates and infants, and in the use of *potent* and *very potent* corticosteroids. Absorption through the skin can rarely cause adrenal suppression and even Cushing's syndrome, depending on the area of the body being treated and the duration of treatment. Absorption of corticosteroid is greatest from severely inflamed skin, thin skin (especially on the face or genital area), from flexural sites (e.g. axillae, groin), and in infants where skin surface area is higher in relation to body-weight; absorption is increased by occlusion.

Compound preparations

The advantages of including other substances (such as antibacterials or antifungals) with corticosteroids in topical preparations are uncertain, but such combinations may have a place where inflammatory skin conditions are associated with bacterial or fungal infection, such as infected eczema. In these cases the antimicrobial drug should be chosen according to the sensitivity of the infecting organism and used regularly for a short period (typically twice daily for 1 week). Longer use increases the likelihood of resistance and of sensitisation.

The keratolytic effect of salicylic acid facilitates the absorption of topical corticosteroids; however, excessive and prolonged use of topical preparations containing salicylic acid may cause salicylism.

Topical corticosteroid preparation potencies

Potency of a topical corticosteroid preparation is a result of the formulation as well as the corticosteroid. Therefore, proprietary names are shown.

Mild

- Hydrocortisone 0.1–2.5%
- Dioderm
- Mildison
- Synalar 1 in 10 dilution

Mild with antimicrobials

- Canesten HC
- Daktacort
- Econacort
- Fucidin H
- Nystaform-HC
- Terra-Cortril
- Timodine

Moderate

- Betnovate-RD
- Eumovate
- Haelan
- Modrasone
- Synalar 1 in 4 Dilution
- Ultralanum Plain

Moderate with antimicrobials

- Trimovate

Moderate with urea:

- Alphaderm

Potent

- Beclometasone dipropionate 0.025%
- Betamethasone valerate 0.1%
- Betacap
- Betesil
- Bettamousse
- Betnovate
- Cutivate
- Diprosone
- Elocon
- Hydrocortisone butyrate
- Locoid
- Locoid Crelo
- Metosyn
- Mometasone furoate 0.1%
- Nerisone
- Synalar

Potent with antimicrobials

- Aureocort
- Betamethasone and clioquinol
- Betamethasone and neomycin
- Fucibet
- Lotriderm
- Synalar C
- Synalar N

Potent with salicylic acid

- Diprosalic

Very potent

- Dermovate
- Nerisone Forte

Very potent with antimicrobials

- Clobetasol propionate 0.05% with neomycin and nystatin

Corticosteroids (topical)

- **CONTRA-INDICATIONS** Acne · perioral dermatitis · potent corticosteroids in widespread plaque psoriasis · untreated bacterial, fungal or viral skin lesions
- **CAUTIONS** Avoid prolonged use (particularly on the face) · cautions applicable to systemic corticosteroids may also apply if absorption occurs following topical and local use · dermatoses of infancy, including nappy rash (extreme caution required—treatment should be limited to 5–7 days) · infection · keep away from eyes · use potent or very potent topical corticosteroids under specialist supervision
- **SIDE-EFFECTS**
  ▸ **Rare** Adrenal suppression · Cushing's syndrome
  ▸ **Frequency not known** Acne · contact dermatitis · hypertrichosis · irreversible striae atrophicae · irreversible telangiectasia · mild depigmentation (may be reversible) ·

perioral dermatitis · side-effects applicable to systemic corticosteroids may also apply if absorption occurs following topical and local use · spread and worsening of untreated infection · thinning of the skin (may be restored over a period after stopping treatment but the original structure may never return) · worsening of acne · worsening of rosacea

SIDE-EFFECTS, FURTHER INFORMATION
In order to minimise the side-effects of a topical corticosteroid, it is important to apply it **thinly** to affected areas **only**, no more frequently than **twice daily**, and to use the least potent formulation which is fully effective.

- DIRECTIONS FOR ADMINISTRATION Topical corticosteroid preparations should be applied no more frequently than twice daily; once daily is often sufficient. Topical corticosteroids should be spread thinly on the skin but in sufficient quantity to cover the affected areas. The length of cream or ointment expelled from a tube may be used to specify the quantity to be applied to a given area of skin. This length can be measured in terms of a *fingertip unit* (the distance from the tip of the adult index finger to the first crease). One fingertip unit (approximately 500 mg from a tube with a standard 5 mm diameter nozzle) is sufficient to cover an area that is twice that of the flat adult handprint (palm and fingers). Mixing topical preparations on the skin should be avoided where possible; several minutes should elapse between application of different preparations.

'Wet-wrap bandaging' increases absorption into the skin, but should be initiated only by a dermatologist and application supervised by a healthcare professional trained in the technique.

- PRESCRIBING AND DISPENSING INFORMATION The potency of each topical corticosteroid should be included on the label with the directions for use. The label should be attached to the container (for example, the tube) rather than the outer packaging.

- PATIENT AND CARER ADVICE Patients or carers should be given advice on how to administer corticosteroid creams and ointments. If a patient is using topical corticosteroids of different potencies, the patient should be told when to use each corticosteroid. Patients and their carers should be reassured that side effects such as skin thinning and systemic effects rarely occur when topical corticosteroids are used appropriately.

F 687

Alclometasone dipropionate

- INDICATIONS AND DOSE
Inflammatory skin disorders such as eczemas
▸ TO THE SKIN
▸ Child: Apply 1–2 times a day, to be applied thinly

POTENCY
Alclometasone dipropionate cream 0.05%: moderate

- UNLICENSED USE Licensed for use in children (age range not specified by manufacturer).

- PATIENT AND CARER ADVICE Patients or carers should be counselled on the application of alclometasone dipropionate cream.

- MEDICINAL FORMS
There can be variation in the licensing of different medicines containing the same drug.
Cream
CAUTIONARY AND ADVISORY LABELS 28
EXCIPIENTS: May contain Cetostearyl alcohol (including cetyl and stearyl alcohol), chlorocresol, propylene glycol
▸ Alclometasone dipropionate (Non-proprietary)
Alclometasone dipropionate 500 microgram per 1 gram Boots Derma Care Eczema & Dermatitis Flare-Up 0.05% cream | 15 gram ℗ no price available

▸ Modrasone (Teva UK Ltd)
Alclometasone dipropionate 500 microgram per 1 gram Modrasone 0.05% cream | 50 gram PoM £2.68 DT price = £2.68

F 687

Beclometasone dipropionate
(Beclomethasone dipropionate)

- INDICATIONS AND DOSE
Severe inflammatory skin disorders such as eczemas unresponsive to less potent corticosteroids | Psoriasis
▸ TO THE SKIN
▸ Child: Apply 1–2 times a day, thin layer to be applied

POTENCY
Beclometasone dipropionate cream and ointment 0.025%: potent.

- UNLICENSED USE Not licensed for use in children under 1 year.

- MEDICINAL FORMS
There can be variation in the licensing of different medicines containing the same drug. Forms available from special-order manufacturers include: cream, ointment
Cream
CAUTIONARY AND ADVISORY LABELS 28
▸ Beclometasone dipropionate (Non-proprietary)
Beclometasone dipropionate 250 microgram per 1 gram Beclometasone 0.025% cream | 30 gram PoM £68.00 DT price = £68.00
Ointment
CAUTIONARY AND ADVISORY LABELS 28
▸ Beclometasone dipropionate (Non-proprietary)
Beclometasone dipropionate 250 microgram per 1 gram Beclometasone 0.025% ointment | 30 gram PoM £68.00 DT price = £68.00

F 687

Betamethasone

- INDICATIONS AND DOSE
Severe inflammatory skin disorders such as eczemas unresponsive to less potent corticosteroids | Psoriasis
▸ TO THE SKIN
▸ Child: Apply 1–2 times a day, to be applied thinly

POTENCY
Betamethasone valerate 0.025% cream and ointment: moderate.
Betamethasone valerate 0.1% cream, lotion, ointment, and scalp application: potent.
Betamethasone valerate 0.12% foam: potent.
Betamethasone dipropionate 0.05% cream, lotion, and ointment: potent.

- UNLICENSED USE *Betacap*®, *Betnovate*® and *Betnovate-RD*® are not licensed for use in children under 1 year. *Bettamousse*® is not licensed for use in children under 6 years.

- CAUTIONS Use of more than 100 g per week of 0.1% preparation likely to cause adrenal suppression

- PATIENT AND CARER ADVICE Patient counselling is advised for betamethasone cream, ointment, scalp application and foam (application).

● **MEDICINAL FORMS**
There can be variation in the licensing of different medicines containing the same drug. Forms available from special-order manufacturers include: cream, ointment

Foam
CAUTIONARY AND ADVISORY LABELS 28, 15
EXCIPIENTS: May contain Cetostearyl alcohol (including cetyl and stearyl alcohol), polysorbates, propylene glycol
▶ Bettamousse (Focus Pharmaceuticals Ltd)
  Betamethasone (as Betamethasone valerate) 1 mg per 1 gram Bettamousse 0.1% cutaneous foam | 100 gram PoM £9.75 DT price = £9.75

Liquid
CAUTIONARY AND ADVISORY LABELS 15 (scalp lotion only), 28
EXCIPIENTS: May contain Cetostearyl alcohol (including cetyl and stearyl alcohol), hydroxybenzoates (parabens)
▶ Betacap (Dermal Laboratories Ltd)
  Betamethasone (as Betamethasone valerate) 1 mg per 1 gram Betacap 0.1% scalp application | 100 ml PoM £3.19 DT price = £3.19
▶ Betnovate (GlaxoSmithKline UK Ltd)
  Betamethasone (as Betamethasone valerate) 1 mg per 1 gram Betnovate 0.1% scalp application | 100 ml PoM £4.99 DT price = £3.19
  Betnovate 0.1% lotion | 100 ml PoM £4.58 DT price = £4.58
▶ Diprosone (Merck Sharp & Dohme Ltd)
  Betamethasone (as Betamethasone dipropionate) 500 microgram per 1 ml Diprosone 0.05% lotion | 30 ml PoM £2.73 DT price = £2.73 | 100 ml PoM £7.80 DT price = £7.80

Cream
CAUTIONARY AND ADVISORY LABELS 28
EXCIPIENTS: May contain Cetostearyl alcohol (including cetyl and stearyl alcohol), chlorocresol
▶ Betamethasone (Non-proprietary)
  Betamethasone (as Betamethasone valerate) 1 mg per 1 gram Betamethasone valerate 0.1% cream | 30 gram PoM £5.99 DT price = £3.31 | 100 gram PoM £12.23 DT price = £11.03
▶ Audavate (Auden McKenzie (Pharma Division) Ltd)
  Betamethasone (as Betamethasone valerate) 250 microgram per 1 gram Audavate RD 0.025% cream | 100 gram PoM £2.52 DT price = £3.15
▶ Betnovate (GlaxoSmithKline UK Ltd)
  Betamethasone (as Betamethasone valerate) 250 microgram per 1 gram Betnovate RD 0.025% cream | 100 gram PoM £3.15 DT price = £3.15
  Betamethasone (as Betamethasone valerate) 1 mg per 1 gram Betnovate 0.1% cream | 30 gram PoM £1.43 DT price = £3.31 | 100 gram PoM £4.05 DT price = £11.03
▶ Diprosone (Merck Sharp & Dohme Ltd)
  Betamethasone (as Betamethasone dipropionate) 500 microgram per 1 gram Diprosone 0.05% cream | 30 gram PoM £2.16 DT price = £2.16 | 100 gram PoM £6.12 DT price = £6.12

Ointment
CAUTIONARY AND ADVISORY LABELS 28
▶ Betamethasone (Non-proprietary)
  Betamethasone (as Betamethasone valerate) 1 mg per 1 gram Betamethasone valerate 0.1% ointment | 30 gram PoM £5.55 DT price = £2.65 | 100 gram PoM £14.99 DT price = £8.83
▶ Audavate (Auden McKenzie (Pharma Division) Ltd)
  Betamethasone (as Betamethasone valerate) 250 microgram per 1 gram Audavate RD 0.025% ointment | 100 gram PoM £2.52 DT price = £3.15
  Betamethasone (as Betamethasone valerate) 1 mg per 1 gram Audavate 0.1% ointment | 30 gram PoM £1.14 DT price = £2.65 | 100 gram PoM £3.24 DT price = £8.83
▶ Betnovate (GlaxoSmithKline UK Ltd)
  Betamethasone (as Betamethasone valerate) 250 microgram per 1 gram Betnovate RD 0.025% ointment | 100 gram PoM £3.15 DT price = £3.15
  Betamethasone (as Betamethasone valerate) 1 mg per 1 gram Betnovate 0.1% ointment | 30 gram PoM £1.43 DT price = £2.65 | 100 gram PoM £4.05 DT price = £8.83

▶ Diprosone (Merck Sharp & Dohme Ltd)
  Betamethasone (as Betamethasone dipropionate) 500 microgram per 1 gram Diprosone 0.05% ointment | 30 gram PoM £2.16 DT price = £2.16 | 100 gram PoM £6.12 DT price = £6.12

Combinations available: *Betamethasone with clioquinol,* p. 694 · *Betamethasone with clotrimazole,* p. 694 · *Betamethasone with fusidic acid,* p. 695 · *Betamethasone with neomycin,* p. 695 · *Betamethasone with salicylic acid,* p. 695

Calcipotriol with betamethasone

The properties listed below are those particular to the combination only. For the properties of the components please consider, calcipotriol p. 704, betamethasone p. 688.

● **INDICATIONS AND DOSE**

DOVOBET® GEL
Scalp psoriasis
▶ TO THE SKIN
▶ Child 12–17 years (specialist use only): Apply 1–4 g once daily usual duration of therapy 4 weeks; if necessary, treatment may be continued beyond 4 weeks or repeated, on the advice of a specialist, shampoo off after leaving on scalp overnight or during day, when different preparations containing calcipotriol used together, maximum total calcipiotriol 3.75 mg in any one week

Mild to moderate plaque psoriasis
▶ TO THE SKIN
▶ Child 12–17 years (specialist use only): Apply once daily usual duration for up to 4 weeks; if necessary treatment should be continued beyond 4 weeks, or repeated, only on the advice of a specialist, apply to maximum 30% on body surface, when different preparations containing calcipotriol used together, max. total calcipotriol 3.75 mg in any one week; maximum 75 g per week

DOVOBET® OINTMENT
Stable plaque psoriasis
▶ TO THE SKIN
▶ Child 12–17 years (specialist use only): Apply once daily for up to 4 weeks; if necessary, treatment may be continued beyond 4 weeks or repeated, on the advice of a specialist, apply to a maximum 30% on body surface, when different preparations containing calcipotriol used together, max. total calcipotriol 3.75 mg in any one week; maximum 75 g per week

● **UNLICENSED USE** *Dovobet*® not licensed for use in children.

● **MEDICINAL FORMS**
There can be variation in the licensing of different medicines containing the same drug.
Ointment
CAUTIONARY AND ADVISORY LABELS 28
EXCIPIENTS: May contain Butylated hydroxytoluene
▶ Dovobet (LEO Pharma)
  Calcipotriol (as Calcipotriol hydrate) 50 microgram per 1 gram, Betamethasone (as Betamethasone dipropionate) 500 microgram per 1 gram Dovobet ointment | 30 gram PoM £19.84 DT price = £19.84 | 60 gram PoM £39.68 | 120 gram PoM £73.86

Gel
CAUTIONARY AND ADVISORY LABELS 28
EXCIPIENTS: May contain Butylated hydroxytoluene
▶ Dovobet (LEO Pharma)
  Calcipotriol (as Calcipotriol monohydrate) 50 microgram per 1 gram, Betamethasone (as Betamethasone dipropionate) 500 microgram per 1 gram Dovobet gel Applicator | 60 gram PoM £37.21 DT price = £37.21
  Dovobet gel | 60 gram PoM £37.21 DT price = £37.21 | 120 gram PoM £69.11

13

Skin

F 687

Clobetasol propionate

● **INDICATIONS AND DOSE**

Short-term treatment only of severe resistant inflammatory skin disorders such as recalcitrant eczemas unresponsive to less potent corticosteroids | **Psoriasis**

▸ TO THE SKIN
▸ **Child:** Apply 1–2 times a day for up to 4 weeks, to be applied thinly

POTENCY
Clobetasol propionate 0.05% cream, foam, ointment, scalp application, and shampoo: very potent.

● **UNLICENSED USE** *Dermovate*® not licensed for use in children under 1 year.

● **PATIENT AND CARER ADVICE** Patients or carers should be given advice on how to administer clobetasol propionate foam, liquid (scalp application), cream, ointment and shampoo.
Scalp application Patients or carers should be advised to apply foam directly to scalp lesions (foam begins to subside immediately on contact with skin).

● **MEDICINAL FORMS**
There can be variation in the licensing of different medicines containing the same drug. Forms available from special-order manufacturers include: cream, ointment, paste

Foam
CAUTIONARY AND ADVISORY LABELS 15, 28
EXCIPIENTS: May contain Cetostearyl alcohol (including cetyl and stearyl alcohol), polysorbates, propylene glycol
▸ Clarelux (Pierre Fabre Dermo-Cosmetique)
  Clobetasol propionate 500 microgram per 1 gram Clarelux 500micrograms/g foam | 100 gram [PoM] £11.06

Liquid
CAUTIONARY AND ADVISORY LABELS 15, 28
▸ Dermovate (GlaxoSmithKline UK Ltd)
  Clobetasol propionate 500 microgram per 1 gram Dermovate 0.05% scalp application | 30 ml [PoM] £3.07 DT price = £3.07 | 100 ml [PoM] £10.42 DT price = £10.42

Cream
CAUTIONARY AND ADVISORY LABELS 28
EXCIPIENTS: May contain Beeswax, cetostearyl alcohol (including cetyl and stearyl alcohol), chlorocresol, propylene glycol
▸ Clobetasol propionate (Non-proprietary)
  Clobetasol propionate 500 microgram per 1 gram Clobetasol 0.05% cream | 30 gram [PoM] no price available DT price = £2.69 | 100 gram [PoM] no price available DT price = £7.90
▸ ClobaDerm (Auden McKenzie (Pharma Division) Ltd)
  Clobetasol propionate 500 microgram per 1 gram ClobaDerm 0.05% cream | 30 gram [PoM] £2.15 DT price = £2.69 | 100 gram [PoM] £6.32 DT price = £7.90
▸ Dermovate (GlaxoSmithKline UK Ltd)
  Clobetasol propionate 500 microgram per 1 gram Dermovate 0.05% cream | 30 gram [PoM] £2.69 DT price = £2.69 | 100 gram [PoM] £7.90 DT price = £7.90

Ointment
CAUTIONARY AND ADVISORY LABELS 28
EXCIPIENTS: May contain Propylene glycol
▸ Clobetasol propionate (Non-proprietary)
  Clobetasol propionate 500 microgram per 1 gram Clobetasol 0.05% ointment | 30 gram [PoM] no price available DT price = £2.69 | 100 gram [PoM] no price available DT price = £7.90
▸ ClobaDerm (Auden McKenzie (Pharma Division) Ltd)
  Clobetasol propionate 500 microgram per 1 gram ClobaDerm 0.05% ointment | 30 gram [PoM] £2.15 DT price = £2.69 | 100 gram [PoM] £6.32 DT price = £7.90
▸ Dermovate (GlaxoSmithKline UK Ltd)
  Clobetasol propionate 500 microgram per 1 gram Dermovate 0.05% ointment | 30 gram [PoM] £2.69 DT price = £2.69 | 100 gram [PoM] £7.90 DT price = £7.90

Shampoo
CAUTIONARY AND ADVISORY LABELS 28
▸ Etrivex (Galderma (UK) Ltd)
  Clobetasol propionate 500 microgram per 1 gram Etrivex 500micrograms/g shampoo | 125 ml [PoM] £10.29 DT price = £10.29

Combinations available: *Clobetasol propionate with neomycin sulfate and nystatin*, p. 696

F 687

Clobetasone butyrate

● **INDICATIONS AND DOSE**

Eczemas and dermatitis of all types | **Maintenance between courses of more potent corticosteroids**

▸ TO THE SKIN
▸ **Child:** Apply 1–2 times a day, to be applied thinly

POTENCY
Clobetasone butyrate 0.05% cream and ointment: moderate.

● **UNLICENSED USE** Licensed for use in children (age range not specified by manufacturer).

● **PATIENT AND CARER ADVICE** Patients or carers should be advised on the application of clobetasone butyrate containing preparations.

● **EXCEPTIONS TO LEGAL CATEGORY** Cream can be sold to the public for short-term symptomatic treatment and control of patches of eczema and dermatitis (but not seborrhoeic dermatitis) in adults and children over 12 years provided pack does not contain more than 15 g.

● **MEDICINAL FORMS**
There can be variation in the licensing of different medicines containing the same drug. Forms available from special-order manufacturers include: cream, ointment

Cream
CAUTIONARY AND ADVISORY LABELS 28
EXCIPIENTS: May contain Cetostearyl alcohol (including cetyl and stearyl alcohol), chlorocresol
▸ Eumovate (GlaxoSmithKline Consumer Healthcare, GlaxoSmithKline UK Ltd)
  Clobetasone butyrate 500 microgram per 1 gram Eumovate Eczema and Dermatitis 0.05% cream | 15 gram [P] £3.57 DT price = £3.57
  Eumovate 0.05% cream | 30 gram [PoM] £1.86 DT price = £1.86 | 100 gram [PoM] £5.44 DT price = £5.44

Ointment
CAUTIONARY AND ADVISORY LABELS 28
▸ Clobavate (Auden McKenzie (Pharma Division) Ltd)
  Clobetasone butyrate 500 microgram per 1 gram Clobavate 0.05% ointment | 30 gram [PoM] £1.49 DT price = £1.86 | 100 gram [PoM] £4.35 DT price = £5.44
▸ Eumovate (GlaxoSmithKline UK Ltd)
  Clobetasone butyrate 500 microgram per 1 gram Eumovate 0.05% ointment | 30 gram [PoM] £1.86 DT price = £1.86 | 100 gram [PoM] £5.44 DT price = £5.44

Combinations available: *Clobetasone butyrate with nystatin and oxytetracycline*, p. 696

F 687

Diflucortolone valerate

● **INDICATIONS AND DOSE**

Severe inflammatory skin disorders such as eczemas unresponsive to less potent corticosteroids (using 0.3% diflucortolone valerate) | **Short-term treatment of severe exacerbations (using 0.3% diflucortolone valerate)** | **Psoriasis (using 0.3% diflucortolone valerate)**

▸ TO THE SKIN
▸ **Child 1 month–3 years:** Apply 1–2 times a day for up to 2 weeks, reducing strength as condition responds, to be applied thinly

13

Skin

▸ Child 4–17 years: Apply 1–2 times a day for up to 2 weeks, reducing strength as condition responds, to be applied thinly; maximum 60 g per week

Severe inflammatory skin disorders such as eczemas unresponsive to less potent corticosteroids (using 0.1% diflucortolone valerate) | Psoriasis (using 0.1% diflucortolone valerate)
▸ TO THE SKIN
▸ Child: Apply 1–2 times a day for up to 4 weeks, to be applied thinly

POTENCY
Diflucortolone valerate 0.1% cream and ointment: potent.
Diflucortolone valerate 0.3% cream and ointment: very potent.

● UNLICENSED USE *Nerisone*® licensed for use in children (age range not specified by manufacturer); *Nerisone Forte*® not licensed for use in children under 4 years.

● PRESCRIBING AND DISPENSING INFORMATION Patients or carers should be advised on application of diflucortolone valerate containing preparations.

● MEDICINAL FORMS
There can be variation in the licensing of different medicines containing the same drug.
Cream
CAUTIONARY AND ADVISORY LABELS 28
EXCIPIENTS: May contain Beeswax, cetostearyl alcohol (including cetyl and stearyl alcohol), disodium edetate, hydroxybenzoates (parabens)
▸ **Nerisone** (Meadow Laboratories Ltd)
  Diflucortolone valerate 1 mg per 1 gram Nerisone 0.1% cream | 30 gram [PoM] £3.98
  Nerisone 0.1% oily cream | 30 gram [PoM] £4.95 DT price = £4.95
  Diflucortolone valerate 3 mg per 1 gram Nerisone Forte 0.3% oily cream | 15 gram [PoM] £4.70 DT price = £4.70
Ointment
CAUTIONARY AND ADVISORY LABELS 28
▸ **Nerisone** (Meadow Laboratories Ltd)
  Diflucortolone valerate 1 mg per 1 gram Nerisone 0.1% ointment | 30 gram [PoM] £3.98
  Diflucortolone valerate 3 mg per 1 gram Nerisone Forte 0.3% ointment | 15 gram [PoM] £4.70

[F 687]

Fludroxycortide

(Flurandrenolone)

● INDICATIONS AND DOSE
Inflammatory skin disorders such as eczemas
▸ TO THE SKIN
▸ Child: Apply 1–2 times a day, to be applied thinly

HAELAN® TAPE
Chronic localised recalcitrant dermatoses (but not acute or weeping)
▸ TO THE SKIN
▸ Child: Cut tape to fit lesion, apply to clean, dry skin shorn of hair, usually for 12 hours daily

POTENCY
Fludroxycortide 0.0125% cream and ointment: moderate

● UNLICENSED USE Licensed for use in children (age range not specified by manufacturer).

● PATIENT AND CARER ADVICE Patients or carers should be counselled on application of fludroxycortide cream and ointment.

● MEDICINAL FORMS
There can be variation in the licensing of different medicines containing the same drug.
Cream
CAUTIONARY AND ADVISORY LABELS 28
EXCIPIENTS: May contain Cetostearyl alcohol (including cetyl and stearyl alcohol), propylene glycol
▸ **Fludroxycortide** (Non-proprietary)
  Fludroxycortide 125 microgram per 1 gram Fludroxycortide 0.0125% cream | 60 gram [PoM] no price available
▸ **Haelan** (Typharm Ltd)
  Fludroxycortide 125 microgram per 1 gram Haelan 0.0125% cream | 60 gram [PoM] £3.26
Ointment
CAUTIONARY AND ADVISORY LABELS 28
EXCIPIENTS: May contain Beeswax, cetostearyl alcohol (including cetyl and stearyl alcohol), polysorbates
▸ **Fludroxycortide** (Non-proprietary)
  Fludroxycortide 125 microgram per 1 gram Fludroxycortide 0.0125% ointment | 60 gram [PoM] no price available
▸ **Haelan** (Typharm Ltd)
  Fludroxycortide 125 microgram per 1 gram Haelan 0.0125% ointment | 60 gram [PoM] £3.26
Impregnated dressing
▸ **Haelan** (Typharm Ltd)
  Fludroxycortide 4 microgram per 1 square cm Haelan 4microgram/square cm tape 7.5cm | 20 cm [PoM] £8.19 | 50 cm [PoM] £9.27 DT price = £9.27

[F 687]

Fluocinolone acetonide

● INDICATIONS AND DOSE
Severe inflammatory skin disorders such as eczemas | Psoriasis
▸ TO THE SKIN
▸ Child 1–17 years: Apply 1–2 times a day, to be applied thinly, reduce strength as condition responds

POTENCY
Fluocinolone acetonide 0.025% cream, gel, and ointment: potent.
Fluocinolone acetonide 0.00625% cream and ointment: moderate.
Fluocinolone acetonide 0.0025% cream: mild.

● UNLICENSED USE Not licensed for use in children under 1 year.

● PRESCRIBING AND DISPENSING INFORMATION Gel is useful for application to the scalp and other hairy areas.

● PATIENT AND CARER ADVICE Patient counselling is advised for fluocinolone acetonide cream, gel and ointment (application).

● MEDICINAL FORMS
There can be variation in the licensing of different medicines containing the same drug.
Cream
CAUTIONARY AND ADVISORY LABELS 28
EXCIPIENTS: May contain Benzyl alcohol, cetostearyl alcohol (including cetyl and stearyl alcohol), polysorbates, propylene glycol
▸ **Synalar** (Derma UK Ltd)
  Fluocinolone acetonide 25 microgram per 1 gram Synalar 1 in 10 Dilution 0.0025% cream | 50 gram [PoM] £4.58 DT price = £4.58
  Fluocinolone acetonide 62.5 microgram per 1 gram Synalar 1 in 4 Dilution 0.00625% cream | 50 gram [PoM] £4.84 DT price = £4.84
  Fluocinolone acetonide 250 microgram per 1 gram Synalar 0.025% cream | 30 gram [PoM] £4.14 DT price = £4.14 | 100 gram [PoM] £11.75 DT price = £11.75

13

Skin

Ointment
CAUTIONARY AND ADVISORY LABELS 28
EXCIPIENTS: May contain Propylene glycol, wool fat and related substances including lanolin
▸ Synalar (Derma UK Ltd)
Fluocinolone acetonide 62.5 microgram per 1 gram Synalar 1 in 4 Dilution 0.00625% ointment | 50 gram $\boxed{\text{PoM}}$ £4.84 DT price = £4.84
Fluocinolone acetonide 250 microgram per 1 gram Synalar 0.025% ointment | 30 gram $\boxed{\text{PoM}}$ £4.14 DT price = £4.14 | 100 gram $\boxed{\text{PoM}}$ £11.75 DT price = £11.75

Gel
CAUTIONARY AND ADVISORY LABELS 28
EXCIPIENTS: May contain Hydroxybenzoates (parabens), propylene glycol
▸ Synalar (Derma UK Ltd)
Fluocinolone acetonide 250 microgram per 1 gram Synalar 0.025% gel | 30 gram $\boxed{\text{PoM}}$ £5.56 DT price = £5.56 | 60 gram $\boxed{\text{PoM}}$ £10.02 DT price = £10.02

Combinations available: *Fluocinolone acetonide with clioquinol*, p. 696 · *Fluocinolone acetonide with neomycin*, p. 697

🌡 687

Fluocinonide

● **INDICATIONS AND DOSE**

Severe inflammatory skin disorders such as eczemas unresponsive to less potent corticosteroids | Psoriasis
▸ TO THE SKIN
▸ Child: Apply 1–2 times a day, to be applied thinly

POTENCY
Fluocinonide 0.05% cream and ointment: potent.

● **UNLICENSED USE** Not licensed for use in children under 1 year.

● **PATIENT AND CARER ADVICE** Patients or carers should be advised on the application of fluocinonide preparations.

● **MEDICINAL FORMS**
There can be variation in the licensing of different medicines containing the same drug.
Cream
CAUTIONARY AND ADVISORY LABELS 28
EXCIPIENTS: May contain Propylene glycol
▸ Metosyn FAPG (Derma UK Ltd)
Fluocinonide 500 microgram per 1 gram Metosyn FAPG 0.05% cream | 25 gram $\boxed{\text{PoM}}$ £3.96 DT price = £3.96 | 100 gram $\boxed{\text{PoM}}$ £13.34 DT price = £13.34

Ointment
CAUTIONARY AND ADVISORY LABELS 28
EXCIPIENTS: May contain Propylene glycol, wool fat and related substances including lanolin
▸ Metosyn (Derma UK Ltd)
Fluocinonide 500 microgram per 1 gram Metosyn 0.05% ointment | 25 gram $\boxed{\text{PoM}}$ £3.50 DT price = £3.50 | 100 gram $\boxed{\text{PoM}}$ £13.15 DT price = £13.15

🌡 687

Fluocortolone

● **INDICATIONS AND DOSE**

Severe inflammatory skin disorders such as eczemas unresponsive to less potent corticosteroids | Psoriasis
▸ TO THE SKIN
▸ Child: Apply 1–2 times a day, to be applied thinly

POTENCY
Fluocortolone hexanoate 0.25% cream and ointment; fluocortolone pivalate 0.25% cream and fluocortolone 0.25% ointment: moderate.

● **UNLICENSED USE** Licensed for use in children (age range not specified by manufacturer).

● **PRESCRIBING AND DISPENSING INFORMATION** Patients or carers should be counselled on the application of fluocortolone preparations.

● **MEDICINAL FORMS**
There can be variation in the licensing of different medicines containing the same drug.
Cream
CAUTIONARY AND ADVISORY LABELS 28
EXCIPIENTS: May contain Cetostearyl alcohol (including cetyl and stearyl alcohol), disodium edetate, fragrances, hydroxybenzoates (parabens)
▸ Ultralanum Plain (Fluocortolone hexanoate / Fluocortolone pivalate) (Meadow Laboratories Ltd)
Fluocortolone hexanoate 2.5 mg per 1 gram, Fluocortolone pivalate 2.5 mg per 1 gram Ultralanum Plain cream | 50 gram $\boxed{\text{PoM}}$ £2.95

Ointment
CAUTIONARY AND ADVISORY LABELS 28
EXCIPIENTS: May contain Fragrances, wool fat and related substances including lanolin
▸ Ultralanum Plain (Fluocortolone / Fluocortolone hexanoate) (Meadow Laboratories Ltd)
Fluocortolone 2.5 mg per 1 gram, Fluocortolone hexanoate 2.5 mg per 1 gram Ultralanum Plain ointment | 50 gram $\boxed{\text{PoM}}$ £2.95

🌡 687

Fluticasone

4.1.2016

● **INDICATIONS AND DOSE**

Severe inflammatory skin disorders such as dermatitis and eczemas unresponsive to less potent corticosteroids | Psoriasis
▸ TO THE SKIN
▸ Child: Apply 1–2 times a day, to be applied thinly

POTENCY
Fluticasone cream 0.05%: potent.
Fluticasone ointment 0.005%: potent.

● **UNLICENSED USE** Not licensed for use in children under 3 months.

● **PATIENT AND CARER ADVICE** Patients or carers should be given advice on application of fluticasone creams and ointments.

● **MEDICINAL FORMS**
There can be variation in the licensing of different medicines containing the same drug.
Cream
CAUTIONARY AND ADVISORY LABELS 28
EXCIPIENTS: May contain Cetostearyl alcohol (including cetyl and stearyl alcohol), imidurea, propylene glycol
▸ Cutivate (GlaxoSmithKline UK Ltd)
Fluticasone propionate 500 microgram per 1 gram Cutivate 0.05% cream | 15 gram $\boxed{\text{PoM}}$ £2.27 DT price = £2.27 | 30 gram $\boxed{\text{PoM}}$ £4.24 DT price = £4.24

Ointment
CAUTIONARY AND ADVISORY LABELS 28
EXCIPIENTS: May contain Propylene glycol
▸ Cutivate (GlaxoSmithKline UK Ltd)
Fluticasone propionate 50 microgram per 1 gram Cutivate 0.005% ointment | 15 gram $\boxed{\text{PoM}}$ £2.27 DT price = £2.27 | 30 gram $\boxed{\text{PoM}}$ £4.24 DT price = £4.24

🌡 687

Hydrocortisone

● **INDICATIONS AND DOSE**

Mild inflammatory skin disorders such as eczemas
▸ TO THE SKIN
▸ Child: Apply 1–2 times a day, to be applied thinly

Nappy rash
▸ TO THE SKIN
▸ Child: Apply as required for no more than 1 week, discontinue as soon as the inflammation subsides

POTENCY
Hydrocortisone cream and ointment 0.5 to 2.5%: mild

- **PRESCRIBING AND DISPENSING INFORMATION** When hydrocortisone cream or ointment is prescribed and no strength is stated, the 1% strength should be supplied. Although *Dioderm*® contains only 0.1% hydrocortisone, the formulation is designed to provide a clinical activity comparable to that of Hydrocortisone Cream 1% BP.
- **PATIENT AND CARER ADVICE** Patient counselling is advised for hydrocortisone cream and ointment (application).
- **PROFESSION SPECIFIC INFORMATION**
  Dental practitioners' formulary
  Hydrocortisone Cream 1% 15 g may be prescribed.
- **EXCEPTIONS TO LEGAL CATEGORY** Skin creams and ointments containing hydrocortisone (alone or with other ingredients) can be sold to the public for the treatment of allergic contact dermatitis, irritant dermatitis, insect bite reactions and mild to moderate eczema in patients over 10 years, to be applied sparingly over the affected area 1–2 times daily for max. 1 week. Over-the-counter hydrocortisone preparations should not be sold without medical advice for children under 10 years or for pregnant women; they should **not** be sold for application to the face, anogenital region, broken or infected skin (including cold sores, acne, and athlete's foot).

- **MEDICINAL FORMS**
  There can be variation in the licensing of different medicines containing the same drug. Forms available from special-order manufacturers include: cream, ointment
  Cream
  CAUTIONARY AND ADVISORY LABELS 28
  EXCIPIENTS: May contain Benzyl alcohol, cetostearyl alcohol (including cetyl and stearyl alcohol), hydroxybenzoates (parabens), propylene glycol
  ▸ Hydrocortisone (Non-proprietary)
  Hydrocortisone 5 mg per 1 gram Hydrocortisone 0.5% cream | 15 gram PoM £4.80 DT price = £1.12 | 30 gram PoM £2.84–£4.90
  Hydrocortisone 10 mg per 1 gram Hydrocortisone 1% cream | 15 gram P £1.64 DT price = £0.94 | 15 gram PoM £11.41 DT price = £0.94 | 30 gram PoM £14.30 DT price = £1.88 | 50 gram PoM £27.75 DT price = £3.13
  Hydrocortisone acetate 10 mg per 1 gram
  Hydrocortisone 25 mg per 1 gram Hydrocortisone 2.5% cream | 15 gram PoM £25.00 DT price = £4.88 | 30 gram PoM £44.00
  ▸ Derma Care Hydrocortisone (The Boots Company Plc)
  Hydrocortisone 10 mg per 1 gram Derma Care Hydrocortisone 1% cream | 15 gram P no price available DT price = £0.94
  ▸ Dermacort (Marlborough Pharmaceuticals Ltd)
  Hydrocortisone 1 mg per 1 gram Dermacort hydrocortisone 0.1% cream | 15 gram P £2.83 DT price = £2.83
  ▸ Dioderm (Dermal Laboratories Ltd)
  Hydrocortisone 1 mg per 1 gram Dioderm 0.1% cream | 30 gram PoM £2.03 DT price = £2.03
  ▸ Hc45 (Reckitt Benckiser Healthcare (UK) Ltd)
  Hydrocortisone acetate 10 mg per 1 gram Hc45 Hydrocortisone 1% cream | 15 gram P £2.58
  ▸ Mildison Lipocream (Astellas Pharma Ltd)
  Hydrocortisone 10 mg per 1 gram Mildison Lipocream 1% cream | 30 gram PoM £1.71 DT price = £1.88
  ▸ Zenoxone (Teva UK Ltd)
  Hydrocortisone 10 mg per 1 gram Zenoxone 1% cream | 15 gram P £1.25 DT price = £0.94
  Ointment
  CAUTIONARY AND ADVISORY LABELS 28
  ▸ Hydrocortisone (Non-proprietary)
  Hydrocortisone 5 mg per 1 gram Hydrocortisone 0.5% ointment | 15 gram PoM £5.55 DT price = £5.55 | 30 gram PoM £11.10–£12.00
  Hydrocortisone 10 mg per 1 gram Hydrocortisone 1% ointment | 15 gram PoM £11.41 DT price = £1.05 | 30 gram PoM £14.30 DT price = £2.10 | 30 gram P £3.31 DT price = £2.10 | 50 gram PoM £27.75 DT price = £3.50
  Hydrocortisone 25 mg per 1 gram Hydrocortisone 2.5% ointment | 15 gram PoM £25.37 DT price = £24.43 | 30 gram PoM £44.86

Combinations available: *Hydrocortisone with benzalkonium chloride, dimeticone and nystatin*, p. 697 · *Hydrocortisone with chlorhexidine hydrochloride and nystatin*, p. 697

⌖ 687
Hydrocortisone butyrate

- **INDICATIONS AND DOSE**
  Severe inflammatory skin disorders such as eczemas unresponsive to less potent corticosteroids | **Psoriasis**
  ▸ TO THE SKIN
  ▸ Child 1–17 years: Apply 1–2 times a day, to be applied thinly
  POTENCY
  Hydrocortisone butyrate 0.1% cream, liquid, and ointment: potent

- **PATIENT AND CARER ADVICE**
  Medicines for Children leaflet: Hydrocortisone (topical) for eczema www.medicinesforchildren.org.uk/hydrocortisone-topical-for-eczema

  Patients or carers should be given advice on how to administer hydrocortisone butyrate lotion, cream, ointment and scalp lotion.

- **MEDICINAL FORMS**
  There can be variation in the licensing of different medicines containing the same drug. Forms available from special-order manufacturers include: ointment
  Liquid
  CAUTIONARY AND ADVISORY LABELS 15 (excluding Locoid Crelo topical emulsion), 28
  EXCIPIENTS: May contain Butylated hydroxytoluene, cetostearyl alcohol (including cetyl and stearyl alcohol), hydroxybenzoates (parabens), propylene glycol
  ▸ Locoid (Astellas Pharma Ltd)
  Hydrocortisone butyrate 1 mg per 1 ml Locoid 0.1% scalp lotion | 100 ml PoM £6.83 DT price = £6.83
  ▸ Locoid Crelo (Astellas Pharma Ltd)
  Hydrocortisone butyrate 1 mg per 1 gram Locoid Crelo 0.1% topical emulsion | 100 gram PoM £5.91
  Cream
  CAUTIONARY AND ADVISORY LABELS 28
  EXCIPIENTS: May contain Benzyl alcohol, cetostearyl alcohol (including cetyl and stearyl alcohol), hydroxybenzoates (parabens)
  ▸ Locoid (Astellas Pharma Ltd)
  Hydrocortisone butyrate 1 mg per 1 gram Locoid 0.1% cream | 30 gram PoM £1.60 DT price = £1.60 | 100 gram PoM £4.93 DT price = £4.93
  ▸ Locoid Lipocream (Astellas Pharma Ltd)
  Hydrocortisone butyrate 1 mg per 1 gram Locoid 0.1% Lipocream | 30 gram PoM £1.69 DT price = £1.60 | 100 gram PoM £5.17 DT price = £4.93
  Ointment
  CAUTIONARY AND ADVISORY LABELS 28
  ▸ Locoid (Astellas Pharma Ltd)
  Hydrocortisone butyrate 1 mg per 1 gram Locoid 0.1% ointment | 30 gram PoM £1.60 DT price = £1.60 | 100 gram PoM £4.93 DT price = £4.93

Hydrocortisone with urea

The properties listed below are those particular to the combination only. For the properties of the components please consider, hydrocortisone p. 692.

- **INDICATIONS AND DOSE**
  Mild inflammatory skin disorders such as eczemas
  ▸ TO THE SKIN
  ▸ Child: To be applied thinly (consult product literature)
  POTENCY
  Hydrocortisone 1% with urea cream: moderate

- **PATIENT AND CARER ADVICE** Patients or carers should be advised on application of hydrocortisone with urea cream.

13

Skin

13

Skin

- **MEDICINAL FORMS**
There can be variation in the licensing of different medicines containing the same drug.

Cream
CAUTIONARY AND ADVISORY LABELS 28
▸ Alphaderm (Alliance Pharmaceuticals Ltd)
**Hydrocortisone 10 mg per 1 gram, Urea 100 mg per
1 gram** Alphaderm 1%/10% cream | 30 gram PoM £2.38 DT price = £2.38 | 100 gram PoM £7.03 DT price = £7.03

⌐ 687

Mometasone furoate

- **INDICATIONS AND DOSE**

Severe inflammatory skin disorders such as eczemas unresponsive to less potent corticosteroids | Psoriasis
▸ TO THE SKIN
▸ Child 1 month-1 year: Apply once daily, to be applied thinly (to scalp in case of lotion)
▸ Child 2-17 years: Apply once daily, to be applied thinly (to scalp in case of lotion)

POTENCY
Mometasone furoate 0.1% cream, ointment, and scalp lotion: potent.

- **UNLICENSED USE** Not licensed for use in children under 2 years.

- **PATIENT AND CARER ADVICE** Patients and carers should be advised on the application of topical mometasone.

- **MEDICINAL FORMS**
There can be variation in the licensing of different medicines containing the same drug. Forms available from special-order manufacturers include: ointment

Liquid
CAUTIONARY AND ADVISORY LABELS 28
EXCIPIENTS: May contain Propylene glycol
▸ Elocon (Merck Sharp & Dohme Ltd)
Mometasone furoate 1 mg per 1 gram Elocon 0.1% scalp lotion | 30 ml PoM £4.36 DT price = £4.36

Cream
CAUTIONARY AND ADVISORY LABELS 28
EXCIPIENTS: May contain Beeswax
▸ Mometasone furoate (Non-proprietary)
Mometasone furoate 1 mg per 1 gram Mometasone 0.1% cream | 30 gram PoM £4.36 DT price = £2.07 | 100 gram PoM £12.58 DT price = £6.90
▸ Elocon (Merck Sharp & Dohme Ltd)
Mometasone furoate 1 mg per 1 gram Elocon 0.1% cream | 30 gram PoM £4.80 DT price = £2.07 | 100 gram PoM £15.10 DT price = £6.90

Ointment
CAUTIONARY AND ADVISORY LABELS 28
EXCIPIENTS: May contain Beeswax, propylene glycol
▸ Mometasone furoate (Non-proprietary)
Mometasone furoate 1 mg per 1 gram Mometasone 0.1% ointment | 15 gram PoM £4.32 | 30 gram PoM £4.45 DT price = £2.18 | 50 gram PoM £12.44 | 100 gram PoM £12.82 DT price = £7.27
▸ Elocon (Merck Sharp & Dohme Ltd)
Mometasone furoate 1 mg per 1 gram Elocon 0.1% ointment | 30 gram PoM £4.32 DT price = £2.18 | 100 gram PoM £12.44 DT price = £7.27

CORTICOSTEROIDS > CORTICOSTEROID COMBINATIONS WITH ANTI-INFECTIVES

Betamethasone with clioquinol

The properties listed below are those particular to the combination only. For the properties of the components please consider, betamethasone p. 688.

- **INDICATIONS AND DOSE**

Severe inflammatory skin disorders such as eczemas unresponsive to less potent corticosteroids | Psoriasis
▸ TO THE SKIN
▸ Child: (consult product literature)
POTENCY
Betamethasone (as valerate) 0.1% with clioquinol cream and ointment: potent.

- **UNLICENSED USE** Betamethasone and clioquinol preparations is not licensed for use in children under 1 year.

- **PATIENT AND CARER ADVICE** Stains clothing. Patients or carers should be counselled on application of betamethasone with clioquinol preparations.

- **MEDICINAL FORMS**
There can be variation in the licensing of different medicines containing the same drug.

Cream
CAUTIONARY AND ADVISORY LABELS 28
EXCIPIENTS: May contain Cetostearyl alcohol (including cetyl and stearyl alcohol), chlorocresol
▸ Betamethasone with clioquinol (Non-proprietary)
Betamethasone (as Betamethasone valerate) 1 mg per 1 gram, Clioquinol 30 mg per 1 gram Betamethasone valerate 0.1% / Clioquinol 3% cream | 30 gram PoM £28.88 DT price = £28.88

Ointment
CAUTIONARY AND ADVISORY LABELS 28
▸ Betamethasone with clioquinol (Non-proprietary)
Betamethasone (as Betamethasone valerate) 1 mg per 1 gram, Clioquinol 30 mg per 1 gram Betamethasone valerate 0.1% / Clioquinol 3% ointment | 30 gram PoM £28.88 DT price = £28.88

Betamethasone with clotrimazole

The properties listed below are those particular to the combination only. For the properties of the components please consider, betamethasone p. 688, clotrimazole p. 481.

- **INDICATIONS AND DOSE**

Severe inflammatory skin disorders such as eczemas unresponsive to less potent corticosteroids | Psoriasis
▸ TO THE SKIN
▸ Child: (consult product literature)
POTENCY
Betamethasone dipropionate 0.064% (=betamethasone 0.5%) with clotrimazole cream: potent.

- **UNLICENSED USE** *Lotriderm* ® not licensed for use in children under 12 years.

- **PATIENT AND CARER ADVICE** Patients or carers should be given advice on how to administer betamethasone with clotrimazole cream.

- **MEDICINAL FORMS**
There can be variation in the licensing of different medicines containing the same drug.

Cream
CAUTIONARY AND ADVISORY LABELS 28
EXCIPIENTS: May contain Benzyl alcohol, cetostearyl alcohol (including cetyl and stearyl alcohol), propylene glycol
▸ Lotriderm (Merck Sharp & Dohme Ltd)
Betamethasone dipropionate 640 microgram per 1 gram, Clotrimazole 10 mg per 1 gram Lotriderm cream | 30 gram PoM £6.34 DT price = £6.34

Betamethasone with fusidic acid

The properties listed below are those particular to the combination only. For the properties of the components please consider, betamethasone p. 688, fusidic acid p. 336.

- **INDICATIONS AND DOSE**

Severe inflammatory skin disorders such as eczemas unresponsive to less potent corticosteroids | Psoriasis
  ▶ TO THE SKIN
  ▶ Child: (consult product literature)

POTENCY
Betamethasone (as valerate) 0.1% with fusidic acid cream: potent.

- **UNLICENSED USE** *Fucibet* ® *Lipid Cream* is not licensed for use in children under 6 years.
- **PATIENT AND CARER ADVICE** Patients or carers should be counselled on application of betamethasone with fusidic acid preparations.

- **MEDICINAL FORMS**
There can be variation in the licensing of different medicines containing the same drug.
Cream
CAUTIONARY AND ADVISORY LABELS 28
EXCIPIENTS: May contain Cetostearyl alcohol (including cetyl and stearyl alcohol), chlorocresol, hydroxybenzoates (parabens)
  ▶ Fucibet (LEO Pharma)
    Betamethasone (as Betamethasone valerate) 1 mg per 1 gram, Fusidic acid 20 mg per 1 gram Fucibet cream | 30 gram [PoM] £6.38 DT price = £6.38 | 60 gram [PoM] £12.76 DT price = £12.76
    Fucibet Lipid cream | 30 gram [PoM] £6.74 DT price = £6.38
  ▶ Xemacort (Mylan Ltd)
    Betamethasone (as Betamethasone valerate) 1 mg per 1 gram, Fusidic acid 20 mg per 1 gram Xemacort cream | 30 gram [PoM] £6.05 DT price = £6.38 | 60 gram [PoM] £12.45 DT price = £12.76

Betamethasone with neomycin

The properties listed below are those particular to the combination only. For the properties of the components please consider, betamethasone p. 688, neomycin sulfate p. 645.

- **INDICATIONS AND DOSE**

Severe inflammatory skin disorders such as eczemas unresponsive to less potent corticosteroids | Psoriasis
  ▶ TO THE SKIN USING OINTMENT, OR TO THE SKIN USING CREAM
  ▶ Child 1–23 months: Apply 1–2 times a day, to be applied thinly
  ▶ Child 2–17 years: Apply 1–2 times a day, to be applied thinly

POTENCY
Betamethasone (as valerate) 0.1% with neomycin cream and ointment: potent.

- **UNLICENSED USE** Betamethasone and neomycin preparations not licensed for use in children under 2 years.
- **PATIENT AND CARER ADVICE** Patient counselling is advised for betamethasone with neomycin cream and ointment (application).

- **MEDICINAL FORMS**
There can be variation in the licensing of different medicines containing the same drug.
Cream
CAUTIONARY AND ADVISORY LABELS 28
EXCIPIENTS: May contain Cetostearyl alcohol (including cetyl and stearyl alcohol), chlorocresol
  ▶ Betamethasone with neomycin (Non-proprietary)
    Betamethasone (as Betamethasone valerate) 1 mg per 1 gram, Neomycin sulfate 5 mg per 1 gram Betamethasone valerate 0.1% / Neomycin 0.5% cream | 30 gram [PoM] £28.88 DT price = £17.74 | 100 gram [PoM] £48.00 DT price = £59.14
Ointment
CAUTIONARY AND ADVISORY LABELS 28
  ▶ Betamethasone with neomycin (Non-proprietary)
    Betamethasone (as Betamethasone valerate) 1 mg per 1 gram, Neomycin sulfate 5 mg per 1 gram Betamethasone valerate 0.1% / Neomycin 0.5% ointment | 30 gram [PoM] £28.88 DT price = £17.74 | 100 gram [PoM] £48.00 DT price = £59.14

Betamethasone with salicylic acid

The properties listed below are those particular to the combination only. For the properties of the components please consider, betamethasone p. 688.

- **INDICATIONS AND DOSE**

DIPROSALIC® OINTMENT

Severe inflammatory skin disorders such as eczemas unresponsive to less potent corticosteroids | Psoriasis
  ▶ TO THE SKIN
  ▶ Child: Apply 1–2 times a day, max. 60 g per week

POTENCY
For *Diprosalic* ® ointment: Betamethasone (as dipropionate) 0.05% with salicylic acid 3%: potent.

DIPROSALIC® SCALP APPLICATION

Severe inflammatory skin disorders such as eczemas unresponsive to less potent corticosteroids | Psoriasis
  ▶ TO THE SKIN
  ▶ Child: Apply 1–2 times a day, apply a few drops

POTENCY
For *Diprosalic* ® scalp application: Betamethasone (as dipropionate) 0.05% with salicylic acid 2%: potent.

- **PATIENT AND CARER ADVICE**

DIPROSALIC® OINTMENT Patients or carers should be counselled on application of betamethasone and salicylic acid preparations.

DIPROSALIC® SCALP APPLICATION Patients or carers should be counselled on application of betamethasone and salicylic acid scalp application.

- **MEDICINAL FORMS**
There can be variation in the licensing of different medicines containing the same drug.
Liquid
CAUTIONARY AND ADVISORY LABELS 28
EXCIPIENTS: May contain Disodium edetate
  ▶ Diprosalic (Merck Sharp & Dohme Ltd)
    Betamethasone (as Betamethasone dipropionate) 500 microgram per 1 ml, Salicylic acid 20 mg per 1 ml Diprosalic 0.05%/2% scalp application | 100 ml [PoM] £10.10 DT price = £10.10
Ointment
CAUTIONARY AND ADVISORY LABELS 28
  ▶ Diprosalic (Merck Sharp & Dohme Ltd)
    Betamethasone (as Betamethasone dipropionate) 500 microgram per 1 gram, Salicylic acid 30 mg per 1 gram Diprosalic 0.05%/3% ointment | 30 gram [PoM] £3.18 DT price = £3.18 | 100 gram [PoM] £9.14 DT price = £9.14

13

Skin

Chlortetracycline with triamcinolone

● **INDICATIONS AND DOSE**

Severe inflammatory skin disorders such as eczemas unresponsive to less potent corticosteroids (associated with infection) | Psoriasis (associated with infection)

▸ TO THE SKIN

▸ Child 1 month–7 years: To be applied thinly (consult product literature)

▸ Child 8–17 years: To be applied thinly (consult product literature)

POTENCY

Triamcinolone acetonide 0.1%, chlortetracycline hydrochloride 3% ointment: potent.

● **UNLICENSED USE** Not licensed for use in children under 8 years.

● **PATIENT AND CARER ADVICE** Stains clothing. Patients or carers should be counselled on the application of chlortetracycline with triamcinolone products.

● **MEDICINAL FORMS**
There can be variation in the licensing of different medicines containing the same drug.

Ointment
CAUTIONARY AND ADVISORY LABELS 28
EXCIPIENTS: May contain Wool fat and related substances including lanolin

▸ Aureocort (AMCo)
Triamcinolone acetonide 1 mg per 1 gram, Chlortetracycline hydrochloride 30.9 mg per 1 gram Aureocort ointment |
15 gram PoM £3.51

Clobetasol propionate with neomycin sulfate and nystatin

The properties listed below are those particular to the combination only. For the properties of the components please consider, clobetasol propionate p. 690, neomycin sulfate p. 645.

● **INDICATIONS AND DOSE**

Short-term treatment only of severe resistant inflammatory skin disorders such as recalcitrant eczemas associated with infection and unresponsive to less potent corticosteroids | Psoriasis associated with infection

▸ TO THE SKIN

▸ Child: (consult product literature)

POTENCY

Clobetasol propionate 0.05% with neomycin sulfate and nystatin cream and ointment: very potent.

● **UNLICENSED USE** Clobetasol with neomycin and nystatin preparations not licensed for use in children under 2 years.

● **PATIENT AND CARER ADVICE** Patients or carers should be advised on application of clobetasol propionate, neomycin sulfate and nystatin containing preparations.

● **MEDICINAL FORMS**
There can be variation in the licensing of different medicines containing the same drug.

Cream
CAUTIONARY AND ADVISORY LABELS 28

▸ Clobetasol propionate with neomycin sulfate and nystatin (Non-proprietary)
Clobetasol propionate 500 microgram per 1 gram, Neomycin sulfate 5 mg per 1 gram, Nystatin 100000 unit per
1 gram Clobetasol 500microgram / Neomycin 5mg / Nystatin 100,000units/g cream | 30 gram PoM £64.00 DT price = £64.00

Ointment
CAUTIONARY AND ADVISORY LABELS 28

▸ Clobetasol propionate with neomycin sulfate and nystatin (Non-proprietary)
Clobetasol propionate 500 microgram per 1 gram, Neomycin sulfate 5 mg per 1 gram, Nystatin 100000 unit per
1 gram Clobetasol 500microgram / Neomycin 5mg / Nystatin 100,000units/g ointment | 30 gram PoM £64.00 DT price = £64.00

Clobetasone butyrate with nystatin and oxytetracycline

The properties listed below are those particular to the combination only. For the properties of the components please consider, clobetasone butyrate p. 690, oxytetracycline p. 334.

● **INDICATIONS AND DOSE**

Steroid-responsive dermatoses where candidal or bacterial infection is present

▸ TO THE SKIN

▸ Child: (consult product literature)

POTENCY

Clobetasone butyrate 0.05% with nystatin and oxytetracyline cream: moderate.

● **PATIENT AND CARER ADVICE** Stains clothing.

● **MEDICINAL FORMS**
There can be variation in the licensing of different medicines containing the same drug.

Cream
CAUTIONARY AND ADVISORY LABELS 28
EXCIPIENTS: May contain Cetostearyl alcohol (including cetyl and stearyl alcohol), chlorocresol, sodium metabisulfite

▸ Trimovate (GlaxoSmithKline UK Ltd)
Clobetasone butyrate 500 microgram per 1 gram, Nystatin 100000 unit per 1 gram, Oxytetracycline (as Oxytetracycline calcium) 30 mg per 1 gram Trimovate cream | 30 gram PoM £3.29

Fluocinolone acetonide with clioquinol

The properties listed below are those particular to the combination only. For the properties of the components please consider, fluocinolone acetonide p. 691.

● **INDICATIONS AND DOSE**

Inflammatory skin disorders such as eczemas associated with infection | Psoriasis associated with infection

▸ TO THE SKIN

▸ Child: Apply 1–2 times a day, to be applied thinly, reducing strength as condition responds

POTENCY

Clioquinol 3% with fluocinolone acetonide 0.025% cream and ointment: potent

● **PATIENT AND CARER ADVICE** Patient counselling is advised for clioquinol with fluocinolone acetonide cream and ointment (application). Ointment stains clothing.

● **MEDICINAL FORMS**
There can be variation in the licensing of different medicines containing the same drug.

Cream
CAUTIONARY AND ADVISORY LABELS 28
EXCIPIENTS: May contain Cetostearyl alcohol (including cetyl and stearyl alcohol), disodium edetate, hydroxybenzoates (parabens), polysorbates, propylene glycol

▸ Synalar C (Derma UK Ltd)
Fluocinolone acetonide 250 microgram per 1 gram, Clioquinol 30 mg per 1 gram Synalar C cream | 15 gram PoM £2.66

Ointment
CAUTIONARY AND ADVISORY LABELS 28
EXCIPIENTS: May contain Propylene glycol, wool fat and related substances including lanolin
▸ Synalar C (Derma UK Ltd)
   Fluocinolone acetonide 250 microgram per 1 gram, Clioquinol 30 mg per 1 gram Synalar C ointment | 15 gram PoM £2.66

Fluocinolone acetonide with neomycin

The properties listed below are those particular to the combination only. For the properties of the components please consider, fluocinolone acetonide p. 691, neomycin sulfate p. 645.

- **INDICATIONS AND DOSE**
  Inflammatory skin disorders such as eczemas associated with infection | Psoriasis associated with infection
  ▸ TO THE SKIN
  ▸ Child 1–11 months: Apply 1–2 times a day, to be applied thinly, reducing strength as condition responds
  ▸ Child 1–17 years: Apply 1–2 times a day, to be applied thinly, reducing strength as condition responds
  POTENCY
  Fluocinolone acetonide 0.025% with neomycin 0.5% cream and ointment: potent.

- **PATIENT AND CARER ADVICE** Patients or carers should be counselled on the application of fluocinolone acetonide with neomycin preparations.

- **MEDICINAL FORMS**
  There can be variation in the licensing of different medicines containing the same drug.
  Cream
  CAUTIONARY AND ADVISORY LABELS 28
  EXCIPIENTS: May contain Cetostearyl alcohol (including cetyl and stearyl alcohol), hydroxybenzoates (parabens), polysorbates, propylene glycol
  ▸ Synalar N (Derma UK Ltd)
     Fluocinolone acetonide 250 microgram per 1 gram, Neomycin sulfate 5 mg per 1 gram Synalar N cream | 30 gram PoM £4.36
  Ointment
  CAUTIONARY AND ADVISORY LABELS 28
  EXCIPIENTS: May contain Propylene glycol, wool fat and related substances including lanolin
  ▸ Synalar N (Derma UK Ltd)
     Fluocinolone acetonide 250 microgram per 1 gram, Neomycin sulfate 5 mg per 1 gram Synalar N ointment | 30 gram PoM £4.36

Hydrocortisone with benzalkonium chloride, dimeticone and nystatin
15.3.2016

The properties listed below are those particular to the combination only. For the properties of the components please consider, hydrocortisone p. 692, dimeticone p. 682.

- **INDICATIONS AND DOSE**
  Mild inflammatory skin disorders such as eczemas associated with infection
  ▸ TO THE SKIN
  ▸ Child: Apply 3 times a day until lesion has healed, to be applied thinly
  POTENCY
  Benzalkonium with dimeticone, hydrocortisone acetate 0.5%, and nystatin cream: mild.

- **PATIENT AND CARER ADVICE** Patients or carers should be advised on application of benzalkonium with dimeticone and hydrocortisone and nystatin preparations.

- **MEDICINAL FORMS**
  There can be variation in the licensing of different medicines containing the same drug.
  Cream
  CAUTIONARY AND ADVISORY LABELS 28
  EXCIPIENTS: May contain Butylated hydroxyanisole, cetostearyl alcohol (including cetyl and stearyl alcohol), hydroxybenzoates (parabens), sodium metabisulfite, sorbic acid
  ▸ Timodine (Alliance Pharmaceuticals Ltd)
     Benzalkonium chloride 1 mg per 1 gram, Hydrocortisone 5 mg per 1 gram, Dimeticone 350 100 mg per 1 gram, Nystatin 100000 unit per 1 gram Timodine cream | 30 gram PoM £3.37

Hydrocortisone with chlorhexidine hydrochloride and nystatin

The properties listed below are those particular to the combination only. For the properties of the components please consider, hydrocortisone p. 692, chlorhexidine p. 656.

- **INDICATIONS AND DOSE**
  Mild inflammatory skin disorders such as eczemas
  ▸ TO THE SKIN
  ▸ Child: To be applied thinly (consult product literature)
  POTENCY
  Hydrocortisone 0.5% with chlorhexidine hydrochloride 1% and nystatin cream: mild
  Hydrocortisone 1% with chlorhexidine hydrochloride 1% and nystatin ointment: mild

- **PATIENT AND CARER ADVICE** Patients or carers should be given advice on application of chlorhexidine hydrochloride with hydrocortisone and nystatin preparations.

- **MEDICINAL FORMS**
  There can be variation in the licensing of different medicines containing the same drug.
  Cream
  CAUTIONARY AND ADVISORY LABELS 28
  EXCIPIENTS: May contain Benzyl alcohol, cetostearyl alcohol (including cetyl and stearyl alcohol), polysorbates
  ▸ Nystaform HC (Typharm Ltd)
     Hydrocortisone 5 mg per 1 gram, Chlorhexidine hydrochloride 10 mg per 1 gram, Nystatin 100000 iu per 1 gram Nystaform HC cream | 30 gram PoM £2.66
  Ointment
  CAUTIONARY AND ADVISORY LABELS 28
  ▸ Nystaform HC (Typharm Ltd)
     Chlorhexidine acetate 10 mg per 1 gram, Hydrocortisone 10 mg per 1 gram, Nystatin 100000 unit per 1 gram Nystaform HC ointment | 30 gram PoM £2.66

Hydrocortisone with clotrimazole

The properties listed below are those particular to the combination only. For the properties of the components please consider, hydrocortisone p. 692, clotrimazole p. 678.

- **INDICATIONS AND DOSE**
  Mild inflammatory skin disorders such as eczemas (associated with fungal infection)
  ▸ TO THE SKIN
  ▸ Child: (consult product literature)
  POTENCY
  Clotrimazole with hydrocortisone 1% cream: mild

- **PATIENT AND CARER ADVICE** Patients or carers should be given advice on how to administer clotrimazole with hydrocortisone cream.

- **EXCEPTIONS TO LEGAL CATEGORY** A 15-g tube is on sale to the public for the treatment of athlete's foot and fungal infection of skin folds with associated inflammation in patients 10 years and over.

13

Skin

● **MEDICINAL FORMS**
There can be variation in the licensing of different medicines containing the same drug.

Cream
CAUTIONARY AND ADVISORY LABELS 28
EXCIPIENTS: May contain Benzyl alcohol, cetostearyl alcohol (including cetyl and stearyl alcohol)

▶ Canesten HC (Bayer Plc)
Clotrimazole 10 mg per 1 gram, Hydrocortisone 10 mg per 1 gram Canesten HC cream | 30 gram PoM £2.42 DT price = £2.42

▶ Canesten Hydrocortisone (Bayer Plc)
Clotrimazole 10 mg per 1 gram, Hydrocortisone 10 mg per 1 gram Canesten Hydrocortisone cream | 15 gram P £3.11 DT price = £3.11

Combinations available: *Hydrocortisone with fusidic acid,* below · *Hydrocortisone with miconazole,* below · *Hydrocortisone with oxytetracycline,* below

Hydrocortisone with fusidic acid

The properties listed below are those particular to the combination only. For the properties of the components please consider, hydrocortisone p. 692, fusidic acid p. 336.

● **INDICATIONS AND DOSE**
Mild inflammatory skin disorders such as eczemas
▶ TO THE SKIN
▶ Child: To be applied thinly (consult product literature)
POTENCY
Hydrocortisone with fusidic acid cream: mild

● **PATIENT AND CARER ADVICE** Patients or carers should be advised on application of hydrocortisone with fusidic acid preparations.

● **MEDICINAL FORMS**
There can be variation in the licensing of different medicines containing the same drug.

Cream
CAUTIONARY AND ADVISORY LABELS 28
EXCIPIENTS: May contain Butylated hydroxyanisole, cetostearyl alcohol (including cetyl and stearyl alcohol), polysorbates, potassium sorbate

▶ Fucidin H (Fusidic acid / Hydrocortisone) (LEO Pharma)
Hydrocortisone acetate 10 mg per 1 gram, Fusidic acid 20 mg per 1 gram Fucidin H cream | 30 gram PoM £6.02 DT price = £6.02 | 60 gram PoM £12.05 DT price = £12.05

Hydrocortisone with miconazole

The properties listed below are those particular to the combination only. For the properties of the components please consider, hydrocortisone p. 692, miconazole p. 679.

● **INDICATIONS AND DOSE**
Mild inflammatory skin disorders such as eczemas associated with infections
▶ TO THE SKIN
▶ Child: (consult product literature)
POTENCY
Hydrocortisone 1% with miconazole cream and ointment: mild

● **INTERACTIONS** → Appendix 1 (antifungals, imidazole).

● **PATIENT AND CARER ADVICE** Patients or carers should be advised on application of hydrocortisone with miconazole preparations.

● **PROFESSION SPECIFIC INFORMATION**
Dental practitioners' formulary
May be prescribed as Miconazole and Hydrocortisone Cream or Ointment for max. 7 days.

● **EXCEPTIONS TO LEGAL CATEGORY** A 15-g tube of hydrocortisone with miconazole cream is on sale to the public for the treatment of athlete's foot and candidal intertrigo in children over 10 years.

● **MEDICINAL FORMS**
There can be variation in the licensing of different medicines containing the same drug.

Cream
CAUTIONARY AND ADVISORY LABELS 28
EXCIPIENTS: May contain Butylated hydroxyanisole, disodium edetate

▶ Daktacort (McNeil Products Ltd, Janssen-Cilag Ltd)
Hydrocortisone 10 mg per 1 gram, Miconazole nitrate 20 mg per 1 gram Daktacort Hydrocortisone cream | 15 gram P £3.17 DT price = £3.17
Daktacort 2%/1% cream | 30 gram PoM £2.49 DT price = £2.49

Ointment
CAUTIONARY AND ADVISORY LABELS 28
▶ Daktacort (Janssen-Cilag Ltd)
Hydrocortisone 10 mg per 1 gram, Miconazole nitrate 20 mg per 1 gram Daktacort ointment | 30 gram PoM £2.50 DT price = £2.50

Hydrocortisone with oxytetracycline

The properties listed below are those particular to the combination only. For the properties of the components please consider, hydrocortisone p. 692, oxytetracycline p. 334.

● **INDICATIONS AND DOSE**
Mild inflammatory skin disorders such as eczemas
▶ TO THE SKIN
▶ Child 12–17 years: (consult product literature)
POTENCY
Hydrocortisone 1% with oxytetracycline ointment: mild.

● **CONTRA-INDICATIONS** Children under 12 years

● **PREGNANCY** Tetracyclines should not be given to pregnant women. Effects on skeletal development have been documented when tetracyclines have been used in the first trimester in animal studies. Administration during the second or third trimester may cause discoloration of the child's teeth.

● **BREAST FEEDING** Tetracyclines should not be given to women who are breast-feeding (although absorption and therefore discoloration of teeth in the infant is probably usually prevented by chelation with calcium in milk).

● **PATIENT AND CARER ADVICE** Patients should be given advice on the application of hydrocortisone with oxytetracycline ointment.

● **MEDICINAL FORMS**
There can be variation in the licensing of different medicines containing the same drug.

Ointment
CAUTIONARY AND ADVISORY LABELS 28
▶ Terra-Cortril (Intrapharm Laboratories Ltd)
Hydrocortisone 10 mg per 1 gram, Oxytetracycline (as Oxytetracycline hydrochloride) 30 mg per 1 gram Terra-Cortril ointment | 30 gram PoM £5.01 DT price = £5.01

DERMATOLOGICAL DRUGS > ANTI-INFECTIVES

Ichthammol

- **INDICATIONS AND DOSE**
Chronic lichenified eczema
▶ TO THE SKIN
▶ Child 1-17 years: Apply 1–3 times a day

- **UNLICENSED USE** No information available.
- **SIDE-EFFECTS** Skin irritation

- **MEDICINAL FORMS**
There can be variation in the licensing of different medicines containing the same drug. Forms available from special-order manufacturers include: ointment, paste
Liquid
▶ Ichthammol (Non-proprietary)
Ichthammol 1 mg per 1 mg Ichthammol liquid | 100 gram GSL
£11.42 DT price = £11.42 | 500 gram GSL £34.27

Ichthammol with zinc oxide

The properties listed below are those particular to the combination only. For the properties of the components please consider, ichthammol above.

- **INDICATIONS AND DOSE**
Chronic lichenified eczema
▶ TO THE SKIN
▶ Child: (consult product literature)

- **MEDICINAL FORMS**
There can be variation in the licensing of different medicines containing the same drug. Forms available from special-order manufacturers include: cream, ointment
Impregnated dressing
▶ Ichthopaste (Smith & Nephew Healthcare Ltd)
Ichthopaste bandage 7.5cm × 6m | 1 bandage £3.68

DERMATOLOGICAL DRUGS > ANTRACEN DERIVATIVES

Dithranol

(Anthralin)

- **INDICATIONS AND DOSE**
Subacute and chronic psoriasis
▶ TO THE SKIN
▶ Child: (consult product literature)
DITHROCREAM®
Subacute and chronic psoriasis
▶ TO THE SKIN
▶ Child: For application to skin or scalp, 0.1–0.5% cream suitable for overnight treatment, 1–2% cream for maximum 1 hour (consult product literature)
MICANOL®
Subacute and chronic psoriasis
▶ TO THE SKIN
▶ Child: Apply once daily, for application to skin or scalp, to be applied for up to 30 minutes, apply 1% cream, if necessary 3% cream can be used under medical supervision

- **UNLICENSED USE**
DITHROCREAM® *Dithrocream®* is licensed for use in children (age range not specified by manufacturer).
MICANOL® *Micanol®* licensed for use in children, but not recommended for infants or young children (age range not specified by manufacturer).

- **CONTRA-INDICATIONS** Acute and pustular psoriasis · hypersensitivity
- **CAUTIONS** Avoid sensitive areas of skin · avoid use near eyes
- **SIDE-EFFECTS** Local burning sensation · local irritation · stains hair · stains skin
- **PREGNANCY** No adverse effects reported.
- **BREAST FEEDING** No adverse effects reported.
- **DIRECTIONS FOR ADMINISTRATION** When applying dithranol, hands should be protected by gloves or they should be washed thoroughly afterwards. Dithranol should be applied to chronic extensor plaques only, carefully avoiding normal skin.
MICANOL® At the end of contact time, use plenty of lukewarm (not hot) water to rinse off cream; soap may be used after the cream has been rinsed off; use shampoo before applying cream to scalp and if necessary after cream has been rinsed off.
- **PRESCRIBING AND DISPENSING INFORMATION** Treatment should be started with a low concentration such as dithranol 0.1%, and the strength increased gradually every few days up to 3%, according to tolerance.
- **PATIENT AND CARER ADVICE** Dithranol can stain the skin, hair and fabrics.
- **EXCEPTIONS TO LEGAL CATEGORY** Prescription only medicine if dithranol content more than 1%, otherwise may be sold to the public.

- **MEDICINAL FORMS**
There can be variation in the licensing of different medicines containing the same drug. Forms available from special-order manufacturers include: ointment
Cream
CAUTIONARY AND ADVISORY LABELS 28
EXCIPIENTS: May contain Cetostearyl alcohol (including cetyl and stearyl alcohol), chlorocresol
▶ Dithrocream (Dermal Laboratories Ltd)
Dithranol 1 mg per 1 gram Dithrocream 0.1% cream | 50 gram P £3.77
Dithranol 2.5 mg per 1 gram Dithrocream 0.25% cream | 50 gram P £4.04
Dithranol 5 mg per 1 gram Dithrocream 0.5% cream | 50 gram P £4.66
Dithranol 10 mg per 1 gram Dithrocream HP 1% cream | 50 gram P £5.42
Dithranol 20 mg per 1 gram Dithrocream 2% cream | 50 gram PoM £5.77
▶ Micanol (Derma UK Ltd)
Dithranol 10 mg per 1 gram Micanol 1% cream | 50 gram P £16.18
Dithranol 30 mg per 1 gram Micanol 3% cream | 50 gram PoM £20.15

Combinations available: *Coal tar with dithranol and salicylic acid,* p. 700

Dithranol with salicylic acid and zinc oxide

The properties listed below are those particular to the combination only. For the properties of the components please consider, dithranol above.

- **INDICATIONS AND DOSE**
Subacute and chronic psoriasis
▶ TO THE SKIN
▶ Child: (consult local protocol)

- **MEDICINAL FORMS**
There can be variation in the licensing of different medicines containing the same drug. Forms available from special-order manufacturers include: ointment, paste

13

Skin

Coal tar

- **INDICATIONS AND DOSE**

Psoriasis | Chronic atopic eczema
▸ TO THE SKIN USING PASTE
▸ Child: Apply 1–3 times a day, start application with low-strength preparations
▸ TO THE SKIN
▸ Child: 100 mL/bath, to be added to an adult sized bath; add proportionally less for a child's bath. Use Coal Tar Solution BP

ALPHOSYL 2 IN 1® SHAMPOO

Psoriasis | Seborrhoeic dermatitis | Scaling | Itching
▸ TO THE SKIN
▸ Child: Apply every 2–3 days

Dandruff
▸ TO THE SKIN
▸ Child: Apply 1–2 times a week as required

EXOREX® LOTION

Psoriasis
▸ TO THE SKIN
▸ Child: Apply 2–3 times a day, to be applied to skin or scalp; can be diluted with a few drops of water before applying

- **CONTRA-INDICATIONS** Avoid broken or inflamed skin · avoid eye area · avoid genital area · avoid mucosal areas · avoid rectal area · infection · sore, acute, or pustular psoriasis
- **CAUTIONS** Application to face · application to skin flexures
- **SIDE-EFFECTS** Acne-like eruptions · photosensitivity · skin irritation
- **PRESCRIBING AND DISPENSING INFORMATION** Coal Tar Solution BP contains coal tar 20%, Strong Coal Tar Solution BP contains coal tar 40%.
- **HANDLING AND STORAGE** Use suitable chemical protection gloves for extemporaneous preparation. May stain skin, hair and fabric.
- **PATIENT AND CARER ADVICE** May stain skin, hair and fabric.
- **MEDICINAL FORMS** There can be variation in the licensing of different medicines containing the same drug. Forms available from special-order manufacturers include: paste

Bath additive
▸ Psoriderm (Dermal Laboratories Ltd)
Coal tar distilled 400 mg per 1 ml Psoriderm Emulsion 40% bath additive | 200 ml P £2.74

Shampoo
EXCIPIENTS: May contain Fragrances, hydroxybenzoates (parabens)
▸ Coal tar (Non-proprietary)
Coal tar extract 20 mg per 1 gram Coal tar extract 2% shampoo | 125 ml GSL no price available DT price = £3.61 | 250 ml GSL no price available DT price = £5.38
▸ Brands may include Alphosyl 2 in 1, Neutrogena T/Gel Therapeutic, Polytar Scalp

Cutaneous emulsion
EXCIPIENTS: May contain Hydroxybenzoates (parabens)
▸ Exorex (Forest Laboratories UK Ltd)
Coal tar solution 50 mg per 1 gram Exorex lotion | 100 ml GSL £8.11 DT price = £8.11 | 250 ml GSL £16.24 DT price = £16.24

Coal tar with arachis oil extract of coal tar, cade oil, light liquid paraffin and tar

The properties listed below are those particular to the combination only. For the properties of the components please consider, coal tar above.

- **INDICATIONS AND DOSE**

Psoriasis | Eczema | Atopic dermatoses | Pruritic dermatoses
▸ TO THE SKIN
▸ Child: 2–4 capfuls/bath, alternatively 15–30 mL, to be added in an adult-size bath and soak for 20 minutes (proportionally less for a child's bath)

- **MEDICINAL FORMS** There can be variation in the licensing of different medicines containing the same drug.
No licensed medicines listed.

Coal tar with coconut oil and salicylic acid

The properties listed below are those particular to the combination only. For the properties of the components please consider, coal tar above.

- **INDICATIONS AND DOSE**

Scaly scalp disorders | Psoriasis | Seborrhoeic dermatitis | Dandruff | Cradle cap
▸ TO THE SKIN USING SHAMPOO
▸ Child: Apply daily as required

- **MEDICINAL FORMS** There can be variation in the licensing of different medicines containing the same drug.
Shampoo
▸ Capasal (Dermal Laboratories Ltd)
Salicylic acid 5 mg per 1 gram, Coal tar distilled 10 mg per 1 gram, Coconut oil 10 mg per 1 gram Capasal Therapeutic shampoo | 250 ml P £4.69

Coal tar with dithranol and salicylic acid

The properties listed below are those particular to the combination only. For the properties of the components please consider, coal tar above, dithranol p. 699.

- **INDICATIONS AND DOSE**

Subacute and chronic psoriasis
▸ TO THE SKIN
▸ Child: Apply up to twice daily

- **UNLICENSED USE** *Psorin®* is licensed for use in children (age range not specified by manufacturer).

- **MEDICINAL FORMS** There can be variation in the licensing of different medicines containing the same drug. Forms available from special-order manufacturers include: ointment

13

Skin

Coal tar with lecithin

The properties listed below are those particular to the combination only. For the properties of the components please consider, coal tar p. 700.

- **INDICATIONS AND DOSE**

PSORIDERM® CREAM

Psoriasis

▸ TO THE SKIN

▸ Child: Apply 1–2 times a day, cream to be applied to the skin or scalp

PSORIDERM® SCALP LOTION

Scalp psoriasis

▸ TO THE SKIN

▸ Child: Apply as required

- **MEDICINAL FORMS**
There can be variation in the licensing of different medicines containing the same drug.

Cream

EXCIPIENTS: May contain Isopropyl palmitate, propylene glycol

▸ Psoriderm (Dermal Laboratories Ltd)
Lecithin 4 mg per 1 gram, Coal tar distilled 60 mg per 1 gram Psoriderm cream | 225 ml ℗ £9.42

Shampoo

EXCIPIENTS: May contain Disodium edetate

▸ Psoriderm (Dermal Laboratories Ltd)
Lecithin 3 mg per 1 ml, Coal tar distilled 25 mg per 1 ml Psoriderm scalp lotion | 250 ml ℗ £4.74

Coal tar with salicylic acid and precipitated sulfur

The properties listed below are those particular to the combination only. For the properties of the components please consider, coal tar p. 700.

- **INDICATIONS AND DOSE**

COCOIS® OINTMENT

Scaly scalp disorders including psoriasis, eczema, seborrhoeic dermatitis and dandruff

▸ INITIALLY TO THE SKIN USING SCALP OINTMENT

▸ Child 6–11 years: Medical supervision required

▸ Child 12–17 years: Apply once weekly as required, alternatively (to the skin) apply daily for the first 3–7 days (if severe), shampoo off after 1 hour

SEBCO® OINTMENT

Scaly scalp disorders including psoriasis, eczema, seborrhoeic dermatitis and dandruff

▸ TO THE SKIN USING SCALP OINTMENT

▸ Child 6–11 years: Medical supervision required

▸ Child 12–17 years: Apply as required, alternatively apply daily for the first 3–7 days (if severe), shampoo off after 1 hour

- **MEDICINAL FORMS**
There can be variation in the licensing of different medicines containing the same drug.

Ointment

EXCIPIENTS: May contain Cetostearyl alcohol (including cetyl and stearyl alcohol)

▸ Cocois (Focus Pharmaceuticals Ltd)
Salicylic acid 20 mg per 1 gram, Sulfur precipitated 40 mg per 1 gram, Coal tar solution 120 mg per 1 gram Cocois ointment | 40 gram GSL £6.22 | 100 gram GSL £11.69

▸ Sebco (Derma UK Ltd)
Salicylic acid 20 mg per 1 gram, Sulfur precipitated 40 mg per 1 gram, Coal tar solution 120 mg per 1 gram Sebco ointment | 40 gram GSL £5.91 | 100 gram GSL £11.11

Coal tar with zinc oxide

The properties listed below are those particular to the combination only. For the properties of the components please consider, coal tar p. 700.

- **INDICATIONS AND DOSE**

Psoriasis | Chronic atopic eczema

▸ TO THE SKIN

▸ Child: Apply 1–2 times a day

- **PRESCRIBING AND DISPENSING INFORMATION** No preparations available—when prepared extemporaneously, the BP states Zinc and Coal Tar Paste, BP consists of zinc oxide 6%, coal tar 6%, emulsifying wax 5%, starch 38%, yellow soft paraffin 45%.

- **MEDICINAL FORMS**
There can be variation in the licensing of different medicines containing the same drug. Forms available from special-order manufacturers include: ointment, paste

Extract of coal tar with arachis oil

The properties listed below are those particular to the combination only. For the properties of the components please consider, coal tar p. 700.

- **INDICATIONS AND DOSE**

Scalp disorders | Psoriasis | Seborrhoea | Eczema | Pruritus | Dandruff

▸ TO THE SKIN

▸ Child: Apply 1–2 times a week, to the scalp

- **MEDICINAL FORMS**
There can be variation in the licensing of different medicines containing the same drug.
No licensed medicines listed.

IMMUNOSUPPRESSANTS ❯ CALCINEURIN INHIBITORS AND RELATED DRUGS

Pimecrolimus

- **INDICATIONS AND DOSE**

Short-term treatment of mild to moderate atopic eczema (including flares) when topical corticosteroids cannot be used (initiated by a specialist)

▸ TO THE SKIN

▸ Child 2–17 years: Apply twice daily until symptoms resolve (stop treatment if eczema worsens or no response after 6 weeks)

- **CONTRA-INDICATIONS** Application to malignant or potentially malignant skin lesions · application under occlusion · congenital epidermal barrier defects · contact with eyes · contact with mucous membranes · generalised erythroderma · immunodeficiency · infection at treatment site

- **CAUTIONS** Alcohol consumption (risk of facial flushing and skin irritation) · avoid other topical treatments except emollients at treatment site · UV light (avoid excessive exposure to sunlight and sunlamps)

- **INTERACTIONS** Concomitant use with drugs that cause immunosuppression is contra-indicated (may be prescribed in exceptional circumstances by specialists).

13

Skin

● SIDE-EFFECTS
▶ **Common or very common** Burning sensation · erythema · folliculitis · pruritus · skin infections
▶ **Uncommon** Herpes simplex · herpes zoster · impetigo · molluscum contagiosum
▶ **Rare** Dryness · local reactions including pain · oedema · papilloma · paraesthesia · peeling · skin discoloration · worsening of eczema
▶ **Frequency not known** Skin malignancy
● PREGNANCY Manufacturer advises avoid; toxicity in *animal* studies following systemic administration.
● BREAST FEEDING Manufacturer advises caution; ensure infant does not come in contact with treated areas.
● NATIONAL FUNDING/ACCESS DECISIONS
NICE technology appraisals (TAs)
▶ **Tacrolimus and pimecrolimus for atopic eczema (August 2004)** NICE TA82
Topical pimecrolimus is an option for atopic eczema not controlled by maximal topical corticosteroid treatment or if there is a risk of important corticosteroid side-effects (particularly skin atrophy).
   Topical pimecrolimus is recommended for moderate atopic eczema on the face and neck of children aged 2–16 years. Pimecrolimus should be used within its licensed indications.
www.nice.org.uk/TA82

● MEDICINAL FORMS
There can be variation in the licensing of different medicines containing the same drug.
Cream
CAUTIONARY AND ADVISORY LABELS 4, 11, 28
EXCIPIENTS: May contain Benzyl alcohol, cetostearyl alcohol (including cetyl and stearyl alcohol), propylene glycol
▶ **Elidel** (Meda Pharmaceuticals Ltd)
Pimecrolimus 10 mg per 1 gram Elidel 1% cream | 30 gram PoM £19.69 DT price = £19.69 | 60 gram PoM £37.41 DT price = £37.41 | 100 gram PoM £59.07 DT price = £59.07

Tacrolimus

● DRUG ACTION Tacrolimus is a calcineurin inhibitor.

● INDICATIONS AND DOSE
Short-term treatment of moderate to severe atopic eczema (including flares) in patients unresponsive to, or intolerant of conventional therapy (initiated by a specialist)
▶ TO THE SKIN
▶ Child 2–15 years: Apply twice daily for up to 3 weeks (consider other treatment if eczema worsens or if no improvement after 2 weeks), 0.03% ointment to be applied thinly, then reduced to once daily until lesion clears
▶ Child 16–17 years: Apply twice daily until lesion clears (consider other treatment if eczema worsens or no improvement after 2 weeks), initially 0.1% ointment to be applied thinly, reduce frequency to once daily or strength of ointment to 0.03% if condition allows

Prevention of flares in patients with moderate to severe atopic eczema and 4 or more flares a year who have responded to initial treatment with topical tacrolimus (initiated by a specialist)
▶ TO THE SKIN
▶ Child 2–15 years: Apply twice weekly, 0.03% ointment to be applied thinly, with an interval of 2–3 days between applications, use short-term treatment regimen during an acute flare; review need for preventative therapy after 1 year
▶ Child 16–17 years: Apply twice weekly, 0.1% ointment to be applied thinly, with an interval of 2–3 days between

applications, use short-term treatment regimen during an acute flare; review need for preventative therapy after 1 year

● CONTRA-INDICATIONS Application to malignant or potentially malignant skin lesions · application under occlusion · avoid contact with eyes · avoid contact with mucous membranes · congenital epidermal barrier defects · generalised erythroderma · immunodeficiency · infection at treatment site
● CAUTIONS UV light (avoid excessive exposure to sunlight and sunlamps)
● INTERACTIONS Interactions do not generally apply to tacrolimus used topically. Concomitant use with drugs that cause immunosuppression (may be prescribed in exceptional circumstances by specialists). Risk of facial flushing and skin irritation with alcohol consumption (does not apply to tacrolimus taken systemically).
● SIDE-EFFECTS
▶ **Common or very common** Application-site infections · application-site reactions · herpes simplex infection · irritation (at application-site) · Kaposi's varicelliform eruption · pain at application-site · rash
▶ **Uncommon** Acne
▶ **Frequency not known** Cutaneous lymphoma · malignancies · other types of lymphomas · rosacea · skin malignancy
● ALLERGY AND CROSS-SENSITIVITY Contra-indicated if history of hypersensitivity to macrolides.
● PREGNANCY Manufacturer advises avoid unless essential; toxicity in *animal* studies following systemic administration.
● BREAST FEEDING Avoid—present in breast milk (following systemic administration).
● PATIENT AND CARER ADVICE Avoid excessive exposure to UV light including sunlight.
● NATIONAL FUNDING/ACCESS DECISIONS
NICE technology appraisals (TAs)
▶ **Tacrolimus and pimecrolimus for atopic eczema (August 2004)** NICE TA82
Topical tacrolimus is an option for atopic eczema not controlled by maximal topical corticosteroid treatment or if there is a risk of important corticosteroid side-effects (particularly skin atrophy). Topical tacrolimus is recommended for moderate to severe atopic eczema in adults and children over 2 years. Tacrolimus should be used within its licensed indications.
www.nice.org.uk/TA82
Scottish Medicines Consortium (SMC) Decisions
The *Scottish Medicines Consortium* has advised (March 2010) that tacrolimus ointment (*Protopic®*) is accepted for restricted use within NHS Scotland for the prevention of flares in patients aged over 2 years with moderate to severe atopic eczema in accordance with the licensed indications; initiation of treatment is restricted to doctors (including general practitioners) with a specialist interest and experience in treating atopic eczema with immunomodulatory therapy.

● MEDICINAL FORMS
There can be variation in the licensing of different medicines containing the same drug.
Ointment
CAUTIONARY AND ADVISORY LABELS 4, 11, 28
EXCIPIENTS: May contain Beeswax
▶ **Protopic** (Astellas Pharma Ltd)
Tacrolimus (as Tacrolimus monohydrate) 300 microgram per 1 gram Protopic 0.03% ointment | 30 gram PoM £19.44 DT price = £19.44 | 60 gram PoM £35.46 DT price = £35.46
Tacrolimus (as Tacrolimus monohydrate) 1 mg per 1 gram Protopic 0.1% ointment | 30 gram PoM £21.60 DT price = £21.60 | 60 gram PoM £39.40 DT price = £39.40

RETINOID AND RELATED DRUGS

Acitretin

● **DRUG ACTION** Acitretin is a metabolite of etretinate.

● **INDICATIONS AND DOSE**

Severe extensive psoriasis resistant to other forms of therapy (under expert supervision) | Palmoplantar pustular psoriasis (under expert supervision) | Severe congenital ichthyosis (under expert supervision)
▸ BY MOUTH
▸ Child 1 month–11 years: 0.5 mg/kg once daily; increased if necessary to 1 mg/kg once daily, to be taken with food or milk, careful monitoring of musculoskeletal development required; maximum 35 mg per day
▸ Child 12–17 years: Initially 25–30 mg daily for 2–4 weeks, then adjusted according to response to 25–50 mg daily, increased to up to 75 mg daily, dose only increased to 75 mg daily for short periods in psoriasis

Severe Darier's disease (keratosis follicularis) (under expert supervision)
▸ BY MOUTH
▸ Child 1 month–11 years: 0.5 mg/kg once daily; increased if necessary to 1 mg/kg once daily, to be taken with food or milk, careful monitoring of musculoskeletal development required; maximum 35 mg per day
▸ Child 12–17 years: Initially 10 mg daily for 2–4 weeks, then adjusted according to response to 25–50 mg daily

Harlequin ichthyosis (under expert supervision)
▸ BY MOUTH
▸ Neonate: 0.5 mg/kg once daily; increased if necessary to 1 mg/kg once daily, to be taken with food or milk, careful monitoring of musculoskeletal development required.

● **CONTRA-INDICATIONS** Hyperlipidaemia
● **CAUTIONS** Avoid excessive exposure to sunlight and unsupervised use of sunlamps · diabetes (can alter glucose tolerance—initial frequent blood glucose checks) · do not donate blood during and for 2 years after stopping therapy (teratogenic risk) · in children use only in exceptional circumstances and monitor growth parameters and bone development (premature epiphyseal closure reported) · investigate atypical musculoskeletal symptoms
● **INTERACTIONS** → Appendix 1 (retinoids). Avoid concomitant use of keratolytics.
● **SIDE-EFFECTS**
▸ **Common or very common** Abdominal pain · abnormal hair texture · alopecia (reversible on withdrawal) · arthralgia · brittle nails · dermatitis · diarrhoea · dryness and inflammation of mucous membranes · dryness of conjunctiva (causing conjunctivitis and decreased tolerance to contact lenses) · epidermal fragility · erythema · headache · myalgia · nausea · paronychia · peripheral oedema · pruritus · reversible increase in serum-cholesterol (with high doses) · reversible increase in serum-triglyceride concentrations (with high doses) · skin exfoliation · sticky skin · vomiting
▸ **Uncommon** Dizziness · hepatitis · photosensitivity · visual disturbances
▸ **Rare** Peripheral neuropathy
▸ **Very rare** Benign intracranial hypertension · bone pain · exostosis · night blindness · ulcerative keratitis
▸ **Frequency not known** Drowsiness · dry skin · flushing · granulomatous lesions · impaired hearing · initial worsening of psoriasis · malaise · rectal haemorrhage · sweating · taste disturbance · tinnitus

SIDE-EFFECTS, FURTHER INFORMATION
▸ Exostosis Skeletal hyperostosis and extra-osseous calcification reported following long-term treatment with etretinate (of which Acitretin is a metabolite) and premature epiphyseal closure in children.
▸ Benign intracranial hypertension Discontinue if severe headache, nausea, vomiting, or visual disturbances occur.
● **CONCEPTION AND CONTRACEPTION** Effective contraception must be used.
Pregnancy prevention In females of child-bearing potential (including those with a history of infertility), exclude pregnancy up to 3 days before treatment, every month during treatment, and every 1–3 months for 3 years after stopping treatment. Treatment should be started on day 2 or 3 of menstrual cycle. Females of child-bearing age must practise effective contraception for at least 1 month before starting treatment, during treatment, and for at least 3 years after stopping treatment. Females should be advised to use at least 1 method of contraception, but ideally they should use 2 methods of contraception. Oral progestogen-only contraceptives are not considered effective. Barrier methods should not be used alone but can be used in conjunction with other contraceptive methods. Females should be advised to seek medical attention immediately if they become pregnant during treatment or within 3 years of stopping treatment. They should also be advised to avoid alcohol during treatment and for 2 months after stopping treatment.
● **PREGNANCY** Avoid—teratogenic.
● **BREAST FEEDING** Avoid.
● **HEPATIC IMPAIRMENT** Avoid in severe impairment—risk of further impairment.
● **RENAL IMPAIRMENT** Avoid in severe impairment; increased risk of toxicity.
● **MONITORING REQUIREMENTS**
▸ Monitor serum-triglyceride and serum-cholesterol concentrations before treatment, 1 month after starting, then every 3 months.
▸ Check liver function at start, at least every 4 weeks for first 2 months and then every 3 months.
● **PRESCRIBING AND DISPENSING INFORMATION**
Prescribing for women of child-bearing potential Each prescription for acitretin should be limited to a supply of up to 30 days' treatment and dispensed within 7 days of the date stated on the prescription.
● **PATIENT AND CARER ADVICE** A patient information leaflet should be provided.
Patient advice required around conception and contraception Females of child-bearing potential must be advised on pregnancy prevention.

● **MEDICINAL FORMS**
There can be variation in the licensing of different medicines containing the same drug. Forms available from special-order manufacturers include: oral suspension, oral solution
Capsule
CAUTIONARY AND ADVISORY LABELS 10, 11, 21
▸ Acitretin (Non-proprietary)
Acitretin 10 mg Acitretin 10mg capsules | 60 capsule [PoM] £23.80 DT price = £23.80
Acitretin 25 mg Acitretin 25mg capsules | 60 capsule [PoM] £55.24 DT price = £55.24
▸ Neotigason (Actavis UK Ltd)
Acitretin 10 mg Neotigason 10mg capsules | 60 capsule [PoM] £17.30 DT price = £23.80 (Hospital only)
Acitretin 25 mg Neotigason 25mg capsules | 60 capsule [PoM] £43.00 DT price = £55.24 (Hospital only)

13

Skin

SALICYLIC ACID AND DERIVATIVES

Salicylic acid with zinc oxide

● **INDICATIONS AND DOSE**

Hyperkeratotic skin disorders

▸ TO THE SKIN

▸ **Child:** Apply twice daily

● **CAUTIONS** Avoid broken skin · avoid inflamed skin

CAUTIONS, FURTHER INFORMATION

▸ **Salicylate toxicity** Salicylate toxicity may occur particularly if applied on large areas of skin or neonatal skin.

● **SIDE-EFFECTS** Excessive drying · irritation · sensitivity · systemic effects (after widespread use)

● **PRESCRIBING AND DISPENSING INFORMATION** Zinc and Salicylic Acid Paste BP is also referred to as Lassar's Paste. When prepared extemporaneously, the BP states Zinc and Salicylic Acid Paste, BP (Lassar's Paste) consists of zinc oxide 24%, salicylic acid 2%, starch 24%, white soft paraffin 50%.

● **MEDICINAL FORMS**

There can be variation in the licensing of different medicines containing the same drug. Forms available from special-order manufacturers include: paste

VITAMINS AND TRACE ELEMENTS ❯ VITAMIN D AND ANALOGUES

Calcipotriol

● **INDICATIONS AND DOSE**

Plaque psoriasis

▸ TO THE SKIN USING OINTMENT

▸ **Child 6–11 years:** Apply twice daily, when preparations used together maximum total calcipotriol 2.5 mg in any one week (e.g. scalp solution 20 mL with ointment 30 g); maximum 50 g per week

▸ **Child 12–17 years:** Apply twice daily, when preparations used together maximum total calcipotriol 3.75 mg in any one week (e.g. scalp solution 30 mL with ointment 45 g); maximum 75 g per week

Scalp psoriasis

▸ TO THE SKIN USING SCALP LOTION

▸ **Child 6–11 years (specialist use only):** Apply twice daily, when preparations used together max. total calcipotriol 2.5 mg in any one week (e.g. scalp solution 20 mL with ointment 30 g); maximum 30 mL per week

▸ **Child 12–17 years (specialist use only):** Apply twice daily, when preparations used together maximum total calcipotriol 3.75 mg in any one week (e.g. scalp solution 30 mL with ointment 45 g); maximum 45 mL per week

● **UNLICENSED USE** Calcipotriol ointment and scalp solution not licensed for use in children.

● **CONTRA-INDICATIONS** Calcium metabolism disorders

● **CAUTIONS** Avoid excessive exposure to sunlight and sunlamps · avoid use on face · erythrodermic exfoliative psoriasis (enhanced risk of hypercalcaemia) · generalised pustular psoriasis (enhanced risk of hypercalcaemia)

● **SIDE-EFFECTS**

▸ **Common or very common** Burning · dermatitis · erythema · itching · local skin reactions · paraesthesia

▸ **Rare** Facial dermatitis · perioral dermatitis

▸ **Frequency not known** Aggravation of psoriasis · dry skin · photosensitivity

● **PREGNANCY** Manufacturers advise avoid unless essential.

● **BREAST FEEDING** No information available.

● **HEPATIC IMPAIRMENT** Manufacturers advise avoid in severe impairment.

● **RENAL IMPAIRMENT** Manufacturers advise avoid in severe impairment.

● **PATIENT AND CARER ADVICE**

Advice on application Patient information leaflet for *Dovonex®* ointment advises liberal application. However, patients should be advised of maximum recommended weekly dose.

Hands should be washed thoroughly after application to avoid inadvertent transfer to other body areas.

● **MEDICINAL FORMS**

There can be variation in the licensing of different medicines containing the same drug. Forms available from special-order manufacturers include: ointment

Liquid

▸ Calcitriol (Non-proprietary)

Calcipotriol (as Calcipotriol hydrate) 50 microgram per 1 ml Calcipotriol 50micrograms/ml scalp solution | 60 ml [PoM] £56.94 DT price = £56.94 | 120 ml [PoM] £113.88 DT price = £113.88

Ointment

EXCIPIENTS: May contain Disodium edetate, propylene glycol

▸ Calcipotriol (Non-proprietary)

Calcipotriol 50 microgram per 1 gram Calcipotriol 50micrograms/g ointment | 30 gram [PoM] £7.37 DT price = £5.78 | 60 gram [PoM] £11.56–£13.86 | 120 gram [PoM] £23.12–£27.72

▸ Dovonex (LEO Pharma)

Calcipotriol 50 microgram per 1 gram Dovonex 50micrograms/g ointment | 30 gram [PoM] £5.78 DT price = £5.78 | 60 gram [PoM] £11.56

Combinations available: *Calcipotriol with betamethasone,* p. 689

Calcitriol

(1,25-Dihydroxycholecalciferol)

● **INDICATIONS AND DOSE**

Mild to moderate plaque psoriasis

▸ TO THE SKIN

▸ **Child 12–17 years:** Apply twice daily, not more than 35% of body surface to be treated daily; maximum 30 g per day

● **CONTRA-INDICATIONS** Do not apply under occlusion · patients with calcium metabolism disorders

● **CAUTIONS** Erythrodermic exfoliative psoriasis (enhanced risk of hypercalcaemia) · generalised pustular psoriasis (enhanced risk of hypercalcaemia)

● **SIDE-EFFECTS**

▸ **Common or very common** Burning · dermatitis · erythema · itching · local skin reactions · paraesthesia

▸ **Frequency not known** Aggravation of psoriasis

● **PREGNANCY** Manufacturer advises use in restricted amounts only if clearly necessary.

Monitor urine- and serum-calcium concentration in pregnancy.

● **BREAST FEEDING** Manufacturer advises avoid.

● **HEPATIC IMPAIRMENT** Manufacturer advises avoid—no information available.

● **RENAL IMPAIRMENT** Manufacturer advises avoid—no information available.

● **HANDLING AND STORAGE** Hands should be washed thoroughly after application to avoid inadvertent transfer to other body areas.

- **MEDICINAL FORMS**
  There can be variation in the licensing of different medicines containing the same drug.
  Ointment
  ‣ Silkis (Galderma (UK) Ltd)
    Calcitriol 3 microgram per 1 gram Silkis ointment | 100 gram [PoM] £18.06 DT price = £18.06

Tacalcitol

- **INDICATIONS AND DOSE**
  Plaque psoriasis
  ‣ TO THE SKIN
  ‣ Child 12–17 years: Apply once daily, preferably at bedtime, maximum 10 g ointment or 10 mL lotion daily, when lotion and ointment used together, maximum total tacalcitol 280 micrograms in any one week (e.g. lotion 30 mL with ointment 40 g)

- **CONTRA-INDICATIONS** Calcium metabolism disorders

- **CAUTIONS** Avoid eyes · erythrodermic exfoliative psoriasis (enhanced risk of hypercalcaemia) · generalised pustular psoriasis (enhanced risk of hypercalcaemia) · if used in conjunction with UV treatment
  CAUTIONS, FURTHER INFORMATION
  ‣ UV treatment If tacalcitol is used in conjunction with UV treatment, UV radiation should be given in the morning and tacalcitol applied at bedtime.

- **SIDE-EFFECTS**
  ‣ **Common or very common** Burning · dermatitis · erythema · itching · local skin reactions · paraesthesia
  ‣ **Frequency not known** Aggravation of psoriasis

- **PREGNANCY** Manufacturer advises avoid unless no safer alternative—no information available.

- **BREAST FEEDING** Manufacturer advises avoid application to breast area; no information available on presence in milk.

- **RENAL IMPAIRMENT** Monitor serum calcium concentration.

- **MONITORING REQUIREMENTS** Monitor serum calcium if risk of hypercalcaemia.

- **PATIENT AND CARER ADVICE** Hands should be washed thoroughly after application to avoid inadvertent transfer to other body areas.

- **MEDICINAL FORMS**
  There can be variation in the licensing of different medicines containing the same drug.
  Liquid
  EXCIPIENTS: May contain Disodium edetate, propylene glycol
  ‣ Curatoderm (Almirall Ltd)
    Tacalcitol (as Tacalcitol monohydrate) 4 microgram per 1 gram Curatoderm 4micrograms/g lotion | 30 ml [PoM] £12.73
  Ointment
  ‣ Curatoderm (Almirall Ltd)
    Tacalcitol (as Tacalcitol monohydrate) 4 microgram per 1 gram Curatoderm 4micrograms/g ointment | 30 gram [PoM] £13.40 DT price = £13.40 | 60 gram [PoM] £23.14 DT price = £23.14 | 100 gram [PoM] £30.86 DT price = £30.86

4   Perspiration

Antiperspirants

Overview

Aluminium chloride hexahydrate p. 706 is a potent antiperspirant used in the treatment of axillary, palmar, and plantar hyperhidrosis. Aluminium salts are also incorporated in preparations used for minor fungal skin infections associated with hyperhidrosis.

In more severe cases specialists use tap water or glycopyrronium bromide below (as a 0.05% solution) in the iontophoretic treatment of hyperhidrosis of palms and soles.

Botox® contains botulinum toxin type A complex p. 243 and is available for use intradermally for severe hyperhidrosis of the axillae unresponsive to topical antiperspirant or other antihidrotic treatment; intradermal treatment is unlikely to be tolerated by most children and should be administered under hospital specialist supervision.

4.1   Hyperhidrosis

ANTIMUSCARINICS

Glycopyrronium bromide
(Glycopyrrolate)

- **INDICATIONS AND DOSE**
  Iontophoretic treatment of hyperhidrosis
  ‣ TO THE SKIN
  ‣ Child: Only 1 site to be treated at a time, maximum 2 sites treated in any 24 hours, treatment not to be repeated within 7 days (consult product literature)

- **UNLICENSED USE** Licensed for use in children (age range not specified by manufacturer).

- **CONTRA-INDICATIONS** Infections affecting the treatment site
  CONTRA-INDICATIONS, FURTHER INFORMATION
  Contra-indications applicable to systemic use should be considered; however, glycopyrronium is poorly absorbed and systemic effects unlikely with topical use.

- **CAUTIONS**
  CAUTIONS, FURTHER INFORMATION
  Cautions applicable to systemic use should be considered; however, glycopyrronium is poorly absorbed and systemic effects unlikely with topical use.

- **SIDE-EFFECTS** Tingling at administration site
  SIDE-EFFECTS, FURTHER INFORMATION
  The possibility of systemic side-effects should be considered; however; glycopyrrhonium is poorly absorbed and systemic effects unlikely with topical use.

- **MEDICINAL FORMS**
  There can be variation in the licensing of different medicines containing the same drug.
  Powder for solution for iontophoresis
  ‣ Glycopyrronium bromide (Non-proprietary)
    Glycopyrronium bromide 1 mg per 1 mg Glycopyrronium bromide powder for solution for iontophoresis | 3 gram [PoM] £313.92

13

Skin

DERMATOLOGICAL DRUGS > ASTRINGENTS

Aluminium chloride hexahydrate

- **INDICATIONS AND DOSE**

Hyperhidrosis affecting axillae, hands or feet
- ▸ TO THE SKIN
- ▸ Child: Apply once daily, apply liquid formulation at night to dry skin, wash off the following morning, reduce frequency as condition improves—do not bathe immediately before use

Hyperhidrosis | Bromidrosis | Intertrigo | Prevention of tinea pedis and related conditions
- ▸ TO THE SKIN
- ▸ Child: Apply powder to dry skin

- **UNLICENSED USE** Licensed for use in children (age range not specified by manufacturer).
- **CAUTIONS** Avoid contact with eyes · avoid contact with mucous membranes · avoid use on broken or irritated skin · do not shave axillae or use depilatories within 12 hours of application
- **SIDE-EFFECTS** Skin irritation
- **PATIENT AND CARER ADVICE** Avoid contact with clothing.
- **EXCEPTIONS TO LEGAL CATEGORY** A 30 mL pack of aluminium chloride hexahydrate 20% is on sale to the public.

- **MEDICINAL FORMS**
There can be variation in the licensing of different medicines containing the same drug.
Liquid
CAUTIONARY AND ADVISORY LABELS 15
- ▸ Aluminium chloride hexahydrate (Non-proprietary)
Aluminium chloride 200 mg per 1 ml Aluminium chloride 20% solution | 60 ml Ⓟ no price available DT price = £2.51
- ▸ Anhydrol (Dermal Laboratories Ltd)
Aluminium chloride 200 mg per 1 ml Anhydrol Forte 20% solution | 60 ml Ⓟ £2.51 DT price = £2.51
- ▸ Driclor (GlaxoSmithKline Consumer Healthcare)
Aluminium chloride 200 mg per 1 ml Driclor 20% solution | 75 ml Ⓟ £3.01 DT price = £3.01

5   Photodamage

Photodamage

Actinic keratoses occur very rarely in healthy children; actinic cheilitis may occur on the lips of adolescents following excessive sun exposure.

Diclofenac gel (Solaraze®) and topical preparations of fluorouracil are licensed for the treatment of actinic keratoses but they are not licensed for use in children.

In children with photosensitivity disorders, such as erythropoietic protoporphyria, specialists may use betacarotene below, mepacrine, chloroquine or hydroxychloroquine to reduce skin reactions.

VITAMINS AND TRACE ELEMENTS > VITAMIN A

Betacarotene

- **DRUG ACTION** Betacarotene is a precursor to vitamin A.

- **INDICATIONS AND DOSE**

Management of photosensitivity reactions in erythropoietic protoporphyria (specialist use only)
- ▸ BY MOUTH
- ▸ Child 1–4 years: 60–90 mg daily, to be given as a single dose or in divided doses
- ▸ Child 5–8 years: 90–120 mg daily, to be given as a single dose or in divided doses
- ▸ Child 9–11 years: 120–150 mg daily, to be given as a single dose or in divided doses
- ▸ Child 12–15 years: 150–180 mg daily, to be given as a single dose or in divided doses
- ▸ Child 16–17 years: 180–300 mg daily, to be given as a single dose or in divided doses

- **UNLICENSED USE** Not licensed.
- **CAUTIONS** Monitor vitamin A intake
CAUTIONS, FURTHER INFORMATION
Protection not total—avoid strong sunlight and use sunscreen preparations; generally 2–6 weeks of treatment (resulting in yellow coloration of palms and soles) necessary before increasing exposure to sunlight; dose should be adjusted according to level of exposure to sunlight.
- **INTERACTIONS** → Appendix 1 (vitamins).
- **SIDE-EFFECTS**
- ▸ **Rare** Arthralgia · bruising
- ▸ **Frequency not known** Loose stools · yellow discoloration of skin
- **PREGNANCY** Partially converted to vitamin A, but does not give rise to abnormally high serum concentration; manufacturer advises use only if potential benefit outweighs risk.
- **BREAST FEEDING** Use with caution—present in milk.
- **HEPATIC IMPAIRMENT** Avoid.
- **RENAL IMPAIRMENT** Use with caution.

- **MEDICINAL FORMS**
There can be variation in the licensing of different medicines containing the same drug. Forms available from special-order manufacturers include: tablet, capsule
Capsule
CAUTIONARY AND ADVISORY LABELS 21
- ▸ Betacarotene (Non-proprietary)
Betacarotene 15 mg Betacarotene 15mg capsules | 90 capsule £5.81 | 100 capsule £13.40
Betacarotene 25 mg Carotaben 25mg capsules | 100 capsule Ⓟ no price available
Betacarotene 30 mg Lumitene 30mg capsules | 100 capsule PoM no price available
- ▸ BetaCare (BioCare Ltd)
Betacarotene 15 mg BetaCare 15mg capsules | 30 capsule £4.55
- ▸ Bio-Carotene (Pharma Nord (UK) Ltd)
Betacarotene 9 mg Bio-Carotene 9mg capsules | 150 capsule no price available
- ▸ Super Betavit (Health+Plus Ltd)
Betacarotene 15 mg Super Betavit 15mg capsules | 30 capsule £3.59

6   Pruritus

Topical local antipruritics

Overview

Pruritus may be caused by systemic disease (such as obstructive jaundice, endocrine disease, chronic renal disease, iron deficiency, and certain malignant diseases), skin disease (such as eczema, psoriasis, urticaria, and scabies), drug hypersensitivity, or as a side-effect of opioid analgesics. Where possible, the underlying cause should be treated. Local antipruritics have a role in the treatment of pruritus in palliative care. Pruritus caused by cholestasis generally requires a bile acid sequestrant.

An **emollient** may be of value where the pruritus is associated with dry skin. Preparations containing calamine or crotamiton below are sometimes used but are of uncertain value.

A topical preparation containing doxepin 5% below is licensed for the relief of pruritus in eczema in children over 12 years; it can cause drowsiness and there may be a risk of sensitisation.

Topical antihistamines and local anaesthetics are only marginally effective and occasionally cause sensitisation. For *insect stings* and *insect bites*, a short course of a topical corticosteroid is appropriate. Short-term treatment with a **sedating antihistamine** may help in insect stings and in intractable where sedation is desirable. Calamine preparations are of little value for the treatment of insect stings or bites.

In *pruritus ani*, the underlying cause such as faecal soiling, eczema, psoriasis, or helminth infection should be treated.

> **Drugs used for Pruritus not listed below** Alimemazine tartrate, p. 167 · Cetirizine hydrochloride, p. 164 · Chlorphenamine maleate, p. 168 · Hydroxyzine hydrochloride, p. 169 · Levocetirizine hydrochloride, p. 166

ANTIPRURITICS

Calamine with zinc oxide

● **INDICATIONS AND DOSE**

Pruritus
▸ TO THE SKIN
▸ Child: (consult product literature)

● **CONTRA-INDICATIONS** Avoid application of preparations containing zinc oxide prior to x-ray (zinc oxide may affect outcome of x-ray)

● **LESS SUITABLE FOR PRESCRIBING** Less suitable for prescribing.

● **MEDICINAL FORMS**
There can be variation in the licensing of different medicines containing the same drug.

Liquid
▸ Calamine with zinc oxide (Non-proprietary)
  Phenol liquefied 5 mg per 1 ml, Sodium citrate 5 mg per 1 ml, Bentonite 30 mg per 1 ml, Glycerol 50 mg per 1 ml, Zinc oxide 50 mg per 1 ml, Calamine 150 mg per 1 ml Numark Calamine lotion | 200 ml GSL £0.81–£0.96 DT price = £0.96
▸ Cala Soothe (Ennogen Healthcare Ltd)
  Phenol liquefied 5 mg per 1 ml, Sodium citrate 5 mg per 1 ml, Bentonite 30 mg per 1 ml, Glycerol 50 mg per 1 ml, Zinc oxide 50 mg per 1 ml, Calamine 150 mg per 1 ml Cala Soothe lotion | 200 ml £19.50 DT price = £0.96

Cream
▸ Calamine with zinc oxide (Non-proprietary)
  Phenoxyethanol 5 mg per 1 gram, Zinc oxide 30 mg per 1 gram, Calamine 40 mg per 1 gram, Cetomacrogol emulsifying wax 50 mg per 1 gram, Self-emulsifying glyceryl monostearate 50 mg per 1 gram, Liquid paraffin 200 mg per 1 gram Aqueous calamine cream | 100 gram GSL £1.29 DT price = £1.29
▸ Cala Soothe (Ennogen Healthcare Ltd)
  Phenoxyethanol 5 mg per 1 gram, Zinc oxide 30 mg per 1 gram, Calamine 40 mg per 1 gram, Cetomacrogol emulsifying wax 50 mg per 1 gram, Self-emulsifying glyceryl monostearate 50 mg per 1 gram, Liquid paraffin 200 mg per 1 gram Cala Soothe cream | 100 ml £18.80

Crotamiton

● **INDICATIONS AND DOSE**

Pruritus (including pruritus after scabies)
▸ TO THE SKIN
▸ Child 1 month–2 years (on doctor's advice only): Apply once daily
▸ Child 3–17 years: Apply 2–3 times a day

● **CONTRA-INDICATIONS** Acute exudative dermatoses

● **CAUTIONS** Avoid use in buccal mucosa · avoid use near eyes · avoid use on broken skin · avoid use on very inflamed skin · use on doctor's advice for children under 3 years

● **PREGNANCY** Manufacturer advises avoid, especially during the first trimester—no information available.

● **BREAST FEEDING** No information available; avoid application to nipple area.

● **MEDICINAL FORMS**
There can be variation in the licensing of different medicines containing the same drug.
Cream
EXCIPIENTS: May contain Beeswax, cetostearyl alcohol (including cetyl and stearyl alcohol), fragrances, hydroxybenzoates (parabens)
▸ Crotamiton (Non-proprietary)
  Crotamiton 100 mg per 1 gram Boots Derma Care Itch Relief cream | 30 gram GSL no price available DT price = £2.50
▸ Brands may include Eurax

Doxepin

● **INDICATIONS AND DOSE**

Pruritus in eczema
▸ TO THE SKIN
▸ Child 12–17 years: Apply up to 3 g 3–4 times a day, apply thinly; coverage should be less than 10% of body surface area; maximum 12 g per day

● **CAUTIONS** Avoid application to large areas · cardiac arrhythmias · mania · severe heart disease · susceptibility to angle-closure glaucoma · urinary retention

● **INTERACTIONS** → Appendix 1 (antidepressants, tricyclic).

● **SIDE-EFFECTS**
▸ **Common or very common** Antimuscarinic effects · dizziness · drowsiness · fever · gastro-intestinal disturbances · headache · irritation · local burning · rash · stinging · tingling

● **PREGNANCY** Manufacturer advises use only if potential benefit outweighs risk.

● **BREAST FEEDING** Manufacturer advises use only if potential benefit outweighs risk.

● **HEPATIC IMPAIRMENT** Manufacturer advises caution in severe liver disease.

13

Skin

- PATIENT AND CARER ADVICE
  Driving and skilled tasks
  Drowsiness may affect performance of skilled tasks (e.g. driving).
  Effects of alcohol enhanced. A patient information leaflet should be provided.

- MEDICINAL FORMS
  There can be variation in the licensing of different medicines containing the same drug.
  Cream
  CAUTIONARY AND ADVISORY LABELS 2, 10
  EXCIPIENTS: May contain Benzyl alcohol
  ▸ Xepin (Cambridge Healthcare Supplies Ltd)
  Doxepin hydrochloride 50 mg per 1 gram Xepin 5% cream |
  30 gram PoM £11.70

7 Rosacea and acne

Rosacea and Acne

Acne vulgaris

Acne vulgaris commonly affects children around puberty and occasionally affects infants. Treatment of acne should be commenced early to prevent scarring; lesions may worsen before improving. The choice of treatment depends on age, severity, and whether the acne is predominantly inflammatory or comedonal.

Mild to moderate acne is generally treated with topical preparations, such as benzoyl peroxide p. 710, azelaic acid p. 711, and retinoids.

For *moderate to severe inflammatory acne* or where topical preparations are not tolerated or are ineffective or where application to the site is difficult, systemic treatment with oral antibacterials may be effective. Co-cyprindiol (cyproterone acetate with ethinylestradiol) p. 709 has anti-androgenic properties and may be useful in young women with acne refractory to other treatments.

Severe acne, acne unresponsive to prolonged courses of oral antibacterials, acne with scarring, or acne associated with psychological problems calls for early referral to a consultant dermatologist who may prescribe oral isotretinoin p. 712.

Neonatal and infantile acne

Inflammatory papules, pustules, and occasionally comedones may develop at birth or within the first month; most neonates with acne do not require treatment. Acne developing at 3–6 months of age may be more severe and persistent; lesions are usually confined to the face. Topical preparations containing benzoyl peroxide (at the lowest strength possible to avoid irritation), adapalene p. 711, or tretinoin p. 514 may be used if treatment for infantile acne is necessary. In infants with inflammatory acne, oral erythromycin p. 310 is used because topical preparations for acne are not well tolerated. In cases of erythromycin-resistant acne, oral isotretinoin can be given on the advice of a consultant dermatologist.

Topical preparations for acne

In mild to moderate acne, comedones and inflamed lesions respond well to benzoyl peroxide or topical retinoids. Alternatively, topical application of an antibacterial such as erythromycin or clindamycin p. 710 may be effective for inflammatory acne. However, topical antibacterials are probably no more effective than benzoyl peroxide and may promote the emergence of resistant organisms. If topical preparations prove inadequate, oral preparations may be needed. The choice of product and formulation (gel, solution, lotion, or cream) is largely determined by skin type, patient preference, and previous usage of acne products.

Benzoyl peroxide and azelaic acid

Benzoyl peroxide is effective in mild to moderate acne. Both comedones and inflamed lesions respond well to benzoyl peroxide. The lower concentrations seem to be as effective as higher concentrations in reducing inflammation. It is usual to start with a lower strength and to increase the concentration of benzoyl peroxide gradually. The usefulness of benzoyl peroxide washes is limited by the short time the products are in contact with the skin. Adverse effects include local skin irritation, particularly when therapy is initiated, but the scaling and redness often subside with a reduction in benzoyl peroxide concentration, frequency, and area of application. If the acne does not respond after 2 months then use of a topical antibacterial should be considered.

Azelaic acid has antimicrobial and anticomedonal properties. It may be used as an alternative to benzoyl peroxide or to a topical retinoid for treating mild to moderate comedonal acne, particularly of the face; azelaic acid is less likely to cause local irritation than benzoyl peroxide.

Topical antibacterials for acne

In the treatment of mild to moderate inflammatory acne, topical antibacterials may be no more effective than topical benzoyl peroxide or tretinoin. Topical antibacterials are probably best reserved for children who wish to avoid oral antibacterials or who cannot tolerate them.

Topical preparations of erythromycin and clindamycin may be used to treat *inflamed lesions* in mild to moderate acne when topical benzoyl peroxide or tretinoin is ineffective or poorly tolerated. Topical benzoyl peroxide, azelaic acid, or retinoids used in combination with an antibacterial (topical or systemic) may be more effective than an antibacterial used alone. Topical antibacterials can produce mild irritation of the skin, and on rare occasions cause sensitisation; gastro-intestinal disturbances have been reported with topical clindamycin.

Antibacterial resistance of *Propionibacterium acnes* is increasing; there is cross-resistance between erythromycin and clindamycin. To avoid development of resistance:

- when possible use non-antibiotic antimicrobials (such as benzoyl peroxide or azelaic acid);
- avoid concomitant treatment with different oral and topical antibacterials;
- if a particular antibacterial is effective, use it for repeat courses if needed (short intervening courses of benzoyl peroxide or azelaic acid may eliminate any resistant propionibacteria);
- do not continue treatment for longer than necessary (but treatment with a topical preparation should be continued for at least 6 months).

Topical retinoids and related preparations for acne

Topical tretinoin, its isomer isotretinoin, and adapalene (a retinoid-like drug), are useful for treating comedones and inflammatory lesions in mild to moderate acne. Patients should be warned that some redness and skin peeling can occur initially but settles with time. If undue irritation occurs, the frequency of application should be reduced or treatment suspended until the reaction subsides; if irritation persists, discontinue treatment. Several months of treatment may be needed to achieve an optimal response and the treatment should be continued until no new lesions develop.

Tretinoin can be used under specialist supervision to treat infantile acne; adapalene can also be used.

Other topical preparations for acne

A topical preparation of nicotinamide p. 714 is available for inflammatory acne.

Oral preparations for acne

Oral antibacterials for acne

Oral antibacterials may be used in *moderate to severe inflammatory acne* when topical treatment is not adequately effective or is inappropriate. Concomitant anticomedonal treatment with topical benzoyl peroxide or azelaic acid may also be required.

Tetracyclines should not be given to children under 12 years. In children over 12 years, either oxytetracycline p. 334 or tetracycline p. 334 is usually given for acne. If there is no improvement after the first 3 months another oral antibacterial should be used. Maximum improvement usually occurs after 4 to 6 months but in more severe cases treatment may need to be continued for 2 years or longer. Doxycycline p. 332 and lymecycline p. 333 are alternatives to tetracycline in children over 12 years.

Although minocycline p. 333 is as effective as other tetracyclines for acne, it is associated with a greater risk of lupus erythematosus-like syndrome. Minocycline sometimes causes irreversible pigmentation.

Erythromycin is an alternative for the management of moderate to severe acne with inflamed lesions, but propionibacteria strains resistant to erythromycin are becoming widespread and this may explain poor response. In cases of erythromycin-resistant *P. acnes* in infants, oral isotretinoin may be used on the advice of a consultant dermatologist.

Concomitant use of different topical and systemic antibacterials is undesirable owing to the increased likelihood of the development of bacterial resistance.

Hormone treatment for acne

Co-cyprindiol (cyproterone acetate with ethinylestradiol) below contains an anti-androgen. It is no more effective than an oral broad-spectrum antibacterial but is useful in females of childbearing age who also wish to receive oral contraception.

Improvement of acne with co-cyprindiol probably occurs because of decreased sebum secretion which is under androgen control. Some females with moderately severe hirsutism may also benefit because hair growth is also androgen-dependent.

Oral retinoid for acne

The retinoid isotretinoin p. 712 reduces sebum secretion. It is used for the systemic treatment of nodulo-cystic and conglobate acne, severe acne, acne with scarring, or for acne which has not responded to an adequate course of a systemic antibacterial. Isotretinoin is used for the treatment of severe infantile acne resistant to erythromycin p. 310.

Isotretinoin is a toxic drug that should be prescribed **only** by, or under the supervision of, a consultant dermatologist. It is given for at least 16 weeks; repeat courses are not normally required. The drug is **teratogenic** and must **not** be given to females of child-bearing age unless they practise effective contraception (oral progestogen-only contraceptives not considered effective) and then only after detailed assessment and explanation by the physician. They must also be registered with a pregnancy prevention programme.

Although a causal link between isotretinoin use and psychiatric changes (including suicidal ideation) has not been established, the possibility should be considered before initiating treatment; if psychiatric changes occur during treatment, isotretinoin should be stopped, the prescriber informed, and specialist psychiatric advice should be sought.

Rosacea

The adult form of rosacea rarely occurs in children. Persistent or repeated use of potent topical corticosteroids may cause periorificial rosacea (steroid acne). The pustules and papules of rosacea may be treated for at least 6 weeks with a topical metronidazole preparation p. 676, or a systemic antibacterial such as erythromycin, or for a child over 12 years, oxytetracycline p. 334. Tetracyclines are **contra-indicated** in children under 12 years of age.

7.1 Acne

ANTI-ANDROGENS

Co-cyprindiol

● **INDICATIONS AND DOSE**

Moderate to severe acne in females of child-bearing age refractory to topical therapy or oral antibacterials | Moderately severe hirsutism

▶ BY MOUTH
▶ Females of childbearing potential: 1 tablet daily for 21 days, to be started on day 1 of menstrual cycle; subsequent courses repeated after a 7-day interval (during which withdrawal bleeding occurs), time to symptom remission, at least 3 months; review need for treatment regularly

● **CONTRA-INDICATIONS** Acute porphyria · gallstones · heart disease associated with pulmonary hypertension or risk of embolus · history during pregnancy of cholestatic jaundice · history during pregnancy of chorea · history during pregnancy of pemphigoid gestationis · history during pregnancy of pruritus · history of breast cancer but can be used after 5 years if no evidence of disease and non-hormonal methods unacceptable · history of haemolytic uraemic syndrome · migraine with aura · personal history of venous or arterial thrombosis · sclerosing treatment for varicose veins · severe or multiple risk factors for arterial disease or for venous thromboembolism · systemic lupus erythematosus with (or unknown) antiphospholipid antibodies · transient cerebral ischaemic attacks without headaches · undiagnosed vaginal bleeding

● **CAUTIONS** Active trophoblastic disease (until return to normal of urine- and plasma-gonadotrophin concentration)—seek specialist advice · arterial disease · gene mutations associated with breast cancer (e.g. BRCA 1) · history of severe depression especially if induced by hormonal contraceptive · hyperprolactinaemia—seek specialist advice · inflammatory bowel disease including Crohn's disease · migraine · personal or family history of hypertriglyceridaemia (increased risk of pancreatitis) · risk factors for venous thromboembolism · sickle-cell disease · undiagnosed breast mass

CAUTIONS, FURTHER INFORMATION
▶ Venous thromboembolism There is an increased risk of venous thromboembolism in women taking co-cyprindiol, particularly during the first year of use. The incidence of venous thromboembolism is 1.5–2 times higher in women using co-cyprindiol than in women using combined oral contraceptives containing levonorgestrel, but the risk may be similar to that associated with use of combined oral contraceptives containing third generation progestogens (desogestrel and gestodene) or drospirenone. Women requiring co-cyprindiol may have an inherently increased risk of cardiovascular disease.

● **INTERACTIONS** → Appendix 1 (oestrogens).

● **SIDE-EFFECTS**
▶ **Rare** Rarely gallstones · systemic lupus erythematosus
▶ **Very rare** Photosensitivity
▶ **Frequency not known** Abdominal cramps · absence of withdrawal bleeding · amenorrhoea after discontinuation · breast enlargement · breast secretion · breast tenderness · cervical erosion · changes in libido · changes in lipid metabolism · changes in vaginal discharge · chloasma · chorea · contact lenses may irritate · depression · fluid retention · headache · hepatic tumours · hypertension · irritability · leg cramps · liver impairment · nausea · nervousness · reduced menstrual loss · skin reactions · thrombosis (more common when factor V Leiden present or

13

Skin

in blood groups A, B, and AB · visual disturbances · vomiting · 'spotting' in early cycles

- **PREGNANCY** Avoid—risk of feminisation of male fetus with cyproterone.
- **BREAST FEEDING** Manufacturer advises avoid; possibility of anti-androgen effects in neonate with cyproterone.
- **HEPATIC IMPAIRMENT** Avoid in active liver disease including disorders of hepatic excretion (e.g. Dubin-Johnson or Rotor syndromes), infective hepatitis (until liver function returns to normal), and liver tumours.
- **PRESCRIBING AND DISPENSING INFORMATION** A mixture of cyproterone acetate and ethinylestradiol in the mass proportions 2000 parts to 35 parts, respectively.
- **MEDICINAL FORMS**
  There can be variation in the licensing of different medicines containing the same drug.
  Tablet
  ▸ **Co-cyprindiol (Non-proprietary)**
  Ethinylestradiol 35 microgram, Cyproterone acetate 2 mg Co-cyprindiol 2000microgram/35microgram tablets | 63 tablet [PoM] £5.70 DT price = £5.56
  ▸ **Clairette** (Stragen UK Ltd) ▼
  Ethinylestradiol 35 microgram, Cyproterone acetate 2 mg Clairette 2000/35 tablets | 63 tablet [PoM] £5.90 DT price = £5.56
  ▸ **Dianette** (Bayer Plc, Mylan Ltd) ▼
  Ethinylestradiol 35 microgram, Cyproterone acetate 2 mg Dianette tablets | 63 tablet [PoM] £7.71–£11.10 DT price = £5.56
  ▸ **Teragezza** (Morningside Healthcare Ltd)
  Ethinylestradiol 35 microgram, Cyproterone acetate 2 mg Teragezza 2000microgram/35microgram tablets | 63 tablet [PoM] £11.10 DT price = £5.56

ANTIBACTERIALS ⟩ LINCOSAMIDES

Clindamycin

- **INDICATIONS AND DOSE**
  DALACIN T® LOTION
  Acne vulgaris
  ▸ TO THE SKIN
  ▸ Child: Apply twice daily, to be applied thinly
  DALACIN T® SOLUTION
  Acne vulgaris
  ▸ TO THE SKIN
  ▸ Child: Apply twice daily, to be applied thinly
  ZINDACLIN® GEL
  Acne vulgaris
  ▸ TO THE SKIN
  ▸ Child 12–17 years: Apply once daily, to be applied thinly

- **MEDICINAL FORMS**
  There can be variation in the licensing of different medicines containing the same drug.
  Liquid
  EXCIPIENTS: May contain Cetostearyl alcohol (including cetyl and stearyl alcohol), hydroxybenzoates (parabens), propylene glycol
  ▸ **Dalacin T** (Pfizer Ltd)
  Clindamycin (as Clindamycin phosphate) 10 mg per 1 ml Dalacin T 1% topical lotion | 30 ml [PoM] £5.08 DT price = £5.08 | 60 ml [PoM] £10.16
  Dalacin T 1% topical solution | 30 ml [PoM] £4.34 DT price = £4.34 | 50 ml [PoM] £7.23
  Gel
  EXCIPIENTS: May contain Propylene glycol
  ▸ **Zindaclin** (Crawford Healthcare Ltd)
  Clindamycin (as Clindamycin phosphate) 10 mg per 1 gram Zindaclin 1% gel | 30 gram [PoM] £8.66 DT price = £8.66

  Combinations available: *Benzoyl peroxide with clindamycin*, p. 711 · *Tretinoin with clindamycin,* p. 713

ANTIBACTERIALS ⟩ MACROLIDES

Erythromycin with zinc acetate

- **INDICATIONS AND DOSE**
  Acne vulgaris
  ▸ TO THE SKIN
  ▸ Child: Apply twice daily

- **CAUTIONS** Some manufacturers advise preparations containing alcohol are not suitable for use with benzoyl peroxide

- **MEDICINAL FORMS**
  There can be variation in the licensing of different medicines containing the same drug.
  Liquid
  ▸ **Zineryt** (Astellas Pharma Ltd)
  Zinc acetate 12 mg per 1 ml, Erythromycin 40 mg per 1 ml Zineryt lotion | 30 ml [PoM] £7.71 DT price = £7.71 | 90 ml [PoM] £16.68 DT price = £16.68

ANTISEPTICS AND DISINFECTANTS ⟩ PEROXIDES

Benzoyl peroxide

- **INDICATIONS AND DOSE**
  Acne vulgaris
  ▸ TO THE SKIN
  ▸ Child 12–17 years: Apply 1–2 times a day, preferably apply after washing with soap and water, start treatment with lower-strength preparations
  Infantile acne
  ▸ TO THE SKIN
  ▸ Child 1 month–1 year: Apply 1–2 times a day, start treatment with lower-strength preparations

- **UNLICENSED USE** Not licensed for use in treatment of infantile acne.

- **CAUTIONS** Avoid contact with broken skin · avoid contact with eyes · avoid contact with mouth · avoid contact with mucous membranes · avoid excessive exposure to sunlight

- **SIDE-EFFECTS** Skin irritation
  SIDE-EFFECTS, FURTHER INFORMATION
  ▸ Skin irritation Reduce frequency or suspend use until irritation subsides and re-introduce at reduced frequency.

- **PATIENT AND CARER ADVICE** May bleach fabrics and hair.

- **MEDICINAL FORMS**
  There can be variation in the licensing of different medicines containing the same drug.
  Cream
  EXCIPIENTS: May contain Cetostearyl alcohol (including cetyl and stearyl alcohol), fragrances, isopropyl palmitate, propylene glycol
  ▸ **Brevoxyl** (GlaxoSmithKline Consumer Healthcare)
  Benzoyl peroxide 40 mg per 1 gram Brevoxyl 4% cream | 50 gram [P] £4.13 DT price = £4.13
  ▸ **PanOxyl** (GlaxoSmithKline Consumer Healthcare)
  Benzoyl peroxide 50 mg per 1 gram PanOxyl 5 cream | 40 gram [P] £1.89 DT price = £1.89
  Gel
  EXCIPIENTS: May contain Fragrances, propylene glycol
  ▸ **Acnecide** (Galderma (UK) Ltd)
  Benzoyl peroxide 50 mg per 1 gram Acnecide 5% gel | 30 gram [P] £5.44 DT price = £5.44 | 60 gram [P] £10.68
  Acnecide Wash 5% gel | 50 gram [P] £5.44
  ▸ **PanOxyl Aquagel** (GlaxoSmithKline Consumer Healthcare)
  Benzoyl peroxide 25 mg per 1 gram PanOxyl 2.5 Aquagel | 40 gram [P] £1.76 DT price = £1.76
  Benzoyl peroxide 50 mg per 1 gram PanOxyl 5 Aquagel | 40 gram [P] £1.92 DT price = £1.92
  Benzoyl peroxide 100 mg per 1 gram PanOxyl 10 Aquagel | 40 gram [P] £2.13 DT price = £2.13

- Panoxyl Acnegel (GlaxoSmithKline Consumer Healthcare)
  Benzoyl peroxide 100 mg per 1 gram PanOxyl 10 Acnegel |
  40 gram P £1.99 DT price = £2.13

Combinations available: *Adapalene with benzoyl peroxide,*
below

Benzoyl peroxide with clindamycin

The properties listed below are those particular to the
combination only. For the properties of the components
please consider, benzoyl peroxide p. 710, clindamycin p. 710.

- **INDICATIONS AND DOSE**
Acne vulgaris
- TO THE SKIN
- Child 12–17 years: Apply once daily, dose to be applied in
  the evening

- **MEDICINAL FORMS**
There can be variation in the licensing of different medicines
containing the same drug.
Gel
EXCIPIENTS: May contain Disodium edetate
- Duac (Stiefel Laboratories (UK) Ltd)
  Clindamycin (as Clindamycin phosphate) 10 mg per 1 gram,
  Benzoyl peroxide 30 mg per 1 gram Duac Once Daily gel (3% and
  1%) | 30 gram PoM £13.14 DT price = £13.14 | 60 gram PoM
  £26.28
  Clindamycin (as Clindamycin phosphate) 10 mg per 1 gram,
  Benzoyl peroxide 50 mg per 1 gram Duac Once Daily gel (5% and
  1%) | 30 gram PoM £13.14 DT price = £13.14 | 60 gram PoM
  £26.28 DT price = £26.28

DERMATOLOGICAL DRUGS > ANTICOMEDONALS

Azelaic acid

- **INDICATIONS AND DOSE**
FINACEA®
Facial acne vulgaris
- TO THE SKIN
- Child 12–17 years: Apply twice daily, discontinue if no
  improvement after 1 month
SKINOREN®
Acne vulgaris
- TO THE SKIN
- Child 12–17 years: Apply twice daily
Acne vulgaris in patients with sensitive skin
- TO THE SKIN
- Child 12–17 years: Apply once daily for 1 week, then
  apply twice daily

- **CAUTIONS** Avoid contact with eyes · avoid contact with
  mouth · avoid contact with mucous membranes
- **SIDE-EFFECTS**
- **Common or very common** Local irritation (reduce frequency
  or discontinue temporarily)
- **Uncommon** Skin discoloration
- **Frequency not known** Worsening of asthma

- **MEDICINAL FORMS**
There can be variation in the licensing of different medicines
containing the same drug.
Cream
EXCIPIENTS: May contain Propylene glycol
- Skinoren (Bayer Plc)
  Azelaic acid 200 mg per 1 gram Skinoren 20% cream |
  30 gram PoM £3.74 DT price = £3.74
Gel
EXCIPIENTS: May contain Disodium edetate, polysorbates, propylene
glycol
- Finacea (Bayer Plc)
  Azelaic acid 150 mg per 1 gram Finacea 15% gel | 30 gram PoM
  £7.48 DT price = £7.48

RETINOID AND RELATED DRUGS

Adapalene

- **INDICATIONS AND DOSE**
Mild to moderate acne vulgaris
- TO THE SKIN
- Child 12–17 years: Apply once daily, apply thinly in the
  evening
Infantile acne
- TO THE SKIN
- Child 1 month–1 year: Apply once daily, apply thinly in
  the evening

- **UNLICENSED USE** Not licensed for use in infantile acne.
- **CAUTIONS** Avoid accumulation in angles of the nose ·
  avoid contact with eyes, nostrils, mouth and mucous
  membranes, eczematous, broken or sunburned skin · avoid
  exposure to UV light (including sunlight, solariums) · avoid
  in severe acne involving large areas · caution in sensitive
  areas such as the neck
- **CONCEPTION AND CONTRACEPTION** Females of childbearing age must use effective contraception (oral
  progestogen-only contraceptives not considered
  effective).
- **PREGNANCY** Avoid.
- **BREAST FEEDING** Amount of drug in milk probably too
  small to be harmful; ensure infant does not come in
  contact with treated areas.
- **PATIENT AND CARER ADVICE** If sun exposure is
  unavoidable, an appropriate sunscreen or protective
  clothing should be used.

- **MEDICINAL FORMS**
There can be variation in the licensing of different medicines
containing the same drug.
Cream
CAUTIONARY AND ADVISORY LABELS 11
EXCIPIENTS: May contain Disodium edetate, hydroxybenzoates
(parabens)
- Adapalene (Non-proprietary)
  Adapalene 1 mg per 1 gram Adapalene 0.1% cream |
  45 gram PoM £19.73 DT price = £16.43
- Differin (Galderma (UK) Ltd)
  Adapalene 1 mg per 1 gram Differin 0.1% cream | 45 gram PoM
  £16.43 DT price = £16.43
Gel
CAUTIONARY AND ADVISORY LABELS 11
EXCIPIENTS: May contain Disodium edetate, hydroxybenzoates
(parabens), propylene glycol
- Adapalene (Non-proprietary)
  Adapalene 1 mg per 1 gram Adapalene 0.1% gel | 45 gram PoM
  £19.73 DT price = £16.43
- Differin (Galderma (UK) Ltd)
  Adapalene 1 mg per 1 gram Differin 0.1% gel | 45 gram PoM
  £16.43 DT price = £16.43

Adapalene with benzoyl peroxide

The properties listed below are those particular to the
combination only. For the properties of the components
please consider, adapalene above, benzoyl peroxide p. 710.

- **INDICATIONS AND DOSE**
Acne vulgaris
- TO THE SKIN
- Child 9–17 years: Apply once daily, to be applied thinly
  in the evening

- **CONCEPTION AND CONTRACEPTION** Females of childbearing age must use effective contraception (oral
  progestogen-only contraceptives not considered
  effective).

13

Skin

13

Skin

- PATIENT AND CARER ADVICE Gel may bleach clothing and hair.
- NATIONAL FUNDING/ACCESS DECISIONS

Scottish Medicines Consortium (SMC) Decisions
The *Scottish Medicines Consortium* has advised (March 2014) that *Epiduo*® should be restricted for use in mild to moderate facial acne when monotherapy with benzoyl peroxide or adapalene is inappropriate.

- MEDICINAL FORMS
There can be variation in the licensing of different medicines containing the same drug.

Gel
CAUTIONARY AND ADVISORY LABELS 11
EXCIPIENTS: May contain Disodium edetate, polysorbates, propylene glycol
- ▸ Adapalene with benzoyl peroxide (Non-proprietary)
Adapalene 1 mg per 1 gram, Benzoyl peroxide 25 mg per 1 gram Adapalene 0.1% / Benzoyl peroxide 2.5% gel | 45 gram [PoM] no price available DT price = £19.05
- ▸ Epiduo (Galderma (UK) Ltd)
Adapalene 1 mg per 1 gram, Benzoyl peroxide 25 mg per 1 gram Epiduo 0.1%/2.5% gel | 45 gram [PoM] £19.05 DT price = £19.05

Isotretinoin

- INDICATIONS AND DOSE
Topical treatment of mild to moderate acne
- ▸ TO THE SKIN
- ▸ Child: Apply 1–2 times a day, to be applied thinly

Severe acne (under expert supervision) | Acne which is associated with psychological problems (under expert supervision) | Acne which has not responded to an adequate course of a systemic antibacterial (under expert supervision) | Acne with scarring (under expert supervision) | Systemic treatment of nodulo-cystic and conglobate acne (under expert supervision)
- ▸ BY MOUTH
- ▸ Child 12-17 years: Initially 500 micrograms/kg daily in 1–2 divided doses, increased if necessary to 1 mg/kg daily for 16–24 weeks, repeat treatment course after a period of at least 8 weeks if relapse after first course; maximum 150 mg/kg per course

Severe infantile acne (under expert supervision)
- ▸ BY MOUTH
- ▸ Child 1 month-1 year: Initially 200 micrograms/kg daily in 1–2 divided doses, increased if necessary to 1 mg/kg daily for 16–24 weeks; maximum 150 mg/kg per course

- UNLICENSED USE
- ▸ With oral use Not licensed for use in infantile acne.
- CONTRA-INDICATIONS
- ▸ With oral use Hyperlipidaemia · hypervitaminosis A
- ▸ With topical use Perioral dermatitis · rosacea
- CAUTIONS
- ▸ With oral use Avoid blood donation during treatment and for at least 1 month after treatment · diabetes · dry eye syndrome (associated with risk of keratitis) · history of depression · monitor for depression
- ▸ With topical use Allow peeling (resulting from other irritant treatments) to subside before using a topical retinoid · alternating a preparation that causes peeling with a topical retinoid may give rise to contact dermatitis (reduce frequency of retinoid application) · avoid accumulation in angles of the nose · avoid contact with eyes, nostrils, mouth and mucous membranes, eczematous, broken or sunburned skin · avoid exposure to UV light (including sunlight, solariums) · avoid in severe acne involving large areas · avoid use of topical retinoids with abrasive cleaners, comedogenic or astringent cosmetics · caution in sensitive

areas such as the neck · personal or familial history of non-melanoma skin cancer
- INTERACTIONS
- ▸ With oral use Appendix 1 (retinoids). Avoid keratolytics.
- SIDE-EFFECTS
- ▸ Common or very common
- ▸ With oral use Anaemia · arthralgia · dryness of eyes (with blepharitis and conjunctivitis) · dryness of lips (sometimes cheilitis) · dryness of nasal mucosa (with epistaxis) · dryness of pharyngeal mucosa (with hoarseness) · dryness of skin (with dermatitis, scaling, thinning, erythema, pruritus) · epidermal fragility (trauma may cause blistering) · haematuria · headache · myalgia · neutropenia · proteinuria · raised blood-glucose concentration · raised plasma-triglyceride concentration · raised serum-cholesterol concentration (with reduced high-density lipoprotein concentration) · raised serum-transaminase concentration · thrombocytopenia · thrombocytosis
- ▸ Rare
- ▸ With oral use Aggressive behaviour · alopecia · anxiety · depression · mood changes · skin reactions
- ▸ Very rare
- ▸ With oral use Acne fulminans · allergic vasculitis · arthritis · benign intracranial hypertension · blurred vision · bone changes following long-term administration · calcification of tendons and ligaments following long-term administration · cataracts · colour blindness · convulsions · corneal opacities · decreased night vision · decreased tolerance to contact lenses · diabetes mellitus · dizziness · drowsiness · early epiphyseal closure following long-term administration · exacerbation of acne · gastrointestinal haemorrhage · glomerulonephritis · Gram-positive infections of skin and mucous membranes · granulomatous lesions · haemorrhagic diarrhoea · hepatitis · hirsutism · hyperuricaemia · impaired hearing · increased sweating · inflammatory bowel disease · keratitis · lymphadenopathy · malaise · nail dystrophy · nausea · papilloedema · paronychia · photophobia · photosensitivity · psychosis · raised serum-creatine kinase concentration · reduced bone density following long-term administration · skeletal hyperostosis following long-term administration · skin hyperpigmentation · suicidal ideation · tendinitis · visual disturbances
- ▸ Frequency not known
- ▸ With oral use Stevens-Johnson syndrome · toxic epidermal necrolysis
- ▸ With topical use Blistering of skin · burning · crusting of skin · dry or peeling skin · erythema · eye irritation · increased sensitivity to UVB light or sunlight · oedema · pruritus · stinging

SIDE-EFFECTS, FURTHER INFORMATION
- ▸ Management of side-effects Risk of pancreatitis if triglycerides above 9 mmol/litre—discontinue if uncontrolled hypertriglyceridaemia or pancreatitis.
Psychiatric side-effects require expert referral.
Discontinue treatment if skin peeling severe or haemorrhagic diarrhoea develops.
Visual disturbances require expert referral and possible withdrawal.

- CONCEPTION AND CONTRACEPTION
Pregnancy prevention
- ▸ With oral use Effective contraception must be used. In women of child-bearing potential, exclude pregnancy up to 3 days before treatment (start treatment on day 2 or 3 of menstrual cycle), every month during treatment (unless there are compelling reasons to indicate that there is no risk of pregnancy), and 5 weeks after stopping treatment—perform pregnancy test in the first 3 days of the menstrual cycle. Women must practise effective contraception for at least 1 month before starting treatment, during treatment, and for at least 1 month after stopping treatment. Women should be advised to use at least 1 method of

contraception, but ideally they should use 2 methods of contraception. Oral progestogen-only contraceptives are not considered effective. Barrier methods should not be used alone, but can be used in conjunction with other contraceptive methods. Each prescription for isotretinoin should be limited to a supply of up to 30 days' treatment and dispensed within 7 days of the date stated on the prescription; repeat prescriptions or faxed prescriptions are not acceptable. Women should be advised to discontinue treatment and to seek prompt medical attention if they become pregnant during treatment or within 1 month of stopping treatment.

‣ With topical use Females of child-bearing age must use effective contraception (oral progestogen-only contraceptives not considered effective).

● PREGNANCY Contra-indicated in pregnancy (teratogenic).

● BREAST FEEDING Avoid.

● HEPATIC IMPAIRMENT
‣ With oral use Avoid—further impairment may occur.

● RENAL IMPAIRMENT
‣ With oral use In severe impairment, reduce initial dose and increase gradually, if necessary, up to 1 mg/kg daily as tolerated.

● MONITORING REQUIREMENTS
‣ With oral use Measure hepatic function and serum lipids before treatment, 1 month after starting and then every 3 months (reduce dose or discontinue if transaminase or serum lipids persistently raised).

● PRESCRIBING AND DISPENSING INFORMATION Isotretinoin is an isomer of tretinoin.

● PATIENT AND CARER ADVICE
‣ With oral use Warn patient to avoid wax epilation (risk of epidermal stripping), dermabrasion, and laser skin treatments (risk of scarring) during treatment and for at least 6 months after stopping; patient should avoid exposure to UV light (including sunlight) and use sunscreen and emollient (including lip balm) preparations from the start of treatment.
‣ With oral use Patients and carers should be told how to recognise signs and symptoms of psychiatric disorders such as depression, anxiety, and rarely suicidal thoughts.
‣ With topical use Patients should be warned that some redness and skin peeling can occur initially but settles with time. If undue irritation occurs, the frequency of application should be reduced or treatment suspended until the reaction subsides; if irritation persists, discontinue treatment. Several months of treatment may be needed to achieve an optimal response and the treatment should be continued until no new lesions develop. If sun exposure is unavoidable, an appropriate sunscreen or protective clothing should be used.

● MEDICINAL FORMS
There can be variation in the licensing of different medicines containing the same drug.
Capsule
CAUTIONARY AND ADVISORY LABELS 10, 11, 21
‣ **Isotretinoin** (Non-proprietary)
Isotretinoin 5 mg Isotretinoin 5mg capsules | 30 capsule [PoM] £10.15 | 56 capsule [PoM] £14.78
Isotretinoin 10 mg Isotretinoin 10mg capsules | 30 capsule [PoM] £15.00 DT price = £14.54
Isotretinoin 20 mg Isotretinoin 20mg capsules | 30 capsule [PoM] £20.00 DT price = £17.08 | 56 capsule [PoM] £37.85
Isotretinoin 40 mg Isotretinoin 40mg capsules | 30 capsule [PoM] £38.98 DT price = £38.98
‣ **Roaccutane** (Roche Products Ltd)
Isotretinoin 10 mg Roaccutane 10mg capsules | 30 capsule [PoM] £14.54 DT price = £14.54
Isotretinoin 20 mg Roaccutane 20mg capsules | 30 capsule [PoM] £20.02 DT price = £17.08

Gel
CAUTIONARY AND ADVISORY LABELS 11
EXCIPIENTS: May contain Butylated hydroxytoluene
‣ **Isotrex** (Stiefel Laboratories (UK) Ltd)
Isotretinoin 500 microgram per 1 gram Isotrex 0.05% gel | 30 gram [PoM] £5.94 DT price = £5.94

Isotretinoin with erythromycin

The properties listed below are those particular to the combination only. For the properties of the components please consider, isotretinoin p. 712, erythromycin p. 310.

● **INDICATIONS AND DOSE**
Topical treatment of mild to moderate acne
‣ TO THE SKIN
  ‣ Child: (consult product literature)

● MEDICINAL FORMS
There can be variation in the licensing of different medicines containing the same drug.
Gel
CAUTIONARY AND ADVISORY LABELS 11
EXCIPIENTS: May contain Butylated hydroxytoluene
‣ **Isotrexin** (Stiefel Laboratories (UK) Ltd)
Isotretinoin 500 microgram per 1 gram, Erythromycin 20 mg per 1 gram Isotrexin gel | 30 gram [PoM] £7.47 DT price = £7.47

Tretinoin with clindamycin

The properties listed below are those particular to the combination only. For the properties of the components please consider, tretinoin p. 514, clindamycin p. 710.

● **INDICATIONS AND DOSE**
Facial acne
‣ TO THE SKIN
  ‣ Child 12–17 years: Apply daily, (to be applied thinly at bedtime)

● CONTRA-INDICATIONS Perioral dermatitis · personal or familial history of non-melanoma skin cancer · rosacea

● CAUTIONS Allow peeling (resulting from other irritant treatments) to subside before using a topical retinoid · alternating a preparation that causes peeling with a topical retinoid may give rise to contact dermatitis (reduce frequency of retinoid application) · avoid accumulation in angles of the nose · avoid contact with eyes, nostrils, mouth and mucous membranes, eczematous, broken or sunburned skin · avoid exposure to UV light (including sunlight, solariums) · avoid in severe acne involving large areas · avoid use of topical retinoids with abrasive cleaners, comedogenic or astringent cosmetics · caution in sensitive areas such as the neck

● SIDE-EFFECTS Blistering of skin · burning · crusting of skin · dry or peeling skin (discontinue if severe) · erythema · eye irritation · increased sensitivity to UVB light or sunlight · oedema · pruritus · stinging · temporary changes of skin pigmentation

● CONCEPTION AND CONTRACEPTION Females of child-bearing age must use effective contraception (oral progestogen-only contraceptives not considered effective).

● PREGNANCY Contra-indicated in pregnancy.

● BREAST FEEDING Amount of drug in milk after topical application probably too small to be harmful; ensure infant does not come in contact with treated areas.

● PATIENT AND CARER ADVICE If sun exposure is unavoidable, an appropriate sunscreen or protective clothing should be used. Patients and carers should be warned that some redness and skin peeling can

13

Skin

13

Skin

occur initially but settles with time. If undue irritation occurs, the frequency of application should be reduced or treatment suspended until the reaction subsides; if irritation persists, discontinue treatment. Several months of treatment may be needed to achieve an optimal response and the treatment should be continued until no new lesions develop.

- MEDICINAL FORMS
  There can be variation in the licensing of different medicines containing the same drug.
  Gel
  CAUTIONARY AND ADVISORY LABELS 11
  EXCIPIENTS: May contain Butylated hydroxytoluene, hydroxybenzoates (parabens), polysorbates
  ▸ Treclin (Meda Pharmaceuticals Ltd)
  Tretinoin 250 microgram per 1 gram, Clindamycin (as Clindamycin phosphate) 10 mg per 1 gram Treclin 1%/0.025% gel | 30 gram PoM £11.94

Tretinoin with erythromycin

The properties listed below are those particular to the combination only. For the properties of the components please consider, tretinoin p. 514, erythromycin p. 310.

- INDICATIONS AND DOSE
  Acne
  ▸ TO THE SKIN
  ▸ Child: Apply 1–2 times a day, apply thinly

- CONTRA-INDICATIONS Perioral dermatitis · personal or familial history of non-melanoma skin cancer · rosacea
- CAUTIONS Allow peeling (resulting from other irritant treatments) to subside before using a topical retinoid · alternating a preparation that causes peeling with a topical retinoid may give rise to contact dermatitis (reduce frequency of retinoid application) · avoid accumulation in angles of the nose · avoid contact with eyes, nostrils, mouth and mucous membranes, eczematous, broken or sunburned skin · avoid exposure to UV light (including sunlight, solariums) · avoid in severe acne involving large areas · avoid use of topical retinoids with abrasive cleaners, comedogenic or astringent cosmetics · caution in sensitive areas such as the neck
- SIDE-EFFECTS Blistering of skin · burning · crusting of skin · dry or peeling skin (discontinue if severe) · erythema · eye irritation · increased sensitivity to UVB light or sunlight · oedema · pruritus · stinging · temporary changes of skin pigmentation
- CONCEPTION AND CONTRACEPTION Females of child-bearing age must use effective contraception (oral progestogen-only contraceptives not considered effective).
- PREGNANCY Contra-indicated in pregnancy.
- BREAST FEEDING Amount of drug in milk after topical application probably too small to be harmful; ensure infant does not come in contact with treated areas.
- PATIENT AND CARER ADVICE Patients and carers should be warned that some redness and skin peeling can occur initially but settles with time. If undue irritation occurs, the frequency of application should be reduced or treatment suspended until the reaction subsides; if irritation persists, discontinue treatment. Several months of treatment may be needed to achieve an optimal response and the treatment should be continued until no new lesions develop. If sun exposure is unavoidable, an appropriate sunscreen or protective clothing should be used.

- MEDICINAL FORMS
  There can be variation in the licensing of different medicines containing the same drug.
  Liquid
  CAUTIONARY AND ADVISORY LABELS 11
  ▸ Aknemycin Plus (Almirall Ltd)
  Tretinoin 250 microgram per 1 gram, Erythromycin 40 mg per 1 gram Aknemycin Plus solution | 25 ml PoM £7.05 DT price = £7.05

VITAMINS AND TRACE ELEMENTS > VITAMIN B GROUP

Nicotinamide

- INDICATIONS AND DOSE
  Inflammatory acne vulgaris
  ▸ TO THE SKIN
  ▸ Child: Apply twice daily, reduced to once daily or on alternate days, dose reduced if irritation occurs

- UNLICENSED USE Licensed for use in children (age range not specified by manufacturer).
- CAUTIONS Avoid contact with eyes · avoid contact with mucous membranes (including nose and mouth) · reduce frequency of application if excessive dryness, irritation or peeling
- SIDE-EFFECTS Burning · dry skin · erythema · irritation · pruritus
- MEDICINAL FORMS
  There can be variation in the licensing of different medicines containing the same drug.
  Gel
  ▸ Freederm (Dendron Ltd)
  Nicotinamide 40 mg per 1 gram Freederm 4% gel | 25 gram P £5.56
  ▸ Nicam (Dermal Laboratories Ltd)
  Nicotinamide 40 mg per 1 gram Nicam 4% gel | 60 gram P £7.10

8   Scalp and hair conditions

Scalp and hair conditions

Overview

The detergent action of shampoo removes grease (sebum) from hair. Prepubertal children produce very little grease and require shampoo less frequently than adults. Shampoos can be used as vehicles for medicinal products, but their usefulness is limited by the short time the product is in contact with the scalp and by their irritant nature.

Oils and ointments are very useful for scaly, dry scalp conditions; if a greasy appearance is cosmetically unacceptable, the preparation may be applied at night and washed out in the morning. Alcohol-based lotions are rarely used in children; alcohol causes painful stinging on broken skin and the fumes may exacerbate asthma.

Itchy, inflammatory, eczematous scalp conditions may be relieved by a simple emollient oil such as **olive oil** or **coconut oil** (arachis oil (ground nut oil, peanut oil) is best avoided in children under 5 years). In more severe cases a topical **corticosteroid** may be required. Preparations containing **coal tar** are used for the common scaly scalp conditions of childhood including seborrhoeic dermatitis, dandruff (a mild form of seborrhoeic dermatitis), and psoriasis; salicylic acid is used as a keratolytic in some scalp preparations.

Shampoos containing antimicrobials such as selenium p. 715 or ketoconazole p. 678 are used for seborrhoeic dermatitis and dandruff in which yeast infection has been implicated, and for tinea capitis (ringworm of the scalp).

Bacterial infection affecting the scalp (usually secondary to eczema, head lice, or ringworm) may be treated with shampoos containing antimicrobials such as **pyrithione zinc**, cetrimide, or povidone-iodine p. 633

In neonates and infants, *cradle cap* (which is also a form of seborrhoeic eczema) can be treated by massaging **coconut oil** or **olive oil** into the scalp; a bland emollient such as **emulsifying ointment** can be rubbed onto the affected area once or twice daily before bathing and a mild shampoo used.

ANTISEPTICS AND DISINFECTANTS >
UNDECENOATES

Cetrimide with undecenoic acid

- ● INDICATIONS AND DOSE

Scalp psoriasis | Seborrhoeic dermatitis | Dandruff
- ▸ TO THE SKIN
- ▸ **Child:** Apply 3 times a week for 1 week, then apply twice weekly

- ● MEDICINAL FORMS
There can be variation in the licensing of different medicines containing the same drug.
Shampoo
- ▸ **Ceanel** (Alliance Pharmaceuticals Ltd)
Undecenoic acid 10 mg per 1 ml, Phenylethyl alcohol 75 mg per 1 ml, Cetrimide 100 mg per 1 ml Ceanel Concentrate shampoo | 150 ml P £3.40 | 500 ml P £9.80

ANTISEPTICS AND DISINFECTANTS > OTHER

Benzalkonium chloride

- ● INDICATIONS AND DOSE

Seborrhoeic scalp conditions associated with dandruff and scaling
- ▸ TO THE SKIN
- ▸ **Child:** Apply as required

- ● MEDICINAL FORMS
There can be variation in the licensing of different medicines containing the same drug.
Shampoo
- ▸ **Dermax** (Dermal Laboratories Ltd)
Benzalkonium chloride 5 mg per 1 ml Dermax Therapeutic 0.5% shampoo | 250 ml P £5.69

VITAMINS AND TRACE ELEMENTS

Selenium

- ● INDICATIONS AND DOSE

Seborrhoeic dermatitis | Dandruff
- ▸ TO THE SKIN USING SHAMPOO
- ▸ **Child 5–17 years:** Apply twice weekly for 2 weeks, then apply once weekly for 2 weeks, then apply as required

Pityriasis versicolor
- ▸ TO THE SKIN USING SHAMPOO
- ▸ **Child 5–17 years:** Apply once daily for 7 days, apply to the affected area and leave on for 10 minutes before rinsing off. The course may be repeated if necessary. Diluting with a small amount of water prior to application can reduce irritation

- ● UNLICENSED USE The use of selenium sulfide shampoo as a lotion for the treatment of pityriasis (tinea) versicolor is an unlicensed indication.

- ● PATIENT AND CARER ADVICE Avoid using 48 hours before or after applying hair colouring, straightening or waving preparations.

- ● MEDICINAL FORMS
There can be variation in the licensing of different medicines containing the same drug.
Shampoo
EXCIPIENTS: May contain Fragrances
- ▸ **Selsun** (Chattem (U.K.) Ltd)
Selenium sulfide 25 mg per 1 ml Selsun 2.5% shampoo | 50 ml P £1.61 DT price = £1.61 | 100 ml P £2.15 DT price = £2.15 | 150 ml P £3.06 DT price = £3.06

9   Skin cleansers, antiseptics and desloughing agents

Skin cleansers, antiseptics and desloughing agents

Skin cleansers and antiseptics

Soap or detergent is used with water to cleanse intact skin but they can irritate infantile skin; emollient preparations such as aqueous cream or emulsifying ointment can be used in place of soap or detergent for cleansing dry or irritated skin.

An antiseptic is used for skin that is infected or that is susceptible to recurrent infection. Detergent preparations containing chlorhexidine p. 717 or povidone-iodine p. 716, which should be thoroughly rinsed off, are used. Emollients may also contain antiseptics.

Antiseptics such as chlorhexidine or povidone-iodine are used on intact skin before surgical procedures; their antiseptic effect is enhanced by an alcoholic solvent. Antiseptic solutions containing cetrimide can be used if a detergent effect is also required.

Preparations containing alcohol, and regular use of povidone-iodine, should be avoided on neonatal skin.

Hydrogen peroxide p. 718, an oxidising agent, is available as a cream and can be used for superficial bacterial skin infections.

For irrigating ulcers or wounds, lukewarm sterile sodium chloride 0.9% solution p. 718 is used but tap water is often appropriate.

Potassium permanganate p. 716 solution 1 in 10 000, a mild antiseptic with astringent properties, can be used as a soak for exudative eczematous areas; treatment should be stopped when the skin becomes dry.

Desloughing agents

Alginate, hydrogel, and hydrocolloid dressings are effective in wound debridement. Sterile larvae (maggots) (available from BioMonde) are also used for managing sloughing wounds and are prescribable on the NHS.

Desloughing solutions and creams are of little clinical value. Substances applied to an open area are easily absorbed and perilesional skin is easily sensitised.

13

Skin

ANTISEPTICS AND DISINFECTANTS

Potassium permanganate

● **INDICATIONS AND DOSE**

Cleansing and deodorising suppurating eczematous reactions and wounds

▸ TO THE SKIN

▸ Child: For wet dressings or baths, use approximately 0.01% (1 in 10 000) solution

● **CAUTIONS** Irritant to mucous membranes

● **DIRECTIONS FOR ADMINISTRATION** Potassium permanganate 0.1% solution to be diluted 1 in 10 to provide a 0.01% (1 in 10 000) solution. With potassium permanganate tablets for solution, 1 tablet dissolved in 4 litres of water provides a 0.01% (1 in 10 000) solution.

● **PATIENT AND CARER ADVICE** Can stain clothing, skin and nails (especially with prolonged use).

● **MEDICINAL FORMS**
There can be variation in the licensing of different medicines containing the same drug. Forms available from special-order manufacturers include: liquid

Tablet for cutaneous solution

▸ Potassium permanganate (Non-proprietary)
Potassium permanganate 400mg Potassium permanganate 400mg tablets for cutaneous solution | 30 tablet no price available DT price = £17.50
EN-Potab 400mg tablets for cutaneous solution | 30 tablet no price available DT price = £17.50

▸ Permitabs (Alliance Pharmaceuticals Ltd)
Potassium permanganate 400 mg Permitabs 400mg tablets for cutaneous solution | 30 tablet £17.50 DT price = £17.50

ANTISEPTICS AND DISINFECTANTS › ALCOHOL DISINFECTANTS

Alcohol

(Industrial methylated spirit)

● **INDICATIONS AND DOSE**

Skin preparation before injection

▸ TO THE SKIN

▸ Child: Apply as required

● **CONTRA-INDICATIONS** Neonates

● **CAUTIONS** Avoid broken skin · flammable · patients have suffered severe burns when diathermy has been preceded by application of alcoholic skin disinfectants

● **INTERACTIONS** For the interactions following the *ingestion* of alcohol, see Appendix 1 (alcohol).

● **SIDE-EFFECTS**

Overdose
Features of acute alcohol intoxication include ataxia, dysarthria, nystagmus, and drowsiness, which may progress to coma, with hypotension and acidosis.
For details on the management of poisoning, see Alcohol, under Emergency treatment of poisoning p. 786.

● **PRESCRIBING AND DISPENSING INFORMATION** Industrial methylated spirits defined by the BP as a mixture of 19 volumes of ethyl alcohol of an appropriate strength with 1 volume of approved wood naphtha.

● **MEDICINAL FORMS**
There can be variation in the licensing of different medicines containing the same drug.

Liquid

▸ Alcohol (Non-proprietary)
Wood naphtha 50 ml per 1 litre, Ethanol 950 ml per 1 litre Industrial methylated spirit 95% | 600 ml £5.04 | 1000 ml £4.42–£6.02
Industrial methylated spirit 70% | 600 ml £6.00

ANTISEPTICS AND DISINFECTANTS › IODINE PRODUCTS

Povidone-iodine

● **INDICATIONS AND DOSE**

Skin disinfection

▸ TO THE SKIN

▸ Child: (consult product literature)

BETADINE® DRY POWDER SPRAY

Skin disinfection, particularly minor wounds and infections

▸ TO THE SKIN

▸ Child 2–17 years: Not for use in serous cavities (consult product literature)

SAVLON® DRY

Skin disinfection of minor wounds

▸ TO THE SKIN

▸ Child: (consult product literature)

VIDENE® SOLUTION

Skin disinfection

▸ TO THE SKIN

▸ Child: Apply undiluted in pre-operative skin disinfection and general antisepsis

VIDENE® SURGICAL SCRUB®

Skin disinfection

▸ TO THE SKIN

▸ Child: Use as a pre-operative scrub for hand and skin disinfection

VIDENE® TINCTURE

Skin disinfection

▸ TO THE SKIN

▸ Child: Apply undiluted in pre-operative skin disinfection

● **CONTRA-INDICATIONS** Concomitant use of lithium · corrected gestational age under 32 weeks · infants body-weight under 1.5 kg · regular use in neonates

VIDENE® TINCTURE Neonates

● **CAUTIONS** Broken skin · large open wounds

CAUTIONS, FURTHER INFORMATION
The application of povidone–iodine to large wounds or severe burns may produce systemic adverse effects such as metabolic acidosis, hypernatraemia and impairment of renal function.

VIDENE® TINCTURE Procedures involving hot wire cautery and diathermy

● **SIDE-EFFECTS**

▸ **Rare** Sensitivity

● **PREGNANCY** Sufficient iodine may be absorbed to affect the fetal thyroid in the second and third trimester.

● **BREAST FEEDING** Avoid regular or excessive use.

● **RENAL IMPAIRMENT** Avoid regular application to inflamed or broken skin or mucosa.

● **EFFECT ON LABORATORY TESTS** May interfere with thyroid function tests.

● **MEDICINAL FORMS**
There can be variation in the licensing of different medicines containing the same drug. Forms available from special-order manufacturers include: liquid

Liquid

CAUTIONARY AND ADVISORY LABELS 15 (Only for use with alcoholic solutions)

▸ Videne (Ecolab Healthcare Division)
Povidone-iodine 75 mg per 1 ml Videne 7.5% surgical scrub solution | 500 ml Ⓟ £7.30
Povidone-iodine 100 mg per 1 ml Videne 10% antiseptic solution | 500 ml GSL £7.30

Spray

▶ Betadine (J M Loveridge Ltd)

Povidone-Iodine 25 mg per 1 gram Betadine 2.5% dry powder spray | 100 ml GSL £9.95 DT price = £9.95

▶ Savlon Dry (Novartis Consumer Health UK Ltd)

Povidone-Iodine 11.4 mg per 1 gram Savlon Dry 1.14% spray | 50 ml GSL £2.51 DT price = £2.51

Impregnated dressing

▶ Povidone-iodine (Non-proprietary)

Povidone-Iodine 100 mg per 1 gram Povitulle dressing 9.5cm × 9.5cm | 1 dressing £0.42 | 10 dressing no price available
Povitulle dressing 5cm × 5cm | 1 dressing £0.28 | 25 dressing no price available

▶ Inadine (Systagenix Wound Management Ltd)

Povidone-Iodine 100 mg per 1 gram Inadine dressing 5cm × 5cm | 1 dressing £0.33 | 25 dressing no price available
Inadine dressing 9.5cm × 9.5cm | 1 dressing £0.49 | 10 dressing no price available

ANTISEPTICS AND DISINFECTANTS ❭ OTHER

| Chlorhexidine

● INDICATIONS AND DOSE

CX ANTISEPTIC DUSTING POWDER

For skin disinfection

▶ TO THE SKIN

▶ Child: (consult product literature)

CEPTON® LOTION

For skin disinfection in acne

▶ TO THE SKIN

▶ Child: (consult product literature)

CEPTON® SKIN WASH

For use as skin wash in acne

▶ TO THE SKIN

▶ Child: (consult product literature)

HIBITANE ® PLUS 5% CONCENTRATE SOLUTION

General and pre-operative skin disinfection

▶ TO THE SKIN

▶ Child: (consult product literature)

HIBISCRUB®

Pre-operative hand and skin disinfection | General hand and skin disinfection

▶ TO THE SKIN

▶ Child: Use as alternative to soap (consult product literature)

HIBITANE OBSTETRIC®

For use in obstetrics and gynaecology as an antiseptic and lubricant

▶ TO THE SKIN

▶ Child: To be applied to skin around vulva and perineum and to hands of midwife or doctor

HIBI® LIQUID HAND RUB+

Hand and skin disinfection

▶ TO THE SKIN

▶ Child: To be used undiluted (consult product literature)

HYDREX® SOLUTION

For pre-operative skin disinfection

▶ TO THE SKIN

▶ Child: (consult product literature)

HYDREX® SURGICAL SCRUB

For pre-operative hand and skin disinfection | General hand disinfection

▶ TO THE SKIN

▶ Child: (consult product literature)

UNISEPT®

For cleansing and disinfecting wounds and burns and swabbing in obstetrics

▶ TO THE SKIN

▶ Child: (consult product literature)

IMPORTANT SAFETY INFORMATION

In preterm neonates, use sparingly, monitor for skin reactions, and do not allow solution to pool—risk of severe chemical burns.

● **CONTRA-INDICATIONS** Alcoholic solutions not suitable before diathermy · alcoholic solutions not suitable for use on neonatal skin · not for use in body cavities

● **CAUTIONS** Avoid contact with brain · avoid contact with eyes · avoid contact with meninges · avoid contact with middle ear

● **SIDE-EFFECTS** Chemical burns in preterm neonates · sensitivity

● **DIRECTIONS FOR ADMINISTRATION**

HIBITANE ® PLUS 5% CONCENTRATE SOLUTION
For pre-operative skin preparation, dilute 1 in 10 (0.5%) with alcohol 70%. For general skin disinfection, dilute 1 in 100 (0.05%) with water. Alcoholic solutions not suitable for use before diathermy or on neonatal skin.

● **MEDICINAL FORMS**
There can be variation in the licensing of different medicines containing the same drug.

Liquid

CAUTIONARY AND ADVISORY LABELS 15 (For ethanolic solutions (e.g. ChloraPrep® and Hydrex® only)
EXCIPIENTS: May contain Fragrances

▶ Cepton (Boston Healthcare Ltd)
Chlorhexidine gluconate 10 mg per 1 ml Cepton 1% medicated skin wash | 150 ml GSL £6.78

▶ HiBiTane Plus (Molnlycke Health Care Ltd)
Chlorhexidine gluconate 50 mg per 1 ml HiBiTane Plus 5% concentrate solution | 5000 ml GSL £14.50

▶ Hibi (Molnlycke Health Care Ltd)
Chlorhexidine gluconate 5 mg per 1 ml HiBi Liquid Hand Rub+ 0.5% solution | 500 ml GSL £5.25

▶ Hibiscrub (Molnlycke Health Care Ltd)
Chlorhexidine gluconate 40 mg per 1 ml Hibiscrub 4% solution | 250 ml GSL £4.25 | 500 ml GSL £5.25 | 5000 ml GSL £24.00

▶ Hydrex (Ecolab Healthcare Division)
Chlorhexidine gluconate 5 mg per 1 ml Hydrex pink chlorhexidine gluconate 0.5% solution | 600 ml GSL £4.50
Hydrex clear chlorhexidine gluconate 0.5% solution | 600 ml GSL £4.50
Chlorhexidine gluconate 40 mg per 1 ml Hydrex 4% Surgical Scrub | 250 ml GSL £4.09 | 500 ml GSL £4.34 | 5000 ml GSL £38.22

▶ Sterets Unisept (Molnlycke Health Care Ltd)
Chlorhexidine gluconate 500 microgram per 1 ml Sterets Unisept 0.05% solution 25ml sachets | 25 sachet P £5.54
Sterets Unisept 0.05% solution 100ml sachets | 10 sachet P £6.83

Cream

EXCIPIENTS: May contain Cetostearyl alcohol (including cetyl and stearyl alcohol)

▶ Hibitane (Derma UK Ltd)
Chlorhexidine gluconate 10 mg per 1 gram Hibitane Obstetric 1% cream | 250 ml GSL £12.00

Powder

▶ CX (Ecolab Healthcare Division)
Chlorhexidine acetate 10 mg per 1 gram CX 1% powder | 15 gram GSL £4.76

Chlorhexidine gluconate with isopropyl alcohol

The properties listed below are those particular to the combination only. For the properties of the components please consider, chlorhexidine p. 717.

● **INDICATIONS AND DOSE**

Skin disinfection before invasive procedures

▸ TO THE SKIN
▸ **Child 2 months-17 years:** (consult product literature)

● **MEDICINAL FORMS**
There can be variation in the licensing of different medicines containing the same drug.

Liquid

CAUTIONARY AND ADVISORY LABELS 15

▸ **ChloraPrep** (CareFusion U.K. Ltd)
Chlorhexidine gluconate 20 mg per 1 ml, Isopropyl alcohol 700 ml per 1 litre ChloraPrep with Tint solution 10.5ml applicators | 25 applicator GSL £76.65
ChloraPrep with Tint solution 26ml applicators | 25 applicator GSL £170.75
ChloraPrep solution 3ml applicators | 25 applicator GSL £21.25
ChloraPrep solution 1.5ml applicators | 20 applicator GSL £11.00
ChloraPrep with Tint solution 3ml applicators | 25 applicator GSL £22.31
ChloraPrep solution 0.67ml applicators | 200 applicator GSL £60.00
ChloraPrep solution 10.5ml applicators | 25 applicator GSL £73.00
ChloraPrep solution 26ml applicators | 25 applicator GSL £162.50

Chlorhexidine with cetrimide

The properties listed below are those particular to the combination only. For the properties of the components please consider, chlorhexidine p. 717.

● **INDICATIONS AND DOSE**

Skin disinfection such as wound cleansing and obstetrics

▸ TO THE SKIN
▸ **Child:** To be used undiluted

● **MEDICINAL FORMS**
There can be variation in the licensing of different medicines containing the same drug.

Liquid

▸ **Savlon disinfectant** (Novartis Consumer Health UK Ltd)
Chlorhexidine gluconate 3 mg per 1 ml, Cetrimide 30 mg per 1 ml Savlon disinfectant liquid | 500 ml £1.32
▸ **Sterets Tisept** (Molnlycke Health Care Ltd)
Chlorhexidine gluconate 150 microgram per 1 ml, Cetrimide 1.5 mg per 1 ml Sterets Tisept solution 25ml sachets | 25 sachet P £5.33
Sterets Tisept solution 100ml sachets | 10 sachet P £6.85

Cream

▸ **Chlorhexidine with cetrimide** (Non-proprietary)
Chlorhexidine gluconate 1 mg per 1 gram, Cetrimide 5 mg per 1 gram Savlon antiseptic cream | 15 gram GSL £0.86 | 30 gram GSL £1.14 | 60 gram GSL £1.82 | 100 gram GSL £2.65

Irrigation solution

▸ **Chlorhexidine with cetrimide** (Non-proprietary)
Chlorhexidine acetate 150 microgram per 1 ml, Cetrimide 1.5 mg per 1 ml Chlorhexidine acetate 0.015% / Cetrimide 0.15% irrigation solution 1litre bottles | 1 bottle P no price available

Diethyl phthalate with methyl salicylate

● **INDICATIONS AND DOSE**

Skin preparation before injection

▸ TO THE SKIN
▸ **Child:** Apply to the area to be disinfected

● **MEDICINAL FORMS**
There can be variation in the licensing of different medicines containing the same drug.

Liquid

CAUTIONARY AND ADVISORY LABELS 15

▸ **Diethyl phthalate with methyl salicylate** (Non-proprietary)
Methyl salicylate 5 ml per 1 litre, Diethyl phthalate 20 ml per 1 litre, Castor oil 25 ml per 1 litre, Industrial methylated spirit 950 ml per 1 litre Surgical spirit | 200 ml GSL £1.06–£1.11 DT price = £1.11 | 500 ml GSL £1.95 | 1000 ml GSL £3.29

Hydrogen peroxide

● **DRUG ACTION** Hydrogen peroxide is an oxidising agent.

● **INDICATIONS AND DOSE**

CRYSTACIDE®

Superficial bacterial skin infection

▸ TO THE SKIN
▸ **Child:** Apply 2–3 times a day for up to 3 weeks

● **UNLICENSED USE** Licensed for use in children (age range not specified by manufacturer).

● **CAUTIONS** Avoid on eyes · avoid on healthy skin · incompatible with products containing iodine or potassium permanganate

● **HANDLING AND STORAGE** Hydrogen peroxide bleaches fabric.

● **MEDICINAL FORMS**
There can be variation in the licensing of different medicines containing the same drug.

Cream

EXCIPIENTS: May contain Edetic acid (edta), propylene glycol

▸ **Crystacide** (Derma UK Ltd)
Hydrogen peroxide 10 mg per 1 gram Crystacide 1% cream | 25 gram P £8.07 DT price = £8.07 | 40 gram P £11.62

Proflavine

● **INDICATIONS AND DOSE**

Infected wounds | Infected burns

▸ TO THE SKIN
▸ **Child:** (consult product literature)

● **PATIENT AND CARER ADVICE** Stains clothing.

● **MEDICINAL FORMS**
There can be variation in the licensing of different medicines containing the same drug. Forms available from special-order manufacturers include: liquid

Irrigation solutions

● **IRRIGATION SOLUTIONS**

Flowfusor sodium chloride 0.9% irrigation solution 120ml bottles (Fresenius Kabi Ltd)
Sodium chloride 9 mg per 1 ml 1 bottle · NHS indicative price = £1.53 · Drug Tariff (Part IXa)

Irriclens sodium chloride 0.9% irrigation solution aerosol spray (ConvaTec Ltd)
Sodium chloride 9 mg per 1 ml 240 ml · NHS indicative price = £3.50 · Drug Tariff (Part IXa)

Normasol sodium chloride 0.9% irrigation solution 100ml sachets (Molnlycke Health Care Ltd)
Sodium chloride 9 mg per 1 ml 10 unit dose · NHS indicative price = £7.83 · Drug Tariff (Part IXa)

13

Skin

Normasol sodium chloride 0.9% irrigation solution 25ml sachets (Molnlycke Health Care Ltd)
   Sodium chloride 9 mg per 1 ml 25 unit dose · NHS indicative price = £6.42 · Drug Tariff (Part IXa)

Sodium chloride 0.9% irrigation solution 20ml Clinipod unit dose (Mayors Healthcare Ltd)
   Sodium chloride 9 mg per 1 ml 25 unit dose · NHS indicative price = £4.80 · Drug Tariff (Part IXa)

Sodium chloride 0.9% irrigation solution 20ml ISO-POD unit dose (St Georges Medical Ltd)
   Sodium chloride 9 mg per 1 ml 25 unit dose · NHS indicative price = £4.95 · Drug Tariff (Part IXa)

Sodium chloride 0.9% irrigation solution 20ml Irripod unit dose (C D Medical Ltd)
   Sodium chloride 9 mg per 1 ml 25 unit dose · NHS indicative price = £5.84 · Drug Tariff (Part IXa)

Sodium chloride 0.9% irrigation solution 20ml Sal-e Pods unit dose (Ennogen Healthcare Ltd)
   Sodium chloride 9 mg per 1 ml 25 unit dose · NHS indicative price = £4.80 · Drug Tariff (Part IXa)

Sodium chloride 0.9% irrigation solution 20ml Steripod unit dose (Molnlycke Health Care Ltd)
   Sodium chloride 9 mg per 1 ml 25 unit dose · NHS indicative price = £7.90 · Drug Tariff (Part IXa)

Sodium chloride 0.9% irrigation solution 20ml Sterowash unit dose (Steroplast Healthcare Ltd)
   Sodium chloride 9 mg per 1 ml 25 unit dose · NHS indicative price = £5.40 · Drug Tariff (Part IXa)

Sodium chloride 0.9% irrigation solution 20ml unit dose (Alissa Healthcare Research Ltd)
   Sodium chloride 9 mg per 1 ml 25 unit dose · NHS indicative price = £7.36 · Drug Tariff (Part IXa)

Sodium chloride 0.9% irrigation solution 20ml unit dose (Crest Medical Ltd)
   Sodium chloride 9 mg per 1 ml 25 unit dose · NHS indicative price = £4.99 · Drug Tariff (Part IXa)

Sodium chloride 0.9% irrigation solution 20ml unit dose (Mylan Ltd)
   Sodium chloride 9 mg per 1 ml 25 unit dose · NHS indicative price = £5.50 · Drug Tariff (Part IXa)

Stericlens sodium chloride 0.9% irrigation solution aerosol spray (C D Medical Ltd)
   Sodium chloride 9 mg per 1 ml 100 ml · NHS indicative price = £2.07 · Drug Tariff (Part IXa)240 ml · NHS indicative price = £3.15 · Drug Tariff (Part IXa)

9.1   Minor cuts and abrasions

Minor cuts and abrasions

Management

Many preparations traditionally used to manage minor burns, and abrasions have fallen out of favour. Preparations containing camphor and sulfonamides should be avoided. Preparations such as magnesium sulfate paste are now rarely used to treat carbuncles and boils as these are best treated with antibiotics.

Cetrimide is used to treat minor cuts and abrasions and proflavine p. 718 may be used to treat infected wounds or burns, but its use has now been largely superseded by other antiseptics or suitable antibacterials. The effervescent effect of hydrogen peroxide p. 718 is used to clean minor cuts and abrasions.

Flexible colloidon (see castor oil with collodion and colophony below) may be used to seal minor cuts and wounds that have partially healed; skin tissue adhesives are used similarly, and also for additional suture support.

DERMATOLOGICAL DRUGS ⟩ COLLODIONS

Castor oil with collodion and colophony

● **INDICATIONS AND DOSE**

Used to seal minor cuts and wounds that have partially healed

▸ TO THE SKIN
   ▸ Child: (consult product literature)

● ALLERGY AND CROSS-SENSITIVITY Contra-indicated if patient has an allergy to colophony in elastic adhesive plasters and tape.

● MEDICINAL FORMS There can be variation in the licensing of different medicines containing the same drug.
   Liquid
   ▸ **Castor oil with collodion and colophony (Non-proprietary)**
      Castor oil 25 mg per 1 ml, Collodion methylated 950 microlitre per 1 ml, Colophony 25 mg per 1 ml Flexible collodion methylated | 100 ml £13.54 | 500 ml £27.52

Skin adhesives

● SKIN ADHESIVES

Derma+Flex skin adhesive (Chemence Ltd)
.5 ml · NHS indicative price = £5.36 · Drug Tariff (Part IXa)

Dermabond ProPen skin adhesive (Ethicon Ltd)
.5 ml · NHS indicative price = £19.26 · Drug Tariff (Part IXa)

Histoacryl L skin adhesive (B.Braun Medical Ltd)
.2 gram · NHS indicative price = £6.20 · Drug Tariff (Part IXa).5 gram · NHS indicative price = £6.72 · Drug Tariff (Part IXa)

Histoacryl skin adhesive (B.Braun Medical Ltd)
.2 gram · NHS indicative price = £6.41 · Drug Tariff (Part IXa).5 gram · NHS indicative price = £6.50 · Drug Tariff (Part IXa)

Indermil skin adhesive (Covidien (UK) Commercial Ltd)
.5 gram · NHS indicative price = £6.50 · Drug Tariff (Part IXa)

LiquiBand flow control tissue adhesive (MedLogic Global Ltd)
.5 gram · NHS indicative price = £5.50 · Drug Tariff (Part IXa)

LiquiBand tissue adhesive (MedLogic Global Ltd)
.5 gram · NHS indicative price = £5.50 · Drug Tariff (Part IXa)

13

Skin

10   Skin disfigurement

Camouflagers

Overview

Disfigurement of the skin can be very distressing to patients and may have a marked psychological effect. In skilled hands, or with experience, camouflage cosmetics can be very effective in concealing scars and birthmarks. The depigmented patches in vitiligo are also very disfiguring and camouflage creams are of great cosmetic value.

Opaque cover foundation or cream is used to mask skin pigment abnormalities; careful application using a combination of dark- and light-coloured cover creams set with powder helps to minimise the appearance of skin deformities.

Borderline substances

The preparations marked 'ACBS' can be prescribed on the NHS for postoperative scars and other deformities and as adjunctive therapy in the relief of emotional disturbances due to disfiguring skin disease, such as vitiligo.

Camouflages

- **CAMOUFLAGES**

  Covermark classic foundation (Derma UK Ltd)
  15 ml(ACBS) · NHS indicative price = £11.86

  Covermark finishing powder (Derma UK Ltd)
  25 gram(ACBS) · NHS indicative price = £11.86

  Dermacolor camouflage creme (Charles H Fox Ltd)
  25 ml(ACBS) · NHS indicative price = £10.52

  Dermacolor fixing powder (Charles H Fox Ltd)
  60 gram(ACBS) · NHS indicative price = £9.05

  Keromask finishing powder (Bellava Ltd)
  20 gram(ACBS) · NHS indicative price = £5.80

  Keromask masking cream (Bellava Ltd)
  15 ml(ACBS) · NHS indicative price = £5.80

  Veil cover cream (Thomas Blake Cosmetic Creams Ltd)
  19 gram(ACBS) · NHS indicative price = £22.4244 gram(ACBS) · NHS
  indicative price = £33.3570 gram(ACBS) · NHS indicative price = £42.10

  Veil finishing powder (Thomas Blake Cosmetic Creams Ltd)
  35 gram(ACBS) · NHS indicative price = £24.58

11 Superficial soft-tissue injuries and superficial thrombophlebitis

Topical circulatory preparations

Overview

These preparations are used to improve circulation in conditions such as bruising and superficial thrombophlebitis but are of little value. First aid measures such as rest, ice, compression, and elevation should be used. Chilblains are best managed by avoidance of exposure to cold; neither systemic nor topical vasodilator therapy is established as being effective.

HEPARINOIDS

Heparinoid

- **INDICATIONS AND DOSE**

  Superficial thrombophlebitis | Bruising | Haematoma
  ▸ TO THE SKIN
  ▸ Child 5–17 years: Apply up to 4 times a day

- **CONTRA-INDICATIONS** Should not be used on large areas of skin, broken or sensitive skin, or mucous membranes
- **LESS SUITABLE FOR PRESCRIBING** Hirudoid® is less suitable for prescribing.

- **MEDICINAL FORMS**
  There can be variation in the licensing of different medicines containing the same drug.

  Cream
  EXCIPIENTS: May contain Cetostearyl alcohol (including cetyl and stearyl alcohol), hydroxybenzoates (parabens)
  ▸ **Hirudoid** (Genus Pharmaceuticals Ltd)
  Heparinoid 3 mg per 1 gram Hirudoid 0.3% cream | 50 gram Ⓟ
  £3.99 DT price = £3.99

  Gel
  EXCIPIENTS: May contain Fragrances, propylene glycol
  ▸ **Hirudoid** (Genus Pharmaceuticals Ltd)
  Heparinoid 3 mg per 1 gram Hirudoid 0.3% gel | 50 gram Ⓟ £3.99
  DT price = £3.99

12 Warts and calluses

Warts and calluses

Overview

Warts (verruca vulgaris) are common, benign, self-limiting, and usually asymptomatic. They are caused by a human papillomavirus, which most frequently affects the hands, feet (plantar warts), and the anogenital region; treatment usually relies on local tissue destruction and is required only if the warts are painful, unsightly, persistent, or cause distress. In immunocompromised children, warts may be more difficult to eradicate.

Preparations of salicylic acid, formaldehyde p. 721, glutaraldehyde p. 721 or silver nitrate p. 721 are used for the removal of warts on hands and feet. Salicylic acid is a useful keratolytic which may be considered first-line in the treatment of warts; it is also suitable for the removal of *corns and calluses*. Preparations of salicylic acid in a collodion basis are available but some patients may develop an allergy to colophony in the formulation; collodion should be avoided in children allergic to elastic adhesive plaster. Cryotherapy causes pain, swelling, and blistering, and may be no more effective than topical salicylic acid in the treatment of warts.

Anogenital warts

Anogenital warts (condylomata acuminata) in children are often asymptomatic and require only a simple barrier preparation. If treatment is required it should be supervised by a hospital specialist. Persistent warts on genital skin may require treatment with cryotherapy or other forms of physical ablation under general anaesthesia.

Podophyllotoxin below (the major active ingredient of podophyllum), or imiquimod p. 722 are used to treat external anogenital warts; these preparations can cause considerable irritation of the treated area and are therefore suitable only for children who are able to co-operate with the treatment.

ANTINEOPLASTIC DRUGS › PLANT ALKALOIDS

Podophyllotoxin

- **INDICATIONS AND DOSE**

  CONDYLINE®

  Condylomata acuminata affecting the penis or the female external genitalia
  ▸ TO THE LESION
  ▸ Child 2–17 years (initiated under specialist supervision):
  Apply twice daily for 3 consecutive days, treatment may be repeated at weekly intervals if necessary for a total of five 3-day treatment courses, direct medical supervision for lesions in the female and for lesions greater than 4 cm^2 in the male, maximum 50 single applications ('loops') per session (consult product literature)

  WARTICON® CREAM

  Condylomata acuminata affecting the penis or the female external genitalia
  ▸ TO THE LESION
  ▸ Child 2–17 years (initiated under specialist supervision):
  Apply twice daily for 3 consecutive days, treatment may be repeated at weekly intervals if necessary for a total of four 3-day treatment courses, direct medical supervision for lesions greater than 4 cm^2

WARTICON® LIQUID

Condylomata acuminata affecting the penis or the female external genitalia
- TO THE LESION
- Child 2–17 years (initiated under specialist supervision): Apply twice daily for 3 consecutive days, treatment may be repeated at weekly intervals if necessary for a total of four 3-day treatment courses, direct medical supervision for lesions greater than 4 cm², maximum 50 single applications ('loops') per session (consult product literature)

- **UNLICENSED USE** Not licensed for use in children.
- **CAUTIONS** Avoid normal skin · avoid open wounds · keep away from face · very irritant to eyes
- **SIDE-EFFECTS** Local irritation
- **PREGNANCY** Avoid.
- **BREAST FEEDING** Avoid.

- **MEDICINAL FORMS**
  There can be variation in the licensing of different medicines containing the same drug.
  Liquid
  CAUTIONARY AND ADVISORY LABELS 15
  - Condyline (Takeda UK Ltd)
    Podophyllotoxin 5 mg per 1 ml Condyline 0.5% solution | 3.5 ml [PoM] £14.49
  - Warticon (Stiefel Laboratories (UK) Ltd)
    Podophyllotoxin 5 mg per 1 ml Warticon 0.5% solution | 3 ml [PoM] £14.86
  Cream
  EXCIPIENTS: May contain Butylated hydroxyanisole, cetostearyl alcohol (including cetyl and stearyl alcohol), hydroxybenzoates (parabens), sorbic acid
  - Warticon (Stiefel Laboratories (UK) Ltd)
    Podophyllotoxin 1.5 mg per 1 gram Warticon 0.15% cream | 5 gram [PoM] £17.83 DT price = £17.83

ANTISEPTICS AND DISINFECTANTS >
ALDEHYDES AND DERIVATIVES

Formaldehyde

- **INDICATIONS AND DOSE**
  Warts, particularly plantar warts
  - TO THE LESION
  - Child: Apply twice daily

- **UNLICENSED USE** Licensed for use in children (age range not specified by manufacturer).
- **CAUTIONS** Impaired peripheral circulation · not suitable for application to anogenital region · not suitable for application to face · not suitable for application to large areas · patients with diabetes at risk of neuropathic ulcers · protect surrounding skin and avoid broken skin · significant peripheral neuropathy
- **SIDE-EFFECTS** Skin irritation · skin ulceration (with high concentrations)

- **MEDICINAL FORMS**
  There can be variation in the licensing of different medicines containing the same drug. Forms available from special-order manufacturers include: liquid
  Liquid
  - Formaldehyde (Non-proprietary)
    Formaldehyde 40 mg per 1 ml Formaldehyde (Buffered) 4% solution | 1000 ml £3.90
  - Formaldehyde (Non-proprietary)
    Formaldehyde 350 mg per 1 gram Formaldehyde solution | 500 ml £5.84 DT price = £5.84 | 2000 ml £9.22–£16.77
  Gel
  - Veracur (Typharm Ltd)
    Formaldehyde 7.5 mg per 1 gram Veracur 0.75% gel | 15 gram [GSL] £2.41

Glutaraldehyde

- **INDICATIONS AND DOSE**
  Warts, particularly plantar warts
  - TO THE LESION
  - Child: Apply twice daily

- **UNLICENSED USE** Licensed for use in children (age range not specified by manufacturer).
- **CAUTIONS** Not for application to anogenital areas · not for application to face · not for application to mucosa · protect surrounding skin
- **SIDE-EFFECTS** Rashes · skin irritation (discontinue if severe) · stains skin brown

- **MEDICINAL FORMS**
  There can be variation in the licensing of different medicines containing the same drug.
  Paint
  - Glutarol (Dermal Laboratories Ltd)
    Glutaraldehyde 100 mg per 1 ml Glutarol 10% cutaneous solution | 10 ml [P] £2.07 DT price = £2.07

ANTISEPTICS AND DISINFECTANTS > OTHER

Silver nitrate

- **INDICATIONS AND DOSE**
  Common warts
  - TO THE LESION
  - Child: Apply every 24 hours for up to 3 applications, apply moistened caustic pencil tip for 1–2 minutes. Instructions in proprietary packs generally incorporate advice to remove dead skin before use by gentle filing and to cover with adhesive dressing after application
  Verrucas
  - TO THE LESION
  - Child: Apply every 24 hours for up to 6 applications, apply moistened caustic pencil tip for 1–2 minutes. Instructions in proprietary packs generally incorporate advice to remove dead skin before use by gentle filing and to cover with adhesive dressing after application
  Umbilical granulomas
  - TO THE SKIN
  - Child: Apply moistened caustic pencil tip (usually containing silver nitrate 40%) for 1–2 minutes, protect surrounding skin with soft paraffin

- **UNLICENSED USE** No age range specified by manufacturer.
- **CAUTIONS** Avoid broken skin · not suitable for application to ano-genital region · not suitable for application to face · not suitable for application to large areas · protect surrounding skin
- **SIDE-EFFECTS** Chemical burns on surrounding skin · stains skin
- **PATIENT AND CARER ADVICE** Patients should be advised that silver nitrate may stain fabric.

13

Skin

13

Skin

- **MEDICINAL FORMS**
  There can be variation in the licensing of different medicines containing the same drug.
  Stick
  ▸ Silver nitrate (Non-proprietary)
    Silver nitrate 400 mg per 1 gram Silver nitrate 40% caustic pencils | 1 applicator P no price available
  ▸ Avoca (Bray Group Ltd)
    Silver nitrate 400 mg per 1 gram Avoca 40% silver nitrate pencils | 1 applicator P £1.03
    Silver nitrate 750 mg per 1 gram Avoca 75% silver nitrate applicators | 100 applicator P £44.48
    Avoca 75% silver nitrate applicators with thick handles | 50 applicator P £43.41
    Silver nitrate 950 mg per 1 gram Avoca 95% silver nitrate applicators | 100 applicator P £44.52
    Avoca 95% silver nitrate pencils | 1 applicator P £1.99 DT price = £2.44

ANTIVIRALS > IMMUNE RESPONSE MODIFIERS

Imiquimod

- **INDICATIONS AND DOSE**
  ALDARA®
  Warts (external genital and perianal)
  ▸ TO THE LESION
  ▸ Child (initiated under specialist supervision): Apply 3 times a week until lesions resolve (maximum 16 weeks), to be applied thinly at night

- **UNLICENSED USE**
  ALDARA® Not licensed for use in children.
- **CAUTIONS** Autoimmune disease · avoid broken skin · avoid normal skin · avoid open wounds · immunosuppressed patients · not suitable for internal genital warts · uncircumcised males (risk of phimosis or stricture of foreskin)
- **SIDE-EFFECTS**
  ▸ **Common or very common** Burning sensation · erosion · erythema · excoriation · headache · influenza-like symptoms · itching · local reactions · myalgia · oedema · scabbing
  ▸ **Uncommon** Alopecia · local ulceration
  ▸ **Rare** Cutaneous lupus erythematosus-like effect · Stevens-Johnson syndrome
  ▸ **Very rare** Dysuria
  ▸ **Frequency not known** Permanent hyperpigmentation · permanent hypopigmentation
- **CONCEPTION AND CONTRACEPTION** May damage latex condoms and diaphragms.
- **PREGNANCY** No evidence of teratogenicity or toxicity in *animal* studies; manufacturer advises caution.
- **BREAST FEEDING** No information available.
- **DIRECTIONS FOR ADMINISTRATION**
  ALDARA® ▸ **Important** Should be rubbed in and allowed to stay on the treated area for 6–10 hours then washed off with mild soap and water (uncircumcised males treating warts under foreskin should wash the area daily). The cream should be washed off before sexual contact.
- **PATIENT AND CARER ADVICE** A patient information leaflet should be provided.

- **MEDICINAL FORMS**
  There can be variation in the licensing of different medicines containing the same drug.
  Cream
  CAUTIONARY AND ADVISORY LABELS 10
  EXCIPIENTS: May contain Benzyl alcohol, cetostearyl alcohol (including cetyl and stearyl alcohol), hydroxybenzoates (parabens), polysorbates
  ▸ Aldara (Meda Pharmaceuticals Ltd)
    Imiquimod 50 mg per 1 gram Aldara 5% cream 250mg sachets | 12 sachet PoM £48.60 DT price = £48.60

SALICYLIC ACID AND DERIVATIVES

Salicylic acid

- **INDICATIONS AND DOSE**
  OCCLUSAL®
  Common and plantar warts
  ▸ TO THE LESION
  ▸ Child: Apply daily, treatment may need to be continued for up to 3 months
  VERRUGON®
  For plantar warts
  ▸ TO THE LESION
  ▸ Child: Apply daily, treatment may need to be continued for up to 3 months

- **UNLICENSED USE** Not licensed for use in children under 2 years.
- **CAUTIONS** Avoid broken skin · impaired peripheral circulation · not suitable for application to anogenital region · not suitable for application to face · not suitable for application to large areas · patients with diabetes at risk of neuropathic ulcers · significant peripheral neuropathy
- **SIDE-EFFECTS** Skin irritation · skin ulceration (with high concentrations)
- **PATIENT AND CARER ADVICE** Advise patient to apply carefully to wart and to protect surrounding skin (e.g. with soft paraffin or specially designed plaster); rub wart surface gently with file or pumice stone once weekly.

- **MEDICINAL FORMS**
  There can be variation in the licensing of different medicines containing the same drug.
  Liquid
  CAUTIONARY AND ADVISORY LABELS 15
  ▸ Occlusal - brand name (Alliance Pharmaceuticals Ltd)
    Salicylic acid 260 mg per 1 ml Occlusal 26% solution | 10 ml P £3.56 DT price = £3.56
  Ointment
  ▸ Verrugon (Optima Consumer Health Ltd)
    Salicylic acid 500 mg per 1 gram Verrugon complete 50% ointment | 6 gram P £3.12

Salicylic acid with lactic acid

- **INDICATIONS AND DOSE**
  CUPLEX®
  Plantar and mosaic warts | Corns | Calluses
  ▸ TO THE LESION
  ▸ Child: Apply twice daily, treatment may need to be continued for up to 3 months
  DUOFILM®
  Plantar and mosaic warts
  ▸ TO THE LESION
  ▸ Child: Apply daily, treatment may need to be continued for up to 3 months
  SALACTOL®
  Warts, particularly plantar warts | Verrucas | Corns | Calluses
  ▸ TO THE LESION
  ▸ Child: Apply daily, treatment may need to be continued for up to 3 months

SALATAC®

Warts | Verrucas | Corns | Calluses

▶ TO THE LESION
▶ **Child:** Apply daily, treatment may need to be continued for up to 3 months

● **PRESCRIBING AND DISPENSING INFORMATION**
Preparations of salicylic acid in a collodion basis (Cuplex® and Salactol®) are available but some patients may develop an allergy to colophony in the formulation.

● **MEDICINAL FORMS**
There can be variation in the licensing of different medicines containing the same drug.

Gel

CAUTIONARY AND ADVISORY LABELS 15

▶ Cuplex (Crawford Healthcare Ltd)
Lactic acid 40 mg per 1 gram, Salicylic acid 110 mg per 1 gram Cuplex Verruca gel | 5 gram GSL £2.88 DT price = £2.88

▶ Salatac (Dermal Laboratories Ltd)
Lactic acid 40 mg per 1 gram, Salicylic acid 120 mg per 1 gram Salatac gel | 8 gram Ⓟ £2.98 DT price = £2.98

Paint

CAUTIONARY AND ADVISORY LABELS 15

▶ Duofilm (GlaxoSmithKline UK Ltd)
Lactic acid 150 mg per 1 gram, Salicylic acid 167 mg per 1 gram Duofilm paint | 15 ml Ⓟ £2.25

▶ Salactol (Dermal Laboratories Ltd)
Lactic acid 167 mg per 1 gram, Salicylic acid 167 mg per 1 gram Salactol paint | 10 ml Ⓟ £1.71 DT price = £1.71

13

Skin

Chapter 14
Vaccines

CONTENTS

1	Immunoglobulin therapy	page 724
2	Post-exposure prophylaxis	730

3	Tuberculosis diagnostic test	page 731
4	Vaccination	731

1   Immunoglobulin therapy

IMMUNE SERA AND IMMUNOGLOBULINS >
IMMUNOGLOBULINS

Immunoglobulins

Passive immunity

Immunity with immediate protection against certain infective organisms can be obtained by injecting preparations made from the plasma of immune individuals with adequate levels of antibody to the disease for which protection is sought. The duration of this passive immunity varies according to the dose and the type of immunoglobulin. Passive immunity may last only a few weeks; when necessary, passive immunisation can be repeated. Antibodies of human origin are usually termed immunoglobulins. The term antiserum is applied to material prepared in animals. Because of serum sickness and other allergic-type reactions that may follow injections of antisera, this therapy has been replaced wherever possible by the use of immunoglobulins. Reactions are theoretically possible after injection of human immunoglobulins but reports of such reactions are very rare.

Two types of human immunoglobulin preparation are available, normal immunoglobulin p. 727 and **disease-specific immunoglobulins.**

Human immunoglobulin is a sterile preparation of concentrated antibodies (immune globulins) recovered from pooled human plasma or serum obtained from outside the UK, tested and found non-reactive for hepatitis B surface antigen and for antibodies against hepatitis C virus and human immunodeficiency virus (types 1 and 2). A global shortage of human immunoglobulin and the rapidly increasing range of clinical indications for treatment with immunoglobulins has resulted in the need for a Demand Management programme in the UK, for further information consult www.ivig.nhs.uk and *Clinical Guidelines for Immunoglobulin Use*, www.gov.uk/dh.

Further information on the use of immunoglobulins is included in Public Health England's *Immunoglobulin Handbook* www.gov.uk/phe, and in the Department of Health's publication, *Immunisation against Infectious Disease*, www.gov.uk/dh.

Availability

Normal immunoglobulin for intramuscular administration is available from some regional Public Health laboratories for protection of contacts and the control of outbreaks of hepatitis A, measles, and rubella only. For other indications, subcutaneous or intravenous normal immunoglobulin should be purchased from the manufacturer.

Disease-specific immunoglobulins are available from some regional Public Health laboratories, with the exception of tetanus immunoglobulin p. 729 which is available from BPL,

hospital pharmacies, or blood transfusion departments. Rabies immunoglobulin p. 729 is available from the Specialist and Reference Microbiology Division, Public Health England, Colindale. Hepatitis B immunoglobulin p. 727 required by transplant centres should be obtained commercially.

In Scotland all immunoglobulins are available from the *Scottish National Blood Transfusion Service* (SNBTS).

In Wales all immunoglobulins are available from the *Welsh Blood Service* (WBS).

In Northern Ireland all immunoglobulins are available from the *Northern Ireland Blood Transfusion Service* (NIBTS).

Normal immunoglobulin

Human normal immunoglobulin ('HNIG') is prepared from pools of at least 1000 donations of human plasma; it contains immunoglobulin G (IgG) and antibodies to hepatitis A, measles, mumps, rubella, varicella, and other viruses that are currently prevalent in the general population.

Uses

Normal immunoglobulin (containing 10–18% protein) is administered by *intramuscular injection* for the protection of susceptible contacts against **hepatitis A** virus (infectious hepatitis), **measles** and, to a lesser extent, **rubella**. Injection of immunoglobulin produces immediate protection lasting for several weeks.

Normal immunoglobulin (containing 3–12% protein) for *intravenous administration* is used as *replacement therapy* for children with congenital agammaglobulinaemia and hypogammaglobulinaemia, and for the short-term treatment of idiopathic thrombocytopenic purpura and Kawasaki disease; it is also used for the prophylaxis of infection following bone-marrow transplantation and in children with symptomatic HIV infection who have recurrent bacterial infections. Normal immunoglobulin for replacement therapy may also be given intramuscularly or subcutaneously, but intravenous formulations are normally preferred. Intravenous immunoglobulin is also used in the treatment of Guillain-Barré syndrome as an alternative to plasma exchange.

The dose of normal immunoglobulin used as replacement therapy in patients with immunodeficiencies is **not the same** as the dose required for treatment of acute conditions. For Kawasaki disease a single dose by intravenous infusion should be given with concomitant aspirin p. 83 within 10 days of onset of symptoms (but children with a delayed diagnosis may also benefit).

For guidance on the use of intravenous normal immunoglobulin and alternative therapies for other conditions, consult *Clinical Guidelines for Immunoglobulin Use* (www.gov.uk/dh).

Hepatitis A

Hepatitis A vaccine p. 749 is preferred for individuals at risk of infection including those visiting areas where the disease is highly endemic (all countries excluding Northern and

Western Europe, North America, Japan, Australia, and New Zealand). In unimmunised individuals, transmission of hepatitis A is reduced by good hygiene. Intramuscular normal immunoglobulin is no longer recommended for routine prophylaxis in travellers, but it may be indicated for immunocompromised patients if their antibody response to the vaccine is unlikely to be adequate.

Intramuscular normal immunoglobulin is recommended for prevention of infection in close contacts (of confirmed cases of hepatitis A) who have chronic liver disease or HIV infection, or who are immunosuppressed; normal immunoglobulin should be given as soon as possible, preferably within 14 days of exposure to the primary case. However, normal immunoglobulin can still be given to contacts at risk of severe disease up to 28 days after exposure to the primary case. Hepatitis A vaccine can be given at the same time, but it should be given at a separate injection site.

Measles

Intravenous or subcutaneous normal immunoglobulin may be given to prevent or attenuate an attack of measles in individuals who do not have adequate immunity. Children with compromised immunity who have come into contact with measles should receive intravenous or subcutaneous normal immunoglobulin as soon as possible after exposure. It is most effective if given within 72 hours but can be effective if given within 6 days.

Subcutaneous or intramuscular normal immunoglobulin should be considered for the following individuals if they have been in contact with a confirmed case of measles or with a person associated with a local outbreak:

- non-immune pregnant women
- infants under 9 months

Further advice should be sought from the Centre for Infections, Public Health England (tel. (020) 8200 6868).

Individuals with normal immunity who are not in the above categories and who have not been fully immunised against measles, can be given measles, mumps and rubella vaccine, live p. 753 for prophylaxis following exposure to measles.

Rubella

Intramuscular immunoglobulin after exposure to rubella does **not** prevent infection in non-immune contacts and is **not** recommended for protection of pregnant women exposed to rubella. It may, however, reduce the likelihood of a clinical attack which may possibly reduce the risk to the fetus. Risk of intra-uterine transmission is greatest in the first 11 weeks of pregnancy, between 16 and 20 weeks there is minimal risk of deafness only, after 20 weeks there is no increased risk. Intramuscular normal immunoglobulin p. 727 should be used only if termination of pregnancy would be unacceptable to the pregnant woman—it should be given as soon as possible after exposure. Serological follow-up of recipients is essential to determine if the woman has become infected despite receiving immunoglobulin.

For routine prophylaxis against Rubella, see measles, mumps and rubella vaccine, live p. 753.

Disease-specific immunoglobulins

Specific immunoglobulins are prepared by pooling the plasma of selected human donors with high levels of the specific antibody required. For further information, see *Immunoglobulin Handbook* (www.gov.uk/phe).

There are no specific immunoglobulins for hepatitis A, measles, or rubella—normal immunoglobulin is used in certain circumstances. There is no specific immunoglobulin for mumps; neither normal immunoglobulin nor measles, mumps and rubella vaccine, live is effective as postexposure prophylaxis.

Hepatitis B immunoglobulin

Disease-specific hepatitis B immunoglobulin ('HBIG') p. 727 is available for use in association with hepatitis B vaccine

p. 750 for the prevention of infection in infants born to mothers who have become infected with this virus in pregnancy or who are high-risk carriers (see hepatitis B vaccine). Hepatitis B immunoglobulin will not inhibit the antibody response when given at the same time as hepatitis B vaccine but should be given at different sites.

An intravenous and preparation of hepatitis B immunoglobulin is licensed for the prevention of hepatitis B recurrence in HBV-DNA negative patients who have undergone liver transplantation for liver failure caused by the virus.

Rabies immunoglobulin

Following exposure of an unimmunised individual to an animal in or from a country where the risk of rabies is high the site of the bite should be washed with soapy water and specific rabies immunoglobulin p. 729 of human origin administered. All of the dose should be injected around the site of the wound; if this is difficult or the wound has completely healed it can be given in the anterolateral thigh (remote from the site used for vaccination).

Rabies vaccine p. 754 should also be given intramuscularly at a different site (for details see rabies vaccine). If there is delay in giving the rabies immunoglobulin, it should be given within 7 days of starting the course of rabies vaccine.

Tetanus immunoglobulin

For the management of tetanus-prone wounds, tetanus immunoglobulin p. 729 should be used in addition to wound cleansing and, where appropriate, antibacterial prophylaxis and a tetanus-containing vaccine. Tetanus immunoglobulin, together with metronidazole p. 313 and wound cleansing, should also be used for the treatment of established cases of tetanus.

Varicella–zoster immunoglobulin

Varicella-zoster immunoglobulin (VZIG) p. 730 is recommended for individuals who are at increased risk of severe varicella *and* who have no antibodies to varicella–zoster virus *and* who have significant exposure to chickenpox or herpes zoster. Those at increased risk include:

- neonates whose mothers develop chickenpox in the period 7 days before to 7 days after delivery;
- susceptible neonates exposed in the first 7 days of life;
- susceptible neonates or infants exposed whilst requiring intensive or prolonged special care nursing;
- susceptible women exposed at any stage of pregnancy (but when supplies of VZIG are short, may only be issued to those exposed in the first 20 weeks' gestation or to those near term) providing VZIG is given within 10 days of contact;
- immunocompromised individuals including those who have received corticosteroids in the previous 3 months at the following dose equivalents of prednisolone; *children* 2 mg/kg daily (or more than 40 mg) for at least 1 week or 1 mg/kg daily for 1 month.

Important: for full details consult *Immunisation against Infectious Disease*. Varicella-zoster vaccine p. 755 is available.

Anti-D (Rh₀) immunoglobulin

● INDICATIONS AND DOSE

To rhesus-negative woman for prevention of Rh₀(D) sensitisation, following birth of rhesus-positive infant

▶ BY DEEP INTRAMUSCULAR INJECTION

▶ Females of childbearing potential: 500 units, dose to be administered immediately or within 72 hours; for transplacental bleed of over 4 mL fetal red cells, extra 100–125 units per mL fetal red cells, subcutaneous route used for patients with bleeding disorders

continued →

14

Vaccines

To rhesus-negative woman for prevention of Rh$_0$(D) sensitisation, following any potentially sensitising episode (e.g. stillbirth, abortion, amniocentesis) up to 20 weeks' gestation
▸ BY DEEP INTRAMUSCULAR INJECTION
▸ Females of childbearing potential: 250 units per episode, dose to be administered immediately or within 72 hours, subcutaneous route used for patients with bleeding disorders

To rhesus-negative woman for prevention of Rh$_0$(D) sensitisation, following any potentially sensitising episode (e.g. stillbirth, abortion, amniocentesis) after 20 weeks' gestation
▸ BY DEEP INTRAMUSCULAR INJECTION
▸ Females of childbearing potential: 500 units per episode, dose to be administered immediately or within 72 hours, subcutaneous route used for patients with bleeding disorders

To rhesus-negative woman for prevention of Rh$_0$(D) sensitisation, antenatal prophylaxis
▸ BY DEEP INTRAMUSCULAR INJECTION
▸ Females of childbearing potential: 500 units, dose to be given at weeks 28 and 34 of pregnancy, if infant rhesus-positive, a further dose is still needed immediately or within 72 hours of delivery, subcutaneous route used for patients with bleeding disorders

To rhesus-negative woman for prevention of Rh$_0$(D) sensitisation, antenatal prophylaxis (alternative NICE recommendation)
▸ BY DEEP INTRAMUSCULAR INJECTION
▸ Females of childbearing potential: 1000–1650 units, dose to be given at weeks 28 and 34 of pregnancy, alternatively 1500 units for 1 dose, dose to be given between 28 and 30 weeks gestation

To rhesus-negative woman for prevention of Rh$_0$(D) sensitisation, following Rh$_0$(D) incompatible blood transfusion
▸ BY DEEP INTRAMUSCULAR INJECTION
▸ Females of childbearing potential: 100–125 units per mL of transfused rhesus-positive red cells, subcutaneous route used for patients with bleeding disorders

RHOPHYLAC®

To rhesus-negative woman for prevention of Rh$_0$(D) sensitisation, following birth of rhesus-positive infant
▸ BY INTRAMUSCULAR INJECTION, OR BY INTRAVENOUS INJECTION
▸ Females of childbearing potential: 1000–1500 units, dose to administered immediately or within 72 hours; for large transplacental bleed, extra 100 units per mL fetal red cells (preferably by intravenous injection), intravenous route recommended for patients with bleeding disorders

To rhesus-negative woman for prevention of Rh$_0$(D) sensitisation, following any potentially sensitising episode (e.g. abortion, amniocentesis, chorionic villous sampling) up to 12 weeks' gestation
▸ BY INTRAMUSCULAR INJECTION, OR BY INTRAVENOUS INJECTION
▸ Females of childbearing potential: 1000 units per episode, dose to be administered immediately or within 72 hours, intravenous route recommended for patients with bleeding disorders, higher doses may be required after 12 weeks gestation

To rhesus-negative woman for prevention of Rh$_0$(D) sensitisation, antenatal prophylaxis
▸ BY INTRAMUSCULAR INJECTION, OR BY INTRAVENOUS INJECTION
▸ Females of childbearing potential: 1500 units, dose to be given between weeks 28–30 of pregnancy; if infant rhesus-positive, a further dose is still needed

immediately or within 72 hours of delivery, intravenous route recommended for patients with bleeding disorders

To rhesus-negative woman for prevention of Rh$_0$(D) sensitisation, following Rh$_0$(D) incompatible blood transfusion
▸ BY INTRAVENOUS INJECTION
▸ Females of childbearing potential: 50 units per mL of transfused rhesus-positive blood, alternatively 100 units per mL of erythrocyte concentrate, intravenous route recommended for patients with bleeding disorders

● CONTRA-INDICATIONS Treatment of idiopathic thrombocytopenia purpura in rhesus negative patients · treatment of idiopathic thrombocytopenia purpura in splenectomised patients

● CAUTIONS Immunoglobulin A deficiency · possible interference with live virus vaccines
CAUTIONS, FURTHER INFORMATION
MMR vaccine may be given in the postpartum period with anti-D (Rh$_0$) immunoglobulin injection provided that separate syringes are used and the products are administered into different limbs. If blood is transfused, the antibody response to the vaccine may be inhibited—measure rubella antibodies after 6–8 weeks and revaccinate if necessary.

● INTERACTIONS → Appendix 1 (immunoglobulins).

● SIDE-EFFECTS
GENERAL SIDE-EFFECTS
▸ **Rare** Anaphylaxis · dyspnoea · hypotension · tachycardia · urticaria
▸ **Frequency not known** Abdominal pain · arthralgia · asthenia · back pain · diarrhoea · dizziness · drowsiness · fever · headache · hypertension · hypotension · injection site pain · malaise · myalgia · nausea · pruritus · rash · sweating · vomiting

SPECIFIC SIDE-EFFECTS
▸ With intravenous use Abdominal distension · blood pressure fluctuations · deep vein thrombosis · haemolytic anaemia · injection site reactions · myocardial infarction · pulmonary embolism · stroke · thromboembolic events

● HANDLING AND STORAGE Care must be taken to store all immunological products under the conditions recommended in the product literature, otherwise the preparation may become ineffective. **Refrigerated storage** is usually necessary; many immunoglobulins need to be stored at 2–8°C and not allowed to freeze. Immunoglobulins should be protected from light. Opened multidose vials must be used within the period recommended in the product literature.

● NATIONAL FUNDING/ACCESS DECISIONS
NICE technology appraisals (TAs)
▸ Routine antenatal anti-D prophylaxis for rhesus-negative women (August 2008) NICE TA156
Routine antenatal anti-D prophylaxis should be offered to all non-sensitised pregnant women who are rhesus negative.
www.nice.org.uk/TA156

● MEDICINAL FORMS
There can be variation in the licensing of different medicines containing the same drug.
Solution for injection
▸ D-Gam (Bio Products Laboratory Ltd)
Anti-D (RHO) immunoglobulin 250 unit D-Gam Anti-D immunoglobulin 250unit solution for injection vials | 1 vial PoM £23.75
Anti-D (RHO) immunoglobulin 500 unit D-Gam Anti-D immunoglobulin 500unit solution for injection vials | 1 vial PoM £33.75

Anti-D (RHO) immunoglobulin 1500 unit D-Gam Anti-D immunoglobulin 1,500unit solution for injection vials | 1 vial [PoM] £58.00

▸ Rhophylac (CSL Behring UK Ltd)
  Anti-D (RHO) immunoglobulin 750 unit per 1 ml Rhophylac 1,500units/2ml solution for injection pre-filled syringes | 1 pre-filled disposable injection [PoM] £39.52

Hepatitis B immunoglobulin

● **INDICATIONS AND DOSE**

Prophylaxis against hepatitis B infection
▸ BY INTRAMUSCULAR INJECTION

▸ Neonate: 200 units, dose to be administered as soon as possible after exposure; ideally within 12–48 hours, but no later than 7 days after exposure.

▸ Child 1 month–4 years: 200 units, dose to be administered as soon as possible after exposure; ideally within 12–48 hours, but no later than 7 days after exposure

▸ Child 5–9 years: 300 units, dose to be administered as soon as possible after exposure; ideally within 12–48 hours, but no later than 7 days after exposure

▸ Child 10–17 years: 500 units, dose to be administered as soon as possible after exposure; ideally within 12–48 hours, but no later than 7 days after exposure

Prevention of transmitted infection at birth
▸ BY INTRAMUSCULAR INJECTION

▸ Neonate: 200 units, dose to be administered as soon as possible after birth; for full details consult Immunisation against Infectious Disease (www.dh.gov.uk).

▸ BY INTRAVENOUS INFUSION

▸ Neonate: (consult product literature).

Prophylaxis against hepatitis B infection, after exposure to hepatitis B virus-contaminated material
▸ BY INTRAVENOUS INFUSION

▸ Child: Dose to be administered as soon as possible after exposure, but no later than 72 hours (consult product literature)

Prophylaxis against re-infection of transplanted liver
▸ BY INTRAVENOUS INFUSION

▸ Child: (consult product literature)

● **CAUTIONS** IgA deficiency · interference with live virus vaccines

● **SIDE-EFFECTS**

GENERAL SIDE-EFFECTS
▸ **Rare** Anaphylaxis · chest tightness · dyspnoea
▸ **Frequency not known** Arthralgia · buccal ulceration · dizziness · facial oedema · glossitis · pain at injection site · swelling at injection site · tremor

SPECIFIC SIDE-EFFECTS
▸ With intravenous use Abdominal distension · blood pressure fluctuations · deep vein thrombosis · haemolytic anaemia · injection site reactions · myocardial infarction · pulmonary embolism · stroke · thromboembolic events

● **PRESCRIBING AND DISPENSING INFORMATION** Vials containing 200 units or 500 units (for intramuscular injection), available from selected Public Health England and NHS laboratories (except for Transplant Centres), also available from BPL.

● **HANDLING AND STORAGE** Care must be taken to store all immunological products under the conditions recommended in the product literature, otherwise the preparation may become ineffective. **Refrigerated storage** is usually necessary; many immunoglobulins need to be stored at 2–8°C and not allowed to freeze.

Immunoglobulins should be protected from light. Opened multidose vials must be used within the period recommended in the product literature.

● **MEDICINAL FORMS**
There can be variation in the licensing of different medicines containing the same drug.

Solution for injection
▸ Hepatitis B immunoglobulin (Non-proprietary)
  Hepatitis B immunoglobulin human 200 unit Hepatitis B immunoglobulin human 200unit solution for injection vials | 1 vial [PoM] £122.44
  Hepatitis B immunoglobulin human 500 unit Hepatitis B immunoglobulin human 500unit solution for injection vials | 1 vial [PoM] £266.33
▸ Zutectra (Biotest (UK) Ltd)
  Zutectra 500units/1ml solution for injection pre-filled syringes | 5 syringe [PoM] £1,275.00

Solution for infusion
▸ Hepatect CP (Biotest (UK) Ltd)
  Hepatitis B immunoglobulin human 50 unit per 1 ml Hepatect CP 100units/2ml solution for infusion vials | 1 vial [PoM] £51.00
  Hepatect CP 2000units/40ml solution for infusion vials | 1 vial [PoM] £935.00
  Hepatect CP 500units/10ml solution for infusion vials | 1 vial [PoM] £255.00
  Hepatect CP 5000units/100ml solution for infusion vials | 1 vial [PoM] £2,550.00
▸ Omri-Hep-B (Imported (Israel))
  Hepatitis B immunoglobulin human 50 unit per 1 ml Omri-Hep-B 5000units/100ml solution for infusion vials | 1 vial [PoM] no price available

---

Normal immunoglobulin

● **INDICATIONS AND DOSE**

To control outbreaks of hepatitis A
▸ BY DEEP INTRAMUSCULAR INJECTION
▸ Child 1 month–9 years: 250 mg
▸ Child 10–17 years: 500 mg

Rubella in pregnancy, prevention of clinical attack
▸ BY DEEP INTRAMUSCULAR INJECTION
▸ Females of childbearing potential: 750 mg

Antibody deficiency syndromes
▸ BY SUBCUTANEOUS INFUSION
▸ Child: (consult product literature)

Kawasaki disease (with concomitant aspirin)
▸ BY INTRAVENOUS INFUSION
▸ Child: 2 g/kg daily for 1 dose, treatment should be given within 10 days of onset of symptom (but children with a delayed diagnosis may also benefit)

SUBGAM®

Hepatitis A prophylaxis in outbreaks
▸ BY INTRAMUSCULAR INJECTION
▸ Child 1 month–9 years: 500 mg
▸ Child 10–17 years: 750 mg

● **UNLICENSED USE**
SUBGAM® *Subgam*® is not licensed for prophylactic use, but due to difficulty in obtaining suitable immunoglobulin products, Public Health England recommends intramuscular use for prophylaxis against Hepatitis A or rubella.

● **CONTRA-INDICATIONS** Patients with selective IgA deficiency who have known antibody against IgA

PRIVIGEN® Hyperprolinaemia (contains -proline)

GAMMAPLEX® Hereditary fructose intolerance (contains sorbitol)

HIZENTRA® Hyperprolinaemia (contains -proline)

FLEBOGAMMA® DIF Hereditary fructose intolerance (contains sorbitol)

14

Vaccines

● **CAUTIONS**

GENERAL CAUTIONS

Agammaglobulinaemia with or without IgA deficiency · hypogammaglobulinaemia with or without IgA deficiency · interference with live virus vaccines

SPECIFIC CAUTIONS

▸ With intravenous use Ensure adequate hydration · obesity · renal insufficiency · risk factors for arterial or venous thromboembolic events · thrombophilic disorders

CAUTIONS, FURTHER INFORMATION

▸ Interference with live virus vaccines Normal immunoglobulin may **interfere with the immune response to live virus vaccines** which should therefore only be given **at least 3 weeks before or 3 months after** an injection of normal immunoglobulin (this does not apply to yellow fever vaccine since normal immunoglobulin does not contain antibody to this virus).

OCTAGAM® Falsely elevated results with blood glucose testing systems (contains maltose)

● **INTERACTIONS** → Appendix 1 (immunoglobulins).

● **SIDE-EFFECTS**

GENERAL SIDE-EFFECTS

▸ **Rare** Acute renal failure · anaphylaxis · aseptic meningitis · cutaneous skin reactions · hypotension

▸ **Frequency not known** Arthralgia · chills · diarrhoea · dizziness · fever · headache · low back pain · muscle spasms · myalgia · nausea

SPECIFIC SIDE-EFFECTS

▸ With intravenous use Abdominal distension · abdominal pain · blood pressure fluctuations · deep vein thrombosis · haemolytic anaemia · injection site reactions · myocardial infarction · pulmonary embolism · stroke · thromboembolic events

SIDE-EFFECTS, FURTHER INFORMATION

Adverse reactions are more likely to occur in patients receiving normal immunoglobulin for the first time, or following a prolonged period between treatments, or when a different brand of normal immunoglobulin is administered.

● **MONITORING REQUIREMENTS** Monitor for acute renal failure; consider discontinuation if renal function deteriorates. Intravenous preparations with added sucrose have been associated with cases of renal dysfunction and acute renal failure.

● **DIRECTIONS FOR ADMINISTRATION**

Preparations for subcutaneous use May be administered by intramuscular injection if subcutaneous route not possible; intramuscular route **not** for patients with thrombocytopenia or other bleeding disorders.

GAMUNEX® Use Glucose 5% intravenous infusion if dilution prior to infusion is required.

KIOVIG® Use Glucose 5% intravenous infusion if dilution prior to infusion is required.

● **PRESCRIBING AND DISPENSING INFORMATION** Antibody titres can vary widely between normal immunoglobulin preparations from different manufacturers—formulations are **not interchangeable**; patients should be maintained on the same formulation throughout long-term treatment to avoid adverse effects.

▸ With intramuscular use Available from the Centre for Infections and other regional Public Health England offices (for contacts and control of outbreaks only).

● **HANDLING AND STORAGE** Care must be taken to store all immunological products under the conditions recommended in the product literature, otherwise the preparation may become ineffective. **Refrigerated storage** is usually necessary; many immunoglobulins need to be stored at 2–8°C and not allowed to freeze. Immunoglobulins should be protected from light. Opened multidose vials must be used within the period recommended in the product literature.

● **MEDICINAL FORMS**

There can be variation in the licensing of different medicines containing the same drug.

Solution for injection

ELECTROLYTES: May contain Sodium

▸ **Gammanorm** (Octapharma Ltd)

Normal immunoglobulin 165 mg per 1 ml Gammanorm 8g/48ml solution for injection vials | 1 vial [PoM] £469.20
Gammanorm 2g/12ml solution for injection vials | 1 vial [PoM] £117.30
Gammanorm 4g/24ml solution for injection vials | 1 vial [PoM] £234.60
Gammanorm 1.65g/10ml solution for injection vials | 1 vial [PoM] £96.77 | 10 vial [PoM] no price available (Hospital only)
Gammanorm 3.3g/20ml solution for injection vials | 1 vial [PoM] £193.55 | 10 vial [PoM] no price available (Hospital only)
Gammanorm 1g/6ml solution for injection vials | 1 vial [PoM] £58.65

▸ **Subcuvia** (Baxalta UK Ltd)

Normal immunoglobulin human 160 mg per 1 ml Subcuvia 800mg/5ml solution for injection vials | 1 vial [PoM] no price available
Subcuvia 1.6g/10ml solution for injection vials | 1 vial [PoM] no price available

▸ **Subgam** (Bio Products Laboratory Ltd)

Normal immunoglobulin human 150 mg per 1 ml Subgam 750mg/5ml solution for injection vials | 1 vial [PoM] £34.20
Subgam 1.5g/10ml solution for injection vials | 1 vial [PoM] £68.40

Powder and solvent for solution for injection

▸ **Gammagard S/D** (Baxalta UK Ltd)

Normal immunoglobulin human 500 mg Gammagard S/D 500mg powder and solvent for solution for injection bottles | 1 bottle [PoM] no price available

Normal immunoglobulin human 2.5 gram Gammagard S/D 2.5g powder and solvent for solution for injection bottles | 1 bottle [PoM] no price available

Normal immunoglobulin human 5 gram Gammagard S/D 5g powder and solvent for solution for injection bottles | 1 bottle [PoM] no price available

Normal immunoglobulin human 10 gram Gammagard S/D 10g powder and solvent for solution for injection bottles | 1 bottle [PoM] no price available

Solution for infusion

EXCIPIENTS: May contain Glucose, maltose, sorbitol, sucrose

▸ Normal immunoglobulin (Non-proprietary)

Normal immunoglobulin human 100 mg per 1 ml Normal immunoglobulin human 5g/50ml solution for infusion vials | 1 vial [PoM] no price available
Normal immunoglobulin human 2.5g/25ml solution for infusion vials | 1 vial [PoM] no price available
Normal immunoglobulin human 20g/200ml solution for infusion vials | 1 vial [PoM] no price available
Normal immunoglobulin human 10g/100ml solution for infusion vials | 1 vial [PoM] no price available
Normal immunoglobulin human 30g/300ml solution for infusion vials | 1 vial [PoM] no price available

▸ **Aragam** (Oxbridge Pharma Ltd)

Normal immunoglobulin human 50 mg per 1 ml Aragam 5g/100ml solution for infusion vials | 1 vial [PoM] no price available
Aragam 2.5g/50ml solution for infusion vials | 1 vial [PoM] no price available

▸ **Flebogammadif** (Grifols UK Ltd)

Normal immunoglobulin human 50 mg per 1 ml Flebogamma DIF 10g/200ml solution for infusion vials | 1 vial [PoM] £510.00
Flebogamma DIF 2.5g/50ml solution for infusion vials | 1 vial [PoM] £127.50
Flebogamma DIF 5g/100ml solution for infusion vials | 1 vial [PoM] £255.00
Flebogamma DIF 500mg/10ml solution for infusion vials | 1 vial [PoM] £30.00
Flebogamma DIF 20g/400ml solution for infusion vials | 1 vial [PoM] £1,020.00

Normal immunoglobulin human 100 mg per 1 ml Flebogamma DIF 10g/100ml solution for infusion vials | 1 vial [PoM] £510.00
Flebogamma DIF 20g/200ml solution for infusion vials | 1 vial [PoM] £1,020.00
Flebogamma DIF 5g/50ml solution for infusion vials | 1 vial [PoM] £255.00

▸ **Gammaplex** (Bio Products Laboratory Ltd)
Normal immunoglobulin human 50 mg per 1 ml Gammaplex 10g/200ml solution for infusion vials | 1 vial PoM £418.00 (Hospital only)
Gammaplex 5g/100ml solution for infusion vials | 1 vial PoM £209.00 (Hospital only)
Gammaplex 20g/400ml solution for infusion vials | 1 vial PoM £660.00 (Hospital only)
Gammaplex 2.5g/50ml solution for infusion vials | 1 vial PoM £104.50 (Hospital only)

▸ **Gamunex** (Grifols UK Ltd)
Normal immunoglobulin human 100 mg per 1 ml Gamunex 10% 1g/10ml solution for infusion vials | 1 vial PoM £42.50
Gamunex 10% 10g/100ml solution for infusion vials | 1 vial PoM £425.00
Gamunex 10% 20g/200ml solution for infusion vials | 1 vial PoM £850.00
Gamunex 10% 5g/50ml solution for infusion vials | 1 vial PoM £212.50

▸ **Hizentra** (CSL Behring UK Ltd)
Normal immunoglobulin human 200 mg per 1 ml Hizentra 2g/10ml solution for infusion vials | 1 vial PoM £91.80
Hizentra 1g/5ml solution for infusion vials | 1 vial PoM £45.90
Hizentra 4g/20ml solution for infusion vials | 1 vial PoM £183.60

▸ **Intratect** (Biotest (UK) Ltd)
Normal immunoglobulin human 50 mg per 1 ml Intratect 5g/100ml solution for infusion vials | 1 vial PoM £191.25
Intratect 1g/20ml solution for infusion vials | 1 vial PoM £38.25
Intratect 2.5g/50ml solution for infusion vials | 1 vial PoM £95.63
Intratect 10g/200ml solution for infusion vials | 1 vial PoM £382.50
Normal immunoglobulin human 100 mg per 1 ml Intratect 10g/100ml solution for infusion vials | 1 vial PoM £382.50
Intratect 20g/200ml solution for infusion vials | 1 vial PoM £765.00
Intratect 5g/50ml solution for infusion vials | 1 vial PoM £191.25
Intratect 1g/10ml solution for infusion vials | 1 vial PoM £38.25

▸ **Kiovig** (Baxalta UK Ltd)
Normal immunoglobulin human 100 mg per 1 ml Kiovig 5g/50ml solution for infusion vials | 1 vial PoM no price available
Kiovig 20g/200ml solution for infusion vials | 1 vial PoM no price available
Kiovig 10g/100ml solution for infusion vials | 1 vial PoM no price available
Kiovig 2.5g/25ml solution for infusion vials | 1 vial PoM no price available
Kiovig 1g/10ml solution for infusion vials | 1 vial PoM no price available

▸ **Octagam** (Octapharma Ltd)
Normal immunoglobulin human 50 mg per 1 ml Octagam 5% 10g/200ml solution for infusion bottles | 1 bottle PoM £408.00 (Hospital only)
Octagam 5% 5g/100ml solution for infusion bottles | 1 bottle PoM £204.00 (Hospital only)
Octagam 5% 2.5g/50ml solution for infusion bottles | 1 bottle PoM £102.00 (Hospital only)
Normal immunoglobulin human 100 mg per 1 ml Octagam 10% 20g/200ml solution for infusion bottles | 1 bottle PoM £1,173.00 (Hospital only)
Octagam 10% 5g/50ml solution for infusion bottles | 1 bottle PoM £293.25 (Hospital only)
Octagam 10% 10g/100ml solution for infusion bottles | 1 bottle PoM £586.50 (Hospital only)
Octagam 10% 2g/20ml solution for infusion vials | 1 vial PoM £117.30 (Hospital only)

▸ **Privigen** (CSL Behring UK Ltd)
Normal immunoglobulin human 100 mg per 1 ml Privigen 5g/50ml solution for infusion vials | 1 vial PoM £229.50
Privigen 10g/100ml solution for infusion vials | 1 vial PoM £459.00
Privigen 20g/200ml solution for infusion vials | 1 vial PoM £918.00
Privigen 2.5g/25ml solution for infusion vials | 1 vial PoM £114.75

▸ **Vigam** (Bio Products Laboratory Ltd)
Normal immunoglobulin human 50 mg per 1 ml Vigam Liquid 5g/100ml solution for infusion vials | 1 vial PoM £209.00
Vigam Liquid 10g/200ml solution for infusion vials | 1 vial PoM £418.00

Rabies immunoglobulin

● **INDICATIONS AND DOSE**

Post-exposure prophylaxis against rabies infection
▸ BY LOCAL INFILTRATION, OR BY INTRAMUSCULAR INJECTION
▸ Child: 20 units/kg, dose administered by infiltration in and around the cleansed wound; if the wound not visible or healed or if infiltration of whole volume not possible, give remainder by intramuscular injection into anterolateral thigh (remote from vaccination site)

● **CAUTIONS** IgA deficiency · interference with live virus vaccines

● **SIDE-EFFECTS**
▸ **Rare** Anaphylaxis · arthralgia · buccal ulceration · chest tightness · dizziness · dyspnoea · glossitis · tremor
▸ **Frequency not known** Facial oedema · injection site pain · injection site swelling

● **PRESCRIBING AND DISPENSING INFORMATION** The potency of individual batches of rabies immunoglobulin from the manufacturer may vary; potency may also be described differently by different manufacturers. It is therefore critical to know the potency of the batch to be used and the weight of the patient in order to calculate the specific volume required to provide the necessary dose.
 Available from Specialist and Reference Microbiology Division, Public Health England (also from BPL).

● **HANDLING AND STORAGE** Care must be taken to store all immunological products under the conditions recommended in the product literature, otherwise the preparation may become ineffective. **Refrigerated storage** is usually necessary; many immunoglobulins need to be stored at 2–8°C and not allowed to freeze. Immunoglobulins should be protected from light. Opened multidose vials must be used within the period recommended in the product literature.

● **MEDICINAL FORMS**
There can be variation in the licensing of different medicines containing the same drug.
Solution for injection
▸ Rabies immunoglobulin (Non-proprietary)
 Rabies immunoglobulin human 500 unit Rabies immunoglobulin human 500unit solution for injection vials | 1 vial PoM £412.13

Tetanus immunoglobulin

● **INDICATIONS AND DOSE**

Post-exposure prophylaxis
▸ BY INTRAMUSCULAR INJECTION
▸ Child: Initially 250 units, then increased to 500 units, dose is only increased if more than 24 hours have elapsed or there is risk of heavy contamination or following burns

Treatment of tetanus infection
▸ BY INTRAMUSCULAR INJECTION
▸ Child: 150 units/kg, dose may be given over multiple sites

● **CAUTIONS** IgA deficiency · interference with live virus vaccines

● **SIDE-EFFECTS**
▸ **Rare** Anaphylaxis · arthralgia · buccal ulceration · chest tightness · dizziness · dyspnoea · glossitis · tremor
▸ **Frequency not known** Facial oedema · injection site swelling · pain at injection site

● **HANDLING AND STORAGE** Care must be taken to store all immunological products under the conditions recommended in the product literature, otherwise the preparation may become ineffective. **Refrigerated storage** is usually necessary; many immunoglobulins need

14

Vaccines

to be stored at 2–8°C and not allowed to freeze. Immunoglobulins should be protected from light. Opened multidose vials must be used within the period recommended in the product literature.

- **MEDICINAL FORMS**
There can be variation in the licensing of different medicines containing the same drug.
Solution for injection
  ▸ Tetanus immunoglobulin (Non-proprietary)
  Tetanus immunoglobulin human 250 unit Tetanus immunoglobulin human 250unit solution for injection vials | 1 vial PoM £45.00

Varicella-zoster immunoglobulin

(Antivaricella-zoster Immunoglobulin)

- **INDICATIONS AND DOSE**
Prophylaxis against varicella infection
  ▸ BY DEEP INTRAMUSCULAR INJECTION

  ▸ Neonate: 250 mg, to be administered as soon as possible—not later than 10 days after exposure, second dose to be given if further exposure occurs more than 3 weeks after first dose, no evidence that effective in severe disease

  ▸ Child 1 month–5 years: 250 mg, to be administered as soon as possible—not later than 10 days after exposure, second dose to be given if further exposure occurs more than 3 weeks after first dose, no evidence that effective in severe disease

  ▸ Child 6–10 years: 500 mg, to be administered as soon as possible—not later than 10 days after exposure, second dose to be given if further exposure occurs more than 3 weeks after first dose, no evidence that effective in severe disease

  ▸ Child 11–14 years: 750 mg, to be administered as soon as possible—not later than 10 days after exposure, second dose to be given if further exposure occurs more than 3 weeks after first dose, no evidence that effective in severe disease

  ▸ Child 15–17 years: 1 g, to be administered as soon as possible—not later than 10 days after exposure, second dose to be given if further exposure occurs more than 3 weeks after first dose, no evidence that effective in severe disease

- **CAUTIONS** IgA deficiency · interference with live virus vaccines
- **SIDE-EFFECTS**
  ▸ **Rare** Anaphylaxis
  ▸ **Frequency not known** Injection site pain · injection site swelling
- **DIRECTIONS FOR ADMINISTRATION** Normal immunoglobulin for intravenous use may be used in those unable to receive intramuscular injections.
- **PRESCRIBING AND DISPENSING INFORMATION** Available from selected Public Health England and NHS laboratories (also from BPL).
- **HANDLING AND STORAGE** Care must be taken to store all immunological products under the conditions recommended in the product literature, otherwise the preparation may become ineffective. **Refrigerated storage** is usually necessary; many immunoglobulins need to be stored at 2–8°C and not allowed to freeze. Immunoglobulins should be protected from light. Opened multidose vials must be used within the period recommended in the product literature.

- **MEDICINAL FORMS**
There can be variation in the licensing of different medicines containing the same drug.
Solution for injection
  ▸ Varicella-Zoster (Bio Products Laboratory Ltd)
  Varicella-Zoster immunoglobulin human 250 mg Varicella-Zoster immunoglobulin human 250mg solution for injection vials | 1 vial PoM £350.00

2   Post-exposure prophylaxis

IMMUNE SERA AND IMMUNOGLOBULINS ›
ANTITOXINS

Botulism antitoxin

- **DRUG ACTION** A preparation containing the specific antitoxic globulins that have the power of neutralising the toxins formed by types A, B, and E of *Clostridium botulinum*.

- **INDICATIONS AND DOSE**
Post exposure prophylaxis of botulism
  ▸ BY INTRAMUSCULAR INJECTION
  ▸ Child: (consult product literature)

- **SIDE-EFFECTS** Hypersensitivity reactions
  SIDE-EFFECTS, FURTHER INFORMATION
  ▸ Hypersensitivity reactions It is essential to read the contra-indications, warnings, and details of sensitivity tests on the package insert. Prior to treatment checks should be made regarding previous administration of any antitoxin and history of any allergic condition, e.g. asthma, hay fever, etc.

- **PRE-TREATMENT SCREENING** All patients should be tested for sensitivity (diluting the antitoxin if history of allergy).

- **PRESCRIBING AND DISPENSING INFORMATION** Available from local designated centres, for details see TOXBASE (requires registration) www.toxbase.org. For supplies outside working hours apply to other designated centres or to the Public Health England Colindale duty doctor (Tel (020) 8200 6868). For major incidents, obtain supplies from the local blood bank.
The BP title Botulinum Antitoxin is not used because the preparation currently in use may have a different specification.

- **MEDICINAL FORMS**
There can be variation in the licensing of different medicines containing the same drug.
Solution for infusion
  ▸ Botulism-antitoxin (Novartis Vaccines and Diagnostics Ltd)
  Botulism antitoxin type E 50 unit per 1 ml, Botulism antitoxin type B 500 unit per 1 ml, Botulinum antitoxin type A 750 unit per 1 ml Botulism-Antitoxin Behring 25g/250ml solution for infusion bottles | 1 bottle PoM no price available

Diphtheria antitoxin

(Dip/Ser)

- **INDICATIONS AND DOSE**
Passive immunisation in suspected cases of diphtheria
  ▸ BY INTRAVENOUS INFUSION
  ▸ Child: Dose should be given without waiting for bacteriological confirmation (consult product literature)

CAUTIONS, FURTHER INFORMATION
▸ Hypersensitivity Hypersensitivity is common after administration; resuscitation facilities should be available. Diphtheria antitoxin is no longer used for prophylaxis because of the risk of hypersensitivity; unimmunised contacts should be promptly investigated and given antibacterial prophylaxis and vaccine.

● **SIDE-EFFECTS**
● Common or very common Hypersensitivity reactions
● **PRE-TREATMENT SCREENING** Diphtheria antitoxin is derived from horse serum and reactions are common; tests for hypersensitivity should be carried out before use.

● **PRESCRIBING AND DISPENSING INFORMATION** Available from Centre for Infections (Tel (020) 8200 6868) or in Northern Ireland from Public Health Laboratory, Belfast City Hospital (Tel (028) 9032 9241).

● **MEDICINAL FORMS**
There can be variation in the licensing of different medicines containing the same drug.

Solution for injection
▸ Diphtheria antitoxin (Non-proprietary)
  Diphtheria antitoxin 1000 unit per 1 ml Antidiphtheria serum 10,000units/10ml solution for injection ampoules | 1 ampoule PoM no price available

---

3   Tuberculosis diagnostic test

DIAGNOSTIC AGENTS

Tuberculin purified protein derivative

(Tuberculin PPD)

● **INDICATIONS AND DOSE**

Mantoux test
▸ BY INTRADERMAL INJECTION
▸ Child: 2 units for one dose

Mantoux test (if first test is negative and a further test is considered appropriate)
▸ BY INTRADERMAL INJECTION
▸ Child: 10 units for 1 dose

DOSE EQUIVALENCE AND CONVERSION
2 units is equivalent to 0.1 mL of 20 units/mL strength.
10 units is equivalent to 0.1 mL of 100 units/mL strength.

● **CAUTIONS**

CAUTIONS, FURTHER INFORMATION
▸ Mantoux test Response to tuberculin may be suppressed by viral infection, sarcoidosis, corticosteroid therapy, or immunosuppression due to disease or treatment and the MMR vaccine. If a tuberculin skin test has already been initiated, then the MMR should be delayed until the skin test has been read unless protection against measles is required urgently. If a child has had a recent MMR, and requires a tuberculin test, then a 4 week interval should be observed. Apart from tuberculin and MMR, all other live vaccines can be administered at any time before or after tuberculin.

● **PRESCRIBING AND DISPENSING INFORMATION** Available from ImmForm (SSI brand). The strength of tuberculin PPD in currently available products may be different to the strengths of products used previously for the Mantoux test; care is required to select the correct strength.

● **MEDICINAL FORMS**
There can be variation in the licensing of different medicines containing the same drug. Forms available from special-order manufacturers include: solution for injection
Solution for injection
▸ Tuberculin purified protein derivative (Non-proprietary)
  Tuberculin purified protein derivative 20 tuberculin unit per 1 ml Tuberculin PPD RT 23 SSI 20 tuberculin units/ml solution for injection 1.5ml vials | 1 vial no price available
  Tuberculin purified protein derivative 100 tuberculin unit per 1 ml Tuberculin PPD RT 23 SSI 100 tuberculin units/ml solution for injection 1.5ml vials | 1 vial no price available

---

4   Vaccination

Vaccines

Active immunity

Active immunity can be acquired by natural disease or by vaccination. **Vaccines** stimulate production of antibodies and other components of the immune mechanism; they consist of either:

- a *live attenuated* form of a virus (e.g. measles, mumps and rubella vaccine) or bacteria (e.g. BCG vaccine), or
- *inactivated* preparations of the virus (e.g. influenza vaccine) or bacteria, or
- *detoxified exotoxins* produced by a micro-organism (e.g. tetanus vaccine), or
- *extracts of* a micro-organism, which may be derived from the organism (e.g. pneumococcal vaccine) or produced by recombinant DNA technology (e.g. hepatitis B vaccine).

Live attenuated vaccines usually produce a durable immunity, but not always as long-lasting as that resulting from natural infection.

Inactivated vaccines may require a primary series of injections of vaccine to produce an adequate antibody response, and in most cases booster (reinforcing) injections are required; the duration of immunity varies from months to many years. Some inactivated vaccines are adsorbed onto an adjuvant (such as aluminium hydroxide) to enhance the antibody response.

Advice reflects that in the handbook *Immunisation against Infectious Disease*, (2013) which in turn reflects the guidance of the Joint Committee on Vaccination and Immunisation (JCVI).

Chapters from the handbook are available at www.immunisation.dh.gov.uk

The advice also incorporates changes announced by the Chief Medical Officer and Health Department Updates.

Children with unknown or incomplete immunisation history

For children born in the UK who present with an inadequate or unknown immunisation history, investigation into immunisations received should be carried out. Outstanding doses should be administered where the routine childhood immunisation schedule has not been completed.

For advice on the immunisation of children coming to the UK, consult the handbook *Immunisation against Infectious Disease* (2006) (available at www.dh.gov.uk).

Immunisation schedule

Vaccines for the childhood immunisation schedule should be obtained from **local health organisations** or from **ImmForm** (www.immform.dh.gov.uk)—not to be prescribed on FP10 (HS21 in Northern Ireland; GP10 in Scotland; WP10 in Wales).

14

Vaccines

Routine immunisation schedule

When to immunise (for preterm infants-see note below)	Vaccine given and dose schedule (for details of dose, see under individual vaccines)
Neonates at risk only	▸ Bacillus calmette-guérin vaccine p. 744 ▸ Hepatitis B vaccine p. 750
2 months	▸ Diphtheria with haemophilus influenzae type b vaccine, pertussis, poliomyelitis and tetanus p. 743 First dose ▸ Meningococcal group B vaccine (rDNA, component, adsorbed) p. 746 First dose ▸ Pneumococcal polysaccharide conjugate vaccine (adsorbed) p. 747 First dose ▸ Rotavirus vaccine p. 754 First dose
3 months	▸ Diphtheria with haemophilus influenzae type b vaccine, pertussis, poliomyelitis and tetanus p. 743 Second dose ▸ Meningococcal group C vaccine p. 746 First dose ▸ Rotavirus vaccine p. 754 Second dose
4 months	▸ Diphtheria with haemophilus influenzae type b vaccine, pertussis, poliomyelitis and tetanus p. 743 Third dose ▸ Meningococcal group B vaccine (rDNA, component, adsorbed) p. 746 Second dose ▸ Pneumococcal polysaccharide conjugate vaccine (adsorbed) p. 747 Second dose
12-13 months	▸ Measles, mumps and rubella vaccine, live p. 753 First dose ▸ Meningococcal group B vaccine (rDNA, component, adsorbed) p. 746 Single booster dose ▸ Pneumococcal polysaccharide conjugate vaccine (adsorbed) p. 747 Single booster dose ▸ Haemophilus influenzae type B with meningococcal group C vaccine p. 745 Single booster dose
2-6 years (including children in school years 1 and 2)	▸ Influenza vaccine p. 752 Each year from September **Note:** Flu nasal spray is recommended (*Fluenz Tetra*®). If contra-indicated and child is in clinical risk group, use inactivated flu vaccine
Between 3 years and 4 months, and 5 years	▸ Diphtheria with pertussis, poliomyelitis vaccine and tetanus p. 743 Single booster dose. **Note:** Preferably allow interval of at least 3 years after completing primary course ▸ Measles, mumps and rubella vaccine, live p. 753 Second dose
11-14 years (females only). First dose of HPV vaccine will be offered to females aged 12-13 years of age in England, Wales, and Northern Ireland, and 11-14 years of age in Scotland.	▸ Human papillomavirus vaccine 2 doses; second dose 12 months after first dose. If a 3-dose course of HPV vaccine has been started under the 2013/2014 programme, where possible, the course should be completed. The two human papillomavirus vaccines are not interchangeable and, ideally, one vaccine product should be used for the entire course. However, for those females who started the schedule with *Cervarix*® under the national immunisation programme, but did not complete the vaccination course, the course can be completed with *Gardasil*®.
13-15 years	▸ Meningococcal groups A with C and W135 and Y vaccine p. 746 Single booster dose
13-18 years	▸ Diphtheria with poliomyelitis and tetanus vaccine p. 744 Single booster dose. **Note:** Can be given at the same time as the booster dose of meningococcal group A with C and W135 and Y vaccine at 13-15 years of age
During adult life, women of child-bearing age susceptible to rubella	▸ Measles, mumps and rubella vaccine, live p. 753 Women of child-bearing age who have not received 2 doses of a rubella-containing vaccine or who do not have a positive antibody test for rubella should be offered rubella immunisation (using the MMR vaccine)—exclude pregnancy before immunisation.

For the most up to date immunisation schedule consult 'The complete routine immunisation schedule', available at www.gov.uk.

Preterm birth
Babies born preterm should receive all routine immunisations based on their actual date of birth. The risk of apnoea following vaccination is increased in preterm babies, particularly in those born at or before 28 weeks postmenstrual age. If babies at risk of apnoea are in hospital at the time of their first immunisation, they should be monitored for 48 hours after immunisation. If a baby develops apnoea, bradycardia, or desaturation after the first immunisation, the second immunisation should also be given in hospital with similar monitoring. Seroconversion may be unreliable in babies born earlier than 28 weeks' gestation or in babies treated with corticosteroids for chronic lung disease; consideration should be given to testing for antibodies against Haemophilus influenzae type b, meningococcal C, and hepatitis B after primary immunisation.

Vaccines and HIV infection
HIV-positive children with or without symptoms can receive the following live vaccines:

- MMR (but avoid if immunity significantly impaired), varicella-zoster vaccine against chickenpox (but avoid if immunity significantly impaired—consult product literature; use of normal immunoglobulin should be considered after exposure to measles and varicella–zoster immunoglobulin considered after exposure to chickenpox or herpes zoster), rotavirus;

and the following inactivated vaccines:

- Anthrax, cholera (oral), diphtheria, haemophilus influenzae type b, hepatitis A, hepatitis B, human papillomavirus, influenza (injection), meningococcal, pertussis, pneumococcal, poliomyelitis (inactivated poliomyelitis vaccine is now used instead of oral poliomyelitis vaccine for routine immunisation of children), rabies, tetanus, tick-borne encephalitis, typhoid (injection).

HIV-positive children should **not** receive:

- BCG, influenza nasal spray (unless stable HIV infection and receiving antiretroviral therapy), typhoid (oral), yellow fever (if yellow fever risk is unavoidable, specialist advice should be sought).

The above advice differs from that for other immunocompromised patients; *Immunisation of HIV infected Children* issued by *Children's HIV Association* (CHIVA) are available at www.chiva.org.uk.

Vaccines and asplenia

The following vaccines are recommended for asplenic patients, those with splenic dysfunction or complement disorders, depending on the age at which their condition is diagnosed:

- Haemophilus influenzae type B with meningococcal group C vaccine;
- Influenza vaccine;
- Meningococcal groups A with C and W135 and Y vaccine;
- pneumococcal polysaccharide vaccine.

Children first diagnosed under 2 years of age should be vaccinated according to the Immunisation Schedule, including the 12 month boosters. If meningococcal group C vaccine p. 746 has not yet been given as part of routine schedule, give one dose of meningococcal groups A with C and W135 and Y vaccine p. 746 followed by a second dose at least one month apart. If meningococcal group C vaccine has already been given as part of routine schedule, then give one additional dose of meningococcal groups A with C and W135 and Y vaccine at least one month later. Following routine 12 month booster vaccines, give a dose of meningococcal groups A with C and W135 and Y vaccine and an additional dose of 13-valent pneumococcal polysaccharide vaccine 2 months later. An additional dose of haemophilus influenzae type B with meningococcal group C vaccine p. 745 and 23-valent pneumococcal polysaccharide vaccine should be given after the second birthday. The influenza vaccine should be administered annually in children aged 6 months or older.

Children first diagnosed over 2 years of age should be vaccinated according to the Immunisation schedule, including the 12 month boosters. The child should receive one additional booster dose of haemophilus influenzae type B with meningococcal group C vaccine along with the 23-valent pneumococcal polysaccharide vaccine, followed by one dose of meningococcal groups A with C and W135 and Y vaccine after 2 months. The influenza vaccine should be administered annually.

Passive immunity

Immunity with immediate protection against certain infective organisms can be obtained by injecting preparations made from the plasma of immune individuals with adequate levels of antibody to the disease for which protection is sought (see under Immunoglobulins). The duration of this passive immunity varies according to the dose and the type of immunoglobulin. Passive immunity may last only a few weeks; when necessary, passive immunisation can be repeated.

Antibodies of human origin are usually termed *immunoglobulins*. The term *antiserum* is applied to material prepared in animals. Because of serum sickness and other allergic-type reactions that may follow injections of antisera, this therapy has been replaced whenever possible by the use of immunoglobulins. Reactions are theoretically possible after injection of human immunoglobulins, but reports of such reactions are very rare.

Vaccines and antisera availability

Anthrax vaccine and yellow fever vaccine, live p. 756, botulism antitoxin p. 730, diphtheria antitoxin p. 730, and snake and spider venom antitoxins are available from local designated holding centres.

For antivenom, see Emergency Treatment of Poisoning.

Enquiries for vaccines not available commercially can also be made to:

Vaccines and Countermeasures Response Department
Public Health England
Wellington House
133–155 Waterloo Road
London
SE1 8UG
vaccinesupply@phe.gov.uk

In Scotland information about availability of vaccines can be obtained from a Specialist in Pharmaceutical Public Health.

In Wales enquiries for vaccines not available commercially should be directed to:

Welsh Medicines Information Centre
University Hospital of Wales
Cardiff
CF14 4XW
(029) 2074 2979

In Northern Ireland:

Pharmacy and Medicines Management Centre
Northern Health and Social Care Trust
Beech House
Antrim Hospital Site
Bush Road
Antrim
BT41 2RL
rphps.admin@northerntrust.hscni.net

For further details of availability, see under individual vaccines.

Anthrax vaccine

Anthrax vaccine is rarely required for children.

BCG vaccine

BCG (bacillus calmette-guérin vaccine p. 744) is a live attenuated strain derived from *Mycobacterium bovis* which stimulates the development of hypersensitivity to *M. tuberculosis*. Bacillus calmette-guérin vaccine should be given intradermally by operators skilled in the technique.

The expected reaction to successful bacillus calmette-guérin vaccine is induration at the site of injection followed by a local lesion which starts as a papule 2 or more weeks after vaccination; the lesion may ulcerate then subside over several weeks or months, leaving a small flat scar. A dry dressing may be used if the ulcer discharges, but air should **not** be excluded.

All children of 6 years and over being considered for bacillus calmette-guérin vaccine must first be given a skin test for hypersensitivity to tuberculoprotein (see under Diagnostic agents). A skin test is not necessary for a child under 6 years, provided that the child has not stayed for longer than 3 months in a country with an incidence of tuberculosis greater than 40 per 100 000 (a list of countries or primary care trusts where the incidence of tuberculosis is greater than 40 cases per 100 000 is available at www.gov.uk/phe), the child has not had contact with a person with tuberculosis, and there is no family history of tuberculosis within the last 5 years.

Bacillus calmette-guérin vaccine is recommended for the following groups of children if BCG immunisation has not previously been carried out and they are negative for tuberculoprotein hypersensitivity:

- neonates with a family history of tuberculosis in the last 5 years;
- all neonates and infants (0–12 months) born in areas where the incidence of tuberculosis is greater than 40 per 100 000;
- neonates, infants, and children under 16 years with a parent or grandparent born in a country with an incidence of tuberculosis greater than 40 per 100 000;
- new immigrants aged under 16 years who were born in, or lived for more than 3 months in a country with an incidence of tuberculosis greater than 40 per 100 000;

- new immigrants aged 16–18 years from Sub-Saharan Africa or a country with an incidence of tuberculosis greater than 500 per 100 000;
- contacts of those with active respiratory tuberculosis;
- children under 16 years intending to live with local people for more than 3 months in a country with an incidence of tuberculosis greater than 40 per 100 000.

Bacillus calmette-guérin vaccine can be given simultaneously with another live vaccine, but if they are not given at the same time, an interval of 4 weeks should normally be allowed between them. When bacillus calmette-guérin vaccine is given to infants, there is no need to delay routine primary immunisations. No further vaccination should be given in the arm used for BCG vaccination for at least 3 months because of the risk of regional lymphadenitis.

For advice on chemoprophylaxis against tuberculosis; for treatment of infection following vaccination, seek expert advice.

Tuberculosis Diagnostic Agents

The *Mantoux test* is recommended for tuberculin skin testing, but no licensed preparation is currently available. Guidance for healthcare professionals is available at www.dh.gov.uk/immunisation.

In the Mantoux test, the diagnostic dose is administered by intradermal injection of Tuberculin Purified Protein Derivative (PPD).

The *Heaf test* (involving the use of multiple-puncture apparatus) is no longer available.

Two interferon gamma release assay (IGRA) tests are also available as an aid in the diagnosis of tuberculosis infection: *QuantiFERON® TB Gold* and *T-SPOT®.TB*. Both tests measure T-cell mediated immune response to synthetic antigens. For further information on the use of interferon gamma release assay tests for tuberculosis, see www.gov.uk/phe.

Botulism antitoxin

A polyvalent botulism antitoxin p. 730 is available for the post-exposure prophylaxis of botulism and for the treatment of persons thought to be suffering from botulism. It specifically neutralises the toxins produced by *Clostridium botulinum* types A, B, and E. It is not effective against infantile botulism as the toxin (type A) is seldom, if ever, found in the blood in this type of infection.

Hypersensitivity reactions are a problem. It is essential to read the contra-indications, warnings, and details of sensitivity tests on the package insert. Prior to treatment checks should be made regarding previous administration of any antitoxin and history of any allergic condition, e.g. asthma, hay fever, etc. All patients should be tested for sensitivity (diluting the antitoxin if history of allergy).

Cholera vaccine

Cholera vaccine p. 745 (oral) contains inactivated Inaba (including El-Tor biotype) and Ogawa strains of *Vibrio cholerae*, serotype O1 together with recombinant B-subunit of the cholera toxin produced in Inaba strains of *V.cholerae*, serotype O1.

Oral cholera vaccine is licensed for travellers to endemic or epidemic areas on the basis of current recommendations. Immunisation should be completed at least 1 week before potential exposure. However, there is no requirement for cholera vaccination for international travel.

Immunisation with cholera vaccine does not provide complete protection and all travellers to a country where cholera exists should be warned that scrupulous attention to food, water, and personal hygiene is **essential**.

Injectable cholera vaccine provides unreliable protection and is no longer available in the UK.

Diphtheria vaccine

Diphtheria vaccines are prepared from the toxin of *Corynebacterium diphtheriae* and adsorption on aluminium hydroxide or aluminium phosphate improves antigenicity. The vaccine stimulates the production of the protective antitoxin. The quantity of diphtheria toxoid in a preparation determines whether the vaccine is defined as 'high dose' or 'low dose'. Vaccines containing the higher dose of diphtheria toxoid are used for primary immunisation of children under 10 years of age. Vaccines containing the lower dose of diphtheria toxoid are used for primary immunisation in adults and children over 10 years. Single-antigen diphtheria vaccine is not available and adsorbed diphtheria vaccine is given as a combination product containing other vaccines.

For primary immunisation *of children aged between 2 months and 10 years* vaccination is recommended usually in the form of 3 doses (separated by 1-month intervals) of **diphtheria, tetanus, pertussis (acellular, component), poliomyelitis (inactivated) and haemophilus type b conjugate vaccine (adsorbed)** (see Immunisation schedule). In unimmunised individuals aged *over 10 years* the primary course comprises of 3 doses of **adsorbed diphtheria** [low dose], **tetanus and poliomyelitis (inactivated) vaccine**.

A booster dose should be given 3 years after the primary course (this interval can be reduced to a minimum of 1 year if the primary course was delayed). Children *under 10 years* should receive *either* **adsorbed diphtheria, tetanus, pertussis (acellular, component) and poliomyelitis (inactivated) vaccine** *or* **adsorbed diphtheria** [low dose], **tetanus, pertussis (acellular, component) and poliomyelitis (inactivated) vaccine**. Individuals aged *over 10 years* should receive **adsorbed diphtheria** [low dose], **tetanus, and poliomyelitis (inactivated) vaccine**.

A second booster dose, of adsorbed diphtheria [low dose], tetanus and poliomyelitis (inactivated) vaccine, should be given 10 years after the previous booster dose (this interval can be reduced to a minimum of 5 years if previous doses were delayed). For children who have been vaccinated following a tetanus-prone wound, see tetanus vaccines.

Travel

Those intending to travel to areas with a risk of diphtheria infection should be fully immunised according to the UK schedule. If more than 10 years have lapsed since completion of the UK schedule, a dose of **adsorbed diphtheria** [low dose], **tetanus and poliomyelitis (inactivated) vaccine** should be administered.

Contacts

Advice on the management of cases of diphtheria, carriers, contacts and outbreaks must be sought from health protection units. The immunisation history of infected children and their contacts should be determined; those who have been incompletely immunised should complete their immunisation and fully immunised individuals should receive a reinforcing dose. Also see advice on antibacterial treatment to prevent a secondary case of diphtheria in a non-immune child.

Haemophilus influenzae type B conjugate vaccine

Haemophilus influenzae type b (Hib) vaccine is made from capsular polysaccharide; it is conjugated with a protein such as tetanus toxoid to increase immunogenicity, especially in young children. Haemophilus influenzae type b vaccine immunisation is given in combination with diphtheria, tetanus, pertussis (acellular, component) and poliomyelitis (inactivated) vaccine, as a component of the primary course of childhood immunisation (see Immunisation schedule) (see under Diphtheria-containing Vaccines). For infants under 1 year, the course consists of 3 doses of a vaccine containing *Haemophilus influenzae* type b component with an interval of 1 month between doses. A booster dose of haemophilus influenzae type b vaccine (combined with meningococcal group C conjugate vaccine) should be given at 12–13 months of age.

Children 1–10 years who have not been immunised against *Haemophilus influenzae* type b need to receive only 1 dose of Haemophilus influenzae type b vaccine (combined with meningococcal group C conjugate vaccine). However, if a primary course of immunisation has not been completed, these children should be given 3 doses of diphtheria with haemophilus influenzae type b vaccine, pertussis, poliomyelitis and tetanus p. 743. The risk of infection falls sharply in older children and the vaccine is not normally required for children over 10 years.

Haemophilus influenzae type b vaccine may be given to those over 10 years who are considered to be at increased risk of invasive *H. influenzae* type b disease (such as those with sickle-cell disease or complement deficiency, or those receiving treatment for malignancy).

Invasive *Haemophilus influenzae* type b disease

After recovery from infection, unimmunised and partially immunised index cases under 10 years of age should complete their age-specific course of immunisation. Previously vaccinated cases under 10 years of age should be given an additional dose of haemophilus influenzae type b vaccine (combined with meningococcal group C conjugate vaccine) if Hib antibody concentrations are low or if it is not possible to measure antibody concentrations. Index cases of any age with asplenia or splenic dysfunction should complete their immunisation according to the recommendations below; fully vaccinated cases with asplenia or splenic dysfunction should be given an additional dose of haemophilus influenzae type b vaccine (combined with meningococcal group C conjugate vaccine) if they received their previous dose over 1 year ago.

Also see use of rifampicin p. 342 in the prevention of secondary cases of *Haemophilus influenzae* type b disease.

Hepatitis A vaccine

Hepatitis A vaccine p. 749 is prepared from formaldehyde-inactivated hepatitis A virus grown in human diploid cells.

Immunisation is recommended for:

- residents of homes for those with severe learning difficulties;
- children with haemophilia or other conditions treated with plasma-derived clotting factors;
- children with severe liver disease;
- children travelling to high-risk areas;
- adolescents who are at risk due to their sexual behaviour;
- parenteral drug abusers.

Immunisation should be considered for:

- children with chronic liver disease including chronic hepatitis B or chronic hepatitis C;
- prevention of secondary cases in close contacts of confirmed cases of hepatitis A, within 14 days of exposure to the primary case (within 8 weeks of exposure to the primary case where there is more than 1 contact in the household).

A booster dose of hepatitis A vaccine is usually given 6–12 months after the initial dose. A second booster dose can be given 20 years after the previous booster dose to those who continue to be at risk. Specialist advice should be sought on re-immunisation of immunocompromised individuals.

In children under 16 years, a single dose of the combined vaccine *Ambirix*® can be used to provide rapid protection against hepatitis A. Intramuscular normal immunoglobulin p. 727 is recommended for use in addition to hepatitis A vaccine for close contacts (of confirmed cases of hepatitis A) who have chronic liver disease or HIV infection, or who are immunosuppressed.

Post-exposure prophylaxis is not required for healthy children under 1 year of age, so long as all those involved in nappy changing are vaccinated against hepatitis A. However, children 2–12 months of age can be given a dose of hepatitis A vaccine if it is not possible to vaccinate their carers, or if the child becomes a source of infection to others [unlicensed use]; in these cases, if the child goes on to require long-term protection against hepatitis A after the first birthday, the full course of 2 doses should be given.

Hepatitis B vaccine

Hepatitis B vaccine p. 750 contains inactivated hepatitis B virus surface antigen (HBsAg) adsorbed on to aluminium hydroxide adjuvant. It is made biosynthetically using recombinant DNA technology. The vaccine is used in individuals at high risk of contracting hepatitis B.

In the UK, high-risk groups include:

- parenteral drug misusers, their sexual partners, and household contacts; other drug misusers who are likely to 'progress' to injecting;
- adolescents who are at risk from their sexual behaviour;
- close family contacts of an individual with chronic hepatitis B infection;
- babies whose mothers have had acute hepatitis B during pregnancy or are positive for hepatitis B surface antigen (regardless of e-antigen markers); hepatitis B vaccination is started immediately on delivery and *hepatitis B immunoglobulin* given at the same time (but at a different site). Babies whose mothers are positive for hepatitis B surface antigen and for e-antigen antibody should receive the vaccine only (but babies weighing 1.5 kg or less should also receive the immunoglobulin regardless of the mother's e-antigen antibody status);
- children with haemophilia, those receiving regular blood transfusions or blood products, and carers responsible for the administration of such products;
- children with chronic renal failure including those on haemodialysis. Children receiving haemodialysis should be monitored for antibodies annually and re-immunised if necessary. Home carers (of dialysis patients) should be vaccinated;
- children with chronic liver disease
- patients of day-care or residential accommodation for those with severe learning difficulties;
- children in custodial institutions;
- children travelling to areas of high or intermediate prevalence who are at increased risk or who plan to remain there for lengthy periods;
- families adopting children from countries with a high or intermediate prevalence of hepatitis B;
- foster carers and their families.

Different immunisation schedules for hepatitis B vaccine are recommended for specific circumstances; an 'accelerated schedule' is recommended for pre-exposure prophylaxis in high–risk groups where rapid protection is required, and for post-exposure prophylaxis. Generally, three or four doses are required for primary immunisation. Immunisation may take up to 6 months to confer adequate protection; the duration of immunity is not known precisely, but a single booster 5 years after the primary course may be sufficient to maintain immunity for those who continue to be at risk.

Immunisation does not eliminate the need for commonsense precautions for avoiding the risk of infection from known carriers by the routes of infection which have been clearly established, consult *Guidance for Clinical Health Care Workers: Protection against Infection with Blood-borne Viruses* (available at www.dh.gov.uk). Accidental inoculation of hepatitis B virus-infected blood into a wound, incision, needle-prick, or abrasion may lead to infection, whereas it is unlikely that indirect exposure to a carrier will do so.

Following significant exposure to hepatitis B, an accelerated schedule, with the second dose given 1 month, and the third dose 2 months after the initial dose, is recommended. For those at continued risk, a fourth dose

14

Vaccines

should be given 12 months after the first dose. More detailed guidance is given in the *Immunisation against Infectious Disease* handbook.

Specific hepatitis B immunoglobulin ('HBIG') p. 727 is available for use with the vaccine in those accidentally inoculated and in neonates at special risk of infection.

A combined hepatitis A and B vaccine p. 748 is also available.

Human papillomavirus vaccine

Human papillomavirus vaccine is available as a bivalent vaccine (*Cervarix*®) or a quadrivalent vaccine (*Gardasil*®). *Cervarix*® is licensed for use in females for the prevention of cervical cancer and other pre-cancerous lesions caused by human papillomavirus types 16 and 18. *Gardasil*® is licensed for use in females for the prevention of cervical and anal cancers, genital warts and pre-cancerous genital (cervical, vulvar, and vaginal) and anal lesions caused by human papillomavirus types 6, 11, 16, and 18. The vaccines may also provide limited protection against disease caused by other types of human papillomavirus. The two vaccines are not interchangeable and one vaccine product should be used for an entire course.

Human papillomavirus vaccine will be most effective if given before sexual activity starts. From September 2014, a 2-dose schedule is recommended, as long as the first dose is received before the age of 15 years. The first dose is given to females aged 11 to 14 years, and the second dose is given 6-24 months after the first dose (for the purposes of planning the national immunisation programme, it is appropriate to give the second dose 12 months after the first—see Immunisation schedule). If the course is interrupted, it should be resumed (using the same vaccine) but not repeated, even if more than 24 months have elapsed since the first dose or if the girl is then aged 15 years or more. Females aged 15 years or older require a 3-dose schedule (see *Cervarix*® and *Gardasil*®), with the second and third doses given 1 and 4–6 months after the first dose; all 3 doses should be given within a 12-month period. If the course is interrupted, it should be resumed (using the same vaccine) but not repeated, allowing the appropriate interval between the remaining doses. If a 3-dose course of vaccination has been started before September 2014, then where possible this should be completed; if the course is interrupted, it should be resumed (using the same vaccine) but not repeated, allowing the appropriate interval between the remaining doses. Under the national programme in England, females remain eligible to receive the vaccine up to the age of 18 years if they did not receive the vaccine when scheduled. Where appropriate, immunisation with human papillomavirus vaccine should be offered to females coming into the UK as they may not have been offered protection in their country of origin. The duration of protection has not been established, but current studies suggest that protection is maintained for at least 6 years after completion of the primary course.

Influenza vaccine

While most viruses are antigenically stable, the influenza viruses A and B (especially A) are constantly altering their antigenic structure as indicated by changes in the haemagglutinins (H) and neuraminidases (N) on the surface of the viruses. It is essential that influenza vaccine p. 752 in use contain the H and N components of the prevalent strain or strains recommended each year by the World Health Organization.

Immunisation is recommended *for persons at high risk*, and to reduce transmission of infection. Annual immunisation is strongly recommended for children (including infants that were preterm or low birth-weight) aged over 6 months with the following conditions:

- chronic respiratory disease (includes asthma treated with continuous or repeated use of inhaled or systemic corticosteroids or asthma with previous exacerbations requiring hospital admission);
- chronic heart disease;
- chronic liver disease;
- chronic renal disease;
- chronic neurological disease;
- complement disorders;
- diabetes mellitus;
- immunosuppression because of disease (including asplenia or splenic dysfunction) or treatment (including prolonged systemic corticosteroid treatment [for over 1 month at dose equivalents of prednisolone: *child under 20 kg*, 1 mg/kg or more daily; *child over 20 kg*, 20 mg or more daily] and chemotherapy);
- HIV infection (regardless of immune status).

Seasonal influenza vaccine is also recommended for all pregnant women, for children living in long-stay facilities, and for carers of children whose welfare may be at risk if the carer falls ill. Influenza immunisation should also be considered for household contacts of immunocompromised individuals.

From September 2015, seasonal influenza vaccine will also be offered to all children aged 2–6 years (including those in school years 1 and 2). Unless contra-indicated, the live influenza vaccine, *Fluenz Tetra*®, is preferred in children aged 2–18 years because it provides a higher level of protection than inactivated influenza vaccine.

Further information on pandemic influenza, avian influenza, and swine influenza may be found at www.dh.gov.uk/pandemicflu and at www.gov.uk/phe.

Japanese encephalitis vaccine

Japanese encephalitis vaccine p. 753 is indicated for travellers to areas in Asia and the Far East where infection is endemic and for laboratory staff at risk of exposure to the virus. The primary immunisation course of 2 doses should be completed at least one week before potential exposure to Japanese encephalitis virus.

Up-to-date information on the risk of Japanese encephalitis in specific countries can be obtained from the National Travel Health Network and Centre (www.nathnac.org).

Management of Measles, Mumps and Rubella

Measles vaccine has been replaced by a combined measles, mumps and rubella vaccine, live (MMR vaccine) p. 753.

A combined measles, mumps and rubella vaccine, live (MMR vaccine) aims to eliminate measles, mumps, and rubella (German measles) and congenital rubella syndrome. Every child should receive two doses of measles, mumps and rubella vaccine, live by entry to primary school, unless there is a valid contra-indication. Measles, mumps and rubella vaccine, live should be given irrespective of previous measles, mumps, or rubella infection or vaccination.

The first dose of measles, mumps and rubella vaccine, live is given to children aged 12–13 months. A second dose is given before starting school at 3 years and 4 months–5 years of age (see Immunisation Schedule).

Children presenting for pre-school booster who have not received the first dose of measles, mumps and rubella vaccine, live should be given a dose of measles, mumps and rubella vaccine, live followed 3 months later by a second dose.

At school-leaving age or at entry into further education, MMR immunisation should be offered to individuals of both sexes who have not received 2 doses during childhood. In those who have received only a single dose of MMR in childhood, a second dose is recommended to achieve full protection. If 2 doses of measles, mumps and rubella vaccine, live are required, the second dose should be given one month after the initial dose.

Measles, mumps and rubella vaccine, live should be used to protect against rubella in *seronegative women of child-bearing age* (see Immunisation Schedule); unimmunised healthcare workers who might put pregnant women and other vulnerable groups at risk of rubella or measles should be vaccinated. Measles, mumps and rubella vaccine, live may also be offered to previously *unimmunised and seronegative post-partum women* (see measles, mumps and rubella vaccine, live)—vaccination a few days after delivery is important because about 60% of congenital abnormalities from rubella infection occur in babies of women who have borne more than one child. Immigrants arriving after the age of school immunisation are particularly likely to require immunisation.

Contacts
Measles, mumps and rubella vaccine, live may also be used in the control of outbreaks of measles and should be offered to susceptible children aged over 6 months who are contacts of a case, within 3 days of exposure to infection. Children immunised before 12 months of age should still receive two doses of measles, mumps and rubella vaccine, live at the recommended ages. If one dose of measles, mumps and rubella vaccine, live has already been given to a child, then the second dose may be brought forward to at least one month after the first, to ensure complete protection. If the child is under 18 months of age and the second dose is given within 3 months of the first, then the routine dose before starting school at 3 years and 4 months–5 years should still be given. Children aged under 9 months for whom avoidance of measles infection is particularly important (such as those with history of recent severe illness) can be given normal immunoglobulin p. 727 after exposure to measles; routine MMR immunisation should then be given after at least 3 months at the appropriate age.

Measles, mumps and rubella vaccine, live p. 753 is **not suitable** for prophylaxis following exposure to mumps or rubella since the antibody response to the mumps and rubella components is too slow for effective prophylaxis.

Children with impaired immune response should not receive live vaccines (for advice on HIV). If they have been exposed to measles infection they should be given normal immunoglobulin p. 727.

Travel
Unimmunised travellers, including children over 6 months, to areas where measles is endemic or epidemic should receive measles, mumps and rubella vaccine, live. Children immunised before 12 months of age should still receive two doses of measles, mumps and rubella vaccine, live at the recommended ages. If one dose of measles, mumps and rubella vaccine, live has already been given to a child, then the second dose should be brought forward to at least one month after the first, to ensure complete protection. If the child is under 18 months of age and the second dose is given within 3 months of the first, then the routine dose before starting school at 3 years and 4 months–5 years should still be given.

Meningococcal vaccine

Almost all childhood meningococcal disease in the UK is caused by *Neisseria meningitidis* serogroups B and C. **Meningococcal group C conjugate vaccine** protects only against infection by serogroup C and **meningococcal group B vaccine** protects only against infection by serogroup B. The risk of meningococcal disease declines with age—immunisation is not generally recommended after the age of 25 years.

Tetravalent meningococcal vaccines that cover serogroups A, C, W135, and Y are available. Although the duration of protection has not been established, the **meningococcal groups A, C, W135, and Y conjugate vaccine** is likely to provide longer-lasting protection than the unconjugated meningococcal polysaccharide vaccine. The antibody response to serogroup C in unconjugated meningococcal polysaccharide vaccines in young children may be suboptimal [not currently available in the UK].

A meningococcal group B vaccine (rDNA, component, adsorbed) p. 746, *Bexsero*®, is licensed in the UK against infection caused by *Neisseria meningitidis* serogroup B and is recommended in the Immunisation Schedule. *Bexsero*® contains 3 recombinant *Neisseria meningitidis* serogroup B proteins and the outer membrane vesicles from the NZ 98/254 strain, in order to achieve broad protection against *Neisseria meningitidis* serogroup B; the proteins are adsorbed onto an aluminium compound to stimulate an enhanced immune response.

Childhood immunisation
Meningococcal group C conjugate vaccine provides long-term protection against infection by serogroup C of *Neisseria meningitidis*. Immunisation consists of 1 dose given at 3 months of age; 2 booster doses are recommended, the first is given at 12–13 months of age (combined with haemophilus influenzae type b vaccine), and the second is given at 13–15 years of age (combined with meningococcal A, W135 and Y vaccine) (see Immunisation Schedule).

Meningococcal group B vaccine provides protection against infection by serogroup B of *Neisseria meningitidis*. Immunisation consists of 1 dose given at 2 months of age, a second dose at 4 months of age, and a booster dose at 12 months of age (see Immunisation Schedule).

Unimmunised children aged under 12 months should be given 1 dose of meningococcal group B and group C conjugate vaccines, followed by a second dose of meningococcal group B vaccine (rDNA, component, adsorbed) two months later. They should then be vaccinated according to the Immunisation Schedule. Unimmunised children aged 12–23 months should be given a single dose of the meningococcal group C vaccine p. 746 and 2 doses of meningococcal group B vaccine (rDNA, component, adsorbed) separated by an interval of two months. Children aged 2–9 years who have not received the meningococcal group C vaccine since 12-13 months should be given a single dose of meningococcal group C vaccine only, followed by a booster dose of meningococcal groups A with C and W135 and Y vaccine p. 746 at 13–15 years of age.

From 2015, unimmunised individuals aged 10–25 years, including those aged under 25 years who are attending university for the first time, should be given a single dose of meningococcal groups A with C and W135 and Y vaccine; a booster dose is not required. All students attending university for the first time who are unvaccinated against meningococcal group C, irrespective of age, should be offered a single dose of meningococcal group C vaccine.

Children with confirmed serogroup C disease, who have previously been immunised with meningococcal group C vaccine, should be offered meningococcal group C conjugate vaccine before discharge from hospital.

Travel
Individuals travelling to countries of risk should be immunised with meningococcal groups A, C, W135, and Y conjugate vaccine, even if they have previously received meningococcal group C conjugate vaccine. If an individual has recently received meningococcal group C conjugate vaccine, an interval of at least 4 weeks should be allowed before administration of the tetravalent (meningococcal groups A, C, W135, and Y) vaccine.

Vaccination is particularly important for those living or working with local people or visiting an area of risk during outbreaks.

Immunisation recommendations and requirements for visa entry for individual countries should be checked before travelling, particularly to countries in Sub-Saharan Africa, Asia, and the Indian sub-continent where epidemics of

14

Vaccines

meningococcal outbreaks and infection are reported. Country-by-country information is available from the National Travel Health Network and Centre (www.nathnac.org).

Proof of vaccination with the tetravalent (meningococcal groups A, C, W135, and Y) vaccine is required for those travelling to Saudi Arabia during the Hajj and Umrah pilgrimages (where outbreaks of the W135 strain have occurred).

Contacts

For advice on the immunisation of *laboratory workers and close contacts* of cases of meningococcal disease in the UK and on the role of the vaccine in the control of *local outbreaks*, consult Guidelines for Public Health Management of Meningococcal Disease in the UK at www.gov.uk/phe. Also see antibacterial prophylaxis for prevention of secondary cases of meningococcal meningitis.

Pertussis vaccine

Pertussis vaccine is given as a combination preparation containing other vaccines. Acellular vaccines are derived from highly purified components of *Bordetella pertussis*. Primary immunisation against pertussis (whooping cough) requires 3 doses of an acellular pertussis-containing vaccine (see Immunisation schedule), given at intervals of 1 month from the age of 2 months.

All children up to the age of 10 years should receive primary immunisation with diphtheria, tetanus, pertussis (acellular, component), poliomyelitis (inactivated) and haemophilus type b conjugate vaccine (adsorbed).

A booster dose of an acellular pertussis-containing vaccine should ideally be given 3 years after the primary course, although, the interval can be reduced to 1 year if the primary course was delayed.

Children aged 1–10 years who have not received a *pertussis-containing* vaccine as part of their primary immunisation should be offered 1 dose of a suitable pertussis-containing vaccine; after an interval of at least 1 year, a booster dose of a suitable pertussis-containing vaccine should be given. Immunisation against pertussis is not routinely recommended in individuals over 10 years of age.

Vaccination of pregnant women against pertussis

In response to the pertussis outbreak, the UK health departments introduced a temporary programme (October 2012) to vaccinate pregnant women against pertussis, and this programme will continue until further notice. The aim of the programme is to boost the levels of pertussis–specific antibodies that are transferred, through the placenta, from the mother to the fetus, so that the newborn is protected before routine immunisation begins at 2 months of age.

Pregnant women should be offered a single dose of acellular pertussis-containing vaccine (as adsorbed diphtheria [low dose], tetanus, pertussis (acellular, component) and poliomyelitis (inactivated) vaccine; *Boostrix-IPV*®) between 28 to 38 weeks of pregnancy; the optimal time for vaccination is between 28–32 weeks of pregnancy. Pregnant women should be offered a single dose of acellular pertussis-containing vaccine up to the onset of labour if they missed the opportunity for vaccination at 28–38 weeks of pregnancy. A single dose of acellular pertussis-containing vaccine may also be offered to new mothers, who have never previously been vaccinated against pertussis, until the child receives the first vaccination.

While this programme is in place, women who become pregnant again should be offered vaccination during each pregnancy to maximise transplacental transfer of antibody.

Contacts

Vaccination against pertussis should be considered for close contacts of cases with pertussis who have been offered antibacterial prophylaxis. Unimmunised or partially immunised contacts under 10 years of age should complete their vaccination against pertussis. A booster dose of an acellular pertussis-containing vaccine is recommended for contacts aged over 10 years who have not received a pertussis-containing vaccine in the last 5 years and who have not received adsorbed diphtheria [low dose], tetanus, and poliomyelitis (inactivated) vaccine in the last month.

Side-effects

Local reactions do not contra-indicate further doses.

The vaccine should not be withheld from children with a history to a preceding dose of:

- fever, irrespective of severity;
- persistent crying or screaming for more than 3 hours;
- severe local reaction, irrespective of extent.

Pneumococcal vaccine

Pneumococcal polysaccharide conjugate vaccine (adsorbed) p. 747 protect against infection with *Streptococcus pneumoniae* (pneumococcus); the vaccines contain polysaccharide from capsular pneumococci, **Pneumococcal polysaccharide vaccine** contains purified polysaccharide from 23 capsular types of pneumococci, whereas **pneumococcal polysaccharide conjugate vaccine** (adsorbed) contains polysaccharide from either 10 capsular types (*Synflorix*®) or 13 capsular types (*Prevenar* 13®) with the polysaccharide being conjugated to protein.

The 13-valent conjugate vaccine is used for childhood immunisation. The recommended schedule consists of 3 doses, the first at 2 months of age, the second at 4 months, and the third at 12–13 months (see Immunisation Schedule).

Pneumococcal vaccination is recommended for individuals at increased risk of pneumococcal infection as follows:

- child under 5 years with a history of invasive pneumococcal disease;
- asplenia or splenic dysfunction (including homozygous sickle cell disease and coeliac disease which could lead to splenic dysfunction);
- chronic respiratory disease (includes asthma treated with continuous or frequent use of a systemic corticosteroid);
- chronic heart disease;
- chronic renal disease;
- chronic liver disease;
- chronic neurological conditions;
- complement disorders;
- diabetes mellitus;
- immune deficiency because of disease (e.g. HIV infection) or treatment (including prolonged systemic corticosteroid treatment for over 1 month at dose equivalents of prednisolone: *child under* 20 *kg*, 1 mg/kg or more daily; *child over* 20 *kg*, 20 mg or more daily);
- presence of cochlear implant;
- conditions where leakage of cerebrospinal fluid could occur.

Where possible, the vaccine should be given at least 2 weeks before splenectomy, cochlear implant surgery, chemotherapy, or radiotherapy; children and carers should be given advice about increased risk of pneumococcal infection. If it is not practical to vaccinate at least 2 weeks before splenectomy, chemotherapy, or radiotherapy, the vaccine should be given at least 2 weeks after the splenectomy or, where possible, at least 3 months after completion of chemotherapy or radiotherapy. Prophylactic antibacterial therapy against pneumococcal infection should not be stopped after immunisation. A patient card and information leaflet for patients with asplenia are available from the Department of Health or in Scotland from the Scottish Government, Health Protection Division (Tel (0131) 244 2879).

Choice of vaccine

Children under 2 years at increased risk of pneumococcal infection (see list above) should receive the 13-valent pneumococcal polysaccharide conjugate vaccine (adsorbed) at the recommended ages, followed by a single dose of the 23-valent pneumococcal polysaccharide vaccine after their second birthday. Children at increased risk of pneumococcal infection presenting late for vaccination should receive 2 doses (separated by at least 1 month) of the 13-valent pneumococcal polysaccharide conjugate vaccine (adsorbed) before the age of 12 months, and a third dose at 12–13 months. Children over 12 months and under 5 years (who have not been vaccinated or not completed the primary course) should receive a single dose of 13-valent pneumococcal polysaccharide conjugate vaccine (adsorbed) 2 doses separated by an interval of 2 months in the immunocompromised or those with asplenia or splenic dysfunction. All children under 5 years at increased risk of pneumococcal infection should receive a single dose of the 23-valent pneumococcal polysaccharide vaccine after their second birthday and at least 2 months after the final dose of the 13- valent pneumococcal polysaccharide conjugate vaccine (adsorbed).

Children over 5 years who are at increased risk of pneumococcal disease should receive a single dose of the 23-valent unconjugated pneumococcal polysaccharide vaccine.

Revaccination

In individuals with higher concentrations of antibodies to pneumococcal polysaccharides, revaccination with the 23-valent pneumococcal polysaccharide vaccine more commonly produces adverse reactions. Revaccination is therefore not recommended, except every 5 years in individuals in whom the antibody concentration is likely to decline rapidly (e.g. asplenia, splenic dysfunction and nephrotic syndrome). If there is doubt, the need for revaccination should be discussed with a haematologist, immunologist, or microbiologist.

Poliomyelitis vaccine

Two types of poliomyelitis vaccines (containing strains of poliovirus types 1, 2, and 3) are available, inactivated poliomyelitis vaccines (for injection) and live (oral) poliomyelitis vaccines. **Inactivated** poliomyelitis vaccines, only available in combined preparation, is recommended for routine immunisation; it is given by injection and contains inactivated strains of human poliovirus types 1, 2 and 3.

A course of primary immunisation consists of 3 doses of a combined preparation containing inactivated poliomyelitis vaccines starting at 2 months of age with intervals of 1 month between doses (see Immunisation schedule). A course of 3 doses should also be given to all unimmunised children; no child should remain unimmunised against poliomyelitis.

Two booster doses of a preparation containing inactivated poliomyelitis vaccines are recommended, the first before school entry and the second before leaving school (see Immunisation schedule). Further booster doses should be given every 10 years only to individuals at special risk.

Live (oral) poliomyelitis vaccines is no longer available for routine use; its use may be considered during large outbreaks, but advice should be sought from Public Health England. The live (oral) vaccine poses a very rare risk of vaccine-associated paralytic polio because the attenuated strain of the virus can revert to a virulent form. For this reason the live (oral) vaccine must **not** be used for immunosuppressed individuals or their household contacts. The use of inactivated poliomyelitis vaccines removes the risk of vaccine-associated paralytic polio altogether.

Travel

Unimmunised travellers to areas with a high incidence of poliomyelitis should receive a full 3–dose course of a preparation containing inactivated poliomyelitis vaccines. Those who have not been vaccinated in the last 10 years should receive a booster dose of **adsorbed diphtheria [low dose], tetanus and poliomyelitis (inactivated) vaccine**. Information about countries with a high incidence of poliomyelitis can be obtained from www.travax.nhs.uk or from the National Travel Health Network and Centre, (www.nathnac.org).

Rabies vaccine

Rabies vaccine p. 754 contains inactivated rabies virus cultivated in either human diploid cells or purified chick embryo cells; vaccines are used for pre- and postexposure prophylaxis.

Pre-exposure prophylaxis

Immunisation should be offered to children at high risk of exposure to rabies—where there is limited access to prompt medical care for those living in areas where rabies is enzootic, for those travelling to such areas for longer than 1 month, and for those on shorter visits who may be exposed to unusual risk. Transmission of rabies by humans has not been recorded but it is advised that those caring for children with the disease should be vaccinated.

Up-to-date country-by-country information on the incidence of rabies can be obtained from the National Travel Health Network and Centre (www.nathnac.org) and, in Scotland, from Health Protection Scotland (www.hps.scot.nhs.uk).

Immunisation against rabies requires 3 doses of rabies vaccine, with further booster doses for those who remain at frequent risk.

Post-exposure management

Following potential exposure to rabies, the wound or site of exposure (e.g. mucous membrane) should be cleansed under running water and washed for several minutes with soapy water as soon as possible after exposure. Disinfectant and a simple dressing can be applied, but suturing should be delayed because it may increase the risk of introducing rabies virus into the nerves.

Post-exposure prophylaxis against rabies depends on the level of risk in the country, the nature of exposure, and the individual's immunity. In each case, expert risk assessment and advice on appropriate management should be obtained from the local Public Health England Centre or Public Health England's Virus Reference Department, Colindale (tel. (020) 8200 4400) or the PHE Colindale Duty Doctor (tel. (020) 8200 6868), in Wales from the Public Health Wales local Health Protection Team or Public Health Wales Virus Reference Laboratory (tel. (029) 2074 7747), in Scotland from the local on-call infectious diseases consultant, and in Northern Ireland from the Public Health Agency Duty Room (tel (028) 9055 3997/(028) 9063 2662) or the Regional Virology Service (tel. (028) 9024 0503).

There are no specific contra-indications to the use of rabies vaccine for post-exposure prophylaxis and its use should be considered whenever a child has been attacked by an animal in a country where rabies is enzootic, even if there is no direct evidence of rabies in the attacking animal. Because of the potential consequences of untreated rabies exposure and because rabies vaccination has not been associated with fetal abnormalities, pregnancy is not considered a contra-indication to post-exposure prophylaxis.

For post-exposure prophylaxis of *fully immunised* individuals (who have previously received pre-exposure or post-exposure prophylaxis with cell-derived rabies vaccine), 2 doses of cell-derived vaccine are likely to be sufficient; the first dose is given on day 0 and the second dose is given between day 3–7. Rabies immunoglobulin p. 729 is not necessary in such cases.

Post-exposure treatment for *unimmunised individuals* (or those whose prophylaxis is possibly incomplete) comprises 5 doses of rabies vaccine given over 1 month (on days 0, 3, 7, 14, and the fifth dose is given between day 28–30); also, depending on the level of risk (determined by factors such as

14

Vaccines

the nature of the bite and the country where it was sustained), rabies immunoglobulin is given to unimmunised individuals on day 0 or within 7 days of starting the course of rabies vaccine. The immunisation course can be discontinued if it is proved that the child was not at risk.

Rotavirus vaccine

Rotavirus vaccine p. 754 is a live, oral vaccine that protects young children against gastro-enteritis caused by rotavirus infection. The recommended schedule consists of 2 doses, the first at 2 months of age, and the second at 3 months of age (see Immunisation schedule). The first dose of rotavirus vaccine must be given between 6–15 weeks of age and the second dose should be given after an interval of at least 4 weeks; the vaccine should not be started in children 15 weeks of age or older. Ideally, the full course should be completed before 16 weeks of age to provide protection before the main burden of disease, and to avoid a temporal association between vaccination and intussusception; the course must be completed before 24 weeks of age.

The rotavirus vaccine virus is excreted in the stool and may be transmitted to close contacts; however, vaccination of those with *immunosuppressed* close contacts may protect the contacts from wild-type rotavirus disease and outweigh any risk from transmission of vaccine virus. Carers of a recently vaccinated baby should be advised of the need to wash their hands after changing the baby's nappies.

Smallpox vaccine

Limited supplies of **smallpox vaccine** are held at the Specialist and Reference Microbiology Division, Public Health England Colindale (Tel. (020) 8200 4400) for the exclusive use of workers in laboratories where pox viruses (such as vaccinia) are handled.

If a wider use of the vaccine is being considered, *Guidelines for smallpox response and management in the post-eradication era* should be consulted at www.gov.uk/phe.

Tetanus vaccine

Tetanus vaccine contains a cell-free purified toxin of *Clostridium tetani* adsorbed on aluminium hydroxide or aluminium phosphate to improve antigenicity.

Primary immunisation for children under 10 years consists of 3 doses of a combined preparation containing adsorbed tetanus vaccine, with an interval of 1 month between doses. Following routine childhood vaccination, 2 booster doses of a preparation containing adsorbed tetanus vaccine are recommended, the first before school entry and the second before leaving school (see Immunisation schedule).

The recommended schedule of tetanus vaccination not only gives protection against tetanus in childhood but also gives the basic immunity for subsequent booster doses. In most circumstances, a total of 5 doses of tetanus vaccine is considered sufficient for long term protection.

For primary immunisation of adults and children over 10 years previously unimmunised against tetanus, 3 doses of **adsorbed diphtheria [low dose], tetanus and poliomyelitis (inactivated) vaccine** are given with an interval of 1 month between doses.

When an individual presents for a booster dose but has been vaccinated following a tetanus-prone wound, the vaccine preparation administered at the time of injury should be determined. If this is not possible, the booster should still be given to ensure adequate protection against all antigens in the booster vaccine.

Very rarely, tetanus has developed after abdominal surgery; patients awaiting elective surgery should be asked about tetanus immunisation and immunised if necessary.

Parenteral drug abuse is also associated with tetanus; those abusing drugs by injection should be vaccinated if unimmunised—booster doses should be given if there is any doubt about their immunisation status.

All laboratory staff should be offered a primary course if unimmunised.

Wounds

Wounds are considered to be tetanus-prone if they are sustained more than 6 hours before surgical treatment or at any interval after injury and are puncture-type (particularly if contaminated with soil or manure) *or* show much devitalised tissue *or* are septic *or* are compound fractures *or* contain foreign bodies. All wounds should receive thorough cleansing.

- For *clean wounds*: fully immunised individuals (those who have received a total of 5 doses of a tetanus-containing vaccine at appropriate intervals) and those whose primary immunisation is complete (with boosters up to date), do not require tetanus vaccine; individuals whose primary immunisation is incomplete or whose boosters are not up to date require a reinforcing dose of a tetanus-containing vaccine (followed by further doses as required to complete the schedule); non-immunised individuals (or those whose immunisation status is not known or who have been fully immunised but are now immunocompromised) should be given a dose of the appropriate tetanus-containing vaccine immediately (followed by completion of the full course of the vaccine if records confirm the need)
- For *tetanus-prone wounds*: management is as for clean wounds with the addition of a dose of tetanus immunoglobulin given at a different site; in fully immunised individuals and those whose primary immunisation is complete (with boosters up to date) the immunoglobulin is needed only if the risk of infection is especially high (e.g. contamination with manure). Antibacterial prophylaxis (with benzylpenicillin, co-amoxiclav, or metronidazole) may also be required for tetanus-prone wounds.

Tick-borne encephalitis vaccine

Tick-borne encephalitis vaccine, inactivated p. 755 contains inactivated tick-borne encephalitis virus cultivated in chick embryo cells. It is recommended for immunisation of those working in, or visiting, high-risk areas (see International Travel). Those working, walking or camping in warm forested areas of Central and Eastern Europe, Scandinavia, Northern and Eastern China, and some parts of Japan, particularly from April to November when ticks are most prevalent, are at greatest risk of tick-borne encephalitis. For full protection, 3 doses of the vaccine are required; booster doses are required every 3–5 years for those still at risk. Ideally, immunisation should be completed at least one month before travel.

Typhoid vaccine

Typhoid vaccine p. 747 is available as Vi capsular polysaccharide (from *Salmonella typhi*) vaccine for injection and as live attenuated *Salmonella typhi* vaccine for oral use.

Typhoid immunisation is advised for children travelling to

- areas where typhoid is endemic, especially if staying with or visiting local people;
- endemic areas where frequent or prolonged exposure to poor sanitation and poor food hygiene is likely;

Typhoid vaccination is not a substitute for scrupulous personal hygiene.

Capsular **polysaccharide typhoid vaccine** is usually given by *intramuscular* injection. Children under 2 years may respond suboptimally to the vaccine, but children aged between 1–2 years should be immunised if the risk of typhoid fever is considered high (immunisation is not recommended for infants under 12 months). Revaccination is needed every 3 years on continued exposure.

Oral typhoid vaccine is a **live attenuated** vaccine contained in an enteric-coated capsule. One capsule taken on alternate days for a total of 3 doses provides protection

7–10 days after the last dose. Protection may persist for up to 3 years in those constantly (or repeatedly) exposed to *Salmonella typhi*, but those who only occasionally travel to endemic areas require further courses at intervals of 1 year.

Varicella-zoster vaccine

Varicella-zoster vaccine (live) p. 755 is licensed for immunisation against varicella (chickenpox) in seronegative individuals. It is not recommended for routine use in children but can be given to seronegative healthy children over 1 year who come into close contact with individuals at high risk of severe varicella infections.

Rarely, the varicella-zoster vaccine virus has been transmitted from the vaccinated individual to close contacts. Therefore, contact with the following should be avoided if a vaccine-related cutaneous rash develops within 4–6 weeks of the first or second dose:

- varicella-susceptible pregnant females;
- individuals at high risk of severe varicella, including those with immunodeficiency or those receiving immunosuppressive therapy.

Varicella-zoster immunoglobulin p. 730 is used to protect susceptible children at increased risk of varicella infection.

Yellow fever vaccine

Live yellow fever vaccine, live p. 756 is indicated for those travelling to or living in areas where infection is endemic. Infants under 6 months of age should not be vaccinated because there is a small risk of encephalitis; infants aged 6–9 months should be vaccinated only if the risk of yellow fever is high and unavoidable (seek expert advice). The immunity which probably lasts for life is officially accepted for 10 years starting from 10 days after primary immunisation and for a further 10 years immediately after revaccination.

Very rarely vaccine-associated adverse effects have been reported, such as viscerotropic disease (yellow fever vaccine, live-associated viscerotropic disease, YEL–AVD) p. 756, a syndrome which may include metabolic acidosis, muscle and liver cytolysis, and multi-organ failure. Neurological disorders (yellow fever vaccine, live-associated neurotropic disease, YEL-AND) such as encephalitis have also been reported. These *very rare* adverse effects have usually occurred after the first dose of yellow fever vaccine, live in those with no previous immunity.

Vaccines for travel

Immunisation

See advice on Malaria, treatment p. 365.

No special immunisation is required for travellers to the United States, Europe, Australia, or New Zealand, although all travellers should have immunity to tetanus and poliomyelitis (and childhood immunisations should be up to date); Tick-borne encephalitis vaccine is recommended for immunisation of those working in, or visiting, high-risk areas. Certain special precautions are required in non-European areas surrounding the Mediterranean, in Africa, the Middle East, Asia, and South America.

Travellers to areas that have a high incidence of **poliomyelitis** or **tuberculosis** should be immunised with the appropriate vaccine; in the case of poliomyelitis previously immunised travellers may be given a booster dose of a preparation containing inactivated poliomyelitis vaccine. BCG immunisation is recommended for travellers aged under 16 years proposing to stay for longer than 3 months (or in close contact with the local population) in countries with an incidence of tuberculosis greater than 40 per 100 000 (list of countries where the incidence of tuberculosis is greater than 40 cases per 100 000 is available

from www.gov.uk/phe); it should preferably be given 3 months or more before departure.

Yellow fever immunisation is recommended for travel to the endemic zones of Africa and South America. Many countries require an International Certificate of Vaccination from individuals arriving from, or who have been travelling through, endemic areas; other countries require a certificate from all entering travellers (consult the Department of Health handbook, *Health Information for Overseas Travel*, www.dh.gov.uk).

Immunisation against **meningococcal meningitis** is recommended for a number of areas of the world.

Protection against **hepatitis A** is recommended for travellers to high-risk areas outside Northern and Western Europe, North America, Japan, Australia and New Zealand. Hepatitis A vaccine is preferred and it is likely to be effective even if given shortly before departure; normal immunoglobulin is no longer given routinely but may be indicated in the immunocompromised. Special care must also be taken with food hygiene.

Hepatitis B vaccine is recommended for those travelling to areas of high or intermediate prevalence who intend to seek employment as healthcare workers or who plan to remain there for lengthy periods and who may therefore be at increased risk of acquiring infection as the result of medical or dental procedures carried out in those countries. Short-term tourists or business travellers are not generally at increased risk of infection but may put themselves at risk by their sexual behaviour when abroad.

Prophylactic immunisation against **rabies** is recommended for travellers to enzootic areas on long journeys or to areas out of reach of immediate medical attention.

Travellers who have not had a **tetanus** booster in the last 10 years and are visiting areas where medical attention may not be accessible should receive a booster dose of adsorbed diphtheria [low dose], tetanus and poliomyelitis (inactivated) vaccine, even if they have received 5 doses of a tetanus-containing vaccine previously.

Typhoid vaccine is indicated for travellers to countries where typhoid is endemic, but the vaccine is no substitute for personal precautions.

There is no requirement for cholera vaccination as a condition for entry into any country, but **oral cholera vaccine** should be considered for backpackers and those travelling to situations where the risk is greatest (e.g. refugee camps). Regardless of vaccination, travellers to areas where cholera is endemic should take special care with food hygiene.

Advice on **diphtheria**, on **Japanese encephalitis**, and on **tick-borne encephalitis** is included in *Health Information for Overseas Travel*.

Food hygiene

In areas where sanitation is poor, good food hygiene is important to help prevent hepatitis A, typhoid, cholera, and other diarrhoeal diseases (including travellers' diarrhoea). Food should be freshly prepared and hot, and uncooked vegetables (including green salads) should be avoided; only fruits which can be peeled should be eaten. Only suitable bottled water, or tap water that has been boiled or treated with sterilising tablets, should be used for drinking.

Information on health advice for travellers

Health professionals and travellers can find the latest information on immunisation requirements and precautions for avoiding disease while travelling from: www.nathnac.org.

The handbook, *Health Information for Overseas Travel* (2010), which draws together essential information *for healthcare professionals* regarding health advice for travellers, can also be obtained from this website.

14

Vaccines

Immunisation requirements change from time to time, and information on the current requirements for any particular country may be obtained from the embassy or legation of the appropriate country or from:

National Travel Health Network and Centre
UCLH NHS Foundation Trust
3rd Floor Central,
250 Euston Road,
London, NW1 2PG
Tel: 0845 602 6712
(8:30–11:45 a.m, 1–3:15 p.m. weekdays for healthcare professionals **only**) www.nathnac.org

Travel Medicine Team
Health Protection Scotland
Meridian Court,
5 Cadogan Street,
Glasgow, G2 6QE
Tel: (0141) 300 1130
(2–4 p.m. Monday to Wednesday, 9:30–11:30 a.m. Friday; for registered TRAVAX users **only**) www.travax.nhs.uk
(free for NHS Scotland users, registration required; subscription fee may be payable for users outside NHS Scotland)

Welsh Assembly Government
Tel (029) 2082 5397
(9 a.m.–5.30 p.m. weekdays)

Department of Health, Social Services and Public Safety
Castle Buildings,
Stormont,
Belfast, BT4 3SQ
Tel: (028) 9052 2118
(9 a.m.–5. p.m. weekdays) www.dhsspsni.gov.uk

VACCINES

Vaccines

> **IMPORTANT SAFETY INFORMATION**
>
> MHRA/CHM ADVICE (APRIL 2016)
> Following reports of death in neonates who received a live attenuated vaccine after exposure to a tumor necrosis factor alpha (TNF-a) inhibitor in utero, the MHRA has issued the following advice:
> - any infant who has been exposed to immunosuppressive treatment from the mother either in utero during pregnancy or via breastfeeding should have any live attenuated vaccination deferred for as long as a postnatal influence on the immune status of the infant remains possible;
> - in the case of infants who have been exposed to TNF-a inhibitors and other biological medicines in utero, any live attenuated vaccination should be deferred until the infant is age 6 months, after which time vaccination should be considered.

● **CONTRA-INDICATIONS**
  CONTRA-INDICATIONS, FURTHER INFORMATION
▸ Impaired immune response Severely immunosuppressed patients should not be given live vaccines (including those with severe primary immunodeficiency).

● **CAUTIONS** Acute illness · minor illnesses
  CAUTIONS, FURTHER INFORMATION
  Vaccination may be postponed if the individual is suffering from an acute illness; however, it is not necessary to postpone immunisation in patients with minor illnesses without fever or systemic upset.
▸ Impaired immune response and drugs affecting immune response Immune response to vaccines may be reduced in immunosuppressed patients and there is also a risk of generalised infection with live vaccines.

Specialist advice should be sought for those being treated with high doses of corticosteroids (dose equivalents of prednisolone: **children**, 2 mg/kg (or more than 40 mg) daily for at least 1 week or 1 mg/kg daily for 1 month), or other immunosuppressive drugs, and those being treated for malignant conditions with chemotherapy or generalised radiotherapy. Live vaccines should be postponed until at least 3 months after stopping high-dose systemic corticosteroids and at least 6 months after stopping other immunosuppressive drugs or generalised radiotherapy (at least 12 months after discontinuing immunosuppressants following bone-marrow transplantation).

The Royal College of Paediatrics and Child Health has produced a statement, *Immunisation of the Immunocompromised Child* (2002) (available at www.rcpch.ac.uk).

▸ Predisposition to neurological problems When there is a personal or family history of *febrile* convulsions, there is an increased risk of these occurring during fever from any cause including immunisation, but this is not a contra-indication to immunisation. In children who have had a seizure associated with fever without neurological deterioration, immunisation is *recommended*; advice on the *management of fever* (see Post-immunisation Pyrexia in Infants) should be given before immunisation. When a child has had a convulsion not associated with fever, and the neurological condition is not deteriorating, immunisation is *recommended*.

Children with stable neurological disorders (e.g. spina bifida, congenital brain abnormality, and peri-natal hypoxic-ischaemic encephalopathy) should be immunised according to the recommended schedule.

When there is a *still evolving neurological problem*, including poorly controlled epilepsy, immunisation should be deferred and the child referred to a specialist. Immunisation is recommended if a cause for the neurological disorder is identified. If a cause is not identified, immunisation should be deferred until the condition is stable.

● **INTERACTIONS** → Appendix 1 (vaccines).

● **SIDE-EFFECTS**
  GENERAL SIDE-EFFECTS
▸ **Common or very common** Fatigue · fever · gastro-intestinal disturbances · headache · irritability · loss of appetite · lymphangitis · malaise · myalgia
▸ **Very rare** Anaphylaxis (can be fatal) · angioedema (can be fatal) · bronchospasm (can be fatal) · hypersensitivity reactions (can be fatal) · urticaria (can be fatal)
▸ **Frequency not known** Arthralgia · asthenia · dizziness · drowsiness · influenza-like symptoms · lymphadenopathy · paraesthesia · rash

  SPECIFIC SIDE-EFFECTS
▸ **Common or very common**
▸ With intradermal or intramuscular or subcutaneous use Induration may develop at the injection site · inflammation · local reactions · pain · redness · sterile abscess may develop at the injection site

  SIDE-EFFECTS, FURTHER INFORMATION
  Occasionally serious adverse reactions can occur—these should always be reported to the CHM.
▸ Post-immunisation pyrexia in infants The parent should be advised that if pyrexia develops after childhood immunisation, and the infant seems distressed, paracetamol can be given. Ibuprofen can be used if paracetamol is unsuitable. The parent should be warned to seek medical advice if the pyrexia persists.

● **ALLERGY AND CROSS-SENSITIVITY** Contra-indicated in patients with a confirmed anaphylactic reaction to a preceding dose of a vaccine containing the same antigens or vaccine component (such as antibacterials in viral vaccines).

- **PREGNANCY** Live vaccines should not be administered routinely to pregnant women because of the theoretical risk of fetal infection but where there is a significant risk of exposure to disease, the need for vaccination usually outweighs any possible risk to the fetus. Termination of pregnancy following inadvertent immunisation is not recommended. There is no evidence of risk from vaccinating pregnant women with inactivated viral or bacterial vaccines or toxoids.

- **BREAST FEEDING** Although there is a theoretical risk of live vaccine being present in breast milk, vaccination is not contra-indicated for women who are breast-feeding when there is significant risk of exposure to disease. There is no evidence of risk from vaccinating women who are breast-feeding, with inactivated viral or bacterial vaccines or toxoids.

- **DIRECTIONS FOR ADMINISTRATION** If alcohol or disinfectant is used for cleansing the skin it should be allowed to evaporate before vaccination to prevent possible inactivation of live vaccines.

  When 2 or more live vaccines are required (and are not available as a combined preparation), they can be administered at any time before or after each other at different sites, preferably in a different limb; if more than one injection is to be given in the same limb, they should be administered at least 2.5 cm apart. See also bacillus calmette-guérin vaccine p. 744.

  Vaccines should not be given intravenously. Most vaccines are given by the intramuscular route, although some are given by either the intradermal, deep subcutaneous, or oral route. The intramuscular route should not be used in patients with **bleeding disorders** such as haemophilia or thrombocytopenia, vaccines usually given by the intramuscular route should be given by deep subcutaneous injection instead.

  The Department of Health has advised *against the use of jet guns* for vaccination owing to the risk of transmitting blood borne infections, such as HIV.

  Particular attention must be paid to instructions on the use of diluents. Vaccines which are liquid suspensions or are reconstituted before use should be adequately mixed to ensure uniformity of the material to be injected.

- **HANDLING AND STORAGE** Care must be taken to store all vaccines under the conditions recommended in the product literature, otherwise the preparation may become ineffective. **Refrigerated storage** is usually necessary; many vaccines need to be stored at 2–8°C and not allowed to freeze. Vaccines should be protected from light. Reconstituted vaccines and opened multidose vials must be used within the period recommended in the product literature. Unused vaccines should be disposed of by incineration at a registered disposal contractor.

VACCINES > BACTERIAL AND VIRAL VACCINES, COMBINED

▶ 742

Diphtheria with haemophilus influenzae type b vaccine, pertussis, poliomyelitis and tetanus

- **INDICATIONS AND DOSE**

Primary immunisation
▶ BY INTRAMUSCULAR INJECTION
▸ Child 2 months–10 years: 0.5 mL every 1 month for 3 doses

- **UNLICENSED USE** *Infanrix-IPV + Hib* ® not licensed for use in children over 36 months; *Pediacel* ® not licensed in children over 4 years. However, the Department of Health recommends that these be used for children up to 10 years.

- **SIDE-EFFECTS** Atopic dermatitis · hypotonia · restlessness · sleep disturbances · unusual crying in infants
  SIDE-EFFECTS, FURTHER INFORMATION
  ▸ Side effects of vaccines containing pertussis The incidence of local and systemic effects is generally lower with vaccines containing acellular pertussis components than with the whole-cell pertussis vaccine used previously. However, compared with primary vaccination, booster doses with vaccines containing acellular pertussis are reported to increase the risk of injection-site reactions (some of which affect the entire limb); local reactions do not contra-indicate further doses.

  The vaccine should not be withheld from children with a history to a preceding dose of:
  - fever, irrespective of severity;
  - persistent crying or screaming for more than 3 hours;
  - severe local reaction, irrespective of extent.

- **PRESCRIBING AND DISPENSING INFORMATION** Available as part of childhood schedule from health organisations or ImmForm.

- **MEDICINAL FORMS**
  There can be variation in the licensing of different medicines containing the same drug.
  Suspension for injection
  EXCIPIENTS: May contain Neomycin, polymyxin b, streptomycin
  ▸ **Pediacel** (sanofi pasteur MSD Ltd)
  Pediacel vaccine suspension for injection 0.5ml vials | 1 vial [PoM] £32.00
  Powder and suspension for suspension for injection
  ▸ **Infanrix-IPV + Hib** (GlaxoSmithKline UK Ltd)
  Infanrix-IPV + Hib vaccine powder and suspension for suspension for injection 0.5ml pre-filled syringes | 1 pre-filled disposable injection [PoM] £27.86

▶ 742

Diphtheria with pertussis, poliomyelitis vaccine and tetanus

- **INDICATIONS AND DOSE**

First booster dose
▶ BY INTRAMUSCULAR INJECTION
▸ Child 3–9 years: 0.5 mL, to be given 3 years after primary immunisation

Vaccination of pregnant women against pertussis (using low dose vaccines)
▶ BY INTRAMUSCULAR INJECTION
▸ Females of childbearing potential: 0.5 mL for 1 dose

- **SIDE-EFFECTS** Restlessness · sleep disturbances · unusual crying in infants
  SIDE-EFFECTS, FURTHER INFORMATION
  ▸ Side effects of vaccines containing pertussis The incidence of local and systemic effects is generally lower with vaccines containing acellular pertussis components than with the whole-cell pertussis vaccine used previously. However, compared with primary vaccination, booster doses with vaccines containing acellular pertussis are reported to increase the risk of injection-site reactions (some of which affect the entire limb); local reactions do not contra-indicate further doses.

  The vaccine should not be withheld from children with a history to a preceding dose of:
  - fever, irrespective of severity;
  - persistent crying or screaming for more than 3 hours;
  - severe local reaction, irrespective of extent.

- **PREGNANCY** Contra-indicated in pregnant women with a history of encephalopathy of unknown origin within 7 days

14

Vaccines

of previous immunisation with a pertussis-containing vaccine. Contra-indicated in pregnant women with a history of transient thrombocytopenia or neurological complications following previous immunisation against diphtheria or tetanus.

- **PRESCRIBING AND DISPENSING INFORMATION** Pregnant women should be vaccinated using low dose vaccines (brands may include *Boostrix-IPV*® or *Repevax*®).

  Available as part of childhood immunisation schedule from health organisations or ImmForm.

  Available for vaccination of pregnant women from ImmForm.

- **MEDICINAL FORMS**
  There can be variation in the licensing of different medicines containing the same drug.

  Suspension for injection
  EXCIPIENTS: May contain Neomycin, polymyxin b, streptomycin
  - Boostrix-IPV (GlaxoSmithKline UK Ltd)
    Boostrix-IPV suspension for injection 0.5ml pre-filled syringes | 1 pre-filled disposable injection [PoM] £22.74
  - Infanrix-IPV (GlaxoSmithKline UK Ltd)
    Infanrix-IPV vaccine suspension for injection 0.5ml pre-filled syringes | 1 pre-filled disposable injection [PoM] £17.56
  - Repevax (sanofi pasteur MSD Ltd)
    Repevax vaccine suspension for injection 0.5ml pre-filled syringes | 1 pre-filled disposable injection [PoM] £20.00

F 742

Diphtheria with poliomyelitis and tetanus vaccine

- **INDICATIONS AND DOSE**
  Primary immunisation
  - BY INTRAMUSCULAR INJECTION
  - Child 10–17 years: 0.5 mL every 1 month for 3 doses

  Booster doses
  - BY INTRAMUSCULAR INJECTION
  - Child 10–17 years: 0.5 mL for 1 dose, first booster dose—should be given 3 years after primary course (this interval can be reduced to a minimum of 1 year if the primary course was delayed), then 0.5 mL for 1 dose, second booster dose—should be given 10 years after first booster dose (this interval can be reduced to a minimum of 5 years if previous doses were delayed), second booster dose may also be used as first booster dose in those over 10 years who have received only 3 previous doses of a diphtheria-containing vaccine

- **SIDE-EFFECTS** Restlessness · sleep disturbances · unusual crying in infants
- **PRESCRIBING AND DISPENSING INFORMATION** Available as part of childhood schedule from health organisations or ImmForm.

- **MEDICINAL FORMS**
  There can be variation in the licensing of different medicines containing the same drug.

  Suspension for injection
  EXCIPIENTS: May contain Neomycin, polymyxin b, streptomycin
  - Revaxis (sanofi pasteur MSD Ltd)
    Revaxis vaccine suspension for injection 0.5ml pre-filled syringes | 1 pre-filled disposable injection [PoM] £6.50

F 742

Bacillus calmette-guérin vaccine

(BCG Vaccine)

- **DRUG ACTION** BCG (Bacillus Calmette-Guérin) is a live attenuated strain derived from *Mycobacterium bovis* which stimulates the development of immunity to *M. tuberculosis*.

- **INDICATIONS AND DOSE**
  Immunisation against tuberculosis
  - BY INTRADERMAL INJECTION
  - Neonate: 0.05 mL, to be injected at insertion of deltoid muscle onto humerus (keloid formation more likely with sites higher on arm); tip of shoulder should be **avoided**.
  - Child 1–11 months: 0.05 mL, to be injected at insertion of deltoid muscle onto humerus (keloid formation more likely with sites higher on arm); tip of shoulder should be **avoided**
  - Child 1–17 years: 0.1 mL, to be injected at insertion of deltoid muscle onto humerus (keloid formation more likely with sites higher on arm); tip of shoulder should be **avoided**

- **CONTRA-INDICATIONS** Generalised septic skin conditions · neonate in household contact with known or suspected case of active tuberculosis

  CONTRA-INDICATIONS, FURTHER INFORMATION
  A lesion-free site should be used to administer BCG vaccine to patients with eczema.

- **CAUTIONS**

  CAUTIONS, FURTHER INFORMATION
  BCG vaccine can be given simultaneously with another live vaccine, but if they are not given at the same time an interval of 4 weeks should normally be allowed. When BCG is given to infants, there is no need to delay routine primary immunisations. No further vaccination should be given in the arm used for BCG vaccination for at least 3 months because of the risk of regional lymphadenitis.

- **SIDE-EFFECTS**
  - **Rare** Disseminated complications · osteitis · osteomyelitis
  - **Frequency not known** Prolonged ulceration at the injection site · subcutaneous abscess at the injection site

- **PRE-TREATMENT SCREENING** Apart from children under 6 years, any person being considered for BCG immunisation must first be given a skin test for hypersensitivity to tuberculoprotein (see tuberculin purified protein derivative p. 731). A skin test is not necessary for a child under 6 years provided that the child has not stayed for longer than 3 months in a country with an incidence of tuberculosis greater than 40 per 100 000, the child has not had contact with a person with tuberculosis, and there is no family history of tuberculosis within the last 5 years.

- **DIRECTIONS FOR ADMINISTRATION**
  Intradermal injection technique Skin is stretched between thumb and forefinger and needle (size 25G or 26G) inserted (bevel upwards) for about 3 mm into superficial layers of dermis (almost parallel with surface). Needle should be short with short bevel (can usually be seen through epidermis during insertion). Tense raised blanched bleb showing tips of hair follicles is sign of correct injection; 7 mm bleb ≡ 0.1 mL injection, 3 mm bleb ≡ 0.05 mL injection; if considerable resistance not felt, needle too deep and should be removed and reinserted before giving more vaccine.

- **PRESCRIBING AND DISPENSING INFORMATION** Available from health organisations or direct from ImmForm www.immform.dh.gov.uk (SSI brand, multidose vial with diluent).

● **MEDICINAL FORMS**
There can be variation in the licensing of different medicines
containing the same drug.
Powder and solvent for suspension for injection
‣ Bacillus calmette-guérin vaccine (Non-proprietary)
   Bacillus Calmette-Guerin vaccine powder and solvent for suspension
   for injection vials | 10 vial [PoM] no price available

Cholera vaccine

● **INDICATIONS AND DOSE**

**Immunisation against cholera (for travellers to endemic
or epidemic areas on the basis of current
recommendations)**
‣ BY MOUTH
‣ Child 2–5 years: 1 dose every 1–6 weeks for 3 doses, if
   more than 6 weeks have elapsed between doses, the
   primary course should be restarted, immunisation
   should be completed at least one week before potential
   exposure
‣ Child 6–17 years: 1 dose every 1–6 weeks for 2 doses, if
   more than 6 weeks have elapsed between doses, the
   primary course should be restarted, immunisation
   should be completed at least one week before potential
   exposure
Booster
‣ BY MOUTH
‣ Child 2–5 years: A single booster dose can be given
   within 6 months after primary course, if more than
   6 months have elapsed since the last vaccination, the
   primary course should be repeated
‣ Child 6–17 years: A single booster dose can be given
   within 2 years after primary course, if more than
   2 years have elapsed since the last vaccination, the
   primary course should be repeated

● **CONTRA-INDICATIONS** Acute gastro-intestinal illness
● **SIDE-EFFECTS**
‣ **Rare** Cough · respiratory symptoms · rhinitis
‣ **Very rare** Insomnia · sore throat
‣ **Frequency not known** Abdominal pain and cramps ·
   diarrhoea · nausea · vomiting

● **DIRECTIONS FOR ADMINISTRATION** Dissolve effervescent
sodium bicarbonate granules in a glassful of water *or*
chlorinated water (approximately 150 mL). For children
over 6 years, add vaccine suspension to make one dose. For
child 2–5 years, discard half (approximately 75 mL) of the
solution, then add vaccine suspension to make one dose.
Drink within 2 hours. Food, drink, and other oral
medicines should be avoided for 1 hour before and after
vaccination.

● **PATIENT AND CARER ADVICE** Counselling on
administration advised. Immunisation with cholera
vaccine does not provide complete protection and all
travellers to a country where cholera exists should be
warned that scrupulous attention to food, water, and
personal hygiene is **essential**.

● **MEDICINAL FORMS**
There can be variation in the licensing of different medicines
containing the same drug.
Oral suspension
‣ Dukoral (Valneva UK Ltd)
   Dukoral cholera vaccine oral suspension | 2 dose [PoM] £23.42

Haemophilus influenzae type B with meningococcal group C vaccine

● **INDICATIONS AND DOSE**

**Booster dose (for infants who have received primary
immunisation with a vaccine containing *Haemophilus
influenzae* type b component)**
‣ BY INTRAMUSCULAR INJECTION
‣ Child 12–13 months: 0.5 mL for 1 dose
**Booster dose (for children who have not been immunised
against *Haemophilus influenza* type b) | Booster dose
after recovery from *Haemophilus influenzae* type b
disease (for index cases previously vaccinated, with low
Hib antibody concentration or if it is not possible to
measure antibody concentration)**
‣ BY INTRAMUSCULAR INJECTION
‣ Child 1–9 years: 0.5 mL for 1 dose
**Booster dose after recovery from *Haemophilus influenzae*
type b disease (for fully vaccinated index cases with
asplenia or splenic dysfunction, if previous dose
received over 1 year ago)**
‣ BY INTRAMUSCULAR INJECTION
‣ Child 1–17 years: 0.5 mL for 1 dose
**Booster dose (for patients diagnosed with asplenia,
splenic dysfunction or complement deficiency at under
2 years of age)**
‣ BY INTRAMUSCULAR INJECTION
‣ Child 12–13 months: 0.5 mL for 1 dose, this booster dose
   should be followed 1 month later by one dose of
   meningococcal A, C, W135, and Y conjugate vaccine,
   followed by 0.5 mL for 1 dose, the second dose should
   be given after the second birthday
**Booster dose (for patients diagnosed with asplenia,
splenic dysfunction or complement deficiency at over
2 years of age)**
‣ BY INTRAMUSCULAR INJECTION
‣ Child 2–17 years: 0.5 mL for 1 dose, this booster dose
   should be followed 1 month later by one dose of
   meningococcal A, C, W135, and Y conjugate vaccine

● **UNLICENSED USE** Not licensed for use in patients over
2 years.
● **SIDE-EFFECTS**
‣ **Rare** Symptoms of meningitis reported (but no evidence
   that the vaccine causes meningococcal C meningitis)
‣ **Frequency not known** Atopic dermatitis · hypotonia
● **PRESCRIBING AND DISPENSING INFORMATION** Available as
part of the childhood immunisation schedule from
ImmForm.

● **MEDICINAL FORMS**
There can be variation in the licensing of different medicines
containing the same drug.
Powder and solvent for solution for injection
‣ Menitorix (GlaxoSmithKline UK Ltd)
   Menitorix vaccine powder and solvent for solution for injection 0.5ml
   vials | 1 vial [PoM] £37.76

14

Vaccines

F 742

Meningococcal group B vaccine (rDNA, component, adsorbed)

- **INDICATIONS AND DOSE**

Immunisation against *Neisseria meningitidis*, primary immunisation
- ▸ BY DEEP INTRAMUSCULAR INJECTION
- ▸ Child 2 months: 0.5 mL for 1 dose, injected preferably into deltoid region (or anterolateral thigh in infants). Three doses of 60 mg prophylactic paracetamol should be given post primary meningococcal B immunisation, at 2 months and 4 months of age. Further information can be found at www.gov.uk.
- ▸ Child 4 months: 0.5 mL for 1 dose, injected preferably into deltoid region (or anterolateral thigh in infants). Three doses of 60 mg prophylactic paracetamol should be given post primary meningococcal B immunisation, at 2 months and 4 months of age. Further information can be found at www.gov.uk.

Immunisation against *Neisseria meningitidis*, primary immunisation booster dose
- ▸ BY DEEP INTRAMUSCULAR INJECTION
- ▸ Child 12-23 months: 0.5 mL for 1 dose, injected preferably into deltoid region (or anterolateral thigh in infants)

Immunisation against *Neisseria meningitidis*, primary immunisation (in unimmunised patients)
- ▸ BY DEEP INTRAMUSCULAR INJECTION
- ▸ Child 6-11 months: 0.5 mL for 2 doses, separated by an interval of at least 2 months; booster dose of 0.5 mL given between 1–2 years of age and at least 2 months after completion of primary immunisation, injected preferably into deltoid region (or anterolateral thigh in infants)
- ▸ Child 12-23 months: 0.5 mL for 2 doses, separated by an interval of at least 2 months; booster dose of 0.5 mL given 12–24 months after completion of primary immunisation, injected preferably into deltoid region (or anterolateral thigh in infants)
- ▸ Child 2-10 years: 0.5 mL for 2 doses, separated by an interval of at least 2 months. Injected preferably into deltoid region (or anterolateral thigh in infants)
- ▸ Child 11-17 years: 0.5 mL for 2 doses, separated by an interval of at least 1 month. Injected preferably into deltoid region

- **SIDE-EFFECTS**
- ▸ **Rare** Kawasaki disease · symptoms of meningitis reported (but no evidence that the vaccine causes meningococcal C meningitis)
- ▸ **Frequency not known** Unusual crying

- **MEDICINAL FORMS**
There can be variation in the licensing of different medicines containing the same drug.
Suspension for injection
EXCIPIENTS: May contain Kanamycin
- ▸ Bexsero (GlaxoSmithKline UK Ltd) ▼
Bexsero vaccine suspension for injection 0.5ml pre-filled syringes | 1 pre-filled disposable injection PoM £75.00

F 742

Meningococcal group C vaccine

- **INDICATIONS AND DOSE**

Primary immunisation against *Neisseria meningitidis*
- ▸ BY INTRAMUSCULAR INJECTION
- ▸ Child 3 months: 0.5 mL for 1 dose, the primary immunisation dose is followed by a booster dose of meningococcal group C conjugate vaccine combined

with haemophilus influenzae type b vaccine at 12–13 months of age

Second booster dose for immunisation against *Neisseria meningitidis*
- ▸ BY INTRAMUSCULAR INJECTION
- ▸ Child 13-15 years: 0.5 mL for 1 dose

Immunisation against *Neisseria meningitidis* in an unimmunised patient
- ▸ BY INTRAMUSCULAR INJECTION
- ▸ Child 4-11 months: 0.5 mL for 1 dose, the primary immunisation dose is followed by a booster dose of meningococcal group C conjugate vaccine combined with haemophilus influenzae type b vaccine at 12–13 months of age, then 0.5 mL for 1 dose, this second booster dose to be given at 13–15 years of age
- ▸ Child 1-9 years: 0.5 mL for 1 dose, then 0.5 mL for 1 dose, this booster dose to be given at 13–15 years of age
- ▸ Child 10-17 years: 0.5 mL for 1 dose, booster dose is not required

Patients with confirmed serogroup C disease (who have previously been immunised)
- ▸ BY INTRAMUSCULAR INJECTION
- ▸ Child 1-17 years: 0.5 mL for 1 dose, dose to be given before discharge from hospital

- **SIDE-EFFECTS**
- ▸ **Rare** Symptoms of meningitis (but no evidence that vaccine causes meningococcal C meningitis)
- **DIRECTIONS FOR ADMINISTRATION** *Menjugate Kit*® may be used via subcutaneous route in children with bleeding disorders.
- **PRESCRIBING AND DISPENSING INFORMATION** Available as part of childhood immunisation schedule from www.immform.dh.gov.uk.

- **MEDICINAL FORMS**
There can be variation in the licensing of different medicines containing the same drug.
Powder and solvent for suspension for injection
- ▸ Menjugate (Novartis Vaccines and Diagnostics Ltd)
Menjugate vaccine powder and solvent for suspension for injection 0.5ml vials | 1 vial PoM no price available | 10 vial PoM no price available
Suspension for injection
- ▸ Meningitec (Nuron Biotech B.V.)
Meningitec vaccine suspension for injection 0.5ml pre-filled syringes | 1 pre-filled disposable injection PoM £4.33 | 10 pre-filled disposable injection PoM £43.30
- ▸ NeisVac-C (Pfizer Ltd)
NeisVac-C vaccine suspension for injection 0.5ml pre-filled syringes | 10 pre-filled disposable injection PoM £187.50

F 742

Meningococcal groups A with C and W135 and Y vaccine

- **INDICATIONS AND DOSE**

MENVEO®

Primary immunisation against *Neisseria meningitidis*
- ▸ BY INTRAMUSCULAR INJECTION
- ▸ Child 13-15 years: 0.5 mL for 1 dose, dose preferably injected into deltoid region

Immunisation against *Neisseria meningitidis* in those at risk of exposure to prevent invasive disease
- ▸ BY INTRAMUSCULAR INJECTION
- ▸ Child 3-11 months: 0.5 mL every 1 month for 2 doses, dose preferably injected into deltoid region
- ▸ Child 1-17 years: 0.5 mL for 1 dose, dose preferably injected into deltoid region

NIMENRIX®

Primary immunisation against *Neisseria meningitidis*

▸ BY INTRAMUSCULAR INJECTION

▸ Child 13-15 years: 0.5 mL for 1 dose, to be injected preferably into deltoid region

Immunisation against *Neisseria meningitidis* in those at risk of exposure

▸ BY INTRAMUSCULAR INJECTION

▸ Child 1-17 years: 0.5 mL for 1 dose, to be injected preferably into deltoid region (or anterolateral thigh in child 12–23 months), then 0.5 mL after 1 year if required for 1 dose, second dose should be considered in those who continue to be at risk of *Neisseria meningitidis* serogroup A infection

● UNLICENSED USE

MENVEO® *Menveo*® is not licensed for use in children under 2 years.

● SIDE-EFFECTS

▸ Rare Symptoms of meningitis reported (but no evidence that the vaccine causes meningococcal C meningitis)

● MEDICINAL FORMS

There can be variation in the licensing of different medicines containing the same drug.

Powder and solvent for solution for injection

▸ Menveo (GlaxoSmithKline UK Ltd)
  Menveo vaccine powder and solvent for solution for injection 0.5ml vials | 1 vial [PoM] £30.00

▸ Nimenrix (Pfizer Ltd) ▼
  Nimenrix vaccine powder and solvent for solution for injection 0.5ml pre-filled syringes | 1 pre-filled disposable injection [PoM] £30.00

F 742

Pneumococcal polysaccharide conjugate vaccine (adsorbed)

● INDICATIONS AND DOSE

PREVENAR 13®

Primary immunisation against pneumococcal infection (first dose)

▸ BY INTRAMUSCULAR INJECTION

▸ Child 2 months: 0.5 mL for 1 dose, anterolateral thigh is preferred site of injection in infants

Primary immunisation against pneumococcal infection (second dose)

▸ BY INTRAMUSCULAR INJECTION

▸ Child 4 months: 0.5 mL for 1 dose, anterolateral thigh is preferred site of injection in infants

Primary immunisation against pneumococcal infection (booster dose)

▸ BY INTRAMUSCULAR INJECTION

▸ Child 12-13 months: 0.5 mL for 1 dose, anterolateral thigh is preferred site of injection in infants

Immunisation against pneumococcal infection (in patients who have not been vaccinated or not completed the primary course)

▸ BY INTRAMUSCULAR INJECTION

▸ Child 12 months-4 years: 0.5 mL for 1 dose, deltoid muscle is preferred site of injection in young children; anterolateral thigh is preferred site in infants

Immunisation against pneumococcal infection, in immunocompromised or asplenic patients or patients with splenic dysfunction (who have not been vaccinated or not completed the primary course)

▸ BY INTRAMUSCULAR INJECTION

▸ Child 12 months-4 years: 0.5 mL every 2 months for 2 doses, deltoid muscle is preferred site of injection in young children; anterolateral thigh is preferred site in infants

SYNFLORIX®

Immunisation against pneumococcal infection

▸ BY INTRAMUSCULAR INJECTION

▸ Child 6 weeks-4 years: Deltoid muscle is preferred site of injection in young children; anterolateral thigh is preferred site in infants (consult product literature)

● UNLICENSED USE

PREVENAR 13® The dose in BNF publications may differ from that in product literature.

● PRESCRIBING AND DISPENSING INFORMATION

PREVENAR 13® Available as part of childhood immunisation schedule from ImmForm www.immform.dh.gov.uk.

● MEDICINAL FORMS

There can be variation in the licensing of different medicines containing the same drug.

Suspension for injection

▸ Prevenar (Pfizer Ltd)
  Prevenar 13 vaccine suspension for injection 0.5ml pre-filled syringes | 1 pre-filled disposable injection [PoM] £49.10 | 10 pre-filled disposable injection [PoM] £491.00

▸ Synflorix (GlaxoSmithKline UK Ltd)
  Synflorix vaccine suspension for injection 0.5ml pre-filled syringes | 1 pre-filled disposable injection [PoM] £27.60

F 742

Pneumococcal polysaccharide vaccine

● INDICATIONS AND DOSE

Immunisation against pneumococcal infection

▸ BY INTRAMUSCULAR INJECTION, OR BY SUBCUTANEOUS INJECTION

▸ Child 2-17 years: 0.5 mL for 1 dose

Immunisation in patients at increased risk of pneumococcal disease

▸ BY INTRAMUSCULAR INJECTION, OR BY SUBCUTANEOUS INJECTION

▸ Child 2-4 years: 0.5 mL for 1 dose, dose should be administered after the second birthday or at least 2 months after the final dose of the 13-valent pneumococcal polysaccharide conjugate vaccine (adsorbed)

▸ Child 5-17 years: 0.5 mL for 1 dose

● MEDICINAL FORMS

There can be variation in the licensing of different medicines containing the same drug.

Solution for injection

▸ Pneumococcal polysaccharide vaccine (Non-proprietary)
  Pneumococcal polysaccharide vaccine solution for injection 0.5ml vials | 1 vial [PoM] £8.32

F 742

Typhoid vaccine

● INDICATIONS AND DOSE

Immunisation against typhoid fever in children at high risk of typhoid fever

▸ BY INTRAMUSCULAR INJECTION

▸ Child 12-23 months: 0.5 mL for 1 dose, dose should be given at least 2 weeks before potential exposure to typhoid infection, response may be suboptimal

Immunisation against typhoid fever

▸ BY INTRAMUSCULAR INJECTION

▸ Child 2-17 years: 0.5 mL for 1 dose, dose should be given at least 2 weeks before potential exposure to typhoid infection

continued →

14

Vaccines

▶ BY MOUTH
- ▶ Child 6–17 years: 1 capsule every 2 days for 3 doses (on days 1, 3, and 5)

● UNLICENSED USE
▶ With intramuscular use Not licensed for use in children under 2 years.

● CONTRA-INDICATIONS
▶ With oral use Acute gastro-intestinal illness

● INTERACTIONS → Appendix 1 (vaccines).
Oral typhoid vaccine is inactivated by concomitant administration of antibacterials or antimalarials:
- ● antibacterials should be avoided for 3 days before and after oral typhoid vaccination;
- ● *Mefloquine* should be avoided for at least 12 hours before or after oral typhoid;
- ● For other antimalarials vaccination with oral typhoid vaccine should be completed at least 3 days before the first dose of the antimalarial (except proguanil hydrochloride with atovaquone, which may be given concomitantly).

● SIDE-EFFECTS
▶ With oral use Abdominal cramps · abdominal pain · diarrhoea · nausea · vomiting

● DIRECTIONS FOR ADMINISTRATION Capsule should be taken one hour before a meal. Swallow as soon as possible after placing in mouth with a cold or lukewarm drink.

● HANDLING AND STORAGE
▶ With oral use It is important to store capsules in a refrigerator.

● PATIENT AND CARER ADVICE
▶ With oral use Patients or carers should be given advice on how to administer and store typhoid vaccine capsules.

● MEDICINAL FORMS
There can be variation in the licensing of different medicines containing the same drug.
Gastro-resistant capsule
CAUTIONARY AND ADVISORY LABELS 25
- ▶ Vivotif (PaxVax Ltd)
Vivotif vaccine gastro-resistant capsules | 3 capsule [PoM] £14.77
Solution for injection
- ▶ Typherix (GlaxoSmithKline UK Ltd)
Salmonella typhi Vi capsular polysaccharide 50 microgram per 1 ml Typherix 25micrograms/0.5ml vaccine solution for injection pre-filled syringes | 1 pre-filled disposable injection [PoM] £9.93 | 10 pre-filled disposable injection [PoM] £99.32
- ▶ Typhim Vi (sanofi pasteur MSD Ltd)
Salmonella typhi Vi capsular polysaccharide 50 microgram per 1 ml Typhim Vi 25micrograms/0.5ml vaccine solution for injection pre-filled syringes | 1 pre-filled disposable injection [PoM] £9.30 | 10 pre-filled disposable injection [PoM] £93.00

Combinations available: *Hepatitis A with typhoid vaccine,* p. 749

VACCINES ❭ VIRAL VACCINES

Hepatitis A and B vaccine

The properties listed below are those particular to the combination only. For the properties of the components please consider, hepatitis A vaccine p. 749, hepatitis B vaccine p. 750.

● INDICATIONS AND DOSE
AMBIRIX®
Immunisation against hepatitis A and hepatitis B infection (primary course)
▶ BY INTRAMUSCULAR INJECTION
- ▶ Child 1–15 years: Initially 1 mL for 1 dose, then 1 mL after 6–12 months for 1 dose, the deltoid region is the preferred site of injection in older children;

anterolateral thigh is the preferred site in infants; not to be injected into the buttock (vaccine efficacy reduced), subcutaneous route used for patients with bleeding disorders (but immune response may be reduced)

TWINRIX® ADULT
Immunisation against hepatitis A and hepatitis B infection (primary course)
▶ BY INTRAMUSCULAR INJECTION
- ▶ Child 16–17 years: Initially 1 mL every 1 month for 2 doses, then 1 mL after 5 months for 1 dose, the deltoid region is the preferred site of injection; not to be injected into the buttock (vaccine efficacy reduced), subcutaneous route used for patients with bleeding disorders (but immune response may be reduced)

Immunisation against hepatitis A and hepatitis B infection—accelerated schedule for travellers departing within 1 month
▶ BY INTRAMUSCULAR INJECTION
- ▶ Child 16–17 years: Initially 1 mL for 1 dose, then 1 mL after 7 days for 1 dose, then 1 mL after 14 days for 1 dose, then 1 mL for 1 dose given 12 months after the first dose, the deltoid region is the preferred site of injection; not to be injected into the buttock (vaccine efficacy reduced), subcutaneous route used for patients with bleeding disorders (but immune response may be reduced)

TWINRIX® PAEDIATRIC
Immunisation against hepatitis A and hepatitis B infection (primary course)
▶ BY INTRAMUSCULAR INJECTION
- ▶ Child 1–15 years: Initially 0.5 mL every 1 month for 2 doses, then 0.5 mL after 5 months for 1 dose, the deltoid region is the preferred site of injection in older children; anterolateral thigh is the preferred site in infants; not to be injected into the buttock (vaccine efficacy reduced), subcutaneous route used for patients with bleeding disorders (but immune response may be reduced)

IMPORTANT SAFETY INFORMATION
Ambirix® and *Twinrix®* are not recommended for post-exposure prophylaxis following percutaneous (needle-stick), ocular, or mucous membrane exposure to hepatitis B virus.

● PRESCRIBING AND DISPENSING INFORMATION
TWINRIX® PAEDIATRIC Primary course should be completed with *Twinrix®* (single component vaccines given at appropriate intervals may be used for booster dose).

AMBIRIX® Primary course should be completed with *Ambirix®* (single component vaccines given at appropriate intervals may be used for booster dose).

TWINRIX® ADULT Primary course should be completed with *Twinrix®* (single component vaccines given at appropriate intervals may be used for booster dose).

● MEDICINAL FORMS
There can be variation in the licensing of different medicines containing the same drug.
Suspension for injection
EXCIPIENTS: May contain Neomycin
- ▶ Ambirix (GlaxoSmithKline UK Ltd)
Ambirix vaccine suspension for injection 1ml pre-filled syringes | 1 pre-filled disposable injection [PoM] £31.18
- ▶ Twinrix (GlaxoSmithKline UK Ltd)
Twinrix Paediatric vaccine suspension for injection 0.5ml pre-filled syringes | 1 pre-filled disposable injection [PoM] £20.79
Twinrix Adult vaccine suspension for injection 1ml pre-filled syringes | 1 pre-filled disposable injection [PoM] £33.31 | 10 pre-filled disposable injection [PoM] £333.13

Hepatitis A vaccine

☞ 742

- **INDICATIONS AND DOSE**

AVAXIM®

Immunisation against hepatitis A infection

▸ BY INTRAMUSCULAR INJECTION

- Child 16–17 years: Initially 0.5 mL for 1 dose, then 0.5 mL after 6–12 months, dose given as booster; booster dose may be delayed by up to 3 years if not given after recommended interval following primary dose, the deltoid region is the preferred site of injection. The subcutaneous route may be used for patients with bleeding disorders; not to be injected into the buttock (vaccine efficacy reduced)

EPAXAL®

Immunisation against hepatitis A infection

▸ BY INTRAMUSCULAR INJECTION

- Child 1–17 years: Initially 0.5 mL for 1 dose, then 0.5 mL after 6–12 months, dose given as booster; booster dose may be delayed by up to 4 years if not given after recommended interval following primary dose. The deltoid region is the preferred site of injection. The subcutaneous route may be used for patients with bleeding disorders

Immunisation against hepatitis A infection (splenectomised patients)

▸ BY INTRAMUSCULAR INJECTION

- Child 1–17 years: Initially 0.5 mL for 1 dose, then 0.5 mL after 1–6 months, dose given as booster; booster dose may be delayed by up to 4 years if not given after recommended interval following primary dose. The deltoid region is the preferred site of injection. The subcutaneous route may be used for patients with bleeding disorders

HAVRIX MONODOSE®

Immunisation against hepatitis A infection

▸ BY INTRAMUSCULAR INJECTION

- Child 1–15 years: Initially 0.5 mL for 1 dose, then 0.5 mL after 6–12 months, dose given as booster; booster dose may be delayed by up to 3 years if not given after recommended interval following primary dose, the deltoid region is the preferred site of injection. The subcutaneous route may be used for patients with bleeding disorders
- Child 16–17 years: Initially 1 mL for 1 dose, then 1 mL after 6–12 months, dose given as booster; booster dose may be delayed by up to 3 years if not given after recommended interval following primary dose, the deltoid region is the preferred site of injection. The subcutaneous route may be used for patients with bleeding disorders

VAQTA® PAEDIATRIC

Immunisation against hepatitis A infection

▸ BY INTRAMUSCULAR INJECTION

- Child 1–17 years: Initially 0.5 mL for 1 dose, then 0.5 mL after 6–18 months, dose given as booster, the deltoid region is the preferred site of injection. The subcutaneous route may be used for patients with bleeding disorders (but immune response may be reduced)

- **ALLERGY AND CROSS-SENSITIVITY** *Epaxal*® contains influenza virus haemagglutinin grown in the allantoic cavity of chick embryos, therefore contra-indicated in those hypersensitive to eggs or chicken protein.

- **MEDICINAL FORMS**
There can be variation in the licensing of different medicines containing the same drug.

Suspension for injection
EXCIPIENTS: May contain Neomycin

▸ Avaxim (sanofi pasteur MSD Ltd)
Avaxim vaccine suspension for injection 0.5ml pre-filled syringes | 1 pre-filled disposable injection [PoM] £18.10 | 10 pre-filled disposable injection [PoM] £181.00

▸ Havrix (GlaxoSmithKline UK Ltd)
Havrix Monodose vaccine suspension for injection 1ml pre-filled syringes | 1 pre-filled disposable injection [PoM] £22.14 | 10 pre-filled disposable injection [PoM] £221.43
Havrix Junior Monodose vaccine suspension for injection 0.5ml pre-filled syringes | 1 pre-filled disposable injection [PoM] £16.77 | 10 pre-filled disposable injection [PoM] £167.68
Havrix Junior Monodose vaccine suspension for injection 0.5ml vials | 1 vial [PoM] £16.77
Havrix Monodose vaccine suspension for injection 1ml vials | 1 vial [PoM] £22.14

▸ VAQTA (sanofi pasteur MSD Ltd)
VAQTA Paediatric vaccine suspension for injection 0.5ml pre-filled syringes | 1 pre-filled disposable injection [PoM] £14.74

Emulsion for injection

▸ Epaxal (Janssen-Cilag Ltd)
Epaxal vaccine emulsion for injection 0.5ml pre-filled syringes | 1 pre-filled disposable injection [PoM] £23.81 | 10 pre-filled disposable injection [PoM] £238.10

Hepatitis A with typhoid vaccine

The properties listed below are those particular to the combination only. For the properties of the components please consider, hepatitis A vaccine above, typhoid vaccine p. 747.

- **INDICATIONS AND DOSE**

HEPATYRIX®

Immunisation against hepatitis A and typhoid infection (primary course)

▸ BY INTRAMUSCULAR INJECTION

▸ Child 15–17 years: 1 mL for 1 dose, the deltoid region is the preferred site of injection; not to be injected into the buttock (vaccine efficacy reduced). The subcutaneous route may be used for patients with bleeding disorders, booster dose given using single component vaccines

VIATIM®

Immunisation against hepatitis A and typhoid infection (primary course)

▸ BY INTRAMUSCULAR INJECTION

▸ Child 16–17 years: 1 mL for 1 dose, the deltoid region is the preferred site of injection; not to be injected into the buttock (vaccine efficacy reduced). The subcutaneous route may be used for patients with bleeding disorders, booster dose given using single component vaccines

- **MEDICINAL FORMS**
There can be variation in the licensing of different medicines containing the same drug.
Suspension for injection
EXCIPIENTS: May contain Neomycin

▸ Hepatyrix (GlaxoSmithKline UK Ltd)
Hepatyrix vaccine suspension for injection 1ml pre-filled syringes | 1 pre-filled disposable injection [PoM] £37.21 | 10 pre-filled disposable injection [PoM] £372.10

▸ ViATIM (sanofi pasteur MSD Ltd)
ViATIM vaccine suspension for injection 1ml pre-filled syringes | 1 pre-filled disposable injection [PoM] £29.80

14

Vaccines

F 742

Hepatitis B vaccine

● **INDICATIONS AND DOSE**

ENGERIX B®

Immunisation against hepatitis B infection
▶ BY INTRAMUSCULAR INJECTION

▸ Neonate: 10 micrograms for 1 dose, then 10 micrograms after 1 month for 1 dose, followed by 10 micrograms after 5 months for 1 dose, anterolateral thigh is preferred site in neonates; not to be injected into the buttock (vaccine efficacy reduced), this dose should not be given to neonates born to hepatitis B surface antigen positive mother.

▸ Child 1 month–15 years: 10 micrograms for 1 dose, then 10 micrograms after 1 month for 1 dose, followed by 10 micrograms after 5 months for 1 dose, deltoid muscle is preferred site of injection in older children; anterolateral thigh is preferred site in infants and young children; not to be injected into the buttock (vaccine efficacy reduced)

▸ Child 16–17 years: 20 micrograms for 1 dose, then 20 micrograms after 1 month for 1 dose, followed by 20 micrograms after 5 months for 1 dose, deltoid muscle is preferred site of injection; not to be injected into the buttock (vaccine efficacy reduced)

Immunisation against hepatitis B infection (accelerated schedule)
▶ BY INTRAMUSCULAR INJECTION

▸ Neonate: 10 micrograms every 1 month for 3 doses, followed by 10 micrograms after 10 months for 1 dose, anterolateral thigh is preferred site in neonates; not to be injected into the buttock (vaccine efficacy reduced), this dose should not be given to neonates born to hepatitis B surface antigen positive mother.

▸ Child 1 month–15 years: 10 micrograms every 1 month for 3 doses, followed by 10 micrograms after 10 months for 1 dose, deltoid muscle is preferred site of injection in older children; anterolateral thigh is preferred site in infants and young children; not to be injected into the buttock (vaccine efficacy reduced)

▸ Child 16–17 years: 20 micrograms every 1 month for 3 doses, followed by 20 micrograms after 10 months for 1 dose, deltoid muscle is preferred site of injection; not to be injected into the buttock (vaccine efficacy reduced)

Immunisation against hepatitis B infection, alternative accelerated schedule
▶ BY INTRAMUSCULAR INJECTION

▸ Child 11–15 years: 20 micrograms for 1 dose, followed by 20 micrograms after 6 months, this schedule is not suitable if high risk of infection between doses or if compliance with second dose uncertain, deltoid muscle is preferred site of injection; not to be injected into the buttock (vaccine efficacy reduced)

Immunisation against hepatitis B infection (for neonates born to hepatitis B surface antigen-positive mother)
▶ BY INTRAMUSCULAR INJECTION

▸ Neonate: 10 micrograms once a month for 3 doses, first dose to be given at birth with hepatitis B immunoglobulin injection (separate site), followed by 10 micrograms after 10 months for 1 dose, anterolateral thigh is preferred site in neonates; not to be injected into the buttock (vaccine efficacy reduced).

Immunisation against hepatitis B infection (in renal insufficiency, including haemodialysis patients)
▶ BY INTRAMUSCULAR INJECTION

▸ Neonate: 10 micrograms every 1 month for 2 doses, followed by 10 micrograms after 5 months for 1 dose, immunisation schedule and booster doses may need to be adjusted in those with low antibody concentration, anterolateral thigh is preferred site in neonates; not to be injected into the buttock (vaccine efficacy reduced), this dose should not be given to neonates born to hepatitis B surface antigen positive mother.

▸ Child 1 month–15 years: 10 micrograms every 1 month for 2 doses, followed by 10 micrograms after 5 months for 1 dose, immunisation schedule and booster doses may need to be adjusted in those with low antibody concentration, deltoid muscle is preferred site of injection in older children; anterolateral thigh is preferred site in infants and young children; not to be injected into the buttock (vaccine efficacy reduced)

▸ Child 16–17 years: 40 micrograms every 1 month for 3 doses, followed by 40 micrograms after 4 months for 1 dose, immunisation schedule and booster doses may need to be adjusted in those with low antibody concentration, deltoid muscle is preferred site of injection; not to be injected into the buttock (vaccine efficacy reduced)

Immunisation against hepatitis B infection (in renal insufficiency, including haemodialysis patients (accelerated schedule))
▶ BY INTRAMUSCULAR INJECTION

▸ Neonate: 10 micrograms every 1 month for 3 doses, followed by 10 micrograms after 10 months for 1 dose, immunisation schedule and booster doses may need to be adjusted in those with low antibody concentration, anterolateral thigh is preferred site in neonates; not to be injected into the buttock (vaccine efficacy reduced), this dose should not be given to neonates born to hepatitis B surface antigen positive mother.

▸ Child 1 month–15 years: 10 micrograms every 1 month for 3 doses, followed by 10 micrograms after 10 months for 1 dose, immunisation schedule and booster doses may need to be adjusted in those with low antibody concentration, deltoid muscle is preferred site of injection in older children; anterolateral thigh is preferred site in infants and young children; not to be injected into the buttock (vaccine efficacy reduced)

FENDRIX®

Immunisation against hepatitis B infection in renal insufficiency (including pre-haemodialysis and haemodialysis patients)
▶ BY INTRAMUSCULAR INJECTION

▸ Child 15–17 years: 20 micrograms every 1 month for 3 doses, followed by 20 micrograms after 4 months for 1 dose, immunisation schedule and booster doses may need to be adjusted in those with low antibody concentration, deltoid muscle is preferred site of injection; not to be injected into the buttock (vaccine efficacy reduced)

HBVAXPRO®

Immunisation against hepatitis B infection
▸ BY INTRAMUSCULAR INJECTION

▸ Neonate: 5 micrograms for 1 dose, followed by 5 micrograms after 1 month for 1 dose, then 5 micrograms after 5 months for 1 dose, booster doses may be required in immunocompromised patients with low antibody concentration, anterolateral thigh is preferred site in neonates; not to be injected into the buttock (vaccine efficacy reduced), dose not to be used for neonate born to hepatitis B surface antigen positive mother.

▸ Child 1 month–15 years: 5 micrograms for 1 dose, followed by 5 micrograms after 1 month for 1 dose, then 5 micrograms after 5 months for 1 dose, booster doses may be required in immunocompromised patients with low antibody concentration, deltoid muscle is preferred site of injection in adults and older children; anterolateral thigh is preferred site in infants; not to be injected into the buttock (vaccine efficacy reduced)

▸ Child 16–17 years: 10 micrograms for 1 dose, followed by 10 micrograms after 1 month for 1 dose, followed by 10 micrograms after 5 months for 1 dose, booster doses may be required in immunocompromised patients with low antibody concentration, deltoid muscle is preferred site of injection in adults and older children; not to be injected into the buttock (vaccine efficacy reduced)

Immunisation against hepatitis B infection (accelerated schedule)
▸ BY INTRAMUSCULAR INJECTION

▸ Neonate: 5 micrograms every 1 month for 3 doses, followed by 5 micrograms after 10 months for 1 dose, booster doses may be required in immunocompromised patients with low antibody concentration, anterolateral thigh is preferred site in neonates; not to be injected into the buttock (vaccine efficacy reduced), dose not to be used for neonate born to hepatitis B surface antigen positive mother.

▸ Child 1 month–15 years: 5 micrograms every 1 month for 3 doses, followed by 5 micrograms after 10 months for 1 dose, booster doses may be required in immunocompromised patients with low antibody concentration, deltoid muscle is preferred site of injection in adults and older children; anterolateral thigh is preferred site in infants; not to be injected into the buttock (vaccine efficacy reduced)

▸ Child 16–17 years: 10 micrograms every 1 month for 3 doses, followed by 10 micrograms after 10 months for 1 dose, booster doses may be required in immunocompromised patients with low antibody concentration, deltoid muscle is preferred site of injection in adults and older children; not to be injected into the buttock (vaccine efficacy reduced)

Neonate born to hepatitis B surface antigen-positive mother
▸ BY INTRAMUSCULAR INJECTION

▸ Neonate: 5 micrograms every 1 month for 3 doses, first dose given at birth with hepatitis B immunoglobulin injection (separate site), followed by 5 micrograms after 10 months for 1 dose, anterolateral thigh is preferred site in neonates; not to be injected into the buttock (vaccine efficacy reduced).

Chronic haemodialysis patients
▸ BY INTRAMUSCULAR INJECTION

▸ Child 16–17 years: 40 micrograms every 1 month for 2 doses, followed by 40 micrograms after 5 months for 1 dose, booster doses may be required in those with low antibody concentration, deltoid muscle is preferred site of injection in adults and older children; not to be injected into the buttock (vaccine efficacy reduced)

● MEDICINAL FORMS
There can be variation in the licensing of different medicines containing the same drug.

Suspension for injection
EXCIPIENTS: May contain Thiomersal

▸ Engerix B (GlaxoSmithKline UK Ltd)
Hepatitis B virus surface antigen 20 microgram per 1 ml Engerix B 20micrograms/1ml vaccine suspension for injection vials | 1 vial PoM £12.34 | 10 vial PoM £123.41
Engerix B 10micrograms/0.5ml vaccine suspension for injection pre-filled syringes | 1 pre-filled disposable injection PoM £9.67
Engerix B 20micrograms/1ml vaccine suspension for injection pre-filled syringes | 1 pre-filled disposable injection PoM £12.99 | 10 pre-filled disposable injection PoM £129.92

▸ Fendrix (GlaxoSmithKline UK Ltd)
Hepatitis B virus surface antigen 40 microgram per 1 ml Fendrix 20micrograms/0.5ml vaccine suspension for injection pre-filled syringes | 1 pre-filled disposable injection PoM £38.10

▸ HBVAXPRO (sanofi pasteur MSD Ltd)
Hepatitis B virus surface antigen 10 microgram per 1 ml HBVAXPRO 10micrograms/1ml vaccine suspension for injection pre-filled syringes | 1 pre-filled disposable injection PoM £12.20
HBVAXPRO 5micrograms/0.5ml vaccine suspension for injection pre-filled syringes | 1 pre-filled disposable injection PoM £8.95
Hepatitis B virus surface antigen 40 microgram per 1 ml HBVaxPRO 40micrograms/1ml vaccine suspension for injection vials | 1 vial PoM £27.60

F 742

Human papillomavirus vaccines

● INDICATIONS AND DOSE

CERVARIX®

Prevention of premalignant genital lesions and cervical cancer
▸ BY INTRAMUSCULAR INJECTION

▸ Child 9–14 years (female): 0.5 mL for 1 dose, followed by 0.5 mL after 5–7 months for 1 dose, if second dose administered earlier than 5 months after the first, a third dose should be administered, dose to be administered into deltoid region, if the course is interrupted, it should be resumed (using the same vaccine) but not repeated, even if more than 24 months have elapsed since the first dose or if the girl is then aged 15 years or more.

▸ Child 15–17 years (female): 0.5 mL for 1 dose, followed by 0.5 mL after 1–2.5 months for 1 dose, then 0.5 mL after 5–12 months from the first dose for 1 dose, dose to be administered into deltoid region, if the course is interrupted, it should be resumed (using the same vaccine) but not repeated, allowing the appropriate interval between the remaining doses.

GARDASIL®

Prevention of premalignant genital (cervical, vulvar and vaginal) and anal lesions, cervical and anal cancers, and genital warts
▸ BY INTRAMUSCULAR INJECTION

▸ Child 9–17 years (female): 0.5 mL for 1 dose, followed by 0.5 mL for 1 dose, second dose to be given at least 1 month after the first dose, then 0.5 mL for 1 dose, third dose to be given at least 3 months after the second dose, schedule should be completed within 12 months of the first dose, dose to be administered preferably into deltoid region or higher anterolateral thigh, if the course is interrupted, it should be resumed (using the same vaccine) but not repeated, allowing the appropriate interval between the remaining doses. continued →

14

Vaccines

Prevention of premalignant genital (cervical, vulvar, and vaginal) and anal lesions, cervical and anal cancers, and genital warts (alternative schedule)
▶ BY INTRAMUSCULAR INJECTION
▶ Child 9-13 years (female): 0.5 mL, for 1 dose, followed by 0.5 mL after 6 months for 1 dose, if the second dose is administered earlier than 6 months after the first dose, a third dose should be administered, dose to be administered preferably into deltoid region or higher anterolateral thigh, if the course is interrupted, it should be resumed (using the same vaccine) but not repeated, even if more than 24 months have elapsed since the first dose or if the girl is then aged 15 years or more.

● PREGNANCY Not known to be harmful, but vaccination should be postponed until completion of pregnancy.

● PRESCRIBING AND DISPENSING INFORMATION To avoid confusion, prescribers should specify the brand to be dispensed.

● MEDICINAL FORMS
There can be variation in the licensing of different medicines containing the same drug.
Suspension for injection
▶ Cervarix (GlaxoSmithKline UK Ltd)
Cervarix vaccine suspension for injection 0.5ml pre-filled syringes | 1 pre-filled disposable injection PoM £80.50
▶ Gardasil (sanofi pasteur MSD Ltd)
Gardasil vaccine suspension for injection 0.5ml pre-filled syringes | 1 pre-filled disposable injection PoM £86.50

⟨ 742

Influenza vaccine

● INDICATIONS AND DOSE
Annual immunisation against seasonal influenza (for children who have not received seasonal influenza vaccine previously)
▶ BY INTRAMUSCULAR INJECTION
▶ Child 6 months-9 years: 0.5 mL for 1 dose, followed by 0.5 mL after at least 4 weeks for 1 dose
▶ BY INTRANASAL ADMINISTRATION
▶ Child 2-9 years: 0.1 mL for 1 dose, followed by 0.1 mL after at least 4 weeks for 1 dose, 0.1 mL dose to be administered into each nostril
Annual immunisation against seasonal influenza
▶ BY INTRAMUSCULAR INJECTION
▶ Child 6 months-17 years: 0.5 mL for 1 dose
▶ BY INTRANASAL ADMINISTRATION
▶ Child 2-17 years: 0.1 mL for 1 dose, dose to be administered into each nostril

● UNLICENSED USE Some products containing inactivated influenza vaccine (surface antigen) are not licensed for use in children under 4 years—check product literature.
FLUVIRIN® Not licensed for use in children under 4 years.
FLUARIX TETRA® Not licensed for use in children under 3 years of age.
OPTAFLU® Not licensed for use in children and adolescents under 18 years.

● CONTRA-INDICATIONS Preparations marketed by Pfizer, or CSL Biotherapies in child under 5 years— increased risk of febrile convulsions
FLUENZ TETRA® Active wheezing · concomitant use with antiviral therapy for influenza · concomitant use with salicylates · severe asthma
CONTRA-INDICATIONS, FURTHER INFORMATION
▶ Concomitant use with antivirals Avoid antivirals for at least 2 weeks after immunisation; avoid immunisation for at least 48 hours after stopping the antiviral.
ENZIRA® Child under 5 years—increased risk of febrile convulsions

● CAUTIONS Increased risk of fever in child 5–9 years with preparations marketed by Pfizer or CSL Biotherapies—use alternative influenza vaccine if available
ENZIRA® Child 5–9 years (increased risk of fever)—use alternative influenza vaccine if available

● SIDE-EFFECTS
GENERAL SIDE-EFFECTS
▶ Uncommon Epistaxis
▶ Frequency not known Febrile convulsions · transient thrombocytopenia
SPECIFIC SIDE-EFFECTS
▶ With intranasal use Rhinorrhoea

● ALLERGY AND CROSS-SENSITIVITY Individuals with a history of egg allergy can be immunised with either an egg free influenza vaccine, if available, or an influenza vaccine with an ovalbumin content less than 120 nanograms/mL (facilities should be available to treat anaphylaxis). Vaccines with an ovalbumin content more than 120 nanograms/mL or where content is not stated should not be used in individuals with egg allergy. If an influenza vaccine containing ovalbumin is being considered in those with a history of anaphylaxis to egg or egg allergy with uncontrolled asthma, these individuals should be referred to a specialist in hospital.

● PREGNANCY Inactivated vaccines not known to be harmful.
FLUENZ TETRA® Avoid in pregnancy.

● BREAST FEEDING Inactivated vaccines not known to be harmful.
FLUENZ TETRA® Avoid in breast-feeding.

● PRESCRIBING AND DISPENSING INFORMATION
FLUARIX TETRA® Ovalbumin content less than 100 nanograms/mL.

● PATIENT AND CARER ADVICE
FLUENZ TETRA® Avoid close contact with severely immunocompromised patients for 1–2 weeks after vaccination.

● MEDICINAL FORMS
There can be variation in the licensing of different medicines containing the same drug.
Suspension for injection
EXCIPIENTS: May contain Gentamicin, kanamycin, neomycin penicillins, polymyxin b, thiomersal
▶ Influenza vaccine (Non-proprietary)
Influenza vaccine (split virion, inactivated) suspension for injection 0.5ml pre-filled syringes | 1 pre-filled disposable injection PoM £5.00-£6.59 | 10 pre-filled disposable injection PoM £65.90
Influenza vaccine (surface antigen, inactivated) suspension for injection 0.5ml pre-filled syringes | 10 pre-filled disposable injection PoM £41.50
▶ Agrippal (Novartis Vaccines and Diagnostics Ltd)
Agrippal vaccine suspension for injection 0.5ml pre-filled syringes | 10 pre-filled disposable injection PoM £58.50
▶ Enzira (Pfizer Ltd)
Enzira vaccine suspension for injection 0.5ml pre-filled syringes | 1 pre-filled disposable injection PoM £5.25 | 10 pre-filled disposable injection PoM £52.50
▶ Fluarix Tetra (GlaxoSmithKline UK Ltd) ▼
Fluarix Tetra vaccine suspension for injection 0.5ml pre-filled syringes | 1 pre-filled disposable injection PoM £9.94 | 10 pre-filled disposable injection PoM £99.40
▶ Imuvac (BGP Products Ltd)
Imuvac vaccine suspension for injection 0.5ml pre-filled syringes | 1 pre-filled disposable injection PoM £6.59 | 10 pre-filled disposable injection PoM £65.90
▶ Influvac Sub-unit (BGP Products Ltd)
Influvac Sub-unit vaccine suspension for injection 0.5ml pre-filled syringes | 1 pre-filled disposable injection PoM £5.22 | 10 pre-filled disposable injection PoM £52.20
▶ Intanza (sanofi pasteur MSD Ltd)
Intanza 15microgram strain vaccine suspension for injection 0.1ml pre-filled syringes | 1 pre-filled disposable injection PoM £9.05 | 10 pre-filled disposable injection PoM £90.50

- Optaflu (Novartis Vaccines and Diagnostics Ltd)
  Optaflu vaccine suspension for injection 0.5ml pre-filled syringes | 1 pre-filled disposable injection PoM £6.59

Spray

EXCIPIENTS: May contain Gelatin, gentamicin

- FluMist Quadrivalent (AstraZeneca UK Ltd)
  FluMist Quadrivalent vaccine nasal suspension 0.2ml unit dose | 10 unit dose PoM £180.00
- Fluenz Tetra (AstraZeneca UK Ltd) ▼
  Fluenz Tetra vaccine nasal suspension 0.2ml unit dose | 10 unit dose PoM £180.00

F 742

Japanese encephalitis vaccine

● INDICATIONS AND DOSE

Immunisation against Japanese encephalitis

▶ BY INTRAMUSCULAR INJECTION

- Child 2 months–2 years: 0.25 mL every 28 days for 2 doses, anterolateral thigh is preferred site of injection in infants, the subcutaneous route may be used for patients with bleeding disorders
- Child 3–17 years: 0.5 mL every 28 days for 2 doses, deltoid muscle is preferred site in older children; anterolateral thigh is preferred in infants, the subcutaneous route may be used for patients with bleeding disorders

● SIDE-EFFECTS
▶ Uncommon Cough

● PREGNANCY Although manufacturer advises avoid because of limited information, miscarriage has been associated with Japanese encephalitis virus infection acquired during the first 2 trimesters of pregnancy.

● MEDICINAL FORMS
There can be variation in the licensing of different medicines containing the same drug.

Solution for injection

▶ Japanese encephalitis vaccine (Non-proprietary)
  Japanese encephalitis GCVC vaccine solution for injection 1ml vials | 1 vial no price available
  Japanese encephalitis GCVC vaccine solution for injection 20ml vials | 1 vial no price available
  Japanese encephalitis GCVC vaccine solution for injection 10ml vials | 1 vial no price available

Suspension for injection

▶ Ixiaro (Valneva UK Ltd)
  Ixiaro vaccine suspension for injection 0.5ml pre-filled syringes | 1 pre-filled disposable injection PoM £59.50

F 742

Measles, mumps and rubella vaccine, live

● INDICATIONS AND DOSE

Primary immunisation against measles, mumps, and rubella (first dose)

▶ BY INTRAMUSCULAR INJECTION, OR BY DEEP SUBCUTANEOUS INJECTION

- Child 12–13 months: 0.5 mL for 1 dose

Primary immunisation against measles, mumps, and rubella (second dose)

▶ BY INTRAMUSCULAR INJECTION, OR BY DEEP SUBCUTANEOUS INJECTION

- Child 40 months–5 years: 0.5 mL for 1 dose

Rubella immunisation (in seronegative women, susceptible to rubella and in unimmunised, seronegative women, post-partum)

▶ BY INTRAMUSCULAR INJECTION, OR BY DEEP SUBCUTANEOUS INJECTION

- Females of childbearing potential: (consult product literature or local protocols)

Children presenting for pre-school booster, who have not received the primary immunisation (first dose) | Immunisation for patients at school-leaving age or at entry into further education, who have not completed the primary immunisation course | Control of measles outbreak | Immunisation for patients travelling to areas where measles is endemic or epidemic, who have not completed the primary immunisation

▶ BY INTRAMUSCULAR INJECTION, OR BY DEEP SUBCUTANEOUS INJECTION

- Child 6 months–17 years: (consult product literature or local protocols)

● UNLICENSED USE Not licensed for use in children under 9 months.

> **IMPORTANT SAFETY INFORMATION**
> MMR VACCINATION AND BOWEL DISEASE OR AUTISM
> Reviews undertaken on behalf of the CSM, the Medical Research Council, and the Cochrane Collaboration, have not found any evidence of a link between MMR vaccination and bowel disease or autism. The Chief Medical Officers have advised that the MMR vaccine is the safest and best way to protect children against measles, mumps, and rubella. Information (including fact sheets and a list of references) may be obtained from www.dh.gov.uk/immunisation.

● CAUTIONS Antibody response to measles component may be reduced after immunoglobulin administration or blood transfusion–leave an interval of at least 3 months before MMR immunisation

CAUTIONS, FURTHER INFORMATION

▶ Administration with other vaccines MMR vaccine should not be administered on the same day as yellow fever vaccine; there should be a 4-week minimum interval between the vaccines. When protection is rapidly required, the vaccines can be given at any interval and an additional dose of MMR may be considered.

  MMR and varicella-zoster vaccine can be given on the same day or separated by a 4-week minimum interval. When protection is rapidly required, the vaccines can be given at any interval and an additional dose of the vaccine given second may be considered.

● SIDE-EFFECTS
▶ Uncommon Parotid swelling (usually in the third week) · sleep disturbances · unusual crying in infants
▶ Rare Arthropathy (2 to 3 weeks after immunisation) · idiopathic thrombocytopenic purpura
▶ Frequency not known Optic neuritis · peripheral neuritis

SIDE-EFFECTS, FURTHER INFORMATION

Malaise, fever, or a rash can occur after the first dose of MMR vaccine–most commonly about a week after vaccination and lasting about 2 to 3 days. Leaflets are available for parents on advice for reducing fever (including the use of paracetamol).

  Febrile seizures–occur rarely 6 to 11 days after MMR vaccination (the incidence is lower than that following measles infection)

▶ Idiopathic thrombocytopenic purpura Idiopathic thrombocytopenic purpura has occurred rarely following MMR vaccination, usually within 6 weeks of the first dose. The risk of idiopathic thrombocytopenic purpura after MMR vaccine is much less than the risk after infection with wild measles or rubella virus. Children who develop idiopathic thrombocytopenic purpura within 6 weeks of the first dose of MMR should undergo serological testing before the second dose is due; if the results suggest incomplete immunity against measles, mumps or rubella then a second dose of MMR is recommended. The Specialist and Reference Microbiology Division, Health Protection Agency offers free serological testing for

14

Vaccines

14

Vaccines

children who develop idiopathic thrombocytopenic purpura *within* 6 *weeks* of the first dose of MMR.

▸ Aseptic meningitis Post-vaccination aseptic meningitis was reported (rarely and with complete recovery) following vaccination with MMR vaccine containing Urabe mumps vaccine, which has now been discontinued; no cases have been confirmed in association with the currently used Jeryl Lynn mumps vaccine. Children with post-vaccination symptoms are not infectious.

▸ Frequency of side effects Adverse reactions are considerably less frequent after the second dose of MMR vaccine than after the first.

● ALLERGY AND CROSS-SENSITIVITY MMR vaccine can be given safely even when the child has had an anaphylactic reaction to food containing egg. Dislike of eggs, refusal to eat egg, or confirmed anaphylactic reactions to egg-containing food is not a contra-indication to MMR vaccination. Children with a confirmed anaphylactic reaction to the MMR vaccine should be assessed by a specialist.

● CONCEPTION AND CONTRACEPTION Exclude pregnancy before immunisation. Avoid pregnancy for at least 1 month after vaccination.

● PRESCRIBING AND DISPENSING INFORMATION Available as part of childhood immunisation schedule from health organisations or ImmForm www.immform.dh.gov.uk.

● MEDICINAL FORMS
There can be variation in the licensing of different medicines containing the same drug.
Powder and solvent for solution for injection
EXCIPIENTS: May contain Neomycin
▸ Priorix (GlaxoSmithKline UK Ltd)
Priorix vaccine powder and solvent for solution for injection 0.5ml vials | 1 vial PoM £7.64
Powder and solvent for suspension for injection
EXCIPIENTS: May contain Gelatin, neomycin
▸ M-M-RVAXPRO (sanofi pasteur MSD Ltd)
M-M-RVAXPRO vaccine powder and solvent for suspension for injection 0.5ml pre-filled syringes | 1 pre-filled disposable injection PoM £11.00

⚑ 742

Rabies vaccine

● INDICATIONS AND DOSE
Pre-exposure prophylaxis
▸ BY INTRAMUSCULAR INJECTION
▸ Child: 1 mL for 2 doses (on days 0 and 7), followed by 1 mL for 1 dose (on day 28), to be administered in deltoid region or anterolateral thigh in infants, for those at continuous risk, measure plasma-concentration of antirabies antibodies every 6 months and give a booster dose if the titre is less than 0.5 units/mL, final dose may be given from day 21, if insufficient time before travel

Pre-exposure prophylaxis booster dose (for patients at frequent risk of exposure)
▸ BY INTRAMUSCULAR INJECTION
▸ Child: 1 mL after 1 year for 1 dose, to be given 1 year after primary course is completed, then 1 mL every 3–5 years, to be administered in deltoid region or anterolateral thigh in infants, the frequency of booster doses may alternatively be determined according to plasma-concentration of antirabies antibodies

Pre-exposure prophylaxis booster dose (for patients at infrequent risk of exposure)
▸ BY INTRAMUSCULAR INJECTION
▸ Child: 1 mL for 1 dose, to be given 10 years after primary course is completed, administered in deltoid region or anterolateral thigh in infants

Post-exposure prophylaxis of fully immunised individuals (who have previously received pre-exposure or post-exposure prophylaxis with cell-derived rabies vaccine)
▸ BY INTRAMUSCULAR INJECTION
▸ Child (administered on expert advice): 1 mL for 1 dose, followed by 1 mL after 3–7 days for 1 dose, to be administered in deltoid region or anterolateral thigh in infants, rabies immunoglobulin is not necessary

Post-exposure treatment for unimmunised individuals (or those whose prophylaxis is possibly incomplete)
▸ BY INTRAMUSCULAR INJECTION
▸ Child (administered on expert advice): 1 mL 5 times a month for 1 month, doses should be given on days 0, 3, 7, 14, and the fifth dose is given between day 28–30, to be administered in deltoid region or anterolateral thigh in infants, depending on the level of risk (determined by factors such as the nature of the bite and the country where it was sustained), rabies immunoglobulin is given to unimmunised individuals on day 0 or within 7 days of starting the course of rabies vaccine, the immunisation course can be discontinued if it is proved that the individual was not at risk

● SIDE-EFFECTS Paresis

● PREGNANCY Because of the potential consequences of untreated rabies exposure and because rabies vaccination has not been associated with fetal abnormalities, pregnancy is not considered a contra-indication to post-exposure prophylaxis. Immunisation against rabies is indicated during pregnancy if there is substantial risk of exposure to rabies and rapid access to post-exposure prophylaxis is likely to be limited.

● MEDICINAL FORMS
There can be variation in the licensing of different medicines containing the same drug.
Powder and solvent for solution for injection
EXCIPIENTS: May contain Neomycin
▸ Rabipur (GlaxoSmithKline UK Ltd)
Rabipur vaccine powder and solvent for solution for injection 1ml vials | 1 vial PoM £34.56
Powder and solvent for suspension for injection
EXCIPIENTS: May contain Neomycin
▸ Rabies vaccine (Non-proprietary)
Verorab powder and solvent for suspension for injection 0.5ml vials | 1 vial PoM no price available
Rabies vaccine powder and solvent for suspension for injection 1ml vials | 1 vial PoM £33.90

⚑ 742

Rotavirus vaccine

● DRUG ACTION Rotavirus vaccine is a live, oral vaccine that protects young children against gastro-enteritis caused by rotavirus infection.

● INDICATIONS AND DOSE
Immunisation against gastro-enteritis caused by rotavirus
▸ BY MOUTH
▸ Child 6–23 weeks: 1.5 mL for 2 doses separated by an interval of at least 4 weeks, first dose must be given between 6–14 weeks of age; course should be completed before 24 weeks of age (preferably before 16 weeks)

● CONTRA-INDICATIONS History of intussusception · predisposition to intussusception · severe combined immunosuppression
CONTRA-INDICATIONS, FURTHER INFORMATION
▸ Immunosuppresion With the exception of severe combined immunodeficiency, rotavirus vaccine is not contra-indicated in immunosuppressed patients—benefit from

vaccination is likely to outweigh the risk, if there is any doubt, seek specialist advice.

- **CAUTIONS** Diarrhoea (postpone vaccination) · immunosuppressed close contacts · vomiting (postpone vaccination)

CAUTIONS, FURTHER INFORMATION

The rotavirus vaccine virus is excreted in the stool and may be transmitted to close contacts; however, vaccination of those with immunosuppressed close contacts may protect the contacts from wild-type rotavirus disease and outweigh any risk from transmission of vaccine virus.

- **SIDE-EFFECTS** Abdominal cramps · abdominal pain · diarrhoea · nausea · vomiting
- **PATIENT AND CARER ADVICE** The rotavirus vaccine virus is excreted in the stool and may be transmitted to close contacts; carers of a recently vaccinated baby should be advised of the need to wash their hands after changing the baby's nappies.

- **MEDICINAL FORMS**
There can be variation in the licensing of different medicines containing the same drug.

Oral suspension
- ▸ Rotarix (GlaxoSmithKline UK Ltd)
Rotarix vaccine live oral suspension 1.5ml pre-filled syringes | 1 unit dose [PoM] £34.76

▶ 742

Tick-borne encephalitis vaccine, inactivated

- **INDICATIONS AND DOSE**

Initial immunisation against tick-borne encephalitis
- ▸ BY INTRAMUSCULAR INJECTION
- ▸ Child 1-15 years: 0.25 mL for 1 dose, followed by 0.25 mL after 1–3 months for 1 dose, then 0.25 mL after further 5–12 months for 1 dose, to achieve more rapid protection, second dose may be given 14 days after first dose, dose to be administered in deltoid region or anterolateral thigh in infants, in immunocompromised patients (including those receiving immunosuppressants), antibody concentration may be measured 4 weeks after second dose and dose repeated if protective levels not achieved
- ▸ Child 16-17 years: 0.5 mL for 1 dose, followed by 0.5 mL after 1–3 months for 1 dose, then 0.5 mL after further 5–12 months for 1 dose, to achieve more rapid protection, second dose may be given 14 days after first dose, dose to be administered in deltoid region, in immunocompromised patients (including those receiving immunosuppressants), antibody concentration may be measured 4 weeks after second dose and dose repeated if protective levels not achieved

Immunisation against tick-borne encephalitis, booster doses
- ▸ BY INTRAMUSCULAR INJECTION
- ▸ Child 1-17 years: First dose to be given within 3 years after initial course completed and then every 3–5 years, dose to be administered in deltoid region or anterolateral thigh in infants (consult product literature)

- **ALLERGY AND CROSS-SENSITIVITY** Individuals with evidence of previous anaphylactic reaction to egg should not be given tick-borne encephalitis vaccine.

- **MEDICINAL FORMS**
There can be variation in the licensing of different medicines containing the same drug.

Suspension for injection
EXCIPIENTS: May contain Gentamicin, neomycin
- ▸ TicoVac (Masta Ltd)
TicoVac Junior vaccine suspension for injection 0.25ml pre-filled syringes | 1 pre-filled disposable injection [PoM] £28.00
TicoVac vaccine suspension for injection 0.5ml pre-filled syringes | 1 pre-filled disposable injection [PoM] £32.00

▶ 742

Varicella-zoster vaccine

- **INDICATIONS AND DOSE**

VARILRIX®

Prevention of varicella infection (chickenpox)
- ▸ BY SUBCUTANEOUS INJECTION
- ▸ Child 1-17 years: 0.5 mL every 4–6 weeks for 2 doses, to be administered preferably into the deltoid region

VARIVAX®

Prevention of varicella infection (chickenpox)
- ▸ BY SUBCUTANEOUS INJECTION, OR BY INTRAMUSCULAR INJECTION
- ▸ Child 1-12 years: 0.5 mL for 2 doses, interval of at least 4 weeks between each dose, to be administered into the deltoid region (or higher anterolateral thigh in young children)
- ▸ Child 13-17 years: 0.5 mL every 4–8 weeks for 2 doses, to be administered preferably into the deltoid region

Prevention of varicella infection (chickenpox) in children with asymptomatic HIV infection
- ▸ BY SUBCUTANEOUS INJECTION, OR BY INTRAMUSCULAR INJECTION
- ▸ Child 1-12 years: 0.5 mL every 12 weeks for 2 doses, to be administered into the deltoid region (or higher anterolateral thigh in young children)

- **CAUTIONS** Post-vaccination close contact with susceptible individuals

CAUTIONS, FURTHER INFORMATION

Rarely, the varicella–zoster vaccine virus has been transmitted from the vaccinated individual to close contacts. Therefore, contact with the following should be avoided if a vaccine-related cutaneous rash develops within 4–6 weeks of the first or second dose:
- varicella-susceptible pregnant women;
- individuals at high risk of severe varicella, including those with immunodeficiency or those receiving immunosuppressive therapy.

Healthcare workers who develop a generalised papular or vesicular rash on vaccination should avoid contact with patients until the lesions have crusted. Those who develop a localised rash after vaccination should cover the lesions and be allowed to continue working unless in contact with patients at high risk of severe varicella.
- ▸ Administration with MMR vaccine Varicella–zoster and MMR vaccines can be given on the same day or separated by a 4-week minimum interval. When protection is rapidly required, the vaccines can be given at any interval and an additional dose of the vaccine given second may be considered.

- **SIDE-EFFECTS**
- ▸ **Rare** Thrombocytopenia
- ▸ **Frequency not known** Conjunctivitis · varicella-like rash

- **CONCEPTION AND CONTRACEPTION** Avoid pregnancy for 3 months after vaccination.

14

Vaccines

Vaccines

14

- **MEDICINAL FORMS**
  There can be variation in the licensing of different medicines
  containing the same drug.
  Powder and solvent for solution for injection
  EXCIPIENTS: May contain Neomycin
  - ► Varilrix (GlaxoSmithKline UK Ltd)
    Varilrix vaccine powder and solvent for solution for injection 0.5ml
    vials | 1 vial [PoM] £27.31
  Powder and solvent for suspension for injection
  EXCIPIENTS: May contain Gelatin, neomycin
  - ► Varivax (sanofi pasteur MSD Ltd)
    Varivax vaccine powder and solvent for suspension for injection 0.5ml
    vials | 1 vial [PoM] £30.28

F 742

Yellow fever vaccine, live

- **INDICATIONS AND DOSE**
  Immunisation against yellow fever
  - ► BY DEEP SUBCUTANEOUS INJECTION
  - ► Child 6–8 months (administered on expert advice): Infants
    under 9 months should be vaccinated only if the risk of
    yellow fever is high and unavoidable (consult product
    literature or local protocols)
  - ► Child 9 months–17 years: 0.5 mL for 1 dose

- **CONTRA-INDICATIONS** Children under 6 months · history of
  thymus dysfunction

- **CAUTIONS**
  CAUTIONS, FURTHER INFORMATION
  - ► Administration with MMR vaccine Yellow fever and MMR
    vaccines should not be administered on the same day;
    there should be a 4-week minimum interval between the
    vaccines. When protection is rapidly required, the vaccines
    can be given at any interval and an additional dose of MMR
    may be considered.

- **SIDE-EFFECTS** Neurotropic disease · viscerotropic disease
  SIDE-EFFECTS, FURTHER INFORMATION
  - ► Vaccine-associated adverse effects *Very rare* adverse effects,
    such as viscerotropic disease (yellow-fever vaccine-
    associated viscerotropic disease, YEL-AVD), a syndrome
    which may include metabolic acidosis, muscle and liver
    cirrhosis, and multi-organ failure. Neurological disorders
    (yellow fever vaccine-associated neurotropic disease, YEL-
    AND) such as encephalitis have also been reported. These
    very rare adverse effects usually occur after the first dose of
    yellow fever vaccine in those with no previous immunity.

- **ALLERGY AND CROSS-SENSITIVITY** Yellow fever vaccine
  should only be considered under the guidance of a
  specialist in individuals with evidence of previous
  anaphylactic reaction to egg.

- **PREGNANCY** Live yellow fever vaccine should not be given
  during pregnancy because there is a theoretical risk of fetal
  infection. Pregnant women should be advised not to travel
  to areas at high risk of yellow fever. If exposure cannot be
  avoided during pregnancy, then the vaccine should be
  given if the risk from disease in the mother outweighs the
  risk to the fetus from vaccination.

- **BREAST FEEDING** Avoid; seek specialist advice if exposure
  to virus cannot be avoided.

- **MEDICINAL FORMS**
  There can be variation in the licensing of different medicines
  containing the same drug.
  Powder and solvent for suspension for injection
  - ► Stamaril (sanofi pasteur MSD Ltd)
    Stamaril vaccine powder and solvent for suspension for injection 0.5ml
    vials | 1 vial [PoM] £33.10

Chapter 15
Anaesthesia

CONTENTS

General anaesthesia	page 757
1 Anaesthesia adjuvants	763
1.1 Neuromuscular blockade	765
1.2 Neuromuscular blockade reversal	770
1.3 Peri-operative analgesia	770

1.4 Peri-operative sedation	page 773
2 Malignant hyperthermia	775
Local anaesthesia	776

General anaesthesia

General anaesthesia

Overview

Several different types of drug are given together during general anaesthesia. Anaesthesia is induced with either a volatile drug given by inhalation or with an intravenously administered drug; anaesthesia is maintained with an intravenous or inhalational anaesthetic. Analgesics, usually short-acting opioids, are also used. The use of neuromuscular blocking drugs necessitates intermittent positive-pressure ventilation. Following surgery, anticholinesterases can be given to reverse the effects of neuromuscular blocking drugs; specific antagonists can be used to reverse central and respiratory depression caused by some drugs used in surgery. A local topical anaesthetic can be used to reduce pain at the injection site.

Individual requirements vary considerably and the recommended doses are only a guide. Smaller doses are indicated in ill, shocked, or debilitated children and in significant hepatic impairment, while robust individuals may require larger doses. The required dose of induction agent may be less if the patient has been premedicated with a sedative agent or if an opioid analgesic has been used.

Intravenous anaesthetics

Intravenous anaesthetics may be used either to induce anaesthesia or for maintenance of anaesthesia throughout surgery. Intravenous anaesthetics nearly all produce their effect in one arm-brain circulation time. Extreme care is required in surgery of the mouth, pharynx, or larynx where the airway may be difficult to maintain (e.g. in the presence of a tumour in the pharynx or larynx).

To facilitate tracheal intubation, induction is usually followed by a neuromuscular blocking drug or a short-acting opioid.

The doses of all intravenous anaesthetic drugs should be titrated to effect (except when using 'rapid sequence induction').

Total intravenous anaesthesia

This is a technique in which major surgery is carried out with all drugs given intravenously. Respiration can be spontaneous, or controlled with oxygen-enriched air. Neuromuscular blocking drugs can be used to provide relaxation and prevent reflex muscle movements. The main problem to be overcome is the assessment of depth of anaesthesia. Target Controlled Infusion (TCI) systems can be used to titrate intravenous anaesthetic infusions to predicted plasma-drug concentrations; specific models with paediatric pharmacokinetic data should be used for children.

Drugs used for intravenous anaesthesia

Propofol p. 759, the most widely used intravenous anaesthetic, can be used for induction or maintenance of anaesthesia in children, but it is not commonly used in neonates. Propofol is associated with rapid recovery and less hangover effect than other intravenous anaesthetics. Propofol can also be used for sedation during diagnostic procedures.

Thiopental sodium p. 209 is a barbiturate that is used for induction of anaesthesia, but has no analgesic properties. Induction is generally smooth and rapid, but dose-related cardiovascular and respiratory depression can occur. Awakening from a moderate dose of thiopental sodium is rapid because the drug redistributes into other tissues, particularly fat. However, metabolism is slow and sedative effects can persist for 24 hours. Repeated doses have a cumulative effect particularly in neonates and recovery is much slower.

Etomidate p. 758 is an intravenous agent associated with rapid recovery without a hangover effect. Etomidate causes less hypotension than thiopental sodium and propofol during induction. It produces a high incidence of extraneous muscle movements, which can be minimised by an opioid analgesic or a short-acting benzodiazepine given just before induction.

Ketamine p. 773 causes less hypotension than thiopental sodium and propofol during induction. It is sometimes used in children requiring repeat anaesthesia (such as for serial burns dressings), however recovery is relatively slow and there is a high incidence of extraneous muscle movements. Ketamine can cause hallucinations, nightmares, and other transient psychotic effects; these can be reduced by a benzodiazepine such as diazepam p. 207 or midazolam p. 210.

Inhalational anaesthetics

Inhalational anaesthetics include gases and volatile liquids. *Gaseous anaesthetics* require suitable equipment for storage and administration. *Volatile liquid anaesthetics* are administered using calibrated vaporisers, using air, oxygen, or nitrous oxide-oxygen mixtures as the carrier gas. To prevent hypoxia, the inspired gas mixture should contain a minimum of 25% oxygen at all times. Higher concentrations of oxygen (greater than 30%) are usually required during inhalational anaesthesia when nitrous oxide p. 762 is being administered.

Volatile liquid anaesthetics

Volatile liquid anaesthetics can be used for induction and maintenance of anaesthesia, and following induction with an intravenous anaesthetic.

Isoflurane p. 761 is a volatile liquid anaesthetic. Heart rhythm is generally stable during isoflurane anaesthesia, but heart-rate can rise. Systemic arterial pressure and cardiac

15

Anaesthesia

output can fall, owing to a decrease in systemic vascular resistance. Muscle relaxation occurs and the effects of muscle relaxant drugs are potentiated. Isoflurane is not recommended for induction of anaesthesia in infants and children of all ages because of the occurrence of cough, breath-holding, desaturation, increased secretions, and laryngospasm. Isoflurane is the preferred inhalational anaesthetic for use in obstetrics.

Desflurane p. 761 is a rapid acting volatile liquid anaesthetic; it is reported to have about one-fifth the potency of isoflurane. Emergence and recovery from anaesthesia are particularly rapid because of its low solubility. Desflurane is not recommended for induction of anaesthesia as it is irritant to the upper respiratory tract.

Sevoflurane p. 762 is a rapid acting volatile liquid anaesthetic and is more potent than desflurane. Emergence and recovery are particularly rapid, but slower than desflurane. Sevoflurane is non-irritant and is therefore often used for inhalational induction of anaesthesia.

Nitrous oxide

Nitrous oxide is used for maintenance of anaesthesia and, in sub-anaesthetic concentrations, for analgesia. For *anaesthesia*, it is commonly used in a concentration of 50 to 66% in oxygen as part of a balanced technique in association with other inhalational or intravenous agents. Nitrous oxide is unsatisfactory as a sole anaesthetic owing to lack of potency, but is useful as part of a combination of drugs since it allows a significant reduction in dosage.

For analgesia (without loss of consciousness), a mixture of nitrous oxide and oxygen containing 50% of each gas (Entonox®, Equanox®) is used. Self-administration using a demand valve may be used in children who are able to self-regulate their intake (usually over 5 years of age) for painful dressing changes, as an aid to postoperative physiotherapy, for wound debridement and in emergency ambulances.

Nitrous oxide may have a deleterious effect if used in children with an air-containing closed space since nitrous oxide diffuses into such a space with a resulting increase in pressure. This effect may be dangerous in conditions such as pneumothorax, which may enlarge to compromise respiration, or in the presence of intracranial air after head injury, entrapped air following recent underwater dive, or recent intra-ocular gas injection.

Malignant hyperthermia

Malignant hyperthermia is a rare but potentially lethal complication of anaesthesia. It is characterised by a rapid rise in temperature, increased muscle rigidity, tachycardia, and acidosis. The most common triggers of malignant hyperthermia are the volatile anaesthetics. Suxamethonium chloride p. 766 has also been implicated, but malignant hyperthermia is more likely if it is given following a volatile anaesthetic. Volatile anaesthetics and suxamethonium chloride should be avoided during anaesthesia in children at high risk of malignant hyperthermia.

Dantrolene sodium p. 775 is used in the treatment of malignant hyperthermia.

Sedation, anaesthesia, and resuscitation in dental practice

Overview

Sedation for dental procedures should be limited to conscious sedation whenever possible. Nitrous oxide p. 762 alone and midazolam p. 210 are effective for many children.

For details of anaesthesia, sedation, and resuscitation in dental practice see *A Conscious Decision: A review of the use of general anaesthesia and conscious sedation in primary dental care*; report by a group chaired by the Chief Medical Officer and Chief Dental Officer, July 2000 and associated documents. Further details can also be found in *Standards for Conscious Sedation in the Provision of Dental Care*; report of an Intercollegiate Advisory Committee for Sedation in Dentistry, 2015 www.rcseng.ac.uk/fds/Documents/dental-sedation-report-2015-web-v2.pdf.

Surgery and long-term medication

Overview

The risk of losing disease control on stopping long-term medication before surgery is often greater than the risk posed by continuing it during surgery. It is vital that the anaesthetist knows about **all** drugs that a patient is (or has been) taking.

Patients with adrenal atrophy resulting from long-term corticosteroid use may suffer a precipitous fall in blood pressure unless corticosteroid cover is provided during anaesthesia and in the immediate postoperative period. Anaesthetists must therefore know whether a patient is, or has been, receiving corticosteroids (including high-dose inhaled corticosteroids).

Other drugs that should normally not be stopped before surgery include drugs for epilepsy, asthma, immunosuppression, and metabolic, endocrine and cardiovascular disorders (but see potassium sparing diuretics). Expert advice is required for children receiving antivirals for HIV infection. See general advice on surgery in children with diabetes in Insulins and anti-diabetic drugs p. 417, Diabetes and surgery.

Children taking antiplatelet medication or an oral anticoagulant present an increased risk for surgery. In these circumstances, the anaesthetist and surgeon should assess the relative risks and decide jointly whether the antiplatelet or the anticoagulant drug should be stopped or replaced with heparin (unfractionated) p. 87 or low molecular weight heparin therapy.

Drugs that should be stopped before surgery include combined oral contraceptives, see Contraceptives, hormonal p. 461. If antidepressants need to be stopped, they should be withdrawn gradually to avoid withdrawal symptoms. Tricyclic antidepressants need not be stopped, but there may be an increased risk of arrhythmias and hypotension (and dangerous interactions with vasopressor drugs); therefore, the anaesthetist should be informed if they are not stopped. Lithium should be stopped 24 hours before major surgery but the normal dose can be continued for minor surgery (with careful monitoring of fluids and electrolytes). Potassium-sparing diuretics may need to be withheld on the morning of surgery because hyperkalaemia may develop if renal perfusion is impaired or if there is tissue damage. Herbal medicines may be associated with adverse effects when given with anaesthetic drugs and consideration should be given to stopping them before surgery.

ANAESTHETICS, GENERAL ⟩ INTRAVENOUS ANAESTHETICS

▎ Etomidate

- ● **INDICATIONS AND DOSE**

Induction of anaesthesia

- ▸ BY SLOW INTRAVENOUS INJECTION
- ▸ Child 1 month–14 years: 150–300 micrograms/kg (max. per dose 60 mg), to be administered over 30-60 seconds (60 seconds for children in whom hypotension might be hazardous), increased if necessary to 400 micrograms/kg

▸ Child 15-17 years: 150–300 micrograms/kg (max. per
  dose 60 mg), to be administered over 30–60 seconds
  (60 seconds for children in whom hypotension might
  be hazardous)

● **UNLICENSED USE** *Hypnomidate* ® licensed for use in
children (age range not specified by manufacturer).
Etomidate-Lipuro ® not licensed for children under
6 months except for imperative indications during
inpatient treatment. Doses in *BNF for Children* may differ
from those in the product literature.

IMPORTANT SAFETY INFORMATION
Etomidate should only be administered by, or under the
direct supervision of, personnel experienced in its use,
with adequate training in anaesthesia and airway
management, and when resuscitation equipment is
available.

● **CAUTIONS** Acute circulatory failure (shock) · Acute
porphyrias p. 562 (avoid) · adrenal insufficiency ·
cardiovascular disease · fixed cardiac output ·
hypovolaemia
CAUTIONS, FURTHER INFORMATION
Adrenal insufficiency Etomidate suppresses adrenocortical
function, particularly during continuous administration,
and it should not be used for maintenance of anaesthesia.
It should be used with caution in patients with underlying
adrenal insufficiency, for example, those with sepsis.

▸ **INTERACTIONS** → Appendix 1 (anaesthetics, general).

▸ **SIDE-EFFECTS**
Common or very common Apnoea · hyperventilation ·
hypotension · nausea · rash · stridor · vomiting
Uncommon Arrhythmias · bradycardia · cough · hiccups ·
hypersalivation · hypertension · phlebitis
Frequency not known AV block · cardiac arrest · extraneous
muscle movement (high incidence) · pain on injection ·
respiratory depression · seizures · shivering · Stevens-
Johnson syndrome
SIDE-EFFECTS, FURTHER INFORMATION
Pain on injection Can be reduced by injecting into a larger
vein or by giving an opioid analgesic just before induction.
Extraneous muscle movement Extraneous muscle movements
can be minimised by an opioid analgesic or a short-acting
benzodiazepine given just before induction.

▸ **PREGNANCY** May depress neonatal respiration if used
during delivery.

▸ **BREAST FEEDING** Breast-feeding can be resumed as soon
as mother has recovered sufficiently from anaesthesia.

▸ **HEPATIC IMPAIRMENT** Reduce dose in liver cirrhosis.

▸ **DIRECTIONS FOR ADMINISTRATION** To be administered
over 30–60 seconds (60 seconds in patients in whom
hypotension might be hazardous).

PATIENT AND CARER ADVICE
Driving and skilled tasks
Patients given sedatives and analgesics during minor
outpatient procedures should be very carefully warned
about the risk of driving or undertaking skilled tasks
afterwards. For a short general anaesthetic the risk extends
to **at least 24 hours** after administration. Responsible
persons should be available to take patients home. The
dangers of taking **alcohol** should also be emphasised.

MEDICINAL FORMS
There can be variation in the licensing of different medicines
containing the same drug.
Solution for injection
EXCIPIENTS: May contain Propylene glycol
▸ Hypnomidate (Janssen-Cilag Ltd)
  Etomidate 2 mg per 1 ml Hypnomidate 20mg/10ml solution for
  injection ampoules | 5 ampoule PoM £6.90

Emulsion for injection
▸ Etomidate-Lipuro (B.Braun Medical Ltd)
  Etomidate 2 mg per 1 ml Etomidate-Lipuro 20mg/10ml emulsion for
  injection ampoules | 10 ampoule PoM £15.62

| Propofol

● **INDICATIONS AND DOSE**
Induction of anaesthesia using 0.5% or 1% injection
▸ BY SLOW INTRAVENOUS INJECTION, OR BY INTRAVENOUS
  INFUSION
▸ Child 1 month-16 years: Usual dose 2.5–4 mg/kg, dose
  adjusted according to age, body-weight and response
▸ Child 17 years: Usual dose 1.5–2.5 mg/kg, to be
  administered at a rate of 20–40 mg every 10 seconds
  until response
Induction of anaesthesia using 2% injection
▸ BY INTRAVENOUS INFUSION
▸ Child 3-16 years: Usual dose 2.5–4 mg/kg, dose adjusted
  according to age, body-weight and response
▸ Child 17 years: Usual dose 1.5–2.5 mg/kg, to be
  administered at a rate of 20–40 mg every 10 seconds
  until response
Maintenance of anaesthesia using 1% injection
▸ BY CONTINUOUS INTRAVENOUS INFUSION
▸ Child 1 month-16 years: Usual dose 9–15 mg/kg/hour,
  dose adjusted according to age, body-weight and
  response
▸ Child 17 years: Usual dose 4–12 mg/kg/hour, adjusted
  according to response
Maintenance of anaesthesia using 2% injection
▸ BY CONTINUOUS INTRAVENOUS INFUSION
▸ Child 3-16 years: Usual dose 9–15 mg/kg/hour, dose
  adjusted according to age, body-weight and response
▸ Child 17 years: Usual dose 4–12 mg/kg/hour, adjusted
  according to response
**Sedation of ventilated patients in intensive care using 1%
or 2% injection**
▸ BY CONTINUOUS INTRAVENOUS INFUSION
▸ Child 16-17 years: Usual dose 0.3–4 mg/kg/hour,
  adjusted according to response
**Induction of sedation for surgical and diagnostic
procedures using 0.5% or 1% injection**
▸ BY SLOW INTRAVENOUS INJECTION
▸ Child 1 month-16 years: Initially 1–2 mg/kg, dose and
  rate of administration adjusted according to desired
  level of sedation and response
▸ Child 17 years: Initially 0.5–1 mg/kg, to be administered
  over 1–5 minutes, dose and rate of administration
  adjusted according to desired level of sedation and
  response
**Maintenance of sedation for surgical and diagnostic
procedures using 0.5% injection**
▸ INITIALLY BY INTRAVENOUS INFUSION
▸ Child 17 years: Initially 1.5–4.5 mg/kg/hour, dose and
  rate of administration adjusted according to desired
  level of sedation and response, followed by (by slow
  intravenous injection) 10–20 mg, (if rapid increase in
  sedation required)
**Maintenance of sedation for surgical and diagnostic
procedures using 1% injection**
▸ INITIALLY BY INTRAVENOUS INFUSION
▸ Child 1 month-16 years: Usual dose 1.5–9 mg/kg/hour,
  dose and rate of administration adjusted according to
  desired level of sedation and response, followed by (by
  slow intravenous injection) up to 1 mg/kg, (if rapid
  increase in sedation required)
▸ Child 17 years: Initially 1.5–4.5 mg/kg/hour, dose and
  rate of administration adjusted according to desired
  level of sedation and response, followed by continued →

(by slow intravenous injection) 10–20 mg, (if rapid increase in sedation required)

Maintenance of sedation for surgical and diagnostic procedures using 2% injection

▸ INITIALLY BY INTRAVENOUS INFUSION

▸ Child 3–16 years: Usual dose 1.5–9 mg/kg/hour, dose and rate of administration adjusted according to desired level of sedation and response

▸ Child 17 years: Initially 1.5–4.5 mg/kg/hour, dose and rate of administration adjusted according to desired level of sedation and response, followed by (by slow intravenous injection) 10–20 mg, using 0.5% or 1% injection (if rapid increase in sedation required)

IMPORTANT SAFETY INFORMATION

Propofol should only be administered by, or under the direct supervision of, personnel experienced in its use, with adequate training in anaesthesia and airway management, and when resuscitation equipment is available.

● CONTRA-INDICATIONS Children under 16 years receiving intensive care

CONTRA-INDICATIONS, FURTHER INFORMATION

Use in intensive care associated with a risk of propofol infusion syndrome (potentially fatal effects, including metabolic acidosis, arrhythmias, cardiac failure, rhabdomyolysis, hyperlipidaemia, hyperkalaemia, hepatomegaly, and renal failure).

● CAUTIONS Acute circulatory failure (shock) · cardiac impairment · cardiovascular disease · epilepsy · fixed cardiac output · hypotension · hypovolaemia · raised intracranial pressure · respiratory impairment

● INTERACTIONS → Appendix 1 (anaesthetics, general).

● SIDE-EFFECTS

▸ **Common or very common** Headache · hypotension · tachycardia · transient apnoea

▸ **Uncommon** Phlebitis · thrombosis

▸ **Rare** Anaphylaxis · arrhythmia · convulsions (onset can be delayed) · delayed recovery from anaesthesia · euphoria

▸ **Very rare** Discoloration of urine · pancreatitis · pulmonary oedema · sexual disinhibition

▸ **Frequency not known** Bradycardia · pain on intravenous injection · propofol infusion syndrome · significant extraneous muscle movements

SIDE-EFFECTS, FURTHER INFORMATION

▸ Bradycardia Bardycardia may be profound and may be treated with intravenous administration of an antimuscarinic drug.

▸ Extraneous muscle movement Extraneous muscle movements can be minimised by an opioid analgesic or a short-acting benzodiazepine given just before induction.

▸ Pain on injection Can be reduced by intravenous lidocaine.

▸ Propofol infusion syndrome Prolonged infusion of propofol doses exceeding 4 mg/kg/hour may result in potentially fatal effects, including metabolic acidosis, arrhythmias, cardiac failure, rhabdomyolysis, hyperlipidaemia, hyperkalaemia, hepatomegaly, and renal failure.

● PREGNANCY Max. dose for maintenance of anaesthesia 6 mg/kg/hour. May depress neonatal respiration if used during delivery.

● BREAST FEEDING Breast-feeding can be resumed as soon as mother has recovered sufficiently from anaesthesia.

● HEPATIC IMPAIRMENT Use with caution.

● RENAL IMPAIRMENT Use with caution.

● MONITORING REQUIREMENTS Monitor blood-lipid concentration if risk of fat overload or if sedation longer than 3 days.

● DIRECTIONS FOR ADMINISTRATION Shake before use; microbiological filter not recommended; may be administered via a Y-piece close to injection site co-administered with Glucose 5% or Sodium chloride 0.9%. 0.5% **emulsion** for injection or intermittent infusion; may be administered undiluted, or diluted with Glucose 5% or Sodium chloride 0.9%; dilute to a concentration not less than 1 mg/mL. 1% **emulsion** for injection or infusion; may be administered undiluted, or diluted with Glucose 5% (*Diprivan®*) or (*Propofol-Lipuro®*) or Sodium chloride 0.9% (*Propofol-Lipuro®* only); dilute to a concentration not less than 2 mg/mL; use within 6 hours of preparation. 2% **emulsion** for infusion; do not dilute.

● PATIENT AND CARER ADVICE

Driving and skilled tasks

Patients given sedatives and analgesics during minor outpatient procedures should be very carefully warned about the risk of driving or undertaking skilled tasks afterwards. For a short general anaesthetic the risk extends to **at least 24 hours** after administration. Responsible persons should be available to take patients home. The dangers of taking **alcohol** should also be emphasised.

● MEDICINAL FORMS

There can be variation in the licensing of different medicines containing the same drug.

Emulsion for injection

▸ Diprivan (AstraZeneca UK Ltd)
Propofol 10 mg per 1 ml Diprivan 1% emulsion for injection 20ml ampoules | 5 ampoule PoM £15.36 (Hospital only)

▸ Propofol-Lipuro (B.Braun Medical Ltd)
Propofol 5 mg per 1 ml Propofol-Lipuro 0.5% emulsion for injection 20ml ampoules | 5 ampoule PoM £14.71

Emulsion for infusion

▸ Diprivan (AstraZeneca UK Ltd)
Propofol 10 mg per 1 ml Diprivan 1% emulsion for infusion 50ml pre-filled syringes | 1 pre-filled disposable injection PoM £10.68
Propofol 20 mg per 1 ml Diprivan 2% emulsion for infusion 50ml pre-filled syringes | 1 pre-filled disposable injection PoM £15.16

ANAESTHETICS, GENERAL > VOLATILE LIQUID ANAESTHETICS

Volatile halogenated anaesthetics

IMPORTANT SAFETY INFORMATION

Should only be administered by, or under the direct supervision of, personnel experienced in their use, with adequate training in anaesthesia and airway management, and when resuscitation equipment is available.

● CONTRA-INDICATIONS Susceptibility to malignant hyperthermia

● CAUTIONS Can trigger malignant hyperthermia · neuromuscular disease (inhalational anaesthetics are very rarely associated with hyperkalaemia, resulting in cardiac arrhythmias and death) · raised intracranial pressure (can increase cerebrospinal pressure)

● SIDE-EFFECTS

▸ **Common or very common** Arrhythmias · cardiorespiratory depression · hypotension

▸ **Frequency not known** Convulsions · mood changes (that can last several days)

● ALLERGY AND CROSS-SENSITIVITY Can cause hepatotoxicity in those sensitised to halogenated anaesthetics.

● DIRECTIONS FOR ADMINISTRATION Volatile liquid anaesthetics are administered using calibrated vaporisers, using air, oxygen, or nitrous oxide-oxygen mixtures as the carrier gas. To prevent hypoxia, the inspired gas mixture should contain a minimum of 25% oxygen at all times.

● PATIENT AND CARER ADVICE

Driving and skilled tasks
Patients given sedatives and analgesics during minor outpatient procedures should be very carefully warned about the risks of driving or undertaking skilled tasks afterwards. For a short general anaesthetic, the risk extends **to at least 24 hours** after administration. Responsible persons should be available to take patients home. The dangers of taking **alcohol** should also be emphasised.

Desflurane

● INDICATIONS AND DOSE

Induction of anaesthesia (but not recommended)
▸ BY INHALATION
▸ Child 12–17 years: 4–11 %, to be inhaled through specifically calibrated vaporiser

Maintenance of anaesthesia (in nitrous oxide–oxygen)
▸ BY INHALATION
▸ Neonate: 2–6 %, to be inhaled through a specifically calibrated vaporiser.
▸ Child: 2–6 %, to be inhaled through a specifically calibrated vaporiser

Maintenance of anaesthesia (in oxygen or oxygen-enriched air)
▸ BY INHALATION
▸ Neonate: 2.5–8.5 %, to be inhaled through a specifically calibrated vaporiser
▸ Child: 2.5–8.5 %, to be inhaled through a specifically calibrated vaporiser

● INTERACTIONS → Appendix 1 (anaesthetics, general).

● SIDE-EFFECTS Apnoea · breath-holding · cough · increased secretions · laryngospasm

● PREGNANCY May depress neonatal respiration if used during delivery.

● BREAST FEEDING Breast-feeding can be resumed as soon as mother has recovered sufficiently from anaesthesia.

● PATIENT AND CARER ADVICE

Driving and skilled tasks
Patients given sedatives and analgesics during minor outpatient procedures should be very carefully warned about the risk of driving or undertaking skilled tasks afterwards. For a short general anaesthetic the risk extends to **at least 24 hours** after administration. Responsible persons should be available to take patients home. The dangers of taking **alcohol** should also be emphasised.

MEDICINAL FORMS
There can be variation in the licensing of different medicines containing the same drug.
Inhalation vapour
▸ **Suprane** (Baxter Healthcare Ltd)
Desflurane 1 ml per 1 ml Suprane volatile liquid | 240 ml PoM no price available (Hospital only)

Isoflurane

● INDICATIONS AND DOSE

Induction of anaesthesia (in oxygen or nitrous oxide-oxygen) (but indication not recommended in infants and children of all ages)
▸ BY INHALATION
▸ Neonate: Initially 0.5 %, increased to 3 %, adjusted according to response, administered using specifically calibrated vaporiser
▸ Child: Initially 0.5 %, increased to 3 %, adjusted according to response, administered using specifically calibrated vaporiser

Maintenance of anaesthesia (in nitrous oxide–oxygen)
▸ BY INHALATION
▸ Neonate: 1–2.5 %, to be administered using specifically calibrated vaporiser; an additional 0.5–1% may be required when given with oxygen alone.
▸ Child: 1–2.5 %, to be administered using specifically calibrated vaporiser; an additional 0.5–1% may be required when given with oxygen alone

Maintenance of anaesthesia in caesarean section (in nitrous oxide–oxygen)
▸ BY INHALATION
▸ Child: 0.5–0.75 %, to be administered using specifically calibrated vaporiser

> IMPORTANT SAFETY INFORMATION
> Isoflurane is not recommended for induction of anaesthesia in infants and children of all ages because of the occurrence of cough, breath-holding, desaturation, increased secretions, and laryngospasm.

● CAUTIONS Children under 2 years—limited experience

● INTERACTIONS → Appendix 1 (anaesthetics, general).

● SIDE-EFFECTS Breath-holding · cough · irritate mucous membrane · laryngospasm

● PREGNANCY May depress neonatal respiration if used during delivery.

● BREAST FEEDING Breast-feeding can be resumed as soon as mother has recovered sufficiently from anaesthesia.

● PATIENT AND CARER ADVICE

Driving and skilled tasks
Patients given sedatives and analgesics during minor outpatient procedures should be very carefully warned about the risk of driving or undertaking skilled tasks afterwards. For a short general anaesthetic the risk extends to **at least 24 hours** after administration. Responsible persons should be available to take patients home. The dangers of taking **alcohol** should also be emphasised.

● MEDICINAL FORMS
There can be variation in the licensing of different medicines containing the same drug.
Inhalation vapour
▸ Isoflurane (Non-proprietary)
Isoflurane 1 ml per 1 ml Isoflurane inhalation vapour | 250 ml PoM £35.29 (Hospital only)
Isoflurane volatile liquid | 250 ml P £47.50 (Hospital only)
▸ **AErrane** (Baxter Healthcare Ltd)
Isoflurane 1 ml per 1 ml AErrane volatile liquid | 250 ml P no price available (Hospital only)

15

Anaesthesia

Nitrous oxide

- **INDICATIONS AND DOSE**

Maintenance of anaesthesia in conjunction with other anaesthetic agents
- ▶ BY INHALATION
  - ▸ Neonate: 50–66 %, to be administered using suitable anaesthetic apparatus in oxygen.
  - ▸ Child: 50–66 %, to be administered using suitable anaesthetic apparatus in oxygen

Analgesia
- ▶ BY INHALATION
  - ▸ Neonate: Up to 50 %, to be administered using suitable anaesthetic apparatus in oxygen, adjusted according to the patient's needs.
  - ▸ Child: Up to 50 %, to be administered using suitable anaesthetic apparatus in oxygen, adjusted according to the patient's needs

IMPORTANT SAFETY INFORMATION
Nitrous oxide should only be administered by, or under the direct supervision of, personnel experienced in its use, with adequate training in anaesthesia and airway management, and when resuscitation equipment is available.

- **CAUTIONS** Entrapped air following recent underwater dive · pneumothorax · presence of intracranial air after head injury · recent intra-ocular gas injection
  CAUTIONS, FURTHER INFORMATION
  Nitrous oxide may have a deleterious effect if used in patients with an air-containing closed space since nitrous oxide diffuses into such a space with a resulting increase in pressure. This effect may be dangerous in conditions such as pneumothorax, which may enlarge to compromise respiration, or in the presence of intracranial air after head injury, entrapped air following recent underwater dive, or recent intra-ocular gas injection.
- **INTERACTIONS** → Appendix 1 (anaesthetics, general).
- **SIDE-EFFECTS** Depression of white cell formation · hypoxia · megaloblastic anaemia · neurological toxic effects
  SIDE-EFFECTS, FURTHER INFORMATION
  - ▸ Hypoxia Hypoxia can occur immediately following the administration of nitrous oxide; additional oxygen should always be given for several minutes after stopping the flow of nitrous oxide.
  - ▸ Prolonged exposure Exposure of patients to nitrous oxide for prolonged periods, either by continuous or by intermittent administration, may result in megaloblastic anaemia owing to interference with the action of vitamin B_{12}; neurological toxic effects can occur without preceding overt haematological changes. Depression of white cell formation may also occur.
- **PREGNANCY** May depress neonatal respiration if used during delivery.
- **BREAST FEEDING** Breast-feeding can be resumed as soon as mother has recovered sufficiently from anaesthesia.
- **MONITORING REQUIREMENTS**
  - ▸ Assessment of plasma-vitamin B_{12} concentration should be considered in those at risk of deficiency, including those who have a poor, vegetarian, or vegan diet, and those with a history of anaemia.
  - ▸ Nitrous oxide should **not** be given continuously for longer than 24 hours or more frequently than every 4 days without close supervision and haematological monitoring.
- **DIRECTIONS FOR ADMINISTRATION** For analgesia (without loss of consciousness), a mixture of nitrous oxide and oxygen containing 50% of each gas (Entonox®, Equanox®) is used.
- **HANDLING AND STORAGE** Exposure of theatre staff to nitrous oxide should be minimised (risk of serious side-effects).
- **PATIENT AND CARER ADVICE**
  Medicines for Children leaflet: Nitrous oxide for pain www.medicinesforchildren.org.uk/nitrous-oxide-for-pain

- **MEDICINAL FORMS**
  There can be variation in the licensing of different medicines containing the same drug.
  Inhalation gas
  - ▸ Nitrous oxide (Non-proprietary)
    Nitrous oxide 1 ml per 1 ml Nitrous oxide cylinders size E | 1800 litre Ⓟ no price available
    Medical Nitrous Oxide cylinders size D | 900 litre Ⓟ no price available
    Medical Nitrous Oxide cylinders size G | 9000 litre Ⓟ no price available
    Nitrous oxide cylinders size F | 3600 litre Ⓟ no price available
    Nitrous oxide cylinders size J | 18000 litre Ⓟ no price available
    Nitrous oxide cylinders size G | 9000 litre Ⓟ no price available
    Nitrous oxide cylinders size C | 450 litre Ⓟ no price available
    Medical Nitrous Oxide cylinders size F | 3600 litre Ⓟ no price available
    Nitrous oxide cylinders size D | 900 litre Ⓟ no price available
    Medical Nitrous Oxide cylinders size E | 1800 litre Ⓟ no price available

Ⓕ 760

Sevoflurane

- **INDICATIONS AND DOSE**

Induction of anaesthesia (in oxygen or nitrous oxide-oxygen)
- ▶ BY INHALATION
  - ▸ Neonate: Up to 4 %, adjusted according to response, to be administered using specifically calibrated vaporiser.
  - ▸ Child: Initially 0.5–1 %, then increased to up to 8 %, increased gradually, according to response, to be administered using specifically calibrated vaporiser

Maintenance of anaesthesia (in oxygen or nitrous oxide-oxygen)
- ▶ BY INHALATION
  - ▸ Neonate: 0.5–2 %, adjusted according to response, to be administered using specifically calibrated vaporiser.
  - ▸ Child: 0.5–3 %, adjusted according to response, to be administered using specifically calibrated vaporiser

- **CAUTIONS** Susceptibility to QT-interval prolongation
- **INTERACTIONS** → Appendix 1 (anaesthetics, general).
  Sevoflurane can interact with carbon dioxide absorbents to form compound A, a potentially nephrotoxic vinyl ether. However, in spite of extensive use, no cases of sevoflurane-induced permanent renal injury have been reported and the carbon dioxide absorbents used in the UK produce very low concentrations of compound A, even in low-flow anaesthetic systems.
- **SIDE-EFFECTS** Agitation · cardiac arrest · dystonia · leucopenia · torsade de pointes · urinary retention
- **PREGNANCY** May depress neonatal respiration if used during delivery.
- **BREAST FEEDING** Breast-feeding can be resumed as soon as mother has recovered sufficiently from anaesthesia.
- **RENAL IMPAIRMENT** Use with caution.
- **PATIENT AND CARER ADVICE**
  Driving and skilled tasks
  Patients given sedatives and analgesics during minor outpatient procedures should be very carefully warned about the risk of driving or undertaking skilled tasks

afterwards. For a short general anaesthetic the risk extends to **at least 24 hours** after administration. Responsible persons should be available to take patients home. The dangers of taking **alcohol** should also be emphasised.

- MEDICINAL FORMS
  There can be variation in the licensing of different medicines containing the same drug.
  Inhalation vapour
  ▸ Sevoflurane (Non-proprietary)
  Sevoflurane 1 ml per 1 ml Sevoflurane volatile liquid | 250 ml [PoM] £123.00 (Hospital only)

1   Anaesthesia adjuvants

Pre-medication and peri-operative drugs

Drugs that affect gastric pH

Regurgitation and aspiration of gastric contents (Mendelson's syndrome) can be a complication of general anaesthesia, particularly in obstetrics and in gastro-oesophageal reflux disease; prophylaxis against acid aspiration is not routinely used in children but may be required in high-risk cases.

An **H$_2$-receptor antagonist** can be used before surgery to increase the pH and reduce the volume of gastric fluid. It does not affect the pH of fluid already in the stomach and this limits its value in emergency procedures; an oral H$_2$-receptor antagonist can be given 1–2 hours before the procedure.

Antimuscarinic drugs

Antimuscarinic drugs are used (less commonly nowadays) as premedicants to dry bronchial and salivary secretions which are increased by intubation, upper airway surgery, or some inhalational anaesthetics. They are also used before or with neostigmine p. 602 to prevent bradycardia, excessive salivation, and other muscarinic actions of neostigmine. They also prevent bradycardia and hypotension associated with drugs such as propofol p. 759 and suxamethonium chloride p. 766.

Atropine sulfate p. 764 is now rarely used for premedication but still has an emergency role in the treatment of vagotonic side-effects. Atropine sulfate may have a role in cardiopulmonary resuscitation.

Hyoscine hydrobromide p. 250 reduces secretions and also provides a degree of amnesia, sedation, and anti-emesis. Unlike atropine sulfate it may produce bradycardia rather than tachycardia.

Glycopyrronium bromide p. 765 reduces salivary secretions. When given intravenously it produces less tachycardia than atropine sulfate. It is widely used with neostigmine for reversal of non-depolarising muscle relaxants.

Glycopyrronium bromide or hyoscine hydrobromide are also used to control excessive secretions in upper airways or hypersalivation in palliative care and in children unable to control posture or with abnormal swallowing reflex; effective dose varies and tolerance may develop. The intramuscular route should be avoided if possible. Hyoscine hydrobromide transdermal patches may also be used.

Sedative drugs

Premedication

Fear and anxiety before a procedure (including the night before) can be minimised by using a sedative drug, usually a **benzodiazepine**. Premedication may also augment the action of anaesthetics and provide some degree of pre-operative amnesia. The choice of drug depends on the individual, the nature of the procedure, the anaesthetic to be used, and other prevailing circumstances such as outpatients, obstetrics, and availability of recovery facilities. The choice also varies between elective and emergency procedures. Oral administration is preferred if possible; the rectal route should only be used in exceptional circumstances.

Premedicants can be given the night before major surgery; a further, smaller dose may be required before surgery. Alternatively, the first dose may be given on the day of the procedure.

Oral midazolam p. 210 is the most common premedicant for children; temazepam p. 774 may be used in older children. The antihistamine alimemazine tartrate p. 167 is occasionally used orally, but when given alone it may cause postoperative restlessness in the presence of pain.

Benzodiazepines

Benzodiazepines possess useful properties for premedication including relief of anxiety, sedation, and amnesia; short-acting benzodiazepines taken by mouth are the most common premedicants. Benzodiazepines are also used for sedation prior to clinical procedures and for sedation in intensive care.

Benzodiazepines may occasionally cause marked respiratory depression and facilities for its treatment are essential; flumazenil p. 794 is used to antagonise the effects of benzodiazepines.

Midazolam, a water-soluble benzodiazepine, is the preferred benzodiazepine for premedication and for sedation for clinical procedures in children. It has a fast onset of action, and recovery is faster than for other benzodiazepines. Recovery may be longer in children with a low cardiac output, or after repeated dosing.

Midazolam can be given by mouth [unlicensed], but its bitter acidic taste may need to be disguised. It can also be given buccally [unlicensed indication] or intranasally [unlicensed]. Midazolam is associated with profound sedation when high doses are given or when it is used with certain other drugs. It can cause severe disinhibition and restlessness in some children. Midazolam is not recommended for prolonged sedation in neonates; drug accumulation is likely to occur.

Temazepam is given by mouth for premedication in older children and has a short duration of action. Anxiolytic and sedative effects last about 90 minutes, although there may be residual drowsiness. Temazepam is rarely used for dental procedures in children.

Lorazepam p. 209 produces more prolonged sedation than temazepam and it has marked amnesic effects.

Peri-operative use of diazepam p. 207 is not recommended in children; onset and magnitude of response are unreliable, and paradoxical effects may occur. Diazepam is not used for dental procedures in children.

Antagonists for central and respiratory depression

Respiratory depression is a major concern with opioid analgesics and it may be treated by artificial ventilation or be reversed by an opioid antagonist. Naloxone hydrochloride p. 796 given intravenously immediately reverses opioid-induced respiratory depression but the dose may have to be repeated because of its **short duration of action**. Intramuscular injection of naloxone hydrochloride produces a more gradual and prolonged effect but absorption may be erratic. Care is required in children requiring pain relief because naloxone hydrochloride also antagonises the analgesic effect of opioids.

Flumazenil is a benzodiazepine antagonist for the reversal of the central sedative effects of benzodiazepines after anaesthetic and similar procedures. Flumazenil has a shorter half-life and duration of action than diazepam or midazolam so patients may become resedated.

15

Anaesthesia

15

Anaesthesia

Neonates

Naloxone hydrochloride is used in newborn infants to reverse respiratory depression and sedation resulting from the use of opioids by the mother, usually for pain during labour. In neonates the effects of opioids may persist for up to 48 hours and in such cases naloxone hydrochloride is often given by intramuscular injection for its prolonged effect. In severe respiratory depression after birth, breathing should first be established (using artificial means if necessary) and naloxone hydrochloride administered only if use of opioids by the mother is thought to cause the respiratory depression; the infant should be monitored closely and further doses of naloxone hydrochloride administered as necessary.

ANTIMUSCARINICS

⬛ 457

▌Atropine sulfate

● **INDICATIONS AND DOSE**

Bradycardia due to acute massive overdosage of beta-blockers

▶ BY INTRAVENOUS INJECTION

▸ Child: 40 micrograms/kg (max. per dose 3 mg)

Treatment of poisoning by organophosphorus insecticide or nerve agent (in combination with pralidoxime chloride)

▶ BY INTRAVENOUS INJECTION

▸ Child: 20 micrograms/kg every 5–10 minutes (max. per dose 2 mg) until the skin becomes flushed and dry, the pupils dilate, and bradycardia is abolished, frequency of administration dependent on the severity of poisoning

Premedication

▶ BY INTRAVENOUS INJECTION

▸ Neonate: 10 micrograms/kg, to be administered immediately before induction of anaesthesia.

▸ Child 1 month-11 years: 20 micrograms/kg, to be administered immediately before induction of anaesthesia (minimum 100 micrograms, max. 600 micrograms)

▸ Child 12-17 years: 300–600 micrograms, to be administered immediately before induction of anaesthesia

▶ BY SUBCUTANEOUS INJECTION, OR BY INTRAMUSCULAR INJECTION

▸ Neonate: 10 micrograms/kg, to be administered 30-60 minutes before induction of anaesthesia.

▸ Child 1 month-11 years: 10–30 micrograms/kg, to be administered 30-60 minutes before induction of anaesthesia (minimum 100 micrograms, max. 600 micrograms)

▸ Child 12-17 years: 300–600 micrograms to be administered 30-60 minutes before induction of anaesthesia

▶ BY MOUTH

▸ Neonate: 20–40 micrograms/kg, to be administered 1–2 hours before induction of anaesthesia.

▸ Child: 20–40 micrograms/kg (max. per dose 900 micrograms), to be administered 1–2 hours before induction of anaesthesia

Intra-operative bradycardia

▶ BY INTRAVENOUS INJECTION

▸ Neonate: 10–20 micrograms/kg.

▸ Child 1 month-11 years: 10–20 micrograms/kg

▸ Child 12-17 years: 300–600 micrograms, larger doses may be used in emergencies

Control of muscarinic side-effects of neostigmine in reversal of competitive neuromuscular block

▶ BY INTRAVENOUS INJECTION

▸ Neonate: 20 micrograms/kg.

▸ Child 1 month-11 years: 20 micrograms/kg (max. per dose 1.2 mg)

▸ Child 12-17 years: 0.6–1.2 mg

● UNLICENSED USE Not licensed for use in children under 12 years for intra-operative bradycardia or by intravenous route for premedication. Not licensed for use by oral route.

> IMPORTANT SAFETY INFORMATION
> Antimuscarinic drugs used for premedication to general anaesthesia should only be administered by, or under the direct supervision of, personnel experienced in their use.

● PREGNANCY Not known to be harmful; manufacturer advises caution.

● BREAST FEEDING May suppress lactation; small amount present in milk—manufacturer advises caution.

● MONITORING REQUIREMENTS
▶ Control of muscarinic side-effects of neostigmine in reversal of competitive neuromuscular block Since atropine has a shorter duration of action than neostigmine, late unopposed bradycardia may result; close monitoring of the patient is necessary.

● DIRECTIONS FOR ADMINISTRATION For administration *by mouth*, injection solution may be given orally.

● EXCEPTIONS TO LEGAL CATEGORY
▶ With intramuscular use or intravenous use or subcutaneous use Prescription only medicine restriction does not apply where administration is for saving life in emergency.

● MEDICINAL FORMS
There can be variation in the licensing of different medicines containing the same drug. Forms available from special-order manufacturers include: oral suspension, oral solution, solution for injection, solution for infusion

Tablet

▶ Atropine sulfate (Non-proprietary)
Atropine sulfate 600 microgram Atropine 600microgram tablets | 28 tablet [PoM] £25.75 DT price = £25.75

Solution for injection

▶ Atropine sulfate (Non-proprietary)
Atropine sulfate 100 microgram per 1 ml Atropine 500micrograms/5ml solution for injection pre-filled syringes | 1 pre-filled disposable injection [PoM] £7.40–£13.00 | 10 pre-filled disposable injection [PoM] £69.00–£130.00
Atropine sulfate 200 microgram per 1 ml Atropine 1mg/5ml solution for injection pre-filled syringes | 1 pre-filled disposable injection [PoM] £7.08–£13.00 | 10 pre-filled disposable injection [PoM] £130.00
Atropine sulfate 300 microgram per 1 ml Atropine 3mg/10ml solution for injection pre-filled syringes | 1 pre-filled disposable injection [PoM] £7.08–£13.00 | 10 pre-filled disposable injection [PoM] £130.00
Atropine sulfate 400 microgram per 1 ml Atropine 400micrograms/1ml solution for injection ampoules | 10 ampoule [PoM] £67.78–£74.56 DT price = £71.17
Atropine sulfate 600 microgram per 1 ml Atropine 600micrograms/1ml solution for injection ampoules | 10 ampoule [PoM] £11.71 DT price = £11.70
Atropine 600micrograms/1ml solution for injection pre-filled syringes | 1 pre-filled disposable injection [PoM] £7.08
Atropine sulfate 1 mg per 1 ml Atropine 1mg/1ml solution for injection ampoules | 10 ampoule [PoM] £57.66–£63.43 DT price = £60.55

Glycopyrronium bromide

▸ 457

(Glycopyrrolate)

● **INDICATIONS AND DOSE**

Premedication at induction

▸ BY INTRAMUSCULAR INJECTION, OR BY INTRAVENOUS INJECTION

- Neonate: 5 micrograms/kg.

- Child 1 month–11 years: 4–8 micrograms/kg (max. per dose 200 micrograms)

- Child 12–17 years: 200–400 micrograms, alternatively 4–5 micrograms/kg (max. per dose 400 micrograms)

Intra-operative bradycardia

▸ BY INTRAVENOUS INJECTION

- Neonate: 10 micrograms/kg, repeated if necessary.

- Child: 4–8 micrograms/kg (max. per dose 200 micrograms), repeated if necessary

Control of muscarinic side-effects of neostigmine in reversal of non-depolarising neuromuscular block

▸ BY INTRAVENOUS INJECTION

- Neonate: 10 micrograms/kg.

- Child 1 month–11 years: 10 micrograms/kg (max. per dose 500 micrograms)

- Child 12–17 years: 10–15 micrograms/kg, alternatively, 200 micrograms per 1 mg of neostigmine to be administered

Control of upper airways secretion | Hypersalivation

▸ BY MOUTH

- Child: 40–100 micrograms/kg 3–4 times a day (max. per dose 2 mg), adjusted according to response

▸ BY SUBCUTANEOUS INFUSION

- Child 1 month–11 years: 12–40 micrograms/kg (max. per dose 1.2 mg) over 24 hours

- Child 12–17 years: 0.6–1.2 mg/24 hours

▸ BY SUBCUTANEOUS INJECTION, OR BY INTRAMUSCULAR INJECTION, OR BY INTRAVENOUS INJECTION

- Child 1 month–11 years: 4–10 micrograms/kg 4 times a day (max. per dose 200 micrograms) as required

- Child 12–17 years: 200 micrograms every 4 hours as required

● **UNLICENSED USE** Not licensed for use in control of upper airways secretion and hypersalivation.

IMPORTANT SAFETY INFORMATION
Antimuscarinic drugs used for premedication to general anaesthesia should only be administered by, or under the direct supervision of, personnel experienced in their use.

● **DIRECTIONS FOR ADMINISTRATION** For administration *by mouth*, injection solution may be given or crushed tablets suspended in water.

● **PRESCRIBING AND DISPENSING INFORMATION** Tablets may be available on a named-patient basis from specialist importing companies.

● **MEDICINAL FORMS**
There can be variation in the licensing of different medicines containing the same drug. Forms available from special-order manufacturers include: capsule, oral suspension, oral solution, liquid

Tablet

▸ Glycopyrronium bromide (Non-proprietary)
Glycopyrronium bromide 1 mg Robinul 1mg tablets | 100 tablet PoM no price available
Glycopyrronium bromide 1mg tablets | 30 tablet PoM £178.50–£216.00 DT price = £197.25

Glycopyrronium bromide 2 mg Robinul Forte 2mg tablets | 100 tablet PoM no price available
Glycopyrronium bromide 2mg tablets | 30 tablet PoM £198.00–£237.60 DT price = £220.80

Solution for injection

▸ Glycopyrronium bromide (Non-proprietary)
Glycopyrronium bromide 200 microgram per 1 ml Glycopyrronium bromide 200micrograms/1ml solution for injection ampoules | 10 ampoule PoM £14.00 DT price = £8.28
Glycopyrronium bromide 600micrograms/3ml solution for injection ampoules | 3 ampoule PoM £8.00–£8.56 | 10 ampoule PoM £11.50

1.1   Neuromuscular blockade

Neuromuscular blockade

Neuromuscular blocking drugs

Neuromuscular blocking drugs used in anaesthesia are also known as **muscle relaxants**. By specific blockade of the neuromuscular junction they enable light anaesthesia to be used with adequate relaxation of the muscles of the abdomen and diaphragm. They also relax the vocal cords and allow the passage of a tracheal tube. Their action differs from the muscle relaxants used in musculoskeletal disorders that act on the spinal cord or brain.

Children who have received a neuromuscular blocking drug should **always** have their respiration assisted or controlled until the drug has been inactivated or antagonised. They should also receive sufficient concomitant inhalational or intravenous anaesthetic or sedative drugs to prevent awareness.

Non-depolarising neuromuscular blocking drugs

Non-depolarising neuromuscular blocking drugs (also known as competitive muscle relaxants) compete with acetylcholine for receptor sites at the neuromuscular junction and their action can be reversed with anticholinesterases such as neostigmine p. 602. Non-depolarising neuromuscular blocking drugs can be divided into the **aminosteroid** group, comprising pancuronium bromide p. 768, rocuronium bromide p. 769, and vecuronium bromide p. 769, and the **benzylisoquinolinium** group, comprising atracurium besilate p. 767, cisatracurium p. 768, and mivacurium p. 768.

Non-depolarising neuromuscular blocking drugs have a slower onset of action than suxamethonium chloride p. 766. These drugs can be classified by their duration of action as short-acting (15–30 minutes), intermediate-acting (30–40 minutes), and long-acting (60–120 minutes), although duration of action is dose-dependent. Drugs with a shorter or intermediate duration of action, such as atracurium besilate and vecuronium bromide, are more widely used than those with a longer duration of action, such as pancuronium bromide.

Non-depolarising neuromuscular blocking drugs have no sedative or analgesic effects and are not considered to trigger malignant hyperthermia.

For patients receiving intensive care and who require tracheal intubation and mechanical ventilation, a non-depolarising neuromuscular blocking drug is chosen according to its onset of effect, duration of action, and side-effects. Rocuronium bromide, with a rapid onset of effect, may facilitate intubation. Atracurium besilate or cisatracurium may be suitable for long-term neuromuscular blockade since their duration of action is not dependent on elimination by the liver or the kidneys.

Atracurium besilate, a mixture of 10 isomers, is a benzylisoquinolinium neuromuscular blocking drug with an intermediate duration of action. It undergoes non-enzymatic metabolism which is independent of liver and kidney function, thus allowing its use in children with hepatic or

15

Anaesthesia

renal impairment. Cardiovascular effects are associated with significant histamine release; histamine release can be minimised by administering slowly or in divided doses over at least 1 minute. Neonates may be more sensitive to the effects of atracurium besilate and lower doses may be required.

Cisatracurium is a single isomer of atracurium besilate. It is more potent and has a slightly longer duration of action than atracurium besilate and provides greater cardiovascular stability because cisatracurium lacks histamine-releasing effects. In children aged 1 month to 12 years, cisatracurium has a shorter duration of action and produces faster spontaneous recovery.

Mivacurium, a benzylisoquinolinium neuromuscular blocking drug, has a short duration of action. It is metabolised by plasma cholinesterase and muscle paralysis is prolonged in individuals deficient in this enzyme. It is not associated with vagolytic activity or ganglionic blockade although histamine release can occur, particularly with rapid injection. In children under 12 years mivacurium has a faster onset, shorter duration of action, and produces more rapid spontaneous recovery.

Pancuronium bromide, an aminosteroid neuromuscular blocking drug, has a long duration of action and is often used in children receiving long-term mechanical ventilation in intensive care units. It lacks a histamine-releasing effect, but vagolytic and sympathomimetic effects can cause tachycardia and hypertension. The half-life of pancuronium bromide is prolonged in neonates; neonates should receive postoperative intermittent positive pressure ventilation.

Rocuronium bromide exerts an effect within 2 minutes and has the most rapid onset of any of the non-depolarising neuromuscular blocking drugs. It is an aminosteroid neuromuscular blocking drug with an intermediate duration of action. It is reported to have minimal cardiovascular effects; high doses produce mild vagolytic activity. In most children, the duration of action of rocuronium bromide may be shorter than in adults; however, in neonates and children under 2 years, usual doses may produce a more prolonged action.

Vecuronium bromide, an aminosteroid neuromuscular blocking drug, has an intermediate duration of action. It does not generally produce histamine release and lacks cardiovascular effects. In most children, the duration of action of vecuronium bromide may be shorter than in adults; however, in neonates and children under 2 years, usual doses may produce a more prolonged action.

Depolarising neuromuscular blocking drugs

Suxamethonium chloride has the most rapid onset of action of any of the neuromuscular blocking drugs and is ideal if fast onset and brief duration of action are required e.g. with tracheal intubation. Neonates and young children are less sensitive to suxamethonium chloride and a higher dose may be required. Unlike the non-depolarising neuromuscular blocking drugs, its action cannot be reversed and recovery is spontaneous; anticholinesterases such as neostigmine potentiate the neuromuscular block.

Suxamethonium chloride should be given after anaesthetic induction because paralysis is usually preceded by painful muscle fasciculations. Bradycardia may occur; premedication with atropine sulfate p. 764 reduces bradycardia as well as the excessive salivation associated with suxamethonium chloride use.

Prolonged paralysis may occur in dual block, which occurs with high or repeated doses of suxamethonium chloride and is caused by the development of a non-depolarising block following the initial depolarising block. Children with myasthenia gravis are resistant to suxamethonium chloride but can develop dual block resulting in delayed recovery. Prolonged paralysis may also occur in those with low or atypical plasma cholinesterase. Assisted ventilation should be continued until muscle function is restored.

NEUROMUSCULAR BLOCKING DRUGS ›
DEPOLARISING

▌Suxamethonium chloride

(Succinylcholine chloride)

- **DRUG ACTION** Suxamethonium acts by mimicking acetylcholine at the neuromuscular junction but hydrolysis is much slower than for acetylcholine; depolarisation is therefore prolonged, resulting in neuromuscular blockade.

- **INDICATIONS AND DOSE**
Neuromuscular blockade (short duration) during surgery
  ▶ **BY INTRAVENOUS INJECTION**
  - Neonate: 2 mg/kg, produces 5–10 minutes neuromuscular blockade.
  - Child 1–11 months: 2 mg/kg
  - Child 1–17 years: 1 mg/kg
  ▶ **BY INTRAMUSCULAR INJECTION**
  - Neonate: Up to 4 mg/kg, produces 10–30 minutes neuromuscular blockade.
  - Child 1–11 months: Up to 5 mg/kg
  - Child 1–11 years: Up to 4 mg/kg (max. per dose 150 mg)
  PHARMACOKINETICS
  ▶ With intramuscular use Intramuscular injection has a duration of onset of 2–3 minutes.

- **IMPORTANT SAFETY INFORMATION**
Should only be administered by, or under the direct supervision of, personnel experienced in its use.

- **CONTRA-INDICATIONS** Duchenne muscular dystrophy · family history of malignant hyperthermia · hyperkalaemia · low plasma-cholinesterase activity (including severe liver disease) · major trauma · neurological disease involving acute wasting of major muscle · personal or family history of congenital myotonic disease · prolonged immobilisation (risk of hyperkalaemia) · severe burns

- **CAUTIONS** Cardiac disease · neuromuscular disease · raised intra-ocular pressure (avoid in penetrating eye injury) · respiratory disease · severe sepsis (risk of hyperkalaemia)

- **INTERACTIONS** → Appendix 1 (muscle relaxants).

- **SIDE-EFFECTS**
  ▶ **Common or very common** Flushing · hyperkalaemia · increased gastric pressure · increased intra-ocular pressure · myoglobinaemia · myoglobinuria · postoperative muscle pain · rash
  ▶ **Rare** Apnoea · arrhythmias · bronchospasm · cardiac arrest · limited jaw mobility · prolonged respiratory depression
  ▶ **Very rare** Anaphylactic reactions · malignant hyperthermia
  ▶ **Frequency not known** Bradycardia (may occur with the first dose) · hypertension · hypotension · rhabdomyolysis · tachycardia (occurs with single use)
  SIDE-EFFECTS, FURTHER INFORMATION
  ▶ **Bradycardia** Premedication with atropine reduces bradycardia as well as the excessive salivation associated with suxamethonium.

- **ALLERGY AND CROSS-SENSITIVITY** Allergic cross-reactivity between neuromuscular blocking drugs has been reported; caution is advised in cases of hypersensitivity to these drugs.

- **PREGNANCY** Mildly prolonged maternal neuromuscular blockade may occur.

- **BREAST FEEDING** Unlikely to be present in breast milk in significant amounts (ionised at physiological pH). Breast-feeding may be resumed once the mother recovered from neuromuscular block.

- **HEPATIC IMPAIRMENT** Prolonged apnoea may occur in severe liver disease because of reduced hepatic synthesis of pseudocholinesterase.

- **DIRECTIONS FOR ADMINISTRATION** For *intravenous injection*, give undiluted or dilute with Glucose 5% or Sodium Chloride 0.9%.

- **MEDICINAL FORMS**
There can be variation in the licensing of different medicines containing the same drug. Forms available from special-order manufacturers include: solution for injection
Solution for injection
  - Suxamethonium chloride (Non-proprietary)
  Suxamethonium chloride 50 mg per 1 ml Suxamethonium chloride 100mg/2ml solution for injection ampoules | 10 ampoule PoM £28.80–£50.00
  - Anectine (GlaxoSmithKline UK Ltd)
  Suxamethonium chloride 50 mg per 1 ml Anectine 100mg/2ml solution for injection ampoules | 5 ampoule PoM £3.57

NEUROMUSCULAR BLOCKING DRUGS > NON-DEPOLARISING

Non-depolarising neuromuscular blocking drugs

IMPORTANT SAFETY INFORMATION
Non-depolarising neuromuscular blocking drugs should only be administered by, or under direct supervision of, personnel experienced in their use, with adequate training in anaesthesia and airway management.

- **CAUTIONS** Burns (resistance can develop, increased doses may be required) · cardiovascular disease (reduce rate of administration) · electrolyte disturbances (response unpredictable) · fluid disturbances (response unpredictable) · hypothermia (activity prolonged, lower doses required) · myasthenia gravis (activity prolonged, lower doses required) · neuromuscular disorders (response unpredictable)
- **INTERACTIONS** → Appendix 1 (muscle relaxants).
- **ALLERGY AND CROSS-SENSITIVITY** Allergic cross-reactivity between neuromuscular blocking drugs has been reported; caution is advised in cases of hypersensitivity to these drugs.
- **PREGNANCY** Non-depolarising neuromuscular blocking drugs are highly ionised at physiological pH and are therefore unlikely to cross the placenta in significant amounts.
- **BREAST FEEDING** Non-depolarising neuromuscular blocking drugs are ionised at physiological pH and are unlikely to be present in milk in significant amounts. Breast-feeding may be resumed once the mother has recovered from neuromuscular block.

⬛ above

Atracurium besilate

(Atracurium besylate)

- **INDICATIONS AND DOSE**
Neuromuscular blockade (short to intermediate duration) for surgery
  - INITIALLY BY INTRAVENOUS INJECTION
  - Neonate: Initially 300–500 micrograms/kg, followed by (by intravenous injection) 100–200 micrograms/kg, repeated if necessary, alternatively (by intravenous infusion) 300–400 micrograms/kg/hour, adjusted according to response.
  - Child: Initially 300–600 micrograms/kg, then (by intravenous injection) 100–200 micrograms/kg,

repeated if necessary, alternatively (by intravenous injection) initially 300–600 micrograms/kg, followed by (by intravenous infusion) 300–600 micrograms/kg/hour, adjusted according to response

Neuromuscular blockade during intensive care
  - INITIALLY BY INTRAVENOUS INJECTION
  - Neonate: Initially 300–500 micrograms/kg, followed by (by intravenous injection) 100–200 micrograms/kg, repeated if necessary, alternatively (by intravenous infusion) 300–400 micrograms/kg/hour, adjusted according to response, higher doses may be necessary.
  - Child: Initially 300–600 micrograms/kg, initial dose is optional, then (by intravenous infusion) 270–1770 micrograms/kg/hour; (by intravenous infusion) usual dose 650–780 micrograms/kg/hour

DOSES AT EXTREMES OF BODY-WEIGHT
To avoid excessive dosage in obese patients, dose should be calculated on the basis of ideal body-weight.

- **UNLICENSED USE** Not licensed for use in neonates.
- **SIDE-EFFECTS**
  - Very rare Anaphylactoid reactions
  - Frequency not known Acute myopathy (after prolonged use in intensive care) · bronchospasm · hypotension · seizures · skin flushing · tachycardia
  SIDE-EFFECTS, FURTHER INFORMATION
  - Cardiovascular effects Cardiovascular effects are associated with significant histamine release; histamine release can be minimised by administering slowly or in divided doses over at least 1 minute. Neonates may be more sensitive to the effects of atracurium and lower doses may be required.

- **DIRECTIONS FOR ADMINISTRATION**
  - With intravenous use For *continuous intravenous infusion*, dilute to a concentration of 0.5–5 mg/mL with Glucose 5% or Sodium Chloride 0.9%; stability varies with diluent.
  - With intravenous use in neonates *Neonatal intensive care*, dilute 60 mg/kg body-weight to a final volume of 50 mL with Glucose 5% or Sodium Chloride 0.9%; minimum concentration of 500 micrograms/mL, maximum concentration of 5 mg/mL; an intravenous infusion rate of 0.1 mL/hour provides a dose of 120 micrograms/kg/hour.

- **MEDICINAL FORMS**
There can be variation in the licensing of different medicines containing the same drug.
Solution for injection
  - Atracurium besilate (Non-proprietary)
  Atracurium besilate 10 mg per 1 ml Atracurium besilate 250mg/25ml solution for injection vials | 1 vial PoM £16.50
  Atracurium besilate 25mg/2.5ml solution for injection ampoules | 5 ampoule PoM £8.50–£9.25
  Atracurium besilate 50mg/5ml solution for injection ampoules | 5 ampoule PoM £15.00–£17.50 | 10 ampoule PoM £35.00
  - Tracrium (GlaxoSmithKline UK Ltd)
  Atracurium besilate 10 mg per 1 ml Tracrium 250mg/25ml solution for injection vials | 2 vial PoM £25.81
  Tracrium 25mg/2.5ml solution for injection ampoules | 5 ampoule PoM £8.28
  Tracrium 50mg/5ml solution for injection ampoules | 5 ampoule PoM £15.02

15

Anaesthesia

Cisatracurium

- **INDICATIONS AND DOSE**

Neuromuscular blockade (intermediate duration) during surgery
▸ INITIALLY BY INTRAVENOUS INJECTION
▸ **Child 1 month–1 year:** Initially 150 micrograms/kg, then (by intravenous injection) 30 micrograms/kg every 20 minutes as required
▸ **Child 2–11 years:** Initially 150 micrograms/kg, 80–100 micrograms/kg if not for intubation, then (by intravenous injection) 20 micrograms/kg every 10 minutes as required, alternatively (by intravenous injection) initially 150 micrograms/kg, followed by (by intravenous infusion) 180 micrograms/kg/hour, (by intravenous infusion) reduced to 60–120 micrograms/kg/hour, adjusted according to response
▸ **Child 12–17 years:** Initially 150 micrograms/kg, then (by intravenous injection) 30 micrograms/kg every 20 minutes as required, alternatively (by intravenous injection) initially 150 micrograms/kg, followed by (by intravenous infusion) 180 micrograms/kg/hour, (by intravenous infusion) reduced to 60–120 micrograms/kg/hour, adjusted according to response

DOSES AT EXTREMES OF BODY-WEIGHT
To avoid excessive dosage in obese patients, dose should be calculated on the basis of ideal body-weight.

- **SIDE-EFFECTS** Acute myopathy (after prolonged use in intensive care) · bradycardia
- **DIRECTIONS FOR ADMINISTRATION** For *continuous intravenous infusion*, dilute to a concentration of 0.1–2 mg/mL with Glucose 5% or Sodium Chloride 0.9%; solutions of 2 mg/mL and 5 mg/mL may be infused undiluted.

- **MEDICINAL FORMS**
There can be variation in the licensing of different medicines containing the same drug.
Solution for injection
▸ Cisatracurium (Non-proprietary)
  Cisatracurium (as Cisatracurium besilate) 2 mg per 1 ml Cisatracurium besilate 20mg/10ml solution for injection ampoules | 5 ampoule PoM £13.03
  Cisatracurium besilate 20mg/10ml solution for injection vials | 5 vial PoM £37.75 (Hospital only) | 5 vial PoM £37.75
  Cisatracurium (as Cisatracurium besilate) 5 mg per 1 ml Cisatracurium besilate 150mg/30ml solution for injection vials | 1 vial PoM £45.00 (Hospital only) | 1 vial PoM £18.66
▸ Nimbex (GlaxoSmithKline UK Ltd)
  Cisatracurium (as Cisatracurium besilate) 2 mg per 1 ml Nimbex 20mg/10ml solution for injection ampoules | 5 ampoule PoM £37.75
  Cisatracurium (as Cisatracurium besilate) 5 mg per 1 ml Nimbex Forte 150mg/30ml solution for injection vials | 1 vial PoM £31.09

Mivacurium

- **INDICATIONS AND DOSE**

Neuromuscular blockade (short duration) during surgery
▸ INITIALLY BY INTRAVENOUS INJECTION
▸ **Child 2–5 months:** Initially 150 micrograms/kg, then (by intravenous injection) 100 micrograms/kg every 6–9 minutes as required, alternatively (by intravenous infusion) 8–10 micrograms/kg/minute, (by intravenous infusion) adjusted in steps of 1 microgram/kg/minute every 3 minutes if required; (by intravenous infusion) usual dose 11–14 micrograms/kg/minute
▸ **Child 6 months–11 years:** Initially 200 micrograms/kg, then (by intravenous injection) 100 micrograms/kg

every 6–9 minutes as required, alternatively (by intravenous infusion) 8–10 micrograms/kg/minute, (by intravenous infusion) adjusted in steps of 1 microgram/kg/minute every 3 minutes if required; (by intravenous infusion) usual dose 11–14 micrograms/kg/minute
▸ **Child 12–17 years:** Initially 70–250 micrograms/kg, then (by intravenous injection) 100 micrograms/kg every 15 minutes as required, alternatively (by intravenous infusion) 8–10 micrograms/kg/minute, (by intravenous infusion) adjusted in steps of 1 microgram/kg/minute every 3 minutes if required; (by intravenous infusion) usual dose 6–7 micrograms/kg/minute

DOSES AT EXTREMES OF BODY-WEIGHT
To avoid excessive dosage in obese patients, dose should be calculated on the basis of ideal bodyweight.

- **CAUTIONS** Burns (low plasma cholinesterase activity; dose titration required)
- **SIDE-EFFECTS**
▸ **Very rare** Anaphylactoid reactions
▸ **Frequency not known** Bronchospasm · hypotension · skin flushing · tachycardia
- **HEPATIC IMPAIRMENT** Reduce dose in severe impairment.
- **RENAL IMPAIRMENT** Clinical effect prolonged in renal failure—reduce dose according to response.
- **DIRECTIONS FOR ADMINISTRATION** For *intravenous injection*, give undiluted or dilute in Glucose 5% or Sodium Chloride 0.9%. Doses up to 150 micrograms/kg may be given over 5–15 seconds, higher doses should be given over 30 seconds. In asthma, cardiovascular disease or in those sensitive to reduced arterial blood pressure, give over 60 seconds.

- **MEDICINAL FORMS**
There can be variation in the licensing of different medicines containing the same drug.
Solution for injection
▸ Mivacron (GlaxoSmithKline UK Ltd)
  Mivacurium (as Mivacurium chloride) 2 mg per 1 ml Mivacron 10mg/5ml solution for injection ampoules | 5 ampoule PoM £13.95
  Mivacron 20mg/10ml solution for injection ampoules | 5 ampoule PoM £22.57

Pancuronium bromide

- **INDICATIONS AND DOSE**

Neuromuscular blockade (long duration) during surgery
▸ BY INTRAVENOUS INJECTION
▸ **Neonate:** Initially 100 micrograms/kg, then 50 micrograms/kg, repeated if necessary.
▸ **Child:** Initially 100 micrograms/kg, then 20 micrograms/kg, repeated if necessary

DOSES AT EXTREMES OF BODY-WEIGHT
To avoid excessive dosage in obese patients, dose should be calculated on the basis of ideal bodyweight.

- **SIDE-EFFECTS** Acute myopathy (after prolonged use in intensive care) · hypertension · tachycardia
SIDE-EFFECTS, FURTHER INFORMATION
Pancuronium lacks histamine-releasing effect, but vagolytic and sympathomimetic effects can cause tachycardia and hypertension.
- **HEPATIC IMPAIRMENT** Possibly slower onset, higher dose requirement, and prolonged recovery time.
- **RENAL IMPAIRMENT** Use with caution; prolonged duration of block.
- **DIRECTIONS FOR ADMINISTRATION** For *intravenous injection*, give undiluted or dilute in Glucose 5% or Sodium Chloride 0.9%.

- **MEDICINAL FORMS**
There can be variation in the licensing of different medicines containing the same drug.
Solution for injection
▸ Pancuronium bromide (Non-proprietary)
Pancuronium bromide 2 mg per 1 ml Pancuronium bromide 4mg/2ml solution for injection ampoules | 10 ampoule [PoM] £50.00

☞ 767

Rocuronium bromide

- **INDICATIONS AND DOSE**
Neuromuscular blockade (intermediate duration) during surgery
▸ INITIALLY BY INTRAVENOUS INJECTION
- Neonate: Initially 600 micrograms/kg, then (by intravenous injection) 150 micrograms/kg, repeated if necessary, alternatively (by intravenous infusion) 300–600 micrograms/kg/hour, adjusted according to response.
- Child: Initially 600 micrograms/kg, then (by intravenous injection) 150 micrograms/kg, repeated if necessary, alternatively (by intravenous infusion) 300–600 micrograms/kg/hour, adjusted according to response

Assisted ventilation in intensive care
▸ INITIALLY BY INTRAVENOUS INJECTION
- Child: Initially 600 micrograms/kg, initial dose is optional, then (by intravenous infusion) 300–600 micrograms/kg/hour for first hour, then (by intravenous infusion), adjusted according to response

DOSES AT EXTREMES OF BODY-WEIGHT
To avoid excessive dosage in obese patients, dose should be calculated on the basis of ideal bodyweight.

- **UNLICENSED USE** Not licensed for use in children for assisted ventilation in intensive care.

- **SIDE-EFFECTS**
▸ **Very rare** Anaphylactoid reactions
▸ **Frequency not known** Acute myopathy (after prolonged use in intensive care) · bronchospasm · hypotension · skin flushing · tachycardia

- **HEPATIC IMPAIRMENT** Reduce dose.

- **RENAL IMPAIRMENT** Reduce maintenance dose; prolonged paralysis.

- **DIRECTIONS FOR ADMINISTRATION** For *continuous intravenous infusion* or via drip tubing, may be diluted with Glucose 5% or Sodium Chloride 0.9%.

- **MEDICINAL FORMS**
There can be variation in the licensing of different medicines containing the same drug.
Solution for injection
▸ Rocuronium bromide (Non-proprietary)
Rocuronium bromide 10 mg per 1 ml Rocuronium bromide 50mg/5ml solution for injection vials | 10 vial [PoM] £28.00–£30.00
Rocuronium bromide 100mg/10ml solution for injection vials | 10 vial [PoM] £57.00–£60.00
▸ Esmeron (Merck Sharp & Dohme Ltd)
Rocuronium bromide 10 mg per 1 ml Esmeron 50mg/5ml solution for injection vials | 10 vial [PoM] £28.92 (Hospital only)
Esmeron 100mg/10ml solution for injection vials | 10 vial [PoM] £57.85 (Hospital only)

☞ 767

Vecuronium bromide

- **INDICATIONS AND DOSE**
Neuromuscular blockade (intermediate duration) during surgery
▸ INITIALLY BY INTRAVENOUS INJECTION
- Neonate: Initially 80 micrograms/kg, then (by intravenous injection) 30–50 micrograms/kg, adjusted according to response.
- Child: Initially 80–100 micrograms/kg, then (by intravenous injection) 20–30 micrograms/kg, repeated if necessary, alternatively (by intravenous infusion) 0.8–1.4 micrograms/kg/minute, adjusted according to response

Assisted ventilation in intensive care
▸ INITIALLY BY INTRAVENOUS INJECTION
- Neonate: Initially 80 micrograms/kg, then (by intravenous injection) 30–50 micrograms/kg, adjusted according to response, alternatively (by intravenous injection) initially 80 micrograms/kg, then (by intravenous infusion) 0.8–1.4 micrograms/kg/minute, adjusted according to response, risk of accumulation—consider interruption of infusion.
- Child: Initially 80–100 micrograms/kg, initial dose is optional, then (by intravenous infusion) 0.8–1.4 micrograms/kg/minute, adjusted according to response, (by intravenous infusion) increased if necessary up to 3 micrograms/kg/minute

DOSES AT EXTREMES OF BODY-WEIGHT
To avoid excessive dosage in obese patients, dose should be calculated on the basis of ideal bodyweight.

- **UNLICENSED USE** Not licensed for assisted ventilation in intensive care.

- **SIDE-EFFECTS**
▸ **Very rare** Anaphylactoid reactions
▸ **Frequency not known** Acute myopathy (after prolonged use in intensive care) · bronchospasm · hypotension · skin flushing · tachycardia

- **HEPATIC IMPAIRMENT** Use with caution in significant impairment.

- **RENAL IMPAIRMENT** Use with caution.

- **DIRECTIONS FOR ADMINISTRATION**
▸ With intravenous use Reconstitute each vial with 5 mL Water for Injections to give 2 mg/mL solution; *alternatively* reconstitute with up to 10 mL Glucose 5% *or* Sodium Chloride 0.9% *or* Water for Injections—unsuitable for further dilution if not reconstituted with Water for Injections. For *continuous intravenous infusion*, dilute reconstituted solution to a concentration up to 40 micrograms/mL with Glucose 5% or Sodium Chloride 0.9%; reconstituted solution can also be given via drip tubing.
▸ With intravenous use in neonates *Neonatal intensive care*, reconstitute each vial with 5 mL Water for Injections to give a 2 mg/mL solution. Dilute 5 mg/kg body-weight to a final volume of 50 mL with Glucose 5% or Sodium Chloride 0.9%; an intravenous infusion rate of 0.5 mL/hour provides a dose of 50 micrograms/kg/hour; minimum concentration of 40 micrograms/mL.

- **MEDICINAL FORMS**
There can be variation in the licensing of different medicines containing the same drug.
Powder and solvent for solution for injection
▸ Norcuron (Merck Sharp & Dohme Ltd)
Vecuronium bromide 10 mg Norcuron 10mg powder and solvent for solution for injection vials | 10 vial [PoM] £33.73 (Hospital only)

15

Anaesthesia

1.2 Neuromuscular blockade reversal

Drugs for reversal of neuromuscular blockade

Anticholinesterases

Anticholinesterases reverse the effects of the non-depolarising (competitive) neuromuscular blocking drugs such as pancuronium bromide but they prolong the action of the depolarising neuromuscular blocking drug suxamethonium chloride.

Neostigmine is used specifically for reversal of non-depolarising (competitive) blockade. It acts within one minute of intravenous injection and its effects last for 20 to 30 minutes; a second dose may then be necessary. Glycopyrronium bromide p. 765 or alternatively atropine sulfate, given before or with neostigmine, prevent bradycardia, excessive salivation, and other muscarinic effects of neostigmine.

Other drugs for reversal of neuromuscular blockade

Sugammadex below is a modified gamma cyclodextrin that can be used in children for the routine reversal of neuromuscular blockade induced by rocuronium bromide.

ANTICHOLINESTERASES

Neostigmine with glycopyrronium bromide

The properties listed below are those particular to the combination only. For the properties of the components please consider, neostigmine p. 602, glycopyrronium bromide p. 765.

- ● INDICATIONS AND DOSE
  Reversal of non-depolarising neuromuscular blockade
  ▶ BY INTRAVENOUS INJECTION
  ▶ Child: 0.02 mL/kilogram, repeated if necessary, alternatively dilute to 1 in 10 solution and give 0.2 mL/kg; maximum 2 mL per course

- ● DIRECTIONS FOR ADMINISTRATION For *intravenous injection,* may be diluted with Sodium Chloride 0.9%, give over 10–30 seconds

- ● MEDICINAL FORMS
  There can be variation in the licensing of different medicines containing the same drug.
  Solution for injection
  ▶ Neostigmine with glycopyrronium bromide (Non-proprietary)
  Glycopyrronium bromide 500 microgram per 1 ml, Neostigmine metilsulfate 2.5 mg per 1 ml Neostigmine 2.5mg/1ml / Glycopyrronium bromide 500micrograms/1ml solution for injection ampoules | 10 ampoule [PoM] £11.50

ANTIDOTES AND CHELATORS

Sugammadex

- ● INDICATIONS AND DOSE
  Routine reversal of neuromuscular blockade induced by rocuronium
  ▶ BY INTRAVENOUS INJECTION
  ▶ Child 2–17 years: 2 mg/kg (consult product literature)

IMPORTANT SAFETY INFORMATION
Should only be administered by, or under the direct supervision of, personnel experienced in its use.

- ● CAUTIONS Cardiovascular disease (recovery may be delayed) · pre-existing coagulation disorders · recurrence of neuromuscular blockade— monitor respiratory function until fully recovered · use of anticoagulants (unrelated to surgery) · wait 24 hours before re-administering rocuronium

- ● INTERACTIONS → Appendix 1 (sugammadex).

- ● SIDE-EFFECTS Bradycardia · bronchospasm · cardiac arrest · hypersensitivity reactions

- ● PREGNANCY Use with caution—no information available.

- ● RENAL IMPAIRMENT Avoid if estimated glomerular filtration rate less than 30 mL/minute/1.73 m².

- ● DIRECTIONS FOR ADMINISTRATION For *intravenous injection* dose may be diluted to a concentration of 10 mg/mL with Sodium Chloride 0.9%.

- ● NATIONAL FUNDING/ACCESS DECISIONS
  Scottish Medicines Consortium (SMC) Decisions
  The *Scottish Medicines Consortium,* has advised (February 2013) that sugammadex (*Bridion* ®) is accepted for restricted use within NHS Scotland for the routine reversal of neuromuscular blockade in high-risk patients only, or where prompt reversal of neuromuscular block is required.

- ● MEDICINAL FORMS
  There can be variation in the licensing of different medicines containing the same drug.
  Solution for injection
  ELECTROLYTES: May contain Sodium
  ▶ Bridion (Merck Sharp & Dohme Ltd)
  Sugammadex (as Sugammadex sodium) 100 mg per 1 ml Bridion 500mg/5ml solution for injection vials | 10 vial [PoM] £1,491.00 (Hospital only)
  Bridion 200mg/2ml solution for injection vials | 10 vial [PoM] £596.40 (Hospital only)

1.3 Peri-operative analgesia

Peri-operative analgesia

Non-opioid analgesics

Since non-steroidal anti-inflammatory drugs (NSAIDs) do not depress respiration, do not impair gastro-intestinal motility, and do not cause dependence, they may be useful alternatives or adjuncts to opioids for the relief of postoperative pain. NSAIDs may be inadequate for the relief of severe pain.

Diclofenac sodium p. 605, diclofenac potassium p. 605, ibuprofen p. 608, paracetamol p. 254, and ketorolac trometamol p. 771 are used to relieve postoperative pain in children; diclofenac sodium and paracetamol can be given parenterally and rectally as well as by mouth. Ketorolac trometamol is given by intravenous injection.

Opioid analgesics

Opioid analgesics are now rarely used as premedicants; they are more likely to be administered at induction. Pre-operative use of opioid analgesics is generally limited to children who require control of existing pain. The main side-effects of opioid analgesics are respiratory depression, cardiovascular depression, nausea, and vomiting; see general notes on opioid analgesics and their use in postoperative pain.

See the management of opioid-induced respiratory depression in Pre-medication and peri-operative drugs p. 763.

Intra-operative analgesia

Opioid analgesics given in small doses before or with induction reduce the dose requirement of some drugs used during anaesthesia.

Alfentanil p. 772, fentanyl p. 262, and remifentanil p. 772 are particularly useful because they act within 1–2 minutes and have short durations of action. The initial doses of alfentanil or fentanyl are followed either by successive intravenous injections or by an intravenous infusion; prolonged infusions increase the duration of effect.

In contrast to other opioids which are metabolised in the liver, remifentanil undergoes rapid metabolism by nonspecific blood and tissue esterases; its short duration of action allows prolonged administration at high dosage, without accumulation, and with little risk of residual postoperative respiratory depression. Remifentanil should not be given by intravenous injection intraoperatively, but it is well suited to continuous infusion; a supplementary analgesic is given before stopping the infusion of remifentanil.

ANALGESICS > NON-STEROIDAL ANTI-INFLAMMATORY DRUGS

Ketorolac trometamol

- ● **INDICATIONS AND DOSE**

  Short-term management of moderate to severe acute postoperative pain only
  - ▶ BY INTRAMUSCULAR INJECTION, OR BY INTRAVENOUS INJECTION
  - ▶ Child 16–17 years (body-weight up to 50 kg): Initially 10 mg, then 10–30 mg every 4–6 hours as required for maximum duration of treatment 2 days, frequency may be increased to up to every 2 hours during initial postoperative period; maximum 60 mg per day
  - ▶ Child 16–17 years (body-weight 50 kg and above): Initially 10 mg, then 10–30 mg every 4–6 hours as required for maximum duration of treatment 2 days, frequency may be increased to up to every 2 hours during initial postoperative period; maximum 90 mg per day
  - ▶ BY INTRAVENOUS INJECTION
  - ▶ Child 6 months–15 years: Initially 0.5–1 mg/kg (max. per dose 15 mg), then 500 micrograms/kg every 6 hours (max. per dose 15 mg) as required for maximum duration of treatment 2 days; maximum 60 mg per day

- ● **UNLICENSED USE** Not licensed for use in children under 16 years.

- ● **CONTRA-INDICATIONS** Active or history of gastro-intestinal bleeding · active or history of gastro-intestinal ulceration · coagulation disorders · complete or partial syndrome of nasal polyps · confirmed or suspected cerebrovascular bleeding · dehydration · following operations with high risk of haemorrhage or incomplete haemostasis · haemorrhagic diatheses · history of gastro-intestinal perforation · hypovolaemia · severe heart failure

- ● **CAUTIONS** Allergic disorders · cardiac impairment (NSAIDs may impair renal function) · cerebrovascular disease ·

coagulation defects · connective-tissue disorders · Crohn's disease (may be exacerbated) · heart failure · ischaemic heart disease · peripheral arterial disease · risk factors for cardiovascular events · ulcerative colitis (may be exacerbated) · uncontrolled hypertension

- ● INTERACTIONS → Appendix 1 (NSAIDs).

- ● SIDE-EFFECTS
  - ▶ **Rare** Alveolitis · aseptic meningitis (patients with connective-tissue disorders such as systemic lupus erythematosus may be especially susceptible) · hepatic damage · interstitial fibrosis associated with NSAIDs can lead to renal failure · pancreatitis · papillary necrosis associated with NSAIDs can lead to renal failure · pulmonary eosinophilia · Stevens-Johnson syndrome · toxic epidermal necrolysis
  - ▶ **Frequency not known** Abnormal dreams · angioedema · asthma · blood disorders · bradycardia · bronchospasm · chest pain · colitis (induction of or exacerbation of) · confusion · convulsions · Crohn's disease (induction of or exacerbation of) · depression · diarrhoea · dizziness · drowsiness · dry mouth · dyspnoea · euphoria · fluid retention (rarely precipitating congestive heart failure) · flushing · gastro-intestinal bleeding · gastro-intestinal discomfort · gastro-intestinal disturbances · gastro-intestinal ulceration · haematuria · hallucinations · headache · hearing disturbances · hyperkalaemia · hyperkinesia · hypersensitivity reactions · hypertension · hyponatraemia · insomnia · malaise · myalgia · nausea · nervousness · optic neuritis · pain at injection site · pallor · palpitation · paraesthesia · photosensitivity · psychosis · purpura · raised blood pressure · rashes · renal failure (especially in patients with pre-existing renal impairment) · sweating · taste disturbances · thirst · tinnitus · urinary frequency · vertigo · visual disturbances

  SIDE-EFFECTS, FURTHER INFORMATION
  - ▶ **Serious side-effects** For information about cardiovascular and gastro-intestinal side-effects, and a possible exacerbation of symptoms in asthma, see Non-steroidal anti-inflammatory drugs p. 604.

- ● **ALLERGY AND CROSS-SENSITIVITY** Contra-indicated in patients with a history of hypersensitivity to aspirin or any other NSAID—which includes those in whom attacks of asthma, angioedema, urticaria or rhinitis have been precipitated by aspirin or any other NSAID.

- ● **PREGNANCY** Avoid unless the potential benefit outweighs the risk. Avoid during the third trimester (risk of closure of fetal ductus arteriosus *in utero* and possibly persistent pulmonary hypertension of the newborn); onset of labour may be delayed and duration may be increased.

- ● **BREAST FEEDING** Amount too small to be harmful.

- ● **HEPATIC IMPAIRMENT** Use with caution; there is an increased risk of gastro-intestinal bleeding and fluid retention. Avoid in severe liver disease.

- ● **RENAL IMPAIRMENT** Avoid if possible or use with caution. Avoid if serum creatinine greater than 160 micromol/litre.
  The lowest effective dose should be used for the shortest possible duration. Max. 60 mg daily by intramuscular injection or intravenous injection.
  Monitor renal function; sodium and water retention may occur and renal function may deteriorate, possibly leading to renal failure.

- ● **DIRECTIONS FOR ADMINISTRATION** For *intravenous injection*, give over at least 15 seconds.

- ● **MEDICINAL FORMS**
  There can be variation in the licensing of different medicines containing the same drug.
  Solution for injection
  - ▶ Ketorolac trometamol (Non-proprietary)
    Ketorolac trometamol 30 mg per 1 ml Ketorolac 30mg/1ml solution for injection ampoules | 6 ampoule [PoM] £6.56

15

Anaesthesia

15

Anaesthesia

ANALGESICS > OPIOIDS

F 256

Alfentanil

- **INDICATIONS AND DOSE**

Assisted ventilation: analgesia and enhancement of anaesthesia for short procedures
▸ BY INTRAVENOUS INJECTION

▸ **Neonate:** Initially 5–20 micrograms/kg, dose to be administered over 30 seconds; supplemental doses up to 10 micrograms/kg.

▸ **Child:** Initially 10–20 micrograms/kg, dose to be administered over 30 seconds; supplemental doses up to 10 micrograms/kg

Assisted ventilation: analgesia and enhancement of anaesthesia during maintenance of anaesthesia for longer procedures
▸ BY INTRAVENOUS INFUSION

▸ **Neonate:** Initially 10–50 micrograms/kg, dose to be administered over 10 minutes, followed by 30–60 micrograms/kg/hour.

▸ **Child:** Initially 50–100 micrograms/kg, dose to be administered over 10 minutes, followed by 30–120 micrograms/kg/hour, usual dose with intravenous anaesthetic, 60 micrograms/kg/hour

DOSES AT EXTREMES OF BODY-WEIGHT
To avoid excessive dosage in obese patients, dose should be calculated on the basis of ideal body-weight.

PHARMACOKINETICS
Half-life is prolonged in neonates and accumulation is likely with prolonged use. Clearance may be increased in children 1 month–12 years and higher infusion doses might be needed.

- **CAUTIONS**

CAUTIONS, FURTHER INFORMATION
▸ Repeated intra-operative doses Repeated intra-operative doses of alfentanil should be given with care since the resulting respiratory depression can persist postoperatively and occasionally it may become apparent for the first time postoperatively when monitoring of the patient might be less intensive.

- **SIDE-EFFECTS**
▸ **Common or very common** Hypertension · myoclonic movements
▸ **Uncommon** Arrhythmias · hiccup · laryngospasm
▸ **Rare** Epistaxis
▸ **Frequency not known** Cardiac arrest · convulsions · cough · muscle rigidity · pyrexia

SIDE-EFFECTS, FURTHER INFORMATION
▸ Muscle rigidity Alfentanil can cause muscle rigidity, particularly of the chest wall or jaw; this can be managed by the use of neuromuscular blocking drugs.

- **BREAST FEEDING** Present in milk—withhold breast-feeding for 24 hours.

- **RENAL IMPAIRMENT** Avoid use or reduce dose; opioid effects increased and prolonged and increased cerebral sensitivity occurs.

- **DIRECTIONS FOR ADMINISTRATION** 5 mg/mL injection to be diluted before use. For *continuous or intermittent intravenous infusion* dilute in Glucose 5% *or* Sodium Chloride 0.9%.

- **MEDICINAL FORMS**
There can be variation in the licensing of different medicines containing the same drug. Forms available from special-order manufacturers include: solution for injection

Solution for injection
▸ Alfentanil (Non-proprietary)
  Alfentanil (as Alfentanil hydrochloride) 500 microgram per 1 ml Alfentanil 1mg/2ml solution for injection ampoules | 10 ampoule [PoM] £7.00 [CD2]
  Alfentanil 5mg/10ml solution for injection ampoules | 5 ampoule [PoM] £16.00 [CD2]
  Alfentanil (as Alfentanil hydrochloride) 5 mg per 1 ml Alfentanil 5mg/1ml solution for injection ampoules | 10 ampoule [PoM] £25.00 [CD2]
▸ Rapifen (Janssen-Cilag Ltd)
  Alfentanil (as Alfentanil hydrochloride) 500 microgram per 1 ml Rapifen 5mg/10ml solution for injection ampoules | 5 ampoule [PoM] £14.50 [CD2]
  Rapifen 1mg/2ml solution for injection ampoules | 10 ampoule [PoM] £6.34 [CD2]
  Alfentanil (as Alfentanil hydrochloride) 5 mg per 1 ml Rapifen Intensive Care 5mg/1ml solution for injection ampoules | 10 ampoule [PoM] £23.19 (Hospital only) [CD2]

F 256

Remifentanil

- **INDICATIONS AND DOSE**

Analgesia and enhancement of anaesthesia at induction (initial bolus injection)
▸ BY INTRAVENOUS INJECTION

▸ **Child 12–17 years:** Initially 0.25–1 microgram/kg, dose to be administered over at least 30 seconds, if child is to be intubated more than 8 minutes after start of intravenous infusion, initial bolus intravenous injection dose is not necessary

Analgesia and enhancement of anaesthesia at induction with or without initial bolus dose
▸ BY INTRAVENOUS INFUSION

▸ **Child 12–17 years:** 30–60 micrograms/kg/hour, if child is to be intubated more than 8 minutes after start of intravenous infusion, initial bolus intravenous injection dose is not necessary

Assisted ventilation: analgesia and enhancement of anaesthesia during maintenance of anaesthesia (initial bolus injection)
▸ BY INTRAVENOUS INJECTION

▸ **Child 1 month–11 years:** Initially 0.1–1 microgram/kg, dose to be administered over at least 30 seconds (omitted if not required)

▸ **Child 12–17 years:** Initially 0.1–1 microgram/kg, dose to be administered over at least 30 seconds (omitted if not required)

Assisted ventilation: analgesia and enhancement of anaesthesia during maintenance of anaesthesia with or without initial bolus dose
▸ BY INTRAVENOUS INFUSION

▸ **Neonate:** 24–60 micrograms/kg/hour, additional doses of 1 microgram/kg can be given *by intravenous injection* during the intravenous infusion.

▸ **Child 1 month–11 years:** 3–78 micrograms/kg/hour, dose to be administered according to anaesthetic technique and adjusted according to response, additional doses can be given *by intravenous injection* during the intravenous infusion

▸ **Child 12–17 years:** 3–120 micrograms/kg/hour, dose to be administered according to anaesthetic technique and adjusted according to response, additional doses can be given *by intravenous injection* during the intravenous infusion

Spontaneous respiration: analgesia and enhancement of anaesthesia during maintenance of anaesthesia
▸ BY INTRAVENOUS INFUSION
▸ Child 12-17 years: Initially 2.4 micrograms/kg/hour, adjusted according to response; usual dose 1.5–6 micrograms/kg/hour

DOSES AT EXTREMES OF BODY-WEIGHT
To avoid excessive dosage in obese patients, dose should be calculated on the basis of ideal body-weight.

● **UNLICENSED USE** Not licensed for use in children under 1 year.
● **CONTRA-INDICATIONS** Analgesia in conscious patients
● **SIDE-EFFECTS**
▸ **Common or very common** Hypertension
▸ **Uncommon** Hypoxia
▸ **Rare** Asystole
▸ **Frequency not known** AV block · convulsions
  SIDE-EFFECTS, FURTHER INFORMATION
▸ Muscle rigidity Alfentanil can cause muscle rigidity, particularly of the chest wall or jaw; this can be managed by the use of neuromuscular blocking drugs.
▸ Respiratory depression In contrast to other opioids which are metabolised in the liver, remifentanil undergoes rapid metabolism by non-specific blood and tissue esterases; its short duration of action allows prolonged administration at high dosage, without accumulation, and with little risk of residual postoperative respiratory depression.
● **PREGNANCY** No information available.
● **BREAST FEEDING** Avoid breast-feeding for 24 hours after administration—present in milk in *animal* studies.
● **RENAL IMPAIRMENT** No dose adjustment necessary in renal impairment.
● **DIRECTIONS FOR ADMINISTRATION** For *intravenous injection*, reconstitute to a concentration of 1 mg/mL; for *continuous intravenous infusion*, dilute further with Glucose 5% or Sodium Chloride 0.9% to a concentration of 20–25 micrograms/mL for child 1–12 years or 20–250 micrograms/mL (usually 50 micrograms/mL) for child 12–18 years.
● **PRESCRIBING AND DISPENSING INFORMATION**
Remifentanil should not be given by intravenous injection intra-operatively, but it is well suited to continuous infusion; a supplementary analgesic is given before stopping the infusion of remifentanil.

● **MEDICINAL FORMS**
There can be variation in the licensing of different medicines containing the same drug.
Powder for solution for injection
▸ Remifentanil (Non-proprietary)
  Remifentanil (as Remifentanyl hydrochloride) 1 mg Remifentanil 1mg powder for concentrate for solution for injection vials | 5 vial PoM £25.58-£25.60 (Hospital only) CD2
  Remifentanil (as Remifentanyl hydrochloride) 2 mg Remifentanil 2mg powder for concentrate for solution for injection vials | 5 vial PoM £51.13-£51.15 (Hospital only) CD2
  Remifentanil (as Remifentanyl hydrochloride) 5 mg Remifentanil 5mg powder for concentrate for solution for injection vials | 5 vial PoM £127.00-£127.90 (Hospital only) CD2
▸ Ultiva (GlaxoSmithKline UK Ltd)
  Remifentanil (as Remifentanyl hydrochloride) 1 mg Ultiva 1mg powder for solution for injection vials | 5 vial PoM £25.58 (Hospital only) CD2
  Remifentanil (as Remifentanyl hydrochloride) 2 mg Ultiva 2mg powder for solution for injection vials | 5 vial PoM £51.15 (Hospital only) CD2
  Remifentanil (as Remifentanyl hydrochloride) 5 mg Ultiva 5mg powder for solution for injection vials | 5 vial PoM £127.88 (Hospital only) CD2

1.4 Peri-operative sedation

Conscious sedation for clinical procedures

Overview
Sedation of children during diagnostic and therapeutic procedures is used to reduce fear and anxiety, to control pain, and to minimise excessive movement. The choice of sedative drug will depend upon the intended procedure and whether the child is cooperative; some procedures are safer and more successful under anaesthesia.
  Midazolam p. 210 and chloral hydrate p. 275 are suitable for sedating children for painless procedures, such as imaging. For painful procedures, alternative choices include nitrous oxide p. 762, local anaesthesia, ketamine below, or concomitant use of sedation with **opioid** or **non-opioid analgesia**.

ANAESTHETICS, GENERAL ❭ NMDA RECEPTOR ANTAGONISTS

Ketamine

● **INDICATIONS AND DOSE**
Induction and maintenance of anaesthesia for short procedures
▸ BY INTRAMUSCULAR INJECTION
▸ Neonate: 4 mg/kg, adjusted according to response, a dose of 4 mg/kg usually produces 15 minutes of surgical anaesthesia.
▸ Child: 4–13 mg/kg, adjusted according to response, a dose of 4 mg/kg sufficient for some diagnostic procedures, a dose of 10 mg/kg usually produces 12–25 minutes of surgical anaesthesia
▸ BY INTRAVENOUS INJECTION
▸ Neonate: 1–2 mg/kg, adjusted according to response, to be given over at least 60 seconds, a dose of 1–2 mg/kg produces 5–10 minutes of surgical anaesthesia.
▸ Child 1 month-11 years: 1–2 mg/kg, adjusted according to response, to be given over at least 60 seconds, a dose of 1–2 mg/kg produces 5–10 minutes of surgical anaesthesia
▸ Child 12-17 years: 1–4.5 mg/kg, adjusted according to response, to be given over at least 60 seconds, a dose of 2 mg/kg usually produces 5–10 minutes of surgical anaesthesia
Induction and maintenance of anaesthesia for long procedures
▸ INITIALLY BY INTRAVENOUS INJECTION
▸ Neonate: Initially 0.5–2 mg/kg, followed by (by continuous intravenous infusion) 8 micrograms/kg/minute, adjusted according to response, doses up to 30 micrograms/kg/minute may be used to produce deep anaesthesia.
▸ Child: Initially 0.5–2 mg/kg, followed by (by continuous intravenous infusion) 10–45 micrograms/kg/minute, adjusted according to response
Sedation prior to invasive or painful procedures
▸ BY INTRAVENOUS INJECTION
▸ Child: 1–2 mg/kg for 1 dose

15

Anaesthesia

15

Anaesthesia

> IMPORTANT SAFETY INFORMATION
> Ketamine should only be administered by, or under the direct supervision of, personnel experienced in its use, with adequate training in anaesthesia and airway management, and when resuscitation equipment is available.

- **CONTRA-INDICATIONS** Acute porphyrias p. 562 · eclampsia · head trauma · hypertension · pre-eclampsia · raised intracranial pressure · severe cardiac disease · stroke
- **CAUTIONS** Acute circulatory failure (shock) · cardiovascular disease · dehydration · fixed cardiac output · hallucinations · head injury · hypertension · hypovolaemia · increased cerebrospinal fluid pressure · intracranial mass lesions · nightmares · predisposition to seizures · psychotic disorders · raised intra-ocular pressure · respiratory tract infection · thyroid dysfunction
- **INTERACTIONS** → Appendix 1 (anaesthetics, general).
- **SIDE-EFFECTS**
  - **Common or very common** Diplopia · hallucinations · hypertension · nausea · nightmares · nystagmus · rash · tachycardia · transient psychotic effects · vomiting
  - **Uncommon** Arrhythmias · bradycardia · hypotension · laryngospasm · respiratory depression
  - **Rare** Apnoea · cystitis · haemorrhagic cystitis · hypersalivation · insomnia
  - **Frequency not known** Raised intra-ocular pressure
  - SIDE-EFFECTS, FURTHER INFORMATION
  - Transient psychotic effects Incidence of hallucinations, nightmares, and other transient psychotic effects can be reduced by a benzodiazepine such as diazepam or midazolam.
- **PREGNANCY** May depress neonatal respiration if used during delivery.
- **BREAST FEEDING** Avoid for at least 12 hours after last dose.
- **HEPATIC IMPAIRMENT** Consider dose reduction.
- **DIRECTIONS FOR ADMINISTRATION** For *intravenous injection*, dilute 10 mg/mL strength to a concentration of not more than 50 mg/mL with Glucose 5% *or* Sodium Chloride 0.9%. For *continuous intravenous infusion*, dilute to a concentration of 1 mg/mL with Glucose 5% *or* Sodium Chloride 0.9%; use microdrip infusion for maintenance of anaesthesia.
- **PATIENT AND CARER ADVICE**
  Driving and skilled tasks
  Patients given sedatives and analgesics during minor outpatient procedures should be very carefully warned about the risk of driving or undertaking skilled tasks afterwards. For a short general anaesthetic the risk extends to **at least 24 hours** after administration. Responsible persons should be available to take patients home. The dangers of taking **alcohol** should also be emphasised.
  For information on 2015 legislation regarding driving whilst taking certain controlled drugs, including ketamine, see *Drugs and driving* under Guidance on prescribing p. 1.
- **MEDICINAL FORMS**
  There can be variation in the licensing of different medicines containing the same drug. Forms available from special-order manufacturers include: solution for injection,
  Solution for injection
  - Ketamine (Non-proprietary)
    Ketamine (as Ketamine hydrochloride) 10 mg per 1 ml Ketamin 10 Curamed 50mg/5ml solution for injection ampoules | 10 ampoule [PoM] no price available [CD2]
    Ketamine (as Ketamine hydrochloride) 50 mg per 1 ml Ketamine 500mg/10ml solution for injection vials | 10 vial [PoM] £87.70 [CD2] Ketamin 100mg/2ml solution for injection ampoules | 10 ampoule [PoM] no price available [CD2]

- Ketalar (Pfizer Ltd)
  Ketamine (as Ketamine hydrochloride) 10 mg per 1 ml Ketalar 200mg/20ml solution for injection vials | 1 vial [PoM] £5.06 (Hospital only) [CD2]
  Ketamine (as Ketamine hydrochloride) 50 mg per 1 ml Ketalar 500mg/10ml solution for injection vials | 1 vial [PoM] £8.77 (Hospital only) [CD2]
  Ketamine (as Ketamine hydrochloride) 100 mg per 1 ml Ketalar 1g/10ml solution for injection vials | 1 vial [PoM] £16.10 (Hospital only) [CD2]

HYPNOTICS, SEDATIVES AND ANXIOLYTICS > BENZODIAZEPINES

⌐ 205

Temazepam

- **INDICATIONS AND DOSE**
  Premedication before surgery or investigatory procedures
  - BY MOUTH
  - Child 12–17 years: 10–20 mg, to be taken 1 hour before procedure
- **UNLICENSED USE** Tablets not licensed for use in children.
- **CONTRA-INDICATIONS** CNS depression · compromised airway · hyperkinesis · obsessional state · phobic states · respiratory depression
- **CAUTIONS** Hypoalbuminaemia · muscle weakness · organic brain changes · personality disorder (within the fearful group—dependent, avoidant, obsessive-compulsive)—may increase risk of dependence
  CAUTIONS, FURTHER INFORMATION
  - Paradoxical effects A paradoxical increase in hostility and aggression may be reported by patients taking benzodiazepines. The effects range from talkativeness and excitement to aggressive and antisocial acts. Adjustment of the dose (up or down) sometimes attenuates the impulses. Increased anxiety and perceptual disorders are other paradoxical effects.
- **SIDE-EFFECTS**
  - **Common or very common** Amnesia · ataxia · confusion · dependence · drowsiness the next day · lightheadedness the next day · muscle weakness · paradoxical increase in aggression
  - **Uncommon** Dizziness · dysarthria · gastro-intestinal disturbances · gynaecomastia · incontinence · salivation changes · tremor · visual disturbances
  - **Rare** Apnoea · blood disorders · changes in libido · headache · hypotension · jaundice · skin reactions · urinary retention · vertigo
  - **Frequency not known** Delusions · excitement · hallucinations · irritability · psychosis · respiratory depression (may be marked when used for sedation; facilities for its treatment are essential) · restlessness
- **BREAST FEEDING** Benzodiazepines are present in milk, and should be avoided if possible during breast-feeding.
- **HEPATIC IMPAIRMENT** Start with smaller initial doses or reduce dose. Can precipitate coma. Avoid in severe impairment.
- **RENAL IMPAIRMENT** Start with small doses in severe impairment.
- **PATIENT AND CARER ADVICE**
  Driving and skilled tasks
  May impair judgement and increase reaction time, and so affect ability to drive or operate machinery; they increase the effects of alcohol. Moreover the hangover effects of a night dose may impair driving on the following day.
  Patients given sedatives and analgesics during minor outpatient procedures should be very carefully warned about the risks of undertaking skilled tasks (e.g. driving) afterwards. Responsible persons should be available to

take patients home afterwards. The dangers of taking **alcohol** should be emphasised.

● PROFESSION SPECIFIC INFORMATION

Dental practitioners' formulary
Temazepam Tablets may be prescribed. Temazepam Oral Solution may be prescribed.

● MEDICINAL FORMS
There can be variation in the licensing of different medicines containing the same drug. Forms available from special-order manufacturers include: oral suspension, oral solution

Tablet
CAUTIONARY AND ADVISORY LABELS 19
▸ Temazepam (Non-proprietary)
Temazepam 10 mg Temazepam 10mg tablets | 28 tablet PoM
£35.00 DT price = £3.80 CD3 | 500 tablet PoM £624.82 CD3
Temazepam 20 mg Temazepam 20mg tablets | 28 tablet PoM
£35.00 DT price = £4.04 CD3 | 250 tablet PoM £307.94 CD3

Oral solution
CAUTIONARY AND ADVISORY LABELS 19
▸ Temazepam (Non-proprietary)
Temazepam 2 mg per 1 ml Temazepam 10mg/5ml oral solution sugar free sugar-free | 300 ml PoM £121.08 DT price = £119.30 CD3

2 Malignant hyperthermia

MUSCLE RELAXANTS ⟩ DIRECTLY ACTING

Dantrolene sodium

● DRUG ACTION Acts on skeletal muscle cells by interfering with calcium efflux, thereby stopping the contractile process.

● INDICATIONS AND DOSE
Malignant hyperthermia
▸ BY RAPID INTRAVENOUS INJECTION
▸ Child: Initially 2–3 mg/kg, then 1 mg/kg, repeated if necessary; maximum 10 mg/kg per course

Chronic severe spasticity of voluntary muscle
▸ BY MOUTH
▸ Child 5–11 years: Initially 500 micrograms/kg once daily for 7 days, then increased to 500 micrograms/kg/dose 3 times a day, then increased in steps of 500 micrograms/kg/dose every 7 days (max. per dose 2 mg/kg 3–4 times a day) until satisfactory response; maximum 400 mg per day
▸ Child 12–17 years: Initially 25 mg once daily for 7 days, then increased to 25 mg 3 times a day, then increased in steps of 500 micrograms/kg/dose every 7 days (max. per dose 2 mg/kg 3–4 times a day) until satisfactory response; maximum 400 mg per day

● UNLICENSED USE Not licensed for use in children.

IMPORTANT SAFETY INFORMATION
Should only be administered by, or under the direct supervision of, personnel experienced in the use of dantrolene when used for malignant hyperthermia.

▸ CONTRA-INDICATIONS
With oral use Acute muscle spasm · avoid when spasticity is useful, for example, locomotion
▸ CAUTIONS
With intravenous use Avoid extravasation (risk of tissue necrosis)
With oral use Females (hepatotoxicity) · history of liver disorders (hepatotoxicity) · if doses greater than 400 mg daily (hepatotoxicity) · impaired cardiac function · impaired pulmonary function · therapeutic effect may take a few weeks to develop— discontinue if no response within 6–8 weeks

● INTERACTIONS → Appendix 1 (muscle relaxants).
▸ With oral use Caution if concomitant use of hepatotoxic drugs.

● SIDE-EFFECTS
▸ Common or very common
▸ With oral use Abdominal pain · anorexia · asthenia · chills · diarrhoea (withdraw if severe, discontinue treatment if recurs on re-introduction) · dizziness · drowsiness · fatigue · fever · headache · hepatotoxicity · nausea · pericarditis · pleural effusion · rash · respiratory depression · seizures · speech disturbances · visual disturbances · vomiting
▸ Uncommon
▸ With oral use Confusion · constipation · crystalluria · depression · dysphagia · dyspnoea · erratic blood pressure · exacerbation of cardiac insufficiency · haematuria · increased sweating · increased urinary frequency · insomnia · nervousness · tachycardia · urinary incontinence · urinary retention
▸ Frequency not known
▸ With intravenous use Dizziness · erythema · hepatotoxicity · injection-site reactions · pulmonary oedema · rash · swelling · thrombophlebitis · weakness
SIDE-EFFECTS, FURTHER INFORMATION
▸ Hepatotoxicity Potentially life-threatening hepatotoxicity reported—discontinue if abnormal liver function tests or symptoms of liver disorder; re-introduce only if complete reversal of hepatotoxicity.

● PREGNANCY
▸ With intravenous use Use only if potential benefit outweighs risk.
▸ With oral use Avoid use in chronic spasticity—embryotoxic in *animal* studies.

● BREAST FEEDING
▸ With intravenous use Present in milk—use only if potential benefit outweighs risk.
▸ With oral use Present in milk—manufacturer advises avoid use in chronic spasticity.

● HEPATIC IMPAIRMENT Avoid—may cause severe liver damage (injection may be used in an emergency for malignant hyperthermia).

● MONITORING REQUIREMENTS
▸ With oral use Test liver function before and at intervals during therapy.

● PATIENT AND CARER ADVICE
Driving and skilled tasks
▸ With oral use Drowsiness may affect performance of skilled tasks (e.g. driving); effects of alcohol enhanced. Hepatotoxicity
▸ With oral use Patients should be told how to recognise signs of liver disorder and advised to seek prompt medical attention if symptoms such as anorexia, nausea, vomiting, fatigue, abdominal pain, dark urine, or pruritus develop.

● MEDICINAL FORMS
There can be variation in the licensing of different medicines containing the same drug. Forms available from special-order manufacturers include: oral suspension, oral solution
Capsule
CAUTIONARY AND ADVISORY LABELS 2
▸ Dantrium (Norgine Pharmaceuticals Ltd)
Dantrolene sodium 25 mg Dantrium 25mg capsules | 100 capsule PoM £16.87 DT price = £16.87
Dantrolene sodium 100 mg Dantrium 100mg capsules | 100 capsule PoM £43.07 DT price = £43.07
Powder for solution for injection
▸ Dantrium (Norgine Pharmaceuticals Ltd)
Dantrolene sodium 20 mg Dantrium Intravenous 20mg powder for solution for injection vials | 12 vial PoM £612.00 (Hospital only) | 36 vial PoM £1,836.00 (Hospital only)

15

Anaesthesia

Local anaesthesia

Local anaesthesia

Local anaesthetic drugs

The use of local anaesthetics by injection or by application to mucous membranes to produce local analgesia is discussed in this section.

Local anaesthetic drugs act by causing a reversible block to conduction along nerve fibres. They vary widely in their potency, toxicity, duration of action, stability, solubility in water, and ability to penetrate mucous membranes. These factors determine their application, e.g. topical (surface), infiltration, peripheral nerve block, intravenous regional anaesthesia (Bier's block), plexus, epidural (extradural), or spinal (intrathecal or subarachnoid) block. Local anaesthetics may also be used for postoperative pain relief, thereby reducing the need for analgesics such as opioids.

Bupivacaine hydrochloride p. 778 has a longer duration of action than other local anaesthetics. It has a slow onset of action, taking up to 30 minutes for full effect. It is often used in lumbar epidural blockade and is particularly suitable for continuous epidural analgesia in labour, or for postoperative pain relief. It is the principal drug used for spinal anaesthesia. Hyperbaric solutions containing glucose may be used for spinal block.

Levobupivacaine p. 779, an isomer of bupivacaine hydrochloride, has anaesthetic and analgesic properties similar to bupivacaine hydrochloride, but is thought to have fewer adverse effects.

Lidocaine hydrochloride p. 780 is effectively absorbed from mucous membranes and is a useful surface anaesthetic in concentrations up to 10%. Except for surface anaesthesia and dental anaesthesia, solutions should **not** usually exceed 1% in strength. The duration of the block (with adrenaline/epinephrine p. 128) is about 90 minutes.

Application of a mixture of lidocaine and prilocaine (*EMLA*®) under an occlusive dressing provides surface anaesthesia for 1–2 hours. *EMLA*® does not appear to be effective in providing local anaesthesia for heel lancing in neonates.

Prilocaine hydrochloride p. 783 is a local anaesthetic of low toxicity which is similar to lidocaine hydrochloride.

Ropivacaine hydrochloride p. 784 is an amide-type local anaesthetic agent similar to bupivacaine hydrochloride. It is less cardiotoxic than bupivacaine hydrochloride, but also less potent.

Tetracaine p. 785, a para-aminobenzoic acid ester, is an effective local anaesthetic for topical application; a 4% gel is indicated for anaesthesia before venepuncture or venous cannulation. Tetracaine is effective for 4–6 hours after a single application in most children. It is not recommended prior to neonatal heel lancing.

Tetracaine is rapidly absorbed from mucous membranes and should never be applied to inflamed, traumatised, or highly vascular surfaces. It should never be used to provide anaesthesia for bronchoscopy or cystoscopy because lidocaine hydrochloride is a safer alternative.

Administration

The dose of local anaesthetic depends on the injection site and the procedure used. In determining the safe dosage, it is important to take account of the rate of absorption and excretion, and of the potency. The child's age, weight, physique, and clinical condition, and the vascularity of the administration site and the duration of administration, must also be considered.

Uptake of local anaesthetics into the systemic circulation determines their duration of action and produces toxicity. Great care must be taken to avoid accidental intravascular injection; local anaesthetic injections should be given slowly in order to detect inadvertent intravascular administration. When prolonged analgesia is required, a long-acting local anaesthetic is preferred to minimise the likelihood of cumulative systemic toxicity. Local anaesthesia around the oral cavity may impair swallowing and therefore increases the risk of aspiration.

Epidural anaesthesia is combined with general anaesthesia for certain surgical procedures in children.

Use of vasoconstrictors

Local anaesthetics cause dilatation of blood vessels. The addition of a vasoconstrictor such as adrenaline/epinephrine to the local anaesthetic preparation diminishes local blood flow, slowing the rate of absorption and thereby prolonging the anaesthetic effect. Great care should be taken to avoid inadvertent intravenous administration of a preparation containing adrenaline/epinephrine, and it is not advisable to give adrenaline/epinephrine with a local anaesthetic injection in digits or appendages because of the risk of ischaemic necrosis.

Adrenaline/epinephrine must be used in a low concentration when administered with a local anaesthetic. Care must also be taken to calculate a safe maximum dose of local anaesthetic when using combination products.

In children with severe hypertension or unstable cardiac rhythm, the use of adrenaline/epinephrine with a local anaesthetic may be hazardous. For these children an anaesthetic without adrenaline/epinephrine should be used.

Dental anaesthesia

Lidocaine hydrochloride is widely used in dental procedures; it is most often used in combination with adrenaline/epinephrine. Lidocaine hydrochloride 2% combined with adrenaline/epinephrine 1 in 80 000 (12.5 micrograms/mL) is a safe and effective preparation; there is no justification for using higher concentrations of adrenaline/epinephrine. The amide-type local anaesthetics articaine and mepivacaine hydrochloride p. 782 are also used in dentistry; they are available in cartridges suitable for dental use. Mepivacaine hydrochloride is available with or without adrenaline/epinephrine, and articaine is available with adrenaline/epinephrine. In children with severe hypertension or unstable cardiac rhythm, mepivacaine hydrochloride without adrenaline/epinephrine may be used. Alternatively, prilocaine hydrochloride with or without felypressin can be used but there is no evidence that it is any safer. Felypressin can cause coronary vasoconstriction when used at high doses; limit dose in children with coronary artery disease.

Toxicity

For management of toxicity see Severe local anaesthetic-induced cardiovascular toxicity below.

Severe local anaesthetic-induced cardiovascular toxicity

Overview

After injection of a bolus of local anaesthetic, toxicity may develop at any time in the following hour. In the event of signs of toxicity during injection, the administration of the local anaesthetic must be stopped immediately.

Cardiovascular status must be assessed and cardiopulmonary resuscitation procedures must be followed

In the event of local anaesthetic-induced cardiac arrest, standard cardiopulmonary resuscitation should be initiated immediately. Lidocaine must not be used as anti-arrhythmic therapy.

If the patient does not respond rapidly to standard procedures, 20% lipid emulsion such as *Intralipid*® [unlicensed indication] should be given intravenously at an initial bolus dose of 1.5 mL/kg over 1 minute, followed by an infusion of 15 mL/kg/hour. After 5 minutes, if cardiovascular stability has not been restored or circulation deteriorates, give a maximum of two further bolus doses of 1.5 mL/kg over 1 minute, 5 minutes apart, and increase the infusion rate to 30 mL/kg/hour. Continue infusion until cardiovascular stability and adequate circulation are restored or maximum cumulative dose of 12 mL/kg is given.

Standard cardiopulmonary resuscitation must be maintained throughout lipid emulsion treatment.

Propofol is not a suitable alternative to lipid emulsion.

Further advice on ongoing treatment should be obtained from the National Poisons Information Service.

Detailed treatment algorithms and accompanying notes are available at www.toxbase.org *or* can be found in the Association of Anaesthetists of Great Britain and Ireland safety guideline, Management of Severe Local Anaesthetic Toxicity and Management of Severe Local Anaesthetic Toxicity – Accompanying notes.

ANAESTHETICS, LOCAL

Adrenaline with articaine hydrochloride

(Carticaine hydrochloride with epinephrine)

- ● **INDICATIONS AND DOSE**

Infiltration anaesthesia in dentistry
- ▶ BY REGIONAL ADMINISTRATION
- ▶ Child 4–17 years: Consult expert dental sources

DOSES AT EXTREMES OF BODY-WEIGHT
To avoid excessive dosage in obese patients, dose should be calculated on the basis of ideal body-weight.

IMPORTANT SAFETY INFORMATION
Should only be administered by, or under the direct supervision of, personnel experienced in their use, with adequate training in anaesthesia and airway management, and should not be administered parenterally unless adequate resuscitation equipment is available.

Adrenaline/epinephrine must be used in a low concentration when administered with a local anaesthetic. The total dose of adrenaline should not exceed 5 micrograms/kg (1 mL/kg of a 1 in 200 000 solution) and it is essential not to exceed a concentration of 1 in 200 000 (5 micrograms/mL) if more than 50 mL of the mixture is to be injected.

- ● **CONTRA-INDICATIONS** Application to damaged skin · application to the middle ear (may cause ototoxicity) · complete heart block · injection into infected tissues · injection into inflamed tissues · preparations containing preservatives should not be used for caudal, epidural, or spinal block, or for intravenous regional anaesthesia (Bier's block)

CONTRA-INDICATIONS, FURTHER INFORMATION
Injection site Local anaesthetics should not be injected into inflamed or infected tissues nor should they be applied to damaged skin. Increased absorption into the blood increases the possibility of systemic side-effects, and the local anaesthetic effect may also be reduced by altered local pH.

- ● **CAUTIONS** Arrhythmias · cardiovascular disease · cerebrovascular disease · children (consider dose reduction) · cor pulmonale · debilitated patients (consider dose reduction) · diabetes mellitus · epilepsy ·

hypercalcaemia · hyperreflexia · hypertension · hyperthyroidism · hypokalaemia · hypovolaemia · impaired cardiac conduction · impaired respiratory function · ischaemic heart disease · myasthenia gravis · obstructive cardiomyopathy · occlusive vascular disease · organic brain damage · phaeochromocytoma · prostate disorders · psychoneurosis · severe angina · shock · susceptibility to angle-closure glaucoma

CAUTIONS, FURTHER INFORMATION
- ▶ Use of vasoconstrictors In patients with severe hypertension or unstable cardiac rhythm, the use of adrenaline with a local anaesthetic may be hazardous. For these patients an anaesthetic without adrenaline should be used.

- ● **INTERACTIONS** → Appendix 1 (sympathomimetics).

- ● **SIDE-EFFECTS** Angina · angle-closure glaucoma · anorexia · anxiety · arrhythmias · blurred vision · cardiac arrest · cold extremities · confusion · convulsions · difficulty in micturition · dizziness · drowsiness · dry mouth · dyspnoea · feeling of inebriation · headache · hyperglycaemia · hypersalavation · hypertension (risk of cerebral haemorrhage) · hypokalaemia · insomnia · lightheadedness · metabolic acidosis · methaemoglobinaemia · muscle twitching · mydriasis · myocardial depression (resulting in hypotension and bradycardia) · myocardial infarction · nausea · numbness of the tongue and perioral region · pallor · palpitation · paraesthesia (including sensations of hot and cold) · peripheral vasodilatation (resulting in hypotension and bradycardia) · psychosis · pulmonary oedema (on excessive dosage or extreme sensitivity) · restlessness · sweating · tachycardia · tinnitus · tissue necrosis at injection site and of extremities, bowel, liver and kidneys · transient excitation (followed by depression with drowsiness, respiratory failure, unconsciousness, and coma) · tremor · urinary retention · vomiting · weakness

SIDE-EFFECTS, FURTHER INFORMATION
- ▶ Toxic effects Toxic effects after administration of local anaesthetics are a result of excessively high plasma concentrations; severe toxicity usually results from inadvertent intravascular injection or too rapid injection.

Following most regional anaesthetic procedures, maximum arterial plasma concentration of anaesthetic develops within about 10 to 25 minutes, so careful surveillance for toxic effects is necessary during the first 30 minutes after injection.

The systemic toxicity of local anaesthetics mainly involves the central nervous and cardiovascular systems.

- ● **ALLERGY AND CROSS-SENSITIVITY**
- ▶ Hypersensitivity and cross-sensitivity Hypersensitivity reactions occur mainly with the ester-type local anaesthetics, such as tetracaine and chloroprocaine; reactions are less frequent with the amide types, such as articaine, bupivacaine, levobupivacaine, lidocaine, mepivacaine, prilocaine, and ropivacaine. Cross-sensitivity reactions may be avoided by using the alternative chemical type.

- ● **PREGNANCY** Use only if potential benefit outweighs risk—no information available.

- ● **BREAST FEEDING** Avoid breast-feeding for 48 hours after administration.

- ● **HEPATIC IMPAIRMENT** Use with caution; increased risk of side-effects in severe impairment.

- ● **RENAL IMPAIRMENT** Manufacturers advise use with caution in severe impairment.

- ● **MONITORING REQUIREMENTS** Consider monitoring blood pressure and ECG (advised with systemic adrenaline/epinephrine).

15

Anaesthesia

● **MEDICINAL FORMS**
There can be variation in the licensing of different medicines containing the same drug.

Solution for injection
EXCIPIENTS: May contain Sulfites
▸ Septanest (Septodont Ltd)
  Adrenaline (as Adrenaline acid tartrate) 10 microgram per 1 ml, Articaine hydrochloride 40 mg per 1 ml Septanest 1 in 100,000 solution for injection cartridges | 50 cartridge PoM no price available

  Adrenaline (as Adrenaline acid tartrate) 5 microgram per 1 ml, Articaine hydrochloride 40 mg per 1 ml Septanest 1 in 200,000 solution for injection cartridges | 50 cartridge PoM no price available

Bupivacaine hydrochloride

● **INDICATIONS AND DOSE**

Surgical anaesthesia | Acute pain
▸ BY REGIONAL ADMINISTRATION
▸ Child: Doses adjusted according to child's physical status and nature of procedure, seek expert advice (consult product literature or local protocols)

DOSES AT EXTREMES OF BODY-WEIGHT
To avoid excessive dosage in obese patients, dose should be calculated on the basis of ideal body-weight.

> **IMPORTANT SAFETY INFORMATION**
> The licensed doses stated may not be appropriate in some settings and expert advice should be sought.
> Should only be administered by, or under the direct supervision of, personnel experienced in their use, with adequate training in anaesthesia and airway management, and should not be administered parenterally unless adequate resuscitation equipment is available.

● **CONTRA-INDICATIONS** Application to the middle ear (can cause ototoxicity) · avoid injection into infected tissues · avoid injection into inflamed tissues · complete heart block · preparations containing preservatives should not be used for caudal, epidural, or spinal block, or for intravenous regional anaesthesia (Bier's block) · should not be applied to damaged skin
CONTRA-INDICATIONS, FURTHER INFORMATION
▸ Injection site Local anaesthetics should not be injected into inflamed or infected tissues nor should they be applied to damaged skin. Increased absorption into the blood increases the possibility of systemic side-effects, and the local anaesthetic effect may also be reduced by altered local pH.

● **CAUTIONS** Cardiovascular disease · cerebral atheroma · children (consider dose reduction) · debilitated patients (consider dose reduction) · epilepsy · hypertension · hypotension · hypovolaemia · impaired cardiac conduction · impaired respiratory function · myasthenia gravis · myocardial depression may be more severe and more resistant to treatment · shock

● **INTERACTIONS** → Appendix 1 (bupivacaine).

● **SIDE-EFFECTS** Arrhythmias · blurred vision · cardiac arrest · convulsions · dizziness · drowsiness · feeling of inebriation · headache · lightheadedness · muscle twitching · myocardial depression (resulting in hypotension and bradycardia) · nausea · numbness of the tongue and perioral region · paraesthesia (including sensations of hot and cold) · peripheral vasodilatation (resulting in hypotension and bradycardia) · restlessness · tinnitus · transient excitation (followed by depression with drowsiness, respiratory failure, unconsciousness, and coma) · tremors · vomiting

SIDE-EFFECTS, FURTHER INFORMATION
▸ Toxic effects Toxic effects after administration of local anaesthetics are a result of excessively high plasma concentrations; severe toxicity usually results from inadvertent intravascular injection or too rapid injection.

Following most regional anaesthetic procedures, maximum arterial plasma concentration of anaesthetic develops within about 10 to 25 minutes, so careful surveillance for toxic effects is necessary during the first 30 minutes after injection.

The systemic toxicity of local anaesthetics mainly involves the central nervous and cardiovascular systems.

● **ALLERGY AND CROSS-SENSITIVITY**
▸ Hypersensitivity and cross-sensitivity Hypersensitivity reactions occur mainly with the ester-type local anaesthetics, such as tetracaine and chloroprocaine; reactions are less frequent with the amide types, such as articaine, bupivacaine, levobupivacaine, lidocaine, mepivacaine, prilocaine, and ropivacaine. Cross-sensitivity reactions may be avoided by using the alternative chemical type.

● **PREGNANCY** Use lower doses for intrathecal use during late pregnancy. Large doses during delivery can cause neonatal respiratory depression, hypotonia, and bradycardia after epidural block.

● **BREAST FEEDING** Amount too small to be harmful.

● **HEPATIC IMPAIRMENT** Use with caution in severe impairment.

● **RENAL IMPAIRMENT** Use with caution in severe impairment.

● **MEDICINAL FORMS**
There can be variation in the licensing of different medicines containing the same drug. Forms available from special-order manufacturers include: solution for injection, infusion, solution for infusion

Solution for injection
▸ Bupivacaine hydrochloride (Non-proprietary)
  Bupivacaine hydrochloride 2.5 mg per 1 ml Bupivacaine 0.25% solution for injection 10ml Sure-Amp ampoules | 20 ampoule PoM £17.50

  Bupivacaine hydrochloride 5 mg per 1 ml Bupivacaine 0.5% solution for injection 10ml Sure-Amp ampoules | 20 ampoule PoM £18.30
  Bupivacaine 50mg/10ml (0.5%) solution for injection ampoules | 10 ampoule PoM no price available
▸ Marcain (AstraZeneca UK Ltd)
  Bupivacaine hydrochloride 2.5 mg per 1 ml Marcain 0.25% solution for injection 10ml Polyamp Steripack ampoules | 5 ampoule PoM £7.92

  Bupivacaine hydrochloride 5 mg per 1 ml Marcain 0.5% solution for injection 10ml Polyamp Steripack ampoules | 5 ampoule PoM £9.25

Infusion
▸ Bupivacaine hydrochloride (Non-proprietary)
  Bupivacaine hydrochloride 1 mg per 1 ml Bupivacaine 100mg/100ml (0.1%) infusion bags | 20 bag PoM no price available
  Bupivacaine 250mg/250ml (0.1%) infusion bags | 20 bag PoM no price available

  Bupivacaine hydrochloride 1.25 mg per 1 ml Bupivacaine 312.5mg/250ml (0.125%) infusion bags | 20 bag PoM no price available

15

Anaesthesia

Bupivacaine with adrenaline

The properties listed below are those particular to the combination only. For the properties of the components please consider, bupivacaine hydrochloride p. 778, adrenaline/epinephrine p. 128.

- **INDICATIONS AND DOSE**
Surgical anaesthesia
▶ BY LUMBAR EPIDURAL, OR BY LOCAL INFILTRATION, OR BY CAUDAL EPIDURAL
▸ Child 12–17 years: (consult product literature)
Acute pain management
▶ BY LUMBAR EPIDURAL, OR BY LOCAL INFILTRATION
▸ Child 1–17 years: (consult product literature)

IMPORTANT SAFETY INFORMATION
Adrenaline/epinephrine must be used in a low concentration when administered with a local anaesthetic. The total dose of adrenaline should not exceed 5 micrograms/kg (1 mL/kg of a 1 in 200 000 solution) and it is essential not to exceed a concentration of 1 in 200 000 (5 micrograms/mL) if more than 50 mL of the mixture is to be injected.

- **CAUTIONS**
CAUTIONS, FURTHER INFORMATION
In patients with severe hypertension or unstable cardiac rhythm, the use of adrenaline with a local anaesthetic may be hazardous. For these patients an anaesthetic without adrenaline should be used.

- **MEDICINAL FORMS**
There can be variation in the licensing of different medicines containing the same drug.
Solution for injection
▶ Bupivacaine with adrenaline (Non-proprietary)
Adrenaline (as Adrenaline acid tartrate) 5 microgram per 1 ml, Bupivacaine hydrochloride 2.5 mg per 1 ml Bupivacaine 25mg/10ml (0.25%) / Adrenaline (base) 50micrograms/10ml (1 in 200,000) solution for injection ampoules | 10 ampoule PoM £40.00
Adrenaline (as Adrenaline acid tartrate) 5 microgram per 1 ml, Bupivacaine hydrochloride anhydrous 2.5 mg per 1 ml Carbostesin-adrenaline 0.25% / 100micrograms/20ml (1 in 200,000) solution for injection ampoules | 1 ampoule PoM no price available
Carbostesin-adrenaline 0.25% / 25micrograms/5ml (1 in 200,000) solution for injection ampoules | 1 ampoule PoM no price available
Adrenaline (as Adrenaline acid tartrate) 5 microgram per 1 ml, Bupivacaine hydrochloride 5 mg per 1 ml Bupivacaine 50mg/10ml (0.5%) / Adrenaline (base) 50micrograms/10ml (1 in 200,000) solution for injection ampoules | 10 ampoule PoM £45.00
Adrenaline (as Adrenaline acid tartrate) 5 microgram per 1 ml, Bupivacaine hydrochloride anhydrous 5 mg per 1 ml Carbostesin-adrenaline 0.5% / 25micrograms/5ml (1 in 200,000) solution for injection ampoules | 1 ampoule PoM no price available
Carbostesin-adrenaline 0.5% / 100micrograms/20ml (1 in 200,000) solution for injection ampoules | 1 ampoule PoM no price available

Levobupivacaine

- **INDICATIONS AND DOSE**
Surgical anaesthesia | Acute pain
▶ BY REGIONAL ADMINISTRATION
▸ Child: Doses adjusted according to child's physical status and nature of procedure, seek expert advice (consult product literature or local protocols)
DOSES AT EXTREMES OF BODY-WEIGHT
To avoid excessive dosage in obese patients, dose should be calculated on the basis of ideal body-weight.

- UNLICENSED USE Not licensed for use in children except for analgesia by ilioinguinal or iliohypogastric block.

IMPORTANT SAFETY INFORMATION
The licensed doses stated may not be appropriate in some settings and expert advice should be sought.
Should only be administered by, or under the direct supervision of, personnel experienced in their use, with adequate training in anaesthesia and airway management, and should not be administered parenterally unless adequate resuscitation equipment is available.

- CONTRA-INDICATIONS Application to the middle ear (can cause ototoxicity) · avoid injection into infected tissues · avoid injection into inflamed tissues · complete heart block · preparations containing preservatives should not be used for caudal, epidural, or spinal block, or for intravenous regional anaesthesia (Bier's block) · should not be applied to damaged skin
CONTRA-INDICATIONS, FURTHER INFORMATION
▸ Injection site Local anaesthetics should not be injected into inflamed or infected tissues nor should they be applied to damaged skin. Increased absorption into the blood increases the possibility of systemic side-effects, and the local anaesthetic effect may also be reduced by altered local pH.

- CAUTIONS Cardiovascular disease · children (consider dose reduction) · debilitated patients (consider dose reduction) · epilepsy · hypovolaemia · impaired cardiac conduction · impaired respiratory function · myasthenia gravis · shock

- INTERACTIONS → Appendix 1 (levobupivacaine).

- SIDE-EFFECTS Anaemia · arrhythmias · blurred vision · cardiac arrest · convulsions · dizziness · drowsiness · feeling of inebriation · headache · lightheadedness · muscle twitching · myocardial depression (resulting in hypotension and bradycardia) · nausea · numbness of the tongue and perioral region · paraesthesia (including sensations of hot and cold) · peripheral vasodilatation (resulting in hypotension and bradycardia) · pyrexia · restlessness · sweating · tinnitus · transient excitation (followed by depression with drowsiness, respiratory failure, unconsciousness, and coma) · tremors · vomiting
SIDE-EFFECTS, FURTHER INFORMATION
▸ Toxic effects Toxic effects after administration of local anaesthetics are a result of excessively high plasma concentrations; severe toxicity usually results from inadvertent intravascular injection or too rapid injection.
Following most regional anaesthetic procedures, maximum arterial plasma concentration of anaesthetic develops within about 10 to 25 minutes, so careful surveillance for toxic effects is necessary during the first 30 minutes after injection.
The systemic toxicity of local anaesthetics mainly involves the central nervous and cardiovascular systems.

- ALLERGY AND CROSS-SENSITIVITY
▸ Hypersensitivity and cross-sensitivity Hypersensitivity reactions occur mainly with the ester-type local anaesthetics, such as tetracaine and chloroprocaine; reactions are less frequent with the amide types, such as articaine, bupivacaine, levobupivacaine, lidocaine, mepivacaine, prilocaine, and ropivacaine. Cross-sensitivity reactions may be avoided by using the alternative chemical type.

- PREGNANCY Large doses during delivery can cause neonatal respiratory depression, hypotonia, and bradycardia after epidural block. Avoid if possible in the first trimester—toxicity in *animal* studies. May cause fetal distress syndrome. Do not use for paracervical block in obstetrics. Do not use 7.5 mg/mL strength in obstetrics.

- BREAST FEEDING Amount too small to be harmful.

15

Anaesthesia

- HEPATIC IMPAIRMENT Use with caution.
- DIRECTIONS FOR ADMINISTRATION For 1.25 mg/mL concentration dilute standard solutions with sodium chloride 0.9%.
- PRESCRIBING AND DISPENSING INFORMATION Levobupivacaine is an isomer of bupivacaine.
- MEDICINAL FORMS
  There can be variation in the licensing of different medicines containing the same drug.

  Solution for injection
  - Chirocaine (AbbVie Ltd)
    Levobupivacaine (as Levobupivacaine hydrochloride) 2.5 mg per 1 ml Chirocaine 25mg/10ml solution for injection ampoules | 10 ampoule [PoM] £14.11 (Hospital only)
    Levobupivacaine (as Levobupivacaine hydrochloride) 5 mg per 1 ml Chirocaine 50mg/10ml solution for injection ampoules | 10 ampoule [PoM] £16.15 (Hospital only)
    Levobupivacaine (as Levobupivacaine hydrochloride) 7.5 mg per 1 ml Chirocaine 75mg/10ml solution for injection ampoules | 10 ampoule [PoM] £24.23 (Hospital only)

  Infusion
  - Chirocaine (AbbVie Ltd)
    Levobupivacaine (as Levobupivacaine hydrochloride) 1.25 mg per 1 ml Chirocaine 125mg/100ml infusion bags | 24 bag [PoM] £174.22
    Chirocaine 250mg/200ml infusion bags | 12 bag [PoM] no price available

Lidocaine hydrochloride
(Lignocaine hydrochloride)

- INDICATIONS AND DOSE
  Infiltration anaesthesia
  ▸ BY LOCAL INFILTRATION
  - Neonate: Up to 3 mg/kg, dose to be given according to patient's weight and nature of procedure, dose may be repeated not more often than every 4 hours, 3 mg/kg equivalent to 0.3 mL/kg of 1% solution.
  - Child 1 month–11 years: Up to 3 mg/kg, dose to be given according to patient's weight and nature of procedure, dose may be repeated not more often than every 4 hours, 3 mg/kg equivalent to 0.3 mL/kg of 1% solution
  - Child 12–17 years: (max. per dose 200 mg), dose to be given according to child's weight and nature of procedure, dose may be repeated not more often than every 4 hours

  DOSES AT EXTREMES OF BODY-WEIGHT
  ▸ When used by local infiltration To avoid excessive dosage in obese patients, dose may need to be calculated on the basis of ideal body-weight.

  Intravenous regional anaesthesia and nerve block
  ▸ BY REGIONAL ADMINISTRATION
  - Child: Seek expert advice

  Dental anaesthesia
  ▸ BY REGIONAL ADMINISTRATION
  - Child: Seek expert advice

  Pain relief (in anal fissures, haemorrhoids, pruritus ani, pruritus vulvae, herpes zoster, or herpes labialis) | Lubricant in cystoscopy | Lubricant in proctoscopy
  ▸ TO THE SKIN USING OINTMENT
  - Child: Apply 1–2 mL as required, avoid long-term use

  LMX 4®
  Anaesthesia before venous cannulation or venepuncture
  ▸ TO THE SKIN
  - Child 1–2 months: Apply up to 1 g, apply thick layer to small area (2.5 cm × 2.5 cm) of non-irritated skin at least 30 minutes before procedure; may be applied under an occlusive dressing; max. application time 60 minutes, remove cream with gauze and perform procedure after approximately 5 minutes

  - Child 3–11 months: Apply up to 1 g, apply thick layer to small area (2.5 cm × 2.5 cm) of non-irritated skin at least 30 minutes before procedure; may be applied under an occlusive dressing; max. application time 4 hours, remove cream with gauze and perform procedure after approximately 5 minutes
  - Child 1–17 years: Apply 1–2.5 g, apply thick layer to small area (2.5 cm × 2.5 cm) of non-irritated skin at least 30 minutes before procedure; may be applied under an occlusive dressing; max. application time 5 hours, remove cream with gauze and perform procedure after approximately 5 minutes

  IMPORTANT SAFETY INFORMATION
  ▸ When used by local infiltration
  The licensed doses stated may not be appropriate in some settings and expert advice should be sought. Should only be administered by, or under the direct supervision of, personnel experienced in their use, with adequate training in anaesthesia and airway management, and should not be administered parenterally unless adequate resuscitation equipment is available.

- CONTRA-INDICATIONS
  ▸ When used by regional administration All grades of atrioventricular block · application to the middle ear (can cause ototoxicity) · avoid injection into infected tissues · avoid injection into inflamed tissues · preparations containing preservatives should not be used for caudal, epidural, or spinal block, or for intravenous regional anaesthesia (Bier's block) · severe myocardial depression · should not be applied to damaged skin · sino-atrial disorders
  CONTRA-INDICATIONS, FURTHER INFORMATION
  ▸ When used by regional administration Local anaesthetics should not be injected into inflamed or infected tissues nor should they be applied to damaged skin. Increased absorption into the blood increases the possibility of systemic side-effects, and the local anaesthetic effect may also be reduced by altered local pH.

- CAUTIONS
  ▸ When used by regional administration Acute porphyria (consider infusion with glucose for its anti-porphyrinogenic effects) · children (consider dose reduction) · congestive cardiac failure (consider lower dose) · debilitated patients (consider dose reduction) · epilepsy · hypovolaemia · impaired cardiac conduction · impaired respiratory function · myasthenia gravis · post cardiac surgery (consider lower dose) · shock

- INTERACTIONS → Appendix 1 (lidocaine). Interactions less likely when lidocaine used topically.

- SIDE-EFFECTS
  ▸ Common or very common
  ▸ When used by regional administration Bradycardia (may lead to cardiac arrest) · confusion · convulsions · hypotension (may lead to cardiac arrest) · respiratory depression
  ▸ Rare
  ▸ When used by regional administration Anaphylaxis
  ▸ Frequency not known
  ▸ When used by regional administration Transient excitation (followed by depression with drowsiness, respiratory failure, unconsciousness, and coma) · arrhythmias · blurred vision · cardiac arrest · feeling of inebriation · headache · hypoglycaemia (following intrathecal or extradural administration) · methaemoglobinaemia · muscle twitching · myocardial depression (resulting in hypotension and bradycardia) · nausea · numbness of the tongue and perioral region · nystagmus · peripheral vasodilatation (resulting in hypotension and bradycardia) · rash · restlessness · tinnitus · tremors · vomiting

SIDE-EFFECTS, FURTHER INFORMATION
▸ Topical application A single application of a topical lidocaine preparation does not generally cause systemic side-effects.
▸ Toxic effects
▸ When used by regional administration Toxic effects after administration of local anaesthetics are a result of excessively high plasma concentrations; severe toxicity usually results from inadvertent intravascular injection or too rapid injection. Following most regional anaesthetic procedures, maximum arterial plasma concentration of anaesthetic develops within about 10 to 25 minutes, so careful surveillance for toxic effects is necessary during the first 30 minutes after injection. The systemic toxicity of local anaesthetics mainly involves the central nervous and cardiovascular systems.
▸ Methaemoglobinaemia
▸ When used by regional administration Methaemoglobinaemia can be treated with an intravenous injection of methylthioninium chloride; neonates and infants under 6 months are particularly susceptible to methaemoglobinaemia.

● ALLERGY AND CROSS-SENSITIVITY
▸ Hypersensitivity and cross-sensitivity Hypersensitivity reactions occur mainly with the ester-type local anaesthetics, such as tetracaine and chloroprocaine; reactions are less frequent with the amide types, such as articaine, bupivacaine, levobupivacaine, lidocaine, mepivacaine, prilocaine, and ropivacaine. Cross-sensitivity reactions may be avoided by using the alternative chemical type.

● PREGNANCY Crosses the placenta but not known to be harmful in *animal* studies—use if benefit outweighs risk. When used as a local anaesthetic, large doses can cause fetal bradycardia; if given during delivery can also cause neonatal respiratory depression, hypotonia, or bradycardia after paracervical or epidural block.

● BREAST FEEDING Present in milk but amount too small to be harmful.

● HEPATIC IMPAIRMENT Caution—increased risk of side-effects.

● RENAL IMPAIRMENT Possible accumulation of lidocaine and active metabolite; caution in severe impairment.

● MONITORING REQUIREMENTS
▸ With systemic use Monitor ECG and have resuscitation facilities available.

● DIRECTIONS FOR ADMINISTRATION For *intravenous infusion*, dilute with Glucose 5% or Sodium Chloride 0.9%.

● MEDICINAL FORMS
There can be variation in the licensing of different medicines containing the same drug.
Solution for injection
▸ Lidocaine hydrochloride (Non-proprietary)
Lidocaine hydrochloride 5 mg per 1 ml Lidocaine 50mg/10ml (0.5%) solution for injection ampoules | 10 ampoule [PoM] £7.00
Lidocaine hydrochloride 10 mg per 1 ml Lidocaine 100mg/10ml (1%) solution for injection Mini-Plasco ampoules | 20 ampoule [PoM] £10.89
Lidocaine 100mg/10ml (1%) solution for injection ampoules | 10 ampoule [PoM] £4.50 DT price = £4.01
Lidocaine 100mg/10ml (1%) solution for injection Sure-Amp ampoules | 20 ampoule [PoM] £8.80
Lidocaine 200mg/20ml (1%) solution for injection vials | 10 vial [PoM] £18.00–£19.00
Lidocaine 200mg/20ml (1%) solution for injection ampoules | 10 ampoule [PoM] £7.00–£8.75 DT price = £8.75
Lidocaine 50mg/5ml (1%) solution for injection ampoules | 10 ampoule [PoM] £2.35–£3.10 DT price = £2.36
Lidocaine 20mg/2ml (1%) solution for injection ampoules | 10 ampoule [PoM] £3.50 DT price = £1.98
Lidocaine 50mg/5ml (1%) solution for injection Sure-Amp ampoules | 20 ampoule [PoM] £6.00

Lidocaine hydrochloride 20 mg per 1 ml Lidocaine 100mg/5ml (2%) solution for injection ampoules | 10 ampoule [PoM] £2.40–£3.80 DT price = £2.41
Lidocaine 400mg/20ml (2%) solution for injection vials | 10 vial [PoM] £18.50–£19.50
Lidocaine 200mg/10ml (2%) solution for injection Mini-Plasco ampoules | 20 ampoule [PoM] £14.52
Lidocaine 40mg/2ml (2%) solution for injection ampoules | 10 ampoule [PoM] £4.00 DT price = £2.11
Lidocaine 100mg/5ml (2%) solution for injection Sure-Amp ampoules | 20 ampoule [PoM] £6.00
Lidocaine 400mg/20ml (2%) solution for injection ampoules | 10 ampoule [PoM] £8.00–£9.00 DT price = £9.00
Cream
EXCIPIENTS: May contain Benzyl alcohol, propylene glycol
▸ LMX 4 (Ferndale Pharmaceuticals Ltd)
Lidocaine 40 mg per 1 gram LMX 4 cream | 5 gram [P] £2.98 DT price = £2.98 | 30 gram [P] £14.90
Ointment
▸ Lidocaine hydrochloride (Non-proprietary)
Lidocaine hydrochloride 50 mg per 1 gram Lidocaine 5% ointment | 15 gram [P] £6.50 DT price = £6.18

Lidocaine with adrenaline

The properties listed below are those particular to the combination only. For the properties of the components please consider, lidocaine hydrochloride p. 780, adrenaline/epinephrine p. 128.

● INDICATIONS AND DOSE
Local anaesthesia
▸ BY LOCAL INFILTRATION
▸ Child 12–17 years: Dosed according to the type of nerve block required (consult product literature)

IMPORTANT SAFETY INFORMATION
Adrenaline/epinephrine must be used in a low concentration when administered with a local anaesthetic. The total dose of adrenaline should not exceed 5 micrograms/kg (1 mL/kg of a 1 in 200 000 solution) and it is essential not to exceed a concentration of 1 in 200 000 (5 micrograms/mL) if more than 50 mL of the mixture is to be injected.

● PROFESSION SPECIFIC INFORMATION
Dental information
A variety of lidocaine injections with adrenaline is available in dental cartridges.
Consult expert dental sources for specific advice in relation to dose of lidocaine for dental anaesthesia.

● MEDICINAL FORMS
There can be variation in the licensing of different medicines containing the same drug. Forms available from special-order manufacturers include: solution for injection
Solution for injection
EXCIPIENTS: May contain Sulfites
▸ Lignospan Special (Kent Pharmaceuticals Ltd)
Adrenaline (as Adrenaline acid tartrate) 12.5 microgram per 1 ml, Lidocaine hydrochloride 20 mg per 1 ml Lignospan Special 2% injection 2.2ml cartridges | 50 cartridge [PoM] £18.11
▸ Rexocaine (Henry Schein Ltd)
Adrenaline (as Adrenaline acid tartrate) 12.5 microgram per 1 ml, Lidocaine hydrochloride 20 mg per 1 ml Rexocaine 2% injection 2.2ml cartridges | 50 cartridge [PoM] no price available
▸ Xylocaine with Adrenaline (AstraZeneca UK Ltd)
Adrenaline (as Adrenaline acid tartrate) 5 microgram per 1 ml, Lidocaine hydrochloride 10 mg per 1 ml Xylocaine 1% with Adrenaline 100micrograms/20ml (1 in 200,000) solution for injection vials | 5 vial [PoM] £9.66 DT price = £9.66
Adrenaline (as Adrenaline acid tartrate) 5 microgram per 1 ml, Lidocaine hydrochloride 20 mg per 1 ml Xylocaine 2% with Adrenaline 100micrograms/20ml (1 in 200,000) solution for injection vials | 5 vial [PoM] £8.85 DT price = £8.85

15

Anaesthesia

Lidocaine with phenylephrine

The properties listed below are those particular to the combination only. For the properties of the components please consider, lidocaine hydrochloride p. 780, phenylephrine hydrochloride p. 116.

- **INDICATIONS AND DOSE**

Anaesthesia before nasal surgery, endoscopy, laryngoscopy, or removal of foreign bodies from the nose
  ‣ BY INTRANASAL ADMINISTRATION
  ‣ Child 12–17 years: Up to 8 sprays

- **MEDICINAL FORMS**
There can be variation in the licensing of different medicines containing the same drug.
Spray
  ‣ Lidocaine with phenylephrine (Non-proprietary)
    Phenylephrine hydrochloride 5 mg per 1 ml, Lidocaine hydrochloride 50 mg per 1 ml Lidocaine 5% / Phenylephrine 0.5% nasal spray | 2.5 ml PoM £11.48 DT price = £11.48

Lidocaine with prilocaine

The properties listed below are those particular to the combination only. For the properties of the components please consider, lidocaine hydrochloride p. 780, prilocaine hydrochloride p. 783.

- **INDICATIONS AND DOSE**
Anaesthesia before minor skin procedures including venepuncture
  ‣ TO THE SKIN

  ‣ Neonate: Apply up to 1 g for maximum 1 hour before procedure, to be applied under occlusive dressing, shorter application time of 15–30 minutes is recommended for children with atopic dermatitis (30 minutes before removal of mollusca); maximum 1 dose per day.

  ‣ Child 1–2 months: Apply up to 1 g for maximum 1 hour before procedure, to be applied under occlusive dressing, shorter application time of 15–30 minutes is recommended for children with atopic dermatitis (30 minutes before removal of mollusca); maximum 1 dose per day

  ‣ Child 3–11 months: Apply up to 2 g for maximum 4 hours before procedure, to be applied under occlusive dressing, shorter application time of 15–30 minutes is recommended for children with atopic dermatitis (30 minutes before removal of mollusca); maximum 2 doses per day

  ‣ Child 1–11 years: Apply 1–5 hours before procedure (2–5 hours before procedures on large areas e.g. split skin grafting), a thick layer should be applied under occlusive dressing, shorter application time of 15–30 minutes is recommended for children with atopic dermatitis (30 minutes before removal of mollusca); maximum 2 doses per day

  ‣ Child 12–17 years: Apply 1–5 hours before procedure (2–5 hours before procedures on large areas e.g. split skin grafting), a thick layer should be applied under occlusive dressing, shorter application time of 15–30 minutes is recommended for children with atopic dermatitis (30 minutes before removal of mollusca)

- **CONTRA-INDICATIONS** Use in child less than 37 weeks corrected gestational age

- **PATIENT AND CARER ADVICE**
Medicines for Children leaflet: EMLA cream for local anaesthesia www.medicinesforchildren.org.uk/emla-cream-for-local-anaesthesia

- **MEDICINAL FORMS**
There can be variation in the licensing of different medicines containing the same drug.
Cream
  ‣ Lidocaine with prilocaine (Non-proprietary)
    Lidocaine 25 mg per 1 gram, Prilocaine 25 mg per 1 gram Lidocaine 2.5% / Prilocaine 2.5% cream | 5 gram P no price available
  ‣ Denela (Auden McKenzie (Pharma Division) Ltd)
    Lidocaine 25 mg per 1 gram, Prilocaine 25 mg per 1 gram Denela 5% cream | 5 gram P £2.84-£3.29 | 25 gram P £12.99 | 30 gram P £14.75 DT price = £12.30
  ‣ Emla (AstraZeneca UK Ltd)
    Lidocaine 25 mg per 1 gram, Prilocaine 25 mg per 1 gram Emla 5% cream | 5 gram P £2.25-£2.99 | 25 gram P £11.70 | 30 gram P £12.30 DT price = £12.30

Mepivacaine hydrochloride

- **INDICATIONS AND DOSE**
Infiltration anaesthesia and nerve block in dentistry
  ‣ Child 3–17 years: Consult expert dental sources
DOSES AT EXTREMES OF BODY-WEIGHT
To avoid excessive dosage in obese patients, dose should be calculated on the basis of ideal body-weight.

> **IMPORTANT SAFETY INFORMATION**
> Should only be administered by, or under the direct supervision of, personnel experienced in their use, with adequate training in anaesthesia and airway management, and should not be administered parenterally unless adequate resuscitation equipment is available.

- **CONTRA-INDICATIONS** Application to the middle ear (can cause ototoxicity) · avoid injection into infected tissues · avoid injection into inflamed tissues · complete heart block · preparations containing preservatives should not be used for caudal, epidural, or spinal block, or for intravenous regional anaesthesia (Bier's block) · should not be applied to damaged skin
CONTRA-INDICATIONS, FURTHER INFORMATION
  ‣ Injection site Local anaesthetics should not be injected into inflamed or infected tissues nor should they be applied to damaged skin. Increased absorption into the blood increases the possibility of systemic side-effects, and the local anaesthetic effect may also be reduced by altered local pH.

- **CAUTIONS** Cardiovascular disease · children (consider dose reduction) · debilitated patients (consider dose reduction) · epilepsy · hypovolaemia · impaired cardiac conduction · impaired respiratory function · myasthenia gravis · shock

- **SIDE-EFFECTS** Arrhythmias · blurred vision · cardiac arrest · convulsions · dizziness · drowsiness · feeling of inebriation · headache · lightheadedness · muscle twitching · myocardial depression (resulting in hypotension and bradycardia) · nausea · numbness of the tongue and perioral region · paraesthesia (including sensations of hot and cold) · peripheral vasodilatation (resulting in hypotension and bradycardia) · restlessness · tinnitus · transient excitation (followed by depression with drowsiness, respiratory failure, unconsciousness, and coma) · tremors · vomiting
SIDE-EFFECTS, FURTHER INFORMATION
  ‣ Toxic effects Toxic effects after administration of local anaesthetics are a result of excessively high plasma

concentrations; severe toxicity usually results from inadvertent intravascular injection or too rapid injection.

Following most regional anaesthetic procedures, maximum arterial plasma concentration of anaesthetic develops within about 10 to 25 minutes, so careful surveillance for toxic effects is necessary during the first 30 minutes after injection.

The systemic toxicity of local anaesthetics mainly involves the central nervous and cardiovascular systems.

- **ALLERGY AND CROSS-SENSITIVITY**
▸ Hypersensitivity and cross-sensitivity Hypersensitivity reactions occur mainly with the ester-type local anaesthetics, such as tetracaine and chloroprocaine; reactions are less frequent with the amide types, such as articaine, bupivacaine, levobupivacaine, lidocaine, mepivacaine, prilocaine, and ropivacaine. Cross-sensitivity reactions may be avoided by using the alternative chemical type.
- **PREGNANCY** Use with caution in early pregnancy.
- **BREAST FEEDING** Use with caution.
- **HEPATIC IMPAIRMENT** Use with caution; increased risk of side-effects in severe impairment.
- **RENAL IMPAIRMENT** Use with caution; increased risk of side-effects.

- **MEDICINAL FORMS**
There can be variation in the licensing of different medicines containing the same drug.
Solution for injection
▸ Scandonest plain (Deproco UK Ltd)
  Mepivacaine hydrochloride 30 mg per 1 ml Scandonest plain 3% solution for injection 2.2ml cartridges | 50 cartridge [PoM] no price available

Mepivacaine with adrenaline

The properties listed below are those particular to the combination only. For the properties of the components please consider, mepivacaine hydrochloride p. 782, adrenaline/epinephrine p. 128.

- **INDICATIONS AND DOSE**
Infiltration anaesthesia and nerve block in dentistry
  ▸ BY LOCAL INFILTRATION
  ▸ Child: (consult product literature)

IMPORTANT SAFETY INFORMATION
Adrenaline/epinephrine must be used in a low concentration when administered with a local anaesthetic. The total dose of adrenaline should not exceed 5 micrograms/kg (1 mL/kg of a 1 in 200 000 solution) and it is essential not to exceed a concentration of 1 in 200 000 (5 micrograms/mL) if more than 50 mL of the mixture is to be injected.

- **MEDICINAL FORMS**
There can be variation in the licensing of different medicines containing the same drug.
Solution for injection
EXCIPIENTS: May contain Sulfites
▸ Scandonest special (Deproco UK Ltd)
  Adrenaline 10 microgram per 1 ml, Mepivacaine hydrochloride 20 mg per 1 ml Scandonest special 2% solution for injection 2.2ml cartridges | 50 cartridge [PoM] no price available

Prilocaine hydrochloride

- **INDICATIONS AND DOSE**
CITANEST 1%®
Infiltration anaesthesia | Nerve block
  ▸ BY REGIONAL ADMINISTRATION
  ▸ Child 6 months–11 years: Up to 5 mg/kg, dose adjusted according to site of administration and response; maximum 400 mg per course
  ▸ Child 12–17 years: 100–200 mg/minute, alternatively, may be given in incremental doses; dose adjusted according to site of administration and response; maximum 400 mg per course
DOSES AT EXTREMES OF BODY-WEIGHT
To avoid excessive dosage in obese patients, dose should be calculated on the basis of ideal body-weight.

IMPORTANT SAFETY INFORMATION
Should only be administered by, or under the direct supervision of, personnel experienced in their use, with adequate training in anaesthesia and airway management, and should not be administered parenterally unless adequate resuscitation equipment is available.

- **CONTRA-INDICATIONS** Acquired methaemoglobinaemia · anaemia · application to the middle ear (can cause ototoxicity) · avoid injection into infected tissues · avoid injection into inflamed tissues · complete heart block · congenital methaemoglobinaemia · preparations containing preservatives should not be used for caudal, epidural, or spinal block, or for intravenous regional anaesthesia (Bier's block) · should not be applied to damaged skin
CONTRA-INDICATIONS, FURTHER INFORMATION
▸ Injection site Local anaesthetics should not be injected into inflamed or infected tissues nor should they be applied to damaged skin. Increased absorption into the blood increases the possibility of systemic side-effects, and the local anaesthetic effect may also be reduced by altered local pH.
- **CAUTIONS** Acute porphyrias p. 562 · cardiovascular disease · children (consider dose reduction) · debilitated patients (consider dose reduction) · epilepsy · hypovolaemia · impaired cardiac conduction · impaired respiratory function · myasthenia gravis · neonates and infants under 6 months are particularly susceptible to methaemoglobinaemia · severe or untreated hypertension · shock
- **INTERACTIONS** → Appendix 1 (prilocaine).
Caution with concomitant use of drugs that cause methaemoglobinaemia.
- **SIDE-EFFECTS** Arrhythmias · blurred vision · cardiac arrest · convulsions · dizziness · drowsiness · feeling of inebriation · headache · hypertension · lightheadedness · methaemoglobinaemia (with high doses) · muscle twitching · myocardial depression (resulting in hypotension and bradycardia) · nausea · numbness of the tongue and perioral region · paraesthesia (including sensations of hot and cold) · peripheral vasodilatation (resulting in hypotension and bradycardia) · restlessness · tinnitus · transient excitation (followed by depression with drowsiness, respiratory failure, unconsciousness, and coma) · tremors · vomiting
SIDE-EFFECTS, FURTHER INFORMATION
▸ Toxic effects Toxic effects after administration of local anaesthetics are a result of excessively high plasma concentrations; severe toxicity usually results from

15

Anaesthesia

inadvertent intravascular injection or too rapid injection.

Following most regional anaesthetic procedures, maximum arterial plasma concentration of anaesthetic develops within about 10 to 25 minutes, so careful surveillance for toxic effects is necessary during the first 30 minutes after injection.

The systemic toxicity of local anaesthetics mainly involves the central nervous and cardiovascular systems.
‣ Methaemoglobinaemia Methaemoglobinaemia can be treated with an intravenous injection of **methylthioninium chloride**.

● ALLERGY AND CROSS-SENSITIVITY
‣ Hypersensitivity and cross-sensitivity Hypersensitivity reactions occur mainly with the ester-type local anaesthetics, such as tetracaine and chloroprocaine; reactions are less frequent with the amide types, such as articaine, bupivacaine, levobupivacaine, lidocaine, mepivacaine, prilocaine, and ropivacaine. Cross-sensitivity reactions may be avoided by using the alternative chemical type.

● PREGNANCY Use lower doses for intrathecal use during late pregnancy. Large doses during delivery can cause neonatal respiratory depression, hypotonia, and bradycardia after epidural block. Avoid paracervical or pudendal block in obstetrics (neonatal methaemoglobinaemia reported).

● BREAST FEEDING Present in milk but not known to be harmful.

● HEPATIC IMPAIRMENT Lower doses may be required for intrathecal anaesthesia. Use with caution.

● RENAL IMPAIRMENT Lower doses may be required for intrathecal anaesthesia. Use with caution.

● MEDICINAL FORMS
There can be variation in the licensing of different medicines containing the same drug.
Solution for injection
‣ Citanest (AstraZeneca UK Ltd)
Prilocaine hydrochloride 10 mg per 1 ml Citanest 1% solution for injection 50ml vials | 1 vial [PoM] £5.06

Prilocaine with felypressin

The properties listed below are those particular to the combination only. For the properties of the components please consider, prilocaine hydrochloride p. 783.

● INDICATIONS AND DOSE
Dental anaesthesia
▸ BY REGIONAL ADMINISTRATION
‣ Child: Consult expert dental sources for specific advice

● MEDICINAL FORMS
There can be variation in the licensing of different medicines containing the same drug.
Solution for injection
‣ Citanest with Octapressin (Dentsply Ltd)
Felypressin .03 unit per 1 ml, Prilocaine hydrochloride 30 mg per 1 ml Citanest 3% with Octapressin Dental 0.054units/1.8ml solution for injection self aspirating cartridges | 100 cartridge [PoM] no price available
Citanest 3% with Octapressin Dental 0.066units/2.2ml solution for injection self aspirating cartridges | 100 cartridge [PoM] no price available

Ropivacaine hydrochloride

● INDICATIONS AND DOSE
Acute pain | Surgical anaesthesia
▸ BY REGIONAL ADMINISTRATION
‣ Child: Adjust according to child's physical status and nature of procedure, seek expert advice
DOSES AT EXTREMES OF BODY-WEIGHT
To avoid excessive dosage in obese patients, dose may need to be calculated on the basis of ideal bodyweight.

● UNLICENSED USE 2 mg/mL strength not licensed for use in children under 12 years except for acute pain management by caudal epidural block and continuous epidural infusion; 7.5 mg/mL and 10 mg/mL strengths not licensed for use in children under 12 years.

IMPORTANT SAFETY INFORMATION
Should only be administered by, or under the direct supervision of, personnel experienced in their use, with adequate training in anaesthesia and airway management, and should not be administered parenterally unless adequate resuscitation equipment is available.

● CONTRA-INDICATIONS Application to the middle ear (can cause ototoxicity) · avoid injection into infected tissues · avoid injection into inflamed tissues · complete heart block · preparations containing preservatives should not be used for caudal, epidural, or spinal block, or for intravenous regional anaesthesia (Bier's block) · should not be applied to damaged skin
CONTRA-INDICATIONS, FURTHER INFORMATION
‣ Injection site Local anaesthetics should not be injected into inflamed or infected tissues nor should they be applied to damaged skin. Increased absorption into the blood increases the possibility of systemic side-effects, and the local anaesthetic effect may also be reduced by altered local pH.

● CAUTIONS Acute porphyrias p. 562 · cardiovascular disease · children (consider dose reduction) · debilitated patients (consider dose reduction) · epilepsy · hypovolaemia · impaired cardiac conduction · impaired respiratory function · myasthenia gravis · shock

● INTERACTIONS → Appendix 1 (ropivacaine).

● SIDE-EFFECTS
▸ **Common or very common** Hypertension · pyrexia
▸ **Uncommon** Hypothermia · syncope
▸ **Frequency not known** Arrhythmias · blurred vision · cardiac arrest · convulsions · dizziness · drowsiness · feeling of inebriation · headache · lightheadedness · muscle twitching · myocardial depression (resulting in hypotension and bradycardia) · nausea · numbness of the tongue and perioral region · paraesthesia (including sensations of hot and cold) · peripheral vasodilatation (resulting in hypotension and bradycardia) · restlessness · tinnitus · transient excitation (followed by depression with drowsiness, respiratory failure, unconsciousness, and coma) · tremors · vomiting
SIDE-EFFECTS, FURTHER INFORMATION
‣ Toxic effects Toxic effects after administration of local anaesthetics are a result of excessively high plasma concentrations; severe toxicity usually results from inadvertent intravascular injection or too rapid injection.

Following most regional anaesthetic procedures, maximum arterial plasma concentration of anaesthetic develops within about 10 to 25 minutes, so careful surveillance for toxic effects is necessary during the first 30 minutes after injection.

The systemic toxicity of local anaesthetics mainly involves the central nervous and cardiovascular systems.

- **ALLERGY AND CROSS-SENSITIVITY**
▸ Hypersensitivity and cross-sensitivity Hypersensitivity reactions occur mainly with the ester-type local anaesthetics, such as tetracaine and chloroprocaine; reactions are less frequent with the amide types, such as articaine, bupivacaine, levobupivacaine, lidocaine, mepivacaine, prilocaine, and ropivacaine. Cross-sensitivity reactions may be avoided by using the alternative chemical type.

- **PREGNANCY** Not known to be harmful. Do not use for paracervical block in obstetrics.

- **BREAST FEEDING** Not known to be harmful.

- **HEPATIC IMPAIRMENT** Use with caution in severe impairment.

- **RENAL IMPAIRMENT** Caution in severe impairment. Increased risk of systemic toxicity in chronic renal failure.

- **MEDICINAL FORMS**
There can be variation in the licensing of different medicines containing the same drug.

Solution for injection
ELECTROLYTES: May contain Sodium
▸ **Ropivacaine hydrochloride (Non-proprietary)**
   Ropivacaine hydrochloride 2 mg per 1 ml Ropivacaine 20mg/10ml solution for injection ampoules | 10 ampoule [PoM] £16.50 (Hospital only)
   Ropivacaine hydrochloride 7.5 mg per 1 ml Ropivacaine 75mg/10ml solution for injection ampoules | 10 ampoule [PoM] £25.00 (Hospital only)
   Ropivacaine hydrochloride 10 mg per 1 ml Ropivacaine 100mg/10ml solution for injection ampoules | 10 ampoule [PoM] £30.00 (Hospital only)
▸ **Naropin (AstraZeneca UK Ltd)**
   Ropivacaine hydrochloride 2 mg per 1 ml Naropin 20mg/10ml solution for injection ampoules | 5 ampoule [PoM] £12.79
   Ropivacaine hydrochloride 7.5 mg per 1 ml Naropin 75mg/10ml solution for injection ampoules | 5 ampoule [PoM] £15.90
   Ropivacaine hydrochloride 10 mg per 1 ml Naropin 100mg/10ml solution for injection ampoules | 5 ampoule [PoM] £19.22

Infusion
ELECTROLYTES: May contain Sodium
▸ **Ropivacaine hydrochloride (Non-proprietary)**
   Ropivacaine hydrochloride 2 mg per 1 ml Ropivacaine 400mg/200ml infusion bags | 5 bag [PoM] £72.25 | 10 bag [PoM] £137.00 (Hospital only)
▸ **Naropin (AstraZeneca UK Ltd)**
   Ropivacaine hydrochloride 2 mg per 1 ml Naropin 400mg/200ml infusion Polybags | 5 bag [PoM] £86.70

Tetracaine

(Amethocaine)

- **INDICATIONS AND DOSE**

Anaesthesia before venepuncture or venous cannulation
▸ TO THE SKIN

▸ **Neonate:** Apply contents of tube (or appropriate proportion) to site of venepuncture or venous cannulation and cover with occlusive dressing; remove gel and dressing after 30 minutes for venepuncture and after 45 minutes for venous cannulation.

▸ **Child 1 month–4 years:** Apply contents of up to 1 tube (applied at separate sites at a single time or appropriate proportion) to site of venepuncture or venous cannulation and cover with occlusive dressing; remove gel and dressing after 30 minutes for venepuncture and after 45 minutes for venous cannulation

▸ **Child 5–17 years:** Apply contents of up to 5 tubes (applied at separate sites at a single time or appropriate proportion) to site of venepuncture or venous cannulation and cover with occlusive dressing; remove gel and dressing after 30 minutes for venepuncture and after 45 minutes for venous cannulation

- **UNLICENSED USE** Not licensed for use in neonates.

- **CONTRA-INDICATIONS** Should not be applied to damaged skin

- **SIDE-EFFECTS** Local skin reactions
SIDE-EFFECTS, FURTHER INFORMATION
The systemic toxicity of local anaesthetics mainly involves the central nervous and cardiovascular systems; systemic side effects unlikely as minimal absorption following topical application.

- **ALLERGY AND CROSS-SENSITIVITY**
▸ Hypersensitivity and cross-sensitivity Hypersensitivity reactions occur mainly with the ester-type local anaesthetics, such as tetracaine and chloroprocaine; reactions are less frequent with the amide types, such as articaine, bupivacaine, levobupivacaine, lidocaine, mepivacaine, prilocaine, and ropivacaine. Cross-sensitivity reactions may be avoided by using the alternative chemical type.

- **BREAST FEEDING** Not known to be harmful.

- **PATIENT AND CARER ADVICE**
Medicines for Children leaflet: Tetracaine gel for local anaesthesia www.medicinesforchildren.org.uk/tetracaine-gel-for-local-anaesthesia

- **MEDICINAL FORMS**
There can be variation in the licensing of different medicines containing the same drug.

Gel
EXCIPIENTS: May contain Hydroxybenzoates (parabens)
▸ **Ametop (Smith & Nephew Healthcare Ltd)**
   Tetracaine 40 mg per 1 gram Ametop 4% gel | 1.5 gram [P] £1.08 | 18 gram [P] no price available

Chapter 16
Emergency treatment of poisoning

CONTENTS

1	**Active elimination from the gastro-intestinal tract**	page 793
2	**Chemical toxicity**	793
2.1	Cyanide toxicity	793
2.2	Organophosphorus toxicity	794
3	**Drug toxicity**	794
3.1	Benzodiazepine toxicity	794

3.2	Digoxin toxicity	page 795
3.3	Heparin toxicity	795
3.4	Opioid toxicity	796
3.5	Paracetamol toxicity	797
4	**Methaemoglobinaemia**	798
5	**Snake bites**	798

Emergency treatment of poisoning

Overview

These notes provide only an overview of the treatment of poisoning, and it is strongly recommended that either **TOXBASE** or the **UK National Poisons Information Service** be consulted when there is doubt about the degree of risk or about management.

Most childhood poisoning is accidental. Other causes include intentional overdose, drug abuse, iatrogenic and deliberate poisoning. The drugs most commonly involved in childhood poisoning are paracetamol p. 254, ibuprofen p. 608, orally ingested creams, aspirin p. 83, iron preparations, cough medicines, and the contraceptive pill.

Hospital admission

Children who have features of poisoning should generally be admitted to hospital. Children who have taken poisons with delayed actions should also be admitted, even if they appear well. Delayed-action poisons include aspirin, iron, paracetamol, tricyclic antidepressants, and co-phenotrope (diphenoxylate with atropine, *Lomotil*®) p. 44; the effects of modified-release preparations are also delayed. A note of all relevant information, including what treatment has been given, should accompany the patient to hospital.

Further information

TOXBASE, the primary clinical toxicology database of the National Poisons Information Service, is available on the internet to registered users at www.toxbase.org (a backup site is available at www.toxbasebackup.org if the main site cannot be accessed). It provides information about routine diagnosis, treatment, and management of patients exposed to drugs, household products, and industrial and agricultural chemicals.

Specialist information and advice on the treatment of poisoning is available day and night from the **UK National Poisons Information Service** on the following number: Tel: 0344 892 0111.

Advice on laboratory analytical services can be obtained from TOXBASE or from the National Poisons Information Service. Help with identifying capsules or tablets may be available from a regional medicines information centre or from the National Poisons Information Service (out of hours).

General care

It is often impossible to establish with certainty the identity of the poison and the size of the dose. This is not usually important because only a few poisons (such as opioids, paracetamol, and iron) have specific antidotes; few patients require active removal of the poison. In most patients, treatment is directed at managing symptoms as they arise. Nevertheless, knowledge of the type and timing of poisoning can help in anticipating the course of events. All relevant information should be sought from the poisoned individual and from carers or parents. However, such information should be interpreted with care because it may not be complete or entirely reliable. Sometimes symptoms arise from other illnesses and patients should be assessed carefully. Accidents may involve domestic and industrial products (the contents of which are not generally known). The **National Poisons Information Service** should be consulted when there is doubt about any aspect of suspected poisoning.

Respiration

Respiration is often impaired in unconscious patients. An obstructed airway requires immediate attention. In the absence of trauma, the airway should be opened with simple measures such as chin lift or jaw thrust. An oropharyngeal or nasopharyngeal airway may be useful in patients with reduced consciousness to prevent obstruction, provided ventilation is adequate. Intubation and ventilation should be considered in patients whose airway cannot be protected or who have respiratory acidosis because of inadequate ventilation; such patients should be monitored in a critical care area.

Most poisons that impair consciousness also depress respiration. Assisted ventilation (either mouth-to-mouth or using a bag-valve-mask device) may be needed. Oxygen is not a substitute for adequate ventilation, although it should be given in the highest concentration possible in poisoning with carbon monoxide and irritant gases.

The potential for pulmonary aspiration of gastric contents should be considered.

Blood pressure

Hypotension is common in severe poisoning with central nervous system depressants; if severe, this may lead to irreversible brain damage or renal tubular necrosis. Hypotension should be corrected initially by raising the foot of the bed and administration of an infusion of either sodium chloride p. 547 or a colloid. Vasoconstrictor sympathomimetics are rarely required and their use may be discussed with the National Poisons Information Service or a paediatric intensive care unit.

Fluid depletion without hypotension is common after prolonged coma and after aspirin poisoning due to vomiting, sweating, and hyperpnoea.

Hypertension, often transient, occurs less frequently than hypotension in poisoning; it may be associated with sympathomimetic drugs such as amfetamines, phencyclidine, and cocaine.

Heart

Cardiac conduction defects and arrhythmias can occur in acute poisoning, notably with tricyclic antidepressants, some antipsychotics, and some antihistamines. Arrhythmias often respond to correction of underlying hypoxia, acidosis, or other biochemical abnormalities, but ventricular arrhythmias that cause serious hypotension require treatment. If the QT interval is prolonged, specialist advice should be sought because the use of some anti-arrhythmic drugs may be inappropriate. Supraventricular arrhythmias are seldom life-threatening and drug treatment is best withheld until the patient reaches hospital.

Body temperature

Hypothermia may develop in patients of any age who have been deeply unconscious for some hours, particularly following overdose with barbiturates or phenothiazines. It may be missed unless core temperature is measured using a low-reading rectal thermometer or by some other means. Hypothermia should be managed by prevention of further heat loss and appropriate rewarming as clinically indicated.

Hyperthermia can develop in patients taking CNS stimulants; children are also at risk when taking therapeutic doses of drugs with antimuscarinic properties. Hyperthermia is initially managed by removing all unnecessary clothing and using a fan. Sponging with **tepid** water will promote evaporation. Advice should be sought from the National Poisons Information Service on the management of severe hyperthermia resulting from conditions such as the serotonin syndrome.

Both hypothermia and hyperthermia require **urgent** hospitalisation for assessment and supportive treatment.

Convulsions

Single short-lived convulsions (lasting less than 5 minutes) do not require treatment. If convulsions are protracted or recur frequently, lorazepam p. 209 or diazepam p. 207 (preferably as emulsion) should be given by slow intravenous injection into a large vein. Benzodiazepines should not be given by the intramuscular route for convulsions. If the intravenous route is not readily available, midazolam oromucosal solution p. 210 can be given by the buccal route or diazepam can be administered as a rectal solution.

Methaemoglobinaemia

Drug- or chemical-induced methaemoglobinaemia should be treated with **methylthioninium chloride** p. 798 if the methaemoglobin concentration is 30% or higher, or if symptoms of tissue hypoxia are present despite oxygen therapy. Methylthioninium chloride p. 798 reduces the ferric iron of methaemoglobin back to the ferrous iron of haemoglobin; in high doses, methylthioninium chloride can itself cause methaemoglobinaemia.

Removal and elimination

Prevention of absorption

Given by mouth, **charcoal, activated** p. 793 can adsorb many poisons in the gastro-intestinal system, thereby reducing their absorption. The **sooner** it is given the **more effective** it is, but it may still be effective up to 1 hour after ingestion of the poison—longer in the case of modified-release preparations or of drugs with antimuscarinic (anticholinergic) properties. It is particularly useful for the prevention of absorption of poisons that are toxic in small amounts, such as antidepressants.

A second dose may occasionally be required when blood-drug concentration continues to rise suggesting delayed drug release or delayed gastric emptying.

Active elimination techniques

Repeated doses of **charcoal, activated** by mouth may *enhance the elimination* of some drugs after they have been absorbed; repeated doses are given after overdosage with:

- Carbamazepine
- Dapsone
- Phenobarbital
- Quinine
- Theophylline

If vomiting occurs after dosing, it should be treated (e.g. with an antiemetic drug) since it may reduce the efficacy of charcoal treatment. In cases of intolerance, the dose may be reduced and the frequency increased but this may compromise efficacy.

Charcoal, activated should **not** be used for poisoning with petroleum distillates, corrosive substances, alcohols, malathion, cyanides and metal salts including iron and lithium salts.

Other techniques intended to enhance the elimination of poisons after absorption are only practicable in hospital and are only suitable for a small number of severely poisoned patients. Moreover, they only apply to a limited number of poisons. Examples include:

- haemodialysis for ethylene glycol, lithium, methanol, phenobarbital, salicylates, and sodium valproate;
- alkalinisation of the urine for salicylates.

Removal from the gastro-intestinal tract

Gastric lavage is rarely required as benefit rarely outweighs risk; advice should be sought from the National Poisons Information Service if a significant quantity of iron or lithium has been ingested within the previous hour.

Whole bowel irrigation (by means of a bowel cleansing preparation) has been used in poisoning with certain modified-release or enteric-coated formulations, in severe poisoning with lithium salts, and if illicit drugs are carried in the gastro-intestinal tract ('body-packing'). However, it is not clear that the procedure improves outcome and advice should be sought from the National Poisons Information Service.

The administration of **laxatives** alone has no role in the management of the poisoned child and is not a recommended method of gut decontamination. The routine use of a laxative in combination with charcoal, activated has mostly been abandoned. Laxatives should not be administered to young children because of the likelihood of fluid and electrolyte imbalance.

Alcohol

Acute intoxication with **alcohol** (ethanol) is common in adults but also occurs in children. The features include ataxia, dysarthria, nystagmus, and drowsiness, which may progress to coma, with hypotension and acidosis. Aspiration of vomit is a special hazard and hypoglycaemia may occur. Patients are managed supportively, with particular attention to maintaining a clear airway and measures to reduce the risk of aspiration of gastric contents. The blood glucose is measured and glucose given if indicated.

Aspirin

The main features of salicylate poisoning are hyperventilation, tinnitus, deafness, vasodilatation, and sweating. Coma is uncommon but indicates very severe poisoning. The associated acid-base disturbances are complex.

Treatment must be in hospital, where plasma salicylate, pH, and electrolytes can be measured; absorption of aspirin may be slow and the plasma-salicylate concentration may continue to rise for several hours, requiring repeated measurement. Plasma-salicylate concentration may not correlate with clinical severity in the young, and clinical and biochemical assessment is necessary. Generally, the clinical

16

Emergency treatment of poisoning

severity of poisoning is less below a plasma-salicylate concentration of 500 mg/litre (3.6 mmol/litre), unless there is evidence of metabolic acidosis. Activated charcoal can be given within 1 hour of ingesting more than 125 mg/kg of aspirin. Fluid losses should be replaced and intravenous sodium bicarbonate may be given (ensuring plasma-potassium concentration is within the reference range) to enhance urinary salicylate excretion (optimum urinary pH 7.5–8.5).

Plasma-potassium concentration should be corrected before giving sodium bicarbonate as hypokalaemia may complicate alkalinisation of the urine.

Haemodialysis is the treatment of choice for severe salicylate poisoning and should be considered when the plasma-salicylate concentration exceeds 700 mg/litre (5.1 mmol/litre) or in the presence of severe metabolic acidosis, convulsions, respiratory failure, pulmonary oedema or persistently high plasma-salicylate concentrations unresponsive to urinary alkalinisation.

Opioids

Opioids (narcotic analgesics) cause varying degrees of coma, respiratory depression, and pinpoint pupils. The specific antidote naloxone hydrochloride p. 796 is indicated if there is coma or bradypnoea. Since naloxone has a shorter duration of action than many opioids, close monitoring and repeated injections are necessary according to the respiratory rate and depth of coma. When repeated administration of naloxone is required, it can be given by continuous intravenous infusion instead and the rate of infusion adjusted according to vital signs. All children should be observed for at least 6 hours after the last dose of naloxone. The effects of some opioids, such as buprenorphine, are only partially reversed by naloxone. Dextropropoxyphene and methadone have very long durations of action; patients may need to be monitored for long periods following large overdoses.

Naloxone reverses the opioid effects of dextropropoxyphene. The long duration of action of dextropropoxyphene calls for prolonged monitoring and further doses of naloxone may be required. Norpropoxyphene, a metabolite of dextropropoxyphene, also has cardiotoxic effects which may require treatment with sodium bicarbonate p. 544 or magnesium sulfate p. 556, or both. Arrhythmias may occur for up to 12 hours.

Paracetamol

In cases of **intravenous** paracetamol poisoning contact the National Poisons Information Service for advice on risk assessment and management.

Toxic doses of paracetamol may cause severe hepatocellular necrosis and, much less frequently, renal tubular necrosis. Nausea and vomiting, the only early features of poisoning, usually settle within 24 hours. Persistence beyond this time, often associated with the onset of right subcostal pain and tenderness, usually indicates development of hepatic necrosis. Liver damage is maximal 3–4 days after paracetamol overdose and may lead to encephalopathy, haemorrhage, hypoglycaemia, cerebral oedema, and death. Therefore, despite a lack of significant early symptoms, children who have taken an overdose of paracetamol should be transferred to hospital urgently.

To avoid underestimating the potentially toxic paracetamol dose ingested by obese children who weigh more than 110 kg, use a body-weight of 110 kg (rather than their actual body-weight) when calculating the total dose of paracetamol ingested (in mg/kg).

Acetylcysteine p. 797 protects the liver if infused up to, and possibly beyond, 24 hours of ingesting paracetamol. It is most effective if given within 8 hours of ingestion, after which effectiveness declines. Very rarely, giving acetylcysteine by mouth [unlicensed route] is an alternative

if intravenous access is not possible—contact the National Poisons Information Service for advice.

Neonates less than 45 weeks corrected gestational age may be more susceptible to paracetamol-induced liver toxicity, therefore, treatment with acetylcysteine should be considered in all paracetamol overdoses, and advice should be sought from the National Poisons Information Service.

Acute overdose

Hepatotoxicity may occur after a single ingestion of more than 150 mg/kg paracetamol taken in less than 1 hour. Rarely, hepatotoxicity may develop with single ingestions as low as 75 mg/kg of paracetamol taken in less than 1 hour.

Children who have ingested 75 mg/kg or more of paracetamol in less than 1 hour should be referred to hospital. Administration of charcoal, activated p. 793 should be considered if paracetamol in excess of 150 mg/kg is thought to have been ingested within the previous hour.

Children at risk of liver damage and, therefore, requiring acetylcysteine, can be identified from a single measurement of the plasma-paracetamol concentration, related to the time from ingestion, provided this time interval is not less than 4 hours; earlier samples may be misleading. The concentration is plotted on a paracetamol treatment graph, with a reference line ('treatment line') joining plots of 100 mg/litre (0.66 mmol/litre) at 4 hours and 3.13 mg/litre (0.02 mmol/litre) at 24 hours. Acetylcysteine treatment should commence immediately in children:

- whose plasma-paracetamol concentration falls on or above the *treatment line* on the paracetamol treatment graph;
- who present 8–24 hours after taking an acute overdose of more than 150 mg/kg of paracetamol, even if the plasma-paracetamol concentration is not yet available; acetylcysteine can be discontinued if the plasma-paracetamol concentration is later reported to be below the *treatment line* on the paracetamol treatment graph, provided that the child is asymptomatic and liver function tests, serum creatinine and INR are normal.

The prognostic accuracy of a plasma-paracetamol concentration taken after 15 hours is uncertain, but a concentration on or above the *treatment line* on the paracetamol treatment graph should be regarded as carrying a serious risk of liver damage. If more than 15 hours have elapsed since ingestion, or there is doubt about appropriate management, advice should be sought from the National Poisons Information Service.

'Staggered' overdose, uncertain time of overdose, or therapeutic excess

A 'staggered' overdose involves ingestion of a potentially toxic dose of paracetamol over more than one hour, with the possible intention of causing self-harm. Therapeutic excess is the inadvertent ingestion of a potentially toxic dose of paracetamol during its clinical use. The paracetamol treatment graph is unreliable if a 'staggered' overdose is taken, if there is uncertainty about the time of the overdose, or if there is therapeutic excess. In these cases, children who have taken more than 150 mg/kg of paracetamol in any 24-hour period are at risk of toxicity and should be commenced on acetylcysteine immediately, unless it is more than 24 hours since the last ingestion, the patient is asymptomatic, the plasma-paracetamol concentration is undetectable, and liver function tests, serum creatinine and INR are normal.

Rarely, toxicity can occur with paracetamol doses between 75–150 mg/kg in any 24-hour period; for some children this may be within the licensed dose, but ingestion of a licensed dose of paracetamol is not considered an overdose. Clinical judgement of the individual case is necessary to determine whether to treat those who have ingested this amount of paracetamol.

Paracetamol overdose treatment graph

Patients whose plasma-paracetamol concentrations are on or above the **treatment line** should be treated with acetylcysteine by intravenous infusion.

The prognostic accuracy after 15 hours is uncertain, but a plasma-paracetamol concentration on or above the treatment line should be regarded as carrying a serious risk of liver damage.

Graph reproduced courtesy of Medicines and Healthcare products Regulatory Agency

Although there is some evidence suggesting that factors such as the use of liver enzyme-inducing drugs (e.g. carbamazepine p. 184, efavirenz p. 388, nevirapine p. 389, phenobarbital p. 203, phenytoin p. 193, primidone p. 204, rifabutin p. 341, rifampicin p. 342, St John's wort), chronic alcoholism, and starvation may increase the risk of hepatotoxicity, the CHM has advised that these should no longer be used in the assessment of paracetamol toxicity.

Significant toxicity is unlikely if, 24 hours or longer after the last paracetamol ingestion, the patient is asymptomatic, the plasma-paracetamol concentration is undetectable, and liver function tests, serum creatinine and INR are normal. Children with clinical features of hepatic injury such as jaundice or hepatic tenderness should be treated urgently with acetylcysteine. If there is uncertainty about a patient's risk of toxicity after paracetamol overdose, treatment with acetylcysteine should be commenced. Advice should be sought from the National Poisons Information Service whenever necessary.

Antidepressants

Tricyclic and related antidepressants

Tricyclic and related antidepressants cause dry mouth, coma of varying degree, hypotension, hypothermia, hyperreflexia, extensor plantar responses, convulsions, respiratory failure, cardiac conduction defects, and arrhythmias. Dilated pupils and urinary retention also occur. Metabolic acidosis may complicate severe poisoning; delirium with confusion, agitation, and visual and auditory hallucinations are common during recovery.

Assessment in hospital is strongly advised in case of poisoning by tricyclic and related antidepressants but symptomatic treatment can be given before transfer. Supportive measures to ensure a clear airway and adequate ventilation during transfer are mandatory. Intravenous lorazepam or intravenous diazepam (preferably in emulsion form) may be required to treat convulsions. Activated charcoal given within 1 hour of the overdose reduces absorption of the drug. Although arrhythmias are worrying, some will respond to correction of hypoxia and acidosis. The use of anti-arrhythmic drugs is best avoided, but intravenous infusion of sodium bicarbonate can arrest arrhythmias or prevent them in those with an extended QRS duration. Diazepam p. 207 given by mouth is usually adequate to sedate delirious patients but large doses may be required.

Selective serotonin re-uptake inhibitors (SSRIs)

Symptoms of poisoning by selective serotonin re-uptake inhibitors include nausea, vomiting, agitation, tremor, nystagmus, drowsiness, and sinus tachycardia; convulsions may occur. Rarely, severe poisoning results in the serotonin syndrome, with marked neuropsychiatric effects, neuromuscular hyperactivity, and autonomic instability; hyperthermia, rhabdomyolysis, renal failure, and coagulopathies may develop.

Management of SSRI poisoning is supportive. Activated charcoal given within 1 hour of the overdose reduces absorption of the drug. Convulsions can be treated with lorazepam p. 209, diazepam p. 207, or buccal midazolam p. 210 (see *Convulsions*). Contact the National Poisons Information Service for the management of hyperthermia or the serotonin syndrome.

Antimalarials

Overdosage with quinine, chloroquine, or hydroxychloroquine is extremely hazardous and difficult to treat. Urgent advice from the National Poisons Information Service is essential. Life-threatening features include arrhythmias (which can have a very rapid onset) and convulsions (which can be intractable).

Antipsychotics

Phenothiazines and related drugs

Phenothiazines cause less depression of consciousness and respiration than other sedatives. Hypotension, hypothermia, sinus tachycardia, and arrhythmias may complicate poisoning. Dystonic reactions can occur with therapeutic doses (particularly with prochlorperazine and trifluoperazine), and convulsions may occur in severe cases. Arrhythmias may respond to correction of hypoxia, acidosis, and other biochemical abnormalities, but specialist advice should be sought if arrhythmias result from a prolonged QT interval; the use of some anti-arrhythmic drugs can worsen such arrhythmias. Dystonic reactions are rapidly abolished by injection of drugs such as procyclidine hydrochloride p. 241 or diazepam (emulsion preferred).

Second-generation antipsychotic drugs

Features of poisoning by second-generation antipsychotic drugs include drowsiness, convulsions, extrapyramidal symptoms, hypotension, and ECG abnormalities (including prolongation of the QT interval). Management is supportive. Charcoal, activated p. 793 can be given within 1 hour of ingesting a significant quantity of a second-generation antipsychotic drug.

Benzodiazepines

Benzodiazepines taken alone cause drowsiness, ataxia, dysarthria, nystagmus, and occasionally respiratory depression, and coma. Charcoal, activated can be given within 1 hour of ingesting a significant quantity of benzodiazepine, provided the patient is awake and the airway is protected. Benzodiazepines potentiate the effects of other central nervous system depressants taken concomitantly. Use of the benzodiazepine antagonist flumazenil p. 794 [unlicensed indication] can be hazardous, particularly in mixed overdoses involving tricyclic antidepressants or in benzodiazepine-dependent patients. Flumazenil may prevent the need for ventilation, particularly in patients with severe respiratory disorders; it should be used on expert advice only and not as a diagnostic test in children with a reduced level of consciousness.

Beta blockers

Therapeutic overdosages with beta-blockers may cause lightheadedness, dizziness, and possibly syncope as a result of bradycardia and hypotension; heart failure may be precipitated or exacerbated. These complications are most likely in children with conduction system disorders or impaired myocardial function. Bradycardia is the most common arrhythmia caused by beta-blockers, but sotalol may induce ventricular tachyarrhythmias (sometimes of the torsade de pointes type). The effects of massive overdosage can vary from one beta-blocker to another; propranolol overdosage in particular may cause coma and convulsions.

Acute massive overdosage must be managed in hospital and expert advice should be obtained. Maintenance of a clear airway and adequate ventilation is mandatory. An intravenous injection of atropine sulfate p. 764 is required to treat bradycardia. Cardiogenic shock unresponsive to atropine sulfate is probably best treated with an intravenous injection of glucagon p. 433 [unlicensed] in glucose 5% (with precautions to protect the airway in case of vomiting) followed by an intravenous infusion. If glucagon is not available, intravenous isoprenaline (available from 'special-

order' manufacturers or specialist importing companies) is an alternative. A cardiac pacemaker can be used to increase the heart rate.

Calcium-channel blockers

Features of calcium-channel blocker poisoning include nausea, vomiting, dizziness, agitation, confusion, and coma in severe poisoning. Metabolic acidosis and hyperglycaemia may occur. Verapamil and diltiazem have a profound cardiac depressant effect causing hypotension and arrhythmias, including complete heart block and asystole. The dihydropyridine calcium-channel blockers cause severe hypotension secondary to profound peripheral vasodilatation.

Charcoal, activated should be considered if the patient presents within 1 hour of overdosage with a calcium-channel blocker; repeated doses of activated charcoal are considered if a modified-release preparation is involved. In patients with significant features of poisoning, calcium chloride p. 553 or calcium gluconate p. 553 is given by injection; atropine sulfate is given to correct symptomatic bradycardia. In severe cases, an insulin and glucose infusion may be required in the management of hypotension and myocardial failure. For the management of hypotension, the choice of inotropic sympathomimetic depends on whether hypotension is secondary to vasodilatation or to myocardial depression—advice should be sought from the National Poisons Information Service.

Iron salts

Iron poisoning in childhood is usually accidental. The symptoms are nausea, vomiting, abdominal pain, diarrhoea, haematemesis, and rectal bleeding. Hypotension and hepatocellular necrosis can occur later. Coma, shock, and metabolic acidosis indicate severe poisoning.

Advice should be sought from the National Poisons Information Service if a significant quantity of iron has been ingested within the previous hour.

Mortality is reduced by intensive and specific therapy with desferrioxamine mesilate p. 536, which chelates iron. The serum-iron concentration is measured as an emergency and intravenous desferrioxamine mesilate given to chelate absorbed iron in excess of the expected iron binding capacity. In severe toxicity intravenous desferrioxamine mesilate should be given immediately without waiting for the result of the serum-iron measurement.

Lithium

Most cases of lithium intoxication occur as a complication of long-term therapy and are caused by reduced excretion of the drug because of a variety of factors including dehydration, deterioration of renal function, infections, and co-administration of diuretics or NSAIDs (or other drugs that interact). Acute deliberate overdoses may also occur with delayed onset of symptoms (12 hours or more) owing to slow entry of lithium into the tissues and continuing absorption from modified-release formulations.

The early clinical features are non-specific and may include apathy and restlessness which could be confused with mental changes arising from the child's depressive illness. Vomiting, diarrhoea, ataxia, weakness, dysarthria, muscle twitching, and tremor may follow. Severe poisoning is associated with convulsions, coma, renal failure, electrolyte imbalance, dehydration, and hypotension.

Therapeutic serum-lithium concentrations are within the range of 0.4–1 mmol/litre; concentrations in excess of 2 mmol/litre are usually associated with serious toxicity and such cases may need treatment with haemodialysis if neurological symptoms or renal failure are present. In acute overdosage much higher serum-lithium concentrations may be present without features of toxicity and all that is usually necessary is to take measures to increase urine output (e.g. by increasing fluid intake but avoiding diuretics). Otherwise, treatment is supportive with special regard to electrolyte balance, renal function, and control of convulsions. Whole-bowel irrigation should be considered for significant ingestion, but advice should be sought from the National Poisons Information Service.

Stimulants

Amfetamines

Amfetamines cause wakefulness, excessive activity, paranoia, hallucinations, and hypertension followed by exhaustion, convulsions, hyperthermia, and coma. The early stages can be controlled by diazepam p. 207 or lorazepam p. 209; advice should be sought from the National Poisons Information Service on the management of hypertension. Later, tepid sponging, anticonvulsants, and artificial respiration may be needed.

Cocaine

Cocaine stimulates the central nervous system, causing agitation, dilated pupils, tachycardia, hypertension, hallucinations, hyperthermia, hypertonia, and hyperreflexia; cardiac effects include chest pain, myocardial infarction, and arrhythmias.

Initial treatment of cocaine poisoning involves cooling measures for hyperthermia (*see Body temperature*); agitation, hypertension and cardiac effects require specific treatment and expert advice should be sought.

Ecstasy

Ecstasy (methylenedioxymethamfetamine, MDMA) may cause severe reactions, even at doses that were previously tolerated. The most serious effects are delirium, coma, convulsions, ventricular arrhythmias, hyperthermia, rhabdomyolysis, acute renal failure, acute hepatitis, disseminated intravascular coagulation, adult respiratory distress syndrome, hyperreflexia, hypotension and intracerebral haemorrhage; hyponatraemia has also been associated with ecstasy use and syndrome of inappropriate antidiuretic hormone secretion (SIADH) can occur.

Treatment of methylenedioxymethamfetamine poisoning is supportive, with diazepam to control persistent convulsions and close monitoring including ECG. For the management of agitation, seek specialist advice. Self-induced water intoxication should be considered in patients with ecstasy poisoning.

'Liquid ecstasy' is a term used for sodium oxybate (gamma-hydroxybutyrate, GHB), which is a sedative.

Theophylline

Theophylline and related drugs are often prescribed as modified-release formulations and toxicity can therefore be delayed. They cause vomiting (which may be severe and intractable), agitation, restlessness, dilated pupils, sinus tachycardia, and hyperglycaemia. More serious effects are haematemesis, convulsions, and supraventricular and ventricular arrhythmias. Severe hypokalaemia may develop rapidly.

Repeated doses of charcoal, activated p. 793 can be used to eliminate theophylline even if more than 1 hour has elapsed after ingestion and especially if a modified-release preparation has been taken (see also under Active Elimination Techniques). Ondansetron p. 248 may be effective for severe vomiting that is resistant to other antiemetics. Hypokalaemia is corrected by intravenous infusion of potassium chloride p. 561 and may be so severe as to require high doses under ECG monitoring. Convulsions should be controlled by intravenous administration of lorazepam or diazepam (see Convulsions). For the management of agitation associated with theophylline overdosage, seek specialist advice.

Provided the child does **not** suffer from asthma, a short-acting beta-blocker can be administered intravenously to reverse severe tachycardia, hypokalaemia, and hyperglycaemia.

Other poisons

Consult either the National Poisons Information Service day and night or TOXBASE, see under the National Poisons Information Service.

Cyanides

Oxygen should be administered to children with cyanide poisoning. The choice of antidote depends on the severity of poisoning, certainty of diagnosis, and the cause. Dicobalt edetate p. 793 is the antidote of choice when there is a strong clinical suspicion of severe cyanide poisoning, but it should **not** be used as a precautionary measure. Dicobalt edetate itself is toxic, associated with anaphylactoid reactions, and is potentially fatal if administered in the absence of cyanide poisoning. A regimen of sodium nitrite p. 793 followed by sodium thiosulfate p. 793 is an alternative if dicobalt edetate is not available.

Hydroxocobalamin p. 534 (*Cyanokit*®—no other preparation of hydroxocobalamin is suitable) can be considered for use in victims of smoke inhalation who show signs of significant cyanide poisoning.

Ethylene glycol and methanol

Fomepizole (available from 'special-order' manufacturers or specialist importing companies) is the treatment of choice for ethylene glycol and methanol (methyl alcohol) poisoning. If necessary, **ethanol** (by mouth or by intravenous infusion) can be used, but with caution. Advice on the treatment of ethylene glycol and methanol poisoning should be obtained from the National Poisons Information Service. It is important to start antidote treatment promptly in cases of suspected poisoning with these agents.

Heavy metals

Heavy metal antidotes include succimer (DMSA) [unlicensed], unithiol (DMPS) [unlicensed], sodium calcium edetate [unlicensed], and dimercaprol. Dimercaprol in the management of heavy metal poisoning has been superseded by other chelating agents. In all cases of heavy metal poisoning, the advice of the National Poisons Information Service should be sought.

Noxious gases

Carbon monoxide

Carbon monoxide poisoning is usually due to inhalation of smoke, car exhaust, or fumes caused by blocked flues or incomplete combustion of fuel gases in confined spaces.

Immediate treatment of carbon monoxide poisoning is essential. The patient should be moved to fresh air, the airway cleared, and high-flow **oxygen** 100% administered as soon as available. Artificial respiration should be given as necessary and continued until adequate spontaneous breathing starts, or stopped only after persistent and efficient treatment of cardiac arrest has failed. The child should be admitted to hospital because complications may arise after a delay of hours or days. Cerebral oedema may occur in severe poisoning and is treated with an intravenous infusion of mannitol p. 133. Referral for hyperbaric oxygen treatment should be discussed with the National Poisons Information Service if the patient is pregnant or in cases of severe poisoning such as if the patient is or has been unconscious, or has psychiatric or neurological features other than a headache or has myocardial ischaemia or an arrhythmia, or has a blood carboxyhaemoglobin concentration of more than 20%.

Sulfur dioxide, chlorine, phosgene, ammonia

All of these gases can cause upper respiratory tract and conjunctival irritation. Pulmonary oedema, with severe breathlessness and cyanosis may develop suddenly up to

36 hours after exposure. Death may occur. Patients are kept under observation and those who develop pulmonary oedema are given oxygen. Assisted ventilation may be necessary in the most serious cases.

CS spray

CS spray, which is used for riot control, irritates the eyes (hence 'tear gas') and the respiratory tract; symptoms normally settle spontaneously within 15 minutes. If symptoms persist, the patient should be removed to a well-ventilated area, and the exposed skin washed with soap and water after removal of contaminated clothing. Contact lenses should be removed and rigid ones washed (soft ones should be discarded). Eye symptoms should be treated by irrigating the eyes with physiological saline (or water if saline is not available) and advice sought from an ophthalmologist. Patients with features of severe poisoning, particularly respiratory complications, should be admitted to hospital for symptomatic treatment.

Nerve agents

Treatment of nerve agent poisoning is similar to organophosphorus insecticide poisoning, but advice must be sought from the National Poisons Information Service. The risk of cross-contamination is significant; adequate decontamination and protective clothing for healthcare personnel are essential. In emergencies involving the release of **nerve agents**, kits ('NAAS pods') containing **pralidoxime chloride** p. 794 can be obtained through the Ambulance Service from the National Blood Service (or the Welsh Blood Service in South Wales or designated hospital pharmacies in Northern Ireland and Scotland—see TOXBASE for list of designated centres).

Pesticides

Organophosphorus insecticides

Organophosphorus insecticides are usually supplied as powders or dissolved in organic solvents. All are absorbed through the bronchi and intact skin as well as through the gut and inhibit cholinesterase activity, thereby prolonging and intensifying the effects of acetylcholine. Toxicity between different compounds varies considerably, and onset may be delayed after skin exposure.

Anxiety, restlessness, dizziness, headache, miosis, nausea, hypersalivation, vomiting, abdominal colic, diarrhoea, bradycardia, and sweating are common features of organophosphorus poisoning. Muscle weakness and fasciculation may develop and progress to generalised flaccid paralysis, including the ocular and respiratory muscles. Convulsions, coma, pulmonary oedema with copious bronchial secretions, hypoxia, and arrhythmias occur in severe cases. Hyperglycaemia and glycosuria without ketonuria may also be present.

Further absorption of the organophosphorus insecticide should be prevented by moving the child to fresh air, removing soiled clothing, and washing contaminated skin. In severe poisoning it is vital to ensure a clear airway, frequent removal of bronchial secretions, and adequate ventilation and oxygenation; gastric lavage may be considered provided that the airway is protected. Atropine sulfate p. 764 will reverse the muscarinic effects of acetylcholine and is given by intravenous injection until the skin becomes flushed and dry, the pupils dilate, and bradycardia is abolished.

Pralidoxime chloride, a cholinesterase reactivator, is used as an adjunct to atropine sulfate in moderate or severe poisoning. It improves muscle tone within 30 minutes of administration. Pralidoxime chloride is continued until the patient has not required atropine sulfate for 12 hours. Pralidoxime chloride can be obtained from designated centres, the names of which are held by the National Poisons Information Service.

Snake bites and animal stings

Snake bites

Envenoming from snake bite is uncommon in the UK. Many exotic snakes are kept, some illegally, but the only indigenous venomous snake is the adder (*Vipera berus*). The bite may cause local and systemic effects. Local effects include pain, swelling, bruising, and tender enlargement of regional lymph nodes. Systemic effects include early anaphylactic symptoms (transient hypotension with syncope, angioedema, urticaria, abdominal colic, diarrhoea, and vomiting), with later persistent or recurrent hypotension, ECG abnormalities, spontaneous systemic bleeding, coagulopathy, adult respiratory distress syndrome, and acute renal failure. Fatal envenoming is rare but the potential for severe envenoming must not be underestimated.

Early anaphylactic symptoms should be treated with adrenaline/epinephrine p. 128. Indications for european viper snake venom antiserum treatment p. 798 include *systemic envenoming*, especially hypotension, ECG abnormalities, vomiting, haemostatic abnormalities, and marked local envenoming such that after bites on the hand or foot, swelling extends beyond the wrist or ankle within 4 hours of the bite. For those children who present with clinical features of *severe envenoming* (e.g. shock, ECG abnormalities, or local swelling that has advanced from the foot to above the knee or from the hand to above the elbow within 2 hours of the bite), a higher initial dose of the european viper snake venom antiserum is recommended; if symptoms of *systemic envenoming* persist contact the National Poisons Information Service.

Adrenaline/epinephrine injection must be immediately to hand for treatment of anaphylactic reactions to the european viper snake venom antiserum.

European viper snake venom antiserum is available for bites by certain foreign snakes and spiders, stings by scorpions and fish. For information on identification, management, and for supply in an emergency, telephone the National Poisons Information Service. Whenever possible the TOXBASE entry should be read, and relevant information collected, before telephoning the National Poisons Information Service.

Insect stings

Stings from ants, wasps, hornets, and bees cause local pain and swelling but seldom cause severe direct toxicity unless many stings are inflicted at the same time. If the sting is in the mouth or on the tongue local swelling may threaten the upper airway. The stings from these insects are usually treated by cleaning the area with a topical antiseptic. Bee stings should be removed as quickly as possible. Anaphylactic reactions require immediate treatment with intramuscular **adrenaline/epinephrine**; self-administered (or administered by a carer) intramuscular adrenaline/epinephrine (e.g. *EpiPen®*) is the best first-aid treatment for patients with severe hypersensitivity. An inhaled bronchodilator should be used for asthmatic reactions, see also the management of anaphylaxis. A short course of an **oral antihistamine** or a **topical corticosteroid** may help to reduce inflammation and relieve itching. A vaccine containing extracts of bee and wasp venom can be used to reduce the risk of anaphylaxis and systemic reactions in patients with systemic hypersensitivity to bee or wasp stings.

Marine stings

The severe pain of weeverfish (*Trachinus vipera*) and Portuguese man-o'-war stings can be relieved by immersing the stung area immediately in uncomfortably hot, but not scalding, water (not more than 45°C). People stung by jellyfish and Portuguese man-o'-war around the UK coast should be removed from the sea as soon as possible. Adherent tentacles should be lifted off carefully (wearing gloves or using tweezers) or washed off with seawater. Alcoholic solutions, including suntan lotions, should **not** be applied because they can cause further discharge of stinging hairs. Ice packs can be used to reduce pain.

Other poisons

Consult either the National Poisons Information Service day and night or TOXBASE.

The **National Poisons Information Service** (Tel: 0344 892 0111) will provide specialist advice on all aspects of poisoning day and night.

1 Active elimination from the gastro-intestinal tract

ANTIDOTES AND CHELATORS > INTESTINAL ADSORBENTS

Charcoal, activated

- **INDICATIONS AND DOSE**

Reduction of absorption of poisons in the gastro-intestinal system
- ▸ BY MOUTH
- ▸ Neonate: 1 g/kg.
- ▸ Child 1 month–11 years: 1 g/kg (max. per dose 50 g)
- ▸ Child 12–17 years: 50 g

Active elimination of poisons
- ▸ BY MOUTH
- ▸ Neonate: 1 g/kg every 4 hours, dose may be reduced and the frequency increased if not tolerated, reduced dose may compromise efficacy.
- ▸ Child 1 month–11 years: 1 g/kg every 4 hours (max. per dose 50 g), dose may be reduced and the frequency increased if not tolerated, reduced dose may compromise efficacy
- ▸ Child 12–17 years: Initially 50 g, then 50 g every 4 hours, reduced if not tolerated to 25 g every 2 hours, alternatively 12.5 g every 1 hour, reduced dose may compromise efficacy

- **CAUTIONS** Comatose patient (risk of aspiration—ensure airway is protected) · drowsy patient (risk of aspiration—ensure airway protected) · reduced gastrointestinal motility (risk of obstruction)
- **SIDE-EFFECTS** Black stools
- **DIRECTIONS FOR ADMINISTRATION** Suspension or reconstituted powder may be mixed with soft drinks (e.g. caffeine-free diet cola) or fruit juices to mask the taste.

- **MEDICINAL FORMS**
There can be variation in the licensing of different medicines containing the same drug.
Granules
- ▸ Carbomix (Beacon Pharmaceuticals Ltd)
Activated charcoal 813 mg per 1 gram Carbomix 81.3% granules sugar-free | 50 gram Ⓟ £11.90
Oral suspension
- ▸ Actidose-Aqua Advance (Alliance Pharmaceuticals Ltd)
Activated charcoal 208 mg per 1 ml Actidose-Aqua Advance 1.04g/5ml oral suspension | 240 ml Ⓟ £12.89
- ▸ Charcodote (Teva UK Ltd)
Activated charcoal 200 mg per 1 ml Charcodote 200mg/ml oral suspension sugar-free | 250 ml Ⓟ £11.88

2 Chemical toxicity

2.1 Cyanide toxicity

ANTIDOTES AND CHELATORS

Dicobalt edetate

- **INDICATIONS AND DOSE**

Severe poisoning with cyanides
- ▸ BY INTRAVENOUS INJECTION
- ▸ Child: Consult the National Poisons Information Service

- **CAUTIONS** Owing to toxicity to be used only for definite cyanide poisoning when patient tending to lose, or has lost, consciousness
- **SIDE-EFFECTS** Anaphylactoid reactions · cardiac abnormalities · facial oedema · hypotension · laryngeal oedema · tachycardia · vomiting
- **EXCEPTIONS TO LEGAL CATEGORY** Prescription only medicine restriction does not apply where administration is for saving life in emergency.

- **MEDICINAL FORMS**
There can be variation in the licensing of different medicines containing the same drug.
Solution for injection
- ▸ Dicobalt edetate (Non-proprietary)
Dicobalt edetate 15 mg per 1 ml Dicobalt edetate 300mg/20ml solution for injection ampoules | 6 ampoule PoM £117.20

Sodium nitrite

- **INDICATIONS AND DOSE**

Poisoning with cyanides (used in conjunction with sodium thiosulfate)
- ▸ BY INTRAVENOUS INJECTION
- ▸ Child: 4–10 mg/kg (max. per dose 300 mg), to be given over 5–20 minutes followed by sodium thiosulphate injection

DOSE EQUIVALENCE AND CONVERSION
4–10 mg/kg equates to 0.13–0.33 mL/kg of a 3% solution. Dose max. of 300 mg equates to 10 mL of a 3% solution.

- **SIDE-EFFECTS** Flushing (due to vasodilatation) · headache (due to vasodilatation)
- **EXCEPTIONS TO LEGAL CATEGORY** Prescription only medicine restriction does not apply where administration is for saving life in emergency.

- **MEDICINAL FORMS**
There can be variation in the licensing of different medicines containing the same drug. Forms available from special-order manufacturers include: solution for injection

Sodium thiosulfate

- **INDICATIONS AND DOSE**

Poisoning with cyanides (used in conjunction with sodium nitrite)
- ▸ BY INTRAVENOUS INJECTION
- ▸ Child: 400 mg/kg (max. per dose 12.5 g), to be given over 10 minutes, dose may be repeated in severe cyanide poisoning if dicobalt edetate not available

DOSE EQUIVALENCE AND CONVERSION
400 mg/kg equates to 0.8 mL/kg of a 50% solution. 12.5 g equates to 25 mL of a 50% solution.

16

Emergency treatment of poisoning

- **EXCEPTIONS TO LEGAL CATEGORY** Prescription only medicine restriction does not apply where administration is for saving life in emergency.

- **MEDICINAL FORMS**
  There can be variation in the licensing of different medicines containing the same drug. Forms available from special-order manufacturers include: solution for injection.

2.2 Organophosphorus toxicity

Drugs used for organophosphorus toxicity not listed below; Atropine sulfate p. 764

ANTIDOTES AND CHELATORS

Pralidoxime chloride

- **INDICATIONS AND DOSE**

  Adjunct to atropine in the treatment of poisoning by organophosphorus insecticide or nerve agent
  - ▶ BY INTRAVENOUS INFUSION
  - ▸ **Child:** Initially 30 mg/kg, to be given over 20 minutes, followed by 8 mg/kg/hour; maximum 12 g per day

- **UNLICENSED USE** Pralidoxime chloride doses may differ from those in product literature. Licensed for use in children (age range not specified by manufacturer).

- **CONTRA-INDICATIONS** Poisoning with carbamates · poisoning with organophosphorus compounds without anticholinesterase activity

- **CAUTIONS** Myasthenia gravis

- **SIDE-EFFECTS** Disturbances of vision · dizziness · drowsiness · headache · hyperventilation · muscular weakness · nausea · tachycardia

- **RENAL IMPAIRMENT** Use with caution.

- **DIRECTIONS FOR ADMINISTRATION** The loading dose may be administered by intravenous injection (diluted to a concentration of 50 mg/mL with water for injections) over at least 5 minutes if pulmonary oedema is present or if it is not practical to administer an intravenous infusion.
  - ▸ With intravenous use For *intravenous infusion*, reconstitute each vial with 20 mL Water for Injections, then dilute to a concentration of 10–20 mg/mL with Sodium Chloride 0.9%.

- **PRESCRIBING AND DISPENSING INFORMATION** Available from designated centres for organophosphorus insecticide poisoning or from the National Blood Service (or Welsh Ambulance Services for Mid West and South East Wales)—see TOXBASE for list of designated centres.

- **EXCEPTIONS TO LEGAL CATEGORY** Prescription only medicine restriction does not apply where administration is for saving life in emergency.

- **MEDICINAL FORMS**
  There can be variation in the licensing of different medicines containing the same drug.
  Powder for solution for injection
  - ▸ Pralidoxime chloride (Non-proprietary)
    Pralidoxime chloride 1 gram Protopam Chloride 1g powder for solution for injection vials | 6 vial [PoM] no price available

3 Drug toxicity
3.1 Benzodiazepine toxicity

ANTIDOTES AND CHELATORS 〉
BENZODIAZEPINE ANTAGONISTS

Flumazenil

- **INDICATIONS AND DOSE**

  Reversal of sedative effects of benzodiazepines
  - ▶ BY INTRAVENOUS INJECTION
  - ▸ **Neonate:** 10 micrograms/kg every 1 minute if required, dose to be administered over 15 seconds.
  - ▸ **Child:** 10 micrograms/kg every 1 minute (max. per dose 200 micrograms) if required, dose to be administered over 15 seconds; maximum 1 mg per course; maximum 50 micrograms/kg per course

  Reversal of sedative effects of benzodiazepines (if drowsiness recurs after injection)
  - ▶ BY INTRAVENOUS INFUSION
  - ▸ **Neonate:** 2–10 micrograms/kg/hour, adjusted according to response.
  - ▸ **Child:** 2–10 micrograms/kg/hour (max. per dose 400 micrograms/hour), adjusted according to response

  Reversal of sedative effects of benzodiazepines in intensive care
  - ▶ BY INTRAVENOUS INJECTION
  - ▸ **Child:** 10 micrograms/kg every 1 minute (max. per dose 200 micrograms) if required, dose to be administered over 15 seconds; maximum 2 mg per course; maximum 50 micrograms/kg per course

- **UNLICENSED USE** Not licensed for use in children under 1 year. Not licensed for use by intravenous infusion in children. Not licensed for use in children in intensive care.

> **IMPORTANT SAFETY INFORMATION**
> Flumazenil should only be administered by, or under the direct supervision of, personnel experienced in its use.

- **CONTRA-INDICATIONS** Life-threatening condition (e.g. raised intracranial pressure, status epilepticus) controlled by benzodiazepines

- **CAUTIONS** Avoid rapid injection following major surgery · avoid rapid injection in high-risk or anxious patients · benzodiazepine dependence (may precipitate withdrawal symptoms) · children · ensure neuromuscular blockade cleared before giving · head injury (rapid reversal of benzodiazepine sedation may cause convulsions) · history of panic disorders (risk of recurrence) · prolonged benzodiazepine therapy for epilepsy (risk of convulsions) · short-acting (repeat doses may be necessary— benzodiazepine effects may persist for at least 24 hours)

- **SIDE-EFFECTS**
  - ▶ **Common or very common** Nausea · vomiting
  - ▶ **Uncommon** Anxiety · fear · palpitation
  - ▶ **Frequency not known** Agitation · chills · convulsions (particularly in those with epilepsy) · dizziness · flushing · sensory disturbance · sweating · tachycardia · transient hypertension

- **PREGNANCY** Not known to be harmful.

- **BREAST FEEDING** Avoid breast-feeding for 24 hours.

- **HEPATIC IMPAIRMENT** Carefully titrate dose.

- **DIRECTIONS FOR ADMINISTRATION**
  - ▶ With intravenous use For *continuous intravenous infusion*, dilute with Glucose 5% or Sodium Chloride 0.9%.

- **MEDICINAL FORMS**
There can be variation in the licensing of different medicines containing the same drug.
Solution for injection
  ‣ Flumazenil (Non-proprietary)
  Flumazenil 100 microgram per 1 ml Flumazenil 500micrograms/5ml solution for injection ampoules | 5 ampoule [PoM] £65.50–£72.46

3.2 Digoxin toxicity

ANTIDOTES AND CHELATORS ⟩ ANTIBODIES

Digoxin-specific antibody

- **INDICATIONS AND DOSE**
Treatment of known or strongly suspected life-threatening digoxin toxicity associated with ventricular arrhythmias or bradyarrhythmias unresponsive to atropine and when measures beyond the withdrawal of digoxin and correction of any electrolyte abnormalities are considered necessary
  ‣ BY INTRAVENOUS INFUSION
  ‣ Child: Serious cases of digoxin toxicity should be discussed with the National Poisons Information Service (consult product literature)

- **MEDICINAL FORMS**
There can be variation in the licensing of different medicines containing the same drug.
Powder for solution for infusion
  ‣ DigiFab (BTG International Ltd)
  Digoxin-specific antibody fragments 40 mg DigiFab 40mg powder for solution for infusion vials | 1 vial [PoM] £750.00 (Hospital only)

3.3 Heparin toxicity

ANTIDOTES AND CHELATORS

Protamine sulfate

- **INDICATIONS AND DOSE**
Overdosage with intravenous injection or intravenous infusion of unfractionated heparin (less than 30 minutes lapsed since overdose)
  ‣ BY INTRAVENOUS INJECTION
  ‣ Child: 1 mg (max. per dose 50 mg), to be administered at a rate not exceeding 5 mg/minute, to neutralise each 100 units of unfractionated heparin
Overdosage with intravenous injection or intravenous infusion of unfractionated heparin (if 30–60 minutes lapsed since overdose)
  ‣ BY INTRAVENOUS INJECTION
  ‣ Child: 500–750 micrograms (max. per dose 50 mg), to be administered at a rate not exceeding 5 mg/minute, to neutralise each 100 units of unfractionated heparin
Overdosage with intravenous injection or intravenous infusion of unfractionated heparin (if 60–120 minutes lapsed since overdose)
  ‣ BY INTRAVENOUS INJECTION
  ‣ Child: 375–500 micrograms (max. per dose 50 mg), to be administered at a rate not exceeding 5 mg/minute, to neutralise each 100 units of unfractionated heparin

Overdosage with intravenous injection or intravenous infusion of unfractionated heparin (if over 120 minutes lapsed since overdose)
  ‣ BY INTRAVENOUS INJECTION
  ‣ Child: 250–375 micrograms (max. per dose 50 mg), to be administered at a rate not exceeding 5 mg/minute, to neutralise each 100 units of unfractionated heparin
Overdosage with subcutaneous injection of unfractionated heparin
  ‣ BY INTRAVENOUS INJECTION, OR BY INTRAVENOUS INFUSION
  ‣ Child: (max. per dose 50 mg), 50–100% of the total dose to be given by intravenous injection (rate not exceeding 5 mg/minute), then give any remainder of dose by intravenous infusion over 8–16 hours, 1 mg neutralises approx. 100 units of unfractionated heparin
Overdosage with subcutaneous injection of low molecular weight heparin
  ‣ BY INTRAVENOUS INJECTION, OR BY CONTINUOUS INTRAVENOUS INFUSION
  ‣ Child: (max. per dose 50 mg), to be administered by intermittent intravenous injection at a rate not exceeding 5 mg/minute or by continuous intravenous infusion, 1 mg neutralises approx. 100 units of low molecular weight heparin, consult product literature of low molecular weight heparin for details

- **CAUTIONS** Excessive doses can have an anticoagulant effect
- **SIDE-EFFECTS** Anaphylaxis · angioedema · back pain · bradycardia · dyspnoea · flushing · hypersensitivity reactions · hypertension · hypotension · lassitude · nausea · pulmonary oedema · rebound bleeding · vomiting
- **ALLERGY AND CROSS-SENSITIVITY** Caution if increased risk of allergic reaction to protamine (includes previous treatment with protamine or protamine insulin, allergy to fish, men who are infertile or who have had a vasectomy and who may have antibodies to protamine).
- **MONITORING REQUIREMENTS** Monitor activated partial thromboplastin time or other appropriate blood clotting parameters.
- **DIRECTIONS FOR ADMINISTRATION**
  ‣ With intravenous use May be diluted if necessary with Sodium Chloride 0.9%.
- **PRESCRIBING AND DISPENSING INFORMATION** The long half-life of low molecular weight heparins should be taken into consideration when determining the dose of protamine sulfate; the effects of low molecular weight heparins can persist for up to 24 hours after administration.

- **MEDICINAL FORMS**
There can be variation in the licensing of different medicines containing the same drug.
Solution for injection
  ‣ Protamine sulfate (Non-proprietary)
  Protamine sulfate 10 mg per 1 ml Protamine sulfate 100mg/10ml solution for injection ampoules | 5 ampoule [PoM] no price available
  Protamine sulfate 50mg/5ml solution for injection ampoules | 10 ampoule [PoM] £49.55

16

Emergency treatment of poisoning

3.4 Opioid toxicity

OPIOID RECEPTOR ANTAGONISTS

Naloxone hydrochloride

- **INDICATIONS AND DOSE**

Overdosage with opioids
- ▸ BY INTRAVENOUS INJECTION, OR BY SUBCUTANEOUS INJECTION, OR BY INTRAMUSCULAR INJECTION
- ▸ Neonate: Initially 100 micrograms/kg, if no response, repeat at intervals of 1 minute to a total max. 2 mg, then review diagnosis; further doses may be required if respiratory function deteriorates.
- ▸ Child 1 month–11 years: Initially 100 micrograms/kg, if no response, repeat at intervals of 1 minute to a total max. 2 mg, then review diagnosis; further doses may be required if respiratory function deteriorates.
- ▸ Child 12–17 years: Initially 400 micrograms, then 800 micrograms for up to 2 doses at 1 minute intervals if no response to preceding dose, then increased to 2 mg for 1 dose if still no response (4 mg dose may be required in seriously poisoned patients), then review diagnosis; further doses may be required if respiratory function deteriorates
- ▸ BY CONTINUOUS INTRAVENOUS INFUSION
- ▸ Neonate: Using an infusion pump, adjust rate according to response (initially, rate may be set at 60% of the initial resuscitative intravenous injection dose per hour). The initial resuscitative *intravenous injection* dose is that which maintained satisfactory ventilation for at least 15 minutes.
- ▸ Child: Using an infusion pump, adjust rate according to response (initially, rate may be set at 60% of the initial resuscitative intravenous injection dose per hour). The initial resuscitative *intravenous injection* dose is that which maintained satisfactory ventilation for at least 15 minutes

Reversal of postoperative respiratory depression
- ▸ INITIALLY BY INTRAVENOUS INJECTION
- ▸ Neonate: 1 microgram/kg, repeated every 2–3 minutes if required.
- ▸ Child 1 month–11 years: 1 microgram/kg, repeated every 2–3 minutes if required
- ▸ Child 12–17 years: Initially 100–200 micrograms, alternatively (by intravenous injection) initially 1.5–3 micrograms/kg, if response inadequate, give subsequent doses, (by intravenous injection) 100 micrograms every 2 minutes, alternatively (by intramuscular injection) 100 micrograms every 1–2 hours

Reversal of respiratory and CNS depression resulting from opioid administration to mother during labour
- ▸ BY INTRAMUSCULAR INJECTION
- ▸ Neonate: 200 micrograms, alternatively 60 micrograms/kg, to be given as a single dose at birth.
- ▸ BY INTRAVENOUS INJECTION, OR BY SUBCUTANEOUS INJECTION
- ▸ Neonate: 10 micrograms/kg, repeated every 2–3 minutes if required.

PHARMACOKINETICS
Naloxone has a short duration of action; repeated doses or infusion may be necessary to reverse effects of opioids with longer duration of action.
Important: Only give by subcutaneous or intramuscular routes if intravenous route is not feasible; intravenous administration has more rapid onset of action.

- **UNLICENSED USE** Naloxone doses in BNF may differ from those in product literature.

> **IMPORTANT SAFETY INFORMATION**
> SAFE PRACTICE
> Doses used in acute opioid overdosage may not be appropriate for the management of opioid-induced respiratory depression and sedation in those receiving palliative care and in chronic opioid use.

- **CAUTIONS** Cardiovascular disease or those receiving cardiotoxic drugs (serious adverse cardiovascular effects reported) · maternal physical dependence on opioids (may precipitate withdrawal in newborn) · pain · physical dependence on opioids (precipitates withdrawal)
  CAUTIONS, FURTHER INFORMATION
- ▸ Titration of dose In postoperative use, the dose should be titrated for each patient in order to obtain sufficient respiratory response; however, naloxone antagonises analgesia.
- **SIDE-EFFECTS**
- ▸ **Common or very common** Cardiac arrest · dizziness · dyspnoea · headache · hypertension · hyperventilation · hypotension · nausea · pulmonary oedema · tachycardia · ventricular fibrilation · vomiting
- ▸ **Uncommon** Agitation · diarrhoea · dry mouth · excitement · paraesthesia · sweating · tremor
- ▸ **Very rare** Erythema multiforme · seizures
- **PREGNANCY** Use only if potential benefit outweighs risk.
- **BREAST FEEDING** Not orally bioavailable.
- **DIRECTIONS FOR ADMINISTRATION** For *continuous intravenous infusion*, dilute to a concentration of up to 200 micrograms/mL with Glucose 5% or Sodium Chloride 0.9%.

- **MEDICINAL FORMS**
There can be variation in the licensing of different medicines containing the same drug.

Solution for injection
- ▸ **Naloxone hydrochloride** (Non-proprietary)
  Naloxone hydrochloride 20 microgram per 1 ml Naloxone 40micrograms/2ml solution for injection ampoules | 10 ampoule [PoM] £55.00
  Naloxone hydrochloride 400 microgram per 1 ml Naloxone 400micrograms/1ml solution for injection Minijet pre-filled syringes | 1 pre-filled disposable injection [PoM] £20.40
  Naloxone 2mg/5ml solution for injection Minijet pre-filled syringes | 1 pre-filled disposable injection [PoM] £20.40
  Naloxone 400micrograms/1ml solution for injection ampoules | 10 ampoule [PoM] £41.00–£53.70
  Naloxone 800micrograms/2ml solution for injection Minijet pre-filled syringes | 1 pre-filled disposable injection [PoM] £20.40
  Naloxone hydrochloride 1 mg per 1 ml Naloxone 2mg/2ml solution for injection pre-filled syringes | 1 pre-filled disposable injection [PoM] £16.80
- ▸ **Prenoxad** (Martindale Pharmaceuticals Ltd)
  Naloxone hydrochloride 1 mg per 1 ml Prenoxad 2mg/2ml solution for injection pre-filled syringes | 1 pre-filled disposable injection [PoM] £15.30

3.5 Paracetamol toxicity

ANTIDOTES AND CHELATORS > ANTIDOTES AND CHELATORS, OTHER

Acetylcysteine

● INDICATIONS AND DOSE

Paracetamol overdosage
▸ BY INTRAVENOUS INFUSION

▸ **Neonate:** Initially 150 mg/kg over 1 hour, dose to be administered in 3 mL/kg glucose 5%, followed by 50 mg/kg over 4 hours, dose to be administered in 7 mL/kg glucose 5%, then 100 mg/kg over 16 hours, dose to be administered in 14 mL/kg glucose 5%.

▸ **Child (body-weight up to 20 kg):** Initially 150 mg/kg over 1 hour, dose to be administered in 3 mL/kg glucose 5%, followed by 50 mg/kg over 4 hours, dose to be administered in 7 mL/kg glucose 5%, then 100 mg/kg over 16 hours, dose to be administered in 14 mL/kg glucose 5%

▸ **Child (body-weight 20–39 kg):** Initially 150 mg/kg over 1 hour, dose to be administered in 100 mL glucose 5%, followed by 50 mg/kg over 4 hours, dose to be administered in 250 mL glucose 5%, then 100 mg/kg over 16 hours, dose to be administered in 500 mL glucose 5%

▸ **Child (body-weight 40 kg and above):** 150 mg/kg over 1 hour, dose to be administered in 200 mL Glucose Intravenous Infusion 5%, then 50 mg/kg over 4 hours, to be started immediately after completion of first infusion, dose to be administered in 500 mL Glucose Intravenous Infusion 5%, then 100 mg/kg over 16 hours, to be started immediately after completion of second infusion, dose to be administered in 1 litre Glucose Intravenous Infusion 5%

Meconium ileus
▸ BY MOUTH

▸ **Neonate:** 200–400 mg up to 3 times a day if required.

Treatment of distal intestinal obstructive syndrome
▸ BY MOUTH

▸ **Child 1 month–1 year:** 0.4–3 g as a single dose
▸ **Child 2–6 years:** 2–3 g as a single dose
▸ **Child 7–17 years:** 4–6 g as a single dose

Prevention of distal intestinal obstruction syndrome
▸ BY MOUTH

▸ **Child 1 month–1 year:** 100–200 mg 3 times a day
▸ **Child 2–11 years:** 200 mg 3 times a day
▸ **Child 12–17 years:** 200–400 mg 3 times a day

● UNLICENSED USE
▸ With oral use Not licensed for use in meconium ileus or for distal intestinal obstructive syndrome in children with cystic fibrosis.

● CAUTIONS
▸ With intravenous use Asthma (see Side-effects for management of asthma but do not delay acetylcysteine treatment) · atopy · may slightly increase INR · may slightly increase prothrombin time
▸ With oral use Asthma · history of peptic ulceration

● SIDE-EFFECTS
▸ With intravenous use Hypersensitivity-like reactions · rashes · slight increase in INR and prothrombin time
▸ With oral use Anaphylaxis · hypersensitivity-like reactions · rashes

SIDE-EFFECTS, FURTHER INFORMATION
▸ Hypersensitivity-like reactions
▸ With intravenous use Hypersensitivity-like reactions managed by reducing infusion rate or suspending until reaction settled (rash also managed by giving antihistamine; acute asthma managed by giving nebulised short-acting beta₂ agonist)—contact the National Poisons Information Service if reaction severe.

● DIRECTIONS FOR ADMINISTRATION
▸ With oral use For *oral* administration, use oral granules, *or* dilute injection solution (200 mg/mL) to a concentration of 50 mg/mL; orange or blackcurrant juice or cola drink may be used as a diluent to mask the bitter taste.
▸ With intravenous use Glucose 5% is preferred fluid; Sodium Chloride 0.9% is an alternative if Glucose 5% unsuitable.

● MEDICINAL FORMS
There can be variation in the licensing of different medicines containing the same drug. Forms available from special-order manufacturers include: tablet, effervescent tablet, capsule, granules, oral solution

Tablet
▸ Acetylcysteine (Non-proprietary)
Acetylcysteine 600 mg Acetylcysteine 600mg tablets | 30 tablet £39.95 | 100 tablet no price available

Effervescent tablet
▸ Acetylcysteine (Non-proprietary)
Acetylcysteine 600 mg Acetylcysteine 600mg effervescent tablets | 10 tablet no price available
Fluimucil 600 effervescent tablets | 10 tablet [PoM] no price available
ACC-600 effervescent tablets | 10 tablet [PoM] no price available

Orodispersible tablet
▸ Acetylcysteine (Non-proprietary)
Acetylcysteine 200 mg Fluimucil 200mg orodispersible tablets | 20 tablet [PoM] no price available

Capsule
▸ Acetylcysteine (Non-proprietary)
Acetylcysteine 600 mg Acetylcysteine 600mg capsules | 30 capsule £39.95 | 60 capsule no price available

Granules
CAUTIONARY AND ADVISORY LABELS 13
▸ Acetylcysteine (Non-proprietary)
Acetylcysteine 100 mg Fluimucil N 100mg granules sachets | 20 sachet [PoM] no price available | 50 sachet [PoM] no price available
Acetylcysteine 200 mg Fluimucil N 200mg granules sachets | 20 sachet [PoM] no price available | 50 sachet [PoM] no price available | 100 sachet [PoM] no price available

Oral solution
▸ Acetylcysteine (Non-proprietary)
Acetylcysteine 20 mg per 1 ml Solmucol 100mg/5ml syrup | 180 ml [PoM] no price available

Solution for infusion
ELECTROLYTES: May contain Sodium
▸ Acetylcysteine (Non-proprietary)
Acetylcysteine 200 mg per 1 ml Acetylcysteine 2g/10ml solution for infusion ampoules | 10 ampoule [PoM] £21.26–£24.99
▸ Parvolex (Phoenix Labs Ltd)
Acetylcysteine 200 mg per 1 ml Parvolex 2g/10ml concentrate for solution for infusion ampoules | 10 ampoule [PoM] £22.50

16

Emergency treatment of poisoning

4 Methaemoglobinaemia

ANTIDOTES AND CHELATORS

Methylthioninium chloride

(Methylene blue)

- **INDICATIONS AND DOSE**

Drug- or chemical-induced methaemoglobinaemia
- ▸ BY SLOW INTRAVENOUS INJECTION
- ▸ **Neonate:** Seek advice from National Poisons Information Service.
- ▸ Child 1-2 months: Seek advice from National Poisons Information Service
- ▸ Child 3 months-17 years: Initially 1–2 mg/kg, then 1–2 mg/kg after 30–60 minutes if required, to be given over 5 minutes, seek advice from National Poisons Information Service if further repeat doses are required; maximum 7 mg/kg per course

Aniline- or dapsone-induced methaemoglobinaemia
- ▸ BY SLOW INTRAVENOUS INJECTION
- ▸ Child 3 months-17 years: Initially 1–2 mg/kg, then 1–2 mg/kg after 30–60 minutes if required, to be given over 5 minutes, seek advice from National Poisons Information Service if further repeat doses are required; maximum 4 mg/kg per course

- **CAUTIONS** Children under 3 months (more susceptible to methaemoglobinaemia from high doses of methylthioninium) · chlorate poisoning (reduces efficacy of methylthioninium) · G6PD deficiency (seek advice from National Poisons Information Service) · methaemoglobinaemia due to treatment of cyanide poisoning with sodium nitrite (seek advice from National Poisons Information Service) · pulse oximetry may give false estimation of oxygen saturation

- **INTERACTIONS** → Appendix 1 (methylthioninium).

- **SIDE-EFFECTS** Abdominal pain · agitation · anxiety · arrhythmia · blue-green discoloration of faeces · blue-green discoloration of skin · blue-green discoloration of urine · chest pain · confusion · dizziness · dyspnoea · fever · haemolytic anaemia · headache · hyperbilirubinaemia (in infants) · hypertension · hypotension · methaemoglobinaemia · mydriasis · nausea · sweating · tachypnoea · tremor · vomiting

- **PREGNANCY** No information available, but risk to fetus of untreated methaemoglobinaemia likely to be significantly higher than risk of treatment.

- **BREAST FEEDING** Manufacturer advises avoid breastfeeding for up to 6 days after administration—no information available.

- **RENAL IMPAIRMENT** Use with caution in severe impairment; dose reduction may be required.

- **DIRECTIONS FOR ADMINISTRATION** For *intravenous injection*, may be diluted with Glucose 5% to minimise injection-site pain; not compatible with Sodium Chloride 0.9%.

- **MEDICINAL FORMS**
There can be variation in the licensing of different medicines containing the same drug. Forms available from special-order manufacturers include: solution for injection
Solution for injection
- ▸ Methylthioninium chloride (Non-proprietary)
Methylthioninium chloride 5 mg per 1 ml Methylthioninium chloride Proveblue 50mg/10ml solution for injection ampoules | 5 ampoule PoM £167.36

5 Snake bites

IMMUNE SERA AND IMMUNOGLOBULINS ›
ANTITOXINS

European viper snake venom antiserum

- **INDICATIONS AND DOSE**

Systemic envenoming from snake bites | Marked local envenoming
- ▸ BY INTRAVENOUS INJECTION, OR BY INTRAVENOUS INFUSION
- ▸ Child: Initially 10 mL for 1 dose, then 10 mL after 1–2 hours if required, the second dose should only be given if symptoms of systemic envenoming persist after the first dose, if symptoms of systemic envenoming persist contact the National Poisons Information Service

Severe systemic envenoming from snake bites in patients presenting with clinical features
- ▸ BY INTRAVENOUS INJECTION, OR BY INTRAVENOUS INFUSION
- ▸ Child: Initially 20 mL for 1 dose, if symptoms of systemic envenoming persist contact the National Poisons Information Service

- **DIRECTIONS FOR ADMINISTRATION** By *intravenous injection* given over 10–15 minutes or by *intravenous infusion* over 30 minutes after diluting in sodium chloride 0.9% (use 5 mL diluent/kg body-weight).

- **PRESCRIBING AND DISPENSING INFORMATION** To order, email immform@dh.gsi.gov.uk.

- **MEDICINAL FORMS**
There can be variation in the licensing of different medicines containing the same drug.
Solution for injection
- ▸ European viper snake venom antiserum (Non-proprietary)
European viper snake venom antiserum 100 mg per 1 ml Viper venom antiserum, European (equine) 1g/10ml solution for injection vials | 1 vial PoM no price available

Appendix 1
Interactions

Two or more drugs given at the same time may exert their effects independently or may interact. The interaction may be potentiation or antagonism of one drug by another, or occasionally some other effect. Adverse drug interactions should be reported to the Medicines and Healthcare products Regulatory Agency (MHRA), through the Yellow Card Scheme (see Adverse Reactions to Drugs), as for other adverse drug reactions.

Drug interactions may be **pharmacodynamic** or **pharmacokinetic**.

Pharmacodynamic interactions

These are interactions between drugs which have similar or antagonistic pharmacological effects or side-effects. They may be due to competition at receptor sites, or occur between drugs acting on the same physiological system. They are usually predictable from a knowledge of the pharmacology of the interacting drugs; in general, those demonstrated with one drug are likely to occur with related drugs. They occur to a greater or lesser extent in most patients who receive the interacting drugs.

Pharmacokinetic interactions

These occur when one drug alters the absorption, distribution, metabolism, or excretion of another, thus increasing or reducing the amount of drug available to produce its pharmacological effects. They are not easily predicted and many of them affect only a small proportion of patients taking the combination of drugs. Pharmacokinetic interactions occurring with one drug cannot be assumed to occur with related drugs unless their pharmacokinetic properties are known to be similar.

Pharmacokinetic interactions are of several types:

Affecting absorption The rate of absorption or the total amount absorbed can both be altered by drug interactions. Delayed absorption is rarely of clinical importance unless high peak plasma concentrations are required (e.g. when giving an analgesic). Reduction in the total amount absorbed, however, may result in ineffective therapy.

Due to changes in protein binding To a variable extent most drugs are loosely bound to plasma proteins. Protein-binding sites are non-specific and one drug can displace another thereby increasing its proportion free to diffuse from plasma to its site of action. This only produces a detectable increase in effect if it is an extensively bound drug (more than 90%) that is not widely distributed throughout the body. Even so displacement rarely produces more than transient potentiation because this increased concentration of free drug results in an increased rate of elimination.

Displacement from protein binding plays a part in the potentiation of warfarin by sulfonamides and tolbutamide but the importance of these interactions is due mainly to the fact that warfarin metabolism is also inhibited.

Affecting metabolism Many drugs are metabolised in the liver. Induction of the hepatic microsomal enzyme system by one drug can gradually increase the rate of metabolism of another, resulting in lower plasma concentrations and a reduced effect. On withdrawal of the inducer plasma concentrations increase and toxicity may occur. Barbiturates, griseofulvin, many antiepileptics, and rifampicin are the most important enzyme inducers. Drugs affected include warfarin and the oral contraceptives.

Conversely when one drug inhibits the metabolism of another higher plasma concentrations are produced, rapidly resulting in an increased effect with risk of toxicity. Some drugs which potentiate warfarin and phenytoin do so by this mechanism.

> Isoenzymes of the hepatic cytochrome P450 system interact with a wide range of drugs. Drugs may be substrates, inducers or inhibitors of the different isoenzymes. A great deal of *in-vitro* information is available on the effect of drugs on the isoenzymes; however, since drugs are eliminated by a number of different metabolic routes as well as renal excretion, the clinical effects of interactions cannot be predicted accurately from laboratory data on the cytochrome P450 isoenzymes. Except where a combination of drugs is specifically contra-indicated, the BNF presents only interactions that have been reported in clinical practice. In all cases the possibility of an interaction must be considered if toxic effects occur or if the activity of a drug diminishes.

Affecting renal excretion Drugs are eliminated through the kidney both by glomerular filtration and by active tubular secretion. Competition occurs between those which share active transport mechanisms in the proximal tubule. For example, salicylates and some other NSAIDs delay the excretion of methotrexate; serious methotrexate toxicity is possible.

Relative importance of interactions

Many drug interactions are harmless and many of those which are potentially harmful only occur in a small proportion of patients; moreover, the severity of an interaction varies from one patient to another. Drugs with a small therapeutic ratio (e.g. phenytoin) and those which require careful control of dosage (e.g. anticoagulants, antihypertensives, and antidiabetics) are most often involved.

Patients at increased risk from drug interactions include those with impaired renal or liver function.

Serious interactions The symbol ● has been placed against interactions that are **potentially serious** and where concomitant administration of the drugs involved should be **avoided** (or only undertaken with caution and appropriate monitoring).

Interactions that have no symbol do not usually have serious consequences.

List of drug interactions

The following is an alphabetical list of drugs and their interactions; to avoid excessive cross-referencing each drug or group is listed twice: in the alphabetical list and also against the drug or group with which it interacts.

Abacavir
▸ Analgesics: abacavir possibly reduces plasma concentration of METHADONE
▸ Antibacterials: plasma concentration of abacavir possibly reduced by RIFAMPICIN
▸ Antiepileptics: plasma concentration of abacavir possibly reduced by FOSPHENYTOIN, PHENOBARBITAL, PHENYTOIN and PRIMIDONE
● Antivirals: abacavir possibly reduces effects of ● RIBAVIRIN; plasma concentration of abacavir reduced by ● TIPRANAVIR
● Orlistat: absorption of abacavir possibly reduced by ● ORLISTAT

Abatacept
● Cytotoxics: increased risk of side-effects when abatacept given with ADALIMUMAB; avoid concomitant use of abatacept with
● CERTOLIZUMAB PEGOL, ● GOLIMUMAB or ● INFLIXIMAB
● Etanercept: avoid concomitant use of abatacept with
● ETANERCEPT
● Vaccines: risk of generalised infections when abatacept given with live ● VACCINES—avoid concomitant use

Abiraterone
▸ Analgesics: abiraterone increases plasma concentration of DEXTROMETHORPHAN
● Antibacterials: plasma concentration of abiraterone possibly reduced by ● RIFABUTIN—manufacturer of abiraterone advises avoid concomitant use; plasma concentration of abiraterone reduced by ● RIFAMPICIN—manufacturer of abiraterone advises avoid concomitant use
● Antidepressants: plasma concentration of abiraterone possibly reduced by ● ST JOHN'S WORT—manufacturer of abiraterone advises avoid concomitant use
● Antiepileptics: plasma concentration of abiraterone possibly reduced by ● CARBAMAZEPINE, ● FOSPHENYTOIN,
● PHENOBARBITAL, ● PHENYTOIN and ● PRIMIDONE— manufacturer of abiraterone advises avoid concomitant use
▸ Diuretics: manufacturer of abiraterone advises avoid concomitant use with SPIRONOLACTONE

Acarbose see Antidiabetics

ACE Inhibitors
▸ Alcohol: enhanced hypotensive effect when ACE inhibitors given with ALCOHOL
▸ Aldesleukin: enhanced hypotensive effect when ACE inhibitors given with ALDESLEUKIN
● Aliskiren: increased risk of hyperkalaemia, hypotension, and impaired renal function when ACE inhibitors given with
● ALISKIREN—avoid concomitant use
▸ Allopurinol: manufacturers state possible increased risk of leucopenia and hypersensitivity reactions when ACE inhibitors given with ALLOPURINOL especially in renal impairment
▸ Alpha-blockers: enhanced hypotensive effect when ACE inhibitors given with ALPHA-BLOCKERS
▸ Anaesthetics, General: enhanced hypotensive effect when ACE inhibitors given with GENERAL ANAESTHETICS
▸ Analgesics: increased risk of renal impairment when ACE inhibitors given with NSAIDs, also hypotensive effect antagonised
● Angiotensin-II Receptor Antagonists: increased risk of hyperkalaemia, hypotension, and impaired renal function when ACE inhibitors given with ● ANGIOTENSIN-II RECEPTOR ANTAGONISTS—avoid concomitant use
▸ Antacids: absorption of ACE inhibitors possibly reduced by ANTACIDS; absorption of captopril, enalapril and fosinopril reduced by ANTACIDS
▸ Antibacterials: plasma concentration of active metabolite of imidapril reduced by RIFAMPICIN (reduced antihypertensive effect); quinapril tablets reduce absorption of TETRACYCLINES (quinapril tablets contain magnesium carbonate); possible increased risk of hyperkalaemia when ACE inhibitors given with TRIMETHOPRIM

ACE Inhibitors (continued)
▸ Anticoagulants: increased risk of hyperkalaemia when ACE inhibitors given with HEPARINS
▸ Antidepressants: hypotensive effect of ACE inhibitors possibly enhanced by MAOIs
▸ Antidiabetics: ACE inhibitors possibly enhance hypoglycaemic effect of INSULIN, METFORMIN and SULFONYLUREAS
▸ Antipsychotics: enhanced hypotensive effect when ACE inhibitors given with ANTIPSYCHOTICS
▸ Anxiolytics and Hypnotics: enhanced hypotensive effect when ACE inhibitors given with ANXIOLYTICS AND HYPNOTICS
▸ Avanafil: hypotensive effect of enalapril possibly enhanced by AVANAFIL
▸ Azathioprine: increased risk of anaemia or leucopenia when captopril given with AZATHIOPRINE especially in renal impairment; increased risk of anaemia when enalapril given with AZATHIOPRINE especially in renal impairment
● Bee Venom Extracts: possible severe anaphylactoid reaction when ACE inhibitors given with ● BEE VENOM EXTRACTS
▸ Beta-blockers: enhanced hypotensive effect when ACE inhibitors given with BETA-BLOCKERS
▸ Calcium-channel Blockers: enhanced hypotensive effect when ACE inhibitors given with CALCIUM-CHANNEL BLOCKERS
▸ Cardiac Glycosides: captopril possibly increases plasma concentration of DIGOXIN
● Ciclosporin: increased risk of hyperkalaemia when ACE inhibitors given with ● CICLOSPORIN
▸ Clonidine: enhanced hypotensive effect when ACE inhibitors given with CLONIDINE; antihypertensive effect of captopril possibly delayed by previous treatment with CLONIDINE
▸ Corticosteroids: hypotensive effect of ACE inhibitors antagonised by CORTICOSTEROIDS
● Cytotoxics: increased risk of angioedema when ACE inhibitors given with ● EVEROLIMUS
▸ Diazoxide: enhanced hypotensive effect when ACE inhibitors given with DIAZOXIDE
▸ Diuretics: enhanced hypotensive effect when ACE inhibitors given with ● DIURETICS; increased risk of severe hyperkalaemia when ACE inhibitors given with ● AMILORIDE, ● POTASSIUM CANRENOATE or ● TRIAMTERENE; increased risk of severe hyperkalaemia when ACE inhibitors given with ● EPLERENONE and ● SPIRONOLACTONE—avoid concurrent use or use lowest possible doses of both drugs
▸ Dopaminergics: enhanced hypotensive effect when ACE inhibitors given with CO-BENELDOPA, CO-CARELDOPA or LEVODOPA
▸ Lithium: ACE inhibitors reduce excretion of ● LITHIUM (increased plasma concentration)
▸ Methyldopa: enhanced hypotensive effect when ACE inhibitors given with METHYLDOPA
▸ Moxisylyte: enhanced hypotensive effect when ACE inhibitors given with MOXISYLYTE
▸ Moxonidine: enhanced hypotensive effect when ACE inhibitors given with MOXONIDINE
▸ Muscle Relaxants: enhanced hypotensive effect when ACE inhibitors given with BACLOFEN or TIZANIDINE
▸ Nitrates: enhanced hypotensive effect when ACE inhibitors given with NITRATES
▸ Oestrogens: hypotensive effect of ACE inhibitors antagonised by OESTROGENS
● Potassium Salts: increased risk of severe hyperkalaemia when ACE inhibitors given with ● POTASSIUM SALTS
▸ Prostaglandins: enhanced hypotensive effect when ACE inhibitors given with ALPROSTADIL
● Sacubitril: manufacturer of sacubitril advises avoid ACE inhibitors for 36 hours before or after ● SACUBITRIL
● Sodium Aurothiomalate: flushing and hypotension reported when ACE inhibitors given with ● SODIUM AUROTHIOMALATE
▸ Vasodilator Antihypertensives: enhanced hypotensive effect when ACE inhibitors given with HYDRALAZINE, MINOXIDIL or SODIUM NITROPRUSSIDE
● Wasp Venom Extracts: possible severe anaphylactoid reaction when ACE inhibitors given with ● WASP VENOM EXTRACTS

Acebutolol see Beta-blockers
Aceclofenac see NSAIDs
Acemetacin see NSAIDs

Acenocoumarol *see* Coumarins

Acetazolamide *see* Diuretics

Aciclovir

NOTE Interactions do not apply to topical aciclovir preparations

▸ Aminophylline: aciclovir possibly increases plasma concentration of AMINOPHYLLINE

▸ Ciclosporin: increased risk of nephrotoxicity when aciclovir given with CICLOSPORIN

▸ Mycophenolate: plasma concentration of aciclovir increased by MYCOPHENOLATE, also plasma concentration of inactive metabolite of mycophenolate increased

▸ Tacrolimus: possible increased risk of nephrotoxicity when aciclovir given with TACROLIMUS

▸ Theophylline: aciclovir possibly increases plasma concentration of THEOPHYLLINE

Acitretin *see* Retinoids

Aclidinium *see* Antimuscarinics

Acrivastine *see* Antihistamines

Adalimumab

▸ Abatacept: increased risk of side-effects when adalimumab given with ABATACEPT

● Anakinra: avoid concomitant use of adalimumab with
  ● ANAKINRA

● Antipsychotics: avoid concomitant use of cytotoxics with
  ● CLOZAPINE (increased risk of agranulocytosis)

● Vaccines: risk of generalised infections when monoclonal antibodies given with live ● VACCINES—avoid concomitant use

Adefovir

▸ Antivirals: avoidance of adefovir advised by manufacturer of TENOFOVIR

▸ Interferons: manufacturer of adefovir advises caution with PEGINTERFERON ALFA

Adenosine

NOTE Possibility of interaction with drugs tending to impair myocardial conduction

▸ Aminophylline: anti-arrhythmic effect of adenosine antagonised by AMINOPHYLLINE—manufacturer of adenosine advises avoid aminophylline for 24 hours before adenosine

▸ Anaesthetics, Local: increased myocardial depression when anti-arrhythmics given with BUPIVACAINE, LEVOBUPIVACAINE, PRILOCAINE or ROPIVACAINE

▸ Anti-arrhythmics: increased myocardial depression when anti-arrhythmics given with other ● ANTI-ARRHYTHMICS

▸ Antipsychotics: increased risk of ventricular arrhythmias when anti-arrhythmics given with ● ANTIPSYCHOTICS that prolong the QT interval

▸ Beta-blockers: increased myocardial depression when anti-arrhythmics given with ● BETA-BLOCKERS

▸ Caffeine citrate: anti-arrhythmic effect of adenosine antagonised by CAFFEINE CITRATE—manufacturer of adenosine advises avoid caffeine citrate for at least 12 hours before adenosine

▸ Dipyridamole: effect of adenosine enhanced and extended by
  ● DIPYRIDAMOLE (important risk of toxicity)—reduce dose of adenosine, see p. 73

▸ Nicotine: effects of adenosine possibly enhanced by NICOTINE

▸ Theophylline: anti-arrhythmic effect of adenosine antagonised by THEOPHYLLINE—manufacturer of adenosine advises avoid theophylline for 24 hours before adenosine

Adrenaline (epinephrine) *see* Sympathomimetics

Adrenergic Neurone Blockers

Alcohol: enhanced hypotensive effect when adrenergic neurone blockers given with ALCOHOL

Alpha-blockers: enhanced hypotensive effect when adrenergic neurone blockers given with ALPHA-BLOCKERS

● Anaesthetics, General: enhanced hypotensive effect when adrenergic neurone blockers given with ● GENERAL ANAESTHETICS

Analgesics: hypotensive effect of adrenergic neurone blockers antagonised by NSAIDs

Angiotensin-II Receptor Antagonists: enhanced hypotensive effect when adrenergic neurone blockers given with ANGIOTENSIN-II RECEPTOR ANTAGONISTS

Adrenergic Neurone Blockers (continued)

▸ Antidepressants: enhanced hypotensive effect when adrenergic neurone blockers given with MAOIs; hypotensive effect of adrenergic neurone blockers antagonised by TRICYCLICS

▸ Antipsychotics: hypotensive effect of adrenergic neurone blockers antagonised by HALOPERIDOL; hypotensive effect of adrenergic neurone blockers antagonised by higher doses of CHLORPROMAZINE; enhanced hypotensive effect when adrenergic neurone blockers given with PHENOTHIAZINES

▸ Anxiolytics and Hypnotics: enhanced hypotensive effect when adrenergic neurone blockers given with ANXIOLYTICS AND HYPNOTICS

▸ Beta-blockers: enhanced hypotensive effect when adrenergic neurone blockers given with BETA-BLOCKERS

▸ Calcium-channel Blockers: enhanced hypotensive effect when adrenergic neurone blockers given with CALCIUM-CHANNEL BLOCKERS

▸ Clonidine: enhanced hypotensive effect when adrenergic neurone blockers given with CLONIDINE

▸ Corticosteroids: hypotensive effect of adrenergic neurone blockers antagonised by CORTICOSTEROIDS

▸ Diazoxide: enhanced hypotensive effect when adrenergic neurone blockers given with DIAZOXIDE

▸ Diuretics: enhanced hypotensive effect when adrenergic neurone blockers given with DIURETICS

▸ Dopaminergics: enhanced hypotensive effect when adrenergic neurone blockers given with CO-BENELDOPA, CO-CARELDOPA or LEVODOPA

▸ Methyldopa: enhanced hypotensive effect when adrenergic neurone blockers given with METHYLDOPA

▸ Moxisylyte: enhanced hypotensive effect when adrenergic neurone blockers given with MOXISYLYTE

▸ Moxonidine: enhanced hypotensive effect when adrenergic neurone blockers given with MOXONIDINE

▸ Muscle Relaxants: enhanced hypotensive effect when adrenergic neurone blockers given with BACLOFEN or TIZANIDINE

▸ Nitrates: enhanced hypotensive effect when adrenergic neurone blockers given with NITRATES

▸ Oestrogens: hypotensive effect of adrenergic neurone blockers antagonised by OESTROGENS

▸ Pizotifen: hypotensive effect of adrenergic neurone blockers antagonised by PIZOTIFEN

▸ Prostaglandins: enhanced hypotensive effect when adrenergic neurone blockers given with ALPROSTADIL

● Sympathomimetics: increased risk of hypertension when guanethidine given with ● ADRENALINE (EPINEPHRINE); hypotensive effect of guanethidine antagonised by
  ● DEXAMFETAMINE and ● LISDEXAMFETAMINE; hypotensive effect of adrenergic neurone blockers antagonised by ● EPHEDRINE,
  ● ISOMETHEPTENE, ● METARAMINOL, ● METHYLPHENIDATE,
  ● NORADRENALINE (NOREPINEPHRINE), ● OXYMETAZOLINE,
  ● PHENYLEPHRINE, ● PSEUDOEPHEDRINE and ● XYLOMETAZOLINE; avoidance of guanethidine advised by manufacturer of MIDODRINE

▸ Vasodilator Antihypertensives: enhanced hypotensive effect when adrenergic neurone blockers given with HYDRALAZINE, MINOXIDIL or SODIUM NITROPRUSSIDE

Adsorbents *see* Kaolin

Afatinib

▸ Anti-arrhythmics: plasma concentration of afatinib possibly increased by AMIODARONE—manufacturer of afatinib advises separating administration of amiodarone by 6 to 12 hours

▸ Antibacterials: plasma concentration of afatinib possibly increased by ERYTHROMYCIN—manufacturer of afatinib advises separating administration of erythromycin by 6 to 12 hours; plasma concentration of afatinib reduced by RIFAMPICIN

▸ Antifungals: plasma concentration of afatinib possibly increased by ITRACONAZOLE and KETOCONAZOLE—manufacturer of afatinib advises separating administration of itraconazole and ketoconazole by 6 to 12 hours

● Antipsychotics: avoid concomitant use of cytotoxics with
  ● CLOZAPINE (increased risk of agranulocytosis)

▸ Antivirals: plasma concentration of afatinib increased by RITONAVIR—manufacturer of afatinib advises separating administration of ritonavir by 6 to 12 hours; plasma

A1

Interactions | Appendix 1

A1

Interactions | Appendix 1

Afatinib

Antivirals (continued)
concentration of afatinib possibly increased by SAQUINAVIR—manufacturer of afatinib advises separating administration of saquinavir by 6 to 12 hours
▸ **Calcium-channel Blockers:** plasma concentration of afatinib possibly increased by VERAPAMIL—manufacturer of afatinib advises separating administration of verapamil by 6 to 12 hours
▸ **Ciclosporin:** plasma concentration of afatinib possibly increased by CICLOSPORIN—manufacturer of afatinib advises separating administration of ciclosporin by 6 to 12 hours
▸ **Tacrolimus:** plasma concentration of afatinib possibly increased by TACROLIMUS—manufacturer of afatinib advises separating administration of tacrolimus by 6 to 12 hours

Agalsidase Alfa and Beta

▸ **Anti-arrhythmics:** effects of agalsidase alfa and beta possibly inhibited by AMIODARONE (manufacturers of agalsidase alfa and beta advise avoid concomitant use)
▸ **Antibacterials:** effects of agalsidase alfa and beta possibly inhibited by GENTAMICIN (manufacturers of agalsidase alfa and beta advise avoid concomitant use)
▸ **Antimalarials:** effects of agalsidase alfa and beta possibly inhibited by CHLOROQUINE and HYDROXYCHLOROQUINE (manufacturers of agalsidase alfa and beta advise avoid concomitant use)

Agomelatine

● **Antibacterials:** manufacturer of agomelatine advises avoid concomitant use with ● CIPROFLOXACIN
● **Antidepressants:** metabolism of agomelatine inhibited by ● FLUVOXAMINE (increased plasma concentration)
● **Antimalarials:** avoidance of antidepressants advised by manufacturer of ● ARTEMETHER WITH LUMEFANTRINE and ● ARTENIMOL WITH PIPERAQUINE
▸ **Atomoxetine:** possible increased risk of convulsions when antidepressants given with ATOMOXETINE

Albendazole

▸ **Anthelmintics:** plasma concentration of both drugs possibly reduced when albendazole given with LEVAMISOLE
● **Antiepileptics:** plasma concentration of albendazole reduced by ● CARBAMAZEPINE, ● FOSPHENYTOIN, ● PHENOBARBITAL, ● PHENYTOIN and ● PRIMIDONE—consider increasing albendazole dose when given for systemic infections
● **Antivirals:** plasma concentration of active metabolite of albendazole reduced by ● RITONAVIR—consider increasing albendazole dose when given for systemic infections
▸ **Corticosteroids:** plasma concentration of active metabolite of albendazole increased by DEXAMETHASONE
▸ **Grapefruit Juice:** plasma concentration of active metabolite of albendazole increased by GRAPEFRUIT JUICE
▸ **Ulcer-healing Drugs:** effects of albendazole possibly enhanced by CIMETIDINE

Albiglutide see Antidiabetics

Alcohol

▸ **ACE Inhibitors:** enhanced hypotensive effect when alcohol given with ACE INHIBITORS
▸ **Adrenergic Neurone Blockers:** enhanced hypotensive effect when alcohol given with ADRENERGIC NEURONE BLOCKERS
▸ **Alpha-blockers:** increased sedative effect when alcohol given with INDORAMIN; enhanced hypotensive effect when alcohol given with ALPHA-BLOCKERS
▸ **Analgesics:** enhanced hypotensive and sedative effects when alcohol given with OPIOID ANALGESICS
▸ **Angiotensin-II Receptor Antagonists:** enhanced hypotensive effect when alcohol given with ANGIOTENSIN-II RECEPTOR ANTAGONISTS
▸ **Anthelmintics:** possibility of disulfiram-like reaction when alcohol given with LEVAMISOLE
▸ **Antibacterials:** disulfiram-like reaction when alcohol given with METRONIDAZOLE; possibility of disulfiram-like reaction when alcohol given with TINIDAZOLE; increased risk of convulsions when alcohol given with ● CYCLOSERINE
● **Anticoagulants:** major changes in consumption of alcohol may affect anticoagulant control with ● COUMARINS or ● PHENINDIONE

Alcohol (continued)

● **Antidepressants:** some beverages containing alcohol and some dealcoholised beverages contain tyramine which interacts with ● MAOIS (hypertensive crisis)—if no tyramine, enhanced hypotensive effect; sedative effects possibly increased when alcohol given with SSRIS; increased sedative effect when alcohol given with ● MIRTAZAPINE, ●TRICYCLIC-RELATED ANTIDEPRESSANTS or ● TRICYCLICS
▸ **Antidiabetics:** alcohol enhances hypoglycaemic effect of ANTIDIABETICS; increased risk of lactic acidosis when alcohol given with METFORMIN
▸ **Antiepileptics:** alcohol possibly increases CNS side-effects of CARBAMAZEPINE; chronic heavy consumption of alcohol possibly reduces plasma concentration of FOSPHENYTOIN and PHENYTOIN; increased sedative effect when alcohol given with PHENOBARBITAL or PRIMIDONE; increased risk of blurred vision when alcohol given with RETIGABINE
▸ **Antifungals:** possibility of disulfiram-like reaction when alcohol given with KETOCONAZOLE; effects of alcohol possibly enhanced by GRISEOFULVIN
▸ **Antihistamines:** increased sedative effect when alcohol given with ANTIHISTAMINES (possibly less effect with non-sedating antihistamines)
▸ **Antimuscarinics:** increased sedative effect when alcohol given with HYOSCINE
▸ **Antipsychotics:** increased sedative effect when alcohol given with ANTIPSYCHOTICS
▸ **Anxiolytics and Hypnotics:** increased sedative effect when alcohol given with ANXIOLYTICS AND HYPNOTICS
▸ **Avanafil:** possible enhanced hypotensive effect when alcohol given with AVANAFIL
▸ **Beta-blockers:** enhanced hypotensive effect when alcohol given with BETA-BLOCKERS
▸ **Calcium-channel Blockers:** enhanced hypotensive effect when alcohol given with CALCIUM-CHANNEL BLOCKERS; plasma concentration of alcohol possibly increased by VERAPAMIL
▸ **Clonidine:** enhanced hypotensive effect when alcohol given with CLONIDINE
● **Cytotoxics:** disulfiram-like reaction when alcohol given with PROCARBAZINE; avoidance of alcohol advised by manufacturer of ● TRABECTEDIN
● **Dapoxetine:** increased sedative effect when alcohol given with ● DAPOXETINE
▸ **Diazoxide:** enhanced hypotensive effect when alcohol given with DIAZOXIDE
▸ **Disulfiram:** disulfiram reaction when alcohol given with DISULFIRAM
▸ **Diuretics:** enhanced hypotensive effect when alcohol given with DIURETICS
▸ **Dopaminergics:** alcohol reduces tolerance to BROMOCRIPTINE
▸ **Guanfacine:** sedative effects possibly increased when alcohol given with GUANFACINE
▸ **Lipid-regulating Drugs:** avoidance of alcohol advised by manufacturer of LOMITAPIDE
▸ **Lofexidine:** increased sedative effect when alcohol given with LOFEXIDINE
▸ **Methyldopa:** enhanced hypotensive effect when alcohol given with METHYLDOPA
▸ **Metoclopramide:** absorption of alcohol possibly increased by METOCLOPRAMIDE
▸ **Moxonidine:** enhanced hypotensive effect when alcohol given with MOXONIDINE
▸ **Muscle Relaxants:** increased sedative effect when alcohol given with BACLOFEN, METHOCARBAMOL or TIZANIDINE
▸ **Nicorandil:** alcohol possibly enhances hypotensive effect of NICORANDIL
▸ **Nitrates:** enhanced hypotensive effect when alcohol given with NITRATES
● **Paraldehyde:** increased sedative effect when alcohol given with ● PARALDEHYDE
▸ **Retinoids:** presence of alcohol causes etretinate to be formed from ● ACITRETIN (increased risk of teratogenicity in women of child-bearing potential)
▸ **Sympathomimetics:** alcohol possibly enhances effects of METHYLPHENIDATE

Alcohol (continued)

▸ Vasodilator Antihypertensives: enhanced hypotensive effect when alcohol given with HYDRALAZINE, MINOXIDIL or SODIUM NITROPRUSSIDE

Aldesleukin

▸ ACE Inhibitors: enhanced hypotensive effect when aldesleukin given with ACE INHIBITORS

▸ Alpha-blockers: enhanced hypotensive effect when aldesleukin given with ALPHA-BLOCKERS

▸ Angiotensin-II Receptor Antagonists: enhanced hypotensive effect when aldesleukin given with ANGIOTENSIN-II RECEPTOR ANTAGONISTS

▸ Antivirals: aldesleukin possibly increases plasma concentration of INDINAVIR

▸ Beta-blockers: enhanced hypotensive effect when aldesleukin given with BETA-BLOCKERS

▸ Calcium-channel Blockers: enhanced hypotensive effect when aldesleukin given with CALCIUM-CHANNEL BLOCKERS

▸ Clonidine: enhanced hypotensive effect when aldesleukin given with CLONIDINE

● Corticosteroids: manufacturer of aldesleukin advises avoid concomitant use with ● CORTICOSTEROIDS

● Cytotoxics: manufacturer of aldesleukin advises avoid concomitant use with ● CISPLATIN, ● DACARBAZINE and ● VINBLASTINE

▸ Diazoxide: enhanced hypotensive effect when aldesleukin given with DIAZOXIDE

▸ Diuretics: enhanced hypotensive effect when aldesleukin given with DIURETICS

▸ Methyldopa: enhanced hypotensive effect when aldesleukin given with METHYLDOPA

▸ Moxonidine: enhanced hypotensive effect when aldesleukin given with MOXONIDINE

▸ Nitrates: enhanced hypotensive effect when aldesleukin given with NITRATES

▸ Vasodilator Antihypertensives: enhanced hypotensive effect when aldesleukin given with HYDRALAZINE, MINOXIDIL or SODIUM NITROPRUSSIDE

Alemtuzumab

● Antipsychotics: avoid concomitant use of cytotoxics with ● CLOZAPINE (increased risk of agranulocytosis)

● Vaccines: risk of generalised infections when monoclonal antibodies given with live ● VACCINES—avoid concomitant use

Alendronic Acid see Bisphosphonates

Alfacalcidol see Vitamins

Alfentanil see Opioid Analgesics

Alfuzosin see Alpha-blockers

Alimemazine see Antihistamines

Aliskiren

● ACE Inhibitors: increased risk of hyperkalaemia, hypotension, and impaired renal function when aliskiren given with ● ACE INHIBITORS—avoid concomitant use

▸ Analgesics: hypotensive effect of aliskiren possibly antagonised by NSAIDs

● Angiotensin-II Receptor Antagonists: increased risk of hyperkalaemia, hypotension, and impaired renal function when aliskiren given with ● ANGIOTENSIN-II RECEPTOR ANTAGONISTS—avoid concomitant use; plasma concentration of aliskiren possibly reduced by IRBESARTAN

▸ Antibacterials: plasma concentration of aliskiren reduced by RIFAMPICIN

● Anticoagulants: increased risk of hyperkalaemia when aliskiren given with HEPARINS

● Antifungals: plasma concentration of aliskiren increased by KETOCONAZOLE; plasma concentration of aliskiren increased by ● ITRACONAZOLE—avoid concomitant use

▸ Calcium-channel Blockers: plasma concentration of aliskiren increased by VERAPAMIL

● Ciclosporin: plasma concentration of aliskiren increased by ● CICLOSPORIN—avoid concomitant use

● Diuretics: aliskiren reduces plasma concentration of FUROSEMIDE; increased risk of hyperkalaemia when aliskiren given with POTASSIUM-SPARING DIURETICS AND ALDOSTERONE ANTAGONISTS

● Grapefruit Juice: plasma concentration of aliskiren reduced by ● GRAPEFRUIT JUICE—avoid concomitant use

Aliskiren (continued)

▸ Potassium Salts: increased risk of hyperkalaemia when aliskiren given with POTASSIUM SALTS

Alitretinoin see Retinoids

Alkylating Drugs see Bendamustine, Busulfan, Carmustine, Cyclophosphamide, Estramustine, Ifosfamide, Lomustine, Melphalan, and Thiotepa

Allopurinol

▸ ACE Inhibitors: manufacturers state possible increased risk of leucopenia and hypersensitivity reactions when allopurinol given with ACE INHIBITORS especially in renal impairment

▸ Aminophylline: allopurinol possibly increases plasma concentration of AMINOPHYLLINE

▸ Antibacterials: increased risk of rash when allopurinol given with AMOXICILLIN, AMPICILLIN or CO-AMOXICLAV

▸ Anticoagulants: allopurinol possibly enhances anticoagulant effect of COUMARINS

● Antivirals: allopurinol increases plasma concentration of ● DIDANOSINE (risk of toxicity)—avoid concomitant use

● Azathioprine: allopurinol enhances effects and increases toxicity of ● AZATHIOPRINE (reduce dose of azathioprine to one quarter of usual dose)

▸ Ciclosporin: allopurinol possibly increases plasma concentration of CICLOSPORIN (risk of nephrotoxicity)

● Cytotoxics: avoidance of allopurinol advised by manufacturer of ● CAPECITABINE; allopurinol enhances effects and increases toxicity of ● MERCAPTOPURINE (reduce dose of mercaptopurine to one quarter of usual dose)

▸ Diuretics: increased risk of hypersensitivity when allopurinol given with THIAZIDES AND RELATED DIURETICS especially in renal impairment

▸ Theophylline: allopurinol possibly increases plasma concentration of THEOPHYLLINE

Almotriptan see 5HT$_1$-receptor Agonists (under HT)

Alogliptin see Antidiabetics

Alpha$_2$-adrenoceptor Stimulants see Apraclonidine, Brimonidine, Clonidine, and Methyldopa

Alpha-blockers

▸ ACE Inhibitors: enhanced hypotensive effect when alpha-blockers given with ACE INHIBITORS

▸ Adrenergic Neurone Blockers: enhanced hypotensive effect when alpha-blockers given with ADRENERGIC NEURONE BLOCKERS

▸ Alcohol: enhanced hypotensive effect when alpha-blockers given with ALCOHOL; increased sedative effect when indoramin given with ALCOHOL

▸ Aldesleukin: enhanced hypotensive effect when alpha-blockers given with ALDESLEUKIN

● Anaesthetics, General: enhanced hypotensive effect when alpha-blockers given with ● GENERAL ANAESTHETICS

▸ Analgesics: hypotensive effect of alpha-blockers antagonised by NSAIDs

▸ Angiotensin-II Receptor Antagonists: enhanced hypotensive effect when alpha-blockers given with ANGIOTENSIN-II RECEPTOR ANTAGONISTS

● Antidepressants: manufacturer of indoramin advises avoid concomitant use with ● MAOIs; enhanced hypotensive effect when alpha-blockers given with MAOIs

● Antifungals: plasma concentration of alfuzosin possibly increased by KETOCONAZOLE; plasma concentration of tamsulosin increased by ● KETOCONAZOLE

▸ Antipsychotics: enhanced hypotensive effect when alpha-blockers given with ANTIPSYCHOTICS

● Antivirals: plasma concentration of doxazosin and tamsulosin possibly increased by BOCEPREVIR—manufacturer of boceprevir advises avoid concomitant use; plasma concentration of alfuzosin possibly increased by ● RITONAVIR—avoid concomitant use; avoidance of alfuzosin advised by manufacturer of ● TELAPREVIR

▸ Anxiolytics and Hypnotics: enhanced hypotensive and sedative effects when alpha-blockers given with ANXIOLYTICS AND HYPNOTICS

● Avanafil: enhanced hypotensive effect when alpha-blockers given with ● AVANAFIL—when patient is stable on the alpha blocker initiate avanafil at the lowest possible dose

A1

Interactions | Appendix 1

Alpha-blockers (continued)
- Beta-blockers: enhanced hypotensive effect when alpha-blockers given with • BETA-BLOCKERS, also increased risk of first-dose hypotension with post-synaptic alpha-blockers such as prazosin
- Calcium-channel Blockers: enhanced hypotensive effect when alpha-blockers given with • CALCIUM-CHANNEL BLOCKERS, also increased risk of first-dose hypotension with post-synaptic alpha-blockers such as prazosin; plasma concentration of tamsulosin increased by VERAPAMIL
▹ Cardiac Glycosides: prazosin increases plasma concentration of DIGOXIN
▹ Clonidine: enhanced hypotensive effect when alpha-blockers given with CLONIDINE
- Cobicistat: plasma concentration of alfuzosin possibly increased by • COBICISTAT—manufacturer of cobicistat advises avoid concomitant use
▹ Corticosteroids: hypotensive effect of alpha-blockers antagonised by CORTICOSTEROIDS
▹ Cytotoxics: avoidance of alfuzosin advised by manufacturer of IDELALISIB
▹ Diazoxide: enhanced hypotensive effect when alpha-blockers given with DIAZOXIDE
• Diuretics: enhanced hypotensive effect when alpha-blockers given with • DIURETICS, also increased risk of first-dose hypotension with post-synaptic alpha-blockers such as prazosin
▹ Dopaminergics: enhanced hypotensive effect when alpha-blockers given with CO-BENELDOPA, CO-CARELDOPA or LEVODOPA
▹ Methyldopa: enhanced hypotensive effect when alpha-blockers given with METHYLDOPA
• Moxisylyte: possible severe postural hypotension when alpha-blockers given with • MOXISYLYTE
▹ Moxonidine: enhanced hypotensive effect when alpha-blockers given with MOXONIDINE
▹ Muscle Relaxants: enhanced hypotensive effect when alpha-blockers given with BACLOFEN or TIZANIDINE
▹ Nitrates: enhanced hypotensive effect when alpha-blockers given with NITRATES
▹ Oestrogens: hypotensive effect of alpha-blockers antagonised by OESTROGENS
▹ Prostaglandins: enhanced hypotensive effect when alpha-blockers given with ALPROSTADIL
• Sildenafil: enhanced hypotensive effect when alpha-blockers given with • SILDENAFIL (avoid alpha-blockers for 4 hours after sildenafil)—when patient is stable on the alpha blocker initiate sildenafil at the lowest possible dose
• Sympathomimetics: avoid concomitant use of tolazoline with • ADRENALINE (EPINEPHRINE) or • DOPAMINE; alpha-blockers possibly antagonise effects of MIDODRINE
• Tadalafil: enhanced hypotensive effect when alpha-blockers given with • TADALAFIL—when patient is stable on the alpha blocker initiate tadalafil at the lowest possible dose; enhanced hypotensive effect when doxazosin given with • TADALAFIL—manufacturer of tadalafil advises avoid concomitant use
• Ulcer-healing Drugs: effects of tolazoline antagonised by • CIMETIDINE and • RANITIDINE
• Vardenafil: enhanced hypotensive effect when alpha-blockers given with • VARDENAFIL—when patient is stable on the alpha blocker initiate vardenafil at the lowest possible dose—separate doses by 6 hours (except with tamsulosin)
▹ Vasodilator Antihypertensives: enhanced hypotensive effect when alpha-blockers given with HYDRALAZINE, MINOXIDIL or SODIUM NITROPRUSSIDE

Alpha-blockers (post-synaptic) see Alpha-blockers
Alprazolam see Anxiolytics and Hypnotics
Alprostadil see Prostaglandins
Aluminium Hydroxide see Antacids
Amantadine
▹ Antimalarials: plasma concentration of amantadine possibly increased by QUININE
▹ Antipsychotics: increased risk of extrapyramidal side-effects when amantadine given with ANTIPSYCHOTICS
▹ Bupropion: increased risk of side-effects when amantadine given with BUPROPION

Amantadine (continued)
• Memantine: increased risk of CNS toxicity when amantadine given with • MEMANTINE (manufacturer of memantine advises avoid concomitant use); effects of dopaminergics possibly enhanced by MEMANTINE
▹ Methyldopa: increased risk of extrapyramidal side-effects when amantadine given with METHYLDOPA; antiparkinsonian effect of dopaminergics antagonised by METHYLDOPA
▹ Tetrabenazine: increased risk of extrapyramidal side-effects when amantadine given with TETRABENAZINE

Ambrisentan
▹ Antibacterials: plasma concentration of ambrisentan possibly increased by RIFAMPICIN
• Ciclosporin: plasma concentration of ambrisentan increased by • CICLOSPORIN (see under Ambrisentan, in BNF)

Amikacin see Aminoglycosides
Amiloride see Diuretics
Aminoglycosides
▹ Agalsidase Alfa and Beta: gentamicin possibly inhibits effects of AGALSIDASE ALFA AND BETA (manufacturers of agalsidase alfa and beta advise avoid concomitant use)
▹ Analgesics: plasma concentration of amikacin and gentamicin in neonates possibly increased by INDOMETACIN
• Antibacterials: neomycin reduces absorption of PHENOXYMETHYLPENICILLIN; increased risk of nephrotoxicity when aminoglycosides given with COLISTIMETHATE SODIUM or POLYMYXINS; increased risk of nephrotoxicity and ototoxicity when aminoglycosides given with CAPREOMYCIN or • VANCOMYCIN; possible increased risk of nephrotoxicity when aminoglycosides given with CEPHALOSPORINS
• Anticoagulants: experience in anticoagulant clinics suggests that INR possibly altered when neomycin (given for local action on gut) is given with • COUMARINS or • PHENINDIONE
▹ Antidiabetics: neomycin possibly enhances hypoglycaemic effect of ACARBOSE, also severity of gastro-intestinal effects increased
▹ Antifungals: increased risk of nephrotoxicity when aminoglycosides given with AMPHOTERICIN
▹ Bisphosphonates: increased risk of hypocalcaemia when aminoglycosides given with BISPHOSPHONATES
▹ Cardiac Glycosides: gentamicin possibly increases plasma concentration of DIGOXIN; neomycin reduces absorption of DIGOXIN
• Ciclosporin: increased risk of nephrotoxicity when aminoglycosides given with • CICLOSPORIN
• Cytotoxics: neomycin possibly reduces absorption of METHOTREXATE; neomycin reduces bioavailability of SORAFENIB; increased risk of nephrotoxicity and possibly of ototoxicity when aminoglycosides given with • PLATINUM COMPOUNDS
• Diuretics: increased risk of ototoxicity when aminoglycosides given with • LOOP DIURETICS
▹ Mannitol: manufacturer of tobramycin advises avoid concomitant use with MANNITOL
• Muscle Relaxants: aminoglycosides enhance effects of • NON-DEPOLARISING MUSCLE RELAXANTS and • SUXAMETHONIUM
▹ Parasympathomimetics: aminoglycosides antagonise effects of • NEOSTIGMINE and • PYRIDOSTIGMINE
• Tacrolimus: increased risk of nephrotoxicity when aminoglycosides given with • TACROLIMUS
▹ Vaccines: antibacterials inactivate ORAL TYPHOID VACCINE—see under Typhoid Vaccine in BNF
▹ Vitamins: neomycin possibly reduces absorption of VITAMIN A

Aminophylline
▹ Allopurinol: plasma concentration of aminophylline possibly increased by ALLOPURINOL
▹ Anaesthetics, General: increased risk of convulsions when aminophylline given with KETAMINE
▹ Anti-arrhythmics: aminophylline antagonises anti-arrhythmic effect of ADENOSINE—manufacturer of adenosine advises avoid aminophylline for 24 hours before adenosine; plasma concentration of aminophylline increased by PROPAFENONE
• Antibacterials: plasma concentration of aminophylline possibly increased by CLARITHROMYCIN and ISONIAZID; plasma concentration of aminophylline increased by • ERYTHROMYCIN (also aminophylline may reduce absorption of *oral*

Aminophylline

- **Antibacterials** (continued)
erythromycin); plasma concentration of aminophylline increased by ● CIPROFLOXACIN and ● NORFLOXACIN; metabolism of aminophylline accelerated by RIFAMPICIN (reduced plasma concentration); possible increased risk of convulsions when aminophylline given with ● QUINOLONES
- **Antidepressants:** plasma concentration of aminophylline increased by ● FLUVOXAMINE (concomitant use should usually be avoided, but where not possible halve aminophylline dose and monitor plasma-aminophylline concentration); plasma concentration of aminophylline possibly reduced by ST JOHN'S WORT
- **Antiepileptics:** metabolism of aminophylline accelerated by CARBAMAZEPINE, ● PHENOBARBITAL and ● PRIMIDONE (reduced effect); plasma concentration of both drugs reduced when aminophylline given with ● FOSPHENYTOIN and ● PHENYTOIN
- **Antifungals:** plasma concentration of aminophylline possibly increased by ● FLUCONAZOLE and ● KETOCONAZOLE
- **Antivirals:** plasma concentration of aminophylline possibly increased by ACICLOVIR and VALACICLOVIR; metabolism of aminophylline accelerated by ● RITONAVIR (reduced plasma concentration)
- **Anxiolytics and Hypnotics:** aminophylline possibly reduces effects of BENZODIAZEPINES
- **Caffeine citrate:** avoidance of aminophylline advised by manufacturer of CAFFEINE CITRATE
- **Calcium-channel Blockers:** plasma concentration of aminophylline possibly increased by ● CALCIUM-CHANNEL BLOCKERS (enhanced effect); plasma concentration of aminophylline increased by DILTIAZEM; plasma concentration of aminophylline increased by ● VERAPAMIL (enhanced effect)
- **Corticosteroids:** increased risk of hypokalaemia when aminophylline given with CORTICOSTEROIDS
- **Cytotoxics:** plasma concentration of aminophylline possibly increased by METHOTREXATE
- **Deferasirox:** plasma concentration of aminophylline increased by ● DEFERASIROX (consider reducing dose of aminophylline)
- **Disulfiram:** metabolism of aminophylline inhibited by DISULFIRAM (increased risk of toxicity)
- **Diuretics:** increased risk of hypokalaemia when aminophylline given with ACETAZOLAMIDE, LOOP DIURETICS or THIAZIDES AND RELATED DIURETICS
- **Doxapram:** increased CNS stimulation when aminophylline given with DOXAPRAM
- **Interferons:** metabolism of aminophylline inhibited by ● INTERFERON ALFA and ● PEGINTERFERON ALFA (consider reducing dose of aminophylline)
- **Leukotriene Receptor Antagonists:** plasma concentration of aminophylline possibly increased by ZAFIRLUKAST, also plasma concentration of zafirlukast reduced
- **Lithium:** aminophylline increases excretion of LITHIUM (reduced plasma concentration)
- **Oestrogens:** plasma concentration of aminophylline increased by OESTROGENS (consider reducing dose of aminophylline)
- **Pentoxifylline:** plasma concentration of aminophylline increased by PENTOXIFYLLINE
- **Roflumilast:** avoidance of aminophylline advised by manufacturer of ROFLUMILAST
- **Sulfinpyrazone:** plasma concentration of aminophylline reduced by SULFINPYRAZONE
- **Sympathomimetics:** manufacturer of aminophylline advises avoid concomitant use with EPHEDRINE in children
- **Sympathomimetics, Beta$_2$:** increased risk of hypokalaemia when aminophylline given with high doses of BETA$_2$ SYMPATHOMIMETICS
- **Ulcer-healing Drugs:** metabolism of aminophylline inhibited by ● CIMETIDINE (increased plasma concentration); absorption of aminophylline possibly reduced by SUCRALFATE (give at least 2 hours apart)
- **Vaccines:** plasma concentration of aminophylline possibly increased by INFLUENZA VACCINE

Aminosalicylates *see* individual drugs

Amiodarone

NOTE Amiodarone has a long half-life; there is a potential for drug interactions to occur for several weeks (or even months) after treatment with it has been stopped

- **Agalsidase Alfa and Beta:** amiodarone possibly inhibits effects of AGALSIDASE ALFA AND BETA (manufacturers of agalsidase alfa and beta advise avoid concomitant use)
- **Anaesthetics, Local:** increased myocardial depression when anti-arrhythmics given with BUPIVACAINE, LEVOBUPIVACAINE, PRILOCAINE or ROPIVACAINE
- **Anti-arrhythmics:** increased myocardial depression when anti-arrhythmics given with other ● ANTI-ARRHYTHMICS; increased risk of ventricular arrhythmias when amiodarone given with ● DISOPYRAMIDE or ● DRONEDARONE—avoid concomitant use; amiodarone increases plasma concentration of ● FLECAINIDE (halve dose of flecainide)
- **Antibacterials:** increased risk of ventricular arrhythmias when amiodarone given with *parenteral* ● ERYTHROMYCIN—avoid concomitant use; increased risk of ventricular arrhythmias when amiodarone given with ● LEVOFLOXACIN or ● MOXIFLOXACIN—avoid concomitant use; possible increased risk of ventricular arrhythmias when amiodarone given with SULFAMETHOXAZOLE and TRIMETHOPRIM (as co-trimoxazole)—manufacturer of amiodarone advises avoid concomitant use of co-trimoxazole; increased risk of ventricular arrhythmias when amiodarone given with ● DELAMANID; avoidance of amiodarone advised by manufacturer of ● FIDAXOMICIN; possible increased risk of ventricular arrhythmias when amiodarone given with ● TELITHROMYCIN
- **Anticoagulants:** amiodarone inhibits metabolism of ● COUMARINS and ● PHENINDIONE (enhanced anticoagulant effect); amiodarone increases plasma concentration of ● DABIGATRAN (see under Dabigatran Etexilate, in BNF)
- **Antidepressants:** avoidance of amiodarone advised by manufacturer of ● CITALOPRAM, ● ESCITALOPRAM and ● VENLAFAXINE (risk of ventricular arrhythmias); increased risk of ventricular arrhythmias when amiodarone given with ● TRICYCLICS—avoid concomitant use
- **Antiepileptics:** amiodarone inhibits metabolism of ● FOSPHENYTOIN and ● PHENYTOIN (increased plasma concentration)
- **Antihistamines:** increased risk of ventricular arrhythmias when amiodarone given with ● MIZOLASTINE—avoid concomitant use
- **Antimalarials:** avoidance of amiodarone advised by manufacturer of ● ARTEMETHER WITH LUMEFANTRINE (risk of ventricular arrhythmias); avoidance of amiodarone advised by manufacturer of ● ARTENIMOL WITH PIPERAQUINE (possible risk of ventricular arrhythmias); increased risk of ventricular arrhythmias when amiodarone given with ● CHLOROQUINE, ● HYDROXYCHLOROQUINE, ● MEFLOQUINE or ● QUININE—avoid concomitant use
- **Antimuscarinics:** increased risk of ventricular arrhythmias when amiodarone given with ● TOLTERODINE
- **Antipsychotics:** increased risk of ventricular arrhythmias when anti-arrhythmics that prolong the QT interval given with ● ANTIPSYCHOTICS that prolong the QT interval; increased risk of ventricular arrhythmias when amiodarone given with ● BENPERIDOL—manufacturer of benperidol advises avoid concomitant use; increased risk of ventricular arrhythmias when amiodarone given with ● AMISULPRIDE, ● DROPERIDOL, ● HALOPERIDOL, ● PHENOTHIAZINES, ● PIMOZIDE or ● ZUCLOPENTHIXOL—avoid concomitant use; increased risk of ventricular arrhythmias when amiodarone given with ● SULPIRIDE
- **Antivirals:** plasma concentration of amiodarone possibly increased by ● ATAZANAVIR; possible increased risk of bradycardia when amiodarone given with ● DACLATASVIR, ● LEDIPASVIR and ● SIMEPREVIR (with sofosbuvir)—see under Amiodarone, in BNF; plasma concentration of amiodarone possibly increased by ● FOSAMPRENAVIR (increased risk of ventricular arrhythmias—avoid concomitant use); plasma concentration of amiodarone possibly increased by ● INDINAVIR—avoid concomitant use; plasma concentration of amiodarone increased by ● RITONAVIR (increased risk of ventricular arrhythmias—avoid concomitant use); increased risk of ventricular arrhythmias when amiodarone given with

A1

Interactions | Appendix 1

Amiodarone

- **Antivirals** (continued)
  - SAQUINAVIR—avoid concomitant use; possible increased risk of bradycardia when amiodarone given with • SOFOSBUVIR— see under Amiodarone, in BNF; avoidance of amiodarone advised by manufacturer of • TELAPREVIR (risk of ventricular arrhythmias)
- **Atomoxetine:** increased risk of ventricular arrhythmias when amiodarone given with • ATOMOXETINE
- **Beta-blockers:** increased risk of bradycardia, AV block and myocardial depression when amiodarone given with • BETA-BLOCKERS; increased myocardial depression when anti-arrhythmics given with • BETA-BLOCKERS; increased risk of ventricular arrhythmias when amiodarone given with • SOTALOL—avoid concomitant use
- **Calcium-channel Blockers:** increased risk of bradycardia, AV block and myocardial depression when amiodarone given with • DILTIAZEM or • VERAPAMIL
- **Cardiac Glycosides:** amiodarone increases plasma concentration of • DIGOXIN (halve dose of digoxin)
- ▸ **Ciclosporin:** amiodarone possibly increases plasma concentration of CICLOSPORIN
- **Cobicistat:** plasma concentration of amiodarone possibly increased by • COBICISTAT—manufacturer of cobicistat advises avoid concomitant use
- **Colchicine:** amiodarone possibly increases risk of • COLCHICINE toxicity
- **Cytotoxics:** amiodarone possibly increases the plasma concentration of AFATINIB—manufacturer of afatinib advises separating administration of amiodarone by 6 to 12 hours; possible increased risk of ventricular arrhythmias when amiodarone given with • BOSUTINIB; amiodarone possibly increases the plasma concentration of • IBRUTINIB—reduce dose of ibrutinib (see under Ibrutinib, in BNF); avoidance of amiodarone advised by manufacturer of IDELALISIB; possible increased risk of ventricular arrhythmias when amiodarone given with • VANDETANIB—avoid concomitant use; increased risk of ventricular arrhythmias when amiodarone given with • ARSENIC TRIOXIDE
- ▸ **Diuretics:** increased cardiac toxicity with amiodarone if hypokalaemia occurs with ACETAZOLAMIDE, LOOP DIURETICS or THIAZIDES AND RELATED DIURETICS; amiodarone increases plasma concentration of EPLERENONE (reduce dose of eplerenone)
- **Fingolimod:** possible increased risk of bradycardia when amiodarone given with • FINGOLIMOD
- ▸ **Grapefruit Juice:** plasma concentration of amiodarone increased by GRAPEFRUIT JUICE
- **Ivabradine:** increased risk of ventricular arrhythmias when amiodarone given with • IVABRADINE
- **Lipid-regulating Drugs:** increased risk of myopathy when amiodarone given with • SIMVASTATIN (see under Simvastatin, p. 125); separating administration from amiodarone by 12 hours advised by manufacturer of LOMITAPIDE
- **Lithium:** manufacturer of amiodarone advises avoid concomitant use with • LITHIUM (risk of ventricular arrhythmias)
- ▸ **Orlistat:** plasma concentration of amiodarone possibly reduced by ORLISTAT
- **Pentamidine Isetionate:** increased risk of ventricular arrhythmias when amiodarone given with • PENTAMIDINE ISETIONATE—avoid concomitant use
- ▸ **Tacrolimus:** amiodarone possibly increases plasma concentration of TACROLIMUS
- ▸ **Thyroid Hormones:** amiodarone can affect serum concentrations of THYROID HORMONES—monitor thyroid function closely
- ▸ **Ulcer-healing Drugs:** plasma concentration of amiodarone increased by CIMETIDINE

Amisulpride see Antipsychotics
Amitriptyline see Antidepressants, Tricyclic
Amlodipine see Calcium-channel Blockers
Amoxicillin see Penicillins
Amphotericin
  NOTE Close monitoring required with concomitant administration of nephrotoxic drugs or cytotoxics

Amphotericin (continued)

- ▸ **Antibacterials:** increased risk of nephrotoxicity when amphotericin given with AMINOGLYCOSIDES or POLYMYXINS; possible increased risk of nephrotoxicity when amphotericin given with VANCOMYCIN
- ▸ **Antifungals:** amphotericin reduces renal excretion and increases cellular uptake of FLUCYTOSINE (toxicity possibly increased); effects of amphotericin possibly antagonised by IMIDAZOLES and TRIAZOLES; plasma concentration of amphotericin possibly increased by MICAFUNGIN
- **Cardiac Glycosides:** hypokalaemia caused by amphotericin increases cardiac toxicity with • CARDIAC GLYCOSIDES
- **Ciclosporin:** increased risk of nephrotoxicity when amphotericin given with • CICLOSPORIN
- **Corticosteroids:** increased risk of hypokalaemia when amphotericin given with • CORTICOSTEROIDS—avoid concomitant use unless corticosteroids needed to control reactions
- **Cytotoxics:** increased risk of ventricular arrhythmias when amphotericin given with • ARSENIC TRIOXIDE
- ▸ **Diuretics:** increased risk of hypokalaemia when amphotericin given with LOOP DIURETICS or THIAZIDES AND RELATED DIURETICS
- ▸ **Pentamidine Isetionate:** possible increased risk of nephrotoxicity when amphotericin given with PENTAMIDINE ISETIONATE
- **Sodium Stibogluconate:** possible increased risk of arrhythmias when amphotericin given after • SODIUM STIBOGLUCONATE— manufacturer of sodium stibogluconate advises giving 14 days apart
- **Tacrolimus:** increased risk of nephrotoxicity when amphotericin given with • TACROLIMUS

Ampicillin see Penicillins
Anabolic Steroids
- **Anticoagulants:** anabolic steroids enhance anticoagulant effect of • COUMARINS and • PHENINDIONE
- ▸ **Antidiabetics:** anabolic steroids possibly enhance hypoglycaemic effect of ANTIDIABETICS

Anaesthetics, General
  NOTE See also Surgery and Long-term Medication, under General Anaesthesia in BNFC

- ▸ **ACE Inhibitors:** enhanced hypotensive effect when general anaesthetics given with ACE INHIBITORS
- **Adrenergic Neurone Blockers:** enhanced hypotensive effect when general anaesthetics given with • ADRENERGIC NEURONE BLOCKERS
- **Alpha-blockers:** enhanced hypotensive effect when general anaesthetics given with • ALPHA-BLOCKERS
- ▸ **Aminophylline:** increased risk of convulsions when ketamine given with AMINOPHYLLINE
- ▸ **Analgesics:** metabolism of etomidate inhibited by FENTANYL (consider reducing dose of etomidate); effects of thiopental possibly enhanced by ASPIRIN; effects of intravenous general anaesthetics and volatile liquid general anaesthetics possibly enhanced by OPIOID ANALGESICS
- ▸ **Angiotensin-II Receptor Antagonists:** enhanced hypotensive effect when general anaesthetics given with ANGIOTENSIN-II RECEPTOR ANTAGONISTS
- ▸ **Antibacterials:** increased risk of hepatotoxicity when isoflurane given with ISONIAZID; effects of thiopental enhanced by SULFONAMIDES; hypersensitivity-like reactions can occur when general anaesthetics given with *intravenous* VANCOMYCIN
- ▸ **Antidepressants:** increased risk of arrhythmias and hypotension when general anaesthetics given with TRICYCLICS
- ▸ **Antipsychotics:** enhanced hypotensive effect when general anaesthetics given with • ANTIPSYCHOTICS; effects of thiopental enhanced by DROPERIDOL
- ▸ **Anxiolytics and Hypnotics:** increased sedative effect when general anaesthetics given with ANXIOLYTICS AND HYPNOTICS
- ▸ **Beta-blockers:** enhanced hypotensive effect when general anaesthetics given with BETA-BLOCKERS
- **Calcium-channel Blockers:** enhanced hypotensive effect when general anaesthetics or isoflurane given with CALCIUM-CHANNEL BLOCKERS; general anaesthetics enhance hypotensive effect of • VERAPAMIL (AV delay)
- ▸ **Clonidine:** enhanced hypotensive effect when general anaesthetics given with CLONIDINE

Anaesthetics, General (continued)

- Cytotoxics: nitrous oxide increases antifolate effect of
  - METHOTREXATE—avoid concomitant use
▹ Diazoxide: enhanced hypotensive effect when general anaesthetics given with DIAZOXIDE
▹ Diuretics: enhanced hypotensive effect when general anaesthetics given with DIURETICS
- Dopaminergics: increased risk of arrhythmias when volatile liquid general anaesthetics given with ● CO-BENELDOPA, ● CO-CARELDOPA or ● LEVODOPA
- Doxapram: increased risk of arrhythmias when volatile liquid general anaesthetics given with ● DOXAPRAM (avoid doxapram for at least 10 minutes after volatile liquid general anaesthetics)
- Memantine: increased risk of CNS toxicity when ketamine given with ● MEMANTINE (manufacturer of memantine advises avoid concomitant use)
▹ Methyldopa: enhanced hypotensive effect when general anaesthetics given with METHYLDOPA
▹ Metoclopramide: effects of thiopental enhanced by METOCLOPRAMIDE
▹ Moxonidine: enhanced hypotensive effect when general anaesthetics given with MOXONIDINE
- Muscle Relaxants: increased risk of myocardial depression and bradycardia when propofol given with ● SUXAMETHONIUM; volatile liquid general anaesthetics enhance effects of NON-DEPOLARISING MUSCLE RELAXANTS and SUXAMETHONIUM; ketamine enhances effects of ATRACURIUM
▹ Nitrates: enhanced hypotensive effect when general anaesthetics given with NITRATES
▹ Oxytocin: oxytocic effect possibly reduced, also enhanced hypotensive effect and risk of arrhythmias when volatile liquid general anaesthetics given with OXYTOCIN
- Sympathomimetics: manufacturer of isoflurane advises avoid concomitant use with ● SYMPATHOMIMETICS (risk of ventricular arrhythmias); increased risk of arrhythmias when volatile liquid general anaesthetics given with ● ADRENALINE (EPINEPHRINE) or ● NORADRENALINE (NOREPINEPHRINE); increased risk of hypertension when volatile liquid general anaesthetics given with ● METHYLPHENIDATE
▹ Theophylline: increased risk of convulsions when ketamine given with THEOPHYLLINE
▹ Vasodilator Antihypertensives: enhanced hypotensive effect when general anaesthetics given with HYDRALAZINE, MINOXIDIL or SODIUM NITROPRUSSIDE

Anaesthetics, General (intravenous) see Anaesthetics, General

Anaesthetics, General (volatile liquids) see Anaesthetics, General

Anaesthetics, Local see Bupivacaine, Chloroprocaine, Levobupivacaine, Lidocaine, Prilocaine, and Ropivacaine

Anagrelide
- Cilostazol: manufacturer of anagrelide advises avoid concomitant use with ● CILOSTAZOL
- Phosphodiesterase Type-3 Inhibitors: manufacturer of anagrelide advises avoid concomitant use with ● ENOXIMONE and ● MILRINONE

Anakinra
- Cytotoxics: avoid concomitant use of anakinra with ● ADALIMUMAB, ● CERTOLIZUMAB PEGOL, ● GOLIMUMAB or ● INFLIXIMAB
- Etanercept: avoid concomitant use of anakinra with ● ETANERCEPT
- Vaccines: risk of generalised infections when anakinra given with live ● VACCINES—avoid concomitant use

Analgesics see Aspirin, Nefopam, NSAIDs, Opioid Analgesics, and Paracetamol

Angiotensin-II Receptor Antagonists
- ACE Inhibitors: increased risk of hyperkalaemia, hypotension, and impaired renal function when angiotensin-II receptor antagonists given with ● ACE INHIBITORS—avoid concomitant use
▹ Adrenergic Neurone Blockers: enhanced hypotensive effect when angiotensin-II receptor antagonists given with ADRENERGIC NEURONE BLOCKERS
▹ Alcohol: enhanced hypotensive effect when angiotensin-II receptor antagonists given with ALCOHOL

Angiotensin-II Receptor Antagonists (continued)

▹ Aldesleukin: enhanced hypotensive effect when angiotensin-II receptor antagonists given with ALDESLEUKIN
- Aliskiren: increased risk of hyperkalaemia, hypotension, and impaired renal function when angiotensin-II receptor antagonists given with ● ALISKIREN—avoid concomitant use; irbesartan possibly reduces plasma concentration of ALISKIREN
▹ Alpha-blockers: enhanced hypotensive effect when angiotensin-II receptor antagonists given with ALPHA-BLOCKERS
▹ Anaesthetics, General: enhanced hypotensive effect when angiotensin-II receptor antagonists given with GENERAL ANAESTHETICS
▹ Analgesics: increased risk of renal impairment when angiotensin-II receptor antagonists given with NSAIDs, also hypotensive effect antagonised
▹ Antibacterials: plasma concentration of losartan and its active metabolite reduced by RIFAMPICIN; possible increased risk of hyperkalaemia when angiotensin-II receptor antagonists given with TRIMETHOPRIM
▹ Anticoagulants: increased risk of hyperkalaemia when angiotensin-II receptor antagonists given with HEPARINS
▹ Antidepressants: hypotensive effect of angiotensin-II receptor antagonists possibly enhanced by MAOIs
▹ Antipsychotics: enhanced hypotensive effect when angiotensin-II receptor antagonists given with ANTIPSYCHOTICS
▹ Antivirals: when given with valsartan manufacturer of PARITAPREVIR advises reduce dose of paritaprevir
▹ Anxiolytics and Hypnotics: enhanced hypotensive effect when angiotensin-II receptor antagonists given with ANXIOLYTICS AND HYPNOTICS
▹ Beta-blockers: enhanced hypotensive effect when angiotensin-II receptor antagonists given with BETA-BLOCKERS
▹ Calcium-channel Blockers: enhanced hypotensive effect when angiotensin-II receptor antagonists given with CALCIUM-CHANNEL BLOCKERS
- Ciclosporin: increased risk of hyperkalaemia when angiotensin-II receptor antagonists given with ● CICLOSPORIN
▹ Clonidine: enhanced hypotensive effect when angiotensin-II receptor antagonists given with CLONIDINE
- Corticosteroids: hypotensive effect of angiotensin-II receptor antagonists antagonised by CORTICOSTEROIDS
▹ Diazoxide: enhanced hypotensive effect when angiotensin-II receptor antagonists given with DIAZOXIDE
▹ Diuretics: enhanced hypotensive effect when angiotensin-II receptor antagonists given with ● DIURETICS; valsartan reduces plasma concentration of FUROSEMIDE; increased risk of severe hyperkalaemia when angiotensin-II receptor antagonists given with ● AMILORIDE, ● POTASSIUM CANRENOATE or ● TRIAMTERENE; increased risk of severe hyperkalaemia when angiotensin-II receptor antagonists given with ● EPLERENONE and ● SPIRONOLACTONE—avoid concurrent use or use lowest possible doses of both drugs
- Dopaminergics: enhanced hypotensive effect when angiotensin-II receptor antagonists given with CO-BENELDOPA, CO-CARELDOPA or LEVODOPA
- Lithium: angiotensin-II receptor antagonists reduce excretion of ● LITHIUM (increased plasma concentration)
▹ Methyldopa: enhanced hypotensive effect when angiotensin-II receptor antagonists given with METHYLDOPA
▹ Moxisylyte: enhanced hypotensive effect when angiotensin-II receptor antagonists given with MOXISYLYTE
▹ Moxonidine: enhanced hypotensive effect when angiotensin-II receptor antagonists given with MOXONIDINE
▹ Muscle Relaxants: enhanced hypotensive effect when angiotensin-II receptor antagonists given with BACLOFEN or TIZANIDINE
▹ Nitrates: enhanced hypotensive effect when angiotensin-II receptor antagonists given with NITRATES
▹ Oestrogens: hypotensive effect of angiotensin-II receptor antagonists antagonised by OESTROGENS
- Potassium Salts: increased risk of hyperkalaemia when angiotensin-II receptor antagonists given with ● POTASSIUM SALTS
▹ Prostaglandins: enhanced hypotensive effect when angiotensin-II receptor antagonists given with ALPROSTADIL

A1

Interactions | Appendix 1

Angiotensin-II Receptor Antagonists (continued)

▸ Tacrolimus: increased risk of hyperkalaemia when angiotensin-II receptor antagonists given with TACROLIMUS

▸ Vasodilator Antihypertensives: enhanced hypotensive effect when angiotensin-II receptor antagonists given with HYDRALAZINE, MINOXIDIL or SODIUM NITROPRUSSIDE

Antacids

NOTE Antacids should preferably not be taken at the same time as other drugs since they may impair absorption

▸ ACE Inhibitors: antacids possibly reduce absorption of ACE INHIBITORS; antacids reduce absorption of CAPTOPRIL, ENALAPRIL and FOSINOPRIL

▸ Analgesics: antacids possibly reduce absorption of ACEMETACIN; alkaline urine due to some antacids increases excretion of ASPIRIN

▸ Anthelmintics: sodium bicarbonate reduces excretion of DIETHYLCARBAMAZINE

▸ Antibacterials: antacids reduce absorption of CEFACLOR, ISONIAZID, NORFLOXACIN and RIFAMPICIN; antacids reduce absorption of AZITHROMYCIN (give at least 2 hours before or 1 hour after antacids); antacids reduce absorption of CIPROFLOXACIN and LEVOFLOXACIN (give at least 2 hours before or 4 hours after ciprofloxacin and levofloxacin); antacids reduce absorption of MOXIFLOXACIN (give at least 6 hours apart); antacids reduce absorption of OFLOXACIN (give at least 2 hours apart); avoid concomitant use of antacids with METHENAMINE; oral magnesium salts (as magnesium trisilicate) reduce absorption of NITROFURANTOIN; antacids possibly reduce absorption of TETRACYCLINES (give at least 2 to 3 hours apart)

▸ Antiepileptics: antacids reduce absorption of FOSPHENYTOIN, GABAPENTIN and PHENYTOIN

▸ Antifungals: antacids reduce absorption of ITRACONAZOLE and KETOCONAZOLE

▸ Antihistamines: antacids reduce absorption of FEXOFENADINE

▸ Antimalarials: antacids reduce absorption of CHLOROQUINE and HYDROXYCHLOROQUINE; oral magnesium salts (as magnesium trisilicate) reduce absorption of PROGUANIL

▸ Antipsychotics: antacids reduce absorption of PHENOTHIAZINES and SULPIRIDE

▸ Antivirals: antacids reduce absorption of ATAZANAVIR (give at least 2 hours before or 1 hour after antacids); aluminium hydroxide reduces absorption of DOLUTEGRAVIR—manufacturer of dolutegravir advises give at least 2 hours before or 6 hours after aluminium hydroxide; oral magnesium salts reduce absorption of DOLUTEGRAVIR—manufacturer of dolutegravir advises give at least 2 hours before or 6 hours after oral magnesium salts; aluminium hydroxide reduces absorption of ELVITEGRAVIR (give at least 4 hours apart); oral magnesium salts reduce absorption of ELVITEGRAVIR (give at least 4 hours apart); separating administration from antacids by 4 hours advised by manufacturer of LEDIPASVIR; oral magnesium salts reduce plasma concentration of RALTEGRAVIR—manufacturer of raltegravir advises avoid concomitant use; aluminium hydroxide reduces plasma concentration of RALTEGRAVIR—manufacturer of raltegravir advises avoid concomitant use; manufacturer of rilpivirine advises give antacids 2 hours before or 4 hours after RILPIVIRINE; antacids reduce absorption of TIPRANAVIR (give at least 2 hours apart)

▸ Bile Acids: antacids possibly reduce absorption of BILE ACIDS; aluminium hydroxide probably reduces effects of CHOLIC ACID (manufacturer of cholic acid advises give at least 5 hours apart)

▸ Bisphosphonates: antacids reduce absorption of BISPHOSPHONATES

▸ Cardiac Glycosides: antacids possibly reduce absorption of DIGOXIN

▸ Corticosteroids: antacids reduce absorption of DEFLAZACORT

● Cytotoxics: aluminium hydroxide and oral magnesium salts possibly reduce absorption of ESTRAMUSTINE—manufacturer of estramustine advises avoid concomitant administration; separating administration with antacids by about 12 hours advised by manufacturer of BOSUTINIB; antacids possibly reduce plasma concentration of ● ERLOTINIB—give antacids at least 4 hours before or 2 hours after erlotinib

Antacids (continued)

▸ Deferasirox: antacids containing aluminium possibly reduce absorption of DEFERASIROX (manufacturer of deferasirox advises avoid concomitant use)

▸ Deferiprone: antacids containing aluminium possibly reduce absorption of DEFERIPRONE (manufacturer of deferiprone advises avoid concomitant use)

▸ Dipyridamole: antacids possibly reduce absorption of DIPYRIDAMOLE

▸ Eltrombopag: antacids reduce absorption of ELTROMBOPAG (give at least 4 hours apart)

▸ Folates: antacids possibly reduce absorption of FOLIC ACID (manufacturer of folic acid advises give at least 2 hours apart)

▸ Iron Salts: oral magnesium salts (as magnesium trisilicate) reduce absorption of *oral* IRON SALTS

▸ Lipid-regulating Drugs: antacids reduce absorption of ROSUVASTATIN

▸ Lithium: sodium bicarbonate increases excretion of LITHIUM (reduced plasma concentration)

▸ Misoprostol: antacids possibly reduce absorption of MISOPROSTOL

▸ Mycophenolate: antacids reduce absorption of MYCOPHENOLATE

▸ Penicillamine: antacids reduce absorption of PENICILLAMINE

▸ Polystyrene Sulfonate Resins: risk of intestinal obstruction when aluminium hydroxide given with POLYSTYRENE SULFONATE RESINS; risk of metabolic alkalosis when oral magnesium salts given with POLYSTYRENE SULFONATE RESINS

▸ Riociguat: antacids reduce absorption of RIOCIGUAT (give at least 2 hours before or 1 hour after riociguat)

▸ Sympathomimetics: aluminium hydroxide possibly increases absorption of PSEUDOEPHEDRINE

▸ Thyroid Hormones: antacids possibly reduce absorption of LEVOTHYROXINE

▸ Ulcer-healing Drugs: antacids possibly reduce absorption of LANSOPRAZOLE

Antazoline *see* Antihistamines

Anthelmintics *see* individual drugs

Anthrax Vaccine *see* Vaccines

Anti-D Immunoglobulins *see* Immunoglobulins

Anti-arrhythmics *see* Adenosine, Amiodarone, Disopyramide, Dronedarone, Flecainide, Lidocaine, and Propafenone

Antibacterials *see* individual drugs

Antibiotics (cytotoxic) *see* Bleomycin, Daunorubicin, Doxorubicin, Epirubicin, Idarubicin, Mitomycin, Mitoxantrone, and Pixantrone

Anticoagulants *see* Apixaban, Argatroban, Bivalirudin, Coumarins, Dabigatran, Danaparoid, Edoxaban, Fondaparinux, Heparins, Phenindione, and Rivaroxaban

Antidepressants *see* Agomelatine; Antidepressants, SSRI; Antidepressants, Tricyclic; Antidepressants, Tricyclic (related); MAOIs; Mirtazapine; Moclobemide; Reboxetine; St John's Wort; Venlafaxine; Vortioxetine

Antidepressants, Noradrenaline Re-uptake Inhibitors *see* Reboxetine

Antidepressants, SSRI

NOTE *see also* Dapoxetine

▸ Alcohol: sedative effects possibly increased when SSRIs given with ALCOHOL

● Aminophylline: fluvoxamine increases plasma concentration of ● AMINOPHYLLINE (concomitant use should usually be avoided, but where not possible halve aminophylline dose and monitor plasma-aminophylline concentration)

▸ Anaesthetics, Local: fluvoxamine inhibits metabolism of ROPIVACAINE—avoid prolonged administration of ropivacaine

● Analgesics: increased risk of bleeding when SSRIs given with ● NSAIDs or ● ASPIRIN; possible increased serotonergic effects when SSRIs given with FENTANYL; fluoxetine, fluvoxamine, paroxetine and sertraline possibly increase plasma concentration of METHADONE; increased risk of CNS toxicity when SSRIs given with ● TRAMADOL

● Anti-arrhythmics: manufacturer of citalopram and escitalopram advises avoid concomitant use with ● AMIODARONE (risk of ventricular arrhythmias); manufacturer of citalopram and escitalopram advises avoid concomitant use with ● DISOPYRAMIDE (risk of ventricular arrhythmias); manufacturer of citalopram and escitalopram advises avoid

Antidepressants, SSRI
- **Anti-arrhythmics** (continued)
  concomitant use with ● DRONEDARONE (risk of ventricular arrhythmias); fluoxetine increases plasma concentration of FLECAINIDE; fluoxetine and paroxetine possibly inhibit metabolism of PROPAFENONE
- **Antibacterials:** manufacturer of citalopram and escitalopram advises avoid concomitant use with *intravenous* ● ERYTHROMYCIN (risk of ventricular arrhythmias); manufacturer of citalopram and escitalopram advises avoid concomitant use with ● MOXIFLOXACIN (risk of ventricular arrhythmias); possible increased risk of ventricular arrhythmias when citalopram given with ● TELITHROMYCIN
- **Anticoagulants:** SSRIs possibly enhance anticoagulant effect of ● COUMARINS; possible increased risk of bleeding when SSRIs given with ● DABIGATRAN
- **Antidepressants:** avoidance of fluvoxamine advised by manufacturer of ● REBOXETINE; possible increased serotonergic effects when SSRIs given with DULOXETINE; fluvoxamine inhibits metabolism of ● DULOXETINE—avoid concomitant use; citalopram, escitalopram, fluvoxamine, paroxetine or sertraline should not be started until 2 weeks after stopping ● MAOIS, also MAOIs should not be started until at least 1 week after stopping citalopram, escitalopram, fluvoxamine, paroxetine or sertraline; fluoxetine should not be started until 2 weeks after stopping ● MAOIS, also MAOIs should not be started until at least 5 weeks after stopping fluoxetine; CNS effects of SSRIs increased by ● MAOIS (risk of serious toxicity); increased risk of CNS toxicity when escitalopram given with ● MOCLOBEMIDE, preferably avoid concomitant use; after stopping citalopram, fluvoxamine, paroxetine or sertraline do not start ● MOCLOBEMIDE for at least 1 week; after stopping fluoxetine do not start ● MOCLOBEMIDE for 5 weeks; increased serotonergic effects when SSRIs given with ● ST JOHN'S WORT—avoid concomitant use; fluvoxamine inhibits metabolism of ● AGOMELATINE (increased plasma concentration); possible increased serotonergic effects when fluoxetine or fluvoxamine given with MIRTAZAPINE; SSRIs increase plasma concentration of some ● TRICYCLICS; manufacturer of citalopram and escitalopram advises avoid concomitant use with ● TRICYCLICS (risk of ventricular arrhythmias); possible increased risk of convulsions when SSRIs given with ● VORTIOXETINE; fluoxetine and paroxetine possibly increase plasma concentration of VORTIOXETINE (consider reducing dose of vortioxetine)
- **Antiepileptics:** SSRIs antagonise anticonvulsant effect of ● ANTIEPILEPTICS (convulsive threshold lowered); fluoxetine and fluvoxamine increase plasma concentration of ● CARBAMAZEPINE; fluoxetine and fluvoxamine increase plasma concentration of ● FOSPHENYTOIN; plasma concentration of sertraline possibly reduced by FOSPHENYTOIN and PHENYTOIN, also plasma concentration of fosphenytoin and phenytoin possibly increased; plasma concentration of paroxetine reduced by FOSPHENYTOIN, PHENOBARBITAL, PHENYTOIN and PRIMIDONE; fluoxetine and fluvoxamine increase plasma concentration of ● PHENYTOIN
- **Antifungals:** plasma concentration of paroxetine possibly increased by TERBINAFINE
- **Antihistamines:** manufacturer of citalopram and escitalopram advises avoid concomitant use with ● MIZOLASTINE (risk of ventricular arrhythmias); antidepressant effect of SSRIs possibly antagonised by CYPROHEPTADINE
- **Antimalarials:** avoidance of antidepressants advised by manufacturer of ● ARTEMETHER WITH LUMEFANTRINE and ● ARTENIMOL WITH PIPERAQUINE; possible increased risk of ventricular arrhythmias when citalopram or escitalopram given with ● ARTEMETHER WITH LUMEFANTRINE—avoid concomitant use; possible increased risk of ventricular arrhythmias when citalopram or escitalopram given with ● ARTENIMOL WITH PIPERAQUINE—avoid concomitant use; possible increased risk of ventricular arrhythmias when citalopram and escitalopram given with ● CHLOROQUINE; possible increased risk of ventricular arrhythmias when citalopram or escitalopram given with ● QUININE—avoid concomitant use

Antidepressants, SSRI (continued)
- **Antimuscarinics:** paroxetine increases plasma concentration of DARIFENACIN and PROCYCLIDINE
- **Antipsychotics:** avoidance of fluoxetine, fluvoxamine and sertraline advised by manufacturer of ● DROPERIDOL (risk of ventricular arrhythmias); manufacturer of citalopram and escitalopram advises avoid concomitant use with ● HALOPERIDOL (risk of ventricular arrhythmias); fluoxetine increases plasma concentration of ● CLOZAPINE, ● HALOPERIDOL and RISPERIDONE; fluvoxamine possibly increases plasma concentration of ASENAPINE and HALOPERIDOL; paroxetine inhibits metabolism of PERPHENAZINE (reduce dose of perphenazine); fluoxetine and paroxetine possibly increase plasma concentration of ● ARIPIPRAZOLE (reduce dose of aripiprazole—consult aripiprazole product literature); plasma concentration of paroxetine possibly increased by ASENAPINE; fluvoxamine, paroxetine and sertraline increase plasma concentration of ● CLOZAPINE; citalopram possibly increases plasma concentration of CLOZAPINE (increased risk of toxicity); fluvoxamine increases plasma concentration of OLANZAPINE; manufacturer of citalopram and escitalopram advises avoid concomitant use with ● PHENOTHIAZINES (risk of ventricular arrhythmias); manufacturer of citalopram and escitalopram advises avoid concomitant use with ● PIMOZIDE (risk of ventricular arrhythmias); SSRIs possibly increase plasma concentration of ● PIMOZIDE (increased risk of ventricular arrhythmias—avoid concomitant use); paroxetine possibly increases plasma concentration of RISPERIDONE (increased risk of toxicity)
- **Antivirals:** plasma concentration of paroxetine and sertraline possibly reduced by DARUNAVIR; plasma concentration of SSRIs possibly increased by ● RITONAVIR; plasma concentration of paroxetine possibly reduced by RITONAVIR
- **Anxiolytics and Hypnotics:** fluoxetine increases plasma concentration of ALPRAZOLAM; fluvoxamine increases plasma concentration of some BENZODIAZEPINES; fluvoxamine increases plasma concentration of ● MELATONIN—avoid concomitant use; sedative effects possibly increased when sertraline given with ZOLPIDEM
- **Atomoxetine:** possible increased risk of convulsions when antidepressants given with ATOMOXETINE; fluoxetine and paroxetine possibly inhibit metabolism of ATOMOXETINE
- **Beta-blockers:** citalopram and escitalopram increase plasma concentration of METOPROLOL; paroxetine possibly increases the plasma concentration of ● METOPROLOL—increased risk of AV block (manufacturer of paroxetine advises avoid concomitant use in cardiac insufficiency); fluvoxamine increases plasma concentration of PROPRANOLOL; increased risk of ventricular arrhythmias when citalopram given with ● SOTALOL—avoid concomitant use; manufacturer of escitalopram advises avoid concomitant use with ● SOTALOL (risk of ventricular arrhythmias)
- **Bupropion:** plasma concentration of citalopram possibly increased by BUPROPION
- **Calcium-channel Blockers:** fluoxetine possibly inhibits metabolism of NIFEDIPINE (increased plasma concentration)
- **Clopidogrel:** fluoxetine and fluvoxamine possibly reduce antiplatelet effect of ● CLOPIDOGREL
- **Dapoxetine:** possible increased risk of serotonergic effects when SSRIs given with ● DAPOXETINE (manufacturer of dapoxetine advises SSRIs should not be started until 1 week after stopping dapoxetine, avoid dapoxetine for 2 weeks after stopping SSRIs)
- **Dopaminergics:** increased risk of CNS toxicity when SSRIs given with ● RASAGILINE; fluvoxamine should not be started until 2 weeks after stopping ● RASAGILINE; fluoxetine should not be started until 2 weeks after stopping ● RASAGILINE, also rasagiline should not be started until at least 5 weeks after stopping fluoxetine; avoidance of citalopram and escitalopram advised by manufacturer of SELEGILINE; increased risk of hypertension and CNS excitation when fluvoxamine or sertraline given with ● SELEGILINE (selegiline should not be started until 1 week after stopping fluvoxamine or sertraline, avoid fluvoxamine or sertraline for 2 weeks after stopping selegiline); increased risk of hypertension and CNS excitation when paroxetine given with ● SELEGILINE (selegiline

Antidepressants, SSRI

● **Dopaminergics** (continued)
should not be started until 2 weeks after stopping paroxetine; avoid paroxetine for 2 weeks after stopping selegiline); increased risk of hypertension and CNS excitation when fluoxetine given with ● SELEGILINE (selegiline should not be started until 5 weeks after stopping fluoxetine, avoid fluoxetine for 2 weeks after stopping selegiline)

▸ Grapefruit Juice: plasma concentration of sertraline possibly increased by GRAPEFRUIT JUICE

● **Hormone Antagonists:** fluoxetine and paroxetine possibly inhibit metabolism of ● TAMOXIFEN to active metabolite (avoid concomitant use)

● **5HT₁-receptor Agonists:** increased risk of CNS toxicity when citalopram given with ● 5HT₁ AGONISTS (manufacturer of citalopram advises avoid concomitant use); fluvoxamine inhibits the metabolism of FROVATRIPTAN; possible increased serotonergic effects when SSRIs given with NARATRIPTAN; CNS toxicity reported when sertraline given with SUMATRIPTAN; increased risk of CNS toxicity when citalopram, escitalopram, fluoxetine, fluvoxamine or paroxetine given with ● SUMATRIPTAN; fluvoxamine possibly inhibits metabolism of ZOLMITRIPTAN (reduce dose of zolmitriptan)

● **5HT₃-receptor Antagonists:** possible increased serotonergic effects when SSRIs given with 5HT₃ ANTAGONISTS

▸ **Lipid-regulating Drugs:** separating administration from fluoxetine and fluvoxamine by 12 hours advised by manufacturer of ● LOMITAPIDE

● **Lithium:** Increased risk of CNS effects when SSRIs given with ● LITHIUM (lithium toxicity reported)

● **Methylthioninium:** risk of CNS toxicity when SSRIs given with ● METHYLTHIONINIUM—avoid concomitant use (if avoidance not possible, use lowest possible dose of methylthioninium and observe patient for up to 4 hours after administration)

▸ **Metoclopramide:** CNS toxicity reported when SSRIs given with METOCLOPRAMIDE

● **Muscle Relaxants:** fluvoxamine increases plasma concentration of ● TIZANIDINE (increased risk of toxicity)—avoid concomitant use

▸ **Parasympathomimetics:** paroxetine increases plasma concentration of GALANTAMINE

● **Pentamidine Isetionate:** manufacturer of citalopram and escitalopram advises avoid concomitant use with ● PENTAMIDINE ISETIONATE (risk of ventricular arrhythmias)

● **Pirfenidone:** fluvoxamine increases plasma concentration of ● PIRFENIDONE—manufacturer of pirfenidone advises avoid concomitant use

▸ **Pomalidomide:** fluvoxamine increases plasma concentration of ● POMALIDOMIDE

▸ **Ranolazine:** paroxetine increases plasma concentration of RANOLAZINE

▸ **Roflumilast:** fluvoxamine inhibits the metabolism of ROFLUMILAST

▸ **Sympathomimetics:** metabolism of SSRIs possibly inhibited by METHYLPHENIDATE

● **Theophylline:** fluvoxamine increases plasma concentration of ● THEOPHYLLINE (concomitant use should usually be avoided, but where not possible halve theophylline dose and monitor plasma-theophylline concentration)

▸ **Ticagrelor:** possible increased risk of bleeding when citalopram, paroxetine or sertraline given with TICAGRELOR

▸ **Ulcer-healing Drugs:** plasma concentration of citalopram, escitalopram and sertraline increased by CIMETIDINE; fluvoxamine possibly increases plasma concentration of LANSOPRAZOLE; plasma concentration of escitalopram increased by OMEPRAZOLE

Antidepressants, SSRI (related) *see* Duloxetine and Venlafaxine

Antidepressants, Tricyclic

▸ **Adrenergic Neurone Blockers:** tricyclics antagonise hypotensive effect of ADRENERGIC NEURONE BLOCKERS

● **Alcohol:** increased sedative effect when tricyclics given with ● ALCOHOL

▸ **Alpha₂-adrenoceptor Stimulants:** avoidance of tricyclics advised by manufacturer of APRACLONIDINE and BRIMONIDINE

● **Anaesthetics, General:** increased risk of arrhythmias and hypotension when tricyclics given with GENERAL ANAESTHETICS

Antidepressants, Tricyclic (continued)

● **Analgesics:** increased risk of CNS toxicity when tricyclics given with ● TRAMADOL; side-effects possibly increased when tricyclics given with NEFOPAM; sedative effects possibly increased when tricyclics given with OPIOID ANALGESICS

● **Anti-arrhythmics:** increased risk of ventricular arrhythmias when tricyclics given with ● AMIODARONE—avoid concomitant use; increased risk of ventricular arrhythmias when tricyclics given with ● DISOPYRAMIDE or ● FLECAINIDE; avoidance of tricyclics advised by manufacturer of ● DRONEDARONE (risk of ventricular arrhythmias); increased risk of arrhythmias when tricyclics given with ● PROPAFENONE

● **Antibacterials:** increased risk of ventricular arrhythmias when tricyclics given with ● MOXIFLOXACIN—avoid concomitant use; possible increased risk of ventricular arrhythmias when tricyclics that prolong the QT interval given with ● DELAMANID; possible increased risk of ventricular arrhythmias when tricyclics given with ● TELITHROMYCIN

● **Anticoagulants:** tricyclics may enhance or reduce anticoagulant effect of ● COUMARINS

● **Antidepressants:** avoidance of tricyclics advised by manufacturer of ● CITALOPRAM and ● ESCITALOPRAM (risk of ventricular arrhythmias); possible increased serotonergic effects when amitriptyline or clomipramine given with DULOXETINE; increased risk of hypertension and CNS excitation when tricyclics given with ● MAOIS, tricyclics should not be started until 2 weeks after stopping MAOIs (3 weeks if starting clomipramine or imipramine), also MAOIs should not be started for at least 1–2 weeks after stopping tricyclics (3 weeks in the case of clomipramine or imipramine); after stopping tricyclics do not start ● MOCLOBEMIDE for at least 1 week; plasma concentration of some tricyclics increased by ● SSRIS; plasma concentration of amitriptyline reduced by ST JOHN'S WORT; possible increased risk of convulsions when tricyclics given with ● VORTIOXETINE

● **Antiepileptics:** tricyclics antagonise anticonvulsant effect of ● ANTIEPILEPTICS (convulsive threshold lowered); metabolism of tricyclics accelerated by ● CARBAMAZEPINE (reduced plasma concentration and reduced effect); plasma concentration of tricyclics possibly reduced by ● FOSPHENYTOIN and ● PHENYTOIN; metabolism of tricyclics possibly accelerated by ● PHENOBARBITAL and ● PRIMIDONE (reduced plasma concentration)

● **Antifungals:** plasma concentration of amitriptyline and nortriptyline possibly increased by FLUCONAZOLE; plasma concentration of tricyclics possibly increased by TERBINAFINE

● **Antihistamines:** increased antimuscarinic and sedative effects when tricyclics given with ANTIHISTAMINES

● **Antimalarials:** avoidance of antidepressants advised by manufacturer of ● ARTEMETHER WITH LUMEFANTRINE and ● ARTENIMOL WITH PIPERAQUINE

▸ **Antimuscarinics:** increased risk of antimuscarinic side-effects when tricyclics given with ANTIMUSCARINICS

● **Antipsychotics:** avoidance of tricyclics advised by manufacturer of ● DROPERIDOL, ● FLUPHENAZINE, ● HALOPERIDOL, ● SULPIRIDE and ● ZUCLOPENTHIXOL (risk of ventricular arrhythmias); possible increased antimuscarinic side-effects when tricyclics given with CLOZAPINE; increased risk of antimuscarinic side-effects when tricyclics given with PHENOTHIAZINES; possible increased risk of ventricular arrhythmias when tricyclics given with ● RISPERIDONE

● **Antivirals:** plasma concentration of tricyclics possibly increased by ● RITONAVIR; increased risk of ventricular arrhythmias when tricyclics given with ● SAQUINAVIR—avoid concomitant use

▸ **Anxiolytics and Hypnotics:** increased sedative effect when tricyclics given with ANXIOLYTICS AND HYPNOTICS

● **Atomoxetine:** increased risk of ventricular arrhythmias when tricyclics given with ● ATOMOXETINE; possible increased risk of convulsions when antidepressants given with ATOMOXETINE

● **Beta-blockers:** plasma concentration of imipramine increased by LABETALOL and PROPRANOLOL; increased risk of ventricular arrhythmias when tricyclics given with ● SOTALOL

▸ **Bupropion:** plasma concentration of tricyclics possibly increased by BUPROPION (possible increased risk of convulsions)

Antidepressants, Tricyclic (continued)

▸ Calcium-channel Blockers: plasma concentration of imipramine increased by DILTIAZEM and VERAPAMIL; plasma concentration of tricyclics possibly increased by DILTIAZEM and VERAPAMIL

▸ Cannabis Extract: possible increased risk of hypertension and tachycardia when tricyclics given with CANNABIS EXTRACT

● Clonidine: tricyclics antagonise hypotensive effect of ● CLONIDINE, also increased risk of hypertension on clonidine withdrawal

● Cytotoxics: increased risk of ventricular arrhythmias when amitriptyline or clomipramine given with ● ARSENIC TRIOXIDE

● Dapoxetine: possible increased risk of serotonergic effects when tricyclics given with ● DAPOXETINE (manufacturer of dapoxetine advises tricyclics should not be started until 1 week after stopping dapoxetine, avoid dapoxetine for 2 weeks after stopping tricyclics)

▸ Disulfiram: metabolism of tricyclics inhibited by DISULFIRAM (increased plasma concentration); concomitant amitriptyline reported to increase DISULFIRAM reaction with alcohol

▸ Diuretics: increased risk of postural hypotension when tricyclics given with DIURETICS

▸ Dopaminergics: caution with tricyclics advised by manufacturer of ENTACAPONE; increased risk of CNS toxicity when tricyclics given with ● RASAGILINE; CNS toxicity reported when tricyclics given with ● SELEGILINE

▸ Histamine: tricyclics theoretically antagonise effects of HISTAMINE—manufacturer of histamine advises avoid concomitant use

▸ Lithium: risk of toxicity when tricyclics given with LITHIUM

▸ Methylthioninium: risk of CNS toxicity when clomipramine given with ● METHYLTHIONINIUM—avoid concomitant use (if avoidance not possible, use lowest possible dose of methylthioninium and observe patient for up to 4 hours after administration)

▸ Moxonidine: tricyclics possibly antagonise hypotensive effect of MOXONIDINE (manufacturer of moxonidine advises avoid concomitant use)

▸ Muscle Relaxants: tricyclics enhance muscle relaxant effect of BACLOFEN

▸ Nicorandil: tricyclics possibly enhance hypotensive effect of NICORANDIL

▸ Nitrates: tricyclics reduce effects of sublingual tablets of NITRATES (failure to dissolve under tongue owing to dry mouth)

● Oestrogens: antidepressant effect of tricyclics antagonised by OESTROGENS (but side-effects of tricyclics possibly increased due to increased plasma concentration)

● Pentamidine Isetionate: increased risk of ventricular arrhythmias when tricyclics given with ● PENTAMIDINE ISETIONATE

● Sodium Oxybate: increased risk of side-effects when tricyclics given with SODIUM OXYBATE

● Sympathomimetics: increased risk of hypertension and arrhythmias when tricyclics given with ● ADRENALINE (EPINEPHRINE) (but local anaesthetics with adrenaline appear to be safe); metabolism of tricyclics possibly inhibited by METHYLPHENIDATE; avoidance of tricyclics advised by manufacturer of MIDODRINE; increased risk of hypertension and arrhythmias when tricyclics given with ● NORADRENALINE (NOREPINEPHRINE) or PHENYLEPHRINE

▸ Thyroid Hormones: effects of tricyclics possibly enhanced by THYROID HORMONES; effects of amitriptyline and imipramine enhanced by THYROID HORMONES

▸ Ulcer-healing Drugs: plasma concentration of tricyclics possibly increased by CIMETIDINE; metabolism of amitriptyline, doxepin, imipramine and nortriptyline inhibited by CIMETIDINE (increased plasma concentration)

Antidepressants, Tricyclic (related)

● Alcohol: increased sedative effect when tricyclic-related antidepressants given with ● ALCOHOL

▸ Alpha$_2$-adrenoceptor Stimulants: avoidance of tricyclic-related antidepressants advised by manufacturer of APRACLONIDINE and BRIMONIDINE

▸ Antibacterials: plasma concentration of trazodone possibly increased by CLARITHROMYCIN

Antidepressants, Tricyclic (related) (continued)

▸ Anticoagulants: trazodone may enhance or reduce anticoagulant effect of WARFARIN

● Antidepressants: tricyclic-related antidepressants should not be started until 2 weeks after stopping ● MAOIS, also MAOIs should not be started until at least 1–2 weeks after stopping tricyclic-related antidepressants; after stopping tricyclic-related antidepressants do not start ● MOCLOBEMIDE for at least 1 week

● Antiepileptics: tricyclic-related antidepressants possibly antagonise anticonvulsant effect of ● ANTIEPILEPTICS (convulsive threshold lowered); plasma concentration of mianserin and trazodone reduced by ● CARBAMAZEPINE; plasma concentration of mianserin reduced by ● FOSPHENYTOIN and ● PHENYTOIN; metabolism of mianserin accelerated by ● PHENOBARBITAL and ● PRIMIDONE (reduced plasma concentration)

▸ Antihistamines: possible increased antimuscarinic and sedative effects when tricyclic-related antidepressants given with ANTIHISTAMINES

● Antimalarials: avoidance of antidepressants advised by manufacturer of ● ARTEMETHER WITH LUMEFANTRINE and ● ARTENIMOL WITH PIPERAQUINE

▸ Antimuscarinics: possible increased antimuscarinic side-effects when tricyclic-related antidepressants given with ANTIMUSCARINICS

● Antivirals: plasma concentration of trazodone increased by ● RITONAVIR (increased risk of toxicity); increased risk of ventricular arrhythmias when trazodone given with ● SAQUINAVIR—avoid concomitant use; plasma concentration of trazodone possibly increased by TELAPREVIR

▸ Anxiolytics and Hypnotics: increased sedative effect when tricyclic-related antidepressants given with ANXIOLYTICS AND HYPNOTICS

▸ Atomoxetine: possible increased risk of convulsions when antidepressants given with ATOMOXETINE

▸ Diazoxide: enhanced hypotensive effect when tricyclic-related antidepressants given with DIAZOXIDE

▸ Nitrates: tricyclic-related antidepressants possibly reduce effects of sublingual tablets of NITRATES (failure to dissolve under tongue owing to dry mouth)

▸ Vasodilator Antihypertensives: enhanced hypotensive effect when tricyclic-related antidepressants given with HYDRALAZINE or SODIUM NITROPRUSSIDE

Antidiabetics

NOTE Other drugs administered orally may need to be taken at least 1 hour before or 4 hours after lixisenatide injection, or taken with a meal when lixisenatide is not administered, to minimise possible interference with absorption

NOTE Other drugs administered orally may need to be taken at least 1 hour before or 4 hours after exenatide injection, or taken with a meal when exenatide is not administered, to minimise possible interference with absorption

▸ ACE Inhibitors: hypoglycaemic effect of insulin, metformin and sulfonylureas possibly enhanced by ACE INHIBITORS

▸ Alcohol: hypoglycaemic effect of antidiabetics enhanced by ALCOHOL; increased risk of lactic acidosis when metformin given with ALCOHOL

▸ Anabolic Steroids: hypoglycaemic effect of antidiabetics possibly enhanced by ANABOLIC STEROIDS

● Analgesics: effects of sulfonylureas possibly enhanced by ● NSAIDS; lixisenatide possibly reduces the absorption of PARACETAMOL when given 1 to 4 hours before paracetamol

▸ Anti-arrhythmics: hypoglycaemic effect of gliclazide, insulin and metformin possibly enhanced by DISOPYRAMIDE

● Antibacterials: hypoglycaemic effect of acarbose possibly enhanced by NEOMYCIN, also severity of gastro-intestinal effects increased; effects of repaglinide enhanced by CLARITHROMYCIN; effects of glibenclamide possibly enhanced by NORFLOXACIN; plasma concentration of canagliflozin and nateglinide reduced by ● RIFAMPICIN; effects of linagliptin possibly reduced by RIFAMPICIN; hypoglycaemic effect of repaglinide possibly antagonised by RIFAMPICIN; effects of sulfonylureas enhanced by ● CHLORAMPHENICOL; metabolism of sulfonylureas possibly accelerated by ● RIFAMYCINS (reduced effect); metabolism of tolbutamide accelerated by

Antidiabetics

- **Antibacterials** (continued)
  - RIFAMYCINS (reduced effect); effects of sulfonylureas rarely enhanced by SULFONAMIDES and TRIMETHOPRIM; hypoglycaemic effect of sulfonylureas possibly enhanced by TETRACYCLINES; hypoglycaemic effect of repaglinide possibly enhanced by TRIMETHOPRIM—manufacturer advises avoid concomitant use
- **Anticoagulants:** exenatide possibly enhances anticoagulant effect of WARFARIN; hypoglycaemic effect of sulfonylureas possibly enhanced by ● COUMARINS, also possible changes to anticoagulant effect
- **Antidepressants:** hypoglycaemic effect of antidiabetics possibly enhanced by MAOIs; hypoglycaemic effect of insulin, metformin and sulfonylureas enhanced by MAOIs
- **Antidiabetics:** manufacturer of dapagliflozin advises avoid concomitant use with PIOGLITAZONE; plasma concentration of dulaglutide increased by SITAGLIPTIN
- **Antiepileptics:** tolbutamide transiently increases plasma concentration of FOSPHENYTOIN and PHENYTOIN (possibility of toxicity); plasma concentration of glibenclamide possibly reduced by TOPIRAMATE; plasma concentration of metformin possibly increased by TOPIRAMATE
- **Antifungals:** plasma concentration of pioglitazone, saxagliptin and tolbutamide increased by KETOCONAZOLE; plasma concentration of sulfonylureas increased by ● FLUCONAZOLE and ● MICONAZOLE; hypoglycaemic effect of gliclazide and glipizide enhanced by ● MICONAZOLE—avoid concomitant use; hypoglycaemic effect of nateglinide possibly enhanced by FLUCONAZOLE; hypoglycaemic effect of repaglinide possibly enhanced by ITRACONAZOLE; hypoglycaemic effect of glipizide possibly enhanced by POSACONAZOLE; plasma concentration of sulfonylureas possibly increased by VORICONAZOLE
- **Antihistamines:** thrombocyte count depressed when metformin given with KETOTIFEN (manufacturer of ketotifen advises avoid concomitant use)
- **Antipsychotics:** hypoglycaemic effect of sulfonylureas possibly antagonised by PHENOTHIAZINES
- **Antivirals:** plasma concentration of metformin increased by DOLUTEGRAVIR—consider reducing dose of metformin; plasma concentration of tolbutamide possibly increased by RITONAVIR; plasma concentration of metformin increased by TELAPREVIR (consider reducing dose of metformin)
- **Aprepitant:** plasma concentration of tolbutamide reduced by APREPITANT
- **Beta-blockers:** warning signs of hypoglycaemia (such as tremor) with antidiabetics may be masked when given with BETA-BLOCKERS; hypoglycaemic effect of insulin enhanced by BETA-BLOCKERS
- **Bosentan:** increased risk of hepatotoxicity when glibenclamide given with ● BOSENTAN—avoid concomitant use
- **Calcium-channel Blockers:** glucose tolerance occasionally impaired when insulin given with NIFEDIPINE
- **Cardiac Glycosides:** canagliflozin and sitagliptin increase plasma concentration of DIGOXIN; acarbose possibly reduces plasma concentration of DIGOXIN
- **Ciclosporin:** hypoglycaemic effect of repaglinide possibly enhanced by CICLOSPORIN
- **Corticosteroids:** hypoglycaemic effect of antidiabetics antagonised by CORTICOSTEROIDS
- **Cytotoxics:** avoidance of repaglinide advised by manufacturer of ● LAPATINIB; plasma concentration of metformin possibly increased by VANDETANIB (consider reducing dose of metformin)
- **Deferasirox:** plasma concentration of repaglinide increased by DEFERASIROX
- **Diazoxide:** hypoglycaemic effect of antidiabetics antagonised by DIAZOXIDE
- **Diuretics:** canagliflozin possibly enhances diuretic effect of DIURETICS; hypoglycaemic effect of antidiabetics antagonised by LOOP DIURETICS and THIAZIDES AND RELATED DIURETICS; dapagliflozin possibly enhances diuretic effect of LOOP DIURETICS and THIAZIDES AND RELATED DIURETICS; manufacturer of canagliflozin advises avoid concomitant use with LOOP DIURETICS

Antidiabetics (continued)

- **Fosaprepitant:** plasma concentration of tolbutamide reduced by FOSAPREPITANT
- **Hormone Antagonists:** requirements for antidiabetics possibly reduced by LANREOTIDE, OCTREOTIDE and PASIREOTIDE
- **Leflunomide:** hypoglycaemic effect of tolbutamide possibly enhanced by LEFLUNOMIDE
- **Lipid-regulating Drugs:** absorption of glibenclamide and glipizide reduced by COLESEVELAM; absorption of glimepiride reduced by COLESEVELAM—manufacturer of glimepiride advises give at least 4 hours before colesevelam; hypoglycaemic effect of acarbose possibly enhanced by COLESTYRAMINE; hypoglycaemic effect of nateglinide possibly enhanced by GEMFIBROZIL; increased risk of severe hypoglycaemia when repaglinide given with ● GEMFIBROZIL—avoid concomitant use; plasma concentration of glibenclamide possibly increased by FLUVASTATIN; manufacturer of canagliflozin advises give at least 1 hour before or 4–6 hours after BILE ACID SEQUESTRANTS; may be improved glucose tolerance and an additive effect when insulin or sulfonylureas given with FIBRATES; separating administration from linagliptin by 12 hours advised by manufacturer of LOMITAPIDE
- **Oestrogens:** hypoglycaemic effect of antidiabetics antagonised by OESTROGENS
- **Orlistat:** avoidance of acarbose advised by manufacturer of ORLISTAT
- **Pancreatin:** hypoglycaemic effect of acarbose antagonised by PANCREATIN
- **Progestogens:** hypoglycaemic effect of antidiabetics antagonised by PROGESTOGENS
- **Sulfinpyrazone:** effects of sulfonylureas enhanced by ● SULFINPYRAZONE
- **Teriflunomide:** plasma concentration of repaglinide increased by TERIFLUNOMIDE
- **Testosterone:** hypoglycaemic effect of antidiabetics possibly enhanced by TESTOSTERONE
- **Ulcer-healing Drugs:** excretion of metformin reduced by CIMETIDINE (increased plasma concentration); hypoglycaemic effect of sulfonylureas enhanced by CIMETIDINE

Antiepileptics see Carbamazepine, Eslicarbazepine, Ethosuximide, Fosphenytoin, Gabapentin, Lacosamide, Lamotrigine, Levetiracetam, Oxcarbazepine, Perampanel, Phenobarbital, Phenytoin, Pregabalin, Primidone, Retigabine, Rufinamide, Sodium valproate, Stiripentol, Tiagabine, Topiramate, Valproic acid, Vigabatrin, and Zonisamide

Antifungals see Amphotericin; Antifungals, Imidazole; Antifungals, Triazole; Caspofungin; Flucytosine; Griseofulvin; Micafungin; Terbinafine

Antifungals, Imidazole

- **Alcohol:** possibility of disulfiram-like reaction when ketoconazole given with ALCOHOL
- **Aliskiren:** ketoconazole increases plasma concentration of ALISKIREN
- **Alpha-blockers:** ketoconazole possibly increases plasma concentration of ALFUZOSIN; ketoconazole increases plasma concentration of TAMSULOSIN
- **Aminophylline:** ketoconazole possibly increases plasma concentration of ● AMINOPHYLLINE
- **Analgesics:** ketoconazole inhibits metabolism of ● BUPRENORPHINE (reduce dose of buprenorphine); possible increased risk of ventricular arrhythmias when ketoconazole given with ● METHADONE—manufacturer of ketoconazole advises avoid concomitant use; ketoconazole increases plasma concentration of OXYCODONE; manufacturer of ketoconazole advises avoid concomitant use with PARACETAMOL
- **Antacids:** absorption of ketoconazole reduced by ANTACIDS
- **Anthelmintics:** ketoconazole increases plasma concentration of PRAZIQUANTEL
- **Anti-arrhythmics:** increased risk of ventricular arrhythmias when ketoconazole given with ● DISOPYRAMIDE—avoid concomitant use; ketoconazole increases plasma concentration of ● DRONEDARONE—avoid concomitant use
- **Antibacterials:** manufacturer of ketoconazole advises avoid concomitant ● CLARITHROMYCIN in severe renal impairment;

Antifungals, Imidazole

- **Antibacterials** (continued)

  metabolism of ketoconazole accelerated by ● RIFAMPICIN (reduced plasma concentration), also plasma concentration of rifampicin may be reduced by ketoconazole; ketoconazole increases plasma concentration of BEDAQUILINE—avoid concomitant use if ketoconazole given for more than 14 days; avoidance of ketoconazole advised by manufacturer of FIDAXOMICIN; plasma concentration of ketoconazole possibly reduced by ISONIAZID; ketoconazole increases the plasma concentration of ● TELITHROMYCIN—avoid in severe renal and hepatic impairment

- **Anticoagulants**: ketoconazole increases plasma concentration of ● APIXABAN—manufacturer of apixaban advises avoid concomitant use; miconazole (including oral gel and possibly vaginal and topical formulations) greatly enhances the anticoagulant effect of ● COUMARINS—avoid concomitant use if possible; ketoconazole enhances anticoagulant effect of ● COUMARINS; ketoconazole increases plasma concentration of ● DABIGATRAN and ● RIVAROXABAN—avoid concomitant use; ketoconazole increases plasma concentration of ● EDOXABAN (reduce dose of Edoxaban—see under Edoxaban, in BNF)

- **Antidepressants**: avoidance of imidazoles advised by manufacturer of ● REBOXETINE; ketoconazole increases plasma concentration of MIRTAZAPINE

- **Antidiabetics**: miconazole enhances hypoglycaemic effect of ● GLICLAZIDE and ● GLIPIZIDE—avoid concomitant use; ketoconazole increases plasma concentration of PIOGLITAZONE, SAXAGLIPTIN and TOLBUTAMIDE; miconazole increases plasma concentration of ● SULFONYLUREAS

- **Antiepileptics**: miconazole possibly increases plasma concentration of CARBAMAZEPINE; plasma concentration of ketoconazole possibly reduced by CARBAMAZEPINE, also plasma concentration of carbamazepine possibly increased; plasma concentration of ketoconazole reduced by ● PHENYTOIN and ● PHENYTOIN; miconazole enhances anticonvulsant effect of ● FOSPHENYTOIN and ● PHENYTOIN (plasma concentration of fosphenytoin and phenytoin increased); ketoconazole increases plasma concentration of PERAMPANEL

▸ **Antifungals**: imidazoles possibly antagonise effects of AMPHOTERICIN

- **Antihistamines**: imidazoles possibly inhibit metabolism of ● MIZOLASTINE (avoid concomitant use)

- **Antimalarials**: avoidance of imidazoles advised by manufacturer of ● ARTEMETHER WITH LUMEFANTRINE; avoidance of imidazoles advised by manufacturer of ● ARTENIMOL WITH PIPERAQUINE (possible risk of ventricular arrhythmias); ketoconazole increases plasma concentration of MEFLOQUINE

- **Antimuscarinics**: absorption of ketoconazole reduced by ANTIMUSCARINICS; ketoconazole increases plasma concentration of DARIFENACIN—avoid concomitant use; manufacturer of fesoterodine advises dose reduction when ketoconazole given with FESOTERODINE—consult fesoterodine product literature; ketoconazole increases plasma concentration of OXYBUTYNIN; ketoconazole increases plasma concentration of ● SOLIFENACIN—see under Solifenacin, in BNF; avoidance of imidazoles advised by manufacturer of ● TOLTERODINE

- **Antipsychotics**: ketoconazole inhibits metabolism of ● ARIPIPRAZOLE (reduce dose of aripiprazole); ketoconazole increases plasma concentration of ● LURASIDONE—avoid concomitant use; increased risk of ventricular arrhythmias when imidazoles given with ● PIMOZIDE—avoid concomitant use; imidazoles possibly increase plasma concentration of ● QUETIAPINE—manufacturer of quetiapine advises avoid concomitant use

- **Antivirals**: ketoconazole increases plasma concentration of ● BOCEPREVIR; ketoconazole increases the plasma concentration of ● DACLATASVIR—reduce dose of daclatasvir (see under Daclatasvir, in BNF); plasma concentration of both drugs increased when ketoconazole given with DARUNAVIR; plasma concentration of both drugs increased when ketoconazole given with ● DASABUVIR and ● PARITAPREVIR—avoid concomitant use; plasma concentration of ketoconazole reduced by ● EFAVIRENZ; plasma concentration of

Antifungals, Imidazole

- **Antivirals** (continued)

  ketoconazole increased by FOSAMPRENAVIR (also plasma concentration of fosamprenavir possibly increased); ketoconazole increases plasma concentration of ● INDINAVIR and ● MARAVIROC (consider reducing dose of indinavir and maraviroc); plasma concentration of ketoconazole reduced by ● NEVIRAPINE—avoid concomitant use; avoidance of ketoconazole advised by manufacturer of OMBITASVIR and ● SIMEPREVIR; plasma concentration of ketoconazole increased by ● RITONAVIR (reduce dose of ketoconazole); imidazoles possibly increase plasma concentration of SAQUINAVIR; ketoconazole increases plasma concentration of ● SAQUINAVIR—manufacturer of ketoconazole advises avoidance of concomitant use; plasma concentration of both drugs possibly increased when ketoconazole given with TELAPREVIR (increased risk of ventricular arrhythmias)—reduce dose of ketoconazole

- **Anxiolytics and Hypnotics**: ketoconazole increases plasma concentration of ● ALPRAZOLAM—manufacturer of ketoconazole advises avoid concomitant use; ketoconazole increases plasma concentration of ● MIDAZOLAM (risk of prolonged sedation—avoid concomitant use of *oral* midazolam); ketoconazole increases plasma concentration of ZOLPIDEM

▸ **Aprepitant**: ketoconazole increases plasma concentration of APREPITANT

- **Avanafil**: ketoconazole increases plasma concentration of ● AVANAFIL—avoid concomitant use

▸ **Beta-blockers**: ketoconazole possibly increases plasma concentration of NADOLOL

- **Bosentan**: ketoconazole increases plasma concentration of BOSENTAN

- **Calcium-channel Blockers**: ketoconazole inhibits metabolism of ● FELODIPINE (increased plasma concentration)—manufacturer of ketoconazole advises avoid concomitant use; avoidance of ketoconazole advised by manufacturer of LERCANIDIPINE; ketoconazole possibly inhibits metabolism of DIHYDROPYRIDINES (increased plasma concentration)

▸ **Cannabis Extract**: ketoconazole increases plasma concentration of CANNABIS EXTRACT

- **Ciclosporin**: ketoconazole inhibits metabolism of ● CICLOSPORIN (increased plasma concentration); miconazole possibly inhibits metabolism of ● CICLOSPORIN (increased plasma concentration)

- **Cilostazol**: ketoconazole increases plasma concentration of ● CILOSTAZOL (see under Cilostazol, in BNF)

▸ **Cinacalcet**: ketoconazole inhibits metabolism of CINACALCET (increased plasma concentration)

- **Clopidogrel**: ketoconazole possibly reduces antiplatelet effect of ● CLOPIDOGREL

▸ **Cobicistat**: plasma concentration of ketoconazole possibly increased by COBICISTAT—manufacturer of cobicistat advises reduce dose of ketoconazole

- **Colchicine**: ketoconazole possibly increases risk of ● COLCHICINE toxicity—suspend or reduce dose of colchicine (avoid concomitant use in hepatic or renal impairment)

- **Corticosteroids**: ketoconazole possibly inhibits metabolism of CORTICOSTEROIDS; ketoconazole increases the plasma concentration of *inhaled* and *oral* (and possibly also *intranasal* and *rectal*) ● BUDESONIDE; ketoconazole increases plasma concentration of active metabolite of ● CICLESONIDE; ketoconazole possibly increases plasma concentration of *inhaled* FLUTICASONE; ketoconazole inhibits the metabolism of METHYLPREDNISOLONE; ketoconazole increases plasma concentration of *inhaled* MOMETASONE

- **Cytotoxics**: ketoconazole inhibits the metabolism of IFOSFAMIDE; possible increased risk of neutropenia when ketoconazole given with ● BRENTUXIMAB VEDOTIN; ketoconazole possibly increases the plasma concentration of AFATINIB—manufacturer of afatinib advises separating administration of ketoconazole by 6 to 12 hours; ketoconazole increases plasma concentration of AXITINIB (reduce dose of axitinib—consult axitinib product literature); ketoconazole increases the plasma concentration of ● BOSUTINIB—manufacturer of bosutinib advises avoid or

Interactions | Appendix 1

A1

Antifungals, Imidazole

- Cytotoxics (continued)

consider reducing dose of bosutinib; ketoconazole increases plasma concentration of BORTEZOMIB, CABOZANTINIB, DABRAFENIB, ETOPOSIDE, IDELALISIB, IMATINIB, NINTEDANIB and PONATINIB; ketoconazole increases plasma concentration of ● CRIZOTINIB, ● LAPATINIB, ● NILOTINIB and ● REGORAFENIB—avoid concomitant use; ketoconazole possibly increases plasma concentration of DASATINIB; ketoconazole inhibits metabolism of ERLOTINIB and SUNITINIB (increased plasma concentration); ketoconazole increases plasma concentration of ● EVEROLIMUS—manufacturer of ketoconazole advises avoid concomitant use; ketoconazole increases plasma concentration of ● IBRUTINIB—reduce dose of ibrutinib (see under Ibrutinib, in BNF); ketoconazole increases plasma concentration of ● PAZOPANIB (reduce dose of pazopanib); manufacturer of ruxolitinib advises dose reduction when ketoconazole given with ● RUXOLITINIB—consult ruxolitinib product literature; ketoconazole increases plasma concentration of active metabolite of ● TEMSIROLIMUS—avoid concomitant use; avoidance of ketoconazole advised by manufacturer of ● CABAZITAXEL; *in vitro* studies suggest a possible interaction between ketoconazole and DOCETAXEL (consult docetaxel product literature); ketoconazole reduces plasma concentration of ● IRINOTECAN (but concentration of active metabolite of irinotecan increased)—avoid concomitant use; ketoconazole increases plasma concentration of ● VINFLUNINE—manufacturer of vinflunine advises avoid concomitant use

- Dapoxetine: ketoconazole increases plasma concentration of ● DAPOXETINE—manufacturer of dapoxetine advises avoid concomitant use
- Diuretics: ketoconazole increases plasma concentration of ● EPLERENONE—avoid concomitant use
- Domperidone: manufacturer of ketoconazole advises avoid concomitant use with ● DOMPERIDONE (risk of ventricular arrhythmias)
- Ergot Alkaloids: manufacturer of ketoconazole advises avoid concomitant use with ● ERGOT ALKALOIDS; increased risk of ergotism when imidazoles given with ● ERGOTAMINE—avoid concomitant use
- Fingolimod: ketoconazole increases plasma concentration of ● FINGOLIMOD
- Fosaprepitant: ketoconazole increases plasma concentration of FOSAPREPITANT
- Guanfacine: ketoconazole increases plasma concentration of ● GUANFACINE (halve dose of guanfacine)
- Hormone Antagonists: manufacturer of ketoconazole advises avoid concomitant use with PASIREOTIDE
- 5HT₁-receptor Agonists: ketoconazole increases plasma concentration of ALMOTRIPTAN (increased risk of toxicity); ketoconazole increases plasma concentration of ● ELETRIPTAN (risk of toxicity)—avoid concomitant use
- Ivabradine: ketoconazole increases plasma concentration of ● IVABRADINE—avoid concomitant use
- Ivacaftor: ketoconazole increases plasma concentration of ● IVACAFTOR (see under Ivacaftor, p. 175)
- Lanthanum: absorption of ketoconazole possibly reduced by LANTHANUM (give at least 2 hours apart)
- Lenalidomide: ketoconazole possibly increases plasma concentration of ● LENALIDOMIDE (increased risk of toxicity)
- Lipid-regulating Drugs: possible increased risk of myopathy when imidazoles given with ATORVASTATIN; possible increased risk of myopathy when ketoconazole given with ● ATORVASTATIN—manufacturer of ketoconazole advises avoid concomitant use; increased risk of myopathy when ketoconazole given with ● SIMVASTATIN (avoid concomitant use); possible increased risk of myopathy when miconazole given with ● SIMVASTATIN; ketoconazole increases plasma concentration of ● LOMITAPIDE—avoid concomitant use
- Macitentan: ketoconazole increases plasma concentration of MACITENTAN
- Mirabegron: when given with ketoconazole avoid or reduce dose of MIRABEGRON in hepatic or renal impairment—see Mirabegron, in BNF

Antifungals, Imidazole (continued)

- Netupitant: ketoconazole possibly increases plasma concentration of NETUPITANT
- Oestrogens: anecdotal reports of contraceptive failure when imidazoles given with OESTROGENS; ketoconazole increases plasma concentration of ETHINYLESTRADIOL
- Parasympathomimetics: ketoconazole increases plasma concentration of GALANTAMINE
- Progestogens: ketoconazole increases plasma concentration of DROSPIRENONE
- Ranolazine: ketoconazole increases plasma concentration of ● RANOLAZINE—avoid concomitant use
- Retinoids: ketoconazole increases plasma concentration of ALITRETINOIN; ketoconazole possibly increases risk of ● TRETINOIN toxicity
- Riociguat: avoidance of ketoconazole advised by manufacturer of RIOCIGUAT
- Sildenafil: ketoconazole increases plasma concentration of ● SILDENAFIL—reduce initial dose of sildenafil for erectile dysfunction and avoid concomitant use of sildenafil for pulmonary hypertension
- Sirolimus: ketoconazole increases plasma concentration of ● SIROLIMUS—avoid concomitant use; miconazole increases plasma concentration of ● SIROLIMUS
- Sympathomimetics, Beta₂: ketoconazole increases plasma concentration of OLODATEROL; ketoconazole inhibits metabolism of ● SALMETEROL (increased plasma concentration)
- Tacrolimus: ketoconazole increases plasma concentration of ● TACROLIMUS (consider reducing dose of tacrolimus); miconazole *oral gel* possibly increases plasma concentration of ● TACROLIMUS
- Tadalafil: ketoconazole increases plasma concentration of ● TADALAFIL—avoid concomitant use of tadalafil for pulmonary hypertension
- Theophylline: ketoconazole possibly increases plasma concentration of ● THEOPHYLLINE
- Ticagrelor: ketoconazole increases plasma concentration of ● TICAGRELOR—manufacturer of ticagrelor advises avoid concomitant use
- Tolvaptan: ketoconazole increases plasma concentration of TOLVAPTAN—manufacturer of ketoconazole advises avoid concomitant use
- Ulcer-healing Drugs: absorption of ketoconazole reduced by HISTAMINE H₂-ANTAGONISTS, PROTON PUMP INHIBITORS and SUCRALFATE
- Ulipristal: ketoconazole increases plasma concentration of *low-dose* ULIPRISTAL—manufacturer of *low-dose* ulipristal advises avoid concomitant use
- Vardenafil: ketoconazole increases plasma concentration of ● VARDENAFIL—avoid concomitant use
- Vitamins: miconazole possibly reduces effects of ALFACALCIDOL, CALCITRIOL, COLECALCIFEROL, ERGOCALCIFEROL, PARICALCITOL and VITAMIN D; ketoconazole possibly increases plasma concentration of PARICALCITOL

Antifungals, Polyene see Amphotericin

Antifungals, Triazole

NOTE In general, fluconazole interactions relate to multiple-dose treatment

- Aliskiren: itraconazole increases plasma concentration of ● ALISKIREN—avoid concomitant use
- Aminophylline: fluconazole possibly increases plasma concentration of ● AMINOPHYLLINE
- Analgesics: fluconazole increases plasma concentration of CELECOXIB (halve dose of celecoxib); voriconazole increases plasma concentration of DICLOFENAC, IBUPROFEN and ● OXYCODONE; fluconazole increases plasma concentration of FLURBIPROFEN, IBUPROFEN and METHADONE; fluconazole increases plasma concentration of PARECOXIB (reduce dose of parecoxib); voriconazole increases plasma concentration of ● ALFENTANIL and ● METHADONE (consider reducing dose of alfentanil and methadone); fluconazole inhibits metabolism of ALFENTANIL (risk of prolonged or delayed respiratory depression); itraconazole possibly inhibits metabolism of ALFENTANIL; triazoles possibly increase plasma concentration of ● FENTANYL; itraconazole possibly increases plasma

Antifungals, Triazole

- **Analgesics** (continued)
  concentration of • METHADONE (increased risk of ventricular arrhythmias); itraconazole increases plasma concentration of OXYCODONE
- **Antacids:** absorption of itraconazole reduced by ANTACIDS
- **Anti-arrhythmics:** manufacturer of itraconazole advises avoid concomitant use with • DISOPYRAMIDE; avoidance of itraconazole, posaconazole and voriconazole advised by manufacturer of • DRONEDARONE
- **Antibacterials:** plasma concentration of itraconazole increased by CLARITHROMYCIN; manufacturer of fluconazole advises avoid concomitant use with ERYTHROMYCIN; triazoles possibly increase plasma concentration of • RIFABUTIN (increased risk of uveitis—reduce rifabutin dose); posaconazole increases plasma concentration of RIFABUTIN (also plasma concentration of posaconazole reduced); voriconazole increases plasma concentration of • RIFABUTIN, also rifabutin reduces plasma concentration of voriconazole (increase dose of voriconazole and also monitor for rifabutin toxicity); fluconazole increases plasma concentration of • RIFABUTIN (increased risk of uveitis—reduce rifabutin dose); plasma concentration of itraconazole reduced by RIFABUTIN and • RIFAMPICIN—manufacturer of itraconazole advises avoid concomitant use; plasma concentration of posaconazole reduced by RIFAMPICIN; plasma concentration of voriconazole reduced by • RIFAMPICIN—avoid concomitant use; metabolism of fluconazole accelerated by • RIFAMPICIN (reduced plasma concentration); fluconazole possibly increases plasma concentration of BEDAQUILINE—avoid concomitant use if fluconazole given for more than 14 days
- **Anticoagulants:** avoidance of itraconazole, posaconazole and voriconazole advised by manufacturer of APIXABAN; fluconazole, itraconazole and voriconazole enhance anticoagulant effect of • COUMARINS; avoidance of itraconazole advised by manufacturer of DABIGATRAN and RIVAROXABAN; avoidance of posaconazole and voriconazole advised by manufacturer of RIVAROXABAN
- **Antidepressants:** avoidance of triazoles advised by manufacturer of • REBOXETINE; fluconazole possibly increases plasma concentration of AMITRIPTYLINE and NORTRIPTYLINE; plasma concentration of voriconazole reduced by • ST JOHN'S WORT—avoid concomitant use
- **Antidiabetics:** posaconazole possibly enhances hypoglycaemic effect of GLIPIZIDE; fluconazole possibly enhances hypoglycaemic effect of NATEGLINIDE; itraconazole possibly enhances hypoglycaemic effect of REPAGLINIDE; voriconazole possibly increases plasma concentration of SULFONYLUREAS; fluconazole increases plasma concentration of • SULFONYLUREAS
- **Antiepileptics:** plasma concentration of itraconazole and posaconazole possibly reduced by • CARBAMAZEPINE; fluconazole possibly increases plasma concentration of CARBAMAZEPINE; plasma concentration of voriconazole possibly reduced by CARBAMAZEPINE, • PHENOBARBITAL and • PRIMIDONE—avoid concomitant use; plasma concentration of itraconazole reduced by FOSPHENYTOIN and • PHENYTOIN—avoid concomitant use; fluconazole increases plasma concentration of • FOSPHENYTOIN and • PHENYTOIN (consider reducing dose of fosphenytoin and phenytoin); voriconazole increases plasma concentration of FOSPHENYTOIN and • PHENYTOIN, also fosphenytoin and phenytoin reduces plasma concentration of voriconazole (increase dose of voriconazole and also monitor for fosphenytoin and phenytoin toxicity); plasma concentration of posaconazole reduced by • FOSPHENYTOIN and • PHENYTOIN; plasma concentration of itraconazole and posaconazole possibly reduced by • PHENOBARBITAL; plasma concentration of itraconazole and posaconazole possibly reduced by • PRIMIDONE
- **Antifungals:** triazoles possibly antagonise effects of AMPHOTERICIN; monitoring for increased voriconazole side effects advised by manufacturer of FLUCONAZOLE if voriconazole given after fluconazole; plasma concentration of itraconazole increased by MICAFUNGIN (consider reducing dose of itraconazole); plasma concentration of fluconazole increased by TERBINAFINE

Antifungals, Triazole (continued)

- **Antihistamines:** itraconazole inhibits metabolism of • MIZOLASTINE—avoid concomitant use
- **Antimalarials:** avoidance of triazoles advised by manufacturer of • ARTEMETHER WITH LUMEFANTRINE; avoidance of triazoles advised by manufacturer of • ARTENIMOL WITH PIPERAQUINE (possible risk of ventricular arrhythmias)
- **Antimuscarinics:** avoidance of itraconazole advised by manufacturer of DARIFENACIN and TOLTERODINE; manufacturer of fesoterodine advises dose reduction when itraconazole given with FESOTERODINE—consult fesoterodine product literature; itraconazole possibly increases plasma concentration of • SOLIFENACIN—see under Solifenacin, in BNF
- **Antipsychotics:** itraconazole possibly increases plasma concentration of HALOPERIDOL; itraconazole possibly increases plasma concentration of • ARIPIPRAZOLE (reduce dose of aripiprazole—consult aripiprazole product literature); itraconazole, posaconazole and voriconazole possibly increase plasma concentration of • LURASIDONE—avoid concomitant use; fluconazole possibly increases the plasma concentration of • LURASIDONE (see under Lurasidone, in BNF); increased risk of ventricular arrhythmias when triazoles given with • PIMOZIDE—avoid concomitant use; triazoles possibly increase plasma concentration of • QUETIAPINE—manufacturer of quetiapine advises avoid concomitant use; itraconazole possibly increases side-effects of RISPERIDONE
- **Antivirals:** posaconazole increases plasma concentration of • ATAZANAVIR; plasma concentration of voriconazole increased or decreased by • ATAZANAVIR and plasma concentration of atazanavir also reduced; itraconazole, posaconazole and voriconazole possibly increase the plasma concentration of • DACLATASVIR—reduce dose of daclatasvir (see under Daclatasvir, in BNF); plasma concentration of voriconazole possibly affected by DARUNAVIR; plasma concentration of both drugs possibly increased when itraconazole and posaconazole given with • DASABUVIR—avoid concomitant use; plasma concentration of voriconazole reduced by • EFAVIRENZ, also plasma concentration of efavirenz increased (increase voriconazole dose and reduce efavirenz dose); plasma concentration of itraconazole and posaconazole reduced by • EFAVIRENZ; plasma concentration of both drugs may increase when itraconazole given with FOSAMPRENAVIR; plasma concentration of posaconazole possibly reduced by FOSAMPRENAVIR; itraconazole increases plasma concentration of • INDINAVIR (consider reducing dose of indinavir); fluconazole increases plasma concentration of • NEVIRAPINE, RITONAVIR and TIPRANAVIR; plasma concentration of itraconazole possibly reduced by NEVIRAPINE—consider increasing dose of itraconazole; plasma concentration of both drugs possibly increased when itraconazole and posaconazole given with • PARITAPREVIR—avoid concomitant use; plasma concentration of voriconazole reduced by • RITONAVIR—avoid concomitant use; combination of itraconazole with • RITONAVIR may increase plasma concentration of either drug (or both); triazoles possibly increase plasma concentration of SAQUINAVIR; fluconazole, itraconazole, posaconazole and voriconazole possibly increase plasma concentration of • SIMEPREVIR—manufacturer of simeprevir advises avoid concomitant use; plasma concentration of voriconazole possibly affected by • TELAPREVIR (possible increased risk of ventricular arrhythmias); plasma concentration of posaconazole possibly increased by • TELAPREVIR (increased risk of ventricular arrhythmias); plasma concentration of itraconazole possibly increased by TELAPREVIR; fluconazole increases plasma concentration of • ZIDOVUDINE (increased risk of toxicity)
- **Anxiolytics and Hypnotics:** itraconazole increases plasma concentration of ALPRAZOLAM; fluconazole and voriconazole increase plasma concentration of • DIAZEPAM (risk of prolonged sedation); fluconazole, itraconazole, posaconazole and voriconazole increase plasma concentration of • MIDAZOLAM (risk of prolonged sedation); itraconazole increases plasma concentration of BUSPIRONE (reduce dose of buspirone)
- **Avanafil:** itraconazole and voriconazole possibly increase plasma concentration of • AVANAFIL—manufacturer of avanafil

A1

Interactions | Appendix 1

Antifungals, Triazole

- Avanafil (continued)
advises avoid concomitant use; fluconazole possibly increases plasma concentration of ● AVANAFIL—see under Avanafil, in BNF
- Bosentan: fluconazole possibly increases plasma concentration of ● BOSENTAN—avoid concomitant use; itraconazole possibly increases plasma concentration of BOSENTAN
- Calcium-channel Blockers: negative inotropic effect possibly increased when itraconazole given with CALCIUM-CHANNEL BLOCKERS; itraconazole inhibits metabolism of ● FELODIPINE (increased plasma concentration); avoidance of itraconazole advised by manufacturer of LERCANIDIPINE; itraconazole possibly inhibits metabolism of DIHYDROPYRIDINES (increased plasma concentration)
- Cardiac Glycosides: itraconazole increases plasma concentration of ● DIGOXIN
- Ciclosporin: fluconazole, itraconazole, posaconazole and voriconazole inhibit metabolism of ● CICLOSPORIN (increased plasma concentration)
- Cilostazol: itraconazole possibly increases plasma concentration of ● CILOSTAZOL (see under Cilostazol, in BNF)
- Clopidogrel: fluconazole, itraconazole and voriconazole possibly reduce antiplatelet effect of ● CLOPIDOGREL
- Cobicistat: plasma concentration of itraconazole possibly increased by COBICISTAT—manufacturer of cobicistat advises reduce dose of itraconazole
- Colchicine: itraconazole possibly increases risk of ● COLCHICINE toxicity—suspend or reduce dose of colchicine (avoid concomitant use in hepatic or renal impairment)
- Corticosteroids: itraconazole possibly inhibits metabolism of CORTICOSTEROIDS and METHYLPREDNISOLONE; itraconazole increases the plasma concentration of *inhaled* and *oral* (and possibly also *intranasal* and *rectal*) ● BUDESONIDE; itraconazole increases plasma concentration of *inhaled* FLUTICASONE
- Cytotoxics: itraconazole inhibits metabolism of BUSULFAN (increased risk of toxicity); fluconazole and itraconazole possibly increase side-effects of CYCLOPHOSPHAMIDE; itraconazole possibly increases the plasma concentration of AFATINIB—manufacturer of afatinib advises separating administration of itraconazole by 6 to 12 hours; itraconazole possibly increases plasma concentration of AXITINIB (reduce dose of axitinib—consult axitinib product literature); fluconazole, itraconazole, posaconazole and voriconazole possibly increase the plasma concentration of ● BOSUTINIB— manufacturer of bosutinib advises avoid or consider reducing dose of bosutinib; itraconazole possibly increases plasma concentration of CABOZANTINIB; itraconazole and voriconazole possibly increase plasma concentration of ● CRIZOTINIB— manufacturer of crizotinib advises avoid concomitant use; avoidance of itraconazole advised by manufacturer of DASATINIB and ● TEMSIROLIMUS (plasma concentration of dasatinib and temsirolimus possibly increased); itraconazole, posaconazole and voriconazole possibly increase plasma concentration of ● EVEROLIMUS—manufacturer of everolimus advises avoid concomitant use; itraconazole increases plasma concentration of GEFITINIB; fluconazole, itraconazole and voriconazole possibly increase the plasma concentration of ● IBRUTINIB—reduce dose of ibrutinib (see under Ibrutinib, in BNF); avoidance of itraconazole, posaconazole and voriconazole advised by manufacturer of ● LAPATINIB; avoidance of itraconazole and voriconazole advised by manufacturer of ● NILOTINIB; itraconazole and voriconazole possibly increase plasma concentration of ● PAZOPANIB (reduce dose of pazopanib); itraconazole and voriconazole possibly increase plasma concentration of PONATINIB— consider reducing initial dose of ponatinib (see under Ponatinib, in BNF); manufacturer of ruxolitinib advises dose reduction when fluconazole, itraconazole, posaconazole and voriconazole given with ● RUXOLITINIB—consult ruxolitinib product literature; itraconazole and voriconazole possibly increase the plasma concentration of ● CABAZITAXEL— manufacturer of cabazitaxel advises avoid or consider reducing dose of cabazitaxel; itraconazole and voriconazole possibly increase plasma concentration of ● DOCETAXEL— manufacturer of docetaxel advises avoid concomitant use or

Antifungals, Triazole

- Cytotoxics (continued)
consider reducing docetaxel dose; increased risk of toxicity when itraconazole given with ● IRINOTECAN—avoid concomitant use; avoidance of itraconazole advised by manufacturer of ● OLAPARIB; posaconazole possibly inhibits metabolism of VINBLASTINE and ● VINCRISTINE (increased risk of neurotoxicity); itraconazole possibly increases risk of ● VINBLASTINE, ● VINDESINE, ● VINFLUNINE and ● VINORELBINE toxicity; itraconazole increases risk of ● VINCRISTINE toxicity
- Dapoxetine: manufacturer of dapoxetine advises dose reduction when fluconazole given with DAPOXETINE (see under Dapoxetine, in BNF); avoidance of itraconazole advised by manufacturer of ● DAPOXETINE (increased risk of toxicity)
- Diuretics: fluconazole increases plasma concentration of EPLERENONE (reduce dose of eplerenone); itraconazole increases plasma concentration of ● EPLERENONE—avoid concomitant use; plasma concentration of fluconazole increased by HYDROCHLOROTHIAZIDE
- Domperidone: possible increased risk of ventricular arrhythmias when itraconazole or voriconazole given with ● DOMPERIDONE—avoid concomitant use
- Ergot Alkaloids: increased risk of ergotism when voriconazole given with ● ERGOMETRINE—avoid concomitant use; manufacturer of itraconazole advises avoid concomitant use with ● ERGOMETRINE (increased risk of ergotism); increased risk of ergotism when triazoles given with ● ERGOTAMINE— avoid concomitant use
- Guanfacine: fluconazole, itraconazole and posaconazole possibly increase the plasma concentration of ● GUANFACINE (halve dose of guanfacine)
- 5HT$_1$-receptor Agonists: itraconazole increases plasma concentration of ● ELETRIPTAN (risk of toxicity)—avoid concomitant use
- Ivabradine: fluconazole increases plasma concentration of IVABRADINE—reduce initial dose of ivabradine; itraconazole possibly increases plasma concentration of ● IVABRADINE— avoid concomitant use
- Ivacaftor: itraconazole, posaconazole and voriconazole possibly increase plasma concentration of ● IVACAFTOR (see under Ivacaftor, p. 175); fluconazole increases plasma concentration of ● IVACAFTOR (see under Ivacaftor, p. 175)
- Lenalidomide: itraconazole possibly increases plasma concentration of ● LENALIDOMIDE (increased risk of toxicity)
- Leukotriene Receptor Antagonists: fluconazole increases plasma concentration of ZAFIRLUKAST
- Lipid-regulating Drugs: increased risk of myopathy when itraconazole, posaconazole or voriconazole given with ● ATORVASTATIN; possible increased risk of myopathy when fluconazole given with ● ATORVASTATIN or ● SIMVASTATIN; fluconazole increases plasma concentration of FLUVASTATIN— possible increased risk of myopathy; itraconazole increases plasma concentration of ROSUVASTATIN—adjust dose of rosuvastatin (consult product literature); increased risk of myopathy when itraconazole or posaconazole given with ● SIMVASTATIN (avoid concomitant use); increased risk of myopathy when voriconazole given with ● SIMVASTATIN; avoidance of triazoles advised by manufacturer of ● LOMITAPIDE (plasma concentration of lomitapide possibly increased)
- Mirabegron: when given with itraconazole avoid or reduce dose of MIRABEGRON in hepatic or renal impairment—see Mirabegron, in BNF
- Oestrogens: plasma concentration of voriconazole increased by OESTROGENS
- Progestogens: plasma concentration of voriconazole possibly increased by PROGESTOGENS
- Ranolazine: itraconazole, posaconazole and voriconazole possibly increase plasma concentration of ● RANOLAZINE— manufacturer of ranolazine advises avoid concomitant use
- Retinoids: fluconazole and voriconazole possibly increase risk of ● TRETINOIN toxicity
- Riociguat: avoidance of itraconazole and voriconazole advised by manufacturer of RIOCIGUAT
- Sildenafil: itraconazole increases plasma concentration of SILDENAFIL—reduce initial dose of sildenafil

Antifungals, Triazole (continued)
- Sirolimus: fluconazole and posaconazole possibly increase plasma concentration of SIROLIMUS; itraconazole and voriconazole increase plasma concentration of • SIROLIMUS—avoid concomitant use
- Tacrolimus: fluconazole, itraconazole, posaconazole and voriconazole increase plasma concentration of • TACROLIMUS (consider reducing dose of tacrolimus)
- Tadalafil: itraconazole possibly increases plasma concentration of TADALAFIL
- Theophylline: fluconazole possibly increases plasma concentration of • THEOPHYLLINE
- Ulcer-healing Drugs: plasma concentration of posaconazole reduced by • CIMETIDINE and • ESOMEPRAZOLE—manufacturer of posaconazole *suspension* advises avoid concomitant use; plasma concentration of posaconazole possibly reduced by • FAMOTIDINE, • LANSOPRAZOLE, • NIZATIDINE, • OMEPRAZOLE, • PANTOPRAZOLE, • RABEPRAZOLE and • RANITIDINE—manufacturer of posaconazole *suspension* advises avoid concomitant use; voriconazole possibly increases plasma concentration of ESOMEPRAZOLE; voriconazole increases plasma concentration of OMEPRAZOLE (consider reducing dose of omeprazole); absorption of itraconazole reduced by HISTAMINE H₂-ANTAGONISTS and PROTON PUMP INHIBITORS
- Uliprital: avoidance of itraconazole advised by manufacturer of ULIPRISTAL
- Vardenafil: itraconazole possibly increases plasma concentration of • VARDENAFIL—avoid concomitant use

Antihistamines
NOTE Sedative interactions apply to a lesser extent to the non-sedating antihistamines. Interactions do not generally apply to antihistamines used for topical action (including inhalation)
- Alcohol: increased sedative effect when antihistamines given with ALCOHOL (possibly less effect with non-sedating antihistamines)
- Analgesics: sedative effects possibly increased when sedating antihistamines given with • OPIOID ANALGESICS
- Antacids: absorption of fexofenadine reduced by ANTACIDS
- Anti-arrhythmics: increased risk of ventricular arrhythmias when mizolastine given with • AMIODARONE, • DISOPYRAMIDE or • FLECAINIDE—avoid concomitant use; manufacturer of mizolastine advises avoid concomitant use with PROPAFENONE (possible risk of ventricular arrhythmias)
- Antibacterials: manufacturer of loratadine advises plasma concentration possibly increased by ERYTHROMYCIN; metabolism of mizolastine inhibited by • ERYTHROMYCIN—avoid concomitant use; increased risk of ventricular arrhythmias when mizolastine given with • MOXIFLOXACIN—avoid concomitant use; effects of fexofenadine possibly reduced by RIFAMPICIN; metabolism of mizolastine possibly inhibited by • MACROLIDES (avoid concomitant use)
- Antidepressants: avoidance of mizolastine advised by manufacturer of • CITALOPRAM and • ESCITALOPRAM (risk of ventricular arrhythmias); increased antimuscarinic and sedative effects when antihistamines given with MAOIs or TRICYCLICS; manufacturer of promethazine advises avoid for 2 weeks after stopping MAOIs; manufacturer of hydroxyzine advises avoid concomitant use with MAOIs; cyproheptadine possibly antagonises antidepressant effect of SSRIs; possible increased antimuscarinic and sedative effects when antihistamines given with TRICYCLIC-RELATED ANTIDEPRESSANTS
- Antidiabetics: thrombocyte count depressed when ketotifen given with METFORMIN (manufacturer of ketotifen advises avoid concomitant use)
- Antifungals: metabolism of mizolastine inhibited by • ITRACONAZOLE—avoid concomitant use; metabolism of mizolastine possibly inhibited by • IMIDAZOLES (avoid concomitant use)
- Antimalarials: avoidance of mizolastine advised by manufacturer of • ARTENIMOL WITH PIPERAQUINE (possible risk of ventricular arrhythmias)
- Antimuscarinics: increased risk of antimuscarinic side-effects when antihistamines given with ANTIMUSCARINICS
- Antivirals: plasma concentration of chlorphenamine possibly increased by LOPINAVIR; plasma concentration of non-

Antihistamines
- Antivirals (continued)
  sedating antihistamines possibly increased by RITONAVIR; increased risk of ventricular arrhythmias when mizolastine given with • SAQUINAVIR—avoid concomitant use
- Anxiolytics and Hypnotics: increased sedative effect when antihistamines given with ANXIOLYTICS AND HYPNOTICS
- Beta-blockers: increased risk of ventricular arrhythmias when mizolastine given with • SOTALOL—avoid concomitant use
- Betahistine: antihistamines theoretically antagonise effect of BETAHISTINE
- Cytotoxics: possible increased risk of ventricular arrhythmias when mizolastine given with • VANDETANIB—avoid concomitant use
- Grapefruit Juice: plasma concentration of bilastine reduced by GRAPEFRUIT JUICE
- Histamine: antihistamines theoretically antagonise effects of HISTAMINE—manufacturer of histamine advises avoid concomitant use
- Sympathomimetics: avoidance of antihistamines advised by manufacturer of MIDODRINE
- Ulcer-healing Drugs: manufacturer of loratadine advises plasma concentration possibly increased by CIMETIDINE; plasma concentration of hydroxyzine increased by CIMETIDINE
- Ulipristal: manufacturer of ulipristal advises give fexofenadine at least 1.5 hours before or after ULIPRISTAL

Antihistamines, Non-sedating *see* Antihistamines
Antihistamines, Sedating *see* Antihistamines
Antimalarials *see* Artemether with Lumefantrine, Artenimol with Piperaquine, Chloroquine, Hydroxychloroquine, Mefloquine, Primaquine, Proguanil, Pyrimethamine, and Quinine
Antimetabolites *see* Capecitabine, Cladribine, Cytarabine, Decitabine, Fludarabine, Fluorouracil, Gemcitabine, Mercaptopurine, Methotrexate, Pemetrexed, Raltitrexed, Tegafur, and Tioguanine

Antimuscarinics
NOTE Many drugs have antimuscarinic effects; concomitant use of two or more such drugs can increase side-effects such as dry mouth, urine retention, and constipation; concomitant use can also lead to confusion in the elderly. Interactions do not generally apply to antimuscarinics used by inhalation
- Alcohol: increased sedative effect when hyoscine given with ALCOHOL
- Analgesics: possible increased risk of antimuscarinic side-effects when antimuscarinics given with CODEINE; increased risk of antimuscarinic side-effects when antimuscarinics given with NEFOPAM
- Anti-arrhythmics: increased risk of ventricular arrhythmias when tolterodine given with • AMIODARONE, • DISOPYRAMIDE or • FLECAINIDE; increased risk of antimuscarinic side-effects when antimuscarinics given with DISOPYRAMIDE
- Antibacterials: manufacturer of fesoterodine advises dose reduction when fesoterodine given with CLARITHROMYCIN and TELITHROMYCIN—consult fesoterodine product literature; manufacturer of tolterodine advises avoid concomitant use with CLARITHROMYCIN and ERYTHROMYCIN; plasma concentration of darifenacin possibly increased by ERYTHROMYCIN; plasma concentration of active metabolite of fesoterodine reduced by • RIFAMPICIN—avoid concomitant use
- Antidepressants: plasma concentration of darifenacin and procyclidine increased by PAROXETINE; increased risk of antimuscarinic side-effects when antimuscarinics given with MAOIs or TRICYCLICS; plasma concentration of active metabolite of fesoterodine possibly reduced by • ST JOHN'S WORT—manufacturer of fesoterodine advises avoid concomitant use; possible increased antimuscarinic side-effects when antimuscarinics given with TRICYCLIC-RELATED ANTIDEPRESSANTS
- Antiepileptics: plasma concentration of active metabolite of fesoterodine possibly reduced by • CARBAMAZEPINE, • PHENOBARBITAL and • PHENYTOIN—manufacturer of fesoterodine advises avoid concomitant use
- Antifungals: antimuscarinics reduce absorption of KETOCONAZOLE; manufacturer of fesoterodine advises dose reduction when fesoterodine given with ITRACONAZOLE and

Antimuscarinics

- **Antifungals** (continued)

KETOCONAZOLE—consult fesoterodine product literature; plasma concentration of darifenacin increased by KETOCONAZOLE—avoid concomitant use; plasma concentration of solifenacin increased by • KETOCONAZOLE—see under Solifenacin, in BNF; plasma concentration of oxybutynin increased by KETOCONAZOLE; manufacturer of tolterodine advises avoid concomitant use with ITRACONAZOLE and • KETOCONAZOLE; manufacturer of darifenacin advises avoid concomitant use with ITRACONAZOLE; plasma concentration of solifenacin possibly increased by • ITRACONAZOLE—see under Solifenacin, in BNF

▸ **Antihistamines:** increased risk of antimuscarinic side-effects when antimuscarinics given with ANTIHISTAMINES

▸ **Antipsychotics:** antimuscarinics possibly reduce effects of HALOPERIDOL; increased risk of antimuscarinic side-effects when antimuscarinics given with CLOZAPINE; antimuscarinics reduce plasma concentration of PHENOTHIAZINES, but risk of antimuscarinic side-effects increased

- **Antivirals:** manufacturer of darifenacin advises avoid concomitant use with ATAZANAVIR, FOSAMPRENAVIR, INDINAVIR, LOPINAVIR, RITONAVIR, SAQUINAVIR and TIPRANAVIR; manufacturer of fesoterodine advises dose reduction when fesoterodine given with ATAZANAVIR, INDINAVIR, RITONAVIR and SAQUINAVIR—consult fesoterodine product literature; manufacturer of tolterodine advises avoid concomitant use with FOSAMPRENAVIR, INDINAVIR, LOPINAVIR, RITONAVIR and SAQUINAVIR; plasma concentration of solifenacin possibly increased by • RITONAVIR—see under Solifenacin, in BNF

- **Beta-blockers:** increased risk of ventricular arrhythmias when tolterodine given with • SOTALOL

▸ **Calcium-channel Blockers:** plasma concentration of solifenacin increased by VERAPAMIL; manufacturer of darifenacin advises avoid concomitant use with VERAPAMIL

▸ **Cardiac Glycosides:** darifenacin possibly increases plasma concentration of DIGOXIN

▸ **Ciclosporin:** manufacturer of darifenacin advises avoid concomitant use with CICLOSPORIN

▸ **Domperidone:** antimuscarinics antagonise effects of DOMPERIDONE on gastro-intestinal activity

▸ **Dopaminergics:** antimuscarinics possibly reduce absorption of CO-BENELDOPA, CO-CARELDOPA and LEVODOPA

▸ **Hormone Antagonists:** possible increased risk of bradycardia when ipratropium or oxybutynin given with PASIREOTIDE

▸ **Memantine:** effects of antimuscarinics possibly enhanced by MEMANTINE

▸ **Metoclopramide:** antimuscarinics antagonise effects of METOCLOPRAMIDE on gastro-intestinal activity

▸ **Nitrates:** antimuscarinics possibly reduce effects of sublingual tablets of NITRATES (failure to dissolve under tongue owing to dry mouth)

▸ **Parasympathomimetics:** antimuscarinics antagonise effects of PARASYMPATHOMIMETICS

Antipsychotics

NOTE Increased risk of toxicity with myelosuppressive drugs

NOTE Avoid concomitant use of clozapine with drugs that have a substantial potential for causing agranulocytosis

▸ **ACE Inhibitors:** enhanced hypotensive effect when antipsychotics given with ACE INHIBITORS

▸ **Adrenergic Neurone Blockers:** enhanced hypotensive effect when phenothiazines given with ADRENERGIC NEURONE BLOCKERS; higher doses of chlorpromazine antagonise hypotensive effect of ADRENERGIC NEURONE BLOCKERS; haloperidol antagonises hypotensive effect of ADRENERGIC NEURONE BLOCKERS

▸ **Adsorbents:** absorption of phenothiazines possibly reduced by KAOLIN

▸ **Alcohol:** increased sedative effect when antipsychotics given with ALCOHOL

▸ **Alpha-blockers:** enhanced hypotensive effect when antipsychotics given with ALPHA-BLOCKERS

- **Anaesthetics, General:** droperidol enhances effects of THIOPENTAL; enhanced hypotensive effect when antipsychotics given with • GENERAL ANAESTHETICS

Antipsychotics (continued)

- **Analgesics:** possible severe drowsiness when haloperidol given with ACEMETACIN or INDOMETACIN; increased risk of ventricular arrhythmias when antipsychotics that prolong the QT interval given with • METHADONE; increased risk of ventricular arrhythmias when amisulpride given with • METHADONE—avoid concomitant use; increased risk of convulsions when antipsychotics given with TRAMADOL; enhanced hypotensive and sedative effects when antipsychotics given with OPIOID ANALGESICS

▸ **Angiotensin-II Receptor Antagonists:** enhanced hypotensive effect when antipsychotics given with ANGIOTENSIN-II RECEPTOR ANTAGONISTS

▸ **Antacids:** absorption of phenothiazines and sulpiride reduced by ANTACIDS

- **Anti-arrhythmics:** increased risk of ventricular arrhythmias when antipsychotics that prolong the QT interval given with • ANTI-ARRHYTHMICS that prolong the QT interval; increased risk of ventricular arrhythmias when amisulpride, droperidol, haloperidol, phenothiazines, pimozide or zuclopenthixol given with • AMIODARONE—avoid concomitant use; increased risk of ventricular arrhythmias when benperidol given with • AMIODARONE—manufacturer of benperidol advises avoid concomitant use; increased risk of ventricular arrhythmias when sulpiride given with • AMIODARONE or • DISOPYRAMIDE; increased risk of ventricular arrhythmias when amisulpride, droperidol, pimozide or zuclopenthixol given with • DISOPYRAMIDE—avoid concomitant use; possible increased risk of ventricular arrhythmias when haloperidol given with • DISOPYRAMIDE—avoid concomitant use; increased risk of ventricular arrhythmias when phenothiazines given with • DISOPYRAMIDE; avoidance of phenothiazines advised by manufacturer of • DRONEDARONE (risk of ventricular arrhythmias); increased risk of arrhythmias when clozapine given with • FLECAINIDE

- **Antibacterials:** plasma concentration of lurasidone possibly increased by • CLARITHROMYCIN and • TELITHROMYCIN—avoid concomitant use; increased risk of ventricular arrhythmias when pimozide given with • CLARITHROMYCIN, • MOXIFLOXACIN or • TELITHROMYCIN—avoid concomitant use; plasma concentration of quetiapine possibly increased by • CLARITHROMYCIN—manufacturer of quetiapine advises avoid concomitant use; plasma concentration of lurasidone possibly increased by • ERYTHROMYCIN (see under Lurasidone, in BNF); increased risk of ventricular arrhythmias when amisulpride given with • ERYTHROMYCIN—avoid concomitant use; plasma concentration of clozapine possibly increased by • ERYTHROMYCIN (possible increased risk of convulsions); possible increased risk of ventricular arrhythmias when pimozide given with • ERYTHROMYCIN—avoid concomitant use; plasma concentration of quetiapine increased by • ERYTHROMYCIN—manufacturer of quetiapine advises avoid concomitant use; increased risk of ventricular arrhythmias when sulpiride given with *parenteral* • ERYTHROMYCIN; increased risk of ventricular arrhythmias when zuclopenthixol given with *parenteral* • ERYTHROMYCIN—avoid concomitant use; plasma concentration of clozapine increased by CIPROFLOXACIN; plasma concentration of olanzapine possibly increased by CIPROFLOXACIN; increased risk of ventricular arrhythmias when droperidol, haloperidol, phenothiazines or zuclopenthixol given with • MOXIFLOXACIN—avoid concomitant use; increased risk of ventricular arrhythmias when benperidol given with • MOXIFLOXACIN—manufacturer of benperidol advises avoid concomitant use; plasma concentration of aripiprazole possibly reduced by • RIFABUTIN and • RIFAMPICIN (avoid concomitant use or consider increasing the dose of aripiprazole—consult aripiprazole product literature); plasma concentration of lurasidone reduced by • RIFAMPICIN—avoid concomitant use; plasma concentration of clozapine possibly reduced by RIFAMPICIN; metabolism of haloperidol accelerated by • RIFAMPICIN (reduced plasma concentration); avoid concomitant use of clozapine with • CHLORAMPHENICOL or • SULFONAMIDES (increased risk of agranulocytosis); increased risk of ventricular arrhythmias when droperidol, haloperidol or pimozide given with • DELAMANID; increased risk of

Antipsychotics

- **Antibacterials** (continued)

ventricular arrhythmias when phenothiazines that prolong the QT interval given with • DELAMANID; manufacturer of droperidol advises avoid concomitant use with • MACROLIDES (risk of ventricular arrhythmias); possible increased risk of ventricular arrhythmias when chlorpromazine given with • TELITHROMYCIN; plasma concentration of quetiapine possibly increased by TELITHROMYCIN

- **Antidepressants**: plasma concentration of clozapine possibly increased by CITALOPRAM (increased risk of toxicity); avoidance of haloperidol, phenothiazines and pimozide advised by manufacturer of • CITALOPRAM (risk of ventricular arrhythmias); avoidance of haloperidol, phenothiazines and pimozide advised by manufacturer of • ESCITALOPRAM (risk of ventricular arrhythmias); plasma concentration of aripiprazole possibly increased by • FLUOXETINE and • PAROXETINE (reduce dose of aripiprazole—consult aripiprazole product literature); plasma concentration of clozapine, haloperidol and risperidone increased by • FLUOXETINE; manufacturer of droperidol advises avoid concomitant use with • FLUOXETINE, • FLUVOXAMINE, • SERTRALINE and • TRICYCLICS (risk of ventricular arrhythmias); plasma concentration of asenapine and haloperidol possibly increased by FLUVOXAMINE; plasma concentration of clozapine and olanzapine increased by • FLUVOXAMINE; asenapine possibly increases plasma concentration of PAROXETINE; plasma concentration of clozapine increased by • PAROXETINE and • SERTRALINE; plasma concentration of risperidone possibly increased by PAROXETINE (increased risk of toxicity); metabolism of perphenazine inhibited by PAROXETINE (reduce dose of perphenazine); plasma concentration of haloperidol increased by VENLAFAXINE; clozapine possibly increases CNS effects of • MAOIS; plasma concentration of pimozide possibly increased by • SSRIS (increased risk of ventricular arrhythmias—avoid concomitant use); plasma concentration of lurasidone possibly reduced by • ST JOHN'S WORT—avoid concomitant use; plasma concentration of aripiprazole possibly reduced by • ST JOHN'S WORT (avoid concomitant use or consider increasing the dose of aripiprazole—consult aripiprazole product literature); manufacturer of fluphenazine, haloperidol, sulpiride and zuclopenthixol advises avoid concomitant use with • TRICYCLICS (risk of ventricular arrhythmias); increased risk of antimuscarinic side-effects when phenothiazines given with TRICYCLICS; possible increased risk of ventricular arrhythmias when risperidone given with • TRICYCLICS; possible increased antimuscarinic side-effects when clozapine given with TRICYCLICS; possible increased risk of convulsions when butyrophenones, phenothiazines or thioxanthenes given with • VORTIOXETINE

- **Antidiabetics**: phenothiazines possibly antagonise hypoglycaemic effect of SULFONYLUREAS

- **Antiepileptics**: antipsychotics antagonise anticonvulsant effect of • ANTIEPILEPTICS (convulsive threshold lowered); metabolism of haloperidol, olanzapine, quetiapine and risperidone accelerated by CARBAMAZEPINE (reduced plasma concentration); metabolism of clozapine accelerated by • CARBAMAZEPINE (reduced plasma concentration), also avoid concomitant use of drugs with substantial potential for causing agranulocytosis; plasma concentration of aripiprazole reduced by • CARBAMAZEPINE (avoid concomitant use or consider increasing the dose of aripiprazole —consult aripiprazole product literature); plasma concentration of paliperidone reduced by CARBAMAZEPINE; plasma concentration of lurasidone possibly reduced by • CARBAMAZEPINE, • FOSPHENYTOIN, • PHENOBARBITAL, • PHENYTOIN and • PRIMIDONE—avoid concomitant use; chlorpromazine possibly increases or decreases plasma concentration of FOSPHENYTOIN and PHENYTOIN; metabolism of clozapine and quetiapine accelerated by FOSPHENYTOIN (reduced plasma concentration); plasma concentration of aripiprazole possibly reduced by • FOSPHENYTOIN, • PHENOBARBITAL, • PHENYTOIN and • PRIMIDONE (avoid concomitant use or consider increasing the dose of

Antipsychotics

- **Antiepileptics** (continued)

aripiprazole—consult aripiprazole product literature); plasma concentration of haloperidol reduced by FOSPHENYTOIN and PHENYTOIN; metabolism of haloperidol accelerated by PHENOBARBITAL and PRIMIDONE (reduced plasma concentration); plasma concentration of both drugs reduced when chlorpromazine given with PHENOBARBITAL and PRIMIDONE; plasma concentration of clozapine possibly reduced by PHENOBARBITAL and PRIMIDONE; metabolism of clozapine and quetiapine accelerated by PHENYTOIN (reduced plasma concentration); increased risk of side-effects including neutropenia when olanzapine given with • SODIUM VALPROATE and • VALPROIC ACID; plasma concentration of clozapine possibly increased or decreased by SODIUM VALPROATE and VALPROIC ACID

- **Antifungals**: plasma concentration of lurasidone increased by • KETOCONAZOLE—avoid concomitant use; metabolism of aripiprazole inhibited by • KETOCONAZOLE (reduce dose of aripiprazole); plasma concentration of lurasidone possibly increased by • FLUCONAZOLE (see under Lurasidone, in BNF); plasma concentration of lurasidone possibly increased by • ITRACONAZOLE, • POSACONAZOLE and • VORICONAZOLE—avoid concomitant use; plasma concentration of aripiprazole possibly increased by • ITRACONAZOLE (reduce dose of aripiprazole—consult aripiprazole product literature); side-effects of risperidone possibly increased by ITRACONAZOLE; plasma concentration of haloperidol possibly increased by ITRACONAZOLE; increased risk of ventricular arrhythmias when pimozide given with • IMIDAZOLES or • TRIAZOLES—avoid concomitant use; plasma concentration of quetiapine possibly increased by • IMIDAZOLES and • TRIAZOLES— manufacturer of quetiapine advises avoid concomitant use

- **Antimalarials**: avoidance of antipsychotics advised by manufacturer of • ARTEMETHER WITH LUMEFANTRINE; avoidance of droperidol, haloperidol, phenothiazines and pimozide advised by manufacturer of • ARTENIMOL WITH PIPERAQUINE (possible risk of ventricular arrhythmias); increased risk of ventricular arrhythmias when droperidol given with • CHLOROQUINE, • HYDROXYCHLOROQUINE or • QUININE—avoid concomitant use; possible increased risk of ventricular arrhythmias when haloperidol given with • MEFLOQUINE or • QUININE—avoid concomitant use; manufacturer of risperidone advises possible risk of ventricular arrhythmias when risperidone given with • MEFLOQUINE; increased risk of ventricular arrhythmias when pimozide given with • MEFLOQUINE or • QUININE—avoid concomitant use; manufacturer of amisulpride advises avoid concomitant use with MEFLOQUINE; possible increased risk of ventricular arrhythmias when risperidone given with • QUININE

- Antimuscarinics: increased risk of antimuscarinic side-effects when clozapine given with ANTIMUSCARINICS; plasma concentration of phenothiazines reduced by ANTIMUSCARINICS, but risk of antimuscarinic side-effects increased; effects of haloperidol possibly reduced by ANTIMUSCARINICS

- **Antipsychotics**: increased risk of ventricular arrhythmias when amisulpride, pimozide or sulpiride given with • DROPERIDOL— avoid concomitant use; increased risk of ventricular arrhythmias when phenothiazines that prolong the QT interval given with • DROPERIDOL—avoid concomitant use; avoid concomitant use of clozapine with depot formulation of • FLUPENTIXOL, • FLUPHENAZINE, • HALOPERIDOL, • RISPERIDONE or • ZUCLOPENTHIXOL as cannot be withdrawn quickly if neutropenia occurs; increased risk of ventricular arrhythmias when sulpiride given with • HALOPERIDOL; chlorpromazine possibly increases plasma concentration of HALOPERIDOL; increased risk of ventricular arrhythmias when droperidol given with • HALOPERIDOL—avoid concomitant use; increased risk of ventricular arrhythmias when pimozide given with • PHENOTHIAZINES—avoid concomitant use; lurasidone possibly increases plasma concentration of PIMOZIDE (increased risk of toxicity); possible increased risk of ventricular arrhythmias when antipsychotics that prolong the QT interval given with • RISPERIDONE; increased risk of ventricular arrhythmias when pimozide given with • SULPIRIDE

Antipsychotics (continued)

- **Antivirals:** plasma concentration of aripiprazole possibly increased by ● ATAZANAVIR, ● DARUNAVIR, ● FOSAMPRENAVIR, ● INDINAVIR, ● LOPINAVIR, ● RITONAVIR, ● SAQUINAVIR and ● TIPRANAVIR (reduce dose of aripiprazole—consult aripiprazole product literature); plasma concentration of quetiapine possibly increased by ● ATAZANAVIR, ● BOCEPREVIR, ● DARUNAVIR, ● FOSAMPRENAVIR, ● INDINAVIR, ● LOPINAVIR, ● RITONAVIR, ● SAQUINAVIR, ● TELAPREVIR and ● TIPRANAVIR— manufacturer of quetiapine advises avoid concomitant use; plasma concentration of pimozide possibly increased by ● ATAZANAVIR—avoid concomitant use; avoidance of pimozide advised by manufacturer of ● BOCEPREVIR and ● TELAPREVIR; plasma concentration of lurasidone possibly increased by ● BOCEPREVIR, ● INDINAVIR, ● RITONAVIR, ● SAQUINAVIR and ● TELAPREVIR—avoid concomitant use; plasma concentration of aripiprazole possibly reduced by ● EFAVIRENZ and ● NEVIRAPINE (avoid concomitant use or consider increasing the dose of aripiprazole—consult aripiprazole product literature); plasma concentration of pimozide possibly increased by ● EFAVIRENZ, ● INDINAVIR and ● SAQUINAVIR (increased risk of ventricular arrhythmias—avoid concomitant use); plasma concentration of pimozide increased by ● FOSAMPRENAVIR and ● RITONAVIR (increased risk of ventricular arrhythmias—avoid concomitant use); plasma concentration of antipsychotics possibly increased by ● RITONAVIR; plasma concentration of olanzapine reduced by RITONAVIR—consider increasing dose of olanzapine; avoidance of clozapine advised by manufacturer of ● RITONAVIR (increased risk of toxicity); increased risk of ventricular arrhythmias when clozapine, haloperidol or phenothiazines given with ● SAQUINAVIR—avoid concomitant use
- **Anxiolytics and Hypnotics:** increased sedative effect when antipsychotics given with ANXIOLYTICS AND HYPNOTICS; plasma concentration of haloperidol possibly increased by ALPRAZOLAM; lurasidone increases plasma concentration of MIDAZOLAM; serious adverse events reported with concomitant use of clozapine and ● BENZODIAZEPINES (causality not established); increased risk of hypotension, bradycardia and respiratory depression when *intramuscular* olanzapine given with *parenteral* ● BENZODIAZEPINES; plasma concentration of haloperidol increased by BUSPIRONE
- **Aprepitant:** avoidance of pimozide advised by manufacturer of ● APREPITANT
- **Atomoxetine:** increased risk of ventricular arrhythmias when antipsychotics that prolong the QT interval given with ● ATOMOXETINE
- **Beta-blockers:** enhanced hypotensive effect when phenothiazines given with BETA-BLOCKERS; plasma concentration of both drugs may increase when chlorpromazine given with ● PROPRANOLOL; increased risk of ventricular arrhythmias when droperidol or zuclopenthixol given with ● SOTALOL—avoid concomitant use; increased risk of ventricular arrhythmias when amisulpride, phenothiazines, pimozide or sulpiride given with ● SOTALOL; possible increased risk of ventricular arrhythmias when risperidone given with ● SOTALOL; possible increased risk of ventricular arrhythmias when haloperidol given with ● SOTALOL—avoid concomitant use
- **Calcium-channel Blockers:** enhanced hypotensive effect when antipsychotics given with CALCIUM-CHANNEL BLOCKERS; plasma concentration of lurasidone increased by ● DILTIAZEM (see under Lurasidone, in BNF); plasma concentration of lurasidone possibly increased by ● VERAPAMIL (see under Lurasidone, in BNF)
- **Clonidine:** enhanced hypotensive effect when phenothiazines given with CLONIDINE
- **Cobicistat:** plasma concentration of lurasidone possibly increased by ● COBICISTAT—avoid concomitant use; plasma concentration of pimozide possibly increased by ● COBICISTAT—manufacturer of cobicistat advises avoid concomitant use
- **Cytotoxics:** avoid concomitant use of clozapine with ● CYTOTOXICS (increased risk of agranulocytosis); possible increased risk of ventricular arrhythmias when haloperidol given with ● BOSUTINIB; caution with pimozide advised by

Antipsychotics

- **Cytotoxics** (continued)
  manufacturer of ● CRIZOTINIB; avoidance of pimozide and quetiapine advised by manufacturer of IDELALISIB; avoidance of pimozide advised by manufacturer of ● LAPATINIB; possible increased risk of ventricular arrhythmias when amisulpride, chlorpromazine, haloperidol, pimozide, sulpiride or zuclopenthixol given with ● VANDETANIB—avoid concomitant use; increased risk of ventricular arrhythmias when antipsychotics that prolong the QT interval given with ● ARSENIC TRIOXIDE; increased risk of ventricular arrhythmias when haloperidol given with ● ARSENIC TRIOXIDE
- **Deferasirox:** avoidance of clozapine advised by manufacturer of DEFERASIROX
- **Desferrioxamine:** manufacturer of levomepromazine advises avoid concomitant use with DESFERRIOXAMINE; avoidance of prochlorperazine advised by manufacturer of DESFERRIOXAMINE
- **Diazoxide:** enhanced hypotensive effect when phenothiazines given with DIAZOXIDE
- **Diuretics:** risk of ventricular arrhythmias with amisulpride increased by hypokalaemia caused by ● DIURETICS; risk of ventricular arrhythmias with pimozide increased by hypokalaemia caused by ● DIURETICS (avoid concomitant use); enhanced hypotensive effect when phenothiazines given with DIURETICS
- **Dopaminergics:** increased risk of extrapyramidal side-effects when antipsychotics given with AMANTADINE; antipsychotics antagonise effects of APOMORPHINE, CO-BENELDOPA, CO-CARELDOPA, LEVODOPA and PERGOLIDE; antipsychotics antagonise hypoprolactinaemic and antiparkinsonian effects of BROMOCRIPTINE and CABERGOLINE; manufacturer of amisulpride advises avoid concomitant use of CO-BENELDOPA, CO-CARELDOPA and LEVODOPA (antagonism of effect); avoidance of antipsychotics advised by manufacturer of PRAMIPEXOLE, ROPINIROLE and ROTIGOTINE (antagonism of effect)
- **Ergot Alkaloids:** lurasidone possibly increases plasma concentration of ERGOT ALKALOIDS (increased risk of toxicity)
- **Fosaprepitant:** avoidance of pimozide advised by manufacturer of ● FOSAPREPITANT
- **Grapefruit Juice:** manufacturer of lurasidone and pimozide advises avoid concomitant use with GRAPEFRUIT JUICE; plasma concentration of quetiapine possibly increased by ● GRAPEFRUIT JUICE—manufacturer of quetiapine advises avoid concomitant use
- **Guanfacine:** sedative effects possibly increased when antipsychotics given with GUANFACINE
- **Histamine:** antipsychotics theoretically antagonise effects of HISTAMINE—manufacturer of histamine advises avoid concomitant use
- **Hormone Antagonists:** manufacturer of droperidol advises avoid concomitant use with ● TAMOXIFEN (risk of ventricular arrhythmias)
- **Ivabradine:** increased risk of ventricular arrhythmias when pimozide given with ● IVABRADINE
- **Lithium:** increased risk of extrapyramidal side-effects and possibly neurotoxicity when clozapine, flupentixol, haloperidol, phenothiazines, risperidone or zuclopenthixol given with ● LITHIUM; possible risk of toxicity when olanzapine given with LITHIUM; extrapyramidal side-effects of quetiapine possibly increased by LITHIUM; increased risk of extrapyramidal side-effects when sulpiride given with LITHIUM
- **Memantine:** effects of antipsychotics possibly reduced by MEMANTINE
- **Methyldopa:** enhanced hypotensive effect when antipsychotics given with METHYLDOPA (also increased risk of extrapyramidal effects)
- **Metoclopramide:** increased risk of extrapyramidal side-effects when antipsychotics given with METOCLOPRAMIDE
- **Moxonidine:** enhanced hypotensive effect when phenothiazines given with MOXONIDINE
- **Muscle Relaxants:** promazine possibly enhances effects of SUXAMETHONIUM
- **Nitrates:** enhanced hypotensive effect when phenothiazines given with NITRATES

Antipsychotics (continued)

- Penicillamine: increased risk of haematological toxicity when clozapine given with ● PENICILLAMINE—manufacturer of penicillamine advises avoid concomitant use
- Pentamidine Isetionate: increased risk of ventricular arrhythmias when amisulpride or droperidol given with ● PENTAMIDINE ISETIONATE—avoid concomitant use; increased risk of ventricular arrhythmias when phenothiazines given with ● PENTAMIDINE ISETIONATE
▸ Sodium Benzoate: haloperidol possibly reduces effects of SODIUM BENZOATE
▸ Sodium Oxybate: antipsychotics possibly enhance effects of SODIUM OXYBATE
▸ Sodium Phenylbutyrate: haloperidol possibly reduces effects of SODIUM PHENYLBUTYRATE
▸ Sympathomimetics: antipsychotics antagonise hypertensive effect of SYMPATHOMIMETICS; antipsychotic effects of chlorpromazine possibly antagonised by DEXAMFETAMINE; chlorpromazine possibly reduces effects of LISDEXAMFETAMINE; side-effects of risperidone possibly increased by METHYLPHENIDATE
- Tacrolimus: manufacturer of droperidol advises avoid concomitant use with ● TACROLIMUS (risk of ventricular arrhythmias)
- Tetrabenazine: increased risk of extrapyramidal side-effects when antipsychotics given with TETRABENAZINE
- Ulcer-healing Drugs: effects of antipsychotics, chlorpromazine and clozapine possibly enhanced by CIMETIDINE; plasma concentration of clozapine possibly reduced by OMEPRAZOLE; absorption of sulpiride reduced by SUCRALFATE
- Vasodilator Antihypertensives: enhanced hypotensive effect when phenothiazines given with HYDRALAZINE, MINOXIDIL or SODIUM NITROPRUSSIDE

Antivirals see individual drugs

Anxiolytics and Hypnotics

- ACE Inhibitors: enhanced hypotensive effect when anxiolytics and hypnotics given with ACE INHIBITORS
- Adrenergic Neurone Blockers: enhanced hypotensive effect when anxiolytics and hypnotics given with ADRENERGIC NEURONE BLOCKERS
- Alcohol: increased sedative effect when anxiolytics and hypnotics given with ALCOHOL
- Alpha-blockers: enhanced hypotensive and sedative effects when anxiolytics and hypnotics given with ALPHA-BLOCKERS
- Aminophylline: effects of benzodiazepines possibly reduced by AMINOPHYLLINE
- Anaesthetics, General: increased sedative effect when anxiolytics and hypnotics given with GENERAL ANAESTHETICS
- Analgesics: metabolism of midazolam possibly inhibited by FENTANYL; increased sedative effect when anxiolytics and hypnotics given with OPIOID ANALGESICS
- Angiotensin-II Receptor Antagonists: enhanced hypotensive effect when anxiolytics and hypnotics given with ANGIOTENSIN-II RECEPTOR ANTAGONISTS
- Antibacterials: metabolism of midazolam inhibited by ● CLARITHROMYCIN, ● ERYTHROMYCIN and ● TELITHROMYCIN (increased plasma concentration with increased sedation); plasma concentration of buspirone increased by ERYTHROMYCIN (reduce dose of buspirone); metabolism of zopiclone inhibited by ERYTHROMYCIN; manufacturer of zolpidem advises avoid concomitant use with CIPROFLOXACIN; metabolism of benzodiazepines possibly accelerated by RIFAMPICIN (reduced plasma concentration); metabolism of diazepam and zaleplon accelerated by RIFAMPICIN (reduced plasma concentration); metabolism of buspirone possibly accelerated by RIFAMPICIN; metabolism of zolpidem accelerated by RIFAMPICIN (reduced plasma concentration and reduced effect); plasma concentration of zopiclone significantly reduced by RIFAMPICIN; metabolism of diazepam inhibited by ISONIAZID
- Anticoagulants: chloral may transiently enhance anticoagulant effect of COUMARINS
- Antidepressants: plasma concentration of alprazolam increased by FLUOXETINE; plasma concentration of melatonin increased by ● FLUVOXAMINE—avoid concomitant use; plasma concentration of some benzodiazepines increased by

Anxiolytics and Hypnotics

- Antidepressants (continued)
FLUVOXAMINE; sedative effects possibly increased when zolpidem given with SERTRALINE; manufacturer of buspirone advises avoid concomitant use with MAOIs; avoidance of buspirone for 14 days after stopping ● TRANYLCYPROMINE advised by manufacturer of tranylcypromine; plasma concentration of *oral* midazolam possibly reduced by ST JOHN'S WORT; increased sedative effect when anxiolytics and hypnotics given with MIRTAZAPINE, TRICYCLIC-RELATED ANTIDEPRESSANTS or TRICYCLICS
▸ Antiepileptics: plasma concentration of midazolam reduced by CARBAMAZEPINE and PERAMPANEL; plasma concentration of clonazepam often reduced by CARBAMAZEPINE, FOSPHENYTOIN, PHENOBARBITAL, PHENYTOIN and PRIMIDONE; benzodiazepines possibly increase or decrease plasma concentration of FOSPHENYTOIN and PHENYTOIN; diazepam increases or decreases plasma concentration of FOSPHENYTOIN and PHENYTOIN; increased sedative effect when anxiolytics and hypnotics given with PHENOBARBITAL or PRIMIDONE; increased risk of side-effects when clonazepam given with SODIUM VALPROATE or VALPROIC ACID; clobazam possibly increases plasma concentration of SODIUM VALPROATE and VALPROIC ACID; plasma concentration of diazepam and lorazepam possibly increased by SODIUM VALPROATE; plasma concentration of clobazam increased by STIRIPENTOL; plasma concentration of diazepam and lorazepam possibly increased by VALPROIC ACID
- Antifungals: plasma concentration of alprazolam increased by ● KETOCONAZOLE—manufacturer of ketoconazole advises avoid concomitant use; plasma concentration of midazolam increased by ● KETOCONAZOLE (risk of prolonged sedation—avoid concomitant use of *oral* midazolam); plasma concentration of zolpidem increased by KETOCONAZOLE; plasma concentration of diazepam and midazolam increased by ● FLUCONAZOLE (risk of prolonged sedation); plasma concentration of alprazolam increased by ITRACONAZOLE; plasma concentration of midazolam increased by ● ITRACONAZOLE, ● POSACONAZOLE and ● VORICONAZOLE (risk of prolonged sedation); plasma concentration of buspirone increased by ITRACONAZOLE (reduce dose of buspirone); plasma concentration of diazepam increased by ● VORICONAZOLE (risk of prolonged sedation)
▸ Antihistamines: increased sedative effect when anxiolytics and hypnotics given with ANTIHISTAMINES
- Antipsychotics: increased sedative effect when anxiolytics and hypnotics given with ANTIPSYCHOTICS; alprazolam possibly increases plasma concentration of HALOPERIDOL; buspirone increases plasma concentration of HALOPERIDOL; serious adverse events reported with concomitant use of benzodiazepines and ● CLOZAPINE (causality not established); plasma concentration of midazolam increased by LURASIDONE; increased risk of hypotension, bradycardia and respiratory depression when *parenteral* benzodiazepines given with *intramuscular* ● OLANZAPINE
- Antivirals: plasma concentration of midazolam possibly increased by ● ATAZANAVIR—avoid concomitant use of *oral* midazolam; plasma concentration of *oral* midazolam increased by ● BOCEPREVIR—manufacturer of boceprevir advises avoid concomitant use; increased risk of prolonged sedation when midazolam given with ● EFAVIRENZ—avoid concomitant use; plasma concentration of midazolam possibly increased by ● FOSAMPRENAVIR, ● INDINAVIR, ● RITONAVIR and ● TELAPREVIR (risk of prolonged sedation—avoid concomitant use of *oral* midazolam); increased risk of prolonged sedation when alprazolam given with ● INDINAVIR—avoid concomitant use; plasma concentration of alprazolam, diazepam, flurazepam and zolpidem possibly increased by ● RITONAVIR (risk of extreme sedation and respiratory depression—avoid concomitant use); plasma concentration of anxiolytics and hypnotics possibly increased by RITONAVIR; plasma concentration of buspirone increased by RITONAVIR (increased risk of toxicity); plasma concentration of midazolam increased by ● SAQUINAVIR (risk of prolonged sedation—avoid concomitant use of *oral* midazolam); plasma concentration of *oral* midazolam increased by SIMEPREVIR

Anxiolytics and Hypnotics (continued)

▸ Aprepitant: plasma concentration of midazolam increased by APREPITANT (risk of prolonged sedation)

▸ Beta-blockers: enhanced hypotensive effect when anxiolytics and hypnotics given with BETA-BLOCKERS

▸ Calcium-channel Blockers: enhanced hypotensive effect when anxiolytics and hypnotics given with CALCIUM-CHANNEL BLOCKERS; midazolam increases absorption of LERCANIDIPINE; metabolism of midazolam inhibited by DILTIAZEM and VERAPAMIL (increased plasma concentration with increased sedation); plasma concentration of buspirone increased by DILTIAZEM and VERAPAMIL (reduce dose of buspirone)

• Cardiac Glycosides: alprazolam increases plasma concentration of DIGOXIN (increased risk of toxicity)

▸ Clonidine: enhanced hypotensive effect when anxiolytics and hypnotics given with CLONIDINE

• Cobicistat: avoidance of *oral* midazolam advised by manufacturer of • COBICISTAT

▸ Cytotoxics: plasma concentration of midazolam increased by • CRIZOTINIB and NILOTINIB; avoidance of *oral* midazolam advised by manufacturer of IDELALISIB

▸ Deferasirox: plasma concentration of midazolam possibly reduced by DEFERASIROX

▸ Diazoxide: enhanced hypotensive effect when anxiolytics and hypnotics given with DIAZOXIDE

▸ Disulfiram: metabolism of benzodiazepines inhibited by DISULFIRAM (increased sedative effects); increased risk of temazepam toxicity when given with DISULFIRAM

▸ Diuretics: enhanced hypotensive effect when anxiolytics and hypnotics given with DIURETICS; administration of chloral with *parenteral* FUROSEMIDE may displace thyroid hormone from binding sites

▸ Dopaminergics: benzodiazepines possibly antagonise effects of CO-BENELDOPA, CO-CARELDOPA and LEVODOPA

▸ Fosaprepitant: plasma concentration of midazolam increased by FOSAPREPITANT (risk of prolonged sedation)

▸ Grapefruit Juice: plasma concentration of *oral* midazolam possibly increased by GRAPEFRUIT JUICE; plasma concentration of buspirone increased by GRAPEFRUIT JUICE

▸ Guanfacine: sedative effects possibly increased when anxiolytics and hypnotics given with GUANFACINE

• Hormone Antagonists: plasma concentration of midazolam reduced by • ENZALUTAMIDE

▸ Ivacaftor: plasma concentration of midazolam increased by IVACAFTOR

▸ Lipid-regulating Drugs: plasma concentration of *intravenous* midazolam increased by ATORVASTATIN; separating administration from alprazolam by 12 hours advised by manufacturer of LOMITAPIDE

• Lithium: increased risk of neurotoxicity when clonazepam given with LITHIUM

• Lofexidine: increased sedative effect when anxiolytics and hypnotics given with LOFEXIDINE

• Methyldopa: enhanced hypotensive effect when anxiolytics and hypnotics given with METHYLDOPA

• Methylthioninium: possible risk of CNS toxicity when buspirone given with • METHYLTHIONINIUM—avoid concomitant use (if avoidance not possible, use lowest possible dose of methylthioninium and observe patient for up to 4 hours after administration)

▸ Moxonidine: enhanced hypotensive effect when anxiolytics and hypnotics given with MOXONIDINE; sedative effects possibly increased when benzodiazepines given with MOXONIDINE

▸ Muscle Relaxants: increased sedative effect when anxiolytics and hypnotics given with BACLOFEN or TIZANIDINE

▸ Netupitant: plasma concentration of midazolam increased by NETUPITANT

▸ Nitrates: enhanced hypotensive effect when anxiolytics and hypnotics given with NITRATES

▸ Oestrogens: plasma concentration of melatonin increased by OESTROGENS; plasma concentration of chlordiazepoxide, diazepam and nitrazepam possibly increased by OESTROGENS; plasma concentration of lorazepam, oxazepam and temazepam possibly reduced by OESTROGENS

▸ Progestogens: plasma concentration of chlordiazepoxide, diazepam and nitrazepam possibly increased by

Anxiolytics and Hypnotics

Progestogens (continued)

PROGESTOGENS; plasma concentration of lorazepam, oxazepam and temazepam possibly reduced by PROGESTOGENS

• Sodium Oxybate: benzodiazepines enhance effects of • SODIUM OXYBATE (avoid concomitant use)

▸ Theophylline: effects of benzodiazepines possibly reduced by THEOPHYLLINE

▸ Ulcer-healing Drugs: plasma concentration of melatonin increased by CIMETIDINE; metabolism of benzodiazepines, clomethiazole and zaleplon inhibited by CIMETIDINE (increased plasma concentration); metabolism of diazepam possibly inhibited by ESOMEPRAZOLE and OMEPRAZOLE (increased plasma concentration)

▸ Vasodilator Antihypertensives: enhanced hypotensive effect when anxiolytics and hypnotics given with HYDRALAZINE, MINOXIDIL or SODIUM NITROPRUSSIDE

Apixaban

• Analgesics: increased risk of haemorrhage when anticoagulants given with *intravenous* • DICLOFENAC (avoid concomitant use, including low-dose heparins); increased risk of haemorrhage when anticoagulants given with • KETOROLAC (avoid concomitant use, including low-dose heparins)

• Antibacterials: manufacturer of apixaban advises avoid concomitant use with CLARITHROMYCIN and TELITHROMYCIN; plasma concentration of apixaban possibly reduced by • RIFAMPICIN—manufacturer of apixaban advises avoid concomitant use when given for treatment of deep-vein thrombosis or pulmonary embolism

• Anticoagulants: increased risk of haemorrhage when apixaban given with other • ANTICOAGULANTS (avoid concomitant use except when switching with other anticoagulants or using heparin to maintain catheter patency); increased risk of haemorrhage when apixaban given with other anticoagulants given with • DABIGATRAN, • EDOXABAN and • RIVAROXABAN (avoid concomitant use except when switching with other anticoagulants or using heparin to maintain catheter patency)

• Antidepressants: plasma concentration of apixaban possibly reduced by • ST JOHN'S WORT—manufacturer of apixaban advises avoid concomitant use when given for treatment of deep-vein thrombosis or pulmonary embolism

• Antiepileptics: plasma concentration of apixaban possibly reduced by • CARBAMAZEPINE—manufacturer of apixaban advises avoid concomitant use when given for treatment of deep-vein thrombosis or pulmonary embolism; plasma concentration of apixaban possibly reduced by • FOSPHENYTOIN, • PHENOBARBITAL, • PHENYTOIN and • PRIMIDONE

• Antifungals: plasma concentration of apixaban increased by • KETOCONAZOLE—manufacturer of apixaban advises avoid concomitant use; manufacturer of apixaban advises avoid concomitant use with ITRACONAZOLE, POSACONAZOLE and VORICONAZOLE

▸ Antivirals: manufacturer of apixaban advises avoid concomitant use with ATAZANAVIR, BOCEPREVIR, DARUNAVIR, FOSAMPRENAVIR, INDINAVIR, LOPINAVIR, RITONAVIR, SAQUINAVIR, TELAPREVIR and TIPRANAVIR

▸ Cobicistat: manufacturer of apixaban advises avoid concomitant use with COBICISTAT

▸ Sulfinpyrazone: increased risk of bleeding when apixaban given with SULFINPYRAZONE

Apomorphine

▸ Antipsychotics: effects of apomorphine antagonised by ANTIPSYCHOTICS

• Domperidone: possible increased risk of ventricular arrhythmias when apomorphine given with • DOMPERIDONE

• Dopaminergics: effects of apomorphine possibly enhanced by ENTACAPONE

• 5HT₃-receptor Antagonists: possible increased hypotensive effect when apomorphine given with • ONDANSETRON—avoid concomitant use

▸ Memantine: effects of dopaminergics possibly enhanced by MEMANTINE

▸ Methyldopa: antiparkinsonian effect of dopaminergics antagonised by METHYLDOPA

Apraclonidine
▸ Antidepressants: manufacturer of apraclonidine advises avoid concomitant use with MAOIS, TRICYCLIC-RELATED ANTIDEPRESSANTS and TRICYCLICS
▸ Sympathomimetics: manufacturer of apraclonidine advises avoid concomitant use with SYMPATHOMIMETICS

Apremilast
● Antibacterials: plasma concentration of apremilast reduced by ● RIFAMPICIN—avoid concomitant use
● Antidepressants: plasma concentration of apremilast possibly reduced by ● ST JOHN'S WORT—avoid concomitant use
● Antiepileptics: plasma concentration of apremilast possibly reduced by ● CARBAMAZEPINE, ● PHENOBARBITAL and ● PHENYTOIN—avoid concomitant use

Aprepitant
● Antibacterials: plasma concentration of aprepitant possibly increased by CLARITHROMYCIN and TELITHROMYCIN; plasma concentration of aprepitant reduced by RIFAMPICIN
● Anticoagulants: aprepitant possibly reduces anticoagulant effect of WARFARIN
● Antidepressants: manufacturer of aprepitant advises avoid concomitant use with ● ST JOHN'S WORT
▸ Antidiabetics: aprepitant reduces plasma concentration of TOLBUTAMIDE
● Antiepileptics: plasma concentration of aprepitant possibly reduced by CARBAMAZEPINE, FOSPHENYTOIN, PHENOBARBITAL, PHENYTOIN and PRIMIDONE
● Antifungals: plasma concentration of aprepitant increased by KETOCONAZOLE
● Antipsychotics: manufacturer of aprepitant advises avoid concomitant use with ● PIMOZIDE
▸ Antivirals: plasma concentration of aprepitant possibly increased by RITONAVIR
▸ Anxiolytics and Hypnotics: aprepitant increases plasma concentration of MIDAZOLAM (risk of prolonged sedation)
▸ Avanafil: aprepitant possibly increases plasma concentration of ● AVANAFIL—see under Avanafil, in BNF
▸ Calcium-channel Blockers: plasma concentration of both drugs may increase when aprepitant given with DILTIAZEM
● Corticosteroids: aprepitant inhibits metabolism of DEXAMETHASONE and METHYLPREDNISOLONE (reduce dose of dexamethasone and methylprednisolone)
● Cytotoxics: aprepitant possibly increases the plasma concentration of ● BOSUTINIB—manufacturer of bosutinib advises avoid or consider reducing dose of bosutinib; aprepitant possibly increases the plasma concentration of ● IBRUTINIB—reduce dose of ibrutinib (see under Ibrutinib, in BNF)
▸ Dapoxetine: manufacturer of dapoxetine advises dose reduction when aprepitant given with DAPOXETINE (see under Dapoxetine, in BNF)
▸ Guanfacine: aprepitant possibly increases plasma concentration of GUANFACINE (halve dose of guanfacine)
● Oestrogens: aprepitant possibly causes contraceptive failure of hormonal contraceptives containing ● OESTROGENS (alternative contraception recommended)
● Progestogens: aprepitant possibly causes contraceptive failure of hormonal contraceptives containing ● PROGESTOGENS (alternative contraception recommended)

Argatroban
● Analgesics: increased risk of haemorrhage when anticoagulants given with *intravenous* ● DICLOFENAC (avoid concomitant use, including low-dose heparins); increased risk of haemorrhage when anticoagulants given with ● KETOROLAC (avoid concomitant use, including low-dose heparins)
● Anticoagulants: increased risk of haemorrhage when other anticoagulants given with ● APIXABAN, ● DABIGATRAN, ● EDOXABAN and ● RIVAROXABAN (avoid concomitant use except when switching with other anticoagulants or using heparin to maintain catheter patency)

Aripiprazole see Antipsychotics

Arsenic Trioxide
● Anti-arrhythmics: increased risk of ventricular arrhythmias when arsenic trioxide given with ● AMIODARONE or ● DISOPYRAMIDE

Arsenic Trioxide (continued)
● Antibacterials: increased risk of ventricular arrhythmias when arsenic trioxide given with ● DELAMANID, ● ERYTHROMYCIN, ● LEVOFLOXACIN or ● MOXIFLOXACIN
● Antidepressants: increased risk of ventricular arrhythmias when arsenic trioxide given with ● AMITRIPTYLINE or ● CLOMIPRAMINE
● Antifungals: increased risk of ventricular arrhythmias when arsenic trioxide given with ● AMPHOTERICIN
● Antimalarials: avoidance of arsenic trioxide advised by manufacturer of ● ARTENIMOL WITH PIPERAQUINE (possible risk of ventricular arrhythmias)
● Antipsychotics: increased risk of ventricular arrhythmias when arsenic trioxide given with ● ANTIPSYCHOTICS that prolong the QT interval; increased risk of ventricular arrhythmias when arsenic trioxide given with ● HALOPERIDOL; avoid concomitant use of cytotoxics with ● CLOZAPINE (increased risk of agranulocytosis)
● Beta-blockers: increased risk of ventricular arrhythmias when arsenic trioxide given with ● SOTALOL
● Cytotoxics: possible increased risk of ventricular arrhythmias when arsenic trioxide given with ● VANDETANIB—avoid concomitant use
● Diuretics: risk of ventricular arrhythmias with arsenic trioxide increased by hypokalaemia caused by ● ACETAZOLAMIDE, ● LOOP DIURETICS or ● THIAZIDES AND RELATED DIURETICS
● Lithium: increased risk of ventricular arrhythmias when arsenic trioxide given with ● LITHIUM

Artemether with Lumefantrine
● Anti-arrhythmics: manufacturer of artemether with lumefantrine advises avoid concomitant use with ● AMIODARONE, ● DISOPYRAMIDE and ● FLECAINIDE (risk of ventricular arrhythmias)
● Antibacterials: manufacturer of artemether with lumefantrine advises avoid concomitant use with ● MACROLIDES and QUINOLONES
● Antidepressants: possible increased risk of ventricular arrhythmias when artemether with lumefantrine given with ● CITALOPRAM or ● ESCITALOPRAM—avoid concomitant use; manufacturer of artemether with lumefantrine advises avoid concomitant use with ● ANTIDEPRESSANTS
● Antifungals: manufacturer of artemether with lumefantrine advises avoid concomitant use with ● IMIDAZOLES and ● TRIAZOLES
● Antimalarials: manufacturer of artemether with lumefantrine advises avoid concomitant use with ● ANTIMALARIALS; increased risk of ventricular arrhythmias when artemether with lumefantrine given with ● QUININE
● Antipsychotics: manufacturer of artemether with lumefantrine advises avoid concomitant use with ● ANTIPSYCHOTICS
● Antivirals: manufacturer of artemether with lumefantrine advises caution with ATAZANAVIR, FOSAMPRENAVIR, INDINAVIR, LOPINAVIR, RITONAVIR, SAQUINAVIR and TIPRANAVIR; avoidance of artemether with lumefantrine advised by manufacturer of ● BOCEPREVIR; plasma concentration of lumefantrine increased when artemether with lumefantrine given with DARUNAVIR; plasma concentration of artemether with lumefantrine reduced by ● EFAVIRENZ and ETRAVIRINE
● Beta-blockers: manufacturer of artemether with lumefantrine advises avoid concomitant use with ● METOPROLOL and ● SOTALOL
● Cytotoxics: possible increased risk of ventricular arrhythmias when artemether with lumefantrine given with ● VANDETANIB—avoid concomitant use
▸ Grapefruit Juice: plasma concentration of artemether with lumefantrine possibly increased by GRAPEFRUIT JUICE
▸ Histamine: avoidance of antimalarials advised by manufacturer of HISTAMINE
▸ Penicillamine: increased risk of haematological toxicity when antimalarials given with PENICILLAMINE—manufacturer of penicillamine advises avoid concomitant use
● Ulcer-healing Drugs: manufacturer of artemether with lumefantrine advises avoid concomitant use with ● CIMETIDINE
▸ Vaccines: antimalarials inactivate ORAL TYPHOID VACCINE—see under Typhoid Vaccine in BNFC

Artenimol with Piperaquine

> NOTE Piperaquine has a long half-life; there is a potential for drug interactions to occur for up to 3 months after treatment has been stopped

- Analgesics: manufacturer of artenimol with piperaquine advises avoid concomitant use with ● METHADONE (possible risk of ventricular arrhythmias)
- Anti-arrhythmics: manufacturer of artenimol with piperaquine advises avoid concomitant use with ● AMIODARONE and ● DISOPYRAMIDE (possible risk of ventricular arrhythmias)
- Antibacterials: manufacturer of artenimol with piperaquine advises avoid concomitant use with ● MACROLIDES and ● MOXIFLOXACIN (possible risk of ventricular arrhythmias); manufacturer of artenimol with piperaquine advises avoid concomitant use with RIFAMPICIN
- Antidepressants: possible increased risk of ventricular arrhythmias when artenimol with piperaquine given with ● CITALOPRAM or ● ESCITALOPRAM—avoid concomitant use; manufacturer of artenimol with piperaquine advises avoid concomitant use with ● ANTIDEPRESSANTS
> Antiepileptics: manufacturer of artenimol with piperaquine advises avoid concomitant use with CARBAMAZEPINE, FOSPHENYTOIN, PHENOBARBITAL, PHENYTOIN and PRIMIDONE
- Antifungals: manufacturer of artenimol with piperaquine advises avoid concomitant use with ● IMIDAZOLES and ● TRIAZOLES (possible risk of ventricular arrhythmias)
- Antihistamines: manufacturer of artenimol with piperaquine advises avoid concomitant use with ● MIZOLASTINE (possible risk of ventricular arrhythmias)
- Antimalarials: avoidance of antimalarials advised by manufacturer of ● ARTEMETHER WITH LUMEFANTRINE
- Antipsychotics: manufacturer of artenimol with piperaquine advises avoid concomitant use with ● DROPERIDOL, ● HALOPERIDOL, ● PHENOTHIAZINES and ● PIMOZIDE (possible risk of ventricular arrhythmias)
- Antivirals: manufacturer of artenimol with piperaquine advises avoid concomitant use with ● SAQUINAVIR (possible risk of ventricular arrhythmias)
- Beta-blockers: manufacturer of artenimol with piperaquine advises avoid concomitant use with ● SOTALOL (possible risk of ventricular arrhythmias)
- Cytotoxics: manufacturer of artenimol with piperaquine advises avoid concomitant use with ● ARSENIC TRIOXIDE (possible risk of ventricular arrhythmias); manufacturer of artenimol with piperaquine advises avoid concomitant use with ● VINBLASTINE, ● VINCRISTINE, ● VINFLUNINE and ● VINORELBINE
- Domperidone: manufacturer of artenimol with piperaquine advises avoid concomitant use with ● DOMPERIDONE (possible risk of ventricular arrhythmias)
> Grapefruit Juice: manufacturer of artenimol with piperaquine advises avoid concomitant use with GRAPEFRUIT JUICE
> Histamine: avoidance of antimalarials advised by manufacturer of HISTAMINE
> Penicillamine: increased risk of haematological toxicity when antimalarials given with PENICILLAMINE—manufacturer of penicillamine advises avoid concomitant use
- Pentamidine Isetionate: manufacturer of artenimol with piperaquine advises avoid concomitant use with ● PENTAMIDINE ISETIONATE (possible risk of ventricular arrhythmias)
> Vaccines: antimalarials inactivate ORAL TYPHOID VACCINE—see under Typhoid Vaccine in BNFC

Ascorbic acid *see* Vitamins

Asenapine *see* Antipsychotics

Aspirin

> Adsorbents: absorption of aspirin possibly reduced by KAOLIN
> Anaesthetics, General: aspirin possibly enhances effects of THIOPENTAL
- Analgesics: avoid concomitant use of aspirin with ● NSAIDS (increased side-effects); antiplatelet effect of aspirin possibly reduced by IBUPROFEN
> Antacids: excretion of aspirin increased by alkaline urine due to some ANTACIDS
- Anticoagulants: increased risk of bleeding when aspirin given with ● COUMARINS or ● PHENINDIONE (due to antiplatelet

Aspirin

- Anticoagulants (continued)
  effect); increased risk of bleeding when high-dose aspirin given with ● EDOXABAN (avoid concomitant use); aspirin enhances anticoagulant effect of ● HEPARINS
- Antidepressants: increased risk of bleeding when aspirin given with ● SSRIS or ● VENLAFAXINE
> Antiepileptics: aspirin enhances effects of FOSPHENYTOIN, PHENYTOIN, SODIUM VALPROATE and VALPROIC ACID
> Clopidogrel: increased risk of bleeding when aspirin given with CLOPIDOGREL
> Corticosteroids: increased risk of gastro-intestinal bleeding and ulceration when aspirin given with CORTICOSTEROIDS, also corticosteroids reduce plasma concentration of salicylate
- Cytotoxics: aspirin reduces excretion of ● METHOTREXATE (increased risk of toxicity); aspirin possibly reduces renal excretion of PEMETREXED—consult product literature
- Diuretics: increased risk of toxicity when high-dose aspirin given with ● ACETAZOLAMIDE; aspirin antagonises diuretic effect of SPIRONOLACTONE; possible increased risk of toxicity when high-dose aspirin given with LOOP DIURETICS (also possible reduced effect of loop diuretics)
- Iloprost: increased risk of bleeding when aspirin given with ILOPROST
> Leukotriene Receptor Antagonists: aspirin increases plasma concentration of ZAFIRLUKAST
> Metoclopramide: rate of absorption of aspirin increased by METOCLOPRAMIDE (enhanced effect)
> Nicorandil: increased risk of gastro-intestinal bleeding and ulceration when aspirin given with NICORANDIL
> Sulfinpyrazone: aspirin antagonises effects of SULFINPYRAZONE

Atazanavir

> Analgesics: atazanavir increases plasma concentration of BUPRENORPHINE
> Antacids: absorption of atazanavir reduced by ANTACIDS (give at least 2 hours before or 1 hour after antacids)
- Anti-arrhythmics: atazanavir possibly increases plasma concentration of ● AMIODARONE and ● LIDOCAINE
- Antibacterials: plasma concentration of both drugs increased when atazanavir given with CLARITHROMYCIN; atazanavir increases plasma concentration of ● RIFABUTIN (reduce dose of rifabutin); plasma concentration of atazanavir reduced by ● RIFAMPICIN—avoid concomitant use; avoidance of concomitant atazanavir in severe renal and hepatic impairment advised by manufacturer of ● TELITHROMYCIN
- Anticoagulants: atazanavir may enhance or reduce anticoagulant effect of WARFARIN; avoidance of atazanavir advised by manufacturer of APIXABAN and RIVAROXABAN
- Antidepressants: plasma concentration of atazanavir reduced by ● ST JOHN'S WORT—avoid concomitant use
- Antifungals: plasma concentration of atazanavir increased by ● POSACONAZOLE; atazanavir increases or decreases the plasma concentration of ● VORICONAZOLE and plasma concentration of atazanavir also reduced
- Antimalarials: caution with atazanavir advised by manufacturer of ARTEMETHER WITH LUMEFANTRINE; atazanavir possibly increases plasma concentration of ● QUININE (increased risk of toxicity)
> Antimuscarinics: avoidance of atazanavir advised by manufacturer of DARIFENACIN; manufacturer of fesoterodine advises dose reduction when atazanavir given with FESOTERODINE—consult fesoterodine product literature
- Antipsychotics: atazanavir possibly increases plasma concentration of ● ARIPIPRAZOLE (reduce dose of aripiprazole—consult aripiprazole product literature); atazanavir possibly increases plasma concentration of ● PIMOZIDE—avoid concomitant use; atazanavir possibly increases plasma concentration of ● QUETIAPINE— manufacturer of quetiapine advises avoid concomitant use
- Antivirals: plasma concentration of atazanavir reduced by ● BOCEPREVIR; atazanavir increases the plasma concentration of ● DACLATASVIR—reduce dose of daclatasvir (see under Daclatasvir, in BNF); absorption of atazanavir reduced by DIDANOSINE *tablets* (give at least 2 hours before or 1 hour after didanosine *tablets*); manufacturer of atazanavir advises avoid concomitant use with ● EFAVIRENZ (plasma concentration of

Atazanavir

- **Antivirals** (continued)
  atazanavir reduced); atazanavir boosted with ritonavir increases plasma concentration of • ELVITEGRAVIR (reduce dose of elvitegravir); avoid concomitant use of atazanavir with • INDINAVIR; atazanavir increases plasma concentration of • MARAVIROC (consider reducing dose of maraviroc); plasma concentration of atazanavir possibly reduced by • NEVIRAPINE—avoid concomitant use; atazanavir increases plasma concentration of • PARITAPREVIR; increased risk of ventricular arrhythmias when atazanavir given with • SAQUINAVIR—avoid concomitant use; atazanavir possibly reduces plasma concentration of TELAPREVIR, also plasma concentration of atazanavir possibly increased; plasma concentration of atazanavir reduced by TENOFOVIR, also plasma concentration of tenofovir possibly increased; atazanavir increases plasma concentration of TIPRANAVIR (also plasma concentration of atazanavir reduced)
- **Anxiolytics and Hypnotics:** atazanavir possibly increases plasma concentration of • MIDAZOLAM—avoid concomitant use of *oral* midazolam
- **Calcium-channel Blockers:** atazanavir increases plasma concentration of • DILTIAZEM (reduce dose of diltiazem); atazanavir possibly increases plasma concentration of VERAPAMIL
- **Ciclosporin:** atazanavir possibly increases plasma concentration of • CICLOSPORIN
- **Colchicine:** atazanavir possibly increases risk of • COLCHICINE toxicity—suspend or reduce dose of colchicine (avoid concomitant use in hepatic or renal impairment)
- **Cytotoxics:** atazanavir possibly increases plasma concentration of AXITINIB (reduce dose of axitinib—consult axitinib product literature); atazanavir possibly increases the plasma concentration of • BOSUTINIB—manufacturer of bosutinib advises avoid or consider reducing dose of bosutinib; atazanavir possibly increases plasma concentration of • CRIZOTINIB and • EVEROLIMUS—manufacturer of crizotinib and everolimus advises avoid concomitant use; atazanavir possibly increases the plasma concentration of • IBRUTINIB—reduce dose of ibrutinib (see under Ibrutinib, in BNF); atazanavir possibly increases plasma concentration of • PAZOPANIB (reduce dose of pazopanib); avoidance of atazanavir advised by manufacturer of • CABAZITAXEL; atazanavir possibly inhibits metabolism of • IRINOTECAN (increased risk of toxicity)
- **Dapoxetine:** avoidance of atazanavir advised by manufacturer of • DAPOXETINE (increased risk of toxicity)
- **Ergot Alkaloids:** atazanavir possibly increases plasma concentration of • ERGOT ALKALOIDS—avoid concomitant use
▹ **Guanfacine:** atazanavir possibly increases plasma concentration of GUANFACINE (halve dose of guanfacine)
- **Lipid-regulating Drugs:** possible increased risk of myopathy when atazanavir given with • ATORVASTATIN or PRAVASTATIN; atazanavir increases plasma concentration of • ROSUVASTATIN—adjust dose of rosuvastatin (consult product literature); increased risk of myopathy when atazanavir given with • SIMVASTATIN (avoid concomitant use)
- **Oestrogens:** atazanavir increases plasma concentration of ETHINYLESTRADIOL
- **Orlistat:** absorption of atazanavir possibly reduced by • ORLISTAT
▹ **Progestogens:** atazanavir increases plasma concentration of NORETHISTERONE
- **Ranolazine:** atazanavir possibly increases plasma concentration of • RANOLAZINE—manufacturer of ranolazine advises avoid concomitant use
- **Sirolimus:** atazanavir possibly increases plasma concentration of • SIROLIMUS
- **Sympathomimetics, Beta₂:** atazanavir possibly increases plasma concentration of SALMETEROL—manufacturer of atazanavir advises avoid concomitant use
- **Tacrolimus:** atazanavir possibly increases plasma concentration of • TACROLIMUS
- **Ticagrelor:** atazanavir possibly increases plasma concentration of • TICAGRELOR—manufacturer of ticagrelor advises avoid concomitant use

Atazanavir (continued)
- **Ulcer-healing Drugs:** manufacturer of atazanavir advises adjust doses of both drugs when atazanavir given with CIMETIDINE and NIZATIDINE—consult atazanavir product literature; plasma concentration of atazanavir reduced by • FAMOTIDINE and • RANITIDINE (adjust doses of both drugs—consult atazanavir product literature); plasma concentration of atazanavir reduced by • PROTON PUMP INHIBITORS—avoid or adjust dose of both drugs (consult product literature)

Atenolol *see* Beta-blockers

Atomoxetine
- **Analgesics:** increased risk of ventricular arrhythmias when atomoxetine given with • METHADONE; possible increased risk of convulsions when atomoxetine given with TRAMADOL
- **Anti-arrhythmics:** increased risk of ventricular arrhythmias when atomoxetine given with • AMIODARONE or • DISOPYRAMIDE
- **Antibacterials:** increased risk of ventricular arrhythmias when atomoxetine given with *parenteral* • ERYTHROMYCIN; increased risk of ventricular arrhythmias when atomoxetine given with • MOXIFLOXACIN
- **Antidepressants:** metabolism of atomoxetine possibly inhibited by FLUOXETINE and PAROXETINE; possible increased risk of convulsions when atomoxetine given with ANTIDEPRESSANTS; atomoxetine should not be started until 2 weeks after stopping • MAOIs, also MAOIs should not be started until at least 2 weeks after stopping atomoxetine; increased risk of ventricular arrhythmias when atomoxetine given with • TRICYCLICS
- **Antimalarials:** increased risk of ventricular arrhythmias when atomoxetine given with • MEFLOQUINE
- **Antipsychotics:** increased risk of ventricular arrhythmias when atomoxetine given with • ANTIPSYCHOTICS that prolong the QT interval
- **Beta-blockers:** increased risk of ventricular arrhythmias when atomoxetine given with • SOTALOL
▹ **Bupropion:** possible increased risk of convulsions when atomoxetine given with BUPROPION
- **Diuretics:** risk of ventricular arrhythmias with atomoxetine increased by hypokalaemia caused by • DIURETICS
▹ **Sympathomimetics, Beta₂:** increased risk of cardiovascular side-effects when atomoxetine given with *parenteral* SALBUTAMOL

Atorvastatin *see* Statins

Atovaquone
- **Antibacterials:** manufacturer of atovaquone advises avoid concomitant use with RIFABUTIN (plasma concentration of both drugs reduced); plasma concentration of atovaquone reduced by • RIFAMPICIN (and concentration of rifampicin increased)—avoid concomitant use; plasma concentration of atovaquone reduced by TETRACYCLINE
- **Antivirals:** plasma concentration of atovaquone reduced by • EFAVIRENZ—avoid concomitant use; atovaquone possibly reduces plasma concentration of INDINAVIR; plasma concentration of atovaquone possibly reduced by RITONAVIR—manufacturer of atovaquone advises avoid concomitant use; atovaquone increases plasma concentration of ZIDOVUDINE (increased risk of toxicity)
▹ **Cytotoxics:** atovaquone possibly increases plasma concentration of ETOPOSIDE
▹ **Histamine:** avoidance of atovaquone advised by manufacturer of HISTAMINE
▹ **Metoclopramide:** plasma concentration of atovaquone reduced by METOCLOPRAMIDE—avoid concomitant use

Atracurium *see* Muscle Relaxants
Atropine *see* Antimuscarinics

Avanafil
▹ **ACE Inhibitors:** avanafil possibly enhances hypotensive effect of ENALAPRIL
▹ **Alcohol:** possible enhanced hypotensive effect when avanafil given with ALCOHOL
- **Alpha-blockers:** enhanced hypotensive effect when avanafil given with • ALPHA-BLOCKERS—when patient is stable on the alpha blocker initiate avanafil at the lowest possible dose
- **Antibacterials:** plasma concentration of avanafil possibly increased by • CLARITHROMYCIN and • TELITHROMYCIN—manufacturer of avanafil advises avoid concomitant use;

Avanafil
- Antibacterials (continued)
  plasma concentration of avanafil increased by
  - ERYTHROMYCIN—see under Avanafil, in BNF; plasma
  concentration of avanafil possibly reduced by RIFAMPICIN—
  manufacturer of avanafil advises avoid concomitant use
- Antiepileptics: plasma concentration of avanafil possibly
  reduced by CARBAMAZEPINE, PHENOBARBITAL and PRIMIDONE—
  manufacturer of avanafil advises avoid concomitant use
- Antifungals: plasma concentration of avanafil increased by
  - KETOCONAZOLE—avoid concomitant use; plasma
  concentration of avanafil possibly increased by
  - FLUCONAZOLE—see under Avanafil, in BNF; plasma
  concentration of avanafil possibly increased by
  - ITRACONAZOLE and - VORICONAZOLE—manufacturer of
  avanafil advises avoid concomitant use
- Antivirals: plasma concentration of avanafil possibly reduced
  by EFAVIRENZ—manufacturer of avanafil advises avoid
  concomitant use; plasma concentration of avanafil possibly
  increased by - FOSAMPRENAVIR—see under Avanafil, in BNF;
  plasma concentration of avanafil possibly increased by
  - INDINAVIR and - SAQUINAVIR—manufacturer of avanafil
  advises avoid concomitant use; plasma concentration of
  avanafil significantly increased by - RITONAVIR—avoid
  concomitant use
- Aprepitant: plasma concentration of avanafil possibly
  increased by - APREPITANT—see under Avanafil, in BNF
- Bosentan: plasma concentration of avanafil possibly reduced
  by BOSENTAN—manufacturer of avanafil advises avoid
  concomitant use
- Calcium-channel Blockers: plasma concentration of avanafil
  possibly increased by - DILTIAZEM and - VERAPAMIL—see under
  Avanafil, in BNF
- Cobicistat: plasma concentration of avanafil possibly increased
  by - COBICISTAT—avoid concomitant use
- Fosaprepitant: plasma concentration of avanafil possibly
  increased by FOSAPREPITANT
- Grapefruit Juice: plasma concentration of avanafil possibly
  increased by GRAPEFRUIT JUICE— manufacturer of avanafil
  advises avoid grapefruit juice for 24 hours before avanafil
- Nicorandil: avanafil significantly enhances hypotensive effect
  of - NICORANDIL (avoid concomitant use)
- Nitrates: avanafil significantly enhances hypotensive effect of
  - NITRATES (avoid concomitant use)
- Riociguat: possible enhanced hypotensive effect when avanafil
  given with - RIOCIGUAT—avoid concomitant use

Axitinib
- Antibacterials: plasma concentration of axitinib possibly
  increased by CLARITHROMYCIN, ERYTHROMYCIN and
  TELITHROMYCIN (reduce dose of axitinib—consult axitinib
  product literature); plasma concentration of axitinib possibly
  decreased by RIFABUTIN (increase dose of axitinib—consult
  axitinib product literature); plasma concentration of axitinib
  decreased by RIFAMPICIN (increase dose of axitinib—consult
  axitinib product literature)
- Antidepressants: plasma concentration of axitinib possibly
  reduced by ST JOHN'S WORT—consider increasing dose of
  axitinib
- Antiepileptics: plasma concentration of axitinib possibly
  decreased by CARBAMAZEPINE, FOSPHENYTOIN, PHENOBARBITAL,
  PHENYTOIN and PRIMIDONE (increase dose of axitinib—consult
  axitinib product literature)
- Antifungals: plasma concentration of axitinib increased by
  KETOCONAZOLE (reduce dose of axitinib—consult axitinib
  product literature); plasma concentration of axitinib possibly
  increased by ITRACONAZOLE (reduce dose of axitinib—consult
  axitinib product literature)
- Antipsychotics: avoid concomitant use of cytotoxics with
  - CLOZAPINE (increased risk of agranulocytosis)
- Antivirals: plasma concentration of axitinib possibly increased
  by ATAZANAVIR, INDINAVIR, RITONAVIR and SAQUINAVIR (reduce
  dose of axitinib—consult axitinib product literature)
- Corticosteroids: plasma concentration of axitinib possibly
  decreased by DEXAMETHASONE (increase dose of axitinib—
  consult axitinib product literature)

Axitinib (continued)
- Grapefruit Juice: plasma concentration of axitinib possibly
  increased by GRAPEFRUIT JUICE

Azathioprine
- ACE Inhibitors: increased risk of anaemia or leucopenia when
  azathioprine given with CAPTOPRIL especially in renal
  impairment; increased risk of anaemia when azathioprine
  given with ENALAPRIL especially in renal impairment
- Allopurinol: enhanced effects and increased toxicity of
  azathioprine when given with - ALLOPURINOL (reduce dose of
  azathioprine to one quarter of usual dose)
- Analgesics: manufacturer of azathioprine advises possible
  increased risk of myelosuppression when azathioprine given
  with INDOMETACIN
- Antibacterials: increased risk of haematological toxicity when
  azathioprine given with - SULFAMETHOXAZOLE (as co-
  trimoxazole); increased risk of haematological toxicity when
  azathioprine given with - TRIMETHOPRIM (also with co-
  trimoxazole)
- Anticoagulants: azathioprine possibly reduces anticoagulant
  effect of - ACENOCOUMAROL; azathioprine reduces
  anticoagulant effect of - WARFARIN
- Antivirals: myelosuppressive effects of azathioprine possibly
  enhanced by - RIBAVIRIN
- Febuxostat: avoidance of azathioprine advised by
  manufacturer of - FEBUXOSTAT
- Ulcer-healing Drugs: manufacturer of azathioprine advises
  possible increased risk of myelosuppression when
  azathioprine given with CIMETIDINE
- Vaccines: risk of generalised infections when azathioprine
  given with live - VACCINES—avoid concomitant use

Azelastine see Antihistamines

Azilsartan see Angiotensin-II Receptor Antagonists

Azithromycin see Macrolides

Aztreonam
- Anticoagulants: aztreonam possibly enhances anticoagulant
  effect of - COUMARINS
- Vaccines: antibacterials inactivate ORAL TYPHOID VACCINE—see
  under Typhoid Vaccine in BNFC

Baclofen see Muscle Relaxants

Bambuterol see Sympathomimetics, Beta$_2$

Basiliximab
- Antipsychotics: avoid concomitant use of cytotoxics with
  - CLOZAPINE (increased risk of agranulocytosis)
- Vaccines: risk of generalised infections when monoclonal
  antibodies given with live - VACCINES—avoid concomitant use

BCG Vaccine see Vaccines

Beclometasone see Corticosteroids

Bedaquiline
- Antibacterials: plasma concentration of bedaquiline possibly
  increased by CIPROFLOXACIN, CLARITHROMYCIN and
  ERYTHROMYCIN—avoid concomitant use if ciprofloxacin,
  clarithromycin and erythromycin given for more than 14 days;
  manufacturer of bedaquiline advises avoid concomitant use
  with MOXIFLOXACIN; plasma concentration of bedaquiline
  possibly reduced by RIFABUTIN—manufacturer of bedaquiline
  advises avoid concomitant use; plasma concentration of
  bedaquiline reduced by - RIFAMPICIN—manufacturer of
  bedaquiline advises avoid concomitant use; possible
  increased risk of ventricular arrhythmias when bedaquiline
  given with - CLOFAZIMINE
- Antidepressants: plasma concentration of bedaquiline possibly
  reduced by ST JOHN'S WORT—manufacturer of bedaquiline
  advises avoid concomitant use
- Antiepileptics: plasma concentration of bedaquiline possibly
  reduced by - CARBAMAZEPINE, - FOSPHENYTOIN and
  - PHENYTOIN—manufacturer of bedaquiline advises avoid
  concomitant use
- Antifungals: plasma concentration of bedaquiline increased by
  KETOCONAZOLE—avoid concomitant use if ketoconazole given
  for more than 14 days; plasma concentration of bedaquiline
  possibly increased by FLUCONAZOLE—avoid concomitant use if
  fluconazole given for more than 14 days
- Antivirals: plasma concentration of bedaquiline possibly
  reduced by EFAVIRENZ and ETRAVIRINE—manufacturer of
  bedaquiline advises avoid concomitant use; plasma

Bedaquiline

Antivirals (continued)
concentration of bedaquiline possibly increased by RITONAVIR—manufacturer of ritonavir advises avoid concomitant use
▸ Vaccines: antibacterials inactivate ORAL TYPHOID VACCINE—see under Typhoid Vaccine in BNFC

Bee Venom Extracts
● ACE Inhibitors: possible severe anaphylactoid reaction when bee venom extracts given with ● ACE INHIBITORS

Belimumab
● Antipsychotics: avoid concomitant use of cytotoxics with ● CLOZAPINE (increased risk of agranulocytosis)
● Vaccines: risk of generalised infections when monoclonal antibodies given with live ● VACCINES—avoid concomitant use

Bendamustine
● Antipsychotics: avoid concomitant use of cytotoxics with ● CLOZAPINE (increased risk of agranulocytosis)

Bendroflumethiazide *see* Diuretics

Benperidol *see* Antipsychotics

Benzodiazepines *see* Anxiolytics and Hypnotics

Benzthiazide *see* Diuretics

Benzylpenicillin *see* Penicillins

Beta-blockers

NOTE Since systemic absorption may follow topical application of beta-blockers to the eye the possibility of interactions, in particular, with drugs such as verapamil should be borne in mind

▸ ACE Inhibitors: enhanced hypotensive effect when beta-blockers given with ACE INHIBITORS
▸ Adrenergic Neurone Blockers: enhanced hypotensive effect when beta-blockers given with ADRENERGIC NEURONE BLOCKERS
▸ Alcohol: enhanced hypotensive effect when beta-blockers given with ALCOHOL
▸ Aldesleukin: enhanced hypotensive effect when beta-blockers given with ALDESLEUKIN
▸ Alpha-blockers: enhanced hypotensive effect when beta-blockers given with ● ALPHA-BLOCKERS, also increased risk of first-dose hypotension with post-synaptic alpha-blockers such as prazosin
● Anaesthetics, General: enhanced hypotensive effect when beta-blockers given with GENERAL ANAESTHETICS
● Anaesthetics, Local: propranolol increases risk of ● BUPIVACAINE toxicity
▸ Analgesics: hypotensive effect of beta-blockers antagonised by NSAIDs; plasma concentration of esmolol possibly increased by MORPHINE
● Angiotensin-II Receptor Antagonists: enhanced hypotensive effect when beta-blockers given with ANGIOTENSIN-II RECEPTOR ANTAGONISTS
● Anti-arrhythmics: increased myocardial depression when beta-blockers given with ● ANTI-ARRHYTHMICS; increased risk of ventricular arrhythmias when sotalol given with ● AMIODARONE, ● DISOPYRAMIDE or ● DRONEDARONE—avoid concomitant use; increased risk of bradycardia, AV block and myocardial depression when beta-blockers given with ● AMIODARONE; plasma concentration of metoprolol and propranolol possibly increased by DRONEDARONE; increased risk of myocardial depression and bradycardia when beta-blockers given with ● FLECAINIDE; nadolol possibly increases risk of LIDOCAINE toxicity; propranolol increases risk of ● LIDOCAINE toxicity; plasma concentration of metoprolol and propranolol increased by PROPAFENONE
● Antibacterials: increased risk of ventricular arrhythmias when sotalol given with ● MOXIFLOXACIN—avoid concomitant use; metabolism of bisoprolol and propranolol accelerated by RIFAMPICIN (plasma concentration significantly reduced); plasma concentration of carvedilol, celiprolol and metoprolol reduced by RIFAMPICIN; plasma concentration of *oral* timolol possibly reduced by RIFAMPICIN; increased risk of ventricular arrhythmias when sotalol given with ● DELAMANID
● Antidepressants: plasma concentration of metoprolol increased by CITALOPRAM and ESCITALOPRAM; increased risk of ventricular arrhythmias when sotalol given with ● CITALOPRAM—avoid concomitant use; avoidance of sotalol advised by manufacturer of ● ESCITALOPRAM and ● VENLAFAXINE (risk of

Beta-blockers
● Antidepressants (continued)
ventricular arrhythmias); plasma concentration of propranolol increased by FLUVOXAMINE; plasma concentration of metoprolol possibly increased by ● PAROXETINE—increased risk of AV block (manufacturer of paroxetine advises avoid concomitant use in cardiac insufficiency); labetalol and propranolol increase plasma concentration of IMIPRAMINE; enhanced hypotensive effect when beta-blockers given with MAOIs; increased risk of ventricular arrhythmias when sotalol given with ● TRICYCLICS
▸ Antidiabetics: beta-blockers may mask warning signs of hypoglycaemia (such as tremor) with ANTIDIABETICS; beta-blockers enhance hypoglycaemic effect of INSULIN
▸ Antiepileptics: plasma concentration of propranolol possibly reduced by PHENOBARBITAL and PRIMIDONE
▸ Antifungals: plasma concentration of nadolol possibly increased by KETOCONAZOLE
● Antihistamines: increased risk of ventricular arrhythmias when sotalol given with ● MIZOLASTINE—avoid concomitant use
● Antimalarials: avoidance of metoprolol and sotalol advised by manufacturer of ● ARTEMETHER WITH LUMEFANTRINE; avoidance of sotalol advised by manufacturer of ● ARTENIMOL WITH PIPERAQUINE (possible risk of ventricular arrhythmias); increased risk of bradycardia when beta-blockers given with MEFLOQUINE
● Antimuscarinics: increased risk of ventricular arrhythmias when sotalol given with ● TOLTERODINE
● Antipsychotics: increased risk of ventricular arrhythmias when sotalol given with ● DROPERIDOL or ● ZUCLOPENTHIXOL—avoid concomitant use; possible increased risk of ventricular arrhythmias when sotalol given with ● HALOPERIDOL—avoid concomitant use; plasma concentration of both drugs may increase when propranolol given with ● CHLORPROMAZINE; increased risk of ventricular arrhythmias when sotalol given with ● AMISULPRIDE, ● PHENOTHIAZINES, ● PIMOZIDE or ● SULPIRIDE; enhanced hypotensive effect when beta-blockers given with PHENOTHIAZINES; possible increased risk of ventricular arrhythmias when sotalol given with ● RISPERIDONE
● Antivirals: increased risk of ventricular arrhythmias when sotalol given with ● SAQUINAVIR—avoid concomitant use; avoidance of sotalol advised by manufacturer of ● TELAPREVIR (risk of ventricular arrhythmias); avoidance of metoprolol for heart failure advised by manufacturer of ● TIPRANAVIR
▸ Anxiolytics and Hypnotics: enhanced hypotensive effect when beta-blockers given with ANXIOLYTICS AND HYPNOTICS
● Atomoxetine: increased risk of ventricular arrhythmias when sotalol given with ● ATOMOXETINE
● Calcium-channel Blockers: enhanced hypotensive effect when beta-blockers given with CALCIUM-CHANNEL BLOCKERS; possible severe hypotension and heart failure when beta-blockers given with ● NIFEDIPINE; increased risk of AV block and bradycardia when beta-blockers given with ● DILTIAZEM; asystole, severe hypotension and heart failure when beta-blockers given with ● VERAPAMIL (see under Verapamil, p. 101)
▸ Cardiac Glycosides: increased risk of AV block and bradycardia when beta-blockers given with CARDIAC GLYCOSIDES
● Ciclosporin: carvedilol increases plasma concentration of ● CICLOSPORIN
● Clonidine: increased risk of withdrawal hypertension when beta-blockers given with ● CLONIDINE (withdraw beta-blockers several days before slowly withdrawing clonidine)
▸ Corticosteroids: hypotensive effect of beta-blockers antagonised by CORTICOSTEROIDS
● Cytotoxics: possible increased risk of ventricular arrhythmias when sotalol given with ● BOSUTINIB; possible increased risk of bradycardia when beta-blockers given with CRIZOTINIB; possible increased risk of ventricular arrhythmias when sotalol given with ● VANDETANIB—avoid concomitant use; increased risk of ventricular arrhythmias when sotalol given with ● ARSENIC TRIOXIDE
▸ Diazoxide: enhanced hypotensive effect when beta-blockers given with DIAZOXIDE
● Diuretics: enhanced hypotensive effect when beta-blockers given with DIURETICS; risk of ventricular arrhythmias with

Beta-blockers

- Diuretics (continued)
  sotalol increased by hypokalaemia caused by ● LOOP DIURETICS or ● THIAZIDES AND RELATED DIURETICS
▹ Dopaminergics: enhanced hypotensive effect when beta-blockers given with CO-BENELDOPA, CO-CARELDOPA or LEVODOPA
▹ Ergot Alkaloids: increased peripheral vasoconstriction when beta-blockers given with ERGOT ALKALOIDS
- Fingolimod: possible increased risk of bradycardia when beta-blockers given with ● FINGOLIMOD
▹ Hormone Antagonists: possible increased risk of bradycardia when carteolol, metoprolol, propranolol or sotalol given with PASIREOTIDE
▹ 5HT₁-receptor Agonists: propranolol increases plasma concentration of RIZATRIPTAN (manufacturer of rizatriptan advises halve dose and avoid within 2 hours of propranolol)
- Ivabradine: increased risk of ventricular arrhythmias when sotalol given with ● IVABRADINE
▹ Methyldopa: enhanced hypotensive effect when beta-blockers given with METHYLDOPA
▹ Mirabegron: plasma concentration of metoprolol increased by MIRABEGRON
- Moxisylyte: possible severe postural hypotension when beta-blockers given with ● MOXISYLYTE
▹ Moxonidine: enhanced hypotensive effect when beta-blockers given with MOXONIDINE
▹ Muscle Relaxants: propranolol enhances effects of MUSCLE RELAXANTS; enhanced hypotensive effect when beta-blockers given with BACLOFEN; possible enhanced hypotensive effect and bradycardia when beta-blockers given with TIZANIDINE
▹ Nitrates: enhanced hypotensive effect when beta-blockers given with NITRATES
▹ Oestrogens: hypotensive effect of beta-blockers antagonised by OESTROGENS
▹ Parasympathomimetics: propranolol antagonises effects of NEOSTIGMINE and PYRIDOSTIGMINE; increased risk of arrhythmias when beta-blockers given with PILOCARPINE
▹ Prostaglandins: enhanced hypotensive effect when beta-blockers given with ALPROSTADIL
- Ranolazine: avoidance of sotalol advised by manufacturer of ● RANOLAZINE
- Sympathomimetics: increased risk of severe hypertension and bradycardia when non-cardioselective beta-blockers given with ● ADRENALINE (EPINEPHRINE), also reponse to adrenaline (epinephrine) may be reduced; increased risk of severe hypertension and bradycardia when non-cardioselective beta-blockers given with ● DOBUTAMINE; possible increased risk of severe hypertension and bradycardia when non-cardioselective beta-blockers given with ● NORADRENALINE (NOREPINEPHRINE)
▹ Thyroid Hormones: metabolism of propranolol accelerated by LEVOTHYROXINE
▹ Ulcer-healing Drugs: plasma concentration of labetalol, metoprolol and propranolol increased by CIMETIDINE; plasma concentration of oral timolol possibly increased by CIMETIDINE
▹ Vasodilator Antihypertensives: enhanced hypotensive effect when beta-blockers given with HYDRALAZINE, MINOXIDIL or SODIUM NITROPRUSSIDE

Betahistine

▹ Antihistamines: effect of betahistine theoretically antagonised by ANTIHISTAMINES

Betamethasone see Corticosteroids

Betaxolol see Beta-blockers

Bethanechol see Parasympathomimetics

Bevacizumab

- Antipsychotics: avoid concomitant use of cytotoxics with ● CLOZAPINE (increased risk of agranulocytosis)
- Cytotoxics: avoidance of bevacizumab advised by manufacturer of ● PANITUMUMAB
- Vaccines: risk of generalised infections when monoclonal antibodies given with live ● VACCINES—avoid concomitant use

Bexarotene

- Antipsychotics: avoid concomitant use of cytotoxics with ● CLOZAPINE (increased risk of agranulocytosis)
- Lipid-regulating Drugs: plasma concentration of bexarotene increased by ● GEMFIBROZIL—avoid concomitant use

Bezafibrate see Fibrates

Bicalutamide

▹ Anticoagulants: bicalutamide possibly enhances anticoagulant effect of COUMARINS
▹ Lipid-regulating Drugs: separating administration from bicalutamide by 12 hours advised by manufacturer of LOMITAPIDE

Biguanides see Antidiabetics

Bilastine see Antihistamines

Bile Acid Sequestrants see Colesevelam, Colestipol, and Colestyramine

Bile Acids

▹ Antacids: absorption of bile acids possibly reduced by ANTACIDS; effects of cholic acid probably reduced by ALUMINIUM HYDROXIDE (manufacturer of cholic acid advises give at least 5 hours apart)
▹ Antiepileptics: manufacturer of cholic acid advises avoid concomitant use with ● PHENOBARBITAL
- Ciclosporin: manufacturer of cholic acid advises avoid concomitant use with CICLOSPORIN; ursodeoxycholic acid increases absorption of ● CICLOSPORIN
▹ Lipid-regulating Drugs: effects of cholic acid probably reduced by COLESEVELAM, COLESTIPOL and COLESTYRAMINE (manufacturer of cholic acid advises give at least 5 hours apart); absorption of bile acids possibly reduced by COLESTIPOL and COLESTYRAMINE

Bisoprolol see Beta-blockers

Bisphosphonates

▹ Antacids: absorption of bisphosphonates reduced by ANTACIDS
▹ Antibacterials: increased risk of hypocalcaemia when bisphosphonates given with AMINOGLYCOSIDES
- Calcium Salts: absorption of bisphosphonates reduced by CALCIUM SALTS
- Cytotoxics: sodium clodronate increases plasma concentration of ● ESTRAMUSTINE
▹ Iron Salts: absorption of bisphosphonates reduced by oral IRON SALTS

Bivalirudin

- Analgesics: increased risk of haemorrhage when anticoagulants given with intravenous ● DICLOFENAC (avoid concomitant use, including low-dose heparins); increased risk of haemorrhage when anticoagulants given with ● KETOROLAC (avoid concomitant use, including low-dose heparins)
- Anticoagulants: increased risk of haemorrhage when other anticoagulants given with ● APIXABAN, ● DABIGATRAN, ● EDOXABAN and ● RIVAROXABAN (avoid concomitant use except when switching with other anticoagulants or using heparin to maintain catheter patency)

Bleomycin

- Antipsychotics: avoid concomitant use of cytotoxics with ● CLOZAPINE (increased risk of agranulocytosis)
▹ Cardiac Glycosides: bleomycin possibly reduces absorption of DIGOXIN tablets
- Cytotoxics: increased risk of pulmonary toxicity when bleomycin given with ● BRENTUXIMAB VEDOTIN—avoid concomitant use; increased pulmonary toxicity when bleomycin given with ● CISPLATIN
- Vaccines: risk of generalised infections when cytotoxic antibiotics given with live ● VACCINES—avoid concomitant use

Boceprevir

▹ Alpha-blockers: boceprevir possibly increases plasma concentration of DOXAZOSIN and TAMSULOSIN—manufacturer of boceprevir advises avoid concomitant use
▹ Analgesics: possible increased risk of prolonged sedation and respiratory depression when boceprevir given with BUPRENORPHINE; boceprevir possibly affects plasma concentration of METHADONE
- Antibacterials: manufacturer of boceprevir advises avoid concomitant use with ● RIFAMPICIN (plasma concentration of boceprevir possibly reduced)
▹ Anticoagulants: avoidance of boceprevir advised by manufacturer of APIXABAN
- Antiepileptics: manufacturer of boceprevir advises avoid concomitant use with ● CARBAMAZEPINE, ● FOSPHENYTOIN, ● PHENOBARBITAL, ● PHENYTOIN and ● PRIMIDONE (plasma concentration of boceprevir possibly reduced)

Boceprevir (continued)

- Antifungals: plasma concentration of boceprevir increased by
  - KETOCONAZOLE
- Antimalarials: manufacturer of boceprevir advises avoid concomitant use with • ARTEMETHER WITH LUMEFANTRINE
- Antipsychotics: boceprevir possibly increases plasma concentration of • LURASIDONE—avoid concomitant use; manufacturer of boceprevir advises avoid concomitant use with • PIMOZIDE; boceprevir possibly increases plasma concentration of • QUETIAPINE—manufacturer of quetiapine advises avoid concomitant use
- Antivirals: boceprevir reduces plasma concentration of • ATAZANAVIR; boceprevir possibly increases the plasma concentration of • DACLATASVIR—reduce dose of daclatasvir (see under Daclatasvir, in BNF); avoid concomitant use of boceprevir with • DARUNAVIR; effects of both drugs possibly reduced when boceprevir given with ETRAVIRINE; avoidance of boceprevir advised by manufacturer of • FOSAMPRENAVIR, NEVIRAPINE and TIPRANAVIR; manufacturers advise avoid concomitant use of boceprevir with • LOPINAVIR; boceprevir increases plasma concentration of MARAVIROC (consider reducing dose of maraviroc); plasma concentration of both drugs reduced when boceprevir given with • RITONAVIR
- Anxiolytics and Hypnotics: boceprevir increases plasma concentration of oral • MIDAZOLAM—manufacturer of boceprevir advises avoid concomitant use
- Cardiac Glycosides: boceprevir possibly increases side-effects of DIGOXIN
- Ciclosporin: boceprevir increases plasma concentration of • CICLOSPORIN
- Cilostazol: boceprevir possibly increases plasma concentration of • CILOSTAZOL (see under Cilostazol, in BNF)
- Cobicistat: avoidance of boceprevir advised by manufacturer of COBICISTAT
- Cytotoxics: boceprevir possibly increases the plasma concentration of • BOSUTINIB—manufacturer of bosutinib advises avoid or consider reducing dose of bosutinib; manufacturer of boceprevir advises avoid concomitant use with • DASATINIB, • ERLOTINIB, • GEFITINIB, • IMATINIB, • LAPATINIB, • NILOTINIB, • PAZOPANIB, • SORAFENIB and • SUNITINIB; manufacturer of ruxolitinib advises dose reduction when boceprevir given with • RUXOLITINIB—consult ruxolitinib product literature; avoidance of boceprevir advised by manufacturer of • OLAPARIB
- Domperidone: possible increased risk of ventricular arrhythmias when boceprevir given with • DOMPERIDONE—avoid concomitant use
- Ergot Alkaloids: manufacturer of boceprevir advises avoid concomitant use with • ERGOT ALKALOIDS
- Guanfacine: boceprevir possibly increases plasma concentration of • GUANFACINE (halve dose of guanfacine)
- Lipid-regulating Drugs: boceprevir increases plasma concentration of ATORVASTATIN (reduce dose of atorvastatin); boceprevir increases plasma concentration of PRAVASTATIN; manufacturers advise avoid concomitant use of boceprevir with • SIMVASTATIN
- Progestogens: boceprevir increases plasma concentration of DROSPIRENONE (increased risk of toxicity)
- Sirolimus: boceprevir increases plasma concentration of • SIROLIMUS (increased risk of toxicity—reduce sirolimus dose)
- Tacrolimus: boceprevir increases plasma concentration of • TACROLIMUS (reduce dose of tacrolimus)

Bortezomib

- Antibacterials: plasma concentration of bortezomib reduced by • RIFAMPICIN—manufacturer of bortezomib advises avoid concomitant use
- Antidepressants: plasma concentration of bortezomib possibly reduced by ST JOHN'S WORT—manufacturer of bortezomib advises avoid concomitant use
- Antiepileptics: plasma concentration of bortezomib possibly reduced by CARBAMAZEPINE, FOSPHENYTOIN, PHENOBARBITAL, PHENYTOIN and PRIMIDONE—manufacturer of bortezomib advises avoid concomitant use
- Antifungals: plasma concentration of bortezomib increased by KETOCONAZOLE

Bortezomib (continued)

- Antipsychotics: avoid concomitant use of cytotoxics with • CLOZAPINE (increased risk of agranulocytosis)

Bosentan

- Antibacterials: plasma concentration of bosentan reduced by • RIFAMPICIN—avoid concomitant use
- Anticoagulants: manufacturer of bosentan recommends monitoring anticoagulant effect of COUMARINS
- Antidiabetics: increased risk of hepatotoxicity when bosentan given with • GLIBENCLAMIDE—avoid concomitant use
- Antifungals: plasma concentration of bosentan increased by KETOCONAZOLE; plasma concentration of bosentan possibly increased by • FLUCONAZOLE—avoid concomitant use; plasma concentration of bosentan possibly increased by ITRACONAZOLE
- Antivirals: avoidance of bosentan advised by manufacturer of ELVITEGRAVIR and TIPRANAVIR; bosentan possibly reduces plasma concentration of INDINAVIR; plasma concentration of bosentan increased by • LOPINAVIR and • RITONAVIR (consider reducing dose of bosentan); bosentan possibly reduces plasma concentration of TELAPREVIR, also plasma concentration of bosentan possibly increased
- Avanafil: bosentan possibly reduces plasma concentration of AVANAFIL—manufacturer of avanafil advises avoid concomitant use
- Ciclosporin: plasma concentration of bosentan increased by • CICLOSPORIN (also plasma concentration of ciclosporin reduced—avoid concomitant use)
- Cobicistat: avoidance of bosentan advised by manufacturer of COBICISTAT
- Cytotoxics: bosentan possibly reduces plasma concentration of • BOSUTINIB—manufacturer of bosutinib advises avoid concomitant use
- Guanfacine: bosentan possibly reduces plasma concentration of • GUANFACINE—increase dose of guanfacine
- Lipid-regulating Drugs: bosentan reduces plasma concentration of SIMVASTATIN
- Oestrogens: bosentan possibly causes contraceptive failure of hormonal contraceptives containing • OESTROGENS (alternative contraception recommended)
- Progestogens: bosentan possibly causes contraceptive failure of hormonal contraceptives containing • PROGESTOGENS (alternative contraception recommended)
- Riociguat: bosentan reduces plasma concentration of RIOCIGUAT
- Sildenafil: bosentan reduces plasma concentration of SILDENAFIL, also plasma concentration of bosentan increased
- Tadalafil: bosentan reduces plasma concentration of TADALAFIL

Bosutinib

- Analgesics: possible increased risk of ventricular arrhythmias when bosutinib given with • METHADONE
- Antacids: manufacturer of bosutinib advises separating administration with ANTACIDS by about 12 hours
- Anti-arrhythmics: possible increased risk of ventricular arrhythmias when bosutinib given with • AMIODARONE and • DISOPYRAMIDE; plasma concentration of bosutinib possibly increased by • DRONEDARONE—manufacturer of bosutinib advises avoid or consider reducing dose of bosutinib
- Antibacterials: plasma concentration of bosutinib possibly increased by • CIPROFLOXACIN, • CLARITHROMYCIN, • ERYTHROMYCIN and • TELITHROMYCIN—manufacturer of bosutinib advises avoid or consider reducing dose of bosutinib; possible increased risk of ventricular arrhythmias when bosutinib given with • MOXIFLOXACIN; plasma concentration of bosutinib possibly reduced by • RIFABUTIN—manufacturer of bosutinib advises avoid concomitant use; plasma concentration of bosutinib reduced by • RIFAMPICIN—manufacturer of bosutinib advises avoid concomitant use
- Antidepressants: plasma concentration of bosutinib possibly reduced by • ST JOHN'S WORT—manufacturer of bosutinib advises avoid concomitant use
- Antiepileptics: plasma concentration of bosutinib possibly reduced by • CARBAMAZEPINE, • FOSPHENYTOIN, • PHENOBARBITAL, • PHENYTOIN and • PRIMIDONE—manufacturer of bosutinib advises avoid concomitant use
- Antifungals: plasma concentration of bosutinib increased by • KETOCONAZOLE—manufacturer of bosutinib advises avoid or

Interactions | Appendix 1

A1

Bosutinib
- Antifungals (continued)
consider reducing dose of bosutinib; plasma concentration of bosutinib possibly increased by ● FLUCONAZOLE, ● ITRACONAZOLE, ● POSACONAZOLE and ● VORICONAZOLE—manufacturer of bosutinib advises avoid or consider reducing dose of bosutinib
- Antimalarials: possible increased risk of ventricular arrhythmias when bosutinib given with ● CHLOROQUINE and ● HYDROXYCHLOROQUINE
- Antipsychotics: possible increased risk of ventricular arrhythmias when bosutinib given with ● HALOPERIDOL; avoid concomitant use of cytotoxics with ● CLOZAPINE (increased risk of agranulocytosis)
- Antivirals: plasma concentration of bosutinib possibly increased by ● ATAZANAVIR, ● BOCEPREVIR, ● DARUNAVIR, ● FOSAMPRENAVIR, ● INDINAVIR, ● RITONAVIR, ● SAQUINAVIR and ● TELAPREVIR—manufacturer of bosutinib advises avoid or consider reducing dose of bosutinib; plasma concentration of bosutinib possibly reduced by ● EFAVIRENZ and ● ETRAVIRINE—manufacturer of bosutinib advises avoid concomitant use
- Aprepitant: plasma concentration of bosutinib possibly increased by ● APREPITANT—manufacturer of bosutinib advises avoid or consider reducing dose of bosutinib
- Beta-blockers: possible increased risk of ventricular arrhythmias when bosutinib given with ● SOTALOL
- Bosentan: plasma concentration of bosutinib possibly reduced by ● BOSENTAN—manufacturer of bosutinib advises avoid concomitant use
- Calcium-channel Blockers: plasma concentration of bosutinib possibly increased by ● DILTIAZEM and ● VERAPAMIL—manufacturer of bosutinib advises avoid or consider reducing dose of bosutinib
- Cytotoxics: plasma concentration of bosutinib possibly increased by ● IMATINIB—manufacturer of bosutinib advises avoid or consider reducing dose of bosutinib
- Domperidone: manufacturer of bosutinib advises avoid concomitant use with ● DOMPERIDONE (risk of ventricular arrhythmias)
- Fosaprepitant: plasma concentration of bosutinib possibly increased by ● FOSAPREPITANT—manufacturer of bosutinib advises avoid or consider reducing dose of bosutinib
- Grapefruit Juice: plasma concentration of bosutinib possibly increased by ● GRAPEFRUIT JUICE—manufacturer of bosutinib advises avoid or consider reducing dose of bosutinib
- Modafinil: plasma concentration of bosutinib possibly reduced by ● MODAFINIL—manufacturer of bosutinib advises avoid concomitant use
▹ Ulcer-healing Drugs: plasma concentration of bosutinib reduced by LANSOPRAZOLE

Brentuximab vedotin
▹ Antibacterials: effects of brentuximab vedotin possibly reduced by RIFAMPICIN
- Antifungals: possible increased risk of neutropenia when brentuximab vedotin given with ● KETOCONAZOLE
- Antipsychotics: avoid concomitant use of cytotoxics with ● CLOZAPINE (increased risk of agranulocytosis)
- Cytotoxics: increased risk of pulmonary toxicity when brentuximab vedotin given with ● BLEOMYCIN—avoid concomitant use
- Vaccines: risk of generalised infections when monoclonal antibodies given with live ● VACCINES—avoid concomitant use

Brimonidine
▹ Antidepressants: manufacturer of brimonidine advises avoid concomitant use with MAOIS, TRICYCLIC-RELATED ANTIDEPRESSANTS and TRICYCLICS

Brinzolamide see Diuretics

Bromocriptine
▹ Alcohol: tolerance of bromocriptine reduced by ALCOHOL
▹ Antibacterials: plasma concentration of bromocriptine increased by ERYTHROMYCIN (increased risk of toxicity); plasma concentration of bromocriptine possibly increased by MACROLIDES (increased risk of toxicity)
▹ Antipsychotics: hypoprolactinaemic and antiparkinsonian effects of bromocriptine antagonised by ANTIPSYCHOTICS

Bromocriptine (continued)
▹ Domperidone: hypoprolactinaemic effect of bromocriptine possibly antagonised by DOMPERIDONE
▹ Hormone Antagonists: plasma concentration of bromocriptine increased by OCTREOTIDE
▹ Memantine: effects of dopaminergics possibly enhanced by MEMANTINE
▹ Methyldopa: antiparkinsonian effect of dopaminergics antagonised by METHYLDOPA
▹ Metoclopramide: hypoprolactinaemic effect of bromocriptine antagonised by METOCLOPRAMIDE
- Sympathomimetics: risk of toxicity when bromocriptine given with ● ISOMETHEPTENE

Buclizine see Antihistamines
Budesonide see Corticosteroids
Bumetanide see Diuretics
Bupivacaine
▹ Anti-arrhythmics: increased myocardial depression when bupivacaine given with ANTI-ARRHYTHMICS
- Beta-blockers: increased risk of bupivacaine toxicity when given with ● PROPRANOLOL

Buprenorphine see Opioid Analgesics
Bupropion
- Antidepressants: bupropion possibly increases plasma concentration of CITALOPRAM; manufacturer of bupropion advises avoid for 2 weeks after stopping ● MAOIS; manufacturer of bupropion advises avoid concomitant use with ● MOCLOBEMIDE; bupropion possibly increases plasma concentration of TRICYCLICS (possible increased risk of convulsions); bupropion increases plasma concentration of VORTIOXETINE (consider reducing dose of vortioxetine)
▹ Antiepileptics: plasma concentration of bupropion reduced by CARBAMAZEPINE, FOSPHENYTOIN and PHENYTOIN; metabolism of bupropion inhibited by SODIUM VALPROATE and VALPROIC ACID
▹ Antivirals: metabolism of bupropion accelerated by EFAVIRENZ (reduced plasma concentration); plasma concentration of bupropion reduced by RITONAVIR
▹ Atomoxetine: possible increased risk of convulsions when bupropion given with ATOMOXETINE
▹ Dopaminergics: increased risk of side-effects when bupropion given with AMANTADINE, CO-BENELDOPA, CO-CARELDOPA or LEVODOPA
- Hormone Antagonists: bupropion possibly inhibits metabolism of ● TAMOXIFEN to active metabolite (avoid concomitant use)
- Methylthioninium: possible risk of CNS toxicity when bupropion given with ● METHYLTHIONINIUM—avoid concomitant use (if avoidance not possible, use lowest possible dose of methylthioninium and observe patient for up to 4 hours after administration)

Buspirone see Anxiolytics and Hypnotics
Busulfan
▹ Analgesics: metabolism of intravenous busulfan possibly inhibited by PARACETAMOL (manufacturer of intravenous busulfan advises caution within 72 hours of paracetamol)
- Antibacterials: plasma concentration of busulfan increased by ● METRONIDAZOLE (increased risk of toxicity)
▹ Antiepileptics: plasma concentration of busulfan possibly reduced by FOSPHENYTOIN and PHENYTOIN
▹ Antifungals: metabolism of busulfan inhibited by ITRACONAZOLE (increased risk of toxicity)
▹ Antipsychotics: avoid concomitant use of cytotoxics with ● CLOZAPINE (increased risk of agranulocytosis)
▹ Cytotoxics: increased risk of hepatotoxicity when busulfan given with TIOGUANINE

Butyrophenones see Antipsychotics
Cabazitaxel
- Antibacterials: plasma concentration of cabazitaxel possibly increased by ● CLARITHROMYCIN and ● TELITHROMYCIN—manufacturer of cabazitaxel advises avoid or consider reducing dose of cabazitaxel; manufacturer of cabazitaxel advises avoid concomitant use with ● RIFABUTIN; plasma concentration of cabazitaxel reduced by ● RIFAMPICIN—manufacturer of cabazitaxel advises avoid concomitant use
- Antidepressants: manufacturer of cabazitaxel advises avoid concomitant use with ● ST JOHN'S WORT

Cabazitaxel (continued)

- Antiepileptics: manufacturer of cabazitaxel advises avoid concomitant use with • CARBAMAZEPINE, • FOSPHENYTOIN, • PHENOBARBITAL, • PHENYTOIN and • PRIMIDONE
- Antifungals: manufacturer of cabazitaxel advises avoid concomitant use with • KETOCONAZOLE; plasma concentration of cabazitaxel possibly increased by • ITRACONAZOLE and • VORICONAZOLE—manufacturer of cabazitaxel advises avoid or consider reducing dose of cabazitaxel
- Antipsychotics: avoid concomitant use of cytotoxics with • CLOZAPINE (increased risk of agranulocytosis)
- Antivirals: manufacturer of cabazitaxel advises avoid concomitant use with • ATAZANAVIR; plasma concentration of cabazitaxel possibly increased by • INDINAVIR, • RITONAVIR and • SAQUINAVIR—manufacturer of cabazitaxel advises avoid or consider reducing dose of cabazitaxel

Cabergoline

▹ Antibacterials: plasma concentration of cabergoline increased by ERYTHROMYCIN (increased risk of toxicity); plasma concentration of cabergoline possibly increased by MACROLIDES (increased risk of toxicity)
▹ Antipsychotics: hypoprolactinaemic and antiparkinsonian effects of cabergoline antagonised by ANTIPSYCHOTICS
▹ Domperidone: hypoprolactinaemic effect of cabergoline possibly antagonised by DOMPERIDONE
▹ Memantine: effects of dopaminergics possibly enhanced by MEMANTINE
▹ Methyldopa: antiparkinsonian effect of dopaminergics antagonised by METHYLDOPA
▹ Metoclopramide: hypoprolactinaemic effect of cabergoline antagonised by METOCLOPRAMIDE

Cabozantinib

- Antibacterials: plasma concentration of cabozantinib possibly increased by CLARITHROMYCIN and ERYTHROMYCIN; plasma concentration of cabozantinib reduced by • RIFAMPICIN—avoid concomitant use
▹ Antidepressants: plasma concentration of cabozantinib possibly reduced by ST JOHN'S WORT—manufacturer of cabozantinib advises avoid concomitant use
- Antiepileptics: plasma concentration of cabozantinib possibly reduced by • CARBAMAZEPINE, • FOSPHENYTOIN, • PHENOBARBITAL, • PHENYTOIN and • PRIMIDONE—avoid concomitant use
▹ Antifungals: plasma concentration of cabozantinib increased by KETOCONAZOLE; plasma concentration of cabozantinib possibly increased by ITRACONAZOLE
- Antipsychotics: avoid concomitant use of cytotoxics with • CLOZAPINE (increased risk of agranulocytosis)
▹ Antivirals: plasma concentration of cabozantinib possibly increased by RITONAVIR
▹ Corticosteroids: plasma concentration of cabozantinib possibly reduced by DEXAMETHASONE—manufacturer of cabozantinib advises avoid concomitant use
▹ Grapefruit Juice: plasma concentration of cabozantinib possibly increased by GRAPEFRUIT JUICE

Caffeine citrate

▹ Aminophylline: manufacturer of caffeine citrate advises avoid concomitant use with AMINOPHYLLINE
▹ Anti-arrhythmics: caffeine citrate antagonises anti-arrhythmic effect of ADENOSINE—manufacturer of adenosine advises avoid caffeine citrate for at least 12 hours before adenosine
▹ Antiepileptics: plasma concentration of caffeine citrate reduced by FOSPHENYTOIN and PHENYTOIN; caffeine citrate possibly antagonises effects of PHENOBARBITAL and PRIMIDONE
▹ Theophylline: manufacturer of caffeine citrate advises avoid concomitant use with THEOPHYLLINE
▹ Ulcer-healing Drugs: plasma concentration of caffeine citrate increased by CIMETIDINE

Calcitriol *see* Vitamins

Calcium Salts

NOTE *see also* Antacids
▹ Antibacterials: calcium salts reduce absorption of CIPROFLOXACIN (give at least 2 hours before or 4 hours after ciprofloxacin); calcium salts possibly reduce absorption of TETRACYCLINES (give at least 2 to 3 hours apart)

Calcium Salts (continued)

▹ Antivirals: calcium salts reduce absorption of DOLUTEGRAVIR—manufacturer of dolutegravir advises give at least 2 hours before or 6 hours after calcium salts; separating administration from calcium salts by 4 hours advised by manufacturer of LEDIPASVIR; manufacturer of rilpivirine advises give calcium salts 2 hours before or 4 hours after RILPIVIRINE
▹ Bisphosphonates: calcium salts reduce absorption of BISPHOSPHONATES
▹ Cardiac Glycosides: large *intravenous* doses of calcium salts can precipitate arrhythmias when given with CARDIAC GLYCOSIDES
▹ Corticosteroids: absorption of calcium salts reduced by CORTICOSTEROIDS
▹ Cytotoxics: calcium salts reduce absorption of ESTRAMUSTINE (manufacturer of estramustine advises avoid concomitant administration)
▹ Diuretics: increased risk of hypercalcaemia when calcium salts given with THIAZIDES AND RELATED DIURETICS
▹ Eltrombopag: calcium salts possibly reduce absorption of ELTROMBOPAG (give at least 4 hours apart)
▹ Fluorides: calcium salts reduce absorption of FLUORIDES
▹ Iron Salts: calcium salts reduce absorption of *oral* IRON SALTS
▹ Thyroid Hormones: calcium salts reduce absorption of LEVOTHYROXINE
▹ Zinc: calcium salts reduce absorption of ZINC

Calcium-channel Blockers

NOTE Dihydropyridine calcium-channel blockers include amlodipine, felodipine, isradipine, lacidipine, lercanidipine, nicardipine, nifedipine, and nimodipine

▹ ACE Inhibitors: enhanced hypotensive effect when calcium-channel blockers given with ACE INHIBITORS
▹ Adrenergic Neurone Blockers: enhanced hypotensive effect when calcium-channel blockers given with ADRENERGIC NEURONE BLOCKERS
▹ Alcohol: enhanced hypotensive effect when calcium-channel blockers given with ALCOHOL; verapamil possibly increases plasma concentration of ALCOHOL
▹ Aldesleukin: enhanced hypotensive effect when calcium-channel blockers given with ALDESLEUKIN
▹ Aliskiren: verapamil increases plasma concentration of ALISKIREN
- Alpha-blockers: verapamil increases plasma concentration of TAMSULOSIN; enhanced hypotensive effect when calcium-channel blockers given with • ALPHA-BLOCKERS, also increased risk of first-dose hypotension with post-synaptic alpha-blockers such as prazosin
- Aminophylline: calcium-channel blockers possibly increase plasma concentration of • AMINOPHYLLINE (enhanced effect); diltiazem increases plasma concentration of AMINOPHYLLINE; verapamil increases plasma concentration of • AMINOPHYLLINE (enhanced effect)
- Anaesthetics, General: enhanced hypotensive effect when calcium-channel blockers given with GENERAL ANAESTHETICS or ISOFLURANE; hypotensive effect of verapamil enhanced by • GENERAL ANAESTHETICS (also AV delay)
▹ Analgesics: hypotensive effect of calcium-channel blockers antagonised by NSAIDs; diltiazem inhibits metabolism of ALFENTANIL (risk of prolonged or delayed respiratory depression)
▹ Angiotensin-II Receptor Antagonists: enhanced hypotensive effect when calcium-channel blockers given with ANGIOTENSIN-II RECEPTOR ANTAGONISTS
- Anti-arrhythmics: increased risk of bradycardia, AV block and myocardial depression when diltiazem or verapamil given with • AMIODARONE; increased risk of myocardial depression and asystole when verapamil given with • DISOPYRAMIDE or • FLECAINIDE; nifedipine increases plasma concentration of • DRONEDARONE; increased risk of bradycardia and myocardial depression when diltiazem and verapamil given with • DRONEDARONE
- Antibacterials: metabolism of calcium-channel blockers possibly inhibited by • CLARITHROMYCIN, • ERYTHROMYCIN and • TELITHROMYCIN (increased risk of side-effects); manufacturer of lercanidipine advises avoid concomitant use with ERYTHROMYCIN; metabolism of diltiazem, nifedipine,

Calcium-channel Blockers

- **Antibacterials** (continued)
nimodipine and verapamil accelerated by ● RIFAMPICIN (plasma concentration significantly reduced); metabolism of isradipine and nicardipine possibly accelerated by ● RIFAMPICIN (possible significantly reduced plasma concentration); plasma concentration of felodipine possibly reduced by RIFAMPICIN; avoidance of verapamil advised by manufacturer of FIDAXOMICIN
- **Anticoagulants**: verapamil possibly increases plasma concentration of ● DABIGATRAN (see under Dabigatran Etexilate, in BNF); verapamil increases plasma concentration of EDOXABAN
- **Antidepressants**: metabolism of nifedipine possibly inhibited by FLUOXETINE (increased plasma concentration); diltiazem and verapamil increase plasma concentration of IMIPRAMINE; enhanced hypotensive effect when calcium-channel blockers given with MAOIs; plasma concentration of amlodipine and felodipine possibly reduced by ST JOHN'S WORT; plasma concentration of verapamil significantly reduced by ● ST JOHN'S WORT; plasma concentration of nifedipine reduced by ST JOHN'S WORT; diltiazem and verapamil possibly increase plasma concentration of TRICYCLICS
- **Antidiabetics**: glucose tolerance occasionally impaired when nifedipine given with INSULIN
- **Antiepileptics**: effects of felodipine and isradipine reduced by CARBAMAZEPINE; effects of dihydropyridines, nicardipine and nifedipine probably reduced by CARBAMAZEPINE; diltiazem and verapamil enhance effects of ● CARBAMAZEPINE; manufacturer of nimodipine advises avoid concomitant use with CARBAMAZEPINE, FOSPHENYTOIN and PHENYTOIN (plasma concentration of nimodipine possibly reduced); effects of felodipine and verapamil reduced by FOSPHENYTOIN; diltiazem increases plasma concentration of ● FOSPHENYTOIN and ● PHENYTOIN but also effect of diltiazem reduced; manufacturer of isradipine advises avoid concomitant use with FOSPHENYTOIN, PHENOBARBITAL, PHENYTOIN and PRIMIDONE; effects of calcium-channel blockers probably reduced by ● PHENOBARBITAL and ● PRIMIDONE; manufacturer of nimodipine advises avoid concomitant use with ● PHENOBARBITAL and ● PRIMIDONE (plasma concentration of nimodipine reduced); effects of felodipine and verapamil reduced by PHENYTOIN
- **Antifungals**: metabolism of dihydropyridines possibly inhibited by ITRACONAZOLE and KETOCONAZOLE (increased plasma concentration); metabolism of felodipine is inhibited by ● KETOCONAZOLE (increased plasma concentration)—manufacturer of ketoconazole advises avoid concomitant use; manufacturer of lercanidipine advises avoid concomitant use with ITRACONAZOLE and KETOCONAZOLE; negative inotropic effect possibly increased when calcium-channel blockers given with ITRACONAZOLE; metabolism of felodipine inhibited by ● ITRACONAZOLE (increased plasma concentration); plasma concentration of nifedipine increased by MICAFUNGIN
- **Antimalarials**: possible increased risk of bradycardia when calcium-channel blockers given with MEFLOQUINE
- **Antimuscarinics**: avoidance of verapamil advised by manufacturer of DARIFENACIN; verapamil increases plasma concentration of SOLIFENACIN
- **Antipsychotics**: enhanced hypotensive effect when calcium-channel blockers given with ANTIPSYCHOTICS; verapamil possibly increases the plasma concentration of ● LURASIDONE (see under Lurasidone, in BNF); diltiazem increases the plasma concentration of ● LURASIDONE (see under Lurasidone, in BNF)
- **Antivirals**: plasma concentration of verapamil possibly increased by ATAZANAVIR; plasma concentration of diltiazem increased by ATAZANAVIR (reduce dose of diltiazem); plasma concentration of diltiazem reduced by EFAVIRENZ; manufacturer of lercanidipine advises avoid concomitant use with RITONAVIR; plasma concentration of amlodipine increased by ● RITONAVIR (reduce dose of amlodipine); plasma concentration of calcium-channel blockers possibly increased by ● RITONAVIR; caution with diltiazem, felodipine, nicardipine, nifedipine and verapamil advised by manufacturer of TELAPREVIR; plasma concentration of

Calcium-channel Blockers

- **Antivirals** (continued)
amlodipine increased by TELAPREVIR (consider reducing dose of amlodipine)
- **Anxiolytics and Hypnotics**: enhanced hypotensive effect when calcium-channel blockers given with ANXIOLYTICS AND HYPNOTICS; diltiazem and verapamil inhibit metabolism of MIDAZOLAM (increased plasma concentration with increased sedation); absorption of lercanidipine increased by MIDAZOLAM; diltiazem and verapamil increase plasma concentration of BUSPIRONE (reduce dose of buspirone)
- **Aprepitant**: plasma concentration of both drugs may increase when diltiazem given with APREPITANT
- **Avanafil**: diltiazem and verapamil possibly increase plasma concentration of ● AVANAFIL—see under Avanafil, in BNF
- **Beta-blockers**: enhanced hypotensive effect when calcium-channel blockers given with BETA-BLOCKERS; increased risk of AV block and bradycardia when diltiazem given with ● BETA-BLOCKERS; asystole, severe hypotension and heart failure when verapamil given with ● BETA-BLOCKERS (see under Verapamil, p. 101); possible severe hypotension and heart failure when nifedipine given with ● BETA-BLOCKERS
- **Calcium-channel Blockers**: plasma concentration of both drugs may increase when diltiazem given with NIFEDIPINE
- **Cardiac Glycosides**: verapamil increases plasma concentration of ● DIGOXIN, also increased risk of AV block and bradycardia; diltiazem, lercanidipine and nicardipine increase plasma concentration of ● DIGOXIN; nifedipine possibly increases plasma concentration of ● DIGOXIN
- **Ciclosporin**: diltiazem, nicardipine and verapamil increase plasma concentration of ● CICLOSPORIN; combination of lercanidipine with ● CICLOSPORIN may increase plasma concentration of either drug (or both)—avoid concomitant use; plasma concentration of nifedipine possibly increased by CICLOSPORIN (increased risk of toxicity including gingival hyperplasia)
- **Cilostazol**: diltiazem increases plasma concentration of CILOSTAZOL (consider reducing dose of cilostazol)
- **Clonidine**: enhanced hypotensive effect when calcium-channel blockers given with CLONIDINE
- **Colchicine**: diltiazem and verapamil possibly increase risk of ● COLCHICINE toxicity—suspend or reduce dose of colchicine (avoid concomitant use in hepatic or renal impairment)
- **Corticosteroids**: hypotensive effect of calcium-channel blockers antagonised by CORTICOSTEROIDS; diltiazem increases plasma concentration of METHYLPREDNISOLONE
- **Cytotoxics**: verapamil possibly increases plasma concentration of DOXORUBICIN; verapamil possibly increases the plasma concentration of AFATINIB—manufacturer of afatinib advises separating administration of verapamil by 6 to 12 hours; diltiazem and verapamil possibly increase the plasma concentration of ● BOSUTINIB—manufacturer of bosutinib advises avoid or consider reducing dose of bosutinib; possible increased risk of bradycardia when diltiazem or verapamil given with CRIZOTINIB; plasma concentration of both drugs may increase when verapamil given with ● EVEROLIMUS (consider reducing the dose of everolimus—consult everolimus product literature); diltiazem and verapamil possibly increase the plasma concentration of ● IBRUTINIB—reduce dose of ibrutinib (see under Ibrutinib, in BNF); nifedipine possibly inhibits metabolism of VINCRISTINE
- **Dapoxetine**: manufacturer of dapoxetine advises dose reduction when diltiazem and verapamil given with DAPOXETINE (see under Dapoxetine, in BNF)
- **Diazoxide**: enhanced hypotensive effect when calcium-channel blockers given with DIAZOXIDE
- **Diuretics**: enhanced hypotensive effect when calcium-channel blockers given with DIURETICS; diltiazem and verapamil increase plasma concentration of EPLERENONE (reduce dose of eplerenone)
- **Dopaminergics**: enhanced hypotensive effect when calcium-channel blockers given with CO-BENELDOPA, CO-CARELDOPA or LEVODOPA
- **Fingolimod**: possible increased risk of bradycardia when diltiazem or verapamil given with ● FINGOLIMOD

Calcium-channel Blockers (continued)

▹ Fosaprepitant: plasma concentration of both drugs may increase when diltiazem given with FOSAPREPITANT

▹ Grapefruit Juice: plasma concentration of felodipine, isradipine, lacidipine, lercanidipine, nicardipine, nifedipine, nimodipine and verapamil increased by GRAPEFRUIT JUICE; plasma concentration of amlodipine possibly increased by GRAPEFRUIT JUICE

▹ Guanfacine: diltiazem and verapamil possibly increase the plasma concentration of GUANFACINE (halve dose of guanfacine)

▹ Hormone Antagonists: diltiazem and verapamil increase plasma concentration of DUTASTERIDE; possible increased risk of bradycardia when diltiazem or verapamil given with PASIREOTIDE

● Ivabradine: diltiazem and verapamil increase plasma concentration of ● IVABRADINE—avoid concomitant use

● Lenalidomide: verapamil possibly increases plasma concentration of ● LENALIDOMIDE (increased risk of toxicity)

● Lipid-regulating Drugs: diltiazem increases plasma concentration of ATORVASTATIN—possible increased risk of myopathy; plasma concentration of verapamil increased by ● ATORVASTATIN, also possible increased risk of myopathy (consider reducing dose of atorvastatin); possible increased risk of myopathy when amlodipine and diltiazem given with ● SIMVASTATIN (see under Simvastatin, p. 125); increased risk of myopathy when verapamil given with ● SIMVASTATIN (see under Simvastatin, p. 125); separating administration from amlodipine and lacidipine by 12 hours advised by manufacturer of LOMITAPIDE; avoidance of diltiazem and verapamil advised by manufacturer of ● LOMITAPIDE (plasma concentration of lomitapide possibly increased)

● Lithium: neurotoxicity may occur when diltiazem or verapamil given with LITHIUM without increased plasma concentration of lithium

● Magnesium (parenteral): profound hypotension reported with concomitant use of nifedipine and ● PARENTERAL MAGNESIUM in pre-eclampsia

▹ Methyldopa: enhanced hypotensive effect when calcium-channel blockers given with METHYLDOPA

▹ Moxisylyte: enhanced hypotensive effect when calcium-channel blockers given with MOXISYLYTE

▹ Moxonidine: enhanced hypotensive effect when calcium-channel blockers given with MOXONIDINE

● Muscle Relaxants: verapamil enhances effects of NON-DEPOLARISING MUSCLE RELAXANTS and SUXAMETHONIUM; enhanced hypotensive effect when calcium-channel blockers given with BACLOFEN or TIZANIDINE; manufacturer of verapamil advises avoid concomitant use of *intravenous* DANTROLENE; possible increased risk of ventricular arrhythmias when diltiazem given with *intravenous* DANTROLENE—manufacturer of diltiazem advises avoid concomitant use; calcium-channel blockers possibly enhance effects of NON-DEPOLARISING MUSCLE RELAXANTS

▹ Nitrates: enhanced hypotensive effect when calcium-channel blockers given with NITRATES

▹ Oestrogens: hypotensive effect of calcium-channel blockers antagonised by OESTROGENS

▹ Prostaglandins: enhanced hypotensive effect when calcium-channel blockers given with ALPROSTADIL

▹ Ranolazine: diltiazem and verapamil increase plasma concentration of RANOLAZINE (consider reducing dose of ranolazine)

● Sildenafil: enhanced hypotensive effect when amlodipine given with SILDENAFIL

● Sirolimus: diltiazem increases plasma concentration of ● SIROLIMUS; plasma concentration of both drugs increased when verapamil given with ● SIROLIMUS; nicardipine possibly increases plasma concentration of SIROLIMUS

▹ Sulfinpyrazone: plasma concentration of verapamil reduced by SULFINPYRAZONE

● Tacrolimus: diltiazem, nicardipine and nifedipine increase plasma concentration of ● TACROLIMUS; felodipine and verapamil possibly increase plasma concentration of TACROLIMUS

Calcium-channel Blockers (continued)

● Theophylline: calcium-channel blockers possibly increase plasma concentration of ● THEOPHYLLINE (enhanced effect); diltiazem increases plasma concentration of THEOPHYLLINE; verapamil increases plasma concentration of ● THEOPHYLLINE (enhanced effect)

▹ Ticagrelor: diltiazem increases plasma concentration of TICAGRELOR

▹ Ulcer-healing Drugs: metabolism of calcium-channel blockers possibly inhibited by CIMETIDINE (increased plasma concentration); plasma concentration of isradipine increased by CIMETIDINE (halve dose of isradipine)

▹ Ulipristal: avoidance of verapamil advised by manufacturer of *low-dose* ULIPRISTAL

▹ Vardenafil: enhanced hypotensive effect when nifedipine given with VARDENAFIL

▹ Vasodilator Antihypertensives: enhanced hypotensive effect when calcium-channel blockers given with HYDRALAZINE, MINOXIDIL or SODIUM NITROPRUSSIDE

Calcium-channel Blockers (dihydropyridines) *see* Calcium-channel Blockers

Canagliflozin *see* Antidiabetics

Canakinumab

● Antipsychotics: avoid concomitant use of cytotoxics with ● CLOZAPINE (increased risk of agranulocytosis)

● Vaccines: risk of generalised infections when monoclonal antibodies given with live ● VACCINES—avoid concomitant use

Candesartan *see* Angiotensin-II Receptor Antagonists

Cannabis Extract

● Antibacterials: plasma concentration of cannabis extract reduced by RIFAMPICIN—manufacturer of cannabis extract advises avoid concomitant use

● Antidepressants: plasma concentration of cannabis extract possibly reduced by ● ST JOHN'S WORT—manufacturer of cannabis extract advises avoid concomitant use; possible increased risk of hypertension and tachycardia when cannabis extract given with TRICYCLICS

● Antiepileptics: plasma concentration of cannabis extract possibly reduced by ● CARBAMAZEPINE, ● FOSPHENYTOIN, ● PHENOBARBITAL, ● PHENYTOIN and ● PRIMIDONE—manufacturer of cannabis extract advises avoid concomitant use

▹ Antifungals: plasma concentration of cannabis extract increased by KETOCONAZOLE

Capecitabine

● Allopurinol: manufacturer of capecitabine advises avoid concomitant use with ● ALLOPURINOL

● Antibacterials: metabolism of capecitabine inhibited by METRONIDAZOLE (increased toxicity)

● Anticoagulants: capecitabine enhances anticoagulant effect of ● COUMARINS

● Antiepileptics: capecitabine possibly inhibits metabolism of FOSPHENYTOIN and PHENYTOIN (increased risk of toxicity)

● Antipsychotics: avoid concomitant use of cytotoxics with ● CLOZAPINE (increased risk of agranulocytosis)

▹ Cytotoxics: capecitabine possibly increases plasma concentration of ERLOTINIB

▹ Filgrastim: neutropenia possibly exacerbated when capecitabine given with FILGRASTIM

● Folates: toxicity of capecitabine increased by ● FOLIC ACID—avoid concomitant use

▹ Lipegfilgrastim: neutropenia possibly exacerbated when capecitabine given with LIPEGFILGRASTIM

▹ Pegfilgrastim: neutropenia possibly exacerbated when capecitabine given with PEGFILGRASTIM

▹ Ulcer-healing Drugs: metabolism of capecitabine inhibited by CIMETIDINE (increased plasma concentration)

Capreomycin

▹ Antibacterials: increased risk of nephrotoxicity when capreomycin given with COLISTIMETHATE SODIUM or POLYMYXINS; increased risk of nephrotoxicity and ototoxicity when capreomycin given with AMINOGLYCOSIDES or VANCOMYCIN

▹ Cytotoxics: increased risk of nephrotoxicity and ototoxicity when capreomycin given with PLATINUM COMPOUNDS

Capreomycin (continued)

▸ Vaccines: antibacterials inactivate ORAL TYPHOID VACCINE—see under Typhoid Vaccine in BNFC

Captopril see ACE Inhibitors

Carbamazepine

▸ Alcohol: CNS side-effects of carbamazepine possibly increased by ALCOHOL

▸ Aminophylline: carbamazepine accelerates metabolism of AMINOPHYLLINE (reduced effect)

● Analgesics: effects of carbamazepine enhanced by
● DEXTROPROPOXYPHENE; carbamazepine possibly accelerates metabolism of FENTANYL (reduced effect); carbamazepine reduces plasma concentration of METHADONE; carbamazepine reduces effects of TRAMADOL; carbamazepine possibly accelerates metabolism of PARACETAMOL (also isolated reports of hepatotoxicity)

● Anthelmintics: carbamazepine reduces plasma concentration of
● ALBENDAZOLE and ● PRAZIQUANTEL—consider increasing albendazole and praziquantel dose when given for systemic infections

● Anti-arrhythmics: carbamazepine possibly reduces plasma concentration of ● DRONEDARONE—avoid concomitant use

● Antibacterials: plasma concentration of carbamazepine increased by CLARITHROMYCIN (consider reducing dose of carbamazepine); plasma concentration of carbamazepine increased by ● ERYTHROMYCIN; plasma concentration of carbamazepine reduced by ● RIFABUTIN; carbamazepine accelerates metabolism of DOXYCYCLINE (reduced effect); carbamazepine possibly reduces plasma concentration of
● BEDAQUILINE—manufacturer of bedaquiline advises avoid concomitant use; avoidance of carbamazepine advised by manufacturer of DELAMANID; plasma concentration of carbamazepine increased by ● ISONIAZID (also possibly increased isoniazid hepatotoxicity); carbamazepine reduces plasma concentration of ● TELITHROMYCIN (avoid during and for 2 weeks after carbamazepine)

● Anticoagulants: carbamazepine possibly reduces plasma concentration of ● APIXABAN—manufacturer of apixaban advises avoid concomitant use when given for treatment of deep-vein thrombosis or pulmonary embolism; carbamazepine accelerates metabolism of ● COUMARINS (reduced anticoagulant effect); carbamazepine possibly reduces plasma concentration of DABIGATRAN—manufacturer of dabigatran advises avoid concomitant use; carbamazepine possibly reduces plasma concentration of ● EDOXABAN; carbamazepine possibly reduces plasma concentration of
● RIVAROXABAN—manufacturer of rivaroxaban advises monitor for signs of thrombosis

● Antidepressants: carbamazepine possibly reduces plasma concentration of REBOXETINE; plasma concentration of carbamazepine increased by ● FLUOXETINE and ● FLUVOXAMINE; carbamazepine reduces plasma concentration of ● MIANSERIN, MIRTAZAPINE and TRAZODONE; anticonvulsant effect of antiepileptics possibly antagonised by MAOIs and ● TRICYCLIC-RELATED ANTIDEPRESSANTS (convulsive threshold lowered); manufacturer of carbamazepine advises avoid for 2 weeks after stopping ● MAOIs, also antagonism of anticonvulsant effect; anticonvulsant effect of antiepileptics antagonised by
● SSRIS and ● TRICYCLICS (convulsive threshold lowered); plasma concentration of carbamazepine possibly reduced by ST JOHN'S WORT; carbamazepine accelerates metabolism of
● TRICYCLICS (reduced plasma concentration and reduced effect); carbamazepine possibly reduces plasma concentration of ● VORTIOXETINE—consider increasing dose of vortioxetine

● Antiepileptics: carbamazepine possibly reduces plasma concentration of ESLICARBAZEPINE but risk of side-effects increased; carbamazepine possibly reduces plasma concentration of ETHOSUXIMIDE and RETIGABINE; plasma concentration of both drugs reduced when carbamazepine given with FOSPHENYTOIN or PHENYTOIN, also plasma concentration of fosphenytoin or phenytoin may be increased; carbamazepine often reduces plasma concentration of LAMOTRIGINE, also plasma concentration of an active metabolite of carbamazepine sometimes raised (but evidence is conflicting); possible increased risk of carbamazepine toxicity when given with LEVETIRACETAM;

Carbamazepine

● Antiepileptics (continued)
plasma concentration of carbamazepine sometimes reduced by OXCARBAZEPINE (but concentration of an active metabolite of carbamazepine may be increased), also plasma concentration of an active metabolite of oxcarbazepine often reduced; carbamazepine reduces plasma concentration of
● PERAMPANEL (see under Perampanel, p. 193); carbamazepine possibly increases plasma concentration of PHENOBARBITAL and PRIMIDONE; plasma concentration of both drugs possibly reduced when carbamazepine given with RUFINAMIDE; carbamazepine reduces plasma concentration of SODIUM VALPROATE and VALPROIC ACID, also plasma concentration of active metabolite of carbamazepine increased; plasma concentration of carbamazepine increased by ● STIRIPENTOL; carbamazepine reduces plasma concentration of TIAGABINE and ZONISAMIDE; carbamazepine often reduces plasma concentration of TOPIRAMATE

● Antifungals: plasma concentration of carbamazepine possibly increased by KETOCONAZOLE, also plasma concentration of ketoconazole possibly reduced; plasma concentration of carbamazepine possibly increased by FLUCONAZOLE and MICONAZOLE; carbamazepine possibly reduces plasma concentration of ITRACONAZOLE and ● POSACONAZOLE; carbamazepine possibly reduces plasma concentration of
● VORICONAZOLE—avoid concomitant use; carbamazepine possibly reduces plasma concentration of CASPOFUNGIN—consider increasing dose of caspofungin

● Antimalarials: avoidance of carbamazepine advised by manufacturer of ARTENIMOL WITH PIPERAQUINE; anticonvulsant effect of antiepileptics antagonised by ● MEFLOQUINE

● Antimuscarinics: carbamazepine possibly reduces plasma concentration of active metabolite of ● FESOTERODINE—manufacturer of fesoterodine advises avoid concomitant use

● Antipsychotics: anticonvulsant effect of antiepileptics antagonised by ● ANTIPSYCHOTICS (convulsive threshold lowered); carbamazepine accelerates metabolism of HALOPERIDOL, OLANZAPINE, QUETIAPINE and RISPERIDONE (reduced plasma concentration); carbamazepine reduces plasma concentration of ● ARIPIPRAZOLE (avoid concomitant use or consider increasing the dose of aripiprazole—consult aripiprazole product literature); carbamazepine accelerates metabolism of ● CLOZAPINE (reduced plasma concentration), also avoid concomitant use of drugs with substantial potential for causing agranulocytosis; carbamazepine possibly reduces plasma concentration of ● LURASIDONE—avoid concomitant use; carbamazepine reduces plasma concentration of PALIPERIDONE

● Antivirals: avoidance of carbamazepine advised by manufacturer of ● BOCEPREVIR and ● RILPIVIRINE (plasma concentration of boceprevir and rilpivirine possibly reduced); carbamazepine possibly reduces plasma concentration of
● DACLATASVIR and ● SIMEPREVIR—manufacturer of daclatasvir and simeprevir advises avoid concomitant use; carbamazepine possibly reduces plasma concentration of DARUNAVIR, FOSAMPRENAVIR, LOPINAVIR, SAQUINAVIR and TIPRANAVIR; carbamazepine reduces plasma concentration of
● DASABUVIR, ● OMBITASVIR and ● PARITAPREVIR—avoid concomitant use; carbamazepine reduces the plasma concentration of ● DOLUTEGRAVIR (see under Dolutegravir, p. 387); plasma concentration of both drugs reduced when carbamazepine given with EFAVIRENZ; avoidance of carbamazepine advised by manufacturer of ● ELVITEGRAVIR, ETRAVIRINE, LEDIPASVIR, SOFOSBUVIR and ● TELAPREVIR; carbamazepine possibly reduces plasma concentration of
● INDINAVIR, also plasma concentration of carbamazepine possibly increased; carbamazepine reduces plasma concentration of NEVIRAPINE; plasma concentration of carbamazepine possibly increased by ● RITONAVIR

▸ Anxiolytics and Hypnotics: carbamazepine often reduces plasma concentration of CLONAZEPAM; carbamazepine reduces plasma concentration of MIDAZOLAM

● Apremilast: carbamazepine possibly reduces plasma concentration of ● APREMILAST—avoid concomitant use

▸ Aprepitant: carbamazepine possibly reduces plasma concentration of APREPITANT

Carbamazepine (continued)

▸ Avanafil: carbamazepine possibly reduces plasma concentration of AVANAFIL —manufacturer of avanafil advises avoid concomitant use

▸ Bupropion: carbamazepine reduces plasma concentration of BUPROPION

● Calcium-channel Blockers: carbamazepine reduces effects of FELODIPINE and ISRADIPINE; carbamazepine probably reduces effects of DIHYDROPYRIDINES, NICARDIPINE and NIFEDIPINE; avoidance of carbamazepine advised by manufacturer of NIMODIPINE (plasma concentration of nimodipine possibly reduced); effects of carbamazepine enhanced by ● DILTIAZEM and ● VERAPAMIL

● Cannabis Extract: carbamazepine possibly reduces plasma concentration of ● CANNABIS EXTRACT—manufacturer of cannabis extract advises avoid concomitant use

● Ciclosporin: carbamazepine accelerates metabolism of ● CICLOSPORIN (reduced plasma concentration)

● Clopidogrel: carbamazepine possibly reduces antiplatelet effect of ● CLOPIDOGREL

● Cobicistat: carbamazepine possibly reduces plasma concentration of ● COBICISTAT—manufacturer of cobicistat advises avoid concomitant use

● Corticosteroids: carbamazepine accelerates metabolism of ● CORTICOSTEROIDS (reduced effect)

● Cytotoxics: carbamazepine possibly decreases plasma concentration of AXITINIB (increase dose of axitinib—consult axitinib product literature); carbamazepine possibly reduces plasma concentration of BORTEZOMIB, ● BOSUTINIB, CRIZOTINIB, ● IBRUTINIB, ● IDELALISIB and PONATINIB—manufacturer of bortezomib, bosutinib, crizotinib, ibrutinib, idelalisib and ponatinib advises avoid concomitant use; carbamazepine possibly reduces plasma concentration of ● CABOZANTINIB— avoid concomitant use; avoidance of carbamazepine advised by manufacturer of ● CABAZITAXEL, DABRAFENIB, GEFITINIB, ● OLAPARIB and VEMURAFENIB; avoidance of carbamazepine advised by manufacturer of DASATINIB, VANDETANIB and ● VISMODEGIB (plasma concentration of dasatinib, vandetanib and vismodegib possibly reduced); carbamazepine reduces plasma concentration of ● IMATINIB and ● LAPATINIB—avoid concomitant use; carbamazepine possibly reduces plasma concentration of ERIBULIN; carbamazepine reduces plasma concentration of IRINOTECAN and its active metabolite; manufacturer of procarbazine advises possible increased risk of hypersensitivity reactions when carbamazepine given with PROCARBAZINE

● Diuretics: increased risk of hyponatraemia when carbamazepine given with DIURETICS; plasma concentration of carbamazepine increased by ● ACETAZOLAMIDE; carbamazepine reduces plasma concentration of ● EPLERENONE—avoid concomitant use

● Fingolimod: carbamazepine reduces plasma concentration of FINGOLIMOD

▸ Fosaprepitant: carbamazepine possibly reduces plasma concentration of FOSAPREPITANT

● Guanfacine: carbamazepine possibly reduces plasma concentration of ● GUANFACINE—increase dose of guanfacine

● Hormone Antagonists: carbamazepine possibly reduces plasma concentration of ● ABIRATERONE—manufacturer of abiraterone advises avoid concomitant use; metabolism of carbamazepine inhibited by ● DANAZOL (increased risk of toxicity); carbamazepine possibly accelerates metabolism of TOREMIFENE (reduced plasma concentration)

● 5HT$_3$-receptor Antagonists: carbamazepine accelerates metabolism of ONDANSETRON (reduced effect)

● Ivacaftor: carbamazepine possibly reduces plasma concentration of ● IVACAFTOR—manufacturer of ivacaftor advises avoid concomitant use

● Lipid-regulating Drugs: carbamazepine reduces plasma concentration of ● SIMVASTATIN—consider increasing dose of simvastatin

▸ Lithium: neurotoxicity may occur when carbamazepine given with LITHIUM without increased plasma concentration of lithium

▸ Macitentan: avoidance of carbamazepine advised by manufacturer of MACITENTAN

Carbamazepine (continued)

▸ Muscle Relaxants: carbamazepine antagonises muscle relaxant effect of NON-DEPOLARISING MUSCLE RELAXANTS (accelerated recovery from neuromuscular blockade)

● Oestrogens: carbamazepine accelerates metabolism of ● OESTROGENS (reduced contraceptive effect with combined oral contraceptives, contraceptive patches, and vaginal rings—see Contraceptive Interactions in BNFC)

● Orlistat: possible increased risk of convulsions when antiepileptics given with ● ORLISTAT

● Progestogens: carbamazepine accelerates metabolism of ● PROGESTOGENS (reduced contraceptive effect with combined oral contraceptives, progestogen-only oral contraceptives, contraceptive patches, vaginal rings, etonogestrel-releasing implant, and emergency hormonal contraception—see Contraceptive Interactions in BNFC)

▸ Retinoids: plasma concentration of carbamazepine possibly reduced by ISOTRETINOIN

▸ Roflumilast: carbamazepine possibly inhibits effects of ROFLUMILAST (manufacturer of roflumilast advises avoid concomitant use)

▸ Theophylline: carbamazepine accelerates metabolism of THEOPHYLLINE (reduced effect)

▸ Thyroid Hormones: carbamazepine accelerates metabolism of THYROID HORMONES (may increase requirements for thyroid hormones in hypothyroidism)

▸ Tibolone: carbamazepine accelerates metabolism of TIBOLONE (reduced plasma concentration)

▸ Ticagrelor: carbamazepine possibly reduces plasma concentration of TICAGRELOR

● Ulcer-healing Drugs: metabolism of carbamazepine inhibited by ● CIMETIDINE (increased plasma concentration)

● Ulipristal: avoidance of carbamazepine advised by manufacturer of ● ULIPRISTAL (contraceptive effect of ulipristal possibly reduced)

▸ Vitamins: carbamazepine increases requirements for ALFACALCIDOL, CALCITRIOL, COLECALCIFEROL, DIHYDROTACHYSTEROL, ERGOCALCIFEROL, PARICALCITOL or VITAMIN D

Carbapenems see Ertapenem, Imipenem with Cilastatin, and Meropenem

Carbimazole

▸ Anticoagulants: carbimazole possibly enhances anticoagulant effect of COUMARINS

Carbonic Anhydrase Inhibitors see Diuretics

Carboplatin see Platinum Compounds

Carboprost see Prostaglandins

Cardiac Glycosides

▸ ACE Inhibitors: plasma concentration of digoxin possibly increased by CAPTOPRIL

▸ Alpha-blockers: plasma concentration of digoxin increased by PRAZOSIN

▸ Aminosalicylates: absorption of digoxin possibly reduced by SULFASALAZINE

▸ Analgesics: plasma concentration of cardiac glycosides possibly increased by NSAIDs, also possible exacerbation of heart failure and reduction of renal function

▸ Antacids: absorption of digoxin possibly reduced by ANTACIDS

● Anti-arrhythmics: plasma concentration of digoxin increased by ● AMIODARONE, ● DRONEDARONE and ● PROPAFENONE (halve dose of digoxin)

▸ Antibacterials: plasma concentration of digoxin possibly increased by GENTAMICIN, TELITHROMYCIN and TRIMETHOPRIM; absorption of digoxin reduced by NEOMYCIN; plasma concentration of digoxin possibly reduced by RIFAMPICIN; plasma concentration of digoxin increased by MACROLIDES (increased risk of toxicity)

● Antidepressants: plasma concentration of digoxin reduced by ● ST JOHN'S WORT—avoid concomitant use

▸ Antidiabetics: plasma concentration of digoxin possibly reduced by ACARBOSE; plasma concentration of digoxin increased by CANAGLIFLOZIN and SITAGLIPTIN

▸ Antiepileptics: plasma concentration of digoxin possibly reduced by FOSPHENYTOIN and PHENYTOIN

Cardiac Glycosides (continued)

- Antifungals: increased cardiac toxicity with cardiac glycosides if hypokalaemia occurs with ● AMPHOTERICIN; plasma concentration of digoxin increased by ● ITRACONAZOLE
- Antimalarials: plasma concentration of digoxin possibly increased by ● CHLOROQUINE and ● HYDROXYCHLOROQUINE; possible increased risk of bradycardia when digoxin given with MEFLOQUINE; plasma concentration of digoxin increased by ● QUININE
- Antimuscarinics: plasma concentration of digoxin possibly increased by DARIFENACIN
- Antivirals: side-effects of digoxin possibly increased by BOCEPREVIR; plasma concentration of digoxin increased by ● DACLATASVIR, ETRAVIRINE, SIMEPREVIR and TELAPREVIR; plasma concentration of digoxin possibly increased by PARITAPREVIR (consider reducing dose of digoxin); plasma concentration of digoxin possibly increased by RITONAVIR
- Anxiolytics and Hypnotics: plasma concentration of digoxin increased by ALPRAZOLAM (increased risk of toxicity)
- Beta-blockers: increased risk of AV block and bradycardia when cardiac glycosides given with BETA-BLOCKERS
- Calcium Salts: arrhythmias can be precipitated when cardiac glycosides given with large *intravenous* doses of CALCIUM SALTS
- Calcium-channel Blockers: plasma concentration of digoxin increased by ● DILTIAZEM, ● LERCANIDIPINE and ● NICARDIPINE; plasma concentration of digoxin possibly increased by ● NIFEDIPINE; plasma concentration of digoxin increased by ● VERAPAMIL, also increased risk of AV block and bradycardia
- Ciclosporin: plasma concentration of digoxin increased by ● CICLOSPORIN (increased risk of toxicity)
- Cobicistat: plasma concentration of digoxin possibly increased by COBICISTAT—reduce initial dose of digoxin
- Colchicine: possible increased risk of myopathy when digoxin given with ● COLCHICINE
- Corticosteroids: increased risk of hypokalaemia when cardiac glycosides given with CORTICOSTEROIDS
- Cytotoxics: absorption of digoxin *tablets* possibly reduced by BLEOMYCIN, CARMUSTINE, CYCLOPHOSPHAMIDE, CYTARABINE, DOXORUBICIN, MELPHALAN, METHOTREXATE, PROCARBAZINE and VINCRISTINE; possible increased risk of bradycardia when digoxin given with CRIZOTINIB; manufacturer of digoxin advises give IBRUTINIB at least 6 hours before or after ibrutinib; plasma concentration of digoxin increased by VANDETANIB—possible increased risk of bradycardia
- Diuretics: increased cardiac toxicity with cardiac glycosides if hypokalaemia occurs with ● ACETAZOLAMIDE, ● LOOP DIURETICS or ● THIAZIDES AND RELATED DIURETICS; plasma concentration of digoxin possibly increased by POTASSIUM CANRENOATE; plasma concentration of digoxin increased by ● SPIRONOLACTONE
- Ivacaftor: plasma concentration of digoxin increased by IVACAFTOR
- Lenalidomide: plasma concentration of digoxin possibly increased by LENALIDOMIDE
- Lipid-regulating Drugs: absorption of cardiac glycosides possibly reduced by COLESTIPOL and COLESTYRAMINE; plasma concentration of digoxin possibly increased by ATORVASTATIN
- Mirabegron: plasma concentration of digoxin increased by MIRABEGRON—reduce initial dose of digoxin
- Muscle Relaxants: risk of ventricular arrhythmias when cardiac glycosides given with SUXAMETHONIUM; possible increased risk of bradycardia when cardiac glycosides given with TIZANIDINE
- Penicillamine: plasma concentration of digoxin possibly reduced by PENICILLAMINE
- Ranolazine: plasma concentration of digoxin increased by RANOLAZINE
- Sympathomimetics: avoidance of digoxin advised by manufacturer of MIDODRINE
- Sympathomimetics, Beta$_2$: plasma concentration of digoxin possibly reduced by SALBUTAMOL
- Ticagrelor: plasma concentration of digoxin increased by ● TICAGRELOR
- Tolvaptan: plasma concentration of digoxin increased by TOLVAPTAN (increased risk of toxicity)
- Ulcer-healing Drugs: plasma concentration of digoxin possibly slightly increased by PROTON PUMP INHIBITORS; absorption of cardiac glycosides possibly reduced by SUCRALFATE

Cardiac Glycosides (continued)

- Ulipristal: manufacturer of ulipristal advises give digoxin at least 1.5 hours before or after ULIPRISTAL

Carmustine

- Antipsychotics: avoid concomitant use of cytotoxics with ● CLOZAPINE (increased risk of agranulocytosis)
- Cardiac Glycosides: carmustine possibly reduces absorption of DIGOXIN *tablets*
- Ulcer-healing Drugs: myelosuppressive effects of carmustine possibly enhanced by CIMETIDINE

Carteolol *see* Beta-blockers
Carvedilol *see* Beta-blockers
Caspofungin

- Antibacterials: plasma concentration of caspofungin initially increased and then reduced by RIFAMPICIN (consider increasing dose of caspofungin)
- Antiepileptics: plasma concentration of caspofungin possibly reduced by CARBAMAZEPINE, FOSPHENYTOIN and PHENYTOIN—consider increasing dose of caspofungin
- Antivirals: plasma concentration of caspofungin possibly reduced by EFAVIRENZ and NEVIRAPINE—consider increasing dose of caspofungin
- Ciclosporin: plasma concentration of caspofungin increased by ● CICLOSPORIN (manufacturer of caspofungin recommends monitoring liver enzymes)
- Corticosteroids: plasma concentration of caspofungin possibly reduced by DEXAMETHASONE—consider increasing dose of caspofungin
- Tacrolimus: caspofungin reduces plasma concentration of ● TACROLIMUS

Catumaxomab

- Antipsychotics: avoid concomitant use of cytotoxics with ● CLOZAPINE (increased risk of agranulocytosis)
- Vaccines: risk of generalised infections when monoclonal antibodies given with live ● VACCINES—avoid concomitant use

Cefaclor *see* Cephalosporins
Cefadroxil *see* Cephalosporins
Cefalexin *see* Cephalosporins
Cefixime *see* Cephalosporins
Cefotaxime *see* Cephalosporins
Cefradine *see* Cephalosporins
Ceftaroline *see* Cephalosporins
Ceftazidime *see* Cephalosporins
Ceftobiprole *see* Cephalosporins
Ceftriaxone *see* Cephalosporins
Cefuroxime *see* Cephalosporins
Celecoxib *see* NSAIDs
Celiprolol *see* Beta-blockers
Cephalosporins

- Antacids: absorption of cefaclor reduced by ANTACIDS
- Antibacterials: possible increased risk of nephrotoxicity when cephalosporins given with AMINOGLYCOSIDES
- Anticoagulants: cephalosporins possibly enhance anticoagulant effect of ● COUMARINS
- Teriflunomide: plasma concentration of cefaclor increased by TERIFLUNOMIDE
- Vaccines: antibacterials inactivate ORAL TYPHOID VACCINE—see under Typhoid Vaccine in BNFC

Certolizumab pegol

- Abatacept: avoid concomitant use of certolizumab pegol with ● ABATACEPT
- Anakinra: avoid concomitant use of certolizumab pegol with ● ANAKINRA
- Antipsychotics: avoid concomitant use of cytotoxics with ● CLOZAPINE (increased risk of agranulocytosis)
- Vaccines: risk of generalised infections when monoclonal antibodies given with live ● VACCINES—avoid concomitant use

Cetirizine *see* Antihistamines
Cetuximab

- Antipsychotics: avoid concomitant use of cytotoxics with ● CLOZAPINE (increased risk of agranulocytosis)
- Vaccines: risk of generalised infections when monoclonal antibodies given with live ● VACCINES—avoid concomitant use

Chenodeoxycholic Acid *see* Bile Acids
Chloral *see* Anxiolytics and Hypnotics

Chloramphenicol
- ▸ Antibacterials: metabolism of chloramphenicol accelerated by RIFAMPICIN (reduced plasma concentration)
- Anticoagulants: chloramphenicol enhances anticoagulant effect of ● COUMARINS
- Antidiabetics: chloramphenicol enhances effects of ● SULFONYLUREAS
- Antiepileptics: chloramphenicol increases plasma concentration of ● FOSPHENYTOIN and ● PHENYTOIN (increased risk of toxicity); metabolism of chloramphenicol possibly accelerated by ● PHENOBARBITAL and ● PRIMIDONE (reduced plasma concentration)
- Antipsychotics: avoid concomitant use of chloramphenicol with ● CLOZAPINE (increased risk of agranulocytosis)
- Ciclosporin: chloramphenicol possibly increases plasma concentration of ● CICLOSPORIN
- Clopidogrel: chloramphenicol possibly reduces antiplatelet effect of ● CLOPIDOGREL
- ▸ Guanfacine: when given with chloramphenicol manufacturer of GUANFACINE advises halve dose
- ▸ Hydroxocobalamin: chloramphenicol reduces response to HYDROXOCOBALAMIN
- ▸ Iron Salts: chloramphenicol possibly inhibits effects of IRON SALTS
- ▸ Tacrolimus: chloramphenicol possibly increases plasma concentration of ● TACROLIMUS
- ▸ Vaccines: antibacterials inactivate ORAL TYPHOID VACCINE—see under Typhoid Vaccine in BNFC

Chlordiazepoxide *see* Anxiolytics and Hypnotics

Chloroprocaine
- Antibacterials: chloroprocaine possibly inhibits effects of ● SULFONAMIDES (manufacturer of chloroprocaine advises avoid concomitant use)

Chloroquine
- ▸ Adsorbents: absorption of chloroquine reduced by KAOLIN
- ▸ Agalsidase Alfa and Beta: chloroquine possibly inhibits effects of AGALSIDASE ALFA AND BETA (manufacturers of agalsidase alfa and beta advise avoid concomitant use)
- ▸ Antacids: absorption of chloroquine reduced by ANTACIDS
- ▸ Anthelmintics: chloroquine reduces plasma concentration of ● PRAZIQUANTEL—consider increasing praziquantel dose when given for systemic infections
- Anti-arrhythmics: increased risk of ventricular arrhythmias when chloroquine given with ● AMIODARONE—avoid concomitant use
- Antibacterials: increased risk of ventricular arrhythmias when chloroquine given with ● MOXIFLOXACIN—avoid concomitant use
- Antidepressants: possible increased risk of ventricular arrhythmias when chloroquine given with ● CITALOPRAM and ● ESCITALOPRAM
- Antimalarials: avoidance of antimalarials advised by manufacturer of ● ARTEMETHER WITH LUMEFANTRINE; increased risk of convulsions when chloroquine given with ● MEFLOQUINE
- Antipsychotics: increased risk of ventricular arrhythmias when chloroquine given with ● DROPERIDOL—avoid concomitant use
- Cardiac Glycosides: chloroquine possibly increases plasma concentration of ● DIGOXIN
- Ciclosporin: chloroquine increases plasma concentration of ● CICLOSPORIN (increased risk of toxicity)
- Cytotoxics: possible increased risk of ventricular arrhythmias when chloroquine given with ● BOSUTINIB
- Histamine: avoidance of antimalarials advised by manufacturer of HISTAMINE
- Lanthanum: absorption of chloroquine possibly reduced by LANTHANUM (give at least 2 hours apart)
- Laronidase: chloroquine possibly inhibits effects of LARONIDASE (manufacturer of laronidase advises avoid concomitant use)
- Parasympathomimetics: chloroquine has potential to increase symptoms of myasthenia gravis and thus diminish effect of NEOSTIGMINE and PYRIDOSTIGMINE
- Penicillamine: increased risk of haematological toxicity when antimalarials given with PENICILLAMINE—manufacturer of penicillamine advises avoid concomitant use
- Ulcer-healing Drugs: metabolism of chloroquine inhibited by CIMETIDINE (increased plasma concentration)

Chloroquine (continued)
- ▸ Vaccines: antimalarials inactivate ORAL TYPHOID VACCINE—see under Typhoid Vaccine in BNFC

Chlorothiazide *see* Diuretics
Chlorphenamine *see* Antihistamines
Chlorpromazine *see* Antipsychotics
Chlortalidone *see* Diuretics
Cholera Vaccine *see* Vaccines
Cholic Acid *see* Bile Acids
Ciclesonide *see* Corticosteroids

Ciclosporin
- ACE Inhibitors: increased risk of hyperkalaemia when ciclosporin given with ● ACE INHIBITORS
- Aliskiren: ciclosporin increases plasma concentration of ● ALISKIREN—avoid concomitant use
- ▸ Allopurinol: plasma concentration of ciclosporin possibly increased by ALLOPURINOL (risk of nephrotoxicity)
- Ambrisentan: ciclosporin increases plasma concentration of ● AMBRISENTAN (see under Ambrisentan, in BNF)
- Analgesics: increased risk of nephrotoxicity when ciclosporin given with ● NSAIDS; ciclosporin increases plasma concentration of ● DICLOFENAC (halve dose of diclofenac)
- Angiotensin-II Receptor Antagonists: increased risk of hyperkalaemia when ciclosporin given with ● ANGIOTENSIN-II RECEPTOR ANTAGONISTS
- ▸ Anti-arrhythmics: plasma concentration of ciclosporin possibly increased by AMIODARONE and PROPAFENONE
- Antibacterials: plasma concentration of ciclosporin increased by ● AZITHROMYCIN; metabolism of ciclosporin inhibited by ● CLARITHROMYCIN and ● ERYTHROMYCIN (increased plasma concentration); metabolism of ciclosporin accelerated by ● RIFAMPICIN (reduced plasma concentration); plasma concentration of ciclosporin possibly reduced by ● SULFADIAZINE; increased risk of nephrotoxicity when ciclosporin given with ● AMINOGLYCOSIDES, ● POLYMYXINS, ● QUINOLONES, ● SULFONAMIDES or ● VANCOMYCIN; plasma concentration of ciclosporin possibly increased by ● CHLORAMPHENICOL and ● TELITHROMYCIN; increased risk of myopathy when ciclosporin given with ● DAPTOMYCIN (preferably avoid concomitant use); avoidance of ciclosporin advised by manufacturer of FIDAXOMICIN; metabolism of ciclosporin possibly inhibited by ● MACROLIDES (increased plasma concentration); ciclosporin increases plasma concentration of ● RIFAXIMIN; increased risk of nephrotoxicity when ciclosporin given with ● TRIMETHOPRIM, also plasma concentration of ciclosporin reduced by *intravenous* trimethoprim
- Anticoagulants: ciclosporin possibly increases plasma concentration of ● DABIGATRAN—manufacturer of dabigatran advises avoid concomitant use; ciclosporin increases plasma concentration of ● EDOXABAN (reduce dose of edoxaban—see under Edoxaban, in BNF)
- Antidepressants: plasma concentration of ciclosporin reduced by ● ST JOHN'S WORT—avoid concomitant use
- ▸ Antidiabetics: ciclosporin possibly enhances hypoglycaemic effect of REPAGLINIDE
- Antiepileptics: metabolism of ciclosporin accelerated by ● CARBAMAZEPINE, ● FOSPHENYTOIN, ● PHENOBARBITAL, ● PHENYTOIN and ● PRIMIDONE (reduced plasma concentration); plasma concentration of ciclosporin possibly reduced by OXCARBAZEPINE
- Antifungals: metabolism of ciclosporin inhibited by ● FLUCONAZOLE, ● ITRACONAZOLE, ● KETOCONAZOLE, ● POSACONAZOLE and ● VORICONAZOLE (increased plasma concentration); metabolism of ciclosporin possibly inhibited by ● MICONAZOLE (increased plasma concentration); increased risk of nephrotoxicity when ciclosporin given with ● AMPHOTERICIN; ciclosporin increases plasma concentration of ● CASPOFUNGIN (manufacturer of caspofungin recommends monitoring liver enzymes); plasma concentration of ciclosporin possibly reduced by GRISEOFULVIN and TERBINAFINE; plasma concentration of ciclosporin possibly increased by MICAFUNGIN
- Antimalarials: plasma concentration of ciclosporin increased by ● CHLOROQUINE and ● HYDROXYCHLOROQUINE (increased risk of toxicity)

Ciclosporin (continued)

▸ Antimuscarinics: avoidance of ciclosporin advised by manufacturer of DARIFENACIN
● Antivirals: increased risk of nephrotoxicity when ciclosporin given with ACICLOVIR OR VALACICLOVIR; plasma concentration of ciclosporin possibly increased by ATAZANAVIR and ● RITONAVIR; plasma concentration of ciclosporin increased by ● BOCEPREVIR, ● FOSAMPRENAVIR and INDINAVIR; plasma concentration of ciclosporin possibly reduced by ● EFAVIRENZ; plasma concentration of both drugs increased when ciclosporin given with ● SAQUINAVIR; plasma concentration of both drugs increased when ciclosporin given with ● TELAPREVIR (reduce dose of ciclosporin)
● Beta-blockers: plasma concentration of ciclosporin increased by ● CARVEDILOL
● Bile Acids: avoidance of ciclosporin advised by manufacturer of CHOLIC ACID; absorption of ciclosporin increased by ● URSODEOXYCHOLIC ACID
● Bosentan: ciclosporin increases plasma concentration of ● BOSENTAN (also plasma concentration of ciclosporin reduced—avoid concomitant use)
● Calcium-channel Blockers: combination of ciclosporin with ● LERCANIDIPINE may increase plasma concentration of either drug (or both)—avoid concomitant use; plasma concentration of ciclosporin increased by ● DILTIAZEM, ● NICARDIPINE and ● VERAPAMIL; ciclosporin possibly increases plasma concentration of NIFEDIPINE (increased risk of toxicity including gingival hyperplasia)
● Cardiac Glycosides: ciclosporin increases plasma concentration of ● DIGOXIN (increased risk of toxicity)
● Colchicine: possible increased risk of nephrotoxicity and myotoxicity when ciclosporin given with ● COLCHICINE—suspend or reduce dose of colchicine (avoid concomitant use in hepatic or renal impairment)
● Corticosteroids: plasma concentration of ciclosporin increased by high-dose ● METHYLPREDNISOLONE (risk of convulsions); ciclosporin increases plasma concentration of PREDNISOLONE
● Cytotoxics: increased risk of nephrotoxicity when ciclosporin given with ● MELPHALAN; increased risk of neurotoxicity when ciclosporin given with ● DOXORUBICIN; ciclosporin increases plasma concentration of ● EPIRUBICIN and ● IDARUBICIN; ciclosporin reduces excretion of MITOXANTRONE (increased plasma concentration); risk of toxicity when ciclosporin given with ● METHOTREXATE; ciclosporin possibly increases the plasma concentration of AFATINIB—manufacturer of afatinib advises separating administration of ciclosporin by 6 to 12 hours; caution with ciclosporin advised by manufacturer of ● CRIZOTINIB; ciclosporin increases plasma concentration of ● EVEROLIMUS (consider reducing the dose of everolimus — consult everolimus product literature); plasma concentration of ciclosporin possibly increased by IMATINIB; in vitro studies suggest a possible interaction between ciclosporin and DOCETAXEL (consult docetaxel product literature); ciclosporin possibly increases plasma concentration of ETOPOSIDE (increased risk of toxicity)
▸ Dexrazoxane: increased risk of immunosupression with ciclosporin advised by manufacturer of DEXRAZOXANE
● Diuretics: plasma concentration of ciclosporin possibly increased by ● ACETAZOLAMIDE; increased risk of hyperkalaemia when ciclosporin given with ● POTASSIUM-SPARING DIURETICS AND ALDOSTERONE ANTAGONISTS; increased risk of nephrotoxicity and possibly hypermagnesaemia when ciclosporin given with THIAZIDES AND RELATED DIURETICS
● Grapefruit Juice: plasma concentration of ciclosporin increased by ● GRAPEFRUIT JUICE (increased risk of toxicity)
● Hormone Antagonists: metabolism of ciclosporin inhibited by ● DANAZOL (increased plasma concentration); plasma concentration of ciclosporin reduced by LANREOTIDE and ● OCTREOTIDE; plasma concentration of ciclosporin possibly reduced by ● PASIREOTIDE
● Lenalidomide: ciclosporin possibly increases plasma concentration of ● LENALIDOMIDE (increased risk of toxicity)
● Lipid-regulating Drugs: absorption of ciclosporin reduced by ● COLESEVELAM; increased risk of renal impairment when ciclosporin given with BEZAFIBRATE OR FENOFIBRATE; increased risk of myopathy when ciclosporin given with

Ciclosporin

● Lipid-regulating Drugs (continued)
● ATORVASTATIN (see under Atorvastatin, p. 123); increased risk of myopathy when ciclosporin given with ● FLUVASTATIN or ● PRAVASTATIN; increased risk of myopathy when ciclosporin given with ● ROSUVASTATIN or ● SIMVASTATIN (avoid concomitant use); plasma concentration of both drugs may increase when ciclosporin given with ● EZETIMIBE; separating administration from ciclosporin by 12 hours advised by manufacturer of LOMITAPIDE
▸ Mannitol: possible increased risk of nephrotoxicity when ciclosporin given with MANNITOL
● Metoclopramide: plasma concentration of ciclosporin increased by ● METOCLOPRAMIDE
● Mifamurtide: avoidance of ciclosporin advised by manufacturer of MIFAMURTIDE
● Modafinil: plasma concentration of ciclosporin reduced by ● MODAFINIL
▸ Oestrogens: plasma concentration of ciclosporin possibly increased by OESTROGENS
● Orlistat: absorption of ciclosporin possibly reduced by ● ORLISTAT
● Potassium Salts: increased risk of hyperkalaemia when ciclosporin given with ● POTASSIUM SALTS
▸ Progestogens: plasma concentration of ciclosporin possibly increased by PROGESTOGENS
▸ Ranolazine: plasma concentration of both drugs may increase when ciclosporin given with RANOLAZINE
● Sevelamer: plasma concentration of ciclosporin possibly reduced by SEVELAMER
▸ Sirolimus: ciclosporin increases plasma concentration of SIROLIMUS
● Sulfinpyrazone: plasma concentration of ciclosporin reduced by ● SULFINPYRAZONE
● Tacrolimus: plasma concentration of ciclosporin increased by ● TACROLIMUS (increased risk of nephrotoxicity)—avoid concomitant use
▸ Ticagrelor: ciclosporin increases plasma concentration of TICAGRELOR
● Ulcer-healing Drugs: plasma concentration of ciclosporin possibly increased by CIMETIDINE; plasma concentration of ciclosporin possibly affected by OMEPRAZOLE
▸ Vitamins: plasma concentration of ciclosporin possibly affected by VITAMIN E

Cilostazol

● Anagrelide: avoidance of cilostazol advised by manufacturer of ● ANAGRELIDE
● Antibacterials: plasma concentration of cilostazol possibly increased by ● CLARITHROMYCIN (see under Cilostazol, in BNF); plasma concentration of cilostazol increased by ● ERYTHROMYCIN (see under Cilostazol, in BNF)
● Antifungals: plasma concentration of cilostazol increased by ● KETOCONAZOLE (see under Cilostazol, in BNF); plasma concentration of cilostazol possibly increased by ● ITRACONAZOLE (see under Cilostazol, in BNF)
● Antivirals: plasma concentration of cilostazol possibly increased by ● BOCEPREVIR, ● RITONAVIR and ● TELAPREVIR (see under Cilostazol, in BNF)
▸ Calcium-channel Blockers: plasma concentration of cilostazol increased by DILTIAZEM (consider reducing dose of cilostazol)
▸ Lipid-regulating Drugs: separating administration from cilostazol by 12 hours advised by manufacturer of LOMITAPIDE
● Ulcer-healing Drugs: plasma concentration of cilostazol increased by ● OMEPRAZOLE (see under Cilostazol, in BNF)

Cimetidine see Histamine H$_2$-antagonists

Cinacalcet

▸ Antifungals: metabolism of cinacalcet inhibited by KETOCONAZOLE (increased plasma concentration)
● Hormone Antagonists: cinacalcet possibly inhibits metabolism of ● TAMOXIFEN to active metabolite (avoid concomitant use)

Cinnarizine see Antihistamines
Ciprofibrate see Fibrates
Ciprofloxacin see Quinolones
Cisatracurium see Muscle Relaxants
Cisplatin see Platinum Compounds
Citalopram see Antidepressants, SSRI

Cladribine

- Antipsychotics: avoid concomitant use of cytotoxics with
  - CLOZAPINE (increased risk of agranulocytosis)
- Antivirals: avoidance of cladribine advised by manufacturer of
  - LAMIVUDINE

Clarithromycin see Macrolides

Clemastine see Antihistamines

Clindamycin

- Muscle Relaxants: clindamycin enhances effects of ● NON-DEPOLARISING MUSCLE RELAXANTS and ● SUXAMETHONIUM
- ▸ Parasympathomimetics: clindamycin antagonises effects of NEOSTIGMINE and PYRIDOSTIGMINE
- ▸ Vaccines: antibacterials inactivate ORAL TYPHOID VACCINE—see under Typhoid Vaccine in BNFC

Clobazam see Anxiolytics and Hypnotics

Clofazimine

- Antibacterials: possible increased risk of ventricular arrhythmias when clofazimine given with ● BEDAQUILINE
- ▸ Vaccines: antibacterials inactivate ORAL TYPHOID VACCINE—see under Typhoid Vaccine in BNFC

Clomethiazole see Anxiolytics and Hypnotics

Clomipramine see Antidepressants, Tricyclic

Clonazepam see Anxiolytics and Hypnotics

Clonidine

- ▸ ACE Inhibitors: enhanced hypotensive effect when clonidine given with ACE INHIBITORS; previous treatment with clonidine possibly delays antihypertensive effect of CAPTOPRIL
- ▸ Adrenergic Neurone Blockers: enhanced hypotensive effect when clonidine given with ADRENERGIC NEURONE BLOCKERS
- ▸ Alcohol: enhanced hypotensive effect when clonidine given with ALCOHOL
- ▸ Aldesleukin: enhanced hypotensive effect when clonidine given with ALDESLEUKIN
- ▸ Alpha-blockers: enhanced hypotensive effect when clonidine given with ALPHA-BLOCKERS
- ▸ Anaesthetics, General: enhanced hypotensive effect when clonidine given with GENERAL ANAESTHETICS
- ▸ Analgesics: hypotensive effect of clonidine antagonised by NSAIDs
- ▸ Angiotensin-II Receptor Antagonists: enhanced hypotensive effect when clonidine given with ANGIOTENSIN-II RECEPTOR ANTAGONISTS
- ▸ Antidepressants: enhanced hypotensive effect when clonidine given with MAOIs; hypotensive effect of clonidine possibly antagonised by MIRTAZAPINE; hypotensive effect of clonidine antagonised by ● TRICYCLICS, also increased risk of hypertension on clonidine withdrawal
- ▸ Antipsychotics: enhanced hypotensive effect when clonidine given with PHENOTHIAZINES
- ▸ Anxiolytics and Hypnotics: enhanced hypotensive effect when clonidine given with ANXIOLYTICS AND HYPNOTICS
- Beta-blockers: increased risk of withdrawal hypertension when clonidine given with ● BETA-BLOCKERS (withdraw beta-blockers several days before slowly withdrawing clonidine)
- ▸ Calcium-channel Blockers: enhanced hypotensive effect when clonidine given with CALCIUM-CHANNEL BLOCKERS
- ▸ Corticosteroids: hypotensive effect of clonidine antagonised by CORTICOSTEROIDS
- ▸ Cytotoxics: possible increased risk of bradycardia when clonidine given with CRIZOTINIB
- ▸ Diazoxide: enhanced hypotensive effect when clonidine given with DIAZOXIDE
- ▸ Diuretics: enhanced hypotensive effect when clonidine given with DIURETICS
- ▸ Dopaminergics: enhanced hypotensive effect when clonidine given with CO-BENELDOPA, CO-CARELDOPA or LEVODOPA
- ▸ Histamine: avoidance of clonidine advised by manufacturer of HISTAMINE
- ▸ Methyldopa: enhanced hypotensive effect when clonidine given with METHYLDOPA
- ▸ Moxisylyte: enhanced hypotensive effect when clonidine given with MOXISYLYTE
- ▸ Moxonidine: enhanced hypotensive effect when clonidine given with MOXONIDINE
- ▸ Muscle Relaxants: enhanced hypotensive effect when clonidine given with BACLOFEN or TIZANIDINE

Clonidine (continued)

- ▸ Nitrates: enhanced hypotensive effect when clonidine given with NITRATES
- ▸ Oestrogens: hypotensive effect of clonidine antagonised by OESTROGENS
- ▸ Prostaglandins: enhanced hypotensive effect when clonidine given with ALPROSTADIL
- Sympathomimetics: possible risk of hypertension when clonidine given with ADRENALINE (EPINEPHRINE) or NORADRENALINE (NOREPINEPHRINE); serious adverse events reported with concomitant use of clonidine and
  - METHYLPHENIDATE (causality not established)
- ▸ Vasodilator Antihypertensives: enhanced hypotensive effect when clonidine given with HYDRALAZINE, MINOXIDIL or SODIUM NITROPRUSSIDE

Clopamide see Diuretics

Clopidogrel

- ▸ Analgesics: increased risk of bleeding when clopidogrel given with NSAIDs or ASPIRIN
- Antibacterials: antiplatelet effect of clopidogrel possibly reduced by ● CHLORAMPHENICOL, ● CIPROFLOXACIN and
  - ERYTHROMYCIN
- Anticoagulants: manufacturer of clopidogrel advises avoid concomitant use with ● WARFARIN; antiplatelet action of clopidogrel enhances anticoagulant effect of ● COUMARINS and
  - PHENINDIONE; increased risk of bleeding when clopidogrel given with HEPARINS
- Antidepressants: antiplatelet effect of clopidogrel possibly reduced by ● FLUOXETINE, ● FLUVOXAMINE and ● MOCLOBEMIDE
- Antiepileptics: antiplatelet effect of clopidogrel possibly reduced by ● CARBAMAZEPINE and ● OXCARBAZEPINE
- Antifungals: antiplatelet effect of clopidogrel possibly reduced by ● FLUCONAZOLE, ● ITRACONAZOLE, ● KETOCONAZOLE and
  - VORICONAZOLE
- Antivirals: antiplatelet effect of clopidogrel possibly reduced by
  - ETRAVIRINE
- ▸ Dipyridamole: increased risk of bleeding when clopidogrel given with DIPYRIDAMOLE
- ▸ Iloprost: increased risk of bleeding when clopidogrel given with ILOPROST
- Lipid-regulating Drugs: clopidogrel increases plasma concentration of ● ROSUVASTATIN—adjust dose of rosuvastatin (consult product literature)
- ▸ Prasugrel: possible increased risk of bleeding when clopidogrel given with PRASUGREL
- ▸ Ulcer-healing Drugs: antiplatelet effect of clopidogrel possibly reduced by ● CIMETIDINE, LANSOPRAZOLE, PANTOPRAZOLE and RABEPRAZOLE; antiplatelet effect of clopidogrel reduced by
  - ESOMEPRAZOLE and ● OMEPRAZOLE

Clotrimazole see Antifungals, Imidazole

Clozapine see Antipsychotics

Co-amoxiclav see Penicillins

Co-beneldopa

- ▸ ACE Inhibitors: enhanced hypotensive effect when co-beneldopa given with ACE INHIBITORS
- ▸ Adrenergic Neurone Blockers: enhanced hypotensive effect when co-beneldopa given with ADRENERGIC NEURONE BLOCKERS
- ▸ Alpha-blockers: enhanced hypotensive effect when co-beneldopa given with ALPHA-BLOCKERS
- Anaesthetics, General: increased risk of arrhythmias when co-beneldopa given with ● VOLATILE LIQUID GENERAL ANAESTHETICS
- ▸ Angiotensin-II Receptor Antagonists: enhanced hypotensive effect when co-beneldopa given with ANGIOTENSIN-II RECEPTOR ANTAGONISTS
- ▸ Antibacterials: effects of co-beneldopa possibly reduced by ISONIAZID
- Antidepressants: risk of hypertensive crisis when co-beneldopa given with MAOIs, avoid co-beneldopa for at least 2 weeks after stopping MAOIs; increased risk of side-effects when co-beneldopa given with MOCLOBEMIDE
- ▸ Antiepileptics: effects of co-beneldopa possibly reduced by FOSPHENYTOIN and PHENYTOIN
- ▸ Antimuscarinics: absorption of co-beneldopa possibly reduced by ANTIMUSCARINICS

Co-beneldopa (continued)

▶ Antipsychotics: effects of co-beneldopa antagonised by ANTIPSYCHOTICS; avoidance of co-beneldopa advised by manufacturer of AMISULPRIDE (antagonism of effect)
▶ Anxiolytics and Hypnotics: effects of co-beneldopa possibly antagonised by BENZODIAZEPINES
▶ Beta-blockers: enhanced hypotensive effect when co-beneldopa given with BETA-BLOCKERS
▶ Bupropion: increased risk of side-effects when co-beneldopa given with BUPROPION
▶ Calcium-channel Blockers: enhanced hypotensive effect when co-beneldopa given with CALCIUM-CHANNEL BLOCKERS
▶ Clonidine: enhanced hypotensive effect when co-beneldopa given with CLONIDINE
▶ Diazoxide: enhanced hypotensive effect when co-beneldopa given with DIAZOXIDE
▶ Diuretics: enhanced hypotensive effect when co-beneldopa given with DIURETICS
▶ Dopaminergics: enhanced effects and increased toxicity of co-beneldopa when given with SELEGILINE (reduce dose of co-beneldopa)
▶ Iron Salts: absorption of co-beneldopa possibly reduced by *oral* IRON SALTS
▶ Memantine: effects of dopaminergics possibly enhanced by MEMANTINE
▶ Methyldopa: enhanced hypotensive effect when co-beneldopa given with METHYLDOPA; antiparkinsonian effect of dopaminergics antagonised by METHYLDOPA
▶ Moxonidine: enhanced hypotensive effect when co-beneldopa given with MOXONIDINE
▶ Muscle Relaxants: possible agitation, confusion and hallucinations when co-beneldopa given with BACLOFEN
▶ Nitrates: enhanced hypotensive effect when co-beneldopa given with NITRATES
▶ Vasodilator Antihypertensives: enhanced hypotensive effect when co-beneldopa given with HYDRALAZINE, MINOXIDIL or SODIUM NITROPRUSSIDE

Cobicistat

● Alpha-blockers: cobicistat possibly increases plasma concentration of ● ALFUZOSIN—manufacturer of cobicistat advises avoid concomitant use
● Anti-arrhythmics: cobicistat possibly increases plasma concentration of ● AMIODARONE—manufacturer of cobicistat advises avoid concomitant use
● Antibacterials: plasma concentration of cobicistat reduced by ● RIFABUTIN (adjust dose—consult product literature); plasma concentration of cobicistat possibly reduced by ● RIFAMPICIN—manufacturer of cobicistat advises avoid concomitant use
● Anticoagulants: avoidance of cobicistat advised by manufacturer of APIXABAN; cobicistat possibly enhances anticoagulant effect of ● RIVAROXABAN—avoid concomitant use
● Antidepressants: plasma concentration of cobicistat possibly reduced by ● ST JOHN'S WORT—manufacturer of cobicistat advises avoid concomitant use
▶ Antiepileptics: plasma concentration of cobicistat possibly reduced by ● CARBAMAZEPINE, ● FOSPHENYTOIN, ● PHENOBARBITAL, ● PHENYTOIN and ● PRIMIDONE—manufacturer of cobicistat advises avoid concomitant use
▶ Antifungals: cobicistat possibly increases plasma concentration of ITRACONAZOLE and KETOCONAZOLE—manufacturer of cobicistat advises reduce dose of itraconazole and ketoconazole
● Antipsychotics: cobicistat possibly increases plasma concentration of ● LURASIDONE—avoid concomitant use; cobicistat possibly increases plasma concentration of ● PIMOZIDE—manufacturer of cobicistat advises avoid concomitant use
● Antivirals: manufacturer of cobicistat advises avoid concomitant use with BOCEPREVIR and RITONAVIR; cobicistat possibly increases the plasma concentration of ● DACLATASVIR—reduce dose of daclatasvir (see under Daclatasvir, in BNF); avoidance of cobicistat advised by manufacturer of DASABUVIR, NEVIRAPINE, OMBITASVIR and PARITAPREVIR; cobicistat possibly increases plasma concentration of ● MARAVIROC (reduce dose of maraviroc);

Cobicistat

● Antivirals (continued)
cobicistat possibly increases plasma concentration of ● SIMEPREVIR—manufacturer of simeprevir advises avoid concomitant use; plasma concentration of both drugs reduced when cobicistat given with ● TIPRANAVIR (avoid concomitant use)
● Anxiolytics and Hypnotics: manufacturer of cobicistat advises avoid concomitant use with *oral* ● MIDAZOLAM
● Avanafil: cobicistat possibly increases plasma concentration of ● AVANAFIL—avoid concomitant use
▶ Bosentan: manufacturer of cobicistat advises avoid concomitant use with BOSENTAN
▶ Cardiac Glycosides: cobicistat possibly increases plasma concentration of DIGOXIN—reduce initial dose of digoxin
● Cytotoxics: cobicistat possibly increases the plasma concentration of ● IBRUTINIB—reduce dose of ibrutinib (see under Ibrutinib, in BNF)
● Domperidone: possible increased risk of ventricular arrhythmias when cobicistat given with ● DOMPERIDONE—avoid concomitant use
● Ergot Alkaloids: cobicistat possibly increases plasma concentration of ● ERGOT ALKALOIDS—manufacturer of cobicistat advises avoid concomitant use
● Lipid-regulating Drugs: cobicistat possibly increases plasma concentration of ATORVASTATIN—manufacturer of cobicistat advises reduce dose of atorvastatin; manufacturer of cobicistat advises avoid concomitant use with ● SIMVASTATIN
● Oestrogens: cobicistat accelerates metabolism of ● OESTROGENS (reduced contraceptive effect with combined oral contraceptives, contraceptive patches, and vaginal rings—see Contraceptive Interactions in BNFC)
▶ Progestogens: cobicistat increases plasma concentration of NORGESTIMATE
● Sildenafil: cobicistat possibly increases plasma concentration of ● SILDENAFIL—manufacturer of cobicistat advises avoid concomitant use of sildenafil for pulmonary arterial hypertension or reduce dose of sildenafil for erectile dysfunction—consult cobicistat product literature
▶ Sympathomimetics, Beta₂: manufacturer of cobicistat advises avoid concomitant use with SALMETEROL
● Tadalafil: cobicistat possibly increases plasma concentration of ● TADALAFIL—manufacturer of cobicistat advises reduce dose of tadalafil (consult cobicistat product literature)
● Vardenafil: cobicistat possibly increases plasma concentration of ● VARDENAFIL—manufacturer of cobicistat advises reduce dose of vardenafil (consult cobicistat product literature)

Co-careldopa

▶ ACE Inhibitors: enhanced hypotensive effect when co-careldopa given with ACE INHIBITORS
▶ Adrenergic Neurone Blockers: enhanced hypotensive effect when co-careldopa given with ADRENERGIC NEURONE BLOCKERS
▶ Alpha-blockers: enhanced hypotensive effect when co-careldopa given with ALPHA-BLOCKERS
● Anaesthetics, General: increased risk of arrhythmias when co-careldopa given with ● VOLATILE LIQUID GENERAL ANAESTHETICS
▶ Angiotensin-II Receptor Antagonists: enhanced hypotensive effect when co-careldopa given with ANGIOTENSIN-II RECEPTOR ANTAGONISTS
▶ Antibacterials: effects of co-careldopa possibly reduced by ISONIAZID
● Antidepressants: risk of hypertensive crisis when co-careldopa given with ● MAOIs, avoid co-careldopa for at least 2 weeks after stopping MAOIs; increased risk of side-effects when co-careldopa given with MOCLOBEMIDE
▶ Antiepileptics: effects of co-careldopa possibly reduced by FOSPHENYTOIN and PHENYTOIN
▶ Antimuscarinics: absorption of co-careldopa possibly reduced by ANTIMUSCARINICS
▶ Antipsychotics: effects of co-careldopa antagonised by ANTIPSYCHOTICS; avoidance of co-careldopa advised by manufacturer of AMISULPRIDE (antagonism of effect)
▶ Anxiolytics and Hypnotics: effects of co-careldopa possibly antagonised by BENZODIAZEPINES
▶ Beta-blockers: enhanced hypotensive effect when co-careldopa given with BETA-BLOCKERS

Co-careldopa (continued)

▸ Bupropion: increased risk of side-effects when co-careldopa given with BUPROPION
▸ Calcium-channel Blockers: enhanced hypotensive effect when co-careldopa given with CALCIUM-CHANNEL BLOCKERS
▸ Clonidine: enhanced hypotensive effect when co-careldopa given with CLONIDINE
▸ Diazoxide: enhanced hypotensive effect when co-careldopa given with DIAZOXIDE
▸ Diuretics: enhanced hypotensive effect when co-careldopa given with DIURETICS
▸ Dopaminergics: enhanced effects and increased toxicity of co-careldopa when given with SELEGILINE (reduce dose of co-careldopa)
▸ Iron Salts: absorption of co-careldopa possibly reduced by *oral* IRON SALTS
▸ Memantine: effects of dopaminergics possibly enhanced by MEMANTINE
▸ Methyldopa: enhanced hypotensive effect when co-careldopa given with METHYLDOPA; antiparkinsonian effect of dopaminergics antagonised by METHYLDOPA
▸ Moxonidine: enhanced hypotensive effect when co-careldopa given with MOXONIDINE
▸ Muscle Relaxants: possible agitation, confusion and hallucinations when co-careldopa given with BACLOFEN
▸ Nitrates: enhanced hypotensive effect when co-careldopa given with NITRATES
▸ Vasodilator Antihypertensives: enhanced hypotensive effect when co-careldopa given with HYDRALAZINE, MINOXIDIL or SODIUM NITROPRUSSIDE

Codeine *see* Opioid Analgesics

Co-fluampicil *see* Penicillins

Colchicine

● Anti-arrhythmics: possible increased risk of colchicine toxicity when given with ● AMIODARONE
● Antibacterials: possible increased risk of colchicine toxicity when given with ● AZITHROMYCIN, ● CLARITHROMYCIN, ● ERYTHROMYCIN and ● TELITHROMYCIN—suspend or reduce dose of colchicine (avoid concomitant use in hepatic or renal impairment)
● Antifungals: possible increased risk of colchicine toxicity when given with ● ITRACONAZOLE and ● KETOCONAZOLE—suspend or reduce dose of colchicine (avoid concomitant use in hepatic or renal impairment)
● Antivirals: possible increased risk of colchicine toxicity when given with ● ATAZANAVIR, ● INDINAVIR, ● RITONAVIR and ● TELAPREVIR—suspend or reduce dose of colchicine (avoid concomitant use in hepatic or renal impairment)
● Calcium-channel Blockers: possible increased risk of colchicine toxicity when given with ● DILTIAZEM and ● VERAPAMIL—suspend or reduce dose of colchicine (avoid concomitant use in hepatic or renal impairment)
● Cardiac Glycosides: possible increased risk of myopathy when colchicine given with ● DIGOXIN
● Ciclosporin: possible increased risk of nephrotoxicity and myotoxicity when colchicine given with ● CICLOSPORIN—suspend or reduce dose of colchicine (avoid concomitant use in hepatic or renal impairment)
● Grapefruit Juice: possible increased risk of colchicine toxicity when given with ● GRAPEFRUIT JUICE
● Lipid-regulating Drugs: possible increased risk of myopathy when colchicine given with ● FIBRATES or ● STATINS
● Netupitant: caution with colchicine advised by manufacturer of NETUPITANT

Colecalciferol *see* Vitamins

Colesevelam

NOTE Other drugs should be taken at least 4 hours before or after colesevelam to reduce possible interference with absorption
▸ Antidiabetics: colesevelam reduces absorption of GLIBENCLAMIDE and GLIPIZIDE; colesevelam reduces absorption of GLIMEPIRIDE—manufacturer of glimepiride advises give at least 4 hours before colesevelam; manufacturer of canagliflozin advises give bile acid sequestrants at least 1 hour after or 4–6 before CANAGLIFLOZIN

Colesevelam (continued)

▸ Antiepileptics: colesevelam possibly reduces absorption of FOSPHENYTOIN and PHENYTOIN
▸ Bile Acids: colesevelam probably reduces effects of CHOLIC ACID (manufacturer of cholic acid advises give at least 5 hours apart)
● Ciclosporin: colesevelam reduces absorption of ● CICLOSPORIN
▸ Lipid-regulating Drugs: bile acid sequestrants possibly reduce absorption of LOMITAPIDE (give at least 4 hours apart)
▸ Oestrogens: colesevelam reduces absorption of ETHINYLESTRADIOL
▸ Thyroid Hormones: colesevelam reduces absorption of LEVOTHYROXINE

Colestipol

NOTE Other drugs should be taken at least 1 hour before or 4–6 hours after colestipol to reduce possible interference with absorption
▸ Antibacterials: colestipol possibly reduces absorption of TETRACYCLINE
▸ Antidiabetics: manufacturer of canagliflozin advises give bile acid sequestrants at least 1 hour after or 4–6 before CANAGLIFLOZIN
▸ Bile Acids: colestipol possibly reduces absorption of BILE ACIDS; colestipol probably reduces effects of CHOLIC ACID (manufacturer of cholic acid advises give at least 5 hours apart)
▸ Cardiac Glycosides: colestipol possibly reduces absorption of CARDIAC GLYCOSIDES
▸ Diuretics: colestipol reduces absorption of THIAZIDES AND RELATED DIURETICS (give at least 2 hours apart)
▸ Lipid-regulating Drugs: bile acid sequestrants possibly reduce absorption of LOMITAPIDE (give at least 4 hours apart)
▸ Thyroid Hormones: colestipol reduces absorption of THYROID HORMONES

Colestyramine

NOTE Other drugs should be taken at least 1 hour before or 4–6 hours after colestyramine to reduce possible interference with absorption
▸ Analgesics: colestyramine increases the excretion of MELOXICAM; colestyramine reduces absorption of PARACETAMOL
▸ Antibacterials: colestyramine possibly reduces absorption of TETRACYCLINE; colestyramine antagonises effects of *oral* VANCOMYCIN
● Anticoagulants: colestyramine may enhance or reduce anticoagulant effect of ● COUMARINS and ● PHENINDIONE
▸ Antidiabetics: colestyramine possibly enhances hypoglycaemic effect of ACARBOSE; manufacturer of canagliflozin advises give bile acid sequestrants at least 1 hour after or 4–6 before CANAGLIFLOZIN
▸ Antiepileptics: colestyramine possibly reduces absorption of SODIUM VALPROATE and VALPROIC ACID
▸ Bile Acids: colestyramine possibly reduces absorption of BILE ACIDS; colestyramine probably reduces effects of CHOLIC ACID (manufacturer of cholic acid advises give at least 5 hours apart)
▸ Cardiac Glycosides: colestyramine possibly reduces absorption of CARDIAC GLYCOSIDES
▸ Diuretics: colestyramine reduces absorption of THIAZIDES AND RELATED DIURETICS (give at least 2 hours apart)
▸ Leflunomide: colestyramine significantly decreases effect of LEFLUNOMIDE (enhanced elimination)—avoid unless drug elimination desired
▸ Lipid-regulating Drugs: bile acid sequestrants possibly reduce absorption of LOMITAPIDE (give at least 4 hours apart)
▸ Mycophenolate: colestyramine reduces absorption of MYCOPHENOLATE
▸ Raloxifene: colestyramine reduces absorption of RALOXIFENE (manufacturer of raloxifene advises avoid concomitant administration)
▸ Teriflunomide: colestyramine significantly decreases effect of TERIFLUNOMIDE (enhanced elimination)—avoid unless drug elimination desired
▸ Thyroid Hormones: colestyramine reduces absorption of THYROID HORMONES
▸ Vitamins: colestyramine possibly reduces absorption of CALCITRIOL (give at least 1 hour before or 4 to 6 hours after colestyramine)

Colistimethate Sodium *see* Polymyxins
Contraceptives, oral *see* Oestrogens and Progestogens
Corticosteroids

NOTE Interactions do not generally apply to corticosteroids used for topical action (including inhalation) unless specified

▸ ACE Inhibitors: corticosteroids antagonise hypotensive effect of ACE INHIBITORS
▸ Adrenergic Neurone Blockers: corticosteroids antagonise hypotensive effect of ADRENERGIC NEURONE BLOCKERS
● Aldesleukin: avoidance of corticosteroids advised by manufacturer of ● ALDESLEUKIN
● Alpha-blockers: corticosteroids antagonise hypotensive effect of ALPHA-BLOCKERS
▸ Aminophylline: increased risk of hypokalaemia when corticosteroids given with AMINOPHYLLINE
▸ Analgesics: increased risk of gastro-intestinal bleeding and ulceration when corticosteroids given with NSAIDs; increased risk of gastro-intestinal bleeding and ulceration when corticosteroids given with ASPIRIN, also corticosteroids reduce plasma concentration of salicylate
▸ Angiotensin-II Receptor Antagonists: corticosteroids antagonise hypotensive effect of ANGIOTENSIN-II RECEPTOR ANTAGONISTS
▸ Antacids: absorption of deflazacort reduced by ANTACIDS
▸ Anthelmintics: dexamethasone increases plasma concentration of active metabolite of ALBENDAZOLE; continuous use of dexamethasone possibly reduces plasma concentration of PRAZIQUANTEL
▸ Antibacterials: plasma concentration of methylprednisolone possibly increased by CLARITHROMYCIN; metabolism of corticosteroids possibly inhibited by ERYTHROMYCIN; metabolism of methylprednisolone inhibited by ERYTHROMYCIN; corticosteroids possibly reduce plasma concentration of ISONIAZID; metabolism of corticosteroids accelerated by ● RIFAMYCINS (reduced effect)
● Anticoagulants: corticosteroids may enhance or reduce anticoagulant effect of ● COUMARINS (high-dose corticosteroids enhance anticoagulant effect); corticosteroids may enhance or reduce anticoagulant effect of PHENINDIONE
▸ Antidiabetics: corticosteroids antagonise hypoglycaemic effect of ANTIDIABETICS
● Antiepileptics: metabolism of corticosteroids accelerated by ● CARBAMAZEPINE, ● FOSPHENYTOIN, ● PHENOBARBITAL, ● PHENYTOIN and ● PRIMIDONE (reduced effect)
● Antifungals: metabolism of corticosteroids possibly inhibited by ITRACONAZOLE and KETOCONAZOLE; plasma concentration of active metabolite of ciclesonide increased by ● KETOCONAZOLE; plasma concentration of *inhaled* mometasone increased by KETOCONAZOLE; plasma concentration of *inhaled* and *oral* (and possibly also *intranasal* and *rectal*) budesonide increased by ● ITRACONAZOLE and ● KETOCONAZOLE; *inhaled* fluticasone plasma concentration is possibly increased by KETOCONAZOLE; metabolism of methylprednisolone inhibited by KETOCONAZOLE; increased risk of hypokalaemia when corticosteroids given with ● AMPHOTERICIN—avoid concomitant use unless corticosteroids needed to control reactions; plasma concentration of *inhaled* fluticasone increased by ITRACONAZOLE; metabolism of methylprednisolone possibly inhibited by ITRACONAZOLE; dexamethasone possibly reduces plasma concentration of CASPOFUNGIN—consider increasing dose of caspofungin
● Antivirals: dexamethasone possibly reduces plasma concentration of DACLATASVIR and SIMEPREVIR—manufacturer of daclatasvir and simeprevir advises avoid concomitant use; dexamethasone possibly reduces plasma concentration of INDINAVIR, LOPINAVIR, SAQUINAVIR and TELAPREVIR; avoidance of dexamethasone (except when given as a single dose) advised by manufacturer of ● RILPIVIRINE; plasma concentration of *inhaled* and *intranasal* fluticasone increased by ● RITONAVIR—increased risk of adrenal suppression; plasma concentration of budesonide (including *inhaled*, *intranasal*, and *rectal* budesonide) possibly increased by ● RITONAVIR—increased risk of adrenal suppresion; plasma concentration of corticosteroids possibly increased by ● RITONAVIR—increased risk of adrenal suppression; plasma concentration of triamcinolone *injection* increased by ● RITONAVIR—increased risk of adrenal suppression; plasma concentration of *inhaled*

Corticosteroids
● Antivirals: (continued)
and *intranasal* budesonide and fluticasone possibly increased by TELAPREVIR
▸ Aprepitant: metabolism of dexamethasone and methylprednisolone inhibited by APREPITANT (reduce dose of dexamethasone and methylprednisolone)
▸ Beta-blockers: corticosteroids antagonise hypotensive effect of BETA-BLOCKERS
▸ Calcium Salts: corticosteroids reduce absorption of CALCIUM SALTS
▸ Calcium-channel Blockers: corticosteroids antagonise hypotensive effect of CALCIUM-CHANNEL BLOCKERS; plasma concentration of methylprednisolone increased by DILTIAZEM
▸ Cardiac Glycosides: increased risk of hypokalaemia when corticosteroids given with CARDIAC GLYCOSIDES
● Ciclosporin: high-dose methylprednisolone increases plasma concentration of ● CICLOSPORIN (risk of convulsions); plasma concentration of prednisolone increased by CICLOSPORIN
● Clonidine: corticosteroids antagonise hypotensive effect of CLONIDINE
▸ Cytotoxics: possible increased risk of hepatoxicity when dexamethasone given with *high-dose* METHOTREXATE; dexamethasone possibly decreases plasma concentration of AXITINIB (increase dose of axitinib—consult axitinib product literature); dexamethasone possibly reduces plasma concentration of CABOZANTINIB—manufacturer of cabozantinib advises avoid concomitant use
▸ Diazoxide: corticosteroids antagonise hypotensive effect of DIAZOXIDE
▸ Diuretics: corticosteroids antagonise diuretic effect of DIURETICS; increased risk of hypokalaemia when corticosteroids given with ACETAZOLAMIDE, LOOP DIURETICS or THIAZIDES AND RELATED DIURETICS
▸ Fosaprepitant: metabolism of dexamethasone and methylprednisolone inhibited by FOSAPREPITANT (reduce dose of dexamethasone and methylprednisolone)
● Grapefruit Juice: plasma concentration of *oral* budesonide increased by ● GRAPEFRUIT JUICE—avoid concurrent use or separate administration by as much as possible and consider reducing *oral* budesonide dose
▸ Histamine: avoidance of corticosteroids advised by manufacturer of HISTAMINE
▸ Methyldopa: corticosteroids antagonise hypotensive effect of METHYLDOPA
▸ Mifamurtide: avoidance of corticosteroids advised by manufacturer of MIFAMURTIDE
▸ Mifepristone: effect of corticosteroids (including *inhaled* corticosteroids) may be reduced for 3–4 days after MIFEPRISTONE
▸ Moxonidine: corticosteroids antagonise hypotensive effect of MOXONIDINE
▸ Muscle Relaxants: corticosteroids possibly antagonise effects of PANCURONIUM and VECURONIUM
● Netupitant: plasma concentration of dexamethasone increased by ● NETUPITANT (halve dose of dexamethasone)
▸ Nicorandil: increased risk of gastro-intestinal bleeding and ulceration when corticosteroids given with NICORANDIL
▸ Nitrates: corticosteroids antagonise hypotensive effect of NITRATES
▸ Oestrogens: plasma concentration of corticosteroids increased by oral contraceptives containing OESTROGENS
▸ Sodium Benzoate: corticosteroids possibly reduce effects of SODIUM BENZOATE
▸ Sodium Phenylbutyrate: corticosteroids possibly reduce effects of SODIUM PHENYLBUTYRATE
▸ Somatropin: corticosteroids may inhibit growth-promoting effect of SOMATROPIN
▸ Sympathomimetics: metabolism of dexamethasone accelerated by EPHEDRINE; possible risk of hypertension when corticosteroids given with MIDODRINE
▸ Sympathomimetics, Beta$_2$: increased risk of hypokalaemia when corticosteroids given with high doses of BETA$_2$ SYMPATHOMIMETICS
▸ Theophylline: increased risk of hypokalaemia when corticosteroids given with THEOPHYLLINE

Corticosteroids (continued)

- Vaccines: high doses of corticosteroids impair immune response to ●VACCINES—avoid concomitant use with live vaccines
- ▸ Vasodilator Antihypertensives: corticosteroids antagonise hypotensive effect of HYDRALAZINE, MINOXIDIL and SODIUM NITROPRUSSIDE

Co-trimoxazole *see* Trimethoprim and Sulfamethoxazole

Coumarins

NOTE Change in patient's clinical condition, particularly associated with liver disease, intercurrent illness, or drug administration, necessitates more frequent testing. Major changes in diet (especially involving salads and vegetables) and in alcohol consumption may also affect anticoagulant control

- Alcohol: anticoagulant control with coumarins may be affected by major changes in consumption of ●ALCOHOL
- ▸ Allopurinol: anticoagulant effect of coumarins possibly enhanced by ALLOPURINOL
- Anabolic Steroids: anticoagulant effect of coumarins enhanced by ●ANABOLIC STEROIDS
- Analgesics: anticoagulant effect of coumarins possibly enhanced by ●NSAIDS; increased risk of haemorrhage when anticoagulants given with *intravenous* ●DICLOFENAC (avoid concomitant use, including low-dose heparins); increased risk of haemorrhage when anticoagulants given with ●KETOROLAC (avoid concomitant use, including low-dose heparins); anticoagulant effect of coumarins enhanced by ●TRAMADOL; increased risk of bleeding when coumarins given with ●ASPIRIN (due to antiplatelet effect); anticoagulant effect of coumarins possibly enhanced by prolonged regular use of PARACETAMOL
- Anthelmintics: anticoagulant effect of coumarins possibly enhanced by IVERMECTIN; anticoagulant effect of warfarin possibly enhanced by ●LEVAMISOLE
- Anti-arrhythmics: metabolism of coumarins inhibited by ●AMIODARONE (enhanced anticoagulant effect); anticoagulant effect of warfarin may be enhanced or reduced by DISOPYRAMIDE; anticoagulant effect of coumarins possibly enhanced by ●DRONEDARONE; anticoagulant effect of coumarins enhanced by ●PROPAFENONE
- Antibacterials: experience in anticoagulant clinics suggests that INR possibly altered when coumarins are given with ●NEOMYCIN (given for local action on gut); anticoagulant effect of coumarins possibly enhanced by ●AZITHROMYCIN, ●AZTREONAM, ●CEPHALOSPORINS, CIPROFLOXACIN, LEVOFLOXACIN, ●TETRACYCLINES, TIGECYCLINE and TRIMETHOPRIM; anticoagulant effect of coumarins enhanced by ●CHLORAMPHENICOL, ●CLARITHROMYCIN, ●ERYTHROMYCIN, ●METRONIDAZOLE, ●NALIDIXIC ACID, ●NORFLOXACIN, ●OFLOXACIN and ●SULFONAMIDES; plasma concentration of warfarin possibly increased by ORITAVANCIN; an interaction between coumarins and broad-spectrum PENICILLINS has not been demonstrated in studies, but common experience in anticoagulant clinics is that INR can be altered; metabolism of coumarins accelerated by ●RIFAMYCINS (reduced anticoagulant effect); anticoagulant effect of warfarin possibly reduced by RIFAXIMIN
- Anticoagulants: increased risk of haemorrhage when other anticoagulants given with ●APIXABAN, ●DABIGATRAN, ●EDOXABAN and ●RIVAROXABAN (avoid concomitant use except when switching with other anticoagulants or using heparin to maintain catheter patency)
- ▸ Antidepressants: anticoagulant effect of warfarin possibly enhanced by ●VENLAFAXINE; anticoagulant effect of warfarin may be enhanced or reduced by TRAZODONE; anticoagulant effect of coumarins possibly enhanced by ●SSRIS; anticoagulant effect of coumarins reduced by ●ST JOHN'S WORT (avoid concomitant use); anticoagulant effect of warfarin enhanced by MIRTAZAPINE; anticoagulant effect of coumarins may be enhanced or reduced by ●TRICYCLICS
- ▸ Antidiabetics: anticoagulant effect of warfarin possibly enhanced by EXENATIDE; coumarins possibly enhance hypoglycaemic effect of ●SULFONYLUREAS, also possible changes to anticoagulant effect

Coumarins (continued)

- Antiepileptics: metabolism of coumarins accelerated by ●CARBAMAZEPINE, ●PHENOBARBITAL and ●PRIMIDONE (reduced anticoagulant effect); plasma concentration of warfarin reduced by ESLICARBAZEPINE; metabolism of coumarins accelerated by ●FOSPHENYTOIN and ●PHENYTOIN (possibility of reduced anticoagulant effect, but enhancement also reported); anticoagulant effect of coumarins possibly enhanced by SODIUM VALPROATE and VALPROIC ACID
- Antifungals: anticoagulant effect of coumarins enhanced by ●FLUCONAZOLE, ●ITRACONAZOLE, ●KETOCONAZOLE and ●VORICONAZOLE; anticoagulant effect of coumarins greatly enhanced by ●MICONAZOLE (including oral gel and possibly vaginal and topical formulations)—avoid concomitant use if possible; anticoagulant effect of coumarins reduced by ●GRISEOFULVIN
- ▸ Antimalarials: isolated reports that anticoagulant effect of warfarin may be enhanced by PROGUANIL; plasma concentration of both drugs increased when warfarin given with QUININE
- Antivirals: anticoagulant effect of warfarin may be enhanced or reduced by ATAZANAVIR, ●NEVIRAPINE and ●RITONAVIR; plasma concentration of coumarins possibly affected by ●EFAVIRENZ; anticoagulant effect of coumarins may be enhanced or reduced by FOSAMPRENAVIR; anticoagulant effect of coumarins possibly enhanced by ●RITONAVIR; anticoagulant effect of warfarin possibly enhanced by SAQUINAVIR; plasma concentration of warfarin possibly affected by ●TELAPREVIR
- ▸ Anxiolytics and Hypnotics: anticoagulant effect of coumarins may transiently be enhanced by CHLORAL
- ▸ Aprepitant: anticoagulant effect of warfarin possibly reduced by APREPITANT
- Azathioprine: anticoagulant effect of acenocoumarol possibly reduced by ●AZATHIOPRINE; anticoagulant effect of warfarin reduced by ●AZATHIOPRINE
- ▸ Bosentan: monitoring anticoagulant effect of coumarins recommended by manufacturer of BOSENTAN
- ▸ Carbimazole: anticoagulant effect of coumarins possibly enhanced by CARBIMAZOLE
- Clopidogrel: anticoagulant effect of coumarins enhanced due to antiplatelet action of ●CLOPIDOGREL; avoidance of warfarin advised by manufacturer of ●CLOPIDOGREL
- Corticosteroids: anticoagulant effect of coumarins may be enhanced or reduced by ●CORTICOSTEROIDS (high-dose corticosteroids enhance anticoagulant effect)
- Cranberry Juice: anticoagulant effect of coumarins possibly enhanced by ●CRANBERRY JUICE—avoid concomitant use
- Cytotoxics: anticoagulant effect of coumarins possibly enhanced by ●ETOPOSIDE, ●IFOSFAMIDE and ●SORAFENIB; anticoagulant effect of coumarins enhanced by ●CAPECITABINE, ●FLUOROURACIL and ●TEGAFUR; anticoagulant effect of warfarin possibly enhanced by GEFITINIB, GEMCITABINE and ●VEMURAFENIB; anticoagulant effect of coumarins possibly reduced by ●MERCAPTOPURINE and ●MITOTANE; plasma concentration of warfarin reduced by DABRAFENIB; increased risk of bleeding when coumarins given with ●ERLOTINIB; avoidance of coumarins advised by manufacturer of IBRUTINIB; replacement of warfarin with a heparin advised by manufacturer of IMATINIB (possibility of enhanced warfarin effect); increased risk of bleeding when warfarin given with ●REGORAFENIB
- Dipyridamole: anticoagulant effect of coumarins enhanced due to antiplatelet action of ●DIPYRIDAMOLE
- Disulfiram: anticoagulant effect of coumarins enhanced by ●DISULFIRAM
- Dopaminergics: anticoagulant effect of warfarin enhanced by ●ENTACAPONE
- Enteral Feeds: anticoagulant effect of coumarins antagonised by vitamin K (present in some ●ENTERAL FEEDS)
- ▸ Fosaprepitant: anticoagulant effect of warfarin possibly reduced by FOSAPREPITANT
- Glucosamine: anticoagulant effect of warfarin enhanced by ●GLUCOSAMINE (avoid concomitant use)
- Hormone Antagonists: anticoagulant effect of coumarins possibly enhanced by BICALUTAMIDE and ●TOREMIFENE; metabolism of coumarins inhibited by ●DANAZOL (enhanced

Coumarins

- Hormone Antagonists (continued)
  anticoagulant effect); plasma concentration of coumarins
  possibly reduced by ● ENZALUTAMIDE; anticoagulant effect of
  coumarins enhanced by ● FLUTAMIDE and ● TAMOXIFEN
- ▹ Iloprost: anticoagulant effect of coumarins possibly enhanced
  by ILOPROST
- ▹ Lactulose: anticoagulant effect of coumarins possibly
  enhanced by LACTULOSE
- ▹ Leflunomide: anticoagulant effect of warfarin possibly
  enhanced by LEFLUNOMIDE
- ▹ Leukotriene Receptor Antagonists: anticoagulant effect of
  warfarin enhanced by ZAFIRLUKAST
- ▹ Levocarnitine: anticoagulant effect of coumarins possibly
  enhanced by LEVOCARNITINE
- Lipid-regulating Drugs: anticoagulant effect of coumarins may
  be enhanced or reduced by ● COLESTYRAMINE; anticoagulant
  effect of warfarin may be transiently reduced by
  ATORVASTATIN; anticoagulant effect of coumarins enhanced by
  ● FIBRATES and ● FLUVASTATIN; anticoagulant effect of
  coumarins possibly enhanced by EZETIMIBE and
  ● ROSUVASTATIN; anticoagulant effect of coumarins can be
  enhanced by SIMVASTATIN; anticoagulant effect of warfarin
  possibly enhanced by LOMITAPIDE
- Memantine: anticoagulant effect of warfarin possibly enhanced
  by MEMANTINE
- Oestrogens: anticoagulant effect of coumarins may be
  enhanced or reduced by OESTROGENS
- ▹ Orlistat: monitoring anticoagulant effect of coumarins
  recommended by manufacturer of ORLISTAT
- ▹ Prasugrel: possible increased risk of bleeding when coumarins
  given with PRASUGREL
- ▹ Progestogens: anticoagulant effect of coumarins may be
  enhanced or reduced by PROGESTOGENS
- ▹ Raloxifene: anticoagulant effect of coumarins antagonised by
  RALOXIFENE
- ▹ Retinoids: anticoagulant effect of coumarins possibly reduced
  by ● ACITRETIN
- Sulfinpyrazone: anticoagulant effect of coumarins enhanced by
  ● SULFINPYRAZONE
- Sympathomimetics: anticoagulant effect of coumarins possibly
  enhanced by ● METHYLPHENIDATE
- Testolactone: anticoagulant effect of coumarins enhanced by
  ● TESTOLACTONE
- Testosterone: anticoagulant effect of coumarins enhanced by
  ● TESTOSTERONE
- Thyroid Hormones: anticoagulant effect of coumarins enhanced
  by ● THYROID HORMONES
- ▹ Ubidecarenone: anticoagulant effect of warfarin may be
  enhanced or reduced by UBIDECARENONE
- Ulcer-healing Drugs: metabolism of coumarins inhibited by
  ● CIMETIDINE (enhanced anticoagulant effect); anticoagulant
  effect of coumarins possibly enhanced by ● ESOMEPRAZOLE and
  ● OMEPRAZOLE; anticoagulant effect of coumarins might be
  enhanced by PANTOPRAZOLE; absorption of coumarins possibly
  reduced by ● SUCRALFATE (reduced anticoagulant effect)
- ▹ Vaccines: anticoagulant effect of warfarin possibly enhanced
  by INFLUENZA VACCINE
- Vitamins: anticoagulant effect of coumarins possibly enhanced
  by ● VITAMIN E; anticoagulant effect of coumarins antagonised
  by ● VITAMIN K

Cranberry Juice

- Anticoagulants: cranberry juice possibly enhances
  anticoagulant effect of ● COUMARINS—avoid concomitant use

Crizotinib

- Analgesics: manufacturer of crizotinib advises caution with
  ● ALFENTANIL and ● FENTANYL
- Antibacterials: plasma concentration of crizotinib possibly
  increased by ● CLARITHROMYCIN and ● TELITHROMYCIN—
  manufacturer of crizotinib advises avoid concomitant use;
  plasma concentration of crizotinib possibly reduced by
  RIFABUTIN—manufacturer of crizotinib advises avoid
  concomitant use; plasma concentration of crizotinib reduced
  by ● RIFAMPICIN—manufacturer of crizotinib advises avoid
  concomitant use

Crizotinib (continued)

- ▹ Antidepressants: plasma concentration of crizotinib possibly
  reduced by ST JOHN'S WORT—manufacturer of crizotinib
  advises avoid concomitant use
- ▹ Antiepileptics: plasma concentration of crizotinib possibly
  reduced by CARBAMAZEPINE, FOSPHENYTOIN, PHENOBARBITAL,
  PHENYTOIN and PRIMIDONE—manufacturer of crizotinib advises
  avoid concomitant use
- Antifungals: plasma concentration of crizotinib increased by
  ● KETOCONAZOLE—avoid concomitant use; plasma
  concentration of crizotinib possibly increased by
  ● ITRACONAZOLE and ● VORICONAZOLE—manufacturer of
  crizotinib advises avoid concomitant use
- ▹ Antimalarials: possible increased risk of bradycardia when
  crizotinib given with MEFLOQUINE
- Antipsychotics: avoid concomitant use of cytotoxics with
  ● CLOZAPINE (increased risk of agranulocytosis); manufacturer
  of crizotinib advises caution with ● PIMOZIDE
- Antivirals: plasma concentration of crizotinib possibly
  increased by ● ATAZANAVIR, ● INDINAVIR, ● RITONAVIR and
  ● SAQUINAVIR—manufacturer of crizotinib advises avoid
  concomitant use
- Anxiolytics and Hypnotics: crizotinib increases plasma
  concentration of ● MIDAZOLAM
- ▹ Beta-blockers: possible increased risk of bradycardia when
  crizotinib given with BETA-BLOCKERS
- ▹ Calcium-channel Blockers: possible increased risk of bradycardia
  when crizotinib given with DILTIAZEM or VERAPAMIL
- ▹ Cardiac Glycosides: possible increased risk of bradycardia when
  crizotinib given with DIGOXIN
- Ciclosporin: manufacturer of crizotinib advises caution with
  ● CICLOSPORIN
- ▹ Clonidine: possible increased risk of bradycardia when
  crizotinib given with CLONIDINE
- Cytotoxics: crizotinib possibly increases the plasma
  concentration of ● IBRUTINIB—reduce dose of ibrutinib (see
  under Ibrutinib, in BNF)
- Ergot Alkaloids: manufacturer of crizotinib advises caution
  with ● ERGOT ALKALOIDS
- Grapefruit Juice: plasma concentration of crizotinib possibly
  increased by ● GRAPEFRUIT JUICE—manufacturer of crizotinib
  advises avoid concomitant use
- ▹ Guanfacine: crizotinib possibly increases plasma concentration
  of GUANFACINE (halve dose of guanfacine)
- Oestrogens: manufacturer of crizotinib advises contraceptive
  effect of ● OESTROGENS possibly reduced
- ▹ Parasympathomimetics: possible increased risk of bradycardia
  when crizotinib given with PILOCARPINE
- Progestogens: manufacturer of crizotinib advises contraceptive
  effect of ● PROGESTOGENS possibly reduced
- Sirolimus: manufacturer of crizotinib advises caution with
  ● SIROLIMUS
- Tacrolimus: manufacturer of crizotinib advises caution with
  ● TACROLIMUS

Cyclizine see Antihistamines

Cyclopenthiazide see Diuretics

Cyclopentolate see Antimuscarinics

Cyclophosphamide

- ▹ Antifungals: side-effects of cyclophosphamide possibly
  increased by FLUCONAZOLE and ITRACONAZOLE
- Antipsychotics: avoid concomitant use of cytotoxics with
  ● CLOZAPINE (increased risk of agranulocytosis)
- ▹ Cardiac Glycosides: cyclophosphamide possibly reduces
  absorption of DIGOXIN tablets
- Cytotoxics: increased toxicity when high-dose
  cyclophosphamide given with ● PENTOSTATIN—avoid
  concomitant use
- Muscle Relaxants: cyclophosphamide enhances effects of
  SUXAMETHONIUM

Cycloserine

- Alcohol: increased risk of convulsions when cycloserine given
  with ● ALCOHOL
- ▹ Antibacterials: increased risk of CNS toxicity when cycloserine
  given with ISONIAZID
- ▹ Vaccines: antibacterials inactivate ORAL TYPHOID VACCINE—see
  under Typhoid Vaccine in BNFC

Cyproheptadine *see* Antihistamines

Cytarabine
- ▸ Antifungals: cytarabine possibly reduces plasma concentration of FLUCYTOSINE
- ● Antipsychotics: avoid concomitant use of cytotoxics with
  - ● CLOZAPINE (increased risk of agranulocytosis)
- ◦ Cardiac Glycosides: cytarabine possibly reduces absorption of DIGOXIN *tablets*
- ▸ Cytotoxics: intracellular concentration of cytarabine increased by FLUDARABINE

Cytotoxics *see* individual drugs

Dabigatran
- ● Analgesics: possible increased risk of bleeding when dabigatran given with ● NSAIDS; increased risk of haemorrhage when anticoagulants given with *intravenous* ● DICLOFENAC (avoid concomitant use, including low-dose heparins); increased risk of haemorrhage when anticoagulants given with ● KETOROLAC (avoid concomitant use, including low-dose heparins)
- ● Anti-arrhythmics: plasma concentration of dabigatran increased by ● AMIODARONE (see under Dabigatran Etexilate, in BNF); plasma concentration of dabigatran increased by ● DRONEDARONE—avoid concomitant use
- ● Antibacterials: possible increased risk of bleeding when dabigatran given with CLARITHROMYCIN; plasma concentration of dabigatran reduced by ● RIFAMPICIN—manufacturer of dabigatran advises avoid concomitant use
- ● Anticoagulants: increased risk of haemorrhage when dabigatran given with other ● ANTICOAGULANTS (avoid concomitant use except when switching with other anticoagulants or using heparin to maintain catheter patency); increased risk of haemorrhage when other anticoagulants given with
  - ● APIXABAN, ● EDOXABAN and ● RIVAROXABAN (avoid concomitant use except when switching with other anticoagulants or using heparin to maintain catheter patency)
- ● Antidepressants: possible increased risk of bleeding when dabigatran given with ● SSRI-RELATED ANTIDEPRESSANTS or
  - ● SSRIS; plasma concentration of dabigatran possibly reduced by ST JOHN'S WORT—manufacturer of dabigatran advises avoid concomitant use
- Antiepileptics: plasma concentration of dabigatran possibly reduced by CARBAMAZEPINE, FOSPHENYTOIN and PHENYTOIN— manufacturer of dabigatran advises avoid concomitant use
- ● Antifungals: plasma concentration of dabigatran increased by
  - ● KETOCONAZOLE—avoid concomitant use; manufacturer of dabigatran advises avoid concomitant use with ITRACONAZOLE
- Antivirals: manufacturers advise avoid concomitant use of dabigatran with DARUNAVIR; plasma concentration of dabigatran possibly increased by RILPIVIRINE and TELAPREVIR
- ◦ Calcium-channel Blockers: plasma concentration of dabigatran possibly increased by ● VERAPAMIL (see under Dabigatran Etexilate, in BNF)
- ● Ciclosporin: plasma concentration of dabigatran possibly increased by ● CICLOSPORIN—manufacturer of dabigatran advises avoid concomitant use
- Netupitant: caution with dabigatran advised by manufacturer of NETUPITANT
- Sulfinpyrazone: possible increased risk of bleeding when dabigatran given with ● SULFINPYRAZONE
- ● Tacrolimus: plasma concentration of dabigatran possibly increased by ● TACROLIMUS—manufacturer of dabigatran advises avoid concomitant use
- ● Ticagrelor: plasma concentration of dabigatran increased by
  - ● TICAGRELOR
- Ulipristal: manufacturer of ulipristal advises give dabigatran at least 1.5 hours before or after ULIPRISTAL

abrafenib
- Antibacterials: manufacturer of dabrafenib advises avoid concomitant use with RIFAMPICIN
- Anticoagulants: dabrafenib reduces plasma concentration of WARFARIN
- Antidepressants: manufacturer of dabrafenib advises avoid concomitant use with ST JOHN'S WORT
- Antiepileptics: manufacturer of dabrafenib advises avoid concomitant use with CARBAMAZEPINE, FOSPHENYTOIN, PHENOBARBITAL, PHENYTOIN and PRIMIDONE

Dabrafenib (continued)
- ▸ Antifungals: plasma concentration of dabrafenib increased by KETOCONAZOLE
- ● Antipsychotics: avoid concomitant use of cytotoxics with
  - ● CLOZAPINE (increased risk of agranulocytosis)
- ▸ Lipid-regulating Drugs: plasma concentration of dabrafenib increased by GEMFIBROZIL
- ● Oestrogens: manufacturer of dabrafenib advises contraceptive effect of hormonal contraceptives containing ● OESTROGENS possibly reduced (alternative contraceptive recommended)
- ● Progestogens: manufacturer of dabrafenib advises contraceptive effect of hormonal contraceptives containing
  - ● PROGESTOGENS possibly reduced (alternative contraceptive recommended)
- ▸ Ulcer-healing Drugs: manufacturer of dabrafenib advises avoid concomitant use with PROTON PUMP INHIBITORS (plasma concentration of dabrafenib possibly reduced)

Dacarbazine
- ● Aldesleukin: avoidance of dacarbazine advised by manufacturer of ● ALDESLEUKIN
- ● Antipsychotics: avoid concomitant use of cytotoxics with
  - ● CLOZAPINE (increased risk of agranulocytosis)

Daclatasvir
- ● Anti-arrhythmics: possible increased risk of bradycardia when daclatasvir (with sofosbuvir) given with ● AMIODARONE—see under Amiodarone, in BNF
- ● Antibacterials: plasma concentration of daclatasvir possibly increased by ● CLARITHROMYCIN and ● TELITHROMYCIN—reduce dose of daclatasvir (see under Daclatasvir, in BNF); plasma concentration of daclatasvir possibly reduced by ● RIFABUTIN— manufacturer of daclatasvir advises avoid concomitant use; plasma concentration of daclatasvir reduced by ● RIFAMPICIN— avoid concomitant use
- ▸ Antidepressants: plasma concentration of daclatasvir possibly reduced by ST JOHN'S WORT—manufacturer of daclatasvir advises avoid concomitant use
- ● Antiepileptics: plasma concentration of daclatasvir possibly reduced by ● CARBAMAZEPINE, ● FOSPHENYTOIN,
  - ● OXCARBAZEPINE, ● PHENOBARBITAL, ● PHENYTOIN and
  - ● PRIMIDONE—manufacturer of daclatasvir advises avoid concomitant use
- ● Antifungals: plasma concentration of daclatasvir increased by
  - ● KETOCONAZOLE—reduce dose of daclatasvir (see under Daclatasvir, in BNF); plasma concentration of daclatasvir possibly increased by ● ITRACONAZOLE, ● POSACONAZOLE and
  - ● VORICONAZOLE—reduce dose of daclatasvir (see under Daclatasvir, in BNF)
- ● Antivirals: plasma concentration of daclatasvir increased by
  - ● ATAZANAVIR and ● TELAPREVIR—reduce dose of daclatasvir (see under Daclatasvir, in BNF); plasma concentration of daclatasvir possibly increased by ● BOCEPREVIR—reduce dose of daclatasvir (see under Daclatasvir, in BNF); manufacturer of daclatasvir advises avoid concomitant use with DARUNAVIR (plasma concentration of daclatasvir possibly increased); plasma concentration of daclatasvir reduced by EFAVIRENZ— increase dose of daclatasvir (see under Daclatasvir, in BNF); manufacturer of daclatasvir advises avoid concomitant use with ETRAVIRINE and NEVIRAPINE (plasma concentration of daclatasvir possibly reduced)
- ● Cardiac Glycosides: daclatasvir increases plasma concentration of ● DIGOXIN
- ● Cobicistat: plasma concentration of daclatasvir possibly increased by ● COBICISTAT—reduce dose of daclatasvir (see under Daclatasvir, in BNF)
- ● Corticosteroids: plasma concentration of daclatasvir possibly reduced by DEXAMETHASONE—manufacturer of daclatasvir advises avoid concomitant use
- ▸ Lipid-regulating Drugs: daclatasvir increases plasma concentration of ROSUVASTATIN

Dactinomycin
- ● Antipsychotics: avoid concomitant use of cytotoxics with
  - ● CLOZAPINE (increased risk of agranulocytosis)
- ● Cytotoxics: increased risk of hepatotoxicity when dactinomycin given with ● VINCRISTINE
- ● Vaccines: risk of generalised infections when cytotoxic antibiotics given with live ● VACCINES—avoid concomitant use

Dactinomycin (continued)
▸ Vitamins: dactinomycin possibly reduces effects of ALFACALCIDOL, CALCITRIOL, COLECALCIFEROL, DIHYDROTACHYSTEROL, ERGOCALCIFEROL, PARICALCITOL and VITAMIN D

Dairy Products
▸ Antibacterials: dairy products reduce absorption of CIPROFLOXACIN (give at least 2 hours apart); dairy products reduce absorption of NORFLOXACIN; dairy products reduce absorption of TETRACYCLINES (except doxycycline and minocycline)
▸ Cytotoxics: dairy products possibly reduce plasma concentration of MERCAPTOPURINE—manufacturer of mercaptopurine advises give at least 1 hour before or 3 hours after dairy products
▸ Eltrombopag: dairy products possibly reduce absorption of ELTROMBOPAG (give at least 4 hours apart)

Dalteparin see Heparins

Danaparoid
● Analgesics: increased risk of haemorrhage when anticoagulants given with *intravenous* ● DICLOFENAC (avoid concomitant use, including low-dose heparins); increased risk of haemorrhage when anticoagulants given with ● KETOROLAC (avoid concomitant use, including low-dose heparins)
● Anticoagulants: increased risk of haemorrhage when other anticoagulants given with ● APIXABAN, ● DABIGATRAN, ● EDOXABAN and ● RIVAROXABAN (avoid concomitant use except when switching with other anticoagulants or using heparin to maintain catheter patency)

Danazol
● Anticoagulants: danazol inhibits metabolism of ● COUMARINS (enhanced anticoagulant effect)
● Antiepileptics: danazol inhibits metabolism of ● CARBAMAZEPINE (increased risk of toxicity)
● Ciclosporin: danazol inhibits metabolism of ● CICLOSPORIN (increased plasma concentration)
● Lipid-regulating Drugs: possible increased risk of myopathy when danazol given with ● SIMVASTATIN—avoid concomitant use
▸ Tacrolimus: danazol possibly increases plasma concentration of TACROLIMUS

Dantrolene see Muscle Relaxants
Dapagliflozin see Antidiabetics
Dapoxetine
● Alcohol: increased sedative effect when dapoxetine given with ● ALCOHOL
● Analgesics: possible increased risk of serotonergic effects when dapoxetine given with ● TRAMADOL (manufacturer of dapoxetine advises tramadol should not be started until 1 week after stopping dapoxetine, avoid dapoxetine for 2 weeks after stopping tramadol)
● Antibacterials: manufacturer of dapoxetine advises dose reduction when dapoxetine given with CLARITHROMYCIN and ERYTHROMYCIN (see under Dapoxetine, in BNF); manufacturer of dapoxetine advises avoid concomitant use with ● TELITHROMYCIN (increased risk of toxicity)
● Antidepressants: possible increased risk of serotonergic effects when dapoxetine given with ● SSRIS, ● ST JOHN'S WORT, ● DULOXETINE, ● TRICYCLICS and ● VENLAFAXINE (manufacturer of dapoxetine advises SSRIs, St John's wort, duloxetine, tricyclics and venlafaxine should not be started until 1 week after stopping dapoxetine, avoid dapoxetine for 2 weeks after stopping SSRIs, St John's wort, duloxetine, tricyclics and venlafaxine); increased risk of serotonergic effects when dapoxetine given with ● MAOIS (MAOIs should not be started until 1 week after stopping dapoxetine, avoid dapoxetine for 2 weeks after stopping MAOIs)
● Antifungals: plasma concentration of dapoxetine increased by ● KETOCONAZOLE—manufacturer of dapoxetine advises avoid concomitant use; manufacturer of dapoxetine advises dose reduction when dapoxetine given with FLUCONAZOLE (see under Dapoxetine, in BNF); manufacturer of dapoxetine advises avoid concomitant use with ● ITRACONAZOLE (increased risk of toxicity)
● Antivirals: manufacturer of dapoxetine advises avoid concomitant use with ● ATAZANAVIR, ● RITONAVIR and

Dapoxetine
● Antivirals (continued)
  ● SAQUINAVIR (increased risk of toxicity); manufacturer of dapoxetine advises dose reduction when dapoxetine given with FOSAMPRENAVIR (see under Dapoxetine, in BNF)
▸ Aprepitant: manufacturer of dapoxetine advises dose reduction when dapoxetine given with APREPITANT (see under Dapoxetine, in BNF)
▸ Calcium-channel Blockers: manufacturer of dapoxetine advises dose reduction when dapoxetine given with DILTIAZEM and VERAPAMIL (see under Dapoxetine, in BNF)
● 5HT₁-receptor Agonists: possible increased risk of serotonergic effects when dapoxetine given with ● 5HT₁ AGONISTS (manufacturer of dapoxetine advises 5HT₁ agonists should not be started until 1 week after stopping dapoxetine, avoid dapoxetine for 2 weeks after stopping 5HT₁ agonists)
● Lithium: possible increased risk of serotonergic effects when dapoxetine given with ● LITHIUM (manufacturer of dapoxetine advises lithium should not be started until 1 week after stopping dapoxetine, avoid dapoxetine for 2 weeks after stopping lithium)
▸ Sildenafil: manufacturer of dapoxetine advises avoid concomitant use with SILDENAFIL
▸ Tadalafil: manufacturer of dapoxetine advises avoid concomitant use with TADALAFIL
▸ Vardenafil: manufacturer of dapoxetine advises avoid concomitant use with VARDENAFIL

Dapsone
● Antibacterials: plasma concentration of dapsone reduced by RIFAMYCINS; plasma concentration of both drugs may increase when dapsone given with TRIMETHOPRIM
● Antivirals: increased risk of ventricular arrhythmias when dapsone given with SAQUINAVIR—avoid concomitant use
▸ Vaccines: antibacterials inactivate ORAL TYPHOID VACCINE—see under Typhoid Vaccine in BNFC

Daptomycin
● Ciclosporin: increased risk of myopathy when daptomycin given with ● CICLOSPORIN (preferably avoid concomitant use)
● Lipid-regulating Drugs: increased risk of myopathy when daptomycin given with ● FIBRATES or ● STATINS (preferably avoid concomitant use)
▸ Vaccines: antibacterials inactivate ORAL TYPHOID VACCINE—see under Typhoid Vaccine in BNFC

Darifenacin see Antimuscarinics
Darunavir
▸ Anti-arrhythmics: darunavir possibly increases plasma concentration of LIDOCAINE—avoid concomitant use
● Antibacterials: darunavir increases plasma concentration of ● RIFABUTIN (reduce dose of rifabutin); plasma concentration of darunavir significantly reduced by ● RIFAMPICIN—avoid concomitant use
● Anticoagulants: avoidance of darunavir advised by manufacturer of APIXABAN and RIVAROXABAN; manufacturers advise avoid concomitant use of darunavir with DABIGATRAN
● Antidepressants: darunavir possibly reduces plasma concentration of PAROXETINE and SERTRALINE; plasma concentration of darunavir reduced by ● ST JOHN'S WORT—avoid concomitant use
▸ Antiepileptics: plasma concentration of darunavir possibly reduced by CARBAMAZEPINE, FOSPHENYTOIN, PHENOBARBITAL, PHENYTOIN and PRIMIDONE
▸ Antifungals: plasma concentration of both drugs increased when darunavir given with KETOCONAZOLE; darunavir possibly affects plasma concentration of VORICONAZOLE
● Antimalarials: plasma concentration of lumefantrine increased when darunavir given with ARTEMETHER WITH LUMEFANTRINE; darunavir possibly increases plasma concentration of ● QUININE (increased risk of toxicity)
● Antipsychotics: darunavir possibly increases plasma concentration of ● ARIPIPRAZOLE (reduce dose of aripiprazole—consult aripiprazole product literature); darunavir possibly increases plasma concentration of ● QUETIAPINE—manufacturer of quetiapine advises avoid concomitant use
● Antivirals: avoid concomitant use of darunavir with ● BOCEPREVIR or ● TELAPREVIR; avoidance of darunavir advised

Darunavir
- **Antivirals** (continued)
  by manufacturer of DACLATASVIR (plasma concentration of daclatasvir possibly increased); manufacturer of darunavir advises take DIDANOSINE 1 hour before or 2 hours after darunavir; plasma concentration of darunavir reduced by ●EFAVIRENZ (adjust dose—consult product literature); plasma concentration of both drugs increased when darunavir given with INDINAVIR; plasma concentration of darunavir reduced by ●LOPINAVIR and SAQUINAVIR—avoid concomitant use; darunavir increases plasma concentration of ●MARAVIROC (consider reducing dose of maraviroc); darunavir increases plasma concentration of ●PARITAPREVIR and plasma concentration of darunavir decreased; increased risk of rash when darunavir given with RALTEGRAVIR; plasma concentration of both drugs increased when darunavir given with ●SIMEPREVIR—manufacturer of simeprevir advises avoid concomitant use
- **Cytotoxics:** darunavir possibly increases the plasma concentration of ●BOSUTINIB—manufacturer of bosutinib advises avoid or consider reducing dose of bosutinib; darunavir possibly increases plasma concentration of ●EVEROLIMUS—manufacturer of everolimus advises avoid concomitant use; darunavir possibly increases the plasma concentration of ●IBRUTINIB—reduce dose of ibrutinib (see under Ibrutinib, in BNF)
- **Ergot Alkaloids:** increased risk of ergotism when darunavir given with ●ERGOT ALKALOIDS—manufacturer of darunavir advises avoid concomitant use
- **Lipid-regulating Drugs:** possible increased risk of myopathy when darunavir given with ATORVASTATIN; darunavir possibly increases plasma concentration of PRAVASTATIN (use lowest possible dose of pravastatin); darunavir increases plasma concentration of ●ROSUVASTATIN—adjust dose of rosuvastatin (consult product literature); avoidance of darunavir advised by manufacturer of ●LOMITAPIDE (plasma concentration of lomitapide possibly increased)
- **Orlistat:** absorption of darunavir possibly reduced by ●ORLISTAT
- **Ranolazine:** darunavir possibly increases plasma concentration of ●RANOLAZINE—manufacturer of ranolazine advises avoid concomitant use

Dasabuvir
- **Antibacterials:** manufacturer of dasabuvir advises avoid concomitant use with CLARITHROMYCIN and TELITHROMYCIN; plasma concentration of dasabuvir possibly reduced by ●RIFAMPICIN—avoid concomitant use
- **Antidepressants:** plasma concentration of dasabuvir possibly reduced by ●ST JOHN'S WORT—manufacturer of dasabuvir advises avoid concomitant use
- **Antiepileptics:** plasma concentration of dasabuvir reduced by ●CARBAMAZEPINE—avoid concomitant use; plasma concentration of dasabuvir possibly reduced by ●FOSPHENYTOIN, ●PHENOBARBITAL, ●PHENYTOIN and ●PRIMIDONE—avoid concomitant use
- **Antifungals:** plasma concentration of both drugs increased when dasabuvir given with ●KETOCONAZOLE—avoid concomitant use; plasma concentration of both drugs possibly increased when dasabuvir given with ●ITRACONAZOLE and ●POSACONAZOLE—avoid concomitant use
- **Antivirals:** manufacturer of dasabuvir advises avoid concomitant use with EFAVIRENZ, ETRAVIRINE and NEVIRAPINE
- **Cobicistat:** manufacturer of dasabuvir advises avoid concomitant use with COBICISTAT
- **Cytotoxics:** manufacturer of dasabuvir advises avoid concomitant use with MITOTANE
- **Diuretics:** dasabuvir increases plasma concentration of ●FUROSEMIDE (reduce dose of furosemide)
- **Hormone Antagonists:** manufacturer of dasabuvir advises avoid concomitant use with ENZALUTAMIDE
- **Lipid-regulating Drugs:** manufacturer of dasabuvir advises avoid concomitant use with ATORVASTATIN, GEMFIBROZIL and ●SIMVASTATIN; dasabuvir increases plasma concentration of ●ROSUVASTATIN (reduce dose of rosuvastatin—see under Rosuvastatin, in BNF)

Dasabuvir (continued)
- **Oestrogens:** manufacturer of dasabuvir advises avoid concomitant use of ●ETHINYLESTRADIOL—use alternative form of contraception

Dasatinib
- **Antibacterials:** manufacturer of dasatinib advises avoid concomitant use with CLARITHROMYCIN, ERYTHROMYCIN and TELITHROMYCIN (plasma concentration of dasatinib possibly increased); metabolism of dasatinib accelerated by ●RIFAMPICIN (reduced plasma concentration—avoid concomitant use)
- **Antiepileptics:** manufacturer of dasatinib advises avoid concomitant use with CARBAMAZEPINE, FOSPHENYTOIN, PHENOBARBITAL, PHENYTOIN and PRIMIDONE (plasma concentration of dasatinib possibly reduced)
▹ **Antifungals:** plasma concentration of dasatinib possibly increased by KETOCONAZOLE; manufacturer of dasatinib advises avoid concomitant use with ITRACONAZOLE (plasma concentration of dasatinib possibly increased)
▹ **Antipsychotics:** avoid concomitant use of cytotoxics with ●CLOZAPINE (increased risk of agranulocytosis)
- **Antivirals:** avoidance of dasatinib advised by manufacturer of ●BOCEPREVIR; manufacturer of dasatinib advises avoid concomitant use with RITONAVIR (plasma concentration of dasatinib possibly increased)
▹ **Grapefruit Juice:** manufacturer of dasatinib advises avoid concomitant use with GRAPEFRUIT JUICE (plasma concentration of dasatinib possibly increased)
▹ **Lipid-regulating Drugs:** dasatinib possibly increases plasma concentration of SIMVASTATIN
▹ **Ulcer-healing Drugs:** plasma concentration of dasatinib possibly reduced by FAMOTIDINE

Daunorubicin
- **Antipsychotics:** avoid concomitant use of cytotoxics with ●CLOZAPINE (increased risk of agranulocytosis)
- **Cytotoxics:** possible increased risk of cardiotoxicity when daunorubicin given with ●TRASTUZUMAB—avoid concomitant use for up to 28 weeks after stopping trastuzumab
- **Vaccines:** risk of generalised infections when cytotoxic antibiotics given with live ●VACCINES—avoid concomitant use

Decitabine
- **Antipsychotics:** avoid concomitant use of cytotoxics with ●CLOZAPINE (increased risk of agranulocytosis)

Deferasirox
- **Aminophylline:** deferasirox increases plasma concentration of ●AMINOPHYLLINE (consider reducing dose of aminophylline)
▹ **Antacids:** absorption of deferasirox possibly reduced by ANTACIDS containing aluminium (manufacturer of deferasirox advises avoid concomitant use)
▹ **Antibacterials:** plasma concentration of deferasirox reduced by RIFAMPICIN
▹ **Antidiabetics:** deferasirox increases plasma concentration of REPAGLINIDE
- **Antipsychotics:** manufacturer of deferasirox advises avoid concomitant use with CLOZAPINE
- **Anxiolytics and Hypnotics:** deferasirox possibly reduces plasma concentration of MIDAZOLAM
▹ **Muscle Relaxants:** manufacturer of deferasirox advises avoid concomitant use with TIZANIDINE
- **Theophylline:** deferasirox increases plasma concentration of ●THEOPHYLLINE (consider reducing dose of theophylline)

Deferiprone
▹ **Antacids:** absorption of deferiprone possibly reduced by ANTACIDS containing aluminium (manufacturer of deferiprone advises avoid concomitant use)

Deflazacort see Corticosteroids

Delamanid
- **Analgesics:** increased risk of ventricular arrhythmias when delamanid given with ●METHADONE
- **Anti-arrhythmics:** increased risk of ventricular arrhythmias when delamanid given with ●AMIODARONE or ●DISOPYRAMIDE
- **Antibacterials:** possible increased risk of ventricular arrhythmias when delamanid given with ●CLARITHROMYCIN and ●ERYTHROMYCIN; increased risk of ventricular arrhythmias when delamanid given with ●MOXIFLOXACIN; plasma

Delamanid
- Antibacterials (continued)
  concentration of delamanid reduced by • RIFAMPICIN; delamanid increases plasma concentration of ETHAMBUTOL
- Antidepressants: possible increased risk of ventricular arrhythmias when delamanid given with • TRICYCLICS that prolong the QT interval
▸ Antiepileptics: manufacturer of delamanid advises avoid concomitant use with CARBAMAZEPINE
- Antipsychotics: increased risk of ventricular arrhythmias when delamanid given with • DROPERIDOL, • HALOPERIDOL or • PIMOZIDE; increased risk of ventricular arrhythmias when delamanid given with • PHENOTHIAZINES that prolong the QT interval
- Antivirals: plasma concentration of delamanid increased by LOPINAVIR and RITONAVIR; increased risk of ventricular arrhythmias when delamanid given with • SAQUINAVIR
- Beta-blockers: increased risk of ventricular arrhythmias when delamanid given with • SOTALOL
- Cytotoxics: increased risk of ventricular arrhythmias when delamanid given with • ARSENIC TRIOXIDE or • VINFLUNINE; possible increased risk of ventricular arrhythmias when delamanid given with • VINBLASTINE, • VINCRISTINE, • VINDESINE and • VINORELBINE
- Domperidone: possible increased risk of ventricular arrhythmias when delamanid given with • DOMPERIDONE
- Pentamidine Isetionate: increased risk of ventricular arrhythmias when delamanid given with • PENTAMIDINE ISETIONATE
▸ Vaccines: antibacterials inactivate ORAL TYPHOID VACCINE—see under Typhoid Vaccine in BNFC

Demeclocycline see Tetracyclines

Desferrioxamine
▸ Antipsychotics: avoidance of desferrioxamine advised by manufacturer of LEVOMEPROMAZINE; manufacturer of desferrioxamine advises avoid concomitant use with PROCHLORPERAZINE

Desflurane see Anaesthetics, General

Desloratadine see Antihistamines

Desmopressin
▸ Analgesics: effects of desmopressin enhanced by INDOMETACIN
▸ Loperamide: plasma concentration of *oral* desmopressin increased by LOPERAMIDE

Desogestrel see Progestogens

Dexamethasone see Corticosteroids

Dexamfetamine see Sympathomimetics

Dexibuprofen see NSAIDs

Dexketoprofen see NSAIDs

Dexrazoxane
- Antiepileptics: dexrazoxane possibly reduces absorption of • FOSPHENYTOIN and • PHENYTOIN
▸ Ciclosporin: manufacturer of dexrazoxane advises increased risk of immunosuppression with CICLOSPORIN
▸ Tacrolimus: manufacturer of dexrazoxane advises increased risk of immunosuppression with TACROLIMUS
- Vaccines: risk of generalised infections when dexrazoxane given with live • VACCINES—avoid concomitant use

Dextromethorphan see Opioid Analgesics

Dextropropoxyphene see Opioid Analgesics

Diamorphine see Opioid Analgesics

Diazepam see Anxiolytics and Hypnotics

Diazoxide
▸ ACE Inhibitors: enhanced hypotensive effect when diazoxide given with ACE INHIBITORS
▸ Adrenergic Neurone Blockers: enhanced hypotensive effect when diazoxide given with ADRENERGIC NEURONE BLOCKERS
- Alcohol: enhanced hypotensive effect when diazoxide given with ALCOHOL
▸ Aldesleukin: enhanced hypotensive effect when diazoxide given with ALDESLEUKIN
▸ Alpha-blockers: enhanced hypotensive effect when diazoxide given with ALPHA-BLOCKERS
▸ Anaesthetics, General: enhanced hypotensive effect when diazoxide given with GENERAL ANAESTHETICS
▸ Analgesics: hypotensive effect of diazoxide antagonised by NSAIDs

Diazoxide (continued)
▸ Angiotensin-II Receptor Antagonists: enhanced hypotensive effect when diazoxide given with ANGIOTENSIN-II RECEPTOR ANTAGONISTS
▸ Antidepressants: enhanced hypotensive effect when diazoxide given with MAOIs or TRICYCLIC-RELATED ANTIDEPRESSANTS
▸ Antidiabetics: diazoxide antagonises hypoglycaemic effect of ANTIDIABETICS
▸ Antiepileptics: diazoxide reduces plasma concentration of FOSPHENYTOIN and PHENYTOIN, also effect of diazoxide may be reduced
▸ Antipsychotics: enhanced hypotensive effect when diazoxide given with PHENOTHIAZINES
▸ Anxiolytics and Hypnotics: enhanced hypotensive effect when diazoxide given with ANXIOLYTICS AND HYPNOTICS
▸ Beta-blockers: enhanced hypotensive effect when diazoxide given with BETA-BLOCKERS
▸ Calcium-channel Blockers: enhanced hypotensive effect when diazoxide given with CALCIUM-CHANNEL BLOCKERS
▸ Clonidine: enhanced hypotensive effect when diazoxide given with CLONIDINE
▸ Corticosteroids: hypotensive effect of diazoxide antagonised by CORTICOSTEROIDS
▸ Diuretics: enhanced hypotensive and hyperglycaemic effects when diazoxide given with DIURETICS
▸ Dopaminergics: enhanced hypotensive effect when diazoxide given with CO-BENELDOPA, CO-CARELDOPA or LEVODOPA
▸ Methyldopa: enhanced hypotensive effect when diazoxide given with METHYLDOPA
▸ Moxisylyte: enhanced hypotensive effect when diazoxide given with MOXISYLYTE
▸ Moxonidine: enhanced hypotensive effect when diazoxide given with MOXONIDINE
▸ Muscle Relaxants: enhanced hypotensive effect when diazoxide given with BACLOFEN or TIZANIDINE
▸ Nitrates: enhanced hypotensive effect when diazoxide given with NITRATES
▸ Prostaglandins: enhanced hypotensive effect when diazoxide given with ALPROSTADIL
▸ Vasodilator Antihypertensives: enhanced hypotensive effect when diazoxide given with HYDRALAZINE, MINOXIDIL or SODIUM NITROPRUSSIDE

Diclofenac see NSAIDs

Dicycloverine see Antimuscarinics

Didanosine
NOTE Antacids in tablet formulation might affect absorption of other drugs—give at least 2 hours apart
- Allopurinol: plasma concentration of didanosine increased by • ALLOPURINOL (risk of toxicity)—avoid concomitant use
▸ Analgesics: plasma concentration of didanosine possibly reduced by METHADONE
▸ Antibacterials: didanosine *tablets* reduce absorption of CIPROFLOXACIN (give at least 2 hours before or 4 hours after ciprofloxacin); manufacturer of levofloxacin advises give didanosine *tablets* at least 2 hours before or after LEVOFLOXACIN; manufacturer of moxifloxacin advises give didanosine *tablets* at least 6 hours before or after MOXIFLOXACIN; manufacturer of norfloxacin advises give didanosine at least 2 hours before or after NORFLOXACIN
- Antivirals: didanosine *tablets* reduce absorption of ATAZANAVIR (give at least 2 hours before or 1 hour after didanosine *tablets*); manufacturer of darunavir advises take didanosine 1 hour before or 2 hours after DARUNAVIR; plasma concentration of didanosine possibly increased by GANCICLOVIR and VALGANCICLOVIR; didanosine *tablets* reduce absorption of INDINAVIR (give at least 1 hour apart); increased risk of side-effects when didanosine given with • RIBAVIRIN—avoid concomitant use; manufacturer of rilpivirine advises give didanosine 2 hours before or 4 hours after RILPIVIRINE; manufacturer of ritonavir advises didanosine and RITONAVIR should be taken 2.5 hours apart; increased risk of side-effects when didanosine given with • STAVUDINE; plasma concentration of didanosine increased by • TENOFOVIR (increased risk of toxicity)—avoid concomitant use; plasma concentration of didanosine reduced by TIPRANAVIR—

Didanosine

- **Antivirals** (continued)
  manufacturer of tipranavir advises tipranavir and didanosine *capsules* should be taken at least 2 hours apart
- **Cytotoxics**: increased risk of toxicity when didanosine given with ● HYDROXYCARBAMIDE—avoid concomitant use
- **Orlistat**: absorption of didanosine possibly reduced by ● ORLISTAT

Dienogest see Progestogens

Diethylcarbamazine

▸ **Antacids**: excretion of diethylcarbamazine reduced by SODIUM BICARBONATE

Digoxin see Cardiac Glycosides

Dihydrocodeine see Opioid Analgesics

Dihydrotachysterol see Vitamins

Diltiazem see Calcium-channel Blockers

Dimethyl sulfoxide

- **Analgesics**: avoid concomitant use of dimethyl sulfoxide with ● SULINDAC

Dinoprostone see Prostaglandins

Diphenoxylate see Opioid Analgesics

Diphtheria Vaccines see Vaccines

Dipipanone see Opioid Analgesics

Dipyridamole

▸ **Antacids**: absorption of dipyridamole possibly reduced by ANTACIDS
- **Anti-arrhythmics**: dipyridamole enhances and extends effect of ● ADENOSINE (important risk of toxicity)—reduce dose of adenosine, see p. 73
- **Anticoagulants**: antiplatelet action of dipyridamole enhances anticoagulant effect of ● COUMARINS and ● PHENINDIONE; dipyridamole enhances anticoagulant effect of HEPARINS
▸ **Clopidogrel**: increased risk of bleeding when dipyridamole given with CLOPIDOGREL
▸ **Cytotoxics**: dipyridamole possibly reduces effects of FLUDARABINE

Disopyramide

- **Anaesthetics, Local**: increased myocardial depression when anti-arrhythmics given with BUPIVACAINE, LEVOBUPIVACAINE, PRILOCAINE or ROPIVACAINE
- **Anti-arrhythmics**: increased myocardial depression when anti-arrhythmics given with other ● ANTI-ARRHYTHMICS; increased risk of ventricular arrhythmias when disopyramide given with ● AMIODARONE or ● DRONEDARONE—avoid concomitant use
- **Antibacterials**: plasma concentration of disopyramide possibly increased by AZITHROMYCIN (increased risk of toxicity); plasma concentration of disopyramide possibly increased by ● CLARITHROMYCIN (increased risk of ventricular arrhythmias); plasma concentration of disopyramide increased by ● ERYTHROMYCIN (increased risk of toxicity); increased risk of ventricular arrhythmias when disopyramide given with ● MOXIFLOXACIN—avoid concomitant use; increased risk of ventricular arrhythmias when disopyramide given with ● DELAMANID; metabolism of disopyramide accelerated by ● RIFAMYCINS (reduced plasma concentration); possible increased risk of ventricular arrhythmias when disopyramide given with ● TELITHROMYCIN
▸ **Anticoagulants**: disopyramide may enhance or reduce anticoagulant effect of WARFARIN
▸ **Antidepressants**: avoidance of disopyramide advised by manufacturer of ● CITALOPRAM and ● ESCITALOPRAM (risk of ventricular arrhythmias); increased risk of ventricular arrhythmias when disopyramide given with ● TRICYCLICS
  Antidiabetics: disopyramide possibly enhances hypoglycaemic effect of GLICLAZIDE, INSULIN and METFORMIN
- **Antiepileptics**: plasma concentration of disopyramide reduced by FOSPHENYTOIN and PHENYTOIN; metabolism of disopyramide accelerated by PHENOBARBITAL and PRIMIDONE (reduced plasma concentration)
- **Antifungals**: increased risk of ventricular arrhythmias when disopyramide given with ● KETOCONAZOLE—avoid concomitant use; avoidance of disopyramide advised by manufacturer of ● ITRACONAZOLE
- **Antihistamines**: increased risk of ventricular arrhythmias when disopyramide given with ● MIZOLASTINE—avoid concomitant use

Disopyramide (continued)

- **Antimalarials**: avoidance of disopyramide advised by manufacturer of ● ARTEMETHER WITH LUMEFANTRINE (risk of ventricular arrhythmias); avoidance of disopyramide advised by manufacturer of ● ARTENIMOL WITH PIPERAQUINE (possible risk of ventricular arrhythmias)
- **Antimuscarinics**: increased risk of antimuscarinic side-effects when disopyramide given with ANTIMUSCARINICS; increased risk of ventricular arrhythmias when disopyramide given with ● TOLTERODINE
- **Antipsychotics**: increased risk of ventricular arrhythmias when anti-arrhythmics that prolong the QT interval given with ● ANTIPSYCHOTICS that prolong the QT interval; increased risk of ventricular arrhythmias when disopyramide given with ● AMISULPRIDE, ● DROPERIDOL, ● PIMOZIDE or ● ZUCLOPENTHIXOL—avoid concomitant use; possible increased risk of ventricular arrhythmias when disopyramide given with ● HALOPERIDOL—avoid concomitant use; increased risk of ventricular arrhythmias when disopyramide given with ● PHENOTHIAZINES or ● SULPIRIDE
- **Antivirals**: plasma concentration of disopyramide possibly increased by ● RITONAVIR (increased risk of toxicity); increased risk of ventricular arrhythmias when disopyramide given with ● SAQUINAVIR—avoid concomitant use; avoidance of disopyramide advised by manufacturer of ● TELAPREVIR (risk of ventricular arrhythmias)
- **Atomoxetine**: increased risk of ventricular arrhythmias when disopyramide given with ● ATOMOXETINE
- **Beta-blockers**: increased myocardial depression when anti-arrhythmics given with ● BETA-BLOCKERS; increased risk of ventricular arrhythmias when disopyramide given with ● SOTALOL—avoid concomitant use
- **Calcium-channel Blockers**: increased risk of myocardial depression and asystole when disopyramide given with ● VERAPAMIL
- **Cytotoxics**: possible increased risk of ventricular arrhythmias when disopyramide given with ● BOSUTINIB; possible increased risk of ventricular arrhythmias when disopyramide given with ● VANDETANIB—avoid concomitant use; increased risk of ventricular arrhythmias when disopyramide given with ● ARSENIC TRIOXIDE
- **Diuretics**: increased cardiac toxicity with disopyramide if hypokalaemia occurs with ● ACETAZOLAMIDE, ● LOOP DIURETICS or ● THIAZIDES AND RELATED DIURETICS
- **Fingolimod**: possible increased risk of bradycardia when disopyramide given with ● FINGOLIMOD
- **Ivabradine**: increased risk of ventricular arrhythmias when disopyramide given with ● IVABRADINE
▸ **Nitrates**: disopyramide reduces effects of sublingual tablets of NITRATES (failure to dissolve under tongue owing to dry mouth)
- **Pentamidine Isetionate**: possible increased risk of ventricular arrhythmias when disopyramide given with ● PENTAMIDINE ISETIONATE
- **Ranolazine**: avoidance of disopyramide advised by manufacturer of ● RANOLAZINE
▸ **Sildenafil**: manufacturer of disopyramide advises avoid concomitant use with SILDENAFIL (risk of ventricular arrhythmias)
▸ **Tadalafil**: manufacturer of disopyramide advises avoid concomitant use with TADALAFIL (risk of ventricular arrhythmias)
▸ **Vardenafil**: manufacturer of disopyramide advises avoid concomitant use with VARDENAFIL (risk of ventricular arrhythmias)

Disulfiram

▸ **Alcohol**: disulfiram reaction when disulfiram given with ALCOHOL
- **Aminophylline**: disulfiram inhibits metabolism of AMINOPHYLLINE (increased risk of toxicity)
- **Antibacterials**: psychotic reaction reported when disulfiram given with METRONIDAZOLE; CNS effects of disulfiram possibly increased by ISONIAZID
- **Anticoagulants**: disulfiram enhances anticoagulant effect of ● COUMARINS

Disulfiram (continued)

▸ Antidepressants: increased disulfiram reaction with alcohol reported with concomitant AMITRIPTYLINE; disulfiram inhibits metabolism of TRICYCLICS (increased plasma concentration)

● Antiepileptics: disulfiram inhibits metabolism of
● FOSPHENYTOIN and ● PHENYTOIN (increased risk of toxicity)

▸ Anxiolytics and Hypnotics: disulfiram increases risk of TEMAZEPAM toxicity; disulfiram inhibits metabolism of BENZODIAZEPINES (increased sedative effects)

● Paraldehyde: risk of toxicity when disulfiram given with
● PARALDEHYDE

▸ Theophylline: disulfiram inhibits metabolism of THEOPHYLLINE (increased risk of toxicity)

Diuretics

NOTE Since systemic absorption may follow topical application of brinzolamide to the eye, the possibility of interactions should be borne in mind

NOTE Since systemic absorption may follow topical application of dorzolamide to the eye, the possibility of interactions should be borne in mind

● ACE Inhibitors: enhanced hypotensive effect when diuretics given with ● ACE INHIBITORS; increased risk of severe hyperkalaemia when amiloride, potassium canrenoate or triamterene given with ● ACE INHIBITORS; increased risk of severe hyperkalaemia when eplerenone and spironolactone given with ● ACE INHIBITORS—avoid concurrent use or use lowest possible doses of both drugs

● Adrenergic Neurone Blockers: enhanced hypotensive effect when diuretics given with ADRENERGIC NEURONE BLOCKERS

● Alcohol: enhanced hypotensive effect when diuretics given with ALCOHOL

● Aldesleukin: enhanced hypotensive effect when diuretics given with ALDESLEUKIN

● Aliskiren: plasma concentration of furosemide reduced by ALISKIREN; increased risk of hyperkalaemia when potassium-sparing diuretics and aldosterone antagonists given with ALISKIREN

● Allopurinol: increased risk of hypersensitivity when thiazides and related diuretics given with ALLOPURINOL especially in renal impairment

● Alpha-blockers: enhanced hypotensive effect when diuretics given with ● ALPHA-BLOCKERS, also increased risk of first-dose hypotension with post-synaptic alpha-blockers such as prazosin

● Aminophylline: increased risk of hypokalaemia when acetazolamide, loop diuretics or thiazides and related diuretics given with AMINOPHYLLINE

● Anaesthetics, General: enhanced hypotensive effect when diuretics given with GENERAL ANAESTHETICS

● Analgesics: diuretics increase risk of nephrotoxicity of NSAIDs, also antagonism of diuretic effect; diuretic effect of potassium canrenoate possibly antagonised by NSAIDs; possible increased risk of hyperkalaemia when potassium-sparing diuretics and aldosterone antagonists given with NSAIDs; furosemide possibly increases the excretion of ACEMETACIN; effects of diuretics antagonised by INDOMETACIN and KETOROLAC; increased risk of hyperkalaemia when potassium-sparing diuretics and aldosterone antagonists given with INDOMETACIN; occasional reports of reduced renal function when triamterene given with ● INDOMETACIN—avoid concomitant use; diuretic effect of spironolactone antagonised by ASPIRIN; possible increased risk of toxicity when loop diuretics given with high-dose ASPIRIN (also possible reduced effect of loop diuretics); increased risk of toxicity with acetazolamide given with high-dose ● ASPIRIN

● Angiotensin-II Receptor Antagonists: enhanced hypotensive effect when diuretics given with ● ANGIOTENSIN-II RECEPTOR ANTAGONISTS; increased risk of severe hyperkalaemia when amiloride, potassium canrenoate or triamterene given with ● ANGIOTENSIN-II RECEPTOR ANTAGONISTS; increased risk of severe hyperkalaemia when eplerenone and spironolactone given with ● ANGIOTENSIN-II RECEPTOR ANTAGONISTS—avoid concurrent use or use lowest possible doses of both drugs; plasma concentration of furosemide reduced by VALSARTAN

● Anti-arrhythmics: hypokalaemia caused by acetazolamide, loop diuretics or thiazides and related diuretics increases cardiac

Diuretics

● Anti-arrhythmics (continued)
toxicity with AMIODARONE; plasma concentration of eplerenone increased by AMIODARONE (reduce dose of eplerenone); hypokalaemia caused by acetazolamide, loop diuretics or thiazides and related diuretics increases cardiac toxicity with ● DISOPYRAMIDE; hypokalaemia caused by acetazolamide, loop diuretics or thiazides and related diuretics increases cardiac toxicity with ● FLECAINIDE; hypokalaemia caused by acetazolamide, loop diuretics or thiazides and related diuretics antagonises action of
● LIDOCAINE

● Antibacterials: plasma concentration of eplerenone increased by ● CLARITHROMYCIN and ● TELITHROMYCIN—avoid concomitant use; plasma concentration of eplerenone increased by ERYTHROMYCIN (reduce dose of eplerenone); plasma concentration of eplerenone reduced by
● RIFAMPICIN—avoid concomitant use; avoidance of diuretics advised by manufacturer of LYMECYCLINE; increased risk of ototoxicity when loop diuretics given with ● AMINOGLYCOSIDES,
● POLYMYXINS or ● VANCOMYCIN; acetazolamide antagonises effects of ● METHENAMINE; increased risk of hyperkalaemia when eplerenone given with TRIMETHOPRIM; possible increased risk of hyperkalaemia when spironolactone given with TRIMETHOPRIM

● Antidepressants: possible increased risk of hypokalaemia when loop diuretics or thiazides and related diuretics given with REBOXETINE; enhanced hypotensive effect when diuretics given with MAOIs; plasma concentration of eplerenone reduced by ● ST JOHN'S WORT—avoid concomitant use; increased risk of postural hypotension when diuretics given with TRICYCLICS

▸ Antidiabetics: loop diuretics and thiazides and related diuretics antagonise hypoglycaemic effect of ANTIDIABETICS; diuretic effect of diuretics possibly enhanced by CANAGLIFLOZIN; avoidance of loop diuretics advised by manufacturer of CANAGLIFLOZIN; diuretic effect of loop diuretics and thiazides and related diuretics possibly enhanced by DAPAGLIFLOZIN

● Antiepileptics: increased risk of hyponatraemia when diuretics given with CARBAMAZEPINE; acetazolamide increases plasma concentration of ● CARBAMAZEPINE; plasma concentration of eplerenone reduced by ● CARBAMAZEPINE, ● FOSPHENYTOIN,
● PHENOBARBITAL, ● PHENYTOIN and ● PRIMIDONE—avoid concomitant use; increased risk of osteomalacia when carbonic anhydrase inhibitors given with FOSPHENYTOIN, PHENOBARBITAL, PHENYTOIN or PRIMIDONE; effects of furosemide antagonised by FOSPHENYTOIN and PHENYTOIN; acetazolamide possibly increases plasma concentration of
● FOSPHENYTOIN and ● PHENYTOIN; hydrochlorothiazide possibly increases plasma concentration of TOPIRAMATE; avoidance of carbonic anhydrase inhibitors in children advised by manufacturer of ZONISAMIDE

● Antifungals: plasma concentration of eplerenone increased by
● ITRACONAZOLE and ● KETOCONAZOLE—avoid concomitant use; increased risk of hypokalaemia when loop diuretics or thiazides and related diuretics given with AMPHOTERICIN; hydrochlorothiazide increases plasma concentration of FLUCONAZOLE; plasma concentration of eplerenone increased by FLUCONAZOLE (reduce dose of eplerenone)

● Antipsychotics: hypokalaemia caused by diuretics increases risk of ventricular arrhythmias with ● AMISULPRIDE; enhanced hypotensive effect when diuretics given with PHENOTHIAZINES; hypokalaemia caused by diuretics increases risk of ventricular arrhythmias with ● PIMOZIDE (avoid concomitant use)

● Antivirals: plasma concentration of furosemide increased by
● DASABUVIR, ● OMBITASVIR and ● PARITAPREVIR (reduce dose of furosemide); plasma concentration of eplerenone increased by ● RITONAVIR—avoid concomitant use; plasma concentration of eplerenone increased by SAQUINAVIR (reduce dose of eplerenone)

▸ Anxiolytics and Hypnotics: enhanced hypotensive effect when diuretics given with ANXIOLYTICS and HYPNOTICS; administration of *parenteral* furosemide with CHLORAL may displace thyroid hormone from binding sites

● Atomoxetine: hypokalaemia caused by diuretics increases risk of ventricular arrhythmias with ● ATOMOXETINE

Diuretics (continued)

- Beta-blockers: enhanced hypotensive effect when diuretics given with BETA-BLOCKERS; hypokalaemia caused by loop diuretics or thiazides and related diuretics increases risk of ventricular arrhythmias with ● SOTALOL
▹ Calcium Salts: increased risk of hypercalcaemia when thiazides and related diuretics given with CALCIUM SALTS
▹ Calcium-channel Blockers: enhanced hypotensive effect when diuretics given with CALCIUM-CHANNEL BLOCKERS; plasma concentration of eplerenone increased by DILTIAZEM and VERAPAMIL (reduce dose of eplerenone)
- Cardiac Glycosides: hypokalaemia caused by acetazolamide, loop diuretics or thiazides and related diuretics increases cardiac toxicity with ● CARDIAC GLYCOSIDES; potassium canrenoate possibly increases plasma concentration of DIGOXIN; spironolactone increases plasma concentration of ● DIGOXIN
- Ciclosporin: increased risk of nephrotoxicity and possibly hypermagnesaemia when thiazides and related diuretics given with CICLOSPORIN; increased risk of hyperkalaemia when potassium-sparing diuretics and aldosterone antagonists given with ● CICLOSPORIN; acetazolamide possibly increases plasma concentration of ● CICLOSPORIN
- Clonidine: enhanced hypotensive effect when diuretics given with CLONIDINE
▹ Corticosteroids: diuretic effect of diuretics antagonised by CORTICOSTEROIDS; increased risk of hypokalaemia when acetazolamide, loop diuretics or thiazides and related diuretics given with CORTICOSTEROIDS
- Cytotoxics: alkaline urine due to acetazolamide increases excretion of METHOTREXATE; hypokalaemia caused by acetazolamide, loop diuretics or thiazides and related diuretics increases risk of ventricular arrhythmias with ● ARSENIC TRIOXIDE; avoidance of spironolactone advised by manufacturer of MITOTANE (antagonism of effect); increased risk of nephrotoxicity and ototoxicity when diuretics given with PLATINUM COMPOUNDS
▹ Diazoxide: enhanced hypotensive and hyperglycaemic effects when diuretics given with DIAZOXIDE
▹ Diuretics: increased risk of hypokalaemia when loop diuretics or thiazides and related diuretics given with ACETAZOLAMIDE; profound diuresis possible when metolazone given with FUROSEMIDE; increased risk of hypokalaemia when thiazides and related diuretics given with LOOP DIURETICS
▹ Dopaminergics: enhanced hypotensive effect when diuretics given with CO-BENELDOPA, CO-CARELDOPA or LEVODOPA
▹ Hormone Antagonists: avoidance of spironolactone advised by manufacturer of ABIRATERONE; increased risk of hypercalcaemia when thiazides and related diuretics given with TOREMIFENE
▹ Lipid-regulating Drugs: absorption of thiazides and related diuretics reduced by COLESTIPOL and COLESTYRAMINE (give at least 2 hours apart)
- Lithium: loop diuretics and thiazides and related diuretics reduce excretion of ● LITHIUM (increased plasma concentration and risk of toxicity)—loop diuretics safer than thiazides; potassium-sparing diuretics and aldosterone antagonists reduce excretion of ● LITHIUM (increased plasma concentration and risk of toxicity); acetazolamide increases the excretion of ● LITHIUM
▹ Methyldopa: enhanced hypotensive effect when diuretics given with METHYLDOPA
▹ Moxisylyte: enhanced hypotensive effect when diuretics given with MOXISYLYTE
▹ Moxonidine: enhanced hypotensive effect when diuretics given with MOXONIDINE
▹ Muscle Relaxants: enhanced hypotensive effect when diuretics given with BACLOFEN or TIZANIDINE
▹ Nitrates: enhanced hypotensive effect when diuretics given with NITRATES
▹ Oestrogens: diuretic effect of diuretics antagonised by OESTROGENS
- Potassium Salts: increased risk of hyperkalaemia when potassium-sparing diuretics and aldosterone antagonists given with ● POTASSIUM SALTS

Diuretics (continued)

▹ Progestogens: risk of hyperkalaemia when potassium-sparing diuretics and aldosterone antagonists given with DROSPIRENONE (monitor serum potassium during first cycle)
▹ Prostaglandins: enhanced hypotensive effect when diuretics given with ALPROSTADIL
▹ Sacubitril: plasma concentration of furosemide reduced by SACUBITRIL
▹ Sympathomimetics, Beta₂: increased risk of hypokalaemia when acetazolamide, loop diuretics or thiazides and related diuretics given with high doses of BETA₂ SYMPATHOMIMETICS
▹ Tacrolimus: increased risk of hyperkalaemia when potassium-sparing diuretics and aldosterone antagonists given with ● TACROLIMUS
▹ Theophylline: increased risk of hypokalaemia when acetazolamide, loop diuretics or thiazides and related diuretics given with THEOPHYLLINE
▹ Vasodilator Antihypertensives: enhanced hypotensive effect when diuretics given with HYDRALAZINE, MINOXIDIL or SODIUM NITROPRUSSIDE
▹ Vitamins: increased risk of hypercalcaemia when thiazides and related diuretics given with ALFACALCIDOL, CALCITRIOL, COLECALCIFEROL, DIHYDROTACHYSTEROL, ERGOCALCIFEROL, PARICALCITOL or VITAMIN D

Diuretics, Loop *see* Diuretics
Diuretics, Potassium-sparing and Aldosterone Antagonists *see* Diuretics
Diuretics, Thiazide and related *see* Diuretics
Dobutamine *see* Sympathomimetics
Docetaxel

- Antibacterials: plasma concentration of docetaxel possibly increased by ● CLARITHROMYCIN and ● TELITHROMYCIN—manufacturer of docetaxel advises avoid concomitant use or consider reducing docetaxel dose
- Antifungals: *in vitro* studies suggest a possible interaction between docetaxel and KETOCONAZOLE (consult docetaxel product literature); plasma concentration of docetaxel possibly increased by ● ITRACONAZOLE and ● VORICONAZOLE—manufacturer of docetaxel advises avoid concomitant use or consider reducing docetaxel dose
- Antipsychotics: avoid concomitant use of cytotoxics with ● CLOZAPINE (increased risk of agranulocytosis)
- Antivirals: plasma concentration of docetaxel possibly increased by ● INDINAVIR, ● RITONAVIR and ● SAQUINAVIR—manufacturer of docetaxel advises avoid concomitant use or consider reducing docetaxel dose
▹ Ciclosporin: *in vitro* studies suggest a possible interaction between docetaxel and CICLOSPORIN (consult docetaxel product literature)
▹ Cytotoxics: possible increased risk of neutropenia when docetaxel given with LAPATINIB; plasma concentration of docetaxel increased by SORAFENIB
▹ Netupitant: plasma concentration of docetaxel increased by NETUPITANT

Dolutegravir

▹ Antacids: absorption of dolutegravir reduced by ALUMINIUM HYDROXIDE and ORAL MAGNESIUM SALTS—manufacturer of dolutegravir advises give at least 2 hours before or 6 hours after aluminium hydroxide and oral magnesium salts
- Antibacterials: plasma concentration of dolutegravir reduced by ● RIFAMPICIN (see under Dolutegravir, p. 387)
- Antidepressants: plasma concentration of dolutegravir possibly reduced by ● ST JOHN'S WORT (see under Dolutegravir, p. 387)
▹ Antidiabetics: dolutegravir increases the plasma concentration of METFORMIN—consider reducing dose of metformin
▹ Antiepileptics: plasma concentration of dolutegravir reduced by ● CARBAMAZEPINE (see under Dolutegravir, p. 387); plasma concentration of dolutegravir possibly reduced by ● FOSPHENYTOIN, ● OXCARBAZEPINE, PHENOBARBITAL, ● PHENYTOIN and ● PRIMIDONE (see under Dolutegravir, p. 387)
▹ Antivirals: plasma concentration of dolutegravir reduced by ● EFAVIRENZ, ● ETRAVIRINE and ● TIPRANAVIR (see under Dolutegravir, p. 387); plasma concentration of dolutegravir reduced by ● FOSAMPRENAVIR; plasma concentration of dolutegravir possibly reduced by ● NEVIRAPINE (see under Dolutegravir, p. 387)

A1

Interactions | Appendix 1

Dolutegravir (continued)
▸ Calcium Salts: absorption of dolutegravir reduced by CALCIUM SALTS—manufacturer of dolutegravir advises give at least 2 hours before or 6 hours after calcium salts
▸ Iron Salts: absorption of dolutegravir reduced by *oral* IRON SALTS—manufacturer of dolutegravir advises give at least 2 hours before or 6 hours after *oral* iron salts

Domperidone
▸ Analgesics: effects of domperidone on gastro-intestinal activity antagonised by OPIOID ANALGESICS
● Antibacterials: possible increased risk of ventricular arrhythmias when domperidone given with ● CLARITHROMYCIN or ● TELITHROMYCIN—avoid concomitant use; plasma concentration of domperidone increased by ● ERYTHROMYCIN (increased risk of ventricular arrhythmias—avoid concomitant use); possible increased risk of ventricular arrhythmias when domperidone given with ● DELAMANID
● Antifungals: avoidance of domperidone advised by manufacturer of ● KETOCONAZOLE (risk of ventricular arrhythmias); possible increased risk of ventricular arrhythmias when domperidone given with ● ITRACONAZOLE or ● VORICONAZOLE—avoid concomitant use
▸ Antimalarials: avoidance of domperidone advised by manufacturer of ● ARTENIMOL WITH PIPERAQUINE (possible risk of ventricular arrhythmias)
▸ Antimuscarinics: effects of domperidone on gastro-intestinal activity antagonised by ANTIMUSCARINICS
● Antivirals: possible increased risk of ventricular arrhythmias when domperidone given with ● BOCEPREVIR, ● RITONAVIR, ● SAQUINAVIR or ● TELAPREVIR—avoid concomitant use
● Cobicistat: possible increased risk of ventricular arrhythmias when domperidone given with ● COBICISTAT—avoid concomitant use
● Cytotoxics: avoidance of domperidone advised by manufacturer of ● BOSUTINIB (risk of ventricular arrhythmias)
● Dopaminergics: possible increased risk of ventricular arrhythmias when domperidone given with ● APOMORPHINE; domperidone possibly antagonises hypoprolactinaemic effects of BROMOCRIPTINE and CABERGOLINE

Donepezil *see* Parasympathomimetics
Dopamine *see* Sympathomimetics
Dopaminergics *see* Amantadine, Apomorphine, Bromocriptine, Cabergoline, Entacapone, Levodopa, Pergolide, Pramipexole, Quinagolide, Rasagiline, Ropinirole, Rotigotine, Selegiline, and Tolcapone
Dopexamine *see* Sympathomimetics
Dorzolamide *see* Diuretics
Dosulepin *see* Antidepressants, Tricyclic
Doxapram
▸ Aminophylline: increased CNS stimulation when doxapram given with AMINOPHYLLINE
● Anaesthetics, General: increased risk of arrhythmias when doxapram given with ● VOLATILE LIQUID GENERAL ANAESTHETICS (avoid doxapram for at least 10 minutes after volatile liquid general anaesthetics)
▸ Antidepressants: effects of doxapram enhanced by MAOIs
▸ Sympathomimetics: increased risk of hypertension when doxapram given with SYMPATHOMIMETICS
▸ Theophylline: increased CNS stimulation when doxapram given with THEOPHYLLINE

Doxazosin *see* Alpha-blockers
Doxepin *see* Antidepressants, Tricyclic
Doxorubicin
● Antipsychotics: avoid concomitant use of cytotoxics with ● CLOZAPINE (increased risk of agranulocytosis)
▸ Antivirals: doxorubicin possibly inhibits effects of STAVUDINE
▸ Calcium-channel Blockers: plasma concentration of doxorubicin possibly increased by VERAPAMIL
▸ Cardiac Glycosides: doxorubicin possibly reduces absorption of DIGOXIN *tablets*
● Ciclosporin: increased risk of neurotoxicity when doxorubicin given with ● CICLOSPORIN
● Cytotoxics: possible increased risk of cardiotoxicity when doxorubicin given with ● TRASTUZUMAB—avoid concomitant use for up to 28 weeks after stopping trastuzumab; plasma concentration of doxorubicin increased by SORAFENIB

Doxorubicin (continued)
▸ Ulcer-healing Drugs: plasma concentration of doxorubicin reduced by CIMETIDINE
● Vaccines: risk of generalised infections when cytotoxic antibiotics given with live ● VACCINES—avoid concomitant use

Doxycycline *see* Tetracyclines
Dronedarone
▸ Anaesthetics, Local: increased myocardial depression when anti-arrhythmics given with BUPIVACAINE, LEVOBUPIVACAINE, PRILOCAINE or ROPIVACAINE
● Anti-arrhythmics: increased myocardial depression when anti-arrhythmics given with other ● ANTI-ARRHYTHMICS; increased risk of ventricular arrhythmias when dronedarone given with ● AMIODARONE or ● DISOPYRAMIDE—avoid concomitant use
● Antibacterials: manufacturer of dronedarone advises avoid concomitant use with ● CLARITHROMYCIN (risk of ventricular arrhythmias); plasma concentration of dronedarone increased by ● ERYTHROMYCIN (increased risk of ventricular arrhythmias—avoid concomitant use); plasma concentration of dronedarone reduced by ● RIFAMPICIN—avoid concomitant use; avoidance of dronedarone advised by manufacturer of FIDAXOMICIN; increased risk of ventricular arrhythmias when dronedarone given with ● TELITHROMYCIN—avoid concomitant use
● Anticoagulants: dronedarone possibly enhances anticoagulant effect of ● COUMARINS and ● PHENINDIONE; dronedarone increases plasma concentration of ● DABIGATRAN—avoid concomitant use; dronedarone increases plasma concentration of ● EDOXABAN (reduce dose of edoxaban—see under Edoxaban, in BNF); avoidance of dronedarone advised by manufacturer of RIVAROXABAN
● Antidepressants: avoidance of dronedarone advised by manufacturer of ● CITALOPRAM and ● ESCITALOPRAM (risk of ventricular arrhythmias); plasma concentration of dronedarone possibly reduced by ● ST JOHN'S WORT—avoid concomitant use; manufacturer of dronedarone advises avoid concomitant use with ● TRICYCLICS (risk of ventricular arrhythmias)
● Antiepileptics: plasma concentration of dronedarone possibly reduced by ● CARBAMAZEPINE, ● FOSPHENYTOIN, ● PHENOBARBITAL, ● PHENYTOIN and ● PRIMIDONE—avoid concomitant use
● Antifungals: plasma concentration of dronedarone increased by ● KETOCONAZOLE—avoid concomitant use; manufacturer of dronedarone advises avoid concomitant use with ● ITRACONAZOLE, ● POSACONAZOLE and ● VORICONAZOLE
● Antipsychotics: increased risk of ventricular arrhythmias when anti-arrhythmics that prolong the QT interval given with ● ANTIPSYCHOTICS that prolong the QT interval; manufacturer of dronedarone advises avoid concomitant use with ● PHENOTHIAZINES (risk of ventricular arrhythmias)
● Antivirals: manufacturer of dronedarone advises avoid concomitant use with ● RITONAVIR; increased risk of ventricular arrhythmias when dronedarone given with ● SAQUINAVIR—avoid concomitant use
● Beta-blockers: increased myocardial depression when anti-arrhythmics given with ● BETA-BLOCKERS; dronedarone possibly increases plasma concentration of METOPROLOL and PROPRANOLOL; increased risk of ventricular arrhythmias when dronedarone given with ● SOTALOL—avoid concomitant use
● Calcium-channel Blockers: plasma concentration of dronedarone increased by ● NIFEDIPINE; increased risk of bradycardia and myocardial depression when dronedarone given with ● DILTIAZEM and ● VERAPAMIL
● Cardiac Glycosides: dronedarone increases plasma concentration of ● DIGOXIN (halve dose of digoxin)
● Cytotoxics: dronedarone possibly increases the plasma concentration of ● BOSUTINIB—manufacturer of bosutinib advises avoid or consider reducing dose of bosutinib; dronedarone possibly increases the plasma concentration of ● IBRUTINIB—reduce dose of ibrutinib (see under Ibrutinib, in BNF)
● Fingolimod: possible increased risk of bradycardia when dronedarone given with ● FINGOLIMOD
● Grapefruit Juice: plasma concentration of dronedarone increased by ● GRAPEFRUIT JUICE—avoid concomitant use

Dronedarone (continued)

- Lipid-regulating Drugs: dronedarone possibly increases plasma concentration of ATORVASTATIN; dronedarone increases plasma concentration of • ROSUVASTATIN—adjust dose of rosuvastatin (consult product literature); increased risk of myopathy when dronedarone given with • SIMVASTATIN; avoidance of dronedarone advised by manufacturer of • LOMITAPIDE (plasma concentration of lomitapide possibly increased)
- ▷ Sirolimus: manufacturer of dronedarone advises caution with SIROLIMUS
- ▷ Tacrolimus: manufacturer of dronedarone advises caution with TACROLIMUS

Droperidol see Antipsychotics

Drospirenone see Progestogens

Dulaglutide see Antidiabetics

Duloxetine

- ▷ Analgesics: possible increased serotonergic effects when SSRI-related antidepressants given with FENTANYL; possible increased serotonergic effects when duloxetine given with PETHIDINE or TRAMADOL
- Antibacterials: metabolism of duloxetine inhibited by • CIPROFLOXACIN—avoid concomitant use
- Anticoagulants: possible increased risk of bleeding when SSRI-related antidepressants given with • DABIGATRAN
- Antidepressants: metabolism of duloxetine inhibited by • FLUVOXAMINE—avoid concomitant use; possible increased serotonergic effects when duloxetine given with SSRIs, ST JOHN'S WORT, AMITRIPTYLINE, CLOMIPRAMINE, • MOCLOBEMIDE or VENLAFAXINE; duloxetine should not be started until 2 weeks after stopping MAOIs, also MAOIs should not be started until at least 5 days after stopping duloxetine; after stopping SSRI-related antidepressants do not start • MOCLOBEMIDE for at least 1 week; possible increased risk of convulsions when SSRI-related antidepressants given with • VORTIOXETINE
- Antimalarials: avoidance of antidepressants advised by manufacturer of • ARTEMETHER WITH LUMEFANTRINE and • ARTENIMOL WITH PIPERAQUINE
- ▷ Atomoxetine: possible increased risk of convulsions when antidepressants given with ATOMOXETINE
- Dapoxetine: possible increased risk of serotonergic effects when duloxetine given with • DAPOXETINE (manufacturer of dapoxetine advises duloxetine should not be started until 1 week after stopping dapoxetine, avoid dapoxetine for 2 weeks after stopping duloxetine)
- ▷ 5HT$_1$-receptor Agonists: possible increased serotonergic effects when duloxetine given with 5HT$_1$ AGONISTS
- ▷ 5HT$_3$-receptor Antagonists: possible increased serotonergic effects when SSRI-related antidepressants given with 5HT$_3$ ANTAGONISTS
- Methylthioninium: risk of CNS toxicity when SSRI-related antidepressants given with • METHYLTHIONINIUM—avoid concomitant use (if avoidance not possible, use lowest possible dose of methylthioninium and observe patient for up to 4 hours after administration)

Dutasteride

- ▷ Calcium-channel Blockers: plasma concentration of dutasteride increased by DILTIAZEM and VERAPAMIL

Dydrogesterone see Progestogens

Edoxaban

- Analgesics: increased risk of bleeding when edoxaban given with • NSAIDS (manufacturer of edoxaban advises avoid long-term NSAIDs); increased risk of haemorrhage when anticoagulants given with intravenous • DICLOFENAC (avoid concomitant use, including low-dose heparins); increased risk of haemorrhage when anticoagulants given with • KETOROLAC (avoid concomitant use, including low-dose heparins); increased risk of bleeding when edoxaban given with high-dose • ASPIRIN (avoid concomitant use)
- ▷ Anti-arrhythmics: plasma concentration of edoxaban increased by • DRONEDARONE (reduce dose of edoxaban—see under Edoxaban, in BNF)
- Antibacterials: plasma concentration of edoxaban increased by • ERYTHROMYCIN (reduce dose of edoxaban—see under Edoxaban, in BNF); plasma concentration of edoxaban reduced by • RIFAMPICIN

Edoxaban (continued)

- Anticoagulants: increased risk of haemorrhage when edoxaban given with other • ANTICOAGULANTS (avoid concomitant use except when switching with other anticoagulants or using heparin to maintain catheter patency); increased risk of haemorrhage when other anticoagulants given with • APIXABAN, • DABIGATRAN and • RIVAROXABAN (avoid concomitant use except when switching with other anticoagulants or using heparin to maintain catheter patency)
- Antidepressants: plasma concentration of edoxaban possibly reduced by • ST JOHN'S WORT
- Antiepileptics: plasma concentration of edoxaban possibly reduced by • CARBAMAZEPINE, • FOSPHENYTOIN, • PHENOBARBITAL, • PHENYTOIN and • PRIMIDONE
- Antifungals: plasma concentration of edoxaban increased by • KETOCONAZOLE (reduce dose of edoxaban—see under Edoxaban, in BNF)
- ▷ Calcium-channel Blockers: plasma concentration of edoxaban increased by VERAPAMIL
- ▷ Ciclosporin: plasma concentration of edoxaban increased by • CICLOSPORIN (reduce dose of edoxaban—see under Edoxaban, in BNF)

Efavirenz

- ▷ Analgesics: efavirenz reduces plasma concentration of METHADONE
- Antibacterials: efavirenz reduces plasma concentration of CLARITHROMYCIN, also plasma concentration of active metabolite of clarithromycin increased; efavirenz reduces plasma concentration of RIFABUTIN—increase dose of rifabutin; plasma concentration of efavirenz reduced by RIFAMPICIN—increase dose of efavirenz; efavirenz possibly reduces plasma concentration of BEDAQUILINE—manufacturer of bedaquiline advises avoid concomitant use
- Anticoagulants: efavirenz possibly affects plasma concentration of • COUMARINS
- Antidepressants: plasma concentration of efavirenz reduced by • ST JOHN'S WORT—avoid concomitant use
- ▷ Antiepileptics: plasma concentration of both drugs reduced when efavirenz given with CARBAMAZEPINE
- Antifungals: efavirenz reduces plasma concentration of ITRACONAZOLE, • KETOCONAZOLE and • POSACONAZOLE; efavirenz reduces plasma concentration of • VORICONAZOLE, also plasma concentration of efavirenz increased (increase voriconazole dose and reduce efavirenz dose); efavirenz possibly reduces plasma concentration of CASPOFUNGIN—consider increasing dose of caspofungin
- Antimalarials: efavirenz reduces plasma concentration of • ARTEMETHER WITH LUMEFANTRINE; efavirenz possibly affects plasma concentration of PROGUANIL
- Antipsychotics: efavirenz possibly reduces plasma concentration of • ARIPIPRAZOLE (avoid concomitant use or consider increasing the dose of aripiprazole—consult aripiprazole product literature); efavirenz possibly increases plasma concentration of • PIMOZIDE (increased risk of ventricular arrhythmias—avoid concomitant use)
- Antivirals: avoidance of efavirenz advised by manufacturer of • ATAZANAVIR (plasma concentration of atazanavir reduced); efavirenz reduces the plasma concentration of • DACLATASVIR—increase dose of daclatasvir (see under Daclatasvir, in BNF); efavirenz reduces plasma concentration of • DARUNAVIR (adjust dose—consult product literature); avoidance of efavirenz advised by manufacturer of • DASABUVIR, ELVITEGRAVIR, OMBITASVIR and PARITAPREVIR; efavirenz reduces the plasma concentration of • DOLUTEGRAVIR (see under Dolutegravir, p. 387); efavirenz possibly reduces plasma concentration of • ETRAVIRINE—avoid concomitant use; efavirenz reduces plasma concentration of INDINAVIR and SIMEPREVIR; efavirenz reduces plasma concentration of • LOPINAVIR—consider increasing dose of lopinavir; efavirenz possibly reduces plasma concentration of • MARAVIROC—consider increasing dose of maraviroc; plasma concentration of efavirenz reduced by • NEVIRAPINE—avoid concomitant use; toxicity of efavirenz increased by • RITONAVIR, monitor liver function tests —manufacturer of Atripla® advises avoid concomitant use with high-dose ritonavir; efavirenz significantly reduces plasma concentration of SAQUINAVIR;

Efavirenz

- **Antivirals** (continued)
  efavirenz reduces plasma concentration of • TELAPREVIR—
  increase dose of telaprevir
- **Anxiolytics and Hypnotics:** increased risk of prolonged sedation
  when efavirenz given with • MIDAZOLAM—avoid concomitant
  use
- **Atovaquone:** efavirenz reduces plasma concentration of
  • ATOVAQUONE—avoid concomitant use
▷ **Avanafil:** efavirenz possibly reduces plasma concentration of
  AVANAFIL—manufacturer of avanafil advises avoid
  concomitant use
▷ **Bupropion:** efavirenz accelerates metabolism of BUPROPION
  (reduced plasma concentration)
▷ **Calcium-channel Blockers:** efavirenz reduces plasma
  concentration of DILTIAZEM
- **Ciclosporin:** efavirenz possibly reduces plasma concentration
  of • CICLOSPORIN
- **Cytotoxics:** efavirenz possibly reduces plasma concentration of
  • BOSUTINIB—manufacturer of bosutinib advises avoid
  concomitant use
- **Ergot Alkaloids:** increased risk of ergotism when efavirenz
  given with • ERGOT ALKALOIDS—avoid concomitant use
▷ **Grapefruit Juice:** plasma concentration of efavirenz possibly
  increased by GRAPEFRUIT JUICE
- **Guanfacine:** efavirenz possibly reduces plasma concentration
  of • GUANFACINE—increase dose of guanfacine
- **Lipid-regulating Drugs:** efavirenz reduces plasma concentration
  of ATORVASTATIN, PRAVASTATIN and SIMVASTATIN
- **Orlistat:** absorption of efavirenz possibly reduced by • ORLISTAT
- **Progestogens:** efavirenz possibly reduces contraceptive effect
  of • PROGESTOGENS
- **Tacrolimus:** efavirenz possibly affects plasma concentration of
  • TACROLIMUS

Eletriptan see 5HT₁-receptor Agonists (under HT)

Eltrombopag

▷ **Antacids:** absorption of eltrombopag reduced by ANTACIDS (give
  at least 4 hours apart)
▷ **Antivirals:** plasma concentration of eltrombopag possibly
  reduced by LOPINAVIR
▷ **Calcium Salts:** absorption of eltrombopag possibly reduced by
  CALCIUM SALTS (give at least 4 hours apart)
▷ **Dairy Products:** absorption of eltrombopag possibly reduced by
  DAIRY PRODUCTS (give at least 4 hours apart)
▷ **Iron Salts:** absorption of eltrombopag possibly reduced by *oral*
  IRON SALTS (give at least 4 hours apart)
- **Lipid-regulating Drugs:** eltrombopag increases plasma
  concentration of • ROSUVASTATIN—adjust dose of rosuvastatin
  (consult product literature)
▷ **Selenium:** absorption of eltrombopag possibly reduced by
  SELENIUM (give at least 4 hours apart)
▷ **Zinc:** absorption of eltrombopag possibly reduced by ZINC (give
  at least 4 hours apart)

Elvitegravir

▷ **Antacids:** absorption of elvitegravir reduced by ALUMINIUM
  HYDROXIDE and ORAL MAGNESIUM SALTS (give at least 4 hours
  apart)
- **Antibacterials:** plasma concentration of elvitegravir reduced by
  • RIFABUTIN also plasma concentration of active metabolite of
  rifabutin increased—reduce dose of rifabutin; manufacturer of
  elvitegravir advises avoid concomitant use with • RIFAMPICIN
- **Antidepressants:** manufacturer of elvitegravir advises avoid
  concomitant use with • ST JOHN'S WORT
- **Antiepileptics:** manufacturer of elvitegravir advises avoid
  concomitant use with • CARBAMAZEPINE, • FOSPHENYTOIN,
  • PHENOBARBITAL, • PHENYTOIN and • PRIMIDONE
- **Antivirals:** plasma concentration of elvitegravir increased by
  • ATAZANAVIR and • LOPINAVIR boosted with ritonavir (reduce
  dose of elvitegravir); manufacturer of elvitegravir advises
  avoid concomitant use with EFAVIRENZ and NEVIRAPINE
▷ **Bosentan:** manufacturer of elvitegravir advises avoid
  concomitant use with BOSENTAN
- **Orlistat:** absorption of elvitegravir possibly reduced by
  • ORLISTAT
▷ **Progestogens:** elvitegravir increases plasma concentration of
  NORGESTIMATE

Empagliflozin see Antidiabetics

Emtricitabine

- **Antivirals:** manufacturer of emtricitabine advises avoid
  concomitant use with LAMIVUDINE
- **Orlistat:** absorption of emtricitabine possibly reduced by
  • ORLISTAT

Enalapril see ACE Inhibitors

Enfuvirtide

- **Orlistat:** absorption of enfuvirtide possibly reduced by
  • ORLISTAT

Enoxaparin see Heparins

Enoximone see Phosphodiesterase Inhibitors

Entacapone

- **Anticoagulants:** entacapone enhances anticoagulant effect of
  • WARFARIN
- **Antidepressants:** manufacturer of entacapone advises caution
  with MOCLOBEMIDE, TRICYCLICS and VENLAFAXINE; avoid
  concomitant use of entacapone with non-selective • MAOIS
▷ **Dopaminergics:** entacapone possibly enhances effects of
  APOMORPHINE; entacapone possibly reduces plasma
  concentration of RASAGILINE; manufacturer of entacapone
  advises max. dose of 10 mg SELEGILINE if used concomitantly
▷ **Iron Salts:** absorption of entacapone reduced by *oral* IRON SALTS
▷ **Memantine:** effects of dopaminergics possibly enhanced by
  MEMANTINE
▷ **Methyldopa:** entacapone possibly enhances effects of
  METHYLDOPA; antiparkinsonian effect of dopaminergics
  antagonised by METHYLDOPA
▷ **Sympathomimetics:** entacapone possibly enhances effects of
  ADRENALINE (EPINEPHRINE), DOBUTAMINE, DOPAMINE and
  NORADRENALINE (NOREPINEPHRINE)

Enteral Feeds

- **Anticoagulants:** the presence of vitamin K in some enteral feeds
  can antagonise the anticoagulant effect of • COUMARINS and
  • PHENINDIONE
▷ **Antiepileptics:** enteral feeds possibly reduce absorption of
  FOSPHENYTOIN and PHENYTOIN

Enzalutamide

- **Anticoagulants:** enzalutamide possibly reduces plasma
  concentration of • COUMARINS
▷ **Antivirals:** avoidance of enzalutamide advised by manufacturer
  of DASABUVIR, OMBITASVIR and PARITAPREVIR
- **Anxiolytics and Hypnotics:** enzalutamide reduces plasma
  concentration of • MIDAZOLAM
- **Lipid-regulating Drugs:** plasma concentration of enzalutamide
  increased by • GEMFIBROZIL—manufacturer of enzalutamide
  advises avoid concomitant use or halve dose of enzalutamide
▷ **Ulcer-healing Drugs:** enzalutamide reduces plasma
  concentration of OMEPRAZOLE

Ephedrine see Sympathomimetics

Epinephrine

  NOTE Epinephrine interactions as for adrenaline, see under
  sympathomimetics

Epirubicin

- **Antipsychotics:** avoid concomitant use of cytotoxics with
  • CLOZAPINE (increased risk of agranulocytosis)
- **Ciclosporin:** plasma concentration of epirubicin increased by
  • CICLOSPORIN
- **Cytotoxics:** possible increased risk of cardiotoxicity when
  epirubicin given with • TRASTUZUMAB—avoid concomitant use
  for up to 28 weeks after stopping trastuzumab
- **Ulcer-healing Drugs:** plasma concentration of epirubicin
  increased by • CIMETIDINE
- **Vaccines:** risk of generalised infections when cytotoxic
  antibiotics given with live • VACCINES—avoid concomitant use

Eplerenone see Diuretics

Eprosartan see Angiotensin-II Receptor Antagonists

Eptifibatide

▷ **Iloprost:** increased risk of bleeding when eptifibatide given
  with ILOPROST

Ergocalciferol see Vitamins

Ergometrine see Ergot Alkaloids

Ergot Alkaloids

- **Antibacterials:** increased risk of ergotism when ergot alkaloids
  given with • CLARITHROMYCIN, • ERYTHROMYCIN or

Ergot Alkaloids

- **Antibacterials** (continued)
  - TELITHROMYCIN—avoid concomitant use; increased risk of ergotism when ergotamine given with TETRACYCLINES
- **Antidepressants:** possible risk of hypertension when ergotamine given with REBOXETINE
- **Antifungals:** avoidance of ergot alkaloids advised by manufacturer of • KETOCONAZOLE; avoidance of ergometrine advised by manufacturer of • ITRACONAZOLE (increased risk of ergotism); increased risk of ergotism when ergometrine given with • VORICONAZOLE—avoid concomitant use; increased risk of ergotism when ergotamine given with • IMIDAZOLES or • TRIAZOLES—avoid concomitant use
- **Antipsychotics:** plasma concentration of ergot alkaloids possibly increased by LURASIDONE (increased risk of toxicity)
- **Antivirals:** plasma concentration of ergot alkaloids possibly increased by • ATAZANAVIR—avoid concomitant use; avoidance of ergot alkaloids advised by manufacturer of • BOCEPREVIR and • TELAPREVIR; increased risk of ergotism when ergot alkaloids given with • DARUNAVIR—manufacturer of darunavir advises avoid concomitant use; increased risk of ergotism when ergot alkaloids given with • EFAVIRENZ or • RITONAVIR— avoid concomitant use; increased risk of ergotism when ergotamine given with • FOSAMPRENAVIR, • INDINAVIR or • SAQUINAVIR—avoid concomitant use; increased risk of ergotism when ergometrine given with INDINAVIR—avoid concomitant use
- **Beta-blockers:** increased peripheral vasoconstriction when ergot alkaloids given with BETA-BLOCKERS
- **Cobicistat:** plasma concentration of ergot alkaloids possibly increased by • COBICISTAT—manufacturer of cobicistat advises avoid concomitant use
- **Cytotoxics:** caution with ergot alkaloids advised by manufacturer of • CRIZOTINIB; avoidance of ergotamine advised by manufacturer of IDELALISIB
- **5HT₁-receptor Agonists:** increased risk of vasospasm when ergotamine given with • ALMOTRIPTAN, • RIZATRIPTAN, • SUMATRIPTAN or • ZOLMITRIPTAN (avoid ergotamine for 6 hours after almotriptan, rizatriptan, sumatriptan or zolmitriptan, avoid almotriptan, rizatriptan, sumatriptan or zolmitriptan for 24 hours after ergotamine); increased risk of vasospasm when ergotamine given with • ELETRIPTAN, • FROVATRIPTAN or • NARATRIPTAN (avoid ergotamine for 24 hours after eletriptan, frovatriptan or naratriptan, avoid eletriptan, frovatriptan or naratriptan for 24 hours after ergotamine)
- **Sympathomimetics:** increased risk of ergotism when ergot alkaloids given with SYMPATHOMIMETICS
- **Ticagrelor:** plasma concentration of ergot alkaloids possibly increased by • TICAGRELOR
- **Ulcer-healing Drugs:** increased risk of ergotism when ergotamine given with • CIMETIDINE—avoid concomitant use

Ergotamine *see* Ergot Alkaloids

Eribulin

- **Antibacterials:** plasma concentration of eribulin possibly reduced by RIFAMPICIN
- **Antidepressants:** plasma concentration of eribulin possibly reduced by ST JOHN'S WORT
- **Antiepileptics:** plasma concentration of eribulin possibly reduced by CARBAMAZEPINE, FOSPHENYTOIN and PHENYTOIN
- **Antipsychotics:** avoid concomitant use of cytotoxics with • CLOZAPINE (increased risk of agranulocytosis)

Erlotinib

- **Analgesics:** increased risk of bleeding when erlotinib given with • NSAIDS
- **Antacids:** plasma concentration of erlotinib possibly reduced by • ANTACIDS—give antacids at least 4 hours before or 2 hours after erlotinib
- **Antibacterials:** plasma concentration of erlotinib increased by CIPROFLOXACIN; metabolism of erlotinib accelerated by RIFAMPICIN (reduced plasma concentration)
- **Anticoagulants:** increased risk of bleeding when erlotinib given with • COUMARINS
- **Antifungals:** metabolism of erlotinib inhibited by KETOCONAZOLE (increased plasma concentration)

Erlotinib (continued)

- **Antipsychotics:** avoid concomitant use of cytotoxics with • CLOZAPINE (increased risk of agranulocytosis)
- **Antivirals:** avoidance of erlotinib advised by manufacturer of • BOCEPREVIR
- **Cytotoxics:** plasma concentration of erlotinib possibly increased by CAPECITABINE
- **Ulcer-healing Drugs:** manufacturer of erlotinib advises avoid concomitant use with • CIMETIDINE, • ESOMEPRAZOLE, • FAMOTIDINE, • LANSOPRAZOLE, • NIZATIDINE, • PANTOPRAZOLE and • RABEPRAZOLE; plasma concentration of erlotinib reduced by • RANITIDINE—manufacturer of erlotinib advises give at least 2 hours before or 10 hours after ranitidine; plasma concentration of erlotinib reduced by • OMEPRAZOLE— manufacturer of erlotinib advises avoid concomitant use

Ertapenem

- **Antiepileptics:** carbapenems reduce plasma concentration of • SODIUM VALPROATE and • VALPROIC ACID—avoid concomitant use
- **Vaccines:** antibacterials inactivate ORAL TYPHOID VACCINE—see under Typhoid Vaccine in BNFC

Erythromycin *see* Macrolides

Escitalopram *see* Antidepressants, SSRI

Eslicarbazepine

- **Anticoagulants:** eslicarbazepine reduces plasma concentration of WARFARIN
- **Antidepressants:** anticonvulsant effect of antiepileptics possibly antagonised by MAOIs and TRICYCLIC-RELATED ANTIDEPRESSANTS (convulsive threshold lowered); anticonvulsant effect of antiepileptics antagonised by • SSRIS and • TRICYCLICS (convulsive threshold lowered)
- **Antiepileptics:** plasma concentration of eslicarbazepine possibly reduced by CARBAMAZEPINE but risk of side-effects increased; plasma concentration of eslicarbazepine reduced by FOSPHENYTOIN and PHENYTOIN, also plasma concentration of fosphenytoin and phenytoin increased; manufacturer of eslicarbazepine advises avoid concomitant use with OXCARBAZEPINE
- **Antimalarials:** anticonvulsant effect of antiepileptics antagonised by • MEFLOQUINE
- **Antipsychotics:** anticonvulsant effect of antiepileptics antagonised by • ANTIPSYCHOTICS (convulsive threshold lowered)
- **Lipid-regulating Drugs:** eslicarbazepine reduces plasma concentration of ROSUVASTATIN; eslicarbazepine reduces plasma concentration of SIMVASTATIN—consider increasing dose of simvastatin
- **Oestrogens:** eslicarbazepine accelerates metabolism of • OESTROGENS (reduced contraceptive effect with combined oral contraceptives, contraceptive patches, and vaginal rings—see Contraceptive Interactions in BNFC)
- **Orlistat:** possible increased risk of convulsions when antiepileptics given with • ORLISTAT
- **Progestogens:** eslicarbazepine accelerates metabolism of • PROGESTOGENS (reduced contraceptive effect with combined oral contraceptives, progestogen-only oral contraceptives, contraceptive patches, vaginal rings, etonogestrel-releasing implant, and emergency hormonal contraception—see Contraceptive Interactions in BNFC)

Esmolol *see* Beta-blockers

Esomeprazole *see* Proton Pump Inhibitors

Estradiol *see* Oestrogens

Estramustine

- **Antacids:** absorption of estramustine possibly reduced by ALUMINIUM HYDROXIDE and ORAL MAGNESIUM SALTS— manufacturer of estramustine advises avoid concomitant administration
- **Antipsychotics:** avoid concomitant use of cytotoxics with • CLOZAPINE (increased risk of agranulocytosis)
- **Bisphosphonates:** plasma concentration of estramustine increased by • SODIUM CLODRONATE
- **Calcium Salts:** absorption of estramustine reduced by CALCIUM SALTS (manufacturer of estramustine advises avoid concomitant administration)

Estriol *see* Oestrogens

Estrone *see* Oestrogens

Etanercept

- Abatacept: avoid concomitant use of etanercept with
  - ● ABATACEPT
- Anakinra: avoid concomitant use of etanercept with
  - ● ANAKINRA
- Vaccines: risk of generalised infections when etanercept given with live ● VACCINES—avoid concomitant use

Ethambutol

- ▷ Antibacterials: plasma concentration of ethambutol increased by DELAMANID
- ▷ Vaccines: antibacterials inactivate ORAL TYPHOID VACCINE—see under Typhoid Vaccine in BNFC

Ethinylestradiol *see* Oestrogens

Ethosuximide

- Antibacterials: metabolism of ethosuximide inhibited by ● ISONIAZID (increased plasma concentration and risk of toxicity)
- Antidepressants: anticonvulsant effect of antiepileptics possibly antagonised by MAOIs and ● TRICYCLIC-RELATED ANTIDEPRESSANTS (convulsive threshold lowered); anticonvulsant effect of antiepileptics antagonised by ● SSRIS and ● TRICYCLICS (convulsive threshold lowered)
- Antiepileptics: plasma concentration of ethosuximide possibly reduced by CARBAMAZEPINE, PHENOBARBITAL and PRIMIDONE; plasma concentration of ethosuximide possibly reduced by ● FOSPHENYTOIN and ● PHENYTOIN, also plasma concentration of fosphenytoin and phenytoin possibly increased; plasma concentration of ethosuximide possibly increased by SODIUM VALPROATE and VALPROIC ACID
- Antimalarials: anticonvulsant effect of antiepileptics antagonised by ● MEFLOQUINE
- Antipsychotics: anticonvulsant effect of antiepileptics antagonised by ● ANTIPSYCHOTICS (convulsive threshold lowered)
- Orlistat: possible increased risk of convulsions when antiepileptics given with ● ORLISTAT

Etodolac *see* NSAIDs

Etomidate *see* Anaesthetics, General

Etonogestrel *see* Progestogens

Etoposide

- Anticoagulants: etoposide possibly enhances anticoagulant effect of ● COUMARINS
- ▷ Antiepileptics: plasma concentration of etoposide possibly reduced by FOSPHENYTOIN, PHENOBARBITAL, PHENYTOIN and PRIMIDONE
- ▷ Antifungals: plasma concentration of etoposide increased by KETOCONAZOLE
- Antipsychotics: avoid concomitant use of cytotoxics with ● CLOZAPINE (increased risk of agranulocytosis)
- ▷ Atovaquone: plasma concentration of etoposide possibly increased by ATOVAQUONE
- ▷ Ciclosporin: plasma concentration of etoposide possibly increased by CICLOSPORIN (increased risk of toxicity)
- ▷ Netupitant: plasma concentration of etoposide increased by NETUPITANT

Etoricoxib *see* NSAIDs

Etravirine

- Antibacterials: etravirine reduces plasma concentration of ● CLARITHROMYCIN (but concentration of an active metabolite increased), also plasma concentration of etravirine increased; plasma concentration of both drugs reduced when etravirine given with ● RIFABUTIN; manufacturer of etravirine advises avoid concomitant use with RIFAMPICIN; etravirine possibly reduces plasma concentration of BEDAQUILINE—manufacturer of bedaquiline advises avoid concomitant use
- ▷ Antidepressants: manufacturer of etravirine advises avoid concomitant use with ST JOHN'S WORT
- ▷ Antiepileptics: manufacturer of etravirine advises avoid concomitant use with CARBAMAZEPINE, FOSPHENYTOIN, PHENOBARBITAL, PHENYTOIN and PRIMIDONE
- Antimalarials: etravirine reduces plasma concentration of ARTEMETHER WITH LUMEFANTRINE
- Antivirals: effects of both drugs possibly reduced when etravirine given with BOCEPREVIR; avoidance of etravirine advised by manufacturer of DACLATASVIR (plasma concentration of daclatasvir possibly reduced); avoidance of

Etravirine

- Antivirals (continued)

  etravirine advised by manufacturer of DASABUVIR, OMBITASVIR, PARITAPREVIR and SIMEPREVIR; etravirine reduces the plasma concentration of ● DOLUTEGRAVIR (see under Dolutegravir, p. 387); plasma concentration of etravirine possibly reduced by ● EFAVIRENZ and ● NEVIRAPINE—avoid concomitant use; etravirine increases plasma concentration of ● FOSAMPRENAVIR (consider reducing dose of fosamprenavir); etravirine possibly reduces plasma concentration of ● INDINAVIR—avoid concomitant use; etravirine possibly reduces plasma concentration of MARAVIROC; plasma concentration of etravirine reduced by ● TIPRANAVIR, also plasma concentration of tipranavir increased (avoid concomitant use)
- ▷ Cardiac Glycosides: etravirine increases plasma concentration of DIGOXIN
- Clopidogrel: etravirine possibly reduces antiplatelet effect of ● CLOPIDOGREL
- Cytotoxics: etravirine possibly reduces plasma concentration of ● BOSUTINIB—manufacturer of bosutinib advises avoid concomitant use
- Guanfacine: etravirine possibly reduces plasma concentration of ● GUANFACINE—increase dose of guanfacine
- ▷ Lipid-regulating Drugs: etravirine possibly reduces plasma concentration of ATORVASTATIN
- Orlistat: absorption of etravirine possibly reduced by ● ORLISTAT
- ▷ Sildenafil: etravirine reduces plasma concentration of SILDENAFIL

Everolimus

- ACE Inhibitors: increased risk of angioedema when everolimus given with ● ACE INHIBITORS
- Antibacterials: plasma concentration of everolimus possibly increased by ● CLARITHROMYCIN and ● TELITHROMYCIN—manufacturer of everolimus advises avoid concomitant use; plasma concentration of everolimus increased by ● ERYTHROMYCIN (consider reducing the dose of everolimus—consult everolimus product literature); plasma concentration of everolimus reduced by ● RIFAMPICIN (avoid concomitant use or consider increasing the dose of everolimus—consult everolimus product literature)
- ▷ Antidepressants: plasma concentration of everolimus possibly reduced by ST JOHN'S WORT—manufacturer of everolimus advises avoid concomitant use
- Antifungals: plasma concentration of everolimus increased by ● KETOCONAZOLE—manufacturer of ketoconazole advises avoid concomitant use; plasma concentration of everolimus possibly increased by ● ITRACONAZOLE, ● POSACONAZOLE and ● VORICONAZOLE—manufacturer of everolimus advises avoid concomitant use
- Antipsychotics: avoid concomitant use of cytotoxics with ● CLOZAPINE (increased risk of agranulocytosis)
- Antivirals: plasma concentration of everolimus possibly increased by ● ATAZANAVIR, ● DARUNAVIR, ● INDINAVIR, ● RITONAVIR and ● SAQUINAVIR—manufacturer of everolimus advises avoid concomitant use
- Calcium-channel Blockers: plasma concentration of both drugs may increase when everolimus given with ● VERAPAMIL (consider reducing the dose of everolimus—consult everolimus product literature)
- Ciclosporin: plasma concentration of everolimus increased by ● CICLOSPORIN (consider reducing the dose of everolimus—consult everolimus product literature)
- Cytotoxics: plasma concentration of everolimus increased by ● IMATINIB (consider reducing the dose of everolimus—consult everolimus product literature)
- ▷ Grapefruit Juice: manufacturer of everolimus advises avoid concomitant use with GRAPEFRUIT JUICE

Exemestane

- ▷ Antibacterials: plasma concentration of exemestane possibly reduced by RIFAMPICIN

Exenatide *see* Antidiabetics

Ezetimibe

- ▷ Anticoagulants: ezetimibe possibly enhances anticoagulant effect of COUMARINS

Ezetimibe (continued)

- Ciclosporin: plasma concentration of both drugs may increase when ezetimibe given with •CICLOSPORIN
- Lipid-regulating Drugs: ezetimibe increases plasma concentration of •ROSUVASTATIN—adjust dose of rosuvastatin (consult product literature); increased risk of cholelithiasis and gallbladder disease when ezetimibe given with FIBRATES—discontinue if suspected

Famotidine see Histamine H₂-antagonists

Fampridine

- Ulcer-healing Drugs: manufacturer of fampridine advises avoid concomitant use with •CIMETIDINE

Febuxostat

- Azathioprine: manufacturer of febuxostat advises avoid concomitant use with •AZATHIOPRINE
- Cytotoxics: manufacturer of febuxostat advises avoid concomitant use with •MERCAPTOPURINE

Felodipine see Calcium-channel Blockers

Fenofibrate see Fibrates

Fenofen see NSAIDs

Fentanyl see Opioid Analgesics

Ferrous Fumarate see Iron salts

Ferrous Gluconate see Iron salts

Ferrous Sulfate see Iron salts

Fesoterodine see Antimuscarinics

Fexofenadine see Antihistamines

Fibrates

- Antibacterials: increased risk of myopathy when fibrates given with •DAPTOMYCIN (preferably avoid concomitant use)
- Anticoagulants: fibrates enhance anticoagulant effect of •COUMARINS and •PHENINDIONE
- Antidiabetics: fibrates may improve glucose tolerance and have an additive effect with INSULIN or SULFONYLUREAS; gemfibrozil possibly enhances hypoglycaemic effect of NATEGLINIDE; increased risk of severe hypoglycaemia when gemfibrozil given with •REPAGLINIDE—avoid concomitant use
- Antivirals: avoidance of gemfibrozil advised by manufacturer of DASABUVIR; gemfibrozil increases plasma concentration of •PARITAPREVIR—manufacturer of paritaprevir advises avoid concomitant use
- Ciclosporin: increased risk of renal impairment when bezafibrate or fenofibrate given with CICLOSPORIN
- Colchicine: possible increased risk of myopathy when fibrates given with •COLCHICINE
- Cytotoxics: gemfibrozil increases plasma concentration of DABRAFENIB; gemfibrozil increases plasma concentration of •BEXAROTENE—avoid concomitant use
- Hormone Antagonists: gemfibrozil increases plasma concentration of •ENZALUTAMIDE—manufacturer of enzalutamide advises avoid concomitant use or halve dose of enzalutamide
- Leukotriene Receptor Antagonists: gemfibrozil increases plasma concentration of MONTELUKAST
- Lipid-regulating Drugs: increased risk of myopathy when gemfibrozil given with •ATORVASTATIN, •FLUVASTATIN or •PRAVASTATIN (preferably avoid concomitant use); increased risk of myopathy when fibrates given with •ROSUVASTATIN (see under Rosuvastatin, p. 124); possible increased risk of myopathy when bezafibrate given with •SIMVASTATIN (see under Simvastatin, p. 125); possible increased risk of myopathy when ciprofibrate given with •SIMVASTATIN (see under Simvastatin, in BNF); increased risk of myopathy when gemfibrozil given with •SIMVASTATIN (avoid concomitant use); increased risk of cholelithiasis and gallbladder disease when fibrates given with EZETIMIBE—discontinue if suspected; increased risk of myopathy when fibrates given with •STATINS; reduce maximum dose of fenofibrate when given with STATINS—see under Fenofibrate, p. 122

Fidaxomicin

  Anti-arrhythmics: manufacturer of fidaxomicin advises avoid concomitant use with AMIODARONE and DRONEDARONE
  Antibacterials: manufacturer of fidaxomicin advises avoid concomitant use with CLARITHROMYCIN and ERYTHROMYCIN
  Antifungals: manufacturer of fidaxomicin advises avoid concomitant use with KETOCONAZOLE

Fidaxomicin (continued)

  ▸ Calcium-channel Blockers: manufacturer of fidaxomicin advises avoid concomitant use with VERAPAMIL
  ▸ Ciclosporin: manufacturer of fidaxomicin advises avoid concomitant use with CICLOSPORIN
  ▸ Vaccines: antibacterials inactivate ORAL TYPHOID VACCINE—see under Typhoid Vaccine in BNFC

Filgrastim

  ▸ Cytotoxics: neutropenia possibly exacerbated when filgrastim given with CAPECITABINE, FLUOROURACIL or TEGAFUR

Fingolimod

- Anti-arrhythmics: possible increased risk of bradycardia when fingolimod given with •AMIODARONE, •DISOPYRAMIDE or •DRONEDARONE
  ▸ Antidepressants: plasma concentration of fingolimod possibly reduced by ST JOHN'S WORT—manufacturer of fingolimod advises avoid concomitant use
  ▸ Antiepileptics: plasma concentration of fingolimod reduced by CARBAMAZEPINE
- Antifungals: plasma concentration of fingolimod increased by •KETOCONAZOLE
- Beta-blockers: possible increased risk of bradycardia when fingolimod given with •BETA-BLOCKERS
- Calcium-channel Blockers: possible increased risk of bradycardia when fingolimod given with •DILTIAZEM or •VERAPAMIL

Flavoxate see Antimuscarinics

Flecainide

  ▸ Anaesthetics, Local: increased myocardial depression when anti-arrhythmics given with BUPIVACAINE, LEVOBUPIVACAINE, PRILOCAINE or ROPIVACAINE
- Anti-arrhythmics: increased myocardial depression when anti-arrhythmics given with other •ANTI-ARRHYTHMICS; plasma concentration of flecainide increased by •AMIODARONE (halve dose of flecainide)
- Antidepressants: plasma concentration of flecainide increased by FLUOXETINE; increased risk of ventricular arrhythmias when flecainide given with •TRICYCLICS
- Antihistamines: increased risk of ventricular arrhythmias when flecainide given with •MIZOLASTINE—avoid concomitant use
- Antimalarials: avoidance of flecainide advised by manufacturer of •ARTEMETHER WITH LUMEFANTRINE (risk of ventricular arrhythmias); plasma concentration of flecainide increased by •QUININE
- Antimuscarinics: increased risk of ventricular arrhythmias when flecainide given with •TOLTERODINE
- Antipsychotics: increased risk of ventricular arrhythmias when anti-arrhythmics that prolong the QT interval given with •ANTIPSYCHOTICS that prolong the QT interval; increased risk of arrhythmias when flecainide given with •CLOZAPINE
- Antivirals: plasma concentration of flecainide possibly increased by •FOSAMPRENAVIR, •INDINAVIR, •LOPINAVIR and •RITONAVIR (increased risk of ventricular arrhythmias—avoid concomitant use); increased risk of ventricular arrhythmias when flecainide given with •SAQUINAVIR—avoid concomitant use; caution with flecainide advised by manufacturer of •TELAPREVIR (risk of ventricular arrhythmias)
- Beta-blockers: increased risk of myocardial depression and bradycardia when flecainide given with •BETA-BLOCKERS; increased myocardial depression when anti-arrhythmics given with •BETA-BLOCKERS
- Calcium-channel Blockers: increased risk of myocardial depression and asystole when flecainide given with •VERAPAMIL
- Diuretics: increased cardiac toxicity with flecainide if hypokalaemia occurs with •ACETAZOLAMIDE, •LOOP DIURETICS or •THIAZIDES AND RELATED DIURETICS
  ▸ Ulcer-healing Drugs: metabolism of flecainide inhibited by CIMETIDINE (increased plasma concentration)

Flucloxacillin see Penicillins

Fluconazole see Antifungals, Triazole

Flucytosine

  ▸ Antifungals: renal excretion of flucytosine decreased and cellular uptake increased by AMPHOTERICIN (toxicity possibly increased)
  ▸ Cytotoxics: plasma concentration of flucytosine possibly reduced by CYTARABINE

Fludarabine
- Antipsychotics: avoid concomitant use of cytotoxics with ● CLOZAPINE (increased risk of agranulocytosis)
- Cytotoxics: fludarabine increases intracellular concentration of CYTARABINE; increased pulmonary toxicity when fludarabine given with ● PENTOSTATIN (unacceptably high incidence of fatalities)
- ▹ Dipyridamole: effects of fludarabine possibly reduced by DIPYRIDAMOLE

Fludrocortisone see Corticosteroids

Fluorides
- ▹ Calcium Salts: absorption of fluorides reduced by CALCIUM SALTS

Fluorouracil
- ▹ Antibacterials: metabolism of fluorouracil inhibited by METRONIDAZOLE (increased toxicity)
- Anticoagulants: fluorouracil enhances anticoagulant effect of ● COUMARINS
- ▹ Antiepileptics: fluorouracil possibly inhibits metabolism of FOSPHENYTOIN and PHENYTOIN (increased risk of toxicity)
- Antipsychotics: avoid concomitant use of cytotoxics with ● CLOZAPINE (increased risk of agranulocytosis)
- Cytotoxics: avoidance of fluorouracil advised by manufacturer of ● PANITUMUMAB
- Filgrastim: neutropenia possibly exacerbated when fluorouracil given with FILGRASTIM
- Folates: toxicity of fluorouracil increased by ● FOLIC ACID—avoid concomitant use
- Lipegfilgrastim: neutropenia possibly exacerbated when fluorouracil given with LIPEGFILGRASTIM
- Pegfilgrastim: neutropenia possibly exacerbated when fluorouracil given with PEGFILGRASTIM
- Temoporfin: increased skin photosensitivity when *topical* fluorouracil used with ● TEMOPORFIN
- Ulcer-healing Drugs: metabolism of fluorouracil inhibited by CIMETIDINE (increased plasma concentration)

Fluoxetine see Antidepressants, SSRI

Flupentixol see Antipsychotics

Fluphenazine see Antipsychotics

Flurazepam see Anxiolytics and Hypnotics

Flurbiprofen see NSAIDs

Flutamide
- Anticoagulants: flutamide enhances anticoagulant effect of ● COUMARINS

Fluticasone see Corticosteroids

Fluvastatin see Statins

Fluvoxamine see Antidepressants, SSRI

Folates
- ▹ Aminosalicylates: absorption of folic acid possibly reduced by SULFASALAZINE
- ▹ Antacids: absorption of folic acid possibly reduced by ANTACIDS (manufacturer of folic acid advises give at least 2 hours apart)
- ▹ Antiepileptics: folates possibly reduce plasma concentration of FOSPHENYTOIN, PHENOBARBITAL, PHENYTOIN and PRIMIDONE
- Cytotoxics: folic acid increases toxicity of ● CAPECITABINE, ● FLUOROURACIL and ● TEGAFUR—avoid concomitant use; avoidance of folates advised by manufacturer of ● RALTITREXED; avoidance of folinic acid advised by manufacturer of ● PANITUMUMAB

Folic Acid see Folates

Folinic Acid see Folates

Fondaparinux
- Analgesics: increased risk of haemorrhage when anticoagulants given with *intravenous* ● DICLOFENAC (avoid concomitant use, including low-dose heparins); increased risk of haemorrhage when anticoagulants given with ● KETOROLAC (avoid concomitant use, including low-dose heparins)
- Anticoagulants: increased risk of haemorrhage when other anticoagulants given with ● APIXABAN, ● DABIGATRAN, ● EDOXABAN and ● RIVAROXABAN (avoid concomitant use except when switching with other anticoagulants or using heparin to maintain catheter patency)

Formoterol see Sympathomimetics, Beta₂

Fosamprenavir
- NOTE Fosamprenavir is a prodrug of amprenavir
- ▹ Analgesics: fosamprenavir reduces plasma concentration of METHADONE

Fosamprenavir (continued)
- Anti-arrhythmics: fosamprenavir possibly increases plasma concentration of ● AMIODARONE, ● FLECAINIDE and ● PROPAFENONE (increased risk of ventricular arrhythmias—avoid concomitant use); fosamprenavir possibly increases plasma concentration of ● LIDOCAINE—avoid concomitant use
- Antibacterials: fosamprenavir increases plasma concentration of ● RIFABUTIN (reduce dose of rifabutin); plasma concentration of fosamprenavir significantly reduced by ● RIFAMPICIN—avoid concomitant use; avoidance of concomitant fosamprenavir in severe renal and hepatic impairment advised by manufacturer of ● TELITHROMYCIN
- Anticoagulants: avoidance of fosamprenavir advised by manufacturer of APIXABAN and RIVAROXABAN; fosamprenavir may enhance or reduce anticoagulant effect of COUMARINS
- Antidepressants: plasma concentration of fosamprenavir reduced by ● ST JOHN'S WORT—avoid concomitant use
- ▹ Antiepileptics: plasma concentration of fosamprenavir possibly reduced by CARBAMAZEPINE, PHENOBARBITAL and PRIMIDONE
- Antifungals: fosamprenavir increases plasma concentration of KETOCONAZOLE (also plasma concentration of fosamprenavir possibly increased); plasma concentration of both drugs may increase when fosamprenavir given with ITRACONAZOLE; fosamprenavir possibly reduces plasma concentration of POSACONAZOLE
- Antimalarials: caution with fosamprenavir advised by manufacturer of ARTEMETHER WITH LUMEFANTRINE; fosamprenavir possibly increases plasma concentration of ● QUININE (increased risk of toxicity)
- ▹ Antimuscarinics: avoidance of fosamprenavir advised by manufacturer of DARIFENACIN and TOLTERODINE
- Antipsychotics: fosamprenavir possibly increases plasma concentration of ● ARIPIPRAZOLE (reduce dose of aripiprazole—consult aripiprazole product literature); fosamprenavir increases plasma concentration of ● PIMOZIDE (increased risk of ventricular arrhythmias—avoid concomitant use); fosamprenavir possibly increases plasma concentration of ● QUETIAPINE—manufacturer of quetiapine advises avoid concomitant use
- Antivirals: manufacturer of fosamprenavir advises avoid concomitant use with ● BOCEPREVIR and ● RALTEGRAVIR; fosamprenavir reduces plasma concentration of ● DOLUTEGRAVIR; plasma concentration of fosamprenavir increased by ● ETRAVIRINE (consider reducing dose of fosamprenavir); plasma concentration of fosamprenavir reduced by LOPINAVIR, effect on lopinavir plasma concentration not predictable—avoid concomitant use; plasma concentration of fosamprenavir reduced by ● MARAVIROC—avoid concomitant use; plasma concentration of fosamprenavir possibly reduced by NEVIRAPINE—avoid unboosted fosamprenavir; manufacturers advise avoid concomitant use of fosamprenavir with ● TELAPREVIR; plasma concentration of fosamprenavir reduced by ● TIPRANAVIR
- Anxiolytics and Hypnotics: fosamprenavir possibly increases plasma concentration of ● MIDAZOLAM (risk of prolonged sedation—avoid concomitant use of *oral* midazolam)
- Avanafil: fosamprenavir possibly increases plasma concentration of ● AVANAFIL—see under Avanafil, in BNF
- Ciclosporin: fosamprenavir increases plasma concentration of ● CICLOSPORIN
- Cytotoxics: fosamprenavir possibly increases the plasma concentration of ● BOSUTINIB—manufacturer of bosutinib advises avoid or consider reducing dose of bosutinib; fosamprenavir possibly increases the plasma concentration of ● IBRUTINIB—reduce dose of ibrutinib (see under Ibrutinib, in BNF)
- ▹ Dapoxetine: manufacturer of dapoxetine advises dose reduction when fosamprenavir given with DAPOXETINE (see under Dapoxetine, in BNF)
- Ergot Alkaloids: increased risk of ergotism when fosamprenavir given with ● ERGOTAMINE—avoid concomitant use
- ▹ Guanfacine: fosamprenavir possibly increases plasma concentration of GUANFACINE (halve dose of guanfacine)
- Lipid-regulating Drugs: possible increased risk of myopathy when fosamprenavir given with ATORVASTATIN; possible increased risk of myopathy when fosamprenavir given with

Fosamprenavir
- **Lipid-regulating Drugs** (continued)
  - ROSUVASTATIN—manufacturer of rosuvastatin advises avoid concomitant use; possible increased risk of myopathy when fosamprenavir given with ● SIMVASTATIN—avoid concomitant use; avoidance of fosamprenavir advised by manufacturer of ● LOMITAPIDE (plasma concentration of lomitapide possibly increased)
- Orlistat: absorption of fosamprenavir possibly reduced by ● ORLISTAT
- Ranolazine: fosamprenavir possibly increases plasma concentration of ● RANOLAZINE—manufacturer of ranolazine advises avoid concomitant use
- Sildenafil: fosamprenavir possibly increases plasma concentration of SILDENAFIL
- Tacrolimus: fosamprenavir increases plasma concentration of ● TACROLIMUS
- Tadalafil: fosamprenavir possibly increases plasma concentration of TADALAFIL
- Vardenafil: fosamprenavir possibly increases plasma concentration of VARDENAFIL

Fosaprepitant
- Antibacterials: plasma concentration of fosaprepitant possibly increased by CLARITHROMYCIN and TELITHROMYCIN; plasma concentration of fosaprepitant reduced by RIFAMPICIN
- Anticoagulants: fosaprepitant possibly reduces anticoagulant effect of WARFARIN
- Antidepressants: manufacturer of fosaprepitant advises avoid concomitant use with ● ST JOHN'S WORT
- Antidiabetics: fosaprepitant reduces plasma concentration of TOLBUTAMIDE
- Antiepileptics: plasma concentration of fosaprepitant possibly reduced by CARBAMAZEPINE, FOSPHENYTOIN, PHENOBARBITAL, PHENYTOIN and PRIMIDONE
- Antifungals: plasma concentration of fosaprepitant increased by KETOCONAZOLE
- Antipsychotics: manufacturer of fosaprepitant advises avoid concomitant use with ● PIMOZIDE
- Antivirals: plasma concentration of fosaprepitant possibly increased by RITONAVIR
- Anxiolytics and Hypnotics: fosaprepitant increases plasma concentration of MIDAZOLAM (risk of prolonged sedation)
- Avanafil: fosaprepitant possibly increases plasma concentration of AVANAFIL
- Calcium-channel Blockers: plasma concentration of both drugs may increase when fosaprepitant given with DILTIAZEM
- Corticosteroids: fosaprepitant inhibits metabolism of DEXAMETHASONE and METHYLPREDNISOLONE (reduce dose of dexamethasone and methylprednisolone)
- Cytotoxics: fosaprepitant possibly increases the plasma concentration of ● BOSUTINIB—manufacturer of bosutinib advises avoid or consider reducing dose of bosutinib; fosaprepitant possibly increases plasma concentration of IBRUTINIB
- Guanfacine: fosaprepitant possibly increases plasma concentration of GUANFACINE (halve dose of guanfacine)
- Lipid-regulating Drugs: separating administration from fosaprepitant by 12 hours advised by manufacturer of LOMITAPIDE
- Oestrogens: fosaprepitant possibly causes contraceptive failure of hormonal contraceptives containing ● OESTROGENS (alternative contraception recommended)
- Progestogens: fosaprepitant possibly causes contraceptive failure of hormonal contraceptives containing ● PROGESTOGENS (alternative contraception recommended)

Foscarnet
- Pentamidine Isetionate: increased risk of hypocalcaemia when foscarnet given with *parenteral* ● PENTAMIDINE ISETIONATE

Fosfomycin
- Metoclopramide: plasma concentration of fosfomycin reduced by METOCLOPRAMIDE
- Vaccines: antibacterials inactivate ORAL TYPHOID VACCINE—see under Typhoid Vaccine in BNFC

Fosinopril *see* ACE Inhibitors

Fosphenytoin
- Alcohol: plasma concentration of fosphenytoin possibly reduced by chronic heavy consumption of ALCOHOL
- Aminophylline: plasma concentration of both drugs reduced when fosphenytoin given with ● AMINOPHYLLINE
- Analgesics: excretion of fosphenytoin possibly reduced by ACEMETACIN (increased risk of toxicity); fosphenytoin possibly accelerates metabolism of FENTANYL (reduced effect); fosphenytoin accelerates metabolism of METHADONE (reduced effect and risk of withdrawal effects); fosphenytoin possibly increases risk of ● PETHIDINE toxicity; effects of fosphenytoin enhanced by ASPIRIN; fosphenytoin possibly accelerates metabolism of PARACETAMOL (also isolated reports of hepatotoxicity)
- Antacids: absorption of fosphenytoin reduced by ANTACIDS
- Anthelmintics: fosphenytoin reduces plasma concentration of ● ALBENDAZOLE and ● PRAZIQUANTEL—consider increasing albendazole and praziquantel dose when given for systemic infections; plasma concentration of fosphenytoin possibly increased by LEVAMISOLE
- Anti-arrhythmics: metabolism of fosphenytoin inhibited by ● AMIODARONE (increased plasma concentration); fosphenytoin reduces plasma concentration of DISOPYRAMIDE; fosphenytoin possibly reduces plasma concentration of ● DRONEDARONE—avoid concomitant use
- Antibacterials: metabolism of fosphenytoin inhibited by CLARITHROMYCIN (increased plasma concentration); metabolism of fosphenytoin possibly inhibited by METRONIDAZOLE (increased plasma concentration); plasma concentration of fosphenytoin increased or decreased by CIPROFLOXACIN; fosphenytoin accelerates metabolism of DOXYCYCLINE (reduced plasma concentration); fosphenytoin possibly reduces plasma concentration of ● BEDAQUILINE—manufacturer of bedaquiline advises avoid concomitant use; plasma concentration of fosphenytoin increased by ● CHLORAMPHENICOL (increased risk of toxicity); metabolism of fosphenytoin possibly inhibited by ISONIAZID (increased risk of toxicity); metabolism of fosphenytoin accelerated by ● RIFAMYCINS (reduced plasma concentration); plasma concentration of fosphenytoin possibly increased by SULFONAMIDES; fosphenytoin reduces plasma concentration of ● TELITHROMYCIN (avoid during and for 2 weeks after fosphenytoin); plasma concentration of fosphenytoin increased by ● TRIMETHOPRIM (also increased antifolate effect)
- Anticoagulants: fosphenytoin possibly reduces plasma concentration of ● APIXABAN and ● EDOXABAN; fosphenytoin accelerates metabolism of ● COUMARINS (possibility of reduced anticoagulant effect, but enhancement also reported); fosphenytoin possibly reduces plasma concentration of DABIGATRAN—manufacturer of dabigatran advises avoid concomitant use; fosphenytoin possibly reduces plasma concentration of ● RIVAROXABAN—manufacturer of rivaroxaban advises monitor for signs of thrombosis
- Antidepressants: plasma concentration of fosphenytoin increased by ● FLUOXETINE and ● FLUVOXAMINE; fosphenytoin reduces plasma concentration of ● MIANSERIN, MIRTAZAPINE and PAROXETINE; plasma concentration of fosphenytoin possibly increased by SERTRALINE, also plasma concentration of sertraline possibly reduced; anticonvulsant effect of antiepileptics possibly antagonised by MAOIs and ● TRICYCLIC-RELATED ANTIDEPRESSANTS (convulsive threshold lowered); anticonvulsant effect of antiepileptics antagonised by ● SSRIS and ● TRICYCLICS (convulsive threshold lowered); plasma concentration of fosphenytoin possibly reduced by ● ST JOHN'S WORT—avoid concomitant use; fosphenytoin possibly reduces plasma concentration of ● TRICYCLICS; fosphenytoin possibly reduces plasma concentration of ● VORTIOXETINE—consider increasing dose of vortioxetine
- Antidiabetics: plasma concentration of fosphenytoin transiently increased by TOLBUTAMIDE (possibility of toxicity)
- Antiepileptics: plasma concentration of both drugs often reduced when fosphenytoin given with CARBAMAZEPINE, also plasma concentration of fosphenytoin may be increased; fosphenytoin reduces plasma concentration of ESLICARBAZEPINE, also plasma concentration of fosphenytoin increased; plasma concentration of fosphenytoin possibly

Fosphenytoin

- **Antiepileptics** (continued)
increased by ● ETHOSUXIMIDE, also plasma concentration of ethosuximide possibly reduced; fosphenytoin reduces plasma concentration of LAMOTRIGINE, TIAGABINE and ZONISAMIDE; plasma concentration of fosphenytoin increased by OXCARBAZEPINE, also plasma concentration of an active metabolite of oxcarbazepine reduced; fosphenytoin reduces plasma concentration of ● PERAMPANEL (see under Perampanel, p. 193); fosphenytoin often increases plasma concentration of PHENOBARBITAL and PRIMIDONE, plasma concentration of fosphenytoin often reduced but may be increased; fosphenytoin possibly reduces plasma concentration of RETIGABINE; fosphenytoin possibly reduces plasma concentration of RUFINAMIDE, also plasma concentration of fosphenytoin possibly increased; plasma concentration of fosphenytoin increased or possibly reduced when given with SODIUM VALPROATE and VALPROIC ACID, also plasma concentration of sodium valproate and valproic acid reduced; plasma concentration of fosphenytoin increased by ● STIRIPENTOL; plasma concentration of fosphenytoin increased by ● TOPIRAMATE (also plasma concentration of topiramate reduced); plasma concentration of fosphenytoin reduced by VIGABATRIN
- **Antifungals:** fosphenytoin reduces plasma concentration of ● KETOCONAZOLE and ● POSACONAZOLE; anticonvulsant effect of fosphenytoin enhanced by ● MICONAZOLE (plasma concentration of fosphenytoin increased); plasma concentration of fosphenytoin increased by ● FLUCONAZOLE (consider reducing dose of fosphenytoin); fosphenytoin reduces plasma concentration of ● ITRACONAZOLE—avoid concomitant use; plasma concentration of fosphenytoin increased by ● VORICONAZOLE, also fosphenytoin reduces plasma concentration of voriconazole (increase dose of voriconazole and also monitor for fosphenytoin toxicity); fosphenytoin possibly reduces plasma concentration of CASPOFUNGIN—consider increasing dose of caspofungin
- **Antimalarials:** avoidance of fosphenytoin advised by manufacturer of ARTENIMOL WITH PIPERAQUINE; anticonvulsant effect of antiepileptics antagonised by ● MEFLOQUINE; anticonvulsant effect of fosphenytoin antagonised by ● PYRIMETHAMINE, also increased antifolate effect
- **Antipsychotics:** anticonvulsant effect of antiepileptics antagonised by ● ANTIPSYCHOTICS (convulsive threshold lowered); fosphenytoin reduces plasma concentration of HALOPERIDOL; plasma concentration of fosphenytoin possibly increased or decreased by CHLORPROMAZINE; fosphenytoin possibly reduces plasma concentration of ● ARIPIPRAZOLE (avoid concomitant use or consider increasing the dose of aripiprazole—consult aripiprazole product literature); fosphenytoin accelerates metabolism of CLOZAPINE and QUETIAPINE (reduced plasma concentration); fosphenytoin possibly reduces plasma concentration of ● LURASIDONE—avoid concomitant use
- **Antivirals:** fosphenytoin possibly reduces plasma concentration of ABACAVIR, DARUNAVIR, LOPINAVIR and SAQUINAVIR; avoidance of fosphenytoin advised by manufacturer of ● BOCEPREVIR and ● RILPIVIRINE (plasma concentration of boceprevir and rilpivirine possibly reduced); fosphenytoin possibly reduces plasma concentration of ● DACLATASVIR and ● SIMEPREVIR—manufacturer of daclatasvir and simeprevir advises avoid concomitant use; fosphenytoin possibly reduces plasma concentration of ● DASABUVIR, ● OMBITASVIR and ● PARITAPREVIR—avoid concomitant use; fosphenytoin possibly reduces the plasma concentration of ● DOLUTEGRAVIR (see under Dolutegravir, p. 387); avoidance of fosphenytoin advised by manufacturer of ● ELVITEGRAVIR, ETRAVIRINE, LEDIPASVIR, SOFOSBUVIR and ● TELAPREVIR; fosphenytoin possibly reduces plasma concentration of ● INDINAVIR, also plasma concentration of fosphenytoin possibly increased; fosphenytoin possibly reduces plasma concentration of RITONAVIR, also plasma concentration of fosphenytoin possibly affected; plasma concentration of fosphenytoin increased or decreased by ZIDOVUDINE
- **Anxiolytics and Hypnotics:** fosphenytoin often reduces plasma concentration of CLONAZEPAM; plasma concentration of

Fosphenytoin

Anxiolytics and Hypnotics (continued)
fosphenytoin increased or decreased by DIAZEPAM; plasma concentration of fosphenytoin possibly increased or decreased by BENZODIAZEPINES
- **Aprepitant:** fosphenytoin possibly reduces plasma concentration of APREPITANT
- **Bupropion:** fosphenytoin reduces plasma concentration of BUPROPION
- **Caffeine citrate:** fosphenytoin reduces plasma concentration of CAFFEINE CITRATE
- **Calcium-channel Blockers:** fosphenytoin reduces effects of FELODIPINE and VERAPAMIL; avoidance of fosphenytoin advised by manufacturer of ISRADIPINE; avoidance of fosphenytoin advised by manufacturer of NIMODIPINE (plasma concentration of nimodipine possibly reduced); plasma concentration of fosphenytoin increased by ● DILTIAZEM but also effect of diltiazem reduced
- **Cannabis Extract:** fosphenytoin possibly reduces plasma concentration of ● CANNABIS EXTRACT—manufacturer of cannabis extract advises avoid concomitant use
- **Cardiac Glycosides:** fosphenytoin possibly reduces plasma concentration of DIGOXIN
- **Ciclosporin:** fosphenytoin accelerates metabolism of ● CICLOSPORIN (reduced plasma concentration)
- **Cobicistat:** fosphenytoin possibly reduces plasma concentration of ● COBICISTAT—manufacturer of cobicistat advises avoid concomitant use
- **Corticosteroids:** fosphenytoin accelerates metabolism of ● CORTICOSTEROIDS (reduced effect)
- **Cytotoxics:** fosphenytoin possibly reduces plasma concentration of BUSULFAN, ERIBULIN and ETOPOSIDE; metabolism of fosphenytoin possibly inhibited by CAPECITABINE, FLUOROURACIL and TEGAFUR (increased risk of toxicity); fosphenytoin increases antifolate effect of METHOTREXATE; plasma concentration of fosphenytoin possibly reduced by CISPLATIN; fosphenytoin possibly decreases plasma concentration of AXITINIB (increase dose of axitinib—consult axitinib product literature); fosphenytoin possibly reduces plasma concentration of BORTEZOMIB, ● BOSUTINIB, CRIZOTINIB, ● IBRUTINIB, ● IDELALISIB and PONATINIB—manufacturer of bortezomib, bosutinib, crizotinib, ibrutinib, idelalisib and ponatinib advises avoid concomitant use; fosphenytoin possibly reduces plasma concentration of ● CABOZANTINIB—avoid concomitant use; avoidance of fosphenytoin advised by manufacturer of ● CABAZITAXEL, DABRAFENIB, GEFITINIB, ● LAPATINIB and VEMURAFENIB; avoidance of fosphenytoin advised by manufacturer of DASATINIB and ● VISMODEGIB (plasma concentration of dasatinib and vismodegib possibly reduced); fosphenytoin reduces plasma concentration of ● IMATINIB—avoid concomitant use; fosphenytoin reduces plasma concentration of IRINOTECAN and its active metabolite; manufacturer of procarbazine advises possible increased risk of hypersensitivity reactions when fosphenytoin given with PROCARBAZINE
- **Dexrazoxane:** absorption of fosphenytoin possibly reduced by ● DEXRAZOXANE
- **Diazoxide:** plasma concentration of fosphenytoin reduced by DIAZOXIDE, also effect of diazoxide may be reduced
- **Disulfiram:** metabolism of fosphenytoin inhibited by ● DISULFIRAM (increased risk of toxicity)
- **Diuretics:** plasma concentration of fosphenytoin possibly increased by ● ACETAZOLAMIDE; fosphenytoin antagonises effects of FUROSEMIDE; fosphenytoin reduces plasma concentration of ● EPLERENONE—avoid concomitant use; increased risk of osteomalacia when fosphenytoin given with CARBONIC ANHYDRASE INHIBITORS
- **Dopaminergics:** fosphenytoin possibly reduces effects of CO-BENELDOPA, CO-CARELDOPA and LEVODOPA
- **Enteral Feeds:** absorption of fosphenytoin possibly reduced by ENTERAL FEEDS
- **Folates:** plasma concentration of fosphenytoin possibly reduced by FOLATES
- **Fosaprepitant:** fosphenytoin possibly reduces plasma concentration of FOSAPREPITANT

Fosphenytoin (continued)

- Hormone Antagonists: fosphenytoin possibly reduces plasma concentration of ● ABIRATERONE—manufacturer of abiraterone advises avoid concomitant use; fosphenytoin possibly accelerates metabolism of TOREMIFENE
- 5HT₃-receptor Antagonists: fosphenytoin accelerates metabolism of ONDANSETRON (reduced effect)
- Ivacaftor: fosphenytoin possibly reduces plasma concentration of ● IVACAFTOR—manufacturer of ivacaftor advises avoid concomitant use
- Leflunomide: plasma concentration of fosphenytoin possibly increased by LEFLUNOMIDE
- Lipid-regulating Drugs: absorption of fosphenytoin possibly reduced by COLESEVELAM; combination of fosphenytoin with FLUVASTATIN may increase plasma concentration of either drug (or both)
- Lithium: neurotoxicity may occur when fosphenytoin given with LITHIUM without increased plasma concentration of lithium
- Macitentan: avoidance of fosphenytoin advised by manufacturer of MACITENTAN
- Modafinil: plasma concentration of fosphenytoin possibly increased by MODAFINIL
- Muscle Relaxants: *long-term use* of fosphenytoin reduces effects of ● NON-DEPOLARISING MUSCLE RELAXANTS (but *acute use* of fosphenytoin might increase effects of non-depolarising muscle relaxants)
- Oestrogens: fosphenytoin accelerates metabolism of ● OESTROGENS (reduced contraceptive effect with combined oral contraceptives, contraceptive patches, and vaginal rings—see Contraceptive Interactions in BNFC)
- Orlistat: possible increased risk of convulsions when antiepileptics given with ● ORLISTAT
- Progestogens: fosphenytoin accelerates metabolism of ● PROGESTOGENS (reduced contraceptive effect with combined oral contraceptives, progestogen-only oral contraceptives, contraceptive patches, vaginal rings, etonogestrel-releasing implant, and emergency hormonal contraception—see Contraceptive Interactions in BNFC)
- Roflumilast: fosphenytoin possibly inhibits effects of ROFLUMILAST (manufacturer of roflumilast advises avoid concomitant use)
- Sulfinpyrazone: plasma concentration of fosphenytoin increased by ● SULFINPYRAZONE
- Sympathomimetics: plasma concentration of fosphenytoin increased by METHYLPHENIDATE
- Tacrolimus: fosphenytoin reduces plasma concentration of TACROLIMUS, also plasma concentration of fosphenytoin possibly increased
- Theophylline: plasma concentration of both drugs reduced when fosphenytoin given with ● THEOPHYLLINE
- Thyroid Hormones: fosphenytoin accelerates metabolism of THYROID HORMONES (may increase requirements in hypothyroidism), also plasma concentration of fosphenytoin possibly increased
- Tibolone: fosphenytoin accelerates metabolism of TIBOLONE
- Ticagrelor: fosphenytoin possibly reduces plasma concentration of TICAGRELOR
- Ulcer-healing Drugs: metabolism of fosphenytoin inhibited by ● CIMETIDINE (increased plasma concentration); effects of fosphenytoin enhanced by ● ESOMEPRAZOLE; effects of fosphenytoin possibly enhanced by OMEPRAZOLE; absorption of fosphenytoin reduced by ● SUCRALFATE
- Uliprostal: avoidance of fosphenytoin advised by manufacturer of ● ULIPRISTAL (contraceptive effect of ulipristal possibly reduced)

Vaccines: effects of fosphenytoin enhanced by INFLUENZA VACCINE

Vitamins: fosphenytoin possibly increases requirements for ALFACALCIDOL, CALCITRIOL, COLECALCIFEROL, DIHYDROTACHYSTEROL, ERGOCALCIFEROL, PARICALCITOL or VITAMIN D

rovatriptan see 5HT₁-receptor Agonists (under HT)
urosemide see Diuretics

Fusidic Acid
- Antivirals: plasma concentration of both drugs increased when fusidic acid given with ● RITONAVIR—avoid concomitant use; plasma concentration of both drugs may increase when fusidic acid given with SAQUINAVIR
- Lipid-regulating Drugs: risk of myopathy and rhabdomyolysis when fusidic acid given with ● STATINS—avoid concomitant use and for 7 days after last fusidic acid dose
- Sugammadex: fusidic acid possibly reduces response to SUGAMMADEX
- Vaccines: antibacterials inactivate ORAL TYPHOID VACCINE—see under Typhoid Vaccine in BNFC

Gabapentin
- Analgesics: bioavailability of gabapentin increased by MORPHINE
- Antacids: absorption of gabapentin reduced by ANTACIDS
- Antidepressants: anticonvulsant effect of antiepileptics possibly antagonised by MAOIs and ● TRICYCLIC-RELATED ANTIDEPRESSANTS (convulsive threshold lowered); anticonvulsant effect of antiepileptics antagonised by ● SSRIS and ● TRICYCLICS (convulsive threshold lowered)
- Antimalarials: anticonvulsant effect of antiepileptics antagonised by ● MEFLOQUINE
- Antipsychotics: anticonvulsant effect of antiepileptics antagonised by ● ANTIPSYCHOTICS (convulsive threshold lowered)
- Orlistat: possible increased risk of convulsions when antiepileptics given with ● ORLISTAT

Galantamine see Parasympathomimetics

Ganciclovir

NOTE Increased risk of myelosuppression with other myelosuppressive drugs—consult product literature
- Antibacterials: increased risk of convulsions when ganciclovir given with ● IMIPENEM with CILASTATIN
- Antivirals: ganciclovir possibly increases plasma concentration of DIDANOSINE; profound myelosuppression when ganciclovir given with ● ZIDOVUDINE (if possible avoid concomitant administration, particularly during initial ganciclovir therapy)
- Mycophenolate: plasma concentration of ganciclovir possibly increased by MYCOPHENOLATE, also plasma concentration of inactive metabolite of mycophenolate possibly increased
- Tacrolimus: possible increased risk of nephrotoxicity when ganciclovir given with TACROLIMUS

Gefitinib
- Antibacterials: plasma concentration of gefitinib reduced by ● RIFAMPICIN—avoid concomitant use
- Anticoagulants: gefitinib possibly enhances anticoagulant effect of ● WARFARIN
- Antidepressants: manufacturer of gefitinib advises avoid concomitant use with ST JOHN'S WORT
- Antiepileptics: manufacturer of gefitinib advises avoid concomitant use with CARBAMAZEPINE, FOSPHENYTOIN, PHENOBARBITAL, PHENYTOIN and PRIMIDONE
- Antifungals: plasma concentration of gefitinib increased by ITRACONAZOLE
- Antipsychotics: avoid concomitant use of cytotoxics with ● CLOZAPINE (increased risk of agranulocytosis)
- Antivirals: avoidance of gefitinib advised by manufacturer of ● BOCEPREVIR
- Ulcer-healing Drugs: plasma concentration of gefitinib reduced by ● RANITIDINE

Gemcitabine
- Anticoagulants: gemcitabine possibly enhances anticoagulant effect of WARFARIN
- Antipsychotics: avoid concomitant use of cytotoxics with ● CLOZAPINE (increased risk of agranulocytosis)

Gemeprost see Prostaglandins
Gemfibrozil see Fibrates
Gentamicin see Aminoglycosides
Gestodene see Progestogens
Glibenclamide see Antidiabetics
Gliclazide see Antidiabetics
Glimepiride see Antidiabetics
Glipizide see Antidiabetics

Glucosamine
- Anticoagulants: glucosamine enhances anticoagulant effect of
  - WARFARIN (avoid concomitant use)

Glyceryl Trinitrate see Nitrates

Glycopyrronium see Antimuscarinics

Gold
  NOTE see Sodium Aurothiomalate

Golimumab
- Abatacept: avoid concomitant use of golimumab with
  - ABATACEPT
- Anakinra: avoid concomitant use of golimumab with
  - ANAKINRA
- Antipsychotics: avoid concomitant use of cytotoxics with
  - CLOZAPINE (increased risk of agranulocytosis)
- Vaccines: risk of generalised infections when monoclonal antibodies given with live • VACCINES—avoid concomitant use

Granisetron see 5HT$_3$-receptor Antagonists (under HT)

Grapefruit Juice
- Aliskiren: grapefruit juice reduces plasma concentration of
  - ALISKIREN—avoid concomitant use
- Anthelmintics: grapefruit juice increases plasma concentration of active metabolite of ALBENDAZOLE; grapefruit juice increases plasma concentration of PRAZIQUANTEL
- Anti-arrhythmics: grapefruit juice increases plasma concentration of AMIODARONE; grapefruit juice increases plasma concentration of • DRONEDARONE—avoid concomitant use
- Antidepressants: grapefruit juice possibly increases plasma concentration of SERTRALINE
- Antihistamines: grapefruit juice reduces plasma concentration of BILASTINE
- Antimalarials: grapefruit juice possibly increases plasma concentration of ARTEMETHER WITH LUMEFANTRINE; avoidance of grapefruit juice advised by manufacturer of ARTENIMOL WITH PIPERAQUINE
- Antipsychotics: avoidance of grapefruit juice advised by manufacturer of LURASIDONE and PIMOZIDE; grapefruit juice possibly increases plasma concentration of • QUETIAPINE—manufacturer of quetiapine advises avoid concomitant use
- Antivirals: grapefruit juice possibly increases plasma concentration of EFAVIRENZ
- Anxiolytics and Hypnotics: grapefruit juice possibly increases plasma concentration of *oral* MIDAZOLAM; grapefruit juice increases plasma concentration of BUSPIRONE
- Avanafil: grapefruit juice possibly increases plasma concentration of • AVANAFIL— manufacturer of avanafil advises avoid grapefruit juice for 24 hours before avanafil
- Calcium-channel Blockers: grapefruit juice possibly increases plasma concentration of AMLODIPINE; grapefruit juice increases plasma concentration of FELODIPINE, ISRADIPINE, LACIDIPINE, LERCANIDIPINE, NICARDIPINE, NIFEDIPINE, NIMODIPINE and VERAPAMIL
- Ciclosporin: grapefruit juice increases plasma concentration of • CICLOSPORIN (increased risk of toxicity)
- Colchicine: grapefruit juice possibly increases risk of
  - COLCHICINE toxicity
- Corticosteroids: grapefruit juice increases plasma concentration of *oral* • BUDESONIDE—avoid concurrent use or separate administration by as much as possible and consider reducing *oral* budesonide dose
- Cytotoxics: grapefruit juice possibly increases plasma concentration of AXITINIB, CABOZANTINIB and PONATINIB; grapefruit juice possibly increases the plasma concentration of • BOSUTINIB—manufacturer of bosutinib advises avoid or consider reducing dose of bosutinib; grapefruit juice possibly increases plasma concentration of CRIZOTINIB and VINFLUNINE—manufacturer of crizotinib and vinflunine advises avoid concomitant use; avoidance of grapefruit juice advised by manufacturer of DASATINIB (plasma concentration of dasatinib possibly increased); avoidance of grapefruit juice advised by manufacturer of EVEROLIMUS, IBRUTINIB, • LAPATINIB, • NILOTINIB and • PAZOPANIB
- Guanfacine: avoidance of grapefruit juice advised by manufacturer of GUANFACINE
- Ivabradine: grapefruit juice increases plasma concentration of IVABRADINE

Grapefruit Juice (continued)
- Ivacaftor: grapefruit juice possibly increases plasma concentration of IVACAFTOR—manufacturer of ivacaftor advises avoid concomitant use
- Lipid-regulating Drugs: grapefruit juice possibly increases plasma concentration of ATORVASTATIN; grapefruit juice increases plasma concentration of • SIMVASTATIN—avoid concomitant use; avoidance of grapefruit juice advised by manufacturer of LOMITAPIDE
- Pirfenidone: avoidance of grapefruit juice advised by manufacturer of PIRFENIDONE
- Ranolazine: grapefruit juice possibly increases plasma concentration of • RANOLAZINE—manufacturer of ranolazine advises avoid concomitant use
- Sildenafil: grapefruit juice possibly increases plasma concentration of SILDENAFIL
- Sirolimus: grapefruit juice increases plasma concentration of • SIROLIMUS—avoid concomitant use
- Tacrolimus: grapefruit juice increases plasma concentration of • TACROLIMUS
- Tadalafil: grapefruit juice possibly increases plasma concentration of TADALAFIL
- Tolvaptan: grapefruit juice increases plasma concentration of • TOLVAPTAN—avoid concomitant use
- Ulipristal: avoidance of grapefruit juice advised by manufacturer of *low-dose* ULIPRISTAL
- Vardenafil: grapefruit juice possibly increases plasma concentration of • VARDENAFIL—avoid concomitant use

Griseofulvin
- Alcohol: griseofulvin possibly enhances effects of ALCOHOL
- Anticoagulants: griseofulvin reduces anticoagulant effect of
  - COUMARINS
- Antiepileptics: absorption of griseofulvin reduced by PHENOBARBITAL and PRIMIDONE (reduced effect)
- Ciclosporin: griseofulvin possibly reduces plasma concentration of CICLOSPORIN
- Oestrogens: anecdotal reports of contraceptive failure and menstrual irregularities when griseofulvin given with OESTROGENS
- Progestogens: anecdotal reports of contraceptive failure and menstrual irregularities when griseofulvin given with PROGESTOGENS

Guanethidine see Adrenergic Neurone Blockers

Guanfacine
- Alcohol: sedative effects possibly increased when guanfacine given with ALCOHOL
- Antibacterials: plasma concentration of guanfacine possibly increased by • CLARITHROMYCIN, ERYTHROMYCIN and • TELITHROMYCIN (halve dose of guanfacine); plasma concentration of guanfacine possibly reduced by • RIFABUTIN—increase dose of guanfacine; plasma concentration of guanfacine reduced by • RIFAMPICIN—increase dose of guanfacine; manufacturer of guanfacine advises halve dose when given with CHLORAMPHENICOL
- Antidepressants: plasma concentration of guanfacine possibly reduced by • ST JOHN'S WORT—increase dose of guanfacine
- Antiepileptics: plasma concentration of guanfacine possibly reduced by • CARBAMAZEPINE, • OXCARBAZEPINE, • PHENOBARBITAL, • PHENYTOIN and • PRIMIDONE—increase dose of guanfacine; guanfacine increases plasma concentration of SODIUM VALPROATE and VALPROIC ACID
- Antifungals: plasma concentration of guanfacine increased by • KETOCONAZOLE (halve dose of guanfacine); plasma concentration of guanfacine possibly increased by FLUCONAZOLE, • ITRACONAZOLE and • POSACONAZOLE (halve dose of guanfacine)
- Antipsychotics: sedative effects possibly increased when guanfacine given with ANTIPSYCHOTICS
- Antivirals: plasma concentration of guanfacine possibly increased by ATAZANAVIR, • BOCEPREVIR, FOSAMPRENAVIR, • INDINAVIR, • RITONAVIR, • SAQUINAVIR and • TELAPREVIR (halve dose of guanfacine); plasma concentration of guanfacine possibly reduced by • EFAVIRENZ, • ETRAVIRINE and • NEVIRAPINE—increase dose of guanfacine
- Anxiolytics and Hypnotics: sedative effects possibly increased when guanfacine given with ANXIOLYTICS AND HYPNOTICS

Guanfacine (continued)
▸ Aprepitant: plasma concentration of guanfacine possibly increased by APREPITANT (halve dose of guanfacine)
● Bosentan: plasma concentration of guanfacine possibly reduced by ● BOSENTAN—increase dose of guanfacine
▸ Calcium-channel Blockers: plasma concentration of guanfacine possibly increased by DILTIAZEM and VERAPAMIL (halve dose of guanfacine)
▸ Cytotoxics: plasma concentration of guanfacine possibly increased by CRIZOTINIB and IMATINIB (halve dose of guanfacine)
▸ Fosaprepitant: plasma concentration of guanfacine possibly increased by FOSAPREPITANT (halve dose of guanfacine)
▸ Grapefruit Juice: manufacturer of guanfacine advises avoid concomitant use with GRAPEFRUIT JUICE
● Modafinil: plasma concentration of guanfacine possibly reduced by ● MODAFINIL—increase dose of guanfacine

Haemophilus Vaccine *see* Vaccines
Haloperidol *see* Antipsychotics
Heparin *see* Heparins
Heparins
▸ ACE Inhibitors: increased risk of hyperkalaemia when heparins given with ACE INHIBITORS
▸ Aliskiren: increased risk of hyperkalaemia when heparins given with ALISKIREN
● Analgesics: possible increased risk of bleeding when heparins given with NSAIDs; increased risk of haemorrhage when anticoagulants given with *intravenous* ● DICLOFENAC (avoid concomitant use, including low-dose heparins); increased risk of haemorrhage when anticoagulants given with ● KETOROLAC (avoid concomitant use, including low-dose heparins); anticoagulant effect of heparins enhanced by ● ASPIRIN
▸ Angiotensin-II Receptor Antagonists: increased risk of hyperkalaemia when heparins given with ANGIOTENSIN-II RECEPTOR ANTAGONISTS
● Anticoagulants: increased risk of haemorrhage when other anticoagulants given with ● APIXABAN, ● DABIGATRAN, ● EDOXABAN and ● RIVAROXABAN (avoid concomitant use except when switching with other anticoagulants or using heparin to maintain catheter patency)
▸ Clopidogrel: increased risk of bleeding when heparins given with CLOPIDOGREL
▸ Dipyridamole: anticoagulant effect of heparins enhanced by DIPYRIDAMOLE
▸ Iloprost: anticoagulant effect of heparins possibly enhanced by ILOPROST
● Nitrates: anticoagulant effect of heparins reduced by *infusion* of ● GLYCERYL TRINITRATE

Hepatitis Vaccines *see* Vaccines
Histamine
▸ Antidepressants: manufacturer of histamine advises avoid concomitant use with MAOIs; effects of histamine theoretically antagonised by TRICYCLICS—manufacturer of histamine advises avoid concomitant use
▸ Antihistamines: effects of histamine theoretically antagonised by ANTIHISTAMINES—manufacturer of histamine advises avoid concomitant use
▸ Antimalarials: manufacturer of histamine advises avoid concomitant use with ANTIMALARIALS
▸ Antipsychotics: effects of histamine theoretically antagonised by ANTIPSYCHOTICS—manufacturer of histamine advises avoid concomitant use
▸ Atovaquone: manufacturer of histamine advises avoid concomitant use with ATOVAQUONE
▸ Clonidine: manufacturer of histamine advises avoid concomitant use with CLONIDINE
▸ Corticosteroids: manufacturer of histamine advises avoid concomitant use with CORTICOSTEROIDS
▸ Ulcer-healing Drugs: effects of histamine theoretically antagonised by HISTAMINE H$_2$-ANTAGONISTS—manufacturer of histamine advises avoid concomitant use

Histamine H$_2$-antagonists
● Alpha-blockers: cimetidine and ranitidine antagonise effects of ● TOLAZOLINE
● Aminophylline: cimetidine inhibits metabolism of ● AMINOPHYLLINE (increased plasma concentration)

Histamine H$_2$-antagonists (continued)
▸ Analgesics: cimetidine inhibits metabolism of OPIOID ANALGESICS (increased plasma concentration)
▸ Anthelmintics: cimetidine possibly enhances effects of ALBENDAZOLE; cimetidine possibly inhibits metabolism of MEBENDAZOLE (increased plasma concentration); cimetidine increases plasma concentration of PRAZIQUANTEL
● Anti-arrhythmics: cimetidine increases plasma concentration of AMIODARONE and ● PROPAFENONE; cimetidine inhibits metabolism of FLECAINIDE (increased plasma concentration); cimetidine increases plasma concentration of ● LIDOCAINE (increased risk of toxicity)
▸ Antibacterials: cimetidine increases plasma concentration of ERYTHROMYCIN (increased risk of toxicity, including deafness); cimetidine inhibits metabolism of METRONIDAZOLE (increased plasma concentration); metabolism of cimetidine accelerated by RIFAMPICIN (reduced plasma concentration)
● Anticoagulants: cimetidine inhibits metabolism of ● COUMARINS (enhanced anticoagulant effect)
▸ Antidepressants: cimetidine increases plasma concentration of CITALOPRAM, ESCITALOPRAM, MIRTAZAPINE and SERTRALINE; cimetidine inhibits metabolism of AMITRIPTYLINE, DOXEPIN, IMIPRAMINE and NORTRIPTYLINE (increased plasma concentration); cimetidine increases plasma concentration of MOCLOBEMIDE (halve dose of moclobemide); cimetidine possibly increases plasma concentration of TRICYCLICS
▸ Antidiabetics: cimetidine reduces excretion of METFORMIN (increased plasma concentration); cimetidine enhances hypoglycaemic effect of SULFONYLUREAS
● Antiepileptics: cimetidine inhibits metabolism of ● CARBAMAZEPINE, ● FOSPHENYTOIN, ● PHENYTOIN, ● SODIUM VALPROATE and ● VALPROIC ACID (increased plasma concentration)
▸ Antifungals: histamine H$_2$-antagonists reduce absorption of ITRACONAZOLE and KETOCONAZOLE; cimetidine reduces plasma concentration of ● POSACONAZOLE—manufacturer of posaconazole *suspension* advises avoid concomitant use; famotidine, nizatidine and ranitidine possibly reduce plasma concentration of ● POSACONAZOLE—manufacturer of posaconazole *suspension* advises avoid concomitant use; cimetidine increases plasma concentration of TERBINAFINE
▸ Antihistamines: manufacturer of loratadine advises cimetidine possibly increases plasma concentration of LORATADINE; cimetidine increases plasma concentration of HYDROXYZINE
● Antimalarials: avoidance of cimetidine advised by manufacturer of ● ARTEMETHER WITH LUMEFANTRINE; cimetidine inhibits metabolism of CHLOROQUINE, HYDROXYCHLOROQUINE and QUININE (increased plasma concentration)
▸ Antipsychotics: cimetidine possibly enhances effects of ANTIPSYCHOTICS, CHLORPROMAZINE and CLOZAPINE
● Antivirals: famotidine and ranitidine reduce the plasma concentration of ● ATAZANAVIR (adjust doses of both drugs—consult atazanavir product literature); manufacturer of atazanavir advises adjust doses of both drugs when cimetidine and nizatidine given with ATAZANAVIR—consult atazanavir product literature; famotidine reduces plasma concentration of LEDIPASVIR; famotidine increases plasma concentration of RALTEGRAVIR; avoidance of histamine H$_2$-antagonists for 12 hours before or 4 hours after RILPIVIRINE advised by manufacturer of rilpivirine—consult product literature; cimetidine possibly increases plasma concentration of SAQUINAVIR
▸ Anxiolytics and Hypnotics: cimetidine inhibits metabolism of BENZODIAZEPINES, CLOMETHIAZOLE and ZALEPLON (increased plasma concentration); cimetidine increases plasma concentration of MELATONIN
▸ Azathioprine: manufacturer of azathioprine advises possible increased risk of myelosuppression when cimetidine given with AZATHIOPRINE
▸ Beta-blockers: cimetidine increases plasma concentration of LABETALOL, METOPROLOL and PROPRANOLOL; cimetidine possibly increases plasma concentration of *oral* TIMOLOL
▸ Caffeine citrate: cimetidine increases plasma concentration of CAFFEINE CITRATE
▸ Calcium-channel Blockers: cimetidine possibly inhibits metabolism of CALCIUM-CHANNEL BLOCKERS (increased plasma

Histamine H$_2$-antagonists

Calcium-channel Blockers (continued)
concentration); cimetidine increases plasma concentration of ISRADIPINE (halve dose of isradipine)
• Ciclosporin: cimetidine possibly increases plasma concentration of • CICLOSPORIN
• Clopidogrel: cimetidine possibly reduces antiplatelet effect of • CLOPIDOGREL
• Cytotoxics: cimetidine possibly enhances myelosuppressive effects of CARMUSTINE and LOMUSTINE; cimetidine reduces plasma concentration of DOXORUBICIN; cimetidine increases plasma concentration of • EPIRUBICIN; cimetidine inhibits metabolism of CAPECITABINE, FLUOROURACIL and TEGAFUR (increased plasma concentration); cimetidine possibly reduces plasma concentration of DASATINIB; avoidance of cimetidine, famotidine and nizatidine advised by manufacturer of • ERLOTINIB; ranitidine reduces plasma concentration of • ERLOTINIB—manufacturer of erlotinib advises give at least 2 hours before or 10 hours after ranitidine; ranitidine reduces plasma concentration of • GEFITINIB; histamine H$_2$-antagonists possibly reduce absorption of LAPATINIB; histamine H$_2$-antagonists possibly reduce absorption of PAZOPANIB—manufacturer of pazopanib advises give at least 2 hours before or 10 hours after histamine H$_2$-antagonists
▸ Dopaminergics: cimetidine reduces excretion of PRAMIPEXOLE (increased plasma concentration)
• Ergot Alkaloids: increased risk of ergotism when cimetidine given with • ERGOTAMINE—avoid concomitant use
• Fampridine: avoidance of cimetidine advised by manufacturer of • FAMPRIDINE
▸ Histamine: histamine H$_2$-antagonists theoretically antagonise effects of HISTAMINE—manufacturer of histamine advises avoid concomitant use
▸ Hormone Antagonists: absorption of cimetidine possibly delayed by OCTREOTIDE
▸ 5HT$_1$-receptor Agonists: cimetidine inhibits metabolism of ZOLMITRIPTAN (reduce dose of zolmitriptan)
▸ Lipid-regulating Drugs: separating administration from cimetidine and ranitidine by 12 hours advised by manufacturer of LOMITAPIDE
▸ Roflumilast: cimetidine inhibits the metabolism of ROFLUMILAST
▸ Sildenafil: cimetidine increases plasma concentration of SILDENAFIL—consider reducing dose of sildenafil for erectile dysfunction
▸ Sympathomimetics: cimetidine possibly inhibits metabolism of DOBUTAMINE
• Theophylline: cimetidine inhibits metabolism of • THEOPHYLLINE (increased plasma concentration)
▸ Thyroid Hormones: cimetidine reduces absorption of LEVOTHYROXINE

Homatropine see Antimuscarinics

Hormone Antagonists see Abiraterone, Bicalutamide, Danazol, Dutasteride, Enzalutamide, Exemestane, Flutamide, Lanreotide, Octreotide, Pasireotide, Tamoxifen, and Toremifene

5HT$_1$-receptor Agonists

• Antibacterials: plasma concentration of eletriptan increased by • CLARITHROMYCIN and • ERYTHROMYCIN (risk of toxicity)—avoid concomitant use; metabolism of zolmitriptan possibly inhibited by QUINOLONES (reduce dose of zolmitriptan)
• Antidepressants: increased risk of CNS toxicity when 5HT$_1$ agonists given with CITALOPRAM (manufacturer of citalopram advises avoid concomitant use); increased risk of CNS toxicity when sumatriptan given with • CITALOPRAM, • ESCITALOPRAM, • FLUOXETINE, • FLUVOXAMINE or • PAROXETINE; metabolism of frovatriptan inhibited by FLUVOXAMINE; metabolism of zolmitriptan possibly inhibited by FLUVOXAMINE (reduce dose of zolmitriptan); CNS toxicity reported when sumatriptan given with SERTRALINE; possible increased serotonergic effects when 5HT$_1$ agonists given with DULOXETINE, VENLAFAXINE or VORTIOXETINE; risk of CNS toxicity when rizatriptan or sumatriptan given with • MAOIS (avoid rizatriptan or sumatriptan for 2 weeks after MAOIs); risk of CNS toxicity when zolmitriptan given with • MAOIS or

5HT$_1$-receptor Agonists

• Antidepressants (continued)
• MOCLOBEMIDE (reduce dose of zolmitriptan); risk of CNS toxicity when rizatriptan or sumatriptan given with
• MOCLOBEMIDE (avoid rizatriptan or sumatriptan for 2 weeks after moclobemide); possible increased serotonergic effects when naratriptan given with SSRIs; increased serotonergic effects when 5HT$_1$ agonists given with • ST JOHN'S WORT—avoid concomitant use
• Antifungals: plasma concentration of eletriptan increased by • ITRACONAZOLE and • KETOCONAZOLE (risk of toxicity)—avoid concomitant use; plasma concentration of almotriptan increased by KETOCONAZOLE (increased risk of toxicity)
• Antivirals: plasma concentration of eletriptan increased by • INDINAVIR and • RITONAVIR (risk of toxicity)—avoid concomitant use
▸ Beta-blockers: plasma concentration of rizatriptan increased by PROPRANOLOL (manufacturer of rizatriptan advises halve dose and avoid within 2 hours of propranolol)
• Dapoxetine: possible increased risk of serotonergic effects when 5HT$_1$ agonists given with • DAPOXETINE (manufacturer of dapoxetine advises 5HT$_1$ agonists should not be started until 1 week after stopping dapoxetine, avoid dapoxetine for 2 weeks after stopping 5HT$_1$ agonists)
▸ Dopaminergics: avoidance of 5HT$_1$ agonists advised by manufacturer of SELEGILINE
• Ergot Alkaloids: increased risk of vasospasm when eletriptan, frovatriptan or naratriptan given with • ERGOTAMINE (avoid ergotamine for 24 hours after eletriptan, frovatriptan or naratriptan, avoid eletriptan, frovatriptan or naratriptan for 24 hours after ergotamine); increased risk of vasospasm when almotriptan, rizatriptan, sumatriptan or zolmitriptan given with • ERGOTAMINE (avoid ergotamine for 6 hours after almotriptan, rizatriptan, sumatriptan or zolmitriptan, avoid almotriptan, rizatriptan, sumatriptan or zolmitriptan for 24 hours after ergotamine)
▸ Lithium: possible risk of toxicity when sumatriptan given with LITHIUM
▸ Ulcer-healing Drugs: metabolism of zolmitriptan inhibited by CIMETIDINE (reduce dose of zolmitriptan)

5HT$_3$-receptor Antagonists

▸ Analgesics: ondansetron possibly antagonises effects of TRAMADOL
▸ Antibacterials: metabolism of ondansetron accelerated by RIFAMPICIN (reduced effect)
▸ Antidepressants: possible increased serotonergic effects when 5HT$_3$ antagonists given with SSRI-RELATED ANTIDEPRESSANTS or SSRIS
▸ Antiepileptics: metabolism of ondansetron accelerated by CARBAMAZEPINE, FOSPHENYTOIN and PHENYTOIN (reduced effect)
• Cytotoxics: increased risk of ventricular arrhythmias when ondansetron given with • VANDETANIB—avoid concomitant use
• Dopaminergics: possible increased hypotensive effect when ondansetron given with • APOMORPHINE—avoid concomitant use

Human papillomavirus Vaccine see Vaccines
Hydralazine see Vasodilator Antihypertensives
Hydrochlorothiazide see Diuretics
Hydrocortisone see Corticosteroids
Hydroflumethiazide see Diuretics
Hydromorphone see Opioid Analgesics
Hydrotalcite see Antacids

Hydroxocobalamin

▸ Antibacterials: response to hydroxocobalamin reduced by CHLORAMPHENICOL

Hydroxycarbamide

• Antipsychotics: avoid concomitant use of cytotoxics with • CLOZAPINE (increased risk of agranulocytosis)
• Antivirals: increased risk of toxicity when hydroxycarbamide given with • DIDANOSINE and • STAVUDINE—avoid concomitant use
• Vaccines: risk of generalised infections when hydroxycarbamide given with live • VACCINES—avoid concomitant use

Hydroxychloroquine

▸ Adsorbents: absorption of hydroxychloroquine reduced by KAOLIN

Hydroxychloroquine (continued)

▸ **Agalsidase Alfa and Beta:** hydroxychloroquine possibly inhibits effects of AGALSIDASE ALFA AND BETA (manufacturers of agalsidase alfa and beta advise avoid concomitant use)
▸ **Antacids:** absorption of hydroxychloroquine reduced by ANTACIDS
● **Anti-arrhythmics:** increased risk of ventricular arrhythmias when hydroxychloroquine given with ● AMIODARONE—avoid concomitant use
● **Antibacterials:** increased risk of ventricular arrhythmias when hydroxychloroquine given with ● MOXIFLOXACIN—avoid concomitant use
● **Antimalarials:** avoidance of antimalarials advised by manufacturer of ● ARTEMETHER WITH LUMEFANTRINE; increased risk of convulsions when hydroxychloroquine given with ● MEFLOQUINE
● **Antipsychotics:** increased risk of ventricular arrhythmias when hydroxychloroquine given with ● DROPERIDOL—avoid concomitant use
● **Cardiac Glycosides:** hydroxychloroquine possibly increases plasma concentration of ● DIGOXIN
● **Ciclosporin:** hydroxychloroquine increases plasma concentration of ● CICLOSPORIN (increased risk of toxicity)
● **Cytotoxics:** possible increased risk of ventricular arrhythmias when hydroxychloroquine given with ● BOSUTINIB
▸ **Histamine:** avoidance of antimalarials advised by manufacturer of HISTAMINE
▸ **Lanthanum:** absorption of hydroxychloroquine possibly reduced by LANTHANUM (give at least 2 hours apart)
▸ **Laronidase:** hydroxychloroquine possibly inhibits effects of LARONIDASE (manufacturer of laronidase advises avoid concomitant use)
▸ **Parasympathomimetics:** hydroxychloroquine has potential to increase symptoms of myasthenia gravis and thus diminish effect of NEOSTIGMINE and PYRIDOSTIGMINE
● **Penicillamine:** increased risk of haematological toxicity when antimalarials given with PENICILLAMINE—manufacturer of penicillamine advises avoid concomitant use
▸ **Ulcer-healing Drugs:** metabolism of hydroxychloroquine inhibited by CIMETIDINE (increased plasma concentration)
▸ **Vaccines:** antimalarials inactivate ORAL TYPHOID VACCINE—see under Typhoid Vaccine in BNFC

Hydroxyzine see Antihistamines
Hyoscine see Antimuscarinics
Ibandronic Acid see Bisphosphonates

Ibrutinib

▸ **Anti-arrhythmics:** plasma concentration of ibrutinib possibly increased by ● AMIODARONE and ● DRONEDARONE—reduce dose of ibrutinib (see under Ibrutinib, in BNF)
▸ **Antibacterials:** plasma concentration of ibrutinib possibly increased by ● CIPROFLOXACIN, ● CLARITHROMYCIN, ● ERYTHROMYCIN and ● TELITHROMYCIN—reduce dose of ibrutinib (see under Ibrutinib, in BNF); plasma concentration of ibrutinib reduced by ● RIFAMPICIN—avoid concomitant use
▸ **Anticoagulants:** manufacturer of ibrutinib advises avoid concomitant use with COUMARINS and PHENINDIONE
▸ **Antidepressants:** plasma concentration of ibrutinib possibly reduced by ● ST JOHN'S WORT—manufacturer of ibrutinib advises avoid concomitant use
▸ **Antiepileptics:** plasma concentration of ibrutinib possibly reduced by ● CARBAMAZEPINE, ● FOSPHENYTOIN and ● PHENYTOIN—manufacturer of ibrutinib advises avoid concomitant use
▸ **Antifungals:** plasma concentration of ibrutinib increased by ● KETOCONAZOLE—reduce dose of ibrutinib (see under Ibrutinib, in BNF); plasma concentration of ibrutinib possibly increased by ● FLUCONAZOLE, ● ITRACONAZOLE and ● VORICONAZOLE—reduce dose of ibrutinib (see under Ibrutinib, in BNF)
▸ **Antipsychotics:** avoid concomitant use of cytotoxics with ● CLOZAPINE (increased risk of agranulocytosis)
▸ **Antivirals:** plasma concentration of ibrutinib possibly increased by ● ATAZANAVIR, ● DARUNAVIR, ● FOSAMPRENAVIR, ● INDINAVIR, ● RITONAVIR and ● SAQUINAVIR—reduce dose of ibrutinib (see under Ibrutinib, in BNF)

Ibrutinib (continued)

● **Aprepitant:** plasma concentration of ibrutinib possibly increased by ● APREPITANT—reduce dose of ibrutinib (see under Ibrutinib, in BNF)
● **Calcium-channel Blockers:** plasma concentration of ibrutinib possibly increased by ● DILTIAZEM and ● VERAPAMIL—reduce dose of ibrutinib (see under Ibrutinib, in BNF)
▸ **Cardiac Glycosides:** manufacturer of ibrutinib advises give DIGOXIN at least 6 hours before or after ibrutinib
● **Cobicistat:** plasma concentration of ibrutinib possibly increased by ● COBICISTAT—reduce dose of ibrutinib (see under Ibrutinib, in BNF)
● **Cytotoxics:** plasma concentration of ibrutinib possibly increased by ● CRIZOTINIB and ● IMATINIB—reduce dose of ibrutinib (see under Ibrutinib, in BNF)
▸ **Fosaprepitant:** plasma concentration of ibrutinib possibly increased by FOSAPREPITANT
▸ **Grapefruit Juice:** manufacturer of ibrutinib advises avoid concomitant use with GRAPEFRUIT JUICE
▸ **Vitamins:** manufacturer of ibrutinib advises avoid concomitant use with VITAMIN E

Ibuprofen see NSAIDs

Idarubicin

● **Antipsychotics:** avoid concomitant use of cytotoxics with ● CLOZAPINE (increased risk of agranulocytosis)
● **Ciclosporin:** plasma concentration of idarubicin increased by ● CICLOSPORIN
● **Cytotoxics:** possible increased risk of cardiotoxicity when idarubicin given with ● TRASTUZUMAB—avoid concomitant use for up to 28 weeks after stopping trastuzumab
● **Vaccines:** risk of generalised infections when cytotoxic antibiotics given with live ● VACCINES—avoid concomitant use

Idelalisib

▸ **Alpha-blockers:** manufacturer of idelalisib advises avoid concomitant use with ALFUZOSIN
▸ **Anti-arrhythmics:** manufacturer of idelalisib advises avoid concomitant use with AMIODARONE
● **Antibacterials:** plasma concentration of idelalisib reduced by ● RIFAMPICIN—avoid concomitant use
● **Antidepressants:** plasma concentration of idelalisib possibly reduced by ● ST JOHN'S WORT—manufacturer of idelalisib advises avoid concomitant use
● **Antiepileptics:** plasma concentration of idelalisib possibly reduced by ● CARBAMAZEPINE, ● FOSPHENYTOIN and ● PHENYTOIN—manufacturer of idelalisib advises avoid concomitant use
▸ **Antifungals:** plasma concentration of idelalisib increased by KETOCONAZOLE
● **Antipsychotics:** avoid concomitant use of cytotoxics with ● CLOZAPINE (increased risk of agranulocytosis); manufacturer of idelalisib advises avoid concomitant use with PIMOZIDE and QUETIAPINE
▸ **Anxiolytics and Hypnotics:** manufacturer of idelalisib advises avoid concomitant use of *oral* MIDAZOLAM
▸ **Ergot Alkaloids:** manufacturer of idelalisib advises avoid concomitant use with ERGOTAMINE
▸ **Lipid-regulating Drugs:** manufacturer of idelalisib advises avoid concomitant use with SIMVASTATIN
▸ **Sildenafil:** manufacturer of idelalisib advises avoid concomitant use of SILDENAFIL for pulmonary arterial hypertension
▸ **Sympathomimetics, Beta₂:** manufacturer of idelalisib advises avoid concomitant use with SALMETEROL

Ifosfamide

● **Anticoagulants:** ifosfamide possibly enhances anticoagulant effect of ● COUMARINS
▸ **Antifungals:** metabolism of ifosfamide inhibited by KETOCONAZOLE
● **Antipsychotics:** avoid concomitant use of cytotoxics with ● CLOZAPINE (increased risk of agranulocytosis)
▸ **Cytotoxics:** increased risk of otoxicity when ifosfamide given with CISPLATIN

Iloprost

▸ **Analgesics:** increased risk of bleeding when iloprost given with NSAIDs or ASPIRIN

Iloprost (continued)

▸ Anticoagulants: iloprost possibly enhances anticoagulant effect of COUMARINS and HEPARINS; increased risk of bleeding when iloprost given with PHENINDIONE
▸ Clopidogrel: increased risk of bleeding when iloprost given with CLOPIDOGREL
▸ Eptifibatide: increased risk of bleeding when iloprost given with EPTIFIBATIDE
▸ Tirofiban: increased risk of bleeding when iloprost given with TIROFIBAN

Imatinib

▸ Analgesics: manufacturer of imatinib advises caution with PARACETAMOL
● Antibacterials: plasma concentration of imatinib reduced by ● RIFAMPICIN—avoid concomitant use
▸ Anticoagulants: manufacturer of imatinib advises replacement of WARFARIN with a heparin (possibility of enhanced warfarin effect)
● Antidepressants: plasma concentration of imatinib reduced by ● ST JOHN'S WORT—avoid concomitant use
● Antiepileptics: plasma concentration of imatinib reduced by ● CARBAMAZEPINE, ● FOSPHENYTOIN, ● OXCARBAZEPINE and ● PHENYTOIN—avoid concomitant use
● Antifungals: plasma concentration of imatinib increased by KETOCONAZOLE
● Antipsychotics: avoid concomitant use of cytotoxics with ● CLOZAPINE (increased risk of agranulocytosis)
● Antivirals: avoidance of imatinib advised by manufacturer of ● BOCEPREVIR
● Ciclosporin: imatinib possibly increases plasma concentration of CICLOSPORIN
● Cytotoxics: imatinib possibly increases the plasma concentration of ● BOSUTINIB—manufacturer of bosutinib advises avoid or consider reducing dose of bosutinib; imatinib increases plasma concentration of ● EVEROLIMUS (consider reducing the dose of everolimus—consult everolimus product literature); imatinib increases the plasma concentration of ● IBRUTINIB—reduce dose of ibrutinib (see under Ibrutinib, in BNF)
▸ Guanfacine: imatinib increases plasma concentration of GUANFACINE (halve dose of guanfacine)
▸ Lipid-regulating Drugs: imatinib increases plasma concentration of SIMVASTATIN
▸ Tacrolimus: imatinib increases plasma concentration of TACROLIMUS
▸ Thyroid Hormones: imatinib possibly reduces plasma concentration of LEVOTHYROXINE

Imidapril see ACE Inhibitors

Imipenem with Cilastatin

● Antiepileptics: carbapenems reduce plasma concentration of ● SODIUM VALPROATE and ● VALPROIC ACID—avoid concomitant use
● Antivirals: increased risk of convulsions when imipenem with cilastatin given with ● GANCICLOVIR or ● VALGANCICLOVIR
▸ Vaccines: antibacterials inactivate ORAL TYPHOID VACCINE—see under Typhoid Vaccine in BNFC

Imipramine see Antidepressants, Tricyclic

Immunoglobulins

● Vaccines: anti-d immunoglobulins and normal immunoglobulin might impair immune response to ● BCG VACCINE—give BCG vaccine at least 3 weeks before or 3 months after anti-d immunoglobulins and normal immunoglobulin; anti-d immunoglobulins and normal immunoglobulin might impair immune response to ● MMR VACCINE—give MMR vaccine at least 3 weeks before or 3 months after anti-d immunoglobulins and normal immunoglobulin; anti-d immunoglobulins and normal immunoglobulin might impair immune response to live ● INFLUENZA VACCINE—give live influenza vaccine at least 3 weeks before or 3 months after anti-d immunoglobulins and normal immunoglobulin; anti-d immunoglobulins and normal immunoglobulin might impair immune response to ● ORAL TYPHOID VACCINE—give oral typhoid vaccine at least 3 weeks before or 3 months after anti-d immunoglobulins and normal immunoglobulin; anti-d immunoglobulins and normal immunoglobulin might impair immune response to

Immunoglobulins

● Vaccines (continued)

oral ● POLIOMYELITIS VACCINE—give oral poliomyelitis vaccine at least 3 weeks before or 3 months after anti-d immunoglobulins and normal immunoglobulin; anti-d immunoglobulins and normal immunoglobulin might impair immune response to ● ROTAVIRUS VACCINE—give rotavirus vaccine at least 3 weeks before or 3 months after anti-d immunoglobulins and normal immunoglobulin; anti-d immunoglobulins and normal immunoglobulin might impair immune response to ● SMALLPOX VACCINE—give smallpox vaccine at least 3 weeks before or 3 months after anti-d immunoglobulins and normal immunoglobulin; anti-d immunoglobulins and normal immunoglobulin might impair immune response to ● VARICELLA-ZOSTER VACCINE—give varicella-zoster vaccine at least 3 weeks before or 3 months after anti-d immunoglobulins and normal immunoglobulin; anti-d immunoglobulins and normal immunoglobulin might impair immune response to ● YELLOW FEVER VACCINE—give yellow fever vaccine at least 3 weeks before or 3 months after anti-d immunoglobulins and normal immunoglobulin

Indacaterol see Sympathomimetics, Beta$_2$

Indapamide see Diuretics

Indinavir

▸ Aldesleukin: plasma concentration of indinavir possibly increased by ALDESLEUKIN
● Anti-arrhythmics: indinavir possibly increases plasma concentration of ● AMIODARONE—avoid concomitant use; indinavir possibly increases plasma concentration of ● FLECAINIDE (increased risk of ventricular arrhythmias—avoid concomitant use)
● Antibacterials: indinavir increases plasma concentration of ● RIFABUTIN, also plasma concentration of indinavir decreased (reduce dose of rifabutin and increase dose of indinavir); metabolism of indinavir accelerated by ● RIFAMPICIN (reduced plasma concentration—avoid concomitant use); avoidance of concomitant indinavir in severe renal and hepatic impairment advised by manufacturer of ● TELITHROMYCIN
▸ Anticoagulants: avoidance of indinavir advised by manufacturer of APIXABAN and RIVAROXABAN
● Antidepressants: plasma concentration of indinavir reduced by ● ST JOHN'S WORT—avoid concomitant use
● Antiepileptics: plasma concentration of indinavir possibly reduced by ● CARBAMAZEPINE, ● FOSPHENYTOIN and ● PHENYTOIN, also plasma concentration of carbamazepine, fosphenytoin and phenytoin possibly increased; plasma concentration of indinavir possibly reduced by ● PHENOBARBITAL and ● PRIMIDONE
● Antifungals: plasma concentration of indinavir increased by ● ITRACONAZOLE and ● KETOCONAZOLE (consider reducing dose of indinavir)
● Antimalarials: caution with indinavir advised by manufacturer of ARTEMETHER WITH LUMEFANTRINE; indinavir possibly increases plasma concentration of ● QUININE (increased risk of toxicity)
▸ Antimuscarinics: avoidance of indinavir advised by manufacturer of DARIFENACIN and TOLTERODINE; manufacturer of fesoterodine advises dose reduction when indinavir given with FESOTERODINE—consult fesoterodine product literature
● Antipsychotics: indinavir possibly increases plasma concentration of ● ARIPIPRAZOLE (reduce dose of aripiprazole—consult aripiprazole product literature); indinavir possibly increases plasma concentration of ● LURASIDONE—avoid concomitant use; indinavir possibly increases plasma concentration of ● PIMOZIDE (increased risk of ventricular arrhythmias—avoid concomitant use); indinavir possibly increases plasma concentration of ● QUETIAPINE—manufacturer of quetiapine advises avoid concomitant use
● Antivirals: avoid concomitant use of indinavir with ● ATAZANAVIR; plasma concentration of both drugs increased when indinavir given with DARUNAVIR; absorption of indinavir reduced by DIDANOSINE tablets (give at least 1 hour apart); plasma concentration of indinavir reduced by EFAVIRENZ and NEVIRAPINE; plasma concentration of indinavir possibly reduced by ● ETRAVIRINE—avoid concomitant use; indinavir increases plasma concentration of ● MARAVIROC (consider

Indinavir

- **Antivirals** (continued)
  reducing dose of maraviroc); avoidance of indinavir advised by manufacturer of PARITAPREVIR; plasma concentration of indinavir increased by RITONAVIR; indinavir increases plasma concentration of SAQUINAVIR
- **Anxiolytics and Hypnotics**: increased risk of prolonged sedation when indinavir given with ● ALPRAZOLAM—avoid concomitant use; indinavir possibly increases plasma concentration of ● MIDAZOLAM (risk of prolonged sedation—avoid concomitant use of *oral* midazolam)
- ▸ **Atovaquone**: plasma concentration of indinavir possibly reduced by ATOVAQUONE
- ▸ **Avanafil**: indinavir possibly increases plasma concentration of ● AVANAFIL—manufacturer of avanafil advises avoid concomitant use
- ▸ **Bosentan**: plasma concentration of indinavir possibly reduced by BOSENTAN
- **Ciclosporin**: indinavir increases plasma concentration of ● CICLOSPORIN
- **Colchicine**: indinavir possibly increases risk of ● COLCHICINE toxicity—suspend or reduce dose of colchicine (avoid concomitant use in hepatic or renal impairment)
- **Corticosteroids**: plasma concentration of indinavir possibly reduced by DEXAMETHASONE
- **Cytotoxics**: indinavir possibly increases plasma concentration of AXITINIB (reduce dose of axitinib—consult axitinib product literature); indinavir possibly increases the plasma concentration of ● BOSUTINIB and ● CABAZITAXEL—manufacturer of bosutinib and cabazitaxel advises avoid or consider reducing dose of bosutinib and cabazitaxel; indinavir possibly increases plasma concentration of ● CRIZOTINIB and ● EVEROLIMUS—manufacturer of crizotinib and everolimus advises avoid concomitant use; indinavir possibly increases the plasma concentration of ● IBRUTINIB—reduce dose of ibrutinib (see under Ibrutinib, in BNF); indinavir possibly increases plasma concentration of ● PAZOPANIB (reduce dose of pazopanib); indinavir possibly increases plasma concentration of ● PONATINIB—consider reducing initial dose of ponatinib (see under Ponatinib, in BNF); manufacturer of ruxolitinib advises dose reduction when indinavir given with ● RUXOLITINIB—consult ruxolitinib product literature; indinavir possibly increases plasma concentration of ● DOCETAXEL—manufacturer of docetaxel advises avoid concomitant use or consider reducing docetaxel dose; avoidance of indinavir advised by manufacturer of ● OLAPARIB
- **Ergot Alkaloids**: increased risk of ergotism when indinavir given with ● ERGOMETRINE or ● ERGOTAMINE—avoid concomitant use
- **Guanfacine**: indinavir possibly increases plasma concentration of ● GUANFACINE (halve dose of guanfacine)
- **5HT₁-receptor Agonists**: indinavir increases plasma concentration of ● ELETRIPTAN (risk of toxicity)—avoid concomitant use
- **Lipid-regulating Drugs**: possible increased risk of myopathy when indinavir given with ATORVASTATIN; possible increased risk of myopathy when indinavir given with ● ROSUVASTATIN—manufacturer of rosuvastatin advises avoid concomitant use; increased risk of myopathy when indinavir given with ● SIMVASTATIN (avoid concomitant use); avoidance of indinavir advised by manufacturer of ● LOMITAPIDE (plasma concentration of lomitapide possibly increased)
- **Orlistat**: absorption of indinavir possibly reduced by ● ORLISTAT
- **Ranolazine**: indinavir possibly increases plasma concentration of ● RANOLAZINE—manufacturer of ranolazine advises avoid concomitant use
- **Sildenafil**: indinavir increases plasma concentration of ● SILDENAFIL—reduce initial dose of sildenafil
- ▸ **Tadalafil**: indinavir possibly increases plasma concentration of TADALAFIL
- **Vardenafil**: indinavir increases plasma concentration of ● VARDENAFIL—avoid concomitant use

Indometacin *see* NSAIDs
Indoramin *see* Alpha-blockers

Infliximab

- **Abatacept**: avoid concomitant use of infliximab with ● ABATACEPT

Infliximab (continued)

- **Anakinra**: avoid concomitant use of infliximab with ● ANAKINRA
- **Antipsychotics**: avoid concomitant use of cytotoxics with ● CLOZAPINE (increased risk of agranulocytosis)
- **Vaccines**: risk of generalised infections when monoclonal antibodies given with live ● VACCINES—avoid concomitant use

Influenza Vaccine *see* Vaccines
Insulin *see* Antidiabetics
Interferon Alfa *see* Interferons
Interferon Gamma *see* Interferons

Interferons

- **Aminophylline**: interferon alfa and peginterferon alfa inhibit metabolism of ● AMINOPHYLLINE (consider reducing dose of aminophylline)
- **Antivirals**: caution with peginterferon alfa advised by manufacturer of ADEFOVIR; increased risk of peripheral neuropathy when interferon alfa and peginterferon alfa given with ● TELBIVUDINE
- **Theophylline**: interferon alfa and peginterferon alfa inhibit metabolism of ● THEOPHYLLINE (consider reducing dose of theophylline)
- ▸ **Vaccines**: manufacturer of interferon gamma advises avoid concomitant use with VACCINES

Ipilimumab

- **Antipsychotics**: avoid concomitant use of cytotoxics with ● CLOZAPINE (increased risk of agranulocytosis)
- ▸ **Cytotoxics**: manufacturer of ipilimumab advises avoid concomitant use with VEMURAFENIB
- **Vaccines**: risk of generalised infections when monoclonal antibodies given with live ● VACCINES—avoid concomitant use

Ipratropium *see* Antimuscarinics
Irbesartan *see* Angiotensin-II Receptor Antagonists

Irinotecan

- **Antidepressants**: metabolism of irinotecan accelerated by ● ST JOHN'S WORT (reduced plasma concentration—avoid concomitant use)
- ▸ **Antiepileptics**: plasma concentration of irinotecan and its active metabolite reduced by CARBAMAZEPINE, FOSPHENYTOIN, PHENOBARBITAL, PHENYTOIN and PRIMIDONE
- **Antifungals**: plasma concentration of irinotecan reduced by ● KETOCONAZOLE (but concentration of active metabolite of irinotecan increased)—avoid concomitant use; increased risk of toxicity when irinotecan given with ● ITRACONAZOLE—avoid concomitant use
- **Antipsychotics**: avoid concomitant use of cytotoxics with ● CLOZAPINE (increased risk of agranulocytosis)
- **Antivirals**: metabolism of irinotecan possibly inhibited by ● ATAZANAVIR (increased risk of toxicity)
- **Cytotoxics**: avoidance of irinotecan advised by manufacturer of ● PANITUMUMAB; plasma concentration of active metabolite of irinotecan increased by ● LAPATINIB—consider reducing dose of irinotecan; plasma concentration of irinotecan increased by REGORAFENIB; plasma concentration of irinotecan possibly increased by SORAFENIB

Iron Salts

- ▸ **Antacids**: absorption of *oral* iron salts reduced by ORAL MAGNESIUM SALTS (as magnesium trisilicate)
- ▸ **Antibacterials**: *oral* iron salts reduce absorption of CIPROFLOXACIN (give at least 2 hours before or 4 hours after ciprofloxacin); *oral* iron salts reduce absorption of LEVOFLOXACIN, NORFLOXACIN and OFLOXACIN (give at least 2 hours apart); *oral* iron salts reduce absorption of MOXIFLOXACIN (give at least 6 hours apart); effects of iron salts possibly inhibited by CHLORAMPHENICOL; *oral* iron salts reduce absorption of tetracyclines, also absorption of *oral* iron salts reduced by TETRACYCLINES (give at least 2 to 3 hours apart)
- ▸ **Antivirals**: *oral* iron salts reduce absoption of DOLUTEGRAVIR—manufacturer of dolutegravir advises give at least 2 hours before or 6 hours after *oral* iron salts
- ▸ **Bisphosphonates**: *oral* iron salts reduce absorption of BISPHOSPHONATES
- ▸ **Calcium Salts**: absorption of *oral* iron salts reduced by CALCIUM SALTS
- ▸ **Dopaminergics**: *oral* iron salts possibly reduce absorption of CO-BENELDOPA, CO-CARELDOPA and LEVODOPA; *oral* iron salts reduce absorption of ENTACAPONE

Iron Salts (continued)
▸ Eltrombopag: *oral* iron salts possibly reduce absorption of ELTROMBOPAG (give at least 4 hours apart)
▸ Methyldopa: *oral* iron salts antagonise hypotensive effect of METHYLDOPA
▸ Mycophenolate: *oral* iron salts reduce absorption of MYCOPHENOLATE
▸ Penicillamine: *oral* iron salts reduce absorption of PENICILLAMINE
▸ Thyroid Hormones: *oral* iron salts reduce absorption of LEVOTHYROXINE (give at least 2 hours apart)
▸ Trientine: absorption of *oral* iron salts reduced by TRIENTINE
▸ Zinc: *oral* iron salts reduce absorption of ZINC, also absorption of *oral* iron salts reduced by zinc

Isocarboxazid *see* MAOIs
Isoflurane *see* Anaesthetics, General
Isometheptene *see* Sympathomimetics
Isoniazid
▸ Aminophylline: isoniazid possibly increases plasma concentration of AMINOPHYLLINE
▸ Anaesthetics, General: increased risk of hepatotoxicity when isoniazid given with ISOFLURANE
▸ Analgesics: avoidance of isoniazid advised by manufacturer of PETHIDINE
● Antacids: absorption of isoniazid reduced by ANTACIDS
● Antibacterials: increased risk of hepatotoxicity when isoniazid given with ● RIFAMPICIN; increased risk of CNS toxicity when isoniazid given with ● CYCLOSERINE
● Antiepileptics: isoniazid increases plasma concentration of ● CARBAMAZEPINE (also possibly increased isoniazid hepatotoxicity); isoniazid inhibits metabolism of ● ETHOSUXIMIDE (increased plasma concentration and risk of toxicity); isoniazid possibly inhibits metabolism of FOSPHENYTOIN and PHENYTOIN (increased risk of toxicity)
▸ Antifungals: isoniazid possibly reduces plasma concentration of KETOCONAZOLE
▸ Anxiolytics and Hypnotics: isoniazid inhibits the metabolism of DIAZEPAM
▸ Corticosteroids: plasma concentration of isoniazid possibly reduced by CORTICOSTEROIDS
▸ Disulfiram: isoniazid possibly increases CNS effects of DISULFIRAM
▸ Dopaminergics: isoniazid possibly reduces effects of CO-BENELDOPA, CO-CARELDOPA and LEVODOPA
● Lipid-regulating Drugs: separating administration from isoniazid by 12 hours advised by manufacturer of LOMITAPIDE
▸ Theophylline: isoniazid possibly increases plasma concentration of THEOPHYLLINE
▸ Vaccines: antibacterials inactivate ORAL TYPHOID VACCINE—see under Typhoid Vaccine in BNFC

Isosorbide Dinitrate *see* Nitrates
Isosorbide Mononitrate *see* Nitrates
Isotretinoin *see* Retinoids
Isradipine *see* Calcium-channel Blockers
Itraconazole *see* Antifungals, Triazole
Ivabradine
● Anti-arrhythmics: increased risk of ventricular arrhythmias when ivabradine given with ● AMIODARONE or ● DISOPYRAMIDE
● Antibacterials: plasma concentration of ivabradine possibly increased by ● CLARITHROMYCIN and ● TELITHROMYCIN—avoid concomitant use; increased risk of ventricular arrhythmias when ivabradine given with ● ERYTHROMYCIN—avoid concomitant use
▸ Antidepressants: plasma concentration of ivabradine reduced by ST JOHN'S WORT—avoid concomitant use
● Antifungals: plasma concentration of ivabradine increased by ● KETOCONAZOLE—avoid concomitant use; plasma concentration of ivabradine increased by FLUCONAZOLE—reduce initial dose of ivabradine; plasma concentration of ivabradine possibly increased by ● ITRACONAZOLE—avoid concomitant use
● Antimalarials: increased risk of ventricular arrhythmias when ivabradine given with ● MEFLOQUINE
● Antipsychotics: increased risk of ventricular arrhythmias when ivabradine given with ● PIMOZIDE

Ivabradine (continued)
● Antivirals: plasma concentration of ivabradine possibly increased by ● RITONAVIR—avoid concomitant use
● Beta-blockers: increased risk of ventricular arrhythmias when ivabradine given with ● SOTALOL
● Calcium-channel Blockers: plasma concentration of ivabradine increased by ● DILTIAZEM and ● VERAPAMIL—avoid concomitant use
▸ Grapefruit Juice: plasma concentration of ivabradine increased by GRAPEFRUIT JUICE
● Pentamidine Isetionate: increased risk of ventricular arrhythmias when ivabradine given with ● PENTAMIDINE ISETIONATE

Ivacaftor
● Antibacterials: plasma concentration of ivacaftor possibly increased by ● CLARITHROMYCIN, ● ERYTHROMYCIN and ● TELITHROMYCIN (see under Ivacaftor, p. 175); plasma concentration of ivacaftor possibly reduced by ● RIFABUTIN—manufacturer of ivacaftor advises avoid concomitant use; plasma concentration of ivacaftor reduced by ● RIFAMPICIN—manufacturer of ivacaftor advises avoid concomitant use
● Antidepressants: plasma concentration of ivacaftor possibly reduced by ● ST JOHN'S WORT—manufacturer of ivacaftor advises avoid concomitant use
● Antiepileptics: plasma concentration of ivacaftor possibly reduced by ● CARBAMAZEPINE, ● FOSPHENYTOIN, ● PHENOBARBITAL, ● PHENYTOIN and ● PRIMIDONE—manufacturer of ivacaftor advises avoid concomitant use
● Antifungals: plasma concentration of ivacaftor increased by ● FLUCONAZOLE and ● KETOCONAZOLE (see under Ivacaftor, p. 175); plasma concentration of ivacaftor possibly increased by ● ITRACONAZOLE, ● POSACONAZOLE and ● VORICONAZOLE (see under Ivacaftor, p. 175)
▸ Anxiolytics and Hypnotics: ivacaftor increases plasma concentration of MIDAZOLAM
▸ Cardiac Glycosides: ivacaftor increases plasma concentration of DIGOXIN
▸ Grapefruit Juice: plasma concentration of ivacaftor possibly increased by GRAPEFRUIT JUICE—manufacturer of ivacaftor advises avoid concomitant use
▸ Lipid-regulating Drugs: separating administration from ivacaftor by 12 hours advised by manufacturer of LOMITAPIDE

Ivermectin
▸ Anthelmintics: plasma concentration of ivermectin possibly increased by LEVAMISOLE
▸ Anticoagulants: ivermectin possibly enhances anticoagulant effect of COUMARINS

Japanese Encephalitis Vaccine *see* Vaccines
Kaolin
▸ Analgesics: kaolin possibly reduces absorption of ASPIRIN
▸ Antibacterials: kaolin possibly reduces absorption of TETRACYCLINES
▸ Antimalarials: kaolin reduces absorption of CHLOROQUINE and HYDROXYCHLOROQUINE
▸ Antipsychotics: kaolin possibly reduces absorption of PHENOTHIAZINES

Ketamine *see* Anaesthetics, General
Ketoconazole *see* Antifungals, Imidazole
Ketoprofen *see* NSAIDs
Ketorolac *see* NSAIDs
Ketotifen *see* Antihistamines
Labetalol *see* Beta-blockers
Lacidipine *see* Calcium-channel Blockers
Lacosamide
● Antidepressants: anticonvulsant effect of antiepileptics possibly antagonised by MAOIs and ● TRICYCLIC-RELATED ANTIDEPRESSANTS (convulsive threshold lowered); anticonvulsant effect of antiepileptics antagonised by ● SSRIS and ● TRICYCLICS (convulsive threshold lowered)
● Antimalarials: anticonvulsant effect of antiepileptics antagonised by ● MEFLOQUINE
● Antipsychotics: anticonvulsant effect of antiepileptics antagonised by ● ANTIPSYCHOTICS (convulsive threshold lowered)
● Orlistat: possible increased risk of convulsions when antiepileptics given with ● ORLISTAT

Lactulose
▸ Anticoagulants: lactulose possibly enhances anticoagulant effect of COUMARINS

Lamivudine
▸ Antibacterials: plasma concentration of lamivudine increased by TRIMETHOPRIM (as co-trimoxazole)—avoid concomitant use of high-dose co-trimoxazole
▸ Antivirals: avoidance of lamivudine advised by manufacturer of EMTRICITABINE
● Cytotoxics: manufacturer of lamivudine advises avoid concomitant use with ● CLADRIBINE
● Orlistat: absorption of lamivudine possibly reduced by ● ORLISTAT

Lamotrigine
● Antibacterials: plasma concentration of lamotrigine reduced by ● RIFAMPICIN
● Antidepressants: anticonvulsant effect of antiepileptics possibly antagonised by MAOIs and ● TRICYCLIC-RELATED ANTIDEPRESSANTS (convulsive threshold lowered); anticonvulsant effect of antiepileptics antagonised by ● SSRIS and ● TRICYCLICS (convulsive threshold lowered)
● Antiepileptics: plasma concentration of lamotrigine often reduced by CARBAMAZEPINE, also plasma concentration of an active metabolite of carbamazepine sometimes raised (but evidence is conflicting); plasma concentration of lamotrigine reduced by FOSPHENYTOIN, PHENOBARBITAL, PHENYTOIN and PRIMIDONE; plasma concentration of lamotrigine increased by ● SODIUM VALPROATE and ● VALPROIC ACID (increased risk of toxicity)—reduce lamotrigine dose)
● Antimalarials: anticonvulsant effect of antiepileptics antagonised by ● MEFLOQUINE
● Antipsychotics: anticonvulsant effect of antiepileptics antagonised by ● ANTIPSYCHOTICS (convulsive threshold lowered)
▸ Antivirals: plasma concentration of lamotrigine possibly reduced by RITONAVIR
▸ Oestrogens: plasma concentration of lamotrigine reduced by ● OESTROGENS—consider increasing dose of lamotrigine
▸ Orlistat: possible increased risk of convulsions when antiepileptics given with ● ORLISTAT
▸ Progestogens: plasma concentration of lamotrigine possibly increased by DESOGESTREL

Lanreotide
▸ Antidiabetics: lanreotide possibly reduces requirements for ANTIDIABETICS
▸ Ciclosporin: lanreotide reduces plasma concentration of CICLOSPORIN

Lansoprazole *see* Proton Pump Inhibitors

Lanthanum
▸ Antibacterials: lanthanum possibly reduces absorption of QUINOLONES (give at least 2 hours before or 4 hours after lanthanum)
▸ Antifungals: lanthanum possibly reduces absorption of KETOCONAZOLE (give at least 2 hours apart)
▸ Antimalarials: lanthanum possibly reduces absorption of CHLOROQUINE and HYDROXYCHLOROQUINE (give at least 2 hours apart)
▸ Thyroid Hormones: lanthanum reduces absorption of LEVOTHYROXINE (give at least 2 hours apart)

Lapatinib
● Antibacterials: manufacturer of lapatinib advises avoid concomitant use with ● RIFABUTIN, ● RIFAMPICIN and ● TELITHROMYCIN
● Antidepressants: manufacturer of lapatinib advises avoid concomitant use with ● ST JOHN'S WORT
● Antidiabetics: manufacturer of lapatinib advises avoid concomitant use with ● REPAGLINIDE
● Antiepileptics: plasma concentration of lapatinib reduced by ● CARBAMAZEPINE—avoid concomitant use; manufacturer of lapatinib advises avoid concomitant use with ● FOSPHENYTOIN and ● PHENYTOIN
● Antifungals: plasma concentration of lapatinib increased by ● KETOCONAZOLE—avoid concomitant use; manufacturer of lapatinib advises avoid concomitant use with ● ITRACONAZOLE, ● POSACONAZOLE and ● VORICONAZOLE

Lapatinib (continued)
● Antipsychotics: avoid concomitant use of cytotoxics with ● CLOZAPINE (increased risk of agranulocytosis); manufacturer of lapatinib advises avoid concomitant use with ● PIMOZIDE
● Antivirals: avoidance of lapatinib advised by manufacturer of ● BOCEPREVIR; manufacturer of lapatinib advises avoid concomitant use with ● RITONAVIR and ● SAQUINAVIR
● Cytotoxics: lapatinib increases plasma concentration of PAZOPANIB; possible increased risk of neutropenia when lapatinib given with DOCETAXEL; increased risk of neutropenia when lapatinib given with ● PACLITAXEL; lapatinib increases plasma concentration of active metabolite of ● IRINOTECAN—consider reducing dose of irinotecan
● Grapefruit Juice: manufacturer of lapatinib advises avoid concomitant use with ● GRAPEFRUIT JUICE
▸ Lipid-regulating Drugs: separating administration from lapatinib by 12 hours advised by manufacturer of LOMITAPIDE
▸ Ulcer-healing Drugs: absorption of lapatinib possibly reduced by HISTAMINE H$_2$-ANTAGONISTS and PROTON PUMP INHIBITORS

Laronidase
▸ Antimalarials: effects of laronidase possibly inhibited by CHLOROQUINE and HYDROXYCHLOROQUINE (manufacturer of laronidase advises avoid concomitant use)

Ledipasvir
▸ Antacids: manufacturer of ledipasvir advises separating administration from ANTACIDS by 4 hours
● Anti-arrhythmics: possible increased risk of bradycardia when ledipasvir (with sofosbuvir) given with ● AMIODARONE—see under Amiodarone, in BNF
▸ Antibacterials: manufacturer of ledipasvir advises avoid concomitant use with RIFABUTIN and RIFAMPICIN
▸ Antidepressants: manufacturer of ledipasvir advises avoid concomitant use with ST JOHN'S WORT
▸ Antiepileptics: manufacturer of ledipasvir advises avoid concomitant use with CARBAMAZEPINE, FOSPHENYTOIN, OXCARBAZEPINE, PHENOBARBITAL, PHENYTOIN and PRIMIDONE
▸ Antivirals: plasma concentration of both drugs increased when ledipasvir given with SIMEPREVIR—manufacturer of ledipasvir advises avoid concomitant use
▸ Calcium Salts: manufacturer of ledipasvir advises separating administration from CALCIUM SALTS by 4 hours
● Lipid-regulating Drugs: possible increased risk of myopathy when ledipasvir given with ● ATORVASTATIN, ● FLUVASTATIN and ● SIMVASTATIN—manufacturer of ledipasvir advises consider reducing dose of atorvastatin, fluvastatin and simvastatin; manufacturer of ledipasvir advises avoid concomitant use with ● ROSUVASTATIN
▸ Ulcer-healing Drugs: plasma concentration of ledipasvir reduced by FAMOTIDINE and OMEPRAZOLE; manufacturer of ledipasvir advises do not take PROTON PUMP INHIBITORS before ledispavir

Leflunomide
NOTE Increased risk of toxicity with other haematotoxic and hepatotoxic drugs
▸ Antibacterials: plasma concentration of active metabolite of leflunomide possibly increased by RIFAMPICIN
▸ Anticoagulants: leflunomide possibly enhances anticoagulant effect of WARFARIN
▸ Antidiabetics: leflunomide possibly enhances hypoglycaemic effect of TOLBUTAMIDE
▸ Antiepileptics: leflunomide possibly increases plasma concentration of FOSPHENYTOIN and PHENYTOIN
● Cytotoxics: risk of toxicity when leflunomide given with ● METHOTREXATE
▸ Lipid-regulating Drugs: the effect of leflunomide is significantly decreased by COLESTYRAMINE (enhanced elimination)—avoid unless drug elimination desired
▸ Vaccines: risk of generalised infections when leflunomide given with live ● VACCINES—avoid concomitant use

Lenalidomide
● Antibacterials: plasma concentration of lenalidomide possibly increased by ● CLARITHROMYCIN (increased risk of toxicity)
● Antifungals: plasma concentration of lenalidomide possibly increased by ● ITRACONAZOLE and ● KETOCONAZOLE (increased risk of toxicity)

Lenalidomide (continued)

- Calcium-channel Blockers: plasma concentration of lenalidomide possibly increased by • VERAPAMIL (increased risk of toxicity)
▸ Cardiac Glycosides: lenalidomide possibly increases plasma concentration of DIGOXIN
- Ciclosporin: plasma concentration of lenalidomide possibly increased by • CICLOSPORIN (increased risk of toxicity)

Lercanidipine see Calcium-channel Blockers

Leukotriene Receptor Antagonists
▸ Aminophylline: zafirlukast possibly increases plasma concentration of AMINOPHYLLINE, also plasma concentration of zafirlukast reduced
▸ Analgesics: plasma concentration of zafirlukast increased by ASPIRIN
▸ Antibacterials: plasma concentration of zafirlukast reduced by ERYTHROMYCIN
▸ Anticoagulants: zafirlukast enhances anticoagulant effect of WARFARIN
▸ Antiepileptics: plasma concentration of montelukast reduced by PHENOBARBITAL and PRIMIDONE
▸ Antifungals: plasma concentration of zafirlukast increased by FLUCONAZOLE
▸ Lipid-regulating Drugs: plasma concentration of montelukast increased by GEMFIBROZIL
▸ Theophylline: zafirlukast possibly increases plasma concentration of THEOPHYLLINE, also plasma concentration of zafirlukast reduced

Levamisole
▸ Alcohol: possibility of disulfiram-like reaction when levamisole given with ALCOHOL
▸ Anthelmintics: plasma concentration of both drugs possibly reduced when levamisole given with ALBENDAZOLE; levamisole possibly increases plasma concentration of IVERMECTIN
- Anticoagulants: levamisole possibly enhances anticoagulant effect of • WARFARIN
▸ Antiepileptics: levamisole possibly increases plasma concentration of FOSPHENYTOIN and PHENYTOIN

Levetiracetam
- Antidepressants: anticonvulsant effect of antiepileptics possibly antagonised by MAOIs and • TRICYCLIC-RELATED ANTIDEPRESSANTS (convulsive threshold lowered); anticonvulsant effect of antiepileptics antagonised by • SSRIS and • TRICYCLICS (convulsive threshold lowered)
- Antiepileptics: levetiracetam possibly increases risk of CARBAMAZEPINE toxicity
- Antimalarials: anticonvulsant effect of antiepileptics antagonised by • MEFLOQUINE
- Antipsychotics: anticonvulsant effect of antiepileptics antagonised by • ANTIPSYCHOTICS (convulsive threshold lowered)
- Cytotoxics: levetiracetam possibly increases plasma concentration of • METHOTREXATE
- Orlistat: possible increased risk of convulsions when antiepileptics given with • ORLISTAT

Levobunolol see Beta-blockers

Levobupivacaine
▸ Anti-arrhythmics: increased myocardial depression when levobupivacaine given with ANTI-ARRHYTHMICS

Levocarnitine
▸ Anticoagulants: levocarnitine possibly enhances anticoagulant effect of COUMARINS

Levocetirizine see Antihistamines

Levodopa
▸ ACE Inhibitors: enhanced hypotensive effect when levodopa given with ACE INHIBITORS
▸ Adrenergic Neurone Blockers: enhanced hypotensive effect when levodopa given with ADRENERGIC NEURONE BLOCKERS
▸ Alpha-blockers: enhanced hypotensive effect when levodopa given with ALPHA-BLOCKERS
- Anaesthetics, General: increased risk of arrhythmias when levodopa given with • VOLATILE LIQUID GENERAL ANAESTHETICS
▸ Angiotensin-II Receptor Antagonists: enhanced hypotensive effect when levodopa given with ANGIOTENSIN-II RECEPTOR ANTAGONISTS

Levodopa (continued)
▸ Antibacterials: effects of levodopa possibly reduced by ISONIAZID
- Antidepressants: risk of hypertensive crisis when levodopa given with • MAOIS, avoid levodopa for at least 2 weeks after stopping MAOIs; increased risk of side-effects when levodopa given with MOCLOBEMIDE
▸ Antiepileptics: effects of levodopa possibly reduced by FOSPHENYTOIN and PHENYTOIN
▸ Antimuscarinics: absorption of levodopa possibly reduced by ANTIMUSCARINICS
▸ Antipsychotics: effects of levodopa antagonised by ANTIPSYCHOTICS; avoidance of levodopa advised by manufacturer of AMISULPRIDE (antagonism of effect)
▸ Anxiolytics and Hypnotics: effects of levodopa possibly antagonised by BENZODIAZEPINES
▸ Beta-blockers: enhanced hypotensive effect when levodopa given with BETA-BLOCKERS
▸ Bupropion: increased risk of side-effects when levodopa given with BUPROPION
▸ Calcium-channel Blockers: enhanced hypotensive effect when levodopa given with CALCIUM-CHANNEL BLOCKERS
▸ Clonidine: enhanced hypotensive effect when levodopa given with CLONIDINE
▸ Diazoxide: enhanced hypotensive effect when levodopa given with DIAZOXIDE
▸ Diuretics: enhanced hypotensive effect when levodopa given with DIURETICS
▸ Dopaminergics: enhanced effects and increased toxicity of levodopa when given with SELEGILINE (reduce dose of levodopa)
▸ Iron Salts: absorption of levodopa possibly reduced by *oral* IRON SALTS
▸ Memantine: effects of dopaminergics possibly enhanced by MEMANTINE
▸ Methyldopa: enhanced hypotensive effect when levodopa given with METHYLDOPA; antiparkinsonian effect of dopaminergics antagonised by METHYLDOPA
▸ Moxonidine: enhanced hypotensive effect when levodopa given with MOXONIDINE
▸ Muscle Relaxants: possible agitation, confusion and hallucinations when levodopa given with BACLOFEN
▸ Nitrates: enhanced hypotensive effect when levodopa given with NITRATES
▸ Vasodilator Antihypertensives: enhanced hypotensive effect when levodopa given with HYDRALAZINE, MINOXIDIL or SODIUM NITROPRUSSIDE
▸ Vitamins: effects of levodopa reduced by PYRIDOXINE when given without dopa-decarboxylase inhibitor

Levofloxacin see Quinolones

Levofolinic Acid see Folates

Levomepromazine see Antipsychotics

Levonorgestrel see Progestogens

Levosimendan
- Nitrates: possible severe postural hypotension when levosimendan given with • ISOSORBIDE MONONITRATE

Levothyroxine see Thyroid Hormones

Lidocaine
  NOTE Interactions less likely when lidocaine used topically
▸ Anaesthetics, Local: increased myocardial depression when anti-arrhythmics given with BUPIVACAINE, LEVOBUPIVACAINE, PRILOCAINE or ROPIVACAINE
- Anti-arrhythmics: increased myocardial depression when anti-arrhythmics given with other • ANTI-ARRHYTHMICS
- Antipsychotics: increased risk of ventricular arrhythmias when anti-arrhythmics that prolong the QT interval given with • ANTIPSYCHOTICS that prolong the QT interval
- Antivirals: plasma concentration of lidocaine possibly increased by ATAZANAVIR and LOPINAVIR; plasma concentration of lidocaine possibly increased by DARUNAVIR and • FOSAMPRENAVIR—avoid concomitant use; increased risk of ventricular arrhythmias when lidocaine given with • SAQUINAVIR—avoid concomitant use; caution with *intravenous* lidocaine advised by manufacturer of TELAPREVIR
- Beta-blockers: increased myocardial depression when anti-arrhythmics given with • BETA-BLOCKERS; possible increased

Lidocaine
- Beta-blockers (continued)
  risk of lidocaine toxicity when given with NADOLOL; increased risk of lidocaine toxicity when given with ● PROPRANOLOL
- Diuretics: action of lidocaine antagonised by hypokalaemia caused by ● ACETAZOLAMIDE, ● LOOP DIURETICS or ● THIAZIDES AND RELATED DIURETICS
▸ Muscle Relaxants: neuromuscular blockade enhanced and prolonged when lidocaine given with SUXAMETHONIUM
▸ Ulcer-healing Drugs: plasma concentration of lidocaine increased by ● CIMETIDINE (increased risk of toxicity)

Linagliptin *see* Antidiabetics
Linezolid *see* MAOIs
Liothyronine *see* Thyroid Hormones
Lipegfilgrastim
▸ Cytotoxics: neutropenia possibly exacerbated when lipegfilgrastim given with CAPECITABINE, FLUOROURACIL or TEGAFUR

Lipid-regulating Drugs *see* Colesevelam, Colestipol, Colestyramine, Ezetimibe, Fibrates, Lomitapide, Nicotinic Acid, and Statins
Liraglutide *see* Antidiabetics
Lisdexamfetamine *see* Sympathomimetics
Lisinopril *see* ACE Inhibitors
Lithium
- ACE Inhibitors: excretion of lithium reduced by ● ACE INHIBITORS (increased plasma concentration)
- Aminophylline: excretion of lithium increased by AMINOPHYLLINE (reduced plasma concentration)
- Analgesics: excretion of lithium reduced by ● NSAIDS (increased risk of toxicity); excretion of lithium reduced by ● KETOROLAC (increased risk of toxicity)—avoid concomitant use
- Angiotensin-II Receptor Antagonists: excretion of lithium reduced by ● ANGIOTENSIN-II RECEPTOR ANTAGONISTS (increased plasma concentration)
- Antacids: excretion of lithium increased by SODIUM BICARBONATE (reduced plasma concentration)
- Anti-arrhythmics: avoidance of lithium advised by manufacturer of ● AMIODARONE (risk of ventricular arrhythmias)
▸ Antibacterials: increased risk of lithium toxicity when given with METRONIDAZOLE
- Antidepressants: possible increased serotonergic effects when lithium given with VENLAFAXINE; increased risk of CNS effects when lithium given with ● SSRIS (lithium toxicity reported); risk of toxicity when lithium given with TRICYCLICS
▸ Antiepileptics: neurotoxicity may occur when lithium given with CARBAMAZEPINE, FOSPHENYTOIN or PHENYTOIN without increased plasma concentration of lithium; plasma concentration of lithium possibly affected by TOPIRAMATE
- Antipsychotics: increased risk of extrapyramidal side-effects and possibly neurotoxicity when lithium given with CLOZAPINE, FLUPENTIXOL, HALOPERIDOL, PHENOTHIAZINES, ● RISPERIDONE or ZUCLOPENTIXOL; possible risk of toxicity when lithium given with OLANZAPINE; lithium possibly increases extrapyramidal side-effects of QUETIAPINE; increased risk of extrapyramidal side-effects when lithium given with SULPIRIDE
▸ Anxiolytics and Hypnotics: increased risk of neurotoxicity when lithium given with CLONAZEPAM
- Calcium-channel Blockers: neurotoxicity may occur when lithium given with DILTIAZEM or VERAPAMIL without increased plasma concentration of lithium
- Cytotoxics: increased risk of ventricular arrhythmias when lithium given with ● ARSENIC TRIOXIDE
- Dapoxetine: possible increased risk of serotonergic effects when lithium given with ● DAPOXETINE (manufacturer of dapoxetine advises lithium should not be started until 1 week after stopping dapoxetine, avoid dapoxetine for 2 weeks after stopping lithium)
- Diuretics: excretion of lithium increased by ● ACETAZOLAMIDE; excretion of lithium reduced by ● LOOP DIURETICS and ● THIAZIDES AND RELATED DIURETICS (increased plasma concentration and risk of toxicity)—loop diuretics safer than thiazides; excretion of lithium reduced by

Lithium
- Diuretics (continued)
  ● POTASSIUM-SPARING DIURETICS AND ALDOSTERONE ANTAGONISTS (increased plasma concentration and risk of toxicity)
▸ 5HT₁-receptor Agonists: possible risk of toxicity when lithium given with SUMATRIPTAN
- Methyldopa: neurotoxicity may occur when lithium given with ● METHYLDOPA without increased plasma concentration of lithium
▸ Muscle Relaxants: lithium enhances effects of MUSCLE RELAXANTS; hyperkinesis caused by lithium possibly aggravated by BACLOFEN
▸ Parasympathomimetics: lithium antagonises effects of NEOSTIGMINE
▸ Theophylline: excretion of lithium increased by THEOPHYLLINE (reduced plasma concentration)

Lixisenatide *see* Antidiabetics
Lofepramine *see* Antidepressants, Tricyclic
Lofexidine
▸ Alcohol: increased sedative effect when lofexidine given with ALCOHOL
▸ Anxiolytics and Hypnotics: increased sedative effect when lofexidine given with ANXIOLYTICS AND HYPNOTICS

Lomitapide
▸ Alcohol: manufacturer of lomitapide advises avoid concomitant use with ALCOHOL
- Anti-arrhythmics: manufacturer of lomitapide advises separating administration from AMIODARONE by 12 hours; manufacturer of lomitapide advises avoid concomitant use with ● DRONEDARONE (plasma concentration of lomitapide possibly increased)
- Antibacterials: manufacturer of lomitapide advises separating administration from AZITHROMYCIN and ISONIAZID by 12 hours; manufacturer of lomitapide advises avoid concomitant use with ● CLARITHROMYCIN, ● ERYTHROMYCIN and ● TELITHROMYCIN (plasma concentration of lomitapide possibly increased)
▸ Anticoagulants: lomitapide possibly enhances anticoagulant effect of WARFARIN
▸ Antidepressants: manufacturer of lomitapide advises separating administration from FLUOXETINE and FLUVOXAMINE by 12 hours
▸ Antidiabetics: manufacturer of lomitapide advises separating administration from LINAGLIPTIN by 12 hours
- Antifungals: plasma concentration of lomitapide increased by ● KETOCONAZOLE—avoid concomitant use; manufacturer of lomitapide advises avoid concomitant use with ● TRIAZOLES (plasma concentration of lomitapide possibly increased)
- Antivirals: manufacturer of lomitapide advises avoid concomitant use with ● DARUNAVIR, ● FOSAMPRENAVIR, ● INDINAVIR, ● LOPINAVIR, ● RITONAVIR, ● SAQUINAVIR, ● TELAPREVIR and ● TIPRANAVIR (plasma concentration of lomitapide possibly increased)
▸ Anxiolytics and Hypnotics: manufacturer of lomitapide advises separating administration from ALPRAZOLAM by 12 hours
- Calcium-channel Blockers: manufacturer of lomitapide advises separating administration from AMLODIPINE and LACIDIPINE by 12 hours; manufacturer of lomitapide advises avoid concomitant use with ● DILTIAZEM and ● VERAPAMIL (plasma concentration of lomitapide possibly increased)
▸ Ciclosporin: manufacturer of lomitapide advises separating administration from CICLOSPORIN by 12 hours
▸ Cilostazol: manufacturer of lomitapide advises separating administration from CILOSTAZOL by 12 hours
▸ Cytotoxics: manufacturer of lomitapide advises separating administration from LAPATINIB, NILOTINIB and PAZOPANIB by 12 hours
▸ Fosaprepitant: manufacturer of lomitapide advises separating administration from FOSAPREPITANT by 12 hours
▸ Grapefruit Juice: manufacturer of lomitapide advises avoid concomitant use with GRAPEFRUIT JUICE
- Hormone Antagonists: manufacturer of lomitapide advises separating administration from BICALUTAMIDE by 12 hours
▸ Ivacaftor: manufacturer of lomitapide advises separating administration from IVACAFTOR by 12 hours
- Lipid-regulating Drugs: lomitapide increases plasma concentration of ATORVASTATIN—manufacturer of lomitapide

Lomitapide
- Lipid-regulating Drugs (continued)
  advises reduce dose of atorvastatin by half or separate administration by 12 hours; lomitapide increases plasma concentration of • SIMVASTATIN (see under Simvastatin, in BNF); absorption of lomitapide possibly reduced by BILE ACID SEQUESTRANTS (give at least 4 hours apart)
- Oestrogens: manufacturer of lomitapide advises separating administration from OESTROGENS by 12 hours
- Ranolazine: manufacturer of lomitapide advises separating administration from RANOLAZINE by 12 hours
- Tacrolimus: manufacturer of lomitapide advises separating administration from TACROLIMUS by 12 hours
- Ticagrelor: manufacturer of lomitapide advises separating administration from TICAGRELOR by 12 hours
- Tolvaptan: manufacturer of lomitapide advises separating administration from TOLVAPTAN by 12 hours
- Ulcer-healing Drugs: manufacturer of lomitapide advises separating administration from CIMETIDINE and RANITIDINE by 12 hours

Lomustine
- Antipsychotics: avoid concomitant use of cytotoxics with
  • CLOZAPINE (increased risk of agranulocytosis)
- Ulcer-healing Drugs: myelosuppressive effects of lomustine possibly enhanced by CIMETIDINE

Loperamide
- Desmopressin: loperamide increases plasma concentration of *oral* DESMOPRESSIN

Lopinavir
  NOTE In combination with ritonavir as *Kaletra*® (ritonavir is present to inhibit lopinavir metabolism and increase plasma-lopinavir concentration)—see also Ritonavir
- Anti-arrhythmics: lopinavir possibly increases plasma concentration of • FLECAINIDE (increased risk of ventricular arrhythmias—avoid concomitant use); lopinavir possibly increases plasma concentration of LIDOCAINE
- Antibacterials: plasma concentration of lopinavir reduced by
  • RIFAMPICIN—avoid concomitant use; lopinavir increases plasma concentration of DELAMANID; avoidance of concomitant lopinavir in severe renal and hepatic impairment advised by manufacturer of • TELITHROMYCIN
- Anticoagulants: avoidance of lopinavir advised by manufacturer of APIXABAN; manufacturers advise avoid concomitant use of lopinavir with RIVAROXABAN
- Antidepressants: plasma concentration of lopinavir reduced by
  • ST JOHN'S WORT—avoid concomitant use
- Antiepileptics: plasma concentration of lopinavir possibly reduced by CARBAMAZEPINE, FOSPHENYTOIN, • PHENOBARBITAL, PHENYTOIN and • PRIMIDONE
- Antihistamines: lopinavir possibly increases plasma concentration of CHLORPHENAMINE
- Antimalarials: caution with lopinavir advised by manufacturer of ARTEMETHER WITH LUMEFANTRINE
- Antimuscarinics: avoidance of lopinavir advised by manufacturer of DARIFENACIN and TOLTERODINE
- Antipsychotics: lopinavir possibly increases plasma concentration of • ARIPIPRAZOLE (reduce dose of aripiprazole—consult aripiprazole product literature); lopinavir possibly increases plasma concentration of
  • QUETIAPINE—manufacturer of quetiapine advises avoid concomitant use
- Antivirals: manufacturers advise avoid concomitant use of lopinavir with • BOCEPREVIR and • TELAPREVIR; lopinavir reduces plasma concentration of • DARUNAVIR—avoid concomitant use; plasma concentration of lopinavir reduced by • EFAVIRENZ—consider increasing dose of lopinavir; lopinavir boosted with ritonavir increases plasma concentration of • ELVITEGRAVIR (reduce dose of elvitegravir); lopinavir reduces plasma concentration of FOSAMPRENAVIR, effect on lopinavir plasma concentration not predictable—avoid concomitant use; lopinavir increases plasma concentration of • MARAVIROC (consider reducing dose of maraviroc); plasma concentration of lopinavir possibly reduced by • NEVIRAPINE—consider increasing dose of lopinavir; lopinavir increases plasma concentration of
  • PARITAPREVIR—manufacturer of paritaprevir advises avoid

Lopinavir
- Antivirals (continued)
  concomitant use; increased risk of ventricular arrhythmias when lopinavir given with • SAQUINAVIR—avoid concomitant use; lopinavir increases plasma concentration of TENOFOVIR; plasma concentration of lopinavir reduced by • TIPRANAVIR
- Bosentan: lopinavir increases plasma concentration of
  • BOSENTAN (consider reducing dose of bosentan)
- Corticosteroids: plasma concentration of lopinavir possibly reduced by DEXAMETHASONE
- Cytotoxics: manufacturer of ruxolitinib advises dose reduction when lopinavir given with • RUXOLITINIB—consult ruxolitinib product literature
- Eltrombopag: lopinavir possibly reduces plasma concentration of ELTROMBOPAG
- Lipid-regulating Drugs: possible increased risk of myopathy when lopinavir given with ATORVASTATIN; lopinavir increases plasma concentration of • ROSUVASTATIN—adjust dose of rosuvastatin (consult product literature); possible increased risk of myopathy when lopinavir given with • SIMVASTATIN—avoid concomitant use; avoidance of lopinavir advised by manufacturer of • LOMITAPIDE (plasma concentration of lomitapide possibly increased)
- Orlistat: absorption of lopinavir possibly reduced by • ORLISTAT
- Ranolazine: lopinavir possibly increases plasma concentration of • RANOLAZINE—manufacturer of ranolazine advises avoid concomitant use
- Sirolimus: lopinavir possibly increases plasma concentration of SIROLIMUS
- Sympathomimetics, Beta$_2$: manufacturer of lopinavir advises avoid concomitant use with SALMETEROL

Loprazolam *see* Anxiolytics and Hypnotics
Loratadine *see* Antihistamines
Lorazepam *see* Anxiolytics and Hypnotics
Lormetazepam *see* Anxiolytics and Hypnotics
Losartan *see* Angiotensin-II Receptor Antagonists
Lurasidone *see* Antipsychotics
Lymecycline *see* Tetracyclines
Macitentan
- Antibacterials: plasma concentration of macitentan reduced by
  • RIFAMPICIN—avoid concomitant use
- Antidepressants: manufacturer of macitentan advises avoid concomitant use with ST JOHN'S WORT
- Antiepileptics: manufacturer of macitentan advises avoid concomitant use with CARBAMAZEPINE, FOSPHENYTOIN and PHENYTOIN
- Antifungals: plasma concentration of macitentan increased by KETOCONAZOLE

Macrogols
  NOTE Some manufacturers suggest taking other oral medication 1 hour before or 1 hour after macrogols to reduce possible interference with absorption

Macrolides
  NOTE *See also* Telithromycin
  NOTE Interactions do not apply to small amounts of erythromycin used topically
- Aminophylline: clarithromycin possibly increases plasma concentration of AMINOPHYLLINE; erythromycin increases plasma concentration of • AMINOPHYLLINE (also aminophylline may reduce absorption of *oral* erythromycin)
- Analgesics: erythromycin increases plasma concentration of ALFENTANIL; clarithromycin possibly increases plasma concentration of FENTANYL
- Antacids: absorption of azithromycin reduced by ANTACIDS (give at least 2 hours before or 1 hour after antacids)
- Anti-arrhythmics: increased risk of ventricular arrhythmias when *parenteral* erythromycin given with • AMIODARONE—avoid concomitant use; erythromycin increases plasma concentration of • DISOPYRAMIDE (increased risk of toxicity); clarithromycin possibly increases plasma concentration of
  • DISOPYRAMIDE (increased risk of ventricular arrhythmias); azithromycin possibly increases plasma concentration of
  • DISOPYRAMIDE (increased risk of toxicity); avoidance of clarithromycin advised by manufacturer of • DRONEDARONE (risk of ventricular arrhythmias); erythromycin increases

Macrolides

- **Anti-arrhythmics** (continued)
  plasma concentration of • DRONEDARONE (increased risk of
  ventricular arrhythmias—avoid concomitant use)
- **Antibacterials:** increased risk of ventricular arrhythmias when
  parenteral erythromycin given with • MOXIFLOXACIN—avoid
  concomitant use; increased risk of side-effects including
  neutropenia when azithromycin given with • RIFABUTIN;
  clarithromycin increases plasma concentration of • RIFABUTIN
  (increased risk of toxicity—reduce rifabutin dose);
  erythromycin possibly increases plasma concentration of
  • RIFABUTIN (increased risk of toxicity—reduce rifabutin dose);
  clarithromycin and erythromycin possibly increase plasma
  concentration of BEDAQUILINE—avoid concomitant use if
  clarithromycin and erythromycin given for more than 14 days;
  possible increased risk of ventricular arrhythmias when
  clarithromycin and erythromycin given with • DELAMANID;
  avoidance of clarithromycin and erythromycin advised by
  manufacturer of FIDAXOMICIN; plasma concentration of
  clarithromycin reduced by RIFAMYCINS
- **Anticoagulants:** avoidance of clarithromycin advised by
  manufacturer of APIXABAN; clarithromycin and erythromycin
  enhance anticoagulant effect of • COUMARINS; azithromycin
  possibly enhances anticoagulant effect of • COUMARINS;
  possible increased risk of bleeding when clarithromycin given
  with DABIGATRAN; erythromycin increases plasma
  concentration of • EDOXABAN (reduce dose of edoxaban—see
  under Edoxaban, in BNF)
- **Antidepressants:** avoidance of macrolides advised by
  manufacturer of • REBOXETINE; avoidance of *intravenous*
  erythromycin advised by manufacturer of • CITALOPRAM and
  • ESCITALOPRAM (risk of ventricular arrhythmias); avoidance of
  erythromycin advised by manufacturer of • VENLAFAXINE (risk
  of ventricular arrhythmias); clarithromycin possibly increases
  plasma concentration of TRAZODONE
- **Antidiabetics:** clarithromycin enhances effects of REPAGLINIDE
- **Antiepileptics:** erythromycin increases plasma concentration of
  • CARBAMAZEPINE; clarithromycin increases plasma
  concentration of • CARBAMAZEPINE (consider reducing dose of
  carbamazepine); clarithromycin inhibits metabolism of
  FOSPHENYTOIN and PHENYTOIN (increased plasma
  concentration); erythromycin possibly inhibits metabolism of
  SODIUM VALPROATE and VALPROIC ACID (increased plasma
  concentration)
- **Antifungals:** avoidance of concomitant clarithromycin in
  severe renal imapirment advised by manufacturer of
  • KETOCONAZOLE; avoidance of erythromycin advised by
  manufacturer of FLUCONAZOLE; clarithromycin increases
  plasma concentration of ITRACONAZOLE
- **Antihistamines:** manufacturer of loratadine advises
  erythromycin possibly increases plasma concentration of
  LORATADINE; macrolides possibly inhibit metabolism of
  • MIZOLASTINE (avoid concomitant use); erythromycin inhibits
  metabolism of • MIZOLASTINE—avoid concomitant use
- **Antimalarials:** avoidance of macrolides advised by
  manufacturer of • ARTEMETHER WITH LUMEFANTRINE; avoidance
  of macrolides advised by manufacturer of • ARTENIMOL WITH
  PIPERAQUINE (possible risk of ventricular arrhythmias)
- **Antimuscarinics:** erythromycin possibly increases plasma
  concentration of DARIFENACIN; manufacturer of fesoterodine
  advises dose reduction when clarithromycin given with
  FESOTERODINE—consult fesoterodine product literature;
  avoidance of clarithromycin and erythromycin advised by
  manufacturer of TOLTERODINE
- **Antipsychotics:** avoidance of macrolides advised by
  manufacturer of • DROPERIDOL (risk of ventricular
  arrhythmias); increased risk of ventricular arrhythmias when
  parenteral erythromycin given with • ZUCLOPENTHIXOL—avoid
  concomitant use; increased risk of ventricular arrhythmias
  when erythromycin given with • AMISULPRIDE—avoid
  concomitant use; erythromycin possibly increases plasma
  concentration of • CLOZAPINE (possible increased risk of
  convulsions); clarithromycin possibly increases plasma
  concentration of • LURASIDONE—avoid concomitant use;
  erythromycin possibly increases the plasma concentration of
  • LURASIDONE (see under Lurasidone, in BNF); increased risk of

Macrolides

- **Antipsychotics** (continued)
  ventricular arrhythmias when clarithromycin given with
  • PIMOZIDE—avoid concomitant use; possible increased risk of
  ventricular arrhythmias when erythromycin given with
  • PIMOZIDE—avoid concomitant use; clarithromycin possibly
  increases plasma concentration of • QUETIAPINE—
  manufacturer of quetiapine advises avoid concomitant use;
  erythromycin increases plasma concentration of
  • QUETIAPINE—manufacturer of quetiapine advises avoid
  concomitant use; increased risk of ventricular arrhythmias
  when *parenteral* erythromycin given with • SULPIRIDE
- **Antivirals:** plasma concentration of both drugs increased when
  clarithromycin given with ATAZANAVIR; clarithromycin
  possibly increases the plasma concentration of
  • DACLATASVIR—reduce dose of daclatasvir (see under
  Daclatasvir, in BNF); avoidance of clarithromycin advised by
  manufacturer of DASABUVIR and PARITAPREVIR; plasma
  concentration of clarithromycin reduced by EFAVIRENZ, also
  plasma concentration of active metabolite of clarithromycin
  increased; plasma concentration of clarithromycin reduced by
  • ETRAVIRINE and NEVIRAPINE (but concentration of an active
  metabolite increased), also plasma concentration of etravirine
  and nevirapine increased; clarithromycin possibly increases
  plasma concentration of • MARAVIROC (consider reducing dose
  of maraviroc); avoidance of clarithromycin and erythromycin
  advised by manufacturer of • RILPIVIRINE (plasma
  concentration of rilpivirine possibly increased); plasma
  concentration of clarithromycin increased by • RITONAVIR
  (reduce dose of clarithromycin in renal impairment); plasma
  concentration of azithromycin and erythromycin possibly
  increased by RITONAVIR; increased risk of ventricular
  arrhythmias when erythromycin given with • SAQUINAVIR—
  avoid concomitant use; plasma concentration of both drugs
  possibly increased when clarithromycin given with
  • SAQUINAVIR and • TELAPREVIR (increased risk of ventricular
  arrhythmias); plasma concentration of both drugs increased
  when erythromycin given with • SIMEPREVIR—manufacturer of
  simeprevir advises avoid concomitant use; clarithromycin
  possibly increases plasma concentration of • SIMEPREVIR—
  manufacturer of simeprevir advises avoid concomitant use;
  plasma concentration of both drugs possibly increased when
  erythromycin given with • TELAPREVIR (increased risk of
  ventricular arrhythmias); plasma concentration of
  clarithromycin increased by • TIPRANAVIR (reduce dose of
  clarithromycin in renal impairment), also clarithromycin
  increases plasma concentration of tipranavir; clarithromycin
  tablets reduce absorption of ZIDOVUDINE (give at least 2 hours
  apart)
- **Anxiolytics and Hypnotics:** clarithromycin and erythromycin
  inhibit metabolism of • MIDAZOLAM (increased plasma
  concentration with increased sedation); erythromycin
  increases plasma concentration of BUSPIRONE (reduce dose of
  buspirone); erythromycin inhibits the metabolism of
  ZOPICLONE
- **Aprepitant:** clarithromycin possibly increases plasma
  concentration of APREPITANT
- **Atomoxetine:** increased risk of ventricular arrhythmias when
  parenteral erythromycin given with • ATOMOXETINE
- **Avanafil:** clarithromycin possibly increases plasma
  concentration of • AVANAFIL—manufacturer of avanafil advises
  avoid concomitant use; erythromycin increases plasma
  concentration of • AVANAFIL—see under Avanafil, in BNF
- **Calcium-channel Blockers:** clarithromycin and erythromycin
  possibly inhibit metabolism of • CALCIUM-CHANNEL BLOCKERS
  (increased risk of side-effects); avoidance of erythromycin
  advised by manufacturer of LERCANIDIPINE
- **Cardiac Glycosides:** macrolides increase plasma concentration
  of DIGOXIN (increased risk of toxicity)
- **Ciclosporin:** macrolides possibly inhibit metabolism of
  • CICLOSPORIN (increased plasma concentration); azithromycin
  increases plasma concentration of • CICLOSPORIN;
  clarithromycin and erythromycin inhibit metabolism of
  • CICLOSPORIN (increased plasma concentration)
- **Cilostazol:** clarithromycin possibly increases plasma
  concentration of • CILOSTAZOL (see under Cilostazol, in BNF);

Macrolides

- Cilostazol (continued)
erythromycin increases plasma concentration of • CILOSTAZOL (see under Cilostazol, in BNF)
- Clopidogrel: erythromycin possibly reduces antiplatelet effect of • CLOPIDOGREL
- Colchicine: azithromycin, clarithromycin and erythromycin possibly increase risk of • COLCHICINE toxicity—suspend or reduce dose of colchicine (avoid concomitant use in hepatic or renal impairment)
- Corticosteroids: erythromycin possibly inhibits metabolism of CORTICOSTEROIDS; erythromycin inhibits the metabolism of METHYLPREDNISOLONE; clarithromycin possibly increases plasma concentration of METHYLPREDNISOLONE
- Cytotoxics: erythromycin possibly increases the plasma concentration of AFATINIB—manufacturer of afatinib advises separating administration of erythromycin by 6 to 12 hours; clarithromycin and erythromycin possibly increase plasma concentration of AXITINIB (reduce dose of axitinib—consult axitinib product literature); clarithromycin and erythromycin possibly increase the plasma concentration of • BOSUTINIB—manufacturer of bosutinib advises avoid or consider reducing dose of bosutinib; clarithromycin and erythromycin possibly increase plasma concentration of CABOZANTINIB; clarithromycin possibly increases plasma concentration of • CRIZOTINIB and • EVEROLIMUS—manufacturer of crizotinib and everolimus advises avoid concomitant use; avoidance of clarithromycin and erythromycin advised by manufacturer of DASATINIB (plasma concentration of dasatinib possibly increased); erythromycin increases plasma concentration of • EVEROLIMUS (consider reducing the dose of everolimus—consult everolimus product literature); clarithromycin and erythromycin possibly increase the plasma concentration of • IBRUTINIB—reduce dose of ibrutinib (see under Ibrutinib, in BNF); avoidance of clarithromycin advised by manufacturer of • NILOTINIB and • OLAPARIB; clarithromycin possibly increases plasma concentration of • PAZOPANIB (reduce dose of pazopanib); clarithromycin possibly increases plasma concentration of • PONATINIB—consider reducing initial dose of ponatinib (see under Ponatinib, in BNF); manufacturer of ruxolitinib advises dose reduction when clarithromycin given with • RUXOLITINIB—consult ruxolitinib product literature; possible increased risk of ventricular arrhythmias when *parenteral* erythromycin given with • VANDETANIB—avoid concomitant use; clarithromycin possibly increases the plasma concentration of • CABAZITAXEL—manufacturer of cabazitaxel advises avoid or consider reducing dose of cabazitaxel; clarithromycin possibly increases plasma concentration of • DOCETAXEL—manufacturer of docetaxel advises avoid concomitant use or consider reducing docetaxel dose; increased risk of ventricular arrhythmias when erythromycin given with • ARSENIC TRIOXIDE; erythromycin increases toxicity of VINBLASTINE—avoid concomitant use; possible increased risk of neutropenia when clarithromycin given with VINORELBINE
- Dapoxetine: manufacturer of dapoxetine advises dose reduction when clarithromycin and erythromycin given with DAPOXETINE (see under Dapoxetine, in BNF)
- Diuretics: clarithromycin increases plasma concentration of • EPLERENONE—avoid concomitant use; erythromycin increases plasma concentration of EPLERENONE (reduce dose of eplerenone)
- Domperidone: possible increased risk of ventricular arrhythmias when clarithromycin given with • DOMPERIDONE—avoid concomitant use; erythromycin increases plasma concentration of • DOMPERIDONE (increased risk of ventricular arrhythmias—avoid concomitant use)
- Dopaminergics: macrolides possibly increase plasma concentration of BROMOCRIPTINE and CABERGOLINE (increased risk of toxicity); erythromycin increases plasma concentration of BROMOCRIPTINE and CABERGOLINE (increased risk of toxicity)
- Ergot Alkaloids: increased risk of ergotism when clarithromycin or erythromycin given with • ERGOT ALKALOIDS—avoid concomitant use
- Fosaprepitant: clarithromycin possibly increases plasma concentration of FOSAPREPITANT

Macrolides (continued)

- Guanfacine: clarithromycin and erythromycin possibly increase the plasma concentration of • GUANFACINE (halve dose of guanfacine)
- 5HT$_1$-receptor Agonists: clarithromycin and erythromycin increase plasma concentration of • ELETRIPTAN (risk of toxicity)—avoid concomitant use
- Ivabradine: clarithromycin possibly increases plasma concentration of • IVABRADINE—avoid concomitant use; increased risk of ventricular arrhythmias when erythromycin given with • IVABRADINE—avoid concomitant use
- Ivacaftor: clarithromycin and erythromycin possibly increase plasma concentration of • IVACAFTOR (see under Ivacaftor, p. 175)
- Lenalidomide: clarithromycin possibly increases plasma concentration of • LENALIDOMIDE (increased risk of toxicity)
- Leukotriene Receptor Antagonists: erythromycin reduces plasma concentration of ZAFIRLUKAST
- Lipid-regulating Drugs: possible increased risk of myopathy when azithromycin or erythromycin given with • ATORVASTATIN; clarithromycin increases plasma concentration of • ATORVASTATIN and PRAVASTATIN; erythromycin increases plasma concentration of PRAVASTATIN; erythromycin reduces plasma concentration of ROSUVASTATIN; possible increased risk of myopathy when azithromycin given with • SIMVASTATIN; increased risk of myopathy when clarithromycin or erythromycin given with • SIMVASTATIN (avoid concomitant use); avoidance of clarithromycin and erythromycin advised by manufacturer of • LOMITAPIDE (plasma concentration of lomitapide possibly increased); separating administration from azithromycin by 12 hours advised by manufacturer of LOMITAPIDE
- Mirabegron: when given with clarithromycin avoid or reduce dose of MIRABEGRON in hepatic or renal impairment—see Mirabegron, in BNF
- Netupitant: plasma concentration of erythromycin increased by NETUPITANT
- Oestrogens: erythromycin increases plasma concentration of ESTRADIOL
- Parasympathomimetics: erythromycin increases plasma concentration of GALANTAMINE
- Pentamidine Isetionate: increased risk of ventricular arrhythmias when *parenteral* erythromycin given with • PENTAMIDINE ISETIONATE
- Progestogens: erythromycin increases plasma concentration of DIENOGEST
- Ranolazine: clarithromycin possibly increases plasma concentration of • RANOLAZINE—manufacturer of ranolazine advises avoid concomitant use
- Sildenafil: clarithromycin increases the plasma concentration of • SILDENAFIL—consider reducing initial dose of sildenafil for erectile dysfunction or reduce sildenafil dose frequency to once daily for pulmonary hypertension; erythromycin increases plasma concentration of SILDENAFIL—reduce initial dose of sildenafil for erectile dysfunction or reduce sildenafil dose frequency to twice daily for pulmonary hypertension
- Sirolimus: clarithromycin increases plasma concentration of • SIROLIMUS—avoid concomitant use; plasma concentration of both drugs increased when erythromycin given with • SIROLIMUS
- Tacrolimus: clarithromycin and erythromycin increase plasma concentration of • TACROLIMUS
- Tadalafil: clarithromycin and erythromycin possibly increase plasma concentration of TADALAFIL
- Theophylline: clarithromycin possibly increases plasma concentration of • THEOPHYLLINE; erythromycin increases plasma concentration of • THEOPHYLLINE (also theophylline may reduce absorption of *oral* erythromycin)
- Ticagrelor: clarithromycin possibly increases plasma concentration of • TICAGRELOR—manufacturer of ticagrelor advises avoid concomitant use; erythromycin possibly increases plasma concentration of TICAGRELOR
- Ulcer-healing Drugs: plasma concentration of erythromycin increased by CIMETIDINE (increased risk of toxicity, including deafness); plasma concentration of both drugs increased when clarithromycin given with OMEPRAZOLE

Macrolides (continued)

▸ Ulipristal: avoidance of clarithromycin advised by manufacturer of *low-dose* ULIPRISTAL; erythromycin increases plasma concentration of *low-dose* ULIPRISTAL—manufacturer of *low-dose* ulipristal advises avoid concomitant use

▸ Vaccines: antibacterials inactivate ORAL TYPHOID VACCINE—see under Typhoid Vaccine in BNFC

▸ Vardenafil: clarithromycin possibly increases plasma concentration of VARDENAFIL (consider reducing initial dose of vardenafil); erythromycin increases plasma concentration of VARDENAFIL (reduce dose of vardenafil)

Magnesium (parenteral)

● Calcium-channel Blockers: profound hypotension reported with concomitant use of parenteral magnesium and ● NIFEDIPINE in pre-eclampsia

▸ Muscle Relaxants: parenteral magnesium enhances effects of NON-DEPOLARISING MUSCLE RELAXANTS and SUXAMETHONIUM

Magnesium Salts (oral) *see* Antacids

Mannitol

▸ Antibacterials: avoidance of mannitol advised by manufacturer of TOBRAMYCIN

▸ Ciclosporin: possible increased risk of nephrotoxicity when mannitol given with CICLOSPORIN

MAOIs

NOTE For interactions of reversible MAO-A inhibitors (RIMAs) see Moclobemide, and for interactions of MAO-B inhibitors see Rasagiline and Selegiline

NOTE Linezolid is a reversible, non-selective MAO inhibitor and an antibacterial

▸ ACE Inhibitors: MAOIs possibly enhance hypotensive effect of ACE INHIBITORS

▸ Adrenergic Neurone Blockers: enhanced hypotensive effect when MAOIs given with ADRENERGIC NEURONE BLOCKERS

● Alcohol: MAOIs interact with tyramine found in some beverages containing ● ALCOHOL and some dealcoholised beverages (hypertensive crisis)—if no tyramine, enhanced hypotensive effect

▸ Alpha₂-adrenoceptor Stimulants: avoidance of MAOIs advised by manufacturer of ● APRACLONIDINE and BRIMONIDINE

● Alpha-blockers: avoidance of MAOIs advised by manufacturer of ● INDORAMIN; enhanced hypotensive effect when MAOIs given with ALPHA-BLOCKERS

● Analgesics: possible increased serotonergic effects when MAOIs given with FENTANYL; CNS excitation or depression (hypertension or hypotension) when MAOIs given with ● PETHIDINE—avoid concomitant use and for 2 weeks after stopping MAOIs; possible increased serotonergic effects and increased risk of convulsions when MAOIs given with ● TRAMADOL—some manufacturers advise avoid concomitant use and for 2 weeks after stopping MAOIs; avoidance of MAOIs advised by manufacturer of ● NEFOPAM; possible CNS excitation or depression (hypertension or hypotension) when MAOIs given with ● OPIOID ANALGESICS—some manufacturers advise avoid concomitant use and for 2 weeks after stopping MAOIs

▸ Angiotensin-II Receptor Antagonists: MAOIs possibly enhance hypotensive effect of ANGIOTENSIN-II RECEPTOR ANTAGONISTS

▸ Antibacterials: plasma concentration of linezolid reduced by RIFAMPICIN (possible therapeutic failure of linezolid)

● Antidepressants: increased risk of hypertension and CNS excitation when MAOIs given with ● REBOXETINE (MAOIs should not be started until 1 week after stopping reboxetine, avoid reboxetine for 2 weeks after stopping MAOIs); after stopping MAOIs do not start ● CITALOPRAM, ● ESCITALOPRAM, ● FLUVOXAMINE, ● PAROXETINE or ● SERTRALINE for 2 weeks, also MAOIs should not be started until at least 1 week after stopping citalopram, escitalopram, fluvoxamine, paroxetine or sertraline; after stopping MAOIs do not start ● FLUOXETINE for 2 weeks, also MAOIs should not be started until at least 5 weeks after stopping fluoxetine; after stopping MAOIs do not start ● DULOXETINE for 2 weeks, also MAOIs should not be started until at least 5 days after stopping duloxetine; enhanced CNS effects and toxicity when MAOIs given with ● VENLAFAXINE (venlafaxine should not be started until 2 weeks after stopping MAOIs, avoid MAOIs for 1 week after stopping venlafaxine); increased risk of hypertension and

MAOIs

● Antidepressants (continued)
CNS excitation when MAOIs given with other ● MAOIS (avoid for at least 2 weeks after stopping previous MAOIs and then start at a reduced dose); after stopping MAOIs do not start ● MOCLOBEMIDE for at least 1 week; MAOIs increase CNS effects of ● SSRIS (risk of serious toxicity); after stopping MAOIs do not start ● MIRTAZAPINE for 2 weeks, also MAOIs should not be started until at least 2 weeks after stopping mirtazapine; after stopping MAOIs do not start ● TRICYCLIC-RELATED ANTIDEPRESSANTS for 2 weeks, also MAOIs should not be started until at least 1–2 weeks after stopping tricyclic-related antidepressants; increased risk of hypertension and CNS excitation when MAOIs given with ● TRICYCLICS, tricyclics should not be started until 2 weeks after stopping MAOIs (3 weeks if starting clomipramine or imipramine), also MAOIs should not be started for at least 1–2 weeks after stopping tricyclics (3 weeks in the case of clomipramine or imipramine); increased risk of hypertension and CNS excitation when MAOIs given with ● VORTIOXETINE (vortioxetine should not be started until 2 weeks after stopping MAOIs, avoid MAOIs for 2 weeks after stopping vortioxetine); avoidance of linezolid advised by manufacturer of ● VORTIOXETINE

▸ Antidiabetics: MAOIs possibly enhance hypoglycaemic effect of ANTIDIABETICS; MAOIs enhance hypoglycaemic effect of INSULIN, METFORMIN and SULFONYLUREAS

● Antiepileptics: MAOIs possibly antagonise anticonvulsant effect of ANTIEPILEPTICS (convulsive threshold lowered); avoidance for 2 weeks after stopping MAOIs advised by manufacturer of ● CARBAMAZEPINE, also antagonism of anticonvulsant effect

▸ Antihistamines: avoidance of MAOIs advised by manufacturer of HYDROXYZINE; avoidance of promethazine for 2 weeks after stopping MAOIs advised by manufacturer of PROMETHAZINE; increased antimuscarinic and sedative effects when MAOIs given with ANTIHISTAMINES

▸ Antimalarials: avoidance of antidepressants advised by manufacturer of ● ARTEMETHER WITH LUMEFANTRINE and ● ARTENIMOL WITH PIPERAQUINE

▸ Antimuscarinics: increased risk of antimuscarinic side-effects when MAOIs given with ANTIMUSCARINICS

● Antipsychotics: CNS effects of MAOIs possibly increased by ● CLOZAPINE

● Anxiolytics and Hypnotics: manufacturer of tranylcypromine advises avoid ● BUSPIRONE for 14 days after stopping tranylcypromine; avoidance of MAOIs advised by manufacturer of BUSPIRONE

● Atomoxetine: after stopping MAOIs do not start ● ATOMOXETINE for 2 weeks, also MAOIs should not be started until at least 2 weeks after stopping atomoxetine; possible increased risk of convulsions when antidepressants given with ATOMOXETINE

▸ Beta-blockers: enhanced hypotensive effect when MAOIs given with BETA-BLOCKERS

● Bupropion: avoidance of bupropion for 2 weeks after stopping MAOIs advised by manufacturer of ● BUPROPION

▸ Calcium-channel Blockers: enhanced hypotensive effect when MAOIs given with CALCIUM-CHANNEL BLOCKERS

▸ Clonidine: enhanced hypotensive effect when MAOIs given with CLONIDINE

● Dapoxetine: increased risk of serotonergic effects when MAOIs given with ● DAPOXETINE (MAOIs should not be started until 1 week after stopping dapoxetine, avoid dapoxetine for 2 weeks after stopping MAOIs)

▸ Diazoxide: enhanced hypotensive effect when MAOIs given with DIAZOXIDE

▸ Diuretics: enhanced hypotensive effect when MAOIs given with DIURETICS

● Dopaminergics: risk of hypertensive crisis when MAOIs given with ● CO-BENELDOPA, ● CO-CARELDOPA or ● LEVODOPA, avoid co-beneldopa, co-careldopa or levodopa for at least 2 weeks after stopping MAOIs; avoid concomitant use of non-selective MAOIs with ● ENTACAPONE; risk of hypertensive crisis when MAOIs given with ● RASAGILINE, avoid MAOIs for at least 2 weeks after stopping rasagiline; enhanced hypotensive effect when MAOIs given with ● SELEGILINE—manufacturer of

A1

MAOIs

- **Dopaminergics** (continued)
  selegiline advises avoid concomitant use; avoid concomitant use of MAOIs with TOLCAPONE
- ▹ Doxapram: MAOIs enhance effects of DOXAPRAM
- ▹ Histamine: avoidance of MAOIs advised by manufacturer of HISTAMINE
- **5HT₁-receptor Agonists**: risk of CNS toxicity when MAOIs given with ● RIZATRIPTAN or ● SUMATRIPTAN (avoid rizatriptan or sumatriptan for 2 weeks after MAOIs); risk of CNS toxicity when MAOIs given with ● ZOLMITRIPTAN (reduce dose of zolmitriptan)
- **Methyldopa**: avoidance of MAOIs advised by manufacturer of ● METHYLDOPA
- **Moxonidine**: enhanced hypotensive effect when MAOIs given with MOXONIDINE
- ▹ Muscle Relaxants: phenelzine enhances effects of SUXAMETHONIUM
- ▹ Nicorandil: enhanced hypotensive effect when MAOIs given with NICORANDIL
- ▹ Nitrates: enhanced hypotensive effect when MAOIs given with NITRATES
- ▹ Pholcodine: avoidance of pholcodine for 2 weeks after stopping MAOIs advised by manufacturer of PHOLCODINE
- **Sympathomimetics**: risk of hypertensive crisis when MAOIs given with ● ADRENALINE (EPINEPHRINE), ● DOBUTAMINE, ● DOPAMINE, ● NORADRENALINE (NOREPINEPHRINE) or ● XYLOMETAZOLINE; risk of hypertensive crisis when MAOIs given with ● DEXAMFETAMINE, ● EPHEDRINE, ● ISOMETHEPTENE, ● LISDEXAMFETAMINE, ● METARAMINOL, ● METHYLPHENIDATE, ● PHENYLEPHRINE or ● PSEUDOEPHEDRINE, avoid dexamfetamine, ephedrine, isometheptene, lisdexamfetamine, metaraminol, methylphenidate, phenylephrine or pseudoephedrine for at least 2 weeks after stopping MAOIs; avoidance of MAOIs advised by manufacturer of MIDODRINE; risk of hypertensive crisis when MAOIs given with ● OXYMETAZOLINE, some manufacturers advise avoid oxymetazoline for at least 2 weeks after stopping MAOIs
- **Tetrabenazine**: risk of CNS toxicity when MAOIs given with ● TETRABENAZINE (avoid tetrabenazine for 2 weeks after MAOIs)
- ▹ Vaccines: antibacterials including linezolid inactivate ORAL TYPHOID VACCINE—see under Typhoid Vaccine in BNFC
- ▹ Vasodilator Antihypertensives: enhanced hypotensive effect when MAOIs given with HYDRALAZINE, MINOXIDIL or SODIUM NITROPRUSSIDE

MAOIs, reversible *see* Moclobemide

Maraviroc

- **Antibacterials**: plasma concentration of maraviroc possibly increased by ● CLARITHROMYCIN and ● TELITHROMYCIN (consider reducing dose of maraviroc); plasma concentration of maraviroc reduced by ● RIFAMPICIN—consider increasing dose of maraviroc
- **Antidepressants**: plasma concentration of maraviroc possibly reduced by ● ST JOHN'S WORT—avoid concomitant use
- **Antifungals**: plasma concentration of maraviroc increased by ● KETOCONAZOLE (consider reducing dose of maraviroc)
- **Antivirals**: plasma concentration of maraviroc increased by ● ATAZANAVIR, BOCEPREVIR, ● DARUNAVIR, ● INDINAVIR, ● LOPINAVIR, ● SAQUINAVIR and TELAPREVIR (consider reducing dose of maraviroc); plasma concentration of maraviroc possibly reduced by ● EFAVIRENZ—consider increasing dose of maraviroc; plasma concentration of maraviroc possibly reduced by ETRAVIRINE; maraviroc reduces plasma concentration of ● FOSAMPRENAVIR—avoid concomitant use; plasma concentration of maraviroc increased by RITONAVIR
- **Cobicistat**: plasma concentration of maraviroc possibly increased by ● COBICISTAT (reduce dose of maraviroc)
- **Orlistat**: absorption of maraviroc possibly reduced by ● ORLISTAT

Mebendazole

- ▹ Ulcer-healing Drugs: metabolism of mebendazole possibly inhibited by CIMETIDINE (increased plasma concentration)

Medroxyprogesterone *see* Progestogens

Mefenamic Acid *see* NSAIDs

Mefloquine

- **Anti-arrhythmics**: increased risk of ventricular arrhythmias when mefloquine given with ● AMIODARONE—avoid concomitant use
- **Antibacterials**: increased risk of ventricular arrhythmias when mefloquine given with ● MOXIFLOXACIN—avoid concomitant use; plasma concentration of mefloquine reduced by ● RIFAMPICIN—avoid concomitant use
- **Antidepressants**: possible increased risk of convulsions when mefloquine given with ● VORTIOXETINE
- **Antiepileptics**: mefloquine antagonises anticonvulsant effect of ● ANTIEPILEPTICS
- ▹ Antifungals: plasma concentration of mefloquine increased by KETOCONAZOLE
- **Antimalarials**: avoidance of antimalarials advised by manufacturer of ● ARTEMETHER WITH LUMEFANTRINE; increased risk of convulsions when mefloquine given with ● CHLOROQUINE or ● HYDROXYCHLOROQUINE; increased risk of convulsions when mefloquine given with ● QUININE (but should not prevent the use of *intravenous* quinine in severe cases)
- **Antipsychotics**: possible increased risk of ventricular arrhythmias when mefloquine given with ● HALOPERIDOL—avoid concomitant use; avoidance of mefloquine advised by manufacturer of AMISULPRIDE; increased risk of ventricular arrhythmias when mefloquine given with ● PIMOZIDE—avoid concomitant use; manufacturer of risperidone advises possible risk of ventricular arrhythmias when mefloquine given with ▹ RISPERIDONE
- ▹ Antivirals: mefloquine possibly reduces plasma concentration of RITONAVIR
- ▹ Atomoxetine: increased risk of ventricular arrhythmias when mefloquine given with ● ATOMOXETINE
- ▹ Beta-blockers: increased risk of bradycardia when mefloquine given with BETA-BLOCKERS
- ▹ Calcium-channel Blockers: possible increased risk of bradycardia when mefloquine given with CALCIUM-CHANNEL BLOCKERS
- ▹ Cardiac Glycosides: possible increased risk of bradycardia when mefloquine given with DIGOXIN
- ▹ Cytotoxics: possible increased risk of bradycardia when mefloquine given with CRIZOTINIB
- ▹ Histamine: avoidance of antimalarials advised by manufacturer of HISTAMINE
- **Ivabradine**: increased risk of ventricular arrhythmias when mefloquine given with ● IVABRADINE
- **Penicillamine**: increased risk of haematological toxicity when antimalarials given with PENICILLAMINE—manufacturer of penicillamine advises avoid concomitant use
- ▹ Vaccines: antimalarials inactivate ORAL TYPHOID VACCINE—see under Typhoid Vaccine in BNFC

Megestrol *see* Progestogens

Melatonin *see* Anxiolytics and Hypnotics

Meloxicam *see* NSAIDs

Melphalan

- ▹ Antibacterials: increased risk of melphalan toxicity when given with NALIDIXIC ACID
- **Antipsychotics**: avoid concomitant use of cytotoxics with ● CLOZAPINE (increased risk of agranulocytosis)
- ▹ Cardiac Glycosides: melphalan possibly reduces absorption of DIGOXIN *tablets*
- ▹ Ciclosporin: increased risk of nephrotoxicity when melphalan given with ● CICLOSPORIN

Memantine

- **Anaesthetics, General**: increased risk of CNS toxicity when memantine given with ● KETAMINE (manufacturer of memantine advises avoid concomitant use)
- **Analgesics**: increased risk of CNS toxicity when memantine given with ● DEXTROMETHORPHAN (manufacturer of memantine advises avoid concomitant use)
- ▹ Anticoagulants: memantine possibly enhances anticoagulant effect of WARFARIN
- ▹ Antimuscarinics: memantine possibly enhances effects of ANTIMUSCARINICS
- ▹ Antipsychotics: memantine possibly reduces effects of ANTIPSYCHOTICS

Memantine (continued)
- Dopaminergics: memantine possibly enhances effects of DOPAMINERGICS and SELEGILINE; increased risk of CNS toxicity when memantine given with ● AMANTADINE (manufacturer of memantine advises avoid concomitant use)
▸ Muscle Relaxants: memantine possibly modifies effects of BACLOFEN and DANTROLENE

Meningococcal Vaccines see Vaccines

Mepacrine
▸ Antimalarials: mepacrine increases plasma concentration of PRIMAQUINE (increased risk of toxicity)

Meprobamate see Anxiolytics and Hypnotics

Meptazinol see Opioid Analgesics

Mercaptopurine
● Allopurinol: enhanced effects and increased toxicity of mercaptopurine when given with ● ALLOPURINOL (reduce dose of mercaptopurine to one quarter of usual dose)
● Antibacterials: increased risk of haematological toxicity when mercaptopurine given with ● SULFAMETHOXAZOLE (as co-trimoxazole); increased risk of haematological toxicity when mercaptopurine given with ● TRIMETHOPRIM (also with co-trimoxazole)
● Anticoagulants: mercaptopurine possibly reduces anticoagulant effect of ● COUMARINS
● Antipsychotics: avoid concomitant use of cytotoxics with ● CLOZAPINE (increased risk of agranulocytosis)
● Dairy Products: plasma concentration of mercaptopurine possibly reduced by DAIRY PRODUCTS—manufacturer of mercaptopurine advises give at least 1 hour before or 3 hours after dairy products
● Febuxostat: avoidance of mercaptopurine advised by manufacturer of ● FEBUXOSTAT

Meropenem
● Antiepileptics: carbapenems reduce plasma concentration of ● SODIUM VALPROATE and ● VALPROIC ACID—avoid concomitant use
▸ Vaccines: antibacterials inactivate ORAL TYPHOID VACCINE—see under Typhoid Vaccine in BNFC

Mestranol see Oestrogens

Metaraminol see Sympathomimetics

Metformin see Antidiabetics

Methadone see Opioid Analgesics

Methenamine
▸ Antacids: avoid concomitant use of methenamine with ANTACIDS
● Antibacterials: increased risk of crystalluria when methenamine given with ● SULFONAMIDES
▸ Diuretics: effects of methenamine antagonised by ● ACETAZOLAMIDE
▸ Potassium Salts: avoid concomitant use of methenamine with POTASSIUM CITRATE
▸ Sodium Citrate: avoid concomitant use of methenamine with SODIUM CITRATE
▸ Vaccines: antibacterials inactivate ORAL TYPHOID VACCINE—see under Typhoid Vaccine in BNFC

Methocarbamol see Muscle Relaxants

Methotrexate
▸ Aminophylline: methotrexate possibly increases plasma concentration of AMINOPHYLLINE
● Anaesthetics, General: antifolate effect of methotrexate increased by ● NITROUS OXIDE—avoid concomitant use
▸ Analgesics: excretion of methotrexate probably reduced by ● NSAIDS (increased risk of toxicity); excretion of methotrexate reduced by ● ASPIRIN, ● DICLOFENAC, ● IBUPROFEN, ● INDOMETACIN, ● KETOPROFEN, ● MELOXICAM and ● NAPROXEN (increased risk of toxicity)
● Antibacterials: absorption of methotrexate possibly reduced by NEOMYCIN; excretion of methotrexate possibly reduced by CIPROFLOXACIN (increased risk of toxicity); increased risk of severe bone marrow depression (fatalities reported) and other haematological toxicities when methotrexate given with ● SULFAMETHOXAZOLE (as co-trimoxazole); increased risk of methotrexate toxicity when given with DOXYCYCLINE, SULFONAMIDES or TETRACYCLINE; excretion of methotrexate reduced by PENICILLINS (increased risk of toxicity); increased risk of severe bone marrow depression (fatalities reported) and other haematological toxicites when

Methotrexate
● Antibacterials (continued)
methotrexate given with ● TRIMETHOPRIM (also with co-trimoxazole)
● Antiepileptics: antifolate effect of methotrexate increased by FOSPHENYTOIN and PHENYTOIN; plasma concentration of methotrexate possibly increased by ● LEVETIRACETAM
● Antimalarials: antifolate effect of methotrexate increased by ● PYRIMETHAMINE
● Antipsychotics: avoid concomitant use of cytotoxics with ● CLOZAPINE (increased risk of agranulocytosis)
▸ Cardiac Glycosides: methotrexate possibly reduces absorption of DIGOXIN *tablets*
● Ciclosporin: risk of toxicity when methotrexate given with ● CICLOSPORIN
● Corticosteroids: possible increased risk of hepatoxicity when *high-dose* methotrexate given with DEXAMETHASONE
● Cytotoxics: increased pulmonary toxicity when methotrexate given with ● CISPLATIN
▸ Diuretics: excretion of methotrexate increased by alkaline urine due to ACETAZOLAMIDE
● Leflunomide: risk of toxicity when methotrexate given with ● LEFLUNOMIDE
● Retinoids: plasma concentration of methotrexate increased by ● ACITRETIN (also increased risk of hepatotoxicity)—avoid concomitant use
▸ Theophylline: methotrexate possibly increases plasma concentration of THEOPHYLLINE
▸ Ulcer-healing Drugs: excretion of methotrexate possibly reduced by PROTON PUMP INHIBITORS (increased risk of toxicity)

Methyldopa
▸ ACE Inhibitors: enhanced hypotensive effect when methyldopa given with ACE INHIBITORS
▸ Adrenergic Neurone Blockers: enhanced hypotensive effect when methyldopa given with ADRENERGIC NEURONE BLOCKERS
▸ Alcohol: enhanced hypotensive effect when methyldopa given with ALCOHOL
▸ Aldesleukin: enhanced hypotensive effect when methyldopa given with ALDESLEUKIN
▸ Alpha-blockers: enhanced hypotensive effect when methyldopa given with ALPHA-BLOCKERS
▸ Anaesthetics, General: enhanced hypotensive effect when methyldopa given with GENERAL ANAESTHETICS
▸ Analgesics: hypotensive effect of methyldopa antagonised by NSAIDs
▸ Angiotensin-II Receptor Antagonists: enhanced hypotensive effect when methyldopa given with ANGIOTENSIN-II RECEPTOR ANTAGONISTS
● Antidepressants: manufacturer of methyldopa advises avoid concomitant use with ● MAOIS
▸ Antipsychotics: enhanced hypotensive effect when methyldopa given with ANTIPSYCHOTICS (also increased risk of extrapyramidal effects)
▸ Anxiolytics and Hypnotics: enhanced hypotensive effect when methyldopa given with ANXIOLYTICS AND HYPNOTICS
▸ Beta-blockers: enhanced hypotensive effect when methyldopa given with BETA-BLOCKERS
▸ Calcium-channel Blockers: enhanced hypotensive effect when methyldopa given with CALCIUM-CHANNEL BLOCKERS
▸ Clonidine: enhanced hypotensive effect when methyldopa given with CLONIDINE
▸ Corticosteroids: hypotensive effect of methyldopa antagonised by CORTICOSTEROIDS
▸ Diazoxide: enhanced hypotensive effect when methyldopa given with DIAZOXIDE
▸ Diuretics: enhanced hypotensive effect when methyldopa given with DIURETICS
▸ Dopaminergics: methyldopa antagonises antiparkinsonian effect of DOPAMINERGICS; increased risk of extrapyramidal side-effects when methyldopa given with AMANTADINE; enhanced hypotensive effect when methyldopa given with CO-BENELDOPA, CO-CARELDOPA or LEVODOPA; effects of methyldopa possibly enhanced by ENTACAPONE
▸ Iron Salts: hypotensive effect of methyldopa antagonised by *oral* IRON SALTS
● Lithium: neurotoxicity may occur when methyldopa given with ● LITHIUM without increased plasma concentration of lithium

Methyldopa (continued)
- Moxisylyte: enhanced hypotensive effect when methyldopa given with MOXISYLYTE
- Moxonidine: enhanced hypotensive effect when methyldopa given with MOXONIDINE
- Muscle Relaxants: enhanced hypotensive effect when methyldopa given with BACLOFEN or TIZANIDINE
- Nitrates: enhanced hypotensive effect when methyldopa given with NITRATES
- Oestrogens: hypotensive effect of methyldopa antagonised by OESTROGENS
- Prostaglandins: enhanced hypotensive effect when methyldopa given with ALPROSTADIL
- Sympathomimetics, Beta$_2$: acute hypotension reported when methyldopa given with *infusion* of ● SALBUTAMOL
- Vasodilator Antihypertensives: enhanced hypotensive effect when methyldopa given with HYDRALAZINE, MINOXIDIL or SODIUM NITROPRUSSIDE

Methylphenidate *see* Sympathomimetics
Methylprednisolone *see* Corticosteroids
Methylthioninium
- Antidepressants: risk of CNS toxicity when methylthioninium given with ● SSRI-RELATED ANTIDEPRESSANTS, ● SSRIS and ● CLOMIPRAMINE—avoid concomitant use (if avoidance not possible, use lowest possible dose of methylthioninium and observe patient for up to 4 hours after administration); possible risk of CNS toxicity when methylthioninium given with ● MIRTAZAPINE—avoid concomitant use (if avoidance not possible, use lowest possible dose of methylthioninium and observe patient for up to 4 hours after administration)
- Anxiolytics and Hypnotics: possible risk of CNS toxicity when methylthioninium given with ● BUSPIRONE—avoid concomitant use (if avoidance not possible, use lowest possible dose of methylthioninium and observe patient for up to 4 hours after administration)
- Bupropion: possible risk of CNS toxicity when methylthioninium given with ● BUPROPION—avoid concomitant use (if avoidance not possible, use lowest possible dose of methylthioninium and observe patient for up to 4 hours after administration)

Metoclopramide
- Alcohol: metoclopramide possibly increases absorption of ALCOHOL
- Anaesthetics, General: metoclopramide enhances effects of THIOPENTAL
- Analgesics: metoclopramide increases rate of absorption of ASPIRIN (enhanced effect); effects of metoclopramide on gastro-intestinal activity antagonised by OPIOID ANALGESICS; metoclopramide increases rate of absorption of PARACETAMOL
- Antibacterials: metoclopramide reduces plasma concentration of FOSFOMYCIN
- Antidepressants: CNS toxicity reported when metoclopramide given with SSRIS
- Antimuscarinics: effects of metoclopramide on gastro-intestinal activity antagonised by ANTIMUSCARINICS
- Antipsychotics: increased risk of extrapyramidal side-effects when metoclopramide given with ANTIPSYCHOTICS
- Atovaquone: metoclopramide reduces plasma concentration of ATOVAQUONE—avoid concomitant use
- Ciclosporin: metoclopramide increases plasma concentration of ● CICLOSPORIN
- Dopaminergics: metoclopramide antagonises hypoprolactinaemic effects of BROMOCRIPTINE and CABERGOLINE; metoclopramide antagonises antiparkinsonian effect of PERGOLIDE; avoidance of metoclopramide advised by manufacturer of ROPINIROLE and ROTIGOTINE (antagonism of effect)
- Muscle Relaxants: metoclopramide enhances effects of SUXAMETHONIUM
- Tetrabenazine: increased risk of extrapyramidal side-effects when metoclopramide given with TETRABENAZINE

Metolazone *see* Diuretics
Metoprolol *see* Beta-blockers
Metronidazole
  NOTE Interactions do not apply to topical metronidazole preparations

Metronidazole (continued)
- Alcohol: disulfiram-like reaction when metronidazole given with ALCOHOL
- Anticoagulants: metronidazole enhances anticoagulant effect of ● COUMARINS
- Antiepileptics: metronidazole possibly inhibits metabolism of FOSPHENYTOIN and PHENYTOIN (increased plasma concentration); metabolism of metronidazole accelerated by PHENOBARBITAL and PRIMIDONE (reduced effect)
- Cytotoxics: metronidazole increases plasma concentration of ● BUSULFAN (increased risk of toxicity); metronidazole inhibits metabolism of CAPECITABINE, FLUOROURACIL and TEGAFUR (increased toxicity)
- Disulfiram: psychotic reaction reported when metronidazole given with DISULFIRAM
- Lithium: metronidazole increases risk of LITHIUM toxicity
- Mycophenolate: metronidazole possibly reduces bioavailability of MYCOPHENOLATE
- Ulcer-healing Drugs: metabolism of metronidazole inhibited by CIMETIDINE (increased plasma concentration)
- Vaccines: antibacterials inactivate ORAL TYPHOID VACCINE—see under Typhoid Vaccine in BNFC

Mianserin *see* Antidepressants, Tricyclic (related)
Micafungin
- Antifungals: micafungin possibly increases plasma concentration of AMPHOTERICIN; micafungin increases plasma concentration of ITRACONAZOLE (consider reducing dose of itraconazole)
- Calcium-channel Blockers: micafungin increases plasma concentration of NIFEDIPINE
- Ciclosporin: micafungin possibly increases plasma concentration of CICLOSPORIN
- Sirolimus: micafungin increases plasma concentration of SIROLIMUS

Miconazole *see* Antifungals, Imidazole
Midazolam *see* Anxiolytics and Hypnotics
Midodrine *see* Sympathomimetics
Mifamurtide
- Analgesics: manufacturer of mifamurtide advises avoid concomitant use with high doses of NSAIDs
- Ciclosporin: manufacturer of mifamurtide advises avoid concomitant use with CICLOSPORIN
- Corticosteroids: manufacturer of mifamurtide advises avoid concomitant use with CORTICOSTEROIDS
- Tacrolimus: manufacturer of mifamurtide advises avoid concomitant use with TACROLIMUS

Mifepristone
- Corticosteroids: mifepristone may reduce effect of CORTICOSTEROIDS (including *inhaled* corticosteroids) for 3–4 days

Milrinone *see* Phosphodiesterase Inhibitors
Minocycline *see* Tetracyclines
Minoxidil *see* Vasodilator Antihypertensives
Mirabegron
- Antibacterials: avoid or reduce dose of mirabegron in hepatic or renal impairment when given with CLARITHROMYCIN—see Mirabegron, in BNF
- Antifungals: avoid or reduce dose of mirabegron in hepatic or renal impairment when given with ITRACONAZOLE and KETOCONAZOLE—see Mirabegron, in BNF
- Antivirals: avoid or reduce dose of mirabegron in hepatic or renal impairment when given with RITONAVIR—see Mirabegron, in BNF
- Beta-blockers: mirabegron increases plasma concentration of METOPROLOL
- Cardiac Glycosides: mirabegron increases plasma concentration of DIGOXIN—reduce initial dose of digoxin

Mirtazapine
- Alcohol: increased sedative effect when mirtazapine given with ● ALCOHOL
- Analgesics: possible increased serotonergic effects when mirtazapine given with TRAMADOL
- Anticoagulants: mirtazapine enhances anticoagulant effect of WARFARIN
- Antidepressants: possible increased serotonergic effects when mirtazapine given with FLUOXETINE, FLUVOXAMINE or

Mirtazapine

- Antidepressants (continued)
  VENLAFAXINE; mirtazapine should not be started until 2 weeks after stopping • MAOIs, also MAOIs should not be started until at least 2 weeks after stopping mirtazapine; after stopping mirtazapine do not start • MOCLOBEMIDE for at least 1 week
- ▸ Antiepileptics: plasma concentration of mirtazapine reduced by CARBAMAZEPINE, FOSPHENYTOIN and PHENYTOIN
- ▸ Antifungals: plasma concentration of mirtazapine increased by KETOCONAZOLE
- • Antimalarials: avoidance of antidepressants advised by manufacturer of • ARTEMETHER WITH LUMEFANTRINE and • ARTENIMOL WITH PIPERAQUINE
- ▸ Anxiolytics and Hypnotics: increased sedative effect when mirtazapine given with ANXIOLYTICS AND HYPNOTICS
- ▸ Atomoxetine: possible increased risk of convulsions when antidepressants given with ATOMOXETINE
- • Clonidine: mirtazapine possibly antagonises hypotensive effect of CLONIDINE
- • Methylthioninium: possible risk of CNS toxicity when mirtazapine given with • METHYLTHIONINIUM—avoid concomitant use (if avoidance not possible, use lowest possible dose of methylthioninium and observe patient for up to 4 hours after administration)
- ▸ Ulcer-healing Drugs: plasma concentration of mirtazapine increased by CIMETIDINE

Misoprostol

- ▸ Antacids: absorption of misoprostol possibly reduced by ANTACIDS

Mitomycin

- • Antipsychotics: avoid concomitant use of cytotoxics with • CLOZAPINE (increased risk of agranulocytosis)
- • Vaccines: risk of generalised infections when cytotoxic antibiotics given with live • VACCINES—avoid concomitant use

Mitotane

- • Anticoagulants: mitotane possibly reduces anticoagulant effect of • COUMARINS
- • Antipsychotics: avoid concomitant use of cytotoxics with • CLOZAPINE (increased risk of agranulocytosis)
- ▸ Antivirals: avoidance of mitotane advised by manufacturer of DASABUVIR, OMBITASVIR and PARITAPREVIR
- ▸ Diuretics: manufacturer of mitotane advises avoid concomitant use of SPIRONOLACTONE (antagonism of effect)

Mitoxantrone

- • Antipsychotics: avoid concomitant use of cytotoxics with • CLOZAPINE (increased risk of agranulocytosis)
- • Ciclosporin: excretion of mitoxantrone reduced by CICLOSPORIN (increased plasma concentration)
- • Vaccines: risk of generalised infections when cytotoxic antibiotics given with live • VACCINES—avoid concomitant use

Mivacurium see Muscle Relaxants
Mizolastine see Antihistamines
MMR Vaccine see Vaccines

Moclobemide

- • Analgesics: possible CNS excitation or depression (hypertension or hypotension) when moclobemide given with • DEXTROMETHORPHAN or • PETHIDINE—avoid concomitant use; possible CNS excitation or depression (hypertension or hypotension) when moclobemide given with • OPIOID ANALGESICS—manufacturer of moclobemide advises consider reducing dose of opioid analgesics
- • Antidepressants: moclobemide should not be started for at least 1 week after stopping • MAOIS, • SSRI-RELATED ANTIDEPRESSANTS, • CITALOPRAM, • FLUVOXAMINE, • MIRTAZAPINE, • PAROXETINE, • SERTRALINE, • TRICYCLIC-RELATED ANTIDEPRESSANTS or • TRICYCLICS; increased risk of CNS toxicity when moclobemide given with • ESCITALOPRAM, preferably avoid concomitant use; moclobemide should not be started until 5 weeks after stopping • FLUOXETINE; possible increased serotonergic effects when moclobemide given with • DULOXETINE; avoidance of moclobemide advised by manufacturer of • VORTIOXETINE
- • Antimalarials: avoidance of antidepressants advised by manufacturer of • ARTEMETHER WITH LUMEFANTRINE and • ARTENIMOL WITH PIPERAQUINE

Moclobemide (continued)

- ▸ Atomoxetine: possible increased risk of convulsions when antidepressants given with ATOMOXETINE
- • Bupropion: avoidance of moclobemide advised by manufacturer of • BUPROPION
- • Clopidogrel: moclobemide possibly reduces antiplatelet effect of • CLOPIDOGREL
- • Dopaminergics: increased risk of side-effects when moclobemide given with CO-BENELDOPA, CO-CARELDOPA or LEVODOPA; caution with moclobemide advised by manufacturer of ENTACAPONE; avoid concomitant use of moclobemide with • SELEGILINE
- • 5HT$_1$-receptor Agonists: risk of CNS toxicity when moclobemide given with • RIZATRIPTAN or • SUMATRIPTAN (avoid rizatriptan or sumatriptan for 2 weeks after moclobemide); risk of CNS toxicity when moclobemide given with • ZOLMITRIPTAN (reduce dose of zolmitriptan)
- • Sympathomimetics: risk of hypertensive crisis when moclobemide given with • SYMPATHOMIMETICS
- ▸ Ulcer-healing Drugs: plasma concentration of moclobemide increased by CIMETIDINE (halve dose of moclobemide)

Modafinil

- ▸ Antiepileptics: modafinil possibly increases plasma concentration of FOSPHENYTOIN and PHENYTOIN
- • Ciclosporin: modafinil reduces plasma concentration of • CICLOSPORIN
- • Cytotoxics: modafinil possibly reduces plasma concentration of • BOSUTINIB—manufacturer of bosutinib advises avoid concomitant use
- • Guanfacine: modafinil possibly reduces plasma concentration of • GUANFACINE—increase dose of guanfacine
- • Oestrogens: modafinil accelerates metabolism of • OESTROGENS (reduced contraceptive effect with combined oral contraceptives, contraceptive patches, and vaginal rings—see Contraceptive Interactions in BNFC)

Moexipril see ACE Inhibitors
Mometasone see Corticosteroids
Monobactams see Aztreonam
Monoclonal antibodies see individual drugs
Montelukast see Leukotriene Receptor Antagonists
Morphine see Opioid Analgesics
Moxifloxacin see Quinolones

Moxisylyte

- ▸ ACE Inhibitors: enhanced hypotensive effect when moxisylyte given with ACE INHIBITORS
- ▸ Adrenergic Neurone Blockers: enhanced hypotensive effect when moxisylyte given with ADRENERGIC NEURONE BLOCKERS
- • Alpha-blockers: possible severe postural hypotension when moxisylyte given with • ALPHA-BLOCKERS
- ▸ Angiotensin-II Receptor Antagonists: enhanced hypotensive effect when moxisylyte given with ANGIOTENSIN-II RECEPTOR ANTAGONISTS
- • Beta-blockers: possible severe postural hypotension when moxisylyte given with • BETA-BLOCKERS
- ▸ Calcium-channel Blockers: enhanced hypotensive effect when moxisylyte given with CALCIUM-CHANNEL BLOCKERS
- ▸ Clonidine: enhanced hypotensive effect when moxisylyte given with CLONIDINE
- ▸ Diazoxide: enhanced hypotensive effect when moxisylyte given with DIAZOXIDE
- ▸ Diuretics: enhanced hypotensive effect when moxisylyte given with DIURETICS
- ▸ Methyldopa: enhanced hypotensive effect when moxisylyte given with METHYLDOPA
- ▸ Moxonidine: enhanced hypotensive effect when moxisylyte given with MOXONIDINE
- ▸ Nitrates: enhanced hypotensive effect when moxisylyte given with NITRATES
- ▸ Vasodilator Antihypertensives: enhanced hypotensive effect when moxisylyte given with HYDRALAZINE, MINOXIDIL or SODIUM NITROPRUSSIDE

Moxonidine

- ▸ ACE Inhibitors: enhanced hypotensive effect when moxonidine given with ACE INHIBITORS
- ▸ Adrenergic Neurone Blockers: enhanced hypotensive effect when moxonidine given with ADRENERGIC NEURONE BLOCKERS

Moxonidine (continued)

▹ Alcohol: enhanced hypotensive effect when moxonidine given with ALCOHOL

▹ Aldesleukin: enhanced hypotensive effect when moxonidine given with ALDESLEUKIN

▹ Alpha-blockers: enhanced hypotensive effect when moxonidine given with ALPHA-BLOCKERS

▹ Anaesthetics, General: enhanced hypotensive effect when moxonidine given with GENERAL ANAESTHETICS

▹ Analgesics: hypotensive effect of moxonidine antagonised by NSAIDs

▹ Angiotensin-II Receptor Antagonists: enhanced hypotensive effect when moxonidine given with ANGIOTENSIN-II RECEPTOR ANTAGONISTS

▹ Antidepressants: enhanced hypotensive effect when moxonidine given with MAOIs; hypotensive effect of moxonidine possibly antagonised by TRICYCLICS (manufacturer of moxonidine advises avoid concomitant use)

▹ Antipsychotics: enhanced hypotensive effect when moxonidine given with PHENOTHIAZINES

▹ Anxiolytics and Hypnotics: enhanced hypotensive effect when moxonidine given with ANXIOLYTICS AND HYPNOTICS; sedative effects possibly increased when moxonidine given with BENZODIAZEPINES

▹ Beta-blockers: enhanced hypotensive effect when moxonidine given with BETA-BLOCKERS

▹ Calcium-channel Blockers: enhanced hypotensive effect when moxonidine given with CALCIUM-CHANNEL BLOCKERS

▹ Clonidine: enhanced hypotensive effect when moxonidine given with CLONIDINE

▹ Corticosteroids: hypotensive effect of moxonidine antagonised by CORTICOSTEROIDS

▹ Diazoxide: enhanced hypotensive effect when moxonidine given with DIAZOXIDE

▹ Diuretics: enhanced hypotensive effect when moxonidine given with DIURETICS

▹ Dopaminergics: enhanced hypotensive effect when moxonidine given with CO-BENELDOPA, CO-CARELDOPA or LEVODOPA

▹ Methyldopa: enhanced hypotensive effect when moxonidine given with METHYLDOPA

▹ Moxisylyte: enhanced hypotensive effect when moxonidine given with MOXISYLYTE

▹ Muscle Relaxants: enhanced hypotensive effect when moxonidine given with BACLOFEN or TIZANIDINE

▹ Nitrates: enhanced hypotensive effect when moxonidine given with NITRATES

▹ Oestrogens: hypotensive effect of moxonidine antagonised by OESTROGENS

▹ Prostaglandins: enhanced hypotensive effect when moxonidine given with ALPROSTADIL

▹ Vasodilator Antihypertensives: enhanced hypotensive effect when moxonidine given with HYDRALAZINE, MINOXIDIL or SODIUM NITROPRUSSIDE

Muscle Relaxants

▹ ACE Inhibitors: enhanced hypotensive effect when baclofen or tizanidine given with ACE INHIBITORS

▹ Adrenergic Neurone Blockers: enhanced hypotensive effect when baclofen or tizanidine given with ADRENERGIC NEURONE BLOCKERS

▹ Alcohol: increased sedative effect when baclofen, methocarbamol or tizanidine given with ALCOHOL

▹ Alpha-blockers: enhanced hypotensive effect when baclofen or tizanidine given with ALPHA-BLOCKERS

● Anaesthetics, General: effects of atracurium enhanced by KETAMINE; increased risk of myocardial depression and bradycardia when suxamethonium given with ● PROPOFOL; effects of non-depolarising muscle relaxants and suxamethonium enhanced by VOLATILE LIQUID GENERAL ANAESTHETICS

▹ Analgesics: excretion of baclofen possibly reduced by NSAIDs (increased risk of toxicity); excretion of baclofen reduced by IBUPROFEN (increased risk of toxicity); increased sedative effect when baclofen given with FENTANYL or MORPHINE

▹ Angiotensin-II Receptor Antagonists: enhanced hypotensive effect when baclofen or tizanidine given with ANGIOTENSIN-II RECEPTOR ANTAGONISTS

Muscle Relaxants (continued)

▹ Anti-arrhythmics: neuromuscular blockade enhanced and prolonged when suxamethonium given with LIDOCAINE

● Antibacterials: effects of non-depolarising muscle relaxants and suxamethonium enhanced by PIPERACILLIN; plasma concentration of tizanidine increased by ● CIPROFLOXACIN (increased risk of toxicity)—avoid concomitant use; plasma concentration of tizanidine possibly increased by NORFLOXACIN (increased risk of toxicity); plasma concentration of tizanidine possibly reduced by RIFAMPICIN; effects of non-depolarising muscle relaxants and suxamethonium enhanced by ● AMINOGLYCOSIDES; effects of non-depolarising muscle relaxants and suxamethonium enhanced by ● CLINDAMYCIN; effects of non-depolarising muscle relaxants and suxamethonium enhanced by ● POLYMYXINS; effects of suxamethonium enhanced by ● VANCOMYCIN

● Antidepressants: plasma concentration of tizanidine increased by ● FLUVOXAMINE (increased risk of toxicity)—avoid concomitant use; effects of suxamethonium enhanced by PHENELZINE; muscle relaxant effect of baclofen enhanced by TRICYCLICS

● Antiepileptics: muscle relaxant effect of non-depolarising muscle relaxants antagonised by CARBAMAZEPINE (accelerated recovery from neuromuscular blockade); effects of non-depolarising muscle relaxants reduced by *long-term use* of ● FOSPHENYTOIN and ● PHENYTOIN (but effects of non-depolarising muscle relaxants might be increased by *acute use* of fosphenytoin and phenytoin)

▹ Antimalarials: effects of suxamethonium possibly enhanced by QUININE

▹ Antipsychotics: effects of suxamethonium possibly enhanced by PROMAZINE

▹ Anxiolytics and Hypnotics: increased sedative effect when baclofen or tizanidine given with ANXIOLYTICS AND HYPNOTICS

▹ Beta-blockers: enhanced hypotensive effect when baclofen or tizanidine given with BETA-BLOCKERS; possible enhanced hypotensive effect and bradycardia when tizanidine given with BETA-BLOCKERS; effects of muscle relaxants enhanced by PROPRANOLOL

▹ Calcium-channel Blockers: enhanced hypotensive effect when baclofen or tizanidine given with CALCIUM-CHANNEL BLOCKERS; effects of non-depolarising muscle relaxants possibly enhanced by CALCIUM-CHANNEL BLOCKERS; possible increased risk of ventricular arrhythmias when *intravenous* dantrolene given with DILTIAZEM—manufacturer of diltiazem advises avoid concomitant use; effects of non-depolarising muscle relaxants and suxamethonium enhanced by VERAPAMIL; avoidance of *intravenous* dantrolene advised by manufacturer of VERAPAMIL

▹ Cardiac Glycosides: possible increased risk of bradycardia when tizanidine given with CARDIAC GLYCOSIDES; risk of ventricular arrhythmias when suxamethonium given with CARDIAC GLYCOSIDES

▹ Clonidine: enhanced hypotensive effect when baclofen or tizanidine given with CLONIDINE

▹ Corticosteroids: effects of pancuronium and vecuronium possibly antagonised by CORTICOSTEROIDS

▹ Cytotoxics: effects of suxamethonium enhanced by CYCLOPHOSPHAMIDE and THIOTEPA

▹ Deferasirox: avoidance of tizanidine advised by manufacturer of DEFERASIROX

▹ Diazoxide: enhanced hypotensive effect when baclofen or tizanidine given with DIAZOXIDE

▹ Diuretics: enhanced hypotensive effect when baclofen or tizanidine given with DIURETICS

▹ Dopaminergics: possible agitation, confusion and hallucinations when baclofen given with CO-BENELDOPA, CO-CARELDOPA or LEVODOPA

▹ Lithium: effects of muscle relaxants enhanced by LITHIUM; baclofen possibly aggravates hyperkinesis caused by LITHIUM

▹ Magnesium (parenteral): effects of non-depolarising muscle relaxants and suxamethonium enhanced by PARENTERAL MAGNESIUM

▹ Memantine: effects of baclofen and dantrolene possibly modified by MEMANTINE

Muscle Relaxants (continued)

‣ Methyldopa: enhanced hypotensive effect when baclofen or tizanidine given with METHYLDOPA

‣ Metoclopramide: effects of suxamethonium enhanced by METOCLOPRAMIDE

‣ Moxonidine: enhanced hypotensive effect when baclofen or tizanidine given with MOXONIDINE

‣ Nitrates: enhanced hypotensive effect when baclofen or tizanidine given with NITRATES

‣ Oestrogens: plasma concentration of tizanidine possibly increased by OESTROGENS (increased risk of toxicity)

‣ Parasympathomimetics: effects of non-depolarising muscle relaxants possibly antagonised by DONEPEZIL; effects of suxamethonium possibly enhanced by DONEPEZIL; effects of suxamethonium enhanced by GALANTAMINE, NEOSTIGMINE, PYRIDOSTIGMINE and RIVASTIGMINE; effects of non-depolarising muscle relaxants antagonised by NEOSTIGMINE, PYRIDOSTIGMINE and RIVASTIGMINE

‣ Progestogens: plasma concentration of tizanidine possibly increased by PROGESTOGENS (increased risk of toxicity)

‣ Sympathomimetics, Beta$_2$: effects of suxamethonium enhanced by BAMBUTEROL

‣ Vasodilator Antihypertensives: enhanced hypotensive effect when baclofen or tizanidine given with HYDRALAZINE; enhanced hypotensive effect when baclofen or tizanidine given with MINOXIDIL; enhanced hypotensive effect when baclofen or tizanidine given with SODIUM NITROPRUSSIDE

Muscle Relaxants, depolarising see Muscle Relaxants

Muscle Relaxants, non-depolarising see Muscle Relaxants

Mycophenolate

‣ Antacids: absorption of mycophenolate reduced by ANTACIDS

● Antibacterials: bioavailability of mycophenolate possibly reduced by METRONIDAZOLE and NORFLOXACIN; plasma concentration of mycophenolate possibly reduced by CO-AMOXICLAV; plasma concentration of active metabolite of mycophenolate reduced by ● RIFAMPICIN

‣ Antivirals: mycophenolate increases plasma concentration of ACICLOVIR and VALACICLOVIR, also plasma concentration of inactive metabolite of mycophenolate increased; mycophenolate possibly increases plasma concentration of GANCICLOVIR and VALGANCICLOVIR, also plasma concentration of inactive metabolite of mycophenolate possibly increased

‣ Iron Salts: absorption of mycophenolate reduced by oral IRON SALTS

‣ Lipid-regulating Drugs: absorption of mycophenolate reduced by COLESTYRAMINE

‣ Sevelamer: plasma concentration of mycophenolate possibly reduced by SEVELAMER

Nabumetone see NSAIDs

Nadolol see Beta-blockers

Nalidixic Acid see Quinolones

Nalmefene

● Analgesics: manufacturer of nalmefene advises avoid concomitant use with ● OPIOID ANALGESICS

Nandrolone see Anabolic Steroids

Naproxen see NSAIDs

Naratriptan see 5HT$_1$-receptor Agonists (under HT)

Natalizumab

● Antipsychotics: avoid concomitant use of cytotoxics with ● CLOZAPINE (increased risk of agranulocytosis)

● Vaccines: risk of generalised infections when monoclonal antibodies given with live ● VACCINES—avoid concomitant use

Nateglinide see Antidiabetics

Nebivolol see Beta-blockers

Nefopam

● Antidepressants: manufacturer of nefopam advises avoid concomitant use with ● MAOIS; side-effects possibly increased when nefopam given with TRICYCLICS

‣ Antimuscarinics: increased risk of antimuscarinic side-effects when nefopam given with ANTIMUSCARINICS

Neomycin see Aminoglycosides

Neostigmine see Parasympathomimetics

Netupitant

● Analgesics: manufacturer of netupitant advises caution with MORPHINE

Netupitant (continued)

● Antibacterials: netupitant increases plasma concentration of ERYTHROMYCIN; plasma concentration of netupitant reduced by ● RIFAMPICIN—avoid concomitant use

‣ Anticoagulants: manufacturer of netupitant advises caution with DABIGATRAN

‣ Antiepileptics: manufacturer of netupitant advises caution with VALPROIC ACID

‣ Antifungals: plasma concentration of netupitant possibly increased by KETOCONAZOLE

‣ Antivirals: manufacturer of netupitant advises caution with ZIDOVUDINE

‣ Anxiolytics and Hypnotics: netupitant increases plasma concentration of MIDAZOLAM

‣ Colchicine: manufacturer of netupitant advises caution with COLCHICINE

● Corticosteroids: netupitant increases plasma concentration of ● DEXAMETHASONE (halve dose of dexamethasone)

‣ Cytotoxics: netupitant increases plasma concentration of DOCETAXEL and ETOPOSIDE

Nevirapine

‣ Analgesics: nevirapine possibly reduces plasma concentration of METHADONE

● Antibacterials: nevirapine reduces plasma concentration of CLARITHROMYCIN (but concentration of an active metabolite increased), also plasma concentration of nevirapine increased; nevirapine possibly increases plasma concentration of RIFABUTIN; plasma concentration of nevirapine reduced by ● RIFAMPICIN—avoid concomitant use

● Anticoagulants: nevirapine may enhance or reduce anticoagulant effect of ● WARFARIN

● Antidepressants: plasma concentration of nevirapine reduced by ● ST JOHN'S WORT—avoid concomitant use

‣ Antiepileptics: plasma concentration of nevirapine reduced by CARBAMAZEPINE

● Antifungals: nevirapine reduces plasma concentration of ● KETOCONAZOLE—avoid concomitant use; plasma concentration of nevirapine increased by ● FLUCONAZOLE; nevirapine possibly reduces plasma concentration of CASPOFUNGIN and ITRACONAZOLE—consider increasing dose of caspofungin and itraconazole

● Antipsychotics: nevirapine possibly reduces plasma concentration of ● ARIPIPRAZOLE (avoid concomitant use or consider increasing the dose of aripiprazole—consult aripiprazole product literature)

● Antivirals: nevirapine possibly reduces plasma concentration of ● ATAZANAVIR and ● ETRAVIRINE—avoid concomitant use; manufacturer of nevirapine advises avoid concomitant use with BOCEPREVIR and RILPIVIRINE; avoidance of nevirapine advised by manufacturer of DACLATASVIR (plasma concentration of daclatasvir possibly reduced); avoidance of nevirapine advised by manufacturer of DASABUVIR, ELVITEGRAVIR, OMBITASVIR and PARITAPREVIR; nevirapine possibly reduces the plasma concentration of ● DOLUTEGRAVIR (see under Dolutegravir, p. 387); nevirapine reduces plasma concentration of ● EFAVIRENZ—avoid concomitant use; nevirapine possibly reduces plasma concentration of FOSAMPRENAVIR—avoid unboosted fosamprenavir; nevirapine reduces plasma concentration of INDINAVIR; nevirapine possibly reduces plasma concentration of ● LOPINAVIR and TELAPREVIR—consider increasing dose of lopinavir and telaprevir; nevirapine possibly reduces plasma concentration of ● SIMEPREVIR—manufacturer of simeprevir advises avoid concomitant use; increased risk of granulocytopenia when nevirapine given with ● ZIDOVUDINE

‣ Cobicistat: manufacturer of nevirapine advises avoid concomitant use with COBICISTAT

‣ Cytotoxics: avoidance of nevirapine advised by manufacturer of ● OLAPARIB

● Guanfacine: nevirapine reduces plasma concentration of ● GUANFACINE—increase dose of guanfacine

● Oestrogens: nevirapine accelerates metabolism of ● OESTROGENS (reduced contraceptive effect with combined oral contraceptives, contraceptive patches, and vaginal rings—see Contraceptive Interactions in BNFC)

Interactions | Appendix 1

A1

Nevirapine (continued)
- Orlistat: absorption of nevirapine possibly reduced by
  - ● ORLISTAT
- Progestogens: nevirapine accelerates metabolism of
  - ● PROGESTOGENS (reduced contraceptive effect with combined oral contraceptives, progestogen-only oral contraceptives, contraceptive patches, vaginal rings, etonogestrel-releasing implant, and emergency hormonal contraception—see Contraceptive Interactions in BNFC)

Nicardipine *see* Calcium-channel Blockers

Nicorandil
- ▸ Alcohol: hypotensive effect of nicorandil possibly enhanced by ALCOHOL
- ▸ Analgesics: increased risk of gastro-intestinal bleeding and ulceration when nicorandil given with NSAIDs OR ASPIRIN
- ▸ Antidepressants: enhanced hypotensive effect when nicorandil given with MAOIs; hypotensive effect of nicorandil possibly enhanced by TRICYCLICS
- ● Avanafil: hypotensive effect of nicorandil significantly enhanced by ● AVANAFIL (avoid concomitant use)
- ▸ Corticosteroids: increased risk of gastro-intestinal bleeding and ulceration when nicorandil given with CORTICOSTEROIDS
- ● Riociguat: possible enhanced hypotensive effect when nicorandil given with ● RIOCIGUAT—avoid concomitant use
- ● Sildenafil: hypotensive effect of nicorandil significantly enhanced by ● SILDENAFIL (avoid concomitant use)
- ● Tadalafil: hypotensive effect of nicorandil significantly enhanced by ● TADALAFIL (avoid concomitant use)
- ● Vardenafil: possible increased hypotensive effect when nicorandil given with ● VARDENAFIL—avoid concomitant use
- ▸ Vasodilator Antihypertensives: possible enhanced hypotensive effect when nicorandil given with HYDRALAZINE, MINOXIDIL OR SODIUM NITROPRUSSIDE

Nicotine
- ▸ Anti-arrhythmics: nicotine possibly enhances effects of ADENOSINE

Nicotinic Acid
- ● Lipid-regulating Drugs: increased risk of myopathy when nicotinic acid given with ● STATINS (applies to lipid regulating doses of nicotinic acid)

Nifedipine *see* Calcium-channel Blockers

Nilotinib
- ● Antibacterials: manufacturer of nilotinib advises avoid concomitant use with ● CLARITHROMYCIN and ● TELITHROMYCIN; plasma concentration of nilotinib reduced by ● RIFAMPICIN—avoid concomitant use
- ● Antifungals: plasma concentration of nilotinib increased by ● KETOCONAZOLE—avoid concomitant use; manufacturer of nilotinib advises avoid concomitant use with ● ITRACONAZOLE and ● VORICONAZOLE
- ● Antipsychotics: avoid concomitant use of cytotoxics with ● CLOZAPINE (increased risk of agranulocytosis)
- ● Antivirals: avoidance of nilotinib advised by manufacturer of ● BOCEPREVIR; plasma concentration of nilotinib possibly increased by RITONAVIR—manufacturer of nilotinib advises avoid concomitant use
- ▸ Anxiolytics and Hypnotics: nilotinib increases plasma concentration of MIDAZOLAM
- ● Grapefruit Juice: manufacturer of nilotinib advises avoid concomitant use with ● GRAPEFRUIT JUICE
- ▸ Lipid-regulating Drugs: separating administration from nilotinib by 12 hours advised by manufacturer of LOMITAPIDE

Nimodipine *see* Calcium-channel Blockers

Nintedanib
- ● Antibacterials: plasma concentration of nintedanib reduced by ● RIFAMPICIN—avoid concomitant use
- ● Antifungals: plasma concentration of nintedanib increased by ● KETOCONAZOLE
- ● Antipsychotics: avoid concomitant use of cytotoxics with ● CLOZAPINE (increased risk of agranulocytosis)

Nitrates
- ▸ ACE Inhibitors: enhanced hypotensive effect when nitrates given with ACE INHIBITORS
- ▸ Adrenergic Neurone Blockers: enhanced hypotensive effect when nitrates given with ADRENERGIC NEURONE BLOCKERS

Nitrates (continued)
- ▸ Alcohol: enhanced hypotensive effect when nitrates given with ALCOHOL
- ▸ Aldesleukin: enhanced hypotensive effect when nitrates given with ALDESLEUKIN
- ▸ Alpha-blockers: enhanced hypotensive effect when nitrates given with ALPHA-BLOCKERS
- ▸ Anaesthetics, General: enhanced hypotensive effect when nitrates given with GENERAL ANAESTHETICS
- ▸ Analgesics: hypotensive effect of nitrates antagonised by NSAIDs
- ▸ Angiotensin-II Receptor Antagonists: enhanced hypotensive effect when nitrates given with ANGIOTENSIN-II RECEPTOR ANTAGONISTS
- ▸ Anti-arrhythmics: effects of sublingual tablets of nitrates reduced by DISOPYRAMIDE (failure to dissolve under tongue owing to dry mouth)
- ● Anticoagulants: *infusion* of glyceryl trinitrate reduces anticoagulant effect of ● HEPARINS
- ▸ Antidepressants: enhanced hypotensive effect when nitrates given with MAOIs; effects of sublingual tablets of nitrates possibly reduced by TRICYCLIC-RELATED ANTIDEPRESSANTS (failure to dissolve under tongue owing to dry mouth); effects of sublingual tablets of nitrates reduced by TRICYCLICS (failure to dissolve under tongue owing to dry mouth)
- ▸ Antimuscarinics: effects of sublingual tablets of nitrates possibly reduced by ANTIMUSCARINICS (failure to dissolve under tongue owing to dry mouth)
- ▸ Antipsychotics: enhanced hypotensive effect when nitrates given with PHENOTHIAZINES
- ▸ Anxiolytics and Hypnotics: enhanced hypotensive effect when nitrates given with ANXIOLYTICS AND HYPNOTICS
- ● Avanafil: hypotensive effect of nitrates significantly enhanced by ● AVANAFIL (avoid concomitant use)
- ▸ Beta-blockers: enhanced hypotensive effect when nitrates given with BETA-BLOCKERS
- ▸ Calcium-channel Blockers: enhanced hypotensive effect when nitrates given with CALCIUM-CHANNEL BLOCKERS
- ▸ Clonidine: enhanced hypotensive effect when nitrates given with CLONIDINE
- ▸ Corticosteroids: hypotensive effect of nitrates antagonised by CORTICOSTEROIDS
- ▸ Diazoxide: enhanced hypotensive effect when nitrates given with DIAZOXIDE
- ▸ Diuretics: enhanced hypotensive effect when nitrates given with DIURETICS
- ▸ Dopaminergics: enhanced hypotensive effect when nitrates given with CO-BENELDOPA, CO-CARELDOPA OR LEVODOPA
- ● Levosimendan: possible severe postural hypotension when isosorbide mononitrate given with ● LEVOSIMENDAN
- ▸ Methyldopa: enhanced hypotensive effect when nitrates given with METHYLDOPA
- ▸ Moxisylyte: enhanced hypotensive effect when nitrates given with MOXISYLYTE
- ▸ Moxonidine: enhanced hypotensive effect when nitrates given with MOXONIDINE
- ▸ Muscle Relaxants: enhanced hypotensive effect when nitrates given with BACLOFEN OR TIZANIDINE
- ▸ Oestrogens: hypotensive effect of nitrates antagonised by OESTROGENS
- ▸ Prostaglandins: enhanced hypotensive effect when nitrates given with ALPROSTADIL
- ● Riociguat: possible enhanced hypotensive effect when nitrates given with ● RIOCIGUAT—avoid concomitant use
- ● Sildenafil: hypotensive effect of nitrates significantly enhanced by ● SILDENAFIL (avoid concomitant use)
- ● Tadalafil: hypotensive effect of nitrates significantly enhanced by ● TADALAFIL (avoid concomitant use)
- ● Vardenafil: possible increased hypotensive effect when nitrates given with ● VARDENAFIL—avoid concomitant use
- ▸ Vasodilator Antihypertensives: enhanced hypotensive effect when nitrates given with HYDRALAZINE, MINOXIDIL OR SODIUM NITROPRUSSIDE

Nitrazepam *see* Anxiolytics and Hypnotics

Nitrofurantoin
- ▸ Antacids: absorption of nitrofurantoin reduced by ORAL MAGNESIUM SALTS (as magnesium trisilicate)

Nitrofurantoin (continued)

▸ Antibacterials: nitrofurantoin possibly antagonises effects of NALIDIXIC ACID

▸ Sulfinpyrazone: excretion of nitrofurantoin reduced by SULFINPYRAZONE (increased risk of toxicity)

▸ Vaccines: antibacterials inactivate ORAL TYPHOID VACCINE—see under Typhoid Vaccine in BNFC

Nitroimidazoles *see* Metronidazole and Tinidazole

Nitrous Oxide *see* Anaesthetics, General

Nizatidine *see* Histamine H₂-antagonists

Nomegestrol *see* Progestogens

Noradrenaline (norepinephrine) *see* Sympathomimetics

Norelgestromin *see* Progestogens

Norepinephrine

NOTE Norepinephrine interactions as for noradrenaline, see under sympathomimetics

Norethisterone *see* Progestogens

Norfloxacin *see* Quinolones

Norgestimate *see* Progestogens

Norgestrel *see* Progestogens

Normal Immunoglobulin *see* Immunoglobulins

Nortriptyline *see* Antidepressants, Tricyclic

NSAIDs

NOTE *See also* Aspirin. Interactions do not generally apply to topical NSAIDs

▸ ACE Inhibitors: increased risk of renal impairment when NSAIDs given with ACE INHIBITORS, also hypotensive effect antagonised

▸ Adrenergic Neurone Blockers: NSAIDs antagonise hypotensive effect of ADRENERGIC NEURONE BLOCKERS

▸ Aliskiren: NSAIDs possibly antagonise hypotensive effect of ALISKIREN

▸ Alpha-blockers: NSAIDs antagonise hypotensive effect of ALPHA-BLOCKERS

● Analgesics: avoid concomitant use of NSAIDs with ● NSAIDs or ● ASPIRIN (increased side-effects); avoid concomitant use of NSAIDs with ● KETOROLAC (increased side-effects and haemorrhage); ibuprofen possibly reduces antiplatelet effect of ASPIRIN

● Angiotensin-II Receptor Antagonists: increased risk of renal impairment when NSAIDs given with ANGIOTENSIN-II RECEPTOR ANTAGONISTS, also hypotensive effect antagonised

▸ Antacids: absorption of acemetacin possibly reduced by ANTACIDS

● Antibacterials: indometacin possibly increases plasma concentration of AMIKACIN and GENTAMICIN in neonates; plasma concentration of celecoxib, diclofenac and etoricoxib reduced by RIFAMPICIN; possible increased risk of convulsions when NSAIDs given with ● QUINOLONES

● Anticoagulants: increased risk of haemorrhage when *intravenous* diclofenac given with ● ANTICOAGULANTS (avoid concomitant use, including low-dose heparins); increased risk of haemorrhage when ketorolac given with ● ANTICOAGULANTS (avoid concomitant use, including low-dose heparins); NSAIDs possibly enhance anticoagulant effect of ● COUMARINS and ● PHENINDIONE; possible increased risk of bleeding when NSAIDs given with ● DABIGATRAN or HEPARINS; increased risk of bleeding when NSAIDs given with ● EDOXABAN (manufacturer of edoxaban advises avoid long-term NSAIDs)

● Antidepressants: increased risk of bleeding when NSAIDs given with ● SSRIs or ● VENLAFAXINE

● Antidiabetics: NSAIDs possibly enhance effects of ● SULFONYLUREAS

● Antiepileptics: acemetacin possibly reduces excretion of FOSPHENYTOIN and PHENYTOIN (increased risk of toxicity)

● Antifungals: plasma concentration of parecoxib increased by FLUCONAZOLE (reduce dose of parecoxib); plasma concentration of celecoxib increased by FLUCONAZOLE (halve dose of celecoxib); plasma concentration of flurbiprofen and ibuprofen increased by FLUCONAZOLE; plasma concentration of diclofenac and ibuprofen increased by VORICONAZOLE

● Antipsychotics: possible severe drowsiness when acemetacin or indometacin given with HALOPERIDOL

● Antivirals: plasma concentration of NSAIDs possibly increased by RITONAVIR; plasma concentration of piroxicam increased by ● RITONAVIR (risk of toxicity)—avoid concomitant use;

NSAIDs

● Antivirals (continued)
increased risk of haematological toxicity when NSAIDs given with ZIDOVUDINE

▸ Azathioprine: manufacturer of azathioprine advises possible increased risk of myelosuppression when indometacin given with AZATHIOPRINE

▸ Beta-blockers: NSAIDs antagonise hypotensive effect of BETA-BLOCKERS

▸ Calcium-channel Blockers: NSAIDs antagonise hypotensive effect of CALCIUM-CHANNEL BLOCKERS

● Cardiac Glycosides: NSAIDs possibly increase plasma concentration of CARDIAC GLYCOSIDES, also possible exacerbation of heart failure and reduction of renal function

● Ciclosporin: increased risk of nephrotoxicity when NSAIDs given with ● CICLOSPORIN; plasma concentration of diclofenac increased by ● CICLOSPORIN (halve dose of diclofenac)

▸ Clonidine: NSAIDs antagonise hypotensive effect of CLONIDINE

▸ Clopidogrel: increased risk of bleeding when NSAIDs given with CLOPIDOGREL

▸ Corticosteroids: increased risk of gastro-intestinal bleeding and ulceration when NSAIDs given with CORTICOSTEROIDS

● Cytotoxics: NSAIDs probably reduce excretion of ● METHOTREXATE (increased risk of toxicity); diclofenac, ibuprofen, indometacin, ketoprofen, meloxicam and naproxen reduce excretion of ● METHOTREXATE (increased risk of toxicity); NSAIDs possibly reduce renal excretion of PEMETREXED—consult product literature; increased risk of bleeding when NSAIDs given with ● ERLOTINIB; avoidance of mefenamic acid advised by manufacturer of REGORAFENIB

▸ Desmopressin: indometacin enhances effects of DESMOPRESSIN

▸ Diazoxide: NSAIDs antagonise hypotensive effect of DIAZOXIDE

● Dimethyl sulfoxide: avoid concomitant use of sulindac with ● DIMETHYL SULFOXIDE

● Diuretics: risk of nephrotoxicity of NSAIDs increased by DIURETICS, also antagonism of diuretic effect; indometacin and ketorolac antagonise effects of DIURETICS; excretion of acemetacin possibly increased by FUROSEMIDE; NSAIDs possibly antagonise diuretic effect of POTASSIUM CANRENOATE; occasional reports of reduced renal function when indometacin given with ● TRIAMTERENE—avoid concomitant use; increased risk of hyperkalaemia when indometacin given with POTASSIUM-SPARING DIURETICS AND ALDOSTERONE ANTAGONISTS; possible increased risk of hyperkalaemia when NSAIDs given with POTASSIUM-SPARING DIURETICS AND ALDOSTERONE ANTAGONISTS

▸ Iloprost: increased risk of bleeding when NSAIDs given with ILOPROST

▸ Lipid-regulating Drugs: excretion of meloxicam increased by COLESTYRAMINE

● Lithium: NSAIDs reduce excretion of ● LITHIUM (increased risk of toxicity); ketorolac reduces excretion of ● LITHIUM (increased risk of toxicity)—avoid concomitant use

▸ Methyldopa: NSAIDs antagonise hypotensive effect of METHYLDOPA

▸ Mifamurtide: avoidance of high doses of NSAIDs advised by manufacturer of MIFAMURTIDE

▸ Moxonidine: NSAIDs antagonise hypotensive effect of MOXONIDINE

▸ Muscle Relaxants: ibuprofen reduces excretion of BACLOFEN (increased risk of toxicity); NSAIDs possibly reduce excretion of BACLOFEN (increased risk of toxicity)

▸ Nicorandil: increased risk of gastro-intestinal bleeding and ulceration when NSAIDs given with NICORANDIL

▸ Nitrates: NSAIDs antagonise hypotensive effect of NITRATES

▸ Oestrogens: etoricoxib increases plasma concentration of ETHINYLESTRADIOL

▸ Penicillamine: possible increased risk of nephrotoxicity when NSAIDs given with PENICILLAMINE

● Pentoxifylline: possible increased risk of bleeding when NSAIDs given with PENTOXIFYLLINE; increased risk of bleeding when ketorolac given with ● PENTOXIFYLLINE (avoid concomitant use)

▸ Prasugrel: possible increased risk of bleeding when NSAIDs given with PRASUGREL

NSAIDs (continued)
- Tacrolimus: possible increased risk of nephrotoxicity when NSAIDs given with TACROLIMUS; increased risk of nephrotoxicity when ibuprofen given with ● TACROLIMUS
▸ Vasodilator Antihypertensives: NSAIDs antagonise hypotensive effect of HYDRALAZINE, MINOXIDIL and SODIUM NITROPRUSSIDE

Obinutuzumab
- Antipsychotics: avoid concomitant use of cytotoxics with ● CLOZAPINE (increased risk of agranulocytosis)
- Vaccines: risk of generalised infections when monoclonal antibodies given with live ● VACCINES—avoid concomitant use

Octreotide
▸ Antidiabetics: octreotide possibly reduces requirements for ANTIDIABETICS
- Ciclosporin: octreotide reduces plasma concentration of ● CICLOSPORIN
▸ Dopaminergics: octreotide increases plasma concentration of BROMOCRIPTINE
▸ Ulcer-healing Drugs: octreotide possibly delays absorption of CIMETIDINE

Oestrogens
▸ ACE Inhibitors: oestrogens antagonise hypotensive effect of ACE INHIBITORS
▸ Adrenergic Neurone Blockers: oestrogens antagonise hypotensive effect of ADRENERGIC NEURONE BLOCKERS
▸ Alpha-blockers: oestrogens antagonise hypotensive effect of ALPHA-BLOCKERS
▸ Aminophylline: oestrogens increase plasma concentration of AMINOPHYLLINE (consider reducing dose of aminophylline)
▸ Analgesics: plasma concentration of ethinylestradiol increased by ETORICOXIB
▸ Angiotensin-II Receptor Antagonists: oestrogens antagonise hypotensive effect of ANGIOTENSIN-II RECEPTOR ANTAGONISTS
▸ Antibacterials: plasma concentration of estradiol increased by ERYTHROMYCIN; metabolism of oestrogens accelerated by ● RIFAMYCINS (reduced contraceptive effect with combined oral contraceptives, contraceptive patches, and vaginal rings—see Contraceptive Interactions in BNFC)
- Anticoagulants: oestrogens may enhance or reduce anticoagulant effect of COUMARINS; oestrogens antagonise anticoagulant effect of ● PHENINDIONE
- Antidepressants: contraceptive effect of oestrogens reduced by ● ST JOHN'S WORT (avoid concomitant use); oestrogens antagonise antidepressant effect of TRICYCLICS (but side-effects of tricyclics possibly increased due to increased plasma concentration)
▸ Antidiabetics: oestrogens antagonise hypoglycaemic effect of ANTIDIABETICS
- Antiepileptics: metabolism of oestrogens accelerated by ● CARBAMAZEPINE, ● ESLICARBAZEPINE, ● FOSPHENYTOIN, ● OXCARBAZEPINE, ● PHENOBARBITAL, ● PHENYTOIN, ● PRIMIDONE, ● RUFINAMIDE and ● TOPIRAMATE (reduced contraceptive effect with combined oral contraceptives, contraceptive patches, and vaginal rings—see Contraceptive Interactions in BNFC); oestrogens reduce plasma concentration of ● LAMOTRIGINE—consider increasing dose of lamotrigine; ethinylestradiol possibly reduces plasma concentration of SODIUM VALPROATE and VALPROIC ACID
▸ Antifungals: plasma concentration of ethinylestradiol increased by KETOCONAZOLE; oestrogens increase plasma concentration of VORICONAZOLE; anecdotal reports of contraceptive failure and menstrual irregularities when oestrogens given with GRISEOFULVIN; anecdotal reports of contraceptive failure when oestrogens given with IMIDAZOLES; occasional reports of breakthrough bleeding when oestrogens (used for contraception) given with TERBINAFINE
- Antivirals: plasma concentration of ethinylestradiol increased by ATAZANAVIR; avoidance of ethinylestradiol advised by manufacturer of ● DASABUVIR, ● OMBITASVIR and ● PARITAPREVIR—use alternative form of contraception; metabolism of oestrogens accelerated by ● NEVIRAPINE and ● RITONAVIR (reduced contraceptive effect with combined oral contraceptives, contraceptive patches, and vaginal rings—see Contraceptive Interactions in BNFC); plasma concentration of ethinylestradiol possibly reduced by ● TELAPREVIR—

Oestrogens
- Antivirals (continued)
manufacturer of telaprevir advises additional contraceptive precautions
▸ Anxiolytics and Hypnotics: oestrogens possibly increase plasma concentration of CHLORDIAZEPOXIDE, DIAZEPAM and NITRAZEPAM; oestrogens possibly reduce plasma concentration of LORAZEPAM, OXAZEPAM and TEMAZEPAM; oestrogens increase plasma concentration of MELATONIN
- Aprepitant: possible contraceptive failure of hormonal contraceptives containing oestrogens when given with ● APREPITANT (alternative contraception recommended)
▸ Beta-blockers: oestrogens antagonise hypotensive effect of BETA-BLOCKERS
- Bosentan: possible contraceptive failure of hormonal contraceptives containing oestrogens when given with ● BOSENTAN (alternative contraception recommended)
▸ Calcium-channel Blockers: oestrogens antagonise hypotensive effect of CALCIUM-CHANNEL BLOCKERS
▸ Ciclosporin: oestrogens possibly increase plasma concentration of CICLOSPORIN
- Clonidine: oestrogens antagonise hypotensive effect of CLONIDINE
- Cobicistat: metabolism of oestrogens accelerated by ● COBICISTAT (reduced contraceptive effect with combined oral contraceptives, contraceptive patches, and vaginal rings—see Contraceptive Interactions in BNFC)
▸ Corticosteroids: oral contraceptives containing oestrogens increase plasma concentration of CORTICOSTEROIDS
- Cytotoxics: possible reduction in contraceptive effect of oestrogens advised by manufacturer of ● CRIZOTINIB and ● VEMURAFENIB; possible reduced contraceptive effect of hormonal contraceptives containing oestrogens advised by manufacturer of ● DABRAFENIB (alternative contraception recommended)
▸ Diuretics: oestrogens antagonise diuretic effect of DIURETICS
- Dopaminergics: oestrogens increase plasma concentration of ROPINIROLE; oestrogens increase plasma concentration of ● SELEGILINE—manufacturer of selegiline advises avoid concomitant use
- Fosaprepitant: possible contraceptive failure of hormonal contraceptives containing oestrogens when given with ● FOSAPREPITANT (alternative contraception recommended)
▸ Lipid-regulating Drugs: absorption of ethinylestradiol reduced by COLESEVELAM; plasma concentration of ethinylestradiol increased by ATORVASTATIN and ROSUVASTATIN; separating administration from oestrogens by 12 hours advised by manufacturer of LOMITAPIDE
▸ Methyldopa: oestrogens antagonise hypotensive effect of METHYLDOPA
- Modafinil: metabolism of oestrogens accelerated by ● MODAFINIL (reduced contraceptive effect with combined oral contraceptives, contraceptive patches, and vaginal rings—see Contraceptive Interactions in BNFC)
- Moxonidine: oestrogens antagonise hypotensive effect of MOXONIDINE
▸ Muscle Relaxants: oestrogens possibly increase plasma concentration of TIZANIDINE (increased risk of toxicity)
▸ Nitrates: oestrogens antagonise hypotensive effect of NITRATES
- Somatropin: oestrogens (when used as oral replacement therapy) may increase dose requirements of SOMATROPIN
▸ Tacrolimus: ethinylestradiol possibly increases plasma concentration of TACROLIMUS
- Teriflunomide: plasma concentration of ethinylestradiol increased by TERIFLUNOMIDE
▸ Theophylline: oestrogens increase plasma concentration of THEOPHYLLINE (consider reducing dose of theophylline)
▸ Thyroid Hormones: oestrogens may increase requirements for THYROID HORMONES in hypothyroidism
▸ Vasodilator Antihypertensives: oestrogens antagonise hypotensive effect of HYDRALAZINE, MINOXIDIL and SODIUM NITROPRUSSIDE

Oestrogens, conjugated see Oestrogens

Ofatumumab
- Antipsychotics: avoid concomitant use of cytotoxics with ● CLOZAPINE (increased risk of agranulocytosis)

Ofatumumab (continued)
- Vaccines: risk of generalised infections when monoclonal antibodies given with live ● VACCINES—avoid concomitant use

Ofloxacin see Quinolones

Olanzapine see Antipsychotics

Olaparib
- Antibacterials: manufacturer of olaparib advises avoid concomitant use with ● CLARITHROMYCIN, ● RIFABUTIN, ● RIFAMPICIN and ● TELITHROMYCIN
- Antidepressants: manufacturer of olaparib advises avoid concomitant use with ● ST JOHN'S WORT
- Antiepileptics: manufacturer of olaparib advises avoid concomitant use with ● CARBAMAZEPINE, ● PHENOBARBITAL and ● PHENYTOIN
- Antifungals: manufacturer of olaparib advises avoid concomitant use with ● ITRACONAZOLE
- Antipsychotics: avoid concomitant use of cytotoxics with ● CLOZAPINE (increased risk of agranulocytosis)
- Antivirals: manufacturer of olaparib advises avoid concomitant use with ● BOCEPREVIR, ● INDINAVIR, ● NEVIRAPINE, ● SAQUINAVIR and ● TELAPREVIR

Olmesartan see Angiotensin-II Receptor Antagonists

Olodaterol see Sympathomimetics, Beta$_2$

Ombitasvir
- Antibacterials: plasma concentration of ombitasvir possibly reduced by ● RIFAMPICIN—avoid concomitant use
- Antidepressants: plasma concentration of ombitasvir possibly reduced by ● ST JOHN'S WORT—manufacturer of ombitasvir advises avoid concomitant use
- Antiepileptics: plasma concentration of ombitasvir reduced by ● CARBAMAZEPINE—avoid concomitant use; plasma concentration of ombitasvir possibly reduced by ● FOSPHENYTOIN, ● PHENOBARBITAL, ● PHENYTOIN and ● PRIMIDONE—avoid concomitant use
- Antifungals: manufacturer of ombitasvir advises avoid concomitant use with KETOCONAZOLE
- Antivirals: manufacturer of ombitasvir advises avoid concomitant use with EFAVIRENZ, ETRAVIRINE and NEVIRAPINE
- Cobicistat: manufacturer of ombitasvir advises avoid concomitant use with COBICISTAT
- Cytotoxics: manufacturer of ombitasvir advises avoid concomitant use with MITOTANE
- Diuretics: ombitasvir increases plasma concentration of ● FUROSEMIDE (reduce dose of furosemide)
- Hormone Antagonists: manufacturer of ombitasvir advises avoid concomitant use with ENZALUTAMIDE
- Lipid-regulating Drugs: manufacturer of ombitasvir advises avoid concomitant use with ● ATORVASTATIN and ● SIMVASTATIN
- Oestrogens: manufacturer of ombitasvir advises avoid concomitant use of ● ETHINYLESTRADIOL—use alternative form of contraception

Omeprazole see Proton Pump Inhibitors

Ondansetron see 5HT$_3$-receptor Antagonists (under HT)

Opioid Analgesics
▹ Alcohol: enhanced hypotensive and sedative effects when opioid analgesics given with ● ALCOHOL
▹ Anaesthetics, General: fentanyl inhibits metabolism of ETOMIDATE (consider reducing dose of etomidate); opioid analgesics possibly enhance effects of INTRAVENOUS GENERAL ANAESTHETICS and VOLATILE LIQUID GENERAL ANAESTHETICS
- Analgesics: possible opioid withdrawal when tapentadol given with ● BUPRENORPHINE and ● PENTAZOCINE; possible opioid withdrawal when buprenorphine given with ● DIAMORPHINE, ● DIPIPANONE, ● HYDROMORPHONE, ● METHADONE, ● MORPHINE, ● OXYCODONE, ● PAPAVERETUM, ● PETHIDINE and ● TRAMADOL; avoidance of buprenorphine advised by manufacturer of FENTANYL; possible opioid withdrawal when diamorphine, dipipanone, hydromorphone, methadone, morphine, oxycodone and papaveretum given with PENTAZOCINE; manufacturer of fentanyl advises avoid concomitant use with PENTAZOCINE; possible opioid withdrawal when pentazocine given with ● PETHIDINE and ● TRAMADOL
- Antibacterials: plasma concentration of fentanyl possibly increased by CLARITHROMYCIN; plasma concentration of alfentanil increased by ERYTHROMYCIN; metabolism of alfentanil, codeine, fentanyl, methadone and morphine

Opioid Analgesics
- Antibacterials (continued)
accelerated by RIFAMPICIN (reduced effect); metabolism of oxycodone possibly accelerated by RIFAMPICIN; increased risk of ventricular arrhythmias when methadone given with ● DELAMANID; manufacturer of pethidine advises avoid concomitant use with ISONIAZID; metabolism of oxycodone inhibited by TELITHROMYCIN; possible increased risk of ventricular arrhythmias when methadone given with ● TELITHROMYCIN
- Anticoagulants: tramadol enhances anticoagulant effect of ● COUMARINS
- Antidepressants: plasma concentration of methadone possibly increased by FLUOXETINE, FLUVOXAMINE, PAROXETINE and SERTRALINE; possible increased serotonergic effects when pethidine or tramadol given with DULOXETINE; possible increased serotonergic effects when tramadol given with MIRTAZAPINE, VENLAFAXINE or VORTIOXETINE; possible increased serotonergic effects and increased risk of convulsions when tramadol given with ● MAOIS—some manufacturers advise avoid concomitant use and for 2 weeks after stopping MAOIs; CNS excitation or depression (hypertension or hypotension) when pethidine given with ● MAOIS—avoid concomitant use and for 2 weeks after stopping MAOIs; possible increased serotonergic effects when fentanyl given with MAOIS, SSRI-RELATED ANTIDEPRESSANTS or SSRIs; possible CNS excitation or depression (hypertension or hypotension) when opioid analgesics given with ● MAOIS—some manufacturers advise avoid concomitant use and for 2 weeks after stopping MAOIs; possible CNS excitation or depression (hypertension or hypotension) when opioid analgesics given with ● MOCLOBEMIDE—manufacturer of moclobemide advises consider reducing dose of opioid analgesics; possible CNS excitation or depression (hypertension or hypotension) when dextromethorphan or pethidine given with ● MOCLOBEMIDE—avoid concomitant use; increased risk of CNS toxicity when tramadol given with ● SSRIS or ● TRICYCLICS; plasma concentration of methadone possibly reduced by ST JOHN'S WORT; sedative effects possibly increased when opioid analgesics given with TRICYCLICS
- Antiepileptics: metabolism of fentanyl possibly accelerated by CARBAMAZEPINE, FOSPHENYTOIN and PHENYTOIN (reduced effect); dextropropoxyphene enhances effects of ● CARBAMAZEPINE; effects of tramadol reduced by CARBAMAZEPINE; plasma concentration of methadone reduced by CARBAMAZEPINE, PHENOBARBITAL and PRIMIDONE; possible increased risk of pethidine toxicity when given with ● FOSPHENYTOIN and ● PHENYTOIN; metabolism of methadone accelerated by FOSPHENYTOIN and PHENYTOIN (reduced effect and risk of withdrawal effects); morphine increases bioavailability of GABAPENTIN
- Antifungals: metabolism of buprenorphine inhibited by ● KETOCONAZOLE (reduce dose of buprenorphine); possible increased risk of ventricular arrhythmias when methadone given with ● KETOCONAZOLE—manufacturer of ketoconazole advises avoid concomitant use; plasma concentration of oxycodone increased by ITRACONAZOLE, KETOCONAZOLE and ● VORICONAZOLE; metabolism of alfentanil inhibited by FLUCONAZOLE (risk of prolonged or delayed respiratory depression); plasma concentration of methadone increased by FLUCONAZOLE; metabolism of alfentanil possibly inhibited by ITRACONAZOLE; plasma concentration of methadone possibly increased by ● ITRACONAZOLE (increased risk of ventricular arrhythmias); plasma concentration of alfentanil and methadone increased by ● VORICONAZOLE (consider reducing dose of alfentanil and methadone); plasma concentration of fentanyl possibly increased by ● TRIAZOLES
- Antihistamines: sedative effects possibly increased when opioid analgesics given with ● SEDATING ANTIHISTAMINES
- Antimalarials: avoidance of methadone advised by manufacturer of ● ARTENIMOL WITH PIPERAQUINE (possible risk of ventricular arrhythmias)
▹ Antimuscarinics: possible increased risk of antimuscarinic side-effects when codeine given with ANTIMUSCARINICS
- Antipsychotics: enhanced hypotensive and sedative effects when opioid analgesics given with ANTIPSYCHOTICS; increased

A1

Interactions | Appendix 1

A1

Interactions | Appendix 1

Opioid Analgesics

● Antipsychotics (continued)
risk of ventricular arrhythmias when methadone given with
● ANTIPSYCHOTICS that prolong the QT interval; increased risk
of convulsions when tramadol given with ANTIPSYCHOTICS;
increased risk of ventricular arrhythmias when methadone
given with ● AMISULPRIDE—avoid concomitant use

● Antivirals: plasma concentration of methadone possibly
reduced by ABACAVIR, NEVIRAPINE and RILPIVIRINE; plasma
concentration of buprenorphine increased by ATAZANAVIR;
plasma concentration of methadone possibly affected by
BOCEPREVIR; possible increased risk of prolonged sedation and
respiratory depression when buprenorphine given with
BOCEPREVIR; methadone possibly reduces plasma
concentration of DIDANOSINE; plasma concentration of
methadone reduced by EFAVIRENZ, FOSAMPRENAVIR and
RITONAVIR; plasma concentration of alfentanil and fentanyl
increased by ● RITONAVIR; plasma concentration of pethidine
reduced by ● RITONAVIR, but plasma concentration of toxic
pethidine metabolite increased (avoid concomitant use);
plasma concentration of morphine possibly reduced by
RITONAVIR; plasma concentration of dextropropoxyphene
increased by ● RITONAVIR (risk of toxicity)—avoid concomitant
use; plasma concentration of buprenorphine possibly
increased by RITONAVIR; increased risk of ventricular
arrhythmias when alfentanil, fentanyl or methadone given
with ● SAQUINAVIR—avoid concomitant use; caution with
methadone advised by manufacturer of ● TELAPREVIR (risk of
ventricular arrhythmias); buprenorphine possibly reduces
plasma concentration of TIPRANAVIR; methadone possibly
increases plasma concentration of ZIDOVUDINE

▹ Anxiolytics and Hypnotics: increased sedative effect when opioid
analgesics given with ANXIOLYTICS AND HYPNOTICS; fentanyl
possibly inhibits metabolism of MIDAZOLAM

● Atomoxetine: increased risk of ventricular arrhythmias when
methadone given with ● ATOMOXETINE; possible increased risk
of convulsions when tramadol given with ATOMOXETINE

▹ Beta-blockers: morphine possibly increases plasma
concentration of ESMOLOL

▹ Calcium-channel Blockers: metabolism of alfentanil inhibited by
DILTIAZEM (risk of prolonged or delayed respiratory
depression)

● Cytotoxics: possible increased risk of ventricular arrhythmias
when methadone given with ● BOSUTINIB; caution with
alfentanil and fentanyl advised by manufacturer of
● CRIZOTINIB; possible increased risk of ventricular
arrhythmias when methadone given with ● VANDETANIB—
avoid concomitant use

● Dapoxetine: possible increased risk of serotonergic effects
when tramadol given with ● DAPOXETINE (manufacturer of
dapoxetine advises tramadol should not be started until
1 week after stopping dapoxetine, avoid dapoxetine for
2 weeks after stopping tramadol)

▹ Domperidone: opioid analgesics antagonise effects of
DOMPERIDONE on gastro-intestinal activity

● Dopaminergics: avoid concomitant use of dextromethorphan
with ● RASAGILINE; risk of CNS toxicity when pethidine given
with ● RASAGILINE (avoid pethidine for 2 weeks after
rasagiline); avoidance of opioid analgesics advised by
manufacturer of SELEGILINE; hyperpyrexia and CNS toxicity
reported when pethidine given with ● SELEGILINE (avoid
concomitant use)

▹ Hormone Antagonists: plasma concentration of
dextromethorphan increased by ABIRATERONE

▹ 5HT₃-receptor Antagonists: effects of tramadol possibly
antagonised by ONDANSETRON

● Memantine: increased risk of CNS toxicity when
dextromethorphan given with ● MEMANTINE (manufacturer of
memantine advises avoid concomitant use)

▹ Metoclopramide: opioid analgesics antagonise effects of
METOCLOPRAMIDE on gastro-intestinal activity

▹ Muscle Relaxants: increased sedative effect when fentanyl or
morphine given with BACLOFEN

● Nalmefene: avoidance of opioid analgesics advised by
manufacturer of ● NALMEFENE

Opioid Analgesics (continued)

▹ Netupitant: caution with morphine advised by manufacturer of
NETUPITANT

● Sodium Oxybate: opioid analgesics enhance effects of ● SODIUM
OXYBATE (avoid concomitant use)

▹ Ulcer-healing Drugs: metabolism of opioid analgesics inhibited
by CIMETIDINE (increased plasma concentration)

Oritavancin

▹ Anticoagulants: oritavancin possibly increases plasma
concentration of WARFARIN

▹ Vaccines: antibacterials inactivate ORAL TYPHOID VACCINE—see
under Typhoid Vaccine in BNFC

Orlistat

▹ Anti-arrhythmics: orlistat possibly reduces plasma
concentration of AMIODARONE

▹ Anticoagulants: manufacturer of orlistat recommends
monitoring anticoagulant effect of COUMARINS

▹ Antidiabetics: manufacturer of orlistat advises avoid
concomitant use with ACARBOSE

● Antiepileptics: possible increased risk of convulsions when
orlistat given with ● ANTIEPILEPTICS

▹ Antivirals: orlistat possibly reduces absorption of ● ABACAVIR,
● ATAZANAVIR, ● DARUNAVIR, ● DIDANOSINE, ● EFAVIRENZ,
● ELVITEGRAVIR, ● EMTRICITABINE, ● ENFUVIRTIDE, ● ETRAVIRINE,
● FOSAMPRENAVIR, ● INDINAVIR, ● LAMIVUDINE, ● LOPINAVIR,
● MARAVIROC, ● NEVIRAPINE, ● RALTEGRAVIR, ● RILPIVIRINE,
● RITONAVIR, ● SAQUINAVIR, ● STAVUDINE, ● TENOFOVIR,
● TIPRANAVIR and ● ZIDOVUDINE

● Ciclosporin: orlistat possibly reduces absorption of
● CICLOSPORIN

▹ Thyroid Hormones: possible increased risk of hypothyroidism
when orlistat given with LEVOTHYROXINE

Orphenadrine *see* Antimuscarinics

Oxaliplatin *see* Platinum Compounds

Oxandrolone *see* Anabolic Steroids

Oxazepam *see* Anxiolytics and Hypnotics

Oxcarbazepine

● Antidepressants: anticonvulsant effect of antiepileptics
possibly antagonised by MAOIs and ● TRICYCLIC-RELATED
ANTIDEPRESSANTS (convulsive threshold lowered);
anticonvulsant effect of antiepileptics antagonised by ● SSRIs
and ● TRICYCLICS (convulsive threshold lowered)

● Antiepileptics: oxcarbazepine sometimes reduces plasma
concentration of CARBAMAZEPINE (but concentration of an
active metabolite of carbamazepine may be increased), also
plasma concentration of an active metabolite of
oxcarbazepine often reduced; avoidance of oxcarbazepine
advised by manufacturer of ESLICARBAZEPINE; oxcarbazepine
increases plasma concentration of FOSPHENYTOIN,
PHENOBARBITAL, PHENYTOIN and PRIMIDONE, also plasma
concentration of an active metabolite of oxcarbazepine
reduced; oxcarbazepine reduces plasma concentration of
● PERAMPANEL, also plasma concentration of oxcarbazepine
increased (see under Perampanel, p. 193); plasma
concentration of an active metabolite of oxcarbazepine
sometimes reduced by SODIUM VALPROATE and VALPROIC ACID

● Antimalarials: anticonvulsant effect of antiepileptics
antagonised by ● MEFLOQUINE

● Antipsychotics: anticonvulsant effect of antiepileptics
antagonised by ● ANTIPSYCHOTICS (convulsive threshold
lowered)

● Antivirals: oxcarbazepine possibly reduces plasma
concentration of ● DACLATASVIR and ● SIMEPREVIR—
manufacturer of daclatasvir and simeprevir advises avoid
concomitant use; oxcarbazepine possibly reduces the plasma
concentration of ● DOLUTEGRAVIR (see under Dolutegravir,
p. 387); avoidance of oxcarbazepine advised by manufacturer
of LEDIPASVIR and SOFOSBUVIR; avoidance of oxcarbazepine
advised by manufacturer of ● RILPIVIRINE (plasma
concentration of rilpivirine possibly reduced)

▹ Ciclosporin: oxcarbazepine possibly reduces plasma
concentration of CICLOSPORIN

● Clopidogrel: oxcarbazepine possibly reduces antiplatelet effect
of ● CLOPIDOGREL

● Cytotoxics: oxcarbazepine reduces plasma concentration of
● IMATINIB—avoid concomitant use

Oxcarbazepine (continued)
- Guanfacine: oxcarbazepine possibly reduces plasma concentration of ● GUANFACINE—increase dose of guanfacine
- Oestrogens: oxcarbazepine accelerates metabolism of ● OESTROGENS (reduced contraceptive effect with combined oral contraceptives, contraceptive patches, and vaginal rings—see Contraceptive Interactions in BNFC)
- Orlistat: possible increased risk of convulsions when antiepileptics given with ● ORLISTAT
- Progestogens: oxcarbazepine accelerates metabolism of ● PROGESTOGENS (reduced contraceptive effect with combined oral contraceptives, progestogen-only oral contraceptives, contraceptive patches, vaginal rings, etonogestrel-releasing implant, and emergency hormonal contraception—see Contraceptive Interactions in BNFC)

Oxprenolol see Beta-blockers
Oxybutynin see Antimuscarinics
Oxycodone see Opioid Analgesics
Oxymetazoline see Sympathomimetics
Oxytetracycline see Tetracyclines
Oxytocin
▸ Anaesthetics, General: oxytocic effect possibly reduced, also enhanced hypotensive effect and risk of arrhythmias when oxytocin given with VOLATILE LIQUID GENERAL ANAESTHETICS
▸ Prostaglandins: uterotonic effect of oxytocin potentiated by PROSTAGLANDINS
▸ Sympathomimetics: risk of hypertension when oxytocin given with vasoconstrictor SYMPATHOMIMETICS (due to enhanced vasopressor effect)

Paclitaxel
- Antipsychotics: avoid concomitant use of cytotoxics with ● CLOZAPINE (increased risk of agranulocytosis)
- Antivirals: plasma concentration of paclitaxel increased by RITONAVIR
- Cytotoxics: increased risk of neutropenia when paclitaxel given with ● LAPATINIB

Paliperidone see Antipsychotics
Palonosetron see 5HT$_3$-receptor Antagonists (under HT)
Pamidronate Disodium see Bisphosphonates
Pancreatin
▸ Antidiabetics: pancreatin antagonises hypoglycaemic effect of ACARBOSE
Pancuronium see Muscle Relaxants
Panitumumab
- Antipsychotics: avoid concomitant use of cytotoxics with ● CLOZAPINE (increased risk of agranulocytosis)
- Cytotoxics: manufacturer of panitumumab advises avoid concomitant use with ● BEVACIZUMAB, ● FLUOROURACIL, ● IRINOTECAN and ● OXALIPLATIN
- Folates: manufacturer of panitumumab advises avoid concomitant use with ● FOLINIC ACID
- Vaccines: risk of generalised infections when monoclonal antibodies given with live ● VACCINES—avoid concomitant use

Pantoprazole see Proton Pump Inhibitors
Papaveretum see Opioid Analgesics
Paracetamol
▸ Anticoagulants: prolonged regular use of paracetamol possibly enhances anticoagulant effect of COUMARINS
▸ Antidiabetics: absorption of paracetamol possibly reduced when given 1 to 4 hours after LIXISENATIDE
▸ Antiepileptics: metabolism of paracetamol possibly accelerated by CARBAMAZEPINE, FOSPHENYTOIN, PHENOBARBITAL, PHENYTOIN and PRIMIDONE (also isolated reports of hepatotoxicity)
▸ Antifungals: avoidance of paracetamol advised by manufacturer of KETOCONAZOLE
▸ Cytotoxics: paracetamol possibly inhibits metabolism of *intravenous* BUSULFAN (manufacturer of *intravenous* busulfan advises caution within 72 hours of paracetamol); caution with paracetamol advised by manufacturer of IMATINIB
▸ Lipid-regulating Drugs: absorption of paracetamol reduced by COLESTYRAMINE
▸ Metoclopramide: rate of absorption of paracetamol increased by METOCLOPRAMIDE
Paraldehyde
- Alcohol: increased sedative effect when paraldehyde given with ● ALCOHOL

Paraldehyde (continued)
- Disulfiram: risk of toxicity when paraldehyde given with ● DISULFIRAM
Parasympathomimetics
▸ Anti-arrhythmics: effects of neostigmine and pyridostigmine possibly antagonised by PROPAFENONE
- Antibacterials: plasma concentration of galantamine increased by ERYTHROMYCIN; effects of neostigmine and pyridostigmine antagonised by ● AMINOGLYCOSIDES; effects of neostigmine and pyridostigmine antagonised by CLINDAMYCIN; effects of neostigmine and pyridostigmine antagonised by ● POLYMYXINS
▸ Antidepressants: plasma concentration of galantamine increased by PAROXETINE
▸ Antifungals: plasma concentration of galantamine increased by KETOCONAZOLE
▸ Antimalarials: effects of neostigmine and pyridostigmine may be diminished because of potential for CHLOROQUINE to increase symptoms of myasthenia gravis; effects of neostigmine and pyridostigmine may be diminished because of potential for HYDROXYCHLOROQUINE to increase symptoms of myasthenia gravis
▸ Antimuscarinics: effects of parasympathomimetics antagonised by ANTIMUSCARINICS
▸ Beta-blockers: increased risk of arrhythmias when pilocarpine given with BETA-BLOCKERS; effects of neostigmine and pyridostigmine antagonised by PROPRANOLOL
▸ Cytotoxics: possible increased risk of bradycardia when pilocarpine given with CRIZOTINIB
▸ Lithium: effects of neostigmine antagonised by LITHIUM
▸ Muscle Relaxants: donepezil possibly enhances effects of SUXAMETHONIUM; galantamine, neostigmine, pyridostigmine and rivastigmine enhance effects of SUXAMETHONIUM; neostigmine, pyridostigmine and rivastigmine antagonise effects of NON-DEPOLARISING MUSCLE RELAXANTS; donepezil possibly antagonises effects of NON-DEPOLARISING MUSCLE RELAXANTS

Parecoxib see NSAIDs
Paricalcitol see Vitamins
Paritaprevir
▸ Angiotensin-II Receptor Antagonists: manufacturer of paritaprevir advises reduce dose when given with VALSARTAN
- Antibacterials: manufacturer of paritaprevir advises avoid concomitant use with CLARITHROMYCIN and TELITHROMYCIN; plasma concentration of paritaprevir possibly reduced by ● RIFAMPICIN—avoid concomitant use
- Antidepressants: plasma concentration of paritaprevir possibly reduced by ● ST JOHN'S WORT—manufacturer of paritaprevir advises avoid concomitant use
- Antiepileptics: plasma concentration of paritaprevir reduced by ● CARBAMAZEPINE—avoid concomitant use; plasma concentration of paritaprevir possibly reduced by ● FOSPHENYTOIN, ● PHENOBARBITAL, ● PHENYTOIN and ● PRIMIDONE—avoid concomitant use
- Antifungals: plasma concentration of both drugs increased when paritaprevir given with ● KETOCONAZOLE—avoid concomitant use; plasma concentration of both drugs possibly increased when paritaprevir given with ● ITRACONAZOLE and ● POSACONAZOLE—avoid concomitant use
- Antivirals: plasma concentration of paritaprevir increased by ● ATAZANAVIR; plasma concentration of paritaprevir increased by ● DARUNAVIR and plasma concentration of darunavir decreased; manufacturer of paritaprevir advises avoid concomitant use with EFAVIRENZ, ETRAVIRINE, INDINAVIR, NEVIRAPINE, SAQUINAVIR and TIPRANAVIR; plasma concentration of paritaprevir increased by ● LOPINAVIR—manufacturer of paritaprevir advises avoid concomitant use
▸ Cardiac Glycosides: paritaprevir possibly increases plasma concentration of DIGOXIN (consider reducing dose of digoxin)
▸ Cobicistat: manufacturer of paritaprevir advises avoid concomitant use with COBICISTAT
▸ Cytotoxics: manufacturer of paritaprevir advises avoid concomitant use with MITOTANE
- Diuretics: paritaprevir increases plasma concentration of ● FUROSEMIDE (reduce dose of furosemide)
▸ Hormone Antagonists: manufacturer of paritaprevir advises avoid concomitant use with ENZALUTAMIDE

Interactions | Appendix 1

Paritaprevir (continued)

- Lipid-regulating Drugs: plasma concentration of paritaprevir increased by ● GEMFIBROZIL—manufacturer of paritaprevir advises avoid concomitant use; manufacturer of paritaprevir advises avoid concomitant use with ● ATORVASTATIN, FLUVASTATIN and ● SIMVASTATIN; paritaprevir increases plasma concentration of ● PRAVASTATIN (reduce dose of pravastatin); paritaprevir increases plasma concentration of ● ROSUVASTATIN (reduce dose of rosuvastatin—see under Rosuvastatin, in BNF)
- Oestrogens: manufacturer of paritaprevir advises avoid concomitant use of ● ETHINYLESTRADIOL—use alternative form of contraception

Paroxetine *see* Antidepressants, SSRI

Pasireotide

▹ Antidiabetics: pasireotide possibly reduces requirements for ANTIDIABETICS
▹ Antifungals: avoidance of pasireotide advised by manufacturer of KETOCONAZOLE
▹ Antimuscarinics: possible increased risk of bradycardia when pasireotide given with IPRATROPIUM or OXYBUTYNIN
▹ Beta-blockers: possible increased risk of bradycardia when pasireotide given with CARTEOLOL, METOPROLOL, PROPRANOLOL or SOTALOL
▹ Calcium-channel Blockers: possible increased risk of bradycardia when pasireotide given with DILTIAZEM or VERAPAMIL
● Ciclosporin: pasireotide possibly reduces plasma concentration of ● CICLOSPORIN

Pazopanib

● Antibacterials: plasma concentration of pazopanib possibly increased by ● CLARITHROMYCIN and ● TELITHROMYCIN (reduce dose of pazopanib); plasma concentration of pazopanib possibly reduced by ● RIFAMPICIN
● Antifungals: plasma concentration of pazopanib increased by ● KETOCONAZOLE (reduce dose of pazopanib); plasma concentration of pazopanib possibly increased by ● ITRACONAZOLE and ● VORICONAZOLE (reduce dose of pazopanib)
● Antipsychotics: avoid concomitant use of cytotoxics with ● CLOZAPINE (increased risk of agranulocytosis)
● Antivirals: plasma concentration of pazopanib possibly increased by ● ATAZANAVIR, ● INDINAVIR and ● RITONAVIR (reduce dose of pazopanib); avoidance of pazopanib advised by manufacturer of ● BOCEPREVIR; increased risk of ventricular arrhythmias when pazopanib given with ● SAQUINAVIR—avoid concomitant use
▹ Cytotoxics: plasma concentration of pazopanib increased by LAPATINIB
● Grapefruit Juice: manufacturer of pazopanib advises avoid concomitant use with ● GRAPEFRUIT JUICE
▹ Lipid-regulating Drugs: separating administration from pazopanib by 12 hours advised by manufacturer of LOMITAPIDE
▹ Ulcer-healing Drugs: absorption of pazopanib possibly reduced by HISTAMINE H$_2$-ANTAGONISTS—manufacturer of pazopanib advises give at least 2 hours before or 10 hours after histamine H$_2$-antagonists; absorption of pazopanib possibly reduced by PROTON PUMP INHIBITORS—manufacturer of pazopanib advises give at the same time as proton pump inhibitors

Pegfilgrastim

▹ Cytotoxics: neutropenia possibly exacerbated when pegfilgrastim given with CAPECITABINE, FLUOROURACIL or TEGAFUR

Peginterferon Alfa *see* Interferons

Pembrolizumab

● Antipsychotics: avoid concomitant use of cytotoxics with ● CLOZAPINE (increased risk of agranulocytosis)
● Vaccines: risk of generalised infections when monoclonal antibodies given with live ● VACCINES—avoid concomitant use

Pemetrexed

▹ Analgesics: renal excretion of pemetrexed possibly reduced by NSAIDs and ASPIRIN—consult product literature
● Antimalarials: antifolate effect of pemetrexed increased by ● PYRIMETHAMINE
● Antipsychotics: avoid concomitant use of cytotoxics with ● CLOZAPINE (increased risk of agranulocytosis)

Penicillamine

▹ Analgesics: possible increased risk of nephrotoxicity when penicillamine given with NSAIDs
▹ Antacids: absorption of penicillamine reduced by ANTACIDS
▹ Antimalarials: increased risk of haematological toxicity when penicillamine given with ANTIMALARIALS—manufacturer of penicillamine advises avoid concomitant use
● Antipsychotics: increased risk of haematological toxicity when penicillamine given with ● CLOZAPINE—manufacturer of penicillamine advises avoid concomitant use
▹ Cardiac Glycosides: penicillamine possibly reduces plasma concentration of DIGOXIN
▹ Iron Salts: absorption of penicillamine reduced by *oral* IRON SALTS
● Sodium Aurothiomalate: increased risk of haematological toxicity when penicillamine given with ● SODIUM AUROTHIOMALATE—see under Penicillamine, in BNF)
▹ Zinc: penicillamine reduces absorption of ZINC, also absorption of penicillamine reduced by zinc

Penicillins

▹ Allopurinol: increased risk of rash when amoxicillin, ampicillin or co-amoxiclav given with ALLOPURINOL
▹ Antibacterials: absorption of phenoxymethylpenicillin reduced by NEOMYCIN; effects of penicillins possibly antagonised by TETRACYCLINES
▹ Anticoagulants: an interaction between broad-spectrum penicillins and COUMARINS and PHENINDIONE has not been demonstrated in studies, but common experience in anticoagulant clinics is that INR can be altered
● Antiepileptics: manufacturer of pivmecillinam advises avoid concomitant use with ● SODIUM VALPROATE and ● VALPROIC ACID
▹ Cytotoxics: penicillins reduce excretion of METHOTREXATE (increased risk of toxicity)
▹ Muscle Relaxants: piperacillin enhances effects of NON-DEPOLARISING MUSCLE RELAXANTS and SUXAMETHONIUM
▹ Mycophenolate: co-amoxiclav possibly reduces plasma concentration of MYCOPHENOLATE
▹ Sulfinpyrazone: excretion of penicillins reduced by SULFINPYRAZONE
▹ Vaccines: antibacterials inactivate ORAL TYPHOID VACCINE—see under Typhoid Vaccine in BNFC

Pentamidine Isetionate

● Anti-arrhythmics: increased risk of ventricular arrhythmias when pentamidine isetionate given with ● AMIODARONE—avoid concomitant use; possible increased risk of ventricular arrhythmias when pentamidine isetionate given with ● DISOPYRAMIDE
● Antibacterials: increased risk of ventricular arrhythmias when pentamidine isetionate given with *parenteral* ● ERYTHROMYCIN; increased risk of ventricular arrhythmias when pentamidine isetionate given with ● MOXIFLOXACIN—avoid concomitant use; increased risk of ventricular arrhythmias when pentamidine isetionate given with ● DELAMANID; possible increased risk of ventricular arrhythmias when *parenteral* pentamidine isetionate given with ● TELITHROMYCIN
● Antidepressants: avoidance of pentamidine isetionate advised by manufacturer of ● CITALOPRAM and ● ESCITALOPRAM (risk of ventricular arrhythmias); increased risk of ventricular arrhythmias when pentamidine isetionate given with ● TRICYCLICS
▹ Antifungals: possible increased risk of nephrotoxicity when pentamidine isetionate given with AMPHOTERICIN
● Antimalarials: avoidance of pentamidine isetionate advised by manufacturer of ● ARTENIMOL WITH PIPERAQUINE (possible risk of ventricular arrhythmias)
● Antipsychotics: increased risk of ventricular arrhythmias when pentamidine isetionate given with ● AMISULPRIDE or ● DROPERIDOL—avoid concomitant use; increased risk of ventricular arrhythmias when pentamidine isetionate given with ● PHENOTHIAZINES
● Antivirals: increased risk of hypocalcaemia when *parenteral* pentamidine isetionate given with ● FOSCARNET; increased risk of ventricular arrhythmias when pentamidine isetionate given with ● SAQUINAVIR—avoid concomitant use

Pentamidine Isetionate (continued)

- Cytotoxics: possible increased risk of ventricular arrhythmias when pentamidine isetionate given with ● VANDETANIB—avoid concomitant use
- Ivabradine: increased risk of ventricular arrhythmias when pentamidine isetionate given with ● IVABRADINE

Pentazocine *see* Opioid Analgesics

Pentostatin

- Antipsychotics: avoid concomitant use of cytotoxics with ● CLOZAPINE (increased risk of agranulocytosis)
- Cytotoxics: increased toxicity when pentostatin given with high-dose ● CYCLOPHOSPHAMIDE—avoid concomitant use; increased pulmonary toxicity when pentostatin given with ● FLUDARABINE (unacceptably high incidence of fatalities)

Pentoxifylline

- ▹ Aminophylline: pentoxifylline increases plasma concentration of AMINOPHYLLINE
- Analgesics: possible increased risk of bleeding when pentoxifylline given with NSAIDs; increased risk of bleeding when pentoxifylline given with ● KETOROLAC (avoid concomitant use)
- ▹ Theophylline: pentoxifylline increases plasma concentration of THEOPHYLLINE

Perampanel

- Antidepressants: anticonvulsant effect of antiepileptics possibly antagonised by MAOIs and ● TRICYCLIC-RELATED ANTIDEPRESSANTS (convulsive threshold lowered); anticonvulsant effect of antiepileptics antagonised by ● SSRIs and ● TRICYCLICS (convulsive threshold lowered)
- Antiepileptics: plasma concentration of perampanel reduced by ● CARBAMAZEPINE, ● FOSPHENYTOIN and ● PHENYTOIN (see under Perampanel, p. 193); plasma concentration of perampanel reduced by ● OXCARBAZEPINE, also plasma concentration of oxcarbazepine increased (see under Perampanel, p. 193); plasma concentration of perampanel reduced by TOPIRAMATE
- ▹ Antifungals: plasma concentration of perampanel increased by KETOCONAZOLE
- Antimalarials: anticonvulsant effect of antiepileptics antagonised by ● MEFLOQUINE
- Antipsychotics: anticonvulsant effect of antiepileptics antagonised by ● ANTIPSYCHOTICS (convulsive threshold lowered)
- ▹ Anxiolytics and Hypnotics: perampanel reduces plasma concentration of MIDAZOLAM
- Orlistat: possible increased risk of convulsions when antiepileptics given with ● ORLISTAT
- Progestogens: perampanel accelerates metabolism of ● PROGESTOGENS (reduced contraceptive effect with combined oral contraceptives, progestogen-only oral contraceptives, contraceptive patches, vaginal rings, etonogestrel-releasing implant, and emergency hormonal contraception—see Contraceptive Interactions in BNFC)

Pergolide

- ▹ Antipsychotics: effects of pergolide antagonised by ANTIPSYCHOTICS
- Memantine: effects of dopaminergics possibly enhanced by MEMANTINE
- ▹ Methyldopa: antiparkinsonian effect of dopaminergics antagonised by METHYLDOPA
- ▹ Metoclopramide: antiparkinsonian effect of pergolide antagonised by METOCLOPRAMIDE

Pericyazine *see* Antipsychotics

Perindopril *See* ACE Inhibitors

Perphenazine *see* Antipsychotics

Pertuzumab

- Antipsychotics: avoid concomitant use of cytotoxics with ● CLOZAPINE (increased risk of agranulocytosis)
- Vaccines: risk of generalised infections when monoclonal antibodies given with live ● VACCINES—avoid concomitant use

Pethidine *see* Opioid Analgesics

Phenelzine *see* MAOIs

Phenindione

NOTE Change in patient's clinical condition particularly associated with liver disease, intercurrent illness, or drug administration, necessitates more frequent testing. Major changes in diet (especially involving salads and vegetables)

Phenindione (continued)

and in alcohol consumption may also affect anticoagulant control

- Alcohol: anticoagulant control with phenindione may be affected by major changes in consumption of ● ALCOHOL
- Anabolic Steroids: anticoagulant effect of phenindione enhanced by ● ANABOLIC STEROIDS
- Analgesics: anticoagulant effect of phenindione possibly enhanced by ● NSAIDs; increased risk of haemorrhage when anticoagulants given with *intravenous* ● DICLOFENAC (avoid concomitant use, including low-dose heparins); increased risk of haemorrhage when anticoagulants given with ● KETOROLAC (avoid concomitant use, including low-dose heparins); increased risk of bleeding when phenindione given with ● ASPIRIN (due to antiplatelet effect)
- Anti-arrhythmics: metabolism of phenindione inhibited by ● AMIODARONE (enhanced anticoagulant effect); anticoagulant effect of phenindione possibly enhanced by ● DRONEDARONE
- Antibacterials: experience in anticoagulant clinics suggests that INR possibly altered when phenindione is given with ● NEOMYCIN (given for local action on gut); anticoagulant effect of phenindione possibly enhanced by LEVOFLOXACIN and ● TETRACYCLINES; an interaction between phenindione and broad-spectrum PENICILLINS has not been demonstrated in studies, but common experience in anticoagulant clinics is that INR can be altered; metabolism of phenindione possibly inhibited by SULFONAMIDES
- Anticoagulants: increased risk of haemorrhage when other anticoagulants given with ● APIXABAN, ● DABIGATRAN, ● EDOXABAN and ● RIVAROXABAN (avoid concomitant use except when switching with other anticoagulants or using heparin to maintain catheter patency)
- Antivirals: anticoagulant effect of phenindione possibly enhanced by ● RITONAVIR
- Clopidogrel: anticoagulant effect of phenindione enhanced due to antiplatelet action of ● CLOPIDOGREL
- ▹ Corticosteroids: anticoagulant effect of phenindione may be enhanced or reduced by CORTICOSTEROIDS
- ▹ Cytotoxics: avoidance of phenindione advised by manufacturer of IBRUTINIB
- Dipyridamole: anticoagulant effect of phenindione enhanced due to antiplatelet action of ● DIPYRIDAMOLE
- Enteral Feeds: anticoagulant effect of phenindione antagonised by vitamin K (present in some ● ENTERAL FEEDS)
- ▹ Iloprost: increased risk of bleeding when phenindione given with ILOPROST
- Lipid-regulating Drugs: anticoagulant effect of phenindione may be enhanced or reduced by ● COLESTYRAMINE; anticoagulant effect of phenindione possibly enhanced by ● ROSUVASTATIN; anticoagulant effect of phenindione enhanced by ● FIBRATES
- Oestrogens: anticoagulant effect of phenindione antagonised by ● OESTROGENS
- ▹ Prasugrel: possible increased risk of bleeding when phenindione given with PRASUGREL
- Progestogens: anticoagulant effect of phenindione antagonised by ● PROGESTOGENS
- Testolactone: anticoagulant effect of phenindione enhanced by ● TESTOLACTONE
- Testosterone: anticoagulant effect of phenindione enhanced by ● TESTOSTERONE
- Thyroid Hormones: anticoagulant effect of phenindione enhanced by ● THYROID HORMONES
- Vitamins: anticoagulant effect of phenindione antagonised by ● VITAMIN K

Phenobarbital

- ▹ Alcohol: increased sedative effect when phenobarbital given with ALCOHOL
- Aminophylline: phenobarbital accelerates metabolism of ● AMINOPHYLLINE (reduced effect)
- ▹ Analgesics: phenobarbital reduces plasma concentration of METHADONE; phenobarbital possibly accelerates metabolism of PARACETAMOL (also isolated reports of hepatotoxicity)
- Anthelmintics: phenobarbital reduces plasma concentration of ● ALBENDAZOLE and ● PRAZIQUANTEL—consider increasing

Phenobarbital

- Anthelmintics (continued)
albendazole and praziquantel dose when given for systemic infections
- Anti-arrhythmics: phenobarbital accelerates metabolism of DISOPYRAMIDE (reduced plasma concentration); phenobarbital possibly reduces plasma concentration of ● DRONEDARONE—avoid concomitant use; phenobarbital possibly accelerates metabolism of PROPAFENONE
- Antibacterials: phenobarbital accelerates metabolism of METRONIDAZOLE (reduced effect); phenobarbital possibly reduces plasma concentration of RIFAMPICIN; phenobarbital accelerates metabolism of DOXYCYCLINE (reduced plasma concentration); phenobarbital possibly accelerates metabolism of ● CHLORAMPHENICOL (reduced plasma concentration); phenobarbital reduces plasma concentration of ● TELITHROMYCIN (avoid during and for 2 weeks after phenobarbital)
- Anticoagulants: phenobarbital possibly reduces plasma concentration of ● APIXABAN and ● EDOXABAN; phenobarbital accelerates metabolism of ● COUMARINS (reduced anticoagulant effect); phenobarbital possibly reduces plasma concentration of ● RIVAROXABAN—manufacturer of rivaroxaban advises monitor for signs of thrombosis
- Antidepressants: phenobarbital possibly reduces plasma concentration of REBOXETINE; phenobarbital reduces plasma concentration of PAROXETINE; phenobarbital accelerates metabolism of ● MIANSERIN (reduced plasma concentration); anticonvulsant effect of antiepileptics possibly antagonised by MAOIs and ● TRICYCLIC-RELATED ANTIDEPRESSANTS (convulsive threshold lowered); anticonvulsant effect of antiepileptics antagonised by ● SSRIS and ● TRICYCLICS (convulsive threshold lowered); plasma concentration of phenobarbital possibly reduced by ● ST JOHN'S WORT—avoid concomitant use; phenobarbital possibly accelerates metabolism of TRICYCLICS (reduced plasma concentration)
- Antiepileptics: plasma concentration of phenobarbital possibly increased by CARBAMAZEPINE; phenobarbital possibly reduces plasma concentration of ETHOSUXIMIDE, RUFINAMIDE and TOPIRAMATE; plasma concentration of phenobarbital often increased by FOSPHENYTOIN and PHENYTOIN, plasma concentration of fosphenytoin and phenytoin often reduced but may be increased; phenobarbital reduces plasma concentration of LAMOTRIGINE, TIAGABINE and ZONISAMIDE; plasma concentration of phenobarbital increased by OXCARBAZEPINE, also plasma concentration of an active metabolite of oxcarbazepine reduced; plasma concentration of phenobarbital increased by SODIUM VALPROATE and VALPROIC ACID (also plasma concentration of sodium valproate and valproic acid reduced); plasma concentration of phenobarbital increased by STIRIPENTOL
- Antifungals: phenobarbital possibly reduces plasma concentration of ITRACONAZOLE and ● POSACONAZOLE; phenobarbital possibly reduces plasma concentration of ● VORICONAZOLE—avoid concomitant use; phenobarbital reduces absorption of GRISEOFULVIN (reduced effect)
- Antimalarials: avoidance of phenobarbital advised by manufacturer of ARTENIMOL WITH PIPERAQUINE; anticonvulsant effect of antiepileptics antagonised by ● MEFLOQUINE
- Antimuscarinics: phenobarbital possibly reduces plasma concentration of active metabolite of ● FESOTERODINE—manufacturer of fesoterodine advises avoid concomitant use
- Antipsychotics: anticonvulsant effect of antiepileptics antagonised by ● ANTIPSYCHOTICS (convulsive threshold lowered); phenobarbital accelerates metabolism of HALOPERIDOL (reduced plasma concentration); plasma concentration of both drugs reduced when phenobarbital given with CHLORPROMAZINE; phenobarbital possibly reduces plasma concentration of ● ARIPIPRAZOLE (avoid concomitant use or consider increasing the dose of aripiprazole—consult aripiprazole product literature); phenobarbital possibly reduces plasma concentration of CLOZAPINE; phenobarbital possibly reduces plasma concentration of ● LURASIDONE—avoid concomitant use
- Antivirals: phenobarbital possibly reduces plasma concentration of ABACAVIR, DARUNAVIR, FOSAMPRENAVIR,

Phenobarbital

- Antivirals (continued)
● INDINAVIR, ● LOPINAVIR and ● SAQUINAVIR; avoidance of phenobarbital advised by manufacturer of ● BOCEPREVIR and ● RILPIVIRINE (plasma concentration of boceprevir and rilpivirine possibly reduced); phenobarbital possibly reduces plasma concentration of ● DACLATASVIR and ● SIMEPREVIR—manufacturer of daclatasvir and simeprevir advises avoid concomitant use; phenobarbital possibly reduces plasma concentration of ● DASABUVIR, ● OMBITASVIR and ● PARITAPREVIR—avoid concomitant use; phenobarbital possibly reduces the plasma concentration of ● DOLUTEGRAVIR (see under Dolutegravir, p. 387); avoidance of phenobarbital advised by manufacturer of ● ELVITEGRAVIR, ETRAVIRINE, LEDIPASVIR, SOFOSBUVIR and ● TELAPREVIR
- Anxiolytics and Hypnotics: increased sedative effect when phenobarbital given with ANXIOLYTICS AND HYPNOTICS; phenobarbital often reduces plasma concentration of CLONAZEPAM
- Apremilast: phenobarbital possibly reduces plasma concentration of ● APREMILAST—avoid concomitant use
- Aprepitant: phenobarbital possibly reduces plasma concentration of APREPITANT
- Avanafil: phenobarbital possibly reduces plasma concentration of AVANAFIL—manufacturer of avanafil advises avoid concomitant use
- Beta-blockers: phenobarbital possibly reduces plasma concentration of PROPRANOLOL
- Bile Acids: avoidance of phenobarbital advised by manufacturer of ● CHOLIC ACID
- Caffeine citrate: effects of phenobarbital possibly antagonised by CAFFEINE CITRATE
- Calcium-channel Blockers: phenobarbital probably reduces effects of ● CALCIUM-CHANNEL BLOCKERS; avoidance of phenobarbital advised by manufacturer of ● ISRADIPINE; avoidance of phenobarbital advised by manufacturer of ● NIMODIPINE (plasma concentration of nimodipine reduced)
- Cannabis Extract: phenobarbital possibly reduces plasma concentration of ● CANNABIS EXTRACT—manufacturer of cannabis extract advises avoid concomitant use
- Ciclosporin: phenobarbital accelerates metabolism of ● CICLOSPORIN (reduced plasma concentration)
- Cobicistat: phenobarbital possibly reduces plasma concentration of ● COBICISTAT—manufacturer of cobicistat advises avoid concomitant use
- Corticosteroids: phenobarbital accelerates metabolism of ● CORTICOSTEROIDS (reduced effect)
- Cytotoxics: phenobarbital possibly decreases plasma concentration of AXITINIB (increase dose of axitinib—consult axitinib product literature); phenobarbital possibly reduces plasma concentration of BORTEZOMIB, ● BOSUTINIB, CRIZOTINIB and PONATINIB—manufacturer of bortezomib, bosutinib, crizotinib and ponatinib advises avoid concomitant use; phenobarbital possibly reduces plasma concentration of ● CABOZANTINIB—avoid concomitant use; avoidance of phenobarbital advised by manufacturer of ● CABAZITAXEL, DABRAFENIB, GEFITINIB and ● OLAPARIB; avoidance of phenobarbital advised by manufacturer of DASATINIB and VANDETANIB (plasma concentration of dasatinib and vandetanib possibly reduced); phenobarbital possibly reduces plasma concentration of ETOPOSIDE; phenobarbital reduces plasma concentration of IRINOTECAN and its active metabolite; manufacturer of procarbazine advises possible increased risk of hypersensitivity reactions when phenobarbital given with PROCARBAZINE
- Diuretics: phenobarbital reduces plasma concentration of ● EPLERENONE—avoid concomitant use; increased risk of osteomalacia when phenobarbital given with CARBONIC ANHYDRASE INHIBITORS
- Folates: plasma concentration of phenobarbital possibly reduced by FOLATES
- Fosaprepitant: phenobarbital possibly reduces plasma concentration of FOSAPREPITANT
- Guanfacine: phenobarbital possibly reduces plasma concentration of ● GUANFACINE—increase dose of guanfacine

Phenobarbital (continued)
- Hormone Antagonists: phenobarbital possibly reduces plasma concentration of ● ABIRATERONE—manufacturer of abiraterone advises avoid concomitant use; phenobarbital accelerates metabolism of TOREMIFENE (reduced plasma concentration)
- Ivacaftor: phenobarbital possibly reduces plasma concentration of ● IVACAFTOR—manufacturer of ivacaftor advises avoid concomitant use
▸ Leukotriene Receptor Antagonists: phenobarbital reduces plasma concentration of MONTELUKAST
- Oestrogens: phenobarbital accelerates metabolism of ● OESTROGENS (reduced contraceptive effect with combined oral contraceptives, contraceptive patches, and vaginal rings—see Contraceptive Interactions in BNFC)
- Orlistat: possible increased risk of convulsions when antiepileptics given with ● ORLISTAT
- Progestogens: phenobarbital accelerates metabolism of ● PROGESTOGENS (reduced contraceptive effect with combined oral contraceptives, progestogen-only oral contraceptives, contraceptive patches, vaginal rings, etonogestrel-releasing implant, and emergency hormonal contraception—see Contraceptive Interactions in BNFC)
▸ Roflumilast: phenobarbital possibly inhibits effects of ROFLUMILAST (manufacturer of roflumilast advises avoid concomitant use)
▸ Sodium Oxybate: avoidance of phenobarbital advised by manufacturer of SODIUM OXYBATE
▸ Sympathomimetics: plasma concentration of phenobarbital possibly increased by METHYLPHENIDATE
- Tacrolimus: phenobarbital reduces plasma concentration of ● TACROLIMUS
- Theophylline: phenobarbital accelerates metabolism of ● THEOPHYLLINE (reduced effect)
▸ Thyroid Hormones: phenobarbital accelerates metabolism of THYROID HORMONES (may increase requirements for thyroid hormones in hypothyroidism)
▸ Ticagrelor: phenobarbital possibly reduces plasma concentration of TICAGRELOR
- Ulipristal: avoidance of phenobarbital advised by manufacturer of ● ULIPRISTAL (contraceptive effect of ulipristal possibly reduced)
- Vitamins: phenobarbital possibly increases requirements for ALFACALCIDOL, CALCITRIOL, COLECALCIFEROL, DIHYDROTACHYSTEROL, ERGOCALCIFEROL, PARICALCITOL or VITAMIN D

Phenothiazines see Antipsychotics
Phenoxybenzamine see Alpha-blockers
Phenoxymethylpenicillin see Penicillins
Phentolamine see Alpha-blockers
Phenylephrine see Sympathomimetics
Phenytoin
▸ Alcohol: plasma concentration of phenytoin possibly reduced by chronic heavy consumption of ALCOHOL
- Aminophylline: plasma concentration of both drugs reduced when phenytoin given with ● AMINOPHYLLINE
- Analgesics: excretion of phenytoin possibly reduced by ACEMETACIN (increased risk of toxicity); phenytoin possibly accelerates metabolism of FENTANYL (reduced effect); phenytoin accelerates metabolism of METHADONE (reduced effect and risk of withdrawal effects); phenytoin possibly increases risk of ● PETHIDINE toxicity; effects of phenytoin enhanced by ASPIRIN; phenytoin possibly accelerates metabolism of PARACETAMOL (also isolated reports of hepatotoxicity)
▸ Antacids: absorption of phenytoin reduced by ANTACIDS
- Anthelmintics: phenytoin reduces plasma concentration of ● ALBENDAZOLE and ● PRAZIQUANTEL—consider increasing albendazole and praziquantel dose when given for systemic infections; plasma concentration of phenytoin possibly increased by LEVAMISOLE
- Anti-arrhythmics: metabolism of phenytoin inhibited by ● AMIODARONE (increased plasma concentration); phenytoin reduces plasma concentration of DISOPYRAMIDE; phenytoin possibly reduces plasma concentration of ● DRONEDARONE—avoid concomitant use

Phenytoin (continued)
- Antibacterials: metabolism of phenytoin inhibited by CLARITHROMYCIN (increased plasma concentration); metabolism of phenytoin possibly inhibited by METRONIDAZOLE (increased plasma concentration); plasma concentration of phenytoin increased or decreased by CIPROFLOXACIN; phenytoin accelerates metabolism of DOXYCYCLINE (reduced plasma concentration); phenytoin possibly reduces plasma concentration of ● BEDAQUILINE—manufacturer of bedaquiline advises avoid concomitant use; plasma concentration of phenytoin increased by ● CHLORAMPHENICOL (increased risk of toxicity); metabolism of phenytoin possibly inhibited by ISONIAZID (increased risk of toxicity); metabolism of phenytoin accelerated by ● RIFAMYCINS (reduced plasma concentration); plasma concentration of phenytoin possibly increased by SULFONAMIDES; phenytoin reduces plasma concentration of ● TELITHROMYCIN (avoid during and for 2 weeks after phenytoin); plasma concentration of phenytoin increased by ● TRIMETHOPRIM (also increased antifolate effect)
- Anticoagulants: phenytoin possibly reduces plasma concentration of ● APIXABAN and ● EDOXABAN; phenytoin accelerates metabolism of ● COUMARINS (possibility of reduced anticoagulant effect, but enhancement also reported); phenytoin possibly reduces plasma concentration of DABIGATRAN—manufacturer of dabigatran advises avoid concomitant use; phenytoin possibly reduces plasma concentration of ● RIVAROXABAN—manufacturer of rivaroxaban advises monitor for signs of thrombosis
- Antidepressants: plasma concentration of phenytoin increased by ● FLUOXETINE and ● FLUVOXAMINE; phenytoin reduces plasma concentration of ● MIANSERIN, MIRTAZAPINE and PAROXETINE; plasma concentration of phenytoin possibly increased by SERTRALINE, also plasma concentration of sertraline possibly reduced; anticonvulsant effect of antiepileptics possibly antagonised by MAOIs and ● TRICYCLIC-RELATED ANTIDEPRESSANTS (convulsive threshold lowered); phenytoin reduces plasma concentration of ● PERAMPANEL; anticonvulsant effect of antiepileptics antagonised by ● SSRIS and ● TRICYCLICS (convulsive threshold lowered); plasma concentration of phenytoin possibly reduced by ● ST JOHN'S WORT—avoid concomitant use; phenytoin possibly reduces plasma concentration of ● TRICYCLICS; phenytoin possibly reduces plasma concentration of ● VORTIOXETINE—consider increasing dose of vortioxetine
▸ Antidiabetics: plasma concentration of phenytoin transiently increased by TOLBUTAMIDE (possibility of toxicity)
- Antiepileptics: plasma concentration of both drugs often reduced when phenytoin given with CARBAMAZEPINE, also plasma concentration of phenytoin may be increased; phenytoin reduces plasma concentration of ESLICARBAZEPINE, also plasma concentration of phenytoin increased; plasma concentration of phenytoin possibly increased by ● ETHOSUXIMIDE, also plasma concentration of ethosuximide possibly reduced; phenytoin reduces plasma concentration of LAMOTRIGINE, TIAGABINE and ZONISAMIDE; plasma concentration of phenytoin increased by OXCARBAZEPINE, also plasma concentration of an active metabolite of oxcarbazepine reduced; phenytoin reduces plasma concentration of ● PERAMPANEL (see under Perampanel, p. 193); phenytoin often increases plasma concentration of PHENOBARBITAL and PRIMIDONE, plasma concentration of phenytoin often reduced but may be increased; phenytoin possibly reduces plasma concentration of RETIGABINE; phenytoin possibly reduces plasma concentration of RUFINAMIDE, also plasma concentration of phenytoin possibly increased; plasma concentration of phenytoin increased or possibly reduced when given with SODIUM VALPROATE and VALPROIC ACID, also plasma concentration of sodium valproate and valproic acid reduced; plasma concentration of phenytoin increased by ● STIRIPENTOL; plasma concentration of phenytoin increased by ● TOPIRAMATE (also plasma concentration of topiramate reduced); plasma concentration of phenytoin reduced by VIGABATRIN
- Antifungals: phenytoin reduces plasma concentration of ● KETOCONAZOLE and ● POSACONAZOLE; anticonvulsant effect of phenytoin enhanced by ● MICONAZOLE (plasma concentration

Phenytoin
- **Antifungals** (continued)
 of phenytoin increased); plasma concentration of phenytoin
 increased by ● FLUCONAZOLE (consider reducing dose of
 phenytoin); phenytoin reduces plasma concentration of
 ● ITRACONAZOLE—avoid concomitant use; plasma
 concentration of phenytoin increased by ● VORICONAZOLE, also
 phenytoin reduces plasma concentration of voriconazole
 (increase dose of voriconazole and also monitor for phenytoin
 toxicity); phenytoin possibly reduces plasma concentration of
 CASPOFUNGIN—consider increasing dose of caspofungin
- **Antimalarials**: avoidance of phenytoin advised by manufacturer
 of ARTENIMOL WITH PIPERAQUINE; anticonvulsant effect of
 antiepileptics antagonised by ● MEFLOQUINE; anticonvulsant
 effect of phenytoin antagonised by ● PYRIMETHAMINE, also
 increased antifolate effect
- **Antimuscarinics**: phenytoin possibly reduces plasma
 concentration of active metabolite of ● FESOTERODINE—
 manufacturer of fesoterodine advises avoid concomitant use
- **Antipsychotics**: anticonvulsant effect of antiepileptics
 antagonised by ● ANTIPSYCHOTICS (convulsive threshold
 lowered); phenytoin reduces plasma concentration of
 HALOPERIDOL; plasma concentration of phenytoin possibly
 increased or decreased by CHLORPROMAZINE; phenytoin
 possibly reduces plasma concentration of ● ARIPIPRAZOLE
 (avoid concomitant use or consider increasing the dose of
 aripiprazole—consult aripiprazole product literature);
 phenytoin accelerates metabolism of CLOZAPINE and
 QUETIAPINE (reduced plasma concentration); phenytoin
 possibly reduces plasma concentration of ● LURASIDONE—
 avoid concomitant use
- **Antivirals**: phenytoin possibly reduces plasma concentration of
 ABACAVIR, DARUNAVIR, LOPINAVIR and SAQUINAVIR; avoidance of
 phenytoin advised by manufacturer of ● BOCEPREVIR and
 ● RILPIVIRINE (plasma concentration of boceprevir and
 rilpivirine possibly reduced); phenytoin possibly reduces
 plasma concentration of ● DACLATASVIR and ● SIMEPREVIR—
 manufacturer of daclatasvir and simeprevir advises avoid
 concomitant use; phenytoin possibly reduces plasma
 concentration of ● DASABUVIR, ● OMBITASVIR and
 ● PARITAPREVIR—avoid concomitant use; phenytoin possibly
 reduces the plasma concentration of ● DOLUTEGRAVIR (see
 under Dolutegravir, p. 387); avoidance of phenytoin advised
 by manufacturer of ● ELVITEGRAVIR, ETRAVIRINE, LEDIPASVIR,
 SOFOSBUVIR and ● TELAPREVIR; phenytoin possibly reduces
 plasma concentration of ● INDINAVIR, also plasma
 concentration of phenytoin possibly increased; phenytoin
 possibly reduces plasma concentration of RITONAVIR, also
 plasma concentration of phenytoin possibly affected; plasma
 concentration of phenytoin increased or decreased by
 ZIDOVUDINE
- ▸ **Anxiolytics and Hypnotics**: phenytoin often reduces plasma
 concentration of CLONAZEPAM; plasma concentration of
 phenytoin increased or decreased by DIAZEPAM; plasma
 concentration of phenytoin possibly increased or decreased
 by BENZODIAZEPINES
- **Apremilast**: phenytoin possibly reduces plasma concentration
 of ● APREMILAST—avoid concomitant use
- ▸ **Aprepitant**: phenytoin possibly reduces plasma concentration
 of APREPITANT
- ▸ **Bupropion**: phenytoin reduces plasma concentration of
 BUPROPION
- ▸ **Caffeine citrate**: phenytoin reduces plasma concentration of
 CAFFEINE CITRATE
- ▸ **Calcium-channel Blockers**: phenytoin reduces effects of
 FELODIPINE and VERAPAMIL; avoidance of phenytoin advised by
 manufacturer of ISRADIPINE; avoidance of phenytoin advised
 by manufacturer of NIMODIPINE (plasma concentration of
 nimodipine possibly reduced); plasma concentration of
 phenytoin increased by ● DILTIAZEM but also effect of diltiazem
 reduced
- **Cannabis Extract**: phenytoin possibly reduces plasma
 concentration of ● CANNABIS EXTRACT—manufacturer of
 cannabis extract advises avoid concomitant use
- ▸ **Cardiac Glycosides**: phenytoin possibly reduces plasma
 concentration of DIGOXIN

Phenytoin (continued)
- **Ciclosporin**: phenytoin accelerates metabolism of ● CICLOSPORIN
 (reduced plasma concentration)
- **Cobicistat**: phenytoin possibly reduces plasma concentration of
 ● COBICISTAT—manufacturer of cobicistat advises avoid
 concomitant use
- **Corticosteroids**: phenytoin accelerates metabolism of
 ● CORTICOSTEROIDS (reduced effect)
- **Cytotoxics**: phenytoin possibly reduces plasma concentration
 of BUSULFAN, ERIBULIN and ETOPOSIDE; metabolism of
 phenytoin possibly inhibited by CAPECITABINE, FLUOROURACIL
 and TEGAFUR (increased risk of toxicity); phenytoin increases
 antifolate effect of METHOTREXATE; plasma concentration of
 phenytoin possibly reduced by CISPLATIN; phenytoin possibly
 decreases plasma concentration of AXITINIB (increase dose of
 axitinib—consult axitinib product literature); phenytoin
 possibly reduces plasma concentration of BORTEZOMIB,
 ● BOSUTINIB, CRIZOTINIB, ● IBRUTINIB, ● IDELALISIB and
 PONATINIB—manufacturer of bortezomib, bosutinib,
 crizotinib, ibrutinib, idelalisib and ponatinib advises avoid
 concomitant use; phenytoin possibly reduces plasma
 concentration of ● CABOZANTINIB—avoid concomitant use;
 avoidance of phenytoin advised by manufacturer of
 ● CABAZITAXEL, DABRAFENIB, GEFITINIB, ● LAPATINIB, ● OLAPARIB
 and VEMURAFENIB; avoidance of phenytoin advised by
 manufacturer of DASATINIB and ● VISMODEGIB (plasma
 concentration of dasatinib and vismodegib possibly reduced);
 phenytoin reduces plasma concentration of ● IMATINIB—avoid
 concomitant use; phenytoin reduces plasma concentration of
 IRINOTECAN and its active metabolite; manufacturer of
 procarbazine advises possible increased risk of
 hypersensitivity reactions when phenytoin given with
 PROCARBAZINE
- **Dexrazoxane**: absorption of phenytoin possibly reduced by
 ● DEXRAZOXANE
- ▸ **Diazoxide**: plasma concentration of phenytoin reduced by
 DIAZOXIDE, also effect of diazoxide may be reduced
- **Disulfiram**: metabolism of phenytoin inhibited by ● DISULFIRAM
 (increased risk of toxicity)
- **Diuretics**: plasma concentration of phenytoin possibly
 increased by ACETAZOLAMIDE; phenytoin antagonises effects
 of FUROSEMIDE; phenytoin reduces plasma concentration of
 ● EPLERENONE—avoid concomitant use; increased risk of
 osteomalacia when phenytoin given with CARBONIC
 ANHYDRASE INHIBITORS
- ▸ **Dopaminergics**: phenytoin possibly reduces effects of CO-
 BENELDOPA, CO-CARELDOPA and LEVODOPA
- ▸ **Enteral Feeds**: absorption of phenytoin possibly reduced by
 ENTERAL FEEDS
- ▸ **Folates**: plasma concentration of phenytoin possibly reduced
 by FOLATES
- **Fosaprepitant**: phenytoin possibly reduces plasma
 concentration of FOSAPREPITANT
- **Guanfacine**: phenytoin possibly reduces plasma concentration
 of ● GUANFACINE—increase dose of guanfacine
- **Hormone Antagonists**: phenytoin possibly reduces plasma
 concentration of ● ABIRATERONE—manufacturer of abiraterone
 advises avoid concomitant use; phenytoin possibly
 accelerates metabolism of TOREMIFENE
- **5HT₃-receptor Antagonists**: phenytoin accelerates metabolism of
 ONDANSETRON (reduced effect)
- **Ivacaftor**: phenytoin possibly reduces plasma concentration of
 ● IVACAFTOR—manufacturer of ivacaftor advises avoid
 concomitant use
- ▸ **Leflunomide**: plasma concentration of phenytoin possibly
 increased by LEFLUNOMIDE
- ▸ **Lipid-regulating Drugs**: absorption of phenytoin possibly
 reduced by COLESEVELAM; combination of phenytoin with
 FLUVASTATIN may increase plasma concentration of either drug
 (or both)
- ▸ **Lithium**: neurotoxicity may occur when phenytoin given with
 LITHIUM without increased plasma concentration of lithium
- ▸ **Macitentan**: avoidance of phenytoin advised by manufacturer
 of MACITENTAN
- ▸ **Modafinil**: plasma concentration of phenytoin possibly
 increased by MODAFINIL

Phenytoin (continued)
- Muscle Relaxants: *long-term use* of phenytoin reduces effects of
  - NON-DEPOLARISING MUSCLE RELAXANTS (but *acute use* of phenytoin might increase effects of non-depolarising muscle relaxants)
- Oestrogens: phenytoin accelerates metabolism of
  - OESTROGENS (reduced contraceptive effect with combined oral contraceptives, contraceptive patches, and vaginal rings—see Contraceptive Interactions in BNFC)
- Orlistat: possible increased risk of convulsions when antiepileptics given with ORLISTAT
- Progestogens: phenytoin accelerates metabolism of
  - PROGESTOGENS (reduced contraceptive effect with combined oral contraceptives, progestogen-only oral contraceptives, contraceptive patches, vaginal rings, etonogestrel-releasing implant, and emergency hormonal contraception—see Contraceptive Interactions in BNFC)
- Roflumilast: phenytoin possibly inhibits effects of ROFLUMILAST (manufacturer of roflumilast advises avoid concomitant use)
- Sulfinpyrazone: plasma concentration of phenytoin increased by ● SULFINPYRAZONE
- Sympathomimetics: plasma concentration of phenytoin increased by METHYLPHENIDATE
- Tacrolimus: phenytoin reduces plasma concentration of TACROLIMUS, also plasma concentration of phenytoin possibly increased
- Theophylline: plasma concentration of both drugs reduced when phenytoin given with ● THEOPHYLLINE
- Thyroid Hormones: phenytoin accelerates metabolism of THYROID HORMONES (may increase requirements in hypothyroidism), also plasma concentration of phenytoin possibly increased
- Tibolone: phenytoin accelerates metabolism of TIBOLONE
- Ticagrelor: phenytoin possibly reduces plasma concentration of TICAGRELOR
- Ulcer-healing Drugs: metabolism of phenytoin inhibited by ● CIMETIDINE (increased plasma concentration); effects of phenytoin enhanced by ● ESOMEPRAZOLE; effects of phenytoin possibly enhanced by OMEPRAZOLE; absorption of phenytoin reduced by ● SUCRALFATE
- Ulipristal: avoidance of phenytoin advised by manufacturer of
  - ULIPRISTAL (contraceptive effect of ulipristal possibly reduced)
- Vaccines: effects of phenytoin enhanced by INFLUENZA VACCINE
- Vitamins: phenytoin possibly increases requirements for ALFACALCIDOL, CALCITRIOL, COLECALCIFEROL, DIHYDROTACHYSTEROL, ERGOCALCIFEROL, PARICALCITOL or VITAMIN D

Pholcodine
- Antidepressants: manufacturer of pholcodine advises avoid for 2 weeks after stopping MAOIs

Phosphodiesterase Type-3 Inhibitors
- Anagrelide: avoidance of enoximone and milrinone advised by manufacturer of ● ANAGRELIDE

Pilocarpine see Parasympathomimetics
Pimozide see Antipsychotics
Pindolol see Beta-blockers
Pioglitazone see Antidiabetics
Piperacillin see Penicillins
Piperaquine see Artenimol with Piperaquine
Pirfenidone
- Antibacterials: plasma concentration of pirfenidone increased by ● CIPROFLOXACIN—see under Pirfenidone, in BNF
- Antidepressants: plasma concentration of pirfenidone increased by ● FLUVOXAMINE—manufacturer of pirfenidone advises avoid concomitant use
- Grapefruit Juice: manufacturer of pirfenidone advises avoid concomitant use with GRAPEFRUIT JUICE

Piroxicam see NSAIDs
Pivmecillinam see Penicillins
Pixantrone
- Antipsychotics: avoid concomitant use of cytotoxics with
  - CLOZAPINE (increased risk of agranulocytosis)
- Vaccines: risk of generalised infections when cytotoxic antibiotics given with live ● VACCINES—avoid concomitant use

Pizotifen
- Adrenergic Neurone Blockers: pizotifen antagonises hypotensive effect of ADRENERGIC NEURONE BLOCKERS

Platinum Compounds
- Aldesleukin: avoidance of cisplatin advised by manufacturer of
  - ALDESLEUKIN
- Antibacterials: increased risk of nephrotoxicity and possibly of ototoxicity when platinum compounds given with
  - AMINOGLYCOSIDES or ● POLYMYXINS; increased risk of nephrotoxicity and ototoxicity when platinum compounds given with CAPREOMYCIN; increased risk of nephrotoxicity and possibly of ototoxicity when cisplatin given with VANCOMYCIN
- Antiepileptics: cisplatin possibly reduces plasma concentration of FOSPHENYTOIN and PHENYTOIN
- Antipsychotics: avoid concomitant use of cytotoxics with
  - CLOZAPINE (increased risk of agranulocytosis)
- Cytotoxics: increased risk of otoxicity when cisplatin given with IFOSFAMIDE; increased pulmonary toxicity when cisplatin given with ● BLEOMYCIN and ● METHOTREXATE; avoidance of oxaliplatin advised by manufacturer of ● PANITUMUMAB
- Diuretics: increased risk of nephrotoxicity and ototoxicity when platinum compounds given with DIURETICS

Pneumococcal Vaccine see Vaccines
Poliomyelitis Vaccine see Vaccines
Polymyxins
- Antibacterials: increased risk of nephrotoxicity when colistimethate sodium or polymyxins given with AMINOGLYCOSIDES; increased risk of nephrotoxicity when colistimethate sodium or polymyxins given with CAPREOMYCIN; increased risk of nephrotoxicity when polymyxins given with VANCOMYCIN; increased risk of nephrotoxicity and ototoxicity when colistimethate sodium given with VANCOMYCIN
- Antifungals: increased risk of nephrotoxicity when polymyxins given with AMPHOTERICIN
- Ciclosporin: increased risk of nephrotoxicity when polymyxins given with ● CICLOSPORIN
- Cytotoxics: increased risk of nephrotoxicity and possibly of ototoxicity when polymyxins given with ● PLATINUM COMPOUNDS
- Diuretics: increased risk of otoxicity when polymyxins given with ● LOOP DIURETICS
- Muscle Relaxants: polymyxins enhance effects of ● NON-DEPOLARISING MUSCLE RELAXANTS and ● SUXAMETHONIUM
- Parasympathomimetics: polymyxins antagonise effects of
  - NEOSTIGMINE and ● PYRIDOSTIGMINE
- Vaccines: antibacterials inactivate ORAL TYPHOID VACCINE—see under Typhoid Vaccine in BNFC

Polysaccharide-iron Complex see Iron salts
Polystyrene Sulfonate Resins
- Antacids: risk of intestinal obstruction when polystyrene sulfonate resins given with ALUMINIUM HYDROXIDE; risk of metabolic alkalosis when polystyrene sulfonate resins given with ORAL MAGNESIUM SALTS
- Thyroid Hormones: polystyrene sulfonate resins reduce absorption of LEVOTHYROXINE

Pomalidomide
- Antidepressants: plasma concentration of pomalidomide increased by ● FLUVOXAMINE

Ponatinib
- Antibacterials: plasma concentration of ponatinib possibly increased by CLARITHROMYCIN and TELITHROMYCIN—consider reducing initial dose of ponatinib (see under Ponatinib, in BNF); plasma concentration of ponatinib possibly reduced by RIFABUTIN—manufacturer of ponatinib advises avoid concomitant use; plasma concentration of ponatinib reduced by ● RIFAMPICIN—manufacturer of ponatinib advises avoid concomitant use
- Antidepressants: plasma concentration of ponatinib possibly reduced by ST JOHN'S WORT—manufacturer of ponatinib advises avoid concomitant use
- Antiepileptics: plasma concentration of ponatinib possibly reduced by CARBAMAZEPINE, FOSPHENYTOIN, PHENOBARBITAL, PHENYTOIN and PRIMIDONE—manufacturer of ponatinib advises avoid concomitant use

Ponatinib (continued)
- ▸ Antifungals: plasma concentration of ponatinib increased by KETOCONAZOLE; plasma concentration of ponatinib possibly increased by ITRACONAZOLE and VORICONAZOLE—consider reducing initial dose of ponatinib (see under Ponatinib, in BNF)
- ● Antipsychotics: avoid concomitant use of cytotoxics with ● CLOZAPINE (increased risk of agranulocytosis)
- ▸ Antivirals: plasma concentration of ponatinib possibly increased by INDINAVIR, RITONAVIR and SAQUINAVIR—consider reducing initial dose of ponatinib (see under Ponatinib, in BNF)
- ▸ Grapefruit Juice: plasma concentration of ponatinib possibly increased by GRAPEFRUIT JUICE

Posaconazole see Antifungals, Triazole

Potassium Canrenoate see Diuretics

Potassium Aminobenzoate
- ▸ Antibacterials: potassium aminobenzoate inhibits effects of SULFONAMIDES

Potassium Bicarbonate see Potassium Salts

Potassium Chloride see Potassium Salts

Potassium Citrate see Potassium Salts

Potassium Salts
NOTE Includes salt substitutes
- ● ACE Inhibitors: increased risk of severe hyperkalaemia when potassium salts given with ● ACE INHIBITORS
- ● Aliskiren: increased risk of hyperkalaemia when potassium salts given with ALISKIREN
- ● Angiotensin-II Receptor Antagonists: increased risk of hyperkalaemia when potassium salts given with ● ANGIOTENSIN-II RECEPTOR ANTAGONISTS
- ▸ Antibacterials: avoid concomitant use of potassium citrate with METHENAMINE
- ● Ciclosporin: increased risk of hyperkalaemia when potassium salts given with ● CICLOSPORIN
- ● Diuretics: increased risk of hyperkalaemia when potassium salts given with ● POTASSIUM-SPARING DIURETICS AND ALDOSTERONE ANTAGONISTS
- ● Tacrolimus: increased risk of hyperkalaemia when potassium salts given with ● TACROLIMUS
- ▸ Ulcer-healing Drugs: avoidance of potassium citrate advised by manufacturer of SUCRALFATE

Pramipexole
- ▸ Antipsychotics: manufacturer of pramipexole advises avoid concomitant use of ANTIPSYCHOTICS (antagonism of effect)
- ▸ Memantine: effects of dopaminergics possibly enhanced by MEMANTINE
- ▸ Methyldopa: antiparkinsonian effect of dopaminergics antagonised by METHYLDOPA
- ▸ Ulcer-healing Drugs: excretion of pramipexole reduced by CIMETIDINE (increased plasma concentration)

Prasugrel
- ▸ Analgesics: possible increased risk of bleeding when prasugrel given with NSAIDs
- ▸ Anticoagulants: possible increased risk of bleeding when prasugrel given with COUMARINS or PHENINDIONE
- ▸ Clopidogrel: possible increased risk of bleeding when prasugrel given with CLOPIDOGREL

Pravastatin see Statins

Praziquantel
- ● Antibacterials: plasma concentration of praziquantel reduced by ● RIFAMPICIN—avoid concomitant use
- ● Antiepileptics: plasma concentration of praziquantel reduced by ● CARBAMAZEPINE, ● FOSPHENYTOIN, ● PHENOBARBITAL, ● PHENYTOIN and ● PRIMIDONE—consider increasing praziquantel dose when given for systemic infections
- ▸ Antifungals: plasma concentration of praziquantel increased by KETOCONAZOLE
- ● Antimalarials: plasma concentration of praziquantel reduced by ● CHLOROQUINE—consider increasing praziquantel dose when given for systemic infections
- ▸ Corticosteroids: plasma concentration of praziquantel possibly reduced by continuous use of DEXAMETHASONE
- ▸ Grapefruit Juice: plasma concentration of praziquantel increased by GRAPEFRUIT JUICE

Praziquantel (continued)
- ▸ Ulcer-healing Drugs: plasma concentration of praziquantel increased by CIMETIDINE

Prazosin see Alpha-blockers

Prednisolone see Corticosteroids

Prednisone see Corticosteroids

Pregabalin
- ● Antidepressants: anticonvulsant effect of antiepileptics possibly antagonised by MAOIs and ● TRICYCLIC-RELATED ANTIDEPRESSANTS (convulsive threshold lowered); anticonvulsant effect of antiepileptics antagonised by ● SSRIs and ● TRICYCLICS (convulsive threshold lowered)
- ● Antimalarials: anticonvulsant effect of antiepileptics antagonised by ● MEFLOQUINE
- ● Antipsychotics: anticonvulsant effect of antiepileptics antagonised by ● ANTIPSYCHOTICS (convulsive threshold lowered)
- ● Orlistat: possible increased risk of convulsions when antiepileptics given with ● ORLISTAT

Prilocaine
- ▸ Anti-arrhythmics: increased myocardial depression when prilocaine given with ANTI-ARRHYTHMICS
- ▸ Antibacterials: increased risk of methaemoglobinaemia when prilocaine given with SULFONAMIDES

Primaquine
- ● Antimalarials: avoidance of antimalarials advised by manufacturer of ● ARTEMETHER WITH LUMEFANTRINE
- ▸ Histamine: avoidance of antimalarials advised by manufacturer of HISTAMINE
- ▸ Mepacrine: plasma concentration of primaquine increased by MEPACRINE (increased risk of toxicity)
- ▸ Penicillamine: increased risk of haematological toxicity when antimalarials given with PENICILLAMINE—manufacturer of penicillamine advises avoid concomitant use
- ▸ Vaccines: antimalarials inactivate ORAL TYPHOID VACCINE—see under Typhoid Vaccine in BNFC

Primidone
- ▸ Alcohol: increased sedative effect when primidone given with ALCOHOL
- ● Aminophylline: primidone accelerates metabolism of ● AMINOPHYLLINE (reduced effect)
- ● Analgesics: primidone reduces plasma concentration of METHADONE; primidone possibly accelerates metabolism of PARACETAMOL (also isolated reports of hepatotoxicity)
- ● Anthelmintics: primidone reduces plasma concentration of ● ALBENDAZOLE and ● PRAZIQUANTEL—consider increasing albendazole and praziquantel dose when given for systemic infections
- ● Anti-arrhythmics: primidone accelerates metabolism of DISOPYRAMIDE (reduced plasma concentration); primidone possibly reduces plasma concentration of ● DRONEDARONE—avoid concomitant use; primidone possibly accelerates metabolism of PROPAFENONE
- ● Antibacterials: primidone accelerates metabolism of METRONIDAZOLE (reduced effect); primidone possibly reduces plasma concentration of RIFAMPICIN; primidone accelerates metabolism of DOXYCYCLINE (reduced plasma concentration); primidone possibly accelerates metabolism of ● CHLORAMPHENICOL (reduced plasma concentration); primidone reduces plasma concentration of ● TELITHROMYCIN (avoid during and for 2 weeks after primidone)
- ● Anticoagulants: primidone possibly reduces plasma concentration of ● APIXABAN and ● EDOXABAN; primidone accelerates metabolism of ● COUMARINS (reduced anticoagulant effect); primidone possibly reduces plasma concentration of ● RIVAROXABAN—manufacturer of rivaroxaban advises monitor for signs of thrombosis
- ● Antidepressants: primidone possibly reduces plasma concentration of REBOXETINE; primidone reduces plasma concentration of PAROXETINE; primidone accelerates metabolism of ● MIANSERIN (reduced plasma concentration); anticonvulsant effect of antiepileptics possibly antagonised by MAOIs and ● TRICYCLIC-RELATED ANTIDEPRESSANTS (convulsive threshold lowered); anticonvulsant effect of antiepileptics antagonised by ● SSRIs and ● TRICYCLICS (convulsive threshold lowered); plasma concentration of

Primidone

- **Antidepressants** (continued)

  primidone possibly reduced by • ST JOHN'S WORT—avoid concomitant use; primidone possibly accelerates metabolism of • TRICYCLICS (reduced plasma concentration)
- **Antiepileptics**: plasma concentration of primidone possibly increased by CARBAMAZEPINE; primidone possibly reduces plasma concentration of ETHOSUXIMIDE, RUFINAMIDE and TOPIRAMATE; plasma concentration of primidone often increased by FOSPHENYTOIN and PHENYTOIN, plasma concentration of fosphenytoin and phenytoin often reduced but may be increased; primidone reduces plasma concentration of LAMOTRIGINE, TIAGABINE and ZONISAMIDE; plasma concentration of primidone increased by OXCARBAZEPINE, also plasma concentration of an active metabolite of oxcarbazepine reduced; plasma concentration of primidone increased by SODIUM VALPROATE and VALPROIC ACID (also plasma concentration of sodium valproate and valproic acid reduced); plasma concentration of primidone increased by • STIRIPENTOL
- **Antifungals**: primidone possibly reduces plasma concentration of ITRACONAZOLE and • POSACONAZOLE; primidone possibly reduces plasma concentration of • VORICONAZOLE—avoid concomitant use; primidone reduces absorption of GRISEOFULVIN (reduced effect)
- **Antimalarials**: avoidance of primidone advised by manufacturer of ARTENIMOL WITH PIPERAQUINE; anticonvulsant effect of antiepileptics antagonised by • MEFLOQUINE
- **Antipsychotics**: anticonvulsant effect of antiepileptics antagonised by • ANTIPSYCHOTICS (convulsive threshold lowered); primidone accelerates metabolism of HALOPERIDOL (reduced plasma concentration); plasma concentration of both drugs reduced when primidone given with CHLORPROMAZINE; primidone possibly reduces plasma concentration of • ARIPIPRAZOLE (avoid concomitant use or consider increasing the dose of aripiprazole—consult aripiprazole product literature); primidone possibly reduces plasma concentration of CLOZAPINE; primidone possibly reduces plasma concentration of • LURASIDONE—avoid concomitant use
- **Antivirals**: primidone possibly reduces plasma concentration of ABACAVIR, DARUNAVIR, FOSAMPRENAVIR, • INDINAVIR, • LOPINAVIR and • SAQUINAVIR; avoidance of primidone advised by manufacturer of • BOCEPREVIR and • RILPIVIRINE (plasma concentration of boceprevir and rilpivirine possibly reduced); primidone possibly reduces plasma concentration of • DACLATASVIR and • SIMEPREVIR—manufacturer of daclatasvir and simeprevir advises avoid concomitant use; primidone possibly reduces plasma concentration of • DASABUVIR, • OMBITASVIR and • PARITAPREVIR—avoid concomitant use; primidone possibly reduces the plasma concentration of • DOLUTEGRAVIR (see under Dolutegravir, p. 387); avoidance of primidone advised by manufacturer of • ELVITEGRAVIR, ETRAVIRINE, LEDIPASVIR, SOFOSBUVIR and • TELAPREVIR
- **Anxiolytics and Hypnotics**: increased sedative effect when primidone given with ANXIOLYTICS AND HYPNOTICS; primidone often reduces plasma concentration of CLONAZEPAM
- **Aprepitant**: primidone possibly reduces plasma concentration of APREPITANT
- **Avanafil**: primidone possibly reduces plasma concentration of AVANAFIL—manufacturer of avanafil advises avoid concomitant use
- **Beta-blockers**: primidone possibly reduces plasma concentration of PROPRANOLOL
- **Caffeine citrate**: effects of primidone possibly antagonised by CAFFEINE CITRATE
- **Calcium-channel Blockers**: primidone probably reduces effects of • CALCIUM-CHANNEL BLOCKERS; avoidance of primidone advised by manufacturer of ISRADIPINE; avoidance of primidone advised by manufacturer of • NIMODIPINE (plasma concentration of nimodipine reduced)
- **Cannabis Extract**: primidone possibly reduces plasma concentration of • CANNABIS EXTRACT—manufacturer of cannabis extract advises avoid concomitant use
- **Ciclosporin**: primidone accelerates metabolism of • CICLOSPORIN (reduced plasma concentration)

Primidone (continued)

- **Cobicistat**: primidone possibly reduces plasma concentration of • COBICISTAT—manufacturer of cobicistat advises avoid concomitant use
- **Corticosteroids**: primidone accelerates metabolism of • CORTICOSTEROIDS (reduced effect)
- **Cytotoxics**: primidone possibly decreases plasma concentration of AXITINIB (increase dose of axitinib—consult axitinib product literature); primidone possibly reduces plasma concentration of BORTEZOMIB, • BOSUTINIB, CRIZOTINIB and PONATINIB—manufacturer of bortezomib, bosutinib, crizotinib and ponatinib advises avoid concomitant use; primidone possibly reduces plasma concentration of • CABOZANTINIB—avoid concomitant use; avoidance of primidone advised by manufacturer of • CABAZITAXEL, DABRAFENIB and GEFITINIB; avoidance of primidone advised by manufacturer of • DASATINIB and VANDETANIB (plasma concentration of dasatinib and vandetanib possibly reduced); primidone possibly reduces plasma concentration of • ETOPOSIDE; primidone reduces plasma concentration of IRINOTECAN and its active metabolite; manufacturer of procarbazine advises possible increased risk of hypersensitivity reactions when primidone given with PROCARBAZINE
- **Diuretics**: primidone reduces plasma concentration of • EPLERENONE—avoid concomitant use; increased risk of osteomalacia when primidone given with CARBONIC ANHYDRASE INHIBITORS
- **Folates**: plasma concentration of primidone possibly reduced by FOLATES
- **Fosaprepitant**: primidone possibly reduces plasma concentration of FOSAPREPITANT
- **Guanfacine**: primidone possibly reduces plasma concentration of • GUANFACINE—increase dose of guanfacine
- **Hormone Antagonists**: primidone possibly reduces plasma concentration of • ABIRATERONE—manufacturer of abiraterone advises avoid concomitant use; primidone accelerates metabolism of TOREMIFENE (reduced plasma concentration)
- **Ivacaftor**: primidone possibly reduces plasma concentration of • IVACAFTOR—manufacturer of ivacaftor advises avoid concomitant use
- **Leukotriene Receptor Antagonists**: primidone reduces plasma concentration of MONTELUKAST
- **Oestrogens**: primidone accelerates metabolism of • OESTROGENS (reduced contraceptive effect with combined oral contraceptives, contraceptive patches, and vaginal rings—see Contraceptive Interactions in BNFC)
- **Orlistat**: possible increased risk of convulsions when antiepileptics given with • ORLISTAT
- **Progestogens**: primidone accelerates metabolism of • PROGESTOGENS (reduced contraceptive effect with combined oral contraceptives, progestogen-only oral contraceptives, contraceptive patches, vaginal rings, etonogestrel-releasing implant, and emergency hormonal contraception—see Contraceptive Interactions in BNFC)
- **Roflumilast**: primidone possibly inhibits effects of ROFLUMILAST (manufacturer of roflumilast advises avoid concomitant use)
- **Sodium Oxybate**: avoidance of primidone advised by manufacturer of SODIUM OXYBATE
- **Sympathomimetics**: plasma concentration of primidone possibly increased by METHYLPHENIDATE
- **Tacrolimus**: primidone reduces plasma concentration of • TACROLIMUS
- **Theophylline**: primidone accelerates metabolism of • THEOPHYLLINE (reduced effect)
- **Thyroid Hormones**: primidone accelerates metabolism of THYROID HORMONES (may increase requirements for thyroid hormones in hypothyroidism)
- **Ticagrelor**: primidone possibly reduces plasma concentration of TICAGRELOR
- **Ulipristal**: avoidance of primidone advised by manufacturer of • ULIPRISTAL (contraceptive effect of ulipristal possibly reduced)
- **Vitamins**: primidone possibly increases requirements for ALFACALCIDOL, CALCITRIOL, COLECALCIFEROL, DIHYDROTACHYSTEROL, ERGOCALCIFEROL, PARICALCITOL or VITAMIN D

Procarbazine
- ▷ Alcohol: disulfiram-like reaction when procarbazine given with ALCOHOL
- ▷ Antiepileptics: manufacturer of procarbazine advises possible increased risk of hypersensitivity reactions when given with CARBAMAZEPINE, FOSPHENYTOIN, PHENOBARBITAL, PHENYTOIN and PRIMIDONE
- • Antipsychotics: avoid concomitant use of cytotoxics with • CLOZAPINE (increased risk of agranulocytosis)
- ▷ Cardiac Glycosides: procarbazine possibly reduces absorption of DIGOXIN *tablets*

Prochlorperazine see Antipsychotics
Procyclidine see Antimuscarinics
Progesterone see Progestogens
Progestogens
- • Antibacterials: plasma concentration of dienogest increased by ERYTHROMYCIN; metabolism of progestogens accelerated by • RIFAMYCINS (reduced contraceptive effect with combined oral contraceptives, progestogen-only oral contraceptives, contraceptive patches, vaginal rings, etonogestrel-releasing implant, and emergency hormonal contraception—see Contraceptive Interactions in BNF)
- • Anticoagulants: progestogens may enhance or reduce anticoagulant effect of COUMARINS; progestogens antagonise anticoagulant effect of • PHENINDIONE
- • Antibacterials: contraceptive effect of progestogens reduced by • ST JOHN'S WORT (avoid concomitant use)
- ▷ Antidiabetics: progestogens antagonise hypoglycaemic effect of ANTIDIABETICS
- • Antiepileptics: metabolism of progestogens accelerated by • CARBAMAZEPINE, • ESLICARBAZEPINE, • FOSPHENYTOIN, • OXCARBAZEPINE, • PERAMPANEL, • PHENOBARBITAL, • PHENYTOIN, • PRIMIDONE, • RUFINAMIDE and • TOPIRAMATE (reduced contraceptive effect with combined oral contraceptives, progestogen-only oral contraceptives, contraceptive patches, vaginal rings, etonogestrel-releasing implant, and emergency hormonal contraception—see Contraceptive Interactions in BNFC); desogestrel possibly increases plasma concentration of LAMOTRIGINE
- ▷ Antifungals: plasma concentration of drospirenone increased by KETOCONAZOLE; progestogens possibly increase plasma concentration of VORICONAZOLE; anecdotal reports of contraceptive failure and menstrual irregularities when progestogens given with GRISEOFULVIN; occasional reports of breakthrough bleeding when progestogens (used for contraception) given with TERBINAFINE
- • Antivirals: plasma concentration of norethisterone increased by ATAZANAVIR; plasma concentration of drospirenone increased by BOCEPREVIR (increased risk of toxicity); contraceptive effect of progestogens possibly reduced by • EFAVIRENZ; plasma concentration of norgestimate increased by ELVITEGRAVIR; metabolism of progestogens accelerated by • NEVIRAPINE (reduced contraceptive effect with combined oral contraceptives, progestogen-only oral contraceptives, contraceptive patches, vaginal rings, etonogestrel-releasing implant, and emergency hormonal contraception—see Contraceptive Interactions in BNFC)
- ▷ Anxiolytics and Hypnotics: progestogens possibly increase plasma concentration of CHLORDIAZEPOXIDE, DIAZEPAM and NITRAZEPAM; progestogens possibly reduce plasma concentration of LORAZEPAM, OXAZEPAM and TEMAZEPAM
- • Aprepitant: possible contraceptive failure of hormonal contraceptives containing progestogens when given with • APREPITANT (alternative contraception recommended)
- • Bosentan: possible contraceptive failure of hormonal contraceptives containing progestogens when given with • BOSENTAN (alternative contraception recommended)
- ▷ Ciclosporin: progestogens possibly increase plasma concentration of CICLOSPORIN
- ▷ Cobicistat: plasma concentration of norgestimate increased by COBICISTAT
- • Cytotoxics: possible reduction in contraceptive effect of progestogens advised by manufacturer of • CRIZOTINIB and • VEMURAFENIB; possible reduced contraceptive effect of hormonal contraceptives containing progestogens advised by

Progestogens
- • Cytotoxics (continued)
  manufacturer of • DABRAFENIB (alternative contraception recommended)
- ▷ Diuretics: risk of hyperkalaemia when drospirenone given with POTASSIUM-SPARING DIURETICS AND ALDOSTERONE ANTAGONISTS (monitor serum potassium during first cycle)
- • Dopaminergics: progestogens increase plasma concentration of • SELEGILINE—manufacturer of selegiline advises avoid concomitant use
- • Fosaprepitant: possible contraceptive failure of hormonal contraceptives containing progestogens when given with • FOSAPREPITANT (alternative contraception recommended)
- ▷ Lipid-regulating Drugs: plasma concentration of norethisterone increased by ATORVASTATIN; plasma concentration of active metabolite of norgestimate increased by ROSUVASTATIN; plasma concentration of norgestrel increased by ROSUVASTATIN
- • Muscle Relaxants: progestogens possibly increase plasma concentration of TIZANIDINE (increased risk of toxicity)
- ▷ Sugammadex: plasma concentration of progestogens possibly reduced by SUGAMMADEX—manufacturer of sugammadex advises additional contraceptive precautions
- ▷ Teriflunomide: plasma concentration of levonorgestrel increased by TERIFLUNOMIDE
- • Ulipristal: contraceptive effect of progestogens possibly reduced by • ULIPRISTAL

Proguanil
- ▷ Antacids: absorption of proguanil reduced by ORAL MAGNESIUM SALTS (as magnesium trisilicate)
- • Anticoagulants: isolated reports that proguanil may enhance anticoagulant effect of WARFARIN
- • Antimalarials: avoidance of antimalarials advised by manufacturer of • ARTEMETHER WITH LUMEFANTRINE; increased antifolate effect when proguanil given with PYRIMETHAMINE
- ▷ Antivirals: plasma concentration of proguanil possibly affected by EFAVIRENZ
- ▷ Histamine: avoidance of antimalarials advised by manufacturer of HISTAMINE
- ▷ Penicillamine: increased risk of haematological toxicity when antimalarials given with PENICILLAMINE—manufacturer of penicillamine advises avoid concomitant use
- ▷ Vaccines: antimalarials inactivate ORAL TYPHOID VACCINE—see under Typhoid Vaccine in BNF

Promazine see Antipsychotics
Promethazine see Antihistamines
Propafenone
- ▷ Aminophylline: propafenone increases plasma concentration of AMINOPHYLLINE
- ▷ Anaesthetics, Local: increased myocardial depression when anti-arrhythmics given with BUPIVACAINE, LEVOBUPIVACAINE, PRILOCAINE or ROPIVACAINE
- • Anti-arrhythmics: increased myocardial depression when anti-arrhythmics given with other • ANTI-ARRHYTHMICS
- • Antibacterials: metabolism of propafenone accelerated by • RIFAMPICIN (reduced effect)
- • Anticoagulants: propafenone enhances anticoagulant effect of • COUMARINS
- • Antidepressants: metabolism of propafenone possibly inhibited by FLUOXETINE and PAROXETINE; increased risk of arrhythmias when propafenone given with • TRICYCLICS
- ▷ Antiepileptics: metabolism of propafenone possibly accelerated by PHENOBARBITAL and PRIMIDONE
- ▷ Antihistamines: avoidance of propafenone advised by manufacturer of MIZOLASTINE (possible risk of ventricular arrhythmias)
- • Antipsychotics: increased risk of ventricular arrhythmias when anti-arrhythmics that prolong the QT interval given with • ANTIPSYCHOTICS that prolong the QT interval
- • Antivirals: plasma concentration of propafenone possibly increased by • FOSAMPRENAVIR (increased risk of ventricular arrhythmias—avoid concomitant use); plasma concentration of propafenone increased by RITONAVIR (increased risk of ventricular arrhythmias—avoid concomitant use); increased risk of ventricular arrhythmias when propafenone given with • SAQUINAVIR—avoid concomitant use; caution with

Propafenone
- Antivirals (continued)
propafenone advised by manufacturer of • TELAPREVIR (risk of ventricular arrhythmias)
- Beta-blockers: increased myocardial depression when anti-arrhythmics given with • BETA-BLOCKERS; propafenone increases plasma concentration of METOPROLOL and PROPRANOLOL
- Cardiac Glycosides: propafenone increases plasma concentration of • DIGOXIN (halve dose of digoxin)
- Ciclosporin: propafenone possibly increases plasma concentration of CICLOSPORIN
- Parasympathomimetics: propafenone possibly antagonises effects of NEOSTIGMINE and PYRIDOSTIGMINE
▸ Theophylline: propafenone increases plasma concentration of THEOPHYLLINE
- Ulcer-healing Drugs: plasma concentration of propafenone increased by • CIMETIDINE

Propantheline *see* Antimuscarinics

Propiverine *see* Antimuscarinics

Propofol *see* Anaesthetics, General

Propranolol *see* Beta-blockers

Prostaglandins
▸ ACE Inhibitors: enhanced hypotensive effect when alprostadil given with ACE INHIBITORS
▸ Adrenergic Neurone Blockers: enhanced hypotensive effect when alprostadil given with ADRENERGIC NEURONE BLOCKERS
▸ Alpha-blockers: enhanced hypotensive effect when alprostadil given with ALPHA-BLOCKERS
▸ Angiotensin-II Receptor Antagonists: enhanced hypotensive effect when alprostadil given with ANGIOTENSIN-II RECEPTOR ANTAGONISTS
▸ Beta-blockers: enhanced hypotensive effect when alprostadil given with BETA-BLOCKERS
▸ Calcium-channel Blockers: enhanced hypotensive effect when alprostadil given with CALCIUM-CHANNEL BLOCKERS
▸ Clonidine: enhanced hypotensive effect when alprostadil given with CLONIDINE
▸ Diazoxide: enhanced hypotensive effect when alprostadil given with DIAZOXIDE
▸ Diuretics: enhanced hypotensive effect when alprostadil given with DIURETICS
▸ Methyldopa: enhanced hypotensive effect when alprostadil given with METHYLDOPA
▸ Moxonidine: enhanced hypotensive effect when alprostadil given with MOXONIDINE
▸ Nitrates: enhanced hypotensive effect when alprostadil given with NITRATES
▸ Oxytocin: prostaglandins potentiate uterotonic effect of OXYTOCIN
▸ Vasodilator Antihypertensives: enhanced hypotensive effect when alprostadil given with HYDRALAZINE, MINOXIDIL or SODIUM NITROPRUSSIDE

Protein Kinase Inhibitors *see* individual drugs

Proton Pump Inhibitors
▸ Antacids: absorption of lansoprazole possibly reduced by ANTACIDS
▸ Antibacterials: plasma concentration of both drugs increased when omeprazole given with CLARITHROMYCIN
- Anticoagulants: pantoprazole might enhance the anticoagulant effect of COUMARINS; esomeprazole and omeprazole possibly enhance anticoagulant effect of • COUMARINS
- Antidepressants: omeprazole increases plasma concentration of ESCITALOPRAM; plasma concentration of lansoprazole possibly increased by FLUVOXAMINE; plasma concentration of omeprazole possibly reduced by ST JOHN'S WORT
- Antiepileptics: esomeprazole enhances effects of
• FOSPHENYTOIN and • PHENYTOIN; omeprazole possibly enhances effects of FOSPHENYTOIN and PHENYTOIN
- Antifungals: proton pump inhibitors reduce absorption of ITRACONAZOLE and KETOCONAZOLE; esomeprazole reduces plasma concentration of • POSACONAZOLE—manufacturer of posaconazole *suspension* advises avoid concomitant use; lansoprazole, omeprazole, pantoprazole and rabeprazole possibly reduce plasma concentration of • POSACONAZOLE—manufacturer of posaconazole *suspension* advises avoid

Proton Pump Inhibitors
- Antifungals (continued)
concomitant use; plasma concentration of esomeprazole possibly increased by VORICONAZOLE; plasma concentration of omeprazole increased by VORICONAZOLE (consider reducing dose of omeprazole)
▸ Antipsychotics: omeprazole possibly reduces plasma concentration of CLOZAPINE
- Antivirals: proton pump inhibitors reduce plasma concentration of • ATAZANAVIR—avoid or adjust dose of both drugs (consult product literature); do not take proton pump inhibitors before LEDIPASVIR advised by manufacturer of ledipasvir; omeprazole reduces plasma concentration of LEDIPASVIR; omeprazole increases plasma concentration of RALTEGRAVIR; omeprazole reduces plasma concentration of • RILPIVIRINE—avoid concomitant use; avoidance of esomeprazole, lansoprazole, pantoprazole and rabeprazole advised by manufacturer of RILPIVIRINE (plasma concentration of rilpivirine possibly reduced); omeprazole increases plasma concentration of • SAQUINAVIR—manufacturer of saquinavir advises avoid concomitant use; esomeprazole, lansoprazole, pantoprazole and rabeprazole possibly increase plasma concentration of • SAQUINAVIR—manufacturer of saquinavir advises avoid concomitant use; plasma concentration of esomeprazole and omeprazole reduced by • TIPRANAVIR
▸ Anxiolytics and Hypnotics: esomeprazole and omeprazole possibly inhibit metabolism of DIAZEPAM (increased plasma concentration)
▸ Cardiac Glycosides: proton pump inhibitors possibly slightly increase plasma concentration of DIGOXIN
▸ Ciclosporin: omeprazole possibly affects plasma concentration of CICLOSPORIN
- Cilostazol: omeprazole increases plasma concentration of • CILOSTAZOL (see under Cilostazol, in BNF)
- Clopidogrel: esomeprazole and omeprazole reduce antiplatelet effect of • CLOPIDOGREL; lansoprazole, pantoprazole and rabeprazole possibly reduce antiplatelet effect of CLOPIDOGREL
- Cytotoxics: proton pump inhibitors possibly reduce excretion of METHOTREXATE (increased risk of toxicity); lansoprazole reduces plasma concentration of BOSUTINIB; avoidance of proton pump inhibitors advised by manufacturer of DABRAFENIB (plasma concentration of dabrafenib possibly reduced); avoidance of esomeprazole, lansoprazole, pantoprazole and rabeprazole advised by manufacturer of • ERLOTINIB; omeprazole reduces plasma concentration of • ERLOTINIB—manufacturer of erlotinib advises avoid concomitant use; proton pump inhibitors possibly reduce absorption of LAPATINIB; proton pump inhibitors possibly reduce absorption of PAZOPANIB—manufacturer of pazopanib advises give at the same time as proton pump inhibitors
▸ Hormone Antagonists: plasma concentration of omeprazole reduced by ENZALUTAMIDE
▸ Tacrolimus: omeprazole possibly increases plasma concentration of TACROLIMUS
▸ Ulcer-healing Drugs: absorption of lansoprazole possibly reduced by SUCRALFATE

Pseudoephedrine *see* Sympathomimetics

Pyrazinamide
▸ Sulfinpyrazone: pyrazinamide antagonises effects of SULFINPYRAZONE
▸ Vaccines: antibacterials inactivate ORAL TYPHOID VACCINE—see under Typhoid Vaccine in BNFC

Pyridostigmine *see* Parasympathomimetics

Pyridoxine *see* Vitamins

Pyrimethamine
- Antibacterials: increased antifolate effect when pyrimethamine given with • SULFONAMIDES or • TRIMETHOPRIM
- Antiepileptics: pyrimethamine antagonises anticonvulsant effect of • FOSPHENYTOIN and • PHENYTOIN, also increased antifolate effect
- Antimalarials: avoidance of antimalarials advised by manufacturer of ARTEMETHER WITH LUMEFANTRINE; increased antifolate effect when pyrimethamine given with PROGUANIL
▸ Antivirals: increased antifolate effect when pyrimethamine given with ZIDOVUDINE

A1

Interactions | Appendix 1

Pyrimethamine (continued)

- Cytotoxics: pyrimethamine increases antifolate effect of ● METHOTREXATE and ● PEMETREXED
- Histamine: avoidance of antimalarials advised by manufacturer of HISTAMINE
- Penicillamine: increased risk of haematological toxicity when antimalarials given with PENICILLAMINE—manufacturer of penicillamine advises avoid concomitant use
- Vaccines: antimalarials inactivate ORAL TYPHOID VACCINE—see under Typhoid Vaccine in BNFC

Quetiapine *see* Antipsychotics

Quinagolide

- Memantine: effects of dopaminergics possibly enhanced by MEMANTINE
- Methyldopa: antiparkinsonian effect of dopaminergics antagonised by METHYLDOPA

Quinapril *see* ACE Inhibitors

Quinine

- Anti-arrhythmics: increased risk of ventricular arrhythmias when quinine given with ● AMIODARONE—avoid concomitant use; quinine increases plasma concentration of ● FLECAINIDE
- Antibacterials: increased risk of ventricular arrhythmias when quinine given with ● MOXIFLOXACIN—avoid concomitant use; plasma concentration of quinine reduced by ● RIFAMPICIN
- Anticoagulants: plasma concentration of both drugs increased when quinine given with WARFARIN
- Antidepressants: possible increased risk of ventricular arrhythmias when quinine given with ● CITALOPRAM or ● ESCITALOPRAM—avoid concomitant use
- Antimalarials: increased risk of ventricular arrhythmias when quinine given with ● ARTEMETHER WITH LUMEFANTRINE; avoidance of antimalarials advised by manufacturer of ● ARTEMETHER WITH LUMEFANTRINE; increased risk of convulsions when quinine given with ● MEFLOQUINE (but should not prevent the use of *intravenous* quinine in severe cases)
- Antipsychotics: increased risk of ventricular arrhythmias when quinine given with ● DROPERIDOL or ● PIMOZIDE—avoid concomitant use; possible increased risk of ventricular arrhythmias when quinine given with ● HALOPERIDOL—avoid concomitant use; possible increased risk of ventricular arrhythmias when quinine given with ● RISPERIDONE
- Antivirals: plasma concentration of quinine possibly increased by ● ATAZANAVIR, ● DARUNAVIR, ● FOSAMPRENAVIR, ● INDINAVIR and ● TIPRANAVIR (increased risk of toxicity); plasma concentration of quinine increased by ● RITONAVIR (increased risk of toxicity); increased risk of ventricular arrhythmias when quinine given with ● SAQUINAVIR—avoid concomitant use
- Cardiac Glycosides: quinine increases plasma concentration of ● DIGOXIN
- Dopaminergics: quinine possibly increases plasma concentration of AMANTADINE
- Histamine: avoidance of antimalarials advised by manufacturer of HISTAMINE
- Muscle Relaxants: quinine possibly enhances effects of SUXAMETHONIUM
- Penicillamine: increased risk of haematological toxicity when antimalarials given with PENICILLAMINE—manufacturer of penicillamine advises avoid concomitant use
- Ulcer-healing Drugs: metabolism of quinine inhibited by CIMETIDINE (increased plasma concentration)
- Vaccines: antimalarials inactivate ORAL TYPHOID VACCINE—see under Typhoid Vaccine in BNFC

Quinolones

- Aminophylline: possible increased risk of convulsions when quinolones given with ● AMINOPHYLLINE; ciprofloxacin and norfloxacin increase plasma concentration of ● AMINOPHYLLINE
- Analgesics: possible increased risk of convulsions when quinolones given with ● NSAIDS
- Antacids: absorption of moxifloxacin reduced by ANTACIDS (give at least 6 hours apart); absorption of ciprofloxacin and levofloxacin reduced by ANTACIDS (give at least 2 hours before or 4 hours after ciprofloxacin and levofloxacin); absorption of norfloxacin reduced by ANTACIDS; absorption of ofloxacin reduced by ANTACIDS (give at least 2 hours apart)

Quinolones (continued)

- Anti-arrhythmics: increased risk of ventricular arrhythmias when levofloxacin or moxifloxacin given with ● AMIODARONE— avoid concomitant use; increased risk of ventricular arrhythmias when moxifloxacin given with ● DISOPYRAMIDE— avoid concomitant use
- Antibacterials: increased risk of ventricular arrhythmias when moxifloxacin given with *parenteral* ● ERYTHROMYCIN—avoid concomitant use; avoidance of moxifloxacin advised by manufacturer of BEDAQUILINE; ciprofloxacin possibly increases plasma concentration of BEDAQUILINE—avoid concomitant use if ciprofloxacin given for more than 14 days; increased risk of ventricular arrhythmias when moxifloxacin given with ● DELAMANID; effects of nalidixic acid possibly antagonised by NITROFURANTOIN; possible increased risk of ventricular arrhythmias when moxifloxacin given with ● TELITHROMYCIN
- Anticoagulants: ciprofloxacin and levofloxacin possibly enhance anticoagulant effect of COUMARINS; nalidixic acid, norfloxacin and ofloxacin enhance anticoagulant effect of ● COUMARINS; levofloxacin possibly enhances anticoagulant effect of PHENINDIONE
- Antidepressants: avoidance of moxifloxacin advised by manufacturer of ● CITALOPRAM, ● ESCITALOPRAM and ● VENLAFAXINE (risk of ventricular arrhythmias); ciprofloxacin inhibits metabolism of ● DULOXETINE—avoid concomitant use; avoidance of ciprofloxacin advised by manufacturer of ● AGOMELATINE; increased risk of ventricular arrhythmias when moxifloxacin given with ● TRICYCLICS—avoid concomitant use
- Antidiabetics: norfloxacin possibly enhances effects of GLIBENCLAMIDE
- Antiepileptics: ciprofloxacin increases or decreases plasma concentration of FOSPHENYTOIN and PHENYTOIN
- Antihistamines: increased risk of ventricular arrhythmias when moxifloxacin given with ● MIZOLASTINE—avoid concomitant use
- Antimalarials: avoidance of quinolones advised by manufacturer of ● ARTEMETHER WITH LUMEFANTRINE; avoidance of moxifloxacin advised by manufacturer of ● ARTENIMOL WITH PIPERAQUINE (possible risk of ventricular arrhythmias); increased risk of ventricular arrhythmias when moxifloxacin given with ● CHLOROQUINE, ● HYDROXYCHLOROQUINE, ● MEFLOQUINE or ● QUININE—avoid concomitant use
- Antipsychotics: increased risk of ventricular arrhythmias when moxifloxacin given with ● BENPERIDOL—manufacturer of benperidol advises avoid concomitant use; increased risk of ventricular arrhythmias when moxifloxacin given with ● DROPERIDOL, ● HALOPERIDOL, ● PHENOTHIAZINES, ● PIMOZIDE or ● ZUCLOPENTHIXOL—avoid concomitant use; ciprofloxacin increases plasma concentration of CLOZAPINE; ciprofloxacin possibly increases plasma concentration of OLANZAPINE
- Antivirals: manufacturer of levofloxacin advises give DIDANOSINE *tablets* at least 2 hours before or after levofloxacin; absorption of ciprofloxacin reduced by DIDANOSINE *tablets* (give at least 2 hours before or 4 hours after ciprofloxacin); manufacturer of moxifloxacin advises give DIDANOSINE *tablets* at least 6 hours before or after moxifloxacin; manufacturer of norfloxacin advises give DIDANOSINE at least 2 hours before or after norfloxacin; increased risk of ventricular arrhythmias when moxifloxacin given with ● SAQUINAVIR—avoid concomitant use
- Anxiolytics and Hypnotics: avoidance of ciprofloxacin advised by manufacturer of ZOLPIDEM
- Atomoxetine: increased risk of ventricular arrhythmias when moxifloxacin given with ● ATOMOXETINE
- Beta-blockers: increased risk of ventricular arrhythmias when moxifloxacin given with ● SOTALOL—avoid concomitant use
- Calcium Salts: absorption of ciprofloxacin reduced by CALCIUM SALTS (give at least 2 hours before or 4 hours after ciprofloxacin)
- Ciclosporin: increased risk of nephrotoxicity when quinolones given with ● CICLOSPORIN
- Clopidogrel: ciprofloxacin possibly reduces antiplatelet effect of ● CLOPIDOGREL
- Cytotoxics: nalidixic acid increases risk of MELPHALAN toxicity; ciprofloxacin possibly reduces excretion of METHOTREXATE (increased risk of toxicity); possible increased risk of

Quinolones

- **Cytotoxics** (continued)
  ventricular arrhythmias when moxifloxacin given with
  ● BOSUTINIB; ciprofloxacin possibly increases the plasma
  concentration of ● BOSUTINIB—manufacturer of bosutinib
  advises avoid or consider reducing dose of bosutinib;
  ciprofloxacin increases plasma concentration of ERLOTINIB;
  ciprofloxacin possibly increases the plasma concentration of
  ● IBRUTINIB—reduce dose of ibrutinib (see under Ibrutinib, in
  BNF); possible increased risk of ventricular arrhythmias when
  moxifloxacin given with ● VANDETANIB—avoid concomitant
  use; increased risk of ventricular arrhythmias when
  levofloxacin or moxifloxacin given with ● ARSENIC TRIOXIDE
- ▸ **Dairy Products:** absorption of ciprofloxacin reduced by DAIRY
  PRODUCTS (give at least 2 hours apart); absorption of
  norfloxacin reduced by DAIRY PRODUCTS
- **Dopaminergics:** ciprofloxacin increases plasma concentration
  of RASAGILINE; ciprofloxacin inhibits metabolism of
  ROPINIROLE (increased plasma concentration)
- **5HT₁-receptor Agonists:** quinolones possibly inhibit metabolism
  of ZOLMITRIPTAN (reduce dose of zolmitriptan)
- **Iron Salts:** absorption of moxifloxacin reduced by *oral* IRON
  SALTS (give at least 6 hours apart); absorption of ciprofloxacin
  reduced by *oral* IRON SALTS (give at least 2 hours before or
  4 hours after ciprofloxacin); absorption of levofloxacin,
  norfloxacin and ofloxacin reduced by *oral* IRON SALTS (give at
  least 2 hours apart)
- **Lanthanum:** absorption of quinolones possibly reduced by
  LANTHANUM (give at least 2 hours before or 4 hours after
  lanthanum)
- **Muscle Relaxants:** ciprofloxacin increases plasma concentration
  of ● TIZANIDINE (increased risk of toxicity)—avoid concomitant
  use; norfloxacin possibly increases plasma concentration of
  TIZANIDINE (increased risk of toxicity)
- **Mycophenolate:** norfloxacin possibly reduces bioavailability of
  MYCOPHENOLATE
- **Pentamidine Isetionate:** increased risk of ventricular
  arrhythmias when moxifloxacin given with ● PENTAMIDINE
  ISETIONATE—avoid concomitant use
- **Pirfenidone:** ciprofloxacin increases plasma concentration of
  ● PIRFENIDONE—see under Pirfenidone, in BNF
- **Sevelamer:** absorption of ciprofloxacin reduced by SEVELAMER
  (give at least 2 hours before or 4 hours after ciprofloxacin)
- **Strontium Ranelate:** absorption of quinolones reduced by
  STRONTIUM RANELATE (manufacturer of strontium ranelate
  advises avoid concomitant use)
- **Theophylline:** possible increased risk of convulsions when
  quinolones given with ● THEOPHYLLINE; ciprofloxacin and
  norfloxacin increase plasma concentration of ● THEOPHYLLINE
- **Ulcer-healing Drugs:** absorption of ciprofloxacin reduced by
  SUCRALFATE (give at least 6 hours apart); absorption of
  levofloxacin, norfloxacin and ofloxacin reduced by SUCRALFATE
  (give at least 2 hours apart); absorption of ciprofloxacin
  reduced by SUCRALFATE (give at least 2 hours before or 4 hours
  after ciprofloxacin)
- **Vaccines:** antibacterials inactivate ORAL TYPHOID VACCINE—see
  under Typhoid Vaccine in BNFC
- **Zinc:** absorption of moxifloxacin reduced by ZINC (give at least
  6 hours apart); absorption of ciprofloxacin, levofloxacin,
  norfloxacin and ofloxacin reduced by ZINC (give at least
  2 hours apart)

Rabeprazole *see* Proton Pump Inhibitors

Rabies Vaccine *see* Vaccines

Raloxifene

- **Anticoagulants:** raloxifene antagonises anticoagulant effect of
  COUMARINS
- **Lipid-regulating Drugs:** absorption of raloxifene reduced by
  COLESTYRAMINE (manufacturer of raloxifene advises avoid
  concomitant administration)

Raltegravir

- **Antacids:** plasma concentration of raltegravir reduced by
  ALUMINIUM HYDROXIDE and ORAL MAGNESIUM SALTS—
  manufacturer of raltegravir advises avoid concomitant use
- **Antibacterials:** plasma concentration of raltegravir reduced by
  ● RIFAMPICIN—consider increasing dose of raltegravir

Raltegravir (continued)

- **Antivirals:** increased risk of rash when raltegravir given with
  DARUNAVIR; avoidance of raltegravir advised by manufacturer
  of ● FOSAMPRENAVIR
- **Orlistat:** absorption of raltegravir possibly reduced by
  ● ORLISTAT
- ▸ **Ulcer-healing Drugs:** plasma concentration of raltegravir
  increased by FAMOTIDINE and OMEPRAZOLE

Raltitrexed

- **Antipsychotics:** avoid concomitant use of cytotoxics with
  ● CLOZAPINE (increased risk of agranulocytosis)
- **Folates:** manufacturer of raltitrexed advises avoid concomitant
  use with ● FOLATES

Ramipril *see* ACE Inhibitors

Ramucirumab

- **Antipsychotics:** avoid concomitant use of cytotoxics with
  ● CLOZAPINE (increased risk of agranulocytosis)
- **Vaccines:** risk of generalised infections when monoclonal
  antibodies given with live ● VACCINES—avoid concomitant use

Ranitidine *see* Histamine H₂-antagonists

Ranolazine

- **Anti-arrhythmics:** manufacturer of ranolazine advises avoid
  concomitant use with ● DISOPYRAMIDE
- **Antibacterials:** plasma concentration of ranolazine possibly
  increased by ● CLARITHROMYCIN and ● TELITHROMYCIN—
  manufacturer of ranolazine advises avoid concomitant use;
  plasma concentration of ranolazine reduced by ● RIFAMPICIN—
  manufacturer of ranolazine advises avoid concomitant use
- **Antidepressants:** plasma concentration of ranolazine increased
  by PAROXETINE
- **Antifungals:** plasma concentration of ranolazine increased by
  ● KETOCONAZOLE—avoid concomitant use; plasma
  concentration of ranolazine possibly increased by
  ● ITRACONAZOLE, ● POSACONAZOLE and ● VORICONAZOLE—
  manufacturer of ranolazine advises avoid concomitant use
- **Antivirals:** plasma concentration of ranolazine possibly
  increased by ● ATAZANAVIR, ● DARUNAVIR, ● FOSAMPRENAVIR,
  ● INDINAVIR, ● LOPINAVIR, ● RITONAVIR, ● SAQUINAVIR and
  ● TIPRANAVIR—manufacturer of ranolazine advises avoid
  concomitant use
- **Beta-blockers:** manufacturer of ranolazine advises avoid
  concomitant use with ● SOTALOL
- ▸ **Calcium-channel Blockers:** plasma concentration of ranolazine
  increased by DILTIAZEM and VERAPAMIL (consider reducing dose
  of ranolazine)
- ▸ **Cardiac Glycosides:** ranolazine increases plasma concentration
  of DIGOXIN
- ▸ **Ciclosporin:** plasma concentration of both drugs may increase
  when ranolazine given with CICLOSPORIN
- **Grapefruit Juice:** plasma concentration of ranolazine possibly
  increased by ● GRAPEFRUIT JUICE—manufacturer of ranolazine
  advises avoid concomitant use
- **Lipid-regulating Drugs:** ranolazine increases plasma
  concentration of ● SIMVASTATIN (see under Simvastatin, in
  BNF); separating administration from ranolazine by 12 hours
  advised by manufacturer of LOMITAPIDE
- **Tacrolimus:** ranolazine increases plasma concentration of
  ● TACROLIMUS

Rasagiline

NOTE Rasagiline is a MAO-B inhibitor

- **Analgesics:** avoid concomitant use of rasagiline with
  ● DEXTROMETHORPHAN; risk of CNS toxicity when rasagiline
  given with ● PETHIDINE (avoid pethidine for 2 weeks after
  rasagiline)
- ▸ **Antibacterials:** plasma concentration of rasagiline increased by
  CIPROFLOXACIN
- **Antidepressants:** after stopping rasagiline do not start
  ● FLUOXETINE for 2 weeks, also rasagiline should not be started
  until at least 5 weeks after stopping fluoxetine; after stopping
  rasagiline do not start ● FLUVOXAMINE for 2 weeks; risk of
  hypertensive crisis when rasagiline given with ● MAOIS, avoid
  MAOIs for at least 2 weeks after stopping rasagiline; increased
  risk of CNS toxicity when rasagiline given with ● SSRIS or
  ● TRICYCLICS; risk of CNS excitation and hypertension when
  rasagiline given with ● VORTIOXETINE

Rasagiline (continued)
- Dopaminergics: plasma concentration of rasagiline possibly reduced by ENTACAPONE
- Memantine: effects of dopaminergics possibly enhanced by MEMANTINE
- Methyldopa: antiparkinsonian effect of dopaminergics antagonised by METHYLDOPA
- Sympathomimetics: avoid concomitant use of rasagiline with ● SYMPATHOMIMETICS

Reboxetine
- Antibacterials: manufacturer of reboxetine advises avoid concomitant use with ● MACROLIDES
- Antidepressants: manufacturer of reboxetine advises avoid concomitant use with ● FLUVOXAMINE; increased risk of hypertension and CNS excitation when reboxetine given with ● MAOIs (MAOIs should not be started until 1 week after stopping reboxetine, avoid reboxetine for 2 weeks after stopping MAOIs)
- Antiepileptics: plasma concentration of reboxetine possibly reduced by CARBAMAZEPINE, PHENOBARBITAL and PRIMIDONE
- Antifungals: manufacturer of reboxetine advises avoid concomitant use with ● IMIDAZOLES and ● TRIAZOLES
- Antimalarials: avoidance of antidepressants advised by manufacturer of ● ARTEMETHER WITH LUMEFANTRINE and ● ARTENIMOL WITH PIPERAQUINE
- Atomoxetine: possible increased risk of convulsions when antidepressants given with ATOMOXETINE
- Diuretics: possible increased risk of hypokalaemia when reboxetine given with LOOP DIURETICS or THIAZIDES AND RELATED DIURETICS
- Ergot Alkaloids: possible risk of hypertension when reboxetine given with ERGOTAMINE

Regorafenib
- Analgesics: manufacturer of regorafenib advises avoid concomitant use with MEFENAMIC ACID
- Antibacterials: plasma concentration of regorafenib reduced by ● RIFAMPICIN—manufacturer of regorafenib advises avoid concomitant use
- Anticoagulants: increased risk of bleeding when regorafenib given with ● WARFARIN
- Antifungals: plasma concentration of regorafenib increased by ● KETOCONAZOLE—avoid concomitant use
- Antipsychotics: avoid concomitant use of cytotoxics with ● CLOZAPINE (increased risk of agranulocytosis)
- Cytotoxics: regorafenib increases plasma concentration of IRINOTECAN

Remifentanil *see* Opioid Analgesics

Repaglinide *see* Antidiabetics

Retigabine
- Alcohol: increased risk of blurred vision when retigabine given with ALCOHOL
- Antidepressants: anticonvulsant effect of antiepileptics possibly antagonised by MAOIs and ● TRICYCLIC-RELATED ANTIDEPRESSANTS (convulsive threshold lowered); anticonvulsant effect of antiepileptics antagonised by ● SSRIS and ● TRICYCLICS (convulsive threshold lowered)
- Antiepileptics: plasma concentration of retigabine possibly reduced by CARBAMAZEPINE, FOSPHENYTOIN and PHENYTOIN
- Antimalarials: anticonvulsant effect of antiepileptics antagonised by ● MEFLOQUINE
- Antipsychotics: anticonvulsant effect of antiepileptics antagonised by ● ANTIPSYCHOTICS (convulsive threshold lowered)
- Orlistat: possible increased risk of convulsions when antiepileptics given with ● ORLISTAT

Retinoids
- Alcohol: etretinate formed from acitretin in presence of ● ALCOHOL (increased risk of teratogenicity in women of child-bearing potential)
- Antibacterials: possible increased risk of benign intracranial hypertension when retinoids given with ● TETRACYCLINES (avoid concomitant use)
- Anticoagulants: acitretin possibly reduces anticoagulant effect of ● COUMARINS
- Antiepileptics: isotretinoin possibly reduces plasma concentration of CARBAMAZEPINE

Retinoids (continued)
- Antifungals: plasma concentration of alitretinoin increased by KETOCONAZOLE; possible increased risk of tretinoin toxicity when given with ● FLUCONAZOLE, ● KETOCONAZOLE and ● VORICONAZOLE
- Cytotoxics: acitretin increases plasma concentration of ● METHOTREXATE (also increased risk of hepatotoxicity)—avoid concomitant use
- Lipid-regulating Drugs: alitretinoin reduces plasma concentration of SIMVASTATIN
- Vitamins: risk of hypervitaminosis A when retinoids given with ● VITAMIN A—avoid concomitant use

Ribavirin
- Antivirals: effects of ribavirin possibly reduced by ● ABACAVIR; increased risk of side-effects when ribavirin given with ● DIDANOSINE—avoid concomitant use; increased risk of toxicity when ribavirin given with ● STAVUDINE; increased risk of anaemia when ribavirin given with ● ZIDOVUDINE—avoid concomitant use
- Azathioprine: ribavirin possibly enhances myelosuppressive effects of ● AZATHIOPRINE

Rifabutin *see* Rifamycins

Rifampicin *see* Rifamycins

Rifamycins

NOTE Interactions do not apply to rifaximin
- ACE Inhibitors: rifampicin reduces plasma concentration of active metabolite of IMIDAPRIL (reduced antihypertensive effect)
- Aliskiren: rifampicin reduces plasma concentration of ALISKIREN
- Ambrisentan: rifampicin possibly increases plasma concentration of AMBRISENTAN
- Aminophylline: rifampicin accelerates metabolism of AMINOPHYLLINE (reduced plasma concentration)
- Analgesics: rifampicin reduces plasma concentration of CELECOXIB, DICLOFENAC and ETORICOXIB; rifampicin accelerates metabolism of ALFENTANIL, CODEINE, FENTANYL, METHADONE and MORPHINE (reduced effect); rifampicin possibly accelerates metabolism of OXYCODONE
- Angiotensin-II Receptor Antagonists: rifampicin reduces plasma concentration of LOSARTAN and its active metabolite
- Antacids: absorption of rifampicin reduced by ANTACIDS
- Anthelmintics: rifampicin reduces plasma concentration of ● PRAZIQUANTEL—avoid concomitant use
- Anti-arrhythmics: rifamycins accelerate metabolism of ● DISOPYRAMIDE (reduced plasma concentration); rifampicin reduces plasma concentration of ● DRONEDARONE—avoid concomitant use; rifampicin accelerates metabolism of ● PROPAFENONE (reduced effect)
- Antibacterials: increased risk of side-effects including neutropenia when rifabutin given with ● AZITHROMYCIN; rifamycins reduce plasma concentration of CLARITHROMYCIN and DAPSONE; plasma concentration of rifabutin increased by ● CLARITHROMYCIN (increased risk of toxicity—reduce rifabutin dose); plasma concentration of rifabutin possibly increased by ● ERYTHROMYCIN (increased risk of toxicity—reduce rifabutin dose); rifampicin possibly reduces plasma concentration of TINIDAZOLE and TRIMETHOPRIM; rifampicin reduces plasma concentration of DOXYCYCLINE—consider increasing dose of doxycycline; rifampicin reduces plasma concentration of ● BEDAQUILINE—manufacturer of bedaquiline advises avoid concomitant use; rifabutin possibly reduces plasma concentration of BEDAQUILINE—manufacturer of bedaquiline advises avoid concomitant use; rifampicin accelerates metabolism of CHLORAMPHENICOL (reduced plasma concentration); rifampicin reduces plasma concentration of ● DELAMANID; increased risk of hepatotoxicity when rifampicin given with ● ISONIAZID; rifampicin reduces plasma concentration of ● TELITHROMYCIN (avoid during and for 2 weeks after rifampicin)
- Anticoagulants: rifampicin possibly reduces plasma concentration of ● APIXABAN—manufacturer of apixaban advises avoid concomitant use when given for treatment of deep-vein thrombosis or pulmonary embolism; rifamycins accelerate metabolism of ● COUMARINS (reduced anticoagulant effect); rifampicin reduces plasma concentration of

Rifamycins

- **Anticoagulants** (continued)
  - • DABIGATRAN—manufacturer of dabigatran advises avoid concomitant use; rifampicin reduces plasma concentration of • EDOXABAN; rifampicin reduces plasma concentration of • RIVAROXABAN—manufacturer of rivaroxaban advises monitor for signs of thrombosis
- **Antidepressants:** rifampicin reduces plasma concentration of LINEZOLID (possible therapeutic failure of linezolid); rifampicin reduces plasma concentration of • VORTIOXETINE—consider increasing dose of vortioxetine
- **Antidiabetics:** rifamycins accelerate metabolism of • TOLBUTAMIDE (reduced effect); rifampicin reduces plasma concentration of • CANAGLIFLOZIN and NATEGLINIDE; rifampicin possibly reduces effects of LINAGLIPTIN; rifampicin possibly antagonises hypoglycaemic effect of REPAGLINIDE; rifampicin possibly accelerate metabolism of • SULFONYLUREAS (reduced effect)
- **Antiepileptics:** rifabutin reduces plasma concentration of • CARBAMAZEPINE; rifamycins accelerate metabolism of • FOSPHENYTOIN and • PHENYTOIN (reduced plasma concentration); rifampicin reduces plasma concentration of • LAMOTRIGINE; plasma concentration of rifampicin possibly reduced by PHENOBARBITAL and PRIMIDONE
- **Antifungals:** rifampicin accelerates metabolism of • KETOCONAZOLE (reduced plasma concentration), also plasma concentration of rifampicin may be reduced by ketoconazole; plasma concentration of rifabutin increased by • FLUCONAZOLE (increased risk of uveitis—reduce rifabutin dose); rifampicin accelerates metabolism of • FLUCONAZOLE (reduced plasma concentration); rifabutin and rifampicin reduce plasma concentration of • ITRACONAZOLE—manufacturer of itraconazole advises avoid concomitant use; plasma concentration of rifabutin increased by • POSACONAZOLE (also plasma concentration of posaconazole reduced); rifampicin reduces plasma concentration of • POSACONAZOLE and • TERBINAFINE; plasma concentration of rifabutin increased by • VORICONAZOLE, also rifabutin reduces plasma concentration of voriconazole (increase dose of voriconazole and also monitor for rifabutin toxicity); rifampicin reduces plasma concentration of • VORICONAZOLE—avoid concomitant use; rifampicin initially increases and then reduces plasma concentration of CASPOFUNGIN (consider increasing dose of caspofungin); plasma concentration of rifabutin possibly increased by • TRIAZOLES (increased risk of uveitis—reduce rifabutin dose)
- **Antihistamines:** rifampicin possibly reduces effects of FEXOFENADINE
- **Antimalarials:** avoidance of rifampicin advised by manufacturer of ARTENIMOL WITH PIPERAQUINE; rifampicin reduces plasma concentration of • MEFLOQUINE—avoid concomitant use; rifampicin reduces plasma concentration of • QUININE
- **Antimuscarinics:** rifampicin reduces plasma concentration of active metabolite of FESOTERODINE—avoid concomitant use
- **Antipsychotics:** rifampicin accelerates metabolism of • HALOPERIDOL (reduced plasma concentration); rifabutin and rifampicin possibly reduce plasma concentration of • ARIPIPRAZOLE (avoid concomitant use or consider increasing the dose of aripiprazole—consult aripiprazole product literature); rifampicin possibly reduces plasma concentration of CLOZAPINE; rifampicin reduces plasma concentration of • LURASIDONE—avoid concomitant use
- **Antivirals:** rifampicin possibly reduces plasma concentration of ABACAVIR; rifampicin reduces plasma concentration of • ATAZANAVIR, • DACLATASVIR, • LOPINAVIR, • NEVIRAPINE and • RILPIVIRINE—avoid concomitant use; plasma concentration of rifabutin increased by • ATAZANAVIR, • DARUNAVIR, • FOSAMPRENAVIR and • TIPRANAVIR (reduce dose of rifabutin); avoidance of rifampicin advised by manufacturer of • BOCEPREVIR (plasma concentration of boceprevir possibly reduced); rifabutin possibly reduces plasma concentration of • DACLATASVIR and SIMEPREVIR—manufacturer of daclatasvir and simeprevir advises avoid concomitant use; rifampicin significantly reduces plasma concentration of • DARUNAVIR, • FOSAMPRENAVIR and • TELAPREVIR—avoid concomitant use; rifampicin possibly reduces plasma concentration of

Rifamycins

- **Antivirals** (continued)
  - • DASABUVIR, • OMBITASVIR, • PARITAPREVIR and • TIPRANAVIR—avoid concomitant use; rifampicin reduces the plasma concentration of • DOLUTEGRAVIR (see under Dolutegravir, p. 387); plasma concentration of rifabutin reduced by EFAVIRENZ—increase dose of rifabutin; rifampicin reduces plasma concentration of • EFAVIRENZ—increase dose of efavirenz; rifabutin reduces plasma concentration of • ELVITEGRAVIR also plasma concentration of active metabolite of rifabutin increased—reduce dose of rifabutin; avoidance of rifampicin advised by manufacturer of • ELVITEGRAVIR, ETRAVIRINE, LEDIPASVIR, SOFOSBUVIR and ZIDOVUDINE; plasma concentration of both drugs reduced when rifabutin given with • ETRAVIRINE; rifampicin accelerates metabolism of • INDINAVIR (reduced plasma concentration—avoid concomitant use); plasma concentration of rifabutin increased by • INDINAVIR, also plasma concentration of indinavir decreased (reduce dose of rifabutin and increase dose of indinavir); avoidance of rifabutin advised by manufacturer of LEDIPASVIR, SOFOSBUVIR and • TELAPREVIR; rifampicin reduces plasma concentration of • MARAVIROC and • RALTEGRAVIR—consider increasing dose of maraviroc and raltegravir; plasma concentration of rifabutin possibly increased by NEVIRAPINE; rifabutin decreases plasma concentration of • RILPIVIRINE (increase dose of rilpivirine—consult rilpivirine product literature); rifampicin reduces plasma concentration of • RITONAVIR; plasma concentration of rifabutin increased by • RITONAVIR (increased risk of toxicity—reduce rifabutin dose); plasma concentration of rifabutin increased by • SAQUINAVIR (also plasma concentration of saquinavir reduced)—reduce rifabutin dose; rifampicin significantly reduces plasma concentration of • SAQUINAVIR, also risk of hepatotoxicity—avoid concomitant use; rifampicin reduces plasma concentration of • SIMEPREVIR—manufacturer of simeprevir advises avoid concomitant use
- **Anxiolytics and Hypnotics:** rifampicin accelerates metabolism of DIAZEPAM and ZALEPLON (reduced plasma concentration); rifampicin possibly accelerates metabolism of BENZODIAZEPINES (reduced plasma concentration); rifampicin possibly accelerates metabolism of BUSPIRONE; rifampicin accelerates metabolism of ZOLPIDEM (reduced plasma concentration and reduced effect); rifampicin significantly reduces plasma concentration of ZOPICLONE
- **Apremilast:** rifampicin reduces plasma concentration of • APREMILAST—avoid concomitant use
- **Aprepitant:** rifampicin reduces plasma concentration of APREPITANT
- **Atovaquone:** avoidance of concomitant rifabutin advised by manufacturer of ATOVAQUONE (plasma concentration of both drugs reduced); rifampicin reduces plasma concentration of • ATOVAQUONE (and concentration of rifampicin increased)—avoid concomitant use
- **Avanafil:** rifampicin possibly reduces plasma concentration of AVANAFIL—manufacturer of avanafil advises avoid concomitant use
- **Beta-blockers:** rifampicin accelerates metabolism of BISOPROLOL and PROPRANOLOL (plasma concentration significantly reduced); rifampicin reduces plasma concentration of CARVEDILOL, CELIPROLOL and METOPROLOL; rifampicin possibly reduces plasma concentration of *oral* TIMOLOL
- **Bosentan:** rifampicin reduces plasma concentration of • BOSENTAN—avoid concomitant use
- **Calcium-channel Blockers:** rifampicin possibly reduces plasma concentration of FELODIPINE; rifampicin possibly accelerates metabolism of • ISRADIPINE and • NICARDIPINE (possible significantly reduced plasma concentration); rifampicin accelerates metabolism of DILTIAZEM, NIFEDIPINE, • NIMODIPINE and • VERAPAMIL (plasma concentration significantly reduced)
- **Cannabis Extract:** rifampicin reduces plasma concentration of • CANNABIS EXTRACT—manufacturer of cannabis extract advises avoid concomitant use
- **Cardiac Glycosides:** rifampicin possibly reduces plasma concentration of DIGOXIN

Rifamycins (continued)

- Ciclosporin: rifampicin accelerates metabolism of ● CICLOSPORIN (reduced plasma concentration)
- Cobicistat: rifabutin reduces plasma concentration of ● COBICISTAT (adjust dose—consult product literature); rifampicin possibly reduces plasma concentration of ● COBICISTAT—manufacturer of cobicistat advises avoid concomitant use
- Corticosteroids: rifamycins accelerate metabolism of ● CORTICOSTEROIDS (reduced effect)
- Cytotoxics: rifampicin possibly reduces effects of BRENTUXIMAB VEDOTIN; rifampicin reduces plasma concentration of AFATINIB, RUXOLITINIB, SORAFENIB and ● TRABECTEDIN; rifabutin possibly decreases plasma concentration of AXITINIB (increase dose of axitinib—consult axitinib product literature); rifampicin decreases plasma concentration of AXITINIB (increase dose of axitinib—consult axitinib product literature); rifabutin possibly reduces plasma concentration of ● BOSUTINIB, CRIZOTINIB and PONATINIB—manufacturer of bosutinib, crizotinib and ponatinib advises avoid concomitant use; rifampicin reduces plasma concentration of ● BORTEZOMIB, ● BOSUTINIB, ● CABAZITAXEL, ● CRIZOTINIB, ● PONATINIB, ● REGORAFENIB and ● VANDETANIB—manufacturer of bortezomib, bosutinib, cabazitaxel, crizotinib, ponatinib, regorafenib and vandetanib advises avoid concomitant use; rifampicin reduces plasma concentration of ● CABOZANTINIB, ● GEFITINIB, ● IBRUTINIB, ● IDELALISIB, ● IMATINIB, ● NILOTINIB and ● NINTEDANIB—avoid concomitant use; avoidance of rifampicin advised by manufacturer of DABRAFENIB, ● LAPATINIB, ● OLAPARIB and VEMURAFENIB; rifampicin accelerates metabolism of ● DASATINIB (reduced plasma concentration—avoid concomitant use); rifampicin accelerates metabolism of ERLOTINIB and SUNITINIB (reduced plasma concentration); rifampicin reduces plasma concentration of ● EVEROLIMUS (avoid concomitant use or consider increasing the dose of everolimus—consult everolimus product literature); avoidance of rifabutin advised by manufacturer of ● CABAZITAXEL, ● LAPATINIB, ● OLAPARIB and VEMURAFENIB; rifampicin possibly reduces plasma concentration of ERIBULIN and ● PAZOPANIB; rifampicin reduces plasma concentration of active metabolite of ● TEMSIROLIMUS—avoid concomitant use; rifampicin possibly reduces plasma concentration of ● VINFLUNINE—manufacturer of vinflunine advises avoid concomitant use; avoidance of rifampicin advised by manufacturer of ● VISMODEGIB (plasma concentration of vismodegib possibly reduced)
- Deferasirox: rifampicin reduces plasma concentration of DEFERASIROX
- Diuretics: rifampicin reduces plasma concentration of ● EPLERENONE—avoid concomitant use
- Fosaprepitant: rifampicin reduces plasma concentration of FOSAPREPITANT
- Guanfacine: rifabutin possibly reduces plasma concentration of ● GUANFACINE—increase dose of guanfacine; rifampicin reduces plasma concentration of ● GUANFACINE—increase dose of guanfacine
- Hormone Antagonists: rifampicin reduces plasma concentration of ● ABIRATERONE—manufacturer of abiraterone advises avoid concomitant use; rifabutin possibly reduces plasma concentration of ● ABIRATERONE—manufacturer of abiraterone advises avoid concomitant use; rifampicin possibly reduces plasma concentration of EXEMESTANE; rifampicin accelerates metabolism of TAMOXIFEN (reduced plasma concentration)
- 5HT₃-receptor Antagonists: rifampicin accelerates metabolism of ONDANSETRON (reduced effect)
- Ivacaftor: rifabutin possibly reduces plasma concentration of ● IVACAFTOR—manufacturer of ivacaftor advises avoid concomitant use; rifampicin reduces plasma concentration of ● IVACAFTOR—manufacturer of ivacaftor advises avoid concomitant use
- Leflunomide: rifampicin possibly increases plasma concentration of active metabolite of LEFLUNOMIDE
- Lipid-regulating Drugs: rifampicin possibly reduces plasma concentration of ATORVASTATIN and SIMVASTATIN; rifampicin accelerates metabolism of FLUVASTATIN (reduced effect)

Rifamycins (continued)

- Macitentan: rifampicin reduces plasma concentration of ● MACITENTAN—avoid concomitant use
- Muscle Relaxants: rifampicin possibly reduces plasma concentration of TIZANIDINE
- Mycophenolate: rifampicin reduces plasma concentration of active metabolite of ● MYCOPHENOLATE
- Netupitant: rifampicin reduces plasma concentration of ● NETUPITANT—avoid concomitant use
- Oestrogens: rifamycins accelerate metabolism of ● OESTROGENS (reduced contraceptive effect with combined oral contraceptives, contraceptive patches, and vaginal rings—see Contraceptive Interactions in BNFC)
- Progestogens: rifamycins accelerate metabolism of ● PROGESTOGENS (reduced contraceptive effect with combined oral contraceptives, progestogen-only oral contraceptives, contraceptive patches, vaginal rings, etonogestrel-releasing implant, and emergency hormonal contraception—see Contraceptive Interactions in BNFC)
- Ranolazine: rifampicin reduces plasma concentration of ● RANOLAZINE—manufacturer of ranolazine advises avoid concomitant use
- Roflumilast: rifampicin inhibits effects of ● ROFLUMILAST (manufacturer of roflumilast advises avoid concomitant use)
- Sirolimus: rifabutin and rifampicin reduce plasma concentration of ● SIROLIMUS—avoid concomitant use
- Tacrolimus: rifabutin possibly reduces plasma concentration of TACROLIMUS; rifampicin reduces plasma concentration of ● TACROLIMUS
- Tadalafil: rifampicin reduces plasma concentration of ● TADALAFIL—manufacturer of tadalafil advises avoid concomitant use
- Teriflunomide: rifampicin reduces plasma concentration of TERIFLUNOMIDE
- Theophylline: rifampicin accelerates metabolism of THEOPHYLLINE (reduced plasma concentration)
- Thyroid Hormones: rifampicin accelerates metabolism of LEVOTHYROXINE (may increase requirements for levothyroxine in hypothyroidism)
- Tibolone: rifampicin accelerates metabolism of TIBOLONE (reduced plasma concentration)
- Ticagrelor: rifampicin reduces plasma concentration of ● TICAGRELOR
- Tolvaptan: rifampicin reduces plasma concentration of TOLVAPTAN
- Ulcer-healing Drugs: rifampicin accelerates metabolism of CIMETIDINE (reduced plasma concentration)
- Ulipristal: avoidance of rifampicin advised by manufacturer of ● ULIPRISTAL (contraceptive effect of ulipristal possibly reduced)
- Vaccines: antibacterials inactivate ORAL TYPHOID VACCINE—see under Typhoid Vaccine in BNFC

Rifaximin

NOTE Rifamycins interactions do not apply to rifaximin

- Anticoagulants: rifaximin possibly reduces anticoagulant effect of WARFARIN
- Ciclosporin: plasma concentration of rifaximin increased by ● CICLOSPORIN
- Vaccines: antibacterials inactivate ORAL TYPHOID VACCINE—see under Typhoid Vaccine in BNFC

Rilpivirine

- Analgesics: rilpivirine possibly reduces plasma concentration of METHADONE
- Antacids: manufacturer of rilpivirine advises give ANTACIDS 2 hours before or 4 hours after rilpivirine
- Antibacterials: manufacturer of rilpivirine advises avoid concomitant use with ● CLARITHROMYCIN and ● ERYTHROMYCIN (plasma concentration of rilpivirine possibly increased); plasma concentration of rilpivirine decreased by ● RIFABUTIN (increase dose of rilpivirine—consult rilpivirine product literature); plasma concentration of rilpivirine reduced by ● RIFAMPICIN—avoid concomitant use
- Anticoagulants: rilpivirine possibly increases plasma concentration of DABIGATRAN

Rilpivirine (continued)
- Antidepressants: manufacturer of rilpivirine advises avoid concomitant use with ● ST JOHN'S WORT (plasma concentration of rilpivirine possibly reduced)
- Antiepileptics: manufacturer of rilpivirine advises avoid concomitant use with ● CARBAMAZEPINE, ● FOSPHENYTOIN, ● OXCARBAZEPINE, ● PHENOBARBITAL, ● PHENYTOIN and ● PRIMIDONE (plasma concentration of rilpivirine possibly reduced)
- Antivirals: manufacturer of rilpivirine advises give DIDANOSINE 2 hours before or 4 hours after rilpivirine; avoidance of rilpivirine advised by manufacturer of NEVIRAPINE
- Calcium Salts: manufacturer of rilpivirine advises give CALCIUM SALTS 2 hours before or 4 hours after rilpivirine
- Corticosteroids: manufacturer of rilpivirine advises avoid concomitant use with ● DEXAMETHASONE (except when given as a single dose)
- Orlistat: absorption of rilpivirine possibly reduced by ● ORLISTAT
- Ulcer-healing Drugs: manufacturer of rilpivirine advises avoid concomitant use with ESOMEPRAZOLE, LANSOPRAZOLE, PANTOPRAZOLE and RABEPRAZOLE (plasma concentration of rilpivirine possibly reduced); plasma concentration of rilpivirine reduced by ● OMEPRAZOLE—avoid concomitant use; manufacturer of rilpivirine advises avoid HISTAMINE H₂-ANTAGONISTS for 12 hours before or 4 hours after rilpivirine—consult product literature

Riociguat
- Antacids: absorption of riociguat reduced by ANTACIDS (give at least 2 hours before or 1 hour after riociguat)
- Antifungals: manufacturer of riociguat advises avoid concomitant use with ITRACONAZOLE, KETOCONAZOLE and VORICONAZOLE
- Antivirals: manufacturer of riociguat advises avoid concomitant use with RITONAVIR
- Avanafil: possible enhanced hypotensive effect when riociguat given with ● AVANAFIL—avoid concomitant use
- Bosentan: plasma concentration of riociguat reduced by BOSENTAN
- Nicorandil: possible enhanced hypotensive effect when riociguat given with ● NICORANDIL—avoid concomitant use
- Nitrates: possible enhanced hypotensive effect when riociguat given with ● NITRATES—avoid concomitant use
- Sildenafil: enhanced hypotensive effect when riociguat given with ● SILDENAFIL—avoid concomitant use
- Tadalafil: possible enhanced hypotensive effect when riociguat given with ● TADALAFIL—avoid concomitant use
- Vardenafil: possible enhanced hypotensive effect when riociguat given with ● VARDENAFIL—avoid concomitant use

Risedronate Sodium *see* Bisphosphonates

Risperidone *see* Antipsychotics

Ritonavir
- Alpha-blockers: ritonavir possibly increases plasma concentration of ● ALFUZOSIN—avoid concomitant use
- Aminophylline: ritonavir accelerates metabolism of ● AMINOPHYLLINE (reduced plasma concentration)
- Analgesics: ritonavir possibly increases plasma concentration of NSAIDs and BUPRENORPHINE; ritonavir increases plasma concentration of ● DEXTROPROPOXYPHENE and ● PIROXICAM (risk of toxicity)—avoid concomitant use; ritonavir increases plasma concentration of ● ALFENTANIL and ● FENTANYL; ritonavir reduces plasma concentration of METHADONE; ritonavir possibly reduces plasma concentration of MORPHINE; ritonavir reduces plasma concentration of ● PETHIDINE, but increases plasma concentration of toxic metabolite of pethidine (avoid concomitant use)
- Anthelmintics: ritonavir possibly reduces plasma concentration of active metabolite of ● ALBENDAZOLE—consider increasing albendazole dose when given for systemic infections
- Anti-arrhythmics: ritonavir increases plasma concentration of ● AMIODARONE and ● PROPAFENONE (increased risk of ventricular arrhythmias—avoid concomitant use); ritonavir possibly increases plasma concentration of ● DISOPYRAMIDE (increased risk of toxicity); avoidance of ritonavir advised by manufacturer of ● DRONEDARONE; ritonavir possibly increases

Ritonavir
- Anti-arrhythmics (continued) plasma concentration of ● FLECAINIDE (increased risk of ventricular arrhythmias—avoid concomitant use)
- Antibacterials: ritonavir possibly increases plasma concentration of AZITHROMYCIN and ERYTHROMYCIN; ritonavir increases plasma concentration of ● CLARITHROMYCIN (reduce dose of clarithromycin in renal impairment); ritonavir increases plasma concentration of ● RIFABUTIN (increased risk of toxicity—reduce rifabutin dose); plasma concentration of ritonavir reduced by RIFAMPICIN; ritonavir possibly increases plasma concentration of BEDAQUILINE—manufacturer of ritonavir advises avoid concomitant use; ritonavir increases plasma concentration of DELAMANID; plasma concentration of both drugs increased when ritonavir given with ● FUSIDIC ACID—avoid concomitant use; avoidance of concomitant ritonavir in severe renal and hepatic impairment advised by manufacturer of ● TELITHROMYCIN
- Anticoagulants: ritonavir may enhance or reduce anticoagulant effect of ● WARFARIN; avoidance of ritonavir advised by manufacturer of APIXABAN; ritonavir possibly enhances anticoagulant effect of ● COUMARINS and ● PHENINDIONE; ritonavir increases plasma concentration of ● RIVAROXABAN—avoid concomitant use
- Antidepressants: ritonavir possibly reduces plasma concentration of PAROXETINE; ritonavir increases plasma concentration of ● TRAZODONE (increased risk of toxicity); ritonavir possibly increases plasma concentration of ● SSRIS and ● TRICYCLICS; plasma concentration of ritonavir reduced by ● ST JOHN'S WORT—avoid concomitant use
- Antidiabetics: ritonavir possibly increases plasma concentration of TOLBUTAMIDE
- Antiepileptics: ritonavir possibly increases plasma concentration of ● CARBAMAZEPINE; plasma concentration of ritonavir possibly reduced by FOSPHENYTOIN and PHENYTOIN, also plasma concentration of fosphenytoin and phenytoin possibly affected; ritonavir possibly reduces plasma concentration of LAMOTRIGINE, SODIUM VALPROATE and VALPROIC ACID
- Antifungals: ritonavir increases plasma concentration of ● KETOCONAZOLE (reduce dose of ketoconazole); plasma concentration of ritonavir increased by FLUCONAZOLE; combination of ritonavir with ● ITRACONAZOLE may increase plasma concentration of either drug (or both); ritonavir reduces plasma concentration of ● VORICONAZOLE—avoid concomitant use
- Antihistamines: ritonavir possibly increases plasma concentration of NON-SEDATING ANTIHISTAMINES
- Antimalarials: caution with ritonavir advised by manufacturer of ARTEMETHER WITH LUMEFANTRINE; plasma concentration of ritonavir possibly reduced by MEFLOQUINE; ritonavir increases plasma concentration of ● QUININE (increased risk of toxicity)
- Antimuscarinics: avoidance of ritonavir advised by manufacturer of DARIFENACIN and TOLTERODINE; manufacturer of fesoterodine advises dose reduction when ritonavir given with FESOTERODINE—consult fesoterodine product literature; ritonavir possibly increases plasma concentration of ● SOLIFENACIN—see under Solifenacin, in BNF
- Antipsychotics: ritonavir possibly increases plasma concentration of ● ANTIPSYCHOTICS; ritonavir possibly increases plasma concentration of ● ARIPIPRAZOLE (reduce dose of aripiprazole—consult aripiprazole product literature); manufacturer of ritonavir advises avoid concomitant use with ● CLOZAPINE (increased risk of toxicity); ritonavir possibly increases plasma concentration of ● LURASIDONE—avoid concomitant use; ritonavir reduces plasma concentration of OLANZAPINE—consider increasing dose of olanzapine; ritonavir increases plasma concentration of ● PIMOZIDE (increased risk of ventricular arrhythmias—avoid concomitant use); ritonavir possibly increases plasma concentration of ● QUETIAPINE—manufacturer of quetiapine advises avoid concomitant use
- Antivirals: plasma concentration of both drugs reduced when ritonavir given with ● BOCEPREVIR; manufacturer of ritonavir advises ritonavir and DIDANOSINE should be taken 2.5 hours apart; ritonavir increases the toxicity of ● EFAVIRENZ, monitor

Ritonavir
- Antivirals (continued)
liver function tests —manufacturer of *Atripla*® advises avoid concomitant use with *high-dose* ritonavir; ritonavir increases plasma concentration of INDINAVIR, MARAVIROC and ● SAQUINAVIR; ritonavir increases plasma concentration of ● SIMEPREVIR—manufacturer of simeprevir advises avoid concomitant use; ritonavir possibly reduces plasma concentration of TELAPREVIR
- Anxiolytics and Hypnotics: ritonavir possibly increases plasma concentration of ● ANXIOLYTICS AND HYPNOTICS; ritonavir possibly increases plasma concentration of ● ALPRAZOLAM, ● DIAZEPAM, ● FLURAZEPAM and ● ZOLPIDEM (risk of extreme sedation and respiratory depression—avoid concomitant use); ritonavir possibly increases plasma concentration of ● MIDAZOLAM (risk of prolonged sedation—avoid concomitant use of *oral* midazolam); ritonavir increases plasma concentration of BUSPIRONE (increased risk of toxicity)
▸ Aprepitant: ritonavir possibly increases plasma concentration of APREPITANT
- Atovaquone: ritonavir possibly reduces plasma concentration of ATOVAQUONE—manufacturer of atovaquone advises avoid concomitant use
- Avanafil: ritonavir significantly increases plasma concentration of ● AVANAFIL—avoid concomitant use
- Bosentan: ritonavir increases plasma concentration of ● BOSENTAN (consider reducing dose of bosentan)
▸ Bupropion: ritonavir reduces plasma concentration of BUPROPION
- Calcium-channel Blockers: ritonavir possibly increases plasma concentration of ● CALCIUM-CHANNEL BLOCKERS; ritonavir increases plasma concentration of ● AMLODIPINE (reduce dose of amlodipine); avoidance of ritonavir advised by manufacturer of LERCANIDIPINE
▸ Cardiac Glycosides: ritonavir possibly increases plasma concentration of DIGOXIN
- Ciclosporin: ritonavir increases plasma concentration of ● CICLOSPORIN
- Cilostazol: ritonavir possibly increases plasma concentration of ● CILOSTAZOL (see under Cilostazol, in BNF)
▸ Cobicistat: avoidance of ritonavir advised by manufacturer of COBICISTAT
- Colchicine: ritonavir possibly increases risk of ● COLCHICINE toxicity—suspend or reduce dose of colchicine (avoid concomitant use in hepatic or renal impairment)
- Corticosteroids: ritonavir possibly increases plasma concentration of ● CORTICOSTEROIDS—increased risk of adrenal supression; ritonavir possibly increases plasma concentration of ● BUDESONIDE (including *inhaled*, *intranasal*, and *rectal* budesonide)—increased risk of adrenal suppresion; ritonavir increases plasma concentration of *inhaled* and *intranasal* ● FLUTICASONE—increased risk of adrenal suppression; ritonavir increases plasma concentration of ● TRIAMCINOLONE *injection*—increased risk of adrenal suppression
- Cytotoxics: ritonavir increases the plasma concentration of AFATINIB—manufacturer of afatinib advises separating administration of ritonavir by 6 to 12 hours; ritonavir possibly increases plasma concentration of AXITINIB (reduce dose of axitinib—consult axitinib product literature); ritonavir possibly increases the plasma concentration of ● BOSUTINIB and ● CABAZITAXEL—manufacturer of bosutinib and cabazitaxel advises avoid or consider reducing dose of bosutinib and cabazitaxel; ritonavir possibly increases plasma concentration of CABOZANTINIB and VINBLASTINE; ritonavir possibly increases plasma concentration of ● CRIZOTINIB, ● EVEROLIMUS, NILOTINIB and ● VINFLUNINE—manufacturer of crizotinib, everolimus, nilotinib and vinflunine advises avoid concomitant use; avoidance of ritonavir advised by manufacturer of DASATINIB (plasma concentration of dasatinib possibly increased); ritonavir possibly increases the plasma concentration of ● IBRUTINIB—reduce dose of ibrutinib (see under Ibrutinib, in BNF); avoidance of ritonavir advised by manufacturer of ● LAPATINIB; ritonavir possibly increases plasma concentration of ● PAZOPANIB (reduce dose of pazopanib); ritonavir possibly increases plasma concentration of PONATINIB—consider reducing initial dose of ponatinib (see

Ritonavir
- Cytotoxics (continued)
under Ponatinib, in BNF); manufacturer of ruxolitinib advises dose reduction when ritonavir given with ● RUXOLITINIB— consult ruxolitinib product literature; ritonavir possibly increases plasma concentration of ● DOCETAXEL— manufacturer of docetaxel advises avoid concomitant use or consider reducing docetaxel dose; ritonavir increases plasma concentration of PACLITAXEL
- Dapoxetine: avoidance of ritonavir advised by manufacturer of ● DAPOXETINE (increased risk of toxicity)
- Diuretics: ritonavir increases plasma concentration of ● EPLERENONE—avoid concomitant use
- Domperidone: possible increased risk of ventricular arrhythmias when ritonavir given with ● DOMPERIDONE—avoid concomitant use
- Ergot Alkaloids: increased risk of ergotism when ritonavir given with ● ERGOT ALKALOIDS—avoid concomitant use
▸ Fosaprepitant: ritonavir possibly increases plasma concentration of FOSAPREPITANT
- Guanfacine: ritonavir possibly increases plasma concentration of ● GUANFACINE (halve dose of guanfacine)
- 5HT$_1$-receptor Agonists: ritonavir increases plasma concentration of ● ELETRIPTAN (risk of toxicity)—avoid concomitant use
- Ivabradine: ritonavir possibly increases plasma concentration of ● IVABRADINE—avoid concomitant use
- Lipid-regulating Drugs: ritonavir possibly increases plasma concentration of ATORVASTATIN (use lowest possible dose of atorvastatin); possible increased risk of myopathy when ritonavir given with ● ROSUVASTATIN—manufacturer of rosuvastatin advises avoid concomitant use; increased risk of myopathy when ritonavir given with ● SIMVASTATIN (avoid concomitant use); avoidance of ritonavir advised by manufacturer of ● LOMITAPIDE (plasma concentration of lomitapide possibly increased)
▸ Mirabegron: when given with ritonavir avoid or reduce dose of MIRABEGRON in hepatic or renal impairment—see Mirabegron, in BNF
- Oestrogens: ritonavir accelerates metabolism of ● OESTROGENS (reduced contraceptive effect with combined oral contraceptives, contraceptive patches, and vaginal rings—see Contraceptive Interactions in BNFC)
- Orlistat: absorption of ritonavir possibly reduced by ● ORLISTAT
- Ranolazine: ritonavir possibly increases plasma concentration of ● RANOLAZINE—manufacturer of ranolazine advises avoid concomitant use
▸ Riociguat: avoidance of ritonavir advised by manufacturer of RIOCIGUAT
- Sildenafil: ritonavir significantly increases plasma concentration of ● SILDENAFIL—avoid concomitant use of sildenafil for pulmonary arterial hypertension or reduce dose of sildenafil for erectile dysfunction (consult sildenafil product literature)
▸ Sympathomimetics: ritonavir possibly increases plasma concentration of DEXAMFETAMINE
- Sympathomimetics, Beta$_2$: manufacturer of ritonavir advises avoid concomitant use with SALMETEROL
- Tacrolimus: ritonavir possibly increases plasma concentration of ● TACROLIMUS
- Tadalafil: ritonavir increases plasma concentration of ● TADALAFIL—avoid concomitant use of tadalafil for pulmonary hypertension
- Theophylline: ritonavir accelerates metabolism of ● THEOPHYLLINE (reduced plasma concentration)
- Ticagrelor: ritonavir possibly increases plasma concentration of ● TICAGRELOR—manufacturer of ticagrelor advises avoid concomitant use
- Ulipristal: avoidance of ritonavir advised by manufacturer of ● ULIPRISTAL (contraceptive effect of ulipristal possibly reduced)
- Vardenafil: ritonavir increases plasma concentration of ● VARDENAFIL—avoid concomitant use

Rituximab
- Antipsychotics: avoid concomitant use of cytotoxics with ● CLOZAPINE (increased risk of agranulocytosis)

Rituximab (continued)
- Vaccines: risk of generalised infections when monoclonal antibodies given with live ● VACCINES—avoid concomitant use

Rivaroxaban
- Analgesics: increased risk of haemorrhage when anticoagulants given with *intravenous* ● DICLOFENAC (avoid concomitant use, including low-dose heparins); increased risk of haemorrhage when anticoagulants given with ● KETOROLAC (avoid concomitant use, including low-dose heparins)
- Anti-arrhythmics: manufacturer of rivaroxaban advises avoid concomitant use with DRONEDARONE
- Antibacterials: plasma concentration of rivaroxaban reduced by ● RIFAMPICIN—manufacturer of rivaroxaban advises monitor for signs of thrombosis
- Anticoagulants: increased risk of haemorrhage when rivaroxaban given with other ● ANTICOAGULANTS (avoid concomitant use except when switching with other anticoagulants or using heparin to maintain catheter patency); increased risk of haemorrhage when other anticoagulants given with ● APIXABAN, ● DABIGATRAN and ● EDOXABAN (avoid concomitant use except when switching with other anticoagulants or using heparin to maintain catheter patency)
- Antidepressants: plasma concentration of rivaroxaban possibly reduced by ● ST JOHN'S WORT—manufacturer of rivaroxaban advises monitor for signs of thrombosis
- Antiepileptics: plasma concentration of rivaroxaban possibly reduced by ● CARBAMAZEPINE, ● FOSPHENYTOIN, ● PHENOBARBITAL, ● PHENYTOIN and ● PRIMIDONE— manufacturer of rivaroxaban advises monitor for signs of thrombosis
- Antifungals: plasma concentration of rivaroxaban increased by ● KETOCONAZOLE—avoid concomitant use; manufacturer of rivaroxaban advises avoid concomitant use with ITRACONAZOLE, POSACONAZOLE and VORICONAZOLE
- Antivirals: manufacturer of rivaroxaban advises avoid concomitant use with ATAZANAVIR, DARUNAVIR, FOSAMPRENAVIR, INDINAVIR, SAQUINAVIR and TIPRANAVIR; manufacturers advise avoid concomitant use of rivaroxaban with LOPINAVIR; plasma concentration of rivaroxaban increased by ● RITONAVIR—avoid concomitant use
- Cobicistat: anticoagulant effect of rivaroxaban possibly enhanced by ● COBICISTAT—avoid concomitant use

Rivastigmine see Parasympathomimetics
Rizatriptan see 5HT₁-receptor Agonists (under HT)
Rocuronium see Muscle Relaxants
Roflumilast
Aminophylline: manufacturer of roflumilast advises avoid concomitant use with AMINOPHYLLINE
Antibacterials: effects of roflumilast inhibited by ● RIFAMPICIN (manufacturer of roflumilast advises avoid concomitant use)
Antidepressants: metabolism of roflumilast inhibited by FLUVOXAMINE
Antiepileptics: effects of roflumilast possibly inhibited by CARBAMAZEPINE, FOSPHENYTOIN, PHENOBARBITAL, PHENYTOIN and PRIMIDONE (manufacturer of roflumilast advises avoid concomitant use)
Theophylline: manufacturer of roflumilast advises avoid concomitant use with THEOPHYLLINE
Ulcer-healing Drugs: metabolism of roflumilast inhibited by CIMETIDINE
opinirole
Antibacterials: metabolism of ropinirole inhibited by CIPROFLOXACIN (increased plasma concentration)
Antipsychotics: manufacturer of ropinirole advises avoid concomitant use of ANTIPSYCHOTICS (antagonism of effect)
Memantine: effects of dopaminergics possibly enhanced by MEMANTINE
Methyldopa: antiparkinsonian effect of dopaminergics antagonised by METHYLDOPA
Metoclopramide: manufacturer of ropinirole advises avoid concomitant use of METOCLOPRAMIDE (antagonism of effect)
Oestrogens: plasma concentration of ropinirole increased by OESTROGENS

Ropivacaine
‣ Anti-arrhythmics: increased myocardial depression when ropivacaine given with ANTI-ARRHYTHMICS
‣ Antidepressants: metabolism of ropivacaine inhibited by FLUVOXAMINE—avoid prolonged administration of ropivacaine
Rosuvastatin see Statins
Rotavirus Vaccine see Vaccines
Rotigotine
‣ Antipsychotics: manufacturer of rotigotine advises avoid concomitant use of ANTIPSYCHOTICS (antagonism of effect)
‣ Memantine: effects of dopaminergics possibly enhanced by MEMANTINE
‣ Methyldopa: antiparkinsonian effect of dopaminergics antagonised by METHYLDOPA
‣ Metoclopramide: manufacturer of rotigotine advises avoid concomitant use of METOCLOPRAMIDE (antagonism of effect)
Rufinamide
● Antidepressants: anticonvulsant effect of antiepileptics possibly antagonised by MAOIs and ● TRICYCLIC-RELATED ANTIDEPRESSANTS (convulsive threshold lowered); anticonvulsant effect of antiepileptics antagonised by ● SSRIS and ● TRICYCLICS (convulsive threshold lowered)
‣ Antiepileptics: plasma concentration of both drugs possibly reduced when rufinamide given with CARBAMAZEPINE; plasma concentration of rufinamide possibly reduced by FOSPHENYTOIN and PHENYTOIN, also plasma concentration of fosphenytoin and phenytoin possibly increased; plasma concentration of rufinamide possibly reduced by PHENOBARBITAL and PRIMIDONE; plasma concentration of rufinamide possibly increased by SODIUM VALPROATE and VALPROIC ACID (reduce dose of rufinamide)
● Antimalarials: anticonvulsant effect of antiepileptics antagonised by ● MEFLOQUINE
● Antipsychotics: anticonvulsant effect of antiepileptics antagonised by ● ANTIPSYCHOTICS (convulsive threshold lowered)
● Oestrogens: rufinamide accelerates metabolism of ● OESTROGENS (reduced contraceptive effect with combined oral contraceptives, contraceptive patches, and vaginal rings—see Contraceptive Interactions in BNFC)
● Orlistat: possible increased risk of convulsions when antiepileptics given with ● ORLISTAT
● Progestogens: rufinamide accelerates metabolism of ● PROGESTOGENS (reduced contraceptive effect with combined oral contraceptives, progestogen-only oral contraceptives, contraceptive patches, vaginal rings, etonogestrel-releasing implant, and emergency hormonal contraception—see Contraceptive Interactions in BNFC)
Ruxolitinib
● Antibacterials: manufacturer of ruxolitinib advises dose reduction when ruxolitinib given with ● CLARITHROMYCIN and ● TELITHROMYCIN—consult ruxolitinib product literature; plasma concentration of ruxolitinib reduced by RIFAMPICIN
● Antifungals: manufacturer of ruxolitinib advises dose reduction when ruxolitinib given with ● FLUCONAZOLE, ● ITRACONAZOLE, ● KETOCONAZOLE, ● POSACONAZOLE and ● VORICONAZOLE— consult ruxolitinib product literature
● Antipsychotics: avoid concomitant use of cytotoxics with ● CLOZAPINE (increased risk of agranulocytosis)
● Antivirals: manufacturer of ruxolitinib advises dose reduction when ruxolitinib given with ● BOCEPREVIR, ● INDINAVIR, ● LOPINAVIR, ● RITONAVIR, ● SAQUINAVIR and ● TELAPREVIR— consult ruxolitinib product literature
Sacubitril
● ACE Inhibitors: manufacturer of sacubitril advises avoid ● ACE INHIBITORS for 36 hours before or after sacubitril
‣ Diuretics: sacubitril reduces plasma concentration of FUROSEMIDE
‣ Lipid-regulating Drugs: sacubitril increases plasma concentration of ATORVASTATIN
St John's Wort
‣ Aminophylline: St John's wort possibly reduces plasma concentration of AMINOPHYLLINE
‣ Analgesics: St John's wort possibly reduces plasma concentration of METHADONE

St John's Wort (continued)
- Anti-arrhythmics: St John's wort possibly reduces plasma concentration of ● DRONEDARONE—avoid concomitant use
- Antibacterials: St John's wort possibly reduces plasma concentration of BEDAQUILINE—manufacturer of bedaquiline advises avoid concomitant use; St John's wort reduces plasma concentration of ● TELITHROMYCIN (avoid during and for 2 weeks after St John's wort)
- Anticoagulants: St John's wort possibly reduces plasma concentration of ● APIXABAN—manufacturer of apixaban advises avoid concomitant use when given for treatment of deep-vein thrombosis or pulmonary embolism; St John's wort reduces anticoagulant effect of ● COUMARINS (avoid concomitant use); St John's wort possibly reduces plasma concentration of DABIGATRAN—manufacturer of dabigatran advises avoid concomitant use; St John's wort reduces plasma concentration of ● EDOXABAN; St John's wort possibly reduces plasma concentration of ● RIVAROXABAN—manufacturer of rivaroxaban advises monitor for signs of thrombosis
- Antidepressants: possible increased serotonergic effects when St John's wort given with DULOXETINE, VENLAFAXINE or VORTIOXETINE; St John's wort reduces plasma concentration of AMITRIPTYLINE; increased serotonergic effects when St John's wort given with ● SSRIs—avoid concomitant use
- Antiepileptics: St John's wort possibly reduces plasma concentration of CARBAMAZEPINE; St John's wort possibly reduces plasma concentration of ● PHENYTOIN, ● PHENOBARBITAL, ● PHENYTOIN and ● PRIMIDONE—avoid concomitant use
- Antifungals: St John's wort reduces plasma concentration of ● VORICONAZOLE—avoid concomitant use
- Antimalarials: avoidance of antidepressants advised by manufacturer of ● ARTEMETHER WITH LUMEFANTRINE and ● ARTENIMOL WITH PIPERAQUINE
- Antimuscarinics: St John's wort possibly reduces plasma concentration of active metabolite of ● FESOTERODINE—manufacturer of fesoterodine advises avoid concomitant use
- Antipsychotics: St John's wort possibly reduces plasma concentration of ● ARIPIPRAZOLE (avoid concomitant use or consider increasing the dose of aripiprazole—consult aripiprazole product literature); St John's wort possibly reduces plasma concentration of ● LURASIDONE—avoid concomitant use
- Antivirals: St John's wort reduces plasma concentration of ● ATAZANAVIR, ● DARUNAVIR, ● EFAVIRENZ, ● FOSAMPRENAVIR, ● INDINAVIR, ● LOPINAVIR, ● NEVIRAPINE, ● RITONAVIR and ● SAQUINAVIR—avoid concomitant use; St John's wort possibly reduces plasma concentration of DACLATASVIR, ● DASABUVIR, ● OMBITASVIR, ● PARITAPREVIR and ● SIMEPREVIR—manufacturer of daclatasvir, dasabuvir, ombitasvir, paritaprevir and simeprevir advises avoid concomitant use; St John's wort possibly reduces the plasma concentration of ● DOLUTEGRAVIR (see under Dolutegravir, p. 387); avoidance of St John's wort advised by manufacturer of ● ELVITEGRAVIR, ETRAVIRINE, LEDIPASVIR, SOFOSBUVIR and ● TELAPREVIR; St John's wort possibly reduces plasma concentration of ● MARAVIROC and ● TIPRANAVIR—avoid concomitant use; avoidance of St John's wort advised by manufacturer of ● RILPIVIRINE (plasma concentration of rilpivirine possibly reduced)
- Anxiolytics and Hypnotics: St John's wort possibly reduces plasma concentration of *oral* MIDAZOLAM
- Apremilast: St John's wort possibly reduces plasma concentration of ● APREMILAST—avoid concomitant use
- Aprepitant: avoidance of St John's wort advised by manufacturer of ● APREPITANT
- Atomoxetine: possible increased risk of convulsions when antidepressants given with ATOMOXETINE
- Calcium-channel Blockers: St John's wort possibly reduces plasma concentration of AMLODIPINE and FELODIPINE; St John's wort reduces plasma concentration of NIFEDIPINE; St John's wort significantly reduces plasma concentration of ● VERAPAMIL
- Cannabis Extract: St John's wort possibly reduces plasma concentration of ● CANNABIS EXTRACT—manufacturer of cannabis extract advises avoid concomitant use

St John's Wort (continued)
- Cardiac Glycosides: St John's wort reduces plasma concentration of ● DIGOXIN—avoid concomitant use
- Ciclosporin: St John's wort reduces plasma concentration of ● CICLOSPORIN—avoid concomitant use
- Cobicistat: St John's wort possibly reduces plasma concentration of ● COBICISTAT—manufacturer of cobicistat advises avoid concomitant use
- Cytotoxics: St John's wort possibly reduces plasma concentration of AXITINIB—consider increasing dose of axitinib; St John's wort possibly reduces plasma concentration of BORTEZOMIB, ● BOSUTINIB, CABOZANTINIB, CRIZOTINIB, EVEROLIMUS, ● IBRUTINIB, ● IDELALISIB, PONATINIB and ● VINFLUNINE—manufacturer of bortezomib, bosutinib, cabozantinib, crizotinib, everolimus, ibrutinib, idelalisib, ponatinib and vinflunine advises avoid concomitant use; avoidance of St John's wort advised by manufacturer of ● CABAZITAXEL, DABRAFENIB, GEFITINIB, ● LAPATINIB, ● OLAPARIB and VEMURAFENIB; St John's wort possibly reduces plasma concentration of ● IMATINIB—avoid concomitant use; avoidance of St John's wort advised by manufacturer of VANDETANIB and VISMODEGIB (plasma concentration of vandetanib and vismodegib possibly reduced); St John's wort possibly reduces plasma concentration of ● ERIBULIN; St John's wort accelerates metabolism of ● IRINOTECAN (reduced plasma concentration—avoid concomitant use)
- Dapoxetine: possible increased risk of serotonergic effects when St John's wort given with ● DAPOXETINE (manufacturer of dapoxetine advises St John's wort should not be started until 1 week after stopping dapoxetine, avoid dapoxetine for 2 weeks after stopping St John's wort)
- Diuretics: St John's wort reduces plasma concentration of ● EPLERENONE—avoid concomitant use
- Fingolimod: St John's wort possibly reduces plasma concentration of FINGOLIMOD—manufacturer of fingolimod advises avoid concomitant use
- Fosaprepitant: avoidance of St John's wort advised by manufacturer of ● FOSAPREPITANT
- Guanfacine: St John's wort possibly reduces plasma concentration of ● GUANFACINE—increase dose of guanfacine
- Hormone Antagonists: St John's wort possibly reduces plasma concentration of ● ABIRATERONE—manufacturer of abiraterone advises avoid concomitant use
- 5HT₁-receptor Agonists: increased serotonergic effects when St John's wort given with ● 5HT₁ AGONISTS—avoid concomitant use
- Ivabradine: St John's wort reduces plasma concentration of IVABRADINE—avoid concomitant use
- Ivacaftor: St John's wort possibly reduces plasma concentration of ● IVACAFTOR—manufacturer of ivacaftor advises avoid concomitant use
- Lipid-regulating Drugs: St John's wort reduces plasma concentration of SIMVASTATIN
- Macitentan: avoidance of St John's wort advised by manufacturer of MACITENTAN
- Oestrogens: St John's wort reduces contraceptive effect of ● OESTROGENS (avoid concomitant use)
- Progestogens: St John's wort reduces contraceptive effect of ● PROGESTOGENS (avoid concomitant use)
- Tacrolimus: St John's wort reduces plasma concentration of ● TACROLIMUS—avoid concomitant use
- Theophylline: St John's wort possibly reduces plasma concentration of THEOPHYLLINE
- Ulcer-healing Drugs: St John's wort possibly reduces plasma concentration of OMEPRAZOLE
- Uliprital: avoidance of St John's wort advised by manufacturer of ● ULIPRISTAL (contraceptive effect of ulipristal possibly reduced)

Salbutamol *see* Sympathomimetics, Beta₂
Salmeterol *see* Sympathomimetics, Beta₂
Saquinavir
- Analgesics: increased risk of ventricular arrhythmias when saquinavir given with ● ALFENTANIL, ● FENTANYL or ● METHADONE—avoid concomitant use
- Anti-arrhythmics: increased risk of ventricular arrhythmias when saquinavir given with ● AMIODARONE, ● DISOPYRAMIDE,

Saquinavir

- **Anti-arrhythmics** (continued)
  - ● DRONEDARONE, ● FLECAINIDE, ● LIDOCAINE or ● PROPAFENONE—avoid concomitant use
- **Antibacterials:** plasma concentration of both drugs possibly increased when saquinavir given with ● CLARITHROMYCIN (increased risk of ventricular arrhythmias); increased risk of ventricular arrhythmias when saquinavir given with ● DAPSONE, ● ERYTHROMYCIN or ● MOXIFLOXACIN—avoid concomitant use; saquinavir increases plasma concentration of ● RIFABUTIN (also plasma concentration of saquinavir reduced)—reduce rifabutin dose; plasma concentration of saquinavir significantly reduced by ● RIFAMPICIN, also risk of hepatotoxicity—avoid concomitant use; increased risk of ventricular arrhythmias when saquinavir given with ● DELAMANID; plasma concentration of both drugs may increase when saquinavir given with FUSIDIC ACID; avoidance of saquinavir advised by manufacturer of ● TELITHROMYCIN (risk of ventricular arrhythmias)
- **Anticoagulants:** saquinavir possibly enhances anticoagulant effect of WARFARIN; avoidance of saquinavir advised by manufacturer of APIXABAN and RIVAROXABAN
- **Antidepressants:** increased risk of ventricular arrhythmias when saquinavir given with ● TRAZODONE or ● TRICYCLICS—avoid concomitant use; plasma concentration of saquinavir reduced by ● ST JOHN'S WORT—avoid concomitant use
- **Antiepileptics:** plasma concentration of saquinavir possibly reduced by CARBAMAZEPINE, FOSPHENYTOIN, ● PHENOBARBITAL, PHENYTOIN and ● PRIMIDONE
- **Antifungals:** plasma concentration of saquinavir increased by ● KETOCONAZOLE—manufacturer of ketoconazole advises avoid concomitant use; plasma concentration of saquinavir possibly increased by IMIDAZOLES and TRIAZOLES
- **Antihistamines:** increased risk of ventricular arrhythmias when saquinavir given with ● MIZOLASTINE—avoid concomitant use
- **Antimalarials:** caution with saquinavir advised by manufacturer of ARTEMETHER WITH LUMEFANTRINE; avoidance of saquinavir advised by manufacturer of ● ARTENIMOL WITH PIPERAQUINE (possible risk of ventricular arrhythmias); increased risk of ventricular arrhythmias when saquinavir given with ● QUININE—avoid concomitant use
- **Antimuscarinics:** avoidance of saquinavir advised by manufacturer of DARIFENACIN and TOLTERODINE; manufacturer of fesoterodine advises dose reduction when saquinavir given with FESOTERODINE—consult fesoterodine product literature
- **Antipsychotics:** increased risk of ventricular arrhythmias when saquinavir given with ● CLOZAPINE, ● HALOPERIDOL or ● PHENOTHIAZINES—avoid concomitant use; saquinavir possibly increases plasma concentration of ● ARIPIPRAZOLE (reduce dose of aripiprazole—consult aripiprazole product literature); saquinavir possibly increases plasma concentration of ● LURASIDONE—avoid concomitant use; saquinavir possibly increases plasma concentration of ● PIMOZIDE (increased risk of ventricular arrhythmias—avoid concomitant use); saquinavir possibly increases plasma concentration of ● QUETIAPINE—manufacturer of quetiapine advises avoid concomitant use
- **Antivirals:** increased risk of ventricular arrhythmias when saquinavir given with ● ATAZANAVIR or ● LOPINAVIR—avoid concomitant use; saquinavir reduces plasma concentration of DARUNAVIR—avoid concomitant use; plasma concentration of saquinavir significantly reduced by EFAVIRENZ; plasma concentration of saquinavir increased by INDINAVIR and ● RITONAVIR; saquinavir increases plasma concentration of ● MARAVIROC (consider reducing dose of maraviroc); avoidance of saquinavir advised by manufacturer of PARITAPREVIR; plasma concentration of saquinavir reduced by TIPRANAVIR
- **Anxiolytics and Hypnotics:** saquinavir increases plasma concentration of ● MIDAZOLAM (risk of prolonged sedation—avoid concomitant use of *oral* midazolam)
- **Avanafil:** saquinavir possibly increases plasma concentration of ● AVANAFIL—manufacturer of avanafil advises avoid concomitant use
- **Beta-blockers:** increased risk of ventricular arrhythmias when saquinavir given with ● SOTALOL—avoid concomitant use

Saquinavir (continued)

- **Ciclosporin:** plasma concentration of both drugs increased when saquinavir given with ● CICLOSPORIN
- **Corticosteroids:** plasma concentration of saquinavir possibly reduced by DEXAMETHASONE
- **Cytotoxics:** saquinavir possibly increases the plasma concentration of AFATINIB—manufacturer of afatinib advises separating administration of saquinavir by 6 to 12 hours; saquinavir possibly increases plasma concentration of AXITINIB (reduce dose of axitinib—consult axitinib product literature); saquinavir possibly increases the plasma concentration of ● BOSUTINIB and ● CABAZITAXEL—manufacturer of bosutinib and cabazitaxel advises avoid or consider reducing dose of bosutinib and cabazitaxel; saquinavir possibly increases plasma concentration of ● CRIZOTINIB and ● EVEROLIMUS—manufacturer of crizotinib and everolimus advises avoid concomitant use; saquinavir possibly increases the plasma concentration of ● IBRUTINIB—reduce dose of ibrutinib (see under Ibrutinib, in BNF); avoidance of saquinavir advised by manufacturer of ● LAPATINIB and ● OLAPARIB; increased risk of ventricular arrhythmias when saquinavir given with ● PAZOPANIB—avoid concomitant use; saquinavir possibly increases plasma concentration of PONATINIB—consider reducing initial dose of ponatinib (see under Ponatinib, in BNF); manufacturer of ruxolitinib advises dose reduction when saquinavir given with ● RUXOLITINIB—consult ruxolitinib product literature; saquinavir possibly increases plasma concentration of ● DOCETAXEL—manufacturer of docetaxel advises avoid concomitant use or consider reducing docetaxel dose
- **Dapoxetine:** avoidance of saquinavir advised by manufacturer of ● DAPOXETINE (increased risk of toxicity)
- **Diuretics:** saquinavir increases plasma concentration of EPLERENONE (reduce dose of eplerenone)
- **Domperidone:** possible increased risk of ventricular arrhythmias when saquinavir given with ● DOMPERIDONE—avoid concomitant use
- **Ergot Alkaloids:** increased risk of ergotism when saquinavir given with ● ERGOTAMINE—avoid concomitant use
- **Guanfacine:** saquinavir possibly increases plasma concentration of ● GUANFACINE (halve dose of guanfacine)
- **Lipid-regulating Drugs:** possible increased risk of myopathy when saquinavir given with ATORVASTATIN; possible increased risk of myopathy when saquinavir given with ● ROSUVASTATIN—manufacturer of rosuvastatin advises avoid concomitant use; increased risk of myopathy when saquinavir given with ● SIMVASTATIN (avoid concomitant use); avoidance of saquinavir advised by manufacturer of ● LOMITAPIDE (plasma concentration of lomitapide possibly increased)
- **Orlistat:** absorption of saquinavir possibly reduced by ● ORLISTAT
- **Pentamidine Isetionate:** increased risk of ventricular arrhythmias when saquinavir given with ● PENTAMIDINE ISETIONATE—avoid concomitant use
- **Ranolazine:** saquinavir possibly increases plasma concentration of ● RANOLAZINE—manufacturer of ranolazine advises avoid concomitant use
- **Sildenafil:** increased risk of ventricular arrhythmias when saquinavir given with ● SILDENAFIL—avoid concomitant use
- **Tacrolimus:** saquinavir increases plasma concentration of ● TACROLIMUS (consider reducing dose of tacrolimus)
- **Tadalafil:** increased risk of ventricular arrhythmias when saquinavir given with ● TADALAFIL—avoid concomitant use
- **Ulcer-healing Drugs:** plasma concentration of saquinavir possibly increased by CIMETIDINE; plasma concentration of saquinavir possibly increased by ● ESOMEPRAZOLE, ● LANSOPRAZOLE, ● PANTOPRAZOLE and ● RABEPRAZOLE—manufacturer of saquinavir advises avoid concomitant use; plasma concentration of saquinavir increased by ● OMEPRAZOLE—manufacturer of saquinavir advises avoid concomitant use
- **Vardenafil:** increased risk of ventricular arrhythmias when saquinavir given with ● VARDENAFIL—avoid concomitant use

Saxagliptin see Antidiabetics

Secukinumab
- Antipsychotics: avoid concomitant use of cytotoxics with • CLOZAPINE (increased risk of agranulocytosis)
- Vaccines: risk of generalised infections when monoclonal antibodies given with live • VACCINES—avoid concomitant use

Selegiline
NOTE Selegiline is a MAO-B inhibitor
- Analgesics: hyperpyrexia and CNS toxicity reported when selegiline given with • PETHIDINE (avoid concomitant use); manufacturer of selegiline advises avoid concomitant use with OPIOID ANALGESICS
- Antidepressants: manufacturer of selegiline advises avoid concomitant use with CITALOPRAM and ESCITALOPRAM; increased risk of hypertension and CNS excitation when selegiline given with • FLUOXETINE (selegiline should not be started until 5 weeks after stopping fluoxetine, avoid fluoxetine for 2 weeks after stopping selegiline); increased risk of hypertension and CNS excitation when selegiline given with • FLUVOXAMINE, • SERTRALINE or • VENLAFAXINE (selegiline should not be started until 1 week after stopping fluvoxamine, sertraline or venlafaxine, avoid fluvoxamine, sertraline or venlafaxine for 2 weeks after stopping selegiline); increased risk of hypertension and CNS excitation when selegiline given with • PAROXETINE (selegiline should not be started until 2 weeks after stopping paroxetine, avoid paroxetine for 2 weeks after stopping selegiline); enhanced hypotensive effect when selegiline given with • MAOIs—manufacturer of selegiline advises avoid concomitant use; avoid concomitant use of selegiline with • MOCLOBEMIDE; CNS toxicity reported when selegiline given with • TRICYCLICS; risk of CNS excitation and hypertension when selegiline given with • VORTIOXETINE
▸ Dopaminergics: selegiline enhances effects and increases toxicity of CO-BENELDOPA, CO-CARELDOPA or LEVODOPA (reduce dose of co-beneldopa, co-careldopa or levodopa); max. dose of 10 mg selegiline advised by manufacturer of ENTACAPONE if used concomitantly
▸ 5HT₁-receptor Agonists: manufacturer of selegiline advises avoid concomitant use with 5HT₁ AGONISTS
▸ Memantine: effects of dopaminergics and selegiline possibly enhanced by MEMANTINE
▸ Methyldopa: antiparkinsonian effect of dopaminergics antagonised by METHYLDOPA
- Oestrogens: plasma concentration of selegiline increased by • OESTROGENS—manufacturer of selegiline advises avoid concomitant use
- Progestogens: plasma concentration of selegiline increased by • PROGESTOGENS—manufacturer of selegiline advises avoid concomitant use
- Sympathomimetics: manufacturer of selegiline advises avoid concomitant use with SYMPATHOMIMETICS; risk of hypertensive crisis when selegiline given with • DOPAMINE

Selenium
▸ Eltrombopag: selenium possibly reduces absorption of ELTROMBOPAG (give at least 4 hours apart)
▸ Vitamins: absorption of selenium possibly reduced by ASCORBIC ACID (give at least 4 hours apart)

Sertraline see Antidepressants, SSRI

Sevelamer
▸ Antibacterials: sevelamer reduces absorption of CIPROFLOXACIN (give at least 2 hours before or 4 hours after ciprofloxacin)
▸ Ciclosporin: sevelamer possibly reduces plasma concentration of CICLOSPORIN
▸ Mycophenolate: sevelamer possibly reduces plasma concentration of MYCOPHENOLATE
▸ Tacrolimus: sevelamer possibly reduces plasma concentration of TACROLIMUS
▸ Thyroid Hormones: sevelamer possibly reduces absorption of LEVOTHYROXINE
▸ Vitamins: sevelamer reduces absorption of CALCITRIOL (give at least 1 hour before or 3 hours after sevelamer)

Sevoflurane see Anaesthetics, General

Sildenafil
- Alpha-blockers: enhanced hypotensive effect when sildenafil given with • ALPHA-BLOCKERS (avoid alpha-blockers for 4 hours after sildenafil)—when patient is stable on the alpha blocker initiate sildenafil at the lowest possible dose

Sildenafil (continued)
▸ Anti-arrhythmics: avoidance of sildenafil advised by manufacturer of DISOPYRAMIDE (risk of ventricular arrhythmias)
- Antibacterials: plasma concentration of sildenafil increased by • CLARITHROMYCIN—consider reducing initial dose of sildenafil for erectile dysfunction or reduce sildenafil dose frequency to once daily for pulmonary hypertension; plasma concentration of sildenafil increased by ERYTHROMYCIN—reduce initial dose of sildenafil for erectile dysfunction or reduce sildenafil dose frequency to twice daily for pulmonary hypertension; plasma concentration of sildenafil possibly increased by • TELITHROMYCIN—consider reducing initial dose of sildenafil for erectile dysfunction or reduce sildenafil dose frequency to once daily for pulmonary hypertension
- Antifungals: plasma concentration of sildenafil increased by • KETOCONAZOLE—reduce initial dose of sildenafil for erectile dysfunction and avoid concomitant use of sildenafil for pulmonary hypertension; plasma concentration of sildenafil increased by ITRACONAZOLE—reduce initial dose of sildenafil
- Antivirals: plasma concentration of sildenafil reduced by ETRAVIRINE; plasma concentration of sildenafil possibly increased by FOSAMPRENAVIR; plasma concentration of sildenafil increased by • INDINAVIR—reduce initial dose of sildenafil; plasma concentration of sildenafil significantly increased by • RITONAVIR—avoid concomitant use of sildenafil for pulmonary arterial hypertension or reduce dose of sildenafil for erectile dysfunction (consult sildenafil product literature); increased risk of ventricular arrhythmias when sildenafil given with • SAQUINAVIR—avoid concomitant use; avoidance of sildenafil advised by manufacturer of • TELAPREVIR; avoidance of sildenafil for pulmonary arterial hypertension advised by manufacturer of TIPRANAVIR
▸ Bosentan: plasma concentration of sildenafil reduced by BOSENTAN, also plasma concentration of bosentan increased
▸ Calcium-channel Blockers: enhanced hypotensive effect when sildenafil given with AMLODIPINE
- Cobicistat: plasma concentration of sildenafil possibly increased by • COBICISTAT—manufacturer of cobicistat advises avoid concomitant use of sildenafil for pulmonary arterial hypertension or reduce dose of sildenafil for erectile dysfunction—consult cobicistat product literature
▸ Cytotoxics: avoidance of sildenafil for pulmonary arterial hypertension advised by manufacturer of IDELALISIB
▸ Dapoxetine: avoidance of sildenafil advised by manufacturer of DAPOXETINE
▸ Grapefruit Juice: plasma concentration of sildenafil possibly increased by GRAPEFRUIT JUICE
- Nicorandil: sildenafil significantly enhances hypotensive effect of • NICORANDIL (avoid concomitant use)
- Nitrates: sildenafil significantly enhances hypotensive effect of • NITRATES (avoid concomitant use)
▸ Riociguat: enhanced hypotensive effect when sildenafil given with • RIOCIGUAT—avoid concomitant use
▸ Ulcer-healing Drugs: plasma concentration of sildenafil increased by CIMETIDINE—consider reducing dose of sildenafil for erectile dysfunction

Siltuximab
- Antipsychotics: avoid concomitant use of cytotoxics with • CLOZAPINE (increased risk of agranulocytosis)
- Vaccines: risk of generalised infections when monoclonal antibodies given with live • VACCINES—avoid concomitant use

Simeprevir
- Anti-arrhythmics: possible increased risk of bradycardia when simeprevir (with sofosbuvir) given with • AMIODARONE—see under Amiodarone, in BNF
- Antibacterials: plasma concentration of simeprevir possibly increased by • CLARITHROMYCIN and • TELITHROMYCIN—manufacturer of simeprevir advises avoid concomitant use; plasma concentration of both drugs increased when simeprevir given with • ERYTHROMYCIN—manufacturer of simeprevir advises avoid concomitant use; plasma concentration of simeprevir possibly reduced by RIFABUTIN—manufacturer of simeprevir advises avoid concomitant use; plasma concentration of simeprevir reduced by • RIFAMPICIN—manufacturer of simeprevir advises avoid concomitant use

Simeprevir (continued)

- Antidepressants: plasma concentration of simeprevir possibly reduced by • ST JOHN'S WORT—manufacturer of simeprevir advises avoid concomitant use
- Antiepileptics: plasma concentration of simeprevir possibly reduced by • CARBAMAZEPINE, • FOSPHENYTOIN, • OXCARBAZEPINE, • PHENOBARBITAL, • PHENYTOIN and • PRIMIDONE—manufacturer of simeprevir advises avoid concomitant use
- Antifungals: plasma concentration of simeprevir advises avoid concomitant use with • KETOCONAZOLE; plasma concentration of simeprevir possibly increased by • FLUCONAZOLE, • ITRACONAZOLE, • POSACONAZOLE and • VORICONAZOLE—manufacturer of simeprevir advises avoid concomitant use
- Antivirals: plasma concentration of both drugs increased when simeprevir given with • DARUNAVIR—manufacturer of simeprevir advises avoid concomitant use; plasma concentration of simeprevir reduced by EFAVIRENZ; manufacturer of simeprevir advises avoid concomitant use with ETRAVIRINE; plasma concentration of both drugs increased when simeprevir given with LEDIPASVIR—manufacturer of ledipasvir advises avoid concomitant use; plasma concentration of simeprevir possibly reduced by • NEVIRAPINE—manufacturer of simeprevir advises avoid concomitant use; plasma concentration of simeprevir increased by • RITONAVIR—manufacturer of simeprevir advises avoid concomitant use
- Anxiolytics and Hypnotics: simeprevir increases plasma concentration of *oral* MIDAZOLAM
- Cardiac Glycosides: simeprevir increases plasma concentration of DIGOXIN
- Cobicistat: plasma concentration of simeprevir possibly increased by • COBICISTAT—manufacturer of simeprevir advises avoid concomitant use
- Corticosteroids: plasma concentration of simeprevir possibly reduced by DEXAMETHASONE—manufacturer of simeprevir advises avoid concomitant use
- Lipid-regulating Drugs: simeprevir increases plasma concentration of ATORVASTATIN, ROSUVASTATIN and SIMVASTATIN (consider reducing dose of atorvastatin, rosuvastatin and simvastatin)

Simvastatin *see* Statins

Sirolimus

- Anti-arrhythmics: caution with sirolimus advised by manufacturer of DRONEDARONE
- Antibacterials: plasma concentration of sirolimus increased by • CLARITHROMYCIN and • TELITHROMYCIN—avoid concomitant use; plasma concentration of both drugs increased when sirolimus given with • ERYTHROMYCIN; plasma concentration of sirolimus reduced by RIFABUTIN and RIFAMPICIN—avoid concomitant use
- Antifungals: plasma concentration of sirolimus increased by • ITRACONAZOLE, • KETOCONAZOLE and • VORICONAZOLE—avoid concomitant use; plasma concentration of sirolimus increased by MICAFUNGIN and MICONAZOLE; plasma concentration of sirolimus possibly increased by FLUCONAZOLE and POSACONAZOLE
- Antivirals: plasma concentration of sirolimus possibly increased by ATAZANAVIR and LOPINAVIR; plasma concentration of sirolimus increased by BOCEPREVIR (increased risk of toxicity—reduce sirolimus dose); plasma concentration of both drugs increased when sirolimus given with TELAPREVIR (reduce dose of sirolimus)
- Calcium-channel Blockers: plasma concentration of sirolimus possibly increased by NICARDIPINE; plasma concentration of sirolimus increased by DILTIAZEM; plasma concentration of both drugs increased when sirolimus given with • VERAPAMIL
- Ciclosporin: plasma concentration of sirolimus increased by CICLOSPORIN
- Cytotoxics: caution with sirolimus advised by manufacturer of CRIZOTINIB
- Grapefruit Juice: plasma concentration of sirolimus increased by • GRAPEFRUIT JUICE—avoid concomitant use

Sitagliptin *see* Antidiabetics

Smallpox Vaccine *see* Vaccines

Sodium Aurothiomalate

- ACE Inhibitors: flushing and hypotension reported when sodium aurothiomalate given with • ACE INHIBITORS
- Penicillamine: increased risk of haematological toxicity when sodium aurothiomalate given with • PENICILLAMINE—see under Penicillamine, in BNF

Sodium Benzoate

▹ Antiepileptics: effects of sodium benzoate possibly reduced by SODIUM VALPROATE and VALPROIC ACID
▹ Antipsychotics: effects of sodium benzoate possibly reduced by HALOPERIDOL
▹ Corticosteroids: effects of sodium benzoate possibly reduced by CORTICOSTEROIDS

Sodium Bicarbonate *see* Antacids

Sodium Citrate

▹ Antibacterials: avoid concomitant use of sodium citrate with METHENAMINE
▹ Ulcer-healing Drugs: avoidance of sodium citrate advised by manufacturer of SUCRALFATE

Sodium Clodronate *see* Bisphosphonates

Sodium Feredetate *see* Iron salts

Sodium Nitroprusside *see* Vasodilator Antihypertensives

Sodium Oxybate

- Analgesics: effects of sodium oxybate enhanced by • OPIOID ANALGESICS (avoid concomitant use)
▹ Antidepressants: increased risk of side-effects when sodium oxybate given with TRICYCLICS
- Antiepileptics: manufacturer of sodium oxybate advises avoid concomitant use with PHENOBARBITAL and PRIMIDONE; plasma concentration of sodium oxybate increased by • SODIUM VALPROATE and • VALPROIC ACID (see under Sodium Oxybate, in BNF)
▹ Antipsychotics: effects of sodium oxybate possibly enhanced by ANTIPSYCHOTICS
- Anxiolytics and Hypnotics: effects of sodium oxybate enhanced by • BENZODIAZEPINES (avoid concomitant use)

Sodium Phenylbutyrate

▹ Antiepileptics: effects of sodium phenylbutyrate possibly reduced by SODIUM VALPROATE and VALPROIC ACID
▹ Antipsychotics: effects of sodium phenylbutyrate possibly reduced by HALOPERIDOL
▹ Corticosteroids: effects of sodium phenylbutyrate possibly reduced by CORTICOSTEROIDS

Sodium Stibogluconate

- Antifungals: possible increased risk of arrhythmias when sodium stibogluconate given before • AMPHOTERICIN—manufacturer of sodium stibogluconate advises giving 14 days apart

Sodium Valproate

▹ Analgesics: effects of sodium valproate enhanced by ASPIRIN
- Antibacterials: metabolism of sodium valproate possibly inhibited by ERYTHROMYCIN (increased plasma concentration); avoidance of sodium valproate advised by manufacturer of • PIVMECILLINAM; plasma concentration of sodium valproate reduced by CARBAPENEMS—avoid concomitant use
▹ Anticoagulants: sodium valproate possibly enhances anticoagulant effect of COUMARINS
- Antidepressants: anticonvulsant effect of antiepileptics possibly antagonised by MAOIs and • TRICYCLIC-RELATED ANTIDEPRESSANTS (convulsive threshold lowered); anticonvulsant effect of antiepileptics antagonised by • SSRIS and • TRICYCLICS (convulsive threshold lowered)
- Antiepileptics: plasma concentration of sodium valproate reduced by CARBAMAZEPINE, also plasma concentration of active metabolite of carbamazepine increased; sodium valproate possibly increases plasma concentration of ETHOSUXIMIDE; sodium valproate increases or possibly decreases plasma concentration of FOSPHENYTOIN and PHENYTOIN, also plasma concentration of sodium valproate reduced; sodium valproate increases plasma concentration of • LAMOTRIGINE (increased risk of toxicity—reduce lamotrigine dose); sodium valproate sometimes reduces plasma concentration of an active metabolite of OXCARBAZEPINE; sodium valproate increases plasma concentration of PHENOBARBITAL and PRIMIDONE (also plasma concentration of sodium valproate reduced); sodium valproate possibly

A1

Interactions | Appendix 1

Sodium Valproate

- Antiepileptics (continued)
increases plasma concentration of RUFINAMIDE (reduce dose of rufinamide); hyperammonaemia and CNS toxicity reported when sodium valproate given with TOPIRAMATE
- Antimalarials: anticonvulsant effect of antiepileptics antagonised by ● MEFLOQUINE
- Antipsychotics: anticonvulsant effect of antiepileptics antagonised by ● ANTIPSYCHOTICS (convulsive threshold lowered); sodium valproate possibly increases or decreases plasma concentration of CLOZAPINE; increased risk of side-effects including neutropenia when sodium valproate given with ● OLANZAPINE
▹ Antivirals: plasma concentration of sodium valproate possibly reduced by RITONAVIR; sodium valproate possibly increases plasma concentration of ZIDOVUDINE (increased risk of toxicity)
▹ Anxiolytics and Hypnotics: plasma concentration of sodium valproate possibly increased by CLOBAZAM; increased risk of side-effects when sodium valproate given with CLONAZEPAM; sodium valproate possibly increases plasma concentration of DIAZEPAM and LORAZEPAM
▹ Bupropion: sodium valproate inhibits the metabolism of BUPROPION
▹ Cytotoxics: sodium valproate increases plasma concentration of TEMOZOLOMIDE
▹ Guanfacine: plasma concentration of sodium valproate increased by GUANFACINE
▹ Lipid-regulating Drugs: absorption of sodium valproate possibly reduced by COLESTYRAMINE
▹ Oestrogens: plasma concentration of sodium valproate possibly reduced by ETHINYLESTRADIOL
▹ Orlistat: possible increased risk of convulsions when antiepileptics given with ● ORLISTAT
▹ Sodium Benzoate: sodium valproate possibly reduces effects of SODIUM BENZOATE
▹ Sodium Oxybate: sodium valproate increases the plasma concentration of ● SODIUM OXYBATE (see under Sodium Oxybate, in BNF)
▹ Sodium Phenylbutyrate: sodium valproate possibly reduces effects of SODIUM PHENYLBUTYRATE
▹ Ulcer-healing Drugs: metabolism of sodium valproate inhibited by ● CIMETIDINE (increased plasma concentration)

Sofosbuvir

- Anti-arrhythmics: possible increased risk of bradycardia when sofosbuvir given with ● AMIODARONE—see under Amiodarone, in BNF
▹ Antibacterials: manufacturer of sofosbuvir advises avoid concomitant use with RIFABUTIN and RIFAMPICIN
▹ Antidepressants: manufacturer of sofosbuvir advises avoid concomitant use with ST JOHN'S WORT
▹ Antiepileptics: manufacturer of sofosbuvir advises avoid concomitant use with CARBAMAZEPINE, FOSPHENYTOIN, OXCARBAZEPINE, PHENOBARBITAL, PHENYTOIN and PRIMIDONE

Solifenacin see Antimuscarinics

Somatropin

▹ Corticosteroids: growth-promoting effect of somatropin may be inhibited by CORTICOSTEROIDS
▹ Oestrogens: increased doses of somatropin may be needed when given with OESTROGENS (when used as oral replacement therapy)

Sorafenib

▹ Antibacterials: bioavailability of sorafenib reduced by NEOMYCIN; plasma concentration of sorafenib reduced by RIFAMPICIN
- Anticoagulants: sorafenib possibly enhances anticoagulant effect of ● COUMARINS
- Antipsychotics: avoid concomitant use of cytotoxics with ● CLOZAPINE (increased risk of agranulocytosis)
- Antivirals: avoidance of sorafenib advised by manufacturer of ● BOCEPREVIR
▹ Cytotoxics: sorafenib increases plasma concentration of DOCETAXEL and DOXORUBICIN; sorafenib possibly increases plasma concentration of IRINOTECAN

Sotalol see Beta-blockers

Spironolactone see Diuretics

Statins

▹ Antacids: absorption of rosuvastatin reduced by ANTACIDS
- Anti-arrhythmics: increased risk of myopathy when simvastatin given with ● AMIODARONE (see under Simvastatin, p. 125); plasma concentration of rosuvastatin increased by ● DRONEDARONE—adjust dose of rosuvastatin (consult product literature); increased risk of myopathy when simvastatin given with ● DRONEDARONE; plasma concentration of atorvastatin possibly increased by DRONEDARONE
- Antibacterials: possible increased risk of myopathy when atorvastatin or simvastatin given with ● AZITHROMYCIN; plasma concentration of atorvastatin and pravastatin increased by ● CLARITHROMYCIN; increased risk of myopathy when simvastatin given with ● CLARITHROMYCIN, ● ERYTHROMYCIN or ● TELITHROMYCIN (avoid concomitant use); plasma concentration of rosuvastatin reduced by ERYTHROMYCIN; possible increased risk of myopathy when atorvastatin given with ERYTHROMYCIN; plasma concentration of pravastatin increased by ERYTHROMYCIN; plasma concentration of atorvastatin and simvastatin possibly reduced by RIFAMPICIN; metabolism of fluvastatin accelerated by RIFAMPICIN (reduced effect); increased risk of myopathy when statins given with ● DAPTOMYCIN (preferably avoid concomitant use); risk of myopathy and rhabdomyolysis when statins given with ● FUSIDIC ACID—avoid concomitant use and for 7 days after last fusidic acid dose; possible increased risk of myopathy when pravastatin given with TELITHROMYCIN; increased risk of myopathy when atorvastatin given with ● TELITHROMYCIN (avoid concomitant use)
- Anticoagulants: atorvastatin may transiently reduce anticoagulant effect of WARFARIN; rosuvastatin possibly enhances anticoagulant effect of ● COUMARINS and ● PHENINDIONE; simvastatin can enhance the anticoagulant effect of COUMARINS; fluvastatin enhances anticoagulant effect of ● COUMARINS
▹ Antidepressants: plasma concentration of simvastatin reduced by ST JOHN'S WORT
▹ Antidiabetics: fluvastatin possibly increases plasma concentration of GLIBENCLAMIDE
- Antiepileptics: plasma concentration of simvastatin reduced by ● CARBAMAZEPINE and ESLICARBAZEPINE—consider increasing dose of simvastatin; plasma concentration of rosuvastatin reduced by ESLICARBAZEPINE; combination of fluvastatin with FOSPHENYTOIN or PHENYTOIN may increase plasma concentration of either drug (or both)
- Antifungals: possible increased risk of myopathy when atorvastatin given with ● KETOCONAZOLE—manufacturer of ketoconazole advises avoid concomitant use; increased risk of myopathy when simvastatin given with ● ITRACONAZOLE, ● KETOCONAZOLE or ● POSACONAZOLE (avoid concomitant use); possible increased risk of myopathy when simvastatin given with ● FLUCONAZOLE or ● MICONAZOLE; possible increased risk of myopathy when atorvastatin given with ● FLUCONAZOLE or IMIDAZOLES; plasma concentration of fluvastatin increased by FLUCONAZOLE—possible increased risk of myopathy; plasma concentration of rosuvastatin increased by ● ITRACONAZOLE—adjust dose of rosuvastatin (consult product literature); increased risk of myopathy when atorvastatin given with ● ITRACONAZOLE, ● POSACONAZOLE or VORICONAZOLE; increased risk of myopathy when simvastatin given with ● VORICONAZOLE
- Antivirals: increased risk of myopathy when simvastatin given with ● ATAZANAVIR, ● INDINAVIR, ● RITONAVIR or ● SAQUINAVIR (avoid concomitant use); possible increased risk of myopathy when atorvastatin or pravastatin given with ● ATAZANAVIR; plasma concentration of rosuvastatin increased by ● ATAZANAVIR, ● DARUNAVIR, ● LOPINAVIR and ● TIPRANAVIR—adjust dose of rosuvastatin (consult product literature); plasma concentration of pravastatin increased by BOCEPREVIR; plasma concentration of atorvastatin increased by BOCEPREVIR (reduce dose of atorvastatin); manufacturers advise avoid concomitant use of simvastatin with ● BOCEPREVIR and ● TELAPREVIR; plasma concentration of rosuvastatin increased by DACLATASVIR; plasma concentration of pravastatin possibly increased by DARUNAVIR (use lowest possible dose of pravastatin); possible increased risk of myopathy when atorvastatin given with DARUNAVIR, FOSAMPRENAVIR,

Statins

- **Antivirals** (continued)
  INDINAVIR, LOPINAVIR or SAQUINAVIR; plasma concentration of rosuvastatin increased by • DASABUVIR and • PARITAPREVIR (reduce dose of rosuvastatin—see under Rosuvastatin, in BNF); avoidance of atorvastatin and simvastatin advised by manufacturer of • DASABUVIR; plasma concentration of atorvastatin, pravastatin and simvastatin reduced by EFAVIRENZ; plasma concentration of atorvastatin possibly reduced by ETRAVIRINE; possible increased risk of myopathy when rosuvastatin given with • FOSAMPRENAVIR, • INDINAVIR, • RITONAVIR and • SAQUINAVIR—manufacturer of rosuvastatin advises avoid concomitant use; possible increased risk of myopathy when simvastatin given with • FOSAMPRENAVIR or • LOPINAVIR—avoid concomitant use; possible increased risk of myopathy when atorvastatin, fluvastatin and simvastatin given with • LEDIPASVIR—manufacturer of ledipasvir advises consider reducing dose of atorvastatin, fluvastatin and simvastatin; avoidance of rosuvastatin advised by manufacturer of • LEDIPASVIR; avoidance of atorvastatin and simvastatin advised by manufacturer of • OMBITASVIR; plasma concentration of pravastatin increased by • PARITAPREVIR (reduce dose of pravastatin); avoidance of atorvastatin, fluvastatin and simvastatin advised by manufacturer of • PARITAPREVIR; plasma concentration of atorvastatin possibly increased by RITONAVIR (use lowest possible dose of atorvastatin); plasma concentration of atorvastatin, rosuvastatin and simvastatin increased by SIMEPREVIR (consider reducing dose of atorvastatin, rosuvastatin and simvastatin); avoidance of atorvastatin advised by manufacturer of • TELAPREVIR; increased risk of myopathy when atorvastatin given with • TIPRANAVIR (see under Atorvastatin, p. 123); plasma concentration of simvastatin possibly increased by • TIPRANAVIR—avoid concomitant use
- **Anxiolytics and Hypnotics:** atorvastatin increases plasma concentration of *intravenous* MIDAZOLAM
- **Bosentan:** plasma concentration of simvastatin reduced by BOSENTAN
- **Calcium-channel Blockers:** possible increased risk of myopathy when simvastatin given with • AMLODIPINE and • DILTIAZEM (see under Simvastatin, p. 125); plasma concentration of atorvastatin increased by DILTIAZEM—possible increased risk of myopathy; atorvastatin increases plasma concentration of • VERAPAMIL, also possible increased risk of myopathy (consider reducing dose of atorvastatin); increased risk of myopathy when simvastatin given with • VERAPAMIL (see under Simvastatin, p. 125)
- **Cardiac Glycosides:** atorvastatin possibly increases plasma concentration of DIGOXIN
- **Ciclosporin:** increased risk of myopathy when rosuvastatin or simvastatin given with • CICLOSPORIN (avoid concomitant use); increased risk of myopathy when atorvastatin given with • CICLOSPORIN (see under Atorvastatin, p. 123); increased risk of myopathy when fluvastatin or pravastatin given with • CICLOSPORIN
- **Clopidogrel:** plasma concentration of rosuvastatin increased by • CLOPIDOGREL—adjust dose of rosuvastatin (consult product literature)
- **Cobicistat:** plasma concentration of atorvastatin possibly increased by COBICISTAT—manufacturer of cobicistat advises reduce dose of atorvastatin; avoidance of simvastatin advised by manufacturer of • COBICISTAT
- **Colchicine:** possible increased risk of myopathy when statins given with • COLCHICINE
- **Cytotoxics:** plasma concentration of simvastatin possibly increased by DASATINIB; avoidance of simvastatin advised by manufacturer of IDELALISIB; plasma concentration of simvastatin increased by IMATINIB
- **Eltrombopag:** plasma concentration of rosuvastatin increased by • ELTROMBOPAG—adjust dose of rosuvastatin (consult product literature)
- **Grapefruit Juice:** plasma concentration of atorvastatin possibly increased by GRAPEFRUIT JUICE; plasma concentration of simvastatin increased by • GRAPEFRUIT JUICE—avoid concomitant use

Statins (continued)

- **Hormone Antagonists:** possible increased risk of myopathy when simvastatin given with • DANAZOL—avoid concomitant use
- **Lipid-regulating Drugs:** possible increased risk of myopathy when simvastatin given with • BEZAFIBRATE (see under Simvastatin, p. 125); possible increased risk of myopathy when simvastatin given with • CIPROFIBRATE (see under Simvastatin, in BNF); when given with statins reduce maximum dose of FENOFIBRATE—see under Fenofibrate, p. 122; increased risk of myopathy when atorvastatin, fluvastatin or pravastatin given with • GEMFIBROZIL (preferably avoid concomitant use); increased risk of myopathy when simvastatin given with • GEMFIBROZIL (avoid concomitant use); plasma concentration of rosuvastatin increased by • EZETIMIBE—adjust dose of rosuvastatin (consult product literature); increased risk of myopathy when statins given with • FIBRATES; increased risk of myopathy when rosuvastatin given with • FIBRATES (see under Rosuvastatin, p. 124); plasma concentration of simvastatin increased by • LOMITAPIDE (see under Simvastatin, in BNF); plasma concentration of atorvastatin increased by LOMITAPIDE—manufacturer of lomitapide advises reduce dose of atorvastatin by half or separate administration by 12 hours; increased risk of myopathy when statins given with • NICOTINIC ACID (applies to lipid regulating doses of nicotinic acid)
- ▹ **Oestrogens:** atorvastatin and rosuvastatin increase plasma concentration of ETHINYLESTRADIOL
- ▹ **Progestogens:** atorvastatin increases plasma concentration of NORETHISTERONE; rosuvastatin increases plasma concentration of active metabolite of NORGESTIMATE; rosuvastatin increases plasma concentration of NORGESTREL
- **Ranolazine:** plasma concentration of simvastatin increased by • RANOLAZINE (see under Simvastatin, in BNF)
- ▹ **Retinoids:** plasma concentration of simvastatin reduced by ALITRETINOIN
- ▹ **Sacubitril:** plasma concentration of atorvastatin increased by SACUBITRIL
- **Teriflunomide:** plasma concentration of rosuvastatin increased by • TERIFLUNOMIDE (consider reducing dose of rosuvastatin)
- **Ticagrelor:** plasma concentration of simvastatin increased by • TICAGRELOR (increased risk of toxicity)

Stavudine

- **Antivirals:** increased risk of side-effects when stavudine given with • DIDANOSINE; increased risk of toxicity when stavudine given with • RIBAVIRIN; effects of stavudine possibly inhibited by • ZIDOVUDINE (manufacturers advise avoid concomitant use)
- **Cytotoxics:** effects of stavudine possibly inhibited by DOXORUBICIN; increased risk of toxicity when stavudine given with • HYDROXYCARBAMIDE—avoid concomitant use
- **Orlistat:** absorption of stavudine possibly reduced by • ORLISTAT

Stiripentol

- **Antidepressants:** anticonvulsant effect of antiepileptics possibly antagonised by MAOIs and • TRICYCLIC-RELATED ANTIDEPRESSANTS (convulsive threshold lowered); anticonvulsant effect of antiepileptics antagonised by • SSRIS and • TRICYCLICS (convulsive threshold lowered)
- **Antiepileptics:** stiripentol increases plasma concentration of • CARBAMAZEPINE, • FOSPHENYTOIN, • PHENOBARBITAL, • PHENYTOIN and • PRIMIDONE
- **Antimalarials:** anticonvulsant effect of antiepileptics antagonised by • MEFLOQUINE
- **Antipsychotics:** anticonvulsant effect of antiepileptics antagonised by • ANTIPSYCHOTICS (convulsive threshold lowered)
- ▹ **Anxiolytics and Hypnotics:** stiripentol increases plasma concentration of CLOBAZAM
- **Orlistat:** possible increased risk of convulsions when antiepileptics given with • ORLISTAT

Streptomycin see Aminoglycosides

Strontium Ranelate
▸ Antibacterials: strontium ranelate reduces absorption of QUINOLONES and TETRACYCLINES (manufacturer of strontium ranelate advises avoid concomitant use)

Sucralfate
▸ Aminophylline: sucralfate possibly reduces absorption of AMINOPHYLLINE (give at least 2 hours apart)
▸ Antibacterials: sucralfate reduces absorption of CIPROFLOXACIN (give at least 2 hours before or 4 hours after ciprofloxacin); sucralfate reduces absorption of LEVOFLOXACIN, NORFLOXACIN and OFLOXACIN (give at least 2 hours apart); sucralfate reduces absorption of MOXIFLOXACIN (give at least 6 hours apart); sucralfate reduces absorption of TETRACYCLINES
● Anticoagulants: sucralfate possibly reduces absorption of ● COUMARINS (reduced anticoagulant effect)
● Antiepileptics: sucralfate reduces absorption of ● FOSPHENYTOIN and ● PHENYTOIN
▸ Antifungals: sucralfate reduces absorption of KETOCONAZOLE
▸ Antipsychotics: sucralfate reduces absorption of SULPIRIDE
▸ Cardiac Glycosides: sucralfate possibly reduces absorption of CARDIAC GLYCOSIDES
● Potassium Salts: manufacturer of sucralfate advises avoid concomitant use with POTASSIUM CITRATE
▸ Sodium Citrate: manufacturer of sucralfate advises avoid concomitant use with SODIUM CITRATE
▸ Theophylline: sucralfate possibly reduces absorption of THEOPHYLLINE (give at least 2 hours apart)
▸ Thyroid Hormones: sucralfate reduces absorption of LEVOTHYROXINE
▸ Ulcer-healing Drugs: sucralfate possibly reduces absorption of LANSOPRAZOLE

Sucroferric Oxyhydroxide *see* Iron Salts

Sugammadex
▸ Antibacterials: response to sugammadex possibly reduced by FUSIDIC ACID
▸ Progestogens: sugammadex possibly reduces plasma concentration of PROGESTOGENS—manufacturer of sugammadex advises additional contraceptive precautions

Sulfadiazine *see* Sulfonamides

Sulfadoxine *see* Sulfonamides

Sulfamethoxazole *see* Sulfonamides

Sulfasalazine
▸ Cardiac Glycosides: sulfasalazine possibly reduces absorption of DIGOXIN
▸ Folates: sulfasalazine possibly reduces absorption of FOLIC ACID

Sulfinpyrazone
▸ Aminophylline: sulfinpyrazone reduces plasma concentration of AMINOPHYLLINE
▸ Analgesics: effects of sulfinpyrazone antagonised by ASPIRIN
▸ Antibacterials: sulfinpyrazone reduces excretion of NITROFURANTOIN (increased risk of toxicity); sulfinpyrazone reduces excretion of PENICILLINS; effects of sulfinpyrazone antagonised by PYRAZINAMIDE
● Anticoagulants: increased risk of bleeding when sulfinpyrazone given with APIXABAN; sulfinpyrazone enhances anticoagulant effect of ● COUMARINS; possible increased risk of bleeding when sulfinpyrazone given with ● DABIGATRAN
● Antidiabetics: sulfinpyrazone enhances effects of ● SULFONYLUREAS
● Antiepileptics: sulfinpyrazone increases plasma concentration of ● FOSPHENYTOIN and ● PHENYTOIN
▸ Calcium-channel Blockers: sulfinpyrazone reduces plasma concentration of VERAPAMIL
● Ciclosporin: sulfinpyrazone reduces plasma concentration of ● CICLOSPORIN
▸ Theophylline: sulfinpyrazone reduces plasma concentration of THEOPHYLLINE

Sulfonamides
▸ Anaesthetics, General: sulfonamides enhance effects of THIOPENTAL
● Anaesthetics, Local: effects of sulfonamides possibly inhibited by ● CHLOROPROCAINE (manufacturer of chloroprocaine advises avoid concomitant use); increased risk of methaemoglobinaemia when sulfonamides given with PRILOCAINE

Sulfonamides (continued)
▸ Anti-arrhythmics: possible increased risk of ventricular arrhythmias when sulfamethoxazole (as co-trimoxazole) given with AMIODARONE—manufacturer of amiodarone advises avoid concomitant use of co-trimoxazole
● Antibacterials: increased risk of crystalluria when sulfonamides given with ● METHENAMINE
● Anticoagulants: sulfonamides enhance anticoagulant effect of ● COUMARINS; sulfonamides possibly inhibit metabolism of PHENINDIONE
▸ Antidiabetics: sulfonamides rarely enhance the effects of SULFONYLUREAS
▸ Antiepileptics: sulfonamides possibly increase plasma concentration of FOSPHENYTOIN and PHENYTOIN
▸ Antimalarials: increased antifolate effect when sulfonamides given with ● PYRIMETHAMINE
● Antipsychotics: avoid concomitant use of sulfonamides with ● CLOZAPINE (increased risk of agranulocytosis)
● Azathioprine: increased risk of haematological toxicity when sulfamethoxazole (as co-trimoxazole) given with ● AZATHIOPRINE
● Ciclosporin: increased risk of nephrotoxicity when sulfonamides given with ● CICLOSPORIN; sulfadiazine possibly reduces plasma concentration of ● CICLOSPORIN
● Cytotoxics: increased risk of haematological toxicity when sulfamethoxazole (as co-trimoxazole) given with ● MERCAPTOPURINE; sulfonamides increase risk of METHOTREXATE toxicity; increased risk of severe bone marrow depression (fatalities reported) and other haematological toxicites when sulfamethoxazole (as co-trimoxazole) given with ● METHOTREXATE
▸ Potassium Aminobenzoate: effects of sulfonamides inhibited by POTASSIUM AMINOBENZOATE
● Tacrolimus: possible increased risk of nephrotoxicity when sulfamethoxazole given with ● TACROLIMUS
▸ Vaccines: antibacterials inactivate ORAL TYPHOID VACCINE—see under Typhoid Vaccine in BNFC

Sulfonylureas *see* Antidiabetics

Sulindac *see* NSAIDs

Sulpiride *see* Antipsychotics

Sumatriptan *see* 5HT$_1$-receptor Agonists (under HT)

Sunitinib
▸ Antibacterials: metabolism of sunitinib accelerated by RIFAMPICIN (reduced plasma concentration)
▸ Antifungals: metabolism of sunitinib inhibited by KETOCONAZOLE (increased plasma concentration)
● Antipsychotics: avoid concomitant use of cytotoxics with ● CLOZAPINE (increased risk of agranulocytosis)
● Antivirals: avoidance of sunitinib advised by manufacturer of ● BOCEPREVIR

Suxamethonium *see* Muscle Relaxants

Sympathomimetics
● Adrenergic Neurone Blockers: ephedrine, isometheptene, metaraminol, methylphenidate, noradrenaline (norepinephrine), oxymetazoline, phenylephrine, pseudoephedrine and xylometazoline antagonise hypotensive effect of ● ADRENERGIC NEURONE BLOCKERS; manufacturer of midodrine advises avoid concomitant use with GUANETHIDINE; dexamfetamine and lisdexamfetamine antagonise hypotensive effect of ● GUANETHIDINE; increased risk of hypertension when adrenaline (epinephrine) given with ● GUANETHIDINE
▸ Alcohol: effects of methylphenidate possibly enhanced by ALCOHOL
▸ Alpha$_2$-adrenoceptor Stimulants: avoidance of sympathomimetics advised by manufacturer of APRACLONIDINE
● Alpha-blockers: effects of midodrine possibly antagonised by ALPHA-BLOCKERS; avoid concomitant use of adrenaline (epinephrine) or dopamine with ● TOLAZOLINE
▸ Aminophylline: avoidance of ephedrine in children advised by manufacturer of AMINOPHYLLINE
● Anaesthetics, General: avoidance of sympathomimetics advised by manufacturer of ● ISOFLURANE (risk of ventricular arrhythmias); increased risk of hypertension when methylphenidate given with ● VOLATILE LIQUID GENERAL ANAESTHETICS; increased risk of arrhythmias when adrenaline

Sympathomimetics

- **Anaesthetics, General** (continued)
  (epinephrine) or noradrenaline (norepinephrine) given with
  ● VOLATILE LIQUID GENERAL ANAESTHETICS
- ▸ **Antacids:** absorption of pseudoephedrine possibly increased by
  ALUMINIUM HYDROXIDE
- ● **Anticoagulants:** methylphenidate possibly enhances
  anticoagulant effect of ● COUMARINS
- ● **Antidepressants:** risk of hypertensive crisis when
  dexamfetamine, ephedrine, isometheptene,
  lisdexamfetamine, metaraminol, methylphenidate,
  phenylephrine or pseudoephedrine given with ● MAOIS, avoid
  dexamfetamine, ephedrine, isometheptene,
  lisdexamfetamine, metaraminol, methylphenidate,
  phenylephrine or pseudoephedrine for at least 2 weeks after
  stopping MAOIS; manufacturer of midodrine advises avoid
  concomitant use with MAOIS and TRICYCLICS; risk of
  hypertensive crisis when adrenaline (epinephrine),
  dobutamine, dopamine or noradrenaline (norepinephrine) or
  xylometazoline given with ● MAOIS; risk of hypertensive crisis
  when oxymetazoline given with ● MAOIS, some manufacturers
  advise avoid oxymetazoline for at least 2 weeks after stopping
  MAOIS; risk of hypertensive crisis when sympathomimetics
  given with ● MOCLOBEMIDE; methylphenidate possibly inhibits
  metabolism of SSRIS and TRICYCLICS; increased risk of
  hypertension and arrhythmias when noradrenaline
  (norepinephrine) or phenylephrine given with ● TRICYCLICS;
  increased risk of hypertension and arrhythmias when
  adrenaline (epinephrine) given with ● TRICYCLICS (but local
  anaesthetics with adrenaline appear to be safe)
- ▸ **Antiepileptics:** methylphenidate increases plasma
  concentration of FOSPHENYTOIN and PHENYTOIN;
  methylphenidate possibly increases plasma concentration of
  PHENOBARBITAL and PRIMIDONE
- ▸ **Antihistamines:** manufacturer of midodrine advises avoid
  concomitant use with ANTIHISTAMINES
- ● **Antipsychotics:** hypertensive effect of sympathomimetics
  antagonised by ANTIPSYCHOTICS; effects of lisdexamfetamine
  possibly reduced by CHLORPROMAZINE; dexamfetamine
  possibly antagonises antipsychotic effects of
  CHLORPROMAZINE; methylphenidate possibly increases side-
  effects of RISPERIDONE
- ▸ **Antivirals:** plasma concentration of dexamfetamine possibly
  increased by RITONAVIR
- ● **Beta-blockers:** increased risk of severe hypertension and
  bradycardia when adrenaline (epinephrine) given with non-
  cardioselective ● BETA-BLOCKERS, also response to adrenaline
  (epinephrine) may be reduced; increased risk of severe
  hypertension and bradycardia when dobutamine given with
  non-cardioselective ● BETA-BLOCKERS; possible increased risk
  of severe hypertension and bradycardia when noradrenaline
  (norepinephrine) given with non-cardioselective ● BETA-
  BLOCKERS
- ▸ **Cardiac Glycosides:** manufacturer of midodrine advises avoid
  concomitant use with DIGOXIN
- ● **Clonidine:** possible risk of hypertension when adrenaline
  (epinephrine) or noradrenaline (norepinephrine) given with
  CLONIDINE; serious adverse events reported with concomitant
  use of methylphenidate and ● CLONIDINE (causality not
  established)
- ▸ **Corticosteroids:** possible risk of hypertension when midodrine
  given with CORTICOSTEROIDS; ephedrine accelerates
  metabolism of DEXAMETHASONE
- ● **Dopaminergics:** risk of toxicity when isometheptene given with
  ● BROMOCRIPTINE; effects of adrenaline (epinephrine),
  dobutamine, dopamine and noradrenaline (norepinephrine)
  possibly enhanced by ENTACAPONE; avoid concomitant use of
  sympathomimetics with ● RASAGILINE; risk of hypertensive
  crisis when dopamine given with ● SELEGILINE; avoidance of
  sympathomimetics advised by manufacturer of SELEGILINE
- ▸ **Doxapram:** increased risk of hypertension when
  sympathomimetics given with DOXAPRAM
- ● **Ergot Alkaloids:** increased risk of ergotism when
  sympathomimetics given with ERGOT ALKALOIDS

Sympathomimetics (continued)

- ▸ **Oxytocin:** risk of hypertension when vasoconstrictor
  sympathomimetics given with OXYTOCIN (due to enhanced
  vasopressor effect)
- ● **Sympathomimetics:** effects of adrenaline (epinephrine) possibly
  enhanced by ● DOPEXAMINE; dopexamine possibly enhances
  effects of ● NORADRENALINE (NOREPINEPHRINE)
- ▸ **Theophylline:** avoidance of ephedrine in children advised by
  manufacturer of THEOPHYLLINE
- ▸ **Thyroid Hormones:** manufacturer of midodrine advises avoid
  concomitant use with THYROID HORMONES
- ▸ **Ulcer-healing Drugs:** metabolism of dobutamine possibly
  inhibited by CIMETIDINE

Sympathomimetics, Beta$_2$

- ▸ **Aminophylline:** increased risk of hypokalaemia when high
  doses of beta$_2$ sympathomimetics given with AMINOPHYLLINE
- ▸ **Antifungals:** plasma concentration of olodaterol increased by
  KETOCONAZOLE; metabolism of salmeterol inhibited by
  ● KETOCONAZOLE (increased plasma concentration)
- ● **Antivirals:** plasma concentration of salmeterol possibly
  increased by ATAZANAVIR—manufacturer of atazanavir advises
  avoid concomitant use; avoidance of salmeterol advised by
  manufacturer of LOPINAVIR, RITONAVIR and TIPRANAVIR;
  avoidance of salmeterol advised by manufacturer of
  ● TELAPREVIR (risk of ventricular arrhythmias)
- ▸ **Atomoxetine:** increased risk of cardiovascular side-effects when
  parenteral salbutamol given with ATOMOXETINE
- ▸ **Cardiac Glycosides:** salbutamol possibly reduces plasma
  concentration of DIGOXIN
- ▸ **Cobicistat:** avoidance of salmeterol advised by manufacturer of
  COBICISTAT
- ▸ **Corticosteroids:** increased risk of hypokalaemia when high
  doses of beta$_2$ sympathomimetics given with CORTICOSTEROIDS
- ▸ **Cytotoxics:** avoidance of salmeterol advised by manufacturer of
  IDELALISIB
- ▸ **Diuretics:** increased risk of hypokalaemia when high doses of
  beta$_2$ sympathomimetics given with ACETAZOLAMIDE, LOOP
  DIURETICS or THIAZIDES AND RELATED DIURETICS
- ● **Methyldopa:** acute hypotension reported when infusion of
  salbutamol given with ● METHYLDOPA
- ▸ **Muscle Relaxants:** bambuterol enhances effects of
  SUXAMETHONIUM
- ▸ **Theophylline:** increased risk of hypokalaemia when high doses
  of beta$_2$ sympathomimetics given with THEOPHYLLINE

Tacrolimus

NOTE Interactions do not generally apply to tacrolimus used
topically; risk of facial flushing and skin irritation with topical
tacrolimus on consumption of alcohol

- ● **Analgesics:** possible increased risk of nephrotoxicity when
  tacrolimus given with NSAIDS; increased risk of nephrotoxicity
  when tacrolimus given with ● IBUPROFEN
- ▸ **Angiotensin-II Receptor Antagonists:** increased risk of
  hyperkalaemia when tacrolimus given with ANGIOTENSIN-II
  RECEPTOR ANTAGONISTS
- ▸ **Anti-arrhythmics:** plasma concentration of tacrolimus possibly
  increased by AMIODARONE; caution with tacrolimus advised by
  manufacturer of DRONEDARONE
- ● **Antibacterials:** plasma concentration of tacrolimus increased
  by ● CLARITHROMYCIN and ● ERYTHROMYCIN; plasma
  concentration of tacrolimus possibly reduced by RIFABUTIN;
  plasma concentration of tacrolimus reduced by ● RIFAMPICIN;
  possible increased risk of nephrotoxicity when tacrolimus
  given with ● SULFAMETHOXAZOLE, ● TRIMETHOPRIM or
  VANCOMYCIN; increased risk of nephrotoxicity when tacrolimus
  given with ● AMINOGLYCOSIDES; plasma concentration of
  tacrolimus possibly increased by ● CHLORAMPHENICOL and
  ● TELITHROMYCIN
- ● **Anticoagulants:** tacrolimus possibly increases plasma
  concentration of ● DABIGATRAN—manufacturer of dabigatran
  advises avoid concomitant use
- ● **Antidepressants:** plasma concentration of tacrolimus reduced
  by ● ST JOHN'S WORT—avoid concomitant use
- ● **Antiepileptics:** plasma concentration of tacrolimus reduced by
  FOSPHENYTOIN and PHENYTOIN, also plasma concentration of
  fosphenytoin and phenytoin possibly increased; plasma

Tacrolimus

- **Antiepileptics** (continued) concentration of tacrolimus reduced by ● PHENOBARBITAL and ● PRIMIDONE
- **Antifungals**: plasma concentration of tacrolimus increased by ● FLUCONAZOLE, ● ITRACONAZOLE, ● KETOCONAZOLE, ● POSACONAZOLE and ● VORICONAZOLE (consider reducing dose of tacrolimus); plasma concentration of tacrolimus possibly increased by ● MICONAZOLE *oral gel*; increased risk of nephrotoxicity when tacrolimus given with ● AMPHOTERICIN; plasma concentration of tacrolimus reduced by ● CASPOFUNGIN
- **Antipsychotics**: avoidance of tacrolimus advised by manufacturer of ● DROPERIDOL (risk of ventricular arrhythmias)
- **Antivirals**: possible increased risk of nephrotoxicity when tacrolimus given with ACICLOVIR, GANCICLOVIR, VALACICLOVIR or VALGANCICLOVIR; plasma concentration of tacrolimus possibly increased by ATAZANAVIR and ● RITONAVIR; plasma concentration of tacrolimus increased by ● BOCEPREVIR (reduce dose of tacrolimus); plasma concentration of tacrolimus possibly affected by ● EFAVIRENZ; plasma concentration of tacrolimus increased by ● FOSAMPRENAVIR; plasma concentration of tacrolimus increased by ● SAQUINAVIR (consider reducing dose of tacrolimus); plasma concentration of both drugs increased when tacrolimus given with ● TELAPREVIR (reduce dose of tacrolimus)
- **Calcium-channel Blockers**: plasma concentration of tacrolimus possibly increased by FELODIPINE and VERAPAMIL; plasma concentration of tacrolimus increased by ● DILTIAZEM, NICARDIPINE and ● NIFEDIPINE
- **Ciclosporin**: tacrolimus increases plasma concentration of ● CICLOSPORIN (increased risk of nephrotoxicity)—avoid concomitant use
- **Cytotoxics**: tacrolimus possibly increases the plasma concentration of AFATINIB—manufacturer of afatinib advises separating administration of tacrolimus by 6 to 12 hours; caution with tacrolimus advised by manufacturer of ● CRIZOTINIB; plasma concentration of tacrolimus increased by IMATINIB
- Dexrazoxane: increased risk of immunosupression with tacrolimus advised by manufacturer of DEXRAZOXANE
- **Diuretics**: increased risk of hyperkalaemia when tacrolimus given with ● POTASSIUM-SPARING DIURETICS AND ALDOSTERONE ANTAGONISTS
- **Grapefruit Juice**: plasma concentration of tacrolimus increased by ● GRAPEFRUIT JUICE
- Hormone Antagonists: plasma concentration of tacrolimus possibly increased by DANAZOL
- Lipid-regulating Drugs: separating administration from tacrolimus by 12 hours advised by manufacturer of LOMITAPIDE
- Mifamurtide: avoidance of tacrolimus advised by manufacturer of MIFAMURTIDE
- Oestrogens: plasma concentration of tacrolimus possibly increased by ETHINYLESTRADIOL
- **Potassium Salts**: increased risk of hyperkalaemia when tacrolimus given with ● POTASSIUM SALTS
- Ranolazine: plasma concentration of tacrolimus increased by ● RANOLAZINE
- Sevelamer: plasma concentration of tacrolimus possibly reduced by SEVELAMER
- Ulcer-healing Drugs: plasma concentration of tacrolimus possibly increased by OMEPRAZOLE

Tadalafil

- **Alpha-blockers**: enhanced hypotensive effect when tadalafil given with ● DOXAZOSIN—manufacturer of tadalafil advises avoid concomitant use; enhanced hypotensive effect when tadalafil given with ● ALPHA-BLOCKERS—when patient is stable on the alpha blocker initiate tadalafil at the lowest possible dose
- Anti-arrhythmics: avoidance of tadalafil advised by manufacturer of DISOPYRAMIDE (risk of ventricular arrhythmias)
- Antibacterials: plasma concentration of tadalafil possibly increased by CLARITHROMYCIN and ERYTHROMYCIN; plasma concentration of tadalafil reduced by ● RIFAMPICIN—manufacturer of tadalafil advises avoid concomitant use

Tadalafil (continued)

- **Antifungals**: tadalafil concentration is increased by ● KETOCONAZOLE—avoid concomitant use of tadalafil for pulmonary hypertension; plasma concentration of tadalafil possibly increased by ITRACONAZOLE
- **Antivirals**: plasma concentration of tadalafil possibly increased by FOSAMPRENAVIR and INDINAVIR; plasma concentration of tadalafil increased by ● RITONAVIR—avoid concomitant use of tadalafil for pulmonary hypertension; increased risk of ventricular arrhythmias when tadalafil given with ● SAQUINAVIR—avoid concomitant use; avoidance of high doses of tadalafil advised by manufacturer of ● TELAPREVIR—consult product literature
- Bosentan: plasma concentration of tadalafil reduced by BOSENTAN
- **Cobicistat**: plasma concentration of tadalafil possibly increased by ● COBICISTAT—manufacturer of cobicistat advises reduce dose of tadalafil (consult cobicistat product literature)
- Dapoxetine: avoidance of tadalafil advised by manufacturer of DAPOXETINE
- Grapefruit Juice: plasma concentration of tadalafil possibly increased by GRAPEFRUIT JUICE
- **Nicorandil**: tadalafil significantly enhances hypotensive effect of ● NICORANDIL (avoid concomitant use)
- **Nitrates**: tadalafil significantly enhances hypotensive effect of ● NITRATES (avoid concomitant use)
- **Riociguat**: possible enhanced hypotensive effect when tadalafil given with ● RIOCIGUAT—avoid concomitant use

Tamoxifen

- Antibacterials: metabolism of tamoxifen accelerated by RIFAMPICIN (reduced plasma concentration)
- **Anticoagulants**: tamoxifen enhances anticoagulant effect of ● COUMARINS
- **Antidepressants**: metabolism of tamoxifen to active metabolite possibly inhibited by ● FLUOXETINE and ● PAROXETINE (avoid concomitant use)
- **Antipsychotics**: avoidance of tamoxifen advised by manufacturer of ● DROPERIDOL (risk of ventricular arrhythmias)
- **Bupropion**: metabolism of tamoxifen to active metabolite possibly inhibited by ● BUPROPION (avoid concomitant use)
- **Cinacalcet**: metabolism of tamoxifen to active metabolite possibly inhibited by ● CINACALCET (avoid concomitant use)

Tamsulosin *see* Alpha-blockers

Tapentadol *see* Opioid Analgesics

Taxanes *see* Cabazitaxel, Docetaxel, and Paclitaxel

Tegafur

- Antibacterials: metabolism of tegafur inhibited by METRONIDAZOLE (increased toxicity)
- **Anticoagulants**: tegafur enhances anticoagulant effect of ● COUMARINS
- **Antiepileptics**: tegafur possibly inhibits metabolism of FOSPHENYTOIN and PHENYTOIN (increased risk of toxicity)
- **Antipsychotics**: avoid concomitant use of cytotoxics with ● CLOZAPINE (increased risk of agranulocytosis)
- Filgrastim: neutropenia possibly exacerbated when tegafur given with FILGRASTIM
- **Folates**: toxicity of tegafur increased by ● FOLIC ACID—avoid concomitant use
- Lipegfilgrastim: neutropenia possibly exacerbated when tegafur given with LIPEGFILGRASTIM
- Pegfilgrastim: neutropenia possibly exacerbated when tegafur given with PEGFILGRASTIM
- Ulcer-healing Drugs: metabolism of tegafur inhibited by CIMETIDINE (increased plasma concentration)

Teicoplanin

- Vaccines: antibacterials inactivate ORAL TYPHOID VACCINE—see under Typhoid Vaccine in BNFC

Telaprevir

- **Alpha-blockers**: manufacturer of telaprevir advises avoid concomitant use with ● ALFUZOSIN
- **Analgesics**: manufacturer of telaprevir advises caution with ● METHADONE (risk of ventricular arrhythmias)
- **Anti-arrhythmics**: manufacturer of telaprevir advises avoid concomitant use with ● AMIODARONE and ● DISOPYRAMIDE (risk of ventricular arrhythmias); manufacturer of telaprevir

Telaprevir

- **Anti-arrhythmics** (continued)
  advises caution with ● FLECAINIDE and ● PROPAFENONE (risk of ventricular arrhythmias); manufacturer of telaprevir advises caution with *intravenous* LIDOCAINE
- **Antibacterials**: plasma concentration of both drugs possibly increased when telaprevir given with ● CLARITHROMYCIN, ● ERYTHROMYCIN and ● TELITHROMYCIN (increased risk of ventricular arrhythmias); manufacturer of telaprevir advises avoid concomitant use with ● RIFABUTIN; plasma concentration of telaprevir significantly reduced by ● RIFAMPICIN—avoid concomitant use
- **Anticoagulants**: telaprevir possibly affects plasma concentration of ● WARFARIN; avoidance of telaprevir advised by manufacturer of APIXABAN; telaprevir possibly increases plasma concentration of DABIGATRAN
- **Antidepressants**: telaprevir possibly increases plasma concentration of TRAZODONE; manufacturer of telaprevir advises avoid concomitant use with ● ST JOHN'S WORT
▹ **Antidiabetics**: telaprevir increases plasma concentration of METFORMIN (consider reducing dose of metformin)
- **Antiepileptics**: manufacturer of telaprevir advises avoid concomitant use with ● CARBAMAZEPINE, ● FOSPHENYTOIN, ● PHENOBARBITAL, ● PHENYTOIN and ● PRIMIDONE
- **Antifungals**: plasma concentration of both drugs possibly increased when telaprevir given with KETOCONAZOLE (increased risk of ventricular arrhythmias)—reduce dose of ketoconazole; telaprevir possibly increases plasma concentration of ITRACONAZOLE; telaprevir possibly increases plasma concentration of ● POSACONAZOLE (increased risk of ventricular arrhythmias); telaprevir possibly affects plasma concentration of ● VORICONAZOLE (possible increased risk of ventricular arrhythmias)
- **Antipsychotics**: telaprevir possibly increases plasma concentration of ● LURASIDONE—avoid concomitant use; manufacturer of telaprevir advises avoid concomitant use with ● PIMOZIDE; telaprevir possibly increases plasma concentration of ● QUETIAPINE—manufacturer of quetiapine advises avoid concomitant use
▹ **Antivirals**: plasma concentration of telaprevir possibly reduced by ATAZANAVIR, also plasma concentration of atazanavir possibly increased; telaprevir increases the plasma concentration of ● DACLATASVIR—reduce dose of daclatasvir (see under Daclatasvir, in BNF); avoid concomitant use of telaprevir with ● DARUNAVIR; plasma concentration of telaprevir reduced by ● EFAVIRENZ—increase dose of telaprevir; manufacturers advise avoid concomitant use of telaprevir with ● FOSAMPRENAVIR and ● LOPINAVIR; telaprevir increases plasma concentration of MARAVIROC (consider reducing dose of maraviroc); plasma concentration of telaprevir possibly reduced by NEVIRAPINE—consider increasing dose of telaprevir; plasma concentration of telaprevir possibly reduced by RITONAVIR; telaprevir increases plasma concentration of TENOFOVIR; avoidance of telaprevir advised by manufacturer of TIPRANAVIR
- **Anxiolytics and Hypnotics**: telaprevir possibly increases plasma concentration of ● MIDAZOLAM (risk of prolonged sedation—avoid concomitant use of *oral* midazolam)
- **Beta-blockers**: manufacturer of telaprevir advises avoid concomitant use with ● SOTALOL (risk of ventricular arrhythmias)
▹ **Bosentan**: plasma concentration of telaprevir possibly reduced by BOSENTAN, also plasma concentration of bosentan possibly increased
- **Calcium-channel Blockers**: telaprevir increases plasma concentration of AMLODIPINE (consider reducing dose of amlodipine); manufacturer of telaprevir advises caution with DILTIAZEM, FELODIPINE, NICARDIPINE, NIFEDIPINE and VERAPAMIL
- **Cardiac Glycosides**: telaprevir increases plasma concentration of DIGOXIN
- **Ciclosporin**: plasma concentration of both drugs increased when telaprevir given with ● CICLOSPORIN (reduce dose of ciclosporin)
- **Cilostazol**: telaprevir possibly increases plasma concentration of ● CILOSTAZOL (see under Cilostazol, in BNF)

Telaprevir (continued)

- **Colchicine**: telaprevir possibly increases risk of ● COLCHICINE toxicity—suspend or reduce dose of colchicine (avoid concomitant use in hepatic or renal impairment)
▹ **Corticosteroids**: telaprevir possibly increases plasma concentration of *inhaled* and *intranasal* BUDESONIDE and FLUTICASONE; plasma concentration of telaprevir possibly reduced by DEXAMETHASONE
- **Cytotoxics**: telaprevir possibly increases the plasma concentration of ● BOSUTINIB—manufacturer of bosutinib advises avoid or consider reducing dose of bosutinib; manufacturer of ruxolitinib advises dose reduction when telaprevir given with ● RUXOLITINIB—consult ruxolitinib product literature; avoidance of telaprevir advised by manufacturer of ● OLAPARIB
- **Domperidone**: possible increased risk of ventricular arrhythmias when telaprevir given with ● DOMPERIDONE—avoid concomitant use
- **Ergot Alkaloids**: manufacturer of telaprevir advises avoid concomitant use with ● ERGOT ALKALOIDS
- **Guanfacine**: telaprevir possibly increases plasma concentration of ● GUANFACINE (halve dose of guanfacine)
- **Lipid-regulating Drugs**: manufacturer of telaprevir advises avoid concomitant use with ● ATORVASTATIN; manufacturers advise avoid concomitant use of telaprevir with ● SIMVASTATIN; avoidance of telaprevir advised by manufacturer of ● LOMITAPIDE (plasma concentration of lomitapide possibly increased)
- **Oestrogens**: telaprevir possibly reduces plasma concentration of ● ETHINYLESTRADIOL—manufacturer of telaprevir advises additional contraceptive precautions
- **Sildenafil**: manufacturer of telaprevir advises avoid concomitant use with ● SILDENAFIL
- **Sirolimus**: plasma concentration of both drugs increased when telaprevir given with ● SIROLIMUS (reduce dose of sirolimus)
- **Sympathomimetics, Beta₂**: manufacturer of telaprevir advises avoid concomitant use with ● SALMETEROL (risk of ventricular arrhythmias)
- **Tacrolimus**: plasma concentration of both drugs increased when telaprevir given with ● TACROLIMUS (reduce dose of tacrolimus)
- **Tadalafil**: manufacturer of telaprevir advises avoid concomitant use with high doses of ● TADALAFIL—consult product literature
- **Vardenafil**: manufacturer of telaprevir advises avoid concomitant use with ● VARDENAFIL

Telavancin

▹ **Vaccines**: antibacterials inactivate ORAL TYPHOID VACCINE—see under Typhoid Vaccine in BNFC

Telbivudine

- **Interferons**: increased risk of peripheral neuropathy when telbivudine given with ● INTERFERON ALFA and ● PEGINTERFERON ALFA

Telithromycin

- **Analgesics**: possible increased risk of ventricular arrhythmias when telithromycin given with ● METHADONE; telithromycin inhibits the metabolism of OXYCODONE
- **Anti-arrhythmics**: possible increased risk of ventricular arrhythmias when telithromycin given with ● AMIODARONE and ● DISOPYRAMIDE; increased risk of ventricular arrhythmias when telithromycin given with ● DRONEDARONE—avoid concomitant use
- **Antibacterials**: possible increased risk of ventricular arrhythmias when telithromycin given with ● MOXIFLOXACIN; plasma concentration of telithromycin reduced by ● RIFAMPICIN (avoid during and for 2 weeks after rifampicin)
▹ **Anticoagulants**: avoidance of telithromycin advised by manufacturer of APIXABAN
- **Antidepressants**: possible increased risk of ventricular arrhythmias when telithromycin given with ● CITALOPRAM and ● TRICYCLICS; plasma concentration of telithromycin reduced by ● ST JOHN'S WORT (avoid during and for 2 weeks after St John's wort)
- **Antiepileptics**: plasma concentration of telithromycin reduced by ● CARBAMAZEPINE, ● FOSPHENYTOIN, ● PHENOBARBITAL, ● PHENYTOIN and ● PRIMIDONE (avoid during and for 2 weeks

Telithromycin
- Antiepileptics (continued)
  after carbamazepine, fosphenytoin, phenobarbital, phenytoin and primidone)
- Antifungals: plasma concentration of telithromycin increased by ● KETOCONAZOLE—avoid in severe renal and hepatic impairment
▸ Antimuscarinics: manufacturer of fesoterodine advises dose reduction when telithromycin given with FESOTERODINE—consult fesoterodine product literature
- Antipsychotics: possible increased risk of ventricular arrhythmias when telithromycin given with ● CHLORPROMAZINE; telithromycin possibly increases plasma concentration of ● LURASIDONE—avoid concomitant use; increased risk of ventricular arrhythmias when telithromycin given with ● PIMOZIDE—avoid concomitant use; telithromycin possibly increases plasma concentration of QUETIAPINE
- Antivirals: manufacturer of telithromycin advises avoid concomitant use with ● ATAZANAVIR, ● FOSAMPRENAVIR, ● INDINAVIR, ● LOPINAVIR, ● RITONAVIR and ● TIPRANAVIR in severe renal and hepatic impairment; telithromycin possibly increases the plasma concentration of ● DACLATASVIR—reduce dose of daclatasvir (see under Daclatasvir, in BNF); avoidance of telithromycin advised by manufacturer of ● DASABUVIR and PARITAPREVIR; telithromycin possibly increases plasma concentration of ● MARAVIROC (consider reducing dose of maraviroc); manufacturer of telithromycin advises avoid concomitant use with ● SAQUINAVIR (risk of ventricular arrhythmias); telithromycin possibly increases plasma concentration of ● SIMEPREVIR—manufacturer of simeprevir advises avoid concomitant use; plasma concentration of both drugs possibly increased when telithromycin given with ● TELAPREVIR (increased risk of ventricular arrhythmias)
- Anxiolytics and Hypnotics: telithromycin inhibits metabolism of ● MIDAZOLAM (increased plasma concentration with increased sedation)
▸ Aprepitant: telithromycin possibly increases plasma concentration of APREPITANT
- Avanafil: telithromycin possibly increases concentration of ● AVANAFIL—manufacturer of avanafil advises avoid concomitant use
- Calcium-channel Blockers: telithromycin possibly inhibits metabolism of ● CALCIUM-CHANNEL BLOCKERS (increased risk of side-effects)
▸ Cardiac Glycosides: telithromycin possibly increases plasma concentration of DIGOXIN
- Ciclosporin: telithromycin possibly increases plasma concentration of ● CICLOSPORIN
- Colchicine: telithromycin possibly increases risk of ● COLCHICINE toxicity—suspend or reduce dose of colchicine (avoid concomitant use in hepatic or renal impairment)
- Cytotoxics: telithromycin possibly increases plasma concentration of ● AXITINIB (reduce dose of axitinib—consult axitinib product literature); telithromycin possibly increases the plasma concentration of ● BOSUTINIB and ● CABAZITAXEL—manufacturer of bosutinib and cabazitaxel advises avoid or consider reducing dose of bosutinib and cabazitaxel; telithromycin possibly increases plasma concentration of ● CRIZOTINIB and ● EVEROLIMUS—manufacturer of crizotinib and everolimus advises avoid concomitant use; avoidance of telithromycin advised by manufacturer of DASATINIB (plasma concentration of dasatinib possibly increased); telithromycin possibly increases the plasma concentration of ● IBRUTINIB—reduce dose of ibrutinib (see under Ibrutinib, in BNF); avoidance of telithromycin advised by manufacturer of ● LAPATINIB, NILOTINIB and ● OLAPARIB; telithromycin possibly increases plasma concentration of PAZOPANIB (reduce dose of pazopanib); telithromycin possibly increases plasma concentration of PONATINIB—consider reducing initial dose of ponatinib (see under Ponatinib, in BNF); manufacturer of ruxolitinib advises dose reduction when telithromycin given with ● RUXOLITINIB—consult ruxolitinib product literature; telithromycin possibly increases plasma concentration of ● DOCETAXEL—manufacturer of docetaxel advises avoid concomitant use or consider reducing docetaxel dose

Telithromycin (continued)
- Dapoxetine: avoidance of telithromycin advised by manufacturer of ● DAPOXETINE (increased risk of toxicity)
- Diuretics: telithromycin increases plasma concentration of ● EPLERENONE—avoid concomitant use
- Domperidone: possible increased risk of ventricular arrhythmias when telithromycin given with ● DOMPERIDONE—avoid concomitant use
- Ergot Alkaloids: increased risk of ergotism when telithromycin given with ● ERGOT ALKALOIDS—avoid concomitant use
▸ Fosaprepitant: telithromycin possibly increases plasma concentration of FOSAPREPITANT
- Guanfacine: telithromycin possibly increases plasma concentration of ● GUANFACINE (halve dose of guanfacine)
- Ivabradine: telithromycin possibly increases plasma concentration of ● IVABRADINE—avoid concomitant use
- Ivacaftor: telithromycin possibly increases plasma concentration of ● IVACAFTOR (see under Ivacaftor, p. 175)
- Lipid-regulating Drugs: increased risk of myopathy when telithromycin given with ● ATORVASTATIN or ● SIMVASTATIN (avoid concomitant use); possible increased risk of myopathy when telithromycin given with PRAVASTATIN; avoidance of telithromycin advised by manufacturer of ● LOMITAPIDE (plasma concentration of lomitapide possibly increased)
- Pentamidine Isetionate: possible increased risk of ventricular arrhythmias when telithromycin given with *parenteral* ● PENTAMIDINE ISETIONATE
- Ranolazine: telithromycin possibly increases plasma concentration of ● RANOLAZINE—manufacturer of ranolazine advises avoid concomitant use
- Sildenafil: telithromycin possibly increases plasma concentration of ● SILDENAFIL—consider reducing initial dose of sildenafil for erectile dysfunction or reduce sildenafil dose frequency to once daily for pulmonary hypertension
- Sirolimus: telithromycin increases plasma concentration of ● SIROLIMUS—avoid concomitant use
- Tacrolimus: telithromycin possibly increases plasma concentration of ● TACROLIMUS
▸ Ulipristal: avoidance of telithromycin advised by manufacturer of *low-dose* ULIPRISTAL
▸ Vaccines: antibacterials inactivate ORAL TYPHOID VACCINE—see under Typhoid Vaccine in BNFC

Telmisartan see Angiotensin-II Receptor Antagonists

Temazepam see Anxiolytics and Hypnotics

Temocillin see Penicillins

Temoporfin
- Cytotoxics: increased skin photosensitivity when temoporfin given with *topical* ● FLUOROURACIL

Temozolomide
▸ Antiepileptics: plasma concentration of temozolomide increased by SODIUM VALPROATE and VALPROIC ACID
- Antipsychotics: avoid concomitant use of cytotoxics with ● CLOZAPINE (increased risk of agranulocytosis)

Temsirolimus
NOTE The main active metabolite of temsirolimus is sirolimus—*see also* interactions of sirolimus and consult product literature
- Antibacterials: plasma concentration of active metabolite of temsirolimus reduced by ● RIFAMPICIN—avoid concomitant use
- Antifungals: plasma concentration of active metabolite of temsirolimus increased by ● KETOCONAZOLE—avoid concomitant use; manufacturer of temsirolimus advises avoid concomitant use with ● ITRACONAZOLE (plasma concentration of temsirolimus possibly increased)
- Antipsychotics: avoid concomitant use of cytotoxics with ● CLOZAPINE (increased risk of agranulocytosis)

Tenofovir
- Antivirals: manufacturer of tenofovir advises avoid concomitant use with ADEFOVIR; tenofovir reduces plasma concentration of ATAZANAVIR, also plasma concentration of tenofovir possibly increased; tenofovir increases plasma concentration of ● DIDANOSINE (increased risk of toxicity)—avoid concomitant use; plasma concentration of tenofovir increased by LOPINAVIR and TELAPREVIR
- Orlistat: absorption of tenofovir possibly reduced by ● ORLISTAT

Tenoxicam see NSAIDs

Terazosin see Alpha-blockers

Terbinafine
- Antibacterials: plasma concentration of terbinafine reduced by ● RIFAMPICIN
- Antidepressants: terbinafine possibly increases plasma concentration of PAROXETINE and TRICYCLICS
- Antifungals: terbinafine increases plasma concentration of FLUCONAZOLE
- Ciclosporin: terbinafine possibly reduces plasma concentration of CICLOSPORIN
- Oestrogens: occasional reports of breakthrough bleeding when terbinafine given with OESTROGENS (when used for contraception)
- Progestogens: occasional reports of breakthrough bleeding when terbinafine given with PROGESTOGENS (when used for contraception)
- Ulcer-healing Drugs: plasma concentration of terbinafine increased by CIMETIDINE

Terbutaline see Sympathomimetics, Beta$_2$

Teriflunomide
- Antibacterials: teriflunomide increases plasma concentration of CEFACLOR; plasma concentration of teriflunomide reduced by RIFAMPICIN
- Antidiabetics: teriflunomide increases plasma concentration of REPAGLINIDE
- Lipid-regulating Drugs: the effect of teriflunomide is significantly decreased by COLESTYRAMINE (enhanced elimination)—avoid unless drug elimination desired; teriflunomide increases plasma concentration of ● ROSUVASTATIN (consider reducing dose of rosuvastatin)
- Oestrogens: teriflunomide increases plasma concentration of ETHINYLESTRADIOL
- Progestogens: teriflunomide increases plasma concentration of LEVONORGESTREL
- Vaccines: risk of generalised infections when teriflunomide given with live ● VACCINES—avoid concomitant use

Testolactone
- Anticoagulants: testolactone enhances anticoagulant effect of ● COUMARINS and ● PHENINDIONE

Testosterone
- Anticoagulants: testosterone enhances anticoagulant effect of ● COUMARINS and ● PHENINDIONE
- Antidiabetics: testosterone possibly enhances hypoglycaemic effect of ANTIDIABETICS

Tetrabenazine
- Antidepressants: risk of CNS toxicity when tetrabenazine given with ● MAOIS (avoid tetrabenazine for 2 weeks after MAOIs)
- Antipsychotics: increased risk of extrapyramidal side-effects when tetrabenazine given with ANTIPSYCHOTICS
- Dopaminergics: increased risk of extrapyramidal side-effects when tetrabenazine given with AMANTADINE
- Metoclopramide: increased risk of extrapyramidal side-effects when tetrabenazine given with METOCLOPRAMIDE

Tetracosactide see Corticosteroids

Tetracycline see Tetracyclines

Tetracyclines
- ACE Inhibitors: absorption of tetracyclines reduced by QUINAPRIL tablets (quinapril tablets contain magnesium carbonate)
- Adsorbents: absorption of tetracyclines possibly reduced by KAOLIN
- Antacids: absorption of tetracyclines possibly reduced by ANTACIDS (give at least 2 to 3 hours apart)
- Antibacterials: plasma concentration of doxycycline reduced by RIFAMPICIN—consider increasing dose of doxycycline; tetracyclines possibly antagonise effects of PENICILLINS
- Anticoagulants: tetracyclines possibly enhance anticoagulant effect of ● COUMARINS and ● PHENINDIONE
- Antidiabetics: tetracyclines possibly enhance hypoglycaemic effect of SULFONYLUREAS
- Antiepileptics: metabolism of doxycycline accelerated by CARBAMAZEPINE (reduced effect); metabolism of doxycycline accelerated by FOSPHENYTOIN, PHENOBARBITAL, PHENYTOIN and PRIMIDONE (reduced plasma concentration)
- Atovaquone: tetracycline reduces plasma concentration of ATOVAQUONE

Tetracyclines (continued)
- Calcium Salts: absorption of tetracyclines possibly reduced by CALCIUM SALTS (give at least 2 to 3 hours apart)
- Cytotoxics: doxycycline or tetracycline increase risk of METHOTREXATE toxicity
- Dairy Products: absorption of tetracyclines (except doxycycline and minocycline) reduced by DAIRY PRODUCTS
- Diuretics: manufacturer of lymecycline advises avoid concomitant use with DIURETICS
- Ergot Alkaloids: increased risk of ergotism when tetracyclines given with ERGOTAMINE
- Iron Salts: absorption of tetracyclines reduced by *oral* IRON SALTS, also absorption of *oral* iron salts reduced by tetracyclines (give at least 2 to 3 hours apart)
- Lipid-regulating Drugs: absorption of tetracycline possibly reduced by COLESTIPOL and COLESTYRAMINE
- Retinoids: possible increased risk of benign intracranial hypertension when tetracyclines given with ● RETINOIDS (avoid concomitant use)
- Strontium Ranelate: absorption of tetracyclines reduced by STRONTIUM RANELATE (manufacturer of strontium ranelate advises avoid concomitant use)
- Ulcer-healing Drugs: absorption of tetracyclines reduced by SUCRALFATE and TRIPOTASSIUM DICITRATOBISMUTHATE
- Vaccines: antibacterials inactivate ORAL TYPHOID VACCINE—see under Typhoid Vaccine in BNFC
- Zinc: absorption of tetracyclines possibly reduced by ZINC (give at least 2 to 3 hours apart)

Theophylline
- Allopurinol: plasma concentration of theophylline possibly increased by ALLOPURINOL
- Anaesthetics, General: increased risk of convulsions when theophylline given with KETAMINE
- Anti-arrhythmics: theophylline antagonises anti-arrhythmic effect of ADENOSINE—manufacturer of adenosine advises avoid theophylline for 24 hours before adenosine; plasma concentration of theophylline increased by PROPAFENONE
- Antibacterials: plasma concentration of theophylline possibly increased by CLARITHROMYCIN and ISONIAZID; plasma concentration of theophylline increased by ● ERYTHROMYCIN (also theophylline may reduce absorption of *oral* erythromycin); plasma concentration of theophylline increased by ● CIPROFLOXACIN and ● NORFLOXACIN; metabolism of theophylline accelerated by RIFAMPICIN (reduced plasma concentration); possible increased risk of convulsions when theophylline given with ● QUINOLONES
- Antidepressants: plasma concentration of theophylline increased by ● FLUVOXAMINE (concomitant use should usually be avoided, but where not possible halve theophylline dose and monitor plasma-theophylline concentration); plasma concentration of theophylline possibly reduced by ST JOHN'S WORT
- Antiepileptics: metabolism of theophylline accelerated by CARBAMAZEPINE, ● PHENOBARBITAL and ● PRIMIDONE (reduced effect); plasma concentration of both drugs reduced when theophylline given with ● FOSPHENYTOIN and ● PHENYTOIN
- Antifungals: plasma concentration of theophylline possibly increased by ● FLUCONAZOLE and ● KETOCONAZOLE
- Antivirals: plasma concentration of theophylline possibly increased by ACICLOVIR and VALACICLOVIR; metabolism of theophylline accelerated by ● RITONAVIR (reduced plasma concentration)
- Anxiolytics and Hypnotics: theophylline possibly reduces effects of BENZODIAZEPINES
- Caffeine citrate: avoidance of theophylline advised by manufacturer of CAFFEINE CITRATE
- Calcium-channel Blockers: plasma concentration of theophylline possibly increased by ● CALCIUM-CHANNEL BLOCKERS (enhanced effect); plasma concentration of theophylline increased by DILTIAZEM; plasma concentration of theophylline increased by ● VERAPAMIL (enhanced effect)
- Corticosteroids: increased risk of hypokalaemia when theophylline given with CORTICOSTEROIDS
- Cytotoxics: plasma concentration of theophylline possibly increased by METHOTREXATE

Theophylline (continued)

- ● Deferasirox: plasma concentration of theophylline increased by ● DEFERASIROX (consider reducing dose of theophylline)
- ▸ Disulfiram: metabolism of theophylline inhibited by DISULFIRAM (increased risk of toxicity)
- ▸ Diuretics: increased risk of hypokalaemia when theophylline given with ACETAZOLAMIDE, LOOP DIURETICS or THIAZIDES AND RELATED DIURETICS
- ▸ Doxapram: increased CNS stimulation when theophylline given with DOXAPRAM
- ● Interferons: metabolism of theophylline inhibited by ● INTERFERON ALFA and ● PEGINTERFERON ALFA (consider reducing dose of theophylline)
- ▸ Leukotriene Receptor Antagonists: plasma concentration of theophylline possibly increased by ZAFIRLUKAST, also plasma concentration of zafirlukast reduced
- ▸ Lithium: theophylline increases excretion of LITHIUM (reduced plasma concentration)
- ▸ Oestrogens: plasma concentration of theophylline increased by OESTROGENS (consider reducing dose of theophylline)
- ▸ Pentoxifylline: plasma concentration of theophylline increased by PENTOXIFYLLINE
- ▸ Roflumilast: avoidance of theophylline advised by manufacturer of ROFLUMILAST
- ▸ Sulfinpyrazone: plasma concentration of theophylline reduced by SULFINPYRAZONE
- ▸ Sympathomimetics: manufacturer of theophylline advises avoid concomitant use with EPHEDRINE in children
- ▸ Sympathomimetics, Beta$_2$: increased risk of hypokalaemia when theophylline given with high doses of BETA$_2$ SYMPATHOMIMETICS
- ● Ulcer-healing Drugs: metabolism of theophylline inhibited by ● CIMETIDINE (increased plasma concentration); absorption of theophylline possibly reduced by SUCRALFATE (give at least 2 hours apart)
- ▸ Vaccines: plasma concentration of theophylline possibly increased by INFLUENZA VACCINE

Thiazolidinediones see Antidiabetics

Thiopental see Anaesthetics, General

Thiotepa

- ● Antipsychotics: avoid concomitant use of cytotoxics with ● CLOZAPINE (increased risk of agranulocytosis)
- ▸ Muscle Relaxants: thiotepa enhances effects of SUXAMETHONIUM

Thioxanthenes see Antipsychotics

Thyroid Hormones

- ▸ Antacids: absorption of levothyroxine possibly reduced by ANTACIDS
- ▸ Anti-arrhythmics: serum concentrations of thyroid hormones can be affected by AMIODARONE—monitor thyroid function closely
- ▸ Antibacterials: metabolism of levothyroxine accelerated by RIFAMPICIN (may increase requirements for levothyroxine in hypothyroidism)
- ● Anticoagulants: thyroid hormones enhance anticoagulant effect of ● COUMARINS and ● PHENINDIONE
- ▸ Antidepressants: thyroid hormones enhance effects of AMITRIPTYLINE and IMIPRAMINE; thyroid hormones possibly enhance effects of TRICYCLICS
- ▸ Antiepileptics: metabolism of thyroid hormones accelerated by CARBAMAZEPINE, PHENOBARBITAL and PRIMIDONE (may increase requirements for thyroid hormones in hypothyroidism); metabolism of thyroid hormones accelerated by FOSPHENYTOIN and PHENYTOIN (may increase requirements in hypothyroidism), also plasma concentration of fosphenytoin and phenytoin possibly increased
- ▸ Beta-blockers: levothyroxine accelerates metabolism of PROPRANOLOL
- ▸ Calcium Salts: absorption of levothyroxine reduced by CALCIUM SALTS
- ▸ Cytotoxics: plasma concentration of levothyroxine possibly reduced by IMATINIB
- ▸ Iron Salts: absorption of levothyroxine reduced by oral IRON SALTS (give at least 2 hours apart)
- ▸ Lanthanum: absorption of levothyroxine reduced by LANTHANUM (give at least 2 hours apart)

Thyroid Hormones (continued)

- ▸ Lipid-regulating Drugs: absorption of levothyroxine reduced by COLESEVELAM; absorption of thyroid hormones reduced by COLESTIPOL and COLESTYRAMINE
- ▸ Oestrogens: requirements for thyroid hormones in hypothyroidism may be increased by OESTROGENS
- ▸ Orlistat: possible increased risk of hypothyroidism when levothyroxine given with ORLISTAT
- ▸ Polystyrene Sulfonate Resins: absorption of levothyroxine reduced by POLYSTYRENE SULFONATE RESINS
- ▸ Sevelamer: absorption of levothyroxine possibly reduced by SEVELAMER
- ▸ Sympathomimetics: avoidance of thyroid hormones advised by manufacturer of MIDODRINE
- ▸ Ulcer-healing Drugs: absorption of levothyroxine reduced by CIMETIDINE and SUCRALFATE

Tiagabine

- ● Antidepressants: anticonvulsant effect of antiepileptics possibly antagonised by MAOIs and ● TRICYCLIC-RELATED ANTIDEPRESSANTS (convulsive threshold lowered); anticonvulsant effect of antiepileptics antagonised by ● SSRIS and ● TRICYCLICS (convulsive threshold lowered)
- ▸ Antiepileptics: plasma concentration of tiagabine reduced by CARBAMAZEPINE, FOSPHENYTOIN, PHENOBARBITAL, PHENYTOIN and PRIMIDONE
- ● Antimalarials: anticonvulsant effect of antiepileptics antagonised by ● MEFLOQUINE
- ● Antipsychotics: anticonvulsant effect of antiepileptics antagonised by ● ANTIPSYCHOTICS (convulsive threshold lowered)
- ● Orlistat: possible increased risk of convulsions when antiepileptics given with ● ORLISTAT

Tiaprofenic Acid see NSAIDs

Tibolone

- ▸ Antibacterials: metabolism of tibolone accelerated by RIFAMPICIN (reduced plasma concentration)
- ▸ Antiepileptics: metabolism of tibolone accelerated by CARBAMAZEPINE (reduced plasma concentration); metabolism of tibolone accelerated by FOSPHENYTOIN and PHENYTOIN

Ticagrelor

- ● Antibacterials: plasma concentration of ticagrelor possibly increased by ● CLARITHROMYCIN—manufacturer of ticagrelor advises avoid concomitant use; plasma concentration of ticagrelor possibly increased by ERYTHROMYCIN; plasma concentration of ticagrelor reduced by ● RIFAMPICIN
- ● Anticoagulants: ticagrelor increases plasma concentration of ● DABIGATRAN
- ▸ Antidepressants: possible increased risk of bleeding when ticagrelor given with CITALOPRAM, PAROXETINE or SERTRALINE
- ▸ Antiepileptics: plasma concentration of ticagrelor possibly reduced by CARBAMAZEPINE, FOSPHENYTOIN, PHENOBARBITAL, PHENYTOIN and PRIMIDONE
- ● Antifungals: plasma concentration of ticagrelor increased by ● KETOCONAZOLE—manufacturer of ticagrelor advises avoid concomitant use
- ● Antivirals: plasma concentration of ticagrelor possibly increased by ● ATAZANAVIR and ● RITONAVIR—manufacturer of ticagrelor advises avoid concomitant use
- ▸ Calcium-channel Blockers: plasma concentration of ticagrelor increased by DILTIAZEM
- ● Cardiac Glycosides: ticagrelor increases plasma concentration of ● DIGOXIN
- ● Ciclosporin: plasma concentration of ticagrelor increased by CICLOSPORIN
- ● Ergot Alkaloids: ticagrelor possibly increases plasma concentration of ● ERGOT ALKALOIDS
- ● Lipid-regulating Drugs: ticagrelor increases plasma concentration of ● SIMVASTATIN (increased risk of toxicity); separating administration from ticagrelor by 12 hours advised by manufacturer of LOMITAPIDE

Ticarcillin see Penicillins

Tick-borne Encephalitis Vaccine see Vaccines

Tigecycline

- ▸ Anticoagulants: tigecycline possibly enhances anticoagulant effect of COUMARINS

Tigecycline (continued)
▸ Vaccines: antibacterials inactivate ORAL TYPHOID VACCINE—see under Typhoid Vaccine in BNFC

Timolol see Beta-blockers

Tinidazole
▸ Alcohol: possibility of disulfiram-like reaction when tinidazole given with ALCOHOL
▸ Antibacterials: plasma concentration of tinidazole possibly reduced by RIFAMPICIN
▸ Vaccines: antibacterials inactivate ORAL TYPHOID VACCINE—see under Typhoid Vaccine in BNFC

Tinzaparin see Heparins

Tioguanine
● Antipsychotics: avoid concomitant use of cytotoxics with ● CLOZAPINE (increased risk of agranulocytosis)
● Cytotoxics: increased risk of hepatotoxicity when tioguanine given with BUSULFAN

Tiotropium see Antimuscarinics

Tipranavir
● Analgesics: plasma concentration of tipranavir possibly reduced by BUPRENORPHINE
● Antacids: absorption of tipranavir reduced by ANTACIDS (give at least 2 hours apart)
● Antibacterials: tipranavir increases plasma concentration of ● CLARITHROMYCIN (reduce dose of clarithromycin in renal impairment), also plasma concentration of tipranavir increased by clarithromycin; tipranavir increases plasma concentration of ● RIFABUTIN (reduce dose of rifabutin); plasma concentration of tipranavir possibly reduced by ● RIFAMPICIN—avoid concomitant use; avoidance of concomitant tipranavir in severe renal and hepatic impairment advised by manufacturer of ● TELITHROMYCIN
● Anticoagulants: avoidance of tipranavir advised by manufacturer of APIXABAN and RIVAROXABAN
● Antidepressants: plasma concentration of tipranavir possibly reduced by ● ST JOHN'S WORT—avoid concomitant use
● Antiepileptics: plasma concentration of tipranavir possibly reduced by CARBAMAZEPINE
● Antifungals: plasma concentration of tipranavir increased by FLUCONAZOLE
● Antimalarials: caution with tipranavir advised by manufacturer of ARTEMETHER WITH LUMEFANTRINE; tipranavir possibly increases plasma concentration of ● QUININE (increased risk of toxicity)
● Antimuscarinics: avoidance of tipranavir advised by manufacturer of DARIFENACIN
● Antipsychotics: tipranavir possibly increases plasma concentration of ● ARIPIPRAZOLE (reduce dose of aripiprazole—consult aripiprazole product literature); tipranavir possibly increases plasma concentration of ● QUETIAPINE—manufacturer of quetiapine advises avoid concomitant use
● Antivirals: tipranavir reduces plasma concentration of ● ABACAVIR, ● FOSAMPRENAVIR, ● LOPINAVIR, ● SAQUINAVIR and ● ZIDOVUDINE; plasma concentration of tipranavir increased by ATAZANAVIR (also plasma concentration of atazanavir reduced); manufacturer of tipranavir advises avoid concomitant use with BOCEPREVIR and TELAPREVIR; tipranavir reduces plasma concentration of DIDANOSINE—manufacturer of tipranavir advises tipranavir and didanosine *capsules* should be taken at least 2 hours apart; tipranavir reduces the plasma concentration of ● DOLUTEGRAVIR (see under Dolutegravir, p. 387); tipranavir reduces plasma concentration of ● ETRAVIRINE, also plasma concentration of tipranavir increased (avoid concomitant use); avoidance of tipranavir advised by manufacturer of PARITAPREVIR
● Beta-blockers: manufacturer of tipranavir advises avoid concomitant use with ● METOPROLOL for heart failure
● Bosentan: manufacturer of tipranavir advises avoid concomitant use with BOSENTAN
● Cobicistat: plasma concentration of both drugs reduced when tipranavir given with ● COBICISTAT (avoid concomitant use)
Lipid-regulating Drugs: increased risk of myopathy when tipranavir given with ● ATORVASTATIN (see under Atorvastatin, p. 123); tipranavir increases plasma concentration of ● ROSUVASTATIN—adjust dose of rosuvastatin (consult product

Tipranavir
● Lipid-regulating Drugs (continued) literature); tipranavir possibly increases plasma concentration of ● SIMVASTATIN—avoid concomitant use; avoidance of tipranavir advised by manufacturer of ● LOMITAPIDE (plasma concentration of lomitapide possibly increased)
● Orlistat: absorption of tipranavir possibly reduced by ● ORLISTAT
● Ranolazine: tipranavir possibly increases plasma concentration of ● RANOLAZINE—manufacturer of ranolazine advises avoid concomitant use
▸ Sildenafil: manufacturer of tipranavir advises avoid concomitant use of SILDENAFIL for pulmonary arterial hypertension
▸ Sympathomimetics, Beta₂: manufacturer of tipranavir advises avoid concomitant use with SALMETEROL
▸ Ulcer-healing Drugs: tipranavir reduces plasma concentration of ● ESOMEPRAZOLE and ● OMEPRAZOLE
▸ Vardenafil: manufacturer of tipranavir advises caution with VARDENAFIL
▸ Vitamins: increased risk of bleeding when tipranavir given with high doses of VITAMIN E

Tirofiban
▸ Iloprost: increased risk of bleeding when tirofiban given with ILOPROST

Tizanidine see Muscle Relaxants

Tobramycin see Aminoglycosides

Tocilizumab
● Antipsychotics: avoid concomitant use of cytotoxics with ● CLOZAPINE (increased risk of agranulocytosis)
● Vaccines: risk of generalised infections when monoclonal antibodies given with live ● VACCINES—avoid concomitant use

Tolazoline see Alpha-blockers

Tolbutamide see Antidiabetics

Tolcapone
▸ Antidepressants: avoid concomitant use of tolcapone with MAOIs
▸ Memantine: effects of dopaminergics possibly enhanced by MEMANTINE
▸ Methyldopa: antiparkinsonian effect of dopaminergics antagonised by METHYLDOPA

Tolfenamic Acid see NSAIDs

Tolterodine see Antimuscarinics

Tolvaptan
▸ Antibacterials: plasma concentration of tolvaptan reduced by RIFAMPICIN
▸ Antifungals: plasma concentration of tolvaptan increased by KETOCONAZOLE—manufacturer of ketoconazole advises avoid concomitant use
▸ Cardiac Glycosides: tolvaptan increases plasma concentration of DIGOXIN (increased risk of toxicity)
● Grapefruit Juice: plasma concentration of tolvaptan increased by ● GRAPEFRUIT JUICE—avoid concomitant use
● Lipid-regulating Drugs: separating administration from tolvaptan by 12 hours advised by manufacturer of LOMITAPIDE

Topiramate
● Antidepressants: anticonvulsant effect of antiepileptics possibly antagonised by MAOIs and ● TRICYCLIC-RELATED ANTIDEPRESSANTS (convulsive threshold lowered); anticonvulsant effect of antiepileptics antagonised by SSRIS and ● TRICYCLICS (convulsive threshold lowered)
▸ Antidiabetics: topiramate possibly increases plasma concentration of METFORMIN; topiramate possibly reduces plasma concentration of GLIBENCLAMIDE
● Antiepileptics: plasma concentration of topiramate often reduced by CARBAMAZEPINE; topiramate increases plasma concentration of ● FOSPHENYTOIN and ● PHENYTOIN (also plasma concentration of topiramate reduced); topiramate reduces plasma concentration of PERAMPANEL; plasma concentration of topiramate possibly reduced by PHENOBARBITAL and PRIMIDONE; hyperammonaemia and CNS toxicity reported when topiramate given with SODIUM VALPROATE and VALPROIC ACID
● Antimalarials: anticonvulsant effect of antiepileptics antagonised by ● MEFLOQUINE

Topiramate (continued)

- Antipsychotics: anticonvulsant effect of antiepileptics antagonised by ● ANTIPSYCHOTICS (convulsive threshold lowered)
- ▸ Diuretics: plasma concentration of topiramate possibly increased by HYDROCHLOROTHIAZIDE
- ▸ Lithium: topiramate possibly affects plasma concentration of LITHIUM
- Oestrogens: topiramate accelerates metabolism of
  ● OESTROGENS (reduced contraceptive effect with combined oral contraceptives, contraceptive patches, and vaginal rings—see Contraceptive Interactions in BNFC)
- Orlistat: possible increased risk of convulsions when antiepileptics given with ● ORLISTAT
- Progestogens: topiramate accelerates metabolism of
  ● PROGESTOGENS (reduced contraceptive effect with combined oral contraceptives, progestogen-only oral contraceptives, contraceptive patches, vaginal rings, etonogestrel-releasing implant, and emergency hormonal contraception—see Contraceptive Interactions in BNFC)

Torasemide see Diuretics

Toremifene

- Anticoagulants: toremifene possibly enhances anticoagulant effect of ● COUMARINS
- Antiepileptics: metabolism of toremifene possibly accelerated by CARBAMAZEPINE (reduced plasma concentration); metabolism of toremifene possibly accelerated by FOSPHENYTOIN and PHENYTOIN; metabolism of toremifene accelerated by PHENOBARBITAL and PRIMIDONE (reduced plasma concentration)
- ▸ Cytotoxics: possible increased risk of ventricular arrhythmias when toremifene given with ● VANDETANIB—avoid concomitant use
- ▸ Diuretics: increased risk of hypercalcaemia when toremifene given with THIAZIDES AND RELATED DIURETICS

Trabectedin

- Alcohol: manufacturer of trabectedin advises avoid concomitant use with ● ALCOHOL
- Antibacterials: plasma concentration of trabectedin reduced by ● RIFAMPICIN
- Antipsychotics: avoid concomitant use of cytotoxics with
  ● CLOZAPINE (increased risk of agranulocytosis)
- Vaccines: risk of generalised infections when trabectedin given with live ● VACCINES—avoid concomitant use

Tramadol see Opioid Analgesics

Trandolapril see ACE Inhibitors

Tranylcypromine see MAOIs

Trastuzumab

- Antipsychotics: avoid concomitant use of cytotoxics with
  ● CLOZAPINE (increased risk of agranulocytosis)
- Cytotoxics: possible increased risk of cardiotoxicity when trastuzumab given with ● DAUNORUBICIN, ● DOXORUBICIN,
  ● EPIRUBICIN and ● IDARUBICIN—avoid concomitant use for up to 28 weeks after stopping trastuzumab
- Vaccines: risk of generalised infections when monoclonal antibodies given with live ● VACCINES—avoid concomitant use

Trazodone see Antidepressants, Tricyclic (related)

Tretinoin see Retinoids

Triamcinolone see Corticosteroids

Triamterene see Diuretics

Trientine

- ▸ Iron Salts: trientine reduces absorption of *oral* IRON SALTS
- ▸ Zinc: trientine reduces absorption of ZINC, also absorption of trientine reduced by zinc

Trifluoperazine see Antipsychotics

Trihexyphenidyl see Antimuscarinics

Trimethoprim

- ▸ ACE Inhibitors: possible increased risk of hyperkalaemia when trimethoprim given with ACE INHIBITORS
- ▸ Angiotensin-II Receptor Antagonists: possible increased risk of hyperkalaemia when trimethoprim given with ANGIOTENSIN-II RECEPTOR ANTAGONISTS
- ▸ Anti-arrhythmics: possible increased risk of ventricular arrhythmias when trimethoprim (as co-trimoxazole) given with AMIODARONE—manufacturer of amiodarone advises avoid concomitant use of co-trimoxazole

Trimethoprim (continued)

- ▸ Antibacterials: plasma concentration of trimethoprim possibly reduced by RIFAMPICIN; plasma concentration of both drugs may increase when trimethoprim given with DAPSONE
- ▸ Anticoagulants: trimethoprim possibly enhances anticoagulant effect of COUMARINS
- ▸ Antidiabetics: trimethoprim possibly enhances hypoglycaemic effect of REPAGLINIDE—manufacturer advises avoid concomitant use; trimethoprim rarely enhances the effects of SULFONYLUREAS
- Antiepileptics: trimethoprim increases plasma concentration of
  ● FOSPHENYTOIN and ● PHENYTOIN (also increased antifolate effect)
- Antimalarials: increased antifolate effect when trimethoprim given with ● PYRIMETHAMINE
- ▸ Antivirals: trimethoprim (as co-trimoxazole) increases plasma concentration of LAMIVUDINE—avoid concomitant use of high-dose co-trimoxazole
- Azathioprine: increased risk of haematological toxicity when trimethoprim (also with co-trimoxazole) given with
  ● AZATHIOPRINE
- ▸ Cardiac Glycosides: trimethoprim possibly increases plasma concentration of DIGOXIN
- Ciclosporin: increased risk of nephrotoxicity when trimethoprim given with ● CICLOSPORIN, also plasma concentration of ciclosporin reduced by *intravenous* trimethoprim
- Cytotoxics: increased risk of haematological toxicity when trimethoprim (also with co-trimoxazole) given with
  ● MERCAPTOPURINE; increased risk of severe bone marrow depression (fatalities reported) and other haematological toxicites when trimethoprim (also with co-trimoxazole) given with ● METHOTREXATE
- ▸ Diuretics: increased risk of hyperkalaemia when trimethoprim given with EPLERENONE; possible increased risk of hyperkalaemia when trimethoprim given with SPIRONOLACTONE
- Tacrolimus: possible increased risk of nephrotoxicity when trimethoprim given with ● TACROLIMUS
- Vaccines: antibacterials inactivate ORAL TYPHOID VACCINE—see under Typhoid Vaccine in BNFC

Trimipramine see Antidepressants, Tricyclic

Tripotassium Dicitratobismuthate

- ▸ Antibacterials: tripotassium dicitratobismuthate reduces absorption of TETRACYCLINES

Tropicamide see Antimuscarinics

Trospium see Antimuscarinics

Typhoid Vaccine (oral) see Vaccines

Typhoid Vaccine (parenteral) see Vaccines

Ubidecarenone

- ▸ Anticoagulants: ubidecarenone may enhance or reduce anticoagulant effect of WARFARIN

Ulcer-healing Drugs see Histamine H_2-antagonists, Proton Pump Inhibitors, Sucralfate, and Tripotassium Dicitratobismuthate

Ulipristal

- Antibacterials: manufacturer of *low-dose* ulipristal advises avoid concomitant use with CLARITHROMYCIN and TELITHROMYCIN; plasma concentration of *low-dose* ulipristal increased by ERYTHROMYCIN—manufacturer of *low-dose* ulipristal advises avoid concomitant use; manufacturer of ulipristal advises avoid concomitant use with ● RIFAMPICIN (contraceptive effect of ulipristal possibly reduced)
- ▸ Anticoagulants: manufacturer of ulipristal advises give DABIGATRAN at least 1.5 hours before or after ulipristal
- Antidepressants: manufacturer of ulipristal advises avoid concomitant use with ● ST JOHN'S WORT (contraceptive effect of ulipristal possibly reduced)
- Antiepileptics: manufacturer of ulipristal advises avoid concomitant use with ● CARBAMAZEPINE, ● FOSPHENYTOIN,
  ● PHENOBARBITAL, ● PHENYTOIN and PRIMIDONE (contraceptive effect of ulipristal possibly reduced)
- ▸ Antifungals: plasma concentration of *low-dose* ulipristal increased by KETOCONAZOLE—manufacturer of *low-dose* ulipristal advises avoid concomitant use; manufacturer of ulipristal advises avoid concomitant use with ITRACONAZOLE

Ulipristal (continued)

▸ Antihistamines: manufacturer of ulipristal advises give FEXOFENADINE at least 1.5 hours before or after ulipristal

● Antivirals: manufacturer of ulipristal advises avoid concomitant use with ● RITONAVIR (contraceptive effect of ulipristal possibly reduced)

▸ Calcium-channel Blockers: manufacturer of *low-dose* ulipristal advises avoid concomitant use with VERAPAMIL

▸ Cardiac Glycosides: manufacturer of ulipristal advises give DIGOXIN at least 1.5 hours before or after ulipristal

▸ Grapefruit Juice: manufacturer of *low-dose* ulipristal advises avoid concomitant use with GRAPEFRUIT JUICE

● Progestogens: ulipristal possibly reduces contraceptive effect of ● PROGESTOGENS

Umeclidinium *see* Antimuscarinics

Ursodeoxycholic Acid *see* Bile Acids

Ustekinumab

● Antipsychotics: avoid concomitant use of cytotoxics with ● CLOZAPINE (increased risk of agranulocytosis)

● Vaccines: risk of generalised infections when monoclonal antibodies given with live ● VACCINES—avoid concomitant use

Vaccines

● Abatacept: risk of generalised infections when live vaccines given with ● ABATACEPT—avoid concomitant use

▸ Aminophylline: influenza vaccine increases plasma concentration of AMINOPHYLLINE

▸ Anakinra: risk of generalised infections when live vaccines given with ● ANAKINRA—avoid concomitant use

▸ Antibacterials: oral typhoid vaccine inactivated by ANTIBACTERIALS—see under Typhoid Vaccine in BNFC

▸ Anticoagulants: influenza vaccine possibly enhances anticoagulant effect of WARFARIN

▸ Antidepressants: oral typhoid vaccine inactivated by antibacterials including LINEZOLID—see under Typhoid Vaccine in BNFC

▸ Antiepileptics: influenza vaccine enhances effects of FOSPHENYTOIN and PHENYTOIN

● Antimalarials: oral typhoid vaccine inactivated by ANTIMALARIALS—see under Typhoid Vaccine in BNFC

● Azathioprine: risk of generalised infections when live vaccines given with ● AZATHIOPRINE—avoid concomitant use

● Corticosteroids: immune response to vaccines impaired by high doses of ● CORTICOSTEROIDS—avoid concomitant use with live vaccines

● Cytotoxics: risk of generalised infections when live vaccines given with ● CYTOTOXIC ANTIBIOTICS, ● HYDROXYCARBAMIDE, ● MONOCLONAL ANTIBODIES or ● TRABECTEDIN—avoid concomitant use

● Dexrazoxane: risk of generalised infections when live vaccines given with ● DEXRAZOXANE—avoid concomitant use

● Etanercept: risk of generalised infections when live vaccines given with ● ETANERCEPT—avoid concomitant use

● Immunoglobulins: impaired immune response to *oral* poliomyelitis vaccine might occur with ● ANTI-D IMMUNOGLOBULINS and ● NORMAL IMMUNOGLOBULIN—give *oral* poliomyelitis vaccine at least 3 weeks before or 3 months after anti-d immunoglobulins and normal immunoglobulin; impaired immune response to BCG vaccine, MMR vaccine, oral typhoid vaccine, rotavirus vaccine, smallpox vaccine, varicella-zoster vaccine and yellow fever vaccine might occur with ● ANTI-D IMMUNOGLOBULINS—give BCG vaccine, MMR vaccine, oral typhoid vaccine, rotavirus vaccine, smallpox vaccine, varicella-zoster vaccine and yellow fever vaccine at least 3 weeks before or 3 months after anti-d immunoglobulins; impaired immune response to live influenza vaccine might occur with ● ANTI-D IMMUNOGLOBULINS and ● NORMAL IMMUNOGLOBULIN—give live influenza vaccine at least 3 weeks before or 3 months after anti-d immunoglobulins and normal immunoglobulin; impaired immune response to BCG vaccine, MMR vaccine, oral typhoid vaccine, rotavirus vaccine, smallpox vaccine, varicella-zoster vaccine and yellow fever vaccine might occur with ● NORMAL IMMUNOGLOBULIN—give BCG vaccine, MMR vaccine, oral typhoid vaccine, rotavirus vaccine, smallpox vaccine, varicella-zoster vaccine and yellow fever vaccine at least 3 weeks before or 3 months after normal immunoglobulin

Vaccines (continued)

▸ Interferons: avoidance of vaccines advised by manufacturer of INTERFERON GAMMA

● Leflunomide: risk of generalised infections when live vaccines given with ● LEFLUNOMIDE—avoid concomitant use

● Teriflunomide: risk of generalised infections when live vaccines given with ● TERIFLUNOMIDE—avoid concomitant use

▸ Theophylline: influenza vaccine possibly increases plasma concentration of THEOPHYLLINE

Valaciclovir

▸ Aminophylline: valaciclovir possibly increases plasma concentration of AMINOPHYLLINE

▸ Ciclosporin: increased risk of nephrotoxicity when valaciclovir given with CICLOSPORIN

▸ Mycophenolate: plasma concentration of valaciclovir increased by MYCOPHENOLATE, also plasma concentration of inactive metabolite of mycophenolate increased

▸ Tacrolimus: possible increased risk of nephrotoxicity when valaciclovir given with TACROLIMUS

▸ Theophylline: valaciclovir possibly increases plasma concentration of THEOPHYLLINE

Valganciclovir

● Antibacterials: increased risk of convulsions when valganciclovir given with ● IMIPENEM WITH CILASTATIN

● Antivirals: valganciclovir possibly increases plasma concentration of DIDANOSINE; profound myelosuppression when valganciclovir given with ● ZIDOVUDINE (if possible avoid concomitant administration, particularly during initial valganciclovir therapy)

▸ Mycophenolate: plasma concentration of valganciclovir possibly increased by MYCOPHENOLATE, also plasma concentration of inactive metabolite of mycophenolate possibly increased

▸ Tacrolimus: possible increased risk of nephrotoxicity when valganciclovir given with TACROLIMUS

Valproic Acid

▸ Analgesics: effects of valproic acid enhanced by ASPIRIN

● Antibacterials: metabolism of valproic acid possibly inhibited by ERYTHROMYCIN (increased plasma concentration); avoidance of valproic acid advised by manufacturer of ● PIVMECILLINAM; plasma concentration of valproic acid reduced by ● CARBAPENEMS—avoid concomitant use

● Anticoagulants: valproic acid possibly enhances anticoagulant effect of COUMARINS

● Antidepressants: anticonvulsant effect of antiepileptics possibly antagonised by MAOIs and ● TRICYCLIC-RELATED ANTIDEPRESSANTS (convulsive threshold lowered); anticonvulsant effect of antiepileptics antagonised by ● SSRIS and ● TRICYCLICS (convulsive threshold lowered)

● Antiepileptics: plasma concentration of valproic acid reduced by CARBAMAZEPINE, also plasma concentration of active metabolite of carbamazepine increased; valproic acid possibly increases plasma concentration of ETHOSUXIMIDE; valproic acid increases or possibly decreases plasma concentration of FOSPHENYTOIN and PHENYTOIN, also plasma concentration of valproic acid reduced; valproic acid increases plasma concentration of ● LAMOTRIGINE (increased risk of toxicity—reduce lamotrigine dose); valproic acid sometimes reduces plasma concentration of an active metabolite of OXCARBAZEPINE; valproic acid increases plasma concentration of PHENOBARBITAL and PRIMIDONE (also plasma concentration of valproic acid reduced); valproic acid possibly increases plasma concentration of RUFINAMIDE (reduce dose of rufinamide); hyperammonaemia and CNS toxicity reported when valproic acid given with TOPIRAMATE

● Antimalarials: anticonvulsant effect of antiepileptics antagonised by ● MEFLOQUINE

● Antipsychotics: anticonvulsant effect of antiepileptics antagonised by ● ANTIPSYCHOTICS (convulsive threshold lowered); valproic acid possibly increases or decreases plasma concentration of CLOZAPINE; increased risk of side-effects including neutropenia when valproic acid given with ● OLANZAPINE

▸ Antivirals: plasma concentration of valproic acid possibly reduced by RITONAVIR; valproic acid possibly increases plasma concentration of ZIDOVUDINE (increased risk of toxicity)

Valproic Acid (continued)

▸ Anxiolytics and Hypnotics: plasma concentration of valproic acid possibly increased by CLOBAZAM; increased risk of side-effects when valproic acid given with CLONAZEPAM; valproic acid possibly increases plasma concentration of DIAZEPAM and LORAZEPAM

▸ Bupropion: valproic acid inhibits the metabolism of BUPROPION

▸ Cytotoxics: valproic acid increases plasma concentration of TEMOZOLOMIDE

▸ Guanfacine: plasma concentration of valproic acid increased by GUANFACINE

▸ Lipid-regulating Drugs: absorption of valproic acid possibly reduced by COLESTYRAMINE

▸ Netupitant: caution with valproic acid advised by manufacturer of NETUPITANT

▸ Oestrogens: plasma concentration of valproic acid possibly reduced by ETHINYLESTRADIOL

● Orlistat: possible increased risk of convulsions when antiepileptics given with ● ORLISTAT

● Sodium Benzoate: valproic acid possibly reduces effects of SODIUM BENZOATE

● Sodium Oxybate: valproic acid increases the plasma concentration of ● SODIUM OXYBATE (see under Sodium Oxybate, in BNF)

▸ Sodium Phenylbutyrate: valproic acid possibly reduces effects of SODIUM PHENYLBUTYRATE

● Ulcer-healing Drugs: metabolism of valproic acid inhibited by ● CIMETIDINE (increased plasma concentration)

Valsartan see Angiotensin-II Receptor Antagonists

Vancomycin

▸ Anaesthetics, General: hypersensitivity-like reactions can occur when *intravenous* vancomycin given with GENERAL ANAESTHETICS

● Antibacterials: increased risk of nephrotoxicity and ototoxicity when vancomycin given with ● AMINOGLYCOSIDES, CAPREOMYCIN or COLISTIMETHATE SODIUM; increased risk of nephrotoxicity when vancomycin given with POLYMYXINS

▸ Antifungals: possible increased risk of nephrotoxicity when vancomycin given with AMPHOTERICIN

● Ciclosporin: increased risk of nephrotoxicity when vancomycin given with ● CICLOSPORIN

▸ Cytotoxics: increased risk of nephrotoxicity and possibly of ototoxicity when vancomycin given with CISPLATIN

● Diuretics: increased risk of otoxicity when vancomycin given with ● LOOP DIURETICS

▸ Lipid-regulating Drugs: effects of *oral* vancomycin antagonised by COLESTYRAMINE

● Muscle Relaxants: vancomycin enhances effects of ● SUXAMETHONIUM

▸ Tacrolimus: possible increased risk of nephrotoxicity when vancomycin given with TACROLIMUS

▸ Vaccines: antibacterials inactivate ORAL TYPHOID VACCINE—see under Typhoid Vaccine in BNFC

Vandetanib

● Analgesics: possible increased risk of ventricular arrhythmias when vandetanib given with ● METHADONE—avoid concomitant use

● Anti-arrhythmics: possible increased risk of ventricular arrhythmias when vandetanib given with ● AMIODARONE or ● DISOPYRAMIDE—avoid concomitant use

● Antibacterials: possible increased risk of ventricular arrhythmias when vandetanib given with *parenteral* ● ERYTHROMYCIN—avoid concomitant use; possible increased risk of ventricular arrhythmias when vandetanib given with ● MOXIFLOXACIN—avoid concomitant use; plasma concentration of vandetanib reduced by ● RIFAMPICIN—manufacturer of vandetanib advises avoid concomitant use

▸ Antidepressants: manufacturer of vandetanib advises avoid concomitant use with ST JOHN'S WORT (plasma concentration of vandetanib possibly reduced)

▸ Antidiabetics: vandetanib possibly increases plasma concentration of METFORMIN (consider reducing dose of metformin)

▸ Antiepileptics: manufacturer of vandetanib advises avoid concomitant use with CARBAMAZEPINE, PHENOBARBITAL and

Vandetanib
Antiepileptics (continued)
PRIMIDONE (plasma concentration of vandetanib possibly reduced)

● Antihistamines: possible increased risk of ventricular arrhythmias when vandetanib given with ● MIZOLASTINE—avoid concomitant use

● Antimalarials: possible increased risk of ventricular arrhythmias when vandetanib given with ● ARTEMETHER WITH LUMEFANTRINE—avoid concomitant use

● Antipsychotics: possible increased risk of ventricular arrhythmias when vandetanib given with ● AMISULPRIDE, ● CHLORPROMAZINE, ● HALOPERIDOL, ● PIMOZIDE, ● SULPIRIDE or ● ZUCLOPENTHIXOL—avoid concomitant use; avoid concomitant use of cytotoxics with ● CLOZAPINE (increased risk of agranulocytosis)

● Beta-blockers: possible increased risk of ventricular arrhythmias when vandetanib given with ● SOTALOL—avoid concomitant use

▸ Cardiac Glycosides: vandetanib increases plasma concentration of DIGOXIN—possible increased risk of bradycardia

● Cytotoxics: possible increased risk of ventricular arrhythmias when vandetanib given with ● ARSENIC TRIOXIDE—avoid concomitant use

● Hormone Antagonists: possible increased risk of ventricular arrhythmias when vandetanib given with ● TOREMIFENE—avoid concomitant use

● 5HT₃-receptor Antagonists: increased risk of ventricular arrhythmias when vandetanib given with ● ONDANSETRON—avoid concomitant use

● Pentamidine Isetionate: possible increased risk of ventricular arrhythmias when vandetanib given with ● PENTAMIDINE ISETIONATE—avoid concomitant use

Vardenafil

● Alpha-blockers: enhanced hypotensive effect when vardenafil given with ● ALPHA-BLOCKERS—when patient is stable on the alpha blocker initiate vardenafil at the lowest possible dose—separate doses by 6 hours (except with tamsulosin)

▸ Anti-arrhythmics: avoidance of vardenafil advised by manufacturer of DISOPYRAMIDE (risk of ventricular arrhythmias)

▸ Antibacterials: plasma concentration of vardenafil possibly increased by CLARITHROMYCIN (consider reducing initial dose of vardenafil); plasma concentration of vardenafil increased by ERYTHROMYCIN (reduce dose of vardenafil)

● Antifungals: plasma concentration of vardenafil increased by ● KETOCONAZOLE—avoid concomitant use; plasma concentration of vardenafil possibly increased by ● ITRACONAZOLE—avoid concomitant use

● Antivirals: plasma concentration of vardenafil possibly increased by FOSAMPRENAVIR; plasma concentration of vardenafil increased by ● INDINAVIR and ● RITONAVIR—avoid concomitant use; increased risk of ventricular arrhythmias when vardenafil given with ● SAQUINAVIR—avoid concomitant use; avoidance of vardenafil advised by manufacturer of ● TELAPREVIR; caution with vardenafil advised by manufacturer of TIPRANAVIR

▸ Calcium-channel Blockers: enhanced hypotensive effect when vardenafil given with NIFEDIPINE

● Cobicistat: plasma concentration of vardenafil possibly increased by ● COBICISTAT—manufacturer of cobicistat advises reduce dose of vardenafil (consult cobicistat product literature)

▸ Dapoxetine: avoidance of vardenafil advised by manufacturer of DAPOXETINE

● Grapefruit Juice: plasma concentration of vardenafil possibly increased by ● GRAPEFRUIT JUICE—avoid concomitant use

● Nicorandil: possible increased hypotensive effect when vardenafil given with ● NICORANDIL—avoid concomitant use

● Nitrates: possible increased hypotensive effect when vardenafil given with ● NITRATES—avoid concomitant use

● Riociguat: possible enhanced hypotensive effect when vardenafil given with ● RIOCIGUAT—avoid concomitant use

Varicella-zoster Vaccine see Vaccines

Vasodilator Antihypertensives

▸ ACE Inhibitors: enhanced hypotensive effect when hydralazine, minoxidil or sodium nitroprusside given with ACE INHIBITORS

▸ Adrenergic Neurone Blockers: enhanced hypotensive effect when hydralazine, minoxidil or sodium nitroprusside given with ADRENERGIC NEURONE BLOCKERS

▸ Alcohol: enhanced hypotensive effect when hydralazine, minoxidil or sodium nitroprusside given with ALCOHOL

▸ Aldesleukin: enhanced hypotensive effect when hydralazine, minoxidil or sodium nitroprusside given with ALDESLEUKIN

▸ Alpha-blockers: enhanced hypotensive effect when hydralazine, minoxidil or sodium nitroprusside given with ALPHA-BLOCKERS

▸ Anaesthetics, General: enhanced hypotensive effect when hydralazine, minoxidil or sodium nitroprusside given with GENERAL ANAESTHETICS

▸ Analgesics: hypotensive effect of hydralazine, minoxidil and sodium nitroprusside antagonised by NSAIDs

▸ Angiotensin-II Receptor Antagonists: enhanced hypotensive effect when hydralazine, minoxidil or sodium nitroprusside given with ANGIOTENSIN-II RECEPTOR ANTAGONISTS

▸ Antidepressants: enhanced hypotensive effect when hydralazine, minoxidil or sodium nitroprusside given with MAOIs; enhanced hypotensive effect when hydralazine or sodium nitroprusside given with TRICYCLIC-RELATED ANTIDEPRESSANTS

▸ Antipsychotics: enhanced hypotensive effect when hydralazine, minoxidil or sodium nitroprusside given with PHENOTHIAZINES

▸ Anxiolytics and Hypnotics: enhanced hypotensive effect when hydralazine, minoxidil or sodium nitroprusside given with ANXIOLYTICS AND HYPNOTICS

▸ Beta-blockers: enhanced hypotensive effect when hydralazine, minoxidil or sodium nitroprusside given with BETA-BLOCKERS

▸ Calcium-channel Blockers: enhanced hypotensive effect when hydralazine, minoxidil or sodium nitroprusside given with CALCIUM-CHANNEL BLOCKERS

▸ Clonidine: enhanced hypotensive effect when hydralazine, minoxidil or sodium nitroprusside given with CLONIDINE

▸ Corticosteroids: hypotensive effect of hydralazine, minoxidil and sodium nitroprusside antagonised by CORTICOSTEROIDS

▸ Diazoxide: enhanced hypotensive effect when hydralazine, minoxidil or sodium nitroprusside given with DIAZOXIDE

▸ Diuretics: enhanced hypotensive effect when hydralazine, minoxidil or sodium nitroprusside given with DIURETICS

▸ Dopaminergics: enhanced hypotensive effect when hydralazine, minoxidil or sodium nitroprusside given with CO-BENELDOPA; enhanced hypotensive effect when hydralazine, minoxidil or sodium nitroprusside given with CO-CARELDOPA; enhanced hypotensive effect when hydralazine, minoxidil or sodium nitroprusside given with LEVODOPA

▸ Methyldopa: enhanced hypotensive effect when hydralazine, minoxidil or sodium nitroprusside given with METHYLDOPA

▸ Moxisylyte: enhanced hypotensive effect when hydralazine, minoxidil or sodium nitroprusside given with MOXISYLYTE

▸ Moxonidine: enhanced hypotensive effect when hydralazine, minoxidil or sodium nitroprusside given with MOXONIDINE

▸ Muscle Relaxants: enhanced hypotensive effect when hydralazine, minoxidil or sodium nitroprusside given with BACLOFEN; enhanced hypotensive effect when hydralazine, minoxidil or sodium nitroprusside given with TIZANIDINE

▸ Nicorandil: possible enhanced hypotensive effect when hydralazine, minoxidil or sodium nitroprusside given with NICORANDIL

▸ Nitrates: enhanced hypotensive effect when hydralazine, minoxidil or sodium nitroprusside given with NITRATES

▸ Oestrogens: hypotensive effect of hydralazine, minoxidil and sodium nitroprusside antagonised by OESTROGENS

▸ Prostaglandins: enhanced hypotensive effect when hydralazine, minoxidil or sodium nitroprusside given with ALPROSTADIL

▸ Vasodilator Antihypertensives: enhanced hypotensive effect when hydralazine given with MINOXIDIL or SODIUM NITROPRUSSIDE; enhanced hypotensive effect when minoxidil given with SODIUM NITROPRUSSIDE

Vecuronium see Muscle Relaxants

Vedolizumab

● Antipsychotics: avoid concomitant use of cytotoxics with ● CLOZAPINE (increased risk of agranulocytosis)

● Vaccines: risk of generalised infections when monoclonal antibodies given with live ● VACCINES—avoid concomitant use

Vemurafenib

▸ Antibacterials: manufacturer of vemurafenib advises avoid concomitant use with RIFABUTIN and RIFAMPICIN

● Anticoagulants: vemurafenib possibly enhances anticoagulant effect of ● WARFARIN

▸ Antidepressants: manufacturer of vemurafenib advises avoid concomitant use with ST JOHN'S WORT

▸ Antiepileptics: manufacturer of vemurafenib advises avoid concomitant use with CARBAMAZEPINE, FOSPHENYTOIN and PHENYTOIN

● Antipsychotics: avoid concomitant use of cytotoxics with ● CLOZAPINE (increased risk of agranulocytosis)

▸ Cytotoxics: avoidance of vemurafenib advised by manufacturer of IPILIMUMAB

● Oestrogens: manufacturer of vemurafenib advises contraceptive effect of ● OESTROGENS possibly reduced

● Progestogens: manufacturer of vemurafenib advises contraceptive effect of ● PROGESTOGENS possibly reduced

Venlafaxine

● Analgesics: increased risk of bleeding when venlafaxine given with ● NSAIDS or ● ASPIRIN; possible increased serotonergic effects when SSRI-related antidepressants given with FENTANYL; possible increased serotonergic effects when venlafaxine given with TRAMADOL

● Anti-arrhythmics: manufacturer of venlafaxine advises avoid concomitant use with ● AMIODARONE (risk of ventricular arrhythmias)

● Antibacterials: manufacturer of venlafaxine advises avoid concomitant use with ● ERYTHROMYCIN and ● MOXIFLOXACIN (risk of ventricular arrhythmias)

● Anticoagulants: venlafaxine possibly enhances anticoagulant effect of ● WARFARIN; possible increased risk of bleeding when SSRI-related antidepressants given with ● DABIGATRAN

● Antidepressants: possible increased serotonergic effects when venlafaxine given with ST JOHN'S WORT, DULOXETINE or MIRTAZAPINE; enhanced CNS effects and toxicity when venlafaxine given with ● MAOIS (venlafaxine should not be started until 2 weeks after stopping MAOIs, avoid MAOIs for 1 week after stopping venlafaxine); after stopping SSRI-related antidepressants do not start ● MOCLOBEMIDE for at least 1 week; possible increased risk of convulsions when SSRI-related antidepressants given with ● VORTIOXETINE

● Antimalarials: avoidance of antidepressants advised by manufacturer of ● ARTEMETHER WITH LUMEFANTRINE and ● ARTENIMOL WITH PIPERAQUINE

● Antipsychotics: venlafaxine increases plasma concentration of HALOPERIDOL

▸ Atomoxetine: possible increased risk of convulsions when antidepressants given with ATOMOXETINE

● Beta-blockers: manufacturer of venlafaxine advises avoid concomitant use with ● SOTALOL (risk of ventricular arrhythmias)

● Dapoxetine: possible increased risk of serotonergic effects when venlafaxine given with ● DAPOXETINE (manufacturer of dapoxetine advises venlafaxine should not be started until 1 week after stopping dapoxetine, avoid dapoxetine for 2 weeks after stopping venlafaxine)

● Dopaminergics: caution with venlafaxine advised by manufacturer of ENTACAPONE; increased risk of hypertension and CNS excitation when venlafaxine given with ● SELEGILINE (selegiline should not be started until 1 week after stopping venlafaxine, avoid venlafaxine for 2 weeks after stopping selegiline)

▸ 5HT$_1$-receptor Agonists: possible increased serotonergic effects when venlafaxine given with 5HT$_1$ AGONISTS

▸ 5HT$_3$-receptor Antagonists: possible increased serotonergic effects when SSRI-related antidepressants given with 5HT$_3$ ANTAGONISTS

● Lithium: possible increased serotonergic effects when venlafaxine given with LITHIUM

Venlafaxine (continued)
- Methylthioninium: risk of CNS toxicity when SSRI-related antidepressants given with ● METHYLTHIONINIUM—avoid concomitant use (if avoidance not possible, use lowest possible dose of methylthioninium and observe patient for up to 4 hours after administration)

Verapamil see Calcium-channel Blockers

Vigabatrin
- Antidepressants: anticonvulsant effect of antiepileptics possibly antagonised by MAOIs and ● TRICYCLIC-RELATED ANTIDEPRESSANTS (convulsive threshold lowered); anticonvulsant effect of antiepileptics antagonised by ● SSRIS and ● TRICYCLICS (convulsive threshold lowered)
▹ Antiepileptics: vigabatrin reduces plasma concentration of FOSPHENYTOIN and PHENYTOIN
- Antimalarials: anticonvulsant effect of antiepileptics antagonised by ● MEFLOQUINE
- Antipsychotics: anticonvulsant effect of antiepileptics antagonised by ● ANTIPSYCHOTICS (convulsive threshold lowered)
- Orlistat: possible increased risk of convulsions when antiepileptics given with ● ORLISTAT

Vilanterol see Sympathomimetics, Beta$_2$

Vildagliptin see Antidiabetics

Vinblastine
- Aldesleukin: avoidance of vinblastine advised by manufacturer of ● ALDESLEUKIN
- Antibacterials: toxicity of vinblastine increased by ● ERYTHROMYCIN—avoid concomitant use; possible increased risk of ventricular arrhythmias when vinblastine given with ● DELAMANID
- Antifungals: possible increased risk of vinblastine toxicity when given with ● ITRACONAZOLE; metabolism of vinblastine possibly inhibited by ● POSACONAZOLE (increased risk of neurotoxicity)
- Antimalarials: avoidance of vinblastine advised by manufacturer of ● ARTENIMOL WITH PIPERAQUINE
- Antipsychotics: avoid concomitant use of cytotoxics with ● CLOZAPINE (increased risk of agranulocytosis)
▹ Antivirals: plasma concentration of vinblastine possibly increased by RITONAVIR

Vincristine
- Antibacterials: possible increased risk of ventricular arrhythmias when vincristine given with ● DELAMANID
- Antifungals: increased risk of vincristine toxicity when given with ● ITRACONAZOLE; metabolism of vincristine possibly inhibited by ● POSACONAZOLE (increased risk of neurotoxicity)
- Antimalarials: avoidance of vincristine advised by manufacturer of ● ARTENIMOL WITH PIPERAQUINE
- Antipsychotics: avoid concomitant use of cytotoxics with ● CLOZAPINE (increased risk of agranulocytosis)
▹ Calcium-channel Blockers: metabolism of vincristine possibly inhibited by NIFEDIPINE
▹ Cardiac Glycosides: vincristine possibly reduces absorption of DIGOXIN tablets
- Cytotoxics: increased risk of hepatotoxicity when vincristine given with ● DACTINOMYCIN

Vindesine
- Antibacterials: possible increased risk of ventricular arrhythmias when vindesine given with ● DELAMANID
- Antifungals: possible increased risk of vindesine toxicity when given with ● ITRACONAZOLE
- Antipsychotics: avoid concomitant use of cytotoxics with ● CLOZAPINE (increased risk of agranulocytosis)

Vinflunine
- Antibacterials: plasma concentration of vinflunine possibly reduced by ● RIFAMPICIN—manufacturer of vinflunine advises avoid concomitant use; increased risk of ventricular arrhythmias when vinflunine given with ● DELAMANID
- Antidepressants: plasma concentration of vinflunine possibly reduced by ● ST JOHN'S WORT—manufacturer of vinflunine advises avoid concomitant use
- Antifungals: plasma concentration of vinflunine increased by ● KETOCONAZOLE—manufacturer of vinflunine advises avoid concomitant use; possible increased risk of vinflunine toxicity when given with ● ITRACONAZOLE

Vinflunine (continued)
- Antimalarials: avoidance of vinflunine advised by manufacturer of ● ARTENIMOL WITH PIPERAQUINE
- Antipsychotics: avoid concomitant use of cytotoxics with ● CLOZAPINE (increased risk of agranulocytosis)
- Antivirals: plasma concentration of vinflunine possibly increased by ● RITONAVIR—manufacturer of vinflunine advises avoid concomitant use
▹ Grapefruit Juice: plasma concentration of vinflunine possibly increased by GRAPEFRUIT JUICE—manufacturer of vinflunine advises avoid concomitant use

Vinorelbine
- Antibacterials: possible increased risk of neutropenia when vinorelbine given with ● CLARITHROMYCIN; possible increased risk of ventricular arrhythmias when vinorelbine given with ● DELAMANID
- Antifungals: possible increased risk of vinorelbine toxicity when given with ● ITRACONAZOLE
- Antimalarials: avoidance of vinorelbine advised by manufacturer of ● ARTENIMOL WITH PIPERAQUINE
- Antipsychotics: avoid concomitant use of cytotoxics with ● CLOZAPINE (increased risk of agranulocytosis)

Vismodegib
- Antibacterials: manufacturer of vismodegib advises avoid concomitant use with ● RIFAMPICIN (plasma concentration of vismodegib possibly reduced)
- Antidepressants: manufacturer of vismodegib advises avoid concomitant use with ● ST JOHN'S WORT (plasma concentration of vismodegib possibly reduced)
- Antiepileptics: manufacturer of vismodegib advises avoid concomitant use with ● CARBAMAZEPINE, ● FOSPHENYTOIN and ● PHENYTOIN (plasma concentration of vismodegib possibly reduced)
- Antipsychotics: avoid concomitant use of cytotoxics with ● CLOZAPINE (increased risk of agranulocytosis)

Vitamin A see Vitamins

Vitamin D see Vitamins

Vitamin E see Vitamins

Vitamin K (Phytomenadione) see Vitamins

Vitamins
▹ Antibacterials: absorption of vitamin A possibly reduced by NEOMYCIN
- Anticoagulants: vitamin E possibly enhances anticoagulant effect of ● COUMARINS; vitamin K antagonises anticoagulant effect of ● COUMARINS and ● PHENINDIONE
▹ Antiepileptics: alfacalcidol, calcitriol, colecalciferol, dihydrotachysterol, ergocalciferol, paricalcitol or vitamin D requirements possibly increased when given with CARBAMAZEPINE; alfacalcidol, calcitriol, colecalciferol, dihydrotachysterol, ergocalciferol, paricalcitol or vitamin D requirements possibly increased when given with FOSPHENYTOIN; alfacalcidol, calcitriol, colecalciferol, dihydrotachysterol, ergocalciferol, paricalcitol or vitamin D requirements possibly increased when given with PHENOBARBITAL; alfacalcidol, calcitriol, colecalciferol, dihydrotachysterol, ergocalciferol, paricalcitol or vitamin D requirements possibly increased when given with PHENYTOIN; alfacalcidol, calcitriol, colecalciferol, dihydrotachysterol, ergocalciferol, paricalcitol or vitamin D requirements possibly increased when given with PRIMIDONE
▹ Antifungals: plasma concentration of paricalcitol possibly increased by KETOCONAZOLE; effects of alfacalcidol, calcitriol, colecalciferol, dihydrotachysterol, ergocalciferol, paricalcitol and vitamin D possibly reduced by MICONAZOLE
▹ Antivirals: increased risk of bleeding when high doses of vitamin E given with TIPRANAVIR
▹ Ciclosporin: vitamin E possibly affects plasma concentration of CICLOSPORIN
▹ Cytotoxics: effects of alfacalcidol, calcitriol, colecalciferol, dihydrotachysterol, ergocalciferol, paricalcitol and vitamin D possibly reduced by DACTINOMYCIN; avoidance of vitamin E advised by manufacturer of IBRUTINIB
▹ Diuretics: increased risk of hypercalcaemia when alfacalcidol, calcitriol, colecalciferol, dihydrotachysterol, ergocalciferol, paricalcitol or vitamin D given with THIAZIDES AND RELATED DIURETICS

Vitamins (continued)

▸ Dopaminergics: pyridoxine reduces effects of LEVODOPA when given without dopa-decarboxylase inhibitor
▸ Lipid-regulating Drugs: absorption of calcitriol possibly reduced by COLESTYRAMINE (give at least 1 hour before or 4 to 6 hours after colestyramine)
● Retinoids: risk of hypervitaminosis A when vitamin A given with ● RETINOIDS—avoid concomitant use
▸ Selenium: ascorbic acid possibly reduces absorption of SELENIUM (give at least 4 hours apart)
▸ Sevelamer: absorption of calcitriol reduced by SEVELAMER (give at least 1 hour before or 3 hours after sevelamer)

Voriconazole see Antifungals, Triazole

Vortioxetine

▸ Analgesics: possible increased serotonergic effects when vortioxetine given with TRAMADOL
● Antibacterials: plasma concentration of vortioxetine reduced by ● RIFAMPICIN—consider increasing dose of vortioxetine
● Antidepressants: plasma concentration of vortioxetine possibly increased by FLUOXETINE and PAROXETINE (consider reducing dose of vortioxetine); increased risk of hypertension and CNS excitation when vortioxetine given with ● MAOIS (vortioxetine should not be started until 2 weeks after stopping MAOIs, avoid MAOIs for 2 weeks after stopping vortioxetine); manufacturer of vortioxetine advises avoid concomitant use with ● LINEZOLID and ● MOCLOBEMIDE; possible increased risk of convulsions when vortioxetine given with ● SSRI-RELATED ANTIDEPRESSANTS, ● SSRIS or ● TRICYCLICS; possible increased serotonergic effects when vortioxetine given with ST JOHN'S WORT
● Antiepileptics: plasma concentration of vortioxetine possibly reduced by ● CARBAMAZEPINE, ● FOSPHENYTOIN and ● PHENYTOIN—consider increasing dose of vortioxetine
● Antimalarials: avoidance of antidepressants advised by manufacturer of ● ARTEMETHER WITH LUMEFANTRINE and ● ARTENIMOL WITH PIPERAQUINE; possible increased risk of convulsions when vortioxetine given with ● MEFLOQUINE
● Antipsychotics: possible increased risk of convulsions when vortioxetine given with ● BUTYROPHENONES, ● PHENOTHIAZINES or ● THIOXANTHENES
● Atomoxetine: possible increased risk of convulsions when antidepressants given with ATOMOXETINE
▸ Bupropion: plasma concentration of vortioxetine increased by BUPROPION (consider reducing dose of vortioxetine)
● Dopaminergics: risk of CNS excitation and hypertension when vortioxetine given with ● RASAGILINE or ● SELEGILINE
▸ 5HT₁-receptor Agonists: possible increased serotonergic effects when vortioxetine given with 5HT₁ AGONISTS

Warfarin see Coumarins

Wasp Venom Extracts

● ACE Inhibitors: possible severe anaphylactoid reaction when wasp venom extracts given with ● ACE INHIBITORS

Xipamide see Diuretics

Xylometazoline see Sympathomimetics

Yellow Fever Vaccine see Vaccines

Zafirlukast see Leukotriene Receptor Antagonists

Zaleplon see Anxiolytics and Hypnotics

Zidovudine

NOTE Increased risk of toxicity with nephrotoxic and myelosuppressive drugs—for further details consult product literature
Analgesics: increased risk of haematological toxicity when zidovudine given with NSAIDS; plasma concentration of zidovudine possibly increased by METHADONE
Antibacterials: absorption of zidovudine reduced by CLARITHROMYCIN tablets (give at least 2 hours apart); manufacturer of zidovudine advises avoid concomitant use with RIFAMPICIN
Antiepileptics: zidovudine increases or decreases plasma concentration of FOSPHENYTOIN and PHENYTOIN; plasma concentration of zidovudine possibly increased by SODIUM VALPROATE and VALPROIC ACID (increased risk of toxicity)
Antifungals: plasma concentration of zidovudine increased by ● FLUCONAZOLE (increased risk of toxicity)
Antimalarials: increased antifolate effect when zidovudine given with PYRIMETHAMINE

Zidovudine (continued)

● Antivirals: profound myelosuppression when zidovudine given with ● GANCICLOVIR or ● VALGANCICLOVIR (if possible avoid concomitant administration, particularly during initial ganciclovir or valganciclovir therapy); increased risk of granulocytopenia when zidovudine given with ● NEVIRAPINE; increased risk of anaemia when zidovudine given with ● RIBAVIRIN—avoid concomitant use; zidovudine possibly inhibits effects of ● STAVUDINE (manufacturers advise avoid concomitant use); plasma concentration of zidovudine reduced by ● TIPRANAVIR
▸ Atovaquone: plasma concentration of zidovudine increased by ATOVAQUONE (increased risk of toxicity)
▸ Netupitant: caution with zidovudine advised by manufacturer of NETUPITANT
● Orlistat: absorption of zidovudine possibly reduced by ● ORLISTAT

Zinc

▸ Antibacterials: zinc reduces absorption of CIPROFLOXACIN, LEVOFLOXACIN, NORFLOXACIN and OFLOXACIN (give at least 2 hours apart); zinc reduces absorption of MOXIFLOXACIN (give at least 6 hours apart); zinc possibly reduces absorption of TETRACYCLINES (give at least 2 to 3 hours apart)
▸ Calcium Salts: absorption of zinc reduced by CALCIUM SALTS
▸ Eltrombopag: zinc possibly reduces absorption of ELTROMBOPAG (give at least 4 hours apart)
▸ Iron Salts: absorption of zinc reduced by oral IRON SALTS, also absorption of oral iron salts reduced by zinc
▸ Penicillamine: absorption of zinc reduced by PENICILLAMINE, also absorption of penicillamine reduced by zinc
▸ Trientine: absorption of zinc reduced by TRIENTINE, also absorption of trientine reduced by zinc

Zoledronic Acid see Bisphosphonates

Zolmitriptan see 5HT₁-receptor Agonists (under HT)

Zolpidem see Anxiolytics and Hypnotics

Zonisamide

● Antidepressants: anticonvulsant effect of antiepileptics possibly antagonised by MAOIS and ● TRICYCLIC-RELATED ANTIDEPRESSANTS (convulsive threshold lowered); anticonvulsant effect of antiepileptics antagonised by ● SSRIS and ● TRICYCLICS (convulsive threshold lowered)
▸ Antiepileptics: plasma concentration of zonisamide reduced by CARBAMAZEPINE, FOSPHENYTOIN, PHENOBARBITAL, PHENYTOIN and PRIMIDONE
● Antimalarials: anticonvulsant effect of antiepileptics antagonised by ● MEFLOQUINE
● Antipsychotics: anticonvulsant effect of antiepileptics antagonised by ● ANTIPSYCHOTICS (convulsive threshold lowered)
▸ Diuretics: manufacturer of zonisamide advises avoid concomitant use with CARBONIC ANHYDRASE INHIBITORS in children
● Orlistat: possible increased risk of convulsions when antiepileptics given with ● ORLISTAT

Zopiclone see Anxiolytics and Hypnotics

Zuclopenthixol see Antipsychotics

Appendix 2
Borderline substances

CONTENTS

Enteral feeds (non-disease specific)	page 928
Enteral feeds (non-disease specific): less than 5 g protein/100 mL	928
Enteral feeds (non-disease specific): 5 g (or more) protein/100 mL	929
Enteral feeds (non-disease specific): Child under 12 years	932
Nutritional supplements (non-disease specific)	936
Nutritional supplements: less than 5 g protein/100 mL	936
Nutritional supplements: 5 g (or more) protein/100 mL	937
Specialised formulas	941
Specialised formulas: Infant and child	941
Specialised formulas for specific clinical conditions	946
Feed supplements	948
High-energy supplements	948
Fibre, vitamin, and mineral supplements	953
Feed additives	954
Special additives for conditions of intolerance	954

Feed thickeners and pre-thickened drinks	page 954
Flavouring preparations	955
Foods for special diets	955
Gluten-free foods	955
Low-protein foods	958
Nutritional supplements for metabolic diseases	959
Glutaric aciduria (type 1)	959
Glycogen storage disease	960
Homocystinuria or hypermethioninaemia	960
Hyperlysinaemia	960
Isovaleric acidaemia	961
Maple syrup urine disease	961
Methylmalonic or propionic acidaemia	962
Other inborn errors of metabolism	962
Phenylketonuria	963
Tyrosinaemia	964

In certain conditions some foods (and toilet preparations) have characteristics of drugs and the Advisory Committee on Borderline Substances (ACBS) advises as to the circumstances in which such substances may be regarded as drugs. Prescriptions issued in accordance with the Committee's advice and endorsed 'ACBS' will normally not be investigated.

Information

General Practitioners are reminded that the ACBS recommends products on the basis that they may be regarded as drugs for the management of specified conditions. Doctors should satisfy themselves that the products can safely be prescribed, that patients are adequately monitored and that, where necessary, expert hospital supervision is available.

Foods which may be prescribed on FP10, GP10 (Scotland), or WP10 (Wales)

All the food products listed in this appendix have ACBS approval. The clinical condition for which the product has been approved is included with each entry.
Note Foods included in this appendix may contain cariogenic sugars and patients should be advised to take appropriate oral hygiene measures.

Enteral feeds and supplements

For most enteral feeds and nutritional supplements, the main source of **carbohydrate** is either maltodextrin or glucose syrup; other carbohydrate sources are listed in the relevant table, below. Feeds containing residual lactose (less than 1 g lactose/100 mL formula) are described as 'clinically lactose-free' or 'lactose-free' by some manufacturers. The presence of lactose (including residual lactose) in feeds is indicated in the relevant table, below. The primary sources of **protein** or **amino acids** are included with each product entry. The **fat** or **oil** content is derived from a variety of sources such as vegetables, soya bean, corn, palm nuts, and seeds; where the fat content is derived from animal or fish sources, this information is included in the relevant table, below. The presence of medium chain triglycerides (MCT) is also noted where the quantity exceeds 30% of the fat content.

Enteral feeds and nutritional supplements can contain varying amounts of **vitamins, minerals**, and **trace elements**—the manufacturer's product literature should be consulted for more detailed information. Feeds containing vitamin K may affect the INR in patients receiving warfarin; see **Interactions:** Appendix 1 (Vitamins).
The suitability of food products for patients requiring a vegan, kosher, halal, or other compliant diet should be confirmed with individual manufacturers.
Note Feeds containing more than 6 g/100 mL protein or 2 g/100 mL fibre should be avoided in children unless recommended by an appropriate specialist or dietician.

Nutritional values

Nutritional values of products vary with flavour and pack size—consult product literature.
Standard ACBS indications: Disease-related malnutrition, intractable malabsorption, pre-operative preparation of malnourished patients, dysphagia, proven inflammatory bowel disease following total gastrectomy, short bowel syndrome, bowel fistula.
Paediatric ACBS indications: Disease-related malnutrition, intractable malabsorption, growth failure, pre-operative preparation of malnourished patients, dysphagia, short bowel syndrome, bowel fistula.

Other conditions for which ACBS products can be prescribed

This is a list of clinical conditions for which the ACBS has approved toilet preparations. For details of the preparations see Chapter 13.

Dermatitis, eczema and pruritis
Aveeno® Bath Oil; *Aveeno*® Cream; *Aveeno*® Lotion; *E45*® Emollient Bath Oil; *E45*® Emollient Wash Cream; *E45*® Lotion

Disfiguring skin lesions (birthmarks, mutilating lesions, scars, vitiligo)

Covermark® classic foundation and finishing powder; *Dermablend*® *Ultra* corrective foundation; *Dermacolor*® Camouflage cream and fixing powder; *Keromask*® masking cream and finishing powder; *Veil*® Cover cream and Finishing Powder. (Cleansing Creams, Cleansing Milks, and Cleansing Lotions are excluded).

Disinfectants (antiseptics)

May be prescribed on an FP10 only when ordered in such quantities and with such directions as are appropriate for the treatment of patients, but not for general hygenic purposes.

Dry mouth (xerostomia)

For patients suffering from dry mouth as a result of having (or having undergone) radiotherapy, or sicca syndrome.

AS Saliva Orthana®; *Biotène Oralbalance*®; *BioXtra*®; *Glandosane*®; *Saliveze*®

Photodermatoses (skin protection in)

Anthelios® XL SPF 50+ Melt-in cream; *Sunsense*® Ultra; *Uvistat*® Lipscreen SPF 50, *Uvistat*® Suncream SPF 30 and 50

Prices quoted in Appendix 2 are basic NHS net prices; for further information see Prices in BNFC.

Borderline substances | **Appendix 2**

A2

Table 1 Enteral feeds (non-disease specific)

Less than 5 g protein/100 mL

Enteral feeds: 1 kcal/mL and less than 5 g protein/100 mL
Not suitable for use in child under 1 year unless otherwise stated; not recommended for child 1–6 years

Product	Formulation	Energy	Protein	Carbohydrate	Fat	Fibre	Special Characteristics	ACBS Indications	Presentation & Flavour
Fresubin® 1500 Complete (Fresenius Kabi Ltd)	Liquid (tube feed) per 100 mL	420 kJ (100 kcal)	3.8 g cows' milk soya	13 g (sugars 0.9 g)	3.4 g	1.5 g	Gluten-free Residual lactose Contains fish oil	Standard p. 926 except bowel fistula and pre-operative preparation of malnourished patients. Not suitable for child under 2 years	Fresubin 1500 Complete liquid: 1.5 litre = £13.28
Fresubin® Original (Fresenius Kabi Ltd)	Liquid (sip or tube feed) per 100 mL	420 kJ (100 kcal)	3.8 g cows' milk soya	13.8 g (sugars 3.5 g)	3.4 g	Nil	Gluten-free Residual lactose Contains fish gelatin Feed in flexible pack contains fish oil and fish gelatin	Standard p. 926	Fresubin Original liquid: blackcurrant, chocolate, nut, peach, vanilla Bottle 200 ml = £2.14, unflavoured 500 ml = £4.17, 1000 ml = £8.26, 1500 ml = £12.39
Fresubin® Original Fibre (Fresenius Kabi Ltd)	Liquid (tube feed) per 100 mL	420 kJ (100 kcal)	3.8 g cows' milk soya	13 g (sugars 0.9 g)	3.4 g	1.5 g	Gluten-free Residual lactose Contains fish oil	Standard p. 926 except bowel fistula and pre-operative preparation of malnourished patients. Not suitable for child under 2 years	Fresubin Original Fibre liquid: 500 ml = £4.72; 1000 ml = £9.42
Jevity® (Abbott Laboratories Ltd)	Liquid (tube feed) per 100 mL	449 kJ (107 kcal)	4 g caseinates	14.1 g (sugars 470 mg)	3.47 g	1.76 g	Gluten-free Residual lactose	Standard p. 926 except bowel fistula. Not suitable for child under 2 years	Jevity liquid: 500 ml = £5.20; 1000 ml = £9.46; 1500 ml = £14.14
Nutrison® (Nutricia Ltd)	Liquid (tube feed) per 100 mL	420 kJ (100 kcal)	4 g cows' milk	12.3 g (sugars 1 g)	3.9 g	Nil	Gluten-free Residual lactose	Standard p. 926	Nutrison liquid: 500 ml = £4.43; 500 ml = £4.92 (bottle); 1000 ml = £8.63; 1500 ml = £12.93
Nutrison® Multi Fibre (Nutricia Ltd)	Liquid (tube feed) per 100 mL	420 kJ (100 kcal)	4 g cows' milk	12.3 g (sugars 1 g)	3.9 g	1.5 g	Gluten-free Residual lactose	Standard p. 926 except bowel fistula	Nutrison Multi Fibre liquid: 500 ml = £5.31 (bottle); 500 ml = £5.31; 1000 ml = £9.99; 1500 ml = £14.97
Osmolite® (Abbott Laboratories Ltd)	Liquid (tube feed) per 100 mL	424 kJ (100 kcal)	4 g caseinates soy isolate	13.6 g (sugars 630 mg)	3.4 g	Nil	Gluten-free Residual lactose	Standard p. 926	Osmolite liquid: 500 ml = £4.65; 1000 ml = £8.46; 1500 ml = £12.65

SOYA PROTEIN FORMULA

Product	Formulation	Energy	Protein	Carbohydrate	Fat	Fibre	Special Characteristics	ACBS Indications	Presentation & Flavour
Fresubin® Soya Fibre (Fresenius Kabi Ltd)	Liquid (tube feed) per 100 mL	420 kJ (100 kcal)	3.8 g soya protein	13.3 g (sugars 4.1 g)	3.6 g	2 g	Gluten-free Lactose-free Contains fish oil	Standard p. 926; *also cows' milk protein intolerance, lactose intolerance*	Fresubin Soya Fibre liquid: 500 ml = £4.88
Nutrison® Soya (Nutricia Ltd)	Liquid (tube feed) per 100 mL	420 kJ (100 kcal)	4 g soy isolate	12.3 g (sugars 1 g)	3.9 g	Nil	Gluten-free Residual lactose Milk protein-free	Standard p. 926; *also cows' milk protein and lactose intolerance*	Nutrison Soya liquid: 500 ml = £5.30; 1000 ml = £10.62

Product	Formulation	Energy	Protein	Carbohydrate	Fat	Fibre	Special Characteristics	ACBS Indications	Presentation & Flavour
Nutrison® Soya Multi Fibre (Nutricia Ltd)	Liquid (tube feed) per 100 mL	420 kJ (100 kcal)	4 g soy isolate	12.3 g (sugars 700 mg)	3.9 g	1.5 g	Gluten-free, Residual lactose, Milk protein-free	Standard p. 926 except bowel fistula; also cows' milk protein and lactose intolerance	Nutrison Soya Multi Fibre liquid: 1.5 litre = £17.66

PEPTIDE-BASED FORMULA

Product	Formulation	Energy	Protein	Carbohydrate	Fat	Fibre	Special Characteristics	ACBS Indications	Presentation & Flavour
Nutrison Peptisorb® (Nutricia Ltd)	Liquid (tube feed) per 100 mL	425 kJ (100 kcal)	4 g whey protein hydrolysate	17.6 g (sugars 1.7 g)	1.7 g (MCT 47 %)	Nil	Gluten-free, Residual lactose	Short bowel syndrome, intractable malabsorption, proven inflammatory bowel disease, bowel fistula	Nutrison Peptisorb liquid: 500 ml = £7.04 (bottle); 500 ml = £7.73; 1000 ml = £13.94
Peptamen® (Nestle Health Science)	Liquid (sip or tube feed) per 100 mL	420 kJ (100 kcal)	4 g whey peptides	12.7 g (sugars 480 mg)	3.7 g (MCT 70 %)	Nil	Gluten-free, Residual lactose	Short bowel syndrome, intractable malabsorption, proven inflammatory bowel disease, bowel fistula	Peptamen liquid: vanilla 800 ml = £12.14 unflavoured 500 ml = £6.66 1000 ml = £12.50
Survimed® OPD (Fresenius Kabi Ltd)	Liquid (tube feed) per 100 mL	420 kJ (100 kcal)	4.5 g whey protein hydrolysate	14.3 g (sugars 1.1 g)	2.8 g (MCT 51 %)	100 mg	Gluten-free, Residual lactose, Contains fish oil	Standard p. 926; also growth failure	Survimed OPD: liquid 500 ml = £6.96 800 ml = £12.84 1000 ml = £13.92 HN liquid 500 ml = £6.70

Enteral feeds: Less than 1 kcal/mL and less than 5 g protein/100 mL

AMINO ACID FORMULA (ESSENTIAL AND NON-ESSENTIAL AMINO ACIDS)
Not suitable for use in child under 1 year unless otherwise stated; not recommended for child 1–6 years

Product	Formulation	Energy	Protein	Carbohydrate	Fat	Fibre	Special Characteristics	ACBS Indications	Presentation & Flavour
Elemental 028® Extra (Nutricia Ltd)	Liquid (sip feed) per 100 mL	360 kJ (86 kcal)	2.5 g (protein equivalent)	11 g (sugars 4.7 g)	3.5 g (MCT 35 %)	Nil		Short bowel syndrome, intractable malabsorption, proven inflammatory bowel disease, bowel fistula	Elemental 028 Extra liquid summer fruits; grapefruit, orange & pineapple 250 ml = £3.68
	Standard dilution (20 %) of powder (sip or tube feed) per 100 mL	374 kJ (89 kcal)	2.5 g (protein equivalent)	11.8 g (sugars 1.8 g)	3.5 g (MCT 35 %)	Nil		Short bowel syndrome, intractable malabsorption, proven inflammatory bowel disease, bowel fistula.	Elemental 028 Extra powder: plain, orange, citrus, banana 100 gram = £7.14 (sachets)

Powder provides protein equivalent 12.5 g, carbohydrate 59 g, fat 17.45 g, energy 1871 kJ (443 kcal)/100 g

Enteral feeds (non-disease specific): 5 g (or more) protein/100 mL

Enteral feeds: 1.5 kcal/mL and 5 g (or more) protein/100 mL
Not suitable for use in child under 1 year unless otherwise stated; not recommended for child 1–6 years

Product	Formulation	Energy	Protein	Carbohydrate	Fat	Fibre	Special Characteristics	ACBS Indications	Presentation & Flavour
Fresubin® 2250 Complete (Fresenius Kabi Ltd)	Liquid (tube feed) per 100 mL	630 kJ (150 kcal)	5.6 g cows' milk	18.8 g (sugars 1.5 g)	5.8 g	2 g	Gluten-free, Residual lactose, Contains fish oil and fish gelatin	Standard p. 926	Fresubin 2250 Complete liquid: 1.5 litre = £14.82

Borderline substances | **Appendix 2**

A2

Enteral feeds: 1.5 kcal/mL and 5 g (or more) protein/100 mL (product list continued)

Not suitable for use in child under 1 year unless otherwise stated; not recommended for child 1–6 years

Product	Formulation	Energy	Protein	Carbohydrate	Fat	Fibre	Special Characteristics	ACBS Indications	Presentation & Flavour
Fresubin® Energy (Fresenius Kabi Ltd)	Liquid (sip feed) per 100 mL	630 kJ (150 kcal)	5.6 g cows' milk	18.8 g (sugars)	5.8 g	Nil	Gluten-free. Residual lactose. Contains fish gelatin. Strawberry flavour may contain traces of wheat starch & egg	Standard p. 926	liquid: 200 ml Fresubin Energy liquid: banana, blackcurrant, cappuccino, chocolate, lemon, strawberry, tropical fruits, vanilla 200 ml = £1.40 (bottle)
	Liquid (tube feed) per 100 mL	630 kJ (150 kcal)	5.6 g cows' milk	18.8 g (sugars 1.4 g)	5.8 g	Nil	Gluten-free. Residual lactose. Contains fish oil and fish gelatin	Standard p. 926	liquid: unflavoured 200 ml = £1.40 500 ml = £5.05 1000 ml = £10.03 1500 ml = £13.45
Fresubin® Energy Fibre (Fresenius Kabi Ltd)	Liquid (sip feed) per 100 mL	630 kJ (150 kcal)	5.6 g cows' milk	18.8 g (sugars)	5.8 g	2 g	Gluten-free. Residual lactose. Contains fish gelatin	Standard p. 926	Fresubin Energy Fibre liquid:banana, caramel, cherry, chocolate, strawberry 200 ml = £2.05
	Liquid (tube feed) per 100 mL	630 kJ (150 kcal)	5.6 g cows' milk	18.8 g (sugars 1.5 g)	5.8 g	2 g	Gluten-free. Residual lactose. Contains fish oil and fish gelatin	Standard p. 926	Fresubin Energy Fibre liquid: unflavoured 500 ml = £5.60 1000 ml = £10.68
Fresubin® HP Energy (Fresenius Kabi Ltd)	Liquid (tube feed) per 100 mL	630 kJ (150 kcal)	7.5 g cows' milk	17 g (sugars 1 g)	5.8 g (MCT 57 %)	Nil	Gluten-free. Residual lactose. Contains fish oil and fish gelatin	Standard p. 926; also CAPD and haemodialysis	Fresubin HP Energy liquid: 500 ml = £5.20; 1000 ml = £10.40
Jevity® 1.5 kcal (Abbott Laboratories Ltd)	Liquid (tube feed) per 100 mL	649 kJ (154 kcal)	6.38 g caseinates and soy protein isolate	20.1 g (sugars 1.47 g)	4.9 g	2.2 g	Gluten-free. Residual lactose	Standard p. 926. Not suitable for child under 2 years; not recommended for child 2–10 years	Jevity 1.5kcal liquid: 500 ml = £6.24; 1000 ml = £11.36; 1500 ml = £16.97
Nutrison® Energy (Nutricia Ltd)	Liquid (tube feed) per 100 mL	630 kJ (150 kcal)	6 g cows' milk	18.5 g (sugars 1.5 g)	5.8 g	Nil	Gluten-free. Residual lactose	Standard p. 926	Nutrison Energy liquid: 500 ml = £5.35 (bottle); 1000 ml = £10.77; 1500 ml = £16.10
Nutrison® Energy Multi Fibre (Nutricia Ltd)	Liquid (tube feed) per 100 mL	630 kJ (150 kcal)	6 g cows' milk	18.5 g (sugars 1.5 g)	5.8 g	1.5 g	Gluten-free. Residual lactose	Standard p. 926	Nutrison Energy Multi Fibre liquid: 500 ml = £5.99; 500 ml = £6.35; 1000 ml = £11.95; 1500 ml = £18.45
Osmolite® 1.5 kcal (Abbott Laboratories Ltd)	Liquid (tube feed) per 100 mL	632 kJ (150 kcal)	6.25 g cows' milk soya protein isolate	20 g (sugars 4.9 g)	5 g	Nil	Gluten-free. Residual lactose	Standard p. 926	Osmolite 1.5kcal tube feed liquid: 500 ml = £5.60; 1000 ml = £10.19; 1500 ml = £15.23
Resource® Energy (Nestle Health Science)	Liquid (sip feed) per 100 mL	630 kJ (150 kcal)	5.6 g cows' milk	21 g (sugars 5.2 g)	5 g	less than 0.5 g	Gluten-free. Residual lactose	Standard p. 926. Not suitable for use in child under 3 years	Resource Energy liquid: apricot, banana, chocolate, coffee, strawberry & raspberry, vanilla 800 ml = £7.67 (bottle) 4 x 200 ml

Enteral feeds: Less than 1.5 kcal/mL and 5 g (or more) protein/100 mL

Not suitable for use in child under 1 year unless otherwise stated; not recommended for child 1-6 years

Product	Formulation	Energy	Protein	Carbohydrate	Fat	Fibre	Special Characteristics	ACBS Indications	Presentation & Flavour
Fresubin® 1000 Complete (Fresenius Kabi Ltd)	Liquid (tube feed) per 100 mL	420 kJ (100 kcal)	5.5 g cows' milk	12.5 g (sugars 1.1 g)	3.1 g	2 g	Gluten-free Residual lactose Contains fish oil	Standard p. 926	Fresubin 1000 Complete liquid: 1 litre = £10.68
Fresubin® 1200 Complete (Fresenius Kabi Ltd)	Liquid (tube feed) per 100 mL	500 kJ (120 kcal)	6 g cows' milk	15 g (sugars 1.22 g)	4.1 g	2 g	Gluten-free Residual lactose Contains fish oil	Standard p. 926	Fresubin 1200 Complete liquid: 1 litre = £13.60
Fresubin® 1800 Complete (Fresenius Kabi Ltd)	Liquid (tube feed) per 100 mL	500 kJ (120 kcal)	6 g cows' milk	15 g (sugars 1.22 g)	4.1 g	2 g	Gluten-free Residual lactose Contains fish oil	Standard p. 926	Fresubin 1800 Complete liquid: 1.5 litre = £13.60
Jevity® Plus (Abbott Laboratories Ltd)	Liquid (tube feed) per 100 mL	514 kJ (122 kcal)	5.5 g caseinates soy isolates	15.1 g (sugars 890 mg)	3.93 g	2.2 g	Gluten-free Residual lactose	Standard p. 926 Not suitable for child under 2 years; not recommended for child 2-10 years	Jevity Plus liquid: 500 ml = £6.20; 1000 ml = £11.28; 1500 ml = £16.86
Jevity® Plus HP (Abbott Laboratories Ltd)	Liquid (tube feed) per 100 mL	551 kJ (131 kcal)	8.13 g cows' milk soy isolates	14.2 g (sugars 950 mg)	4.33 g	1.5 g	Gluten-free Residual lactose	Standard p. 926; also CAPD, haemodialysis Not suitable for child under 2 years; not recommended for child 2-10 years	Jevity Plus HP gluten free liquid: 500 ml = £6.20
Jevity® Promote (Abbott Laboratories Ltd)	Liquid (tube feed) per 100 mL	434 kJ (103 kcal)	5.55 g caseinates soy isolates	12 g (sugars 670 mg)	3.32 g	1.7 g	Gluten-free Residual lactose	Standard p. 926 Not suitable for child under 2 years; not recommended for child 2-10 years	Jevity Promote liquid: 1 litre = £10.80
Nutrison® 800 Complete Multi Fibre (Nutricia Ltd)	Liquid (tube feed) per 100 mL	345 kJ (83 kcal)	5.5 g cows' milk pea protein soya protein	8.8 g (sugars 600 mg)	2.5 g	1.5 g	Gluten-free Residual lactose Contains fish oil	Standard p. 926 except bowel fistula Not suitable for child under 6 years; not recommended for child 6-12 years	Nutrison 800 Complete Multi Fibre liquid: 1 litre = £10.27
Nutrison® 1000 Complete Multi Fibre (Nutricia Ltd)	Liquid (tube feed) per 100 mL	420 kJ (100 kcal)	5.5 g cows' milk	11.3 g (sugars 700 mg)	3.7 g	2 g	Gluten-free Residual lactose	Disease related malnutrition in patients with low energy and/or low fluid requirements	Nutrison 1000 Complete Multi Fibre liquid: 1 litre = £11.08
Nutrison® 1200 Complete Multi Fibre (Nutricia Ltd)	Liquid (tube feed) per 100 mL	505 kJ (120 kcal)	5.5 g cows' milk	15 g (sugars 1.2 g)	4.3 g	2 g	Gluten-free Residual lactose	Standard p. 926 except bowel fistula	Nutrison 1200 Complete Multi Fibre liquid: 1000 ml = £11.73; 1500 ml = £17.61
Nutrison® MCT (Nutricia Ltd)	Liquid (tube feed) per 100 mL	420 kJ (100 kcal)	5 g cows' milk	12.6 g (sugars 1 g)	3.3 g (MCT 61%)	Nil	Gluten-free Residual lactose	Standard p. 926	Nutrison MCT liquid: 1000 ml = £9.98
Nutrison® Protein Plus (Nutricia Ltd)	Liquid (tube feed) per 100 mL	525 kJ (125 kcal)	6.3 g cows' milk	14.2 g (sugars 1.1 g)	4.9 g	Nil	Gluten-free Residual lactose	Standard p. 926	Nutrison Protein Plus liquid: 1 litre = £10.25
Nutrison® Protein Plus Multi Fibre (Nutricia Ltd)	Liquid (tube feed) per 100 mL	525 kJ (125 kcal)	6.3 g cow's milk	14.1 g (sugars 1.1 g)	4.9 g	1.5 g	Gluten-free Residual lactose	Disease related malnutrition	Nutrison Protein Plus Multifibre liquid: 1 litre = £11.42

Borderline substances | Appendix 2

A2

Enteral feeds: Less than 1.5 kcal/mL and 5 g (or more) protein/100 mL (product list continued)

Not suitable for use in child under 1 year unless otherwise stated; not recommended for child 1-6 years

Product	Formulation	Energy	Protein	Carbohydrate	Fat	Fibre	Special Characteristics	ACBS Indications	Presentation & Flavour
Osmolite® Plus (Abbott Laboratories Ltd)	Liquid (tube feed) per 100 mL	508 kJ (121 kcal)	5.55 g caseinates	15.8 g (sugars 730 mg)	3.93 g	Nil	Gluten-free Residual lactose	Standard p. 926 Not suitable for child under 10 years	Osmolite Plus liquid: 500 ml = £5.20; 1000 ml = £9.46; 1500 ml = £14.15
Peptamen® HN (Nestle Health Science)	Liquid (tube feed) per 100 mL	556 kJ (133 kcal)	6.6 g whey protein hydrolysates	15.6 g (sugars 1.4 g)	4.9 g (MCT 70%)	Nil	Gluten-free Residual lactose Hydrolysed with pork trypsin	Short bowel syndrome, intractable malabsorption, proven inflammatory bowel disease, bowel fistula Not suitable for child under 3 years	Peptamen HN liquid: 500 ml =£7.34
Perative® (Abbott Laboratories Ltd)	Liquid (sip or tube feed) per 100 mL	552 kJ (131 kcal)	6.7 g caseinate whey protein hydrolysates	17.7 g (sugars 660 mg)	3.7 g (MCT 42%)	Nil	Gluten-free Residual lactose	Standard p. 926 Not suitable for child under 5 years	Perative liquid: 500 ml = £7.50; 1000 ml = £13.66

Enteral feeds: More than 1.5 kcal/mL and 5 g (or more) protein/100 mL

Not suitable for use in child under 1 year unless otherwise stated; not recommended for child 1-6 years

Product	Formulation	Energy	Protein	Carbohydrate	Fat	Fibre	Special Characteristics	ACBS Indications	Presentation & Flavour
Ensure® Twocal (Abbott Laboratories Ltd)	Liquid (sip or tube feed) per 100 mL	838 kJ (200 kcal)	8.4 g cows' milk	21 g (sugars 4.5 g)	8.9 g	1 g	Gluten-free Residual lactose	Standard p. 926; also haemodialysis and CAPD	Ensure TwoCal liquid: banana, neutral, strawberry, vanilla 200 ml = £2.22 (bottle)

Enteral feeds (non-disease specific): Child under 12 years

Enteral feeds, Child: Less than 1 kcal/mL and less than 4 g protein/100 mL

Product	Formulation	Energy	Protein	Carbohydrate	Fat	Fibre	Special Characteristics	ACBS Indications	Presentation & Flavour
Nutrini® Low Energy Multi Fibre (Nutricia Ltd)	Liquid (tube feed) per 100 mL	315 kJ (75 kcal)	2.1 g whey protein and caseinate	9.3 g (sugars 600 mg)	3.3 g	800 mg	Gluten-free Residual lactose Contains fish oil	Paediatric p. 926 except bowel fistula, in child 1-6 years, body-weight 8-20 kg	Nutrini Low Energy Multifibre liquid: 200 ml = £2.64 (bottle); 500 ml = £6.69
Nutriprem® 1 (Cow & Gate Ltd)	Liquid (sip feed) per 100 mL	335 kJ (80 kcal)	2.5 g whey protein and casein	7.6 g (lactose 6.3 g)	4.4 g	0.8 g	Contains soya fish oil and egg lipid	Low birth-weight formula	Nutriprem 1: bottle 70 ml = Hospital supply only
Nutriprem® 2 (Cow & Gate Ltd)	Liquid (sip feed) per 100 mL	310 kJ (75 kcal)	2 g whey protein and casein	7.4 g (lactose 5.8 g)	4 g	600 mg	Contains soya fish oil and egg lipid	Catch-up growth in pre-term infants (less than 35 weeks at birth) and small for gestational-age infants up to 6 months corrected age.	Nutriprem 2: liquid 200 ml = £1.74
	Standard dilution (15.3%) of powder (sip feed) per 100 mL	315 kJ (75 kcal)	2 g whey protein and casein	7.4 g (lactose 5.9 g)	4 g (including MCT oil)	600 mg			Nutriprem 2: powder 900 gram = £11.67 (5.1 g measuring scoop provided)
SMA® Gold Prem 2 (SMA Nutrition)	Standard dilution (14%) of powder (sip feed) per 100 mL	305 kJ (73 kcal)	1.9 g cows' milk	7.5 g sugars 6.4 g	3.9 g	Nil	Contains lactose	Catch-up growth in preterm and small for gestational age infants on discharge from hospital, up to 6 months corrected age.	SMA Gold Prem 2: powder 400 gram = £4.92 (4.7 g measuring scoop provided)
SMA® High Energy (SMA Nutrition)	Liquid (sip feed) per 100 mL	382 kJ (91 kcal)	2 g whey protein and casein	9.8 g lactose	4.9 g	Nil	Contains lactose	Disease related malnutrition and malabsorption, and growth failure in child from birth to 18 months	SMA High Energy milk: 250 ml = £2.46

AMINO ACID FORMULA (ESSENTIAL AND NON-ESSENTIAL AMINO ACIDS)

Product	Formulation	Energy	Protein	Carbohydrate	Fat	Fibre	Special Characteristics	ACBS Indications	Presentation & Flavour
Emsogen® (SHS)	Standard dilution (20 %) of powder (sip or tube feed) per 100 mL	368 kJ (88 kcal)	2.5 g protein equivalent (essential and non-essential amino acids)	12 g (sugars 1.6 g)	3.3 g (MCT 83 %)	Nil	Lactose-free	Short-bowel syndrome, intractable malabsorption, proven inflammatory bowel disease, bowel fistula Not suitable for child under 1 year or as sole source of nutrition in child 1–5 years	Emsogen powder, unflavoured: 100 gram = £7.36

Powder provides: protein equivalent 12.5 g, carbohydrate 60 g, fat 16.4 g, energy 1839 kJ (438 kcal)/100 g

Enteral feeds, Child: 1 kcal/mL and less than 4 g protein/100 mL
Not suitable for use in child under 1 year unless otherwise stated

Product	Formulation	Energy	Protein	Carbohydrate	Fat	Fibre	Special Characteristics	ACBS Indications	Presentation & Flavour
Fortini® 1.0 Multi Fibre (Nutricia Ltd)	Liquid (sip feed) per 100 mL	420 kJ (100 kcal)	2.4 g cows' milk	11.8 g (sugars 4.7 g)	4.5 g	1.5 g	Gluten-free Residual lactose	Disease-related malnutrition and growth failure in child 1–6 years, body-weight 8–20 kg	Fortini 1.0 Multi Fibre liquid: banana, chocolate, strawberry, vanilla 200 ml = £2.52
Frebini® Original (Fresenius Kabi Ltd)	Liquid (tube feed) per 100 mL	420 kJ (100 kcal)	2.5 g cows' milk	12.5 g (sugars 700 mg)	4.4 g	Nil	Gluten-free Residual lactose Contains fish oils and fish gelatin	Standard p. 926 and growth failure in child 1–10 years, body-weight 8–30 kg	Frebini Original liquid: 500 ml = £6.16
Frebini® Original Fibre (Fresenius Kabi Ltd)	Liquid (tube feed) per 100 mL	420 kJ (100 kcal)	2.5 g cows' milk	12.5 g (sugars 700 mg)	4.4 g	0.75 g	Gluten-free Residual lactose Contains fish oils and fish gelatin	Standard p. 926 and growth failure in child 1–10 years, body-weight 8–30 kg	Frebini Original Fibre liquid: 500 ml = £6.85
Infatrini® (Nutricia Ltd)	Liquid (sip or tube feed) per 100 mL	415 kJ (100 kcal)	2.6 g cows' milk	10.3 g (lactose 5.2 g)	5.4 g	0.8 g	Gluten-free Contains fish oil	Failure to thrive, disease-related malnutrition and malabsorption, in child from birth up to body-weight 8 kg	Infatrini liquid: 125 ml = £1.43; 200 ml = £2.27; 500 ml = £6.16
Nutrini® (Nutricia Ltd)	Liquid (tube feed) per 100 mL	420 kJ (100 kcal)	2.8 g cows' milk	12.3 g (sugars 1 g)	4.4 g	Nil	Gluten-free Residual lactose	Standard p. 926 and growth failure in child 1–6 years, body-weight 8–20 kg	Nutrini liquid: 200 ml = £2.75; 500 ml = £6.83
Nutrini® Multi Fibre (Nutricia Ltd)	Liquid (tube feed) per 100 mL	420 kJ (100 kcal)	2.8 g whey protein and caseinate	12.3 g (sugars 800 mg)	4.4 g	800 mg	Gluten-free Residual lactose Contains fish oil	Standard p. 926 and growth failure in child 1–6 years, body-weight 8–20 kg	Nutrini Multifibre liquid: 200 ml = £3.04; 500 ml = £7.58
Paediasure® (Abbott Laboratories Ltd)	Liquid (sip or tube feed) per 100 mL	422 kJ (100 kcal)	2.8 g cows' milk	11.2 g (sugars 3.92 g)	4.98 g	Nil	Gluten-free Residual lactose	Paediatric p. 926 in child 1–10 years, body-weight 8–30 kg	PaediaSure liquid: vanilla 200 ml = £2.37 500 ml = £6.55 banana, chocolate, strawberry 200 ml = £2.37 Nutritional values may vary with flavour—consult product literature
Paediasure® Fibre (Abbott Laboratories Ltd)	Liquid (sip or tube feed) per 100 mL	424 kJ (101 kcal)	2.8 g caseinates and whey protein	10.9 g (sugars 3.84 g)	4.98 g	730 mg	Gluten-free Residual lactose	Paediatric p. 926 in child 1–10 years, body-weight 8–30 kg	PaediaSure fibre liquid: vanilla 200 ml = £2.60 500 ml = £7.30 banana, strawberry 200 ml = £2.60 Nutritional values may vary with flavour consult product literature

Borderline substances | **Appendix 2**

A2

Enteral feeds, Child: 1 kcal/mL and less than 4 g protein/100 mL (product list continued)

Not suitable for use in child under 1 year unless otherwise stated

Product	Formulation	Energy	Protein	Carbohydrate	Fat	Fibre	Special Characteristics	ACBS Indications	Presentation & Flavour
Paediasure® Peptide (Abbott Laboratories Ltd)	Liquid (sip or tube feed) per 100 mL	420 kJ (100 kcal)	3 g whey protein and caseinate	13 g (sugars 2.98 g)	4 (MCT 50%) g	Nil	Gluten-free Residual lactose	Standard p. 926 and growth failure in child 1-10 years, body-weight 8-30 kg	PaediaSure Peptide liquid vanilla: 200 ml = £3.82; vanilla 500 ml = £10.20
Similac® High Energy (Abbott Laboratories Ltd)	Liquid (sip or tube feed) per 100 mL	419 kJ (100 kcal)	2.6 g cows' milk and whey protein	10.1 g (sugars 5.6 g)	5.2 g	400 mg	Gluten-free Contains lactose and soy oil	Increased energy requirements, faltering growth, and/or need for fluid restriction, in child body-weight up to 8 kg	Similac High Energy liquid: 60 ml = £0.66; 200 ml = £2.13
Tentrini® (Nutricia Ltd)	Liquid (tube feed) per 100 mL	420 kJ (100 kcal)	3.3 g whey protein and caseinate	12.3 g (sugars 800 mg)	4.2 g	Nil	Gluten-free Residual lactose Contains fish oil	Standard p. 926 and growth failure in child 7-12 years, body-weight 21-45 kg	Tentrini liquid: 500 ml = £6.02
Tentrini® Multi Fibre (Nutricia Ltd)	Liquid (tube feed) per 100 mL	420 kJ (100 kcal)	3.3 g whey protein and caseinate	12.3 g (sugars 800 mg)	4.2 g	1.1 g	Gluten-free Residual lactose Contains fish oil	Standard p. 926 except bowel fistula, and growth failure in child 7-12 years body-weight 21-45 kg	Tentrini Multifibre liquid: 500 ml = £6.61

HYDROLYSATE FORMULA

Product	Formulation	Energy	Protein	Carbohydrate	Fat	Fibre	Special Characteristics	ACBS Indications	Presentation & Flavour
Nutrini® Peptisorb (Nutricia Ltd)	Liquid (tube feed) per 100 mL	420 kJ (100 kcal)	2.8 g whey protein hydrolysate	13.7 g (sugars 800 mg)	3.9 g (MCT 46 %)	Nil	Gluten-free Residual lactose	Standard p. 926 and growth failure in child 1-6 years, body-weight 8-20 kg	Nutrini Peptisorb liquid: 500 ml = £10.66
Peptamen® Junior (Nestle Health Science)	Liquid (tube feed) per 100 mL	420 kJ (100 kcal)	3 g whey protein hydrolysate	13.2 g	4 g (MCT 60 %)	Nil	Gluten-free Residual lactose Hydrolysed with pork trypsin	Short bowel syndrome, intractable malabsorption, proven inflammatory bowel disease, bowel fistula, in child 1-10 years	Peptamen Junior: liquid 500 ml = £6.81
	Standard dilution (22%) of powder (sip or tube feed) per 100 mL	420 kJ (100 kcal)	3 g whey protein hydrolysate	13.8 g	3.85 g (MCT 60 %)	Nil	Gluten-free Residual lactose Hydrolysed with bacterial trypsin		Peptamen Junior: powder 400 gram = £17.86 (7.86 g measuring scoop provided)

Powder provides: protein 13.7 g, carbohydrate 62.9 g, fat 17.5 g, energy 1910 kJ (457 kcal)/100 g

Enteral feeds, Child: More than 1 kcal/mL and less than 4 g protein/100 mL

Not suitable for use in child under 1 year unless otherwise stated

Product	Formulation	Energy	Protein	Carbohydrate	Fat	Fibre	Special Characteristics	ACBS Indications	Presentation & Flavour
Fortini® (Nutricia Ltd)	Liquid (sip feed) per 100 mL	630 kJ (150 kcal)	3.4 g cows' milk	18.8 g (sugars 7.4 g)	6.8 g	Nil	Gluten-free Residual lactose	Disease-related malnutrition and growth failure in child 1-6 years, body-weight 8-20 kg	Fortini liquid: strawberry, vanilla 200 ml = £3.27
Fortini® Multifibre (Nutricia Ltd)	Liquid (sip feed) per 100 mL	630 kJ (150 kcal)	3.4 g cows' milk	18.8 g (sugars 7.4 g)	6.8 g	1.5 g	Gluten-free Residual lactose	Disease-related malnutrition and growth failure in child 1-6 years, body-weight 8-20 kg	Fortini Multi Fibre liquid: banana, chocolate, strawberry, unflavoured, vanilla 200 ml = £3.43
Fortini® Smoothie Multifibre (Nutricia Ltd)	Liquid (sip feed) per 100 mL	625 kJ (150 kcal)	3.4 g cows' milk	19 g (sugars 11.5 g)	6.4 g	1.4 g	Gluten-free Residual lactose	Disease-related malnutrition and growth failure in child 1-6 years, body-weight 8-20 kg	Fortini Smoothie Multi Fibre liquid: berry fruit, summer fruit 200 ml = £3.43

Product	Formulation	Energy	Protein	Carbohydrate	Fat	Fibre	Special Characteristics	ACBS Indications	Presentation & Flavour
Frebini® Energy (Fresenius Kabi Ltd)	Liquid (tube feed) per 100 mL	630 kJ (150 kcal)	3.75 g cows' milk	18.75 g (sugars 830 mg)	6.7 g	Nil	Gluten-free Residual lactose Contains fish oil and fish gelatin	Standard p. 926 and growth failure in child 1-10 years, body-weight 8-30 kg	Frebini Energy: 500 ml = £7.22
Frebini® Energy Drink (Fresenius Kabi Ltd)	Liquid (sip feed) per 100 mL	630 kJ (150 kcal)	3.8 g cows' milk	18.7 g (sugars 4.5 g)	6.7 g	Nil	Gluten-free Residual lactose	Disease-related malnutrition and growth failure in child 1-10 years, body-weight 8-30 kg	Frebini Energy Drink: banana, strawberry 200 ml = £2.92
Frebini® Energy Fibre (Fresenius Kabi Ltd)	Liquid (tube feed) per 100 mL	630 kJ (150 kcal)	3.75 g cows' milk	18.75 g (sugars 830 mg)	6.7 g	1.13 g	Gluten-free Residual lactose Contains fish oils and fish gelatin	Standard p. 926 and growth failure in child 1-10 years, body-weight 8-30 kg	Frebini Energy Fibre liquid unflavoured: 500 ml = £8.27
Frebini® Energy Fibre Drink (Fresenius Kabi Ltd)	Liquid (sip feed) per 100 mL	630 kJ (150 kcal)	3.8 g cows' milk	18.75 g (sugars 4.5 g)	6.7 g	1.1 g	Gluten-free Residual lactose	Disease-related malnutrition and growth failure in child 1-10 years, body-weight 8-30 kg	Frebini Energy Fibre liquid: chocolate, vanilla 200 ml = £2.98
Resource® Junior (Nestle Health Science)	Liquid (sip feed) per 100 mL	630 kJ (150 kcal)	3 g cows' milk	20.6 g (sugars 4.9 g)	6.2 g	Nil	Gluten-free Residual lactose	Standard p. 926 in child 1-10 years. Not suitable for use in child under 1 year	Resource Junior complete sip feed: chocolate, strawberry, vanilla 200 ml = £2.14

Enteral feeds, Child: 1.5 kcal/mL and more than 4 g protein/100 mL

Not suitable for use in child under 1 year unless otherwise stated

Product	Formulation	Energy	Protein	Carbohydrate	Fat	Fibre	Special Characteristics	ACBS Indications	Presentation & Flavour
Nutrini® Energy (Nutricia Ltd)	Liquid (tube feed) per 100 mL	630 kJ (150 kcal)	4.1 g caseinate whey protein	18.5 g (sugars 1.1 g)	6.7 g	Nil	Gluten-free Residual lactose Contains fish oil	Standard p. 926 and growth failure in child 1-6 years, body-weight 8-20 kg	Nutrini Energy liquid: 200 ml = £3.35; 500 ml = £8.57
Nutrini® Energy Multi Fibre (Nutricia Ltd)	Liquid (tube feed) per 100 mL	630 kJ (150 kcal)	4.1 g caseinate whey protein	18.5 g (sugars 1.1 g)	6.7 g	800 mg	Gluten-free Residual lactose Contains fish oil	Paediatric p. 926 except bowel fistula; also total gastrectomy, in child 1-6 years, body-weight 8-20 kg	Nutrini Energy Multifibre liquid: 200 ml = £3.53; 500 ml = £8.85
Paediasure® Plus (Abbott Laboratories Ltd)	Liquid (sip or tube feed) per 100 mL	632 kJ (151 kcal)	4.2 g caseinates whey protein	16.7 g	7.47 g	Nil	Gluten-free Residual lactose	Paediatric p. 926 in child 1-10 years, body-weight 8-30 kg	PaediaSure Plus liquid: banana, strawberry, unflavoured 200 ml = £2.89 vanilla 200 ml = £2.89 500 ml = £8.25 Sugar content varies with presentation
Paediasure® Plus Fibre (Abbott Laboratories Ltd)	Liquid (sip or tube feed) per 100 mL	635 kJ (152 kcal)	4.2 g caseinates whey protein	16.4 g (sugars 5.3 g)	7.47 g	1.1 g	Gluten-free Residual lactose	Paediatric p. 926 in child 1-10 years, body-weight 8-30 kg. Not suitable for use in child under 1 year.	PaediaSure Plus fibre liquid: banana, strawberry 200 ml = £3.14 vanilla 200 ml = £3.14 500 ml = £8.45 Nutritional values vary with flavour–consult product literature Sugar content varies with presentation
Peptamen® Junior Advance (Nestle Health Science)	Liquid (tube feed) per 100 mL	630 kJ (150 kcal)	4.5 g whey protein	18 g (sugars 2.1 g)	6.6 g (MCT 61%)	540 mg	Gluten-free Residual lactose Hydrolysed with pork trypsin Contains fish oil	Intractable malabsorption, short-bowel syndrome, bowel fistula, and proven inflammatory bowel disease in child 1-10 years	Peptamen Junior Advance gluten free liquid: 500 ml = £7.77
Tentrini® Energy (Nutricia Ltd)	Liquid (tube feed) per 100 mL	630 kJ (150 kcal)	4.9 g whey protein and caseinate	18.5 g (sugars 1.1 g)	6.3 g	Nil	Gluten-free Residual lactose Contains fish oil	Standard p. 926 and growth failure, in child 7-12 years, body-weight 21-45 kg	Tentrini Energy liquid: 500 ml = £7.43

Borderline substances | **Appendix 2**

A2

Enteral feeds, Child: 1.5 kcal/mL and more than 4 g protein/100 mL (product list continued)

Not suitable for use in child under 1 year unless otherwise stated

Product	Formulation	Energy	Protein	Carbohydrate	Fat	Fibre	Special Characteristics	ACBS Indications	Presentation & Flavour
Tentrini® Energy Multi Fibre (Nutricia Ltd)	Liquid (tube feed) per 100 mL	630 kJ (150 kcal)	4.9 g whey protein and caseinate	18.5 g (sugars 1.1 g)	6.3 g	1.1 g	Gluten-free Residual lactose Contains fish oil	Paediatric p. 926 and proven inflammatory bowel disease, in child 7–12 years, body-weight 21–45 kg	Tentrini Energy Multifibre liquid: 500 ml = £8.18

Table 2 Nutritional supplements (non-disease specific)

Less than 5 g protein/100 mL

Nutritional supplements: 1 kcal/mL and less than 5 g protein/100 mL

Not suitable for use in child under 1 year; use with caution in child 1–5 years unless otherwise stated

Product	Formulation	Energy	Protein	Carbohydrate	Fat	Fibre	Special Characteristics	ACBS Indications	Presentation & Flavour
Ensure® (Abbott Laboratories Ltd)	Liquid (sip or tube feed) per 100 mL	423 kJ (100 kcal)	4 g caseinates soy isolate	13.6 g (sugars 3.93 g)	3.36 g	Nil	Gluten-free Residual lactose	Standard p. 926	Ensure liquid: vanilla, chocolate, coffee 250 ml = £2.26

Nutritional supplements: More than 1 kcal/mL and less than 5 g protein/100 mL

Not suitable for use in child under 1 year; use with caution in child 1–5 years unless otherwise stated

Product	Formulation	Energy	Protein	Carbohydrate	Fat	Fibre	Special Characteristics	ACBS Indications	Presentation & Flavour
AYMES® Shake (Aymes International Ltd)	Standard dilution of powder (57 g in 200 mL water) (sip feed) per 100 mL	530.5 kJ (126 kcal)	4.5 g cows' milk	17.5 g (sugars 8.4 g)	4.2 g	Nil	Gluten-free Contains lactose	Standard p. 926. Use with caution in child 1–6 years. Not suitable for child under 1 year.	Aymes Shake Sample Pack powder: 285 gram = £4.78 Aymes Shake powder: banana, chocolate, neutral, strawberry, vanilla 57 gram 399 gram = £4.90
	Powder 57 g reconstituted with 200 ml whole milk provides: protein 15.8 g, carbohydrate 44.1 g, fat 16.4, energy 1625 kJ (388 kcal)								
Ensure® Plus Juce (Abbott Laboratories Ltd)	Liquid (sip feed) per 100 mL	638 kJ (150 kcal)	4.8 g whey protein isolate	32.7 g (sugars 9.4 g)	Nil	Nil	Gluten-free Residual lactose Non-milk taste	Standard p. 926	Ensure Plus Juce liquid: assorted 880 ml apple, fruit punch, lemon & lime, orange, peach 220 ml = £1.97
Fortijuce® (Nutricia Ltd)	Liquid (sip feed) per 100 mL	640 kJ (150 kcal)	4.0 g cows' milk	33.5 g (sugars 13.1 g)	Nil	Nil	Gluten-free Residual lactose Non-milk taste	Standard p. 926 Not suitable for child under 3 years	Fortijuce Starter Pack liquid: 800 ml = £8.08 Fortijuce liquid: apple, blackcurrant, forest fruits, lemon, orange, strawberry, tropical 200 ml = £2.02 assorted 800 ml. Sugar content varies with flavour.
Fresubin® Jucy Drink (Fresenius Kabi Ltd)	Liquid (sip feed) per 100 mL	630 kJ (150 kcal)	4 g whey protein	33.5 g (sugars 8 g)	Nil	Nil	Gluten-free Residual lactose	Standard p. 926; also CAPD, haemodialysis	Fresubin Jucy drink: apple, blackcurrant, cherry, orange, pineapple 800 ml = £7.80 (4 x 200 ml bottles)
Paediasure® Plus Juce (Abbott Laboratories Ltd)	Liquid (sip feed) per 100 mL	638 kJ (150 kcal)	4.2 g cows' milk	33.3 g (sugars 9.4 g)	Nil	Nil	Gluten-free Residual lactose Non-milk taste	Nutritional supplement in child 1–10 years, body-weight 8–30 kg with disease-related malnutrition and, or growth failure	PaediaSure Plus Juce liquid: apple, very berry 200 ml = £3.03

Product	Formulation	Energy	Protein	Carbohydrate	Fat	Fibre	Special Characteristics	ACBS Indications	Presentation & Flavour
Resource® Dessert Energy (Nestle Health Science)	Semi-solid per 100 g	671 kJ (160 kcal)	4.8 g cows' milk	21.2 g (sugars 9.9 g)	6.2 g	Nil	Gluten-free Contains lactose	Standard p. 926; also CAPD, haemodialysis.	Resource Dessert Energy semi-solid food: caramel, chocolate, vanilla 125 gram = £1.63. Sugar content varies with flavour.
Resource® Fruit (Nestle Health Science)	Liquid (sip feed) per 100 mL	520 kJ (125 kcal)	4 g whey protein hydrolysate	27 g (sugars 9.5 g)	less than 0.2 g	less than 0.2 g	Gluten-free Residual lactose Non-milk taste	Standard p. 926 Not suitable for child under 3 years.	Resource Fruit liquid: apple, orange, pear & cherry, raspberry & blackcurrant 800 ml = £7.35 (4 x 200 ml bottles). Sugar and fibre content varies with flavour.

Nutritional supplements: 5 g (or more) protein/100 mL

Not suitable for use in child under 1 year; use with caution in child 1-5 years unless otherwise stated.

Nutritional supplements: 1.5 kcal/mL and 5 g (or more) protein/100 mL

Product	Formulation	Energy	Protein	Carbohydrate	Fat	Fibre	Special Characteristics	ACBS Indications	Presentation & Flavour
Altraplen® Protein (Nualtra Ltd)	Liquid (sip feed) per 100 mL	632 kJ (150 kcal)	10 g cows' milk soya protein	15 g (sugars 4.6 g)	5.6 g	Nil	Gluten-free Residual lactose	Standard p. 926 Not suitable for child under 3 years; use with caution in child 3-6 years	Altraplen Protein liquid: strawberry, vanilla 800 ml = £8.00 (4 x 200 ml bottles)
Ensure® Plus Commence (Abbott Laboratories Ltd)	Starter pack (5–10 days supply), contains: Ensure® plus milkshake style (various flavours), 1 pack (10 x 220 ml) = £14.00								
Ensure® Plus Fibre (Abbott Laboratories Ltd)	Liquid (sip or tube feed) per 100 mL	652 kJ (155 kcal)	6.25 g cows' milk soya protein isolate	20.2 g (sugars 5.5 g)	4.92 g	2.5 g	Gluten-free Residual lactose	Standard p. 926; also CAPD, haemodialysis.	Ensure Plus Fibre liquid: banana, chocolate, raspberry, strawberry, vanilla 200 ml = £2.02. Nutritional values vary with flavour—consult product literature.
Ensure® Plus Milkshake style (Abbott Laboratories Ltd)	Liquid (sip or tube feed) per 100 mL	632 kJ (150 kcal)	6.25 g cows' milk soya protein isolate	20.2 g (sugars 6.89 g)	4.92 g	Nil	Gluten-free Residual lactose	Standard p. 926; also CAPD, haemodialysis	Ensure Plus milkshake style liquid: banana, chocolate, coffee, fruits of the forest, neutral, orange, peach, raspberry, strawberry, vanilla 220 ml = £1.40. Nutritional values vary with flavour—consult product literature.
Ensure® Plus Savoury (Abbott Laboratories Ltd)	Liquid (sip or tube feed) per 100 mL	632 kJ (150 kcal)	6.25 g cows' milk soy protein isolate	20.2 g (sugars 1.13 g)	4.92 g	Nil	Gluten-free Residual lactose	Standard p. 926; also CAPD, haemodialysis.	Ensure Plus savoury liquid: chicken, mushroom 220 ml = £1.40
Ensure® Plus Yoghurt style (Abbott Laboratories Ltd)	Liquid (sip feed) per 100 mL	632 kJ (150 kcal)	6.25 g cows' milk	20.2 g (sugars 11.7 g)	4.92 g	Nil	Gluten-free Residual lactose	Standard p. 926; also CAPD, haemodialysis	Ensure Plus yoghurt style liquid: orchard peach, strawberry swirl 220 ml = £1.40
Fortisip® Bottle (Nutricia Ltd)	Liquid (sip feed) per 100 mL	630 kJ (150 kcal)	6 g cows' milk	18.4 g	5.8 g	Nil	Gluten-free Residual lactose	Standard p. 926 Not suitable for child under 3 years; use with caution in child 3-5 years.	Fortisip Bottle: banana, caramel, chocolate, neutral, orange, strawberry, tropical fruit, vanilla 200 ml = £1.40 assorted 800 ml. Sugar content varies with flavour.

Borderline substances | **Appendix 2**

A2

Nutritional supplements: 1.5 kcal/mL and 5 g (or more) protein/100 mL (product list continued)

Not suitable for use in child under 1 year; use with caution in child 1-5 years unless otherwise stated.

Product	Formulation	Energy	Protein	Carbohydrate	Fat	Fibre	Special Characteristics	ACBS Indications	Presentation & Flavour
Fortisip® Yoghurt Style (Nutricia Ltd)	Liquid (sip feed) per 100 mL	630 kJ (150 kcal)	6 g cows' milk	18.7 g (sugars 10.8 g)	5.8 g	200 mg	Gluten-free Contains lactose	Standard p. 926 Not suitable for child under 3 years	Fortisip Yogurt Style liquid vanilla & lemon: 200 ml = £2.02
Fortisip® Range (Nutricia Ltd)	Starter pack contains 4 x Fortisip® Bottle, 4 x Fortijuice® 2 x Fortisip® Yogurt Style, 1 pack (10 x 200 ml) = £20.20								
Fresubin® Protein Energy Drink (Fresenius Kabi Ltd)	Liquid (sip feed) per 100 mL	630 kJ (150 kcal)	10 g cows' milk	12.4 g (sugars 6.4 g)	6.7 g	Nil	Gluten-free Residual lactose Contains fish gelatin	Standard p. 926; also CAPD, haemodialysis.	Fresubin Protein Energy drink: cappuccino, chocolate, tropical fruits, vanilla, wild strawberry 200 ml = £2.04. Sugar content varies with flavour. Fibre content varies with flavour.
Fresubin® Thickened (Fresenius Kabi Ltd)	Liquid (sip feed) per 100 mL	630 kJ (150 kcal)	10 g cows' milk	12.2 g (sugars 7.1 g)	6.7 g	480 mg	Gluten-free Residual lactose	Dysphagia or disease-related malnutrition. Not suitable for child under 3 years; use with caution in child 3-5 years.	Fresubin Thickened Stage 1 syrup: vanilla, wild strawberry 800 ml = £9.12 Fresubin Thickened Stage 2 custard: vanilla, wild strawberry 800 ml = £9.24. Sugar content varies with consistency. Fibre content varies with consistency.
Fresubin® YOCréme (Fresenius Kabi Ltd)	Semi-solid per 100 g	630 kJ (150 kcal)	7.5 g whey protein	19.5 g (sugars 16.8 g)	4.7 g	Nil	Gluten-free Contains lactose	Dysphagia, or presence or risk of malnutrition Not suitable for child under 3 years	Fresubin YOcreme dessert: apricot-peach, biscuit, lemon, raspberry 500 gram = £8.00 (4 x 125 ml pots)

Nutritional supplements: Less than 1.5 kcal/mL and 5 g (or more) protein/100 mL

Not suitable for use in child under 1 year; use with caution in child 1-5 years unless otherwise stated.

Product	Formulation	Energy	Protein	Carbohydrate	Fat	Fibre	Special Characteristics	ACBS Indications	Presentation & Flavour
Ensure® Plus Crème (Abbott Laboratories Ltd)	Semi-solid per 100 g	574 kJ (137 kcal)	5.68 g cow's milk soy protein isolates	18.4 g (sugars 12.4 g)	4.47 g	Nil	Gluten-free Residual lactose Contains soya	Standard p. 926; also CAPD, haemodialysis. Not suitable for child under 3 years; use with caution in child 3-5 years.	Ensure Plus Creme: chocolate, neutral, vanilla 500 gram = £7.51. Nutritional values vary with flavour—consult product literature.
Nutilis® Fruit Stage 3 (Nutricia Ltd)	Semi-Solid per 100 g	560 kJ (133 kcal)	7 g whey isolate	16.7 g (sugars 11.3 g)	4 g	2.6 g	Gluten-free Residual lactose	Standard p. 926 except bowel fistula; also CAPD, haemodialysis. Not suitable for child under 3 years; use with caution in child 3-5 years.	Nutilis Fruit Stage 3: apple, strawberry 450 gram = £7.08
Oral Impact® (Nestle Health Science)	Standard dilution of powder (74 g in 250 mL water) (sip feed) per 100 mL	425 kJ (101 kcal)	5.6 g cows' milk	13.4 g (sugars 7.4 g)	2.8 g	1 g	Residual lactose Contains fish oil	Pre-operative nutritional supplement for malnourished patients or patients at risk of malnourishment Not suitable for child under 3 years; use with caution in child 3-5 years.	Oral Impact oral powder 74g sachets: citrus, coffee, tropical 5 sachet = £16.93

Nutritional supplements: More than 1.5 kcal/mL and 5 g (or more) protein/100 mL

Not suitable for use in child under 1 year; use with caution in child 1-5 years unless otherwise stated.

Product	Formulation	Energy	Protein	Carbohydrate	Fat	Fibre	Special Characteristics	ACBS Indications	Presentation & Flavour
Altraplen Compact® (Nualtra Ltd)	Liquid (sip feed) per 100 mL	1008 kJ (240 kcal)	9.6 g cows' milk soya protein	28.8 g (sugars 11.6 g)	9.6 g	Nil	Gluten-free Residual lactose	Standard p. 926 Not suitable for child under 3 years; use with caution in child 3-6 years.	Altraplen Compact: strawberry, vanilla 500 ml = £5.80
Complan® Shake (Nutricia Ltd)	Powder per 57 g	1057 kJ (251 kcal)	8.8 g cows' milk	35.2 g (sugars 22.7 g)	8.4 g	Trace g	Gluten-free Contains lactose	Standard p. 926	Complan Shake Starter Pack sachets: 5 sachet = £4.79 Complan Shake oral powder 57 g sachets: banana, chocolate, milk, strawberry, vanilla 1 sachet 4 sachet = £3.12

Powder 57 g reconstituted with 200 ml whole milk provides: protein 15.6 g, carbohydrate 44.5 g, fat 16.4 g, energy 1612 kJ (387 kcal)

Product	Formulation	Energy	Protein	Carbohydrate	Fat	Fibre	Special Characteristics	ACBS Indications	Presentation & Flavour
Foodlink® Complete (Nualtra Ltd)	Powder per 100 g	1826 kJ (434 kcal)	21.3 g cows' milk	56.7 g	13.5 g	Nil	Contains lactose	Standard p. 926	Foodlink Complete powder: banana, chocolate, natural, strawberry 399 gram = £4.27. Nutritional values vary with flavour—consult product literature.

Recommended serving = 4 heaped dessertspoonfuls in 200 ml full cream milk provides: protein 18.9 g, carbohydrate 41.8 g, fat 15.7 g, energy 1605 kJ (383 kcal)

Product	Formulation	Energy	Protein	Carbohydrate	Fat	Fibre	Special Characteristics	ACBS Indications	Presentation & Flavour
Foodlink® Complete with Fibre (Nualtra Ltd)	Powder per 100 g	1683 kJ (400 kcal)	19.4 g cows' milk	52.7 g (sugars 27.3 g)	12.4 g	7.2 g	Contains lactose	Standard p. 926	Foodlink Complete powder with fibre vanilla: 441 gram = £4.69. Nutritional values vary with flavour—consult product literature.

Recommended serving = 4 heaped dessertspoonfuls (or the contents of a 63 g sachet) in 200 ml full cream milk provides: protein 19.0 g, carbohydrate 42.7 g, fat 15.8 g, fibre 4.5 g, energy 1624 kJ (388 kcal)

Product	Formulation	Energy	Protein	Carbohydrate	Fat	Fibre	Special Characteristics	ACBS Indications	Presentation & Flavour
Forticreme® Complete (Nutricia Ltd)	Semi-solid per 100 g	675 kJ (160 kcal)	9.5 g cows' milk	19.2 g (sugars 10.6 g)	5 g	0.1 g	Gluten-free Residual lactose	Standard p. 926; also CAPD, haemodialysis. Not suitable for child under 3 years; use with caution in child 3-5 years.	Forticreme Complete dessert: banana, chocolate, forest fruits, vanilla 500 gram = £7.84
Fortisip® Compact (Nutricia Ltd)	Liquid (sip feed) per 100 mL	1010 kJ (240 kcal)	9.6 g cows' milk	29.7 g (sugars 15 g)	9.3 g	Nil	Residual lactose	Standard p. 926 Not suitable for child under 3 years; use with caution in child 3-5 years.	Fortisip Compact liquid: apricot, banana, forest fruit, mocha, strawberry, vanilla 125 ml 500 ml = £5.80 chocolate 500 ml = £5.80
Fortisip® Compact Fibre (Nutricia Ltd)	Liquid (sip feed) per 100 mL	1000 kJ (240 kcal)	9.4 g cows' milk	25.2 g (sugars 13.9 g)	10.4 g	3.6 g	Gluten-free Residual lactose	Standard p. 926 Not suitable for child under 3 years; use with caution in child 3-5 years.	Fortisip Compact Fibre Starter Pack liquid: 500 ml = £8.36 Fortisip Compact Fibre liquid: mocha, strawberry, vanilla 500 ml = £8.36
Fortisip® Compact Protein (Nutricia Ltd)	Liquid (sip feed) per 100 mL	1010 kJ (240 kcal)	14.4 g cows' milk	24.4 g (sugars 13.3 g)	9.4 g	Nil	Gluten-free Residual lactose	Standard p. 926 Not suitable for child under 3 years; use with caution in child 3-5 years.	Fortisip Compact Protein Starter Pack liquid: 500 ml = £8.00 Fortisip Compact Protein liquid: banana, mocha, strawberry, vanilla 125 ml 500 ml = £8.00. Nutritional values vary with flavour—consult product literature.

Borderline substances | **Appendix 2**

A2

Nutritional supplements: More than 1.5 kcal/mL and 5 g (or more) protein/100 mL (product list continued)
Not suitable for use in child under 1 year; use with caution in child 1-5 years unless otherwise stated.

Product	Formulation	Energy	Protein	Carbohydrate	Fat	Fibre	Special Characteristics	ACBS Indications	Presentation & Flavour
Fortisip® Extra (Nutricia Ltd)	Liquid (sip feed) **per 100 mL**	675 kJ (160 kcal)	10 g cows' milk	18.1 g (sugars 9 g)	5.3 g	Nil	Gluten-free Contains lactose	Standard p. 926 Not suitable for child under 3 years.	Fortisip Extra Starter Pack liquid: 800 ml = £8.72 Fortisip Extra liquid: chocolate, forest fruits, mocha, strawberry, vanilla 200 ml = £2.18
Fresubin® 2 kcal Drink (Fresenius Kabi Ltd)	Liquid (sip feed) **per 100 mL**	840 kJ (200 kcal)	10 g cows' milk	22.5 g (sugars 5.8 g)	7.8 g	Nil	Gluten-free Residual lactose	Standard p. 926; also CAPD, haemodialysis. Not suitable for use in child under 1 year; use with caution in child 1-5 years.	Fresubin 2kcal drink: apricot-peach, cappuccino, fruits of the forest, neutral, toffee, vanilla 200 ml = £1.98
Fresubin® 2 kcal Fibre Drink (Fresenius Kabi Ltd)	Liquid (sip feed) **per 100 mL**	840 kJ (200 kcal)	10 g cows' milk	22.5 g (sugars 5.8 g)	7.8 g	1.6 g	Gluten-free Residual lactose	Standard p. 926; also CAPD, haemodialysis. Not suitable for use in child under 1 year; use with caution in child 1-5 years.	Fresubin 2kcal Fibre drink: apricot-peach, cappuccino, chocolate, lemon, neutral 200 ml = £1.98 Nutritional values vary with flavour—consult product literature.
Fresubin® Powder Extra (Fresenius Kabi Ltd)	Powder **per 100 g**	1764 kJ (420 kcal)	17.5 g cows' milk whey protein	63 g (sugars 24.7 g)	10.9 g	Nil	Gluten-free Contains lactose	Standard p. 926 Not suitable for child under 1 year; use with caution in child 1-5 years.	Fresubin Powder Extra oral powder 62g sachets: chocolate, neutral, strawberry, vanilla 7 sachet = £5.32. Nutritional values vary with flavour—consult product literature.
Powder 62 g reconstituted with 200 ml whole milk provides: protein 17.7 g, carbohydrate 48.5 g, fat 14.8 g, energy 1658 kJ (397 kcal)									
Nutilis® Complete Stage 1 (Nutricia Ltd)	Liquid (pre-thickened) **per 100 mL**	1010 kJ (240 kcal)	9.6 g cows' milk	29.1 g (sugars 5.4 g)	9.3 g	3.2 g	Residual lactose	Standard p. 926 Not suitable for child under 3 years; use with caution in child 3-5 years.	Nutilis Complete Stage 1 liquid: strawberry, vanilla 500 ml = £8.84
Nutilis® Complete Stage 2 (Nutricia Ltd)	Semi-solid **per 100 g**	1030 kJ (245 kcal)	9.6 g cows' milk	29.1 g (sugars 11.8 g)	9.4 g	3.2 g	Gluten-free Residual lactose	Standard p. 926 Not suitable for child under 3 years; use with caution in child 3-6 years.	Nutilis Complete Stage 2 custard: chocolate, strawberry, vanilla 500 gram = £8.84. Nutritional values vary with flavour—consult product literature.
Nutricrem® (Nualtra Ltd)	Semi-solid **per 100 g**	756 kJ (180 kcal)	10 g cows' milk soya protein	18.8 g (sugars 9.7 g)	7.2 g	Nil	Gluten-free Residual lactose	Standard p. 926 Not suitable for child under 3 years; use with caution in child 3-6 years.	Nutricrem dessert: strawberry, vanilla 500 gram = £5.60

Product	Formulation	Energy	Protein	Carbohydrate	Fat	Fibre	Special Characteristics	ACBS Indications	Presentation & Flavour
Renilon® 7.5 (Nutricia Ltd)	Liquid (sip feed) per 100 mL	840 kJ (200 kcal)	7.5 g cows' milk	20 g (sugars 4.8 g)	10 g	Nil	Gluten-free Residual lactose	Standard p. 926 Not suitable for child under 3 years; use with caution in child 3-5 years.	Renilon 7.5 liquid: apricot, caramel 500 ml = £8.64
Resource® 2.0 Fibre (Nestle Health Science)	Liquid (sip feed) per 100 mL	836 kJ (200 kcal)	9 g cows' milk	21.4 g (sugars 5.5 g)	8.7 g	2.5 g	Gluten-free Residual lactose	Standard p. 926 Not suitable for child under 6 years; caution in child 6-10 years.	Resource Fibre 2.0 liquid: apricot, coffee, neutral, strawberry, summer fruit, vanilla 200 ml = £1.88
Resource® Dessert Fruit	Semi-solid per 100 g	678 kJ (160 kcal)	5 g cows' milk	24 g (sugars 16.4 g)	5 g	1.4 g	Gluten-free Residual lactose	Standard p. 926; also CAPD, haemodialysis.	

Table 3 Specialised formulas

Specialised formulas: Infant and child

Specialised formulas: Infant and child: Amino acid-based formula

Specialised formulas are suitable for infants from birth unless otherwise indicated.

Product	Formulation	Energy	Protein	Carbohydrate	Fat	Fibre	Special Characteristics	ACBS Indications	Presentation & Flavour
Alfamino® (Nestle Health Science)	Standard dilution (13.8 %) of powder per 100 mL	291 kJ (69 kcal)	1.8 g protein equivalent (essential and non-essential amino acids)	7.9 g (sugars 2.2 g)	3.4 g	Nil		Severe cows' milk allergy and or multiple food allergies	SMA Alfamino powder: 400 gram = £23.00
Neocate® Active (Nutricia Ltd)	Standard dilution (21 %) of powder per 300 mL serving (63-g sachet made up to 300 mL with water)	1255 kJ (300 kcal)	8.3 g protein equivalent (essential and non-essential amino acids)	34 g (sugars 3.1 g)	14.5 g	Nil	Milk protein-free	Proven whole protein intolerance, short bowel syndrome, intractable malabsorption, or other gastro-intestinal disorders where an elemental diet is indicated. Nutritional supplement only. Not suitable for child under 1 year.	Neocate Active powder: blackcurrant, unflavoured 945 gram = £66.60

Powder provides: protein equivalent 13.1 g, carbohydrate 54 g, fat 23 g, energy 1992 kJ (475 kcal)/100 g

Product	Formulation	Energy	Protein	Carbohydrate	Fat	Fibre	Special Characteristics	ACBS Indications	Presentation & Flavour
Neocate® Advance (Nutricia Ltd)	Standard dilution (25 %) of powder per 100 mL	420 kJ (100 kcal)	2.5 g protein equivalent (essential and non-essential amino acids)	14.6 g (sugars 1.3 g)	3.5 g (MCT 35 %)	Nil	Milk protein-free	Proven whole protein intolerance, short bowel syndrome, intractable malabsorption, or other gastro-intestinal disorders where an elemental diet is indicated. Not suitable for child under 1 year	Neocate Advance powder: banana & vanilla 750 gram = £46.35

Powder provides: protein equivalent 10 g, carbohydrate 58.5 g, fat 14 g, energy 1683 kJ (400 kcal)/100 g

A2

Borderline substances | **Appendix 2**

Borderline substances | **Appendix 2**

A2

Specialised formulas: Infant and child: Amino acid-based formula (product list continued)

Specialised formulas are suitable for infants from birth unless otherwise indicated.

Product	Formulation	Energy	Protein	Carbohydrate	Fat	Fibre	Special Characteristics	ACBS Indications	Presentation & Flavour
Neocate® LCP (Nutricia Ltd)	Standard dilution (13.8%) of powder per 100 mL	279 kJ (67 kcal)	1.8 g protein equivalent (essential and non-essential amino acids)	7.2 g (sugars 650 mg)	3.4 g	Nil	Milk protein-free	Cows' milk allergy, multiple food protein intolerance, and conditions requiring an elemental diet	Neocate LCP powder: 400 gram = £28.30

Powder provides protein equivalent 8.2 g, carbohydrate 67.4 g, fat 18.8 g, energy 1981 kJ (472 kcal)/100 g

Product	Formulation	Energy	Protein	Carbohydrate	Fat	Fibre	Special Characteristics	ACBS Indications	Presentation & Flavour
Neocate® Spoon (Nutricia Ltd)	Standard dilution (38%) of powder per 97 g serving (37-g sachet diluted with 60 mL water)	733 kJ (175 kcal)	3 g protein equivalent (essential and non-essential amino acids)	24.9 g (sugars 4.6 g)	7 g	Nil	Milk protein-free	Cows' milk allergy, multiple food protein intolerance, and conditions requiring an elemental diet. Not suitable for child under 6 months.	Neocate Spoon powder: 555 gram = £39.30

Powder provides protein 13.9 g, carbohydrate 53 g, fat 26 g, energy 2100 kJ (500 kcal)/100 g

Product	Formulation	Energy	Protein	Carbohydrate	Fat	Fibre	Special Characteristics	ACBS Indications	Presentation & Flavour
Nutramigen® Puramino (Mead Johnson Nutrition (UK) Ltd)	Standard dilution (13.6 %) of powder per 100 mL	290 kJ (68 kcal)	1.89 g essential and non-essential amino acids	7.2 g	3.6 g	Nil	Gluten-free Lactose-free	For use in the management of severe protein intolerance, multiple food intolerance and other gastro-intestinal disorders where an amino acid based diet is specifically indicated for infants and young children.	Nutramigen PurAmino powder: 400 gram = £27.09

Specialised formulas: Infant and child: Hydrolysate formula

Product	Formulation	Energy	Protein	Carbohydrate	Fat	Fibre	Special Characteristics	ACBS Indications	Presentation & Flavour
Althéra® (Nestle Health Science)	Standard dilution (13.2%) of powder per 100 mL	280 kJ (67 kcal)	1.7 g whey hydrolysed	7.3 g (sugars 4 g)	3.4 g	Nil	Contains lactose	Complete nutritional support from birth to 3 years or supplementary feeding from 6 months to 3 years, in cow's milk protein allergy or multiple food protein allergies	Althéra can: 450 g = £10.68

Powder provides: protein 12.5 g, carbohydrate 55.5 g, fat 26 g, energy 2117 kJ (506 kcal)/100 g

Product	Formulation	Energy	Protein	Carbohydrate	Fat	Fibre	Special Characteristics	ACBS Indications	Presentation & Flavour
Aptamil Pepti® 1 (Allergy) (Milupa Ltd)	Standard dilution (13.6 %) of powder per 100 mL	280 kJ (67 kcal)	1.6 g whey hydrolysed	7.1 g (sugars 3.5 g)	3.5 g	0.6 g	Contains lactose and fish oil	Established cows' milk protein intolerance, with or without secondary lactose intolerance	Milupa Aptamil Pepti 1 (Allergy) powder: 400 gram = £9.74; 800 gram = £19.48

Formerly Aptamil Pepti® Powder provides: protein 11.6 g, carbohydrate 52 g, fat 25.6 g, energy 2025 kJ (484 kcal)/100 g

Product	Formulation	Energy	Protein	Carbohydrate	Fat	Fibre	Special Characteristics	ACBS Indications	Presentation & Flavour
Aptamil Pepti® 2 (Allergy) (Milupa Ltd)	Standard dilution (14.3 %) of powder per 100 mL	285 kJ (68 kcal)	1.6 g	8 g (sugars 3.6 g)	3.1 g	0.6 g	Contains lactose and fish oil	Established cows' milk protein allergy or intolerance. Not suitable for child under 6 months.	Milupa Aptamil Pepti 2 (Allergy) powder: 400 gram = £9.29; 800 gram = £18.58

Powder provides: protein 11.2 g, carbohydrate 56.1 g, fat 21.8 g, energy 1985 kJ (473 kcal)/100 g

Product	Standard dilution / preparation	Energy	Protein	Carbohydrate	Fat		Notes	Indication	Pack / price
Cow & Gate Pepti-Junior® (Cow & Gate Ltd)	Standard dilution (12.8 %) of powder **per 100 mL**	275 kJ (66 kcal)	1.8 g whey hydrolysed	6.8 g (sugars 1.1 g)	3.5 g	Nil	Residual lactose. Contains fish oil	Disaccharide and/or whole protein intolerance, or where amino acids and peptides are indicated in conjunction with medium chain triglycerides.	Pepti-Junior powder: 450 gram = £13.06
Powder provides: protein 14 g, carbohydrate 53.4 g, fat 27.3 g, energy 2155 kJ (515 kcal)/100 g									
Infatrini® Peptisorb (Nutricia Ltd)	Liquid (sip or tube feed) **per 100 mL**	420 kJ (100 kcal)	2.6 g whey protein hydrolysate	10.3 g (sugars 2.7 g)	5.4 g (MCT 50%)	Nil	Gluten-free. Residual lactose. Contains fish oil	Disease-related malnutrition, intractable malabsorption, proven inflammatory bowel disease, short bowel syndrome, bowel fistula, and intolerance to whole protein feeds in child from birth to 18 months or body-weight up to 9 kg	Infatrini Peptisorb liquid: 200 ml = £3.47
Nutramigen 1 with LGG® (Mead Johnson Nutrition (UK) Ltd)	Standard dilution (13.5 %) of powder **per 100 mL**	280 kJ (68 kcal)	1.9 g casein hydrolysed	7.5 g	3.4 g	Nil	Gluten-free. Lactose-free	For the dietary management of cow's milk allergy with / or without lactose intolerance	Nutramigen 1 with LGG powder: 400 gram = £10.87
Powder provides: protein 14 g, carbohydrate 55 g, fat 25 g, energy 2100 kJ (500 kcal)/100 g									
Nutramigen 2 with LGG® (Mead Johnson Nutrition (UK) Ltd)	Standard dilution (14.1 %) of powder **per 100 mL**	285 kJ (68 kcal)	1.7 g casein hydrolysed	8.8 g	2.8 g	Nil	Gluten-free. Lactose-free	For the dietary management of cow's milk allergy with / or without lactose intolerance	Nutramigen 2 with LGG powder: 400 gram = £10.99
Powder provides: protein 12 g, carbohydrate 62 g, fat 20 g, energy 2000 kJ (480 kcal)/100 g									
Pepdite® (Nutricia Ltd)	Standard dilution (15 %) of powder **per 100 mL**	297 kJ (71 kcal)	2.1 g protein equivalent (non-milk hydrolysate)	7.8 g (sugars 700 mg)	3.5 g	Nil	Lactose-free. Contains meat (pork) and soya derivatives	Disaccharide and/or whole protein intolerance	Pepdite powder: 400 gram = £18.78
Powder provides: protein equivalent 13.8 g, carbohydrate 52 g, fat 23.2 g, energy 1977 kJ (472 kcal)/100 g									
Pepdite® 1+ (Nutricia Ltd)	Standard dilution (22.8 %) of powder **per 100 mL**	423 kJ (100 kcal)	3.1 g protein equivalent (non-milk hydrolysate essential amino acids)	13 g (sugars 1.2 g)	3.9 g (MCT 35%)	Nil	Lactose-free. Contains meat (pork) and soya derivatives	Disaccharide and/or whole protein intolerance, or where amino acids or peptides are indicated in conjunction with medium chain triglycerides. Not suitable for child under 1 year.	Pepdite 1+ powder: 400 gram = £19.71
Powder provides: protein equivalent 13.8 g, carbohydrate 57 g, fat 17.3 g, energy 1844 kJ (439 kcal)/100 g									
Pregestimil® Lipil (Mead Johnson Nutrition (UK) Ltd)	Standard dilution (13.5 %) of powder **per 100 mL**	280 kJ (68 kcal)	1.89 g casein hydrolysed	6.9 g	3.8 g (MCT 54%)	Nil	Gluten-free. Lactose-free	Disaccharide and/or whole protein intolerance, or where amino acids or peptides are indicated in conjunction with medium chain triglycerides.	Pregestimil LIPIL powder: 400 gram = £12.19
Powder provides: protein 14 g, carbohydrate 51 g, fat 28 g, energy 2100 kJ (500 kcal)/100 g									
Similac® Alimentum (Abbott Laboratories Ltd)	Standard dilution (14%) of powder **per 100 mL**	283 kJ (67.6 kcal)	1.86 g casein hydrolysed	6.62 g (sugars 1.5 g)	3.75 g (MCT 33%)	Nil	Gluten-free. Lactose-free. Contains meat derivatives	Cows' milk protein allergy and other conditions where an extensively hydrolysed formula is indicated.	Similac Alimentum powder: 400 gram = £9.10
Powder provides: protein equivalent 14.4 g, carbohydrate 51.4 g, fat 29.1 g, energy 2196 kJ (525 kcal)/100 g									

Borderline substances | **Appendix 2**

Specialised formulas: Infant and child: Residual lactose formula

Product	Formulation	Energy	Protein	Carbohydrate	Fat	Fibre	Special Characteristics	ACBS Indications	Presentation & Flavour
Enfamil® O-Lac (Mead Johnson Nutrition (UK) Ltd)	Standard dilution (13%) of powder per 100 mL	280 kJ (68 kcal)	1.42 g cows' milk	7.2 g	3.7 g	Nil	Gluten-free Residual lactose	Proven lactose intolerance	Enfamil O-Lac powder: 400 gram = £4.98

Powder provides: protein 10.9 g, carbohydrate 55 g, fat 28 g, energy 2200 kJ (524 kcal)/100 g

Product	Formulation	Energy	Protein	Carbohydrate	Fat	Fibre	Special Characteristics	ACBS Indications	Presentation & Flavour
Galactomin 17® (Nutricia Ltd)	Standard dilution (13.6%) of powder per 100 mL	295 kJ (70 kcal)	1.7 g protein equivalent (cows' milk)	7.5 g (sugars 1.4 g)	3.7 g	Nil	Residual lactose	Proven lactose intolerance in pre-school children, galactosaemia, and galactokinase deficiency.	Galactomin 17 powder: 400 gram = £16.80

Powder provides: protein equivalent 12.3 g, carbohydrate 55.3 g, fat 27.2 g, energy 2155 kJ (515 kcal)/100 g

Product	Formulation	Energy	Protein	Carbohydrate	Fat	Fibre	Special Characteristics	ACBS Indications	Presentation & Flavour
SMA® LF (SMA Nutrition)	Standard dilution (13 %) of powder per 100 mL	281 kJ (67 kcal)	1.5 g casein whey	7.2 g (sugars 2.6 g)	3.6 g	Nil	Residual lactose	Proven lactose intolerance	SMA LF powder: 430 gram = £5.34

Powder provides: protein 12 g, carbohydrate 55.6 g, fat 28 g, energy 2185 kJ (522 kcal)/100 g

Specialised formulas: Infant and child: MCT-enhanced formula

Product	Formulation	Energy	Protein	Carbohydrate	Fat	Fibre	Special Characteristics	ACBS Indications	Presentation & Flavour
Lipistart® (Vitaflo International Ltd)	Standard dilution (15%) of powder per 100 mL	282 kJ (68 kcal)	2.1 g protein equivalent (whey soya)	8.3 g (sugars 700 mg)	3.1 g (MCT 81%)	Nil	Residual lactose	Dietary management of fat malabsorption, long-chain fatty acid oxidation disorders, and other disorders requiring a high MCT, low LCT formula.	Lipistart powder: 400 gram = £19.37
MCT Pepdite® (Nutricia Ltd)	Standard dilution (15 %) of powder per 100 mL	286 kJ (68 kcal)	2 g protein equivalent (non-milk peptides essential amino acids)	8.8 g (sugars 1.2 g)	2.7 g (MCT 75 %)	Nil	Gluten-free Lactose-free Contains meat (pork) and soya derivatives	Disorders in which a high intake of MCT is beneficial	MCT Pepdite powder: 400 gram = £20.43

Powder provides: protein equivalent 13.8 g, carbohydrate 59 g, fat 18 g, energy 1903 kJ (453 kcal)/100 g

Product	Formulation	Energy	Protein	Carbohydrate	Fat	Fibre	Special Characteristics	ACBS Indications	Presentation & Flavour
MCT Pepdite® +1 (Nutricia Ltd)	Standard dilution (20 %) of powder per 100 mL	381 kJ (91 kcal)	2.8 g protein equivalent (non-milk peptides essential amino acids)	11.8 g (sugars 1.6 g)	3.6 g (MCT 75 %)	Nil	Gluten-free Lactose-free Contains meat (pork) and soya derivatives	Disorders in which a high intake of MCT is beneficial Not suitable for child under 1 year.	MCT Pepdite 1+ powder: 400 gram = £20.43

Powder provides: protein equivalent 13.8 g, carbohydrate 59 g, fat 18 g, energy 1903 kJ (453 kcal)/100 g

Product	Formulation	Energy	Protein	Carbohydrate	Fat	Fibre	Special Characteristics	ACBS Indications	Presentation & Flavour
Monogen® (Nutricia Ltd)	Standard dilution (17.5%) of powder per 100 mL	310 kJ (74 kcal)	2.2 g protein equivalent (whey)	12 g (sugars 1.2 g)	1.9 g (MCT 80 %)	Nil	Residual lactose Supplementation with essential fatty acids may be needed	Long-chain acyl-CoA dehydrogenase deficiency (LCAD), carnitine palmitoyl transferase deficiency (CPTD), primary and secondary lipoprotein lipase deficiency, chylothorax, and lymphangiectasia	Monogen powder: 400 gram = £20.31

Powder provides: protein equivalent 12.5 g, carbohydrate 68 g, fat 11 g, energy 1769 kJ (420 kcal)/100 g

Specialised formulas: Infant and child: Soya-based formula

Product	Formulation	Energy	Protein	Carbohydrate	Fat	Fibre	Special Characteristics	ACBS Indications	Presentation & Flavour
Wysoy® (SMA Nutrition)	Standard dilution (13.2%) of powder per 100 mL	280 kJ (67 kcal)	1.8 g soya protein isolate	6.9 g (sugars 2.5 g)	3.6 g	Nil	Lactose-free	Proven lactose and associated sucrose intolerance in pre-school children, galactokinase deficiency, galactosaemia, and proven whole cows' milk sensitivity.	SMA Wysoy powder: 860 gram = £9.91

Powder provides: protein 14 g, carbohydrate 54 g, fat 27 g, energy 2155 kJ (515 kcal)/100 g

Specialised formulas: Infant and child: Low calcium formula

Product	Formulation	Energy	Protein	Carbohydrate	Fat	Fibre	Special Characteristics	ACBS Indications	Presentation & Flavour
Locasol® (Nutricia Ltd)	Standard dilution (13.1%) of powder per 100 mL	278 kJ (66 kcal)	1.9 g protein equivalent (cows' milk)	7 g (sugars 6.9 g)	3.4 g	Nil	Contains lactose Calcium less than 7 mg/100 mL No added vitamin D	Conditions of calcium intolerance requiring restriction of calcium and vitamin D intake	Locasol powder: 400 gram = 23.36

Powder provides: protein 14.6 g, carbohydrate 53.7 g, fat 26.1 g, energy 2125 kJ (508 kcal)/100 g

Specialised formulas: Infant and child: Fructose-based formula

Product	Formulation	Energy	Protein	Carbohydrate	Fat	Fibre	Special Characteristics	ACBS Indications	Presentation & Flavour
Galactomin 19® (Nutricia Ltd)	Standard dilution (12.9%) of powder per 100 mL	288 kJ (69 kcal)	1.9 g protein equivalent (cows' milk)	6.4 g (fructose 6.3 g)	4 g	Nil	Residual lactose galactose and glucose	Conditions of glucose plus galactose intolerance	Galactomin 19 powder: 400 gram = £44.23

Powder provides: protein equivalent 14.6 g, carbohydrate 49.7 g, fat 30.8 g, energy 2233 kJ (534 kcal)/100 g

Specialised formulas: Infant and child: Pre-thickened infant feeds
Not to be used for a period of more than 6 months; not to be used in conjunction with any other feed thickener or antacid products.

Product	Formulation	Energy	Protein	Carbohydrate	Fat	Fibre	Special Characteristics	ACBS Indications	Presentation & Flavour
Enfamil® AR (Mead Johnson Nutrition (UK) Ltd)	Standard dilution (13.5%) of powder per 100 mL	285 kJ (68 kcal)	1.7 g cows' milk	7.6 g (lactose 4.6 g)	3.5 g	Nil	Contains lactose pregelatinised rice starch	Significant gastro-oesophageal reflux	Enfamil AR powder: 400 gram = £3.73

Powder provides: protein 12.5 g, carbohydrate 56 g, fat 26 g, energy 2093 kJ (500 kcal)/100 g

Product	Formulation	Energy	Protein	Carbohydrate	Fat	Fibre	Special Characteristics	ACBS Indications	Presentation & Flavour
SMA® Staydown (SMA Nutrition)	Standard dilution (12.9%) of powder per 100 mL	279 kJ (67 kcal)	1.6 g casein whey	7 g (lactose 5 g)	3.6 g	Nil	Contains lactose pre-cooked corn starch	Significant gastro-oesophageal reflux	SMA Staydown powder: 900 gram = £7.80

Powder provides: protein 12.4 g, carbohydrate 54.3 g, fat 28 g, energy 2166 kJ (518 kcal)/100 g

Borderline substances | **Appendix 2**

A2

Specialised formulas for specific clinical conditions

Product	Formulation	Energy	Protein	Carbohydrate	Fat	Fibre	Special Characteristics	ACBS Indications	Presentation & Flavour
Alicalm® (Nutricia Ltd)	Standard dilution (30%) of powder per 100 mL	567 kJ (135 kcal)	4.5 g caseinate whey	17.4 g (sugars 3.2 g)	5.3 g	Nil	Residual lactose	Crohn's disease Not suitable for child under 1 year; use as nutritional supplement only in children 1–6 years.	Alicalm oral powder: 400 gram = £21.49
Powder provides: protein 15 g, carbohydrate 58 g, fat 17.5 g, energy 1889 kJ (450 kcal)/100 g									
Forticare® (Nutricia Ltd)	Liquid (sip feed) per 100 mL.	675 kJ (160 kcal)	9 g cows' milk	19.1 g (sugars 13.6 g)	5.3 g	2.1 g	Gluten-free Residual lactose Contains fish oil	Nutritional supplement in patients with lung cancer undergoing chemotherapy, or with pancreatic cancer Not suitable in child under 3 years	Forticare liquid: cappuccino, orange & lemon, peach & ginger 500 mL = £8.92
Heparon® Junior (Nutricia Ltd)	Standard dilution (18%) of powder per 100 mL	363 kJ (86 kcal)	2 g cows' milk	11.6 g (sugars 2.9 g)	3.6 g	Nil	Contains lactose Electrolytes/100 mL: Na⁺ 0.56 mmol K⁺ 1.9 mmol Ca²⁺ 2.3 mmol P⁺ 1.6 mmol	Enteral feed or nutritional supplement for children with acute or chronic liver failure	Heparon Junior powder: 400 gram = £21.65
Powder provides: protein 11.1 g, carbohydrate 64.2 g, fat 19.9 g, energy 2016 kJ (480 kcal)/100 g									
KetoCal® (Nutricia Ltd)	Standard dilution (20 %) of powder per 100 mL	602 kJ (146 kcal)	3.1 g cows' milk with additional amino acids	600 mg (sugars 120 mg)	14.6 g (LCT 100 %)	Nil	Electrolytes/100 mL: Na⁺ 4.3 mmol K⁺ 4.1 mmol Ca²⁺ 2.15 mmol P⁺ 2.77 mmol	Enteral feed or nutritional supplement as part of ketogenic diet in management of epilepsy resistant to drug therapy, in children over 1 year, only on the advice of secondary care physician with experience of ketogenic diet.	KetoCal 4:1 powder: unflavoured, vanilla 300 gram = £30.48
Powder provides: protein 15.25 g, carbohydrate 3 g, fat 73 g, energy 3011 kJ (730 kcal)/100 g									
KetoCal® 3:1 (Nutricia Ltd)	Standard dilution (9.5%) of powder per 100 mL	276 kJ (66 kcal)	1.5 g	680 mg (sugars 570 mg)	6.4 g	Nil	Electrolytes/100 mL: Na⁺ 1.3 mmol K⁺ 2.4 mmol Ca²⁺ 2 mmol P⁺ 1.7 mmol	Enteral feed or nutritional supplement as part of ketogenic diet in management of drug resistant epilepsy or other conditions for which a ketogenic diet is indicated in children from birth to 6 years; as a nutritional supplement in children over 6 years.	KetoCal 3:1 powder: 300 gram = £29.50
Powder provides: protein 15.3 g, carbohydrate 7.2 g, fat 67.7 g, energy 2927 kJ (699 kcal)/100 g									
KetoCal® 4:1 LQ (Nutricia Ltd)	Liquid (sip or tube feed) per 100 mL	620 kJ (150 kcal)	3.09 g casein and whey with additional amino acids	610 mg (sugars 230 mg)	14.8 g (LCT 100 %)	1.12 g	Residual lactose Electrolytes/100 mL: Na⁺ 4.9 mmol K⁺ 4.7 mmol Ca²⁺ 2.4 mmol P⁺ 3.1 mmol	Enteral feed or nutritional supplement as part of ketogenic diet in management of drug resistant epilepsy or other conditions for which a ketogenic diet is indicated in children 1–10 years; as a nutritional supplement in children over 10 years.	KetoCal 4:1 LQ liquid: unflavoured, vanilla 200 ml = £4.35

Product	Presentation	Energy	Protein	Carbohydrate	Fat	Fibre	Special characteristics	Indications	Price
Kindergen® (Nutricia Ltd)	Standard dilution (20%) of powder per 100 mL	421 kJ (101 kcal)	1.5 g whey protein	11.8 g (sugars 1.2 g)	5.3 g (LCT 93%)	Nil	Electrolytes/100 mL: Na⁺ 2 mmol, K⁺ 0.6 mmol, Ca²⁺ 2.8 mmol, P⁻ 3 mmol, Low Vitamin A	Enteral feed or nutritional supplement for children with chronic renal failure receiving peritoneal rapid overnight dialysis.	Kindergen powder: 400 gram = £29.06

Powder provides: protein 7.5 g, carbohydrate 59 g, fat 26.3 g, energy 2104 kJ (504 kcal)/100 g

Product	Presentation	Energy	Protein	Carbohydrate	Fat	Fibre	Special characteristics	Indications	Price
Modulen IBD® (Nestle Health Science)	Standard dilution (20%) of powder (sip or tube feed) per 100 mL	420 kJ (100 kcal)	3.6 g casein	11 g (sugars 3.98 g)	4.7 g	Nil	Gluten-free, Residual lactose	Crohn's disease active phase, and in remission if malnourished	Modulen IBD powder: 400 gram = £15.06 (8.3 g measuring scoop provided)

Powder provides: protein 18 g, carbohydrate 54 g, fat 23 g, energy 2070 kJ (500 kcal)/100 g

Product	Presentation	Energy	Protein	Carbohydrate	Fat	Fibre	Special characteristics	Indications	Price
Nepro® (Abbott Laboratories Ltd)	Liquid (sip or tube feed) per 100 mL	838 kJ (200 kcal)	7 g cows' milk	20.6 g (sugars 3.26 g)	9.6 g	1.56 g	Gluten-free, Residual lactose, Electrolytes/100 mL: Na⁺ 3.67 mmol, K⁺ 2.72 mmol, Ca²⁺ 3.43 mmol, P⁻ 2.23 mmol	Enteral feed or nutritional supplement in patients with chronic renal failure who are on haemodialysis or CAPD, or with cirrhosis, or other conditions requiring a high energy, low fluid, low electrolyte diet. Not suitable for child under 1 year; use with caution in child 1–5 years.	Nepro HP liquid: strawberry 220 ml = £2.98 vanilla 220 ml = £2.98 500 ml = £6.80
ProSure® (Abbott Laboratories Ltd)	Liquid (sip or tube feed) per 100 mL	536 kJ (127 kcal)	6.65 g cows' milk	18.3 g (sugars 2.95 g)	2.56 g	2.07 g	Gluten-free, Residual lactose, Contains fish oil	Nutritional supplement for patients with pancreatic cancer. Not suitable for child under 1 year; use with caution in child 1–4 years.	ProSure liquid: 240 ml = £3.34
Renamil® (Stanningley Pharma Ltd)	Powder (sip or tube feed when reconstituted) per 100 g	2003 kJ (477 kcal)	4.6 g cows' milk	70.8 g	19.3 g	Nil	Contains lactose, Gluten-free, Electrolytes/100 g: Na⁺ 1.04 mmol, K⁺ 0.13 mmol, Ca²⁺ 10.22 mmol, P⁻ 1.06 mmol, Contains no vitamin A or vitamin D	Enteral feed or nutritional supplement for adults and children over 1 year with chronic renal failure.	Renamil powder: 1000 gram = £25.40
Renapro® (Stanningley Pharma Ltd)	Powder per 100 g	1580 kJ (372 kcal)	90 g whey protein	0.8 g	1 g	Nil	Gluten-free, Residual lactose, Electrolytes/100 g: Na⁺ 23 mmol, K⁺ 2 mmol, Ca²⁺ 4.99 mmol, P⁻ 4.84 mmol	Nutritional supplement for biochemically proven hypoproteinaemia and patients undergoing dialysis. Not suitable for child under 1 year.	Renapro powder: 600 gram = £69.60

Powder provides: protein 18 g, energy 316 kJ (74 kcal)/20 g sachet

Product	Presentation	Energy	Protein	Carbohydrate	Fat	Fibre	Special characteristics	Indications	Price
Renastart® (Vitaflo International Ltd)	Standard dilution (20%) of powder per 100 mL	414 kJ (99 kcal)	1.5 g cows' milk soya	12.5 g (sugars 1.3 g)	4.8 g	Nil	Contains lactose, Electrolytes/100 mL: Na⁺ 2.1 mmol, K⁺ 0.6 mmol, Ca²⁺ 0.6 mmol, P⁻ 0.6 mmol	Dietary management of renal failure in child from birth to 10 years.	Renastart powder: 400 gram = £26.37

Powder provides: protein 7.5 g, carbohydrate 62.5 g, fat 23.8 g, energy 2071 kJ (494 kcal)/100 g

Borderline substances | **Appendix 2**

A2

Borderline substances | **Appendix 2**

Table 4 Feed supplements

High-energy supplements

High-energy supplements: carbohydrate

Flavoured carbohydrate supplements are not suitable for child under 1 year; liquid supplements should be diluted before use in child under 5 years.

Product	Formulation	Energy	Protein	Carbohydrate	Fat	Fibre	Special Characteristics	ACBS Indications	Presentation & Flavour
Caloreen® (Nestlé Health Science)	Powder per 100 g	1640 kJ (390 kcal)	Nil	96 g Maltodextrin	Nil	Nil	Gluten-free Lactose-free	Disease-related malnutrition, malabsorption states, or other conditions requiring fortification with a high or readily available carbohydrate supplement. Not suitable for child under 3 years.	Caloreen powder: 500 gram = £3.69
Maxijul® Super Soluble (Nutricia Ltd)	Powder per 100 g	1615 kJ (380 kcal)	Nil	95 g Glucose polymer (sugars 8.6 g)	Nil	Nil	Gluten-free Lactose-free	Disease-related malnutrition, malabsorption states, or other conditions requiring fortification with a high or readily available carbohydrate supplement.	Maxijul Super Soluble powder: 200 gram = £2.60; 528 gram = £6.48; 25000 gram = £155.56
Polycal® (Nutricia Ltd)	Liquid per 100 mL	1050 kJ (247 kcal)	Nil	61.9 g Maltodextrin (sugars 12.2 g)	Nil	Nil		Disease-related malnutrition, malabsorption states, or other conditions requiring fortification with a high or readily available carbohydrate supplement. Not suitable for child under 3 years.	Polycal liquid: neutral, orange 200 ml = £1.72
	Powder per 100 g	1630 kJ (384 kcal)	Nil	96 g Maltodextrin (sugars 6 g)	Nil	Nil	Gluten-free Lactose-free	Disease-related malnutrition, malabsorption states, or other conditions requiring fortification with a high or readily available carbohydrate supplement.	powder: 400 gram = £4.28
S.O.S.® (Vitaflo International Ltd)	Powder per 100 g	1590 kJ (380 kcal)	Nil	95 g (sugars 9 g)	Nil	Nil		For use as an emergency regimen in the dietary management of inborn errors of metabolism in adults and children from birth.	S.O.S.: 15 oral powder 31g sachets 30 sachet =£10.79; S.O.S. 10 oral powder 21g sachets 30 sachet = £7.31; S.O.S. 20 oral powder 42g sachets 30 sachet = £14.62; S.O.S. 25 oral powder 52g sachets 30 sachet = £18.09

Contents of each sachet should be reconstituted with water to a total volume of 200 mL

| Vitajoule® (Vitaflo International Ltd) | Powder per 100 g | 1590 kJ (380 kcal) | Nil | 95 g Dried glucose syrup (sugars 9 g) | Nil | Nil | Gluten-free Lactose-free | Disease-related malnutrition, malabsorption states, or other conditions requiring fortification with a high or readily available carbohydrate supplement. Flavoured carbohydrate supplements are not suitable for child under 1 year; liquid supplements should be diluted before use in child under 5 years. | Vitajoule powder: 500 gram = £4.38 |

High-energy supplements: fat

Liquid supplements should be diluted before use in child under 5 years

Product	Formulation	Energy	Protein	Carbohydrate	Fat	Fibre	Special Characteristics	ACBS Indications	Presentation & Flavour
Calogen® (Nutricia Ltd)	Liquid (emulsion) per 100 mL	1850 kJ (450 kcal)	Nil	0.1 g	50 g (LCT 100 %)	Nil	Gluten-free Lactose-free	Disease-related malnutrition, malabsorption states, or other conditions requiring fortification with a high fat (or fat and carbohydrate) supplement. Liquid supplements should be diluted before use in child under 5 years.	Calogen emulsion: banana 500 ml = £10.72 neutral, strawberry 200 ml = £4.36 500 ml = £10.72
Fresubin® 5 kcal Shot (Fresenius Kabi Ltd)	Liquid (emulsion) per 100 mL	2100 kJ (500 kcal)	Nil	4.0 g (sucrose)	53.8 g	0.4 g	Gluten-free Lactose-free	Disease-related malnutrition, malabsorption states, or other conditions requiring fortification with a high fat (or fat and carbohydrate) supplement. Liquid supplements should be diluted before use in child under 5 years.	Fresubin 5kcal shot drink neutral: 480 ml = £11.20
Liquigen® (Nutricia Ltd)	Liquid (emulsion) per 100 mL	1850 kJ (450 kcal)	Nil	Nil	50 g (MCT 97 %) Fractionated coconut oil	Nil	Gluten-free Lactose-free	Steatorrhoea associated with cystic fibrosis of the pancreas, intestinal lymphangiectasia, intestinal surgery, chronic liver disease, liver cirrhosis, other proven malabsorption syndromes, ketogenic diet in epilepsy, and in type 1 lipoproteinaemia Not suitable for child under 3 years.	Liquigen emulsion: 250 ml = £9.26
Medium-chain Triglyceride (MCT) Oil (Nutricia Ltd)	Liquid per 100 mL	3515 kJ (855 kcal)	Nil	Nil	MCT 100 %	Nil		Nutritional supplement for steatorrhoea associated with cystic fibrosis of the pancreas, intestinal lymphangiectasia, intestinal surgery, chronic liver disease and liver cirrhosis, other proven malabsorption syndromes, ketogenic diet in management of epilepsy, type 1 hyperlipoproteinaemia	MCT oil: 500 ml = £14.68

FAT AND CARBOHYDRATE

Product	Formulation	Energy	Protein	Carbohydrate	Fat	Fibre	Special Characteristics	ACBS Indications	Presentation & Flavour
Duocal® Super Soluble (Nutricia Ltd)	Powder per 100 g	2061 kJ (492 kcal)	Nil	72.7 g (sugars 6.5 g)	22.3 g (MCT 35 %)	Nil	Gluten-free Lactose-free	Disease-related malnutrition, malabsorption states, or other conditions requiring fortification with a high fat (or fat and carbohydrate) supplement.	Duocal Super Soluble powder: 400 gram = £18.09
Energivit® (Nutricia Ltd)	Standard dilution (15%) of powder per 100 mL	309 kJ (74 kcal)	Nil	10 g (sugars 900 mg)	3.75 g	Nil	Lactose-free With vitamins minerals and trace elements	For children requiring additional energy, vitamins, minerals, and trace elements following a protein-restricted diet	Energivit powder: 400 gram = £21.99

High-energy supplements: protein

Product	Formulation	Energy	Protein	Carbohydrate	Fat	Fibre	Special Characteristics	ACBS Indications	Presentation & Flavour
ProSource® Jelly (Nutrinovo Ltd)	Semi-solid per 100 mL	315 kJ (75 kcal)	16.9 g collagen protein hydrolysate whey protein isolate	Less than 1 g	Nil	Less than 1 g	Gluten-free Lactose-free Contains porcine derivatives	Hypoproteinaemia Not recommended for child under 3 years	ProSource jelly: fruit punch, orange 118 ml = £1.80
Protifar® (Nutricia Ltd)	Powder per 100 g	1580 kJ (373 kcal)	88.5 g cows' milk	less than 1.5 g	1.6 g	Nil	Gluten-free Residual lactose Electrolytes/100 mL: Na⁺ 1.3 mmol K⁺ 1.28 mmol Ca²⁺ 33.75 mmol P⁻ 22.58 mmol	Nutritional supplement for use in biochemically proven hypoproteinaemia.	Protifar powder: 225 gram = £8.69

Powder provides: protein 2.2 g per 2.5 g scoopful

PROTEIN AND CARBOHYDRATE

Product	Formulation	Energy	Protein	Carbohydrate	Fat	Fibre	Special Characteristics	ACBS Indications	Presentation & Flavour
Dialamine® (Nutricia Ltd)	Standard dilution (20%) of powder per 100 mL	264 kJ (62 kcal)	4.3 g protein equivalent (essential and non-essential amino acids)	11.2 g (sugars 10.2 g)	Nil	Nil	Contains vitamin C	Hypoproteinaemia, chronic renal failure, wound fistula leakage with excessive protein loss, conditions requiring a controlled nitrogen intake, and haemodialysis. Not suitable for child under 6 months.	Dialamine powder: 400 gram = £73.46
								Powder provides: protein equivalent 25 g, carbohydrate 65 g, vitamin C 125 mg, energy 1530 kJ (360 kcal)/100 g	
ProSource® liquid (Nutrinovo Ltd)	Liquid per 30 mL	420 kJ (100 kcal)	10 g collagen protein whey protein isolate	15 g (sugars 8 g)	Nil	Nil	Gluten-free Lactose-free May contain porcine derivatives	Biochemically proven hypoproteinaemia Not recommended for child under 3 years.	ProSource liquid 30ml sachets: citrus berry, lemon, orange creme, original 100 sachet = £97.23
ProSource® Plus (Nutrinovo Ltd)	Liquid per 30 mL	420 kJ (100 kcal)	15 g collagen protein whey protein isolate	11 g (sugars 10 g)	Nil	Nil	Gluten-free Lactose-free May contain porcine derivatives	Hypoproteinaemia Not recommended for child under 3 years	ProSource Plus liquid sachet: 100 x 30 mL = £140.53 unflavoured

PROTEIN, FAT, AND CARBOHYDRATE

Product	Formulation	Energy	Protein	Carbohydrate	Fat	Fibre	Special Characteristics	ACBS Indications	Presentation & Flavour
Calogen® Extra (Nutricia Ltd)	Liquid per 100 mL	1650 kJ (400 kcal)	5 g cows' milk	4.5 g (sugars 3.5 g)	40.3 g	Nil	Gluten-free Residual lactose Contains vitamins and minerals	Disease-related malnutrition, malabsorption states, or other conditions requiring fortification with a high fat or carbohydrate (with protein) supplement. Not suitable for child under 3 years; use with caution in child 3–6 years. May require dilution for child 3–5 years.	Calogen Extra emulsion: neutral, strawberry 200 ml = £4.98
Calogen® Extra Shots (Nutricia Ltd)	Liquid per 100 mL	1650 kJ (400 kcal)	5 g cows' milk	4.5 g (sugars 3.5 g)	40.3 g	Nil	Gluten-free Residual lactose With vitamins and minerals	Disease-related malnutrition, malabsorption states, or other conditions requiring fortification with a high fat or carbohydrate (with protein) supplement. Not suitable for child under 3 years; use with caution in child 3–6 years. May require dilution for child 3–5 years.	Calogen Extra Shots emulsion: neutral, strawberry 240 ml = £5.75
Calshake® (Fresenius Kabi Ltd)	Powder per 87 g	1841 kJ (439 kcal)	4.1 g cows' milk	56.4 g (sugars 20 g)	22 g	Nil	Contains lactose Gluten-free	Disease-related malnutrition, malabsorption states, or other conditions requiring fortification with a high fat or carbohydrate (with protein) supplement. Not suitable for child under 1 year.	Calshake powder: chocolate 630 gram = £16.73 banana, neutral, strawberry, vanilla 609 gram = £16.73

Powder: one sachet reconstituted with 240 mL whole milk provides approx. 2 kcal/ml & protein 12 g

Product	Formulation	Energy	Protein	Carbohydrate	Fat	Fibre	Special Characteristics	ACBS Indications	Presentation & Flavour
Enshake® (Abbott Laboratories Ltd)	Powder per 100 g	1893 kJ (450 kcal)	8.4 g cows' milk soy protein isolate	69 g (sugars 14.5 g)	15.6 g	Nil	Residual lactose Contains vitamins and minerals	Disease-related malnutrition, malabsorption states, or other conditions requiring fortification with a high fat or carbohydrate (with protein) supplement. Not suitable for child under 1 year; use with caution in child 1–6 years.	Enshake oral powder 96.5g sachets: banana, chocolate, strawberry, vanilla 6 sachet = £12.93

Powder: 96.5 g reconstituted with 240 mL whole milk provides approx. 2 kcal/ml & protein 16 g

Product	Formulation	Energy	Protein	Carbohydrate	Fat	Fibre	Special Characteristics	ACBS Indications	Presentation & Flavour
MCT Procal® (Vitaflo International Ltd)	Powder per 100 g	2742 kJ (657 kcal)	12.5 g cows' milk	20.6 g (sugars 3.1 g)	63.1 g (MCT 99%)	Nil	Contains lactose	Dietary management of disorders of long-chain fatty acid oxidation, fat malabsorption, and other disorders requiring a low LCT, high MCT supplement. Not suitable for child under 1 year.	MCT Procal oral powder 16g sachets: 30 sachet = £23.76

Powder 16 g provides: protein 2 g, carbohydrate 3.3 g, fat 10.1 g, energy 439 kJ (105 kcal)

High-energy supplements: protein (product list continued)

PROTEIN, FAT, AND CARBOHYDRATE

Product	Formulation	Energy	Protein	Carbohydrate	Fat	Fibre	Special Characteristics	ACBS Indications	Presentation & Flavour
Pro-Cal® (Vitaflo International Ltd)	Powder per 100 g	2787 kJ (667 kcal)	13.6 g cows' milk	28.2 g (sugars 16 g)	55.5 g	Nil	Contains lactose Gluten-free	Disease-related malnutrition, malabsorption states, or other conditions requiring fortification with a high fat or carbohydrate with protein) supplement. Not suitable for child under 1 year; use with caution in child 1–5 years.	Pro-Cal powder: 375 gram = £15.83; 510 gram = £14.67; 1500 gram = £29.88; 3000 gram =£70.54; 12500 gram = £212.37

Powder 15 g provides: protein 2 g, carbohydrate 4.2 g, fat 8.3 g, energy 418 kJ (100 kcal)

Product	Formulation	Energy	Protein	Carbohydrate	Fat	Fibre	Special Characteristics	ACBS Indications	Presentation & Flavour
Pro-Cal® Shot (Vitaflo International Ltd)	Liquid per 100 mL	1385 kJ (334 kcal)	6.7 g cows' milk	13.4 g (sugars 13.3 g)	28.2 g	Nil	Contains lactose Gluten-free Contains soya	Disease-related malnutrition, malabsorption states, or other conditions requiring fortification with a high fat or carbohydrate (with protein) supplement. Not suitable for child under 3 years.	Pro-Cal: shot starter pack 360 ml = £7.23; neutral, shot strawberry 120 ml 720 ml = £14.44 banana 720 ml = £14.44
Scandishake® Mix (Nutricia Ltd)	Powder per 100 g	2099 kJ (500 kcal)	4.7 g cows' milk	65 g (sugars 14.3 g)	24.7 g	Nil	Gluten-free Contains lactose	Disease-related malnutrition, malabsorption states, or other conditions requiring fortification with a high fat or carbohydrate (with protein) supplement. Not suitable for child under 3 years.	Scandishake Mix oral powder 85g sachets: banana, caramel, chocolate, strawberry, unflavoured, vanilla 6 sachet = £14.70

Powder, 85 g reconstituted with 240 mL whole milk provides: protein 11.7 g, carbohydrate 66.8 g, fat 30.4 g, energy 2457 kJ (588 kcal)

Product	Formulation	Energy	Protein	Carbohydrate	Fat	Fibre	Special Characteristics	ACBS Indications	Presentation & Flavour
Vitasavoury® (Flavour Not Specified)	Powder per 100 g	2562 kJ (619 kcal)	12 g cows' milk	22.5 g (sugars 1.4 g)	52 g	6.4 g	Contains lactose Contains soya (chicken flavour)	Disease-related malnutrition, malabsorption states, or other conditions requiring fortification with a high fat or carbohydrate (with protein) supplement. Not suitable for child under 3 years.	Vitasavoury powder: chicken, golden vegetable, leek & potato, mushroom 500 g = £18.97 Vitasavoury powder starter pack: 400g = £15.18

Fibre, vitamin, and mineral supplements

High-fibre supplements

Product	Formulation	Energy	Protein	Carbohydrate	Fat	Fibre	Special Characteristics	ACBS Indications	Presentation & Flavour
Resource® Optifibre® (Nestle Health Science)	Powder per 100 g	323 kJ (76 kcal)	Nil	19 g guar gum partially hydrolysed	Nil	78 g	Gluten-free Lactose-free	Standard p. 926 except dysphagia Not suitable for child under 5 years	Resource Optifibre powder: 80 gram = £4.18; 250 gram = £10.28

Vitamin and Mineral supplements

Product	Formulation	Energy	Protein	Carbohydrate	Fat	Fibre	Special Characteristics	ACBS Indications	Presentation & Flavour
FruitiVits® (Vitaflo International Ltd)	Powder per 100 g	133 kJ (33 kcal)	Nil	8.3 g (sugars 400 mg)	0.1 g	3.3 g		Vitamin, mineral, and trace element supplement in children 3–10 years with restrictive therapeutic diets	Sachets: 30 x 6 g = £64.23
Paediatric Seravit® (Nutricia Ltd)	Powder per 100 g	1275 kJ (300 kcal)	Nil	75 g (sugars 6.75 g)	Nil	Nil	Pineapple flavour. Not suitable for child under 6 months	Vitamin, mineral, and trace element supplement in infants and children with restrictive therapeutic diets.	Seravit Paediatric powder: pineapple 200 gram = £19.08 unflavoured 200 gram = £17.91

Feed additives

Special additives for conditions of intolerance

Colief®
► For the relief of symptoms associated with lactose intolerance in infants, provided that lactose intolerance is confirmed by the presence of reducing substances and/or excessive acid in stools, a low concentration of the corresponding disaccharide enzyme on intestinal biopsy or by breath hydrogen test or lactose intolerance test. For dosage and administration details, consult product literature.
LIQUID, lactase 50 000 units/g

Colief 50,000units/g infant drops (Forum Health Products Ltd)
7 ml (ACBS) · NHS indicative price = £8.40

Fructose
► (Laevulose) For proven glucose/galactose intolerance

Glucose
► (Dextrose monohydrate) For use as an energy supplement in sucrose-isomaltase deficiency

VSL#3®
► Nutritional supplement for use under the supervision of a physician, for the maintenance of remission of ileoanal pouchitis induced by antibacterials in adults. For dosage and administration details, consult product literature.
POWDER, containing 8 strains of live, freeze-dried, lactic acid bacteria. Contains traces of soya, gluten, and lactose.

VSL#3 Probiotic Food Supplement oral powder 4.4g sachets (Ferring Pharmaceuticals Ltd)
10 sachet (ACBS) · NHS indicative price = £14.64 | 30 sachet (ACBS) · NHS indicative price = £41.66

Feed thickeners and pre-thickened drinks

Carobel, Instant®
► For thickening feeds in the treatment of vomiting.
POWDER, carob seed flour.

Instant Carobel powder (Cow & Gate Ltd)
135 gram (ACBS) · NHS indicative price = £2.80

Multi-thick®
► For thickening of liquids and foods in dysphagia. Not suitable for children under 1 year except in cases of failure to thrive.
POWDER, modified maize starch, gluten- and lactose-free.

Multi-thick powder (Abbott Laboratories Ltd)
250 gram (ACBS) · NHS indicative price = £4.83

Nutilis® Clear
► For thickening of liquids or foods in dysphagia. Not suitable for children under 3 years.
POWDER, maltodextrin, xanthan gum, guar gum, gluten- and lactose-free.

Nutilis Clear powder (Nutricia Ltd)
175 gram (ACBS) · NHS indicative price = £8.46

Nutilis® Powder
► For thickening of foods in dysphagia. Not suitable for child under 3 years.
POWDER, carbohydrate 86 g, energy 1520 kJ (358 kcal)/100 g, modified maize starch, gluten- and lactose-free.

Nutilis powder (Nutricia Ltd)
240 gram (ACBS) · NHS indicative price = £6.40 | 300 gram (ACBS) · NHS indicative price = £5.01

Resource® ThickenUp Clear
► For thickening of liquids or foods in dysphagia. Not suitable for children under 3 years.
POWDER, maltodextrin, xanthum gum, gluten- and lactose-free.

Resource ThickenUp Clear powder (Nestle Health Science)
28.8 gram (ACBS) · NHS indicative price = £5.28 | 125 gram (ACBS) · NHS indicative price = £8.46

Resource® ThickenUp®
► For thickening of foods in dysphagia. Not suitable for children under 1 year.
POWDER, modified maize starch. Gluten- and lactose-free.

Resource ThickenUp powder (Nestle Health Science)
227 gram (ACBS) · NHS indicative price = £4.55 | 337.5 gram (ACBS) · NHS indicative price = £17.44

Resource® Thickened Drink
► For dysphagia. Not suitable for children under 1 year.
LIQUID, carbohydrate 22 g, energy: orange 382 kJ (90 kcal); apple 376 kJ (89 kcal)/100 mL. Gluten- and lactose-free.

Resource Thickened Drink custard (Nestle Health Science)
apple, orange 114 ml (ACBS) · NHS indicative price = £0.73

Resource Thickened Drink syrup (Nestle Health Science)
apple, orange 114 ml (ACBS) · NHS indicative price = £0.73

SLO Drinks®
► Nutritional supplement for patient hydration in the dietary management of dysphagia. Not suitable for children under 3 years.
POWDER, carbohydrate content varies with flavour and chosen consistency (3 consistencies available), see product literature.

SLO Drink 1 oral powder (SLO Drinks Ltd)
lemon, orange, hot chocolate, white coffee, white tea 25 cup (ACBS) · NHS indicative price = £7.50

SLO Drink 2 oral powder (SLO Drinks Ltd)
hot chocolate, lemon, orange, white tea 25 cup (ACBS) · NHS indicative price = £7.50

SLO Drink 3 oral powder orange (SLO Drinks Ltd)
25 cup (ACBS) · NHS indicative price = £7.50

SLO Milkshakes+®
► Nutritional supplement in the dietary management of dysphagia. Not suitable for children under 3 years.
POWDER, carbohydrate content varies with flavour and chosen consistency (2 consistencies available), see product literature.

SLO Milkshake+ 1 oral powder chocolate (SLO Drinks Ltd)
7 x 50 gram (ACBS) · NHS indicative price = £5.88

SLO Milkshake+ 1 oral powder strawberry (SLO Drinks Ltd)
7 x 50 gram (ACBS) · NHS indicative price = £5.88

SLO Milkshake+ 2 oral powder chocolate (SLO Drinks Ltd)
7 x 50 gram (ACBS) · NHS indicative price = £5.88

SLO Milkshake+ 2 oral powder strawberry (SLO Drinks Ltd)
7 x 50 gram (ACBS) · NHS indicative price = £5.88

Thick and Easy®
► For thickening of foods in dysphagia. Not suitable for children under 1 year except in cases of failure to thrive.
POWDER Modified maize starch

Thick & Easy powder (Fresenius Kabi Ltd)
225 gram (ACBS) · NHS indicative price = £5.12 | 900 gram (ACBS) · NHS indicative price = £31.00 | 4540 gram (ACBS) · NHS indicative price = £85.64

Thicken Aid®
► For thickening of foods in dysphagia. Not suitable for children under 1 year.
POWDER, modified maize starch, maltodextrin, gluten- and lactose-free.

Thicken Aid powder (M & A Pharmachem Ltd)
225 gram (ACBS) · NHS indicative price = £3.71 | 900 gram (ACBS) · NHS indicative price = £22.40

Thixo-D®
► For thickening of foods in dysphagia. Not suitable for children under 1 year except in cases of failure to thrive.
POWDER, modified maize starch, gluten-free.

Thixo-D (Sutherland Health Ltd)
Cal-Free powder 30 gram · NHS indicative price = £2.85 | powder 375 gram (ACBS) · NHS indicative price = £7.15

Vitaquick®
► For thickening of foods in dysphagia. Not suitable for children under 1 year except in cases of failure to thrive.
POWDER. Modified maize starch.

Vitaquick powder (Vitaflo International Ltd)
300 gram (ACBS) · NHS indicative price = £7.13

Flavouring preparations

Flavour Mix®
POWDER

Nestle Nutrition Flavour (Nestle Health Science)
Mix banana, Mix chocolate 60 gram (ACBS) · NHS indicative price = £7.17

flavourPac®
For use with Vitaflo's range of unflavoured protein substitutes for metabolic diseases; not suitable for child under 3 years.
POWDER

flavourPac oral powder 4g sachets (Vitaflo International Ltd)
Blackcurrant, lemon, orange, raspberry, tropical 30 sachet (ACBS) · NHS indicative price = £13.79 | 120 sachet (ACBS) No NHS indicative price available

---

Foods for special diets

Gluten-free foods

ACBS indications: established gluten-sensitive enteropathies including steatorrhoea due to gluten sensitivity, coeliac disease, and dermatitis herpetiformis.

Bread

LOAVES

Barkat® Loaf
GLUTEN-FREE

Barkat gluten free (Gluten Free Foods Ltd)
wholemeal bread sliced 500 gram (ACBS) · NHS indicative price £3.98
brown rice bread, wheat free multigrain bread, white rice bread 500 gram (ACBS) · NHS indicative price = £5.73
par baked white bread sliced 300 gram (ACBS) · NHS indicative price = £4.13
home fresh country loaf 250 gram (ACBS) · NHS indicative price £4.35

Ener-G® Loaves
GLUTEN-FREE

Ener-G gluten free (General Dietary Ltd)
Seattle brown loaf 454 gram · NHS indicative price = £6.22
rice loaf 612 gram (ACBS) · NHS indicative price = £5.41
white rice bread 456 gram (ACBS) · NHS indicative price = £5.41
tapioca bread 480 gram (ACBS) · NHS indicative price = £5.41
brown rice bread 474 gram (ACBS) · NHS indicative price = £5.41

Genius Gluten Free® Loaf
GLUTEN-FREE

Genius gluten free brown bread (Genius Foods Ltd)
unsliced 400 gram (ACBS) · NHS indicative price = £2.67
sliced 400 gram (ACBS) · NHS indicative price = £2.77

Genius gluten free brown sandwich bread sliced (Genius Foods Ltd)
535 gram (ACBS) · NHS indicative price = £3.59

Genius gluten free white bread (Genius Foods Ltd)
unsliced 400 gram (ACBS) · NHS indicative price = £2.67
sliced 400 gram (ACBS) · NHS indicative price = £2.77

Genius gluten free white sandwich bread sliced (Genius Foods Ltd)
535 gram (ACBS) · NHS indicative price = £3.59

Glutafin® Loaves
GLUTEN-FREE

Glutafin gluten free (Dr Schar UK Ltd)
fibre loaf sliced, white loaf sliced 400 gram (ACBS) · NHS indicative price = £3.85

Glutafin® Select Loaves
GLUTEN-FREE

Glutafin gluten free Select fibre loaf sliced (Dr Schar UK Ltd)
400 gram (ACBS) · NHS indicative price = £3.43

Glutafin gluten free Select fresh (Dr Schar UK Ltd)
brown loaf sliced, white loaf sliced 400 gram (ACBS) · NHS indicative price = £3.43

Glutafin gluten free Select seeded loaf sliced (Dr Schar UK Ltd)
400 gram (ACBS) · NHS indicative price = £3.72

Glutafin gluten free Select white loaf sliced (Dr Schar UK Ltd)
400 gram (ACBS) · NHS indicative price = £3.43

Juvela® Loaf
GLUTEN-FREE

Juvela gluten free fibre loaf (Hero UK Ltd)
sliced, unsliced 400 gram (ACBS) · NHS indicative price = £3.54

Juvela gluten free fresh (Hero UK Ltd)
fibre loaf sliced 400 gram (ACBS) · NHS indicative price = £3.39
white loaf sliced 400 gram (ACBS) · NHS indicative price = £3.69

Juvela gluten free loaf unsliced (Hero UK Ltd)
400 gram (ACBS) · NHS indicative price = £3.43

Juvela gluten free part baked (Hero UK Ltd)
fibre loaf 400 gram (ACBS) · NHS indicative price = £3.80
loaf 400 gram (ACBS) · NHS indicative price = £3.95

Lifestyle® Loaf
GLUTEN-FREE

Lifestyle gluten free (Ultrapharm Ltd)
high fibre bread sliced 400 gram · NHS indicative price = £2.82
brown bread sliced, white bread sliced 400 gram (ACBS) · NHS indicative price = £2.82

Livwell® Loaf
GLUTEN-FREE

Livwell gluten free (Livwell Ltd)
multi grain bread sliced 200 gram · NHS indicative price = £2.25
white bread sliced 200 gram (ACBS) · NHS indicative price = £2.25

Warburtons® Loaf
GLUTEN-FREE

Warburtons gluten free (Warburtons Ltd)
brown bread sliced, white bread sliced 400 gram (ACBS) · NHS indicative price = £3.06

Wellfoods® Loaf
GLUTEN-FREE

Wellfoods gluten free loaf (Wellfoods Ltd)
unsliced 600 gram (ACBS) · NHS indicative price = £4.85
sliced 600 gram (ACBS) · NHS indicative price = £4.95

BAGUETTES, BUNS AND ROLLS

Barkat® Baguettes and rolls
GLUTEN-FREE

Barkat gluten free par baked (Gluten Free Foods Ltd)
baguettes 200 gram (ACBS) · NHS indicative price = £4.35
rolls 200 gram (ACBS) · NHS indicative price = £3.98

Ener-G® Rolls
GLUTEN-FREE

Ener-G gluten free (General Dietary Ltd)
white round rolls, white long rolls 220 gram (ACBS) · NHS indicative price = £2.95
dinner rolls 280 gram (ACBS) · NHS indicative price = £3.67

Glutafin® Baguettes and rolls
GLUTEN-FREE

Glutafin gluten free (Dr Schar UK Ltd)
4 white rolls, part baked 4 fibre rolls 200 gram (ACBS) · NHS indicative price = £3.68
baguettes 350 gram (ACBS) · NHS indicative price = £3.51

Glutafin® Select Rolls
GLUTEN-FREE

Glutafin gluten free part baked (Dr Schar UK Ltd)
2 long white rolls 150 gram (ACBS) · NHS indicative price = £2.81
4 white rolls 200 gram (ACBS) · NHS indicative price = £3.68

Juvela® Rolls
GLUTEN-FREE

Juvela gluten free bread rolls (Hero UK Ltd)
425 gram (ACBS) · NHS indicative price = £4.77

Juvela gluten free fibre bread rolls (Hero UK Ltd)
425 gram (ACBS) · NHS indicative price = £4.77

Juvela gluten free fresh (Hero UK Ltd)
fibre rolls, white rolls 425 gram (ACBS) · NHS indicative price = £4.42

Juvela gluten free part baked (Hero UK Ltd)
fibre bread rolls, white bread rolls 375 gram (ACBS) · NHS indicative price = £4.94

Lifestyle® Rolls
GLUTEN-FREE

Lifestyle gluten free (Ultrapharm Ltd)
brown bread rolls, high fibre bread rolls, white bread rolls 400 gram (ACBS) · NHS indicative price = £2.82

Livwell® Baguettes, buns and rolls
GLUTEN-FREE

Livwell gluten free (Livwell Ltd)
toasting bread buns 180 gram (ACBS) · NHS indicative price = £2.40
white baguettes 140 gram (ACBS) · NHS indicative price = £2.15
part baked square dinner rolls 160 gram (ACBS) · NHS indicative price = £2.09

Proceli® Baguettes, buns and rolls
GLUTEN-FREE

Proceli gluten free (Ambe Ltd)
part baked baguettes 250 gram (ACBS) · NHS indicative price = £3.24

Warburtons® Baguettes and rolls
GLUTEN-FREE

Warburtons gluten free (Warburtons Ltd)
brown rolls, white rolls 220 gram (ACBS) · NHS indicative price = £2.55
baguettes 150 gram (ACBS) · NHS indicative price = £2.86

Wellfoods® Buns and rolls
GLUTEN-FREE

Wellfoods gluten free (Wellfoods Ltd)
burger buns 380 gram (ACBS) · NHS indicative price = £3.95
rolls 360 gram (ACBS) · NHS indicative price = £3.65

SPECIALITY BREADS

Livwell® Flat bread
GLUTEN-FREE

Livwell gluten free (Livwell Ltd)
tear drop flat bread 180 gram (ACBS) · NHS indicative price = £3.00
flat bread 220 gram (ACBS) · NHS indicative price = £3.00

Cereals

Juvela® Fibre flakes and oats
GLUTEN-FREE

Juvela gluten free (Hero UK Ltd)
fibre flakes, flakes 300 gram (ACBS) · NHS indicative price = £2.78
pure oats 500 gram (ACBS) · NHS indicative price = £2.78

Nairns® Porridge
GLUTEN-FREE

Nairn's gluten free oat porridge (Nairn's Oatcakes Ltd)
500 gram (ACBS) · NHS indicative price = £3.05

Cookies and biscuits

Barkat® Biscuits
GLUTEN-FREE

Barkat gluten free (Gluten Free Foods Ltd)
digestive biscuits 175 gram (ACBS) · NHS indicative price = £2.61
coffee biscuits 200 gram (ACBS) · NHS indicative price = £3.38

Ener-G® Cookies
GLUTEN-FREE

Ener-G gluten free vanilla cookies (General Dietary Ltd)
435 gram

Glutafin® Cookies and biscuits
GLUTEN-FREE

Glutafin gluten free (Dr Schar UK Ltd)
digestive biscuits, sweet biscuits 150 gram (ACBS) · NHS indicative price = £2.13
tea biscuits 150 gram (ACBS) · NHS indicative price = £2.09
biscuits 200 gram (ACBS) · NHS indicative price = £4.14
savoury short biscuits 130 gram (ACBS) · NHS indicative price = £2.80
shortbread biscuits 100 gram (ACBS) · NHS indicative price = £1.73

Juvela® Biscuits
GLUTEN-FREE

Juvela gluten free (Hero UK Ltd)
sweet biscuits 150 gram (ACBS) · NHS indicative price = £2.88
digestive biscuits, tea biscuits 150 gram (ACBS) · NHS indicative price = £3.05
savoury biscuits 150 gram (ACBS) · NHS indicative price = £3.82

Crackers, crispbreads, and breadsticks

Barkat® Crackers
GLUTEN-FREE

Barkat gluten free matzo crackers (Gluten Free Foods Ltd)
200 gram (ACBS) · NHS indicative price = £3.52

Glutafin® Crackers
GLUTEN-FREE

Glutafin gluten free (Dr Schar UK Ltd)
mini crackers 175 gram (ACBS) · NHS indicative price = £2.96
crackers 200 gram (ACBS) · NHS indicative price = £3.46
high fibre crackers 200 gram (ACBS) · NHS indicative price = £2.90

Juvela® Crispbread
GLUTEN-FREE

Juvela gluten free crispbread (Hero UK Ltd)
200 gram (ACBS) · NHS indicative price = £4.64

Warburtons® Crackers
GLUTEN-FREE

Warburtons gluten free bran crackers (Warburtons Ltd)
150 gram (ACBS) · NHS indicative price = £2.34

Flour mixes and xanthan gum

FLOUR MIXES

Barkat® Flour mix
GLUTEN-FREE

Barkat gluten free (Gluten Free Foods Ltd)
bread mix 500 gram (ACBS) · NHS indicative price = £6.81
flour mix 500 gram (ACBS) · NHS indicative price = £4.65

Finax® Flour mix
GLUTEN-FREE

Finax gluten free (Drossa Ltd)
coarse flour mix, flour mix 900 gram (ACBS) · NHS indicative price = £8.66
fibre bread mix 1000 gram (ACBS) · NHS indicative price = £9.9

Glutafin gluten free multipurpose white mix (Dr Schar UK Ltd)
500 gram (ACBS) · NHS indicative price = £6.66

Glutafin Select® Flour mix
GLUTEN-FREE

Glutafin gluten free Select bread mix (Dr Schar UK Ltd)
500 gram (ACBS) · NHS indicative price = £6.66

Glutafin gluten free Select fibre bread mix (Dr Schar UK Ltd)
500 gram (ACBS) · NHS indicative price = £6.66

Glutafin gluten free Select multipurpose (Dr Schar UK Ltd)
fibre mix, white mix 500 gram (ACBS) · NHS indicative price = £6.66

Heron Foods® Flour mix
GLUTEN-FREE

Heron Hi-Fibre gluten free (Gluten Free Foods Ltd)
organic bread mix, wheat free organic bread mix 500 gram (ACBS) · NHS indicative price = £8.96

Juvela® Flour mix
GLUTEN-FREE

Juvela gluten free (Hero UK Ltd)
fibre mix, harvest mix, mix 500 gram (ACBS) · NHS indicative
price = £7.35

Mrs Crimbles® Flour mixes
GLUTEN-FREE

Mrs Crimble's gluten free (Stiletto Foods (UK) Ltd)
pastry mix 200 gram (ACBS) · NHS indicative price = £1.09
bread mix 275 gram (ACBS) · NHS indicative price = £1.09

Orgran® Flour mix
GLUTEN-FREE

Orgran gluten free (Naturally Good Food Ltd)
pizza & pastry mix 375 gram (ACBS) · NHS indicative price =
£3.80
self-raising flour 500 gram (ACBS) · NHS indicative price =
£3.10
all purpose plain flour 500 gram · NHS indicative price = £3.10

Proceli® Flour mix
GLUTEN-FREE

Proceli gluten free white plain flour (Ambe Ltd)
1000 gram (ACBS) · NHS indicative price = £9.95

Pure® Flour mix
GLUTEN-FREE

Innovative Solutions Pure gluten free blended flour (Innovative
Solutions (UK) Ltd)
1000 gram (ACBS) . NHS indicative price = £4.23

Innovative Solutions Pure gluten free brown rice flour (Innovative
Solutions (UK) Ltd)
500 gram (ACBS) . NHS indicative price = £1.58

Innovative Solutions Pure gluten free white rice flour (Innovative
Solutions (UK) Ltd)
500 gram (ACBS) . NHS indicative price = £1.68

Innovative Solutions Pure gluten free potato flour (Innovative
Solutions (UK) Ltd)
500 gram (ACBS) . NHS indicative price = £1.68

Innovative Solutions Pure gluten free tapioca flour (Innovative
Solutions (UK) Ltd)
500 gram (ACBS) . NHS indicative price = £2.26

Innovative Solutions Pure gluten free brown teff flour (Innovative
Solutions (UK) Ltd)
1000 gram (ACBS) . NHS indicative price = £4.77

Innovative Solutions Pure gluten free white teff flour (Innovative
Solutions (UK) Ltd)
1000 gram (ACBS) . NHS indicative price = £4.77

Tobia® Flour mix
GLUTEN-FREE

Tobia Teff gluten free (Tobia Teff UK Ltd)
brown teff flour, white teff flour 1000 gram (ACBS) · NHS
indicative price = £3.35

Tritamyl® Flour mix
GLUTEN-FREE

Tritamyl gluten free (Gluten Free Foods Ltd)
brown bread mix 1000 gram (ACBS) · NHS indicative price =
£7.10
flour mix, white bread mix 2000 gram (ACBS) · NHS indicative
price = £14.26

Wellfoods® Flour mix
GLUTEN-FREE

Wellfoods gluten free flour alternative (Wellfoods Ltd)
1000 gram (ACBS) · NHS indicative price = £7.65

XANTHAN GUM

Ener-G® Xanthan gum
GLUTEN-FREE

Ener-G xanthan gum (General Dietary Ltd)
170 gram (ACBS) · NHS indicative price = £8.53

Pure® Xanthan gum
GLUTEN-FREE

Innovative Solutions Pure xanthan gum (Innovative Solutions (UK)
Ltd)
200 gram (ACBS) · NHS indicative price = £6.85

Pasta

Barkat® Pasta
GLUTEN-FREE

macaroni (Gluten Free Foods Ltd)
500 gram (ACBS) · NHS indicative price = £5.88

spaghetti (Gluten Free Foods Ltd)
500 gram (ACBS) · NHS indicative price = £5.88

spirals (Gluten Free Foods Ltd)
500 gram (ACBS) · NHS indicative price = £5.88

tagliatelle (Gluten Free Foods Ltd)
500 gram (ACBS) · NHS indicative price = £5.88

Barkat gluten free pasta animal shapes (Gluten Free Foods Ltd)
500 gram (ACBS) · NHS indicative price = £5.88

Barkat gluten free pasta buckwheat (Gluten Free Foods Ltd)
penne, spirals 250 gram (ACBS) · NHS indicative price = £2.93

BiAlimenta® Pasta
GLUTEN-FREE

BiAlimenta gluten free pasta (Drossa Ltd)
tubetti 500 gram (ACBS) · NHS indicative price = £5.90
acini di pepe, penne, sagnette, spirali, tubetti 500 gram (ACBS) ·
NHS indicative price = £5.97

Glutafin® Pasta
GLUTEN-FREE

Glutafin gluten free pasta (Dr Schar UK Ltd)
lasagne, tagliatelle nests 250 gram (ACBS) · NHS indicative price
= £3.53
fibre spaghetti 500 gram (ACBS) · NHS indicative price = £5.74
macaroni penne, shells, spirals, long-cut spaghetti 500 gram
(ACBS) · NHS indicative price = £6.73

Juvela® Pasta
GLUTEN-FREE

Juvela gluten free fibre penne (Hero UK Ltd)
500 gram (ACBS) · NHS indicative price = £6.61

Juvela gluten free pasta (Hero UK Ltd)
tagliatelle 250 gram (ACBS) · NHS indicative price = £3.47
fusilli, macaroni, spaghetti 500 gram (ACBS) · NHS indicative
price = £7.21
lasagne 250 gram (ACBS) · NHS indicative price = £3.68

Orgran® Pasta
GLUTEN-FREE

Orgran gluten free pasta brown rice spirals (Naturally Good Food
Ltd)
250 gram (ACBS) · NHS indicative price = £2.42

Orgran gluten free pasta buckwheat spirals (Naturally Good Food
Ltd)
250 gram (ACBS) · NHS indicative price = £2.42

Orgran gluten free pasta corn spirals (Naturally Good Food Ltd)
250 gram (ACBS) · NHS indicative price = £2.42

Orgran gluten free pasta rice & corn (Naturally Good Food Ltd)
macaroni, spirals 250 gram (ACBS) · NHS indicative price =
£2.42
lasagne 200 gram (ACBS) · NHS indicative price = £3.13

Orgran gluten free pasta rice & millet spirals (Naturally Good Food
Ltd)
250 gram (ACBS) · NHS indicative price = £2.42

Rizopia® Pasta
GLUTEN-FREE

Rizopia gluten free organic brown rice pasta (PGR Health Foods Ltd)
lasagne 375 gram (ACBS) · NHS indicative price = £2.72
fusilli, penne, spaghetti 500 gram (ACBS) · NHS indicative price
= £2.72

Pizza bases

Barkat®, Pizza crust
GLUTEN-FREE

Barkat gluten free (Gluten Free Foods Ltd)
brown rice pizza crust, white rice pizza crust 150 gram (ACBS) ·
NHS indicative price = £5.00

Glutafin® Pizza base
GLUTEN-FREE

Glutafin gluten free pizza base (Dr Schar UK Ltd)
300 gram (ACBS) · NHS indicative price = £6.56

Juvela® Pizza base
GLUTEN-FREE

Juvela gluten free pizza base (Hero UK Ltd)
360 gram (ACBS) · NHS indicative price = £8.78

Proceli® Pizza base
GLUTEN-FREE

Proceli gluten free pizza base (Ambe Ltd)
250 gram (ACBS) · NHS indicative price = £3.90

Wellfoods® Pizza base
GLUTEN-FREE

Wellfoods gluten free pizza base (Wellfoods Ltd)
600 gram (ACBS) · NHS indicative price = £8.95

Gluten- and wheat-free foods

ACBS indications: established gluten-sensitive enteropathies with coexisting established wheat sensitivity only.

Ener-G® (General Dietary Ltd)
Gluten-free, wheat-free. Rolls, Seattle brown, round (hamburger) 4 x 80 gram (ACBS) · NHS indicative price = £4.08
long (hot dog) 4 x 80 gram (ACBS) · NHS indicative price = £4.08
Pizza base 3 x 124 gram (ACBS) · NHS indicative price = £4.74

Glutafin® (Dr Schar UK Ltd)
Gluten-free. Flour mix, bread, fibre 500 gram (ACBS) · NHS indicative price = £6.66
Crispbread 150 gram (ACBS) · NHS indicative price = £3.25

Heron Foods® (Gluten Free Foods Ltd)
Gluten-free, wheat-free. Flour mix, organic, bread, fibre 500 gram (ACBS) · NHS indicative price = £8.96
Bread and cake mix 500 gram (ACBS) · NHS indicative price = £8.96

Low-protein foods

ACBS indications: inherited metabolic disorders, renal or liver failure, requiring a low-protein diet

Bread

Ener-G® Rice bread
LOW PROTEIN

Ener-G low protein rice bread (General Dietary Ltd)
600 gram (ACBS) · NHS indicative price = £5.54

Juvela® Loaf and rolls
LOW PROTEIN

Juvela gluten free loaf sliced (Hero UK Ltd)
400 gram (ACBS) · NHS indicative price = £3.54

Juvela low protein (Hero UK Ltd)
loaf sliced 400 gram (ACBS) · NHS indicative price = £3.64
bread rolls 350 gram (ACBS) · NHS indicative price = £4.52

Loprofin® Bread
LOW-PROTEIN

Loprofin low protein part baked (Nutricia Ltd)
loaf sliced 400 gram (ACBS) · NHS indicative price = £3.98
bread rolls 260 gram (ACBS) · NHS indicative price = £4.20

PK Foods® Loaf
LOW PROTEIN

PK Foods low protein white bread sliced (Gluten Free Foods Ltd)
550 gram (ACBS) · NHS indicative price = £4.75

Cake, biscuits, and snacks

Juvela® Cookies
LOW-PROTEIN

Juvela low protein (Hero UK Ltd)
chocolate chip cookies 110 gram (ACBS) · NHS indicative price = £7.62

cinnamon cookies, orange cookies 125 gram (ACBS) · NHS indicative price = £7.62

Loprofin® Wafers
LOW-PROTEIN

Loprofin low protein (Nutricia Ltd)
chocolate cream wafers, vanilla cream wafers 100 gram (ACBS) · NHS indicative price = £2.58
crackers, herb crackers 150 gram (ACBS) · NHS indicative price = £3.62

PK Foods® Biscuits
LOW-PROTEIN

PK Foods Aminex low protein (Gluten Free Foods Ltd)
biscuits, rusks 200 gram (ACBS) · NHS indicative price = £5.04
cookies 150 gram (ACBS) · NHS indicative price = £5.04

PK Foods low protein (Gluten Free Foods Ltd)
crispbread 75 gram (ACBS) · NHS indicative price = £2.42
chocolate chip cookies, cinnamon cookies, orange cookies 150 gram (ACBS) · NHS indicative price = £5.04

Promin® Cooked and flavoured pasta snax
LOW-PROTEIN

Promin low protein (Firstplay Dietary Foods Ltd)
Snax salt & vinegar 25g sachets, Snax ready salted 25g sachets, Snax cheese & onion 25g sachets 3 sachet No NHS indicative price available

Taranis® Cake bars
LOW-PROTEIN

Taranis low protein (Firstplay Dietary Foods Ltd)
apricot cake, lemon cake, pear cake 240 gram (ACBS) · NHS indicative price = £6.08

Vita Bite®
▶ Not recommended for any child under 1 year.
LOW PROTEIN.Bar, protein 30 mg (less than 2.5 mg phenylalanine), carbohydrate 15.35 g, fat 8.4 g, energy 572 kJ (137 kcal)/25 g.

VitaBite bar (Vitaflo International Ltd)
175 gram (ACBS) · NHS indicative price = £8.61

Vitaflo Choices® Mini crackers
LOW-PROTEIN

Vitaflo Choices mini crackers (Vitaflo International Ltd)
40 gram (ACBS) · NHS indicative price = £0.85

Cereals

Loprofin® Breakfast cereal
LOW-PROTEIN

loops (Nutricia Ltd)
375 gram (ACBS) · NHS indicative price = £8.12

Loprofin low protein breakfast cereal flakes (Nutricia Ltd)
apple, chocolate, strawberry 375 gram (ACBS) · NHS indicative price = £7.98

Promin® Hot breakfast
LOW-PROTEIN

Promin low protein hot breakfast powder sachets (Firstplay Dietary Foods Ltd)
apple & cinnamon, banana, chocolate 342 gram (ACBS) · NHS indicative price = £8.09
original 336 gram (ACBS) · NHS indicative price = £8.09

Desserts

Loprofin® Powder
LOW-PROTEIN

Loprofin low protein dessert (Nutricia Ltd)
mix chocolate, mix strawberry, mix vanilla 150 gram (ACBS) · NHS indicative price = £4.88

PK Foods® Jelly
LOW-PROTEIN

PK Foods low protein jelly mix dessert (Gluten Free Foods Ltd)
cherry, orange 320 gram (ACBS) · NHS indicative price = £8.03

Promin® Desserts
LOW-PROTEIN

Promin low protein imitation rice pudding (Firstplay Dietary Foods
td)
pple, banana, original, strawberry 276 gram (ACBS) · NHS
ndicative price = £6.33

Flour mixes and egg substitutes

ner-G® Egg replacer
LOW-PROTEIN

ner-G low protein egg replacer (General Dietary Ltd)
54 gram (ACBS) · NHS indicative price = £5.11

ate® Flour mix
LOW PROTEIN

ate low protein (Fate Special Foods)
ll purpose mix, chocolate cake mix, plain cake mix 500 gram
ACBS) · NHS indicative price = £6.97

uvela® Mix
LOW-PROTEIN

uvela low protein mix (Hero UK Ltd)
00 gram (ACBS) · NHS indicative price = £7.79

oprofin® Flour mixes and egg substitutes
OW-PROTEIN

ix (Nutricia Ltd)
00 gram

oprofin low protein cake (Nutricia Ltd)
ix lemon, mix chocolate 500 gram (ACBS) · NHS indicative
rice = £8.76

oprofin low protein egg (Nutricia Ltd)
hite replacer 100 gram (ACBS) · NHS indicative price = £9.98
eplacer 500 gram (ACBS) · NHS indicative price = £15.51

K Foods® Flour mix and egg substitute
OW-PROTEIN

K Foods low protein (Gluten Free Foods Ltd)
gg replacer 200 gram (ACBS) · NHS indicative price = £4.08
our mix 750 gram (ACBS) · NHS indicative price = £10.71

asta

oprofin® Pasta
OW-PROTEIN

ce (Nutricia Ltd)
00 gram

oprofin low protein pasta (Nutricia Ltd)
enne, long cut spaghetti 500 gram (ACBS) · NHS indicative
ice = £8.82
nimal shapes 500 gram (ACBS) · NHS indicative price = £8.49
gliatelle, macaroni elbows 250 gram (ACBS) · NHS indicative
ice = £4.24
sagne 250 gram (ACBS) · NHS indicative price = £4.29

omin® Pasta
OW-PROTEIN

omin Plus low protein pasta (Firstplay Dietary Foods Ltd)
acaroni, flat noodles 500 gram (ACBS) · NHS indicative price =
.99

omin low protein imitation rice (Firstplay Dietary Foods Ltd)
00 gram (ACBS) · NHS indicative price = £6.99

omin low protein lasagne sheets (Firstplay Dietary Foods Ltd)
00 gram (ACBS) · NHS indicative price = £3.03

omin low protein pasta (Firstplay Dietary Foods Ltd)
phabets, shells, short cut spaghetti, spirals 500 gram (ACBS) ·
HS indicative price = £6.99

omin low protein tricolour pasta (Firstplay Dietary Foods Ltd)
irals, alphabets, shells 500 gram (ACBS) · NHS indicative price
£6.99

izza bases

vela® Pizza base
W-PROTEIN

vela low protein pizza base (Hero UK Ltd)
0 gram (ACBS) · NHS indicative price = £8.61

Savoury meals and mixes

Promin® Savoury meals and mixes
LOW-PROTEIN

pastameal (Firstplay Dietary Foods Ltd)
500 gram (ACBS) · NHS indicative price = £6.99

elbows (Firstplay Dietary Foods Ltd)
500 gram (ACBS) · NHS indicative price = £6.99

macaroni (Firstplay Dietary Foods Ltd)
500 gram (ACBS) · NHS indicative price = £6.99

Promin Plus low protein pasta spirals (Firstplay Dietary Foods Ltd)
500 gram (ACBS) · NHS indicative price = £6.99

Promin low protein X-Pot (Firstplay Dietary Foods Ltd)
all day scramble, beef & tomato, chip shop curry, rogan style
curry 240 gram (ACBS) · NHS indicative price = £20.94

Promin low protein burger mix (Firstplay Dietary Foods Ltd)
124 gram (ACBS) · NHS indicative price = £6.36

Promin low protein cous cous (Firstplay Dietary Foods Ltd)
500 gram (ACBS) · NHS indicative price = £6.99

Promin low protein lamb and mint burger mix (Firstplay Dietary
Foods Ltd)
124 gram (ACBS) · NHS indicative price = £6.36

Promin low protein pasta in (Firstplay Dietary Foods Ltd)
cheese and broccoli sauce 264 gram (ACBS) · NHS indicative
price = £8.31
tomato, pepper and herb sauce 288 gram (ACBS) · NHS
indicative price = £8.31

Promin low protein pasta spirals in Moroccan sauce (Firstplay
Dietary Foods Ltd)
288 gram (ACBS) · NHS indicative price = £8.31

Promin low protein potato pot (Firstplay Dietary Foods Ltd)
onion, cabbage & bacon, sausage 200 gram (ACBS) · NHS
indicative price = £16.40

Promin low protein sausage (Firstplay Dietary Foods Ltd)
mix apple and sage, mix original, mix tomato and basil
120 gram (ACBS) · NHS indicative price = £7.15

Spreads

Taranis® Spread
LOW-PROTEIN

Taranis low protein hazelnut spread (Firstplay Dietary Foods Ltd)
230 gram (ACBS) · NHS indicative price = £7.87

Nutritional supplements for metabolic diseases

GA1 Anamix® Infant
▸ Nutritional supplement for the dietary management of proven
glutaric aciduria (type 1) in children from birth to 3 years.
POWDER, protein equivalent (essential and non-essential amino
acids except lysine, and low tryptophan) 13.1 g, carbohydrate
49.5 g, fat 23 g, fibre 5.3 g, energy 1915 kJ (457 kcal)/100 g, with
vitamins, minerals, and trace elements; standard dilution (15%)
provides protein equivalent 2 g, carbohydrate 7.4 g, fat 3.5 g,
fibre 800 mg, energy 287 kJ (69 kcal)/100 mL.

Glutaric aciduria (type 1)

GA Gel®
▸ Nutritional supplement for dietary management of type 1
glutaric aciduria in children 6 months–10 years.
GEL, protein equivalent (essential and non-essential amino
acids except lysine, and low tryptophan) 10 g, carbohydrate
10.3 g, fat trace, energy 339 kJ (81 kcal)/24 g, with vitamins,
minerals, and trace elements.

GA gel oral powder 24g sachets (Vitaflo International Ltd)
30 sachet (ACBS) · NHS indicative price = £212.44

XLYS, Low TRY, Maxamaid®
▸ Nutritional supplement for the dietary management of type 1
glutaric aciduria.

POWDER, protein equivalent (essential and non-essential amino acids except lysine, and low tryptophan) 25 g, carbohydrate 51 g, fat less than 500 mg, energy 1311 kJ (309 kcal)/100 g, with vitamins, minerals, and trace elements.

XLYS LOW TRY Maxamaid powder (Nutricia Ltd)
500 gram (ACBS) · NHS indicative price = £98.23

XLYS, TRY Glutaridon®
▸ Nutritional supplement for the dietary management of type 1 glutaric aciduria in children and adults; requires additional source of vitamins, minerals, and trace elements.
POWDER, protein equivalent (essential and non-essential amino acids except lysine and tryptophan) 79 g, carbohydrate 4 g, energy 1411 kJ (332 kcal)/100 g.

XLYS TRY Glutaridon powder (Nutricia Ltd)
500 gram (ACBS) · NHS indicative price = £186.08

Glycogen storage disease

Corn flour and corn starch

For glycogen storage disease

Glycosade®
▸ A nutritional supplement for use in the dietary management of glycogen storage disease and other metabolic conditions where a constant supply of glucose is essential. Not suitable for use in children under 2 years.
POWDER, protein 200 mg, carbohydrate (maize starch) 47.6 g, fat 100 mg, fibre less than 600 mg, energy 803 kJ (192 kcal)/60 g.

Glycosade oral powder 60g sachets (Vitaflo International Ltd)
30 sachet (ACBS) · NHS indicative price = £111.65

Homocystinuria or hypermethioninaemia

HCU Anamix® Infant
▸ Nutritional supplement for the dietary management of proven vitamin B6 non-responsive homocystinuria or hypermethioninaemia in children from birth to 3 years.
POWDER, protein equivalent (essential and non-essential amino acids except methionine) 13.1 g, carbohydrate 49.5 g, fat 23 g, fibre 5.3 g, energy 1915 kJ (457 kcal)/100 g, with vitamins, minerals, and trace elements; standard dilution (15%) provides protein equivalent 2 g, carbohydrate 7.4 g, fat 3.5 g, fibre 800 mg, energy 287 kJ (69 kcal)/100 mL.

HCU Anamix Infant powder (Nutricia Ltd)
400 gram (ACBS) · NHS indicative price = £38.91

HCU cooler® 15
▸ A methionine-free protein substitute for use as a nutritional supplement in children over 3 years with homocystinuria.
LIQUID, protein (essential and non-essential amino acids except methionine) 15 g, carbohydrate 7 g, fat 500 mg, energy 393 kJ (92 kcal)/130 mL, with vitamins, minerals, and trace elements.

HCU orange cooler 15 liquid (Vitaflo International Ltd)
130 ml (ACBS) · NHS indicative price = £11.21

HCU Express® 15
▸ A methionine-free protein substitute for use as a nutritional supplement in children over 8 years with homocystinuria.
POWDER, protein (essential and non-essential amino acids except methionine) 15 g, carbohydrate 3.8 g, fat 30 mg, energy 315 kJ (75.3 kcal)/25 g with vitamins, minerals, and trace elements.

HCU express 15 oral powder 25g sachets (Vitaflo International Ltd)
30 sachet (ACBS) · NHS indicative price = £329.89

HCU Express® 20
▸ A methionine-free protein substitute for use as a nutritional supplement in children over 8 years with homocystinuria.
POWDER, protein (essential and non-essential amino acids except methionine) 20 g, carbohydrate 4.7 g, fat 70 mg, energy 416 kJ (99 kcal)/34 g with vitamins, minerals, and trace elements.

HCU express 20 oral powder 34g sachets (Vitaflo International Ltd)
30 sachet (ACBS) · NHS indicative price = £426.21

HCU gel®
▸ A methionine-free protein substitute for use as a nutritional supplement for the dietary management of children 1–10 years with homocystinuria.
POWDER, protein (essential and non-essential amino acids except methionine) 10 g, carbohydrate 10.3 g, fat 20 mg, energy 339 kJ (81 kcal)/24 g with vitamins, minerals, and trace elements.

HCU gel oral powder 24g sachets (Vitaflo International Ltd)
30 sachet (ACBS) · NHS indicative price = £212.38

HCU Lophlex® LQ 20
▸ Nutritional supplement for the dietary management of homocystinuria in children over 3 years.
LIQUID, protein equivalent (essential and non-essential amino acids except methionine) 20 g, carbohydrate 8.8 g, fat 440 mg, energy 509 kJ (120 kcal)/125 mL, with vitamins, minerals, and trace elements.

HCU Lophlex LQ 20 liquid (Nutricia Ltd)
125 ml (ACBS) · NHS indicative price = £16.05

HCU LV®
▸ Nutritional supplement for the dietary management of hypermethioninaemia or vitamin B6 non-responsive homocystinuria in children over 8 years.
POWDER, protein (essential and non-essential amino acids except methionine) 2.5 g, carbohydrate 34 g, fat 190 mg, energy 390 kJ (92 kcal)/27.8-g sachet, with vitamins, minerals, and trace elements.

HCU-LV oral powder 27.8g sachets (Nutricia Ltd)
tropical, unflavoured 30 sachet (ACBS) · NHS indicative price = £493.20

XMET Homidon®
▸ Nutritional supplement for the dietary management of hypermethioninaemia or homocystinuria in children and adults.
POWDER, protein equivalent (essential and non-essential amino acids, except methionine) 77 g, carbohydrate 4.5 g, fat nil, energy 1386 kJ (326 kcal)/100 g.

XMET Homidon powder (Nutricia Ltd)
500 gram (ACBS) · NHS indicative price = £186.08

XMET Maxamaid®
▸ Nutritional supplement for the dietary management of hypermethioninaemia or homocystinuria.
POWDER, protein equivalent (essential and non-essential amino acids except methionine) 25 g, carbohydrate 51 g, fat less than 500 mg, energy 1311 kJ (309 kcal)/100 g, with vitamins, minerals, and trace elements.
Maxamaid products are generally intended for use in children 1–8 years.

XMET Maxamaid powder (Nutricia Ltd)
500 gram (ACBS) · NHS indicative price = £98.23

XMET Maxamum®
▸ Nutritional supplement for the dietary management of hypermethioninaemia or homocystinuria.
POWDER, protein equivalent (essential and non-essential amino acids except methionine) 39 g, carbohydrate 34 g, fat less than 500 mg, energy 1260 kJ (297 kcal)/100 g, with vitamins, minerals, and trace elements.
Maxamum products are generally intended for use in children over 8 years.

XMET Maxamum powder (Nutricia Ltd)
500 gram (ACBS) · NHS indicative price = £157.46

Hyperlysinaemia

HYPER LYS Anamix® Infant
▸ Nutritional supplement for the dietary management of proven hyperlysinaemia in children from birth to 3 years.
POWDER, protein equivalent (essential and non-essential amino acids except lysine) 13.1 g, carbohydrate 49.5 g, fat 23 g, fibre 5.3 g, energy 1915 kJ (457 kcal)/100 g, with vitamins, minerals, and trace elements; standard dilution (15%) provides protein

equivalent 2 g, carbohydrate 7.4 g, fat 3.5 g, fibre 800 mg, energy 287 kJ (69 kcal)/100 mL.

HYPER LYS Anamix Infant powder (Nutricia Ltd)
400 gram (ACBS) · NHS indicative price = £38.91

XLYS Maxamaid®
Nutritional supplement for the dietary management of hyperlysinaemia.

POWDER, protein equivalent (essential and non-essential amino acids except lysine) 25 g, carbohydrate 51 g, fat less than 500 mg, energy 1311 kJ (309 kcal)/100 g with vitamins, minerals, and trace elements.

XLYS Maxamaid powder (Nutricia Ltd)
500 gram (ACBS) · NHS indicative price = £98.23

Isovaleric acidaemia

IVA Anamix® Infant
Nutritional supplement for the dietary management of proven isovaleric acidaemia or other proven disorders of leucine metabolism in children from birth to 3 years.
POWDER, protein equivalent (essential and non-essential amino acids except leucine) 13.1 g, carbohydrate 49.5 g, fat 23 g, fibre 5.3 g, energy 1915 kJ (457 kcal)/100 g, with vitamins, minerals, and trace elements; standard dilution (15%) provides protein equivalent 2 g, carbohydrate 7.4 g, fat 3.5 g, fibre 800 mg, energy 287 kJ (69 kcal)/100 mL.

IVA Anamix Infant powder (Nutricia Ltd)
400 gram (ACBS) · NHS indicative price = £38.91

XLEU Faladon®
Nutritional supplement for the dietary management of isovaleric acidaemia.
POWDER, protein equivalent (essential and non-essential amino acids except leucine) 77 g, carbohydrate 4.5 g, fat nil, energy 1386 kJ (326 kcal)/100 g.

XLEU Maxamaid®
Nutritional supplement for the dietary management of isovaleric acidaemia.
POWDER, protein equivalent (essential and non-essential amino acids except leucine) 25 g, carbohydrate 51 g, fat less than 500 mg, energy 1311 kJ (309 kcal)/100 g with vitamins, minerals, and trace elements.

XLEU Maxamaid powder (Nutricia Ltd)
500 gram (ACBS) · NHS indicative price = £98.23

Maple syrup urine disease

MSUD Aid III®
Nutritional supplement for the dietary management of maple syrup urine disease and related conditions in children and adults where it is necessary to limit the intake of branched chain amino acids.
POWDER, protein equivalent (essential and non-essential amino acids except leucine, isoleucine, and valine) 77 g, carbohydrate 4.5 g, fat nil, energy 1386 kJ (326 kcal)/100 g.

MSUD Aid 111 powder (Nutricia Ltd)
500 gram (ACBS) · NHS indicative price = £186.08

MSUD Anamix® Infant
Nutritional supplement for the dietary management of proven maple syrup urine disease in children from birth to 3 years.
POWDER, protein equivalent (essential and non-essential amino acids except isoleucine, leucine, and valine) 13.1 g, carbohydrate 49.5 g, fat 23 g, fibre 5.3 g, energy 1915 kJ (457 kcal)/100 g, with vitamins, minerals, and trace elements; standard dilution (15%) provides protein equivalent 2 g, carbohydrate 7.4 g, fat 3.5 g, fibre 800 mg, energy 287 kJ (69 kcal)/100 mL.

MSUD Anamix Infant powder (Nutricia Ltd)
400 gram (ACBS) · NHS indicative price = £38.91

MSUD Anamix® Junior
Nutritional supplement for the dietary management of maple syrup urine disease in children 1–10 years.

POWDER, protein equivalent (essential and non-essential amino acids except isoleucine, leucine, and valine) 8.4 g, carbohydrate 11 g, fat 3.9 g, energy 474 kJ (113 kcal)/29-g sachet, with vitamins, minerals, and trace elements.

MSUD Anamix Junior oral powder 36g sachets (Nutricia Ltd)
30 sachet (ACBS) · NHS indicative price = £207.90

MSUD Anamix® Junior LQ
▶ Nutritional supplement for the dietary management of maple syrup urine disease in children 1–10 years.
LIQUID, protein equivalent (essential and non-essential amino acids except isoleucine, leucine, and valine) 10 g, carbohydrate 8.8 g, fat 4.8 g, fibre 310 mg, energy 497 kJ (118 kcal)/125 mL, with vitamins, minerals, and trace elements. Lactose-free.

MSUD Anamix Junior LQ liquid (Nutricia Ltd)
125 ml (ACBS) · NHS indicative price = £9.02

MSUD cooler® 15
▶ Nutritional supplement for the dietary management of maple syrup urine disease in children over 3 years and adults.
LIQUID, protein equivalent (essential and non-essential amino acids except leucine, isoleucine, and valine) 15 g, carbohydrate 7 g, fat 500 mg, energy 393 kJ (92 kcal)/130-mL pouch, with vitamins, minerals, and trace elements.

MSUD (Vitaflo International Ltd)
orange cooler 15 liquid, red cooler 15 liquid 130 ml (ACBS) · NHS indicative price = £11.21

MSUD express® 15
▶ Nutritional supplement for the dietary management of maple syrup urine disease in children over 8 years and adults.
POWDER, protein equivalent (essential and non-essential amino acids except leucine, isoleucine, and valine) 15 g, carbohydrate 3.8 g, fat less than 100 mg, energy 315 kJ (75 kcal)/25 g, with vitamins, minerals, and trace elements.

MSUD express 15 oral powder 25g sachets (Vitaflo International Ltd)
30 sachet (ACBS) · NHS indicative price = £329.89

MSUD express® 20
▶ Nutritional supplement for the dietary management of maple syrup urine disease in children over 8 years and adults.
POWDER, protein equivalent (essential and non-essential amino acids except leucine, isoleucine, and valine) 20 g, carbohydrate 4.7 g, fat less than 100 mg, energy 416 kJ (99 kcal)/34 g, with vitamins, minerals, and trace elements.

MSUD express 20 oral powder 34g sachets (Vitaflo International Ltd)
30 sachet (ACBS) · NHS indicative price = £426.21

MSUD Gel®
▶ Nutritional supplement for the dietary management of maple syrup urine disease in children 1–10 years.
POWDER, protein equivalent (essential and non-essential amino acids except leucine, isoleucine, and valine) 10 g, carbohydrate 10.3 g, fat less than 100 mg, energy 339 kJ (81 kcal)/24 g, with vitamins, minerals, and trace elements.

MSUD gel 24g sachets (Vitaflo International Ltd)
30 sachet (ACBS) · NHS indicative price = £214.88

MSUD Lophlex® LQ 20
▶ Nutritional supplement for the dietary management of maple syrup urine disease in children over 3 years.
LIQUID, protein equivalent (essential and non-essential amino acids except isoleucine, leucine, and valine) 20 g, carbohydrate 8.8 g, fat less than 500 mg, energy 509 kJ (120 kcal)/125 mL, with vitamins, minerals, and trace elements.

MSUD Lophlex LQ 20 liquid (Nutricia Ltd)
125 ml (ACBS) · NHS indicative price = £16.05

MSUD Maxamaid®
▶ Nutritional supplement for the dietary management of maple syrup urine disease.
POWDER, protein equivalent (essential and non-essential amino acids except isoleucine, leucine, and valine) 25 g, carbohydrate 51 g, fat less than 500 mg, energy 1311 kJ (309 kcal)/100 g, with vitamins, minerals, and trace elements.
Maxamaid products are generally intended for use in children 1–8 years.

MSUD Maxamaid powder (Nutricia Ltd)
500 gram (ACBS) · NHS indicative price = £98.23

MSUD Maxamum®
▸ Nutritional supplement for the dietary management of maple syrup urine disease.
POWDER, protein equivalent (essential and non-essential amino acids except isoleucine, leucine, and valine) 39 g, carbohydrate 34 g, fat less than 500 mg, energy 1260 kJ (297 kcal)/100 g, with vitamins, minerals, and trace elements.
Maxamum products are generally intended for use in children over 8 years.

MSUD Maxamum powder (Nutricia Ltd)
orange, unflavoured 500 gram (ACBS) · NHS indicative price = £157.46

Methylmalonic or propionic acidaemia

MMA/PA Anamix® Infant
▸ Nutritional supplement for the dietary management of proven methylmalonic acidaemia or propionic acidaemia in children from birth to 3 years.
POWDER, protein equivalent (essential and non-essential amino acids except methionine, threonine, and low isoleucine) 49.5 g, carbohydrate 49.5 g, fat 23 g, fibre 5.3 g, energy 1915 kJ (457 kcal)/100 g, with vitamins, minerals, and trace elements; standard dilution (15%) provides protein equivalent 2 g, carbohydrate 7.4 g, fat 3.5 g, fibre 800 mg, energy 287 kJ (69 kcal)/100 mL.

MMA PA Anamix Infant powder (Nutricia Ltd)
400 gram (ACBS) · NHS indicative price = £38.91

XMTVI Asadon®
▸ Nutritional supplement for the dietary management of methylmalonic acidaemia or propionic acidaemia in children and adults.
POWDER, protein equivalent (essential and non-essential amino acids except methionine, threonine, and valine, and low isoleucine) 77 g, carbohydrate 4.5 g, fat nil, energy 1386 kJ (326 kcal)/100 g.

XMTVI Asadon powder (Nutricia Ltd)
200 gram (ACBS) · NHS indicative price = £74.43

XMTVI Maxamaid®
▸ Nutritional supplement for the dietary management of methylmalonic acidaemia or propionic acidaemia.
POWDER, protein equivalent (essential and non-essential amino acids except methionine, threonine, and valine, and low isoleucine) 25 g, carbohydrate 51 g, fat less than 500 mg, energy 1311 kJ (309 kcal)/100 g, with vitamins, minerals, and trace elements.

XMTVI Maxamaid powder (Nutricia Ltd)
500 gram (ACBS) · NHS indicative price = £98.23

XMTVI Maxamum®
▸ Nutritional supplement for the dietary management of methylmalonic acidaemia or propionic acidaemia.
POWDER, protein equivalent (essential and non-essential amino acids except methionine, threonine, and valine, and low isoleucine) 39 g, carbohydrate 34 g, fat less than 500 mg, energy 1260 kJ (297 kcal)/100 g, with vitamins, minerals, and trace elements.

XMTVI Maxamum powder (Nutricia Ltd)
500 gram (ACBS) · NHS indicative price = £157.46

Other inborn errors of metabolism

Cystine500®
▸ Nutritional supplement for the dietary management of inborn errors of amino acid metabolism in adults and children from birth.
POWDER, cystine 500 mg, carbohydrate 3.3 g, fat nil, energy 63 kJ (15 kcal)/4 g

DocOmega®
▸ Nutritional supplement for the dietary management of inborn errors of metabolism for adults and children from birth.

POWDER, protein (cows' milk, soya) 100 mg, carbohydrate 3.2 g, fat 500 mg (of which docosahexaenoic acid 200 mg), fibre nil, energy 74 kJ (18 kcal)/4 g, with minerals

DocOmega oral powder 4g sachets (Vitaflo International Ltd)
30 sachet (ACBS) · NHS indicative price = £39.06

EAA® Supplement
▸ Nutritional supplement for the dietary management of disorders of protein metabolism including urea cycle disorders in children over 3 years.
POWDER, protein equivalent (essential amino acids) 5 g, carbohydrate 4 g, fat nil, energy 151 kJ (36 kcal)/12.5 g, with vitamins, minerals, and trace elements.

EAA Supplement oral powder 12.5g sachets (Vitaflo International Ltd)
50 sachet (ACBS) · NHS indicative price = £203.64

Isoleucine50®
▸ Nutritional supplement for use in the dietary management of inborn errors of amino acid metabolism in adults and children from birth.
POWDER, isoleucine 50 mg, carbohydrate 3.8 g, fat nil, energy 63 kJ (15 kcal)/4 g

Isoleucine50 oral powder 4g sachets (Vitaflo International Ltd)
30 sachet (ACBS) · NHS indicative price = £53.97

KeyOmega®
▸ Nutritional supplement for the dietary management of inborn errors of metabolism.
POWDER, protein (cows' milk, soya) 170 mg, carbohydrate 2.8 g, fat 800 mg (of which arachidonic acid 200 mg, docosahexaenoic acid 100 mg), energy 80 kJ (19 kcal)/4 g.

KeyOmega oral powder 4g sachets (Vitaflo International Ltd)
30 sachet (ACBS) · NHS indicative price = £39.94

Leucine100®
▸ Nutritional supplement for the dietary management of inborn errors of amino acid metabolism in adults and children from birth.
POWDER, leucine 100 mg, carbohydrate 3.7 g, fat nil, energy 63 kJ (15 kcal)/4 g

Leucine100 oral powder sachets (Vitaflo International Ltd)
30 sachet (ACBS) · NHS indicative price = £53.97

Low protein drink
▸ Nutritional supplement for the dietary management of inborn errors of amino acid metabolism in adults and children over 1 year.
POWDER, protein (cows' milk) 4.5 g (phenylalanine 100 mg), carbohydrate 59.5 g, fat 29.9 g, fibre nil, energy 2194 kJ (528 kcal)/100 g, with vitamins, minerals, and trace elements. Contains lactose.

Milupa LP drink (Nutricia Ltd)
400 gram (ACBS) · NHS indicative price = £9.23

Phenylalanine50®
▸ Nutritional supplement for use in the dietary management of inborn errors of metabolism in adults and children from birth.
POWDER, phenylalanine 50 mg, carbohydrate 3.8 g, fat nil, energy 63 kJ (15 kcal)/4 g

Phenylalanine50 oral powder sachets (Vitaflo International Ltd)
30 sachet (ACBS) · NHS indicative price = £52.40

ProZero®
▸ A protein-free nutritional supplement for the dietary management of inborn errors of metabolism in children over 6 months and adults.
LIQUID, carbohydrate 8.1 g (of which sugars 3.5 g), fat 3.8 g, energy 278 kJ (66 kcal)/100 mL. Contains lactose.

ProZero liquid (Vitaflo International Ltd)
250 ml (ACBS) · NHS indicative price = £1.44 | 1000 ml (ACBS) · NHS indicative price = £5.75

Tyrosine1000®
▸ Nutritional supplement for the dietary management of inborn errors of metabolism in adults and children from birth.
POWDER, tyrosine 1 g, carbohydrate 2.9 g, fat nil, energy 63 kJ (15 kcal)/4-g sachet.

Tyrosine1000 oral powder 4g sachets (Vitaflo International Ltd)
30 sachet (ACBS) · NHS indicative price = £4.95

Valine50®
Nutritional supplement for the dietary management of inborn errors of amino acid metabolism in adults and children from birth.
POWDER, valine 50 mg, carbohydrate 3.8 g, fat nil, energy 63 kJ (15 kcal)/4 g

Valine50 oral powder 4g sachets (Vitaflo International Ltd)
30 sachet (ACBS) · NHS indicative price = £53.97

Phenylketonuria

Add-Ins®
Nutritional supplement for the dietary management of proven phenylketonuria in children over 4 years.
POWDER, protein equivalent (containing essential and non-essential amino acids except phenylalanine) 10 g, carbohydrate nil, fat 5.1 g, energy 359 kJ (86 kcal)/18.2-g sachet, with vitamins, minerals, and trace elements.

Add Ins oral powder 18.2g sachets (Nutricia Ltd)
60 sachet (ACBS) · NHS indicative price = £375.60

Easiphen®
Nutritional supplement for the dietary management of proven phenylketonuria in children over 8 years.
LIQUID, protein equivalent (containing essential and non-essential amino acids except phenylalanine) 6.7 g, carbohydrate 5.1 g, fat 2 g, energy 275 kJ (65 kcal)/100 mL with vitamins, minerals, and trace elements.

Easiphen liquid (Nutricia Ltd)
250 ml (ACBS) · NHS indicative price = £9.65

L-Tyrosine
Nutritional supplement for the dietary management of phenylketonuria in pregnant women with low plasma tyrosine concentrations.
POWDER, L-tyrosine 20 g, carbohydrate 76.8 g, fat nil, energy 1612 kJ (379 kcal)/100 g.

L-Tyrosine powder (Nutricia Ltd)
100 gram (ACBS) · NHS indicative price = £21.91

Lophlex®
Nutritional supplement for the dietary management of proven phenylketonuria in children over 8 years and adults including pregnant women.
POWDER, protein equivalent (essential and non-essential amino acids except phenylalanine) 20 g, carbohydrate 2.5 g, fat 60 mg, fibre 220 mg, energy 385 kJ (91 kcal)/27.8-g sachet, with vitamins, minerals, and trace elements.

Lophlex powder 27.8g sachets (Nutricia Ltd)
berry, orange, unflavoured 30 sachet (ACBS) · NHS indicative price = £289.80

Loprofin® PKU Drink
Nutritional supplement for the dietary management of phenylketonuria in children over 1 year and adults.
LIQUID, protein (cows' milk) 400 mg (phenylalanine 10 mg), lactose 9.4 g, fat 2 g, energy 165 kJ (40 kcal)/100 mL.

Loprofin PKU drink (Nutricia Ltd)
200 ml (ACBS) · NHS indicative price = £0.75

Loprofin® Sno-Pro
Nutritional supplement for the dietary management of phenylketonuria, chronic renal failure and other inborn errors of amino acid metabolism.
LIQUID, protein (cows' milk) 220 mg (phenylalanine 12.5 mg), carbohydrate 8 g, fat 3.8 g, energy 273 kJ (65 kcal)/100 mL. Contains lactose.

Loprofin SNO-PRO drink (Nutricia Ltd)
200 ml (ACBS) · NHS indicative price = £1.25

Phlexy-10® Exchange System
Nutritional supplement for the dietary management of phenylketonuria.
CAPSULES, protein equivalent (essential and non-essential amino acids except phenylalanine) 416.5 mg/capsule.

Phlexy-10 500mg capsules (Nutricia Ltd)
200 capsule (ACBS) · NHS indicative price = £42.80
TABLETS, protein equivalent (essential and non-essential amino acids except phenylalanine) 833 mg tablet.

Phlexy-10 tablets (Nutricia Ltd)
75 tablet (ACBS) · NHS indicative price = £27.00
DRINK MIX, powder, protein equivalent (essential and non-essential amino acids except phenylalanine) 8.33 g, carbohydrate 8.8 g/20-g sachet.

Phlexy-10 drink (Nutricia Ltd)
mix apple & blackcurrant, mix citrus burst, mix tropical surprise 600 gram (ACBS) · NHS indicative price = £128.40

Phlexy-Vits®
▸ For use as a vitamin and mineral component of restricted therapeutic diets in children over 11 years adults with phenylketonuria and similar amino acid abnormalities.
POWDER, vitamins, minerals, and trace elements

Phlexy-Vits (Nutricia Ltd)
powder 210 gram (ACBS) · NHS indicative price = £71.40
TABLETS, vitamins, minerals, and trace elements

Phlexy-Vits (Nutricia Ltd)
tablets 180 tablet (ACBS) · NHS indicative price = £81.00

PK Aid 4®
▸ Nutritional supplement for the dietary management of phenylketonuria in children and adults.
POWDER, protein equivalent (essential and non-essential amino acids except phenylalanine) 79 g, carbohydrate 4.5 g, fat nil, energy 1420 kJ (334 kcal)/100 g.

PK Aid 4 powder (Nutricia Ltd)
500 gram (ACBS) · NHS indicative price = £143.04

PKU Anamix® First Spoon
▸ Nutritional supplement for the dietary management of proven phenylketonuria in children from 6 months to 5 years.
POWDER, protein equivalent (essential and non-essential amino acids except phenylalanine) 5 g, carbohydrate 4.8 g, fat 150 mg, fibre nil, energy 168 kJ (41 kcal)/12.5-g sachet, with vitamins, minerals, and trace elements

PKU Anamix First Spoon oral powder 12.5g sachets (Nutricia Ltd)
30 sachet (ACBS) · NHS indicative price = £91.80

PKU Anamix® Infant
▸ Nutritional supplement for the dietary management of proven phenylketonuria in children from birth to 3 years.
POWDER, protein equivalent (essential and non-essential amino acids except phenylalanine) 13.1 g, carbohydrate 49.5 g, fat 23 g, fibre 5.3 g, energy 1915 kJ (457 kcal)/100 g, with vitamins, minerals, and trace elements; standard dilution (15%) provides protein equivalent 2 g, carbohydrate 7.4 g, fat 3.5 g, fibre 800 mg, energy 287 kJ (69 kcal)/100 mL

PKU Anamix Infant powder (Nutricia Ltd)
400 gram (ACBS) · NHS indicative price = £35.36

PKU Anamix® Junior
▸ Nutritional supplement for the dietary management of phenylketonuria in children 1–10 years.
POWDER, protein equivalent (essential and non-essential amino acids except phenylalanine) 8.4 g, carbohydrate 9.9 g, fat 3.9 g, energy 455 kJ (108 kcal)/29-g sachet, with vitamins, minerals, and trace elements

PKU Anamix Junior powder (Nutricia Ltd)
chocolate, neutral 870 gram (ACBS) · NHS indicative price = £123.90 | 1080 gram (ACBS) · NHS indicative price = £126.30

PKU Anamix® Junior LQ
▸ Nutritional supplement for the dietary supplement of phenyketonuria in children 1–10 years.
LIQUID, protein equivalent (essential and non-essential amino acids except phenylalanine) 10 g, carbohydrate 8.8 g, fat 4.8 g, fibre 310 mg, energy 497 kJ (118 kcal)/125 mL, with vitamins, minerals, and trace elements. Lactose-free. Flavours: Berry, orange, or unflavoured, net price 125-mL carton = £5.61

PKU Anamix Junior LQ liquid (Nutricia Ltd)
berry, orange 125 ml (ACBS) · NHS indicative price = £5.51

PKU cooler10®

▸ Nutritional supplement for the dietary management of phenylketonuria in children over 3 years.
LIQUID, protein equivalent (essential and non-essential amino acids except phenylalanine) 10 g, carbohydrate 5.1 g, energy 258 kJ (62 kcal)/87-mL pouch, with vitamins, minerals, and trace elements.

PKU (Vitaflo International Ltd)
orange cooler 10 liquid, purple cooler 10 liquid, red cooler 10 liquid, white cooler 10 liquid 87 ml (ACBS) · NHS indicative price = £4.56

PKU cooler15®

▸ Nutritional supplement for the dietary management of phenylketonuria in children over 3 years.
LIQUID, protein equivalent (essential and non-essential amino acids except phenylalanine) 15 g, carbohydrate 7.8 g, energy 386 kJ (92 kcal)/130-mL pouch, with vitamins, minerals, and trace elements.

PKU (Vitaflo International Ltd)
orange cooler 15 liquid, purple cooler 15 liquid, red cooler 15 liquid, white cooler 15 liquid 130 ml (ACBS) · NHS indicative price = £6.80

PKU cooler20®

▸ Nutritional supplement for the dietary management of phenylketonuria in children over 3 years.
LIQUID, protein equivalent (essential and non-essential amino acids except phenylalanine) 20 g, carbohydrate 10.2 g, energy 517 kJ (124 kcal)/174-mL pouch, with vitamins, minerals, and trace elements.

PKU (Vitaflo International Ltd)
orange cooler 20 liquid, purple cooler 20 liquid, red cooler 20 liquid, white cooler 20 liquid 174 ml (ACBS) · NHS indicative price = £9.12

PKU express15®

▸ Nutritional supplement for the dietary management of phenylketonuria. Not recommended for children under 3 years.
POWDER, protein equivalent (essential and non-essential amino acids except phenylalanine) 15 g, carbohydrate 2.4 g, energy 293 kJ (70 kcal)/25 g, with vitamins, minerals, and trace elements.

PKU express 15 powder (Vitaflo International Ltd)
lemon, orange, tropical, unflavoured 750 gram (ACBS) · NHS indicative price = £200.00

PKU express20®

▸ Nutritional supplement for the dietary management of phenylketonuria. Not recommended for children under 3 years.
POWDER, protein equivalent (essential and non-essential amino acids except phenylalanine) 20 g, carbohydrate 3.3 g, energy 389 kJ (93 kcal)/34 g, with vitamins, minerals, and trace elements.

PKU express 20 powder (Vitaflo International Ltd)
lemon, orange, tropical, unflavoured 1020 gram (ACBS) · NHS indicative price = £258.39

PKU gel®

▸ For use as part of the low-protein dietary management of phenylketonuria in children 1–10 years
POWDER, protein equivalent (essential and non-essential amino acids except phenylalanine) 10 g, fat less than 100 mg, energy 318 kJ (76 kcal)/24 g, with vitamins, minerals, and trace elements.

PKU gel powder (Vitaflo International Ltd)
orange, orange, raspberry, unflavoured 720 gram (ACBS) · NHS indicative price = £138.36

PKU Lophlex® LQ 10

▸ Nutritional supplement for the dietary management of phenylketonuria in children over 4 years and adults including pregnant women.
LIQUID, protein equivalent (essential and non-essential amino acids except phenylalanine) 10 g, carbohydrate 4.4 g, fibre 250 mg, energy 245 kJ (58 kcal)/62.5 mL, with vitamins, minerals, and trace elements.

PKU Lophlex LQ 10 liquid juicy (Nutricia Ltd)
berries, orange 62.5 ml (ACBS) · NHS indicative price = £5.18

PKU Lophlex® LQ 20

▸ Nutritional supplement for the dietary management of phenylketonuria in children over 4 years and adults including pregnant women.
LIQUID, protein equivalent (essential and non-essential amino acids except phenylalanine) 20 g, carbohydrate 8.8 g, fibre 340 mg, energy 490 kJ (115 kcal)/125 mL, with vitamins, minerals, and trace elements.

PKU Lophlex LQ 20 liquid (Nutricia Ltd)
berry, juicy berries, orange 125 ml (ACBS) · NHS indicative price = £10.33

PKU Lophlex® Sensation 20

▸ Nutritional supplement for the dietary management of phenylketonuria in children over 4 years and adults including pregnant women.
SEMI-SOLID, protein equivalent (containing essential and non-essential amino acids except phenylalanine) 20 g, carbohydrate 20.2 g, fibre 1 g, energy 706 kJ (166 kcal)/109 g, with vitamins, minerals, and trace elements.

PKU Lophlex Sensation 20 (Nutricia Ltd)
berries, orange 327 gram (ACBS) · NHS indicative price = £33.00

PKU squeezie®

▸ Nutritional supplement for the dietary management of phenylketonuria in children from 6 months to 10 years.
LIQUID, protein equivalent (essential and non-essential amino acids except phenylalanine) 22.5 g, fat 500 mg, energy 565 kJ (135 kcal)/85 g, with vitamins, minerals, and trace elements.

PKU squeezie liquid (Vitaflo International Ltd)
2550 gram (ACBS) · NHS indicative price = £132.27

XP Maxamaid®

▸ Nutritional supplement for the dietary management of phenylketonuria in children 1–8 years.
POWDER, protein equivalent (essential and non-essential amino acids except phenylalanine) 25 g, carbohydrate 51 g, fat less than 500 mg, energy 1311 kJ (309 kcal)/100 g, with vitamins, minerals, and trace elements.

XP Maxamaid powder (Nutricia Ltd)
orange, unflavoured 500 gram (ACBS) · NHS indicative price = £58.11

XP Maxamum®

▸ Nutritional supplement for the dietary management of phenylketonuria in children over 8 years and adults.
POWDER, protein equivalent (essential and non-essential amino acids except phenylalanine) 39 g, carbohydrate 34 g, fat less than 500 mg, energy 1260 kJ (297 kcal)/100 g, with vitamins, minerals, and trace elements.

XP Maxamum oral powder 50g sachets (Nutricia Ltd)
orange, unflavoured 30 sachet (ACBS) · NHS indicative price = £269.40

XP Maxamum powder (Nutricia Ltd)
orange, unflavoured 500 gram (ACBS) · NHS indicative price = £89.88

Tyrosinaemia

Methionine-free TYR Anamix® Infant

▸ Nutritional supplement for the dietary management of proven tyrosinaemia type 1 in children from birth to 3 years.
POWDER, protein equivalent (essential and non-essential amino acids except methionine, phenylalanine, and tyrosine) 13.1 g, carbohydrate 49.5 g, fat 23 g, fibre 5.3 g, energy 1915 kJ (457 kcal)/100 g, with vitamins, minerals, and trace elements; standard dilution (15%) provides protein equivalent 2 g, carbohydrate 7.4 g, fat 3.5 g, fibre 800 mg, energy 287 kJ (69 kcal)/100 mL.

TYR Anamix Infant methionine free powder (Nutricia Ltd)
400 gram (ACBS) · NHS indicative price = £38.91

TYR Anamix® Infant

Nutritional supplement for the dietary management of proven tyrosinaemia where plasma-methionine concentrations are normal in children from birth to 3 years.

POWDER, protein equivalent (essential and non-essential amino acids except phenylalanine and tyrosine) 13.1 g, carbohydrate 49.5 g, fat 23 g, fibre 5.3 g, energy 1915 kJ (457 kcal)/100 g, with vitamins, minerals, and trace elements; standard dilution (15%) provides protein equivalent 2 g, carbohydrate 7.4 g, fat 3.5 g, fibre 800 mg, energy 287 kJ (69 kcal)/100 mL.

TYR Anamix Infant (Nutricia Ltd)
methionine free powder, powder 400 gram (ACBS) · NHS indicative price = £38.91

TYR Anamix® Junior

Nutritional supplement for the dietary management of proven tyrosinaemia in children 1–10 years.

POWDER, protein equivalent (essential and non-essential amino acids except phenylalanine and tyrosine) 8.4 g, carbohydrate 11 g, fat 3.9 g, energy 475 kJ (113 kcal)/29-g sachet, with vitamins, minerals, and trace elements.

TYR Anamix Junior oral powder 29g sachets (Nutricia Ltd)
30 sachet (ACBS) · NHS indicative price = £206.40

TYR Anamix® Junior LQ

Nutritional supplement for the dietary management of tyrosinaemia type 1 (when nitisinone (NTBC) is used, see), type II, and type III, in children over 1 year.

LIQUID, protein equivalent (essential and non-essential amino acids except phenylalanine and tyrosine) 10 g, carbohydrate 8.8 g, fat 4.8 g, fibre 310 mg, energy 500 kJ (119 kcal)/125 mL, with vitamins, minerals, and trace elements.

TYR Anamix Junior LQ liquid (Nutricia Ltd)
125 ml (ACBS) · NHS indicative price = £9.02

TYR cooler® 15

Nutritional supplement for the dietary management of tyrosinaemia in children over 3 years and adults.

LIQUID, protein equivalent (essential and non-essential amino acids except tyrosine and phenylalanine) 15 g, carbohydrate 7 g, fat 500 mg, energy 393 kJ (92 kcal)/130 mL, with vitamins, minerals, and trace elements.

TYR orange cooler 15 liquid (Vitaflo International Ltd)
130 ml (ACBS) · NHS indicative price = £11.21

TYR red cooler (Vitaflo International Ltd)
20 liquid 174 ml (ACBS) · NHS indicative price = £14.84
15 liquid 130 ml (ACBS) · NHS indicative price = £11.21
10 liquid 87 ml (ACBS) · NHS indicative price = £7.10

TYR express15®

Nutritional supplement for the dietary management of tyrosinaemia in children over 8 years and adults.

POWDER, protein equivalent (essential and non-essential amino acids except tyrosine and phenylalanine) 15 g, carbohydrate 5.4 g, fat less than 100 mg, energy 310 kJ (74 kcal)/25 g, with vitamins, minerals, and trace elements.

TYR express 15 oral powder 25g sachets (Vitaflo International Ltd)
30 sachet (ACBS) · NHS indicative price = £329.89

TYR express20®

Nutritional supplement for the dietary management of tyrosinaemia in children over 8 years.

POWDER, protein equivalent (essential and non-essential amino acids except tyrosine and phenylalanine) 20 g, carbohydrate 7.7 g, fat less than 100 mg, energy 416 kJ (99 kcal)/34 g, with vitamins, minerals, and trace elements.

TYR express 20 oral powder 34g sachets (Vitaflo International Ltd)
30 sachet (ACBS) · NHS indicative price = £426.21

TYR Gel®

Nutritional supplement for the dietary management of tyrosinaemia in children 1–10 years.

GEL, protein equivalent (essential and non-essential amino acids except tyrosine and phenylalanine) 10 g, carbohydrate 10.3 g, fat less than 100 mg, energy 339 kJ (81 kcal)/24 g, with vitamins, minerals, and trace elements.

TYR gel oral powder 24g sachets (Vitaflo International Ltd)
30 sachet (ACBS) · NHS indicative price = £212.38

TYR Lophlex® LQ 20

▸ Nutritional supplement for the dietary management of tyrosinaemia in children over 3 years and adults.

LIQUID, protein equivalent (essential and non-essential amino acids except phenylalanine and tyrosine) 20 g, carbohydrate 8.8 g, fat less than 500 mg, fibre 500 mg, energy 509 kJ (120 kcal)/125 mL, with vitamins, minerals, and trace elements.

TYR Lophlex LQ 20 liquid (Nutricia Ltd)
125 ml (ACBS) · NHS indicative price = £16.05

XPHEN TYR Maxamaid®

▸ Nutritional supplement for the dietary management of tyrosinaemia in children 1–8 years.

POWDER, protein equivalent (essential and non-essential amino acids except phenylalanine and tyrosine) 25 g, carbohydrate 51 g, fat less than 500 mg, energy 1311 kJ (309 kcal)/100 g, with vitamins, minerals, and trace elements.

XPHEN TYR Maxamaid powder (Nutricia Ltd)
500 gram (ACBS) · NHS indicative price = £98.23

XPHEN TYR Tyrosidon®

▸ Nutritional supplement for the management of tyrosinaemia in children and adults where plasma-methionine concentrations are normal.

POWDER, protein equivalent (essential and non-essential amino acids except phenylalanine and tyrosine) 77 g, carbohydrate 4.5 g, fat nil, energy 1386 kJ (326 kcal)/100 g.

XPHEN TYR Tyrosidon Free AA Mix powder (Nutricia Ltd)
500 gram (ACBS) · NHS indicative price = £186.08

XPTM Tyrosidon®

▸ Nutritional supplement for the dietary management of tyrosinaemia type 1 in children and adults where plasma-methionine concentrations are above normal.

POWDER, protein equivalent (essential and non-essential amino acids except methionine, phenylalanine, and tyrosine) 77 g, carbohydrate 4.5 g, fat nil, energy 1386 kJ (326 kcal)/100 g.

XPTM Tyrosidon powder (Nutricia Ltd)
500 gram (ACBS) · NHS indicative price = £91.31

A2

Borderline substances | Appendix 2

Appendix 3
Cautionary and advisory labels for dispensed medicines

Guidance for cautionary and advisory labels

Medicinal forms within BNF publications include code numbers of the cautionary labels that pharmacists are recommended to add when dispensing. It is also expected that pharmacists will counsel patients and carers when necessary.

Counselling needs to be related to the age, experience, background, and understanding of the individual patient or carer. The pharmacist should ensure understanding of how to take or use the medicine and how to follow the correct dosage schedule. Any effects of the medicine on co-ordination, performance of skilled tasks (e.g. driving or work), any foods or medicines to be avoided, and what to do if a dose is missed should also be explained. Other matters, such as the possibility of staining of the clothes or skin, or discolouration of urine or stools by a medicine should also be mentioned.

For some medicines there is a special need for counselling, such as an unusual method or time of administration or a potential interaction with a common food or domestic remedy, and this should be mentioned where necessary.

Original packs

Most preparations are dispensed in unbroken original packs that include further advice for the patient in the form of patient information leaflets. The advice in patient information leaflets may be less appropriate when the medicine is for a child, particularly for unlicensed medicines or indications. Pharmacists should explain discrepancies to carers, if necessary. The patient information leaflet should only be withheld in exceptional circumstances because it contains other information that should be provided. Label 10 may be of value where appropriate. More general leaflets advising on the administration of preparations such as eye drops, eye ointments, inhalers, and suppositories are also available.

Scope of labels

In general no label recommendations have been made for injections on the assumption that they will be administered by a healthcare professional or a well-instructed patient. The labelling is not exhaustive and pharmacists are recommended to use their professional discretion in labelling new preparations and those for which no labels are shown.

Individual labelling advice is not given on the administration of the large variety of antacids. In the absence of instructions from the prescriber, and if on enquiry the patient has had no verbal instructions, the directions given under 'Dose' should be used on the label.

It is recognised that there may be occasions when pharmacists will use their knowledge and professional discretion and decide to omit one or more of the recommended labels for a particular patient. In this case counselling is of the utmost importance. There may also be an occasion when a prescriber does not wish additional cautionary labels to be used, in which case the prescription should be endorsed 'NCL' (no cautionary labels). The exact wording that is required instead should then be specified on the prescription.

Pharmacists label medicines with various wordings in addition to those directions specified on the prescription. Such labels include 'Shake the bottle', 'For external use only', and 'Store in a cool place', as well as 'Discard.... days after opening' and 'Do not use after....', which apply particularly to antibiotic mixtures, diluted liquid and topical preparations, and to eye-drops. Although not listed in the *BNF for Children* these labels should continue to be used when appropriate; indeed, 'For external use only' is a legal requirement on external liquid preparations, while 'Keep out of the reach of children' is a legal requirement on all dispensed medicines. Care should be taken not to obscure other relevant information with adhesive labelling.

It is the usual practice for patients to take standard tablets with water or other liquids and for this reason no separate label has been recommended.

The label wordings recommended by the *BNF for Children* apply to medicines dispensed against a prescription. Children and carers should be aware that a dispensed medicine should never be taken by, or shared with, anyone other than for whom the prescriber intended it. Therefore, the *BNF for Children* does not include warnings against the use of a dispensed medicine by persons other than for whom it was specifically prescribed.

The label or labels for each preparation are recommended after careful consideration of the information available. However, it is recognised that in some cases this information may be either incomplete or open to a different interpretation. The *BNF for Children* will therefore be grateful to receive any constructive comments on the labelling suggested for any preparation.

Recommended label wordings

For *BNF for Children* 2011–2012, a revised set of cautionary and advisory labels were introduced. All of the existing labels were user-tested, and the revised wording selected reflects terminology that is better understood by patients.

Wordings which can be given as separate warnings are labels 1–19, 29–30, and 32. Wordings which can be incorporated in an appropriate position in the directions for dosage or administration are labels 21–28. A label has been omitted for number 20; labels 31 and 33 no longer apply to any medicines in the *BNF for Children* and have therefore been deleted.

If separate labels are used it is recommended that the wordings be used without modification. If changes are made to suit computer requirements, care should be taken to retain the sense of the original.

Welsh labels

Comprehensive Welsh translations are available for each cautionary and advisory label. These appear directly under the English label.

Labels

1 **Warning: This medicine may make you sleepy**
Rhybudd: Gall y feddyginiaeth hon eich gwneud yn gysglyd
To be used on *preparations for children* containing antihistamines, or other preparations given to children where the warnings of label 2 on driving or alcohol would not be appropriate.

2 **Warning: This medicine may make you sleepy. If this happens, do not drive or use tools or machines. Do not drink alcohol**
Rhybudd: Gall y feddyginiaeth hon eich gwneud yn gysglyd. Peidiwch â gyrru, defnyddio offer llaw neu beiriannau os yw hyn yn digwydd. Peidiwch ag yfed alcohol
To be used on *preparations for adults that can cause drowsiness*, thereby affecting coordination and the ability to drive and operate hazardous machinery; label 1 is more appropriate for children. *It is an offence to drive while under the influence of drink or drugs.*

Some of these preparations only cause drowsiness in the

first few days of treatment and some only cause drowsiness in higher doses.

In such cases the patient should be told that the advice applies until the effects have worn off. However many of these preparations can produce a slowing of reaction time and a loss of mental concentration that can have the same effects as drowsiness.

Avoidance of alcoholic drink is recommended because the effects of CNS depressants are enhanced by alcohol. Strict prohibition however could lead to some patients not taking the medicine. Pharmacists should therefore explain the risk and encourage compliance, particularly in patients who may think they already tolerate the effects of alcohol (see also label 3). Queries from patients with epilepsy regarding fitness to drive should be referred back to the patient's doctor.

Side-effects unrelated to drowsiness that may affect a patient's ability to drive or operate machinery safely include *blurred vision, dizziness,* or *nausea.* In general, no label has been recommended to cover these cases, but the patient should be suitably counselled.

3 **Warning: This medicine may make you sleepy. If this happens, do not drive or use tools or machines**
Rhybudd: Gall y feddyginiaeth hon eich gwneud yn gysglyd. Peidiwch â gyrru, defnyddio offer llaw neu beiriannau os yw hyn yn digwydd
To be used on *preparations containing monoamine-oxidase inhibitors;* the warning to avoid alcohol and dealcoholised (low alcohol) drink is covered by the patient information leaflet.

Also to be used as for label 2 but where alcohol is not an issue.

4 **Warning: Do not drink alcohol**
Rhybudd: Peidiwch ag yfed alcohol
To be used on *preparations where a reaction such as flushing may occur if alcohol is taken* (e.g. metronidazole). Alcohol may also enhance the hypoglycaemia produced by some oral antidiabetic drugs but routine application of a warning label is not considered necessary.

Patients should be advised not to drink alcohol for as long as they are receiving/using a course of medication, and in some cases for a period of time after the course is finished.

5 **Do not take indigestion remedies 2 hours before or after you take this medicine**
Peidiwch â chymryd meddyginiaethau camdreuliad 2 awr cyn neu ar ôl y feddyginiaeth hon
To be used with label 25 on *preparations coated to resist gastric acid* (e.g. enteric-coated tablets). This is to avoid the possibility of premature dissolution of the coating in the presence of an alkaline pH.

Label 5 also applies to drugs such as gabapentin *where the absorption is significantly affected by antacids.* Pharmacists will be aware (from a knowledge of physiology) that the usual time during which indigestion remedies should be avoided is at least 2 hours before and after the majority of medicines have been taken; when a manufacturer advises a different time period, this can be followed, and should be explained to the patient.

6 **Do not take indigestion remedies, or medicines containing iron or zinc, 2 hours before or after you take this medicine**
Peidiwch â chymryd meddyginiaethau camdreuliad neu feddyginiaethau sy'n cynnwys haearn neu sinc, 2 awr cyn neu ar ôl y feddyginiaeth hon
To be used on *preparations containing ofloxacin and some other quinolones, doxycycline, lymecycline, minocycline, and penicillamine.* These drugs chelate calcium, iron, and zinc and are less well absorbed when taken with calcium-containing antacids or preparations containing iron or zinc. Pharmacists will be aware (from a knowledge of physiology) that these incompatible preparations should be taken at least 2 hours apart for the majority of medicines; when a manufacturer advises a different time period, this can be followed, and should be explained to the patient.

7 **Do not take milk, indigestion remedies, or medicines containing iron or zinc, 2 hours before or after you take this medicine**
Peidiwch â chymryd llaeth, meddyginiaethau camdreuliad, neu feddyginiaeth sy'n cynnwys haearn neu sinc, 2 awr cyn neu ar ôl cymryd y feddyginiaeth hon
To be used on *preparations containing ciprofloxacin, norfloxacin, or tetracyclines that chelate calcium, iron, magnesium, and zinc,* and are thus less available for absorption. Pharmacists will be aware (from a knowledge of physiology) that these incompatible preparations should be taken at least 2 hours apart for the majority of medicines; when a manufacturer advises a different time period, this can be followed, and should be explained to the patient. Doxycycline, lymecycline, and minocycline are less liable to form chelates and therefore only require label 6 (see above).

8 **Warning: Do not stop taking this medicine unless your doctor tells you to stop**
Rhybudd: Peidiwch â stopio cymryd y feddyginiaeth hon, oni bai fod eich meddyg yn dweud wrthych am stopio
To be used on *preparations that contain a drug which is required to be taken over long periods without the patient necessarily perceiving any benefit* (e.g. antituberculous drugs).

Also to be used on *preparations that contain a drug whose withdrawal is likely to be a particular hazard* (e.g. clonidine for hypertension). Label 10 (see below) is more appropriate for corticosteroids.

9 **Space the doses evenly throughout the day. Keep taking this medicine until the course is finished, unless you are told to stop**
Gadewch yr un faint o amser rhwng pob dôs yn ystod y dydd. Parhewch i gymryd y feddyginiaeth nes bod y cyfan wedi'i orffen, oni bai eich bod yn cael cyngor i stopio
To be used on *preparations where a course of treatment should be completed* to reduce the incidence of relapse or failure of treatment.

The preparations are antimicrobial drugs given by mouth. Very occasionally, some may have severe side-effects (e.g. diarrhoea in patients receiving clindamycin) and in such cases the patient may need to be advised of reasons for stopping treatment quickly and returning to the doctor.

10 **Warning: Read the additional information given with this medicine**
Rhybudd: Darllenwch y wybodaeth ychwanegol gyda'r feddyginiaeth hon
To be used particularly on *preparations containing anticoagulants, lithium, and oral corticosteroids.* The appropriate treatment card should be given to the patient and any necessary explanations given.

This label may also be used on other preparations to remind the patient of the instructions that have been given.

11 **Protect your skin from sunlight—even on a bright but cloudy day. Do not use sunbeds**
Diogelwch eich croen rhag golau'r haul, hyd yn oed ar ddiwrnod braf ond cymylog. Peidiwch â defnyddio gwely haul
To be used on *preparations that may cause phototoxic or photoallergic reactions* if the patient is exposed to ultraviolet radiation. Many drugs other than those listed in Appendix 3 (e.g. phenothiazines and sulfonamides) may, on rare occasions, cause reactions in susceptible patients. Exposure to high intensity ultraviolet radiation from sunray lamps and sunbeds is particularly likely to cause reactions.

12 **Do not take anything containing aspirin while taking this medicine**
Peidiwch â chymryd unrhyw beth sy'n cynnwys aspirin gyda'r feddyginiaeth hon
To be used on *preparations containing sulfinpyrazone* whose activity is reduced by aspirin.

Label 12 should not be used for anticoagulants since label 10 is more appropriate.

13 **Dissolve or mix with water before taking**
Gadewch i doddi mewn dŵr cyn ei gymryd
To be used on *preparations that are intended to be dissolved in water* (e.g. soluble tablets) or *mixed with water* (e.g. powders,

granules) before use. In a few cases other liquids such as fruit juice or milk may be used.

14 **This medicine may colour your urine. This is harmless**
Gall y feddyginiaeth hon liwio eich dŵr. Nid yw hyn yn arwydd o ddrwg
To be used on *preparations that may cause the patient's urine to turn an unusual colour*. These include triamterene (blue under some lights), levodopa (dark reddish), and rifampicin (red).

15 **Caution: flammable. Keep your body away from fire or flames after you have put on the medicine**
Rhybudd: Fflamadwy. Ar ôl rhoi'r feddyginiaeth ymlaen, cadwch yn glir o dân neu fflamau
To be used on *preparations containing sufficient flammable solvent to render them flammable if exposed to a naked flame.*

16 **Dissolve the tablet under your tongue—do not swallow. Store the tablets in this bottle with the cap tightly closed. Get a new supply 8 weeks after opening**
Rhowch y dabled i doddi dan eich tafod - peidiwch â'i lyncu. Cadwch y tabledi yn y botel yma gyda'r caead wedi'i gau yn dynn. Gofynnwch am dabledi newydd 8 wythnos ar ôl ei hagor
To be used on *glyceryl trinitrate tablets* to remind the patient not to transfer the tablets to plastic or less suitable containers.

17 **Do not take more than... in 24 hours**
Peidiwch â chymryd mwy na... mewn 24 awr
To be used on *preparations for the treatment of acute migraine* except those containing ergotamine, for which label 18 is used. The dose form should be specified, e.g. tablets or capsules.
    It may also be used on preparations for which no dose has been specified by the prescriber.

18 **Do not take more than... in 24 hours. Also, do not take more than... in any one week**
Peidiwch â chymryd mwy na... mewn 24 awr. Hefyd, peidiwch â chymryd mwy na... mewn wythnos
To be used on preparations containing ergotamine. The dose form should be specified, e.g. tablets or suppositories.

19 **Warning: This medicine makes you sleepy. If you still feel sleepy the next day, do not drive or use tools or machines. Do not drink alcohol**
Rhybudd: Bydd y feddyginiaeth hon yn eich gwneud yn gysglyd. Os ydych yn dal i deimlo'n gysglyd drannoeth, peidiwch â gyrru, defnyddio offer llaw neu beiriannau. Peidiwch ag yfed alcohol
To be used on *preparations containing hypnotics (or some other drugs with sedative effects)* prescribed to be taken at night. On the rare occasions when hypnotics are prescribed for daytime administration (e.g. nitrazepam in epilepsy), this label would clearly not be appropriate. Also to be used as an *alternative to the label 2 wording* (the choice being at the discretion of the pharmacist) *for anxiolytics prescribed to be taken at night.*
    It is hoped that this wording will convey adequately the problem of residual morning sedation after taking 'sleeping tablets'.

21 **Take with or just after food, or a meal**
Cymerwch gyda neu ar ôl bwyd
To be used on *preparations that are liable to cause gastric irritation*, or those that are better absorbed with food.
    Patients should be advised that a *small amount of food is sufficient.*

22 **Take 30 to 60 minutes before food**
Cymerwch 30 i 60 munud cyn bwyd
To be used on some preparations *whose absorption is thereby improved.*
    Most oral antibacterials require label 23 instead (see below).

23 **Take this medicine when your stomach is empty. This means an hour before food or 2 hours after food**
Cymerwch y feddyginiaeth hon ar stumog wag. Mae hyn yn golygu awr cyn, neu 2 awr ar ôl bwyd
To be used on *oral antibacterials whose absorption may be reduced by the presence of food and acid in the stomach.*

24 **Suck or chew this medicine**
Bydd angen cnoi neu sugno'r feddyginiaeth hon
To be used on *preparations that should be sucked or chewed.*
    The pharmacist should use discretion as to which of these words is appropriate.

25 **Swallow this medicine whole. Do not chew or crush**
Llyncwch yn gyfan. Peidiwch â chnoi neu falu'n fân
To be used on *preparations that are enteric-coated or designed for modified-release.*
    Also to be used on *preparations that taste very unpleasant or may damage the mouth* if not swallowed whole.
    Patients should be advised (where relevant) that some modified-release preparations can be broken in half, but that the halved tablet should still be swallowed whole, and not chewed or crushed.

26 **Dissolve this medicine under your tongue**
Gadewch i'r feddyginiaeth hon doddi o dan y tafod
To be used on *preparations designed for sublingual use.* Patients should be advised to hold under the tongue and avoid swallowing until dissolved. The buccal mucosa between the gum and cheek is occasionally specified by the prescriber.

27 **Take with a full glass of water**
Cymerwch gyda llond gwydr o ddŵr
To be used on *preparations that should be well diluted* (e.g. chloral hydrate), *where a high fluid intake is required* (e.g. sulfonamides), or *where water is required to aid the action* (e.g. methylcellulose). The patient should be advised that 'a full glass' means at least 150 mL. In most cases fruit juice, tea, or coffee may be used.

28 **Spread thinly on the affected skin only**
Taenwch yn denau ar y croen sydd wedi'i effeithio yn unig
To be used on *external preparations* that should be applied sparingly (e.g. corticosteroids, dithranol).

29 **Do not take more than 2 at any one time. Do not take more than 8 in 24 hours**
Peidiwch â chymryd mwy na 2 ar unrhyw un adeg. Peidiwch â chymryd mwy nag 8 mewn 24 awr
To be used on containers of dispensed *solid dose preparations containing paracetamol for adults when the instruction on the label indicates that the dose can be taken on an 'as required' basis.* The dose form should be specified, e.g. tablets or capsules.
    This label has been introduced because of the serious consequences of overdosage with paracetamol.

30 **Contains paracetamol. Do not take anything else containing paracetamol while taking this medicine. Talk to a doctor at once if you take too much of this medicine, even if you feel well**
Yn cynnwys paracetamol. Peidiwch â chymryd unrhyw beth arall sy'n cynnwys paracetamol tra'n cymryd y feddyginiaeth hon. Siaradwch gyda'ch meddyg ar unwaith os ydych yn cymryd gormod, hyd yn oed os ydych yn teimlo'n iawn
To be used on all containers of dispensed *preparations containing paracetamol.*

32 **Contains aspirin. Do not take anything else containing aspirin while taking this medicine**
Yn cynnwys aspirin. Peidiwch â chymryd unrhyw beth arall sy'n cynnwys aspirin tra'n cymryd y feddyginiaeth hon
To be used on containers of dispensed *preparations containing aspirin when the name on the label does not include the word 'aspirin'.*

Dental Practitioners' Formulary

List of Dental Preparations

The following list has been approved by the appropriate Secretaries of State, and the preparations therein may be prescribed by dental practitioners on form FP10D (GP14 in Scotland, WP10D in Wales).

Licensed **sugar-free** versions, where available, are preferred.
Licensed **alcohol-free** mouthwashes, where available, are preferred.

Aciclovir Cream, BP
Aciclovir Oral Suspension, BP, 200 mg/5 mL
Aciclovir Tablets, BP, 200 mg
Aciclovir Tablets, BP, 800 mg
Amoxicillin Capsules, BP
Amoxicillin Oral Powder, DPF
Amoxicillin Oral Suspension, BP
Artificial Saliva Gel, DPF
Artificial Saliva Oral Spray, DPF
Artificial Saliva Pastilles, DPF
Artificial Saliva Protective Spray, DPF
Artificial Saliva Substitutes as listed below (to be prescribed only for indications approved by ACBS (patients suffering from dry mouth as a result of having or, having undergone, radiotherapy or sicca syndrome):
  BioXtra® Gel Mouthspray
  BioXtra® Moisturising Gel
  Glandosane®
  Saliveze®
Artificial Saliva Substitute Spray, DPF
Aspirin Tablets, Dispersible, BP
Azithromycin Capsules, 250 mg, DPF
Azithromycin Oral Suspension, 200 mg/5 mL, DPF
Azithromycin Tablets, 250 mg, DPF
Azithromycin Tablets, 500 mg, DPF
Beclometasone Pressurised Inhalation, BP, 50 micrograms/metered inhalation, CFC-free, as:
  Clenil Modulite®
Benzydamine Mouthwash, BP 0.15%
Benzydamine Oromucosal Spray, BP 0.15%
Betamethasone Soluble Tablets, 500 micrograms, DPF
Carbamazepine Tablets, BP
Cefalexin Capsules, BP
Cefalexin Oral Suspension, BP
Cefalexin Tablets, BP
Cefradine Capsules, BP
Cetirizine Oral Solution, BP, 5 mg/5 mL
Cetirizine Tablets, BP, 10 mg
Chlorhexidine Gluconate Gel, BP
Chlorhexidine Mouthwash, BP
Chlorhexidine Oral Spray, DPF
Chlorphenamine Oral Solution, BP
Chlorphenamine Tablets, BP
Choline Salicylate Dental Gel, BP
Clarithromycin Oral Suspension, 125 mg/5 mL, DPF
Clarithromycin Oral Suspension, 250 mg/5 mL, DPF
Clarithromycin Tablets, BP
Clindamycin Capsules, BP
Co-amoxiclav Tablets, BP, 250/125 (amoxicillin 250 mg as trihydrate, clavulanic acid 125 mg as potassium salt)
Co-amoxiclav Oral Suspension, BP, 125/31 (amoxicillin 125 mg as trihydrate, clavulanic acid 31.25 mg as potassium salt)/5 mL
Co-amoxiclav Oral Suspension, BP, 250/62 (amoxicillin 250 mg as trihydrate, clavulanic acid 62.5 mg as potassium salt)/5 mL
Diazepam Oral Solution, BP, 2 mg/5 mL

Diazepam Tablets, BP
Diclofenac Sodium Tablets, Gastro-resistant, BP
Dihydrocodeine Tablets, BP, 30 mg
Doxycycline Tablets, Dispersible, BP
Doxycycline Capsules, BP, 100 mg
Doxycycline Tablets, 20 mg, DPF
Ephedrine Nasal Drops, BP
Erythromycin Ethyl Succinate Oral Suspension, BP
Erythromycin Ethyl Succinate Tablets, BP
Erythromycin Stearate Tablets, BP
Erythromycin Tablets, Gastro-resistant, BP
Fluconazole Capsules, 50 mg, DPF
Fluconazole Oral Suspension, 50 mg/5 mL, DPF
Hydrocortisone Cream, BP, 1%
Hydrocortisone Oromucosal Tablets, BP
Hydrogen Peroxide Mouthwash, BP, 6%
Ibuprofen Oral Suspension, BP, sugar-free
Ibuprofen Tablets, BP
Lansoprazole Capsules, Gastro-resistant, BP
Lidocaine Ointment, BP, 5%
Lidocaine Spray 10%, DPF
Loratadine Syrup, 5 mg/5 mL, DPF
Loratadine Tablets, BP, 10 mg
Menthol and Eucalyptus Inhalation, BP 1980
Metronidazole Oral Suspension, BP
Metronidazole Tablets, BP
Miconazole Cream, BP
Miconazole Oromucosal Gel, BP
Miconazole and Hydrocortisone Cream, BP
Miconazole and Hydrocortisone Ointment, BP
Nystatin Oral Suspension, BP
Omeprazole Capsules, Gastro-resistant, BP
Oxytetracycline Tablets, BP
Paracetamol Oral Suspension, BP
Paracetamol Tablets, BP
Paracetamol Tablets, Soluble, BP
Phenoxymethylpenicillin Oral Solution, BP
Phenoxymethylpenicillin Tablets, BP
Promethazine Hydrochloride Tablets, BP
Promethazine Oral Solution, BP
Saliva Stimulating Tablets, DPF
Sodium Chloride Mouthwash, Compound, BP
Sodium Fluoride Mouthwash, BP
Sodium Fluoride Oral Drops, BP
Sodium Fluoride Tablets, BP
Sodium Fluoride Toothpaste 0.619%, DPF
Sodium Fluoride Toothpaste 1.1%, DPF
Sodium Fusidate Ointment, BP
Temazepam Oral Solution, BP
Temazepam Tablets, BP
Tetracycline Tablets, BP

Nurse Prescribers' Formulary

Nurse Prescribers' Formulary for Community Practitioners

List of preparations approved by the Secretary of State which may be prescribed on form FP10P (form HS21(N) in Northern Ireland, form GP10(N) in Scotland, forms WP10CN and WP10PN in Wales) by Nurses for National Health Service patients.

Community practitioners who have completed the necessary training may only prescribe items appearing in the nurse prescribers' list set out below. Community Practitioner Nurse Prescribers are recommended to prescribe generically, except where this would not be clinically appropriate or where there is no approved generic name.

Medicinal Preparations

Preparations on this list which are not included in the BP or BPC are described under Details of NPF preparations (p. 971).

Almond Oil Ear Drops, BP
Arachis Oil Enema, NPF
Aspirin Tablets, Dispersible, 300 mg, BP (max. 96 tablets; max. pack size 32 tablets)
Bisacodyl Suppositories, BP (includes 5-mg and 10-mg strengths)
Bisacodyl Tablets, BP
Catheter Maintenance Solution, Sodium Chloride, NPF
Catheter Maintenance Solution, 'Solution G', NPF
Catheter Maintenance Solution, 'Solution R', NPF
Chlorhexidine Gluconate Alcoholic Solutions containing at least 0.05%
Chlorhexidine Gluconate Aqueous Solutions containing at least 0.05%
Choline Salicylate Dental Gel, BP
Clotrimazole Cream 1%, BP
Co-danthramer Capsules, NPF
Co-danthramer Capsules, Strong, NPF
Co-danthramer Oral Suspension, NPF
Co-danthramer Oral Suspension, Strong, NPF
Co-danthrusate Capsules, NPF
Co-danthrusate Oral Suspension, NPF
Crotamiton Cream, BP
Crotamiton Lotion, BP
Dimeticone barrier creams containing at least 10%
Dimeticone Lotion, NPF
Docusate Capsules, BP
Docusate Enema, NPF
Docusate Oral Solution, BP
Docusate Oral Solution, Paediatric, BP
Econazole Cream 1%, BP
Emollients as listed below:
   Aquadrate® 10% w/w Cream
   Arachis Oil, BP
   Balneum® Plus Cream
   Cetraben® Emollient Cream
   Dermamist®
   Diprobase® Cream
   Diprobase® Ointment
   Doublebase®
   Doublebase® Dayleve Gel
   E45® Cream
   E45® Itch Relief Cream
   Emulsifying Ointment, BP
   Eucerin® Intensive 10% w/w Urea Treatment Cream
   Eucerin® Intensive 10% w/w Urea Treatment Lotion
   Hydromol® Cream

   Hydromol® Intensive
   Hydrous Ointment, BP
   Lipobase®
   Liquid and White Soft Paraffin Ointment, NPF
   Neutrogena® Norwegian Formula Dermatological Cream
   Nutraplus® Cream
   Oilatum® Cream
   Oilatum® Junior Cream
   Paraffin, White Soft, BP
   Paraffin, Yellow Soft, BP
   Ultrabase®
   Unguentum M®
Emollient Bath and Shower Preparations as listed below:
   Aqueous Cream, BP
   Balneum® (except pack sizes that are not to be prescribed under the NHS (see Part XVIIIA of the Drug Tariff, Part XI of the Northern Ireland Drug Tariff))
   Balneum Plus® Bath Oil (except pack sizes that are not to be prescribed under the NHS (see Part XVIIIA of the Drug Tariff, Part XI of the Northern Ireland Drug Tariff))
   Cetraben® Emollient Bath Additive
   Dermalo® Bath Emollient
   Doublebase® Emollient Bath Additive
   Doublebase® Emollient Shower Gel
   Doublebase® Emollient Wash Gel
   Hydromol® Bath and Shower Emollient
   Oilatum® Emollient
   Oilatum® Gel
   Oilatum® Junior Bath Additive
   Zerolatum® Emollient Medicinal Bath Oil
Folic Acid Tablets 400 micrograms, BP
Glycerol Suppositories, BP
Ibuprofen Oral Suspension, BP (except for indications and doses that are prescription-only)
Ibuprofen Tablets, BP (except for indications and doses that are prescription-only)
Ispaghula Husk Granules, BP
Ispaghula Husk Granules, Effervescent, BP
Ispaghula Husk Oral Powder, BP
Lactulose Solution, BP
Lidocaine Ointment, BP
Lidocaine and Chlorhexidine Gel, BP
Macrogol Oral Liquid, Compound, NPF
Macrogol Oral Powder, Compound, NPF
Macrogol Oral Powder, Compound, Half-strength, NPF
Magnesium Hydroxide Mixture, BP
Magnesium Sulfate Paste, BP
Malathion aqueous lotions containing at least 0.5%
Mebendazole Oral Suspension, NPF
Mebendazole Tablets, NPF
Methylcellulose Tablets, BP
Miconazole Cream 2%, BP
Miconazole Oromucosal Gel, BP
Mouthwash Solution-tablets, NPF
Nicotine Inhalation Cartridge for Oromucosal Use, NPF
Nicotine Lozenge, NPF
Nicotine Medicated Chewing Gum, NPF
Nicotine Nasal Spray, NPF
Nicotine Oral Spray, NPF
Nicotine Sublingual Tablets, NPF
Nicotine Transdermal Patches, NPF
Nystatin Oral Suspension, BP
Olive Oil Ear Drops, BP
Paracetamol Oral Suspension, BP (includes 120 mg/5 mL and 250 mg/5 mL strengths—both of which are available as sugar-free formulations)

Paracetamol Tablets, BP (max. 96 tablets; max. pack size 32 tablets)

Paracetamol Tablets, Soluble, BP (includes 120-mg and 500-mg tablets; max. 96 tablets; max. pack size 32 tablets)

Permethrin Cream, NPF

Phosphates Enema, BP

Povidone–Iodine Solution, BP

Senna Oral Solution, NPF

Senna Tablets, BP

Senna and Ispaghula Granules, NPF

Sodium Chloride Solution, Sterile, BP

Sodium Citrate Compound Enema, NPF

Sodium Picosulfate Capsules, NPF

Sodium Picosulfate Elixir, NPF

Spermicidal contraceptives as listed below:
   Gygel® Contraceptive Jelly

Sterculia Granules, NPF

Sterculia and Frangula Granules, NPF

Titanium Ointment, BP

Water for Injections, BP

Zinc and Castor Oil Ointment, BP

Zinc Oxide and Dimeticone Spray, NPF

Zinc Oxide Impregnated Medicated Bandage, NPF

Zinc Oxide Impregnated Medicated Stocking, NPF

Zinc Paste Bandage, BP 1993

Zinc Paste and Ichthammol Bandage, BP 1993

Appliances and Reagents (including Wound Management Products)

Community Practitioner Nurse Prescribers in England, Wales and Northern Ireland can prescribe any appliance or reagent in the relevant Drug Tariff. In the Scottish Drug Tariff, Appliances and Reagents which may **not** be prescribed by nurses are annotated **Nx**.

Appliances (including Contraceptive Devices) as listed in Part IXA of the Drug Tariff (Part III of the Northern Ireland Drug Tariff, Part 3 (Appliances) and Part 2 (Dressings) of the Scottish Drug Tariff). (Where it is not appropriate for nurse prescribers in family planning clinics to prescribe contraceptive devices using form FP10(P) (forms WP10CN and WP10PN in Wales), they may prescribe using the same system as doctors in the clinic.)

Incontinence Appliances as listed in Part IXB of the Drug Tariff (Part III of the Northern Ireland Drug Tariff, Part 5 of the Scottish Drug Tariff).

Stoma Appliances and Associated Products as listed in Part IXC of the Drug Tariff (Part III of the Northern Ireland Drug Tariff, Part 6 of the Scottish Drug Tariff).

Chemical Reagents as listed in Part IXR of the Drug Tariff (Part II of the Northern Ireland Drug Tariff, Part 9 of the Scottish Drug Tariff).

   The Drug Tariffs can be accessed online at:
   National Health Service Drug Tariff for England and Wales: www.ppa.org.uk/ppa/edt_intro.htm
   Health and Social Care, Business Services Organisation, Northern Ireland Drug Tariff:
   http://www.hscbusiness.hscni.net/services/2034.htm
   Scottish Drug Tariff: www.isdscotland.org/Health-topics/Prescribing-and-Medicines/Scottish-Drug-Tariff/

Details of NPF preparations

Preparations on the Nurse Prescribers' Formulary which are not included in the BP or BPC are described as follows in the Nurse Prescribers' Formulary. Although brand names have sometimes been included for identification purposes, it is recommended that non-proprietary names should be used for prescribing medicinal preparations in the NPF except where a non-proprietary name is not available.

Arachis Oil Enema
arachis oil 100%

Catheter Maintenance Solution, Sodium Chloride
(proprietary products: *OptiFlo S; Uro-Tainer Sodium Chloride; Uriflex-S*), sodium chloride 0.9%

Catheter Maintenance Solution, 'Solution G'
(proprietary products: *OptiFlo G; Uro-Tainer Suby G; Uriflex G*), citric acid 3.23%, magnesium oxide 0.38%, sodium bicarbonate 0.7%, disodium edetate 0.01%

Catheter Maintenance Solution, 'Solution R'
(proprietary products: *OptiFlo R; Uro-Tainer Solution R; Uriflex R*), citric acid 6%, gluconolactone 0.6%, magnesium carbonate 2.8%, disodium edetate 0.01%

Chlorhexidine gluconate alcoholic solutions
(proprietary products: *ChloraPrep; Hydrex Solution; Hydrex spray*), chlorhexidine gluconate in alcoholic solution

Chlorhexidine gluconate aqueous solutions
(proprietary product: *Unisept*), chlorhexidine gluconate in aqueous solution

Co-danthramer Capsules [PoM]
co-danthramer 25/200 (dantron 25 mg, poloxamer '188' 200 mg)

Co-danthramer Capsules, Strong [PoM]
co-danthramer 37.5/500 (dantron 37.5 mg, poloxamer '188' 500 mg)

Co-danthramer Oral Suspension [PoM]
(proprietary product: *Codalax*), co-danthramer 25/200 in 5 mL (dantron 25 mg, poloxamer '188' 200 mg/5 mL)

Co-danthramer Oral Suspension, Strong [PoM]
(proprietary product: *Codalax Forte*), co-danthramer 75/1000 in 5 mL (dantron 75 mg, poloxamer '188' 1 g/5 mL)

Co-danthrusate Oral Suspension [PoM]
(proprietary product: *Normax*), co-danthrusate 50/60 (dantron 50 mg, docusate sodium 60 mg/5 mL)

Dimeticone barrier creams
(proprietary products *Conotrane Cream*, dimeticone '350' 22%; *Siopel Barrier Cream*, dimeticone '1000' 10%), dimeticone 10–22%

Dimeticone Lotion
(proprietary product: *Hedrin*), dimeticone 4%

Docusate Enema
(proprietary product: *Norgalax Micro-enema*), docusate sodium 120 mg in 10 g

Liquid and White Soft Paraffin Ointment
liquid paraffin 50%, white soft paraffin 50%

Macrogol Oral Liquid, Compound
(proprietary product: *Movicol Liquid*), macrogol '3350' (polyethylene glycol '3350') 13.125 g, sodium bicarbonate 178.5 mg, sodium chloride 350.7 mg, potassium chloride 46.6 mg/25 mL

Macrogol Oral Powder, Compound
(proprietary products: *Laxido Orange, Molaxole, Movicol*), macrogol '3350' (polyethylene glycol '3350') 13.125 g, sodium bicarbonate 178.5 mg, sodium chloride 350.7 mg, potassium chloride 46.6 mg/sachet; (amount of potassium chloride varies according to flavour of *Movicol*® as follows: plain-flavour (sugar-free) = 50.2 mg/sachet; lime and lemon flavour = 46.6 mg/sachet; chocolate flavour = 31.7 mg/sachet. 1 sachet when reconstituted with 125 mL water provides K^+ 5.4 mmol/litre)

Macrogol Oral Powder, Compound, Half-strength
(proprietary product: *Movicol-Half*), macrogol '3350' (polyethylene glycol '3350') 6.563 g, sodium bicarbonate 89.3 g, sodium chloride 175.4 mg, potassium chloride 23.3 mg/sachet

Malathion aqueous lotions
(proprietary products: *Derbac-M Liquid*), malathion 0.5% in an aqueous basis

Mebendazole Oral Suspension [PoM]
(proprietary product: *Vermox*), mebendazole 100 mg/5 mL

Mebendazole Tablets PoM
(proprietary products: *Ovex, Vermox*), mebendazole 100 mg
(can be supplied for oral use in the treatment of enterobiasis
in adults and children over 2 years provided its container or
package is labelled to show a max. single dose of 100 mg and
it is supplied in a container or package containing not more
than 800 mg)

Mouthwash Solution-tablets
consist of tablets which may contain antimicrobial,
colouring and flavouring agents in a suitable soluble
effervescent basis to make a mouthwash

Nicotine Inhalation Cartridge for Oromucosal Use
(proprietary products: *NicAssist Inhalator, Nicorette
Inhalator*), nicotine 15 mg (for use with inhalation
mouthpiece; to be prescribed as either a starter pack
(6 cartridges with inhalator device and holder) or refill pack
(42 cartridges with inhalator device)

Nicotine Lozenge
nicotine (as bitartrate) 1 mg or 2 mg (proprietary product:
Nicorette Mint Lozenge, Nicotinell Mint Lozenge), or nicotine
(as resinate) 1.5 mg, 2 mg, or 4 mg (proprietary product:
NiQuitin Lozenges, NiQuitin Minis, NiQuitin Pre-quit)

Nicotine Medicated Chewing Gum
(proprietary products: *NicAssist Gum, Nicorette Gum,
Nicotinell Gum, NiQuitin Gum*), nicotine 2 mg or 4 mg

Nicotine Nasal Spray
(proprietary product: *NicAssist Nasal Spray, Nicorette Nasal
Spray*), nicotine 500 micrograms/metered spray

Nicotine Oral Spray
(proprietary product: *Nicorette Quickmist*), nicotine
1 mg/metered spray

Nicotine Sublingual Tablets
(proprietary product: *NicAssist Microtab, Nicorette Microtab*),
nicotine (as a cyclodextrin complex) 2 mg (to be prescribed
as either a starter pack (2 × 15-tablet discs with dispenser)
or refill pack (7 × 15-tablet discs))

Nicotine Transdermal Patches
releasing in each 16 hours, nicotine approx. 5 mg, 10 mg, or
15 mg (proprietary products: *Boots NicAssist Patch, Nicorette
Patch*), or releasing in each 16 hours approx. 10 mg, 15 mg, or
25 mg (proprietary products: *NicAssist Translucent Patch,
Nicorette Invisi Patch*), or releasing in each 24 hours nicotine
approx. 7 mg, 14 mg, or 21 mg (proprietary products:
Nicopatch, Nicotinell TTS, NiQuitin, NiQuitin Clear)
(prescriber should specify the brand to be dispensed)

Permethrin Cream
(proprietary product: *Lyclear Dermal Cream*), permethrin 5%

Senna Oral Solution
(proprietary product: *Senokot Syrup*), sennosides 7.5 mg/5 mL

Senna and Ispaghula Granules
(proprietary product: *Manevac Granules*), senna fruit 12.4%,
ispaghula 54.2%

Sodium Citrate Compound Enema
(proprietary products: *Micolette Micro-enema; Micralax
Micro-enema; Relaxit Micro-enema*), sodium citrate 450 mg
with glycerol, sorbitol and an anionic surfactant

Sodium Picosulfate Capsules
(proprietary products: *Dulcolax Perles*), sodium picosulfate
2.5 mg

Sodium Picosulfate Elixir
(proprietary product: *Dulcolax Liquid*), sodium picosulfate
5 mg/5 mL

Sterculia Granules
(proprietary product: *Normacol Granules*), sterculia 62%

Sterculia and Frangula Granules
(proprietary product: *Normacol Plus Granules*), sterculia 62%,
frangula (standardised) 8%

Zinc Oxide and Dimeticone Spray
(proprietary product: *Sprilon*), dimeticone 1.04%, zinc oxide
12.5% in a pressurised aerosol unit

Zinc Oxide Impregnated Medicated Bandage
(proprietary product: *Steripaste*), sterile cotton bandage
impregnated with paste containing zinc oxide 15%

Zinc Oxide Impregnated Medicated Stocking
(proprietary product: *Zipzoc*), sterile rayon stocking
impregnated with ointment containing zinc oxide 20%

Non-medical prescribing

Overview

A range of non-medical healthcare professionals can prescribe medicines for patients as either Independent or Supplementary Prescribers.

Independent prescribers are practitioners responsible and accountable for the assessment of patients with previously undiagnosed or diagnosed conditions and for decisions about the clinical management required, including prescribing. They are recommended to prescribe generically, except where this would not be clinically appropriate or where there is no approved non-proprietary name.

Supplementary prescribing is a partnership between an independent prescriber (a doctor or a dentist) and a supplementary prescriber to implement an agreed Clinical Management Plan for an individual patient with that patient's agreement.

Independent and Supplementary Prescribers are identified by an annotation next to their name in the relevant professional register.

Information and guidance on non-medical prescribing is available on the Department of Health website at www.dh.gov.uk/health/2012/04/prescribing-change.

For information on the mixing of medicines by Independent and Supplementary Prescribers, see *Mixing of medicines prior to administration in clinical practice—responding to legislative changes*, National Prescribing Centre, May 2010 (available at www.npc.nhs.uk/improving_safety/mixing_meds/resources/mixing_of_medicines.pdf).

For information on the supply and administration of medicines to groups of patients using Patient Group Directions see Guidance on prescribing p. 1.

Nurses

Nurse Independent Prescribers (formerly known as Extended Formulary Nurse Prescribers) are able to prescribe any medicine for any medical condition.

Nurse Independent Prescribers are able to prescribe, administer, and give directions for the administration of Schedule 2, 3, 4, and 5 Controlled Drugs. This extends to diamorphine, dipipanone, or cocaine for treating organic disease or injury, but not for treating addiction.

Nurse Independent Prescribers must work within their own level of professional competence and expertise.

The Nurse Prescribers' Formulary for Community Practitioners p. 970 provides information on prescribing.

Pharmacists

Pharmacist Independent Prescribers can prescribe any medicine for any medical condition.

They are also able to prescribe, administer, and give directions for the administration of Schedule 2, 3, 4, and 5 Controlled Drugs. This extends to diamorphine, dipipanone, or cocaine for treating organic disease or injury, but not for treating addiction.

Pharmacist Independent Prescribers must work within their own level of professional competence and expertise.

Optometrists

Optometrist Independent Prescribers can prescribe any licensed medicine for ocular conditions affecting the eye and the tissues surrounding the eye, except Controlled Drugs or medicines for parenteral administration. Optometrist Independent Prescribers must work within their own level of professional competence and expertise.

Index of proprietary manufacturers

Alphabetical list of manufacturers and other companies

The following is an alphabetical list of manufacturers and other companies referenced in the BNF, with their medicines information or general contact details. For information on 'special-order' manufacturers and specialist importing companies see 'Special-order manufacturers'.

3M Health Care Ltd, Tel: (01509) 611 611

Allen & Hanburys Ltd, Tel: 0800 221 441, customercontactuk@gsk.com

A1 Pharmaceuticals Plc, Tel: (01708) 528 900, sales@a1plc.co.uk

Abbott, Tel: (01628) 773 355

Abbott Healthcare Products Ltd, Tel: (01628) 773 355, medinfo.shl@abbott.com

AbbVie Ltd, Tel: (01628) 561 090, ukmedinfo@abbvie.com

Abraxis BioScience Ltd, Tel: (020) 7081 0850, abraxismedical@idispharma.com

Acorus Therapeutics Ltd, Tel: (01244) 625 152

Actavis UK Ltd, Tel: (01271) 311 257, medinfo@actavis.co.uk

Actelion Pharmaceuticals UK Ltd, Tel: (020) 8987 3333, medinfo.uk@actelion.com

Activa Healthcare, Tel: 0845 060 6707, advice@activahealthcare.co.uk

Adienne Pharma and Biotech, Tel: 0039 (0) 335 873 8731

ADI Medical UK, Tel: (01628) 485159, info@adimedical.co.uk

Advanced Medical Solutions Group Plc, Tel: (01606) 863 500

Advancis Medical Ltd, Tel: (01623) 751 500, info@advancis.co.uk

Advantech Surgical Ltd, Tel: 0845 130 5866, customerservice@newgel.co.uk

Aegerion Pharmaceuticals Ltd, Tel: 00800 2343 7466, medinfo.emea@aegerion.com

AgaMatrix Europe Ltd, Tel: (01235) 838 639, info@wavesense.co.uk

Agepha GmbH, Tel: (020) 3239 6241, uk@agepha.com

Aguettant Ltd, Tel: (01934) 835 694, info@aguettant.co.uk

Air Products plc, Tel: 0800 373 580

Alan Pharmaceuticals, Tel: (020) 7284 2887, info@alanpharmaceuticals.com

Alcon Laboratories (UK) Ltd, Tel: 0345 266 9363, gbmedicaldepartment@alcon.com

Alexion Pharma UK Ltd, Tel: (01932) 359 220, alexion.uk@alxn.com

Alimera Sciences Limited, Tel: 0800 019 1253, medicalinformation@alimerasciences.com

Alissa Healthcare, Tel: (01489) 80 759, enquiries@alissahealthcare.com

ALK-Abelló (UK) Ltd, Tel: (0118) 903 7940, info@uk.alk-abello.com

Alkopharma Sarl, Tel: (0041) 277 206 969, regulatory@alkopharma.com

Allergan Ltd, Tel: (01628) 494 026

Allergy Therapeutics Ltd, Tel: (01903) 844 702

Alliance Pharmaceuticals Ltd, Tel: (01249) 466 966, info@alliancepharma.co.uk

Almirall Ltd, Tel: 0800 008 7399, medinfouk@almirall.com

Altacor Ltd, Tel: (01223) 421 411, info@altacor-pharma.com

Amdipharm Mercury Company Ltd, Tel: 08700 70 30 33, medicalinformation@amcolimited.com

Amgen Ltd, Tel: (01223) 420 305, gbinfoline@amgen.com

Abbot Medical Optics, Tel: 0800 376 7950

Amred Healthcare Ltd, Tel: (0330) 333 0079, info@amredhealthcare.com

Apollo Medical Technologies Ltd, Tel: (01636) 831 201, supercheck2@btinternet.com

Archimed, Tel: 0800 756 9951, enquiries@archimed.co.uk

Archimedes Pharma UK Ltd, Tel: (0118) 931 5094, medicalinformationuk@archimedespharma.com

Arctic Medical Ltd, Tel: (01303) 277 751, sales@arcticmedical.co.uk

Ardana Bioscience Ltd, Tel: (0131) 226 8550

ARIAD Pharma UK Ltd, Tel: 0800 0002 7423, eumedinfo@ariad.com

Ark Therapeutics Group Plc, Tel: (020) 7388 7722, info@arktherapeutics.com

Aspen, Tel: 0800 008 7392, aspenmedinfo@professionalinformation.co.uk

Aspen Medical Europe Ltd, Tel: (01527) 587 728, customers@aspenmedicaleurope.com

AS Pharma Ltd, Tel: 0870 066 4117, info@aspharma.co.uk

Aspire Pharma Ltd, Tel: (01730) 231 148, info@aspirepharma.co.uk

Astellas Pharma Ltd, Tel: (020) 3379 8000, medinfo.gb@astellas.com

AstraZeneca UK Ltd, Tel: 0800 783 0033, medical.informationuk@astrazeneca.com

Auden Mckenzie (Pharma Division) Ltd, Tel: (01895) 627 420

Auxilium, Tel: 0845 017 2315, auxilium@pilglobal.com

Axcan Pharma SA, Tel: (0033) 130 461 900

AYMES International Ltd, Tel: 0845 6805 496, info@aymes.com

Ayrton Saunders Ltd, Tel: (0151) 709 2074, info@ayrtons.com

BAP Medical UK Ltd, Tel: 0844 879 7689

Bard Ltd, Tel: (01293) 527 888

Basilea Pharmaceuticals Ltd, Tel: (01483) 790 023, ukmedinfo@basilea.com

Bausch & Lomb UK Ltd, Tel: (01748) 828 864, medicalinformationuk@bausch.com

Baxter Healthcare Ltd, Tel: (01635) 206 345, surecall@baxter.com

Bayer Healthcare Pharmaceuticals, Tel: (01635) 563 000, medical.information@bayer.co.uk

BBI Healthcare, Tel: (01792) 229 333, info@bbihealthcare.com

B. Braun Medical Ltd, Tel: (0114) 225 9000, info.bbmuk@bbraun.com

Beacon Pharmaceuticals Ltd, Tel: (01892) 600 930, info@beaconpharma.co.uk

Beiersdorf UK Ltd, Tel: (0121) 329 8800

Besins Healthcare (UK) Ltd, Tel: (01748) 828 789, information@besins-healthcare.com

BHR Pharmaceuticals Ltd, Tel: (024) 7637 7210, info@bhr.co.uk

Biogen Idec Ltd, Tel: 0800 008 7401

Biolitec Pharma Ltd, Tel: (00353) 1463 7415

BioMarin Europe Ltd, Tel: (020) 7420 0800, biomarin-europe@bmrn.com

BioMonde, Tel: 0845 230 1810, info@biomonde.com

Biotest (UK) Ltd, Tel: (0121) 733 3393, medicinesinformation@biotestuk.com

Blackwell Supplies Ltd, Tel: (01634) 877 620

BOC Medical, Tel: 0800 111 333

Boehringer Ingelheim Ltd, Tel: (01344) 424 600, medinfo@bra.boehringer-ingelheim.com

The Boots Company Plc, Tel: (0115) 959 5165

BPC 100 Ltd, Tel: 01942 852085

Bio Products Laboratory Ltd, Tel: (020) 8957 2255, medinfo@bpl.co.uk

Bray Healthcare, Tel: (01367) 240 736, info@bray-healthcare.com

Bristol-Myers Squibb Pharmaceuticals Ltd, Tel: (01895) 523 000, medical.information@bms.com

Britannia Pharmaceuticals, Tel: 0870 851 0207, enquiries@medinformation.co.uk

BSN Medical Ltd, Tel: 0845 122 3600

BTG International Ltd, Tel: (0207) 575 0000, medical.services@btgplc.com

Bullen Healthcare, Tel: 0800 269 327

Cambridge Medical Aesthetics Ltd, Tel: (01733) 396171, info@cambridgemedicalaesthetics.com

Cambridge Sensors Ltd, Tel: (01480) 482 920, sales-orders@cs-limited.co.uk

CareFusion UK 244 Ltd, Tel: 0800 043 7546, enquiries@chloraprep.co.uk

Casen-Fleet, Tel: (0034) 913 518 800

C D Medical Ltd, Tel: (01942) 816 184

Celgene Ltd, Tel: 0844 801 0045, medinfo.uk.ire@celgene.com

Chanelle Medical UK Ltd, Tel: (01233) 822 297

Chattem UK Ltd, Tel: (01256) 844 144

Chefaro UK Ltd, Tel: (01748) 828 860, info@omegapharma.co.uk

Chemidex Pharma Ltd, Tel: (01784) 477 167, info@chemidex.co.uk

Chiesi Ltd, Tel: (0161) 488 5555, medinfo.uk@chiesi.com

C. H. Fox Ltd, Tel: (020) 7240 3111

Cambridge Healthcare Supplies Ltd, Tel: (01953) 607 856, customerservices@cambridge-healthcare.co.uk

Chugai Pharma UK Ltd, Tel: (020) 8987 5680

Clement Clarke International Ltd, Tel: (01279) 414 969, resp@clement-clarke.com

Clinigen Group Plc, Tel: (01748) 828 375, clinigeneu@professionalinformation.co.uk

CliniMed Ltd, Tel: (01628) 535 250

Clinisupplies Ltd, Tel: (020) 8863 4168, info@clinisupplies.co.uk

Colgate-Palmolive, Tel: (01483) 302 222

Coloplast Ltd, Tel: (01733) 392 000

Community Foods Ltd, Tel: (020) 8450 9411, email@communityfoods.co.uk

Complan Foods Ltd, Tel: (020) 7395 7565

Consilient Health UK Ltd, Tel: (020) 8956 2310, drugsafety@consilienthealth.com

ConvaTec Ltd, Tel: (01895) 628 400

Co-Pharma Ltd, Tel: 0870 851 0207

Correvio GmbH, Tel: (020) 3002 8114, info@correvio.com

Covidien UK Commercial Ltd, Tel: (01329) 224 226

Cow & Gate, Tel: 0845 762 3624

Cranage Healthcare Ltd, Tel: (01477) 549 392, db@cranagehealth.com

Crawford Healthcare Ltd, Tel: (01565) 654 920

Crescent Pharma, Tel: (01256) 772 730, info@crescentpharma.com

Crucell (UK) Ltd, Tel: 0844 800 3907, info@crucell.co.uk

CSL Behring UK Ltd, Tel: (01444) 447 400, medinfo@cslbehring.com

CTI Life Sciences Ltd, Tel: (01628) 643 974

Daiichi Sankyo UK Ltd, Tel: (01753) 482 771, medinfo@daiichi-sankyo.co.uk

Danetre Health Products Ltd, Tel: (01327) 310 909, enquiries@danetrehealthproducts.com

DDD Ltd, Tel: (01923) 229 251

Dee Pharmaceuticals, Tel: (01978) 661993, enquiries@deepharmaceuticalsltd.co.uk

Dental Health Products Ltd, Tel: (01622) 749 222

Dentsply Ltd, Tel: (01932) 837 279

Dermal Laboratories Ltd, Tel: (01462) 458 866

Dermato Logical Ltd, Tel: (0208) 449 2931, enquiries@aqua-max.co.uk

Dermatonics Ltd, Tel: (01480) 462 910, sales@dermatonics.co.uk

Derma Sciences Europe Ltd, Tel: (01628) 625 916, cs@dermasciences.com

Derma UK Ltd, Tel: (01462) 733 500, info@dermauk.co.uk

Desitin Pharma Ltd, Tel: (01483) 688 240, medinfo@desitin.co.uk

DeVilbiss Healthcare UK Ltd, Tel: (01384) 446 688

Dexcel-Pharma Ltd, Tel: (01327) 312 266, office@dexcelpharma.co.uk

DHP Healthcare Ltd, Tel: (01622) 749 222, sales@dhphealthcare.co.uk

DiME, Tel: (01483) 715 008, info@dime-med.com

Dreamskin Health Ltd, Tel: (01707) 228 688

Dr Falk Pharma UK Ltd, Tel: (01628) 536 600

Drossa Ltd, Tel: (020) 3393 0859, info@drossa.co.uk

Durbin plc, Tel: (020) 8869 6500, info@durbin.co.uk

T G Eakin, Tel: (028) 9187 1000, mail@eakin.co.uk

Easigrip Ltd, Tel: (01926) 497 108, enquiry@easigrip.co.uk

Ecolab UK, Tel: (0113) 232 0066, info.healthcare@ecolab.co.uk

Egis Pharmaceuticals UK Ltd, Tel: (020) 7266 2669, enquiries@medimpexuk.com

Eisai Ltd, Tel: (020) 8600 1400, eumedinfo@eisai.net

Encysive (UK) Ltd, Tel: (01895) 876 168

Entra Health Systems, Tel: (0113) 815 5108

Espere Healthcare Ltd, Tel: (01462) 346 100, info@esperehealth.co.uk

Essential Pharmaceuticals Ltd, Tel: (01784) 477 167, info@essentialpharmaceuticals.com

Ethicon Ltd, Tel: (01506) 594 500

Eumedica S.A., Tel: (020) 8444 3377, enquiries@eumedica.com

European Pharma Group, Tel: 0031 (0) 20 316 0140, info@insujet.com

EUSA Pharma (Europe) Ltd, Tel: (01438) 740 720, medinfo-uk@eusapharma.com

Pierre Fabre Ltd, Tel: (01962) 874 435, medicalinformation@pierre-fabre.co.uk

Fate Special Foods, Tel: (01215) 224 433

Fenton Pharmaceuticals Ltd, Tel: (020) 7224 1388, mail@fent-pharm.co.uk

Ferndale Pharmaceuticals Ltd, Tel: (01937) 541 122, info@ferndalepharma.co.uk

Ferring Pharmaceuticals (UK), Tel: 0844 931 0050, medical@ferring.com

Finox Biotech AG, Tel: 00 800 3466 9246, finoxEY@piglobal.cpm

Firstplay Dietary Foods Ltd, Tel: (0161) 474 7576

Flynn Pharma Ltd, Tel: (01438) 727 822, medinfo@flynnpharma.com

Focus Pharmaceuticals Ltd, Tel: (01283) 495 280, medinfo@focuspharma.co.uk

Foodlink (UK) Ltd, Tel: (01752) 344 544, info@foodlinkltd.co.uk

Ford Medical Associates Ltd, Tel: (01233) 633 224, enquiries@fordmedical.co.uk

Forest Laboratories UK Ltd, Tel: (01322) 421 800, medinfo@forest-labs.co.uk

Forum Health Products Ltd, Tel: (01737) 857 700, enquiries@forumgroup.co.uk

Fresenius Biotech GmbH, Tel: 0049 (0) 893 065 9311, med.info@fresenius-biotech.com

Fresenius Kabi Ltd, Tel: (01928) 533 533, med.info-uk@fresenius-kabi.com

Fresenius Medical Care UK Ltd, Tel: (01623) 445 171, medinfo-uk@fmc-ag.com

Frontier Multigate, Tel: (01495) 233 050, multigate@frontier-group.co.uk

Fyne Dynamics Ltd, Tel: (01279) 423 423, info@fyne-dynamics.com

Galderma (UK) Ltd, Tel: (01923) 208 950, medinfo.uk@galderma.com

Galen Ltd, Tel: (028) 3833 4974, customer.services@galen.co.uk

Gedeon Richter UK Ltd, Tel: (020) 7604 8806, drugsafety.uk@gedeonrichter.eu

GE Healthcare, Tel: (01494) 544 000

Geistlich Pharma, Tel: (01244) 347 534

General Dietary Ltd, Tel: (0203) 044 2933, info@generaldietary.com

Mylan, Tel: (01707) 853 000, info@mylan.co.uk

Genius Foods Ltd, Tel: 0845 874 4000, info@geniusglutenfree.com

Laboratoires Genopharm, Tel: (0808) 234 2664, info@genopharm.eu

Genus Pharmaceuticals, Tel: (01635) 568 400, info@genuspharma.com

Genzyme Therapeutics, Tel: (01865) 405 200, ukmedinfo@genzyme.com

GF Foods Ltd, Tel: (01757) 289 207, admin@gffdirect.co.uk

Gilead Sciences Ltd, Tel: 0800 011 3700, ukmedinfo@gilead.com

Glenwood GmbH, Tel: (0049) 815 199 8790, info@glenwood.de

GlucoRx Ltd, Tel: (01483) 755 133, info@glucorx.co.uk

Gluten Free Foods Ltd, Tel: (020) 8953 4444, info@glutenfree-foods.co.uk

Derma Pharma Ltd, Tel: (01462) 733 500, info@dermauk.co.uk

Grifols Ltd, Tel: (01223) 395 700, medinfo.uk@grifols.com

Grünenthal Ltd, Tel: 0870 351 8960, medicalinformationuk@grunenthal.com

GlaxoSmithKline, Tel: 0800 221 441, customercontactuk@gsk.com

GlaxoSmithKline Consumer Healthcare, Tel: (020) 8047 2500, customer.relations@gsk.com

H&R Healthcare Ltd, Tel: (01482) 631 606, info@hrhealthcare.co.uk

Paul Hartmann Ltd, Tel: (01706) 363 200, info@uk.hartmann.info

Henleys Medical Supplies Ltd, Tel: (01707) 333 164

Hennig Arzneimittel GmbH & Co., Tel: 0844 504 0866

HFA Healthcare Ltd, Tel: 0844 335 8270

HK Pharma Ltd, Tel: 0845 519 1609

Hollister Ltd, Tel: (0118) 989 5000

Hospira UK Ltd, Tel: 0800 088 5133, hospirami@pi-arm.co.uk

HRA Pharma UK & Ireland Ltd, Tel: 0800 917 9548, med.info.uk@hra-pharma.com

Huntleigh Healthcare Ltd, Tel: (01582) 413 104

Huxley Europe Ltd, Tel: (0161) 773 0485

Idis Ltd, Tel: (01932) 824 000, mi@idispharma.com

iMed Systems Ltd, Tel: (0203) 397 8020, emerade@imed-systems.com

INCA-Pharm UK, Tel: (01748) 828 812, info@inca-pharm.com

Infai UK Ltd, Tel: (01904) 435 228, info@infai.co.uk

Injex UK Ltd, Tel: 0845 126 8900, enquiries@injexuk.com

Innovative Solutions UK Ltd, Tel: (01706) 746 713, enquiries@innovative-solutions.org.uk

Insight Medical Products Ltd, Tel: (01666) 500 055, info@insightmedical.ne

InterMune, Tel: (03308) 080 960, med-info@intermune.co.uk

Internis Pharmaceuticals Ltd, Tel: (020) 8346 5588, regulatory@jensongroup.com

Intrapharm Laboratories Ltd, Tel: (01628) 771 800, sales@intrapharmlabs.com

Ipsen Ltd, Tel: (01753) 627 777, medical.information.uk@ipsen.com

Iroko Cardio GmbH, Tel: (020) 3002 8114, info@irokocardio.com

Johnson & Johnson Ltd, Tel: (01628) 822 222, medinfo@congb.jnj.com

Janssen-Cilag Ltd, Tel: 0800 731 8450, medinfo@its.jnj.com

Jobskin Ltd, Tel: (0115) 973 4300, dw@jobskin.co.uk

Juvela (Hero UK) Ltd, Tel: (0151) 432 5300, info@juvela.co.uk

K/L Pharmaceuticals Ltd, Tel: (01294) 215 951

KCI Medical Ltd, Tel: (01865) 840 600

Kestrel Ophthalmics Ltd, Tel: (01202) 658 444, info@kestrelophthalmics.co.uk

King Pharmaceuticals Ltd, Tel: (01438) 356 924

KoRa Healthcare Ltd, Tel: 0845 303 8631, info@kora.ie

Labopharm Europe Ltd, Tel: 0800 028 0037, medinfo@paladin-labs.com

Laboratoires CTRS, ctrsgb@pi-arm.co.uk

LaCorium Health (UK) Ltd, Tel: 0800 158 8233, ukinfo@flexitol.com

Lantor UK Ltd, Tel: (01204) 855 000, help@lantor.co.uk

LEO Laboratories Ltd, Tel: (01844) 347 333, medical-info.uk@leo-pharma.com

LifeScan, Tel: 0800 001 210

Eli Lilly & Co Ltd, Tel: (01256) 315 000, ukmedinfo@lilly.com

Lincoln Medical Ltd, Tel: (01722) 742 900, info@lincolnmedical.co.uk

Linderma Ltd, Tel: (01942) 816 184, linderma@virgin.ne

Lipomed GmbH, Tel: (0041) 6170 20200, save@lipomed.com

Livwell Ltd, Tel: 0845 120 0038, info@livwell.eu

LogixX Pharma Solutions Ltd, Tel: (01189) 011 747, medinfo@logixxpharma.com

Lornamead UK Ltd, Tel: (01276) 674000, lornamead@dhl.com

LPC Pharmaceuticals Ltd, Tel: (01582) 560 393, info@lpcpharma.com

Lucane Pharma, Tel: 0033 (0) 153 868 750, info@lucanepharma.com

Lundbeck Ltd, Tel: (01908) 649 966, ukmedicalinformation@lundbeck.com

L'Oréal Active Cosmetics UK, Tel: 0800 055 6822

M & A Pharmachem Ltd, Tel: (01942) 816 184

Manuka Medical Ltd, Tel: (01623) 600 669

Manx Healthcare, Tel: (01926) 482 511, info@manxhealthcare.com

Marlborough Pharmaceuticals, Tel: (01279) 406 759, info@marlborough-pharma.co.uk

Martindale Pharma, Tel: (01277) 266 600, medinfo@martindalepharma.co.uk

MASTA, Tel: (0113) 238 7500, medical@masta.org

McNeil Products Ltd, Tel: (01628) 822 222

Medical Diagnostics Europe Ltd, Tel: 0845 370 8077, info@mdediagnostic.co.uk

Mead Johnson Nutritionals, Tel: (01895) 230 575

Meadow Laboratories Ltd, Tel: (020) 8597 1203

Meda Pharmaceuticals Ltd, Tel: (01748) 828 810, meda@professionalinformation.co.uk

Medac (UK), Tel: (01786) 458 086, info@medac-uk.co.uk

Medical Developments UK Ltd, Tel: 0870 850 1234, enquiries@ashfieldin2focus.com

Medicare Plus International Ltd, Tel: (020) 8810 8811, info@medicare-plus.com

Medicom Healthcare Ltd, Tel: (01489) 574 119, info@medicomhealthcare.com

Medihoney (Europe) Ltd, Tel: 0800 071 3912 0

Medisana, Tel: +49 (0) 2131/36 68 0

Medlock Medical Ltd, Tel: (0161) 621 2100

MedLogic Global Ltd, Tel: (01752) 209 955, enquiries@mlgl.co.uk

A. Menarini Farmaceutica Internazionale SRL, Tel: (01628) 856 400, menarini@medinformation.co.uk

A. Menarini Diagnostics, Tel: (0118) 944 4100

Merck Serono Ltd, Tel: (020) 8818 7200, medinfo.uk@merckserono.net

Merus Labs, Tel: 00352 (0) 2637 5878, qchs.mi@quintiles.com

Merz Pharma UK Ltd, Tel: (020) 8236 0000, info@merzpharma.co.uk

Micro Medical Ltd, Tel: (01634) 893 500

Milupa Aptamil, Tel: 0845 762 3676, careline@aptamil4hcps.co.uk

Mitsubishi Pharma, Tel: (0207) 382 9000, medinfo@mitsubishi-pharma.eu

Mölnlycke Health Care Ltd, Tel: (0161) 777 2628, info.uk@molnlycke.net

Moorfields Pharmaceuticals, Tel: (020) 7684 9090

Morningside Healthcare Ltd, Tel: (0116) 204 5950

Movianto UK, Tel: (01234) 248 500, movianto.uk@movianto.com

Merck Sharp & Dohme Ltd, Tel: (01992) 467 272, medicalinformationuk@merck.com

Mylan, Tel: (01707) 853 000, info@mylan.co.uk

Nagor Ltd, Tel: (01624) 625 556, enquiries@nagor.com

Nairn's Oatcakes Ltd, Tel: (0131) 620 7000

Napp Pharmaceuticals Ltd, Tel: (01223) 424 444

Neoceuticals Ltd, Tel: (01748) 828 865

Neolab Ltd, Tel: (01256) 704 110, info@neolab.co.uk

Neomedic Ltd, Tel: (01923) 836 379, marketing@neomedic.co.uk

Neon Diagnostics Ltd, Tel: (01376) 500 720

Nestlé Nutrition, Tel: 00800 6887 4846, nestlehealthcarenutrition@uk.nestle.com

Newport Pharmaceuticals Ltd, Tel: (00353) 1890 3011

Nicox Pharma, Tel: (01483) 549 211, ukmedicalinformation@nicox.com

Northern Ireland Blood Transfusion Service, Tel: (028) 9032 1414, inet@nibts.hscni.net

Nipro Diagnostics (UK) Ltd, Tel: (01489) 569 469, info@homediagnostics-uk.com

Nordic Pharma UK Ltd, Tel: (0118) 929 8233, info@nordicpharma.co.uk

Norgine Pharmaceuticals Ltd, Tel: (01895) 826 600, medinfo@norgine.com

Nova Laboratories Ltd, Tel: 08707 120 655, xaluprine@aptivsolutions.com

Novartis Pharmaceuticals UK Ltd, Tel: (01276) 692 255, medinfo.uk@novartis.com

Novartis Consumer Health, Tel: (01276) 687 202, medicalaffairs.uk@novartis.com

Novartis Vaccines Ltd, Tel: 0845 745 1500, service.uk@novartis.com

Novo Nordisk Ltd, Tel: (01293) 613 555

nSPIRE Health Ltd, Tel: (01992) 526 300, info@nspirehealth.com

Nualtra Ltd, Tel: 0808 101 0926, support@nualtra.co.uk

Nutricia, Tel: (01225) 751 098, resourcecentre@nutricia.com

Nutrinovo Ltd, Tel: (01304) 829 068, info@nutrinovo.com

Nutrition Point Ltd, Tel: (07041) 544 044, info@nutritionpoint.co.uk

Nycomed UK Ltd, Tel: (01628) 646 4397, medinfo@nycomed.com

OakMed Ltd, Tel: 0800 592 786, orders@oakmed.co.uk

Octapharma Ltd, Tel: (0161) 837 3770, octapharma@octapharma.co.uk

Omega Pharma, Tel: (01748) 828 860, omega@professionalinformation.co.uk

Omron Healthcare (UK) Ltd, Tel: 0870 750 2771, info.omronhealthcare.uk@eu.omron.com

Merck Sharp & Dohme Ltd, Tel: (01992) 467 272, medicalinformationuk@merck.com

Orion Pharma (UK) Ltd, Tel: (01635) 520 300, medicalinformation@orionpharma.com

Orphan Europe (UK) Ltd, Tel: (01491) 414 333, infouk@orphan-europe.com

Otsuka Pharmaceuticals (UK) Ltd, Tel: (020) 3747 5300, ukmedinfo@otsuka.co.uk

Otsuka Novel Products GmbH, Tel: (0049) 892 0602 0500, medical@otsuka-onpg.com

Ovation Healthcare International Ltd, Tel: (00353) 1613 9707

Owen Mumford Ltd, Tel: (01993) 812 021, customerservices@owenmumford.co.uk

Oxbridge Pharma Ltd, Tel: (020) 8335 4110, enquiries@oxbridgepharma.com

Oxford Nutrition Ltd, Tel: (01626) 832 067, info@nutrinox.com

PARI Medical Ltd, Tel: (01932) 341 122, infouk@pari.de

Parkside Healthcare, Tel: (0161) 795 2792

Peckforton Pharmaceuticals Ltd, Tel: (01270) 582 255, info@peckforton.com

Penn Pharmaceuticals Services Ltd, Tel: (01495) 711 222, penn@pennpharm.co.uk

Pfizer Ltd, Tel: (01304) 616 161, eumedinfo@pfizer.com

PGR Health Foods Ltd, Tel: (01992) 581 715, info@pgrhealthfoods.co.uk

Pharmacosmos UK Ltd, Tel: (01844) 269 007, info@vitalineuk.co.uk

Idis Ltd, Tel: (01932) 824 000, mi@idispharma.com

Pharma Nord (UK) Ltd, Tel: (01670) 519 989, uksales@pharmanord.co.uk

Pharmasure Ltd, Tel: (01923) 233 466, info@pharmasure.co.uk

Pharmaxis Pharmaceuticals Ltd, Tel: (01628) 902 053, med.info@pharmaxis.com.au

PharSafer Associates Ltd, Tel: 01483 212151, medinfoenquiries@pharsafer.com

Phoenix Labs, Tel: (00353) 1468 8917, medicalinformation@phoenixlabs.ie

Pinewood Healthcare, Tel: (00353) 523 6253, info@pinewood.ie

Pinnacle Biologics Inc., Tel: 1-866-248-2039, pinnaclemedinfo@optum.com

Potters Herbal Medicines, Tel: (01942) 219 960

Proceli, Tel: (01226) 713 044, admin@ proceli.co.uk

Procter & Gamble (Health and Beauty Care) Ltd, Tel: (0191) 297 5000

Profile Pharma Ltd, Tel: 0800 1300 855, info@ profilepharma.com

ProStrakan Ltd, Tel: (01896) 664 000, medinfo@prostrakan.com

Protex Healthcare (UK) Ltd, Tel: 0870 011 4112, orders@protexhealthcare.co.uk

Qdem, Tel: (01223) 426 929, medicalinformationukqdem@qdem.co.uk

Ranbaxy UK Ltd, Tel: (020) 8280 1986, medinfoeurope@ranbaxy.com

Ransom Consumer Healthcare, Tel: (01462) 437 615, info@williamransom.com

Ratiopharm UK Ltd, Tel: (023) 9231 3592, info@ratiopharm.co.uk

Reckitt Benckiser Healthcare, Tel: (01482) 326 151, info.miu@reckittbenckiser.com

Recordati Pharmaceuticals Ltd, Tel: (01491) 576 336, medinfo@recordati.co.uk

ReSource Medical UK Ltd, Tel: (01484) 531 489, info@resource-medical.co.uk

Philips Respironics (UK) Ltd, Tel: 0800 130 0840, rukmarketing@respironics.com

RF Medical Supplies Ltd, Tel: (0151) 493 1473, enquiries@rfmedicalsupplies.co.uk

Richardson Healthcare Ltd, Tel: 0800 170 126, info@richardsonhealthcare.com

Riemser Arzneimittel AG, Tel: (0049) 383 517 9679, info@riemser.de

RIS Products Ltd, Tel: (01438) 840 135

Robinson Healthcare Ltd, Tel: (01909) 735 964, enquiry@robinsonhealthcare.com

Roche Products Ltd, Tel: 0800 328 1629, medinfo.uk@roche.com

Roche Diagnostics Ltd, Tel: (01444) 256 000

Rosemont Pharmaceuticals Ltd, Tel: 0800 919 312, infodesk@rosemontpharma.com

Rowa Pharmaceuticals Ltd, Tel: (00353) 275 4077, rowa@rowa-pharma.ie

RPH Pharmaceuticals, Tel: (01483) 212 151, medinfoenquiries@pharsafer.com

Smith & Nephew Healthcare Ltd, Tel: (01482) 222 200, advice@smith-nephew.com

Sallis Healthcare Ltd, Tel: (0115) 978 7841

Sandoz Ltd, Tel: (01276) 698 020, sandoz@ professionalinformation.co.uk

Sanochemia Diagnostics UK Ltd, Tel: (0117) 906 3562

Sanofi-Aventis Ltd, Tel: 0845 372 7101, uk-medicalinformation@sanofi-aventis.com

Sanofi Pasteur MSD Ltd, Tel: (01628) 785 291

SanoMed Manufacturing bv, Tel: +32 503 3627, info@sanomed.nl

Merck Sharp & Dohme Ltd, Tel: (01992) 467 272, medicalinformationuk@merck.com

Schuco International Ltd, Tel: (020) 8368 1642, sales@schuco.co.uk

Schülke UK, Tel: (0114) 254 3500, mail.uk@ schuelke.com

Scope Ophthamics Ltd, Tel: (01293) 897 209, info@scopeophthalmics.com

SD Biosensor, Inc., Tel: 0082 31 300 0475, sales@sdbiosensor.com

SD Healthcare, Tel: (0161) 776 7626, sales@ sdhealthcare.com

Seahorse Laboratories Ltd, Tel: (020) 8257 8412, info@seahorse-labs.com

Septodont Ltd, Tel: (01622) 695 520

Servier Laboratories Ltd, Tel: (01753) 666 409, medical.information@uk.netgrs.com

Seven Seas Ltd, Tel: (01482) 375 234

Shermond, Tel: 0870 242 7701, sales@ shermond.com

Shire Pharmaceuticals Ltd, Tel: 0800 055 6614, medinfouk@shire.com

Shire Human Genetic Therapies, Tel: (01256) 894 000, hgtmedcomm@shire.com

SHS International Ltd, Tel: (0151) 228 8161

Siemens Healthcare Diagnostics Ltd, Tel: 0845 600 1966, dx-diag sales-uk.med@ siemens.com

Sigma-Tau Pharma Ltd (UK), Tel: 0800 043 1268, medical.information@sigma-tau.co.uk

SilDerm Ltd, Tel: (01260) 271 666

Sinclair IS Pharma, Tel: (01244) 625 152, enquiries@ispharma.plc.uk

Skinnies UK, Tel: (01562) 546 123, info@ skinniesuk.com

SLO Drinks Ltd, Tel: 03452 222 205, info@ slodrinks.com

Scottish National Blood Transfusion Service, Tel: (0131) 536 5700, contact.pfc@ snbts.csa.scot.nhs.uk

Sound Opinion, Tel: 0870 192 3283, enquiries@medinformation.co.uk

Speciality European Pharma Ltd, Tel: (020) 7421 7400, info@spepharma.com

Spectrum Thea Pharmaceuticals, Tel: 0870 192 3283, theasupport@spectrum-thea.co.uk

SpePharm UK Ltd, Tel: 0844 800 7579, medinfo.uk@spepharm.com

Spirit Healthcare Ltd, Tel: 0800 881 5423, cs@ spirit-healthcare.co.uk

SSL International plc, Tel: 0870 122 2690

Stanningley Pharma Ltd, Tel: (01159) 124 253, medinfo@stanningleypharma.co.uk

STD Pharmaceutical Products Ltd, Tel: (01432) 373 555, enquiries@stdpharm.co.uk

Steraid (Gainsborough) Ltd, Tel: (01427) 677 559

St George's Medical, Tel: (020) 7582 1015

Stiefel (a GSK company), Tel: 0800 221 441

Stiletto Foods UK Ltd, Tel: 0845 130 0869

Stragen UK Ltd, Tel: 0870 351 8744, info@ stragenuk.com

Sucampo Pharma, Tel: 0800 756 3416, infoeu@sucampo.com

Su-Med International UK Ltd, Tel: (01457) 890 980, sales@sumed.co.uk

Sunovion Pharmaceuticals Europe Ltd, Tel: (020) 7821 2840, medinfo@sunovion.eu

Sutherland Health Ltd, Tel: (01635) 874 488

Swedish Orphan Biovitrum Ltd, Tel: (01638) 722 380, medical.info@sobi.com

Synergy Healthcare (UK) Ltd, Tel: (0161) 624 5641, healthcaresolutions@ synergyhealthplc.com

Syner-Med (Pharmaceutical Products) Ltd, Tel: 0845 634 2100, mail@syner-med.com

Systagenix Wound Management, Tel: (01293) 842 000

Takeda UK Ltd, Tel: (01628) 537 900, medinfo@takeda.co.uk

Talley Group Ltd, Tel: (01794) 503 500

Taro Pharmaceuticals (UK) Ltd, Tel: 0870 736 9544, customerservice@taropharma.co.uk

Teofarma S.r.l., servizioclienti@teofarma.it

TEVA UK Ltd, Tel: (020) 7540 7117, medinfo@ tevauk.com

The Medicines Company, Tel: 00800 8436 3326, medical.information@themedco.com

The Skin Camouflage Company Ltd, Tel: (01507) 343 091, smjcovermark@aol.com

Therabel Pharma UK Ltd, Tel: 0800 066 5446, info@therabel.co.uk

The Urology Company Ltd, Tel: (020) 3077 5411, info@theurologyco.com

Thomas Blake Cosmetic Creams Ltd, Tel: (01207) 272 311, sales@veilcover.com

Thornton & Ross Ltd, Tel: (01484) 842 217

Tillomed Laboratories Ltd, Tel: (01480) 402 400, info@tillomed.co.uk

Tillotts Pharma UK Ltd, Tel: 0845 034 4476

TMC Pharma Services Ltd, Tel: (01252) 842 255, info@tmcpharma.com

Tobia Teff UK Ltd, Tel: (020) 7328 2045, info@ tobiateff.co.uk

Torbet Laboratories Ltd, Tel: (01953) 607 856, customerservices@cambridge-healthcare.co.uk

Transdermal Ltd, Tel: (020) 8654 2251, info@ transdermal.co.uk

TRB Chemedica (UK) Ltd, Tel: 0845 330 7556

Typharm Ltd, Tel: (01603) 722 480, customerservices@typharm.com

UCB Pharma Ltd, Tel: (01753) 534 655, medicalinformationuk@ucb.com

Ultrapharm Ltd, Tel: (01491) 578 016

Univar Ltd, Tel: (01908) 362 200, trientine@ univareurope.com

Unomedical Ltd, Tel: (01527) 587 700

Urgo Ltd, Tel: (01509) 502 051, woundcare@ uk.urgo.com

Vertex Pharmaceuticals (UK) Ltd, Tel: 0800 028 2616, eumedicalinfo@vrtx.com

Vifor Pharma UK Ltd, Tel: (01276) 853 633, medicalinfo_uk@viforpharma.com

ViiV Healthcare UK Ltd, Tel: 0800221441, customercontactuk@gsk.com

Viridian Pharma Ltd, Tel: (01633) 400 335, info@viridianpharma.co.uk

ViroPharma Ltd, Tel: (020) 7572 1222

Vitaflo International Ltd, Tel: (0151) 709 9020, vitaflo@vitaflo.co.uk

Vitalograph Ltd, Tel: (01280) 827 110, sales@ vitalograph.co.uk

Wallace Cameron Ltd, Tel: (01698) 354 600, sales@wallacecameron.com

Wallace Manufacturing Chemists Ltd, Tel: (01235) 538 700, info@alinter.co.uk

Warburtons, Tel: (01204) 513 004

Warner Chilcott UK Ltd, Tel: (01932) 824 700

Welsh Blood Service, Tel: (01443) 622 000, donor.care@wales.nhs.uk

Wellfoods Ltd, Tel: (01226) 381 712, wellfoods@wellfoods.co.uk

Williams Medical Supplies Ltd, Tel: (01685) 844 739

Wockhardt UK Ltd, Tel: (01978) 661 261

Wyeth Pharmaceuticals, Tel: (01628) 604 377, eumedinfo@pfizer.com

Wynlit Laboratories, Tel: (07903) 370 130

Wyvern Medical Ltd, Tel: (01531) 631 105

Zentiva, Tel: (01483) 554 101, gb-zentivamedicalinformation@sanofi.com

Zeroderma Ltd, Tel: (01858) 525 643

Special-order manufacturers

Unlicensed medicines are available from 'special-order' manufacturers and specialist-importing companies; the MHRA maintains a register of these companies at tinyurl.com/cdslke.

Licensed **hospital manufacturing units** also manufacture 'special-order' products as unlicensed medicines, the principal NHS units are listed below. A database (*Pro-File*; www.pro-file.nhs.uk) provides information on medicines manufactured in the NHS; access is restricted to NHS pharmacy staff.

The Association of Pharmaceutical Specials Manufacturers may also be able to provide further information about commercial companies (www.apsm-uk.com).

The MHRA recommends that an unlicensed medicine should only be used when a patient has special requirements that cannot be met by use of a licensed medicine.

As well as being available direct from the hospital manufacturer(s) concerned, many NHS-manufactured Specials may be bought from the Oxford Pharmacy Store, owned and operated by Oxford Health NHS Foundation Trust.

England

London

Barts and the London NHS Trust
Mr J. A. Rickard, Head of Barts Health Pharmaceuticals
Barts Health NHS Trust
The Royal London Hospital
Pathology and Pharmacy Building
80 Newark St
Whitechapel
London
E1 2ES
(020) 3246 0394 (order/enquiry)
barts.pharmaceuticals@bartshealth.nhs.uk

Guy's and St. Thomas' NHS Foundation Trust
Mr P. Forsey, Associate Chief Pharmacist
Guy's and St. Thomas' NHS Foundation Trust
Guy's Hospital
Pharmacy Department
Great Maze Pond
London
SE1 9RT
(020) 7188 4992 (order)
(020) 7188 5003 (enquiry)
Fax: (020) 7188 5013
paul.forsey@gstt.nhs.uk

Moorfields Pharmaceuticals
Mr. T. Record, Technical Director
Moorfields Pharmaceuticals
25 Provost St
London
N1 7NH
(020) 7684 9090 (order/enquiry)
Fax: (020) 7502 2332

London North West Healthcare NHS Trust
Mr K. Wong,
London North West Healthcare NHS Trust
Northwick Park Hospital
Watford Rd
Harrow
Middlesex
HA1 3UJ
(020) 8869 2295 (order)
(020) 8869 2204/2223 (enquiry)
kwong@nhs.net

Royal Free Hampstead NHS Trust
Ms C. Trehane, Production Manager
Royal Free Hampstead NHS Trust
Pond St
London
NW3 2QG
(020) 7830 2424 (order)
(020) 7830 2282 (enquiry)
Fax: (020) 7794 1875
christine.trehane@nhs.net

St George's Healthcare NHS Trust
Mr V. Kumar, Assistant Chief Pharmacist
St George's Hospital
Technical Services
Blackshaw Rd
Tooting
London
SW17 0QT
(020) 8725 1770/1768
Fax: (020) 8725 3947
vinodh.kumar@stgeorges.nhs.uk

University College Hospital NHS Foundation Trust
Mr T. Murphy, Production Manager
University College Hospital
235 Euston Rd
London
NW1 2BU
(020) 7380 9723 (order)
(020) 7380 9472 (enquiry)
Fax: (020) 7380 9726
tony.murphy@uclh.nhs.uk

Midlands and Eastern

Barking, Havering and Redbridge University Trust
Mr N. Fisher, Senior Principal Pharmacist
Queen's Hospital
Pharmacy Department
Romford
Essex
RM7 0AG
(01708) 435 463 (order)
(01708) 435 042 (enquiry)
neil.fisher@bhrhospitals.nhs.uk

Burton Hospitals NHS Foundation Trust
Mr D. Raynor, Head of Pharmacy Manufacturing Unit
Queens Hospital
Burton Hospitals NHS Foundation Trust
Pharmacy Manufacturing Unit
Belvedere Rd
Burton-on-Trent
DE13 0RB
(01283) 511 511 ext: 5275 (order/enquiry)
Fax: (01283) 593 036
david.raynor@burtonft.nhs.uk

Colchester Hospital University NHS Foundation Trust
Mr S. Pullen, Pharmacy Production Manager
Colchester General Hospital
Main Pharmacy
Turner Rd
Colchester
Essex
CO4 5JL
(01206) 742 007 (order)
(01206) 744 208 (enquiry)
Fax: (01206) 841 249
pharmacy.stores@colchesterhospital.nhs.uk (order)
psu.enquiries@colchesterhospital.nhs.uk (enquiry)

Ipswich Hospital NHS Trust
Dr J. Harwood, Production Manager
Ipswich Hospital NHS Trust
Pharmacy Manufacturing Unit
Heath Rd
Ipswich
IP4 5PD
(01473) 703 440 (order)
(01473) 703 603 (enquiry)
Fax: (01473) 703 609
john.harwood@ipswichhospital.nhs.uk

Nottingham University Hospitals NHS Trust
Mr J. Graham, Senior Pharmacist, Production
Nottingham University Hospitals NHS Trust
Pharmacy Production Units
Queens Medical Centre Campus
Nottingham
NG7 2UH
(0115) 924 9924 ext: 66521 (enquiry/order)
Fax: (0115) 970 9780
jeff.graham@nuh.nhs.uk

University Hospital of North Staffordshire NHS Trust
Ms K. Ferguson, Chief Technician
University Hospital of North Staffordshire NHS Trust
Pharmacy Technical Services
City General Site
Stoke-on-Trent
ST4 6QG
(01782) 674 568 (order)
(01782) 674 568 (enquiry)
Fax: (01782) 674 575
caroline.ferguson@uhns.nhs.uk

North East

The Newcastle upon Tyne Hospitals NHS Foundation Trust
Mr Y. Hunter-Blair, Production Manager
Royal Victoria Infirmary
Newcastle Specials
Pharmacy Production Unit
Queen Victoria Rd
Newcastle-upon-Tyne
NE1 4LP
(0191) 282 0395 (order)
(0191) 282 0389 (enquiry)
Fax: (0191) 282 0469
yan.hunter-blair@nuth.nhs.uk

North West

Preston Pharmaceuticals
Ms A. Bolch, Deputy Chief Pharmacist (PMU)
Preston Pharmaceuticals
Royal Preston Hospital
Fulwood
Preston
PR2 9HT
(01772) 523 617 (order)
(01772) 522 593 (enquiry)
Fax: (01772) 523 645
angela.bolch@lthtr.nhs.uk

Stockport Pharmaceuticals
Mr A. Singleton, Head of Production
Stepping Hill Hospital
Stockport NHS Foundation Trust
Stockport Pharmaceuticals
Stockport
SK2 7JE
(0161) 419 5666 (order)
(0161) 419 5657 (enquiry)
Fax: (0161) 419 5426
andrew.singleton@stockport.nhs.uk

South

Portsmouth Hospitals NHS Trust
Mr R. Lucas, Product Development Manager
Portsmouth Hospitals NHS Trust
Pharmacy Manufacturing Unit
Unit D2, Railway Triangle Industrial Estate
Walton Road
Farlington
Portsmouth
PO6 1TF
(02392) 389 078 (order)
(02392) 316 312 (enquiry)
Fax: (02392) 316 316
robert.lucas@porthosp.nhs.uk

South East

East Sussex Healthcare NHS Trust
Mr P. Keen, Business Manager
Eastbourne District General Hospital
East Sussex Hospitals NHS Trust
Eastbourne Pharmaceuticals
Kings Drive
Eastbourne
BN21 2UD
(01323) 414 906 (order)
(01323) 417 400 ext: 3076 (enquiry)
Fax: (01323) 414 931
paul.keen@esht.nhs.uk

South West

Torbay PMU
Mr P. Bendell, Pharmacy Manufacturing
Services Manager
South Devon Healthcare NHS Foundation Trust
Torbay PMU
Kemmings Close, Long Rd
Paignton
TQ4 7TW
(01803) 664 707
Fax: (01803) 664 354
phil.bendell@nhs.net

Yorkshire

Calderdale and Huddersfield NHS Foundation Trust
Dr B. Grewal, Managing Director
Calderdale and Huddersfield NHS Foundation
Trust
Huddersfield Pharmacy Specials
Gate 2 - Acre Mills, School St West
Huddersfield
HD3 3ET
(01484) 355 388 (order/enquiry)
info.hps@cht.nhs.uk

Northern Ireland

Victoria Pharmaceuticals
Mr S. Cameron, Production Manager - Pharmacy
Victoria Pharmaceuticals
Royal Hospitals
Plenum Building
Grosvenor Road
Belfast
BT12 6BA
(028) 9063 0070 (order/enquiry)
Fax: (028) 9063 5282 (order/enquiry)
samuel.cameron@belfasttrust.hscni.net

Scotland

NHS Greater Glasgow and Clyde
Mr G. Conkie, Production Manager
Western Infirmary
Dumbarton Rd
Glasgow
G11 6NT
(0141) 211 2754 (order)
(0141) 211 2882 (enquiry)
Fax: (0141) 211 1967
graham.conkie@ggc.scot.nhs.uk

Tayside Pharmaceuticals
Mr S. Bath, Production Manager
Ninewells Hospital
Tayside Pharmaceuticals
Dundee
DD1 9SY
(01382) 632 052 (order)
(01382) 632 273 (enquiry)
Fax: (01382) 632 060
sbath@nhs.net

Wales

Cardiff and Vale University Health Board
Mr P. Spark, Principal Pharmacist (Production)
Cardiff and Vale University Health Board
20 Fieldway
Cardiff
CF14 4HY
(029) 2074 8120
Fax: (029) 2074 8130
paul.spark@wales.nhs.uk

Index

A

A2A Spacer, 161
Abacavir, **390**
‣ With dolutegravir and lamivudine, **391**
‣ With lamivudine, **391**
‣ With lamivudine and zidovudine, **391**
Abasaglar preparations, 425
Abatacept, **598**
Abbreviations and Symbols, *inside back cover*
Abelcet, 352
Abidec Multivitamin, 583
Abilify, 235
Able Spacer, 161
Absence seizures, 182
Abtard, 268
Accofil, 538
Accolate, 157
Accrete D3, 590
Acea, 676
ACE inhibitors, 103
Acetaminophen, *see* Paracetamol
Acetazolamide, **638**
Acetic acids, 572
Acetylcholine chloride, **634**
Acetylcysteine, **625**, **797**
Acetylsalicylic Acid, *see* Aspirin
Aciclovir, **381**, **632**, **683**
Acid-base imbalance, 540
Acitretin, **703**
Acnamino MR, 334
Acne, 709
Acnecide, 710
Acne vulgaris, 708
Acondro, 468
Acrivastine, **163**
Actidose-Aqua Advance, 793
Actilyse, 126
Actilyse Cathflo, 126
Actinomycin D, *see* Dactinomycin
Actiq, 263
Activated dimeticone, *see* Simeticone
Active, 428
Active elimination from the gastro-intestinal tract, 793
Active immunity, 731
Actonel, 438
Actrapid, 426
Acular, 636
Acute diarrhoea, 43
‣ Adsorbents and bulk-forming drugs, 43
‣ Antibacterial drugs, 43
‣ Antimotility drugs, 43
‣ Antispasmodics, 44
‣ Enkephalinase inhibitors, 44
‣ Management of acute diarrhoea, 43
Acute porphyrias, 562
‣ Drugs unsafe for use in acute porphyrias, 562
Acyclovir, *see* Aciclovir
Adalat, 101
Adalimumab, **598**

Adapalene, **711**
‣ With benzoyl peroxide, **711**
Adcal, 552
Adcal-D3, 590, 591
Adcortyl Intra-articular / Intradermal, 617
Add Ins, 963
Additrace, 578
Adenocor, 74
Adenoscan, 74
Adenosine, **73**
Adoport, 491
Adrenaline/epinephrine, **128**
Adrenaline with articaine hydrochloride, **777**
Adrenaline with bupivacaine, *see* Bupivacaine with adrenaline
Adrenaline with lidocaine, *see* Lidocaine with adrenaline
Adrenergic neurone blocking drugs, 91
Adrenocortical function testing, 441
Advate, 78
Adverse reactions to drugs, 11
Adverse reactions to medical devices, 12
Advocate Redi-Code+, 428
AeroChamber Plus, 161
AErrane, 761
Agalsidase alfa, **565**
Agalsidase beta, **565**
Agrippal, 752
Aidulan, 469
Airomir preparations, 147
AirSalb, 147
Airways disease, obstructive, 138
Airways disease, use of corticosteroids, 149
AirZone, 160
Aizea, 474
Aknemin, 334
Aknemycin Plus, 714
Albendazole, **360**
Albumin solution, **554**
Albunorm, 554
Alburex, 554
Albustix, 432
Albutein, 554
Albuterol, *see* Salbutamol
Alclometasone dipropionate, **688**
Alcohol, **716**, 787
Aldactone, 118
Aldara, 722
Aldehydes and derivatives, 721
Aldosterone antagonists, 117
Aldurazyme, 568
Alendronate, *see* Alendronic acid
Alendronic acid, **436**
Alenini, 467
Alenvona, 467
Alfacalcidol, **588**
Alfentanil, **772**
Alginates, 46
Alginic acid, **46**
Alglucosidase alfa, **570**
Alicalm, 946
Alimemazine tartrate, **167**
Alkalising drugs, 460, 540

Alkylating agents, 497
Allergen immunotherapy, 162
Allergen-type vaccines, 172
Allergic and inflammatory eye conditions, 620
Allergic conditions, 162
Allergic conjunctivitis, 620
Allergic emergencies, 162
Allerief, 169
Alli, 63
Allopurinol, **516**
Almond oil, **647**
Alomide, 622
Alopecia, 496
Alpha-adrenoceptor blocking drugs, 91, 458
Alphaderm, 694
AlphaNine, 78
Alpha$_2$-adrenoceptor agonists, 217, 641
Alpha tocopherol, **592**
Alpha tocopheryl acetate, **592**
Alprostadil, **135**
Altacite Plus, 47
Altargo, 678
Alteplase, **126**
Altraplen preparations, 937, 939
Alu-Cap, 558
Aluminium, 558
Aluminium acetate, **647**
Aluminium chloride hexahydrate, **706**
Aluminium hydroxide, **558**
Aluminium hydroxide with dicycloverine hydrochloride, magnesium oxide and simeticone, *see* Dicycloverine hydrochloride with aluminium hydroxide, magnesium oxide and simeticone
Aluminium hydroxide with magnesium hydroxide and simeticone, *see* Simeticone with aluminium hydroxide and magnesium hydroxide
Aluminium hydroxide with magnesium hydroxide, *see* Co-magaldrox
Alvedon, 256
Alverine citrate, **58**
Alvesco, 152
Ambirix, 748
AmBisome, 352
Ambulatory oxygen therapy, 142
Amethocaine, *see* Tetracaine
Ametop, 785
Amfetamines, 791
Amfexa, 216
Amias, 107
Amikacin, **292**
Amikin, 292
Amilamont, 134
Amiloride hydrochloride, **133**
Amino acid formula (essential and non-essential amino acids), 929, 933
Amino acids and derivatives, 564, 569, 571
Aminoglycosides, 291, 630, 644, 650, 675
‣ Cystic fibrosis, 291
‣ Neonates, 291
‣ Once daily dosage, 291

Serum concentrations, 291
Aminoglycosides (by injection), **291**
Aminophylline, **158**
Aminosalicylates, **25**
Amiodarone hydrochloride, **72**
Amisulpride, **234**
Amitriptyline hydrochloride, **224**
Amlodipine, **99**
Amlostin, 100
Ammonaps, 573
Ammonia lowering drugs, 573
Amoebicides, 362
Amoebic infection, 281
Amorolfine, **680**
Amoxicillin, **320**
Amoxicillin with clavulanic acid, *see* Co-amoxiclav
Amoxil, 321
Amoxycillin, *see* Amoxicillin
Amphotericin, **351**
Amphotericin B, *see* Amphotericin
Ampicillin, **321**
Ampicillin with flucloxacillin, *see* Co-fluampicil
Anabact, 676
Anabolic steroids, 449, 522
Anaemia, iron deficiency, 527
- Compound preparations, 528
- Oral iron, 528
- Parenteral iron, 528
- Prophylaxis of iron deficiency, 528
- Treatment and prophylaxis, 527
- Treatment of iron-deficiency anaemia, 528
Anaemia, megaloblastic, 532
Anaemias, 521
- Drugs used in hypoplastic, haemolytic, and renal anaemias, 522
- Drugs with definite risk of haemolysis in most G6PD-deficient individuals, 522
- Erythropoietins, 522
- G6PD deficiency, 521
- Initiation of treatment, 521
- Sickle-cell anaemia, 521
Anaesthesia adjuvants, 763
Anaesthetics, general, 758, 773
Anaesthetics, local, 634, 659, 777
Anagrelide, **540**
Anal fissures, 64
Analgesics, 67, 252, 605, 635, 660, 771
- Compound analgesic preparations, 253
- Dental and orofacial pain, 252
- Drugs used for pain, 252
- Dysmenorrhoea, 253
- Non-opioid analgesics and compound analgesic preparations, 253
- Opioid analgesics, 253
- Pain in sickle-cell disease, 252
- Pain management and opioid dependence, 254
- Postoperative analgesia, 254
- Strong opioids, 253
- Weak opioids, 254
Analgesics, non-opioid, 254
Anaphylaxis, 162
Ancotil, 356
Androcur, 451
Androgens, 449, **450**

Androgens, anti-androgens and anabolic steroids, 449
Androstan derivatives, 449, 522
Anectine, 767
Angioedema, 163, 174
Angiotensin-converting enzyme inhibitors, 92, **103**
Angiotensin II receptor antagonists, **106**
Angular cheilitis, 662, 674
Anhydrol, 706
Anogenital warts, 720
Antacids, 46, 67
- Antacids, alginate, 46, 56
- Antacids, aluminium and magnesium, 47
- Antacids, magnesium, 48
- Alginates, 46
- Simeticone, 46
Antazoline with xylometazoline, **620**
Anterior pituitary hormones, 441
Anterior uveitis, 624
Anthelmintics, 360
Anthracyclines and related drugs, 501
Anthralin, *see* Dithranol
Anthrax, 339
- Treatment and post-exposure prophylaxis, 339
Anthrax vaccine, 733
Anti-androgens, 450, 709
Anti-androgens and precocious puberty, 449
Antiarrhythmics, 70
Antibacterial drugs
- Acute diarrhoea, 43
- Eye infections, 629
- Oral bacterial infections, 289
- Skin infections, 673
Antibacterials, 291
Antibacterials, principles of therapy, 281
- Antibacterial policies, 281
- Before starting therapy, 281
- Choice of a suitable drug, 281
- Notifiable diseases, 282
- Prophylaxis, 282
- Superinfection, 282
- Switching from parenteral to oral treatment, 282
- Therapy, 282
Antibacterials that do not induce liver enzymes, 464
Antibacterials, use for prophylaxis, 282
- Animal and human bites, 283
- Endocarditis, 284
- Gastro-intestinal procedures, 283
- Immunosuppression and indwelling intraperitoneal catheters, 285
- Joint prostheses and dental treatment, 285
- Obstetric surgery, 284
- Orthopaedic surgery, 284
- Pertussis, 283
- Pneumococcal infection in asplenia or in patients with sickle-cell disease, 283
- Recurrence of rheumatic fever, 282
- Secondary case of diphtheria in non-immune patient, 283
- Secondary case of *Haemophilus influenzae* type b disease, 283

- Secondary case of invasive group A streptococcal infection, 282
- Secondary case of meningococcal meningitis, 282
- *Staphylococcus aureus* lung infection in cystic fibrosis, 283
- Tuberculosis in susceptible close contacts or those who have become tuberculin positive, 283
- Urinary-tract infection, 283
Antibacterial therapy for
- Blood infections, 285
- Cardiovascular system infections, 285
- Central nervous system infections, 286
- Ear infections, 287
- Eye infections, 287
- Gastro-intestinal system infections, 287
- Genital system infections, 288
- Musculoskeletal system infections, 288
- Nose infections, 289
- Oral infections, 289
- Respiratory system infections, 290
- Skin infections, 290
Antibody responsive malignancy, 493
Anticholinesterases, **601**, 770
Anticoagulants, 83, 365
Anticomedonals, 711
Antidepressant drugs, 221
- Anxiety, 221
- Choice, 221
- Dosage, 221
- Hyponatraemia and antidepressant therapy, 221
- Important safety information: Depressive illness in children and adolescents, 221
- Serotonin syndrome, 221
- Suicidal behaviour and antidepressant therapy, 221
Antidepressants, emergency treatment of poisoning, 789
Antidiabetic drugs, 419
Antidiarrhoeal drugs, 44, 67
Antidiuretic hormone disorders, 403
Anti-doping, 22
Antidotes and chelators, 535, 559, 573, 770, 793, 794, 795, 797, 798
Anti-D (Rh$_0$) immunoglobulin, **725**
Antiemetics and antinauseants, 244, 272
Antiepileptic drugs, 183
Antiepileptic hypersensitivity syndrome, 181
Antiepileptics, 184, 208
- Barbiturates, 203, 209
Antifibrinolytic drugs and haemostatics, 76
Antifoaming drugs, 48
Antifungal preparations, 674
Antifungals, 629
Antifungals, systemic use, 348
- Aspergillosis, 348
- Candidiasis, 348
- Common fungal infections, 348
- Cryptococcosis, 348
- Echinocandin antifungals, 349
- Histoplasmosis, 349
- Imidazole antifungals, 349

▸ Immunocompromised children, 349
▸ Other antifungals, 349
▸ Polyene antifungals, 349
▸ Skin and nail infections, 349
▸ Triazole antifungals, 349
Antigiardial drugs, 362
Antihaemorrhagics, 76
Antihistamines, 162, 244, 249, 275, 620
Antihistamines, allergen immunotherapy and allergic emergencies, 162
▸ Allergen immunotherapy, 162
▸ Allergic emergencies, 162
▸ Anaphylaxis, 162
▸ Angioedema, 163
▸ Antihistamines, 162
▸ Hereditary angioedema, 163
▸ Intramuscular adrenaline (epinephrine), 163
▸ Intravenous adrenaline (epinephrine), 163
▸ Treatment of anaphylaxis, 162
Antihypertensive drugs, 91
▸ Adrenergic neurone blocking drugs, 91
▸ Alpha-adrenoceptor blocking drugs, 91
▸ Centrally acting antihypertensive drugs, 91, 93
▸ Vasodilator antihypertensive drugs, 91
Anti-lymphocyte monoclonal antibodies, **493**
Antimalarials, 363, 370, 595, 596, 790
▸ Artemether with lumefantrine, 363
▸ Chloroquine, 363
▸ Mefloquine, 363
▸ Piperaquine with artenimol, 363
▸ Primaquine, 363
▸ Proguanil, 363
▸ Pyrimethamine, 364
▸ Quinine, 364
▸ Tetracyclines, 364
Antimetabolites, 485, 497, 504
Antimuscarinic bronchodilators, 141
Antimuscarinic drugs
▸ Anaesthesia adjuvants, 763
▸ Dystonias, 240
▸ Gastro-intestinal, 56
▸ Other, 250, 624, 633, 651, 705, 764
Antimuscarinics (eye), **624**
Antimuscarinics (inhaled), **143**
Antimuscarinics (systemic), **457**
Antimycobacterials, 341, 344
Antineoplastics, 497, 512, 720
Antiperspirants, 705
Antiplatelet drugs, 83
▸ Kawasaki disease, 83
Antiproliferative immunosuppressants, 483
Antiprotozoal drugs, 362
▸ Amoebicides, 362
▸ Antigiardial drugs, 362
▸ Drugs for toxoplasmosis, 362
▸ Leishmaniacides, 362
▸ Trichomonacides, 362
▸ Trypanocides, 362
Antiprotozoals, 281, 358, 363, 370, 632
Antipruritics, 707
Antipseudomonal penicillins, 316

Antipsychotics, 218, **230**, 227, 251, 790
▸ First-generation, 230
▸ Second-generation, 234
▸ Depot injections, 229
▸ Emergency treatment of poisoning, 790
Antisecretory drugs, 67
Antiseptic mouthwashes, 659
Antiseptics and disinfectants, 633, 710, 716
▸ Alcohol disinfectants, 716
▸ Iodine products, 716
▸ Other antiseptics and disinfectants, 656, 681, 715, 717, 719, 721
Antispasmodics, 31, 44, 56, 58
▸ Antimuscarinics, 56
▸ Motility stimulants, 56
▸ Other antispasmodics, 56
Antithrombotic drugs, 81, 110, 125, 540
Antithymocyte immunoglobulin (rabbit), **484**
Antithyroid drugs, 451
▸ Neonates, 452
▸ Pregnancy, 452
Antitoxins, 730, 798
Antituberculosis drugs, 341
Antivaricella-zoster Immunoglobulin, *see* Varicella-zoster immunoglobulin
Antivirals, 378, 384, 386, 399, 629, 632, 674, 683, 722
Antracen derivatives, 699
Anugesic-Hc, 64
Anusol-Hc, 64
Anxiety, 221
Anxiolytics, 275
Apidra, 427
Apidra SoloStar, 427
Approximate Conversions and Units, 1026
Apraclonidine, **641**
Apresoline, 108
Aprinox, 102
Aptivus, 398
Aquadrate, 673
Aquamax, 669, 671
Aquamol, 671
Arachis oil, **43**
Arachis oil with chlorobutanol, **647**
Arachis oil with extract of coal tar, *see* Extract of coal tar with arachis oil
Aragam, 728
Aranesp, 524
Aranesp SureClick, 524
Arcoxia, 608
Arginine, **571**
Aripiprazole, **234**
Arjun, 647
Arkolamyl, 237
Aromatase inhibitors, 451
Aromatic inhalations, 176
Aromatic inhalations, cough preparations and systemic nasal decongestants, 176
Arpicolin, 241
Arrhythmias, 69, 94, 555
▸ Atrial fibrillation, 69
▸ Atrial flutter, 69
▸ Bradycardia, 69
▸ Drugs for arrhythmias, 69
▸ Ectopic tachycardia, 69
▸ Supraventricular tachycardia, 69

▸ Syndromes associated with accessory conducting pathways, 69
▸ Torsade de pointes, 69
▸ Ventricular tachycardia and ventricular fibrillation, 69
Artelac, 625, 627, 628
Artemether with lumefantrine, 363, **370**
Artenimol with piperaquine phosphate, **371**
Arthritis, 595
Articaine hydrochloride with adrenaline, *see* Adrenaline with articaine hydrochloride
Artificial saliva products, 654, 655
Artificial tears, 626
Asacol preparations, 28
Ascaricides (common roundworm infections), 359
Ascites, 134
Ascorbic acid, 582, **587**
Ascur, 587
Asmabec Clickhaler, 151
Asmanex Twisthaler, 154
Asmavent, 147
Asparaginase, 497
Aspergillosis, 348
Aspirin, **83**, 787
Asplenia, 364
AS Saliva Orthana, 654
Asthma, 138, 149, 604
▸ Aims of treatment, 139
▸ Description of condition, 138
▸ Follow up in all cases, 140
▸ Lifestyle changes, 139
▸ Management of acute asthma, 140
▸ Management of chronic asthma, 139
▸ Pregnancy and breast-feeding, 141
Astringents, 647, 706
Atarax, 170
Atazanavir, **396**
Atenolol, **97**
Atimos Modulite, 145
Ativan, 210
Atomoxetine, **212**
Atorvastatin, **123**
Atovaquone, **358**
Atovaquone with proguanil hydrochloride, **371**
Atracurium besilate, **767**
Atracurium besylate, *see* Atracurium besilate
Atrial fibrillation, 69
Atrial flutter, 69
Atriance, 508
Atrolak XL, 238
Atropine sulfate, **624**, **764**
Atropine sulfate with diphenoxylate hydrochloride, *see* Co-phenotrope
Atrovent preparations, 144
Attention deficit hyperactivity disorder, 212
Atypical haemolytic uraemic syndrome and paroxysmal nocturnal haemoglobinuria, 527
Audavate, 689
Audmonal, 58
Augmentin preparations, 324
Aureocort, 696
Autopen products, 432
AutoSense, 428

Avamys, 653
Avaxim, 749
Aveeno, 668, 671
Aviticol, 589
Aviva, 428
Avloclor, 373
Avoca, 722
Avomine, 250
Axorid, 612
Ayendi, 261
Aymes Shake, 936
Azactam, 313
Azapress, 485
Azathioprine, **485**
Azelaic acid, **711**
Azelastine hydrochloride, **621**
Azelastine with fluticasone, *see*
  Fluticasone with azelastine
Azidothymidine, *see* Zidovudine
Azithromycin, **308**, **630**
Azopt, 639
Aztreonam, **313**
AZT, *see* Zidovudine
Azyter, 630
Azzalure, 243

B

Babyhaler, 161
Bacillus calmette-guérin vaccine, **744**
Bacitracin with polymyxin B, **677**
Baclofen, **603**
Bacterial eye infection, 630
Bacterial infection, 281
Bacterial skin infections, 675
Bactroban, 651, 678
Balance Activ, 481
Balneum products, 670, 673
Balsalazide sodium, **26**
Barkat products, 955, 956, 957
Barrier creams and ointments, **667**
Barrier preparations, 666, 667
Basiliximab, **492**
BCG Vaccine, *see* Bacillus calmette-
  guérin vaccine
Beacita, 63
Beclometasone dipropionate, **150**, **652**,
  688
Beclometasone dipropionate, *see*
  Beclometasone dipropionate
Beconase, 652
Bedranol SR, 97
Bee Venom, 172
Bee venom extract, **172**
Benadryl products, 164, 165
Bendrofluazide, *see* Bendroflumethiazide
Bendroflumethiazide, **102**
BeneFIX, 78
Benepali, 601
Benoxinate hydrochloride, *see*
  Oxybuprocaine hydrochloride
Benzalkonium chloride, **715**
Benzhexol hydrochloride, *see*
  Trihexyphenidyl hydrochloride
Benzoates, 572, 682
Benzodiazepine antagonists, 794
Benzodiazepines, 184, **205**, 209, 212, 218,
  763, 774, 790
Benzodiazepine toxicity, 794
Benzoic acid with salicylic acid, **682**
Benzoin tincture, **177**

Benzoyl peroxide, **710**
  ⊳ With clindamycin, **711**
Benzoyl peroxide and azelaic acid, 708
Benzoyl peroxide with adapalene, *see*
  Adapalene with benzoyl peroxide
Benzydamine hydrochloride, **660**
Benzyl benzoate with bismuth oxide,
  bismuth subgallate, hydrocortisone
  acetate, peru balsam and zinc oxide, **64**
Benzyl benzoate with bismuth oxide,
  hydrocortisone acetate, peru balsam,
  pramocaine hydrochloride and zinc
  oxide, **64**
Benzylpenicillin sodium, **318**
Beractant, **178**
Berinert P, 171
Beta-adrenoceptor blockers (systemic),
  95
  ⊳ Alpha- and beta-adrenoceptor
    blockers, 116
  ⊳ Arrhythmias, 94
  ⊳ Heart failure, 94
  ⊳ Hypertension, 94
  ⊳ Other uses, 94
  ⊳ Thyrotoxicosis, 94
Beta-blockers (eye), 636
Beta-blocker toxicity, 790
Betacap, 689
Beta-Cardone, 75
BetaCare, 706
Betacarotene, **706**
Betachek products, 428
Betadine, 717
Betagan, 637
Betaine, **566**
Beta₂ agonists, 141
Betamethasone, **409**, **622**, **645**, **652**, **660**,
  688
  ⊳ With clioquinol, **694**
  ⊳ With clotrimazole, **694**
  ⊳ With fusidic acid, **695**
  ⊳ With neomycin, **623**, **646**, **651**, **695**
  ⊳ With salicylic acid, **695**
Betamethasone with calcipotriol, *see*
  Calcipotriol with betamethasone
Beta-Prograne, 97
Beta-₂-adrenoceptor agonists, selective,
  144
  ⊳ Selective beta₂-agonists (long-acting),
    144
  ⊳ Selective beta₂-agonists (short-
    acting), 146
Betaxolol, **637**
Betnesol preparations, 622, 623, 645, 646,
  651, 652
Betnovate, 689
Betoptic, 637
Bettamousse, 689
Bexsero, 746
Bezafibrate, **121**
Bezalip preparations, 121
BGStar, 428
Bicarbonate, 544, 647
Bicarbonate and trometamol, 543
Biguanides, 419, 420
Bilastine, **164**
Bile acids, 59
Biliary disorders, 59
  ⊳ Bile acid sequestrants, 59, **120**

  ⊳ Drugs affecting biliary composition
    and flow, 59
  ⊳ Pancreatin, 59
  ⊳ Smith-Lemli-Opitz syndrome, 59
Bimizza, 467
Binosto, 437
Bio-Carotene, 706
Biosimilar medicines, 2
Biotene Oralbalance, 654
Biotest, 554
Biotin, **584**
BioXtra, 654
Biphasic insulin
  ⊳ Aspart, **423**
  ⊳ Lispro, **423**
  ⊳ Isophane, **422**
Bipolar disorder and mania, 217
Biquelle XL, 238
Bisacodyl, **40**
Bisphosphonates, **435**
Bladder and urinary disorders, 456
Bladder instillations and urological
  surgery, 460
  ⊳ Bladder infection, 460
  ⊳ Dissolution of blood clots, 460
  ⊳ Maintenance of indwelling urinary
    catheters, 461
Bleeding disorders, 76
Bleo-Kyowa, 509
Bleomycin, **509**
Blephagel, 626
Blerone XL, 458
Blink Intensive, 628
Blood and blood-forming organs, 521
Blood and related products, 77, 554, 564
Blood clots, 81
Blood dyscrasias, 229
Blood glucose lowering drugs, 420
Blood infections, bacterial, 285
  ⊳ Antibacterial therapy for septicaemia
    community-acquired, 285
  ⊳ Antibacterial therapy for septicaemia
    hospital-acquired, 285
  ⊳ Antibacterial therapy for septicaemia
    in neonates, 285
  ⊳ Meningococcal septicaemia, 285
  ⊳ Septicaemia related to vascular
    catheter, 285
Blood monitoring, 428
Blood monitoring test strips, 428
Blood pressure conditions, 90
Bocouture, 243
Body surface area in children (image),
  inside back cover
Bonefos, 438
Bone-marrow suppression, 496
Bone metabolism, 435
  ⊳ Bisphosphonates, 435
  ⊳ Calcitonin, 435
  ⊳ Corticosteroid-induced osteoporosis,
    435
  ⊳ Disorders of bone metabolism, 435
  ⊳ Osteoporosis, 435
Bone metastases, 18
Bone resorption inhibitors, 439
Bonjela, 661
Boostrix-IPV, 744
Borderline substances, 666, 719
Boric acid with salicylic acid and tannic
  acid, **682**

Bosentan, **111**
Botox, 243
Botulinum toxin type A, **243**
Botulism antitoxin, **730**, 734
Bowel cleansing, 32
Bowel cleansing preparations, 35
Bowel colic and excessive respiratory secretions, 21
Bradycardia, 69
Bramitob, 295
Breeze 2, 428
Brevibloc, 98
Brevinor, 471
Brevoxyl, 710
Bricanyl preparations, 148
Bridion, 770
Brinzolamide, **639**
Broad-spectrum penicillins, 289, 316
Brochlor, 632
Brolene products, 627, 632
Bronchodilators, 141
▸ Antimuscarinic bronchodilators, 141
▸ Beta₂ agonists, 141
▸ Compound bronchodilator preparations, 141
▸ Long-acting beta2 agonists, 141
▸ Oral, 141
▸ Parenteral, 141
▸ Short-acting beta₂ agonists, 141
▸ Theophylline, 141
Brufen preparations, 610
Buccastem, 252
Buccolam, 212
Buclizine hydrochloride with codeine phosphate with paracetamol, see Paracetamol with buclizine hydrochloride and codeine phosphate
Budelin Novolizer, 151
Budenofalk, 30
Budesonide, 30, **151**, **652**
▸ With formoterol, **152**
Bulk-forming laxatives, 35, 36
Bumetanide, **132**
Bupivacaine hydrochloride, **778**
Bupivacaine with adrenaline, **779**
Buprenorphine, **257**
Buscopan, 58
Busilvex, 497
Buspirone, 275
Busulfan, **497**
Busulphan, see Busulfan

C

Cacit preparations, 552, 591
Caelyx, 502
Caffeine citrate, **179**
Calamine with zinc oxide, **707**
Cala Soothe, 707
Calceos, 590
Calcichew products, 552, 590
Calci-D, 590
Calciferol, see Ergocalciferol
Calcineurin inhibitors and related drugs, 486, 701
Calcipotriol, **704**
▸ With betamethasone, **689**
Calcitonin (salmon), **439**
Calcitriol, **588**, **704**
Calcium, 551, 552, 558
Calcium acetate, **558**

Calcium and vitamin D, see Ergocalciferol with calcium lactate and calcium phosphate
Calcium carbonate, **552**
▸ With calcium lactate gluconate, **552**
Calcium carbonate with colecalciferol, see Colecalciferol with calcium carbonate
Calcium carbonate with sodium alginate and sodium bicarbonate, see Sodium alginate with calcium carbonate and sodium bicarbonate
Calcium-channel blockers, 80, 98, **99**, 136, 790
Calcium chloride, **553**
Calcium chloride with potassium chloride, sodium chloride and sodium lactate, see Potassium chloride with calcium chloride and sodium chloride and sodium lactate
Calcium gluconate, **553**
Calcium imbalance, 551
Calcium lactate, **554**
Calcium lactate gluconate with calcium carbonate, see Calcium carbonate with calcium lactate gluconate
Calcium lactate with calcium phosphate and ergocalciferol, see Ergocalciferol with calcium lactate and calcium phosphate
Calcium phosphate, **554**
Calcium phosphate with calcium lactate and ergocalciferol, see Ergocalciferol with calcium lactate and calcium phosphate
Calcium phosphate with colecalciferol, see Colecalciferol with calcium phosphate
Calcium polystyrene sulfonate, **559**
Calcium regulating drugs, 439
Calcium Resonium, 560
Calcium salts, **552**
Calcium supplements, 551
Calcort, 410
Calfovit D3, 591
Calmurid, 673
Calogen products, 949, 951
Caloreen, 948
Calpol preparations, 256
Calprofen, 610
Calshake, 951
Camcolit, 220
Camouflagers, 719
Canakinumab, **491**
Cancidas, 350
Candesartan cilexetil, **106**
Candidiasis, 348, 674
Canesten (clotrimazole), 481, 645, 678
Canesten (fluconazole), 353
Canesten HC, 698
Canesten Hydrocortisone, 698
Cannibinoids, 245
Capasal, 700
Capexion, 491
Capimune, 487
Capoten, 104
Capsorin, 487
Captopril, **103**
Carbagen, 186
Carbaglu, 572
Carbamazepine, **184**, 218

Carbamazepine and related antiepileptics, 183
Carbapenems, 295
Carbidopa with levodopa, see Co-careldopa
Carbimazole, **452**
Carbocisteine, **175**
Carbomers, **625**
Carbomix, 793
Carbonic anhydrase inhibitors, 638
Carbonic anhydrase inhibitors and systemic drugs, 636
Carbon monoxide, 791
Carboplatin, **509**
Carboxylic acids, 481
Cardene preparations, 100
Cardiac arrest, 128
Cardiac glycosides, 75
▸ Digoxin, 75
▸ Digoxin-specific antibody, 75
Cardiac prostheses, 285
Cardiopulmonary resuscitation, 128
▸ Paediatric advanced life support, 128
Cardiovascular system infections, antibacterial therapy, 285
▸ Endocarditis caused by enterococci (e.g. Enterococcus faecalis), 286
▸ Endocarditis caused by Haemophilus, Actinobacillus, Cardiobacterium, Eikenella, and Kingella species ('HACEK' micro-organisms), 286
▸ Endocarditis caused by staphylococci, 285
▸ Endocarditis: initial 'blind' therapy, 285
▸ Native-valve endocarditis caused by fully-sensitive streptococci (e.g. viridans streptococci), 285
▸ Native-valve endocarditis caused by less-sensitive streptococci, 286
▸ Prosthetic valve endocarditis caused by streptococci, 286
Cardozin XL, 459
Cardura preparations, 459
Care of stoma, 68
CareSens N, 428
Carexil, 268
Carglumic acid, **571**
Carmeleze, 626
Carmellose, 626
Carmellose sodium, **626**
Carmize, 626
Carnitine deficiency, 564
Carnitine, see Levocarnitine
Carnitor, 565
Carteolol hydrochloride, **637**
Carvedilol, **116**
Caspofungin, **350**
Castor oil with collodion and colophony, **719**
Catacrom, 622
Catapres, 94
Catheter maintenance solutions, 461
▸ OptiFlo products, 461
▸ Uro-Tainer products, 461
Cautionary and advisory labels for dispensed medicines, 966
Cayston, 313
Ceanel, 715
Cefaclor, **299**

Cefadroxil, **298**
Cefalexin, **298**
Cefixime, **300**
Cefotaxime, **301**
Cefradine, **299**
Ceftazidime, **301**
Ceftriaxone, **302**
Cefuroxime, **300**
Celevac, 36
CellCept, 493
Cellusan, 626
Celluvisc, 626
Celsentri, 399
Centrally acting antihypertensive drugs, 91
Centrally acting sympathomimetics, 212
 ‣ Amfetamines, 215
Central nervous system infections, bacterial, 286
 ‣ Antibacterial therapy for meningitis caused by group B streptococcus, 286
 ‣ Antibacterial therapy for meningitis caused by Listeria, 287
 ‣ Antibacterial therapy for meningitis caused by Haemophilus influenzae, 286
 ‣ Antibacterial therapy for meningitis caused by meningococci, 286
 ‣ Antibacterial therapy for meningitis caused by pneumococci, 286
 ‣ Antibacterial therapy for meningitis: initial empirical therapy, 286
Cephalexin, see Cefalexin
Cephalosporins, 289, **297**
 ‣ Cephalosporins, first-generation, 298
 ‣ Cephalosporins, second-generation, 299
 ‣ Cephalosporins, third-generation, 300
Cephradine, see Cefradine
Ceporex, 298
Ceprotin, 80
Cepton, 717
Cerazette, 474
Cerelle, 474
Cerezyme, 566
Cernevit, 578
Cerumol (olive oil), 647
Cervarix, 752
C1-esterase inhibitor, **174**
Cetirizine hydrochloride, **164**
Cetraben, 669, 671
Cetrimide with chlorhexidine, see Chlorhexidine with cetrimide
Cetrimide with undecenoic acid, **715**
Changes, xix
Charcoal, activated, **793**
Charcodote, 793
Chelates and complexes, 50
 ‣ Sucralfate, 50
Chenodeoxycholic acid, **59**
Childhood immunisation, 737
Children with unknown or incomplete immunisation history, 731
Chirocaine, 780
Chloral and derivatives, 275
Chloral hydrate, **275**
Chlorambucil, **498**
Chloramphenicol, **334**, **631**, **645**
ChloraPrep, 718
Chlorhexidine, **656**, **717**
 ‣ Gluconate with isopropyl alcohol, **718**

 ‣ With cetrimide, **718**
 ‣ With chlorobutanol, **656**
Chlorhexidine hydrochloride with hydrocortisone and nystatin, see Hydrocortisone with chlorhexidine hydrochloride and nystatin
Chlorhexidine with neomycin, **650**
Chlorhexidine with nystatin, **681**
Chlorobutanol and arachis oil, see Arachis oil with chlorobutanol
Chlorobutanol with chlorhexidine, see Chlorhexidine with chlorobutanol
Chloromycetin, 632
Chloroquine, 363, **372**
 ‣ With proguanil, **373**
Chlorothiazide, **103**
Chlorphenamine maleate, **168**
Chlorpheniramine maleate, see Chlorphenamine maleate
Chlorpromazine hydrochloride, **230**
Chlortalidone, **134**
Chlortetracycline with triamcinolone, **696**
Chlorthalidone, see Chlortalidone
Cholecalciferol, see Colecalciferol
Cholera vaccine, 734, **745**
Cholesterol, **61**
Cholesterol absorption inhibitors, 121
Cholestyramine, see Colestyramine
Cholic acid, **60**
Choline salicylate, **661**
Choragon, 443
Chorionic gonadotrophin, **443**
Chronic bowel disorders, 24
 ‣ Irritable bowel syndrome, 24
 ‣ Clostridium difficile infection, 24
 ‣ Malabsorption syndromes, 24
Chronic constipation, 35
Chronic facial pain, 275
Chronic hepatitis B, 377
Chronic hepatitis C, 378
Chronic hypoglycaemia, 433, 434
Chronic otitis media, 644
Ciclesonide, **152**
Ciclosporin, **486**
Cidomycin, 293
Cilastatin with imipenem, see Imipenem with cilastatin
Cilest, 471
Cilique, 471
Ciloxan, 631
Cimizt, 467
Cinchocaine hydrochloride with fluocortolone caproate and fluocortolone pivalate, **64**
Cinchocaine with hydrocortisone, **65**
Cinchocaine with prednisolone, **65**
Cinnarizine, **249**
Cinryze, 174
Cipramil, 223
Ciprofloxacin, **328**, **630**
Ciproxin, 329
Circadin, 276
Cisatracurium, **768**
Cisplatin, **510**
Citalopram, **222**
Citanest, 784
 ‣ With Octapressin, 784
Citramag, 33
Citric acid, **177**
 ‣ With magnesium carbonate, **33**

 ‣ Potassium citrate, **460**
Citrulline, **572**
Clairette, 710
Clarelux, 690
Clarie XL, 310
Clarithromycin, **309**
Clarityn (Loratadine), 167
Clasteon, 438
Clavulanic acid with amoxicillin, see Co-amoxiclav
Clavulanic acid with ticarcillin, see Ticarcillin with clavulanic acid
Clenil Modulite, 150
Cleosensa, 468
Clexane, 87
ClikSTAR, 432
Clindamycin, 289, **307**, **480**, **710**
Clindamycin with benzoyl peroxide, see Benzoyl peroxide with clindamycin
Clindamycin with tretinoin, see Tretinoin with clindamycin
Clinipod, 719
Clinitas, 628
Clinitas Carbomer, 626
Clioquinol with betamethasone, see Betamethasone with clioquinol
Clioquinol with flumetasone pivalate, **646**
Clioquinol with fluocinolone acetonide, see Fluocinolone acetonide with clioquinol
ClobaDerm, 690
Clobavate, 690
Clobazam, **205**
Clobetasol propionate, **690**
 ‣ With neomycin sulfate and nystatin, **696**
Clobetasone butyrate, **690**
 ‣ With nystatin and oxytetracycline, **696**
Clofarabine, **504**
Clonazepam, **206**
Clonidine hydrochloride, **93**
Closure of the ductus arteriosus, 134
Clotrimazole, **481**, **645**, **678**
Clotrimazole with betamethasone, see Betamethasone with clotrimazole
Clotrimazole with hydrocortisone, see Hydrocortisone with clotrimazole
Clozapine, **235**
Clozaril, 236
Cluster headache and the trigeminal autonomic cephalalgias, 272
Coagulation factor deficiencies, 77
Coagulation proteins, 77
Coal tar, **700**
 ‣ With arachis oil extract of coal tar, cade oil, light liquid paraffin and tar, **700**
 ‣ With coconut oil and salicylic acid, **700**
 ‣ With dithranol and salicylic acid, **700**
 ‣ With lecithin, **701**
 ‣ With salicylic acid and precipitated sulfur, **701**
 ‣ With zinc oxide, **701**
Co-amoxiclav, **323**
Cobalin, 535
Cocaine, 791
Co-careldopa, **242**
Co-codamol, **258**

Cocois, 701
Co-cyprindiol, **709**
Co-danthramer, **40**
Co-danthrusate, **41**
Codeine phosphate, **259**
Codeine phosphate with buclizine hydrochloride and paracetamol, *see* Paracetamol with buclizine hydrochloride and codeine phosphate
Codeine phosphate with paracetamol, *see* Co-codamol
Codipar, 259
Co-dydramol, **260**
Coeliac disease, 580
Co-enzyme Q10, *see* Ubidecarenone
Co-fluampicil, **322**
Colazide, 26
Colecalciferol, **589**
  › With calcium carbonate, **590**
  › With calcium phosphate, **591**
Colestid, 120
Colestipol hydrochloride, **120**
Colestyramine, **120**
Colgate products, 658, 659
Colief, 954
Colifoam, 412
Colistimethate sodium, **326**
Colistin sulfomethate sodium, *see* Colistimethate sodium
Collodions, 719
Collodion with castor oil and colohony, *see* Castor oil with collodion and colophony
Colofac, 58
Colofac MR, 59
Colomycin, 327
Colpermin, 32
Co-magaldrox, **47**
Combined hormonal contraceptives, 461, **465**
Combivir, 395
Compact, 428
Complan Shake, 939
Complement regulatory proteins, 174
Compound analgesic preparations, 253
Compound bronchodilator preparations, 141
Compound, Hartmann's Solution for Injection, *see* Potassium chloride with calcium chloride and sodium chloride and sodium lactate
Compound topical preparations, 674
Concerta XL, 215
Condyline, 721
Conotrane, 667
Conscious sedation for clinical procedures, 773
Constipation, 34
  › Bowel cleansing preparations, 35
  › Bulk-forming laxatives, 35
  › Chronic constipation, 35
  › Faecal softeners, 35
  › Laxatives drugs, 35
  › Osmotic laxatives, 35
  › Pregnancy, 35
  › Stimulant laxatives, 35
Constipation and bowel cleansing, 32
Contact lenses and drug treatment, 620
Contiflo XL, 460
Contour products, 428

Contraception, 461
  › Combined, 465
  › Devices, 471
  › Emergency, 473
  › Oral progestogen-only, 474
  › Parenteral progestogen-only, 477
  › Spermicidal, 479
Contraceptive devices, 471
Contraceptives, hormonal, 461
  › Choice, 462
  › Combined hormonal contraceptives, 461
  › Emergency contraception, 463
  › Hormonal methods, 463
  › Intra–uterine device, 463
  › Intra-uterine progestogen-only device, 463
  › Oral progestogen-only contraceptives, 463
  › Parenteral progestogen-only contraceptives, 463
  › Progestogen-only contraceptives, 463
  › Reason to stop immediately, 462
  › Surgery, 463
Contraceptives, interactions, 464
  › Antibacterials that do not induce liver enzymes, 464
  › Combined hormonal contraceptives interactions, 464
  › Hormonal emergency contraception interactions, 464
  › Oral progestogen-only contraceptives interactions, 464
  › Parenteral progestogen-only contraceptives interactions, 464
Controlled drugs and drug dependence, 8
Control of microbial contamination, 619
Control of the epilepsies, 180
Convulex, 201
Convulsions, 20, 787
Convulsive status epilepticus, 184
Co-phenotrope, **44**
Copper absorption inhibitors, 573
Copper chelators, 574
Cordarone X, 73
Corsodyl, 656
Corticorelin, **442**
Corticosteroid combinations with anti-infectives, 651
Corticosteroid-induced osteoporosis, 435
Corticosteroid responsive conditions, 405
Corticosteroids, 30, 64, 149, 340, 405, 616, 620, 622, 645, 648, 651, 659, 660, 686
  › Corticosteroid combinations with anti-infectives, 623, 646, 694
Corticosteroids and other immunosuppressants, 483
Corticosteroids, general use, 405
  › Glucocorticoid side effects, 406
  › Managing side-effects, 406
  › Mineralocorticoid side effects, 406
  › Side-effects, 406
Corticosteroids, inflammatory disorders, 616
  › Local corticosteroid injections, 616
  › Systemic corticosteroids, 616
Corticosteroids (inhaled), **149**
Corticosteroids (intranasal), **651**
Corticosteroids, replacement therapy, 407
Corticosteroids (systemic), **407**

Corticosteroids (topical), **687**
Corticotrophin-releasing hormone, *see* Corticorelin
Corticotrophins, 441
Co-simalcite, **47**
Cositam XL, 459
Cosmegen, 509
CosmoCol, 39
CosmoFer, 529
Cosopt, 640
Co-trimoxazole, **330**
Cough preparations, 176, 177
Cough suppressants, 176
Covermark products, 720
Cozaar, 107
Crab lice, 675
Crackers, crispbreads, and breadsticks (ACBS), 956
Creon, 67
Crestor, 125
CRH, *see* Corticorelin
Crisantaspase, **512**
Cromoglicate and related therapy, 157
Cromolux, 622
Crotamiton, **707**
Croup, 142
Cryptococcosis, 348
Crystacide, 718
CS spray, 792
Cuplex, 723
Cuprofen, 610
Curasept, 656
Curatoderm, 705
Curosurf, 178
Cushing's Syndrome, 414
Cushing's syndrome and disease, 414
Cutivate, 692
CX, 717
Cyanides, 791
Cyanide toxicity, 793
Cyanocobalamin, **534**
Cyanokit, 535
Cyclic AMP phosphodiesterase III inhibitors, 540
Cyclimorph, 267
Cyclizine, **244**
Cyclizine with morphine, *see* Morphine with cyclizine
Cyclopentolate hydrochloride, **625**
Cyclophosphamide, **498**
Cycloserine, **344**
Cyclosporin, *see* Ciclosporin
Cyklokapron, 77
Cymevene, 384
Cyprostat, 451
Cyproterone acetate, **450**
Cyproterone acetate with ethinylestradiol, *see* Co-cyprindiol
Cystadane, 567
Cystagon, 569
Cysteamine, *see* Mercaptamine
Cystic fibrosis, 175, 291
Cysticide, 362
Cystinuria, 574
Cystrin, 457
Cytacon, 534
Cytarabine, **504**
Cytokine modulators, 25, 595
Cytomegalovirus infection, 381, 383
Cytotoxic antibiotics, 497

Cytotoxic antibiotics and related substances, 509
Cytotoxic chemotherapy, palliative care, and migraine, 244
Cytotoxic drug-induced side effects, 515
Cytotoxic drugs, 494
 ‣ Alopecia, 496
 ‣ Antimetabolites, 497
 ‣ Asparaginase, 497
 ‣ Bone-marrow suppression, 496
 ‣ Cytotoxic antibiotics, 497
 ‣ Doses, 495
 ‣ Gastro-intestinal effects, 495
 ‣ Guidelines for handling cytotoxic drugs, 494
 ‣ Hyperuricaemia, 496
 ‣ Important safety information, 495
 ‣ Intrathecal chemotherapy, 495
 ‣ Long-term and delayed toxicity, 496
 ‣ Methotrexate-induced mucositis and myelosuppression, 496
 ‣ Nausea and vomiting, 495
 ‣ Oral mucositis, 495
 ‣ Other antineoplastic drugs, 497
 ‣ Pregnancy and reproductive function, 495
 ‣ Risks of incorrect dosing of oral anti-cancer medicines, 495
 ‣ Safe systems for cytotoxic medicines, 495
 ‣ Side-effects of cytotoxic drugs and their management, 495
 ‣ Thromboembolism, 496
 ‣ Treatment for cytotoxic-induced side effects, 496
 ‣ Tumour lysis syndrome, 496
 ‣ Urothelial toxicity, 496
 ‣ Vinca alkaloids, 497
Cytotoxic responsive malignancy, 494
Cytoxan, 499

D

Dacarbazine, **499**
Dactinomycin, **509**
Daktacort, 698
Daktarin preparations, 663, 679
Dalacin preparations, 307, 480, 710
Dalivit, 584
Dalteparin sodium, **86**
Danaparoid sodium, **85**
Dandrazol, 679
Dantrium, 775
Dantrolene sodium, **775**
Dantron with docusate sodium, *see* Co-danthrusate
Dantron with poloxamer 188, *see* Co-danthramer
Dapsone, **358**
Daraprim, 375
Darbepoetin alfa, **523**
Dario, 428
Dario Lite, 428
Darunavir, **396**
Daunorubicin, **501**
DaunoXome, 502
Daylette, 468
DDAVP, 405
Decapeptyl SR, 441
Defective medicines, 13
Deferasirox, **535**

Deferiprone, **536**
Deferoxamine Mesilate, *see* Desferrioxamine mesilate
Deflazacort, **409**
Deltacortril Enteric, 414
Demeclocycline hydrochloride, **332**
Demorem, 249
Demulcent and expectorant cough preparations, 176
Denela, 782
Dental anaesthesia, 776
Dental and orofacial pain, 252, 604
Dental caries, 657
Dental Practitioners' Formulary, 969
Dentinox Infant, 48
Denzapine, 236
DepoCyte, 504
Depolarising neuromuscular blocking drugs, 766
Depo-Medrone, 412, 617
Depo-Provera, 479
Depression, 221
Derbac-M, 683
Dermabond, 719
Derma Care Hydrocortisone, 693
Dermacolor products, 720
Dermacort, 693
Derma+Flex, 719
Dermalo, 669
Dermamist, 672
Dermatological drugs, 667
Dermatonics once, 673
Dermatophytoses, 674
Dermax, 715
Dermol preparations, 667, 668, 671
Dermovate, 690
Desferal, 537
Desflurane, **761**
Desitrend, 192
Desloratadine, **165**
Desloughing agents, 715
DesmoMelt, 405
Desmopressin, **403**
Desmospray, 405
Desmotabs, 405
Desogestrel, **474**
Desogestrel with ethinylestradiol, *see* Ethinylestradiol with desogestrel
Desomono, 474
Desorex, 474
Desserts, 958
Destolit, 61
Desunin, 589
Detoxifying drugs, 515
Detrusitol preparations, 458
Dexafree, 623
Dexamethasone, **410**, **623**
 ‣ With framycetin sulfate and gramicidin, **624**, **646**
 ‣ With glacial acetic acid and neomycin sulfate, **646**
 ‣ With hypromellose, neomycin and polymyxin B sulfate, **624**
Dexamfetamine sulfate, **215**
Dexamphetamine sulfate, *see* Dexamfetamine sulfate
Deximune, 487
Dexsol, 410

Dextran 70 with hypromellose, *see* Hypromellose with dextran 70
Dextrogel, 550
Dextrose Monohydrate, *see* Glucose
DF 118, 262
D-Gam, 726
DHC Continus, 262
Diabact UBT, 56
Diabetes, 229, 415
 ‣ Diabetic nephropathy, 416
 ‣ Diabetic neuropathy, 416
 ‣ Driving, 416
 ‣ Measurement of HbA$_{1c}$, 416
 ‣ Prevention of diabetic complications, 416
 ‣ Treatment of diabetes, 416
Diabetes and surgery, 418
Diabetes, diagnosis and monitoring, 428
Diabetes insipidus, 403
Diabetes mellitus, 415
Diabetes mellitus and hypoglycaemia, 415
Diabetes mellitus, diagnostic and monitoring devices, 428
 ‣ Blood monitoring, 428
 ‣ Oral glucose tolerance test, 428
 ‣ Urinalysis, 428
Diabetic ketoacidosis, 416
Diacomit, 198
Dialamine, 950
Dialysis, 16
Diamicron, 421
Diamorphine hydrochloride, **261**
Diamox preparations, 639
Dianette, 710
Diarrhoea, 43
Diastix, 428, 432
Diatrizoates, *see* Meglumine amidotrizoate with sodium amidotrizoate
Diazemuls, 208
Diazepam, **207**
Diazoxide, **434**
Diclofenac potassium, **605**
Diclofenac sodium, **605**, **635**
Dicloflex preparations, 607
Diclomax preparations, 607
Dicobalt edetate, **793**
Dicyclomine hydrochloride, *see* Dicycloverine hydrochloride
Dicycloverine hydrochloride, **57**
 ‣ With aluminium hydroxide, magnesium oxide and simeticone, **57**
Didanosine, **392**
Dienogest with estradiol valerate, **467**
Dietary supplements for oral use, 579
Diethylcarbamazine, **360**
Diethyl phthalate with methyl salicylate, **718**
Differin, 711
Difflam, 660
Diffundox XL, 460
Diflucan, 353
Diflucortolone valerate, **690**
DigiFab, 795
Digoxin, 68, **75**
Digoxin-specific antibody, 75, **795**
Digoxin toxicity, 795
Dihydrocodeine tartrate, **262**
Dihydrocodeine with paracetamol, *see* Co-dydramol

1,25-Dihydroxycholecalciferol, *see* Calcitriol
Dilacort, 414
Diloxanide furoate, **281**
Diltiazem hydrochloride, **136**
Dimeticone, **682**
Dinoprostone, **135**
Dioctyl, 43
Dioctyl sodium sulphosuccinate, *see* Docusate sodium
Dioderm, 693
Dioralyte preparations, 551
Diovan, 108
Dipeptiven, 578
Diphenoxylate hydrochloride with atropine sulfate, *see* Co-phenotrope
Diphtheria antitoxin, **730**
Diphtheria vaccine, 734
Diphtheria with haemophilus influenzae type b vaccine, pertussis, poliomyelitis and tetanus, **743**
Diphtheria with pertussis, poliomyelitis vaccine and tetanus, **743**
Diphtheria with poliomyelitis and tetanus vaccine, **744**
Diprivan, 760
Diprobase, 671, 672
Diprosalic, 695
Diprosone, 689
Dip/Ser, *see* Diphtheria antitoxin
Dipyridamole, **84**
Disease-modifying anti-rheumatic drugs, 596
Disease-specific immunoglobulins, 725
Disodium hydrogen citrate with glucose, potassium chloride and sodium chloride, **550**
Disorders of bone metabolism, 435
Disorders of gastric acid and ulceration, 46
Dissolution of blood clots, 460
Distaclor, 299
Distaclor MR, 299
Distamine, 574
Dithranol, **699**
▸ With salicylic acid and zinc oxide, **699**
Dithranol with coal tar and salicylic acid, *see* Coal tar with dithranol and salicylic acid
Dithrocream, 699
Ditropan, 457
Diuresal, 133
Diuretics, 68, 130
▸ Heart failure, 130
▸ Loop diuretics, 131
▸ Potassium-sparing diuretics and aldosterone antagonists, 131
▸ Potassium-sparing diuretics with other diuretics, 131
▸ Thiazides and related diuretics, 130
▸ With potassium, 131
▸ Other diuretics, 131
Dixarit, 94
Dobutamine, **113**
DocOmega, 962
Docusate sodium, **43**, **647**
Docusate sodium with dantron, *see* Co-danthrusate
Docusol, 43
Dolmatil, 233

Dolutegravir, **387**
Dolutegravir with abacavir and lamivudine, *see* Abacavir with dolutegravir and lamivudine
Domiciliary oxygen, 142
Domperidone, **245**
Dopamine hydrochloride, **114**
Dopamine precursors, 242
Dopamine receptor antagonists, 245
Dopaminergic drugs used in dystonias, 240
Dorisin XL, 124
Dornase alfa, **175**
Dorzolamide, **639**
▸ With timolol, **640**
Dose of intramuscular injection of adrenaline (epinephrine) for the emergency treatment of anaphylaxis by healthcare professionals, 163
Doublebase preparations, 669
Dovobet, 689
Dovonex, 704
Doxadura preparations, 459
Doxazosin, **458**
Doxepin, **225**, **707**
Doxorubicin hydrochloride, **502**
Doxorubin, 502
Doxycycline, **332**, **662**
Doxzogen XL, 459
Drapolene, 667
Dravet syndrome, 182
Dretine, 468
Driclor, 706
Dried prothrombin complex, **77**
Droperidol, **251**
Dropodex, 623
Drospirenone with ethinylestradiol, *see* Ethinylestradiol with drospirenone
Droxia, 513
Drug class monographs, xviii
Drug toxicity, 794
Drugs acting on the renin-angiotensin system, 103
Drugs affecting biliary composition and flow, 59
Drugs affecting the ductus arteriosus, 134
▸ Closure of the ductus arteriosus, 134
▸ Maintenance of patency, 134
Drugs affecting the immune response, 25, 595
Drugs affecting the renin-angiotensin system, 92
▸ ACE inhibitors in combination with other drugs, 92
▸ Angiotensin-converting enzyme inhibitors, 92
▸ Angiotensin-II receptor antagonists, 92
▸ Concomitant diuretics, 92
▸ Diabetic nephropathy, 92
▸ Heart failure, 92
▸ Hypertension, 92
▸ Initiation under specialist supervision, 92
▸ Neonates, 92
▸ Renal effects, 92
Drugs and driving, 2
Drugs and sport, 22
Drugs for mania and hypomania, 217
▸ Antipsychotic drugs, 218

▸ Benzodiazepines, 218
▸ Carbamazepine, 218
▸ Lithium, 218
▸ Valproate, 218
Drugs for reversal of neuromuscular blockade, 770
Drugs for urinary retention, 458
▸ Alpha-blockers, 458
Drugs that affect gastric pH, 763
Drugs that enhance neuromuscular transmission, 601
Drugs unsafe for use in acute porphyrias, 562
Dry and scaling skin disorders, 666
Dry eye, 625
▸ Tear deficiency, ocular lubricants, and astringents, 625
Dry mouth, 654
Drytec saline, 548
D4T, *see* Stavudine
Duac, 711
Dukoral, 745
Dulco-Lax (sodium picosulfate), 43
Duocal Super Soluble, 949
Duofilm, 723
Duphalac, 37
Durogesic DTrans, 264
Dyes, 633
Dymista, 653
Dysmenorrhoea, 253
Dysport, 243
Dyspepsia, 46
Dysport, 243
Dystonias and related disorders, 240
▸ Antimuscarinic drugs used in dystonias, 240
▸ Dopaminergic drugs used in dystonias, 240
▸ Drugs used in essential tremor, chorea, tics, and related disorders, 240
▸ Dystonias, 240

E

E45 preparations, 671
EAA®, 962
Ear, 643
▸ Administration, 644
▸ Otitis externa, 643
▸ Otitis media, 643
▸ Removal of ear wax, 644
Ear infections, bacterial, 287
▸ Antibacterial therapy for otitis externa, 287
▸ Antibacterial therapy for otitis media, 287
Earol, 647
Easiphen, 963
Easyhaler preparations (beclometasone), 151
Easyhaler (budesonide), 151
Easyhaler (formoterol), 145
Easyhaler (salbutamol), 147
EBchek, 432
Ebesque XL, 238
E-Caps, 593
Echinocandin antifungals, 349, 350
Eciferol, 591
Econac preparations, 607
Econazole nitrate, **481**, **678**
Ecopace, 105
Eculizumab, **527**

Eczema, 683
▸ Infection, 684
▸ Management of other features of eczema, 684
▸ Medicated bandages, 684
▸ Seborrhoeic dermatitis, 684
▸ Types and management, 683
Eczema and psoriasis, 683
Eczmol, 671
EEA and Swiss prescriptions, 3
Efavirenz, **388**
Efflosomyl XL, 458
Eformoterol fumarate, *see* Formoterol fumarate
Elaprase, 568
Electrolyte replacement therapy, 541
Electrolytes and minerals, 545
Electrolytes and water, 544
Element, 428
Elemental 028 Extra, 929
Elevin, 470
Elidel, 702
Ellaone, 473
Elocon, 694
Elocta, 79
ELOINE, 468
Eltroxin, 454
Elvanse, 216
Emadine, 621
Emedastine, **621**
Emelpin, 672
Emerade, 130
Emergency contraception, 463
Emergency supply of medicines, 7
Emergency treatment of poisoning, 786
▸ Active elimination techniques, 787
▸ Acute overdose, 788
▸ Alcohol, 787
▸ Amfetamines, 791
▸ Antidepressants, 789
▸ Antimalarials, 790
▸ Antipsychotics, 790
▸ Aspirin, 787
▸ Benzodiazepines, 790
▸ Beta blockers, 790
▸ Blood pressure, 786
▸ Body temperature, 787
▸ Calcium-channel blockers, 790
▸ Carbon monoxide, 791
▸ Cocaine, 791
▸ Convulsions, 787
▸ CS spray, 792
▸ Cyanides, 791
▸ Ecstasy, 791
▸ Ethylene glycol and methanol, 791
▸ Further information, 786
▸ General care, 786
▸ Heavy metals, 791
▸ Hospital admission, 786
▸ Insect stings, 792
▸ Iron salts, 790
▸ Lithium, 790
▸ Marine stings, 792
▸ Methaemoglobinaemia, 787
▸ Nerve agents, 792
▸ Noxious gases, 791
▸ Opioids, 788
▸ Organophosphorus insecticides, 792
▸ Other poisons, 793
▸ Paracetamol, 788

▸ Pesticides, 792
▸ Phenothiazines and related drugs, 790
▸ Prevention of absorption, 787
▸ Removal and elimination, 787
▸ Removal from the gastro-intestinal tract, 787
▸ Respiration, 786
▸ Second-generation antipsychotic drugs, 790
▸ Selective serotonin re-uptake inhibitors (SSRIs), 789
▸ Snake bites, 792
▸ Snake bites and animal stings, 792
▸ 'Staggered' overdose, uncertain time of overdose, or therapeutic excess, 788
▸ Stimulants, 791
▸ Sulfur dioxide, chlorine, phosgene, ammonia, 791
▸ Theophylline, 791
▸ Tricyclic and related antidepressants, 789
Emerres, 477
Emeside, 187
Emla, 782
Emollient and barrier preparations, 666
▸ Barrier preparations, 666
▸ Borderline substances, 666
▸ Emollient bath and shower preparations, 666
▸ Emollients, 666
▸ Nappy rash (Dermatitis), 666
Emollient bath and shower products, antimicrobial-containing, **667**
Emollient bath and shower products, colloidal oatmeal-containing, **668**
Emollient bath and shower products, paraffin-containing, **668**
Emollient bath and shower products, soya-bean oil-containing, **670**
Emollient bath and shower products, tar-containing, **670**
Emollient creams and ointments, antimicrobial-containing, **670**
Emollient creams and ointments, colloidal oatmeal-containing, **671**
Emollient creams and ointments, paraffin-containing, **671**
Emollients, urea-containing, **672**
Emollin, 672
Emozul, 53
Emsogen, 939
Emtricitabine, **392**
Emtriva, 392
Emulsiderm, 668
Enalapril maleate, **105**
Enbrel, 601
Enbrel MyClic, 601
Endekay, 658, 659
Endoscopic retrograde cholangiopancreatography, 284
Endothelin receptor antagonists, 111
Energivit, 949
Ener-G products, 955, 956, 957, 958, 959
Enfamil products, 944, 945
Enfuvirtide, **386**
Engerix B, 751
Enkephalinase inhibitors, 44
Enopen, 671
Enoxaparin sodium, **86**

Enoximone, **118**
Enshake, 951
Ensure products, 932, 936, 937, 938
Enteral nutrition, 578
▸ Clearing blockages, 580
▸ Dietary supplements for oral use, 579
▸ Enteral feeding tubes, 580
▸ Enteral feeds, 579
▸ Feed thickeners, 579
▸ Infant formula feeds, 578
▸ Products for metabolic diseases, 580
▸ Specialised formula, 579
Entocort preparations, 30
E numbers, *inside back cover*
Enzira, 752
Epaderm, 671, 672
Epanutin (Phenytoin), 194, 195
Epanutin (Phenytoin sodium), 195
Epaxal, 749
Ephedrine hydrochloride, **114**, **649**
Epiduo, 712
Epilepsy, 180, 364
▸ Absence seizures, 182
▸ Antiepileptic drugs, 183
▸ Antiepileptic hypersensitivity syndrome, 181
▸ Benzodiazepines, 184
▸ Breast-feeding, 182
▸ Carbamazepine and related antiepileptics, 183
▸ Convulsive status epilepticus, 184
▸ Dravet syndrome, 182
▸ Driving, 181
▸ Epilepsy and Pregnancy Register, 182
▸ Epilepsy syndromes, 182
▸ Ethosuximide, 183
▸ Febrile convulsions, 184
▸ Focal seizures with or without secondary generalisation, 182
▸ Gabapentin, 183
▸ Generalised seizures, 182
▸ Infantile spasms, 182
▸ Interactions, 181
▸ Lamotrigine, 183
▸ Landau-Kleffner syndrome, 183
▸ Lennox-Gastaut syndrome, 182
▸ Levetiracetam, 183
▸ MHRA/CHM advice: Antiepileptic drugs: new advice on switching between different manufacturers' products for a particular drug (November 2013), 180
▸ Monitoring, 181
▸ Myoclonic seizures, 182
▸ Neonatal seizures, 183
▸ Non-convulsive status epilepticus, 184
▸ Phenobarbital and primidone, 183
▸ Phenytoin, 183
▸ Pregnancy, 181
▸ Rufinamide, 183
▸ Status epilepticus, 184
▸ Tonic and atonic seizures, 182
▸ Tonic-clonic seizures, 182
▸ Topiramate, 183
▸ Valproate, 183
▸ Zonisamide, 184
Epilepsy and other seizure disorders, 180
Epilepsy and Pregnancy Register, 182
Epilim preparations, 197

Epinastine hydrochloride, **621**
EpiPen, 130
Epirubicin hydrochloride, **502**
Episenta, 198
Epival CR, 197
Epivir, 393
Epoetin alfa, **524**
Epoetin beta, **525**
Epoetins, **522**
Epoetin zeta, **526**
Epoprostenol, 83, **110**
Eposin, 511
Eprex, 525
Eptacog alfa (activated), *see* Factor VIIa (recombinant)
Equasym XL, 215
Equivalent doses
  ‣ Anti-inflammatory doses of corticosteroids, 407
  ‣ Antipsychotics, oral, 229
  ‣ Opioid analgesics, 19
Erectile dysfunction, 479
Ergamisol, 361
Ergocalciferol, **591**
  ‣ With calcium lactate and calcium phosphate, **591**
Ergoral, 591
Erlibelle, 470
Ertapenem, **295**
Erwinase, 512
Erymax, 312
Erythrocin, 311
Erythrolar, 311
Erythromycin, **310**
Erythromycin with isotretinoin, *see* Isotretinoin with erythromycin
Erythromycin with tretinoin, *see* Tretinoin with erythromycin
  ‣ with zinc acetate, **710**
Erythroped preparations, 311, 312
Erythropoietins, 522
Esmeron, 769
Esmolol hydrochloride, **98**
Esmya, 473
Esomeprazole, **52**
Essential thrombocythaemia, 539, 540
Estradiol with nomegestrol, **467**
Estradiol valerate with dienogest, *see* Dienogest with estradiol valerate
E-Tabs, 592
Etanercept, **600**
Ethambutol hydrochloride, **345**
Ethinylestradiol, **446**
  ‣ With desogestrel, **467**
  ‣ With drospirenone, **468**
  ‣ With etonogestrel, **468**
  ‣ With gestodene, **469**
  ‣ With levonorgestrel, **469**
  ‣ With norelgestromin, **470**
  ‣ With norethisterone, **471**
  ‣ With norgestimate, **471**
Ethinylestradiol with cyproterone acetate, *see* Co-cyprindiol
Ethinyloestradiol, *see* Ethinylestradiol
Ethosuximide, 183, **186**
Ethylene glycol and methanol, 791
Etomidate, **758**
Etomidate-Lipuro, 759
Etonogestrel, **477**

Etonogestrel with ethinylestradiol, *see* Ethinylestradiol with etonogestrel
Etopophos, 511
Etoposide, **510**
Etoricoxib, **607**
Etravirine, **389**
Etrivex, 690
Eucalyptus with menthol, **177**
Eucerin, 673
Eudemine, 434
Eumovate, 690
Eurartesim, 371
European viper snake venom antiserum, **798**
Evacal D3, 590
Everolimus, **519**
Evidence grading, *see* How BNF Publications are constructed
Evoltra, 504
Evolve HA, 628
Evra, 470
Exjade, 536
Exocin, 631
Exorex, 700
Extemporaneous preparation, 6
Exterol, 648
Extract of coal tar with arachis oil, **701**
Extrapyramidal side-effects, 229
Extravasation, 617
Eye, 619
  ‣ Administration of drugs to the eye, 619
  ‣ Contact lenses, 620
  ‣ Contact lenses and drug treatment, 620
  ‣ Control of microbial contamination, 619
  ‣ Eye drops and eye ointments, 619
  ‣ Eye lotions, 619
  ‣ Ophthalmic Specials, 619
  ‣ Other preparations administered to the eye, 619
  ‣ Preservatives and sensitisers, 619
Eye, allergy and inflammation, 620
  ‣ Corticosteroids, 620
  ‣ Other anti-inflammatory preparations, 620
Eye infections, 629
  ‣ With corticosteroids, 629
Eye infections, bacterial, 287
  ‣ Antibacterial therapy for congenital chlamydial conjuctivitis, 287
  ‣ Antibacterial therapy for congenital gonococcal conjunctivitis, 287
  ‣ Antibacterial therapy for purulent conjuctivitis, 287
Eye lotions, 619
Eye procedures, 633
Eye, surgical and peri-operative drug use, 634
  ‣ Local anaesthetics, 634
  ‣ Ocular peri-operative drugs, 634
Eytazox, 639
Ezetimibe, **121**
Ezetimibe with simvastatin, *see* Simvastatin with ezetimibe
Ezetrol, 121

F

Fabrazyme, 565

Fabry's disease, 565
Factor IX fraction, dried, **78**
Factor VIIa (recombinant), **78**
Factor VIII fraction, dried, **78**
Factor VIII inhibitor bypassing fraction, **80**
Factor XIII fraction, dried, **79**
Faecal softeners, 35
Falciparum malaria (treatment), 365
Fanhdi, 79
Faramsil, 459
Fasigyn, 315
Fasturtec, 516
Fate, 959
Faverin, 223
Feanolla, 474
Febrile convulsions, 184
Feed additives, 954
Feed supplements, 948
Feed thickeners, 579
Feed thickeners and pre-thickened drinks, 954
FEIBA Imuno, 80
Feldene, 616
Feldene Melt, 616
Felypressin with prilocaine, *see* Prilocaine with felypressin
Female sex hormone responsive conditions, 446
FemCap, 473
Femodene, 469
Femodette, 469
Fenactol preparations, 607
Fencino, 264
Fendrix, 751
Fenofibrate, **122**
Fentalis, 264
Fentanyl, **262**
Fenticonazole nitrate, **482**
Feospan Spansules, 531
Ferinject, 529
Ferric carboxymaltose, **529**
Ferriprox, 536
Ferrograd preparations, 531, 532
Ferrous fumarate, **530**
Ferrous gluconate, **531**
Ferrous sulfate, **531**
  ‣ With folic acid, **531**
Fersaday, 531
Fexofenadine hydrochloride, **165**
Fibrates, 121
Fibre, vitamin, and mineral supplements, 953
Fibrinogen, dried, **79**
Fibrinolytic drugs, 125
Fibrinolytics, **126**
Fibrogammin P, 79
Fifty:50, 672
Filaricides, 360
Filgrastim, **538**
Finacea, 711
Fistulating Crohn's disease, 25
Flagyl, 315
Flamazine, 677
Flavouring preparations, 955
Flavour Mix, 955
FlavourPac, 955
Flebogammadif, 728
Flecainide acetate, **71**

Flectone XL, 460
Fleet Ready-to-use, 40
Flexbumin, 554
Flexitol, 673
Flixonase, 653
Flixotide preparations, 153
Flolan, 110
Flomax MR, 460
Flomaxtra XL, 460
Flour mixes, 956
Flour mixes and egg substitutes, 959
Flour mixes and xanthan gum, 956
Flowfusor, 718
Fluarix Tetra, 752
Flucloxacillin, **325**
Flucloxacillin with ampicillin, see Co-
    fluampicil
Fluconazole, **352**
Flucytosine, **356**
Fludara, 505
Fludarabine phosphate, **505**
Fludrocortisone acetate, **411**
Fludroxycortide, **691**
Fluenz Tetra, 753
Fluid and electrolyte imbalances, 541
Fluid overload, 130
Fluid requirements for children, 542
Fluids and electrolytes, 541
  ▸ Bicarbonate and trometamol, 543
  ▸ Electrolyte replacement therapy, 541
  ▸ Electrolytes and water, 544
  ▸ Intravenous glucose, 542
  ▸ Intravenous potassium, 543
  ▸ Intravenous sodium, 544
  ▸ Management of hyperkalaemia, 541
  ▸ Oral bicarbonate, 542
  ▸ Oral potassium, 541
  ▸ Oral preparations for fluid and
    electrolyte imbalance, 541
  ▸ Oral rehydration therapy (ORT), 541
  ▸ Oral sodium and water, 541
  ▸ Parenteral preparations for fluid and
    electrolyte imbalance, 544
  ▸ Plasma and plasma substitutes, 543
  ▸ Plasma substitutes, 543
Flumazenil, **794**
Flumetasone pivalate with clioquinol, see
    Clioquinol with flumetasone pivalate
FluMist Quadrivalent, 753
Fluocinolone acetonide, **691**
  ▸ With clioquinol, **696**
  ▸ With neomycin, **697**
Fluocinonide, **692**
Fluocortolone, **692**
Fluocortolone caproate with cinchocaine
    hydrochloride and fluocortolone
    pivalate, see Cinchocaine hydrochloride
    with fluocortolone caproate and
    fluocortolone pivalate
Fluocortolone hexanoate with
    fluocortolone pivalate, **692**
Fluor-a-day, 658
Fluorescein sodium, **633**
Fluorescein with lidocaine, **634**
Fluoride, 657
Fluorometholone, **623**
Fluoxetine, **223**
Flurandrenolone, see Fludroxycortide
Flurbiprofen, **608, 636, 660**

Fluticasone, **152, 652, 692**
  ▸ With azelastine, **653**
  ▸ With formoterol, **153**
  ▸ With salmeterol, **153**
  ▸ With vilanterol, **154**
Flutiform, 153
Fluvastatin, **124**
Fluvoxamine maleate, **223**
FML Liquifilm, 623
Focal seizures with or without secondary
    generalisation, 182
Folates, 515, 533
Folic acid, **533**
Folic acid with ferrous sulphate, see
    Ferrous sulfate with folic acid
Folinic acid, **515**
Fomicyt, 336
Food allergy, 56
Food hygiene, 741
Foodlink Complete, 939
Foods for special diets, 955
Foradil, 145
Forceval, 587
Formaldehyde, **721**
Formoterol fumarate, **144**
Formoterol with budesonide, see
    Budesonide with formoterol
Formoterol with fluticasone, see
    Fluticasone with formoterol
Forticare, 946
Forticreme Complete dessert, 939
Fortijuce, 936
Fortini preparations, 933, 934
Fortisip preparations, 937, 938, 939, 940
Fortum, 302
Fosamax, 437
Fosamprenavir, **397**
Foscarnet sodium, **384**
Foscavir, 384
Fosfomycin, **335**
Fosphenytoin sodium, **187**
Fragmin, 86
Framycetin sulfate, **644**
Framycetin sulfate with dexamethasone
    and gramicidin, see Dexamethasone
    with framycetin sulfate and gramicidin
Frangula with sterculia, see Sterculia with
    frangula
Frebini preparations, 933, 935
Freederm, 714
FreeStyle products, 431
Fresh frozen plasma, **80**
Fresubin products, 928, 929, 930, 931, 936,
    938, 940, 949
Friars' Balsam, see Benzoin tincture
Frisium, 206
FruitiVits, 953
Frusemide, see Furosemide
Frusol, 133
FTC, see Emtricitabine
Fucibet, 695
Fucidin (Fusidic acid), 337
Fucidin H (Fusidic acid / Hydrocortisone),
    698
Fucidin (Sodium fusidate), 337
Fultium-D3, 589, 590
Fungal infections (skin), 678
Fungal infection (systemic), 348
Fungal infections (vulvovaginal), 480
Fungating tumours in palliative care, 20

Fungizone, 352
Furosemide, **132**
Fusidic acid, **336, 632**
Fusidic acid with betamethasone, see
    Betamethasone with fusidic acid
Fusidic acid with hydrocortisone, see
    Hydrocortisone with fusidic acid
Fuzeon, 386
Fybogel preparations, 32, 36
Fycompa, 193
Fyne Dynamics Pinnacle, 161

G

Gabapentin, 183, **187**
Gabitril, 199
GA gel, 959
Galactomin 17, 944
Galactomin 19, 945
Galcodine, 260
Galebon, 460
Galenphol, 177
Galfer, 531
Galpseud, 650
Galsulfase, **567**
Gammagard S/D, 728
Gammanorm, 728
Gammaplex, 729
Gamunex, 729
Ganciclovir, **383**
Gardasil, 752
Gastric and duodenal ulceration, 49
Gastrografin, 32
Gastro-intestinal smooth muscle spasm,
    56
Gastro-intestinal system infections,
    antibacterial therapy, 287
  ▸ Campylobacter enteritis, 287
  ▸ Clostridium difficile infection, 287
  ▸ Gastro-enteritis, 287
  ▸ Necrotising enterocolitis in neonates,
    288
  ▸ Peritonitis, 288
  ▸ Peritonitis: peritoneal dialysis-
    associated, 288
  ▸ Salmonella (non-typhoid), 287
  ▸ Shigellosis, 287
  ▸ Typhoid fever, 287
Gastro-oesophageal reflux disease, 55
  ▸ Pregnancy, 55
Gastroprotective complexes and
    chelators, 50
Gaucher's disease, 566
Gaviscon products, 46, 47
G-CSF, see Filgrastim
Gedarel, 467
Gelaspan, 555
Gelatin, **555**
Gelofusine, 555
Geloplasma, 555
GelTears, 626
General anaesthesia, 757
  ▸ Drugs used for intravenous
    anaesthesia, 757
  ▸ Inhalational anaesthetics, 757
  ▸ Intravenous anaesthetics, 757
  ▸ Malignant hyperthermia, 758
  ▸ Nitrous oxide, 758
  ▸ Total intravenous anaesthesia, 757
  ▸ Volatile liquid anaesthetics, 757
Generalised seizures, 182

Genfura, 348
Genital system infections, antibacterial
therapy, 288
▸ Asymptomatic contacts of patients
with infectious syphilis, 288
▸ Early syphilis (infection of less than
2 years), 288
▸ Gonorrhoea: uncomplicated, 288
▸ Late latent syphilis (asymptomatic
infection of more than 2 years), 288
▸ Neonatal congenital syphilis, 288
▸ Pelvic inflammatory disease, 288
▸ Syphilis, 288
▸ Uncomplicated genital chlamydial
infection, non-gonococcal urethritis,
and non-specific genital infection, 288
Genius products, 955
Genotropin preparations, 444
Gentamicin, 293, 630, **644**
Gentamicin with hydrocortisone, **645**
Gestodene with ethinylestradiol, *see*
Ethinylestradiol with gestodene
Glandosane, 655
Glaucoma, 636
▸ Beta-blockers, 636
▸ Carbonic anhydrase inhibitors and
systemic drugs, 636
▸ Miotics, 636
▸ Prostaglandin analogues, 636
▸ Sympathomimetics, 636
Glaucoma and ocular hypertension, 636
Glibenclamide, **421**
Gliclazide, **421**
Glivec, 520
GlucaGen Hypokit, 434
Glucagon, **433**
GlucoBoost, 550
Glucocorticoid and mineralocorticoid
activity, 407
Glucocorticoid side effects, 406
Glucocorticoid therapy, 407
GlucoDock, 431
Glucoflex-R, 431
GlucoGel, 550
GlucoLab, 431
GlucoMen products, 431, 432
Glucophage, 420
GlucoRx products, 431, 432, 433
Glucose, **549**
Glucose with disodium hydrogen citrate
with potassium chloride and sodium
chloride, *see* Disodium hydrogen citrate
with glucose, potassium chloride and
sodium chloride
Glucose with potassium chloride, sodium
bicarbonate and sodium chloride, **551**
Glucose with sodium chloride, *see* Sodium
chloride with glucose
Glucosylceramide synthase inhibitors,
569
GlucoZen.auto, 431
GluNEO, 431
Glutafin products, 955, 956, 957, 958
Glutaraldehyde, **721**
Glutaric aciduria (type 1), 959
Glutarol, 721
Gluten- and wheat-free foods, 958
Gluten-free foods, 955
Glycerin, *see* Glycerol
Glycerol, **41**

Glyceryl trinitrate, **127**
Glycogenolytic hormones, 433, 434
Glycogen storage disease, 960
Glycopeptide antibacterials, 305
Glycopyrrolate, *see* Glycopyrronium
bromide
Glycopyrronium bromide, **705**, **765**
Glycopyrronium bromide with
neostigmine, *see* Neostigmine with
glycopyrronium bromide
Glycosade, 960
Glypressin, 62
GnRH, *see* Gonadorelin
Golden eye, 632
Gonadorelin, **442**
Gonadotrophin-releasing hormone, *see*
Gonadorelin
Gonadotrophin replacement therapy, 443
Gonadotrophin responsive conditions,
439
Gonadotrophins, 441, 443
Gonadotropin-releasing hormones, 439,
442
Gonapeptyl Depot, 441
Goserelin, **439**
G6PD deficiency, 521
Granisetron, **247**
Granocyte, 539
Griseofulvin, **357**
Grifols, 554
Granulocyte-colony stimulating factors,
537
Grass pollen extract, **172**
Grazax, 173
Grifols, 554
Griseofulvin, **357**
Growth hormone, 441
Growth hormone disorders, 443
Guanfacine, **217**
Guidance
▸ for handling cytotoxic drugs, 494
▸ on intravenous infusions, 14
▸ on prescribing, 1
▸ on treatment of drug misuse, 276
Gygel, 479
Gyno-Daktarin, 482, 679
Gyno-Pevaryl, 482
Gynoxin, 482

H

Haelan, 691
Haem arginate, **564**
Haem derivatives, 564
Haemoctin, 79
Haemonine, 78
Haemophilus influenzae type B conjugate
vaccine, 734
Haemophilus influenzae type B with
meningococcal group C vaccine, **745**
Haemophilus influenza with diphtheria
with pertussis with poliomyelitis and
tetanus, *see* Diphtheria with
haemophilus influenzae type b vaccine,
pertussis, poliomyelitis and tetanus
Haemorrhage, 82
Haemorrhoids, 64
Haldol, 232
Haleraid products, 161
Half Beta-Prograne, 97
Haloperidol, **231**
Havrix, 749
Hayleve, 169

HBVAXPRO, 751
Hc45, 693
HCG, *see* Chorionic gonadotrophin
HCU products, 960
Head lice, 675
Healthy Start Children's Vitamin, 584
Heavy metals poisoning, 791
Hedrin Products, 682
Helicobacter pylori diagnosis, 56
Helicobacter Test INFAI, 56
Helixate NexGen, 79
Helminth infections, 359
▸ Ascaricides (common roundworm
infections), 359
▸ Drugs for cutaneous larva migrans
(creeping eruption), 360
▸ Drugs for hookworms, 360
▸ Drugs for strongyloidiasis, 360
▸ Drugs for tapeworm infections, 359
▸ Drugs for threadworms, 359
▸ Filaricides, 360
▸ Hydatid disease, 359
▸ Schistosomicides (bilharziasis), 360
▸ Specialist centres, 359
▸ Taenicides, 359
Heparin, 83, **85**
▸ Flushes, 83
▸ Toxicity, 795
▸ Unfractionated, **87**
Heparinoid, 83, 85, **720**
Heparon Junior, 946
Hepatect CP, 727
Hepatitis, 377
▸ Chronic hepatitis B, 377
▸ Chronic hepatitis C, 377
▸ Hepatitis A, 724
▸ Hepatitis A and B vaccine, **748**
▸ Hepatitis A vaccine, 735, **749**
▸ Hepatitis A with typhoid vaccine, **749**
▸ Hepatitis B and A vaccine, *see*
Hepatitis A and B vaccine
▸ Hepatitis B immunoglobulin, 725, **727**
▸ Hepatitis B vaccine, 735, **750**
Hepatyrix, 749
Hereditary angioedema, 163
Heroin hydrochloride, *see* Diamorphine
hydrochloride
Heron Foods, 956, 958
Herpes labialis, 674
Herpesvirus infections, 380
▸ Choice, 380
▸ Cytomegalovirus infection, 381
▸ Herpes simplex and varicella–zoster
infection, 380
▸ Herpes simplex infections, 380
▸ Varicella-zoster infections, 380
Hexetidine, **657**
Hibi products, 717
Hiccup in palliative care, 20
Hidrasec, 45
High-energy supplements, 948
▸ Carbohydrate, 948
▸ Fat, 949
▸ Protein, 950
High-fibre supplements, 953
Hirudoid, 720
Histoacryl preparations, 719
Histoplasmosis, 349
HIV-fusion inhibitors, 386

HIV infection, 385
▸ Breast-feeding, 385
▸ Drugs used for HIV infection, 385
▸ Immune reconstitution syndrome, 386
▸ Initiation of treatment, 385
▸ Lipodystrophy syndrome, 386
▸ Neonates, 386
▸ Osteonecrosis, 386
▸ Post-exposure prophylaxis, 385
▸ Pregnancy, 385
▸ Principles of treatment, 385
▸ Switching therapy, 385
HIV-integrase inhibitors, 387
Hizentra, 729
H$_2$-receptor antagonists, 50
Homatropine hydrobromide, **625**
Homocystinuria, 566
Homocystinuria or hypermethioninaemia, 960
Hormonal emergency contraception, 463
Hormone antagonists and related agents, 451
Hormone replacement therapy, 445
Hormone responsive malignancy, 517
Hormone treatment for acne, 709
How BNF Publications are constructed, ix
How to use BNF Publications, xii
H$_2$-receptor antagonists, **50**
5HT1-receptor agonists, 272
Humalog preparations, 424
Human Albumin Solution, *see* Albumin solution
Human chorionic gonadotrophin, *see* Chorionic gonadotrophin
Human coagulation factor VIII, dried, *see* Factor VIII fraction, dried
Human fibrinogen, *see* Fibrinogen, dried
Human fibrin-stabilising factor, dried, *see* Factor XIII fraction, dried
Human growth hormones, 443
Human hemin, *see* Haem arginate
Human papillomavirus vaccines, 736, **751**
Human prothrombin complex, *see* Dried prothrombin complex
HumaPen Luxura HD, 432
Humatrope, 445
Humira, 599
Humulin preparations, 422, 423, 426
Hyabak, 628
Hyaluronidase, **618**
Hycosan, 628
Hydatid disease, 359
Hydralazine hydrochloride, **108**
HydraMed, 628
Hydrea, 513
Hydrex, 717
Hydrocortisone, **411, 616, 661, 692**
▸ With benzalkonium chloride, dimeticone and nystatin, **697**
▸ With chlorhexidine hydrochloride and nystatin, **697**
▸ With clotrimazole, **697**
▸ With fusidic acid, **698**
▸ With miconazole, **698**
▸ With oxytetracycline, **698**
▸ With urea, **693**
Hydrocortisone acetate with benzyl benzoate, bismuth oxide, bismuth subgallate, peru balsam and zinc oxide, *see* Benzyl benzoate with bismuth oxide, bismuth subgallate, hydrocortisone acetate, peru balsam and zinc oxide
Hydrocortisone acetate with benzyl benzoate, bismuth oxide, peru balsam, pramocaine hydrochloride and zinc oxide, *see* Benzyl benzoate with bismuth oxide, hydrocortisone acetate, peru balsam, pramocaine hydrochloride and zinc oxide
Hydrocortisone butyrate, **693**
Hydrocortisone with cinchocaine, *see* Cinchocaine with hydrocortisone
Hydrocortisone with gentamicin, *see* Gentamicin with hydrocortisone
Hydrocortisone with lidocaine, **65**
Hydrocortisone with pramocaine, **66**
Hydrocortistab, 616
Hydrogen peroxide, **657, 718**
Hydrolysate Formula, 934
Hydromol products, 669, 672, 673
Hydromoor, 628
Hydromorphone hydrochloride, **265**
Hydrotalcite with simeticone, *see* Co-simalcite
Hydroxocobalamin, **534**
Hydroxycarbamide, **512**
Hydroxychloroquine sulfate, **596**
1α-Hydroxycholecalciferol, *see* Alfacalcidol
Hydroxyethylcellulose, **626**
Hydroxypropyl guar with polyethylene glycol and propylene glycol, **626**
Hydroxyzine hydrochloride, **169**
Hylo-Comod, 628
Hylo-fresh, 628
Hy-Opti, 628
Hyoscine butylbromide, **57**
Hyoscine hydrobromide, **250**
Hypercalciuria, 552
Hyperhidrosis, 705
Hyperkalaemia, 559
▸ Management of, 541
Hyperlipidaemia, 119
HYPER LYS Anamix Infant, 960
Hyperlysinaemia, 960
Hyperphosphataemia, 558
Hyperprolactinaemia, 228
Hypersal, 628
Hypertension, 90, 92, 94
▸ Hypertension in diabetes, 90
▸ Hypertension in pregnancy, 90
▸ Hypertension in renal disease, 90
▸ Hypertensive emergencies, 90
▸ Other measures to reduce cardiovascular risk, 90
▸ Phaeochromocytoma, 90
▸ Pulmonary hypertension, 90
Hypertensive crises, 109
Hyperthyroidism, 451
Hyperuricaemia, 496
Hyperuricaemia associated with cytotoxic drugs, 516
Hypnomidate, 759
Hypnotics, 275
Hypnotics and anxiolytics, 275
▸ Antihistamines, 275
▸ Anxiolytics, 275
▸ Buspirone, 275
▸ Chloral and derivatives, 275
▸ Dental procedures, 275
▸ Hypnotics, 275
▸ Melatonin, 275
Hypnotics, sedatives and anxiolytics, 205, 209, 275, 774
Hypnovel, 212
Hypocalcaemia, 552
Hypodermic equipment, 419
Hypodermic insulin injection pens, 432
Hypoglycaemia, 418, 433
▸ Chronic hypoglycaemia, 433
▸ Neonatal hypoglycaemia, 433
▸ Treatment of hypoglycaemia, 433
Hypokalaemia, 561
Hypomagnesaemia, 555, 556
Hyponatraemia and antidepressant therapy, 221
Hypophosphataemia, 559
Hypoplastic, haemolytic, and renal anaemias, 522
Hypotension and interference with temperature regulation, 229
Hypotension and shock, 112
Hypothalamic and anterior pituitary hormones, 441
▸ Corticotrophins, 441
▸ Gonadotrophins, 441
▸ Growth hormones, 441
▸ Hypothalamic hormones, 441
Hypothyroidism, 119, 453
Hypovase, 93
Hypromellose, **626**, 627
Hypromellose with dexamethasone, neomycin and polymyxin B sulfate, *see* Dexamethasone with hypromellose, neomycin and polymyxin B sulfate
Hypromol, 627
Hypurin preparations, 423, 425, 426

I

Ibucalm, 610
Ibuprofen, **608**
ICare Advanced products, 432
Ichthammol, **699**
▸ With zinc oxide, **699**
Ichthopaste, 699
Idiopathic thrombocytopenic purpura, 539
Idursulfase, **568**
Ifosfamide, **499**
IHealth, 432
Ilaris, 492
Iloprost, **110**
Ilube, 625
Imatinib, **519**
IME-DC, 431
Imidazole antifungals, 349, 481, 645, 663, 678
Imiglucerase, **566**
Imigran preparations, 274
Imipenem with cilastatin, **295**
Imipramine hydrochloride, **226**
Imiquimod, **722**
Immukin, 518
Immune interferon, *see* Interferon gamma-1b
Immune reconstitution syndrome, 386

Immune response, 483
▸ Antiproliferative immunosuppressants, 483
▸ Corticosteroids and other immunosuppressants, 483
▸ Immunosuppressant therapy, 483
▸ Impaired immune responsiveness, 483
▸ Inflammatory bowel disease, 483
Immune response modifiers, 722
Immune sera and immunoglobulins, 484, 724, 730, 798
Immune system, 483
Immune system disorders and transplantation, 483
Immunisation for travel, 741
Immunisation schedule, 732
Immunocompromised children, 349
Immunocompromised patients, 340, 662
Immunoglobulins, 484, 724
▸ Availability, 724
▸ Disease-specific immunoglobulins, 725
▸ Hepatitis A, 724
▸ Hepatitis B immunoglobulin, 725
▸ Measles, 725
▸ Normal immunoglobulin, 724
▸ Passive immunity, 724
▸ Rabies immunoglobulin, 725
▸ Rubella, 725
▸ Tetanus immunoglobulin, 725
▸ Uses, 724
▸ Varicella–zoster immunoglobulin, 725
Immunostimulants, 379, 517, 537
Immunosuppressant therapy, 483, 601
Immunosuppressants, 30, 485, 527, 597, 701
Immunosuppression and indwelling intraperitoneal catheters, 285
Immunotherapy responsive malignancy, 517
Imodium preparations, 45
Impaired immune responsiveness, 483
Impetigo: widespread infection, 290
Imuran, 485
Imuvac, 752
Inadine, 717
Inconex XL, 458
Increlex, 445
Indermil, 719
Index of proprietary manufacturers, 974
Indometacin, **611**
Indomethacin, *see* Indometacin
Industrial methylated spirit, *see* Alcohol
Inegy, 125
Infacol, 48
Infanrix-IPV, 744
Infanrix-IPV + Hib, 743
Infantile spasms, 182
Infatrini preparations, 933, 943
Inflammatory bowel disease, 24, 483
▸ Adjunctive treatment of inflammatory bowel disease, 25
▸ Aminosalicylates, 25
▸ Cytokine modulators, 25
▸ Drugs affecting the immune response, 25
▸ Drugs used in inflammatory bowel disease, 25
▸ Fistulating Crohn's disease, 25

▸ Maintenance of remission of acute ulcerative colitis and Crohn's disease, 25
▸ Management of acute ulcerative colitis and Crohn's disease, 24
▸ Treatment of acute ulcerative colitis and Crohn's disease, 24
Inflammatory eye conditions, 622
Inflammatory skin conditions, 683
Inflectra, 31
Infliximab, **30**
Influenza, 399
Influenza vaccine, 736, **752**
Influvac Sub-unit, 752
Inhalational anaesthetics, 757
Inhaled corticosteroids, 149
Inhaler devices, 137
Innovace, 105
Inovelon, 195
Insect stings, 792
Insomnia, 20, 275
Instant Carobel, 954
InsuJet, 432
Insulatard preparations, 423
Insulin, 417, **425**
Insulin and glucose, 420
Insulin aspart, **426**
Insulin degludec, **424**
Insulin detemir, **424**
Insulin glargine, **424**
Insulin glulisine, **427**
Insulin Injection, *see* Insulin
Insulin-like growth factor-I deficiency, 445
Insulin lispro, **427**
Insulin requirements, 417
Insulins, **422**
▸ Intermediate-acting, 422
▸ Intermediate-acting combined with rapid-acting, 423
▸ Long-acting, 424
▸ Rapid-acting, 425
Insulins and anti-diabetic drugs, 417
▸ Antidiabetic drugs, 419
▸ Biguanides, 419
▸ Biphasic insulins, 419
▸ Diabetes and surgery, 418
▸ Elective surgery, 418
▸ Emergency surgery, 418
▸ Examples of insulin regimens, 417
▸ Hypodermic equipment, 419
▸ Hypoglycaemia, 418
▸ Insulin, 417
▸ Insulin and glucose, 420
▸ Insulin requirements, 417
▸ Intermediate- and long-acting insulins, 418
▸ Intravenous fluids and continuous insulin infusion, 418
▸ Management of diabetes with insulin, 417
▸ Neonatal diabetes, 420
▸ Neonatal hyperglycaemia, 420
▸ Other antidiabetic drugs, 419
▸ Pregnancy and breast-feeding, 419
▸ Safe and Effective Use of Insulin in Hospitalised Patients (March 2010), 417
▸ Short-acting insulins, 418

▸ Sulfonylureas, 419
Insulin zinc suspension, **425**
Insuman preparations, 423, 426
Intal, 158
Intanza, 752
Intelence, 389
Interactions, 799
Interferon alfa, **517**
Interferon gamma-1b, **518**
Interleukin inhibitors, 597
Intermediate-acting insulin, *see* Biphasic insulin aspart
Intermediate-acting insulin, *see* Biphasic insulin lispro
Intermediate- and long-acting insulins, 418
Intestinal adsorbents, 793
Intractable cough, 20
Intramuscular adrenaline (epinephrine), 163
Intra-operative analgesia, 771
Intratect, 729
Intrathecal chemotherapy, 495
Intra-uterine contraceptive devices (copper), **471**
Intra-uterine progestogen-only device, 463
Intravenous adrenaline (epinephrine), 163
Intravenous anaesthetics, 757, 758
Intravenous fat emulsions, 14
Intravenous fluids and continuous insulin infusion, 418
Intravenous glucose, 542
Intravenous nutrition, 575
▸ Administration, 577
Intravenous potassium, 543
Intravenous sodium, 544
IntronA, 517
Intuniv, 217
Invanz, 295
Invasive Haemophilus influenzae type b disease, 735
InVita D3, 590
Invodol SR, 270
Iodide with iodine, **453**
Iodine products, 633
Iodine with iodide, *see* Iodide with iodine
Iopidine, 642
Ipocol, 28
Ipratropium bromide, **143, 651**
Iron chelators, 535
Iron deficiency anaemia, 527
Iron dextran, **529**
Iron (injectable), **528**
Iron (oral), **530**
Ironorm, 531
Iron overload, 535
Iron sucrose, **529**
Irriclens, 657, 718
Irrigation solutions, 718
▸ *Clinipod*, 719
Irripod, 719
Irritable bowel syndrome, 24, 31
Isentress, 388
Isoflurane, **761**
Isoleucine50, 962
Isoniazid, **345**
Isoniazid and rifampicin, *see* Rifampicin with isoniazid

Isoniazid with pyrazinamide and rifampicin, *see* Rifampicin with isoniazid and pyrazinamide
Isophane insulin, **423**
Isoplex, 555
ISO-POD, 719
Isopropyl alcohol with chlorhexidine gluconate, *see* Chlorhexidine gluconate with isopropyl alcohol
Isopto preparations, 627
Isotretinoin, **712**
  ‣ With erythromycin, **713**
Isotrex, 713
Isotrexin, 713
Isovaleric acidaemia, 961
Isovorin, 516
Ispagel, 36
Ispaghula husk, **36**
Ispaghula husk with mebeverine, *see* Mebeverine with ispaghula husk
Ispaghula husk with senna, *see* Senna with ispaghula husk
Isteranda, 477
Istin, 100
Itraconazole, **353**
IVA Anamix Infant, 961
Ivacaftor, **175**
Ivermectin, **361**
Ixiaro, 753

J

Japanese encephalitis vaccine, 736, **753**
Jaydess, 477
Jet nebulisers, 138
Jevity products, 928, 930, 931
Jext, 130
Joint prostheses and dental treatment, 285
Joy-Rides, 251
Juliperla, 469
Junior Parapaed, 257
Juvela products, 955, 956, 957, 958, 959
Juvenile idiopathic arthritis, 595

K

Kalcipos-D, 590
Kaletra, 397
Kalydeco, 176
Kapake, 259
Katya, 469
Kawasaki disease, 83
Kay-Cee-L, 562
Keflex, 298
Keftid, 299, 300
Kemadrin, 241
Kemicetine, 335
Kenalog, 617
Keppra, 191
Ketalar, 774
Ketamine, **773**
KetoCal, 946
Ketoconazole, **414**, **678**
Ketoprofen, **612**
  ‣ With omeprazole, **612**
Ketorolac trometamol, **636**, **771**
Ketostix, 433
Ketotifen, **170**, **621**
Ketovite, 587
KeyOmega, 962
Kindergen, 947

Kiovig, 729
Kivexa, 391
Klaricid, 310
Klaricid XL, 310
Klean-Prep, 34
Klorafect, 632
Kogenate, 79
Kolanticon, 57
Kolbam, 60
Konakion MM, 594
Kuvan, 581
Kwells, 251
Kytril, 247

L

Labelling of prescribed medicines, 6
Labetalol hydrochloride, **95**
Lacosamide, **188**
Lacri-Lube, 627
Lactic acid, **481**
Lactic acid with salicylic acid, *see* Salicylic acid with lactic acid
Lactugal, 37
Lactulose, **37**
Lamictal, 190, 191
Lamisil, 681
Lamivudine, **393**
Lamivudine with abacavir and dolutegravir, *see* Abacavir with dolutegravir and lamivudine
Lamivudine with abacavir and zidovudine, *see* Abacavir with lamivudine and zidovudine
Lamivudine with abacavir, *see* Abacavir with lamivudine
Lamivudine with zidovudine, *see* Zidovudine with lamivudine
Lamotrigine, 183, **189**
Landau-Kleffner syndrome, 183
Lanoxin, 76
Lansoprazole, **53**
Lantus preparations, 425
Larbex XL, 459
Largactil, 231
Lariam, 374
Laronidase, **568**
Lasix, 133
Latanoprost, **641**
Latin abbreviations, *inside back cover*
Laxatives, 33, 35
Laxido, 39
Leishmaniacides, 362
Leishmaniasis, 363
Lennox-Gastaut syndrome, 182
Lenograstim, **539**
Lescol preparations, 124
Lestramyl, 468
Leucine100, 962
Leukotriene receptor antagonists, 155
Leuprorelin acetate, **440**
Levamisole, **361**
Levemir preparations, 424
Levest, 470
Levetiracetam, 183, **191**
Levobunolol hydrochloride, **637**
Levobupivacaine, **779**
Levocarnitine, **564**
Levocetirizine hydrochloride, **166**
Levodopa with carbidopa, *see* Co-careldopa

Levofloxacin, **631**
Levofolinic acid, **516**
Levomepromazine, **251**
Levonelle, 477
Levonorgestrel, **475**
Levonorgestrel with ethinylestradiol, *see* Ethinylestradiol with levonorgestrel
Levosert, 477
Levothyroxine sodium, **454**
Lexpec, 534
LH–RH, *see* Gonadorelin
Lidocaine hydrochloride, **70**, **659**, **780**
Lidocaine with adrenaline, **781**
Lidocaine with fluorescein, *see* Fluorescein with lidocaine
Lidocaine with hydrocortisone, *see* Hydrocortisone with lidocaine
Lidocaine with phenylephrine, **782**
Lidocaine with prilocaine, **782**
Lifestyle Products, 955, 956
Life support algorithm (image), *inside back cover*
Lignocaine hydrochloride, *see* Lidocaine hydrochloride
Lignospan Special, 781
Li-Liquid, 221
Lincosamides, 307, 480, 710
Linezolid, **337**
Lioresal, 603, 604
Liothyronine sodium, **455**
Lipantil Micro, 122
Lipase inhibitors, 63
Lipid-regulating drugs, 119
  ‣ Choice of drugs, 119
  ‣ Drug treatment in heterozygous familial hypercholesterolaemia, 119
  ‣ Drug treatment in secondary hypercholesterolaemia, 119
  ‣ Hypothyroidism, 119
  ‣ Risk factors for cardiovascular disease, 119
Lipistart, 944
Lipitor, 123, 124
Lipobase, 672
Lipodystrophy syndrome, 386
LiquaMag GP, 556
LiquiBand, 719
Liquid paraffin with retinol palmitate with white soft paraffin with light liquid paraffin and wool, *see* Retinol palmitate with white soft paraffin and light liquid paraffin and liquid paraffin and wool fat
Liquid paraffin with white soft paraffin and wool alcohols, **627**
Liquifilm Tears, 627
Liquigen, 949
Liquivisc, 626
Lisdexamfetamine mesilate, **216**
Lisinopril, **106**
Liskonum, 220
Lithium carbonate, **219**
Lithium citrate, **220**
Lithium salts, **218**
Liver disorders and related conditions, 59
Livwell Products, 955, 956
Lizinna, 471
LMX 4, 781
Loaves (ACBS), 955

Local anaesthesia, 776
  ▸ Administration, 776
  ▸ Dental anaesthesia, 776
  ▸ Local anaesthetic drugs, 776
  ▸ Toxicity, 776
  ▸ Use of vasoconstrictors, 776
Local anaesthetics, 634
Local analgesics, 659
Local corticosteroid injections, 616
Local inflammation of joints and soft tissue, 616
Locasol, 945
Loceryl, 680
Locoid preparation, 693
Lodoxamide, **622**
Loestrin preparations, 471
Long-acting beta2 agonists, 141
Longtec, 268
Long-term oxygen therapy, 142
Loniten, 109
Loop diuretics, **131**
Loperamide hydrochloride, **44**
  ▸ With simeticone, **45**
Lophlex, 963
Lopinavir with ritonavir, **397**
Lopresor preparations, 98
Loprofin products, 958, 959, 963
Loratadine, **166**
Lorazepam, **209**
Loron, 438
Losartan potassium, **107**
Losec, 55
Losinate MR, 460
Lotriderm, 694
Low blood volume, 554
Low molecular weight heparins, 83
Low-protein foods, 958
LPL, 669
L-Tri-iodothyronine sodium, *see* Liothyronine sodium
L-Tyrosine, 963
Lubristil, 628
Lucette, 468
Lumecare preparations, 626, 627
Lumefantrine with artemether, *see* Artemether with lumefantrine
Lustral, 224
Luvinsta XL, 124
Lyclear, 683
Lyflex, 603
Lymecycline, **333**
Lyme disease, 339
Lynlor, 268
Lyrinel XL, 457
Lysodren, 514

M

Maalox preparations, 47, 48
Mabron, 271
MabThera, 494
Macilax, 39
Macrobid, 348
Macrogol 3350 with anhydrous sodium sulfate, potassium chloride, sodium bicarbonate and sodium chloride, **33**
Macrogol 3350 with potassium chloride, sodium bicarbonate and sodium chloride, **37**
Macrolides, 289, 307, **308**, 377, 630, 710

Maexeni, 470
MagnaPhate, 556
Magnesium, 555, 556
Magnesium aspartate, **556**
Magnesium carbonate with citric acid, *see* Citric acid with magnesium carbonate
Magnesium carbonate with magnesium trisilicate and sodium bicarbonate, *see* Magnesium trisilicate with magnesium carbonate and sodium bicarbonate
Magnesium citrate with sodium picosulfate, **34**
Magnesium glycerophosphate, **556**
Magnesium hydroxide, **39**
Magnesium hydroxide with aluminium hydroxide and simeticone, *see* Simeticone with aluminium hydroxide and magnesium hydroxide
Magnesium hydroxide with aluminium hydroxide, *see* Co-magaldrox
Magnesium imbalance, 555
Magnesium oxide with aluminium hydroxide, dicycloverine hydrochloride and simeticone, *see* Dicycloverine hydrochloride with aluminium hydroxide, magnesium oxide and simeticone
Magnesium sulfate, **556**
Magnesium trisilicate with magnesium carbonate and sodium bicarbonate, **48**
Malabsorption syndromes, 24
Malaria, 363
Malaria, prophylaxis, 364
  ▸ Anticoagulants, 365
  ▸ Asplenia, 364
  ▸ Breast-feeding, 365
  ▸ Epilepsy, 364
  ▸ Length of prophylaxis, 364
  ▸ Pregnancy, 364
  ▸ Protection against bites, 364
  ▸ Renal impairment, 364
  ▸ Return from malarial region, 364
  ▸ Specific recommendations, 365
  ▸ Standby treatment, 365
Malaria, treatment, 365
  ▸ Advice for healthcare professionals, 365
  ▸ Advice for travellers, 365
  ▸ Falciparum malaria (treatment), 365
  ▸ Non-falciparum malaria (treatment), 365
  ▸ Parenteral, 370
  ▸ Pregnancy, 370
Malarivon, 373
Malarone, 372
Malathion, **682**
Male sex hormone antagonism, 450
Male sex hormone responsive conditions, 449
Malignant disease, 493
Malignant hyperthermia, 758, 775
Mandafen, 610
Mandanol preparations, 255, 256, 549, 627
Maneo, 271
Manevac, 42
Mannitol, **133**
Mantoux test, *see* Tuberculin purified protein derivative
Maple syrup urine disease, 961
Maraviroc, **399**

Marcain, 778
Marevan, 89
Marine stings, 792
Mariosea XL, 458
Marol, 271
Martapan, 410
Marvelon, 468
Mast-cell stabilisers, 157, 622, 654
Matever, 192
Matrifen, 264
Maxidex, 623
Maxijul Super Soluble, 948
Maxitram SR, 271
Maxitrol, 624
Maxolon, 247
Maxtrex, 507
MCT products, 576, 931, 944, 949, 951
Measles, 725
Measles, mumps and rubella vaccine, live, **753**
Mebendazole, **361**
Mebeverine hydrochloride, **58**
  ▸ With ispaghula husk, **31**
Mecasermin, **445**
Mecillinams, 316
Medi, 160
Medical emergencies in dental practice, *see* BNF
Medical emergencies in the community, *inside back cover*
Medicines Information Services, *inside back cover*
Medikinet preparations, 214
MediSense SoftSense, 431
Medi-Test products, 431, 432
MediTouch, 431
Medrone, 412
Medroxyprogesterone acetate, **478**
Mefenamic acid, **612**
Mefloquine, 363, **373**
Megaloblastic anaemia, 532
Meglumine amidotrizoate with sodium amidotrizoate, **32**
Melatonin, 275, **276**
Meloxicam, **613**
Melphalan, **500**
Menadiol sodium phosphate, **593**
Mendor Discreet, 431
Meningitec, 746
Meningococcal group B vaccine (rDNA, component, adsorbed), **746**
Meningococcal group C vaccine, **746**
Meningococcal group C vaccine with haemophilus influenzae type B, *see* Haemophilus influenzae type B with meningococcal group C vaccine
Meningococcal groups A with C and W135 and Y vaccine, **746**
Meningococcal septicaemia, 285
Meningococcal vaccine, 737
Menitorix, 745
Menjugate, 746
Mental health disorders, 212
Menthol and derivatives, 177
Menthol with eucalyptus, *see* Eucalyptus with menthol
Menveo, 747
Mepact, 518
Meperidine, *see* Pethidine hydrochloride

Mepivacaine hydrochloride, **782**
▸ With adrenaline, **783**
Mepradec, 55
Mercaptamine, **569**
Mercaptopurine, **505**
6-Mercaptopurine, *see* Mercaptopurine
Mercilon, 468
Meronem, 297
Meropenem, **296**
Mesalazine, **26**
Mesna, **515**
Mestinon, 602
Mestranol with norethisterone, *see*
Norethisterone with mestranol
Metabolic acidosis, 540
Metabolic disorders, 562
Metaraminol, **115**
Meters and test strips, 429
Metformin hydrochloride, **420**
Methadone hydrochloride, **279**
Methaemoglobinaemia, 787, 798
Metharose, 280
Methicillin-resistant staphylococcus
aureus, 339
Methotrexate, **506**
Methotrimeprazine, *see*
Levomepromazine
Methylcellulose, **36**
Methyl donors, 566
Methylene blue, *see* Methylthioninium
chloride
Methylmalonic or propionic acidaemia,
962
Methylphenidate hydrochloride, **213**
Methylprednisolone, **412, 617**
Methylthioninium chloride, **798**
Metoclopramide hydrochloride, **246**
Metoject PEN, 507
Metolazone, **134**
Metopirone, 415
Metoprolol tartrate, **98**
Metosyn preparations, 692
Metrogel, 676
Metronidazole, **313, 480, 676**
Metronidazole and tinidazole, 289
Metrosa, 676
Metyrapone, **415**
Mezolar Matrix, 264
Mezzopram, 55
MHRA Drug Safety Update, 11
Miacalcic, 439
Micafungin, **350**
Micanol, 699
Micolette Micro-enema, 40
Miconazole, **482, 663, 679**
Miconazole with hydrocortisone, *see*
Hydrocortisone with miconazole
Micralax Micro-enema, 40
Microdot+, 431
Microgynon 30, 470
Micronor, 448
MicroPeak, 160
Micropirin, 84
Midazolam, **210**
Mifamurtide, **518**
Miglustat, **569**
Migraine, 272
▸ Antiemetics, 272
▸ Cluster headache and the trigeminal
autonomic cephalalgias, 272

▸ 5HT1-receptor agonists, 272
▸ Prophylaxis of migraine, 272
▸ Treatment of acute migraine, 272
Migraitan, 274
Migraleve preparations, 259, 272
Mildison Lipocream, 693
Milex, 473
Millinette, 469
Milrinone, **118**
Milupa lpd, 962
Mineral and trace elements deficiencies,
575
Mineralocorticoid side effects, 406
Minerals with vitamins and trace
elements, *see* Vitamins with minerals
and trace elements
Mini-Wright, 160
Minocin MR, 334
Minocycline, **333**
Minor cuts and abrasions, 719
Minoxidil, **108**
Mintreleq XL, 238
Miochol-E, 634
Miotics, 636
Miphtel, 634
Mirena, 477
Mission products, 431, 432
Mitochondrial disorders, 567
Mitotane, **513**
Mitoxantrone, **503**
Mitozantrone, *see* Mitoxantrone
Mivacron, 768
Mivacurium, **768**
Mizolastine, **167**
Mizollen, 167
MMA PA Anamix Infant, 962
M-M-RVAXPRO, 754
Modigraf, 491
Modrasone, 688
Modulen IBD, 947
MODZ, 431
Molaxole, 39
Molcer, 647
Mometasone furoate, **154, 653, 694**
Monoamine-oxidase inhibitors, **221**
Monobactams, 313
Monoclonal antibodies, 154, 402, 491, 493,
527
▸ Monoclonal antibodies, anti-
lymphocyte, 492
Monogen, 945
Monographs, xii
▸ Typical layout, xiv
Mononine, 78
Monopost, 641
Monotrim, 339
Montelukast, **155**
Morphgesic SR, 266
Morphine, **265**
▸ With cyclizine, **267**
Motifene, 607
Motility stimulants, 56
Motilium, 246
Motion sickness, 244
Mouthwashes and other preparations for
oropharyngeal use, 655
▸ Lozenges and sprays, 655
▸ Mouthwashes and gargles, 655
Movement disorders, 240
Movicol, 39

Moxifloxacin, **631**
Moxivig, 631
MRSA, 339
Mrs Crimbles products, 957
MST Continus, 266, 267
MSUD products, 961
MucoClear, 160
Mucodyne, 175
Mucogel, 47
Mucolytics, 175
Mucolytics for cystic fibrosis, 174
Mucopolysaccharidosis, 567
Multi-thick, 954
Multivitamins, 583
Munalea, 468
Mupirocin, **650, 677**
Muscle relaxants, 601, 765
Muscle relaxants, centrally acting, 603
Muscle relaxants, directly acting, 775
Muscle relaxants, peripherally acting, 243
Muscle spasm in palliative care, 20
MXL, 266
Myasthenia gravis, 601
Mycamine, 351
Mycobutin, 342
Mycophenolate mofetil, **492**
Mydriacyl, 633
Mydriatics and cycloplegics, 633
Mydrilate, 625
Myfenax, 493
Myfortic, 493
Myglucohealth, 431
Mylafent, 264
Mylan, 249
Mylife Pura, 431
Mylife Unio, 431
Myocardial ischaemia, 125
Myocet, 502
Myoclonic seizures, 182
Myozyme, 570

N

Nabilone, **245**
Nacrez, 474
Naglazyme, 568
Nairns products, 956
Nalcrom, 158
Nalidixic acid, **329**
Naloxone hydrochloride, **796**
Nandovar XL, 124
Nappy rash (Dermatitis), 666
Naproxen, **614**
Naropin, 785
Nasacort, 654
Nasal congestion, 649
Nasal infection, 650
Nasal inflammation, nasal polyps and
rhinitis, 651
Nasal polyps, 648
Naseptin, 650
Nasobec, 652
Nasofan, 653
Nasonex, 653
Natecal, 590
Nausea and labyrinth disorders, 243
▸ Cytotoxic chemotherapy, palliative
care, and migraine, 244
▸ Drug treatment, 243
▸ Motion sickness, 244

▸ Opioid-induced nausea and vomiting, 244
▸ Other vestibular disorders, 244
▸ Postoperative nausea and vomiting, 244
▸ Vomiting during pregnancy, 244
Nebcin, 295
Nebuliser diluent, 138
Nebulisers, 137
Nebuliser solutions, 160
Nebusal, 160
Neditol XL, 458
Nedocromil sodium, **157, 622**
Needle free Insulin delivery systems, 432
NeisVac-C, 746
Nelarabine, **508**
Neocate products, 941, 942
Neoclarityn, 165
Neo-Cytamen, 535
Neokay, 594
Neomycin sulfate, **645, 675**
Neomycin sulfate with clobetasol propionate and nystatin, see Clobetasol propionate with neomycin sulfate and nystatin
Neomycin sulfate with dexamethasone and glacial acetic acid, see Dexamethasone with glacial acetic acid and neomycin sulfate
Neomycin with betamethasone, see Betamethasone with neomycin
Neomycin with chlorhexidine, see Chlorhexidine with neomycin
Neomycin with dexamethasone, hypromellose and polymyxin B sulfate, see Dexamethasone with hypromellose, neomycin and polymyxin B sulfate
Neomycin with fluocinolone, see Fluocinolone acetonide with neomycin
Neo-Naclex, 102
Neoral, 487
NeoRecormon, 526
Neostigmine, **602**
▸ With glycopyrronium bromide, **770**
Neostigmine methylsulfate, see Neostigmine
Neotigason, 703
Neovent, 146
Nephropathic cystinosis, 569
Nepro HP, 947
Nerisone, 691
Nerve agents, 792
Neupogen preparations, 538, 539
Neural tube defects (prevention in pregnancy), 594
Neuraminidase inhibitors, 399
Neuroleptic malignant syndrome, 229
Neuromuscular blockade, 765
▸ Anticholinesterases, 770
▸ Depolarising neuromuscular blocking drugs, 766
▸ Drugs for reversal of neuromuscular blockade, 770
▸ Neuromuscular blocking drugs, **765**
▸ Non-depolarising neuromuscular blocking drugs, 765
▸ Other drugs for reversal of neuromuscular blockade, 770
Neuromuscular blockade reversal, 770

Neuromuscular disorders, 601
▸ Anticholinesterases, 601
▸ Drugs that enhance neuromuscular transmission, 601
▸ Immunosuppressant therapy, 601
▸ Skeletal muscle relaxants, 601
Neurontin, 188
Neuropathic pain, 275
▸ Chronic facial pain, 275
▸ Overview and management, 275
Neuropathy, 416
Neurotoxins (botulinum toxins), 243
Neutral Insulin, see Insulin
Neutropenia, 537
▸ Neonatal neutropenia, 537
Neutropenia and stem cell mobilisation, 537
Nevirapine, **389**
Nexium, 53
Nexplanon, 478
Nicam, 714
Nicardipine hydrochloride, **100**
Nicef, 299
Nicotinamide, **714**
Nicotine, **277**
Nicotine dependence, 276, 277
Nicotine replacement therapy, 277
Nicotinic receptor agonists, 277
Niemann-pick type c disease, 569
Nifedipine, **100**
Niferex, 532
Nimbex, 768
Nimenrix, 747
Nimodipine, **80**
Nimotop, 81
NiQuitin, 279
Nitisinone, **570**
Nitrates, **127**
Nitrocine, 127
Nitrofurantoin, **347**
Nitroimidazole derivatives, 313, 480, 676
Nitronal, 127
Nitrous oxide, 758, **762**
Nivestim, 539
Nizoral, 679, 715
NMDA receptor antagonists, 773
Nocturnal enuresis in children, 456
Nomegestrol with estradiol, see Estradiol with nomegestrol
Non-benzodiazepine hypnotics and sedatives, 275
Non-convulsive status epilepticus, 184
Non-depolarising neuromuscular blocking drugs, 765, **767**
Non-falciparum malaria (treatment), 365
Non-medical prescribing, 973
Non-nucleoside reverse transcriptase inhibitors, 388
Non-opioid analgesics, 770
Nonoxinol, **479**
Non-sedating antihistamines, 163
Non-steroidal anti-inflammatory drugs, 604, 605, 635, 660, 771
▸ Asthma, 604
▸ Choice, 604
▸ Dental and orofacial pain, 604
▸ NSAIDs and cardiovascular events, 604
▸ NSAIDs and gastro-intestinal events, 604

▸ Therapeutic effects, 604
Noradrenaline/norepinephrine, **115**
Norcuron, 769
Norditropin preparations, 444
Norelgestromin with ethinylestradiol, see Ethinylestradiol with norelgestromin
Norethisterone, **447**
▸ With mestranol, **471**
Norethisterone with ethinylestradiol, see Ethinylestradiol with norethisterone
Norgalax, 43
Norgestimate with ethinylestradiol, see Ethinylestradiol with norgestimate
Norgeston, 477
Noriday, 448
Norimin, 471
Norimode, 45
Norinyl-1, 471
Noristerat, 448
Normacol preparations, 37
Normal immunoglobulin, 724, **727**
Normaloe, 45
Normasol, 718, 719
Normosang, 564
Nortriptyline, **227**
Norvir, 398
Nose, 648
▸ Corticosteroids, 648
▸ Drugs used in nasal allergy, 648
▸ Nasal polyps, 648
▸ Nasal preparations for infection, 649
▸ Nasal staphylococci, 649
▸ Pregnancy, 648
▸ Rhinitis and bacterial sinusitis, 648
▸ Sinusitis and oral pain, 648
▸ Topical nasal decongestants, 648
Nose infections, bacterial, 289
▸ Antibacterial therapy for sinusitis, 289
Notifiable diseases, 282
NovoMix preparations, 423
NovoPen 4, 432
NovoRapid preparations, 427
NovoSeven, 78
Noxious gases, 791
Noyada, 105
Nozinan, 252
NSAID-associated ulcers, 49
NSpire products, 160, 161
NTBC, see Nitisinone
Nucleoside reverse transcriptase inhibitors, **390**
Nuelin SA, 160
Nurofen preparations, 610
Nurse Prescribers' Advisory Group 2015-2016, viii
Nurse Prescribers' Formulary, 970
Nu-Seals, 84
Nutilis products, 938, 940, 954
Nutramigen products, 942, 943
Nutraplus, 673
Nutricrem, 940
Nutrini products, 932, 933, 934, 935
Nutriprem 2, 932
Nutrison products, 928, 929, 930, 931
Nutrition in special diets, 580
▸ Coeliac disease, 580
▸ Phenylketonuria, 580
Nutrition (intravenous), 575
Nutrition (oral), 578
Nutrizym, 67

NutropinAq, 444
NuvaRing, 469
Nuwiq, 79
Nystaform preparations, 681, 697
Nystan, 663
Nystatin, **663**
Nystatin with benzalkonium chloride,
    dimeticone and hydrocortisone, *see*
    Hydrocortisone with benzalkonium
    chloride, dimeticone and nystatin
Nystatin with chlorhexidine
    hydrochloride and hydrocortisone, *see*
    Hydrocortisone with chlorhexidine
    hydrochloride and nystatin
Nystatin with chlorhexidine, *see*
    Chlorhexidine with nystatin
Nystatin with clobetasol propionate and
    neomycin sulfate, *see* Clobetasol
    propionate with neomycin sulfate and
    nystatin
Nystatin with clobetasone butyrate and
    oxytetracycline, *see* Clobetasone
    butyrate with nystatin and
    oxytetracycline

O

Obesity, 62
Occlusal, 722
Octagam, 729
Octasa MR, 28
Octim, 405
Octreotide, **434**
Ocufen, 636
Ocular peri-operative drugs, **634**
Ocu-Lube, 627
Ocusan, 628
ODM5, 628
Oedema, 130
Oesophageal varices, 61
Oestrogens, 446
Oestrogens combined with progestogens,
    465
Ofloxacin, **631**
Oftaquix, 631
Oilatum products, 668, 669, 672
Olanzapine, **236**
Oldaram, 271
Oleax, 647
Olena, 223
Olive oil, **647**
Olopatadine, **621**
Olsalazine sodium, **28**
Omalizumab, **154**
Omeprazole, **54**
Omeprazole with ketoprofen, *see*
    Ketoprofen with omeprazole
Omicur, 680
Omnitest 3, 431
Omnitrope preparations, 444
Omri-Hep-B, 727
Ondansetron, **248**
Ondemet, 248
One-Alpha, 588
OneTouch products, 431
Onkotrone, 503
Opatanol, 621
Ophthalmic herpes simplex, 632
Opiodur, 264
Opioid analgesics, 253, 771
Opioid dependence, 279

Opioid-induced nausea and vomiting, 244
Opioid receptor antagonists, 796
Opioids, **256**, 279, 772, 788
Opioid toxicity, 796
Optaflu, 753
OptiChamber products, 161
Opticrom, 622
OptiFlo products, 461
Optilast, 621
Optive preparations, 626, 628
Optometrists, 973
Optrex preparations, 622, 632
Oral anticoagulants, 82
  ▹ Dose, 82
  ▹ Haemorrhage, 82
  ▹ Target INR, 82
  ▹ Uses, 82
Oral bacterial infections, 289
  ▹ Antibacterial drugs, 289
  ▹ Broad-spectrum penicillins, 289
  ▹ Cephalosporins, 289
  ▹ Clindamycin, 289
  ▹ Macrolides, 289
  ▹ Metronidazole and tinidazole, 289
  ▹ Penicillins, 289
  ▹ Tetracyclines, 289
Oral bicarbonate, 542
Oraldene, 657
Oral glucose tolerance test, 428
Oral hygiene, 655
Oral Impact, 938
Oral iron, 528
Oral mucositis, 495
Oral preparations for fluid and electrolyte
    imbalance, 541
Oral rehydration therapy (ORT), 541
Oral ulceration and inflammation, 659
  ▹ Antiseptic mouthwashes, 659
  ▹ Corticosteroids, 659
  ▹ Local analgesics, 659
  ▹ Other preparations, 659
  ▹ Periodontitis, 659
  ▹ Simple mouthwashes, 659
  ▹ Ulceration and inflammation, 659
Oramorph, 267
Orap, 233
Orbifen, 610
Orencia, 598
Orfadin, 570
Organophosphorus insecticides, 792
Organophosphorus toxicity, 794
Orgran products, 85, 957
Orlistat, **63**
Oropharyngeal bacterial infections, 661
  ▹ Antibacterial therapy for gingivitis:
    acute necrotising ulcerative, 661
  ▹ Antibacterial therapy for periapical or
    periodontal abscess, 661
  ▹ Antibacterial therapy for
    pericoronitis, 661
  ▹ Antibacterial therapy for
    periodontitis, 662
  ▹ Antibacterial therapy for throat
    infections, 662
Oropharyngeal fungal infections, 662
  ▹ Acute erythematous candidiasis, 662
  ▹ Angular cheilitis, 662
  ▹ Drugs used in oropharyngeal
    candidiasis, 662
  ▹ Immunocompromised patients, 662

  ▹ Thrush, 662
Oropharyngeal viral infections, 663
Oropharynx, 654
Orphacol, 60
Ortho products, 473
Oseltamivir, **399**
Osmanil, 264
Osmolite preparations, 928, 930, 932
Osmotic diuretics, 133
Osmotic laxatives, 33, 35, 37
Osteonecrosis, 386
Osteoporosis, 435
Otex, 648
Otitis externa, 643, 644
Otitis media, 643
Otitis media with effusion, 644
Otomize, 646
Otrivine preparations, 621, 650
Ovex, 362
Ovranette, 470
Oxactin, 223
Oxandrolone, **449**
Oxcarbazepine, **192**
Oxeltra, 268
Oxis Turbohaler, 145
Oxyal, 628
Oxybuprocaine hydrochloride, **635**
Oxybutynin hydrochloride, **457**
Oxycodone hydrochloride, **267**
OxyContin, 268
Oxygen, 142
  ▹ Ambulatory oxygen therapy, 142
  ▹ Arrangements for supplying oxygen,
    143
  ▹ Domiciliary oxygen, 142
  ▹ Long-term oxygen therapy, 142
  ▹ Oxygen therapy equipment, 142
  ▹ Short-burst oxygen therapy, 142
Oxylan, 268
Oxymetholone, **522**
OxyNorm, 269
Oxytetracycline, **334**
Oxytetracycline with clobetasone
    butyrate and nystatin, *see* Clobetasone
    butyrate with nystatin and
    oxytetracycline
Oxytetracycline with hydrocortisone, *see*
    Hydrocortisone with oxytetracycline

P

Paediasure products, 933, 934, 935, 936
Paediatric advanced life support, *inside
    back cover*
Paediatric Formulary Committee, vii
Pain, 252
Pain and inflammation in
    musculoskeletal disorders, 604
Palivizumab, **402**
Palladone preparations, 265
Paludrine, 375
Paludrine/Avloclor, 373
Pamidronate disodium, **437**
Pamsvax XL, 460
Panadol, 256
Pancrease, 67
Pancreatic enzymes, 66
Pancreatin, 59, **66**
Pancreatin preparations, 59
Pancrex, 67
Pancuronium bromide, **768**

PanOxyl preparations, 710, 711
Papaveretum, **269**
Paracetamol, **254**, 788
▸ With buclizine hydrochloride and codeine phosphate, **272**
▸ With tramadol, **256**
Paracetamol overdose treatment graph, 789
Paracetamol toxicity, 797
Paracetamol with codeine phosphate, *see* Co-codamol
Paracetamol with dihydrocodeine, *see* Co-dydramol
Paracodol, 259
Paraffin, yellow, soft, **627**
Paraldehyde, **208**
Parasiticidal preparations, 675
Parasiticides, 682
Parasitic skin infections, 682
Parasympathomimetics, 634, 640
Parenteral anticoagulants, 83
▸ Anticoagulants, 83
▸ Epoprostenol, 83
▸ Heparin, 83
▸ Heparin flushes, 83
▸ Heparinoids, 83
▸ Low molecular weight heparins, 83
Parenteral nutrition supplements, **577**
Parvolex, 797
Passive immunity, 724, 733
Pasta (ACBS), 957, 959
Patent ductus arteriosus, 134
Pavacol-D, 177
Peak flow meters, 138, 160
PecFent, 265
Pedea, 610
Pediacel, 743
Peditrace, 578
Pegasys, 380
Peginterferon alfa, **379**
Penbritin, 322
Penicillamine, **574**
Penicillinase-resistant penicillins, 316
Penicillin G, *see* Benzylpenicillin sodium
Penicillins, 289, **316**
▸ Antipseudomonal with beta-lactamase inhibitor, 317
▸ Antipseudomonal penicillins, 316
▸ Beta-lactamase sensitive, 318
▸ Benzylpenicillin and phenoxymethylpenicillin, 316
▸ Broad-spectrum, 320
▸ Broad-spectrum penicillins, 316
▸ Broad-spectrum with beta-lactamase inhibitor, 323
▸ Mecillinams, 316
▸ Mecillinam-type, 324
▸ Penicillinase-resistant, 325
▸ Penicillinase-resistant penicillins, 316
Penicillin V, *see* Phenoxymethylpenicillin
Pentacarinat, 359
Pentamidine isetionate, **358**
Pentasa, 28
Pentostam, 363
Pepdite preparations, 943
Peppermint oil, **32**
Peptamen products, 929, 932, 934, 935
Peptic ulceration, 49
▸ *Helicobacter pylori* infection, 49
▸ NSAID-associated ulcers, 49

▸ Test for Helicobacter pylori, 49
Peptide-based formula, 929
Pepti-Junior, 943
Peptisorb, 929, 934, 943
Perampanel, **193**
Perative, 932
Percutaneous endoscopic gastrostomy or jejunostomy, 284
Perfalgan, 256
Perfan, 118
Performa, 431
Periciazine, *see* Pericyazine
Pericyazine, **232**
Perinal, 66
Periodontitis, 659
Peri-operative analgesia, 770
▸ Intra-operative analgesia, 771
▸ Non-opioid analgesics, 770
▸ Opioid analgesics, 771
Peri-operative sedation, 773
Perioral lesions, 686
Periostat, 333
Peripheral vascular disease, 135
Peripheral vasodilators, 109, 112
Peripherally acting antiobesity products, 63
Perizam, 206
Permethrin, **683**
Permitabs, 716
Peroxides, 711
Peroxyl, 657
Perphenazine, **232**
Persantin preparations, 84
Pertussis with diphtheria with haemophilus influenza with poliomyelitis and tetanus, *see* Diphtheria with haemophilus influenzae type b vaccine, pertussis, poliomyelitis and tetanus
Pertussis with diphtheria with poliomyelitis and tetanus, *see* Diphtheria with pertussis, poliomyelitis vaccine and tetanus
Pesticides, 792
Pethidine hydrochloride, **269**
Petyme MR, 460
Pevanti, 414
Pevaryl, 678
Peyona, 179
Phaeochromocytoma, 90
Pharmorubicin, 503
Pheburane, 573
Phenergan, 171
Phenobarbital, **203**
Phenobarbital and primidone, 183
Phenobarbitone, *see* Phenobarbital
Phenothiazines and related drugs, 790
Phenoxybenzamine hydrochloride, **109**
Phenoxymethylpenicillin, **319**
Phenylalanine50, 962
Phenylephrine hydrochloride, **116**, **634**
Phenylephrine with lidocaine, *see* Lidocaine with phenylephrine
Phenylketonuria, 580, 963
Phenytoin, 183, **193**
Phlexy products, 963
Pholcodine, **176**
Phosex, 558
Phosphate, **559**
Phosphate binders, 558

Phosphate-binding agents, 558
Phosphate imbalance, 557
Phosphate Sandoz, 559
Phosphate supplements, 557
Phosphodiesterase type-5 inhibitors, 111
Phosphodiesterase type-3 inhibitors, 118
Phosphorylated glycosylated recombinant human deoxyribonuclease 1 (rhDNase), *see* Dornase alfa
Photodamage, 706
Phototherapy, 685
Phyllocontin Continus, 159
Physeptone, 280
Phytomenadione, **593**
Picolax, 34
Pilocarpine, **640**
Pilocarpine nitrate, 640
Pimecrolimus, **701**
Pimozide, **232**
Pinexel PR, 460
Pinmactil, 124
Piperacillin with tazobactam, **317**
Piperaquine phosphate with artenimol, *see* Artenimol with piperaquine phosphate
Piperaquine tetraphosphate with dihydroartemisinin, *see* Artenimol with piperaquine phosphate
Piperaquine with artenimol, 363
Pirinase Hayfever, 653
Piriton, 169
Piroxicam, **615**
Pituitary and hypothalamic hormones and analogues, 61, 403, 434, 439
Pityriasis versicolor, 674
Pivmecillinam hydrochloride, **324**
Pizotifen, **272**
Pizza bases, 957, 959
PK Aid 4, 963
PK Foods products, 958, 959
PKU products, 963, 964
Plant alkaloids, 720
Plaquenil, 596
Plasma and plasma substitutes, 543, 555
Platelet disorders, 539
▸ Essential thrombocythaemia, 539
▸ Idiopathic thrombocytopenic purpura, 539
Platinum compounds, 509
Plenachol, 589
Pneumococcal polysaccharide conjugate vaccine (adsorbed), **747**
Pneumococcal polysaccharide vaccine, **747**
Pneumococcal vaccine, 738
Pneumocystis pneumonia, 357
▸ Adjunctive therapy, 357
▸ Mild to moderate disease, 357
▸ Prophylaxis, 357
▸ Severe disease, 357
▸ Treatment, 357
Pocket Chamber, 161
Podophyllotixin derivatives, 510
Podophyllotoxin, **720**
Poisoning *see* Emergency treatment of poisoning
Poisons information services, *inside front cover*
Poliomyelitis vaccine, 739

Poliomyelitis with diphtheria with haemophilus influenza with pertussis and tetanus, *see* Diphtheria with haemophilus influenzae type b vaccine, pertussis, poliomyelitis and tetanus
Poliomyelitis with diphtheria with pertussis and tetanus, *see* Diphtheria with pertussis, poliomyelitis vaccine and tetanus
Poliomyelitis with diptheria and tetanus, *see* Diphtheria with poliomyelitis and tetanus vaccine
Pollenase preparations, 169, 622, 652
Pollenshield, 165
Pollinex preparations, 173
Polyacrylic acid, *see* Carbomers
Polycal, 948
Polyene antifungals, 349, 351, 663
Polyethylene glycol with hydroxypropyl guar and propylene glycol, *see* Hydroxypropyl guar with polyethylene glycol and propylene glycol
Polyfax, 677
Polymyxin B sulfate with dexamethasone, hypromellose and neomycin, *see* Dexamethasone with hypromellose, neomycin and polymyxin B sulfate
Polymyxin B with bacitracin, *see* Bacitracin with polymyxin B
Polymyxins, 326, **676**
Polysaccharide-iron complex, **532**
Polyvinyl alcohol, **627**
Pompe disease, 570
Ponstan, 613
Poractant alfa, **178**
Posterior pituitary hormones, 403
Posterior pituitary hormones and antagonists, 403
 ‣ Diabetes insipidus, 403
 ‣ Other uses, 403
 ‣ Posterior pituitary hormones, 403
Post-exposure prophylaxis, 385, 730
Post-operative pain and inflammation, 634
Potassium bicarbonate with potassium acid tartrate, **561**
Potassium bicarbonate with potassium chloride, *see* Potassium chloride with potassium bicarbonate
Potassium bicarbonate with sodium alginate, *see* Sodium alginate with potassium bicarbonate
Potassium canrenoate, **117**
Potassium chloride, **561**
 ‣ With calcium chloride and sodium chloride and sodium lactate, **545**
 ‣ With calcium chloride dihydrate and sodium chloride, **545**
 ‣ With glucose, **545**
 ‣ With glucose and sodium chloride, **546**
 ‣ With potassium bicarbonate, **546**
 ‣ With sodium chloride, **546**
Potassium chloride with calcium chloride dihydrate and sodium chloride, *see* Potassium chloride with calcium chloride dihydrate and sodium chloride
Potassium chloride with disodium hydrogen citrate with glucose and sodium chloride, *see* Disodium

hydrogen citrate with glucose, potassium chloride and sodium chloride
Potassium chloride with glucose with sodium bicarbonate and sodium chloride, *see* Glucose with potassium chloride, sodium bicarbonate and sodium chloride
Potassium chloride with rice powder, sodium chloride and sodium citrate, **551**
Potassium citrate with citric acid, *see* Citric acid with potassium citrate
Potassium imbalance, 559
Potassium permanganate, **716**
Potassium-sparing diuretics, 117, 133
Potassium-sparing diuretics with other diuretics, 131
Povidone-iodine, **633**, **716**
Pralidoxime chloride, **794**
Pramocaine with hydrocortisone, *see* Hydrocortisone with pramocaine
Pravastatin sodium, **124**
Praziquantel, **362**
Prazosin, **92**
Preblacon XL, 458
Precocious puberty, 451
Pred Forte, 623
Prednisolone, **413**, **623**, **646**
Prednisolone with cinchocaine, *see* Cinchocaine with prednisolone
Predsol, 623, 646
Pregestimil, 943
Pregnancy, *see* Prescribing in pregnancy
Pregnyl, 443
Pre-medication and peri-operative drugs, 763
 ‣ Antagonists for central and respiratory depression, 763
 ‣ Antimuscarinic drugs, 763
 ‣ Benzodiazepines, 763
 ‣ Drugs that affect gastric pH, 763
 ‣ Neonates, 764
 ‣ Premedication, 763
 ‣ Sedative drugs, 763
Prenoxad, 796
Preparations for vaginal and vulval changes, 479
Prescribing
 ‣ Drugs likely to cause dependence or misuse, 9
 ‣ for children: weight, height, and gender, 1026
 ‣ in breast-feeding, 17
 ‣ in dental practice, 23
 ‣ in hepatic impairment, 15
 ‣ in palliative care, 18
 ‣ in pregnancy, 17
 ‣ in renal impairment, 15
 ‣ unlicensed medicines, 6
Prescriptions, 8
 ‣ Prescription-event monitoring, 11
 ‣ Prescription writing, 4
 ‣ Private prescriptions, 9
 ‣ Requirements, 4
 ‣ Sample, 4
 ‣ Security and validity, 3
 ‣ Writing, 4
Preservatives and sensitisers, 619
Prevenar, 747

Prezista, 396
Priadel preparations, 220
Prilocaine hydrochloride, **783**
 ‣ With felypressin, **784**
Prilocaine with lidocaine, *see* Lidocaine with prilocaine
Primacor, 119
Primaquine, 363, **374**
Primaxin I.V., 296
Primidone, **204**
Primolut N, 448
Priorix, 754
Privigen, 729
Pro-Banthine, 58
Pro-cal products, 952
Procarbazine, **514**
Proceli products, 956, 957
Prochlorperazine, **252**
Proctofoam HC, 66
Proctosedyl, 65
Procyclidine hydrochloride, **241**
Procysbi, 569
Pro-Epanutin, 187
Proflavine, **718**
Progesterone receptor modulators, 473
Progestogen-only contraceptives, 463
Progestogens, 446, 447, 474, 477
Prograf, 491
Proguanil, 363
Proguanil hydrochloride, **375**
Proguanil hydrochloride with atovaquone, *see* Atovaquone with proguanil hydrochloride
Proguanil with chloroquine, *see* Chloroquine with proguanil
Promethazine hydrochloride, **171**
Promethazine teoclate, **249**
Prominproducts, 958, 959
Promixin, 327
Propamidine isetionate, **632**
Propantheline bromide, **58**
Propofol, **759**
Propofol-Lipuro, 760
Propranolol hydrochloride, **96**
Proprietary infusion fluids for parenteral feeding, 576
Propylene glycol with hydroxypropyl guar and polyethylene glycol, *see* Hydroxypropyl guar with polyethylene glycol and propylene glycol
Propylthiouracil, **452**
Prosource, 950
Prostacyclin, *see* Epoprostenol
Prostaglandin analogues, 636
Prostaglandin analogues and prostamides, 641
Prostaglandins, cardiovascular, 110
Prostap preparations, 440
Prostin preparations, 135
ProSure, 947
Prosurin XL, 460
Protamine sulfate, **795**
Protamine zinc insulin, **425**
Protamine zinc insulin injection—long acting, *see* Protamine zinc insulin
Protease inhibitors, **395**
Protein C concentrate, **79**
Protein kinase inhibitors, 519
Protifar, 950

Proton pump inhibitors, 51, **52**
Protopic, 702
Protozoal infection, 362
Provera, 479
Proxymetacaine, 635
Proxymetacaine hydrochloride, **635**
Prozac, 223
Prozep, 223
ProZero, 962
Pruritus, 20, 707
Pseudoephedrine hydrochloride, **649**
Psoriasis, 685
▸ Phototherapy, 685
▸ Systemic treatment, 686
▸ Topical treatment, 686
Psoriderm, 670, 700, 701
Psychoses and related disorders, 227
▸ Antipsychotic drugs, 227
▸ Equivalent doses of oral
  antipsychotics, 229
▸ Neuroleptic malignant syndrome, 229
▸ Schizophrenia, 228
▸ Sexual dysfunction, 228
▸ Sexual dysfunction and prolactin, 229
▸ Side effects of antipsychotic drugs,
  228
Psychoses and schizophrenia, 227
Psyquet XL, 238
Pulmicort products, 152
Pulmonary hypertension, 90, 110
Pulmonary surfactants, 178
Pulmozyme, 175
Pure, 957
Purine synthesis inhibitors, 492
PVA, 627
Pylobactell, 56
Pyralvex, 661
Pyrazinamide, **346**
Pyrazinamide with rifampicin and
  isoniazid, *see* Rifampicin with isoniazid
  and pyrazinamide
Pyridostigmine bromide, **602**
Pyridoxine hydrochloride, **585**
Pyrimethamine, 364, **375**
▸ With sulfadoxine, **375**

Q

Qlaira, 467
Questran preparations, 121
Quetiapine, **238**
Quinine, 364, **376**
Quinolones, 327, **328**, 630
Quinoric, 596
Qvar preparations, 151
QV preparations, 669, 672

R

Rabies immunoglobulin, 725, **729**
Rabies vaccine, 739, **754**
Rabipur, 754
Racecadotril, **45**
Raised intracranial pressure in palliative
  care, 20
Raltegravir, **387**
Ranitidine, **50**
Ranitil, 51
Rapamune, 488
Rapifen, 772
Rapilose products, 550
Rapitil, 622

Raporsin XL, 459
Rasburicase, **516**
Rebetol, 379
Recombinant human granulocyte-colony
  stimulating factor, *see* Filgrastim and
  Lenograstim
Recombinant Human Growth Hormone,
  see Somatropin
Recombinant human insulin analogue—
  long acting, *see* Insulin degludec,
  Insulin detemir and Insulin glargine
Recombinant human insulin analogue—
  short acting, *see* Insulin aspart, Insulin
  glulisine and Insulin lispro
Recombinant human insulin-like growth
  factor-I, *see* Mecasermin
Recommended regimens for *Helicobacter
  pylori* eradication, 49
Recommended regimens for prophylaxis
  against malaria, 366
Rectal and anal disorders, 63
▸ Anal fissures, 64
▸ Soothing anal and rectal preparations,
  63
Recurrent vulvovaginal candidiasis, 480
Reduced exocrine secretions, 66
Refolinon, 515
Refresh Ophthalmic, 628
Relaxit, 40
Relenza, 402
Relestat, 621
Reltebon, 268
Relvar Ellipta, 154
Remicade, 31
Remifentanil, **772**
Removal of earwax, 644, 647
Remsima, 31
Renacet, 558
Renagel, 559
Renamil, 947
Renapro, 947
Renastart, 947
Renilon, 941
Repevax, 744
Replagal, 565
Replenine-VF, 78
Resins, 177
Resonium A, 560
Resource products, 930, 954
Respiratory depression, respiratory
  distress syndrome and apnoea, 178
Respiratory stimulants, 178
▸ Pulmonary surfactants, 178
Respiratory syncytial virus, 402
Respiratory system, drug delivery, 137
▸ Inhalation, 137
▸ Inhaler devices, 137
▸ Jet nebulisers, 138
▸ Nebuliser diluent, 138
▸ Nebulisers, 137
▸ Oral, 138
▸ Parenteral, 138
▸ Peak flow meters, 138
▸ Spacer devices, 137
▸ Use and care of spacer devices, 137
Respiratory system infections,
  antibacterial therapy, 290
▸ For *haemophilus influenzae*
  epiglottitis, 290

▸ For *Haemophilus influenzae* lung
  infection in cystic fibrosis, 290
▸ For pneumonia, 290
▸ For pseudomonal lung infection in
  cystic fibrosis, 290
▸ For staphylococcal lung infection in
  cystic fibrosis, 290
Respontin, 144
Restandol, 450
Retacrit, 526
Retapamulin, **678**
Retinoid and related drugs, 514, 703, 711
Retinol palmitate with white soft paraffin
  and light liquid paraffin and liquid
  paraffin and wool fat, **628**
Retinol, *see* Vitamin A
Retrovir, 395
Revatio, 112
Revaxis, 744
Rexocaine, 781
Reyataz, 396
Rheumatic disease, suppressing drugs,
  595
▸ Antimalarials, 595
▸ Cytokine modulators, 595
▸ Drugs affecting the immune response,
  595
▸ Sulfasalazine, 596
RhIGF-I, *see* Mecasermin
Rhinitis and bacterial sinusitis, 648
Rhinocort, 652
Rhophylac, 727
RHuG-CSF, *see* Lenograstim
Riamet, 371
Riastap, 79
Ribavirin, **378**
Riboflavin, **585**
Riboflavine, *see* Riboflavin
Rifabutin, **341**
Rifadin, 343
Rifampicin, **342**
▸ With isoniazid, **344**
▸ With isoniazid and pyrazinamide, **344**
Rifamycins, 341
Rifater, 344
Rifinah, 344
Rigevidon, 470
Rimactane, 343
Rinatec, 651
Ringer-Lactate Solution for Injection, *see*
  Potassium chloride with calcium
  chloride and sodium chloride and
  sodium lactate
Ringer's solution, *see* Potassium chloride
  with calcium chloride dihydrate and
  sodium chloride
Risedronate sodium, **437**
Risk factors for cardiovascular disease,
  119
Risks of incorrect dosing of oral anti-
  cancer medicines, 495
Risperdal preparations, 240
Risperidone, **239**
Ritalin preparations, 214
Ritonavir, **397**
Ritonavir with lopinavir, *see* Lopinavir
  with ritonavir
Rituximab, **494**
Rizopia products, 957
Roaccutane, 713

INDEX

RoActemra, 597
Rocaltrol, 589
Rocephin, 304
Rocuronium bromide, **769**
Roferon-A, 517
Ropivacaine hydrochloride, **784**
Rosacea, 709, 714
Rosacea and acne, 708
 ‣ Acne vulgaris, 708
 ‣ Benzoyl peroxide and azelaic acid, 708
 ‣ Hormone treatment for acne, 709
 ‣ Neonatal and infantile acne, 708
 ‣ Oral antibacterials for acne, 708
 ‣ Oral preparations for acne, 708
 ‣ Oral retinoid for acne, 709
 ‣ Other topical preparations for acne, 708
 ‣ Rosacea, 709
 ‣ Topical antibacterials for acne, 708
 ‣ Topical preparations for acne, 708
 ‣ Topical retinoids and related preparations for acne, 708
Rosiced, 676
Rosuvastatin, **124**
Rotarix, 755
Rotavirus vaccine, 740, **754**
Routine immunisation schedule, 732
Rozex, 676
Rt-PA, see Alteplase
Rubella, 725
Rufinamide, 183, **195**

S

Sabril, 202
Saizen, 444, 445
Salactol, 723
Salamol preparations, 147, 148
Salatac, 723
Salazopyrin preparations, 29
Salbulin Novolizer, 147
Salbutamol, **146**
Salcatonin, see Calcitonin (salmon)
Sal-e Pods, 549, 719
Salicylic acid, **722**
 ‣ With benzoic acid, **682**
 ‣ With lactic acid, **722**
 ‣ With rhubarb extract, **661**
 ‣ With zinc oxide, **704**
Salicylic acid and derivatives, 661, 682, 704, 722
Salicylic acid with benzoic acid, see Benzoic acid with salicylic acid
Salicylic acid with betamethasone, see Betamethasone with salicylic acid
Salicylic acid with boric acid and tannic acid, see Boric acid with salicylic acid and tannic acid
Salicylic acid with coal tar and coconut oil, see Coal tar with coconut oil and salicylic acid
Salicylic acid with coal tar and dithranol, see Coal tar with dithranol and salicylic acid
Salicylic acid with coal tar and precipitated sulfur, see Coal tar with salicylic acid and precipitated sulfur
Salicylic acid with dithranol and zinc oxide, see Dithranol with salicylic acid and zinc oxide
Saline, 628

Saliveze, 655
Salivix, 655
Salmeterol, **145**
Salmeterol with fluticasone, see Fluticasone with salmeterol
Salofalk, 28
Sample prescription, 4
Sandimmun, 487
Sandocal, 553
Sando-K, 546
Sandostatin preparations, 435
Santizor XL, 458
Sapropterin dihydrochloride, **580**
Savlon preparations, 717, 718
Sayana Press, 479
Scabies, 675
Scalp and hair conditions, 714
Scandishake, 952
Scandonest preparations, 783
Scheriproct, 65
Schistosomicides (bilharziasis), 360
Schizophrenia, 228
Scopoderm, 251
Scopolamine hydrobromide, see Hyoscine hydrobromide
SD CodeFree, 431
Sebco, 701
Seborrhoeic dermatitis, 684
Second-generation antipsychotic drugs, 228, 790
Security and validity of prescriptions, 3
Securon preparations, 102
Sedating antihistamines, 167, 249, 272
Sedation, anaesthesia, and resuscitation in dental practice, 758
Selective serotonin re-uptake inhibitors, **222**
Selective serotonin re-uptake inhibitors, emergency treatment of poisoning, 789
Selenium, **715**
Selexid, 325
Selsun, 715
Senna, **42**
 ‣ With ispaghula husk, **42**
Senokot, 42
Sensocard, 432
Septanest, 778
Septicaemia related to vascular catheter, 285
Septrin, 331
Seravit, 953
Serenace, 232
Seretide preparations, 154
Serevent preparations, 146
Seroquel preparations, 238
Serotonin (5HT$_3$) receptor antagonists, 247
Serotonin syndrome, 221
Sertraline, **224**
Setofilm, 248
Sevelamer, **558**
Sevoflurane, **762**
Sevredol, 266
Sex hormone responsive conditions, 445
Sex hormones, 445
 ‣ Female sex hormones, 446
 ‣ Hormone replacement therapy, 445
 ‣ Oestrogens, 446
 ‣ Progestogens, 446
Sexual dysfunction, 228

Short-acting beta$_2$ agonists, 141
Short-acting insulins, 418
Short-burst oxygen therapy, 142
Shortec, 269
Sickle-cell anaemia, 521
Siklos, 513
Sildenafil, **111**
Silkis, 705
Silver nitrate, **721**
Silver sulfadiazine, **677**
Simeticone, 46, **48**
 ‣ With aluminium hydroxide and magnesium hydroxide, **48**
Simeticone with aluminium hydroxide, dicycloverine hydrochloride and magnesium oxide, see Dicycloverine hydrochloride with aluminium hydroxide, magnesium oxide and simeticone
Simeticone with hydrotalcite, see Co-simalcite
Simeticone with loperamide, see Loperamide with simeticone
Similac preparations, 934, 943
Simple mouthwashes, 659
Simulect, 492
Simvador, 125
Simvastatin, **125**
 ‣ With ezetimibe, **125**
Sinemet preparations, 242
Singulair, 156
Sinusitis and oral pain, 648
Siopel, 667
Sirolimus, **487**
Skeletal muscle relaxants, 601
Skin adhesives, 719
Skin and nail infections, 349
Skin cleansers, antiseptics and desloughing agents, 715
Skin conditions, management, 665
 ‣ Dilution, 665
 ‣ Excipients and sensitisation, 666
 ‣ Neonates, 666
 ‣ Suitable quantities for prescribing, 665
 ‣ Topical preparations, 665
 ‣ Vehicles, 665
Skin disfigurement, 719
Skin infections
 ‣ Angular cheilitis, 674
 ‣ Antibacterial preparations, 673
 ‣ Antibacterial preparations also used systemically, 674
 ‣ Antifungal preparations, 674
 ‣ Antiviral preparations, 674
 ‣ Candidiasis, 674
 ‣ Compound topical preparations, 674
 ‣ Crab lice, 675
 ‣ Dermatophytoses, 674
 ‣ Head lice, 675
 ‣ Herpes labialis, 674
 ‣ Itching, 675
 ‣ Parasiticidal preparations, 675
 ‣ Pityriasis versicolor, 674
 ‣ Scabies, 675
 ‣ Wet combing methods, 675
Skin infections, antibacterial therapy for,
 ‣ Animal and human bites, 291
 ‣ Cellulitis, 290
 ‣ Erysipelas, 290

‣ Impetigo: small areas of skin infected, 290
‣ Impetigo: widespread infection, 290
‣ Paronychia or 'septic spots' in neonate, 291
‣ Staphylococcal scalded skin syndrome, 291
‣ Surgical wound infection, 291
Skinoren, 711
Sleep disorders, 275
Slocinx XL, 459
SLO preparations, 954
Slo-Phyllin, 160
Slow Sodium, 548
Smallpox vaccine, 740
Smith-Lemli-Opitz syndrome, 59
Snake bites and animal stings, 792
Sno-Pro, 963
Sno Tears, 628
Sodiofolin, 515
Sodium acid phosphate with sodium phosphate, **39**
Sodium alginate with calcium carbonate and sodium bicarbonate, **56**
Sodium alginate with potassium bicarbonate, **47**
Sodium benzoate, **572**
Sodium bicarbonate, **544**, **647**
‣ With sodium chloride, **657**
Sodium bicarbonate with calcium carbonate and sodium alginate, *see* Sodium alginate with calcium carbonate and sodium bicarbonate
Sodium bicarbonate with glucose with potassium chloride and sodium chloride, *see* Glucose with potassium chloride, sodium bicarbonate and sodium chloride
Sodium bicarbonate with magnesium carbonate and magnesium trisilicate, *see* Magnesium trisilicate with magnesium carbonate and sodium bicarbonate
Sodium chloride, **547**, **625**, **628**, **657**
Sodium chloride with calcium chloride dihydrate and potassium chloride, *see* Potassium chloride with calcium chloride dihydrate and sodium chloride
Sodium chloride with sodium bicarbonate, *see* Sodium bicarbonate with sodium chloride
Sodium citrate, **40**
Sodium citrate with potassium chloride, rice powder and sodium chloride, *see* Potassium chloride with rice powder, sodium chloride and sodium citrate
Sodium clodronate, **438**
Sodium cromoglicate, **157**, **622**, **654**
Sodium cromoglycate, *see* Sodium cromoglicate
Sodium dichloroacetate, **572**
Sodium feredetate, **532**
Sodium fluoride, **658**
Sodium hyaluronate, **628**
Sodium ironedetate, *see* Sodium feredetate
Sodium Lactate Intravenous Infusion, Compound, *see* Potassium chloride with calcium chloride and sodium chloride and sodium lactate

Sodium lactate with calcium chloride, potassium chloride and sodium chloride, *see* Potassium chloride with calcium chloride and sodium chloride and sodium lactate
Sodium nitrite, **793**
Sodium nitroprusside, **109**
Sodium phenylbutyrate, **573**
Sodium phosphate with sodium acid phosphate, *see* Sodium acid phosphate with sodium phosphate
Sodium picosulfate, **42**
Sodium picosulfate with magnesium citrate, *see* Magnesium citrate with sodium picosulfate
Sodium picosulphate, *see* Sodium picosulfate
Sodium polystyrene sulfonate, **560**
Sodium stibogluconate, **363**
Sodium thiosulfate, **793**
Sodium valproate, **195**
Soffen, 672
Sofiperla, 469
Sofradex, 646
SoftDrops, 627
Softening drugs, 43, 647
Soft tissue and joint disorders, 616
Soft-tissue disorders, 617
‣ Enzymes, 618
‣ Extravasation, 617
‣ Management of extravasation, 618
‣ Prevention of extravasation, 618
‣ Soft-tissue and musculoskeletal disorders, 617
Solian, 234
Soliris, 527
Solivito N, 578
Solpadol, 259
Soluble Insulin—short acting, *see* Insulin
Solu-Cortef, 412
Solu-Medrone, 412
Solvazinc, 575
Somatomedins, 445
Somatostatin analogues, **434**
Somatropin, **443**
Sondate XL, 238
Soothing anal and rectal preparations, 63
S.O.S., 948
Sotacor, 75
Sotalol hydrochloride, **74**
Sources of BNFC information, ix
Soya protein formula, 928
Soybean oil, **629**
Space Chamber Plus, 161
Spacers, 137, 161
Spasmonal, 58
Spasticity, 603
Special diets, 580
Specialised formulas, 941, 946
Speciality breads (ACBS), 956
Special-order manufacturers, 979
Spermicidals, 479
Spiramycin, **377**
Spironolactone, **117**
Sporanox, 355
Spreads, 959
Sprilon, 667
SST - brand name, 655
Stamaril, 756
Statins, **122**

Status epilepticus, 184, 208
Stavudine, **393**
Stemetil, 252
Sterculia, **36**
‣ With frangula, **37**
Sterets preparations, 717, 718
Stericlens, 719
Steripod, 719
Sterols, 61
Sterowash, 719
Stesolid, 208
Stexerol-D3, 589
Stimulant laxatives, 34, 35, 40
Stiripentol, **198**
Stirlescent, 615
Stoma care, 67
‣ Analgesics, 67
‣ Antacids, 67
‣ Antidiarrhoeal drugs, 67
‣ Antisecretory drugs, 67
‣ Care of stoma, 68
‣ Description of condition, 67
‣ Digoxin, 68
‣ Diuretics, 68
‣ Iron preparations, 68
‣ Laxatives, 68
Strattera, 213
Strefen, 660
Streptokinase, **126**
Streptomycin, **293**
Strivit-D3, 589
Stugeron, 249
Subarachnoid haemorrhage, 80
Subcuvia, 728
Subgam, 728
Sublimaze, 264
Substance dependence, 276
‣ Choice, 277
‣ Concomitant medication, 277
‣ Guidance on treatment of drug misuse, 276
‣ Neonatal abstinence syndrome, 277
‣ Nicotine dependence, 276
‣ Nicotine replacement therapy, 277
‣ Side-effects of specific nicotine preparations, 277
Succinylcholine chloride, *see* Suxamethonium chloride
Sucralfate, **50**
Sudafed preparations, 650
Sudocrem, 667
Sugammadex, **770**
Sugars, 549
Suicidal behaviour and antidepressant therapy, 221
Suitable quantities for specific areas of the body
‣ of dermatological preparations, 665
‣ of parasiticidal preparations, 675
Sulazine EC, 29
Sulfadiazine, **331**
Sulfadoxine and pyrimethamine, *see* Pyrimethamine with sulfadoxine
Sulfamethoxazole with trimethoprim, *see* Co-trimoxazole
Sulfasalazine, **29**, 596
Sulfonamides, 330, 677
Sulfonylureas, 419, **420**
Sulfur-containing imidazoles, 452

Sulfur dioxide, chlorine, phosgene, ammonia, 791
Sulphadiazine, *see* Sulfadiazine
Sulphasalazine, *see* Sulfasalazine
Sulpiride, **233**
Sulpor, 233
Sumatriptan, **273**
Sunya, 469
Super Betavit, 706
Super Bio-Quinone, 567
SuperCheck products, 432
Superficial soft-tissue injuries and superficial thrombophlebitis, 720
Superinfection, 282
Supply of medicines, 6
Suprane, 761
Supraventricular tachycardia, 69
Suprax, 301
SURESIGN Resure, 432
Survanta, 178
Survimed OPD, 929
Sustiva, 388
Suxamethonium chloride, **766**
Symbicort Turbohaler, 152
Sympathomimetics, 112, 636
‣ Inotropic sympathomimetics, 112, 113
‣ Shock, 113
‣ Vasoconstrictor sympathomimetics, 113, 114, 128, 634, 649
Synacthen preparations, 442
Synagis, 402
Synalar preparations, 691, 692, 697
Syndromes associated with accessory conducting pathways, 69
Synflorix, 747
Syprol, 97
Syringe driver rate settings, 21
Systane, 626
Systemic corticosteroids, 616
Systemic nasal decongestants, 176
Systemic treatment, 686
Sytron, 532

T

Tabphyn MR, 460
Tacalcitol, **705**
Tacrolimus, **488**, **702**
Taenicides, 359
Tambocor preparations, 72
Tamfrex XL, 460
Tamiflu, 400
Tamsulosin hydrochloride, **459**
Tamurex, 460
Tapclob, 206
Taranis products, 958, 959
Targeted therapy responsive malignancy, 519
Target INR, 82
Targocid, 305
Tars, 700
Tazobactam with piperacillin, *see* Piperacillin with tazobactam
Tazocin, 317
T-cell activation inhibitors, 598
3TC, *see* Lamivudine
Tear deficiency, ocular lubricants, and astringents, 625
Tear-Lac, 627
Tears Naturale, 627
TEE2, 432

Tegretol preparations, 186
Teicoplanin, **305**
Telfast, 166
Telithromycin, **312**
Telzir, 397
Temazepam, **774**
Temgesic, 258
Temodal, 501
Temomedac, 501
Temozolomide, **500**
Tenofovir disoproxil, **394**
Tenormin, 98
Tenprolide XL, 239
Tentrini products, 934, 936
Teoptic, 637
Tepadina, 501
Tephine, 258
Teragezza, 710
Terbinafine, **680**
Terbutaline sulfate, **148**
Terlipressin acetate, **61**
Termination of pregnancy, 284
Terra-Cortril, 698
Test for *Helicobacter pylori*, 49
Testolactone, **451**
Testosterone enantate, **450**
Testosterone propionate, **450**
Testosterone undecanoate, **450**
Tetanus and diphtheria with poliomyelitis, *see* Diphtheria with poliomyelitis and tetanus vaccine
Tetanus immunoglobulin, 725, **729**
Tetanus vaccine, 740
Tetanus with diphtheria with haemophilus influenza with pertussis and poliomyelitis, *see* Diphtheria with haemophilus influenzae type b vaccine, pertussis, poliomyelitis and tetanus
Tetanus with diphtheria with pertussis and diptheria, *see* Diphtheria with pertussis, poliomyelitis vaccine and tetanus
Tetracaine, **635**, **785**
Tetracosactide, **441**
Tetracosactrin, *see* Tetracosactide
Tetracycline, **334**
Tetracyclines, 289, 331, **332**, 364
Tetracyclines and related drugs, 331, 662
Tetrahydrobiopterin, **581**
Tetrahydrobiopterin and derivatives, 580
Tetralysal, 333
Thamicarb, 545
TheiCal-D3, 590
Theophylline, 141, **159**, 791
Thiamine, **586**
Thiazides and related diuretics, **102**, 130, 134
Thick & Easy, 954
Thicken Aid, 954
Thioguanine, *see* Tioguanine
Thiopental sodium, **209**
Thiopentone sodium, *see* Thiopental sodium
Thiotepa, **501**
Thiouracils, 452
Thirty:30, 672
Thixo-D products, 954
Thorens, 590
Thromboembolism, 81, 496
Thrush, 662

Thymoglobulin, 484
Thyroid disorders, 451
Thyroid hormones, 453, 454
Thyrotoxicosis, 94
Thyroxine sodium, *see* Levothyroxine sodium
Tiagabine, **199**
Ticarcillin with clavulanic acid, **318**
Tick-borne encephalitis vaccine, 740
Tick-borne encephalitis vaccine, inactivated, **755**
TicoVac, 755
Tilade, 157
Tildiem preparations, 136
Tilodol SR, 271
Tilofyl, 264
Tiloryth, 312
Timentin, 318
Timodine, 697
Timolol and dorzolamide, *see* Dorzolamide with timolol
Timolol maleate, **638**
Timoptol preparations, 638
Tinidazole, **315**
Tinzaparin sodium, **88**
Tioconazole, **679**
Tioguanine, **508**
Tiopex, 638
Tipranavir, **398**
Tissue plasminogen activators, 81, 125
Tissue-type plasminogen activator, *see* Alteplase
Tivicay, 387
TOBI, 295
Tobia products, 957
Tobi Podhaler, 295
Tobramycin, **294**, **630**
Tobravisc, 630
Tocilizumab, **597**
Tocopherol, *see* Alpha tocopherol
Tolazoline, **112**
Tolbutamide, **421**
Tolterodine tartrate, **458**
Tonic and atonic seizures, 182
Tonic-clonic seizures, 182
Topamax, 200
Topical antibacterials for acne, 708
Topical circulatory preparations, 720
Topical corticosteroids, 686
‣ Absorption through the skin, 687
‣ Choice, 686
‣ Compound preparations, 687
‣ Perioral lesions, 686
‣ Topical corticosteroid preparation potencies, 687
Topical local antipruritics, 707
Topical nasal decongestants, 648
Topical preparations for acne, 708
Topical retinoids and related preparations for acne, 708
Topiramate, 183, **199**
Torsade de pointes, 69
Total intravenous anaesthesia, 757
Toujeo, 425
Toxoplasmosis, 377
Trace elements with vitamins and minerals, *see* Vitamins with minerals and trace elements
Tracleer, 111

Tracrium, 767
Tracutil, 578
Tradorec XL, 271
Tramacet, 256
Tramadol hydrochloride, **270**
Tramadol with paracetamol, see
  Paracetamol with tramadol
Tramquel SR, 271
Tramulief SR, 271
Trandate, 96
Tranexamic acid, **76**
Tranquilyn, 214
Travel, 739
Treclin, 714
Tree pollen extract, **173**
Tresiba preparations, 424
Tretinoin, **514**
  ▸ With clindamycin, **713**
  ▸ With erythromycin, **714**
Triamcinolone acetonide, **617, 653**
Triamcinolone hexacetonide, **617**
Triamcinolone with chlortetracycline, see
  Chlortetracycline with triamcinolone
Triazole antifungals, 349, 352
Tribavirin, see Ribavirin
Trichomonacides, 362
Tricyclic and related antidepressants, 789
Tricyclic antidepressants, 224
Trientine dihydrochloride, **574**
Trifluoperazine, **233**
Trihexyphenidyl hydrochloride, **241**
Trileptal, 193
Trimeprazine tartrate, see Alimemazine
  tartrate
Trimethoprim, **338**
Trimethoprim with sulfamethoxazole, see
  Co-trimoxazole
Trimovate, 696
Triptans, 273
Triptorelin, **440**
Tris(hydroxymethyl)aminomethane,
  THAM, see Trometamol
Tritamyl products, 957
Triumeq, 391
Trizivir, 391
Trometamol, **540**
Tropicamide, **633**
Trosyl, 679
TRUEone, 432
TRUEresult, 432
TrueTrack System, 432
TRUEyou, 432
Trusopt, 640
Trypanocides, 362
Tuberculin PPD, see Tuberculin purified
  protein derivative
Tuberculin purified protein derivative,
  731
Tuberculosis, 340
  ▸ Antituberculosis drugs, 341
  ▸ Continuation phase, 340
  ▸ Corticosteroids, 340
  ▸ Immunocompromised patients, 340
  ▸ Initial phase, 340
  ▸ Neonates, 340
  ▸ Pregnancy and breast-feeding, 340
  ▸ Prevention of tuberculosis, 340
  ▸ Supervised treatment, 340
  ▸ Treatment failure, 340
  ▸ Unsupervised treatment, 340

Tumor necrosis factor alpha (TNF-α)
  inhibitors, 598
Tumour lysis syndrome, 496
Twinrix, 748
Tylex, 259
Tymbrineb, 295
Typherix, 748
Typhim Vi, 748
Typhoid vaccine, 740, **747**
Typhoid with hepatitis A vaccine, see
  Hepatitis A with typhoid vaccine
Tyrosinaemia, 964
Tyrosinaemia type I, 570
Tyrosine1000, 962
TYR preparations, 965
Tyvera, 586

U

Ubidecarenone, **567**
Ubiquinone, see Ubidecarenone
UK Drugs in Lactation Advisory Service
  (UKDILAS), inside front cover
Ulceration and inflammation, 659
Ulipristal acetate, **473**
Ultiva, 773
Ultralanum Plain preparations, 692
Ultraproct, 65
Undecenoates, 681, 715
Undecenoic acid with cetrimide, see
  Cetrimide with undecenoic acid
Undecenoic acid with zinc undecenoate,
  681
Unguentum M, 672
Uniphyllin Continus, 160
Uniroid HC, 65
Upostelle, 477
Urate oxidases, 516
Urea (13C), **56**
Urea cycle disorders, 562, 571
Urea hydrogen peroxide, **648**
Urea with hydrocortisone, see
  Hydrocortisone with urea
Uricto, 517
Urinalysis, 428
Urinalysis reagent strips, 432
Urinary frequency, enuresis and
  incontinence, 456
  ▸ Nocturnal enuresis in children, 456
  ▸ Urinary incontinence, 456
Urinary retention, 458
Urinary-tract infections, 347
  ▸ Antibacterial prophylaxis, 347
  ▸ Antibacterial therapy for urinary-tract
    infections, 347
  ▸ Pregnancy, 347
  ▸ Renal impairment, 347
  ▸ Resistant infections, 347
Urokinase, **81**
Urological pain, 460
  ▸ Alkalinisation of urine, 460
Uroprotective drugs, 515
Uro-Tainer products, 461, 656
Urothelial toxicity, 496
Ursodeoxycholic acid, **60**
Ursofalk, 61
Utovlan, 448

V

Vaccines, 731, **742**
  ▸ Bacterial and viral vaccines,
    combined, 743
  ▸ Bacterial vaccines, 744
  ▸ Viral vaccines, 748
  ▸ Active immunity, 731
  ▸ Anthrax vaccine, 733
  ▸ BCG vaccine, 733
  ▸ Botulism antitoxin, 734
  ▸ Childhood immunisation, 737
  ▸ Children with unknown or incomplete
    immunisation history, 731
  ▸ Choice of vaccine, 738
  ▸ Cholera vaccine, 734
  ▸ Diphtheria vaccine, 734
  ▸ Haemophilus influenzae type B
    conjugate vaccine, 734
  ▸ Hepatitis A vaccine, 735
  ▸ Hepatitis B vaccine, 735
  ▸ Human papillomavirus vaccine, 736
  ▸ Immunisation schedule, 731
  ▸ Influenza vaccine, 736
  ▸ Invasive Haemophilus influenzae type
    B disease, 735
  ▸ Japanese encephalitis vaccine, 736
  ▸ Management of Measles, Mumps and
    Rubella, 736
  ▸ Meningococcal vaccine, 737
  ▸ Passive immunity, 733
  ▸ Pertussis vaccine, 738
  ▸ Pneumococcal vaccine, 738
  ▸ Poliomyelitis vaccine, 739
  ▸ Post-exposure management, 739
  ▸ Pre-exposure prophylaxis, 739
  ▸ Preterm birth, 732
  ▸ Rabies vaccine, 739
  ▸ Revaccination, 739
  ▸ Rotavirus vaccine, 740
  ▸ Side-effects, 738
  ▸ Smallpox vaccine, 740
  ▸ Tetanus vaccine, 740
  ▸ Tick-borne encephalitis vaccine, 740
  ▸ Travel, 739
  ▸ Tuberculosis Diagnostic Agents, 734
  ▸ Typhoid vaccine, 740
  ▸ Vaccination of pregnant women
    against pertussis, 738
  ▸ Vaccines and antisera availability, 733
  ▸ Vaccines and asplenia, 733
  ▸ Vaccines and HIV infection, 732
  ▸ Varicella-zoster vaccine, 741
  ▸ Wounds, 740
  ▸ Yellow fever vaccine, 741
Vaccines for travel, 741
  ▸ Food hygiene, 741
  ▸ Immunisation, 741
  ▸ Information on health advice for
    travellers, 741
Vaginal and vulval conditions, 479
  ▸ Preparations for vaginal and vulval
    changes, 479
  ▸ Recurrent vulvovaginal candidiasis,
    480
  ▸ Vaginal and vulval infections, 480
  ▸ Vulvovaginal candidiasis in
    pregnancy, 480
Vaginal contraceptives, 473
Valaciclovir, **383**
Valine50, 963

Valproate, 183, 218
Valproic acid, **200**
Valsartan, **107**
Valtrex, 383
Vancocin preparations, 307
Vancomycin, **305**
Vanquoral, 487
VAQTA, 749
Varicella-Zoster, 730
Varicella-zoster immunoglobulin, 725, **730**
Varicella-zoster infections, 380
Varicella-zoster vaccine, 741, **755**
Varilrix, 756
Variquel, 62
Varivax, 756
Vascular disease, 135
Vaseline, 672
Vasoconstrictor sympathomimetics, 113
Vasodilator antihypertensives, 91, 108, 109
Vasodilators, 109, 112
Vasopressin, **62**
Vasopressin and analogues, 61, 403
Vecuronium bromide, **769**
Vedrop, 592
Vehicles (skin), 665
Velaglucerase alfa, **566**
Veletri, 110
Venofer, 530
Venous thromboembolism, 81
 ‣ Extracorporeal circuits, 81
 ‣ Haemorrhage, 82
 ‣ Management of venous thromboembolism in pregnancy, 81
 ‣ Prophylaxis of venous thromboembolism, 81
 ‣ Treatment of venous thromboembolism, 81
Ventavis, 111
Ventolin preparations, 147, 148
Ventricular tachycardia and ventricular fibrillation, 69
Vepesid, 511
Veracur, 721
Verapamil hydrochloride, **101**
Vermox, 362
Verrugon, 722
Vertine, 146
VFEND, 356
ViATIM, 749
Vibramycin-D, 333, 662
Vibrox, 333
Victanyl, 264
Videne, 716
Videx preparations, 392
Vigabatrin, **201**
Vigam, 729
Vigranon-B, 586
Vilanterol with fluticasone, see Fluticasone with vilanterol
Vimpat, 189
Vinblastine sulfate, **511**
Vinca alkaloids, 497, 511
Vincristine sulfate, **511**
ViraferonPeg preparations, 380
Viral eye infection, 632
Viral infection, 377
Viral skin infections, 683
Viramune, 390

Viread, 394
Viscotears, 626
Vismed, 628
Vistamethasone, 622, 646, 652
VitaBite, 958
Vita-E, 592
Vitaflo Choices, 958
Vitajoule, 948
Vitalograph, 161
Vitamin A, 581, **584**, 706
Vitamin and Mineral supplements, 953
Vitamin B complex, **586**
Vitamin B group, 534, 581, 584, 714
Vitamin B$_6$, see Pyridoxine hydrochloride
Vitamin B$_2$, see Riboflavin
Vitamin B$_1$, see Thiamine
Vitamin C, see Ascorbic acid
Vitamin D, 582
Vitamin D and analogues, 588, 704
Vitamin D and analogues (systemic), **588**
Vitamin deficiency, 581
Vitamin D$_3$, see Colecalciferol
Vitamin D$_2$, see Ergocalciferol
Vitamin E, 582, 592
Vitamin H, see Biotin
Vitamin K, 583, 593
Vitamin K antagonists, **88**
Vitamin K deficiency bleeding, 583
Vitamin K$_1$, see Phytomenadione
Vitamins, 581
 ‣ Dental patients, 581
 ‣ Multivitamins, 583
 ‣ Vitamin A, 581
 ‣ Vitamin B group, 581
 ‣ Vitamin C, 582
 ‣ Vitamin D, 582
 ‣ Vitamin E, 582
 ‣ Vitamin K, 583
Vitamins A and D, **583**
Vitamins A, B group, C and D, **583**
Vitamins A, C and D, **584**
Vitamins and trace elements, 453, 515, 533, 583, 592, 658, 704, 714, 715
Vitamins with minerals and trace elements, **586**
VitA-POS, 628
Vitaquick, 954
Vitasavoury, 952
Vitlipid N preparations, 578
Vividrin, 622
Vivotif, 748
Volatile halogenated anaesthetics, **760**
Volatile liquid anaesthetics, 757, 760
Volplex, 555
Voltarol Ophtha preparations, 621, 633, 635
Voltarol preparations, 605, 606, 607
Volumatic, 161
Vomiting during pregnancy, 244
Voriconazole, **355**
Vortex products, 161
Votubia, 519
VPRIV, 566
VSL#3, 954

W

Warburtons products, 955, 956
Warfarin sodium, **89**
Warticon, 721

Warts and calluses, 720
 ‣ Anogenital warts, 720
Wasp venom extract, **173**
WaveSense JAZZ Products, 432
Waxsol, 647
Wellfoods products, 955, 956, 957, 958
Wellvone, 358
White soft paraffin with liquid paraffin and wool alcohols, see Liquid paraffin with white soft paraffin and wool alcohols
White soft paraffin with retinol palmitate with light liquid with liquid paraffin and wool, see Retinol palmitate with white soft paraffin and light liquid paraffin and liquid paraffin and wool fat
Wilson's disease, 573
Wilzin, 574
Wounds, 740

X

Xagrid, 540
Xailin preparations, 626
Xalatan, 641
Xaluprine, 506
Xanthan gum, 957
Xanthine oxidase inhibitors, 516
Xanthines, 158, 179
Xemacort, 695
Xenical, 63
Xeomin, 243
Xepin, 708
Xerotin, 655
XLEU Maxamaid, 961
XLYS products, 959, 961
XMET products, 960
XMTVI products, 962
Xolair, 155
Xomolix, 251
XPHEN TYR products, 965
XP preparations, 964
XPTM Tyrosidon, 965
Xylocaine, 660
Xylocaine with adrenaline, 781
Xylometazoline hydrochloride, **650**
Xylometazoline with antazoline, see Antazoline with xylometazoline
Xyloproct, 65
Xyzal, 166

Y

Yacella, 468
Yasmin, 468
Yellow card scheme, 11
Yellow fever vaccine, 741
Yellow fever vaccine, live, **756**
Yemex, 264

Z

Zaditen, 170, 621
Zafirlukast, **156**
Zalasta, 237
Zaluron XL, 239
Zamadol Products, 271
Zanamivir, **401**
Zantac, 51
Zapain, 259

Zaponex, 236
Zarontin, 187
Zarzio, 539
Zavesca, 570
Zeffix, 393
Zelleta, 474
Zenalb, 554
Zenoxone, 693
Zeridame SR, 271
Zerit, 394
ZeroAQS, 672
Zerobase, 672
Zerocream, 672
Zeroguent, 672
Zerolatum preparations, 669
Zeroneum, 670
Zestril, 106
Ziagen, 391
Zicron, 421
Zidoval, 481
Zidovudine, **394**
  ▸ With lamivudine, **395**
Zidovudine with abacavir and lamivudine,
  see Abacavir with lamivudine and
  zidovudine
Zinacef, 300
Zinamide, 347
Zinc, 575
Zinc acetate, **573**
Zinc acetate with erythromycin, see
  Erythromycin with zinc acetate
Zinc deficiency, 575
Zinc oxide with benzyl benzoate, bismuth
  oxide, bismuth subgallate,
  hydrocortisone acetate and peru
  balsam, see Benzyl benzoate with
  bismuth oxide, bismuth subgallate,
  hydrocortisone acetate, peru balsam
  and zinc oxide
Zinc oxide with benzyl benzoate, bismuth
  oxide, hydrocortisone acetate, peru
  balsam and pramocaine hydrochloride,
  see Benzyl benzoate with bismuth
  oxide, hydrocortisone acetate, peru
  balsam, pramocaine hydrochloride and
  zinc oxide
Zinc oxide with calamine, see Calamine
  with zinc oxide
Zinc oxide with coal tar, see Coal tar with
  zinc oxide
Zinc oxide with dithranol and salicylic
  acid, see Dithranol with salicylic acid
  and zinc oxide
Zinc oxide with ichthammol, see
  Ichthammol with zinc oxide
Zinc oxide with salicyclic acid, see
  Salicylic acid with zinc oxide
Zinc sulfate, **575**
Zinc undecenoate with undecenoic acid,
  see Undecenoic acid with zinc
  undecenoate
Zindaclin, 710
Zineryt, 710
Zinnat, 300
Zirtek, 165
Zithromax, 309
Zlatal, 508
Zocor, 125
Zoely, 467
Zofran preparations, 248, 249

Zoladex preparations, 439
Zolmitriptan, **274**
Zolvera, 102
Zomacton, 445
Zomestine, 268
Zomig preparations, 274
Zomorph, 267
Zonegran, 203
Zonisamide, 184, **202**
Zoton FasTab, 53
Zovirax, 382, 632, 683
Zumenon, 468
Zutectra, 727
Zyclara, 723
Zydol preparations, 270, 271
Zyloric, 517
Zyomet, 676
Zyprexa preparations, 237
Zyvox, 338